W9-BUA-454

HIV Infection, 1232
Hordeolum, 337
Hypercalcemia, 1104, 1332
Hyperhidrosis, 288
Hyperkalemia, 1108
Hyperlipidemia, 128
Hypernatremia, 1112
Hyperparathyroidism, 1131
Hypertension, 128, 569
Hyperthyroidism, 1141
Hyperuricemia, 1333
Hypocalcemia, 1104, 1331
Hypokalemia, 1108
Hyponatremia, 1114
Hypoparathyroidism, 1131
Hypotension, 221
Hypothyroidism, 1145
Immunizations, 145, 155, 173
Immunodeficiency, 1200
Incontinence, 731
Infections
  Abdominal, 623
  Breast, 807
  Central Nervous System, 1037
  Fungal, 279
  Oral, 406
  Urinary Tract, 777
Infectious Disease, 1225
Infertility, 845
Inflammatory Bowel Disease, 692
Influenza, 1241
Insect Bites and Stings, 197
Insomnia, 1210
Intertrigo, 290
Irritable Bowel Syndrome, 699
Jaundice, 705
Labyrinthitis, 367
Leukemias, Acute and Chronic, 1307
Leukostasis, 1131
Lichen Planus, 1198
Lichen Sclerosis, 883
Lipid Disorders, 1120
Lyme Disease, 1254
Lymphadenopathy, 1204
Lymphomas, 1314
  Hodgkin's Lymphoma, 1314
  Non-Hodgkin's Lymphoma, 1315
Meniere's Disease, 368
Meniscus Injuries, 949
Menopause, 850
Metabolic Syndrome, 129, 1126
Mitral Regurgitation, 617
Mitral Stenosis, 620
Mitral Valve Prolapse, 619
Mononucleosis, Infectious, 1251
Morton's Neuroma, 902
Movement Disorders, 1040
  Sleep-Related, 1215
Multiple Sclerosis, 1044
Myelodysplastic Syndromes, 1320
Myocarditis, 567
Myofascial Pain Syndrome, 924
Nail Disorders, 292
  Herpetic Whitlow, 292
  Onychomycosis and Tinea Unguium, 294
  Paronychial Infections, 293
Nasal Congestion and Discharge, Chronic, 3378
Nasal Polyps, 394
Nasal Trauma, 382
Nasolacrimal Duct Obstruction, 349
Nausea and Vomiting, 709
Nipple Discharge, 811
Non-Neoplastic Epithelial Disorders, 885
Obesity, 109
Obstructive Uropathy, 794
Ocular Burns, 355
Ocular Surface Foreign Bodies, 343
Ocular Trauma, 355
Onychomycosis, 294
Osteoarthritis, 976
Osteochondritis Dissecans, 901
Osteomyelitis, 980
Osteoporosis, 960
Otitis Externa,371
Otitis Media, 373
Paget's Disease
  of the Bone, 960
  of the Nipple, 813
Pain
  Chronic, 1186
  Elbow, 920
  Hand and Wrist, 932
  Hip, 936
  Knee, 946
  Neck, 970
  Oncology, 1335
  Pelvic, Chronic, 817
  Shoulder, 985
  Vulvar, 889
Pancreatic Pseudocyst, 720
Pancreatitis, 713
  Acute, 713
  Chronic, 717
Pancytopenia, 1311
Pap Test Abnormalities, 868
Paraneoplastic Syndromes, 1330
Parasomnias, 1217
Parathyroid Gland Disorders, 1131
Parkinson's Disease, 1050
Paronychial Infections, 293
Parotitis, 409
Pelvic Inflammatory Disease, 871
Peptic Ulcer Disease, 728
Peptic Ulcer, Perforated, 626
Peripheral Arterial Insufficiency, 599
Peripheral Venous Insufficiency, 605
Peritonitis, 628
Pharyngitis, 413
Pheochromocytoma, 1074
Pigmentation Changes (Vitiligo), 296
Pinguecula, 353
Plantar Fasciitis, 901
Pleural Effusions, 479
Pleurisy, 483
Pneumonia, 485
Pneumothorax, 491
Poisoning, 224
Polymyalgia Rheumatica, 1159
Popliteal (Baker's) Cysts, 952
Posttraumatic Stress Disorder, 1349
Prenatal Care, 65
Pregnancy, 65
Ectopic, 828
Thyroid Disease, 1150
Unplanned, 879
Prostatic Hyperplasia, Benign, 738
Prostatitis, 741
Proteinuria, 743
Pruritus, 299
  Ani, 633
  Cutaneous, 269
  Vulvar, 883
Psoriasis, 301, 888
Psychotic Disorders, 1377
Pterygium, 353
Pulmonary Hypertension, 496
Purpura, 304
Raynaud's Phenomenon, 1164
Reactive Arthritis, 1152
Renal Failure, 749
Reptile Bites and Scorpion Stings, 200
Respiratory Disease, Occupational, 166
Rhinitis
  Allergic, 384
  Idiopathic/Vasomotor, 387
  Other Causes, 388
Salivary Gland Disease, 399
Sarcoidosis, 500
Scabies, 307
Seizure Disorder, 1054
Sexual Assault, 227
Sexual Dysfunction
  Disorders of Orgasm, 758
  Erectile Dysfunction, 756
  Female, 875
  Male, 756
Sexually Transmitted Infections, 782
  Chancroid, 793
  Chlamydia, 790
  Genital Herpes, 792
  Gonorrhea, 784
  Human Immunodeficiency Virus, 782
  Human Papillomavirus, 782
  Other Ulcerative, 793
  Syphilis, 791
Sinusitis, 389
Sleep
  Apnea, 1213
  Nonrestorative, 1210
Small Bowel Obstruction, 625
Smell and Taste Disturbances, 392
Spider Bites, 198
Spinal Cord Compression, Malignant, 1331
Sprains, 897, 994
  Ankle, 897
  Knee, 994
Squamous Cell Hyperplasia, 886
Strains, 994
Stroke
  Hemorrhagic, 1011
  Ischemic, 1010
Substance Abuse, 1370
Superior Vena Cava Syndrome, 1330
Syncope, 230
Syndrome of Inappropriate Antidiuretic Hormone, 1334
Systemic Lupus Erythematosus, 1170
Tachyarrhythmia, 515
Tachycardia, 201
Testicular Disorders, 763
Thermal Injuries, 233
  Cold-Related, 235
  Heat-Related, 233

Continued

Table of Contents by Disorder—Cont'd

Thrombophilia, 1303
Thyroid Nodule, 1139
Tinnitus, 369
Tonsillitis, 413
Trauma
  Eye, 355
  Head, 218
  Nasal, 382
Trichomoniasis, 893
Trigeminal Neuralgia, 1063
Tuberculosis, 1262
Tumor Lysis Syndrome, 1311, 1333
Tumors
  Bone, 906
  Colon, 726
  Esophageal, 722
  Gastrointestinal, 722
  Genitourinary Tract, 794
  Intracranial, 1066
  Nasal, 394
  Of Unknown Origin, 1345
  Small Intestine, 725
  Stomach, 723
Tympanic Membrane Perforation, 377
Urinary Calculi, 771
Urticaria, 312
Vaginitis/Vaginosis, 892
Valvular Heart Disease, 611
Varicose Veins, 5609
Vasculitis, 1176
Venous Stasis
  Chronic, 608
  Ulceration, 609
Vertigo, 1024
von Willebrand Disease, 1302
Vulvar Eczema, 888
Vulvar Pain, 889
Warts
  Cutaneous, 314
  Genital, 885
Wegener's Granulomatosis, 396
Weight Loss, Unintended, 1218
West Nile Virus, 1271
Wound Management, 317

PRIMARY CARE

A Collaborative Practice

EDITION

5

Terry Mahan Buttaro, PhD, AGPCNP-BC, FAANP, DPNAP
Assistant Clinical Professor
University of Massachusetts Boston
Coastal Medical Associates
Salisbury, Massachusetts

JoAnn Trybulski, PhD, ARNP, FNAP
Director, DNP Program
Chamberlain College of Nursing
Miami, Florida

Patricia Polgar-Bailey, PsyD, MPH, FNP-BC, CDE, BC-ADM
Family Nurse Practitioner
Pediatric Hematology/Oncology
University of Virginia Medical Center
Charlottesville, Virginia;
Clinical Psychologist
Rational-Therapeutics, LLC
Charlottesville, Virginia

Joanne Sandberg-Cook, MS, APRN, ANP/GNP-BC
Adult/Gerontologic Nurse Practitioner (retired)
Dartmouth-Hitchcock Medical Center
Lebanon, New Hampshire;
Dartmouth Medical School
Hanover, New Hampshire

ELSEVIER

ELSEVIER

3251 Riverport Lane
St. Louis, Missouri 63043

BUTTARO: PRIMARY CARE: A COLLABORATIVE PRACTICE, FIFTH EDITION

ISBN: 978-0-323-35501-8

Copyright © 2017 by Elsevier, Inc. All rights reserved.

No part of this publication may be reproduced or transmitted in any form or by any means, electronic or mechanical, including photocopying, recording, or any information storage and retrieval system, without permission in writing from the publisher. Details on how to seek permission, further information about the Publisher's permissions policies and our arrangements with organizations such as the Copyright Clearance Center and the Copyright Licensing Agency, can be found at our website: www.elsevier.com/permissions.

This book and the individual contributions contained in it are protected under copyright by the Publisher (other than as may be noted herein).

Details on how to seek permission, further information about the Publisher's permissions policies and our arrangements with organizations such as the Copyright Clearance Center and the Copyright Licensing Agency, can be found at our website: www.elsevier.com/permissions.

This book and the individual contributions contained in it are protected under copyright by the Publisher (other than as may be noted herein).

Notices

Knowledge and best practice in this field are constantly changing. As new research and experience broaden our understanding, changes in research methods, professional practices, or medical treatment may become necessary.

Practitioners and researchers must always rely on their own experience and knowledge in evaluating and using any information, methods, compounds, or experiments described herein. In using such information or methods they should be mindful of their own safety and the safety of others, including parties for whom they have a professional responsibility.

With respect to any drug or pharmaceutical products identified, readers are advised to check the most current information provided (i) on procedures featured or (ii) by the manufacturer of each product to be administered, to verify the recommended dose or formula, the method and duration of administration, and contraindications. It is the responsibility of practitioners, relying on their own experience and knowledge of their patients, to make diagnoses, to determine dosages and the best treatment for each individual patient, and to take all appropriate safety precautions.

To the fullest extent of the law, neither the Publisher nor the authors, contributors, or editors, assume any liability for any injury and/or damage to persons or property as a matter of products liability, negligence or otherwise, or from any use or operation of any methods, products, instructions, or ideas contained in the material herein.

Previous editions copyrighted 2013, 2008, 2003, and 1999.

International Standard Book Number: 978-0-323-35501-8

Executive Content Strategist: Lee Henderson
Content Development Manager: Laurie Gower
Content Development Specialist: Rebecca Corradetti
Publishing Services Manager: Julie Eddy
Book Production Specialist: Celeste Clingan
Design Direction: Amy Buxton

Printed in Canada

Last digit is the print number: 9 8 7 6 5 4 3

ELSEVIER Book Aid International
Working together to grow libraries in developing countries
www.elsevier.com • www.bookaid.org

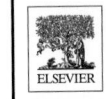

This book is dedicated to Maria Melkis, JD, BSN, RN, our friend and colleague. Maria embodied empathy, kindness, generosity, and passion for our profession. She is deeply loved and sadly missed.

Contributors

Karen S. Abate, PhD, FNP-BC
Nurse Practitioner
One Medical Group
New York City, New York

Lisa V. Adams, MD
Associate Dean for Global Health Medicine
Director, Center for Health Equity
Geisel School of Medicine at Dartmouth
Hanover, New Hampshire

Imatullah Akyar, PhD, MsN, RN
Visiting Scholar
School of Nursing
University of Alabama at Birmingham
Birmingham, Alabama;
Assistant Professor
Faculty of Nursing
Hacettepe University
Ankara, Turkey

Traci L. Alberti, PhD, FNP-BC
Assistant Professor & Coordinator
Family Nurse Practitioner Program
Graduate School of Nursing
University of Massachusetts
Worcester, Massachusetts

Deborah C. Allen, PhD, FNP-C, BC
Associate Professor,
Graduate Program Director
School of Nursing
Georgia Southern University
Statesboro, Georgia

Sharon Alzner, MPT, OCS
Clinical Specialist
Department of Rehabilitation Services
Brigham and Women's Hospital
Boston, Massachusetts

Patricia Polgar-Bailey, MS, MA, MPH
Family Nurse Practitioner
Pediatric Hematology/Oncology
University of Virginia
Charlottesville, Virginia

Marie A. Bakitas, DNSc, NP-C, FAAN
Professor, Marie O'Koren Endowed Chair
School of Nursing;
Associate Director,
Center for Palliative and Supportive Care
University of Alabama at Birmingham
Birmingham, Alabama

James T. Banta, MD
Associate Professor of Clinical Ophthalmology
Bascom Palmer Eye Institute
Miller School of Medicine
University of Miami
Miami, Florida

Jodie Barkin, MD
Division of Gastroenterology
Leonard W. Miller School of Medicine
University of Miami
Miami, Florida

María I. Bascarán, MD
Physical Medicine/Rehab
Partners HealthCare System, Inc
Boston, Massachusetts

Theresa A. Bedford, BSN, MSN
Family Nurse Practitioner
Family Health Clinic
Mike O'Callaghan Federal Medical Center
Nellis AFB, Nevada

Virginia L. Beggs, MSc, APRN, BC, CHFN
Heart and Vascular Center
Dartmouth-Hitchcock Medical Center
Lebanon, New Hampshire

Jillian C. Belmont, MSN, FNP-BC, SCRN
Advanced Practice Nurse Practitioner
Neurology
Dartmouth-Hitchcock Medical Center
Lebanon, New Hampshire;
Instructor in Neurology
Geisel School of Medicine at Dartmouth
Hanover, New Hampshire

Courtney L. Betts, MSN, ANP-BC
Adult Nurse Practitioner
New England Community Medical Services
North Andover, Massachusetts

Wendy L. Biddle, PhD, MSN, RN, FNP-BC
Program Director
MSN-FNP Program
South University
Virginia Beach, Virginia;
Nurse Practitioner
Gastroenterology LTD
Virginia Beach, Virginia

Barbara S. Bishop, MS, ANP-C, MSCN, CNRN
Adult Nurse Practitioner
Virginia Beach Neurology
Virginia Beach, Virginia

Margaret Firer Bishop, MSN, ANP-BC, ACHPN
Nurse Practitioner
Palliative Care Medicine
Sentara Martha Jefferson Hospital
Charlottesville, Virginia

Glen Blair, BS, MSN
Program Coordinator
Department of Dermatology
Harvard Vanguard Medical Associates
Boston, Massachusetts;
Lecturer
Graduate School of Nursing and Health Professions
University of Massachusetts
Boston, Massachusetts

Daniel Blaz, DNP, FNP-C
Assistant Professor
Graduate School of Nursing
Uniformed Services University of the Health Sciences
Bethesda, Maryland

Nathan Blessing, MD
Resident Physician
Bascom Palmer Eye Institute
University of Miami
Miami, Florida

Maureen Bell Boardman, BSN, MSN
Clinical Assistant Professor of Community and Family Medicine
Community and Family Medicine
Geisel School of Medicine at Dartmouth
Hanover, New Hampshire;
ARNP/Director of Clinical Quality
Little Rivers Healthcare
Bradford, Vermont

William A. Boller, MD, MS
Family Physician
Flight Line Clinic;
Chair
Pharmacy and Therapeutics Committee
Naval Hospital Sigonella
Sigonella, Catania, Italy

Marie Elena Botte, MSN, FNP-BC, CDE
Family Nurse Practitioner;
Diabetes Educator
Davis Square Family Practice
Somerville, Massachusetts

Nicole C. Bove, PCT
Virtua Health System
New Jersey

Susan E. Bove, MSN, APRN
Family Nurse Practitioner
Family Care Center
Stoneham, Massachusetts

Jennifer C. Braimon, MD
Endocrinologist;
Assistant Clinical Professor
Department of Endocrinology
Lahey Hospital and Medical Center
Tufts University School of Medicine
Peabody, Massachusetts

Susan Culbertson Brighton, MS, APRN, AOCMP
Nurse Practitioner
Hematology and Oncology
Dartmouth-Hitchcock Medical Center
Lebanon, New Hampshire

Lin A. Brown, MD
Clinical Professor of Medicine
Geisel School of Medicine at Dartmouth
Hanover, New Hampshire;
Staff Rheumatologist
New London Hospital
New London, New Hampshire

Ann S. Bruner-Welch, PA-C, DFAAPA, AS
Physician Assistant—Board Certified
Preoperative Medicine and Orthopedics
Kaiser Permanente
Santa Rosa, California

Jacqueline Rosenjack Burchum, DNSc, FNP-BC, CNE
Associate Professor
College of Nursing
Department of Advanced Practice and Doctoral Studies
University of Tennessee Health Science Center
Memphis, Tennessee

Terry Mahan Buttaro, PhD, ANP-BC, GNP-BC, FAANP, DPNAP
Assistant Clinical Professor
College of Nursing and Health Sciences
University of Massachusetts Boston
Boston, Massachusetts;
Nurse Practitioner
Coastal Medical Associates
Salisbury, Massachusetts

John R. Butterly, AB, MA, MD
Professor of Medicine
Geisel School of Medicine at Dartmouth
Hanover, New Hampshire;
Adjunct Professor, Geography
Dartmouth College
Hanover, New Hampshire

Virginia Curtin Capasso, PhD, ANP-BC, ACNS-BC, CWS, FACCWS
Nurse Practitoner
Wound Care Center;
Nurse Scientist
Munn Center for Nursing Research
Massachusetts General Hospital
Boston, Massachusetts;
Instructor in Surgery
Harvard Medical School
Boston, Massachusetts

Natalie N. Carrier, BA, MSN
Family Nurse Practitioner
Orthopaedics Surgery
Beth Israel Deaconess Medical Center
Boston, Massachusetts

Stephanie Cassone, MSN, FNP-BC, ACHPN
Nurse Practitioner
Palliative Care
Cedars Sinai Medical Center
Los Angeles, California

Barbara B. Chase, RN, MSN, ANP-C, CDE
Nurse Practitioner
MGH Chelsea Health Center
Massachusetts General Hospital
Chelsea, Massachusetts

Daniel S. Churgin, BS, MD
Resident Physician/Ophthalmologist
Bascom Palmer Eye Institute
Miami, Florida

Emma Virginia Clark, MHS, MSN
Certified Nurse Midwife
Community of Hope's Family Health and Birth Center
Washington, District of Columbia

Cara B. Cohen, MS, BS
Nurse Practitioner
Student Health Services
Assumption College,
Worcester, Massachusetts;
Instructor, Nursing
Simmons College
Boston, Massachusetts;
Instructor, Nursing
Worcester State University
Worcester, Massachusetts

Kathryn Colcher, MSN, FNP-BC
Family Nurse Practitioner
Private Practice
Herndon, Virginia;
Adjunct Instructor
School of Nursing and Health Studies
Georgetown University
Washington, District of Columbia

Michelle Collins, PhD, MSN, BSN
Professor, Director
Nurse-Midwifery Program
Vanderbilt University School of Nursing
Nashville, Tennessee

Kathleen M. Craig, MSN
Director
Women's and Children's Services
Rutland Regional Medical Center
Rutland, Vermont

Cathleen Crowley-Koschnitzki, DNP, CNM, WHNP, FNP
Assistant Professor
Family Nurse Practitioner Track
Chamberlain College of Nursing
Downers Grove, Illinois

Jennifer Culgin, BSN, MA
Hospice and Palliative Care Nurse Practitioner
Care Dimensions
Danvers, Massachusetts

Lauren Curtis, BSN, MSN
Nurse Practitioner
TAVR Program
Hartford Hospital
Hartford, Connecticut

Constance Dahlin, MSN, AB, ANP-BC, ACHPN, FPCN, FAAN
Director of Professional Practice
Hospice and Palliative Nurses Association
Pittsburgh, Pennsylvania;
Co-Director APRN Externship
Massey Cancer Center
Virginia Commonwealth University
Richmond, Virginia;
Consultant
Center to Advance Palliative Care
New York, New York;
Palliative Nurse Practitioner
Palliative Care Service
North Shore Medical Center
Salem, Massachusetts

Melissa C. Davis, MSN
Nurse Practitioner
Hematology/Oncology
Dartmouth-Hitchcock Medical Center
Lebanon, New Hampshire

Keith A. Deardorff, BSN, MA, MSN
Family Nurse Practitioner—Certified
Family Health Clinic
Mike O'Callaghan Federal Medical Center
Nellis Air Force Base, Nevada

Kerry A. Decker, MSN
Nurse Practitioner
UCSF Medical Center
San Francisco, California

Henry DeGroot III, MD
Instructor in Orthopedic Surgery
Tufts University Medical School
Medford, Massachusetts;
Clinical Associate Professor
Orthopedic Surgery
University of Massachusetts
Amherst, Massachusetts;
Staff Orthopedic Surgeon
Newton Wellesley Hospital
Newton, Massachusetts

Karen Dick, PhD, GNP-BC, FAANP
Associate Dean for Advanced Practice Programs
Graduate School of Nursing
University of Massachusetts Medical School
Worcester, Massachusetts;
Nurse Practitioner
Hebrew Senior Life
Boston, Massachusetts

Mary DiGiulio, DNP, ANP-BC, GNP-BC
Director of Clinical Practice
School of Nursing
Rutgers, the State University of New Jersey
Newark, New Jersey;
Nurse Practitioner
Bergen Volunteer Medical Initiative
Hackensack, New Jersey

Jodie Dionne-Odom, MD
Assistant Professor
Medicine, Division of Infectious Diseases
University of Alabama at Birmingham
Birmingham, Alabama

John Distler, DPA, MBA, MS, FNP-C, FAANP
Dean, Nurse Practitioner Tracks
Chamberlain College of Nursing
Downers Grove, Illinois

Evelyn Duffy, BS, MS, DNP
Associate Professor
Bolton School of Nursing
Case Western Reserve University
Cleveland, Ohio;
Adult Gerontology Nurse Practitioner
Geriatric Medicine
University Hospitals of Cleveland
Cleveland, Ohio

Catherine Marie Duffy, MSN, APRN-BC, ACHPN
Nurse Practitioner
Palliative Care
Care Dimensions
Danvers, Massachusetts

Joel Dulaigh, MSN, ACNP-BC
NOAA Diving Medical Officer
NOAA Diving Program
National Oceanic and Atmospheric Administration
Seattle, Washington

Quannetta Tucker Edwards, BSN, MSN, MS, PhD
Dr (PhD) Professor
College of Graduate Nursing
Western University of Health Sciences
Pomona, California

Andrea Efre, DNP, ARNP, ANP-BC
Owner, Nurse Practitioner and Educator
Healthcare Education Consultants
Tampa, Florida

Kathryn K. Ellis, DNP, ANP-BC, FNP-BC
Assistant Professor
School of Nursing & Health Studies
Georgetown University
Washington, District of Columbia

Sabine Eustache, DrPH, MBA, MPH
Public Health Consultant
SEJ Associates, Inc.
Jenkintown, Pennsylvania

Kathy J. Fabiszewski, PhD, RN, BC
Adult/Gerontological Nurse Practitioner
Harvard Vanguard Medical Associates
Peabody, Massachusetts

Camilo E. Fadul, MD, FAAN
Professor of Neurology
University of Virginia School of Medicine
Charlottesville, Virginia

Heidi Collins Fantasia, PhD, RN, WHNP-BC
Assistant Professor
College of Health Sciences, School of Nursing
University of Massachusetts Lowell
Lowell, Massachusetts;
Women's Health Nurse Practitioner
Health Quarters
Beverly, Massachusetts

Mary E. Farrell, RN, PhD, CCRN
Professor Emerita
School of Nursing
Salem State University
Salem, Massachusetts

Matthew Favazza, MSN, FNP-BC
Family Nurse Practitioner
Internal Medicine
Seacoast Medical Associates
Newburyport, Massachusetts;
Associative Consultant
Integrative & Complementary Medicine
Summit Health Products
Tampa, Florida;
Clinical Preceptor
Simmons College
Boston, Massachusetts

Henrique J. Fernandez, MD, FACP
Director, Gastroenterology Fellowship
Gastroenterology
Parkview Medical Center
Pueblo, Colorado

Carey J. Field, MD
Staff Rheumatologist
Rheumatology
Dartmouth-Hitchcock Medical Center
Lebanon, New Hampshire

Jane Flanagan, PhD, ANP-BC
Associate Professor, Program Director
William F. Connell School of Nursing
Boston College
Chestnut Hill, Massachusetts

Brad E. Franklin, DNP, RN, FNP-C
Officer in Charge, Byrd Medical Home
Blanchfield Army Community Hospital
Fort Campbell, Kentucky

Catherine M. Franklin, NP, DNP
Family Nurse Practitioner
East Boston Neighborhood Health Center
Boston, Massachusetts

Michelle Freshman, MPH, MSN, APRN, FNP-BC
Nurse Practitioner
Department of Medicine
Newton-Wellesley Hospital
Newton, Massachusetts

Alexander Fuld, MD, MS
Section of Hematology/Oncology
White River Junction Veterans Affairs Medical Center
White River Junction, Vermont;
Assistant Professor of Medicine
Department of Medicine
Geisel School of Medicine at Dartmouth
Hanover, New Hampshire

Anthony S. Gemignani, MD
Cardiologist
Cardiology
White River Junction Veterans Affairs Medical Center
White River Junction, Vermont;
Assistant Professor
Geisel School of Medicine at Dartmouth
Dartmouth, New Hampshire

Maryjane Giacalone, MS
ANP, ACNP-BC
Cardiology
Massachusetts General Hospital
Boston, Massachusetts

Cene' L. Gibson, DNP, APRN, FNP-C, CNE
Assistant Professor of Nursing
Kramer School of Nursing
Oklahoma City University
Oklahoma City, Oklahoma

Meghan Glynn, MSN, FNP-BC
Family Nurse Practitioner
Francisan Hospital for Children
Brighton, Massachusetts

Donna M. Glynn, PhD, RN, ANP-BC
Assistant Professor of Nursing Practice
School of Nursing and Health Sciences
Simmons College
Boston, Massachusetts;
Nurse Scientist
Nursing Administration
VA Boston Healthcare System
West Roxbury, Massachusetts

Randy Michael Gordon, DNP, FNP-BC
Assistant Professor
Graduate Program, Family Nurse Practitioner Track
Chamberlain College of Nursing
Downers Grove, Illinois

Sharon L. Grantham, MSN, DNP
Advanced Registered Nurse Practitioner
Family Practice
Dr. Grantham & Associates, LLC
Fort Myers, Florida

John J. Graykoski, MPAS
Instructor
Emergency Medicine
Mayo Clinic Medical School
Rochester, Minnesota;
Staff Emergency Medicine
Physician Assistant
Community Emergency Medicine
Mayo Clinic Health System
Barron, Wisconsin

Glen P. Greenough, MD
Assistant Professor
Psychiatry and Neurology
Geisel School of Medicine at Dartmouth
Lebanon, New Hampshire

Ann Guttendorf, MS, NP-C
Nurse Practitioner
Interventional Cardiology/Interventional Vascular
Massachusetts General Hospital
Boston, Massachusetts

Patricia Hadidian, NP
Nurse Practitioner – Gerontology
Edith Nourse Rogers Memorial Veterans Memorial Hospital
Bedford, Massachusetts

Mellisa A. Hall, DNP, AGNP-BC, FNP-BC
Associate Professor of Nursing
University of Southern Indiana
Evansville, Indiana

Wendy Halm, DNP, FNP-BC
Clinical Assistant Professor
School of Nursing
University of Wisconsin Madison
Madison, Wisconsin

Wanda J. Handel, MSN, RN, ACCNS-AG, CNRN
Clinical Nurse Specialist—Neuroscience
Office of Professional Nursing
Dartmouth-Hitchcock Medical Center
Lebanon, New Hampshire

Eric Hansen, MD
Ophthalmology
Bascom Palmer Eye Institute
Miami, Florida

Margaret Thorman Hartig, PhD, APRN-BC, FAANP
Professor
Advanced Practice and Doctoral Studies
College of Nursing
University of Tennessee Health Science Center
Memphis, Tennessee

Jean P. Hartin del Castillo, MSN, ARNP, FNP-BC
Nurse Practitioner
Cardiology
University of Miami Health System
Miami, Florida

Simon M. Helfgott, MD, CM
Director
Education and Fellowship Training
Division of Rheumatology
Brigham and Women's Hospital
Boston, Massachusetts;
Associate Professor of Medicine
Harvard Medical School
Boston, Massachusetts

Michael Huang, MD
Fellow
Gastroenterology
Miller School of Medicine
University of Miami
Miami, Florida

Zacharia Isaac, MD
Director, Interventional Physical Medicine and Rehabilitation
Physical Medicine and Rehabilitation
Harvard Medical School
Boston, Massachusetts;
Medical Director, Comprehensive Spine Care Center
Brigham and Women's Hospital
Boston, Massachusetts

Brian Jennings, MD
Resident Physician
University of Connecticut School of Medicine
Farmington, Connecticut

Robyn Meredith Jennings, MD, MPH
Family Medicine Resident
North Colorado Family Medicine Residency Program
Greeley, Colorado

Dorothy K. Johnson, FNP, PhD
Nurse Practitioner
Rheumatology
LAC/USC Healthcare Network
Los Angeles, California

Brenda L. Jordan, MSN, APRN,
Nurse Practitioner
Dartmouth-Hitchcock Medical Center—Kendal
Lebanon, New Hampshire;
Clinical Instructor
Department of Community & Family Medicine
Dartmouth Medical School
Hanover, New Hampshire

Patricia Jordano, BS, MS, ANP, ACNP
Nurse Practitioner
Cardiology
Massachusetts General Hospital
Boston, Massachusetts

Brooke G. Judd, MD
Section Chief, Sleep Medicine
Dartmouth-Hitchcock Medical Center
Lebanon, New Hampshire;
Assistant Professor of Psychiatry, Sleep Medicine
Geisel School of Medicine at Dartmouth
Hanover, New Hampshire

Daniel E. Kane, MEd, BSN, CEN, CCRN, CFRN, EMT-P
Assistant Professor
Clinical Simulation Lab Coordinator
School of Nursing
MGH Institute of Health Professions
Boston, Massachusetts

Elaine D. Kauschinger, PhD, MS, ARNP, FNP-BC
Assistant Professor of Nursing
School of Nursing
Duke University
Durham, North Carolina

Marilyn Juliette Kenebrew, BSN, MSN, RN, APP
Advanced Practice Nurse
Integrative Medicine
MD Anderson Cancer Center
Houston, Texas

Lori Keough, PhD, MEd, FNP-BC, PMHNP-BC
Assistant Professor
School of Nursing
University of Massachusetts, Lowell
Lowell, Massachusetts;
Nurse Practitioner
Adolescent Medicine
Boston Children's Hospital
Boston, Massachusetts

Kevin D. Kerin, MD
Physician, Rheumatology
University of Vermont Health Network
Central Vermont Medical Center
Berlin, Vermont

David H. Kerman, MD
Assistant Professor, Clinical Medicine
Division of Gastroenterology
Leonard W. Miller School of Medicine
University of Miami
Miami, Florida

Elizabeth Kimtis, BA, BSN, MSN, APRN
Nurse Practitioner
Hematology/Oncology
Dartmouth-Hitchcock Medical Center
Lebanon, New Hampshire

Audrey C. Ko, MD
Physician
Department of Ophthalmology
Bascom Palmer Eye Institute
Miami, Florida

Seth Kolkin, MD
Service Chief
Neurology, Physiatry and Rehabilitation
White River Junction VA Medical Center
White River Junction, Vermont

Nancy Kuemmerle, DO, PhD
Staff Physician
Medicine, Section of Hematology/Oncology
Veterans Affairs Medical Center
White River Junction, Vermont;
Assistant Professor of Medicine
Geisel School of Medicine at Dartmouth
Hanover, New Hampshire

Elissa Ladd, PhD, FNP-BC
Associate Professor, Nursing
MGH Institute of Health Professions
Boston, Massachusetts

Lindsey Law, BS, MPAS, PA-C
Physician Assistant
Gastrointestinal Medical Oncology
UT MD Anderson Cancer Center
Houston, Texas

Nancy McQueen Le, MSN, GNP, CNRN
Gerentologic Nurse Practitioner
Boston University School of Medicine
Department of Neurology
Braintree Rehabilitation Hospital
Braintree, Massachusetts

Renato Lenzi, MD
Associate Professor
Department of GI Medical Oncology
University of Texas MD Anderson Cancer Center
Houston, Texas

V. Ted Leon, MD, MPH
Assistant Clinical Professor
Department of Family and Community Medicine
John A. Burns School of Medicine
University of Hawaii
Honolulu, Hawaii;
Director
Cardiac Exercise Stress Laboratory
The Queens Medical Center
Honolulu, Hawaii;
Attending Physician
University of Hawaii Student Health Services
University of Hawaii, Manoa
Honolulu, Hawaii

JoAnn Lepke, MSN, FNP-BC, RN, MBA, BSE
Nurse Practitioner
Dr. George Martin Dermatology Associates
Kihei, Hawaii;
Family Nurse Practitioner
North Shore Medical Center
Kilauea, Hawaii

Leslie Levitan, NP
Nurse Practitioner
Palliative Care
Danvers, Massachusetts

Catherine G. Ling, PhD, FNP-BC, FAANP
Assistant Professor
Daniel K. Inouye Graduate School of Nursing
Uniformed Services University of the Health Sciences
Bethesda, Maryland

Magen Lorenzi, MSN, FNP-BC
Family Nurse Practitioner
Primary Care
Upham's Corner Health Center
Boston, Massachusetts

Rene Love, DNP, PMHNP
DNP Director, Clinical Associate Professor
Nursing
University of Arizona
Tucson, Arizona

Patricia Lowry, BS, MS
Acute Care Nurse Practitioner
Cardiology
Massachusetts General Hospital
Boston, Massachusetts

Jason R. Lucey, MSN, FNP-BC
Assistant Professor
School of Nursing
MGH Institute of Health Professions
Boston, Massachusetts

Erin Lyden, MSN, BSN, BS, FNP-C
North Port, Florida

Margaret Ann Mahoney, PhD, ANP
Assistant Professor
School of Nursing
MGH Institute of Health Professions
Charlestown, Massachusetts

Alan Ona Malabanan, MD
Staff Physician
Endocrinology, Diabetes and Metabolism
Beth Israel Deaconess Medical Center
Boston, Massachusetts

Maura A. Malone, MSN, RN
Clinical Nurse Specialist
Hemophilia and Thrombosis
Hematology
Dartmouth-Hitchcock Medical Center
Lebanon, New Hampshire

Ann H. Maradiegue, PhD, BC-FNP, FAANP
Nurse Practitioner Consultant
Department of Nursing
James Madison University
Harrisonburg, Virginia

Bryan J. Marsh, MD
Associate Professor of Medicine
Section of Infectious Disease
Dartmouth-Hitchcock Medical Center
Lebanon, New Hampshire;
Associate Professor of Medicine
Section of Infectious Disease
Geisel School of Medicine at Dartmouth
Hanover, New Hampshire

Christina F. Martin, MSN, APRN, FNP-BC
Clinical Specialist, Nurse Practitioner
Dartmouth-Hitchcock Medical Center
Lebanon, New Hampshire

Varghese Mathai, MPAS, MDiv
Physician Assistant
Lymphoma/Myeloma
MC Anderson Cancer Center
Houston, Texas

Kathleen Rose Golden McAndrew, DNP, ANP, COHN-S, CCM, FAAOHN, FAANP
Adult Nurse Practitioner, Occupational and Environmental Health
University of Massachusetts Boston
Boston, Massachusetts

Elizabeth B. McCabe, MS, APRN
Nurse Practitioner, Surgical Oncology
Dartmouth-Hitchcock Medical Center
Lebanon, New Hampshire

Katherine McCube, MSN, FNP-BC
Family Nurse Practitioner
Plymouth Heart Center
Plymouth, Massachusetts

Talli McCormick, BS, MSN, GNP
Clinical Assistant Professor
School of Nursing
MGH Institute of Health Professions
Boston, Massachusetts

Annette McDonough, PhD, CNS
Assistant Professor
Nursing
University of Massachusetts
Lowell, Massachusetts;
Faculty Scientist
Munn Center for Nursing Research
Massachusetts General Hospital
Boston, Massachusetts

Laurel McKernan, MSN, RN
Hemophilia Clinical Specialist
Section of Hematology
Dartmouth-Hitchcock Medical Center
Lebanon, New Hampshire

MAJ Sheila Ann Medina, DNP, FNP-C, MBA
Family Nurse Practitioner
Chief, Soldier Center Medical Home
Bassett Army Community Hospital (BACH)
Fort Wainwright, Alaska

Maria Meklis, JD, BSN, RN
Patient Safety Risk Specialist
Boston Medical Center
Boston, Massachusetts

Ashley Moore-Gibbs, MSN, AGPCNP-BC, CHFN
Nurse Practitioner
Adult Cardiology
Sanger Heart & Vascular Institute
Charlotte, North Carolina

Deanne Munroe, JD, MSN
Director, Ambulatory Risk Management
Enterprise Risk Managemnet
PIH Health Hospital—Whittier
Whittier, California;
Lecturer
School of Nursing
California State University, Los Angeles
Los Angeles, California

David Patrick Murphy, MD, FCCP
Head, Pulmonary/Critical Care Medicine
Internal Medicine
Naval Hospital Camp Pendleton
Camp Pendleton, California

Jennifer A. Neves, BSN, MSN
Nurse Practitioner
Hospitalist Service
Massachusetts Eye and Ear
Boston, Massachusetts

Thuy Dang Nguyen, MD
Medical Resident
Internal Medicine
Dartmouth-Hitchcock Medical Center
Lebanon, New Hampshire

Patrice K. Nicholas, DNSc, DHL (Hon.), MPH, MS, RN, ANP, FAAN
Professor
School of Nursing
MGH Institute of Health Professions
Boston, Massachusetts;
Director and Senior Nurse Scientist
Division of Global Health Equity and Center for Nursing Excellence
Brigham and Women's Hospital
Boston, Massachusetts

Neda Nikpoor, MD
Resident
Opthalmology
Bascom Palmer Eye Institute
Miami, Florida

Michael L. Norris, MS, AuD
Clinical Audiologist (Retired)
Otolaryngology/Audiology Section
Dartmouth-Hitchcock Medical Center
Louisville, Kentucky

Peter Oates, RN, MSN, NP-C, ACRN
Director, Health Care Services
François-Xavier Bagnoud Center
Rutgers School of Nursing
Newark, New Jersey

Lisa O'Neal, MSN, MS, BSN, BA, ACNP-BC, ANP-BC
Charlotte, North Carolina

Daniel W. O'Neill, MD
Assistant Professor
Clinical Family Medicine
University of Connecticut School of Medicine
Farmington, Connecticut;
Physician
Family Medicine
Day Kimball Medical Group
Putnam, Connecticut

Deborah L. Ornstein, MD
Associate Professor
Medicine and Pathology
Dartmouth Medical School
Hanover, New Hampshire;
Medical Director
Hemophilia and Thrombosis Center
Dartmouth-Hitchcock Medical Center
Lebanon, New Hampshire

Diane Todd Pace, PhD, APRN, FNP-BC, NCMP, FAANP
Associate Professor/Director
DNP Program
College of Nursing
University of Tennessee Health Science Center
Memphis, Tennessee

Vincent Pair, DNP, MSN, MS, BSN, BS, BA
US Army
Active Duty Clinic
Kenner Army Health Clinic
Fort Lee, Virginia

Donna Jenell Pease, BSN, MSN, ANP, GNP, CDE, BC-ADM
Diabetes Nurse Practitioner
Gold Medical Home
Blanchfield Army Community Hospital
Fort Campbell, Kentucky

Kenneth Scott Peterson, PhD, FNP-BC
Assistant Professor
Graduate School of Nursing
University of Massachusetts
Worcester, Massachusetts;
Family Nurse Practitioner
Plumley Village Health Services
UMass Memorial Medical Center
Worcester, Massachusetts

Stephen Pixley, RN, BS
Emergency Preparedness Coordinator
Emergency Management
Dartmouth-Hitchcock Medical Center
Lebanon, New Hampshire;
Staff RN
Emergency Department
Alice Peck Day Memorial Hospital
Lebanon, New Hampshire

Richard M. Prior, DNP, MSN, FNP-BC, FAANP
Chief Nursing Officer
Ireland Army Community Hospital
Fort Knox, Kentucky

Francisco P. Quismorio, Jr., MD, MACR, FACP
Professor of Medicine and Pathology
Keck School of Medicine
University of Southern California
Los Angeles, California

Laura A. Rabin, PhD
Professor
Department of Psychology
Brooklyn College and the Graduate Center
The City University of New York, Brooklyn
New York, New York

Lindsay N. Ramey, MD
Resident Physician
Physical Medicine and Rehabilitation
Spaulding Rehabilitation Hospital
Charlestown, Massachusetts

Sarah Read, MD, PhD
Department of Ophthalmology
Bascom Palmer Eye Institute
Miami, Florida

Geri Cage Reeves, MSN, PhD
Program Director, FNP Program
Nursing
Vanderbilt University School of Nursing
Nashville, Tennessee

Patricia A. Reidy, DNP, FNP-BC
Clinical Associate Professor
School of Nursing
Institute of Health Professions
Massachusetts General Hospital
Boston, Massachusetts;
Family Nurse Practitioner
Family Health Center of Worcester
Worcester, Massachusetts

Suzanne Rieke, MD
Endocrinologist, Assistant Clinical Professor
Tufts University School of Medicine
Department of Endocrinology
Lahey Hospital and Medical Center
Peabody, Massachusetts

Wendy A. Ritch, MA, MTS
Doctoral Student
Urban Systems Joint PhD Program
Rutgers University and NJIT
Newark, New Jersey

Marylou Virginia Robinson, PhD, FNP-C
Associate Professor
College of Nursing
University of Colorado Denver
Aurora, Colorado

Maria Isabel Romano, MSN, NP-C, ARNP
Family Nurse Practitioner
Kendall Medical Center
Miami, Florida

Isabella Rosa-Cunha, MD
Associate Professor of Clinical Medicine
Medicine/Division of Infectious Diseases
Miller School of Medicine
University of Miami
Miami, Florida
Charlottesville, Virginia

Joanne Sandberg-Cook, MS, APRN, ANP, GNP-BC
Adult/Gerontological Nurse Practitioner
Dartmouth-Hitchcock Medical Center, Kendal (Retired)
Hanover, New Hampshire

Susan Sanner, PhD, APRN, FNP-BC
Associate Professor of Nursing
MSN FNP Program
Chamberlain College of Nursing
Downer's Grove, Illinois

Anna D. Schaal, RN, MS, APRN
Nurse Practitioner
Hematology
Norris Cotton Cancer Center
Dartmouth-Hitchcock Medical Center
Lebanon, New Hampshire

Naomi Schlesinger, MD
Chief, Division of Rheumatology
Department of Medicine
Rutgers—Robert Wood Johnson Medical School
New Brunswick, New Jersey

Terri Schmitt, PhD, ARNP, FNP-BC, CDE
Associate Professor
Family Nurse Practitioner Track
Chamberlain College of Nursing
Jacksonville, Florida;
Nurse Practitioner
Pediatric Diabetes and Endocrine
Palm Beach Gardens, Florida

Karen L. Secore, MS, APRN, CNRN
Nurse Practitioner/Coordinator
Dartmouth-Hitchcock Epilepsy Center
Dartmouth-Hitchcock Medical Center
Lebanon, New Hampshire

Diane C. Seibert, PhD, MSN, BSN
Interim Associate Dean for Academic Affairs
Graduate School of Nursing
Uniformed Services University
Bethesda, Maryland

Margaret Sennett, RN, MS, CPNP
Pediatric Nurse Practitioner
Pediatric Hematology & Oncology
University of Virginia Children's Hospital
Charlottesville, Virginia

Ruta M. Shah, MD, PhD
Attending Physician
Infectious Diseases
North Shore Medical Center
Salem, Massachusetts

Laura Elyse Shevy, MD
Internist, Hospital Medicine
Dartmouth-Hitchcock Medical Center
Lebanon, New Hampshire

Rebecca Shields, MD
Resident Physician
Bascom Palmer Eye Institute
University of Miami Health System
Miami, Florida

Emily Karwacki Sheff, MS, RN, CMSRN, FNP-BC
Clinical Instructor
Institute of Health Professions
Massachusetts General Hospital
Boston, Massachusetts;
Nursing Practice and Standards Coordinator
Catholic Medical Center
Manchester, New Hampshire

Pamela Slaven-Lee, DNP, FNP-C, CHSE
Assistant Professor
Graduate School of Nursing
The George Washington University
Washington, District of Columbia

Laurie Soroken, MS, ANP-BC
Clinical Assistant Professor
School of Nursing
University of Massachusetts at Lowell
Lowell, Massachusetts

Julie G. Stewart, DNP, MPH, MSN, FNP-BC
Associate Professor
College of Nursing
Sacred Heart University
Fairfield, Connecticut

Jack D. Stringham, MD
Resident Physician
Bascom Palmer Eye Institute
University of Miami Health System
Miami, Florida

Kathryn D. Swartwout, PhD, APN, FNP-BC
Assistant Professor
Community Systems and Mental Health Nursing
Rush University
Chicago, Illinois

Elizabeth A. Talbot, MD
Associate Professor
Medicine
Geisel School of Medicine at Dartmouth
Hanover, New Hampshire;
Deputy State Epidemiologist
New Hampshire Department of Health and Human Services
Concord, New Hampshire

Ashley Taylor, MSN, FNP-C
Urgent Care and Convenient Care
Augusta Health, Augusta Medical Group
Fisherville, Virginia

Thomas H. Taylor, MD
Chief of Infectious Diseases and Rheumatology
Medicine
White River Junction VA Hospital
White River Junction, Vermont;
Associate Professor of Medicine
Geisel School of Medicine at Dartmouth
Hanover, New Hampshire

Derrick J. Todd, MD, PhD
Staff Physician,
Rheumatology, Immunology, & Allergy
Brigham & Women's Hospital
Boston, Massachusetts

JoAnn Trybulski, PhD, MSN, BS
Director
DNP Program
Chamberlain College of Nursing
Chicago, Illinois

Nena Tucker, DNP, MBA, FNP-C
Assistant Professor
Nursing
Southeastern Louisiana University
Hammond, Louisiana

Denise A. Vanacore-Chase, PhD, CRNP, ANP-BC, PMHNP
Director, DNP & NP Programs
Graduate Nursing
Gwynedd Mercy University
Gwynedd Valley, Pennsylvania

Rose Vick, MSN
Faculty Instructor
Psychiatric Mental Health Nurse
Practitioner Program
Vanderbilt University School of Nursing
Nashville, Tennessee

J. Nile Wagley, PhD
Founder
Rational Therapeutics, PLC
Charlottesville, Virginia;
Visiting Assistant Professor
Psychiatry and Neurobehavioral Sciences
The University of Virginia
Charlottesville, Virginia

Scott D. Walter, MD, MSc
Resident Physician
Ophthalmology
Bascom Palmer Eye Institute
Miller School of Medicine
University of Miami
Miami, Florida;
Vitreoretinal Surgery Fellow
Ophthalmology
Duke University Eye Center
Durham, North Carolina

Kevin Wei, MD, PhD
Fellow, Medicine
Division of Rheumatology, Immunology, and Allergy
Brigham and Women's Hospital
Boston, Massachusetts

Alicia Wierenga, MSN, NP
Nurse Practitioner
Vascular Surgery
UMASS Memorial Hospital
Worcester, Massachusetts

Alexandra Wilder, MSN, ANP-BC
Nurse Practitioner
Cambridge, Massachusetts

Jane Taylor Williams, MSN, RN, FNP-BC
Advanced Practice Nurse
Integrative Medicine Program
MD Anderson Cancer Center
Houston, Texas

Christine Wilson, PhD, ANP-BC, FNP-BC
Medical Affairs
Omeros Corporation
Seattle, Washington

Diane Wink, EdD, FNP-BC
Professor Emerita
Graduate Department College of Nursing
University of Central Florida
Orlando, Florida

Chris Winkelman, RN, PhD, CCRN, ACNP, FAANP, FCCM
Associate Professor
Frances Payne Bolton School of Nursing
Case Western Reserve University
Cleveland, Ohio

Mary E. Wood, RN, MS, CDE, BC-ADM
Diabetes Clinical Nurse Specialist
Nursing Practice
Dartmouth-Hitchcock Medical Center
Lebanon, New Hampshire;
Instructor, Community and Family Medicine
The Geisel School of Medicine at Dartmouth
Hanover, New Hampshire

Ryan Young, MD
Fellow
Bascom Palmer Eye Institute
University of Miami Health System
Miami, Florida

Mary Young-Breuleux, MSN, APRN, BC, CNE
Adult Nurse Practitioner
Good Neighbor Health Clinic
White River Junction, Vermont

Leo R. Zacharski, MD
Active Emeritus Professor of Medicine
Geisel School of Medicine
Dartmouth College
Hanover, New Hampshire

Elke Jones Zschaebitz, DNP, FNP-BC
Nurse Practitioner
General Medicine
University of Virginia
Charlottesville, Virginia;
Faculty
Department of Nusting and Health Science
Georgetown University
Washington, District of Columbia

Randall M. Zusman, MD, BS
Associate Professor of Medicine
Harvard Medical School;
Director, Section of Hypertension and Vascular Medicine
Massachusetts General Hospital;
Consultant (Cardiology)
Massachusetts Institute of Technology
Boston, Massachusetts

Reviewers

Diane Daddario, MSN, ANP-C, ACNS-BC, RN-BC CMSRN
Certified Registered Nurse Practitioner
Geisinger Medical Center
Danville, Pennsylvania
Pennsylvania State University
University Park, Pennsylvania

Janice B., Foust, PhD, RN
Associate Professor
Department of Nursing
University of Massachusetts—Boston
Boston, Massachusetts

LaWanda Herron, PhD, MSA, MSN, FNP-BC
Director of the Associate Degree Nursing Program
Holmes Community College
Grenada, Mississippi

Tamara Kear, PhD, RN, CNS, CNN
Assistant Professor of Nursing
Villanova Nursing
Villanova, Pennsylvania

Cathy R. Kessenich, PhD, ARNP, FAANP
Professor of Nursing
University of Tampa
Tampa, Florida

Susanne Quallich, ANP-BC, NP-C, CUNP, FAANP
Andrology Nurse Practitioner
University of Michigan Medical Center
Department of Urology
Ann Arbor, Michigan

Preface

Since the very first edition of *Primary Care: A Collaborative Practice*, our vision has been to emphasize the value of professionals working together to improve patient care and well-being. In the past twenty years, hundreds of healthcare professionals from a wide geographic range have shared that vision and worked jointly with us and others in this intellectual endeavor. We, the editors, work together respecting one another's unique talents and strengths, solving problems together, just as you as healthcare professionals do each day. In the clinical setting collaboration is the essence of interprofessional care, and team-based care is a fundamental component of complex care management. Most important, though, is the collaborative partnership between patient and provider. These relationships are the foundation of high-performing primary care practices.

NEW CHAPTERS

In the fifth edition of *Primary Care: A Collaborative Practice* we introduce several new chapters to our readers. Each of these chapters recognizes aspects of clinical practice that are fundamental yet at times perhaps not fully considered. In **Transitional Care (Chapter 2)**, we explore the increasing responsibilities of caring for patients across the continuum of care. Our hope in providing this chapter is that understanding the challenges that patients and families face when entering or leaving a healthcare facility will aid in preventing adverse events, stress, and re-hospitalizations. Because many of our patients prefer a more holistic approach to health and well-being, **The Patient, The Provider and Primary Care: An Integrated Perspective** examines Western and Eastern healthcare practices in providing patient-centered care. Information about alternative therapies in which many patients and caregivers are interested enables nurse practitioners and other primary care providers to more fully understand the risks and benefits of the supplements that patients are using. **Minimizing Clinical Risk in the Primary Care Setting** identifies the attitudes and relationship skills in healthcare settings that can positively or negatively impact the patient's perceptions of the patient-provider relationship. The chapter authors address the legal risks inherent in practice and recommend strategies to improve care, patient satisfaction, and risk management. **LGBTQ Patient Care** reflects the editors' concern about disparities in healthcare, with the hope that the information in this chapter will aid all of us in improving care for all patients. The impetus for the **Pulmonary Embolism** chapter is that an estimated 60,000 to 100,000 people in the United States die each year from pulmonary embolisms, in part because the associated signs and symptoms can be nonspecific. We hope that raised awareness of the risk factors and clinical presentation variables will decrease this morbidity and mortality.

FORMAT

The format of the fifth edition of *Primary Care: A Collaborative Practice* purposefully is similar to the systematic approach used in primary care practice. The **Evaluation** and **Management** sections are organized to promote improved clinical reasoning skills. Understanding the **Epidemiology** and **Pathophysiology** of illness is integral to understanding a patient's symptoms and the consideration of possible causes. The **Clinical Presentation** and **Physical Examination** sections in each chapter address the cognitive, physical, or psychosocial features and physical exam findings that can be associated with the patient's complaint. Attention to the patient's concerns and detection of pertinent positive and negative findings are the clues that create the list of possible **Differential Diagnoses.** "Differentials" require clinical reasoning, a decision-making process that helps determine the most likely diagnosis and necessary **Diagnostics.** To aid in this process, the Differential Diagnosis boxes list possible differentials, and the Diagnostics boxes list appropriate tests that can be considered. These include initial tests (tests that may be performed in the office setting, such as peak flow measurement or pulse oximetry), laboratory tests, imaging studies (radiographic, ultrasound, nuclear, or magnetic resonance imaging), or other miscellaneous studies that may be necessary in the evaluation of the disorder (such as EEGs or biopsies). Because the clinical presentation differs with each patient, not all diagnostic tests listed may be necessary in each circumstance. An asterisk is placed beside those tests that may be indicated by clinical presentation and physical examination findings. For more detailed information, the reader should refer to the "Diagnostics" and "Differential Diagnosis" sections included with each disorder.

The **Management** section of each chapter addresses goals of treatment and therapeutic interventions based on current evidence and guidelines. Pharmacologic agents are included, as are recommendations for non-pharmacologic therapies. The management sections make every attempt to incorporate the research contributions that create an evidence base for practice. Authoritative management guidelines, as well as current ongoing research findings, are incorporated whenever available. As with any evolving science, recommendations can be in a state of flux. Management recommendations may change, and new recommendations for practice supersede the management recommendations presented in this textbook. In addition, the reader is directed to check drug indications, dosages, and potential drug-drug interactions in medication product information before prescribing or administering any medication.

Complications associated with the disease and treatments are described, and clear recommendations for **Patient and Family Education** are included throughout the textbook. This information is crucial in promoting health literacy and assisting healthcare providers in interpreting information about the illness and management to patients and caregivers.

This edition continues to provide clear guidelines for referrals, and the **Emergency and Physician Referral Icons** highlight conditions that may require immediate consultation. The reader should be aware that more comprehensive referral or consultation criteria are contained in the text of the chapters that contain these special icons. The reader should also realize that the emergency icons might not represent all of the conditions requiring emergency referral. The editors are also aware that experienced providers may not require consultation for all the specified circumstances. In addition, state practice regulations may mandate referral under certain circumstances; these regulations supersede any consultation recommendations detailed in this text.

New to the 5th edition is a collection of Instructor Resources on an Evolve website (http://evolve.elsevier.com/Buttaro), available via your Elsevier Education Solutions Consultant for programs adopting classroom quantities of the book. The Instructor Resources consist of a Test Bank, PowerPoint Collection, and Image Collection. The Test Bank includes approximately 685 test items delivered in Evolve Assessment Manager for easy exam construction and administration. The PowerPoint Collection consists of approximately 685 slides for classroom or online instruction. The Image Collection includes all original images from the textbook. We trust that these frequently requested resources will help to facilitate high-quality instruction of Nurse Practitioner students.

THE FUTURE

It is evident that an aging population, globalization, science, and technology will impact healthcare and clinical practice in the future. An aging population with multiple co-morbidities is likely to result in increased healthcare expenditures unless we are able to identify and control these diseases early and effectively. Global travel and an increase in transnational businesses have increased the risk of disease spread and the importance of vigilant awareness of global threats to the public health. Every day, scientific breakthroughs affect disease management, healthcare quality, and health information management. It is clear that to meet the healthcare needs of the future, innovative technology will be needed to relieve the cognitive burden created by these new discoveries. According to Dr. Yuri Ostrovsky, a Boston neuroscientist, "Digitized data collected from patients can identify relevant knowledge from the scientific literature[,] alerting healthcare providers to warning signs, common or obscure, and freeing up valuable time to focus on the personal and emotional needs of patients." It is the editors' hope that *Primary Care: A Collaborative Practice,* fifth edition, will provide a solid foundation on which tomorrow's primary care providers can help patients to lead increasingly healthy lives.

ACKNOWLEDGMENTS

This textbook represents a strong collaborative effort. We remain indebted to our contributors, past and present. They generously provided their time and expertise to make this textbook the trusted resource that it is. We welcome and are appreciative of the contributions made by our patients, students, and colleagues. We continue to try to incorporate their suggestions to make this book a useful one for students and practicing clinicians alike.

We greatly appreciate the support of everyone at Elsevier. Still, we are particularly thankful for the guidance of Celeste Clingan, Laurie Gower, and Rebecca Corradetti throughout the editing and production process, and for Lee Henderson, who encouraged us through both the fourth and fifth editions.

Our families and friends deserve our eternal thanks.

TRANSITIONS

Finally, we are especially thankful to Joanne Sandberg-Cook, our esteemed colleague and friend, who will be retiring from the book upon the publication of this fifth edition. Joanne writes, "Working on this text has been an incredible experience which has broadened my sense of collaboration and improved my clinical practice. It has been a great privilege to work with my fellow authors and understand that my part in the text has contributed to the practice of many nurse practitioners and, by extension, improved the lives of thousands of patients." Through five editions, the four editors have continued to work together, respecting each other's unique talents and strengths without sacrificing the expectation of individual accountability and high standards. We have met the challenges imposed by rapid changes in the U.S. healthcare system and the continuous scientific achievements of science and medicine. Our collaborative work reflects our individual practices, which have remained focused on our patients and our relationships with our colleagues and communities. We have faced professional, personal, and family challenges by supporting each other in spite of the many miles between us."

We wish Joanne all the best in her retirement and thank her for her many contributions. We hope that this edition of the textbook reflects all of this and continues to be a useful academic and clinical asset to this generation of primary care healthcare providers.

Contributors to Previous Edition

Julio C. Albornoz; Joanne Aldrich; Antonia Altomare; Marjorie S. Bernice; Mary Ann Best; Sharon M. Bouvier; Matthew S. Bowdish; Christell O. Bray; David R. Campbell; Raymond J. Carlson, Jr.; Trisha Carlson; Diana Hey Cauley; Jonathan S. Chang; Erin Cox; Patricia D. Cunningham; Susan M. DeNisco; Avnish Arvind Deobhakta; Susan DiMattia; Wendy DiSalvo; John E. Duffy, Jr.; Maura Malone Dumas; Melissa Edwards; Walter Elias III; Debra Fournier; Bridget R. Franciose; Kelli Gershon; Oscar K. Gibbs; Roger A. Goldberg; Clara M. Gona; Spencer Gould; Katherine P. Griffis; Brenda L. Hage; Linda A. Hagemann; Farah Hameed; Diane Hislop-Chestnut; Susan Hoch; Connie Hutson; David C. Jimerson; Irma O. Jordan; Nancy W. Knee; William J. Koopman; Andrea Lora Kossler; Marisaa L. LaHaie; Noreen M. Leahy; Kelley Hamill Lemay; Zita D. Lim; Ahila Lingappan; Vivian McGhee; Eran D. Metzger; Catharine Moffett; Allison Barker Morse; Stephanie Moss; Debra S. Munsell; Nancy C. O'Rourke; D. Wilkin Parke III; Michael Brandon Parrott; Jill M. Paulson; Joanne M. Petrelli; William R. Prebloa, Jr.; Carmen Rose Presti; Judy Ptak; Joseph Rampulla; Nancy Faye Rogers; Mayola Rowser; Nathan W. Samuels; Michael J. Sateia; Somal Shah; Roberta A. Silveira; Cathy J. Sizer; Margaret M. Sullivan; Sara M. Tinsley; Elizabeth C. Todd; Justin H. Townsend; Susan R. Tussey; Gretchen Van Buren; Carol A. Whelan; Patricia A. White; Alexis E. Whittaker; Barbara E. Wolfe; Kathleen Wright.

Contents

PART 1 Introduction

1 The Changing Landscape of Collaborative Practice, 1
2 Transitional Care, 3
3 Translating Research into Clinical Practice, 6
4 The Patient, the Provider, and Primary Care: An Integrated Perspective, 15
5 Population-Based Care for Primary Care Providers, 19
6 Health Literacy, Health Care Disparities, and Culturally Responsive Primary Care, 27
7 Genetic Considerations in Primary Care, 30
8 Risk Management, 43

PART 2 Primary Care: Adolescence Through Adulthood

9 Adolescent Issues, 54
10 LGBTQ Patient Care, 59
11 Pregnancy and Prenatal Care, 65
12 Lactation Guidance, 78
13 Aging and Common Geriatric Syndromes, 84
14 Palliative and End-of-Life Care, 94

PART 3 Health Maintenance

15 Obesity and Weight Management, 109
16 Lifestyle Management, 125
17 Routine Health Screening and Immunizations, 145
18 Principles of Occupational and Environmental Health in Primary Care, 163
19 College Health, 170
20 Health Care of the International Traveler, 173
21 Presurgical Clearance, 181
22 Preparticipation Sports Physical, 185

PART 4 Office Emergencies

23 Disaster and Emergency Preparedness and Response in Primary Care, 188
24 Acute Bronchospasm, 192
25 Anaphylaxis, 194
26 Bites and Stings, 197
27 Bradycardia and Tachycardia, 201
28 Cardiac Arrest, 205
29 Chemical Exposure, 208
30 Electrical Injuries, 211
31 Environmental and Food Allergies, 213
32 Head Trauma, 218
33 Hypotension, 221
34 Poisoning, 224
35 Sexual Assault, 227
36 Syncope, 230
37 Thermal Injuries, 233

PART 5 Evaluation and Management of Skin Disorders

38 Examination of the Skin and Approach to Diagnosis of Skin Disorders, 237
39 Surgical Office Procedures, 240
40 Principles of Dermatologic Therapy, 243
41 Screening for Skin Cancer, 245
42 Acne Vulgaris, 249
43 Alopecia, 252
44 Animal and Human Bites, 255
45 Bullous Pemphigoid, 258
46 Burns (Minor), 259

47 Cellulitis, 261

48 Contact Dermatitis, 266

49 Corns and Calluses, 268

50 Cutaneous Herpes, 269

51 Dermatitis Medicamentosa (Drug Eruption), 273

52 Dry Skin, 275

53 Eczematous Dermatitis (Atopic Dermatitis), 277

54 Fungal Infections (Superficial), 279

55 Herpes Zoster (Shingles), 284

56 Hidradenitis Suppurativa (Acne Inversa), 286

57 Hyperhidrosis, 288

58 Intertrigo, 290

59 Nail Disorders, 292

60 Pigmentation Changes (Vitiligo), 296

61 Pruritus, 299

62 Psoriasis, 301

63 Purpura, 304

64 Scabies, 307

65 Seborrheic Dermatitis, 309

66 Stasis Dermatitis, 310

67 Urticaria, 312

68 Warts, 314

69 Wound Management, 317

PART 6 Evaluation and Management of Eye Disorders

70 Evaluation of the Eyes, 326

71 Cataracts, 335

72 Blepharitis, Hordeolum, and Chalazion, 337

73 Conjunctivitis, 339

74 Corneal Surface Defects and Ocular Surface Foreign Bodies, 343

75 Dry Eye Syndrome, 345

76 Nasolacrimal Duct Obstruction and Dacryocystitis, 349

77 Preseptal and Orbital Cellulitis, 350

78 Pinguecula and Pterygium, 353

79 Traumatic Ocular Disorders, 355

PART 7 Evaluation and Management of Ear Disorders

80 Auricular Disorders, 359

81 Cerumen Impaction, 361

82 Cholesteatoma, 362

83 Impaired Hearing, 364

84 Inner Ear Disturbances, 367

85 Otitis Externa, 371

86 Otitis Media, 373

87 Tympanic Membrane Perforation, 377

PART 8 Evaluation and Management of Nose Disorders

88 Chronic Nasal Congestion and Discharge, 378

89 Epistaxis, 380

90 Nasal Trauma, 382

91 Rhinitis, 384

92 Sinusitis, 389

93 Smell and Taste Disturbances, 392

94 Tumors and Polyps of the Nose, 394

PART 9 Evaluation and Management of Oropharyynx Disorders

95 Dental Abscess, 398

96 Diseases of the Salivary Gland, 399

97 Epiglottitis, 403

98 Oral Infections, 406

99 Parotitis, 409

100 Peritonsillar Abscess, 411

101 Pharyngitis and Tonsillitis, 413

PART 10 Evaluation and Management of Pulmonary Disorders

102 Acute Bronchitis, 417

103 Asthma, 421

104 Chest Pain (Noncardiac), 445

105 Chronic Cough, 451

106 Chronic Obstructive Pulmonary Disease, 457

107 Dyspnea, 467

108 Hemoptysis, 471

109 Lung Cancer, 474

110 Pleural Effusions and Pleurisy, 479

111 Pneumonia, 485

112 Pneumothorax, 491

113 Pulmonary Embolism, 493

114 Pulmonary Hypertension, 496

115 Sarcoidosis, 500

PART 11 Evaluation and Management of Cardiovascular Disorders

116 Cardiac Diagnostic Testing: Noninvasive Assessment of Coronary Artery Disease, 504

117 Abdominal Aortic Aneurysm, 510

118 Cardiac Arrhythmias, 515

119 Carotid Artery Disease, 529

120 Chest Pain and Coronary Artery Disease, 536

121 Heart Failure, 554

122 Hypertension, 569

123 Infective Endocarditis, 584

124 Myocarditis, 597

125 Peripheral Arterial and Venous Insufficiency, 599

126 Valvular Heart Disease and Cardiac Murmurs, 611

PART 12 Evaluation and Management of Gastrointestinal Disorders

127 Abdominal Pain and Infections, 623

128 Anorectal Complaints, 630

129 Cholelithiasis and Cholecystitis, 635

130 Cirrhosis, 639

131 Constipation, 644

132 Diarrhea, Noninfectious, 647

133 Diverticular Disease, 657

134 Dysphagia, 663

135 Gastroesophageal Reflux Disease, 669

136 Gastrointestinal Hemorrhage, 677

137 Hepatitis, 683

138 Inflammatory Bowel Disease, 692

139 Irritable Bowel Syndrome, 699

140 Jaundice, 705

141 Nausea and Vomiting, 709

142 Pancreatitis, 713

143 Tumors of the Gastrointestinal Tract, 722

144 Peptic Ulcer Disease, 728

PART 13 Evaluation and Management of Genitourinary Disorders

145 Incontinence, 731

146 Prostate Cancer, 736

147 Prostatic Hyperplasia (Benign), 738

148 Proteinuria and Hematuria, 743

149 Renal Failure, 749

150 Sexual Dysfunction (Male), 756

151 Testicular Disorders, 763

152 Urinary Calculi, 771

153 Urinary Tract Infections and Sexually Transmitted Infections, 777

154 Uropathies (Obstructive) and Tumors of the Genitourinary Tract (Kidneys, Ureters, and Bladder), 794

PART **14** Evaluation and Management of Gynecologic Concerns

155 Amenorrhea, 799

156 Bartholin Gland Cysts and Abscesses, 803

157 Breast Disorders, 806

158 Chronic Pelvic Pain, 817

159 Dysmenorrhea, 821

160 Dyspareunia, 825

161 Ectopic Pregnancy, 828

162 Fertility Control, 831

163 Genital Tract Cancers, 837

164 Infertility, 845

165 Menopause, 850

166 Pap Test Abnormalities, 868

167 Pelvic Inflammatory Disease, 871

168 Sexual Dysfunction (Female), 875

169 Unplanned Pregnancy, 879

170 Vulvar and Vaginal Disorders, 883

PART **15** Evaluation and Management of Musculoskeletal and Arthritic Disorders

171 Ankle and Foot Pain, 897

172 Bone Tumors, 906

173 Bursitis, 913

174 Elbow Pain, 920

175 Fibromyalgia and Myofascial Pain Syndrome, 924

176 Gout, 928

177 Hand and Wrist Pain, 932

178 Hip Pain, 936

179 Infectious Arthritis, 940

180 Knee Pain, 946

181 Low Back Pain, 952

182 Metabolic Bone Disease: Osteoporosis and Paget Disease of Bone, 960

183 Neck Pain, 970

184 Osteoarthritis, 976

185 Osteomyelitis, 980

186 Shoulder Pain, 985

187 Sprains, Strains, and Fractures, 994

PART **16** Evaluation and Management of Neurologic Disorders

188 Neuropsychological Evaluation, 999

189 Amyotrophic Lateral Sclerosis, 1005

190 Bell Palsy, 1008

191 Cerebrovascular Events, 1010

192 Delirium, 1016

193 Dementia, 1019

194 Dizziness and Vertigo, 1024

195 Guillain-Barré Syndrome, 1028

196 Headache, 1030

197 Infections of the Central Nervous System, 1037

198 Movement Disorders and Essential Tremor, 1040

199 Multiple Sclerosis, 1044

200 Parkinson Disease, 1050

201 Seizure Disorder, 1054

202 Trigeminal Neuralgia, 1063

203 Intracranial Tumors, 1066

PART **17** Evaluation and Management of Endocrine and Metabolic Disorders

204 Acromegaly, 1071

205 Adrenal Gland Disorders, 1074

206 Diabetes Mellitus, 1077

207 Hirsutism, 1096

208 Hypercalcemia and Hypocalcemia, 1104

209 Hyperkalemia and Hypokalemia, 1108

210 Hypernatremia and Hyponatremia, 1112

211 Lipid Disorders, 1120

212 Metabolic Syndrome, 1126

213 Parathyroid Gland Disorders, 1131

214 Thyroid Disorders, 1135

PART 18 Evaluation and Management of Rheumatic Disorders

215 Ankylosing Spondylitis and Related Disorders, 1152

216 Polymyalgia Rheumatica and Giant Cell Arteritis, 1159

217 Raynaud Phenomenon, 1164

218 Rheumatoid Arthritis, 1166

219 Systemic Lupus Erythematosus, 1170

220 Vasculitis, 1176

PART 19 Evaluation and Management of Multisystem Disorders

221 Barotrauma and Other Diving Injuries, 1181

222 Chronic Pain, 1186

223 Fatigue, 1189

224 Fever, 1196

225 Immunodeficiency, 1200

226 Lymphadenopathy, 1204

227 Sleep Disorders, 1209

228 Unintended Weight Loss, 1218

PART 20 Evaluation and Management of Infectious Diseases

229 Emerging and Reemerging Infectious Diseases, 1225

230 HIV Infection, 1232

231 Influenza, 1241

232 Infectious Diarrhea, 1243

233 Infectious Mononucleosis, 1251

234 Tick-Borne Illnesses, 1254

235 Tuberculosis, 1262

236 West Nile Virus, 1271

PART 21 Evaluation and Management of Hematologic Disorders

237 Anemia, 1278

238 Blood Coagulation Disorders, 1297

239 Leukemias, 1307

240 Lymphomas, 1314

241 Myelodysplastic Syndromes, 1320

PART 22 Evaluation and Management of Oncologic Disorders

242 Collaborative Management of the Oncology Patient, 1325

243 Basic Principles of Oncology Treatment, 1326

244 Oncology Complications and Paraneoplastic Syndromes, 1330

245 Oncology Pain and Symptom Management in Primary Care, 1335

246 Unknown Primary Carcinoma, 1345

PART 23 Evaluation and Management of Mental Health Disorders

247 Anxiety Disorders, 1349

248 Mood Disorders, 1354

249 Substance Use Disorders, 1369

250 Other Mental Health Disorders, 1377

PART 1

Introduction

CHAPTER 1

THE CHANGING LANDSCAPE OF COLLABORATIVE PRACTICE

JoAnn Trybulski • Terry Mahan Buttaro

We are living in a world of *VUCA*—volatility, uncertainty, complexity, and ambiguity. Used by Robert Johansen to characterize the world at large, VUCA is certainly applicable to the current state of collaborative practice and primary care.[1] The former state of primary care practice with well-defined rules and roles has been replaced by new rules and new types of health care professionals. There is unchallenged recognition of the importance of an evidence base for practice decisions, disease prevention, health promotion, maintenance of well-being, involvement of patients in their health decisions, and coordination of care given by a team of health care providers. With the institution of provisions of the Affordable Care Act, the type of insurance and policy level chosen by a patient shapes the providers and hospitals from which a patient may receive care and dictates the cost of medications and treatments for each patient. The landscape of collaborative practice is in a constant state of evolution, with patients and purchasers of health care at the center.

CURRENT FORCES SHAPING THE PRIMARY CARE LANDSCAPE

Evidence-Based Practice

The evidence-based practice movement continues to shape the landscape of primary care. Best practices and clinical care guidelines are updated at an increasingly rapid pace. Insurers use this information to create reimbursement structures, driving providers and patients to treatments that have been found to be efficacious and cost-effective, based on available evidence. See Chapter 3, Translating Research into Clinical Practice, for background on how clinical evidence is created, evaluated, and disseminated.

Value-Based Purchasing

Value-Based Purchasing (VBP) is an initiative that affects all providers who practice in or admit patients to a hospital setting. VBP is part of the Affordable Care Act of 2009; its goal is improving care quality by linking payment by the Centers for Medicare and Medicaid Services (CMS) for inpatient services to successful outcome measures.[2] VBP uses hospital quality metrics in the five domain areas of processes of care (core measure compliance), experience of care (Hospital Consumer Assessment of Healthcare Providers and Systems [HCAHPS] scores), outcomes of care (in patient mortality rates for specific conditions such as heart failure, myocardial infarction [MI], and pneumonia and rates of hospital-acquired conditions), efficiency of care (Medicare per-case cost), and safety (rates of hospital-acquired infections such as central line–associated bloodstream infections, catheter-associated urinary tract infections, and surgical site infections).[3] Private insurers are using similar metrics when negotiating contracts with institutions and primary care providers. We have entered a "pay for performance" world where contracts are negotiated based on quality metrics. As a result, the field of practice analytics has arisen. There are now sophisticated computer programs modeling financial opportunities for hospital service lines and individual health care practices based on payer mix per-case cost and contribution margin. Primary care providers now have a crucial opportunity with inpatient care management to affect not only the quality of care delivered to their patients but also the financial state of organizations in which their patients receive care, as well as their own financial opportunities.

Management of Care Transitions

The new reality of VBP is further shaping primary care delivery by reducing Medicare payments for all patients by a small percentage in a hospital where the unplanned readmission rate within 30 days of discharge exceeds the hospital's expected rate for patients with the selected conditions of acute MI, heart failure, coronary artery bypass graft surgery, pneumonia, chronic obstructive pulmonary disease (COPD), hip arthroplasty, and knee arthroplasty.[4] This reality highlights the importance of managing care transitions, particularly the transition from inpatient care to home. Many institutions have created transitional care teams; nurse practitioners are critical members of these transitional care teams. See Chapter 2, Transitional Care, for an in-depth exploration.

Accountable Care Organizations

The vision of primary care as a collaborative practice is realized with the advent of accountable care organizations (ACOs), which form the centerpiece of health care reform efforts. There are multiple models for ACOs; the concept of an ACO is a comprehensive health care delivery system that has real or virtual integration of individual caregivers and hospital-based systems, connected in a reimbursement system that contains performance measures to ensure accountability.[5] There are three levels, or tiers, of an ACO, each with its distinct requirements for organizational structure, performance measures, information technology (IT) requirements, and payment models.

Level 1 ACOs have the least amount of financial risk and fewest requirements. The organization's structure may be just a legal entity, and the ACO may have the IT capability to track a limited number of performance measures. Level 1 ACOs receive shared savings bonuses based on achievement of benchmarks for quality measures and expenditures.[5,6]

Level 2 ACOs have the potential to capture a greater portion of below-target spending amounts but have accountability for above-budget spending. The Level 2 ACO has an evolved infrastructure, with advanced IT systems and care coordination for chronic diseases such as asthma, diabetes, and heart failure. Performance measures are linked to outcomes for chronic diseases and reduction in health risks. These organizations must make financial projections and have minimum cash reserve standards.[5,6]

Level 3 ACOs offer a full range of services and have the infrastructure to provide comprehensive health care services. They have electronic medical records (EMRs) linking all components and report on health-related outcomes, care experiences, and quality of life in multiple patient populations in the system. Level 3 ACOs have strict requirements for financial reporting and maintain larger cash reserves.[5,6]

High-quality primary care is essential to the successful formation of ACOs. In addition, there must be sufficient technical capability and support, innovation in payment and reimbursement systems (bundled payments), and establishment of performance measures using practice analytics that reflect improved health state in patients. In the ACOs, there are care navigators to assist patients with care access and sophisticated technology to communicate with and monitor patients. Nurses have various roles—system administrators, service line managers, practice managers, primary care providers, educators, and home health providers.

We are now seeing the advent of the "super ACO"—alliances of two or more successful health systems.[7] The super ACO alliance is created to expand the reach of the systems in the alliance to create initiatives that enhance the care experience for patients and providers, control costs, and maximize reimbursement potential.[7]

THE NEW LOOK OF PRIMARY CARE

In a 2014 survey conducted by the Advisory Board Company, 4000 consumers were asked questions about primary care preferences. Patients' preferences for low-acuity complaints in primary care included "24/7" access to care, a walk-in setting with the ability to be seen within 30 minutes, and close proximity to home.[8] The retail health movement, with urgent care walk-in clinics associated with pharmacy chains and department stores, is now an accepted component of the health care delivery system and is part of the new look of primary care. Retail clinics have expanded services beyond minor acute emergencies and now include several components of primary care (e.g., annual physicals, some chronic disease management, and medispa services) in response to documented patient preferences for close proximity to home and readily accessible primary care.[8] Primary care practices are responding to this emerging trend by opening urgent care centers, some in and near retail locations that are linked to the primary care practices, providing needed care continuity while meeting patient preferences. Other previously traditional primary care practices have turned into concierge practices, where patients pay an additional yearly fee for 24/7 rapid access to primary care, sometimes with home visits (house calls by a provider).

The new look of primary care has spawned new collaborative health care partner roles. Many health care systems have community health resource specialists who assist patients with obtaining a variety services, care navigators who help patients with coordinating care appointments and services, and practice-based clinical pharmacists who assist both providers and patients with medication regimens. Emergency medical services (EMS) providers now participate in the delivery of high-quality primary care. Many communities are pioneering the concept of community paramedics. These EMS providers have access to community demographics. Community paramedics not only monitor patients identified as high risk by hospitals and medical practices, but also in turn assist with getting patients known to them into care provision and coordination services.

OPPORTUNITIES TO SHAPE THE LANDSCAPE

APRN Compact License Movement

In May, 2015, the National Council of State Boards of Nursing (NCSBN) took an unprecedented step forward in potentially shaping the landscape of primary care. The NCSBN created rules and a model for the APRN Compact legislation, modeled after the successful nurse compact model, now in effect in 25 states.[9] The purpose of the APRN Compact is to allow advanced practice registered nurses (APRNs) within the compact states who meet the compact requirements to obtain a multistate license, thereby expanding advanced nursing practice and mobility for APRNs, fostering the use of technologies to monitor and communicate with patients, and increasing the safety of and access to health care.[9] The proposed legislation under the compact mode includes provisions for independent APRN practice and prescriptive authority for controlled substances.[9] There is ongoing discussion about a similar compact model for medical licenses. Primary care providers interested in fostering collaborative efforts to increase access to high-quality health care should advocate for legislation to make the APRN Compact license a reality.

Building Collaborative Practice Initiatives

Collaboration is a crucial element in today's changing landscape. Collaboration is a requirement for funding in research and program support. Collaborative research is exponentially productive because it combines resources, expertise, and thinking in the creation of knowledge for practice and should include a focus on patient outcomes. Collaborative leadership of health care initiatives allows more individuals to participate, and the outcome derives from a collective of minds. Collaboration in clinical practice offers improved quality of care for patients and significant others as professionals share expertise.

The Interprofessional Education Collaborative (IPEC), composed of representatives from the major care delivery disciplines in health care, models collaboration that is advancing the practice.[10] An IPEC expert panel produced guidelines for collaborative practice core competencies that begin with interprofessional education to enable collaboration and improve outcomes.[10] The IPEC report advocates for components of professional education of the various disciples to occur together, in interprofessional teams, to build the core collaboration competencies of values and ethics needed for interprofessional practice, roles and responsibilities in collaborative practice, interprofessional team communication, and knowledge of teams and teamwork.[10] The interprofessional educational efforts should instill the core competencies by following guiding principles of being patient centered; having a community or population focus; emphasizing relationships and processes; containing developmentally appropriate activities and assessments; and being outcome driven.[10]

A recent study, with results published in 2015, explored the experiences of collaboration among physicians, nurses, and unlicensed assistive personnel.[11] Findings from this qualitative exploration indicate that we have much work to do in the area of collaboration. Most participants in this study indicated that they experienced a hierarchical feel to communication and decision-making. When there was collaboration between physicians and nurses, they failed to solicit input from unlicensed assistive personnel.[11] Patient care involves activities apportioned among physicians, nurses, and unlicensed assistive personnel; seamless coordination is required to prevent errors and a siloed experience for the patients and their families.[11] Creating a model without a hierarchical structure requires that members of the team understand the roles and expected contributions of each member, encourage one another to meet team expectations, and make the outcomes desired for patients and families the center of focus.[11]

CONCLUSION

The landscape of the health care system is ever changing. Primary care providers are delivering care in new venues with new technologies, with new types of collaborators, and in new types of health care systems. Health care reform continues to evolve and shape the vision for primary care. In this world of VUCA, there are some aspects of primary care that will remain time tested and will form the cornerstone of health care into the future. Health promotion and wellness is now and will be a critical component in health care systems. The current focus on wellness and primary care continues to provide opportunities for nurse practitioners, particularly Doctor of Nursing Practice (DNP)–prepared nurse practitioners, to shape the direction and structures of health care delivery systems. Although there is continued focus on interdisciplinary collaboration, we still have many challenges and opportunities before collaborative practice reaches its potential.

The vision of primary care as a collaborative practice remains timely and important. Collaborative practice represents the best response that a group of interdisciplinary expert clinicians can offer patients and their families as we move forward in the evolving landscape of primary care.

CHAPTER 2

TRANSITIONAL CARE

Terry Buttaro

Transitions of care occur at many points during health care delivery: from primary care provider to hospitalist, from hospitalist to consultants, from consultants to hospitalists, and from hospitalists to health care providers in primary care or in rehabilitation or long-term care facilities or to home care. At each of these junctures, provider communication can result in one of the recognized complications associated with poor care transitions: adverse events (e.g., laboratory abnormalities), adverse drug events (ADEs), infections, injuries, surgical complications, and rehospitalizations. These unfavorable events occur in patients of all ages and for a variety of reasons, but often occur across these transitions of care: when patients enter or leave a health care facility or see their primary care or other health care provider. ADEs after hospitalization are particularly problematic and often related to cardiovascular medications, corticosteroids, antibiotics, anticoagulants, and analgesics.[1] Many of these events can be prevented with careful patient education before hospital discharge and with careful monitoring after discharge.[1] In children, adverse events are frequently associated with complex chronic conditions, whereas in older adults unintended drug overdoses and high-risk medications (e.g., insulin, warfarin, oral antiplatelet and oral hypoglycemic medications) are the most common causes.[1-3] Factors associated with patient-provider communication issues during care transitions include health literacy, cognitive impairment, and cultural and linguistic differences between patient and provider.

The period after hospital discharge is particularly problematic for patients. Discharge instructions across the transitions of care are unclear for many patients and their families, particularly concerning medication management.[3] The effects are costly in terms of both patient harm and hospital readmissions, with estimated Medicare costs of approximately $26 million annually as well as substantial penalties.[4,5]

Although challenging, it is possible to improve care and decrease adverse events, emergency room visits, and hospitalizations.[6] Researchers have identified some of the factors that contribute to medication and health management misunderstandings, although more studies are necessary.[4,7] Health literacy; cognitive impairment; medication complexity; inclusive discharge planning; prompt discharge follow-up; improved patient and family education; and enhanced communication among care providers and patients and their families are concepts that can be addressed to improve patient safety.

HEALTH LITERACY

Health literacy is defined by the Institute of Medicine as "the degree to which individuals have the capacity to obtain, process, and understand basic health information and services needed to make appropriate health decisions."[8] Age, race, ethnicity, culture, education, language, and socioeconomic factors are all associated with low health literacy, which in turn is a factor in medication nonadherence, adverse health outcomes, and increased hospitalizations, rehospitalizations, and mortality.[9-12] The costs associated with low health literacy are estimated to be $106 billion to $238 billion each year.[13]

Ninety million Americans lack health literacy skills, meaning that their ability to access health care and communicate with health care providers can be affected.[10] In addition, their ability to find health care information, understand diagnostic test results, calculate medication doses, understand and implement health care instructions (e.g., diet, activity), and evaluate the risks and benefits of treatment can be affected.[13] There are other impediments to health literacy: fear of disclosing an inability to read or understand directions; patients' inability to explain symptoms to their health care providers; and lack of numeric, visual, and computer skills. Whatever the cause(s), the goal of health literacy is not only to improve health, but also to aid patient comprehension of health and the health care system. Because health literacy can be unrecognized, it is important to assess every patient's health literacy.[14] There are varied tools to assess health literacy, including the Rapid Estimate of Adult Literacy in Medicine (REALM) tool, Test of

Functional Health Literacy in Adults (TOFHLA), and the Newest Vital Sign tool, which is quite easy to use in primary care and involves having the patient read and interpret a nutrition label.[15] Another helpful resource is the North Carolina Health Literacy Universal Precautions Toolkit, available at www.nchealthliteracy.org/toolkit.

For providers, the Agency for Healthcare Research and Quality recommends "a health literacy affects all approach" for all health care practices.[14] Their recommendations include (1) using clear, simple-to-understand language, (2) highlighting three to five key points, (3) using pictures or visual tools to enhance understanding, (4) repeating the instructions, (5) using the teach-back method, and (6) empowering patients.[14] This approach plus easy-to-follow instructions, handouts, and telephone follow-up can aid in addressing health literacy.[14] Identifying health literacy is especially important during care transitions when any patient, but particularly an older adult, is receiving important new information that he or she is then responsible to implement. Interventions to improve patient understanding of health care instructions are essential to improve health care outcomes and aid in engaging patients in their own health care.

COGNITIVE IMPAIRMENT

Cognitive impairment is associated with health literacy, yet cognitive changes are not always easily recognized.[16] Cognitive impairment may be notable in older patients and in patients with mental illness, Parkinson disease, cardiovascular disease, or other illnesses. These changes in understanding and memory can be subtle, occurring years before diagnosis and affecting a patient's decision-making ability, although even adults without cognitive decline may make poor decisions.[13] People with mild cognitive impairment (MCI) can function independently without problems. They are able to perform activities of daily living without difficulty and may or may not have a memory problem. Their cognitive impairment may or may not progress to Alzheimer disease or another type of dementia, conditions that affect memory, executive function, and the ability to function independently. Illness can also affect cognition, yet cognitive defects are easily missed by health care providers. At times, it is families that first report patient memory changes, but providers may note that the patient is not focused, seems unable to follow directions, or asks the same question repeatedly. Recognizing cognitive impairment is important because it can affect patient health and well-being. Memory impairment, attention deficit, word-finding difficulties, and disturbances in executive functioning are cues suggesting MCI in a patient. Some of these changes may be related to a medication effect, anxiety, depression, or a medical condition, but MCI is also an early sign of dementia. Varied tools (e.g., General Practitioner Assessment of Cognition, eight-item Ascertain Dementia screen, Montreal Cognitive Assessment, Folstein Mini-Mental State Examination, six-item screen, Mini-Cog, and Memory Impairment Screen) are available for use in primary care and should be used if cognitive impairment is suspected. Early identification of cognitive impairment is important because in some instances treatment is possible. Involving family members is helpful in determining if there has been a concerning change in the patient's memory or functioning. A careful patient and family history is essential and should include a medication review. Screening for alcohol, anxiety, depression, drugs, thyroid disorders, or vitamin B_{12} or folic acid deficiency is also necessary because these are potential contributors to cognitive impairment. A complete physical and neurological examination may identify visual or hearing deficits that affect cognition; memory problems; gait disturbances; frailty; weight loss; and decreased psychomotor speed associated with dementia.[17] Computed tomography or magnetic resonance imaging of the brain and neuropsychological testing are also recommended. And as noted earlier, an older adult's ability to understand health care instructions is critical during care transitions when new medications, diet, or follow-up care is prescribed.

MEDICATION SAFETY

Medication safety is profoundly affected by health literacy and cognitive impairment, but alcohol, aging changes, comorbidity, and drug-drug interactions are additional factors to consider. Hospital-based medication reconciliation across transitions in care is a mandate, but postdischarge follow-up is an equally essential intervention.[11] Primary care providers play an important role in coordinating post-transition interventions. A timely follow-up appointment after discharge is one element that can improve medication safety; it is an opportunity to assess patient understanding, as is a telephone call or house call within 48 hours of hospital discharge to determine the need for expedited follow-up and patient comprehension of medication changes.[18]

A "brown-bag" medication review at each office visit is also very helpful in identifying patients' medication understanding and adherence. It is an opportunity to review new medications prescribed by other health care providers, prior medication dose or frequency changes, and discontinuation of prior medications and to assess potential drug-drug interactions, polypharmacy risks, and the complexity of medication instructions. Revisiting the necessity of continued drug therapy for some conditions (e.g., proton pump inhibitor therapy for gastroesophageal reflux disease [GERD]) is also beneficial. For older adults, the STOPP and START criteria (i.e., the Screening Tool of Older Persons' Potentially Inappropriate Prescriptions [STOPP] and Screening Tool to Alert Doctors to Right Treatment [START]) are tools that can increase provider awareness of potentially dangerous medications for elders, but also remind us of potential treatment omissions.[19]

In addition, all patients should receive a printed medication list at the end of each office visit. A current medication list can help the patient but is also important for other providers caring for patients. For many patients and especially older adults, medication instructions need to be presented in a specific, organized way using a patient-centered approach. Providing clear printed information using large print at a third- to sixth-grade reading level is helpful. Patients should be encouraged to bring their medication lists to all health care provider appointments.

CULTURAL COMPETENCE AND LANGUAGE

Concerns about health care disparities were the initial impetus for improving cultural competence in health care providers.[20] However, language differences, social issues, attitudes, biases, and other factors are also identified as barriers to improving health care for all patients. Awareness of culture is an important consideration for health care providers because there are obvious health care disparities affecting minority populations as evidenced by a higher incidence of diabetic complications and mortality in African Americans, Mexican Americans, American

Indians, and Hispanics/Latinos than in non-Hispanic whites throughout the United States.[21] Achieving cultural competence in a multicultural society is challenging, but self-awareness, self-reflection, and learning about a patient's health beliefs are components of cultural humility that all providers can attain. Recognizing that cultural humility is important allows providers the opportunity to acknowledge each patient's values and perspectives, but cultural humility is an ongoing process requiring continued training and practice. Organizational support is also necessary.[22] Awareness and maintenance of cultural and linguistic competencies require a sustained, systematic team approach that includes patient, provider, and community participation; a more diverse health care workforce; bilingual staff; regular cultural competence assessments; and qualified, available interpreters.[22]

TRANSITIONAL CARE

The risks in transitions of care include medication changes, the complexity of medication instructions, and polypharmacy. Provider role ambiguity has also been identified as an impediment to patient safety during transitions of care, particularly during the post–hospital discharge period.[23] The reasons are multifactorial but include communication, one of the most persistent problems identified as contributing to ADEs and rehospitalizations.[24] Personal communication is essential in caring for patients across the life span and throughout the transitions of care. This requires communication not only between the primary care provider and other health care specialists but also among providers, patients, and family members involved in the patient's safety and well-being.[23] When patients are admitted to or discharged from the hospital, rehabilitation service, long-term care facility, or home care services, ongoing personal communication with the primary care provider and receiving health care provider is essential. In the past, this communication was provided by the discharge summary. Discharge summaries and medical reconciliation forms remain a vital component of communication, but improving care requires more timely communication among health care providers. Primary care providers should contact the hospitalist or other health care provider when patients are admitted to a health care facility to provide pertinent information about the patient's past medical history and to stay apprised of ongoing medical problems.[23] Visiting the patient in the hospital or other health care facility is also recommended.

There are now penalties associated with inadequate care transitions that result in complications and rehospitalizations. The component of the Affordable Care Act that resulted in the Readmissions Reduction Program requires that the Centers for Medicare and Medicaid Services (CMS) reduce payments to Acute Care Hospital Inpatient Prospective Payment System (IPPS) hospitals for readmission hospitalizations to the same hospital or another IPPS-associated acute care hospital within 30 days of discharge.[25] Initially, this policy was associated with readmissions related to acute myocardial infarction, pneumonia, and heart failure.[25] Readmissions related to chronic obstructive pulmonary disease (COPD) and elective hip and knee arthroplasties were added in 2015.

Transitions in care can be especially problematic for older adults. The challenge for any health care provider treating older adults is to recognize the individual aging process of each older adult, promote optimum health and functioning, provide care and comfort during illness, minimize the length and severity of the premorbid illness and disability period, and, finally, ensure a comfortable and dignified death.

Several models of care proposed over the past decade were designed to shorten or avoid hospital admission, avoid hospital readmission after discharge, reduce overtreatment, provide older adults and their families with information specific to their individual situation and preferences, and provide care in the preferred setting, allowing aging in place. The most studied and successful are transitional care models designed to help older adults with multiple comorbidities transition from hospital to home or nursing home or from nursing home to home. The American Geriatrics Society describes the transitional care model as a "set of actions designed to ensure the coordination and continuity of health care as patients transfer between different locations or different levels of care within the same location. Representative locations include (but are not limited to) hospitals, sub-acute and post-acute nursing facilities, the patient's home, primary and specialty care offices, and long-term care facilities. Transitional care is based on a comprehensive plan of care and the availability of health care practitioners who are well-trained in chronic care and have current information about the patient's goals, preferences, and clinical status. It includes logistical arrangements, education of the patient and family, and coordination among the health professionals involved in the transition. Transitional care, which encompasses both the sending and the receiving aspects of the transfer, is essential for persons with complex care needs."[26]

One example is Eric Coleman's Care Transitions Intervention, which enlists nurses or social workers to follow hospitalized patients from an initial meeting in the hospital though a 4-week period of home visits and phone calls to promote patient understanding of medications as well as signs of deteriorating health.[27] Mary Naylor's Transitional Care Model provided evidence that high-risk older patients with posthospital coordinated care by advanced practice nurses (APNs) would result in reduced rehospitalizations as well as costs.[28] Naylor's model provided patients with a weekly APN visit, telephone availability every day, and coordinated care with the patient's primary care physician.[28] Since the Affordable Care Act was established in 2010, a variety of transitional care programs have been designed to improve quality and reduce costs. Often these services are managed by an APN and frequently include discharge planning, case management services, counseling or coaching, and assistance with navigating the health care system.[22] Basic primary care services delivered to people at home as well as restorative services such as physical and occupational therapy can also be features.[29] House call programs are gaining in popularity and availability because care delivered at home is timely, less expensive, and more acceptable to frail elders.[30] Town or parish nurses are becoming more common as communities look for better ways to care for their aging population. The value of caring for vulnerable older adults in their homes is substantiated in multiple studies and is confirmed as preferable in most surveys of older adults.[31] These varied transitional care models provide essential continuity and individualized care that is more likely to improve patient outcomes and reduce complications.

Concerns about patient safety mandate improved health literacy assessment, uncomplicated medication instructions, and safer transitions for patients from hospital to home as well as from primary care office to home. Improved medication reconciliation and more expedient follow-up after hospitalization may promote improved care transitions, but primary care providers need to take a more proactive role in promoting coordinated care for patients across the health care continuum regardless of setting. Identifying at-risk patients (e.g., those with cognitive deficits, frailty, or multiple comorbidities) and communicating closely with other health care providers as well as with patients and, when possible, families are important first steps.

CHAPTER 3

TRANSLATING RESEARCH INTO CLINICAL PRACTICE

Sabine Eustache

Collaborative practice models among clinicians have succeeded because they benefit from the synergy among all medical professionals' unique skills. Similarly, collaborations between clinicians and academic researchers maximize the expertise of each partner in producing timely and effective clinical research and in translating research into clinical practice. Given the significant impact that collaborative research results have on clinical care, it is imperative that clinicians recognize the importance of research design, understand the process of translating research findings into clinical practice, and work collaboratively with researchers to determine the direction and practice of clinical care. In this chapter, the research designs and data analysis methods commonly used in clinical research are reviewed; important considerations in determining the significance of research findings are identified; the process and importance of translating research findings into clinical practice are described; strategies used to establish and strengthen successful collaborations between clinicians and researchers are explored; and the research process is reviewed.

RESEARCH DESIGNS AND DATA ANALYSIS METHODS

Level I Research: Descriptive Studies

Described as the first scientific "toe in the water,"[1] descriptive research is a simple descriptive account of interesting characteristics observed in a group of patients.[2] The purpose of Level I research is to describe the pertinent characteristics of the phenomenon of interest.[3] The question usually includes the stem "What is ...?"; for example, "What is the average age at which children learn to crawl?" or "What is the experience of individuals diagnosed with human immunodeficiency virus (HIV) infection?"

Investigators may apply qualitative methods, such as observations, structured interviews, and focus groups, while conducting descriptive studies. Qualitative data may be analyzed with a variety of techniques that help the investigators to identify ranges of typical responses. Alternatively, investigators may use quantitative methods, such as a survey. Analysis of the quantitative data generated in descriptive studies includes nonparametric statistics, which generate measures of central tendency and dispersion. These measures indicate typical responses by determining the average response (mean, mode, median) and variability of responses (range of responses, standard deviation, other measures of dispersion). Clinicians may use descriptive study results to expand the usual assessment parameters but should not use these findings to guide the selection of an intervention or a treatment.

During descriptive studies, patients are typically seen for a relatively short time. Whereas these studies produce accurate and objective data, descriptive research does not establish causality, in which one variable affects another. However, they can emphasize features of a new disease, which may become the precursor to more rigorous studies.

Level II Research: Relationships Between or Among Variables

Once the fundamental characteristics of a phenomenon have been described, the next logical step is to describe the relationships between and among characteristics or variables. The purpose of Level II research questions is to establish associations or differences between variables. Level II questions include the stem "What is the relationship between ...?" or "What are the differences between ...?"; for example, "What is the association between a history of cigarette smoking and the incidence of heart disease in women older than 40 years?"

Research Methods for Level II Questions. Researchers may use several approaches to investigate Level II questions. For example, investigators may carry out epidemiologic studies in large data sets. This approach has been taken to identify the risk factors commonly used to assess patients, to gather specific diagnostic data, and to counsel persons to change behavior. Investigators may also design research to compare the differences between two or more groups of variables. For example, an investigator may measure selected variables in a group of persons with HIV infection and a group of matched persons without HIV infection to determine associations between CD4 counts and fatigue levels. The results of these studies simply describe the associations and differences between the groups and suggest that the differences may be associated with group membership.

Data analysis techniques used in Level II studies are measures of association (e.g., correlation coefficients) and differences between the means of the study groups (e.g., *t* tests and analysis of variance).[3,4] Level II study findings are usually insufficient to demonstrate a mechanistic cause-and-effect relationship between variables. Demonstration of such a relationship requires more rigorous control of extraneous variables and active manipulation of the independent variable (the variable thought to be the causal variable). The clinician may use Level II study results to suggest a change in behavior, but the results do not guide methods to change those behaviors, nor do they explain how the behavioral change will be effective.

Level III Research: Cause and Effect

Armed with the results of level II studies, investigators can design Level III studies. The purpose of Level III studies is to identify the mechanistic relationships among characteristic variables associated with the phenomenon of interest.[1] Level III research questions are more complicated because the investigator has a hypothesis about the nature of the relationships among variables (i.e., which is the causal variable and which is the effect variable). Rather than a research question, the putative relationship tested in the study is often stated as a hypothesis. A hypothesis is a declarative sentence that asserts a relationship:

changes in A (the independent variable) cause changes in B (the dependent variable). Depending on the amount of preliminary evidence or the theoretical model proposed by the investigator, the investigator might suggest a directional relationship (e.g., as A increases, B decreases). The design applied to this level of question is either experimental or quasi-experimental.

Experimental Design. To demonstrate a causal relationship, investigators must exercise maximum control over the study. In an experimental design, the investigator controls the conditions under which the study is to be conducted.[5] A true experiment provides this level of maximum control. A true experiment is characterized by random selection of participants and manipulation of the independent or causal variable. In its strictest sense, an experimental design has three essential characteristics: a treatment or experimental group and a control group; random selection of large groups with randomly assigned members; and control of extraneous variables.

The experimental design consists of two groups: an experimental (also termed treatment) group and a control group. The experimental group is exposed to the independent variable or the treatment, but the control group is not.[6] Hence, the control group serves as a baseline measure or a measure of comparison when treatment results are evaluated.

Random selection is the method used to draw a study sample from a population in such a way that the data from the sample can be extrapolated to the general population.[7] A population is defined as all units targeted by the study. A sample is the percentage of units selected for study that represent the population. Random selection ensures that the study sample is representative of a population.[1] Several strategies may be used to ensure a representative sample, with each strategy engineered such that each eligible member of the population has an equal chance of being included in the study.[1] Random assignment, on the other hand, refers to how the investigator assigns members of the sample to the experimental and control groups in the study.[7] Random assignment of the study sample ensures that the groups are comparable or that every patient has an equal chance of being placed in either the experimental or the control group. Without random assignment, individuals who are significantly better or worse may be disproportionately represented in one of the groups.

When human subjects are used in Level III studies, investigators must take considerable care to control extraneous variables. Extraneous variables are those characteristics of the subject or setting that may influence the behavior of the dependent variable. Random selection of participants and random assignment to the experimental or control group provide control of extraneous variables. For example, if the study's purpose is to demonstrate that slow and rhythmic breathing by persons with essential hypertension results in lower systolic blood pressure, investigators may send a letter asking for volunteers to all persons being treated at a specific clinic. Because participation in a research study must be voluntary, it is safe to assume that participants "self-select" the study. Willingness to participate in a study may differentiate study participants from the overall population. Therefore, random assignment to either the experimental or control group helps ensure that the sampling methods did not contribute to errors.

Similarly, the investigator may consider other inclusion and exclusion criteria to guide subject recruitment. For example, the investigator may specify that subjects must be following a specific pharmacologic treatment regimen. Because these types of controls increase the complexity of recruitment, the investigator may select persons who are newly diagnosed with hypertension and test them before they begin rhythmic breathing treatments and again after a specified period of treatment. The study may include a control group of newly diagnosed persons who are monitored in exactly the same way as the experimental group but do not change their respiratory pattern. One way to ensure that environmental stimulation is the same for all subjects is to conduct the experimental sessions in the same laboratory setting. Subjects return at the same time after the initiation of treatment. By contrasting the blood pressure measures of the experimental group with those of the control group, the investigator is able to differentiate the effects of changes in breathing patterns alone from the effects of pharmacologic treatment alone, as well as the effects of changes in both breathing patterns and pharmacologic treatment (Table 3-1).

TABLE 3-1 True Experimental Design

Group	Baseline	Treatment
Control	No treatment	Pharmacologic treatment
Experimental	Rhythmic breathing treatment	Rhythmic breathing treatment *and* pharmacologic treatment

The purpose of this study is to evaluate the effectiveness of intermittent rhythmic breathing exercises to control hypertension in newly diagnosed persons. During the baseline period, the control group receives no treatment, whereas the experimental group practices the rhythmic breathing treatment. During the treatment period, the control group receives the usual treatment—pharmacologic treatment. The experimental group also receives the usual pharmacologic treatment because it would be unethical to withhold treatment, given the complications of untreated hypertension. A comparison of data from each cell reveals the effects of no treatment, pharmacologic treatment alone,.rhythmic breathing treatment alone, and rhythmic breathing with pharmacologic intervention.

Quasi-Experimental Design. When the three essential factors of an experimental design are not possible, investigators rely on a quasi-experimental design. In many cases, it is not possible to randomly select participants or to randomly assign them to experimental and control groups. For example, if an investigator is interested in the effects of a disease, it would not be possible to assign some subjects to have the disease and others to be free of the disease. In such cases, the disease would be the treatment variable. Suppose, for instance, an investigator is interested in understanding the pathology of HIV infection in the immune system. Clearly, it would be unethical to randomly assign persons to be infected with HIV to be in the experimental group. Instead, the investigator monitors persons diagnosed with HIV infection at baseline and at regular intervals thereafter.

The comparison of baseline data with subsequent observations allows the investigator to characterize the causal relationship between HIV infection and changes in immune parameters. This design is referred to as quasi-experimental because there is no random assignment to the experimental condition. This type of design is sometimes called a repeated-measures design, and it is argued that the subject serves as his or her own control.[2] In some ways, quasi-experimental designs ensure better control of extraneous variables associated with the constitution of individual subjects. However, the investigator should demonstrate with some assurance that every subject is representative of the general population. For example, if the sample lacks diversity of gender, age, and ethnicity, one would wonder to what degree the sample represents the overall population. The results can be applied only to those individuals represented in the sample. In other words, if the sample is not representative of the target population, the results may not be extrapolated to the population.

Level III data analysis tests hypothesize relationships between independent and dependent variables. For example, regression techniques generate a mathematical model to predict the change in dependent variables in response to changes in the independent variable. Level III studies may provide clinicians a degree of confidence in their prediction of outcomes. Clinicians may use results from a Level III study to anticipate the clinical course of a disease state.

Level IV Research: Randomized Clinical Trials

Level IV studies demonstrate the effectiveness of an intervention or treatment. The mechanistic relationships among variables, which are identified in Level III studies, support the proposition of the interventions and treatments tested in Level IV research. The randomized, placebo-controlled, double-blind clinical trial is the definitive way of conducting randomized clinical trials because it provides the researcher maximum control of the sources of error inherent in human clinical investigations.

Random Selection and Random Assignment. As with Level III studies, random selection and random assignments are required in a randomized clinical trial. Investigators use several methods to ensure that eligible subjects are randomly selected. When the availability of subjects is limited, investigators may conduct the study at a variety of sites. Within each site, the research team informs potential subjects about the study and offers them the opportunity to participate. Casting the widest possible net helps ensure that the investigators recruit a representative sample. Random assignment minimizes the likelihood that individuals who are significantly better or worse will be assigned to a specific group. If an investigator were free to assign the treatment group, he or she might inadvertently assign those most likely to respond to the new treatment group. There might also be a bias toward one treatment over another. For example, a surgeon participating in a study that tests the effectiveness of a lumpectomy in comparison with the usual treatment of mastectomy may prefer to assign young women to the lumpectomy group because of the disfigurement associated with mastectomy.

Placebos. Placebos, or sham interventions or treatments, exclude the possibility that changes in patient behavior are the result of a desire to please a researcher. The Hawthorne effect must also be acknowledged in any research. The Hawthorne effect produces improvements in performance because subjects are aware that they are being observed. Observation of the placebo control group permits investigators to demonstrate effects such as accelerated resolution of symptoms or palliative effects rather than curative effects. For conditions in which an effective treatment exists for the targeted population, those in the placebo group receive the usual treatment rather than a placebo because, in most cases, it would be unethical to withhold treatment.

Blinding of the Subject and Researcher. Blinding of the subject, researchers, and caregivers as to group membership (control group or experimental group) prevents personal biases from contaminating the study results. Investigators who are invested in obtaining positive results may be biased in their observations. In the case of pharmaceuticals, only the pharmacist may know which patient is receiving the investigational treatment. Patients who enroll in studies may do so simply because there is no alternative therapy. Hope for a positive effect could bias their reports of effects.

In a study of female cigarette smokers, researchers used a randomized, placebo-controlled, double-blinded clinical trial to compare the efficacy of varenicline tablets versus transdermal nicotine patches on smoking cessation. Researchers screened women ages 18 to 45 years who smoked an average of 10 or more cigarettes per day for at least 6 months with a desire to quit. The 140 eligible research subjects were then randomly assigned to receive a 4-week course of either varenicline tablets and placebo patches (case group) or placebo tablets and nicotine patches (control group).[8] Neither the patient nor the clinician knew to which group the patient was assigned. The double-blind study design helped reduce researcher bias and decrease the likelihood of any other types of human error.

Analysis of Level IV data reveals whether there are group-wise differences in treatment effects. Analysis of variance methods or *t* tests are most often used; however, regression analysis may also be done. The quandary investigators face is how to treat the numbers relative to subjects who do not complete a study. Obviously, it is essential to know if significantly more subjects died in the treatment group, but what about subjects who withdrew from the study?

One of the important aspects to be evaluated in any new treatment is patient preference and a tolerance for side effects. Some have argued that an intent-to-treat approach to these data ought to be used. In this approach, subjects who withdraw or die are counted as treatment failures, thus raising the standard for significant results. Consider a case in which 100 subjects are recruited for a study (Table 3-2). Fifty subjects are randomly assigned to the usual treatment, and 50 are assigned to the new treatment. At the end of the study, 10 in each group have died. No subjects withdrew from the usual treatment, but 10 withdrew from the new treatment group. At the end of the study, 20 subjects "got better" with the usual treatment, and 20 subjects showed improvement with the new treatment. When investigators calculate success rates, if the number of persons completing the study is used as the denominator, the success rate is 20 of 40 (50%) for the usual treatment group compared with 20 of 30 (66%) for the new treatment or experimental group. The experimental treatment would appear to be superior. However, if instead the number who began the study is used as the denominator, the success rate is 20 of 50 (40%) in the usual treatment group compared with 20 of 50 (40%) in the new treatment group, which suggests no difference between the groups. Thus, with the intent-to-treat approach, one would conclude no difference in success rate between the two treatments and a twofold increase in the failure rate for the new treatment.

WEIGHING THE EVIDENCE: EVALUATING KEY STUDY PARAMETERS

Identifying the level of research simply informs the clinician of the possible usefulness of the results. The decision to actually modify clinical practices on the basis of research findings must also include some evaluation of the design, subject selection, methods, data analysis scheme, and resultant conclusions. Table 3-3 summarizes some of these elements as they relate to each level of the research question. Inherent in the progression from the description of the phenomenon to a randomized

TABLE 3-2 Intent-to-Treat Table

	Usual Treatment			Experimental Treatment		
Participants	**N**	**Total Intent-to-Treat (%)**	**Complete (%)**	**N**	**Total Intent-to-Treat (%)**	**Complete (%)**
Admitted	50	100	80	50	100	60
Died	10	20	NA	10	20	NA
Withdrew	0	0	NA	10	20	NA
Completed, improved	20	40	50	20	40	66
Completed, did not improve	20	40	50	10	20	33
Total completing	40	80	100	30	60	100

The analysis of data from a clinical trial may be carried out in several ways. Of main concern is how investigators handle participant attrition. The inclusion of participants who begin a study but do not complete it is referred to as the intent-to-treat approach. This table illustrates the difference in results with an intent-to-treat scheme versus an approach that disregards attrition.

TABLE 3-3 Summary of Study Parameters

Level of Question	Purpose	Methods	Analysis	Application
I. What is it?	To describe or to define a phenomenon of interest To identify pertinent variables or characteristics	Qualitative methods Structured interviews Questionnaires Surveys	Content analysis Ethnography Nonparametric statistics Measures of central tendency	May suggest assessment parameters (Do you experience ...?)
II. What is happening here?	To identify relationships between variables—associations and differences	Epidemiologic studies Cross-sectional studies Correlational studies Studies of group-wise differences	Correlations among variables Differences between variables or groups Mann-Whitney *U* test; analysis of variance; *t* test	Suggests avenues of further assessment (If you observe *x*, what is the likelihood that *y* will occur?)
III. What is the nature of the relationship among variables (cause-and-effect relationship)?	To determine cause-and-effect relationships among variables To explicate mechanisms mediating the phenomenon of interest	Experimental designs Quasi-experimental designs	Analysis of variance Regression analysis	Suggests underlying pathologic conditions that may be treated
IV. What is the therapeutic effect of a proposed intervention? What is the proper dose of a treatment to achieve a predictable outcome?	To determine predictability of hypothesized outcome at specific dose in selected population	Randomized clinical trial	Intent-to-treat analysis Analysis of variance Regression analysis	Demonstrates usefulness of particular treatment for patient population; with sufficient replication, clinician may be reasonably sure that treatment will be effective

clinical trial is an increasing amount of control that the investigator can exert over the study's conduct, which allows the investigator to control error. Error is that portion of the measurement that cannot be explained. A simplistic way of describing a statistic is the ratio between the effect of the experiment and the error.

Although it is beyond the scope of this chapter to fully explore statistical methods, it may be helpful to review some basic statistical principles. The purpose of any statistic is to provide a mathematic measure of the effects of study variables while accounting for error. At the core of statistical analysis is the assumption that variance is normally distributed within a given population.

Type I and Type II Errors

One significant source of error in any study is an investigator's failure to include samples that represent all characteristics of the population. As discussed previously, one way to avoid this error is to select study participants carefully. A basic rule of thumb for selection of representative samples is to accrue a sufficient sample size, ensuring that all characteristic elements of the population are represented. If a sample is insufficiently representative of a population, the investigator may report false results and may erroneously conclude that the research hypothesis is supported—that is, the investigator may find that the effect of the study is sufficiently robust to conclude that differences or associations exist between baseline and outcome, or between the experimental and control groups, when in fact there is no difference. This type of error is a type I error. The investigator also risks what is known as a type II error, or failure to detect significant associations or differences when they are present. During the study design, the investigator may protect the study from these errors by conducting a power analysis.[3]

Power Analysis

Simply defined, *power* is an estimate of the likelihood of detecting significant effects at a given probability of a type II error.[3] In other words, power is an indication of the confidence one may have that the results are true. Research reports discuss power analysis as a way of calculating the sample size needed to adequately represent the target population. In general, the proportional risk of a type II error is set at 0.80; that is, the investigator estimates that the risk of failure to detect significant results is 2 in 10. If a power analysis has been done, clinicians can feel confident about the study findings because the investigator took care to ensure that the sample was representative of the target population.

Description of Data and Measures of Central Tendency

The first step in analyzing study results is usually describing the sample. Descriptive statistics, which summarize data, include measures of central tendency, dispersion, and association. The simplest descriptive statistic is graphic representation of the data. Pie charts, bar graphs, and line graphs are pictorial representations of the distribution of the data.

Measures of central tendency indicate the "typicalness" of the data set. The three most common measures of central tendency are the mode, median, and mean. The appropriate measure is determined by the way the variable of interest is scaled. When the variable of interest may have three or more possible responses, the appropriate measure of central tendency is the mode.[2] The mode is the category most frequently selected. For example, suppose the variable of interest is the effectiveness of an educational program for newly diagnosed diabetic patients. The evaluation tool consists of a list of statements attached to a scale with five possible responses: 1 represents strongly agree; 2, agree; 3, neutral; 4, disagree; and 5, strongly disagree. These responses represent categories with unknown relationships. Therefore the appropriate measure of central tendency for these questions is the mode, or the category with the most responses.

The median is the measure of central tendency used for rank order data, such as income.[2] Study participants are often asked to indicate their annual income by selecting from a range of incomes. The median is the point on the scale with 50% of the responses below and 50% above.

The mean, which is simply the arithmetic mean, is the measure used for discrete data.[4] For example, a study of the effects of stress on systolic blood pressure might indicate the mean, or average baseline, systolic blood pressure for the sample.

Standard Deviation

Dispersion is a measure of the variability of the data, or the degree to which data deviate from one another. The range is the difference between the highest score and the lowest score. Standard deviation is a measure of dispersion commonly reported for discrete data. The standard deviation is a summary of the average amount of difference among the data points.[4] A complete description of discrete data would include the mean plus or minus the standard deviation. Assuming that the study group is truly representative of the population, the mean, plus and minus the standard deviation, may represent the "normal" range of responses the clinician may expect to see.

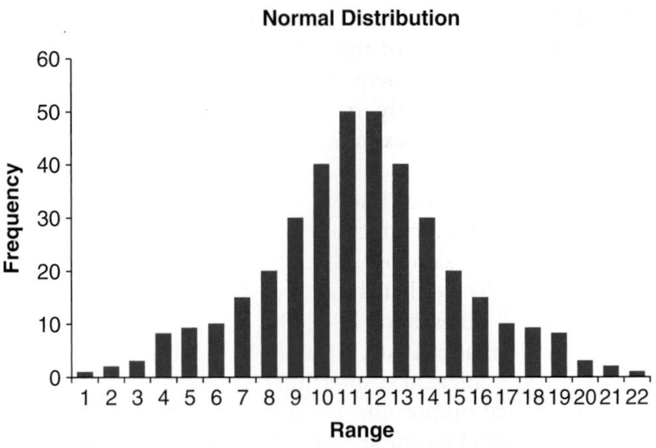

FIGURE 3-1 A graph of a theoretical normal distribution. The x-axis represents all possible responses, and the y-axis is simply the number of responses. This graph demonstrates that the majority of responses cluster in the middle range of possible responses and that the rest are evenly distributed above and below the middle.

Distribution and Error

If the responses from everyone in a population across the range of possible responses are counted and graphed, the majority of responses fall in the middle, with the rest evenly distributed above and below the middle (Figure 3-1). This sort of distribution is referred to as normal distribution. Underlying the parametric statistics is the assumption that all responses to an experimental condition are normally distributed.[3] If participants have been truly selected at random from the same population, then the sum of responses should be normally distributed. Individual responses are therefore a result of chance. By randomly sampling from a population, the investigator assumes that the sample is representative of the overall population. The distribution of the sample's responses should therefore mirror the distribution of the population's responses. Deviation from a normal distribution model is assumed to be a result of error. A well-designed study, engineered to reduce error, uses instruments with demonstrated validity and reliability. Subject selection is based on clear and reasoned inclusion and exclusion criteria so that only members of the targeted population are included. Data collection protocols are rigorously followed. Despite these best practice methods, however, some error is inevitable.

Statistical Significance (Alpha Values)

The purpose of statistical analysis is to estimate the amount of error. Because error is inevitable, the investigator decides before data are collected how much error can be tolerated and still demonstrate significant effects. The amount of tolerable error is defined as the *alpha* (α) *value*. The alpha value is expressed as a decimal representation of the proportional risk for error. An alpha value of 0.05 is interpreted as 5 chances in 100 that an error may occur. Similarly, $\alpha = .01$ is interpreted as 1 in 100 chance of error. The maximum risk for error is generally set at .05.[3]

The more rigorous or lower the alpha value, the less likelihood the study will incorrectly demonstrate positive or significant results. For example, an investigator evaluating a new therapy might decide that the risk of the therapy's being ineffective 5 of 100 times is too high. The alpha value could be set at 0.01, or 1 chance in 100. If that is done, the results are reported as not significant if statistical analysis demonstrates a *P* value (the actual proportion of error) of .05 at the completion of the study. The clinician may use the strength of the statistical significance to determine the robustness of the effect of the intervention when deciding to change a therapeutic routine. Suppose a study is conducted to compare the usual treatment (drug A) with a new treatment (drug B). The alpha value has been set a priori (beforehand) at .05. The reported *P* values at the end of the study are .05, which suggest that the new treatment is better than the old. The clinician must decide whether the 5% risk of a false conclusion is sufficiently low to change the usual prescription.

Statistics of Differences and Associations

Statistics measure associations among variables or differences between variables. During the design of a study, the investigator plans to demonstrate that participants behave in similar or different ways. Association statistics evaluate the similarities among the data. Association statistics compare the distribution of the variables of interest and evaluate whether they are consistently similar enough to conclude that they are related. The appropriate association statistic depends on the way the variables are scaled. For example, associations between two categorical variables (the values of the variables are not on a numeric continuum) are evaluated by use of a goodness-of-fit statistic, whereas associations between two ranked variables (the values of these variables are in hierarchical order) are evaluated by use of a rank order correlation statistic. Associations among continuous data are determined by calculating correlation coefficients.[4] Strong correlations among variables may indicate to clinicians that if one symptom is observed, a second may also be present.

Many times, an investigator is interested in discerning the differences among variables or groups. For example, if the purpose of the study were to evaluate the effects of a treatment, the investigator would be interested in demonstrating that a significant difference has occurred. Therefore, difference statistics compare the distribution of variables to determine if they are sufficiently different. Because an assumption that all data are normally distributed is central to statistics, difference statistics evaluate the difference between the appropriate measure of central tendency and dispersion to ensure that the distributions are actually independent. In the case of categorical data, differences are determined by the chi-square (χ^2) statistic.[4] For continuous data, a comparison between two variables is evaluated by a *t* test. More than two discrete variables are evaluated with some type of analysis of variance (ANOVA).[4]

The appropriateness of analytic methods is an essential element that the clinician needs to consider when using specific research findings. In general, if the results are consistent across several studies and the analytic methods are similar, the clinician may feel comfortable that the conclusions are correct.

Clinical Significance Versus Statistical Significance

The definitive method to determine the correctness of a research finding is whether the statistical analysis yields significant results. However, an investigator will occasionally report the results to be clinically significant despite no statistical significance. Such an assertion is usually made when the level of significance has approached the 0.05 level. Hence, if the alpha value is the minimally acceptable risk that a false report is made, then this argument is for increasing that risk. A slightly lower significance is usually the result of small sample sizes. Pragmatically speaking, the time, energy, and resources needed to gather some clinical data may preclude increases in sample size. Therefore the clinician must be careful in considering the usefulness of such data, particularly when translating data to justify changes in usual clinical practice.

CROSSING THE DIVIDE: TRANSLATING RESEARCH RESULTS INTO CLINICAL PRACTICE

Translational research is the dynamic and fluid exchange of scientific and clinical knowledge.[9] Generally speaking, the goal of translational research is to make new scientific discoveries useful in clinical care. Referencing the 1979 publication entitled *Translating Research into Practice,* Mitchell[10] pointed out that translational research has been part of the nursing research mission since its inception. Although the profession has shifted its language since the 1970s, using *research translation* in the 1970s, *research utilization* in the 1980s, *evidence-based practice* in the 1990s, and *translation* again after 2000, nurses have not wavered in their commitment to move research knowledge into clinical practice. Whereas translational research has been the topic of discussion among researchers and clinicians for more than 30 years, an increasing number of publications on the concept have emerged during the past decade.

What Is Translational Research?

In "The Meaning of Translational Research and Why It Matters," Steven H. Woolf acknowledged that *translational research* means different things to different people.[11] Whereas we have traditionally heard translational research defined as "from bench to bedside," a different definition, "translating research into practice," has emerged. The traditional classification, from bench to bedside, specifically refers to the transfer of new understandings of disease mechanisms gained in the laboratory to the development of new methods for diagnosis, therapy, and prevention and their first testing in humans.[12] Other researchers and clinicians have delineated translational research as the translation of results from clinical studies into everyday clinical practice and health decision-making.[13,14]

Recent definitions have acknowledged the continuum from *bench to bedside* to *clinical practice.* The National Institutes of Health (NIH) defined translational research as "research that translates scientific discoveries and advances from the bench or laboratory into a clinically germane application."[15] The NIH classifies translational research into type 1 and type 2 translations. Type 1 translation applies basic scientific discoveries to human health care under controlled conditions. Type 2 translation promotes the adoption of the outcomes of promising clinical research by community-based health care under uncontrolled and often uncontrollable conditions.[15] Whereas there is growing consensus on a continuum of translation that moves from basic biomedical research to clinical research to clinical practice and a collective push to accelerate the rate in which this translation occurs, there remains a lack of clarity and consistency on how to move new scientific knowledge into clinical practice.[16,17]

Various terms have been used to label the study and practice of adopting and implementing research findings into clinical practice. Among the terms are *knowledge translation, knowledge transfer, dissemination, implementation research, uptake, diffusion,* and *dissemination.*[18-20] In addition, although some researchers and practitioners have offered implementation strategies for translating research into practice, these strategies are often inadequately defined and poorly described.[21] The use of multiple terms and the absence of widely accepted and used methodologies for bridging research findings to the health care setting hinder progress toward the modification of clinical practices in response to available scientific evidence and health care knowledge. Among the models proposed in the literature to guide the field of translational research are Thornicroft's translational medicine continuum and the translational science spectrum.

Thornicroft's Translational Medicine Continuum

Thornicroft and coworkers proposed a comprehensive five-phase translational continuum for moving research findings into clinical practice (Figure 3-2).[22]

Basic science research is the basis of new discoveries that can significantly influence clinical practice. Phase 0 of the translational medicine continuum, called *basic science discovery,* refers to basic laboratory research, which includes understanding of therapeutic mechanisms of action, identification of promising molecule or gene targets and protein biomarkers, selection of candidate drugs, and animal and laboratory (preclinical) studies.[22] Phase 1 (early human studies) determines safety, tolerability, dose-effect relationships, and early adverse effects in healthy human volunteers. Phase 2 (early clinical trials) uses early exploratory clinical studies to test efficacy in the target population—namely, individuals with the disorder to be treated. During the early trials, scientists can determine optimal doses, determine treatment duration, and compare the safety profiles of the treatment under study with existing treatment options.[22]

The final phases focus on the effectiveness, safety, and implementation of new discoveries in clinical practice. Phase 3 (late clinical trials) refers to clinical studies of effectiveness and safety conducted for a longer time in populations with the condition to be treated.[22] During this stage of clinical discovery, researchers can identify less frequent and longer-term side effects and compare a fully defined replicable intervention with an appropriate alternative under everyday clinical conditions.[23] Phase 4 (implementation) focuses on implementation of scientific discoveries into clinical practice, one of the challenges of translational research. It is not clear who bears the responsibility of implementing evidence-based practices in clinical settings. Researchers disseminate new scientific findings, primarily through peer-reviewed journals, which are most often read by their scientific peers.[24,25] There are relatively few publications on how to implement new clinical guidelines as cost-effective, routine practice in clinical settings.[22,26] Addressing this gap is critical if clinical practice is to efficiently benefit from new scientific advances.

The translational medicine continuum includes three "translational blocks," areas along the continuum that may obstruct the flow of knowledge. The first translational block (T1) is at the interface between animal and early human trials. T1 mediates the transfer of new understandings of disease mechanisms and drug actions gained in the laboratory into the development of new methods for diagnosis, therapy, and prevention and their first testing in humans.[11,22] Translational block 2 (T2) references the interface between efficacy and effectiveness trials. Efficacy studies determine whether an intervention produces the expected result under highly controlled experimental conditions; effectiveness trials examine how well a treatment works under routine clinical conditions.[23] Finally, translational block 3 (T3) refers to the gap between scientifically proven treatments and interventions and knowledge on hand during everyday clinical encounters.[27,28] Dissemination gaps between researchers and clinicians hinder the translation of clinical study results into everyday clinical practice. Collaborative research may help close

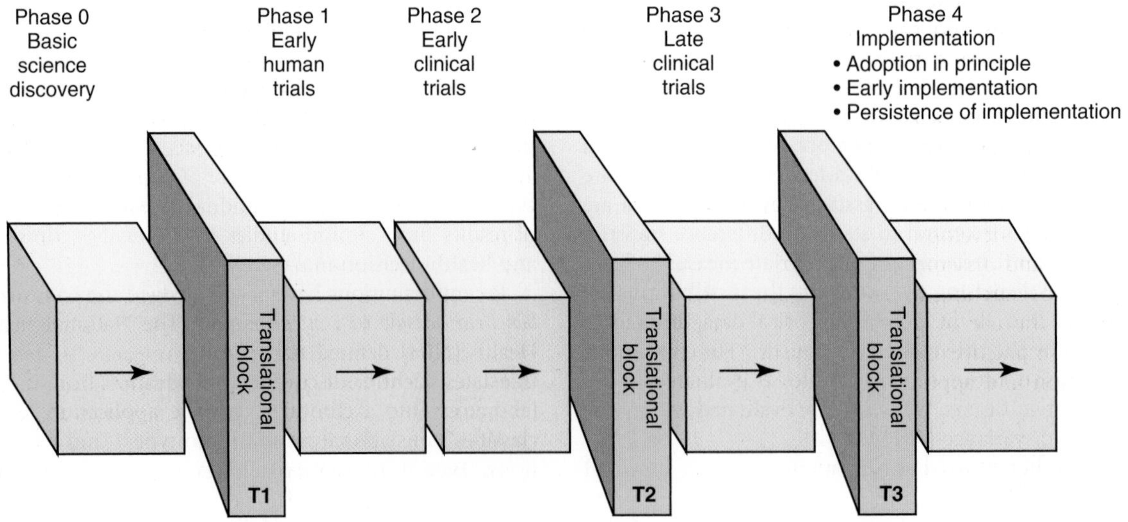

FIGURE 3-2 Five phases and three blocks in the translational medicine continuum. (From Thornicroft G, Lempp H, Tansella M: The place of implementation science in the translational medicine continuum, *Psychol Med* Feb 15:1-7, 2011.)

the gap between researchers and clinicians and facilitate the translation of research findings into clinical practice.

Translational Science Spectrum

Over the past decade, the NIH has introduced several programs and initiatives aimed at advancing clinical treatments and innovating strategies for disease management and health promotion through the application of translational sciences. These programs have been designed to overcome historical barriers to collaborations between academic researchers and clinicians and facilitate greater cooperation between these two groups.[29,30] Among the NIH's more recent endeavors is the National Center for Advancing Translational Sciences (NCATS). Established in 2011, the mission of the Center is "to catalyze the generation of innovative methods and technologies that will enhance the development, testing and implementation of diagnostics and therapeutics across a wide range of human diseases and conditions."[31] NCATS promotes and supports efforts that enable researchers across different sectors to more efficiently develop clinical treatments, demonstrate the treatments' effectiveness in improving health, and accelerate the pace at which new treatments are delivered to patients.[31] In the short time since it was established, NCATS has launched several major research initiatives that support effective strategic partnerships. NCATS primarily supports research to identify and test promising translational innovations and develop, demonstrate, and disseminate advances in medicine, health care, and public health across the clinical phases of the translational science spectrum.[32]

The translational science spectrum represents five stages of research along the path from basic research to public health. The basic research stage involves scientific exploration that can reveal fundamental mechanisms of biology, disease, or behavior. During the preclinical research stage, scientists apply fundamental discoveries made in the laboratory to understand the basis of diseases and uncover treatment options. Clinical research includes clinical trials with human subjects to examine intervention safety and effectiveness, behavioral and observational studies, outcomes and health services research, and the efficacy of new technologies. Clinical implementation refers to the adoption of interventions, technology, and clinical practices into routine clinical care. This stage also includes implementation research to evaluate clinical trial results and identify new clinical questions and gaps in care. Finally, during the public health stage of the spectrum, researchers investigate health outcomes to determine the effects of diseases at the population level and approaches to prevent, diagnose and treat them. Findings help guide scientists working to improve interventions or develop new ones. The translational science spectrum is a not linear model; each stage builds on and informs the others. NCATS develops new approaches, demonstrates their usefulness, and disseminates the findings at each of the five stages. One overarching strategy across the field of translation research is the use of strategic collaborations to ensure the application in practice. Collaboration is essential to ensuring dissemination and application of scientific discoveries in practice.

STRATEGIES TO FORM RESEARCH COLLABORATIONS

Collaborations between clinicians and researchers maximize the expertise of each partner to yield timely and effective clinical research. In addition, clinical and academic research affiliations help translate new discoveries into clinical practice. Such collaborations have been rare, as clinicians and academics often work in orbits that seldom intersect. The climate is changing, however, as we race to treat serious threats to health, such as diabetes, hypertension, HIV/AIDS, and cancer. Given the importance of collaborative research, this section presents strategies to encourage new partnerships between clinicians and researchers and to accelerate those that already exist.

Forming Research Partnerships Between Clinicians and Researchers

Research partnerships form for a variety of reasons. In general, each partner brings a unique research perspective or skill to the research question. Collaborations among researchers are common and are often limited to a specific experiment or set of experiments. Team approaches to investigations of health issues will likely be enduring partnerships, perhaps lasting for the researchers' entire careers. This section offers some general observations about the nature of the processes governing interdisciplinary teams.

Initiating Collaborations. Initial contacts among investigators often begin in a social setting. Once individuals establish that they are comfortable with one another's communication styles, they begin to ascertain the scientific expertise, intellectual characteristics, and technical skills of potential collaborators. This stage of exploration can be stimulating and interesting but also challenging, depending on the styles of the participants. The critical outcome of this exploration is establishing the strengths and weaknesses of the team members. Optimally, the strengths of the whole balance the deficiencies of individual potential team members.

Another important outcome of these early formative interactions is a new articulation of the theoretical focus of the research collaboration. Investigators come together initially because of some common interest. The common interest may be a particular disease or patient population. Each investigator may represent a particular discipline (e.g., medicine, nursing, molecular biology). Whereas each potential collaborator may be an expert investigator within his or her discipline, most likely each approaches the research question in a different way and perhaps conceptualizes the question differently. If the team is to investigate the problem from a truly interdisciplinary perspective, the question must be reframed to incorporate the unique points of view of each discipline represented.

Merging Perspectives. Practicing clinicians can bring an orientation to the research enterprise that reflects the "real world" of health care. Targeting the most relevant aspects of the clinical research problem under investigation will likely result in findings that are more directly relevant to clinical solutions. Investigators may experience some angst in accommodating the clinical perspective because it may mean leaving some pertinent but perhaps less germane questions unanswered. In some cases, for example, a clinician may be more interested in finding a solution that works and be less interested in why it works. This pragmatic approach to scientific development is not the norm and may not be the most intriguing to investigators motivated by the search for knowledge. However, both perspectives must be incorporated because the how and the why—the mechanisms of the intervention—are essential building blocks of clinical diagnosis and treatment. Treatment outcome variables are, in fact, measures of the mechanistic elements of disease or healthy life processes. The merger of the two perspectives will achieve an efficient research enterprise.

UNDERSTANDING THE RESEARCH PROCESS

Developing the Research Question, Proposal, and Research Protocol

During the application process, applicants focus on formulating the research questions and producing a strong proposal. Researchers will discuss and begin to develop the research protocol, which is used to generate data and to delineate the responsibilities of the various team members. In large projects, researchers often engage advisory groups to help refine the protocol, ensuring that the positions of constituencies, including the target population, are adequately considered in the design and implementation of the project.

The time between submission of the application and the award of a grant may be as long as 1 year. During this time, the team may find it useful to continue to meet and work on the project. For example, if the team generated pilot data as part of the preparation process, team meetings could focus on data analysis and interpretation. Such discussions will help solidify the intellectual connections among team members, further clarifying each member's contributions to the project. In addition, team meetings will facilitate regular communication among the team members, helping to strengthen team dynamics. Failure to maintain regular communication will mean that team building will coincide with implementation of the protocol, an inopportune time for team building. Furthermore, without regular communication, individuals may accept other responsibilities and be unavailable to participate. All team members, including clinician and novice researchers, should be included in grant preparation deliberations, as well, and in meetings after the grant submission. Failure to engage all members may gravely affect team dynamics.

Role of the Team Leader. Team building is a crucial step in collaborative research, whether the collaboration is between scientists and clinicians or among a diverse group of scientists. It is essential that all team members feel they are integral to the project's success. The team leader must be extremely attentive to communication among team members. Open communication is essential. Co-investigators should not be excluded from administrative meetings by design or accident. Leaders should not assume that a named investigator is "not interested" in any element of the project's implementation. Leaders should provide feedback on the effectiveness of each member and should elicit feedback about his or her communication and leadership style. Team leaders must also follow the progress of each investigator's activities and ensure proper and adequate resource allocations, as delineated in the grant application.

Resource Issues. As part of the grant application process, many funders, including the NIH, allow administrative cost allocations to cover expenses associated with managing grant funds. These indirect costs are allocated in different ways within institutions, although the indirect cost allocation in part or in whole is usually given to the department of the principal investigator. In the case of team research, this arrangement may be a barrier to interdepartmental cooperation. In rare instances, it could lead to infighting about the lead investigator position. Administrators must address solutions to abate this potential issue of contention; the potential co-investigators should consult with department leaders early in the process.

Other resource concerns in collaborative research include resource allocations, typically negotiated during the application process. Departmental or organizational resources often differ across disciplines and clinical settings. In general, departmental resources are greater in departments with several successful investigators. Nevertheless, all investigators should be provided similar support services. For example, if the research team is participating in professional meetings, the grant should cover travel and registration costs for each investigator. Support from statisticians, research coordinators, and editors should also be available for each team member. Team leaders need to assess the needs of each investigator and secure the resources required for the whole team to be successful. As we continue to move in the direction of collaborative interdisciplinary research, academic health centers and universities may begin to reconsider current policies on resource distribution, such as indirect cost allocations.

Enhancing the Research Infrastructure: Interdisciplinary Team Building. The push toward translational research, and the corresponding reform of the research enterprise supported by agencies such as the NIH, will affect and perhaps restructure the research enterprises of academic health centers and universities. Many such institutions are organized around disciplinary lines, making it difficult to meet or to become acquainted with scientists and clinicians affiliated with other organizational units. There may also be barriers to cross-departmental collaboration. Consequently, research administrators may need to devise strategies to encourage and to support interdisciplinary research activities.

Administrators may need to be proactive in encouraging interdisciplinary team building to promote and support such collaborations across the institution. Many academic organizations are structured in disciplinary silos. For example, in the past, it was atypical for the faculty of medical schools and nursing schools to co-teach classes or to share research space; fortunately, this situation is changing. Sharing research space and co-teaching classes are natural venues for each specialist to become familiar with the other's work. Organizing seminars that bring together investigators from throughout the organization helps assemble interdisciplinary teams. These seminars focus on an area of research or process elements of collaborative research. Searchable databases of researcher interests and expertise are also useful tools for those seeking research partnerships. Incentives, such as seed funding for new research partnerships, provide the impetus to forge partnerships and may be required to generate preliminary data to support research grant applications.

Challenges of Research Collaboration on Career Development. Academic health centers and universities have established criteria to evaluate career development and scholarly achievement. To progress through the ranks to tenured professor, the faculty member must be recognized as a national or international leader in his or her field of research. If team research is to become a norm, how will career development and achievement be judged? Proposing strategies for this go beyond the scope of this chapter; however, it is noteworthy that we frame the question.

In institutions with tenure, faculty members must complete promotion criteria in an established time frame. If the criteria require that the individual be the principal recipient of a research grant, participation in team research may jeopardize his or her career. On the other hand, the ability to join an accomplished investigator who is willing to serve as a mentor may result in rapid significant research experience and even selection as the lead investigator in subsequent team research. As we move closer to the collaborative clinical research enterprises, academic institutions are likely to change the promotion and tenure criteria to recognize the necessity of the team in translating research into clinical practice.

Collaborative Research as a Strategy for Career Development. Although the efforts of the NIH and others have become a stimulus for collaborative research, the concept of partnering on research projects, particularly partnerships between scientists, is not new. In fact, collaborative research has been used successfully to launch research careers in resource-limited organizations. Rarely is an investigator successful in obtaining grant funding without providing some evidence that he or she can generate the proposed data. This evidence usually requires submission of pilot or feasibility data, which ordinarily cannot be generated without cost. A new investigator may negotiate to assist a senior investigator with his or her research in exchange for amending the protocol to include needed pilot data.

In negotiating this relationship, the researchers must consider similar concerns previously discussed, including the nature of the relationship, communication, access to resources, and data ownership. In addition, the junior researcher should discern that he or she and the principal investigator have compatible management and communication styles.

Benefits of Having a Mentor. In academic centers and universities, senior investigators usually hold teaching or mentoring roles. Most embrace them and see them as a contributing factor to their job satisfaction. Hence, a successful collaboration, which may have helped launch an academic career, may, in fact, have long-term benefits. Often, a senior investigator within an organization has knowledge of the bureaucracy associated with the research enterprise. Navigating that bureaucracy is rarely simple for anyone, especially new investigators. Having an experienced researcher to "show you the ropes" can be invaluable. Senior investigators also know how to access support services that may not be readily apparent. These resources are often oversubscribed, making the experience and leadership of an experienced investigator particularly useful in accessing these services.

Seasoned investigators have knowledge of the personal characteristics required to succeed as a scientist. If a mentor is willing and the novice investigator is amenable, the junior researcher will be able to progress rapidly and develop the skills required to be a successful investigator and professor. A successful collaborative research experience is a win-win situation for all concerned, including the affiliated organization.

SUMMARY

Collaborative research is not a new phenomenon. Teams of investigators coalesce around common research interests. Each member of the team brings unique skills to the research process and is integral to the project's success. Successful collaborative research teams are based on clear and accurate communication of the roles and responsibilities of each member and respect for the perspective each discipline brings to the collaboration. Successful translational research efforts also require administrative support from both the academic and clinical partners to foster and to support building of research teams. In translational research, as in other areas of clinical practice, collaboration is the essential element linking researchers and clinicians from multiple disciplines as they translate research into clinical practice.

CHAPTER 4

THE PATIENT, THE PROVIDER, AND PRIMARY CARE: AN INTEGRATED PERSPECTIVE

Matthew Favazza

During the past two decades, we have experienced remarkable societal and health care changes. In recent years, health care providers have recognized the value of the shared relationship between provider and patient. Careful listening in a supportive environment can help identify the unique health care needs of each patient. Because many patients are from diverse cultural and ethnic backgrounds as well as varied age groups, it is necessary for primary health care providers to recognize that most patients are using alternative therapies and to work collaboratively with integrative health practitioners to deliver culturally sensitive, holistic care.

INTEGRATIVE HEALTH CARE AND ALTERNATIVE THERAPIES

Integrative health care recognizes the biologic, psychological, sociologic, and spiritual dimensions inherent in every patient encounter. This integrative approach combines Western and Eastern health practices, energy therapies, nutritional approaches, dietary supplements, and environmental health recommendations in health care management decisions for patients who are viewed to be part of a larger whole. Integrative health providers acknowledge each individual's reality of health, health beliefs, health practices, and values. The Bravewell Collaborative, a nationally recognized resource for integrative health, defines integrative medicine as patient-centered care that does the following:

- Focuses on healing the whole person—mind, body, and spirit—in the context of community
- Educates and empowers people to be active participants in their own care and to take responsibility for their own health and wellness
- Integrates the best of Western scientific medicine with a broader understanding of the nature of illness, healing, and wellness
- Makes use of all appropriate therapeutic approaches and evidenced-based global medical modalities to achieve optimal health and healing
- Encourages healing partnerships between the provider and patient
- Supports the individualization of care
- Creates a culture of wellness[1]

Effective primary care providers recognize that their patients may use integrative health practices, including nutritional supplements, in their personal health care and may be reluctant to discuss this with the health care provider. A careful history of all supplements and health practices is imperative for a safe and collaborative approach that fosters a trusting relationship.

Alternative Therapies for Common Chronic Conditions

Nonvitamin, nonmineral oral supplements, which include herbs and other dietary supplements, are the most commonly used alternative therapies in the United States, accounting for approximately 17.9% of complementary health approaches. This greatly surpasses other complementary treatment modalities by more than double the percentage of those who try yoga, massage, or osteopathic manipulation.[2] Approximately one half to three fourths of American adults use such dietary supplements with ambitions to promote a healthier lifestyle or ameliorate various health conditions.[2] With such a large number of Americans using over-the-counter dietary supplements, it not only is important for providers to take a careful history of all supplements used by patients, but it also is crucial for providers to have a general understanding of commonly used dietary supplements available and the data behind their clinical use and safety profiles. Even though a large number of Americans are using dietary supplements, only about one fourth of those alternative therapies were recommended by a health care provider.[3] It is imperative that providers understand patient motivations to use dietary supplements because it will allow for safe, effective care and potentially build trust and open attitudes to foster a better relationship between patient and provider. With such a sizeable proportion of the American population using dietary supplements to help improve comorbidities, it is in the best interest of providers to consider the use of integrative medicine to encourage patients to take initial steps toward achieving their health goals.

Dietary supplements are not currently approved by the U.S. Food and Drug Administration (FDA); however, per federal mandate, these products must be safe and cannot make misleading or false claims with regard to their use in various health conditions.[2] Because these supplements are not FDA regulated, safety and efficacy become a priority when choosing dietary supplementation. To deliver holistic care, providers need to have an open attitude toward the use of dietary supplements, understand patient motivation to use such products, and identify safe and effective indications to integrate into current health care practices. Many dietary supplements lack clinical evidence to support their use in current health problems; however, it is at the discretion of the provider to assess the current data regarding a particular supplement's use in any one condition, as well as the safety and risk for any given patient.[4] With the increasing use of dietary supplements, patients are more frequently preferring supplement use over that of commonly used medications. This desire for alternative therapies arises from the notion that dietary supplements are safer than most pharmacologic interventions.[5] Because nurse practitioners are holistic providers, it is of the utmost importance that they broaden their knowledge base regarding dietary supplements to build patient relationships, provide education regarding supplement safety to those who are receiving care, offer various alternative therapies for patients to choose from, and create a stepping stone for more traditional therapies when indicated.

Many patients can be found to have borderline dyslipidemia, prehypertension, or glucose intolerance or impaired fasting glucose in which medications are not indicated per recommended guidelines but morbidity and mortality pose a risk. The following recommendations have varying strengths of evidence and continue to require further research to determine efficacy, dosage, and medication interactions. When recommending nutraceuticals, dietary supplements, and herbal remedies, nurse practitioners should use their best clinical judgment based on current research. Providers should remain vigilant in their clinical practice by employing evidence-based alternative therapies.

Prehypertension and Hypertension. Because prehypertension can be associated with a higher risk of mortality, it is important to reduce risk factors through diet and other lifestyle modifications. However, for those unwilling to make changes or start a new medication for their prehypertension, dietary supplementation may be a viable option. L-Arginine supplementation has been shown in some studies to provide a mild reduction in both systolic and diastolic blood pressure.[6] L-Arginine is an amino acid and nitric oxide synthesis substrate.[6] It is important to note that caution should be exercised when L-arginine is used in conjunction with other pharmacologic antihypertensive agents, erectile dysfunction medications, and nitrates, because this can result in an unsafe drop in blood pressure.[6]

Another commonly used dietary supplement is garlic extract, which is still debated because of varying evidence.[7] Although the current data regarding the efficacy of garlic in hypertension are still under investigation, clinical understanding of the effects of garlic's polysulfides and their upregulation of hydrogen sulfide on vasodilation as well as on endothelial oxidative stress can suggest some benefit.[7] Just as with any other antihypertensive, caution should be exercised when recommending the concomitant use of garlic with other antihypertensive agents.

Most providers have encountered patients using coenzyme Q10 (CoQ10) or a supplement also known as *ubiquinone* for various reasons.[8] This supplement has shown promise as an alternative therapy for prehypertension or hypertension; it has been studied in various trials demonstrating a 17-mm Hg systolic and 10-mm Hg diastolic reduction in blood pressure.[8] In a meta-analysis evaluating the use of CoQ10 in hypertension, it was found that CoQ10 can be used safely and can result in a significant decrease in blood pressure without significant adverse reactions.[8] Dosage is still debated; however, doses varying from 75 to 360 mg/day have been used in studies with reported effects.[8]

Glucose Intolerance and Impaired Fasting Glucose. Glucose intolerance and impaired fasting glucose pose significant cardiovascular risks, and their incidence is on the rise.[9] Because dysglycemia (glucose intolerance or impaired fasting glucose) is different from overt type 2 diabetes mellitus, it is important to treat it before the disease process advances.[9] As with most metabolic conditions, an integral part of prevention and treatment is modification of diet and lifestyle.[9] To supplement these dietary and lifestyle modifications, herbal and dietary supplements may be used to help improve glycemic control in these individuals.

Two different supplements whose role in diabetes have been studied with controversial evidence are chromium picolinate and chromium yeast.[10] A meta-analysis of multiple trials showed equivocal evidence that both refutes the efficacy of chromium and possibly supports a mild reduction in hemoglobin A_{1c} (HbA_{1c}).[10] With such conflicting evidence, it is difficult to determine whether or not chromium has a role in treatment of insulin resistance and glycemic control.[10] Chromium, however, has potential use in treatment of diabetes and insulin resistance because of its role on a molecular level and according to current scientific understanding.[11] Through in vitro and in vivo studies, chromium was found to potentiate insulin, inhibit negative regulators of insulin signaling, and enhance the glucose metabolism effects of adenosine monophosphate–activated protein kinase (AMPK), which in theory has the potential to lower HbA_{1c} levels and fasting glucose.[11]

Many small studies suggest that bitter melon may have glucose-lowering effects. Although the bitter melon did have a reported glucose-lowering effect in that particular study, metformin was still superior.[12] Bitter melon acts by inhibiting protein tyrosine phosphatase 2, which is found in skeletal muscle and antagonizes insulin activity, resulting in improved insulin sensitivity.[13] Because of this, bitter melon has a theoretical use in the treatment of glucose intolerance and type 2 diabetes mellitus. However, as with most alternative therapies, further research is needed to determine its efficacy.[13]

Berberine is a compound extracted from Rhizoma coptidis, which has been used in the treatment of diabetes.[14] Just as chromium enhances the effects of AMPK, berberine activates this AMPK pathway and increases insulin sensitivity while inhibiting mitochondrial activity, which increases glycolysis.[14] Another small study provided some insight that 500 mg of berberine three times a day had a significant impact on lowering HbA_{1c} levels and postprandial glucose.[15] For those who experienced gastrointestinal symptoms such as bloating and diarrhea, a decreased dose of 300 mg three times a day was used.[15] Other than gastrointestinal side effects, berberine has a fairly wide safety profile and has not demonstrated any significant renal or hepatic adverse reactions.[15] Also of note was a lipid-lowering effect triggered by berberine; this is covered later in the chapter.[14,15]

Cinnamon has long been used in supporting healthy glucose levels in those with glucose intolerance and type 2 diabetes mellitus.[16] In in vitro and in vivo studies, cinnamon was found to activate insulin receptor kinase and inhibit dephosphorylation of insulin receptors, which ultimately results in increased insulin sensitivity.[16] A dose of 1 to 6 g was used in a particular trial, which showed significant reductions in fasting glucose and HbA_{1c} levels after 40 days.[16] A comparison with placebo also showed that cinnamon resulted in statistically significant reduction in fasting triglyerides.[16] A meta-analysis and systematic review showed that cinnamon lowered fasting glucose, total cholesterol, triglycerides, and low-density lipoprotein (LDL) cholesterol but did not have any statistically significant impact on HbA_{1c}.[17] As with other glucose-lowering medications, cinnamon does pose the risk of lowering sugars too much, causing symptoms of hypoglycemia; therefore caution should be exercised when cinnamon is used with other antidiabetic agents.[16]

Reportedly, the use of fenugreek can decrease fasting glucose and in a small way affects HbA_{1c}. In various trials a dose of 2 to 5 g has been used with only mild, self-limited side effects of gastrointestinal upset, diarrhea, and changes in urine odor. Fenugreek was also found to remain renal and hepatic neutral.[18]

Dyslipidemia. Dyslipidemia, a major cardiovascular risk factor, is becoming a widespread problem among Americans because of a worsening obesity epidemic.[19] Plant sterols and β-sitosterol have been studied in the setting of hyperlipidemia.[20] The most common stanols and sterols found in the modern diet are β-sitosterol and campesterol.[20] The average individual consumes 300 mg of plant sterols daily and about 17 to 24 mg of plan stanols.[20] Such plant stanols and sterols inhibit intraluminal cholesterol absorption.[20] Although researchers have reported that increased dietary intake of plant stanols and sterols did not provide any significant LDL-lowering effects, absence of stanols and sterols in the diet resulted in increased low-density lipoprotein cholesterol (LDL-C).[20] A suggested supplementation of 1 to 2 g of plant stanols and sterols has been found to have some lipid-lowering effects with a fairly wide safety profile.[20] Of note, increased intake of plant stanols and sterols has been associated with poor absorption of carotenoids and vitamin E, which may require supplementation.[20]

As mentioned previously, berberine has been associated with not only improved fasting glucose levels but also improved LDL and triglyceride levels.[14] It is postulated that berberine lowers cholesterol through its metabolites jatrorrhizine, columbamine, berberrubine, and demethyleneberberine, which upregulate low-density lipoprotein receptor (LDLR) mRNA and protein expression, thus inhibiting cellular lipid buildup.[21] When 500 mg of berberine was combined with 200 mg of red yeast rice and 10 mg of policosanols in a specific trial, LDL-C and total cholesterol were found to be lowered over a 24-week period without adverse reactions.[21] In a separate study, berberine did provide improved lowering effects on total cholesterol and LDL-C when compared with diet alone as well as with oral lipid-lowering agents and berberine in combination.[22] Although berberine had a statistically significant impact on these lipid levels, tolerability was also noted during this study.[22]

Red yeast rice is one of the most well-known herbal supplements used by individuals for lipid management owing to its long-time use in Eastern medicine and its similarity to statin therapy. The functional component of red yeast rice is monacolin K, which is naturally occurring lovastatin.[23] Because of varying concentrations of monacolin K in over-the-counter products, red yeast rice supplementation and its efficacy in lipid management are difficult to truly assess.[23] Monacolin K, because of its similarity to statin medications, has effects on total cholesterol and LDL-C levels that resemble the effects of statin therapy.[24] Multiple studies, albeit small, show significant improvements in LDL-C and total cholesterol with a wide safety profile.[24] Unfortunately, many studies do not show any statistically significant increase in high-density lipoprotein cholesterol (HDL-C).[24] With varying results, some studies suggest a 20% to 26% reduction in LDL-C. Although some studies show that this medication has not had a significant impact on creatine kinase, transaminases, or renal function and has reported benefits in lowering total cholesterol and LDL-C, patients should avoid using red yeast rice supplements with statin therapy.[24] Also, caution should be exercised when recommending the use of certain medications such as cyclosporine, azole antifungals, erythromycin, and clarithromycin with red yeast rice because they may increase serum levels just as these medications do with synthetic statins.[25] A small study in mice suggests that red yeast rice used in combination with CoQ10 supplementation may provide an alternative to atorvastatin if that drug is not tolerated owing to myopathies and myalgias.[26] Recent studies have proposed that vitamin D deficiency plays a small role in statin-induced myopathy as well, and vitamin D supplementation may help reduce muscle cramps.

Neuropathy. Some individuals experience chronic pain and paresthesias as a result of neuropathy. Although there are many pharmacologic therapies approved for the treatment of neuropathy, most commonly a complication of diabetes, alternative supplementation can provide improvement in pain with superior tolerability as compared with traditional medications.

A supplement known as *α-lipoic acid* (ALA) has been studied for its role in the support of those with neuropathy. It is a coenzyme found in the Krebs cycle and known to be a potent antioxidant that can protect microvessels in the setting of diabetes mellitus. A study using intravenous ALA, 600 mg/day, over a 3-week course showed significant improvement in neuropathic pain.[18] It was well tolerated, and oral supplementation did not show clinical significance within this particular study.[18]

A long-term trial over 4 years showed improvement in diabetic neuropathy pain with use of ALA, 600 mg orally, without serious adverse reactions that were directly attributed to the use of ALA.[27] From the evidence presented by multiple studies, ALA can be considered an effective adjuvant therapy for diabetic polyneuropathy at either 600 mg given intravenously over a 3-week period or 600 mg given orally, with a wide safety profile and tolerability.[28,29]

Another supplement studied in the treatment of neuropathy is acetyl-L-carnitine (ALC). The use of ALC has been implicated as an adjuvant therapy in chemotherapy-induced polyneuropathy; however, some studies have suggested that it has benefits in improving nerve conduction and neuropathic pain in those with diabetic neuropathy.[30] One particular review of two randomized, placebo-controlled studies involving a large population over 1 year in which ALC was used at 1000 mg three times daily reported significant improvement in diabetic neuropathic pain as well as vibratory sense. In recommending the use of ALC to patients with diabetic polyneuropathy, the provider can be assured of a wide safety profile with limited adverse reactions including paresthesia and pain.[30-32] A dose of 1000 to 3000 mg/day can be used, as suggested by multiple studies.[30-32]

There are multiple proposed beneficial supplements in the adjuvant treatment of diabetic peripheral neuropathy; however, further studies need to be conducted to determine efficacy and dosage. One particular study found that a fixed dose of methylcobalamin, benfotiamine, biotin, folic acid, pyridoxine, ALA, myo-inositol, omega fatty acids, and glutathione provided dramatic improvement of neuropathy symptoms.[33] Such a well-tolerated, relatively safe combination of inexpensive nutraceutical components could provide a better-tolerated alternative therapy for diabetic polyneuropathy.[33]

Insomnia. Insomnia is a common complaint that is multifactorial and usually a result of the culmination of stress, anxiety, depression, and environmental factors. Once dietary and lifestyle modifications have been made, most providers rely on pharmacologic agents to treat those with insomnia. Before using medications such as benzodiazepines, many individuals may explore use of alternative therapies.

Commonly used in the treatment of insomnia, melatonin has been used with mixed evidence. Melatonin is secreted by the pineal gland and regulates the sleep-wake cycle.[34] Because of a short half-life of approximately 45 minutes, most individuals fail to maintain sleep after taking the recommended dose of melatonin (2 to 3 mg).[34] This, however, may prove useful for those who are traveling across time zones, have difficulty initiating sleep, or work overnight shifts with an alternating sleep-wake schedule.[34] It is suggested by some studies that melatonin may provide adequate improvement in sleep cycles in older adults because it provides a better safety profile than most other sleep aids, which are associated with delirium, drowsiness, and memory loss.[34-36]

Another alternative remedy for insomnia that has improved sleep is valerian, with minimal side effects of drowsiness.[37,38] Sleep latency and quality of sleep were found to be improved in some small studies.[37] Valerian acts as a partial 5-HT_{5A} receptor agonist, which has been associated with improved sleep patterns.[39] Because of varying formulations and inconsistencies among valerian products, efficacy is left to particular products with superior purity.[40] As with any sleep aid, caution should be exercised with regard to the individual patient's age and concurrent medications that may cause drowsiness.[37,38,40]

Joint Pain. Chronic pain, especially related to osteoarthritis (OA) and overuse, is another complaint commonly encountered in primary care. Most patients rely on nonsteroidal anti-inflammatory drugs (NSAIDs) for their joint pain; however, this can result in gastrointestinal upset or bleeding and, in some extreme cases, renal injury. Also, because of their availability over the counter, many patients tend to take more than the recommended amounts, causing unfortunate adverse reactions.[41]

Most health care providers are familiar with the use of glucosamine chondroitin in OA pain. This is a commonly used supplement that can help those with mild to moderate OA.[42] It has been shown to help reduce joint space narrowing and hip and knee pain in most studies; however, some studies do not show significant improvement in overall symptoms.[42] This compound is safe when taken at recommended doses; only minor side effects of gastrointestinal symptoms have been reported. However, it can prolong bleeding if taken with other blood-thinning agents.[43-45] A recommended dose of 1200 to 1500 mg/day has been used in studies that support its use.[42,44]

Bromelain is a compound that is extracted from pineapple; it has been shown to act as an anti-inflammatory compound and implied to provide pain relief in those with inflammatory joint pain.[46] Doses as high as 800 mg have been used in various studies with equivocal evidence but limited side effects including gastrointestinal upset.[46,47] Turmeric with its active component, curcumin, is another alternative therapy to help improve joint pain; its anti-inflammatory properties result from its inhibition of the proinflammatory cytokines.[48] Some small studies with both human and rat trials attempted to compare traditional NSAIDs such as indomethacin or diclofenac with alternative therapies such as bromelain or turmeric.[48] Curcumin has been found to be effective in the treatment of inflammatory joint pain in some studies, with significantly limited side effects.[49] Molecular and cytologic research has shown the use of curcumin to result in inhibition of prostaglandin synthesis in rheumatoid arthritis patients, which shows promise for further adjuvant treatments.[50] Curcumin has been well tolerated at doses as high as 12 g for 3 months without adverse reactions; however, doses of 1200 mg/day have been used in some studies.[51,52]

Another frequently used over-the-counter product some patients find useful for their OA pain is capsaicin, a compound isolated from chili peppers. Studies indicate that capsaicin, when topically applied, is well tolerated, with only minor adverse reactions of localized erythema and burning.[53] It is recommended to be used up to four times daily and applied to affected joints; this causes defunctionalization of nociceptors, resulting in reduced pain.[53] Topical capsaicin has been associated with pain relief in not only OA joint pain but also postherpetic neuralgia.[54]

CONCLUSION

Providing education about all medications is necessary so that patients and families understand the risks and benefits of both prescribed medications and alternative therapies. Acknowledging and accepting that patients may be consulting integrative health providers or using alternative therapies is important in guiding patients to care that is safe and effective.

CHAPTER 5

POPULATION-BASED CARE FOR PRIMARY CARE PROVIDERS

Barbara B. Chase

This chapter aims to increase the reader's appreciation of how population management is used to improve practice in primary care. It invites the reader to apply a systems approach to care while simultaneously remembering that each patient is an individual with distinct needs, beliefs, and values. To this end, it describes the chronic care model (CCM) and its relation to the patient-centered medical home (PCMH); discusses population management in the primary care setting; and suggests skills that are useful to design and lead health care teams, quality initiatives, and practice innovations. A case study gives concrete examples of what 1 day in a nurse practitioner's practice might look like in this model.

CURRENT CHALLENGES

In recent years, with decreasing reimbursements and increasing regulatory requirements, too few young physicians have entered primary care, and many older ones have given up their practices, leaving many areas in the United States with not enough primary care providers to handle the growing burden of chronic disease and an aging population. Meanwhile, there is mounting pressure to increase access to care, to improve outcomes, to enhance patient satisfaction, and to reduce costs.[1,2]

SOLUTIONS TO CURRENT CHALLENGES

To avert a looming crisis, policy experts have called for a radical transformation of primary care.[2-4] Population management activities are integral to the implementation of the CCM and the PCMH, both paradigms for primary care transformation. Therefore, population-based practice must be understood in this context.[1,5,6] Although population research results are variable, the results show that the impact of quality and efficiency interventions is directly related to the proven effectiveness and wide adoption of successful interventions.[3,4,7]

Another important proposal to improve quality and access to care is the increased use of nurse practitioners as primary care providers and practice leaders.[2,8,9-12] Supporting nurse practitioner practice, numerous studies during the past 40 years have demonstrated that nurse practitioner care meets or exceeds the quality of physician care and often does so at a lower cost.[8-12] Furthermore, in 2009 the American College of Physicians encouraged nurse practitioner–led PCMH projects.[13] It would seem that in this transformative environment, nurse practitioners have a rare opportunity both to reach their potential as primary care providers and to influence health care policy.

The overall goal of primary care transformation is the creation of an environment that puts patients at the center of care while improving quality and efficiency. The use of a multidisciplinary systems approach to clinician-patient collaboration could meet this end while generating positive experiences for both patients and clinicians. Collaboration among disciplines is integral to primary care practice, but the most important partnership that takes place in a primary care setting is between patient and clinician. The ideal care partnership is characterized by good communication, shared purpose, mutual trust and understanding, beneficial to each individual as well as to health outcomes.

CHRONIC CARE MODEL

The World Health Organization reports that chronic noncommunicable diseases cause nearly two thirds of all premature deaths and disability worldwide and accrue disproportionate costs. The organization recommends that prevention and management of these diseases be addressed with multifaceted interventions at every level of the care delivery system.[14] Nevertheless, much of the ambulatory care in the United States is still delivered in a traditional model that has not changed for decades.[2,15] In response, Wagner and colleagues designed the CCM to help clinicians manage the routine delivery of ambulatory care in a more effective way, placing patients at the center of care and making quality improvement integral to office practice. The CCM offers guidelines for the development of patient, clinician, and organizational systems to successfully improve patient care.[6]

The CCM was first developed by the Group Health Cooperative of Puget Sound, Washington, in response to their recognition that the traditional acute care model does not effectively meet the longitudinal health care needs of patients and populations with complicated chronic conditions. Their aim was to change care from acute and reactive to proactive, planned, and population based. Group Health based the CCM on strong evidence suggesting that four interventions led to the greatest improvements in health outcomes: increased provider expertise and skill; educated and supported patients; planned, team-based care; and better use of registry-based information systems.[6] The evidence on the CCM, widely used and studied for well over a decade, suggests that its use leads to both improved processes of care and better health outcomes.[2,6,16-21]

The CCM is made up of six components that address chronic care management and practice improvement.[6] They are discussed briefly here.

Organizational Support

For the CCM to be optimized, top organizational leadership must create a culture that expects and supports evidence-based practice, enhanced chronic care processes, care coordination, and innovative practice improvement. For improved chronic disease management outcomes to become a reality on the ground, leaders not only must value the results but also must show that they understand the process of change and support it with incentives and access to resources that will make things happen. The best organizations openly and systematically use quality initiatives as a way to teach and to reinforce the culture of excellence.[6,16,17]

Clinical Information Systems

Clinical information systems organize data to make efficient, safe, and effective care possible. Population quality and practice improvement cannot realistically be done without sophisticated data systems. Practice analytics have become a staple of health care systems administration; they are used to track resource use and per-case care delivery cost by provider and diagnosis and to compare outcomes by both individual providers and provider groups. An electronic medical record is a start, but to understand the health of a population, systems must be in place that are capable of showing trends for individual patients, groups of patients, providers, and whole practices. Registries, really better described as population management tools, should be embedded within the electronic record; but if that is not possible, they must at least be linked to it. Registry lists determined by risk stratification and disease that show process and outcome data are essential to identify and to engage patients who are overdue for care, to track patient self-care progress, to discover patient care needs, and to evaluate the results of care interventions. Registries should also be able to track immunizations, recommend routine screenings, and stratify risk identification of patients needing preventive care and counseling to prevent disease onset. Reminders of care guidelines, performance targets, immunizations, and medication interactions and administration can be generated by the registry or electronic record. As electronic messaging to patients has become more mainstream, voice mail, e-mail, and text messages are also used to enhance care. Electronic transmission of information can also include clinical data such as blood pressures, heart rates, electrocardiogram tracings, weights, and blood glucose readings.[2,17,18,22,23]

Delivery System Design

Delivery system design refers to the roles and tasks of each individual participating in patient care, the way these individuals work together, the structure of visits, and the management of ongoing follow-up. The CCM promotes care teams, with an emphasis on all team members working collaboratively with one another and the patient, within their scope but to the highest level of their training—the right person doing the right job in the right amount at the right time. For the team to work efficiently and safely, roles and tasks must be well defined, training must be ongoing, communication among members must be frequent, and leadership must be strong. The care team is simultaneously focused on the health of individuals and on the health of the practice. Population management to promote healthy habits and to support ongoing chronic problems is at the foundation of care.[2,10,24,25]

Physicians may not need to know each healthy patient in the practice and may simply collaborate with nurse practitioners as needed in this population. At the other end of the spectrum, patients with complicated needs may have planned visits with nurse practitioners between physician visits to improve their self-care skills and for adjustment of their treatment plans. Nurse practitioners and physicians may work in tandem with nurses, coaches, medical assistants, navigators, and others to facilitate various population functions, such as phone follow-up, medication adjustment, refills, immunizations, referrals, and triage.[10,11,24,26]

A clear definition of visit types should be considered. Whereas schedules should be designed to adequately accommodate urgent access, most visits should be planned visits either for health promotion and screening or for follow-up of ongoing problems. Regularly scheduled follow-up through planned interactions has been shown to have a positive effect on chronic disease outcomes and should be a mainstay of chronic care system design. However, follow-up need not be limited to traditional office visits. Multidisciplinary shared medical appointments, individual and group education visits, support groups, health coach or navigator outreach, and phone, e-mail or other virtual contacts show promise.[2,10,24,26-30] A caveat noted in the research is that as practices change from physician-centric to team-based care, patients must be included in the process so that they understand each team member's function and feel confident that the collaboration improves their care rather than diminishes or fragments it. Thus practices should consider effective ways to educate patients not only about the health care team but also about the patient's role in his or her own health.[3,4,29,31]

Decision Support

Evidence-based practice guidelines as well as the opportunity to consult with clinical experts should be embedded in primary care practice to support care. Clinical guidelines can be integrated into the electronic medical record locally; Web-based products, such as *Essential Evidence Plus, DXplain, UpToDate, Harrison's Online,* and others, can facilitate daily practice. Electronic access to a network of clinician colleagues makes phone calls and face-to-face meetings less necessary. Strong clinical information systems can streamline most improvements in decision support by automatically placing information on the desktop or other electronic device.[23,32,33]

Self-Management Support

Self-management support is a crucial component of the CCM and is effectively implemented by use of a population approach. The goal of self-management support is to engage patients in their own care and to empower them to reach their full potential as self-advocates and partners in care. For many patients and providers alike, this patient-centered practice is a new method. In the acute care model, clinicians prescribe and patients comply. Self-management support in the CCM requires different assumptions, processes, and skills.[2,6,21,34,35]

Before patients can begin self-management, they must have access to information that is appropriate for how they learn and who they are—cognitively, emotionally, culturally, and experientially. Clinical information systems can be invaluable in making a variety of written and Web-based materials easily accessible to those who can use them. In-person education can take the form of one-on-one visits, but shared medical appointments and education or support groups are becoming increasingly common.[34-37] Although education alone does not ensure improved self-management, education programs that emphasize patient empowerment, recognize and work with the patient's readiness for change, and use techniques such as motivational interviewing (MI) have been shown to improve patient self-management behaviors and outcomes.[19,21,28,31,34-37]

Once patients have knowledge and skills, they are better prepared to make informed health care choices for themselves based on the facts of their situation, their personal values, and their goals. Unfortunately, many patients lack problem-solving skills. These patients benefit from help in setting SMART (specific, measurable, attainable, realistic, and timely) goals, making an action plan, and anticipating and addressing problems or barriers.[21,28,34-37]

After a specific period of trying out a plan, patients should evaluate what went well and what did not and make new choices as they move forward with the evolution of their self-care skills. Most patients need guidance and support as they learn self-management, and because of psychological and social barriers, many need intensive interventions to help them adapt to living with a chronic disease. These activities can be facilitated by individual clinicians but are very effectively managed by a population approach and multidiscipline health care

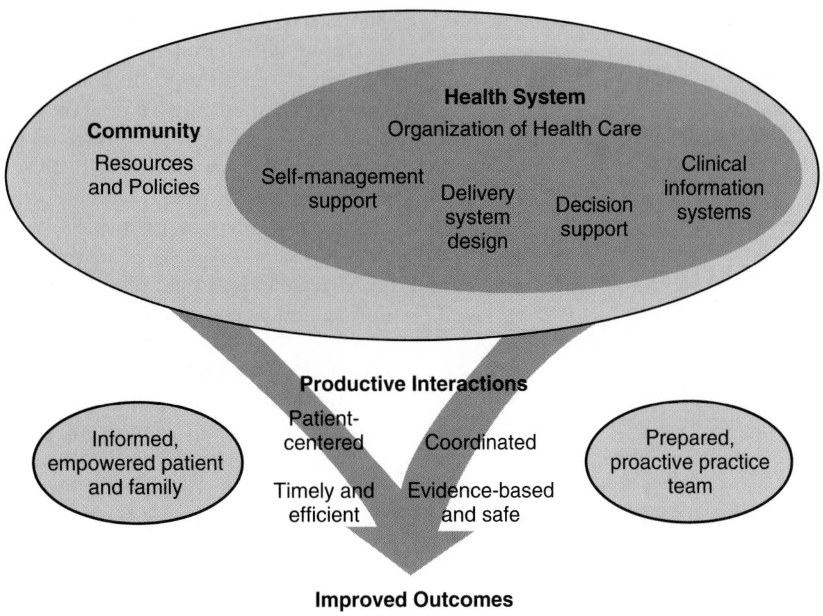

FIGURE 5-1 Chronic care model. (From Wagner EH: Chronic disease management: what will it take to improve chronic illness? *Effect Clin Pract* 1:2-4, 1998.)

teams.[19,28,29,34-37] Specific assessment and counseling skills needed to work with patients struggling with adjustment to living with a chronic disease are discussed later in this chapter.

Community Resources

Relationships with community-based programs can support or expand organization and practice resources and should be encouraged (Fig. 5-1). Neighborhood, government, insurance, and specialty organization programs can at times be more convenient for patients. Peer-to-peer support groups, church groups, wellness programs, education programs, elder services, pharmacies, visiting nurses, social workers, physical therapists, home health aides, and homemaker services may be available, depending on the community. As with other components of the CCM, further research must be done to better understand both the concepts and their effect on health care processes and outcomes.[38-40]

THE PATIENT-CENTERED MEDICAL HOME

The PCMH is at the center of primary care redesign. The term *medical home* was introduced in 1967 by the American Academy of Pediatrics to indicate where a child's medical information was archived. After several years of discussion about how to improve primary care, in 2007 the American College of Physicians, American Academy of Family Physicians, American Academy of Pediatrics, and American Osteopathic Association together published the joint principles of a new medical home model, the PCMH, describing it as an approach to providing comprehensive primary care for both children and adults.[5] Two years later, the American College of Physicians published a monograph that discussed the role of nurse practitioners in the PCMH, acknowledging that nurse practitioners are qualified to serve as primary care providers.[13] Ongoing demonstration projects throughout the United States are implementing the PCMH model and measuring the effects on care quality and cost. Health care organizations and insurers are increasingly encouraging and supporting application for PCMH recognition by the National Committee for Quality Assurance (NCQA) and other accreditation organizations such as URAC (formerly the Utilization Review Accreditation Commission), the Joint Commission (TJC), and the Accreditation Association for Ambulatory Health Care (AAAHC). Nurse practitioners are taking leadership roles in team care in all states, and nurse practitioner–led PCMHs are recognized in all states that allow advanced practice registered nurses (APRNs) to practice independently.[3,4,9,11,12,41]

The seven principles underlying the PCMH build directly on the CCM framework of chronic care management and practice improvement (Box 5-1). They address patient access to longitudinal, comprehensive, coordinated, high-quality, team-based care.[5] The PCMH also addresses compensation in the principles. This subject is critically important to primary care redesign because without fundamental changes in the fee-for-service model or the development of a hybrid model, multidisciplinary population-based care cannot be adequately reimbursed and therefore will not be viable.[2-5] Wagner's early concept figure of the CCM has been updated at the McColl center to include the principles of the PCMH and is now called the *care model* (see Fig. 5-1).

Whether serving as primary care providers leading teams or participating as team members in physician-led practices, nurse practitioners must understand and implement new models of care. They must learn to collaborate in innovative ways with both patients and colleagues to optimize the nurse practitioner role in the delivery of high-quality, cost-effective primary care.[8,9]

POPULATION MANAGEMENT

Population management is an integral component of the CCM and PCMH. Not a new concept, it has been a public health model used in communities for decades to prevent and to control infectious diseases. More recently, the government, insurers, and large health care organizations have used population management to encourage healthy behaviors that modify risk in the populations they serve. In fact, until recent years, government and large health care organizations have been the only entities

BOX 5-1

Seven Principles of the Patient-Centered Medical Home

- Personal physician: ongoing relationship, first contact, continuous, comprehensive care
- Physician-directed medical practice: leads team responsible for ongoing care
- Whole-person orientation: responsible for all health care needs for all stages of life
- Care coordinated and integrated: prevention and chronic care facilitated by information technology
- Quality and safety: decision support, performance feedback, active quality improvement, patient experience
- Enhanced access: timely and varied types of appointments and communications
- Payment reform: hybrid structure that compensates for care coordination and quality

Data from Rittenhouse D, Thom D, Schmittdiel J: Developing a policy-relevant research agenda for the patient centered medical home: a focus on outcomes, *J Gen Intern Med* 6:593-600, 2010.

with the data management infrastructure capable of creating the efficiency of electronic registries to engage in large-scale population management activities. Individual primary care practices wanting to stratify patients by various characteristics and to analyze data did paper chart reviews and created manual spreadsheets. Fortunately, electronic medical records and clinical informatics seem to be overwhelmingly accepted as necessary as we move forward with health care reform.[2,3,23] Although the number of practices with electronic medical records is still not optimal, the Patient Protection and Affordable Care Act (PPACA) promotes and supports widespread use of clinical information systems that will make practice-level population management activities more achievable.[2,3,23,40]

A clear understanding of what population management entails, how it is used in the primary care setting, and what interventions yield the best results in various situations would be helpful; however, a review of the evidence on population management in the primary care setting is limited by multiple factors. The most daunting is the inconsistent use of terminology. Several terms are used to discuss different activities of population management, a consensus on clear definitions of them does not seem to exist, and different authors use the terms interchangeably.[16,20,25,38,40,42] Closely following confusing terminology is the wide-ranging intensity and duration of various population interventions that do not take into consideration the complexity of chronic diseases or the time needed to track the process of change.* At one end of the spectrum are studies that identify a population and introduce a single intervention for a short duration and then measure outcomes, often with minimal effect. At the other end are programs that introduce more comprehensive, longitudinal activities but evaluate all of them as one measure without investigating which individual interventions might be more powerful than others.*

In addition to inconsistent use of population terminology and varied levels of intervention intensity and duration, population studies were often limited by the use of subjective or ambiguous measures, lack of controls, and small sample size. Significant variations in the training of those implementing the interventions also caused difficulty in interpreting results.[16,42-52] For example, patient encounters with medical assistants who were trained for a few hours in MI did not significantly effect patient behavior change, whereas interactions with professionally trained behavioral clinicians produced better results.[50] For the purpose of this discussion, patient populations are stratified by increasing risk, using the terms *population health, population disease,* and *case or care management.*

Population Health

The term *population health* emphasizes wellness and is often used by large health care organizations or communities to describe activities to promote healthy habits and risk reduction in otherwise healthy, low-risk groups. These activities might include mailed or electronic communication that suggests opportunities such as smoking cessation programs, diet education, or gym memberships.[40] Sometimes *population management* is used to convey the same meaning as *population health.* Used in primary care, the terms emphasize the care and prevention activities required to improve the health of the overall practice rather than thinking solely in terms of individual patient needs. Population management can be applied at the primary care practice level by risk stratifying the population on the basis of criteria such as age, gender, habits, and personal and family history and by determining the most effective, evidence-based interventions to promote routine screenings and healthy habits.[40,42,49] In so doing, practices aim to decrease the number of patients who will go on to become higher risk and eventually develop chronic and life-threatening diseases. An example would be the use of a population registry to generate a list of patients due for routine screenings, such as colorectal cancer screening or mammography, and then activate the practice team to promote completion of the desired screenings.

Population Disease Management

Population disease management is a term used to describe activities targeted toward patients with specific high-prevalence diseases, such as diabetes, hypertension, asthma, and congestive heart failure. The aim of these activities is to engage patients in their own care and help them to improve their self-management skills, follow their process measures, and ultimately improve outcomes. As reported, population disease management activities have a particularly wide range of intensity and duration. Everything from single events, such as a reminder letter that an appointment or hemoglobin A_{1c} test is due, to high-intensity, multifaceted, ongoing activities that might include previsit laboratory tests, postvisit phone follow-up, and group visits has been reported. Another potentially confounding factor in this population stratification is that a subset of the population more appropriate for case management is often included in the data. For example, patients who are not otherwise medically complex but who struggle with behavioral, literacy, and other social challenges, who often miss appointments, discontinue their medication, or have the most hospital admissions, make their care plans more difficult to implement and therefore make midlevel interventions appear less effective.[43] Thus the evidence on population disease management is abundant, but our understanding of best practices is incomplete, and therefore further study is needed to improve our knowledge base.[16,20,21,28-30,35,37,42-47,51]

*See references 16, 20, 21, 25, 28, 30, 31, 35, 37, 38, 43-50.

Case and Care Management

Case management and *care management*, sometimes used interchangeably, are population management terms used with the most complicated patients. They both include intensive activities and involve the sickest patients who have the most complex health needs.[42,43,48,53] Case management is a concept closely associated with managed care organizations, insurers, hospital systems, employers, Medicaid, and Medicare. Case managers, usually nurses but in some settings social workers, work to coordinate care to improve quality and to lower costs.[43,48,53] Some case management programs are evolving into care management programs because the increased efficacy of care management is becoming evident. Population care management is more expansive than case management and more comprehensive than disease management. Most patients included in this population have several ongoing chronic diseases or unusual barriers to self-care.[42] According to Goodell, care management is "a set of activities designed to assist patients and their support systems in managing medical conditions and related psychosocial problems more effectively with the aim of improving patients' health status and reducing the need for medical services."[42] The key components or steps of care management are often carried out by a multidisciplinary team and include (1) patient identification (who would most benefit?), (2) risk and needs assessment (what do they need?), (3) collaborative care planning (who has the most appropriate skill set?), (4) patient and family education (how can the patient and support system participate?), (5) anticipatory coaching (how do we head off problems?), (6) tracking (how well are we doing?), and (7) care plan revision (how can we improve?). This intense ongoing level of care management has been shown to significantly improve cost and outcomes in this population.[42,43,53]

Conclusions

In spite of many limitations, the large body of work on the subject shows increasing evidence on the patient side that population management activities can improve process and outcome measures as well as patient satisfaction. On the practice side, these activities have been shown to improve practice efficiency and reduce cost, to enhance provider satisfaction, and to reduce provider stress. Moreover, when population management is considered integral to and inseparable from the other elements of the CCM and PCMH, the evidence for its efficacy mounts considerably.* Practice-based, team-implemented, longitudinal, multifaceted, patient-directed interventions appear to be significantly more effective compared with off-site, short-interval, single-intervention, insurance, disease management company, or isolated phone, e-mail, text, or letter activities.* Personal collaboration—good communication, shared purpose, and mutual trust and understanding—does seem to make a difference in working with large groups of patients or with individuals. Thus organizations could test a range of possible population management interventions and over time adopt the most effective.

PREPARING FOR THE PRIMARY CARE PRACTICE OF THE FUTURE

The radical transformation of primary care is proving to be a challenging endeavor requiring innovation and new skill acquisition for all members of the health care team. When it comes to implementing population management strategies, ongoing research must be done to clarify questions such as the following: Should we focus on prevention, disease, and case management equally? How do we know what patients in a given population will respond to? How do we measure success? Who should train and lead the team? To prepare for this challenge, advanced practice nurses need to hone their skills to design and to lead care initiatives, quality innovations, and health care teams.

Design of Clinical Information Systems

Nurse practitioners should become informed consumers and active participants when practices make decisions about clinical information system design. Because nurse practitioners are accustomed to working in collaborative relationships, they are well suited to advise practices about electronic features that will enhance communication and teamwork among team members. For example, embedded electronic decision support resources could decrease the need for provider consultations. When necessary, specialty consultations could be made more efficient with the use of electronic messaging that is part of the patient record and automatically attaches the pertinent patient information to the message. Templated notes that reflect the processes of care and patient education and behavior change, as well as the outcomes, could facilitate standardization of care as well as document it, making high-quality measurement more reliable. Multilingual information for patients regarding common problems could be available on the desktop so that materials could be printed or electronically transmitted and at the same time be documented in the record.

Because they may work directly with the population management tools or may be coordinators, supervising registry work done by other team members, nurse practitioners have a vested interest in the optimal integration of medical record and population registries. Therefore their input should be sought when registries are designed.[23,54] Registries should be more than lists of patients by demographics or disease. Registry windows could contain elements including identification and contact information, insurance, primary care and specialty providers, diagnoses, medication, allergies, test results and measurements, screenings, last appointment, next appointments, self-management education status, and virtual encounters. Ideally, registries for patients with multiple chronic diseases should be linked so the team can see the whole picture at one time and avoid duplication of effort. The system must be able to compile lists of patients and create reports according to multiple criteria by request and be able to automatically generate electronic notifications when results are overdue or outside of preset parameters. Features such as pop-up balloons, dual screens, and expansion and compression of screen information and messaging ability all make registries easier to use.[23,54]

Leading Teams

Population management is a team activity, and when it comes to leading teams, nurse practitioners have an opportunity to excel. The CCM and PCMH promote care teams with an emphasis on all team members working collaboratively with one another and the patient, within their scope but to the highest level of their training. To work efficiently and safely, roles and tasks must be well defined, training must be ongoing, communication among members must be frequent, and leadership

*See references 3, 4, 6, 16, 19-21, 25, 26, 28, 29, 37, 39, 42, 44.

must be strong.[10,11,29,45,55] As collaborators, nurse practitioners are ideally trained to lead teams because of their history. As nurses advancing their own scope of practice, they are aware of issues related to scope of practice in a way that unlicensed team members and physicians may not be.[9,11,12]

A comprehensive review of the literature regarding the factors influencing interprofessional teams in primary care identified two themes that significantly affect teamwork: team structure and team process. The authors defined three categories associated with each theme. Team co-location, controlled team size and composition, and strong organizational support were associated with successful team structure. Regular team meetings, consistently clear goals and objectives, and ongoing assessment or audit were categories important to an effective team process. Understanding these concepts is key when implementing teamwork in the PCMH.[55]

Teams that occupied the same geographic space functioned more productively than did those that were on different floors or buildings. Teams that were too large became unwieldy, whereas teams of fewer than 10 or 12 invited more vigorous participation by members. The role groups composing a team also influenced the success of teamwork. Increased diversity stimulated higher effectiveness and innovation; decreased diversity or including too many representatives from one role group, especially physicians, tended to disempower members and to advance a top-down mentality. The establishment of a clear leader also enhanced team effectiveness, as did the stability of team membership. The final category under team structure was organizational support. It appeared that team effectiveness naturally decreased with time, but with ongoing recognition and reward for innovation and change from the organization, teamwork quality remained high.[55]

On the subject of team process, regular team meetings were associated with several positive influences on teamwork. Meeting on a regular basis improved communication among individuals and role groups, improved understanding of each group's skill set, and increased respect and trust among team members. One of the most important factors for the optimal effectiveness of teamwork was clear, shared objectives. If the structure of a team did not include unambiguous leadership and the goals and objectives were not well defined, effective teamwork was difficult to promote, and both conflict and misunderstanding increased. Written position or role descriptions were shown to help clarify each member's place on the team, and education updates were suggested to ensure that each team member's competencies remained current.[55] "Clear goals and objectives facilitate good team functioning as they help to clarify each professional's roles and responsibilities and provide the team with a vision so that individual creativity can be pooled to produce creative team outcomes."[55]

The final process theme is the need for teamwork assessment or audit. In a review of the current literature, feedback to teams regarding their effectiveness was very often absent, and this omission was found to be damaging to team performance. This omission was found to cause frustration in team members because they were offered no incentive to do better or corrective feedback about where to improve. Team members reported feeling let down, undervalued, and disrespected if no feedback was given about their work. Furthermore, the lack of regular quality improvement reviews precluded an opportunity to problem solve, to recognize hard work, and to offer support to one another.[55] Therefore the team design prototype should aim for small, diverse, well-trained teams that share geography, purpose, and trust; have a defined leader; and enjoy organizational support, recognition, and feedback.

Self-Management Support and Delivery System Design

One of the definitive skills that nurse practitioners historically bring to primary care is their health promotion and patient education expertise.[8,9,10,12] Because self-management support interventions show positive results, it would seem wise to invest in expanding the skills that support these activities. Without access to information that is tailored to all their needs, patients do not have the opportunity to make informed decisions about their care and about their self-care behaviors. Health promotion and education activities open the door for patients to reflect on what is right for them and to make decisions that are consistent with their values and goals. Group education and shared medical appointments are two team-based, population-focused innovations that have been shown to improve efficiency, patient satisfaction, and outcomes.[28,51,52,56]

The most widespread group education program and a good model to learn about conducting educational groups is the diabetes self-management education (DSME) model. Diabetes education has evolved from a content-driven, didactic-style curriculum to a patient-centered approach more consistent with adult learning theory and the CCM. Patients discover new information, process what it means to live with a chronic disease, learn to self-manage, problem solve, and also gain support from one another in the group setting.[28,34,36,51,57] If programs are designed to meet the Centers for Medicare and Medicaid Services criteria for reimbursement, DSME may be covered by insurance. The American Diabetes Association (ADA) and American Association of Diabetes Educators (AADE) offer recognition or accreditation programs that qualify DSME for reimbursement. Nurses and nurse practitioners participating in DSME who want to expand their skill set may become a certified diabetes educator (CDE) or receive a Board Certified–Advanced Diabetes Management (BC-ADM) certification. Information can be accessed at the organizations' websites. The DSME model can be used in one-on-one visits and could be modified for use with other chronic disease education. However, education groups for other problems are often not usually covered by insurance at this time. In future practice models, accommodations must be made for time spent developing self-management skills with patients. For now, nurses and nurse practitioners are encouraged to seek research grants to study the efficacy of group education visits as a way of strengthening the evidence and improving the opportunity for reimbursement.

Meanwhile, nurse practitioners are well suited to lead shared medical appointments or medical group visits, which in the current reimbursement system are more cost-effective than education-only groups. In medical group visits, the same group dynamics are used to engage patients as in education-only groups, but because a diagnosing and prescribing provider is part of the team, visits include integrated medical management, making them more comprehensive.[28,52,56] Shared medical appointments often use one clinician as the "behaviorist" and another as the expert or guest speaker. Either a physician or a nurse practitioner is used to do the medical management, and support staff are used for previsit preparation and clerical and administrative tasks and sometimes act as scribes to document the visits. There are no hard and fast rules except that the criteria for evaluation and management billing must be met. Providers and patients seem to both enjoy and benefit from the format. To learn more about getting started with shared medical appointments, an excellent reference is *Running Group Visits in Your Practice* by Edward Noffsinger.[52]

What about the many "struggling," "difficult," or "noncompliant" patients, the patients who seem to have different priorities? We know our goals are to help all patients become knowledgeable, gain skills, develop positive adaptations, and optimize self-care; but we also know that education alone does not ensure that patients will make healthy choices. Therefore, to become more effective, clinicians should reflect on the philosophy of patient empowerment, increase their understanding of behavior change, and consider improving their general counseling skills.[34,36,58,59]

The philosophy of empowerment is straightforward, but it can become overshadowed in the acute care medical model. Put simply, patient empowerment recognizes that the patient is always the expert on himself or herself, defining the problems, identifying feelings surrounding them, developing long- and short-term goals, and implementing and evaluating a plan.[34,36] Patient centeredness is at the heart of the CCM and PCMH, but if one has been practicing in the acute care model, it may take time to internalize this point of view.

Techniques to Encourage Patient Self-Management: the Transtheoretical Model and Motivational Interviewing

A well-accepted change theory is the transtheoretical model (TTM), which conceptualizes the process of change in five stages: precontemplation—no desire to change; contemplation—thinking about it; preparation—making plans; action—doing it; and maintenance—keeping it going.[36,58,59] Many clinicians are familiar with the model as long used in smoking cessation, but have not known how it could apply to general practice. The model has gained prominence in recent years as it has been linked with MI, and the two have been used together by clinicians to help patients to self-manage chronic medical conditions.[36,58,59]

Primary care clinicians may be less familiar with MI. MI is used with the TTM and is described as a directive, person-centered counseling style for increasing intrinsic motivation and helping patients explore and resolve ambivalence.[36,58] When using MI, clinicians explore the patient's values and wishes, look for discrepancies between them and their health behaviors, and listen for verbal hints that they may wish to make changes. Instead of making recommendations that are sure to prompt resistance, the clinician uses techniques such as reflective listening, affirmation, summarizing, and asking questions to guide patients to generate solutions that are feasible and workable given their personal situation. In this process, patients' ambivalence about their situations decrease and their conviction to succeed in being consistent with what they believe strengthens. MI can be used in education or support encounters with individuals or in groups. MI creates relationships that are more like partnerships than top-down connections and decreases the frustration both patients and clinicians sometimes feel when clinicians try to "fix" the patient or see the patient as noncompliant. Many resources are available to help clinicians expand their counseling knowledge and skills. A good place to start is *Motivational Interviewing in Health Care* by Rollnick, Miller, and Butler[58] or the MI website at *www.motivationalinterviewing.org/*.

SUMMARY

Whether as team leaders or team members, nurse practitioners are poised to play a significant role in the design and delivery of primary care as we move forward with health care reform. Using the CCM and the principles of the PCMH as guides, nurse practitioners must create innovative patient-centered systems to safely and efficiently improve the health of whole practices as well as the health of individual patients. (Box 5-2 features a case study that illustrates what a nurse practitioner's PCMH practice might look like.) For the evidence on the efficacy of nurse practitioners as primary care providers and practice leaders to be advanced, nurse practitioners must seek opportunities to publish results of their practice innovations. The skills mastered in the achievement of this goal could benefit not only the health of the populations we serve but also the health of the profession.

BOX 5-2

A Day with Lisa, Primary Care Nurse Practitioner

Lisa works in a large, urban, hospital-based adult primary care practice that is part of a health center. The health center population is about 50% recent immigrants, mostly from Central America. The poverty level is high, and cultural, literacy, and language challenges abound, but almost everyone has some kind of health insurance.

The hospital provides abundant resources, including sophisticated clinical information systems and ongoing education and support for practice innovation. An electronic population management tool is linked to the electronic record. Hospital leadership also encourages and financially supports clinical and clerical staff continuing education as well as self-management education groups and shared medical appointments. Billing and administration are managed centrally by the hospital. Employees are salaried, but everyone receives bonuses when the team produces high-quality outcomes.

Lisa works in one of four geographic practice teams. Support staff includes bilingual patient care assistants, who are cross-trained to perform both clerical and medical assistant functions; one registered nurse (RN), who does phone triage and patient education and oversees care coordination; and a licensed practical nurse (LPN), who manages prescription authorizations and prior approvals and works on care coordination under the direction of the RN. In addition, the pod shares an RN who is a certified diabetes educator (CDE), a dietitian, a pharmacist, a physical therapist, a social worker, and a bilingual community outreach worker, called a navigator. To accommodate patients who find it difficult to travel

Continued

BOX 5-2

A Day with Lisa, Primary Care Nurse Practitioner—cont'd

to the main hospital campus, several specialists from the main campus come to the health center to see scheduled patients one or more times a month, and an urgent care center is open after practice office hours to provide access so that patients can avoid going to the emergency department.

Lisa is considered a full-time provider, along with the two full-time physicians on the team.

She works in a state where nurse practitioners are authorized to practice independently, so she does not legally need a supervising or collaborating physician. However, the team members work together in a very collaborative way, often reviewing cases with one another. One physician is credentialed in addictions treatment, the other is certified in geriatrics, and Lisa's CDE, BC-ADM credential makes her the diabetes resource for the team. Each provider takes a leadership role on the team by coordinating various aspects of population management. Lisa sees patients by appointment the equivalent of 3 days a week and is responsible for leading and evaluating population-based initiatives: preventative care; screening tests; immunizations; and longitudinal disease management of diabetes, hypertension, and congestive heart failure. Everyone on the team is engaged in population management initiatives and participates in these activities.

Lisa starts her day with a brief team meeting. Together the team members review the electronic record and population management registry to plan for a smooth-running session. Lisa has a shared medical appointment scheduled from 9:00 to 11:00 AM with 10 to 12 confirmed Spanish-speaking patients. All the patients have diabetes, and she knows all of them because she has seen them in individual intake visits, which were prompted by a weekly registry report identifying patients who had not yet participated in basic education. As patients arrive, their vital signs are checked; home testing data are downloaded, and their medications, which they always bring with them, are reviewed and reconciled in the electronic record. Because prompts show up on the laptop screen, the patient care assistants know when a blood pressure or cholesterol level is not at goal or if the patient is due for immunizations, eye examinations, or laboratory studies. Lisa reviews the list and signs off on any needed referrals or requisitions, and the data are entered electronically. Because orders are in the electronic record, the team LPN automatically gets an electronic message and meets the patients in the onsite laboratory to give the immunizations while they have other tests done. Most of the patients know to come in for testing a few days before an appointment, so few laboratory tests need to be done at the time of the visit unless the patient has a new problem.

Lisa greets the assembled patients; reviews the idea of shared medical appointments, including confidentiality; and begins by addressing the concerns expressed at check-in, which have been entered on a whiteboard along with the patients' most recent laboratory test results. Lisa asks patients to share what has been going well for them. The previous group visit had included time with the dietitian, so some participants have stories to share about what they have done differently, or not, with food since the last visit. Inevitably, some things come up that have not been going as well, and the patients work together, with Lisa's facilitation, on problem solving and goal setting. Lisa uses motivational interviewing to encourage the patients' movement to the next stage of change by helping them to resolve their ambivalence about their behavior choices. As the conversation continues, the patient care assistant takes cues from Lisa to document the patient history and educational content of the conversation on a templated note. After about 45 minutes, Sally, the pod RN CDE, arrives as the guest speaker. She has come to discuss barriers to physical activity and to teach the group an exercise routine that can be done anywhere and requires no equipment. She brings a Latin dance CD to make it more fun.

During this time, Lisa and a patient care assistant take individual patients to a private examination room for a few minutes, where Lisa does any physical assessment that is needed, makes any medication adjustments that are indicated, and discusses any issues the patient is not comfortable raising in the group. The medical assistant documents the examination using the templated note, and Lisa signs off on any prescription changes and e-faxes the prescriptions directly to the pharmacy. Each patient receives a printed update of the prescribed medications and any recommended changes in treatment at the end of this encounter as a visit summary.

After all the patients have been seen individually, Lisa returns to the group. Everyone participates in summing up what has happened in the visit. Lisa asks each participant to share what he or she got out of the meeting and encourages the patients to move forward with their goals and self-management "experiments." Everyone in the group agrees that the theme for today has been the emotional struggles each individual encounters in coping with ongoing self-management. Lisa asks if it would be helpful to have Estela, the team social worker, join them for the next appointment. The patient care assistant makes sure everyone has their next appointment, and any orders for laboratory studies to be done before the next visit are entered into the electronic system. Lisa meets briefly with the care team to debrief. She then checks over the notes, makes any corrections or additions, and signs off on them, electronically messaging the patient's primary care provider as she does so. She electronically messages a request to the LPN that one of the patients needs a prior approval for an insulin pen and sends Estela a message that she has been invited to the next shared medical visit. She also electronically messages the outreach navigator that one of the patients is struggling with depression, and although she is in treatment and taking medication, she could use a bit more attention and suggests a phone, office, or home visit with the navigator.

Today is weekly team meeting day, so the whole team gathers in the conference room for lunch. Everyone reports on how the practice is functioning from his or her perspective and participates in problem solving. Lisa electronically opens the population reports for discussion with the group and shares that routine health care monitoring continues to show improved results. Registry reports confirm ongoing improved documentation of 21 screenings, including alcohol or substance use, bone density, breast cancer, cervical cancer, colorectal cancer, dental, depression, diabetes, diet, domestic violence, exercise, firearms, hypertension, immunizations, lipids, prostate cancer, sexually transmitted infections, smoking, vision, seat belt, and weight screenings. The providers agree that initiation of two automated reminders has helped them stay on track. One reminder, which includes education materials and a checklist, goes to the patient as part of the previsit preparation packet that is automatically mailed out to each patient before an upcoming planned health maintenance visit. Patient care assistants are trained to explain the screening tests in a general way to supplement the mailed patient education materials. The second reminder pops up at the top of the page when the provider opens a patient's chart at the time of the visit, thereby cueing the provider if the patient does not bring up the health maintenance topics. To ensure that patients stay on track, planned visits for the next routine health monitoring visit are scheduled as the patient leaves the current visit. One month before the upcoming appointment, the previously mentioned reminder packet is automatically sent to help the patient organize and prepare for the visit. One to 2 days before the visit, a reminder phone call is made by the patient care assistants. If a patient misses or cancels a health monitoring visit, the system generates a letter. If a patient does not respond by making an appointment, the patient care assistant calls. If there is still no response, the nurse practitioner or physician is notified. Meanwhile, if the

BOX 5-2

A Day with Lisa, Primary Care Nurse Practitioner—cont'd

patient comes in for an acute visit, the electronic record prompts the provider that the patient needs routine care. Disease management is more cumbersome. Currently, the patient care assistants review the registry by disease with the physicians. Patients who are flagged as overdue for testing or a visit are called to come in and offered appointments. Patients who do not come in are called by the navigator, who educates about the reasons for planned follow-up, assesses for barriers to care, and refers any patient with symptoms or resistance to making an appointment to one of the nurses. If the nurse is not successful in arranging a patient visit, the nurse practitioner or physician is notified. Patients who have unstable or multiple system diseases in spite of regular follow-up are stratified into the care management group. Their status is reviewed weekly, and individual care plans are devised according to their needs.

After the meeting, Lisa takes a few minutes to check any unacknowledged results of laboratory tests on her computer's results manager page. She acknowledges results and sends computer-generated letters to patients with just a few clicks. She checks her electronic messages from the triage nurses. Two patients have been put into her open access schedule with notes from triage regarding the nature of the urgent visit. One patient is an elderly woman with a cough and fever. Lisa arranges for the patient to have a chest x-ray examination before her appointment. The other is a young woman with acute back pain after lifting her 3-year-old child. Lisa has six planned visits. Three are healthy young women for routine examinations and contraception follow-up. Each has been mailed one of the previsit packets, and Lisa uses a templated note for their visits. One appointment is with a 57-year-old male patient with newly diagnosed diabetes who was referred by one of Lisa's physician colleagues. Using a templated note to prompt and document, Lisa does a complete assessment and begins education, testing, referrals, and medication titration. She makes sure the patient has a secure portal e-mail account so he can share home test results and she can respond with appropriate medication titration between office visits. The final two patients are elderly patients with multiple chronic illnesses with whom she alternates primary care physician visits. One is a patient with congestive heart failure who had been having frequent emergency department visits because of fluid overload. She has been set up with electronic monitoring of her weight, blood pressure, heart rate, and medication use. This visit is to check her status and to see how the new system is working for her. The second patient is a patient who struggles with depression, diabetes, peripheral neuropathy, coronary artery disease, hyperlipidemia, hypertension, and chronic renal failure. After many years of dropping in and out of care at multiple practices, she is now observed closely by Lisa and her primary care physician, who help her manage her many tests and medications and whose visits are interspersed with calls from the navigator. Lisa finishes up notes within a half-hour of her last patient and leaves knowing that if she has any seriously abnormal laboratory results, she will receive a text.

CONCLUSION

The literature abounds with articles on population management and ideas for health care delivery reform. Lisa illustrates an efficient, patient-centered model of primary care that maximizes provider resources while enhancing patient access to care and ensuring care quality.

CHAPTER 6

HEALTH LITERACY, HEALTH CARE DISPARITIES, AND CULTURALLY RESPONSIVE PRIMARY CARE

Catherine Ling

The power and impact of social factors on health behaviors and outcomes has become an increasingly critical part of primary care delivery. Social determinants of health are individual and societal factors, including race, socioeconomic status, gender, education, occupation, and sexual orientation.[1] These factors are integral to delivery of holistic care. Failure to integrate all factors that affect health care behaviors and health care decisions creates a significant cost, both for the individual and for society as a whole. Three specific social determinants of concern for providers are health literacy, disparities, and culturally responsive care.

HEALTH LITERACY

Health literacy is the capacity of a person to find, discuss, and comprehend health information and systems and to be able to use that knowledge to make informed decisions about all aspects of his or her health.[2-4] *Healthy People 2020* has a goal focused on improving health communication that addresses the need to "increase the proportion of the people who report that their health care providers always explain things so they can understand them".[5] The financial costs of inadequate health literacy have been estimated at $106 to $238 billion annually.[6] The Health Literacy of America's Adults report from the National Assessment of Adult Literacy survey (NAAL) stated that only 12% of Americans had a proficient level of health literacy, with 53% having an intermediate level.[7] This leaves approximately 88 million Americans with a basic or below-basic level of health literacy. Factors associated with high health literacy included being female, having an education beyond high school, and speaking primarily English, whereas low health literacy was associated with belonging to an ethnic minority, living in poverty, and being older than age 65.[7,8]

HEALTH LITERACY AND HEALTH CARE OUTCOMES

Patients with low health literacy are at risk for myriad poor health outcomes and increased costs (Box 6-1).[9,10] These poor outcomes start in childhood. Children with parents who have low health literacy are more prone to be seen in the emergency department, have increased severity of conditions such as asthma, and are less likely to be fully immunized.[11-13] Adolescents have not been as thoroughly studied, but it stands to reason that this is a dynamic life stage and presents an opportunity to improve health literacy.[14] During adulthood, low health literacy is related to inadequately treated conditions such as hypertension, influenza, and mental health issues, which, in turn, lead to increased morbidity.[9,10,15] Findings from two systematic reviews were increased emergency department use and hospitalizations, inappropriate use of medications, misunderstanding

BOX 6-1

Risks Associated with Low Health Literacy

- Misunderstood forms
- Missed appointments
- Limited use of preventive health measures, including screenings and immunizations
- Limited knowledge about personal health conditions
- Higher hospitalization rates
- Higher emergency department use
- Misunderstanding of treatment options and medications
- Limited self-management skills
- Misunderstanding of follow-up recommendations

of follow-up instructions, and decreased use of preventative services such as mammograms.[9,10] Older adults are particularly vulnerable to poor health outcomes related to low health literacy and have a higher risk of all-cause mortality even when lower cognition is not a consideration.[9]

HEALTH LITERACY COMPONENTS

Health literacy does not refer solely to the general ability to read and write. However, those with low general literacy rates will often have low health literacy rates. Conversely, the ability to understand physiology and pathology is a key component of health literacy; even patients who are highly literate and educated can have low health literacy. During the course of caring for a patient, key pieces of information are given verbally (requires adequate hearing and language comprehension); in written format (requires adequate eyesight and reading comprehension, including numeracy); and now via technology (requires ability to use and understand technology). Examining these components identifies strategies for improving communication with patients and can have a positive impact on health outcomes.

Oral Communication

Oral communication (sending and receiving) is the cornerstone of health care delivery. Conversations with patients with low literacy can be affected by four different qualities: (1) use of medical terminology, (2) complex speech content, (3) abstract context, and (4) dense rapid discussion.[16] Providers need to use plain speech and avoid cramming multiple abstract and complex concepts into a fast-paced discussion.

Reading Comprehension

Every handout, prescription, or written referral is provided with the assumption of a certain level of patient reading comprehension. The average American has a ninth-grade reading level; the suggested reading level for health information is fifth grade.[17] There are several tools for determining the reading level expectation of written material. Two that are integrated into Microsoft Word are the Flesch Reading Ease test and the Flesch Kincaid Reading Ease level. The Centers for Medicare and Medicaid Services has an 11-part toolkit for gauging the reading comprehension level of a provider's written materials, along with tools and tips to clarify those materials and make them more user-friendly for patients (www.cms.gov/Outreach-and-Education/Outreach/WrittenMaterialsToolkit).

Numeracy

Numeric literacy is the capacity to comprehend quantitative data in all forms and use it to make health care decisions.[18] Data forms range from statistical to epidemiologic to simple number use and include numeric data that is presented graphically.[18,19] There is a preponderance of health education literature containing graphs and percentages; gauging a patient's interpretation of numeric data is a key component in individually tailoring oral and written communication when delivering health care education to a patient.

Technology

Educational materials are now often delivered electronically and involve literacy expectations that transcend reading comprehension. The patient must know how to use technology devices and navigate through virtual materials.

Electronic health or eHealth materials that have successfully reached individuals with low health literacy through a number of different platforms include audio files, videos, and voiceover slides, along with read-only materials and non–Internet-dependent DVDs.[20] It will become more and more critical to gauge the patient's technologic literacy as electronic health records and communication via smart phones and computers become more integrated into health care delivery.[21]

HEALTH LITERACY ASSESSMENT

A health literacy assessment is the first step in addressing the needs of low–health literacy patients. Although there are a variety of tools for gauging health literacy, we will be looking at three that are readily translatable into primary care settings: the Rapid Estimate of Adult Literacy in Medicine–Short Form (REALM-SF); Ask Me 3; and the Newest Vital Sign or ice cream label assessment.

REALM-SF

The REALM-SF is a seven-item instrument that has been validated and used with a variety of populations.[22] It is easy and fast to administer; a drawback is that it looks only at medical word recognition—not comprehension or numeracy. The full instrument and instructions on how to administer it can be found on the Agency for Healthcare Research and Quality (AHRQ) website (www.ahrq.gov/professionals/quality-patient-safety/quality-resources/tools/literacy/indes.html).

Ask Me 3

Another tool, Ask Me 3, encourages patients to ask the health care provider three primary questions to enhance patient-provider communication:

1. What is my main problem?
2. What do I need to do?
3. Why is it important for me to do this?

This simple yet effective framework helps patients and caregivers initiate communication with the health care provider about health concerns. These are great prompts to start dialogue but do not help to gauge the health literacy of the patient—that is, his or her understanding of the answers that providers will give to those questions.

Newest Vital Sign

The Newest Vital Sign instrument, distributed by Pfizer, is also known as the ice cream label test.[23] A patient is asked to look

BOX 6-2

Measures to Reduce Health Literacy Impact

1. Assess patients for health literacy level.
2. Provide written patient education materials at reading level appropriate for every patient.
3. Use pictographs and symbols to convey information in patient education materials.
4. Minimize the use of text in written materials.
5. Provide alternative formats of information (e.g., audio, video).

at the nutrition label from a container of ice cream and answer six questions. These questions include numeracy skills (calculating the number of calories in the container) and general knowledge (should a patient who is allergic to peanuts eat this ice cream?). In validity testing it was found to be more sensitive than other measures of health literacy and easy to administer in clinical settings.[24] The toolkit containing the instrument and administration and scoring instructions can be found on the Pfizer website (www.pfizer.com/health/literacy/public_policy_researchers/nvs_toolkit).

HEALTH LITERACY INTERVENTIONS

Patient-Centered Interventions

To effectively meet the needs of patients with less-than-optimal health literacy, providers must develop the awareness, knowledge, and interventions required to address low or inadequate health literacy. Patients should be assessed for health literacy levels. Research has found that using images and symbols and decreasing the overall amount of text broaden the health literacy scope of materials.[25] In addition, use of alternate formats to print only (podcasts, videos, tables) can help to address information needs of patients with low health literacy.[3,25] Box 6-2 provides measures to reduce health literacy impact.

Organization Centered Interventions

It is not the job of the provider alone to do the work of reducing low health literacy's barrier to optimal care. Organizations should systematically review materials and navigation procedures to gauge the health literacy expectation of users and then involve employees and community members in planning, implementing, and evaluating steps to address health literacy needs.[26] The Centers for Disease Control and Prevention provides health literacy toolkits emphasizing the use of plain language in all written, audio, video, and virtual materials; these toolkits can be found by accessing www.cdc.gov/healthliteracy. The Ask Me 3 website (www.npsf.org/?page=askme3) offers helpful resources for providers and ideas for making primary care settings more user-friendly for patients with lower health literacy. Box 6-3 has a list of some additional resources for individual providers and organizations.

BOX 6-3

Health Literacy Resources

Agency for Healthcare Research and Quality's Health Literacy Universal Precautions Toolkit provides a plethora of resources for improving health literacy communication. Available at www.ahrq.gov/professionals/quality-patient-safety/quality-resources/tools/literacy-toolkit/index.html.

Centers for Disease Control and Prevention's Health Literacy website provides tools and information for providers and organizations. Available at www.cdc.gov/healthliteracy.

Institute of Medicine: Roundtable on Health Literacy (2014). Provides updates on the latest discussions and reports from the Institute of Medicine examining health literacy. Available at www.iom.edu/Activities/PublicHealth/HealthLiteracy.aspx.

National Action Plan to Improve Health Literacy is an initiative from the Department of Health and Human Services to assist health care systems, organizations, and providers in reducing the barrier to care posed by health literacy issues. Available at www.health.gov/communication/hlactionplan/pdf/Health_Literacy_Action_Plan.pdf.

HEALTH CARE DISPARITIES

The presence of health care disparities is a key social determinant affecting health outcomes. Disparities occur when one group has barriers to the standard of care and poorer health outcomes than another group.[27] The inability to access high-quality and timely care leads to increased morbidity and mortality, and it has been estimated that the direct cost of disparities is over $229 million.[28] Specific populations are particularly vulnerable to disparities in accessing adequate care and resources. The poor, people of color, those with activity-limiting conditions, and those in certain geographic regions face ongoing or worsening health care disparities.[27] Lesbian, gay, bisexual, and transgendered persons also face disparities.[29,30] The Office of the Surgeon General, Department of Health and Human Services Office of Minority Health, National Partnership for Action to End Health Disparities, and Centers for Disease Control and Prevention are just a few of the federal agencies involved in addressing health care disparities.

At first glance, this would appear to be a system- or organizational-level concern. Health care providers must know who the vulnerable populations are in their communities, identify the disparities those patients face, and implement programs to address those disparities. Examples include examining the application of national standards for hypertension control in a minority Medicare population in the Midwest or implementing an automobile safety program in a Native American community.[31,32] The initial efforts providers can make to address disparities are through self-examination for personal biases. Unintended or implicit biases in a health care professional affect clinical decision-making.[33]

CULTURALLY RESPONSIVE CARE

Like disparities and health literacy, an individual's cultural context determines how, when, and to what degree he or she will seek care and what interventions are considered acceptable. Cultural context determines what is considered to be health, what are normative treatments, and what is illness behavior. Providers must provide culturally responsive care in patient-centered environments, maximizing communication and minimizing bias.

OBLIGATIONS IN CULTURALLY RESPONSIVE PRIMARY CARE

Address Cultural Variations among Diverse Patient Groups

With increases in globalization and increasing access to health care services, the diversity of patient populations in the United

States has increased. Health care professionals might not be familiar with all the cultural views represented in a practice; however, this knowledge is essential to provide high-quality care. In a patient-centered environment, health care professionals inquire about patient beliefs regarding illness and treatment, are responsive to individual patient preferences, and work with patients and their families to devise treatment plans that are acceptable and therefore have an increased likelihood of adherence.[34]

Create a Patient-Centered Environment

Clinicians must always ask and not assume a patient's cultural, race, ethic, or gender context. A discussion of health concerns should include the patient's perspective because that perspective factors greatly into the approach to and success of the treatment plan. That plan should be negotiated within the framework of the patient's worldview. Culturally responsive patient-centered environments seek a culturally relevant understanding of health from the patient and other sources.[35]

Minimize Clinician Bias

The personal views and professional and personal experiences of health care providers can also create bias and impede culturally responsive care. Provider bias (e.g., regarding race, ethnicity, size, socioeconomic class, gender, age, physical disabilities, sexual orientation) can be an unconscious influence on a provider's plan of care. Clinicians need to recognize and address personal bias. Patient care decisions should be evidence based and individualized and not based on supposition or assumption. Available treatment options should also be openly discussed with patients. Clinicians may share a preferred treatment but need to decipher if this is a personal preference or if the treatment decision is based on evidence-based practice principles.

Overcome Patient Barriers: Language Environment

Increasingly, health care providers deliver care to culturally diverse populations of individuals who are not native language speakers. Only approved, professional interpreters experienced in health care interpretation should be allowed to interpret for patients. Family members or friends should *not* be used as interpreters. Use of family members or friends may create misinterpretation or misunderstanding between the clinician and the patient. Family members may not understand medical terms or may interpret only what they feel is important, or patients might feel uncomfortable divulging personal information to the person interpreting.

Every effort should be made to use a certified, professional interpreter, with bilingual staff members used as interpreters only in emergency situations. When interacting with a patient through an interpreter, clinicians should still speak directly to the patient and refrain from discussing the patient in the third person with the interpreter. The patient should feel that the clinician is directly interacting with him or her and not with the interpreter. Pausing every two or three sentences, especially in discussing or describing complex diseases or treatments, will ensure that the interpreter is able to correctly interpret all of the information discussed with the patient. Disease information, brochures, and consent for treatment and procedures should be printed in the patient's language. Federal law regarding Medicaid and Medicare federally funded programs mandates access to linguistic services. Certified translation services are available by phone 24 hours a day from multiple vendors.

CONCLUSION

In today's changing and challenging health care environment, primary care providers are called to improve health care literacy, to reduce health care disparities, and to deliver care to culturally diverse populations. This challenge is accomplished by assessing and improving health care literacy, delivering culturally responsive primary care, and closing disparities. Key components of culturally responsive primary care include addressing cultural variations among diverse patient groups, creating patient-centered friendly environments, recognizing clinician bias, and overcoming patient language and social barriers.

CHAPTER 7

GENETIC CONSIDERATIONS IN PRIMARY CARE

Quannetta Tucker Edwards • Ann H. Maradiegue • Diane C. Seibert

The health/illness continuum encompasses genes, environmental exposures, and the interaction of genes with the environment. Although the term *genetics* has been around for a long time, this term is quite narrow in focus, examining the influence of individual genes on health and disease (i.e., single-gene disorders). The more recent term, *genomics,* coined in 1987,[1] describes the interaction of many genes and reflects the influence of the psychosocial, cultural, and physical environments in which humans live.[2] Genomic concepts must be used when assessing an individual's disease risk because humans interact in highly complex ways with one another and with their environments. Perhaps the clearest example of how much is known about genetics is to look inside an online resource known as *OMIM* (Online Mendelian Inheritance in Man). OMIM is a comprehensive, authoritative compendium of human genes and genetic disorders and traits that focuses on molecular relationships between genetic variations and phenotypic expression; it is available online and updated daily.[3] As of January 2015, OMIM included 22,747 genetic entry statistics entailing descriptions of individual genes, combined genes and phenotype, phenotype description, molecular basis known, phenotype description or locus, molecular basis unknown, and other, mainly phenotypes with suspected mendelian basis.[3] Although a tremendously valuable resource, OMIM is focused primarily on inherited genetic diseases, not on the interaction of multiple genes or on gene-environment interactions. Although much remains to be learned about the genetics of complex diseases such as cancer, heart disease, diabetes, hypertension, and psychiatric disorders, as well as behavioral conditions associated with tobacco and drug addiction,[4] new information is emerging in this area every day.

Since Dr. Francis Collins and his colleagues announced the complete sequencing of the human genome on April 24, 2003 at the National Institutes of Health,[5] advances in technology for genomic health care continue to evolve, moving beyond the genetics of single-gene disorders to the use of genomic technologies to address chronic diseases. Clinicians are already seeing the effects of genomics throughout the spectrum of nursing and medicine to address the needs and challenges of a complex health care system. *Genomics,* unlike the study of single genes *(genetics)* entails all genes and their interrelationships and how they influence growth and development.[6] The emphasis of genomic health is the movement toward understanding that an individual's genes themselves are not acting in isolation; many factors affect overall health of an individual. The term *genomic assessment* captures not only the evaluation of single-gene disorders, but also an individual's overall health including diseases throughout the life cycle spanning infancy to old age. Single-gene disorders are rare and play a small role in the health of the public; thus expansion of the science to genomic discoveries is being applied to more common complex diseases such as heart disease, mental health and behavioral disorders, cancer, and diabetes.[7] Understanding both single-gene disorders (e.g., sickle cell anemia, breast and ovarian cancer syndrome, Lynch syndrome, cystic fibrosis, hereditary hemochromatosis) as well as the impact of genomics on chronic diseases is essential for all health care providers including advanced practice nurses (APNs) to appropriately assess risk, diagnose, manage, refer, and educate patients and families in today's health care system. This understanding includes knowledge of current genetic disorders and genetic testing as well as the implication of genomics with regard to personalized and precision medicine.

Today's health care, as well as future health care, is moving toward personalized or precision medicine. *Personalized medicine* involves the use of genetic or genomic information to guide decision-making with regard to prevention, diagnosis, and treatment of disease.[8] Personalized medicine can already be seen in clinical settings, particularly in oncology (e.g., molecular tumor testing for breast and colon cancers) and in the management of disease through pharmacogenomics (e.g., warfarin dose indication by pharmacogenetic testing). The future movement toward *precision medicine* further expands the concept of personalized medicine in the realm of molecular causes incorporating genomic, epigenomic, exposure, and behavioral factors and additional information.[9,10] Genomic testing strategies (e.g., exome sequencing) that are faster, cheaper, and more accurate also have the potential to change health care delivery.[11] Whole genome sequencing (WGS) and exome sequencing are currently being studied for use in the clinical setting to uncover disease predisposition in healthy individuals.[12,13] WGS and exome sequencing are next-generation technology to determine the variations of coding regions or exomes of the gene. Whole exome sequencing (WES) can revolutionize personalized or precision health care because it has the ability to provide coverage of more than 95% of the exons of genes, which contain 85% of disease-causing mutations in mendelian disorders, as well as identifying variants in the genome that can predispose to other diseases.[14] WES may have future clinical use in genetic or genomic diagnosis, disease treatment, screening, disease management, drug discovery, and prenatal diagnosis.[14] This is in contrast to most genetic testing today, which focuses on a single-gene disorder and testing one gene at a time.

Already today, advances in genetic testing have come to the forefront of health care. Multigene panel tests are now available that can provide genetic sequencing for more than one disease or syndrome or multiple genes. For example, panel tests are now available for individuals suspected to have such disorders as hereditary breast cancer syndromes, hereditary colon cancer syndromes, and cardiomyopathy, offering testing for a number of genes associated with the disease and enabling clinical genetic testing for multiple disorders or syndromes[15]—thus providing a more cost-effective strategy for the testing process. This approach can be beneficial when compared with that of a stepwise approach for those who may initially test negative for a single gene but in whom suspicion for an inherited disorder is high, warranting multiple testing. However, panel testing may identify variants of uncertain clinical significance rather than a deleterious mutation, often making clinical interpretation and management challenging[15]; thus use of multigene panel testing should be left to individuals with expertise in the area.

Implications of genomic technologies are many and cannot be fully appreciated at this time. As genomic technology continues to advance, many health care providers admit to feeling poorly prepared to provide genomic health care.[2,16] Because genomic content is not adequately emphasized in basic clinical preparation programs, the ability to integrate medical findings into the family medical history and physical examination and to account for the cultural preferences and psychological state of the patient is more important than ever.[17,18] Clinicians need to be familiar with the attributes and limitations of genomic sequencing so that they can give guidance at the point of care. Information for clinicians includes understanding the testing options, facilitating informed decision-making by patients and providers to identify the best test, communicating the test results to the patient and at-risk family members, facilitating the referrals, formulating a plan for future disclosure of additional or secondary findings, and reanalyzing genomic data when appropriate.[19] Although WGS can provide valuable information, there are often secondary or incidental findings that will need to be addressed and will require interpretation.

The American Nurses Association (ANA)[20] issued a competency document outlining essential genomic competencies for graduate nurses. The document was established by an expert consensus panel in genetics and genomics. The document contains 38 competencies under seven major categories that include risk assessment and interpretation; genetic education, counseling, testing, and results interpretation; clinical management; ethical, legal, and social implications; professional role; leadership; and research. In *professional practice,* the essential competencies of the ANA document require nurses with graduate level education to be competent in risk assessment and interpretation; genetic education, counseling, testing, and results interpretation; clinical management; and ethical, legal, and social implications as they relate to genetics and genomics.[20] A detailed discussion of genetic and genomic principles and disorders is beyond the scope of this chapter, but two key principles—risk assessment and family history collection—are discussed in this chapter in detail because they form the foundation for providing genomic health care in the practice setting and are part of the ANA genetic and genomic competencies. Two other important genomic issues, the 2008 passage of the Genetic Information Nondiscrimination Act (GINA) and direct-to-consumer (DTC) genetic testing are discussed at the end of this chapter because they have the potential to profoundly change the way genomic health care is perceived and/or delivered as well as to affect the ethical, legal, and social implications of genetics and genomics in today's health care.

If genomics is to take its rightful place in health care, clinicians must be prepared to look at both health and illness through a genomic lens. Nurses are the largest group of health care professionals in the United States, and nurse practitioners are on the front line of health care. Collectively, nurses have the power to change health care in powerful ways.

RISK ASSESSMENT

If optimal outcomes are to be achieved, clinicians must be prepared to assess and identify patients at increased risk for gene-gene and gene-environment interactions.[21]

Analysis of a patient's risk for developing a disease, or *risk assessment,* is essential in health care. Broadly defined, risk assessment is a systematic process used to determine whether a potential hazard exists and/or to evaluate the extent of possible risk to human health, safety, or the environment. Risk assessment incorporates the nature, duration, intensity, and frequency of the hazard or exposure.[22] Risk assessment has been used for many years in a variety of disciplines, including business, the insurance industry, law, government agencies, and organizations that focus on assessing risk for natural disasters, epidemic disease, and pollution.[23] Risk assessment in health care is different in that it includes more than a potential environmental hazard or external factor(s). In assessing risk in a health care setting, genetic and biologic factors (e.g., age, race, ethnic background, ancestry, country of origin), individual behaviors (e.g., smoking, alcohol abuse), and environmental factors (e.g., radiation exposure, dietary preferences) must all be combined to accurately evaluate an individual's risk for developing a particular disease, disability, or behavior.[24] Health care risk assessment includes gathering data about the patient, his or her immediate and multigenerational family members,[21] and their environmental exposures. These data are then evaluated in the context of emerging research and epidemiologic studies to predict the likelihood that an adverse event or illness will occur.[25] Risk assessment therefore is a process used to assist clinicians in making a medical decision.[24,26] Assessment of risk may also involve the use of empirical and/or probability risk assessment models—tools that can provide valuable information in the form of a risk estimate because they compare an individual's risk with the population risk. Two commonly used empirical risk models are the Gail model,[27] used to calculate breast cancer risk, and the Framingham model,[28] used to predict heart disease. Other probability models—for example, BRCAPRO, the Breast and Ovarian Analysis of Disease Incidence and Carrier Estimation Algorithm (BOADICEA), and PENN II—are used in genetic specialty clinics by trained professionals to assess a individuals risk for having an inherited predisposition to a genetic condition such as breast and/or ovarian cancer.[29-31]

The overarching goal of risk assessment is to recognize disease early or identify asymptomatic individuals at increased risk, so that appropriate preventative measures (e.g., chemoprevention, prophylactic medications), enhanced surveillance (e.g., more frequent mammograms for individuals at high risk for breast cancer), or risk-reduction surgery (e.g., bilateral mastectomy or oophorectomy for individuals at high risk for breast or ovarian cancer) can be initiated to improve health care outcomes. If an individual is suspected to be at high risk for a particular genetic condition, collaboration with another health professional is often indicated. For example, a genetic specialist (e.g., geneticist, genetic counselor, APN trained in genetics) should be consulted if the personal or family history is suspicious for an inherited cancer predisposition syndrome, such as that of hereditary breast and ovarian cancer (HBOC) syndrome. These specialists will often perform additional risk assessment and will gather and interpret personal and family histories, offer education about disease inheritance, discuss risks and benefits of genetic testing, discuss management and prevention strategies, and provide resources, information, and counseling.[21] These genetic counseling services are used to help both the individuals and their families understand and adapt to the stressful medical, psychological, and familial issues[21] that often arise during the process of testing for or diagnosing a genetic disorder.

Although risk assessment is a process involving numerous dimensions and elements for identifying patients who may be a risk for a particular disease (Fig. 7-1), the most valuable components of risk assessment are thorough personal and family histories. The personal history and family histories can assist a clinician in recognizing: (1) single-gene or chromosomal disorders, (2) susceptibilities that may pose future risk for health problems because of increased familial risk of common chronic disorders (e.g., diabetes, hypertension); (3) increased susceptibility to cancers; and (4) "red flags" that warrant referral, consultation, or genetic testing, all important toward personalized care.[32,33] See Box 7-1 for an example of how family and personal medical histories influence risk assessment.

FAMILY HISTORY

A first step to assessing risk for the individual and family members is to take a good family history. Family history is so important that it has often been called the "first genetic test," because when done correctly it can highlight common diseases and disease clusters within a family. This information can then be used to guide the kind of genetic or diagnostic testing that might be needed for clinical decision-making.[21]

Personal and Family History

A personal history should include the current age of the patient, their race and/or ethnicity, a history of their current concern or problem, and any pertinent past medical, surgical, or ancillary history. A detailed reproductive and obstetric or infertility history should also be collected from female patients. Confirmatory documentation of medical, laboratory, or ancillary tests should be obtained if possible,[21] and a focused physical examination should be conducted based on the physical, laboratory, and family history findings.[33]

Family history, collected in the form of at least a three-generation pedigree on both the maternal and paternal lineage, may reveal critical information that can be ascertained visibly, including pertinent personal health history, size of the family, possible familial or genetic predisposition to disease based on patterns suggestive of a mode of inheritance as well as denoting familial members at increased disease risk[34-36]; in addition, the pedigree may include environmental (e.g., asbestos) and behavioral (e.g., alcohol; tobacco) risk factors. Once the family history has been obtained, it can be used to determine the correct category of risk and appropriate screening interventions and surveillance to prevent disease and/or disease progression, as well as provide a measure for diagnosis.

Assessment of health risks in primary care settings is used to improve individual and population outcomes. Categories of risk include average or population risk, moderate risk, and increased or high risk.[21] Prevention guidelines were developed with the average or population risk in mind. For example, using the U.S. Preventive Services Task Force (USPSTF) guidelines, an

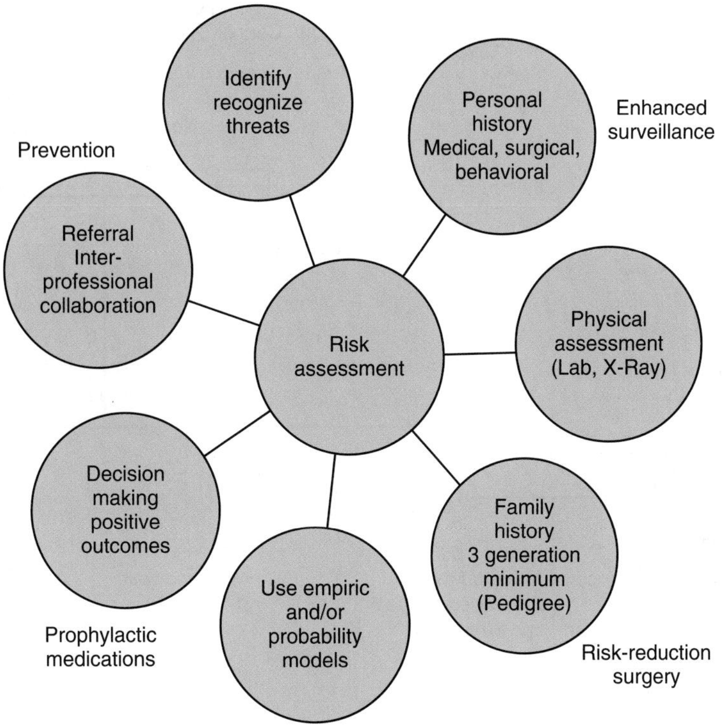

FIGURE 7-1 Risk assessment model denoting important elements in the process of analyzing patients' disease risk, including factors associated with decision-making and need for interprofessional collaboration.

BOX 7-1

Case Scenario

J.D. is a 34-year-old white man of Northern European descent on both the maternal and paternal lineage. He comes to the primary care clinic with a 3-month history of a facial lesion that he is afraid may be skin cancer. His medical history is unremarkable, but his family history is significant, for a 43-year-old brother who was diagnosed a year ago with colon cancer and a father who was diagnosed with colon cancer twice—at ages 45 and 49—and who died of the disease at age 51. His paternal grandparents' histories are unknown; and his maternal lineage is uneventful (Fig. 7-2). The nurse practitioner (NP) suspects that the facial lesion is a sebaceous adenoma, which, when combined with the "red flags" in the family history (i.e., early-age onset of colon cancer; two first-degree relatives with colon cancer), raises the suspicion for Muir-Torre syndrome (MTS), a subtype of a familial hereditary colon cancer syndrome known as Lynch syndrome.[34] The facial lesion was biopsied with a confirmatory diagnosis of sebaceous adenoma, and further testing revealed microsatellite high lesion (MSI-H) and absence of MutS Homolog 2 (MSH2) protein staining consistent with a history of Muir-Torre syndrome.[34] A colonoscopy was performed on J.D., and two benign adenomatous polyps were found in the right colon. The patient and his brother went for genetic counseling on advice of the NP and both tested positive for Lynch syndrome caused by a deleterious mutation in the *MSH2* gene. Additional interprofessional collaboration with the surgeon, genetic counselor, gastrointestinal specialists, oncologists, and mental health counselors, based on the patient's history, is now in progress. Sebaceous adenomas, particularly with this pattern of genetic changes, are often found in individuals with Lynch syndrome.[35]

In this example, the NP integrated the patient's personal and family histories, his physical examination findings, his ancillary test results, and the NP's knowledge of hereditary syndromes to identify the genetic red flags in the scenario. The NP suspected that J.D. might be at increased risk for a high-risk cancer syndrome, and initiated appropriate early colon cancer screening and initiated referral for additional genetic counseling and consultation.

individual with no personal or family history of colorectal cancer would be considered to be at average or population risk for colon cancer and should begin screening for the disease at age 50[37]; guidelines from the American Cancer Society are similar.[38] Earlier routine colorectal cancer screening beginning at age 45 years for African Americans is recommended by the American College of Gastroenterology.[39] Individuals with a personal or family history of colon cancer are not at average risk, and screening recommendations are significantly different. Individuals at increased colon cancer risk may warrant earlier or more frequency screening based on a history of one of the following: personal history of adenomatous polyp(s) or sessile serrated polyp(s); personal history of inflammatory bowel disease; family history of colorectal cancer; and/or a first-degree relative with advanced adenomas.[40] Recommended criteria for colorectal cancer screening and frequency related to family history are based on the family member with colorectal cancer (i.e., first-degree, second-degree) and his or her age at diagnosis and/or the presence of a first-degree relative with advanced adenoma(s).[40] Individuals at high risk for colon cancer, such as

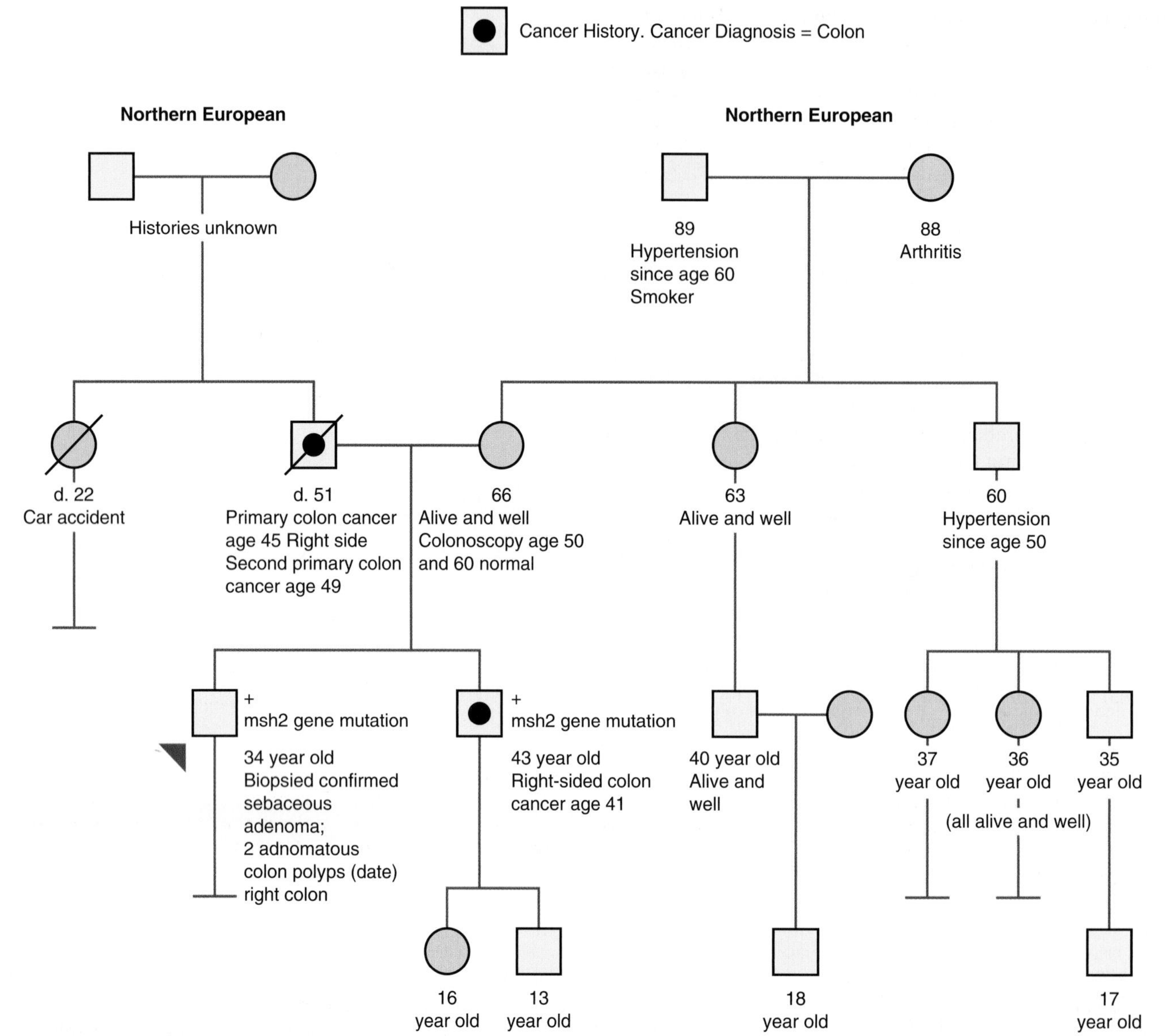

FIGURE 7-2 Four-generation pedigree of fictitious patient J.D. (arrowhead), with biopsied confirmed facial sebaceous adenoma, two adenomatous right colon polyps, and deleterious *MSH2* gene mutation.

those with a history of Lynch syndrome or polyposis syndromes (i.e., classic familial adenomatous polyposis [FAP]; attenuated FAP; *MUTYH*-associated polyposis; Peutz-Jeghers syndrome; juvenile polyposis syndrome; serrated polyposis syndrome), warrant enhanced colorectal surveillance as well as other management of care and surveillance depending on the syndrome.[41] Enhanced surveillance may also be warranted for those with no inherited syndromes but the presence of significant personal or familial risk. Referral to a genetic specialist should be considered for individuals with a strong personal and/or family history or a genetic predisposition to the disease.

Gathering a Family History

For appropriate assessment of risk, the family history has to be taken in a systematic fashion. Although clinicians are usually taught to take a family history and how to record it in the form of a pedigree, more often they ask a single question: "Do you have a family history of heart disease, cancer, or diabetes?" Although all these are important health care concerns, gathering information in this way is not systematic; there is no information about who has had the disease, how many people have been affected, at what age the disease manifested, or whether a family member has died from the disease. In addition, by merely asking about a specific disorder, the clinician may miss pertinent conditions that may be caused by an inherited syndrome. Completing a family history by using a pedigree provides a means to ensure that all members in both lineages are included in the assessment and that the pattern of disease(s), if present, can be identified.[42]

Drawing a pedigree is not a difficult process, and several tools are available to assist in gathering and recording an accurate pedigree. For example, asking patients to complete the Surgeon General's family history tool online and to bring the pedigree with them to an appointment greatly facilitates both the collection process (saves time) and accuracy (they can call family members for additional information) of this critical information. It also involves patients in the process, which may illuminate familial patterns that were not visible to them before, and may encourage adherence to lifestyle recommendations (e.g., smoking cessation) once the patient sees the impact of shared genetic and lifestyle factors in disease(s) affecting the family.

The systematic nature of a pedigree collection facilitates the gathering of complete information, and recording that information in a systematic manner is critical. Standard pedigree figures have been developed and should be used so that other health professionals can quickly interpret the pedigree (Fig. 7-3).[21] When drawing a pedigree, the affected individual (the proband)[43] is identified by an arrow. If the person reporting the family history is not the proband (e.g., a parent of an affected child), then the proband is identified on the pedigree and a note is made on the form regarding the individual who provided the history. The term "consultand" is also used when conducting a pedigree when the individual is not affected with a disorder of concern but is undergoing history taking or seeking medical attention or has other family members with a specific disorder(s).[43] Information on all of the proband's or consultand's first-degree (i.e., parents, siblings, children, stillborn fetuses, and miscarriages) and second-degree (i.e., grandparents, aunt and uncles, and cousins) relatives, both living and deceased, should be collected and recorded (Fig. 7-4). At a minimum, each family member's information should include significant health history, the age of disease onset, and the cause and age of death (Box 7-2). Environmental exposures (e.g., smoking) should also be included. For example, if a first-degree relative died of lung cancer at a young age, the interviewer would want to establish whether or not this relative was a smoker.

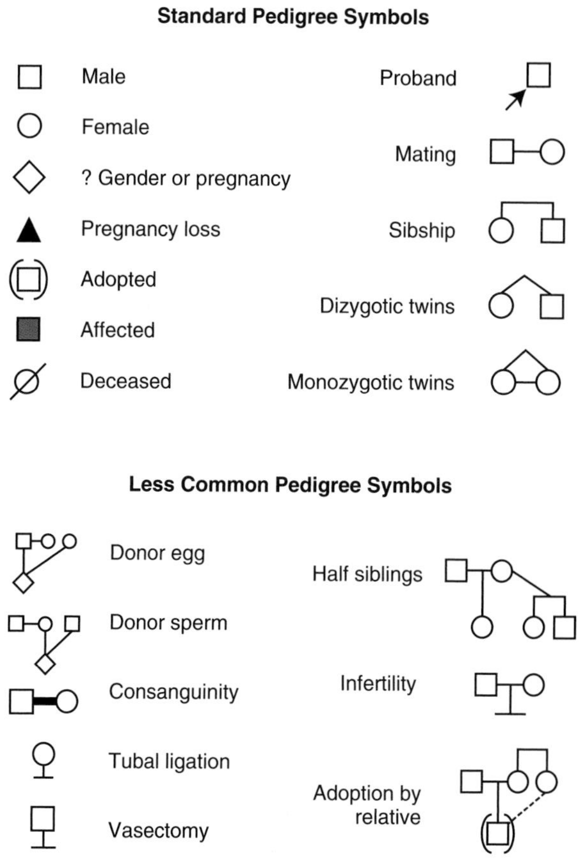

FIGURE 7-3 Example of commonly used standardized pedigree symbols. (With permission from Bennett R: *The practical guide to the genetic family history*, ed 2, Malden, MA, 2010, Wiley-Blackwell.)

BOX 7-2

"Red Flags" and Collection Guidelines

INDIVIDUAL MEDICAL HISTORY

Dysmorphic features (especially with a learning disorder)
Learning disabilities or behavioral problems
Movement disorders—hypotonia, ataxia
Unexplained infertility
Congenital or juvenile deafness, blindness or cataracts
Environmental or lifestyle risk factors (smoking, alcohol use, and dietary preferences)
Patient's occupation and the occupation of relatives with chronic conditions
Protective environmental or lifestyle modifications, such as regular exercise

FAMILY MEDICAL HISTORY

Multiple affected family members with same or related conditions
Earlier age at onset than expected (e.g., myocardial infarction age 40)
Condition in the less-often-affected sex (breast cancer in a male)
Disease in the absence of a known risk factors (hyperlipidemia in a young, athletic, normal-weight individual)
Ethnic predisposition to certain diseases (Tay-Sachs in an Ashkenazi Jewish infant)
Close biologic relationship between parents (consanguinity)
Three or more pregnancy losses

PEDIGREE SHOULD INCLUDE

Legend

- Pedigree key (e.g. darkened circle indicates breast cancer)
- Date recorded or updated
- Name of the person reviewing the history with the patient

Race or ethnicity; country or countries of family origin for maternal and paternal lineage
Gender
Age, and age at diagnosis
Age and cause of death
Primary site for any cancer
Pregnancy losses
Chronic or long-term conditions (noting the condition[s] of interest)
Surgical history and/or relevant interventions or procedures
Increased risk, or unusual diagnosis: validate by reviewing medical records, pathology reports, death certificates
Surgical history

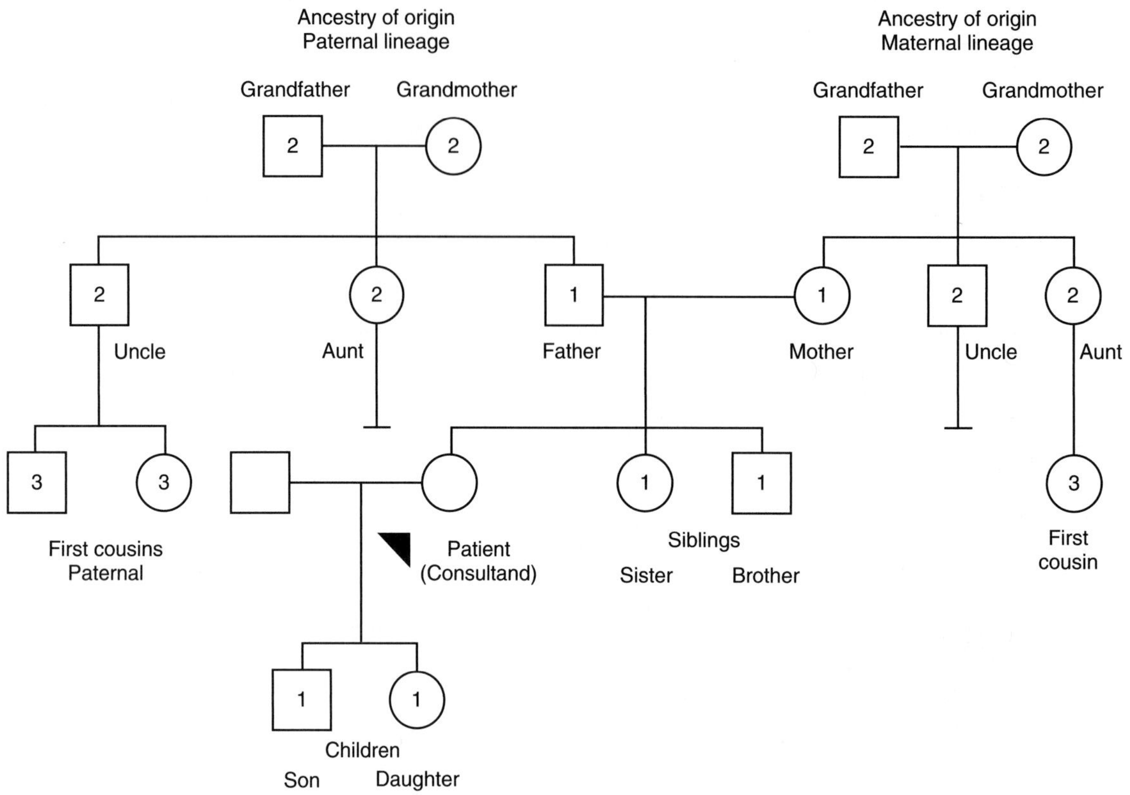

FIGURE 7-4 A four-generation pedigree depicting first-, second-, and third-degree relatives of the consultand (unaffected individual or patient seeking care as noted per arrowhead).

It is important to indicate how family members are related to one another, whether the relatives are in the maternal or paternal lineage, and what other type of relationships exist in the family, such as adoption (in or out), half-siblings, and twins, either dizygotic (fraternal) or monozygotic (identical). These relationships may have a significant impact (monozygotic twins) or no impact at all (nonbiologic adopted sibling). It is also important to recognize that some family histories are limited in structure because of few family members by history, early-age onset of death among family members, limited number or few members of a specific gender, or lack of information from birth parents (e.g., adoption). This limited structure may result in interpretation of the pedigree as challenging because of difficulty in identifying patterns when there are few or no informative family members to evaluate. For example, an autosomal dominant (AD) pattern of inheritance for breast cancer may be masked when assessing a patient for a hereditary breast cancer syndrome such as that of HBOC resulting from a deleterious mutation in the *BRCA* genes because of a small family size or transmission through males via sex-limited expression.[44]

Pertinent family health information, when possible, should be verified through medical records, pathology reports, and/or laboratory results. Verification is an important part of the risk assessment process because family members do not always have accurate health information (e.g., reported history of prostate cancer, but medical record reveals benign prostatic hypertrophy). In addition, family history is a living document that needs to be updated regularly. Family health history is dynamic process, and regular updating is required to annotate births, deaths, and change in health status of individuals as well as family members.

Interpreting a Family History

Once the three-generation pedigree has been collected, interpretation can begin. Interpretation is done by identifying patterns and red flags in the pedigree as shown in Figures 7-5 and 7-6. Red flags include early age of disease onset (e.g., colon cancer at age 38); disease across multiple generations; disorders occurring predominantly in one gender (only males affected); disease in the absence of known risk factors (e.g., hyperlipidemia in an individual of normal weight, adequate diet and exercise) or uncommon disease presentation (e.g., breast cancer in a male).[45] The acronym *GENES* may be useful in identifying red flags. For this acronym, *G* = groups of anomalies; *E* = early or extreme presentation of common diseases; *N* = neurodevelopmental or neurodegenerative conditions; *E* = exception or unusual pathology; and *S* = surprising laboratory findings—any of which may be indicative of an underlying genetic condition.[46] In addition, some genetic disorders are more common among certain ethnic groups (e.g., sickle cell anemia and African Americans), and families with a history of consanguinity among members are at increased risk for autosomal recessive (AR) conditions.[45] Often pedigrees are complex and may be difficult to interpret. Consultation and/or referral to experts in genetics should be sought if interpretation of the pedigree is uncertain and there is a potential for a disease or syndrome. Important online resources such as for locating a genetic counselor for high-risk patients are listed in Table 7-1.

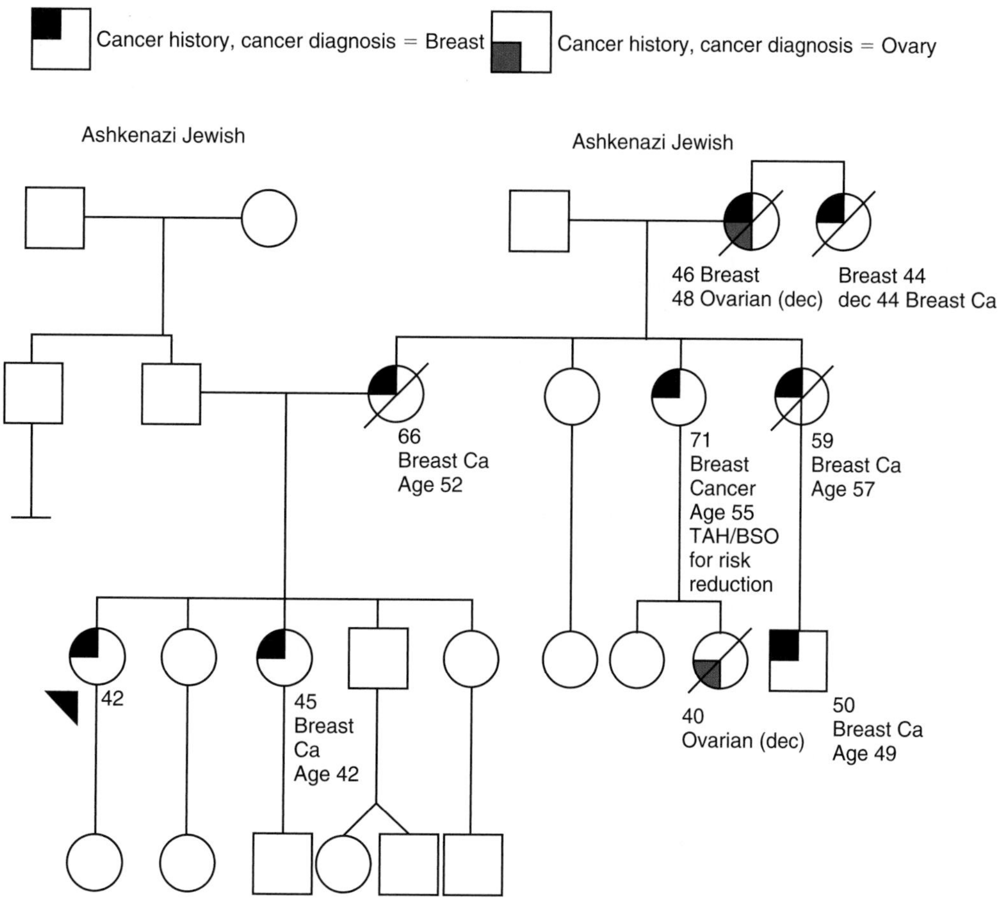

FIGURE 7-5 Fictitious four-generation pedigree of family members with inherited breast and ovarian cancer (positive for deleterious *BRCA1* mutation, an autosomal inherited syndrome). Pedigree displays "red flags" including early age of onset of breast and ovarian cancer among family members; male breast cancer; multiple generations affected with breast cancer; and breast and ovarian cancer in a family in the same lineage (maternal), raising suspicion for an inherited breast cancer syndrome.

Common Inheritance Patterns

Interpretation of a pedigree requires that the clinician be knowledgeable of inheritance patterns. In an AD disorder, only one parent has to have a gene mutation to pass on the disease to the next generation. These mutations are carried on autosomes (chromosomes 1 to 22) not on the sex chromosomes (X and Y), so both genders are equally affected. Examples of AD disorders include many of the hereditary cancer syndromes (e.g., Lynch Syndrome, HBOC), Marfan syndrome, familial hypercholesterolemia, polycystic kidney disease, and Huntington disease. Features of AD inheritance include individuals affected in each generation (with the exception of some families with limited structure) and males and females equally affected. The usual pattern of inheritance seen on the pedigree is one of vertical transmission (see Fig. 7-6). At conception there is a 50% chance of the infant inheriting the condition when the gene mutation has an AD pattern.

A genetic disease that appears to emerge suddenly in one generation raises suspicion for an AR disorder. The pedigree in AR disorders usually has a horizontal pattern of inheritance (Fig. 7-7) rather than the vertical pattern of transmission found frequently in AD disorders. Like AD disorders, AR disorders are also carried on autosomes (chromosomes 1 to 22), so they affect both sexes equally. In the case of a recessive disorder, however, both parents are typically unaffected carriers. Children of two carrier parents fall into one of three categories: (1) they receive two normal genes, one from each parent, and are not carriers, nor are they affected; (2) they receive one copy of the mutation from one parent and a normal gene from the other and are carriers like their parents; or (3) they receive a two copies of the mutation, one from each parent, and are affected. In many AR disorders, carrier frequencies (individuals in the population who carry a copy of the mutation) can be high, but the number of affected individuals (people with two copies of a mutation) can be relatively low. In certain cultural and ethnic groups, however, AR disorders may be more common because marriages to close relatives (consanguineous relationships) are sanctioned, increasing the likelihood that both parents carry the same AR mutation. Examples of AR disorders include sickle cell disease, cystic fibrosis, and thalassemia disorders.

Another form of genetic inheritance is X-linked disorders. X-linked disorders should be ruled out if the disease appears to manifest exclusively in male family members (Fig. 7-8). Men are affected by mutations on the X chromosome because they have only one copy of the X chromosome, and there is no "backup" X chromosome to produce even a little normal gene product. Depending on the type of X-linked mutation, female carriers may be asymptomatic or may have very mild symptoms because their other X chromosome is producing normal gene products. Males with an X-linked gene disorder do not pass the

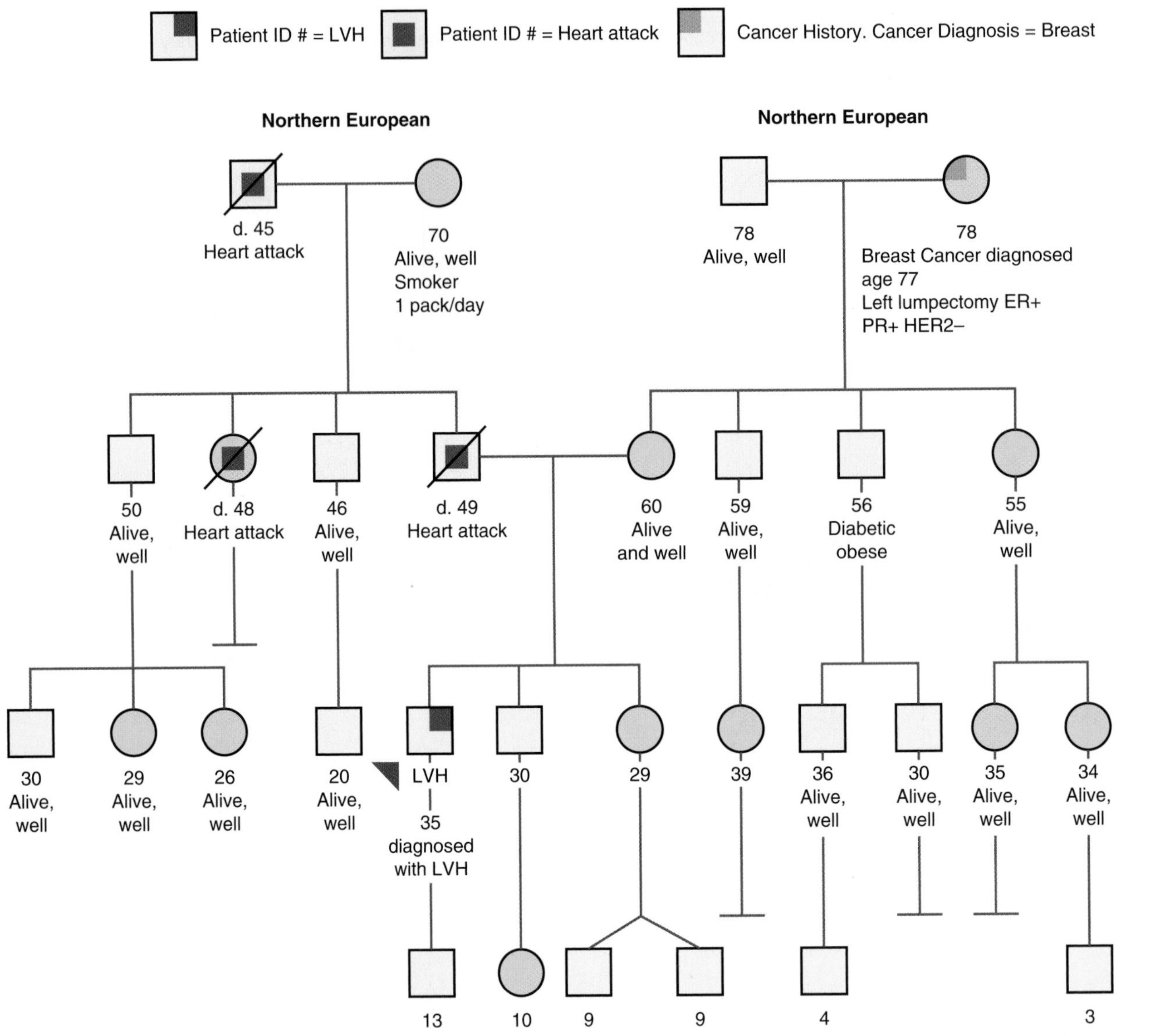

FIGURE 7-6 Fictitious four-generation pedigree of proband (noted with arrowhead) diagnosed with early-age onset of left ventricular hypertrophy and family history of early-age sudden cardiac death in father, paternal uncle, and paternal grandfather, raising suspicion for hypertrophic cardiomyopathy.

mutation on to any of their sons because their sons get only the Y chromosome from the male parent. Fathers will, however, pass the mutation along to each of their daughters. Daughters of men with X-linked diseases are therefore considered "obligate carriers" (one normal X and one affected X chromosome), and every one of their children has a 50% chance of inheriting the affected X chromosome. If the carrier female passes the affected X chromosome along to her daughter, the daughter, like her mother, will be a carrier. If the carrier female passes the affected X chromosome along to her son, however, he will be affected with the disease. Examples of X-linked disorders include hemophilia, fragile X syndrome, red-green color blindness, and Duchenne muscular dystrophy.

GENETIC INFORMATION NONDISCRIMINATION ACT

Gathering a complete health history, recognizing genetic red flags, and referring patients to appropriate genomics resources is essential, but it is only the beginning for many patients and their families. As part of a genomics workup, genetic testing may be recommended and concerns may arise about who will have access to the results and how those results will be used. Individuals have a legitimate concern about employment or health insurance discrimination. It is one thing to have a genetic disorder but another to be asymptomatic and know that one might be at increased risk because of a strong family history of a genetic disease. When someone has a genetic disease, health insurance companies usually know about it because these individuals use specific health care resources (e.g., children with cystic fibrosis are typically hospitalized once a year and their medications are expensive). These individuals often pay higher insurance premiums; however, under the Affordable Care Act, people with preexisting health conditions cannot be denied health insurance.[47] For otherwise healthy individuals considering genetic testing based solely on a strong family history, misuse of genetic information is a significant concern.

TABLE 7-1 Examples of Online Genetic Resources[57,58]

Genetics clinics and clinical genetics specialists	GeneTests (select "Clinics"): www.genetests.org or www.genetests.org/clinics American College of Medical Genetics (select "Find a Geneticist"): www.acmg.net National Society of Genetic Counselors: www.nsgc.org American Society of Human Genetics: www.ashg.org Cancer Genetics Services Directory: www.cancer.gov/cancertopics/genetics/directory Genetic and Rare Diseases Information Center: http://rarediseases.info.nih.gov/resources/pages/25/how-to-find-a-disease-specialist
Disease-specific information for health care professionals	GeneTests (select "Disorders"): www.genetests.org OMIM (Online Mendelian Inheritance in Man): www.ncbi.nlm.nih.gov/sites/entrez?db=OMIM Genes and Disease (NCBI) (organized by parts of the body affected): www.ncbi.nlm.nih.gov/books/bv.fcgi?rid=gnd Chromosomal Variation in Man online database: www.wiley.com/legacy/products/subject/life/borgaonkar/access.html
Patient information and support groups	FORCE—Facing Our Risk of Cancer Empowered (information regarding hereditary breast and ovarian cancer): www.facingourrisk.org/index.php National Organization for Rare Disorders: www.rarediseases.org/patients-and-families/patient-assistance GeneTests (select "Resources" link): www.genetests.org Genetic and Rare Diseases Information Center: http://rarediseases.info.nih.gov/resources/5/support-for-patients-and-families March of Dimes "Family Teams": www.marchforbabies.org/FamilyTeams?intnav=MFB_PUB_HDR_FAMTEAMS
Pregnancy, birth defects	March of Dimes: www.marchforbabies.org/Why?intnav=MFB_PUB_HDR_WHY Organization of Teratology Information Specialists (select "Fact Sheets" for medication information): www.otispregnancy.org
Family history tools	U.S. Surgeon General's Family History Initiative: www.hhs.gov/familyhistory Centers for Disease Control and Prevention (family history fact sheet, tools, resources): www.cdc.gov/genomics/famhistory/index.htm American Medical Association (brochure and questionnaires for prenatal, pediatric, and adult patients): www.ama-assn.org/ama/pub/physician-resources/medical-science/genetics-molecular-medicine/family-history.shtml National Society of Genetic Counselors: http://nsgc.org/p/cm/ld/fid=52
Genetic tests	GeneTests (select "Laboratory Directory"; for DNA banking, select "Services"): www.genetests.org National Newborn Screening and Genetics Resource Center (newborn screening tests, state newborn screening, and genetics programs): http://genes-r-us.uthscsa.edu American Medical Association—DNA banking information, ethical consideration: http://virtualmentor.ama-assn.org/2012/08/ecas2-1208.html
Genetic information—implications for insurance and employment	National Human Genome Research Institute—Issues in Genetics: www.genome.gov/PolicyEthics National Conference of State Legislatures—Genetics Laws and Legislative Activity: www.ncsl.org/research/health/genetic-nondiscrimination-in-health-insurance-laws.aspx
General genetics resources	National Human Genome Research Institute: www.genome.gov/Education Dolan DNA Learning Center: www.dnalc.org Genetic Science Learning Center: http://learn.genetics.utah.edu Genetics Education Center: www.kumc.edu/gec
Resources to help clinicians integrate genetics into patient care	National Coalition for Health Professional Education in Genetics: www.nchpeg.org GeneTests (select "Educational Materials" and "Genetic Tools"): www.genetests.org March of Dimes Genetics and Your Practice: www.marchofdimes.com/professionals/pregnancy-and-health-profile.aspx National Cancer Institute: Prevention, Genetics, Causes: www.cancer.gov/cancerinfo/prevention/genetics
Clinical genetics specialist professional organizations	American College of Medical Genetics: www.acmg.net National Society of Genetic Counselors: www.nsgc.org International Society of Nurses in Genetics: www.isong.org American Board of Medical Genetics: www.abmg.org American Board of Genetic Counseling: www.abgc.net (Can be searched by name, city, or state but does not currently differentiate genetics researchers from clinicians, unless one cross-checks individual entries with certification status.)

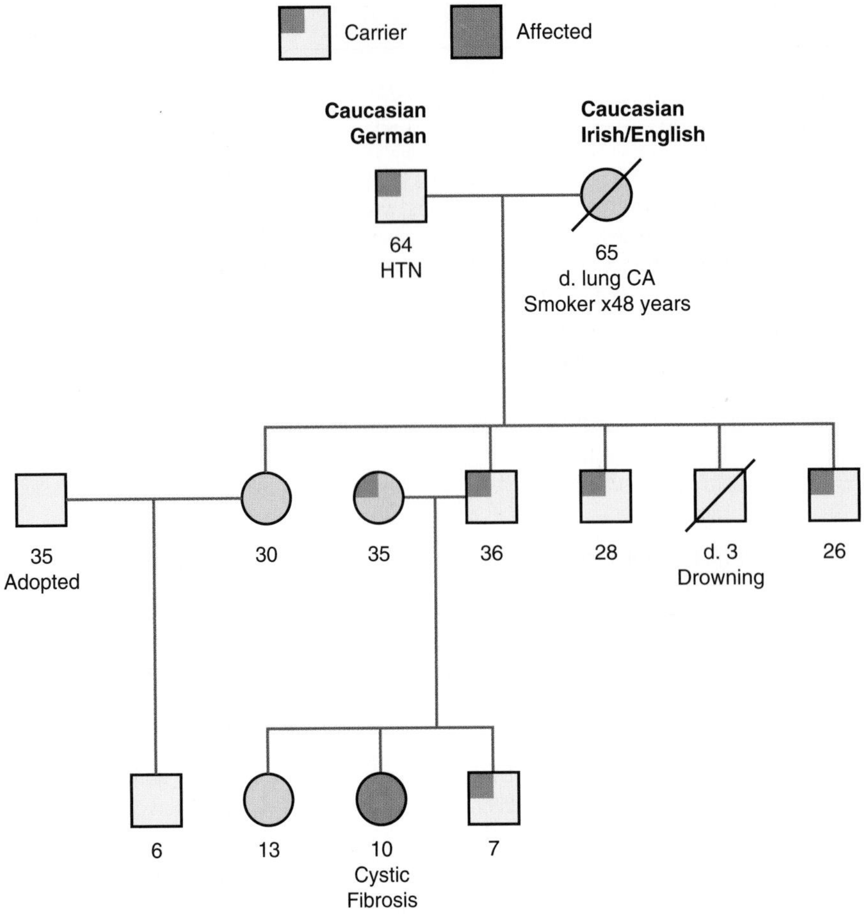

FIGURE 7-7 Example of a fictitious three-generation pedigree of a 10-year-old girl with cystic fibrosis and family members who are carriers of the disease. A horizontal pattern of inheritance is revealed, consistent with autosomal recessive genetic disorders.

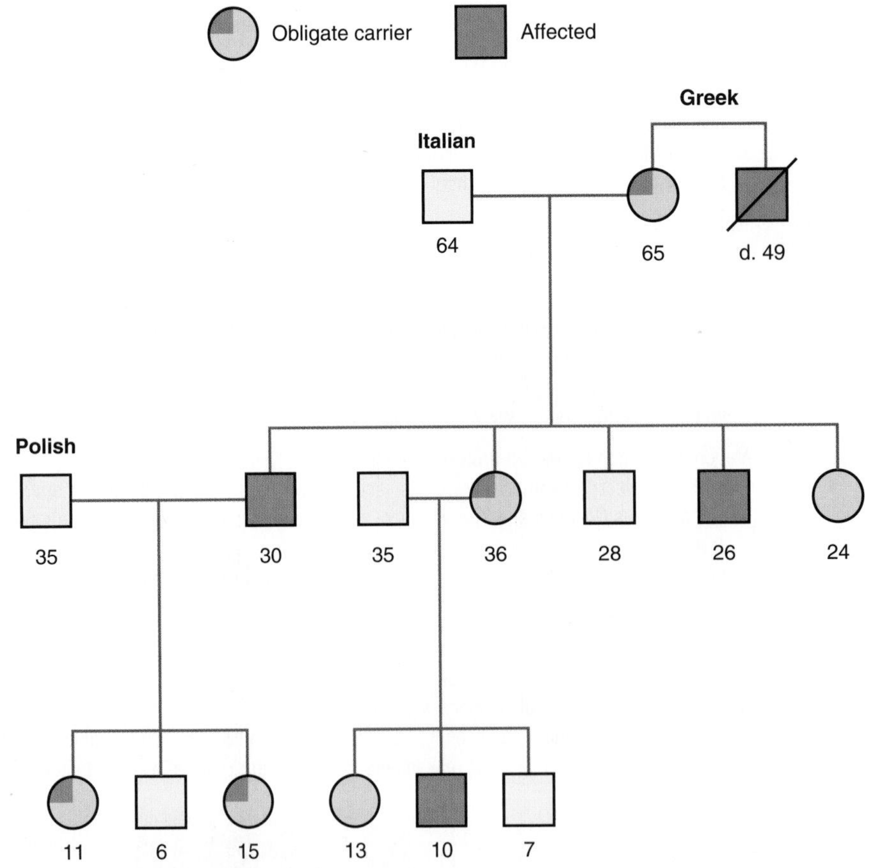

FIGURE 7-8 Example of a three-generation pedigree depicting an X-linked genetic disorder with female carriers and affected males.

Legal protections from genetic discrimination took a long time to secure. Genetic nondiscrimination language was first proposed in the U.S. House of Representatives in 1995 and in the U.S. Senate the following year. Neither bill passed, but advocates were persistent, and the bills were brought forward every year for over a decade. Finally, in April 2007 GINA passed in the House and in April 2008 the legislation passed in the Senate. GINA was signed into law by President George W. Bush on May 21, 2008, and all aspects of GINA went into effect on November 21, 2009.[48,49]

All health care providers should be knowledgeable about GINA and its prohibitions related to discrimination in health coverage and employment based on genetic information. Table 7-2 provides a summary of important information about GINA pertaining to health insurance and employment. For additional information on GINA, a resource pertaining to case studies involving GINA in clinical settings can also be found on the National Coalition for Health Professional Education in Genetics (NCHPEG) website at www.nchpeg.org/index.php?option=com_content&view=article&id=97&Itemid=120&limitstart=3.[50]

Direct-to-Consumer Genetic Testing

Clinicians should be aware that several companies are marketing genetic testing services directly to consumers, providing individuals the opportunity to order and receive genetic test results without involving a health care provider or insurance company. As the cost for DTC testing continues to decline, this may be a viable option for many consumers. Supporters of DTC testing believe this is part of the consumer's right to exercise autonomy in health care decisions. The benefits of DTC genetic testing include the private nature of the testing (e.g., insurance companies will not find out the results), an increased awareness of genetic diseases, and the ability of interested consumers to take a test to explore their ancestral origins.

TABLE 7-2 Overview of the Genetic Information Nondiscrimination Act (GINA)

HEALTH INSURANCE PROTECTIONS	
General protections	Genetic information regarding an individual and his or her family members. DOES NOT cover an individual who is symptomatic, is being treated for, or has been diagnosed with a genetic condition.
Health insurers may NOT:	Require an individual to provide genetic information about himself or herself or a family member for eligibility, coverage, underwriting, or premium-setting decisions. • An insurer may *request* genetic information if coverage may be appropriate only if there is a known genetic risk. Use genetic information to make enrollment or coverage decisions. Request or require a genetic test. Use genetic information as a preexisting condition in the Medicare supplemental and individual health insurance markets.
Research exceptions	For research activities conducted jointly by health insurers and external research entities, a health insurer may request, but not require, in writing that an individual undergo a genetic test. The individual may voluntarily choose to undergo such genetic testing, but noncompliance will not have a negative effect on his or her premium or enrollment status. This information may be used only for research and not for underwriting purposes.
EMPLOYMENT PROTECTIONS	
General protections	Covers genetic information of an individual and his or her family members. DOES NOT cover an individual who is symptomatic, is being treated for, or has been diagnosed with a genetic condition.
Employers and/or unions may NOT:	Use genetic information in making decisions regarding hiring, promotion, terms or conditions, privileges of employment, compensation, or termination. Limit, segregate, or classify an employee or member or deprive that employee or member of employment opportunities on the basis of genetic information. Request, require, or purchase genetic information about the individual or a family member of the individual, except when: • Inadvertently provided as part of the medical history. • Information is publicly available. • Obtained as part of an occupational assessment. • Employer offers health or genetic services, including services offered as part of a wellness program. • Employer operates as a law enforcement entity and requires the individual's DNA for quality control purposes in the forensic laboratory or human remains identification settings. Fail or refuse to refer an individual for employment on the basis of genetic information. Use genetic information in making decisions regarding admission to or employment in any program for apprenticeship or training and retraining, including on-the-job training. Exclude or expel from membership, or otherwise discriminate against, an individual because of genetic information.

Despite these benefits, professional groups have raised concerns about the type of genetic information that is provided by DTC testing companies and the lack of counseling for consumers.[51,52] DTC testing encompasses a wide variety of genetic testing including both single-gene disorders and susceptibility to common complex disorders based on genome-wide association study (GWAS) data, which provide relatively small contributions to disease prediction[53] including results of studies that still need to be confirmed by the scientific community. Because much of the evidence provided for the markers tested is inconclusive at this time, interpretation of the DTC results is difficult[54] and does not necessarily signify that those markers are the strongest indicators for a disease or that patients who have the same mutations will manifest the same health condition clinically. For complex diseases, the family history in the form of a three-generation pedigree provides a first-line measure to evaluate potential risk based on first-degree relatives (parents and siblings), which is not part of most DTC testing processes. Although some DTC testing centers reportedly offer to consumers the assistance of a genetic counselor for an additional fee to assist with understanding of the results, most do not provide any form of genetic counseling.[55]

Concerns about the genetic risk information being provided to consumers by one DTC center, as well as the validity and usefulness of their platform and risk algorithms, came to the attention of the U.S. Food and Drug Administration (FDA), which is responsible for DTC testing oversight. This prompted a letter to be issued in 2013, requiring the DTC site to stop dispensing genetic health risk reports to consumers until the company complied with an order to provide FDA-requested materials.[56] It is anticipated that this DTC site will be authorized to reinstate the health risks portion of its platform in the near future, but there are still issues that need to be addressed in DTC testing. For example, most U.S. states and European countries require a physician's order for genetic testing, and as genetic and genomic technologies evolve (e.g., WGS), the usefulness of DTC testing remains controversial.

Additional information regarding genetic testing can be found on the U.S. National Library of Medicine Genetics Home Reference website at http://ghr.nlm.nih.gov/handbook/testing/directtoconsumer.

CONCLUSION

This introductory chapter sets the stage for thinking about health and disease through a genomics lens. The important role that genomics play in overall health and illness provides a means for personalized health care. The most important first step in genomic health care is to assess an individual's risk by obtaining a structured, complete personal and family history, looking for genetic red flags, and referring to an appropriate genetics consultant if indicated. Risk assessment and interpretation are part of the ANA's genetic core competencies for nurses with graduate degrees. Although advanced technologies in genomics including molecular profiles and genetic testing enable clinicians to accurately diagnose and classify diseases as well as provide personalized management of care, health care providers must first be able to identify individuals at risk. Identification of risk entails not only assessment and interpretation of the potential for disease or injury, but competency in providing genetic education, counseling, testing, and interpretation of results to appropriately refer and provide management of care. As genetic knowledge continues to expand through the use of powerful genomic tools such as next-generation sequencing and GWAS, the term *genomics* will gradually replace the word *genetics* in the clinician's lexicon. Chronic diseases such as diabetes, hypertension, arthritis, Parkinson disease, and mental health disorders that have both genomic and environmental components will become more understood in relation to factors that alter gene expression resulting in disease development and how this information may affect disease prevention or diagnosis and treatment. As scientists learn more about basic biologic processes, they will have more accurate diagnostic tools, drugs targeting specific diseases, and new treatments—ultimately moving toward the promise of precision medicine based on an individual patient's genomic profile.

RESOURCES

Genetic Alliance
www.geneticalliance.org
A national, nonprofit health advocacy organization committed to transforming health through genetics and promoting an environment of openness centered on the health of individuals, families, and communities. The Alliance chaired the Coalition for Genetic Fairness, a multistakeholder coalition of more than 500 organizations committed to passing federal genetic nondiscrimination legislation.

National Coalition for Health Professional Education in Genetics (NCHPEG)
www.nchpeg.org
A nonprofit organization founded in 1996 whose mission was to promote genetics education for all health professionals. NCHPEG's membership represented a broad range of professional societies, advocacy groups, corporate entities, and government agencies dedicated to the integration of genetically based health care into mainstream practice. The Jackson Laboratory signed an agreement with NCHPEG to acquire its website, content and other assets; the Jackson Laboratory and NCHPEG are attempting to expand health care provider education (www.jax.org/news/archives/2013/healthcare-education.html).

Genetics and Public Policy Center
www.dnapolicy.org/policy.privacy.php
Created to help policymakers, the press, and the public understand and respond to the challenges and opportunities of genetic medicine and it potential to transform global public health.

National Institutes of Health, National Human Genome Research Institute (NHGRI)
www.genome.gov
Supports the development of resources and technology that will accelerate genome research and its application to human health. A critical part of the NHGRI mission is the study of the ethical, legal, and social implications of genome research. NHGRI also supports the training of investigators and the dissemination of genome information to the public and to health professionals. Website includes information on research and research funding; health information for patients and the public and for professionals; a calendar of events and media information; information on education, issues in genetics, and careers and training; and specialized information for students, educators, patients, health professionals, grant applicants, and news media.

CHAPTER 8

RISK MANAGEMENT

Deanne C. Munroe • Maria Meklis

Useful practice principle: refer any patient seen twice for the same complaints without resolution to a physician provider.

As primary care providers, nurse practitioners (NPs) and other health care providers need to understand the malpractice risks inherent in caring for patients in office practices, nursing homes, hospitals, and the community. Unfortunately, despite the best of intentions, health care providers sometimes do not understand how easily a simple error or omission can negatively affect a career as well as professional and personal relationships or lead to substance abuse or suicide. Not every patient concern or unexpected or adverse patient outcome is related to a practitioner error. However, if a patient care error or unexpected patient outcome occurs, risk management team members should be notified as soon as possible The purpose of this chapter is to introduce the NP to risks associated with clinical practice, provide knowledge that will empower the NP, and improve patient care.

NURSE PRACTITIONER MALPRACTICE CLAIMS

Data related to claims asserted against NPs are difficult to determine. Malpractice carriers possess the best information and statistics on malpractice claims and the factors involved in those cases. A malpractice claim is the "tip of the iceberg." Each malpractice claim contains multiple diagnostic process failures that culminate in the malpractice claim. In outpatient care, the primary allegations are associated with diagnosis, medications, and medical and surgical treatment.[1,2] Handoff communication and electronic health records play a role in cases with adverse patient outcomes and are discussed later.

A report published by CNA HealthPro and Nurses Service Organization (CNA/NSO) analyzed NP claims from January 1, 2007 to December 31, 2011. Their assessment determined that the most frequently asserted malpractice claims against NPs were related to diagnosis, treatment, or prescription of medications.[2] The following are examples of the types of malpractice claims associated with NP practice:

- Diagnosis-related allegations involved a failure or delay in the diagnosis of an infection, abscess, sepsis, or cancer. Case claims included failure to order appropriate tests or obtain consultations and delay in obtaining (or failure to obtain) diagnostic test results or acting on them. These account for the most frequent causes of failure or delay in diagnosis. CNA/NSO claims data analysis found that lung cancer was the most often missed diagnosis, but there was also a delay in diagnosing breast cancer.[1,2]
- Treatment-related malpractice claims most frequently asserted involved (1) failure to establish or order proper treatment appropriately or in a timely manner, (2) the improper or negligent performance of a treatment or test, (3) the improper or untimely management of an elderly resident, a medical patient, or a medical complication.[1,2]
- Medication-prescribing allegations involved failure to recognize a known complication or adverse interaction of prescribed medications. Improper prescription or management of an anticoagulant also was associated with monitoring for patient compliance (to be discussed later).[2,3]
- Multiple diagnostic failures. When a patient sees multiple providers, there is an increased risk that the health care provider(s) will fail to identify the patient's problem and an even greater possibility that the patient's problem will be overlooked or mismanaged. This type of episodic patient care increases the risk of a malpractice claim for all providers. Some of the factors involved in these types of diagnostic failures include (1) failure to update the family history or to indicate a recent treatment or preexisting disease, (2) failure to make a referral or ensure patient follow-through with a referral or a diagnostic test, and (3) failure to require a different evaluation.[3] Multiple diagnostic process failures frequently culminate in a multiple claim.
- Patient injuries. Diederich Healthcare's 2015 medical malpractice payout analysis, derived from the National Practitioner Data Bank Public Use Data File, found that 30% of all payouts were related to patient deaths and 48% of payouts were related to major permanent injury.[1] Similarly, unexpected death unrelated to the normal course of the patient's illness was the most common injury related to NP claims. The cause of death was related to infection, abscess or sepsis, cancer, cardiopulmonary arrest, myocardial infarction, bleeding or hemorrhage, or a medication prescribing error.[1,2] The next most common patient injuries were related to cerebral vascular accidents, undiagnosed cancer or delay in cancer diagnosis, and infection, abscess, or sepsis.[1,2]

DISCLOSURE OF ERRORS AND ADVERSE MEDICAL EVENTS

In 2002, the University of Michigan Health System adopted a policy of sharing investigative findings of adverse events with patients and families. A process of apologizing and offering compensation was initiated when deemed appropriate based on the organization's inquiry. The University of Michigan Health System has reported that this policy succeeded in decreasing litigation costs by half, and new claims fell by more than 40%.[4]

To ensure that the patient and family will receive a consistent message, one person on the health care team is designated as spokesperson to be certain that one message is communicated. Mistrust of the health care team can occur when patients and families hear different information from multiple providers or spokespersons.

Determining the root cause of an adverse event requires effort and time. The Harvard School of Medicine's affiliated teaching hospitals developed the following approach for communicating adverse events to patients and families immediately after the occurrence of the adverse event[5,6]:

- Acknowledge that the event occurred.
- Express regret and empathize with the patient's situation.
- Apologize if appropriate.
- Take appropriate steps to minimize further harm.
- Explain to the patient and family what will happen next.
- Communicate that an investigation will commence to determine how the adverse event occurred.

Discussion of the results of the internal investigation includes the following:

- Disclose the results of the internal investigation.
- Apologize if there has been an error or systems failure.
- Make changes to prevent the failure from recurring.

- Provide continuing emotional support to the patients and health professionals involved.[5,6]

In a situation involving an adverse event, the practitioner may assume an adverse outcome was the result of an error on his or her part and may feel guilt or overwhelming shock. The provider should avoid blaming another practitioner, blaming a piece of equipment, or blaming the system. An appropriate response to patient or family is "I am sorry for your loss. We are doing everything in our power to investigate the facts surrounding this event." The practitioner should continue to demonstrate appropriate empathy when a family's grief or fear manifests as anger or threats of legal action.[6]

Many states have enacted "I'm sorry" laws that bar the admissibility of statements, writings, or gestures expressing apology or condolences. Communication protected by law differs from state to state. "I'm sorry" laws allow the practitioner to apologize without fear of legal repercussions.[7,8] The provider should know his or her state law; some practitioner statements are admissible in malpractice claims.

THE "SECOND VICTIM"

Practitioners are often the overlooked second victim of a serious medical error that results in in permanent serious injury or patient death. The practitioner experiences stress related psychological and physical reactions. Emotions can range from sadness to anger to despair. Practitioners may fear losing their job; a medical malpractice claim; loss of licensure; and being viewed as incompetent by colleagues, their family, and the patient's family.[9-11] A wide range of emotions include self-doubt, loss of professional confidence, intrusive thoughts, and embarrassment in the weeks after an event.[9-13]

Signs of post-traumatic stress disorder may develop in the months after an adverse event and manifest as sleep disturbances, flashbacks, insecurity, and thoughts of suicide.[14] Immediate intervention after an event includes debriefing and counseling and is proactive in preventing post-traumatic stress disorder. Some organizations also have informal peer support networks that can be helpful. Potential consequences to the practitioner include leaving the profession,[10] isolation, and deterioration of professional and personal relationships, which may lead to divorce, substance misuse, and suicide.[13,14]

THE NATIONAL PRACTITIONER DATA BANK

The National Practitioner Data Bank collects information disclosed by state boards against NP licensure and certification. Medical malpractice payouts, judgments, and negative actions by peer review and private accreditation organizations are also collected and reported. Also reported are adverse actions taken by state Medicaid fraud units, state agencies administering or supervising the administration of state health care programs, and state law enforcement agencies; civil judgments; and criminal convictions. The preceding reportable information is disclosed on initial credentialing and at each credentialing cycle thereafter. Information reported by the National Practitioner Data Bank can potentially affect employment.[15]

DEFENDING AGAINST A BOARD OF NURSING COMPLAINT

If an NP receives a letter from the board of nursing advising of a complaint, the NP should immediately contact his or her malpractice insurance carrier and then contact an attorney experienced in administrative law. Board of nursing complaints usually involve a violation of the nurse practice act related to incompetent, unsafe, or negligent nursing practice that places the patient at risk. Violations include but are not limited to practicing under the influence of drugs or alcohol, practicing beyond the NP's scope of practice, falsifying records, engaging in criminal conduct, or crossing professional boundaries, including emotional, physical, or sexual abuse of a patient. NPs have been falsely accused of misconduct by patients, families of patients, and employers.[16]

Filing a board of nursing complaint against an NP is not complicated. Many websites of boards of nursing contain a link for submitting a complaint online. The name of the complainant is kept confidential in most cases to protect his or her identity unless the complainant is a key witness to the conduct of the NP. When the board of nursing complaint is unfounded, the complainant is protected from civil liability in most states if the complaint was made in good faith.[16]

The board of nursing will notify the NP in writing of a complaint and the commencement of an investigation. If an investigator or attorney for the board contacts the NP, it is best, from a risk perspective, to obtain that person's contact information, because any statement made by the NP can be used against him or her. The primary role of the board of nursing is to protect the public through regulation of nursing practice, and the board's formal inquiry is analogous to a criminal investigation. A board of nursing complaint may result in the loss of licensure, loss of a career, and fines.[16]

The NP should carry his or her own malpractice insurance with a provision for licensure defense of at least $25,000. An employer may provide malpractice insurance; however, a conflict of interest may arise, and the NP could then be unprotected.[16] In this situation, the following questions should be asked and answered in writing by any attorney the employer retains to represent the NP in a matter:

- "Who are you working for, me or my employer?"
- "If there is a conflict between my defense and my employer's defense, will you continue to represent me or will you represent my employer?"

The American Association of Nurse Attorneys (TAANA), the American Health Lawyers Association (AHLA), or the state bar association referral service can assist with an appropriate attorney referral. Representing oneself before the board of nursing may result in an unfavorable outcome for the practitioner.[16]

TELEMEDICINE

The American Telemedicine Association defines telemedicine as "the use of medical information exchanged from one site to another via electronic communications to improve a patient's clinical health status." Telemedicine has been available for decades formally and informally and includes a growing variety of applications and services using two-way video, e-mail, smart phones, wireless tools, and other forms of telecommunications technology.[17]

Telemedicine is used to improve access to care and the health of patients in rural and underserved communities. Practitioners must be licensed in the state in which the patient is located; the state of California criminally prosecuted a Colorado practitioner who prescribed medications over the Internet to a patient in California.[18] The primary care practitioner who dispenses advice over the phone or receives a picture of a wound or rash via cellular phone or by electronic mail is participating in telemedicine. Devices other than traditional landline telephones must meet the compliance requirements of Health Insurance Portability and Accountability Act (HIPAA) and the Health Information Technology for Economic and Clinical Health (HITECH) Act, including the security of point-to-point contact and the use of encryption-protected devices.[19,20] Protocols and guidelines for telemedicine patient encounters are required.

Professional liability may not cover the exposures inherent to telemedicine: (1) privacy breaches; (2) disruption of telemedicine communication; and (3) errors and omissions of telemedicine practice. Product liability insurance must be considered for equipment failures. Good communication between the practitioner and patient are imperative because breakdowns in communication can lead to patient claims of abandonment.

MEDICAL MALPRACTICE RISK MANAGEMENT STRATEGIES

Patients First

"Patients first" is a value espoused by many organizations emphasizing patient-centered care. However, unless this value is embraced and modeled by health care providers and administrators, patients may not experience the compassionate care and service that strengthens the provider-patient relationship.

Ambulatory medicine should be "customer-centric," emphasizing patient experience and satisfaction. Risk management begins with the patient's first interaction with office staff. The patient should feel valued with his or her initial experience, whether it is a phone call to a receptionist or to a call-center operator to schedule an appointment. Policies and procedures for triaging urgent matters requiring a same-day appointment are essential to ensure patient safety and satisfaction. Then, when a patient arrives in the office, front office staff should acknowledge the patient, smile, make eye contact, and maintain a welcoming, professional demeanor.

The patient's experience with office personnel affects the patient's perception of the clinician. Their interpersonal skills and ability to work together as a team decrease liability risk. Treating patients with empathy and kindness is always important. The acronym *SHARE*[21] encompasses the attitude and skill set that each office staff member should possess:

*S*ense patients' needs before they ask (initiative)
*H*elp one another (teamwork)
*A*cknowledge people's feelings (empathy)
*R*espect the dignity and privacy of everyone (courtesy)
*E*xplain what is happening (communication)

Patient Communication

First Impressions. Communication with patients in all health care settings is an important factor in patient satisfaction and safe care. In ambulatory care, patients should be informed when the practitioner is running behind—ideally at the time of check-in—and then given the option to reschedule the appointment with another provider or for another date and time. This practice communicates respect for the patient's time. Once a patient is roomed, practitioner delays should be communicated to the patient at least every 15 minutes. Staff can use a variety of means to track patient communication about practitioner delays (e.g., a sticky note with the patient's rooming time placed on the door or on a wall-mounted whiteboard or medical chart holder outside the patient's room).

The first few seconds a provider spends with a patient are crucial and are the cornerstone of the patient-practitioner relationship. The first impression made by a health care professional should communicate professionalism and genuine regard for the patient. It is important to recognize that greetings in some cultures may vary. The provider should smile, make eye contact, extend his or her hand, and as a rule shake the patient's hand firmly and confidently. It is important to be aware, however, that handshake culture around the world can vary. For example, in some cultures a gentler handshake is indicated or it might not be appropriate at all. If the patient has been waiting, apologize and thank the patient for his or her patience.

Although it is important that patients have a favorable experience, patient satisfaction can have unfavorable consequences. We want patients to be happy with the care provided, but patient satisfaction should not override evidence-based practice. For example, taking time to explain to patients why they do not need an antibiotic for acute bronchitis and making an effort to manage patient expectations are important.[22] A prescription for an antibiotic in this example might produce high patient satisfaction scores on a survey; however, prescribing antibiotics inappropriately is not proper and does not aid the patient or society.

Communication Issues. The patient-provider relationship and patient-provider communication are often cited as factors in litigation claims. Having good interpersonal skills and establishing effective communication with the patient and family are paramount in providing safe and effective patient care. More than 20 years ago, Beckmam (1994) found that the patient or family decision to sue was based on problematic physician-patient communication issues that fell into four categories: (1) deserting the patient; (2) devaluing patient and/or family views; (3) poor delivery of information; and (4) failure to recognize or understand the patient and/or family views.[23] Despite this knowledge, there continues to be a positive correlation between patient complaints and malpractice claims.[24]

A review of malpractice claims asserted against CRICO-insured health care providers and the Harvard Medical Institutions from 2006 to 2010 revealed that ineffective communication among practitioners, nurses, residents, or specialists about patients occurred in 42% of cases.[24] Half of these litigation claims involved outpatient cases. Patient communication included issues surrounding informed consent.[24]

Similarly, Levinson and colleagues identified communication behaviors of primary care physicians without malpractice claims. Positive behaviors included managing patients' expectations, using humor and laughter, actively seeking the patients' opinion, encouraging a dialogue with the patient, and confirming patients' understanding of their care. In addition, the length of time spent with the patient during routine visits was a positive predictor of malpractice claims. Physicians without malpractice claims spent more time with their patients.[25]

Listening to patients and families is integral to assessing the patient's clinical condition as well as meeting the patient's needs and expectations. Meeting, anticipating, and managing patient expectations are basic risk management skills and are essential elements in patient satisfaction and patient safety.

In addition, effective patient communication should be stated in a positive manner. For example, the provider should state, "It's my pleasure" or "You're welcome" rather than "It's not a problem." This change may seem small but is significant in setting a positive tone for communication with the patient.

Patient Concerns. Referring to a patient complaint as a *concern* has a more positive connotation. Patient concerns are a great opportunity to view an experience through a patient's eyes, then review and improve processes. In general, patient concerns are handled from an administrative perspective, but there are a variety of ways to review a clinical concern (e.g., a quality-of-care perspective or peer review). A referral to risk management specialists is appropriate when a patient requests a refund or waiver of a balance owed or insurance copayment.

Acknowledging the patient's concern in a positive manner is important—for example, by saying, "I understand that we did not meet your needs with ..." or "I am sorry that we did not meet your expectations." Do not assume blame or liability, but emphasize that all patient concerns are taken seriously.[26]

Every patient concern should be entered into an event report or an electronic event reporting system designed to track patient concerns and trends over time. Box 8-1 is a checklist for use in addressing a patient concern.

BOX 8-1

Checklist for Handling Patient Concerns

- ☐ By phone: Instruct staff to prioritize patients calling and asking for the manager. If the manager is unavailable to take the call, ask staff to document the best time to return the call and the phone number.
- ☐ **INTRODUCTION:** In person—Introduce yourself.
  - ☐ Discuss the patient's concerns in a private area.
  - ☐ Sit down—this communicates to the patient that you are not in a hurry and the conversation can take as long as the patient needs.
- ☐ **ACKNOWLEDGE/DESCRIBE:** "I understand we did not meet your needs with _______ (e.g., returning phone calls, scheduling an appointment, getting back to you with your test results). Can you tell me about it?" Take notes as necessary. Listen to the patient until the patient has finished speaking.
- ☐ **APOLOGIZE:** "I would like to apologize on behalf of the practice and the staff that we did not meet your needs. This is not the experience we want for our patients."
- ☐ **EXPECTATIONS:** Review the patient's concerns and ask questions to ensure you understand what happened. "We take your concerns seriously. If possible, what do you think could be done ...?"
- ☐ **REVIEW CONCERNS:** Tell the patient you will review his or her concerns, and ask what form of response the patient would like. Document this information in an event report.
  ☐ Letter ☐ Phone call ☐ None
- ☐ **INTERVIEW:** Talk to all staff and physicians involved in the incident. Take notes, update the RDE with either staff or physician statements or results of your interviews.
- ☐ **FOLLOW-UP:** Contact the patient in the manner in which the patient previously stated. Most patients will be satisfied to receive a call back and hear that their complaint has been discussed.
  - ☐ Offer your direct phone number to patients and invite them to call you if they have any further concerns.
  - ☐ If the concern is taken over the phone, tell the patient to ask for you when they come in next for an appointment so you can meet them face to face.
- ☐ **EVENT REPORT DOCUMENTATION:** All patient concerns should be entered into an event report.
- ☐ **REFER** any patient concern that cannot be addressed immediately to Patient Services if that is an option.[26]

Informed Consent

Informed consent is based on the ethical principle of autonomy and is required for any invasive patient procedure done in an office or health care facility (e.g., joint aspiration, joint injection, biopsy, or lesion excision; may be appropriate for complex medical treatment plans as well). Every competent adult has the fundamental right to self-determination over his or her body.[27] Minors or incompetent adults have the right to be represented by a competent adult who will protect their interests and preserve their basic rights. Informed consent applies to one practitioner and the patient unless otherwise stated and documented. A well-written, signed informed consent form serves as evidence that the patient received the appropriate information and is crucial to defending a malpractice claim. Informed consent is just as important in managing the patient's expectations. Malpractice claims may arise when the patient's expectations do not align with treatment outcomes.[28]

A certified medical interpreter should be used for non–English-speaking patients for the informed consent discussion.[29] There is no guarantee that a family member is interpreting correctly. Avoid assumptions of medical literacy based on language fluency. There may be cultural barriers or family dynamics that prevent a family member from interpreting certain medical diagnoses or treatment options. Documentation of the interpreter's name is included either on the informed consent form or in the medical record.

Documentation of informed consent includes the following elements as well as the patient's understanding of the procedure. Procedure-specific informed consent forms can be used that include (1) the nature of the procedure; (2) risks, complications, and expected benefits or effects of the procedure; and (3) reasonable alternatives and relevant risks, benefits, and side effects related to such alternatives, including the possible results of receiving no care or treatment; and (4) disclosure of potential conflicts of interest such as financial or research interests.

Excision, shave, and punch biopsies of lesions should be documented with photographs of the marked sites. Photographs should be taken from a distance to give context to the location of a lesion. If a biopsy is positive and requires a referral to a dermatologist or plastic surgeon, the picture taken in the primary care office provides an extra layer of safety in confirming the site for further treatment.

Universal protocols or "time-outs" serve to maximize patient safety and minimize clinical risk. Elements include use of two patient identifiers, involvement of the patient in confirming the correct site, and confirmation of the procedure.[30]

The procedure note contains the following elements:

- Name of procedure
- Location of the procedure
- Skin preparation
- Anesthesia
- Description of the procedure
- Medications used
- How the patient tolerated the procedure

Informed consent is effective until the patient revokes it or until the patient's circumstances materially change. A material change can be a new diagnosis, decompensation in physical status, or a recent update in family history. The material change may alter the risks of the procedure and/or the alternatives to the procedure to which the patient initially consented. Material patient changes require a new informed consent discussion with the patient along with documention.[28] Informed consent may be done once for a series of injections—for example, as in a planned series of joint injections.

Informed Refusal. Informed refusal is a concept built on informed consent. A patient may not initially fully comprehend the consequences of his or her decision. The health care provider has a duty to discuss the medical consequences of treatment refusal with the patient. Documentation of the informed refusal discussion should include the specific clinical consequences disclosed to the patient. A treatment refusal form confirms that the patient acknowledges the medical consequences of refusing treatment and is aware of the risks of not proceeding with the proposed treatment.[31]

Patient Adherence and Compliance

Missed appointments, failure to follow up with a referral or a diagnostic test, and failure to comply with dietary, medication, or exercise recommendations are all obstacles to improved patient health and safety. When appropriate, missed appointments should be followed up with a letter to the patient that summarizes the clinical consequences of follow-up failure. Concerns regarding patient lifestyle or medication recommendations require exploration to determine factors that may be a barrier to compliance. Patient discussions require specific documentation in the medical record and should include the clinical consequences of continued nonadherence. These discussions should be followed up with a letter describing the clinical consequences of continued noncompliance.

From a medicolegal perspective, the ordering practitioner is responsible for patient completion of referrals, laboratory testing, and diagnostic studies. The practitioner needs to develop a suitable system of monitoring referrals, tests, and other diagnostic studies to be certain they are completed. Each type of health record system, whether paper, electronic, or a hybrid (paper and electronic), poses its own challenges in terms of monitoring when patients complete provider recommendations. The electronic health record can be optimized to monitor for ordered referrals and tests.[32]

These recommendations are important because in the event of a poor patient outcome, the practitioner's failure to address a patient's noncompliance may be construed by a plaintiff's attorney as condoning the behavior. Patient letters should be sent with a Return Receipt requested and via First Class Mail. Sending a letter by First Class Mail creates a legal presumption that the patient received it.

Patient letters should be written at a Flesch-Kincaid level as close to grades 6 to 8 as possible. Grade level can be checked with Microsoft Word under "Review," then click on "ABC Spelling and Grammar." The ease with which a letter can be read should be considered and checked in Word simultaneously with grade level.[33]

Patient Dismissal. Allegations of abandonment can result when a patient is dismissed. To avoid the allegation, certain rules are followed. Patient dismissals may be regulated by the board of medicine, the state department of public health, or individual health plans. It is important to develop an office policy that incorporates applicable regulations and contractual health plan agreements.

Dismissal of patients is done for defined patient behaviors that result in undermining the patient-practitioner relationship. Behavior ranges from chronic tardiness for appointments that inconveniences other patients and upsets the workflow of staff and practitioners to missed appointments or disruptive behavior. All patient noncompliance and disruptive behavior is documented in an objective manner in the medical record. Documentation supports the practitioner's dismissal decision and is the best evidence to protect against charges of abandonment or medical malpractice.[34]

From a risk perspective, a patient dismissed from one practitioner in a practice is dismissed from the entire practice or group, whichever the circumstances dictate. Otherwise, there is the likelihood that the practitioner will encounter the dismissed patient in the future while covering for another provider within the group practice.

The patient dismissal letter is sent with a Return Receipt requested and by First Class Mail and should include the following information:

- The last day the practitioner will be available to render emergency medical care, ensuring that the patient will receive emergency care for 30 days
- Indication that medication refills will be provided during this period
- Alternative sources of medical care (e.g., refer to a local medical society's referral service if available)
- Information necessary to obtain the medical records

Patient Handoffs. Patient handoff is the transfer of care of a patient from one practitioner to another. Handoff is a vulnerable time for patients as well as practitioners. Inadequate assessment or communication can result in a poor patient outcome.[35-37] Checklists help ensure that all pertinent patient information is communicated correctly. Checklists should be standardized and include major diagnoses, recent hospitalizations, procedures, medications, allergies, and pending laboratory and diagnostic studies with the facilities' contact information.[35]

Interruptions should be limited during handoff. Tools such as *SBAR* (situation, background, assessment, recommendations) should be used to keep the communication focused. A "read-back" to confirm that the correct information was received and understood is necessary.[36,37]

ELECTRONIC MEDICAL RECORDS

Offices and other health care facilities may have paper medical records, electronic medical records (EMRs), or a combination of both. Computerized EMRs were developed in part for patient continuity of care and patient safety. There are differences in EMR software depending on the vendor. Unfortunately, there are possible inherent risks in software that can limit the tasks that can be completed electronically (e.g., entering patient information electronically on a laboratory or pathology order form versus a paper form). The more steps needed to complete a task, the more likely an error can occur. In addition, medical information in the ambulatory or inpatient medical record may not be available because of a lack of an interface or because the information entered is incorrect.

The ECRI Institute Patient Safety Organization (formerly the Emergency Care Research Institute) ranked electronic data hazards as the No. 2 patient safety concern in 2015. The Pennsylvania-based nonprofit identified the following as factors voluntarily reported that caused patient harm or "near misses":

- Appearance of one patient's data in another patient's record—patient-data mismatch
- Missing data or delayed data delivery caused by network limitations, configuration errors, or data entry delays
- Clock synchronization errors between different medical devices and systems
- Default values used in error or prepopulated fields containing erroneous data
- Inconsistencies in patient information between paper and electronic records
- Outdated information being copied and pasted into a new encounter[38]

Similarly, in addition to the factors reported by ECRI, CRICO identified the following factors in its malpractice claims:

- The electronic system failed to meet the need of the practitioner
- Inadequate training
- Incompatibility of system or lack of integration
- User error not related to data entry[39]

Another risk is the overreliance on system alerts, resulting in alert fatigue from the false-positive warnings and missing real warnings requiring action. "Overlays" may exist between two separate systems that may or may not interface. The expectation of toggling back and forth between systems increases the likelihood of missing information germane to the care of the patient.

The autofill capability of the EMR system should be used cautiously. Bringing all available patient information into a note and not addressing each item is also done at the practitioner's peril. This practice results in "note bloat" and the presumption that everything in the note was acknowledged and addressed by the practitioner.

EMRs have produced challenges and opportunities to effectively communicate with the patient during an office visit, over the telephone, or through a patient portal. Facing the patient with both provider and patient at eye level is essential to frame and sustain the provider-patient relationship. Providing the patient undivided attention when communicating over the telephone or electronically is a practice that improves patient safety.

Release of Information

Release of information (ROI) to third parties requires authorization by the patient or his or her legal representative. Specially protected information, such as information related to drug and alcohol abuse, mental health, and human immunodeficiency virus (HIV) and acquired immunodeficiency syndrome (AIDS), requires specific authorization by the patient or legal representative before release.

Reasonable efforts must be taken to limit the use or disclosure of, and requests for, protected health information to the minimum amount necessary to fulfill the authorized request.[40] The Minimum Necessary standard does not apply to the following:

- Disclosures to or requests by a health care practitioner for treatment purposes
- Disclosures to the individual who is the subject of the information
- Uses or disclosures made with the individual's authorization
- Uses or disclosures required for compliance with HIPAA Administrative Simplification Rules
- Disclosures to the Department of Health and Human Services (HHS) when disclosure of information is required under the Privacy Rule for enforcement purposes
- Uses or disclosures required by other law[40]

Patient Portals

Patient portals offer secure non-urgent, non-emergency communication between the practitioner and the patient. Depending on the size of the practice or group, a staff member or department may be assigned to follow up on prescription refills and to triage appropriate communication, thus freeing up the practitioner. Consequences regarding patient abuse of the portal should be included in the office or organizational policy.

Patient Request to Amend or Make an Addendum to the Medical Record. Many portals allow patients access to their problem list and the health information contained in their medical records. Patient access has led to an increase in the number of requests for amendments to the medical record or addendums. Aside from the organization's policy and procedures, there may be laws regarding medical record amendment and addendums. Changes should be made based on the presence of an error in the record and not because the patient disagrees with what is written.

Meaningful Use and Automatic Technology. Some organizations are using automatic technology to communicate with patients through voice calls, e-mails, and text messages. An entry is automatically made into the patient's medical record after delivery of the communication. Documentation serves as an attestation for the Preventative Care Reminders measure for both Stage 1 and Stage 2 Meaningful Use. The measure states that reminders for follow-up and preventative care are to be sent to patients by the mechanism the patient chooses, including but not limited to telephone, mail, and secure messaging.[41]

The preceding paragraph sets the stage for the potential risk with the expanded use of this automatic technology for appointment reminders, referral reminders, laboratory reminders, and any other order. The NP is ultimately responsible for anything he or she orders and therefore should be notified of missed appointments and patient failure to follow through on laboratory orders, diagnostic studies, and referrals. It is imperative that the NP be notified of missed appointments, laboratory tests, referrals, and other diagnostic evaluations.

Electronic Mail Communication with Patients. Private electronic mail does not afford the security mandated by HIPAA to transmit personal health information. Electronic mail communication must be secure. An alternative method of communication with the patient must be established—for instance, a telephone number or address.[42,43]

The practitioner should refrain from giving medical advice through electronic mail. This recommendation is based on the following scenario: Consider the patient who customarily communicates with the practitioner via private electronic mail. One day the patient e-mails complaining of chest discomfort, but the practitioner is on vacation with no one monitoring his or her private electronic mail. The patient dies 2 days later from a myocardial infarction.[42]

Discovery is the phase of a lawsuit in which each party asks for information to build their case. Practitioners are responsible for preserving e-mail communication with or regarding their patients. Electronic mail is electronically stored information (ESI) and as such is subject to discovery. An obligation to retain electronic mail may be triggered by an adverse event, by a notice of a malpractice claim against the practitioner, or in some states by a notice of intent to sue. The practitioner has an obligation to preserve evidence as spelled out in the Federal Rules of Civil Procedure. One must ask, who has control over the practitioner's electronic mail (e.g., Google, Yahoo, or other internet provider)?[43]

SOCIAL MEDIA

Many office practices have an Internet presence for marketing purposes. It is important that the website not contain false advertisements. Disclaimers are necessary when any medical information appears on the website. The disclaimer must specify that the information posted does not constitute medical advice, nor is the accuracy of the information guaranteed. Users are advised to seek medical attention in the event of a medical emergency.

As data become transparent and more accessible to the public, plaintiff's attorneys will use these data along with The Joint Commission's standards to support allegations and theories of malpractice claims.

Removal of Social Media Posts

The majority of social media sites have a privacy complaint process. The individual whose recognizable appearance is posted is the one who can make the request to have the image removed from the site. An organization cannot ask to have an image removed on behalf of an individual because the organization does not have the same standing.

Threats on Social Media

All threats should be taken seriously. Local law enforcement should be notified, as well as the individual targeted in the threat. A duty to protect or to warn the intended victim has been established by case law and by statute that varies from state to state.[44]

Responding to Negative Comments

Negative comments should be addressed with the individual who posted, if appropriate. The practitioner should not respond publicly to a negative post, nor should protected health information be divulged publicly to answer a post. Avoid responding publicly by attacking the negative poster. Do not ask patients to sign an agreement not to post on social media.

SURREPTITIOUS RECORDING BY PATIENTS

The patient is required to obtain authorization to record an office visit before recording any interaction. Thorough clinical summaries provided to the patient negate the need to tape an office visit. If a staff member believes he or she is being recorded, it is within his or her rights to ask the patient directly, "Are you recording this conversation?" If the patient responds yes, then the staff member may ask the patient to stop and tell the patient, "I do not authorize you to record my conversation with you." If the patient refuses to stop, then the staff member should leave the situation and find the manager. It would be helpful to have staff practice this dialogue ahead of time so that if the situation arises the words will flow easily.[45]

Documentation of the patient recording without permission and the practitioner's discussion with the patient should be placed in the medical record. A follow-up letter sent to the patient reiterating the discussion serves as notice to the patient that the behavior will not be tolerated and evidence for dismissal if needed. Secretly recording is not legal; individual staff members have to consent to having their images or voice recorded. Secret recording makes staff feel uncomfortable and undermines the patient-practitioner relationship. The patient may be made aware of office policies regarding photography and recording via posted signage and through the notice of Patient's Rights and Responsibilities.

SCOPE OF PRACTICE

NPs are nationally certified health care providers licensed by the state in which they practice. As a health care provider caring for patients in a nursing home or in primary, acute, or specialty care, NPs are accountable for patients' well-being and health care outcomes. The scope of practice for NPs varies from state to state. In some states, NPs can practice independently without physician oversight. In most states, but not all, NPs are recognized as primary care providers; however, in many states, NPs do not have independent prescribing privileges. Knowing the scope of practice as prescribed by the board of nursing in the state in which he or she practices is each NP's responsibility.

Ancillary staff mix is a consideration when assessing any practitioner's medical legal risk. NPs work with individuals with a variety of clinical and nonclinical training in the ambulatory setting and need to be aware if staff are practicing within their scope of practice.[46,47] Scope of practice for licensed personnel is defined by the appropriate state board. Medical assistants are not licensed; however, the board of medicine defines the scope of practice for medical assistants in many states.

NPs in independent practice who employ staff may be responsible for the negligent acts or omissions of employees based on the legal theory of *respondeat superior.* The employee must be acting within the course and scope of his employment. The finding of liability is based on the concept of *vicarious liability,* which states that the employer is responsible for the employee's acts of negligence or omissions and not based on anything the employer may have done improperly. Liability attaches to the employer regardless of employee hiring, training, or proof of competencies.[48]

From a risk management perspective, professional liability insurance should cover the NP as well as nursing and all staff in the office. An example of a malpractice claim arising from nonclinical staff is a scheduler failing to recognize the urgency of the patient's stated reason for the appointment, resulting in a delay in care and patient injury. Additional examples include misfiled laboratory and diagnostic study results and failure to communicate patient complaints to the practitioner.

Employees must be held accountable for their actions and behavior. Employee issues must be addressed in a timely manner and documented in the employee file. Problematic employees should not be retained.

LEGAL DOCUMENTS

Legal documents are time sensitive. Subpoenas or letters of intent to sue should be served directly to the named practitioner. Legal documents may also be served by First Class Mail. There is no prerequisite for them to arrive in an envelope with an attorney's return address. Patients may become plaintiffs, or the party who sues, in a medical malpractice action. When the patient (plaintiff) sues without retaining an attorney, he or she is referred to as a *pro se litigant.* A pro se litigant may download a legal document from the Internet and serve the notice of intent to sue or the subpoena by First Class Mail, giving the recipient no indication as to the contents of the envelope.

Open all mail immediately. Notify the malpractice carrier and/or risk management at once on receipt of any legal document involving professional practice.

THIRD-PARTY CASES

Third-party cases are those cases in which the NP is not a named party in the lawsuit but cared for one of the parties in the legal case who was a patient. The patient may be either the plaintiff—the party bringing the legal action—or the defendant—the party defending against the legal action. Examples of third-party cases include employment discrimination, workers' compensation, motor vehicle liability, and slip and fall cases. Although the NP is not a party to these cases, it is advisable to have an attorney prepare the NP for the deposition.

A plaintiff's attorney may name the treating NP as a nonretained expert witness in a third-party case. The NP forms his or her opinion based on the injured party's medical history, independent physical examination, diagnostic studies, and so on. A treating NP is not hired specifically to testify regarding the injured party's injuries, but was sought by the injured party or patient to treat his or her injuries at the time.

In contrast, a retained expert witness is hired by the attorney of the injured party to examine the injured party or other documents and deposition testimony to form opinions outside the realm of the treating NP, such as rendering an opinion in response to the other party's retained expert witness.

AGAINST MEDICAL ADVICE

Occasionally a patient has a clinical condition that warrants a transfer to an emergency department by emergency medical services. A patient with the capacity to make medical decisions who has all the information needed to make an informed decision to go against sound medical advice may do so. However, each situation is different. The patient's decision does not relieve the practitioner from the duty of contacting emergency services when the patient is driving himself or herself. The patient cannot refuse to have the NP call emergency services; rather, the patient must refuse emergency services once they arrive on scene. The NP has a duty to a third party in the event that the patient crashes a car and injures someone else or destroys property.

A patient with capacity may leave against medical advice (AMA) when accompanied by someone to drive. The practitioner has an obligation to discuss the risks of leaving AMA. Documentation of the patient's decision should include specific risks, either on an AMA form or in the medical record.[49]

HIGH-LIABILITY CLINICAL AREAS

Medications

Medication was cited in 17.7% of malpractice claims against NPs in the CNA's Nurse Practitioner Claims Study (1998 to 2008). The most common errors were prescribing the wrong medication, prescribing the wrong dose, failing to properly discontinue a medication, and prescribing an incompatible, contraindicated, or interactive medication.[2]

Reconciliation. Patients receive health care from various practitioners. One of the biggest risks to patient safety is multiple prescribers. The primary care NP is expected to coordinate care and is responsible for reconciling medications.[50,51]

Medication Samples and Dispensing. A system of accounting for medication samples and controlling staff access is required. Each sample dispensed should be tracked in a log or documented in the medical record; otherwise there is no way of accounting for patients who may have been given medication that has been recalled by the manufacturer. The NP is responsible for educating the patient and explaining the risks and benefits of medications he or she is dispensing.[52] Documentation of the specific education provided is required by many states that place the duty of educating patients about medications with the pharmacist.

Office Medication Administration Safety. The Joint Commission has identified improving medication safety as an Ambulatory National Patient Safety Goal for 2015. Medications should be labeled when withdrawn from the original packaging. Single-dose vials should be used whenever possible.[53] In spite of "the five rights of medication administration," medication administration errors continue to occur. Each wrong medication, wrong dose, wrong route, or wrong patient error should be reviewed from a process standpoint rather than a punitive provider perspective. This perspective advocated by the Institute of Medicine in its 1999 report "To Err Is Human" does not eliminate personal responsibility for errors.[54] Each situation is unique and requires a thoughtful approach to preventing the same error from coming close to or reaching the patient.

Prescription Pad Security. The NP is responsible for the security of his or her prescription pads. The pads should be secured at all times when not in use. Patients and staff should not have free access to a prescription pad. Practitioner identity theft as evidenced by fraudulently obtained controlled substances is reportable to the Drug Enforcement Administration (DEA).[55]

Chronic Pain Management

Accidental overdose has become a leading cause of death in the United States, prompting the DEA to reschedule hydrocodone and hydrocodone-containing drugs from Schedule III to Schedule II on October 6, 2014.[48] The Centers for Disease Control and Prevention (CDC) reports an annual increase in drug overdose deaths involving opioids; since 1999, there has been a 400% increase in prescription opioid overdose deaths in women, and 265% in men. Women aged 45 to 54 are at the highest risk of dying from too many narcotics. Ten percent of suicides in females are accomplished with prescribed narcotics.[56]

Practitioner's Duty to Prescribe Responsibly. The DEA relegates pain management to the practitioner's judgment, cautioning about prescribing for a "legitimate medical purpose" and in the "usual course of professional practice." The DEA revokes prescribers' registrations for "failure to conform to minimal standards of care of similar practitioners."[57] The DEA's guidance is vague and open to interpretation. The Department of Justice has been active in recent years in shutting down "pill mills"—health care providers or clinics that prescribe opioids without supporting documentation of medical need.

Evaluation of the Patient in Chronic Pain. Several professional organizations have issued guidelines for prescribing in the setting of chronic pain (Table 8-1).The guidelines present a challenge in defending a malpractice claim or criminal charge, particularly when state boards of medicine have issued chronic pain management guidelines.[58] These guidelines can potentially transform the standard of care when a plaintiff's attorney enters settlement negotiations or argues before a jury.

TABLE 8-1 Pain Management Guidelines

Year	Organization
2014	California Board of Medicine Guidelines for Prescribing Controlled Substances for Pain
2014	Opioids for Chronic Noncancer Pain: American Academy of Neurology position paper
2014	Oklahoma Opioid Prescribing Guidelines
2014	North Carolina Medical Board Policy for the Use of Opiates for Treatment of Pain
2013	Model Policy on the Use of Opioid Analgesics in the Treatment of Chronic Pain—Federation of State Medical Boards
2012	American Society of Interventional Pain Physicians Guidelines for Responsible Opioid Prescribing in Chronic Non-Cancer Pain
2011	Canadian Guideline for Safe and Effective Use of Opioids for Chronic Non-Cancer Pain
2010	Veterans Affairs—Department of Defense Management of Opioid Therapy for Chronic Pain
2009	American Pain Society—American Academy of Pain Medicine Guidelines for the Use of Chronic Opioid Therapy in Chronic Noncancer Pain

Establish a Chronic Pain Diagnosis and Medical Necessity. A diagnosis with documentation of medical necessity for chronic pain management must exist for malpractice claims or criminal prosecution to be avoided. The diagnosis is established with a thorough patient assessment, the administration of appropriate risk tools, a careful review of past medical records, and the ordering of new diagnostic studies as appropriate. Nonopioid treatment options must be considered in addition to opioid therapy in developing a treatment plan. Regular reviews of goals, determination of whether goals are met, and therapy adjustment to meet the patient's needs are required. Elements of documentation follow in the next section.[59]

Risk assessment tools predict opioid abuse and the extent of the substance abuse problem. Screener and Opioid Assessment for Patients with Pain–Revised (SOAPP-R) predicts possible opioid abuse in chronic pain patients. The Opioid Risk Tool (ORT) predicts aberrant behavior in patients receiving chronic pain management. The CAGE questionnaire evaluates the extent of substance misuse. A patient experienced in diversion will complete the tools without raising a "red flag" with the practitioner.[52]

Similarly, it is just as important to gain insight into how the patient measures his or her own pain and its impact on daily living (see Chapter 222). There are numerous patient-rated measurement scales—for example, the Wong-Baker Faces Pain Rating Scale, the 0-to-10 numeric pain rating scale, and the Sheehan Disability Scale.[59]

A pain management agreement between the practitioner and the patient establishes documented expectations of opiate use. Pain management agreements should be employed at the third visit within 2 months, for all long-acting opiates, and for pain management that is anticipated to be required for more than 2 to 3 months.[59]

The pain management agreement includes but is not limited to addressing safe medication use, frequency of refills, establishment of the one pharmacy that will be used for medication refills, random toxicology screens, and the patient's obligation to inform all health care providers of the medication agreement. From a risk management perspective, the agreement should be formatted to allow the patient to initial each element of the agreement. Patient violation of the pain management agreement provides documentation and establishes the foundation for patient dismissal.

The practitioner has a duty to counsel patients on the risk of overdose. Family members and friends should be involved in education to recognize the signs of overdose. This counseling equates to the patient's informed consent for treatment and should be documented thoroughly.[59]

Medical Record Documentation. Medical record documentation of chronic pain assessment and treatment should include the following elements:

- Patient's medical history
- Physical examination findings
- Results of laboratory and diagnostic tests
- Pain management agreement
- Risk assessment results, including screening tools used
- Treatments provided, including medications prescribed or administered (date, type, dose, and quantity)
- Instructions to patients, including discussions of risks and benefits with patient and significant others
- Results of ongoing monitoring of patient progress (or lack of) in terms of pain management and functional improvement
- Consultations
- Any other information used to support initiation, continuation, revision, or termination of treatment and the steps taken in response to aberrant medication use behavior
- Authorization for ROI to other treatment providers
- Results from the Prescription Drug Monitoring Program (PDMP), a statewide database that collects information pertaining to controlled substances
- Treatment plan and objectives, with regular reviews
- Patient consent form
- Patient management agreement
- Documentation of counseling on overdose risk[59]

Patient compliance tools are essential to patient safety, as well as practitioner protection should a malpractice claim arise. Compliance tools include (1) random pill counts; (2) random urine toxicology screens; and (3) use of the PDMP. Compliance applies to *all* patients, not just patients thought to have a drug problem. All patients must be treated in the same way to avoid claims of discrimination.[59]

The Anesthesia Closed Claims Project evaluated 10,367 claims and found that chronic pain management claims increased from 3% in 1980 to 18% in 2012. Overdose deaths accounted for 17% of patient complications. Major neurologic injury from cervical neuraxial injections accounted for 27% of asserted malpractice claims.[60]

Falls

The consequences of a patient fall can be devastating. Up to 30% of falls result in moderate to severe injuries such as lacerations, hip fracture, and head trauma. In older individuals, the results of a fall may lead to permanent disability or death. A fall may result in a loss of independence or in self-limitation of

BOX 8-2

Falls

Factors That Increase Risk of a Fall	Fall Prevention Methods
Use of an assistive device—for example, walker, cane	Remove obstacles in the waiting and patient care areas
Sensory deficits—poor vision, hearing loss	Offer a wheelchair if appropriate
Impaired judgment	Education of staff on identification of individuals at risk for fall
Altered mental status—confusion, anxiety	Alert in the scheduling or EMR
Medications—narcotics, benzodiazepines, diuretics, stool softeners	Assist patients with transfers into and out of chairs and onto and off of examination tables
History of previous fall[53,54]	

activity, leading to decreased physical fitness and thus increasing the risk of another fall (see Chapter 13).[61]

A fall in the outpatient setting may result in a general liability claim for injuries to either a patient or visitor. A fall prevention program identifies individuals at risk for a fall. Risk reduction includes employing interventions for high-risk fall patients and educating staff, patients, and families on falls and injury prevention (Box 8-2).[62]

Managing Risk in the Nursing Home

Risk management in the nursing home is complicated by the pervasive cognitive deficits and complex medical problems of the patients. Patients are very frail and are often taking multiple medications, which increase the risk of adverse events. Areas of concern include preventing falls (see earlier); decreasing use of restraints, both chemical and mechanical; ensuring adequate nutrition and hydration; preventing pressure sores; preventing medication errors and overuse, especially of antipsychotic medication; monitoring residents who are prone to wandering or elopement; and addressing medical concerns on a timely basis. These are the most vulnerable of patients, who are often living in these facilities for extended periods of time. Staff turnover is high, and there is often no medical provider on site. This combination of circumstances requires open and honest communication with residents and families regarding the current condition and concerns as well as solid policies in place to ensure a culture of safety.[63]

CURBSIDE CONSULTATIONS

A curbside consultation is an informal discussion between practitioners regarding a patient. The curbside "consultant" must be clear in his or her communication that opinions rendered are general and not based on a review of the patient's medical record or an examination of the patient. Therefore the practitioner seeking advice should not rely on the consultant's opinion for a treatment decision. The name of any curbside consultant is not be entered into the medical record. If the practitioner insists on the consultant rendering a treatment decision, then a request for a formal consultation is necessary.[64,65]

It is important to understand the risks inherent in curbside consultations: a plaintiff's attorney may be able to establish a duty to the patient through a curbside consultation when an audit of the EMR reveals the electronic footprint of the practitioner. A plaintiff must prove four elements in a malpractice claim. First, was there a duty to the patient? Was a practitioner-patient relationship established? Second, was the duty breached? Third, was the patient harmed? And last, was the practitioner the proximate cause of the patient's harm?

STAFF AS PATIENTS

Before a provider makes the decision of whether or not to accept as a patient an employee who works in the same office, the provider should consider the following from a risk perspective:

- Patient privacy and HIPAA and confidentiality concerns may be issues.
- Roles may blur between the NP (or any health care provider) and the employee/patient.
- Basic rules should be established to prevent certain circumstances (e.g., an employee approaching a prescriber with a request for a prescription without the expectation of a proper assessment).
- Any medical care or advice rendered to an employee/patient must be documented in the medical record.
- The practitioner may be placed in an uncomfortable situation that affects the practitioner's ability to maintain a professional work relationship with the employee/patient.

PATIENT REQUESTS FOR WAIVER, WRITE-OFF, OR REIMBURSEMENT OF FEES FOR SERVICES

There are occasions when the NP will be asked to write off, waive, or reimburse the fee for their services. There are many reasons for this type of patient request. The practitioner's rationale for considering the patient's request is often based on a patient outcome or the fear of being sued. However, a patient's decision to sue will not be negated by the waiving of a $10.00 insurance copayment; the patient will sue regardless.

From a risk perspective, the routine waiver of copayments may (1) constitute violation of Medicare and Medicaid antikickback statutes, false claims, or abuse; (2) expose the organization as well as the practitioner to potential charges of fraud, jeopardizing nonprofit status; and (3) affect contractual obligations with the insurer to collect copayments, as well as the contractual obligation between the insurer and the insured to pay the copayment. In addition, there is no guarantee that the patient will not file a formal complaint or file legal action. Waiver of copayments may be construed by a plaintiff's (patient's) attorney as an indication that an error or mistake was made by the practitioner (i.e., an admission of guilt). Some insurance companies require explanation of why the copayment was waived. An expectation can be created that the patient is entitled to reimbursement of other monies paid for related hospital or outpatient services.

CHAPERONES

Chaperones should be available to make the patient feel comfortable during examinations. The practitioner shows respect for a patient's dignity by providing a comfortable atmosphere as well as appropriate gowns and drapes. Female breast, genital, or anorectal examinations and male genital and anorectal examinations call for the use of a chaperone. Each aspect of an examination should be explained to the patient before any of these physical examinations. Discussions of a sensitive nature should be done privately outside the presence of the chaperone.[66]

Signage displayed prominently in the examination room communicates the policy of providing chaperones. Health care professionals rather than friends or family members should serve as chaperones; this practice helps to protect the practitioner against accusations of physical, emotional, or sexual abuse.[66]

Chaperones should be available to patients of both genders and not withheld because the practitioner is the same gender as the patient. Documentation of the examination includes the presence of and the full name of the chaperone. The offer of a chaperone, any refusal of a chaperone, and subsequent informed refusal discussion should be documented in the patient's record.[66,67]

POLICIES

Office policies provide guidance for the operation of an office, whereas procedures outline steps in carrying out tasks in the most efficient manner. Procedures create consistency and uniformity in the way that tasks are carried out—for example, answering the telephone or filing. The Joint Commission's Ambulatory Health Care National Patient Safety Goals should be incorporated into office policies and procedures regardless of whether the office is accredited through The Joint Commission.[49] Policies and procedures should be reviewed annually. Revised policies are to be archived and retained. Policies and procedures are retained for the purpose of discovery should a malpractice or general liability suit occur. Policy and procedure retention periods vary. The following is a list of basic policies for the medical office:

- Medical emergency action plan
- Office safety precautions
- HIPAA policies and procedures
- ROI
- Scheduling policy
- No shows and cancelled appointments
- Billing and collection policies
- Tracking and filing incoming laboratory and diagnostic study results
- Abnormal laboratory and diagnostic study results—patient notification
- General consent to treat
- Informed consent—for all invasive procedures
- Patient portal
- Disclosure
- Chaperones
- Patient complaints or grievances
- Securing prescription pads
- Medication refills
- Telephone guidelines for issues that require immediate notification of the practitioner
- Chronic pain management guidelines
- Counseling and dismissal of patients
- Medical record retention policy
- Business record retention policy
- Patient request to amend the medical record
- Workplace violence

REFERENCES

For a full list of references, scan the QR code or visit http://booksite.elsevier.com/9780323355018

PART 2

Primary Care: Adolescence Through Adulthood

CHAPTER 9

ADOLESCENT ISSUES

Lori Keough

There is no standard definition of adolescence and no precise chronological age at which it begins and ends. It is a period of rapid growth and physical, cognitive, emotional, and psychosocial development and is generally accepted to occur between 11 and 21 years of age.[1] Despite some of the challenges associated with this life stage, most adolescents develop normally without major difficulties; however, there are certain subgroups of the population that are at high risk for alterations in expected growth and development trajectories, such as those of low socioeconomic status, those with untreated mental health conditions, and those with special health care needs.

Transition from adolescence to adulthood results in a firmer sense of identity and emotional stability and involves the attainment of economic and emotional independence from parents. As adolescents transition into adulthood, they have established sexual identity and the development of meaningful relationships. This life stage often culminates with a concern for the future and interest in moral reasoning and the hallmark milestones of the adolescent period: an increased capacity for abstract thinking.[2]

Adolescence is also a time when individuals may engage in intentional or unintentional risky behaviors that can lead to significant consequences and complicate their future care.[1] There are several theories as to why adolescents engage in risky behaviors—for example, peer involvement and acceptance, the need for excitement, the modeling of adult behaviors, or some combination thereof. It is important to note that although most youths do engage in some risk taking and problematic behavior, the youths at highest risk are those who engage in multiple high-risk behaviors.[1] Some of the safety issues faced by adolescents are substance use and abuse, cigarette smoking, homicide, suicide, and firearms.[1]

The transformation in adolescence is gradual, occurs over time, and is often delineated by three stages: early (ages 11 to 14), middle (15 to 17), and late (18 to 21), with each stage having physical, emotional, cognitive, and psychosocial-emotional developmental milestones that vary with each individual.

Individuals in early adolescence challenge authority, experience wide mood swings, reject the activities and ideation of childhood, can be argumentative or disobedient, and desire more privacy. This period is marked by tremendous physical growth that is rapid ("growth spurt"). Secondary sex characteristics and puberty accompany preoccupation with normal body changes such as menses or nocturnal emissions ("wet dreams"). Greater sexual interest occurs during this stage. An imaginary audience may influence behavior and increase insecurities. Peer groups, manifested by close friendships with those of the same sex along with contact with members of the opposite sex in groups, may become more important than parental influence. These adolescents may express future plans and an emerging value system; although these ideations are initially idealistic, they may change frequently. During this stage, health promotion should focus on the immediate impact of behaviors. Priorities for health promotion in this age group include evaluating physical growth and development, social and academic connectedness, and emotional well-being. Risk reduction with regard to substance use, tobacco use, and sexual activity (pregnancy and sexually transmitted infections [STIs]), along with violence and injury prevention, is important.[1]

Individuals in middle adolescence (those aged 15 to 17 years) are strongly influenced, positively or negatively, by peer groups. Physical growth slows for females but continues for males, and puberty is typically completed during this stage. In addition, the "tired teenager" surfaces, sexual drive heightens, and fad behavior predominates. This is the age of experimentation with sex, drugs, different types of friends, and risk-taking behaviors. However, as abstract thought continues to develop, consideration of the future and goal setting increase, as does intellectual ability. Health promotion goals outside of physical growth and development continue to include risk reduction related to tobacco and substance use, with an increased focus on sexual activity.[3] As youths spend more time away from their families and develop more independence, an increased emphasis on injury prevention, texting while driving, substance use, and interpersonal (dating) violence are of utmost importance

As they become emancipated from the nuclear family, individuals in late adolescence (those aged 18 to 21 years) begin to assimilate adult roles. At this age, adolescents are usually comfortable with their body image, and abstract thinking matures. Peer influences remain important and become more serious with increased emotional stability. Physical growth and development are complete in females; however, males continue to gain height, muscle mass, and body hair. Adolescents pursue realistic goals, understand the consequences of their behavior, and may be able to delay gratification by the end of this period. However, parts of the brain develop at different times, in particular the prefrontal cortex, and impulse control may not fully developed until young adulthood.[4] Priorities for this stage include evaluation of physical growth and development, use of substances, reproductive health, and transitions to adult care.

PHYSICAL DEVELOPMENT

Although growth occurs over a continuum, adolescence is marked by a 15% to 18% growth spurt, during which time about 95% of the adult size is reached.[1] Before that growth spurt occurs, other specific pubertal physical changes take place. These changes are regulated by the endocrine feedback systems, including the somatotropic, the adrenal, and the hypothalamic-pituitary-gonadal axes, as well as by interplay with the thyroid axis. For girls, physical changes usually begin with breast development or breast buds around the age of 10 years. For boys, testicular enlargement at an average age of 11.5 years marks the initiation of puberty.[5]

The average age at menarche, which follows a growth spurt, is 12.5 years, with more than 95% of girls experiencing menarche between 10.5 and 14.5 years of age.[5] African-American girls may experience an earlier menarche. Dysmenorrhea is rare because the first few periods are usually anovulatory. Girls acquire fat during puberty because a body fat composition of at least 17% is needed for menarche, and 22% to maintain regular ovulatory cycles.[5] Girls may have asymmetric breast development in the early stages. Physiologic leukorrhea, which begins several months before menarche, may continue for several years. Puberty for female adolescents is completed with the sculpting of the body resulting in the familiar adult shape.

For boys, the first sign of puberty is around age 11 and begins with testicular enlargement.[5] Nocturnal emissions begin after testicular and penile growth is under way and dreams become more sexual in nature under the influence of hormones. Male adolescents may have tender or nontender gynecomastia or unilateral breast buds, which may be present for about 1 year. Testicular asymmetry is also common. These adolescents may need reassurance that the size of the penis is not an indication of sexual functioning, and they should be made aware that impregnation is a possibility because the testicles are probably capable of producing a few sperm at ejaculation. The remaining male physical developmental changes include voice deepening, axillary hair, and facial hair.

Pubertal changes in adolescents should be tracked with each physical examination by use of the Sexual Maturation Scale (SMS) or Tanner stages. The family history will often dictate the timing of puberty, but it is worrisome for boys when testicular enlargement occurs before the age of 9.5 to 10 years (precocious) or when no changes have occurred by the age of 13.5 years (delayed). It is equally worrisome for girls when breast buds appear before the age of 8 to 8.5 years (precocious) or when no breast buds have appeared by the age of 13 years (delayed).[5] An easy and inexpensive intervention to evaluate these variations is the bone age radiograph. If the bone age (wrist) is less than the chronologic age but is still appropriate for height, no further diagnostic testing is necessary. For adolescents who have not reached puberty and for whom an evaluation of the hypothalamic-pituitary-gonadal axis is being considered, referral to a pediatric endocrinologist is warranted because interpretation of hormone test results and treatment require a specialist.

COGNITIVE DEVELOPMENT

A distinguishing feature of adolescent thought is abstract reasoning. By late adolescence, many adolescents can understand and create general principles or formal rules to explain many aspects of human experience. Piaget called this last stage of cognitive development, which is ideally attained by approximately 15 years of age, formal operational thought. However, many adolescents arrive at this cognitive stage later than the age of 15 years. One of the qualities of adolescence that is most exasperating to parents is that adolescents are able to reason well in academic subjects but at the same time exhibit illogical thinking about their own lives.[6] It is normal for youths to argue and go on tangents, jump to conclusions, and be self-centered and dramatic. It is important for caregivers and clinicians to understand this as a normal part of growth and development, which may help them to understand adolescent behavior. Simply listening and not correcting is the best approach to use with adolescents.

The capacity of a person to learn will never be greater than during adolescence.[4] However, with increasing sophistication and mental agility, an egocentric attitude emerges and peaks at about 13 years of age. The belief that they can handle anything and that adults do not understand them can lead adolescents to engage in risk-taking behaviors such as drug use and unprotected sex. It is important to note that despite this higher level of thinking, adolescents continue to need guidance from adults to develop and make rational decisions.[7] Adults can also assist adolescents to make better decisions by helping them to weigh their options and consider consequences, as opposed to telling them which decision is the correct one.

EMOTIONAL DEVELOPMENT

Throughout adolescence, the parts of the brain involved in keeping emotional, impulsive responses under control are still reaching maturity.[4] A major task for youths is to learn to manage their emotions and cope with common emotions such as disappointment, stress, and anger. The quest for identity, a major task of adolescence, is accomplished in part by the development of new goals and the abandonment of childhood aspirations. The successful managing of emotions combined with increased moral development is referred to as an individual's "emotional intelligence" (EI). A high degree of EI helps the adolescent master skills in building relationships and getting along well with others.[7]

Each adolescent develops uniquely, although, as with physical development, there are gender-related patterns that emerge. For example, males tend toward higher self-esteem than females, and higher self-esteem is important to identity formation. Other gender differences include that females need to be more assertive and males more cooperative when forming relationships.[7]

SOCIAL DEVELOPMENT

Successful identity formation depends on the support of family and friends. Peer groups are important not only to social development, but also to development of the transition between childhood dependency and adult independence. This is a period of heightened self-consciousness, and adolescents are often preoccupied with other people's thoughts and opinions of them. This has been termed *egocentrism* and was described as the "imaginary audience" and the "personal fable" by psychologist David Elkind (1967) and is a normal part of adolescent development.[8]

Given the developmental tasks of increasing independence, some parental conflict is inevitable. A consistent and fair parenting style can help alleviate the ongoing conflict. Parents can be influential, especially if family members respect one another and engage in rational discussion. If parents recognize and become more comfortable with the growing autonomy of their adolescent, the difficulties will usually diminish with time. Adults can engage adolescents with questions that are nonthreatening and open ended. It is essential to be nonjudgmental and refrain from asking "why," which can put adolescents on the defensive. Neighborhoods, faith institutions, school, and work are also important influences on development. "Rites of passage" such as bar or bat mitzvahs, achievement awards, proms, parties, driver's licenses, voter registration, and graduations foster, focus, celebrate, and further the attainment of adult identity.[9]

THE ADOLESCENT HEALTH VISIT

A comprehensive health history should be taken. The Guidelines for Adolescent Preventive Services (GAPS) consist of 24 recommendations (Table 9-1) that have been developed by the American Medical Association and provide a framework for a complete screening history, physical assessment, appropriate testing, and immunization update.[6] Anticipatory guidance for health promotion, safety, and risk issues is also addressed. The focus of these guidelines varies with each stage of adolescence. Therefore, modifications based on variations of patient populations are recommended. The American Academy of Pediatrics has also published tools for purchase for adolescent preventive health care that include screening cards with the appropriate actions and adolescent visit protocols by age (early, middle, and late adolescence) (available at www.aap.org). Finally, the provider must take into account the socioeconomic and cultural background of the family.

The comprehensive adolescent health visit should begin with the parent present with an interview to assess the family and patient medical, mental health, and surgical history. Family practices such as household smoking, rules, meals, and safety are discussed in addition to routine health screening questions. The parent's presence at the beginning of the adolescent interview affords the opportunity to observe the relationship between the adolescent and the parent. The adolescent should remain dressed at this stage of the visit. Careful explanation of the changing provider-patient relationship for adolescents and the safeguarding of their privacy are stressed. At this time, parents should be asked about their current concerns or stressors. Once these have been addressed, parents should leave the room.

Adolescents may delay medical care if privacy is not ensured,[10] so the interview continues in private with the adolescent. The format of the visit should also be explained, and confidentiality should be maintained. Before proceeding, inform adolescent patients of what the limits of confidentiality are, such as not sharing answers to personal questions unless someone is hurting them or they are hurting themselves.[10] After information about the patient's diet, elimination, and sleep

TABLE 9-1 Current U.S. Preventive Services Task Force (USPSTF) Recommendations for Children and Adolescents

Recommendation	Grade	Recommendation	Grade
Cervical cancer (Papanicolaou test) screening (2003)	A	Alcohol misuse (drinking, risky or hazardous): screening and counseling (2004)	I
Gonococcal ophthalmic neonatorum: preventive medication (newborns) (2005)	A	Family violence: screening (2004)	I
Human immunodeficiency virus (HIV) infection: screening (2005)	A	Speech and language delay: screening (2006)	I
Chlamydial infection: screening (2007)	A	Lipid disorders in children (cholesterol abnormalities, dyslipidemia): screening (2007)	I
High blood pressure: screening (2007) (18 years and older)	A	Motor vehicle occupant restraints: counseling (2007)	I
Sickle cell disease: screening (2007)	A	Illicit drug use: screening (2008)	I
Hypothyroidism, congenital: screening (2008)	A	Smoking (tobacco use): counseling (children and adolescents) (2003)	I
Phenylketonuria: screening (2008)	A	Suicide risk: screening (2004)	I
Visual impairment in children ages 0-5: screening (2004)	B	Dental caries in preschool children: screening (2004)	I
Gonorrhea: screening (2005)	B	Prophylaxis with oral fluoride supplementation at currently recommended doses to preschool children older than 6 mo whose primary water source is deficient in fluoride	B
Hearing loss, newborn: screening (2008)	B	Exercise (physical activity): counseling (2002)	I
Sexually transmitted infections		Healthy diet (nutrition): counseling (2003)	I
Counseling for sexually active adolescents (2008)	B	Hyperbilirubinemia in infants: screening (2009)	I
Counseling for nonsexually active adolescents (2008)	I	Iron deficiency anemia (anemia): screening (2006)	I
Depression in children and adolescents: screening (2009)	B	Lead levels in childhood and pregnancy: screening (2006)	I
Obesity in children and adolescents: screening (2010)	B	Hip, developmental dysplasia: screening (2006)	I
Idiopathic scoliosis in adolescents (scoliosis): screening (2004)	D		
Testicular cancer: screening (2004)	D		
Herpes simplex, genital: screening (2005)	D		
Skin cancer: counseling (2003)	I		

A and B grade recommendations: discuss these services with eligible patients and offer them as a priority. D grade recommendations: discourage the use of the services unless there are unusual additional considerations. I grade recommendations: current evidence is insufficient to assess benefits.
From Melnyk BM, Grossman DC, Chou R, et al: USPSTF perspective on evidence-based preventive recommendations for children. *Pediatrics* 130(2):e399-407, 2012.

BOX 9-1

CRAFFT Screening Questions[11]

- Ever ridden in a car driven by someone who was high or had been using drugs (including yourself)?
- Ever use alcohol or drugs to relax, feel better about yourself, or fit in?
- Ever use alcohol or drugs while you are alone?
- Ever forget things you did while using alcohol or drugs?
- Do family or friends ever tell you to cut down on your drinking or drug use?
- Ever in trouble while using alcohol or drugs?

BOX 9-3

Violence Screening Questions

- How many fights have you been in during the past year?
- How many of those fights were serious?
- How do you get out of a fight?
- Have you ever been threatened with a weapon?
- Have you ever carried a weapon?
- Does anyone in your family carry a weapon?
- Do your parents physically fight in front of you?
- What is your favorite television show or movie?

BOX 9-2

Suicide Risk Factors

- Recent loss of a family member
- Social isolation
- Family history of affective disorders
- Interpersonal problems with peers
- Sexual identity concerns
- Abuse or neglect
- Exposure to suicide
- Prior attempts
- Suicidal ideation
- Physical illness or injury
- Intense life stresses
- Poor coping skills

habits has been elicited and screening has been done for hearing and vision, the remainder of the health history can be organized around the mnemonic *HEADSS FIRST.* In this assessment, adolescents are asked about home, education, activities, drugs, sexual activity, suicide or depression, friends, image, recreation, safety issues, and threats.[6]

Research has shown that approximately 46% of middle school and 77% of senior year high school adolescents have used alcohol.[1] Affirmative answers to questions concerning the use of street drugs or alcohol can be further explored with a useful mnemonic: *CRAFTT* (cars, relax, alone, forget, friends, trouble) (Box 9-1).[1,11]

ADOLESCENT MENTAL HEALTH

Mental health problems affect a sizable proportion of adolescents.[12] As with adult depression, depression in adolescents involves multiple factors (see Chapter 248). Adolescents tend to mask their depression and to exhibit behavioral symptoms such as anger and self-destructive activities. These behaviors are used as a defense mechanism to protect the adolescent from feeling or appearing vulnerable or dependent.[12]

A referral for immediate psychiatric assessment is indicated if the adolescent has made a suicide plan or has actually attempted suicide. Suicide risk factors are listed in Box 9-2.

ADOLESCENTS AND VIOLENCE

Youth violence refers to being a victim of, perpetrator of, or witness to harmful behaviors that are physical or emotional and can start early and continue into adulthood.[13] This includes behaviors that range from bullying, slapping, or hitting to robbery and assault, which are dangerous. Often, youth violence can cause more emotional than physical harm, although it is the second leading cause of death in those 15 to 24 years of age.[13] The prevalence of violence in society necessitates a violence risk screening (Box 9-3).[13] Affirmative answers to any of the questions in Box 9-3 suggest the need for further intervention. A referral to appropriate professionals for conflict resolution, anger management, or assertiveness training should be considered. A suspicion of abuse mandates reporting according to the laws in each state.

With the need to belong so prevalent during adolescence, joining a gang may inappropriately fulfill that need. There are various reasons that adolescents choose to join a gang; these may include the opportunity to make money, thrill seeking, protection from bullies or other gangs, desire for prestige, and a chance to belong. Gang members are 60 times more likely than the general population to experience death by homicide. One fourth are aged 15 to 17 years; the average age is 17 to 18 years; and more males than females join gangs, although the female numbers keep increasing.[14] Warning signs that suggest gang involvement include sudden changes in the wearing of clothing with the same color schemes, a desire to hide activities, changes in who the adolescent's friends are, a loss of interest in family activities, declining interest in school, declining grades, possession of relatively large amounts of money without a clear explanation, run-ins with the police, and known gang symbols on belongings including clothing.[14]

Teen bullying is a major societal issue and, in the wake of school-related violence, warrants screening and intervention efforts. About 30% of teenagers in the United States have been involved in bullying, either as a bully or as a victim of teenage bullying; this is more common among younger teens.[13] However, it may be that older teens are also subject to bullying but may be better at hiding it.[15] Bullying is the use of power to cause distress to another.[15] There are associations between involvement in bullying and physical and psychosocial health problems. Both teens who bully and those who are victims are more likely to experience physical and psychosomatic symptoms such as headache, stomach ache, sleep disturbances, or bed wetting and are also more prone to substance abuse.[15] Screening can be incorporated as assessment for bullying indicators or bullying involvement. Once bullying has been identified, management solutions and resources can be identified and shared with the adolescent and parents (Table 9-2).

TABLE 9-2 Assess Bullying Involvement

	Child Who Is Being Bullied	Child Who Bullies Others
Frequency	How often are you bullied?	How frequently do you bully?
Length of time	How long have you been bullied?	How long have you bullied others?
Location	Where are you bullied?	Where do you bully?
Methods	How are you bullied? (e.g., cyberbullying, hitting)	How do you bully?
Feelings associated with bullying	How do you feel when bullied?	How do you feel when bullying?
Indicators of bully involvement	Physical symptoms Anxiety Depression Absenteeism from school Drop in performance or motivation Suicidal thoughts	Physical symptoms Anxiety Depression Alcohol and substance use Poor school performance Suicidal thoughts
Behavioral signs	Losing things, money Injuries, broken belongings Threatens to hurt self or others	Has unexplained money or items Aggressive with animals, parents, siblings Little concerns for others

Modified from Lamb J, Pepler DJ, Craig W: Approach to bullying and victimization. *Can Fam Physician* 55:356-360, 2009.

ADOLESCENTS AND SEXUAL ACTIVITY

Sexually active adolescents need counseling concerning the risks of sexual activity and the benefits of delaying future sexual encounters. In particular, the risks of sexually transmitted infections and human immunodeficiency virus (HIV) infection as well as the necessity for screening are discussed. The use and limitations of condoms should be explained. Contraception options are also addressed during this discussion. All 50 states and the District of Columbia have confidentiality laws regarding sexual health in teens. Adolescents should be made aware that they are able to seek care without parental consent and should be informed about confidentiality laws as they pertain to sexual health.[10]

PHYSICAL EXAMINATION

Annual adolescent preventive visits continue to the age of 21 years and include appropriate anticipatory guidance and a complete physical examination.[6] It is important to note that although many of the problems in this age group are social, not physical, adolescents are still at risk for physical issues as well. Height, weight, vital signs (including blood pressure), and body mass index are obtained and graphed appropriately for age and gender. The findings from these examinations should be explained to the patient. Privacy should be respected to the extent possible, and parents should remain out of the room. At a minimum, an examination should include evaluation of the head, ears, eyes, nose, and throat (HEENT) and the integumentary, cardiovascular, and respiratory systems. An abdominal examination and musculoskeletal examination should also be performed.

For males, the American Academy of Family Physicians recommends against routine screening for testicular cancer in asymptomatic adolescents, as does the American Academy of Pediatrics; similarly, the American Cancer Society does not recommend testicular self-examination.

Gynecologic examinations are necessary for female adolescents once they become sexually active. The initial reproductive visit is important because it sets the tone for future visits. The components of the examination vary by patient; however, it should include screening for STIs annually or more frequently, depending on risk. Also, a Papanicolaou (Pap) cytology smear screening should be initiated at age 21 and every 3 years thereafter, depending on results.[16]

The Preparticipation Physical Evaluation (PPE) is an important part of the adolescent health evaluation and is required for all school-sponsored sports.[17] Many youths participate in activities that do not require a physical examination but are also at the same risk for the health problems that are screened for in the PPE. Therefore it is recommended that the PPE be incorporated into the annual health visit for all children and adolescents regardless of current or anticipated athletic participation (www.aap.org and Chapter 22).[17] Precollege visits are an opportune time to update the adolescent's records, including immunization status, and to offer anticipatory guidance regarding sexuality (e.g., contraception, risks and prevention of STIs and HIV infection, responsible sexual behavior, prevention of sexual assault), cardiovascular health (e.g., nutrition, exercise, smoking), injury prevention (e.g., automobile and campus safety), obesity prevention, and mental health (e.g., stress, substance abuse, eating disorders). Patient education should occur at each visit, and the transition to adult care is an essential component of this visit.[18] Box 9-4 lists some available resources.

HEALTH MAINTENANCE AND HEALTH PROMOTION

Because of the rapid physical and behavioral changes that occur during adolescence, the Advisory Committee on Immunization Practices and GAPS recommend a routine comprehensive adolescent visit beginning at the age of 11 years to lay the groundwork for future annual visits. Unlike for younger children, health promotion as a focus of anticipatory guidance should shift from the parent to the adolescent.[6] Although working with parents is also essential, it is important to build autonomy in the adolescent patient and to address risk factors in balance with strengths and assets. Furthermore, as adolescents begin to be more independent in many areas of their lives, this is an

BOX 9-4

Resources for Caring for Adolescents

American Academy of Child and Adolescent Psychiatry
3615 Wisconsin Ave., NW
Washington, DC 20016-3007
800-333-7636
www.aacap.org

American Academy of Pediatrics
141 Northwest Point Blvd.
Elk Grove Village, IL 60007
847-434-4000
www.aap.org

American Psychological Association Parenting
http://www.apa.org/topics/parenting/

Bright Futures
Family Tip Sheets
www.brightfutures.org/TipSheets/index.html

Center for Young Women's Health, Boston Children's Hospital
333 Longwood Ave., 5th Floor
Boston, MA 02115
617-355-2994
www.youngwomenshealth.org

Department of Child and Adolescent Health and Development, World Health Organization
20 Avenue Appia
1211 Geneva 27
Switzerland
+41-22-791-3281
www.who.int/child_adolescent_health/en

PFLAG: Parents, Families, and Friends of Lesbians and Gays
1726 M St., NW, Suite 400
Washington, DC 20036
202-467-8180
www.pflag.org

Society for Adolescent Health and Medicine (SAHM)
www.adolescenthealth.org

Suicide Prevention Hotline
800-621-4000

opportune time to begin a gradual transition from adolescent to adult care.[18]

Immunizations are an important part of health promotion and should be reviewed and updated at these annual visits. Chapter 17, Routine Health Screening and Immunizations, contains important information. The American Academy of Pediatrics (www.aap.org), the American Academy of Family Physicians (www.aafp.org), and the CDC (www.cdc.gov) publish annual immunization schedules.

Routine tuberculosis (TB) screening (with use of purified protein derivative [PPD]) is not usually performed unless the patient has risk factors for TB or the test is required for college admission or employment. High-risk groups include close contacts of a person with infectious disease, foreign-born persons from areas where TB is common, and persons from medically underserved and low-income populations, including certain racial and ethnic groups.

Adolescence is a challenging time for providers, parents, and adolescents themselves. However, this is an important transitional period of rapid growth and development; health habits, attitudes, and beliefs can carry into adulthood, and the provider's role should not be underestimated. Providers are in an opportune place to provide comprehensive health promotion, education, and care to youths and to have a positive impact and influence on the emerging adult during this important life stage.

CHAPTER 10

LGBTQ PATIENT CARE

Mary DiGiulio • Wendy A. Ritch • Peter Oates

Structural inequalities and health inequities are inextricably related.[1] Although, even in 2016, health inequities based on race, ethnicity, gender, income, employment, education, physical ability, mental capacity, and other characteristics continue to thrive in the United States, there are federal, state, and local laws that prohibit discrimination against members of "protected classes." Discrepancy between federal and state legislation has resulted in a patchwork of laws, from relationship recognition to antidiscrimination and hate crimes legislation, which vary from one state to another and in many cases have left LGBTQ populations vulnerable to health care inequities. Members of sexual and gender minorities (SGMs) are socially, politically, and economically vulnerable; these individuals may experience discrimination in health care settings at the hands of practitioners and staff who do not provide culturally competent care. Over the course of the life spans of these individuals, structural inequalities combined with health inequities result in poor health outcomes for LGBTQ elders, which are compounded even further by intersectionality.[2]

In 2015 the U. S. Supreme Court upheld the decision that a marriage between individuals of the same sex must be recognized in all states if the two individuals are lawfully married in any state.[3] Even after the implementation of the Affordable Care Act, which prohibits health insurers from discriminating against LGBTQ patients, most Americans younger than 65 years are insured either by their employer or by their spouse's employer. Employers operating in states that do not offer full marriage equality can deny the extension of all types of benefits to same-sex partners of their employees, which can result in both health and economic insecurity. SGMs can experience significantly greater disparities of many types and have correspondingly worse health outcomes than the general population.

Health authorities within and outside of the federal government do recognize that health disparities exist for LGBTQ people. In 1999 the Institute of Medicine (IOM) published a report on lesbian health that indicated that certain negative health outcomes were more prevalent among lesbians; lesbians experienced financial and cultural barriers to accessing health care. The report called for more population-based research on lesbian health and the funding to conduct these studies.[4] *Healthy People 2010* did not include LGBTQ health as a topic in its main volume, but there was a companion volume created, in large part because of the advocacy of a group of SGM health experts who were instrumental in writing it. The *Healthy People 2010* companion volume identified seven of the country's 10 leading health indicators as areas in need of special attention for SGMs.[5]

Unlike *Healthy People 2010*, *Healthy People 2020* includes LGBTQ health as a topic with a single objective: "increase the number of population-based data systems used to monitor *Healthy People 2020* objectives that include in their core a standardized set of questions that identify LGBTQ populations."[6] The 2011 release of the IOM report on the health of LGBTQ populations, 12 years after the report on lesbian health, still said the same things: disparities exist, but their causes are complex and poorly understood; researchers need more data about the demographics of these populations; improved methods for collecting and analyzing data are necessary; and increased participation of SGMs in research as well as funding for these studies are required.[1] Although identification of LGBTQ people in national population and health surveillance surveys will go a long way toward building national data sets on these groups, it will take years before researchers have substantial longitudinal data on which to draw.

As with any group that experiences discrimination throughout the life course, LGBTQ populations are at an increased risk of morbidity and mortality. Some of the causes are shared with the general population, as well as with other oppressed groups, whereas other causes are specific to SGMs, including stigma, stress, financial and employment insecurity, fear, risky coping behaviors, lack of social and familial support, aging, poor cultural competence among health care providers, and genetics. Health care providers who are well-versed in culturally competent care of LGBTQ populations can go a long way toward countering some of the obstacles created by health inequities that contribute to poor health outcomes for SGMs.

The relationship between different U.S. states' LGBTQ policies and the mental health of LGBTQ people in those states was well documented in a 2011 study.[7] The researchers found that LGB respondents in states without LGBTQ protective policies were almost five times more likely than those in states with protections to have two or more mental disorders; and when states passed constitutional bans on same sex marriage, mood disorders increased by one third among their LGB populations, whereas there was no increase among non-LGB people.[7] Although there have not yet been similar studies linking physical health of LGBTQ populations with policies that positively and negatively affect SGMs, it seems to follow logically, particularly given the relationship between mental and physical well-being, that findings would be similar to those of the study by Haas[7] and colleagues.

The IOM reports in 1999 and 2011 as well as the *Healthy People 2010* companion volume and *Healthy People 2020* state that LGBTQ health disparities exist. *Healthy People 2020* specifically identifies social determinants related to oppression and discrimination, such as those mentioned earlier in this chapter, and problems with the physical environment, such as safe schools, neighborhoods, and housing, as factors that contribute to LGBTQ health disparities.[6]

The IOM's 2011 report on LGBTQ health recognized that SGM populations had special health needs, but because of the dearth of funding devoted to research in this area, the absence of demographic information about these groups, and the negligible participation of LGBTQ people in research studies, the report authors could not identify those needs.[9] Given the challenges that LGBTQ individuals can face with health care, it is essential for health care professionals to become familiar with the general and special health needs of their LGBTQ patients and to ensure that their practice sites are welcoming to LGBTQ populations.

DEFINITIONS

LGBTQ is a common acronym that typically refers to lesbian, gay, bisexual, transgender, and queer or questioning. The acronym LGBTQIA is also used and refers to lesbian, gay, bisexual, transgender, queer or questioning, intersex, and ally. These terms are defined as follows:

- *Lesbian* refers to a woman who has a physical, romantic, and/or emotional attraction toward other women.
- *Gay* refers to a man who has a physical, romantic, and/or emotional attraction toward other men.
- *Bisexual* refers to an individual who is attracted to both men and women.
- *Transgender* refers to individuals who identify or express themselves as the opposite of their birth gender or those for whom their gender and sex are not necessarily evident or do not conform to the conventional expectations for male or female. Patients may identify as male to female (MTF) or female to male (FTM). Some individuals in this group consider themselves to be gender nonconforming. Approximately 5% of the LGBTQ population primarily identifies as transgender.
- *Queer* is currently a term used by an individual to self-identify. It is also sometimes used by patients who feel that their gender identity or expression is outside of societal norms. Many older individuals still find this term pejorative.
- *Questioning* may be used by those who are still discovering their true sexual orientation, identity, or expression.
- *Intersex* refers to those individuals with a disorder related to fetal sexual development resulting in a chromosomal anomaly or ambiguous genitalia. Many adults underwent surgical intervention as infants that resulted in an assigned sex that may or may not coincide with the person's gender identity.
- *Ally* refers to an individual who is supportive of SGMs.[8]

Gender identity refers to a person's individual association gender—whether they feel primarily male, female, or a combination of both or do not identify with either. *Gender expression* refers to the way in which a person communicates gender identity. This may be expressed through appearance (e.g., clothing, accessories) or through actions (e.g., mannerisms). *Gender role conformity* refers to the degree to which a person's outward appearances and mannerisms are consistent with the accepted cultural norms for an individual of that gender.[9]

GOALS OF CARE

The goal of health care for LGBTQ patients is really no different from the goal of health care for any population of patients. It is to treat the patient in the manner in which we would want our family members or ourselves to be treated. The provision of care should be holistic and occur in an inclusive and culturally sensitive environment that enhances the health and well-being of the patient. LGBTQ patients share many of the same risk factors and health concerns of the general population. LGBTQ patients may also have specific risk factors or health concerns that are specific to their personal history.

The provider should be aware if the patient is gay, lesbian, bisexual, or transgender to provide appropriate care and health screening for the individual. Health care needs to be individualized appropriately for each patient, to provide the best care possible.

ACCESS TO CARE

Sexual identity can change depending on a variety of factors, including context, culture, geography, and the progression through life's journey. A person's sexual identity, sexual behavior, and feelings of attraction all contribute to sexual orientation. There is a large variety of words that LGBTQ patients may use to describe themselves. Be respectful of patients' choice of language in describing themselves.[10]

Patients will assess the practice environment and personnel for signs of acceptance or affirmation. A rainbow flag posted on the window in the reception area or patient education materials with positive images of LGBTQ people can signal that a practice or provider is accepting of LGBTQ patients. Subtle visual cues can be provided within the waiting area, such as a small rainbow emblem or pictures of same-sex couples. Something as simple as unisex bathrooms can also make a difference.[11] Patient intake forms should include an area that allows the patient to self-identify. The term "spouse/partner" can be used on intake forms, and the provider might consider renaming *marital status* to *relationship status.* A statement about nondiscrimination based on sexual or gender identity can be included on forms.

Providers should be sensitive to the needs of the patient.[11] Professional relationships between providers and patients are dependent on confidentiality, trust, respect for the individual, and active listening. Clinical competence or expertise may not be able to overcome the insensitivity of the provider.

Patients should feel included and accepted during all interactions with health care staff. All staff members should be aware of their attitudes and speech choices (e.g., language, tone) when interacting with patients, whether in person or via electronic means. An office would be considered to be user-friendly when interaction with staff (both professional and support) members is respectful of the individual. Patients may need to overcome prior negative experiences with health care staff.

The Gay and Lesbian Medical Association (GLMA) offers a provider listing service. LGBTQ-friendly practices or providers can enter their information into the site, and patients can search for providers using location, specialty, or community partnerships as a guide. Regional groups also offer mapping of providers who are deemed to be competent in LGBTQ care.

The Joint Commission (2011)[23] published a field guide to help inform practice and offer guidance in identification of quality improvement areas regarding patient safety and compliance with expected regulations. The Joint Commission established the requirements for LGBTQ patient-centered care in facilities that receive accreditation from the organization.

In 2013, the U.S. Supreme Court ruled that Section 3 of the Defense of Marriage Act (DOMA) was unconstitutional. This ruling allowed Medicare to recognize same-sex marriages when determining eligibility for Medicare. As long as the couple is married and resides in a state that recognizes same-sex marriage, the spouse should be eligible for Medicare.

Medicaid is a state-run program to provide health insurance coverage to those who qualify. Some funding for Medicaid is provided by the federal government. Individuals in a civil union or registered domestic partnership recognized by the state may be considered to be married for Medicaid eligibility purposes. In states that do not recognize a legal relationship for the same sex couple, the spouse will not be eligible for Medicaid coverage.

Gender dysphoria is the medical diagnostic terminology used to identify transgender patients. It is listed in the *Diagnostic and Statistical Manual of Mental Disorders,* Fifth Edition (2013)[10A] as a psychiatric diagnosis. This is a change from gender identity disorder, which was used in prior editions. The diagnosis is currently used to justify the medical necessity of treatments for transgender patients. Proof of medical necessity is necessary for payment from health insurance companies.

BARRIERS TO CARE

Some LGBTQ patients have had prior experiences with health care providers that have left them feeling marginalized or stigmatized. Patients may have a fear of stigma in future health care encounters. In some patients, the past experiences with stigmatization are enough to cause avoidance of health care providers altogether. LGBTQ patients may feel discriminated against because of either interpersonal interactions or institutional policies or practices, which may be unintentionally discriminatory in nature. This is particularly true for transgender patients, who may have had prior problems with health care providers being able to adequately meet their needs. Even in practices that self-identify as being LGBTQ-friendly, providers may not be knowledgeable enough about hormonal therapies to offer comprehensive care to transgender patients. Transgender health care needs are not often covered within the curriculum at many institutions of higher learning.[12]

Consider your own feelings about sexual identity and sexual expression. Are you comfortable discussing sexuality or gender roles? Transgender patients experience mistreatment from health care providers in the forms of gender insensitivity, lack of consideration of health care needs, discrimination, and use of improper terminology.

Don't assume that all patients are heterosexual. Don't assume that there has been no change in a patient's behavior or identity since the last visit. Patients may be in long-term, committed same-sex relationships and still identify as bisexual. Gay or lesbian patients may have been in previous heterosexual relationships and may have children regardless of current or prior relationship status.

Encourage all patients to define themselves, or self-identify. Ask patients what terminology they prefer. Most patients are not offended when asked what their preference is but may be offended if assumptions are made.

Be aware of the language that you chose. Asking the patient, "Do you have sex with men, women, or both?" is very different than asking, "You don't have sex with men (or women, depending on the patient's gender), do you?" Providers who make a habit of asking all patients this question have found that the practice normalized the question as part of a routine. Some patients may answer the question in a manner that the provider was not initially expecting. This can open the door to further communication and allow the provider to personalize the health screenings and education regarding the patient's actual risk profile.

When asking about sexual behavior, the provider should not assume to know the patient's preferences. All patients should be asked if they are attracted to men, women, or both. Many providers and health care facility forms limit the options for patients and, sometimes unknowingly, decrease the comfort of the patient to discuss concerns or provide a complete health history. Health forms in use should be checked for noninclusive language.

During patient interviews, the questions that are asked should have medical relevance. The information being sought should have medical relevance. Asking about a patient's sexual practices (e.g., oral; vaginal and/or anal penetration) is appropriate when calculating overall health risk and necessary health screenings, but not necessary information when treating a simple laceration on a hand. It is equally important to consider context of information when treating a transgender patient. Hormonal therapy is important to be aware of when prescribing. Surgical intervention is not always relevant to the care being sought. It is relevant in determining health screenings. Does the MTF transgender patient still have a prostate gland than needs to be evaluated? Keep the information about the patient's sexual orientation private. It is protected health information under the Health Insurance Portability and Accountability Act of 1996 (HIPAA) in the same way that a diagnosis of diabetes is protected health information.

As with all patients, a good place to start on the first encounter is to give patients an opportunity to tell you a little bit about themselves, and see where it leads. If needed, direct questions may be asked to obtain a brief overview of the current lifestyle or to elicit further clarification—questions such as "Where is home?" "What kind of work do you do?" "Are you in a relationship?" "Do you have a significant other, partner, or spouse?" "Do you have children?" Asking these generic-type questions normalizes the encounter, gives patients the opportunity to tell their story, and allows them to define themselves.

Because of varied social pressures, some LGBTQ patients have followed societal expectations—for example, a gay man may have a wife or girlfriend and a male sexual partner. Assumptions about a patient's sexual orientation should not be made based on the current relationship status.

Men who have sex with men are still prohibited from donating blood. This lifelong ban preventing donation of blood or blood products was instituted in 1983, when acquired immunodeficiency syndrome (AIDS) was epidemic and there was no ability to test for presence of the virus.

CHALLENGES IN PRIMARY CARE

A thorough history and physical examination should be undertaken for all new patients. This includes information on social history, including sexual activity. Some patients will not disclose their sexual orientation or gender identity at an initial visit, unless it is pertinent to the reason they are being seen (known as their chief complaint). It may take several visits to a practice or particular provider before the patient feels comfortable enough to disclose. In contrast, other patients will disclose immediately. Almost 40% of LGBTQ people have experienced the rejection of a close friend or family member as a result of their sexual orientation or gender identity.[13] It is important to ensure that each patient is getting a personalized plan of care with consideration for screenings that are appropriate for age and gender (both biologic and identified).

Some of the unique challenges for LGBTQ patients include coming out as lesbian, gay, bisexual, or transgender; long-term partnerships and marriage; reproduction and adoption; parenting; adolescent and aging issues; and legal rights as both partners and parents. Patients who are working with an adoption agency typically need to have a comprehensive physical examination. The provider needs to assert that the applicant in question is mentally and physically fit for parenthood. It is important for the provider to be aware of any potential personal bias before agreeing to complete those forms.

Risky Behavior

Patients who engage in high-risk sexual behavior increase their risk for certain diseases. Health risk is associated with engaging in risky behaviors, not the patient's sexual orientation. High-risk sexual contact increases the risk for sexually transmitted diseases, such as chlamydia or herpes, as well as systemic disease, such as human immunodeficiency virus (HIV). Rates of sexually transmitted infections vary geographically. It is important for providers to familiarize themselves with current rates in their locales. Screening for sexually transmitted infections, such as syphilis, chlamydia, gonorrhea, and HIV, is recommend for patients with higher-risk sexual practices.[15]

Increased rates of smoking, drinking alcohol, and substance abuse are found in LGBTQ youths compared with their heterosexual peers. Gay, bisexual, and transgender men were found to smoke tobacco more than heterosexual men, and lesbian women smoked almost more than their peers.[17] Increased personal stress has been associated with increased use of tobacco, alcohol and drug use. This stress has also been found to affect the patient's perceived body image, activity levels, and eating patterns.[5] There are also increased rates of eating disorders, anxiety, depression, and suicidal thoughts among LGBTQ youths.[9] Transgender patients may become disenfranchised and experience intermittent employment and subsequently intermittent health insurance. Some transgender patients will seek alternatives to conventional medical care, including silicone injections (also known as "pumping") to create changes in body contour.[5] These interventions are typically not provided by health care professionals and are therefore unregulated, which can increase health risks for the patient.

SPECIFIC HEALTH SCREENINGS

The GLMA has compiled a list of the top 10 health issues for gay, lesbian, or transgender individuals to consider when going to see a provider. These health issues should be considered when the provider is taking a medical history (Box 10-1).

A number of these health issues are related to psychosocial or behavioral health and may possibly be associated with stigma, negative societal attitudes, and internalized homophobia (social learning to reject one's basic personal preferences).[15]

A thorough mental health assessment should therefore be a part of the comprehensive medical assessment. This may not take place on the first encounter but should be a part of the continuity of care within the primary care setting.

Tobacco use, alcohol consumption, and drug use are considerably greater in the LGBTQ community. Smoking rates in the LGBTQ population reach up to 50%, which is significantly higher than in the rest of the population. This behavior increases the risk of cardiovascular disease, lung disorders such as chronic obstructive pulmonary disease (COPD), and lung cancer. LGBTQ patients are more likely to engage in drug use and continue its use later in life. The incidence of substance abuse is two to three times greater in the LGBTQ community compared with the general population. The use of drugs and/or consumption of alcohol can impair decision-making and increase the risky behaviors in which the patient engages.[16,17]

Depression occurs at higher rates in the LGBTQ population. This may be partly because of the increased rates of harassment and physical violence encountered or lack of social support for

BOX 10-1

Top 10 Issues for LGBTQ Patients to Discuss with Health Care Providers

GAY
- Disclose to your health care provider
- HIV/AIDS, safer sex
- Hepatitis screening and immunization
- Diet and exercise
- Substance use, alcohol use
- Depression and anxiety
- Sexually transmitted infection
- Cancer screening for prostate, testicular, and colon cancers
- Tobacco
- Human papillomavirus (HPV) and anal papilloma

LESBIAN
- Breast cancer screening
- Depression and anxiety
- Cardiovascular health
- Gynecologic cancer screening
- Diet and exercise
- Tobacco use
- Alcohol use
- Substance use
- Intimate partner violence
- Sexual health

BISEXUAL
- Disclose to your health care provider
- HIV/AIDS, safer sex
- Hepatitis screening and immunization
- Diet and exercise
- Substance use, alcohol use
- Depression and anxiety
- Sexually transmitted infections
- Cancer screening for colon, prostate, and testicular cancers, or breast and cervical cancers
- Tobacco
- HPV

TRANSGENDER
- Access to health care
- Health history
- Hormones
- Cardiovascular health
- Cancer screening
- Sexually transmitted infections and safer sex
- Alcohol and tobacco use
- Depression and anxiety
- Injectable silicone
- Diet and exercise

Data from Gay and Lesbian Medical Association (GLMA): *Top ten issues to discuss with your healthcare provider,* 2012. Available at www.glma.org/index.cfm?fuseaction=Page.viewPage&pageId=947&grandparentID=534&parentID=938. Accessed September 12, 2014.

those who have experienced rejection by their family. Gay teenagers are much more likely to have considered or attempted suicide than their heterosexual counterparts.[8] Providers should screen for depression and ask about suicidal ideation. Patients may experience a personal crisis related to sexual orientation. In adolescent males, this has been associated with almost one third of the suicide attempts.[10]

Sexual harassment has also been associated with increased rates of attempted suicide. There is a correlation among depression, higher-risk sexual contact, and attempted suicide with patients who are victims of sexual assault. Sexual violence directed toward LGBTQ individuals may be a bias or hate-based crime.

Intimate partner violence (IPV) is non-discriminatory and touches the lives of the rich and the poor; men and women; the well-educated and the illiterate; and heterosexual, homosexual and bisexual individuals. The actual rates of IPV and sexual violence appear to be similar in same-sex couples as in the population overall; however, individuals involved in a same-sex relationship are less likely to be screened by health care providers.[10,18] LGBTQ patients in abusive relationships may be fearful of being exposed or "outed" and therefore not report the violence they are experiencing.

LGBTQ patients may also be victims of violence or harassment. Almost one third of LGBTQ adults reported being physical threatened or attacked in the past because of their sexual orientation or gender identity.[13] This is especially true for transgender patients who appear to be gender variant, with just over three quarters of transgender survey participants noting harassment and over one third experiencing sexual assault.[19] Patients who have experienced repeated violence may also experience post-traumatic stress disorder (PTSD).[5]

Vaccinations are often not up-to-date. Patients need to be aware of age-appropriate vaccination recommendations, such as diphtheria and tetanus boosters, as well as vaccinations that are related to individual health risks, such as hepatitis. Some LGBTQ patients mistakenly believe that human papillomavirus (HPV) is not a concern in same-sex physical relationships.

Both hepatitis A and hepatitis B are vaccine preventable. The vaccine should be offered to patients who are engaging in sexual contact, regardless of the patient's sexual orientation. The provider should ask the patient about the type of sexual activity (oral, vaginal, rectal) to ascertain the individual's risk of exposure. Hepatitis A is transmitted via a fecal-oral route, whereas hepatitis B is transmitted via body fluids (blood, semen),

Cancer Screening

Appropriate cancer screenings should be offered to all patients, regardless of sexual orientation or sexual behaviors. Some patients will have more risk factors for certain cancer types. Patients with a history of HPV exposure have a higher risk of cervical, anal, penile, and certain oral cancers.[14] Screening for breast and gynecologic cancers in lesbian patients is important because they may have higher risks for these cancers. Risk for breast, endometrial, and ovarian cancers is increased when a woman has never been pregnant. Delays in diagnosis because of avoidance of health care providers or missed opportunities for screening can have a pronounced negative impact on disease outcome.[14]

Human Papillomavirus

Patients with HPV exposure have increased risks for cervical, oral, anal, and penile cancers. Vaccination for HPV is recommended for both boys and girls at age 11 or 12. The vaccines are approved for use in females aged 9 to 26 and males aged 9 to 21 and up to age 26 for MSM or those with compromised immune systems. Screening for HPV can help to identify patients at higher risk.

Patients may have had sexual partners of both genders during their lifetime. Some patients mistakenly believe that their personal risk of sexually transmitted diseases, including HPV, is lower because they are in same-sex relationships. HPV can be transmitted between any two individuals, regardless of gender or sexual orientation. It can also be transmitted by sharing sex toys. Teaching patients to properly clean sex toys between use or between partners can help to decrease disease transmission in all patient populations.

Human Immunodeficiency Virus

The fastest growing populations of those newly diagnosed with HIV include young adults, adolescents, and MSM. Gay and bisexual MSM comprise the group that is most affected by HIV, accounting for 78% of newly diagnosed cases of HIV in men in 2010. The rates of new HIV infection are increasing in MSM and decreasing in females. Less than half of those diagnosed with HIV are engaged in care.[20] HIV screening is recommended for all pregnant women and patients aged 15 to 65 years old. Patients younger than 15 or older than 65 who engage in high-risk behavior should also be screened.[21]

ISSUES WITH HEALTH SCREENING

Creating a positive, therapeutic relationship with your patient can help alleviate some of the concerns the patient has regarding trusting the health care provider. Patients may be unaware of screening tests that are needed. Some lesbian patients are unaware that the risk for sexually transmitted disease exists with the use of sex toys if they are not properly cleaned after use. They consider the risk to be associated with heterosexual interactions.

SEXUAL REASSIGNMENT INTERVENTION

The World Professional Association for Transgender Health publishes Standards of Care in 10 languages. It is a valuable resource for care of patients, currently in its seventh edition.[22]

Transgender patients identify or express themselves as the opposite of their biologic birth gender. Hormonal therapy and surgical intervention may be sought by some of these patients. Many transgender patients do not have surgery. Support of the patient and the patient's evolving medical needs is a necessary component of this process.

Before the initiation of any therapy or intervention, the patient should be made aware of the options available as well as the likelihood of health care insurance covering the expenses. There are stages to transition. A social transition may help to decrease the disconnect or dysphoria patients feel between their gender appearance and their gender identity. Social transition can be more easily achieved before puberty.

Mental health professionals can assist in the determination that the patient is ready to transition before the initiation of hormonal treatments, regardless of the patient's age. Consideration of the ramifications of transitioning need to be explored, and the patient can be assisted in developing strategies for coping with potential problem areas, especially if family or social supports are not strong.

Sexual reassignment is a long process involving hormonal therapy and multiple surgical procedures. Hormonal blockers can be used to prevent or minimize the development of secondary sexual characteristics. Not all patients have self-identified by the onset of adolescence, and not all families are supportive of a child's assertion that the child is transgender. A male child's ongoing declaration that "I am a girl" is very different from a young boy who occasionally engages in play traditionally considered female (e.g., playing with dolls, dressing up in "girly" clothes, wearing make-up). Cross-sex hormones are given to begin development of the identified gender's secondary sexual characteristics. Regardless of the age at which hormonal therapy begins, hormonal levels need to be monitored regularly by a provider who is familiar with the necessary hormonal regimens. Long-term use of cross-sex hormones, especially those started during or before adolescence, will make the possibility of biologic children unlikely. Some patients are able to have a biologic child, which requires cessation of the cross-sex hormones. These patients often start hormonal therapy well after the onset of puberty.

Medical risks for hormonal therapy need to be considered. Feminizing hormonal therapy has an increased risk of thrombus formation, cardiovascular events, and impaired lipid metabolism. Masculinizing hormone therapy has an increased risk of polycythemia, weight gain, and mania or hypomania in patients with comorbid or occult psychiatric disorders. Hormonal therapy needs to be tailored for the patient based on need and potential risks, considering both personal and family medical history.

By the time a patient is scheduling a transitional surgical procedure, the patient should be quite ready, both emotionally and physically. The patient has undergone a social transition and hormonal therapy and is now ready for the next phase of transition. General preoperative care is the same as for any patient undergoing a planned surgical intervention. Evaluation is made by a provider who will not be involved in the surgical procedure that the patient is indeed physically fit for the stress of surgery, based on history, physical examination, and diagnostic test results.

Postoperative care in the first few days after surgery is no different from other postoperative care. The patient is monitored for complications of the surgical intervention such as signs of infection, as well as assessing for adequate pain control. The more extensive the surgical intervention, the longer the recovery will take. Some patients undergo multiple surgical procedures. Patients who have transformative surgery will also have body image alterations. These physical changes are better aligned with the gender identity of the individual.

It is important for both the patient and caregiver to understand what surgical procedures have occurred. Male-to-female transitions often leave the female patient with an intact prostate gland. Appropriate screening for prostate cancer must still occur in these patients. Female-to-male transitions continue to involve risk for breast cancer, and patients may have risk for cervical or ovarian cancer if those organs remain intact.

Referrals to specialists, including surgeons, may occur during the physical transition process for a transgender patient. Patients may benefit from a referral to a mental health provider or social worker to help in managing the stress associated with specific adjustment periods. Patients should never be referred to a mental health provider to "fix" their sexual orientation or gender identity.

LIFE SPAN CONSIDERATIONS

Adolescence can be a difficult time for any person as the physical and emotional development of the person changes the status quo. The addition of questions about one's gender identity or sexual orientation can add significantly to the stresses of adolescence. Some adolescents may experiment sexually, engaging in risky practices, as they struggle to determine their own sexual orientation. Adolescents may experience pressure to fit in with their peers. LGBTQ teenagers may not have the support of their peer group, or even their close friends from childhood, as they begin to express their sexual orientation. Some will actually face rejection by friends and/or family members. The individual may be the victim of bullying, threats, or physical violence.[23]

LGBTQ seniors face many of the same challenges as they age. In addition, they may be concerned about lack of acceptance, discrimination, or stigma. These seniors are less likely to have children or grandchildren. LGBTQ seniors who live in residential facilities, such as long-term care or assisted living facilities, may experience harassment from other residents who may not be comfortable with LGBTQ people. For partners who are unmarried, there may be loss of financial stability for the surviving partner after death, because many pension plans, including

Social Security, do not continue payments to the surviving, but unmarried, partner.[23]

PATIENT EDUCATION AND HEALTH PROMOTION

Health education and screenings should be relevant to the individual's actual needs. This is true for all patients, not only LGBTQ patients. Age-appropriate screenings are the appropriate starting point for all patients. Care should include mitigation of risks based on lifestyle behaviors, such as high-risk sexual practices or avoidance of health care. Patients should be encouraged to have screenings that they may have thought were unnecessary, such as Pap tests or screening for sexually transmitted diseases in lesbian patients or prostate screening in an MTF transgender patient.

Provider and support staff education is also necessary to ensure that patients are getting the appropriate health care and health screenings necessary.

CHAPTER 11

PREGNANCY AND PRENATAL CARE

Emma Clark

Pregnancy, beginning at conception, moving through embryologic and fetal development to parturition, is a period of dynamic change for both mother and baby.[1] The U.S. Public Health Service (USPHS) and the World Health Organization (WHO) have identified pregnancy as a time to identify and minimize health risks, to promote health, and to provide medical follow-up with psychosocial support for a woman and her family.[2,3]

At the turn of the 20th century, high rates of infant and maternal mortality were associated with poor nutrition, inadequate sanitation, limited access to care, and low education levels. In response to these concerns, the provision of prenatal care moved from the hand of lay midwives to nurse midwives and physicians,[4] and delivery moved out of the home and into the more clinical but sometimes more hazardous hospital setting. In the decades that followed, medical advancements brought about a decline in infant and maternal mortality rates, and, for the first time, maternal and fetal health and well-being could be closely observed many months before delivery.

By the 1980s, a plethora of agencies offered a variety of prenatal services; although they differed in scope, they shared the same goal of improving prenatal outcomes.[4] In 1985, the Institute of Medicine (IOM) acknowledged the relationship between low birth weight and infant mortality.[5] Four years later, the USPHS released a landmark report defining the number of visits and the content of each visit, and it was recommended that women be offered preconception counseling before pregnancy.[2] In the 1990s, additional social programs were created, increasing services to address health care disparities for women of lower socioeconomic status.[4] Broad social goals from the *Healthy People* initiatives have provided continued maternal and child health surveillance. *Healthy People 2020* has retained many of the maternal-child care objectives of *Healthy People 2010*, continuing to emphasize a reduction in infant and maternal mortality, early and adequate prenatal care for all pregnant women, and the reduction of both preterm births and infants of low and very low birth weight.[6]

In recent years, some of the emphasis on the role of prenatal care in improving fetal and maternal outcomes has shifted to the role that preconception and interconception care can play. This has occurred at a time when women around the world are increasingly facing chronic health conditions during their childbearing years and has been driven by a slowing of progress in improvement of pregnancy outcomes, particularly the key indicators of low birth weight, premature birth, and infant mortality, and an improvement in understanding of the way that chronic diseases contribute to these.[7] Although a woman's health in and of itself should be the primary goal of prepregnancy health care, there is little doubt that improving her prepregnancy health has a great deal of potential to improve her reproductive health. In general, preconception care that focuses on reducing unintended pregnancies, reducing risky behavior (drinking, smoking), and controlling chronic conditions is likely to have the greatest impact on pregnancy outcomes.[8] However, awareness of need for this type of care remains low, and there are many opportunities to improve preconception care and access.

GOALS OF PRENATAL CARE

Ultimately, the goal of prenatal care is to provide primary preventive care to pregnant women and identify the small but critical subgroup of women who will have pregnancy-related complications that affect fetal or maternal health.[9] A major goal of prenatal care is to reduce the number of premature and low-birth-weight infants. Research results have not been uniform; some studies show that prenatal care reduces premature delivery,[9,10] whereas others have not shown a positive relationship between prenatal care and the number of preterm deliveries.[11,12] The Central Intelligence Agency's *World Factbook* reports that the United States ranks 55th in infant mortality in the world (6.17 of every 1000 live births), behind countries often perceived as "less developed," including Cuba, Greece, Hungary, and Slovenia.[13] It is believed that preterm births and low-birth-weight deliveries account for approximately 35% of these deaths.[14]

Another primary goal of prenatal care has been to reduce maternal mortality. Whereas maternal death remains relatively rare in the United States (12.7 per 100,000 live births),[15] disparities exist across ethnic and economic groups, and the United States continues to lag behind other developed countries here as well. The maternal mortality rate for non-Hispanic black women is almost three times the rate (28.4 versus 10.5 per 100,000) for non-Hispanic white women.[15] Evidence does not support a greater prevalence of preeclampsia or eclampsia, presence of placenta previa or abruption, and postpartum hemorrhage between black and white women, so it has been hypothesized that the severity of maternal conditions, comorbidities, or the quality or timing of prenatal care may explain the disparity.[16]

During the past 100 years, prenatal outcomes have improved significantly in the United States, but much work remains. It has been suggested that there is a need to determine which components of care are most beneficial for a targeted outcome and to clearly evaluate current practices through evidence-based research to establish a future course for prenatal care.[17]

USE OF PRENATAL CARE

Use of prenatal care can be broken down into two concepts: motivation to use services and facilitation of service providers in helping women access prenatal care.[18] Facilitation of access can improve motivation and ultimately improve use of prenatal care, resulting in the improved maternal and fetal outcomes associated with prenatal care use. This is especially critical given that women with the lowest motivation to seek care are highly correlated with those at risk for poor outcomes, such as those with unplanned pregnancies. Facilitation of access by clinics and providers includes making facilities physically accessible (e.g., located on bus routes, no parking fees), financially accessible (e.g., acceptance of a variety of payment options, low out-of-pocket costs for care), culturally accessible (e.g., immigration status blind, multiple languages spoken), temporally accessible (e.g., evening appointments, reasonable wait times, initial appointments soon after first contact), and practically accessible (e.g., safe play areas for children).

DELIVERY OF PRENATAL CARE

In the United States, a number of different organizations have published recommendations for the delivery of prenatal care, although it has received little attention or updating in recent years. Perhaps the most traditional format for care begins with an initial visit at 8 to 10 weeks or earlier if patient is at risk, every 4 weeks until 28 weeks, every 2 to 3 weeks until 36 weeks, and weekly visits until delivery, totaling 13 visits.[1,19] The USPHS diverged from this recommendation in its outdated but unfortunately not updated 1989 report, suggesting that nine visits are adequate, omitting weeks 20 and 28 in an uncomplicated pregnancy. The USPHS expert panel also recommended bimonthly instead of weekly appointments beginning at 36 weeks until delivery.[2] Internationally, the prenatal picture is more complicated. Infrastructure is poor in many undeveloped nations, and it is not feasible to support the same prenatal care rendered in developed nations. WHO found that four goal-directed prenatal visits are just as effective as more frequent visits in optimizing pregnancy outcomes.[3,20]

In an effort to improve access to and quality of prenatal care, an innovative model called CenteringPregnancy was initiated in 1993. In CenteringPregnancy, a woman attends 10 2-hour group sessions with the same cohort, assuming responsibility for self-monitoring of blood pressure, weight, and fundal height and participating in group discussion and education.[21] This method has been shown to increase the satisfaction with and use of prenatal care, improve perinatal knowledge, decrease preterm birth rates, and promote higher breastfeeding initiation rates.[21] Providers are also more satisfied. It is important to note that when compared with standard prenatal care, CenteringPregnancy is notable for its ability to recruit and retain a demographic of women who have historically had the poorest pregnancy and birth outcomes and to improve not only outcomes but overall mental health and well-being of participants.[22]

CONTENT OF PRENATAL VISIT

Standard components of an initial prenatal visit are a complete history, a comprehensive physical examination including ensuring that clinical information correlates to dating of the pregnancy, baseline laboratory and diagnostic tests, and educational and anticipatory guidance about the expected pregnancy course. Subsequent visits are to track progress of the pregnancy and to assess gestational milestones, to follow up on tests, and to provide ongoing education and support both about the pregnancy and in preparation for the postpartum period and parenthood. Table 11-1 details the content and timing of prenatal care.

Diagnosis of Pregnancy

The diagnosis of pregnancy is the gateway to initiation of prenatal care. For the diagnosis of pregnancy to be made, either a urine or serum pregnancy test or ultrasound study may be

TABLE 11-1 Content and Timing of Routine Prenatal Care

Prenatal Care	First Trimester (6-12 wk)	Second Trimester (13-27 wk)	Third Trimester (28-39 wk)	Post Dates (40-42 wk)
HISTORY				
Menstrual, establish gestational age	X			
Obstetric (complications)	X			
Medical and surgical	X			
Medications and immunizations (influenza, tetanus, and diphtheria)	X	X	X	X
Family and genetics	X			
Social (habits, abuse, stress, work)	X			
PHYSICAL EXAMINATION				
Periodontal	X			
Blood pressure	X	X	X	X
Weight, body mass index	X	X	X	X
Pelvic	X			
Fundal height	X*	X	X	X
Fetal heart tone, position	X*	X	X	X

TABLE 11-1 **Content and Timing of Routine Prenatal Care—cont'd**

Prenatal Care	First Trimester (6-12 wk)	Second Trimester (13-27 wk)	Third Trimester (28-39 wk)	Post Dates (40-42 wk)
LABORATORY AND DIAGNOSTIC TESTS				
Pregnancy test	X			
Ultrasound examination	X*	X*	X*	X*
Blood type, Rh	X			
Antibody screen	X		X*	
Hemoglobin and hematocrit	X		X*	
Glucose tolerance test			X	
Urine	X			
Urine culture	X			
Pap smear	X*			
Chlamydia and gonorrhea, if indicated	X		X*	
RPR, VDRL (syphilis screen)	X		X*	
Hepatitis B surface antigen	X			
HIV infection	X†			
Herpes simplex	X			
Rubella	X			
Varicella	X			
Tuberculosis	X*			
Group B *Streptococcus*			X	
Fetal aneuploidy screen		X‡		
Neural tube defect screen		X‡		
Cystic fibrosis screen	X†			
COUNSELING, EDUCATION, AND SCREENING				
Physical and emotional changes, self-care	X	X	X	X
Preterm labor, blood pressure precautions	X	X	X	X
Fetal movement		X*	X	X
Nutrition and exercise	X	X	X	X
Tobacco, alcohol, drug use	X	X	X	X
Safety (seat belt, avoid teratogens)	X	X	X	X
Domestic violence	X	X	X	X
Depression, social	X	X	X	X
Breastfeeding	X	X	X	X
Sexuality	X	X	X	X
Family planning			X	X
Labor preparation			X	X

*If indicated.
†Offer or counsel.
‡Offer or counsel early in trimester.
HIV, human immunodeficiency virus; RPR, rapid plasma reagin; VDRL, Venereal Disease Research Laboratory.
Data from Cunningham FG, Leveno KJ, Bloom SL, et al: *Williams obstetrics,* ed 23, New York, 2009, McGraw-Hill; Callahan TL, Caughey AB: *Obstetrics and gynecology,* ed 5, Philadelphia, 2009, Lippincott Williams & Wilkins/Wolters Kluwer Health; U.S. Public Health Service: *Caring for our future: the content of prenatal care,* Washington, DC, 1989, U.S. Government Printing Office; American College of Obstetricians and Gynecologists (ACOG), American Association of Pediatrics: *Guidelines for perinatal care,* ed 6, Washington, DC, 2009, ACOG; U.S. Department of Veterans Affairs and Department of Defense: *VA/DoD clinical practice guideline: management of pregnancy,* Washington, DC, 2009, available at www.healthquality.va.gov/up/mpg_v2_1_sumc.pdf; and U.S. Department of Health and Human Services, Centers for Disease Control and Prevention: Sexually transmitted diseases treatment guidelines, 2010, *MMWR Recomm Rep* 59(RR-12):1-110, 2010, available at www.cdc.gov/std/treatment/2010/STD-Treatment-2010-RR5912.pdf.

used. Serum pregnancy tests can detect human chorionic gonadotropin (β-hCG) levels as low as 1.0 mIU/mL as early as 8 to 9 days after ovulation and before the onset of menses. Urine pregnancy tests are also highly accurate but are not as sensitive as serum tests, and very few can detect β-hCG levels lower than 12.5 mIU/mL, making them subject to a higher false-negative rate.[1] In experienced hands, a pelvic ultrasound study (ideally with a vaginal probe) can detect a pregnancy as early as 4 to 5 weeks of gestation, with β-hCG levels as low as 1500 to 2000 mIU/mL.[1,23]

Assumptions should not be made about a woman's desire for or plans for pregnancy. A woman with an unplanned pregnancy should be offered unbiased, nonjudgmental, direct information regarding her reproductive options, tailored to her stage of gestation at diagnosis of pregnancy.[24] These include medical or surgical elective termination of pregnancy or continuation of pregnancy with plans to either keep the baby or place it up for adoption. Appropriate referrals should be given as necessary.

Estimated Date of Delivery

An accurate menstrual history assists in determining the estimated due (delivery) date (EDD), which facilitates clinical decision-making, particularly determining viability or post dates.[23] In addition, trimester of first visit is a standard, if incomplete, clinical quality indicator of access to prenatal care and requires accurate calculation of pregnancy dates.[17] An EDC is calculated based on the first day of the last normal menstrual period (LNMP). A traditional way to calculate the EDD is called the Nägele's rule, which is done by subtracting 3 months and adding 7 days to the LNMP. If the LNMP is unsure or unknown, an ultrasound study may be used to determine EDC. As a last resort, clinical data such as fundal height can be used to provide a rough estimate of pregnancy dating. As a word of caution, ultrasound dating becomes increasingly less accurate as the pregnancy advances and the fetus becomes susceptible to genetic and environmental influences.[1,23]

Gravidity and Parity

Gravidity and *parity* are terms used to describe a woman's obstetric history. *Gravidity* describes the total number of pregnancies (including the current one) that a woman has experienced in her lifetime. *Parity* is the total number of pregnancies that have progressed beyond 20 gestational weeks in a woman's lifetime. Parity is about the uterus being empty; it is not about the number of babies born (i.e., in the situation of multifetal deliveries [twins, triplets], parity is still a single event).

Gravidity and parity are often strung together as a form of obstetric shorthand to communicate a woman's obstetric history. Gravidity, G, is usually listed first, followed by a series of four numbers (TPAL) to communicate what happened during each pregnancy: T, the number of term (>37 completed gestational weeks) deliveries; P, the number of preterm (20 to $36\frac{6}{7}$ completed gestational weeks) deliveries; A, abortion (elective or spontaneous delivery before 20 completed gestational weeks); and L, living children.[1,23]

As an example, a woman arrives for prenatal care and reports that she has had four previous pregnancies: one delivery at 38 weeks (child is living), one miscarriage at 9 weeks, one elective termination at 10 weeks, and a delivery of twins at 36 weeks (both living). Her G/TPAL is G5 and P:1123 (one delivery at 38 weeks, one preterm delivery, two abortions, and three living children).

Health History

In addition to the menstrual and obstetric history, thorough medical, surgical, family, and social histories are vital to prenatal care.[25] A medication history identifies therapies that should be changed to reduce risk of teratogenicity.[26] All women should be screened for use of tobacco, alcohol, and illicit substances (see Chapters 16 and 249). Studies indicate that the rate of domestic violence may increase during pregnancy; a woman's current safety and abuse history should be evaluated at her initial visit, at least once per trimester, and as indicated by behavioral and physical signs throughout pregnancy, using direct, specific questions about abuse (see Chapter 16).[26] Weight gain goals for pregnancy should be set at the initial visit based on prepregnancy body mass index (BMI); dietary and exercise patterns should be reviewed regularly, especially if excessive or insufficient weight gain is noted.[27] An awareness of preexisting physical and mental health conditions, such as depression, helps tailor management during the prenatal and postpartum period (see Chapter 248 for depression screening). If there is a personal or family history of genetic disease, the pregnant woman can be offered individual counseling and testing (Table 11-2).[1,23,26] With recognized safety of vaginal birth after cesarean

TABLE 11-2 Considerations for Genetic Counseling or Testing

Chromosomal abnormalities	Trisomy 21 Trisomy 18 Trisomy 13
Sex chromosomal abnormalities	Turner syndrome Klinefelter syndrome
Autosomal dominant disease	Achondroplasia Polycystic kidney disease Huntington chorea Marfan syndrome Neurofibromatosis types 1 and 2
Autosomal recessive disease	Cystic fibrosis Sickle cell disease Tay-Sachs disease Thalassemia syndrome
X-linked disease	Duchenne and Becker muscular dystrophy Hemophilia A and B Fragile X syndrome
Congenital anomalies	Neural tube defect (spina bifida, anencephaly) Cardiac defects Potter syndrome
Other conditions	Advanced maternal or paternal age Abnormal genetic screening, ultrasound abnormalities Consanguinity Stillbirth or neonatal death Mental retardation Ambiguous genitalia, dysmorphic disease

Data from Cunningham FG, Leveno KJ, Bloom SL et al: *Williams obstetrics,* ed 23, New York, 2009, McGraw-Hill; Callahan TL, Caughey AB: *Obstetrics and gynecology,* ed 5, Philadelphia, 2009, Lippincott Williams & Wilkins/Wolters Kluwer Health; and Fortner KB, Szymanski LM, Fox H, et al: *The Johns Hopkins manual of gynecology and obstetrics,* ed 3, Philadelphia, 2009, Lippincott Williams & Wilkins/Wolters Kluwer Health.

section, a woman with a previous cesarean section should be counseled on vaginal as well as repeated cesarean delivery options, depending on the indications for previous cesarean sections, type of uterine incision, coexisting medical conditions, and plans for future pregnancies.[28]

Oral health should also be assessed, including presence of swollen or bleeding gums or other mouth problems and date of last dental visit.[29] Periodontal infection has been linked in some studies to preterm birth, although dental treatment has not been shown to improve outcomes. Pregnancy does, however, represent an important time to initiate and maintain good oral health practices. Any woman who has oral health problems or has not had a dental examination in more than 6 months should be encouraged to schedule a visit and should receive reassurance that diagnosis and treatment of dental conditions, including radiographs with shielding of abdomen and use of local anesthesia (lidocaine with or without epinephrine), are safe.[29]

A vaccination history can help determine if any immunizations will be required during pregnancy. Common vaccinations not recommended during pregnancy include measles, mumps, and rubella (MMR), varicella, herpes zoster, live attenuated influenza, and human papillomavirus (HPV).[30] The inactivated influenza vaccine is not only safe but strongly recommended to receive at any point in pregnancy.[31] The tetanus, diphtheria, and acellular pertussis (Tdap) vaccine is similarly safe, and pregnant women should receive a Tdap vaccine in every pregnancy, optimally between 27 and 36 weeks' gestation.[32] Family members and others who will have close contact with the newborn should also be counseled to receive the flu vaccine annually and be up to date on their Tdap vaccine.[30] Women who are at risk for hepatitis B (have had more than one sex partner during the previous 6 months, have been evaluated or treated for a sexually transmitted infection [STI], have a history of recent or current injection drug use, or have a sex partner with hepatitis B) should receive the hepatitis B vaccine.[30] If a pregnant woman has been exposed to varicella, varicella-zoster immune globulin is recommended. For additional information on administration schedules for other vaccinations, see Chapter 17.

Nutrition and Weight Gain in Pregnancy

Nutritional requirements during pregnancy range from 1800 to 2400 kcal/day, and daily protein intake increases to 60 to 75 g/day,[23,33] depending on the physical stature and exercise habits of an individual woman. Most women overestimate the number of additional calories. Dietary recommendation must be personalized to the woman's age, her prepregnant BMI, and her rate of weight gain.[33] Women are encouraged to eat a variety of foods to ensure adequate intake of folic acid, vitamin B_{12}, iron, calcium, and vitamin D.[33]

Women with inadequate weight gain should be evaluated for food security and, as necessary, referred to food assistance programs (such as the Special Supplemental Nutrition Program for Women, Infants, and Children [WIC]), many of which target pregnant women. Thyroid-stimulating hormone (TSH) levels, toxicology, serum albumin, and hepatitis screening should be considered as clinically indicated, as well as ultrasound to evaluate for intrauterine growth restrictrion.[24] Poor maternal weight gain is associated with fetal undernutrition, which affects fetal survival and poor health outcomes later in life.[33]

On the flip side, excessive weight gain in pregnancy and being overweight or obese before the start of pregnancy are also associated with a number of health problems and poor outcomes, including miscarriage, preeclampsia, gestational diabetes mellitus (GDM), perinatal depression, large-for-gestational age fetus, further excess weight gain, risk of preterm birth, stillbirth, birth injury, neural tube defects, postpartum hemorrhage, delayed lactogenesis, and need for labor induction and operative birth.[24,34] In addition, pregnancy can worsen preexisting diabetes and hypertension (HTN), and obesity can complicate surgical interventions such as cesarean section.[34] Because of the significant risks associated with obesity in pregnancy, the IOM revised its recommendations for weight gain in pregnancy (Table 11-3). Overweight and obese women should undergo a 1-hour oral glucose tolerance test (OGTT) at their first visit and a repeat OGTT at 24 to 28 weeks, a urine dipstick at every visit for glucose and protein related to the increased risk of GDM and preeclampsia, and monitoring of fetal growth and should receive careful nutritional counseling and support.[24]

TABLE 11-3 Recommendations for Total and Rate of Weight Gain During Pregnancy, by Prepregnancy Body Mass Index (BMI)

Prepregnancy BMI	BMI* (kg/m²)	Total Weight Gain Range (lb)	Rates of Gain† in Second and Third Trimesters (mean range in lb/wk)
Underweight	<18.5	28-40	1 (1-1.3)
Normal weight	18.5-24.9	25-35	1 (0.8-1)
Overweight	25.0-29.9	15-25	0.6 (0.5-0.7)
Obese (includes all classes)	≥30.0	11-20	0.5 (0.4-0.6)

*Based on the World Health Organization cutoff points. To calculate body mass index (BMI), go to www.nhlbisupport.com/bmi/.

†Calculations assume a 0.5- to 2-kg (1.1- to 4.4-lb) weight gain in the first trimester.

From Rasmussen KM, Yaktine AL, editors; Committee to Reexamine IOM Pregnancy Weight Guidelines; Institute of Medicine; National Research Council: *Weight gain during pregnancy: reexamining the guidelines*, Washington, DC, 2009, National Academies Press.

Women who have undergone malabsorptive or restrictive gastric bypass surgeries, such as Roux-en-Y and laparoscopic gastric banding, could experience micronutrient deficiencies, and close monitoring and supplementation with micronutrients may be indicated. Band adjustment may be necessary if decreased oral intake negatively affects the pregnancy.

Iron deficiency anemia (IDA) is very common in pregnancy—approximately 20% of pregnant women are affected in industrialized countries. IDA increases risks of preterm labor, low birth weight, and infant mortality.[33] It is usually detected through routine complete blood count (CBC) testing at the initial visit and repeat testing early in the third trimester, although a woman may also be symptomatic with fatigue, dizziness, pica (eating of nonfood items such as starch or clay or ice chewing), dyspnea, or tachycardia or palpitations, depending on severity and maternal tolerance.[24] Iron replacement therapy with 60 to 120 mg of elemental iron daily is indicated if hemoglobin is less than 11 g/dL, along with an increase in iron-rich food intake.

Activity in Pregnancy

According to the *2008 Physical Activity Guidelines for Americans,* moderate-intensity activity by healthy women during pregnancy does not increase risk of low birth weight, preterm delivery, or early pregnancy loss.[35] Vigorous-intensity physical activity (e.g., running), particularly for women who were already engaged in these activities before pregnancy, is also not associated with problems, although helping these women transition to more moderate physical activity may be more sustainable throughout pregnancy.[36] Physical activity for healthy pregnant women should be encouraged for 30 minutes or more, broken up into 10-minute chunks as necessary, most days of the week, as should "active living" (walking, gardening, household activities).[36] Those beginning physical activity for the first time during pregnancy should be encouraged to start slowly and gradually increase over time, with activities such as swimming. Although it is not conclusive, some research indicates that physical activity during pregnancy can reduce the risk of preeclampsia, GDM, and excessive gestational weight gain and may decrease labor length.[33,35-37]

The American College of Obstetricians and Gynecologists (ACOG) advises a clinical evaluation before initiation of an exercise regimen and provides guidelines for absolute and relative contraindications to aerobic exercise in pregnancy. Certain activities (scuba diving; activities that increase the risk for trauma, such as mountain climbing) should be avoided during pregnancy. Women should be instructed to stop exercising if they experience preterm labor signs (contractions, bleeding, leakage of amniotic fluid), chest or head pain, calf pain, or decreased fetal movement. Women should also be reminded that they need to take into account their shifting center of gravity, the additional effort that the extra weight of pregnancy requires, and the effect of pregnancy hormones on relaxing all ligaments, especially in later pregnancy.[38]

Sexual activity in pregnancy is considered safe. Anticipatory guidance should be offered to women about physical changes and sexual positions that may influence sexual comfort during pregnancy. Women at risk for preterm labor, placenta previa, or recurrent pregnancy loss may be advised to avoid sexual activity.[1]

Physical Examination and Laboratory and Diagnostic Tests

The purpose of the physical examination and laboratory and diagnostic tests is to establish baselines, to detect abnormalities, and to monitor underlying chronic conditions.[25] The pelvic examination should evaluate the cervix and uterus, and the remainder of the physical examination (heart, lungs, thyroid, abdomen) is focused on identification of any previously unrecognized disorders.[23] Although no randomized controlled trials have been conducted to determine efficacy or timing of screening laboratory tests or tests for at-risk populations, they have become a routine part of pregnancy care.[19]

Whereas ultrasound imaging has a place in obstetric care, commercial ultrasound examinations used for the specific purpose of imaging to "see the baby," to preserve keepsakes, or to determine the sex of the unborn child are increasing in popularity. The American Institute of Ultrasound in Medicine and ACOG advise that fetal ultrasound examinations be conducted only by trained professionals and be based on medical necessity.[1,19]

Counseling and Education

Counseling and education are fundamental components of prenatal care. Counseling and education should be individualized and timely and should empower the woman and her family to make healthy decisions.[19] Historically, the primary focus of education and counseling in pregnancy has been the prenatal course and preparation for labor and delivery. However, this focus misses critical opportunities to prepare a woman for the postpartum period and motherhood, including breastfeeding education and postpartum birth control options. There is increasing evidence that prenatal education and support for breastfeeding by clinicians increases breastfeeding rates.[39] The prevalence of postpartum contraceptive use is highest when both prenatal and postpartum counseling is done.[40]

COMMON PROBLEMS IN PREGNANCY

Infections

Some infections may occur more frequently or pose increased risk during pregnancy. See Table 11-4 for an overview of the important infections in pregnancy.[1,23,25,41]

Urinary Tract Infections. Pregnant women are at increased risk for urinary tract infections (UTIs), which are the most common bacterial infection in pregnancy[1,23] and are implicated in premature deliveries and low birth weight. UTIs are also much more likely to progress to pyelonephritis in pregnant women. Asymptomatic bacteriuria occurs in 8% of pregnant women, but if it is identified and treated early, the risk of pyelonephritis can be reduced by 40%, thus reducing premature births twofold.[42] Pregnant women should have a urine culture (ideally including sensitivity of any identified bacteria to various antibiotics) at 12 to 16 weeks' gestation, or at the first prenatal visit if later, to screen for asymptomatic bacteriuria, and should be treated with antibiotics if colony counts are 100,000 or higher.[42] Screening for asymptomatic bacteriuria has consistently been shown to significantly reduce the number of symptomatic maternal UTIs as well as the incidence of preterm birth, low birth weight, and perinatal mortality. Nitrofurantoin and sulfonamides are the first-line agents for treatment and prevention of UTI in the second and third trimesters and are appropriate for use in the first trimester if no alternative antibiotics are available.[43] Women should undergo a test of cure after treatment and have a repeat urine culture every 6 to 12 weeks for the remainder of the pregnancy, and a urine dipstick should be performed at every visit to evaluate for blood, nitrites, and leukocytes.[24] After two positive cultures, suppressive therapy should be given.

Vaginitis. Vaginitis can be caused by yeast, bacteria, or protozoa, and symptoms may vary by the cause; common symptoms are itching, burning, and/or increased or malodorous discharge. Vaginitis can be a common but often overlooked cause of mild bleeding in pregnancy, particularly after intercourse, because vaginal infections can cause the cervix to become friable.[24] Diagnosis is generally by pelvic examination confirmed with microscopic evaluation using a wet preparation with saline and 10% KOH (yeast) and a whiff test (bacteria, protozoa) (a fishy amine odor when 10% KOH is added).

Seventy-five percent of all females will experience a vaginal yeast infection (vulvovaginal candidiasis [VVC]) at least once in their lifetime and therefore may be more familiar with this infection than they are with other types of vaginitis.[24] VVC manifests most commonly with thick, curdlike vaginal discharge and severe vaginal itching. A wet preparation will generally show

TABLE 11-4 Infections in Pregnancy

Infection	Organism	Symptoms	Diagnostics	Treatment Options
Urinary tract infection	*Escherichia coli* *Klebsiella pneumoniae* *Enterococcus* *Proteus* *Staphylococcus* Group B *Streptococcus*	May be absent Dysuria Frequency Urgency	Suprapubic tenderness Urinalysis Culture Repeat 1-2 wk after treatment	Amoxicillin Ampicillin Nitrofurantoin Trimethoprim-sulfamethoxazole* Cephalexin
Vulvovaginal candidiasis	*Candida albicans* *Candida* species Yeast	Pruritus Dyspareunia Abnormal vaginal discharge	Wet mount Hyphae or buds Normal pH	Topical azoles only
Bacterial vaginosis	*Gardnerella vaginalis* *Mobiluncus* species *Bacteroides* *Mycoplasma hominis* *Prevotella* species *Ureaplasma* *Mycoplasma*	May be absent Odor Irritation	Wet mount Clue cells Whiff pH > 4.5	Metronidazole (oral)† Clindamycin (oral) Avoid douching
Trichomoniasis	*Trichomonas vaginalis*	Odor Yellow-green discharge Irritation	Wet mount *T. vaginalis* Whiff *Trichomonas* rapid test Culture	Metronidazole (oral)† Counseling for sexually transmitted disease

*Avoid in first and third trimesters.
†Use with consultation only.
Data from Cunningham FG, Leveno KJ, Bloom SL, et al: *Williams obstetrics,* ed 23, New York, 2009, McGraw-Hill; U.S. Department of Health and Human Services, Centers for Disease Control and Prevention: Sexually transmitted diseases treatment guidelines, 2010, *MMWR Recomm Rep* 59(RR-12):1-110, 2010, available at www.cdc.gov/std/treatment/2010/STD-Treatment-2010-RR5912.pdf; Callahan TL, Caughey AB: *Obstetrics and gynecology,* ed 5, Philadelphia, 2009, Lippincott Williams & Wilkins/Wolters Kluwer Health; and Lyons P: *Obstetrics in family medicine: a practical guide,* Totowa, NJ, 2006, Humana.

branching hyphae and budding yeast, with a negative whiff test. Although new evidence suggests that short-term use of low-dose (150 mg) oral azole antifungal agents (fluconazole) in pregnancy is not associated with birth defects, the most appropriate first-line treatment of VVC in pregnancy remains topical vaginal azole cream.[47] A 7-day treatment is recommended owing to improved treatment success.[41] In the case of complicated VVC (severe symptoms, recurrence more than four times per year), extended treatment (2 to 3 weeks) or use of fluconazole (150 mg PO once) is advised.[23,42] Women should be advised to consult their providers before beginning self-treatment with an over-the-counter preparation. A low-potency topical corticosteroid may be used for a limited time if symptomatic relief of itchiness is required. If antibiotics are given for a UTI or other infections, a prescription for yeast treatment to be taken as needed at completion of antibiotic treatment may also be given, particularly for women who are prone to yeast infections.[24]

Women are less familiar with bacterial vaginosis (BV) and may not be aware that it is the most common cause of vaginal discharge and malodor.[48] Symptoms of BV include thin, grayish vaginal discharge that coats the walls of the vagina and may be associated with redness and irritation. A common complaint from women with BV is a fishy odor after sexual intercourse or during menses. This odor arises from exposure of the amines produced by the anaerobic bacteria common with BV to alkaline blood and sperm. Diagnosis is made by the character of discharge; presence of clue cells, vaginal epithelial cells with adherent coccobacilli on their borders, on a wet preparation; a vaginal pH above 4.5; and a positive whiff test. BV is correlated with adverse pregnancy outcomes because if it is left untreated, bacteria can ascend into the uterus, inducing preterm labor, preterm premature rupture of membranes (PPROM), intrauterine infection, and postpartum endometritis. Despite this association, current recommendations do not support routine screening for BV, because this approach has not consistently yielded a reduction in preterm births.[41,48] There is some increasing evidence that if treatment of BV is given early in pregnancy (<22 completed weeks' gestation), the rate of preterm birth decreases, presumably because treatment prevents irreversible inflammatory damage, but there is currently lack of consensus regarding this.[49] Treatment with 500 mg of oral metronidazole (Flagyl) twice a day for 7 days has been shown to be safe in pregnancy and is recommended over vaginal regimens because of the possible presence of subclinical upper genital tract infection.[41,48]

Vaginitis caused by the protozoan *Trichomonas vaginalis* manifests similarly to BV in pregnancy, although the symptoms may be much more severe and discharge may be more diffuse and yellowish-green. Impact on pregnancy outcomes is similar to BV as well. On a wet preparation, motile trichomonads will be seen, along with numerous leukocytes; a positive whiff test and a vaginal pH above 5.4 will also be present.[48] Alternatively, or if a microscopic evaluation is equivocal, a vaginal culture may be done. Trichomoniasis is an STI, and the woman and her partner should both be treated. The pregnant woman receives a single 2 gm oral dose and her partner can be treated with either a single 2 gm oral dose or 500 mg of oral metronidazole twice daily for 7 days.[41]

With all of the aforementioned vaginal infections, patients should be counseled to refrain from douching, frequently wash hands with soap and water, wear cotton underwear and loose clothing, keep underwear dry, promptly change wet underwear, avoid scented panty liners and pads, avoid wearing panty liners or pads every day, avoid the use of scented products on the vaginal area, and eat yogurt or use probiotics to promote the growth of "good bacteria" that keep yeast in check.[50] In addition, women should avoid scratching, which can make symptoms worse and introduce infection. Cold yogurt or petroleum jelly or a freezer gel pack can soothe itchy, irritated areas, as can a tepid bath.

Group B *Streptococcus*

Approximately 25% of pregnant women are colonized with group B *Streptococcus* (GBS) in their rectum and/or vagina and are considered GBS positive.[44] Universal screening of pregnant women at 35 to 37 weeks' gestation by sterile rectovaginal swab is used to identify GBS in pregnant women.[45] Although not generally considered clinically significant for women, they are at risk for passing the GBS bacteria to their babies during birth, causing neonatal GBS disease—commonly sepsis, pneumonia, or meningitis. Antibiotic treatment for GBS positive women during labor is highly effective, reducing the chances of a GBS-positive woman delivering a baby with GBS disease from 1 in 200 to 1 in 4000.

If GBS is identified in urine in any number, a woman should be considered GBS positive.[24,46] As with bacteriuria caused by other organisms, pregnant women who have GBS colony counts below 100,000 colony-forming units (CFU) per milliliter and are asymptomatic should not receive antibiotics at time of culture.[46] However, treatment with antibiotics in labor or after rupture of membranes to prevent early-onset neonatal GBS disease is indicated, and additional vaginal and rectal screening at 35 to 37 weeks' gestation is not necessary. Women who have previously given birth to an infant with GBS disease should automatically be given antibiotics in labor and do not need the vaginal and rectal screening at 35 to 37 weeks.

Nausea and Vomiting

Approximately 75% of women experience some nausea and/or vomiting in pregnancy, and 1% will develop hyperemesis gravidarum, which may require evaluation for underlying causes (e.g., a hydatidiform mole, metabolic or gastrointestinal disorders) and hospitalization for rehydration therapy and parenteral nutrition.[51] Although usually not life-threatening and usually self-limiting by 12 to 16 weeks of pregnancy, nausea and vomiting can negatively affect a woman's quality of life. Initial treatment consists of emotional support and reassurance of normalcy. Recommend dietary changes include small, frequent meals (with food eaten first thing in the morning before rising), bland foods high in carbohydrates and low in fat, high-protein foods that promote level blood sugar, avoidance of "trigger" or strong-smelling foods and sour foods; carbonated beverages can bring relief in some women. If nausea or vomiting persists, ginger, acupressure, and vitamin B_6 (25 mg PO q8h) may be introduced.[19,52]

If nonpharmacologic treatment is not effective, a combination of doxylamine and pyridoxine (vitamin B_6) is the first-line pharmacologic treatment. A medication combining 10 mg of doxylamine and 10 mg of pyridoxine (Bendectin) was pulled from the market in 1983 owing to safety concerns despite multiple studies showing no increased risk of birth defects but remained on the market in Canada. This combination was reintroduced in 2013 in the United States as Diclegis, a U.S. Food and Drug Administration (FDA)–approved Category A drug for the management of nausea and vomiting (2 tablets PO hs for mild symptoms; up to 4 tablets PO hs for more severe symptoms).[51] Alternatively, the combination can be replicated with an over-the-counter histamine H_1 blocker (Unisom) and vitamin B_6 (25 mg PO q8h B_6 plus 12.5 mg Unisom PO hs). If this is not adequate, antiemetics are the second-line treatment, including prochlorperazine (Compazine), chlorpromazine (Thorazine), trimethobenzamide (Tigan), or ondansetron (Zofran).[39,51] Other H_1 blockers that have been used include diphenhydramine (Benadryl), hydroxyzine, and meclizine. If a patient reports that she has been unable to eat or drink for more than 24 hours or has signs of dehydration or significant weight loss, evaluation of the urine for ketones and specific gravity and blood tests for electrolytes, blood urea nitrogen (BUN), and creatinine can provide valuable information about the need for further intervention.[24]

Gastroesophageal Reflux

High progesterone levels, which relax the gastroesophageal sphincter, and pressure on the diaphragm from an enlarging uterus combine to cause reflux of hydrochloric acid into the esophagus. This gastroesophageal reflux produces an unpleasant, midsternal burning sensation. Raising the head of the bed; eating small, bland meals; and avoiding lying flat after eating can reduce symptoms.[53] If lifestyle changes are inadequate, antacids are first-line treatment, but bicarbonate-containing antacids should be avoided to reduce the risk of metabolic acidosis and fluid overload. Antacids containing aluminum, calcium, and magnesium are recommended, but women should be counseled to limit intake to 1.0 g because doses higher than 1.4 g of calcium carbonate have been associated with an increase in milk-alkali syndrome. The H_2 blockers cimetidine and ranitidine and the proton pump inhibitor omeprazole have been shown to be safe and effective in pregnancy.[1,23] For women hoping to avoid medication, papaya enzymes may be suggested as an herbal alternative.[24]

Constipation and Hemorrhoids

Approximately one third of women will experience constipation during pregnancy, with the worst symptoms occurring during the third trimester. This is believed to result from a combination of hormonal and metabolic changes, the relaxation effect of progesterone on bowel motility, the increasing compression of the bowel as the fetus enlarges, dehydration, decreased physical activity, and dietary changes (small, more frequent meals with inadequate fiber intake).

Management of constipation begins with dietary and behavioral changes, starting with increased water and fiber intake, intake of foods with laxative properties (e.g., prunes, decaffeinated coffee), and moderate physical activity. Bulking agents (psyllium, methylcellulose) have been shown to be safe in pregnancy and are first-line treatments, usually 1 tablespoon in 8 ounces of fluid one to three times a day. Polyethylene glycol is not approved by the FDA for use in pregnancy, but toxicity is unlikely because of its reduced absorption. Stimulant laxatives such as anthraquinones, senna, and cascara are safe to use intermittently but not routinely in pregnancy. Although there is no evidence to support the use of docusate sodium for constipation in pregnancy, the drug does permit fluid to be absorbed into the stool, which can soften the stool and make it easier to pass through the colon. Mineral oil, castor oil, and saline should be avoided during pregnancy.

Straining to pass bowel movements when constipated combined with increased pressure on the rectum and perineum can lead to hemorrhoids in pregnant women. If this occurs, the woman should be counseled in the aforementioned measures to prevent constipation. Cold witch hazel compresses, sitz baths with baking soda, and Tucks pads can be used for symptomatic relief as needed.[24] Topical anesthetics may be used unless otherwise contraindicated, although evidence regarding the efficacy of these is lacking.[54] Hemorrhoids typically resolve spontaneously postpartum.

OBSTETRIC COMPLICATIONS

Bleeding in Pregnancy

Twenty percent to 25% of women will experience bleeding during the first trimester, and only half of these pregnancies will result in a live infant.[1] First-trimester bleeding may be caused by cervical or uterine abnormalities, chromosomal abnormalities, ectopic implantation, hormonal or nutritional imbalance, maternal infection, substance use, poorly controlled diabetes, or trauma.[1,24] Assessment of pregnancies with first-trimester bleeding includes ultrasound examination to evaluate viability, ruling out ectopic or trophoblastic pregnancy, and laboratory studies. The laboratory tests ordered include serial β-hCG measurements 48 hours apart, CBC with platelets, blood type and Rh, antibody screen, coagulation studies if a missed abortion is suspected, and type and crossmatch if surgery is being considered.[24] To reduce risk of isoimmunization, women who are Rh negative should receive RhoGAM.[1,24]

If a nonviable pregnancy is located within the uterus and there are no signs of infection, a woman may be offered expectant, medical, or surgical management. With expectant management, the expulsion of the uterine contents can be allowed to proceed spontaneously. A woman should be counseled to maintain pelvic rest; be prepared for significant bleeding lasting up to 7 to 10 days; return for care if uterine contents have not passed within 7 days; and call if bleeding increases or is accompanied by pain, adnexal pain or fever occurs, or heavy bleeding with pain lasts for longer than 1 hour.[24] Medical management with 800 μg of vaginal or 600 μg of oral misoprostol is very safe for incomplete spontaneous abortion (SAB) at less than 13 weeks' gestation and results in less pain, but more bleeding, than surgical intervention.[24,55] If expulsion of uterine contents has not occurred by day 3, the dose should be repeated, and if it has still not occurred by day 8, surgical management is indicated. Surgical intervention (dilation and curettage) may be necessary if the products of conception are not completely evacuated (incomplete) or are not evacuated at all (missed) or the woman develops sepsis, or if desired by the woman at any point.[1] Antibiotics are not indicated unless there are signs of sepsis. A repeat β-hCG measurement should be done 4 to 6 weeks after an SAB to ensure that β-hCG has returned to nonpregnant levels.[24]

An ectopic pregnancy, or pregnancy with implantation outside of the uterus, should be suspected with slowly rising or continued positive β-hCG levels after no intrauterine pregnancy is seen on an ultrasound.[24] The ultrasound should be repeated in 2 to 7 days to confirm. Transvaginal ultrasound may be more accurate in diagnosing ectopic pregnancy than transabdominal ultrasound, particularly if β-hCG levels are below 1500 to 2000 mIU/mL.[1] An ectopic pregnancy may or may not be accompanied by severe lower abdominal pain, spotting, and diaphragmatic irritation, particularly with rupture. Management of ectopic pregnancy is very different from management of SAB; watchful waiting is not an option in this case. Medical management with methotrexate can be offered, but surgical intervention for an ectopic pregnancy is often used, depending on the location of the ectopic products of conception and the hemodynamic status of the woman.[1]

Bleeding in the second and third trimesters may be related to benign causes such as bloody show in term labor, postcoital or postexamination spotting, or vaginal or cervical infection or to more serious conditions such as placenta previa, preterm labor, or placental abruption.[24] For benign causes, reassurance, review of danger signs, and treatment of any underlying causes (e.g., BV) should be provided. Placenta previa is caused by implantation of the placenta near or across the cervical os, and although it typically occurs early in gestation, serial ultrasound examinations are important because the condition often resolves as the uterus enlarges. Although complete previa occurs in a very small (0.5%) number of pregnancies, it contributes to 20% of all antepartum hemorrhages. Bleeding is painless and usually occurs after the 28th week.[1] If previa is suspected, vaginal examination should be delayed until location of the placenta has been confirmed.[24] If bleeding stops and the fetus is not compromised, delivery may be delayed until the pregnancy reaches term with bed and strict pelvic rest. For complete previa, a cesarean section is scheduled at term; for marginal previa with minimal or no bleeding and if the fetus remains healthy, a vaginal birth can be attempted, with monitoring of the fetus. If the fetus status becomes compromised and bleeding continues, immediate delivery by cesarean section is indicated.

Placental abruption occurs when part of or the entire placenta separates inappropriately from the uterine wall. Abruption occurs in approximately 0.5% to 1.5% of pregnancies and accounts for up to 25% of third-trimester bleeding.[56] Risk factors that have been associated with abruption include increased age and parity, maternal HTN, PPROM, multiple gestation, smoking, and cocaine use.[1,24,56] Diagnosis is clinical, with the classic presentation including blackish metrorrhagia with severe abdominal and/or back pain and uterine hypertonia, although in reality this "classic" triad was found to be present in only 9.7% of abruption cases.[56] Symptoms can vary by the degree of placental separation, and the bleeding can be concealed and discovered only on examination of the placenta after delivery. Bleeding was the only clinical presenting sign in 60% of cases in one study.[56] If the placental separation is abrupt and complete or nearly complete, hemorrhage and hypovolemic shock can occur.[56] Abruption significantly increases the risk for fetal hypoxia and is the underlying cause in 15% of perinatal mortality.[56]

Emotional support is critical, regardless of the trimester in which unexpected bleeding occurs. Exploring all options with the pregnant woman and her family can assist them in making informed, empowered decisions for the best physiologic and psychological outcomes.[24,55]

Preterm Labor

Preterm labor, defined as spontaneous rupture of membranes and/or uterine contractions that cause cervical change and dilation before 37 weeks of gestation, is a serious pregnancy complication that often (45% of the time) leads to premature delivery.[1] Approximately 70% of neonatal deaths are related to prematurity, and those infants who survive face potential lifetime consequences including 50% of the long-term neurologic disabilities in the United States.[57] Factors associated with preterm labor include socioeconomic status, genetic conditions, periodontal disease, uterine or cervical abnormalities, multiple gestation, substance use, maternal infections, and diseases such as preeclampsia.[1,24]

Of women with preterm labor, only about 10% will give birth within 7 days.[58] Fetal fibronectin (fFN) testing and cervical length assessment can help predict which women with premature uterine contractions are the most likely to progress to premature delivery, with positive fFN and cervical length below 25 mm being strong predictors of preterm birth,[24] although they should be used in conjunction with other information to direct management.[55] fFN testing must be done before digital examination of the cervix and can be affected by recent sexual activity or bleeding.[24] Taking fFN, gestational age, fetal status, and cervical length variables into account, timely identification and treatment of high-risk women including cerclage or tocolytics (beta-mimetics, calcium channel blockers, magnesium sulfate, or prostaglandin inhibitors) can prolong pregnancy and reduce morbidity and mortality associated with preterm birth.[1,24,58] Tocolytics are effective for only 48 hours and are thus usually reserved for cases in which the fetus is viable and would benefit from an additional 48 hours, such as for the administration of corticosteroids.[58] They are not indicated after 34 weeks' gestation or if contractions are not leading to cervical change, and are not recommended for maintenance therapy to prevent preterm birth. Vaginal progesterone gel may delay preterm birth in women with a short cervix.[59]

If delivery appears possible in the next 7 days, injectable steroids (betamethasone, dexamethasone) should be used at 24 to 34 weeks' gestation to mature fetal lungs and to prevent neurologic and gastrointestinal complications associated with extreme prematurity.[1,55] Antibiotics are recommended only to prevent GBS infection and to conservatively manage PPROM when the fetus is very immature.[55] Women with a history of preterm birth may be candidates for treatment with 17-hydroxyprogesterone to prevent preterm birth in subsequent pregnancies.[57]

OTHER MEDICAL CONDITIONS IN PREGNANCY

Physician consultation, collaborative management, or referral is indicated for many preexisting and emergent disorders associated with pregnancy. Common conditions that may indicate the need for this include severe HTN, preeclampsia, or eclampsia; gestational, type 1, or type 2 diabetes; new-onset hyperthyroidism; vaginal bleeding; pyelonephritis; congenital or suspected heart disease; renal disease; ectopic pregnancy; or asthma exacerbation. The initial visit should include screening for prepregnancy conditions that could affect pregnancy, and a plan of care with appropriate levels of care should be developed and put into action as soon as possible to ensure adequate management.

Asthma

Given that the prevalence of asthma continues to increase in the United States, it is critical to understand asthma in pregnancy.[60] Approximately 4% to 8% of women have a history of asthma when they become pregnant, and some additional women will first receive an asthma diagnosis during pregnancy.[61] Of these women, approximately one third will have their asthma improve, one third will have no change, and one third will have their asthma worsen, and there is no good way of predicting which will occur with any given woman.[60] However, it is clear that women with mild or well-controlled moderate asthma are not at increased risk for adverse pregnancy outcomes, but women with poorly controlled or severe disease are likely to have more exacerbations[1] and are at increased risk for premature delivery, preeclampsia, intrauterine growth restriction (IUGR), and cesarean section. Thus, to reduce maternal and fetal morbidity and mortality, preconception care should focus on ensuring that women with asthma enter pregnancy with well-controlled disease and prenatal care should focus on closely monitoring asthma and taking necessary steps to maintain control to reduce maternal and fetal morbidity and mortality.[61]

Diagnosis and monitoring of asthma are done through tracking of symptom frequency, timing, and severity (such as by using a daily asthma symptom diary) and spirometry to measure peak expiratory flow rate twice daily, with a goal range of 380 to 550 L/min.[1] Management goals are reinforced through education, reduction of environmental triggers, routine monitoring of pulmonary function, and use of pharmacologic management as indicated.[1] A stepwise approach to management of asthma medication is listed in Table 11-5.[61] The most commonly used classes of asthma medications in pregnancy are inhaled corticosteroids, long-acting beta-2 agonists, a combination of these two, and short-acting $beta_2$ agonists.[60] According to the National Asthma Education and Prevention Program, albuterol is the short-acting $beta_2$ agonist drug of choice, and the preferred

TABLE 11-5 Stepwise Therapy for Chronic Asthma During Pregnancy

Asthma Severity	Medication
Mild intermittent	No daily medications Short-acting $beta_2$ agonist (if needed)
Mild persistent	Low-dose inhaled corticosteroid Alternative: cromolyn, leukotriene receptor antagonist, or theophylline*
Moderate persistent	Low-dose inhaled corticosteroid and salmeterol; *or* Medium-dose inhaled corticosteroid; *or* Medium-dose inhaled corticosteroid and salmeterol† Alternative: low- or medium-dose inhaled corticosteroid + leukotriene receptor antagonist or theophylline*
Severe persistent	High-dose inhaled corticosteroid and salmeterol† and (if needed) oral corticosteroid Alternative: high-dose inhaled corticosteroid + theophylline* and oral corticosteroid (if needed)

*Check therapeutic level, 5 to 12 μg/mL.
†Add-on use of salmeterol is preferred to add-on use of leukotriene receptor antagonist or theophylline.
From American College of Obstetricians and Gynecologists: Practice bulletin no. 90: asthma in pregnancy, *Obstet Gynecol* 111:457-464, 2008.

inhaled corticosteroid is budesonide. However, a woman should continue taking the same inhaled corticosteroid used before pregnancy if possible. Pregnant women should be counseled that use of asthma medications during pregnancy is safer for both the woman and the fetus than are the consequences of uncontrolled asthma and exacerbations.[24] ACOG recommends fetal surveillance for women with poorly controlled, moderate, or severe asthma or women recovering from a severe exacerbation, with serial ultrasound examinations and antenatal fetal testing beginning at 32 weeks' gestation.[61] Stepdown of corticosteroid inhalers should only be done postpartum.[60]

Hypertension

There are four categories of HTN in pregnancy: chronic HTN, gestational HTN, and, most dangerous, preeclampsia and eclampsia, and preeclampsia superimposed on chronic HTN.[1,24] Collectively, these conditions affect 5% to 10% of pregnancies, making HTN the most common medical condition in pregnancy.[1] Diagnostic criteria are outlined in Table 11-6.[23,62]

Risk factors for the development of preeclampsia are preexisting HTN, chronic renal disease, multiple gestations, molar pregnancy, African or Asian race, maternal age younger than 20 years or older than 35 years), nulliparity, previous preeclampsia, new paternal partner, obesity, pregestational diabetes, and antiphospholipid antibody syndrome.[1,23,63] Uteroplacental insufficiency can result in fetal consequences, including fetal distress, IUGR, and iatrogenic prematurity. Maternal consequences of HTN include increased risk for preterm labor, placental abruption, disseminated intravascular coagulopathy, and HELLP syndrome (hemolytic anemia, elevated liver enzymes, low platelet count), making HTN one of the leading causes of maternal mortality worldwide.[24] Given the tremendous potential for devastating effects, careful antenatal surveillance, evaluation of symptoms, and prompt treatment are indicated.

For women with chronic HTN, baseline laboratory testing includes urine dipstick for proteinuria, hematocrit and hemoglobin, platelet count, serum creatinine, and electrolytes; liver function tests may be useful in later differentiation of onset of preeclampsia.[24] Chronic HTN is associated with increased risk of cesarean section, postpartum hemorrhage, GDM, preeclampsia, and increased severity of HTN during pregnancy. Home monitoring of BP is recommended for women with chronic HTN.[63] Treatment of mild to moderate chronic HTN in pregnancy does not appear to decrease fetal risk or prevent development of preeclampsia, so management remains controversial, but antihypertensive treatment is recommended if maternal blood pressure is higher than 160/105 mm Hg.[63] Nifedipine is the recommended antihypertensive, although labetalol and methyldopa are reasonable second-line alternatives.[64] Consultation is recommended if use of one of these is not effective. BP levels should be maintained in the range of 120 to 160/80 to 105 to prevent compromised uteroplacental flow with pharmacologically induced low BP levels.[64] Ultrasonography to screen for fetal growth restriction is recommended, and antenatal fetal testing should be performed if there is evidence of growth restriction.[63]

Management of gestational HTN and mild preeclampsia (including superimposed preeclampsia) is expectant management, with delivery at 37 weeks' gestation recommended if mother and fetus are stable. Antenatal testing for the fetus should be performed twice weekly for preeclampsia and once weekly for gestational HTN.[63] The fetus is monitored by daily kick counts,

TABLE 11-6 Diagnostic Criteria for Hypertension in Pregnancy

Classification	Blood Pressure*	Laboratory Values†	Symptoms
Chronic	BP >140/90 mm Hg <20 wk Persistent >12 wk PP	No urine protein	Asymptomatic
Gestational	BP >149/90 mm Hg >20 wk Normal by 12 wk PP	No urine protein	Asymptomatic
Preeclampsia‡§	Mild: ≥140/90 mm Hg Severe: ≥160/110 mm Hg Normal by 12 wk PP	Mild: urine protein >2 g/24 hr or ≥1+ dipstick Severe: urine protein ≥5 g/24 hr or ≥3+ dipstick Platelets <100,000 mm^3 AST and ALT elevated LDH elevated Serum creatinine >1.2 mg/dL	Altered mental status Headaches Visual disturbances Pulmonary edema Epigastric pain <500 mL urine output per day Thrombocytopenia Hemolytic anemia
Superimposed preeclampsia	BP ≥140/90 mm Hg <20 wk Persistent >12 wk PP	New onset: urine protein ≥2 g (300 mg)/24 hr >20 wk Sudden increase in BP Sudden increase in urine protein Low platelet count <20 wk	Same as preeclampsia
Eclampsia			Seizures (other causes ruled out)

*To reduce artifact, take BP on two separate occasions no more than 7 days apart.
†Use 24-hour urine protein for diagnosis.
‡May progress to HELLP (hemolytic anemia, elevated liver enzymes, low platelet count), a subcategory of preeclampsia.
§Unless previously elevated.
ALT, alanine transaminase; AST, aspartate transaminase; BP, blood pressure; LDH, lactate dehydrogenase; PP, postpartum.
Data from Callahan TL, Caughey AB: *Obstetrics and gynecology*, ed 5, Philadelphia, 2009, Lippincott Williams & Wilkins/Wolters Kluwer Health; and National Institutes of Health, National High Blood Pressure Education Program: *Working group report on high blood pressure in pregnancy*, U.S. Department of Health and Human Services, National Heart, Lung, and Blood Institute, 2000, available at www.nhlbi.nih.gov/guidelines/archives/hbp_preg/hbp_preg_archive.pdf.

ultrasonography to assess growth every 3 weeks, and amniotic fluid assessment weekly. The mother is monitored by BP assessment twice weekly and CBC and liver enzyme and serum creatinine levels once a week. Women with gestational HTN should also be evaluated for proteinuria at each visit. Women should be counseled to report immediately symptoms of severe preeclampsia: severe headaches that do not resolve with rest, acetaminophen, fluids, and food; right upper quadrant pain; visual changes; or shortness of breath.

If severe features are present or develop, expectant management beyond 34 weeks is not recommended and referral is indicated. Parenteral magnesium sulfate for seizure prevention is recommended, as are antenatal corticosteroids for fetal lung development if less than 34 weeks' gestation, and delivery is deferred for 48 hours if the fetus is viable and the mother and fetus are stable. Eclampsia (status epilepticus) requires emergent delivery, regardless of the age of the fetus.[1,63,65]

Pharmacologic management of gestational HTN and preeclampsia is the same as for chronic HTN. Low-dose aspirin (75 mg/day) for women at high risk of developing preeclampsia is recommended, as is calcium supplementation (1.5 to 2.0 g of elemental calcium per day) to increase placental blood flow in pregnancies complicated by preeclampsia.[65] However, calcium supplementation appears to decrease risk only in women with poor dietary calcium intake.[65] Bed rest; restricted salt intake; supplementation with vitamins C, D, and/or E; diuretics; magnesium; omega-3 fatty acids; and antioxidants have not proved to be effective in reducing maternal blood pressure or improving fetal outcomes.[1,65]

Diabetes

Diabetes mellitus (DM) is classified as type 1 diabetes (insulin deficiency), type 2 diabetes (decreased insulin secretion and insulin resistance), diabetes from other causes including cystic fibrosis and medication therapy, or GDM (diabetes diagnosed during pregnancy).[66] Approximately 6% to 7% of pregnancies are complicated by DM, 90% of them by GDM, although with global increases in obesity and sedentary lifestyles, the number of women with DM is growing.[67]

In addition to women who have been diagnosed with DM before pregnancy, some women will be diagnosed with overt (nongestational) DM at their first prenatal visit based on high plasma glucose levels (>200 mg/dL random plus classic signs and symptoms, or >126 mg/dL fasting), glucosuria, and ketoacidosis.[1] Women with a high risk of overt DM (strong family history, history of large-for-gestational age infant, current obesity) may be screened at their first prenatal visit and diagnosed with overt diabetes if the aforementioned are noted. Given a lack of evidence regarding this type of screening, providers must use their clinical judgment to determine who requires first-trimester or early pregnancy screening.[68] The American Diabetes Association (ADA) supports diagnosis of women with pregestational (overt) diabetes rather than GDM when they meet diagnostic criteria at the initial prenatal visit.[66]

The risks to a fetus of a mother who has been diagnosed with DM (type 1 or type 2) vary greatly depending on how well controlled her sugars are in the first trimester, which underscores the need for preconception counseling and care for women with diabetes and early identification of previously undiagnosed diabetes whenever possible.[69] Even mild levels of hyperglycemia have the potential to cause fetal malformations (particularly cardiac and skeletal), with the risk of a major birth defect directly proportional to the degree of blood sugar control in the first trimester. In caring for the patient with preexisting diabetes, a clinician should carefully evaluate the patient for use of drugs commonly prescribed for patients with diabetes including statins, angiotensin-converting enzyme inhibitors, and angiotensin receptor antagonists, all of which are contraindicated and should be discontinued during pregnancy.[66]

GDM is typically diagnosed at 24 to 28 weeks' gestation. Risk factors for GDM include race (i.e., Hispanic/Latino, Asian/Pacific Islander, Native American), obesity, sedentary lifestyle, family history, previous history of GDM, delivery of a macrosomic infant, polycystic ovarian syndrome or other signs of insulin resistance, and history of cardiovascular disease. If a woman has HTN, high-density lipoprotein level below 35 mg/dL, triglyceride level above 250 mg/dL, hemoglobin A_{1c} (HbA_{1c}) above 5.7%, signs of impaired glucose tolerance, or impaired fasting glucose on a previous test, she is also at risk for GDM during pregnancy.[66]

Like pregestational DM, GDM is associated with poor maternal and fetal outcomes. Although congenital malformations are less common in pregnancies complicated by GDM, adverse maternal and fetal effects similar to those seen in pregnancies complicated by pregestational diabetes do occur. Fetal effects of GDM include macrosomia, IUGR, preterm delivery, operative delivery, shoulder dystocia birth trauma, and stillbirth; maternal complications include miscarriage, polyhydramnios, increased risk of infection, gestational HTN, preeclampsia, cesarean section, and, of greatest concern, an increased risk of developing diabetes later in life.[1] Neonates born from pregnancies complicated by uncontrolled diabetes can experience hypoglycemia, hypocalcemia, polycythemia, jaundice, and respiratory distress. Interestingly, maternal hyperglycemia during pregnancy is a risk factor for fetal hyperinsulinemia, childhood obesity, and later development of type 2 diabetes.

Given all of the aforementioned, it is paramount that women with diabetes of any type be identified in a timely manner and receive extensive counseling regarding how to maintain glycemic control before conception, prenatally, and throughout pregnancy to avoid short-term and long-term consequences of the disease.[67-69] And yet, a great deal of controversy exists over who, how, and when women should be screened for GDM. Some organizations support universal screening; others encourage selective screening based on risk, either at the time of pregnancy or at 24 to 28 weeks' gestation.[1,66,67] Given that only about 10% of women meet the low-risk criteria that would opt them out of risk-based screening, many health care providers find it more practical to simply screen all women rather than introduce complexity and risk missing higher-risk women.[66] The U.S. Preventive Task Force reported insufficient evidence in support of or against screening before 24 weeks and a moderate net benefit for screening after 24 weeks to prevent maternal and neonatal complications.[68] Equally controversial are whether to use a single- or two-step screening test and what glucose load (50, 75, or 100 g) will offer the most accurate assessment of glucose tolerance. An increasing number of health care providers are using the single 75-g, 2-hour glucose tolerance test proposed by the Fifth International Workshop-Conference on Gestational Diabetes Mellitus, but many continue to use the 50-g, 1-hour test, with those who exceed the screening threshold undergoing a diagnostic 100-g, 3-hour test.[67]

To reduce the development of fetal and maternal complications, women are counseled to maintain tight glycemic control without becoming hypoglycemic during pregnancy. For women diagnosed with GDM, the initial strategy should be achievement of normoglycemia through dietary management and moderate exercise.[67] If possible, dietary counseling with a registered dietitian and development of a personalized nutrition plan should occur shortly after diagnosis. The focus of nutritional counseling is total caloric allotment (30 to 35 kcal/kg/day), carbohydrate intake as 33% to 40% of calories, and remaining calories distributed between protein (20%) and fat (40%). Complex carbohydrates rather than simple carbohydrates should be eaten when possible, and caloric intake should be spread over three meals and two snacks to reduce glucose fluctuations. Continued surveillance of blood glucose levels is necessary to ensure that glycemic control is consistently achieved with diet management alone. Daily fasting and 2-hour postprandial testing can be used for this, with the goal to have 75% of glucose readings (no more than one abnormal value per day) within normal range of fasting glucose of 95 or less and 2-hour postprandial glucose of 120 or less.[66]

If dietary management of GDM to control hyperglycemia is inadequate, pharmacologic management is indicated. Pharmacologic management is adjusted to the type of diabetes and level of disease. Whereas insulin has historically been the preferred treatment option for all women in pregnancy, oral medications (glyburide, metformin) are equally effective, may be used as first-line therapy and are not associated with increased short-term adverse maternal and neonatal outcomes as compared with insulin.[67] Insulin is required for all type 1 diabetes patients, although their levels may require adjustment in pregnancy. Women with preexisting type 2 diabetes may continue to use any oral medications they were using before pregnancy.

Women with preexisting diabetes and GDM with poor glycemic control may benefit from antenatal fetal testing related to the increased risk of fetal demise. However, there is little agreement on the role of fetal surveillance for women with well-controlled GDM. The type, timing, and requirements of fetal surveillance may largely be dictated by local practice at this stage, given the current lack of consensus. Evaluation for fetal macrosomia, particularly in women with uncontrolled gestational diabetes, may prevent fetal complications related to shoulder dystocia and its sequelae through induction of labor at 38 to 39 weeks or scheduled cesarean.[67,68]

Thyroid Disease

Thyroid disease is increasingly being seen in women of childbearing age. When left undiagnosed or untreated, it is associated with increased risk of miscarriage, placental abruption, hypertensive disorders, and growth restriction of the fetus.[70] However, identification of thyroid disorders in pregnancy can be challenging; symptoms can mimic those of pregnancy itself, and significant metabolic changes occur very early in pregnancy.[71] Typically, as early as 4 weeks' gestation, total thyroxine (T_4) and triiodothyronine (T_3) levels have increased significantly and plateau through the remainder of pregnancy, whereas TSH has decreased.[70] Even with increased thyroid hormone levels, no physiologic hyperthyroid state occurs because thyroxine-binding globulin also increases significantly in pregnancy. Abnormal thyroid hormone levels complicate 0.5% to 2.5% of all pregnancies, and subclinical disease affects even more, at 4.6% to 11.8% of pregnancies.[72]

Universal screening for thyroid disease in pregnancy remains controversial because of a lack of large, conclusive clinical trials. Current practice is to screen on the basis of an individual woman's risk for thyroid disease, although there appears to be some shift of consensus toward universal screening, especially as our knowledge of the impact of thyroid disorders on pregnancy outcomes grows.[72] However, to date, universal screening recommendations remain to screen only women at high risk for thyroid disease. Risk factors include personal or family history of thyroid disease, history of type 1 diabetes, history of infertility or preterm delivery, and symptoms of thyroid disease.[73] Diagnosis is made through interpretation of a TSH level and, if it is abnormal, the results of a free T_4 (fT_4) level or fT_4 index. Trimester-specific reference ranges are needed to accurately interpret laboratory values.[73] Antibody testing should be considered because the majority of prenatal thyroid abnormalities are the result of autoimmune thyroiditis, and even in a euthyroid state, the presence of antibodies has been found to influence perinatal outcomes.[73]

Hyperthyroid disease in pregnancy is typically the result of Graves disease, which predisposes the woman to hyperemesis gravidarum, preeclampsia, and heart failure and the fetus to goitrous thyrotoxicosis, nonimmune hydrops, hypothyroidism related to maternal treatment, and possible death. Subclinical hyperthyroid disease, estimated to affect 1.7% of pregnancies, contributes minimally to adverse maternal or neonatal effects.[1] The diagnosis of hyperthyroidism is made when TSH levels are low and fT_4 levels are high. If antithyroid therapy is initiated in pregnancy, propylthiouracil (PTU) is preferred in the first trimester, because methimazole is associated with birth defects, but should be switched to methimazole after the first trimester when the risk of liver failure associated with PTU outweighs the risk of congenital anomalies.[70] The goal of PTU therapy is to maintain a serum fT_4 level in the upper one third level of normal. Serum TSH and fT_4 levels are evaluated every 2 weeks until the woman is on a stable dose to achieve this. Monthly sonographs from 20 weeks should be done for women on antithyroid medication or with poorly controlled hyperthyroidism to assess fetal thyroid dysfunction, as well as weekly fetal testing from 32 to 34 weeks.[70] Surgical management is indicated when pharmacotherapy is ineffective.[73] The use of radioactive iodine is contraindicated in pregnancy because it can cross the placenta and destroy the fetal thyroid as well.[1,73] Subclinical hyperthyroidism is diagnosed when the TSH level is low but the fT_4 remains within normal limits. No treatment is currently recommended because the risks of adverse effects to the fetus outweigh the benefits of treatment; these women require regular monitoring for thyroid function throughout the pregnancy and postpartum.[1,73]

Hypothyroidism and subclinical hypothyroidism can have a more profound impact on outcomes than hyperthyroid disease. Hypothyroidism increases the risk of preterm labor, anemia, and low birth weight and is associated with miscarriage[70,71,73]; maternal hypothyroidism, particularly in the first trimester, has been associated with negative neurologic effects on the infant later in life.[70] Many studies have also shown a relationship among thyroid antibodies, PPROM, and placental abruption.[1]

Hypothyroidism is characterized by high TSH and low fT_4 levels. If hypothyroidism predates the pregnancy, it is important to achieve and to maintain a euthyroid state (<2.5 ng/dL) within the first trimester. Higher doses (30% to 50%) are likely to be required to match the physiologic increase in thyroid hormone requirements with pregnancy; women are reevaluated every 4 to 6 weeks until 20 weeks' gestation and they achieve a stable dosage, then at 24 to 28 weeks and 32 to 34 weeks' gestation.[70,73] Levothyroxine 1.8 to 2 μg/kg/day for overt disease and 75 to 100 μg/day for mild disease are typical dosage regimens.[71] Subclinical hypothyroidism is diagnosed when TSH is elevated but fT_4 remains within normal limits. Although some professional organizations do not recommend treatment, the Endocrine Society recommends that hormone therapy be initiated for subclinical hypothyroidism.[73]

Gallbladder Disease

Approximately 1 of 1000 women will develop cholecystitis in pregnancy. During the first trimester, women experience an increased residual volume of bile in the gallbladder, which leads to incomplete emptying of the cystic duct and the formation of biliary sludge. This increases susceptibility to gallstone formation. Most pregnant women are asymptomatic, and the condition resolves after pregnancy.[1] When the gallbladder becomes inflamed or a stone lodges in the cystic duct, women become nauseated, begin vomiting, and experience loss of appetite. Upper right quadrant pain can be intermittent or persist, depending on whether the cystic duct is partially or completely obstructed.

Women are instructed to eat a balanced diet, to consume adequate amounts of vitamin C and iron, and to avoid processed or fatty foods. Weight management has been shown to help manage gallbladder disease.[74] Surgery is indicated if the woman is symptomatic and conservative management is not helpful. Cholecystectomy during pregnancy is associated with a low complication rate; overall morbidity is reduced when surgery is not delayed,[1,75] because a delay in surgery is associated with recurrent symptoms and increased hospitalizations.[76]

Integrated Health Care for Women

Rapidly expanding research in the area of epigenetics is unveiling reasons for and reinforcing the importance of preconception care. *Healthy People 2020* is reshaping the current prenatal care model by placing greater emphasis on preconception and intraconception health,[6] highlighting the important role of genetics and genomics, removing barriers to care, and emphasizing the importance of evidence-based care for ideal pregnancy outcomes for both mothers and their babies.

CHAPTER 12

LACTATION GUIDANCE

Kathleen M. Craig

The evidence in support of breastfeeding as a primary health practice for both mother and baby is strong. Research into the human microbiome and epigenetics shows that breastfeeding increases physical and emotional well-being across the life span.[1] With childhood obesity rates increasing, nutrition counseling will focus on consumption of whole foods and avoidance of processed foods, a lifelong effort that can begin with breastfeeding. Optimal breastfeeding duration has been defined by the World Health Organization (WHO) and the American Academy of Pediatrics (AAP) as exclusive breastfeeding for 6 months and continued breastfeeding for a year or longer.[2]

Social support from family members has the most significant influence on breastfeeding initiation and duration, but professional support consistently increases women's engagement in breastfeeding as either an exclusive or a supplemented feeding practice. Pregnancy presents an opportunity for health care professionals to inform the decisions a woman makes for herself and for her family. It is important for primary care providers to develop skill in client-centered communication techniques, such as motivational interviewing or cognitive behavioral counseling, to have effective conversations about change or to shift strongly held beliefs or values that negatively affect health.[3-5]

Breastfeeding is both simple and complex. Nelson describes breastfeeding as "a method of infant feeding that involves an intimate, vulnerable relationship between a mother and infant that is personal, engrossing, and physical, and that requires commitment, adaptation, and support from a variety of networks, and presents a need for resolution, whether positive or negative, upon discontinuation."[6] The health care professional promotes and supports lactation, engages in open dialogue with the patient or family, provides information based on clinical assessment and knowledge, and coordinates care appropriately. Health care professionals consider cultural and situational contexts for each family while eliminating barriers to breastfeeding whenever possible. The AAP has developed a free online learning program to increase breastfeeding knowledge for healthcare providers: www2.aap.org/breastfeeding/curriculum. The Academy of Breastfeeding Medicine provides evidence-based protocols for use by primary care providers: www.bfmed.org

PRENATAL PREPARATION FOR BREASTFEEDING

Prenatal Lactation Counseling

Health care providers promote and support exclusive breastfeeding for the first 6 months and continued breastfeeding for at least 1 year.[2] Lactation counseling begins with the first prenatal or pediatric office visit and includes both verbal and written education about breastfeeding. During subsequent visits, the health care provider reinforces the value of exclusive breastfeeding for both short-term and long-term health (Box 12-1), explores social supports for breastfeeding as well as barriers and concerns, and begins a discussion about what to expect in the immediate postpartum period. Pregnant women should be educated about the value of early skin-to-skin contact, early initiation of breastfeeding, rooming in, baby-led feeding, and the relationship between these practices and successful breastfeeding. During prenatal care, mothers will learn about the relationship between feeding frequency and establishing an adequate milk supply and learn effective positioning and latch techniques.

Common hospital practices may interfere with breastfeeding. The Baby-Friendly Hospital Initiative serves to promote evidence-based practices in hospitals and birth centers. The Ten Steps to Successful Breastfeeding are evidence-based practices that increase breastfeeding initiation and duration (Box 12-2). A mother should be advised to keep her newborn close in the first 2 weeks, as the infant learns to nurse, and encouraged to sleep when the baby sleeps. Mothers should be taught to nurse frequently in the first days after birth to minimize breast engorgement and optimize milk supply. Breastfeeding mothers should avoid bottles and supplements unless their use is medically indicated.[7]

Breastfeeding has been associated with a decreased risk of sudden infant death syndrome (SIDS). Mothers should be

BOX 12-1

Significant Maternal and Infant Health Benefits Associated with Breastfeeding

BENEFITS OF BREASTFEEDING FOR INFANT

- Optimal immune system development and establishment of gut health
- Decreased risk of hospitalization in first year of life
- Decreased frequency and severity of communicable diseases: diarrhea, otitis media, and respiratory tract infections
- Decreased risk of chronic noncommunicable disease including respiratory and gastrointestinal allergies, obesity, diabetes, hypertension, cancer, and Crohn disease.
- Improved motor and intellectual development

BENEFITS OF BREASTFEEDING FOR MOTHER

- Decreased risk of ovarian cancer
- Decreased risk of osteoporosis
- Decreased blood loss in the postpartum period
- Decreased risk of some types of breast cancers
- Promotion of postpartum weight loss

Data from Lutter C, Ross J, Martin L: *Quantifying the benefits of breastfeeding: a summary of the evidence.* Washington, DC, 2002, Pan American Health Organization (PAHO).

BOX 12-2

Ten Steps to Successful Breastfeeding

Every facility providing maternity services and care for newborn infants should:

1. Have a written breastfeeding policy that is routinely communicated to all health care staff.
2. Train all health care staff in skills necessary to implement this policy.
3. Inform all pregnant women about the benefits and management of breastfeeding.
4. Help mothers initiate breastfeeding within half an hour of birth.
5. Show mothers how to breastfeed, and how to maintain lactation even if they should be separated from their infants.
6. Give newborn infants no food or drink other than breast milk, unless medically indicated.
7. Practice rooming-in—allow mothers and infants to remain together—24 hours a day.
8. Encourage breastfeeding on demand.
9. Give no artificial nipples or pacifiers to breastfeeding newborns.
10. Foster the establishment of breastfeeding support groups and refer mothers to them on discharge from hospital or clinic.

informed about this association, as well as the AAP recommendation that infants sleep on their backs on a firm mattress in separate beds or bassinets in the mother's room. Close sleeping arrangements have been shown to increase breastfeeding satisfaction for mothers and breastfeeding duration for babies, and many breastfeeding mothers fall asleep while breastfeeding in bed. The AAP recommends that babies brought to bed to nurse should be returned to a separate sleep surface when the mother is ready for sleep. Soft objects and loose bedding should always be kept out of the infant's crib or bed, and babies should not be placed prone or on their sides. The AAP SIDS reduction

BOX 12-3

Provider Checklist for Patient Education in Prenatal Care

Pregnant women are educated on the following topics:

- Benefits of breastfeeding for mother and child
- The importance of exclusive breastfeeding for the first 6 months
- Early initiation of breastfeeding
- Early skin-to-skin contact
- Rooming-in on a 24-hour basis
- Baby-led feeding
- Promotion of milk supply through frequent feeding
- Effective positioning and latch techniques
- Continuation of breastfeeding after introduction of appropriate complementary foods

recommendations also advise that once breastfeeding is well established, infants 1 month of age should be offered a pacifier when laid down to sleep.[8]

Mothers should be informed that they can breastfeed even if they are returning to work. Laws that support breastfeeding in the workplace aim to decrease early weaning. When women return to work after the birth of a child, employers must offer reasonable break time to pump or express milk for at least a year. Women should discuss their plans with their employer prenatally.[9]

Health care providers can use the Checklist for Patient Education in Prenatal Care to guide mothers in thorough planning for successful breastfeeding (Box 12-3).

Breast and Nipple Evaluation for Breastfeeding

Assessment of breast and nipple is best done during the first trimester of prenatal care. Breasts generally increase by about one bra cup size, and nipples and areola typically darken. These are indications that the mother's body is preparing to breastfeed. No other breast or nipple preparation is necessary. Lack of changes in the breasts may be an indication of primary lactation insufficiency. Women with primary hypoplasia of the breasts require close follow-up during the early postpartum period.[10]

Women who have had breast augmentation can generally breastfeed without difficulty unless the indication was severe glandular hypoplasia. In general, breast reduction leads to problems with milk extraction because of interrupted ductal pathways. Breast surgeons have developed nipple-sparing breast reduction surgical techniques, but breastfeeding outcomes for women who have had reduction mammoplasty continue to be individual and highly variable.[11]

Nipples come in a variety of configurations of size, depth, and breadth. There is no evidence that nipple preparation devices improve breastfeeding outcomes for women with dimpled, flat, or inverted nipples. Health care providers concerned about the presentation of a woman's breasts or nipples prenatally may refer to a lactation consultant or plan for close follow-up in the early postpartum period.

THE FIRST FEW DAYS

During the day or two after birth, mothers are taught to position the baby for correct latching and to assess whether the baby is getting enough milk. Mothers learn about the immunologic benefits of colostrum and the transition to lactogenesis, or full milk production, which occurs in general between the second and fifth day. A feeding log will help mothers record feeding frequency and understand stooling and voiding patterns. Mothers are encouraged to feed the baby on demand and to wake a sleepy baby to ensure that the newborn has 8 to 12 good feedings in 24 hours. Mothers learn that an infant feeds frequently in the first 2 weeks and, in general, will begin to space out feedings thereafter.[12]

The first few weeks are very demanding for new mothers, whether they are breastfeeding or not. Mothers should be supported during this transition and reassured that mother-infant dyads sustained through the first 2 weeks of breastfeeding typically go on to meet the mother's breastfeeding goals.[13]

DISCHARGE INSTRUCTIONS

Discharge plans are based on AAP recommendations and the baby's progress with feedings. Discharge instructions should be provided in writing and reviewed with the mother to assess her understanding. Health care providers should teach mothers about expected feeding and voiding patterns and the normal progression of the stool. Expected goals for feeding and elimination are reviewed, and mothers are taught to report concerns, rather than being taught "danger" signs. Use of language that associates breastfeeding with danger should be avoided. A mother should be taught to recognize and to report when her infant is not meeting the standard for a "good" intake, because early intervention is critical.[13]

To help the parents determine whether the infant is feeding well, a feeding log is recommended for the first week or so to track the number and quality of feedings and the number of stools and voids.

Feeding requirements for breastfed infants depend on many factors, such as gestational age, size for gestational age, birth history, and early adaptation to extrauterine life. Preterm infants have fewer reserves and are vulnerable to complications, such as hypoglycemia and low weight gain.[14] Infants who are large for gestational age or small for gestational age require careful observation of feeding as well.

In general, newborns feed at least 8 to 12 times per day. With an optimum feeding pattern, the infant should latch on securely to the breast and suck and swallow rhythmically and vigorously. Suckling time at the breast should not be limited because some babies are less efficient than others. Signs of good feeds include the mother's breasts softening after feeding; the infant is satisfied and may fall asleep after suckling. The second breast should be offered, but in the early days, the baby may fall asleep after one breast and feed at more frequent intervals. As the baby becomes accustomed to larger milk volumes, feeding on both sides is more common, as are longer feeding intervals.[13]

The stool initially will be meconium, dark and tarry. Transitional stool is brown, and after the milk comes in, usually by day 3 or 4, the stools will become yellow with milk curds. For the first week of life, the number of stools and the number of voids should approximately match the infant's age in days. The infant will then develop a personal pattern of elimination that may change again at 1 month of age. Any changes in an infant's established pattern should be evaluated.

Infants should be evaluated 1 to 3 days after discharge to assess weight and check for jaundice. Mothers should be instructed to call the provider before the scheduled visit if the infant develops jaundice or has difficulty feeding. Infants may lose up to 8% to 10% of their birth weight during the first week of life. A supplemental feeding plan should be initiated for infants who lose more than 10% of their birth weight (Box 12-4).[15]

BOX 12-4

Components of a Plan to Improve Breast Milk Intake

- Evaluate the breastfeeding and correct any problems with attachment technique or positioning.
- Suggest the appropriate feeding frequency and duration based on individual assessment.
- Use a hospital-grade breast pump with a double-pump setup (pumping both sides at once) to increase breast emptying and stimulation. Use the pumped milk to supplement breastfeeding.
- Assess adequacy of feeding by closely following weight gain. If the maternal supply is adequate, weight gain should be about 1 oz/day. If the supply is less than required, supplemental feedings of formula or banked human milk may be required temporarily. Taper supplemental volumes as soon as the supply is increased and weight gain is improved.
- Slowly taper the pumping sessions after the infant has gained the appropriate weight and is breastfeeding without supplement.
- If the breastfeeding problem is not resolved by improving technique and supply, contact the referral network for expert help. Continue to maintain contact with the mother and specialists.

Mothers should be provided with a list of community-based lactation resources; problems that threaten continued lactation should be referred to lactation consultants.[16,17]

NEONATAL JAUNDICE

Physiologic Jaundice

Most newborns become mildly jaundiced during the third to fifth days of life. Breastfed babies commonly appear jaundiced into the third or fourth week of life, and less commonly for 8 to 12 weeks. Bilirubin levels decrease as the endocrine and digestive systems mature. Hyperbilirubinemia, or persistent or excessive jaundice, may be a result of inadequate fluid intake or complicating conditions.[18]

Newborn care providers must familiarize themselves with AAP neonatal jaundice guidelines and develop follow-up plans to assess the baby during the most vulnerable period, 3 to 5 days of age. The AAP has developed hyperbilirubinemia phototherapy treatment guidelines based on the rate of rise of the bilirubin levels plotted against the baby's age in hours. See http://bilitool.org.

All newborns will be assessed for risk of hyperbilirubinemia before hospital discharge. Risk factors for hyperbilirubinemia include jaundice that develops in the first 24 hours, blood group incompatibility, and gestational age less than 37 weeks. Other risk factors are cephalohematoma, significant bruising, excessive weight loss, difficulty establishing breastfeeding, East Asian race, and a previous sibling requiring phototherapy.

The most common cause of indirect or unconjugated hyperbilirubinemia in the first 5 to 10 days of life is infrequent feeding and low milk intake, resulting in an exaggerated physiologic jaundice. Frequent feedings usually result in frequent stools, and bowel movements are the primary excretion route for bilirubin. When feedings and associated stools are infrequent, the bilirubin in the meconium stool is reabsorbed into the bloodstream, which raises the serum bilirubin level and results in clinical jaundice. Suboptimal breastfeeding can lead to starvation jaundice. This condition responds to increased breastfeeding, which may require the use of a breast pump to increase the mother's supply. Supplementation with water and sugar water is not recommended. Frequent breastfeeding, once the mother's milk is in, will usually improve the jaundice. Formula supplementation may be required in cases of low milk supply. If the baby is lethargic, the mother may extract the milk with a breast pump and feed it to the baby with a supplemental nursing system, cup, or bottle until the baby regains the vigor to extract milk directly from the breast.[19]

Pathologic Jaundice

Babies with high direct or conjugated hyperbilirubinemia need to be evaluated for biliary obstruction or hepatitis. Babies with high levels of unconjugated bilirubin who meet criteria established by AAP guidelines are treated with phototherapy to prevent kernicterus, also called chronic bilirubin encephalopathy. Bilirubin encephalopathy occurs when bilirubin level are high enough to cross the blood-brain barrier and damage basal ganglia and brainstem nuclei. Discharge screening for predictive risk of hyperbilirubinemia aims to eliminate the preventable condition by treating bilirubin levels before they are high enough to risk toxicity.[18,19]

Breast Milk Jaundice

The cause of breast milk jaundice is unknown. It usually occurs after 1 to 2 weeks of age, after breastfeeding is well established, and in the setting of appropriate weight gain. Laboratory results reveal late-onset, prolonged, unconjugated hyperbilirubinemia. The infant with true breast milk jaundice is typically thriving, gaining weight, and producing four or more milk curd stools per day. There is no need to interrupt breastfeeding. Bilirubin levels drop gradually over 8 to 12 weeks. The bilirubin level may rise slightly, but not usually to clinically significant levels.[19]

MANAGING CHALLENGES TO BREASTFEEDING SUCCESS

Attachment and Latch-on in Newborns

Most newborns, given the opportunity for 1 to 2 hours of interrupted skin-to-skin contact with their mothers immediately after birth, will latch on and begin suckling with very little assistance. Hospital policies should be designed to facilitate early attachment. Sometimes there are delays in early attachment, or the baby may have structural problems, such as a short frenulum that limits tongue mobility and the ability to suckle effectively. Babies with ankyloglossia should be evaluated for frenuloplasty if attachment and milk extraction are impaired.[20]

If the baby is having difficulty latching on, positioning strategies can improve comfort for the mother and milk transfer for the baby. Mothers should be taught how to bring the baby to the breast to prevent the infant from sucking on the nipple tip. Shallow latch causes pain and poor let-down.[21] It is important that the mother be positioned comfortably. A seated, cross-legged position with pillows for back and thigh support is comfortable for most women, even those who have had a cesarean section. An upright seated position may require a stool under the feet to create some hip flexion. The infant should be positioned at the breast in an open position, so that the upper body is slightly extended. The infant's head should not be cradled in the crook of her arm or cupped in the mother's hand if doing so causes the baby's head to be flexed forward with the chin tucked in. Instead, the infant is held in the cradle position with the head allowed to fall over mother's arm, so the baby is looking up to the breast. The baby is held very close to the mother's body, tucked under the opposite breast.

For women with sore nipples, the cross-cradle position provides more control of attachment. In the cross-cradle position, the mother holds the baby in the arm opposite the breast by grasping the baby's shoulders and upper back and tucking the baby closely under both breasts; this allows the head to fall through the web space in her hand. The baby's head will tip back, creating plenty of room between the chin and chest so that the mouth can gape. The baby will be able to open the mouth widely if the mother entices him or her by moving the baby, not the breast. The mother's hand should grasp the breast well behind the areola, compressing and projecting the breast forward so that when the infant latches on with flanged lips, he or she connects deeply with the tissue behind the areola to extract colostrum or milk. The infant should be attached asymmetrically, with more of the underside of the breast laid on the baby's gaping lower jaw and the nipple tucked into the baby's mouth last, disappearing just under the upper gum line. The baby is drawn into the mother's body deeply. Latching asymmetrically allows the baby to strip the breast effectively, minimizing nipple trauma and maximizing colostrum or milk transfer.[22] Helpful materials for health care providers, mothers, and families are available at Coffective.com.

Every mother-infant pair should have frequent assessment of latch-on during the early postpartum period. This is an opportunity to teach parents about their infant's unique characteristics and to practice good attachment techniques. If the mother is still hospitalized, skilled personnel should work with the mother and infant to improve latch-on and to assess colostrum or milk transfer. Sustained suckling with deep attachment promotes effective colostrum and milk extraction. If the mother reports poor feeding after the infant has been discharged, the infant should be evaluated. An infant who is consistently unsatisfied after feeding for long periods is probably not getting enough to eat at the breast and may not be latched on correctly. Babies who are suckling intermittently should be assessed for deep latch.

After the baby has attained deep latch, the mother may improve feeding with facilitated feeding techniques, such as breast compression to encourage swallowing. The mother may also massage the baby to encourage active, wakeful feeding.

The mother will not need to provide as much structure and guidance for the baby after breastfeeding is established. Lactogenesis can be adversely affected by hormones of the stress response, so it is important to offer the mother reassurance and to assess her general well-being during a time that is often quite fraught, especially for first-time parents in an increasingly mobile society. Lack of close-relationship social support is the primary cause of early breastfeeding cessation.[22,23]

Breast Engorgement

Breast engorgement may occur on the third or fourth postpartum day in first-time mothers and sooner in women who have had previous births. It can usually be minimized by feeding the infant 8 to 12 times each day in the days leading up to the milk coming in. Mothers should be taught to evaluate the difference between sustained and intermittent suckling, grazing at breast, and milk or colostrum removal. A feeding log helps the mother assess whether she needs to wake her baby. Babies who are gulping with feeds and having copious wet diapers with yellow stools do not need to be awakened to feed to meet their own needs but may be awakened after 2 to 3 hours to assist the mother to manage engorgement. Some women with engorgement may need to express some milk manually or with a pump to soften the areola enough to allow the infant to latch on. When an engorged breast is not well emptied, the resulting backpressure on the milk glands can result in decreased milk production.[24] Treatment of engorgement benefits from mothers and providers understanding breastfeeding as a dynamic and interdependent relationship.

Some mothers develop sore nipples as a result of difficulty with latch-on during engorgement. To prevent nipple damage and extract milk, infants need to latch deeply onto engorged breasts. A mother with engorgement may need to compress the breast manually to form it for the infant's mouth.

Deep asymmetric latch-on and sustained suckling will resolve most engorgement. If engorgement persists, ice packs may be applied to the breasts between feedings to reduce edema, and hot packs may be applied right before feedings to soften the areola. Pumping for a minute or two before latch-on may also help. If the mother cannot get her infant to latch on, direct observation of feeding is required. The mother with engorgement at discharge should have a breastfeeding support plan. This may include breast pump rental and follow-up with a visiting nurse, a lactation nurse, or other health care providers. Obstetric nurses can provide 24-hour phone support and triage for breastfeeding mothers.[25]

Coffective.com has resources for breastfeeding families. The U.S. Department of Health and Human Services also maintains an evidence-based information site for breastfeeding women at http://womenshealth.gov/breastfeeding.

Delayed Let-Down

Let-down, or milk ejection, results from smooth muscle contraction of the myoepithelial cells surrounding the secretory alveoli of the breast. Oxytocin produced in response to the infant's suckling as well as to the sight, sound, and smell of the infant causes this contraction and the resultant milk flow. Uterine cramping signals early oxytocin production, and the presence of these cramps is a good predictor of ultimate breastfeeding success. The cramping is usually more pronounced with second and subsequent infants. Mothers may need analgesics in the early postpartum period to manage the "afterpains." After a few weeks, the let-down response may be sensed as a tingling sensation throughout the breasts, followed by leaking of milk from the nipple.

Stress, pain, and alcohol inhibit let-down. The let-down response is enhanced through thoughts about the infant, breast massage, and relaxation. Although all mothers should be informed about inhibiting and enhancing factors for let-down, this information may be especially important for mothers who need to pump milk from their breasts, including mothers of premature infants or mothers returning to work.[26]

Low Milk Production. Low milk supply is the most common reason for discontinuing breastfeeding. Lactogenesis is a complex and not completely understood biochemical and psychosocial process. Mothers who have suboptimal milk production must be assessed for physiologic, psychological, and social support variables that may be influencing milk supply.[25]

Low milk production usually results from inadequate suckling and breast emptying, low prolactin levels, inadequate mammary glandular tissue, delayed or inadequate lactogenesis, or undetermined causes. Medications or herbs to increase milk supply do not produce consistent results. Double pumping in addition to nursing produces the best results for increasing supply.

Prolactin levels measured in mothers before and after breastfeeding show a threefold increase after suckling. A similar increase in prolactin levels occurs after the mother pumps her breasts. Uniformly low prolactin levels suggest an endocrine basis for low milk supply.

Inadequate mammary glandular tissue can result in low milk production despite normal prolactin levels. Breast glandular tissue should be assessed prenatally and may also be assessed during the breastfeeding newborn's first office visit, if the health care provider has any concern about milk supply. The mother should report that the areola darkened and the breasts increased by one cup size during pregnancy.

If lactogenesis is delayed or inadequate, the infant should receive supplemental feedings while breast stimulation is increased with a breast pump.[25] Close follow-up of mother and baby is required.

Lactogogues or galactogogues are medications or herbs believed to improve milk production. In small randomized controlled studies, lactogogues had no statistically significant effect when compared with placebo. The Academy of Breastfeeding Medicine recommends caution when considering medication or herbs to enhance milk production, because neither pharmaceutical nor herbal lactogogues have produced consistent results.[25]

Low Infant Weight Gain

Low infant weight gain in the first few weeks after birth is usually caused by inappropriate breastfeeding management in the hospital and during the immediate postdischarge period. Infants who have lost 8% or more of their birth weight must be closely monitored to prevent problems. Infants who are feeding well should have four or more milk curd stools per day by the fourth day and at least six wet diapers per day.

To assess an infant with low weight gain, providers must observe a breastfeeding session. Strategies to increase success include breast pumping to increase the milk supply and increased feeding frequency. Mothers may also use techniques to arouse sleepy infants, such as stroking the infant's back, talking softly to the infant, stroking the feet, rocking the baby from sitting position to lying (supported baby sit-ups), changing the diaper, and placing the infant on the mother in skin-to-skin contact.

A supplemental nursing system can deliver supplemental formula or pooled pasteurized human milk while the infant is breastfeeding. Supplemental nursing systems offer an important alternative to bottles; breastfed babies who are offered bottles sometimes have difficulty returning to the breast, especially when the mother's milk supply is low. The supplemental nursing system offers increased flow at the breast to keep the baby interested and engaged while increasing stimulation and extraction at the breast.

Significant infant weight loss or difficult management problems require careful evaluation and follow-up. Health care providers should consider consultation with lactation consultants or physicians experienced with breastfeeding management and care of infants with failure to thrive.[17]

Cracked Nipples

Cracked nipples are usually caused by attachment or latch-on problems. The nipple becomes abraded when the infant latches only to the tip of the nipple, instead of to the underside of the breast followed by the nipple. Mothers should be taught the asymmetric latch-on technique. Treatment of cracked nipples includes correcting the attachment and supporting milk extraction.

Nipple damage and pain are sometimes so severe that mothers temporarily stop breastfeeding and maintain lactation by pumping or hand expression. Twenty-four hours of nipple rest and pumping may allow enough healing of the irritated nipples for breastfeeding to be resumed. Close-interval assessment of mother-infant dyad breastfeeding sessions will limit the need for nipple rest.

Sore nipples can heal while the baby is breastfeeding if the attachment is corrected. The mother should be taught to listen for audible swallowing to determine when the infant is actively feeding. She can remove the infant from the breast after the nursing rhythm changes from active deep suckling that removes milk to leisurely comfort sucking. The mother should be taught to use her finger to detach the baby by sliding her finger over the baby's lips, over the gum line, all the way back to the hinge of the baby's jaw. This will protect the nipple from further damage.

Medical-grade lanolin may improve breastfeeding comfort if the nipples are dry and cracked. For severely damaged nipples, hydrogel dressings are useful to maintain a moist wound healing environment. In addition, mothers must avoid overdrying their nipples and should apply warm, moist compresses after feedings to soothe and promote healing. Nipple soreness typically improves after a rest from breastfeeding for 24 hours and institution of the correct attachment position. Mothers will need to pump every 3 hours while not breastfeeding. In general, it takes 10 days for sore nipples to heal completely. If improvement is not progressive, the health care provider should reevaluate the breastfeeding technique and treatment plan. A referral to a lactation specialist may be indicated. Bacterial infection or yeast overgrowth should be considered and treated appropriately with topical or oral antibiotics or antifungal medication.[26,27]

Mastitis

Mastitis, or cellulitis of the interlobular connective tissue of the breast, is often a marker of breastfeeding problems. Mastitis usually manifests with fever, generalized malaise, influenza-like symptoms, local erythema, and breast warmth and tenderness. Bacteria often gain entry to breast tissue through a combination of unrelieved breast engorgement with cracked or abraded nipples.

Treatment of mastitis includes the application of warm packs to the breast and frequent breastfeeding or pumping. In addition to these nonpharmacologic interventions, the infection is treated with antibiotics such as amoxicillin-clavulanate, dicloxacillin, or a broad-spectrum cephalosporin to cover a probable staphylococcal or streptococcal infection. The infant's sucking technique and the mother's breastfeeding pattern and support system should also be evaluated. Mastitis can progress to abscess if early intervention is not instituted. Therefore, any occurrence of influenza-like symptoms in a breastfeeding mother requires an evaluation for mastitis.[27]

Referrals

Expectant and new mothers may be referred to breastfeeding support groups such as La Leche League International, Nursing Mothers Council, and Women, Infants, and Children (WIC) services. Patients who need additional assistance or specialized help during prenatal or postpartum periods should be referred to breastfeeding or lactation specialists. Lactation consultants can be found through the International Lactation Consultant Association. The AAP, Academy of Breastfeeding Medicine, La Leche League International Medical Associates, and International Board of Lactation Consultant Examiners are resources for health care providers.

OTHER CONSIDERATIONS

Breast Pumps and Hand Expression

Breast milk can be expressed by hand or by use of a breast pump. Hand expression is a learned skill that can easily be taught. Many different types of manual and electric pumps are available. Hospital-grade electric pumps are available for rent, and effective single-user pumps can be purchased from vendors specializing in breastfeeding support. A mother should choose the pump designed for her needs. Mothers should be provided with written instructions about milk storage and handling. Women may be directed to the Centers for Disease Control and Prevention (CDC) website for specific information about human milk storage and handling.

Working Mothers

Mothers who must return to work or school or be separated from their infants for regular periods can usually continue breastfeeding. The milk supply will adjust to the demands. Depending on the mother and the child's age, the mother may need to pump the breasts two or three times per day to maintain a milk supply for the infant's bottle feeding by a caretaker.[28]

Multiple Births

Twins or triplets can breastfeed successfully. With proper support and management, many mothers will have a sufficient supply. Initially, twins may need to be breastfed separately until they learn how to nurse, progressing to breastfeeding simultaneously. The need for supplemental feedings depends on both the mother's milk supply and the infants' needs.

Weaning

Weaning is a natural process. It is physically and emotionally less painful when it is done gradually and the infant leads the process. As the infant grows, other activities and other foods often replace the need to breastfeed. Babies who wean before 1 year of age should continue to use formula until their first birthday. Weaning may happen as late as 2 or 3 years of age. Some mothers and infants choose to breastfeed into the toddler years, and there is no reason to oppose a continuation of this bond. The ethnographic literature suggests that before the widespread use of artificial infant formulas, children were traditionally nursed for 3 to 4 years.[29]

When mothers desire to wean, feedings should be replaced by supplemental milk or formula (depending on the infant's age), one feeding at a time, for a period of a few weeks until all feedings have been replaced. Cow's milk should be withheld until infants are older than 1 year. When weaning toddlers, mothers may replace some feedings with activities instead of food.

SUMMARY

Breastfeeding is the optimal health care practice in infant feeding. Primary care providers are in a unique position to protect, support, and promote breastfeeding. There are many resources to assist the health care provider in this work.

CHAPTER 13

AGING AND COMMON GERIATRIC SYNDROMES

Joanne Sandberg-Cook • Patricia Hadidian

Demographic predictions for society are for both greater numbers of older adults and increased longevity of the population. By 2020, one in six Americans will be elderly, and by 2050, one in five. The fastest-growing cohort in the late 20th century was the group identified as "old old" (over age 85 years), and the number of centenarians increased the fastest.[1]

Because of this anticipated increase in numbers of older adults, as well as their ethnic diversity, this age group will have an unprecedented need for services and goods. Heart disease, cancer, and cerebrovascular disease continue to be the chief causes of death and disability among older adults. However, Alzheimer disease (AD) now ranks as the fifth leading cause of death in the United States in adults older than 65, with one in three people older than 85 having the disease.[2,3] The most common chronic conditions in addition to AD include arthritis, cardiovascular disease, hypertension, diabetes, and hearing and vision impairment.[2]

CHALLENGES IN PRIMARY CARE

The goal of geriatric primary care is to maximize independence and functional status and shorten the morbidity period in the life of each older adult. The challenges in achieving this goal include ageism, the paucity of geriatric education in the nation's health professional schools, the low numbers of health care providers choosing geriatrics, the complexity of illness in older adults, the increasing numbers of older adults, and cost.

Robert Butler coined the term *ageism* in 1965 to describe the culturally rooted discomfort with growing older. He observed not only revulsion on the part of young people but also fear of losses associated with aging.[4] Neither older adults nor health care providers are immune to ageism. Older adults and their families often determine when to seek screening or treatment and are known to assume that many symptoms of disease are a result of advanced age and therefore have no effective treatment.

Health care providers continue to receive minimum education in gerontology and geriatrics, in spite of the fact that more than 50% of hospitalized patients are older than 65, and a much higher proportion of the office practice is elderly.[5] Recently proposed curricula based on a consensus of minimum geriatric competencies are a start; however, more aggressive interdisciplinary geriatric specific education is crucial.[4-6] Research demonstrates that the presentation of disease is often atypical in an aging patient. Treatment must be based on an understanding of the body's ability to adapt to aging and the effect of aging on pharmacokinetics. Although the human body demonstrates remarkable resiliency with aging, physiologic and psychological stress disrupts this adaptation.

An individual experiencing the usual aging pattern is increasingly vulnerable to multiple health problems and experience losses that affect stamina, motivation for self-care, and the ability to function effectively. Functional problems affecting the older adult's mental and physical status and care are aggravated by many factors, including a lack of exercise, nutritional deficiencies, constipation, infection, sleep disturbances, failing cognition, social isolation, and depression. Nonprescription drugs and prescriptions from multiple medical specialists can result in a dangerous mix of medications, which must be identified to avoid adverse reactions and interactions. Reduced memory, slowed mental processing of new information, and impaired sensory input further complicate diagnosis and treatment plans. Additional challenges arise from the use of alcohol and tobacco.

MENTAL STATUS AND FUNCTIONAL ASSESSMENTS

Geriatric specialists have multiple assessment tools, such as the Folstein Mini-Mental State Examination, the Mini-Cog screen for dementia, the Short Portable Mental Status Questionnaire, the AD8 Dementia Screening Interview, and the Montreal Cognitive Assessment (MoCa), to differentiate short-term memory loss from dementia and to observe the progression of cognitive impairment. These tools are screening tools at best and can be misleading in individuals with higher educational levels, lower socioeconomic levels, or vision, hearing, or speech impairments.[7] A detailed history of cognitive change and lifelong habits is a vital element in the differential diagnosis of cognitive impairment and often necessitates an interview with an observant family member or friend. Maintaining a record of the patient's baseline mental status, ruling out depression as a factor in impaired mental status, and tracking the results of subsequent mental status testing are helpful for accurate diagnosis and management.[8] Screening for cognitive impairment is a required part of the Medicare Annual Wellness visit.

Tools for the assessment of functional status, including the Barthel Index, the Physical Self-Maintenance Scale, and the Katz Index, are also well developed, validated, and easily administered. Function is addressed on two levels: (1) basic activities of daily living, including feeding, bathing, dressing, ambulation, and toileting; and (2) the more complex, instrumental activities of daily living, including cooking, shopping, using the telephone, reading, writing, and managing money. Poor performance on functional or mental status testing might explain a failure to respond to medications, noncompliance with exercise or diet recommendations, falls and injuries, or the occurrence of depression or anxiety.[8] The provider should never rely solely on assessment tools to determine an older adult's functional or cognitive capacity because many older adults, even those with impairment, can do very well on testing or are only partially truthful, therefore skewing the results in their favor. Researchers are questioning the use of mental status tests during routine screening and advise their use only after concern for cognitive impairment is raised.

HEALTH SCREENING

Routine screening of older adults for disease remains controversial simply because few outcome data exist for this population. Guidelines for cutoff ages for various screenings vary among entities (Table 13-1). For example, the U.S. Preventive Services Task Force (USPSTF) recommends mammograms only to the age of 75, whereas the American Cancer Society recommends no upper age limit. More recently, the American Board of Internal Medicine Choosing Wisely initiative lists evidence-based recommendations for tests and screenings to help providers and patients make decisions on appropriate care based on the individual's general health, predicted longevity, and personal and family history.[9] These tests should focus on the function, comfort, and safety of the individual. It is reasonable to assess and discuss with the older adult his or her anticipated life expectancy, considering all comorbidities, and his or her personal preferences before embarking on routine screening. Many older patients refuse invasive and even routine screening or treatment regimens, choosing comfort and quality of life over longevity. Explanation to older adults who are accustomed to years of routine screening for issues that are no longer of concern must be carefully undertaken and can be difficult. Annual examinations should be comprehensive, are necessarily time-consuming, and should include responsible family members; however, time should be set aside to discuss care preferences and current recommendations and when to stop screening, especially for cancer.

COUNSELING ELDER DRIVERS

Providing useful assessment and counseling to the older adult driver often falls to primary health care providers. Driving helps older adults remain mobile and independent. However, the incidence of crashes, especially fatal ones, is high among elder

TABLE 13-1 Recommended Screening and Immunizations

Service	USPSTF Rating	CDC	Medicare Benefit
IMMUNIZATIONS			
Pneumovax: one time after age 65	B	Y	Y
Influenza: annually	B	Y	Y
Hepatitis B: annually	A	Y	Y
Herpes zoster: one time after ago 60	NR	Y	Y
Tetanus: every 10 years	B	Y	Y
CARDIOVASCULAR SCREENING			
Abdominal aorta ultrasound: once in every smoking man			
Hypertension: at each office visit, no age restriction			
CANCER SCREENING			
Colonoscopy: every 10 years after age 50, stopping at age 74	A	Y	Y
Fecal occult blood slides: annually until age 74	A	Y	Y
Breast: every 2 years until age 74	B	Y	Y
Prostate: insufficient evidence for age >75	D		
BONE MASS			
Once at age 65	B	Y	
Other Screenings			
Diabetes	B	Y	Y
Dementia	I		Y
Hearing	I		
Vision	I		
Glaucoma	I		

Y means yes.
Ratings:
A: Recommended service—usually covered by Medicare.
B: Recommended service—usually covered by Medicare.
C: USPSTF recommends against routine use of this service.
D: USPSTF discourages the use of this service.
I: Insufficient evidence for recommendations.
NR: No recommendations.
CDC, Centers for Disease Control and Prevention; USPSTF, U.S. Preventive Services Task Force.
Modified from Reuben D, Herr, K, Pacala J, et al: *Geriatrics at your fingertips*, ed 16, New York, 2014, American Geriatrics Society; and Nichols J, Hall W: Screening and preventive services for older adults. *Mt Sinai J Med* 78(4):498-508, 2011.

drivers.[10] Older adults will comfortably report difficulty with selected driving situations, including driving in bright sunlight or at dusk or transitions from light to darkness (e.g., driving into a parking garage, driving in bad weather, and driving at night). These situations are often easy to avoid, and many older adults will voluntarily give up driving in these situations. Older adults may also avoid interstate driving or driving over long distances. However, some older adults may lack insight into the extent of their driving impairment as related to information processing, memory, and visual-spatial orientation, thereby putting themselves and others at great risk.[11] The incidence of traffic accidents begins to increase in this population around the age of 75 and increases with age. On average, there are 500 motor vehicle injuries and 15 deaths daily involving older adults.[12] Assessment of cardiovascular status, mental and cognitive status, vision, hearing, balance, gait, range of motion, and strength of hips and knees can provide information regarding the older adult's ability to drive. Reports from family members or friends are very informative. Those drivers judged at risk should be referred to the registry of motor vehicles for a road test or to a private rehabilitation facility where trained screeners, usually occupational therapists, can test the older adult's driving skills in a safe environment. Frank discussions with patients, families, and supportive peers that elaborate the risks of driving can be difficult, especially if the recommendation is to discontinue driving, but are essential to protect the safety of the elder driver and the public at large. Mandatory reporting of unsafe drivers is the law in many states.

IMPORTANCE OF ADVANCE DIRECTIVES

The primary care of older adults includes a discussion of advance directives and the identification of a health care proxy or durable power of attorney for health care. A living will or similar document, which describes in detail the patient's wishes with regard to resuscitation, hospitalization, treatment goals and limits, and a health care proxy, should be part of each patient's health care record. The goal in completion of advance directives is to provide the individual autonomy in decisions regarding his or her manner and location of death as well as relieving family burden and conflict while the older individual is mentally competent to do so.

Silveira and colleagues in two retrospective cohort studies measured trends over time of advance directive completion and compared hospitalizations before death and death in hospital. They found an increase in completion of advance directives from 47% in 2000 to 72% in 2010. There was also a coincident finding of a decrease in the proportion of patients dying in the hospital from 45% to 35%, although it is difficult to prove completion of an advance directive as a causative factor.[13]

Time to discuss choices and offer explanations of terminology can be set aside in an office visit; ideally, the named health care proxy is included. Individual states are now offering forms online and are keeping this information in statewide registries. A lawyer is usually not necessary for the completion of these documents; witnesses and notarization are all that are typically required. Typically emergency medical technicians are unable to implement advance directives. Once emergency services are called, stabilization and transport to the nearest hospital are required. Once the patient has been evaluated, advance directives can be activated.

The Physician Orders for Life-Sustaining Treatment (POLST) or Medical Orders for Life-Sustaining Treatment (MOLST) Paradigm programs are designed to improve the quality of care people receive at the end of life. These programs are based on effective communication of patient wishes, documentation of medical orders, and a promise by health care professionals to honor these wishes. Recent studies confirm that patients with POLST Paradigm instructions were less likely to die in the hospital and more likely to receive the care specified than those without such orders.[14] These are typically printed on a brightly colored form, often pink, as well as on wallet-sized cards for portability. The existence and regulation of POLST Paradigm programs vary from state to state. The website www.polst.org can be used to check for a local POLST Paradigm program.

THE CHALLENGE OF GERIATRICS

The challenge for any health care provider who treats older adults is to recognize the individual aging process, promote optimum health and functioning, provide care and comfort during illness, minimize the length and severity of the premorbid illness and disability period, and finally, ensure a comfortable and dignified death

To this end, several models of care have been proposed over the past decade designed to shorten or avoid hospital admission, avoid hospital readmission after discharge, reduce overtreatment, provide older adults and their families with information specific to their individual situation and preferences, and provide care in the preferred setting, allowing aging in place. The most studied and successful are transitional care models designed to help older adults with multiple comorbidities transition from hospital to home or nursing home or from nursing home to home (see Chapter 2). The 2010 Affordable Care Act established a variety of transitional care programs designed to improve quality and reduce costs. Often these services are managed by an advanced practice nurse and frequently include discharge planning, case management services, counseling or coaching, and assistance with navigating the health care system.[15] Basic primary care services delivered to individuals at home as well as restorative services such as physical and occupational therapy can also be features.[16] House-call programs are gaining in popularity and availability because care delivered at home is timely, less expensive, and more acceptable to frail elders.[17] Town or parish nurses are becoming more common as communities look for better ways to care for their aging population. The value of caring for vulnerable older adults in their homes is substantiated in multiple studies and is confirmed as preferable in most surveys of older adults.[18]

Continuity of primary care services as the end of life approaches is the key to avoiding overdiagnosis, unnecessary hospitalizations, and overtreatment of acute problems when the outcome is generally acknowledged as death regardless of the intensity of treatment.

COMMON GERIATRIC SYNDROMES

Primary care, including health promotion and disease prevention, as well as the prevention of disease exacerbation, complications, and disability, must continue in all settings in which older adults live and is ideally provided by a coordinated team of health care professionals. Geriatric syndromes are complex, multicausal entities that test the diagnostic prowess of the health care provider. Chaos may reign, but therein lies the challenge in meeting the primary care needs of older patients. This section discusses six common syndromes seen in older adults: polypharmacy, cognitive impairment, dehydration, falls, failure to thrive (FTT), and elder abuse.

POLYPHARMACY

Definition and Etiology

Polypharmacy is the use or misuse of multiple drugs (usually defined as more than five per person or any not medically indicated), both prescription and nonprescription, and their interaction with one another. It is a common cause of iatrogenic illness in older adults, including a higher risk of falls and drug-related changes in mental status.[19] Polypharmacy arises from many sources, including multiple comorbidities, multiple prescribers for the same patient, fear of accusation of ageism or cultural bias, changing medical guidelines for treatment of specific conditions, medication advertising, and good intentions to treat the side effects of one medication with another.[20]

Pathophysiology

Drug distribution and clearance are affected by normal aging changes, including a reduction in lean body mass and blood flow to the kidney and liver and an increase in body fat. These issues are compounded in frail older adults because, in addition to normal aging changes, disease alters the function of specific organ systems and affects pharmacokinetics. Abnormalities in the cardiac conduction system, decreased gastric acid production, decreased total body water, and increased total body fat all affect drug absorption and metabolism. Age-related renal changes lead to increased drug levels and potentially toxic effects of renally excreted drugs.[20]

Consequences of Polypharmacy

The most prevalent consequence of polypharmacy is adverse drug reaction leading to change in mental status, sedation, falls, and other serious outcomes (Box 13-1). The risk of adverse drug reactions increases precipitously as the number of medications an individual takes increases.[21] A drug-related side effect should be considered for any presenting symptom until proven otherwise. Drug-drug interactions and poor adherence because of the complexity of a medication regimen or cost are other consequences of polypharmacy.

BOX 13-1

Medication Analysis: General Considerations

DRUG ISSUES RELATED TO DRUG CLASS

1. Pharmacokinetic properties of class (e.g., ACE inhibitors affect renal excretion)
2. Common side effects (e.g., ACE = hyperkalemia)

PATIENT ISSUES

1. Common adverse effects in older adults:
   - Anticholinergic effects
   - Constipation or diarrhea
   - Indigestion
   - Delirium
   - Dizziness
   - Depression
   - Dermatologic effects
2. Specific prior problems in older adults that affect medication risks:
   - Dehydration
   - Drug cost
   - Malnutrition
   - Poor compliance
   - Renal failure

ACE, angiotensin-converting enzyme.

Management

To avoid the negative consequences of polypharmacy, it is important to review all medications at each patient contact and to maintain good communication with consultants. There are a number of tools available to assist with evaluating for polypharmacy. The Beers list is the most familiar for practicing providers in the United States.[22] It provides a list of potentially inappropriate medications in all patients age 65 and older as well as a list of potentially inappropriate medications for those older adults with specific conditions. Although not 100% foolproof, this tool enables providers to plan interventions that may minimize drug-related problems and reduce costs.

Other tools, more often used in Europe and Canada, are the Improved Prescribing in the Elderly Tool (IPET), Screening Tool to Alert Doctors to the Right Treatment (START), Screening Tool of Older Persons' Potentially Inappropriate Prescriptions (STOPP), McLeod criteria, and Medication Appropriateness Index (MAI).[23]

Patients should be encouraged to carry an up-to-date list of their medications and have one readily available to give emergency medical providers in the event of an emergency. Patients should be encouraged to order drugs from a pharmacy with computerized drug data whenever possible. As an educator for both the patient and the health care provider, the pharmacist plays an important role in preventing poor outcomes from polypharmacy. In fact, most pharmacies are equipped with programs that can review a list of medications and immediately detect potential drug-drug interactions and alert prescribers. Providers also can subscribe to affordable, point-of-care, technologic clinical tools that aid in identifying potential drug-drug interactions and safety concerns.

The drug risk/benefit ratio should be determined when considering the use of any new drug. The general principles of drug therapy in geriatrics are first considered, such as the pharmacodynamics of the drug class and common adverse effects experienced by older adults (see Box 13-1). For example, older adults are more susceptible than younger adults to the anticholinergic effects of drugs. Second, the specific side effect profiles of a drug class and a patient's history of previous adverse effects, morbidity, and general nutritional state are considered. The known or suspected risk is weighed against the presumed benefit of administering the drug. "Start low and go slow" is common advice when prescribing for older adults. The prescription of any drug regardless of clinical indication must be balanced against the patient's functional and cognitive capacity as well as predicted longevity. The ongoing medical necessity of all drugs should be reviewed at each visit, with strong consideration given to discontinuing those that are marginally effective, may be causing an adverse effect, and are poorly tolerated by the patient or being administered to a patient with a limited life span.

COGNITIVE IMPAIRMENT

Definition and Etiology

The most common and feared cause of a decline in cognition is dementia, and the most prevalent form of dementia is AD (see Chapter 193). The cost of treating AD approaches $100 billion annually in the United States. The incidence of AD doubles every 5 years after age 65, approaching 30% by age 85 and 50% by age 90.[13,24]

Clinical Presentation

AD is a chronic, irreversible illness with a gradual onset and a steady decline in cognition. Short-term memory loss is the primary symptom in AD, along with one or more of the following: disorientation; disturbance in executive functioning (planning, organizing, and abstract thinking); problems with activities of daily living; and one of three common neurologic disorders—aphasia, apraxia, or agnosia. Day-night sleep cycles are often reversed; consciousness and psychomotor changes are not evident until late in the disease. Irritability, withdrawal, and apathy may be exhibited in the early stages of the disease. Psychotic symptoms such as paranoia and agitation can be seen later in the disease (see Chapter 193).

Delirium, a common cause of cognitive change in the sick or hospitalized elder, is a transient waxing and waning level of consciousness. It is characterized by acute onset and fluctuations in orientation and attention. The incidence in hospitalized elders is high and associated with longer lengths of stay and increased rates of admission to nursing homes. Delirium is more likely seen in the hospitalized cognitively impaired older adult. Some providers believe that in-hospital delirium may actually be the unmasking of a previously undiagnosed dementia (see Chapter 192).

DEHYDRATION

Definition and Etiology

Dehydration is more prevalent in older adults and has a greater likelihood of a negative outcome than in younger adults. It is defined as a state of fluid intake deprivation and/or excess fluid loss. Accompanying electrolyte imbalances may ensue (see Chapter 210). The most significant electrolyte abnormality is sodium imbalance. Because of this, dehydration is further categorized by the associated relationship between free water and sodium.[25]

In older adults, dehydration is often multifactorial (Box 13-2 and Table 13-2). Environmental issues, polypharmacy, and diseases prevalent in older adults predispose this group to dehydration, as do age-related changes in plasma osmolality and thirst response.

TABLE 13-2 Dehydration Management

	Low Risk*		High Risk*	
Setting	**Treatment**	**Comfort**	**Treatment**	**Comfort**
Office practice	OR[†]	OR	NA	OR
Home	OR, clysis	OR	NA	OR
Nursing home	OR, clysis	OR	Clysis, intravenous	OR
Hospital	OR	OR	IV	OR

*Risk is defined by clinical parameters and may include severity of electrolyte imbalance. High risk may be defined as a serum sodium ≥150 mEq/L, an inability to take sufficient fluids by mouth, or comorbid conditions that increase the risk of complications from rehydration (e.g., congestive heart failure). This definition of risk is not research based.
[†]OR is used when fluids by mouth are possible.
NA, not applicable; OR, oral rehydration.

BOX 13-2

Common Causes of Dehydration

INTAKE (FLUID DEPRIVATION)

Environmental Factors
- Restricted ambulation
- Decreased hearing or vision

Increased Metabolic Demands
- Infections (resulting in malaise, reduced appetite, and poor intake)

Dehydration
- Poorly fitting dentures
- Esophageal lesions
- Neurologic disease

Pharmacologic Factors
- Narcotics
- Sedatives
- Neuroleptics
- Anticholinergics

Normal Aging Changes
- Ineffective water conservation
- Decreased thirst drive

Poor Appetite
- Fatigue
- Constipation
- Depression

Fluid Limitations
- Before a procedure or operation
- Prevention of urinary incontinence
- Management of heart failure
- Management of hyponatremia

OUTPUT (FLUID EXCESS)

Environmental Factors
- Hot weather
- Alcohol intake

Increased Metabolic Demands
- Infections (resulting in tachypnea and sweating)
- Diarrhea
- Vomiting
- Sweating

Endocrine Disorders
- Diabetes insipidus
- Hyperglycemia or glycosuria

Pharmacologic Factors
- Diuretics
- Laxatives

Normal Aging Changes
- Ineffective salt conservation

Pathophysiology

Three principal changes in the homeostatic mechanism that controls the volume and osmolality of extracellular fluids occur in older adults. These normal changes result in a reduced adaptability and reserve to deal with system stressors. First, the thirst response, which is stimulated by dehydration, is diminished and results in an increased solute/water ratio. Second, decreased renal plasma flow may be responsible for a decline in the body's ability to concentrate urine. The inability to concentrate urine prevents the body from retaining enough fluid to avert dehydration. Finally, vasopressin release stimulated by low fluid volume is diminished. Therefore the inherent homeostatic mechanism that prevents the sequelae of hypovolemia is blunted.[25]

Clinical Presentation

The presenting symptoms of dehydration are often vague and nonspecific. These include confusion, lethargy, rapid weight loss, and functional decline. Dehydration is often a feature of FTT. The history should include an assessment of fluid intake, functional status, weight, and cognition. The presence of constipation may indicate a lack of water intake (see Box 13-2).

Physical Examination

The physical examination includes a cardiovascular assessment and may reveal an orthostatic drop in blood pressure and a rise in pulse, indicating volume depletion. Temperature may be elevated as a result of dehydration or an inflammatory or infectious process. Mucous membranes are often not noticeably dry until severe dehydration is present. Because of changes in skin collagen, poor skin turgor, often used as a sign of dehydration in younger individuals, is unreliable in older adults. The tongue may be swollen and furrowed.

Diagnostics

Laboratory data include a review of serum electrolytes, blood urea nitrogen (BUN)/creatinine ratio, osmolality, hematocrit and hemoglobin, and glucose. A BUN/creatinine ratio of 25:1 or more suggests dehydration. Dehydration is present when the sodium level is greater than 148 mEq/L.[25] However, with isotonic or hypotonic dehydration, serum sodium is normal or low, respectively. Hematocrit is elevated compared with the level of hematocrit when the patient is well hydrated. Respiratory and genitourinary infections are common, and a urinalysis and chest x-ray studies may be appropriate.

Differential Diagnosis

Fever, poor fluid intake, iatrogenic drug use, and gastrointestinal fluid losses are the most common causes of dehydration in older adults. Other causes of dehydration should be pursued if electrolyte imbalances persist after treatment, with a focus on the endocrine system (see Chapter 210). However, older adults respond slowly to the treatment of severe electrolyte abnormalities.

Management

Management is determined by the severity of the electrolyte imbalance, the treatment setting, and the patient's treatment goals. Fluid deficit is determined by establishing the pre-illness weight minus the current weight.

$$\text{Pre-illness weight (kg)} - \text{Current weight (kg)} = \text{Fluid deficit (L)}^{26}$$

A "prescription" for oral fluid replacement can then be recommended to include half of the calculated fluid deficit plus ongoing losses in the first 24 hours, totaling at least 1500 mL/day.[13] Although oral hydration may be the preferred route, patients who are vomiting, drowsy, or cognitively impaired may not be able to comply. In that case, especially if the patient resides in a nursing facility, hypodermoclysis (clysis) may be a good alternative.[27] This is a subcutaneous administration of fluid into the upper arm or abdomen using a standard subcutaneous needle or "button." Maximum volume of (isotonic) fluid administered subcutaneously is 1500 mL per site per 24 hours. There are many advantages to the subcutaneous route for hydration. The cost is substantially lower, there are fewer side effects, it can be administered in a variety of settings including the office or nursing facility, and it may result in avoidance of hospital admission. Clysis should not be used in an emergency situation.

Intravenous administration of fluid remains the fastest method for rehydration, but comes with a cost. The fluid type used depends on the serum sodium level, which depends on the availability of a laboratory. The administration and monitoring of the fluid and intravenous site requires specialized training often not available outside the hospital setting. It is often difficult and painful to insert a cannula into dehydrated, older patients, and the process may not be consistent with the patient's advance directives.

Complications include fluid overload, heart failure, or cerebral edema; there can be pain or infection or infiltration of fluid at the insertion site. After dehydration has been treated, it may take weeks or months for the older adult to regain functional or cognitive losses.

Education

Education focuses on the prevention of dehydration (Box 13-3). When it occurs, the amounts and types of fluids to ingest are included in the educational plan. Fluids high in sodium (e.g., tomato juice, bouillon, or sports drinks) are appropriate for those with low sodium levels, whereas water is appropriate for those with high sodium levels. Caffeinated and alcoholic beverages, especially beer, have a mild diuretic effect and should be avoided.

FALLS

Definition and Etiology

Falling is an unintentional loss of balance that results in a position change and contact with the ground. The most feared sequela of a fall is a fracture. Quality of life may also be severely affected by a "fear of falling," with self-imposed isolation and immobility causing a vicious cycle of risk. Fall assessment

BOX 13-3

Dehydration Prevention

- Drink six to eight 8-ounce glasses of water or juice daily.
- Take a full glass of water or juice with medications.
- Drink more than usual in hot weather or when you have a fever.
- Keep a fluid intake record for 2 days.
- Poor dental hygiene, missing teeth, or poorly fitting dentures will interfere with food and fluid intake.
- People with memory problems need fluid monitoring.

focuses on known risk factors, including sensory abnormalities and abnormalities of the central and peripheral nervous system, musculoskeletal system, and cognition.[28,29]

In a community sample, one third to one half of older adults fell each year. The probability of falling increases with age. In long-term care, the annual fall incidence per resident is greater than 50%. Approximately 20% to 30% of falls result in major injuries, including lacerations, contusions, and head injuries; 3% to 5% result in fractures. Falls are a major contributor to death in the older population and contribute to 40% of nursing home admissions.[30]

Pathophysiology

Falls are multifactorial in origin. The majority occur during walking, stepping, or position changes and not during more hazardous activities. Contributing factors are lower extremity weakness, poor balance, orthostatic hypotension, central nervous system disease, cognition and sensory abnormalities, and unsafe environments. The role of lower extremity weakness as a marker of preclinical disability has been well demonstrated.

Sensory input from vision, hearing, vestibular function, and proprioception is important in preventing falls. Visual impairment increases as a result of normal age-related changes and the increased prevalence of ocular diseases. Normal age-related changes cause glare intolerance and slower adaptation to changes in light levels than in younger adults.

Balance depends on sensory cues and vestibular function, both peripheral and central. Disequilibrium and unsteadiness are common in older adults and are related to aging changes and disease of the inner ear, as well as to changes in the transmission of signals from the periphery. Acute and chronic changes in mental status and depression contribute to falls, but the mechanism of action is unclear. Drugs causing sedation, postural hypotension, and electrolyte imbalance have been implicated in the risk for falls. The use of four or more medications increases the risk for falls, regardless of the type of medication.[29]

Normal aging changes in the cardiovascular system blunt the homeostatic mechanisms that maintain adequate organ perfusion and blood pressure control, causing hypotension and threatening the ability to maintain balance. Musculoskeletal and joint diseases affect balance and gait, as do environmental factors, such as loose rugs, cords, and clutter in the home. A fall erodes the self-confidence of older adults and intensifies their fear of dependence and loss of control over their lives. This may result in more cautious behavior and reduced activity and ambulation because of a fear of falling again. Ironically, the fear of falling is an independent risk factor for further falls.

Clinical Presentation

The clinical presentation of falling is varied. The health history should focus on previous falls and events surrounding a fall, including episodes of syncope, unsteadiness, and dizziness. The mnemonic *DDROPP* (diseases, drugs, recovery, onset, prodrome, and precipitants) helps ensure a complete postfall assessment. The assessment should also focus on any history of coronary artery disease or arrhythmias, vision and hearing problems, neurologic dysfunction, lower extremity joint pain or foot problems, fractures, cognitive changes, and medications.

Self-reported functional scales quickly supplement the history with information on mobility, self-care abilities, mood, hospitalizations, and nutrition. It is important to ask questions in reference to current activities. The reply to "How did you get to this appointment?" is immensely informative, as is simply watching how a patient enters the examination room and with whom.

Physical Examination

A complete physical examination with a focus on postural vital signs is necessary and should include a cardiovascular and neurologic examination, including Romberg test with a sternal nudge and a check for nystagmus. Mobility (including gait and balance), upper extremity function and strength, cognition, vision, and hearing are also examined. Quick and easy mobility and gait tests are now available and correlate positively with the risk for falls and a decline in self-care ability. With the "get up and go" test, the patient is timed as he or she gets up from a chair with his or her arms folded across the chest, walks 10 feet, returns to the chair, and sits down using regular footwear and any regular walking aid.[31] The ease of gait, balance, position change, and turning are evaluated. Completion of the task in 20 seconds or less correlates with functional independence; those taking 30 seconds or more are considered at high risk of falling.

Lower extremity balance is tested by evaluating the patient standing with the feet side by side, semi-tandem and tandem, and balancing for 10 seconds. The functional reach test for balance is completed by asking the individual to reach forward in a parallel plane without taking a step.[32] Patients with a reach of less than 17.8 cm (7 inches) are considered very frail and at higher risk of falling. Patients should be closely monitored by a member of the clinical team while performing any activity that may be associated with falling.

Diagnostics

Most falls are mechanical, but frequent fallers may benefit from additional testing including complete blood count (CBC) (to rule out anemia and infections), electrolytes, BUN, creatinine (to look for dehydration and electrolyte imbalance), serum glucose, and a stool occult blood test. An electrocardiogram (ECG) can help rule out rhythm disturbances. If syncope and ECG abnormalities are present, a myocardial infarction must be excluded, and a careful examination and diagnostic workup for ischemic disease are indicated. If the neurologic examination is positive, magnetic resonance imaging (MRI) will rule out brain or spinal cord lesions or other abnormalities. The patient with true vertigo is most likely to have inner ear disease. Benign positional vertigo (BPV) is common in older adults. The vertigo of BPV is episodic and is provoked by position changes (see Chapter 194).

Management

The goal of treatment and education is to alter modifiable risk factors (Box 13-4). The American Geriatrics Society and the British Geriatrics Society have collaborated on the development of evidence-based fall prevention guidelines.[21,22,33] If lower extremity weakness is present, a referral to a physical therapist for strength training is recommended. Resistance training benefits even those of advanced age and frailty.[33] If balance is altered, balance training consists of having the patient stand on one foot for 10 seconds and gradually increase the time and frequency. Low-intensity tai chi has been demonstrated to improve balance.[34] Balance may also be improved by proper footwear and the use of assistive devices including canes, walking sticks, or walkers. Medication reduction and the avoidance of alcohol are important if hypotension is present. A home safety evaluation or checklist is indicated if trips and falls are prevalent (Figure 13-1).

Complications

Serious complications of falls (e.g., subdural hematoma, hip fracture, or cervical fracture) occur 3% to 5% of the time. Because of the high incidence of osteoporosis in older adults, fractures requiring surgical intervention occur with falls. The most feared fractures are of the hip, but wrist, humerus, and compression fractures of the spine are common and disabling. Soft tissue injury is a more common outcome. Consultation should be considered if complications are suspected, particularly if fracture, syncope, true vertigo, or abnormal cardiovascular or neurologic findings are present.

BOX 13-4

Fall Prevention

- Evaluate the home to eliminate loose cords, clutter, trip hazards, and slippery surfaces.
- Install and use bathroom and stair rails.
- Change position slowly.
- Treat foot problems and wear well-fitting, low-heeled footwear.
- Light the environment well.
- Exercise to maintain lower leg strength.
- Join a tai chi class for balance training.
- Bring all medications, including nonprescription medications, to your health care provider at each visit.
- Have regular hearing and vision testing.

Fall prevention is an excellent example of success through the collaborative effort of a multidisciplinary team.[35] Physical and occupational therapists provide appropriate exercise, balance, and gait-training programs and teach patients about environmental hazards. Physicians, nurse practitioners, and physician assistants assess medication usage and monitor the treatment of orthostatic hypotension, peripheral vascular disease, and incontinence (a few of the immediate causes of falls). Nutritionists prevent dehydration and anemia through teaching sessions. Community exercise and educational programs are fun and effective at improving strength and balance. When falls are prevented, pain, disability, and hospitalization with iatrogenic complications are also prevented.

FAILURE TO THRIVE (FRAILTY)

Definition and Etiology

FTT is a syndrome described as a progressive loss of energy, strength, and stamina leading to decreased function and general physical and cognitive deterioration. A physiologic vulnerability results from reduced reserve and capacity to withstand stress. Patients exhibit signs of anorexia, weight loss, skeletal muscle loss (sarcopenia), and functional decline. There may be

Check Your Risk for Falling

Please circle "Yes" or "No" for each statement below.			Why it matters
Yes (2)	No (0)	I have fallen in the last 6 months.	People who have fallen once are likely to fall again.
Yes (2)	No (0)	I use or have been advised to use a cane or walker to get around safely.	People who have been advised to use a cane or walker may already be more likely to fall.
Yes (1)	No (0)	Sometimes I feel unsteady when I am walking.	Unsteadiness or needing support while walking are signs of poor balance.
Yes (1)	No (0)	I steady myself by holding onto furniture when walking at home.	This is also a sign of poor balance.
Yes (1)	No (0)	I am worried about falling.	People who are worried about falling are more likely to fall.
Yes (1)	No (0)	I need to push with my hands to stand up from a chair.	This is a sign of weak leg muscles, a major reason for falling.
Yes (1)	No (0)	I have some trouble stepping up onto a curb.	This is also a sign of weak leg muscles.
Yes (1)	No (0)	I often have to rush to the toilet.	Rushing to the bathroom, especially at night, increases your chance of falling.
Yes (1)	No (0)	I have lost some feeling in my feet.	Numbness in your feet can cause stumbles and lead to falls.
Yes (1)	No (0)	I take medicine that sometimes makes me feel light-headed or more tired than usual.	Side effects from medicines can sometimes increase your chance of falling.
Yes (1)	No (0)	I take medicine to help me sleep or improve my mood.	These medicines can sometimes increase your chance of falling.
Yes (1)	No (0)	I often feel sad or depressed.	Symptoms of depression, such as not feeling well or feeling slowed down, are linked to falls.
Total______		Add up the number of points for each "yes" answer. If you scored 4 points or more, you may be at risk for falling. Discuss this brochure with your doctor.	

FIGURE 13-1 Algorithm for fall risk assessment and interventions. (From CDC.org, *Stay Independent* brochure. Available at http://www.cdc.gov/homeandrecreationalsafety/pdf/steadi-2015.04/Stay_Independent_brochure-a.pdf accessed Oct 26, 2015.)

accompanying depression and impaired immune function. The results of these signs can be weakness, osteopenia, balance and gait disorders, undernutrition, deconditioning, and slow gait speed.[36]

The diagnostic evaluation of FTT seeks to differentiate reversible from irreversible causes. Because of inconsistent definitions of the syndrome, its incidence is unknown. Approximately 15% of hospitalized older adults with FTT die during hospitalization, and 30% of the survivors are discharged to nursing homes.[37]

Pathophysiology

FTT, also known as *frailty*, is strongly associated with age and is seen in the late stages of decline. Weight loss and sarcopenia are strongly associated with age and undernutrition. The results are decreased strength and endurance, weakness, and fatigue. Loss of muscle mass may result in decreased bone density and slowing of metabolic rate, thereby disrupting thermoregulation and leading to heat and cold intolerance. Age-related changes in lean body mass are partially caused by changes in growth hormone, estrogen, and androgen secretion. Administering these hormones increases lean body mass but does not necessarily improve functional capacity and strength, and the associated risks of lower high-density lipoprotein (HDL), metabolic syndrome, and possibly prostate cancer seem to outweigh the potential benefit.[37] The immune system changes with age, including an overall decline in T cells and decreased effectiveness of T memory cells. This decline may explain the shorter duration of effectiveness of immunizations in older individuals and their increased vulnerability to infections.[38] End-stage chronic diseases (e.g., heart failure, pulmonary disease, renal disease) and malignancy cause weight loss, general weakness, and debility.

Clinical Presentation

Patients with FTT may be seen by their health care provider with any of the following symptoms: weakness, inability to care for self, dizziness, weight and memory loss, and depression. Weight loss in FTT is often gradual. The health history focuses on chronic diseases with signs of organ failure, the presence of gastrointestinal malabsorption, cancer risk factors, infection, thyroid abnormalities, depression, and changes in memory. Nutritional intake and the progression of weight loss are calculated. Adverse reactions to medications, including confusion or anorexia, may be partially responsible for FTT. A history of smoking and alcohol use may be helpful in discovering cause. Reversible causes of FTT are sought (Box 13-5).[39]

BOX 13-5

Failure-to-Thrive Causes

DISEASE
- Organ failure
- Metastases
- Infection
- Stroke
- Thyroid disease
- Fractures

MEDICATION
- Cognitive changes
- Anorexia
- Dehydration

ENVIRONMENTAL CAUSES
- Isolation
- Neglect
- Poverty

PSYCHIATRIC CAUSES
- Depression
- Dementia
- Psychosis
- Delirium

GASTROINTESTINAL CAUSES
- Malabsorption
- Dysphagia
- Dental problems
- Diarrhea
- Vitamin deficiency

Physical Examination and Diagnostics

An unplanned loss of 10% or more of body weight in less than a year requires a search for a reversible cause. A complete physical examination should focus on symptoms, organ failure, infections, and malignancy. A skin, mucous membrane, and eye examination may reveal muscle wasting; ulcerative lesions; and signs of vitamin deficiency, anemia, and dehydration. A complete oral examination, including an evaluation of the dentition and denture fit, is necessary. Tests of swallowing ability and the gag reflex are included in the neurologic examination. Many older women have not had a vaginal or breast examination for years, if ever; thus it is important to consider these as indicated by symptoms to rule out malignancy. Mammography continues to be recommended by the American Cancer Society as long as a woman is in reasonable health and a good candidate for treatment.[40] Pap smears are generally discontinued after age 65, especially if previously screened and negative. Bimanual pelvic examination may be indicated.

Screening tests should include a CBC, electrolytes, kidney and thyroid studies, fasting blood glucose, liver function tests, calcium levels, urinalysis, stool for occult blood × 3, and possibly a chest x-ray examination. Additional diagnostics may be indicated, depending on initial testing, examination, and patient preference.[36]

Any discovered explanation for FTT, such as malignancy or end-stage organ disease, should prompt careful discussion with the older adult and family. The patient, family, or both need to be involved in any decision to perform further or invasive diagnostic testing. The patient or proxy may not always desire treatment of potentially life-threatening conditions, making expensive and invasive diagnostic testing moot. End-of-life support and comfort may be a reasonable approach after discussion and preliminary evaluation.

A lifelong history of anorexia because of body image concerns has been reported in the literature. Older adults may have lifelong patterns of dieting and anorexia nervosa–like symptoms, which can be overlooked as a cause of weight loss in this population.[41]

Management

Adequate protein and caloric intake is mandatory. Meals on Wheels and other community support organizations may be necessary if isolation or functional decline is present. High-calorie and high-protein supplements may be beneficial.[42,43] A daily multivitamin supplement and 800 IU of vitamin D is recommended. Appetite stimulants are not recommended.[9] Depression can be treated with antidepressants and counseling for the older adult and/or caregivers.

Creative solutions to prevent malnutrition in nursing home residents have been proposed and include small group dining for dementia patients, the use of volunteer or family assistants at dinner time, and ethnically appropriate foods.[29]

Regular exercise is possible and helpful in building strength in even the very old, deconditioned nursing home patient. In one study, weight training coupled with nutritional supplements over a 10-week period in nursing home patients ages 85 and older improved muscle strength by more than 125% compared with 3% in the control group.[44-46]

Families need to be included in education and support measures when older adults begin to fail. Often families are the first ones to urge patients to seek health care when the patients themselves are reluctant to do so. Concerned families can be encouraged to set up appointments with health care providers and accompany the older adult to these appointments as a witness and provider of information that may not otherwise be revealed. Patient autonomy can be preserved as long as dementia and depression are not found to be contributing to the frailty. If explanations for FTT are not found, it may be the natural course of life's end.

ELDER ABUSE

Definition

Recent studies indicate that 1 in 10 adults over the age of 60 have experienced abuse for more than 1 year.[47] Elder abuse is defined by the Centers for Disease Control and Prevention (CDC) as "any abuse and neglect of persons age 60 and older by a caregiver or another person in a relationship involving expectation of trust." *Self-neglect* refers to the behavior of an older person that results in being unable to provide for his or her needs. There are seven kinds of elder abuse: physical, sexual, psychological, financial, neglect, abandonment, and self-neglect.[48] Elders with disabilities and dementia are at particular risk. It is believed that close to 50% of elders with dementia experience some type of abuse at the hands of their caregivers.[48] One literature review concluded that 26% to 90% of adult men and women with disabilities experience abuse in their lifetime.[49,50] The vast majority of abusers are family members.[48] Elders whose family members are overwhelmed by caregiving responsibilities or who have problems with mental illness or substance abuse are at higher risk for abuse.[51-53]

Clinical Presentation

Older adults who come into the health care provider's office or hospital with bruises, pressure or rope marks, broken bones, or burns may be suffering physical abuse. Bruising of the breasts or genital area may indicate sexual abuse.[49] Sudden withdrawal from usual activities or a change in behavior or alertness may indicate psychological abuse. A change in financial situation or checks signed by unauthorized persons raises suspicions of financial exploitation. Bedsores, unattended medical needs, poor hygiene or nutritional status, hoarding, or inappropriate clothing for the weather can be signs of neglect or self-neglect.[52] The suffering is often in silence, but an alert health care provider will notice subtle changes and start to question causes.

Management

In the home setting, any suspicion of abuse is reported to the state adult protective services. Concern for abuse in the long-term setting is reported to the long-term care ombudsman, or, if the risk is immediate, the police. Older adults and their caregivers can reduce the risk of abuse by seeking professional help for medical, psychological, and substance abuse problems. Residents of long-term care facilities, knowing their rights as patients and individuals, can report abuse either personally experienced or witnessed to the state long-term care ombudsman. Choosing a trusted person to hold durable power of attorney or to be a guardian reduces the risk of financial abuse. Unfortunately, many older adults in abusive situations are cognitively impaired or mentally ill and often cannot advocate for themselves. In this case, concerned families or friends, health care providers, or religious or community organizations should call state adult protective services. The Elder Justice Act (EJA) was passed into law as part of the Affordable Care Act in 2010.[54] Features of this law include penalties to long-term care facilities that punish whistle-blowers, increased funding for adult protective services, grants for long-term care staff training, and civil and monetary consequences for failing to report abuse in long-term care facilities.

More information on elder abuse can be found on the National Center on Elder Abuse website (www.ncea.aoa.gov/Library/Data); on the American Bar Association Commission on Law and Aging website (www.americanbar.org/groups/law_aging.html); and through adult protective services and long-term care ombudsman program laws by state.

SUMMARY

Comprehensive assessment of geriatric syndromes by an interdisciplinary team may be the preferred approach to problems that clearly involve medical, mental, and social disability (Box 13-6). Annual examinations should be comprehensive, are necessarily time-consuming, and should include responsible family members. Time should be set aside to discuss care preferences

BOX 13-6

Components of a Comprehensive Outpatient Geriatric Evaluation

1. Medical history and physical examination
2. Medication and supplement review
3. General assessment of dentition, hearing, and vision
4. Pain assessment
5. Bowel and bladder function
6. Nutritional status
7. Frequency of falls
8. Cognitive status
9. Emotional status
10. Functional status (activities of daily living [ADLs]; instrumental activities of daily living [IADLs])
11. Balance and gait
12. Social history, alcohol use, home environment (living situation, safety, financial)
13. Advance directive, health care proxy
14. Care preferences

Modified from Reuben D, Herr, K, Pacala J, et al: *Geriatrics at your fingertips*, ed 16, New York, 2014, American Geriatrics Society.

and when to stop screening, especially for cancer. Patients and families should be asked to bring all medications and supplements to the examination and to be prepared with a list of concerns. Please see Box 13-6 for a list of elements included in a comprehensive geriatric evaluation.

Specialized geriatric assessment focuses on prioritizing problems and approaches, improving functional capacity, and minimizing invasive and expensive medical care, with goals focused on high quality of life with the very shortest premorbid period possible and a comfortable, dignified death.

CHAPTER 14

PALLIATIVE AND END-OF-LIFE CARE

Marie A. Bakitas • Constance Dahlin • Margaret Firer Bishop • Imatullah Akyar

Palliative care has long been associated only with hospice care provided at the end of life. Such beliefs by health care providers have limited this care to patients who are dying. However, a preponderance of evidence now demonstrates that this care should begin at the time of any serious or life-limiting illness so that patients and their families can experience the full spectrum of benefits to quality of life, improved symptom control, less depression, reduced family burden, and possibly reduced health care costs.[1-5] Health care consumers may be equally uninformed or misinformed about the range of services offered in palliative care. An opinion poll found that 70% of the general public were "not at all knowledgeable" about palliative care.[6] Subsequent focus groups with consumers resulted in a definition that was found to be informative and to clearly communicate the holistic nature of these services in a nonthreatening fashion. This new definition reads as follows: "Palliative care is specialized medical care for people with serious illness. This type of care is focused on providing patients with relief from the symptoms, pain, and stress of a serious illness—whatever the diagnosis. The goal is to improve quality of life for both the patient and the family. Palliative care is provided by a team of doctors, nurses, and other specialists who work with a patient's other doctors to provide an extra layer of support. Palliative care is appropriate at any age and at any stage in a serious illness, and can be provided together with curative treatment."[6]

PALLIATIVE CARE

DEFINITION AND EPIDEMIOLOGY

In 2004 the National Consensus Project for Quality Palliative Care (NCP) first released *Clinical Practice Guidelines for Quality Palliative Care,* with subsequent editions released in 2009 and 2013.[12] These nationally recognized standards guide the development of palliative care programs in all settings and offer a benchmark for established programs. The NCP endorses the definition put forth by the Centers for Medicare and Medicaid Services: "Palliative care means patient and family-centered care that optimizes quality of life by anticipating, preventing, and treating suffering. Palliative care throughout the continuum of illness involves addressing physical, intellectual, emotional, social, and spiritual needs and [facilitating] patient autonomy, access to information, and choice."[13,14]

Palliative care is operationalized through effective management of pain and other distressing symptoms while incorporating psychosocial and spiritual care with consideration of patient and family needs, preferences, values, beliefs, and culture. Evaluation and treatment should be comprehensive and patient centered with a focus on the central role of the family unit in decision making. Palliative care affirms life by supporting the patient and family's goals for the future, including their hopes for cure or prolongation of life, as well as their hopes for peace and dignity throughout the course of illness, the dying process, and death.[12]

Moreover the NCP expanded the reach of palliative care to include the spectrum of neonates to adults who have progressive, chronic conditions and life-limiting diseases or trauma, congenital issues, and conditions in which individuals are supported by others for their activities of daily living, with a focus on underserved and under-resourced populations.[12]

The goals of palliative care are listed in Box 14-1.[15]

BOX 14-1

Underlying Tenets of Palliative Care

- Care is provided and services are coordinated by an interdisciplinary team.
- Patients, families, and palliative and nonpalliative health care providers collaborate and communicate about care needs.
- Services are available concurrently with or independent of curative or life-prolonging care.
- Patient and family hopes for peace and dignity are supported throughout the course of illness, during the dying process, and after death.
- There is emphasis on coordinated assessment and continuity of care across health care settings. There should be an interdisciplinary team with specialty education, training, and certification.
- Management of physical and psychological symptoms is multidimensional with pharmacologic, interventional, behavioral, and complementary interventions.
- Bereavement is a necessary aspect of every palliative care program.
- Interdisciplinary engagement and collaboration with patients and families to identify, support, and capitalize on patient and family strengths are essential to social support.
- Spiritual care includes exploration, assessment, and attention to spiritual issues of the patient and family, including spiritual and religious rituals and practices for comfort and relief.
- Culture is recognized as a source of resilience and strength for the patient and family, with particular attention to cultural and linguistic competence including plain language, literacy, and linguistically appropriate service delivery.
- Care of the patient at the end of life focuses on the meticulous assessment and management of pain and other symptoms; family guidance as to what to expect during the dying process and the postdeath period is emphasized.
- It is recognized that palliative care includes advance care planning, ethics, and legal aspects of care.

From National Consensus Project for Quality Palliative Care: *Clinical practice guidelines for quality palliative care,* ed 3, Pittsburgh, PA, 2013, National Consensus Project.

ACCESS TO CARE

Most Americans express a wish to spend their final days in their own home, surrounded by loved ones. The reality of dying in the United States in the 21st century is very different; currently 28% of patients die in a hospital and 28% die in nursing homes. Only 30% of those dying patients received hospice services.[19] A recent Institute of Medicine (IOM) report, *Dying in America*, suggests that palliative care offers patients and families the best possible quality of life. This is achieved through patient-centered care, optimal communication with health care professionals, education and professional development of all health care providers, policies and payment systems that support end-of-life care, and public engagement.[19] Resources for learning about palliative care approaches and specialists are listed in Box 14-2.

ADVANCE CARE PLANNING

In primary care, the first step of providing palliative care support is by understanding patients' preferences and helping them to identify goals of care, recognizing that such goals may change as the disease status changes. Health care providers should initiate such discussions as a component of the initial history of all adults, regardless of age or health status, as an important aspect of preventive care.[19] This advance care planning process is ongoing and needs to be revisited whenever a patient's health status or life goals change.[20] It includes discussion and documentation of the patient's values and care preferences through the completion of advance directives. To be complete, it should include the type of care the patient does or does not wish at the end of life and should name a proxy decision maker who can express the

BOX 14-2

Palliative Care Web Resources

American Academy of Hospice and Palliative Medicine (www.aahpm.org) is a national professional organization dedicated to promoting palliative medicine. Services include publications, education, competencies, and certification. Nurses may be nonvoting members.

Americans for Better Care of the Dying (www.abcd-caring.org) is dedicated to social, professional, and policy reform aimed at improving the care system for patients with serious illness and for their families.

Center to Advance Palliative Care (CAPC) (www.capc.org) is a membership organization that provides technical assistance needed to establish palliative care programs as well as opportunities to network with colleagues in the palliative care community. CAPC publications, education calendar, and information about advocacy activities are offered.

Education in Palliative and End-of-Life Care (EPEC) (www.epec.net) is a program with the mission to educate all health care professionals on the essential clinical competencies in palliative care.

End-of-Life Nursing Education Consortium (ELNEC) (www.aacn.nche.edu/ELNEC/about.htm) is a national education initiative to improve end-of-life care in the United States. The project provides training for undergraduate and graduate nursing faculty, continuing education providers, staff development educators, pediatric and oncology specialty nurses, and other nurses in end-of-life care so that they can teach this essential information to nursing students and practicing nurses. Current curricula include ELNEC-Advanced Practice Registered Nurse (APRN), ELNEC-Critical Care, ELNEC-Core, ELNEC-Pediatric Palliative Care, ELNEC-Geriatric, ELNEC-For Veterans, and ELNEC-International programs.

End of Life/Palliative Education Resource Center (EPERC) (www.eperc.mcw.edu) is a site intended to support individuals involved in the design, implementation, or evaluation of end-of-life and palliative education for physicians, nurses, and other health care professionals. More specifically, the site has been designed for use by medical school course and clerkship directors, residency and continuing education program directors, medical faculty, community preceptors, and other professionals who are (or will be) involved in providing end-of-life instruction to health care professionals in training. Major content areas in end-of-life and palliative education include pain, nonpain symptoms, communications skills, ethics, terminal care, and clinical interventions used near the end of life.

Growth House (www.growthhouse.org) is a search engine that offers access to the Internet's most comprehensive collection of reviewed resources for end-of-life care.

Hospice and Palliative Nurses Association (HPNA) (www.hpna.org) fosters exchange of information, experiences, and ideas; promotes understanding of the specialties of hospice and palliative nursing; and studies and promotes hospice and palliative nursing research. It also sets the standards for palliative nursing. Current resources include Palliative Nursing: Scope and Standards of Practice, Competencies for the Hospice and Palliative APN, Core Curriculum for the Advanced Practice Hospice and Palliative Registered Nurse, and a certification review course for APRNs. There is also a social community available for advanced practice nurses.

Hospice Foundation of America (www.hospicefoundation.org) provides education and information about death and dying in America.

Innovations in End-of-Life Care (www.edc.org/lastacts) is an online journal featuring peer-reviewed examples of promising practices in end-of-life care. Each bimonthly issue focuses on a different theme.

National Board for Certification of Hospice and Palliative Nurses (www.nbchpn.org) promotes a certification process that advances quality in the provision of end-of-life care. The advanced practice examination results in the following credential: ACHPN (Advanced Certified Hospice and Palliative Nurse).

National Consensus Project for Quality Palliative Care (www.nationalconsensusproject.org) promotes the implementation of clinical practice guidelines that ensure care of consistent and high quality and that guide the development and structure of new and existing palliative care services.

National Hospice and Palliative Care Organization (www.nhpco.org) is the industry's largest association and leading resource for professionals and volunteers committed to and providing service to patients and their families during end of life.

National Palliative Care Research Center (NPCRC) (www.npcrc.org) is committed to stimulating, developing, and funding research directed at improving care for seriously ill patients and their families. The mission of the NPCRC is to improve care for patients with serious illness and meet the needs of their families by promoting palliative care research. In partnership with the Center to Advance Palliative Care, the NPCRC will rapidly translate these findings into clinical practice.

BOX 14-3

Five Wishes

- The person I want to make care decisions for me when I can't
- The kind of medical treatment I want or don't want
- How comfortable I want to be
- How I want people to treat me
- What I want my loved ones to know

From *Five wishes: an advance directives document.* Available from Aging with Dignity, 888-594-7437 or www.agingwithdignity.org.

patient's goals and care preferences if the patient loses the capacity to express these preferences. Easy-to-use approaches to advance care planning that are tailored to low-literacy populations are now available. These approaches use video representations[21] or websites (e.g., prepareforyourcare.org) based on behavior change theory.[22]

Most standardized advance directive forms are written in a defensive tone, indicating the type of care a patient does not want. Another, more comprehensive approach to this type of documentation, called *Five Wishes,* addresses the type of care a patient *does* want as disease progresses (Box 14-3). For example, patients can describe their wish to shift the focus of medical interventions to "comfort care" when they are very near death. This type of care involves minimizing procedures that do not contribute to comfort. Some common medical procedures may be "invisible" to the provider but uncomfortable for the patient (e.g., daily weights, laboratory tests, vital signs) and hence not appropriate at the very end of life.[23]

Health care providers should ensure that patients' wishes are carried out even when they are not able to speak for themselves.[19] For example, for patients wishing to die at home, it is critical that the proxy decision maker (usually a family member) be prepared to anticipate symptom crises or the moment of natural death. Unprepared family members may panic in such circumstance and call 911. Most do not realize that when the 911 system is activated, emergency medical personnel are obligated by law to perform life-sustaining measures, including cardiopulmonary resuscitation (CPR) and intubation, unless a do-not-resuscitate (DNR) order is written for the home. Many states have provisions for "no code," DNR orders, or out-of-hospital medical orders for life-sustaining treatment for patients at home; such provisions allow emergency personnel to provide comfort care rather than CPR if they are called to the home by family members or if patients are brought to an emergency department with a need for symptom control. A Physician (or Provider) Orders for Life-Sustaining Treatment (POLST) program, available in many states, is useful in identifying ambulatory or outpatient wishes outside of the hospital. More information on individual state efforts regarding POLST-type programs is available at www.ohsu.edu/polst.

SYMPTOM MANAGEMENT IN PALLIATIVE CARE

Palliative care addresses physical, psychological, social, and spiritual distress of the patient and the family. This section describes common symptoms and palliative care management strategies that can be applied by health care providers who care for patients with life-limiting illnesses.

ANOREXIA AND CACHEXIA

Definition and Epidemiology

Anorexia is the reduced desire to eat or reduced calorie intake. Because food is the essence of life and often represents love, a loss of interest in food can be upsetting to families. Anorexia is characterized by a loss of appetite and a loss of interest in food associated with a decrease in food and calorie intake. Food is not appealing, and the patient may be too tired or lose the desire to eat. Eating may cause increased shortness of breath or increased secretions. Cachexia is a state of general malnutrition marked by weight loss, malnutrition, weakness, and emaciation. It can be induced by anorexia and is marked by an equal loss of fat, muscle, and bone mineral content. There is often no improvement with nutritional supplements or increased intake.[24,25]

Anorexia is common in patients with human immunodeficiency virus (HIV) infection and is the second most common symptom in patients with cancer.[25] Anorexia is also common in chronic diseases such as chronic kidney disease, heart failure, and chronic obstructive pulmonary disease (COPD).[26] Adults age 65 to 84 have been found to be significantly more likely to report anorexia than younger adults.[27]

Patients who have advanced dementia may experience loss of appetite and decreasing oral intake as a marker of the transition to end-stage disease. Progressive anorexia occurs as the patient nears death and is a natural part of the dying process.[24]

Similarly, cachexia prevalence varies widely because of various diagnostic criteria and according to the disease and disease state. Prevalence ranges from 12% to 85% mostly in cancer, chronic infections (acquired immunodeficiency syndrome [AIDS], tuberculosis), and other chronic illnesses (rheumatoid arthritis; renal, heart, and liver failure; COPD).[26]

Pathophysiology

Anorexia and cachexia are complex problems associated with a multifactorial combination or cascade of contributing problems. Research has focused on varied and complex interactions that can trigger a chronic inflammatory state resulting in abnormal metabolic functioning. Classically, cachexia is known to be a combination of reduced caloric intake and increased catabolism, which is associated with negative protein and energy balance and results in accelerated weight loss.[28,29]

Anorexia and cachexia can be related to physical, psychological, or physiologic factors, including the following[26,30]:

- Metabolic abnormalities: cytokine production, chronic inflammation, tumor-produced peptides, mechanical obstruction, altered carbohydrate (insulin resistance, glucose intolerance), protein (decreased synthesis), and fat (lipolysis) metabolism
- Gastrointestinal disorders: impaired gastric emptying, constipation, stomatitis, nausea and vomiting, altered smell and taste perceptions, xerostomia
- Systemic infections; oral, pharyngeal, or esophageal infections
- Medications, treatment side effects (amphetamines, antibiotics, opioids, cancer treatments)
- Physical symptoms: pain, fatigue, increased resting energy expenditure

- Psychological symptoms: stress, anxiety, impaired situational coping, and depression
- Learned food aversions, dentition problems

Clinical Presentation and Physical Examination

Comprehensive assessment of anorexia is important. Completing a careful history focused on nutritional issues and a physical examination focused on loss of subcutaneous fat, muscle wasting, edema, or ascites can reveal potentially reversible physiologic and psychological causes that can guide management strategies.[26,30]

An international consensus group has recommended the following domains in cachexia assessment: catabolic drivers, muscle mass and strength, anorexia or reduced food intake, and functional and psychological impairments.[31] The assessment should include appetite, satiety level, problems with taste or smell, dry mouth (xerostomia), mouth sores, chewing and swallowing difficulties, food preferences, aversions and intolerances, nutritional intake track, energy expenditure assessment, pain, dyspnea, anxiety, depression symptoms, performance and functionality, and social history including the impact of, meaning of, perspective on, and anxieties and fears of patient and family about the patient's condition.[23,26,28]

Physical examination should include observation of general appearance; anthropometric measures including current weight, weight changes, height, body mass index, mid-upper arm circumference, and skin fold thickness measurement; bioelectrical impedance analysis; skin turgor and muscle strength examination; cognition level assessment; oral examination that looks for dryness (xerostomia) or lesions, infections, stomatitis, and mucositis; and abdominal examination including rectal examination for masses and bowel sounds.[23,28,29]

Diagnostics

Blood studies may sometimes be appropriate during the diagnostic phase. Serum albumin, prealbumin, transferrin, triglycerides, total lymphocytes, hemoglobin, and electrolytes (sodium, potassium, magnesium, and calcium) can be used for diagnosis. An indicator for the presence of a cachectic state is C-reactive protein, a marker for systemic inflammation is appropriate. Radiologic investigations can be used to rule out treatable problems such as bowel obstruction and constipation.[26]

Differential Diagnosis

Primary care providers should appreciate the palliative care approach to these patients. End-of-life anorexia or cachexia is not typically worked up because these conditions are treated symptomatically.

Management

Physician consultation may be indicated for the presence of uncomfortable symptoms that require hospitalization for relief to be obtained (diarrhea, nausea and vomiting, mucositis, xerostomia).

Immediate emergency department referral is indicated for no oral intake for 24 hours, signs of dehydration, and sudden, severe decrease in functional or performance status if these are considered reversible and if this is consistent with the patient's goals of care.

Management is aimed at minimizing symptoms that affect appetite, implementing measures to improve appetite, and educating patients and families about treatment interventions.

An appetite stimulant may be offered if the patient wishes. A progesterone steroid such as megestrol (Megace), 200 to 800 mg/day, or cannabinoids such as dronabinol (Marinol), 2.5 mg twice daily, can be helpful.[32] Corticosteroids (e.g., dexamethasone) can be used to improve appetite as well, because they are used to treat various symptoms such as pain and nausea.[26] Also, short-term symptom relief medications for depression (e.g., methylphenidate [Ritalin]) can have the added benefit of increasing appetite.[32] Eliminating blood glucose monitoring and evaluating the need for other diet-related medications (e.g., cholesterol-lowering agents) reduce the burden of treatment at this time.[32]

Prokinetic agents (e.g., metoclopramide) can be used before meals to improve gastric emptying and decrease nausea.[30] The efficacy of other nonspecific agents such as mirtazapine and olanzapine (antidepressants), anabolic steroids (testosterone and its derivatives), melatonin, amino acids and peptide hormones (L-carnitine, ghrelin), thalidomide, and anti-inflammatory therapies are still being studied.[26]

A glass of beer, sherry, or wine may stimulate the appetite, particularly if this has been a part of the patient's established routine.[29] Supportive measures including good mouth care, maintaining pleasant surroundings, supporting oral support instead of parenteral intervention, and encouraging patients and families can aid coping.[30]

Thirst is best relieved by keeping the mouth moist (see the section on dry mouth [xerostomia]) rather than by administering intravenous fluids.[25] Enteral and parenteral feeding is incapable of reversing cachexia.[5,28]

Education and Health Promotion

Intensive and ongoing communication and education are the cornerstones of care. Realistic goals of nutritional intake (e.g., relief of hunger or thirst, socialization at mealtimes) should be encouraged. The focus should be on giving patients preferred foods that improve their quality of life, offering welcome relief from lifelong dietary restrictions (e.g., diabetic, low-salt, or low-cholesterol diets).[32]

Patients and families should be encouraged to eat at the dining table with other family members; the pleasure of tasting food should be emphasized over total caloric intake. Patients who have anorexia or cachexia are recommended to have small, frequent meals dense in calories. Also, patients and family members can be encouraged to offer meals that require little preparation, and patients can be encouraged to rest before meals.[26,30]

A loss of appetite is common in dying patients because they cannot tolerate premorbid calorie intake, nor do they want to eat. Anorexia usually generates many issues because food is seen as the sustenance and essence of life. Family and friends may not understand the patient's inability to eat and should be counseled about the pros and cons of artificial (or medically provided) nutrition and hydration.[23,24] In discussing medically provided nutrition and hydration, it is important to avoid using the terms *food* and *water*. Rather, use of the terms *medically provided nutrition* and *hydration* helps define these as medical interventions, different from the natural impulse of eating and drinking.

As nutritional intake declines, ketones that promote a sense of well-being are released.[25] In particular, family members must be informed that anorexia and cachexia are a natural part of the dying process. The administration of intravenous fluids or feedings by means of total parenteral nutrition or a nasogastric or gastrostomy tube may cause discomfort. The dying patient may experience fluid overload from such strategies because the body is unable to metabolize fluids and proteins in the same way as a "normal, healthy" person. This can result in edema in the arms, legs, and abdomen; incontinence and skin breakdown; and pulmonary congestion and ascites, causing dyspnea as the abdomen pushes up on the diaphragm.

ANXIETY AND FEAR

Definition and Epidemiology

Anxiety is a sense of deep unease, distress, or tension with an unknown stimulus.[33] It is related to fear and is characterized by a constellation of signs and symptoms, including insomnia, headache, shortness of breath, weakness, chest pain, palpitations, sensation of butterflies in the stomach, urinary frequency, pallor, restlessness, tremor, and sweating. The difference between fear and anxiety is that fear has a definable quality or cause.[34]

Pathophysiology

Causes of anxiety for the patient with a serious, life-limiting illness include situational issues (e.g., financial or family worries, unfinished business, fears, and adjustment to disease) and organic causes (e.g., uncontrolled pain or dyspnea, psychiatric causes, medications, existential distress, altered physiologic status, addictive substance withdrawal, endocrine disorders, pheochromacytoma and islet tumors, and lack of control).[24] The newest *Diagnostic and Statistical Manual of Mental Disorders,* Fifth Edition (DSM-5) offers a new category of anxiety labeled *anxiety from another condition,* which may be particularly relevant to patients with serious advanced illness as well as progressive chronic conditions.[35,36] This term may capture the stressors in dealing with such illnesses, particularly loss of normalcy, continued surveillance of a condition, ongoing worry about diagnostic testing, the wait for disease progression, and end-stage disease.

Clinical Presentation and Physical Examination

Assessment of anxiety begins with understanding of the patient's knowledge of his or her disease, specifically if there are any fears about dying or death.[37,38] The patient should be asked about troubling symptoms, previous stressful incidents, and his or her previous coping style with stress and illness. Complaints of tremors, weakness, agitation, limb numbness, or shortness of breath should be noted. The patient may also complain of gastrointestinal upset, palpitations, muscle aches, and sleep disorders.

The physical assessment includes vital signs, noting rapid pulse, high blood pressure, or hyperventilation. Generalized signs, including flushing, wheezing, sweating, and tremor, may be found on examination. Muscle tightness, nausea, or vomiting can also occur.

Diagnostics[33,35,36]

The following laboratory and imaging studies may be appropriate: complete blood count (CBC) to assess hemoglobin and potential infections, chemistry profile to assess for electrolyte abnormality, glucose level to detect hypoglycemia or hyperglycemia, thyroid-stimulating hormone level to detect thyroid abnormalities, folate level, ferritin level, vitamin B_{12} measurement to detect nutrition deficiencies, and drug screening for drugs that have anxiety as a side effect, such as cocaine.

Oxygen saturation should be measured to detect hypoxia.

Chest x-ray study may be performed to rule out pneumonia, pleural effusion, and pulmonary embolus.

An electrocardiogram (ECG) may be obtained to evaluate for dysrhythmia as a causative factor.

Differential Diagnosis

See the differential diagnosis box.

Management

Physician consultation is indicated for complex medication conditions that are causes of anxiety.

Treatment focuses on both pharmacologic interventions and nonpharmacologic strategies to alleviate, if possible, the specific problem.[33,35,36] Pharmacologic interventions include the use of anxiolytics for short-term therapy (e.g., benzodiazepines such as lorazepam, 0.5 to 2 mg orally for a maximal dose of 2 to 8 mg/day, or diazepam, 2.5 to 10 mg for a maximal dose of 10 to 60 mg/day, as well as alprazolam, oxazepam, or temazepam as a second choice. Selective serotonin reuptake inhibitors (SSRIs) may also be prescribed for long-term anxiety (e.g., fluoxetine, 10 to 80 mg once daily [qd]; sertraline, 25 to 20 mg qd; paroxetine, 10 to 160 mg qd; citalopram, 10 to 60 mg qd). Because anxiety and depression are often seen together, it may be necessary to treat both. Thus the dosage of SSRIs will be important.

Nonpharmacologic management includes psychotherapy. Factual information should be provided when the services of psychosocial or spiritual therapists are used. Such services can include counseling, spiritual care, cognitive behavioral therapy, and hypnotherapy to focus on recognizing anxiety and taking control of it. Stress management can be essential in promoting wellness and discharging the anxiety; this includes exercise, relaxation, massage, distraction, music and art therapy, yoga, and visualization. These activities are often available at community centers or YMCAs or YWCAs. Environmental manipulation may afford a measure of control; a home safety evaluation, treatment schedule control, or control over any other part of the daily schedule may offer normalcy. Dietary modifications such as decreasing caffeine-containing products such as soda, coffee, and/or chocolate along with nicotine products in tobacco can reduce anxiety. Alcohol reduction may also help reduce anxiety. Alleviation of anxiety may also require relief of a symptom cluster, such as the cycle of pain, dyspnea, and anxiety. In such cases, it may be impossible to separate and to treat the "initiating event." The selection of agents that treat multiple symptoms (e.g., morphine, which can relieve pain and dyspnea and provide a calming effect) is often the best approach.

Complications

If anxiety becomes severe, the patient may experience panic attacks. If the anxiety is produced by trauma, post-traumatic stress disorder (PTSD) may ensue. There may also be medication side effects; therefore, judicious prescribing is necessary.

Indications for Referral or Hospitalization

- Severe anxiety escalating into panic attacks
- Suicidal thoughts

Education and Health Promotion

Information in and of itself is useful for patients. It alleviates elements of surprise about the patient's condition, treatment, and the future. Patient and family education should be provided to aid in understanding of the nature of anxiety and related manifestations; how anxiety interferes with the ability to learn, communicate, and solve problems; and the safe use of medications and medication side effects.

DELIRIUM

Definition and Epidemiology

Delirium is a reversible, sudden, and acute confusional state. It is characterized by sudden changes in mental status, a mental status that waxes and wanes, a reduced attention span, and hyperactivity or hypoactivity (see Chapter 192).

Pathophysiology

Delirium is common in patients with advanced disease. It may be caused by tumor pressure in the brain; medication side effects, withdrawal, or overdose; uncontrolled pain; metabolic changes; liver or kidney dysfunction; infections; or nutritional deficiencies. More than half of all dying patients experience delirium as they approach death.[39] This may be attributed to the actual dying process or to one of the previously listed causes.

Clinical Presentation and Physical Examination

Delirium often occurs suddenly and may fluctuate during the course of the day. It often worsens in the late afternoon or at night, disturbing the patient's sleep-wake cycle. Speech may be incoherent or inappropriate to the situation. The patient may have altered perceptions that manifest as hallucinations or delusions. Disorientation to person, place, date, and time as well as agitation, restlessness, aggressiveness, and paranoia are also possible.[40]

The Folstein Mini-Mental State Examination and the Confusion Assessment Method (CAM) are both simple and reliable initial assessments of cognitive function. These tests typically include questions that evaluate orientation to person, place, date, and residence; memory and recall; attention and calculation; language; response to commands; and spatial relationships. These assessments can begin to define the degree of disturbance and are best used when symptoms are first noted. A thorough neurologic examination may provide further clues to the cause.

Diagnostics

Diagnostic studies should be undertaken only if death is not imminent and the results are likely to change patient management (e.g., correct dehydration, metabolic abnormalities, or hypercalcemia). Blood chemistries and metabolic measurements may reveal easily reversible causes of delirium. Serum glucose, serum electrolytes, liver function, urea, calcium, blood urea nitrogen (BUN) concentration, creatinine level urinalysis, urine sodium, urine osmolality, arterial blood gas, and pulse oximetry should be assessed. Because infection is a common cause of altered mental status, a CBC, white blood cell (WBC) count differential, urinalysis, and urine culture should be obtained if an infection is suspected.

Differential Diagnosis

See the differential diagnosis box.

Management

Physician consultation is indicated for an acute, unexpected, potentially reversible cause that is consistent with the patients' goals of care.

Immediate emergency department referral is indicated only after assessment of the patients' advance directives for goals of care.

First and foremost, education of the family about delirium, its causes (if known or suspected), and its prognosis is critical. If otherwise beneficial medications are the cause, the family needs to assist in identifying the patient's priorities for comfort. Older adults are particularly sensitive to medications for pain and symptom control and hence are at high risk for delirium.[40]

The provider should identify and treat the reversible causes while keeping the patient in a safe and comfortable environment. Stimuli should be reduced and the patient reoriented (if possible). Neuroleptics are administered. Neuroleptic medications such as haloperidol are the drugs of choice for patients who are delirious in the last few days of life (Table 14-1).[39] These medications may be given to help calm the patient and to ease fear and panic. Intravenous administration (in an appropriate setting) is recommended to initially provide rapid relief and to minimize the extrapyramidal symptoms. Once a dose has been established, converting to an equivalent oral administration regimen (whenever possible) on a scheduled basis can maintain a calm state. If the delirium is a result of opioid or benzodiazepine withdrawal, the tapering process is slowed. Treatment of delirium with a benzodiazepine alone can result in paradoxical effects and actually worsen the delirium. Hence, this often-prescribed approach to calm or quiet a delirious patient is discouraged in the dying patient.[25] However, for some patients with intractable delirium, palliative sedation (described later) may be necessary.

Long-term, high-dose opioids may cause delirium because of the accumulation of metabolites.[32] Meperidine should not be

TABLE 14-1 Medications Used for Terminal Delirium and Palliative Sedation at End of Life

Generic Name	Approximate Daily Dose	Route
NEUROLEPTICS		
Haloperidol	0.5-5 mg q2-12h not to exceed 100 mg/day PO	PO, IV, SC, IM
Chlorpromazine	12.5-50 mg q4-12h	PO, IV, IM
Droperidol	0.5-5 mg q12h	PO
BENZODIAZEPINES		
Lorazepam	0.5-2.0 mg q1-4h up to 10 mg/day PO	PO, IV, IM
Midazolam	30-100 mg/24 hr for sedation	IV, SC

used for pain management in any seriously ill or elderly patient for this reason. Opioid delirium is especially common in patients who were previously stable with a particular dose and experience acute dehydration or renal insufficiency. However, opioids should not be discontinued in a dying patient. If the current opioid regimen is believed to be the cause of delirium; a different opioid in an equianalgesic dose may provide pain relief without delirium. For example, fentanyl, hydromorphone, and oxycodone may be less deliriogenic than morphine; these agents lack the metabolites that can accumulate and cause delirium.

For the patient who is close to death, the family needs to be counseled that delirium may signal impending death.[41] This subtlety is often missed, resulting in missed opportunity for closure.

BOX 14-4

SIGECAPS Mnemonic to Assess Depression

S	Sleep changes—either increased or decreased sleep
I	Interest changes—increased or decreased interest in the activities of daily living
G	Guilt—feelings of guilt for any number of circumstances
E	Energy changes—either fatigue or loss of energy
C	Concentration changes—inability to focus or think
A	Appetite—either decreased or increased food intake
P	Psychomotor agitation
S	Suicidal thoughts

From Carlat D: The psychiatric review of systems: a screening tool for family physicians. *Am Fam Physician* 58(7):1617-1624, 1998.

Life Span Considerations

Older adults will be more sensitive to all medications, so dosage considerations are imperative both in treating delirium and in prescribing deliriogenic medications.

Education and Health Promotion

Educating family members about the features of delirium is key because patient behaviors can be extremely upsetting, particularly if the delirium causes the patient to lash out. Family will also need to be instructed about safety measures because the patient may be at greater risk for falls or other harms while not fully aware.

DEPRESSION

Definition and Epidemiology

Depression is a mood disorder with both somatic and psychological symptoms, affecting mood, affect, and personality.[33,36,42] Somatic symptoms include altered sleep, fatigue, slowed movements, and decreased energy. Psychological symptoms include low mood and altered decision-making or cognition. It is defined as a depressive episode when it last 2 weeks or longer and is accompanied by lack of pleasure or interest in most other activities. It may be situational in the case of a diagnosis of a serious or advanced illness.[33] Depressive disorders are illnesses that affect mood and result in a variety of symptoms, including anhedonia, helplessness, hopelessness, worthlessness, and guilt. Feelings of personal failure are strong.

Diagnosis of depression in patients with advanced disease can be a challenge because the neurovegetative signs that are typically part of the diagnostic criteria of depression are often normally present in such patients, particularly patients with advanced cancer. Observing the patient for psychological and cognitive symptoms of worthlessness, hopelessness, excessive guilt, and suicidal ideation may be more diagnostic.[36,42] Box 14-4 provides a helpful acronym for diagnosis.

Depression with serious or terminal illness should not be considered a normal symptom. Although sadness and grief may be anticipated in patients with advanced illness, a mood of total despair can lead to a request for assisted suicide, attempts to hasten death, or suicide. The desire for a hastened death is highly linked to depression and unmanaged symptoms.[37,43] Treatment of depression in seriously ill patients can allow patients to experience some psychological healing. Through the ability to achieve psychosocial and spiritual closure and to make meaning in life, patients may also experience pleasure in their time remaining.

Causes include physical, psychological, social, genetic, and medication induced. See Chapter 248.[36,42]

Clinical Presentation and Physical Examination

The assessment of depression in the patient with serious illness is multifaceted, with particular sensitivity to culture and religion. The advanced practice registered nurse (APRN) must assess for a triad of symptoms including change in mood, disturbances in self-perception of the environment and the future, and regulative physical and behavioral symptoms. The patient's appearance, including dress and grooming, is an important indicator of the presence of depression, in addition to affect, speech, and orientation. Obtaining a history with attention to substance abuse and previous depressive or bipolar episodes is critical. Assessment also includes mood and lifestyle changes. A history of sleep disturbances, weight loss, impaired concentration, psychomotor changes, loss of interest in life, feelings of guilt, loss of energy, fatigue, and suicidal thoughts should be noted. Patients must be asked directly about whether they feel depressed, whether they have contemplated taking their own lives, and if they have a plan for doing so. The most effective question is "Are you depressed?"

Diagnostics[36,42]

Diagnostic testing is indicated to exclude other causes of mood disorders and includes laboratory studies, radiology, electrocardiography, and tests for oxygenation. Laboratory testing includes a CBC to evaluate for dehydration and anemia, a glucose level to evaluate for hyperglycemia suggestive of diabetes, a thyroid profile to evaluate for hypothyroidism, vitamin B_{12} and folate levels to evaluate for vitamin deficiencies, liver function tests to evaluate for liver dysfunction, and BUN and creatinine to evaluate for kidney dysfunction. Serology testing should include a Venereal Disease Research Laboratory (VDRL) test in older adults to evaluate for syphilis, enzyme-linked immunosorbent assay (ELISA) or Western blot for HIV testing, and Epstein-Barr nuclear antigen for Epstein-Barr virus.

An ECG should be ordered to evaluate the presence of a dysrhythmia. If the patient is short of breath, a chest x-ray study is obtained to evaluate for infection and lung masses, and O_2 saturation is measured; O_2 saturation will allow evaluation for hypoxia indicative of other respiratory disorders such as COPD. If indicated, a CT scan of the head is ordered to evaluate for cerebrovascular accident, tumor, or other brain disorders.

Management

Physician consultation is indicated for intractable moderate to severe depression and/or poor response to pharmacologic treatment.

Immediate emergency department referral is indicated for suicidal ideation and suicidal gestures.

Treatment includes pharmacologic and psychotherapeutic modalities. Pharmacologic treatment depends on the prognosis of the patient.

When death is anticipated to occur within 1 month, a psychostimulant[44] or steroid may be the drug of choice. Methylphenidate is rapid acting and may reduce pain. It can be started at 2.5 to 5 mg/day and increased to 10 to 20 mg/day.[41,42,44] This medication is given early in the morning, with the same dose repeated at noon to allow the peak effect to wear off by bedtime. Administration later in the day may cause insomnia, although some patients may do better with more frequent administration. Both psychostimulants and steroids may help improve multiple common end-of-life symptoms, including depression, loss of appetite, and sedation.

When death is anticipated to occur within 3 to 6 months, a trial of SSRIs is appropriate. SSRIs are often considered a first-line choice because of an improved side effect profile over antidepressant medications.

Some antidepressant medications can also help with neuropathic pain (duloxetine), appetite, and insomnia (mirtazapine). See Table 14-2.

Indications for Referral or Hospitalization

Substantial literature documents that the best treatment of depression includes both pharmacologic interventions and counseling. Referrals for the patient and family members to a psychiatrist, psychologist, social worker, pastoral counselor, or hospice worker can help in the understanding and management of depression at the end of life. Psychotherapeutic approaches can encourage the patient to talk about past and present experiences as well as the dying experience. Behavioral interventions and cognitive restructuring may also be helpful. A formal psychiatric evaluation may be used to determine the appropriateness of antidepressant medications for patients with comorbid conditions and for stoic patients who may not be willing to admit depression to their family or health care provider for fear of causing disappointment or appearing weak.

A multidisciplinary approach may be helpful in engaging the patient and acknowledging his or her feelings. Reiteration of the goals of pain and symptom management may provide reassurance and promote feelings of support.

TABLE 14-2 Selected Medications Used for Depression Management

PSYCHOSTIMULANTS	
Dextroamphetamine	2.5-5 mg qd/bid
Methylphenidate	2.5-5 mg qd/bid
SELECTIVE SEROTONIN REUPTAKE INHIBITORS (SSRIS)	
Citalopram	10-40 mg qd
Sertraline	12.5-50 mg qd
Fluoxetine	5-10 mg qd
Paroxetine	5-20 mg qd
Nefazodone	100-500 mg qd
Fluvoxamine	50-300 mg qd
Mirtazapine	15-45 mg qd
SEROTONIN–NOREPINEPHRINE REUPTAKE INHIBITORS (SNRIS)	
Venlafaxine	37.5 mg qd
Duloxetine	20-60 mg qd
Bupropion	75-450 mg qd

Data from Blatt, 2012[96]; Pasacreta et al, 2010[97]; and Candy et al, 2009.[98]

Life Span Considerations

It may be difficult to recognize depression in the older adult. Many older adults do not perceive that they are depressed or may be of a generation in which psychological problems were not discussed. In addition, there is the misperception that all elders become depressed as part of the aging process, including changes that occur in appetite, sleep-wake cycles, and the inability to continue previous life pursuits.[45]

Education and Health Promotion

Patients and families should be educated about depression and its causes. This includes risk factors such as cancer, heart disease, and other chronic illnesses. Education should include medications, their intended effect, and side effects. Combined cognitive behavioral therapy and pharmacologic management produce the best results. Finally, it is critical to identify an ongoing safety plan for emergency assistance if the patient is suicidal.

DYSPNEA

Definition and Pathophysiology

Dyspnea is defined by the American Thoracic Society as an experience of breathing discomfort that consists of qualitatively distinct sensations that vary in intensity. The experience of dyspnea derives from interactions among multiple physiologic, psychological, social, and environmental factors and may induce secondary physiological and behavioral responses.[46] It is a subjective symptom that may not correlate with findings of hypoxia, hypercarbia, or tachypnea.[47] It is felt by the patient but may not be seen by the clinician. It generally results from three main abnormalities: increased load requiring greater respiratory effort (e.g., obstruction), an increase in the proportion of respiratory muscle required to maintain a normal workload (e.g., weakness), or an increase in ventilatory requirements (e.g., fever, anemia).[47] The most common causes of dyspnea tend to be pulmonary pathologies related to cancer, such as tumor obstruction and malignant pleural effusion; pathologies related to cancer treatments, such as chemotherapy and/or radiation; and nonmalignant causes such as COPD, congestive heart failure, and anxiety. Up to 30% of patients may have no identifiable cause of dyspnea.[48]

Clinical Presentation and Physical Examination

A patient's self-report of dyspnea is the most important assessment criterion.[49] The patient may appear short of breath but may deny it, or may report being short of breath without appearing so. Although subjective report of dyspnea is the gold standard of measurement, the numeric rating scale (NRS) is the most practical and feasible for use in the clinical setting. The NRS is a 0-to-10 scale, with 0 being no problem and 10 being the worst trouble breathing the patient can imagine. Because the NRS measures only severity, it is important for the provider to ask patients the extent to which dyspnea disrupts normal activities and inhibits functioning, the level of distress it causes, the impact it has on family members and social interactions, and the meaning that is tied to the experience of the symptom.[50] A history of shortness of breath, including onset, frequency, and contributing factors, should be obtained.

In addition to subjective reporting, objective examination includes chest auscultation, observations of the patient's breathing, and oxygen saturation. Pulse oximetry should be obtained with the patient at rest, during activity, and in different positions. However, oxygen levels may not correlate with degree or even presence of dyspnea. The objective criteria may not correlate with the subjective report of dyspnea, particularly if dyspnea is chronic.

Diagnostics

The recommended examinations and tests should be performed only if the data would change treatment and the patient is not actively dying, because these examinations and tests can be exhausting for the patient and do not alter treatment decisions. For example, chest radiographs are used for acute exacerbations to determine presence of pneumothorax, pneumonia, and pleural effusions. CT scans are reserved for possible disease progression, and high-resolution spiral CT for pulmonary embolism. CBCs are useful to identify anemia. Pulmonary function tests to measure lung volumes may indicate potentially reversible obstruction.

Differential Diagnosis

Determining the underlying cause of the dyspnea may help guide treatment, but even without a known cause, dyspnea can be and should be aggressively treated. The following may be origins of dyspnea in palliative care patients: progressive primary or metastatic cancer, pleural effusion, pneumonia, COPD, pulmonary embolus, anemia, pneumothorax, congestive heart failure, pericardial effusion with or without tamponade, ascites, and anxiety.

Management

Desired goals of care drive both diagnostic and management choices. All management is dependent on goals of care. Goals must be clarified before diagnostics or management interventions are considered.

Physician consultation is indicated for uncontrolled dyspnea. If a comfort-oriented approach is desired, diagnostic workup would be kept to a minimum and subjective report would direct therapies.

Immediate emergency department referral is indicated for uncontrolled dyspnea. If patient is home with hospice support, emergency department referral would be avoided and the emergency call would be directed to the hospice team. If goals of care are comfort oriented, the provider should call the emergency department before sending to inform the emergency department staff that this is a comfort care situation.

Morphine is used most commonly, but any opioid can have the desired effect. It can be given orally or parenterally, but there has been no evidence that nebulized opioids are of value.[51] In the opioid-naive patient, the oral route is preferred when possible, and recommendations would be to start low with oral doses of 2.5 to 10 mg every 3 hours as needed (prn). Parenterally, morphine, 1 to 3 mg, can be given intravenously or subcutaneously every hour prn. If the patient is already on regular doses of opioid, higher doses may be needed.[52] If dyspnea is not relieved by opioids and there is accompanying anxiety, lorazepam, 0.5 to 1.0 mg orally every hour prn, may be tried.[52] If there is an inflammatory component to dyspnea, steroids may be of use. The provider may consider decreasing or stopping fluids if contributing to volume overload and dyspnea. Oxygen may or may not be of value. It is reasonable to perform a trial and determine usefulness. Oxygen may be used even in the event of adequate oxygenation. Respiratory and cardiac optimization should be achieved with bronchodilators, diuretics, and appropriate cardiac medications. Mechanical ventilation and or noninvasive ventilator support often is not useful. Benefit versus the burden of intervention needs to be explored fully in the setting of prognosis and expected versus desired outcomes. Therapeutic procedures for cardiac, pleural, or abdominal fluid removal may be indicated. Anticoagulants for pulmonary embolus may be used if consistent with goals of care. Blood transfusions are usually not recommended for end-of-life dyspnea. Blood transfusions have some value if the prognosis is thought to be several months.

The loss of the ability to swallow and control airway secretions is common in the dying process and can add to patients' anxiety. Glycopyrrolate (Robinul), scopolamine patch, or atropine 1% ophthalmic solution given buccally are commonly used to help control increase oral-pharyngeal secretions associated with the "death rattle."[53] Oral cavity suctioning may help, but secretions will reaccumulate. Deep suctioning is rarely effective and may cause more distress than benefit in the dying person.

Anxious patients should be placed in the upright position. Environmental measures include cooling patients' rooms and enhancing airflow with fans. Relaxation techniques, breathing techniques, guided imagery, and music may be used.

Complications

Dyspnea is a very distressing symptom that can cause fear and panic in the patient and family if not addressed. Feeling oneself or fearing a loved one is "suffocating" is a frightening experience and can leave a horrible memory in the minds of loved ones.

Indications for Referral or Hospitalization

For palliative and end-of-life care, patients and families may opt to avoid rehospitalization. Therefore reviewing goals of care is essential. If hospital-level interventions are congruent with goals of care (e.g., patient is full code and desirous of intubation) then nonreversible hypoxemia would be an indication for hospitalization. In general, uncontrolled symptoms will be what drive admission.

Life Span Considerations

As the population continues to age, myriad comorbidities are common and may contribute to the experience of dyspnea. Therefore, multimodal approaches will be necessary. Because of diminished drug clearance in the elderly, a low starting dose of opioid in opioid-naive elders is recommended.

Education and Health Promotion

Patient and family education should include a physiologic description of the cause of dyspnea and the prognosis and thorough discussion of goals of care including benefit versus burden of interventions and therapy.

Use of opioids for dyspnea will likely be a novel idea to the patient and family, and there may be a fear of addiction. Allaying fears and encouraging trials of small doses may be helpful.

Teaching relaxation techniques to both patient and family can help reduce potential escalation of accompanying anxiety.

Explanation and reassurance to families regarding irregular, gasping, and agonal-appearing respirations during the dying process is important. It helps the family to understand that the irregular breathing is involuntary, brainstem driven, and not an indicator of suffering.[53]

DRY MOUTH (XEROSTOMIA)[54]

Definition and Epidemiology

Dry mouth, or xerostomia, is the sensation of oral dryness, often accompanied by decreased salivary secretions.[55] It may be difficult to identify the exact underlying cause and contributing factors. Decreased salivary function and prolonged xerostomia cause significant oral symptoms, including pain; gum, tongue, and mucosal irritations and lesions; mouth infections; taste changes; and bad breath as well as dental caries.[55] Esophageal symptoms include swallowing issues and altered speech and voice. However, treatment offers much comfort and relief to patients.

Pathophysiology

Well described in the cancer literature, xerostomia has been described in other conditions, including diabetes, end-stage renal failure, end-stage cardiac disease, and end-stage liver disease.[56-58] Common causes of dry mouth in terminally ill patients include medication side effects; mouth breathing; side effects of oxygen administration; infection; ulcers; and treatments such as surgery, chemotherapy, and radiotherapy.[55]

Clinical Presentation and Physical Examination

Assessment begins with a thorough oral examination that includes inspection for mucosal and buccal dryness; pallor; dry mucosal and buccal areas; dry, raw, or fissured tongue or cracked lips; absence of salivary pooling; and oral ulcerations, gingivitis, or candidiasis.[54,55,58]

Diagnostics

Two quick bedside tests are the cracker biscuit test and the tongue blade test. The cracker biscuit test involves giving the patient a dry cracker or biscuit. If the patient cannot eat it, xerostomia is present. The tongue blade test is an extension of the mouth examination. After inspection is complete, the tongue blade is placed on the tongue. If it sticks, xerostomia is present.[55]

Management

Meticulous mouth care with dental care should be provided, including use of dentifrices and nonalcoholic mouthwashes and dental appliance cleaning.

Physician consultation may be indicated for dry mouth that does not respond to treatment.

Stepwise Process for Xerostomia Management[55]

1. Treat underlying infections such as thrush.
2. Review and alter current medications as appropriate.
3. Stimulate salivary flow through both nonpharmacologic and pharmacologic interventions.
4. Replace lost secretions with saliva substitutes.
5. Protect teeth and mouth through meticulous mouth care and fluoride rinses.
6. Rehydrate with plenty of liquids.
7. Avoid mouth pain through diet modification with attention to acidic foods and hard foods.

Pharmacologic Interventions[58,59]

Pilocarpine, 2.5 to 5 mg orally three times daily, slowly titrated, may be used. Saliva production is greatest after a dose, and the response lasts for approximately 4 hours and varies with severity of xerostomia. Cevimeline increases saliva by inhibiting acetylcholinesterase. This agent is given in a mouthwash or mouth gargle every 6 hours. Lost secretions are replaced with water and artificial saliva if necessary. An inexpensive spritzer filled with nine parts water and one part fine oil (e.g., grapeseed oil) can be helpful. The teeth should be protected with frequent oral hygiene, and the lips should be lubricated with lip balm. Topical rehydration with water or ice chips is a more subjectively effective remedy to dry mouth and thirst than is intravenous hydration. Dietary modifications, such as the avoidance of spicy or salty foods, may help.

Complications

Pilocarpine[60] should not be used in patients with COPD, asthma, bradycardia, renal or hepatic impairment, glaucoma, or bowel obstruction. Side effects include mild to moderate sweating, visual disturbances, nausea, rhinitis, chills, flushing, sweating, dizziness, increased urinary frequency, abdominal cramping, and asthenia.[60] Side effects can be lessened if the drug is taken with milk.

Indications for Referral or Hospitalization

Nutrition referral for meal preparation guidance may be considered. A dentist may be consulted for progressive oral ulcers and pain.

Life Span Considerations

Mouth care is important across all the life span, no matter what the age. It may be more challenging in patients with complex medical histories as well as cognitive impairment.

Education and Health Promotion

Education focuses on proactive management and clear explanation of oral care.

NAUSEA AND VOMITING

Definition and Epidemiology

Nausea is an unpleasant subjective experience and feeling of queasiness or a need or desire to vomit. Nausea manifests in a wavelike sensation and can be accompanied by autonomic symptoms such as cold sweat, fast heart rate, salivation, or diarrhea. Vomiting (emesis) is the physical event of the rapid forceful expulsion of the contents of the stomach, duodenum, or jejunum through the mouth.[25,61,62]

Despite methodologic issues with epidemiologic studies of nausea and vomiting, these symptoms seem to be less common and less bothersome than pain, breathlessness, and fatigue. Nausea and vomiting were reported by 16% to 68% of patients and were most common in patients with AIDS (43%), end-stage renal failure (30%), and cancer (6%).[62] Prevalence of nausea and vomiting is higher in women and in patients younger than age 65[63] and appears to increase as the disease progresses, rising as high as 70% in the last week of life.[61]

Pathophysiology

The pathophysiology of nausea and vomiting is complex. Successful treatment requires an understanding of underlying processes involved.

The chemoreceptor trigger zone and vomiting centers located in the brainstem receive input from vagus, vestibular, cerebral cortex, hypothalamus, glossopharyngeal, and splenic nerves, which are stimulated by activation of mechanoreceptors and dopamine, serotonin, acetylcholine, histamine, and opioid receptors.[61,64]

Causes of nausea and vomiting can be divided into six categories[61,65]:

- Chemical (medications, metabolic disturbances, toxins)
- Gastrointestinal stretch or irritation (constipation, bowel obstruction, metastases)
- Gastric stasis (medications, gastritis, autonomic failure, ascites)
- Increased intracranial pressure
- Movement-related causes (opioids, gastroparesis, cerebellar tumors)
- Anxiety-related causes (anxiety, anticipatory vomiting)

Clinical Presentation and Physical Examination

Understanding the cause of nausea and vomiting is critical to facilitate treatment. The causes of nausea and vomiting can be found through a detailed history and physical examination.

The history should include onset (when did it start?); pattern (specific time during day?); duration (continuous or intermittent?); intensity (how bothersome on a scale of 0 to 10, with 0 being not bothersome and 10 being most bothersome?); association between nausea and vomiting (nausea precedes vomiting, or vomiting occurs suddenly?); content of vomiting (food, bile, or feces?); volume of vomiting (small or large?); color, force, and timing of vomiting; other symptoms (epigastric pain, pain on swallowing, thirst, hiccups, heartburn); aggravating factors (what makes nausea and vomiting better or worse?); medical history (along with presence of peptic ulcer disease, constipation, intracranial pressure, nausea-inducing medications, surgical procedures); and treatment history (pharmacologic, nonpharmacologic interventions).[61-63]

Physical examination includes weight change (note any recent loss), signs of dehydration (assess hydration status by examining mucous membranes and skin turgor), oral intake (assess past 24-hour intake and output), oral examination (check for hygiene, signs of infection or irritation), abdominal examination (auscultate bowel sounds; palpate for organomegaly, ascites, masses; check for distention, pain, discomfort), rectal examination (check for constipation or impaction), neurologic examination (identify orientation and consciousness level), and other signs (check for sepsis, liver failure, kidney failure signs).

Diagnostics

If there is concern about other issues (such as bowel obstruction, gastroenterologic conditions) based on the physical examination, the following diagnostic studies are considered[61-63]:

- Laboratory studies: renal and hepatic function tests, electrolytes (sodium—dehydration; calcium—hypercalcemia), therapeutic drug level monitoring (digoxin, theophylline), blood and other body fluid cultures (sepsis, infection)
- Radiographic studies: x-ray studies, brain scanning, CT, magnetic resonance imaging (obstruction, abdominal pathologies)
- Endoscopic evaluation: to assess reflux, esophagitis, obstruction

Management

Physician consultation is indicated if surgical management or hospitalization is needed. Patients with bowel obstructions can have acute symptoms of vomiting, colicky abdominal pain, constipation, or diarrhea with a slow, insidious onset. These patients should be referred for surgical consultation.[63]

Immediate emergency department referral is indicated for vomiting of bright red blood, uncontrolled vomiting for 4 to 5 hours, vomiting accompanied by diarrhea and/or fever, and also severe abdominal pain, lethargy, and mental confusion.[66]

General principles of management include a comprehensive and regular assessment; consideration of multiple causes of symptoms, some of which are reversible; administration of drugs regularly by the appropriate route; and consideration of nonpharmacologic measures.[67]

Treatment of nausea and vomiting depends on the cause. Reversible causes of nausea and vomiting should be corrected first.

Different classes of antiemetics, alone or in combination, can be administered orally, subcutaneously, intravenously, or by a suppository for symptomatic relief.[65] Phenothiazines (prochlorperazine, chlorpromazine), butyrophenones (haloperidol), serotonin receptor antagonists (ondansetron, dolasetron), histamine receptor blockers (diphenhydramine), acetylcholine antagonist (scopolamine), steroids, prokinetic agents (metoclopramide), benzodiazepines (lorazepam), and cannabinoids provide a vast array of choices, combinations, and costs.[25]

Nonpharmacologic therapy includes relaxation, distraction, imagery, acupuncture or acupressure, cold therapy, aromatherapy, and music therapy. Diet modifications include eating dry crackers on awakening and eating fewer spicy and greasy foods. Both ginger and peppermint can be helpful.[23] Offering small, simple meals can make person feel less overwhelmed; cool fizzy drinks, cool tempered foods, and carbohydrate-based meals are often better tolerated.[63] Holding or slowing down tube feedings may eliminate nausea induced by bloating.[25] If nausea and vomiting are caused by an obstruction that cannot be relieved, placement of a venting gastrostomy rather than a nasogastric tube may decrease these symptoms, allow the patient the pleasure of eating, and increase the patient's overall quality of life.[25]

Regular mouth care should be offered (especially after vomiting episodes); eating slowly and sitting up or reclining with the head raised for a least 1 hour after eating helps to eliminate nausea and vomiting.[64] Environmental modifications include elimination of strong smells, sights, and use of air fresheners.[64]

Indications for Referral or Hospitalization

See the earlier information regarding physician consultation and immediate emergency department referral.

Life Span Considerations

Nausea and vomiting are more common in women and in patients younger than 65 years of age[63] and increase by the last weeks of life.[61] Use of histaminic antagonists in older adults results in especially high risk for severe adverse outcome according to the Beers criteria.[62]

Education and Health Promotion

Providing education and information to patients and family members can enhance their ability to cope with this distressing experience and also can help to decrease the incidence and to increase the effectiveness of treatment. Patients and family members should be encouraged to monitor the nausea and vomiting pattern, duration, and frequency. They should be informed to notify the health care provider when vomiting occurs after oral administration of medication and when more than three episodes of vomiting occur in a day.[62,64]

Also, patients and family members should be taught to avoid spicy, fatty, and salty foods and foods with strong odors; mixing liquids and solids and not lying flat after eating as well as to use small frequent meals and drinking cool and fizzy drinks.

They need to be aware of mouth care and importance. Patients and family members must be educated to restrict intake when gastric distention is a factor. They should be taught to start with sips, then ice chips, gradually increasing from fluids to semisolid to fully solid foods, and to step back if nausea recurs.[61,67]

CONSTIPATION

Definition and Epidemiology

Constipation is infrequent (relative to a patient's normal bowel habits) rectal emptying (usually defined as less frequently than every 3 days) or physical difficulty in emptying the rectum. The difficulty will vary according to the patient's usual elimination pattern. Constipation is also characterized by hard or infrequent stools.[68]

Pathophysiology

In advanced illness, constipation is a common problem resulting from opioid analgesics, immobility, and decreased fluid and food intake. However, constipation may also be age related, neurologically induced, endocrine disorder related, or associated with colorectal tumors or lesions such as fissures or hemorrhoids.[25,69]

Clinical Presentation and Physical Examination

A bowel history is essential in assessing constipation and includes the patient's usual pattern, day of last bowel movement, laxative use or other interventions in an effort to move the bowels, and current drug regimen with special attention to the use of opioids. Physical assessment includes bowel sounds, inspection and palpation of the abdomen, and rectal examination to check for stool.

Diagnostics

Diagnostic evaluation is limited. Tests such as a serum calcium level, CBC, and abdominal flat plate radiographs may be used to identify any intestinal obstruction.[68]

Management

Physician consultation is indicated for suspected bowel obstruction or a reversible cause requiring hospitalization.

Immediate emergency department referral is indicated for obstipation, uncontrolled emesis, uncontrolled pain, passage of bright red blood per rectum, or concern for bowel obstruction.

Patients' dignity, individual preferences, and cultural sensitivities must be considered before the provider proceeds with any intervention.[68] If possible and appropriate, the patient's fluid intake should be increased and a bowel regimen with a stimulant initiated (e.g., senna 1 to 4 tablets once or twice daily). Table 14-3 provides a comprehensive list of oral and rectal laxative choices. An aggressive prophylactic bowel regimen needs to be prescribed concomitantly when opioids are initiated or increased. Alternative stimulants if senna is not adequate include lactulose, 15 to 30 mL one to three times daily; polyethylene glycol (MiraLax) 17 g daily; milk of magnesia, 15 to 30 mL twice daily; and citrate of magnesia. A senna-based tea such as Smooth Move tea each day is also beneficial. An enema or disimpaction may be necessary if there is no stool for several days.[25,69]

An opioid antagonist, methylnaltrexone (Relistor), given subcutaneously is indicated for the treatment of opioid-induced constipation in patients with advanced illness. It usually produces results in 4 hours, and, unlike other opioid antagonists, it less readily crosses the blood-brain barrier, so it is less likely to reverse opioid analgesia.[69,70]

Relief of constipation remains a major comfort measure even toward the very end of life. Constipation can exacerbate lower abdominal pain, nausea, and restlessness, affecting patient rest and comfort.

TABLE 14-3 Recommended Laxatives*

Type of Laxative	Examples
Bulking agents	Dietary fiber, bran, psyllium, methylcellulose, polycarbophil
Stimulant (irritant) laxatives	Senna, bisacodyl (oral and suppository)
Osmotic laxatives	Lactulose, sorbitol, glycerin suppository
Saline laxatives	Magnesium hydroxide, magnesium sulfate, magnesium citrate, phosphate enema
Lubricant laxatives*	Mineral oil enema,* vegetable oil enema
Polyethylene glycol—PEG 3350 (with and without electrolytes)	

Docusate sodium has been found to be ineffective, and oral mineral oil may interfere with absorption of other medications and nutrients, so these laxatives are not recommended.[68,99]

Indications for Referral or Hospitalization

See the earlier information regarding physician consultation and immediate emergency department referral.

Life Span Considerations

Older adults may have long-standing bowel habits that may be difficult to change, so it is important to educate the patient on the appropriate use and misuse of laxatives.

Education and Health Promotion

A prophylactic bowel regimen should always be prescribed whenever an opioid analgesic is ordered. Prevention of constipation is a key comfort measure in the palliative care setting.

BOWEL OBSTRUCTION

Definition and Epidemiology

Bowel obstruction is the total or partial occlusion of the bowel lumen or the alteration of normal peristaltic motion.[69] An obstruction can occur in the small or large intestine, and distinguishing features and outcomes will vary. It is most likely to occur with advanced abdominal or pelvic cancers, such as ovarian, colorectal, and pancreatic cancers.[71] Symptoms can be mild to severe and intermittent or continuous and include distention, intractable nausea and vomiting, and a colicky pain.

Clinical Presentation and Physical Examination

Assessment includes an abdominal examination. Bowel sounds may be normal or absent and hyperactive or hypoactive, depending on the location, cause, and degree of obstruction. Distention will be noted. An abdominal x-ray study and a CT scan will reveal the obstruction.

Diagnostics

Patient evaluation includes laboratory studies such as CBC, electrolytes, BUN, creatinine, arterial blood gases, and blood cultures. Plain radiographs and CT of the abdomen can aid in the diagnosis.

Management

Physician consultation is indicated for a reversible cause that may require hospitalization, nasogastric tube placement, or surgical intervention.

Immediate emergency department referral is indicated for uncontrolled nausea and vomiting or a suspected reversible cause.

Treatment depends in part on the patient's prognosis. Acute management is aimed at the immediate relief of symptoms and includes stopping of oral intake and insertion of a nasogastric tube to alleviate gastric distention. This is the treatment of choice for patients who have a longer prognosis and are able to withstand surgery. Endoscopically placed stents can provide relief. A venting gastrostomy can provide decompression of gas and fluids.[41]

Conservative management is aimed at providing comfort for very ill patients. This can be accomplished through the use of subcutaneously or intravenously administered agents (e.g., analgesics, somatostatin analogues). Analgesics reduce the pain of abdominal distention. Morphine, started at 1 mg/hr and titrated to the appropriate level to treat the pain, is effective. Antiemetics such as prochlorperazine orally or per rectum and haloperidol, 0.5 to 1.5 mg/24 hr, can help. Prokinetic agents such as metoclopramide can help in partial obstructions by increasing peristalsis but should be avoided if complete obstruction is suspected. Anti-inflammatories (e.g., corticosteroids) help reduce the inflammatory response and may partially alleviate the obstruction. Dexamethasone, 8 to 20 mg/24 hr, can reduce inflammatory edema and also help decrease nausea. Somatostatin analogues such as octreotide, 300 to 500 µg one to three times every 24 hours, are thought to inhibit the cascade effect of the glandular secretions and to inhibit peristalsis and blood flow to the splanchnic area.[69] The use of total parenteral nutrition is rarely if ever indicated, and the goals of this therapy should be carefully considered in patients with an obstruction.[71]

Complications

Bowel obstructions can be a life-ending event in patients with advanced illness.

Indications for Referral or Hospitalization

See the earlier information regarding physician consultation and immediate emergency department referral.

Life Span Considerations

Outcomes of surgical treatment for geriatric patients with bowel obstructions are poor, particularly for those who have DNR orders.[72] Thirty-day mortality (30%) and postoperative complications (47%) were quite high in a large series. Based on these data, it was recommended that patients, families, and physicians be counseled on surgical expectations preoperatively when emergency surgical management of bowel obstruction in the older adult is being considered.[72]

Education and Health Promotion

Patients and family should be aware of the patients' overall prognosis and the potential outcomes for various treatments in specific disease states (e.g., benign versus malignant disease) before a treatment decision is reached.[73]

PAIN

Definition and Epidemiology

Pain at the end of life is one of the most feared symptoms. It can be present with many disease conditions, including heart failure and cancer, and in hospice patients, nursing home residents, and community-dwelling elders.[74] Pain is highly prevalent, especially in the 4 months before death.[75] The International Association for the Study of Pain (IASP) defines pain as an unpleasant sensory and emotional experience associated with actual or potential tissue damage.[76] Dame Cicely Saunders, key contributor to the modern hospice movement, coined the term *total pain* and suggested that pain be understood as having physical, psychological, social, emotional, and spiritual components.[77] Margo McCaffrey developed the classic definition of pain as "whatever the experiencing person says it is, existing whenever the experiencing person says it does."[78] Hospitalized patients who continue to follow normal routines and undergo unnecessary procedures such as daily weights, laboratory tests, vital signs, and prescribed position changes may also experience unnecessary discomfort. Essential to good pain assessment is providing comfort to family members and eliciting their assessment of the patient's comfort when the patient cannot communicate. The following section briefly addresses pain issues specific to the end of life. (Chapter 19 provides a comprehensive review of many similar principles of pain management.)

Diagnostics

Radiographic imaging at the site of pain can be considered, particularly if fracture is a concern and if radiography is in alignment with goals of care. For patients with goals of care focused on quality of life, if imaging will not change the course of treatment, it may be superfluous.

Differential Diagnosis

Differentiating between nociceptive and neuropathic pain can affect management strategies (see Chapter 222).

Management

Physician consultation is indicated for uncontrolled intractable pain.

Immediate emergency department referral is indicated for uncontrolled intractable pain. If patient is on hospice, hospice should be called before emergency room referral. It is important to communicate patients' goals of care to the emergency department and all other treating health care providers.

Unrelieved pain at the end of life is unnecessary and with few exceptions is treatable. Practical issues can be the most challenging, including the loss of the oral route for medication administration, a wish to die at home, non–opioid-responsive total pain or suffering, and fear that pain treatment may hasten death. With the skill and expertise of hospice or home care support, all of the previously mentioned issues can be overcome and expert pain relief can occur at home or in long-term care settings.

Loss of Oral Route. There are many alternatives to oral opioid administration, and routes of administration should be modified as needed.[79] Medications can be provided rectally (including enteric-coated tablets or suppositories), transdermally, sublingually (by high-concentrate solutions administered to the oral cavity), or subcutaneously (continuously, intermittently, or by a patient-controlled pump). Given these options, there rarely is a need for intravenous catheters, which can be painful to insert and provide interrupted analgesia when infiltrated. There is no ceiling dose of opioids. Balancing analgesia against reduced level of consciousness can be based on patient preference.[79]

Fear of Hastening Death. There is great fear that the administration of opioids at the end of life will hasten death. This has resulted in inadequate pain management at the end of life. The American Society for Pain Management Nursing has a position statement regarding pain management at the end of life.[80] It refers to the American Nurses Association position regarding the nurse's roles and responsibilities in providing expert care at the end of life, noting that nurses must use effective doses of medications prescribed for symptom control.[81] A retrospective study of patients cared for at home found that the use of opioids, even high-dose opioids or escalating doses, did not shorten survival.[82] Patients develop enormous tolerance to the respiratory depressant effects of opioids, and high doses of opioids can be both appropriate and safe in terminally ill patients with pain.[78] Patients who have a life-limiting illness should continue to receive opioids for pain relief or dyspnea until the time of death. Respiratory depression from opioids can occur but is most often noted in the opioid-naive person. Careful upward titration in response to pain rarely causes respiratory depression because pain is a natural stimulant to the respiratory center. Patients, families, and nursing staff should be educated about the appropriate use of pain medications for symptom control.

Complications

Complications included here are adverse effects of opioids. Constipation is an expected side effect of opioid use. Stimulants should be started concurrently with standing opioid regimens with a note to hold for diarrhea. Senna with docusate, 1 to 4 tablets twice daily and titrated to effect, is commonly used.

Usually opioid tolerance develops. If patients experience nausea and vomiting, antiemetics are prescribed on a schedule for the first 3 to 5 days after opioid use is initiated. Undesirable sedation can be managed with low-dose methylphenidate (Ritalin), which can be rapidly tapered when no longer needed.

Life Span Considerations

Pain in older patients is often undertreated with patterns of low doses of analgesics or the use of only nonopioids. Guidelines from the APS, the National Comprehensive Cancer Network (NCCN), and the American Geriatric Society recommend application of the same pharmacologic approaches as for younger adults, with the direction to "start low and go slow" as the general rule of opioid titration and to compensate for potentially diminished drug metabolism. Geriatric oncologists emphasize the importance of individual assessment rather than treatment based solely on age.[83]

Education and Health Promotion

Pain at the end of life is a commonly held fear by both patients and families. Reassurance needs to be provided that pain will be managed.

SPIRITUAL DISTRESS

Spirituality has been found to be one of the most important components of quality of life, at the end of life.[84] Greater spiritual quality at life's end is associated with higher overall quality of life, greater coping with disease-related symptoms, better psychosocial well-being, and dignified dying.[85,86] Enhanced spirituality may result in fewer symptoms of anxiety and depression,[87] and a belief in God has been associated with overall better coping.[88] Recognizing and supporting the spiritual aspect of patients can help mitigate the experience of loss and suffering.

Spirituality can be difficult for patients to describe.[89,90] It is a broad concept, and there are many ways to be spiritual. Connectedness is one of the core components of spirituality.[90] If relationships are fractured or if individuals are physically, emotionally, and spiritually preparing to disconnect from their families, the sense of connectedness may take on even greater importance.[91]

Under the strain of life-threatening illness, patients can develop spiritual distress. This distress is heard in questions such as "Why me?" or "What did I do to deserve this?" Such questions reflect a search for meaning in the experience, an effort to make sense of the incomprehensible. Patients may begin to question their sense of connectedness to a higher power or to relationships that they consider important. The health care provider can act as an intuitive listener who remains present with the patient. The healing begins in the telling of the story.[92] Many health care providers instinctively know that their most meaningful interventions involve the simplest gestures: the touch of a hand, a nod of affirmation, and a look of full and complete attention that exudes presence.

If a sense of hopelessness emerges in the patient, it is incumbent on the health care provider to determine meaningful, empowering interventions. Assessment of prior coping strategies provides a basis for intervening. Such assessment must include examination of the family, social, and community support available to the patient. These connections with others provide a basis for new hope. Patients who have relied more on cognitive coping strategies often find information or anticipatory guidance useful in alleviating anxiety and finding a new source of hope. Patients and families may wish to know what to expect as they approach the end of life and to have their decisions and beliefs regarding end-of-life experiences validated. Strategies for intervention that intentionally include spiritual care encourage the patient's own search for meaning. As body, mind, and spirit are bound together, spiritual care can take the form of relaxation, allowing the patient to exercise some control over his or her body and its sensory experiences. Relaxation and comfort can quickly be attained through hands-on physical interventions. Therapies such as acupuncture, therapeutic touch, biofeedback, reiki, reflexology, aromatherapy, chiropractic therapy, and massage serve as physical forms of care and pain relief for the whole patient. Guided imagery can draw on music, voices, images, scents, and color to induce a period of helpful relaxation and meditation. Use of these interventions helps promote a peaceful environment, can reduce anxiety and fear, and facilitates a patient's own sense of the spiritual. This approach can be as nourishing to the provider as it is to the patient.

Exploring ways to integrate a patient's own sense of spirituality into his or her ongoing plan of care is likely to improve quality of life, enhance a sense of control, and fortify a sense of connectedness.

PALLIATIVE SEDATION FOR MANAGEMENT OF INTRACTABLE SYMPTOMS IN PATIENTS NEAR DEATH

The term *palliative sedation* includes three primary aspects: (1) pharmacologic agents used to reduce consciousness, (2) use that is reserved for the treatment of intolerable and refractory symptoms, and (3) consideration only for a patient who has been diagnosed with an advanced progressive illness.[93] A hospital policy should be in place for palliative sedation, and it must incorporate an interdisciplinary team including nurses, physicians, social worker, and chaplains.[94] Palliative sedation is an intervention of last resort when all other aggressive attempts to relieve symptomatic suffering have been exhausted. Before the initiation of palliative sedation, interdisciplinary team discussions are recommended; the ethics committees of the institutions can be involved in the team discussions. These discussions are efforts to clarify issues in the decision to initiate palliative sedation. Involving the family and other people close to the patient in decision-making is important.[93] Patient or family informed consent is obtained.

In clinical practice, palliative sedation does not alter the timing or the mechanism of a patient's death because refractory symptoms are most often associated with very advanced terminal illness. The possibility that palliative sedation might hasten death as an unintended consequence should be assessed by the health care team in its consideration of palliative sedation and addressed directly in the process of informed consent. Institutional bioethics teams should be consulted in cases wherein there is disagreement regarding the provision of palliative sedation.[95]

REFERENCES

For a full list of references, scan the QR code or visit http://booksite.elsevier.com/9780323355018

PART 3

Health Maintenance

CHAPTER 15

OBESITY AND WEIGHT MANAGEMENT

Sharon L. Grantham

EPIDEMIOLOGY

Obesity is a worldwide problem of epidemic proportions. Globally, nearly 2.5 billion adults are affected by overweight or obesity (body mass index [BMI] of 25 kg/m^2 or greater). It is associated with an estimated 3.4 million deaths, 3.9% of years of life lost, and 3.8% of disability-adjusted life-years (DALYs). From 1980 to 2013, the global prevalence of overweight and obesity increased from 28.8% to 36.9% in men and from 29.8% to 38.0% in women. Estimated prevalence is over 50% in men in Tonga and women in Kuwait, Kiribati, Federated States of Micronesia, Libya, Qatar, Tonga, and Samoa. In developed countries, the increase in adult obesity has slowed. However, no country has made progress in reducing obesity in the past 30 years.[1]

In the United States, the estimated prevalence of overweight adults is 68.5%; obesity, 34.9%; and class 3 obesity (BMI >40 kg/m^2), 6.4%.[2] The pattern is widely variable across populations. Over 50% of U.S. non-Hispanic black women older than 40 years are obese compared with 40% of Hispanic and 33% of non-Hispanic white women.[3] Food insecurity is modestly associated with higher obesity rates in U.S. women but not in men, and the relationship is stronger in nonwhite women.[4] Level of education is inversely related to obesity and overweight.[4] In immigrant adults born outside the United States, obesity rates increase with time lived in the United States and vary among countries of origin. U.S. adults born in Mexico, South America, Europe, Russia, Africa, and the Middle East have a three-times-higher odds ratio (OR) of being overweight after 15 years compared with their counterparts who have resided less than 5 years in the United States. Among immigrants from the Indian subcontinent and Southeast Asia, weight increases begin earlier. In young women migrants from Africa and the Indian subcontinent, the OR of being overweight is higher than in those from Europe.[5] Of U.S. military veterans, 78% are obese or overweight.[6]

Obesity-related deaths account for 5% to 15% of deaths in the United States. Spending for obesity-related illness costs are estimated at $150 million per year in 2013 dollars and $821 million in 2017 dollars for Medicare, Medicaid, and private insurance payers. Medical spending per year was 42%, or $1429, greater in obese than in normal-weight people in 2008 dollars and accounts for 16.5% of U.S. national health expenditures.[7] Another research method estimated these costs to be $2826 per year.[8] The costs related to obesity-related illness may increase to $344 billion per year by 2018 if current obesity trends continue.[9] Understanding, treating, and preventing obesity has a substantial economic impact for the country.

DEFINITION

Obesity is a chronic condition in which the body's homeostatic balance between energy intake and energy expenditure is dysfunctional, resulting in excess energy stored in adipose tissue to the extent that this excess adipose negatively affects health with signs, symptoms, harm, and morbidity An obesogenic environment has myriad contributors, including genetic factors, excess calorie intake, reduced physical activity, increased sedentary behavior, environmental contributions, and food industry promotion to increase consumption. Obesity is considered a chronic disorder because it requires perpetual care, support, and follow-up.[10,11]

Adipose tissue is composed of adipocytes (fat cells that store energy as triglycerides plus glycerol), preadipocytes, vascular structures, fibroblasts, endothelial cells, and macrophages.[12] The size and number of adipocytes vary across body regions; more deleterious health consequences are linked with fat cells in the intra-abdominal area visceral fat depots compared with subcutaneous or femoral-hip fat deposits. Adipose tissue functions include energy storage, body structure cushioning, and complex endocrine, exocrine, paracrine, and immune roles. Adipose tissue has embryonic origins and may contain only one lipid droplet in the immature state.

Body Mass Index and Waist Circumference

BMI is a proxy measure of body fatness, more accurate than weight alone, and is easy and inexpensive to use in clinical settings. It is a simple numeric calculation of weight in kilograms divided by height in meters squared (BMI = kg/m^2). English measurement conversion involves a multiplier of 703: BMI = ($pounds/inches^2$) × 703.

BMI is a screening tool, with low specificity, and to be used as a screening tool rather than a definitive diagnostic standard. There are limitations in using BMI as a standard for determining excess body fat in association with increased disease risk, overweight, and obesity. The BMI measurement does not account for body fat percentage, body fat distribution, body frame size, capacity for metabolic activity, and amount of lean tissue, such as muscle and bone. The BMI calculation does not account for muscularity resulting from physical training, puberty or menopause status, race or ethnicity, gender, limb length, limb amputations, spinal deformities, or sarcopenia related to aging.[10] For example, physically fit individuals with increased muscle mass may have a high BMI measurement indicating erroneously that they are overweight and at risk for the complications of obesity. Patients with BMI under 25, especially when accompanied by excess abdominal fat and enlarged waist circumference, may have obesity-associated metabolic disturbances. Screening for obesity through use of BMI is recommended for all adults.[6,10]

Waist circumference as a reliable surrogate adipose measure is clinically practical because of its low cost, portability, and ease of use. Even with variable user techniques and guideline differences about tape measure locations for waist circumference, the strong association of central adiposity with higher morbidity and mortality is maintained. This waist circumference relationship is strongest for adverse cardiovascular and cancer outcomes and is more robust in women than in men. Waist-to-hip ratios indicate increasing cardiometabolic disease risk as the ratio increases in men and women (larger waist compared with smaller hips), and the risk increases with circumference. In North American adults with BMI between 25 and 35 kg/m^2, waist measurement circumference of 102 cm (40 inches) or greater in men and 102 cm (35 inches) or greater in women indicates increased cardiometabolic risk. These cutoff values are lower in individuals of European, South Asian, Chinese, or Japanese origin as compared with North American cutoffs with regard to cardiometabolic disease risks.[13] Annual measurement is indicated. However, in individuals with BMI above 35, elevated waist circumference is not likely to provide additional information regarding disease risk.[13]

Reliable measures of adiposity include hydrodensitometry (underwater weighing), air displacement plethysmography, dual-energy x-ray absorptiometry (DXA), computed tomography (CT) scan, and magnetic resonance imaging (MRI), which are used in research settings but are not practical in routine clinical use.

Bioimpedance Analysis

Bioimpedance analysis (BIA) predicts body fat and lean mass by use of alternating current that passes through the body. BIA is noninvasive, portable, safe, and inexpensive. It allows practitioners to estimate body fat in a clinic setting and is often used in weight loss research; patients may be familiar with it because BIA instruments are present in some fitness centers and available for consumer home use. Results are comparable to those of DXA and hydrostatic weighing and are reliable. BIA has disadvantages that include variable results according to hydration status and recent physical activity. Its use in elders, children, and those with high levels of physical fitness are not as reliable. Men with body fat higher than 25% and women with higher than 30% are considered obese.[14] Guidelines for treatment of overweight and obesity do not recommend the use of BIA in routine clinical application, because it adds no more information than BMI and waist circumference and requires additional resources.[13]

PATHOPHYSIOLOGY

The causes of common obesity are multifactorial with two commonalities: increased energy intake and reduced energy expenditure. These obesogenic factors, kilocalorie abundance in a sedentary environment, interact with genetic predispositions in complex obesogenic systems favoring increasing adiposity storage. Excess body weight and obesity result when the energy intake and conserving energy expenditure forces are greater than the opposing forces. Determinants of energy balance and obesity are many, complex, interrelated, and not fully elucidated; determinants alone do not fully explain obesity's prevalence, severity, or unequal distribution.

Individual appetite, satiety, and meal size are driven by neuroendocrine factors, adipocyte size and number, gut factors, food availability, and nutrient interactions that occur in the context of social, economic, and genetic environments. An abundance of food is needed for obesity to develop, but variations occur across genotypes, age at exposure, source and quality of food, conscious efforts to control calorie intake, hormone status, endocrine disruptors, and as yet undefined environmental interactions. An extra 100 kcal/day taken in or not expended can result in a gain of 4.5 kg (10 pounds) per year.

Individual energy intake and output balance factors are of great interest to obesity researchers. The central nervous system (CNS) controls energy intake through appetite, hunger, and satiety; the drive for energy expenditure occurs mainly in the hypothalamus, with feedback from adipose tissue, muscle, liver, pancreas, and gut signals. Insulin and leptin signal adequacy of food and adipose tissue; gut hormones send satiety signals during meals. A competing system between anorexic neuron and orexigenic neuron activity controls in the arcuate nucleus of the hypothalamus regulates food intake, energy expenditure, and glucose homeostasis. The orexin pathway is mediated by agouti-related protein/neuropeptide Y (AgRP/NPY) neurons; they promote hunger and increased food intake and conserve energy by inhibiting activities that use energy. Anorexic neurons, pro-opiomelanocortin (POMC) and cocaine-amphetamine–regulated transcript (CART), drive anorexia and energy-expending, catabolic processes. Both neuron populations signal alternatively through the melanocortin receptors (MC4R and MC3R).

The competing systems are asymmetric, with redundancy in the mechanisms regulating hunger and conservation of energy as well as stronger drivers in the orexigenic hunger and energy-conserving pathways. Overriding of the satiety system's homeostasis can be accomplished with hedonic foods, those that have high neurally mediated rewarding properties. Highly rewarding sights and sounds and palatable layering of flavors contribute to hedonic rewards of food. The hedonic pathway is especially activated with the combination of sweet plus fatty foods. Hedonic hunger occurs when there is no physiologic basis for perceived energy needs. The amount of work needed to obtain food, the food's hedonic qualities, and the quantity of food available override homeostatic energy balance mechanisms.[15,16] Dopamine- and opioid-mediated pleasure and reward pathways in the brain can become fixed and hardwired to crave sweet plus high-fat foods. Hyperinsulinemia, common in obesity and metabolic syndrome, prevents dopamine clearance from the pleasure centers, so pleasure from food is enhanced and intake continues beyond energy needs.[17] Obese persons also have lower dopamine D_2 receptor activity in negative correlation with BMI when it is measured by positron emission tomography. Motivation to eat and pleasure or reward may be dysfunctional, inhibitory satiety processes may be disrupted, and increased eating and obesity may result.

Lesions—chemically caused, inherited, or arising from structural damage to the hypothalamus—can induce hyperphagia by suppressing POMC and CART neurons and MC3R and MC4R, so satiety signaling is impaired, energy output is reduced, and hunger increases. Causes of hypothalamic obesity include head trauma, cranial surgery, ventriculoperitoneal shunt placement, hypothalamic radiation therapy, antipsychotic medications, and tumors; they are associated with rapid weight gain, uncontrolled eating, reduced energy expenditure, and hyperinsulinemia.[18]

Adipocytes in white adipose tissue store extra energy through insulin, affecting lipid and glucose uptake by glucose transporter type 4 (GLUT4) and other transporters. Insulin is the central controller of energy balance. Higher insulin levels, whether endogenous or exogenous, promote greater uptake of energy (glucose) in fat and muscle cells and inhibit lipolysis, or fat breakdown. Pancreatic beta cells secrete insulin in response to food intake, glucose and fatty acid uptake is facilitated, and glycogenesis (glucose storage in muscle or hepatic tissue) is inhibited. In a fasted state, glucagon is released from pancreatic alpha cells to maintain euglycemia by stimulating hepatic gluconeogenesis and glycogenolysis.[19] Insulin, whether it is endogenous or exogenous, not only inhibits lipolysis (the use of stored lipids), but also stimulates de novo free fatty acid synthesis.[19] Decreased pancreatic insulin secretion occurs in the absence of carbohydrates, and lower insulin levels will increase the use of stored fat.[20] Insulin, along with leptin, crosses the blood-brain barrier and signals satiety in the lateral hypothalamus.[19] Central, CNS administration of insulin antibodies results in increased food intake and weight gain, and inactivated insulin receptors plus excess food results in obesity. In addition to lower insulin levels, adrenal epinephrine and norepinephrine released during exercise promote use of stored fat.[20]

Leptin, a hormone secreted by adipocytes, acts as a long-term "lipostat"; it communicates the amount of stored body fat to the hypothalamus. Leptin secretion by adipocytes increases in parallel with increases in fat mass. Leptin and insulin receptors in the hypothalamus are saturable, contributing to central leptin and insulin resistance in obesity. In leptin resistance, higher levels fail to initiate an anorectic plus increased energy expenditure effect that should follow an overabundance of stored energy. Leptin is also secreted by gastric mucosa, along with cholecystokinin, and relays gut information to the CNS that results in satiety and controls meal size.[19] Leptin levels reflect subcutaneous fat more than visceral adipose tissue and are higher in women. Adipokines are cytokines of adipose tissue origin and include leptin, adiponectin, and tumor necrosis factor-α (TNF-α) among others.[12] Adiponectin secreted by adipocytes is inversely proportionate to fat mass; higher fat masses are associated with lower serum levels. Adiponectin has beneficial effects on glycemic control, insulin sensitivity, and nonatherogenic lipid profiles and has anti-inflammatory properties. Visceral adipose tissue secretes less adiponectin than subcutaneous depots do. TNF-α is an inflammatory cytokine secreted from resident macrophages of adipose tissues in proportion to BMI.[12]

Gut hormones involved with energy homeostasis include ghrelin, a potent gastric orexigen that signals hunger through arcuate nucleus–released AgRP/NPY to drive increased food intake. Cholecystokinin, in response to protein and fat ingestion, is secreted from the small bowel; it stimulates pancreatic digestive enzymes and gallbladder contraction and sends satiety signals through the vagus nerve to the hindbrain. Glucagon-like peptide 1 (GLP-1) from the bowel also acts as a CNS satiety signal, slows gastric emptying, and regulates glucose by alternating insulin and glucagon activity.[19]

Energy Output

Energy is needed for physical activity, digestion of food, heat liberation from brown adipose tissue, and maintenance of the minimal essential functions of body organs. These essential energy needs constitute 50% to 70% of a sedentary person's energy output and collectively make up the basal metabolic rate (BMR). BMR varies according to gender, thyroid activity, smoking status, growth hormone levels, skeletal muscle mass, and fever. The remaining energy output is expended in purposeful physical activity (25%), nonexercise activity (7%), and the thermic effect of food (8%).[20] Processing, digesting, absorbing, and storing of food after meals raise the metabolic rate. This increased metabolic, thermogenic effect of food can be about 4% after a high-carbohydrate meal and as much as 30% after ingestion of a high-protein meal.[20]

Insufficient Physical Activity

Lack of physical activity is risk factor for obesity and its related comorbidities, type 2 diabetes mellitus (T2DM), cardiovascular disease, hypertension, stroke, breast and colon cancer, and other health concerns.[21] Moderate to vigorous levels of recommended activity are based on promotion and maintenance of health. Recommended endurance (aerobic) exercise minimums are 30 minutes per day for moderate-intensity or 20 minutes per day for vigorous-intensity physical activity, in bouts of 10 minutes or more. Brisk walking at 3 mph, bicycling at 10 to 12 mph, and dancing are moderate, expending 3.0 to 6.0 metabolic equivalents (METs). Jogging, shoveling, and bicycling at 12 to 16 mph are vigorous activities that expend more than 6.0 METs. The health benefits of physical activity are dose dependent. For preventing weight gain, maintaining weight loss, or relying on physical activity as a primary means to weight loss, more than the minimum (150 minutes of moderate or 60 to 75 minutes of vigorous physical activity accumulated per week) may be necessary. Most studies and recommendations support as much as 300 minutes of moderate-intensity activity per week, or about 1 hour per day, to avoid weight gain or to prevent regain after weight loss.[22] Less than half of U.S. adults get the recommended minimum level of physical activity, and more than one in five have no leisure-time activity.[21] Physical activity energy expenditure is frequently distorted, and even among adults educated in guidelines, distortions persist about actual activity performed. It is common to overestimate the relative kilocalories expended in various physical activities and also to overestimate the amount of one's physical activity.[3]

Energy Intake

Energy intake has increased by 150 to 300 kcal/day during the last 30 years, with about half of these calories from sugar-sweetened beverages. Liquid kilocalories do not have the stronger satiety signaling properties of solid foods, and sugar-sweetened beverages may contribute to hedonic rewards that mediate greater kilocalorie ingestion.[3] Factors contributing to this include media consumption, food exposure, more food-efficient consumption, nutritional quality of food and drink, variety, and grazing habits. Observation of the proximate and conventional approaches to obesity management and those links that promote greater intake of energy highlights the pressing number of factors to be overcome in managing obesity.

Genetics

Obesity genes are those that influence BMI, waist-to-hip ratio, eating behaviors, energy expenditure, and abdominal fat, with overlap for genes that influence lipids, blood pressure, insulin, and nutrient partitioning. Putative loci are on all chromosomes except Y. The understanding of gene-environment contributions to obese phenotypes is continuing to expand, as is discovery of how genes can be silenced or activated by environmental triggers. Genome-wide association studies support theories that interactions of multiple genes contribute to obesity.[23]

Adiposity is a heritable, quantitative trait. BMI, as a measure of adiposity, can vary quantitatively. For example, a 5-foot, 8-inch person's BMI can range from 16 to 60 kg/m^2 (105 to 400 pounds). Gene pool shifts cannot account for the sharp increase in global obesity; a gene-environment effect offers more likely explanations, with abundant food supply a necessary component. Family and twin studies have confirmed strong heritable factors in BMI, accounting for as much as 45% to 75% variance. Maternal obesity has a stronger effect than paternal obesity, perhaps from the prenatal and postnatal environment, with sex difference correlations in offspring obesity. Genetic bases for macronutrient preferences, restrained and binge eating, meal size, and activity levels have been studied.[24]

Monogenic causes of obesity are rare and are associated with MC4R-mediated appetite control center disruption involving satiety and energy expenditure signaling dysfunctions. Normally, adiposity increases coincide with increased circulating leptin from adipose tissue, which signals satiety. In *MC4R* mutations, rising leptin levels fail to signal satiety by MC4R mechanisms. More than 130 *MC4R* mutations are known; most confer extra obesity risk.

Inborn leptin deficiency is rare, but treatment with recombinant leptin results in substantial fat loss as hyperphagic, all-day eating patterns cease. Mutations for leptin, leptin receptor, and prohormone convertase 1 and *POMC* genes result in early, severe obesity, along with specific phenotype characteristics. The two most common syndrome obesities are Prader-Willi and Bardet-Biedl.[25]

Polygenic obesity, the most common type, is caused by expression of additive and nonadditive effects of multiple alleles that control the quantitative BMI phenotype. Perhaps 100 polygenic variants, each with small effect sizes of less than 100 g, are present uniquely in obese individuals.[24,25] The fat mass and obesity gene, *FTO*, is recognized as the strongest obesity signaling gene; yet the *FTO* BMI effects are small, accounting for less than 0.5% variance, about 6 pounds.[23]

Maternal Influences

Metabolic programming begins at least in utero and probably sooner, in the preconception period. The hypothalamic appetite center, adipocytes, and insulin-glucose homeostasis are sensitive to the gestational environment. High maternal glucose concentration—130 mg/dL or higher—even in healthy BMI mothers without gestational diabetes, is associated with a doubled risk for overweight or obesity in toddlers compared with gestational glucose concentration below 100 mg/dL.[26] Excessive weight during pregnancy is associated with higher childhood and adult obesity in the offspring.[4] After birth, early feeding practices continue to influence BMI. Breastfeeding seems to confer a decreased risk for childhood, adolescent, and adult obesity and reduces maternal cardiometabolic risks decades later,[27] during the mother's menopause years. Breastfeeding infants are self-regulators of their intake and do not ingest more even when supplies are intentionally increased. Leptin from maternal mammary secretion may signal infant satiety and affect hypothalamic appetite. In addition to leptin, the hormones adiponectin, insulin-like growth factor 1, resistin, and obestatin are found in human milk and may be part of early nutritional programming in developing hypothalamic appetite and energy output control centers. These human milk peptides could have effects beyond the time of lactation. Formula-fed infants have higher serum ghrelin (hunger hormone) levels.[4] Timing of solid food introduction may have variable effects on weight gain based on formula feeding versus breastfeeding. Formula-fed infants had greater odds of obesity at the age of 3 years when solid foods were introduced before 4 months of age compared with breastfed infants.[28]

Famine, resulting from natural causes or war, has given evidence of long-lasting effects on offspring obesity that manifest in toddlerhood and midlife, preferentially in female children, from poorly nourished mothers during gestation. These children are shorter and, as adults, remain short with a greater risk of obesity 50 years later.[29] Maternal smoking during pregnancy is associated with 50% increased odds of obesity in children and young adults, ages 3 to 33 years.[30]

Smoking Status and Smoking Cessation

The BMIs of cigarette smokers tend to be lower than those of nonsmokers, but their visceral fat stores are greater even without increased waist circumferences. Weight gain related to smoking cessation occurs in the majority of quitters, occurs mostly in the early months after cessation, and is typically 10 pounds or less. Weight gain predictors after cessation include younger age, higher baseline BMI, smoking more than 25 cigarettes per day, African-American race, pregnancy, and genetic predisposition. Weight gain concerns can be barriers to smoking cessation, especially in women. Nicotine also acts as an appetite suppressant, more so when it is combined with caffeine.[31] Further effects of nicotine include increased metabolic rate, about 200 kcal/25 cigarettes, decreased neuropeptide Y and orexin (both increase food intake), suppression of fat storage effects from adipose tissue protein lipase, and changes in leptin levels. Weight gain from smoking cessation tends to involve visceral, centrally located adipose tissue and is accompanied by worsening of other metabolic syndrome components, except high-density lipoprotein cholesterol (HDL-C). The risk for diabetes increases in early years after smoking cessation, and this seems to be associated with weight gain. However, diabetes risk drops significantly in subsequent years. Nicotine replacement therapy with bupropion or varenicline may delay weight gain associated with smoking cessation, but the gain typically occurs when these therapies are discontinued. Some individuals use cigarette smoking, and possibly electronic e-cigarettes, as a means of weight control. In past years the tobacco industry promoted smoking as "slimming" and as an alternative to snacking.[32] The health benefits of smoking cessation greatly exceed the short-term metabolic weight gain and in general take priority over weight concerns. Use of other nicotine delivery methods, such as the increasingly popular electronic e-cigarettes can be expected to play a role in undesirable weight control strategies used by individuals.

Pharmaceuticals Associated with Weight Gain

Genetic variations contribute to different metabolic responses to the weight gain effects of pharmaceuticals. CNS-mediated weight gain is associated with antidepressants, antipsychotics, anticonvulsants, mood stabilizers, and migraine prophylaxis agents. Many antidiabetic medications are associated with significant weight gain, which compromises health and increases risk factors for cardiovascular disease and mortality.[33,34]

Diabetes Medications. Insulin and insulin analogues increase weight more than other antidiabetic drugs, through multiple means. Glycosuria calories are recovered, lipolysis is inhibited, triglyceride and glucose storage in adipocytes is upregulated, appetite increases, and anabolic protein and adipose synthesis increases. Expected weight gain follows expected improvement in hemoglobin A_{1c} (HbA_{1c}): additional 2 to 10 kg for 1.5% to 2.5% improvements. Insulin secretagogues—sulfonylureas especially, but also meglitinides—have a similar effect; as insulin levels increase, the anabolic effects result from more insulin. Thiazolidinediones increase appetite, fat mass through the adipogenic effects of peroxisome proliferator-activated receptor γ (PPAR-γ), and fluid retention and may cause 0.5 to 1.4 kg weight gain. Metformin may be weight negative (−0.5 to −4.5 kg) initially because of gastrointestinal (GI) side effects, but also because of reduced hepatic glucose output and stimulation of GLP-1 endogenous release without an increase in insulin output. GLP-1 receptor agonists and amylin analogues are associated with weight loss. Dipeptidyl peptidase 4 inhibitors and α-glucosidase inhibitors are weight neutral.[33]

Antidepressants, Neuroleptic and Seizure Medications. Tricyclic antidepressants (TCAs) are hypothesized to increase carbohydrate craving because of antihistaminergic effects, altering hypothalamic neuromodulated food-energy balance toward increasing fat stores and decreasing energy expenditures. Resting metabolic rate decreases during TCA treatment. Irreversible monoamine oxidase inhibitors (MAOIs) are also associated with weight gain. Selective serotonin reuptake inhibitors (SSRIs) are commonly prescribed. SSRIs disrupt appetite stimulation through changes in 5-hydroxytryptamine type 2 C and histamine H_1 receptors and may induce carbohydrate cravings. These agents may result in an initial weight loss, followed by weight gain. Paroxetine is the most weight-positive SSRI, especially in women. Mirtazapine has been associated with 11% weight gain, mostly in the early time period. Lithium weight gain tends to peak within the first 2 years and is greater in those with greater baseline BMI. Lithium's weight gain effects possibly result from increased carbohydrate craving, increased storage of carbohydrates and lipids, and lower BMR from reduced thyroid function. The antidepressant venlafaxine is weight neutral, and bupropion is associated with 1.0- to 4.4-kg weight loss.[33,34]

Atypical antipsychotics have potent orexigenic effects of reversing leptin's hypothalamic anorectic effect, upregulating adenosine monophosphate-activated protein kinase, blocking a histamine receptor, stimulating appetite, and causing central insulin resistance, all of which contribute to weight gain of 2 to 17 kg, impaired glucose handling, diabetes, and dyslipidemia. Clozapine and olanzapine cause the greatest weight gains, which tend to be dose dependent. Risperidone and quetiapine weight gains are more modest and possibly dose dependent. Aripiprazole, olanzapine, and zotepine are associated with less weight gain.[33,34]

Valproic acid elevates leptin and insulin levels and decreases gluconeogenesis, beta-oxidation of fatty acids, albumin binding with long-chain fatty acids, and energy expenditure, all of which contribute to weight gain that continues even after years of treatment. Carbamazepine, pregabalin, and gabapentin are associated with weight gain. Lamotrigine, levetiracetam, and oxcarbazepine are weight neutral, whereas topiramate and zonisamide promote weight loss.[33,34]

Antihistamines. The weight gain effects of antihistamines are mediated by blockade of H_1 receptors. H_1 activity promotes satiety; hence, blockade increases appetite with possible increased carbohydrate cravings. Antihistamine users have higher BMIs, waist circumferences and insulin levels. Cyproheptadine is especially appetite stimulating. Loratadine and desloratadine are associated with little or no weight gain.[33,34]

The metabolic effects of antiretrovirals lead to redistribution of fat from subcutaneous to visceral depots, insulin resistance, and weight gain.[34]

Hormonal Preparations. Combined hormone contraceptives and menopause hormone replacement are not associated with weight gain in population studies, but individual responses could vary. Progesterone-only contraceptive medroxyprogesterone injections may increase fat gains without increasing appetite, but the effect may be limited to adolescents with preexisting overweight condition.[33] The levonorgestrel-releasing intrauterine system also lists weight gain as a side effect in its provider information. Megestrol stimulates appetite. Tamoxifen and aromatase inhibitors have mixed reports about weight gain. Corticosteroids increase weight, especially centrally located fat, by impairing glucose tolerance. All administration routes, including inhaled corticosteroids, have been implicated in weight gains.[33]

Cardiac Medications. Beta blockade inhibits beta-adrenergic satiety effects and lipolysis, reduces thermogenic responses to food, reduces BMR, and reduces energy expenditure. Beta blockers also increase insulin resistance and serum triglycerides, and because visceral fat depots have more beta-adrenergic receptors, visceral fat could increase.[33] Blockade of sympathetic activity was researched in hypertensive, beta blocker–treated participants compared with weight-matched controls. Results demonstrated that treated individuals had higher BMI, 50% lower thermogenic responses to food, 32% lower fat oxidation rate, and 30% lower energy expenditure from physical activity.[35] Calcium channel blockers can increase edema but not fat gains. Central-acting alpha$_2$-adrenergic receptor agonists can decrease metabolic rate and increase appetite.[33]

Environmental Factors

An endocrine-disrupting substance is defined by the U.S. Environmental Protection Agency as "an exogenous agent that interferes with synthesis, secretion, transport, metabolism, binding action, or elimination of natural hormones that are present in the body and are responsible for homeostasis, reproduction, and developmental process."[36] Endocrine disrupters acting as obesogens may be pharmaceuticals, environmental toxins, and food components that promote fat accumulation through several pathways. The disruptions can occur in metabolic sensing, sex steroid regulation, central (hypothalamic) energy balance, adipogenesis, and metabolic set-points.[37] The exposure effects vary according to timing of exposure (perinatal and developmental periods), levels of exposure, and synergistic interactions with multiple endocrine disrupters; the effects may have latent expression and in some cases be transmitted across multiple generations. Adipose tissue stores and concentrates many fat-soluble compounds, and a positive correlation exists between BMI and endocrine disrupter burden. Environmental estrogens can affect lipogenesis, lipolysis, adipocyte production of leptin, and estrogen receptors. Genistein, found in soy, in low concentrations seems to inhibit lipogenesis through its binding with estrogen receptors, but in high concentrations, genistein promotes lipogenesis through PPAR-γ receptors. Bisphenol A (BPA) has an impact on pancreatic beta cell function, is associated with hyperinsulinemia, inhibits adiponectin (thus reducing insulin sensitivity), and increases susceptibility to obesity comorbidities, metabolic syndrome, and T2DM. BPA may increase estrogen receptor expression in the hypothalamus, and it is highly concentrated in amniotic fluid. Endocrine disrupters appear in the food supply, including human milk, which concentrates substances, and soy-based formulas that are packaged in BPA-lined cans.[36] The effects may be synergistic because endocrine-disrupting substances act as obesogens, interacting with other genetic and behavioral factors and a food supply rich in highly palatable, rewarding foods to disrupt regulation of energy balance.[37]

Sleep Factors

Inadequate sleep is associated with increased ghrelin, decreased leptin, disturbed glucose-insulin homeostasis, increased appetite with preference for high-carbohydrate foods, and more opportunities for food intake, which may contribute to its association with obesity in many populations.[38,39] Sleep habits may be an overlooked factor in weight gain and weight loss efforts. A small study of short duration reported better fat loss and sparing of lean tissue and better fat oxidation in those sleeping 8.5 hours compared with those with short sleep conditions (5.5 hours) during a kilocalorie-restricted diet.[40]

Gut Microbiota

Intestinal flora, or gut microbiota, in obese persons tends toward a greater proportion of gram-negative Firmicutes and fewer gram-negative Bacteroidetes compared with lean individuals. These differences may provide a gut environment that favors greater calorie extraction from carbohydrates ingested, enhances lipogenic effects favoring fat storage, and provides a source of endotoxins that support a chain of events involving low-grade inflammation, insulin resistance, adverse atherosclerotic environments, and nonalcoholic fatty liver disease (NAFLD).[41] Gut microbiota changes may predate or be the result of obesity, and alterations are associated with antibiotics, non-nutritive artificial sweeteners, and cesarean section birth methods that bypass the vaginal flora exposure for neonates.[42]

Psychosocial Stress

Stress is a risk factor for modest adiposity gains, but the effect size was small in meta-analysis of 14 longitudinal cohort studies. Men experiencing major life events and acute stressors showed a greater effect, possibly related to the higher cardiovascular, neuroendocrine, and elevated cortisol responses to stressors compared with women. Studies with follow-up of 5 years or longer showed stronger effects than those with follow-up of less than 5 years.[43]

Food Quality, Nutrients, and Availability

The nutritional content or lack of nutritional content of food affects weight status. Nutrient-poor but energy-dense foods are less expensive than nutrient-rich foods and more abundant in most settings.[4] Deficiencies in micronutrients are common in obesity. In preoperative nutritional evaluations, bariatric surgery patients commonly have deficiencies of vitamins D, A, E, and C and some B vitamins as well as calcium, iron and ferritin, zinc, and selenium.[44] Deficiencies occur across countries of varying income status, and although the relationship between cause and effect is not solid, the deficiencies seem to precede obesity in populations with greater deficiencies. U.S. families with food insecurity eat foods that are less nutrient rich, get less dietary calcium, and eat fewer vegetables and consume more kilocalories from nutrient-poor foods, have greater access to market outlets for such foods ("food swamps"), and may have less access to market outlets for nutrient-rich foods ("food deserts").[4]

A report to Congress examined availability and affordability of nutritious food—such as access to fruits, vegetables, whole grains, and milk and grocery stores—in relation to their impact on health, including obesity. Food deserts are areas of low access to nutritional high-quality food,[45] and food swamps are areas replete with energy-dense food of low nutritional value. Food swamps seem to have a greater association with increased energy intake and obesity than food deserts do.[4,45]

Food pricing and government policy have both short- and long-term effects on food choices, and future policy decisions propose greater integration of health outcomes.[4] If the nation's individuals decided to follow nutrition guidelines, there would be a shortfall in fruits, vegetables, whole grains, and milk. A national mismatch occurs between what is produced and what is recommended.[46]

Food density—the proportion of nutrients to water and air—is correlated with greater BMI in population studies, and lower–food density diets have been shown to be effective in weight loss.[47]

Differences in food quality can have variable effects on metabolic health, weight gain, and fat gain. For example, recent trends indicate that monounsaturated fats, such as those found in peanuts and olives, may increase metabolism and assist weight loss.

Complications, Social Stigma, and Discrimination

Significant social stigma and discrimination affect obese persons. The stigma of obesity is pervasive and may profoundly affect many individuals. Obesity stigma is the devaluation of obese individuals as members of a group. It can manifest externally as weight-based discrimination or internally as prejudice. Stigma can also be self-directed as devaluation, guilt, and shame. Discrimination based on weight status affects opportunities for housing, career, education, and parental support; it is associated with bullying and harassment, and it contributes to health care disparities in provider expectations, recommendations, and preventive screenings ordered by practitioners.

Increased Morbidity and Mortality

Compared with a reference BMI of 22 to 24.9, mortality increases as BMI increases in nonsmoking adults without prevalent disease. This relationship is strongest when the higher BMI is noted before age 79 years. Significant health consequences associated with excess adiposity include increased mortality, chiefly from cardiovascular disease and cancers, but also from all other causes.[47] Cancers of the uterus, gallbladder, kidney, cervix, thyroid, liver, colon, and ovaries, leukemia, and postmenopausal breast cancer are associated with BMIs above 22 kg/m^2.[48] Other obesity-related conditions are gallbladder disease, NAFLD and nonalcoholic steatohepatitis (NASH), dyslipidemias, hypertension, atrial fibrillation, infertility, erectile dysfunction, asthma, chronic back pain, eye diseases (cataracts, glaucoma, age-related maculopathy, and retinopathy), osteoarthritis, decreased functioning in elderly, obstructive sleep apnea (OSA), and pulmonary embolism.

Relative risk for death from respiratory, cardiovascular, and cancer causes increased as waist circumferences increased above

90 cm in men and 75 cm in women. NAFLD represents the liver's response to obesity and is a hepatic component of metabolic syndrome. Steatosis, increased liver fat, begins the process of inflammation, hepatic cell death, and fibrotic scarring, leading to end-stage liver disease or hepatic cancer. Excess liver fat is an independent cardiovascular disease risk factor.[49]

Obesity and insulin resistance occur in half of women with polycystic ovary syndrome (PCOS); obese women overall have a 12% PCOS prevalence.[36] Fertility is impaired with obesity, mainly from oligo-ovulation and anovulation, and there is a reduced response to gonadotropin ovulation therapy. When pregnancy occurs in obese women, risks for miscarriage, spontaneous preterm birth, gestational diabetes, preeclampsia, cesarean delivery, and infectious complications are greater. Vaginal birth after cesarean delivery is less likely to be successful in obese women. Surgical times are increased, recovery from anesthesia is longer, greater blood loss occurs, and incidence of thromboembolism is higher in obese maternal surgeries. Labor is more likely to be prolonged. Fetal risks for congenital anomalies, growth abnormalities, defects of the neural tube and cardiac system, and cleft palate are increased. Stillbirth rates can be two to four times greater in obese mothers compared with normal-weight mothers.[50] Infants small and large for gestational age are associated with maternal obesity, and these children face an increased risk of childhood obesity.

Osteoarthritis risk is increased, not only in the weight-bearing joints of obese persons, but also in non–weight-bearing joints. Disability and reduced quality-adjusted life-years in obese persons with knee osteoarthritis are much higher than in nonobese individuals with this condition. Obese black and Hispanic women experience even greater reduced quality-adjusted life-years because of knee osteoarthritis than white obese women.[51] A dose-dependent response between BMI above 22.5 kg/m^2 and knee osteoarthritis was noted in a meta-analysis of studies from seven countries. BMIs at 25, 30, and 35 kg/m^2 were associated with increased relative risks of 1.59, 3.55, and 7.45, respectively.[52]

OSA prevalence in obesity is 41% to 58% and markedly higher when BMI is above 40 kg/m^2.[38] Chest wall compliance is reduced, work of breathing is increased, a higher minute ventilation accommodates a higher metabolic rate, and reduced lung volumes lend mechanical contributions to obesity hypoventilation. Insulin resistance with an altered hypothalamic response to orexins may contribute to neuroendocrine components of OSA in obese persons. In obese women with PCOS, OSA prevalence may be as high as 44% to 70%.[38]

Obesity-related impaired immunity function creates increased susceptibility for infectious disease from tuberculosis, influenza, coxsackievirus, *Helicobacter pylori,* and encephalomyocarditis virus and reduces antibody responses to vaccinations.[12] Risks for surgical wound infection, community-acquired pneumonia and other respiratory tract infections, in-hospital septicemia, and severe H1N1 influenza outcomes, including death, are increased.[12]

CLINICAL PRESENTATION

Overweight and obesity affect more U.S. adults than are not affected, and measurement of BMI is indicated in all adults. Obesity comorbidities are major (increased waist circumference, established coronary artery disease [history of myocardial infarction, angioplasty, coronary artery bypass graft surgery, or acute coronary event], peripheral vascular disease, abdominal aortic aneurysm, symptomatic carotid artery disease, T2DM, and OSA) or minor (cigarette smoking, hypertension or use of antihypertensives, dyslipidemia, elevated glucose concentration or impaired glucose handling, and family history of premature coronary artery disease). Osteoarthritis, gallbladder disease, gout, PCOS, stress incontinence, and fatty liver diseases are common, less life-threatening conditions. Direct specific OSA queries about loud snoring, witnessed periods of apnea, morning headache, and daytime sleepiness should be asked. Depression and eating disorder screening is indicated. Beliefs about healthy weight, food, and physical activity and health consequences of obesity are diverse and need to be queried with open-ended questions. Current nutrition and physical activity levels need to be quantified as part of the assessment, including portions, nutrients overconsumed or underconsumed, meal replacements, supplements, timing of meals and snacks, and eating disorder behaviors. All medications, including supplements, should be reviewed. Attend to sleep patterns, shift work, current smoking status or other nicotine use, country of birth, and support system information gathered in the social history. Medical and surgical history, patterns of weight gain, associations with childbirth, life-changing events, smoking and tobacco cessation history, and medications must be thoroughly investigated. Any previous attempts to lose weight, diets, medications, supplements, and surgeries should be investigated from the patient's perspective, clarifying details and perceptions as needed. Permit the patient to identify anything that is perceived to contribute to the weight (food intake, physical activity level, weight-based discrimination or stigma, and weight-associated comorbidities) without judgment. A questionnaire can facilitate the history gathering and can be completed before the appointment. Determine readiness for change in areas of weight loss, prevention of weight gain, physical activity, and dietary improvements.

Treatment of comorbidities may not improve weight status but must be addressed. If the history reveals more pressing concerns, such as bulimia with purging or substance abuse, these take priority. Smoking cessation is also considered a priority over weight loss.

PHYSICAL EXAMINATION

Every encounter should be nonjudgmental, nonbiased, and free of stereotypes. Language and other communications by staff should have no negative connotations. Weighing can be sensitive for many and should be private, with efforts made to avoid embarrassment. Medical equipment must be size appropriate, including armless, wide chairs; sturdy examination tables; step stools to approach examination tables; gowns; blood pressure cuffs; and speculums. The waiting room environment, including reading material, should reflect the needs of every size patient. All office processes, protocols, and standards should incorporate a team approach that is therapeutic. The provider must accept the task of treating patients who are overweight and obese with no condemnation, judgment, or weight-based stereotypes.

Weight status is categorized by obtaining an accurate height (measured, not stated), weight, and abdominal circumference (Box 15-1). Abdominal girth is measured above the iliac crest, with an inelastic tape placed parallel to the ground. Hip circumference is measured at the widest area across the gluteus, but this measurement is not necessary according to some guidelines. Comfort should be facilitated as much as possible by ensuring adequate lighting, warmth, and draping.

BOX 15-1

BMI Calculations and Classification

METRIC

Weight in kilograms/(height in meters)^2

AMERICAN STANDARD

Weight in pounds/(height in inches)^2 × 703

CLASSIFICATION

Underweight: BMI less than 18.5 kg/m^2
Normal weight: BMI 18.5 to 24.9 kg/m^2
Overweight: BMI 25 to 29.9 kg/m^2
Obesity class 1: BMI 30 to 34.9 kg/m^2
Obesity class 2: BMI 35 to 39.9 kg/m^2
Obesity class 3: BMI ≥40 kg/m^2 (formerly *morbid obesity*)
Obesity class 4: BMI 50 to 59.9 kg/m^2
Obesity class 5: BMI 60 kg/m^2 and above

Intertriginous areas susceptible to maceration should be inspected—under breasts, under an abdominal pannus (apron), in the groin, between buttocks, and between toes. Acanthosis nigricans, a velvety maculopapular condition, occurs mostly in the neck, axilla, and groin. It indicates insulinemia and insulin resistance and is more prevalent in black and Hispanic populations. Skin tags are common. Acne, male pattern hirsutism, and linea nigra may indicate PCOS. Carotenemia noted on the palms or soles may indicate low thyroid hormone level, as can absent eyebrows in the lateral third margin.[53] An obese abdomen is evaluated no differently from a nonobese abdomen.

A neck circumference of more than 17 inches in men or 16 inches in women increases the risk of OSA and may also be associated with scleral injection and leg edema. Leg edema may also be related to a large pannus or right-sided heart congestion. An upper back fat pad indicates hypercortisolism. Rectal examination is best approached from the left Sims position, with the patient's assistance in holding up the upper buttock, or the lithotomy position. Search for indications of other common obesity-related conditions: osteoarthritis, mobility limitations, gout, and diabetic neuropathies.

DIAGNOSTICS

Common tests for all obese individuals are urinalysis; serum glucose, uric acid, blood urea nitrogen, and creatinine concentrations; complete blood count (CBC); thyroid-stimulating hormone level; lipid profile (total cholesterol, low-density lipoprotein [LDL], high-density lipoprotein [HDL], triglycerides); liver function tests (alanine aminotransferase, aspartate aminotransferase, total and direct bilirubin); alkaline phosphatase level; and, if hyperinsulinemia or insulin resistance is considered, a 2-hour oral glucose tolerance test with insulin levels. Diagnostic studies depend on findings of the history and physical examination: polysomnography for OSA; gallbladder ultrasonography for gallstones; ultrasound or hepatic CT or MRI if hepatomegaly is found or NASH or NAFLD is suspected.[53] Other tests are listed in Table 15-1. Indications for electrocardiography are coronary disease risk factors, T2DM, family history of cardiovascular disease, and consideration of anorectic medications.[53] Routine mammography and colorectal screenings are often done less often in obese individuals, even though obesity increases breast and colon cancer risk, and should be scheduled.

DIFFERENTIAL DIAGNOSIS

Sedentary lifestyle, changes in diet, nutritional supplements with increased energy, smoking cessation, and pharmaceuticals associated with weight gain (discussed earlier) are commonly associated with increased weight. Others diagnoses must be considered, explored, and based on history, physical examination findings, and index of suspicion (see Table 15-1).[54]

MANAGEMENT

Motivational Interviewing and the Transtheoretical Model for Change

The five As of motivational interviewing (MI), adapted from smoking cessation counseling, are useful for providers who may feel unprepared to give obesity counseling.

Ask: Ask permission to discuss weight in a nonjudgmental manner and explore readiness for change.

Assess: Assess the person's BMI and obesity stage, waist circumference, and contributing factors of excess weight.

Advise: Advise on the individual health risks of obesity and the benefits of modest weight loss, and set the stage for long-term treatment strategy.

Agree: Agree on realistic goals and specific treatment options.

Assist: Assist in locating resources, addressing barriers, making consultations, and arranging follow-up.

Principles and strategies of MI incorporate resisting directing of the patient; understanding the individual's motivation; listening with empathy; asking open-ended questions that lead to improved understanding and change talk; and using affirmations, reflections, and summaries that foster a therapeutic relationship while supporting motivation to change.[6,54A]

Identification of the individual's stage of change, according to the transtheoretical model, can help integrate MI with patients at any level of motivation. The stages of change are precontemplation; contemplation; preparation; action; and maintenance, relapse, or recycling. The stages are nonlinear, tend to cycle, and do not necessarily predict behavior changes.[55]

Strategies for Weight Loss

Three components—an energy deficit from reduced kilocalories, physical activity, and behavioral changes—are interrelated for all weight loss and management efforts. The trio combined is known as *lifestyle intervention.* Individualization of the right strategy depends on assessment of contributing components, willingness to change, and derivation of patient-centered goals. A decrease in energy intake is needed to create a deficit sufficient for weight loss efforts to succeed; behavioral and lifestyle changes and physical activity together may be insufficient to achieve weight loss when energy intake is not also reduced. Typically, a 500- to 1000-kcal deficit must be created through a combination of decreased intake and increased physical activity for excess weight to be lost. Intentional weight loss success definitions vary and are not concrete or consistent historically. Recent guidelines advocate using percent body weight lost from the initial starting weight. Clinical benefits begin at 5% weight loss, especially in patients with greater cardiometabolic risk factors. Improvements are noted specifically in blood pressure, blood lipid profiles, waist circumference, glycemic control, and reduced cardiovascular events. Nonsurgical weight loss is based

TABLE 15-1 Differential Diagnoses to Consider in Obese Patients

Disorder	Clinical Presentation	Diagnostics
Hyperinsulinemia	Exogenous insulin Insulin secretagogue therapy Diet high in simple carbohydrates Little physical activity Hyperglycemia or hypoglycemia Exogenous steroid therapy Insulinoma Acanthosis nigricans PCOS	Serum glucose concentration OGTT Serum insulin, proinsulin, and C-peptide Endoscopic pancreatic ultrasound
Hypothyroidism	Mild weight gain Fatigue, lethargy, weakness, slow speech, slow cerebration, cold intolerance Skin: dryness, carotenemia, nonpitting edema in hands and eyelids (myxedema) Hair: brittle, coarse; loss of lateral eyebrows Dull facies, thick tongue, coarse speech Distant heart sounds; bradycardia Delayed DTR relaxation, cerebellar ataxia, peripheral neuropathies with paresthesia Musculoskeletal weakness, stiffness, carpal tunnel syndrome History of hyperthyroidism treatment Menorrhagia, secondary amenorrhea Decreased libido Hyponatremia Mild anemia	TSH, free T_4, free T_3 Serum TBG Lipid profile Serum electrolytes CBC
PCOS	Oligomenorrhea, amenorrhea (or menses may be regular) Infertility Hirsutism, acne (androgen excess) Insulin resistance	Fasting glucose and insulin LH/FSH ratio Prolactin Testosterone, DHEA-S Ultrasound of pelvis
Binge eating disorder (BED)—DSM-5	Recurrent binge episodes; occurs discretely; lack of control, rapid eating, eating discomfort, eating alone, guilt and/or distress about binge eating Occurs >1/wk for 3 mo Absence of compensation or purging	Occurs >1/wk for 3 mo
Eating disorder not otherwise specified (EDNOS), BED—DSM-IV	Binge eating ≥2/wk for past 6 mo in the absence of inappropriate compensatory behaviors characteristic of bulimia nervosa (see DSM-5, BED)	Number of binge eating episodes per week Eating disorder screening tools (SCOFF, EAT-26)
Hypothalamic obesity	Growth hormone deficiency (decreased muscle mass and obesity) History of pituitary resection or dysfunction Dwarfism History of cranial surgery or irradiation	Insulin-induced hypoglycemia stimulation test Serum insulin-like growth factor 1 MRI, head Growth hormone, with provocation or serial levels

DHEA-S, dehydroepiandrosterone sulfate; DSM-5, *Diagnostic and Statistical Manual of Mental Disorders,* Fifth Edition; DSM-IV, *Diagnostic and Statistical Manual of Mental Disorders,* Fourth Edition; DTR, deep tendon reflex; FSH, follicle-stimulating hormone; LH, luteinizing hormone; OGTT, oral glucose tolerance test; T_3, triiodothyronine; T_4, thyroxine; TBG, thyroxine-binding globulin; TSH, thyroid-stimulating hormone.

on percentage difference from beginning weight, with the initial target set at 10% or more. A 10% weight loss, with 7% kept off during maintenance, is associated with decreased risk of morbidity and mortality, especially for cardiovascular disease and T2DM.[56] The clinical benefits begin at 5% and increase as weight losses become more dramatic.[57] Successful weight loss maintenance, according to the 1998 National Heart, Lung, and Blood Institute (NHLBI) guideline, is weight regain of less than 6.6 pounds in 2 years and a sustained reduction in waist circumference of 4 cm (1⅗ inches). When an initial weight loss goal is not agreeable to an individual, an alternative goal is avoidance of weight gain.[58]

Weight loss resulting from bariatric surgery approaches success differently and is based on excess body weight (the amount of weight above a BMI of 25). Surgically achieved success is the loss of more than 50% of excess body weight.

Successful maintenance after bariatric surgery is a minimum of 80% loss kept off 3 to 5 years after loss stabilizes. Surgical weight loss failure is weight loss that is less than 50% of excess body weight.

Reducing Energy Intake

Reducing energy intake is primary among the three components for weight loss. Kilocalories or calories are supplied mainly by three macronutrients: protein, carbohydrates, and fats.

Proteins. Protein provides 4 kcal/g. Essential amino acids are the protein building blocks that must be ingested, as the body cannot synthesize them. Major protein sources are animal (meat, poultry, fish, milk) and nonanimal (legumes, nuts and seeds). U.S. Department of Agriculture (USDA) 2010 guidelines recommend that men and women consume 56 g and 46 g of protein per day, respectively, and typically represent the need as a percentage of kilocalories.[46] However, protein needs are unchanged when kilocalories are reduced, and protein intake should not be lowered. Rather, protein needs during weight loss should be met first, with fats and carbohydrates added to meet calorie needs.[59] Weight loss recommendations suggest protein's primacy to protect lean body mass, to help stabilize blood glucose concentration, to improve lipid profile, to provide greater satiety properties (compared with carbohydrates or fats), and to increase postmeal thermogenic effects.[59] Breakfast protein intake is especially important after an overnight fast, with optimal benefits from 30 g. Other protein intake suggested is 20 to 30 g per meal spread over the day to prevent sarcopenia.[60] Post-bariatric surgery protein intake is recommended as a minimum of 60 to 120 g/day for the short and long term to prevent loss of lean body tissue and to avoid protein malnutrition, with supplements used if dietary sources are not tolerated.[59] Protein supplements and meal replacement package labeling should indicate protein sources, not just total grams. High-quality protein sources supply all essential amino acids and may come from eggs, whey, or soy. Collagen sources are inferior sources and should not be solely relied on to supply protein needs. Protein ingestion is associated with improved weight loss maintenance, and a combination of protein sources (low-fat animal and nonanimal) may have the best effects when protein sources are low in saturated fat.[61]

Carbohydrates. Carbohydrates supply 4 kcal/g, are a major energy source, and may come from simple or complex glucose polymers. Plants are the major carbohydrate source, except for lactose from dairy.[62] A *simple carbohydrate* refers to a monosaccharide or a disaccharide. Simple carbohydrates occur in fruit, milk, beets, and honey naturally and in processed added sugar products, table sugar, and corn syrup. Americans average more than 22 teaspoons of added sugars, or 355 kcal, per day. Added sugars supply no nourishment with their energy and are associated with dyslipidemias (low HDL, high triglycerides), insulin-glucose disruption, higher blood pressure, T2DM, and poorer overall nutrition.[17] Complex carbohydrates are larger polymers, an important fiber source, and are mainly supplied by cereal grains. Other sources are legumes, fruits, and vegetables. Whole grains are associated with lower BMI and other long-term health benefits compared with refined grains.[63] Whole grains supply 1.1 g fiber per 10 g carbohydrates. Reducing simple carbohydrate sugar energy intake is appropriate for people of all ages and is a general recommendation in the 2010 USDA guidelines. The American Heart Association (AHA) recommendations are more specific: maximum added sugar intake for men is 150 kcal/day and for women is 100 kcal/day. These should be lower to meet weight loss goals.[17]

Fats. Fats are the most energy dense among the macronutrients, supplying 9 kcal/g. They supply essential fatty acids and the fat-soluble vitamins A, D, E, and K; they slow gastric emptying and can reduce satiety, leading to more intake. About one third of Americans' energy intake is from fats. Sources include animal products, grain oils, vegetable oils, seeds, and nuts. Alpha-linolenic and linoleic acids must be obtained from the diet to avoid deficiency. Reduced-fat diets are considered conventional for weight loss.[62] The Mediterranean diet pattern is moderate in fat content, supplied mostly from olive oil. Preferred sources of monounsaturated and polyunsaturated fats are olive oil, nuts, seeds, and fatty fish.[62]

Alcohol. Although it is not considered a macronutrient, alcohol has 7 kcal/g and is a large energy source for some adults. It is not an important source of nutrients and may be combined with sugar-sweetened mixers and contribute to greater kilocalorie intake. Moderate alcohol use is defined as two to one drinks per day for men and women, respectively. And is a component of the Mediterranean dietary pattern. About half of Americans do not drink alcohol. For those who do not drink, it is not recommended that alcohol consumption be initiated for health benefits.

Weight Loss Diets

Dietary patterns for weight loss have one commonality: reduced kilocalories to create an energy deficit. The macronutrient proportions used in achieving the kilocalorie deficit are variable, and these variable proportions are debated. Discretionary calories in excess from sugar, solid fats, and alcohol should be limited for general and cardiovascular health benefits across most populations, regardless of weight status, and are generally agreed to be the starting point for creating an energy deficit to treat (or to prevent) obesity.

Balanced energy deficit diets reduce overall kilocalories by approximately 500 to 1000 across all macronutrients and follow USDA nutrition guidelines for macronutrient percentages. They are low in fat (<30%), high in carbohydrates (>55%), moderate in protein (10% to 15%), high in fiber (25 to 30 g/day), and very low in alcohol. Weight loss is slow, about 1 and 2 pounds per week in women and men, respectively.[64]

Low-calorie diets are similar to balanced energy deficits but supply only 1000 to 1500 kcal/day, which creates a greater energy deficit. They are considered traditional weight loss diets.[62]

Portion-controlled servings and meal replacement facilitate weight loss by providing individuals with predetermined foods having a known kilocalorie and nutrient content. Low-fat diets have been a traditional approach for decades and guide the preponderance of weight loss intervention studies. Reducing fat intake alone is not sufficient for clinically significant weight loss without reducing overall kilocalories.[64]

Low-carbohydrate diets have variable carbohydrate restrictions, some as low as 20 g/day, typically supplied from green vegetables. The remaining macronutrient percentages are high for protein, and the fat content varies according to protein sources. A popular low-carbohydrate diet is the Atkins diet. Low-carbohydrate intervention studies have used the Atkins protocol and found the weight loss method safe in adults and adolescents, with supervision.[65] Older versions of Atkins diets were high in saturated fat, but newer protocols have modified the protein sources to be leaner. There are also vegetarian Atkins variations. Low-carbohydrate diets produce rapid weight loss in the early months. Non–weight loss uses of low-carbohydrate diets are higher in kilocalories and useful in treatment of PCOS, resistant epilepsy in children, and some glycolytic cancers.

Very-low-calorie diets (VLCDs) typically contain approximately 800 kcal/day and 70 to 100 g of protein; they use meal replacement products solely or in combination with lean protein sources. Vitamin and mineral supplementation is essential, and health care supervision is warranted. Weight loss is rapid with VLCDs. They may be used preoperatively for bariatric surgery patients.[64]

The Mediterranean diet is plant based and composed of fruits, vegetables, whole grains, nuts, and legumes; it has olive oil for its main source of fat. Animal protein sources are low-fat fish and poultry consumed in low to moderate amounts. Red meat consumption is low, and wine intake is moderate. When this diet is used along with exercise, it is effective as a weight loss method, even though its fat content is much higher than that of conventional weight loss diets. The carbohydrate proportion is lower at 45%, fat is 35% to 40%, and protein is 15% to 20% of kilocalories. The Mediterranean diet is associated with treatment and reduction of the risk for development of metabolic syndrome.[66]

Dansinger and coworkers[65] compared the Atkins, Ornish, Weight Watchers, and Zone diets for weight loss and heart disease risk factor reduction in a 1-year, random assignment study. Because of high attrition rates and waning adherence to assigned dietary patterns, the 12-month comparisons were similar across all groups. Those who adhered to their diet assignment had better weight loss and improvements in cardiovascular risk factors.

Look AHEAD

Look AHEAD (Actions in Health and Diabetes) was an ongoing study that observed 5145 obese diabetic participants who were randomly assigned to intensive lifestyle intervention (with goals of at least 10% weight loss and at least 175 minutes of moderate physical activity per week) or to diabetic support and education as the control. Diabetes Prevention Program (DPP) materials were adapted for the group delivery format of Look AHEAD. Primary outcomes included cardiovascular deaths, nonfatal myocardial infarctions, and hospitalizations for cardiac events during a prolonged follow-up after intensive weight loss and other intensive lifestyle intervention.[67] The study was stopped after 9.6 years. Although weight loss was greater in the intervention group, cardiovascular events were not decreased in overweight or obese adults with T2DM.[68] Participants in the Look AHEAD study are still being followed, so more information about this project should be available in the future. The objective of the Look AHEAD participant to achieve weight loss is addressed in group meetings and reinforced with homework and handouts. MI and cognitive restructuring guide the weight loss coaches. Weight loss topics fall into five categories: knowledge (nutrition, safe exercise, controlling kilocalories); motivation (increasing self-efficacy built on successes); self-regulatory skills (keys to weight loss and long-term success, self-monitoring, cognitive restructuring, relapse plans); group and individual experience (social support); and environmental factors (overcoming barriers with practical advice). All critical components within an individual's control to succeed at weight loss and long-term management within the current obesogenic system are addressed.[67] The length of the intervention, 4 years, helps establish new behaviors that develop into new neurally reinforced habits.

The diet chosen for the Look AHEAD study is low fat, 1200 to 1800 kcal/day or less if necessary; it supplies a minimum of 15% calories from protein and provides meal replacements three times per day during the first 6 months. Meal replacement continues for one meal and one snack per day for 4 years. If weight loss is not realized after 6 months of participation, orlistat may be used by those who choose. Both exercise and increasing lifestyle physical activity are priorities in the weight loss intervention. A weekly goal of at least 175 minutes of moderate-intensity physical activity is set as a means of improving cardiovascular risk factors, improving lipids, reducing blood glucose and serum insulin levels, and facilitating maintenance of weight loss. It is not the primary means of creating a kilocalorie deficit for weight loss.[67]

Side Effects of Weight Loss

Side effects of weight loss are generally mild and self-limited.[65] However, iatrogenic effects from diabetic medications are more serious, and reduction or discontinuation of insulin and insulin secretagogues (sulfonylureas, repaglinide, and nateglinide) should be done preemptively before weight loss. Home glucose monitoring is expected. Antihypertensives and diuretics likewise require astute blood pressure monitoring and appropriate medication alterations.[56] It is the responsibility of the provider to anticipate and prevent dangerous episodes of hypoglycemia, hypovolemia, and hypotension from prescribed medications when patients are losing weight, especially in the early days and weeks of rapid weight loss.[6,69]

Patients with a history of gout may experience an increase in uric acid during early weight loss, and prophylactic prescription of allopurinol may be appropriate. Cholestasis can be prevented by ensuring that dietary fat is at least 20 g/day. Prophylactic use of ursodeoxycholic acid may be considered in those predisposed to gallstones. Side effects from VLCDs tend be greater than in patients reducing carbohydrates while keeping calorie restriction to 1200 to 1500 kcal/day.

Resources for Weight Loss, Physical Activity, and Overweight and Obesity

A useful resource for all providers comes from the Department of Veterans Affairs (VA) and Department of Defense clinical practice guideline for screening and management of overweight and obesity, version 2.0 2014,[6] and is accessible by providers outside the VA system. It contains a provider guideline, including obesity screening, MI information, dietary approaches, physical activity approaches, behavioral change components, pharmacotherapy, bariatric surgery, evidence for interventions, treatment cards, evidence ratings for approaches, and research summaries in about 200 pages that clinicians may find valuable. In addition to this, more than 100 patient handouts for group or individual counseling cover standard components: food and activity diaries, setting goals, and cognitive changes; nutrition components (30 handouts); and physical activity components (38 handouts).[6] An additional helpful resource is available from the American Society of Bariatric Physicians (www.asbp.org/obesityalgorithm.html). Available materials include an obesity algorithm, fact sheets, patient information, and PowerPoint presentation.[32]

Exercise and physical activity counseling from a health care provider has a dose-dependent effect. The website

ExerciseIsMedicine.org has public access resources from the American College of Sports Medicine for providers; these resources include exercise prescriptions, a readiness for change overview, office brochures on myriad exercise-related topics, fliers, patient handouts for physical activity in specific health conditions, and the Physical Activity Readiness Questionnaire (PAR-Q). The website's patient information is also comprehensive but requires high literacy ability for patients (http://exerciseismedicine.org/physicians.htm). The AHA website has strength and balance and stretching and flexibility exercise handouts to download for use as handouts. Writing of a prescription for physical activity (and other lifestyle changes) reinforces the desired activity.

Materials, protocols, manuals (English and Spanish), and publications related to the DPP are accessible. The Look AHEAD protocol, leader and participant manuals, and publications are also still available. DPP handout materials were modified for the Look AHEAD study. They are evidence-based intervention tools to help individuals successfully navigate an obesogenic environment. The Look AHEAD publication topics relate aggressive weight loss as part of an intensive lifestyle intervention to reduce cardiovascular events and deaths and to improve physical functioning.[70] The intervention methods and materials can be appropriated in the health care and larger community settings.

The NHLBI National Institutes of Health (NIH) website has materials for its Aim for a Healthy Weight available to download, or hardcopies can be purchased. Information is accessible for both patients and providers.[71]

MOVE! is the Veterans Health Administration's weight management program, available at the Administration's website. The materials consider health needs unique to older veteran populations, address issues not relevant in Look AHEAD research protocols (pain and physical activity, psychiatric diagnoses, smoking cessation), and require less-demanding reading skills.[72] The materials are comprehensive for weight loss, physical activity, modifying behavior, and cognitive restructuring. Group application is intended, but it can be adopted for individuals.

Group weight loss is an effective and economical format. The MOVE! and Look AHEAD materials can also guide weight loss in groups with obesity-related comorbidities. Cardiovascular diseases, T2DM, hypertension, OSA, stress incontinence, osteoarthritis, and menopause symptom reduction improve with weight loss interventions. Diagnosis, gender, ethnicity, culture, and language should be considered in forming weight loss groups because the social interaction is part of the therapeutic milieu.

Pharmaceutical Options

In 2015, a consensus process among members of the Endocrine Society, the European Society of Endocrinology, and the Obesity Society produced a clinical practice guideline on the pharmacologic management of obesity. A summary of the recommendations for management of obesity includes the following:

1. Work with all patients to reduce food intake, increase physical activity, and engage in behavior modification techniques.
2. For patients with BMI of 25 kg/m^2 or higher, use diet, exercise, and behavior modification techniques alone.
3. Reserve pharmacotherapy for weight loss in patients with BMI of 27 kg/m^2 or higher with comorbidity, or BMI of 30 kg/m^2 or higher.
4. Consider bariatric surgery as an adjunct in patients with BMI of 35 kg/m^2 or higher with comorbidity, or BMI of 40 kg/m^2 or higher.
5. Patients may be candidates for weight loss medications if they have a history of lack of success with weight loss and maintenance of the weight loss and if they meet medication label requirements.
6. Consider use of weight loss medications to promote long-term weight maintenance in patients with a BMI of 30 kg/m^2 or higher, or a BMI of 27 kg/m^2 or higher with one comorbidity such as hypertension, dyslipidemia, T2DM, or OSA.
7. Assess patients monthly for the first 3 months, then reassess need for medication every 3 months.
8. In patients with an adequate response (weight loss of 5% body weight or more in 3 months), continue weight loss medication. If response is not adequate or if safety or tolerability concerns arise, discontinue medication and consider alternative medications or referral for alternative therapies.
9. Start medication at a low dose and escalate while monitoring for side effects; do not exceed recommended doses.
10. Do not use sympathomimetic agents such as phentermine and diethylpropion in patients with a history of heart disease or uncontrolled hypertension; consider lorcaserin or orlistat.
11. In overweight patients with T2DM, choose oral antidiabetic medications that are weight neutral or promote weight loss (GLP-1 analogues or sodium-glucose linked transporter-2 inhibitors) in addition to metformin.
12. If obese T2DM patients require insulin therapy, add at least one of the following: metformin, pramlintide, or GLP-1 agonists to offset insulin-induced weight gain. Use basal (long-acting) insulin instead of insulin alone or in combination with sulfonylurea.
13. For obese patients with T2DM and hypertension, angiotensin-converting enzyme inhibitors, angiotensin receptor blockers, and calcium channel blockers are preferred over beta-adrenergic blockers for first-line therapy.
14. Always consider a medication's effect on weight, and select medications that do not have weight gain as a side effect, whenever possible.

Pharmaceutical treatment can target centrally mediated appetite, satiety, neural pathways of reward, and peripheral gastric absorption of nutrients. All agents are associated with weight loss plateaus; none is indicated as monotherapy without lifestyle changes, and all are associated with weight regain on discontinuation if lifestyle changes are not adopted. Several pharmaceuticals have been approved and labeled for long-term maintenance, in keeping with the chronic disease model because obesity is a chronic condition.[73]

The sympathomimetic monotherapy drugs phentermine, 15 to 30 mg/day; diethylpropion (Tenuate), 25 mg three times per day or sustained release (SR) 75 mg/day; benzphetamine (Didrex), 25 to 50 mg one to three times a day; and phendimetrazine (Bontril), 17.5 to 70 mg three times per day, inhibit norepinephrine and dopamine uptake at nerve endings, resulting in hypothalamically mediated anorexia. Bontril dose is 25 mg two to three times a day. The sustained release form of phendimetrazine (Bontril) is 105 mg, once a day, taken 30-60 minutes before breakfast. These medications are Schedule III and IV drugs because of U.S. Drug Enforcement Administration (DEA) concerns regarding abuse. The medications were labeled for short-term use for weight loss, probably because they were approved before obesity was recognized as a chronic condition, but they have not demonstrated drug-dependence properties such as withdrawal symptoms or escalating doses needed for weight loss effects. Abrupt withdrawal is associated with increased appetite. Some providers prescribe them intermittently, or alternatively, because of concerns about short-term use.[56] There exists a possibility for dependence and withdrawal. The most widely prescribed sympathomimetic agent, phentermine, is indicated for exogenous obesity in adults or children older than 16 years, with BMI of 30 kg/m^2 or higher, or 27 kg/m^2 or higher with comorbidities.[57,73,74]

Common side effects of sympathomimetic weight loss drugs are CNS stimulation, insomnia, and nervousness, which may abate with use. Tremor and dry mouth are common. Other adverse effects are pulmonary hypertension, valvular heart disease, psychosis, tachyarrhythmias, euphoria, dysphoria, GI complaints, and blood marrow suppression (diethylpropion). As a precaution, baseline cardiac evaluation, including echocardiogram, may be warranted in some patients. These agents are not recommended in patients with valvular heart disease or heart murmur. Diabetic medications and antihypertensives require astute monitoring. Phentermine is contraindicated in patients with glaucoma, or within 14 days of MAOI agents. None are to be used in pregnancy.[57,69]

Orlistat (Xenical, 120 mg, by prescription and Alli, 60 mg, over the counter [OTC]), is an irreversible pancreatic lipase inhibitor than prevents dietary fat from hydrolysis and absorption. Fecal fat loss, as undigested triglycerides, occurs in a dose-dependent manner, with up to 30% of dietary fat not absorbed. It was approved in 1999 as an adjunct to a low-fat diet (30% kilocalories from fat) for weight loss and has shown minimal benefit in weight maintenance. The indication is BMI of 30 kg/m^2 or higher, or 27 kg/m^2 or higher with comorbidities. Dose is 60 mg (OTC) or 120 mg (by prescription) taken with a fat-containing meal (about 15 g) or up to 1 hour after meal ingestion. Orlistat raises GLP-1 and C-peptide but lowers an acute cholecystokinin response to meals. It has been implicated in rare cases of liver-related adverse events in reports to the U.S. Food and Drug Administration (FDA). Patients may develop increased urinary oxalate; use cautiously in patients with a history of calcium oxalate kidney stone. It must be accompanied by vitamin supplementation containing fat-soluble vitamins A, D, E, and K and beta carotene, given at bedtime or a minimum of 2 hours before or after the medication, to reduce fat-soluble vitamin deficiency risks. Weight loss results with orlistat peak at about 8% to 9% after 35 weeks when it is combined with dietary restrictions, followed by partial weight regain. Final weight reductions are approximately 7%, compared with approximately 5% for placebo, after 2 years. Mean weight loss in three 1-year studies was 3.45 kg more than placebo at 120 mg three times per day. GI side effects are common and include defecation urgency, flatus with discharge, diarrhea, abdominal discomfort, and oily fecal leakage. These GI side effects are reduced when dietary fat intake is restricted to less than 50 to 60 g/day or 30% of the dietary kilocalories distributed over 3 meals. Drug interactions include the need to separate doses of orlistat and levothyroxine by 4 hours and orlistat and cyclosporine by 3 hours. Warfarin and anticonvulsant drug monitoring is recommended.[10,69,74,75]

Cetilistat is a lipase inhibitor, similar to orlistat, currently under investigation. It may have a better side effect profile than orlistat; the gastrointestinal GI side effects of orlistat are not acceptable to many patients.[6]

Lorcaserin (Belviq) was approved by the FDA in 2012 as an adjunct to a reduced calorie diet and exercise for chronic weight management in adults with initial BMI of 30 kg/m^2 or higher, or BMI 27 kg/m^2 or higher with at least one weight-related condition. Dose is 10 mg PO twice daily, without regard to food. It is contraindicated in pregnancy (FDA Category X). Clinical trials included only 2.5% (135 participants) adults older than age 65, and it was not determined if dose or response was different from that in younger subjects. Dosage used in those older than 65 years should be based on renal function. No dose adjustment for mild renal impairment; use lorcaserin with caution in patients with moderate renal impairment. Lorcaserin is not recommended for patients with severe renal impairment or in end stage renal disease. No dose adjustment is required in patients with mild hepatic impairment (Child-Pugh score 5 or 6) to moderate hepatic impairment (Child-Pugh 7 to 9). Use lorcaserin with caution in patients with severe hepatic impairment. Discontinue lorcaserin after 12 weeks if 5% weight loss is not achieved.[76]

Common adverse effects in nondiabetic patients include nausea, diarrhea, constipation, dry mouth, vomiting, fatigue, headache, and dizziness; and in diabetic patients, hypoglycemia, headache, back pain, cough, and fatigue. Suspected adverse drug reactions should be reported (Eisai, 1-888-274-2378; FDA, 1-800-FDA-1088 or www.fda.gov/medwatch).[76]

Monitoring includes weight; blood pressure (especially in patients taking antihypertensive medication); pregnancy tests in women of childbearing potential if deemed appropriate; glucose and hypoglycemia in diabetics; signs and symptoms of valvulopathy; signs and symptoms of depression or suicidal thought or behavior; prolactin excess; pulmonary hypertension; CBC changes; and cognitive impairment or mood changes. Heart rate may be decreased, and hence this medication should be used with caution in patients with a history of bradycardia or heart block greater than first degree.[76]

Warnings and precautions include possible serotonin syndrome (agitation, hallucinations, coma, autonomic instability, hyperreflexia, incoordination, and/or GI symptoms) or neuroleptic malignant syndrome–like reactions. Valvulopathy has been reported with other 5-HT_{2B} receptor agonists, because these receptors are located on cardiac interstitial cells, and is theoretically possible with lorcaserin, a 5-HT_{2C} agonist. In clinical trials, 2.4% of patients taking lorcaserin and 2.0% receiving placebo developed echocardiographically determined changes, with none noted to be symptomatic. The drug should be discontinued if any valvular heart disease signs or symptoms develop, including dyspnea, dependent edema, congestive heart failure (CHF), or a new cardiac murmur, and the appropriate evaluations should be performed. Lorcaserin is used with caution in combination with other serotonergic or antidopaminergic drugs or MAOIs.[76]

Priapism is a potential result of 5-HT_{2C} receptor agonism, and lorcaserin should be used with caution in men with predisposition to priapism (e.g., those with sickle cell anemia, multiple myeloma, or penile anatomic deformations). Lorcaserin is used with caution when combined with phosphodiesterase type 5 inhibitors. Moderate prolactin level elevations occurred in clinical trials in a subset of patients; serum prolactin should be measured when prolactin excess is suspected or if patients develop galactorrhea or gynecomastia.[76]

Lorcaserin is a serotonergic agonist that activates the 5-HT_{2C} receptors. It is believed to decrease food intake and promote satiety by activation of these receptors, creating an anorexigenic effect via opiomelanocortin neurons located in the hypothalamus.[77] It is a DEA Schedule IV controlled substance with low incidence of euphoria and hallucination in obese patients. Clinical trial weight loss in nondiabetic patients taking lorcaserin was 3.3% greater than with placebo, with 47.1% of patients losing 5% or more of their initial body weight compared with 22.6% in the placebo group. Mean weight loss at 52 weeks for lorcaserin-treated patients was 7.9 kg compared with 3.7-kg weight loss in the placebo group.[76]

Phentermine combined with topiramate SR (P/T), branded as Qsymia, received approval in 2012 for long-term use in obesity or overweight with weight-related complications. P/T capsules come in formulations of 3.75 mg/23 mg, 7.5 mg/46 mg, 11.25 mg/69 mg, and 15 mg/92 mg to titrate upward during initiation; titration should be used during discontinuation as well, to prevent possible seizures from sudden withdrawal of topiramate. Administration is begun with 3.75 mg/23 mg in the morning for 14 days; the dosage is increased to 7.5 mg/46 mg each morning for 12 weeks. If a 3% weight loss is not achieved with the 7.5 mg/46 mg formulation, the dose is increased to 11.25 mg/69 mg. If the patient is not responding and if the drug is to be withdrawn, alternate-day administration for a minimum of 1 week is used to avoid precipitation of seizures. Maximum dose is 15 mg/92 mg. Use in older adult patients should begin with a low doses and increased cautiously.[78]

P/T (Qsymia) is DEA Schedule C-IV because of the phentermine component. Teratogenicity—topiramate's association with cleft lip and cleft palate in infants born to mothers taking the drug during pregnancy—is a safety risk for which a Risk Evaluation and Mitigation Strategy (REMS) has been required by the FDA. Provider training is available on the website http://qsymiarems.com, along with downloadable files, including a dose-management chart; full prescribing information; a patient brochure on the risk of birth defects; and links to certified pharmacies participating in Qsymia's REMS program. If a patient becomes pregnant while using P/T, this should be reported by the patient and the provider to the Qsymia pregnancy surveillance program.

P/T warnings and precautions include the risk of fetal toxicity in females of reproductive potential. A negative pregnancy test result should be obtained before initiation of therapy and monthly during therapy, and effective contraception use should be assessed. Heart rate may increase. The possibility of suicidal behavior and ideation necessitate close monitoring for depression or suicidal thoughts. If acute myopia and secondary angle-closure glaucoma occur, the drug should be discontinued; if mood and sleep disorders occur, the dose should be reduced or the drug discontinued. Cognitive impairment including disturbed attention or memory can occur, so patients should be cautioned. Metabolic acidosis and elevated creatinine may occur, requiring monitoring before and during treatment. The most common adverse reactions are paresthesia, dizziness, dysgeusia (altered taste), insomnia, constipation, and dry mouth. Patients taking oral contraceptives may experience irregular bleeding or spotting, but the risk of pregnancy is not increased. Combination with alcohol should be avoided because of CNS depressant effect. Hypokalemia may occur when used with non–potassium-sparing diuretics. Reduced urinary citrate excretion and elevated urinary pH may promote kidney stone formation, and the risk may increase with a diet-induced ketogenic environment. P/T is contraindicated in pregnant patients, in those with glaucoma or hyperthyroidism, during or with MAOI use, and in those with known hypersensitivities to sympathomimetic amine drugs.[76]

Phentermine's known anorectic properties reduce appetite and food consumption. Topiramate's mechanism of action is not known, but the drug has been shown to reduce appetite and enhance satiety. These effects may be the result of the central augmentation of neurotransmitter γ-aminobutyric acid (GABA); topiramate is associated with weight loss when used as monotherapy.[69,77]

The combination agent containing of SR bupropion and naltrexone (Contrave)[79] was approved in 2014 for chronic weight management. It is indicated for treatment of obese patients or overweight patients with weight-related comorbidities. A boxed warning includes increased risk of suicidal thinking and behavior; the provider should monitor for worsening and emergence of depression or other psychic disorders. Serious neuropsychiatric events have been associated with use of bupropion for smoking cessation, and study data in pediatric patients are lacking. Contraindications include uncontrolled hypertension; seizure disorders; anorexia nervosa or bulimia; abrupt alcohol cessation; use of benzodiazepines, barbiturates, and/or antiepileptic drugs; use with other bupropion-containing products; chronic opioid use; use of MAOIs currently or within previous 14 days; known allergies to ingredients; and pregnancy. Tablets are a combination of extended-release naltrexone 8 mg and bupropion 90 mg to be administered incrementally over 4 weeks: 1 tablet in the morning during week 1, adding a second tablet in the evening in week 2, increase to 2 tablets in the morning during week 3, and from week 4 onward, 2 tablets twice daily, morning and evening.[79]

Drugs metabolized by CYP2D6 (SSRIs, TCAs, antipsychotics, beta blockers, propafenone) may have increased concentration owing to bupropion's action and require dose reduction. Drugs metabolized by CYP2B6 (ticlopidine or clopidogrel) (CYP2B6 inhibitors) may increase bupropion's concentration; hence bupropion/naltrexone should be given at the lower dose, 1 tablet twice per day (bid). CYP2B6 inducers (ritonavir, carbamazepine, phenobarbital, phenytoin) may reduce bupropion effect and should not be used with bupropion/naltrexone.[79]

The GLP-1 receptor agonists exenatide and liraglutide, currently used in treatment of T2DM, are associated with weight loss independent of their side effect of nausea. They have boxed warnings for an increased pancreatitis and thyroid tumor risk. Liraglutide, under the name Saxenda (Novo Nordisk), is a GLP-1 receptor agonist given by subcutaneous injection for the chronic treatment of obesity in nondiabetics.[6,69] Weight loss should be monitored and liraglutide discontinued if a minimum of 4% weight loss has not occurred. Liraglutide is contraindicated in pregnancy (Category X) and in patients with multiple endocrine neoplasia syndrome.

Pharmacologic agents that are approved for indications other than weight loss but are associated with weight loss include bupropion, extended-release exenatide, pramlintide, metformin, topiramate, and zonisamide. Agents under investigation include bupropion SR combined with zonisamide SR; cetilistat (see discussion on orlistat); pramlintide with metreleptin; and tesofensine.[6,57,69]

Sibutramine (Meridia) was voluntarily removed from U.S. and Canadian markets in 2010 for adverse cardiovascular risk associations.[74] Rimonabant (Acomplia) blocks endocannabinoid receptors but has been associated with neuropsychiatric side effects, including suicide, and has never been approved for use in the United States.[80] Fenfluramine-phentermine ("fen-phen") combination therapy and dexfenfluramine were voluntarily withdrawn in 1997 after cardiac valvulopathy side effects were attributed to fenfluramine.[74] Human chorionic gonadotropin (hCG) injections have been prescribed with a 500-kcal diet (i.e., Dr. Simeon's protocol) but are not FDA approved for weight loss and have not been shown to benefit weight loss, fat redistribution, appetite suppression, or improvement in mood when compared with placebo injections.[81,82]

Other pharmaceutical options not recommended for inducing weight loss include testosterone replacement in hypogonadal obese men; cyanocobalamin (vitamin B_{12}); and levothyroxine or liothyronine thyroid use in euthyroid patients.[69]

Dietary Supplements

Dietary supplements during weight loss are commonly used to replace missing dietary vitamins and minerals. However, some supplements are also proposed to contribute to weight loss as an intended effect above that attributed to reduced kilocalories and increased energy expenditure. They may be viewed as more "natural" than pharmaceuticals. Nutraceuticals, botanicals, amino acids, and trace elements have been marketed for weight loss effects. A systematic review of weight loss supplements found that clinical studies are small, are of poor quality, have variable measurements that are not consistent, and do not control for covariables. No weight loss above 5% was achieved. Nine supplements, their associated weight loss findings, and some proposed mechanisms of actions were reviewed and reported on by Onakpoya and colleagues.[83] Ephedrine is associated with significant short-term weight loss effects but can have serious side effects. It works by enhancing thermogenesis. Glucomannan studies showed significant weight loss in obese persons; the proposed effect is by increasing satiety through slowing of gastric emptying. *Camellia sinensis* (green tea) demonstrated efficacy for weight loss and maintenance by fat oxidation stimulus and increased energy expenditure. Chromium picolinate was associated with a relatively small weight loss effect by increasing BMR and insulin sensitivity. Chitosan had inconclusive short-term weight loss effects. The authors concluded that conjugated linoleic acid, calcium supplements, *Citrus aurantium* (bitter orange), and guar gum were not efficacious for weight loss.[74,83]

Weight loss supplements are frequently a target of FDA actions. Supplements for weight loss have been tainted with many ingredients, including sibutramine (the appetite-suppressant drug removed in 2010 from the U.S. market), the diuretic bumetanide, rimonabant, phenytoin, and the suspected carcinogen phenolphthalein.[84]

Bariatric Surgery

Reduced food energy intake, being central in all obesity treatment, is achieved mechanically by bariatric surgery. Approximately 179,000 bariatric surgeries were performed in 2013, and primary care, endocrine, and gastroenterology providers follow many patients for decades after surgery.[85] Bariatric surgery does not cure obesity or guarantee weight loss results. Weight regain is a common problem, and nutritional and metabolic complications routinely occur.[59]

Indications and Contraindications. Indications for bariatric surgery are BMI of 40 kg/m^2 or higher, or 35 kg/m^2 or higher with obesity-associated comorbidity; failure of previous weight loss attempts; commitment to postoperative care, supplements, and testing; and exclusion of reversible endocrine or other causes of obesity. In 2011 the FDA approved use of the Lap-Band for those with BMIs of 30 to 40 kg/m^2 or higher with one obesity-related comorbidity.[86] Suggested contraindications are current substance abuse; uncontrolled, severe psychiatric illness; lack of understanding of surgical risks and benefits, expected outcomes, alternative weight loss options, and lifestyle changes required after bariatric surgery; and extremely high operative risk.[87]

Surgical Techniques and Outcomes. Surgically induced weight loss is rapid. Comorbidities improve or may be resolved. Mortality from all causes is reduced, with reductions greatest in cardiovascular deaths.[88] Weight loss is more durable in bariatric surgery compared with no treatment or presently available nonsurgical treatments. Current primary surgical options restrict food volume capacity or reduce food nutrient absorption in the GI tract. Procedures are performed laparoscopically most often. Secondary procedures are for bariatric surgery reversal, revision, or conversion to another surgical weight loss technique. Vagal nerve blocking (vBloc) was recently approved for weight loss by the FDA and is available soon to help reduce hunger and stimulate satiety.[87]

Restrictive bariatric procedures restrict food intake and intend early satiety. They include adjustable gastric banding and fixed gastric banding by vertical banded gastroplasty (VBG). Laparoscopically performed adjustable gastric banding (LAGB) is less invasive than VBG, the band can be removed, and the procedure has better outcomes than VBG and is thus performed more often. LAGB creates an upper stomach pouch at the end of the esophagus that holds 15 to 45 mL and has an outlet stoma of 10 to 11 mm that connects the pouch to the stomach. A port is implanted in the abdominal wall that is accessed percutaneously to adjust the saline volume of the band. Compared with Roux-en-Y gastric bypass (RYGB), weight loss from LAGB is less and control of T2DM less dramatic, but LAGB results in fewer long-term nutritional and metabolic complications and is associated with less lean tissue loss during weight loss. LAGB is more likely to need reversal because of complications, and it may require conversion to a more malabsorptive procedure. Complications include band slippage, band erosion, balloon failure, port dilation, and port infections. Regurgitation, vomiting, and gastric dysmotility may occur.[59] Weight loss success with LAGB is associated with a starting BMI of 45 or higher, postprandial satiety after placement, and frequent band adjustments in the first year.[87] Long-term LAGB outcomes of 12 years or longer in 151 Belgium patients were 0% operative mortality and 3.7% long-term mortality (not surgically related); 22% had minor complications, and 39% experienced major complications, including 28% with band erosions. Seventeen percent had the LAGB converted to RYGB, and 51% retained their band. A bariatric surgery meta-analysis found that excess body weight loss was 50% after LAGB and 76% after RYGB.[59]

RYGB is a commonly performed bariatric procedure in the United States. The upper section of the stomach is transected, creating a small 10- to 30-mL pouch. The gastric pouch is attached to the proximal jejunum, leaving some of the jejunum, the duodenum, and the remaining stomach "bypassed" and not available for nutrient absorption. The length of the limb determines the extent of malabsorption. RYGB results in greater loss of excess body weight, faster weight loss, and quicker

T2DM improvements and resolution compared with LAGB.[87] RYGB is considered by some bariatric providers to be a metabolic surgery. In addition to its mechanical restrictive and malabsorptive properties, it is associated with changes in gut hormones GLP-1, ghrelin, and peptide YY and improvements in T2DM independent of weight loss.[89]

Laparoscopic vertical sleeve gastrectomy (VSG) reduces the stomach size by 85% and has a complication rate of less than 1%. In this procedure, the greater curvature of the stomach is stapled and removed, resulting in anatomic and physiologic changes to the alimentary canal. This is a restrictive, irreversible procedure involving a distinct anatomic change to the alimentary canal with associated physiologic implications.[90] The surgical resection of the greater curvature of the stomach results in a lack of ghrelin hormone, causing increased satiety.

Operative mortality varies from 0.1% to 2% after RYGB.[91] Complications are related to complexity of the surgical procedure, surgeon experience, bariatric center experience, number of comorbidities, higher BMIs, and size of visceral fat stores.[91] Early perioperative complications include thromboembolism, pulmonary insufficiency, hemorrhage, peritonitis, postoperative leaks, and wound infection. Nutritional deficiencies, anastomotic stenosis, internal hernia, diarrhea, bacterial overgrowth, and dumping syndrome may follow RYGB later. Dumping syndrome symptoms include abdominal pain, cramping, lightheadedness, flushing tachycardia, and syncope. It is commonly related to ingestion of simple carbohydrates and occurs in as many as three of four patients after RYGB. It typically improves with time and can be mitigated with small, slow meals (30 minutes' duration), avoiding liquids with meals, avoiding simple carbohydrates, and increasing protein intake.[59]

Nutritional Supplementation. In addition to a chewable multivitamin, vitamin B_{12} (by various routes), folate, iron as ferrous sulfate with vitamin C, calcium as calcium citrate, and vitamin D supplementation are needed lifelong. Thiamine supplementation may be indicated for some patients, particularly if neuropathy occurs, or for patients with significant emesis or weight loss after bariatric surgery surgery.[92] For post–bariatric surgery patients with thinning hair, zinc is a supplement consideration.[92] Prenatal vitamins, products from bariatric suppliers, and specially compounded medications may be combined to meet individual needs. Therapy changes are based on laboratory analysis, physical signs of deficiency, dietary shortfalls, and nutritionist recommendations.[59]

Monitoring. Lifelong testing after bariatric surgery includes vitamin D, calcium, phosphorus, parathyroid hormone (PTH); alkaline phosphatase levels and bone density DXA every 6 months until weight is stable; and perhaps urinary C-peptide for bone health monitoring. A full annual mandatory test list includes these in addition to CBC, liver function tests, glucose, creatinine, electrolytes, iron, vitamin B_{12}, folate, calcium, intact PTH, 25-hydroxyvitamin D, and optionally albumin or prealbumin, vitamin A, zinc, and vitamin B_1.[59] Testing is more frequent in the first 24 postoperative months.

Obesity is a risk factor for gallstones and gout, and any rapid weight loss may incite acute gout attacks and cholelithiasis. During early postsurgical weight loss months, prophylactic therapy may be indicated.[87]

Medications. Medications to avoid after bariatric surgery are nonsteroidal anti-inflammatory drugs, salicylates, corticosteroids, oral bisphosphonates, ethanol, and extended-release formulations, which can irritate the GI tract, injure the pouch, or result in altered absorption. To minimize dumping syndrome, medications with sucrose, corn syrup, maltose, and sorbitol should be avoided. Calcium channel blockers, beta blockers, nitrates, anticholinergics, and some antihistamines may increase gastroesophageal reflux and thus should be avoided if possible. Pills and tablets may not be tolerated; liquid or nonenteric delivery options may be pursued. Diuretics should be held any time liquids are not tolerated and if vomiting or diarrhea persists.[87] Tobacco should also be avoided.[91]

Pregnancy. Women should delay pregnancy 12 to 24 months after bariatric surgery but may have variable responses to oral contraceptives and should consider nonhormonal or nonoral hormone delivery methods. Gestational diabetes and preeclampsia are reduced in post–bariatric surgery pregnancies in comparison to presurgery pregnancies. Rates of cesarean delivery and premature rupture of membranes may be higher in comparison to nonsurgical obese women. Bariatric surgery is not an indication for cesarean delivery. The bariatric surgeon should be consulted if adjustment to the LAGB is indicated. Nutritional evaluation must be thorough, with parenteral supplementation if deficiencies are not responsive to oral replacements. Common GI complaints of pregnancy, such as nausea and vomiting, may warrant investigation for anastomotic leaks, bowel obstructions, internal or ventral hernias, and band migration or erosion. Dumping syndrome may preclude tolerance of oral glucose tolerance testing. Consider home glucose monitoring.[50]

Weight Gain. Weight regain is common after any weight loss, but special considerations after surgical weight loss include evaluation for GI anastomosis, fistula, or loss of band integrity in LAGB.[59] Expected weight regain 10 years after bariatric surgery is commonly 20% to 25% of weight lost, but the true prevalence is not known because patients are not typically followed up long term or are lost to follow-up.[59]

Psychological Results. Improved health-related quality of life is typically expected after bariatric surgery. Body image, sexual functioning, and marital relationships have been reported to improve. Not all enjoy these benefits, and some may find the life-changing experience negative and the nutritional and GI side effects problematic; overall, they may perceive themselves as being greatly restricted because of these changes. In a qualitative study, participants' concerns, chronic pain, low energy levels, and lower social functioning were dismissed by practitioners, and patients reported feeling shame and stigma because of their less-than-ideal responses to surgery.[93] In Pennsylvania, the suicide risk among post–bariatric surgery individuals was alarmingly high compared with the state average. The first 3 years after surgery were found to be the most critical period; 70% of the suicides occurred in this time frame.[94] Lifelong caring for the whole person requires understanding of these possibilities and appropriate intervention after astute assessment for depression and suicide ideation.

Preoperative Management. Preoperative management includes optimization of nutritional status, a psychological evaluation with clearance, initiation of a physical activity program, and control of comorbidities. Weight loss before surgery improves operative risks and comorbidity management and aids in the technical aspects of the procedure. A VLCD may be used to reduce liver volume. Patients requiring coronary artery bypass grafting or stent placement before surgery may also require an aggressive VLCD before the needed cardiac intervention.[87] Some third-party insurance payers require preoperative weight loss.

LIFE SPAN CONSIDERATIONS

Obesity has perinatal and multigenerational origins. Maternal health and nutrition, gestational weight gain, cigarette smoking, environmental toxin exposures, exercise, and early infant feedings affect short- and long-term energy balance in offspring, with durable manifestations spanning developmental phases from birth weight to midlife weight. Appropriate BMI during preconception, limiting of pregnancy weight gain to less than 40 pounds, promotion of breastfeeding, and delay of food introduction in formula-fed infants are early preventive measures. In adults, prevention applies to a minority, because two thirds of U.S. adults are above a healthy BMI. Avoiding future weight gain, improving dietary intake, and increasing physical activity are minimal goals for populations and individuals.

Older adults can increase physical activity and reduce weight safely. Nearly 300 older adults—with an average age of 67 years, obesity, cardiovascular or cardiometabolic disease, and limitations in mobility and who were not physically active—were assigned to successful aging education, physical activity, or weight loss plus physical activity intervention groups for 18 months in a community center. The weight loss and physical activity treatment group had clinically significant improvements in physical walking performance, decreased weight by 8.5%, and maintained a weight loss of 7.7% at 18 months. The successful aging and physical activity groups had similar but minimal improvement in walking performance scores, with weight decreases about 1% from baseline after 18 months. The greatest treatment effects were in those with poorest baseline mobility. The side effects were mostly minor, temporary musculoskeletal effects with two serious side effects (not specified) and not statistically significant between groups.[95]

Individuals with sarcopenia, muscle loss occurring after the age of 30 years, can accumulate a 30% reduced muscle mass by the age of 60 years. Sarcopenia may be mitigated by physical activity and adequate protein ingestion. Protein synthesis, which contributes to gains in muscle mass, immune components, and wound healing, may be maximized by sufficient high-quality dietary protein intake of 25 to 30 g at each meal combined with resistance training.[96] Weight loss in older adults is associated with body composition changes comparable to changes in younger weight loss individuals. Typically, losses consist of about 25% lean and 75% fat tissue. Metabolic abnormalities and cardiac risk factors improve with intentional weight loss in older adults, and physical function is best improved in combination with physical activity.

INDICATIONS FOR REFERRAL OR HOSPITALIZATION

Obese patients may be referred to sleep specialists for OSA or obesity hypoventilation syndrome evaluations. Binge eating does not always require a referral, but patients with other eating disorders, such as bulimia, should be referred to an experienced provider.

When bariatric surgery is considered, evaluation by a nutritionist is suggested. A referral should be made to a bariatric center of excellence that performs large numbers of bariatric procedures. Specific performance data should be reviewed. Preoperative and postoperative involvement with a full bariatric surgical team is correlated with success, and the primary care provider should encourage full engagement. An ongoing relationship with the primary care provider and experienced bariatric surgeons begins before referrals are made and continues long term.[59] The American Society for Metabolic and Bariatric Surgery website (www.asmbs.org) and the Obesity Society website (www.obesity.org) can facilitate locating bariatric surgery providers.

A post–bariatric surgery complication that requires inpatient treatment is severe protein deficiency, which requires hospitalization for parenteral nutrition in about 1% of malabsorption cases.[59] Surgical revision may be indicated if weight loss is inadequate, significant weight regain occurs, or malnutrition therapy is not amenable to medical intervention. Reversal is considered after medical options have failed.[87] Frequent vomiting should be evaluated with a contrast study before an endoscopic examination. A radionuclide gastric emptying study should be ordered if gastroparesis is suspected. Other indications for endoscopic examination include stoma stricture, reflux, inflammation, and stoma erosion. Outpatient management is indicated for dilation of strictures.[59]

EDUCATION AND HEALTH PROMOTION

Patients and families should be educated about the benefits of maintaining ideal weight and engaging in regular exercise (see Chapter 16). Obesity by its chronic nature is difficult to treat and presents a lifelong struggle for many adults. Early diagnosis and aggressive treatment are essential. Ideal intervention programs incorporate all family members and include education about healthy eating and the importance of daily physical activity.

Practitioners should include questions on dietary habits and physical activity in routine health assessments. The key to effective obesity prevention and treatment is open discussion, combined with support and resources for education.

CHAPTER 16

LIFESTYLE MANAGEMENT

Kenneth Peterson

LIFESTYLE MANAGEMENT

Dietary deficiencies or excesses, inactivity, and stress often promote disease in contemporary society. Nearly half of the U.S. population has at least one chronic condition traceable to lifestyle factors.[1A] Inappropriate nutrition, inadequate physical activity, and a lack of stress management are dominant lifestyle factors that contribute to leading causes of death in the United States. Heart disease, cancer, and stroke persisted as the top five leading causes of death from 1935 to 2010.[1] Weight, physical activity, diet, obesity, and stress remain high on lists of independent risk factors for morbidity and mortality.[2,3] Substantial gains have been made in reducing death rates and improving the health and well-being of the U.S. population.[1] Implementation of public health initiatives to improve health and well-being and national goal setting to reduce the burden of morbidity continue to be top priorities.[1]

The U.S. Department of Health and Human Services (HHS) examines evidence-based studies and national health trends on an ongoing basis. The Office of Disease Prevention and Health Promotion communicates these data as well as the national health improvement objectives via the federal prevention initiative *Healthy People.* Overarching goals of the *Healthy People* initiative are to increase quality and length of life, free of preventable disease, disability, injury, and premature death; to achieve health equality by eliminating disparities; to create social and physical environments that promote proper health; and to promote increased quality of life, healthy development, and healthy behaviors across all life stages.

Healthy People offers a plan to enhance health through health promotion, disease prevention efforts, and increasing access to health services. Major goals for *Healthy People 2020* are to identify nationwide health improvement priorities; to increase public awareness and understanding of the determinants of health, disease, and disability; to provide measurable objectives and goals that are applicable at the national, state, and local levels; to engage multiple sectors to take actions to strengthen evidence-based policies and practices; and to identify critical research, evaluation, and data collection needs.[4] *Healthy People 2020* can be accessed online at www.healthypeople.gov. *Healthy People 2020* identifies 42 topic areas with over 1200 corresponding objectives. The Leading Health Indicators section presents a smaller set of objectives, which emphasize 26 high-priority health issues including nutrition, physical activity, and obesity.[4]

INTERCONNECTION AMONG LIFESTYLE COMPONENTS

Lifestyle influences are not mutually exclusive but are interconnected in ways that affect health and well-being. The epidemiology of chronic disease refers to this interconnection as a "web of causation," or multifactorial causation. Nutrition and stress are interrelated in that poor nutritional status may be a stressor. For example, a diet lacking in calcium is likely to lead to osteoporosis. Conversely, states of stress may influence eating behaviors. Some individuals consume greater quantities of food when they are under stress, whereas others lose their appetites. Food intake and exercise are linked through metabolic processes. Exercise enhances the effectiveness of metabolic processes, and food is the necessary fuel. Exercise and levels of stress are connected. On one hand, exercise is an effective means to diffuse the tension associated with stress. Conversely, humans need some stress to perform at peak levels, and exercise affords an opportunity to experience positive stress through the exhilaration of engaging in physical activity.

Overweight and obesity are linked to cardiovascular problems and some forms of cancer. An imbalance in lifestyle influences is associated with a multitude of medical conditions, including type 2 diabetes, sleep apnea, gallbladder disease, hypertension, musculoskeletal injuries, and psychiatric illnesses.

Obesity

The Centers for Disease Control and Prevention (CDC) reported that for 2011 and 2012 the prevalence of obesity was 16.9% in youths and 34.9% in adults.[5] The prevalence of overweight and obesity among U.S. adults 20 years of age and older is 68.8%.[6] There was no significant change in the overall prevalence of obesity in youths compared with 2009 and 2010 data.[5] Also, no significant change was identified in obesity prevalence among adults.[5] See Chapter 15 for a more complete discussion of obesity.

Sedentary Lifestyle

Sedentary lifestyle worsens the problem of overweight for the majority of Americans. Data collected by the National Center for Health Statistics indicate that 49.6% of adults 18 years of age or older met the physical activity guidelines for aerobic physical activity.[7] Of adults 18 years of age or older, 23.6% met the physical activity guidelines for muscle-strengthening activity.[7] National Health Interview Survey data from 2012 indicate that 20.6% of adults age 18 years and older have met the *Healthy People 2020* physical activity and muscle-strengthening activity objectives set for 2020. Although this is slightly above the *Healthy People 2020* target of 20.1%, it suggests that individuals in the United States should continue to work toward increasing their physical activity potential.[7]

Stress

The pioneering work of Hans Selye, with his General Adaptation Syndrome (GAS) model, helped to establish the relationship of stress and illness. Stress and subsequent physiologic responses can lead to a variety of health conditions including but not limited to hypertension, cardiovascular disease, arthritis, kidney disease, and some allergic reactions. Knowledge of the role of stress in health and illness is essential for all. The American Institute of Stress (AIS) is a nonprofit clearinghouse for stress-related information. Goals of the AIS include dissemination of innovative stress research to help build resilience among the global community.[8] AIS emphasizes priority for matters related to reducing overall stress, workplace stress, and stress related to military service and the health considerations associated with long-term, unmanaged stress.[8]

LIFESTYLE ASSESSMENT

A comprehensive assessment of lifestyle includes screening for and assisting patients with nutritional status, weight management, stress management, wellness promotion across the life span, safety issues, and substance use. Most negative effects of poor lifestyle choices are cumulative. Providers must recognize that patients are not always forthcoming in their discussion of personal lifestyle matters. Primary care providers often need to use their history taking and physical examination skills to identify lifestyle factors needing further elaboration. Detailed family history taking may uncover health problems responsive to lifestyle management. Observant providers can uncover clues throughout the interview and physical examination encounter, which may help to identify lifestyle concerns needing additional attention. For example, cigarette smoke odor often lingers on a patient's clothing. Also, tobacco-stained fingertips or other signs of substance use such as additional skin integrity manifestations or altered affect may be observed while conversing with the patient. Providers who prioritize lifestyle factors in the overall assessment of their patients are more likely to have an impact on negative health consequences, which occur over time.

Nutrition

The comprehensive patient history will provide important clues to lifestyle, including those related to cultural and religious practices that influence food preparation and consumption. Eating habits such as frequency of eating and types of food consumed should be identified. For an individual with weight management problems, the provider should evaluate dietary intake of sugar and fats, high-fiber foods including fruits and

BOX 16-1

Dietary CAGE Questions for Assessment of Intake of Saturated Fat and Cholesterol

C—Cheese (and other sources of dairy fats—whole milk, 2% milk, ice cream, cream, whole-fat yogurt)
A—Animal fats (hamburger, ground meat, frankfurters, bologna, salami, sausage, fried foods, fatty cuts of meat)
G—Got it away from home (high-fat meals either purchased and brought home or eaten in restaurants)
E—Eat (extra) high-fat commercial products: candy, pastries, pies, doughnuts, cookies

Courtesy U.S. Department of Health and Human Services: *Third report of the National Cholesterol Education Program on Detection, Evaluation, and Treatment of High Blood Cholesterol in Adults*, Washington, DC, 2001, U.S. Government Printing Office.

vegetables, overall caloric intake, and consumption of alcohol and caffeinated products.

The National Cholesterol Education Program, under the auspices of the National Heart, Lung, and Blood Institute (NHLBI) of the National Institutes of Health, has established a dietary CAGE questionnaire for providers to use in assessing the fat and cholesterol consumption of patients (Box 16-1).[9] This measure enables the diagnostician to quickly identify potentially detrimental fat consumption.

Exercise

Physical activity must also be considered a part of the lifestyle assessment. Insufficient exercise produces harmful consequences, not only for cardiovascular health and flexibility but also for psychological well-being. Sedentary lifestyle predisposes individuals to fatigue, low self-esteem, and a host of health problems including sleep disorders, obesity, prediabetes and metabolic syndrome. The lifestyle assessment should include information about the type, frequency, and duration of physical activity.

Stress

An individual's response to stress has the potential to produce detrimental effects on cardiovascular health and other organ systems. Understanding the nature of a particular stressor is an important process that can assist both patients and providers to plan more effective interventions. The provider should explore attributes of stress with the patient. What is the source of the stress? Is there a single stressor, or are there multiple stressors? What is the acuity level of the stress? Some stressors are chosen, whereas others present themselves. Is the stress long-standing or newly acquired? Does the patient have prior experience in coping with the particular stressor? How effective are the patient's usual means of managing stress?

Behavioral signs of stress manifest physically by rigidity and tightness of the body, such as folded or crossed arms or legs. Fists may be clenched to indicate anxiety, or the forehead may be furrowed to signify worry. Direct behavioral distress symptoms reflect internal states and include teeth grinding, irritability, compulsiveness, rapid speech, stuttering, verbal aggression, a withdrawn demeanor, and crying spells. Indirect symptoms encompass addictive and escape behaviors. An elevated level of stress can increase the frequency of unhealthy behaviors. Addictions may be observed in increased smoking, alcohol consumption, use of drugs to mitigate tension or to induce sleep, excessive sleep or television use, and excessive consumption of caffeinated products.

Signs of stress may be apparent in the patient's self-report or in distracting mannerisms, such as agitation. When questioned about stress in their lives, patients are often forthcoming with evidence and usually can identify their most significant stressors. Stress related to overload is common and is characterized by an urgency about time. Other common sources of stress are interpersonal relationships, relationships within social or work domains, financial worries, and major life changes.

In general, stress is associated with distress. However, happy events and occasions can create a type of stress known as eustress. These events may include a wedding, the birth of a baby, or winning the lottery. The stress accompanies the modifications in behavior required to adapt and to adjust to the change. However, the stress associated with the changes accompanying these pleasant events is often not acknowledged.

PHYSICAL EXAMINATION

Assessment of the patient's overall appearance when he or she is first examined is an important preliminary diagnostic activity. Measurement of vital signs as well as height, weight, and waist circumference should be taken into account. A well-nourished patient is alert, has good color and smooth skin, stands erect, and is of normal weight for body build and age. A poorly nourished patient is languid with pale, dry skin and poor posture; weighs more or less than normal for body build; and may appear to be high-strung. Ease of movement can be observed to indicate body flexibility. Conversely, limited movement may be apparent. A patient under great stress may have signs such as agitation, excessive perspiration, impatience, anxiety, and perhaps even mental dullness.

Established guidelines from the Obesity Education Initiative (OEI) of the NHLBI recommend the use of surrogate measures to assess body fat.[10] Although technologically sophisticated measures exist, they are expensive and unavailable to many providers; therefore, body mass index (BMI) and waist circumference should be used. For a discussion of how to calculate BMI, see Chapter 15. The expert panel has defined overweight as a BMI ranging from 25 to 29.9 kg/m^2,[10] and obesity as a BMI of more than 30 kg/m^2.[10]

In addition, the OEI recommends use of waist circumference to measure abdominal fat. A measuring tape is placed on the upper hip bone and at the top of the right iliac crest so it is horizontal and parallel with the floor. The tape measure is extended around the waist in a snug manner but not so as to compress the skin. The measure is made at the end of a normal expiration. For men, a high-risk value is 102 cm or more (≥40 inches). A measure of more than 89 cm (>35 inches) is considered high risk for women.

The physical examination should include evaluation of cardiovascular fitness, musculature, and flexibility. Heart rate is one indicator of cardiovascular fitness. A fit person will have a lower heart rate, greater endurance, greater muscle strength, and full range of motion. Patients who are not fit may have dyspnea or chest pain with exertion, be unable to participate in activities for extended periods, have less muscle tone and mass, and have limited range of motion.

DIAGNOSTICS

Identification of individuals at risk for health problems is key. Evaluation of blood glucose concentration will identify those with type 2 diabetes. Lipid profile testing is important to detect individuals at risk for coronary artery disease. Lipoprotein analysis includes the measurement of concentrations of triglycerides, total cholesterol, α-lipoproteins (high-density lipoproteins [HDLs]), β-lipoproteins (low-density lipoproteins [LDLs]), and pre-β-lipoproteins (very-low-density lipoproteins [VLDLs]). Epidemiologic investigations suggest that HDL cholesterol is inversely related to coronary disease, with high levels offering protection and lower levels increasing risk.[9] High cholesterol levels may be caused by some drugs, such as corticosteroids, and by diseases such as hypothyroidism, biliary obstruction, and pancreatic dysfunction.

An at-risk individual older than 35 years who plans to begin an exercise program should undergo stress electrocardiography as a precautionary measure. Patients younger than 35 years with abnormal blood chemistry values and blood pressure readings indicating risk for metabolic or cardiopulmonary disease also require a complete physical examination and stress electrocardiography. Bone density studies should be conducted for postmenopausal women to ascertain their risk for fracture and to diagnose osteopenia and osteoporosis.

LIFESTYLE-RELATED MEDICAL PROBLEMS

Hypertension

A diagnosis of hypertension can be linked to lifestyle factors such as nutrient-deficient diet, alcohol intake, overweight or obesity, lack of exercise, and stress. Guidelines from the American Heart Association state that a diagnosis of hypertension is based on blood pressure readings taken over time after the initial measurement.[11] To ensure a more accurate reading, patients should not consume caffeine for 1 hour or smoke for 30 minutes before having a blood pressure reading. An optimum reading is less than 120 mm Hg for systolic blood pressure and less than 80 mm Hg for diastolic blood pressure. Prehypertension is systolic blood pressure in the range of 120 to 139 mm Hg and diastolic blood pressure in the range of 80 to 89 mm Hg. These ranges may differ slightly when the patient has other cardiac risk factors, such as diabetes. Patients managing diabetes should maintain a blood pressure reading of less than 140 mm Hg for systolic and less than 90 mm Hg for diastolic pressure. Patients with chronic hypertension should monitor their blood pressure on a regular basis.

Hyperlipidemia

Hyperlipidemia, elevated lipids in the blood, can develop in response to poor lifestyle factors. Cholesterol is a sterol that is synthesized in the liver from fats consumed in the diet and endogenously within body cells. Cholesterol is essential for the production of bile acids, steroids, cell membranes, and sex hormones. Cholesterol enters the bloodstream by lipoproteins, with almost 75% being bound to LDLs. Normally, a value of less than 200 mg/dL is considered an acceptable cholesterol level. Table 16-1 presents the normal ranges of total cholesterol, HDL, and LDL for men and women per the NHLBI. The U.S. Preventive Services Task Force (USPSTF) recommends beginning routine screening of cholesterol levels at the age of 35 years for men and 45 years for women. If other risks for cardiac disease are present, such as increased weight and insulin resistance, screening should begin sooner.[9]

TABLE 16-1 Adult Treatment Panel III Classification of LDL, Total, and HDL Cholesterol

Cholesterol Level	Cholesterol Category
TOTAL CHOLESTEROL	
<200 mg/dL	Desirable
200-239 mg/dL	Borderline high
≥240 mg/dL	High
LDL CHOLESTEROL	
<100 mg/dL	Optimal
100-129 mg/dL	Near optimal or above optimal
130-159 mg/dL	Borderline high
160-189 mg/dL	High
≥190 mg/dL	Very high
HDL CHOLESTEROL	
<40 mg/dL	A major risk factor for heart disease
40-59 mg/dL	The higher, the better
≥60 mg/dL	Considered protective against heart disease

Data from National Heart, Lung, and Blood Institute: *How is high blood cholesterol diagnosed?* September 19, 2012. Available at www.nhlbi.nih.gov/health/health-topics/topics/hbc/diagnosis. Accessed June 5, 2015.

Diabetes

Hyperglycemia, or blood glucose that is higher than normal, often results from poor lifestyle management and may be the precursor to diabetes. Approximately 29.1 million people in the United States have diabetes, with another 86 million being in the prediabetes stage.[12] Diabetes mellitus is a metabolic disease characterized by impaired insulin secretion and insulin resistance resulting in hyperglycemia. If it is uncontrolled, diabetes can lead to a number of complications including retinopathy, peripheral vascular disease, coronary artery disease, renal disease, and neuropathy that result in blindness, sexual impotence, myocardial infarction, stroke, renal failure, and amputation of extremities.[12] Diabetes is one of the leading contributors to the development of blindness, kidney failure, and amputations in the United States.

The concentration of blood glucose varies by the time since and the contents of the last meal. The American Diabetes Association (ADA) recognizes fasting glucose levels of 100 to 125 mg/dL or a blood glucose level of 140 to 199 mg/dL 2 hours after an oral glucose tolerance test as impaired glucose tolerance; such patients are at increased risk for development of overt diabetes and atherosclerotic vascular disease. Fasting blood glucose levels of 126 mg/dL or higher are diagnostic of overt diabetes. The fasting blood glucose level is used as a screening test, and the 75-g glucose tolerance test is recommended for the diagnosis of type 1 and gestational diabetes.[13] A 2-hour plasma glucose concentration of more than 200 mg/dL after an oral glucose tolerance test or a random plasma glucose level of more than 200 mg/dL in a patient with classic symptoms of hyperglycemic crisis is now also considered diagnostic.

Hemoglobin A_{1c} (HbA_{1c}) values to diagnose type 2 diabetes and prediabetes values are used. An HbA_{1c} value of 5.7% to 6.4% demonstrates impaired glucose tolerance; an HbA_{1c} value of 6.5% or higher demonstrates a diagnosis of diabetes.[13,14]

Metabolic Syndrome

The suggestion of the existence of a "metabolic syndrome" originated from the co-occurrence of metabolic risk factors for both type 2 diabetes and coronary vascular disease. These include central adiposity, hyperglycemia, dyslipidemia, and hypertension. Family history and genetic predisposition for insulin resistance, decreased physical activity, and fat distribution all affect the likelihood of an overweight patient's developing diabetes or cardiac disease.

The International Diabetes Federation, the NHLBI, the American Heart Association, the World Heart Federation, the International Atherosclerosis Society, and the International Association for the Study of Obesity have standardized the diagnostic criteria for the metabolic syndrome.[15] The criteria are as follows:

- Elevated waist circumference: population- and country-specific definitions
- Elevated triglyceride levels: 150 mg/dL (1.7 mmol/L) or higher, or specific treatment for this lipid abnormality
- Reduced HDL cholesterol: below 40 mg/dL (1.0 mmol/L) in males and below 50 mg/dL (1.3 mmol/L) in females, or specific treatment for this lipid abnormality
- Elevated blood pressure: systolic 130 mm Hg or higher or diastolic 85 mm Hg or higher, or drug treatment of previously diagnosed hypertension
- Elevated fasting plasma glucose of 100 mg/dL or higher, or drug treatment for elevated glucose[15]

LIFE SPAN ISSUES

Adverse health consequences from lifestyle influences evolve over long periods of time, ranging up to several decades. It follows that interventions for risk factors at an early age will produce better health outcomes later in life. Risk factors that can be modified are dietary habits, physical activity, and stress management. In addition, methods to intervene in addictions, such as smoking and alcohol consumption, will result in a longer life with more healthy years.

In general, it is not until the middle years of life that problems rooted in earlier patterns of health behaviors begin to arise; these problems include hyperlipidemia, hypertension, and type 2 diabetes, which are currently seen at increasingly early ages. Men are more likely than women to have coronary problems, although postmenopausal women have risks similar to those of men. The incidence of lung cancer has increased among women, who are more likely to begin smoking at younger ages. Postmenopausal women are also at risk for calcium deficiency and decreased physical activity, both of which contribute to osteopenia or osteoporosis.

Older persons are particularly susceptible to malnutrition because of decreased physiologic functioning and changes associated with social factors, such as living alone. Osteoporosis, iron deficiency anemia, weight management issues, and constipation are often manifestations of suboptimum nutrition. Because malnutrition in the older patient is difficult to remedy, early detection is imperative. Older persons often erroneously believe that they have less need for physical activity. In reality, however, moderate to high levels of exercise boost their physiologic functioning and improve muscle strength.

COMPONENTS OF A HEALTHY LIFESTYLE

Lifestyle counseling is essential to the prevention of disease and disability. At the level of primary prevention, health education and counseling about nutrition, physical activity, and stress management are likely to produce positive results for patients. This approach is key to affecting the many modifiable risk factors associated with diseases such as hypertension and hyperlipidemia.

Although essential to the prevention of disease and disability, lifestyle-counseling interventions may be arduous to initiate. Lifestyle behavior change is often difficult for patients, and the process toward change can be challenging. Setbacks frequently occur. Patients lose motivation easily, and momentum toward adopting healthy lifestyle choices and balance may be reduced. Patient-centered approaches such as relationship-based care and motivational interviewing will be helpful to both patients and providers throughout the process of lifestyle behavior change.

Nutrition

The American diet has changed substantially during the past few decades. More meals are consumed on the run, away from home and family. Much of the food consumed is fast food, which is usually high in saturated fats, calories, and sodium. The cumulative effects of poor dietary intake combined with an increasingly sedentary lifestyle may result in overweight, obesity, and other comorbidities. Patients need support, encouragement and teaching to improve decision-making around dietary needs.

The U.S. Department of Agriculture (USDA) revises the Dietary Guidelines for Americans every 5 years. The 2015 key recommendations made by the Dietary Guidelines Advisory Committee (DGAC) emphasize improved intake of underconsumed vitamins (A, E, D, and C) and essential nutrients (folate, calcium, magnesium, fiber, and potassium) and the overconsumed nutrients of sodium and fat.[16] The DGAC suggests that nutritional and dietary considerations be approached from a lifespan perspective. For example, providers caring for adolescent girls and premenopausal women should take into consideration the potential risk of deficiency in iron intake.[16] They advise improvements in diet quality, given the U.S. population's current preference for solid fats, added sugar, and refined grains over nutritious alternatives such as vegetables, fruits, dairy products, and whole grains.

Several key components of the 2015 recommendations are consistent with prior dietary guidelines including reducing sodium intake, consuming moderate amounts of alcohol, and maintaining dietary practices that are low in saturated fat and added sugar.[16] DGAC goals for the general population include consuming less than 2300 mg of dietary sodium per day, getting less than 10% of total calories per day from saturated fat, and getting a maximum of 10% of total calories per day from added sugars.[16] Dietary recommendations to address underconsumption of essential nutrients are discussed in detail in the 2015 report. The shortfall nutrients receiving highest priority, given their association with adverse health outcomes, are calcium, vitamin D, fiber, and potassium.[16] The current recommendations for intake of specific nutrients and food groups are based on analysis of national trends of various dietary patterns and eating behaviors shown to have health benefits.[16] The report references the Mediterranean-style diet, the Healthy U.S.-style diet, and the Healthy Vegetarian-style diet as examples of dietary patterns with potential health benefits. Practical application of the recommendations made in the 2015 DGAC scientific report can be found in the eighth edition of the USDA *Dietary Guidelines for Americans.* This publication can be found in its entirety at www.cnpp.usda.gov/DietaryGuidelines.[17]

Eating well has multiple benefits: providing a sense of vitality; maintaining a healthy weight; decreasing depression and anxiety; decreasing the risk of diabetes, hypertension, heart disease, and cancer; and increasing self-confidence and energy levels. Identification of factors that influence food consumption behaviors will enable the health care provider to adapt health counseling to the patient's circumstances. Motives that influence food selection and consumption may relate to culture, habit, or convenience. Cultural practices must be acknowledged and accommodated in health counseling. Negative habits related to food intake, such as binge and comfort eating, are best addressed through behavioral change programs. Food consumption behaviors born out of convenience, such as reaching for chips when hunger is felt, may be amenable to health education.

Adequacy of nutritional intake should be ensured. Sufficient intake of daily dietary fiber is often neglected. Fiber in the form of whole-grain foods, fruits, and vegetables is essential to proper health and aids in reducing heart disease and cancer. Fiber-rich foods are often neglected because of increased cleaning and preparation times. These nutrients are often replaced with prepackaged snack foods that have increased saturated fats and sodium. One technique to avoid convenience foods is having clean fruits and vegetables prepared in advance and stored so they are ready to eat when a quick snack is desired. The NHLBI offers an online interactive menu planner to assist people in meal planning (www.nhlbi.nih.gov/health/educational/lose_wt/menuplanneir.html). Middle-aged women may be at risk for hypocalcemia resulting from a diet that lacks calcium-rich foods. The ingestion of calcium-enriched orange juice, almonds, spinach, broccoli, kale, turnip greens, milk, cheese, and yogurt should be encouraged.

Caffeine has been classified as a drug because of its effects on the body. Caffeine is used for its stimulating effect, which increases alertness. Excess caffeine, however, can induce headaches, irritability, anxiety, insomnia, and heart palpitations. Studies suggest that moderate intake of caffeine may not have the detrimental consequences once associated with its use. Some studies have even demonstrated that a moderate intake of caffeine might decrease the risk for Parkinson and Alzheimer diseases, type 2 diabetes, and some cancers. Low to moderate coffee consumption (up to three to five cups per day) may also protect against myocardial infarctions. However, heavy coffee intake might trigger coronary or arrhythmic events in individuals with preexisting cardiac disease or risk factors and is associated with lower bone mineral density. Moderate use is generally considered to be approximately 400 mg/day, or the equivalent of not more than five cups of coffee per day.[16] Percolated coffee has 64 to 124 mg of caffeine per 5 ounces, whereas drip-brewed coffee has 110 to 150 mg of caffeine per 5 ounces. Coca-Cola has 46 mg of caffeine in a 12-ounce can, and Mountain Dew has 54 mg.[18]

The Vegetarian Diet. Many individuals choose to become vegetarians. Reasons for this include personal life philosophy, concern about excess consumption of saturated fat in beef products, concern about food-borne illnesses associated with meat consumption, and a desire for a healthier lifestyle. Vegetarians should follow the principle of complementation in selecting foods. To ensure that the required amino acids are supplied, complementation combines a grain with legumes or a dairy product (for lactovegetarians). Possible combinations include a peanut butter and jelly sandwich, beans and corn, brown bread and baked beans, a flour tortilla and beans, macaroni and cheese, and rice and milk. A major health concern is the adequacy of vitamin B intake because meats are the major source of this nutrient. Because vegetarians may not deliberately plan their meals to incorporate essential nutrients, they should be advised to take a daily multivitamin.

Weight Management. Management of overweight and obesity has many components, including behavioral, dietary, physical, and pharmacologic. From a behavioral perspective, the provider must communicate with the patient in a nonjudgmental manner. Some individuals are exceptionally sensitive about weight and likely to have a long history of frustration and trouble with weight control. In addition, providers need to examine their own attitudes toward the condition.[10]

Obesity is a chronic disease that requires changes in behavior and lifestyle management to produce positive results. Lifestyle management and behavior change are difficult for individuals. Patient-centered strategies to engage patients in long-term behavior change and improved self-management are required. Providers are advised to build a partnership with the patient, taking into account the patient's weight management goals. Individual care planning should include counseling on how to set appropriate long- and short-term goals. An action plan including a discussion of possible barriers and solutions should be discussed. Goal setting should be specific, yet achievable. Most weight loss plans recommend 1 to 2 pounds of weight loss per week. Frequent contact with the health care provider is beneficial to the patient for continued support and encouragement. This can be achieved through frequent monitoring of weight, which has the advantage of being an effective motivator.[10]

Dietary Considerations. There is evidence to support the energy balance perspective on weight loss. The perspective contends that for weight loss to occur, individuals must consume less energy than is expended or must expend more energy than is consumed.[19] Strategies that will reduce food and calorie intake have been suggested. These effective strategies include any of the following: "prescription for women 1200 to 1500 kcal/day, prescription for men 1500 to 1800 kcal/day, prescription for 500 kcal/day or 750 kcal/day energy deficit, or prescription of an evidence-based diet that restricts certain food types and produces energy deficit and food reduction."[19] Total calorie recommendations are usually individualized based on the patient's weight, energy demands, and specified weight loss goals.

The patient's motivation or inclination toward weight loss is a primary concern. Diet is an essential element of a weight management program. There are numerous topics for care providers to consider and integrate in a patient education program. The patient needs basic instructions on the composition of foods, including information on calorie content, how to read food labels, and what constitutes a serving size. In addition, the patient may need coaching on how to make wise food purchases and techniques for low-calorie food preparation. The patient should understand the value of adequate water intake and the importance of limiting alcohol consumption.

Eating well and making the appropriate behavior changes in lifestyle practices are key factors to individual health and weight management. However, evidence suggests that a multicomponent approach involving environmental and policy factors is required to create significant impact for reducing obesity and related chronic diseases.[16] A population-based approach may be required. Efforts to improve diet and weight status should take into consideration a broader perspective for the food environment, which includes settings such as child care organizations, schools, worksites, and community food access sites and operations. The DGAC contends that health care delivery practices should incorporate multicomponent obesity prevention and solution-oriented strategies. This approach is likely to reduce existing nutrition-related health issues and improve disparity gaps.[16]

Dietary Influences on Heart Health

The American Heart Association has publically supported the current USDA Dietary Guidelines for Americans, with the exception of the sodium recommendation. The current guidelines recommend less than 2300 mg of sodium for the general population and less than 1500 mg for those who have or are at risk for hypertension. The American Heart Association recommends that following a sodium restriction of less than 1500 mg daily of sodium will contribute to overall blood reduction. Rees and colleagues[20] reviewed the scientific literature on the effects of dietary advice given to healthy adults to assess the consequences of diet on cardiovascular health. They concluded that changes to diet and cardiovascular risk factors continue to be of benefit for a period of at least 12 months. They are uncertain of the longer-term benefits.

The American Heart Association has published the dietary factors associated with hypertension treatment and control: less dietary salt; alcohol use in moderation; weight loss; increased potassium; and adherence to a food plan based on the Dietary Approaches to Stop Hypertension eating plan, also known as the DASH diet.[21] The authors concluded that in particular, African Americans and older adults benefit from the diet. The DASH diet is within the current dietary guidelines published by the USDA. It is presented in Table 16-2 from the National Institutes of Health.[22]

Exercise

Patients who do not participate in any type of physical activity may have a plethora of excuses. The most familiar excuses include pain, limited time, fatigue, and an overall dislike of exercise. Older adults often use age to justify a lack of physical activity. However, physical activity has been called a "magic bullet" that can ward off heart disease and should be encouraged. Studies have also demonstrated that increased physical activity improves depression and anxiety.

Before encouraging any type of exercise program, the health care provider must be aware of the patient's current level of fitness. A patient wishing to exercise who is in midlife or sedentary and significantly overweight may need medical clearance before engaging in aggressive exercise.

For the sedentary patient, it is extremely important to begin a physical fitness program slowly so that the body can acclimate to the new demands. Moreover, a slow start safeguards against injury, especially to lower extremities and joints. An overzealous exercise program is likely to have a negative impact on motivation (i.e., the exercise prescription may serve as a deterrent if it is too rigorous early on). The patient must be committed to carrying out the program. Most individuals are aware of the value of incorporating exercise into their daily schedules, yet many do not. Exercise requires a personal commitment, and individuals need to be deliberate about making time for exercise in their daily lives. Thirty to 40 minutes of moderate activity 3 to 5 days a week is recommended.[10] Good results can be achieved through a program of walking. Many fitness experts suggest that individuals should engage in physical activities that are enjoyable and group oriented. Individuals are more likely to initiate and sustain exercise in those activities that produce pleasurable emotional states. Table 16-3 provides a suggested plan.

Aerobic activity is particularly recommended for cardiac health because it strengthens the heart muscle. Aerobic endurance training consists of three phases: the warm-up, aerobics, and the cool-down. Warming up for the intensity of aerobic training begins to raise the pulse rate and prepares the muscles and joints. This generally takes 3 to 5 minutes but may take longer in lower temperatures. Often, the warm-up activity is a gentler motion of the same type of physical activity that is part of the aerobic exercise and may involve stretching. The aerobic portion encompasses the dimensions of frequency, intensity, and time (known by the acronym *FIT*). The recommended frequency is three to five times per week.

Heart rate is a measure of intensity. Resting heart rate can be calculated by counting the number of beats during a minute when the patient is most relaxed; this is best done in the morning after an adequate night's sleep. Average resting heart rate is 60 to 80 beats per minute, but it may be lower for those who are in better physical condition. Resting heart rate also generally increases with age. The maximum heart rate, calculated by subtracting one's age from 220, represents the heart rate that should not be exceeded during exercise. For example, an individual who is 55 years of age should not have a pulse rate in excess of 165 beats per minute during training. The target heart rate is recommended for maximum effectiveness of aerobic activity and is represented by a range of values between 50% and 80% of the maximum heart rate. Thus, the 55-year-old individual is well advised to keep the pulse rate between 83 beats per minute (165 maximum heart rate × 50% = 83) and 132 beats per minute (165 × 80% = 132). The aerobic portion of activity should be at least 20 minutes long, with the heart beating within the range of the target heart rate. Conditioned individuals may extend their workouts to up to 1 hour.

Any activity that requires rhythmic, continuous movement and the use of the large muscles of the arms and legs may be selected. Bicycling, cross-country skiing, and some forms of dancing are examples of aerobic activities. The final component of the workout is the cool-down, during which the heart rate gradually returns to normal. Because the muscles are warm, stretching exercises may be incorporated to enhance flexibility.

The benefits of strength training are well documented for individuals of all ages. Several disease states may be improved through engagement in regular strength or resistance training sessions, including arthritis, cardiovascular disease, and diabetes. Strength training reduces falls and improves bone health. This type of exercise is known to improve emotional states and aid in weight reduction through body fat loss. Resistance training for muscle strength and endurance may be performed before aerobic activity, as part of a high-intensity endurance session, or as an isolated physical activity. The frequency of

TABLE 16-2 The DASH Diet

Food Group	Daily Servings	Serving Sizes	Examples and Notes	Significance of Each Food Group to DASH Food Group Diet Pattern
Grains and grain products	7-8	1 slice bread ½ cup dry cereal ½ cup cooked rice, pasta, or cereal	Whole-wheat bread, English muffin, pita bread, bagel, cereals, grits, oatmeal	Major sources of energy and fiber
Vegetables	4-5	1 cup raw leafy vegetable ½ cup cooked vegetable 6 oz vegetable juice	Tomatoes, potatoes, carrots, peas, squash, broccoli, turnip greens, collards, kale, spinach, artichokes, sweet potatoes, beans	Rich sources of potassium, magnesium, and fiber
Fruits	4-5	6 oz fruit juice 1 medium fruit ¼ cup dried fruit ½ cup fresh, frozen, or canned fruit	Apricots, bananas, dates, oranges, orange juice, grapefruit, grapefruit juice, mangoes, melons, peaches, pineapples, prunes, raisins, strawberries, tangerines	Important sources of potassium, magnesium, and fiber
Low-fat or nonfat dairy foods	2-3	8 oz milk 1 cup yogurt 1½ oz cheese	Skim or 1% milk, skim or low-fat buttermilk, nonfat or low-fat yogurt, part skim mozzarella cheese, nonfat cheese	Major sources of calcium and protein
Meats, poultry, and fish	2 or fewer	3 oz cooked meats, poultry, or fish	Select only lean; trim away visible fats; broil, roast, or boil, instead of frying; remove skin from poultry	Rich sources of protein and magnesium
Nuts, seeds, and legumes	4-5/wk	1½ oz or ⅓ cup nuts ½ oz or 2 Tbsp seeds ½ cup cooked legume	Almonds, filberts, mixed nuts, peanuts, walnuts, sunflower seeds, kidney beans, lentils	Rich sources of energy, magnesium, potassium, protein, and fiber

THE DASH DIET SAMPLE MENU*

Food	Amount	Servings Provided
Breakfast		
Orange juice	6 oz	1 fruit
1% Low-fat milk	8 oz (1 cup)	1 dairy
Corn flakes (with 1 tsp sugar)	1 cup	2 grains
Banana	1 medium	1 fruit
Whole-wheat bread (with 1 Tbsp jelly)	1 slice	1 grain
Soft margarine	1 tsp	1 fat
Lunch		
Chicken salad	¾ cup	1 poultry
Pita bread	½, large	1 grain
Raw vegetable medley:		1 vegetable
Carrot and celery sticks	3-4 sticks each	
Radishes	2	
Loose-leaf lettuce	2 leaves	
Part-skim mozzarella cheese	1½ slice (1½ oz)	1 dairy
1% Low-fat milk	8 oz (1 cup)	1 dairy
Fruit cocktail in light syrup	½ cup	1 fruit

TABLE 16-2 The DASH Diet—cont'd

Food	Amount	Servings Provided
Dinner		
Herbed baked cod	3 oz	1 fish
Scallion rice	1 cup	2 grains
Steamed broccoli	½ cup	1 vegetable
Stewed tomatoes	½ cup	1 vegetable
Spinach salad:	½ cup	1 vegetable
Raw spinach	½ cup	
Cherry tomatoes	2	
Cucumber	2 slices	
Light Italian salad dressing	1 Tbsp	½ fat
Whole-wheat dinner roll	1 small	1 grain
Soft margarine	1 tsp	1 fat
Melon balls	½ cup	1 fruit
Snacks		
Dried apricots	1 oz (¼ cup)	1 fruit
Mini-pretzels	1 oz (¾ cup)	1 grain
Mixed nuts	1½ oz (⅓ cup)	1 nuts
Diet ginger ale	12 oz	—

TOTAL NUMBER OF SERVINGS IN 2100 CALORIES/DAY MENU

Food Group	Servings
Grains	6-8
Vegetables	4-5
Fruits	4-5
Dairy foods	2-3
Meats, poultry, and fish	6 oz
Nuts, seeds, and legumes	4-5/wk
Fats and oils	2-3

TIPS ON EATING THE DASH WAY

- Start small. Make gradual changes in your eating habits.
- Center your meal around carbohydrates, such as pasta, rice, beans, or vegetables.
- Treat meat as one part of the whole meal, instead of the focus.
- Use fruits or low-fat, low-calorie foods such as sugar-free gelatin for desserts and snacks.

REMEMBER!

If you use the DASH diet to help prevent or control high blood pressure, make it part of a lifestyle that includes choosing foods lower in salt and sodium, keeping a healthy weight, being physically active, and, if you drink alcohol, doing so in moderation.

*Based on 2100 calories/day.

From National Heart, Lung, and Blood Institute (NHLBI): *Your guide to lowering your blood pressure with DASH*, Bethesda, Md, 1998, revised 2006, NHLBI Information Center.

TABLE 16-3 Sample Walking Program

	Warm-Up	Exercising	Cool-Down	Total Time
Week 1				
Session A	Walk 5 minutes.	Then walk briskly 5 minutes.	Then walk more slowly 5 minutes.	15 minutes
Session B	Repeat above pattern.			
Session C	Repeat above pattern.			
Continue with at least three exercise sessions during each week of the program.				
Week 2	Walk 5 minutes.	Walk briskly 7 minutes.	Walk 5 minutes.	17 minutes
Week 3	Walk 5 minutes.	Walk briskly 9 minutes.	Walk 5 minutes.	19 minutes
Week 4	Walk 5 minutes.	Walk briskly 11 minutes.	Walk 5 minutes.	21 minutes
Week 5	Walk 5 minutes.	Walk briskly 13 minutes.	Walk 5 minutes.	23 minutes
Week 6	Walk 5 minutes.	Walk briskly 15 minutes.	Walk 5 minutes.	25 minutes
Week 7	Walk 5 minutes.	Walk briskly 18 minutes.	Walk 5 minutes.	28 minutes
Week 8	Walk 5 minutes.	Walk briskly 20 minutes.	Walk 5 minutes.	30 minutes
Week 9	Walk 5 minutes.	Walk briskly 23 minutes.	Walk 5 minutes.	33 minutes
Week 10	Walk 5 minutes.	Walk briskly 26 minutes.	Walk 5 minutes.	36 minutes
Week 11	Walk 5 minutes.	Walk briskly 28 minutes.	Walk 5 minutes.	38 minutes
Week 12	Walk 5 minutes.	Walk briskly 30 minutes.	Walk 5 minutes.	40 minutes
Week 13 on	Gradually increase your brisk walking time to 30 to 60 minutes, three or four times a week. Remember that your goal is to get the benefits you are seeking and enjoy your activity.			

From National Heart, Lung, and Blood Institute (NHLBI): *The practical guide: identification, evaluation, and treatment of overweight and obesity in adults*, Bethesda, Md, 2000, NHLBI Information Center.

strength training is recommended to occur a few times a week. Many new fitness opportunities are available for individuals in which strength training or resistance training techniques are incorporated.

The American Heart Association advises that individuals be aware of any sensation of pressure or pain in the middle or left chest area and of pallor, cold sweat, sudden lightheadedness, or fainting during a workout.[11] The patient should be advised that if any of these events occur, he or she needs to stop exercising and to call the health care provider. If symptoms are not alleviated with rest, the patient should seek emergency services.

Physical Activity and Chronic Illness

Evidence strongly suggests that physical activity has a significant positive effect on patients with chronic diseases.[23] Osteoporosis, a disease that affects not only postmenopausal women but also female athletes who are amenorrheic or who lack sufficient calcium in their diet, is linked to a low bone mineral density. The condition is averted through impact and weight-bearing exercises. For those with fibromyalgia, cardiovascular conditioning enhances fitness and elevates the pain threshold. Arthritic patients benefit both physically and psychologically. Muscle strength and joint flexibility are improved, and morning stiffness is decreased; psychologically, anxiety and depression are decreased. Exercise regimens that are particularly effective with arthritic patients are water-based exercises and modified dance exercises. However, with any chronic illness or condition, proper clinical evaluation must be done to evaluate the safety of the exercise program.

Stress Management

Avoidance of stress produces benefits to physiologic wellness similar to the lifestyle behaviors of engaging in physical activity and eating a healthy diet. Excessive stress is harmful because it interferes with the function of the immune system, and high levels of stress can impede disease protection. Fortunately, there are many ways to minimize the detrimental consequences, including adequate amounts of sleep, cultivation of interpersonal relationships, relaxation techniques, time management skills, prayer, a good perspective on life, and a sense of humor.

Sleep. Impairment secondary to insufficient sleep is in itself a common health problem that increases the risk for errors in performance and problem solving. Originally, it was believed that sleep was essential to rejuvenate the body physically. Current interest in sleep research centers on the effect of sleep on the prefrontal cerebral cortex, the part of the brain associated with higher-level thinking abilities. For many, sleep is a low priority and is often sacrificed to make time for other activities. Sleep-deprived individuals are more at risk for automobile accidents, anxiety, and depression; they are less productive and are poorer at problem solving. To operate at peak performance, most individuals require 7 to 8 hours of sleep each day. Some individuals can manage with fewer than 5 hours of sleep, but they represent the exception.

To guarantee adequate time for sleep, patients can use time management techniques to deliberately block out the time needed for adequate rest. The sleep schedule should be regular, which means arising at the same time daily. Caffeinated products should be avoided for a minimum of 6 and up to 11 hours before retiring. Sleeping pills and alcohol should be avoided as aids to sleep. A glass of warm milk or a slice of turkey may be helpful because these foods contain the amino acid tryptophan, which is a natural sedative. Daily exercise is also an effective sleep inducer, although it should be avoided before bedtime, when it may have a stimulating effect. Life stressors and concerns should not preoccupy the patient during the time before dozing off. Instead, noting concerns and planning courses of action before going to bed may be helpful to alleviate anxiety before sleep. Bedtime rituals are also effective for sleep preparation. These may include reading, praying, preparing for the next day, and bathing. Watching television should not be considered part of a normal bedtime ritual, because television watching can hinder sleep. Televisions and workspaces should not be included in the sleeping area when possible. Associating the sleeping space only with sleep will also help the body relax and prepare for sleep.

Interpersonal Relationships. Healthy and satisfying personal relationships not only are rewarding but also buffer some of the stressors in life. Encouraging patients to nurture, maintain, and cherish relationships with family and friends is beneficial. In addition, patients need to have realistic expectations of what to expect from their relationships with others. The quality of relationships takes precedence over quantity; therefore a few good friends confer greater resistance to stress than do many superficial ones.

Relaxation. The relaxation response is an antidote to the physiologic alterations triggered by exposure to a stressor. Blood glucose levels decrease with relaxation, as do the heart rate, respiration rate, and blood pressure. Muscles relax as well. Psychological advantages may include decreased anxiety and an enhanced ability to cope with fearful situations.

Napping, walking, stroking a pet, participating in a hobby, listening to soothing music, and other activities can elicit the relaxation response. Breathing techniques are also effective for decreasing stress. Deep breathing involves two steps: (1) inhaling through the nose with the intention of inflating the lungs and (2) exhaling through the mouth at a slower rate than inhaling. This is the "cleansing breath" many individuals learn in Lamaze classes. Another technique involves diaphragmatic breathing (i.e., using the diaphragm to regulate respiration). This is sometimes called "belly breathing," which can be observed in the way an infant breathes. The belly is thrust outward as a long, deep breath is taken. Because the relaxation occurs on exhalation, the exhalation should be long and slow.

Time Management. Time is a precious commodity and must be managed wisely. Americans are overextended by the sheer volume of tasks they hope to complete daily. Even youths are beginning to complain of not having enough time in the day, a phenomenon previously reserved for adulthood and its concomitant responsibilities. A common time management technique is to apply an *A, B, C* format to the list of tasks that need to be achieved on a given day. *A* represents what must be achieved during the day, *B* signifies an important task, and *C* means that the activity can wait for another day. The goal is to achieve tasks assigned to the *A* group, to make progress on those in the *B* group, and possibly to begin the tasks in the *C* group. To ensure successful completion of required and important tasks, individuals should schedule themselves at 75% capacity. Inevitably, tasks, projects, and assignments consume more time than originally allocated. "Underscheduling" will probably convert to a full, rather than overloaded, slate of activities. As the day progresses, it is helpful to ask the question, "What is the best use of my time right now?" Breaks are important and can be used during transition times between activities. A break may be filled by having a meal, engaging in a physical activity (e.g., walking around the block, jumping rope), or calling a friend on the telephone. In the long run, continuously working without a break will diminish productivity and may lead to psychological burnout.

Prayer. Many people respond to adversity by becoming more spiritual and turning to a higher power for assistance. Overall, those with an active prayer life tend to be more optimistic in their outlook. Certainly, the spiritual domain of health must be acknowledged and faith practices encouraged.

Perspective on Life. Optimists seem to fare better than do pessimists. Patients can be encouraged and supported in their attempts to keep a positive perspective. Care needs to be taken with unduly upset patients or with those who are experiencing a significant personal loss. To coach these individuals in optimism would be to trivialize their needs. These patients could be better served by identifying a source of hope for them, such as local community resources and support groups.

Safety

Home Safety. Many regard home as a "safe" haven, yet it is the scene for most accidents and injuries. Falls result from navigating cluttered rooms and steps. Kitchen fires can arise from cooking fats and improperly using small appliances. Poisonings occur from chemicals commonly found in household cleaning solutions. In addition, toxic fumes in the form of carbon monoxide or radon may be emitted within homes. Larger appliances, power tools, and electrical cords also pose potential dangers. The use of goggles or safety glasses and ear plugs may be warranted with some types of tools.

Safety at home requires knowledge of potential sources of trauma and injury. Smoke detectors are recommended for each level of the house. If the smoke detectors are battery powered, batteries should be checked twice a year and replaced as necessary. The schedule should coincide with an event, such as resetting of the clock for daylight saving time in spring and for standard time in fall. Carbon monoxide detectors may be useful for detection of carbon monoxide leaks. Radon, another poisonous gas, can also be detected with a home testing kit. Ventilation systems also need to be checked.

Lighting needs to be assessed for adequacy. In dark homes and in homes with small children or older adults, nightlights may prevent injury from tripping or falling. Floor rugs need to be anchored securely to prevent falls, and stairs should be free of clutter. Slippery floors may also cause household accidents. Electrical cords should not be frayed and should be out of the path of normal daily activity.

Hazardous cleaning supplies need to be stored safely, and toxic supplies disposed of properly. Medications should be labeled and kept out of the reach of children. If firearms are kept in the home, extra care needs to be exercised to reduce the risk of injury. Guns should be stored unloaded and be secured under lock and key. Ammunition should be stored away from the firearm, preferably in a locked compartment or container.

Personal Preparedness. The incidence of natural disasters, such as flooding, earthquakes, and storms, has increased. Thus, it is important for families to have mapped out emergency plans. Important papers and documents, such as birth certificates and Social Security cards for all family members, should be kept in a central place so they are available in case household members need to evacuate quickly. Moreover, a supply of any necessary medications should be on hand. A central meeting place should be designated, or an extended family member or representative away from the residence should be identified as a communication link should household members become separated in an emergency.

Biologic Threats and Epidemics. Biologic threats to health such as the H1N1 influenza virus, which caused an outbreak in 2010, exist. This virus, which causes acute respiratory infection and illness, originated from swine and was discovered in the spring of 2009 in Mexico. The global spread of the virus in 2010 resulted in the first influenza pandemic since 1968. A large number of countries reported influenza cases in March 2010, with more than 17,700 cases confirmed through laboratory samples taken by the World Health Organization (WHO). However, according to the Writing Committee of the WHO Consultation on Clinical Aspects of Pandemic (H1N1) 2009 Influenza, an estimated 59 million illnesses, 265,000 hospitalizations, and 12,000 deaths were caused in the United States by H1N1. The threat of a virulent, infectious disease with the potential for high mortality rates and widespread social disruption has prompted the federal government to develop guidelines for the general population. More information is available at www.flu.gov/pandemic/about/index.html. See Chapter 23 for a discussion of emergency preparedness.

Sports and Vehicular Safety. Seat belts should always be worn in vehicles. Although some may argue that seat belt use may be responsible for some injuries or deaths by trapping individuals in the vehicle, this is the rare exception. In most cases, seat belts save lives. Drivers need to be alert to the possibility of "road rage" or aggression by other drivers on the road. When encountering an enraged individual, one should avoid eye contact and be alert for opportunities for safety, such as escape routes. Hands-free driving should be taken seriously. New driving laws mandate text-free driving and limited or no cellular phone use. Patients, especially younger or new drivers, should be educated on these evolving driver safety concerns.

Eye protection should be worn to prevent unintentional injuries to the eyes during sporting activities. Mouth guards are advised when participating in upper body contact sports, such as soccer, basketball, and football. If there is any possibility of being forcefully thrown in a sport, such as horseback riding or bicycling, a helmet should be worn. Patients should be advised that additional protective devices, such as wrist guards and elbow and knee protectors, prevent traumatic injuries during in-line skating.

SMOKING CESSATION

Cigarette smoking is the single most preventable cause of premature death in the United States. More than 480,000 Americans die annually as a result of cigarette smoking.[24] Of these deaths, 41,000 are attributed to exposure from secondhand smoke. The costs associated with smoking are estimated to be over $300 billion a year.[24] Direct medical care for adult smokers is estimated to cost $170 billion a year, and $156 billion a year is associated with lost productivity. The number of current adult cigarette smokers in the United States is estimated to be 42.1 million.[24]

The causes of smoking are varied; the appeal is different for each smoker. Smoking is pleasurable for some and a habit for others. Tobacco has more than 4000 components, many of which have biologic activity. Nicotine, a vasoconstrictor, is the most widely known component of cigarette smoke. With inhalation of cigarette smoke, nicotine is distributed throughout the body within 10 seconds. At high exposure levels, nicotine is a potentially lethal poison that may cause intoxication in young children who ingest cigarettes. Long-term nicotine exposure affects many organ systems and has been associated with cancer, hypertension, cardiovascular disease, and gastrointestinal and reproductive disorders.

EFFECTS OF NICOTINE

Most smokers use tobacco products regularly because they are addicted to nicotine. Health care providers should remember that approximately 70% of adult cigarette smokers want to quit and that over 50% of current smokers try quitting each year.[25] Cigarettes are efficient and highly engineered drug delivery systems. Because a typical smoker inhales an average of 10 puffs per cigarette, if that person smokes one and a half packs a day, there will be on average 300 hits a day, which strongly reinforces the habit.[25]

Neurochemical Effects of Nicotine

Nicotine affects how a person feels and thinks by activating nicotine receptor sites in the brain. These receptors affect both the mesolimbic dopaminergic pathway and the locus coeruleus. Dopamine causes cognitive arousal, which leads to feeling alert and vigorous as well as the perception of pleasure. Activation of the locus coeruleus causes the smoker to feel more alert and cognitively aroused, which leads to memory formation, storage, retention, and recall. Analytical thinking, arithmetic, and verbal skills may be enhanced as a result of the release of epinephrine from the adrenal glands.[25] The number of nicotine receptor sites is increased by two or three times in as little as 3 to 6 weeks of regular cigarette smoking. Unfortunately, this is not reversible.

Nicotine Withdrawal

When a smoker stops "cold turkey," he or she may experience one or more withdrawal symptoms from the sudden removal of nicotine from the receptor sites. The most common are dysphoria and difficulty thinking. This usually occurs 1 or 2 days after stopping of smoking. These symptoms can be ameliorated by the use of nicotine replacement therapy (NRT).

Genetics of Nicotine Addiction

Central nervous system sensitivity and response to nicotine are genetically determined. If a smoker does not have the proper genetic substrate, he or she cannot become addicted to nicotine.[25] About 10% of smokers lack the genes for nicotine dependence and can smoke rarely without having withdrawal symptoms. These individuals are social smokers and are able to control when and where they smoke.

STRATEGIES TO HELP PATIENTS QUIT SMOKING

In the early 1980s, psychologists James Prochaska and Carlo DiClemente sought to understand how people can change behavior, with or without professional intervention. They theorized that patients' willingness to change addictive behavior

TABLE 16-4 Six Stages of Change

Stage of Change	Description	Intervention Strategies
Precontemplation	Patient is not considering change.	Raise doubts; increase perception of risks.
Contemplation	Patient shows awareness of a problem.	Evoke reasons to change; list risks of not changing.
Determination	Patient says, "I've got to do something."	Help patient determine steps to take (if no intervention in this stage, patient may slip back to precontemplation stage).
Action	Patient stops smoking.	Help patient take steps toward change.
Maintenance	Patient sustains change.	Help patient identify strategies to prevent relapse (self-efficacy is important).
Relapse	"Slips" occur.	Help patient avoid demoralization and discouragement (sends him or her back to contemplation).

Data from DiClemente CC, Prochaska JO, Fairhurst SK, et al: The process of smoking cessation: an analysis of precontemplation and preparation stages of change, *J Consult Clin Psychol* 59:295-304, 1991.

depended on their state of readiness. There are six distinct phases of change that patients must experience to stop smoking (Table 16-4).[26]

The first stage is precontemplation, in which the patient is not considering change. If a patient is not considering change, the health care provider must be careful not to argue or to defend a position on smoking. Arguments are counterproductive, and resistance is a signal to change strategies. Patients should be asked if they smoke and are thinking of quitting. If they say that they smoke and are not thinking of quitting, they should be advised to quit and given some literature to read "in case they change their mind." The subject is not pursued at this visit.

Patients may be in denial. Patients who are in denial will disagree with the provider, will express no need for help, and will not accept help if it is offered. Patients who are in denial may perceive further advice as nagging, which may trigger a paradoxical response. If their anxiety levels are increased and they perceive that their freedom is being threatened, they may respond to this threat by increasing smoking.[26]

This does not mean that the provider never brings up the subject again. Patients should be questioned about smoking and offered help at each visit, but the provider's response should be determined by the patient's response. The provider can look for a "teaching moment," raise doubts about smoking, and help the patient increase his or her understanding of the risks of smoking. The provider can point out links between smoking and specific health concerns of the patient (e.g., the number of colds this year).

Awareness of a problem is the next step toward changing behavior. Once a patient admits there is a problem, he or she is in the contemplation stage of change. The provider must "tip the balance" at this point by evoking reasons to change and pointing out the risks of not changing behavior.

When a patient makes statements such as "I've got to do something," he or she has entered the determination stage. The best course of action should be planned together with the patient. This is the crucial point in the stages of change model. If there is no intervention at this stage, the patient will return to the precontemplation stage. Any barriers to treatment should be explored and removed if possible. Self-efficacy is an important tool for patients to become successful in their goal. The provider should give the patient information and determine the patient's reaction. Patients should be asked to list the rewards and problems of smoking and to identify any past unsuccessful attempts; they should be asked why they thought they did not succeed and what they would do differently this time.

Patients have reached the action phase of the model when they have smoked their last cigarette. The patient must have a specific plan by this stage and should have a follow-up visit scheduled so that there is something invested in the smoking cessation attempt.

Maintenance is the phase in which patients must sustain change. The patient needs help identifying strategies to make this a success. The patient needs to be encouraged to find other ways to deal with the urge to smoke, such as taking a walk or doodling, and should be warned of the inherent dangers in thinking of smoking and the importance of substituting alternative behaviors at those times.

Unfortunately, many patients relapse. DiClemente and colleagues found that smokers ordinarily went around the wheel of change three or four times before a stable change was effected. If the patient relapses, the provider should point out that a coping behavior is learned on each attempt. This can lessen the feeling of failure.

Patients should be continually moved toward their goal and counseled to quit on every visit. This does not need to be a formal counseling session; a brief talk should suffice. The American Cancer Society advises health care providers to cover the "five As":

- *Ask* about tobacco use: Identify and document tobacco use status at every visit.
- *Advise* to quit: Use direct, patient-centered communication to urge the tobacco user to quit.
- *Assess* willingness to make a quit attempt: Is the user willing to make a quit attempt at this time?
- *Assist* in the quit attempt: Offer interventions now and/or provide others to increase future quit attempts.
- *Arrange* a follow-up visit: Begin within the first week after the quit date and/or establish a plan for future willingness assessment.

When patients discover what drives them to smoke, interventions can be designed to help meet those needs. By determining the patient's specific motivators for smoking, the health care provider can assist patients in designing a program that is tailored to them (Table 16-5).

TABLE 16-5 **Smoking Motivation and Strategies for Cessation**

Motivations for Smoking	Strategies for Cessation
To keep from slowing down; to perk up; to get a lift	Change activity with urge to smoke; stimulate mouth with mouthwash or brush teeth; avoid fatigue.
Enjoys handling cigarettes; enjoys steps in lighting up; enjoys watching exhaled smoke	Doodle; do crossword puzzles; handle a small object.
Because smoking is pleasant, relaxing; because smoking is pleasurable; to relax	List pleasures of not smoking; contemplate harmful effect of smoking; go to a movie or read to substitute.
When upset; when uncomfortable; when "blue"	Identify what is needed when upset; do deep breathing or relaxation exercises; take up hobby or sport.

Modifying the Approach

Patients have different smoking issues that vary by age and gender. The message that the patient is given has greater impact if it is directed toward his or her needs and drives. Women often worry about weight gain after quitting. They should be encouraged to have low-calorie snacks on hand (e.g., carrot sticks) to substitute for handling a cigarette. If it is medically appropriate, women should also incorporate an exercise program into their quitting plan to increase their metabolic rate and make up for the lowered metabolism that results from the drop in nicotine levels.

Moreover, women who are at different stages of their life need different approaches. A young mother should be warned of the dangers to her born and unborn children. Smoking is one of the most modifiable risk factors associated with adverse pregnancy outcomes. Smoking during pregnancy is associated with 5% of infant deaths, 10% of preterm births, and 30% of small-for-gestational age infants. Smoking also increases the risk of infertility, placental abruption, preterm premature rupture of membranes, and placenta previa. Pregnant women should be advised to stop smoking and to avoid secondhand smoke exposure.

Health care providers have an obligation to inform patients that any maternal smoking also increases the danger of fetal congenital heart anomalies. Nicotine is contained in breast milk, and infants who breathe environmental tobacco smoke are more prone to otitis media and upper respiratory tract infections. Parents of asthmatic children should be advised to never allow them to be in an environment with tobacco smoke. Infants are at greater risk than older children are because their systems are more immature and they are less able to independently escape a smoky environment.

On the other hand, young men may be more interested in the image they convey by smoking. Professional athletes are often shown using smokeless tobacco. Young men should be encouraged to make their own decisions about nicotine use in any form and to not rely on marketing information to make this important health decision.

In addition, adolescents are not convinced of their own mortality; therefore, health concerns associated with smoking have a lesser impact on their smoking decisions. Instead, counseling highlights nicotine's effect on appearance (e.g., yellow teeth and fingers, hair and clothes that smell like smoke, bad breath). Factors associated with the initiation of adolescent smoking include poor academic performance in middle or high school and prior smoking behavior. Other predictors are a younger age than grade cohorts, an intention to smoke in the following 6 months, and underage drinking. Adults are more receptive to the messages about health concerns with smoking. Counseling should include the effects on blood pressure, the cardiovascular system, and the lungs. The encouragement to stop or to refrain from smoking can be individualized according to the patient's personal and family medical history. Other health implications of smoking are its effect on mood and affect. Patients with depression or anxiety disorders are at particular risk for nicotine addiction. With these patients, it may be helpful to augment therapy with an antidepressant, such as bupropion (Wellbutrin). If the patient has a personal or family history of a psychiatric disorder, nicotine withdrawal may exacerbate symptoms of depression or anxiety. Many of these patients require more extensive psychiatric treatment, behavioral therapy, and support.

Pharmacologic Interventions

Health care providers should remember that pharmacologic adjuncts are most successful when they are combined with behavior modification strategies or a formalized smoking cessation class. Classes are usually offered at area hospitals or through the American Cancer Society or American Lung Association.

There are basically two types of pharmacologic interventions: one aimed at nicotine replacement and the other aimed at neurochemical mechanisms of the brain pathways. There are numerous commercially available NRT products including gum, transdermal patch, nasal spray, inhaler, and sublingual tablets or lozenges. NRT products are known to increase the rate of quitting by 50% to 70%.[27] Nicotine gum is available in 2- or 4-mg doses. The patient must refrain from smoking while using NRT. With cardiovascular disease patients, nicotine gum should be used only after consideration of the risk/benefit ratio because nicotine is a potent vasoconstrictor and can precipitate arrhythmias. Other adverse effects include mouth soreness, hiccups, dyspepsia, and jaw ache; these are usually mild and transient.

In general, when commencing NRT, the patient initially uses the 2-mg dose. Patients using the 2-mg dose should have a maximum of 24 pieces per day, and patients using the 4-mg dose should have a maximum of 20 pieces per day.[27] The gum is chewed until a peppery taste emerges and then is held between the cheek and gum. The patient is instructed to chew and hold intermittently for 30 minutes and to avoid eating or drinking anything but water for 15 minutes beforehand; this prevents any interference with buccal absorption.

Nicotine patches are available in varying doses, depending on the manufacturer. Most manufacturers recommend using the higher dose for the first 4 weeks and then switching to lower doses at 2-week intervals. Evidence suggests that use of an NRT patch in combination with a rapid form of NRT is more effective than use of only a single NRT treatment.[27] An interval of 8 weeks has been found to be the most effective length of treatment.[27] Light smokers may experience more side effects and may need to begin at a lower dose. The patient must refrain from smoking while using the patch. The same precautions as with the gum apply to patients with cardiovascular disease.

The patch is placed on a relatively hairless location between the neck and waist. Patients should be advised to place the patch on awakening on their quit day. The location should be changed daily. Up to 50% of patients may experience a localized skin reaction, which is usually mild and self-limited.[27] The reaction can be treated locally with 5% hydrocortisone cream or 0.5% triamcinolone cream if necessary. Rotating patch sites will decrease the likelihood of a rash.

The dose for a nicotine nasal spray begins at 1 to 2 sprays per hour, which may be increased to a maximum of 5 doses per hour and 40 sprays daily. Treatment is recommended for 8 weeks, followed by gradual tapering during 4 to 6 weeks. Proper technique for use of nicotine nasal spray begins by gently blowing the nose, then tilting the head back slightly and spraying the nares. The spray should be aimed toward the center of the nasal opening while avoiding direct spraying of the nasal septum. Sniffing, swallowing, or inhaling of the spray should be avoided. Side effects include nasal irritation, blisters or tingling, watery eyes, sneezing, coughing, and change in taste or smell. Additional rarely reported side effects are chest pain, muscle weakness, speech problems, dyspnea, and rash.

The dose for nicotine inhalers is 6 to 16 cartridges daily. This dose is maintained for 3 months and gradually tapered during the next 6 to 12 weeks. Maximum treatment duration is 6 months. Side effects include headache; mouth, tooth, or throat irritation; cough; nasal congestion; change in taste; dyspepsia; and diarrhea. Rarely reported side effects are tachycardia and chest pain.

NRT alone has been proven to double the quit rate of smokers. However, even with this increase, only 10% to 30% of smokers remain continuously abstinent for 1 year.[27] There are two hypotheses for low success rates. The first is that "no current formulation mimics the extremely rapid, rewarding high arterial nicotine concentrations from inhaled tobacco smoke." The second possible explanation is underdosage of NRT by the user. All standard NRT therapies average half the plasma nicotine concentrations of a heavy smoker. Underdosage is thought to result either from incorrect technique or from the user's finding the side effects unpleasant.

Bupropion has been found to be an aid in smoking cessation. Initially marketed and formulated as an antidepressant, bupropion has the unexpected result of enabling patients to quit smoking. The drug has been remarketed under the name Zyban. The efficacy of bupropion may be explained in part by its effect on the neural uptake of dopamine, prolonging the action of this neurotransmitter. Nicotine, like all addictive drugs, is believed to stimulate increases in the neurotransmitter dopamine. Bupropion should not be prescribed for patients with a seizure disorder, patients with an eating disorder, or patients who are concurrently taking Wellbutrin or any other medication containing bupropion. The dose may need to be reduced for patients with liver or renal dysfunction. The most common side effect is insomnia. The usual dose is 150 mg twice daily. Therapy should begin at 150 mg every day for the first 3 days and then be increased to 150 mg twice daily. Patients may smoke while taking bupropion, and it is recommended that the patient start bupropion 1 to 2 weeks before the intended quit date to allow stabilization of blood levels. A combination of bupropion and NRT was found to be more effective than bupropion alone.[27]

U.S. Food and Drug Administration (FDA) approval was also granted for varenicline (Chantix). The mechanism of action is similar to that of NRT (i.e., nicotine receptors are bound and thus deactivated). Varenicline is designed to bind potently with the nicotine receptors that stimulate the mesolimbic dopamine system, which is believed to be the neuronal mechanism underlying reinforcement and reward experienced on smoking.

Treatment length in the six reported phase II clinical trials varied from 9 to 52 weeks. By weeks 9 through 12, 45% had carbon monoxide–confirmed abstinence in the group randomized to Chantix versus 12% in the placebo group. The numbers of subjects who remained abstinent with Chantix by week 40 dropped to 29% versus 9% of the placebo subjects. By 52 weeks, 23% of subjects taking Chantix had carbon monoxide–confirmed abstinence versus 8% of subjects taking placebo and 16% of subjects taking bupropion sustained release (SR). In addition, on the basis of responses to the Brief Questionnaire of Smoking Urges and the Minnesota Nicotine Withdrawal Scale "Urge to Smoke" item, patients treated with Chantix had a reduced urge to smoke compared with patients taking placebos in all studies.[28]

Administration of Chantix should be initiated 1 week before the target quit date, beginning with a single 0.5-mg tablet daily for the first 3 days, and then twice daily for the next 4 days. On day 8, dosage is increased to 1 mg twice daily. Nausea was the most commonly reported adverse event. Most of the nausea was described as mild or moderate and was often transient. The incidence was dose dependent; nausea was reported by 30% in the group treated with the 1-mg dose and 16% in the group treated with the 0.5-mg dose.[28]

Both of these medications have been shown to assist in smoking cessation; however, prescribers must use caution when ordering them. In 2011 the FDA warned that Chantix may increase the risk of heart attacks, and in July 2009 the FDA placed a "black box" warning and asked for the development of medication guidelines highlighting the risk of serious neuropsychiatric symptoms in patients using these products.[29] Prescribers should note that the FDA has also included a new warning regarding the potential interaction between Chantix and alcohol and a rare risk of seizure.[29] Neuropsychiatric symptoms include changes in behavior, hostility, agitation, depressed mood, suicidal thoughts and behavior, and attempted suicide. Clinicians should advise patients to contact a health care provider immediately if they experience any chest discomfort or any of the described neuropsychiatric symptoms, any changes in behavior that are not typical of nicotine withdrawal, or suicidal thoughts or behavior. If medication is discontinued because of neuropsychiatric symptoms, patients should be monitored until symptoms resolve.[29]

Nicotine vaccines for smoking cessation are under development. At this time no vaccines are licensed for public use. Nicotine vaccine research emphasizes mechanisms to help reduce the amount of nicotine reaching the brain. The NicVAX vaccine facilitates nicotine antibody development. The antibody binds to nicotine in the blood and prevents nicotine from reaching the brain, thus reducing nicotine's pleasurable sensation. Four key trials have been performed. Evidence that nicotine vaccines enhance long-term smoking cessation has not been established.[30]

Incorporation of Smoking Cessation with Primary Care Strategies

Health care providers should remember that it is possible to incorporate basic, brief primary care interventions into a busy practice setting. The first step to treating tobacco use and dependence is to identify the patient's use of the substance.[31] Providers should intervene with behaviors such as the Screening, Brief Intervention, and Referral for Treatment (SBIRT) approach for tobacco use and nicotine addiction. The "five As" approach to smoking cessation intervention discussed previously is a routine practice behavior clinicians should adopt. Providers should also keep in mind five essential elements when dealing with smoking cessation intervention: (1) offer a strong message to quit smoking, (2) provide self-help motivational quitting techniques and relapse materials, (3) provide brief counseling that includes a quit date, (4) use pharmacologic interventions when indicated, and (5) offer follow-up support.

Adopting an intensive intervention approach may be required. This approach is often appropriate for tobacco users who have expressed a willingness to quit or interest in quitting. In this case health care providers may need to expand their practice behavior to introduce other individuals in the care and management of the patient, such as smoking cessation experts and behavioral health care providers.[31] The provider should keep in mind that interventions for successful smoking cessation often require endeavors beyond the patient level of care. Appreciating a health care systems approach, including the awareness of the policy perspectives involved in a tobacco-using society, is key to increasing successful outcomes.[31]

Deciding on the most efficacious therapeutic regimen can increase the chances of the successful transition from smoker to ex-smoker. Use of one NRT product alone has only a 20% success rate; a combination of different NRT products and/or a combination of NRT products with other pharmacologic agents may be more efficacious.[27]

A valuable smoking cessation resource for primary care providers is the Clinical Practice Guideline *Treating Tobacco Use and Dependence: 2008 Update.*[31] It available at www.ncbi.nlm.nih.gov/books/NBK63952.

The Office of the Surgeon General provides many other resources and materials for smoking cessation at www.surgeongeneral.gov/priorities/tobacco.

Additional resources are available through many organizations, including the following:

- American Cancer Society: 1-800-ACS-2345; www.cancer.org/healthy/stayawayfromtobacco/guidetoquittingsmoking/guide-to-quitting-smoking-toc
- American Lung Association: 1-800-LUNG-USA; www.lung.org/stop-smoking/tobacco-control-advocacy
- National Cancer Institute: 1-800-4-CANCER; www.cancer.gov/about-cancer/causes-prevention/risk/tobacco
- Office on Smoking and Health, National Center for Chronic Disease Prevention and Health Promotion, Centers for Disease Control and Prevention: 1-800-CDC-INFO; www.cdc.gov/tobacco

INTIMATE PARTNER VIOLENCE

DEFINITION AND EPIDEMIOLOGY

Intimate partner violence (IPV) is defined as a pattern of coercive and controlling behavior exercised by one partner over the other. Behaviors can range from economic control, social isolation, emotional abuse, and stalking to sexual assault and threats of or actual physical violence and death. IPV occurs in all age, racial, socioeconomic, and sexual orientation groups. IPV is a significant public health care problem with widespread and devastating effects for patients, their children, their families, and their communities. Individuals who experience these types of violent insults are at significant risk for physical injury, poor mental health, and chronic physical health problems.[32] All patients seen in primary care should be screened for IPV, and help should be offered to address this growing threat.

IPV epidemiologic data are often described in three distinct categories, which include (1) sexual violence (rape); (2) stalking; and (3) IPV (physical harm and psychological aggression). One in three women and one in four men have experienced the physical forms of IPV (rape, physical violence, and stalking), and more than 48% of both men and women will experience a form of IPV, psychological aggression, in their lifetimes.[32,33]

The prevalence of sexual violence victimization in the United States is estimated at 19.3% for women and 1.7% for men. This accounts for more than 23 million women and more than 2 million men raped in their lifetime.[32,33] IPV involving rape has become a staggering issue; one in four women report having been raped at some point in their lives; over 50% of these women were raped by a partner, and 40% of the time by an acquaintance.[32,33] For men, the figures differ: 1 in 71 men have been raped at some point in their lives, but over 50% of the time an acquaintance was involved.[32,33] Of women, 43.9% experience sexual violence other than rape, compared with 23.4% of men[32,33]; 32.3% of multiracial women, 27.5% of American Indian/Alaskan Native women, 21.2% of non-Hispanic black women, 20.5% of non-Hispanic white women, and 13.5% of Hispanic women report having been raped during their lifetime.[32,33] Of multiracial men, 39.5% report having experienced sexual violence other than rape in their lifetime.[32,33] Men are most often described as the perpetrators of sexual violence acts with women who are raped (99%) and with the majority of males who experienced sexual victimization.[32,33]

Stalking and cyberstalking are recognized legally as crimes of power and control. Stalking behaviors vary but are recognized as any and all behaviors that may cause fear and victimization in others. In the United States it is estimated that 15.2% of women and 5.7% of men have experienced stalking victimization in their lifetimes.[32,33] The highest prevalence rates of stalking for racial or ethnic minorities occur in American Indian/Alaskan Native women and non-Hispanic black men.[32,33] Of female stalking victims, 61.7% were unwillingly approached in their work or home environments, and 55.3% received unwanted calls and messages.[32,33] Male stalking victims report having received unwanted calls and messages at rates similar to women victims (58.2%).[32,33] Males and females are identified as stalking perpetrators. The gender of the perpetrator varies with the gender of the victim. For example, for female stalking victims, 88.3% were stalked by only male perpetrators.[32,33] Technologic advances such as the Internet and social media provide stalkers with easier access to potential victims' locations and patterns and provide communication avenues. Recent data indicate that of the women and men who have been stalked, 20% of these women and 7% of the men experienced being stalked for the first time at ages 11 to 17.[32]

Physical violence other than sexual victimization occurs often for both women and men. Acts of physical violence range from slapping, shoving, and pushing to more severe acts of choking or suffocation; victims may be beaten, burned, knifed, or gunned. Psychological aggressive acts include actual expressive aggression and coercive control. Of women, 31.5% report having experienced physical violence by an intimate partner during their lifetime[32,33]; 27.5% of men have experienced physical violence by an intimate partner.[32,33] In their lifetime, 22.3% of women and 14.0% of men have experienced an act of severe physical violence[32,33]; 47.1% of women and 46.5% of men have experienced psychological aggression by an intimate partner during their lifetime.[32,33] The prevalence of physical violence by an intimate partner for racial or ethnic minority women ranges from 15.3% in Asian or Pacific Islanders to as high as 51.7% in American Indian/Alaskan Natives.[32,33] Rates of physical violence by an intimate partner are slightly lower for racial or ethnic minority men.[32,33]

The impact of IPV (contact sexual violence, physical violence, and stalking) is significant. Both female and male victims experience negative impacts of IPV.[32,33] Reports of negative impacts are somewhat higher from women than from men.[32,33] Victims of IPV identify having experienced fear and concern for their safety. Twenty percent of women and 5.2% of men identify having experienced one or more post-traumatic stress disorder (PTSD) symptoms.[32,33] Physical injury and the need for medical attention occur most often for women. Resources including housing support, victim advocacy, legal services, and crisis hotline support are often required by victims of IPV. School and work attendance is affected by IPV. As a result of IPV, 1.3% of women contract sexually transmitted infections (STIs) and 1.7% of women become pregnant.[32,33]

Victims experience IPV at varying ages; however, the majority of IPV victimizations occur before the age of 25 years. Of women who reported having been raped, 78.7% were first victimized before age 25 years[32,33]; 12.1% of women reporting rape experienced the violence before age 10 years.[32,33] Of men who were made to penetrate a perpetrator, 71.0% first experienced this violence before age 25 years.[32,33] More than half of the women (53.8%) who reported being stalked experienced an event before age 25 years.[32,33] Nearly 50% of men who reported being stalked experienced it before the age of 25 years.[32,33]

There are significant health care costs associated with IPV. Annual health care costs are highest among victims who have experienced physical types of IPV.[34] Costs are even greater in victims who experienced ongoing or recent physical abuse.[34] Use of health care services, particularly mental health services, is higher in women who have been abused compared with women who have never experienced abuse.[34] Data examined from a nationwide emergency department sample (2006 to 2009) identify that 5% of victims of IPV are hospitalized.[35] These data report that the mean charge for treat-and-release visits was $1904.69; and for those individuals who were hospitalized, the mean charge was $27,068.00.[35] Findings from this analysis identified common diagnoses requiring treatment, including superficial injuries; contusions; skull and face fractures; open wounds of the head, neck, trunk, and extremities; and complications of pregnancy.[35]

In 2007, intimate partners committed 14% of all homicides in the United States; 70% of victims killed by intimate partners in 2007 were female.[36] Females experiencing IPV are killed by their intimate partners at twice the rate of males.[36] African-American females are four times more likely to be killed by a boyfriend or girlfriend than are white females.[36] Abusive behavior by the perpetrator may be sporadic but generally is cyclic and usually escalates in terms of frequency and severity.

Violence Perspectives

Violence is expressed in multiple ways. IPV is one expression. More effective approaches for addressing the problem of IPV will be developed when primary care providers consider additional perspectives on violence.

Violence occurs at an individual level, a community level, and at societal and structural levels. Much of the knowledge surrounding IPV takes into consideration perspectives on violence at the individual level. This level emphasizes psychological and relationship-based notions of violence. It is most reflective of the psychosocial impacts that influence individual behavior. This perspective often lacks an explanation of violent behavior, which might arise from particular biologic, neurochemical, or developmental processes. The violent acts or behaviors that occur between and among individuals in two-person relationships and families are an expression of violence at the individual level. The domestic violence literature and the IPV literature describe violence at this level.

Community-level perspectives on violence consider group-level characteristics or a population lens to determine influences on violent actions or behavior. Determinants of violence at this level include aspects of individuals or groups such as socioeconomic status, which includes income, occupation, and education. Communities composed of individuals of mostly lower socioeconomic status experience more violence. Gang violence is an expression of community-level violence. Violence exhibited by gangs is motivated by negative group-level dynamics such as poor social cohesion, limited social and economic opportunity, and sociopolitical unrest and may be directed toward individuals or groups. Individuals engaged in gang-related violence have a greater propensity for engaging in acts such as sexual aggression and assault.[37]

Societal or structural violence is expressed when social institutions limit, restrict, or prevent individuals or groups from access or receipt of privileges, rights, or basic needs. Acts of social injustice and oppression are common in organized societies. When conditions perpetuate unequal opportunities for people and unequal distribution to key social resources and liberties, then societal or structural violence can occur. Inequities in health care, such as unequal access to health care services for certain racial or ethnic populations in the United States, are considered the outcomes of structural violence. The effects of societal violence manifest in many ways. Acts of violence within families, including physical and psychological harm to children, have been attributed to sociocultural contextual factors. Perpetrators of IPV are considered to have a higher propensity for child maltreatment.[38]

Current perspectives on IPV follow from a more than 30-year history of comprehending domestic violence. Key lines of thought established from appreciating domestic violence include considerations from feminism and psychology. Feminist thought supports the precepts in which a patriarchal system perpetuates violence against women.[39] Victimization of women occurs as a result of male domination and control.[39] Psychological views propose that particular background and personality attributes of individuals may contribute to the risk of becoming perpetrators of violence against others.[39]

Power and Control. Interpersonal control and associated abusive behavior is exercised in different ways. Perpetrators of violence may use abusive behaviors such as coercion and threats of physical, psychological, or economic harm; intimidation; and physical or sexual violence to victimize others. Partners who abuse may exert psychological, emotional, and financial control over their partners through verbal degradation, isolation, and economic manipulation. Perpetrators often minimize or deny their abusive behaviors. They may shift the responsibility for their abusive behavior and blame the victim. In family environments the abuser may use children to create guilt or to manipulate the victim. The abuser may threaten to harm the children or have them taken away in an effort to control the victim's emotional reaction and response. In violence against women, male perpetrators dominate and claim male privilege to define and devalue women's household roles. The fear that ensues from this type of behavior is often a powerful deterrent to individual's care-seeking and treatment behavior.

Cycle of Abuse. Violence in relationships often develops into ongoing patterns of abuse. This is commonly referred to as the cycle of abuse or violence. Within relationships a systematic pattern of dominance, control, and violence occurs. This cyclic process is said to occur in three or four stages (tension building; acute violence; reconciliation or honeymoon; and calm). During the first stage the relationship becomes tenser as stress and conflict erupt. This phase may wax and wane over extended periods, with the victim working to reduce tension and prevent violence. In the second stage, violence develops. The perpetrator seeks to give the victim "what they deserve," as a means of relieving the tension and stress. Violent actions vary during this stage depending on the context of the relationship. The third stage is characterized by feelings of guilt or responsibility for actions. In this stage the perpetrator often gives the victim a false sense of remorse. There may be subtle behaviors of control and dominance disguised in what appears to be regretful action. The fourth stage is recognized as a period of calm. This phase is sometimes considered a component of the third stage. In this stage the perpetrator offers to obtain help and promises to stop violent behavior and aggression.

Relationship dynamics inherent in partner violence create significant challenges for victims. Perpetrators of violence engage in behaviors to maintain an imbalance of power over their victims and to exert interpersonal control. Victims are challenged by these oppressive behaviors, which often produce serious emotional and psychological distress. Victims of violence will often develop symptoms of post-traumatic stress or depression and exhibit their own behaviors of fear, guilt, shame, self-blame, and social withdrawal. The negative effects of this behavior profoundly alter the victim's life circumstances. These effects also challenge primary care providers, given that victims of violence have a tendency to avoid or delay seeking care and treatment, deny violence in their lives, and neglect chronic health conditions.[40]

Barriers to Identification and Treatment

The health consequences related to intimate partner victimization are well documented. A primary health care environment is the most appropriate location for the assessment and management of IPV. Primary care providers should be cognizant of missed opportunities to identify and treat IPV and its sequelae.

Patient Barriers. Numerous challenges and effects of violence affect patients' disclosure and health care–seeking behavior. Patients are often reluctant to disclose information about victimization or ongoing abuse because of shame and embarrassment. Certain cultural or religious beliefs may interfere with the disclosure of violence. Negative interactions or responses from past encounters with care providers and health care agencies may prevent individuals from seeking care. Victims are often reluctant to seek care for fear of a repeated unpleasant experience or poor treatment. A victim's impaired insight or ability to be fully aware of the violence and abuse inflicted on them may present a barrier to adequate identification. Individuals experiencing ongoing patterns of violent behavior (domination, control, emotional and psychological threats) from a perpetrator may lack the ability to adequately recognize their victimized state or the potential threat of severe violent action.

Health Care Barriers. The health care environment inclusive of care provider behavior and assessment pose significant barriers to care access and effective treatment. Victims of violence may experience difficulties in access to needed care. Individuals without health insurance benefits or those who have limited resources to pay for out-of-pocket medical expenses may not seek care or receive the necessary follow-up and referrals. Illegal immigration status poses a significant barrier to accessing of required health care services. The fear of retribution or escalation in violent behavior from a perpetrator may influence a victim from engaging in care and social services. Victims of violence may be reluctant to use their health insurance or seek required help at a particular agency or care environment for fear of alerting the perpetrator.

Provider Barriers. Health care provider actions are often barriers to the effective assessment and management required in IPV encounters. The greatest barrier to the identification of violence in patient's lives is that providers often fail to screen for it. Explanations for ineffective screening vary and often include provider knowledge deficit regarding IPV and its impact and misconceptions about risks in certain patient populations. Some care providers may feel powerless to address the problem or lack resources to deal with adequate intervention and counseling. IPV is now recognized as a significant public health concern, yet it often remains undetected in health care settings. Health care providers should play an active role in screening for IPV and its required treatment.

CLINICAL PRESENTATION

Victims of IPV often seek care first in emergency departments.[35] Therefore a history of recent visits to the emergency department for repeated physical injuries should alert care providers to a potential violence problem. Repeated office visits for either physical injuries or complaints should suggest to the provider the possibility of ongoing violence in the life of the patient. A patient who has been victimized may show obvious signs of abuse, or the symptoms may be more obscure. In general, clinical indicators of IPV may be categorized into physical complaints, psychosocial indicators, or a combination of the two.

Physical Complaints

Injuries to the head and neck are the most common injuries in partner abuse situations, followed by upper extremity, breast, back, and buttock injuries. Some of the less obvious signs and symptoms include loss of appetite, eating binges and self-induced vomiting, vaginal discharge, diarrhea or constipation, fainting, difficulty passing urine, hyperventilation, and headaches. Other indicators of partner violence include injuries in various stages of healing, repeated office visits, delayed treatment for an injury, reluctance to talk about an injury, and explanations that are inconsistent with the type of injury.

Sexual assault can occur with the physical or emotional abuse, or it can be the only form of abuse in the relationship.

Intimate partner sexual assault includes any forced sex acts that occur within the context of any intimate relationship, and it may include the use of objects, rape, or uncomfortable or embarrassing sexual experiences. Men who sexually abuse their partners are particularly dangerous, which means that women are at greater risk of death. Evidence of sexual assault should automatically prompt further exploration by providers. This form of violence can result in problems such as pelvic inflammatory disease, STIs, human immunodeficiency virus (HIV) infection and acquired immunodeficiency syndrome (AIDS), vaginal or anal tearing, urinary tract infections, dysmenorrhea, unexplained vaginal bleeding, or pelvic pain. The male partner may exert control over his partner by not using a condom, thereby increasing her risk for STIs and an unintended pregnancy. In 2009 the rate of intimate partner victimizations for females was 4.3 victimizations per 1000 females age 12 years or older versus a rate of 0.8 victimizations per 1000 males age 12 years or older.[36] This disparity supports the critical role of health care providers in identifying IPV and offering support and resources to their patients.

Physical abuse during pregnancy poses a significant health risk for mother and fetus; therefore assessment for abuse during pregnancy should be part of routine prenatal care. For some relationships, violence may begin when a woman becomes pregnant; if violence is already occurring, it may escalate during pregnancy. The American College of Obstetricians and Gynecologists (ACOG) has acknowledged the increased risk of abuse in pregnancy and has responded with recommendations for more comprehensive screening methods. Studies on patterns of abuse during pregnancy suggest that violence occurs in up to 15% of pregnancies.[41] The prevalence of physical abuse during pregnancy is often higher than the prevalence of gestational diabetes or preeclampsia. Adolescent women or those with an unintended pregnancy are at higher risk.[41]

Possible complications of victimization during pregnancy include low birth weight, miscarriage, and maternal death. These symptoms could result from abdominal trauma, inadequate prenatal care, suboptimal weight gain, an unhealthy diet, or severe stress. Because pregnancy may be the only time healthy women come in frequent contact with health care providers, an important opportunity exists to ask about IPV.

Psychosocial Indicators

In addition to physical injuries and complaints, patients may experience a variety of psychosocial problems. A study supports the need for better understanding of the effects of nonphysical forms of abuse. Women may be treated for symptoms of depression or anxiety without assessment for IPV; if these symptoms are taken out of context of the abuse, treatment may be ineffective. Psychologically, the patient can experience a complex traumatic stress response, which includes the symptoms of post-traumatic stress disorder—intrusive thoughts, nightmares, dissociative flashbacks, psychic numbness, hypervigilance, and exaggerated startle response. Victims commonly experience depression, anxiety, and their related symptoms, including anhedonia, difficulty concentrating, changes in sleep and eating patterns, depressed mood, somatization, decreased self-esteem, and suicidal ideations. There may be an alteration in affect (predominantly depressed or restricted), an alteration in perceptions of the perpetrator (seeing the abuser as omnipotent), and an alteration in the sense of self (disappearance of self and increased feelings of self-blame). This complex traumatic response can be immobilizing and can prevent the victim from escaping the abusive relationship or seeking help.

PHYSICAL EXAMINATION

It is important to address patients' urgent and nonurgent health care needs at the time of the visit. Some victims of partner violence may have difficulty returning to the health care provider's office for follow-up. Patients who report partner violence and who are not ready to leave the abusive relationship may benefit from education and services targeting the prevention of unintended pregnancy. When treating the patient's illness or injuries, the provider must take care not to prescribe any medication that could impair the patient's judgment or ability to respond because this would place her at increased risk for further harm. If necessary, the patient can be referred to a specialist for additional health care needs.

The documentation of the patient's visit is important and may be needed for legal proceedings. The patient's account of IPV should be documented in the medical record with use of the patient's own words, when possible. It is advisable to avoid use of the term *alleges*. An appropriate substitute is "patient reports" or "patient states." Caution should be used in documenting the patient's demeanor. Because the patient's medical record may be used in legal proceedings, accuracy is important. Documentation should also indicate the patient's report on when and how the patient sustained the injuries. It should include the identity of the person who caused the injury. It is important that the health care provider stick to his or her area of expertise. Documented inferences that are out of the provider's area of expertise may create legal difficulties for a patient who pursues legal action against the abuser. Documentation should include a detailed description of the injuries and a body map to identify the location of injuries. Care should be taken not to attempt to date the injuries on the basis of appearance; rather, the provider should document objective data, such as color and size of bruises. Dating of injuries can create complications with legal proceedings.

If possible, the provider should offer to photograph the patient's injuries. The patient's written consent is required before pictures are taken, and all pictures must be labeled with the patient's name and medical record number. When appropriate, an object of standard size (e.g., a tape measure or coin) can be placed in the picture, near the injury, to illustrate size. This will aid in providing an accurate perspective of the injuries should the patient need the photographs as evidence of the assault for legal purposes. Care should be taken to preserve the patient's dignity during photographing, and the patient should not be asked to remove more clothing than is necessary. Some of the photographs of the injuries should include the patient's face, when possible, to protect against a possible dispute over the identity of the person photographed.

If a patient was recently sexually assaulted, before beginning the physical examination the provider should consider referring the patient to an emergency department that has a program to assist victims of sexual assault. Personnel there can assist in securing evidence that may be lost during a regular physical examination. This referral should be encouraged even if the patient is not considering notifying law enforcement at the time of disclosure of sexual assault. There are time restrictions on these types of services; therefore, providers should check with the local hospital for service guidelines.

MANAGEMENT

Clinical Intervention

The health care provider can assist the patient who admits to being a victim of partner violence by assessing and treating medical problems, educating about the dynamics of violence, discussing safety issues, and providing referrals.

Universal Screening. All patients seen in primary care settings should be routinely screened for IPV. However, special attention and additional screening should be considered in interacting with female trauma victims, emergency department patients, women with chronic abdominal pain, women with chronic headaches, women with STIs, and especially pregnant women with injuries. Because many patients are reluctant to disclose that they are being abused the first time that the subject is raised, they may be more likely to disclose information after they have developed some level of trust with the provider. Therefore, screening should not be limited to the first visit; providers should continue to screen at subsequent visits. Research with survivors of domestic violence revealed that with or without direct disclosure and identification, compassionate asking from health care professionals provided validation and helped victims change their situations and move toward safety.[42]

Framing the Question. When screening or interviewing a patient about IPV, the provider must remember that privacy and confidentiality are essential. The patient's partner or a third party should never be informed that the patient is being screened for violence because this may place the patient and provider at risk for retaliation. Providers should use their own style of communication to introduce the subject and convey the need for screening because of the seriousness and prevalence of domestic violence. It may be helpful to normalize the process for patients by using statements such as "Since IPV is so prevalent, I have started screening all my patients." It is usually most beneficial to ask direct questions when screening, such as the following:

- Have you ever been hit, slapped, kicked, or otherwise physically hurt by someone? If yes, by whom?
- Have you ever been threatened, controlled, or forced to do things you did not want to do? If yes, by whom?
- Are you afraid of your partner or anyone else?

The provider's demeanor when screening a patient can negatively influence the patient's willingness to disclose his or her victimization. If the provider is not comfortable with the subject matter and the screening process, it is advisable to have an appropriate staff member screen patients. It is essential that the provider be aware of not only how to appropriately interview patients to screen for IPV but also how to respond to them when the screening has been completed. It is recommended that the provider compile a list of resources and related brochures and have them available to aid in the education of the patient regarding IPV.

Patient Denial of Victimization. If the patient denies being victimized, the provider should document in the patient's chart that the screening was completed. If the patient has injuries that are inconsistent with the explanation as to how they occurred and denies violence or abuse, the provider documents in the patient's chart that the "injury is inconsistent with explanation." There is generally no therapeutic benefit in challenging the patient's explanation. Consider the need to report to appropriate authorities if the patient is a minor or a dependent adult. Providers should acquaint themselves with the mandatory reporting laws in the state in which they practice because the laws vary greatly from state to state. Even when a patient denies abuse and is well known to the provider, the patient should be rescreened at subsequent visits. Providers should continue to convey to the patient that they are available to assist, if needed.

Patient Disclosure of Victimization. When a patient discloses that she or he is being victimized, the provider can use the opportunity to convey concern, to educate, and to provide information on available resources. The patient should be assured that the patient is not at fault for the violence, regardless of what he or she may or may not have done. The provider should not try to verify the patient's report with the partner or other family members. The primary focus should be on the patient's safety and the provision of appropriate referrals. Victims of IPV will react in many different ways. If the victim does not cry or appear distraught when disclosing incidents of abuse or violence, it does not mean that she or he has not been victimized.

Psychosocial Intervention

Repeated abuse can have a monumental psychological impact on the victim. Care should be taken to discuss the patient's psychological well-being. Patients may experience feelings of intense fear and helplessness. Some victims may develop PTSD. Victims of chronic abuse should be screened for suicidal and homicidal ideations because they may feel that there is no way out of the abusive relationship other than death. If appropriate, the patient should be referred for crisis intervention. Referrals to individual counseling and support groups specific to IPV are also appropriate. However, couples counseling is highly discouraged because of the potential for further harm to the patient. The provider should inform the patient about how to access emergency shelters and financial and legal assistance.

Children who are exposed to family violence should be referred to age-appropriate counseling. Many organizations that provide services to adult victims of IPV also have services for children. Victims should be encouraged to have a pediatrician examine their children to assess their well-being, physically and psychologically. Many people mistakenly think that if a child was not physically assaulted, he or she is not in need of services. Children who are exposed to violence are at significant risk for using violence themselves, becoming delinquent, experiencing school and behavioral problems, and having serious and possibly lifelong mental health problems.[43]

Safety Assessment and Planning. On identification and discussion of a violence situation, the provider should perform a thorough assessment and discuss a safety plan. The provider should obtain information on the history of the violence, including when the violence first occurred, types of incidents, whether weapons were used, and frequency of assaults. This will assist in determining whether the violence is escalating and in raising the victim's awareness of the progression of violence. The presence of weapons in the home increases the potential lethality of the situation. Patients need to make their own decisions about their safety and whether they should leave the abusive relationship. Violence often escalates when the victim attempts to leave; as a result, patients should be advised to take extra precautions to protect their safety when leaving a relationship.

If the patient is in immediate danger while in the clinical setting, immediately contact the appropriate security services.

The health care provider should not attempt to mediate between the victim and their partner.

The safety plan should consider various scenarios that the patients may find themselves in and need to escape from. It may include having the patient develop a code with someone she or he trusts who lives in the home, or next door, that would indicate the patient needs help and that the police should be notified. Details should be discussed about where the patient would go if the home is not safe. Patients should be encouraged to use emergency shelters to protect their safety, rather than going to family or friends' homes where the abuser may be able to locate them. Providers should encourage patients to compile important documents such as birth certificates and photo identification, an address book, checkbook, bank cards, medical cards, Social Security cards, chronic medication, and clothing. The patient's safety is of the utmost importance, so if compiling documents places her at greater risk, she should be advised not to do so. Providers should help the patient identify people and agencies that are able to assist. A follow-up appointment, as appropriate, should be scheduled before the patient leaves. Furthermore, the health care provider should inquire about whether the patient can be contacted through the mail or on the phone. The provider's good intention of calling the patient later to inquire about her or his well-being may actually further jeopardize the patient's safety.

A determination of the success of an intervention should not hinge on whether the patient leaves the abusive relationship. A successful intervention is one in which the provider has acknowledged and validated the situation and offered appropriate referrals. The patient may decide at a later date to seek services on the basis of the groundwork that was laid at a previous visit.

LIFE SPAN CONSIDERATIONS

IPV occurs across the life span, and therefore health care practitioners must maintain the same standards of screening and identification of all patients. The USPSTF recommends screening for family violence and IPV. The most recent guideline emphasizes screening for asymptomatic women (women who do not have evidence of abuse) of childbearing years, elders, and vulnerable adults.[44]

A further consideration regarding life span issues is the impact of IPV on children. Findings from report of the National Task Force on Children Exposed to Violence indicate that children who are exposed to violence of any form have the potential for lifelong negative impacts.[43] Children who experience IPV within their family are at significant risk for developing problems with their physical and mental health, school, and peer relationships including disruptive behavior disorders.[43]

PATIENT AND FAMILY EDUCATION

Patients and their families are often unaware of the prevalence of this issue. The isolative nature of IPV results in a lack of awareness of this problem among patients and their families. Individuals are frequently unaware that their own maladaptation with these issues and can gain support from others who have survived similar experiences. Educating patients and their families about controlling behaviors that often escalate into violence may prompt change before the violence occurs. Health care providers should offer additional education about community programs and resources to further support victims of violence. Finally, because most victimizations are perpetrated against women by current and former intimate partners and because women are more likely to be injured if their assailant is a current or former partner, violence prevention strategies for women that focus on how they can protect themselves from perpetrators are needed.

HEALTH PROMOTION

IPV and the consequences associated with it are preventable problems. Health care activities that support its prevention potential are essential to positively affect the health of individuals, children, and families. Screening and counseling for interpersonal violence and domestic violence are current priorities of the HHS and the Institute of Medicine (IOM). These recommendations for implementation of IPV screening mechanisms coincide with the National Health Policy commitment of the Affordable Care Act, which emphasizes prevention efforts and health promotion. Implementation of simple screening and counseling approaches in health care settings and within the patient-provider relationship is essential to the goal of effective identification and treatment of IPV.[40] However, effective IPV screening requires a comprehensive approach. Evidence from a 2011 systematic review of the literature suggests that screening programs achieve the greatest success (increased IPV screening and disclosure and identification rates) when there is integration of multiple program components including institutional support.[45] Findings revealed that the program components of institutional support, effective screening protocols, thorough initial and ongoing trainings, and immediate access or referrals to onsite and/or offsite support services produce the best increase in provider self-efficacy for screening.[45]

CHAPTER 17

ROUTINE HEALTH SCREENING AND IMMUNIZATIONS

Elaine D. Kauschinger • Joanne Sandberg-Cook

Achieving and maintaining optimum health for each individual patient is the goal of high-quality primary care. Primary disease prevention and health promotion are critical elements of comprehensive health care that must be addressed by primary care providers. Health screenings and immunizations along with health risk assessment and education about a healthy lifestyle form the cornerstone for primary prevention and health promotion activities in primary care. Each visit with a patient provides the opportunity to offer appropriate health screening and to ensure that an individual's immunization status meets age-recommended guidelines.

ROUTINE HEALTH SCREENINGS

Which health screenings are considered routine varies with the agency making the recommendations and health care insurers. In most countries, government agencies publish guidelines for overall health promotion and disease prevention that include recommendations for specific health screenings. In addition, specialty organizations such as the American Cancer Society make recommendations for health care screenings pertaining to their specialty focus. Although there may be some variation in recommendations, all agencies base recommendations on evaluation of the evidence and comparative effectiveness parameters; these recommendations are considered to be guidelines, not prescriptions, and primary care providers are encouraged to evaluate what may be appropriate for the individual patient based on the patient's family history, personal health history, and individual concerns. Health care insurers make determinations about which tests they will cover and how often they will pay for the test to be performed, depending on levels of purchased insurance coverage. The decision to recommend a test to an individual patient should not depend solely on whether the individual patient's insurer will pay for the test to be performed; instead, the national specialty organization and government recommendations should be consulted in making these decisions.

Overall Health Evaluation and Screening

The U.S. Department of Health and Human Services (HHS) guidelines recommend that in all adult age categories, patients should have a full health evaluation that includes measurement of height and weight, skin examination for lesions and moles, and appropriate evaluation for heart health, bone health, diabetes, breast health, reproductive health, colon and rectal health, eye and ear health, and oral health. Tables 17-1 and 17-2 provide these recommendations for women and men,

TABLE 17-1 Screening Tests for Women

Screening Tests	Ages 18-39	Ages 40-49	Ages 50-64	Ages 65 and Older
Blood pressure test	Get tested at least every 2 years if you have normal blood pressure (lower than 120/80). Get tested once a year if you have blood pressure between 120/80 and 139/89. Discuss treatment with your doctor or nurse if you have blood pressure 140/90 or higher.	Get tested at least every 2 years if you have normal blood pressure (lower than 120/80). Get tested once a year if you have blood pressure between 120/80 and 139/89. Discuss treatment with your doctor or nurse if you have blood pressure 140/90 or higher.	Get tested at least every 2 years if you have normal blood pressure (lower than 120/80). Get tested once a year if you have blood pressure between 120/80 and 139/89. Discuss treatment with your doctor or nurse if you have blood pressure 140/90 or higher.	Get tested at least every 2 years if you have normal blood pressure (lower than 120/80). Get tested once a year if you have blood pressure between 120/80 and 139/89. Discuss treatment with your doctor or nurse if you have blood pressure 140/90 or higher.
Bone mineral density test (osteoporosis screening)			Discuss with your doctor or nurse if you are at risk of osteoporosis.	Get this test at least once at age 65 or older. Talk to your doctor or nurse about repeat testing.
Breast cancer screening (mammogram)		Discuss with your doctor or nurse.	Starting at age 50, get screened every 2 years.	Get screened every 2 years through age 74. Age 75 and older, ask your doctor or nurse if you need to be screened.
Cervical cancer screening (Pap test)	Get a Pap test at least every 3 years if you are 21 or older or are younger than 21 and have been sexually active for at least 3 years.	Get a Pap test at least every 3 years.	Get a Pap test at least every 3 years.	Ask your doctor or nurse if you need to get a Pap test.
Chlamydia test	Get tested for chlamydia yearly through age 24 if you are sexually active or pregnant. Age 25 and older, get tested for chlamydia if you are at increased risk, pregnant or not pregnant.	Get tested for chlamydia if you are sexually active and at increased risk, pregnant or not pregnant.	Get tested for chlamydia if you are sexually active and at increased risk.	Get tested for chlamydia if you are sexually active and at increased risk.
Cholesterol test	Starting at age 20, get a cholesterol test regularly if you are at increased risk for heart disease. Ask your doctor or nurse how often you need your cholesterol tested.	Get a cholesterol test regularly if you are at increased risk for heart disease. Ask your doctor or nurse how often you need your cholesterol tested.	Get a cholesterol test regularly if you are at increased risk for heart disease. Ask your doctor or nurse how often you need your cholesterol tested.	Get a cholesterol test regularly if you are at increased risk for heart disease. Ask your doctor or nurse how often you need your cholesterol tested.

TABLE 17-1 Screening Tests for Women—cont'd

Screening Tests	Ages 18-39	Ages 40-49	Ages 50-64	Ages 65 and Older
Colorectal cancer screening (using fecal occult blood testing, sigmoidoscopy, or colonoscopy)			Starting at age 50, get screened for colorectal cancer. Talk to your doctor or nurse about which screening test is best for you and how often you need it.	Get screened for colorectal cancer through age 75. Talk to your doctor or nurse about which screening test is best for you and how often you need it.
Diabetes screening	Get screened for diabetes if your blood pressure is higher than 135/80 or if you take medicine for high blood pressure.	Get screened for diabetes if your blood pressure is higher than 135/80 or if you take medicine for high blood pressure.	Get screened for diabetes if your blood pressure is higher than 135/80 or if you take medicine for high blood pressure.	Get screened for diabetes if your blood pressure is higher than 135/80 or if you take medicine for high blood pressure.
Gonorrhea test	Get tested for gonorrhea if you are sexually active and at increased risk, pregnant or not pregnant.	Get tested for gonorrhea if you are sexually active and at increased risk, pregnant or not pregnant.	Get tested for gonorrhea if you are sexually active and at increased risk.	Get tested for gonorrhea if you are sexually active and at increased risk.
Human immunodeficiency virus (HIV) test	Get tested if you are at increased risk for HIV. Discuss your risk with your doctor or nurse. All pregnant women need to be tested for HIV.	Get tested if you are at increased risk for HIV. Discuss your risk with your doctor or nurse. All pregnant women need to be tested for HIV.	Get tested if you are at increased risk for HIV. Discuss your risk with your doctor or nurse.	Get tested if you are at increased risk for HIV. Discuss your risk with your doctor or nurse.
Syphilis test	Get tested for syphilis if you are at increased risk or pregnant.	Get tested for syphilis if you are at increased risk or pregnant.	Get tested for syphilis if you are at increased risk.	Get tested for syphilis if you are at increased risk.

From U.S. Department of Health and Human Services (HHS), Office on Women's Health (OWH): *Screening tests for women,* June 25, 2013. Available at www.womenshealth.gov/publications/our-publications/screening-tests-for-women.pdf. Accessed May 30, 2015.

respectively. In the HHS full health evaluation guidelines, there is the recommendation that primary providers assess for obesity, tobacco use, alcohol use, drug use, and mental health issues, such as stress and depression. In addition, providers should screen for violence, including exposure to firearms; use of safety devices such as helmets and seat belts; relationship issues; potential work and recreational exposures to chemicals, noise, and equipment; and skin cancer prevention.

U.S. Preventive Services Task Force Recommendations. The U.S. Preventive Services Task Force (USPSTF) is a panel of nongovernment primary care providers and health behavior providers considered to be experts in health promotion and disease prevention and in the evaluation of evidence for health-related research. The USPSTF is supported by a U.S. government agency, the Agency for Healthcare Research and Quality (AHRQ). With the administrative and research support of the AHRQ, the USPSTF experts periodically review available scientific evidence and make screening, counseling, and prevention recommendations for primary care providers and health care systems.[1]

The USPSTF has made and maintained recommendations on dozens of clinical preventive services that are intended to prevent or reduce the risk for heart disease, cancer, infectious diseases, and other conditions and events that affect the health of children, adolescents, adults, and pregnant women.[2] USPSTF recommendations for care and screening of adults can be found online (www.uspreventiveservicestaskforce.org). USPSTF recommendations are graded from A (offer or provide this service) to I (read the clinical considerations section of the USPSTF Recommendation Statement). If the service is offered, patients should understand the uncertainty about the balance of benefits and harms. In preparation for health care reform efforts, the USPSTF panel has compiled a list of A (USPSTF recommends; high certainty that the net benefit is substantial—offer or provide) and B (USPSTF recommends; high certainty that net benefit is moderate to substantial) recommendations (Table 17-3).

Tools for Health Risk Assessment

There are multiple tools to assess an individual lifetime risk for certain diseases such as heart disease and breast cancer. These are used as an adjunct to making health screening decisions, indicating whether the patient is at high, medium, or low risk for the condition.

AHRQ's Electronic Preventive Services Selector (ePSS) is a quick, hands-on tool designed to help primary care clinicians and health care teams identify, prioritize, and offer the screening, counseling, and preventive medication services that are appropriate for their patients. The ePSS is based on the current, evidence-based recommendations of the USPSTF and can be searched by specific patient characteristics, such as age, sex, and selected behavioral risk factors. Available both as a Web-based selector and as a downloadable PDA application, the ePSS brings information on clinical preventive services that clinicians need—recommendations, clinical considerations, and selected practice tools—to the point of care (available at http://epss.ahrq.gov).[3]

TABLE 17-2 Screening Tests for Men

Screening Tests	Ages 18-39	Ages 40-49	Ages 50-64	Ages 65 and Older
Abdominal aortic aneurysm screening				Get this one-time screening if you are age 65 to 75 and have ever smoked.
Blood pressure test	Get tested at least every 2 years if you have normal blood pressure (lower than 120/80). Get tested once a year if you have blood pressure between 120/80 and 139/89. Discuss treatment with your doctor or nurse if you have blood pressure 140/90 or higher.	Get tested at least every 2 years if you have normal blood pressure (lower than 120/80). Get tested once a year if you have blood pressure between 120/80 and 139/89. Discuss treatment with your doctor or nurse if you have blood pressure 140/90 or higher.	Get tested at least every 2 years if you have normal blood pressure (lower than 120/80). Get tested once a year if you have blood pressure between 120/80 and 139/89. Discuss treatment with your doctor or nurse if you have blood pressure 140/90 or higher.	Get tested at least every 2 years if you have normal blood pressure (lower than 120/80). Get tested once a year if you have blood pressure between 120/80 and 139/89. Discuss treatment with your doctor or nurse if you have blood pressure 140/90 or higher.
Cholesterol test	Starting at age 20 until age 35, get a cholesterol test if you are at increased risk for heart disease. Starting at age 35 and older, get a cholesterol test regularly. Ask your doctor or nurse how often you need your cholesterol tested.	Get a cholesterol test regularly. Ask your doctor or nurse how often you need your cholesterol tested.	Get a cholesterol test regularly. Ask your doctor or nurse how often you need your cholesterol tested.	Get a cholesterol test regularly. Ask your doctor or nurse how often you need your cholesterol tested.
Colorectal cancer screening (using fecal occult blood testing, sigmoidoscopy, or colonoscopy)			Starting at age 50, get screened for colorectal cancer. Talk to your doctor or nurse about which screening test is best for you and how often you need it.	Get screened for colorectal cancer through age 75. Talk to your doctor or nurse about which screening test is best for you and how often you need it.
Diabetes screening	Get screened for diabetes if your blood pressure is higher than 135/80 or if you take medicine for high blood pressure.	Get screened for diabetes if your blood pressure is higher than 135/80 or if you take medicine for high blood pressure.	Get screened for diabetes if your blood pressure is higher than 135/80 or if you take medicine for high blood pressure.	Get screened for diabetes if your blood pressure is higher than 135/80 or if you take medicine for high blood pressure.
Human immunodeficiency virus (HIV) test	Get tested if you are at increased risk for HIV. Discuss your risk with your doctor or nurse.	Get tested if you are at increased risk for HIV. Discuss your risk with your doctor or nurse.	Get tested if you are at increased risk for HIV. Discuss your risk with your doctor or nurse.	Get tested if you are at increased risk for HIV. Discuss your risk with your doctor or nurse.
Syphilis screening	Get tested for syphilis if you are at increased risk.	Get tested for syphilis if you are at increased risk.	Get tested for syphilis if you are at increased risk.	Get tested for syphilis if you are at increased risk.

From U.S. Department of Health and Human Services (HHS), Office on Women's Health (OWH): *Screening tests for men*, July 8, 2011. Available at www.womenshealth.gov/publications/our-publications/screening-tests-for-men.pdf. Accessed May 30, 2015.

In the United States, for heart disease, clinicians use the Framingham risk score. Currently, the Framingham risk score uses age, gender, total and high-density lipoprotein (HDL) cholesterol, smoking history, systolic blood pressure, and use of medication for hypertension to calculate a 10-year risk for coronary artery disease (see http://cvdrisk.nhlbi.nih.gov/calculator.asp for an electronic tool to calculate 10-year risk for coronary artery disease). In 2013, the National Heart, Lung, and Blood Institute's expert panel published updated guidelines on cholesterol, hypertension, and obesity (see www.nhlbi.nih.gov/health-pro/guidelines for links to these guidelines). The recommendations in these guidelines were used to develop an integrated set of new cardiovascular risk reduction guidelines.[4]

The Breast Cancer Risk Assessment tool is based on the statistical Gail model and was developed for use by health professionals by experts at the U.S. National Cancer Institute (NCI)

TABLE 17-3 **USPSTF A and B Recommendations**

Topic	Description	Grade	Release Date of Current Recommendation
Abdominal aortic aneurysm screening: men	The USPSTF recommends one-time screening for abdominal aortic aneurysm by ultrasonography in men ages 65 to 75 years who have ever smoked.	B	June 2014*
Alcohol misuse: screening and counseling	The USPSTF recommends that clinicians screen adults age 18 years or older for alcohol misuse and provide persons engaged in risky or hazardous drinking with brief behavioral counseling interventions to reduce alcohol misuse.	B	May 2013*
Anemia screening: pregnant women	The USPSTF recommends routine screening for iron deficiency anemia in asymptomatic pregnant women.	B	May 2006
Aspirin to prevent cardiovascular disease: men	The USPSTF recommends the use of aspirin for men ages 45 to 79 years when the potential benefit from a reduction in risk of myocardial infarction outweighs the potential harm from an increase in risk of gastrointestinal hemorrhage.	A	March 2009
Aspirin to prevent cardiovascular disease: women	The USPSTF recommends the use of aspirin for women ages 55 to 79 years when the potential benefit of a reduction in risk of ischemic strokes outweighs the potential harm of an increase in risk of gastrointestinal hemorrhage.	A	March 2009
Bacteriuria screening: pregnant women	The USPSTF recommends screening for asymptomatic bacteriuria with urine culture in pregnant women at 12 to 16 weeks' gestation or at the first prenatal visit, if later.	A	July 2008
Blood pressure screening in adults	The USPSTF recommends screening for high blood pressure in adults age 18 years and older.	A	December 2007
BRCA risk assessment and genetic counseling and testing	The USPSTF recommends that primary care providers screen women who have family members with breast, ovarian, tubal, or peritoneal cancer with one of several screening tools designed to identify a family history that may be associated with an increased risk for potentially harmful mutations in breast cancer susceptibility genes (*BRCA1* or *BRCA2*). Women with positive screening results should receive genetic counseling and, if indicated after counseling, *BRCA* testing.	B	December 2013*
Breast cancer preventive medications	The USPSTF recommends that clinicians engage in shared, informed decision-making with women who are at increased risk for breast cancer about medications to reduce their risk. For women who are at increased risk for breast cancer and at low risk for adverse medication effects, clinicians should offer to prescribe risk-reducing medications, such as tamoxifen or raloxifene.	B	September 2013*
Breast cancer screening	The USPSTF recommends screening mammography for women, with or without clinical breast examination, every 1 to 2 years for women age 40 years and older.	B	September 2002†
Breastfeeding counseling	The USPSTF recommends interventions during pregnancy and after birth to promote and support breastfeeding.	B	October 2008
Cervical cancer screening	The USPSTF recommends screening for cervical cancer in women ages 21 to 65 years with cytology (Pap smear) every 3 years or, for women ages 30 to 65 years who want to lengthen the screening interval, screening with a combination of cytology and human papillomavirus (HPV) testing every 5 years.	A	March 2012*
Chlamydia screening: women	The USPSTF recommends screening for chlamydia in sexually active women age 24 years or younger and in older women who are at increased risk for infection.	B	September 2014*
Cholesterol abnormalities screening: men 35 and older	The USPSTF strongly recommends screening men age 35 years and older for lipid disorders.	A	June 2008

Continued

TABLE 17-3 USPSTF A and B Recommendations—cont'd

Topic	Description	Grade	Release Date of Current Recommendation
Cholesterol abnormalities screening: men younger than 35	The USPSTF recommends screening men ages 20 to 35 years for lipid disorders if they are at increased risk for coronary heart disease.	B	June 2008
Cholesterol abnormalities screening: women 45 and older	The USPSTF strongly recommends screening women age 45 years and older for lipid disorders if they are at increased risk for coronary heart disease.	A	June 2008
Cholesterol abnormalities screening: women younger than 45	The USPSTF recommends screening women ages 20 to 45 years for lipid disorders if they are at increased risk for coronary heart disease.	B	June 2008
Colorectal cancer screening	The USPSTF recommends screening for colorectal cancer using fecal occult blood testing, sigmoidoscopy, or colonoscopy in adults beginning at age 50 years and continuing until age 75 years. The risks and benefits of these screening methods vary.	A	October 2008
Dental caries prevention: infants and children up to age 5 years	The USPSTF recommends the application of fluoride varnish to the primary teeth of all infants and children starting at the age of primary tooth eruption in primary care practices. The USPSTF recommends primary care clinicians prescribe oral fluoride supplementation starting at age 6 months for children whose water supply is fluoride deficient.	B	May 2014*
Depression screening: adolescents	The USPSTF recommends screening adolescents (ages 12-18 years) for major depressive disorder when systems are in place to ensure accurate diagnosis, psychotherapy (cognitive behavioral; interpersonal), and follow-up.	B	March 2009
Depression screening: adults	The USPSTF recommends screening adults for depression when staff-assisted depression care supports are in place to ensure accurate diagnosis, effective treatment, and follow-up.	B	December 2009
Diabetes screening	The USPSTF recommends screening for type 2 diabetes in asymptomatic adults with sustained blood pressure (either treated or untreated) greater than 135/80 mm Hg.	B	June 2008
Fall prevention in older adults: exercise or physical therapy	The USPSTF recommends exercise or physical therapy to prevent falls in community-dwelling adults age 65 years and older who are at increased risk for falls.	B	May 2012
Fall prevention in older adults: vitamin D	The USPSTF recommends vitamin D supplementation to prevent falls in community-dwelling adults age 65 years and older who are at increased risk for falls.	B	May 2012
Folic acid supplementation	The USPSTF recommends that all women planning or capable of pregnancy take a daily supplement containing 0.4-0.8 mg (400-800 μg) of folic acid.	A	May 2009
Gestational diabetes mellitus screening	The USPSTF recommends screening for gestational diabetes mellitus in asymptomatic pregnant women after 24 weeks of gestation.	B	January 2014
Gonorrhea prophylactic medication: newborns	The USPSTF recommends prophylactic ocular topical medication for all newborns for the prevention of gonococcal ophthalmia neonatorum.	A	July 2011*
Gonorrhea screening: women	The USPSTF recommends screening for gonorrhea in sexually active women age 24 years or younger and in older women who are at increased risk for infection.	B	September 2014*
Healthy diet and physical activity counseling to prevent cardiovascular disease: adults with cardiovascular risk factors	The USPSTF recommends offering or referring adults who are overweight or obese and have additional cardiovascular disease (CVD) risk factors to intensive behavioral counseling interventions to promote a healthful diet and physical activity for CVD prevention.	B	August 2014*
Hearing loss screening: newborns	The USPSTF recommends screening for hearing loss in all newborn infants.	B	July 2008

TABLE 17-3 USPSTF A and B Recommendations—cont'd

Topic	Description	Grade	Release Date of Current Recommendation
Hemoglobinopathies screening: newborns	The USPSTF recommends screening for sickle cell disease in newborns.	A	September 2007
Hepatitis B screening: nonpregnant adolescents and adults	The USPSTF recommends screening for hepatitis B virus infection in persons at high risk for infection.	B	May 2014
Hepatitis B screening: pregnant women	The USPSTF strongly recommends screening for hepatitis B virus infection in pregnant women at their first prenatal visit.	A	June 2009
Hepatitis C virus (HCV) infection screening: adults	The USPSTF recommends screening for HCV infection in persons at high risk for infection. The USPSTF also recommends offering one-time screening for HCV infection to adults born between 1945 and 1965.	B	June 2013
Human immunodeficiency virus (HIV) screening: nonpregnant adolescents and adults	The USPSTF recommends that clinicians screen for HIV infection in adolescents and adults ages 15 to 65 years. Younger adolescents and older adults who are at increased risk should also be screened.	A	April 2013*
HIV screening: pregnant women	The USPSTF recommends that clinicians screen all pregnant women for HIV, including those in labor who are untested and whose HIV status is unknown.	A	April 2013*
Hypothyroidism screening: newborns	The USPSTF recommends screening for congenital hypothyroidism in newborns.	A	March 2008
Intimate partner violence screening: women of childbearing age	The USPSTF recommends that clinicians screen women of childbearing age for intimate partner violence, such as domestic violence, and provide or refer women who screen positive to intervention services. This recommendation applies to women who do not have signs or symptoms of abuse.	B	January 2013
Iron supplementation in children	The USPSTF recommends routine iron supplementation for asymptomatic children ages 6 to 12 months who are at increased risk for iron deficiency anemia.	B	May 2006
Lung cancer screening	The USPSTF recommends annual screening for lung cancer with low-dose computed tomography in adults ages 55 to 80 years who have a 30 pack-year smoking history and currently smoke or have quit within the past 15 years. Screening should be discontinued once a person has not smoked for 15 years or develops a health problem that substantially limits life expectancy or the ability or willingness to have curative lung surgery.	B	December 2013
Obesity screening and counseling: adults	The USPSTF recommends screening all adults for obesity. Clinicians should offer or refer patients with a body mass index of 30 kg/m^2 or higher to intensive, multicomponent behavioral interventions.	B	June 2012*
Obesity screening and counseling: children	The USPSTF recommends that clinicians screen children age 6 years and older for obesity and offer them or refer them to comprehensive, intensive behavioral interventions to promote improvement in weight status.	B	January 2010
Osteoporosis screening: women	The USPSTF recommends screening for osteoporosis in women age 65 years and older and in younger women whose fracture risk is equal to or greater than that of a 65-year-old white woman who has no additional risk factors.	B	January 2012*
Phenylketonuria screening: newborns	The USPSTF recommends screening for phenylketonuria in newborns.	B	March 2008
Preeclampsia prevention: aspirin	The USPSTF recommends the use of low-dose aspirin (81 mg/day) as preventive medication after 12 weeks of gestation in women who are at high risk for preeclampsia.	B	September 2014

Continued

TABLE 17-3 USPSTF A and B Recommendations—cont'd

Topic	Description	Grade	Release Date of Current Recommendation
Rh incompatibility screening: first pregnancy visit	The USPSTF strongly recommends Rh (D) blood typing and antibody testing for all pregnant women during their first visit for pregnancy-related care.	A	February 2004
Rh incompatibility screening: 24-28 weeks' gestation	The USPSTF recommends repeated Rh(D) antibody testing for all unsensitized Rh(D)-negative women at 24 to 28 weeks' gestation, unless the biologic father is known to be Rh(D)-negative.	B	February 2004
Sexually transmitted infection counseling	The USPSTF recommends intensive behavioral counseling for all sexually active adolescents and for adults who are at increased risk for sexually transmitted infections.	B	September 2014*
Skin cancer behavioral counseling	The USPSTF recommends counseling children, adolescents, and young adults ages 10 to 24 years who have fair skin about minimizing their exposure to ultraviolet radiation to reduce risk for skin cancer.	B	May 2012
Syphilis screening: nonpregnant persons	The USPSTF strongly recommends that clinicians screen persons at increased risk for syphilis infection.	A	July 2004
Syphilis screening: pregnant women	The USPSTF recommends that clinicians screen all pregnant women for syphilis infection.	A	May 2009
Tobacco use counseling and interventions: nonpregnant adults	The USPSTF recommends that clinicians ask all adults about tobacco use and provide tobacco cessation interventions for those who use tobacco products.	A	April 2009
Tobacco use counseling: pregnant women	The USPSTF recommends that clinicians ask all pregnant women about tobacco use and provide augmented, pregnancy-tailored counseling to those who smoke.	A	April 2009
Tobacco use interventions: children and adolescents	The USPSTF recommends that clinicians provide interventions, including education or brief counseling, to prevent initiation of tobacco use in school-aged children and adolescents.	B	August 2013
Visual acuity screening in children	The USPSTF recommends vision screening for all children at least once at ages 3 to 5 years to detect the presence of amblyopia or its risk factors.	B	January 2011*

*Previous recommendation was an "A" or "B."

†The Department of Health and Human Services (HHS), in implementing the Affordable Care Act under the standard it sets out in revised Section 2713(a)(5) of the Public Health Service Act, uses the 2002 recommendation on breast cancer screening of the USPSTF. To see the USPSTF 2009 recommendation on breast cancer screening, go to www.uspreventiveservicestaskforce.org/Page/Topic/recommendation-summary/breast-cancer-screening.

Data from U.S. Preventive Services Task Force (USPSTF): *USPSTF A and B recommendations*, October 2014. Available at www.uspreventiveservicestaskforce.org/Page/Name/uspstf-a-and-b-recommendations. Accessed October 31, 2015.

(see http://dceg.cancer.gov/tools/risk-assessment for links to this tool). The tool is designed to yield the estimate of the invasive breast cancer risk for a woman in the next 5-year period and estimates her lifetime risk (up to the age of 90 years) as well; for comparison, the tool generates the 5-year and lifetime risk for the same-age woman with average breast cancer risk.[5] This tool has the advantage of periodic updates based on evolving research and data.

In addition, there are many global assessments of health. Many of these global assessments are proprietary and are offered as a component of employee health services packages and can be found online from government sources or on health system websites.

Cancer Screening

Cancer is the second overall cause of death in the United States, accounting for one in every four deaths. Internal and external factors combine to make an individual susceptible to the uncontrolled proliferation and spread of dysplastic or abnormal cells. Some cancers can be prevented. Preventable cancers fall into two categories. One category is those associated with specific lifestyle factors, such as tobacco use, obesity, physical inactivity, poor nutrition, and excessive alcohol use; eliminating tobacco and excessive alcohol, engaging in regular exercise, and following healthy eating habits can reduce the occurrence of some cancers. Other cancers result or are associated with infectious agents such as hepatitis B virus (HBV), human papillomavirus (HPV), and *Helicobacter pylori;* vaccines and antibiotics can reduce or eliminate the occurrence of cancers associated with these agents. Regular screening can detect certain precancerous tissue changes and certain cancers at earlier stages, when treatment is more likely to be successful. Screening has been demonstrated to reduce mortality for cancers of the breast, cervix, colon, and rectum.[6] A comparison of American Cancer Society and USPSTF recommendations for cancer screening can be found in Table 17-4.

TABLE 17-4 Comparison of American Cancer Society and USPSTF Screening Guidelines for the Early Detection of Cancer in Asymptomatic Individuals

Site	American Cancer Society Screening Recommendations	USPSTF Screening Recommendations
Breast	*Women:* Yearly mammogram at age 40, then yearly as long as a woman is in good health; women who are at high risk for breast cancer based on certain factors should undergo magnetic resonance imaging (MRI) and get a mammogram every year.* Clinical breast examination (CBE) early starting at 40, at least every 3 years when women are in their 20s and 30s. Women should be encouraged to know how their breasts look and feel and report any changes to their provider. Breast self-examination (BSE) is an option starting at age 20. *Men:* Mammography along with careful breast examinations might be useful for screening men with a strong family history of breast cancer and/or with *BRCA* mutations found by genetic testing. Men with such a history should discuss this with their provider.	*Women:* Every-other-year mammogram ages 50 to 74. The decision to start regular, biennial screening mammography before the age of 50 years should be an individual one and take patient context into account, including the patient's values regarding specific benefits and harms. Insufficient evidence to: • Assess the additional benefits and harms of screening mammography in women 75 years or older • Assess the additional benefits and harms of CBE beyond screening mammography in women 40 years or older • Assess the additional benefits and harms of either digital mammography or MRI instead of film mammography as screening modalities for breast cancer Recommends against teaching BSE for all women.
Colon and rectum (men and women)	Beginning at age 50, follow one of these testing schedules: *Tests that find polyps and cancer:* • Flexible sigmoidoscopy every 5 years†, or • Colonoscopy every 10 years, or • Double-contrast barium enema every 5 years†, or • Computed tomography (CT) colonography (virtual colonoscopy) every 5 years† *Tests that primarily find cancer:* • Yearly fecal occult blood test (gFOBT),† or • Yearly fecal immunochemical test (FIT) every year‡, or • Stool DNA test (sDNA), interval uncertain† For positive family history, schedule is developed by provider.	Screening for colorectal cancer (CRC) using fecal occult blood testing, sigmoidoscopy, or colonoscopy, in adults, beginning at age 50 years and continuing until age 75 years. The risks and benefits of these screening methods vary. Evidence is insufficient to assess the benefits and harms of CT colonography and fecal DNA testing as screening modalities for colorectal cancer.
Cervical (women)	Cervical cancer testing should start at age 21. Women younger than 21 should not be tested. Women aged 21 to 29 should have a Pap test done every 3 years. Human papillomavirus (HPV) testing should not be used in this age group unless it is needed after an abnormal Pap test result. Women aged 30 to 65 should undergo a Pap test plus an HPV test (called "co-testing") every 5 years. This is the preferred approach, but it is acceptable to have a Pap test alone every 3 years. Women older than 65 who have had regular cervical cancer testing with normal results should not be tested for cervical cancer. Once testing is stopped, it should not be started again. Women with a history of a serious cervical precancer should continue to be tested for at least 20 years after that diagnosis, even if testing continues past age 65. A woman who has had her uterus removed (and also her cervix) for reasons not related to cervical cancer and who has no history of cervical cancer or serious precancer should not be tested. A woman who has been vaccinated against HPV should still follow the screening recommendations for her age group.	Evidence can be accessed at www.uspreventiveservicestaskforce.org/uspstf11/cervcancer/cervcanceres.pdf

Continued

TABLE 17-4 Comparison of American Cancer Society and USPSTF Screening Guidelines for the Early Detection of Cancer in Asymptomatic Individuals—cont'd

Site	American Cancer Society Screening Recommendations	USPSTF Screening Recommendations
Prostate (men)	Starting at age 50, discuss risks and benefits of screening. For African-American patients or those who have a father or brother who had prostate cancer before age 65, initiate screening discussion at age 45. Screening consists of a prostate-specific antigen (PSA) blood test with or without a rectal examination. Frequency of screening is determined by PSA level; see www.cancer.org/Cancer/ProstateCancer/MoreInformation/ProstateCancerEarlyDetection/prostate-cancer-early-detection-tests.	Recommends against PSA-based screening for prostate cancer. Contemporary recommendations for prostate cancer screening all incorporate the measurement of serum PSA levels; other methods of detection, such as digital rectal examination or ultrasonography, may be included. There is convincing evidence that PSA-based screening programs result in the detection of many cases of asymptomatic prostate cancer, and that a substantial percentage of men who have asymptomatic cancer detected by PSA screening have a tumor that either will not progress or will progress so slowly that it would have remained asymptomatic for the man's lifetime (i.e., PSA-based screening results in considerable overdiagnosis). Management strategies for localized prostate cancer include watchful waiting, active surveillance, surgery, and radiation therapy. There is no consensus regarding optimal treatment. The reduction in prostate cancer mortality 10 to 14 years after PSA-based screening is, at most, very small, even for men in the optimal age range of 55 to 69 years. The harms of screening include pain, fever, bleeding, infection, and transient urinary difficulties associated with prostate biopsy, psychological harm of false-positive test results, and overdiagnosis. Harms of treatment include erectile dysfunction, urinary incontinence, bowel dysfunction, and a small risk for premature death. Because of the current inability to reliably distinguish tumors that will remain indolent from those destined to be lethal, many men are being subjected to the harms of treatment for prostate cancer that will never become symptomatic. The benefits of PSA-based screening for prostate cancer do not outweigh the harms.
Endometrium (women)	At the time of menopause, all women should be informed about the risks and symptoms of endometrial cancer. Women should report any unexpected bleeding or spotting to their doctors. Based on history, some women should have a yearly endometrial biopsy.	
Cancer-related checkup (men and women)	Starting at age 20, in conjunction with periodic health examinations, a cancer-related checkup includes health counseling and, depending on a person's age and gender, examinations for cancers of the thyroid, oral cavity, skin, lymph nodes, testes, and ovaries as well as for some nonmalignant (noncancerous) diseases.	Additional recommendations can be found in the USPSTF topic index www.uspreventiveservicestaskforce.org/uspstopics.htm#AZ

*Women at high risk: those with known *BRCA1* or *BRCA2* gene mutation; with a first-degree relative (parent, brother, sister, or child) with a *BRCA1* or *BRCA2* gene mutation, and who have not had genetic testing themselves; with a lifetime risk of breast cancer of 20% to 25% or greater, according to risk assessment tools that are based mainly on family history; who had radiation therapy to the chest when they were aged 10 to 30 years; who have Li-Fraumeni syndrome, Cowden syndrome, or hereditary diffuse gastric cancer syndrome, or have first-degree relatives with one of these syndromes.

†If the test result is positive, a colonoscopy should be done.

‡The multiple stool take-home test should be used. One test done by the doctor in the office is not adequate for testing. A colonoscopy should be done if the test result is positive.

Data from American Cancer Society: *American Cancer Society guidelines for the early detection of cancer,* 2011, available at www.cancer.org/healthy/findcancerearly/cancerscreeningguidelines/american-cancer-society-guidelines-for-the-early-detection-of-cancer, accessed July 30, 2015 American Cancer Society: *Breast cancer: early detection,* 2011, available at www.cancer.org/Cancer/BreastCancer/MoreInformation/BreastCancerEarlyDetection/breast-cancer-early-detection-acs-recs, accessed July 30, 2015; U.S. Preventive Services Task Force (USPSTF): *Screening for breast cancer,* 2009, available at www.uspreventiveservicestaskforce.org/uspstf/uspsbrca.htm, accessed July 30, 2015; USPSTF: *Screening for colorectal cancer,* 2008, available at www.uspreventiveservicestaskforce.org/uspstf/uspscolo.htm, accessed July 30, 2015; USPSTF: *Screening for prostate cancer,* 2008, available at www.uspreventiveservicestaskforce.org/uspstf/uspsprca.htm, accessed July 30, 2015.

Genetic Testing. Genetic testing for cancer risk is recommended for patients with several first-degree relatives with the same type of cancer; family history of breast, ovarian, or pancreatic cancer linked to a single-gene mutation; multiple family members with cancers at a young age; relatives with cancers linked to hereditary cancer syndromes; known cancer-linked gene mutation in a family member; or personal physical finding, such as colon polyps, linked to hereditary cancers.[7] Consultation or referral to a genetics counselor is indicated when genetics testing is being considered to guide test selection and interpretation (see Chapter 7).

Screening for Coronary Artery Disease

The American College of Cardiology (ACC) guidelines have as a Class I recommendation (suggested) based on Class B evidence (limited populations studied) that health care providers ascertain risk for cardiovascular disease in asymptomatic individuals by use of a global assessment tool such as the Framingham score (see Chapter 116 for a discussion of cardiac testing).[8] The recent ACC guidelines use the level of risk determined by these scores to evaluate the evidence and to classify recommendations for the use of various testing modalities in the investigation and determination of subclinical cardiovascular disease. For example, the ACC guidelines suggest that C-reactive protein can be used in asymptomatic men older than 50 years and women older than 60 years with low-density lipoprotein (LDL) cholesterol below 160 mg/dL to determine if statin therapy is indicated and in asymptomatic intermediate-risk men older than 50 years and women older than 60 years to assess risk of cardiovascular disease.[8] Ankle-brachial index assessment is acceptable for intermediate-risk individuals to determine their risk for subclinical cardiovascular disease.[8] For European countries, the European Society of Cardiology members have developed a risk score system to estimate the risk of cardiovascular disease called HeartScore. The HeartScore risk charts can be found online at www.heartscore.org.

Screening for Tuberculosis

Screening for tuberculosis (TB) is recommended for asymptomatic individuals for whom new infection is suspected, individuals who are close contacts of patients with active TB, those who inject street drugs, patients who are from countries where TB is common (the countries of the former Soviet Republics, Latin America, the Caribbean, Africa, Asia, and Eastern Europe), and those who spend time in settings where active TB is common, such as nursing homes, migrant camps, or institutional settings.[9] There are two major tests for identification of latent TB infection: the tuberculin skin test (TST) and the interferon-γ release assay (IGRA)[10] (see Chapter 235).

IMMUNIZATIONS

At the beginning of the new millennium, the Centers for Disease Control and Prevention (CDC) listed immunization as one of the top 10 public health achievements of the 20th century.[11] Along with other public health measures, the control of infectious diseases, primarily by vaccines, doubled the life span during the 20th century.[12] Despite this great accomplishment, people in the United States continue to be susceptible to diseases that are vaccine preventable. Although childhood vaccination rates are relatively high, most adults are not vaccinated as recommended, leaving them needlessly vulnerable to illness, long-term suffering, and even death.[13] A major goal of *Healthy People 2020* is to reduce, to eliminate, or to maintain elimination of cases of vaccine-preventable disease (VPD).[14]

About 95% of the 50,000 Americans who die every year of VPD are adults.[15] Viral hepatitis, influenza, and TB remain among the leading causes of illness and death in the United States and account for substantial spending on the related consequences of infection.[14] According to the National Vaccine Advisory Committee, evidence to date indicates that adult immunization is highly cost-effective,[16] and it is a core component of any preventive services.

Standards for Adult Immunization Practice

The Standards for Adult Immunization Practice have been widely endorsed by major professional organizations and are recommended for use by all health care professionals and payers in the public and private sectors who provide immunizations for adults.[17] All individuals involved in adult immunization should strive to follow these standards. Since the Standards were first published in 1990, health care researchers and providers have learned important lessons on how better to achieve and to maintain high vaccination rates in adults.[17] The revised 15 Standards for Adult Immunization Practice provide a concise, convenient summary of the most desirable immunization practices.[17] These standards are grouped into general recommendations: make vaccines available, assess patients' vaccination status, communicate effectively with patients, administer and document vaccinations properly, implement strategies to improve vaccination rates, and partner with the community (Box 17-1).

Vaccine Acronyms

A table of standardized vaccine acronyms for immunization schedules for children, adolescents, and adults can be found at www.cdc.gov/vaccines/acip/committee/guidance/vac-abbrev.pdf.[18]

Vaccine Information Statements

Vaccine information statements (Vases) are information sheets produced by the CDC that explain to vaccine recipients, their parents, or their legal representatives both the benefits and risks of a vaccine. Federal law requires that VISs be handed out whenever (before each dose) certain vaccinations are given. VISs are available from the CDC at http://www.cdc.gov/vaccines/hcp/vis/index.html.

Issues with Vaccine Administration

Decision-Making. In the United States, the CDC makes recommendations about vaccination schedules based on age; these recommendations are updated annually and are available at www.cdc.gov/vaccines/schedules/index.html. Deciding which vaccine an individual requires should also include a HALO assessment:

- *H*ealth factors: presence of chronic disease, pregnancy, sexually transmitted disease history, or immunosuppression
- *A*ge factors: adolescents and young adults, age 50 years and older, age 65 years and older
- *L*ifestyle factors: born outside the United States, men having sex with men, more than one sex partner in 6 months, injection drug use, international travel
- *O*ccupational factors: college student, daycare worker, sanitation worker, prisoner, nursing home resident[19]

Safe Administration. Some vaccines are recommended to be administered intramuscularly. For the deltoid muscle to be

BOX 17-1

Standards for Adult Immunization Practices

MAKE VACCINATIONS AVAILABLE

Standard 1: Adult vaccination services are readily available (should be included as part of primary care; may refer to another provider for travel vaccines or meningococcal vaccine).

Standard 2: Barriers to receiving vaccines are identified and minimized.

Standard 3: Patient "out-of-pocket" vaccination costs are minimized (advocacy for vaccines to be included in health care benefits package; fees should be cost of vaccine and administration).

ASSESS PATIENTS' VACCINATION STATUS

Standard 4: Health care professionals routinely review the vaccination status of patients.

Standard 5: Health care professionals assess and differentiate between valid and invalid contraindications (consult current Advisory Committee on Immunization Practices [ACIP] recommendations found at http://cdc.gov/vaccines).

COMMUNICATE EFFECTIVELY WITH PATIENTS

Standard 6: Patients are educated about risks and benefits of vaccination in easy-to-understand language (consult Vaccine Information Statements found at http://cdc.gov/vaccines, or call the CDC information hotline at 1-800-232-4636).

ADMINISTER AND DOCUMENT VACCINATIONS PROPERLY

Standard 7: Written vaccination protocols are available at all locations where vaccines are administered (vaccination protocol should detail procedures for vaccine storage and handling, vaccine schedules, contraindications, administration techniques, management and reporting of adverse events, and record maintenance and accessibility).

Standard 8: People who administer vaccines are properly trained.

Standard 9: Health care professionals recommend simultaneous administration of all indicated vaccine doses.

Standard 10: Vaccination records for patients are accurate and easily accessible.

Standard 11: All personnel who have contact with patients are appropriately immunized.

IMPLEMENT STRATEGIES TO IMPROVE VACCINATION RATES

Standard 12: Systems are developed and used to remind patients and health care professionals when vaccinations are due and to recall patients who are overdue.

Standard 13: Standing orders for vaccinations are employed.

Standard 14: Regular assessments of vaccination coverage rates are conducted in a provider's practice.

PARTNER WITH THE COMMUNITY

Standard 15: Patient-oriented and community-based approaches are used to reach target populations.

From National Vaccine Advisory Committee: Recommendations from the National Vaccine Advisory Committee: Standards for Adult Immunization Practice. *Public Health Rep* 129(2):115-123, 2014.

TABLE 17-5 **Needle Length and Injection Site of Intramuscular Injections**

Sex and Weight	Needle Length	Injection Site
Male and female <60 kg (130 lb)	1 inch (25 mm)	Deltoid muscle of the arm
Female 60-90 kg (130-200 lb)	1 inch-1½ inches (25-38 mm)	
Male 60-118 kg (130-260 lb)	1 inch-1½ inches (25-38 mm)	
Female >90 kg (200 lb)	1½ inches (38 mm)	
Male >118 kg (260 lb)	1½ inches (38 mm)	

Modified from Kroger AT, Atkinson WL, Marcuse EK, et al: General recommendations on immunization: recommendations of the Advisory Committee on Immunization Practices (ACIP), *MMWR Recomm Rep* 55(RR-15):1-48, 2006.

reached, proper needle length is essential. Table 17-5 lists the recommended needle lengths for intramuscular injections, based on gender and weight.

Recognition and Management of Anaphylaxis to Vaccines. Anaphylaxis after immunization is very rare—about one case per 1.5 million doses of vaccine.[20] Vaccines are complex biologic preparations, and allergies may be caused by an ingredient in the vaccine rather than by the antigen itself.[20] Anaphylaxis is not always easy to recognize clinically because the patterns of target organ involvement are variable and may differ among individuals, as well as among episodes in the same individual.[21] Anaphylaxis typically occurs within minutes of exposure to the allergen. Signs and symptoms include flushing, facial edema, urticaria, itching, swelling of the mouth or throat, wheezing, difficulty breathing, and gastrointestinal symptoms.[20] Skin symptoms and signs (such as hives, itching, flushing, and angioedema), which are helpful in making the diagnosis, are absent or unrecognized in up to 20% of all episodes.[21] Health care providers should ensure appropriate screening for any history of vaccine allergy before administration. A VIS should be provided to and reviewed with each patient before vaccine administration. In the event of adverse events after vaccination, appropriate measures are to be taken (i.e., 0.2 to 0.5 mg intramuscularly in the lateral aspect of the thigh as the preferred site repeat every 5 minutes as needed to a maximum dose of 1 mg if indicated for adult patients, cardiopulmonary resuscitation, and transfer to the nearest emergency room) by the health care provider to guarantee the safety and care of the patient.

Vaccine Adverse Event Reporting System. Clinically significant adverse events that follow vaccination should be reported to the Vaccine Adverse Event Reporting System (VAERS) at http://vaers.hhs.gov/esub/index. Reports can be filed securely online, by mail, or by fax. A VAERS form can be downloaded from the VAERS website or requested by sending an e-mail message to info@vaers.org, by calling 1-800-822-7967, or by sending a faxed request to 1-877-721-0366. Additional information on VAERS or vaccine safety is available at http://vaers.hhs.gov/about/index or by calling 1-800-822-7967.

Vaccine-Specific Information

Hepatitis A Vaccine. Hepatitis A vaccination is recommended for all children at age 1 year, for persons who are at increased risk for infection, for persons who are at increased risk for complications from hepatitis A, and for any person wishing to obtain immunity. In the United States, two single-antigen inactivated hepatitis A vaccines are commercially available, Havrix and Vaqta. Both vaccines are licensed for persons 12 months of age and older. A combination inactivated vaccine, Twinrix, which contains both hepatitis A virus (HAV) and HBV antigens, is also available for use in persons aged 18 years and older.[22] Persons traveling to or working in countries that have high or intermediate endemicity of infection, men who have sex with men, users of injection and noninjection illegal drugs, persons working with nonhuman primates or with HAV in a research laboratory, persons with clotting factor disorders, and persons who have chronic liver disease should be vaccinated against hepatitis.[22] These vaccines should be administered by intramuscular injection in the deltoid muscle or lateral thigh, with a needle length appropriate for the person's age and size. Serologic testing after vaccination is not required, given the high rate of vaccine response among adults and children.[23] A recent review by an expert panel, which evaluated the projected duration of immunity from vaccination, concluded that protective levels of antibody to HAV could be present for at least 25 years in adults and at least 14 to 20 years in children.[22]

Hepatitis B Vaccine.[7] In 2013 an estimated 19,764 persons in the United States were newly infected with HBV; rates are highest among adults, particularly men aged 25 to 44 years. An estimated 700,000 to 1.4 million persons in the United States have chronic HBV infection.[24] In primary care settings, targeting vaccination to persons at risk is an efficient approach to prevention of HBV infection.[25] The rate of new HBV infections has declined by approximately 82% since 1991, when a national strategy to eliminate HBV infection was implemented in the United States; in 2013 the overall incidence of reported acute hepatitis B was 0.9 cases per 100,000 population.[24]

Populations that are at increased risk of becoming infecting with HBV include infants born to infected mothers, sex partners of infected persons, health care and public safety workers at risk for occupational exposure to blood or blood-contaminated body fluids, travelers to countries with intermediate or high prevalence of HBV infection, hemodialysis patients, and men who have sex with men.[24]

Two single-antigen vaccines and three combination vaccines are currently licensed in the United States.[24]

Of the three licensed combination vaccines, one (Twinrix) is used for vaccination of persons 18 years or older with risk factors for both hepatitis A and hepatitis B; it contains recombinant hepatitis B surface antigen (HBsAg) and inactivated HAV.[24] The dose of the hepatitis A component in the combined vaccine is lower than that in the single-antigen hepatitis A vaccine, allowing it to be administered in a three-dose schedule instead of the two-dose schedule used for the single-antigen vaccine. An immune response against hepatitis A and B was observed and maintained over the long term in a high percentage of vaccines.[26] The hepatitis B three-dose vaccine series administered intramuscularly at 0, 1, and 6 months produces a protective antibody response in approximately 30% to 55% of healthy adults 40 years of age and younger after the first dose, 75% after the second dose, and more than 90% after the third dose.[25] In addition to age, other host factors (e.g., smoking, obesity, genetic factors, and immune suppression) contribute to decreased vaccine response.[25]

It is well known that HBV vaccination provides effective defense against the disease. A positive immune response to the vaccine is defined as the development of hepatitis B surface antibody (anti-HBs) at a titer of greater than 10 mIU/mL. The overall seroconversion rate is about 95% in healthy adults. Although anti-HBs titers decrease with time, the duration of protection is long; protection has been estimated to persist for up to 22 years after the primary vaccination schedule. Most studies suggest that routine booster injections are not required (although there have been exceptions).[26]

The other combination vaccines currently licensed in the United States are Comvax—combined hepatitis B–*Haemophilus influenzae* type b (Hib) conjugate vaccine, which cannot be administered before age 6 weeks or after age 71 months—and Pediatix, combined hepatitis B, diphtheria, tetanus, acellular pertussis (DTaP), and inactivated poliovirus (IPV) vaccine, which cannot be administered before age 6 weeks or after age 7 years.

Herpes Zoster (Shingles) Vaccine. A vaccine to prevent herpes zoster and its associated complications, primarily postherpetic neuralgia, was licensed for use in the United States in May 2007.[27] Appropriate vaccination remains a serious concern in the United States. In 2013, only 24% of adults aged 60 years and older reported having received herpes zoster vaccination to prevent shingles.[28] This vaccine is a live attenuated virus vaccine indicated for prevention of herpes zoster.[29] A single dose of herpes zoster vaccine is recommended for individuals 50 years or older, including those who previously had herpes zoster.[30,31] Persons with chronic medical conditions may be vaccinated unless their condition constitutes a contraindication.[30] Compared with placebo, the vaccine reduced the incidence of herpes zoster by 51.3% and incidence of postherpetic neuralgia by 66.5%; when herpes zoster did develop, burden of illness was reduced by 61.1% with vaccination.[32] This vaccine is not indicated for the treatment of zoster and postherpetic neuralgia and is not indicated for prevention of primary varicella infection (chickenpox).

Herpes zoster vaccine should not be provided to individuals who have ever had a life-threatening allergic reaction to gelatin, the antibiotic neomycin, or any other component of shingles vaccine or to individuals who have a weakened immune system because of the following current conditions: AIDS or another disease that affects the immune system; treatment with drugs that affect the immune system, such as prolonged use of high-dose steroids; cancer treatment, such as radiation or chemotherapy; and cancer affecting the bone marrow or lymphatic system, such as leukemia or lymphoma.[29] This vaccine should not be provided to pregnant patients or patients who might be pregnant.[29] Women should not become pregnant until at least 4 weeks after receiving the shingles vaccine.[29] Adults with a minor acute illness, such as a cold, may be vaccinated; however, patients with a moderate or severe acute illness should usually wait until they recover before receiving the vaccine.[29]

Human Papillomavirus Vaccine. Three different vaccines, which vary in the number of HPV types they contain, are available in the United States:

- Gardasil, a quadrivalent HPV vaccine, targets HPV types 6, 11, 16, and 18
- Gardasil 9, a 9-valent vaccine, targets the same HPV types as the quadrivalent vaccine (6, 11, 16, and 18) as well as types 31, 33, 45, 52, and 58
- Cervarix, a bivalent vaccine, targets HPV types 16 and 18

Various guideline committees have made recommendations regarding the use of HPV vaccine, including the U.S. Advisory

Committee on Immunization Practices (ACIP), the American Academy of Pediatrics (AAP), and the American Cancer Society. The ACIP recommends the bivalent, quadrivalent, or 9-valent HPV vaccine for girls ages 11 or 12 for the prevention of cervical, vaginal, and vulvar cancer and the related precursor lesions caused by the HPV types targeted by these vaccine. The ACIP also recommends the quadrivalent or 9-valent HPV vaccine for the prevention of anal cancer and its precursor lesions, and genital warts in females.[32]

The ACIP recommends the routine use of quadrivalent or 9-valent HPV vaccine in boys aged 11 or 12 years. The vaccination series can be administered to individuals as young as 9 years. Vaccination is also recommended for males aged 13 to 21 years who have not been vaccinated previously or who have not completed the three-dose series. For males who have sex with males (MSM) and for males who are immunocompromised (including those with human immunodeficiency virus [HIV] infection), ACIP recommends vaccination through age 26 for those not previously vaccinated.[32] The CDC initially did not add this vaccine to the recommended immunization schedules for males in these age groups because early studies suggested that the best way to prevent the most disease from HPV was to vaccinate as many girls and women as possible; however, in 2011 the CDC recommended that young males also receive the vaccine.[33]

Clinical trial data of vaccine efficacy in males and females suggest that immunization with HPV vaccine is most effective among individuals who have not been infected with HPV (i.e., patients who are HPV naive). Thus, the optimal time for HPV immunization is before an individual's sexual debut. Neither vaccine treats nor accelerates the clearance of preexisting vaccine-type HPV infections or related disease. Males who are sexually active may still be vaccinated consistent with age-specific recommendations. A history of anal intraepithelial neoplasia, genital warts, or HPV infection is *not* a contraindication to HPV immunization. However, immunization is less beneficial for males who have already been infected with one or more of the HPV vaccine types.[32]

HPV vaccine can be administered at the same visit with other recommended vaccinations. Vaccination may be given even in patients with equivocal or abnormal Pap test result, positive HPV DNA test result (HC2 high risk), genital warts, and immunosuppression and patients who are breastfeeding.[33]

Syncope can occur after vaccination and has been observed among adolescents and young adults.[34] For avoidance of serious injury related to a syncopal episode, vaccine providers should consider observing patients for 15 minutes after they have been vaccinated.

Influenza Vaccine. The majority of deaths attributed to VPDs are associated with influenza. Ninety percent of influenza-related deaths are in persons older than 65 years.[35] Adults older than 75 years have significantly higher mortality rates from influenza than younger persons.[36]

Since 1945, influenza vaccines have been in use. Each year, the vaccines contain three virus strains that are expected to affect the United States in the upcoming winter. Influenza virus is remarkable for its high rate of mutation, compromising the ability of the immune system to protect against new variants; as a consequence, new vaccines are produced each year to match circulating viruses.[37] Health care providers are required to remind patients that timely, yearly influenza vaccination is essential.

In 2010, a new high-dose formulation of trivalent inactivated influenza vaccine was made available for use in people aged 65 years and older.[35] This Fluzone High-Dose vaccine contains four times the amount of influenza antigens than the other TIVs to induce a higher immune response in older people who are most susceptible to the complications of seasonal influenza but who respond less well to the vaccine.[35] It appears that this vaccine preparation provides greater protection for the elderly population but is also associated with a slightly higher rate of local reactions.

Since 2001, a live, attenuated, cold-adapted, temperature-sensitive, trivalent influenza virus vaccine (LAIV, FluMist) was licensed in the United States. The temperature-sensitive type A and B strains of influenza virus contained in LAIV replicate (multiply) in the nasal passages but not in the lower respiratory tract.[35] Healthy, nonpregnant adults younger than 50 years without high-risk medical conditions can receive FluMist intranasally.

Annual vaccination against influenza is recommended for all persons aged 6 months and older, including all adults.[38] Before 2010, the ACIP had recommended focused seasonal influenza vaccination for higher-risk persons, children 6 months to 18 years of age, and close contacts of higher-risk persons; these recommendations applied to about 85% of the U.S. population. The CDC recommends administration of seasonal influenza vaccine as soon as the vaccine becomes available in the community.[30] Vaccination before December is optimal because this timing ensures protective antibody levels before the onset of "flu" season, which peaks in late December through March.[30] The peak of influenza activity can occur as late as April or May.[38] Influenza vaccination should be encouraged throughout the flu season.[30]

Because of the changing nature of influenza and vaccinations, the HHS has a dedicated website at http://flu.gov. It is highly recommended that health care providers review the updated vaccination information annually in order to select the most appropriate type of immunization for each patient.

Measles, Mumps, Rubella Vaccine. Before the introduction of the measles vaccine in 1963, roughly a half-million cases were reported each year in the United States.[39] The measles, mumps, and rubella (MMR) II vaccine, which effectively protects against these diseases, is available as a combination of components.

There have been four outbreaks (three or more cases linked in time or place), and 804 of the 911 cases from 2001 to 2011 were associated with importation of measles. In 2015 a major outbreak in California resulted in 131 cases. As of August, 2015, there have been 183 cases in the United States, making 2015 the worst outbreak since measles was declared eradicated in the United States in 2000.[40] Health care providers should remain mindful that the overall number of cases of U.S. measles is low because of continuous vaccination of the population.

Mumps vaccine was licensed in the United States in 1967.[39] Live attenuated mumps virus vaccine is incorporated with combined MMR vaccine.[39] For prevention of mumps, two doses of MMR vaccine are recommended for adults at high risk, including international travelers, college students, and health care workers born during or after 1957; all other adults born during or after 1957 without other evidence of mumps immunity should be vaccinated with one dose of MMR vaccine.[39]

In 1969, live attenuated rubella vaccines were licensed in the United States.[39] After vaccine licensure, the number of reported cases of rubella in the United States has declined more than 99%, from 57,686 cases in 1969 to 10 cases or fewer annually since 2005.[39] Even though rubella has been considered to be eradicated in the United States since 2004, from 2005 to 2011 a total of 67 rubella cases were reported and 4 congenital rubella syndrome cases; close to half (42%) were imported.[39] Health care providers who treat women of childbearing age should routinely determine rubella immunity and vaccinate those who are susceptible and not pregnant. Women found to be susceptible during pregnancy should be vaccinated immediately postpartum. The ACIP recommends that pregnancy be avoided for 28 days after receipt of a rubella-containing vaccine instead of 3 months, as previously recommended.[39]

Meningococcal Vaccine. There are several different meningococcal vaccines available in the United States:

- A meningococcal polysaccharide vaccine (Menomune, MPSV4) has been available in the United States for several decades.
- A quadrivalent meningococcal polysaccharide vaccine conjugated to diphtheria toxoid (Menactra, MenACWY-D) became available in 2005.
- Another quadrivalent meningococcal polysaccharide vaccine conjugated to a mutant diphtheria toxin, CRM197 (Menveo, MenACWY-CRM), was approved in 2010.
- A combination conjugate vaccine against *Neisseria meningitidis* serogroups C and Y and *H. influenzae* type b (MenHibrix, Hib–MenCY) was approved in 2012 for infants and children aged 6 weeks to 18 months
- Two serogroup B meningococcal vaccines (Trumenba, MenB-FHbp; and Bexsero, MenB-4C) were approved in late 2014 and early 2015 for use in individuals 10 through 25 years of age.[41]

In the United States, either formulation of the quadrivalent meningococcal conjugate vaccine (Menactra or Menveo) is recommended for all individuals 11 to 18 years of age, and for individuals 2 to 10 years of age and 19 to 55 years of age who are at increased risk for invasive meningococcal disease.[41] For vaccine recommendations for individuals at increased risk for meningococcal disease who are younger than 2 years and older than 55 years, health care providers should review the recommendations of the AAP and ACIP.

Pertussis Vaccination. In the prevaccine era, pertussis was a common childhood disease and a major cause of child and infant mortality in the United States.[42] From 2001 through 2003, persons older than 10 years accounted for 56% of reported cases, more than double the 24% they accounted for from 1990 to 1993.[42]

An acellular vaccine to prevent pertussis in adults was licensed in 2006.[43] Currently, the pertussis vaccines available in the United States are found in combination with diphtheria and tetanus toxoids (DTaP, combination vaccines, Tdap).[43] A pertussis-only vaccine is not available in the United States.[43] Tdap is the pertussis-containing vaccine for adolescents and adults.[43]

Pneumococcal Vaccination. The *Healthy People 2020* national health target is to achieve at least 90% vaccination coverage among persons aged 65 years and older who receive a pneumonia vaccination.[14] In 2008, only 60% of persons aged 65 years and older reported ever having received a pneumococcal vaccination.[14]

The pneumococcal conjugate vaccine, PCV13 or Prevnar 13, is currently recommended for all children younger than 5 years, all adults 65 years or older, and people 6 through 64 years old with certain medical conditions.[44]

Pneumovax is a 23-valent pneumococcal polysaccharide vaccine (PPSV23) that is currently recommended for use in all adults 65 years or older and for people who are 2 years or older and at high risk for pneumococcal disease (e.g., those with sickle cell disease, HIV infection, or other immunocompromising conditions). PPSV23 is also recommended for use in adults 19 through 64 years old who smoke cigarettes or who have asthma.[44]

Tetanus, Diphtheria, and Acellular Pertussis (Td/Tdap) Vaccination. Currently, there is only one Tdap product (Adacel) licensed for use in adults.[27] Coverage with any tetanus vaccination among U.S. adults was similar in 2008 compared with 1999 (61.6% versus 60.4%); coverage with the newly licensed Tdap vaccine was suboptimal among adults aged 18 to 64 years (5.9%), including health care personnel (HCP) (15.9%) and persons with infant contact (5.0%), two populations at increased risk for transmission of pertussis to susceptible contacts.[43]

In October 2010, the ACIP issued a permissive recommendation for use of tetanus, diphtheria, and acellular pertussis (Tdap) vaccine in adults aged 65 years and older and approved the recommendation that Tdap vaccine be administered regardless of how much time has elapsed since the most recent tetanus and diphtheria toxoid (Td)–containing vaccine.

The experts at the CDC made the following recommendations for Td/Tdap vaccinations[45]:

- All age groups are currently recommended to receive one dose of Tdap (tetanus diphtheria toxoids combined with acellular pertussis vaccine). Tdap can be administered without regard for the time since the last vaccination with tetanus- or diphtheria-containing vaccine. Once an adult has received one dose of Tdap, immunization with tetanus diphtheria toxoid is recommended for all patients with tetanus-prone wounds (including all contaminated wounds) if the previous immunization was more than 5 years ago.
- Adults with an uncertain or incomplete history of completing a three-dose primary vaccination series with Td-containing vaccines should begin or complete a primary vaccination series. For unvaccinated adults, the first two doses are administered at least 4 weeks apart, and the third dose 6 to 12 months after the second. If the individual was incompletely vaccinated (i.e., fewer than three doses), the remaining doses are administered. A one-time dose of Tdap is substituted for one of the doses of Td, either in the primary series or for the routine booster, whichever comes first.[46]
- If a woman is pregnant and received the most recent Td vaccination 10 or more years previously, Td is administered during the second or third trimester. If the woman received the most recent Td vaccination less than 10 years previously, Tdap is administered during the immediate postpartum period. At the clinician's discretion, Td may be deferred during pregnancy and Tdap substituted in the immediate postpartum period, or Tdap may be administered instead of Td to a pregnant woman after an informed discussion with the woman.

The ACIP statement for recommendations for administering Td as prophylaxis in wound management is available at http://www.cdc.gov/vaccines/hcp/acip-recs/index.html.

Extensive information on adult immunization schedule is available at www.cdc.gov/vaccines/schedules/hcp/adult.html.

General Administration Considerations. All vaccines used for routine vaccination in the United States can be given simultaneously (i.e., at the same visit, not in the same syringe).[19] If two live vaccines are not given simultaneously, the provider must wait at least 4 weeks before administering the second live vaccine. Inactivated vaccines can be given at any time before or after one another and live vaccines.[19] A guide to the contraindications to and precautions for the commonly used vaccines can be found in Table 17-6.

Vaccine Recommendations for Health Care Personnel

General recommendations regarding immunization of immunocompetent health care providers have been published by the CDC, the Association for Professionals in Infection Control and Epidemiology, the APIC, the American College of Physicians (ACP), and infectious diseases experts. The general approach is as follows:

- All health care providers should be immune to measles, mumps, rubella, and varicella.
- All health care providers with potential exposure to blood or body fluids should be immune to hepatitis B.
- All health care providers should be offered annual immunization with influenza vaccine.
- All health care workers should receive a one-time dose of Tdap as soon as possible, unless they are certain that they have received Tdap.
- All health care providers should either be offered immunizations that are routinely recommended for adults, such as tetanus, diphtheria, and pneumococcal vaccine, or be referred to their primary care provider.
- At-risk health care providers and laboratory personnel should be offered the following vaccines: polio, meningococcal, bacillus Calmette-Guérin (BCG), rabies, plague, typhoid, and hepatitis A.[47]

Influenza. Influenza (the flu) can cause disease among health care personnel (HCP) and their patients. Significant changes have taken place in influenza vaccination of HCP. The responsibility for increasing the rates of HCP influenza vaccination is rapidly shifting from the employee to the employer.[34] Flu vaccination has been shown to reduce the risk of flu and absenteeism in vaccinated adults, and HCP vaccination in particular has been shown to reduce the risk of respiratory illness and deaths in nursing home residents.[49] Flu vaccination coverage among HCP has improved but remains below the national *Healthy People 2020* target for flu vaccination among HCP, which is 90%.[14] In the 2010-2011 period, HCP vaccination coverage was 56% to 64%, and in the 2011-2012 period, it was 62% to 67%.

Because influenza infection in staff and patients is common, ranging from 25% to 80%, the CDC has published extensive guidelines for the prevention and control of nosocomial influenza. The AAP, American College of Physicians, American Public Health Association, Infectious Diseases Society of America, and Society for Healthcare Epidemiology of America have all endorsed mandatory influenza vaccination for all health care workers. A central part of the prevention strategy is annual immunization (between mid-October and mid-November) of health care providers, particularly clinicians, nurses, employees of nursing homes or other long-term health facilities who have contact with patients or residents, and providers of home care to high-risk patients.[49]

Additional information about HCP vaccination recommendations is available at www.cdc.gov/flu/fluvaxview/hcp-ips-nov2012.htm#ref7.

Hepatitis B. HCP who perform tasks that may involve exposure to blood or body fluids should receive a three-dose series of hepatitis B vaccine at 0-, 1-, and 6-month intervals and should be tested for anti-HBs to document immunity 1 to 2 months after the third dose.[48] Further recommendations from the CDC are as follows[48]:

- If anti-HBs is at least 10 mIU/mL (positive), the patient is immune. No further serologic testing or vaccination is recommended.
- If anti-HBs is less than 10 mIU/mL (negative), the patient is unprotected from HBV infection; revaccinate with a three-dose series. Retest anti-HBs 1 to 2 months after third dose.
- If anti-HBs is positive, the patient is immune. No further testing or vaccination is recommended.
- If anti-HBs is negative after six doses of vaccine, the patient is a nonresponder and should be considered susceptible to HBV and should be counseled about precautions to prevent HBV infection and the need to obtain hepatitis B immune globulin (HBIG) prophylaxis for any known or probable parenteral exposure to HBsAg-positive blood. It is also possible that nonresponders are persons who are HBsAg positive. Testing should be considered. HCP found to be HBsAg positive should be counseled and medically evaluated.

"CDC Guidance for Evaluating Health-Care Personnel for Hepatitis B Virus Protection and for Administering Postexposure Management" (2013) can be accessed at www.cdc.gov/mmwr/preview/mmwrhtml/rr6210a1.htm.

Measles, Mumps, Rubella. HCP who work in medical facilities should be immune to measles, mumps, and rubella.[47] HCP born in 1957 or later can be considered immune to measles, mumps, or rubella only if they have documentation of (1) laboratory confirmation of disease or immunity (HCP who have an "indeterminate" or "equivocal" level of immunity on testing should be considered nonimmune) or (2) appropriate vaccination against measles, mumps, and rubella (i.e., two doses of live measles and mumps vaccines given on or after the first birthday, separated by 28 days or more, and at least one dose of live rubella vaccine).

Although birth before 1957 generally is considered acceptable evidence of measles, mumps, and rubella immunity, health care facilities should consider recommending two doses of MMR vaccine routinely to unvaccinated HCP born before 1957 who do not have laboratory evidence of disease or immunity to measles, mumps, and rubella. For these same HCP who do not have evidence of immunity, health care facilities should recommend two doses of MMR vaccine during an outbreak of measles or mumps and one dose during an outbreak of rubella.

Varicella. It is recommended that all HCP be immune to varicella. Evidence of immunity in HCP includes documentation of two doses of varicella vaccine given at least 28 days apart, history of varicella or herpes zoster based on physician diagnosis, laboratory evidence of immunity, or laboratory confirmation of disease.[47]

Tetanus, Diphtheria, Pertussis. All adults who have completed a primary series of a tetanus/diphtheria-containing product (DTP, DTaP, DT, Td) should receive Td boosters every 10 years. HCP of all ages with direct patient contact should be

TABLE 17-6 Guide to Contraindications to and Precautions for Commonly Used Vaccines in Adults

Vaccine	Contraindications	Precautions[a]
Hepatitis A (HepA) Havrix Vaqta Twinrix (A and B)	Severe allergic reaction (e.g., anaphylaxis) after a previous dose or to a vaccine component	Moderate or severe acute illness with or without fever Pregnancy
Hepatitis B (HepB) Recombivax HB Engerix-B Twinrix (A and B)	Severe allergic reaction (e.g., anaphylaxis) after a previous dose or to a vaccine component	Moderate or severe acute illness with or without fever
HPV Gardasil	Severe allergic reaction (e.g., anaphylaxis) after a previous dose or to a vaccine component	Moderate or severe acute illness with or without fever Pregnancy
Influenza, injectable trivalent (TIV) Afluria Fluvirin Fluarix FluLaval Fluzone	Severe allergic reaction (e.g., anaphylaxis) after a previous dose or to a vaccine component, including egg protein	Moderate or severe acute illness with or without fever History of Guillain-Barré syndrome (GBS) within 6 weeks of previous influenza vaccine
Diphtheria, tetanus, pertussis (DTaP) Tetanus, diphtheria, pertussis (Tdap) Adacel Boostrix	Severe allergic reaction (e.g., anaphylaxis) after a previous dose or to a vaccine component Encephalopathy (e.g., coma, decreased level of consciousness, prolonged seizures) not attributable to another identifiable cause within 7 days of administration of previous dose of DTP or DTaP (for DTaP) or of previous dose of DTP, DTaP, or Tdap (for Tdap)	Moderate or severe acute illness with or without fever GBS within 6 weeks after a previous dose of tetanus toxoid–containing vaccine History of Arthus-type hypersensitivity reactions after a previous dose of tetanus toxoid–containing vaccine; defer vaccination until at least 10 years have elapsed since the last tetanus toxoid–containing vaccine Progressive or unstable neurologic disorder (including infantile spasms for DTaP), uncontrolled seizures, or progressive encephalopathy: defer vaccination with DTaP or Tdap until a treatment regimen has been established and the condition has stabilized *For DTaP only:* Temperature of 105° F or higher (40.5° C or higher) within 48 hours after vaccination with a previous dose of DTP/DTaP Collapse or shocklike state (i.e., hypotonic hyporesponsive episode) within 48 hours after receipt of a previous dose of DTP/DTaP Seizure within 3 days after receipt of a previous dose of DTP/DTaP Persistent, inconsolable crying lasting 3 hours or more within 48 hours after receipt of a previous dose of DTP/DTaP
Tetanus, diphtheria (DT, Td)	Severe allergic reaction (e.g., anaphylaxis) after a previous dose or to a vaccine component	Moderate or severe acute illness with or without fever GBS within 6 weeks after a previous dose of tetanus toxoid–containing vaccine History of Arthus-type hypersensitivity reactions after a previous dose of tetanus toxoid–containing vaccine; defer vaccination until at least 10 years have elapsed since the last tetanus toxoid–containing vaccine
Pneumococcal (PCV or PPSV) Pneumovax 23	For PCV13, severe allergic reaction (e.g., anaphylaxis) after a previous dose (of PCV7, PCV13, or any diphtheria toxoid–containing vaccine) or to a vaccine component (of PCV7, PCV13, or any diphtheria toxoid–containing vaccine) For PPSV, severe allergic reaction (e.g., anaphylaxis) after a previous dose or to a vaccine component	Moderate or severe acute illness with or without fever

Continued

TABLE 17-6 Guide to Contraindications to and Precautions for Commonly Used Vaccines in Adults—cont'd

Vaccine	Contraindications	Precautions[a]
Measles, mumps, rubella (MMR)[b] MMR II	Severe allergic reaction (e.g., anaphylaxis) after a previous dose or to a vaccine component Pregnancy Known severe immunodeficiency (e.g., from hematologic and solid tumors; receiving chemotherapy; congenital immunodeficiency; or long-term immunosuppressive therapy[c]; or patients with HIV infection who are severely immunocompromised)	Moderate or severe acute illness with or without fever Recent (within 11 months) receipt of antibody-containing blood product (specific interval depends on product)[d] History of thrombocytopenia or thrombocytopenic purpura Need for tuberculin skin testing[e]
Varicella (Var)[b] Varivax	Severe allergic reaction (e.g., anaphylaxis) after a previous dose or to a vaccine component Known severe immunodeficiency (e.g., from hematologic and solid tumors, receiving chemotherapy, congenital immunodeficiency, or long-term immunosuppressive therapy[c] or patients with HIV infection who are severely immunocompromised) Pregnancy	Moderate or severe acute illness with or without fever Recent (within 11 months) receipt of antibody-containing blood product (specific interval depends on product)[d] Receipt of specific antivirals (i.e., acyclovir, famciclovir, or valacyclovir) 24 hours before vaccination; if possible, delay resumption of these antiviral drugs for 14 days after vaccination
Influenza, live attenuated (LAIV)[b] FluMist	Severe allergic reaction (e.g., anaphylaxis) after a previous dose or to a vaccine component, including egg protein Possible reactive airway disease in a child aged 2 through 4 years (e.g., history of recurrent wheezing or a recent wheezing episode) Pregnancy Immunosuppression Certain chronic medical conditions[f]	Moderate or severe acute illness with or without fever History of GBS within 6 weeks of previous influenza vaccine Receipt of specific antivirals (i.e., amantadine, rimantadine, zanamivir, or oseltamivir) 48 hours before vaccination. Avoid use of these antiviral drugs for 14 days after vaccination.
Meningococcal, conjugate (MCV4) Menactra Meningococcal, polysaccharide (MPSV4) Menomune	Severe allergic reaction (e.g., anaphylaxis) after a previous dose or to a vaccine component	Moderate or severe acute illness with or without fever
Zoster (Zos) Zostavax	Severe allergic reaction (e.g., anaphylaxis) after a previous dose or to a vaccine component Substantial suppression of cellular immunity Pregnancy	Moderate or severe acute illness with or without fever Receipt of specific antivirals (i.e., acyclovir, famciclovir, or valacyclovir) 24 hours before vaccination; if possible, delay resumption of these antiviral drugs for 14 days after vaccination

[a]Events or conditions listed as precautions should be reviewed carefully. Benefits of and risks for administering a specific vaccine to a person under these circumstances should be considered. If the risk from the vaccine is believed to outweigh the benefit, the vaccine should not be administered. If the benefit of vaccination is believed to outweigh the risk, the vaccine should be administered. Whether and when to administer DTaP to children with proven or suspected underlying neurologic disorders should be decided on a case-by-case basis.
[b]LAIV, MMR, and varicella vaccines can be administered on the same day. If not administered on the same day, these vaccines should be separated by at least 28 days.
[c]Substantially immunosuppressive steroid dose is considered to be 2 weeks or more of daily receipt of 20 mg (or 2 mg/kg body weight) of prednisone or equivalent.
[d]Vaccine should be deferred for the appropriate interval if replacement immune globulin products are being administered (see Table 5 in CDC "General Recommendations on Immunization: Recommendations of the Advisory Committee on Immunization Practices [ACIP]" at http://www.cdc.gov/vaccines/hcp/acip-recs/index.html).
[e]Measles vaccination might suppress tuberculin reactivity temporarily. Measles-containing vaccine can be administered on the same day as tuberculin skin testing. If testing cannot be performed until after the day of MMR vaccination, the test should be postponed for at least 4 weeks after the vaccination. If an urgent need exists to skin test, do so with the understanding that reactivity might be reduced by the vaccine.
[f]For details, see CDC "Prevention and Control of Influenza: Recommendations of the Advisory Committee on Immunization Practices [ACIP], 2010" at http://www.cdc.gov/vaccines/hcp/acip-recs/index.html.
Modified from National Center for Immunization and Respiratory Diseases: General recommendations on immunization: recommendations of the Advisory Committee on Immunization Practices (ACIP), *MMWR Recomm Rep* 60(RR-2):1-64, 2011.

given a one-time dose of Tdap, with priority given to those having contact with infants younger than 12 months.[47]

According to the Immunization Action Coalition (IAC) 2011 recommendations, Tdap may be used to protect against pertussis even when more than 10 years has passed since the most recent tetanus vaccination.

In 2011, revised language on the use of tetanus, diphtheria, and pertussis (Tdap) vaccination in HCP was approved by the ACIP.[50] The wording states that HCP, regardless of age, should receive a single dose of Tdap as soon as feasible if they have not previously received Tdap and regardless of time since their last dose of tetanus and diphtheria toxoid (Td) vaccine.[50]

Meningococcal. Vaccination is recommended for microbiologists who are routinely exposed to isolates of *N. meningitidis.*[47] Use of MCV4 is preferred for persons younger than 56 years; it should be given intramuscularly. MPSV4 is used only if there is a permanent contraindication or precaution to MCV4.[47] Use of MPSV4 (not MCV4) is recommended for HCP older than 55 years; it should be given subcutaneously.

ADDITIONAL RESOURCES

Information can be obtained by calling the CDC-INFO contact center at 800-232-4636 or 800-CDC-INFO or by sending e-mail to nipinfo@cdc.gov. Free mobile and desktop applications are available at www.immunizationed.org/Default.aspx.

CDC Vaccine Schedules App for Clinicians and Other Immunization Providers, 2015

This free tool provides the most current version of the following:

- Child and adolescent schedules with immunization recommendations from birth through age 18
- Catch-up schedule for children 4 months through 18 years
- Adult schedule, including recommended vaccines for adults by age group and by medical condition
- Contraindications and precautions table, with all footnotes that apply to schedules

Features of the app include the following:

- Color coding coordinates with printed schedules are included.
- Hyperlinked vaccine name opens as a pop-up with dose specifics.
- Catch-up schedule for children shows minimum dosage intervals.
- Related vaccine resources and websites are included.
- Any changes in the schedules will be released through app updates.

Popular Websites

Handouts for Patients and Staff

www.immunize.org/handouts

- Includes more than 250 information sheets for health care professionals and the public. All are free, ready to copy, and reviewed for technical accuracy by experts at the CDC. Many are available in translation.

Vaccine Information Statements

www.immunize.org/vis

- The VIS section includes all VISs published in the United States and offers VISs in more than 35 languages.

State Information

www.immunize.org/stateinfo

- Direct links to state immunization websites, tables and maps of state immunization mandates, and contact information for local, state, and territory immunization coordinators.

Ask the Experts

www.immunize.org/askexperts

- Experts from the CDC answer challenging and timely questions about vaccines and their administration.

Practical Resources for Vaccinating Health Care Personnel Against Influenza

Centers for Disease Control and Prevention

- Access CDC's influenza web page: www.cdc.gov/flu.

National Adult and Influenza Immunization Summit (NAIIS)

www.izsummitpartners.org

- The NAIIS is dedicated to addressing and resolving adult and influenza immunization issues. The NAIIS consists of over 700 partners, representing more than 130 public and private organizations.

Adult Vaccination Resources Library

www.immunize.org/adult-vaccination/resources.asp

- The Adult Vaccination Resources Library (AVRL) gathers adult immunization resources into one location, allowing health care providers and the general public to pinpoint adult immunization resources that can be used in a clinic setting or for individual education.

Immunization Action Coalition (IAC). The following IAC print materials are available online:

- Standing Orders for Administering Influenza Vaccine to Adults: www.immunize.org/catg.d/p3074.pdf
- Screening Checklist for Contraindications to Inactivated Injectable Influenza Vaccination: www.immunize.org/catg.d/p4066.pdf
- Screening Checklist for Contraindications to Live Attenuated Intranasal Influenza Vaccination: www.immunize.org/catg.d/p4067.pdf
- Declination of Influenza Vaccination form: www.immunize.org/catg.d/p4068.pdf

CHAPTER 18

PRINCIPLES OF OCCUPATIONAL AND ENVIRONMENTAL HEALTH IN PRIMARY CARE

Kathleen Golden McAndrew

Occupational and environmental medicine is a specialty focused on the overall health and wellness of workers in relation to the workplace, the home environment, and the community.[1,2] Occupational and environmental health services emphasize health promotion, wellness, and injury prevention strategies as a focus in maintaining the health and safety of workers. To provide occupational and environmental health services to their patients, providers must have current knowledge of state and federal regulations and laws. In addition, occupational and environmental health providers must meet the changing expectations of society, employers, and workers that affect workers' health, safety, and performance.[1]

Occupational and environmental medicine provides a variety of health care–related services, from on-site business and manufacturing facilities to independently owned occupational and environmental medicine clinics and wellness centers, to consulting services. The scope of services offered through occupational and environmental health programs and centers may vary according to the training, education, and experience of the provider delivering these services as well as the needs and desires of the client requesting these programs.[2]

PRIMARY CARE ROLE IN OCCUPATIONAL AND ENVIRONMENTAL HEALTH

Primary health care providers play an important role in off-site occupational and environmental health care through evaluation and treatment of workers' compensation injuries, identification of workplace hazards, provision of regulatory agency–required medical evaluations and health screenings, and treatment of employees' illnesses. They may assist occupational and environmental health professionals with evaluation of employees for fitness-for-duty or return-to-work issues. Primary care providers may also initially diagnose signs and symptoms of acute or chronic illness or reactions that could be caused or triggered by work-related exposures manifesting as respiratory irritation or illness, dermatitis, allergy, or chemical sensitivity.

Any complete health evaluation of a patient should include an occupational and environmental health history and assessment for risks associated with a patient's occupation. A thorough occupational and environmental health history should include at least the following[2,3]:

- Current and past positions held
- Previous employers; years employed; type of industry or employer; and products manufactured, developed, or used in production process
- A brief description of the position requirements
- Known health hazards in the workplace
- Any current or past exposure to chemicals or other hazardous substances, noise, radiation, heat, vibration, or repetitive motion
- Use of personal protective equipment
- Significant time off work for a health problem or injury
- Changed residence because of health problems
- Household member with dust or chemical contact at work
- Use of pesticides in gardens or around the home
- Recreational activities and exposure to noise, radiation, repetitive motion, heat, vibration, and chemicals in these activities

WORKPLACE HEALTH PROTECTION AND PROMOTION

Workplace health protection and promotion programs are developed and offered to "enhance the overall health and well-being of the workforce while decreasing the likelihood of workplace injuries and illness."[4,5] These programs, which are focused on integrating health promotion activities and safety and environmental health programs and interventions,[4] are important for the maintenance of a healthy, engaged, productive, creative workforce. A healthy workforce results in reduced risk of work-related injuries, less sick time usage, and improved employee morale.[4] To assist with improving the health and well-being of their employees, many companies offer health promotion programs and wellness initiatives at the worksite, which may include on-site fitness centers and organized exercise programs, health risk assessments for high-risk indicators, and health education programs that are aimed at improving health-related behaviors and that cover topics including smoking cessation, nutrition, exercise, stress reduction, and personal safety.[4,5] Medical clearance from the worker's personal health care provider is sometimes requested before the employee may participate in programs that involve strenuous physical activity.

Health risk assessments offered at the work site often include screening for chronic illnesses such as diabetes, hypertension, and obesity by measuring hemoglobin A_{1c} (HbA_{1c}), blood glucose concentration, cholesterol and triglyceride levels, blood pressure, weight, and body mass index. Health screenings are used as part of a health promotion effort that most often includes educational programs for employees on health risk reduction strategies through lifestyle changes, as well as offering onsite programs that target promotion of healthy living. Test results that require medical intervention or monitoring should be referred to the employee's health care provider for further evaluation and treatment. Work site health risk appraisals and other screening programs serve as an adjunct to primary care services, the role of which is to function as the central player in the employee's medical home model of health care delivery.[2]

PREPLACEMENT HEALTH EVALUATION

Some employers require some form of preplacement screening or a physical examination before an employee may begin work. Health care providers who offer preplacement evaluations as part of their practice must understand the purpose and focus of these examinations.

The provider's focus in a preplacement evaluation is to ensure that the employee is free from any medical condition that may preclude him or her from performing the duties required by the position, to determine if the condition could be aggravated during performance of job duties, and to determine if the individual has a condition that negatively affects the health or safety of others.[1,3] During the evaluation, the health care provider establishes a baseline health status for comparison when work-related injuries, illnesses, or exposures occur. In addition, the provider can include worker health protection promotion education and recommend updates on any outstanding health maintenance needs such as immunizations.[2]

Employees who are required to perform certain functions as part of their job duties, such as truck drivers or airline pilots, are required to have specific tests and rigid physical examinations per Department of Transportation (DOT) or other federal agency laws and regulations, as part of their pre-employment evaluations.[6] These examinations must be performed only by physicians and other health care providers who have achieved board certification and are listed on national registries. These tight restrictions are in place to ensure that the providers are familiar with the job duty requirements and the employee's work environment and to ensure public and worker safety when the worker is performing his or her job duties.

Components of a preplacement evaluation should include a position-specific physical examination with appropriate ancillary testing.[1,7] Position-specific ancillary testing can include spirometry, audiometry, vision screening, baseline chest radiography, various blood studies, and urinalysis, depending on job demands and potential exposure risk. Drug testing or other regulatory agency–required testing may be required for certain licenses or certificates, as well.[7,8]

After completion of the preplacement evaluation, any recommendations, restrictions, abnormal findings, identified special protective measures, or other issues should be discussed with the employee. Recommendations for periodic screening should also be brought to the employee's attention. In addition, the health care provider should emphasize the need to use appropriate protective equipment and review proper body mechanics as they relate to the employee's position requirements.

During the preplacement evaluation, health findings can be discovered that do not affect the ability of the individual to perform the position requirements. Although these findings need to be addressed and plans for follow-up discussed, the findings should not be included in the clearance or report to the employer. Only those findings that pertain to the employee's ability to perform his or her job should be included in the report to the employer. The report is a written evaluation for work fitness—whether the employee is cleared for full work duty and any work restrictions for the individual. Documentation of restrictions should be specific and described by function. In addition, restrictions are reported without including the underlying medical reason, because medical information should not be provided to the employer without the employee's written consent.

WORKPLACE SURVEILLANCE

Potential workplace hazards encountered by employees can be biologic, chemical, physical, or ergonomic.[3] The person responsible for Occupational Safety and Health Administration (OSHA) and other regulatory agency compliance at the work site performs a needs assessment to determine whether a surveillance program is necessary. Occupational and environmental health care providers are often requested to provide some of the components of workplace surveillance programs, such as medical examinations, biologic testing, or other health screenings.[3]

Both the nature and the frequency of workplace surveillance are determined by national or state OSHA requirements as well as by individual employers. The purpose of OSHA surveillance evaluations is to collect, to analyze, and to disseminate data on groups of workers and workplaces to prevent illness and injury.[9] Standards are available for each hazard (e.g., lead, asbestos, noise) to which workers are exposed.[10] These standards detail the specifics of both routine medical surveillance (e.g., for workers requiring respiratory protection) and surveillance after exposure (e.g., exposure to noise or blood-borne pathogens).[3,9,10] Specific requirements are listed in each code and should be referenced before evaluations are performed.

DRUG AND ALCOHOL TESTING

Drug and alcohol testing is required of employees who work for companies covered by agencies of the DOT and Federal Aviation Administration and employees in other positions identified as safety sensitive.[3,7,8] In addition, companies or contractors whose federal grants exceed $25,000 are required to establish a drug-free workplace policy that includes drug screening. Individual companies also may choose to implement their own drug-free workplace requirements.[8]

Drug and alcohol testing may be performed at the time of preplacement screening, at random intervals, after accidents, and when there is suspicion of impairment from substances (or "for cause").[7,8] The most common drugs tested for include the panel required by the DOT and other federal agencies. This panel includes marijuana (tetrahydrocannabinol [THC] metabolite), cocaine, amphetamines, opiates, and phencyclidine (PCP). Private companies may screen for other drugs, such as barbiturates, hallucinogens, inhalants, or designer drugs.[7,8] Special panels are sometimes used that include multiple drugs with potential for abuse among those with specific occupations.

Most drug testing programs adopt federal drug testing regulations, including levels for positive results and chain-of-custody procedures for specimen collection. Guidelines must be strictly followed with every specimen collection, and facilities must be set up to meet the specifications for collection (e.g., chain of custody during collection, dry bathrooms). Because of the strict guidelines by which specimens must be collected, tested, and interpreted, drug and alcohol testing should be performed by occupational medicine programs or private laboratories that offer drug collection as part of their services and are certified and expert in this area.

Specimens are analyzed by laboratories certified by the Substance Abuse and Mental Health Services Administration. Results of the substance testing are sent to a designated medical review officer, whose role is to interpret drug screen results and to determine whether there is a medical or other explanation for positive results before the employer is contacted.[7]

WORKERS' COMPENSATION TREATMENT AND CASE MANAGEMENT

The treatment, evaluation, and management of workers' compensation cases involve collaboration among multiple disciplines.[2,3] The number of professionals and their titles vary according to the nature and severity of the injury or exposure and with the employer's insurance. There are forms and reports of the injured employee's status that must be completed within defined time frames. With certain insurers, the health care provider needs preauthorization before referring the patient to specialty or adjunct treatment modalities or before ordering certain diagnostic tests.

Requirements governing workers' compensation certification vary by employer and state. Health care providers who are interested in providing workers' compensation as part of their practice should ensure that they and their support staff have a basic understanding of what is required with each patient interaction. They must review the pertinent state regulations and employer requirements for workers' compensation with each case. Conferences, webinars, or presentations pertaining to workers' compensation give primary care providers assistance with remaining current in this important area.

After each workers' compensation visit, the treating health care provider's office is required to provide work status and treatment plan updates to the case manager and/or the insurance plan representative concerning medical treatment and recommended work restrictions, if any.

With contact to the worker's manager or supervisor, it is vital to understand and adhere to patient confidentiality rules and regulations that safeguard information related to work-related injuries and illness.[1,3] These regulations limit the information employers receive about the exact nature of the occupational illness or injury, specifics of treatment, reasons for restrictions and limitations, and details of the plan for continual care.[1,3] Reports are limited to the diagnosis, approximate length of disability, and any recommendations for restrictions or limitations.

Many companies have developed modified-duty programs to address situations in which the injured employee may not be able to perform his or her complete duties but may be able to perform parts of the position or other tasks in an organization. In these cases, the health care provider works with the employer to identify what temporary accommodation of these employees can be provided through modified or light duty or temporary assignment to a different task. In these cases, employers must provide information concerning physical job demands. Once they understand the physical position requirements, providers describe limitations or restrictions by function and qualify and quantify restrictions in as much detail as possible to assist the employer in accommodating these restrictions.

TREATMENT OF WORK-RELATED INJURIES, ILLNESSES, AND EXPOSURES

Workers' compensation is a system that provides medical care, wage replacement, and rehabilitation for workers who incur injuries or illnesses as a result of workplace exposure or activity. Most programs are regulated by the individual states; there are some workers' compensation programs that are administered by the federal government.

Many potential hazards in the workplace can cause a work-related injury, illness, or exposure. Some of these injuries are similar to those already encountered within a primary care practice and are managed in the same manner as non–work-related injuries. For example, poor ergonomics is the cause of a large number of work-related injuries, including back injuries and injuries caused by repetitive motion or cumulative trauma. Individuals with musculoskeletal pain from repetitive trauma are managed with rest, anti-inflammatory medications, ice, or heat. The differences in managing work-related injuries are (1) injury documentation and reporting requirements; (2) more frequent status evaluations; (3) specific recommendations about returning to work, including what activities the individual may undertake at given intervals; and (4) recommendations for appropriate ergonomic devices.

Chemical exposures may occur when employees work around potentially toxic chemicals or biologic agents. Chemical-related injury, illness, or exposure may occur as a result of normal working conditions or through accidents. For chemical injuries and exposures, primary care providers consult Material Safety Data Sheets (MSDSs), databases, or poison control centers for guidance with specific treatments and for managing the exposure.

Workers such as health care facility employees, public health workers, emergency or first responders, university researchers and professors, and employees in laboratory and research facilities may encounter biologic hazards and exposures. For biologic exposures, primary care providers must know the epidemiology of the biologic agent, including mode of transmission, incubation, employee's immunity status, and appropriate or required follow-up testing.[3,11]

OCCUPATIONAL RESPIRATORY DISEASES

DEFINITION AND SCOPE OF THE PROBLEM

Occupational respiratory disease results from work-related exposure to inhaled dusts, powders, solvents, gases, or fumes that adversely affect the upper and lower respiratory tract. Because many exposures do not result in acute symptoms, workers may be unaware that they have been exposed to potentially hazardous materials. The challenge for health care providers, especially those unfamiliar with occupational medicine, is to maintain a high index of suspicion that a symptom or cluster of symptoms may have a connection with a patient's job or work history. Work-related exposures do occur in occupations other than the obvious.[12]

Although the true scope of occupational lung disease is difficult to quantify, it is recognized that a small percentage of chronic occupational respiratory diseases is correctly associated with work-related exposures. Asthma is the most common type of occupational pulmonary disease in the industrialized world; up to 15% of all asthma cases in adults are work related or are associated with an increase in asthma symptoms at work.[13] Occupational asthma may be related to specific antigens in the workplace (e.g., psyllium or latex) or to chemical irritants.[13] Interstitial pulmonary fibrosis, which results from workplace exposure to asbestos and silica, persists throughout the world despite knowledge of the potential hazards of these substances and effective means for prevention. The death rate for silicosis declined by approximately 70% from 1982 to 2000, but it has increased nearly 400% for asbestosis, which is the only major pneumoconiosis to demonstrate increased mortality.[14] Approximately 65,000 workers in the United States have asbestosis; it is estimated that occupational asbestos exposure will continue to rise 19,000 cases of mesothelioma and 55,000 cases of lung cancer by 2009. In the United States, 85,000 cotton mill workers are permanently or partially disabled as a result of exposure to cotton dust.[15] The prevalence of latex hypersensitivity, including latex-induced asthma, is as high as 14% among some groups of health care workers.[16]

Despite these significant statistics, the number of affected individuals captured in any occupational surveillance system remains a gross underestimate because the majority of cases are undiagnosed or are not attributed to workplace exposure.[14] Preventing the transmission of infectious diseases and mitigating the risk of other occupational illnesses pose a significant challenge. Incorporating the latest information of infection control and other work-related exposure and implementing the most effective and proven methods for prevention should be a high priority in all workplaces.

Military Personnel and Veterans: Overlooked Populations

The short- and long-term health effects of war-related exposures on military service personnel are a growing concern. Exposures to toxins during the past two decades have been different from those of previous wars. The Centers for Disease Control and Prevention and other organizations, such as the Agency for Toxic Substances and Disease Registry, have been studying the postservice morbidity and mortality of veterans who have served in the Vietnam, Gulf, and Iraq wars as well as in the conflict in Afghanistan. There is some evidence that Gulf War veterans with previous respiratory illnesses, such as asthma, experienced more respiratory symptoms than did veterans without a history of illness. However, this may not be unique to Gulf War veterans and may be similar to the experience of veterans of other wars, despite the exposure to spilled oil and smoke plumes unique to Gulf War veterans. At this point, it is unclear whether there is a connection between war-related exposures and specific health outcomes that remain long after the exposure.[16,17]

PATHOPHYSIOLOGY

Inhaled noxious substances affect the respiratory tract in several ways. Direct irritation results in increased mucus production, cough, and airway hyperreactivity that may cause bronchospasm, chest tightness or pain, dyspnea, pneumonitis, or pulmonary edema. The full effect of certain irritants may not be realized until 12 to 24 hours after the exposure. Small particles (≤5 mm) may remain in the lung to induce a fibrotic or granulomatous response. A latency period of 15 to 20 years between exposure and onset of clinical disease often obscures the causal relationship, which makes the diagnosis of occupational lung disease more difficult. Hypersensitivity and abnormal functioning of the immune system may contribute to the development of certain occupational respiratory diseases, including asthma, hypersensitivity pneumonitis, asbestosis, and chronic beryllium disease. The presence of certain host factors, such as cigarette smoking and exposure in the home environment (e.g., proximity to sources of pollutants), plays a role in the development of work-related lung disease. Data for 2004 to 2011 from the National Health Interview Survey suggested that workplace exposures may contribute to chronic obstructive pulmonary disease (COPD).[18]

Occupational respiratory diseases include obstructive airway diseases (asthma, byssinosis), interstitial lung disease (coal workers' pneumoconiosis, asbestosis, silicosis, acute and chronic beryllium disease, hypersensitivity pneumonitis), industrial bronchitis, cancer, and noncardiogenic pulmonary edema. Asthma, one of the most common types of occupational respiratory disease, has been associated with at least 250 specific workplace exposures. In comparison to many other occupational illnesses, asthma produces more persistent, even permanent, effects.[19] Byssinosis is another obstructive airway disease; it is associated with exposure to cotton, hemp, and flax processing and is characterized by shortness of breath and chest tightness. Prolonged exposure can cause irreversible byssinosis, which is associated with fixed airway obstruction. Cigarette smoking significantly increases the risk of irreversible byssinosis.[15]

Many occupational toxins, including coal dust, asbestos, silica, and beryllium, contribute to the development of interstitial lung disease. The occurrence and extent of disease often depend on the level and chronicity of the exposure. Depending on the specific disease, fibrosis of the lung parenchyma, pleural thickening, and formation of pleural plaques contribute to respiratory failure and increase the risk for the subsequent development of lung cancer and mesothelioma. Occupational exposures are associated with different types of pleuropulmonary malignant neoplasms, including laryngeal, bronchogenic, and oat cell carcinomas, as well as with mesothelioma, a tumor of the pleura and peritoneum.

Bronchitis is a common manifestation of airway irritation and inflammation that is associated with many occupational exposures, including irritant gases, welding fumes, and coal dust. Chronic bronchitis is defined as the presence of cough and sputum on most days for 3 months or longer per year and for 2 or more consecutive years.

Certain groups of health care professionals are at increased risk for occupational respiratory problems as a result of their exposure to specific pathogens and toxins. Occupational asthma (as well as latex-related dermatitis and life-threatening anaphylaxis) resulting from latex allergy is becoming an increasing problem among health care workers. Establishing a diagnosis of latex-related asthma is essential to avoid permanent respiratory compromise. With the resurgence of tuberculosis (TB) in this decade, increasing numbers of health care workers have become infected with TB. The risk for infection is compounded by the convergence of immunocompromised individuals in various settings staffed by health care workers, including long-term care facilities, hospitals, homeless shelters, correctional facilities, and drug treatment centers. Since 1990, a number of TB outbreaks have occurred in these settings, resulting in approximately 300 cases of TB. These outbreaks were characterized by transmission of both isoniazid-resistant TB and, in many cases, multidrug-resistant TB.[20]

HISTORY AND CLINICAL PRESENTATION

A thorough history should be obtained from patients; this includes environmental and occupational exposure, smoking habits, and careful review of respiratory symptoms. The review of symptoms should include questions about onset of symptoms (rhinitis, conjunctivitis, cough, sputum production, wheezing, dyspnea, chest tightness or pain) and a history of allergies, asthma, and respiratory infections. In addition, it is important to elicit the temporal relationship of symptoms to time spent at work. For example, an improvement of symptoms during periods away from work or intensification during periods at work might suggest an occupational exposure. An accurate diagnosis of occupational asthma is imperative. If this diagnosis is overlooked, continued exposure to precipitants at work can increase asthma symptoms and contribute to persistent asthma, even when exposure to precipitants has been eliminated.[13] Conversely, making the diagnosis of occupational disease in error has serious implications for workers; removal of the worker from the workplace has psychological and economic consequences.[13]

To accurately diagnose and manage occupational disease, health care providers must familiarize themselves with their patients' social and occupational environments. However, much more is involved than simply knowing an individual's work history. Detailed information about the jobs performed (including an outline of a typical workday), work habits, materials used (dyes, solvents, dusts, powders, acids, alkalis, gases, metals), and use of protective equipment must be elicited. All workers should be asked about any safety or health concerns they might have. For many providers, some investigation and research are necessary before an accurate assessment of exposures is possible.

Exposure to noxious substances can cause various types of reactions in both the upper and lower respiratory tract. Acute symptoms of upper respiratory tract irritation include nasal and paranasal sinus irritation, sinus congestion, frontal headaches, rhinorrhea, and occasionally epistaxis. A dry cough and hoarseness may indicate pharyngeal and laryngeal inflammation, respectively. Mid–respiratory tract irritation and inflammation often result in bronchospasm, of which asthma is an example. Acute irritation of the deep respiratory tract causes pulmonary edema and pneumonitis.

Chronic respiratory exposure can result in various permanent pulmonary reactions. Chronic bronchitis is one of the most common pulmonary responses to long-term occupational exposure and results from excessive mucus production in the bronchi. Toxic workplace substances that can cause chronic bronchitis include mineral dusts and fumes (e.g., from coal, fibrous glass, asbestos, metal, and oils), organic dusts (e.g., from cotton, grains, and wood), gases (e.g., ozone and nitrous oxide), plastic compounds (isocyanates), acids, and smoke. Fibrosis or pneumoconiosis (localized and nodular) is usually caused by small particles of inorganic dust and produces symptoms that initially include a nonproductive cough and shortness of breath; in the later stages, there is a productive cough, distant breath sounds, and right-sided heart failure. Pleural plaques and diffuse pleural thickening are manifestations of asbestos exposures. Emphysema-related changes, which include destruction of alveolar walls and air trapping, result from chronic exposure to coal dust or cadmium. The formation of pulmonary granulomas is a less common response to inhaled work-related exposures but can occur from chronic exposure to metal dust.[15] In addition, catastrophic exposures, such as occurred during the World Trade Center collapse, have been implicated in the development of granulomatous pulmonary disease.[20A]

PHYSICAL EXAMINATION

Many workplace exposures do not cause acute respiratory symptoms, and therefore the physical examination findings may be entirely normal. The physical examination is most helpful when the results are abnormal because normal physical examination findings do not negate the possibility of work-related respiratory disease. In fact, once an occupational exposure results in obvious acute symptoms, the disease may have already progressed to the point that symptomatic relief, rather than a cure, is all that is possible. However, it is important always to consider occupational asthma when an adult suddenly develops asthma.

A thorough physical examination with special attention to the respiratory system is necessary. Auscultation can provide helpful diagnostic clues. Fine basilar crackles and a pleural friction rub are more common in certain interstitial lung diseases such as asbestosis. Wheezes, especially in association with a temporal relationship to work exposures, may suggest asthma. Digital clubbing in a worker with a history of asbestos exposure might suggest asbestosis, especially if other manifestations of the disease have already become apparent.

A cardiac examination is important; ventricular failure may reflect underlying lung disease; left ventricular failure may manifest as dyspnea, and right ventricular failure may denote severe and advanced lung disease.[19] In addition to assessing the respiratory and cardiac systems, the health care provider must perform a complete physical examination to identify manifestations of chronic or acute occupational exposure and to provide clues to the cause of the specific respiratory syndrome being evaluated.

DIAGNOSTICS

Important diagnostic studies include chest radiography and pulmonary function tests (PFTs). A chest x-ray examination can help identify early evidence and progression of parenchymal and pleural disease, including opacities, calcifications, and pleural thickening. In addition to a standard reading, chest radiographs should be interpreted according to the International Labour Organization (ILO) nomenclature and classification system. The ILO system provides a standardized set of comparison radiographs that can be used to classify x-ray films at one point in time or to observe an individual or group for changes over time.[19] Although chest radiographs do reveal evidence of abnormalities, they do not provide information about the degree of disability or impairment, nor do they provide an accurate assessment of lung function.

PFTs are used to assess lung function. They are of value in determining the type and extent of lung disease, observing the progression of disease for changes in severity or response to therapy, and fulfilling legal and compensatory purposes. The basic tests of ventilatory function can be performed with a spirometer, which can provide an accurate assessment of the relationship between chronic respiratory symptoms and diminished ventilatory capacity.[21] Although spirometry provides many measures, the most useful for evaluation of work-related respiratory disease are forced vital capacity (FVC), forced expiratory volume in 1 second (FEV_1), and the ratio of these two measurements (FEV_1/FVC). FVC refers to the maximum volume of air that is exhaled after a maximum inspiration. FEV_1 is an estimate of the flow rate and is obtained by measuring the volume exhaled during the first second. Results are compared with expected values, which are derived from a healthy population of nonsmoking adults, and are expressed as a percentage of the expected value.[19]

Obstructive diseases such as asthma involve an obstruction in airflow without a reduction in lung volume. Therefore measurements of FVC remain within 80% to 120% of the population standard and are considered normal. However, measurements of both FEV_1 and FEV_1/FVC are decreased in asthma and other obstructive diseases. In contrast, restrictive disease, including silicosis, asbestosis, and coal workers' pneumoconiosis, is characterized by reductions in both FEV_1 and FVC, resulting in a normal or greater ratio of FEV_1/FVC. Mixed pulmonary conditions may also be present; this occurs when cigarette smoking or multiple environmental exposures coexist with a given occupational exposure and may confuse the results of the PFTs. Nonetheless, PFTs are a useful instrument for considering the general characteristics of work-related lung disease. The response to bronchodilator inhalation is another method for differentiating between obstructive and restrictive airway disease.[19]

DIAGNOSTICS

Occupational Respiratory Diseases

IMAGING

Chest x-ray studies
CT scan*

OTHER DIAGNOSTICS

PFTs
ABGs*
Skin testing*
Sputum cytology for eosinophils

*If indicated.
ABGs, arterial blood gases; CT, computed tomography.

Additional PFTs include the measurement of residual volume, pulmonary diffusion lung capacity, and arterial blood gases (PaO_2, PCO_2, and pH) and exercise testing. Pulmonary compliance measures the distensibility of the lungs, which is reduced when lungs stiffen.

Skin testing can be helpful in identifying specific antigens. A diagnosis of occupational asthma is a strong consideration if the result of skin testing is positive and the patient has been having bronchospasms. The addition of sputum cytology eosinophil counts to serial peak expiratory flow (PEF) measurement can enhance the diagnosis of occupational asthma.[13] In one study, sputum eosinophil counts were found to increase by 1 % to 2% when subjects with occupational asthma were at work.[22]

MANAGEMENT

The management of occupational respiratory diseases is a multifaceted process and should include general guidelines and specific instructions for modifying hazardous work conditions. Important steps include elimination of the exposure source, referral to a specialist, early diagnosis, effective treatment, and workers' compensation (if indicated).[21]

It is useful to distinguish among exposures that cause acute symptoms, those that may produce irreversible symptoms after prolonged exposure, and those that produce disease that manifests only after a long latency period. Workers whose exposure produces airway changes that are acute or reversible once the exposure has been removed benefit the most from environmental controls (e.g., an exhaust system), alteration of work practices (e.g., wetting asbestos before removing it), and substitution of a nonhazardous substance for a hazardous one. Other preventive measures that benefit workers to a lesser extent include education about specific work hazards, use of personal protective equipment, administrative measures (e.g., job rotation), and screening for early detection of disease.

The management of occupational respiratory disease depends on the specific respiratory illness treated. It is essential that the patient be removed from the exposure as promptly as possible after symptoms have developed. For many occupational respiratory diseases, the most important prognostic determinant is the length of exposure before diagnosis. The principles of managing occupational symptomatic asthma are the same as for nonoccupational asthma.[23] Treatment modalities specific to the disease and close monitoring of symptoms and lung function must be maintained for every individual with an occupational respiratory disease.

LIFE SPAN CONSIDERATIONS

Certain occupational respiratory toxins affect both the female and male reproductive processes, compromising the health of both the workers and their children. Information about pregnant women's work activities and those of their partner (including work done at home) and all related exposures should be obtained as part of the perinatal history. Although household work is performed by more women in American society than in any other, it is often forgotten as a source of potential respiratory toxins. Products used routinely in the home—including scouring powders, chlorine bleaches, furniture polish, drain cleaners, furniture or paint strippers containing organic solvents, glues, paints, epoxies, and pesticides—are all potential hazards, especially when they are used in a small or poorly ventilated area.[24]

Another important life span consideration related to occupational respiratory disease involves latency and older adults. Many occupational respiratory diseases are characterized by long asymptomatic periods from the time of exposure to clinical evidence of disease. The manifestation of certain cancers may not appear for 10 to 20 years or even longer after an occupational exposure. The screening of workers at risk for certain diseases such as cancer must take into consideration such latency issues. In addition, the differential diagnosis for a constellation of signs and symptoms must reflect occupational exposure that may have occurred many years before.

COMPLICATIONS

Complications of occupational respiratory disease depend on the specific disease process. TB or a fungal infection is a complication peculiar to silica pneumoconiosis. The increased risk of mortality associated with certain chronic respiratory exposures is now well recognized. For example, asbestos-related pleural thickening can cause respiratory failure. Multiple occupational exposures, including those to arsenic, chromium, vinyl chloride monomer, asbestos, and radiation, have been causally identified with respiratory tract cancers.

INDICATIONS FOR REFERRAL OR HOSPITALIZATION

Most health care providers are unfamiliar with occupational medicine. Patients should be referred to an occupational medicine specialist if a diagnosis is not clear or if symptoms are unresponsive to treatment. Chronic work-related respiratory tract illnesses are often best managed by an occupational medicine or pulmonary specialist. This includes the management of many respiratory diseases resulting from chronic exposures (e.g., asbestosis or byssinosis) and may also include the management of acute problems, such as silicosis-related TB.

PATIENT AND FAMILY EDUCATION

Education must include an explanation of diagnostic tests and the specific treatment modalities being considered and used. The specifics depend on the specific respiratory disease involved. Occupational medicine is at its best preventive health care. Patients need to be educated about the relationship of their symptoms to workplace exposure, the consequences of continued exposure, and their rights and responsibilities as employees. Employers are required by law to maintain MSDSs, which describe toxic substances, their proper handling, and the symptoms that may arise from contact with them. However, many workers are unaware of the existence of MSDSs and need to be encouraged to read those that are relevant to their jobs. Education needs to include information about the importance of personal protective equipment and workplace hygiene. A list of resources, such as those offered through OSHA and the National Institute for Occupational Safety and Health (NIOSH), should be made available to the patient.

REGULATORY AGENCY AND OTHER REQUIREMENTS IN OCCUPATIONAL AND ENVIRONMENTAL HEALTH

Primary health care providers who choose to provide evaluation for employment and other occupational health–related issues need to be familiar with other regulations and recommendations for screening and treatment. Copies of these regulations can be obtained through the respective agency responsible for the regulation, or they can be found on the Internet. There are several sources to consult when primary care providers include occupational or environmental health issues as part of their practice. The major agencies with regulations affecting workplace surveillance and workers' compensation are OSHA and NIOSH. In addition, the Americans with Disabilities Act has provisions that apply to workers disabled in the workplace. Finally, many professional organizations have specific recommendations for maintaining the health of their members in the workplace.

OCCUPATIONAL SAFETY AND HEALTH ADMINISTRATION

Created by Congress in 1970, OSHA requires each employer to provide "a place of employment, which is free from recognized hazards that are causing or are likely to cause death or serious physical harm to employees."[9] OSHA functions under the Department of Labor. It has the authority to fine or to imprison employers who are found to be in violation of its regulations. Although most of OSHA's regulations deal with safety-related concerns, this organization has also issued a number of standards that specify medical evaluations and the testing of employees who may be exposed to certain workplace hazards.[9] Testing is required when exposures meet or exceed a certain level. Other standards require that employees receive medical clearance before using required protective equipment. Providers granting medical clearance for the use of protective equipment must be familiar with these standards.

National Institute for Occupational Safety and Health

NIOSH was established under the Occupational Safety and Health Act of 1970 and is part of the U.S. Department of Health and Human Services. Its function is to conduct research and to advise OSHA on issues about hazards in the workplace. NIOSH provides educational information to health care providers, employers, and employees.

Americans with Disabilities Act

Congress enacted the Americans with Disabilities Act in 1990 to protect disabled workers from discrimination in the workplace. This act must be considered in offering many occupational health–related evaluations. The Act requires that an employer make reasonable accommodations so that the disabled employee is able to perform those job functions considered essential to the position.[25] In addition, it is necessary to determine whether disabled employees can perform the job without posing a "direct threat" to the health and safety of themselves or others.[25]

Professional Organizations

Professional organizations such as the American College of Occupational and Environmental Medicine,[3] the American Association of Occupational Health Nurses,[26] and the American Conference of Governmental Industrial Hygienists[27] offer texts, guidelines, and other information that can assist the health care provider with occupational health–related cases.

CHAPTER 19

COLLEGE HEALTH

Terri Schmitt

Over 20 million persons are enrolled in college in the United States.[1] Considering that half of all adults in the United States have one or more chronic conditions or disabilities,[2] the unique developmental challenges of adolescence, young adulthood, communal living, campus population issues and the importance of college health services are undeniable. College health services are essentially primary care for the young adult, within the framework of a culture of peer living and learning. Because of this contextual difference, care of the college student must be considered with variables not usually encountered in a public health setting.

College health services often reflect the campus culture and are varied in composition and services. A large university with a medical center can offer a wider variety of providers and specialists than can a small rural college health center. However, one nurse working collaboratively with a local physician at a small college may be acquainted with every student.

The mission of college health services is to provide primary care for the student, to promote the well-being of the institution's citizens through health education and illness prevention programs, and to contribute ultimately to the academic success of the college's students.[3] The student health service may also position itself as the student's "interim" health care provider, with the understanding that communication with the student's provider at home will be ongoing. College health services are important enough to warrant their own oversight body, the American College Health Association (ACHA), which offers a wide variety of information, recommendations, guidelines, and resources.

Student health services must also be in the position to advise or to create the institution's emergency preparedness plan or health policy, particularly concerning infectious disease issues such as pandemic flu or bioterrorism.

ROLES OF COLLEGE HEALTH CARE PROVIDERS

In college health services, the health care provider has an ideal opportunity to affect the young adult at a critical time of development. The college years are a transitional stage between the end of adolescence and the beginning of adulthood. A college health care provider can assist in that transition by explaining issues of confidentiality (often a new concept to the student), modeling the practice of partnership between provider and patient in treatment or care decisions, and instructing a student in the often confusing world of health insurance. In such encounters, a college health care provider can positively influence the student's developmental transition from dependent living at home to independent living and from pediatric to adult health care.

Health education plays a critical role in the services offered to students. Some institutions have separate wellness programs that may be housed in athletic facilities, student unions, or health or counseling services. Ideally, health education programs result from collaboration among the college health services, counseling services, athletics department, health educators, Alcohol and Other Drug (AOD) counselors, peer educators, and residential life staff. With these various talents and teaching skills, programs can target the current trends on campus, including popular health issues or risk-taking behaviors, and tailor programs to specific issues and audiences.[4]

TOPICS IN COLLEGE HEALTH

Confidentiality

For some students, the college setting marks the first time they receive health care without a parent present. If the student is older than 18 years, he or she is legally able to make a health care decision without parental involvement. Explaining the right to confidentiality to the student can foster more open communication with the provider. Obtaining a student's written permission to discuss a specific illness episode with a parent, professor, or administrator confirms the legal nature of the information in the student's medical chart. However, parents often need the reassurance that although their over-18-year-old child may desire privacy regarding visits to the college health center, serious or life-threatening illnesses can and will be made known to parents at the discretion of the professional staff.

Access to care is a national issue as well as a critical issue in college health. Each institution has its own method of financing student health (by per-capita fee or as a part of the general funds) with the ultimate goal of providing free access to preventive care and basic primary care services. Outreach to students regarding these services (and possible fees) should be a priority in the long list of outreach messages to students. Student health insurance is one way to provide for students who are not covered by their family's plan or who have inadequate coverage. The student health insurance should be affordable yet adequate for a student's needs.

If a student is covered by a parent's medical insurance plan, confidential information may be inadvertently revealed to the policyholder (parent) as a result of routine billing procedures and documents. When students have the privacy of their own policy, they may be less hesitant in seeking gynecologic care, contraception, or treatment for sexually transmitted diseases (STDs). Costs of these services should never be a barrier.

Health Care Issues: Female College Students

For some young women, being away from home provides an opportunity for more intimate sexual relationships and lack of daily parental oversight; these new experiences come with concomitant responsibilities. A first well-woman visit to the student health services should include a thorough lifestyle assessment and enough time for a first pelvic examination (if appropriate), a thorough sexual history, STD education, and contraceptive counseling. Some institutions schedule this as a two-part visit.

Reproductive, Substance, and Safety Issues. Appointments requested specifically for STD screening or emergency contraception create opportunities for the provider to explore the college woman's sense of control in a sexual situation, the impact of drug or alcohol use on her decisions, and any sense of guilt or regret connected to her sexual experience. Although sexual assault is covered elsewhere (see Chapter 35), it must be noted here that research suggests that college women are at greater risk for sexual assault than are women of a comparable age in the general population.[5] In a survey conducted by the ACHA, 5% of college women reported an attempted or completed rape in 2009.[6] Other studies put the annual (9-month) incidence at 3%.[5] Discrepancies in numbers may be based on underreporting resulting from certain barriers, such as fears about confidentiality; fear of sanction and guilt over alcohol use; cultural differences in definitions of dating violence, sexual assault, or rape; or institutional misunderstanding or ignorance about the guidelines for reporting the data. Several legislative acts (1990 to 1998), including the Clery Act, have mandated that colleges and universities make available statistics on campus crime, including sexual assault, and that schools have policies to address sexual assault.[7] The student health services are an active participant in reporting such crimes and in preventive programs related to sexual assault. As a supportive member of the community, student health services must have a thorough understanding of the institution's policies and procedures for reporting rape, sexual misconduct, and sexual harassment.

Understanding the student's level of risk-taking behavior enables the provider to guide the student in contraceptive care, to provide a referral to student counseling services or alcohol or drug programs, or to schedule a follow-up appointment at student health services to continue in the educational and supportive aspect of her care. Unplanned pregnancies can require the collaboration of student health services, student counseling services, and other appropriate community services.

Eating Disorders and Weight Management. All students, particularly women, who visit student health services should be observed for evidence of an eating disorder. Diagnosis and management of anorexia nervosa or bulimia are addressed elsewhere in this text; however, diagnosis and treatment in the college setting have some unique aspects. Female students are acutely aware of the myth of the "freshman 15," which purports that women will gain 15 pounds during their first year on campus.[8] Students with an eating disorder in remission who find college life stressful are prone to regression. Women pressured to compete socially or athletically may respond with disordered eating at college, which can progress to a full eating disorder.

Students living in dorms or sororities and students participating in activities such as athletic teams, dance, or theater groups may notice fellow students exhibiting behavior indicative of an eating disorder. These students as well as coaches, professors, or student leaders should be encouraged to approach student health services to seek advice concerning treatment for a friend or classmate. Whether working alone or in concert with student counseling services, the student health services staff must proceed carefully to protect the individual while also reassuring the group concerned about their friend or classmate. Depending on the clinical situation, remaining in treatment and meeting established goals to remain in college can serve as strong motivating factors for the student with an eating disorder. Unfortunately, health services personnel are powerless if the student never seeks treatment on her own. Mandated visits have limited value beyond possible diagnosis and can sabotage future treatment.

Health Care Issues: Male College Students

Males 16 to 20 years of age have far fewer health care visits than younger males (11 to 15 years old) or their female contemporaries.[9] Male college students visit the health center only episodically for sick visits or injuries. Therefore there are fewer opportunities for health education or risk-reduction counseling than for college-age women. Efforts to reach this population through outreach programs in dormitories, fraternities, or athletic teams can help bridge this gap.

Reproductive, Substance, and Safety Issues. Young men also come to the health center for STD screening. This occasion provides the opportunity to screen for high-risk behaviors, including drug and alcohol use, violence, nonrelational sexual activity, and condom use. The STD screening visit is an excellent opportunity for one-on-one teaching of college men. Because testicular cancer is more prevalent in this age group, education about testicular cancer and self-examination should be offered to the individual and promoted in wellness efforts. The proper use of condoms can also be taught at an STD screening visit.

Injuries related to violence as a result of male clubs, organizations, or initiation rites are a cause for concern and must be discussed with the student, particularly if coupled with substance use. However, the student may be conflicted about giving information, particularly if the student took an oath of confidentiality. Understanding the institution's policies about these activities will help guide the provider's response. All forms of campus violence or abuse—sexual, psychological, physical, or verbal—impede the educational mission of the college campus. Providers in college health have a critical role in prevention, reporting, and care for the victims of violence. Likewise, in recent years the risk of students to be the perpetrator of violence to others has become a national issue. Reporting these risks to the appropriate persons and organizations while keeping the health of the patient in mind is key. Campuses should have not only a plan for mass acts of violence, but clear policies and guidelines for handling situations of risk within the student population.

Lesbian, Gay, Bisexual, and Transgender Students

Lesbian, gay, bisexual, and transgender (LGBT) students face multiple challenges on college campuses. Student health services must initiate outreach to the LGBT student communities because these students may be hesitant to have contact with student health services. Student health services must be visible to these communities and understand their special needs by speaking with student LGBT organizations and requesting feedback on the health services and programs. Specific health concerns of LGBT students include but are not limited to human immunodeficiency virus, STD prevention, identifying and reducing suicide risk, help in "coming out," school antibullying policies, smoking prevention and cessation, and culturally competent care.[10]

Mental Health Issues

As a result of advancements in pharmacologic treatment, increasing numbers of college students have complex psychiatric diagnoses and need various types of on-campus support.[11] Student health services can be involved in medical maintenance, treatment, referral, or co-management of students with mental health needs. The relationship of student health services with student counseling services can range from a merged, fully integrated center to separate services with shared administration to completely independent services. Regardless of the structure, health services and counseling services must collaborate when necessary for optimum care for the student while maintaining confidentiality.

Transfer or coordination of mental health care from home to the college setting can cause concerns. As with any chronic illness, students may have established a therapeutic relationship with their mental health provider and may be reluctant to establish a new relationship with an unfamiliar therapist. Outreach to students who may benefit from on-site counseling services is crucial. Students with mental health needs may be identified through information on their health form, which should record chronic psychiatric medications. Health care providers in student health services should note medications and inquire as to on-site treatment. Student health services can serve as a conduit to campus counseling services when asked by the athletic or dance department to evaluate a student with a potential eating disorder, substance abuse disorder, or other mental health issue. The academic or student life department may also refer a student with a potential mood, thought, or adjustment disorder. Health care providers must be sensitive to the fact that the possible perception of a stigma in seeking mental health services can be a barrier to care for some, and access through a medical service for a mental health–related complaint can be more acceptable. Students should be encouraged to sign a release when the referral is made to allow a collaborative approach to treatment.

The college years are acutely stressful and accompanied by periods of hopelessness for some students. It is essential that college and university health providers and counselors maintain a high level of vigilance for suicide or depression risk in assessing all students.

Sleep

Whether a result of academic, social, athletic, or work schedules or for psychological or pharmacologic reasons, college students are notorious for not getting adequate sleep.[12] Sleeping problems can be a symptom of depression or a precipitant of depression. By resetting their biologic clocks, sleep-deprived students can develop concentration difficulties, impaired immune systems, anxiety, irritability, and possibly increased drug or alcohol abuse.[13] Consideration of sleep habits and sleep disorders must be included in a clinical visit for fatigue, illness, or depression.

Alcohol and Tobacco

Alcohol use in the college population continues to be a problem despite institutional efforts to curb it.[14] Secondary effects of binge drinking include academic failure, sexual assault, violence, property damage, motor vehicle accidents, and death. Among the strategies most often used to curb alcohol consumption are alternative late-night alcohol-free events, increased sanctions, student involvement in campus policies and adjudication, and peer education. Student health services treat both the acute and secondary effects of alcohol intoxication. This encounter affords the opportunity to educate the student on issues connected with alcohol use. In addition, referrals to counseling services, on-campus alcohol education programs, or community alcohol treatment programs may be appropriate.

Tobacco use on college campuses continues to be an issue. Almost 19% of college students smoke, with new opportunities arising in hooka and e-cigarette use and risks relating to parties, socializing, and weekend use.[15,16] College health care providers have a role both in advocating for policies that restrict smoking and in promoting smoking prevention and cessation. Tobacco use should be the "fifth vital sign" in student sick visit encounters to initiate the opportunity to discuss smoking cessation. Even when there is little student demand for formal cessation programs, these programs must remain part of the wellness armamentarium for the student health center.

Other Drugs of Abuse and Prescription Abuse

College health providers will encounter students who abuse prescription or illicit drugs. Educating the student on the health, mental health, and academic consequences of drug abuse may be beyond the scope of the provider and merit a referral to a specialist. Students who are prescribed neurostimulants must be advised of the consequences of giving or selling prescription medication to others (a felony) and, if these medications are prescribed by the college health center, must engage in some sort of written or verbal contract regarding their safekeeping. Legalization of substances, such as marijuana in some states, warrants knowledge of school polices and health concerns for use of those substances related to school performance and overall health risks.

SCREENINGS AND IMMUNIZATIONS

Evidence of immunity or current immunization to measles and rubella is usually required for college enrollment. Immunization or evidence of immunity to hepatitis B, chickenpox, meningococcal disease, and tetanus is recommended. Prematriculation immunizations are mandated by colleges and universities and by state law. Student health services are responsible for ensuring student compliance with these mandates, including documentation of students who are not immunized because of religious beliefs. The most recent recommendations by the Centers for Disease Control and Prevention Advisory Committee on Immunization Practices as well as by the ACHA advise students and parents to be educated about the risks of meningococcal disease in the college population and encourage vaccination.[17] Students arriving from tuberculosis-endemic countries within the past 5 years must typically receive tuberculin skin testing before enrollment.[18] Current meningococcal prevention mandates for colleges and universities state by state can be found at the Immunization Action Coalition website at www.immunize.org/laws/menin.asp.

Students studying abroad during college need advice on travel immunizations and information on infectious disease prevention. After returning from a tuberculosis-endemic country, students should be rescreened.

CULTURAL ISSUES

Cultural competency is crucial to the success of student health services in caring for a diverse student population. Cultural competency is more than cultural awareness (knowledge) and cultural sensitivity (knowledge plus some experience with the culture). Cultural competency encompasses the ability to think about power differentials in relationships and respond with varied skills to establish rapport with diverse individuals.[19] Student health care providers must be sensitive to voice, body language, and gestures as they communicate with patients. There may be culture-specific meanings in populations of patients for aspects of health care such as pain and reproductive issues. College health providers can expect to experience multiple cultures on their campus and must be leaders in modeling and fostering cultural competency.

RESOURCES

A student health advisory committee is a useful tool for student feedback on student perception of services, cultural competency, sponsored insurance plans, and other issues related to delivery of service. A reasonable representation should include athletes, LGBT students, underrepresented minority students, users of student health insurance, and student government members. Students not only can provide critical feedback on health services, but also can advocate to the administration for needed funding for improvements.

The ACHA, with membership representing more than 2500 health care providers and 920 institutions of higher education, provides useful standards and guidelines for college health programs and services. Its website can be accessed at www.acha.org.

CHAPTER 20

HEALTH CARE OF THE INTERNATIONAL TRAVELER

V. Ted Leon

According to the World Tourism Organization, the number of worldwide travelers who crossed an international border rose from 565 million persons in 1995 to 1.1 billion persons in 2014, and it is expected to rise further to 1.8 billion persons by the year 2030. This number does not include migrants, refugees, or persons traveling within their own country. Of the 1.1 billion international travelers in 2014, about 52% traveled for leisure, 27% were visiting friends and relatives, and 14% were traveling for business purposes.

The demand for travel medicine services in Western Europe and North America is expected to rise with increased globalization. The proportion of travelers to an "emerging region" outside of North America and Western Europe had increased from 31% in the 1990s to 47% in 2013 and is projected to rise to 57% of all international arrivals by 2030, with over 1 billion travelers to an emerging nation anticipated by the year 2030.[1]

A total of 62 million trips across an international border were taken by U.S. citizens in 2013, with 20 million trips to Mexico, 12 million to Canada, 11 million to Europe, 6.5 million to the Caribbean, 4.2 million to Central or South America, and 351,000 to Africa.[2] Some of these countries or regions are associated with higher risk for infectious diseases and environmentally acquired illnesses. Many of these destinations are also less capable of providing adequate hospital services for major injuries or illnesses when they do occur. Even where medical care is generally excellent, as in Japan, Canada, or Western Europe, the idea of hospitalization in a foreign country remains a discomforting thought for most Americans.

It has been estimated that approximately 1300 Americans die while traveling abroad each year. Some inexperienced travelers are surprised to learn that the leading causes of death for the international traveler are not rare and exotic infectious diseases, but rather accidents and underlying chronic diseases.[3,4] About 50% of deaths are the result of cardiovascular events, mostly in elderly travelers, who presumably might have had the same problems at home. Another 25% of the deaths are caused by motor vehicle accidents, and 15% by other accidents, including falls and drownings. The remaining 10% of deaths are from infectious causes, but even these are often caused by ordinary pathogens such as the influenza virus or the pneumococcus bacterium, which are prevalent throughout the world. It is thought that only 1% to 4% of all deaths that occur while traveling can be attributed to a uniquely tropical infectious disease.[5,6]

A great amount of media attention has been devoted to Ebola virus. As of January 2015, there had been a total of 21,206 cases and 8386 deaths, mostly in the three countries of Guinea, Sierra Leone, and Liberia. Another very important emerging infectious disease in the Western Hemisphere is chikungunya fever, a debilitating mosquito-borne illness with the same insect vector and a similar clinical presentation as dengue fever. In October 2013, there was an epidemic in the Caribbean with rapid spread to Central and South America. As of November 2014, there had been 875,000 suspected cases of chikungunya, and 153 confirmed deaths, in those regions. Moreover, 1616 cases had been imported to the United States, and in July 2014 transmission to a nontraveling resident in Florida was documented.[7]

Although new and emerging diseases are likely to be a topic of discussion at the initial travel medicine consultation, other tropical diseases are much more prevalent and of greater importance for the international traveler. The World Health Organization[7] has estimated that as of 2014 there were still 128 million new cases of malaria each year, 240 million individuals infected with schistosomiasis, 50 to 100 million new cases of dengue fever, and 200,000 new cases of yellow fever, to highlight just a few of the major tropical pathogens that cause enormous morbidity and mortality in the developing world. Travelers to regions where these and other diseases are endemic need to be aware of these diseases and take appropriate precautions and preventive measures.

Despite recent trends toward more international travel, more adventure travel, more travel to developing countries, and more travel by older adults with significant underlying chronic illness, studies have shown that many European and American travelers are not seeking pre-travel advice, nor are they carrying antimalarials or being vaccinated appropriately. A European study looked at 5465 travelers about to depart from nine major European airports to areas known to be high-risk locations for hepatitis A or malaria.[8] Only 52% had sought any pre-travel health advice, and just 42% had been vaccinated against hepatitis A and 31% against hepatitis B. Although 84% of travelers to high-risk malaria zones were carrying antimalarial medications, just 22% of travelers to areas with at least some malaria risk carried antimalarials. To further demonstrate the disconnect between perceived and actual risk, about 13% of the travelers to countries with no malaria risk were planning to take malaria prophylaxis.

A similar American study of 404 travelers from John F. Kennedy International Airport in New York to high-risk areas for hepatitis A and malaria found that only 36% had sought pre-travel health advice of any kind.[9] Only 14% had been vaccinated against hepatitis A, only 13% had been vaccinated against hepatitis B, and just 11% of adults had received a tetanus booster in the previous 10 years as routinely recommended. Moreover, only 46% of U.S. travelers to malarial regions were carrying antimalarial prophylaxis, and of the travelers to sub-Saharan Africa, where chloroquine is not recommended because of widespread drug resistance, 42% were carrying only chloroquine—the wrong medication. Because 57% of the Europeans and 60% of the Americans who sought pre-travel advice stated that they obtained their information from their primary care physician, it is evident that primary care providers have an important role in education and provision of services.

Travelers who need pretravel advice, vaccines, or medications have a wide choice of both location and providers. Many will visit their primary care provider, but others will go to their employee health or student health clinic, or to an urgent care clinic. Only a minority of travelers will seek care in a specialized travel medicine clinic. In a primary care office, it can be difficult to offer a full range of services because of the logistics of maintaining a complete stock of all the recommended travel vaccines. In addition, some health care providers understandably do not feel comfortable prescribing medications or giving advice for prevention of diseases that they have never had to treat. In an employee health, student health, or urgent care clinic, there is a greater economy of scale in terms of vaccine supply, and the provision of vaccines is often more efficient than in a private office, but the level of interest in and knowledge of travel medicine among the providers are variable. In a travel clinic, on the other hand, the vaccines are readily available, and the providers are more likely to be interested, knowledgeable, and experienced with some of the travel-related health problems and country-specific diseases that are likely to arise on an international trip (Box 20-1).

Unfortunately, the patient who comes for travel medicine services is not always well known to the provider. It is therefore very important to assess the patient's expectations and to discover whether he or she is coming just to get "pills and shots" or also for travel health education, advice, and consultation. An intake form (Fig. 20-1) can help clarify these expectations. Unless the patient is coming strictly for a particular vaccine that his or her primary care physician has recommended but was unable to provide, it is important to learn more about the traveler and the details of the planned trip. In addition to the usual questions about itinerary and duration of stay, it is important to know if the traveler is experienced and to ask if he or she has traveled with this particular itinerary before. Will the patient be traveling alone, with family and friends, or on an organized tour? Does he or she have any chronic medical conditions that could worsen on this trip? Does the traveler already have an established relationship with a primary care provider? What are the traveler's occupation and marital status? If the patient is traveling for work reasons, what are the job demands and

BOX 20-1

Providers of Travel Medicine Services

Travel medicine services are usually provided by nurse practitioners or by physicians trained in family medicine or internal medicine. Some physicians who practice travel medicine are also board certified in preventive medicine, occupational medicine, or infectious disease. Although there is no board certification in either travel medicine or tropical medicine, some providers receive a Certificate of Knowledge in Travel Health from the International Society of Travel Medicine (www.istm.org), and some physicians who have international experience take an 8- to 12-week course in tropical medicine, pass a written examination, and receive a Certificate of Knowledge in Clinical Tropical Medicine and Travelers' Health from the American Society of Tropical Medicine and Hygiene (www.astmh.org).

occupational exposures related to this trip? Although privacy may be a concern for some, most patients will welcome the provider's interest in these aspects of their life.

A detailed initial consultation before international travel is typically a very worthwhile experience for the traveler. The consultation is not usually covered by insurance, however, so some patients will request to just come in for certain vaccinations, without incurring the cost of an office visit. For a seasoned traveler with no medical problems going to a low-risk country, it is reasonable to administer an immunization without a formal travel medicine consultation. However, for any traveler who has questions and concerns or underlying health problems or has travel planned anywhere to the developing regions of Asia, Africa, or South America, a full pre-travel consultation is more appropriate.

As the purpose and details of the trip are described, it is the health care provider's duty to anticipate the various problems that are likely to arise. Discussion should include accident prevention; secondary prevention of any worsening of the underlying health problems; and reduction of physical hazards and chemical or infectious exposures through the judicious use of personal protective devices, behavior change, or medications and vaccines.

Most noxious chemicals and infectious agents enter the human body through the respiratory or gastrointestinal tract, or through the skin and mucous membranes. Many environmental and infectious illnesses can therefore be avoided with personal protective devices, such as gloves or masks. Gastrointestinal illnesses are more difficult to prevent entirely. (See the later section on food and water precautions.)

Initial Travel Medicine Consultation

Name: ____________________ Age: __________ Male/Female *(circle one)*

Height: __________ Weight: __________

Today's date: __________ Departure date: __________ Trip duration: __________

- Do you need pretravel vaccines? Yes No Not sure
- Do you need pretravel medications? Yes No Not sure
- Do you need any travel-related medical advice? Yes No Not sure
- Do you have any travel-related health questions? Yes No

Itinerary: City/province/country → Duration (days/weeks)

1. ____________________
2. ____________________
3. ____________________
4. ____________________

- Have you ever traveled to these countries on this itinerary before? Yes No

We are eager to help you have a safe trip and to avoid any health problems along the way. Please take a moment to answer the following questions regarding your upcoming trip and your general health history so that we may give you all the necessary vaccines, medications, and relevant health information. Please circle all that apply; you may leave a question blank if privacy is a concern.

Type of trip

1. Business
2. Visiting family/friends
3. Studying, teaching, or missions
4. Vacation, cruise, or relaxation
5. Adventure travel: trek, raft, or bike
6. Safari

How are you traveling?

1. Alone
2. With spouse or partner
3. With children
4. With friends
5. With work colleagues
6. With an organized group tour

Mode of transport

Airplane Ship or ferry Rail Bus Taxi Car Motorbike

Lodging

Tent Local hotel Western-style hotel Ship cabin Private home

Travel health risks: Will you be...

Climbing about 8000 feet/2500 meters?	Yes	No
Exposed to insects or other pests?	Yes	No
Swimming in freshwater lakes?	Yes	No
Eating at local restaurants and from street vendors?	Yes	No

FIGURE 20-1 Form for initial travel medicine consultation.

Continued

Your medical history

1. Who is your primary care physician? ____________________
2. Please list any medications you are taking (prescription, over the counter, herbal)
____
3. Please list medication allergies: ____________________
Are you allergic to eggs, neomycin/streptomycin/polymyxin B, or any foods? Yes No
Have you ever had measles? Yes No Chickenpox? Yes No
4. If you have had any of the following vaccines, please list the most recent dates:
Tetanus ______ Measles ______ Polio ______ Influenza ______ Pneumococcal pneumonia ______
Varicella ______ Hepatitis A ______ Hepatitis B ______ Typhoid ______ Rabies ______
Japanese encephalitis ______ Meningococcal pneumonia ______ Yellow fever ______
5. Have you ever been tested for HIV? Yes No If yes, date of last test: ______
6. Have you been tested for exposure to tuberculosis (PPD test)? Yes No If yes, date: ______
7. Could you be pregnant? Yes Maybe No, impossible
8. What form of contraception do you use? *(circle all that apply)* None Condom Pills Other: ______
9. Are you often troubled by motion sickness or jet lag? Yes No

Do you have a personal history of any of the following medical problems? *(circle all that apply)*

Heart disease	Diabetes	Digestive problems
Lung disease	High blood pressure	Joint problems
Liver disease	High cholesterol	Skin problems
Kidney disease	Seizures	Depression or anxiety
Obesity	Asthma	Cancer or decreased immunity
Sleep apnea	Ulcers	Other major medical problems

Work status *(circle one)*
Student Unemployed Self-employed Employed Homemaker Disabled Retired
Current/former occupation(s): ____________________

Marital status *(circle all that apply)*
Single Married Have partner Separated Divorced Widowed

Family history *(circle all that apply)*
Diabetes Heart disease or stroke Cancer Psychiatric problems

Habits

What is your tobacco history?	Never used	Quit	Current
How many days per week do you drink alcohol currently?	0 1 2 3 4 5 6 7		
How many days per week do you exercise currently?	0 1 2 3 4 5 6 7		
How many days per week will you exercise while on this trip?	0 1 2 3 4 5 6 7		

Thank you! We look forward to helping you with your travel health needs.

FIGURE **20-1,** cont'd

It is important to anticipate the special category of sexually transmitted infections and to be prepared to answer questions about transmission of disease. Most sexually transmitted infections can be prevented with a properly used condom or female condom.

Travelers to the tropics should have a solid understanding of the various diseases transmitted by insect vectors (e.g., malaria, dengue, yellow fever, chikungunya fever, Japanese encephalitis) and should be able to make informed choices about prevention and vaccination options. Travelers also need to be aware of the zoonotic diseases, such as rabies, avian influenza, and leptospirosis, which cause disease in humans because of proximity to diseased animals or their secretions.

Travelers should be given the relevant patient education brochures and be directed toward relevant resources in print or on the Internet (Box 20-2). Above all, they should be given ample time to have all their travel health questions answered.

PRE-TRAVEL PREPARATION AND PATIENT EDUCATION

Some health insurance plans do not provide coverage for health care services obtained outside of the United States. Medicare, for example, will not provide coverage for illness or accidents occurring outside the United States, including in Canada.[5] Thus all travelers should be encouraged to closely examine their health care policies and consider purchasing a short-term policy if necessary to cover any episodic medical needs that could occur while traveling. Any traveler to the developing world and all travelers with serious preexisting medical conditions who might require hospitalization should be encouraged to purchase air

BOX 20-2

Resources for Travel Health

INTERNET SITES

International Society of Travel Medicine (ISTM) (www.istm.org) lists courses, conferences, and travel medicine providers around the world. ISTM has an excellent link to news from the World Health Organization and Centers for Disease Control and Prevention, which is updated monthly, and publishes *Journal of Travel Medicine.*

American Society of Tropical Medicine and Hygiene (www.astmh.org) is similar to the ISTM. Its website includes several publications and a travel clinic directory focused on infectious and communicable diseases commonly seen in the tropics.

Centers for Disease Control and Prevention (CDC) (www.cdc.gov) has a wide range of information available by clicking on "Travelers' health."

World Health Organization (www.who.int) has an excellent online publication, *International Travel and Health,* which was updated in 2015. Click on "Health topics," then "Travel."

PRINT RESOURCES

The CDC's *Health Information for International Travel,* known as the Yellow Book, is a valuable resource that is updated biannually.

The Travel and Tropical Medicine Manual is a popular and concise textbook by Elaine Jong (Elsevier, 2008).

HOTLINES

CDC public inquiries: 404-639-3534 or 800-311-3435

The CDC Malaria Hotline: 855-856-4713 during business hours and 770-488-7100 after hours and weekends

TRAVEL EVACUATION INSURANCE

International SOS: www.internationalsos.com

Medex Assistance Corporation: www.medexassist.com

MedicAlert Foundation: www.medicalert.org

MedjetAssist: www.medjetassistance.com

Travelex: www.travelex.com

Travel Guard: www.travelguard.com

International Medical Group (IMG): *www.imglobal.com*

evacuation insurance, unless they are comfortable with the quality of hospital services in the countries they plan to visit.[10]

Travelers with chronic health conditions should carry a written summary of their health problems, a list of current medications and allergies, and a copy of a recent electrocardiogram if they have any cardiac history. A complete list of suggested travel documents is shown in Box 20-3. Travelers who use inhalers (which may arouse suspicion), require needles or syringes (e.g., for insulin administration), or use controlled substances may find it worthwhile to carry a letter from their physician certifying their diagnosis and need for treatment in case of customs or security questions.

At the pretravel visit, travelers should be reminded to bring an adequate supply of their routine medications and keep them in clearly labeled bottles. Some travelers may also want to wear an identification bracelet listing major allergies or important medical conditions. All travelers should carry a backup pair of eyeglasses.

BOX 20-3

Travel Documentation

- Passport and visa information
- International driver's permit and photo identification
- Emergency contact information for family, health care provider, and any other specialists you may need to contact from overseas
- List of physicians and hospitals in the host countries where you intend to travel
- Evidence of yellow fever vaccination, if traveling to countries where yellow fever is present or that require evidence of vaccination, recorded on the Traveler's International Certificate of Vaccination or Prophylaxis (yellow passport insert)
- Complete and up-to-date list of all routine and travel immunizations, including recent PPD (purified protein derivative [tuberculin]) results, recorded on the yellow passport insert
- Copy of recent human immunodeficiency virus (HIV) test results (may be needed for entry to some countries)
- Copy of current electrocardiogram if any relevant cardiac history
- Physician's letter listing traveler's specific health needs, including all prescription medications, syringes, and exemption from vaccines with reason for exemption

IMMUNIZATIONS

The pretravel visit is an ideal time to update all routine immunizations and to provide all the required and recommended immunizations (Table 20-1). The only vaccines that are currently "required" and would block the traveler's entry to certain countries if documentation were absent are yellow fever and meningococcal vaccines, but many more vaccines are frequently "recommended" to protect the traveler. These may include hepatitis A and B, typhoid fever, polio, Japanese encephalitis, and rabies. The traveler's decision to be vaccinated should be an informed choice based on the destination, length of stay, current disease outbreaks, and other factors. Immunization requirements should be reviewed at least 6 to 8 weeks before travel commences to ensure adequate time for antibody response as well as sufficient time to complete certain vaccines that need to be administered as a two- or three-dose series. Country-specific guidelines for recommended and required immunizations are found in the Centers for Disease Control and Prevention documents (see Box 20-2).

MEDICATIONS AND PRESCRIPTIONS

Malaria

Malaria is the most deadly parasitic disease in the world and the fifth leading infectious cause of death overall, trailing only lower respiratory tract infections, diarrheal diseases, human immunodeficiency virus (HIV) and acquired immunodeficiency syndrome (AIDS), and complications of tuberculosis (Table 20-2). The malaria parasite is considered one of the "big three" pathogens in terms of global importance, along with HIV and the tuberculosis bacillus.

Malaria is transmitted from human to human, primarily through the bite of an infected female *Anopheles* mosquito. Malaria is currently present in more than 100 countries, including almost all countries in the tropics. An estimated 128 million cases and 627,000 deaths occur annually because of the malaria parasite. Malaria vaccines are in development; however, these reduce rather than eliminate the risk of malaria. Unfortunately,

TABLE 20-1 Vaccine Information

Vaccine	Dosing
ROUTINE IMMUNIZATIONS	
Tetanus, diphtheria, and pertussis (Tdap) or tetanus and diphtheria (Td)	Booster every 10 yr
Measles, mumps, and rubella (MMR)	1 dose for adults born after 1957 if not immune
Chickenpox (varicella)	2 doses to all >13 yr old if there is no history of varicella or evidence of immunity
Flu shot (influenza)	Annually for all >50 yr old or earlier if there is a history of chronic disease
Pneumococcal	Once at age 65 yr or earlier if there is a history of chronic disease
Hepatitis B	0-, 1-, 6-mo series
TRAVEL VACCINES AND BOOSTERS	
Polio (inactivated polio vaccine)	One booster if primary series >10-15 yr ago
Hepatitis A	2 doses at 0, 6-12 mo
Hepatitis B	3 doses at 0, 1, 6 mo
Hepatitis A and B (Twinrix)	3 doses at 0, 1, 6-12 mo (booster after 10 yr?)
Typhoid Ty21a (oral live attenuated)	1 capsule on day 0, 2, 4, 6; booster every 5 yr
Typhoid Vi (capsular polysaccharide)	1 dose intramuscularly; booster every 2 yr
Rabies	3 doses at 0, 7, 21-28 days
Japanese encephalitis	Age 1-16 yr: use Je-Vax, 3 doses at 0, 7, 30 days Age >17 yr: use Ixiaro, 2 doses at 0 and 28 days
Meningococcal conjugate	1 dose intramuscularly
Yellow fever	1 dose subcutaneously; booster every 10 yr

Modified from Centers for Disease Control and Prevention: *Health information for international travel 2014,* Atlanta, 2014, U.S. Department of Health and Human Services, Public Health Service.

TABLE 20-2 Death from Infectious Diseases (Worldwide)

Cause of Death	Number of Deaths (Millions)
Lower respiratory tract infection	3.1
Diarrheal diseases	1.5
HIV/AIDS	1.5
Tuberculosis	0.9
Malaria	0.6
Measles	0.4

From World Health Organization: *The global burden of disease,* 2012 update, Geneva, 2012, World Health Organization.

malaria will remain a scourge, especially in Africa, for years to come.

For the traveler, most cases of malaria can be prevented by avoiding mosquito bites with protective clothing, mosquito netting, and diethyltoluamide (DEET)-containing insect repellants and by taking a prophylactic medication before, during, and after travel to the malaria-endemic region. Medication options include chloroquine, mefloquine, Malarone (atovaquone and proguanil), and doxycycline. Chloroquine is useful in only a few areas (e.g., Central America, Haiti, Dominican Republic, Iraq, Egypt, Turkey, northern Argentina, and Paraguay). For most malarial regions, travelers are advised to take one of the other three medications as prophylaxis. Mefloquine has the advantage of weekly administration, but its use has been limited by severe neuropsychiatric side effects in some patients. Malarone, a combination of atovaquone and proguanil, has fewer side effects, but it is expensive and must be taken daily. Doxycycline is inexpensive and effective and is the first-line drug in the Thai-Cambodia border areas where mefloquine resistance has emerged. Doxycycline cannot be taken by pregnant women or preteen children, however. It can also cause some photosensitivity and gastrointestinal upset. Regardless of which antimalarial is used, the traveler needs to be educated about fever and other symptoms of malaria and encouraged to seek medical treatment promptly should such symptoms occur.

Any fever in a returned traveler from a malaria-endemic region must be considered suggestive of malaria until proven otherwise. Thin and thick blood smears should be taken to look for evidence of the parasite. In a European study of 147 consecutive febrile hospitalized patients who had a history of travel to the tropics in the previous 6 months, malaria was the most common diagnosis.[11] In that study, 70 of the 147 admissions (47.6%) were attributed to malaria. The other common causes of fever in that study included 13 admissions for viral hepatitis (8.8%), 7 cases of gastroenteritis (4.8%), 7 cases of schistosomiasis (4.8%), 6 cases of typhoid fever (4.1%), and 5 cases of dengue fever (3.4%). The majority of these illnesses and hospital admissions would be preventable with a judicious combination of vaccination, malaria prophylaxis, and food and water precautions.

Food and Water Precautions and Traveler's Diarrhea

Diarrhea is the most common health problem among travelers to underdeveloped and tropical countries. Although it is rarely life-threatening if it is properly treated, traveler's diarrhea is notorious for causing many lost work days and lost vacation days.

Diarrhea is spread through contaminated food and water that carry pathogenic bacteria, parasites, and viruses. The most common cause of traveler's diarrhea is the bacterium *Escherichia coli.* Other common bacterial causes include *Salmonella, Shigella,* and *Campylobacter* organisms.

It is important for the traveler to note if the diarrhea is watery, contains any blood or pus, or is associated with fever or abdominal pain. Watery diarrhea is often caused by intestinal viruses such as the rotavirus or Norwalk virus and responds primarily to oral rehydration solution or intravenous fluids. Bloody diarrhea, on the other hand, is more commonly caused by bacteria or parasites. Simple dysentery without fever is often caused by the parasite *Entamoeba histolytica* (amebiasis), which is treatable with metronidazole (Flagyl). Dysentery can also be caused by other parasites, including *Cryptosporidium, Schistosoma,* and *Cyclospora* organisms. Bloody diarrhea with fever or abdominal pain is typically bacterial. However, it may also be seen in viral hemorrhagic fevers such as dengue or Ebola. Either way, bloody diarrhea with fever requires immediate medical attention.

A small number of travelers develop chronic diarrhea during or after travel, often caused by the *Giardia lamblia* parasite. In its classic presentation, the *Giardia* parasite causes bloating and belching or flatulence with a characteristic "rotten egg" or sulfur smell. It is usually treated with metronidazole. Among expatriates and long-term travelers, chronic diarrhea can also be caused by a condition called *tropical sprue.*

Because most cases of traveler's diarrhea are caused by bacteria, antibiotics are often indicated. For a mild case of traveler's diarrhea caused by *E. coli,* one or two doses of a quinolone such as ciprofloxacin or levofloxacin is sufficient. For the sicker traveler with *Salmonella* or *Shigella* infection, a 5-day course of ciprofloxacin, 500 mg twice a day, may be necessary. For patients thought to have *Campylobacter* infection, the macrolide azithromycin should be used, 500 mg/day for 3 days. Because of increasing resistance to trimethoprim-sulfamethoxazole, sulfa drugs such as Bactrim are no longer the drug of choice.

In addition to antibiotics, travelers may use bismuth subsalicylate (Pepto-Bismol) or antimotility drugs such as loperamide (Imodium) to treat diarrhea. Both these medications reduce the number of unformed stools and usually make the patient feel better. Some providers believe that loperamide and other antimotility drugs may actually prolong the duration of illness, but this has not been observed in most cases of travel-related watery diarrhea. However, antimotility drugs are contraindicated if the patient has a fever or blood in the stool.

In 2004 the Food and Drug Administration approved the antibiotic rifaximin for the prevention and treatment of uncomplicated traveler's diarrhea caused by noninvasive strains of *E. coli.* Rifaximin is not systemically absorbed and carries few side effects. It has been approved for use in Europe since 1987. A study of travelers to Mexico showed that only 20% of travelers who used rifaximin as prophylaxis developed traveler's diarrhea, compared with 48% of travelers who took a placebo.[12] Another randomized study showed that rifaximin was safe and effective as a treatment of traveler's diarrhea. Resolution of symptoms was slightly slower than with ciprofloxacin but still much faster than with placebo.[13] The major limiting factors for rifaximin are that it is expensive, is not approved for individuals younger than 12 years, and should not be used when fever or bloody diarrhea is present.

There is also a vaccine, Dukoral, that has been approved in the United State since late 2006 as a vaccine against traveler's diarrhea. Dukoral is used, with modest effectiveness, in more than 50 countries as a cholera vaccine, but it has also been shown to provide some protection against enterotoxigenic *E. coli.* The Dukoral vaccine is expensive, and therefore several cost-effectiveness studies have been done. One study[14] estimated that Dukoral is cost-effective only where the attack rates for enterotoxigenic *E. coli* are greater than 9% to 13%.

A major limitation of both the rifaximin antibiotic and the Dukoral oral vaccine is that each is effective only against *E. coli.* Neither offers any protection against the other bacterial causes or the viral causes of traveler's diarrhea.

Education about proper food and water precautions is therefore imperative. The adage "boil it, cook it, peel it, or forget it" is helpful to pass on to travelers: Eat well-cooked foods served hot, or peeled fruits and vegetables, and drink only bottled beverages or hot tea or hot coffee that was made with boiled water. Travelers should avoid milk and milk products that have not been pasteurized, ice that was not made from previously boiled water, and uncapped or locally bottled water. Even clear wilderness stream and lake water can be contaminated with *Giardia* or *Campylobacter* organisms. Travelers should try to avoid eating food from street vendors and choose to eat in restaurants where the kitchen and restrooms are known to be clean.

AIR TRAVEL RISKS

Air travel of more than 6 hours' duration increases the risk of deep venous thrombosis and peripheral edema. To minimize this risk, travelers should be encouraged to get out of their seats and walk around every 1 to 2 hours. On most flights, cabin pressure is maintained at a level equivalent to that of altitudes of about 8000 feet, which does result in some reduction in available oxygen. As a result, travelers with chronic pulmonary or cardiac disease may require supplemental oxygen. Travelers should wait at least 3 weeks after a myocardial infarction to fly and should be aware that supplemental oxygen may be needed for up to 4 months after the event.[15] Air travel during pregnancy is generally considered safe until about 36 weeks' gestation.

Travelers with diabetes must monitor their serum glucose levels more closely because changes in time zone, food choices, and exercise routines will affect glucose levels, even among diabetics who normally have excellent glucose control. Travelers with recently diagnosed and unstable diabetes should be advised to wait until glycemic control is stabilized before traveling. Stuart Rose's *International Travel Health Guide* includes protocols for adjustment of insulin doses across multiple time zones based on the direction and duration of travel.[5]

TRAVEL SAFETY

All travelers should be aware of safety risks while traveling and take appropriate measures to reduce those risks. Crime is a problem in most parts of the world, and travelers should take precautions to avoid being robbed. Travelers should keep valuables in a hotel safe if one is available, refrain from wearing expensive jewelry, minimize the amount of cash carried, use traveler's checks where possible, and dress modestly and inconspicuously.

The most common cause of death while overseas for most healthy travelers is a motor vehicle accident. Motor vehicle accidents rank above all other accidents, including falls, drownings, burns, gunshot wounds, and plane and boating accidents. Only heart attacks kill more travelers, and these are typically among the subset of elderly travelers with known coronary artery disease. Worldwide, approximately 1.2 million people are killed, and another 20 to 50 million are severely injured or disabled in motor vehicle accidents, on an annual basis. Motor vehicle accidents represent about 2.1% of total global mortality[16] and are ranked as the ninth leading cause of death worldwide, just below lung cancer and just above complications of prematurity and neonatal infections. Moreover, despite many fewer average road miles per person per year in the developing world, about 85% of the global motor vehicle deaths occur in low- and middle-income countries, where roads and vehicles are less safe. Compared with road travel in the United States, seat belts are rarely used or available, and traffic is less regulated. Moreover, when a major accident does occur, the hospital and trauma services are often lacking, and there may be insufficient time to evacuate the traveler to a major trauma center. As a result, the relative risk of actually dying in a motor vehicle accident is considerably higher when driving overseas than it is in the United States.[16] The magnitude of that increased risk can be as high as 40 to 1, depending on the country studied. Even in Europe, the risk of death per mile driven is 5.4 to 1, as compared with driving in the United States.

Travelers should be advised that air travel is still the safest mode of transport, followed by rail, ship, and finally travel by road. Travelers to the developing world need to actively seek out vehicles with seat belts and should avoid traveling by road at night if possible. Depending on the length of stay and the countries visited and whether a major trauma center with a safe blood supply exists, even young healthy travelers to urban areas should consider obtaining medical evacuation insurance, known as *SOS insurance,* mostly because of this risk of death or serious injury in a major motor vehicle accident. For older travelers or travelers to rural areas with more infectious disease, the argument for SOS insurance is even more compelling. Several companies are listed in Box 20-2.

SUMMARY

As international travel becomes more common, health care providers will need to become more knowledgeable about travel medicine and the relevant health care issues for international travel. At the very least, providers should have fully explored the health care options around them and should be prepared to make referrals for travelers who require additional services. Travelers with any underlying or chronic illness should be well prepared to manage the common minor complications or manifestations of their illness for themselves and should know which signs and symptoms should prompt them to seek professional medical care. All travelers should attend to their routine health care maintenance needs before travel and should be educated about how to improve their personal safety and reduce their risk from injury in a motor vehicle accident. Travelers should receive the vaccines that are required (e.g., yellow fever or meningococcal vaccine) or recommended (e.g., hepatitis A and B, typhoid fever, rabies, Japanese encephalitis) for their particular itinerary, preferably 4 to 6 weeks before departure. They also must be offered appropriate malaria prophylaxis and malaria education if there is any risk of malaria at their destination. Travelers should also clearly understand basic food and water

BOX 20-4

Provider Toolbox for Travelers: Brochures, Vaccines, and Medications

BROCHURES

Vaccine safety and indications
Malaria prevention
Traveler's diarrhea
Dengue fever and chikungunya fever
Ebola fever
Food and water safety
Insect and sun avoidance
First aid kit
Personal and transport safety
Evacuation insurance
Sexually transmitted disease and HIV infection prevention
Animals and rabies risk
Fresh water and schistosomiasis risk
High-altitude sickness
Jet lag and motion sickness
Exercise and travel

VACCINES

Tdap (tetanus, diphtheria, pertussis) or Td (tetanus and diphtheria)
MMR (measles, mumps, rubella)
Varicella
Influenza
Pneumococcal
Hepatitis A
Hepatitis B
Typhoid
Polio
Rabies
Japanese encephalitis
Yellow fever
PPD (purified protein derivative [tuberculin]) testing

MEDICATIONS (USES)

Chloroquine (malaria)
Doxycycline (malaria)
Mefloquine (malaria)
Atovaquone and proguanil (malaria)
Primaquine (malaria)
Bismuth subsalicylate (traveler's diarrhea, gastrointestinal upset)
Loperamide (traveler's diarrhea)
Ciprofloxacin (traveler's diarrhea)
Azithromycin (*Campylobacter* infection)
Rifaximin (traveler's diarrhea)
Metronidazole (*E. histolytica* or *Giardia* infection)
Meclizine (motion sickness)
Scopolamine (motion sickness)
Acetaminophen (pain or fever)
Ibuprofen (pain or fever)

precautions and how to manage traveler's diarrhea if it occurs. They should know how to protect themselves against sexually transmitted infections and pathogens spread person to person through the respiratory tract. Finally, travelers should be advised to research the best sources of medical care in the countries they will be visiting and to make an informed decision about whether they will obtain medical evacuation insurance before departure.

An example of a travel medicine "toolbox" is shown in Box 20-4. It lists commonly used medications, vaccines, and patient education brochures or handouts. Many of the vaccines and medications have already been discussed. However, it is equally important to create or to collect good patient education materials and to be prepared to discuss these materials and answer questions. General and country-specific travel education should include clearly written patient education handouts about jet lag, motion sickness, altitude sickness, urban air quality, traveler's diarrhea, hepatitis A and B, typhoid fever, and prevention of sexually transmitted diseases. Travelers will also appreciate well-written handouts about the diseases spread by insect vectors (e.g., malaria, dengue fever, chikungunya fever, yellow fever, Japanese encephalitis) as well as the important zoonotic diseases, such as rabies, avian influenza, and leptospirosis.

CHAPTER 21

PRESURGICAL CLEARANCE

Jane Flanagan • Jennifer A. Neves

DEFINITION AND EPIDEMIOLOGY

Before the late 1980s, patients were hospitalized at least 1 day before surgery for presurgical clearance, during which time they were assessed by a surgical team that included anesthesiologists, surgeons, and nurses. As a result of improvements in surgical technology, anesthesia delivery, and patient demand, along with financial restrictions, ambulatory surgery clinics were instituted to ensure that ambulatory patients would continue to receive that same level of assessment and preparation.[1,2] These clinics were originally intended to serve only a same-day outpatient (ambulatory) and healthy population of patients. Continued financial demands were placed on hospitals to reduce costs, however, and presurgery evaluation clinics were viewed as a cost-effective way to provide comprehensive presurgery assessment and care to patients requiring inpatient admissions after surgery. As a result, these clinics evolved to serve a growing population of patients.[3] Presurgical clinics are evolving to embrace the conceptual framework of a "surgical home." The intended outcome of these recent initiatives is that all surgical patients should be cleared in clinics with an affiliation to the institution where anesthesia will be administered and the surgical procedure will occur.

Although surgical and anesthesia advances and refinement have resulted in less invasive procedures, they have paradoxically led to an availability of more surgeries that are performed on an older and medically complex group of patients.[3-5] As the population in the United States grows, it also ages, primarily because life expectancy has increased and "baby boomers" are fast approaching the age bracket of 65 years and above. The U.S. Census Bureau projects that the percentage of Americans 65 and older will increase from 13% to more than 20% by 2030. Individuals 85 and older will comprise the fastest-growing segment of the elderly, tripling in number over the next four decades.[6] Surgical trends from 2012 indicate that the most common surgical procedure was total knee replacement, with more than 671,374 being performed in 2012 compared with 533,216 in 2005. In 2012 the mean age for any major joint replacement was 67.[7] Overall, the number of older adults having surgery continues to rise at an unprecedented rate as the population in the United States ages.

PATHOPHYSIOLOGY

Advanced practice nurses in presurgery settings must be aware of the pathophysiologic changes of the underlying and concurrent medical problems and the effect that surgery and anesthesia will have on these problems. One common characteristic of all surgical patients is that their surgeries and hospitalizations are considered elective, nonemergent admissions. It is this characteristic that serves as a basis for classifying these patients from an anesthesia risk perspective.

CLINICAL PRESENTATION

The types of adult patients entering a presurgical clinic vary greatly by age, medical condition, and diagnosis, but as noted, the population of patients undergoing elective surgery continues to trend toward being older and potentially more medically complex.[3-5] Overall, patients may be young and healthy or older with varied comorbid conditions. All patients who are admitted to a presurgical clinic are considered outpatients. They can come from home, rehabilitation centers, nursing facilities, or other extended care environments. The intent is that these patients will return to these environments after clearance.

There are no evidence-based guidelines indicating the appropriate leeway in terms of days needed for presurgical clearance, but typically the evaluation occurs 1 to 30 days before surgery. It is important that the visit occur enough in advance of the surgical procedure to allow necessary consultations with and referrals to other appropriate health care providers as indicated. For example, if a patient scheduled for an open, elective abdominal aortic aneurysm repair develops new-onset angina, it is important that there be enough time to schedule cardiac stress testing and to review the results with the anesthesia team. The anesthesiologists will then determine the appropriate anesthetic plan for this patient based on the cardiac stress test results.

Important information and history to determine appropriateness for surgery include the following:

- The type of surgical procedure and expected date, as well as social supports for the patient after surgery and the possible need for rehabilitation or home services
- A thorough medication list including any over-the-counter and herbal products
- A detailed list of allergic reactions and adverse effects to any medications
- Personal and family history of adverse reactions to anesthesia (e.g., malignant hyperthermia) or bleeding problems
- Past medical history and patient comorbidities and status (e.g., previous history of myocardial infarction, uncontrolled diabetes, asthma, chronic lung disease, hypertension, hypothyroidism, malignancy)

TABLE 21-1 Tests for Presurgical Clearance

Test	Indications for Performing Test
Chest radiograph	Patient older than 60 yr; smoking history of >20 pack-years; history of cardiovascular or pulmonary diseases, having thoracic procedure, or presence of malignant disease
Electrocardiography	Men >45 yr of age, women >55 yr of age; history or symptoms of cardiac disease, diabetes, morbid obesity, significant pulmonary disease, and cocaine abuse
Pulmonary function testing	All patients undergoing major thoracic surgery; history of severe chronic obstructive pulmonary disease
Complete blood count	Patient older than 60 yr; history of pulmonary, cardiovascular, or renal disease; smoking history of >20 pack-years; history of radiation therapy, chemotherapy, or bleeding disorder; symptoms of infectious process (increased temperature and cough)
Coagulation studies	Patient currently receiving coagulation therapy; history of alcohol abuse, hepatic disease, easy bruising (family or personal history), bleeding disorders, or malignant disease; undergoing procedures with associated blood loss or postoperative coagulation therapy
Pregnancy test	All women of childbearing age except those who have had oophorectomy
Electrolyte values	Patient on dialysis; diabetes; hypertension or heart disease; potential for alterations in electrolytes because of other disease processes or medications
Liver function tests	Patient with history of alcohol abuse, hepatitis, or known hepatic disease
Urinalysis or urine culture and sensitivity	Patient undergoing urologic procedure who has a history of frequent urinary tract infections or is receiving a graft, prosthetic, or implantable device
Albumin level	Patient who is malnourished or has a history of alcohol abuse or hepatic or malignant disease

- Past surgical history
- Quantification of daily intake of alcohol, tobacco, marijuana, or other substances of abuse

PHYSICAL EXAMINATION

The physical examination focuses on the presenting surgical problem and expected type of anesthesia. The general examination should include generalized appearance, height, weight, and baseline vital signs, including oxygen saturation. Evaluation of mental status, airway, dentition, and range of motion of the head and neck is necessary. Note should be made of abnormalities in the appearance of neck veins or of the presence of bruits, and abnormalities on auscultation of the heart, lungs, and abdomen are noted. Further evaluation for abdominal masses, genitourinary or rectal problems, peripheral pulses, and cranial nerve and neurologic changes may also be warranted, depending on the reason for presentation, the medical history, and the anesthetic plan. For example, the physical examination of a healthy 32-year-old man with a herniated lumbar disc should include all of these evaluations because this patient may manifest neurologic or peripheral vascular changes or these changes could occur postoperatively. In addition, sexual, urinary, and bowel function may be a presenting symptom associated with his back problem or may develop postoperatively as a complication of the surgery.

DIAGNOSTICS

Diagnostic testing for presurgical clearance is variable and depends on several factors: (1) the presenting diagnosis, (2) the patient's age, (3) the patient's comorbidities, (4) the type of anesthetic agent planned, and (5) the surgeon's preference. Surgeons and anesthesiologists do sometimes vary in their opinion of what testing is necessary, but in general, much of what was once considered necessary preoperative testing in preparation for surgery has been modified. Guidelines for patients' presurgical testing is often based on risk stratification[8] as determined by American Society of Anesthesiologists (ASA) anesthesia classification. The ASA[8] anesthesia classifications and guidelines for preoperative testing[9,10] in the presurgical period for inpatients are outlined in Tables 21-1 and 21-2.

TABLE 21-2 Anesthesia Classification in Presurgery Setting*

ASA Class	Criteria
1	Healthy, normal patient
2	Patient with mild systemic disease
3	Patient with severe systemic disease
4	Patient with severe systemic disease that is a threat to life

*American Society of Anesthesiologists (ASA) class 5 and class 6 patients are not seen in presurgical clinics or in primary care providers' offices.

DIFFERENTIAL DIAGNOSIS

Patients who come into a presurgical clinic have a known diagnosis requiring surgery. Most patients are referred by their health care provider to a surgical specialist, who performs appropriate and specific diagnostic testing before determining the exact diagnosis and referring the patient to the presurgical clinic. Therefore there are few if any instances when a differential diagnosis is necessary with regard to the surgical procedure. There are, however, patients who come to the presurgery clinic who do not have regular primary care. In these cases, no prior or recent physical examination findings are available. This absence of data is often coupled with the person's being a poor historian, and the medical history and medication use can be vague. In these patients, there can be countless differential diagnoses. Management of this is discussed in the next section.

MANAGEMENT

Patients who come into a presurgical clinic will ideally be well known to a primary care provider (PCP) and will have underlying medical conditions well managed on presentation. In two instances, the PCP must provide management of comorbid disease processes: (1) when a patient does not have appropriate primary care and (2) when a patient does have good primary care but needs further testing because of the anesthesia plan and comorbid diseases.

When the patient does not have a PCP, it is important that the person performing the presurgical clearance determine the need for a preoperative evaluation by a primary care health care provider. If a primary care evaluation is not indicated before the surgical procedure, the patient progresses through presurgical clearance. However, the patient is educated about the importance of primary care. If the patient needs evaluation by a PCP before surgery, the surgeon is contacted by the person performing the presurgical clearance, and the patient is referred to a PCP before surgery.

At other times, a patient has been well managed by a PCP but the PCP is uncertain about appropriate diagnostic testing for surgery. In these instances, the health care provider in the presurgical clinic makes recommendations for the appropriate diagnostic testing and refers the patient to the PCP. For example, a patient scheduled for general anesthesia for a total hip replacement with a history of well-managed angina but who has not had a recent stress test will need a stress test before surgery. This may be arranged in collaboration with the PCP, or the patient may be referred back to the PCP, who will order the test and send the results to the presurgical clinic. Other diagnostic tests that may be required because of the anesthesia plan include echocardiography for patients with known cardiac valve disease and pulmonary function testing in patients with severe chronic obstructive pulmonary disease (COPD).

Medication and Fasting Guidelines

Medication and fasting requirements are other management issues addressed in the presurgical clinic. The American Association of Nurse Anesthetists[11] and the ASA[12] recommend that all herbal medicines be stopped 2 weeks before surgery. Medications used to control medical conditions such as hypertension, heart disease, eye problems, anxiety, pain, and COPD should be continued and taken on the morning of surgery.

Oral agents to treat type 2 diabetes should be withheld the morning of surgery.[13] Patients on injectable insulin including type 1 diabetics will follow an algorithm based on the type of insulin typically used (e.g., basal versus intermediate acting), time of day for surgery, and potential for hypoglycemia, which should be assessed preoperatively. In addition, blood glucose concentration should be monitored carefully both before and after surgery.[13]

Despite evidence supporting fairly standard fasting guidelines preoperatively, the actual practice continues to be quite variable. Evidence supports that patients may have clear fluids until 2 hours before surgery and solid foods until 6 hours before surgery.[14] The exceptions to this are people who have gastroesophageal reflux disease (GERD) and those who are scheduled to have surgery requiring a prone position. These patients need to fast from both food and fluids for 8 hours before surgery.[14] Because the presence of upper gastrointestinal disease (including GERD) can predispose a patient to aspiration of stomach contents during intubation, current guidelines suggest that patients should take an H_2 receptor antagonist the night before and the morning of surgery to diminish the risk of aspiration.[14]

The 2007 guidelines on perioperative cardiovascular evaluation and care for noncardiac surgery[15] recommended the use of beta blockers before surgery for many patients. The evidence for routine beta blocker use before surgery has since been discredited. Current guidelines recommend that for noncardiac patients, beta blockers should be prescribed only preoperatively and only after careful considerations of the benefit to each individual patient. In patients with a history of a myocardial infraction, beta blocker therapy is still considered beneficial.[16]

COMPLICATIONS

Complications related to anesthesia are multiple and range from major life-threatening (rare) to the more benign and easily resolved (more common) events. Complications vary by anesthetic type, but comorbid conditions can increase risk. For general anesthesia, complications include nausea, vomiting, sore throat, fatigue, stroke, myocardial infarction, allergic reaction, and death. For spinal or other regional anesthesia, complications can include headache, nerve damage, infection, and limb loss.[7A] All potential complications are considered in the presurgical clinic to stratify risk and to minimize perioperative morbidity and mortality.[7A] The potential risks and complications are readdressed by the anesthesiologist or anesthetist providing care on the day of surgery before consent is obtained.

INDICATIONS FOR REFERRAL OR HOSPITALIZATION

The health care provider in the presurgical clinic collaborates with the PCP, the surgeon, and the anesthesiologist who will be providing anesthesia to establish the appropriate care plan for the patient. In conjunction with the PCP and surgeon, referrals to cardiologists and other specialists are provided as needed to determine the safest anesthesia plan. The presurgical clinic health care provider and anesthesiologist will review the results of any diagnostic tests and discuss with the surgeon the proposed anesthesia plan. The proposed plan is then communicated to the PCP.

Patients in presurgical clinics should have their general health managed in the primary care setting, but in some instances this is not the case. If this is so, the presurgical visit provides the nurse practitioner with an excellent opportunity to review the importance of good primary care and refer the patient to a PCP in a convenient location.

The American College of Cardiology and American Heart Association[15] have established clinical predictors of increased perioperative cardiac risk. The clinical predictors are divided into three categories: major, intermediate, and minor predictors (Table 21-3). Consideration of five other factors in addition to these clinical predictors helps determine whether preoperative cardiac evaluation is required. A decision tree related to these five factors is shown in Table 21-4.

LIFE SPAN CONSIDERATIONS

Patients coming to the hospital for surgery are unique, and the ways in which they cope cannot be predicted or assumed.

Although providers might expect that an older, more medically complex patient undergoing a life-threatening surgery could be anxious and that a younger healthy patient undergoing a minor surgery would be calm, the opposite may in fact be the case. Anxiety level and coping style are not predictable in this setting and are often related to current life stresses, perceived level of support, and psychosocial development issues more than to age or illness. Studies examining patients' postoperative experience indicate that younger patients who did not perceive a "need for help" postoperatively experienced more distress than older, frail patients who had planned to have help available postoperatively.[1,2] Therefore a careful assessment of these factors is necessary to accurately evaluate and plan for each individual's care.

TABLE 21-3 Clinical Predictors of Increased Perioperative Cardiac Risk

Type of Clinical Predictors	Specific Predictors That Increase Risk
Major	Myocardial infarction within past 30 days Unstable angina Decompensated heart failure High-grade atrioventricular block Symptomatic ventricular arrhythmia Supraventricular arrhythmias with uncontrolled ventricular rate Severe valvular disease
Intermediate	Mild angina Previous myocardial infarction by history or pathologic Q waves, compensated or previous heart failure Diabetes (especially type 1) Renal insufficiency
Minor	Advanced age Abnormal electrocardiogram Rhythm other than sinus Low functional capacity History of stroke Uncontrolled hypertension

Age alone does not increase the risk for a person undergoing surgery; rather, the number and type of chronic diseases an individual has and how optimized the disease state is will have an effect on the morbidity and mortality in the postoperative period. Overall, the more chronic the disease and the older the individual, the more likely that life expectancy will be negatively affected.[17]

Because older adults may be at increased risk for changes in cognition, delirium, functional decline, polypharmacy, and comorbid illness, the optimum preoperative evaluation as suggested by the American College of Surgeons (ACS) National Surgical Quality Improvement Program (NSQIP) and the American Geriatrics Society (AGS)[18] is a comprehensive presurgical evaluation designed to capture issues specific to the more medically complex older adult. In addition to a complete history and physical examination and other screens already mentioned, the optimum care guidelines suggest that the following be screened for and assessed:

1. Cognition, ability to understand the surgery and recovery, decision-making capacity
2. Depression
3. Risk factors for developing postoperative delirium
4. Risk factors for postoperative pulmonary complications
5. Functional status and history of falls
6. Baseline frailty score
7. Nutritional status and possible preoperative interventions
8. Polypharmacy[18]

EDUCATION AND HEALTH PROMOTION

Education of the patient and family in the presurgical clinic is related to the surgical and anesthesia care plan. Studies indicate that patients forget much of the material taught to them individually during the presurgical evaluation.[1,2] Therefore after the patient has been assessed individually, the family should be brought into the setting to discuss preoperative and postoperative teaching and expectations about the patient's care on discharge either to home or to another facility. Teaching about the anesthesia care plan is also completed by the nurse practitioner or other health care provider in this setting and includes possible complications as well as effects of anesthesia and pain management concerns during and after surgery. The individual

TABLE 21-4 Factors to Consider for Preoperative Cardiac Evaluation

Question	If "Yes"	If "No"
Is surgery emergent?	Proceed to surgery.	Obtain cardiac evaluation.
Has the patient undergone coronary revascularization in the past 5 yr and currently is without cardiac-related symptoms?	Proceed to surgery.	Obtain cardiac evaluation.
Has the patient had a recent favorable cardiac evaluation?	Proceed to surgery.	Obtain cardiac evaluation.
Can the patient climb two flights of stairs (as one measure of functional capacity)?	Proceed to surgery.	Obtain cardiac evaluation.
Is the level of risk for the surgery low?	Proceed to surgery.	If no, as in surgeries such as abdominal aortic aneurysm repair, obtain cardiac evaluation.
Are any of the clinical predictors listed in Table 23-3 present?	If intermediate or major, obtain cardiac evaluation; if minor, proceed to surgery.	Proceed to surgery.

learning style should be assessed, and teaching should be done accordingly.

Lifestyle issues can promote or exacerbate disease processes. The presurgical clinic setting provides the health care provider an opportunity to encourage lifestyle changes and appropriately refer the patient to programs that address alcohol or drug abuse, smoking cessation, stress management, nutritional counseling, exercise, home safety, or domestic violence. The advanced practice nurse in a presurgery setting should advocate for a caring, holistic, patient- and family-centered environment that creates a safe space for patients to share their concerns about the surgery and other life stresses that may have an impact on healing.[3]

SURGICAL OR PERIOPERATIVE HOME

Traditional presurgical clinics are evolving to incorporate the surgical or perioperative home as a conceptual framework for perioperative care. Advanced by literature from the ASA, the surgical home reduces the fragmentation of care across the perioperative continuum, providing seamless care using standard protocols for each phase of the surgical experience: presurgical, intrasurgical, postoperative, and postdischarge.[19] The role of anesthesia providers has changed with the surgical home model to include oversight of the entire perioperative process. Benefits include tailored optimization for medical conditions; early identification of risk for surgical complications; initiation of evidence-based practice EBP protocols to address delirium risk and venous thromboembolism (VTE) risk; initiation and oversight of quality metrics (Surgical Care Improvement Project [SCIP] measures, methicillin-resistant *Staphylococcus aureus* [MRSA] precautions, first case starts); and individually tailored patient recovery plans leading to reduction in length of stay with reduction of emergency department visits and readmission by early remote monitoring using teletechnology.[19] The surgical home approach offers exciting opportunities for health care providers to collaborate across the care continuum.

CHAPTER 22

PREPARTICIPATION SPORTS PHYSICAL

Cené L. Gibson

The American Heart Association (AHA) recommends cardiovascular preparticipation screening with a history and physical examination for all athletes participating in high school and college sports.[1] However, the AHA also states that these recommendations are applicable to other populations (i.e., children younger than 12 years and those older than 30 years participating in masters sports).[1] For secondary school and college athletes, an annual sports physical is a prerequisite for student participation in school-related sports, but sports medicine physicians recommend that middle school and junior high school students also have a physical examination for school-related sports activities. Despite the recommendations to screen athletes, the actual requirements of this examination remain controversial and are not clearly defined. The primary purpose of the sports physical is to determine the patient's health status and physical fitness for participation in sports; yet the concerns about cardiovascular death among young athletes heighten concerns about the consistency of these examinations. Nurse practitioners should be aware of their state's requirements and be attentive to emerging research and recommendations related to preparticipation physical examinations.[4,5]

The primary goal for these examinations is to identify athletes at risk for an adverse event (e.g., cardiovascular event), but it is also necessary to identify other medical problems and to provide appropriate treatment before the athlete participates in any athletics. Determining the athlete's overall health, providing counseling, and strengthening the provider-patient relationship are other objectives. The preparticipation sports physical is an excellent opportunity to provide education related to healthy behaviors and injury prevention, in addition to identifying risk factors that affect well-being.[2,4,7] Still, the importance of the sports preparticipation examination cannot be overstated. The examiner must be skilled and have significant experience in performing both cardiovascular and musculoskeletal examinations to identify any condition that would prohibit participation in the chosen sport. Despite these screening precautions, it is not possible to completely eliminate injuries, particularly in contact or collision sports.

It is preferable to perform the examination in the office so that adequate time can be spent ascertaining the personal and family health history and performing the examination. If possible, the examination should be performed at least 6 weeks before the beginning of the sports activity.[3,6] For student athlete sports physicals, it is essential that a parent accompany the student to the examination to fully establish the family history and cardiovascular risk factors.[5,6] It is often helpful to have the student and parent complete and sign a preparticipation health history form before the examination. It is then necessary that the provider review the form with the student and parent and specifically question the parent and student about each item on the health history form.

HISTORY

Allergies, current and past medications, and the personal and family history should be carefully assessed. Answers to the following questions should be determined before the examination commences.[6]

1. Medical history, including the following:
   - Anaphylaxis or allergic or untoward reactions to exercise, medications, pollens, foods, and stinging insects (including the specific nature of the reaction)
   - Current medications, including vitamins or herbal supplements, prescribed or over-the-counter medications, and nutritional supplements
   - Habits such as smoking, caffeine, and alcohol or drug use
   - Immunization history: tetanus status, hepatitis, chickenpox, and MMR (measles, mumps, rubella)
   - Previous surgeries (particularly orthopedic, genital, kidney, or eye surgeries)
   - Previous hospitalizations
   - Loss of an organ such as eye, kidney, or testicle
2. Present or past illness, including the following:
   - Recent viral illness, such as mononucleosis or myocarditis

- Recent weight loss or gain
- Previous sports restriction
- History of heat-related illness
- Skin piercings or reactions (hives, rashes, infections)
- Head injury, neck injury, loss of consciousness, fainting, concussion, dizziness, headaches, seizures
- Visual problems, such as blurred vision or a history of detached retina; whether the patient wear glasses or contacts
- History of heart surgery, hypertrophic cardiomyopathy, myocarditis, mitral valve prolapse, prior embolic event, commotio cordis, or coronary artery abnormalities; history of chest pain, dizziness, fatigue or weakness, syncope, near syncope, or palpitations (heart racing or skipped heart beats) with or after exercise; history of hypertension; history of heart murmur[1,2,5]
- Breathing problems, such as wheezing, coughing, excessive exertional and unexplained dyspnea associated with exercise; history of asthma[5]
- History of musculoskeletal injury, such as fracture or dislocation; injury or pain in neck, shoulder, back, elbow, hand, finger, knee, ankle, foot, or toe that caused missed work, school, or practice
- History of use of special equipment for sports-related activities
- History of numbness or tingling in the upper or lower extremities
- History of "burners" or "stingers" (injury to arm nerve supply) caused by contact or collision sport activity[7]
- History of eating disorder, excessive fatigability, diabetes, bleeding problems, anemia, hepatitis, mononucleosis
- History of stress, anxiety, or depression
- Menstrual history: menarche, last menstrual period, frequency of menses (number of menstrual periods in the past year), history of amenorrhea or other menstrual dysfunction
- History of anemia or sickle cell disease

3. Family history, including the following:
   - History of premature or sudden death before the age of 50 years, ion channelopathies, short QT syndrome,* long QT syndrome, Wolff-Parkinson-White syndrome, arrhythmias, hypertrophic or dilated cardiomyopathy, Marfan syndrome, or Brugada syndrome†
   - Family history of coronary artery disease
   - Disabling heart disease in a close relative

PHYSICAL EXAMINATION

The physical examination should be focused and thorough to determine the presence of an acute infection or any impairment that would prohibit participation in the selected sport. General appearance, posture, overall health, height, weight, and percentage of body fat should be determined. It is vital to note congenital deformities, such as arachnodactyly or other signs of Marfan syndrome. Additional components of the physical examination include the following:

1. Visual acuity with Snellen chart (Corrected visual acuity should be 20/40 or better.)
2. Vital signs including bilateral brachial blood pressure and heart rate sitting at rest, 3 minutes after exercise, and again 6 minutes after exercise
3. Skin evaluation for signs of fungal, candidal, scabies, or other infection
4. Head, eye (including documentation of pupil reactivity or anisocoria), ear, nose, and throat (HEENT) evaluation to determine infectious processes and to evaluate any lymphadenopathy
5. Cardiovascular examination
   - Pectus deformity of the anterior chest; evaluate for Marfan syndrome.
   - Assess the heart sounds with the patient in the supine, standing, and squatting positions with a Valsalva maneuver. Special emphasis is necessary to determine the presence of any murmurs or arrhythmias. Arrhythmias, extra heart sounds (S_3, S_4), a new murmur, a diastolic murmur, a systolic murmur grade 3/6 or higher, a left sternal border systolic murmur that increases in intensity with standing or Valsalva maneuver, or a mitral valve click accompanied by a murmur requires further evaluation before clearance for sports participation can be given.[1,5]
   - Radial and femoral pulses should be symmetric to exclude coarctation of the aorta.
   - Blood pressure must be compared with age-adjusted tables. Elevated blood pressure requires treatment, and it must be within the accepted range before medical clearance is given. The use of beta blockers, which can be considered to be performance enhancers, or diuretics may preclude athletic participation in some states.
6. Pulmonary examination; an assessment of lung sounds anteriorly and posteriorly
7. Abdominal examination; further evaluation if organomegaly is detected‡
8. Genitourinary examination
   - Tanner staging.
   - The testes must be descended.
   - The presence of inguinal hernias must be determined.
9. Musculoskeletal examination
   - Is there neck pain on examination or with range of motion (ROM)?‡
   - With the patient standing, the back should be evaluated for scoliosis, flexibility, and pain with ROM.‡
   - All extremities, muscles, and joints, including the shoulders and arms, elbow and forearm, wrist and hand, hip and thigh, knee, leg and ankle, foot, and acromioclavicular joint, must be evaluated for muscle atrophy, flexibility, symmetry, tenderness, and full ROM. Resisted shoulder shrug plus shoulder abduction, internal and external rotation, and resisted flexion and extension must be determined.‡ Heel-toe walking, knee extension, and patellar tracking should be assessed. Asymmetry or pain with ROM requires further evaluation.
   - The physical signs of Marfan syndrome should be excluded.
   - Can the patient "duck walk" at least four steps?
   - Can the patient hop on each foot several times?

*Sudden death in individuals with structurally normal hearts associated with short QT interval.[5]

†Sudden death in individuals with normal hearts associated with ST-segment elevation in right precordial leads.[5]

‡Any pain or deficit requires further evaluation before medical clearance is given for sports participation.

10. Neuromuscular examination
    - Cranial and sensory nerves
    - Deep tendon reflexes
    - Cerebellar function

DIAGNOSTICS

Diagnostics are not usually necessary for student preparticipation sports physicals, although some states require urinalysis to determine the presence of protein or glucose in the urine. Further diagnostics are dependent on the history and physical examination findings. In some countries, a 12-lead electrocardiogram (ECG) is a routine part of the diagnostic evaluation. ECG screening is not currently recommended by the AHA.[1,4,5] An ECG is warranted to determine QT prolongation when the patient is taking a medication known to prolong the QT and for patients who note palpitations. If an arrhythmia is not identified on ECG, a Holter monitor, event recorder, or continuous telemetry ambulatory cardiac event monitor is indicated with a history of palpitations.[5] A complete blood count with differential, electrolyte determinations, and thyroid-stimulating hormone level are also necessary for patients who note palpitations.[5] Other diagnostics, such as exercise stress testing, echocardiography, lipid panel, or fasting glucose concentration, are necessary if the history and physical examination suggest that there is risk of coronary artery disease or cardiac abnormalities. Hemoglobin and hematocrit should be determined as necessary in female athletes.

MEDICAL CLEARANCE

Physician consultation or referral is indicated and medical clearance deferred if there is a family history of the following:

- Sudden or unexpected death before the age of 50 years[1,5]
- Disabling cardiac disease in a family member younger than 50 years[1,5]
- Cardiomyopathy, long QT syndrome or ion channelopathies, Marfan syndrome, significant arrhythmias (e.g., Wolff-Parkinson-White syndrome)[1,5]

Physician consultation or referral is indicated and medical clearance deferred if there is a personal history or physical finding of the following:

- Abdominal organomegaly
- Absence of an eye, kidney, or testicle (These conditions usually prohibit participation in any contact sport.)
- Acute systemic infection
- Asthma, uncontrolled
- Asymmetric femoral pulses[1,5]
- Atlantoaxial instability[1]
- Audible heart murmur in standing position or with Valsalva maneuver[1,5]
- Bleeding disorder[1]
- Cardiac history of hypertension,[1] heart murmur,[1] structural heart disease
- Detached retina or visual acuity less than 20/40 in both eyes
- Diabetes, uncontrolled
- Down syndrome
- Eating disorder[5]
- Exercise-related chest discomfort, dyspnea,[1,5] pain, or fatigue[1,5]
- Fever
- Hypertension[1,2]
- Inability to perform duck walk maneuvers
- Lymphadenopathy (significant)
- Marfan syndrome stigmata[1,5]
- Neck pain or cervical stenosis
- Neurologic deficit
- Obesity
- Palpitations or dysrhythmias
- Previous history of hypertension,[1,5] heart murmur,[1,5] structural heart disease
- Post-traumatic convulsive disorder
- Shoulder asymmetry, joint tenderness, or pain with ROM
- Unexplained syncope or near-syncope[1,5]

Physician consultation or referral is indicated if the athlete or athlete's family refuses diagnostic testing and specialist referral or does not understand the risk of sports participation.[6]

PATIENT AND FAMILY EDUCATION

Students, parents, and coaches can exert considerable pressure on the health care provider to provide medical clearance for the athlete. However, the health care provider's fundamental responsibility is to protect the student from harm. Any concerns elicited during the history or physical examination must be carefully explained to both the parent and the student. It is important that both the parent and student understand that medical clearance cannot be given until the results of diagnostic testing and specialist evaluation are known. The parent and student should also understand that a preparticipation sports physical examination has limitations and cannot completely eliminate the risks inherent in any athletic activity.

REFERENCES

For a full list of references, scan the QR code or visit http://booksite.elsevier.com/9780323355018

PART 4

Office Emergencies

CHAPTER 23

DISASTER AND EMERGENCY PREPAREDNESS AND RESPONSE IN PRIMARY CARE

Stephen Pixley

THE EVOLUTION OF EMERGENCY AND DISASTER PREPAREDNESS EFFORTS IN HEALTH CARE

Disaster preparedness has evolved dramatically over the past two decades. Before 2001, disaster preparedness in many hospitals was often little more than the development of a single all-or-nothing mass casualty plan. Collaboration, coordination, or joint planning seldom took place among hospitals, or among hospitals and other health care entities such as public health, extended care facilities, clinics, or other entities.[1] Fortunately, disaster planning in U.S. health care has changed; unfortunately, the major drivers for change were actual disasters. After the attack on the World Trade Center on September 11, 2001, then-President George Bush signed Presidential Directive 5, which directed the development of the National Response Framework and the National Incident Management System, both of which were efforts to standardize our response to large-scale threats. During any large-scale disaster, all agencies and efforts are now coordinated through the use of the Incident Command System (ICS), which is used by all governmental agencies and reflected at federal, state, and municipal levels. In addition, the Hospital Preparedness Program (HPP) was initiated; this program has used grant funding to encourage preparedness efforts in specific categories such as communications, decontamination, evacuation planning, and training, and requires a participating hospital to use a standardized incident command system to respond to emergencies. After Hurricane Katrina, the Joint Commission (TJC) revised and augmented its emergency management guidelines, offering significantly more detail and placing greater emphasis on the emergency management section. Accreditation requirements for preparedness for the Centers for Medicare and Medicaid Services (CMS) have recently been revised also and now more closely resemble those of TJC and other Homeland Security and HPP guidance—the goal being to move standards for all individual facilities toward uniformity regardless of accreditation agency. Preparedness and standardization efforts are also encouraged and guided by state and regional entities such as departments of health and state hospital associations. Hospitals are pulled toward preparedness by the desire to be prepared for emergencies and by HPP grant funding, and they are pushed toward preparedness by requirements outlined in accreditation standards (noting that reimbursement for care delivered is contingent on accreditation).

DISASTER PREPAREDNESS IN THE PRIMARY CARE SETTING

Unlike hospitals, primary care practice settings are not generally moved toward disaster preparedness. Practices that are connected to hospitals may fall under hospital requirements and hence have specific guidelines, and some primary care practices are reviewed and guided by TJC's Standards for Ambulatory Care, but stand-alone office practices and health centers often have little requirement or financial incentive to undertake formal preparedness efforts. Although a survey of primary care physicians has indicated that they are willing to serve during a disaster,[2] it is not clear how they can best serve, and most feel that they are too busy to train or to participate in planning or other preparations.[3] Is it reasonable to ask all health care entities, to include primary care, to prepare for disasters? In short, yes. It is virtually certain that our nation will encounter major catastrophic events in the future, whether from terrorism, from natural events such as Hurricane Katrina, or from a variety of other man-made or natural causes. In other words, it is highly probable that every health care practitioner, regardless of work setting, will ultimately be affected by a disaster of some sort. In addition, as probable as a major large-scale event might be, we are also nearly certain to experience one of the less dramatic events that happen every day somewhere, including information systems (computer) outages, severe weather, extended power outages, loss of water supply or septic system, flooding, or fire. Several of these might necessitate building evacuation or the salvaging of patient records, medical equipment, computers, and other office equipment. Consider the financial impact of a few days or weeks of business loss, or the practical challenge of losing all patient records! Less dramatic than a full-scale disaster, these are events that we also need to prepare for because they are far more likely to happen and because we may not receive much support during the response and recovery phases. These threats also provide practice in planning and preparing for a larger disaster. Although plans do not have to be elegant, the planning process itself makes us better prepared for *any* event than we were. Dwight David Eisenhower, a general in the U.S. Army before his presidency, is credited with saying that "Plans are nothing; planning is everything."

PREPARING THE PRIMARY CARE OFFICE FOR SMALL-SCALE EMERGENCIES AND DISASTERS

In the esoteric realm of emergency management, the cycle of emergency management is broken down into four phases: mitigation, preparedness, response, and recovery.

In the *mitigation* phase, risks are first identified. Many hospitals use complex hazard vulnerability assessment tools to weight probability, impact, and preparedness. This process may be more than the average office practice really needs. A primary care practice group might achieve the same objective by simply sitting down with office staff to assess events that have actually happened (e.g., severe weather) and events that might happen (e.g., a violent patient). What possibilities make the staff nervous? Other sources might be emergency preparedness personnel at the local hospital or officials from municipal or city services (e.g., fire chief), who can indicate what they have identified as top risks. Once specific risks have been identified, the practice can begin to either reduce the likelihood of the event happening (e.g., develop data system backup or emergency power generation) or reduce the impact of the event (e.g., add hurricane-resistant shutters). It may be possible to consider risks when designing new structures (e.g., restricting access) or to change existing structures (e.g., by moving generators out of low-lying areas that could flood).

In the *preparedness* phase, preparing or updating plans for specific events and training personnel through drills and exercises make staff as ready as possible. Top risks can be addressed by developing a very simple plan and then conducting a short drill after office hours in which the staff "walks through" the event detail by detail. Is the response realistic? For example, if the decision is made to call someone in particular, is the telephone number available? Contact information for staff and for outside agencies such as local emergency services and vendors should be updated frequently and kept in hard copy as well as in the office computer system. Stockpiling resources that might be in short supply is not always easy with today's cost constraints, but keeping a few critical items on hand, such as personal protective equipment (PPE), potable water, and flashlights, might be lifesaving.

In the *response* phase, hospitals and governmental agencies are required to use an incident command system. Although the practice may not use a formal Federal Emergency Management Agency (FEMA)–style ICS in the office, the designation of one clear commander and delineation of other specific roles, regardless of what they are called, will save time and prevent confusion during an urgent response. All staff members should know their own individual role during a crisis (e.g., leadership, patient care and movement, communications, logistics); preplanning ensures that the response will focus on the most critical tasks without duplication of effort and without wasted time.

During the *recovery* phase, while returning to "normal," a debriefing and review of the event is undertaken to gather feedback from participants at all levels. In the quality improvement process that follows, suggestions for improvement are channeled into corrective actions that are tracked for completion, and the cycle of four phases begins again.

THE CRITICAL ROLE OF PRIMARY CARE PRACTICES IN LARGE-SCALE DISASTERS

There is no well-defined or standard role for primary care practices during disasters as yet; defining that role is a process that may ultimately be left to community-level planners. What is clear is that the basic health care needs of patients do not stop during a disaster. Primary care is often likely to be a critical component in meeting the majority of patient health care needs, at times even more so than acute care (as in the case study on Hurricane Katrina later in this chapter). However, primary care is typically the least planned; the majority of planning efforts and resources focus on acute care needs. Community health centers are probably not well prepared yet and are often not part of community plans.[4] The U.S. in general is probably not prepared for a catastrophic event that would require a coordinated health care system response, and the development of health care coalitions has been described as the single most important step in preparing the U.S. health care system to respond more effectively.[5] Grant monies have been designated to support development of community planning efforts, and it is suggested that coalitions should include not only hospitals and extended care facilities, but community health centers and physician office practices as well.[1] Health care coalitions should also include health departments, emergency management agencies, and emergency medical services as well as community responders such as Medical Reserve Corps. In many locations the inclusion of additional health care entities such as specialty hospitals, long-term care facilities, dialysis centers, freestanding clinics, and surgical centers has been valuable.[1] Because of the relatively autonomous nature of their practices, it is unlikely that primary care providers will respond in a uniform way. Federal planning is far more likely to address aggregate organizations such as medical societies or associations than individual primary care practitioners, and the conclusion of one study was that full coordination of physicians is not possible under the current U.S. health care system.[2] However, community planners may be able to consider the resource of primary care physicians, nurses, and practices more effectively than the federal government, and community planners are more likely to incorporate them into a coherent and realistic plan. Primary care providers will almost certainly continue to address a variety of primary care needs to their own patients, to vulnerable populations, and to patients with specific needs.

PRIMARY PATIENT CARE CONTINUES DURING A DISASTER

Primary care is a relationship that is familiar and trusted to most people, and community health centers may be the only health care link with hard-to-reach populations such as homeless individuals, undocumented immigrants, and people engaged in illegal activities. Several studies have suggested that individuals from populations that are socially marginalized, have limited proficiency in English, and include diverse cultures may be reluctant to seek medical care or to report disease to sites viewed as government based or related to public health.[6-8] In general, the relationship established during routine primary care is likely to carry into times of increased stress and anxiety, and patients may continue to seek care through established and trusted pathways even in the face of disaster or terrorism.[9] Older adults, and in particular frail elders, individuals with chronic conditions, and those who live in long-term care facilities, are disproportionately affected by disaster,[10] and all of these individuals rely heavily on primary care. In addition to apparent core missions such as family practice, prenatal care, or pediatric practice, some practices may serve less obvious subpopulations of patients who require specific and critically important elements of care. Patients whose safety might be threatened by service interruption include juvenile diabetic patients identified as "brittle," patients receiving anticoagulant therapy, and other patients who are closely monitored, tracked, and advised by the primary care office practice on a near-daily basis. In addition to physical support, behavioral support offered by primary care can also be important, whether it is in the form of information for those who do not seek care from public health,[6] simple human empathy, or screening for inappropriate coping. Children in particular may need information and reassurance when affected by the fear and uncertainty surrounding a disaster event. Even if individuals are not physically traumatized, adverse effects may last for years afterward,[11] and such problems as cardiovascular morbidity and mortality may be increased for years after a major catastrophic event.[12] Unfortunately, individuals with chronic conditions are often not well prepared for adverse situations, having neither an evacuation plan nor even a 3-day supply of prescription medications.[13]

PRIMARY CARE AND SURGE CAPACITY

Facilitating surge capacity is also a role for primary care in most disaster scenarios, whether directly or indirectly. Although primary care providers will not usually be first responders in a disaster area (unless they are on site already), the primary care system will absolutely be affected in some manner by an overall surge in patient volumes during a disaster, and the response of primary care providers will in turn affect hospital surge capacity. Primary care, and particularly the primary care safety net, may have the capacity to provide health care surge capacity to prevent the overwhelming of hospital emergency departments.[14] Surge capacity—the ability to absorb large numbers of casualties during a catastrophic event—presents a critical challenge to hospitals, which are often near their maximum staffed capacity during normal operations. This may be particularly true for critical (intensive) care and acute (emergency) care capacities. During any widespread surge challenge, hospital patient flow or throughput can slow as discharges fail because of receiving bed shortage or illness in the receiving home. As discharges slow, admission beds decrease in number and patients await hospital admission in emergency departments or outpatient settings. If tertiary care centers fill, community and critical access hospitals have to hold patients who cannot be transferred; this is a significant problem in the event of critical care needs such as ventilation.

However, during large-scale events such as pandemic influenza, ambulatory patient surge occurs as well; many of these patients will visit primary care practices. As with hospitals, many primary care practices routinely operate near maximum capacity, in part because of the shortage of primary care providers. Although a primary care practice can refuse to see patients (i.e., turn away nonscheduled patients), a hospital emergency department may not turn patients away because of the Emergency Medical Treatment and Active Labor Act (EMTALA). If ambulatory care patients overwhelm emergency departments because primary care is not available in the community, capacity for true emergency care at the hospital will be reduced.

Community (municipal, city, or region) plans may include setting up points of distribution for medications, such as the H1N1 vaccination sites that were implemented in many communities during the fall of 2009. Communities may also have plans for setting up triage or screening clinics in the community, which may help to lessen the volume of patients seeking care in both hospitals and primary care practices. Many communities also have plans in place for setting up 24-hour care centers in which minimal supportive care such as fluid or oxygen administration can be administered.

Unfortunately, all these options, which are designed to reduce congestion, promote flow, and avoid surge, may prove very difficult to staff in a disaster or pandemic situation. Regardless of the availability of community care sites, primary care will likely continue to be used by many patients and victims as part of the screening, regardless of the availability of community-supported and community-coordinated sites. It is also likely that office practice personnel may be recruited to work with such emergency-focused response groups as the Medical Reserve Corps, whose mission is usually centered around disaster medical needs within the community (such as the community screening clinics or alternate care sites described earlier). Unfortunately, this could remove staff from the primary care practices themselves. At some point in a surge event, if hospital beds are simply no longer available (as in the 1918 pandemic influenza), primary care providers may be tasked with helping to develop community-based management plans for treatment and monitoring of their patients in the home.[15] In summary, patient surge during a disaster will affect all the health care entities within a community, including primary care, and how each responds will affect the others.

CASE STUDY 1: H1N1—PRIMARY CARE DURING A PANDEMIC INFLUENZA EVENT

In 2009, an outbreak of H1N1 afforded a glimpse of some of the primary care issues that arise during a surge of patients in an epidemic or pandemic situation. Correcting for under-ascertainment, a study estimated the following numbers of U.S. cases for the period from April 12, 2009 to April 10, 2010[16]:

- About 60.8 million people were infected with H1N1.
- About 274,304 H1N1-related hospitalizations occurred.
- About 12,469 H1N1-related deaths occurred.

In a widespread event of this nature and in particular during a more lethal pandemic or a biologic terrorism event, coordination among the many affected agencies will be extremely difficult. The resources of the federal government may not be sufficient to prevent the spread of a pandemic across the nation, and communities cannot automatically assume the availability of federal or state assistance.[17] At the peak of the H1N1 pandemic, much of the response effort did indeed fall to communities, some of which set up community screening clinics, and many of which set up points of distribution for administration of vaccine. Difficult issues such as dissemination of information, availability of pharmaceuticals, protection of staff and safety training, and staffing in general all pointed to the need for coordination and established working relationships among the various providers of health care at the community and regional levels, to include primary care. Although information was widely available from CDC and state websites and via Health Alert Network bulletins, active communication to primary care providers was often sparse and sometimes confusing as guidelines changed rapidly. PPE and training for primary care personnel were also limited in many areas, again demonstrating the need for community networking, planning, and operational support.

Despite activation of state medication caches and the Strategic National Stockpile, shortages of antivirals occurred and vaccine was slow in getting to the public despite the best efforts of the pharmaceutical industry. Consequently, it became necessary to prioritize the use of limited stores of vaccines and antivirals. Instead of distributing on a "first-come, first-served" basis, or worse yet on the basis of perceived social worth or the ability to pay, prioritized categories of recipients were proposed at a national level, based on the impact of influenza (degree of risk) and the likelihood of acquiring or spreading the virus. Health care personnel were declared a critical resource in order to maintain their ability to care for patients and hence were among the top tiers of that list.

Availability of PPE, specifically masks and respirators and gloves, was limited, and "just-in-time" training of personnel was instituted wherever and whenever possible. Difficulty in acquiring staff for community clinics, primary care, and hospital units was clearly seen, although most of these settings were able to maintain essential services throughout. The ability to maintain adequate staff levels over a prolonged period of surge was a crucial consideration.

Although H1N1 did not push us to the point of degradation of services, many hospitals began to plan for limiting services and for the reallocation of available (and healthy) staff to mission-critical beds. Primary care, however, has little ability to shut down services to reallocate staff. The H1N1 outbreak supported the concept that a large-scale event such as a pandemic will force us to view all health care resources as community resources and to use them in a coordinated and efficient manner. Only through proper planning at the community level will the United States be truly prepared for the next public health emergency.[18]

CASE STUDY 2: HURRICANE KATRINA—PRIMARY CARE DURING THE POSTDISASTER PERIOD

Hurricane Katrina destroyed several hospitals in New Orleans. Primary care practices in New Orleans, including safety net clinics, were also devastated; 1.1 million persons were displaced and 450,000 persons were evacuated from the Gulf region to safety in shelters in 27 states across the nation. Disaster medical assistance teams (DMATs) were moved in to provide acute and emergency care to survivors who remained in New Orleans. The key role of community health centers and primary care in postdisaster health care quickly became evident, in most cases far from the flooded city. Most evacuees arrived without prescription medications and health records, often unable to provide information, and most health records were inaccessible.[19] As evacuees surged into shelters, the ability of receiving communities to provide routine health care was challenged.

Initial screening and first aid were offered at several locations by the American Red Cross, which is tasked by the federal government with assisting in mass care and sheltering. Care needs of sheltered patients demonstrated that most needs were for primary care or very low-level acute care, most commonly for ongoing care of chronic medical conditions. A survey of 30,000 sheltered persons showed that 36% required acute care, 33% required preventive or chronic care, and 31% required both acute and preventive or chronic care. In addition, prescriptions were given to 29% of this sample group; of note, only 4% of those seen for initial (primary) care were referred to the emergency department or hospital for further care,[20] a testament to the ability of primary care to prevent hospital emergency department surge.

Chronic diseases identified as medical management priorities by key informants were mental health disorders, diabetes mellitus, hypertension, respiratory illness, end-stage renal disease, cardiovascular disease, and cancer.[19] The most frequent barrier to providing care for chronic disease was maintaining continuity of medications or medication procurement, and contributing factors were inadequate information (inaccessible medical records and poor patient knowledge) and financial constraints.[19] In a study of 12,000 evacuees to San Antonio, evacuees seeking care for chronic medical complaints accounted for only 15% of encounters, but their medication needs constituted 69% of all medications dispensed.[21] Cardiovascular medications were most commonly dispensed, but specific problem areas noted were highly patient-specific pharmaceutical treatments for chronic ailments such as depression and human immunodeficiency virus (HIV). DMATs were often unable to provide these specific medications, being armed more for acute and short-term care. Mental health needs also increased, in particular both anxiety and depression, and existing conditions were exacerbated. As temporary shelters in Louisiana's capitol of Baton Rouge began to close, emergency department visits increased, often because it was difficult for evacuees to obtain routine health care, which was often for chronic illnesses and often because of the need for medications—in other words, primary care.

SUMMARY

Emergency management, defined here as preparing for, responding to, and recovering from large-scale events that have the potential to overwhelm health care systems, has evolved dramatically over the past several years, initially in response to such events as the attack on the World Trade Center on September 11, 2001 and Hurricane Katrina in 2005. Current standards for accreditation, federal grants, and federal and state initiatives encourage the evolution of preparedness, and future plans are expected to involve all health care resources, including primary care.

Primary care plays a critical role during any large-scale emergency or disaster, and the primary care needs of victims will continue beyond the initial disaster period. Therefore, primary care should be included in plans that will likely be formed at the community level. As participants in a disaster effort, primary care providers should prepare for their own individual response (how their practice will continue to do business during both small- and large-scale events), but should also participate in and become familiar with the planning process for the larger overall response. How effectively primary care responds to the challenge of surge will ultimately affect the rest of the health care system, and an effective response to ambulatory care surge may prevent hospital emergency services from being overwhelmed, hence enabling them to remain available for the surge of acute care needs.

RESOURCES

Adalja AA, Toner E, Inglesby TV: Clinical management of potential bioterrorism-related conditions. *N Engl J Med* 372: 954-962, 2015. Available at www.nejm.org/doi/full/10.1056/NEJMra1409755?query=pfw&.

CHAPTER 24

ACUTE BRONCHOSPASM

Laurie Soroken • Annette McDonough

DEFINITION AND EPIDEMIOLOGY

Asthma that is not appropriately managed may lead to exacerbations requiring emergent care.[1] Bronchospasm, a symptom of asthma, is also referred to as *bronchial spasm. Bronchospasm* is defined as a sudden constriction of the muscles of the bronchial walls that leads to a temporary narrowing of the bronchi. When muscle tightening and inflammation occur, coughing, wheezing, shortness of breath, and thicker mucus production develop.[2]

The actual incidence of bronchospasm is difficult to determine because many cases are intermittent and the conditions that cause bronchospasm are multiple. It is estimated that 39.5 million Americans have been diagnosed with asthma. Females have higher prevalence rates than males, by 14%. The 2011 prevalence rate for blacks was higher than for whites by 36.9%.[3] Acute bronchospasm is responsible for an estimated 10.6 million physician office visits, 1.2 million hospital outpatient department visits, 2.1 million emergency department visits, 500,000 hospital admissions, and 4000 deaths annually.[3-6] In addition, young adults have been identified as a population at risk, because these individuals are reported to have a high incidence of asthma and less access to primary and preventive care and are most likely not to fill their asthma medication prescriptions.[1]

Bronchospasm usually occurs as a response to a specific trigger, the most common being identified as asthma. Clinical conditions that are associated with bronchospasm include anaphylactic reactions to medications or other allergens, asthma, chronic obstructive pulmonary disease, congestive heart failure, exercise, lower respiratory tract infection, mechanical airway obstruction by anatomic changes or tumor, pulmonary embolism, and vocal cord dysfunction.[4,6] Allergic triggers include "pet dander, dust mites, pollen or mold."[2] Exposures to smoke, pollution, cold air, and changes in weather are examples of nonallergic triggers.[2]

Immediate emergency department referral or physician consultation is indicated for patients in acute respiratory distress. During a severe exacerbation, arterial blood gases (ABGs) need to be monitored for hypoxemia, hypercapnia, and respiratory acidosis. Recommendations are that Pao_2 be kept above 60 mm Hg. An arterial saturation greater than 90% is needed to prevent tissue hypoxia and to preserve tissue cellular oxygenation.[6]

Physician consultation is indicated for patients with an Sao_2 of less than 92% on room air and failure to improve with nebulizer treatment given three times or epinephrine injection administered three times or to a peak flow of greater than 80% of predicted.

PATHOPHYSIOLOGY

Bronchospasm results when hyperreactivity of the airways, caused by inflammatory substances, produces airway bronchoconstriction, edema, and obstruction. On exposure to causative agents, substances that are released from basophils or mast cells lead to an allergic reaction that causes constriction and inflammation.[7] Airway hyperresponsiveness (AHR) occurs along with inflammation. AHR is the contraction of small muscles surrounding the airways, and this can limit the individual's ability to move air throughout the lungs.[8] The bronchospasm may be intermittent and resolve without treatment, or the obstruction may progress to respiratory arrest, with its potential for death.

CLINICAL PRESENTATION

Patient presentations can vary from mild anxiety to acute respiratory distress. Symptoms may occur spontaneously or be precipitated by a trigger.[5,6] The most common symptom of bronchospasm is wheezing. However, the patient with acute bronchospasm may have breathlessness, chest tightness, and coughing. Symptoms may vary in degree of severity.

A repetitive, spasmodic cough may be the only sign of bronchospasm. The patient's inability to speak a full sentence without pausing to breathe indicates severe bronchospasm. Patients' psychological states vary according to their previous experience with this condition and the severity of symptoms. Patients with a history of asthma may have experienced bronchospasm frequently and may even have come to accept this as a usual daily pattern, whereas patients who experience their first episode or a severe episode may understandably be anxious.

PHYSICAL EXAMINATION

The skin color of a patient with acute bronchospasm may be normal, flushed, or pale. The presence of pruritus or a rash suggests an allergic cause. In addition, the patient may have tachypnea, tachycardia, and a normal or slightly elevated blood pressure. Hypotension occurs in an allergic reaction with anaphylaxis. Pulsus paradoxus of greater than 25 mm Hg is a uniform indicator of severe respiratory compromise.[7]

The use of accessory muscles is noted as a sign of more severe bronchospasm. Wheezing may be audible or detected during auscultation on inspiration or expiration. The finding of a silent chest indicates severe spasm and is an ominous sign. With audible wheezing, the trachea should be auscultated to discern whether these sounds are indicative of laryngospasm or partial airway obstruction with a foreign body.

DIAGNOSTICS

Peak flow measurements will be less than expected for the patient's age and height or reduced from the patient's baseline. Pulse oximetry values below 90% in adults indicate more severe bronchospasm. ABG analysis is best performed in an emergency department.

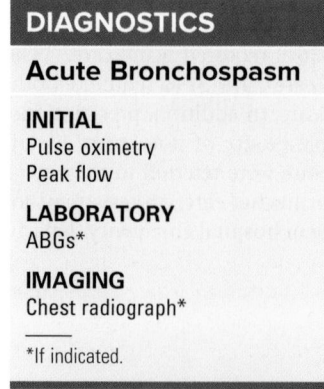

Chest radiographs may assist in determining the cause of the bronchospasm. With asthma or allergy, the chest radiograph can be normal or show hyperinflation. Serology may reveal eosinophilia and elevated immunoglobulin E levels, suggesting an allergic cause.

DIAGNOSTICS

Acute Bronchospasm

INITIAL
Pulse oximetry
Peak flow

LABORATORY
ABGs*

IMAGING
Chest radiograph*

*If indicated.

DIFFERENTIAL DIAGNOSIS

The history and clinical presentation indicate the origin of the respiratory failure. Potentially fatal conditions require immediate exclusion. The presence of a urticarial rash with decreasing blood pressure is a sign of anaphylaxis, necessitating immediate treatment with supplemental oxygen through nasal cannula or mask and diphenhydramine (Benadryl), 25 or 50 mg intravenously or intramuscularly; or epinephrine, 0.3 to 0.5 mg of a 1:1000 solution intramuscularly in the middle aspect of the thigh, anterolateral aspect for the adult patient.

Cardiac failure may manifest as bronchospasm in the setting of known cardiac disease. A history of paroxysmal nocturnal dyspnea associated with distended neck veins or pedal edema on examination confirms the diagnosis. Vascular redistribution or pleural effusion may be seen on chest radiographs, but treatment for cardiac failure should not be delayed to obtain chest radiographic studies.

Bronchospasm with acute dyspnea may herald impending respiratory failure in patients with chronic lung disease. Other causes of respiratory failure include depressed respiratory drive, pneumonia, atelectasis, asthma, airway obstruction, pulmonary edema, pulmonary hemorrhage, pulmonary contusion, and acute respiratory distress syndrome. Bronchospasm is also a potential complication of intubation during general anesthesia.

DIFFERENTIAL DIAGNOSIS

Acute Bronchospasm

- Airway obstruction
- Anaphylaxis
- Congestive heart failure
- Respiratory failure
- Pulmonary embolism
- Tremor
- Vocal cord dysfunction

Pulmonary embolization should be suspected when bronchospasm occurs in a patient at risk for a pulmonary embolus (i.e., smokers and patients with signs of vascular thrombosis, a history of atrial fibrillation, a history of oral contraceptive use, or other risk factors).

Recurrent bronchospasm or a poor response to bronchodilation medication indicates the need for reassessment and thorough evaluation for mechanical airway obstruction caused by anatomic changes or tumor as well as for vocal cord dysfunction, a missed case of heart failure, or pulmonary embolus.

INITIAL STABILIZATION AND MANAGEMENT

The ultimate goal of both expert care and patient self-management is to reduce the impact of acute bronchospasm and asthma on related morbidity, functional ability, and quality of life. Treatment goals include facilitating expectoration, eliminating airway irritation, and suppressing the stimulation of cough receptors.[9,10] Acute bronchospasm occurring in the setting of lower respiratory tract infection, asthma, or chronic obstructive pulmonary disease is initially managed by supplemental oxygen through nasal cannula or mask and inhalation of a beta agonist through a metered dose inhaler (MDI) or nebulizer. Short-acting beta$_2$ agonists include medications such as albuterol, levalbuterol (Xopenex), metaproterenol (Alupent), and pirbuterol (Maxair). Other medications include anticholinergics, such as ipratropium bromide (Atrovent), and systemic corticosteroids, such as methylprednisolone, prednisolone, and prednisone.

There are several delivery device mechanisms: MDIs, dry powdered inhalers, and spacer or valved holding chambers and nebulizers.[5] Treatment to reverse bronchospasm by an MDI (90 μg/puff) consists of 4 to 8 puffs of albuterol every 20 minutes up to 4 hours as long as tachycardia does not increase or palpitations are not precipitated by the treatments.[9] As an alternative, nebulizer treatments with 2.5 to 5 mg of albuterol can be administered every 20 minutes for up to three treatments, and then 2.5 to 10 mg every 1 to 4 hours as needed.[9] Alternatively, a continuous nebulizer treatment with albuterol at a rate of 10 to 15 mg/hr can be used.[8] For best results, the albuterol should be diluted with saline to a volume of at least 3 mL and delivered at an oxygen flow rate of 6 to 8 L/min.[9] Ipratropium bromide 0.5 mg may be added to the nebulizer solution with saline for administration every 30 minutes for three doses, then given every 2 to 4 hours as needed to augment and to prolong bronchodilation.

Investigations have centered on the alternative routes and procedures for albuterol administration. Endotracheal administration of albuterol has been used successfully in two case reports involving children.[11] Use of a resuscitator bag device as a spacer device for albuterol has been reported.[10] A continuous nebulizer treatment using albuterol at a rate of 7.5 mg/hr was found to be as effective as a rate of 15 mg/hr in cases of moderate to severe bronchospasm in one study.[11]

Worsening respiratory status, increased respiratory difficulty, decreasing pulse oximetry values, and failure to respond to beta agonist therapy indicate impending respiratory failure. The health care provider should be prepared to support respiration by intubation and mechanical ventilation while transferring the patient to the nearest emergency facility for other therapeutic modalities. Once acute bronchospasm is resolved, oral prednisone 60. No advantage has been found for the intravenous administration of steroids over oral administration, provided gastrointestinal transit time is not increased or absorption is not impaired.[5] Studies point to the efficacy of magnesium sulfate intravenously as an adjunct to treat acute bronchospasm.[6] Doses for intravenous magnesium sulfate reported in a meta-analysis ranged from 10 to 25 mg/kg with infusion during 20 minutes.[6] Studies also using nebulizer-administered lidocaine have shown it to be safe and effective in treating refractory cough.[10]

DISPOSITION AND REFERRAL

The health care provider should be acquainted with the capabilities of the local emergency medical services (EMS) system and have a plan for the emergency transport of patients. Patients who fail to respond to treatment or who do not improve with initial therapy should be transported to an emergency treatment facility.

PREVENTION AND PATIENT EDUCATION

Clinicians should take every opportunity to reinforce the patient's understanding of bronchospasm. Patient education should include reinforcing the difference between quick-release medications and long-term control medications, reviewing how to take medications correctly, reviewing device usage, and advising on how to avoid environmental exposures that trigger bronchospasm. Review of self-monitoring and an action plan benefits the patient's self-management skills to prevent or to control exacerbations and to reduce urgent care visits, hospitalizations, and health care costs.[9] In addition to regular assessment by a consistent clinician, a written action plan should be provided. Written action plans can be based on either symptoms or peak flow measurements when asthma is the cause of the bronchospasm. These written action plans should include three important concepts: (1) management of daily medications; (2) actions to control environmental factors that trigger bronchospasm; and (3) how to recognize symptoms and necessary actions to take when rescue medications fail. Several action plans are available from professional sources such as the National Institutes of Health and the American Lung Association.

The health care provider needs to be prepared to manage acute bronchospasm in the office setting and must have a plan for emergency medical support. Equipment and supplies needed in initial management of the patient include pulse oximetry, peak flow meters (disposable or capable of being decontaminated), beta-agonist inhalers (albuterol), anticholinergic medication (ipratropium), epinephrine, and oxygen. If an emergency department is not readily available, additional recommended supplies include a handheld nebulizer, parenteral steroids, intravenous access capability, and intubation equipment.

When evaluating the patient in primary care, the clinician should also address preventive health care measures. Patient and family education includes the importance of yearly influenza vaccination, good handwashing practice, avoidance of those who are sick, maintenance of optimal weight, and smoking cessation if indicated. In addition, for those patients taking corticosteroids, bone density measurement should be performed, and calcium with vitamin D supplementation should be prescribed.[5]

CHAPTER 25

ANAPHYLAXIS

Karen S. Abate

DEFINITION AND EPIDEMIOLOGY

Anaphylaxis is an acute life-threatening systemic event associated with exposure to an allergen. Manifestations of a hypersensitive anaphylactic reaction occur across multiple organ systems, including the cardiovascular, respiratory, integumentary, gastrointestinal, and central nervous systems. Reactions may occur within seconds to days after exposure to the offending allergen.[1,2] It is imperative that an anaphylactic reaction be immediately recognized and treated appropriately to prevent an untoward outcome. It is estimated that in the United States the prevalence of anaphylaxis is 1.6% or greater.[3] Common offending allergens include food, medication, insect venom, latex, occupational or inhaled allergens, radiocontrast media, cold air, exercise, heat, blood products, and potentially any substance (Box 25-1).[1-3]

BOX 25-1

Potential Anaphylaxis-Inducing Allergens

Foods
- Peanuts
- Tree nuts (walnuts, almonds, hazelnuts, Brazil nuts)
- Shellfish (lobster, shrimp)
- Fin fish (tuna, salmon, cod)
- Cow milk
- Eggs
- Soy
- Wheat
- Preservatives

Drugs
- β-Lactam antibiotics
- Penicillin
- Cephalosporin
- Vancomycin
- Ciprofloxacin
- Angiotensin-converting enzyme inhibitors
- Insulin
- Nonsteroidal anti-inflammatory drugs
- Vaccines (rare)
- Aspirin
- Vitamin K
- Ibuprofen
- Anesthetics
- Oversulfated chondroitin sulfate–contaminated heparin
- Contrast media (iodine, fluorescein)
- Blood products

Insect venom
- Bees
- Wasps
- Hornets
- Yellow jackets
- Fire ants

Latex

Allergen immunotherapy injections

Occupational allergens (various chemicals, hair dye)

Red meat

Inhaled allergens (animal dander, grass, pollen)

Nonimmunologic triggers
- Cold air
- Cold water
- Exercise
- Heat
- Radiation
- Ethanol
- Exercise

No known cause

PATHOPHYSIOLOGY

An anaphylactic reaction occurs when there is a rapid release of immunoglobulin E in an immune hypersensitivity reaction, resulting in the activation of mast cells and basophils.[4,5] On activation, histamine, platelet-activating factor, prostaglandins, leukotriene, and heparin are released.[4-6] The clinical presentation is reflective of the systemic effects of these inflammatory mediators. The release of histamine stimulates vasodilation, increases vascular permeability, increases heart rate and force of contraction, and increases glandular secretions.[5] The release of prostaglandins results in bronchoconstriction, coronary vasoconstriction, and peripheral vasodilation.[5] Leukotriene release further stimulates bronchoconstriction and increases vascular permeability.[5] The result can be a potentially life-threatening upper or lower airway obstruction causing bronchospasm, hypoxemia, or respiratory distress. All of these, as well as vascular collapse and angioedema (Fig. 25-1), are indicative of a severe reaction.

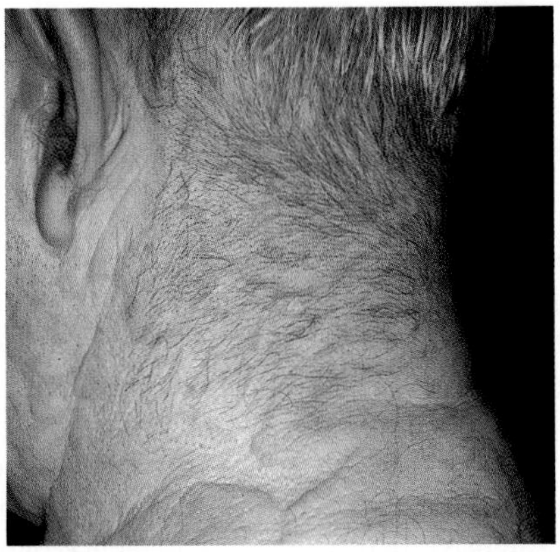

FIGURE 25-1 Angioedema affects the face, lips, palms, soles, or a portion of the extremity. It may become confluent and cover wide areas. The color is uniform. Hives vary in color. (From Habif TP, Campbell JL, Chapman MS, et al: *Skin disease: diagnosis and treatment*, ed 3, St Louis, 2011, Saunders.)

PHYSICAL EXAMINATION AND CLINICAL PRESENTATION

Anaphylactic reactions differ in how long they take to manifest. Uniphasic and biphasic reactions can occur anywhere from minutes to up to 10 hours after exposure.[1,2] Protracted reactions can be severe, lasting from 24 to 32 hours.[1,2] The intensity of previous hypersensitivity reactions is not an indication of intensity of subsequent occurrences.[1] In addition, clinical presentation may vary in severity from pruritic dermal rashes to more severe systemic manifestations. A comprehensive history and physical examination are invaluable. This information should be obtained from the patient as well as the family and those who have witnessed an anaphylactic event whenever possible.[2] The clinician must determine the following:

- History of past reactions
- Significant past medical history
- Travel history
- Detailed past and current exposure history
- Presence of risk factors
- Onset and severity of presenting symptoms
- Medications or herbal supplements used
- Alternative or home remedies implemented
- Recent activities
- Food and drug consumption over last several hours

PHYSICAL EXAMINATION

The rapid and accurate identification of anaphylaxis is imperative. The presentation of an individual having an anaphylactic reaction depends on the organ system affected. Physical findings related to the cardiovascular system and associated increases in vascular permeability may include tachycardia, hypotension, arrhythmias, or cardiopulmonary arrest. Pulmonary examination may reveal bronchospasm, hoarseness, wheezing, dyspnea, or nasal congestion. The oropharynx should be examined for edema, itchy throat, or stridor.[1,2,7] Common findings include the presence of angioedema, erythema, pruritus, and cutaneous wheals.[1,2,7] These cutaneous manifestations can be localized or systemic; therefore the entire body surface area should be examined. Angioedema, coryza, syncope, nausea, cramping, vomiting, vertigo, flushing, and weakness may also occur.[1,2,7] Central nervous system manifestations can include headache, confusion, and a sense of unease.[7] Any of these manifestations can occur at various times after allergen exposure based on whether the reaction is uniphasic, biphasic, or protracted.[1,2]

DIAGNOSTICS

Diagnostics should be used to monitor as well as to eliminate any other conditions that may mimic this presentation.

DIAGNOSTICS

Anaphylaxis

INITIAL
Pulse oximetry
Electrocardiogram (ECG)

LABORATORY
ABGs
24-Hour urine specimen for *N*-methylhistamine*
Plasma histamine level*: to confirm anaphylaxis
Serum or urinary tryptase level*: to confirm anaphylaxis

IMAGING
Chest radiograph

*If indicated.

- Cardiac monitoring and pulse oximetry should be used to monitor cardiopulmonary status.
- Analysis of arterial blood gases (ABGs) can be used to exclude a pulmonary embolism, foreign body obstruction, or acute asthma attack.
- Chest x-ray examination is indicated for patients with underlying pathologic processes or respiratory compromise.
- Electrocardiography is beneficial for individuals with chest pain or cardiac symptoms.
- Common laboratory tests are not helpful in the diagnosis of anaphylaxis except as indicated.[2]

DIFFERENTIAL DIAGNOSIS

The diagnosis of anaphylaxis is based on clinical presentation, history, and physical examination. In children, clinicians should consider foreign body aspiration, congenital malformations, or sudden infant death syndrome. Acute asthma, syncope, panic or anxiety attack, pulmonary embolism, and vasovagal reaction should be considered. Inflammatory mediators can cause coronary artery spasms that can resemble a myocardial infarction.

MANAGEMENT

Immediate emergency department referral or physician consultation is indicated for patients with angioedema, respiratory distress, and vascular collapse.

In an emergent anaphylactic reaction, it is imperative to assess and to maintain airway patency. Continuous maintenance of airway, breathing, circulation, and level of consciousness is vital. Monitoring of vital signs and mental status is essential. Individuals experiencing an anaphylactic event must be immediately transported to a local emergency facility, and physician consultation should be obtained. Intravenous access must be promptly established and isotonic saline administered to support volume expansion. If it is not contraindicated,

DIFFERENTIAL DIAGNOSIS

Anaphylaxis

- Asthma
- Syncope
- Panic attack or anxiety
- Pulmonary embolism
- Vasovagal reaction
- Myocardial infarction
- Metastatic carcinoid
- Postprandial syndromes
- Hyperventilation syndromes
- Hypoglycemia
- Seizure disorders
- Septic shock
- Cardiogenic shock
- Hypovolemic shock
- Foreign body aspiration, acute poisoning, congenital malformation, and sudden infant death syndrome in children

supplemental oxygen should be administered, and preparation should be made for potential endotracheal intubation as warranted.

Epinephrine is always first-line treatment of choice in an anaphylactic event because of the maximum pharmacodynamic effect that occurs within 10 minutes of administration in the lateral aspect of the thigh.[1,2,7]

Epinephrine dose for adults:

- Aqueous epinephrine: 1:1000 dilution (1 mg/mL), 0.2 to 0.5 mg intramuscularly in the anterolateral aspect of the mid thigh as the preferred site. Repeat every 5 minutes as needed to a maximum dose of 1 mg.

Epinephrine dose for children and infants:

- Aqueous epinephrine: 1:1000 dilution (1 mg/mL), 0.01 mg/kg per dose in children, maximum of 0.3 mg, intramuscularly or subcutaneously; repeat every 5 to 20 minutes as needed with a maximum dose of 0.3 mg.[2]
- The maximum dose for adolescents is 0.5 mg.[7]

Intramuscular injection in the mid-anterolateral thigh (vastus lateralis) is preferred. The vastus lateralis provides for faster absorption and less variability than a subcutaneous injection. Endotracheal epinephrine administration can be used if intravenous access is unattainable.

H_1 and H_2 antagonists are commonly used as a second line of treatment for less severe or cutaneous anaphylactic reactions but should not ever be used as a first-line modality.[2] For adults, diphenhydramine 25 to 50 mg may be given parenterally; the dose for children would be 1 to 2 mg/kg.[2]

The use of ranitidine as a second-line agent may be considered, as well. Ranitidine 50 mg for adults and 1 mg/kg for children intravenously over 5 minutes is appropriate.[2] The use of ranitidine and diphenhydramine in combination has demonstrated improved efficacy over stand-alone therapy. Once again, this would be a second-line therapy and should not be used alone in the treatment of anaphylaxis.[2]

If respiratory symptoms persist after administration of epinephrine, the administration of inhaled $beta_2$ agonists may be useful.[2] These will not have any effect on obstruction or shock; however, they can be useful with bronchospasm. Identification and removal of the offending allergen are imperative.

COMPLICATIONS

Most individuals recover from an anaphylactic event without incident; however, monitoring for sequelae is warranted.

INDICATIONS FOR REFERRAL OR HOSPITALIZATION

Any individual having an anaphylactic reaction should be immediately transported to an emergency facility for treatment monitoring and should be observed for 6 to 8 hours relative to the reaction type to monitor for additional incidents or complications.[1] Individuals with severe anaphylactic reactions or cardiovascular or respiratory compromise should be observed for a more extensive period in the emergency department or admitted to the hospital as warranted.

Follow-up with a primary care provider is recommended. In addition, referral to an allergist or immunologist is warranted for potential identification of triggers and the development of appropriate treatment plans.[1,2]

LIFE SPAN CONSIDERATIONS

Vigilant lifetime avoidance of the precipitating allergen is the primary goal. Management of comorbid disorders is advisable.

EDUCATION AND HEALTH PROMOTION

All individuals who have experienced or are at risk for anaphylaxis should wear a medical identification bracelet. Printed information should be provided about trigger identification and avoidance.[2] Instruction should be provided surrounding reading food labels to determine potential allergen exposures in processed food. Children should have an emergency action plan in place in schools, camps, and other regularly attended places. In addition, individuals attending college should be in close contact with campus health services, staff, and faculty to develop an emergency treatment plan.[7]

All at-risk individuals should be equipped with at least two epinephrine auto-injectors.[1,2,7] Epinephrine auto-injectors are commercially available devices that provide a single premeasured epinephrine dose; they should be prescribed for individuals with a known history of allergen sensitivity or past anaphylactic reaction. Instruction in proper use is key. It is imperative that patients, friends, family, coworkers, and others understand that epinephrine auto-injectors should be used without delay before emergency personnel assistance arrive on the scene.[1,2,7]

Epinephrine auto-injectors come in two fixed doses: 0.15 mg and 0.3 mg. The 0.15-mg dose is appropriate for use in young children weighing 15 to 30 kg.[7] For children weighing 30 kg or more, the 0.3-mg auto-injector should be prescribed.[7] Injection can be repeated with one additional dose. There is no commercially available auto-injector preparation for children weighing less than 10 kg.[8]

For adults, the 0.3-mg auto-injector should be prescribed for one-time use intramuscularly. Injection can be repeated with one dose.

Most states allow students and children to self-carry an epinephrine auto-injector with proper consent and a prescription.[7] It is recommended that providers and patients check their own state regulations.

The American Academy of Allergy, Asthma, and Immunology recommends the development of an individual emergency action plan for those at risk for anaphylaxis.[1]

CHAPTER 26

BITES AND STINGS

Joanne Sandberg-Cook

INSECT BITES AND STINGS

DEFINITION AND EPIDEMIOLOGY

More species of insects are in existence than any other form of multicellular life. Insects that bite and infest include mosquitoes, flies, bedbugs, kissing bugs, fleas, lice, blister beetles, centipedes, millipedes, scabies, chiggers, and ticks. Stinging insects include vespids, bees, and ants. The medical importance of insects is that they bite, sting, and envenomate; they are vectors for infectious pathogens, and they cause hypersensitivity reactions. Insect bites and stings can cause toxic reactions that range from local and mild to life-threatening.

Immediate emergency department referral or physician consultation is indicated for anaphylaxis and suspected black widow or brown recluse spider bites.

PATHOPHYSIOLOGY AND CLINICAL PRESENTATION

Although many insect bites and stings are simply a nuisance, some patients can have severe skin or systemic reactions. Vespids (yellow jackets, hornets, and wasps), bees (honeybees and bumblebees), and ants inject venom with a stinger. The sting results in immunoglobulin E–mediated systemic reactions that cause the release of mediators (histamines, the slow-reacting substance of anaphylaxis, and eosinophil chemotactic factors of anaphylaxis)[1] from mast cells, culminating in local inflammation involving many cell types and numerous mechanisms.[2]

These stings induce local, toxic, systemic, and delayed reactions. A local reaction consists of erythema, edema, and pruritus at the sting site. A toxic reaction is initially seen as gastrointestinal distress, lightheadedness, syncope, headache, fever, drowsiness, muscle spasms, edema, and occasionally seizures. A systemic reaction is anaphylaxis, which initially manifests as itchy eyes, facial flushing, generalized urticaria, and dry cough. Anaphylaxis can quickly intensify to respiratory distress, and it may deteriorate to respiratory or cardiovascular failure. A delayed reaction can occur 10 to 14 days after the sting and cause fever, malaise, headache, urticaria, lymphadenopathy, polyarthritis, or more systemic autoimmune illnesses (i.e., leukocytoclastic vasculitis or Henoch-Schönlein purpura).[2] Table 26-1 describes the pathophysiology and clinical presentation of other insect bites and stings.

PHYSICAL EXAMINATION

The initial assessment of bites and stings should determine any compromise in airway, breathing, and circulation (i.e., evidence of anaphylaxis). A thorough examination of the bite or sting and surrounding area should be made to determine the extent of envenomation and any associated infection.

TABLE 26-1 Summary of Insect Bites and Stings

Insect	Clinical Presentation	Pathophysiology
Wasps, bees, ants, hornets, yellow jackets	Local reaction Toxic reaction Systemic reaction Delayed reaction	Inject venom with stinger
Fire ants	Papule progressing to sterile pustule in 6-24 hours	Inject venom with stinger
Mosquitoes, flies	Pruritic, painful papule Secondary infection common	Inject salivary material
Bedbugs, kissing bugs	Clustered, erythematous, pruritic nodules	Painlessly suck blood
Fleas	Pruritic grouped welts, papules, vesicles Secondary infection common	Deposit saliva in bite
Lice	Pruritus Nits in scalp, body, or pubic hair	Deposit saliva in bite
Blister beetles	Large blisters	Release hemolymph
Centipedes	Pain and itching with local necrosis	Inject venom with fangs
Millipedes	Brown-stained area with blistering	Excrete toxic chemicals
Scabies	Burrow lesion with pruritus Secondary infection common	Burrow in epidermis
Chiggers	Pruritic papules or vesicles Secondary infection common	Release digestive substances in bite
Ticks	Pruritic papule with tick present Secondary infection common	Attach to victim with painless bite

DIAGNOSTICS

Adults with systemic allergic reactions should be considered for venom immunotherapy, which is successful in virtually all patients. The diagnosis of insect sting allergy can be made on the basis of a history of anaphylaxis with a sting and/or positive skin test results.[1] Otherwise, no specific laboratory evaluation is required unless it is indicated by the clinical course.

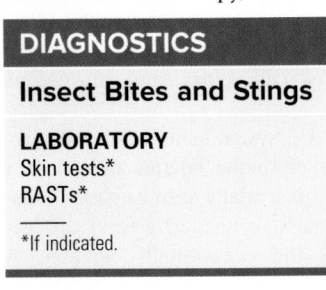

DIAGNOSTICS

Insect Bites and Stings

LABORATORY
Skin tests*
RASTs*

*If indicated.

DIFFERENTIAL DIAGNOSIS

The diagnosis of all insect bites and stings is made by obtaining a careful history. It is helpful if the patient brings in the insect. Insect bites are commonly confused with contact dermatitis and viral exanthems. Flea bites may resemble varicella. Reactions to blister beetles may resemble bullous impetigo and burns. Because of such similarities, a history of exposure may be the only diagnostic clue.[3]

DIFFERENTIAL DIAGNOSIS

Insect Bites and Stings

- Contact dermatitis
- Varicella
- Viral exanthems
- Bullous impetigo
- Burns

INITIAL STABILIZATION AND MANAGEMENT

The management of all insect bites and stings begins with local wound care, including removal of the stinger and the use of ice packs, antihistamines (H_1 and H_2 blockers) for itching, topical steroids for inflammation, topical or systemic antibiotics for secondary infection, and nonsteroidal anti-inflammatory drugs to relieve discomfort.[3] Any evidence of a systemic reaction must be treated as anaphylaxis.

Management also includes eradication of the insect. For flea infestation, it is necessary to vacuum thoroughly, treat pets, wash the rugs and beds, and use an insecticide. Lice and scabies are eradicated by applying 1% lindane lotion or shampoo (Kwell, Scabene) on two consecutive nights. Permethrin (Nix, Elimite) is another effective scabies treatment. Longstanding or crusted scabies infestation may require oral Ivermectin.

Bedbugs have become an increasingly prevalent problem in institutional settings including dormitories, assisted-living and nursing home facilities, and hotels. These pests are difficult to eradicate and travel easily, "hitching" rides in suitcases and sleeping bags. Although their bites do not carry disease and often go unnoticed, they can cause significant psychological and economic distress.[4]

Ticks are effectively removed with blunt, angled, medium-tipped forceps or a specific tick-removal instrument. The tick should be removed as soon as possible by grasping it close to the mouth, flipping the tick so the backside is closest to the skin, and pulling the tick straight up.[5] After removal of the tick, the health care provider should inspect the bite area for retained mouth parts, remove if possible, then carefully clean the area with an antiseptic.[5] Antibiotic prophylaxis may be indicated where Lyme disease is endemic or if the length of time the tick has been imbedded is not known. A tick needs to be embedded and feeding for more than 36 hours to infect with Lyme disease (see Chapter 234).

DISPOSITION AND REFERRAL

Systemic reactions to bites and stings may be life-threatening. Thus, any systemic or anaphylactic reaction requires a referral to the emergency department for definitive management including epinephrine and antihistamines and possible hospitalization.

PREVENTION AND PATIENT EDUCATION

Preventive management against bites and stings includes avoidance and protective clothing. Repellents can be used, including diethyltoluamide (DEET), dimethyl phthalate, dimethyl carbate, ethyl hexanediol, butopyronoxyl (Indalone), and benzyl benzoate.[6] Any person with a history of anaphylaxis from wasp or bee stings should be given medical warning tags, epinephrine injector kits, and a referral to an allergist or immunologist for venom immunotherapy.[1,7,8]

Bedbugs are becoming a more serious problem worldwide, probably because of increasing global travel and resistance to insecticides. Bedbugs are not known to carry any pathogen but cause significant emotional and psychological distress, qualifying them as serious pests. Sleeplessness is a common problem for people in known infested settings. Because bedbugs are visible, travelers should be advised to look for them in the crevices of mattresses, behind headboards, and in the folds of bed linens and curtains. Luggage should be thoroughly vacuumed and cleaned if it is suspected of being infested. Clothing and bed linens are washed in hot water and dried on the hottest setting the fabric can withstand to eradicate the bedbugs. Serious infestations should be managed by professional exterminators.[4]

SPIDER BITES

DEFINITION AND EPIDEMIOLOGY

More than 45,000 species of spiders, very few of which are medically important to humans, are found worldwide.[9] In the United States, problems are caused by the bites of only two spiders: brown recluse spiders and black widow spiders.[9] Most bites thought to be spider bites are actually caused by other insects. However, urticating hairs of the tarantula can be associated with stinging, inflammation, and even anaphylaxis.[10]

The brown recluse spider is a six-eyed nocturnal spider that avoids people. Its bite is always unintentional. It is yellow, brown, or black with thin legs that are five times the body length; the entire spider is approximately the size of a quarter. It has a violin-shaped marking on its back. A native of the United States, it is commonly found in the central Midwest south to the Gulf of Mexico. These spiders do travel in boxes and packages, exposing people in other parts of the country to potential bites. In its natural environment, the brown recluse spider is found in warm, dry areas such as abandoned buildings, woodpiles, and cellars.[1]

The female black widow spider is the most venomous of all spiders and has a body size of approximately 1.5 cm.[1] This spider is found in temperate climates all over the world. In the

United States, although they are seen everywhere, they are most common in the South and West. Despite the name *black widow,* these spiders may be black, brown, tan, or variegated.[9] The classic orange-red, hourglass-shaped marking is actually found on only one species *(Latrodectus mactans)* and may be merely an indistinct yellow or orange spot. The male spider is only one third the size of the female; its bite cannot penetrate human skin. Black widow spiders are aggressive toward other insects; humans are not their usual prey, and bites tend to be defensive only. They tend to live in basements, gardens, woodpiles, and garages.[1]

PATHOPHYSIOLOGY AND CLINICAL PRESENTATION

The venom of the brown recluse spider is chemotactic, which results in endothelial injury and subsequent thrombosis.[9] It is a neurotoxin that causes the release of acetylcholine and norepinephrine at the neurosynaptic junction.[2] The bite of the brown recluse spider is almost painless and most commonly manifests as a mild, erythematous lesion that may become firm and then heal during several days to weeks. The bite can also be more severe, causing erythema, blistering, and a bluish discoloration within 24 hours and possibly becoming necrotic within 3 to 4 days. The lesions can vary in size from 1 to 30 cm and take 6 weeks to 4 months to heal. The victim may have a systemic response and experience fevers, chills, nausea, vomiting, myalgia, arthralgia, petechiae, hemolysis, or seizures within 24 to 48 hours of the bite. Severe systemic manifestations can lead to hemoglobinuria, renal failure, disseminated intravascular coagulation, and death.[9]

The bite of the black widow spider is mildly to moderately painful; erythema, swelling, and muscle cramps begin at the site within 30 minutes to 12 hours. The muscle cramping progresses to large muscle groups and the abdomen and can mimic peritonitis. The muscle pain can subside in a few hours but can flare during the following 2 to 3 days, with muscle weakness and intermittent spasms persisting for weeks to months. Hypertension can be a serious complication. Anxiety or confusion can also occur. Severe envenomation may lead to shock, coma, or respiratory failure secondary to muscle paralysis. The bite is fatal only to small children or frail elders.[9]

HISTORY AND PHYSICAL EXAMINATION

The history and physical examination of the patient should be thorough. The history is important to elicit associated symptoms such as fever, nausea, or pain in addition to information on when and where the suspected bite occurred. In areas where spider bites are not endemic, a recent history of travel should be determined if a spider bite is suspected. It is most helpful if the actual spider is captured and brought for identification.

The primary survey should determine any compromise of the airway, breathing, or circulation (i.e., evidence of anaphylaxis). Assessment of vital signs and a thorough examination, including a careful evaluation of the bite and surrounding area, are then necessary to determine the extent of envenomation and any associated infection.

DIAGNOSTICS

If a brown recluse spider bite is suspected, complete blood count (CBC), blood urea nitrogen (BUN), electrolytes, blood glucose, creatinine, coagulation profile, and urinalysis (for hemoglobinuria) should be ordered. No specific laboratory tests are indicated for a suspected black widow spider bite.[1] However, CBC, urinalysis, BUN, creatinine, glucose, electrolytes, and an acute abdominal series may be indicated because the presentation may mimic an acute abdomen.

DIAGNOSTICS

Spider Bites

LABORATORY (BROWN RECLUSE)
CBC and differential
Serum electrolytes
BUN
Serum glucose
Creatinine
Coagulation profile
Urinalysis

LABORATORY (BLACK WIDOW) (TO DISTINGUISH BITE FROM ACUTE ABDOMEN)
CBC and differential
Serum electrolytes
BUN
Creatinine
Serum glucose
Urinalysis

DIFFERENTIAL DIAGNOSIS

Brown recluse and black widow spider bites should be included in the differential diagnosis of any spider bite. However, the diagnosis of either of these spider bites can be difficult, especially in the absence of the actual spider. Very few necrotic skin lesions are the result of a spider bite. The unusual presentation of acute abdominal pain requires that all causes of acute abdomen be considered in the differential diagnosis.

DIFFERENTIAL DIAGNOSIS

Spider Bites

- All spider bites
- All causes of acute abdominal pain

INITIAL STABILIZATION AND MANAGEMENT

The bite of the brown recluse spider requires no medications, and no antivenom is currently available. Tetanus prophylaxis and supportive measures should be provided. Antibiotics are indicated only if infection is suspected. Pain relief may be required in some cases. Daily wound care is important for necrotic lesions, and surgical debridement may be required for necrotic lesions larger than 2 cm.[1]

The initial therapy for black widow spider bites is basic supportive care—airway, breathing, and circulation. Local wound care and tetanus prophylaxis should always be provided. Narcotic analgesics, benzodiazepines, and calcium gluconate are all effective means of pain relief and muscle relaxation. Antivenom is available and reasonably safe but only moderately effective.[9] Antivenom is indicated only for a confirmed severe bite because of the risk of anaphylaxis and serum sickness, and it can be given only to patients who have not previously had exposure to horse serum.[9]

The wolf spiders, of which the tarantula is the most common, cause bites the equivalent of a wasp sting without necrosis. These bites usually require only supportive care.[3]

DISPOSITION AND REFERRAL

Adults and children with evidence of significant systemic reactions should be referred for hospitalization and close observation. Patients with black widow spider bites that require antivenom should always be referred to the emergency department or for hospital admission.

PREVENTION AND PATIENT EDUCATION

Everyone in endemic areas should be taught to recognize the brown recluse spider and to avoid its habitats. Clothing, bed linens, attics, closets, and woodpiles should be examined closely in endemic areas because the spider is aggressive only if it is forced into contact with humans.[9]

Black widow spiders are more commonly found in their webs at night. Therefore, the webs should be cleaned cautiously at night and the spider mechanically destroyed. Professional exterminators are indicated for heavy infestations. Everyone in endemic areas should be taught to recognize the black widow spider. Protective sleeves and gloves are recommended in handling wood and brush in infested areas.[11]

REPTILE BITES AND SCORPION STINGS

DEFINITION AND EPIDEMIOLOGY

In the United States, the venomous snakes include the pit vipers and coral snakes. Pit vipers include rattlesnakes, copperheads, cottonmouths (water moccasins), and bushmasters. Worldwide, 100,000 to 125,000 deaths occur each year from snake bites, but in the United States, 5000 snakebites are reported annually.[12] Only one third to one half of these are caused by venomous snakes. The most severe envenomations tend to occur with rattlesnakes, but copperheads, coral snakes, and snakes imported from other countries and kept as pets are other causes of snakebites. Of the venomous snakebites, 20% result in no envenomation and 40% result in only mild envenomation.[13]

Other reptiles to consider are Gila monsters, which are slow-moving lizards in the deserts of the southwestern United States. Medically significant scorpion stings also occur in the southwestern United States from the bark scorpion (so named because it often lives under the bark of trees).[14]

PATHOPHYSIOLOGY

The venom of the pit viper is a complex mixture of cytotoxic, hemotoxic, and neurotoxic enzymes that cause local tissue injury, systemic vascular damage, hemolysis, fibrinolysis, and neuromuscular dysfunction.[12] Coral snake venom is neurotoxic.[12] Gila monster venom is as toxic as rattlesnake venom, but Gila monsters lack the apparatus to effectively inject it; they have short, grooved teeth, and therefore a prolonged bite is required for envenomation.[12] Scorpion venom is primarily neurotoxic and is composed of proteins and polypeptides that activate sodium channels to produce a hyperadrenergic state.[14]

CLINICAL PRESENTATION

The history is particularly important in identifying the type of bite. An attempt should be made to determine whether the bite is venomous. Venomous rattlesnakes have fangs, whereas nonvenomous rattlesnakes do not.[12,13] Poisonous coral snakes also have fangs and are easily identified by their red and yellow bands.[12] Information about associated symptoms, such as pain, dizziness, nausea, vomiting, or paresthesias, is important to elicit.

For the bites in which there is no envenomation, the only clinical finding is the puncture wound. The clinical picture of patients who are envenomated depends on several factors: the amount of venom introduced; the anatomic location of the bite; and the patient's size, age, and overall health. The bites are classified by the degree of envenomation: none, minimum, moderate, or severe. The presentation of no envenomation is minimum pain and no significant swelling. Minimum envenomation manifests as local swelling of less than 15 cm (6 inches) from the bite wound and no systemic manifestations. Moderate envenomation has local swelling of 15 to 30 cm (6 to 12 inches) with systemic signs and symptoms. Severe envenomation has local swelling of more than 30 cm with severe systemic signs and symptoms, including coagulation abnormalities.[13]

Coral snake bites resemble scratch marks and are somewhat painful. Patients are initially seen with neurologic symptoms such as tremors, salivation, dysarthria, diplopia, dysphagia, dyspnea, and seizures. These symptoms, which are usually delayed 1 to 6 hours or even up to 12 hours, may progress to respiratory muscle paralysis and death.[13] In most cases, the bite of the Gila monster causes only local pain and swelling that worsens during several hours and then subsides in the next several hours. Only occasionally will a systemic reaction occur, with weakness, lightheadedness, paresthesias, diaphoresis, or hypertension.[2] Scorpion stings may cause mild symptoms with only local pain or paresthesias, or they may progress to somatic or cranial nerve dysfunction. Cardiovascular dysfunction including conduction abnormalities can be seen. Autonomic nervous system symptoms including hypersalivation, hypotension, and diaphoresis can occur. Motor nerve effects include roving eye movements, fasciculations, dysphagia, and the autonomic effects of tachycardia and excessive secretions.[14]

PHYSICAL EXAMINATION

The physical examination of the patient should be thorough. First, any compromise of the airway, breathing, or circulation (i.e., anaphylaxis) should be determined. This is followed by assessment of vital signs; evaluation of the patient for bleeding; and thorough examination of the bite and surrounding area to determine the extent of envenomation, tissue damage, and associated lymphadenopathy. A careful neurologic examination and documentation are necessary initially and should be routinely repeated to assess for neurologic involvement.

DIAGNOSTICS

Several corroborating laboratory studies are needed, including CBC, coagulation studies, fibrinogen level, electrolytes, BUN, creatinine, and urinalysis. A type and crossmatch for blood, an arterial blood gas analysis, and an electrocardiogram are needed if the envenomation is severe.[14]

DIFFERENTIAL DIAGNOSIS

The diagnosis is made on the basis of a history of a snakebite or scorpion bite, with a clinical presentation consistent with envenomation. It is helpful if the victim can identify the snake or scorpion with use of a picture or photograph. Patients should

DIAGNOSTICS

Reptile Bites and Scorpion Stings

LABORATORY
CBC and differential
Coagulation studies: PT/PTT, clotting time
Fibrinogen level
Serum electrolytes
BUN
Creatine kinase
Creatinine
Urinalysis

PT, prothrombin time; PTT, partial thromboplastin time.

be discouraged from bringing the actual snake in for identification as snakes can reflexively bite immediately after death.

INITIAL STABILIZATION AND MANAGEMENT

First aid measures must be instituted first, but all patients bitten by venomous snakes or scorpions must be taken to a health care facility. First aid measures include retreating beyond striking range, remaining calm, immobilizing the extremity involved, minimizing physical activity, wiping the bite site, identifying the snake if it can be done safely, and closely observing the patient's respiratory status.[15] Incision of the wound, suction of the wound, and tourniquets are not recommended.[12] The limb should not be elevated above the level of the heart. In the prehospital or office setting, management includes providing advanced cardiac life support as appropriate, immobilizing the limb, establishing intravenous access, and administering oxygen. The wound should be cleaned and tetanus prophylaxis administered.[12]

The major determinant of the required therapy is the degree of envenomation; the mainstay of therapy for moderate to severe venomous snakebites is antivenom.[13] For Gila monsters, local wound care is probably sufficient and must include the removal of any teeth in the wound; no antivenom is available.[1] For scorpion bites, management is supportive with analgesics and wound care; there is antivenom for severe bites, but it is available only in Arizona and is rarely used.[14]

DISPOSITION AND REFERRAL

Because the clinical symptoms can be delayed, all bites by venomous snakes and scorpions need to be observed for a minimum of 12 hours. The patient must be in an emergency department or hospital setting in which antivenom is available. For snakebites, consultation with a physician or poison control center familiar with envenomation is always recommended.

PREVENTION AND PATIENT EDUCATION

Most snakebites occur in April through October when outdoor activities are popular. Snakes are most often found in tall grass or brush, rocky outcrops, fallen logs, swamps, and deep holes. Patients should be given the following advice:

- In an area where snakes are likely to live, walk with a stick tapping ahead of you to scare the snakes away.
- Watch where you step, swim, and sit when outdoors.
- Wear loose, long pants and high, thick leather or rubber boots.
- Shine a flashlight on your path when walking outside at night.
- Never handle a snake, even if you think it is dead. Recently killed snakes may still bite by reflex.
- Regularly trim hedges, keep your lawn mowed, and remove brush from your yard and any nearby vacant lots. This will reduce the number of places where snakes like to live.
- Don't allow children to play in vacant lots with tall grass and weeds.
- Always use tongs when moving firewood, brush, or lumber. This will safely expose any snakes that may be hidden underneath.
- Always sleep on a cot when camping.
- Be aware of snakes if you are swimming or wading in rivers, lakes, or other bodies of water (this includes areas covered with water because of flooding).
- Learn to identify poisonous snakes and avoid them.[16]

CHAPTER 27

BRADYCARDIA AND TACHYCARDIA

Terry Mahan Buttaro

BRADYCARDIA

DEFINITION AND EPIDEMIOLOGY

Absolute bradycardia is defined as a heart rate of less than 60 beats per minute. Athletes, older adults, and other individuals may have normally slow heart rates, and bradycardia may not be pathologic during sleep or after a Valsalva maneuver or other vagal stimulation.[1] Relative bradycardia occurs when the heart does not respond as expected to trauma, hypovolemia, or an infectious process.[1] Lyme borreliosis, malaria, and dengue fever are other possible causes.[2]

Numerous medications, cardiac disease, hypothyroidism, electrolyte abnormalities, sleep apnea, infections, increased intracranial pressure, hypothermia, hypoxemia, acidemia, and other disease states can also produce bradycardia. Asymptomatic bradycardia does not require urgent intervention. However, careful monitoring and therapy are indicated if the bradycardia causes symptoms (e.g., angina, change in mental status, dizziness associated with hypotension, hypertension, heart failure, or syncope) or if the bradycardia is related to type II second-degree (Mobitz type II) or third-degree atrioventricular (AV) block.

Immediate emergency department referral or physician consultation is indicated for patients with symptomatic bradycardia or Mobitz type II or third-degree heart block.

PATHOPHYSIOLOGY

Bradycardia may result from sinus node dysfunction or AV block.[3] Sinus node dysfunction can be a result of increased vagal tone, as seen in athletes or conditioned young people or in older adults as the result of underlying disease processes, medications, or toxicity.[4] AV block is also associated with various disease processes, including myocardial infarction, coronary artery spasm, digitalis toxicity, cardiac mesotheliomas, and infectious processes. Medications, particularly beta blockers and calcium channel blockers, may induce either sinus node or AV dysfunction.

CLINICAL PRESENTATION

Some symptoms may be nonspecific, but dizziness, fatigue, and syncope are complaints commonly identified with bradycardia.[3] Nausea, vomiting, and confusion have also been correlated with bradycardia. Any bradyarrhythmia associated with chest pain, shortness of breath, exercise intolerance, decreased level of consciousness, hypotension, seizure, congestive heart failure, or myocardial infarction is considered a prearrest condition. A careful symptom analysis and review of the patient's medical history, including allergies and prescribed and over-the-counter medications, is necessary to discern the cause of the bradycardia so that appropriate treatment can be initiated.

PHYSICAL EXAMINATION

Although associated symptoms will often guide the physical examination, a focused history and physical examination are necessary. The patient's level of responsiveness and vital signs (including temperature, blood pressure, pulse, respiratory rate, and oxygen saturation) are significant and should be continually reassessed. Hypotension, ventricular arrhythmias, and pulmonary congestion are serious signs indicating the need to identify the cardiac rhythm and to institute rapid, appropriate treatment.

DIAGNOSTICS

An electrocardiogram (ECG) is necessary for rhythm analysis and appropriate management. Further diagnostics are guided by the history and physical examination but can include drug levels, electrolyte values, glucose concentration, blood urea nitrogen (BUN) level, creatinine concentration, complete blood count (CBC), creatine kinase muscle-brain (CK-MB) fraction, troponin T or troponin I level, thyroid studies, and chest x-ray studies.

DIAGNOSTICS

Bradycardia

INITIAL
ECG

LABORATORY
Drug levels*
Serum electrolytes*
BUN*
Creatinine*
CK-MB*
Troponin T or I*
Serum glucose*
CBC and differential*
TSH*

OTHER
Chest radiograph*

*If indicated.
TSH, thyroid stimulating hormone.

DIFFERENTIAL DIAGNOSIS

Determination of the bradyarrhythmia and associated disease is essential for treatment. Herbals and medications can be a common cause of bradycardia, but infections, vasovagal syncope, myocardial infarction, digitalis toxicity, sick sinus syndrome, bradycardia-tachycardia syndrome, hypothyroidism, and other disease states are also possible reasons.[3]

DIFFERENTIAL DIAGNOSIS

Bradycardia

- Medication induced
- Infection
- Vasovagal syncope
- Myocardial ischemia or infarction
- Digitalis toxicity
- Sick sinus syndrome
- Hypothyroidism
- Bradycardia-tachycardia syndrome

INITIAL STABILIZATION AND MANAGEMENT

The American Heart Association recommends cardiac monitoring, intravenous access, and continuous assessment of the patient (including airway, breathing, vital signs, oxygen saturation, and supplementary oxygen) when indicated It is crucial to differentiate the symptoms caused by the bradycardia from those not related to the slow rate. No intervention is necessary if the patient is stable and asymptomatic, but continued monitoring is indicated to ensure the patient's well-being.

For correct identification of the cardiac rhythm, a 12-lead ECG is necessary. Patients with suspected myocardial infarction should be treated for acute coronary syndrome according to the 2010-2015 American Heart Association guidelines (with oxygen, if indicated; aspirin [162 to 325 mg chewed, if not aspirin allergic]; nitroglycerin; morphine; and, if appropriate, reperfusion therapy).[5]

Symptomatic patients with worsening clinical symptoms or prearrest conditions related to the bradycardia may require urgent intervention before a definitive underlying condition is identified. For adult patients with symptomatic bradycardia, especially if the bradycardia is associated with Mobitz type II second-degree heart block or third-degree heart block, the American Heart Association recommends atropine, 0.5 mg intravenously every 3 to 5 minutes (up to a total dose 3 mg), until a transcutaneous or transvenous pacer (class I intervention) is available.[5] However, atropine can induce cardiac ischemia, precipitate ventricular tachycardia (VT) or fibrillation, and be deleterious for patients with a history of cardiac transplantation.[5] In the presence of Mobitz type II second-degree heart block or third-degree heart block associated with wide-complex ventricular escape beats, atropine should be avoided and treatment with a transcutaneous or transvenous pacer applied as soon as possible.[5] Some defibrillator monitors may also have a transcutaneous pacer component.

If the bradycardia is drug induced (e.g., beta blocker or calcium channel blocker overdose), a pacer is not available, atropine is contraindicated, or the patient is unresponsive to atropine or pacing, intravenous epinephrine 2 to 10 μg/min can be used to treat critical bradycardia.[5] A dopamine infusion of 2 to 10 μg/kg/min can also improve cardiac output and increase blood pressure and may be used alone or in conjunction with an epinephrine infusion.[5]

DISPOSITION AND REFERRAL

Patients experiencing signs and symptoms related to bradyarrhythmias require constant reassessment and definitive management in an emergency department. Immediate transfer to an emergency center is required.

PREVENTION

Prevention, when possible, may avert complications or serious injury. Patients who complain of syncope, fatigue, or other symptoms that may be related to bradycardia require diagnostic assessment. A permanent pacemaker may be indicated for bradycardia associated with sinus node dysfunction and certain heart blocks (e.g., fascicular block or acquired AV block).[3,5,6]

PATIENT AND FAMILY EDUCATION

Patients should understand the importance of calling their health care provider if they experience syncope, lightheadedness, or a slow heart rate that hinders activities. In addition, patients and caregivers should know how to activate the emergency medical system (911) if these symptoms occur with chest discomfort or shortness of breath.

Careful explanation and supportive therapy will enhance patient and family understanding. These measures will also help allay the anxiety inherent in an emergent situation. Medication regimens, if associated with the bradyarrhythmias, should be reviewed to prevent misinterpretation.

TACHYCARDIA

DEFINITION AND EPIDEMIOLOGY

Tachycardia is described as a heart rate exceeding 100 beats per minute. Normal sinus tachycardia does not usually require medical intervention, but other tachyarrhythmias can result in hemodynamic compromise and warrant urgent treatment. A rapid assessment of airway, breathing, and circulation and a complete history, physical examination, and 12-lead ECG are indicated.

Asymptomatic individuals with tachycardia can have stable cardiac rhythms that do not require emergent treatment. Fever, nicotine, exercise, stimulants, medications, and anxiety can precipitate normal sinus tachycardia. Pregnancy, coronary heart disease, congestive heart failure, valvular heart disease, pulmonary embolus, pericardial disease, valvular disorders, ischemia, metabolic and electrolyte abnormalities, medications, toxins, infection, and volume depletion should be considered possible precipitants identified with atrial and ventricular arrhythmias as well as tachycardia.

Emergency department referral or physician consultation is indicated for new-onset atrial fibrillation, atrial flutter, sick sinus syndrome, VT, or supraventricular tachycardia (SVT).

PATHOPHYSIOLOGY

The pathology of tachycardia is varied. Sinus tachycardia is a normal physiologic response and should not be considered pathologic. Atrial fibrillation and flutter, the narrow-complex tachycardias (ectopic atrial tachycardia, multifocal atrial tachycardia, junctional tachycardia, and paroxysmal SVT), the stable wide-complex tachycardias of unknown type, and monomorphic-polymorphic VT are tachyarrhythmias that can cause hemodynamic instability (see Chapter 118). In narrow-complex tachycardia, such as paroxysmal tachycardia, the heart rate increases suddenly and rapidly and then decreases suddenly. The attack may last seconds or days, during which time the ventricular rate is rapid and regular, usually between 150 and 225 beats per minute. This pathologic condition is most likely related to an aberrant reentry involving the AV node, although an obscure bypass tract near the AV node may cause the aberrant conduction (as in Wolff-Parkinson-White syndrome).

Atrial fibrillation and atrial flutter are rhythm disturbances characterized by rapid atrial stimulation and varied ventricular response. In flutter, this can be a fleeting phenomenon. In fibrillation, it can be related to stress. However, atrial arrhythmias are commonly related to varied disease states. These include coronary heart disease, rheumatic fever, mitral stenosis, thyrotoxicosis, infection, metabolic abnormalities, pulmonary embolism, and chronic lung disease.

Whether monomorphic or polymorphic, VT is a rhythm disturbance that arises in the ventricles. The arrhythmia is life-threatening if the patient is pulseless, but the patient can be hemodynamically stable when VT is associated with a pulse.

CLINICAL PRESENTATION

Some tachyarrhythmias are well tolerated, but chest discomfort, anxiety, restlessness, shortness of breath, weakness, fatigue, dizziness, and palpitations are common presenting symptoms.[5] Any tachycardia associated with chest pressure, acute myocardial infarction or cardiac ischemia, alteration in consciousness, hypotension or shock, shortness of breath, dyspnea on exertion, heart failure, or dizziness requires emergency care and urgent synchronized cadioversion.[5] A careful history of the presenting event; past medical history; and review of allergies, medications, and excessive use of caffeine, alcohol, or stimulants can help determine whether an underlying pathologic condition is causing the tachycardia and will facilitate appropriate treatment.

PHYSICAL EXAMINATION

An ECG or "quick look" with a conventional or external defibrillator is necessary to determine the cardiac rhythm and presence of arrhythmias or ischemia. Because tachycardia can precipitate hemodynamic instability, cardiac monitoring and assessment of vital signs (including temperature, blood pressure, heart rate, respirations, and oxygen saturation) should be continuous. The physical examination should be focused and exact with particular attention to the patient's respiratory and oxygenation status, as tachycardia is frequently related to hypoxemia.[5] The assessment will help determine the precipitating pathologic condition, establish whether the patient is stable or unstable, and determine whether the tachycardia has precipitated serious signs and symptoms.

DIAGNOSTICS

Continuous assessment, cardiac monitoring, and a 12-lead ECG are necessary to identify the tachyarrhythmia and any deterioration in the patient's condition. A chest x-ray study and laboratory studies, including drug levels, electrolyte values, CBC, and thyroid studies, may also be indicated but are usually deferred to emergency department evaluation.

DIFFERENTIAL DIAGNOSIS

Atrial fibrillation, atrial flutter, narrow-complex tachycardias, stable wide-complex tachycardia of uncertain type, and VT are tachyarrhythmias with potentially serious consequences. The 2010–2015 American Heart Association guidelines for emergency cardiovascular care recommend classifying patients

DIAGNOSTICS

Tachycardia

INITIAL
ECG
Laboratory
Drug levels*
Serum electrolytes (serum sodium, potassium, chloride, CO_2, and magnesium), BUN, and creatinine*
CBC and differential*
TSH*

IMAGING
Chest radiograph*

*If indicated.

DIFFERENTIAL DIAGNOSIS

Tachycardia

- Alcohol abuse
- Anxiety
- Cocaine abuse
- Drug induced
- Energy drinks
- Hyperthyroidism
- Acute myocardial infarction
- Congestive heart failure
- Pulmonary embolus
- Hypotension
- Hypoxia
- Hypovolemia
- Infection
- Electrolyte disturbance
- Structural cardiac issues: Wolff-Parkinson-White syndrome

BOX 27-1

Cardioversion and Defibrillation of Unstable Patients with Tachycardia

ATRIAL FIBRILLATION
- Synchronized cardioversion with monophasic waveform: 100-200 J.*
- Synchronized cardioversion with biphasic waveform: 120-200 J.

ATRIAL FLUTTER
- Synchronized cardioversion with monophasic waveform: 200 J.* Increase as necessary in step increments.
- Synchronized cardioversion with biphasic waveform: 50 J.* Increase as necessary in step increments.

MONOMORPHIC VENTRICULAR TACHYCARDIA
- Synchronized cardioversion with monophasic waveform: 100 J.* Increase as necessary in step increments.
- Synchronized cardioversion with biphasic waveform: 100 J. Increase as necessary in step increments.

POLYMORPHIC VENTRICULAR TACHYCARDIA
- Treat as ventricular fibrillation with unsynchronized shocks.
- If monophasic defibrillator: one shock at 360 J, then resume chest compressions and CPR for five cycles before checking rhythm and delivering a repeated shock.
- If biphasic defibrillator: one shock at 120-200 J, then resume chest compressions and CPR for five cycles before checking rhythm and delivering a repeated shock.†

*If second shock is necessary, the number of joules can be increased as needed.
†The effective electrical dose for monophasic and biphasic defibrillators is unclear. With biphasic defibrillators, the effective waveform dose can vary from manufacturer to manufacturer.
CPR, cardiopulmonary resuscitation.
Data from Neumar RW, Otto CW, Link MS, et al: Part 8: adult advanced cardiovascular life support: 2010 American Heart Association guidelines for cardiopulmonary resuscitation and emergency cardiovascular care., *Circulation* 122(183):S729-S767, 2010.

as stable or unstable, identifying whether serious signs and symptoms are present, and determining whether the arrhythmia has caused these signs and symptoms.[5] Patients with unstable tachycardia may complain of chest discomfort, be hypotensive, or display cognitive changes or signs of shock.[5]

Identification of the tachycardia and its related pathologic condition is essential for appropriate treatment. For prevention of inappropriate therapy, the patient's condition and the etiology of the tachycardia should be carefully considered before treatment is initiated. Medications, pregnancy, hyperthyroidism, acute myocardial infarction, congestive heart failure, pulmonary embolus, hypotension, hypoxia, hypovolemia, infection, electrolyte abnormalities, and other disorders may precipitate a rapid heart rate and its resultant symptoms. Treatment of the specific disorder may result in resolution of the tachycardia.

INITIAL STABILIZATION AND MANAGEMENT

A 12-lead ECG, oxygen when indicated, and continuous monitoring of the patient's oxygen saturation and vital signs are critical. The ECG will permit identification of the tachycardia and enable appropriate treatment. Intravenous access with a large-bore catheter and isotonic normal saline solution (with the intravenous fluid running at "keep open rate" to maintain catheter patency) is recommended. Suction, intubation, and defibrillation equipment should be readily available.

In healthy patients, urgent cardioversion is rarely necessary when the heart rate is less than 150 beats per minute; but for patients with coronary artery disease or other comorbid illnesses, an elevated heart rate may cause significant compromise. Immediate synchronized cardioversion is indicated if the patient is unstable because of the tachycardia.[5] Consult with a physician experienced in advanced cardiac life support for synchronized cardioversion of unstable reentry SVT, unstable atrial flutter or fibrillation, unstable monomorphic VT, and polymorphic (irregular) tachycardia (Box 27-1). If the patient is stable, certain medications can also be used to treat specific tachyarrhythmias (Box 27-2).

The advanced cardiovascular life support guidelines do not recommend treatment of tachycardia if the patient is stable and does not have chest pressure, acute myocardial infarction, change in mental status, hypotension, shortness of breath, congestive heart failure, or other signs and symptoms indicating instability.[5] The underlying precipitant of the tachycardia should be determined and appropriate treatment initiated.

BOX 27-2

Medication Therapy for Patients with Stable Tachycardia

SINUS TACHYCARDIA

Treat underlying precipitant.

NARROW-COMPLEX QRS TACHYCARDIA

Reentry supraventricular rhythm; narrow-complex QRS (<0.12 sec) with or without P waves.

If vagal maneuvers are unsuccessful, consider adenosine 6 mg rapid intravenous (IV) push. If rhythm continues, give adenosine 12 mg IV rapid push. Reentry SVT is probable rhythm if the rhythm converts to normal sinus rhythm (patient will require monitoring for recurrence). If rhythm does not convert with adenosine by rapid IV push, reevaluate rhythm (consider atrial flutter, ectopic atrial tachycardia, or junctional tachycardia and treat with nondihydropyridine calcium channel blocker or beta blocker [use cautiously if patient has history of lung disease or congestive heart failure]). Amiodarone (150 mg IV over 10 min; can repeat every 10 min to maximum dose of 2.2 g) is also recommended for narrow-complex QRS tachycardias (reentry SVT rhythms) unresponsive to vagal maneuvers or adenosine.

IRREGULAR NARROW QRS TACHYCARDIA

Atrial fibrillation, atrial flutter, or multifocal atrial tachycardia.

Control rate with nondihydropyridine calcium channel blocker (diltiazem 0.25 mg/kg IV over 2 min [may repeat 0.35 mg/kg in 15 min if necessary]. The AHA/ACC/HRS 2014 guidelines for treatment of atrial fibrillation recommend a verapamil bolus 0.075 to 0.15 mg/kg IV over 2 minutes [may repeat with10 mg in -30 mg if necessaryfollowed by verapamil infusion 0.005 mg/kg/minute or metoprolol 2.5 TO 5 mg IV every 2 to 5 minutes. Maximum dose in 10 to 15 minutes is 15 mg.[9]). Beta blockers should be used cautiously if there is a history of lung disease or congestive heart failure.

REGULAR STABLE WIDE-COMPLEX TACHYCARDIA

QRS >0.12 sec.

This is most likely VT or SVT. If SVT, treat with adenosine (as in narrow-complex QRS tachycardia). If monomorphic, stable VT, treat with synchronized cardioversion or procainamide 20-50 mg/min. Procainamide therapy is discontinued if the arrhythmia resolves, the QRS is prolonged more than 50% compared with the original QRS, the patient develops hypotension, or the maximum dose is given (17 mg/kg). Amiodarone 150 mg IV over 10 min (may repeat if needed up to 2.2 g/24 hr) is an alternative antiarrhythmic, as is sotalol 1.5 mg/kg IV over 5 min. Sotalol is not appropriate for patients with QT prolongation.

POLYMORPHIC (IRREGULAR) VENTRICULAR TACHYCARDIA

Immediate defibrillation. Consider cause of polymorphic VT (e.g., ischemia, Brugada syndrome, torsades de pointes, or long QT syndrome) and treat appropriately.

Data from Neumar RW, Otto CW, Link MS, et al: Part 8: adult advanced cardiovascular life support: 2010 American Heart Association guidelines for cardiopulmonary resuscitation and emergency cardiovascular care. *Circulation* 122(183):S729-S767, 2010; and: January, CT, Wann, LS, Alpert, JS et al, AHA/ACC/HRS Guideline for the management of atrial fibrillation: A Report of the American College of Cardiology/American Heart Association Task Force on Practice Guidelines and the Heart Rhythm Society. 2014.

DISPOSITION AND REFERRAL

Ideally, symptomatic patients with tachycardia should be stabilized with initial management and transferred to the nearest emergency department. Immediate transfer by ambulance to an emergency department is indicated for patients requiring continued assessment and management.

PREVENTION AND PATIENT EDUCATION

Tachyarrhythmias often recur. Careful explanation of the specific disorder and how to recognize untoward symptoms is an important part of patient education. Because electrolyte disturbances and medications can precipitate some tachyarrhythmias, it is important that health care providers consider and review medication therapies regularly. Amiodarone or other antiarrhythmic medications, wearable defibrillators, implantable cardioverter-defibrillators, pacemakers, or ablation therapy may be indicated for the prevention of recurrent symptomatic tachycardia.[4-8]

CHAPTER 28

CARDIAC ARREST

Terry Mahan Buttaro

DEFINITION AND EPIDEMIOLOGY

According to the American Heart Association (AHA), 17.3 million people in the world die each year from heart disease.[1] In the United States, cardiovascular disease is the cause of one of three deaths annually, and it is important to realize that out-of-hospital sudden deaths affect children as well as adults and elders.[1] What is startling is that most sudden deaths in young athletes are related to cardiovascular disease.[1] The majority of these events (82%) in young athletes occur during physical exertion while training or participating in competitive sports.[1] Unfortunately, despite the important research and information available about coronary artery disease (CAD), our efforts to combat this disease and provide education on cardiopulmonary resuscitation (CPR), sudden cardiac death remains a significant cause of cardiac-related death. Only 10.6 % of those who have an out-of-hospital cardiac arrest survive, and only 8.3% have good neurologic outcomes.[1] If the event is witnessed, one of three victims of sudden cardiac arrest survives.[1] Equally concerning is the awareness that the incidence of out-of-hospital arrest and survival is less for blacks and Hispanics than for whites.[1]

Many out-of-hospital cardiac arrest victims seem symptom free before the event occurs, and, surprisingly, only 23% have a shockable cardiac rhythm (i.e., ventricular tachycardia, ventricular fibrillation) when the cardiac arrest occurs.[2] The importance of immediate cardiac resuscitation is evident, particularly because survival rates for out-of-hospital arrests continue to be low.[2]

Whether cardiac arrest occurs in the hospital, in the office, or in the community, resuscitative efforts should be initiated immediately.[3] Trained health care professionals should immediately initiate resuscitation to maintain circulation, airway, and

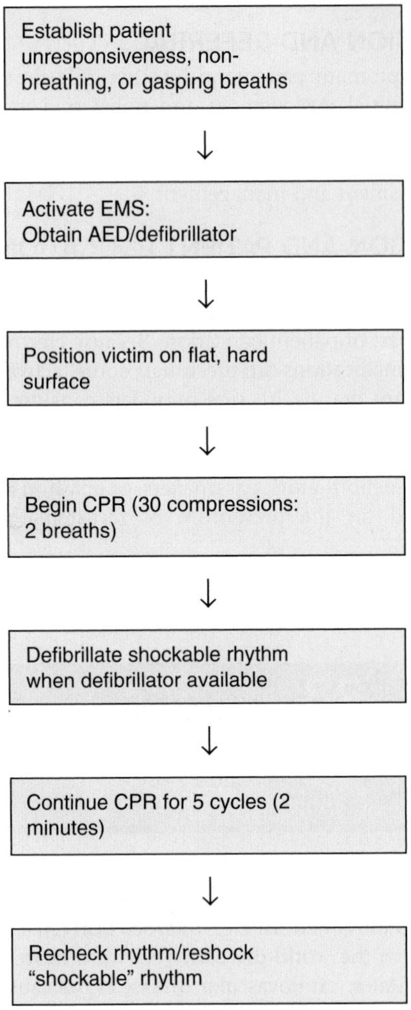

Establish patient unresponsiveness, non-breathing, or gasping breaths
Activate EMS: Obtain AED/defibrillator
Position victim on flat, hard surface
Begin CPR (30 compressions: 2 breaths)
Defibrillate shockable rhythm when defibrillator available
Continue CPR for 5 cycles (2 minutes)
Recheck rhythm/reshock "shockable" rhythm

FIGURE 28-1 Adult cardiopulmonary resuscitation.

breathing (CAB) until advanced life support (ALS) is available (Fig. 28-1).[3] Preplanning is essential. Health care providers should be trained in basic CPR as well as in acute life support. In addition, each member of the office team should have a specified role if a cardiac arrest occurs in the office or clinic setting.

Immediate emergency department referral or physician consultation is indicated for cardiac arrest.

If available, intramuscular or intranasal naloxone is appropriate if an unresponsive victim is not breathing, has a pulse, and is suspected to be opiate addicted.

PATHOPHYSIOLOGY

Cardiac arrest may result from either cardiac causes or extraneous circumstances. The net effect is the cessation of cardiac rhythm and the resultant tissue hypoxia and acidosis. Biologic death will occur if resuscitative measures are not instituted immediately.

CLINICAL PRESENTATION

There may be no warning that an acute event is about to occur. Presentation can include the classic midsternal, crushing, viselike chest pressure with radiation to the arm, neck, or jaw and accompanying diaphoresis, or it may consist of vague, nonspecific symptoms that include chest tightness, discomfort, nausea, shortness of breath, palpitations, lightheadedness, or syncope. A recent history of angina, fatigue, and other nonspecific complaints is also frequently reported. A medical history of smoking, hypertension, elevated cholesterol level, diabetes, sedentary lifestyle, and family history of CAD are significant risk factors for cardiac arrest; therefore it is beneficial to obtain this information.[2] If information cannot be elicited from the patient, family members or others should be questioned to determine the patient's medical history and details of the circumstances surrounding the event.

PHYSICAL EXAMINATION

Assessing unresponsiveness in a calm but efficient manner is critical in the initial management of cardiac arrest. Determining breathlessness and pulselessness in less than 10 seconds is crucial. Once breathlessness and/or pulselessness is confirmed, the resuscitation team or emergency medical services (EMS) system should be activated to enable rapid procurement of an automated external defibrillator (AED) or a conventional defibrillator. If a second person is available to activate the EMS system, the primary provider should place the victim in a supine position on a hard, firm surface. The AHA recommends ensuring scene safety, determining if the victim is not breathing, has "gasping" breaths, or no pulse and then calling for help and activating the Emergency Response System (using a mobile phone is rapid and efficient), simultaneously with beginning CPR.[3] A search for a pulse should not exceed 10 seconds to avoid delaying chest compressions.[4] If the victim has a pulse, but is not breathing, a rescue breath every 5 to 6 seconds is indicated. If there is no pulse, begin CPR. The compression rate should be 100 to 120 compressions per minute, the compression depth for an adult patient should be 2 inches, but not more than 2.4 inches, and interruptions to compressions must be minimumized (<10 seconds) throughout the resuscitation effort.[3] The chest should be allowed to fully recoil between compressions. Health care professionals and trained rescuers should provide two ventilations for every 30 compressions, but rescuers who are not trained are encouraged to provide chest compressions only.

For trained rescuers, ventilations can be started after chest compressions have been initiated, although the time interval without chest compressions should be minimal.[3] After the initial 30 chest compressions have been performed, the approach to providing ventilations to the victim consists of opening and inspecting the airway with the head tilt–chin lift or jaw thrust (if trauma is suspected) maneuver. The rescuer will use mouth to mask or a bag mask device to provide ventilation and oxygen to the victim. The breath is given during 1 second and should have enough volume to make the chest rise. The chest should be allowed to recoil completely after the compression. Once the chest recoils, the second breath is given. If the chest does not rise, the rescuer should reposition the victim's head and attempt another breath. The resuscitation effort is continued with at least 100 to 120 compressions per minute, and a compression depth of (2 to 2.4 inches, 30 compressions to two breaths). The AHA recommends minimal interruptions to CPR and that victims of a witnessed arrest be defibrillated as soon as possible (preferably within 3 to 5 minutes),[3] but CPR is administered until the AED or defibrillator is available and ready. As soon as an AED or conventional defibrillator is available, the leads are attached to the victim, the rhythm is assessed, and, if appropriate, the victim is defibrillated according to AHA standards (see Fig. 28-1).[3] For victims with an implantable pacemaker or implantable cardioverter-defibrillator (ICD), the recommendation is to not place the AED or defibrillator pads or paddles over the device.[4] If a monophasic defibrillator is used, the recommended energy level is 360 J for all shocks.[5] If a biphasic defibrillator is used, the recommendation is 120 to 200 joules.[4] Once the defibrillator is attached, one shock should be given if the rhythm is a shockable rhythm. CPR should then immediately commence again and continue for five cycles of CPR (about 2 minutes).[4] At the end of each five-cycle sequence (after the 30 compressions), the rhythm should be reassessed and the patient again defibrillated for a shockable rhythm.[4] Pulse checks by health care providers should not exceed 10 seconds.

If the arrest was not witnessed, a precordial thump is not recommended.[6] As soon as an AED or conventional defibrillator is available, the leads are attached to the victim, the rhythm is assessed, and, if appropriate, the victim is defibrillated according to AHA standards (see Fig. 28-1).[3]

If the patient's own defibrillator is activated, the rescuers should wait 30 to 60 seconds before the AED is placed on the patient and activated.[4] In a witnessed arrest, the AHA considers the precordial thump to be a "consideration" for health care providers if the victim is monitored and in unstable ventricular tachycardia and if a defibrillator or AED is not available.[6]

Continued assessment of the resuscitation efficacy—compression rate and depth, airway maintenance, and the need for defibrillation—is ongoing. At frequent intervals, the provider should reassess heart rate, blood pressure, oxygen saturation, and effectiveness of CPR and defibrillation.

DIAGNOSTICS

An electrocardiogram (ECG), a defibrillator monitor, or an AED is needed to determine cardiac rhythm, which indicates the necessity of defibrillation and appropriate ALS intervention. Once the patient is intubated, quantitative waveform capnography is recommended to ensure appropriate endotracheal tube placement. Serum electrolytes, drug levels, cardiac enzymes, and arterial blood gases (ABGs) are required for more definitive diagnosis but are deferred to emergency department management.

> **DIAGNOSTICS**
>
> **Cardiac Arrest**
>
> **INITIAL**
> Pulse oximetry
> ECG
>
> **LABORATORY**
> Serum electrolytes
> Drug levels*
> Cardiac enzymes
> ABGs
>
> *If indicated.

DIFFERENTIAL DIAGNOSIS

Sudden cardiac death is often associated with ventricular fibrillation. Other emergency situations associated with cardiac arrest include significant but nonlethal arrhythmias, coronary thrombosis, electrolyte abnormalities, hypovolemia, hypoxia, pulmonary edema, pulmonary embolus, toxicologic cardiac emergencies, metabolic imbalance, near-drowning, hypothermia, cardiac tamponade, tension pneumothorax, electrical shock, and lightning strike. It is important to consider, determine, and treat reversible causes of the arrest.

> **DIFFERENTIAL DIAGNOSIS**
>
> **Cardiac Arrest**
>
> - Arrhythmias
> - Cardiac tamponade
> - Coronary thrombosis
> - Electrical shock
> - Electrolyte abnormality (hypokalemia or hyperkalemia)
> - Hypothermia
> - Hypovolemia
> - Hypoxia
> - Lightning strike
> - Metabolic abnormality
> - Near drowning
> - Pulmonary edema
> - Pulmonary embolus
> - Tension pneumothorax
> - Toxicologic cardiac emergencies

INITIAL STABILIZATION AND MANAGEMENT

Management should follow the guidelines of the AHA (see Fig. 28-1).[3] If the patient's collapse may have caused trauma, the head, neck, and spine must be maintained in a straight line to stabilize the cervical spine. After activation of the EMS system, the patient should be positioned on a flat, firm surface, and basic life support (BLS) should be initiated. The cause of the cardiac arrest should be considered throughout the resuscitative effort to facilitate appropriate interventions and to promote successful resuscitation.

Because most victims of cardiac arrest are in ventricular fibrillation, the AHA still considers early defibrillation the most effective treatment of adult victims of cardiac arrest.[3] There is evidence suggesting the benefit of early CPR and defibrillation; therefore defibrillation with a biphasic defibrillator, a conventional defibrillator, or an AED should occur as soon as the defibrillator is available. Defibrillation consists of one shock, with chest compressions restarted immediately after defibrillation. After five cycles (or 2 minutes) of CPR, the cardiac rhythm should be reanalyzed. If a shockable rhythm is present, the victim should be defibrillated again and CPR immediately restarted after the defibrillation. Minimal interruptions to CPR ensure oxygenation to the myocardium. As soon as possible, the patient should be transported to the nearest emergency facility by trained EMS personnel.

COMPLICATIONS

Death will ensue rapidly if adequate CPR, defibrillation, and treatment are not immediately initiated; few victims will survive if CPR is not started within 4 minutes. Those who do survive cardiac arrest may sustain central nervous system injury, hemodynamic instability, and arrhythmias.

DISPOSITION AND REFERRAL

Circulation has been restored if a pulse is present. ABCs should be supported and the patient transported to the nearest emergency department. Emergency department personnel should be advised of pertinent medical information.

PREVENTION

Primary prevention of cardiac arrest is the ultimate goal. Patients with dyspnea, lightheadedness, angina, palpitations, or fatigue should be evaluated for underlying CAD. The identification of risk factors for CAD and the appropriate interventions are indicated to decrease the number of sudden cardiac deaths. In addition, community programs enhance the understanding of coronary disease, reinforce early management of chest pain, and promote early access to the EMS system.

Training in CPR and emergency cardiac care is essential for any health care provider. Caregivers of patients with CAD should also be trained in BLS and understand the warning signs associated with sudden cardiac death.

If the cardiac arrest was the result of sustained ventricular tachycardia, the victim will need therapy to reduce the chance of future events. An automated ICD or cardiac surgery may be indicated.

PATIENT AND FAMILY EDUCATION

Patients and caregivers should be aware that chest discomfort that increases in intensity or is associated with sweating, palpitations, irregular heartbeat, shortness of breath, lightheadedness, nausea or vomiting, loss of consciousness, or discomfort that radiates to the jaw and neck or arm necessitates calling 911 or other emergency service immediately. It is important to explain that presentation can be atypical, particularly in women, diabetic persons, and older adults. Everyone should be encouraged to learn BLS, but families who have loved ones with CAD should know how to perform CPR. In addition, patients with risk factors for CAD should be constantly encouraged to make lifestyle changes to reduce the risk of cardiac arrest.

CHAPTER 29

CHEMICAL EXPOSURE

Terry Mahan Buttaro

DEFINITION AND EPIDEMIOLOGY

Chemical exposures can occur by inhalation, ingestion, injection, or absorption through the skin and mucous membranes. Although a chemical exposure can be related to a biologic, radioactive, or chemical toxin, harmful chemicals are ubiquitous and occur at home, at work, and at play. Smoke, pesticides, lead, mercury, phthalates, bisphenol A, and frequently used household and beauty products all have potential long-term health ramifications.[1,2]

Common household chemicals that are a more immediate concern include shoe polishes, cosmetics, over-the-counter and prescription medications, alcohols (isopropyl alcohol, methanol, and ethanol), detergents, cleaning products (especially chlorine, ammonia, and lye-containing cleaners), rodent and insect poisons, common yard chemicals, and paints and paint products. Household chemicals are often associated with poisonings in children, but chemical exposures in the home affect people of all ages. Exposure to wood or cigarette smoke, fumes, or other compounds can cause nausea, dizziness, cough, difficulty concentrating, and other symptoms that cause patients to seek care.[3]

Chemicals also abound in the workplace, and many of these cause irritation or toxicity if the human body is exposed to them. The Occupational Safety and Health Administration (OSHA) requires that all employers and employees be advised of chemical hazards by means of a hazards communication program, which includes having a Material Safety Data Sheet (MSDS) for each chemical used in the workplace. The employer must ensure that MSDSs are readily accessible to employees during each work shift when they are in the work area.[4] MSDSs are fact sheets provided by chemical manufacturers that list chemical, physical, and health hazard data for a particular substance.[4] Health hazard data include routes of entry, acute and chronic effects, signs and symptoms of exposure, and emergency and first aid procedures.[5] For safety reasons and because federal law requires accurate labeling on chemical containers, it is wise to avoid the unnecessary transfer of potentially dangerous chemicals into any other containers. If transfer to another container is necessary, OSHA labeling requirements must be followed.[4]

In 2010, 42,917 people died from poisoning. Many of the deaths were related to opioids, which are increasingly related to overdoses and deaths.[6] Medication-related poisonings in adults were related to prescription medications (pain medications, sedatives, antipsychotics, hypnotics, antidepressants, cardiac medications, stimulants) and cosmetics and personal care products.[7] In young children the causes were different; the primary cause of poisoning was related to cosmetics and personal care products, followed by cleaners and pain medications.[7] Carbon monoxide poisoning is another common cause of poisoning in the United States.[8,9] Newer sources of concern in poison control centers are the growing use of e-cigarettes and the potential for nicotine toxicity, the use of synthetic cannabinoids, the risk of poisoning in children by ingestion of laundry detergent packs, and energy drink toxicity.[10-13]

The poisoning statistics are alarming and demonstrate the need for increased patient education by primary care providers to help prevent poisonings and other accidental exposures, because the majority of poisonings are accidental. Prevention is best achieved by keeping cosmetics, personal care products, medications, and cleaners out of the sight and reach of children and by keeping any hazardous material clearly labeled and out of children's reach.[4] Parents, grandparents, caregivers, and primary care offices should always have the telephone number of the poison control center readily available.

Immediate emergency department referral, physician consultation, and contact with a poison control center are indicated for chemical exposure.

PATHOPHYSIOLOGY

The pathophysiologic and systemic effects of a chemical exposure depend on the characteristics and effects of the substance, the degree and route of exposure, and the patient's comorbidities.

CLINICAL PRESENTATION

For poisoning, the history should address the five *W*s: who—the patient's age, weight, sex, and relationship to others present; what—the name and dose of the substance, co-ingestants, and amount ingested; when—the time and date of ingestion; where—both the route of poisoning and the geographic location in which the poisoning occurred; and why—whether the ingestion was intentional or unintentional, plus associated details. A detailed medical history should be obtained, including previous poisonings, comorbid medical conditions, and concurrent medications that might affect the patient's response to and the metabolism or elimination of ingestants. Additional information should include a history of psychiatric illness, alcohol or substance abuse, and presence of hepatic or renal disease.

The patient who has had a toxic exposure may be affected in many different ways. The presentation of chemical exposures is varied and can be particularly challenging, ranging from a headache to coma or death. With children, there often is physical evidence (e.g., a smell of cleaning products, pill or plant fragments, nonfood stains, open bottles or containers). In acute chemical exposures, adults commonly know the type of exposure unless they are incapacitated by it, in which case witnesses may be able to identify the exposure. If the exposure is occupational, the chemical may be readily identifiable. Review of the MSDS for pertinent information after an occupational exposure may also be helpful.

The clinical presentations of chemical exposures are related to the specific toxins involved. Medications such as dimenhydrinate, diphenhydramine, astemizole, loratadine, meclizine, promethazine, and tricyclic antidepressants and household and wild plants such as mandrake, jimsonweed ("loco weed"), and nightshade are anticholinergics. Anticholinergics cause a syndrome that is best remembered by the mnemonic "hot as Hades, blind as a bat, red as a beet, dry as a bone, mad as a hatter," which describes, respectively, the following effects: hyperthermia, mydriasis, flushed skin, dry mucous membranes, urinary retention, decreased bowel motility, and hallucinations or frank psychosis.[14]

Alkalis are found in numerous household cleaning products (e.g., detergents, drain cleaners, dishwashing fluids), batteries, and other substances and cause irritation to the oral mucosa, esophagus, and stomach. This irritation ranges from mild to extremely severe. Both acids and alkalis cause extensive tissue damage to mucous membranes and the gastric system. The alkalis, however, are associated with a much more serious prognosis because they tend to penetrate tissues more deeply and rapidly than do the acids, particularly if the eye is involved.[14,15]

Hydrocarbons and metals are potential toxins that can cause poisoning acutely or chronically. Hydrocarbons are the basis of many industrial chemicals, yet they are also often found in products in many garages and sheds. These substances cause a host of reactions, including coughing, vomiting, a chemical odor to the breath, and, in severe exposure, unconsciousness and coma. Metals such as iron, arsenic, aluminum, lead, mercury, and cadmium also cause poisoning. Aluminum poisoning can affect welders; lead and cadmium are sometimes found in jewelry. Arsenic, mercury, and lead are found almost everywhere in the environment.

Patients with chronic chemical exposure may visit the primary care provider with a variety of complaints, and the cause of the patient's concerns may not be obvious. Because chemical exposure can be so pervasive, it is always important to consider heavy metals and other sources of poisoning as a potential cause of the patient's symptoms.

PHYSICAL EXAMINATION

In acute situations, the initial physical examination for chemical exposure must be rapid, focused, but also comprehensive. Airway, breathing, and circulation must be supported and cardiac function monitored. Temperature, heart and respiratory rates, blood pressure, oxygen saturation, blood glucose concentration, and cardiopulmonary function should be assessed and then frequently reassessed, and a possible deterioration in the patient's status should be anticipated. The examination must focus on systems (e.g., cognitive status, responsiveness, restlessness, agitation, or seizure activity), skin appearance (e.g., needle marks, contusions, petechiae, bullae, skin color, flushed appearance, or diaphoresis), pupil appearance and reactivity, nares, mucous membranes (odor, excessive salivation), cardiac rhythm and rate, pulmonary congestion, bowel sounds or abdominal rigidity, and motor tone to help determine clues to the chemical exposure and on adjuvant diagnostic laboratory studies.[16-18]

DIAGNOSTICS AND DIFFERENTIAL DIAGNOSIS

Useful diagnostic studies in the evaluation of a chemical exposure include complete blood count (CBC), serum glucose, electrolyte panel to calculate the anion gap, liver function tests (LFTs), blood urea nitrogen (BUN), and creatinine. If an inhalation injury is suspected, analysis of arterial blood gases (ABGs) is indicated to assess ventilation or perfusion problems related to the possible exposure. Other diagnostics should be ordered as the history warrants. These may include drug and alcohol levels; methemoglobin level for possible carbon monoxide toxicity; blood serum measurements of specific chemicals, such as lead, arsenic, or mercury; and, if indicated, serum levels of acetaminophen, aspirin, or other drugs.[18] An electrocardiogram (ECG) is necessary, as is urinalysis for drug screening.

The differential diagnosis depends on the type, length, and route of exposure as well as on the patient's presenting signs and symptoms. Causes not related to the exposure (e.g., head trauma in a patient with altered mental status) and comorbid conditions should be considered in the differential diagnosis.

DIAGNOSTICS

Chemical Exposure

INITIAL
Pulse oximetry, if inhalation exposure

LABORATORY
CBC and differential
Serum electrolytes
Serum glucose
BUN
Creatinine
Anion gap
LFTs
ABGs, if inhalation exposure
Methemoglobin for carbon monoxide
Ethylene glycol test*
Serum lead, arsenic, mercury, or other specific chemical tests*
Blood and urine toxicology (alcohol and drug levels)*

IMAGING
Chest radiograph for inhalation exposure*

OTHER
ECG

*If indicated.

The poison control center and appropriate references should be consulted for specific recommendations.

INITIAL STABILIZATION AND MANAGEMENT

The initial objective in the treatment of any chemical exposure or poisoning is to ensure circulation and protect or establish an airway and breathing for adequate oxygenation. Oxygenation and intubation are recommended for obtunded or comatose patients if gastric lavage is considered.[16] Once circulation, airway, and breathing have been established, it is important to consult the nearest poison control center, to examine the patient carefully (including a cautious search of clothing and belongings), and to arrange transfer to the nearest emergency department.[16] Poison control center personnel are able to help identify the chemical and guide appropriate treatment. The main poison control telephone number (800-222-1222) will direct callers to their specific regional centers, and all health care providers should be aware of the location of the main telephone number or the number to their regional poison control center.

Intravenous access should be obtained as soon as possible.[16] Naloxone and thiamine are usually given immediately. Intravenous dextrose is administered if the patient is hypoglycemic.[16] Physical examination findings may indicate the type of toxicologic emergency and expedite appropriate treatment. Vital signs and an ECG are particularly important because poisonings may cause significant hypertension, hemodynamic instability, cardiac arrhythmias, conduction defects, respiratory depression, or coronary ischemia.[14,16,17] It is essential to determine state of consciousness and presence of agitation, ocular or facial burns, and cardiopulmonary status. Toxin decontamination depends on the type of exposure and should be expeditious.

Ingestions

For ingestions, therapy depends on the material ingested. It is essential to check toxicologic clinical guidelines and poison control for specific recommendations based on the substance. Although not always recommended, possible therapeutic modalities can include gastrointestinal decontamination through gastric lavage or with activated charcoal.[14,16] All decontamination procedures are associated with potentially serious complications, and in some instances there are no studies to prove efficacy.[16] Orogastric lavage (accomplished by insertion of an orogastric tube through the mouth to the stomach) may be acceptable for some ingestions (e.g., a potentially life-threatening amount of poison) and should be initiated within 60 minutes of ingestion and only by a provider skilled in the procedure.[16] The procedure often initiates vomiting in the victim; thus, adequate airway protection must always be ensured. Orogastric lavage also has been associated with aspiration, esophageal or gastric perforation and hypoxemia.[16]

Ipecac should not be administered routinely in the management of poisoned patients and should be avoided in patients with a decreased level of consciousness.[14,16] Ipecac is contraindicated in patients who have ingested a corrosive substance or hydrocarbon with high aspiration potential.[14] However, in specific situations with poison control guidance, ipecac may be an option.

Activated charcoal is still used for gastrointestinal decontamination in specific situations.[18] It can be taken orally or administered through a nasogastric tube and must be given within an hour of ingestion of the toxin.[16,18] The charcoal absorbs ingested substances, thereby reducing absorption by the gastrointestinal tract.[18] However, it is also associated with vomiting and aspiration and is not helpful for caustic acids and alkalis, alcohols, petroleum distillates, lithium, iron, potassium, or heavy metals and may cause bowel obstruction.[16,18]

In specific circumstances, enhancing bowel motility to reduce the body's absorption of specific toxins (e.g., medications or metals not absorbed with activated charcoal) may be indicated.[18] Sorbitol (70%) or magnesium citrate can be coadministered with the activated charcoal, although evidence of efficacy is unclear.[16] Whole bowel irrigation with polyethylene glycol administered through a feeding tube may be helpful in selected poisonings (e.g., medications that are enteric coated or prepared for sustained release, alcohols, acids, alkalis, heavy metals, and body packer ingestions).[16]

Agitated patients with anticholinergic exposure will require sedation (e.g., lorazepam) to prevent rhabdomyolysis and hyperthermia.[14,18] Medications with anticholinergic effects should be avoided.[14] Used in the past, treatment with physostigmine is now used less frequently, although it is appropriate if supportive therapies are not successful.[18]

Other treatments can include antidotes for specific poisons (e.g., acetylcysteine for acetaminophen) or hemodialysis, which is beneficial for some drug overdoses (e.g., salicylate poisoning).[18] Salicylate intoxication is also treated with urinary alkalinization, although this procedure is contraindicated for patients with renal failure or hypokalemia.[16,18]

Age is an important consideration in toxicologic emergencies because the treatment for an infant or child can differ from that for an adult. In addition, specific toxins have specific antidotes. The poison control center is the single best source to quickly determine these antidotes.

Skin Exposure

Most skin exposure to chemicals must be treated immediately with copious irrigation with water (i.e., "dilution is the solution to pollution"). Removal of saturated clothing and vigorous showering to wash the chemical off the skin with large quantities of water are essential to prevent further damage to the patient. Exposed areas should be irrigated for at least 15 to 30 minutes. This minimizes the time the offending agent is in direct contact with the skin, thus limiting the damage caused by the chemical agent. Provider caution during any decontamination procedure is strongly advised.

DISPOSITION AND REFERRAL

Once a patient's condition has been initially stabilized, he or she should be referred for definitive care. If the exposure has been minimal, follow-up with the health care provider may be all that is necessary. Severe intoxication may warrant admission to the intensive care unit. Hospital admission should be considered if the extent of exposure is unknown or significant; this is especially true for older adults and the very young.

PREVENTION AND PATIENT EDUCATION

Toxic and chemical exposure can be easily prevented by correctly labeling, storing, and locking up potentially harmful agents and by using appropriate protective measures, such as wearing appropriate personal protective equipment. Patients should be reminded to handle and to dispose of hazardous chemicals appropriately, and they should be able to recognize the signs and symptoms of chemical exposure: dizziness, headache, blurred vision, unsteady gait, clumsiness, poor coordination, difficulty breathing, nausea, abdominal cramping, skin discoloration or irritation, and eye or mucous membrane irritation. MSDSs are available online.

The telephone number for the local poison control center should be posted in every primary care office and near every home and business telephone for ready access if required. The U.S. national Poison Help line is 1-800-222-1222.

RESOURCES

U.S. Environmental Protection Agency: *Integrated risk information system.* Available at www.epa.gov/IRIS/.

CHAPTER 30

ELECTRICAL INJURIES

Terry Mahan Buttaro • Joanne Sandberg-Cook

DEFINITION AND EPIDEMIOLOGY

Injuries from an electrical accident can be minor or can involve severe damage, electrocution, and even death from an electrical fire or cardiopulmonary arrest.[1] In the United States, there are approximately 400 deaths and 4000 electrical injuries yearly, with an additional 140,000 electricity-related fires accounting for an additional 400 deaths and 4000 injuries.[2] Each year, 1000 people are killed in electrical accidents. Although the actual number of accidental and environmental electrical injuries is uncertain, electrical injuries are the fourth leading cause of death in the workplace, the result of electricity-related trauma, burns, or shock.[3] In addition to the aforementioned injuries, electrical injuries can also cause cardiac arrhythmias and respiratory arrest as well as seizures.[4]

Electrical injuries caused by low-voltage current account for 60% to 70% of reported electrical injury and have been responsible for nearly half of deaths from electrical shock and 1% of accidental deaths in the home.[5] This number is declining, likely because of the widespread use of grounded plugs. The majority of household electrocutions involve 110- or 220-V current and are usually the result of failure to ground tools or appliances or the use of hair dryers or other electrical devices near water. Contact with low- and high-voltage electrical current is responsible for a significant number of hand and oral injuries in children.[5] The most common cause of electrical injury in children younger than 6 years is oral contact with electrical cords or wall sockets and the placement of conductive bodies in wall sockets. Adolescent boys 11 to 18 years of age often sustain high-voltage injuries in tree- or pole-climbing accidents.

Lightning is a common but rarely fatal natural phenomenon. In recent years, fatalities related to lightning strikes have decreased to fewer than 50 each year.[6] Seventy to 90% of people struck by lightning survive but will have permanent sequelae.[7]

Immediate emergency department referral or physician consultation is indicated for patients with electrical injuries.

PATHOPHYSIOLOGY

Electrical injuries result from the direct effects of current and from the conversion of electrical energy into thermal energy as current passes through body tissues. Factors that determine the severity and distribution of injury include the type of current, voltage, amperage, tissue resistance, surface contacted, pathway of current, duration of contact, and other associated trauma.[8] Alternating current (AC), the more common cause of electrical injuries, is more dangerous than direct current (DC) because it can produce tetanic skeletal muscle contractions and prevent the victim from letting go of the energized source, thus increasing current delivery to the victim. AC voltage at 25 to 300 Hz and 25 to 220 V, the common household current level, can easily cause ventricular fibrillation if the pathway of the current includes the heart. Low-voltage contact, although potentially lethal, does not result in the magnitude of tissue necrosis seen with high-voltage injury. The voltage in a lightning strike is in the range of 10 million to 2 billion volts, but the duration of a lightning strike is short.

Heat generation is responsible for most burns seen with electrical injuries. Heat damage is proportional to tissue resistance. Tissues with high fluid and electrolyte content conduct electrical current better than others do. Listed in decreasing order of magnitude of tissue necrosis are nerves, blood vessels, muscle, skin, tendon, fat, and bone. Nerve tissue has the least resistance to direct flow and therefore is most easily damaged.[8] Electrical current passing through the head or crossing the thorax is more likely to cause respiratory arrest or ventricular fibrillation than is current passing through the leg. Skin, the initial barrier to current flow, is an effective insulator to deeper tissues. As current flows from the contact point, tissue with the least electrical resistance sustains the greatest current density and destructive injury. The most severe cutaneous and deep injuries are adjacent to contact sites, and the damage decreases with increasing distance from damage points.

CLINICAL PRESENTATION

The spectrum of electrical injury ranges from a transient unpleasant sensation to instantaneous death. Injuries from electricity occur by three mechanisms: (1) the direct effect of current on tissue; (2) the conversion of electrical energy to heat, causing burns; and (3) a mechanical injury caused by muscle contraction, falling, or a direct lightning strike. Cardiopulmonary arrest is the primary cause of immediate fatalities from electrical injury and is common in patients with high-voltage electrical and lightning injury. In lightning injuries, cardiac activity can spontaneously return, but the associated respiratory arrest often continues, causing death.[9] Common sequelae include hypertension; tachycardia; cardiac muscle necrosis; respiratory paralysis; burns; fractures; ruptured tympanic membrane; hyphema; vitreous hemorrhage; and injuries to the spinal cord, peripheral nervous system, and vascular systems.[10] Oliguria or anuria from deep tissue damage and rhabdomyolysis can cause acute renal failure. Visible myoglobinuria indicates massive acute muscle necrosis and impending renal failure. Disseminated intravascular coagulation can result from massive trauma. Neurologic deficits are sometimes evident immediately after the current exposure. However, complications such as reflex sympathetic dystrophy and motor neuron disease may not become apparent for days to months after the electrical trauma.[11] Long bone fracture often occurs with falls, and fractures (particularly of the vertebral column) can result from tetanic muscle contraction at the time of electrocution.[11] Cataracts can form up to 2 years after such injury.[11] Direct injury to internal organs is uncommon.

PHYSICAL EXAMINATION

When evaluating a victim with an electrical injury, the health care provider should always completely undress the patient to determine entry and exit wounds and associated injuries. Patients should be assessed for associated cranial, spinal, or other trauma, and the neck should initially be treated as being unstable, particularly with DC injuries. Arrhythmic conduction disturbances and infarct patterns can be present on the electrocardiogram (ECG). Cardiopulmonary presentations vary, and most patients lack the characteristic chest discomfort indicative of myocardial ischemia. Transient, mild paresthesias and complete and irreversible impairment of sensory or motor function, or both, can be present in patients with electrical injuries. Absent pulses, decreased peripheral perfusion, and impaired neurologic function are also seen in patients with acute vascular complications from electrical trauma.

Injuries consistent with findings of blunt trauma to the head, spinal cord, and musculoskeletal, intrathoracic, and intra-abdominal areas can be present in patients who were thrown from the energized current source, had forceful tetanic muscle contractions associated with AC injuries, or fell after losing consciousness and muscle control. Skin wounds are typically leathery or charred areas of full-thickness skin loss. The patient with lightning injury may have linear, punctate, feathery burns that often are referred to as *Lichtenberg flowers*.[12] The entry and exit sites are usually depressed, giving the appearance that current exploded the tissue. Underlying injury to a major muscle compartment is accompanied by edema formation. Circulatory integrity is best judged with Doppler ultrasound of distal pulses.

DIAGNOSTICS

Initial studies include complete blood count (CBC), electrolytes, glucose, blood urea nitrogen (BUN), creatinine, coagulation profile, arterial blood gas (ABG) analysis, creatine kinase level, creatine kinase muscle-brain (CK-MB) fraction, and myoglobin level.[4] A 12-lead ECG and continuous cardiac monitoring are necessary for all patients with electrical injury. Fetal monitoring is necessary if the victim is pregnant. Patients with suspected spinal injuries should undergo cervical spine radiography. Other x-ray studies are indicated to exclude fracture if localized edema and pain are present. Consideration of other diagnostic studies should be coordinated with the consulting specialists.

DIAGNOSTICS

Electrical Injuries

INITIAL
ECG

LABORATORY
CBC and differential
Serum electrolytes
BUN
Creatinine
Serum glucose
Coagulation studies
ABGs
Creatine kinase level
CK-MB fraction
Myoglobin

DIFFERENTIAL DIAGNOSIS

The diagnosis of electrical injury may be unclear, particularly in unwitnessed cases in which the victim is confused, amnestic, or unconscious or if external signs of injury are absent. In these cases, several conditions should be considered as part of the differential diagnosis: cardiopulmonary arrest, arrhythmias, peripheral neuropathies, seizures, cerebral vascular accident, syncope, and nonelectrical trauma or burns. Circumstances surrounding the electrical injuries should also be sought to determine the possible mechanism of the injury. Precipitating factors such as intoxication, suicidal intention, or foul play should be considered.

A person struck by lightning may appear to be comatose or dead and have no physical injury.[7] Other lightning victims may be close by with a similar appearance.[7] After ensuring that the environment is safe (e.g., no downed power lines), immediate resuscitation is advised because the person likely is in respiratory or cardiac arrest.[7]

The Taser is a conducted electrical weapon used by law enforcement to subdue violent or dangerous individuals. Injuries associated with the use of Tasers are generally mild skin burns, but serious injuries, including fractures, injuries to the face or eyes, head injuries related to falls, and even death from cardiac arrest are also seen.[13] The use of conducted electrical weapons is not recommended for pregnant women, individuals with low body weight, or those with obvious medical issues such as seizures.

DIFFERENTIAL DIAGNOSIS

Electrical Injuries

- Cardiopulmonary arrest
- Arrhythmias
- Peripheral neuropathies
- Seizures
- Nonelectrical trauma

INITIAL STABILIZATION AND MANAGEMENT

Patients who have experienced an electrical injury are treated as trauma patients. Immediate priorities include restoration of circulation, airway, and breathing as taught in basic life support and advanced cardiac life support classes.[14] The cervical spine should be immobilized and the airway secured while respiration is supported, with adequate oxygenation and stabilization of circulation if required. Cardiopulmonary resuscitation must be initiated, and the emergency medical services system should be activated.[14] Defibrillation is indicated for ventricular tachycardia or ventricular fibrillation, and early intubation is recommended for patients with facial or neck burns.[14] Continued thermal damage can be limited by removal of affected clothing. Intravascular volume is initially managed per the Parkland formula. Increased intravenous fluid resuscitation, osmotic diuretics, and alkalinization of the urine with the addition of sodium bicarbonate to the intravenous fluids (i.e., 44 to 50 mEq of bicarbonate to 1 L of lactated Ringer's or normal saline solution) is recommended if myoglobinuria develops.[4,18]

Wound care involves treatment of both cutaneous and deep soft tissue injuries with a saline dressing. Consultation with a surgeon is recommended to evaluate the need for formal wound exploration, debridement, and, if compartment syndrome is suspected, fasciotomy.[18] Tetanus prophylaxis should be updated. Prophylactic antibiotics have not been shown to decrease episodes of infection and usually are not indicated. Management of other complications resulting from electrical trauma generally follows standard emergency therapy.[15]

DISPOSITION AND REFERRAL

Prompt specialty consultation is required in addition to the liberal involvement of surgical specialists. All patients who have lost consciousness or sustained cardiac or respiratory arrest as well as those with ischemic chest pain, myoglobinuria, or significant burn wounds should be hospitalized. Referral to a burn center is often necessary for electrical burns because considerable injury to deeper neurovascular and musculoskeletal structures may not be obvious until several days after the injury.

PREVENTION AND PATIENT AND FAMILY EDUCATION

All discharged patients should have reliable home support. Patients should be advised to return immediately to their health care provider if any symptoms occur. A specific follow-up visit should be arranged with a health care provider familiar with electrical injuries, and patients should receive careful explanation of the injury and recuperative process.

Open sockets and outlets must be covered with childproof devices, and children must be watched carefully. Older children should be aware of the dangers of climbing near high-tension wires. Plug-in electrical appliances should be kept away from water sources. Community education programs, particularly at school and at work, are necessary to help prevent accidents. Safety standards in industry and in the community must be constantly updated and enforced.[16,17]

CHAPTER 31

ENVIRONMENTAL AND FOOD ALLERGIES

John W. Distler

ENVIRONMENTAL ALLERGIES

DEFINITION AND EPIDEMIOLOGY

Environmental allergens are responsible for a wide range of signs and symptoms ranging from rhinitis, eczema, urticaria, and bronchospasm to anaphylaxis. With repeated exposure, immediate type 1 hypersensitivity reactions may occur through the development of immunoglobulin E (IgE). Allergens can be found both indoors and outdoors and fluctuate among households, with the change of seasons, by weather patterns including heat and humidity, and by the area in which one lives in the United States. Common indoor allergens include dust mites, indoor molds, and animal dander. The more common outdoor allergens are pollen (i.e., grass, trees, and weeds) and outdoor molds, including mold smuts in wheat, corn, oat, and barley fields.[1] The incidence of environmental allergies with subsequent symptom development has been on the rise.[2] Allergic rhinitis may affect up to 20% of the U.S. population and up to 40% of children.[1] Atopic dermatitis was found to have a direct cost to the U.S. health care system ranging from $1 billion to $4 billion, with an average cost per patient of approximately $609.[3] The potential psychosocial effects of atopic dermatitis are also staggering.

Allergic rhinitis may be considered the first step in the development of allergic asthma.[4] The Centers for Disease Control and Prevention (CDC) reported a steady increase in the development of asthma in both adults and children from 1996 to 2007.[5] However, symptom development may be secondary to other non–IgE-mediated environmental factors, such as urbanization, toxins, air pollution, and tobacco smoke exposure.[1] Occupational exposure has also become an increasingly important patient consideration.[6] It is important to make the clinical distinction between a true IgE-mediated cause and those symptoms that result in irritation and subsequent inflammation of the mucous membranes in the nose, lungs, and skin.[7]

COMMON ENVIRONMENTAL ALLERGENS

Recurrent exposure to an environmental allergen and subsequent sensitization result in the typical presenting signs and symptoms of patients with a genetically determined atopic disorder. Environmental allergens may be either indoor or outdoor and are influenced by a variety of factors.

Common indoor allergens include molds, dust mites, cockroaches, and animal dander. Prominent indoor molds include *Penicillium, Alternaria, Cladosporium,* and *Aspergillus.* Indoor molds are fungi and are found in warm, moist, and humid environments of bathrooms, basements, and laundry rooms.[8] Molds thrive in these conditions and spread through the production of spores. The mold spores become airborne in certain conditions, resulting in exposure to the host. Molds are hearty in that they can survive environmental conditions adverse to their growth, such as dry air and exposure to sunshine. No growth occurs under these conditions, but molds also do not die. Dust mites are microscopic relatives of the spider and are common in all households. Two common dust mites responsible for triggering of an atopic reaction are *Dermatophagoides pteronyssinus* and *Dermatophagoides farinae.* Like molds, dust mites also thrive in warm, moist environments; they survive through the ingestion of flakes of skin from humans and live in bedding, mattresses, carpets, curtains, and upholstered furniture.[8] The total eradication of dust mites from the home is impossible. Pet dander is created by the oil glands, saliva, and urine of animals, not the fur. In combination, these excreted substances become allergenic to some individuals. An important consideration for patients with animal dander allergy is that dander is a sticky allergen and may remain in the home weeks or months after an animal has been removed. Cat dander and dog dander are among the most common allergens in schools, brought in by students with an animal in their home.[8] Animals such as rabbits, gerbils, hamsters, guinea pigs, horses, and cows are also potentially allergenic, depending on exposure. Cockroaches are another indoor allergen and can cause severe asthma reactions in children living in crowded urban environments and older dwellings. The allergenic protein that cockroaches create is from their saliva and feces.[8]

Outdoor allergens consist mainly of pollen from trees, grass, and weeds in addition to molds and mold smuts. Tree pollen, grass pollen, and weed pollen are the only seasonal environmental allergens. The pollination season varies from one area of the United States to another. In the spring, trees are typically the first to shed their pollen. Southern states may have detectable levels of tree pollen as early as late January, whereas northern states may not have measurable levels until May or June. Not all tree pollen is allergenic. Trees that release allergenic pollen include oak, elm, maple, hickory, poplar, willow, box elder, and walnut.[8] As with trees, only a small number of the many species of grass are allergenic. For the most part, grass pollen season tends to follow tree season, and again the variability is dependent on the area of the United States. Some common grasses that release allergic pollen are Kentucky bluegrass, Johnson grass, Bermuda grass, orchard grass, sweet vernal grass, and timothy. Grass pollen levels are affected by temperature, moisture, humidity, and time of day. Weeds are typically fall pollen producers and may begin to pollinate as early as August and into November, depending on the type of weed and location in the United States. Common allergenic weeds include ragweed, pigweed, plantain, sheep's sorrel, sagebrush, and lamb's quarters. Like grass pollen counts, weed pollen counts are higher at dawn and dusk and also on hot, dry, windy days.[8] Flower pollens are rarely allergenic because their pollen is heavier and is dispersed by insects that carry the pollen from plant to plant.[9] Outdoor molds tend to be more allergenic than indoor molds. Common outdoor molds include *Alternaria* and *Hormodendrum* (i.e., *Cladosporium*). *Alternaria* is a common mold that can be brought indoors by humans and pets. Like indoor molds, outdoor molds produce spores for growth and are found commonly on fallen leaves and rotting vegetation. Mold smuts grow in the soil and roots of wheat, corn, oat, and barley fields. Mold counts tend to be higher from July into late summer, depending on the geographic location. In the colder months, mold becomes dormant but does not die with snow or frost. When it is covered with snow or ice, mold is less likely to release its spores into the wind.[8] Therefore a warmer, more humid late fall and early winter may produce more mold spores.

PATHOPHYSIOLOGY

With repeated exposure to an environmental allergen through the respiratory tract, genetically predisposed people begin to develop IgE as an inappropriate means to protect the body from the protein allergen (antigen). Antigen-specific T cells are activated through the lymphatic system in response to the antigen. The activated antigen-specific T cells then activate B cells, and IgE is created in lymphoid tissue or at local tissue sites.[3,10] The newly created antigen-specific IgE is released by plasma cells and binds to high-affinity IgE receptors located on the basophils and mast cells. This leads to the sensitization of the cells in the tissues of the nose, lung, or skin.[4,10]

Although other immunoglobulins, such as IgG, IgA, and IgM, are produced to appropriately protect the body, circulating levels of IgE and the attachment to the allergen are responsible for the atopic reaction.[10] With repeated exposure and further sensitization, IgE binds with the antigen protein, and degranulation of the mast cells and basophils begins, starting the allergic cascade. Mediators, including histamine, proteoglycans, enzymes, cytokines, and many others, are released as a result of the degranulation. The chain in the release of mediators is responsible for the immediate and late-phase responses of the cells. Histamine may be fully released within 30 minutes of degranulation, whereas cytokines may be released over many hours.[1,9,10]

Atopic diseases are typically genetically determined, yet individual responses to antigen exposure are also based on environmental factors and susceptibility of the host as well. For instance, the timing of the exposure to an allergen may affect the exposure response. High-level exposure to allergens early on may predispose a person to develop a more severe atopic response. The period of sensitivity is highly variable among people. In addition, exposure to cigarette smoke and pathogens may also alter the body's immune response, modifying the level of IgE activation.

CLINICAL PRESENTATION AND PHYSICAL EXAMINATION

Patients with environmental allergies may have a variety of signs and symptoms. Typical presenting signs and symptoms include rhinitis, eczema, urticaria, bronchospasm, and anaphylaxis.[1] Exposure to environmental allergens may also exacerbate other non–IgE-mediated symptoms.

A cause-and-effect relationship must be determined; a patient may have rhinitis because of grass pollen, bronchospasm from cat exposure, or urticaria from dust mite sensitivity.[11] An important diagnostic consideration is to determine whether a patient's symptoms are seasonal or perennial or both. A patient may live with dust mite sensitivity and have subclinical symptoms, yet the symptoms become bothersome only during the spring when the seasonal flare results in further IgE activation. Similarly, patients may become symptomatic only in the winter when doors and windows are closed and their exposure to dust mites and animal dander increases. Understanding of the patient's individualized IgE activation triggers and the environmental timing is essential in helping patients control their symptoms.

A detailed history is required to determine a cause-and-effect relationship of environmental allergen exposure and the development of symptoms. Standard history questions include current medications, medication allergies, past medical history, family history, and surgeries and hospitalizations. In addition, further atopy, including the potential for stinging insect venom allergy and food allergies, must be understood; the presence of these conditions may trigger further IgE activation, potentially increasing a patient's physical response.

To understand the entire allergic presentation, additional questions must be asked about the environment. The type of home in which one lives and the age of the dwelling may indicate the potential for mold or cockroaches. Heating and cooling sources must be identified because the use of forced hot air may add to the disbursement of dust mite and animal dander. Radiant heat may increase the humidity of the home, resulting in an increase in mold spore production and dust mites. The presence of a crawl space or unfinished damp basement may also increase the potential for indoor mold. Dust mites may be present in bed linens, older pillows, mattresses, and stuffed animals. The frequency of laundering of bed linens must also be recorded. Determination of the number and type of animals in the home and the area of the house in which they are allowed is essential. Recent renovations to the home could modify mold or dust mite exposure. Ideally, the humidity in the home should be 35% to 40% to decrease indoor mold spore growth and to control dust mite propagation.

A thorough physical examination must be performed after the environmental allergy history. The examination should always include a careful head, eyes, ears, nose, and throat (HEENT) examination to look for allergic symptoms of the nose and eyes, including sclera erythema and injection, allergic shiners from venous engorgement, swollen pink nasal turbinates, and tonsillar enlargement. Small, nontender movable posterior cervical nodes in the neck are a common finding in children. Direct visualization of the skin with ambient lighting should be performed to look for cutaneous symptoms of urticaria and eczema. Encouraging the patient and parents to take pictures of the cutaneous response would also be helpful in cases of intermittent symptoms. Pulmonary function tests (PFTs) should be performed, if they are available, to look for reversibility of symptoms and PFT results after bronchodilation. A heart and abdominal examination should also be conducted for each patient, looking for other diagnostic clues.

DIAGNOSTICS

History and physical examination includes the following.

- Skin testing
  - A skin prick test (SPT) can be performed by either the scratch or intradermal method. Both histamine and normal saline controls are placed on patients at the time of testing. The reaction to histamine must be positive and the reaction to saline negative to ensure reliability of the test results.[12]
  - Certain medications, such as antihistamines, H_2 blockers, and tricyclic antidepressants, must be discontinued for up to 5 days before skin testing because these may interfere with test result reliability.
  - Skin tests are placed on the back, upper arm, or ventral surface of the forearms, depending on the amount of testing to be performed and the age of the patient.[13] The use of the back in children is recommended because pruritus from a positive test result may make the patient scratch the area. Scratching of the area may mix allergens placed on the skin, interfering with evaluation of the results. Results are read within 15 to 20 minutes.
  - Scratch testing involves scratching the surface of the skin with a single stylus for each allergen.[12] This form of allergy testing is safer, more rapid, and less uncomfortable to patients than intradermal testing but is not as sensitive as intradermal testing. Depending on the practice, providers may begin with scratch testing and proceed to intradermal testing if the results are negative.[13] Scratch testing is also associated with a lower potential for anaphylaxis than intradermal testing.
  - Intradermal testing is more sensitive and reproducible than scratch testing. This test involves the use of a 25-gauge needle with a small drop of allergen (0.02 to 0.05 mL) placed beneath the skin.[9] Depending on the practice and the type of allergen, the concentration placed beneath the skin may be 1:10 or as high as 1:1000.[12] If the patient reacts to the allergen, that particular allergen (e.g., grass pollen) is not tested further, and the test result is considered positive. If the test result is negative, higher concentrations are used. A stepwise approach to intradermal testing should be taken to ensure safe patient outcomes. All providers and staff must be trained to handle any potential systemic reactions, including urticaria, bronchospasm, and full anaphylaxis.
- Serum IgE levels

DIFFERENTIAL DIAGNOSIS

The differential diagnoses for rhinitis, eczema, urticaria, bronchospasm, and anaphylaxis are extensive and may require additional referrals to a dermatologist, otolaryngologist, or pulmonologist for further workup. Some of the more common differential diagnoses include vasomotor rhinitis, type IV delayed hypersensitivity reactions, idiopathic urticaria, nonallergic asthma, and food or stinging insect anaphylaxis. The diagnosis can be determined by the history, the causal relationship, and the results of SPTs. PFTs will aid in the diagnosis of reversible bronchospasm but not allergic or nonallergic triggers. Urticaria or eczema may be more difficult to diagnose, and biopsy may be indicated to confirm the diagnosis. Discontinuation of the potential offending agent (e.g., removal of animals and other control measures) is also diagnostic. Depending on the results of the workup, allergy immunotherapy may be indicated.

DIFFERENTIAL DIAGNOSIS

- Vasomotor rhinitis
- Type IV delayed hypersensitivity reactions
- Idiopathic urticaria
- Nonallergic asthma
- Food allergy

MANAGEMENT

Specialist Consultation

When environmental control and medications are not controlling a patient's symptoms, a referral to an allergy practice may be indicated.[14] This is especially true if the patient has more than one atopic disorder, such as allergic rhinitis and allergic asthma, or if there is also the potential for food or stinging insect sensitivity.

Skin testing can be performed in patients with atopic disorders. However, desensitization can be performed only in patients with environmental allergies and stinging insect sensitivity, not food allergies.

Subcutaneous injections to desensitize patients to environmental allergies (allergy immunotherapy) began in 1911.[14] Before that, an oral route was used. Desensitization may prevent the development of allergic asthma in patients with allergic rhinitis.[14] Allergy immunotherapy is proposed to work through the lymphocyte response by decreasing the T-cell response to the allergen. Mast cell and eosinophil responses are decreased by upregulation of antigen-specific T-regulatory cells. IgG4 antibodies that are protective to the body may be produced and inhibit basophil histamine release. The result is a decrease in the binding mechanism of the antigen to IgE and therefore the inhibition of the allergic cascade.

Allergy immunotherapy is started with weekly injections of allergens according to the results of skin testing. Depending on the practice, dilutions of either 1:1000 or 1:10,000 are given in minute quantities (e.g., 0.05 mL). The amount is increased weekly until the patient reaches the maintenance dose, typically within 4 to 6 months.[14] If a patient has a reaction to the dose, the next dose is typically decreased, and it is only increased once the patient tolerates it without reaction. Once this dose is reached, maintenance continues for 4 to 6 years on an every 2- to 3-week schedule. Patients must remain in the office for 20 minutes after their allergy injection to be sure that they do not have a significant reaction. Patients must also be advised that there is a potential for delayed reactions and must be given instructions for intervention should this occur.[15]

Rush schedules are also used in some settings; however, the probability of systemic reactions is much greater than with standard therapy.

Allergy immunotherapy is contraindicated in patients with poorly controlled, severe persistent asthma and in those with comorbid conditions, such as unstable angina or uncontrolled hypertension. Patients taking beta blockers are also not candidates for allergy immunotherapy because these medications can block the effect of epinephrine if it is given as a result of a systemic side effect.

Sublingual therapy, another form of allergy immunotherapy, has been used in Europe with some documented positive results.[14] Data available in the United States on the efficacy of sublingual therapy show mixed results and are limited in terms of patient outcomes. There is less standardization of sublingual extract than of intradermal extract.[16] Therefore, results of studies cannot be used for extracts manufactured in the United States. The Food and Drug Administration has approved two forms of sublingual tablets as immunotherapy to treat both grass and ragweed pollen allergic rhinitis symptoms with or without conjunctivitis. Treatment is initiated at least 12 weeks before the expected onset of the pollen season and continues throughout the season. The dose is 1 tablet daily under the tongue. The initial dose of the sublingual tablet must be given under the supervision of trained medical personnel, and patients must remain in the practice for 30 minutes after the initial dose.[16]

Management of environmental allergies depends on the patient's presenting signs and symptoms in addition to the results of the allergy workup. In the primary care practice, management begins with environmental control and appropriate medications. Antihistamines including the nonsedating forms, steroid nasal sprays, topical steroids for skin reactions, and oral steroids for severe reactions are commonly used medications. Asthma may need to be diagnosed and treated (see Chapter 103). Patients whose symptoms are not controlled with these initial actions may need to be referred to an allergy practice for consideration of allergy immunotherapy, especially if perennial or seasonal flares are severe.

Control of reactions to seasonal pollen from trees and grass in the spring and weeds in the summer and fall can be effective with use of simple measures. It is essential that patients keep their windows closed and air conditioning on during periods of high pollen counts, especially from 5 AM to 10 AM.[8] Pollen easily enters the screens of windows and is deposited on furniture and bedding.[15] Therefore, bed linens should be changed weekly and washed in hot water.

High-efficiency particulate air (HEPA) filters can be used in bedrooms and living areas. Patients should also be encouraged to shower and change their clothes when coming in from the outside. Clothes should be dried in an automatic dryer, not outdoors.

Outdoor mold exposure can be decreased by avoiding areas of decaying plants, rotting leaves, and other debris. Wearing a mask when working outside might also be of benefit. Indoor mold can best be controlled by increasing light and ventilation in damp areas of the home and by keeping the humidity levels between 35% and 40%. This also helps control dust mite growth. Diluted bleach can be used in bathrooms to remove mold and mildew from surfaces.

Dehumidifiers in the basement and other potentially moist areas of the home help remove dampness.[15] Indoor plants may also contain mold in the soil, but the spores become airborne only if the soil is disturbed.

The control of dust mite sensitivity is focused on the bedroom because of the time spent in that room. Hardwood floors are best, with no scatter rugs or clutter. Carpets should be vacuumed routinely with use of a HEPA cleaner. Pillows should be hypoallergenic and both the pillow and mattress covered with hypoallergenic covers. Stuffed animals and books should be covered in the room in storage bins.

Homes with forced hot air and central air conditioning should have the filters changed every 2 to 3 weeks.

Patients with animal dander sensitivity can be more difficult to treat if the family's decision is to keep the pet. Pets must be kept out of the patient's room at all times, and a HEPA filter should be run in the bedroom. Because animal dander is sticky, bedclothes should be clean before entering the bedroom. Washing the hands and face after pet exposure is also advised.[8]

It is imperative to control a patient's exposure to environmental allergens that cause an atopic reaction, but nonallergic triggers can also add to the clinical picture. Exposure to cigarette smoke in the home or vehicle can cause exacerbations of rhinitis or asthma and should be prohibited. Air pollution including perfumes, paints, carpet off-gassing, diesel or other industrial fumes, or woodsmoke can cause reactions. Weather conditions, such as hot, humid days or extremes of cold temperatures, can also exacerbate symptoms.[9] Patients should be advised of these nonallergic triggers and their potential for increasing symptoms. Finally, viral syndromes can also exacerbate symptoms of rhinorrhea and asthma.

COMPLICATIONS

Complications of allergy immunotherapy are cause for concern and must be treated appropriately. Allergy extract must be checked for its expiration date as well as to make certain that the right patient is receiving the correct dose. Documentation of reactions to allergy immunization must be performed routinely, and patients must be given clear instructions on what to expect from their allergy immunotherapy as well as potential side effects and systemic reactions. Providers and staff must be thoroughly trained to effectively deal with systemic reactions in their practices.

PATIENT EDUCATION

Much of what has been discussed in the section on management must be given to the patient in written format, and the patient should verbalize understanding of these avoidance modalities. Medications used in the treatment of rhinitis, eczema, urticaria, bronchospasm, and anaphylaxis must be reviewed at each visit. Emergency action plans in the case of systemic reactions must be reviewed and documented at each patient visit. Those in allergy specialty practices must be certain that communication with the primary care provider is ongoing and up to date to prevent duplicate services.

FOOD ALLERGIES

DEFINITION AND EPIDEMIOLOGY

The incidence of food allergies in children has risen dramatically over the past decade. In 2010, the CDC reported that 5 of every 100 children in the Unites States had some form of food allergy. An 18% increase was reported from 1997 to 2007 for children younger than 18 years. From 2006 to 2008, hospital discharge rates for children with a food allergy–related diagnosis were nearly 9500 per year. In addition, children with food allergies were also more likely to have other IgE-mediated disorders such as asthma, allergic rhinitis, and eczema.[17]

Although an allergy may develop to a wide variety of foods, 90% of all allergic reactions occur from the ingestion of just eight foods. These foods are cow's milk, hen eggs, peanuts, tree nuts, fish, shellfish, soy, and wheat.[18] Whereas these eight foods are responsible for the majority of reactions, cow's milk, hen eggs, and peanuts account for nearly 80% of these reactions.[3] In adults, shellfish, peanuts, tree nuts, and fish are the more common allergens.[19]

The allergic reactions patients may exhibit range from rhinorrhea to full anaphylaxis.[20] Other possible reactions include asthma exacerbations, eczema, urticaria, gastrointestinal pain, and possibly nausea and vomiting. Patients may also exhibit a combination of symptoms caused by specific foods (e.g., eczema to milk and anaphylaxis to peanuts). Adults are less likely to develop food allergies in comparison to children. Many children tend to outgrow their allergic reactions to some foods within the first decade of life. Nearly two thirds of children with egg allergy will outgrow the allergy by 5 years of age. With milk allergy, 85% to 90% will no longer have an allergic response after 3 years of age.[17] In children, only 20% tend to outgrow their allergy to peanuts by 6 years of age. Peanuts, tree nuts, and shellfish have a higher incidence of lifetime allergy.[21]

PATHOPHYSIOLOGY

The development of food sensitivity is dependent on many factors. After ingestion of the food, the body undergoes an abnormal response through the mucosal immune system. The mucosal immune system "sees" a large quantity of food and in genetically predisposed people develops an inappropriate immune response to the protein antigens present in foods.[22] The breakdown or lack of development of oral tolerance starts the sensitivity process, resulting in food-specific IgE production. IgE-mediated interactions occur with mast cells and basophils on target organs.

Once stimulated by further food protein ingestion, IgE antibodies bind the food protein antigen to high-affinity FcεRI receptors on mast cells and basophils and low-affinity FcεRII receptors on macrophages, monocytes, lymphocytes, eosinophils, and platelets.[23] As in other IgE-mediated disorders, inflammatory mediators are released including histamine, prostaglandins, leukotrienes, and cytokines. The inflammatory cascade continues with vasodilatation, smooth muscle contraction, mucus secretion, and potential for petechial hemorrhage. Specific symptoms result depending on the target organ affected.[22]

This period of increasing sensitivity is highly variable among patients. Reactions do not occur until the immune response has developed to a degree that the IgE levels are elevated sufficiently to cause some form of allergic reaction. In some patients, a reaction may occur after the second ingestion; others may need 100 or more exposures to develop an allergic response.[23]

DIAGNOSTICS

Prior to age 5 or 6, in most pediatric patients with persistent rhinorrhea, eczema, or urticaria, the condition is secondary to food allergies. At this age, asthma is commonly caused by nonallergic triggers such as viral syndrome. The diagnosis is based on the patient's history of food ingestion and the subsequent field reaction, skin prick testing, and the results of ImmunoCAP laboratory testing.[20,21]

Skin prick testing is performed at the scratch level (i.e., the strongest dilution scratched on the skin). A positive SPT results in erythema, pruritus, and elevation at the test site with both a flare and wheal.[24] Histamine and saline controls are placed simultaneously on another area of the body (e.g., the back or upper arms). Readings of SPTs are done 15 minutes after placement. The histamine should cause a positive reaction and the saline should cause no reaction for the results to be considered reliable.

It is important that patients be reminded to stop all antihistamines, H_2 blockers, and tricyclic antidepressants before testing, because these will interfere with the allergic response.

Negative SPT reactions are most likely accurate, and skin prick testing is more sensitive than serum IgE ImmunoCAP testing. Positive results may be falsely positive, indicating patient tolerance. IgE levels may also be elevated because of a cross-reactivity of environmental pollen and food proteins.

An important clinical pearl is that patients are allergic to a food only if they develop symptoms after ingestion. If the skin test and/or ImmunoCAP indicates a positive result and the patient eats the food routinely without reaction, then this indicates clinical tolerance.[24]

When testing for potential food allergies, it is essential that a careful dietary history be obtained. If the patient rarely or never ingests a particular food, it is highly unlikely that he or she is allergic to the food protein. The body must "see" the food in sufficient quantity to build up the IgE–food protein response.

Component-resolved diagnostics (CRD) testing can also be considered in the diagnosis of food allergies. This serum blood test provides a molecular view of the individual protein components of an allergenic source. This allows valuable knowledge of IgE sensitization patterns to specific allergen components and cross-reactive allergen components.[25]

DIFFERENTIAL DIAGNOSES

Nearly 20% to 25% of parents believe that their child has a food allergy based on observed signs and symptoms. However, the actual prevalence is much lower, with approximately 4% of adults and 6% to 8% of children affected. Therefore it is important to distinguish a true IgE-mediated allergic reaction from adverse food reactions.[20,21]

DIFFERENTIAL DIAGNOSIS

- Cell-mediated food hypersensitivities include food-induced enterocolitis and colitis, malabsorption syndrome, and celiac disease.
- Dietary protein–induced enterocolitis or colitis is seen in infants from 1 week to 3 months of age after milk and soy ingestion. Symptoms typically resolve by 1 to 2 years of age as the child develops tolerance.
- Malabsorption syndrome is also self-limited but may result in failure to thrive (FTT). In addition to milk and soy, wheat is also commonly implicated in this disorder. Resolution is typical by 6 to 18 months of age.[22]
- Celiac disease results in FTT and is often lifelong. The offending foods with celiac disease include wheat, rye, and barley.
- Other non–IgE-mediated food intolerances include lactase deficiency, psychological aversions to particular foods, and toxic reactions to foods (e.g., sulfites, aspartame).[22,27]

MANAGEMENT AND PATIENT AND FAMILY EDUCATION

Once the diagnosis of food allergy has been made, the mainstay of therapy involves strict removal of all foods causing allergic reactions. The majority of patients have an IgE-mediated allergy to one food. In others, multiple foods may be allergenic, especially in patients younger than 5 years. The literature also makes note of food families—for example, legumes include peanuts, string beans, and peas. Although a patient may develop an allergy to one food in the food family, it is unlikely that one would be allergic to all foods in the same family.

Two exceptions to food family allergies include tree nuts and crustaceans (i.e., shrimp, crab, and lobster). Patients may react clinically to only one food in the family; however, because of the high allergenicity of these foods and potential for anaphylaxis, patients should be advised to avoid all foods in the family. It is also imperative to point out that the protein in tree nuts is entirely different from the protein in peanuts. An allergic response to one does not indicate an allergy to both foods.[19]

Strict avoidance of foods must be considered a therapeutic intervention. When recommending the avoidance of a food, it is imperative that an alternative be recommended.[26] In children, coordinated efforts must be in place with the patient's primary care provider to be certain that there is appropriate height and weight gain. The nutritional requirements for patients with food allergies are not different from those without food allergies. When withholding foods as a result of an allergy, one must consider total calories, carbohydrates, fat, and protein requirements, as well as minerals and vitamins. Consultation with a registered dietitian may be required.[26]

The length of time a food must be avoided to produce tolerance is dependent on the severity of the reaction, the patient's age, and the results of skin prick testing and serum IgE testing. In children with milk, egg, or wheat allergy who have rhinorrhea or eczema, withholding the food for 3 to 6 months may result in clinical tolerance. Reintroduction of foods one at a time is required as parents monitor symptoms. The return of symptoms necessitates further food avoidance. With egg allergy, it is best to have the patient eat egg in cooked and baked products as a means of developing tolerance.[21]

Patients who have more severe symptoms such as urticaria, facial swelling, or anaphylaxis may require a longer length of time for avoidance and may require lifelong avoidance as discussed earlier. The results of IgE testing become important in this clinical situation. A patient with a peanut IgE of less than 2.0 may safely undergo a food challenge to test for food tolerance or sensitivity. Any IgE result above this level is not considered safe for food challenge, especially in light of past anaphylaxis. Oral food challenge (OFC) remains the gold standard in the evaluation of food allergies.[26]

In the case of true anaphylaxis, parents must undergo substantial education regarding accidental ingestion and the need for a written emergency action plan. Parents need to be encouraged to have a healthy respect for the food allergy, not a fear of the reaction. Parents who are adequately prepared can educate the child about reading food labels and checking food content when eating out or at a friend's house. Accidental ingestions can occur even in the most vigilant families. This is an important period of time for patient education because those with a lifelong allergy will need to be prepared to handle accidental ingestion once they leave the home.

Oral diphenhydramine in either tablet, dissolvable, or liquid form is the preferred antihistamine used in cases of accidental ingestion and the development of symptoms. Diphenhydramine is used with symptoms of pruritus, urticaria, or eczema.

The development of respiratory compromise, facial flushing, abdominal pain, and nausea and vomiting indicate the possibility of impending anaphylaxis. Most cases of anaphylaxis occur within 1 hour of ingestion, but latent reactions up to 4 hours after ingestion are possible.[26] Epinephrine (1:1000 solution) is given immediately via the subcutaneous route. Doses may be repeated at 5- to 15-minute intervals two or three times.[17] The emergency management system is also activated.

One important clinical pearl is that the only way to predict anaphylaxis is to have had prior anaphylaxis. Patients with a past history of pruritus, urticaria, or facial swelling may progress to anaphylaxis with future ingestions. Finally, death is most frequent in the late teenage years, after the individual has left the home, when epinephrine is not given rapidly with the onset of early signs of anaphylaxis.

CHAPTER 32

HEAD TRAUMA

Terry Mahan Buttaro

DEFINITION AND EPIDEMIOLOGY

Each year, up to 2.5 million people in the United States sustain a traumatic brain injury (TBI).[1] This number can be deceiving, however, because many individuals who incur a sports or recreational brain injury are not hospitalized, nor do they seek emergency department treatment.[2] Falls are the number one cause of TBI in children younger than age 14 and in adults older than age 65.[1] Unintentional blunt trauma and motor vehicle accidents are the second and third most common causes of TBI with motor vehicle crashes the second most common cause of TBI death.[1] Older adults require more hospitalizations and have a higher mortality rate than other age groups for TBI. In elders, morbidity and mortality are related to an increased fall risk as well as increased brain tissue fragility and age-related changes.[3] The costs nationwide are significant: 76.5 billion dollars per year.[1]

TBI is also a common injury for active duty military personnel and can range from mild to severe depending on the type of injury.[4] There is increased concern about the number of mild traumatic brain injuries (MTBIs) and undiagnosed TBIs that occur not only in combat but also in sports and recreational activities.[2] In MTBI, imaging studies may be normal, but patients may complain of a variety of symptoms that affect daily work and life activities for weeks to months after the injury.[2]

Repetitive brain trauma or chronic traumatic encephalopathy is usually related to repeated injuries and is often associated with sports. Although chronic head trauma does not result in immediate death, there are chronic brain changes that cause depression and other personality changes, as well as Alzheimer or Parkinson disease.[2] The injury can be mild or severe enough to dramatically affect a patient's intellectual and physical capacity as well as his or her psychological, social, and economic well-being.

Loss of consciousness has always been considered one of the most significant indicators of brain injury.[5] However, patients with MTBI may not lose consciousness, and patients with epidural bleeding may have only brief loss of consciousness, then be alert and behave appropriately before clinical deterioration rapidly ensues.[2] It is essential that health care providers be aware of the "talk and deteriorate" syndrome. Patients with this

TABLE 32-1 Glasgow Coma Scale

Sign	Score
EYE OPENING	
Spontaneous	4
To verbal command	3
To pain	2
No response	1
BEST MOTOR RESPONSE	
Obeys verbal commands	6
Localizes pain	5
Movement or withdrawal to pain	4
Flexion response to pain (decorticate)	3
Extension response to pain (decerebrate)	2
No response	1
BEST VERBAL RESPONSE	
Alert and oriented	5
Converses but confused or disoriented	4
Nonsensical or inappropriate words	3
Nonspecific sounds	2
No response	1

Modified from Quality Standards Subcommittee of the American Academy of Neurology: *American Academy of Neurology practice handbook,* St Paul, MN, 1997, American Academy of Neurology.

syndrome utter recognizable words after the head injury and then deteriorate to a severe, brain-injured condition within 48 hours. The most common neurologic findings are altered mental status and focal hemispheric deficits. For these patients, early and appropriate use of computed tomography (CT) scanning is helpful in detecting significant intracranial lesions before clinical neurologic deterioration occurs.

Older patients can also incur serious injury even when the head injury is minor. In general, however, patients who lose consciousness for more than 10 minutes or have a focal neurologic deficit are considered to have a major brain injury, whereas those who are unconscious for less than 10 minutes and have no neurologic deficit are classified as having a minor TBI.[3] In acute injury, the severity of damage can be described by an injury-rating system such as the Glasgow Coma Scale (GCS) score (Table 32-1).[6] The GCS assesses eye opening responses, motor responses, and verbal responses. Numbers are assigned for the level of function attained in each category and then totaled. A normal patient has a score of 15, whereas a patient who is brain dead has a score of 3. Minor head trauma is defined as an initial GCS score of 13 to 15 and a period of unconsciousness of less than 20 minutes. Moderate head injury refers to an initial GCS score of 9 to 12 with or without loss of consciousness. Severe head trauma is defined as an initial GCS score of less than 8 or a comatose state for 6 hours or more.[6]

PATHOPHYSIOLOGY

The cranial vault is a fixed space that contains the brain, cerebrospinal fluid (CSF), and blood. Because the skull limits intracranial volume, neurologic damage after head injury can be directly related to cerebral edema that causes increased intracranial pressure (ICP), which in turn decreases cerebral blood flow and causes cerebral ischemia. Head trauma can consist of soft tissue injury, skull fracture, and/or hemorrhage. Brain injury from trauma can occur in two stages: primary and secondary. Primary injury is sustained in the initial insult and may result from blunt trauma, penetrating injury, coup-contrecoup lacerations or contusions of the brain, or direct disruption of brain tissue by the shearing of axons. Secondary injury may occur from increased ICP, cerebral hypoxia, systemic hypotension, decreased cerebral blood flow, and oxygen free radicals resulting in cellular death. The secondary sequelae may cause further neuronal damage, which can compromise an already injured brain. In mild TBI, the primary cause of injury is the dysfunction of brain metabolism rather than structural injury.[7]

CLINICAL PRESENTATION

It is important to establish the mechanism of the trauma, the stability or progression of the patient's symptoms, the patient's prior condition, and the patient's significant medical history including current medications (especially antiplatelet or anticoagulant therapy) and allergies. The cause and exact location of the injury should be determined: Was it accidental or intentional? Changes in mentation and any loss or change in level of consciousness should be determined and elicited not only from the patient, when possible, but also from witnesses. A history of amnesia (retrograde or anterograde) concerning the traumatic event, even if fleeting, often indicates altered consciousness and needs to be quantified.[2] It is also necessary to ascertain consciousness before the head injury to identify other pathologic conditions, such as stroke, myocardial infarction, or respiratory distress. Additional causes of altered mental status, such as hypoglycemia, drug overdose, hyperthermia, or arrhythmias, must also be investigated. Alcohol intoxication can mask the signs and symptoms of a head injury; therefore it is important to determine if alcohol was involved. The history should also elicit previous history of concussion or other brain trauma, complaints of seizure activity, confusion, drowsiness, dizziness, headache, visual changes, blurred vision, tinnitus, slurred speech, neck pain, nausea, vomiting, upper or lower extremity weakness, difficulty concentrating, and emotional lability such as increased irritability or other change in behavior.[2]

In older patients, the first sign of brain injury may be confusion or a change in behavior rather than a reported fall or other injury. The patient may not remember a fall or injury or may believe that the injury was insignificant. Family members or caregivers may also not be aware that an event occurred.

PHYSICAL EXAMINATION

The patient with head trauma can fluctuate from being awake and alert to being comatose and in respiratory distress. The initial evaluation should follow the standard protocol developed for all trauma patients. The patient's circulation, airway, and breathing and the cervical spine must be evaluated and stabilized. The initial observation should focus on the patient's level of consciousness, oxygen saturation, vital signs, and determination of GCS score. The extremities should be examined for injuries and symmetric movement. A quick but thorough neurologic examination is necessary to assess brain injury, focal deficits, and stability of the patient. The neurologic examination should include mental status, memory, concentration, cranial nerves, motor strength and tone, deep tendon reflexes, and, when possible, finger-to-nose test, deep tendon reflexes gait, and Romberg test. The skull must also be examined for fractures, penetrating injuries, lacerations, or CSF drainage. Clinical signs of skull fracture include raccoon sign (bruising around the orbit), Battle sign, and blood in the external auditory canal. It is also important to perform repeated neurologic examinations to determine whether the patient's condition is stable, improving, or deteriorating. *However, normal neurologic examination findings do not eliminate the possibility of brain injury.* The severity of injury and prognosis are indicated by the amount of retrograde or post-traumatic amnesia.

DIAGNOSTICS

- Pulse oximetry and continuous vital signs.
- Cervical spine x-ray examination, because patients with head injury can have an associated cervical spine fracture.
- Non-enhanced head CT scan or x-ray study is indicated for:
  - Patients with a depressed or deteriorating level of consciousness, skull fracture, neurologic deficit, open head wound, penetrating head injury, amnesia, or high risk of intracranial injury
  - Older patients and patients who are receiving anticoagulants or antiplatelet therapy
  - Patients with MTBI (loss of consciousness for less than 5 minutes or amnesia accompanied by GCS score <15, headache, post-traumatic seizure, focal neurologic deficit, impaired short-term memory, depressed skull fracture, trauma above clavicle, age older than 60 years, or presence of alcohol or drug intoxication)[8,9]
- Repeated head CT scans may be necessary if neurologic deficits develop.[10]
- Magnetic resonance imaging has a limited role in head injury but may be indicated after CT scan in some instances for more specific anatomic detail and identification of diffuse axonal injury.
- Laboratory studies.
  - Complete blood count (CBC)
  - Electrolytes, magnesium, serum glucose, blood urea nitrogen (BUN), creatinine
  - Urinalysis, arterial blood gases (ABGs)
  - Coagulation panel
  - Blood alcohol level and drug screen, if indicated
  - Type and crossmatch for blood transfusion in cases of severe trauma

DIFFERENTIAL DIAGNOSIS

> **DIFFERENTIAL DIAGNOSIS**
>
> **Head Trauma**
>
> - Skull fracture, concussion, or contusion
> - Epidural or subdural hematoma
> - Subarachnoid bleed
> - Cerebral edema
> - Penetrating injuries

The differential diagnosis must include skull fracture, concussion, cerebral contusion, epidural hematoma, subdural hematoma, subarachnoid bleeding, cerebral edema, and penetrating injuries. Cerebral concussion is defined as the loss of consciousness without significant anatomic damage to the brain. The severity of the injury is quantified by the duration of amnesia—the length of amnesia concerning the time before impact (antegrade amnesia) plus the length of amnesia after impact (retrograde amnesia). It is usually helpful to determine the time interval between the first thing and the last thing remembered. Cerebral contusions usually occur on the undersurface of the poles of the frontal lobes or on the poles of the temporal lobes. The patient is typically awake and alert after the initial injury, but increasing ICP, decreased level of consciousness, and focal neurologic deficits may develop as the contusion mass increases in size.

INITIAL STABILIZATION AND MANAGEMENT

Traumatic Brain Injury

- First priority for patient with traumatic head injury: Manage circulation, airway, breathing, and cervical spine.
- Second priority: Correct hypoxia with 100 % high flow oxygen (in adults, PaO_2 <60 mm Hg) and hypotension (in adults, systolic blood pressure <90 mm Hg) because of associated morbidity and mortality.[11]
- Third priority: Assess primary injury and rapidly recognize surgically correctable lesion.
- Further evaluation for evidence of lacerations and other trauma (e.g. depressed skull fracture) is necessary.

Minor Head Trauma

- Diagnostic testing is dependent on the patient's history and physical examination findings. In general, it is important to assess and treat for alcohol ingestion, hypoglycemia, hypothermia, and/or narcotic overdose.
  - CT scans are not indicated for most patients with minor head trauma or a GCS score of 15.
  - Patients *without* the following do not require a CT scan:
    - Loss of consciousness
    - Confusion
    - Agitation
    - Behavior change
    - Drowsiness
    - Seizures
    - Amnesia
    - Worsening headache
    - Continued nausea or vomiting
    - Weakness
    - Slurred speech
    - Focal neurologic deficits
    - Depressed skull fracture[12]
- Patients may be discharged home if observation is available and instructions are given on proper patient evaluation.
- Patients with mild TBI and a negative head CT are also able to be discharged home with appropriate discharge instructions.
- In the future, laboratory biomarkers (e.g., plasma total tau) may be able to predict which patients with a concussion will require specific clinical therapy.[13]

DISPOSITION AND REFERRAL

- Patients may be discharged home with proper instructions if the CT scan is normal and if a family member or friend can provide close observation for 24 hours.
- If no one is available to monitor the patient or if there is evidence of a pathologic condition, the patient should be admitted to the hospital for observation.
- A patient who has had more than 5 minutes of unconsciousness, post-traumatic seizures, a GCS score of 12 to 14, focal neurologic deficits, a lesion on the CT scan, or a moderate

head injury (a GCS score of 9 to 12) should be hospitalized, stabilized, and closely observed for any neurologic deterioration; a neurosurgical evaluation is also indicated.
- Patients with severe head trauma (a GCS score of 8 or less, penetrating skull injuries, or compound skull fractures) should be evaluated at the nearest hospital and have a neurosurgical evaluation.

Immediate emergency department referral or physician consultation is indicated for head trauma with alteration in level of consciousness, paralysis, paresthesia, rhinorrhea, raccoon sign (ecchymosis beneath both eyes), Battle sign, otorrhea, and hemotympanum.

PATIENT AND FAMILY EDUCATION

Specific instructions must be provided to those who will be observing the patient who is discharged home. The patient should remain in the care of a competent caregiver and rest in a quiet environment for the first 24 hours after discharge, because the first 24 hours after the injury are the most important. The patient should return for treatment if any of the following develop: drowsiness or difficulty awakening (the patient should be awakened every 2 hours during sleep), continuous nausea, vomiting more than twice, seizures or convulsions, visual disturbances or pupillary changes, slurred speech, new-onset weakness or an inability to move body parts, severe headache, confusion, personality changes, unusual restlessness, difficulty breathing, dizziness, or difficulty walking.[4,14] Aspirin (and medications that contain aspirin), alcohol, and narcotics should not be taken for 1 week after the injury.

Patients should also be informed about the post-traumatic or postconcussion syndrome, which is not life-threatening but may disable a patient for weeks to months to even years. Symptoms may include headache, tinnitus, memory loss, dizziness, giddiness, poor concentration, emotional lability, irritability, nervousness, disturbed sleep, fatigue, and decreased libido. Symptoms last for 2 to 6 weeks in most cases but can be present for longer. Treatment consists of rest, reassurance, and analgesics. It is also extremely important that patients return to work as soon as possible, even if a reduced workload is necessary. Athletes who are diagnosed with a concussion, however, should not be permitted to return to physical activity until the concussion has resolved (Level B evidence).[14] Neurocognitive testing or other evidence of concussion resolution is necessary before these patients return to practice or play sports (Level B evidence).[14] Physical therapy, occupational therapy, psychotherapy, and speech therapy may benefit some patients, whereas others may require cognitive behavioral therapy if anxiety is a concern.[15] If the injury was related to substance abuse, the patient is encouraged to seek treatment.[15] Patients and families should understand that a potential complication is the development of post-traumatic epilepsy, which is defined as two or more seizures after head trauma.[7]

Patients must be educated about safety issues, such as the proper use of bicycle helmets, seat belts, and car seats for infants and children. Safety issues in the home should also be reviewed (e.g., staircases, gates, throw rugs, cluttered environment, and lighting) in an attempt to reduce falls in children and older adults.

CHAPTER 33

HYPOTENSION

Ashley Moore-Gibbs

DEFINITION AND EPIDEMIOLOGY

Hypotension, or low blood pressure, is defined as a systolic blood pressure of 90 mm Hg or less. Blood pressure readings should always be interpreted in the context of the patient's prior measurements. In patients with preexisting hypertension, a significant reduction from baseline with accompanying symptoms may represent relative hypotension, despite a reading above 90 mm Hg. The causes of hypotension are numerous, ranging from relatively benign to life-threatening. It is important for health care providers in the ambulatory setting to develop a methodical approach to the evaluation, treatment, and referral of patients with hypotension.

Orthostatic hypotension is defined by a sustained reduction in systolic blood pressure of more than 20 mm Hg or in diastolic blood pressure of more than 10 mm Hg within 3 minutes of standing.[1] Orthostatic hypotension is common in older adults, and its incidence is highest in those with Parkinson disease and those taking vasoactive medications.[2]

PATHOPHYSIOLOGY

When hypotension occurs, there is an alteration in one or more of the three components necessary for the maintenance of normal blood pressure. The first component is the state of contraction of the muscles in the blood vessel wall. Vasodilator medications, sepsis, anaphylaxis, autonomic nervous system dysfunction, and certain endocrine disorders may cause abnormal blood vessel relaxation and a decrease in blood pressure. The second component is intravascular volume. When intravascular volume is reduced as a result of bleeding, vomiting, diarrhea, or inadequate fluid intake, hypotension may result. The third component is the adequacy of cardiopulmonary function. A decrease in cardiac function resulting from pump failure or dysrhythmia will cause a reduction in cardiac output and blood pressure. Understanding of these three fundamental mechanisms of hypotension will help generate a differential diagnosis. Abnormalities of more than one of these three components may occur simultaneously in the same patient.

Orthostatic hypotension is a sustained reduction in systolic blood pressure of more than 20 mm Hg or in diastolic blood pressure of more than 10 mm Hg within 3 minutes of standing.[1] Common in older adults, orthostatic hypotension occurs most frequently in those with Parkinson disease and those taking vasoactive medications.[2]

Orthostatic hypotension may result from either neurogenic or non-neurogenic causes. In turn, neurogenic orthostatic hypotension can be caused by abnormalities of either the central or peripheral nervous system. Peripheral autonomic dysfunction is the most frequent cause of orthostatic hypotension in the elderly.[3] With aging, there is a decrease in baroreflex sensitivity. This blunts the normal physiologic response to standing (i.e., vasoconstriction and a modest increase in heart rate), with a resultant drop in blood pressure. In addition to decreased baroreflex sensitivity, older individuals have diminished heart rate responses and impaired $alpha_1$-adrenergic vasoconstriction.[2] Age-related reductions in parasympathetic tone also occur and result in less cardioacceleration during vagal withdrawal on standing.[2] Orthostatic hypotension is more common in patients with degenerative neurologic diseases and some peripheral neuropathic syndromes.[2] Medications, including diuretics, antihypertensives, alpha blockers, nitrates, calcium channel blockers, antidepressants, and opiates, may provoke or worsen orthostatic hypotension.[2]

Neurogenic orthostatic hypotension involves the central nervous system and is well associated with increased mortality rates in patients with diabetes, hypertension, or Parkinson disease and those receiving dialysis.[4] Patients with neurogenic orthostatic hypotension may be symptomatic or asymptomatic during episodes of orthostatic hypotension. Symptoms emerge during postural changes, after prolonged standing, with dehydration, after alcohol ingestion, after carbohydrate-heavy meals, with heat exposure or fever, during stressful events, or with Valsalva maneuvers from straining.[4]

Non-neurogenic causes of orthostatic hypotension include cardiac functional impairment, dehydration, and vasodilation. A transient drop in blood pressure occurring with an abrupt change in position and resolving rapidly suggests a non-neurogenic cause.[1]

Postprandial hypotension is another potential cause of hypotension in the elderly. It should be suspected when there is a decrease in blood pressure within 2 hours after eating.[3] The mechanism of postprandial hypotension is poorly understood. Current evidence suggests that the cause of postprandial hypotension is multifactorial, including autonomic and neural dysfunction, changes in gastrointestinal hormones, meal composition, gastric distention, and the rate of delivery of nutrients to the small intestine.[3] Multiple factors contribute to a postprandial fall in blood pressure, and this manifests with inadequate cardiovascular compensation for meal-induced splanchnic blood pooling.[3] Postprandial changes in diastolic blood pressure are not as marked as systolic blood pressure changes. Typically there is a fall in systolic blood pressure of more than 20 mm Hg, or a decrease to 90 mm Hg or lower when the preprandial blood pressure is 100 mm Hg or higher within 2 hours of a meal.[3]

CLINICAL PRESENTATION AND PHYSICAL EXAMINATION

Although the symptoms of hypotension vary greatly, those related to the brain and heart predominate. Lightheadedness and dizziness are common symptoms of orthostatic hypotension. In addition, some individuals may experience blurred or tunnel vision and a dull pain in the back of the neck and shoulders.[1] Symptoms are more pronounced with positional changes such as standing and do not occur while the patient is supine.[1] Neurologic symptoms of hypotension include lightheadedness, dizziness, confusion, focal neurologic deficits, and loss of consciousness.[4] Cardiopulmonary symptoms of hypotension include shortness of breath, dyspnea on exertion, chest pain, palpitations, and syncope.[1]

In addition to identification of the physical symptoms that result from hypotension, careful attention should be paid to symptoms that may reveal the underlying cause. Inquiry should be made about fluid intake, nausea and vomiting, diarrhea, rectal bleeding or melena, polyuria, and any antecedent cardiopulmonary symptoms.

DIAGNOSTICS

Hypotension may be evident on simple blood pressure measurement or after an assessment of orthostatic vital signs. A decrease in systolic blood pressure of 20 mm Hg and/or a decrease in diastolic blood pressure of 10 mm Hg when the patient changes position from lying to standing is diagnostic of orthostatic hypotension.[1]

Pulse and blood pressure measurements are performed with the patient in the supine, sitting, and standing positions (if the patient's response allows for this) when the patient has been supine at least 5 minutes and ideally at both 1 and 3 minutes of standing.[1] Detection of orthostatic hypotension may require multiple measurements performed on different days and at different times. Orthostatic measurements are more sensitive early in the morning when the patient awakens, because of nighttime pressure natriuresis.[1] Ambulatory automated blood pressure monitors may be useful in detecting orthostatic changes, but the patient must be able to recall specific times symptoms were noted with a change in posture. A low blood pressure, absolute or in comparison with the patient's normal pressure when the patient is supine, confirms the diagnosis, particularly if the decrease is associated with dizziness, lightheadedness, or tachycardia when the patient is in the standing position.[1] In those with hypertension, a reduction of systolic blood pressure readings of 30 mm Hg may be more appropriate when determining a diagnosis of orthostatic hypotension, depending on the patient's baseline.[1] Prospective studies have demonstrated that a reduction in systolic blood pressure of more than 20 mm Hg is a risk factor for falls, especially in older patients with hypertension.[1]

Measurement of heart rate concomitantly with blood pressure is important because failure of the pulse to increase with a decrease in blood pressure is indicative of neurogenic hypotension or central or peripheral nervous system diseases resulting in autonomic failure.[1] Tachycardic heart rates that are exaggerated suggest underlying volume depletion such as dehydration.[1] In elders, age-related reduction in baroreflex sensitivity decreases the ability for an appropriate heart rate response and is less useful as a diagnostic tool for measurement of heart rate.[1]

However, younger patients experiencing symptoms concerning for hypotension may maintain their systolic blood pressure and exhibit an increased pulse with a position change in conjunction with symptoms of cerebral hypoperfusion (fatigue, lightheadedness, exercise intolerance, or cognitive impairment); this represents postural orthostatic tachycardia syndrome (POTS).[5] There is an absence of orthostatic hypotension; however, the standing heart rate is often 120 beats per minute or higher.[5] POTS is more common in women aged 15 to 25 years. Up to half of those diagnosed with POTS have antecedent viral illness, and 25% have a family history of similar complaints.[5] Pathophysiologic mechanisms of POTS are multifactorial and include hypovolemia, venous pooling, hyperadrenergic states, and restricted adrenergic neuropathies in the lower limbs.[5]

When hypotension is identified, diagnostic testing is guided by the patient's history and physical examination findings. Relatively simple bedside tests with a high diagnostic yield include electrocardiography (ECG), serum hemoglobin, serum electrolytes, stool testing for occult blood, and urine pregnancy test in women of childbearing age. A careful review of the patient's medical regimen is fundamental because numerous drugs may cause or worsen hypotension. Additional testing should be based on the differential diagnosis. If cardiac dysfunction is suspected, additional studies (e.g., echocardiography, cardiac monitoring) may be indicated. When a pulmonary embolus is suspected, a D-dimer test and, if positive, a computed tomography (CT) scan of the chest should be performed. If intra-abdominal bleeding is the presumed cause, a CT scan of the abdomen may be required.

DIAGNOSTICS

Hypotension

INITIAL

ECG
Hemoglobin
Serum electrolytes, BUN and creatinine, glucose
Stool testing for occult blood
Urine pregnancy test (all women of childbearing age)

TARGETED

Echocardiography, cardiac monitoring (when cardiac dysfunction is suspected)
CT imaging of the chest (when pulmonary embolus is suspected)
CT imaging of the abdomen (when intra-abdominal bleeding is suspected)
Chest x-ray study, urinalysis, and blood cultures (when sepsis is suspected)
Endocrine studies (when adrenal insufficiency is suspected)

OTHER TESTS AS INDICATED

Tilt-table testing
Ambulatory blood pressure monitoring

BUN, blood urea nitrogen.

DIFFERENTIAL DIAGNOSIS

See the differential diagnosis box for possible causes of hypotension.

MANAGEMENT

The patient with hypotension should initially be placed in a recumbent position. Supplemental oxygen is essential for those patients in whom bleeding, myocardial infarction or failure, arrhythmia, or pulmonary embolus is suspected or for any patient with difficulty breathing. If hypovolemia is suspected, a fluid challenge of 250 to 500 mL of normal saline solution is administered intravenously, and its effect on the blood pressure is assessed.

The suspected cause of the hypotension guides further diagnostic evaluation and management. Patients should be educated about simple nonpharmacologic interventions for orthostatic hypotension. These include performance of gradual staged movements with postural change; avoidance of coughing, straining, and other maneuvers that increase intrathoracic pressure; and elevation of the head of the bed 6 to 9 inches, decreasing nocturnal diuresis.[1] Additional interventions include the use of custom-fitted elastic stockings (although these may not be tolerated by patients with motor dysfunction or neuropathies); physical activity and exercise to avoid deconditioning, which is known to exacerbate orthostatic intolerance; and increase in fluid and salt intake.[1] Physical countermaneuvers, such as crossing the legs to stand and performing dorsiflexion of the feet and toe crunches several times before arising, reduce peripheral pooling and increase venous return to the heart.[1] Treatment recommendations for postprandial hypotension include eating frequent small meals, avoiding sitting for prolonged periods after a meal, and, unless it is contraindicated, and ensuring adequate fluid consumption.[3]

DIFFERENTIAL DIAGNOSIS

Hypotension

CARDIOVASCULAR

- Cardiac pump failure (e.g., myocardial infarction, heart failure)
- Dysrhythmia
- Inadequate cardiopulmonary function
- Inadequate intravascular volume
- Inadequate vascular tone
- Pericardial tamponade
- Negative inotropic medications
- Vasodilator medications
- Vasovagal reaction

ENDOCRINOLOGIC

- Adrenal insufficiency

GASTROINTESTINAL

- Gastrointestinal bleeding
- Poor fluid intake
- Volume loss: vomiting and/or diarrhea

IMMUNOLOGIC

- Anaphylaxis

INFECTIOUS DISEASE

- Sepsis

NEUROLOGIC

- Autonomic dysfunction

PULMONARY

- Inadequate cardiopulmonary function
- Pulmonary embolus

RENAL

- Volume loss: diuresis

VASCULAR

- Ruptured abdominal aortic aneurysm
- Ruptured ectopic pregnancy

TRAUMATIC

- Intracavitary bleeding (chest, abdomen, pelvis)
- Long bone fracture
- Pericardial tamponade
- Tension pneumothorax

Pharmacologic therapy is instituted in conjunction with physician consultation. Medications used in the normotensive patient include fludrocortisone, which acts as a volume expander; or a sympathomimetic such as midodrine may be tried.[1] Short-acting pressor agents such as midodrine, an $alpha_1$-adrenergic agonist, are preferred in those with supine hypertension or heart failure.[1] Another potential agent is pyridostigmine, a cholinesterase inhibitor that increases blood pressure preferentially on standing. The use of pyridostigmine is limited by side effects that include nausea, vomiting, loose stools, and urinary urgency and frequency.[1]

Patients with a history of hypertension and who also have orthostatic hypotension should continue on antihypertensive medications. Withholding antihypertensive treatment often worsens orthostatic hypotension.[1] Older adult patients may receive benefit by taking angiotensin-converting enzyme inhibitors or angiotensin receptor blockers because of improved blood pressure regulation and cerebral blood flow.[1]

Those with neurogenic orthostatic hypotension may experience severe hypertension in the supine position. Raising the head of the bed 6 to 9 inches and/or taking a short-acting antihypertensive drug at bedtime may be needed in the management of these patients.[1]

LIFE SPAN CONSIDERATIONS

Postural and postprandial hypotension are both common in older adults for a number of reasons. Postural hypotension is potentiated by an impaired compensatory mechanisms to rapid changes in position (i.e., vascular tone and increases in heart rate), limited cardiovascular reserve, poor fluid intake, and concomitant use of vasoactive medication.[6] Postprandial hypotension is more likely a result of autonomic and neural dysfunction, changes in gastrointestinal hormones, gastric distention, and the use of antihypertensive medications before eating a high-carbohydrate meal. Both postural and postprandial hypotension care have serious consequences in older adults, including syncope, cardiovascular complications, and injuries secondary to falls.[6]

INDICATIONS FOR REFERRAL OR HOSPITALIZATION

Patients with hypotension as a result of dehydration may be rehydrated on an outpatient basis. Those with a poor response to a fluid challenge and those with signs of an acutely precipitated bout of hypotension need rapid transport to an emergency facility for further diagnosis, consultation, and treatment.

PATIENT AND FAMILY EDUCATION

Patient education is essential in the prevention and control of hypotension. Patients should be educated to recognize the factors that precipitate low blood pressure, such as prolonged standing, alcohol consumption (causing vasodilation), heat exposure (hot weather or hot bath or shower), sudden postural changes, prolonged recumbency, early morning orthostatic hypotension related to nocturnal diuresis and arising from bed, and high-carbohydrate meals (causing postprandial orthostatic hypotension). Patients taking medications that cause orthostasis should be taught to change positions slowly.

To maintain adequate plasma volume during warm weather and when vomiting or diarrhea occurs, patients should understand the importance of drinking five to eight 8-ounce glasses of fluid daily as well as having an adequate salt intake (i.e., intake should be 10 to 20 g of salt daily to help with retention of ingested fluids).[2] Instruction on nonpharmacologic management strategies for hypotensive episodes reviewed in the Management section should be discussed with the patient. Instructing patients to keep a log of supine and upright blood pressures during symptomatic episodes can aid in identifying whether worsening symptoms are related to a mechanism other than orthostatic hypotension.[1]

CHAPTER 34

POISONING

John J. Graykoski

DEFINITION

Poison is defined as a chemical capable of causing illness that enters the body through ingestion, transdermal absorption, intravenous administration, radiation, inhalation, or venom transmitted by stings or bites. Poisonings can be accidental (e.g., contact with concentrated chemicals or industrial agents, taking the wrong medication) or intentional (e.g., illicit drug use). Poisonings can also be industrial (e.g., spraying field workers with pesticides) or an act of war or terrorism (e.g., chemical weapons).

By any means or by any cause, poisoning represents a life-threatening situation until proven otherwise. It will always be best treated in an emergency department that has decontamination and isolation resources (if required), diagnostic laboratory services immediately available, and intensive care monitoring.

EPIDEMIOLOGY

The United States has a system of 57 regional poison control centers that upload all contacts in real time, providing a rapid threat assessment for clusters of poisoning as well as a major database for understanding of poisoning trends. In 2013, more than 3,060,122 calls were fielded by the centers; 48% of the cases involved children younger than 6 years.[1] Eighty percent of exposures were determined to be accidental, whereas suicide was suspected in 10.5%. Therapeutic errors and unintentional misuse represented 18.1% of cases[1]. A total of 2477 fatalities occurred[1]. Of particular concern is the fact that drug overdose is the second leading cause of injury-related death in this country.[2] The data from the American Association of Poison Control Centers represent an important window into the substances involved in poisoning as well as trends analyzed yearly since 1983.

PATHOPHYSIOLOGY

The pathophysiologic process depends on the poisonous substance and on the route, duration, and amount of exposure. The patient's underlying physical condition and initial first aid measures will also affect the impact of the toxin.

CLINICAL PRESENTATION

The presentation of poisoning can have differing signs and symptoms depending on the patient and type of poisoning. In an ideal scenario, the patient or patient's family can provide accurate information about the situation. However, in many cases the poisoning is assumed based on circumstantial findings, such as a sleeping person who will not wake and empty acetaminophen bottles found in the room.

The provider should suspect poisoning in patients with unexplained and sudden respiratory wheezing or dyspnea, acute agitation, somnolence that is progressive, hallucinations or delusions, areas of erythema or rash that appear suddenly, acute onset of epigastric pain, vomiting, diarrhea, hypertension and hyperthermia, and sudden and unexplained loss of consciousness. The provider should be particularly alert to situations in which a number of people show similar symptoms within a short time, especially if they were in a common area. A low threshold of suspicion for a common source of poisoning requires action to prevent additional casualties—for example, several people with vomiting and diarrhea who report having eaten potato salad at the volunteer fire department picnic, or a group of postal workers who develop worsening cough and shortness of breath after coming in contact with a package. An early call to the local health department is indicated to report such cases so that further investigation may be implemented. In cases involving exposure of a group of people to a toxic substance, such as the release of refrigerant in cold processing plants, the fire department should be called to the scene before transport to a health facility so that appropriate decontamination can occur.

PHYSICAL EXAMINATION

The clinical evaluation begins with a detailed history. Special attempts are made to obtain information from family and first responders. Attempts must be made to recover medication bottles and over-the-counter medicines. Recovery of any chemicals used at the site of overdose or exposure is important. Material Safety Data Sheets should be available at any site where chemicals are in use. These provides vital information on the chemicals' composition and phone numbers for additional information.

Previous exposures, medical conditions including chronic illnesses, and current medications should be obtained. Psychiatric issues will be important in assessment of stress reaction to the poisoning as well as previous suicide attempts, mental health interventions, and hospitalizations. The physical examination should assess mood and emotions. Issues of depression, anxiety, sleep disturbance, substance abuse, and hallucinatory or delusional processes must be explored. An assessment of suicidal risk should be undertaken.

The neurologic examination should note pupillary reaction, nystagmus, deep tendon reflexes, gait, station, Romberg test result, and pronator drift. The Glasgow Coma Scale score is recorded on arrival and monitored for change (see Table 32-1). Skin temperature and color are noted. The body must be exposed, looking for rashes, burns or irritations, bruising, and needle marks suggestive of injection drug use. The provider must observe for areas of discoloration or frank necrosis as well as blistering. Cardiovascular considerations include tachycardia, bradycardia, and peripheral circulation. The respiratory system must be evaluated for good air movement and oxygen saturation; carbon monoxide and carbon dioxide should be tested at bedside; and secretions, color, retractions, rales, and wheezing should be noted. Gastrointestinal examination includes observation of vomitus and feces, watching especially for bleeding. Guaiac testing of stool and vomitus should be done. Bowel sounds must be noted and their character reported.

DIAGNOSTICS

In addition to vital signs and physical findings, laboratory values can be an important aspect of the diagnostic evaluation and aid in management. Diagnostic tests should be dictated by the toxicologic exposure. Some substances, including alcohol, aspirin, acetaminophen, illicit drugs, iron, lead, mercury, carboxyhemoglobin, and ethylene glycol, can be measured directly. Assessment of arterial blood gases, the anion gap, the osmolar gap, and the oxygen saturation gap may provide additional information.

DIAGNOSTICS
Poisoning

INITIAL
- Pulse oximetry
- ECG
- Capnography

LABORATORY
- CBC
- Serum electrolytes
- BUN
- Creatinine
- AST, ALT, GGT
- Serum ammonia
- Serum lactate
- Blood gases (arterial if respiratory distress)*
- Acetaminophen level (if ingestion)
- Salicylate level (if ingestion)
- Ethanol level
- Toxicology (urine or blood)
- Serum hCG (female patients)*
- INR, PTT

OTHER DIAGNOSTICS
- Phenytoin*
- Digoxin*
- T_4*
- Lithium*
- Valproic acid*
- Iron*
- Carboxyhemoglobin (carbon monoxide)*
- Methemoglobin*

*If indicated.
AST, aspartate aminotransferase; ALT, alanine transaminase; GGT, γ-glutamyl transpeptidase; hCG, human chorionic gonadotropin; INR, international normalized ratio; PTT, partial thromboplastin time.

Other laboratory studies are helpful in assessing end-organ involvement. These should include electrolyte values; glucose, blood urea nitrogen (BUN), and creatinine concentrations; and liver function tests. Urine screens may be indicated if cocaine, opiates, or marijuana is suspected. A pregnancy test should be obtained, if indicated. An electrocardiogram (ECG) is necessary with specific poisons, and assessment will need to be repeated in some instances.[3] Further evaluation is indicated if abnormalities such as acidosis and hypoxia are discovered.

DIFFERENTIAL DIAGNOSIS

Poisoning can manifest with symptoms that can represent many other disease processes. The history is essential in arriving at the proper diagnosis.

DIFFERENTIAL DIAGNOSIS
Poisoning

NEUROLOGIC
- Stroke or acute cerebrovascular syndrome
- Seizure

ENDOCRINE
- Hypoglycemia

PSYCHIATRIC
- Alcohol intoxication
- Other drug use or abuse syndromes
- Suicidality

IMMUNOLOGIC
- Infectious disease
- Sepsis

INITIAL STABILIZATION AND MANAGEMENT

Immediate emergency department referral is indicated for victims of poisoning.

- Mobilize the emergency medical services (EMS) system (911).

- Contact the U.S. national Poison Help line for treatment guidance: 1-800-222-1222.
- The initial assessment and frequent reassessment of the poisoned patient require attention to airway, breathing, and circulation (ABC).[4]
- Oxygen and continuous airway maintenance are critical. The patient should be evaluated for intubation, and the provider should be ready to secure the airway with an endotracheal tube.
- Intravenous access is also necessary.
- Transport must be arranged to the closest appropriate facility by use of transport ambulance capable of critical care intervention.
- Determine the identity of the poison or substance, how it entered the person's system, why it was used or encountered, and when the contact was made. Transmit the substance with the patient to the emergency department if the patient has stable vital signs and is alert and oriented, and if this information is believed to be reliable. The provider can initiate a call to the poison control center for further instruction. The national Poison Help line can be reached at 1-800-222-1222. Any volatile or toxic chemical exposure requires decontamination of the patient and the patient's EMS caregivers. The patient should not be allowed into a hospital or clinic without decontamination. The facility should have in place a system for avoiding contact with the patient and isolating the patient until decontamination can be set up. This is vitally important in mass casualties. Workers trained in decontamination technique are appropriately garbed in self-contained breathing apparatus and protective clothing. The water used to decontaminate must be segregated and not allowed to enter public drainage systems. All of these issues are addressed in training of the decontamination team. The goal is to prevent rescuers from becoming victims and extension of the contamination to others. The next steps will occur simultaneously in the emergency department. In an unconscious or obtunded patient, a standard cocktail will be given to treat hypoglycemia, Wernicke encephalopathy, and opioid overdose: glucose, 25 to 50 g intravenously; thiamine, 100 mg intravenously; and naloxone, 2 mg intravenously, intramuscularly, or subcutaneously.[4] In general, this is done immediately on arrival. Immediate contact is made with poison control for expert guidance in management. Poison control should be alerted at the first notice of the arrival of a potential poisoning patient.
- If the airway is not secured, endotracheal intubation and ventilation will occur. After the ABCs are managed, attention returns to reversal of the poison's effect. For ingested components, activated charcoal, the usefulness of which is dependent on the length of time since ingestion (within one hour of poison ingestion is recommended), may be indicated for patients whose airway is intact or protected.[4,5] Considering the large number of substances that could potentially act as toxins, a relatively small number of antidotes are available. Some commonly used antidotes include the following:
  - *N*-acetylcysteine for acetaminophen. *N*-acetylcysteine is administered at an initial dose of 140 mg/kg by a standard protocol based on a nomogram to determine the necessity of treatment for acetaminophen overdoses.
  - Flumazenil for benzodiazepines. Flumazenil administered intravenously in 0.2-mg doses every minute to a maximum of 1 to 3 mg reverses the effects of benzodiazepines but could be detrimental if it is given to patients with benzodiazepine dependence, mixed substance overdose, alcohol overdose, or seizure history.[3,4,5]
  - Naloxone for opioids. Naloxone is an opiate antagonist and is given in doses of 0.4 mg intravenously, repeated every 2 to 3 minutes in the non–opiate-dependent patient, and 0.1 to 0.2 mg every 2 to 3 minutes in the opiate-dependent patient.[6]

TERRORISM

Biologic and chemical weapons remain a threat. State and national planning efforts are attempting to prepare an emergency response. Information systems are being developed to alert health care providers when a crisis occurs, and training programs in managing poisonings are under way. At this time, the existing systems for hazardous materials decontamination and basic and advanced life support measures remain the standard of care. Although all health care providers must maintain vigilance for suspicious presentations and clusters of patients with the same toxidrome, it will remain a complex system of identification of the chemical or biologic used and dissemination of antidotes, vaccines, and response plans. The first priority is to contain the exposures and to prevent expansion of the event; the second priority is basic life support; and the third priority is close communication with authorities charged with managing such emergencies.

PREVENTION AND PATIENT EDUCATION

With the majority of poisonings occurring in children younger than 6 years, prenatal and well-child counseling is an excellent opportunity to provide education and prevention advice. Families with young children need to survey their home for chemicals and medications. All need to be stored in areas inaccessible to children (with the caveat that few areas remain inaccessible to determined and curious children). These visits also provide the opportunity to discuss home and over-the-counter medications and treatments. Acetaminophen, a common fever and pain reliever, is a valuable medication, but dangerous at improper doses. A careful review of age-appropriate dosage and when to use acetaminophen can help parents prevent accidents. Increasing attention must also be addressed to various forms of nicotine and caffeine ingestion, as well as an awareness that marijuana is now legally available in many jurisdictions. Alerting parents to the effects of these drugs and substances should be part of early childhood counseling. In addition, many homes have other "recreational" drugs, from which children must also be protected.

Time spent with adults in reviewing potentially dangerous substances (e.g., energy drinks), new prescriptions, and proper scheduling is important to prevent poisoning or drug overdose. Equipping patients with a basic understanding of each drug's intended effect, the expected outcome, and symptoms or reaction of toxicity is valuable.

Education becomes increasingly important with older patients. Confusion in taking medication can result in accidental overdose. Helping to set up a system or engaging family, pharmacist, or caregivers in organizing medications is invaluable.

CHAPTER 35

SEXUAL ASSAULT

Julie G. Stewart

DEFINITION AND EPIDEMIOLOGY

Sexual violence consists of a variety of crimes including rape, sexual assault, and sexual harassment.[1] Sexual harassment includes many types of unwelcome sexual advances, remarks, and gestures. The legal definition of rape according to the Federal Bureau of Investigation (FBI) is "penetration, no matter how slight, of the vagina or anus with any body part or object, or oral penetration by a sex organ of another person, without the consent of the victim." The National Incident-Based Reporting System (NIBRS) defines rape as "The carnal knowledge of a person, without the consent of the victim, including instances where the victim is incapable of giving consent because of his/her age or because of his/her temporary or permanent mental or physical incapacity."[2] Sexual assault has a much broader definition. It is defined as any sexual act that is forced or coerced without the consent of the victim, not including penetration.[3] Rape and sexual assault are not sexually motivated acts; rather, they are motivated by rage, aggression, and the determination to dominate another human being.

In the United States, a person is a victim of sexual assault every 2 minutes.[4] According to the National Crime Victimization Survey, 346,830 rapes and sexual assaults of persons aged 12 years or older were reported in 2012.[5] Further surveys indicate that 1 of 5 women and 1 of 71 men in the United States experience a completed rape at some point in their lifetime.[6] Despite the general belief that the vast majority of perpetrators are male, a survey of 1058 14- to 21-year-old youths in the United States found that 9% reported having engaged in some form of sexual perpetration; rates of perpetration were similar between males and females by late adolescence.[7] The rates of sexual assault are higher for female college students, with validated reports of 18% to 20% experiencing some form of sexual assault during their years in college.[8] These statistics reflect only reported incidents. Sixty percent of sexual assaults are not reported to the police.[4] The incidence of rape is about 10 times higher for women than for men, although men are less likely to report the occurrence. (For the purpose of this chapter, the term *she* is used, although this information can also apply to men who have been victims of sexual assault.)

There are no known absolute risk factors for becoming a victim of sexual assault. In fact, anyone can be a victim regardless of age, race, gender, or socioeconomic status. However, sexual assault victims are predominantly female, and the perpetrators are almost always heterosexual males. Female victims are more likely to be assaulted by someone they know, and reports indicate that 63% of sexual assault victimizations involve offenders with whom the victim had a relationship as a family member, intimate, or acquaintance.[4] Among developmentally disabled adults, up to 83% of women and 32% of men are victims of sexual violence; of these victims of sexual violence, 49% will experience 10 or more abusive incidents.[9]

Sexual assault can also occur in the context of any intimate partner relationship. This includes marital, nonmarital, gay, lesbian, or past relationships. However, these sexual assaults are often recurring and one of the symptoms of a larger domestic violence problem that needs to be addressed. Consequences for ongoing sexual violence by an intimate partner are severe and require ongoing monitoring and attention by the health care provider.

CLINICAL PRESENTATION

The physical presentation of a patient in the clinic or office setting who has been sexually assaulted is immensely varied. Some patients may report a chief complaint of sexual assault to their health care provider, whereas others may not mention that a sexual assault has occurred. Likewise, the presentation of psychological effects of trauma also varies among victims, ranging from visibly shaken and crying to appearing calm. Some patients may choose to disclose that a sexual assault occurred if they are asked by a trusted health care provider. However, other patients may deny that violence occurred despite evidence of trauma. Whatever the reasons for the patient's denial, the health care provider must respect it and offer compassionate support. Reassuring the patient that sexual assault is always an act of control and violence and is never something anyone "deserves" or "asked for" is crucial for emotional support.

The health care provider does not need to make a final determination whether sexual assault has occurred; that must be left to the court to decide if the patient opts to report the assault. However, reporting to the police should be encouraged. It is helpful for the provider to let the patient know that sexual assault is, unfortunately, a common experience and that it is a problem the provider may be able to assist with. This may leave the door open should the patient decide in the future to disclose what happened. Unfortunately, in a national study, most rape and sexual assault victims were not treated for their injuries.[5] According to this study, only approximately 30% of victims received treatment, with 20% of this total receiving care at a physician's office or clinic.[5] Health care providers are mandated to report sexual assault of children (state laws vary on age limit), the elderly, and the disabled.

PHYSICAL EXAMINATION

If the patient does disclose a sexual assault, the provider should defer a physical examination and refer the patient to the emergency department if the sexual assault occurred within the past 5 days, preferably within 72 hours. A referral to the emergency department will ensure that the appropriate measures are taken to collect evidence and to comply with standardized protocol. This is essential to support the patient's current or future desire for legal pursuits, because some patients may decide later to report the incident to the police. This specialized forensic examination should be free of charge because federal and state funds are available. Having this examination and collection of evidence completed does not require the patient to press criminal charges or to report the incident to law enforcement. Testing for drugs that might have been used to render the patient unaware of what was happening can also be done at no cost to the patient. Furthermore, the emergency department will also be able to provide the patient with comprehensive and compassionate services, including crisis intervention, rape counseling, and referrals to appropriate community agencies. In many emergency departments, there are specially trained nurses (sexual assault nurse examiners [SANEs] and sexual assault forensic examiners) who help provide the patient with appropriate sensitive care.

The health care provider can prepare the patient for what to expect in the emergency department. It is not important that the provider request specific information about the assault; this information will be gathered in the emergency department. Retelling of the story can be traumatizing for the patient. Rather, providers can attentively listen and document what the patient desires to express, using exact quotes whenever possible. The health care provider should carefully note emotional responses (e.g., crying, restlessness, anxious behavior, shaking, withdrawal) because this would be useful in court as an adjunct to the emergency department records. It is important to advise the patient not to shower, urinate, brush teeth, or wash clothing that might contain evidence.

If the patient does not desire to pursue an examination in the emergency department or if more than 5 days have passed since the assault, medical care can be managed in the office setting. The provider needs to obtain a detailed history and perform a full physical examination and gynecologic examination. About 40% of rape victims sustained a collateral injury; 5% sustained a major injury, such as severe lacerations, fractures, internal injuries, or unconsciousness.[10] Injuries are most common among victims aged 30 years or older.[10] Possible gynecologic injuries include vaginal or anal tearing, rectal bleeding, bruising, and soreness. Other physical symptoms associated with trauma include gastrointestinal irritability, dysmenorrhea, pelvic pain, and urinary tract infection. (For specific treatment considerations, see chapters that address the specific injury, infection, and medical disorder.)

When the patient prefers to have a physical examination in the primary care office, the provider should assure her that the examination can stop at any time and that there is time to take a break if needed. The examination that should be performed is a complete head-to-toe examination observing for any injuries, because the patient may not be aware of abrasions or bruising in areas not visible to her. If any injuries are discovered, it is important to measure them with a ruler for documentation. Using the face of a clock to reference areas in the genitalia with the clitoris at the 12-o'clock position and the anus at the 6-o'clock position, the provider documents any abnormal findings. In particular, one should closely examine the posterior fourchette because it is frequently an area in which injuries such as lacerations and abrasions occur.[10,11] Culture specimens are obtained for gonorrhea and chlamydia testing; serum testing for syphilis, hepatitis B and C, and human immunodeficiency virus (HIV) infection and pregnancy is discussed as appropriate (see later).

DIAGNOSTICS

Potential consequences of sexual assault include the risk of pregnancy and sexually transmitted diseases (STDs), including HIV infection. If it has been more than 72 hours since the sexual assault, it is not feasible to offer pregnancy or STD prophylactics or antiretroviral therapy for postexposure prophylaxis.[12] A pregnancy test should be completed, with appropriate counseling pending the results. Testing for STDs should be determined individually. If the patient seeks treatment within 72 hours after the assault, the presence of an infection may indicate that the STD was present before the assault, even though laws in the United States limit the use of prior infections and sexual history as evidence in court. The patient may express fears about having contracted HIV infection; testing should be done 6 weeks and 3 and 6 months after the assault because of the length of time for seroconversion to occur. If the appropriate time has passed, patients should have pretest and post-test education and counseling. Education should include risks of acquiring the infection, potential transmission of the virus, and instruction about safe sex practices at least until testing is complete or longer if the results are positive.

Documentation

Accurate and precise documentation of the patient's physical and emotional signs and symptoms of sexual assault are always necessary, but especially so when there is a possibility that the documentation will corroborate the patient's testimony in court. It is essential that health care providers use medical rather than legal terminology. For example, calling the assault the "alleged rape" should be avoided; rather, it should be described as the "reported sexual assault." Likewise, the word "patient" should be used rather than "victim." The connotation of words must be considered. *Penetration* is a better word than *intercourse* because the latter may sound as though the act were consensual. If the patient does not wish to have a certain part of the examination completed, it should not be documented as "refused" because this makes the patient sound uncooperative; rather, the provider should write that the patient "declined" the examination. Use of the patient's own words in quotation marks whenever possible best captures the description of the incident and is extremely helpful in court. The provider should avoid writing "no weapons used" but should describe exactly what happened because there may have been verbal or implied threats. It is also important to be wary of using medical terminology that could be misinterpreted. For example, if the patient appears calm and collected, it is better to document that than to say "no apparent distress." Documentation of unnecessary history that is not related to the chief complaint (e.g., psychiatric history, substance abuse history) could be used in court to discredit the patient's testimony.[11]

Primary Care Management

When a patient reports that she has been a victim of sexual assault and it has been determined that she will be treated in the primary care setting, it is important to assess more than the patient's physical well-being. Patients may seek care soon after the assault or after an extended period. The patient's account of the assault will aid the provider in understanding the patient's experience and what type of services may be of benefit.

Patients who seek care shortly after the assault may display a range of emotions or may show a lack of emotions. Some may appear frightened, shocked, or angry. Regardless of their demeanor, they are in need of understanding and support. The patient's emotional presentation is not indicative of the level of trauma that has been experienced. A review of the patient's home environment and support system is appropriate. Because of the stigma associated with sexual assault, it is sometimes difficult for victims to inform significant people in their life about their victimization. Some fear that their intimate partner or parent may seek physical revenge against the perpetrator, if the perpetrator is known to them. As a result, they may be reluctant or unwilling to disclose information in an effort to protect their partner or parent from potential legal problems. Unfortunately, some patients are afraid to inform someone about the assault because they think that no one will believe them or that they are to blame for the assault. This is especially true if the patient consumed alcohol or drugs before the assault or if she thought she was dressed in provocative attire. As a result, the patient may not receive adequate support.

The provider can assist patients in identifying people in their lives to whom they can disclose the assault and who can provide support. Patients may also benefit from a discussion of the various ways in which to talk with their family or partner about the assault. Patients may experience a high degree of fear over the potential for further harm and may be afraid to be alone or to return home. They must be assisted in determining how to appropriately address their fears.

Patients who initially seek care a while after the assault may be prompted to do so because of physical complaints, such as STDs or pregnancy, or because of psychological difficulties. Some patients may experience symptoms of distress consistent with post-traumatic stress disorder. One study revealed that almost one third of rape victims develop post-traumatic stress disorder at some point after the rape; this rate is six times higher than the rate for women who have not been raped.[13]

Reactions of people who have been sexually assaulted vary according to a variety of factors, including age, gender, ethnicity, and circumstances surrounding the assault. Regardless of when the patient seeks care after a sexual assault, it is important for the provider to gain an accurate understanding of the patient's concerns, level of functioning, and support system before developing an appropriate treatment plan. The health care provider's comfort level with the subject matter may affect the patient's willingness to disclose information that would provide insight into the patient's needs. The provider is in a pivotal role to aid the patient in identifying the need for additional services, including mental health services.

INDICATIONS FOR REFERRAL OR HOSPITALIZATION

- *Emergency department:* It is strongly advised that the patient be treated in a specially equipped emergency department by trained sexual assault nurse examiners (SANE), sexual assault forensic examiners (SAFEs), or other appropriate health care providers if the examination occurs within several days of the assault.
- *Mental health services:* The patient should always be referred to mental health services that explicitly address issues surrounding sexual assault. Most areas have sexual assault crisis services available 24 hours per day, 7 days per week.
- *Legal services or police:* If the patient is treated in the primary care setting, an assessment must be made to determine her or his legal needs, level of functioning, and willingness to pursue additional services.
- *Other services:* Clearly, appropriate referral needs to be made for any symptoms, illnesses, or injuries for which treatment is beyond the scope of the office setting.
- *Mandated reporting:* Any sexual assault perpetrated on a victim who is younger than 18 years or on any adult who is physically dependent or cognitively impaired must be reported to the local child or adult protective agency as well as to law enforcement. Health care providers are mandated to report any suspicion of sexual assault in these populations, regardless of whether the patient reports that sexual assault has occurred. Although it is not the provider's responsibility to prove that the violence occurred, it is his or her responsibility to act on the clinical evidence presented. Because laws vary among states, providers should become familiar with the laws within their area.

LIFE SPAN CONSIDERATIONS

Children and Adolescents

Sexual abuse of children and adolescents is a serious and complicated issue that requires specialized training in interviews and physical examinations whenever abuse is suspected. Guidelines for caring for children and adolescents and collaboration with agencies that are child and adolescent specific should be the goal for this population in an effort to avoid lifelong complications related to the abuse.

Older Adults

Older patients are particularly vulnerable because of age-related illness and an overall decrease in physical strength. In fact, people over the age of 60 account for 18% of sexual assault victims.[14,15] In a study of elderly female sexual abuse victims, 81% of abuse was perpetrated by the victim's primary caregiver.[14] Seventy-eight percent was perpetrated by family members, of whom 39% were sons.[14]

Older adults may sustain more injuries and specifically more genital injuries. Older women are also unlikely to report being sexually assaulted; they may feel extreme embarrassment, humiliation, and shame because they were raised during a time when issues related to sex were not discussed. Some patients may be concerned that reporting the assault will result in a loss of their independence. Risk factors for being sexually assaulted include impaired hearing, diminished physical strength, limited mobility, reliance on others for help, and memory issues.

SPECIFIC POPULATIONS

Male Patients

Although male victims represent a minority of sexual assault victims, it is critical that they be treated the same as female patients. Male victims may experience rectal or penile trauma, bleeding or discharge, infection, or trauma to the mouth and pharynx. The patient may receive frontal injuries from being in a prone position during the assault. Men are usually assaulted by other men. For many reasons, men are less likely than women to seek services after being sexually assaulted, although they commonly experience similar physical and emotional reactions. Men may feel that they are "less of a man," may experience shame about not being able to defend themselves, and may be confused about their sexuality. If the assailant was a woman, the patient may feel particularly weak or inferior. Anxiety, depression, alienation, and insomnia are some of the psychological effects for men who have been sexually assaulted. As with all victims of sexual assault, it is important for the patient to receive mental health services.

Disabled Adults

Among the most vulnerable populations are individuals who are developmentally and/or physically disabled. Interpersonal violence against women and men with disabilities ranges from 26% to 90%.[16] Among developmentally disabled adults, up to 83% of women and 32% of men are victims of sexual violence.[16] Of those victims of sexual violence, 49% will experience 10 or more abusive incidents.[16] From 97% to 99% of their attackers are known to the victims.[16] Health care providers who provide medical services to the developmentally disabled need to assess for any signs and/or symptoms of abuse (physical and/or sexual). Examples of signs and symptoms include unexplained bruises, genital lacerations, STDs, regression, acting out, sleep disturbances, and depression.

Homeless or Marginally Housed

The intersection between lack of adequate housing and sexual violence occurs on a variety of levels. It is vital for the health care provider to be sensitive and to assess for any history of sexual assault in patients who are either homeless or living in inadequate housing. Being homeless or marginally housed increased the risk for being sexually assaulted, particularly for lesbian, gay, bisexual, and/or transgendered (LGBT) youth. According to data from the National Sexual Violence Resource Center, over 60% of young women left their homes because they had been sexually abused, and LGBT youths were either forced out of their homes or ran away because of rejection related to their sexual orientation.[17] For those youths and adults who sought to relocate after being abused by their landlords or whose perpetrator lived nearby, over 70% to 80% were unable to move because of lease or legal issues or a lack of housing options.[17]

Immigrants

Many immigrants have difficulty accessing care because of limited resources, language barriers, and lack of awareness about how to access services; however, additional concerns arise with respect to receiving services for sexual assault. Some patients may be afraid to report the sexual assault to authorities because they are concerned that it may have a negative impact on their immigration status, especially if the patient is an undocumented alien. They also may not understand that it is illegal for them to be assaulted and that they have a right to report the crime. Another significant factor for immigrants in accessing services to address sexual assault is their cultural beliefs. Some may think it is inappropriate for them to discuss intimate matters with a professional, although they may not have the means or methods to address their issues within a cultural context. It is important for health care providers to be aware of cultural factors when providing care, to modify their treatment to the extent that they are able, and to ensure that the patient is aware of his or her rights and the availability of services.

PATIENT EDUCATION AND HEALTH PROMOTION

Sexual assault occurs in a variety of settings and may victimize people of all ages, races, religions, and socioeconomic backgrounds. Providers can give patients various tips to promote their general safety; however, there is no known prevention for sexual assault. All health care providers should assess every patient for any history of sexual abuse and assault; should educate their patients about the dynamics of sexual assault, including the fact that it is an act of violence; and should encourage patients to seek mental health services if a positive history is uncovered.

CHAPTER 36

SYNCOPE

Magen M. Lorenzi

DEFINITION AND EPIDEMIOLOGY

Syncope is defined as a temporary loss of consciousness and postural tone that is followed by spontaneous complete recovery and does not require resuscitation. Presyncope or near-syncope is a sensation of lightheadedness or faintness in which the patient senses that true syncope may be imminent but complete loss of consciousness never occurs.

The true incidence of syncope in the general population is not well known owing to differences in definition, underreporting, and variations within age groups or special populations. There is a similar incidence for men and women until 70 years of age, after which there is a sharp increase in incidence that favors women.[1] Women are therefore twice as likely as men to experience syncope during their lifetime.[2] Syncope is more common in older patients than in other age groups and is often associated with falls and greater risk for adverse outcomes.[3] The increase in syncopal events is likely to be related to the number of comorbidities and prescribed medications in this cohort.[4] In addition, the physiologic changes of aging increase an elder's risk for syncope.[4]

PATHOPHYSIOLOGY

Syncope is a symptom of an underlying process or processes (Box 36-1). These processes result in syncope by one of two pathophysiologic mechanisms: deprivation of nutrients to the brain or deprivation of oxygen to the brain. Deprivation of nutrients most often results from decreased blood flow secondary to hypovolemia, cardiac outflow obstruction, cardiac arrhythmias, or neurovascular causes. Deprivation of oxygen is most often associated with hypoxia or anemia. It is important to distinguish true syncope from seizure disorders or other conditions that might result in altered levels of consciousness, such as iatrogenic syncope from medication therapy, drug or alcohol intoxication, concussions, amnesia, or metabolic causes such as hypoglycemia. Seizure-like activity may be present with syncope; this is secondary to generalized cerebral hypoxia.

There are three main classifications of syncope: (1) neurally mediated or reflex, (2) orthostatic hypotensive, and (3) cardiac.[5] A review of the literature cites a fourth classification, neurogenic, which includes stroke.[6] The most common cause of syncope is vasovagal; however, cardiac causes have an increased incidence of sudden death and must be evaluated early.[5] In general, cardiac syncope is seen in older adults.[6] The cardiac causes consist of two major categories: (1) mechanical or ventricular outflow obstructive processes and, more common, (2) arrhythmias. Possible mechanical or obstructive processes responsible for syncope include cerebrovascular disease, cardiac valvular disease, atrial myxoma, hypertrophic or obstructive cardiomyopathy, pulmonary hypertension, pulmonary embolism, pericardial disease or tamponade, acute myocardial infarction or ischemia, and possible prosthetic valve malfunction. Possible rhythm disturbances include sick sinus syndrome, atrioventricular conduction disturbances, supraventricular and ventricular tachycardias, long QT syndrome, and pacemaker system malfunction. Tachycardias can also trigger vasovagal syncope.[5]

BOX 36-1

Causes of Syncope

CARDIAC

Mechanical or Obstructive Processes

- Cardiac valvular diseases
- Atrial myxoma
- Hypertrophic or obstructive cardiomyopathy
- Pulmonary hypertension
- Pulmonary embolism
- Pericardial disease
- Cardiac tamponade
- Myocardial infarction or ischemia

Arrhythmias

- Sick sinus syndrome
- Atrioventricular conduction disturbances
- Supraventricular or ventricular tachycardia
- Prolonged or shortened QT syndrome
- Pacemaker malfunction

NEUROLOGIC

Reflex or Neuromediated

- Autonomic failure
- Vasovagal (common faint)
- Situational (micturition, cough, swallow, defecation)
- Carotid sinus hypersensitivity (primarily found in older adults)

Cerebrovascular

- Vertebrovascular transient ischemic attack

MISCELLANEOUS

- Hypoglycemia
- Hypovolemia (especially in older patients who are taking antihypertensive medications)
- Postprandial hypotension
- Psychiatric disease (panic disorder, hysteria, depression)

Neurally mediated syncope is the most common type of syncope and is primarily seen in young adults.[2,6] Situational syncope, carotid sinus syncope, and others are also classified as neurally mediated. Although different in their provocation, these disorders share a reflex response that causes vasodilation, bradycardia, and paradoxical systemic hypotension, eventually leading to decreased blood flow to the brain.[5,6] In carotid sinus syncope, the trigger sites are thought to be peripheral receptors that respond to mechanical stimuli (such as neck stretching or tight collars); this type of syncope occurs most often in older adults.[5]

Finally, orthostatic stress can cause insufficient peripheral vasoconstriction, leading to syncope. Orthostatic hypotension is rare in patients younger than 40 years, yet is one of the most common causes of syncope in patients older than 70 years.[6] Classic orthostatic hypotension is defined as a drop in systolic blood pressure (BP) of greater than 20 mm Hg or of diastolic BP of greater than 10 mm Hg within 3 minutes of transition from supine to standing.[7] This can be triggered by blood loss, dehydration, or autonomic dysfunction. In the elderly population, syncope is often reported in the morning after taking medications.[6] It is important to note that orthostatic stress can be present with both cardiac and neurally mediated syncope.[5]

Several miscellaneous causes of syncope are not easily classified into any of the previously mentioned categories. Hypoglycemia is a possible metabolic case of syncope and is usually found in individuals with diabetes who have taken too much of a particular hypoglycemic agent. Hyperventilation is another possible cause. Several psychiatric causes, including depression, hysteria, and panic attacks, may subsequently result in hyperventilation, which can lead to hypocapnia and cerebral vasoconstriction compounded by possible peripheral vasodilation.

CLINICAL PRESENTATION

The patient's past medical history, family history, and history of present illness are essential in determining the cause of the event and whether the patient requires hospitalization. The history needs to detail the syncopal episode, including presyncopal and postsyncopal signs and symptoms.[1,8] In many cases, a witness is needed for the specific details of the event to be determined. It should be established what the patient was doing before the syncopal episode and whether there were any preceding symptoms.

A history of syncope during exercise should raise concern for a cardiac cause such as an arrhythmia or hypertrophic cardiomyopathy, especially in patients younger than 40 years.[5,6] In addition, abrupt syncope without warning, the presence of chest pain or palpitations, or a positive family history of sudden death, coronary artery disease, arrhythmias, Wolff-Parkinson-White syndrome, prolonged QT, or Brugada syndrome also necessitates exclusion of a cardiac cause.[8]

A report of defecating, swallowing, coughing, shaving, neck straining or pressure, pain, or stressful event before syncope is suggestive of a form of neurally mediated syncope. However, older patients may have difficulty recalling any presyncopal symptoms, in part because of retrograde amnesia, which is common with vasovagal syncope.[5] If the provider is unable to evoke an accurate presyncopal history, postsyncopal symptoms can aid in differentiation of cardiac and vasovagal episodes. Patients with cardiac syncope may experience a rapid recovery, whereas vasovagal syncope often results in fatigue and nausea for up to several hours after consciousness is regained.[5]

If the patient is able to relate the presyncopal or syncopal episode to a change from a horizontal to a vertical position, the episode may be a result of hypovolemia or orthostatic hypotension. Numbness and tingling in the face and hands suggest hyperventilation.

The patient may also have noted nausea, diaphoresis, or warmth just before losing consciousness; however, the presence of an aura, such as a peculiar smell, might be a clue to an underlying seizure disorder. Differentiation among a seizure, post-syncope symptoms, and seizure-like activity can be difficult. Therefore, determining how the patient acted while unconscious is important. Signs most suggestive of a seizure include tongue laceration, head turning, and abnormal posturing. Signs less likely to indicate seizure include presyncope spells, diaphoresis, and loss of consciousness after an extended period of standing or sitting.[6] Most syncopal events are brief; patients often recover once they are in the horizontal position, which allows the resumption of blood flow to the brain. Postictal symptoms during the recovery phase are more consistent with seizures.

Younger patients who report frequent syncopal episodes with vague symptoms and no injury history should be evaluated by a specialist for psychiatric disorders.[6] Certain medications may be the underlying or contributing cause. Antihypertensive medications may aggravate orthostatic symptoms, especially in older adults. Antiarrhythmic drugs may have proarrhythmic side effects. It is important to know if the patient is being treated for a seizure disorder, any psychiatric disorders, or diabetes and if the patient has been taking medications as prescribed.

The importance of thoroughly reviewing the patient's past medical history and current medications, especially recently prescribed medications, herbals, and over-the-counter medications, cannot be overstated. The social history should include alcohol use, possible illicit drug use, and the patient's occupation. In patients suspected of having an underlying cardiac problem, the presence of any cardiac risk factors for coronary artery disease should be determined. Risk factors include male gender, a family history of premature coronary artery disease or sudden death, hypercholesterolemia, hypertension, smoking, and diabetes.

PHYSICAL EXAMINATION

After it is established that the patient is stable, the initial physical evaluation needs to focus on the cardiovascular system. The presence of bruits indicates cardiovascular disease.[5] Cardiac auscultation may reveal murmurs (e.g., a midsystolic ejection murmur radiating to the right side of the neck suggests aortic stenosis), gross rhythm disturbances, or extra heart sounds such as an S_3 or S_4. The pulmonary evaluation might indicate heart failure, possibly secondary to an acute myocardial infarction or pulmonary disease. Other signs of heart failure include jugular venous distention, hepatojugular reflux, and edema.

Orthostatic BP should be measured to determine the presence of hypovolemia.[5] These measurements are obtained by having the patient lie in the supine position for at least 5 minutes and then measuring the BP and pulse. The BP and pulse are checked while the patient is sitting up and then on standing. A drop in systolic pressure by at least 20 mm Hg, a drop in diastolic pressure by at least 10 mm Hg, or an increase in the pulse rate by at least 20 beats per minute within the first 3 minutes of assuming a more upright position is considered a positive test result.[7]

In patients older than 40 years with an unknown cause of syncope, carotid sinus massage can assist with diagnosis.[5] Carotid sinus massage should not be performed in patients with carotid bruits, or within 3 months after myocardial infarction or stroke. Massage is ideally performed with continuous electrocardiogram (ECG) monitoring and beat-to-beat BP monitoring. It should be initiated in the supine position, with gentle rhythmic massage to the right and then to the left of the carotid body for 5 to 10 seconds each.[5] The current diagnostic criteria for carotid sinus hypersensitivity require an asystolic pause of 3 seconds or more or a fall in systolic BP of 50 mm Hg or more; however, suggested revisions to these criteria recommend diagnosis if asystole exceeds 6 seconds or if systolic BP falls below 60 mm Hg.[5] Carotid sinus massage in older patients without history of syncope has a 39% false-positive rate.[6]

A complete neurologic examination, including a funduscopic examination, is necessary to determine focal deficits indicating a neurologic cause. A rectal examination will help determine if gastrointestinal bleeding is present.

DIAGNOSTICS

Initial evaluation for all patients reporting syncope should include a standard 12-lead ECG and QT interval monitoring.[5,6] An electroencephalogram (EEG) should be obtained if there is concern for seizure disorder.[6] Broad-panel laboratory testing is not recommended because less than 2% to 3% of patients reporting syncope will have abnormal results.[6] Initial evaluation should include a serum glucose test, complete blood count (CBC), and pregnancy test for women of childbearing age.[6]

An ECG is necessary to detect ischemia, arrhythmias, pacemaker failure, prolonged QT, or other congenital cardiac syndromes. Cardiac enzyme levels should be measured if the patient has cardiac risk factors, if the patient has a history of chest pain, or if physical findings are consistent with heart failure. A chest radiograph and brain natriuretic peptide level will help determine the presence of heart failure or cardiomegaly (i.e., a heart shadow that takes up more than half of the chest cavity on the posteroanterior view). If a cardiac obstructive cause is suspected, echocardiography may be indicated.[6] Further diagnostics may also be indicated because the cause of the event can be difficult to determine. These include an exercise stress test, ECG monitoring (i.e., Holter, event, or implantable loop monitoring), electrophysiologic studies, tilt-table testing, EEG, head computed tomography (CT) or magnetic resonance imaging (MRI), and carotid Doppler evaluation.[5,6]

DIAGNOSTICS

Syncope

INITIAL	**IMAGING**
ECG	Echocardiography*
Orthostatic BP	CT scan or MRI of head*
Pulse oximetry	
	OTHER
LABORATORY	Holter monitor, event monitor, or implantable loop monitor*
CBC and differential	Tilt-table test*
Serum glucose	Exercise testing*
Urine hCG	EEG*
Cardiac isoenzymes if cardiac cause suspected	Electrophysiologic studies*
Brain natriuretic peptide*	

*If indicated.
hCG, human chorionic gonadotropin.

DIFFERENTIAL DIAGNOSIS

The differential diagnosis of syncope includes vasovagal syncope, orthostatic hypotension, seizure disorder, autonomic failure, alcohol abuse, cardiovascular disease with obstruction, cardiac arrhythmias, transient ischemic attack, concussion, hypovolemia, hypoglycemia, anemia, pulmonary emboli, and hypoxia. In addition, syncope may be related to medication therapy or an anxiety attack.

INITIAL STABILIZATION AND MANAGEMENT

During a witnessed event, the patient should be placed in a supine position. Tight clothing should be loosened and the patient's head turned to the side. If the history and diagnostic testing indicate that an initial episode of syncope was not secondary to a cardiac pathologic condition, therapy can be directed at the underlying disorder. Low-risk patients can be evaluated safely in an outpatient setting.[6] If the patient's condition is unstable, the appropriate advanced cardiac life support and advanced trauma life support protocols need to be followed.

Immediate emergency department referral or physician consultation is indicated for syncope in a patient with a family history of sudden death or for syncope associated with exercise, chest pain, congestive heart failure, palpitations, acute hemorrhage, trauma, transient ischemic attacks, seizures, or abnormal ECG recording or chest x-ray study. Patients with syncope and a medical history of anatomic heart disease or previous surgical repair of a cardiac lesion also require emergency department referral or physician consultation. Patients who may have new-onset seizure disorder should be considered for hospital admission to a unit with appropriate monitoring capabilities.

DISPOSITION AND REFERRAL

In older patients, a thorough history should be taken to determine whether some other problem in their home environment is preventing them from staying hydrated or taking their medications properly. These patients may need a visiting nurse, a social worker, or a health benefits adviser. For neurally mediated syncope, and especially with recurring episodes, the patient should be referred to a neurologist for possible tilt-table testing and if indicated tilt-training treatment.[5] Other therapies that may be helpful for patients with recurrent syncope include compression stockings, isometric physical counterpressure maneuvers, or treatment with salt tablets, fludrocortisones, desmopressin, or pressor agents.

All patients need to understand the importance of adequate hydration and need to avoid circumstances that might precipitate syncope. They should be told to return to the clinic if the syncope recurs. Depending on the suspected underlying cause, a referral to either a neurologist or a cardiologist is appropriate at this time.

PREVENTION AND PATIENT EDUCATION

Patients and families should receive a careful explanation regarding the cause of the syncopal event. Prevention of injury is an important goal for older adults because many falls are related to a syncopal event.[3] In the case of vasovagal, carotid sinus, and situational syncope, patients need to be made aware of the particular behaviors, activities, or circumstances that might result in syncopal episodes, and they should be given adequate avoidance strategies. Prevention of orthostatic changes necessitates that patients learn to rise slowly from the bed or chair, exercising the leg muscles before standing. Although syncope is often not recurrent, patients with syncope should be advised not to operate motorized equipment until the cause of the event has been determined and treated.

CHAPTER 37

THERMAL INJURIES

Karen S. Abate

HEAT-RELATED ILLNESS

DEFINITION AND EPIDEMIOLOGY

Heat-related illnesses are a continuum of conditions related to sensitivity and acclimation to heat. In all heat-related illnesses, there is an acute inability to adjust to elevations in the core temperature.[1] The manifestations of this inability vary with the type of heat-related condition. Heat stroke is an emergent medical condition in which the core body temperature exceeds above 104° F and in which central nervous system (CNS) abnormalities occur.[1-4] Heat exhaustion is a less severe condition that is the result of excessive sweating and sodium and water loss.[1] Heat exhaustion can rapidly progress to the more severe and potentially fatal heat stroke. Heat syncope is dizziness or fainting that occurs with standing for long periods or on sudden rising during heat exposure.[2] Heat cramps are muscle pains or spasms occurring in individuals performing physical activity and result from low sodium levels and volume loss.[5] It is imperative that heat-related illnesses be properly recognized and treated to prevent additional complications.

The Centers for Disease Control and Prevention (CDC) estimates that more than 7000 heat-related deaths occurred from 1999 to 2010.[3] The majority of these deaths occurred in males.

PATHOPHYSIOLOGY

The body maintains homeostasis by efficiently balancing heat gains and losses. Thermoregulatory centers of the CNS, including the hypothalamus and spinal cord, address heat gains by increasing blood flow to the skin, dilating peripheral blood vessels, increasing eccrine gland production, and increasing heart rate and cardiac output.[3] Ineffective heat regulation can be caused by numerous factors, resulting in the core temperature being elevated beyond the capabilities of the thermoregulatory compensatory systems.[1] Escalating ambient environmental temperatures and humidity can overwhelm the body's natural ability to dissipate heat. Increases in internal heat production related to disease processes or hypothermic dysfunction, as well as impaired heat dissipation caused by medications or age, can result in deficient heat regulation.[1]

In heat stroke, an extremely elevated core body temperature can result in cerebellar and liver dysfunction. Heat exhaustion, heat syncope, and heat cramps are caused by dehydration and electrolyte depletion associated with heat exposure.[1,4]

CLINICAL PRESENTATION

Heat-related illnesses can develop rapidly or over a period of several days. Physical symptoms may differ in the amount of time they take to manifest. Rapid diagnosis and treatment are imperative. A comprehensive history and physical examination are invaluable. The clinician must determine the following:

- Significant past medical history
- Travel history
- Onset of presenting symptoms
- Medications or herbal supplements that can contribute
- Alternative or home remedy exposure history and severity

Heat stroke is considered a medical emergency in which core body temperature exceeds above 104° F.[5,6] Patients with heat stroke will have CNS abnormalities, which can include hallucinations, confusion, slurred speech, and headache.[1,6] Dehydration, tachycardia, and hypotension can occur. Red, hot, dry skin is a key characteristic of heat stroke. Heat stroke can rapidly deteriorate to hepatocellular damage or multiorgan system failure.[1,5]

Symptoms are milder in patients with heat exhaustion. These patients may have generalized fatigue, weakness, profuse sweating, nausea, vomiting, diarrhea, irritability, and potentially hypotension, but no CNS involvement.[1-6] Skin will be pale and flushed, which is significantly different from the red, hot, dry skin of patients experiencing heat stroke.[1,6] Patients with heat exhaustion will have a pulse that is fast and breathing that is rapid and shallow.[1]

The presentation of patients with heat syncope will involve vertigo, lightheadedness, and syncope.[1,4-6] Heat cramps will involve pain or spasms in muscles of the abdomen, arms, or legs.[2,5,6] These symptoms are caused by dehydration and electrolyte depletion.

PHYSICAL EXAMINATION

Rapid identification of heat stroke and heat exhaustion is imperative to prevent complications and untoward outcomes. A complete comprehensive physical examination including past extent and severity of exposure is required.[1] Evaluation of airway, breathing, and circulation (*ABCs*) is warranted. Physical examination findings related to the neurologic system include inappropriate behavior, impaired judgment, vertigo, delirium, seizures, and other symptoms of CNS dysfunction.[1,2,6] A baseline Glasgow Coma Scale score should be obtained and reassessed throughout treatment.

Cardiovascular findings may include tachycardia, and hypotension may occur because of vasodilation and dehydration. Patients with a heat-related illness could manifest symptoms associated with decreased preload, decreased peripheral vascular resistance, increased stroke volume, and increased cardiac output.[1] It is possible to have normotensive findings in some patients as well because of compensatory mechanisms.[3] Musculoskeletal examination may demonstrate muscle tenderness, cramping, or weakness.

DIAGNOSTICS

Diagnostics should be based on the patient's exposure and severity history, the clinical presentation, and past medical history. Testing should be used in conjunction with physical examination findings. Diagnostics should be used to monitor treatment as well as to determine the presence of associated complications. Cardiac monitoring and pulse oximetry may be indicated to obtain baseline and monitor hemodynamic status. Arterial blood gas (ABG) analysis and chest x-ray examination can be beneficial for patients with shallow breathing. Computed tomography may be indicated for patients with altered mental status. A urine sample should be obtained to monitor kidney function. Laboratory tests that may be indicated include a complete blood count (CBC) and differential, coagulation studies and an electrolyte panel, blood urea nitrogen (BUN), and creatinine. The following values should be obtained to assess for progression of disease or complications: BUN, creatinine, sodium, potassium, calcium, lactate dehydrogenase, aspartate aminotransferase, alanine aminotransferase, creatine kinase, and bilirubin. Liver function test (LFT) results can be elevated, in some cases, 12 hours after initial injury.[1] Creatine kinase should be measured if there are concerns surrounding potential rhabdomyolysis.[1]

DIAGNOSTICS

Heat-Related Injuries

INITIAL	Serum glucose
Electrocardiography (ECG)	LFTs
LABORATORY	Coagulation studies (prothrombin time/partial thromboplastin time [PT/PTT])
Serum electrolytes	Urinalysis
BUN	CBC and differential
Creatinine	
Creatine kinase	

DIFFERENTIAL DIAGNOSIS

The diagnosis of heat-related illness is based on clinical presentation, history, and physical examination. The differential should include infections, head trauma or CNS injury, epilepsy, thyroid storm, acute cocaine intoxication, malignant hyperthermia, pheochromocytoma, anticholinergic poisoning, serotonin syndrome, drug-associated toxicity, and environmental exposure.[1]

MANAGEMENT

Immediate emergency department referral or specialist referral is indicated for individuals with any thermal injuries.

- In an emergent heat-related illness, it is imperative to assess and to maintain airway patency. Continuous maintenance of the ABCs is vital. Monitoring of vital signs and mental status is essential.
- Individuals experiencing heat stroke or heat exhaustion must be immediately transported to a local emergency facility, and physician consultation should be obtained. Intravenous access must be promptly established and intravenous solutions administered to rehydrate. If it is not contraindicated, supplemental oxygen should be administered, and preparation should be made for potential endotracheal intubation as warranted.
- The goals of treatment are lowering of core body temperature, rehydration, and electrolyte replenishment. Patients with any heat-related illness should be moved to a cool, well-ventilated area with most clothing removed to allow for increased surface area exposure. This will facilitate heat evaporation.[1,4,6] Increased air flow can be provided with fans and a cool mist. Shivering can occur when some rapid cooling techniques are implemented. Shivering is the result of peripheral vasoconstriction and heat production; therefore caution must be used with cooling. Antipyretics are ineffective in heat stroke. Core temperature should be regularly monitored. Complications and sequelae should be treated accordingly. Electrolytes such as sodium and potassium should be replenished as warranted.

DIFFERENTIAL DIAGNOSIS

Heat-Related Injuries

- Systemic infection
- Head trauma
- CNS injury
- Thyroid storm
- Myocardial infarction
- Acute cocaine intoxication
- Malignant hyperthermia
- Pheochromocytoma
- Anticholinergic poisoning

COMPLICATIONS

Complications related to heat stroke include rhabdomyolysis and renal, hepatic, or cardiac failure.[4] There is potential for the occurrence of multiorgan dysfunction syndrome, which includes disseminated intravascular coagulation, encephalopathy, acute respiratory distress syndrome, myocardial injury, intestinal ischemia or injury, pancreatic injury, and thrombocytopenia.[1,4]

INDICATIONS FOR REFERRAL OR HOSPITALIZATION

Any individual having a heat stoke or heat exhaustion should be immediately transported to an emergency facility for treatment.

- Individuals with heat syncope or heat cramps who are not responding to treatment should also be reassessed at an emergency facility.
- Referral to specialists will be required on the basis of the patient's response to treatment and long-term sequelae.

LIFE SPAN CONSIDERATIONS

Select populations are more prone to heat-related injury. The elderly and those with hypertension or poor cardiac function are prone to heat exhaustion.[2] This includes people who regularly take beta blocker medications because of an inability to increase cardiac output relative to the demands in a heat-related illness.[1] Individuals on diuretics are at risk for dehydration, and those on anticholinergics have diminished capacity to perspire, putting them at higher risk for thermal illness.[1] Outdoor workers, those without air conditioning, and patients with obesity, mental illness, or sickle cell trait are also at risk.[6]

PATIENT EDUCATION AND HEALTH PROMOTION

All heat-related illnesses are preventable. Education to increase awareness and early identification of heat-related conditions is invaluable. Individuals who are at risk for heat-related illnesses should be instructed in how to properly maintain hydration. Strenuous outdoor activities and exercise should be monitored and limited. Heat-related prevention plans should be developed and implemented during heat waves. The consumption of alcohol should be deterred, whereas the use of fans or air conditioning should be encouraged.

COLD INJURY

DEFINITION AND EPIDEMIOLOGY

Cold injuries can range from minor to life-threatening. In thermal injuries related to cold, transitional physiologic changes occur as the patient's core body temperature progressively decreases. Decreases in core body temperature can be caused by environmental cold exposure or abnormal thermoregulation.

Frostbite is tissue injury caused by direct and indirect cellular damage that occurs with crystallization of fluids on exposure to freezing temperatures.[7] Frostbite may potentially occur on any exposed area; however, the majority of frostbite injuries occur on the fingers, toes, nose, and ears.[7-9] Frostbite can be classified as grade I to IV on the basis of severity or simply as superficial or deep.[10] Superficial frostbite is limited to the skin, either partial- or full-thickness freezing of dermis and subcutaneous tissue.[9,10] Deep frostbite involves the skin, subcutaneous tissue, muscle, tendon, bone, and deep tissue.[9,10]

PATHOPHYSIOLOGY

The pathophysiologic process associated with frostbite involves the freezing of exposed tissues. Ice crystals form in the intracellular and extracellular tissue, which is followed by intracellular dehydration and microvascular occlusion.[7] Peripheral vasoconstriction and decreased blood flow occur. These progressive changes ultimately can result in ischemic changes and tissue necrosis.[7,9]

As the core body temperature decreases, progressive changes associated with hypothermia occur. These changes vary in severity by the extent of core body temperature reduction. Cardiovascular response is initially tachycardia followed by atrial fibrillation, bradycardia, ventricular dysrhythmia, and ultimately asystole. Cardiac output and blood pressure gradually diminish. Respiratory response to the hypothermic state involves increased oxygen consumption, depressed respiratory drive, and, ultimately, acidosis. Ataxia, slurred speech, loss of deep tendon reflexes, loss of consciousness, and coma are neurologic occurrences for hypothermic patients.

CLINICAL PRESENTATION

Presentation of the individual with frostbite will vary according to the severity of exposure. Hypothermia presentation also corresponds to the extreme lowering of core body temperatures. Severity can range from ataxia and slurred speech to absent reflexes and asystole. Hypothermia can be life-threatening.

A comprehensive history and physical examination are imperative for any patient with a potential cold-related injury. The clinician must determine the following:

- Exposure history, including length and severity
- Significant past medical history
- Presence of risk factors
- Current medications taken

PHYSICAL EXAMINATION

Rapid identification of cold-related injuries is imperative. The presentation of an individual having a cold-related injury depends on the severity of core body temperature drop. Core temperature should be accurately measured on initial presentation and at regular intervals during treatment. Physical findings related to the integumentary system vary according to exposure and severity. In superficial frostbite, the affected area will demonstrate erythema, blistering, edema, and potentially desquamation.[9]

Blistering can occur within 24 to 48 hours if there is partial-thickness frostbite.[7] With rewarming, the area will appear mottled and swollen, with superficial blisters developing within 6 to 24 hours.[4]

Deep frostbite manifests as skin that is blueish grey in appearance with hemorrhagic blisters and potential necrosis to underlying structures.[9] During the course of several days, there is a progression from edema, nonblanching surface, cyanosis, and hemorrhagic blisters to tissue necrosis. It is important for the clinician to examine all limbs and the entire surface for affected areas.

Cardiovascular effects may include arrhythmias, dysrhythmias, hypotension, fibrillation, and asystole. Neurologic examination may reveal sensory changes, ataxia, progressive loss of deep tendon reflexes, changes in level of consciousness, and decreased response to noxious stimuli. Respiratory drive will be steadily diminished as core temperature is lowered in hypothermia.

DIAGNOSTICS

Diagnostics are not warranted in frostbite. In patients with hypothermia, diagnostics are warranted to assess the severity of hypothermia and subsequent response to ongoing treatment. Cardiac monitoring and pulse oximetry may be indicated. Arterial blood gas analysis can be used to assess for acidosis. Chest x-ray examination is indicated for patients with underlying pathologic changes or respiratory compromise. Electrocardiography (ECG) is beneficial for individuals with cardiac symptoms. Blood work should include a CBC, electrolytes, BUN, creatinine, and clotting factors.

DIAGNOSTICS

Cold-Related Injuries

INITIAL
ECG, cardiac monitoring

LABORATORY
CBC and differential
Serum electrolytes
BUN
Creatinine
Serum glucose
Coagulation studies (prothrombin time/partial thromboplastin time [PT/PTT])
Cardiac isoenzymes
ABGs

DIFFERENTIAL DIAGNOSIS

The diagnosis of cold-related conditions is based on clinical presentation, history, and physical examination. The differential diagnosis of individuals with frostbite should include frostnip and chilblains, commonly known as trench foot.[8,9] The differential diagnosis of individuals with hypothermia should include hypoglycemia, drug intoxication, myxedema, coma, cerebral vascular attack, allergic reactions, and compartment syndrome.[7,9]

DIFFERENTIAL DIAGNOSIS

Cold-Related Injuries

- Frostnip
- Chilblains

HYPOTHERMIA
- Hypoglycemia
- Drug intoxication
- Myxedema
- Coma
- Cerebral vascular attack
- Allergic reactions
- Compartment syndrome

MANAGEMENT (INCLUDING INTERDISCIPLINARY MANAGEMENT)

- Any individual with a cold-related injury should immediately be removed from the cold exposure.
- In the case of frostbite, management focuses on stabilization of the patient and rewarming of the affected area. Wet or constrictive clothing should be removed once the individual is out of the cold environment. Rewarming can be achieved with warm blankets or immersion in a warm water bath for repeated short periods.[10] Spontaneous rewarming once the patient has been removed from the cold exposure might be sufficient; however, he or she should be assessed relative to the extent of the injury.[10] The affected area can be elevated or splinted as needed, but it should not be massaged or rubbed.[8,10] Pain control may be needed.[10] Antibiotics are needed only for contaminated areas.
- Post-thaw management follows traditional principles of wound management. It is imperative to use nonadherent dressings on the affected areas to prevent maceration.[10] Debridement, physical therapy, or amputation may be needed.
- In patients with hypothermia, it is imperative to assess and to maintain airway patency. Continuous maintenance of the ABCs is vital, and monitoring of vital signs and mental status is essential. In the severely hypothermic individual, peripheral pulses may not be palpable; therefore the cardiac electrical rhythm should be obtained before chest compressions are initiated. Individuals experiencing hypothermia must be immediately transported to a local emergency facility, and physician consultation should be obtained. Intravenous access must be promptly established. If it is not contraindicated, supplemental oxygen should be administered, and preparation should be made for potential endotracheal intubation as warranted.

COMPLICATIONS

In the case of superficial frostbite, there may be long-term neuropathic pain, sensory deficits, edema, or hair and nail deformities. Tissue necrosis can occur with deep frostbite.[9,10]

INDICATIONS FOR REFERRAL OR HOSPITALIZATION

Any individual having frostbite or hypothermia should be immediately transported to an emergency facility for evaluation and treatment. Hospitalization may be warranted for deep frostbite or hypothermia patients. Referral to a surgeon can be advantageous for possible amputation.

LIFE SPAN CONSIDERATIONS

Individuals who have experienced a cold-related thermal injury may maintain lifetime sensitivity to cold.

EDUCATION AND HEALTH PROMOTION

Awareness of weather conditions to avoid illness or injury should be encouraged in all populations. Individuals who have experienced a cold-related injury should be instructed in the proper identification of cold-related conditions. Patients should be advised to stop smoking because of the vasoconstrictive effects. In addition, patients should refrain from alcohol intake, especially with exposure to cold conditions. The use of protective clothing in cold environments should be stressed. Clothing should be well ventilated and loose to limit perspiration during activity.

REFERENCES

For a full list of references, scan the QR code or visit http://booksite.elsevier.com/9780323355018

PART 5

Evaluation and Management of Skin Disorders

CHAPTER 38

EXAMINATION OF THE SKIN AND APPROACH TO DIAGNOSIS OF SKIN DISORDERS

Maria Isabel Romano

DEFINITION AND EPIDEMIOLOGY

Skin problems occur often in the general population and are the presenting complaint in many primary care patients.[1] A large number of skin diseases manifest in similar ways. Factors such as age, ethnic and genetic makeup, risk factors, body habitus, skin surface, and self-care practices may complicate a diagnosis by altering the appearance and distribution of lesions that are characteristic of the skin disorder. Underlying systemic pathologic conditions may also contribute to the difficulty of making a definitive diagnosis of skin lesions.

OVERVIEW OF SKIN FUNCTION, ANATOMY, AND STRUCTURES

The primary functions of the skin are protection of the underlying body structures from the entrance of microorganisms, control of body heat and elimination of body waste through perspiration, and prevention of injury to core body structures. The skin protects the body from infectious agents; protects against loss of body heat through conduction, convection, and radiation; and provides a first-line defense against mechanical, chemical, and thermal injury. Glands in the dermal layer of the skin secrete a substance that lubricates the body surface and assists with a variety of body functions. The peripheral sense receptors contained in the skin alert the body to pain, temperature changes, pressure, and touch.

The skin is composed of three layers: the epidermis, the dermis, and the hypodermis or subcutis. The outer epidermal, or cuticle, layer is avascular and is divided into an outer horny layer (the stratum corneum) and an underlying horny layer (the stratum mucosum). The stratum corneum consists of keratinocytes—cells that originate in the basal cell layer of the epidermis and migrate upward to the stratum corneum and slough off as dead cells, called *squames*. As long as the stratum corneum (the outer horny layer) is intact, normal skin bacteria are prevented from invading deeper skin and gaining access to the bloodstream. The lower layer of the epidermis contains the Langerhans cells, which function as antigen-presenting cells that migrate to the lymph nodes and play an important role in the allergic skin response. Melanocytes found in the basal layer of the epidermis constitute the body's principal protection against ultraviolet (UV) radiation.[2]

The second layer of the skin, the dermis (also termed the *cutis, corneum,* or *true skin*), holds the epidermis in place. The dermis is composed of an outer papillary layer and an inner reticular layer that contains connective tissue and the blood supply as well as lymphatic vessels, peripheral nerves, elastic tissue, and a reservoir of water and electrolytes. The dermal appendages are contained within the reticular layer and include the eccrine sweat glands that serve to control body temperature by evaporation, the sebum-producing sebaceous glands that lubricate the stratum corneum through openings in the skin (called *pores*), the hair follicles, and the nail bed. Other appendages include apocrine glands attached to hair shafts located in the axillary, perianal, and genital areas. These glands respond to the increased hormone levels associated with puberty, adolescence, and young adulthood and decrease their activity with normal aging. A variation of the apocrine gland is the cerumen-producing glands lining the external auditory canal. The oily substance, cerumen, serves to protect the skin lining the ear canal from bacterial invasion.

A third layer of the skin, the hypodermis or subcutis, functions to store fat, to insulate the body from extremes in temperature, and to provide a cushion against injury. It also contributes to the skin's mobility over underlying body parts.

CHANGES IN THE SKIN ASSOCIATED WITH AGING

With age, both structural and functional changes occur in the skin. These changes include decrease in the number of Langerhans cells; variation in size, shape, and staining of the keratinocytes; decrease in the thickness of the dermis; and loss of elastic tissue. There is a decrease in the number of sweat glands, hair follicles, and specialized nerve endings as well as decreased vascularity and increased fragility of existing capillaries. Functional changes in the skin include a decreased inflammatory response; increased time for wound healing; thinning of the skin, resulting in increased fragility and risk of injury; decreased sweat capacity; and increased dryness secondary to reduced sebum production.[3]

ASSESSMENT

Formulation of a differential diagnosis for skin lesions is based on an in-depth knowledge of various common skin disorders and their characteristic physical properties, including location and morphologic appearance. In addition, knowledge of the associated history typical of common rashes is essential. Variations in color, texture, and continuity of a patient's skin may be a normal genetic or ethnic variant, an indicator of a local skin pathologic condition, or an indicator of an underlying systemic disease process. A proper assessment forms the basis for an appropriate care plan, patient education for self-care of acute and

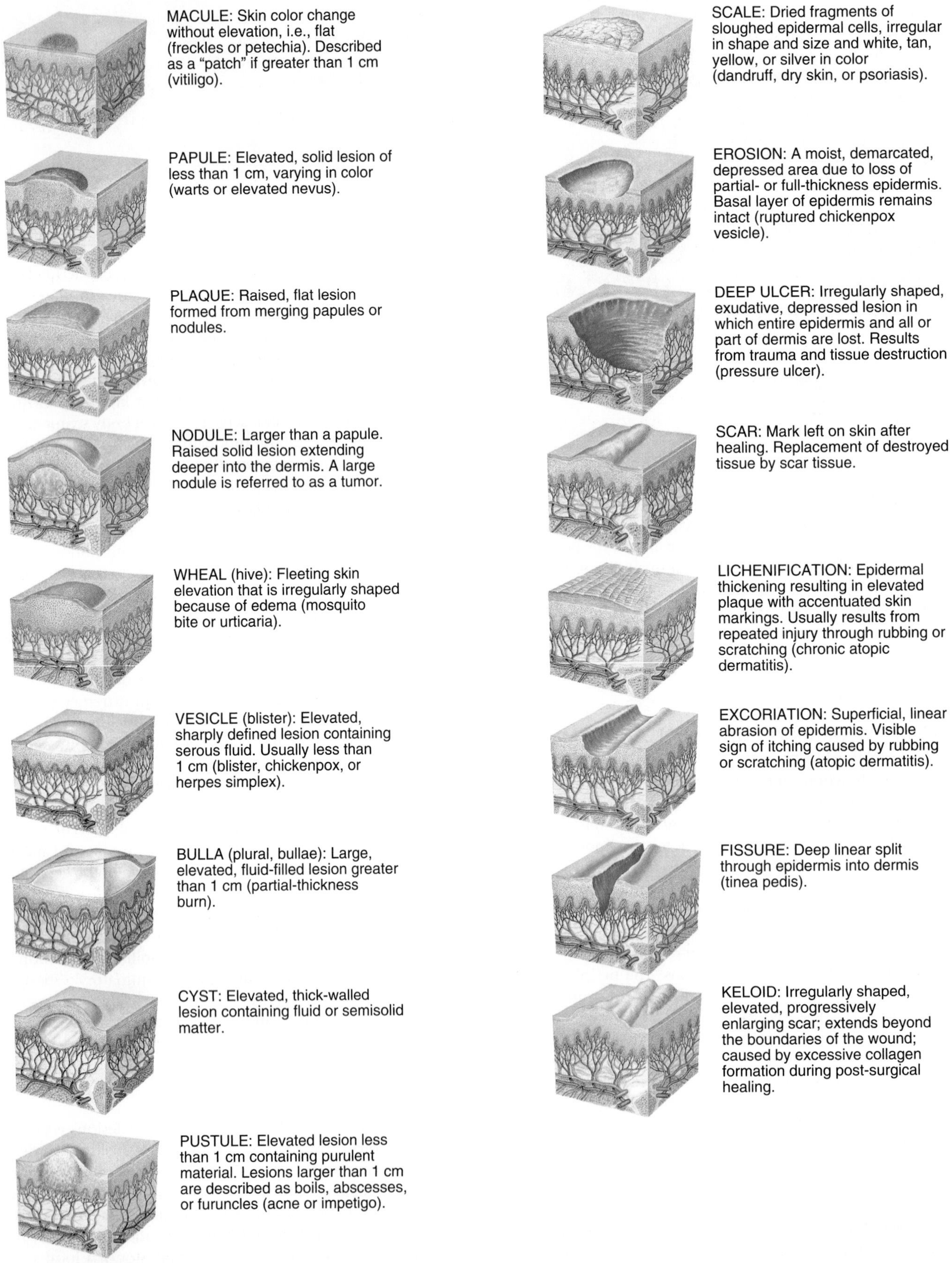
MACULE: Skin color change without elevation, i.e., flat (freckles or petechia). Described as a "patch" if greater than 1 cm (vitiligo).
PAPULE: Elevated, solid lesion of less than 1 cm, varying in color (warts or elevated nevus).
PLAQUE: Raised, flat lesion formed from merging papules or nodules.
NODULE: Larger than a papule. Raised solid lesion extending deeper into the dermis. A large nodule is referred to as a tumor.
WHEAL (hive): Fleeting skin elevation that is irregularly shaped because of edema (mosquito bite or urticaria).
VESICLE (blister): Elevated, sharply defined lesion containing serous fluid. Usually less than 1 cm (blister, chickenpox, or herpes simplex).
BULLA (plural, bullae): Large, elevated, fluid-filled lesion greater than 1 cm (partial-thickness burn).
CYST: Elevated, thick-walled lesion containing fluid or semisolid matter.
PUSTULE: Elevated lesion less than 1 cm containing purulent material. Lesions larger than 1 cm are described as boils, abscesses, or furuncles (acne or impetigo).
SCALE: Dried fragments of sloughed epidermal cells, irregular in shape and size and white, tan, yellow, or silver in color (dandruff, dry skin, or psoriasis).
EROSION: A moist, demarcated, depressed area due to loss of partial- or full-thickness epidermis. Basal layer of epidermis remains intact (ruptured chickenpox vesicle).
DEEP ULCER: Irregularly shaped, exudative, depressed lesion in which entire epidermis and all or part of dermis are lost. Results from trauma and tissue destruction (pressure ulcer).
SCAR: Mark left on skin after healing. Replacement of destroyed tissue by scar tissue.
LICHENIFICATION: Epidermal thickening resulting in elevated plaque with accentuated skin markings. Usually results from repeated injury through rubbing or scratching (chronic atopic dermatitis).
EXCORIATION: Superficial, linear abrasion of epidermis. Visible sign of itching caused by rubbing or scratching (atopic dermatitis).
FISSURE: Deep linear split through epidermis into dermis (tinea pedis).
KELOID: Irregularly shaped, elevated, progressively enlarging scar; extends beyond the boundaries of the wound; caused by excessive collagen formation during post-surgical healing.

FIGURE 38-1 *Left,* Primary lesions: visually recognizable structural changes in the skin that have specific characteristics. *Right,* Secondary lesions: primary lesions that have changed because of the natural progression of the lesion or because of physical change (scratching, irritation, or secondary infection). (From Black JM, Hawks JH: Medical-surgical nursing: clinical management for positive outcomes, ed 8, St Louis, 2008, Saunders.)

chronic skin lesions, and prevention of recurrence. Assessment begins with a careful history and physical examination of basic features, including skin turgor, pigmentation, and degree of photodamage to sun-exposed surfaces.[2] Additional investigative techniques, such as Wood light examination, laboratory data, and microscopic skin scraping examination, may be necessary to ensure a definitive diagnosis.

History

Subjective components of a dermatologic history include taking a history from the patient or caregiver regarding the onset and progression of the rash, associated symptoms, any prior skin disorder, medications, travel history, lesions in close contacts, social and occupational factors, and dietary practices. The health care provider inquires about self-care practices, such as homeopathic remedies, lotions, soaps, any change in laundry products, new clothing or fabrics, use of rubber gloves, cosmetics, sunbathing, tanning salons, and the humidity of the patient's typical ambient environment. In addition, a family history or self-history of skin disorders, allergy, atopy, asthma, or eczema in childhood is reviewed.

Physical Examination

The use of a contact dermatoscope or a noncontact microscope that uses cross-polarized light is an important adjunct to the objective examination of skin lesions. Dermoscopy affords the examiner the advantage of visualizing the epidermis and superficial dermis and can reveal changes in pigmentation throughout the lesion, such as in a melanoma.[4] It can also be used to determine whether the lesion's borders are regular or irregular. When a contact dermatoscope is used, the application of immersion oil or ultrasound gel to the skin further enhances the translucency of the stratum corneum and permits better visualization of skin fissures, hair follicles, and pores in the lesion.[4] The presence of scaling and inflammation can also be determined. A listing of primary and secondary lesions is provided in Figure 38-1.

A freestanding light that can be adjusted to provide direct or oblique lighting is a necessary adjunct. Darkening of the ambient lighting allows greater illumination and contrast of the involved lesion. Overillumination, however, may wash out important details of a lesion. Direct lighting with an intense penlight or the ophthalmoscope head with a halogen light permits visualization of closed vesicles or pustules and differentiation of fluid or cystic masses.

Another form of lighting is the Wood light, or black light, which emits long wavelengths (>365 nm) of UV rays through a filter made of nickel oxide and silica, rendering UV rays harmless to the skin. The advantage is that under this lighting method, skin diseases such as tinea versicolor fluoresce white to yellow, and erythrasma, a scaly skin condition caused by *Corynebacterium minutissimum,* fluoresces a bright coral red.[5] Even small amounts of decreased melanin, such as vitiligo, are accentuated under Wood light and appear stark white. *Pseudomonas* infections appear pale blue, and the presence of dermatophytes such as *Microsporum canis* will appear yellow.[6]

Palpation of skin lesions provides information on the extent of the lesion below the skin surface, its consistency, its exact size, and associated pain. Certain lesions, such as dermatofibromas, will indent with lateral palpation, a distinguishing

BOX 38-1

Skin Examination Technique

Diascopy can be performed with use of a flat microscope slide or other clear instrument, such as a magnifying glass. Blanching of blue to red lesions followed by a gradual refilling indicates blood in the capillaries; absence of blanching indicates blood leaching outside of the capillaries, as in petechiae.

Gram stain of exudates from lesions is helpful in distinguishing the cause as either a gram-positive or gram-negative organism.

The Tzanck test with Wright or Giemsa stain can uncover multinucleated giant cells that are typical of herpes simplex or varicella-zoster virus. The top of the vesicle must be removed to obtain fresh fluid from the base of the lesion.

A 10% to 30% potassium hydroxide (KOH) stain determines the presence of hyphae and spores consistent with candidiasis or uncovers the spaghetti-and-meatball appearance of tinea versicolor, caused by the skin fungus *Malassezia furfur* or *Malassezia ovalis.* Attempts should be made to obtain scrapings from the top of a lesion or from the advancing edge of a lesion. The skin lesion is aligned vertical to the microscopic slide, and a gentle scraping of the lesion with the side of a slide or a scalpel loosens skin debris, collected on the slide below. KOH is applied directly to the scale debris, and a coverslip is placed over the skin scraping; or the KOH is applied alongside the edge of the coverslip, and the KOH then gravitates to cover the specimen by capillary action. Heating of the preparation over a low flame will allow the hyphae to separate from the epithelial cells. The specimen is then set under the microscope for examination, first using 10× power and then proceeding to 40× for finer detail. The examiner must be certain to close the condenser diaphragm and turn the condenser down to enhance the detail of hyphae that are embedded in the scaly debris.

Culture for herpesvirus, *Streptococcus, Staphylococcus,* or *Pseudomonas* organisms requires removal of the outer crust or cuticle of the lesion to obtain fluid for culture. The fluid at the base of the lesion is most likely to be positive for the contributing organisms and free of contamination from the skin surface. A special collecting device for a viral culture specimen must be used in accordance with laboratory specifications. Bacterial culture specimens for streptococci and staphylococci can be collected with a regular throat culture–collecting swab. *Candida* organisms can be grown on Sabouraud agar in a 2- to 6-day period, whereas dermatophytes take up to 2 to 4 weeks to grow on the same agar. The organisms of tinea versicolor grow only on special media.

In *scabies preparation,* a superficial skin shaving from a skinfold area is obtained from the top of a burrow and examined under oil immersion. Oil or KOH solution should be placed on the lesion first. With a scalpel, the top is shaved off the lesion, and the debris is placed on a microscopic slide. Additional oil and a coverslip are added, and the specimen is examined under 10× magnification. The presence of adult mites, eggs, or feces in the burrows is sufficient in the diagnosis of scabies.

Data from Habif TP: Clinical dermatology: a color guide to diagnosis and therapy, ed 5, St Louis, 2010, Mosby; and Klauss W, Johnson RA, Saavedra AP: Fitzpatrick's color atlas and synopsis of clinical dermatology, ed 7, New York, 2013, McGraw-Hill.

characteristic known as the *Fitzpatrick sign*. Dermatographism is a phenomenon that occurs when the skin of a person with urticaria is lightly rubbed with a pointed object, such as the back of a fingernail; histamine is released under the skin surface, and the skin becomes raised and red where the object touched it.

Diagnosis involves a close evaluation of the lesion's distribution or location, configuration, borders, size, shape, color, and surface characteristics or appearance. A cluster of lesions may appear in various stages of evolution, as with varicella and dermatitis herpetiformis, whereas others, such as warts, will remain the same for the duration of their existence.[7] Documentation includes a description of the lesion's size, color, shape, surface characteristics, distribution, and configuration. A discussion of skin examination techniques is provided in Box 38-1.

Quality of care is enhanced when providers develop strong interpersonal relationships with patients who come to see them with dermatologic problems. The patient's satisfaction has been shown to be related to the provider's ability to teach patients about their condition and to show concern and caring for their problem. This, in turn, may lead to enhanced compliance and better treatment outcomes.[8]

CHAPTER 39

SURGICAL OFFICE PROCEDURES

Glen Blair

The skin is the largest organ of the human body and the only organ that is nearly completely visible to examination by the naked eye. Cutaneous diseases such as rashes, infections, benign and malignant tumors, and lesions represent a sizeable portion of the skin complaints of patients seen in primary care, yet many providers are not comfortable with diagnosis or treatment of cutaneous disease.[1]

Concurrently, multiple forces are at work that will influence the provision of dermatologic care in the future. Demand for dermatology services is predicted to increase but the supply of dermatology providers is predicted to remain low, despite the influx of nonphysician providers.[2,3] The need to restrain the growth of health care spending is likely to place greater pressures on primary care providers to treat common dermatologic issues in the office rather than to refer patients for more expensive specialty services. Providers of primary care services will be challenged to be selective in which patients to refer and which patients to treat. Dermatologists delivering telemedicine can work with primary care providers to determine whether dermatology services are needed or to assist with diagnosis. Education of primary care providers to perform skin biopsies for diagnosis in primary care could conceivably help prioritize requests for high-demand specialty services, especially in the early age of teledermatology.[4-6]

Performance of office-based procedures for the treatment of benign lesions such as warts, skin tags, and irritated seborrheic keratoses is one way to try to meet this challenge while also reducing the cost to the patient. Cryosurgery, electrocautery, curettage, punch biopsy, shave biopsy, and scissor excision are common dermatology office procedures. Primary care providers can safely perform these procedures with proper education and training.

A note on the treatment of benign lesions: Patients may request treatment of benign lesions that are painful or irritating, such as plantar warts, but at times they may seek treatment because they find the lesion unattractive. Although treatment of benign lesions that are causing physical discomfort is usually a covered expense, patients are often distressed to discover that many insurance carriers do not cover dermatology treatment performed for cosmetic concerns.

CRYOSURGERY

Cryosurgery or cryotherapy is the application of cold, such as nitrogen in its liquid state, to produce therapeutic tissue necrosis. Liquid nitrogen is the most common cryogenic agent because of its low boiling point (−196° C). It is administered with a cryosurgical canister with a spray tip attachment or sometimes manually with a cotton-tipped applicator. Tissue injury results from the direct effects of the freeze on intracellular and extracellular components and from vascular stasis.[7] Further destruction occurs during the thaw phase. Maximum destruction occurs with repeated freeze-thaw cycles.

Cryosurgery is indicated in the treatment of myriad skin conditions, and its use is ubiquitous in dermatology. In primary care, it is used typically in the destruction of benign lesions that are easily recognizable, such as acrochorda (skin tags), warts, and seborrheic keratosis. It is also used for the treatment of actinic keratosis—gritty, erythematous patches on typically sun-exposed surfaces that are considered precancerous. Cold intolerance, cold urticaria, and cryoglobulinemia are relative contraindications to cryosurgery, as is treatment of digits in patients with a history of Raynaud disease. Patients who are darkly pigmented are at risk for depigmentation resulting from destruction of melanocytes or postinflammatory hyperpigmentation after tissue injury. Alternative treatments should be considered. Use at the vermilion border of the lips, oral commissures, eyebrows, canthi, and nasal ala is avoided because of the risk of scarring.[7]

Freeze time, the duration of cooling, varies from lesion to lesion. For some lesions, complete freezing may take only a few seconds; but for mosaic-type plantar warts, freeze time may be considerably longer. The freeze should spread laterally 2 to 3 mm from the edge of the lesion. For skin tags, flat warts, genital warts, and molluscum contagiosum, one freeze-thaw cycle is generally sufficient. For thicker, more keratotic lesions such as plantar warts and large seborrheic keratosis, two freeze-thaw cycles are recommended.

Patients are counseled to expect some redness and swelling during the healing process. Bullae, sometimes hemorrhagic, can develop; patients should be advised to protect the bullae from trauma until healing is complete, but they can be drained if uncomfortable.[8] Scarring can occur if damage is sustained in the dermis. Post-treatment care includes keeping the area clean with soap and water and using petrolatum if the patient desires. Unless patients use them routinely and without issue, topical antibiotic ointments such as bacitracin should be avoided owing to the high incidence of contact dermatitis.[9]

ELECTROCAUTERY

Electrocautery is the delivery of direct current through a heated metal wire to cause local tissue destruction or hemostasis. Small wall-mounted units (hyfrecators) are available that deliver variable amounts of electricity. The electrode used for electrocautery is monopolar, meaning that it has only one tip to make contact with the skin, and no indifferent electrode (ground plate) is required.[7] Bipolar or biterminal electrodes are used in electrosurgery when deeper levels of tissue destruction are needed; this procedure is not discussed here.

In primary care, electrocautery can be used for the treatment of acrochorda, actinic keratosis, small angiomata, compound nevi, warts, and seborrheic keratoses. There are no absolute contraindications to the use of electrocautery, and it can be used in patients with pacemakers or implantable cardioverter-defibrillators when appropriate precautions are taken (i.e., lower voltage, shorter bursts).

The area to be treated is cleaned with a non–alcohol-based skin cleanser. Alcohol wipes are avoided because of concerns of the alcohol's igniting on the skin.[7] One percent or 2% lidocaine, with or without epinephrine, can be used in those cases when significant pain is anticipated. Treatment of small lesions without anesthesia is often preferable to the discomfort of the anesthesia itself. Vascular lesions may become less identifiable because of the vascular effects of the anesthetic agent, so they are best treated without local anesthesia. Electrodesiccation is the direct application of the tip to the skin or lesion surface to deliver the current and is the preferred method for treatment of most lesions. Electrofulguration, the delivery of the current from a small distance above the surface, is used for very small, superficial lesions. Current and power settings are determined by the lesion to be treated and the specifications of the device being used and are influenced by the knowledge that deeper tissue injury results in greater risk of scarring. When it is ready, the tip is passed lightly and repeatedly over the treatment surface until the degree of desired tissue destruction has been achieved.

Electrocautery is an attractive alternative to cryotherapy when pigmentation issues are of concern and is more useful in the treatment of vascular lesions. Complications are rare. In combination with curettage (i.e., electrodesiccation and curettage), it is one of several standard treatment options available for nodular basal cell and invasive squamous cell carcinomas.

CURETTAGE

Curettage is a technique that uses a scraping instrument, a curet, to remove soft and superficial skin lesions. These include seborrheic keratoses, some warts, and molluscum as well as some types of skin cancers. The curet has a sharp oval ring that separates the lesion from the dermis. The area is cleaned. Local anesthesia is usually required. The skin is stabilized with the nondominant hand. The curet is pressed against the skin until firm resistance is met, and the soft area is removed with multiple strokes of the curet. The specimen is placed in a fixative and submitted to the pathology laboratory to confirm its histologic nature. Local hemostasis is achieved with electrocautery or the application of a hemostatic solution such as aluminum chloride. Curets come in various sizes, and single-use, sharp disposables are available.

BIOPSY

A biopsy is appropriate when the nature of the lesion or dermatitis is in question. Primary care offices are seeing increasing numbers of patients with suspicious melanocytic lesions, and some practices have begun to perform skin biopsies if the provider has education in this procedure.[10] In addition, the provider performing the biopsy must be able to establish a differential diagnosis, be prepared to interpret the pathology report, be able to recognize whether the pathologic process is consistent with the clinical presentation, and be able to arrange for appropriate treatment.[10] With a federal push toward computerized medical records and the advent of teledermatology, it is conceivable that images will be shared more routinely with specialists who will be available for consultation from remote sites.

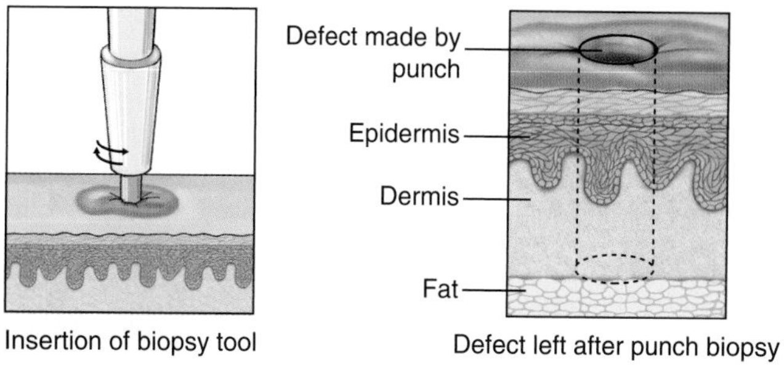

FIGURE 39-1 Punch biopsy. With the use of a punch, living tissue is removed for microscopic examination. (From Leonard PC: Building a medical vocabulary: with Spanish translations, ed 7, St Louis, 2009, Saunders.)

A punch biopsy (Fig. 39-1) is performed when knowledge of the depth of the lesion is required, such as with pigmented lesions, for which the depth of the lesion is one of the most important prognostic indicators of malignant melanoma. Punches are also useful when the lesion is small and can be entirely removed. They are available as single-use, disposable tools that are fitted with a sharp, round blade and come in various sizes, 2 to 8 mm in diameter. When removal cannot be accomplished with a punch, an elliptical excision of the entire lesion with a 1- to 3-mm border is recommended.[10] Referral is recommended for large lesions. For those occasions when options are limited, multiple smaller samples can be obtained from the most unusual portions of the lesion, knowing that a negative finding on pathologic examination is not necessarily a negative diagnosis.

To perform a punch biopsy procedure, the provider measures the pigmented lesion to choose the appropriate diameter of the biopsy punch; the punch should remove the lesion with at least a 1-mm margin, because any portion of a lesion that remains as well as the adjacent skin may contain pathologic changes. First, the provider dons clean gloves and prepares the area with an alcohol wipe before infiltrating with the appropriate local anesthesia; in general, 1% to 2% lidocaine with or without epinephrine is used. Lidocaine should not be used with epinephrine at the tips of the digits and nose and the glans penis. A small-volume syringe (1 to 3 mL) and a small-gauge needle (e.g., 31 gauge) are used to inject the anesthetic into the dermis by producing a wheal. A visible wheal indicates that the anesthetic has been deposited into the dermis. The area intended to be sampled should be draped, and the provider should don sterile gloves and position the punch over the lesion. The punch is pushed into the skin as the provider rotates it between thumb and forefingers. The punch is inserted until resistance eases, indicating that the punch has reached the subcutaneous fat. The provider must ensure that the punch is inserted into the subcutaneous fat layer; this ensures that the entire lesion is sampled. The cylinder of skin is gently removed with forceps without crushing the sample. The specimen is cut with sterile scissors

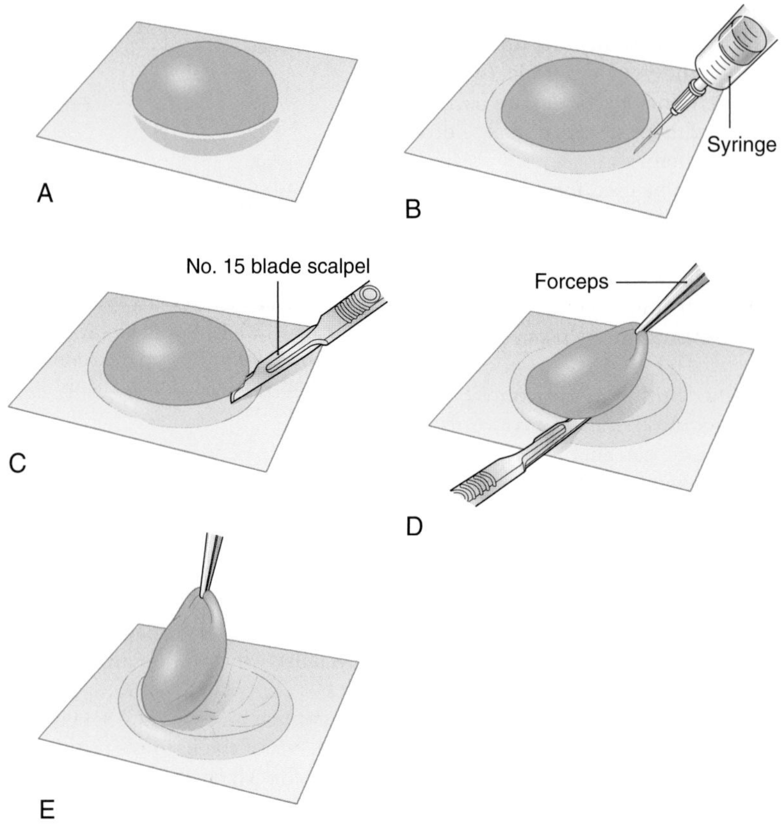

FIGURE 39-2 Shave biopsy. **A,** Skin lesion. **B,** Raised wheal created by infiltration of local anesthetic. **C,** Horizontal section by scalpel. **D,** Continue horizontal section. **E,** Biopsy specimen removed. (From Nouri K, Leal-Khouri S: *Techniques in dermatologic surgery,* St Louis, 2003, Mosby.)

deep enough to include subcutaneous fat, and the sample is placed in a container with a standard fixative. The defect is closed with suture material suitable for the area of the body and the strength of the surrounding tissue: 5.0 or 6.0 for the face and genitalia; 5.0 for the dorsa of the hands, ventral forearms, and breasts; 4.0 or 5.0 for the torso and extremities; and 3.0 or 4.0 for the scalp, palms, and soles. The wound is dressed with petrolatum and a dry sterile bandage. The patient should be instructed to keep the area clean with soap and water, to monitor the wound for signs of infection, and to change the bandage daily until the sutures are removed. As general guidelines, suture removal occurs typically after 3 to 5 days for the face and neck; 7 days for the scalp, chest, abdomen, and upper extremities; 10 days for the back; and 10 to 14 days for the lower extremities and the feet.

A shave biopsy (Fig. 39-2) is used when a full-thickness specimen is not required for diagnosis. This includes nonmelanocytic lesions such as actinic keratoses, basal and squamous cell carcinomas, warts, and seborrheic keratosis. To perform a shave biopsy, the provider cleans the skin area with an alcohol wipe and anesthetizes as described previously. A No. 15 scalpel is selected; razor blades are also used. The blade is obliquely pressed through the skin to remove all or part of the lesion. If the lesion is small, the lesion can sometimes be removed entirely. Removal of larger lesions through a shave, though, is likely to leave a visible scar. The goal of a shave biopsy is to produce a saucer-shaped skin defect that has smooth edges.[11] The specimen is removed with forceps and placed into a container with fixative. Bleeding can be controlled with direct pressure, light electrocautery, or hemostatic solutions such as aluminum chloride. The biopsy site is dressed with a small amount of petrolatum and a bandage. The patient should be instructed to clean the wound daily with soap and water, to monitor for signs of infection, and to apply a small amount of petrolatum and a clean bandage daily for 2 or 3 days.

Scissor excision should be performed on pedunculated lesions such as skin tags. With these lesions, anesthesia is rarely needed. The area should be cleaned with an alcohol wipe. The lesion should be grasped with forceps by the nondominant hand while the base is snipped with sterile iris scissors held in the dominant hand. Bleeding can be controlled by direct pressure, light electrocautery, or hemostatic solutions such as aluminum chloride. The biopsy site should be dressed with a small amount of petrolatum and a bandage. The patient should be instructed to clean the wound daily with soap and water, to monitor for signs of infection, and to apply a small amount of petrolatum and a clean bandage daily for 2 or 3 days.

SUMMARY

Cryosurgery, curettage, electrocautery, punch biopsy, shave biopsy, and scissor excision are common office procedures used in the diagnosis and treatment of dermatologic conditions. Primary care providers can safely perform these procedures with proper education and training. Referral to or consultation with a dermatology specialist is indicated for large lesions, lesions that do not respond to treatment, malignant lesions, lesions whose diagnosis cannot be established, and lesions for which the provider has not received education to manage.

CHAPTER 40

PRINCIPLES OF DERMATOLOGIC THERAPY

Kathryn K. Ellis • Kathryn R. Colcher

DEFINITION AND EPIDEMIOLOGY

The critical first step in treating any dermatologic condition is accurate diagnosis. Other important components are the type of lesion to be treated, the medication, the vehicle of the active medication, and the method used to apply the medication. A thorough history is the most important step in the assessment of dermatologic problems.

In dermatologic therapy, the type of lesion guides therapy. Moist, weeping lesions are treated with Burow solution to hasten drying while providing soothing relief. Wet dressings are beneficial when treating exudative skin diseases because they help to suppress inflammation through vasoconstriction of superficial vessels as well as promote drying of lesions and wound debridement.[1] In dry dermatitis, therapeutic agents incorporated into creams or ointments increase moisture in the skin and provide relief from pruritus.

SKIN STRUCTURE

The skin is the largest organ of the body. The primary function of the skin is to provide a barrier to passage of substances into the body and to maintain internal homeostasis.[2] Three main layers form this barrier.[2] The stratum corneum is the most superficial section of the epidermis, or outer layer. The stratum corneum consists of enucleated keratinocytes, which are filled with keratin and an interfilamentous matrix. The middle layer is the vascularized dermis, which contains connective tissue and skin appendages. The innermost layer is the hypodermis, or subcutaneous layer, composed of adipose tissue.

The thickness and permeability of the stratum corneum vary on different areas of the body. When the stratum corneum is irritated and inflamed, the protective skin barrier is interrupted. These characteristics have clinical implications for dermatologic therapy because they affect drug absorption. The skin structure in older adults is dryer, thinner, and less elastic, which needs to be considered in prescribing for the elderly population.

MEDICATIONS

Variables to Consider in Prescribing

Several variables affect the pharmacologic response when dermatologic agents are applied to the skin.[2,3] The first variable is the regional variation in drug penetration, which is based on the thickness of the stratum corneum. There is an inverse relationship between the thickness of the stratum corneum and drug concentration. Therefore in areas such as the face, scalp, axilla, and scrotum, the stratum corneum is more permeable. There is also increased permeability when the skin is broken down by disease, trauma, and chemicals (soaps and detergents).[2] In addition, the concentration of the dermatologic medication affects its absorption in the skin. Finally, because the principal transport mechanism is passive diffusion, increasing the concentration gradient increases absorption. Because of the physiology of the skin, the local half-life of a topical medication is extended to allow once-daily administration.

TABLE 40-1 **Fingertip Units (FTUs) Needed to Treat Different Body Parts**

Body Part	FTUs for One Application	Weight of Ointment Required for One Application	Tube Size to Dispense for Complete Coverage of Area for bid Application over 10 days
Face and neck	2.5 FTUs	1.25 g	30 g
Trunk (front or back)	7 FTUs	3.5 g	60 g
One arm	3 FTUs	1.5 g	30 g
One hand (both sides)	1 FTUs	0.5 g	15 g
One leg	6 FTUs	3 g	60 g
One foot	2 FTUs	1 g	30 g

Modified from From Habif TP: *Clinical dermatology*, ed 5, St Louis, 2009, Mosby.

In addition to the type of medication, important elements to include in topical prescription writing are the vehicle, concentration, amount, and application instructions.[2] Consideration needs to be given to the size of the area to be treated, frequency of application, and expected time to healing. One gram typically covers an area of 10 × 10 cm; ointments cover a slightly larger area.[2] For example, the amount needed for a single application for the entire body is approximately 30 g. Another practical way to measure topical application is the fingertip unit (FTU). A FTU is defined as the amount of ointment expressed from a tube with a 5-mm nozzle to cover from the tip of the index ringer to the distal skin crease. This is approximately 0.5 g.[1] Table 40-1 contains additional information about the number of FTUs needed to treat a particular body part. Prescribing the appropriate amount of medication will prevent unnecessary cost, waste, and inconvenience to the patient.

Dermatologic Vehicles

The base in which the active medication is delivered (the vehicle) affects the drug's ability to permeate the skin. The vehicle may also provide important therapeutic effects to the skin, such as hydration. Drug absorption may be enhanced up to 10 times with the application of occlusive dressings.

The most common vehicles are combinations of powders, oils, and liquids in varying proportions. Powders aid in absorbing moisture, decrease friction, and help cover wide areas. Oils provide an emollient function and, because of their occlusive properties, often enhance drug absorption. Liquids provide a cooling, soothing sensation by evaporation while helping exudative lesions to dry. With variations in skin thickness, body hair, and type of lesion, it is important to choose the most appropriate vehicle. Table 40-2 contains additional information.

All types of dermatologic medications are applied in a single thin layer; thicker applications do not increase skin penetration or effectiveness of the medication.[1]

Ointments. Ointments consist mainly of water suspended in oil and are excellent lubricants. In general, ointments are the most potent vehicles because of their increased occlusive effect; however, they are not useful in hairy areas, and the greasiness of the product is not aesthetically acceptable to many patients.

TABLE 40-2 Common Vehicles for Topical Pharmacotherapeutic Preparations

Type of Preparation	Properties
Lotion	Cools and dries as it evaporates; useful for treating moist or pruritic skin.
Cream	Helps retain water; cosmetically appealing; useful in high-humidity environments; easily washed off.
Gel	Becomes liquid on contact; cosmetically appealing; avoid on acutely inflamed skin because alcohol base may cause stinging.
Ointment	Helps retain water, hydrating; avoid use in exudative, infected lesions; may be greasy; complications include folliculitis, maceration, and miliaria.
Emulsion	Water-in-oil preparation that is less occlusive than ointment.
Paste	Less greasy than ointment, with some drying action; good as protective barrier.
Wet dressing	
Open	Anti-inflammatory action and vasoconstriction helpful in decreasing edema and removing crust; offers relief of pruritus through evaporation and cooling.
Closed	Retains heat and causes maceration.
Bath soaks	Temperature should be lukewarm, not hot; limit to 20-30 minutes; oils may make tub slippery.
Powder	Promotes drying; increases surface area; decreases maceration and moisture; avoid in open wounds.
Fixed	Proper application aids in decreasing edema; leave the dressing in place for 1 week, then remove by soaking in warm water.

TABLE 40-3 Topical Corticosteroids Ranked by Potency

Class	Concentration and Generic Name (Selected Brand Names and Vehicle)
Class 1—Superpotent	0.05% Clobetasol propionate (Clobex lotion, spray, shampoo) 0.05% Halobetasol propionate (Ultravate cream) 0.1% Fluocinonide (Vanos cream)
Class 2—Potent	0.05% Diflorasone diacetate (ApexiCon E cream) 0.1% Mometasone furoate (Elocon ointment) 0.1% Halcinonide (Halog ointment) 0.25% Desoximetasone (Topicort cream, ointment)
Class 3—Upper midstrength	0.05% Fluocinonide (Lidex-E cream) 0.05% Desoximetasone (Topicort LP cream)
Class 4—Midstrength	0.05% Clocortolone pivalate (Cloderm cream) 0.1% Mometasone furoate (Elocon ointment) 0.1% Triamcinolone acetonide (Aristocort A cream, Kenalog ointment) 0.1% Betamethasone valerate (Valisone ointment) 0.025% Fluocinolone acetonide (Synalar ointment)
Class 5—Lower midstrength	0.05% Fluticasone propionate (Cutivate cream, lotion) 0.1% Prednicarbate (Dermatop cream) 0.1% Hydrocortisone probutate (Pandel cream) 0.1% Triamcinolone acetonide (Kenalog lotion) 0.025% Fluocinolone acetonide (Synalar cream)
Class 6—Mild	0.05% Alclometasone dipropionate (Aclovate cream, ointment) 0.05% Desonide (Verdeso foam, Desonate gel) 0.025% Triamcinolone acetonide (Aristocort A cream, Kenalog lotion) 0.1% Hydrocortisone butyrate (Locoid cream, ointment) 0.01% Fluocinolone acetonide (Derma-Smoothe/FS scalp oil, Synalar topical solution)
Class 7—Least potent	2%-2.5% Hydrocortisone (Nutracort lotion, Synacort cream) 0.1%-0.5% Hydrocortisone (Cortaid cream, spray, lotion)

Modified from Weston WL, Lane AT, Morelli JG: *Color textbook of pediatric dermatology,* ed 4, St Louis, 2007, Mosby/Elsevier.

Ointments are best for dry, lichenified lesions because of the effects of lubrication and heat retention through decreased transepidermal water loss.

Creams. Creams are less potent than ointments but stronger than lotions. They consist of a semisolid emulsion of oil in water. Creams are a cosmetically appealing vehicle that can be washed off with water. They are used on nonhairy areas such as the palms and soles.[4]

Lotions. Lotions consist of a powder-in-water preparation and are a less potent vehicle.[4] Indications for the use of lotions include moist areas, dermatoses, pruritus, hairy areas, and large treatment areas. Lotions are commonly used to provide a cooling effect on the skin.

Solutions. Solutions consist of water in combination with various medications or substances. When used as bath soaks, solutions provide coolness and aid in drying of exudative lesions.[4] Solutions are best for open or closed dressings, infected dermatoses, or hairy areas.

Gels. A gel is an oil-in-water, semisolid emulsion with alcohol in the base; it is transparent and colorless and liquefies on contact with the skin. Gels are an excellent vehicle for use on hairy body areas, and they combine the therapeutic advantages of ointments with the cosmetic advantages of creams.[4]

TABLE 40-4 Suggested Strength of Topical Steroids to Initiate Treatment*

Groups I and II	Groups III to V	Groups VI and VII
Psoriasis	Atopic dermatitis	Dermatitis (eyelids)
Lichen planus	Nummular eczema	Dermatitis (diaper area)
Discoid lupus†	Asteatotic eczema	Mild dermatitis (face)
Severe hand eczema	Stasis dermatitis	Mild anal inflammation
Poison ivy (severe)	Seborrheic dermatitis	Mild intertrigo
Lichen simplex chronicus	Lichen sclerosus et atrophicus (vulva)	
Hyperkeratotic eczema	Intertrigo (brief course)	
Chapped feet	Tinea (brief course to control inflammation)	
Lichen sclerosus et atrophicus (skin)	Scabies (after scabicide)	
Alopecia areata	Intertrigo (severe cases)	
Nummular eczema (severe)	Anal inflammation (severe cases)	
Atopic dermatitis (resistant adult cases)	Severe dermatitis (face)	

*Stop treatment, change to less potent agent, or use intermittent treatment once inflammation is controlled.
†Use on the face may be justified.
From Habif TP: *Clinical dermatology*, ed 5, St Louis, 2009, Mosby.

Topical Corticosteroids

Some of the most useful topical agents for treatment of a variety of dermatologic conditions are corticosteroids. The major effects of corticosteroids are the reduction of inflammatory response, vasoconstriction, and decrease in collagen synthesis.[5] They are available in several classes based on potency (Table 40-3), and they come in a variety of strengths and vehicles. The suggested potencies for specific diagnoses are listed in Table 40-4.

Topical corticosteroids are exceptionally useful in treating various dermatologic diseases, but they are not without potential adverse effects. The higher the potency and the more prolonged the use, the higher the chance for development of adverse effects. Collagen synthesis is affected, which results in striae and tissue atrophy. These effects may be reversible when the drug is discontinued. Visible distended capillaries (telangiectasia) and purpura may result from a thinning of the epidermis. Systemic side effects are rare when topical corticosteroids are prescribed and used appropriately.[1]

Corticosteroids in classes I to IV should never be used on the face or genitals. The health care provider should use caution in prescribing classes I, II, and III and should consider consultation with a physician. The health care provider should be familiar with several medication types in each class of corticosteroid for ease in prescribing.

When corticosteroids are used with occlusive dressings, there is an increase in drug penetration in the skin and an increased potential for adverse reactions. Learning a few drugs in each class will benefit the health care provider in prescribing topical corticosteroids.

PATIENT AND FAMILY EDUCATION

The first guideline of dermatologic therapy is to keep the treatment as simple as possible. Health care providers should prescribe enough medication to complete therapy, and the patient should discard any left over after the treatment.

The provider should write out application procedures and ensure that the patient fully understands the instructions. Important information to review with the patient includes whether to moisten the skin first, how much topical medication to apply and where to apply it, and whether the area can be occluded by a dressing. Patients should be instructed not to apply the dermatologic medication to areas other than where instructed. In addition, patients should be aware of possible adverse reactions and should know when to call the office and return for follow-up evaluation.

CHAPTER 41

SCREENING FOR SKIN CANCER

Randy M. Gordon

DEFINITION AND EPIDEMIOLOGY

Although early detection and treatment of skin cancer can improve patient outcomes, evidence is insufficient to recommend for or against routine screening for early detection of skin cancer by a total-body skin examination (TBSE) during a routine office visit.[1] The U.S. Preventive Services Task Force (USPSTF) based this decision in part on poor and inconsistent research methodology in the literature. Nevertheless, one significant purpose of the skin cancer screening is to educate both the patient and the provider to identify the characteristic changes associated with skin cancer. The USPSTF agreed there is fair evidence that supports screening for skin cancer by clinicians to be moderately accurate in detecting melanoma. The USPSTF offered the following recommendations regarding skin cancer screening research: (1) standardizing skin cancer screening research methodology, (2) modeling studies based on the available indirect evidence, and (3) targeting high-risk patient populations for screening.[1]

The American Cancer Society (ACS) recommends skin cancer screening every 3 years for people aged 20 to 40 and annually for people older than 40.[2] The American College of Preventive Medicine recommends a TBSE for patients at high risk for malignant melanoma (MM). The American College of Obstetricians and Gynecologists recommends screenings for females aged 13 years or older with a history of habitual exposure to sunlight, a family or personal history of skin cancer, or clinical evidence of precursor lesions (actinic keratosis).[3] These cancers include nonmelanomatous skin cancers (NMSCs), such as basal cell carcinoma (BCC) and squamous cell carcinoma (SCC), and melanomatous skin cancers, such as MM.

Researchers estimate that one in five Americans will develop skin cancer at least once in their lifetime.[2] The most recent research suggests that approximately 3.5 million cases of BCC or SCC are diagnosed each year. Although BCC is the most common form of skin cancer, MM is by far the most fatal. Based on reports from 2008 to 2012, the age-adjusted incidence rate of melanoma is 21.6 per 100,000 men and women per year according to the national Surveillance, Epidemiology, and End Results (SEER) database.[4] Of the estimated 73,870 new cases of melanoma of the skin that occur annually, 9940 deaths are expected.[4] Overall MM incidence rates are higher in women than in men before age 50. However, MM incidence rates in men versus women are twice as high by age 65, and nearly triple by age 80.[2] The differences in risk by age and sex primarily reflect differences in occupational and recreational sun exposure, which have changed over time. The rising incidence of skin cancer during the past several decades may also be attributed to increased sun exposure associated with societal and lifestyle shifts in the U.S. population and to depletion of the protective ozone layer.[3]

Ninety percent of all skin cancers are caused by the sun.[5] Acute sunburns place the patient at increased risk, and the effects of sun damage are cumulative. Second-degree burns before the age of 18 years can double the incidence of NMSC and greatly increase the risk for MM.[6] Fair-skinned men and women older than 65 years, patients with atypical moles, and those with more than 50 nevi constitute known groups at substantially increased risk for development of melanoma.[2] In addition, skin cancers appear to have a hereditary component. Xeroderma pigmentosum is the prototype syndrome of genetically determined increased skin cancer risk.[3]

Multiple risk factors exist for all types of skin cancer, including endogenous factors (phototype, skin and eye color, number of melanocytic nevi, presence of dysplastic nevi, and individual or family history of skin cancer), and exogenous factors (type and degree of cumulative sun exposure, history of sunburn, and sun protection behavior).[2-3,5] Primary care providers should devote more time to screening patients with multiple risk factors. Providers must learn to identify high-risk patients for targeted assessment by incorporating patient risk assessment tools into their practice.[3]

PATHOPHYSIOLOGY

The pathogenesis of skin cancer is multifactoral.[3] Heavy sun exposure is a significant risk factor for MM.[3] Ultraviolet radiation (UVR) in sunlight is the main causative agent in the development of MM and NMSC. UVR produces DNA damage, gene mutations, immunosuppression, oxidative stress, and inflammatory responses, all of which play a pivotal role in photoaging of the skin and skin cancer genesis. Researchers have suggested an association between skin cancer genesis and UVR-induced immunosuppression. UVR is a complete carcinogen in that it not only initiates tumorigenesis by inducing mutations in tumor suppressor genes, but also promotes tumor development. When UVR penetrates the skin, much of its energy is absorbed by the DNA of epidermal keratinocytes. Another major mechanism of carcinogenesis is UVR-induced free radical damage, and genetically determined ability to metabolize free radicals may also predispose patients to skin cancer.[3] Repeated and unprotected exposure to ultraviolet light causes photoaging of the skin over time.

Normal skin aging begins by 30 to 35 of age and is characterized by thinning, atrophy, decreased elasticity, and fragility that lead to wrinkling. Skin that is photoaged from sun damage may be coarse with yellow discoloration (solar elastosis), irregularly pigmented, rough, or atrophic with deep wrinkling. Reactive hyperplasia of melanocytes results in persistent hyperpigmentation or hypopigmentation of the hands, forearms, legs, chest, and back.[3] Chronic exposure disrupts the maturation of the outer layer of the epidermis, resulting in scaling, roughness, seborrheic keratoses, actinic keratoses, and NMSCs.[6-8] Tanning beds and sun lamps provide additional sources of ultraviolet light exposure and should be avoided.[2] The International Agency for Research on Cancer has classified indoor tanning devices as "carcinogenic to humans" based on an extensive review of scientific evidence.[2]

CLINICAL PRESENTATION

Primary care providers must solicit a detailed patient history, including a social, family, and UVR-exposure history, to identify patients with the highest risk of developing skin cancer. Questions about the patient's use of sunscreens, repeated sun exposure without protection, tendency to burn, outdoor employment, or family history of melanoma are beneficial to estimate the risk for NMSC and MM.[3,6] Patients scheduled for routine physical examinations should be queried about any changes in the appearance or size of skin lesions (Table 41-1). Warning signs for skin cancer include (1) an open sore that does not heal for 3 weeks; (2) a spot or sore that burns, itches, stings, crusts, or bleeds; and (3) any mole or spot that changes in size or texture, develops irregular borders, or appears pearly, translucent, or multicolored. Important clinical signs of cutaneous carcinoma include changes in size, shape, color, or texture of a mole or other skin lesion or the appearance of a new growth on the skin. Changes that occur over a few days are usually not cancer, but changes that progress over a month or more should be evaluated by a health care provider.[3]

PHYSICAL EXAMINATION

The most commonly advocated screening test for skin cancer is a complete and thorough TBSE. With the patient disrobed, the examiner must systematically inspect the entire skin surface, including the scalp, nails, and palms of the hands and the soles of the feet.[1] Detection of a suspicious skin lesion, such as BCC, warrants biopsy or referral. NMSC lesions such as BCC may vary from a normal flesh-colored lesion to a slightly pigmented lesion (Fig. 41-1). These are characterized by a raised, shiny appearance, often with pearly borders. An SCC lesion is a roughened, scaling area that does not heal and readily bleeds when scraped (Fig. 41-2). Keratinization of these can lead to a heaped-up appearance that flakes. MM is characterized by a lesion that is best described by the *ABCDE*s of MM (Fig. 41-3).[1-3] These include *a*symmetry (of the entire lesion), *b*order (irregularities), *c*olor (variability within the lesion from a brown to black discoloration), *d*iameter (>6 mm [¼ inch]), and *e*levation (recently raised). As mentioned, other symptoms suggestive of skin cancer include nonhealing skin areas, ulceration, bleeding, and weeping sores. In African Americans, Asian Americans, and dark-skinned individuals, abnormal lesions of the nails, hands, or feet should also be evaluated because these are common sites for melanomas in these populations (Fig. 41-4).

DIAGNOSTICS

Skin biopsy is the definitive diagnostic test and is best performed by an experienced heath care provider. A shave or punch biopsy technique is appropriate for diagnostic evaluation of

TABLE 41-1 Signs Suggesting Malignant Transformation in Pigmented Lesions

Sign	Implication
CHANGE IN COLOR	
Sudden darkening; brown, black	Increased number of tumor cells, the density of which varies within the lesion, creating irregular pigmentation
Spread of color into previously normal skin	Tumor cells migrating through epidermis at various speeds and in different directions (horizontal growth phase)
Red	Vasodilation and inflammation
White	Areas of regression or inflammation
Blue	Pigment deep in dermis; sign of increasing depth of tumor
CHANGE IN CHARACTERISTICS OF BORDER	
Irregular outline	Malignant cells migrating horizontally at different rates
Satellite pigmentation	Cells migrating beyond confines of primary tumor
Development of depigmented halo	Destruction of melanocytes by possible immunologic reaction and inflammation
CHANGES IN SURFACE CHARACTERISTICS THAT SHOULD PROMPT EVALUATION FOR SKIN CANCER	
Scaliness	
Erosion	
Oozing	
Crusting	
Bleeding	
Ulceration	
Elevation	
Loss of normal skin lines	
DEVELOPMENT OF SYMPTOMS THAT SHOULD PROMPT EVALUATION FOR SKIN CANCER	
Pruritus	
Tenderness	
Pain	

From Habif TP: *Clinical dermatology*, ed 5, St Louis, 2010, Mosby.

suspected NMSC (see Chapter 40). Excisional biopsy (total removal) of suspicious MM lesions should be followed by a wider excision if MM is diagnosed.

DIAGNOSTICS
Skin Cancer
Skin biopsy (shave, punch, or excisional)

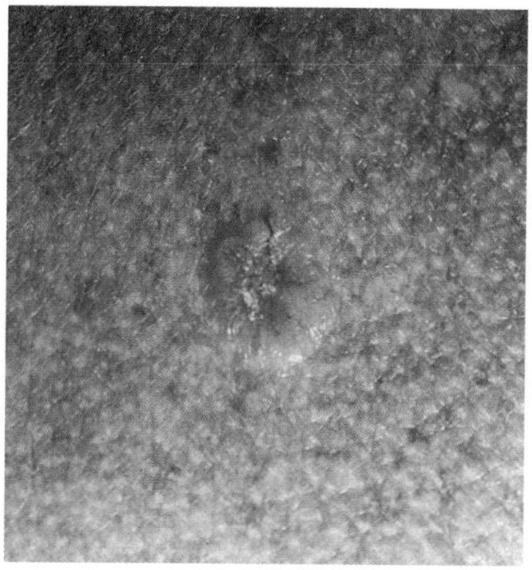

FIGURE 41-1 Nodular basal cell carcinoma. (From Ignatavicius DD, Workman ML, *Medical-Surgical Nursing: Patient Centered Collaborative Care,* ed 8, St. Louis, 2016, Mosby.)

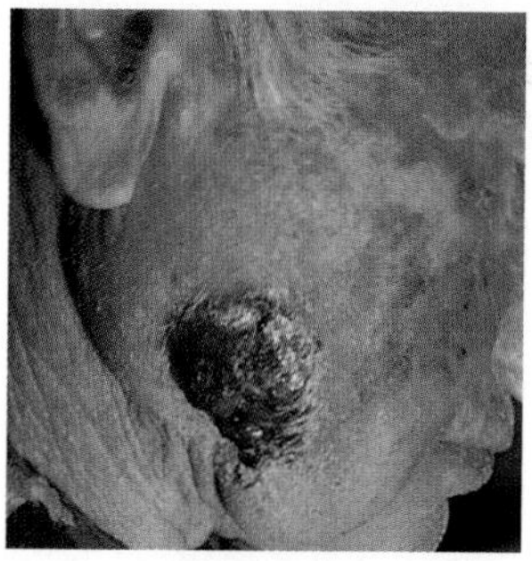

FIGURE 41-2 Squamous cell cancer. (From Ignatavicius DD, Workman ML, *Medical-Surgical Nursing: Patient Centered Collaborative Care,* ed 8, St. Louis, 2016, Mosby.)

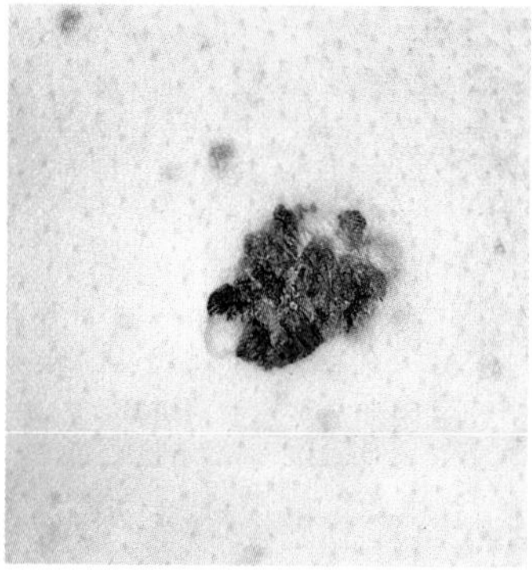

FIGURE 41-3 Superficial spreading melanoma. (From Ignatavicius DD, Workman ML, *Medical-Surgical Nursing: Patient Centered Collaborative Care,* ed 8, St. Louis, 2016, Mosby.)

DIFFERENTIAL DIAGNOSIS

Screening for skin cancer includes the evaluation of skin for all atypical-appearing lesions. Skin lesions may range from a seborrheic keratosis (Fig. 41-5) to a premalignant solar (actinic) keratosis to BCC, SCC, or MM. An actinic keratosis is a persistent

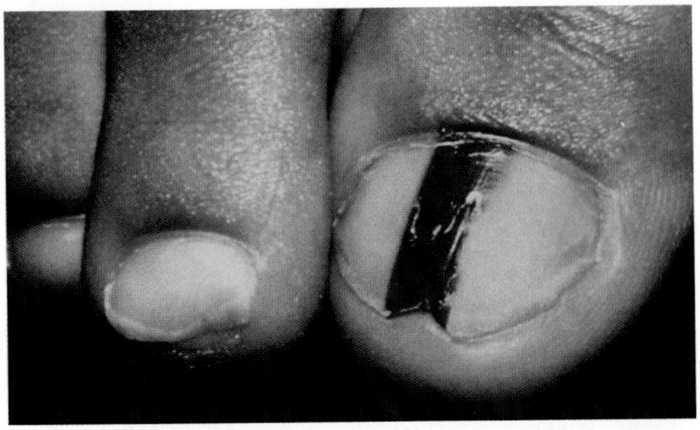

FIGURE 41-4 Acral-lentiginous melanoma. It occurs most often on hands, feet, or nail beds of dark-skinned individuals. Very common in African Americans and Asian Americans. (From Habif TP, Campbell JL, Chapman MS, et al: *Skin disease: diagnosis and treatment*, ed 3, St Louis, 2011, Saunders.)

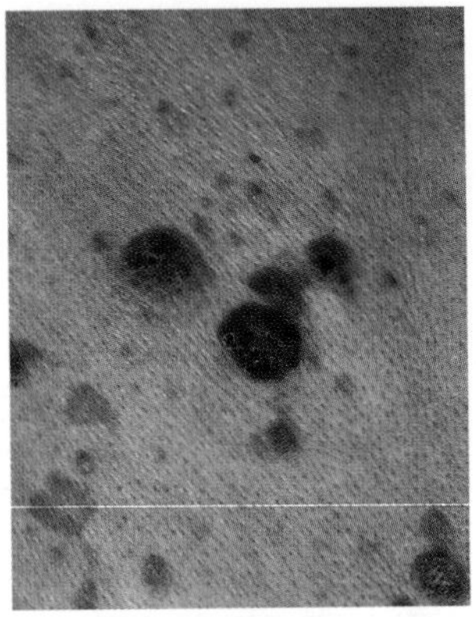

FIGURE 41-5 Seborrheic keratosis (mimicking melanoma). (From Kumar V, Cotran RS, Robbins SL, *Robbins Basic Pathology*, ed 7, Philadelphia, 2003, Saunders.)

DIFFERENTIAL DIAGNOSIS

Skin Cancer

- Actinic keratoses
- BCC
- SCC
- MM
- Dysplastic nevi

or recurrent reddened and roughened area that scales or crusts. These lesions are effectively treated with liquid nitrogen by a freeze-thaw technique to obtain a 1- to 3-mm (0.04- to 0.12-inch) rim of freeze, which allows appropriately slow thawing during 20 to 40 seconds.[7]

MANAGEMENT

Treatment

BCC is treated with electrodessication and curettage. Definitive treatment of SCC is total excision. An experienced dermatologist or surgeon is best equipped to treat an MM lesion based on the stage of the disease with a wide excision. If an NMSC or MM is recognized early by the patient or provider, surgical cure is close to 100%.

Interdisciplinary Management

An annual skin examination of sun-exposed areas is recommended for patients with the diagnosis of BCC or SCC. A primary care provider or dermatology specialist can accomplish this. A total body skin examination by an experienced clinician is recommended for patients diagnosed with MM lesions.

Complications and Life Span Considerations

Despite the tendency of NMSC lesions to grow slowly, failure to diagnose them can result in disfigurement. There is indirect evidence that the shift to screening and recognition of melanoma at earlier tumor stages may be associated with better clinical outcomes.[1] The survival rate at 5 years is inversely proportional to the depth of the MM at the time of diagnosis—the deeper the lesion at diagnosis, the lower the survival rate at 5 years. There are minimum risks from TBSE; however, the examination may be embarrassing to some patients and could lead to unnecessary treatment as a result of misdiagnosis or detection of lesions that might not have caused clinical consequences but were sampled by biopsy.[1,3]

INDICATIONS FOR REFERRAL OR HOSPITALIZATION

The identification of atypical-appearing skin lesions warrants referral or a biopsy. If the biopsy reveals an NMSC or MM, a trained primary care provider, dermatology specialist, or surgeon should provide the definitive treatment.

PATIENT EDUCATION AND HEALTH PROMOTION

Overall, MM incidence rates have risen rapidly over the past 30 years, with an average rise of 1.4% each year over the last 10 years.[4] In 2014, the U.S. Surgeon General released *Call to Action to Prevent Skin Cancer*, citing the elevated and growing burden of this disease.[2] The purpose of this initiative is to increase awareness and encourage all Americans to engage in behaviors that reduce the risk of skin cancer. Knowing that damage to the skin caused by the sun is cumulative may help patients take precautions against sun exposure and thereby reduce their risk; 80% of lifetime sun exposure occurs before the age of 18 years.[1] Precautions include avoiding the sun, wearing protective clothing, and using sunscreens to prevent solar damage to the skin, both for young children and for adults. Prevention of sunburns, which carry a high risk of malignant transformation over time, is paramount. Education of patients at higher risk is crucial. (See the Clinical Presentation section for factors that place patients at higher risk.)

Sun exposure for longer than 15 minutes requires protection with a sunscreen that has a sun protection factor (SPF) of at least 15. Sunscreens should be applied before sun exposure and reapplied every 2 hours or after swimming.

It is important for patients to know that they should seek medical attention for nonhealing sores (sores usually heal within 4 to 6 weeks) or for any lesion that changes in size, shape, texture, or color. Early identification of atypical-appearing skin lesions results in timely referral and effective treatment.

Strategies to improve skin cancer screening by health care providers in the primary care setting include (1) increasing clinicians' skin cancer awareness and understanding, (2) training providers to target high-risk patient populations for screening, and (3) empowering nonphysician providers to gain confidence and competence in their screening skills. By increasing skin cancer and screening comprehension, clinicians can improve screening practices and promote early detection.[2,9]

CHAPTER 42

ACNE VULGARIS

Theresa A. Bedford

DEFINITION AND EPIDEMIOLOGY

Acne vulgaris is the most common dermatologic disorder in the United States. Although first observed in the pediatric age group, the condition can persist well into the adult years. Whereas it is not usually a serious medical problem, acne should never be dismissed as a minor condition that will eventually be outgrown. The psychological effects of prolonged acne and scars include poor confidence, impaired social contact, embarrassment, shame, anxiety, and difficulty with employment.[1] Advances in acne treatment enable management of this disease for many patients.

Acne vulgaris is a disorder of the pilosebaceous follicles resulting in increased sebum production, altered keratinization, inflammation, and bacterial colonization. Acne is characterized by the formation of comedones, erythematous papules and pustules, and nodules.[1]

Up to 80% of individuals with a first-degree relative with acne may have acne.[2] Acne affects nearly all people 15 to 17 years of age.[2,3] Up to 85% of people aged 12 to 24 have acne. Severity has been correlated to pubertal maturity. Of adults in their 20s and 30s, respectively, up to 64% and 43% of individuals have acne. Women beyond the age of 25 tend to have acne related to circulating androgens.[2] Although acne is not clearly associated with ethnicity, black individuals are more prone to postinflammatory hyperpigmentation.[3]

PATHOPHYSIOLOGY

There are four key processes in the development of acne: inflammation (inflammatory mediators are released into the skin); abnormal desquamation of keratinocytes, which plugs the pilosebaceous follicles; increased or altered sebum production; and colonization with *Propionibacterium acnes.*[2,4] Before and during puberty, hormonal stimulation increases production of the sebaceous glands in the pilosebaceous follicles. Abnormally adherent keratinocytes cause plugging of the pilosebaceous follicles, which contributes to the formation of the primary lesion (the comedone). The open comedone (blackhead) is an obstruction at the follicular mouth, which is filled with a plug of stratum corneum cells. The black color is a result of compacted follicular cells, not dirt.[5] Closed comedones (whiteheads) are a result of cystic swelling of the follicular duct below the epidermis. These closed comedones are the precursors of inflammatory papules and pustules (Fig. 42-1). Inflammation, increased sebum production, altered keratinization, and bacterial colonization with *P. acnes* lead to production of chemotactic factors and proinflammatory cytokines.[3] Inflammatory material around the comedone creates inflammatory papules and pustules.

Self-inflicted trauma such as scratching and squeezing of the lesions may result in scars, appearing as pits or hypopigmented spots. Furthermore, the rupture of cystic acne lesions may also result in scar formation without any manipulation of the lesions. Another potential aftereffect of acne is the formation of keloids, especially over the sternum and upper back. In patients with darker skin, inflammatory lesions often resolve with postinflammatory hyperpigmentation. Patients can be reassured that this "staining" is not scarring and usually clears spontaneously after several months.[3,4,6]

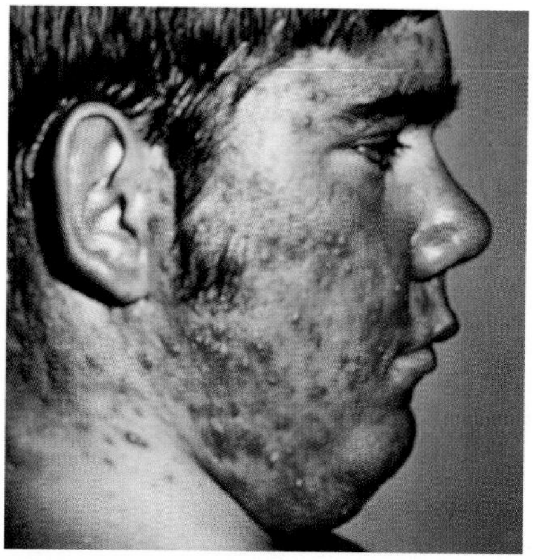

FIGURE **42-1** Pustular acne. (From Weston WL, Lane AT, Morelli JG, *Color Textbook of Pediatric Dermatology,* ed 4, St. Louis, 2008, Mosby.)

CLINICAL PRESENTATION AND PHYSICAL EXAMINATION

The duration of acne, past treatments, use of topical products for acne, menstrual history and contraceptive method, family history of acne, allergies, past medical history and review of systems, and current medications should be included in the patient's history. It is important to document how long previous treatments were used and any side effects. One frustrating fact of acne therapy is that most treatments require 6 to 12 weeks to take effect; shorter treatment therapies may not have been given an adequate trial.[4]

While obtaining the history, the provider must consider that seasonal and hormonal factors may affect acne flares. More severe lesions occur during the winter months when there is less sunlight because acne is an inflammatory condition that improves with exposure to ultraviolet light.[7]

A careful history should include an inquiry about exposure to cosmetic and hair styling products. Cosmetic acne can result from oil-based cosmetics, lotions, and hair products. It is usually worse in the areas in contact with the cosmetic. Pomade acne is seen on the forehead and neck as the result of oily lotions and creams used to style the hair.[2,4]

Mechanical acne can result from friction from headbands, hats, helmets, chin straps, collars, and tight bras. This presentation typically demonstrates acneiform lesions in the area where these devices contact the body, whereas other locations are spared. Acne excoriée is a subtype of acne in which the primary lesions have been scratched. Patients with acne excoriée must be encouraged to stop manipulating or scratching these lesions as an important part of successful therapy for this acne condition.[8]

Certain medications can induce or aggravate acne (Box 42-1).[9] Typically, drug-induced acne has a rapid onset and may involve the usual acne areas as well as unusual areas, such as the postauricular area, upper arms, lower back, abdomen, and legs.[8]

Lifestyle factors may play a role in acne exacerbations. Although diet has not been shown to cause acne, diets with high

BOX 42-1

Drugs That Induce or Aggravate Acne

Anabolic steroids
Androgens
Adrenocorticotropic hormone
Bromides
Dehydroepiandrosterone (DHEA)
Glucocorticoids
Oral and fluorinated topical corticosteroids
Hydantoins
Iodides
Isoniazid
Lithium
Phenobarbital
Phenytoin
Rifampin
Trimethadione

glycemic loads and dairy have been associated with an increase in acne exacerbations.[10] In addition, stress has been to be a major trigger for exacerbations. Although smoking and poor hygiene have not been shown to cause or worsen acne, clinicians are encouraged to promote a healthy lifestyle for their patients.[3]

A physical examination should include the type, location, and extent of acne lesions.[4] The highest concentration of sebaceous glands occurs on the face, chest, back, and shoulders. Patients may be seen with a variety of lesions, including comedones, papules, pustules, and nodules. Surprisingly, the skin of a patient with acne will not necessarily be oily.[2] Mild acne covers less than a fourth of the face without the presence of nodules or scarring. Moderate acne involves half of the face with some nodules and few scars. Severe acne involves at least three quarters of the face with multiple nodules and scars.[4]

DIAGNOSTICS AND DIFFERENTIAL DIAGNOSIS

Acne is diagnosed by physical examination. Laboratory blood testing is necessary only if adrenal or gonadal dysfunction is a possible cause.[4] Other conditions may be misdiagnosed as acne. These include milia, rosacea (Fig. 42-2), the adenoma sebaceum lesions of tuberous sclerosis, nevus comedonicus, miliaria of the newborn, flat warts, and molluscum contagiosum.

DIAGNOSTICS

Acne Vulgaris

LABORATORY
Adrenal or gonadal testing*

*If indicated.

DIFFERENTIAL DIAGNOSIS

Acne Vulgaris

- Tuberous sclerosis
- Nevus comedonicus
- Flat warts
- Molluscum contagiosum
- Acne rosacea
- Steatocystoma multiplex
- Adnexal tumors
- Favre-Racouchot syndrome
- Keratosis pilaris
- Folliculitis
- Acne keloidalis nuchae
- Pseudofolliculitis barbae
- Periorbital dermatitis
- Sebaceous hyperplasia

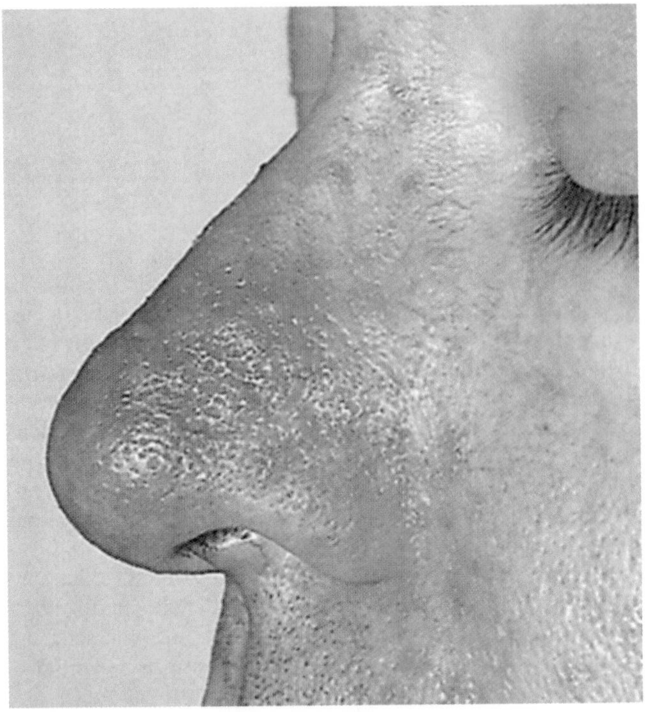

FIGURE 42-2 Rosacea. (From White GM, *ColorAtlas of Regional Dermatology*, St. Louis, 1994, Mosby.)

MANAGEMENT

Therapy should be individualized according to the severity of acne. Goals of treatment include normalizing keratinization of the follicular epithelium, decreasing sebum production, reducing *P. acnes* proliferation, reducing inflammation, and minimizing scarring.[11]

Mild cleansers and cleansing bars are helpful to remove sebum from the surface of the skin. They do not alter sebum production. Harsh soaps, astringents, "buff puffs," and grainy washes should be avoided because they may dry the skin or aggravate inflammatory lesions. Moisturizers, makeup, and hair products should be water based and labeled noncomedogenic or nonacnegenic.[4]

Topical therapy is considered first-line therapy. Topical medications reduce inflammation, inhibit the growth of *P. acnes*, and regulate keratinocyte desquamation to prevent comedone formation, reduce existing lesions, and decrease formation of new lesions. Topical preparations include tretinoin (Retin-A), adapalene (Differin), tazarotene (Tazorac), azelaic acid (Azelex), benzoyl peroxide, and salicylic acid. These agents are applied to clean skin once daily, usually before bedtime. Side effects include erythema, dryness, and sun sensitivity. Patients should be warned that acne may worsen before skin clears. Patients should continue to use a noncomedogenic moisturizer and sunblock.[4]

Several topical agents are available to decrease *P. acnes* proliferation and inhibit the production of inflammatory mediators. These agents include erythromycin, clindamycin, metronidazole, sulfonamide, azelaic acid, and benzoyl peroxide. Topical antibiotics are not recommended in monotherapy. There are combination products with benzoyl peroxide and erythromycin or clindamycin. These are usually applied once or twice a day after cleansing. Although these agents may be used alone, they also work synergistically with keratolytics.[4]

Oral antibiotics are effective in treating inflammatory acne by decreasing *P. acnes* and by reducing the concentration of free fatty acids, thereby inhibiting comedogenesis. Oral antibiotics are reserved for severe cases, lesions unresponsive to topical therapy, patients at risk for scarring, and lesions on the trunk or back.[2] Treatment is necessary for a minimum of 6 to 8 weeks for improvement to be shown and may continue for several months with a reevaluation period at 12 to 18 weeks. Antibiotic therapy should include the use of benzoyl peroxide to reduce resistance.[4] The most commonly used oral antibiotics include erythromycin, tetracycline, doxycycline, and minocycline.[2] Minocycline may be more effective than doxycycline.[1] Less commonly used antibiotics include clindamycin, trimethoprim-sulfamethoxazole, azithromycin, cephalexin, ampicillin, and amoxicillin.[2] Once acne improvement is achieved, antibiotics should be discontinued and retinoids should be continued for maintenance.[4]

Androgen induces sebum production, which in combination with keratin leads to comedone formation. Antiandrogen medications that cause sebaceous gland suppression include combined oral contraceptives, spironolactone, and drospirenone.[2]. A Cochrane review found that combined oral contraceptives (COCs) were effective in reducing inflammatory and noninflammatory acne. Yaz (drospirenone and ethinyl estradiol), Ortho Tri-Cyclen (ethinyl estradiol and norgestimate), and Estrostep (norethindrone acetate and ethinyl estradiol) are the only COCs with a labeled use for acne treatment.[12] Progesterone-only contraceptives may worsen acne.[2] Spironolactone and drospirenone are additional antiandrogens that reduce sebum production. Drospirenone is available as a combination oral contraceptive pill. According to the U.S. Food and Drug Administration (FDA), patients taking drospirenone may have an increased risk of blood clots.[13] Combination oral contraceptives and spironolactone are contraindicated in pregnant and lactating women and in the presence of thromboembolic disorders, renal impairment, and hyperkalemia.

Isotretinoin is restricted to the treatment of recalcitrant nodulocystic acne that has been unresponsive to standard therapies. Its use is best managed by a dermatologist or dermatology nurse practitioner. It is thought to inhibit sebum production, to decrease follicular obstruction, and to have an anti-inflammatory effect. Patients need monthly monitoring of triglyceride levels and hepatic function. Isotretinoin is teratogenic, and careful contraceptive measures should be taken. Sexually active women of childbearing age must use two forms of birth control and be monitored for pregnancy monthly. Treatment usually lasts 4 to 6 months. Approximately 60% of patients who complete a course of isotretinoin therapy will experience a long-term remission. Of the other 40%, some require further courses of isotretinoin, but some have acne that is controllable with simpler forms of acne therapy.[1,2,4]

Patients with skin of color pose a challenge because of their increased tendency to develop postinflammatory hyperpigmentation. Keloid formation is also more prevalent in blacks compared with other ethnicities. Concomitant therapy is important in patients with skin of color to reduce the risk of permanent skin alterations from acne.[14]

Rosacea

Rosacea often coexists with acne vulgaris and may closely mimic it. Sometimes called *acne rosacea* (see Fig. 42-2), this condition is rare in adolescents and occurs most often between the ages of 30 and 50 years.[15] The primary distinction between acne vulgaris and rosacea, however, is that comedones do not occur in rosacea. Rosacea may arise de novo or may follow acne, sometimes by years. On occasion, rosacea is confused with perioral dermatitis, which is much more common in the younger population. Hallmark characteristics of rosacea include flushing, facial erythema, inflammatory papules and pustules, telangiectasia, edema, and watery or irritated eyes.[15]

To date there is no cure for rosacea. Treatment is aimed managing the signs and symptoms and improving the patient's quality of life.[15] Proper skin care has been shown to improve symptoms.[16] Mild emollient-based cleansers along with light nongreasy facial moisturizers promote health and repair of the skin through gentle cleansing and hydration without further aggravating the inflamed and sensitive skin. Cleansers and moisturizers should have a neutral pH; surfactants that do not strip the natural lipids, proteins, and moisture from the skin barrier; and formulas without potential irritants or allergens.[16,17] Oil-based products are to be avoided.[17] Patients do not need to avoid makeup. Persistent erythema and edema are difficult to treat but may be improved with lasers or intense pulsed light. Transient flushing, especially of the central face, is also difficult to treat.[17] Avoidance of trigger factors (e.g., alcohol, hot fluids, spicy foods) is essential.[15] Papules and pustules are best treated with topical or oral antibiotics or topical azelaic acid. These medications help disrupt the link between flushing and papules.[17]

Metronidazole, azelaic acid, and sodium sulfacetamide and sulfur are the three topical medications approved for the treatment of rosacea by the FDA.[15] Both metronidazole and azelaic acid have been shown to be effective in treating the erythema associated with rosacea. Metronidazole 1% or 0.75% gel, cream, or lotion is applied twice daily for an average of 3 to 4 months and up to 2 years; treatment should be stopped if there is no clinical improvement. Topical azelaic acid 15% gel or cream (depending on patient preference) is applied twice a day for 2 months. If there is no clinical improvement within 4 weeks, the medication should be discontinued. Plexion cleanser (sodium sulfacetamide 10% and sulfur 5%) has also been shown to help reduce erythema, as well as papules.[18] Oral antibiotics are commonly used in refractory cases of rosacea. Tetracycline, 250 to 500 mg twice daily; doxycycline, 100 to 200 mg/day; or minocycline, 50 to 100 mg/day is typically prescribed for 3 months but may continue long term.[17] Isotretinoin is occasionally used, under the care of a dermatologist, in recalcitrant or severe cases and is effective in low doses.[19] Diffuse erythema with minimal inflammatory lesions and telangiectasis, often the result of constant flushing, responds to a series of intense pulsed light or laser treatments.[20] Medications to reduce flushing associated with rosacea include oral contraceptives, beta blockers, clonidine, spironolactone, naloxone, ondansetron, aspirin, and selective serotonin reuptake inhibitors. None of these products has evidence-based data to support its use in this manner.[21] Sun exposure should be avoided, especially midday. Topical steroids should not be used for the treatment of rosacea.[19]

COMPLICATIONS

Scarring, hyperpigmentation, and keloids are complications associated with acne. Complications can also result from therapy. Serious side effects are associated with some systemic therapies, particularly isotretinoin, which not only is teratogenic but may also cause hypertriglyceridemia and hepatic dysfunction. Serious social and psychological effects are associated with severe acne and rosacea.[1]

The most serious medical complication of rosacea is the ocular form, which causes watery eyes, telangiectasia of the conjunctiva and lid margin, and periocular erythema. Blepharitis, conjunctivitis, and keratitis are common presentations. Ocular rosacea can cause patients to have light sensitivity, blurred vision, and foreign body sensation.[15] In addition to the dermatologist, an ophthalmologist consultation should be sought for ocular symptoms that are not responsive to treatment in primary care.[17] If corneal ulcers are suspected, the patient should be referred to an ophthalmologist immediately.

INDICATIONS FOR REFERRAL OR HOSPITALIZATION

All patients with recalcitrant or severe nodulocystic acne should be referred to a dermatologist for treatment. Considering that suicide is one of the five leading causes of death in the adolescent population, patients with issues related to depression and self-esteem should be referred to a mental health professional.

Patients with severe rosacea not responsive to topical or oral antibiotics should also be referred to a dermatologist. Complications such as rhinophyma, lymphedema, or ocular involvement should be managed by a dermatologist. Rosacea cases causing psychological distress should also be considered for referral.[17]

PATIENT AND FAMILY EDUCATION

Acne treatment may take several weeks to months before improvement is appreciated. Patience and understanding of the prescribed treatment regimen are crucial. Phone contact and periodic office visits will help evaluate improvement and compliance. This type of support is often important for this frustrating and often long-term or recurrent disorder. Patients with rosacea can contact the National Rosacea Society at www.rosacea.org for more information.

HEALTH PROMOTION

Patients are encouraged to gently wash the involved skin once or twice a day. Increasing patient awareness that non–water-based cosmetic and hair products may cause acne is important. Patients may have jobs that require them to wear protective headgear and should be encouraged to maintain a careful face cleansing routine to minimize the occurrence of mechanical acne.

CHAPTER 43

ALOPECIA

Terry Mahan Buttaro

DEFINITION AND EPIDEMIOLOGY

Alopecia is a term used to describe abnormal hair loss. There are varied causes of hair loss. Medications, chemotherapy, radiation therapy, diabetes, trichotillomania, and hair loss from hair dyes or hairdos are possible causes, but alopecia is also related to congenital hair abnormalities and the more commonly observed alopecia from androgenetic or pattern hair loss. Whatever the cause, hair loss is a disturbing and highly emotional issue for many patients.

PATHOPHYSIOLOGY

Alopecia, except for congenital alopecia, can be divided into two types of alopecia: scarring (cicatricial alopecia) and nonscarring (noncicatricial alopecia).[1] In noncicatricial alopecia, the hair follicles are still present and there is no sign of inflamed tissue, scarring, or atrophy.[1] Alopecia areata, androgenetic alopecia, lupus erythematosus, syphilis, telogen effluvium, and tinea capitus are all potential causes of noncicatricial alopecia.[2] Cicatricial alopecia—scarring alopecia—is usually the result of an intense inflammatory process of the scalp, with resultant skin atrophy and scarring.[1] Chronic cutaneous discoid lupus, folliculitis decalvans, lichen planus, linear scleroderma, sarcoidosis, and cutaneous metastasis are potential causes of scarring alopecia.[2]

Each hair follicle goes through a highly programmed cycle over and over again throughout its life. The cycle of hair growth involves three phases: anagen, catagen, and telogen, which represent the growth, involution, and rest phases.[1] The anagen (growth) phase varies according to the location of the follicle on the body. This phase is longest on the scalp (producing long hairs) and much shorter on the eyebrows (producing short hairs). During the catagen phase, the hair involutes. This is the shortest of the three stages. During the telogen phase, the mature hair is shed, resulting in the loss of 50 to 150 scalp hairs each day.

Anagen Phase Disturbances

Three common types of hair loss are a result of anagen phase disturbance: androgenetic alopecia, anagen effluvium, and alopecia areata. Androgenetic alopecia, the most common type of hair loss, is the hereditary thinning of hair in susceptible men and women, and is related to an androgen receptor variation.[3] This condition results from the sensitivity of hair on certain portions of the scalp to androgens. Testosterone, an androgen, is converted to dihydrotestosterone (DHT) peripherally. DHT binds to receptors on scalp hair follicles, causing a series of events that leads to the shortening of the anagen or growth part of the cycle. As a result, hair follicles that previously produced thick, pigmented terminal hairs begin to make thin vellus hairs. This process, called miniaturization, produces the fine hair seen in androgenetic alopecia, or pattern hair loss.

Anagen effluvium is the term used to describe the alopecia from the diffuse, rapid, and dramatic loss of anagen hairs.

The most common cause is chemotherapy. Chemotherapeutic agents prevent the rapid division of the hair matrix cells. Hair production stops, and the hairs that are already present become frail, break off, and are shed. Normal hair production resumes when the antineoplastic medication is stopped.

Alopecia areata is fairly common and is often an autoimmune condition that results in well-demarcated areas of alopecia on the scalp or body. T-cell–mediated alopecia areata causes a chronic idiopathic inflammatory response around the hair bulb at the base of the hair.[3] The inflammation results in hair that that is not well developed and as it hits the surface easily breaks or is shed.[3] Stress may be a contributory factor in alopecia areata, but other conditions are also associated with this type of hair loss and include Addison disease, lupus erythematosus, and thyroid disease.[3]

Telogen Phase Disturbance

The transient shedding of telogen phase hairs is termed *telogen effluvium.* In this condition, the hair prematurely enters the telogen phase, resulting in a sudden onset of hair loss.[4] Multiple factors, including high fever, certain medications, endocrine abnormalities, anemia, childbirth, and malnutrition, can cause telogen effluvium.[5] Telogen effluvium affects men, women, and even infants and can persist for several months after the precipitating event.

CLINICAL PRESENTATION

The history is a critical part of the evaluation of a person with alopecia. The provider should inquire about the onset, duration, and rapidity of the hair loss; any acute or chronic illnesses; current and past medications; and any symptoms that may be related to trichotillomania. It is important to determine whether the patient has had this type of hair loss before. Long and insidious hair loss is more indicative of androgenetic alopecia. Alopecia areata is often recurrent. An acute illness, such as a high fever, can trigger telogen effluvium, as can hyperthyroidism or hypothyroidism. A family history of hair loss may represent a clue for androgenetic alopecia, sometimes a hereditary disorder.

It is also important to inquire about associated symptoms. Scalp itching, pain, or flaking can suggest an inflammation of the scalp from psoriasis or contact dermatitis from hair dye. These conditions inflame the scalp and can cause hair breakage with resultant alopecia. In addition, symptoms of scalp itching and flaking can indicate tinea capitis, a fungal infection of the scalp that weakens the hairs and produces alopecia.

PHYSICAL EXAMINATION

The physical examination begins with an evaluation of the pattern of hair loss. Androgenetic alopecia in men usually is seen as recession of the hairline at the temples and thinning in the frontal areas and the vertex. Women with androgenetic alopecia usually have diffuse thinning that is most pronounced in the frontal and parietal areas. A rim of hair along the frontal hairline is usually preserved.

Alopecia areata usually is initially seen as well-demarcated patches of hair loss on the scalp, eyebrows, and eyelashes. Singular, "exclamation point" hairs are sometimes visible. These exclamation point hairs are normal distally but are thinned proximal to the scalp. The scalp is not inflamed in alopecia areata. Men may experience alopecia areata in the beard area. When the whole scalp is affected, the process is called alopecia totalis.[5] If the whole body is involved, the process is called alopecia universalis.[5,6]

Anagen effluvium tends to result in a diffuse loss of hair, as does telogen effluvium. Scarring of the scalp suggests an inflammatory process, such as lupus or lichen planus follicularis. Scaling on the scalp may suggest psoriasis or tinea capitis. Patchy hair loss with regrowing hairs of multiple lengths suggests trichotillomania, a condition in which the patient pulls or twists the hair.

DIAGNOSTICS

Findings from the history and physical examination guide diagnostic testing. If there is scaling on the scalp that is suggestive of tinea capitis, a sample of several hairs or a scalp scraping is examined after preparation with potassium hydroxide (KOH). The presence of hyphae in the KOH preparation confirms the fungal cause of the alopecia.

A hair pull test, in which a few dozen hairs are grasped (with the patient's permission) firmly at the base and pulled, can help determine a telogen or anagen effluvium. A positive test result is noted when five or more hairs that include anagen hairs (with the follicle sheath) are pulled.[7] The hair bulb from these pulled hairs is examined with a magnifying glass or under the microscope to identify the characteristic appearance of anagen and telogen hairs.

If telogen effluvium is suspected and there is no obvious cause, an underlying illness should be considered (e.g., a thyroid disorder or iron deficiency anemia). If anemia is considered, iron studies should include serum iron, iron-binding capacity, and ferritin in addition to a complete blood count (CBC).[4] A scalp biopsy and trichogram may also be of benefit.[4]

A hormonal evaluation of a woman with androgenetic alopecia is not necessary unless she has other signs of a hormonal imbalance, such as irregular menses, infertility, hirsutism, cystic acne, virilization, or galactorrhea. In these women, evaluation for alopecia may include testosterone or dehydroepiandrosterone-5 (DHEA-5) levels in addition to the other hormonal tests indicated by their symptoms.

Secondary syphilis is a cause of patchy alopecia. Patients suspected of having secondary syphilis should have a Venereal Disease Research Laboratory (VDRL) test performed. Finally, a scalp biopsy is sometimes helpful when the cause of the alopecia is not clear.

DIAGNOSTICS

Alopecia

LABORATORY

KOH preparation	TIBC*
TSH*	TSH*
CBC*	VDRL test*
Serum glucose or hemoglobin A_{1c}*	DHEA-5 level*
Ferritin level*	Testosterone level*
Serum iron*	Trichogram*
	Biopsy*

*If indicated.
TIBC, total iron-binding capacity; TSH, thyroid-stimulating hormone.

TABLE 43-1 **Diagnosis of Alopecia**

Disease	Duration (yr)	Scalp	Pattern	Pull Test
Alopecia areata	<1	Normal	Patchy; "exclamation point" hairs*	±
Anagen effluvium	Duration of chemotherapy	Normal	Diffuse	Hair breakage
Tinea capitis	<1	Scale, crust	Patchy	Hair breakage
Trichotillomania	>1	Normal to scarring	Patchy with stubble	—
Telogen effluvium	<1	Normal	Diffuse	Telogen
Androgenetic alopecia	>1	Normal	Pattern baldness	—
Systemic disease	<1	Normal	Diffuse	Normal/↑ telogen
Hair breakage	<1	Normal	Patchy	Age appropriate

*Short, stubby, straight hairs.

DIFFERENTIAL DIAGNOSIS

Alopecia

GENERALIZED HAIR LOSS

- Telogen effluvium
- Acute blood loss
- Childbirth
- Inadequate protein intake
- High fever
- Medications (heparin, propranolol, vitamin A, warfarin, propylthiouracil, isotretinoin, lithium, beta blockers, amphetamines, acitretin)
- Stress
- Metabolic abnormalities (hypothyroidism, hyperthyroidism, diabetes)
- Severe illness
- Anemia
- Anagen effluvium
- Cancer therapy (chemotherapy, radiation therapy)
- Poisoning (arsenic, thallium)
- Generalized patchy hair loss
- Secondary syphilis

LOCALIZED HAIR LOSS

- Androgenic alopecia (male or female pattern)
- Alopecia areata
- Atopic dermatitis
- Anemia
- Diabetes
- Pregnancy
- Thyroid disease
- Infection
- Stress
- Tick bite
- Lupus erythematosus
- Myasthenia gravis
- Vitiligo
- Hirsutism
- Scarring alopecia
- Developmental defects (aplasia cutis)
- Physical injury (burns, pressure)
- Infection (bacterial [folliculitis, furuncle], fungal [kerion], viral [herpes zoster])
- Neoplasms (metastatic cancer, sclerosing basal cell carcinoma)
- Lupus
- Lichen planus follicularis
- Cicatricial pemphigoid
- Scleroderma
- Traction alopecia
- Trichotillomania

DIFFERENTIAL DIAGNOSIS

The differential diagnosis of hair loss is extensive. Table 43-1 can be used to differentiate among these conditions. The cause can usually be isolated with a careful history, physical examination, and some diagnostic tests.

MANAGEMENT

The role of the primary care provider is to distinguish normal hair loss from hair loss associated with illness or another disorder.[5] When an external factor is found with anagen or telogen effluvium, the key to the management of alopecia is removal of this causative factor. Anagen effluvium as a result of chemotherapy will be reversed when the medication is stopped and the hair matrix is allowed to mature again. Telogen effluvium will also be reversed when the causative factor or event is over or corrected and the hair cycle is allowed to return to normal.

Only two medications, minoxidil (Rogaine) and finasteride (Propecia), are currently approved by the U.S. Food and Drug Administration (FDA) to treat androgenetic alopecia.[4] Finasteride is Pregnancy Category X, so Minoxidil is the only medication approved by the FDA for use by women.[4] Applied twice a day to the dry scalp, minoxidil side effects include dryness and irritation of the scalp. Finasteride, an oral medication, inhibits the change of testosterone to DHT, the hormone responsible for causing the miniaturization of hairs in androgenetic alopecia. Both minoxidil and finasteride should be used for 8 to 12 months to determine efficacy, and require continued treatment to maintain hair growth.[5]

Alopecia areata can spontaneously resolve, but if it does not, treatment options are available (although not FDA approved). Therapies include ultraviolet B light, cyclosporine, and topical and intralesional corticosteroids.[4] Anthralin, an antipsoriatric agent, and minoxidil are two topical agents that can be effective treatments.[4] Topical immunotherapy, or contact sensitization, is also very effective.[4]

COMPLICATIONS

Some types of hair loss are the result of systemic illness. Complications can result from these illnesses. In addition, complications can occur as a result of the psychological effects that patients may experience with hair loss.

INDICATIONS FOR REFERRAL OR HOSPITALIZATION

Alopecia without a timely response to standard management options or in cases in which the cause is unclear requires consultation with a dermatologist. Patients should also be referred to a dermatologist or surgeon for consideration of hair transplantation. Patients with suspected trichotillomania may benefit from treatment with a selective serotonin reuptake inhibitor (SSRI) and a mental health referral.

PATIENT AND FAMILY EDUCATION

Patients with androgenetic alopecia may be reassured to know that this is a common disorder. They should be reminded that there are no restrictions on types of grooming products that they use. In addition, the frequency of hair washing will not affect the hair loss process.[5]

Patients with alopecia areata should know that spontaneous remissions and recurrences are common. They should also know that vitiligo, atopy (eczema, asthma, and hay fever), and thyroid disease are more common in people with alopecia areata.[8]

CHAPTER 44

ANIMAL AND HUMAN BITES

Daniel W. O'Neill • Brian Jennings

DEFINITION AND EPIDEMIOLOGY

Every year there are millions of people throughout the world who sustain bite wounds. Although many of these bites are minor, there is significant risk of injury and infection. In the United States, there is an annual incidence of 2 million to 5 million occurrences, which account for about 1% of all visits to emergency departments. Animal and human bites have a large health care cost, with dog bites alone estimated to cost $165 million dollars per year.[1]

Domestic animals inflict the majority of bite wounds. Dog bites account for 80% to 90% of those bites that require medical care, yet have the lowest incidence of wound infection (2% to 13%).[2,3] Even though the majority of injuries that are caused by dog bites are relatively minor, severe injuries can occur. These can include destructive soft tissue injuries, neurovascular injuries, orthopedic injuries, and even death.[4] Severe dog bite wounds most commonly affect the extremities, are seen more often in children and young adults, and are more frequent when the animal is provoked. Cat bites are the second most common type of mammalian bite, accounting for 3% to 15% of bite wound cases per year. However, the infection rate is much higher (30% to 50%) as a result of the deep puncture wounds from the animal's sharp teeth.[1] The most common sites of injury are the arm, forearm, and hand.

Human bites can occur from physical altercations, often with closed-fist injuries, in the setting of alcohol ingestion. These can also occur accidentally during sexual activity, or from self-inflicted causes such as nail biting. Human bites have overall infection rates of around 10%.[5] The most common sites of infection are the nose, lip, and ear. Bites not located on the hand have an infection rate similar to that of routine lacerations, but the clenched-fist injury, or "fight bite," has a much higher complication rate because of the high penetrating force causing local tissue destruction and potentially osteomyelitis, tendinitis, and septic arthritis.

Physician consultation is indicated for suspected rabid animal bites; facial, hand, or extensive bites; tendon, bone, or joint involvement; or significant infectious complications.

PATHOPHYSIOLOGY

The morbidity and mortality associated with mammalian bites are mostly related to tissue injury or, more accurately, polymicrobial infection near the bite site. The pathogens involved reflect the oral flora of the culprit, the skin flora of the victim, and the environment in which the bite took place. Infections involving aerobes alone (24% to 44%) or mixed aerobes and anaerobes (54% to 66%) are the most common.[2] The risk factors for infection are listed in Box 44-1.

Animal bites can contain a variety of pathogens, both bacterial and viral. The most common aerobic bacteria are *Pasteurella, Streptococcus, Staphylococcus,* and *Corynebacterium* species.[1-3,5] *Bacteroides, Actinomyces, Porphyromonas,* and *Fusobacterium* species are common anaerobic isolates and may produce β-lactamase.[1-3,5] A rare but serious bacterial infection caused by *Capnocytophaga canimorsus* causes overwhelming sepsis and disseminated intravascular coagulation with mortality rates from 25% to 30%. It is more common in patients with predisposing conditions, such as asplenia, liver disease, or immunosuppressive therapy.[6]

Among viral diseases, rabies is the most common and well known. The rabies virus infects the central nervous system of the bite victim, which eventually leads to disease in the brain

BOX 44-1

Risk Factors for Bite Wound Infection

- Location on the hand or foot
- Puncture wounds
- Crush injuries
- Injuries that may have penetrated the periosteum or joint capsule
- Advanced liver disease
- Treatment delay of more than 12 hours
- Failure to irrigate and to debride wound during initial management
- Age older than 50 years
- Asplenia
- Alcoholism
- Diabetes mellitus
- Preexisting or resulting edema at the bite site
- Peripheral vascular disease

and death. Animals such as bats, raccoons, skunks, and foxes are the most common carriers in the United States, whereas dogs and cats are the most predominant carriers in other countries. Other pathogens rarely transmitted through animal bites include those that cause tularemia, leptospirosis, cat-scratch disease, rat-bite fever, tetanus, plague, sporotrichosis, and blastomycosis.

Human bites are also polymicrobial, with similar pathogens; however, there are some important differences. *Staphylococcus aureus* is the organism most often isolated in human bite cases if the studies did not use anaerobic methodology. Methicillin-resistant *Staphylococcus aureus* (MRSA) is an increasingly recognized pathogen in bite wounds.[7] Penicillin-resistant gram-negative rods have been reported in 24% to 43% of human bite cultures. *Streptococcus pyogenes* is also generally found in human bites.[8] *Pasteurella* and *Capnocytophaga* species are not transmitted through humans, but *Eikenella corrodens* is present in 30% of infected human bite injuries (particularly clenched-fist injuries), is often resistant to certain antibiotics, and can lead to a serious indolent infection.[2] Many of the isolates (24% to 43%) produce β-lactamase. Rare organisms from humans include herpes simplex virus types 1 and 2, hepatitis B and C viruses, and *Mycobacterium tuberculosis*. Human immunodeficiency virus (HIV) has a biologic possibility of transmission through a bite wound, but the risk of transmission is extremely low.[9]

CLINICAL PRESENTATION

The history must include the location and time of the bite; the breed and behavior of the animal; the domestication and rabies vaccine status of the animal; whether the animal was provoked; drug allergies; current immunization status for tetanus and rabies; alcohol use; current medications; and past medical history with an emphasis on immunocompetence, history of splenectomy, chronic edema, or liver disease. With human bites, the presence of infectious diseases in the attacker should be investigated. Patients may be unwilling to admit to human bite wounds, particularly in a clenched-fist injury.

PHYSICAL EXAMINATION

Physical examination should document the location, extent, and depth of the wound; type of wound (puncture, scratch, tear, or avulsion); and tenderness and other signs of infection (e.g., erythema, streaking, warmth, fluctuation, adenopathy, purulent discharge). There should be careful testing for involvement of underlying tendons, joints (range of motion), and nerves and for signs of compartment syndrome (disproportionate pain, paresthesia, pallor, paralysis).

DIAGNOSTICS

Culture of uncomplicated fresh bite wounds is rarely beneficial, but wounds with signs of infection should be cultured for aerobic and anaerobic bacteria.[1] Blood cultures and complete blood count (CBC) may be indicated if there are signs of systemic infection, but they have a low sensitivity.[10] C-reactive protein level and erythrocyte sedimentation rate (ESR) can be used to monitor response to treatment.[11] In cases of bites that occur near joints, or those that look severely infected, radiographs should be obtained to look for fractures, the presence of foreign bodies, soft tissue injury, subcutaneous gas, and osteomyelitis.[8] Careful examination is warranted to assess the extent of the injury, which may include tendon laceration or joint space penetration.[12]

MANAGEMENT

After assessing for and treating life-threatening injuries, the provider should irrigate the wound and treat the the patient in accordance with the following management principles:

- Irrigate the wound with at least 150 mL of sterile saline solution.[8] Devitalized tissue, foreign bodies, and clots are cautiously debrided. Aggressive drainage, irrigation, and wound packing are necessary if cultures reveal an established wound infection. Most wounds do not develop signs of infection until 24 to 72 hours after the bite.[2]
- Bites to the face, whether of animal or human origin, should be managed with extensive irrigation, cautious debridement, preemptive antibiotics, and primary closure.[10]
- It is generally accepted that most cat and human bites, deep puncture wounds, clinically infected wounds, wounds more than 6 to 12 hours old, and bites to the hand should be left open because of the high risk of infection.[1-5] These wounds can be closed by delayed primary closure or by secondary intention.
- Wounds involving the hand or foot should be immobilized and elevated for 1 to 3 days.[12] Close outpatient follow-up monitoring is recommended to track complications or treatment failures.
- For fresh bites, prophylactic therapy is most effective with amoxicillin–clavulanic acid, 875 mg/125 mg twice daily for 5 to 7 days as the regimen of choice, or cefoxitin, 1000 mg (1 g) intravenously twice daily.[12]
- Older infected bites require 7 to 14 days of targeted antibiotic therapy when soft tissue is involved. In bone or joint infections, longer courses of antibiotics are needed and referral to a specialist is indicated.[10] The selection of antibiotics is based on knowledge of the most common microorganisms encountered and on susceptibility testing of cultured microorganisms from infected wounds.
- In patients who are allergic to penicillin, a combination of clindamycin, 300 mg orally three times daily, plus doxycycline, 100 mg orally twice daily, may be used. Double-strength trimethoprim-sulfamethoxazole may be taken twice daily or ciprofloxacin can be used.[12] Later-generation quinolones (e.g., moxifloxacin) are active against all major bite wound pathogens.[8] Agents such as dicloxacillin, cephalexin, erythromycin, and clindamycin should not be used alone because they lack activity against *Pasteurella* species.[12] Macrolides should be reserved for pregnant patients allergic to β-lactamase.[13]
- The incidence of MRSA colonization in domestic animals has been found to be increasing. One retrospective study examined *S. aureus* isolates taken from domestic cats and

DIAGNOSTICS

Animal and Human Bites

LABORATORY

Aerobic and anaerobic cultures of infected wounds only
Hepatitis, HIV, and other transmissible disease status of the perpetrator if a human bite

IMAGING

X-ray studies for any bone or joint involvement or foreign body dogs. Of the 139 samples, 35% were found to be MRSA.[7] Coverage can be considered in regions in which the incidence of community-acquired MRSA incidence is high. Trimethoprim-sulfamethoxazole should be considered if MRSA contact is suspected, or doxycycline can be used, except for children younger than 8 years. Clindamycin can also be used in areas that do not have clindamycin-resistant MRSA strains. Oral linezolid can be used in more severe cases that do not require hospitalization. Parenteral vanomycin, daptomycin, linezolid, tigecycline, or quinupristin-dalfopristin can be considered in more complicated or systemic infections for MRSA coverage.[7]

- Antimicrobial therapy is obviously indicated in infected wounds, but treatment of fresh, uninfected wounds is still controversial. Prophylaxis is indicated in high-risk bites and in high-risk patients (see Box 44-1). Patients with cat bites and hand bites from any animal, including humans, should receive 3- to 5-day prophylaxis. Some recommend that antibiotic prophylaxis be given for all bite wounds except for patients who are seen 72 hours after injury with no signs of infection.[2]
- Tetanus toxoid and diphtheria (Td) or tetanus, diphtheria toxoid, and acellular pertussis (Tdap), 0.5 mL intramuscularly, should be administered to those who have not had a Td booster within the past 5 years.[4] Patients who have not completed a full primary series of three injections or whose vaccination status is unknown will require tetanus immune globulin, 250 to 500 units intramuscularly, with the first of three monthly doses of tetanus toxoid.[4] For more information, see Chapter 17.
- Rabies prevention: The decision to provide postexposure antirabies treatment should be based on the guidelines of city or state public health departments, the Centers for Disease Control and Prevention, and the Advisory Committee on Immunization Practices (ACIP).[14] The most common vectors in the United States are bats, with cases found in every state except Hawaii. It can sometimes be difficult to assess for wounds after a bat exposure, and there have been multiple cases of people getting rabies when no bite wound was noted on examination.
- With these considerations, the ACIP recommends postexposure prophylaxis for any direct contact between human and bat unless the person is fairly certain that a bite, scratch, or mucous membrane exposure did not occur, or if the offending bat can be captured.[14]
- Every effort must be made with the help of public health authorities to make a decision regarding quarantine (isolation and observation) or sacrifice of the biting animal for pathologic brain examination. Animals that can be quarantined should be watched for 10 days, as studies have shown that animals with rabies present in the saliva will begin to sicken and die within this time frame.[15] If the animal shows signs of becoming sick, prophylaxis should be started for the victim.
- Prophylaxis should always be started immediately in bite wounds to the head or neck because the incubation period can be shorter.[16] In these cases if the animals are well after 10 days of observation the prophylaxis can be stopped.
- Prophylaxis should be considered in appropriate cases even when the bite happened in the distant past. One case report describes a patient who developed rabies 8 years after having been bitten.[17]
- If rabies is suspected in the animal, the wound must be immediately washed with soap and water or 1% povidone-iodine solution, which significantly lowers transmission rates.[4]
- Postexposure prophylaxis consists of passive immunization with 20 IU/kg of human rabies immune globulin (HRIG) or purified chick embryo cell vaccine (PCECV) per kilogram, with half the dose injected around the wound and half given intramuscularly (gluteal or deltoid).[18] In addition, active immunization with 1 mL of human diploid cell vaccine (HDCV) or PCECV given intramuscularly (deltoid) on days 0, 3, 7, and 14 is indicated. Individuals with a history of pre-exposure immunization with HDCV should receive an HDCV booster on days 0 and 3 but do not require HRIG.[18]

COMPLICATIONS

Infection is the most serious complication of bite wounds, resulting in cellulitis, lymphangitis, tenosynovitis, septic arthritis, and osteomyelitis. Rare complications include meningitis and death from sepsis. Patients with human bite and clenched-fist injuries are at particular risk for these complications. Other potential complications include hemorrhage, disfigurement, and decreased motor function or compartment syndrome. Hepatitis B or other systemic disease from human bites is an additional concern.

INDICATIONS FOR REFERRAL OR HOSPITALIZATION

Although most bite wounds can be handled on an outpatient basis, hospitalization is indicated in a few cases (1% to 2% of patients):

- Patients with systemic manifestations of infection (fever and chills)
- Severe cellulitis
- Suspicion of nonadherence to therapy
- Infected bites refractory to oral or outpatient therapy

Referrals would be necessary for the following:

- Involvement of a joint, nerve, bone, or tendon or compartment syndrome (orthopedic referral)
- Underlying illness, such as poorly controlled diabetes, peripheral vascular disease, or an immunocompromised state (internal medicine or infectious disease referral)
- Significant hand bites (hand surgery referral)
- Extensive wounds requiring reconstructive surgery (plastic surgery referral)
- Head injuries (otolaryngologic or neurosurgery referral)[2,4]

PATIENT EDUCATION AND HEALTH PROMOTION

All patients should be encouraged not to provoke domestic animals or to handle wild animals, especially raccoons, skunks, foxes, and bats. A rabies vaccine for pets (both dogs and cats) is mandatory in the United States but not in many foreign countries, including Mexico. Nervousness, aggressiveness, excessive drooling or foaming at the mouth, or fearlessness should raise the suspicion of rabid animals and prompt notification of the animal warden or health authorities.

Preventive measures include teaching children about safe play with pets. Parents can also be educated about supervisory practices while their children play with pets and selection factors in choosing pets. In addition, they can be taught the benefits of spaying or neutering their pets.[19] On a broader level, legislative efforts such as control of high-risk breeds can also help in prevention. A review done in Canadian municipalities showed decreased bite rates in areas with higher ticketing rates by animal control.[20]

Pre-exposure immunization with HDCV should be considered for high-risk groups, such as animal handlers, veterinarians, certain laboratory workers, and persons living in or visiting countries with a significant rabies risk. The regimen would be 1 mL intramuscularly on days 0, 7, and 21 or 28 and a booster every 2 years.[6] A good source of patient education is http://pier.acponline.org/physicians/public/d267/d267-pi.html.

Td or Tdap boosters should be given every 10 years routinely in all patients. Instructions to clean all bite wounds and to seek medical care immediately should be given, especially for fight bites to the hand.

CHAPTER 45

BULLOUS PEMPHIGOID

Kathryn K. Ellis • Kathryn R. Colcher

DEFINITION AND EPIDEMIOLOGY

Bullous pemphigoid (BP) is the most common of the autoimmune blistering diseases affecting primarily the elderly population.[1,2] It belongs to the group of pemphigoid diseases characterized by the presence of circulating immunoglobulin G (IgG) autoantibodies against structural proteins of the dermal-epidermal junction leading to tissue damage and blister formation.[3] Incidence increases in older adults, with the majority of patients diagnosed older than 70 years.[1,3-5] Males and females are equally affected, and there is no apparent racial predilection. Childhood-onset BP has been reported in the literature; however, is it generally self-limited.[6]

PATHOPHYSIOLOGY

The hallmark of BP is the presence of circulating and tissue-bound IgG autoantibodies specific for the hemidesmosomal BP antigens BP230 and BP180.[1,7] These autoantibodies along with complement components bind to the basement membrane at the dermal-epidermal junction of the perilesional skin. Complement activation attracts inflammatory cells (lymphocytes, histiocytes, eosinophils) to the skin basement membrane, initiating release of proteolytic enzymes that lead to degradation of the hemidesmosomal proteins, resulting in blister formation.[7]

CLINICAL PRESENTATION AND PHYSICAL EXAMINATION

Patients with BP often experience a nonbullous prodromal phase characterized by mild to severe pruritus accompanied by erythematous, eczematous papules and/or urticarial lesions. These nonspecific skin eruptions lasting several weeks to months may be the only early signs of the disease and often delay the diagnosis of BP.[3,4] Constitutional symptoms are absent except in severe widespread disease.

The bullous phase may appear suddenly with intense pruritus and widespread blister formation symmetrically distributed primarily on the abdomen and the flexor aspects of the extremities (axillae, medial aspects of groin, thighs, flexor aspects of forearms and lower legs). The tense oval or round blisters are filled with either clear or hemorrhagic exudate erupting on either normal or erythematous skin accompanied by urticarial plagues and papules. Blisters may persist for several days, either rupturing or collapsing, resulting in oozing erosions and crusts.[7] Oral lesions develop in 10% to 20% of patients; however, eyes, nose, esophagus, and anogenital areas are rarely affected.[1,3]

Triggers that have been reported to precipitate the onset of BP include traumatic, pharmacologic, or infectious agents. Trauma to the skin such as burns, radiotherapy, and ultraviolet radiation can trigger BP. Drugs associated with the onset of BP include furosemide, phenacetin, enalapril, ibuprofen, influenza vaccine, and several antibiotics (penicillamine, ampicillin, penicillin, and cephalexin).[1,3,7] Infections such as human herpesvirus (HHV), Epstein-Barr virus, cytomegalovirus, and hepatitis B and C may contribute to the induction of BP.[7]

Physical examination begins with general appearance and vital signs, observing for signs of discomfort or toxicity. Although skin lesions may involve any part of the body in BP, inspection of the skin should focus on the axillae, groin, and flexor aspects of the extremities and lower legs for papular or urticarial lesions, excoriations, hemorrhagic crusts, vesicles, and erosions. Mucous membranes must be inspected for blisters or erosions in the oropharynx, conjunctiva, and genitalia. Nikolsky sign (ability to split or dislodge the epidermis from the dermis by applying lateral pressure with a finger resulting in an erosion) is negative in patients with BP.[2,8]

DIAGNOSTICS

The diagnosis of BP relies on both evaluation of clinical features and immunopathologic findings. Direct immunofluorescence (DIF) microscopy of a skin biopsy specimen obtained from perilesional skin remains the gold standard for the diagnosis of BP, demonstrating the presence of IgG and/or C3 deposits along the dermal-epidermal border.[1]

Indirect immunofluorescence microscopy studies can be used to document the presence of IgG autoantibodies in the serum that target the skin basement membrane. Circulating autoantibodies that bind to the split skin can be found in 80% to 85% of patients with BP.

Emerging procedures are now available including enzyme-linked immunosorbent assay (ELISA), which analyzes the BP antigen–specific IgG autoantibodies in the patient's serum.[1]

Immunoblotting or Western blotting shows varying sensitivity in the diagnosis of BP. In 75% of patients a reaction occurs with BP230 antigen, and in 50% of patients a reaction occurs with BP 180 antigen.[1,5] Peripheral blood smear may show the presence of eosinophilia in some patients.

DIAGNOSTICS

Immunofluorescence, both direct and indirect	Immunoblotting
ELISAs	CBC and differential

CBC, complete blood count.

DIFFERENTIAL DIAGNOSIS

BP often imitates other conditions. In either the nonbullous prodromal stage or in an atypical presentation, it is often confused with a variety of inflammatory dermatoses including drug reactions, contact or allergic dermatitis, urticaria, arthropod reactions, scabies, or pityriasis lichenoides.[1] To distinguish BP from these other disorders, a detailed history, clinical evaluation, histopathologic features, and direct immunology immunofluorescence microscopy are essential.

DIFFERENTIAL DIAGNOSIS

Dermatologic Conditions

- Localized or generalized drug reaction
- Contact or allergic dermatitis
- Urticaria
- Arthropod reaction
- Pityriasis lichenoides
- Dermatitis herpetiformis
- Hereditary epidermolysis bullosa
- Pemphigoid gestationis
- Other bullous diseases (pemphigus vulgaris, pemphigus foliaceus, paraneoplastic pemphigus)

MANAGEMENT

The goal of treatment for BP is to reduce the formation of blisters, promote the healing of erosions, decrease itching, and prevent secondary infection. Topical steroids (class 1) are effective in treating limited or regional disease and are applied twice daily until lesions are healed.[3,5]

Systemic oral corticosteroids remain the treatment of choice and should be initiated and continued until the skin is clear. Prednisone doses in the range of 0.5 to 0.75 mg/kg/day have proven to be as effective as higher doses.[3,5] Immunosuppressive drugs such as azathioprine can be combined with systemic prednisone to induce remission.[2] Low dose oral pulse methotrexate is effective and safe therapy for the elderly.[2] Treatment with an anti-CD20 antibody (rituximab) should be considered in difficult-to-control cases.[9] Hydroxyzine may be prescribed to control itching; however, it should be used with caution in older adults because of risks of sedation.

LIFE SPAN CONSIDERATIONS

PB is a disease affecting primarily older adults and has been associated with significant morbidity. Living with chronic PB can lead to isolation, anxiety, and depression. Special consideration needs to address coping strategies for elders with BP. Involvement of family members and caregivers in the management plan will help to ensure adherence to the treatment regimen and prevention of complications.

COMPLICATIONS

Secondary infections can occur as a result of the presence of skin erosions and the use of immunosuppressive medications to treat the disease process. Infections may be localized or systemic, resulting in sepsis. Prolonged use of corticosteroids can lead to osteoporosis and bone fractures and potentially to adrenal insufficiency. Immunosuppressive medications may result in bone marrow suppression.

INDICATIONS FOR REFERRAL OR HOSPITALIZATION

The management of BP requires a team approach with a dermatologist, the patient's primary care provider, and in-home nursing services if indicated. A referral to a dermatologist should be made to confirm the diagnosis and manage the disease process. A consultation with a dentist and/or otolaryngologist is required for patients with oropharyngeal lesions. Debilitated older patients with BP vulnerable to secondary infections as well as the adverse effects of high-dose corticosteroids and immunosuppressive medications may require hospitalization owing to treatment complications.

PATIENT AND FAMILY EDUCATION

Education about skin care is essential for patients with BP to prevent further skin breakdown and secondary infection. Patients should avoid excessive rubbing, and trauma to already fragile skin resulting from the disease and use of topical and oral corticosteroids. Patients must have an understanding of the disease process and treatment in order to know when to alert their health care provider about adverse effects.

CHAPTER 46

BURNS (MINOR)

Randy M. Gordon

DEFINITION AND EPIDEMIOLOGY

The skin is the largest organ of the body and functions as an excellent barrier against external injury. A burn can disturb this barrier function as a result of trauma from electrical, thermal, or chemical agents. Thermal burns constitute a large majority of these injuries.[1]

According to the American Burn Association, an estimated 486,000 burns are treated annually.[1] This figure was compiled by combining data on visits to hospital emergency departments and outpatient clinics, freestanding urgent care centers, and private physician offices. Over 60% of the estimated U.S. acute hospitalizations related to burn injury involve patients who are admitted to 128 burn centers.[1] Such centers now average over 200 annual admissions for burn injury and skin disorders requiring similar treatment. This percentage has increased steadily in recent decades as emergency care and transportation have improved. The most common burns occur in the home secondary to fire or flame and scalding or hot object contact; industrial accidents occur more often than electrical and chemical injuries.[1] Statistically, males are more than twice as likely as females to sustain injury from burns, and Caucasians account for more injuries than patients of African-American, Hispanic, and other races combined.

Immediate emergency department referral or specialist referral is indicated for burns that cause respiratory injury (inhalation or facial burns); burns of the hands, feet, genitals, or perianal area; full-thickness burns of more than 2% of the total body surface area (TBSA); minor burns of more than 10% TBSA in patients older than 50 years; or burns of more than 15% TBSA in patients 10 to 50 years of age.

PATHOPHYSIOLOGY

The temperature or heat content of the burning agent and the duration of exposure determine the extent of burn injury. A burn wound is best described by the zones of injury. Typically, three zones exist, with the innermost zone (zone of coagulation) representing the most damaged area. Cellular death and thrombosis of the blood vessels occur in this zone. The area of tissue adjacent to this zone is the zone of stasis, where blood flow is compromised. This zone may quickly progress to ischemia or may return to normal, depending on several factors related to resuscitation. The outermost zone is the zone of hyperemia. This zone has received minimum damage, is characterized by increased blood flow, and will fully recover.[2]

A burn wound is defined by the size and depth of the wound. The size of the burn is quantified by the percentage of the TBSA burned. This percentage can be estimated in several ways. A quick method assumes that the back of the patient's hand is approximately 1% of the patient's TBSA. Therefore, the percentage of TBSA burned is the number of "hands" equal to the size of the burn.[3]

The depth of a burn is measured by the skin layers injured, and nonprofessionals still refer to depth of injury as first, second, or third degree. Clinicians more commonly define burns by partial-thickness or full-thickness depth of injury. First-degree (superficial or partial-thickness) burns involve only the epidermis, which with the injury becomes glossy, red, and painful, such as a sunburn. Second-degree (partial-thickness) burns involve the dermis, which may present as dull or glossy with pink, red, or white pigmentation. The area may blister and be severely painful. Third-degree burns are full-thickness burns that extend to the subcutaneous fat. The area appears matte and may be white, brown, red, or black. The hallmark of the third-degree burn is that the burn site is insensate.[4-5]

CLINICAL PRESENTATION

The health care provider must obtain a full history of the mechanism of injury. The type of thermal or chemical exposure, the duration of exposure, and the time since the injury are important details. This history will help determine any risk for associated traumatic, pulmonary, or ocular injury. In assessing a patient with even a minor burn, any preexisting health condition is noted; some, such as diabetes or an immunocompromised status, affect the prognosis and disposition.[6-7]

PHYSICAL EXAMINATION

The physical examination of the burn victim should be methodic and thorough. Initial general patient assessment should include evaluation for adequacy of airway, breathing, and circulation. The clinician should be alert for circumferential burns on a limb because the injury may compromise perfusion to the involved appendage. The depth, extent (percentage of TBSA burned), and location of the burn must be accurately determined and recorded. The examination should also include evaluation for any associated injuries.[7]

DIAGNOSTICS

The skin is a significant protective physiologic barrier; infection and metabolic abnormalities can result when this barrier is disrupted. Simple thermal burns do not require diagnostic testing. For more serious injuries, a complete blood count (CBC), glucose, electrolytes, blood urea nitrogen (BUN), creatinine, and urinalysis may be necessary. Amino acid catabolism and fluid or protein loss through burn wound exudate may create increased metabolic needs and thus require laboratory evaluation for adequacy of hydration and protein stores.[8]

A chest x-ray study is indicated for a suspected inhalation injury. Wound sites with delayed healing may require cultures to determine if infection is a factor. If wounds are not healing, wound biopsy may also be indicated to facilitate detection of any underlying comorbidities or malignant neoplasms.

In the case of a chemical burn, the local poison control center can assist in determining toxicity of and antidote for the chemical. If possible, the patient should provide the chemical container or a complete description of the substance to aid in identification.[9]

DIAGNOSTICS

Burns

LABORATORY (FOR SERIOUS BURNS)	Urinalysis
CBC and differential	Tissue cultures
Serum electrolyte	Imaging
Serum glucose	Chest x-ray studies*
BUN	Electrocardiogram, urine myoglobin, creatine kinase isoenzymes if electrical burn*
Creatinine	

*If indicated.

DIFFERENTIAL DIAGNOSIS

The differential diagnosis is determined primarily by history. Certain skin conditions (e.g., staphylococcal scalded skin syndrome, toxic epidermal necrolysis) can resemble a generalized burn.

DIFFERENTIAL DIAGNOSIS

Burns

- Chemical burns
- Electrical burns
- Thermal burns
- Ritter disease
- Scalded skin
- Toxin epidermal necrolysis
- Stevens-Johnson syndrome
- Epidermolysis bullosa

MANAGEMENT

The severity, extent, and location of the burn guide the clinician's decisions for patient management. The American Burn Association classifies burn risk levels as major/high, moderate, and minor/low. Low-risk patients are those aged 10 to 50 years. High-risk patients are those younger than 10 years and older than 50 years or those with underlying medical conditions, such as heart disease, diabetes, or pulmonary problems. Minor burns involve less than 15% of TBSA in the 10- to 50-year age group or less than 10% of TBSA in patients younger than 10 years or older than 50 years. Minor full-thickness burns are less than 2% of TBSA in all age groups.[1]

Minor burns having no associated injuries can be managed in the clinician's office or outpatient setting. The goal of initial treatment for a partial-thickness thermal burn is to reduce heat and tissue injury by irrigation with cool tap water. Similarly, initial therapy for a chemical burn is to remove the offending chemical and garments, and then begin aggressive irrigation. In rare cases involving certain industrial chemicals (e.g., metal sodium), water should not be used because it can actually worsen the burn; it is important to identify the source of the chemical burn when treatment is initiated. Information as to appropriate management of a topical chemical exposure may be found in the industrial facility's Material Safety Data Sheet (MSDS) manual.

Intact blisters in burn injuries should not be ruptured because they maintain a physiologic protection function while underlying tissues begin the healing process.[4] The burn wound needs to be cleaned with mild soap and water or saline; unroofed blisters and devitalized tissue should be debrided.

Finally, a dressing must be applied. There are several ways to dress minor burns. First, the burn is covered with a thin layer of antimicrobial cream or ointment; the most common topical therapy used is silver sulfadiazine cream (Silvadene). Silvadene cannot be used on patients with sulfa allergy and should be used cautiously on patients with significant pain. This product may cause tattooing or staining and may not be appropriate for use on facial burns. When Silvadene is used, the wound should be washed and redressed twice daily. A nonadherent secondary dressing is used to protect the burn from contamination until the site is healed. Advances in wound technology now provide silver in various delivery forms, including gels, hydrocolloids, and nonadherent dressing sheets; the slow release of silver in these formulations lengthens the time between dressing changes from 2 to 7 days, thus promoting patient comfort and decreasing trauma to the healing wound.

Some burns may require open dressings, in which a topical agent is applied without a covering. The most common sites for open dressings are the face, neck, and perineum. The wound should be thoroughly washed two or three times a day and the topical agent reapplied. Aloe vera in a gel, cream, or ointment formulation may promote healing and soothe painful areas.[10]

Minor burns are painful, and treatment should include analgesics as needed. Ibuprofen, with its antiprostaglandin properties, is an effective anti-inflammatory and analgesic medication. Naproxen and narcotic agents, such as codeine, are also appropriate analgesics. Tetanus prophylaxis should be given as indicated.

COMPLICATIONS

Most partial-thickness burns heal within several days to a week without complications. Some swelling may occur in extremities affected by burns, which can be diminished by elevation of the limb above heart level. Some minor burns may become infected. Infections may require systemic antibiotic therapy or a change in topical therapy to manage bioburden or bacteria in the wound. Burns occurring over a joint may require a splint to promote comfort and wound healing.

INDICATIONS FOR REFERRAL OR HOSPITALIZATION

Any burn injury larger than the American Burn Association's criteria for minor burns (see Management) should be referred to the nearest emergency department for further evaluation and hospitalization as necessary. Burns that may result in functional or cosmetic impairment, have an associated injury, or involve high-risk patients require a referral for emergency evaluation. Burns that fail to heal within 2 to 3 weeks require further evaluation with a wound specialist. Consultation with a physiatrist or physical or occupational therapist should be considered when appropriate to initiate gentle range-of-motion exercises and to prevent localized contractures.

PATIENT AND FAMILY EDUCATION

All burn patients should be seen as soon as possible after injury for a clinical assessment of the depth and extent of the burn along with evaluation for additional injuries. Patients should be given clear discharge instructions that explain topical wound care. They also should be alerted to any signs and symptoms of infection or vascular compromise. If an extremity is involved, it should be elevated for control of pain and swelling. Pain medications may be required; if one is prescribed, an explanation of how to use the analgesic and of the potential side effects is also necessary.

HEALTH PROMOTION

Home and work safety is the cornerstone of burn prevention. Manufacturer recommendations for protective equipment such as gloves, protective eyewear, and ventilation with certain household cleaning products and at the work site can prevent chemical and inhalation burns. To prevent electrical burns, the electrical current must be turned off before any electrical repairs are attempted, electrical outlets should have covers, and frayed electrical cords should be repaired or the fixture discarded. A listing of chemicals used in the workplace, including product ingredients and treatment indicated for accidental exposures, should be accessible to all employees.

In the home, a working smoke alarm and fire extinguisher are key to early fire detection and intervention. Lowering of hot water temperatures will reduce the risk of scald injuries, the most common source of burn injury in children. Pot and pan handles should be turned over the cooktop, away from the reach of children. Loose clothing should be restricted when cooking or when around open flames. Everyone should be familiar with the "stop, drop, and roll" technique to control or to extinguish fire if their clothes ignite, and children should be taught about the hazards of matches and fireworks. Similarly, education should be provided about the importance of wearing sunscreen and the damaging effects of the sun's rays.

CHAPTER 47

CELLULITIS

Elizabeth Talbot • Laura Elyse Shevy

DEFINITION AND EPIDEMIOLOGY

Skin and soft tissue infections (SSTIs) are among the most common reasons for which patients seek outpatient care and require antibiotics. Such visits have increased over the last several years to now exceed 6.3 million annually.[1] Health care providers who know the clinical presentation of SSTIs, their causative pathogens, and local antibiotic susceptibility patterns will maximize treatment efficacy and avoid inducing resistance to the limited armamentarium of antimicrobial therapies available.

The management of SSTIs is best conceptualized on the basis of the presence or absence of pus. Purulent SSTIs include abscesses, furuncles, and carbuncles; nonpurulent SSTIs include erysipelas and necrotizing fasciitis.[1] Cellulitis may cross these categories because it may be secondary to skin ulcers or other lesions that themselves produce pus, and so cellulitis is further subdivided into purulent and non-purulent types. This chapter reviews all the SSTIs, although emphasis is placed on the diagnosis and management of cellulitis.

PATHOPHYSIOLOGY

Purulent Skin and Soft Tissue Infections

Purulent SSTIs include abscesses, furuncles, and carbuncles. *Abscesses* are collections of pus that may be within the dermis or deeper layers. Typically they are painful or tender to palpation and appear as raised lesions that may be fluctuant, red, and/or nodular. There is often a central pustule with erythematous margins, which represents inflammation rather than spreading infection (i.e., cellulitis). *Epidermoid cysts* are collections of keratinous material and usually contain skin flora; these may also become inflamed and rupture into the dermal layer. *Furuncles*, commonly known as boils, are infections that arise at the hair follicle and extend deep into the dermis, where an abscess forms. This is distinguished from folliculitis, which extends only as deep as the epidermis. A *carbuncle* forms when several adjacent furuncles coalesce, forming an inflammatory mass with pus draining from multiple follicles. These are seen more frequently in persons with diabetes.

Most often, skin abscesses are polymicrobial infections, consisting of bacteria from local skin flora and the adjacent mucous membranes. Approximately 25% of the time, *Staphylococcus aureus* may occur as a mono-pathogen. Furuncles and carbuncles are most commonly caused by *S. aureus*. Community-acquired (CA) methicillin-resistant *S. aureus* (MRSA) rates are dependent on local resistance patterns.

In the setting of severe immunocompromise, such as patients with neutropenic fever or human immunodeficiency virus (HIV) or acquired immunodeficiency syndrome (AIDS) with depressed CD4 count, or among patients with tropical travel, animal bites, and other exposures, the differential diagnosis of these SSTIs is extensively expanded, and consideration should be given to involving infectious disease specialists.[2]

Nonpurulent Skin and Soft Tissue Infections

Nonpurulent SSTIs include impetigo, ecthyma, erysipelas, and cellulitis; cellulitis is discussed later. *Impetigo* is a toxin-mediated skin infection caused by *S. aureus* or *Streptococcus* causing dermal-epidermal junction cleavage. *Ecthyma* is a deeper infection, also typically caused by *S. aureus* and *Streptococcus* species. Initially, vesicular lesions rupture and form round erythematous crusting ulcers that often are surrounded by erythema and edema. Owing to the depth of these lesions, a scar forms.

Erysipelas is an SSTI limited to the superficial dermis including lymphatics, whereas *cellulitis* involves the deeper dermis and subcutaneous fat. These terms are often used interchangeably, especially in Europe, but erysipelas is most correctly distinguished from cellulitis by the former's restriction to the superficial dermis and lymphatics.[1] In contrast, cellulitis rapidly spreads and extends deeply from the dermis to the subcutaneous tissue. When it is left untreated, cellulitis may progress to more severe soft tissue infection and osteomyelitis and may even become limb- or life-threatening.[2]

Cellulitis typically begins when pathogens find a portal of entry through nonintact skin, as is seen after traumatic laceration; at sites of diabetic, vascular, or other types of skin ulceration; in chronic dermatoses with skin breakdown such as macerated tinea pedis; surgical wound infections; or even at sites of insect bites. Cellulitis may, however, develop with no recognized trauma in otherwise normal-appearing skin. Predisposing risk factors for cellulitis include venous or lymphatic compromise from previous episodes of cellulitis, peripheral edema, previous radiation to an affected area, history of lymph node resection, lymphedema such as occurs after radical mastectomy and lymph node dissection in the upper extremity, and obesity.

Most cases of cellulitis and erysipelas in adults are caused by group A β-hemolytic streptococci. Non–group A streptococci are more likely pathogens in patients with underlying abnormalities of the lymphatic system, such as lymphedema. *S. aureus* is less likely to be causal but should be considered in the setting of penetrating trauma, sites of injection drug use, surgical site infections, indwelling catheter skin infections, or other preexisting open wounds.[1] Other pathogens may also be implicated in cellulitis, when cellulitis occurs as a complication of animal bites, with injuries occurred in fresh water or saltwater, or in immunocompromised hosts.

CLINICAL PRESENTATION AND PHYSICAL EXAMINATION

Purulent Skin and Soft Tissue Infections

The Infectious Diseases Society of America classifies the severity of SSTIs into mild, moderate, and severe.[1] A mild SSTI is defined as occurring in an immunocompetent patient with hemodynamic stability who appears nontoxic: patients with these infections can typically be treated on an outpatient basis with appropriate incision and drainage, and often without need for antibiotics. Moderate SSTIs are those occurring in an immunocompetent patient with systemic symptoms and signs. Severe SSTIs are defined as those (1) refractory to oral antibiotics and, if purulent, refractory to incision and drainage; (2) in patients demonstrating hemodynamic alteration including temperature higher than 38 °C, heart rate greater than 90, respiratory rate greater than 24, leukocytosis greater than 12,000 or leukopenia below 400 cells/μL; and (3) in immunocompromised patients. In general, moderate and severe SSTIs require admission for management.

Nonpurulent Skin and Soft Tissue Infections

The common initial presentation of impetigo is vesiculopustular or even bullous lesions. When the lesions rupture and exude their contents, they create the classic honey-colored crusts.

Clinically, erysipelas tends to have more clearly demarcated borders of inflammation than cellulitis. Either may have lymphangitic streaking present. The most commonly affected areas in erysipelas include the lower legs, face, and ears (the ears have no dermis; therefore, superficial infection of the ears is erysipelas by default). Facial erysipelas may follow a streptococcal infection of the upper respiratory tract.[3]

The lower extremity is the most common site of cellulitis, although it can occur anywhere. The initial clinical presentation of cellulitis is characterized by spreading erythema, induration, warmth, and pain and may be associated with systemic symptoms such as fevers, chills, and malaise.[1,2] Bullae, abscesses, erosions, necrosis, and even focal areas of hemorrhage manifesting as ecchymosis or petechiae may develop within cellulitis. The site of entry of the bacteria may be evident as breaks in the skin or ulcerations. Careful inspection of the interdigital areas is crucial in the physical examination for lower extremity cellulitis, because macerated tinea pedis may have provided the portal of entry for bacteria. Left untreated, this predisposes to recurrent cellulitis. Regional lymph nodes may be enlarged and tender, a condition called *lymphadenitis*. Lymphangitic streaking may occur in the direction of a regional lymph node. Edema of the area can manifest as dimpling of the overlying skin, called *peau d'orange* (orange peel).

DIAGNOSTICS

Purulent Skin and Soft Tissue Infections

For mild and apparently uncomplicated infections, only Gram stain and culture of the drained purulent material need be performed. In typical cases of SSTIs, empirical treatment may also be tried without such data. Epidermoid cysts need not be cultured.

Microbiologic diagnosis should be undertaken in moderate or severe infections, for those refractory to current antibiotic treatment,[1] and in cases involving multiple sites of infection, cutaneous gangrene, or extensive surrounding cellulitis. Appropriate additional laboratory investigations include complete blood count (CBC) with differential, creatinine, bicarbonate, creatine phosphokinase, and blood cultures.[1] If a definitive microbiologic diagnosis is not readily evident from the Gram stain and cultures of purulent material or via blood cultures, other potential methods for identifying the pathogen(s) include needle aspirate, punch biopsy, and material sent from intraoperative procedures, should surgical consultation be necessary.

Nonpurulent Skin and Soft Tissue Infections

Diagnosis is largely by clinical recognition. The causal pathogen may be determined by culturing any existing vesicular fluid, pus, ulcer, or erosions; this is indicated to evaluate bacteriology and susceptibility patterns. If no obvious cultivable source is present, however, empirical treatment is pursued. Punch biopsy for pathology may be necessary if noninfectious causes are in the differential diagnosis.

Laboratory investigations are not warranted in otherwise healthy children and adults with cellulitis. Blood cultures have been found to be of low yield, identifying the causal organism 5% or less of the time.[4,5] The yield of skin biopsy for culture is also low in nonpurulent SSTIs (around 20%), so isolation of the causative agent is usually not attempted in otherwise healthy adults, and treatment is empirical (see later).

However, blood cultures and cultures of any pus or bullae are more useful and should be performed in patients with moderate to severe nonpurulent SSTI, extensive body surface involvement, underlying comorbidities including immunodeficiencies, previous splenectomy, diabetes, lymphedema, malignancy, neutropenia, specific exposures such as animal bites or water-associated injuries, and recurrent or refractory cellulitis.

In patients with longer-standing disease or in whom more deep-seated infection is suspected, radiography may be helpful to evaluate for underlying osteomyelitis and even occult abscess. Although radiographs may delineate subcutaneous emphysema in gas-producing infections, they do not have sufficient sensitivity to reliably detect necrotizing fasciitis or gas gangrene and should not delay emergent surgical management of such clinically apparent infections.

DIFFERENTIAL DIAGNOSIS

Purulent Skin and Soft Tissue Infections

Because SSTIs have a variety of causes and corresponding management, a detailed history of exposures and comorbidities is key for developing a pathogenic differential diagnosis. Such history includes areas of residence, detailed travel history, immune status, recent surgeries, trauma, antimicrobial therapy, hobbies, lifestyle, and animal and animal bite exposures. Mimics of purulent SSTIs (i.e., abscesses, furuncles, and carbuncles) include bursitis (infectious or inflammatory), inflamed epidermoid cyst, tophaceous gout, and other inflammatory processes.

Nonpurulent Skin and Soft Tissue Infections

The differential diagnosis of erysipelas and cellulitis includes other infections such as bursitis, osteomyelitis, erythema migrans, and herpes zoster, as well as inflammatory conditions including eczema, psoriasis, contact dermatitis, urticaria, and erythema nodosum. Other potential noninfectious mimics include stasis dermatitis, deep venous thrombosis, thrombophlebitis, acute gout, drug reactions, insect bite or sting hypersensitivity, and neoplastic changes.[1] More severe, life-threatening infections, such as necrotizing fasciitis, gas gangrene, staphylococcal scalded skin syndrome, and toxic epidermal necrolysis, must also be differentiated from cellulitis. Cellulitis may also be superimposed on concurrent skin disease, such as stasis dermatitis, hemosiderin staining, and lipodermatosclerosis associated with venous insufficiency.

The purulent skin infections as well as purulent bursitis may manifest with surrounding inflammatory changes clinically reminiscent of cellulitis. However, these infections are primarily purulent SSTIs, and the local erythema is more likely a result of inflammation than active infection.

DIFFERENTIAL DIAGNOSIS

Cellulitis

INFECTIOUS
- Bursitis
- Osteomyelitis
- Erythema migrans
- Herpes zoster

CONNECTIVE TISSUE, RHEUMATOLOGIC, IMMUNOLOGIC
- Psoriasis
- Erythema nodosum
- Acute gout
- Urticaria

DERMATOLOGIC
- Eczema
- Contact dermatitis
- Drug reactions

VASCULAR
- Stasis dermatitis
- Deep venous thrombosis
- Thrombophlebitis

OTHER
- Insect bite or sting hypersensitivity
- Neoplastic

TREATMENT

Purulent Skin and Soft Tissue Infections

In purulent SSTIs, incision and drainage is key to treatment. Small furuncles often spontaneously drain with application of moist heat. Larger furuncles, carbuncles, and skin abscesses, however, require incision and drainage with focus on adequate debridement of any septations or loculations.

For moderate or severe purulent SSTIs, systemic antibiotics that primarily target *S. aureus* are required. The decision to empirically cover MRSA (rather than methicillin-sensitive *S. aureus* [MSSA]) while awaiting culture and sensitivity results can be challenging. If the patient has failed initial non-MRSA antibiotic treatment, is critically ill, has had previous MRSA infections, or is known to be MRSA colonized, empirical antibiotics should target MRSA pending culture and susceptibility results. If the patient can take oral therapy, possible antibiotics for MRSA include trimethoprim-sulfamethoxazole (TMP-SMX) or doxycycline (or others depending on local antibiogram). If the purulent SSTIs is eventually determined to be caused by MSSA, an oral cephalosporin such as cephalexin or an antistaphylococcal penicillin such as dicloxacillin is appropriate, according to the full laboratory-reported susceptibilities.

For severe purulent SSTIs, empirical intravenous antimicrobial options for MRSA include vancomycin, daptomycin, linezolid, telavancin, and ceftaroline. Vancomycin is the preferred agent for severe infections in children. If the pathogen is confirmed as MSSA, therapy can be more directed, using nafcillin, cefazolin, or clindamycin (depending on susceptibility pattern).

Outbreaks of furunculosis occur in families and those with close contact (e.g., sports teams) and have most often been caused by MSSA or MRSA. Control of such infections may require that all contacts use antibacterial soaps such as chlorhexidine and that laundering of all soiled clothing, bedsheets, towels, and so on, is ensured. Older studies demonstrated benefit with clindamycin, 150 mg orally [PO] daily for 3 months, or twice daily mupirocin, 5 days per month, although efficacy of these empirical regimens for MRSA is unclear.[1]

Nonpurulent Skin and Soft Tissue Infections

For nonpurulent SSTIs, clinicians should choose empirical antimicrobials that are active against both *S. aureus* and *Streptococcus* species. An oral penicillinase-resistant penicillin or first-generation cephalosporin is sufficient therapy, because the *S. aureus* causing impetigo or ecthyma typically is methicillin sensitive. For penicillin-allergic patients or those with MRSA, TMP-SMX, doxycycline, and clindamycin may be alternatives depending on local susceptibility patterns. If *Streptococcus* is isolated as a monopathogen, penicillin is the drug of choice, with macrolides or clindamycin employed as alternatives for penicillin-allergic patients.

The management of cellulitis involves both nonpharmacologic and pharmacologic therapies.

Nonpharmacologic management of cellulitis involves postural drainage (i.e., elevation of the infected limb if possible) and compression when not contraindicated (e.g., in the setting of vascular compromise). These will allow drainage of the inflammatory milieu and help to decrease peripheral edema. Management should also address the underlying and precipitating disease(s). This may include management of systemic causes of underlying peripheral edema, venous insufficiency, peripheral vascular disease, lymphedema, tinea pedis, obesity, chronic dermatoses, and so on. In patients with cellulitis arising from ulcerative lesions, sharp debridement of necrotic or devitalized tissue should be performed to remove this nidus for infection and to reinitiate the wound-healing cascade. There is some weak evidence that NSAIDs or steroids hasten clinical improvement if not otherwise contraindicated.[1] Steroids should be avoided if severe or deeper infection is possible (e.g., necrotizing fasciitis).

With respect to antimicrobial therapy for otherwise healthy adults with mild cellulitis, antibiotics effective against streptococci and staphylococci should be used. Penicillin, amoxicillin, amoxicillin-clavulanate, a penicillinase-resistant penicillin such as dicloxacillin, a cephalosporin such as cephalexin, or clindamycin for 5 days is usually sufficient, but treatment may be extended if symptoms have not resolved within that time.[6] Care must be taken to ensure adequate doses (especially in the obese), and the dose should be appropriately adjusted for elderly patients and those with renal or hepatic impairment.

It is important to note that cutaneous inflammation and systemic signs and symptoms often paradoxically worsen briefly after initiation of appropriate antimicrobial therapy. This may be a result of bacterial cell death, lysis, and release of proinflammatory compounds contributing to local inflammation.

NEW ANTIBIOTICS

Several new antibiotics are worth mentioning because of their activity against MRSA and, in the case of the lipoglycopeptides, for their remarkably convenient administration.

Ceftaroline (Teflaro)

Ceftaroline is a cephalosporin with activity against gram-positive bacteria including MRSA, as well as some aerobic gram-negative bacteria, and was approved by the U.S. Food and Drug Administration (FDA) for treatment of acute bacterial skin and skin structure infections (ABSSSIs) in May 2010. It is typically administered intravenously (IV) at 600 mg q8h and requires adjustment for renal dysfunction or severe infection.[7-9]

Dalbavancin (Dalvance)

Dalbavancin is a lipoglycopeptide with activity against gram-positive organisms, including MSSA and MRSA, and *Streptococcus pyogenes,* the major pathogens in cellulitis.[10] Dalbavancin was approved by the FDA in May 2014 for treatment of acute bacterial skin and skin structure infections.[11] It has a long half-life, which allows once-weekly administration at 1 g IV over 30 minutes on day 1 and 500 mg IV over 30 minutes on day 8.[10]

Tedizolid (Sivextro)

Tedizolid is an oxazolidinone with activity against both methicillin-sensitive and methicillin-resistant strains of *S. aureus,* as well as various *Streptococcus* species and *Enterococcus faecalis*. Tedizolid was approved by the FDA in June 2014 to treat patients with ABSSSIs. It is available in both oral and intravenous forms.[12,13]

Oritavancin (Orbactiv)

Oritavancin, another lipoglycopeptide, was approved by the FDA in August 2014 to treat patients with ABSSSIs caused by *S. aureus* (including methicillin-susceptible and methicillin-resistant strains), various *Streptococcus* species, and *E. faecalis*. Like its predecessor, dalbavancin, it is administered IV, although the dose is 1200 mg IV once.[14,15]

INDICATIONS FOR REFERRAL OR HOSPITALIZATION

The following patients warrant consideration for inpatient admission for management including intravenous antibiotics and possible consultations with infectious disease and/or dermatology specialists:

- Severely immunocompromised patients
- Patients with poor clinical response to outpatient management
- Patients with severe infections including hemodynamic compromise
- Patients in whom there is concern for necrotizing fasciitis
- Patients with diabetes mellitus
- Patients with ischemic vascular disease or other pathology of circulation affecting the ability of a wound or infection to heal
- Patients with periorbital cellulitis
- Patients with hand infections
- Patients with infections of animal or human bite wounds

SPECIAL CIRCUMSTANCES

Skin and Soft Tissue Infections in Diabetic Patients

Patients with diabetes mellitus need to be monitored closely, particularly when cellulitis involves the feet or hands. As a result of decreased circulation in the extremities from microvascular compromise, persons with diabetes are at a greater risk for development of ulcerations and osteomyelitis. Radiographs of the affected extremity are indicated to evaluate for bony involvement or the presence of air in soft tissues. Uncomplicated cases of nonulcerative cellulitis in patients with diabetes can be treated with amoxicillin-clavulanate or quinolones. These antibiotics are chosen because they cover gram-negative organisms and anaerobes that may infect patients with diabetes. For mild cases of infected diabetic ulcers, ciprofloxacin plus either clindamycin or metronidazole may be used.[1,3,16] More severe ulcerative infections or cases of osteomyelitis require intravenous antibiotics and consultation with a surgeon for debridement. Hyperbaric oxygen therapy has also been found to be effective in the treatment of chronic refractory osteomyelitis and chronic nonhealing wounds related to tissue hypoxia, such as diabetic lower extremity ulcers.[17]

Periorbital Cellulitis

Periorbital cellulitis must be distinguished from the far less common and more serious orbital cellulitis.

Orbital cellulitis clinically manifests with exophthalmos, orbital pain, restricted eye movement, and occasionally visual disturbance. Orbital cellulitis often stems from ethmoid or maxillary sinusitis, and left untreated may lead to blindness, diplopia, brain abscess, and meningitis. Orbital cellulitis is a medical emergency and must be treated as such, including prompt evaluation with a computed tomography scan and intravenous antibiotics. Referral to an otolaryngologist is recommended for closer evaluation.

Periorbital cellulitis typically follows sinusitis, upper respiratory tract infection, or eye trauma and is more common in children. Symptoms typically include erythema and edema of the eyelid, conjunctivitis, and chemosis (conjunctival edema). This condition is treated with warm soaks and aggressive antibiotic therapy, such as intravenous nafcillin or oxacillin.[1,16]

Skin and Soft Tissue Infections of the Hands

Soft tissue infections of the hands must be carefully evaluated to determine whether tendon sheaths or joint or muscle spaces are involved. Necrotizing soft tissue infections are a surgical emergency. The condition starts with redness and painful swelling of the deep tissues. A black eschar rapidly develops with necrosis of the underlying tissues. If necrotizing fasciitis, cellulitis, or myonecrosis is suspected, immediate referral is indicated for prompt surgical debridement, intravenous antibiotics, and hyperbaric oxygen treatment if it is locally available.[1,16,17]

Animal and Human Bites and Closed Fist Injuries

The causative pathogens of bite infections depend on the mouth and host skin flora, and such infections are often polymicrobial. *Pasteurella* species are classically involved in dog and cat bites, but the more familiar streptococci and staphylococci are most often identified. *Capnocytophaga, Moraxella, Corynebacterium, Neisseria,* and anaerobic bacteria are also implicated with some frequency in dog and cat bites.[18] *Eikenella corrodens* is a pathogen commonly associated with human bites or closed fist injuries (CFIs). CFIs, also sometimes called clenched fist injuries, occur when a person's closed fist strikes the teeth of another person, usually in the course of a fight. CFIs are at high risk for infection because of wound contamination with human saliva.

Bite injuries can also be classified as high risk or low risk depending on wound and host factors. High-risk injuries include puncture wounds, multiple injuries, injuries in immunocompromised patients (e.g., drug-mediated immunocompromise, liver disease, asplenic patients), injuries that violated the periosteum or joint capsule, and bites that involve the face, hand, or foot.

In patients with low-risk injuries who are seen within 12 to 24 hours of the trauma, without the aforementioned characteristics and for whom close follow-up can be ensured, preemptive antibiotic therapy has been demonstrated to provide only marginal benefit, and may be avoided.[1]

In patients with high-risk injuries, however, evaluation including blood cultures, cultures of any available pus or exudate, consultation with an appropriate surgical specialist, and consideration of admission for intravenous antibiotics are all recommended depending on wound location and severity and patient factors. Early preemptive antibiotic therapy for a minimum of 3 to 5 days is recommended, with antibiotic regimens that cover both aerobic and anaerobic bacteria, including *Staphylococcus and Streptococcus.* For animal and human bites and CFIs, amoxicillin-clavulanate is the preferred oral therapy unless there is cause to suspect MRSA. There are multiple alternative regimens, but because of resistance patterns, routine use of macrolides and clindamycin should be avoided.[1]

Depending on the animal, postexposure prophylaxis for rabies may also be indicated; consultation with an infectious disease specialist or local health official is recommended. Tetanus toxoid should be given to those patients without toxoid vaccination in the past 10 years, or for dirty wounds if more than 5 years have passed since the last booster.

EDUCATION AND HEALTH PROMOTION

Patients and families should be educated about the importance of preventing skin infections. With thorough routine hygiene and standard first aid of any skin wounds including careful cleaning and appropriate dressings, many skin infections can be prevented. Patients with diabetes should be educated about the importance of consistently wearing well-fitted protective shoes and encouraged to make a daily visual inspection of their feet to evaluate for wounds or breaks in skin integrity. Furthermore, they should be encouraged to regularly visit a podiatrist for nail care and callus removal, avoiding self-treatment of these conditions with over-the-counter products.[11] Underlying dermatoses such as tinea pedis, stasis dermatitis, and lymphedema should be treated promptly and aggressively, particularly in patients with diabetes, so the skin does not become a portal of entry for secondary infections.

CHAPTER 48

CONTACT DERMATITIS

Glen Blair

DEFINITION AND EPIDEMIOLOGY

Contact dermatitis is a type of rash that falls under the umbrella diagnosis of eczematous dermatitis, one of several types of dermatitis that share a similar "ill-defined scaling"[1] and histology. Others in the category include atopic dermatitis, nummular and dyshidrotic eczema, and id reactions. On histologic examination, they are characterized by spongiosis (intercellular edema). Contact dermatitis is further classified as irritant or allergic type.

Irritant contact dermatitis (ICD) is caused by the direct cytotoxic action of an agent on the cells of the epidermis and dermis. Cellular destruction and injury of the epidermal barrier result in inflammation and the nonimmunologic release of vasoactive peptides and proinflammatory cytokines. ICD is responsible for 80% of occupational contact dermatitis, most commonly on the hands. Irritants are mostly chemical in nature and include soaps, detergents, acids, and alkalis. Dermatitis may not develop until a threshold of exposure has been reached. Itching may be present, but the predominant symptoms are of pain and burning.

Allergic contact dermatitis (ACD) is a type 4 delayed hypersensitivity reaction, requiring prior sensitization for symptoms to be induced. After contact, the allergen combines with epidermal proteins that are taken up by Langerhans cells. T cells and macrophages then relay this information to precursor T cells in the lymph nodes, where sensitized T cells are produced.[2] Sensitization takes 10 to 15 days. Once an individual is sensitized, the dermatitis begins to erupt in 8 to 48 hours and, untreated, can persist for days or weeks.[3] The most common allergens according to the North American Contact Dermatitis Group[4] analysis of pooled data from January 1, 2009 to December 31, 2010 include substances such as nickel, neomycin, and bacitracin. In this report, the incidences of skin reactions to substances such as nickel and neomycin decreased, but reactions to allergens such as fragrances, propylene glycol, and benzocaine were reported more frequently. Workers in specific occupations associated with higher-than-average rates of ACD included hairdressers, printers, cement workers, painters, mechanics, food processors, and florists, among others.[5]

CLINICAL PRESENTATION AND PHYSICAL EXAMINATION

The distribution of the dermatitis is an important clue to the diagnosis. Both ICD and ACD cause a rash on the surface of the skin that was exposed. In ICD, symptoms may develop minutes to hours after exposure, or they may develop months after chronic exposure. A well-demarcated area of erythema, scaling, or crusting will occur at the site of the exposure. The hands are the most common area affected, followed by wrists and forearms.[3] Contact dermatitis of the hand is more likely to be of the irritant than allergic type.[6]

Cumulative ICD is more common than the acute form and is characterized by hyperkeratosis (thickening), lichenification (accentuation of skin lines as a result of scratching), scaling, and fissuring. Weak irritants produce cumulative ICD, which may develop after months of continual exposure.[5] Most reactions to cosmetics are of the irritant type. The dermatitis may occur on the face, eyelids, lips, and neck, often having been exposed by hand-to-face contact. Patients report burning and stinging sensations associated with the application of cosmetics.[7]

ACD is identified by its distribution, the acute nature of the symptoms, the complaint of itch, and the development of inflammation and vesicles. Rhus dermatitis (poison ivy or oak) is caused by a plant resin called urushiol. Exposure results in vesicles and bullae that develop for up to 2 weeks after contact and can last for up to 8 weeks if treatment is insufficient.[8] To the patient, the dermatitis may seem to be spreading because it may not show up all at once. Once the resin is washed off, however, no further spread should occur, although full presentation may take several days.

Sensitivity to nickel can manifest as dermatitis around the neck from jewelry, around the umbilicus from metal waist fasteners, or under the breasts from bras with underwires. ACD of the hand can occur on the dorsum from allergy to rubber or gloves and on the palm from solid objects such as the leather grip of a tennis racket. Dermatitis that affects the hands and feet together may indicate an endogenous cause, such as a dietary metal sensitivity, but it could also represent other disorders, such as psoriasis or dermatomyositis.[9] Pedal involvement without hand involvement suggests an ACD reaction to footwear, often resulting from allergy to the resins used in the leather tanning process. Table 48-1 lists possible irritants or allergens by anatomic location.

DIAGNOSTICS AND DIFFERENTIAL DIAGNOSIS

Diagnosis relies on a careful history—including occupation, hobbies, topical pharmaceutical or cosmetic products, type of clothing and footwear, and contact with plants or foliage[10]—and an analysis of lesion morphology and rash distribution. ICD may resemble atopic dermatitis or nummular dermatitis. Bullous diseases such as impetigo, herpetic infection such as herpes zoster (shingles), and dermatophyte infections may be

DIFFERENTIAL DIAGNOSIS

Contact Dermatitis

- Atopic dermatitis
- Dyshidrotic eczema
- Bacterial infections
- Candidal infections
- Phytophotodermatitis
- Herpes zoster

DIAGNOSTICS

Contact Dermatitis

LABORATORY

KOH preparation (to exclude tinea)*
Culture*
Patch testing to identify contact allergen*

*If indicated.

TABLE 48-1 Contact Dermatitis: Distribution Diagnosis

Location	Material
Scalp and ears	Shampoo, hair dyes, topical medicines, metal earrings, eyeglasses
Eyelid	Nail polish (transferred by rubbing), cosmetics, contact lens solution, metal eyelash curlers
Face	Airborne allergens (poison ivy from burning leaves, ragweed), cosmetics, sunscreens, acne medications (e.g., benzoyl peroxide), aftershave lotion
Neck	Necklaces, airborne allergens (ragweed), perfumes, aftershave lotion
Trunk	Topical medication, sunscreens, poison ivy, plants (phototoxic reactions), clothing, undergarments (e.g., spandex bra, elastic waistband), metal belt buckles
Axillae	Deodorant (axillary vault), clothing (axillary folds)
Arms	Same as hand; watch and watchband
Hands	Soaps and detergents, foods, poison ivy, industrial solvents and oils, cement, metal (pots, rings), topical medications, rubber gloves in surgeons
Genitals	Poison ivy (transferred by hand), rubber condoms
Anal region	Hemorrhoid preparations (benzocaine, dibucaine [Nupercaine]), nystatin and triamcinolone (Mycolog II) cream
Lower legs	Topical medication (benzocaine, lanolin, neomycin), dye in socks
Feet	Shoes (rubber or leather), cement spilling into boots

From Habif TP: *Clinical dermatology,* ed 6, Philadelphia, 2012, Elsevier.

confused with ACD. A potassium hydroxide (KOH) slide can rule out dermatophyte infection; bacterial or viral cultures may be indicated when diagnosis is in doubt.

MANAGEMENT

Treatment of both ICD and ACD involves avoidance of the offending agents. Acutely, patients should be advised not to use any self-applied personal care skin products until the dermatitis is healed to avoid further inflaming the dermatitis. Patients should be directed to use products of low irritation and allergy potential, such as petrolatum. Domeboro solution is soothing for acutely inflamed and crusting lesions.

Handwashing should be kept to a minimum, with use of warm, not hot, water and a gentle cleanser. Alcohol-based hand cleansers have been repeatedly shown to cause less irritant hand dermatitis than soap and water.[5] Use of barriers such as gloves is vital for hand protection. Liberal use of emollients is encouraged.[2]

The mainstay of treatment of ACD is topical application of medium- to high-potency corticosteroids. The choice is based on the thickness of the skin and the surface area involved. Ointments are often preferred because they tend to have fewer preservatives and are less likely to sting when applied. The clinician must also be mindful of the fact that some patients may be sensitive to the topically applied vehicle as well as to the steroid itself. Topical calcineurin inhibitors are effective alternatives to steroids.[5]

When the periorbital or genital regions are affected or more than 20% of the body surface area is involved, the use of an oral steroid such as prednisone is appropriate. For rhus dermatitis, a 2- to 3-week taper can prevent the rebound that sometimes develops from more rapid steroid discontinuation. Whereas antihistamines may produce relaxation and improve sleep as a side effect, they have not been shown to reduce the pruritus associated with contact dermatitis.

Because ACD is a type 4 hypersensitivity reaction, the use of antihistamines may be of benefit. ICD, not being an allergic type of eczema, will not directly respond to the antipruritic effects of antihistamines, but they may produce sedative effects that may help in some cases.

COMPLICATIONS

Uncontrolled scratching can cause excoriations, impetigo eruptions, and cellulitis. Chronic scratching results in continued pruritus, scarring, and thickening of the skin, resulting in a condition called lichen simplex chronicus.

INDICATIONS FOR REFERRAL OR HOSPITALIZATION

Referral to a dermatology provider is indicated for refractory cases or cases in which the diagnosis is in question. Patch testing, provided by a dermatologist or an allergist, can assist in the precise diagnosis of the offending agent(s).

PATIENT AND FAMILY EDUCATION

Patients and family need to be educated about the nature of their dermatitis and how to avoid re-exposure. Urushiol resin, for instance, can remain allergenic on garden gloves and tools for months, waiting for its next opportunity to cause misery in some unsuspecting person.

For some patients, avoidance of contact could mean simply changing soaps or wearing gloves. For others, this could mean more significant lifestyle modifications. When the dermatitis is an occupational issue, patients may be eligible for Family Medical Leave Act (FMLA) benefits or short-term disability. Referral to a dermatology, allergy, or occupational health specialist is helpful in many cases.

Patients should know how to safely use topical or enteral steroids, tapering the dose to avoid rebound. Short courses of high-potency corticosteroids may be needed to control the itch and to prevent the scratching that causes infection, scarring, and chronic dermatitis. Antihistamines may be helpful for sleeping but are not helpful for the pruritus and should be used cautiously in select patients.

CHAPTER 49

CORNS AND CALLUSES

Maria Isabel Romano

DEFINITION

Corns and calluses are a painful reaction to pressure or friction on the underlying dermis covering the digital and plantar surfaces of the feet. Areas of excessive pressure or friction lead to hyperkeratotic, thickened skin that forms a padded area of protection for underlying skin structures. Corns, also termed *helomas,* are of two kinds: soft (heloma molle) and the more common hard (heloma durum). Calluses *(tylomas),* although unsightly, are less bothersome than corns and are usually a reaction to friction on the metatarsal heads or other bone prominences and may be a response to body weight distribution.[1] Calluses are not well circumscribed and lack the central hyperkeratotic painful core that is found in corns.

PATHOPHYSIOLOGY

Soft corns stem from hyperkeratotic development in response to excessive pressure or friction. A soft corn is a spongy hyperkeratosis usually found in the interdigital areas of the fourth and fifth toes. The pain associated with soft corns is often extreme because the inflammation excites pressure on the nerve receptors in the dermis. Pressure on the skin over the heads and bases of the condyles of the metatarsals and phalanges results from extrinsic factors, including an improperly fitting toe box, short shoes, and shoes with stiff soles, or from intrinsic factors, such as arthritic changes, fractures, and congenital foot deformity. Both intrinsic and extrinsic factors contribute to the development of a compensatory response of the foot and toes. Downward pressure on the metatarsal heads and contracture of the phalanges set the stage for friction and pressure, leading to corn and callus formation. Both are hard and produce pain as the conical keratin points into the dermis, stimulating painful sensory nerve endings.[2] Pain is triggered by development of an underlying bursitis or adventitious bursa that acts as a buffer of protection for the underlying bone.[1]

CLINICAL PRESENTATION

Corns typically produce problems when symptoms interfere with the performance of daily activities. Obtaining a good occupational history and inspecting the style and fit of the patient's customary shoe are important. Inability to move the toes in the toe box or wearing of pointed-toe or high-heeled shoes is frequently reported. Self-treatment by cutting or using over-the-counter plasters to remove the outer horny layer of tissue is common. Soft corns can be extremely painful and are characterized by their white, macerated appearance, which is a result of the absorption of perspiration.[3] Secondary infections of interdigital soft corns are common and painful and will often cause additional oozing and inflammation.

PHYSICAL EXAMINATION

Corns appear as well-circumscribed, translucent formations of keratin derived from the stratum corneum of the epidermis. Corns and calluses are located in areas of mechanical trauma. The dorsolateral aspect of the fifth toe and the dorsal surface of the distal interphalangeal joints of the second, third, and fourth toes are the areas most commonly affected by pressure. Seed corns are small, localized lesions anywhere on the plantar surface; hard corns are located over bone prominences; soft corns occur between the toes, most often in the fourth web space; and a "pump bump" or Haglund deformity is a bony enlargement on the back of the calcaneus resulting from high arches, a tight Achilles tendon, or walking on the lateral foot aspect.[4]

DIAGNOSTICS AND DIFFERENTIAL DIAGNOSIS

Inspection and examination are the only diagnostics generally indicated. Sometimes x-ray studies may be ordered to examine the bony structures of the feet. Hard corns are distinguished from warts by their slow onset, location over bone prominences, and painful response to direct pressure. Other factors include the lack of punctate bleeding when the corn is pared with a No. 15 blade surgical scalpel as well as evidence of furrowed skin lines on magnification that are not present in warts.[2] In some instances, radiographs of the bony structures of the feet may be necessary to determine the intrinsic cause of corn and callus formation, such as arthritis, bone prominences, condylar projections, and malunion of an old fracture.[5]

DIAGNOSTICS

Corns and Calluses

IMAGING
X-ray studies*

*If indicated.

DIFFERENTIAL DIAGNOSIS

Corns and Calluses

- Plantar warts
- Foreign body granuloma
- Porokeratosis plantaris discreta

MANAGEMENT

In general, patients should not apply caustic over-the-counter solutions to corns or calluses. An educated provider, however, can treat troublesome corns and calluses. Treatment begins by decreasing the size of the callus or corn by gently paring the skin with a No. 15 scalpel blade. After the paring, the provider applies a 40% salicylic acid plaster cut to fit the size of the remaining lesion. Instructions to the patient after paring include keeping the area dry and leaving the acid plaster undisturbed for 48 to 72 hours. At the next visit, the provider pares the remaining skin and repositions the plaster patch. Tape is useful for keeping the patch positioned clear of normal skin. After the second paring, patients can use a metal nail file or a pumice stone to carefully remove the white "dead" skin before replacing the salicylic acid plaster themselves. Other instructions to the patient include discontinuing the patch once the lesion has cleared and returning to the provider should lesions fail to resolve within 1 to 2 weeks of treatment.

Providers should assess all patients for peripheral neuropathies and avoid the application of plasters in those affected with neuropathies because of risk for damage to normal skin if patients cannot feel foot pain that results from slippage of the patch onto normal skin. In lesions not amenable to the use of a plaster patch, providers can prescribe salicylic acid 10% to 20% in petrolatum (available in 30- to 45-g tubes). Patients for whom treatment fails should be referred for foot x-ray studies to determine whether underlying bone abnormalities exist.[5]

Soft corn infections can be treated by twice-daily warm soaks and application of a topical antibiotic, such as mupirocin, which is effective against gram-positive organisms. If signs of cellulitis are present, additional oral medication should be started in the form of penicillinase-resistant penicillin, a first-generation cephalosporin, or erythromycin. After healing, the patient should be instructed to wear lamb's wool between the affected toes. The lamb's wool should be thick enough to prevent pain when the toes are juxtaposed. The patient also should be instructed to wear open-toed shoes if possible and to purchase shoes that promote proper foot alignment plus provide room for movement of the toes in the toe box.

Treatment of calluses includes regular sanding with a pumice stone after softening of the callus in warm water. Proper footwear, posture, and body habitus are further considerations in managing calluses.

General principles of treatment and prevention of corns and calluses are (1) to provide pain relief, (2) to discover and to correct the cause of increased mechanical stress, (3) to recommend appropriate footwear and orthotic devices, and (4) to recommend surgery if conservative approaches fail.[1,6] Patients should be advised to wear shoes with extra depth to increase room for their toes. Padding may prove helpful in the form of toe crests and metatarsal pads that redistribute weight from the metatarsal head to the pad. Toe crests work well for patients with painful hammertoes but must be worn in conjunction with shoes with a sufficiently wide toe box. Other, more recent advances include a variety of shoe pads.

Co-Management with Specialists

Patients should be referred to a podiatrist or orthopedic surgeon who specializes in the care of feet if conservative treatments fail to relieve pressure and to restore foot health. Patients with arthritis or hip deformities, those who bear weight on only one foot, and those who use assistive devices for ambulation are at greater risk for severe corns and calluses that do not respond to conservative treatment because intrinsic factors are the underlying cause of the mechanical stress. These individuals are also more likely to develop painful hammertoes. Surgical remodeling of the toes can provide the patient with marked relief from painful pressure spots and enhance quality of life. Custom shoes are also a helpful adjunct.

LIFE SPAN CONSIDERATIONS

Adolescents and young adults are more likely to wear shoes that fit improperly to be fashionable or to make their feet look smaller. Foot inspection during annual physical examinations should focus on early detection of corns, calluses, and bunions that result from short, tight-fitting footwear. Studies indicate that women more commonly develop corns, calluses, bunions, and foot deformities than men do.[7] Patients older than 65 years have more foot problems than the general population.[7,8] Foot pain associated with corns and calluses may prevent older adults from performing instrumental activities of daily living, such as standing, shopping, and walking.[9] Improperly fitted shoes are common in the elderly. Narrow shoes contribute to the development of toe corns, hallux valgus deformity, and foot pain in older patients.[9] Older adults are at increased risk for foot infections secondary to corn and callus formation coupled with an increased incidence of poor circulation.

Working men and women who stand for long hours on the job are at greater risk for foot problems. Efforts should be made to assess their feet frequently and to determine the adequacy of shoe fit for comfort and prevention of pressure points. Foot assessment should be included in the comprehensive physical examination of all patients as a means to evaluate foot health and to provide necessary preventive education.

COMPLICATIONS

Secondary infections often occur in soft corns. Other complications are primarily in the form of irritation, self-inflicted injury from paring down the corns, and chemical burns from use of caustic over-the-counter keratolytic solutions.

INDICATIONS FOR REFERRAL OR HOSPITALIZATION

Hospitalization is generally not warranted except in cases of serious infection or when surgery is indicated for corns that fail to respond to conservative treatment. Diabetic patients with infected corns may require intravenous antibiotic treatment. Other indications for referral include custom fitting for orthotic shoes.[2,6] Patients with severe foot deformity who are unable to purchase commercially available shoes that do not put pressure on the feet and toes may benefit from custom-fit shoes; these are expensive but worth the investment for comfort and freedom from pressure-induced pain. Custom-fit shoes promote optimum balance and assist in the prevention of falls.

PATIENT EDUCATION AND HEALTH PROMOTION

Education focuses on prevention and treatment with properly fitting footwear that allows sufficient toe space and an even distribution of body weight over the plantar surface of the foot.[7] Shoes should provide a shock-absorbing quality that absorbs pressure and friction rather than creating it. Gait and body habitus are other considerations.

CHAPTER 50

CUTANEOUS HERPES

Keith A. Deardorff • Theresa A. Bedford

DEFINITION AND EPIDEMIOLOGY

Cutaneous infections caused by the herpes simplex virus (HSV) can be of two serologic types: HSV-1, primarily oral lesions; and HSV-2, mainly genital infections. However, either virus can cause infection at either site. Oral HSV-1 infection recurs more frequently and earlier than oral HSV-2 infection; likewise, genital HSV-2 infection recurs more frequently than genital HSV-1 infection.[1,2] Both HSV-1 and HSV-2 are DNA viruses. Clinically, the lesions produced by each strain of the virus are indistinguishable.

There is a high prevalence of HSV-1 and HSV-2 throughout the world. Infection with the virus shows no seasonal variation, and there are no known animal vectors. By the fifth decade of life, 90% of adults have antibodies to HSV-1. In the United States alone, at least 50 million people have genital HSV infection.[1] One third to one half of infected individuals lack clinical manifestations of infection and can shed the virus in the absence of symptoms. HSV-2 antibodies start to develop during puberty and correlate with the onset of sexual activity.[3]

PATHOPHYSIOLOGY

Transmission of HSV occurs by direct contact with active lesions or with secretions containing the virus. HSV is a double-stranded DNA virus that may enter the host through a skin disruption (e.g., small crack in the skin) or intact mucous membranes (e.g., oropharynx, cervix, conjunctiva). The virus attaches itself to epithelial cells, enters, and replicates, exploiting cellular components. Once infected, cells die and release clear fluid, causing the formation of vesicles, which can fuse to form multinucleated giant cells. During the infection process the virus gains access to and infects regional, sensory, or autonomic nerves. The virus travels through the nerve axon to the ganglion, where it establishes a latent infection. Subsequently, the virus can reactivate and travel down the axon, where it causes a recurrent infection in the cutaneous area innervated by the affected root.[3,4]

CLINICAL PRESENTATION

HSV infection has three distinct phases: primary, latent, and recurrent infection. An outbreak is considered to be a primary occurrence if the patient was found to be both HSV-1 and HSV-2 seronegative before the outbreak of genital lesions.[5] A person's first occurrence of HSV infection is usually the most severe and may start after an incubation period of 4 to 6 days; however, the incubation period may range anywhere from 1 to 26 days after initial exposure.[6] Patients frequently report a prodrome of burning or tenderness at the site. Multiple painful round vesicles then appear at the site of infection and may be accompanied by tender lymphadenopathy in regional nodes. Fever, dysuria, vaginal discharge, or malaise may accompany the primary infection. Ulceration subsequently occurs, and lesions crust over and heal in immunocompetent patients within 2 to 3 weeks.

During the latent phase, the virus remains dormant in the ganglion of the nerve that serves the affected dermatome. The recurrent phase is characterized by virus reactivation and the reappearance of lesions in the dermatome affected during the primary infection. The outbreak may not occur at exactly the same site. Reactivation of either HSV type can be caused by local or systemic stimuli, such as immunodeficiency, trauma to mucosa, stress, depression, chronic anxiety, and poor sleep. HSV-1–specific triggers include ultraviolet light, cold weather, hot foods, lip biting, food allergy, and fever. HSV-2–specific triggers are noted to be food allergy and menses (usually 5 to 12 days before onset).[5] The primary infection may last 10 to 14 days, whereas recurrent infections are shorter and usually less severe, with markedly fewer lesions.

PHYSICAL EXAMINATION

The lesions of HSV infection are distinct. Grouped round vesicles on an erythematous base appear on the lips, facial area, throat, or genital area (Fig. 50-1). The fluid contained in the vesicles turns cloudy. Vesicles rupture, leaving erosions that subsequently crust over. Regional lymphadenopathy may be associated with primary or recurrent infections but is more common with primary infections. The various stages of lesions can often make diagnosis challenging.

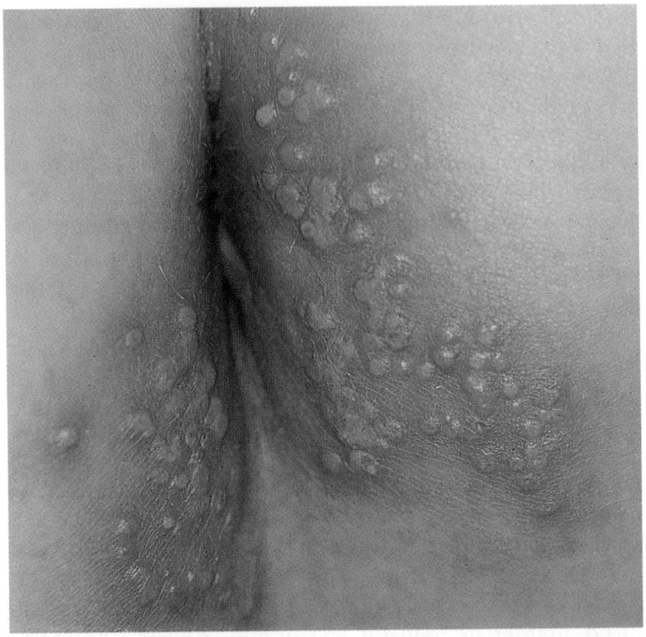

FIGURE 50-1 Primary herpes simplex on the perineum and buttocks with groups of vesicles on a red base. (From Fisher BK, Margesson LJ: *Genital skin disorders: diagnosis and treatment,* St Louis, 1998, Mosby.)

DIAGNOSTICS

A diagnosis of HSV infection can be made clinically with a thorough history and physical examination. However, laboratory confirmation should be considered in patients with a newly diagnosed primary infection. In addition, it is important to elicit any history of HSV infection, human immunodeficiency virus (HIV) infection, or pregnancy. The definitive test for the diagnosis of cutaneous herpes simplex infections remains viral culture. Viral cultures can take 2 to 7 days to achieve maximum sensitivity. Diagnosis may also be made with use of fluid obtained from a freshly unroofed vesicle for Tzanck preparation or by a direct fluorescent antibody (DFA) test. Both tests have lower sensitivity rates than culture. Cultures are most likely to be positive for virus when fresh, moist lesions exist; however, the DFA test result may still be positive in crusted, healing lesions.[1,7]

Serologic testing is available but often does not differentiate HSV-1 from HSV-2 and may only reveal previous exposure. Antigen detection tests are also of limited usefulness in primary infections because antibody development may be delayed.[1,4] Polymerase chain reaction (PCR) tests are extremely sensitive and specific but are expensive and are not indicated for mucocutaneous infections. Serologic tests assessing for the specific

DIAGNOSTICS

Cutaneous Herpes

LABORATORY

Viral cultures (90% sensitivity on vesicular lesion)
PCR (not approved by the FDA for genital swabs)
Tzanck smear (not effectively sensitive)
Serologic tests (sensitive and specific)

FDA, U.S. Food and Drug Administration

immunoglobulin to HSV are available and are much more sensitive than viral cultures, PCR testing, and Tzanck smears.[8]

DIFFERENTIAL DIAGNOSIS

The differential diagnosis of suspected HSV infections is varied. Varicella, herpangina, aphthous stomatitis, erythema multiforme, impetigo, Vincent angina, infectious mononucleosis, coxsackievirus infection, and Stevens-Johnson syndrome should be considered. Primary genital herpes can mimic Behçet syndrome, syphilis, candidiasis, infectious balanitis, erosive lichen planus, atopic dermatitis, and urethritis.[2,9] A thorough health history, the appearance of lesions, and the results of appropriate laboratory testing help with the differentiation among these diagnoses.

DIFFERENTIAL DIAGNOSIS

Cutaneous Herpes

- Erythema multiforme
- Impetigo
- Varicella
- Herpes zoster
- Behçet syndrome
- Herpes zoster
- Syphilis
- Coxsackievirus infection
- Herpangina
- Stevens-Johnson syndrome
- Aphthous stomatitis
- Ulcerative balanitis

MANAGEMENT

Immediate physician or obstetrician consultation is indicated for pregnant women.

Physician or specialist consultation for HIV co-infected patients is indicated.

Prevention is key in the management of HSV infections. Examples of prevention strategies include widespread public education about the nature of the disease and its spread, urging the use of barrier methods for prevention of sexually transmitted infections with all sexual contact and prophylactic antiviral therapy.[2] According to the 2010 Centers for Disease Control and Prevention guidelines for the treatment of sexually transmitted diseases, the recommendation is to treat all patients who are experiencing initial genital herpes infections, regardless of severity, presentation, timing, or duration of symptoms, to reduce complications and possibly recurrences.[1]

The treatment of choice for most HSV infections remains acyclovir (Zovirax), 400 mg, given orally three times a day for 7 to 10 days; acyclovir, 200 mg, given orally five times a day for 7 to 10 days; famciclovir (Famvir), 250 mg, given orally three times a day for 7 days; or valacyclovir, 1 g, given orally twice daily for 7 to 10 days and with dosage, frequency, or duration reduced with renal impairment. It is also recommended that therapy be extended longer if indicated by incomplete healing despite treatment (Table 50-1).

Primary Herpes Labialis

Evidence suggests that most cases of mild herpes labialis are self-limiting and do not require treatment. Topical medications have been shown to reduce the duration of pain; however, they may not affect the healing time. Oral medications are most likely to have an impact on healing when started during the prodromal period. Acyclovir, 400 mg orally five times daily for 5 days, may reduce pain with eating and drinking; however, the healing period may not be reduced. On the other hand, valacyclovir—2000 mg two times a day for day 1, repeated with 1000 mg two times a day for day 2—may shorten the period to healing and reduce pain.[10] Combining topical acyclovir with hydrocortisone in medications such as topical Xerese, Xerclear, and Denavir has been shown to be more effective at reducing the progression to ulcerative lesions in up to 35% of patients.[11] Penciclovir cream (Denavir) is applied at the first sign of symptoms (e.g., tingling, itching, burning, swelling) and thereafter every 2 hours (while awake) for 4 days.[12] Xerese is applied five times a day for five day.[13] Pain and discomfort can be treated with applications of over-the-counter analgesics or anesthetics such as camphor, benzyl alcohol, pramoxine, phenol, menthol, tetracaine, or benzocaine. Protectants including petroleum jelly, lip balms, calamine, zinc oxide, allantoin, and cocoa butter may also be used. Patients should avoid products with salicylic acid, which can erode the compromised skin.[14]

TABLE 50-1 Medication Schedule for Herpes Simplex Virus (HSV) Infections

Drug	Dosage
INITIAL EPISODE	
Acyclovir	400 mg PO 3 times daily for 7-10 days
Acyclovir	200 mg PO 5 times daily for 7-10 days
Famciclovir	250 mg PO 3 times daily for 7-10 days
Valacyclovir	1 g PO twice daily for 7-10 days 2000 mg PO every 12 hr for 1 day for herpes labialis (cold sore); begin treatment within 48 hr of symptom onset
RECURRENT EPISODES	
Acyclovir	400 mg PO twice daily for 5 days 800 mg PO twice daily for 5 days 800 mg PO 3 times daily for 2 days
Valacyclovir	500 mg PO twice daily for 3 days; or 1 g PO per day for 5 days
Famciclovir	125 mg PO twice daily for 5 days 1000 mg PO twice daily for 1 day 500 mg once, followed by 250 mg twice daily for 2 days
SUPPRESSION	
Acyclovir	400 mg PO twice daily
Valacyclovir	500 or 1000 mg PO per day (higher dose for those with more than 10 recurrences per year) For cold sores, reassess treatment need at 4 months For genital HSV suppression, reassess treatment need at 6 months
Famciclovir	250 mg PO twice daily

Recurrent Herpes Labialis

Recurrent episodes of orofacial herpes tend to be milder and shorter in duration than the primary infection.[2] Persons without a prodromal period with multiple painful or disfiguring lesions or more than four episodes should consider suppressive therapy. Most immunocompetent individuals with recurrent herpes labialis do not require treatment other than over-the-counter topical anesthetics for pain control. Also to be considered is the patient's ability to cope with the outbreaks. Both acyclovir and valacyclovir (Valtrex) may prevent recurrent episodes. Although the literature is lacking strong randomized controlled trials to fully support and define suppressive therapy, acyclovir, 800 to 1600 mg daily, and valacyclovir, 500 mg once a day, have been shown to be effective in studies with a low risk of bias. Their use was studied for up to 1 year.[15,16]

Primary Genital Herpes

The incubation period is 2 to 14 days with an average duration of symptoms of 22 to 28 days. Persons with a different HSV type may have milder symptoms. Genital lesions are often painful.[17] Acyclovir, valacyclovir, and famciclovir have been shown to effectively treat primary genital herpes. Antiviral therapy should be initiated within the first 6 days. Patients may be treated with one of the following regimens: (1) 400 mg orally three times daily for 5 days; or (2) 200 mg orally five times daily for 5 days. Valacyclovir, 500 mg two times day, or famciclovir, 250 mg three times a day, can also be used.[17,18] The duration of therapy should be extended if new lesions develop or systemic symptoms are present.[17] Although valacyclovir and famciclovir may also be used, there is no evidence to suggest that they are any more effective clinically, and they cost considerably more. They do offer the benefit of easier administration if compliance or ease of dosage schedule is an important consideration.[18]

Recurrent Genital Herpes

Depending on the patient's desire, tolerance, and other presenting symptoms, outbreaks of genital herpes that are mild and infrequent may not need to be treated, Acyclovir, valacyclovir, and famciclovir can be chosen as oral treatment regimens for recurrent outbreaks to assist in aborting the development of lesions, reducing viral shedding, and limiting the extent of the outbreak while speeding the healing of lesions.[2] Therapy for recurrences should be initiated within the first 24 to 48 hours of the repeat episode.[17] Treatment with acyclovir, 400 mg orally three times daily for 5 days, 800 mg orally twice daily for 5 days, or 200 mg orally five times daily for 5 days is appropriate.[2,19]

Suppression of Frequent Recurrences

Some evidence indicates that patients with frequently recurring HSV infections (more than six per year) can benefit from suppression with acyclovir, famciclovir, or valacyclovir.[2] Patients may be treated with one of the following long-term suppressive therapy regimens: (1) acyclovir, 400 mg orally twice daily; (2) valacyclovir, 500 to 1000 mg orally every day; or (3) famciclovir, 250 mg orally twice daily.[1] This reduces the number of recurrences and the frequency of asymptomatic shedding. It is important to understand that famciclovir and valacyclovir are no more effective than acyclovir for treatment of recurrent HSV infections and are more costly. Valacyclovir and famciclovir find greatest usefulness when compliance or convenience of administration is an issue.[2,18]

COMPLICATIONS

Complications of HSV infection are rare and typically occur in those who are already immunocompromised. Possible complications include aseptic meningitis, urinary retention, cutaneous dissemination, bacterial superinfection, erythema multiforme, and spontaneous abortion.[17] A cesarean section is usually performed if the mother has active herpes lesions at or around the time of delivery. Women who contract genital HSV-1 or HSV-2 infection in their third trimester of pregnancy are at high risk of infecting their newborns (30% to 50%).[17,21,22] Routine screening during pregnancy is not recommended by the American College of Obstetricians and Gynecologists.[19]

INDICATIONS FOR REFERRAL OR HOSPITALIZATION

Patients for whom a diagnosis of HSV is in question, who have superimposed HIV infection, who are receiving long-term suppressive therapy, or in whom routine therapy fails should be referred to a physician or specialist. Pregnant women also represent a special population and should be referred for evaluation by their obstetrician or family physician immediately.[17]

Patients requiring large amounts of pain medication or patients who have severe disseminated infections, severe superimposed bacterial infections, inability to void, or inability to take anything by mouth should be considered for hospitalization.

LIFE SPAN CONSIDERATIONS

Patients should understand that infection with HSV is lifelong and that there is no cure.[1] There is currently no vaccination available; however, many vaccines are currently in different stages of development. These include vaccines made from proteins, peptides, or chains of amino acids and the DNA virus itself.[21] In most individuals, the frequency and severity of attacks diminish with time.[17]

PATIENT AND FAMILY EDUCATION

Patients must be made aware of their ability to transmit HSV even when they have no apparent lesions or when using suppressive therapy.[23] Encouraging safe sexual practices, including the use of latex condoms and dental dams, is essential.[19] The risk of neonatal transmission during pregnancy must be explained to both male and female patients. Patients should be encouraged to use lip balm with sunscreen when exposed to ultraviolet light to avoid precipitation of an outbreak.

Two types of counseling are required for those newly diagnosed with genital herpes: (1) medical counseling, dealing with clinical issues; and (2) emotional counseling concerning the impact of herpes on self-esteem, sexuality, and social interactions.[2,19] Patients may experience shame or depression because of their infection with HSV and should be referred to the National Herpes Hotline at 919-361-8488 for available resources.[11] The National Herpes Hotline is operated by the American Social Health Association as part of the Herpes Resource Center. The hotline, which receives more than 60,000 calls a year, provides accurate information and appropriate referrals to anyone concerned about herpes.[1]

HEALTH PROMOTION

Patients can reduce their risk of acquiring genital herpes by limiting their lifetime number of sexual partners, by using condoms, and by becoming educated about transmission and shedding so they can avoid high-risk situations.[1,19] The risk of orolabial herpes infection can also be reduced by limiting sexual partners, incorporating the use of a dental dam, and avoiding direct contact with individuals with cold sores. Patients with orolabial and genital herpes must be counseled not to excoriate or to rub the herpes lesions because of the risk for autoinoculation of other parts of the body. Routine screening for HSV is not recommended by the U.S. Preventive Services Task Force and the Centers for Disease Control and Prevention.[19,20]

CHAPTER 51

DERMATITIS MEDICAMENTOSA (DRUG ERUPTION)

Nancy W. Knee • Joanne Sandberg-Cook

DEFINITION AND EPIDEMIOLOGY

Dermatitis medicamentosa (drug eruption) is an eruption of the skin or mucous membranes that can occur within 1 hour and up to 2 weeks after drug administration. These eruptions imitate almost all of the morphologic variations in dermatology, including exanthems, urticaria, photosensitivity, fixed drug reactions, palpable purpura, bullae, alopecia, onycholysis, acral erythema, lichenoid and acneiform lesions, lupus erythematosus–like lesions, toxic epidermal necrolysis, and erythema multiforme syndrome. Maculopapular exanthema is the skin eruption that is most commonly induced by a wide range of drugs.[1]

Drug eruptions may occur at any age, are more common in women, and are the most common form of drug sensitivity reactions.[2] Three percent of hospitalized patients experience a drug reacton,[3] with elders at increased risk because of the high number of medications typically taken by individuals in this age group.[4] There is a concern about underdiagnosis because of under-reporting, and also over-reporting because of the overuse of the term *allergy*. Specific skin testing, often not available or necessary, is the only way to distinguish a true allergy from a drug reaction, so the most recent terminology refers to both as drug hypersensitivity reactions (DHRs).

Immediate emergency department referral or physician consultation is indicated for anaphylaxis, severe erythema multiforme, or Stevens-Johnson syndrome.

PATHOPHYSIOLOGY

Drug eruptions are hypersensitivity manifestations of immunologic (immunoglobulin E–dependent) or nonimmunologic (T-cell–mediated) mechanisms stimulated by oral, topical, or parenteral drug administration.[5] Immunologic responses (true allergies) occur when specific antibodies or specifically sensitized lymphocytes to a drug develop during the sensitization period, which may be 4 or 5 days after initial exposure. Subsequent exposure to the drug results in a reaction that may occur within minutes, hours, or days.

Nonimmunologic responses, the most commonly occurring condition, may be caused by cumulative accumulation of a drug, pharmacologic action of a drug, individual genetic predisposition, drug sensitization of the skin producing reaction with exposure to ultraviolet light, increased sensitivity to irritating topical solutions, and other factors, such as individual immune status.[5] Hypersensitivity reactions to antibacterial agents (mostly penicillin), aspirin or nonsteroidal anti-inflammatory drugs (NSAIDs), and protease inhibitors are examples of the last, involving maculopapular rashes and urticaria.[5]

Protease inhibitors, antibiotics, and chloroquine may cause acute generalized exanthematous pustulosis (AGEP). A very rare reaction, AGEP manifests with onset of acute clinical symptoms, including temperature higher than 38° C (100.4° F) and widespread exfoliative dermatitis after a pustular, morbilliform eruption that heals within 15 days of discontinuation of the medication.[6]

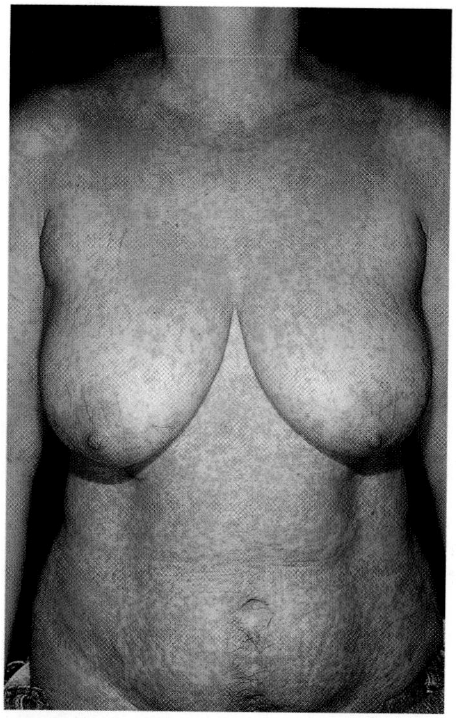

FIGURE 51-1 Cutaneous drug reaction. (From Habif TP, Campbell JL, Chapman MS, et al: *Skin disease: diagnosis and treatment*, St Louis, 2001, Mosby.)

CLINICAL PRESENTATION

Patients may come in for an office visit with a variety of skin reactions (itching, burning, pain), with or without rash (Table 51-1). The most common is a confluent, maculopapular rash that may be pruritic (Fig. 51-1). Knowledge about onset, progression of symptoms, fever, recent medication change, and family history is essential. Onset can occur 7 to 10 days after the drug is started but may not occur until the course of medication is finished. The rash can last 1 to 2 weeks and then fade. The rash may also be urticarial (always highly suggestive of drug reaction) or a fixed drug reaction that occurs in the same area each time the drug is taken.[7]

PHYSICAL EXAMINATION

Careful skin examination is indicated. The category of lesions and distribution should be noted. Further examination of the head, eyes, ears, nose, throat, and cardiopulmonary status may be necessary to exclude viral exanthems or anaphylaxis, a more severe, systemic reaction.

DIAGNOSTICS

No laboratory tests are available that can establish the diagnosis, although a complete blood count (CBC) may occasionally reveal eosinophilia. Skin tests can evaluate sensitivity to penicillin only at this point. Diagnosis depends on a thorough drug history, including known allergies or hypersensitivities to all oral, topical, parenteral, over-the-counter, prescription, vitamin, and "natural" preparations and duration of symptoms.[3] Serum

TABLE 51-1 Skin Reactions

Dermatologic Types	Causative Agents	Manifestations
Exanthems	Cillins, sulfonamides, barbiturates, aspirin, NSAIDs, protease inhibitors	Bright red scarlatiniform lesions, usually on trunk
Urticaria	Cillins, salicylates, erythromycin, carbamazepine, NSAIDs, radiocontrast material, bupropion	Typical, well-defined wheals on hands, feet, lips; generalized
Angioedema	Angiotensin-converting enzyme inhibitors, angiotensin II antagonists, chemotherapeutic agents	Skin-colored or pink asymmetric areas of swelling on eyelids, lips, tongue, and extremities
Photosensitivity	Phenothiazines, tetracyclines, sulfonamides, fluoroquinolones, NSAIDs, artificial sweeteners	Dermatitis or gray-blue hyperpigmented areas on skin exposed to sun
Fixed drug reactions	Phenolphthalein (in laxatives), pseudoephedrine, tetracycline, sulfonamides, anticonvulsants	Dusky red or purple lesions that reappear in same area with repeated drug exposure
Purpura (see Chapter 63)	Chlorothiazide, meprobamate, anticoagulants	Nonblanching purple lesions, usually generalized and on lower extremities
Bullae (part of erythema multiforme group)	Cillins, barbiturates, iodines, sulfonamides, vancomycin, carbamazepine, anticonvulsants, allopurinol	Symmetric, erythematous, edematous, bullous lesions
Lichenoid lesions	Antimalarials, gold, thiazides, chlorpromazine, proton pump inhibitors, hepatitis B immunization, NSAIDs, aspirin	Angular papules that turn into scaly patches
Acneiform lesions	Corticosteroids, iodines, bromides, hydantoins, epidermal growth factor receptor inhibitors, diuretics	Acne-like but no comedones and with sudden onset
Toxic epidermal necrolysis (part of erythema multiforme group)	Barbiturates, hydantoins, cillins, sulfonamides	Areas of loosened, easily detached epidermis with a scalded appearance
Erythema multiforme	Cillins, barbiturates, sulfonamides	Vary from small vesicles or ulcers to widespread bullous lesions (Stevens-Johnson syndrome)

Data from James WD, Berger TG, Elston DM: *Andrews' diseases of the skin: clinical dermatology,* ed 11, Philadelphia, 2011, Elsevier.

DIAGNOSTICS

Dermatitis Medicamentosa

LABORATORY
CBC and differential (to exclude eosinophilia)*
Skin testing (for suspected penicillin allergy)*
Serum tryptase*

*If indicated.

DIFFERENTIAL DIAGNOSIS

Dermatitis Medicamentosa

- Urticaria
- Purpura
- Photosensitivity
- Bullous impetigo
- Contact or irritant dermatitis
- Acne vulgaris
- Rosacea
- Scarlet fever
- Staphylococcal infection
- Secondary syphilis
- Viral rashes: herpes simplex virus, mycoplasma, human immunodeficiency virus (HIV), Epstein-Barr virus, cytomegalovirus, Kawasaki syndrome
- Still disease

tryptase is a marker of the release of mast cell granules, which signals an allergic reaction. It can be used to verify an anaphylactic event caused by an allergen or a drug reaction.[3]

DIFFERENTIAL DIAGNOSIS

The sudden onset and symmetric nature of the eruptions (except in cases of topical administration of the offending product) usually establish the diagnosis as a DHR. For example, urticaria-related drug reactions are seen as transient wheals in the skin caused by acute dermal edema. The more sudden and explosive the appearance of the urticaria, the more likely that a potent, life-threatening anaphylaxis may occur. Immediate discontinuation of the drug is imperative. Urticaria lesions are distinguished from erythema multiforme by the pruritic nature of urticaria, and the lesions will often "move" during 1 to 2 hours. Erythema multiforme lesions are not pruritic, are often painful, and may last 1 to 4 weeks.[3] Readministration of the pharmacologic preparation will confirm sensitivity (drug provocation test); however, even though this can confirm the hypersensitivity, it can be life-threatening, especially in immunologic responses. For a list of possible causes of DHRs, see Table 51-1.

MANAGEMENT

Identification of the offending preparation and its removal will usually resolve the drug reaction, although the course of the reaction may progress for several days until the preparation is eliminated from the body. Close monitoring for the first 48 hours to check for progression or systemic involvement is the standard of care for any drug eruption.

Symptomatic treatment and hydration are advised. Cool compresses and tepid baths (e.g., Aveeno) may be soothing. Nonacute eruptions with dry, scaly, nonpruritic lesions will benefit from cooling lotions or topical antihistamine gels or creams (e.g., Sarna Anti-Itch).[8] Topical high-potency corticosteroid ointment can be applied to a small area for more pruritic eruptions, although data documenting its effectiveness are lacking.[8] Oral antihistamines should also be administered to manage pruritus. Oral corticosteroids may be indicated for refractory cases. Patients with severe reactions, including anaphylaxis, will require epinephrine 1:1000 (0.2 to 0.5 mL subcutaneously) in addition to oral antihistamines.

Epidermal growth factor receptor inhibitors, only one of a class of drugs commonly used in oncology, can cause follicular and pustular skin reactions. The treatment for epidermal growth factor receptor inhibitor–induced eruptions is topical antibiotics (e.g., clindamycin 1% gel and erythromycin 4% solution) for mild reactions, along with low-potency topical steroids; systemic antibiotics (e.g., minocycline or doxycycline) may be used for more severe rash.[4]

COMPLICATIONS

Anaphylaxis is a potentially life-threatening, immune-mediated complication of first exposure or, more commonly, re-exposure to the offending preparation. Immunologic responses vary and may progress to Stevens-Johnson syndrome (epidermis peeling off in sheets), erythema multiforme (eruption of symmetric erythematous and edematous lesions of the skin or mucous membranes), myocarditis (inflammation of the myocardium), serum sickness, or other life-threatening conditions.

INDICATIONS FOR REFERRAL OR HOSPITALIZATION

Patients with erythema multiforme, Stevens-Johnson syndrome, toxic epidermal necrolysis, AGEP, and drug reaction with eosinophilia and systemic symptoms (DRESS) or anaphylaxis require immediate referral. Any patient whose symptoms do not resolve in a timely manner should be referred for confirmation of the diagnosis and additional consultation.

CLINICAL INFORMATION RESOURCES

Online and other resources for DHRs include www.pdr.net, www.nlm.nih.gov/medlineplus/drugreactions.html, and Jerome Litt's Drug Eruption and Reaction Database (www.drugeruptiondata.com).

PATIENT AND FAMILY EDUCATION AND HEALTH PROMOTION

Health care providers must give careful instructions to patients who have had reactions to medication. First, these patients are encouraged to wear medical alert bracelets or devices that list medication allergies. Next, patients are encouraged to add the new allergy to an up-to-date list of allergies that they carry in their wallet, along with the list of current medications they take. Patients who have had a severe or anaphylactic reaction to a drug should be educated on the importance of carrying an epinephrine pen at all times, and knowing how and when to use it. In addition, health care providers should flag the patient's record to alert other health care providers of the allergy. Other instructions include reminding allergic patients to tell providers about their allergy before they accept a prescription for any antibiotics or other medications.

CHAPTER 52

DRY SKIN

Cené L. Gibson

DEFINITION AND EPIDEMIOLOGY

Dry skin (xerosis) is literally skin that lacks moisture or water. It is often characterized as rough or xerotic. Dry skin is common in dry climates and during the winter months. It is especially prevalent in older adults.

Older skin (older than 60 years) is affected by physiologic changes, the wear and tear of aging, hormone deficits, and the cumulative effect of years of sun exposure. By the age of 70 years, nearly all adults are affected with dry skin, resulting in significant morbidity and reduction in quality of life.[1]

Teenage skin is susceptible to drying because of the hormonal changes of puberty. Teens are also susceptible because of application of chemical preparations, such as makeup and cleansers.

Obesity, now an epidemic in the Western world, is also responsible for changes in skin barrier function. Studies suggest that obese individuals have increased transdermal water loss and erythema compared with control subjects, resulting in an altered epidermal barrier.[2]

Environments in which the humidity is below 30% cause dehydration of the stratum corneum layer of the skin. Cold air and heat in buildings, cars, and homes contribute to skin dehydration, especially during the winter.

PATHOPHYSIOLOGY

The moisture content of the skin contributes to its overall elasticity, tone, smoothness, and softness. Dysfunction of the epidermis can allow water to be lost, resulting in drying.

The stratum corneum of the epidermis is the primary protective layer of the skin. The thickness of the stratum corneum varies with location on the body. It averages 0.1 mm in thickness and is made up of flattened keratinocytes. These cells originate below the epidermal layer and migrate to the surface, where they die and slough in the continual process of desquamation. The process of migration (from below the corneum) to the surface takes 28 days.

The stratum corneum layer is composed of lipids, water, proteins, and salts. Lipids come from sebaceous gland secretions in the form of sebum; the salts come from the sweat or apocrine glands. This lipid layer forms a natural emulsion of lipid and water. Depending on genetics and subject to age, climate, and time of year, this layer can be either more oil-in-water emulsion or water-in-oil emulsion.[1,2]

Hormones also play a role in this layer. Androgenic hormones tend to stimulate the layer, whereas estrogen, progesterone, and the corticosteroids tend to inhibit production of this layer.[3] Hormone production is relatively low during childhood, peaks during adolescence, decreases after the age of 35 years, and dramatically decreases after the age of 60 years. In older adults, the decrease in sweat and sebum production from glandular tissue leads to water loss through the skin, resulting in a decreased ability to repair skin defects.[1]

If the skin is working properly, the lipid layer and lower water barrier maintain the skin in a supple state. The lipid layer prevents water absorption by acting as a repellent. The lower water barrier prevents drying out and potential damage to lower skin structures in the dermis and subcutaneous layers. Repeated exposure to solvents and soaps removes lipids from the skin. Loss of water, lipids, or proteins alters overall skin integrity.

CLINICAL PRESENTATION AND PHYSICAL EXAMINATION

Some patients report having dry skin most of their lives; in others, the problem developed with aging. Typically, patients with dry skin will experience skin changes with the seasons or after an illness. Initially, dry skin appears as a rough patch that itches. Pruritus is worse on the lower extremities, which have less fat and muscle mass and therefore less ability to replace the lipid layer elements. The hands and face are also common sites for dry skin because of exposure to wind or air and handwashing.

Dry skin has a rough appearance and is not supple. The presence of cracks and fissures indicates a severe condition. Eczema craquelé is a condition that develops on lower legs or arms when skin is dry; the skin will have an uneven diamond pattern with erythema at the edges (Figure 52-1).

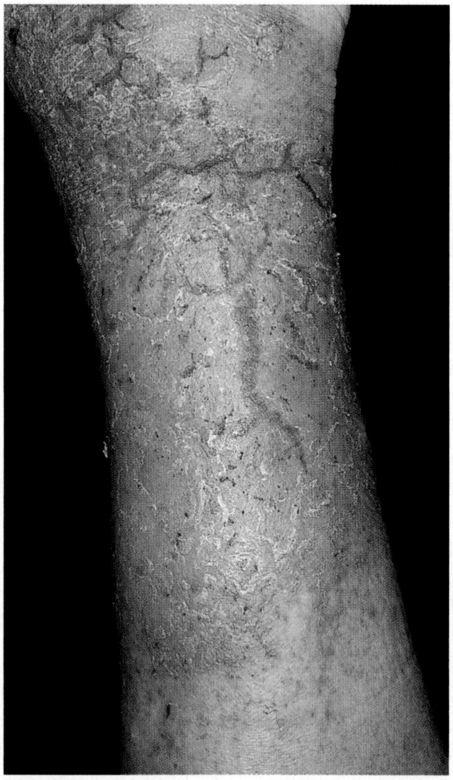

FIGURE 52-1 Asteatotic eczema. (From Habif TP, Campbell JL, Chapman MS, et al: *Skin disease: diagnosis and treatment,* St Louis, 2001, Mosby.)

DIAGNOSTICS AND DIFFERENTIAL DIAGNOSIS

DIFFERENTIAL DIAGNOSIS

Dry Skin

- Eczema
- Ichthyosis vulgaris
- Scabies

Dry skin is a visual diagnosis. The differential diagnosis includes all other forms of dermatitis, including eczema, ichthyosis vulgaris, and scabies. Secondary skin changes including lichenification as a result of scratching can complicate the appearance of the skin, making accurate diagnosis difficult.

MANAGEMENT

Xerotic skin is dry because of a lack of water. Treatment with lubricants and water-in-oil emulsions two or three times daily will restore moisture. Patients should be advised to take short baths with tepid water. For some older adults, bathing every other day and spot washing the axilla and groin can help minimize moisture loss. When toweling, the patient should pat the skin dry. Oils can be applied to the skin immediately after rinsing or within 2 to 3 minutes after drying to prevent further loss of moisture. Patients should be cautioned about the risk for falls with oil preparations because these preparations make the skin slippery. The application of emollients (white petrolatum or products containing 10% urea or 5% lactic acid)[3] to the skin after rinsing is a safe, effective alternative.

Antihistamines should be prescribed to minimize scratching. However, patients should be reminded that the sedative effects of traditional antihistamines are potentially problematic (e.g., raising the risk for falls and impaired driving). The primary care provider must be alert for the interactions of the antihistamines with other medications or other disease entities, such as urinary retention that can occur with antihistamines in older men who have benign prostatic hypertrophy. Creams and lotions containing the chemicals menthol and phenol can often help in the relief of pruritus and may be tried before antihistamines are used.

Dry skin should be treated early with moisturizers and emollients to prevent the development of secondary skin lesions from scratching and irritation. Topical steroid creams can be applied to dry, itching skin for a limited time. Topical steroid creams help treat the pruritus and resulting inflammation. The carrier cream in these preparations adds additional emollient to the skin to help retard further moisture loss. Steroid creams should be used with caution to prevent thinning of the skin. Patients should be instructed to use them for no more than a week and to use them cautiously on the face, breasts, or genital areas. Good hygiene practices and attention to skin care with moisturizing agents are the mainstays in the management and prevention of dry skin.[4]

COMPLICATIONS

Infections and even cellulitis are complications produced by scratching. Scratching disrupts the protective epidermal barrier. Once the epidermal barrier is disrupted, penetration by exogenous toxins from surface staphylococci can occur. In allergic patients, reactions with pruritic lesions exacerbate dry skin conditions. Other complications seen with dry skin are typically secondary to treatment. Local reactions to perfumes in moisturizers as well as atrophy from long-term use of topical steroids can occur.

INDICATIONS FOR REFERRAL OR HOSPITALIZATION

A dermatologic referral and hospitalization are not usually indicated. A referral to a dermatologist is warranted if the diagnosis is unclear or if the condition persists despite treatment.

PATIENT EDUCATION AND HEALTH PROMOTION

Good skin care programs help control and prevent dry skin and its complications. Patients with dry skin should understand the importance of consistent efforts to maintain skin hydration and have a clear plan of care in case there is an exacerbation. The patient should be cautioned against scratching; scratching leads to complications and exacerbates the skin irritation.

Humidifiers can replenish moisture in the air and maintain the humidity at the 60% ideal. Bath water should be tepid. Moisturizers should be applied just before rinsing or immediately after drying. Patients are cautioned about the risk of slipping when moisturizing agents are used. Mild soaps or cleansers should be used sparingly. Laundry detergents should be fragrance free. Topical corticosteroid ointments of low (hydrocortisone) to medium (betamethasone) potency provide rapid relief for extreme eczematous changes but should be discontinued when symptoms have resolved.

Travel increases during the winter and holiday months. Because air travel can significantly pull moisture from the air and lead to drying of the skin, patients should be instructed to keep well hydrated and to use moisturizers as necessary when flying.

Soups and stews help replace water in the diet and are good sources of nutrients during the winter months. Older adults should be cautioned to limit sodium consumption; however, the need for adequate hydration both externally and internally is important. Vitamins can be added to the daily regimen for patients who are not already taking a multivitamin or whose nutritional balance is of concern. This will help promote good skin integrity through overall nutritional health.

CHAPTER 53

ECZEMATOUS DERMATITIS (ATOPIC DERMATITIS)

Cené L. Gibson

DEFINITION AND EPIDEMIOLOGY

Eczematous dermatitis, or atopic dermatitis (AD), is a pruritic inflammatory skin disorder characterized by exacerbations and remissions of dry, itchy red skin. Onset of the disorder is most common at 3 to 6 months of age, affecting 1 in 10 children and 1 in 10 to 14 adults in the United States.[1] AD is also associated with other atopic (immunoglobulin E [IgE]) diseases (e.g., asthma, allergic rhinitis, urticaria, or acute reactions to foods).[1-3] AD affects persons of all races, with the international prevalence on the rise.[4] Patients with a tendency to develop these conditions are referred to as atopics. Many atopic patients also have a family history of atopy.

AD is often called "the itch that rashes." Patients initially are bothered by incessant itching, scratch an area, and then develop a rash at the site of scratching. Eventually, lichenification may develop at the site if it remains untreated.

PATHOPHYSIOLOGY

The primary cause of AD continues to be poorly understood. Primary immune dysfunction resulting in IgE sensitization and/or a primary defect in the epithelial barrier with resultant secondary immunologic dysregulation have been proposed as potential underlying causes of AD.[4]

CLINICAL PRESENTATION AND PHYSICAL EXAMINATION

AD is characterized by pruritic, erythematous, dry patches of skin, often with scale. Linear excoriations may be seen as a secondary change (Fig. 53-1). The borders of eczematous lesions are not initially well defined. Crusting and oozing are common. Thickened skin with well-defined skin markings (lichenification) may develop in long-standing lesions as the result of scratching. In infants, eruption may involve the cheeks, scalp, forehead, and extensor extremities.[1] In adults, eczema or AD may be generalized, with a tendency to develop lesions on the face, neck, flexural folds, wrists, and dorsa of the feet.

DIAGNOSTICS AND DIFFERENTIAL DIAGNOSIS

AD is a clinical diagnosis that is based on a careful history and examination. Seborrheic dermatitis can be differentiated from AD by its presentation and distribution. Seborrheic dermatitis typically manifests as nonpruritic, mildly erythematous plaques with waxy, yellow scale on the face, postauricular area, and scalp.

Psoriasis is characterized by well-demarcated, intensely erythematous plaques with characteristic overlying silvery scale, usually located on the scalp, elbows, and knees.

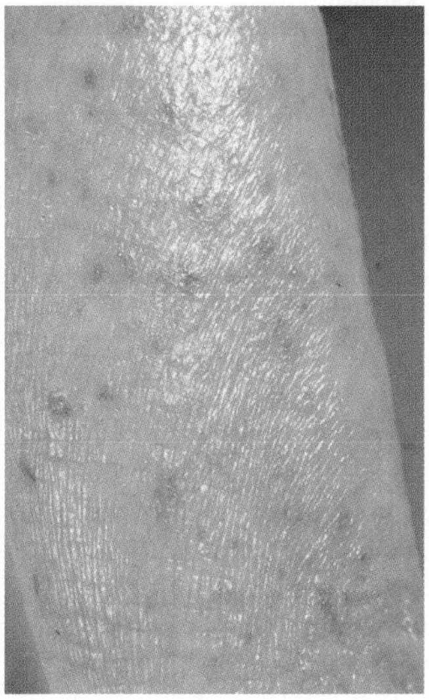

FIGURE 53-1 Atopic dermatitis. Note the erythema, excoriation, and lichenification. (From Goldman L, Scafer AI: *Goldman's Cecil medicine*, ed 24, Philadelphia, 2012, Saunders.)

Scabies typically is a poorly defined pruritic eruption, often with linear burrows in the web spaces of the fingers. The breasts and genital areas are also often involved. The condition is commonly complicated by eczematous changes from nocturnal scratching and rubbing. The diagnosis is confirmed by scraping of a burrow and microscopic identification of mites, eggs, or feces.

Molluscum contagiosum lesions are small, dome-shaped papules with central umbilication. They are not easily confused with AD, but patients with molluscum often develop dermatitis at the site of the lesions.

Tinea (or superficial fungal infection) lesions have a sharply demarcated border with scale at the edge and central clearing. They are usually limited in number and sometimes form an arciform array. A scraping of the border of the lesion and treatment of the removed sample with potassium hydroxide (KOH) reveal hyphae on microscopic evaluation. The diagnosis of AD is differentiated on the basis of the presence of xerosis, age at presentation, history of atopic diseases, early onset, and a chronic relapsing course.[4]

The presentation of allergic contact dermatitis depends on the offending substance. The severity of inflammation associated with contact dermatitis is dependent on the concentration of the irritant and the length of exposure.[4] Careful patient history will often reveal potential exposures.

Immunodeficiency should be considered in infants with severe itching in the setting of recurrent infection.

Mycosis fungoides manifests as hypopigmentation with dermatitis.

DIAGNOSTICS

Atopic Dermatitis

LABORATORY
KOH preparation (to exclude other disorders)

DIFFERENTIAL DIAGNOSIS

Atopic Dermatitis

- Seborrheic dermatitis
- Psoriasis
- Scabies
- Molluscum contagiosum
- Tinea or other fungal infection
- Allergic contact dermatitis

MANAGEMENT

Patient education is the cornerstone of AD treatment. Patients must be encouraged to avoid rubbing and scratching the involved areas because this exacerbates the condition. The goals of treatment are management of pruritus to prevent scratching, moisturization for dryness, and control of inflammation of the eczematous lesions to maintain a healthy skin barrier.[2,3]

Antihistamines can control itching, allay anxiety, and induce sleep. Diphenhydramine (Benadryl) and hydroxyzine (Atarax) are the drugs of choice, although nonsedating antihistamines such as cetirizine (Zyrtec) and loratadine (Claritin) may be preferred for daytime use.

Hydration with a tepid water bath can be soothing during an acute flare of AD. The bath should be immediately followed by the application of a bland emollient such as hydrated petrolatum or Aquaphor. Other measures that may improve symptoms include wearing soft cotton clothing, maintaining cool temperatures, using a cool mist humidifier, and washing with mild detergents.[4,5]

Topical corticosteroid ointments are usually necessary to alleviate inflammation during an acute flare. Hydrocortisone ointment 1% (Cortaid), a mild steroid, can be applied sparingly to affected areas two or three times daily for both adult and pediatric patients.[5] Use of topical steroids is limited by the wide distribution of steroid-responsive elements found in various cells and tissues. Long-term use may lead to skin atrophy such as striae, telangiectasis, and systemic side effects including growth restriction in children and glaucoma.[4] Topical corticosteroids should be discontinued when the inflammation has subsided, whereas the use of lubricants and emollients should be continued.

The nonsteroidal calcineurin inhibitor topical medications such as tacrolimus (Protopic) and pimecrolimus (Elidel) can be helpful for managing chronic moderate to severe AD. These medications are not indicated for patients younger than 2 years.

Atopic patients are predisposed to skin infections. Only overt secondary bacterial, fungal, or viral infections should be treated with appropriate topical and systemic antibiotics.[5] *Staphylococcus aureus* is a common colonizer of the skin in AD and is thought to trigger multiple inflammatory cascades.[4]

Systemic corticosteroids are seldom used in the treatment of AD and should be reserved for extreme cases that are not controlled with topical treatments. Phototherapy with narrow-band ultraviolet B light and photochemotherapy with psoralen plus ultraviolet A light may be helpful when standard therapies have failed.

COMPLICATIONS

Secondary microbial infections are common from chronic excoriations and defects in innate immunity.

Group A β-hemolytic streptococci and staphylococci are the most common bacterial organisms. Bacterial secondary infection should be suspected, cultured for, and treated in patients with purulent or weepy lesions and in cases of AD that are slow to respond to standard therapies. Cephalexin (Keflex) is effective and well tolerated. It has been found that dilute bleach baths consisting of ½ cup regular strength bleach per 1 full bathtub of water (except on face and neck) twice weekly and intranasal mupirocin (Bactroban) for 3 months led to reduction in bacterial superinfections of the skin.[5]

Patients with AD have a higher incidence of herpes simplex virus infection, molluscum contagiosum, and warts. These infections can be more frequent and widespread in patients with AD. Increases in cutaneous viral infections are related to defective cell-mediated immunity in the skin as well as to the use of topical steroids.

A particularly serious viral complication of AD is eczema herpeticum. A patient with this condition has an underlying skin disorder (usually AD) and develops a widespread eruption of vesicles and erosions when experiencing a primary herpes infection or herpes infection reactivation. A Giemsa-stained scraping of the base of a vesicle will reveal multinucleated giant cells. Eczema herpeticum should be treated with oral antiviral medications (e.g., valacyclovir [Valtrex]) and supportive care.

INDICATIONS FOR REFERRAL OR HOSPITALIZATION

Failure to respond to topical treatments requires referral to a dermatologist or dermatology nurse practitioner for management. An eruption that is recalcitrant to treatment may resemble AD but actually be another disorder. For example, bullous pemphigoid, cutaneous T-cell lymphoma, and allergic or irritant contact dermatitis can sometimes resemble AD in their early stages.

In addition, evaluation and management by an allergist or allergy nurse practitioner may be needed for optimum care of a patient with known allergies or when an allergic role is suspected in the disease.

Hospitalization may be required for intensive topical or systemic treatments. Hospitalization is also indicated for patients with secondary infection who are unresponsive to outpatient therapies.

LIFESPAN CONSIDERATIONS

Use of high-potency topical corticosteroids should be minimized with the very young and very old. Long-term use of topical corticosteroids should be avoided, if possible, for all age groups.

EDUCATION AND HEALTH PROMOTION

Patients with AD should understand that the goal is diligent avoidance of known triggers and, if a flare occurs, timely management of symptoms. Weeks or months of control will be followed by sudden exacerbations. Patients should understand the proper use of antihistamines to control itching and the continuous use of lubricants and emollients to moisturize the skin. Patients require careful education on proper bathing and moisturizing and their role in decreasing the need for topical corticosteroids.

Patients should use a humidifier year-round to avoid dryness induced by winter dry air and air conditioning. People with AD should be aware of the drying effect of soaps. Mild soaps can be used to wash the body folds and genital area but should be avoided on other body parts. Laundry detergents (e.g., All Free and Clear) should also be mild to prevent irritation.

Identification of individually specific aggravating factors, such as stress, infections, perspiration, weather change, dry skin, and contact sensitivity, will aid in management.

CHAPTER 54

FUNGAL INFECTIONS (SUPERFICIAL)

Melissa A. Hall

Superficial fungal infections are common problems. Greater exposure to fungal pathogens is occurring in the health and fitness–minded population, in debilitated patients using systemic antibiotics, in diabetics, and in other patients who are immunocompromised. These fungal infections can cause a primary or secondary infection of the skin that complicates accurate diagnosis of the precipitating condition. Fungal infections are caused typically by dermatophytes or yeast organisms.

DERMATOPHYTE INFECTIONS

DEFINITION AND EPIDEMIOLOGY

Dermatophytes, the most common fungi that invade the skin and nails, proliferate within the nonviable keratinized tissues—the stratum corneum of the skin, hair, and nails. Three of the most common pathologic dermatophytes are *Trichophyton*, *Microsporum*, and *Epidermophyton* organisms. The infections produced by these dermatophytes are known as *tinea*, *dermatophytosis*, *or ringworm*. The term *tinea* is derived from the Latin word for worm and was probably chosen because of the common presence of a migrating, circular pattern with the infection. The tinea infection is named by the part of the body that is affected by the dermatophyte.[1]

PATHOPHYSIOLOGY

Fungal infections are usually acquired through inhalation of endemic fungi in the environment, with soil being the natural reservoir.[1] They are also transmitted through close contact with an infected person or animal. Tinea corporis is the second most common infection passed from dogs and cats to humans.[2] Indirect contact with fomites (infected towels, hats, upholstery, and hairbrushes) may also cause dermatophyte infections. Infections of scalp hair and body surfaces are most frequent during childhood; hand, foot, or nail infections are much more common after puberty.[3]

CLINICAL PRESENTATION AND PHYSICAL EXAMINATION

Dermatophyte infections are characterized and named according to their location. Tinea capitis (head or scalp) can be seen initially as patchy, scaly, nonscarring areas of hair loss (Fig. 54-1). Depending on the infectious organism, the lesions may become inflamed, boggy, and pustular. Tinea corporis (body)

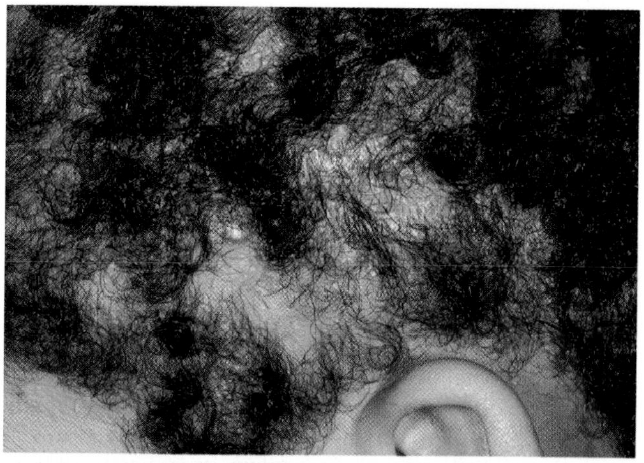

FIGURE 54-1 Tinea capitis. (Paller, SA, *Hurwitz Clinical Pediatric Dermatology: A Textbook of Skin Disorders of Childhood and Adolescence,* ed 4, Philadelphia, 2012, Saunders.)

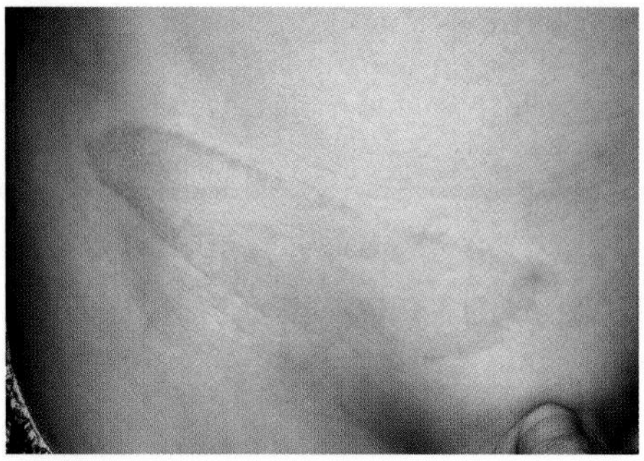

FIGURE 54-2 Tinea corporis (ringworm of the body). (Paller, SA, *Hurwitz Clinical Pediatric Dermatology: A Textbook of Skin Disorders of Childhood and Adolescence,* ed 4, Philadelphia, 2012, Saunders.)

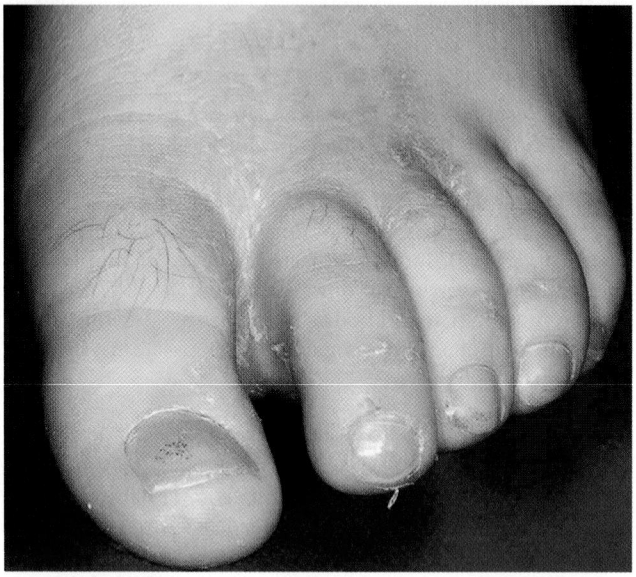

FIGURE 54-3 Tinea pedis. (Paller SA, *Hurwitz Clinical Pediatric Dermatology: A Textbook of Skin Disorders of Childhood and Adolescence,* ed 4, Philadelphia, 2012, Saunders.)

appears on skin as erythematous plaques and papules in an annular or arciform pattern. Lesions often have slightly elevated borders with central clearing (Fig. 54-2). Tinea cruris (jock itch) appears on the groin and upper inner thigh and extends to the gluteal folds as erythematous scaling patches with raised borders. The scrotum is often spared. Tinea pedis (athlete's foot) can occur as interdigital scaling, maceration, and fissuring (Fig. 54-3). It can also appear as a mild erythematous scaling eruption that involves the sole and sides of the foot (moccasin distribution). Tinea manus (hand) is often a dry, diffuse, scaly eruption of the palms, with sharply marginated plaques on the dorsum of the hands. The feet are often also involved. Tinea unguium (nail), also called *onychomycosis,* most commonly manifests as the distal subungual type. The infection begins in the distal nail bed and spreads to infect the nail plate, causing the nail to appear thickened and yellowed, with subungual keratinous debris. Onychomycosis appears on lateral nail margins as a yellow discoloration. Increased nail thickness and distortion usually occur over time.[4]

DIAGNOSTICS

The diagnosis of all fungal infections is based on clinical features and simple diagnostic procedures. The potassium hydroxide (KOH) microscopy preparation is a valuable, cost-effective tool that provides rapid confirmation of many types of fungal infections.[5] The key to a reliable KOH preparation is properly obtaining an adequate specimen by scraping the active, leading border of a lesion. The provider should use a No. 15 blade to scrape the lesion gently, collecting the scrapings on a glass slide, and then place several drops of a 10% to 20% solution of KOH directly on the collected scale and apply a coverslip. Next, the provider should gently heat the sample and examine it under a microscope, looking for the diagnostic branching appearance typically seen with these organisms, which indicates a positive result. The provider should note that a negative KOH result does not exclude dermatophyte infections.

Fungal cultures can help detect infection in the absence of a positive KOH result. Dermatophytes can take a few weeks to grow in fungal cultures. A Wood lamp can be used to screen for tinea capitis caused by certain fungal species; these species fluoresce in the long-wave ultraviolent light produced by the Wood lamp. However, *Trichophyton tonsurans,* the most common cause of tinea capitis in the United States, does not fluoresce.[5]

DIAGNOSTICS

Dermatophyte Infections

LABORATORY
- KOH preparation of nail scraping
- Skin culture on Sabouraud medium*
- Wood lamp examination*
- Skin or nail biopsy*

*If indicated.

DIFFERENTIAL DIAGNOSIS

See the Differential Diagnosis box.

DIFFERENTIAL DIAGNOSIS

Dermatophyte Infections

- Atopic dermatitis
- Figurate erythemas
- Granulomatous dermatoses
- Papulosquamous eruptions
- Psoriasis
- Skin cancer
- Urticaria
- Alopecia areata
- Impetigo
- Pediculosis
- Cutaneous lupus erythematosus
- Erythema multiforme
- Pityriasis rosea
- Secondary syphilis
- Candidal intertrigo
- Contact dermatitis
- Dyshidrosis

MANAGEMENT

The treatment of tinea infections consists of removal of the infecting organisms. Acute, exudative lesions are treated with drying agents such as aluminum sulfate (Domeboro) soaks. Topical antifungal solutions and creams reduce superficial scaling and organisms; keratolytic agents remove the thick scales on the hands and feet, allowing topical antifungal agents to penetrate better. Topical applications are available to treat dermatophyte infections (Table 54-1); these medications include terbinafine

TABLE 54-1 Examples of Treatments

Recommended Application to Affected Areas		Indicated for				
		Tinea (Pedis Cruris, or Corporis)	Candidiasis	Tinea Versicolor	Tinea Unguium	Tinea Capitis
Clotrimazole (Lotrimin)	Twice daily	X	X	X		
Miconazole (Monistat-Derm)	Once to twice daily	X	X	X		
Ketoconazole (Nizoral)	Once daily	X	X	X		X
Oxiconazole (Oxistat)	Once daily	X				
Ciclopirox (Loprox)	Twice daily	X	X	X		
Nystatin (Mycostatin)	Twice daily		X			
Butenafine (Mentax)	Once daily	X		X		
Econazole (Spectazole)	Once to twice daily	X	X	X		
Itraconazole (Sporanox)	Once daily	X			X	X
Griseofulvin	Once daily	X			X	X
Luliconazole (Luzu)	Once daily	X				
Fluconazole (Diflucan)	Weekly		X		X	X
Terbinafine (Lamisil)	Once to twice daily	X		X	X	X

GENERAL CONSIDERATIONS

Clinical improvement may be seen fairly soon after initiation of treatment. Twice-daily applications, when indicated, should be done morning and evening. In general, all infections should be treated for 2 weeks after infection has resolved to reduce the possibility of recurrence. Tinea pedis, tinea unguium, and tinea capitis require 6 weeks or more of treatment.

Data from Topical antifungal agents for tinea infections, *Pharm Lett Prescr Lett* 30(5), 2014.

(Lamisil), naftifine (Naftin), butenafine (Mentax), clotrimazole (Lotrimin), econazole (Ecoza), ketoconazole (Nizoral), luliconazole (Luzu), miconazole OTC, oxiconazole (Oxistat), sertaconazole (Ertaczo), ciclopirox (Penlac), and tolnaftate (Tinactin). The products should be continued 1 week after clearing of the lesions to discourage recurrence; however, recurrence of tinea infections is common.[6] Oral ketoconazole (Nizoral) should be avoided because of risks of hepatotoxicity and serious drug interations.[7] Multiple randomized controlled trials provide evidence that tinea pedis (athlete's foot) can be treated successfully with over-the-counter terbinafine.[8]

Oral Medications

Systemic antifungal medications are used for widespread tinea or infections that involve the nails or scalp. A long-standing treatment of tinea capitis is griseofulvin for 2 to 4 months or for 2 weeks after negative KOH or culture results are obtained. Griseofulvin needs to be taken with high-fat food for complete absorption. Antifungal agents such as terbinafine and fluconazole (Diflucan) are effective within 2 to 4 weeks of therapy.[8] The use of oral medications requires careful dosage calculation and monitoring for potential side effects. Again, oral ketoconazole should not be considered because of the risk of serious drug interactions and hepatotoxicity.[7] Treatment should not be considered complete until a follow-up negative fungal culture is obtained.[5]

Onychomycosis may be treated with oral terbinafine or with oral itraconazole (Sporanox). The oral dose of terbinafine is 250 mg daily, 6 weeks for fingernail onychomycosis and 12 weeks for toenail involvement.[8] Terbinafine is not recommended for patients with a history of renal or liver dysfunction. Monitoring of liver function is required every 6 weeks or if the patient experiences nausea, anorexia, or fatigue during therapy. Neutropenia has been reported as a side effect of terbinafine therapy; therefore a complete blood count should be performed every 6 weeks or if there are symptoms suggestive of neutropenia.[8]

Varied dosage regimens are used with oral itraconazole. One regimen is 200 mg daily for 12 weeks for toenail involvement and 200 mg twice daily for 1 week, then 3 weeks off, and then 200 mg daily for 1 additional week for fingernail involvement.[8] The provider should monitor the patient for any hepatic dysfunction. A careful and complete drug history should be taken before therapy is initiated with itraconazole; itraconazole is metabolized by the cytochrome P-450 3A4 (CYP3A4) system and affects the cytochrome P-450 enzyme system, creating many drug interactions.[9] Note that topical therapy for onychomycosis is relatively ineffective. Neither the oral nor the topical form of oral terbinafine or oral itraconazole is recommended for pregnant or nursing women. Unfortunately, the recurrence of onychomycosis is high, even with compliant therapy.

Herbal therapies for onychomycosis have little evidence of effectiveness. Oral herbal therapies may also cause unknown drug interactions or side effects. A few natural antifungals include Mycozil, olive leaf oil, pau d'arco oregano oil, garlic, horopito, lemongrass, and *Bacillus laterosporus*.[10]

COMPLICATIONS

An uncommon complication of tinea capitis is the formation of a kerion, a boggy, exudative area on the scalp, caused by a hypersensitivity reaction to the fungus. Kerion formations (tinea capitis) may result in permanent hair loss and scarring.[5] Fungal infections can also be complicated by bacterial superinfections.

Other complications are associated with side effects and drug interactions with oral antifungal medications.

INDICATIONS FOR REFERRAL OR HOSPITALIZATION

Dermatophyte infections usually respond at least partially to treatment. Severe infections or infections that do not respond to treatment require a referral to a dermatologist. A referral to a dermatologist or dermatology nurse practitioner is recommended for treatment with oral antifungal medications.

PATIENT AND FAMILY EDUCATION

Patients should be cautioned about the use of over-the-counter steroid creams for tinea infections because prolonged use of topical steroids may cause thinning of the skin or striae.[5] Absorbent powders help reduce moisture and prevent reinfection. Tinea of the scalp requires cleaning of combs, towels, and bedding to prevent reinfection. These items should not be shared. Patients should be encouraged to take antifungals for the duration as directed to prevent recurrence.[5]

TINEA VERSICOLOR

DEFINITION AND EPIDEMIOLOGY

Tinea versicolor is a chronic, asymptomatic, and superficial fungal infection. Tinea versicolor is more common during the years of high sebaceous gland activity (teens and young adults).

PATHOPHYSIOLOGY

The causative organism of tinea versicolor is *Malassezia furfur*. *Pityrosporum orbiculare* is the yeast form of the organism. The fungus is found on normal skin, and the infection is caused by a change in the host's resistance to this organism. Tinea versicolor causes lesions in some individuals during periods of high heat and humidity. Thus the condition is more prevalent during the summer and in hot, humid regions. Exposure to sunlight often initiates an episode.[11,12]

CLINICAL PRESENTATION AND PHYSICAL EXAMINATION

Lesions vary in color and are either white or light pink in the hypopigmented version or tan or brown in the hyperpigmented version. They are slightly scaly and are round or oval coalescing papules and plaques. The usual sites for these lesions are the sternal region; the sides of the chest, abdomen, or back; the pubis; and the intertriginous areas. Hypopigmented lesions are more noticeable in darkly pigmented skin. Patients should be reassured that repigmentation will occur after treatment and with exposure to natural sunlight. However, this process can take several months.

DIAGNOSTICS

DIAGNOSTICS

Tinea Versicolor

LABORATORY
KOH preparation
Skin culture*

*If indicated.

Diagnosis is by KOH examination, which reveals numerous short, straight hyphae and clusters of round, budding yeast; this configuration is commonly referred to as "spaghetti and meatballs." A KOH examination may be falsely negative if the patient has just showered. If the diagnosis is still in question, skin scrapings may be obtained for fungal culture on lipid-containing medium.[5]

DIFFERENTIAL DIAGNOSIS

Vitiligo, pityriasis alba, pityriasis rosea, and small plaque parapsoriasis should be considered in the differential diagnosis. Lesions may resemble seborrheic dermatitis, but tinea versicolor most commonly affects the trunk, neck, and upper extremities, whereas seborrheic dermatitis affects hairy body areas. Although it is uncommon, secondary syphilis should be considered in the differential diagnosis.[5]

DIFFERENTIAL DIAGNOSIS

Tinea Versicolor

- Pityriasis alba
- Pityriasis rosea
- Vitiligo
- Seborrheic dermatitis
- Secondary syphilis
- Viral exanthem

MANAGEMENT

Common antifungal creams, such as the imidazoles, are useful in treating tinea versicolor (see Table 54-1). Medication is applied to the entire torso during active infections to eliminate subclinical lesions. Oral antifungal agents can also be used. Topical shampoos or suspensions containing selenium sulfide or pyrithione zinc are affordable and effective in treatment or prophylaxis. Shampoos are applied to affected areas, allowed to dry, and rinsed away after remaining in place approximately 10 minutes. This treatment is repeated for 7 to 14 consecutive days during active infections, followed by periodic use of these shampoos or soaps if the patient is prone to frequent infections. Specific instructions should be reviewed with patients with every product or drug. Perspiration may improve the distribution of oral medications on the skin surface, and refraining from bathing for at least 12 hours is recommended.[5]

COMPLICATIONS

Complications are unusual, although drug-drug interactions are possible with the systemic antifungal medications.[9] Careful review of the patient's current medications is essential, particularly if fluconazole will be prescribed. Some patients may develop *Malassezia* folliculitis, although this disorder usually resolves with topical therapy.

INDICATIONS FOR REFERRAL OR HOSPITALIZATION

A referral is not usually necessary. Rashes recalcitrant to treatment require a dermatology referral for reconsideration of the diagnosis.

PATIENT AND FAMILY EDUCATION

Patients should understand that tinea versicolor commonly recurs but is not a serious disorder. It is more common in warmer climates and often flares during summer months. The regular use of any selenium sulfide shampoo for 10 minutes each day for a week followed by consistent biweekly treatments will often prevent recurrences.[13]

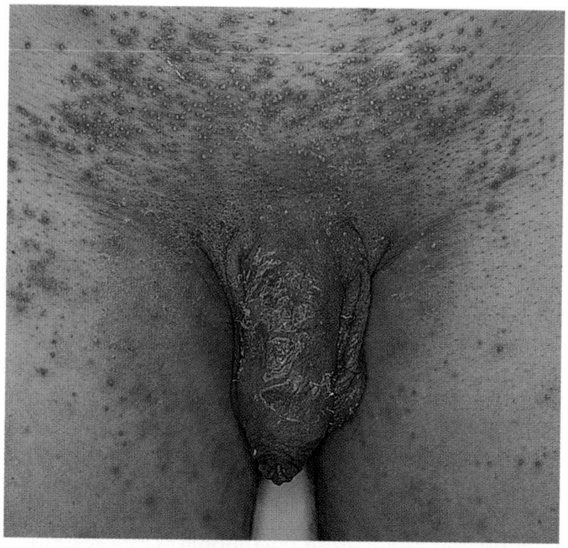

FIGURE 54-4 Moniliasis (candidiasis). (From Fisher BK, Margesson LJ: *Genital skin disorders: diagnosis and treatment,* St Louis, 1998, Mosby.)

CANDIDIASIS

PATHOPHYSIOLOGY

Candida albicans, a yeast, can normally be found on mucous membranes, in the gastrointestinal tract, in the vagina, and on the skin (Fig. 54-4). Candida is usually an opportunistic organism. It is able to behave like a pathogen usually only in the presence of immunosuppression or in intertriginous areas. Predisposing factors to candidal infection include obesity, medications such as antibiotics and corticosteroids, malnutrition, diabetes and other endocrine diseases, and immunosuppressed conditions including HIV and acquired immunodeficiency syndrome (AIDS). A local environment that is warm, moist, macerated, or occluded favors the growth of this organism.[14]

CLINICAL PRESENTATION AND PHYSICAL EXAMINATION

The clinical appearance of candidiasis depends on its location. Candidiasis of the mucous membranes is called *thrush.* Thrush appears as white or gray membranous plaques that are adherent to the buccal mucosa. If the plaques are scraped away, the base is macerated and brightly erythematous. The lesions can extend down the esophagus and to the lips and corners of the mouth. Perlèche, or angular cheilitis, is a fissuring and maceration of the corners of the mouth. The common causes of perlèche include candidal infection, bacterial infection, and irritant dermatitis.[5]

Common sites of skin infection with *Candida* organisms are axillary, gluteal, interdigital, perianal or diaper region, beneath pendulous breasts and panniculus folds, shaved areas (e.g., folliculitis of the beard), vagina, and glans penis (see Fig. 54-4). These intertriginous candidiasis lesions are usually pink or red moist patches bordered by a thin collarette of scale. They are sometimes surrounded by characteristic satellite pustules. Vaginal thrush causes intense itching and often a "cheesy" vaginal discharge. Candidal paronychia, or nail fold infection, is an inflammation of the nail fold. There is rounding and lifting of the nail fold, sometimes with a pus discharge. The nail can become thickened and discolored over time. Untreated severe candidiasis in any location has the potential to cause fungal septicemia in an immunocompromised patient.[14] Older persons are especially susceptible to fungal infection including vulvovaginal infection, cutaneous candidiasis, and balanitis.[15] Elderly persons experience a higher risk of morbidity, including systemic fungal infections. Systemic candidiasis in the elderly may cause vague symptomology and progress to multisystem organ failure, making diagnosis vital yet challenging.[14]

DIAGNOSTICS

The diagnosis of candidiasis is based on clinical appearance, microscopic evaluation with a KOH preparation to look for budding yeast with or without hyphae, or fungal culture. Positive skin or mucous membrane cultures are not diagnostic if not confirmed by microscopic evaluation.[5]

DIAGNOSTICS

Candidiasis

LABORATORY	Skin culture*
KOH preparation	Skin biopsy*

*If indicated.

DIFFERENTIAL DIAGNOSIS

The differential diagnosis depends on the affected area.[14]

DIFFERENTIAL DIAGNOSIS

Candidiasis

ORAL PHARYNX
- Aphthous ulcers, geographic tongue
- Leukoplakia

INTERTRIGINOUS AREAS
- Miliaria
- Bacterial infection (erysipelas or cellulitis)
- Erythrasma
- Seborrheic dermatitis
- Atopic dermatitis
- Tinea cruris
- Inverse psoriasis
- Mycosis fungoides
- Scabies

FEMALE GENITALS
- Bacterial vaginosis
- Trichomoniasis
- Allergic contact dermatitis
- Pediculosis pubis

MALE GENITALS
- Bacterial infection
- Psoriasis
- Tinea

NAILS
- Bacterial infection
- Tinea

MANAGEMENT

The treatment of candidiasis is aimed at elimination of both the predisposing factors and the organism. In the elderly, avoiding hyperglycemia and maintaining skin integrity is important for prevention. A variety of agents—powders, vaginal douches, oral suspensions, creams, and tablets—are commonly used for the treatment of candidal infections (see Table 54-1). Superficial infections should usually be treated with topical therapy. If the infection is so widespread that the use of topical agents is impractical or too expensive, oral fluconazole is appropriate and has received a high level of support from evidence-based research.[15]

COMPLICATIONS

The most serious complication of candidiasis is fungal septicemia, which may be seen in immunocompromised patients. Candidal esophagitis is a potential complication of antibiotic therapy or may be noted in patients who are severely immunocompromised, particularly patients with AIDS.

INDICATIONS FOR REFERRAL OR HOSPITALIZATION

Treatment is usually effective, and a referral is not indicated. The differential diagnosis of candidal infection is large, however. Therefore, infections recalcitrant to treatment require a physician or dermatologist referral to look for other causes of the eruption. Patients with yeast septicemia or other systemic manifestations of infection also require a physician consultation.

PATIENT AND FAMILY EDUCATION

Methods for reducing environmental factors that encourage heat, moisture, maceration, and trauma should be emphasized: drying thoroughly after bathing (especially in the axillae and toe webs and between and under the breasts), wearing absorbent materials such as cotton underwear and socks, changing socks frequently, avoiding constrictive clothing, not wearing the same shoes each day, and wearing sandals in warm weather to promote air exposure to the affected skin.

During active infections or in the hope of preventing recurrence, a simple talc powder or antifungal powder (tolnaftate or miconazole) should be applied to intertriginous or interdigital areas twice daily. Aluminum sulfate (Domeboro solution) is an over-the-counter product and helps with drying of excessively moist areas. With the reintroduction of many powders that contain cornstarch, it is extremely important to inform patients who are prone to fungal infections to avoid cornstarch-containing products because this substance encourages fungal growth.

Patients using oral steroid inhalers should understand the importance of rinsing the oral cavity after use of these inhalers.[9] Yogurt with live cultures, or other sources of probiotics daily, help prevent vaginal or oral yeast infections.[16]

CHAPTER 55

HERPES ZOSTER (SHINGLES)

Glen Blair

DEFINITION AND EPIDEMIOLOGY

Herpes zoster (shingles) is a dermatologic eruption caused by reactivation of the varicella-zoster virus (VZV) that follows, sometimes by decades, a primary varicella-zoster (chickenpox) infection. A prodrome of pain or dysesthesia may precede by several days a vesicular eruption that typically occurs in a unilateral dermatomal distribution. Vesicular lesions appear during several days and may last for 7 to 10 days or more, although they can last for more than 4 weeks on rare occasions. The eruption can be extremely painful, and 5% to 20% of patients go on to develop a protracted pain syndrome called postherpetic neuralgia (PHN).[1]

One in three persons will develop zoster during their lifetime, roughly 1 million Americans per year.[2] After primary infection, VZV lies dormant in the sensory root ganglion, kept in check by the host's acquired cell-mediated immunity. The zoster eruption results from reactivation of the latent varicella infection in the dorsal root or cranial nerve ganglion cells, a process that is thought to be caused by an age-related decline in cell-mediated immunity.[3] Zoster incidence is seen to increase with age and immune suppression.

Zoster is common and usually self-limited in adults, but serious complications can occur that may require consultation. Involvement of the ophthalmic branch of the trigeminal nerve can result in ocular keratitis, scarring, and loss of vision. Patients who are immunocompromised may have a disseminated infection that can result in a diffuse varicella-like eruption, neurologic complications, or visceral involvement that can cause death, most commonly from pneumonia.[2]

PATHOPHYSIOLOGY

After initial varicella infection, the virus lies dormant in the dorsal root ganglia. Once it is reactivated, the virus replicates and travels through the axons, spreading from cell to cell until it penetrates the epidermis. Reactivation is likely to be multifactorial, age being the most important risk factor. Immunosuppressed individuals of all types are at increased risk, as are some populations with chronic comorbid diseases, such as rheumatoid arthritis and inflammatory bowel disease. Trauma, surgery, and a recent cancer diagnosis have also been linked to zoster reactivation. Anecdotal references to stress as a cause have not been supported by research, but those with severe physical limitations as well as older women are certainly at higher risk.[2]

Herpes zoster lesions contain high concentrations of virus that can be spread by contact and by air but are less contagious than primary infection. Contagion is possible once the rash has appeared and continues until the lesions have crusted.

CLINICAL PRESENTATION AND PHYSICAL EXAMINATION

Zoster classically is seen as a unilateral eruption within one dermatome; however, 20% of the time, an adjacent dermatome will be involved. The eruption is often preceded by a prodrome of pain, dysesthesia, or pruritus in the affected dermatome. Pain can be described as stabbing, burning, aching, or excruciating. The eruption is initially erythematous and maculopapular and becomes clusters of clear vesicles during the course of several hours (Fig. 55-1). New lesions may continue to develop for several days. Low-grade fever and lymphadenopathy may be present. The most common areas of involvement are the thoracic, cranial (especially the trigeminal), and lumbar nerves. On the rare occasion that there is no visible eruption, a condition called zoster sine herpete, the pain is sometimes attributed to other causes (e.g., angina, renal colic, pleural pain, sciatica, or migraine), depending on the dermatome affected. There is lack of consensus as to how long after rash resolution the pain needs to persist to be considered PHN. Regardless, pain can exist in varying degrees for many years.

DIAGNOSTICS

Diagnosis is based on the clinical presentation of a vesicular eruption in a unilateral, dermatomal distribution. Without the

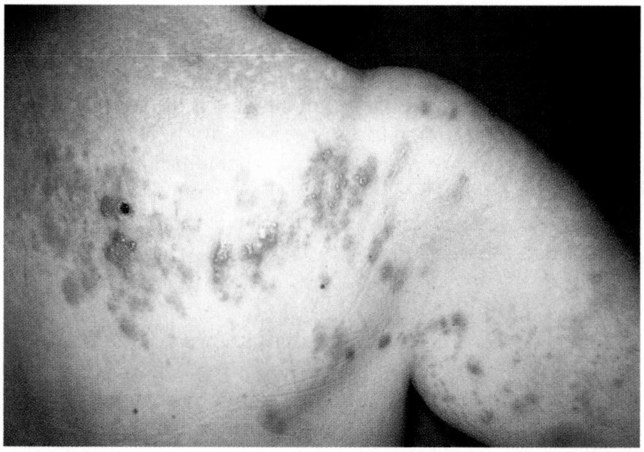

FIGURE 55-1 Herpes zoster. (From Ignatavicius DD, Workman ML, *Medical-Surgical Nursing: Patient Centered Collaborative Care*, ed 8, St. Louis, 2016, Mosby.)

skin eruption, zoster is a diagnosis of exclusion. Disseminated herpes zoster is a generalized eruption of lesions along with the typical segmental distribution and occurs primarily in immunocompromised individuals.

DIAGNOSTICS

Herpes Zoster

Tzanck preparation
DFA test
PCR analysis
Culture

A Tzanck test is a rapid way to confirm the diagnosis of zoster in the provider's office but does not distinguish between VZV and herpes simplex virus. The direct fluorescent antibody (DFA) test is another rapid test that is available in some settings. Polymerase chain reaction (PCR) analysis, although not available in all settings, is rapid and sensitive. All of these tests are preferred to viral culture because they are more rapid and often more sensitive.[4]

DIFFERENTIAL DIAGNOSIS

The pain associated with zoster can precede the eruption by 4 or 5 days. Depending on the distribution, the pain may mimic angina, renal colic, or pleuritic pain. Once the eruption is present, the cause of the pain is more obvious. The presentation of primary varicella can be similar to that of disseminated zoster, and serologic testing may be needed in the absence of a known history of chickenpox. Eczema herpeticum is an infection of herpes simplex virus inoculated into a patch of eczema, resulting in a more widely distributed herpes simplex virus infection. A DFA test, PCR analysis, or viral culture will differentiate the two.[4] Any of the numerous other vesicle-producing dermatoses, such as coxsackievirus infection, impetigo, contact dermatitis, and dermatitis herpetiformis, should be considered in the differential diagnosis.[5]

DIFFERENTIAL DIAGNOSIS

Herpes Zoster

- Coxsackievirus infection
- Contact dermatitis
- Dermatitis herpetiformis
- Eczema herpeticum
- Impetigo
- Varicella

MANAGEMENT

The treatment of uncomplicated herpes zoster is symptomatic treatment of lesions and prevention of secondary infection. Antiviral therapy is an important part of zoster therapy. Studies have shown that initiation of antiviral therapy (acyclovir, famciclovir, and valacyclovir) within 72 hours of rash onset reduces the duration and severity of both the rash and the pain and reduces the risk for PHN for localized and disseminated disease. Each of these medications is effective; the choice is often based on cost and convenience of administration. Dosages may need to be adjusted for renal impairment.[2,5]

The use of prophylactic oral corticosteroids has not been shown to prevent the development of PHN, although a 3-week tapering course may modestly reduce the duration and severity of pain and could be considered on a case-by-case basis.[5]

Analgesic agents may be administered if necessary. Narcotics may be required. Topical cool moist compresses and agents, such as calamine and aluminum sulfate (Domeboro) soaks, are soothing and will help dry vesicles. Other topical treatments including lidocaine patches, nonsteroidal anti-inflammatories patches, and capsaicin creams can also be helpful.[5] Patients should be instructed to keep the area clean and dry, to avoid the topical antibiotics bacitracin and neomycin because of the high incidence of allergic contact dermatitis,[6] and, if possible, to keep the rash covered.

COMPLICATIONS

Herpes zoster lesions on the tip of the nose, around the eyes, and on the forehead require immediate ophthalmology consultation and evaluation. These findings signal possible involvement of the branch of the trigeminal nerve that innervates the cornea, which may cause ulceration on the cornea and result in permanent damage. Motor paralysis and facial palsy (Ramsay Hunt syndrome) may follow herpes zoster. Immunosuppressed individuals may develop dissemination, pneumonia, hepatitis, meningoencephalitis, and purpura fulminans.[3,5] Patients with disseminated zoster should be evaluated for malignant disease, immunodeficiency, or acquired immunodeficiency syndrome (AIDS).

PHN is the most common complication of zoster. Numerous treatments are available to manage the pain associated with PHN, including oral analgesics such as acetaminophen, nonsteroidal anti-inflammatory drugs, and opiates. Topically applied lidocaine and capsaicin have been used successfully to reduce the pain of PHN. Anticonvulsants such as gabapentin and pregabalin are effective for treatment of neuropathic pain and have a more favorable side effect profile than their older predecessors carbamazepine and valproic acid. The tricyclic antidepressants nortriptyline and amitriptyline are also effective, but their use is limited by side effects.

LIFE SPAN CONSIDERATIONS

In 2006, the Food and Drug Administration approved Zostavax, a live, attenuated vaccine for the prevention of zoster in patients older than 60 years. (Zostavax is a higher-potency form of Varivax vaccine.) The Advisory Committee on Immunization Practices at the Centers for Disease Control and Prevention issued the recommendation in 2008 (and updated it in 2013) dose of VZV vaccine regardless of chickenpox history.[7] The vaccination appears to be most effective in the 60- to 69-year age group; a significant reduction in incidence of zoster (54%) and PHN was realized (61% measured at 30 days).[8] In patients older than 80 years, protection against zoster occurrence was not as high (18% reduction), but efficacy against PHN was better preserved (39%).[8]

INDICATIONS FOR REFERRAL OR HOSPITALIZATION

Immediate referral to an ophthalmologist is indicated for herpes zoster lesions on the tip of the nose, around the eyes, and on the forehead.

Hospitalization may be necessary for evaluation and treatment of complications.

PATIENT AND FAMILY EDUCATION

Lesions of herpes zoster may contain VZV, enabling transmission to susceptible individuals (including infants and women of childbearing age who have not had the varicella vaccine or previous varicella infection). Herpes zoster itself is not transmissible, but VZV-naive patients are at risk for primary varicella (chickenpox) infection. Patients should avoid direct contact with susceptible persons and cover active lesions until they have crusted over, indicating that the lesions are no longer contagious. Patients and family must be alerted to the possibility of PHN and be advised to seek appropriate medical attention if pain persists after the rash has cleared.

Anyone older than 60 years with no contraindications to live vaccines should be considered for VZV vaccination during routine health maintenance visits. The vaccine has been approved by the U.S. Food and Drug Administration for patients 50 to 59 years of age, but it is currently not recommended that these patients be routinely vaccinated.[7] Individual consideration must be used in this population.

CHAPTER 56

HIDRADENITIS SUPPURATIVA (ACNE INVERSA)

Maria Isabel Romano

DEFINITION AND EPIDEMIOLOGY

Hidradenitis suppurativa, also referred to as *acne inversa* or *cicatrizing perifolliculitis,* has long been considered a disease of the apocrine glands. Histopathologic research indicates that the primary lesion is infundibular hyperkeratosis of sebaceous gland follicles with secondary infection of the apocrine glands.[1] The presence of inflamed perifollicular and subepidermal CD3, CD4, CD68, CD79, and CD8 lymphocytes indicates a cell-mediated cause of this disorder.[1] This chronic disease is characterized by recurrent abscesses, draining sinus tracts, and comedones and may be found in association with severe nodulocystic acne and pilonidal sinuses.[2] The prevalence of hidradenitis is greater in females, with genitofemoral lesions being most common; axillary lesions are found equally in males and females, and anogenital lesions are found more commonly in males.[3,4] Case studies indicate that the onset of hidradenitis is associated with the production of adrenal androgens, dehydroepiandrosterone, and androstenedione at the time of adrenarche.[2] All ethnic groups are affected. A hereditary predisposition has been noted in females, with mother-daughter transmission being most common, and a familial autosomal dominant tendency exists.[2]

PATHOPHYSIOLOGY

The exact cause of hidradenitis is not known and is controversial. Theories of causation include keratin plugging of the apocrine ducts and a primary failure of the apocrine glands to drain effectively. An association with immunosuppression is cited in the literature.[2,3] With keratin plugging, the apocrine duct and hair follicle are occluded by keratin, which causes increased ductal pressure and inflammation. Bacteria cause the ducts to rupture and, with extension of infection, lead to cyst, sinus tract, and fistula formation. *Acne inversa* is proposed as a more appropriate name for this disease because in the early stages, the pathogenic change occurs in the pilosebaceous ducts, similar to the pathogenesis of acne.[2] Deep cultures of active lesions in hidradenitis suppurativa are often polymicrobial. The most commonly isolated bacteria are *Staphylococcus aureus, Staphylococcus epidermidis,* and *Staphylococcus hominis.*[5,6] Other organisms implicated include *Escherichia coli, Proteus mirabilis, Pseudomonas aeruginosa,* and streptococci.[6]

CLINICAL PRESENTATION

The hallmarks of hidradenitis suppurativa are single or multiple areas of swelling, pain, and erythema accompanied by acute abscess formation. The active phase of the disease is preceded by the appearance of double or triple black comedones on the affected skin surface (Fig. 56-1). The condition often progresses to a chronic state of pain, sepsis, sinus tract and fistula formation, purulent discharge, and keloids. Disfiguring scar formation marks long-standing hidradenitis. Patients usually give a history of multiple episodes of repeated abscesses that have been drained and treated with antibiotic medications for a period of years. Unlike acne, the disease is unrelenting and often

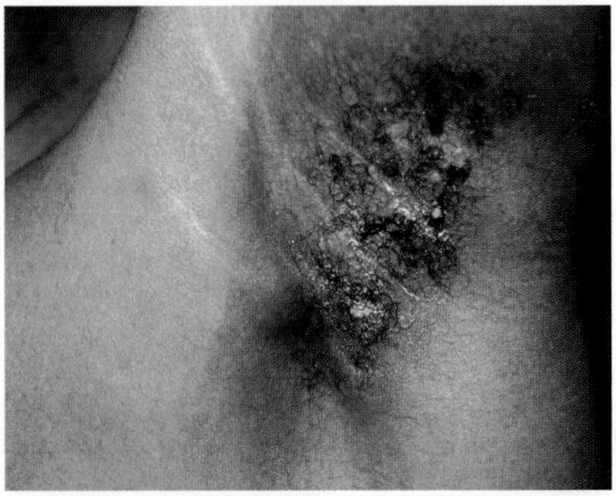

FIGURE 56-1 Hidradenitis suppurative (acne inversa). Erythematous papules, cysts, nodules, and sinus tracts are seen in the axilla of this adolescent boy. (From Paller AS, Mancini AJ: *Hurwitz clinical pediatric dermatology,* ed 4, St Louis, 2011, Elsevier.)

BOX 56-1

Hurley Stages

Stage I: Abscess formation (single or multiple) without sinus tracts and cicatrization
Stage II: One or more widely separated recurrent abscesses with tract formation and scars
Stage III: Multiple interconnected tracts and abscesses throughout an entire area

progressive, leaving hypertrophic scars that form a basket-weave configuration accented by marked erythema beneath the breast and in the axillary, suprapubic, groin, and anogenital regions. Sinus tracts form under the skin in which connecting, inflamed, and plugged glands drain into one another and trap bacteria. Patients are concerned about the cause of the problem and may fear they have a malignant disease. Predisposing factors include obesity, dissecting cellulitis of the scalp, smoking, hirsutism, history of acne, use of lithium, and hyperandrogenism.[3,5] Remissions of a spontaneous nature are noted in patients older than 35 years.[6]

PHYSICAL EXAMINATION

The lesions are palpated to determine their readiness for incision and drainage. The axillae, groin, perianal region, buttocks, chest, inframammary area, and back are examined to determine the involvement and extent of the disease. Hurley stages are used to classify the severity of the disease (Box 56-1).[2,3]

DIAGNOSTICS

The initial diagnosis is based on clinical observation. Lesions that are actively discharging are cultured, and sensitivity tests are performed. A skin biopsy is performed for patients with stubborn cases or suspicious lesions. Laboratory tests may be needed to exclude other, more serious underlying diseases.

DIAGNOSTICS

Hidradenitis Suppurativa

LABORATORY
Culture and sensitivity of lesions with discharge

OTHER
Skin biopsy

DIFFERENTIAL DIAGNOSIS

The differential diagnosis for early-stage hidradenitis suppurativa includes furuncle, carbuncle, lymphadenitis, bacterial folliculitis, inclusion cyst, and cat-scratch disease. In the later stages, the differential diagnosis includes granuloma inguinale, lymphogranuloma venereum, squamous cell carcinoma, regional enteritis, cutaneous tuberculosis, sinus tracts, and fistulas associated with ulcerative colitis.[3,5,6]

DIFFERENTIAL DIAGNOSIS

Hidradenitis Suppurativa

- Bacterial folliculitis
- Bacterial furunculosis
- Cat-scratch disease
- Lymphadenitis
- Scrofuloderma
- Granuloma inguinale
- Lymphogranuloma venereum
- Squamous cell carcinoma
- Cutaneous tuberculosis
- Regional enteritis

MANAGEMENT

There are a variety of treatment measures, including the following topical, oral, and surgical interventions. A combination approach to treatment is advocated, including steroids, antibiotics, traditional surgery, carbon dioxide (CO_2) laser surgery, monoclonal antibody therapy, and isotretinoin.

Fluctuant abscesses in which the skin has become thin and the underlying mass is soft can be surgically incised and drained in the health care provider's office. A local anesthetic with 1% to 2% lidocaine with or without epinephrine is provided through a 30-gauge needle and a 1- to 3-mL syringe. The sting of lidocaine can be buffered by preparing a mixture of 1 mL of sodium bicarbonate with 9 mL of lidocaine. A pointed, lance-shaped No. 11 surgical blade is recommended for incision. The blade is inserted parallel to the skin lines, cutting across the thin area of skin and creating an opening through which purulent material can drain. Pressure is applied to the surrounding tissue to facilitate drainage. A curet drawn back and forth through the abscess will loosen adhesions and aid in the removal of necrotic material. A semiocclusive sterile dressing with a thin film of topical bacitracin should then be applied. Care must be taken to cleanse the area daily with soap and water; the dressing is reapplied for 3 to 5 days.

Smaller nodules can be injected with triamcinolone acetonide, 3 to 5 mg/mL diluted with lidocaine, followed by a course of oral antibiotics. Larger cysts can be injected with triamcinolone, 3 to 5 mg/mL, directly into the wall of the lesion, and later incised. Low-grade inflammation is responsive to oral antibiotics, but long-term treatment is necessary before clinical remission is evident. Erythromycin (250 to 500 mg four times a day), tetracycline (250 to 500 mg four times a day), or minocycline (100 mg twice a day) should be considered. Higher doses of antibiotics should be used during an active flare; lower doses can be used long term to maintain control.[7] Remission of up to 4 years has been achieved with a 10-week course of rifampin, 300 mg twice daily, and clindamycin, 300 mg twice daily.[7] Topical isotretinoin cream 0.05% may be efficacious in relieving keratin plugging of the apocrine glands.[7] Isotretinoin, 1 mg/kg/day for 20 weeks, may be tried under co-management with a physician in the early stages of the disease or as an adjunct to surgical intervention, although it has a very limited therapeutic effect when it is used as monotherapy.[7] Because of the teratogenic effects of this medication, all women must be screened for pregnancy before taking isotretinoin and protected against pregnancy while taking the medication. For severe pain and inflammation, a tapering dose of 70 mg of prednisone for 2 or 3 days and tapered during a 14-day period is prescribed.[6] Finasteride, 5 mg daily, has also been used as an effective monotherapy in men and postmenopausal women; women of childbearing age can be treated with dapsone.[5,7]

Co-Management with Specialists

A referral to a dermatologist is recommended for patients with hidradenitis that is recalcitrant to traditional oral therapy or for patients with recurrent lesions after incision and drainage. Newer treatment approaches used by these specialists include CO_2

and infliximab (Remicade), a chimeric monoclonal antibody with high affinity for tumor necrosis factor-α. Laser treatment of moderate-stage hidradenitis suppurativa is an effective noninvasive alternative for patients who wish to avoid systemic therapies.[8] Patients treated with oral isotretinoin, 1 mg/kg/day for 20 weeks, may be co-managed with a nurse practitioner or physician assistant for the purposes of determining treatment response and monitoring side effects (see Chapter 43 for precautions regarding isotretinoin therapy).

LIFE SPAN CONSIDERATIONS

Onset of hidradenitis suppurativa is usually between the second and fifth decades, with onset as early as puberty in some individuals.[2,3] Many cases of hidradenitis disappear after patients reach 35 years of age.

COMPLICATIONS

The health care provider should be aware of the impact of body image changes on patients with this disease, especially young adolescents. As with any chronic illness, an assessment for clinical depression and threats to self-esteem should be included as part of the ongoing care. Patients may become progressively less social in moderate to severe disease because of embarrassment, foul odor, and chronic pain.[9] Complications other than chronicity are rare, but fistulas from the groin area to the urethra and bladder have been reported.[2,3] Cases of reactive arthritis have been identified in the literature.[10] Vigilant follow-up monitoring is necessary to uncover those patients who fail to respond to treatment. Cases of anogenital squamous cell carcinoma have been diagnosed in patients with long-term hidradenitis.[3] Other complications are related to the treatment regimen. Patients taking large doses of erythromycin may experience damage to their auditory nerve and deafness.

INDICATIONS FOR REFERRAL OR HOSPITALIZATION

Surgical excision is recommended for patients with chronic, recurrent hidradenitis suppurativa that involves sinus tracts and fibrotic scarring. Complete excision of the involved glands and skin grafting may be necessary. CO_2 laser treatments can be performed by a qualified dermatologist skilled in this technique. If surgery will involve extensive surgical resection and reconstruction of the female genitals, the services of a gynecologic oncologist may be required.[11]

PATIENT EDUCATION

Patient education should explain that a clear cause of the disease is not known. Hypothetical causes of the disease process should be discussed. Patients should be reassured that antiperspirants, shaving, underarm deodorants, and depilatories are not implicated as a cause. Topical isotretinoin may cause skin irritation, and caution should be exercised to avoid excessive use. The provider should stress sun sensitivity with the use of isotretinoin and encourage patients to wear appropriate protective clothing while in the sun. Patients should be educated on the side effects of the prescribed antibiotics, including photosensitivity and interaction with oral contraceptives. Patients taking erythromycin must be advised to avoid concurrent ingestion of terfenadine, astemizole, and ketoconazole.

CHAPTER 57

HYPERHIDROSIS

Maria Isabel Romano

DEFINITION AND EPIDEMIOLOGY

Hyperhidrosis is a condition of excessive sweating marked by abnormal wetness, sweaty palms, excessive axillary sweating, gustatory-stimulated sweating, wet shoes, and offensive body odor. Most cases are idiopathic or primary in nature and only rarely indicate an underlying secondary pathologic condition.[1-3]

PATHOPHYSIOLOGY

Perspiration is one of the body's mechanisms for thermal regulation and fluid and electrolyte balance. The center for body temperature regulation is located in the hypothalamus. Cooling perspiration is under hypothalamic control, whereas emotional perspiration is under cerebral control.[4] Sweat glands are located in the hypodermis of the skin. The eccrine duct opens directly onto the surface of the skin. Millions of sweat glands are located in the hypodermis throughout the body, with the largest concentration in the palms, soles, and axillae. Secretions from the eccrine glands function to cool the body. Neural control is anatomically sympathetic. However, sweating is subject to cholinergic control mediated by acetylcholine, not epinephrine.[2] Overactivity of the thoracic sympathetic ganglion may be the underlying cause of non–medically related excessive sweating.

The most common cause of generalized increased sweating is a decline in ovarian function. Changes in neurohumoral function lead to increased stimulation of the hypothalamic thermal regulatory center, leading to the hot flashes associated with menopause. Other factors include fever, underlying infection or malignant disease, peripheral neuropathy or surgical damage to the autonomic nervous system, thyrotoxicosis, Parkinson disease, a variety of medications (including insulin, meperidine, and pilocarpine), and alcohol abuse.[2]

CLINICAL PRESENTATION

The presentation of primary hyperhidrosis is excessive sweating unrelated to ambient heat or humidity. Areas most commonly affected include the palms, soles, and axillae, but the condition may involve any body surface or may take on a unilateral distribution. Concern about the social consequences of this disorder (and its resulting body odor) and embarrassment may create a barrier to intimate relationships or affect the patient's choice of occupation. When the soles are involved, widespread fungal infections of the skin and nails are accompanied by foot odor. More generalized body sweating is associated with an underlying condition, whereas localized sweating confined to the palms, soles, and axillae is more often a response to anxiety or heat or is idiopathic. Episodic sweating may be associated with hypoglycemia. A history of medications, including oral hypoglycemic agents and selective serotonin reuptake inhibitors (SSRIs), and alcohol intake is an important consideration.

PHYSICAL EXAMINATION

Based on the history and presenting complaint, the health care provider should try to locate evidence of any underlying disease process. A complete history is taken and a thorough physical assessment is performed, searching for signs and symptoms of hyperthyroidism. Blood pressure should be measured to exclude high blood pressure associated with pheochromocytoma.[2] Heat intolerance associated with sweating in the upper half of the body and absence of sweating in the lower half of the body is evidence of diabetic peripheral autonomic neuropathy.[5]

In assessing the patient with generalized sweating, the examiner should look for miliaria rubra, an abnormal blocking of the sweat ducts. In this condition, sweat is trapped in the stratum corneum, creating tiny, pinpoint, clear papules that with pressure rupture the sweat ducts, creating an erythematous maculopapular rash. Other associated presentations include dyshidrotic eczema. This is a simple eczema promoted by the retention of sweat in the stratum corneum.

DIAGNOSTICS AND DIFFERENTIAL DIAGNOSIS

Thyroid and fasting blood glucose studies are indicated to exclude thyroid disease and diabetes. If night sweats are present, a purified protein derivative test or interferon-γ release assay (QuantiFERON-TB Gold In-Tube [QFT-GIT] test; T-SPOT) is necessary to exclude tuberculosis. For perimenopausal women with hyperhidrosis, tests for follicle-stimulating hormone and luteinizing hormone are recommended to document menopause and to provide reassurance to the patient. SSRIs may provoke night sweats. A different SSRI should be considered before the drug class is changed.

The most common cause of excessive perspiration is a sympathetic-mediated response to stress. A careful history and examination will indicate the necessity to exclude hyperthyroidism with an ultrasensitive test for thyroid-stimulating hormone (TSH) and thyroxine (T_4). A patient symptom diary of provoking factors, response to foods, body temperature, and amount and location of perspiration is a helpful adjunct in determining the cause of sweating. If infection or malignant disease is suspected, a thorough evaluation is mandated. A tuberculin skin test should be performed for those with complaints of night sweats. A fasting blood glucose study is performed to exclude diabetes mellitus. In women with variations in the length and amount of menses, a search for accompanying symptoms of vasomotor hot flashes and objective evidence of ovarian failure is necessary. Symptoms of sweating and flushing accompanied by marked hypertension require an evaluation for pheochromocytoma. Evidence of central nervous system disease or autonomic peripheral neuropathy warrants referral to a neurologist.

DIAGNOSTICS

Hyperhidrosis

LABORATORY

- TSH, T_4
- Purified protein derivative*
- Fasting blood glucose
- Follicle-stimulating hormone, luteinizing hormone*
- Other tests as indicated to exclude systemic conditions

*If indicated.

DIFFERENTIAL DIAGNOSIS

Hyperhidrosis

- Hyperthyroidism
- Infection
- Malignant disease
- Tuberculosis
- Diabetes mellitus
- Pheochromocytoma
- Alcoholism
- Central nervous system diseases
- Autonomic peripheral neuropathy
- Other hormonal imbalances

MANAGEMENT

Topical applications of a 20% alcoholic solution of aluminum chloride hexahydrate (Drysol, Keralyt) can be effective in decreasing excessive perspiration on the hands, soles, and axillae. These treatments provide for a chemodenervation of the eccrine sweat glands.[3] A less potent solution of 6.25% aluminum chloride hexahydrate (Xerac) can be prescribed for patients who have more sensitive skin. The perspiring area is coated lightly with the solution and allowed to dry. An occlusive wrap is then applied, or vinyl gloves can be worn on the hands and left on for 8 hours, followed by a complete soap-and-water wash of the affected areas. Applications are repeated every 2 or 3 days as tolerated. With satisfactory dryness, maintenance requires a once-weekly application.[2,6]

Liposuction of the axillary sweat glands has been effective,[7,8] as has surgical excision of axillary tissue.[7] Persistent primary palmar hyperhidrosis has shown a positive response to thoracic endoscopic surgery. Bilateral interruption of the upper dorsal sympathetic chain of D2 and D3 can provide a cure for primary hyperhidrosis.[9] Oral medications such as anticholinergic agents, antihypertensive agents, anxiolytics, and antidepressants are rarely used in the management of primary hyperhidrosis and should be used only as a second- or third-line therapy.[10] More recently, a practice guideline was released stating there was minimal compelling evidence that would support the use of systemic anticholinergic agents in a safe and efficacious manner.[10]

Co-Management with Specialists

Consultation with a dermatologist may be useful for patients with hyperhidrosis that is refractory to topical treatments. The dermatologist may try a number of other remedies, including iontophoresis, in which an electrical current may be used to obstruct the sweat ducts.[2,6,10] Botulinum toxin has been found to be effective for hyperhidrosis affecting the axillae and palms and for gustatory sweating.[6] Liposuction has been shown to be effective for axillary hyperhidrosis.[7,8,10] Consideration of these and other treatments warrants consultation with an appropriate specialist. Sweating associated with anxiety or panic attacks warrants co-management with a mental health specialist or neuropsychiatrist.

COMPLICATIONS

Patients with hyperhidrosis may experience difficulty functioning in social or occupational situations as a result of this disorder, significantly affecting their quality of life. Other complications are rare, although patients with sensitive skin may develop reactions to the topical solutions prescribed for treatment. In most instances, decreasing the concentration of the solution will decrease skin irritation. Patients who undergo sympathectomy may experience compensatory sweating.

INDICATIONS FOR REFERRAL OR HOSPITALIZATION

Evidence of an underlying medical condition leading to secondary hyperhidrosis, such as pheochromocytoma, warrants referral. Patients with primary hyperhidrosis refractory to topical treatments are referred for evaluation to a surgeon experienced in thoracoscopic sympathicolysis,[9] liposuction,[6-8] or axillary dissection.[6-8] Patients with excessive perspiration associated with anxiety or panic disorders can benefit from mental health counseling.

PATIENT AND FAMILY EDUCATION

Education is critical to assist patients in coping with and understanding this socially stigmatizing condition. A complete explanation of the etiology of primary hyperhidrosis and an explanation of sympathetic overactivity are provided. Patients need assurance that a search has been conducted for an underlying pathologic reason for the disorder. Results of laboratory tests must be provided. Support in the form of education for family members and significant others is an important aspect of comprehensive care. Good personal hygiene is encouraged for those with axillary sweating. Both open-toe and canvas shoes with cotton socks promote evaporation of foot perspiration while decreasing foot odor and preventing fungal infections of the feet. Occupational environments should be well ventilated and include air conditioning.

CHAPTER 58

INTERTRIGO

JoAnn D. Lepke

DEFINITION AND EPIDEMIOLOGY

Intertrigo is a superficial inflammatory skin disorder that occurs in the setting of persistent skin-to-skin contact, friction, moisture, warmth, and inadequate ventilation. It is usually characterized by varying degrees of erythema, peripheral scaling, and macerated erythematous plaques. Common intertriginous sites include inframammary and abdominal folds, inner thighs, and axillary, interdigital, and perianal areas. Sweat retention, incontinence, immobility, alterations in systemic immunity, systemic antibiotic therapy, and overgrowth of resident microorganisms are related factors. If intertrigo is not treated, affected areas with impaired skin integrity can become secondarily infected with *Candida* (most common), *Staphylococcus aureus, Pseudomonas aeruginosa*, group A β-hemolytic streptococci, or *Corynebacterium minutissimum*.[1,2]

Patients are susceptible to intertrigo at any age, but it is more common in the young and in older adults. Women with vulvovaginitis, men with balanitis, individuals infected with human immunodeficiency virus (HIV), and prolonged steroid users are particularly susceptible.[1] Other predisposing conditions and factors include diaper use, psoriasis, eczema, diabetes, obesity, pregnancy, oral contraceptive use, chemotherapy, and living in hot and humid climates.[2] Obesity is associated with larger skinfolds with thick layers of subcutaneous brown fat, increasing the risk of overheating, friction, and moisture.[1]

PATHOPHYSIOLOGY

Intertrigo is a skin disorder resulting in altered barrier function, which allows opportunistic infections such as yeast, bacteria, or fungi to infiltrate the skin. Moisture and friction are present, causing maceration in the stratum corneum, leading to erosion and skin breakdown and thus creating an opportunity for primary and secondary infections.[3]

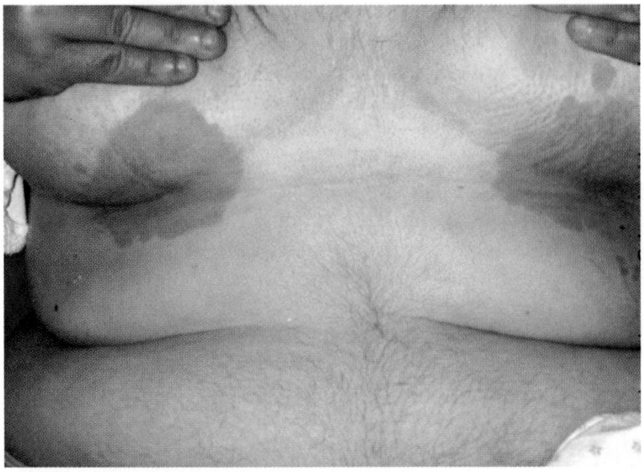

FIGURE 58-1 Intertrigo in inframammary folds without evidence of bacterial infection. (Copyright © Logical Images, Inc.)

Skin in elders and in diabetic and obese individuals has a higher skin surface pH than in other individuals.[3,4] The skin's barrier function may be more easily compromised in this situation, making it more vulnerable to organisms such as yeasts, bacteria, and other pathogens.[1,3,4]

CLINICAL PRESENTATION AND PHYSICAL EXAMINATION

Intertrigo is initially seen as mildly erythematous, moist, glistening plaques, patches, papules, and/or pustules. The borders are well defined, with areas of epidermal erosion and scaling. See Figure 58-1 for an example of inframammary intertrigo without fungal or bacterial infection. Pinpoint pustules outside the border are diagnostically important in candidal infections.[3] Initial symptoms usually include itching, burning, and stinging.[1-3] Odor, copious discharge, severe erythema, acute discomfort, fever, and abscesses may signal secondary infection.[1,2]

DIAGNOSTICS

Diagnosis is typically based on clinical appearance. Scrapings from the lesion may be examined via potassium hydroxide (KOH) wet mount and/or Gram stain.[5] A KOH preparation that is positive for pseudohyphae and budding spores confirms the diagnosis of *Candida* infection. Bacterial or fungal superinfection (e.g., *Staphylococcus*, group A β-hemolytic streptococci, *P. aeruginosa, Proteus mirabilis*) may be identified by culture. Examination with a Wood lamp may indicate erythrasma

DIAGNOSTICS

Intertrigo

LABORATORY
KOH wet mount
Gram stain*
Culture*
Wood lamp examination

*If indicated.

(coral-red fluorescence) or *Pseudomonas* infection (yellow-green fluorescence).[1,3]

DIFFERENTIAL DIAGNOSIS

It is important to determine the underlying cause(s) of the skin eruption, because treatment options vary accordingly.

DIFFERENTIAL DIAGNOSIS

Intertrigo

INFECTIOUS DISEASES
- Candidiasis
- Dermatophytosis
- Erythrasma
- Pyoderma
- Scabies
- Seborrheic dermatitis
- Syphilis
- Cellulitis
- Granuloma inguinale
- Lymphogranuloma venereum

NONINFECTIOUS INFLAMMATORY DISEASES
- Atopic dermatitis
- Contact dermatitis (allergic, irritant)
- Pemphigus vulgaris
- Familial benign pemphigus (Hailey-Haley Disease)
- Granuloma gluteale infantum
- Psoriasis
- Acrodermatitis enteropathica
- Keratosis follicularis

NONINFLAMMATORY DISEASES
- Acanthosis nigricans
- Hidradenitis suppurativa
- Intertrigo
- Lichen sclerosis

NEOPLASMS
- Bowen disease
- Paget disease
- Superficial basal cell carcinoma

Data from Kalra MG, Higgins KE, Kinney BS: Intertrigo and secondary skin infections. *Am Fam Physician* 89(7):569-573, 2014; and Selden ST. Intertrigo. Mar 27, 2012. Available at http://emedicine.medscape.com/article/1087691-overview#showall. Accessed July 17, 2014.

MANAGEMENT

The treatment of uninfected intertrigo involves keeping the skinfolds cool and dry so healing can occur. Principles of management include minimizing skin-to-skin friction, removing irritants, wicking moisture away, minimizing the source of moisture, and preventing secondary infection. Skin should be cleansed with pH balanced, rinseless cleanser, then patted dry. Clothing should be made of either lightweight natural fibers or wicking material; textiles made with a moisture-wicking silver compound have been found to be effective. Women should wear brassieres to reduce skin-to-skin friction.[3]

Compresses with Burrow solution may be soothing.[5] Use of drying agents containing aluminum sulfate and calcium acetate solution is recommended. Cornstarch is ineffective and may result in fungal growth.[3]

For intertrigo associated with fungal infections (including *Candida* and tinea), clotrimazole, ketoconazole, oxiconazole, or econazole may be applied two times daily until the rash resolves. Nystatin is effective only for candidal intertrigo.[1] In cases of recalcitrant or recurrent fungal infections, systemic antifungal therapy with agents such as oral fluconazole should be used, with careful monitoring of the patient for drug interactions or hepatic impairment. The suggested dosage is 100 to 200 mg daily for 7 days, but obese individuals may need an increased dose.[1]

When persistent redness is present, secondary infections with *S. aureus*, group A β-hemolytic streptococci, *P. aeruginosa*, *P. mirabilis*, or *Proteus vulgaris* should be considered. In patients with secondary infections, topical treatment with mupirocin, erythromycin, or clindamycin should be used. If an oral agent is required, the lesions should be cultured and the results used to determine the selection of an antibiotic. Cephalexin, ceftriaxone, cefazolin, clindamycin, erythromycin, and sulfamethoxazole-trimethoprim are typically used for oral therapy.[1]

Patients with frequent candidal infections should be evaluated for HIV infection, diabetes mellitus, or other immunocompromised states.

COMPLICATIONS

A secondary bacterial infection may develop if intertrigo is left untreated or if behaviors such as scratching impair skin integrity. Aggressive infections such as with β-hemolytic streptococci may lead to considerable complications; systemic involvement must also be considered.

INDICATIONS FOR REFERRAL OR HOSPITALIZATION

Immediate emergency department referral should be considered for rapidly progressing infections or suspicion of serious systemic involvement.

Physician consultation is indicated for symptoms including fever, systemic involvement, or significant evidence of nonhealing or worsening erosions. Any patient who does not experience a resolution of symptoms within 2 weeks should be referred to a dermatologist. Immunocompromised patients require consultation with the appropriate specialist.

LIFE SPAN CONSIDERATIONS

Women of childbearing age should be informed of the risk of *Candida* infections while taking oral contraceptives and during pregnancy.

The growing population of older adults presents significant challenges to the provider regarding skin disorders including intertrigo. Physiologic changes of aging skin include the thinning of dermis and epidermis, which increases the risk for mechanical trauma, and an impaired immune response that increases the risk of infection.[6] The development of incontinence and immobility increases the risk for skin breakdown.[1] A thorough skin examination performed routinely could reveal early stages of intertrigo, thus reducing the risk for infection.

PATIENT AND FAMILY EDUCATION AND HEALTH PROMOTION

Patients with intertrigo need assistance with weight reduction if they are overweight and close monitoring of comorbidities (e.g., diabetes mellitus). Affected areas need to be exposed to light and air several times daily. Once the affected epidermis has healed, patients should be encouraged to keep susceptible areas clean and dry. Intertrigo in itself is not contagious, but infections resulting from impaired skin integrity may be transferable. Cornstarch-containing powders should be avoided. Patients will benefit from use of a balanced pH, nonrinsing cleanser and a handheld hair dryer with a cool setting to dry the area. Women should wear bras with good support to reduce skin friction.[3] Wearing of lightweight, natural-fiber clothing or clothing made of wicking material will reduce recurrence rates.

CHAPTER 59

NAIL DISORDERS

Kathryn D. Swartwout

HERPETIC WHITLOW

DEFINITION AND EPIDEMIOLOGY

Herpetic whitlow is a self-limited viral infection of the area between the fascial planes of the distal finger, usually surrounding the nail. This infection is most often seen in patients with gingivostomatitis caused by herpes simplex, in patients with genital herpes, and in health care workers.[1,2] Symptoms develop 2 to 14 days after exposure and generally resolve in about 3 weeks. The patient is infectious until lesions are healed.[2] Autoinfection from nail biting[1] and recurrences can occur.[2]

PATHOPHYSIOLOGY

The infecting pathogen is herpes simplex virus (HSV-1 or HSV-2). Transmission may occur from a primary herpetic lesion or infected body fluids. The virus remains dormant in the nerve ganglia; secondary eruptions may be related to stress, certain foods, sun exposure, and unknown precipitants.

CLINICAL PRESENTATION

Herpetiform vesicles or blisters erupt on the distal phalanx, sometimes after a short prodromal period of flulike symptoms (particularly in the primary infection) and throbbing, tingling, numbness, or pruritus in the area of the eruption. Painful vesicles can be singular or coalescent, resemble a group of warts or a bacterial infection, and persist for 8 to 12 days; lesions then begin to dry, forming crusted fissures.[3] The course of the eruptions can persist for 21 days until resolution; healing may take longer in areas that remain moist. In addition to the vesicles, the fingertip may be edematous, erythematous streaking may be evident on the forearm, and the axillary lymph nodes may become enlarged.

PHYSICAL EXAMINATION

The nails should be inspected for shape, configuration, texture, and herpetiform vesicles. Axillary and epitrochlear nodes should be examined for lymphadenopathy. Examination for genital herpes should be considered if there are genital symptoms.

DIAGNOSTICS

DIAGNOSTICS

Herpetic Whitlow

LABORATORY
Tzanck test*
HSV culture*
Serum antibody titers*

*If indicated.

Diagnosis is typically established based on history and physical examination findings. If warranted, viral culture of vesicular fluid, Tzanck smear, or serum titer may be used to confirm the diagnosis.[2] If secondary bacterial infection is suspected, bacterial culture may be indicated.

DIFFERENTIAL DIAGNOSIS

See differential diagnosis box.

DIFFERENTIAL DIAGNOSIS

Herpetic Whitlow

DERMATOLOGIC
- Bacterial infection
- Candidal infection
- Felon (painful abscess in digital pulp)
- Paronychia
- Warts

MANAGEMENT

Immediate emergency department–surgical referral is indicated for paronychial infection of the tendon sheath.

Use of incision and drainage (I&D) is avoided because it may lead to superinfection[2] or longer duration of healing.[1] Cool compresses can be used to decrease erythema and to debride crusts, thus promoting healing.[3] The area should be covered with gauze to prevent transmission. The area is kept dry because moisture may prolong healing and promote superinfection. Analgesics are used at doses appropriate for the patient's age and medical history. Oral antivirals (acyclovir, famciclovir, valacyclovir) may be considered for severe cases, management of recurrences, during the prodromal period, and in patients with acquired immunodeficiency syndrome (AIDS).[2] Creatinine clearance should be checked and the dose adjusted according to the creatinine clearance values if they are abnormal. L-Lysine is ineffective.[3]

COMPLICATIONS

Secondary bacterial infection in conjunction with the viral syndrome is possible. Transmission to others during viral shedding is possible.

INDICATIONS FOR REFERRAL OR HOSPITALIZATION

Physician referral is necessary if the virus is recalcitrant to treatment after 3 weeks. Hospitalization should not be required.

LIFESPAN CONSIDERATIONS

Herpetic whitlow is generally more common in young children and young adults. Atypical presentations and more severe infection can occur in immunocompromised individuals.

EDUCATION AND HEALTH PROMOTION

Patients require education about the risk of infecting others and medication administration. If used in recurrences, antivirals should be administered within 48 hours of the first prodromal signs. Patients should be advised to keep their infected digits away from the mouth and eyes to prevent inoculation of these surfaces with the virus. If patients work in occupations in which they could infect other persons (e.g., health care providers, dental providers, manicurists), they should be advised to wear gloves when working. The provider should carefully explain signs and symptoms of infection and encourage the patient to call if complications develop.

PARONYCHIAL INFECTIONS

DEFINITION AND EPIDEMIOLOGY

Paronychial infections manifest as acute or chronic inflammation of the tissues surrounding the nail, usually with an underlying bacterial or fungal infection. Other noninfectious causes are possible and include "chemical irritants, excessive moisture, systemic conditions and medications".[4] Most commonly a microorganism penetrates the tissue after breakdown between the nail plate and nail fold. A split in the epidermis from trauma, nail biting, a hangnail, irritation, or chronic exposure to water (such as with dishwashing) or irritants can precede the development of a paronychia. Symptoms typically develop 2 to 5 days after trauma.[4]

Paronychial infections may be seen more often in women than in men; this may be related to manicures or the application of acrylic nails. Patients who work with chemicals are more at risk for infections because of the irritant nature of these substances and the risk of trauma. Patients who have their hands in water frequently are also at risk.

PATHOPHYSIOLOGY

There are numerous possible causative organisms for acute paronychial infections. Some organisms include *Pseudomonas, Proteus, Streptococcus, Staphylococcus, Candida albicans,* and HSV.[4,5] A paronychial infection results when periungual tissue is inoculated by trauma, inert vehicles such as water, or soluble chemicals. The resulting infection follows the nail margin or the infection penetrates under the nail.

If paronychial inflammation is present for longer than 6 weeks, the condition is considered a chronic paronychia. Chronic paronychia is primarily an inflammatory disorder, but *C. albicans* is also often present. It is most commonly present in workers with frequent exposure to environmental irritants (such as cooks, dishwashers, and nurses).[4]

Medications can cause chronic paronychia, increasing the risk for infection. Retinoids and protease inhibitors (e.g., lamivudine [Epivir], darunavir [Prezista], and fosamprenavir [Lexiva]) affect nail fold integrity, setting the stage for a paronychia.[6,7] An antiretroviral, indinavir (Crixivan), is associated with paronychias as a result of interference with retinoid metabolism.[8] Chemotherapeutic selective inhibition of the epidermal growth factor receptor (EGFR; e.g., cetuximab) is increasingly used to treat solid organ malignant neoplasms in patients whose standard chemotherapeutic regimens have failed. Tenderness, swelling, and pain in both fingers and toes occur after 2 weeks to months of therapy. Anatomic predisposition may increase risk in the development of paronychias.[9]

CLINICAL PRESENTATION AND PHYSICAL EXAMINATION

Symptoms are usually localized to one finger, and patients report throbbing pain of the nail fold, nail, and even adjacent portions of the finger. The affected nail may display distal onycholysis, discoloration, distortion, and ridging; the affected nail folds have erythema and edema. When the examiner applies force to the affected area, there can be a release of purulent, often foul-smelling discharge.[5] Pyogenic granuloma–like lesions and granulation tissue are seen in the nail sulci in paronychias associated with indinavir and anti-EGFR agents.[8]

DIAGNOSTICS

Skin scrapings can be combined with potassium hydroxide (KOH) preparation on a glass slide and viewed under a microscope. Pseudohyphae and spores indicate candidal infection. Any exudate from the nail can be cultured to determine the pathogen and to guide treatment.

DIFFERENTIAL DIAGNOSIS

The differential diagnosis of paronychial infections includes bacterial origin, herpetic whitlow, onychomycosis, circulatory changes, and irritation from environmental causes (such as nail products).[10] Malignancies of the area are possible and should be considered, especially in patients with persistent paronychia or those with a cancer history.[4] However, paronychial infection is usually readily recognized by its appearance and absence of medication history preceding the infection.

DIAGNOSTICS

Paronychial Infections

LABORATORY

KOH preparation

CBC and differential (if infection is suspected or if the patient is immunocompromised)

Culture and sensitivity*

*If indicated.
CBC, complete blood count.

DIFFERENTIAL DIAGNOSIS

Paronychial Infections

DERMATOLOGIC
- Herpetic whitlow
- Onychomycosis
- Psoriasis
- Tic deformity
- Lichen planus
- Eczema
- Bacterial infections

ENDOCRINE
- Diabetes

IMMUNE
- Immunocompromised state

MANAGEMENT

Immediate emergency department–surgical referral is indicated for paronychial infection of the tendon sheath. Specialist consultation is indicated if a provider skilled in I&D is not available.

Acute Paronychia

Treatment of minor acute paronychial infection includes warm water soaks or warm compresses four times a day. A topical antibiotic may be added for minor cases. Topical neomycin is indicated for pseudomonal infection.[11]

Oral antibiotic therapy is indicated for more substantial infection. Antibiotic choice depends on the suspected organism. Considerations could include trimethoprim-sulfamethoxazole (good if methicillin-resistant *Staphylococcus aureus* [MRSA] is suspected), clindamycin, amoxicillin-clavulanate, and cephalexin.[4] Appropriate analgesics and dosages are based on patient age and medical history.

For all cases, the area is kept dry because moisture may prolong healing and cause further irritation. I&D is considered if abscess is suspected or infection is not responding to noninvasive care. Complete removal of the nail plate is sometimes necessary in situations in which the nail plate has separated from the underlying tissue. Oral antibiotics may be used in conjunction with I&D.

Chronic Paronychia

Treatment of chronic paronychia includes identification and elimination of causative irritants. Topical steroids have been shown to be most often superior to topical antifungals in treating chronic paronychia. Topical betamethasone is the recommended preparation.[4]

For persistent or nonresponsive cases, use of oral antifungal preparations is considered. A short course of oral corticosteroids may be considered for severe cases with multiple fingers involved.[4] I&D is reserved for severe persistent cases.

COMPLICATIONS

Serious complications of paronychia include loss of the nail or spread of the infection into the bloodstream, deeper tissue, or bone. If it is untreated or in patients with immunosuppression or diabetes, the paronychial infection can invade deep into the digit, infecting the tendon and tendon sheaths. Infection along the tendon sheath requires immediate surgical intervention. Chronic mucocutaneous candidiasis can cause hyperkeratosis of the entire nail plate. These chronically infected nails can become distorted and may require excision.

INDICATIONS FOR REFERRAL OR HOSPITALIZATION

Patients are referred to a physician if there is continued infection after 2 weeks of treatment. Suspected infection of the tendons or tendon sheaths requires immediate referral to a physician or surgeon. Hospitalization may be required for surgical intervention.

LIFE SPAN CONSIDERATIONS

Postmenopausal women may be at greater risk for chronic candidal paronychial infections because of diminished estrogen levels.

EDUCATION AND HEALTH PROMOTION

It is imperative that patients understand the importance of keeping hands and nails as clean and dry as possible. Patient education should address the individual patient's causative factors including their environmental and work exposures. Patients who have manicures or who wear acrylic nails should be advised to rest their nails and hands for 1 week every month.[5] Patients who deal with caustic chemicals and irritants should be advised to wear protective gloves. In addition, patients should be instructed to wear waterproof gloves when washing dishes or clothing by hand and to keep the nails trimmed and dry to prevent further infections.

ONYCHOMYCOSIS

DEFINITION AND EPIDEMIOLOGY

Onychomycosis (or *tinea unguium*) refers to any infection of the nails caused by a dermatophyte, yeast, or sometimes mold.[10] Onychomycosis is the most common nail condition, most frequently occurs in the toenails (great toe is often first), is classified based on nail bed location of the infection, and has a reputation for being quite difficult to resolve. These infections cause nail discoloration, thickening, roughness, splitting of the nail, and sometimes onycholysis (a painful separation of the nail from the nail bed). Onychomycosis is common in patients of advancing age as a result of a reduction in blood flow.[5] Other risk factors include swimming, nail trauma, diabetes, tinea pedis, psoriasis, and immunodeficiency.[11,12] Onycholysis has a significant incidence of pain and can affect patients' lives physically and psychologically, interfering with walking, exercise, and social interaction.

PATHOPHYSIOLOGY

The most common pathogens associated with tinea unguium are *Trichophyton rubrum* and *Trichophyton interdigitale.*[12] *Candida* organisms are rarer and may be associated with immunosuppression. A nail can be infected by multiple organisms.[3] The infection is located inside the nail. Distal subungual onychomycosis, the most common presentation, begins with discoloration in the distal portion of the nail partially caused by the accumulation of keratinous debris under the nail.[12] Proximal subungual onychomycosis, the rarest presentation, begins deeper near the cuticle and occurs mostly in immunocompromised patients. White superficial onychomycosis has a flaky white appearance and affects the nail surface.[11,12]

CLINICAL PRESENTATION

Table 59-1 describes the physical presentation of onychomycosis nail dystrophies. Pain rating and any interference with daily activities should be assessed.

PHYSICAL EXAMINATION

Careful examination of the toes and fingers is essential. Typically, the nail is white or yellowed, with a powdery or thickened nail texture. The nail surface typically has a greenish tinge with bacterial infections. The examiner should assess for onycholysis (disassociation of the nail from the nail bed). The condition of the subungual nail bed should be noted—that is, the degree of elevation and separation of the nail from the nail bed and surrounding tissue.

DIAGNOSTICS

Confirmation of the diagnosis is made by microscopic examination of nail scrapings with a KOH preparation or culture of nail debris. It is essential to identify the invading organism as a dermatophyte or *Candida* to guide treatment. Histologic tests and periodic acid–Schiff staining are reliable for an accurate diagnosis to identify organisms susceptible to specific therapeutic agents.[3]

DIAGNOSTICS

Onychomycosis and Tinea Unguium

LABORATORY	CBC and differential
KOH smear and culture	LFTs*

*If indicated.
CBC, complete blood count; LFTs, liver function tests.

TABLE 59-1 Nail Dystrophies

Nail Disorder	Clinical Presentation	Manifestations
Distal or lateral subungual onychomycosis	White to brownish-yellow discoloration of nail	Subungual hyperkeratosis; separation of nail plate and nail bed lineal channels
White superficial onychomycosis	White, sharply outlined area on nail plate; nail surface soft, dry, and friable	Common in fingernails and toenails of HIV-infected patients Nail plate not thick; no separation of nail plate and nail bed
Proximal subungual onychomycosis (rare), candidal infections	Leukonychia on proximal aspect of nail plate Thickening of nail plate Yellowish-brown discoloration	Patient may be immunosuppressed Chronic mucocutaneous candidiasis Involves all nails Eventual disintegration of nail

HIV, human immunodeficiency virus.

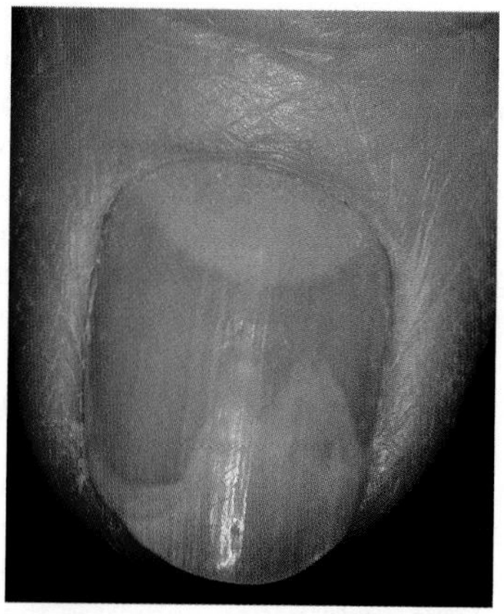

FIGURE 59-1 Psoriasis of nails. (Bolognia JL, Schaffer JV, Duncan KO, Ko CJ, *Dermatology Essentials,* ed 1, St Louis, 2015, Saunders.)

DIFFERENTIAL DIAGNOSIS

Onychomycosis accounts for about 50% of nail abnormalities, so consideration should be given to other causes. Psoriasis, not fungal infection, causes pitting of the nail surface. Psoriasis is often mistaken for dermatophyte and fungal infections, but the two may coexist (Fig. 59-1).[3] Leukonychia, white spots or bands that appear proximally, is most likely caused by minor trauma and may be mistaken for proximal subungual onychomycosis.[13] Other conditions that cause nail findings similar to onychomycosis include eczema, trauma, lichen planus, and leukonychia.[3] Onychomycosis should not be confused with onychogryphosis, which is a nail hypertrophy sometimes caused by trauma but more often caused by neglecting to trim the nails for a long period. Subungual malignant melanoma is a nail cancer. Subungual malignant melanoma can manifest as a dark stripe discoloration and requires urgent referral for evaluation.

DIFFERENTIAL DIAGNOSIS

Onychomycosis

DERMATOLOGIC
- Bacterial infection
- Psoriasis
- Eczema
- Lichen planus
- Herpetic whitlow
- Subungual malignant melanoma
- Trophic changes
- Black nail paronychia
- Darier disease

OTHER
- Trauma
- Medications
- Onychogryposis

MANAGEMENT

Confirmed onychomycosis is most effectively treated systemically. Ciclopirox, a nail lacquer applied to the nail over an extended period of time, maybe be considered in a patient for whom oral therapy is contraindicated. Topical antifungal creams rarely penetrate deeply enough to be effective. Onychomycosis may be treated with terbinafine (Lamisil) orally and daily for 12 weeks for toenails, 6 weeks for fingernails. This medication has a low incidence of side effects. Liver function tests should be performed at baseline and 6 weeks after starting terbinafine. The drug should not be used in patients with abnormal creatinine clearance and is Pregnancy Category B. Other oral medications that may be used are fluconazole, itraconazole, and griseofulvin. Indications and contraindications for all oral antifungal medications should be reviewed carefully before prescribing. Consistent, prolonged application of a topical antifungal agent after clinical response to an oral agent may prevent nail reinfection. Removal of the infected nail affords better cure rates and longer remissions.[3] *Candida* onychomycosis is a sign of depressed immune function; topical amorolfine and two pulse doses with itraconazole are effective, low-cost treatments.[14] Trials of various phototherapy methods for treatment of *T. rubrum* infection are promising and ongoing.

COMPLICATIONS

The result of chronic inflammation and infection is nail bed cornification (formation of a granular layer) causing permanent separation of the nail plate from the underlying supporting structures (onycholysis).[15] Patients with diabetes or peripheral neuropathy may be at higher risk for complications and need aggressive diagnosis and treatment of onychomycosis and tinea unguium.[14]

INDICATIONS FOR REFERRAL OR HOSPITALIZATION

Patients with combinations of infection and underlying disease (e.g., psoriasis) would benefit from a dermatology referral. Patients with nail stripe discolorations or persistent subungual discolorations should be referred to rule out subungual malignant melanoma. Discussion with the physician regarding recurrence and surgical or nonsurgical avulsion of nail dystrophy is also a consideration for a referral.

PATIENT AND FAMILY EDUCATION AND HEALTH PROMOTION

The health care provider should review information concerning medication administration and instructions regarding signs of liver toxicity. In many cases, nails do not appear clear after the recommended course of treatment and it may take 12 to 18 months after treatment for the patient to visually see improvement.[11] Patients should be assured that the medication remains in the nail plate for months and will continue to kill fungus.[3] These infections can be recalcitrant to treatment; it may take months or even years for complete resolution of the pathogens. To prevent recurrences, the patient can apply ciclopirox two or three times a week, apply terbinafine cream in the nail area weekly, and avoid trauma to the tip of the nails from tight-fitting shoes.

It is imperative that patients keep their hands and nails as dry as possible and avoid recurrence of tinea pedis. Nails should be trimmed, and chewing or picking at nails avoided. Footwear should be evaluated annually for size and suitability. Patients should powder toe webs and soles, not shoes; avoid going barefoot in communal showers; wear sweat-wicking socks; and alternate several pairs of shoes for daily wear that maintain a dry, roomy environment for the feet. Using an antifungal spray in shoes may be helpful.

CHAPTER 60

PIGMENTATION CHANGES (VITILIGO)

Maria Isabel Romano

DEFINITION AND EPIDEMIOLOGY

Vitiligo is a skin disorder characterized by either a lifelong or a rapid disappearance of pigment-producing melanocytes in the epidermis and hair follicle. Lack of melanin leads to the appearance of progressive, symmetrically patterned, milky-white macules that merge to form larger depigmented areas. The macules give a variegated appearance to the skin that is similar to the white patches on a Holstein calf, hence the origin of the word from the Greek *vitellius,* which means "calf." The disease is psychologically troublesome, affecting the patient's self-esteem and interpersonal relationships. Although the disease shows no increased prevalence among dark-skinned racial groups, the variegated appearance of the skin proves to be especially traumatic for dark-pigmented patients. The appearance of vitiligo resembles leprosy, but the lesions of vitiligo do not have the anesthetic property of leprosy. However, the similarity in appearance to leprosy presents a social stigma for those patients with vitiligo living in leprosy-affected areas of the world.[1] The disease manifests in two forms: type A, a nondermatomal distribution; and type B, a segmental or dermatomal distribution (zosteriform) characterized by rapid spread.[2]

Vitiligo is seen in 1% to 2% of the general population without regard to race, ethnic origin, or gender.[2,3] Although some patients have no vitiligo in their family history, the condition has an inherited tendency; in 30% of cases, a family history of vitiligo in parents, offspring, or siblings is reported.[2] Familial cases of vitiligo have been associated with autoimmune endocrine disorders; studies indicate that there is a genetic locus in affected individuals, and a possible pathogenic connection between vitiligo and oxidative damage exists.[4] A family history of thyroid disease, pernicious anemia, systemic lupus erythematosus, inflammatory bowel disease, and vitiligo is associated with a risk for development of the condition.[6] Disease onset occurs between 10 and 30 years of age; 50% of the cases occur before the age of 20 years, and fewer cases are reported in infancy and old age.[2,5,6,7]

PATHOPHYSIOLOGY

The exact cause of vitiligo is not known. Multiple pathogenic theories exist and are under investigation, including autoimmune involvement, viral causes, decreased melanocyte survival, genetic defects in the structure of melanocytes, and neurochemical destruction of melanocytes.[8,9] Except for the absence of melanocytes, skin function is normal. There is a progressive destruction of pigment-producing cells at the border of the dermis and epidermis. The nonsegmental (nondermatomal) variety of vitiligo is associated with a small risk of autoimmune-related disorders, such as type 1 diabetes mellitus and thyroid disease.[2]

Several theories exist to explain the phenomenon of vitiligo. The autoimmune theory proposes that there is a destruction of the cutaneous melanocytes with loss of the melanin-producing pigment. Histologic examination indicates that lymphocytes build up within the dermis and are involved in the destruction of the melanocytes. Coexisting diseases such as alopecia areata, autoimmune thyroid disorders, Addison disease, atrophic gastritis, pernicious anemia, and type 1 diabetes underscore the relationship of dermatomal vitiligo to autoimmunity. Serum autoimmune antibodies against melanocytes, thyroid and adrenal tissue, islet cells, gastric parietal cells, and intrinsic factors have been demonstrated.

A second explanation, the neurogenic theory, supposes that a toxic substance is released by the peripheral nerve endings and interferes with the production of melanin. A third theory suggests a defect in the natural protective mechanism of melanin synthesis by melanocytes. Toxic substances accumulate during normal melanin production and later precipitate the destruction of the melanocytes.[7-9] The variation in presentation and progression of the two types of vitiligo indicates that the underlying pathologic condition for the two forms of disease may be distinctly different.

CLINICAL PRESENTATION

Vitiligo is characterized by a progressive and invasive hypopigmentation of the skin that is found on sun-exposed areas and extensor surfaces of the upper body. Most patients have no other clinical findings.[2] Vitiligo manifesting with well-defined areas of white hair is referred to as poliosis.[8] In general, the onset of vitiligo may follow stress; an injury to the skin, such as a burn, bruise, or contusion (Koebner phenomenon); and sunburn.[8] Vitiligo should not be confused with postinflammatory hypopigmentation, in which the skin has a faded pigment appearance rather than an absence of pigment.[10] Chemicals,

BOX 60-1

Common Locations for Hypopigmented Vitiligo Lesions

Bony surfaces: back of hands and fingers, elbows and knees
Body orifices: around the eyes, mouth, and nose
Body folds: armpits and groin
Other areas: legs, wrists, nipples, and genitals
Hair: area within the affected path turning white

including phenols and catechols, may cause depigmentation of the skin; therefore any history of a patient with vitiligo should include questions about chemical exposure.[6] In fair-skinned individuals, the disease may go undetected until summer, when the sun-exposed areas tan and the melanin-free areas appear a contrasting chalky white.

PHYSICAL EXAMINATION

The extensor surfaces may have been traumatized previously; depigmentation first appears here in a symmetric fashion typical of the more common nondermatomal variety. The segmental variety is more often seen in children and follows a dermatomal distribution that progresses more rapidly. The dermatomal variety is not likely to be associated with autoimmune disorders or Koebner phenomenon.[2] The border is not sharply demarcated but instead exhibits a tricolored, uneven appearance.[8] Box 60-1 indicates the usual locations of the hypopigmented lesions of vitiligo. Because melanocytes are located in the eyes, ocular changes, such as uveitis and pigmentary changes in the fundus, can occur; other findings may include healed chorioretinitis and iritis.[2,8]

Vitiligo can best be described as a white, flat macule within the epidermis that varies in size from 5 mm to 5 cm (1/5 to 1 1/5 inches) with a convex outer edge. In the common nonsegmental variety, the lesion is initially seen in a symmetric distribution on the body parts. Macules may eventually merge to cover the entire body in a condition termed vitiligo universalis. Variations of the disease presentation include smaller confetti-like lesions mixed with larger ones and the less common presentation of elevated, erythematous, pruritic lesions known as inflammatory vitiligo.[2,7] The segmental variety occurs in a band-type distribution on one side of the body. Confetti-sized hypomelanotic macules are common on sun-exposed surfaces of the arms.

DIAGNOSTICS

The clinical presentation and physical examination are generally sufficient for a diagnosis to be made. In some instances, in lighter-skinned individuals and in underarm and genital regions, Wood light examination is necessary for the diagnosis. The Wood light will illuminate depigmented areas as chalky white. A skin scraping for a potassium hydroxide (KOH) examination fails to demonstrate hyphae or spores consistent with tinea versicolor, another common depigmenting lesion. Although it is not usually necessary, a skin biopsy will show an absence of melanocytes and melanin in the epidermis.

Vitiligo patients show an increased frequency of autoimmune disorders, such as thyroid disease, type 1 diabetes, and pernicious anemia.[2] The patient should be assessed for signs and symptoms of thyroid disease; screening for thyroid-stimulating hormone (TSH) and thyroxine (T_4) is recommended. However, the treatment of thyroid disease has no impact on the progression of vitiligo because this skin condition does not occur as a result of an increase or reduction of thyroid hormone but rather exists as one of several components of autoimmune polyendocrine syndromes.[11] A fasting blood glucose concentration is included in the initial diagnostic evaluation. A complete blood count (CBC) with indexes is performed to detect the presence of macrocytosis, followed by an evaluation for vitamin B_{12} deficiency if indicated.

DIAGNOSTICS

Vitiligo

LABORATORY
Wood lamp examination
KOH preparation
TSH, T_4
Fasting blood glucose
CBC and differential
Vitamin B_{12}

OTHER
Skin biopsy*

*If indicated.

DIFFERENTIAL DIAGNOSIS

Early or atypical lesions often require the exclusion of other hypopigmented conditions, including albinism, piebaldism, tuberous sclerosis, nevus anemicus, tinea, pityriasis alba, chemical skin exposure, and lichen sclerosus. Some of these disorders are associated with patchy depigmentation with inflammation and scaling or atrophy induration. A biopsy may be indicated to differentiate the underlying cause of depigmentation associated with these disorders.[8]

DIFFERENTIAL DIAGNOSIS

Vitiligo

- Albinism
- Piebaldism
- Tuberous sclerosis
- Nevus anemicus
- Chemical leukoderma
- Tinea versicolor
- Leprosy
- Pityriasis alba
- Lichen sclerosus
- Psoriasis
- Eczema

MANAGEMENT

Care of the patient with vitiligo involves the use of sunscreens (sun protection factor [SPF] 15 to 30) to protect the depigmented skin from burning and to reduce the tanning of melanin-producing areas of the adjacent skin. Extensive sunburn can produce a response similar to Koebner phenomenon (trauma to the skin) and stimulate the depigmentation process to extend farther. Cosmetic cover-ups assist the patient in managing the psychological aspects of the disease and improve body image and coping mechanisms. A variety of cosmetic substances are commercially available, marketed under the names Covermark (Lydia O'Leary), Dermablend (Flori Roberts), Dermage, and C-ESTA Make-Up for Vitiligo. These products can be customized to match individual skin tones and are used by both sexes. Although these products do not come off in water, they do rub off and therefore may not be sustained for long periods of wear.

Tanning creams containing dihydroxyacetone may be applied to induce the tanning of affected areas; these substances can be used for eyelids. Some patients desire no treatment aside from cosmetics and prefer to allow the disease to progress until all body parts are depigmented. However, it is difficult to judge how long this will take, which limits the usefulness of this approach in the treatment regimen.

After coexistent autoimmune disorders have been excluded, patients with vitiligo are usually referred to a dermatologist for treatment options. Therapy is directed toward either repigmentation therapy of the affected areas or depigmentation therapy of the unaffected areas. Repigmentation involving the use of high- to mid-potency class 3 and class 4 steroid creams applied twice a day to the affected areas is usually the first approach for patients with depigmentation involving less than 10% of the body and not involving the face. Another treatment approach with proven efficacy for patients with lesser involvement or more generalized vitiligo is treatment with narrow-band ultraviolet B (UVB) light; this approach, which involves the use of psoralens, has been found to be just as effective as psoralens plus ultraviolet A (PUVA) light.[3,12] Recently occurring lesions and those of the facial and neck areas are the most responsive to topical steroid treatment.[3] Patients must be monitored every 2 months for evidence of skin atrophy. A response to treatment is indicated by the development of follicular pigmented spots that widen with time and persist. Areas with minimum hair follicles are slower to repigment. Oral corticosteroids have shown promise in patients with more aggressive forms of the disease; referral to a dermatologist is recommended.[6]

Efforts are in progress to develop guidelines in the management of vitiligo.[4] Meta-analysis of studies using multiple treatment modalities including class 3 corticosteroids, topical calcineurin inhibitors, topical and systemic photochemotherapy, and narrow-band UVB have shown these methods to be largely effective and safe for localized and generalized vitiligo. However, comprehensive randomized clinical trials are still necessary to establish safety and efficacy profiles for many of the treatments being used to treat vitiligo at this time.[4] Steroid treatment failure is seen in nearly 20% of cases; failure is likely if no response is seen by the end of 2 months.[2,8] If treatment failure should occur, the patient should be referred to the specialist for further evaluation and for treatment with PUVA, either topical or systemic. PUVA treatments should be performed only by a qualified specialist. Close monitoring of the patient for response to treatment is necessary. Prevention of eye exposure to UV light must be strictly enforced by making certain that the patient wears glasses that filter all UV light. Up to 2 years of treatment may be necessary before repigmentation occurs.[12]

Another technique is chemical depigmentation to produce an artificially induced vitiligo universalis if more than 50% to 80% of the body is affected. Studies indicate that depigmentation treatments using a combination therapy of mequinol, a Q-switched ruby laser, and cryotherapy show promising results.[4] Monobenzone hydroquinone 20% (MEH) cream applied twice daily produces an irreversible depigmentation that takes up to 2 to 3 months to begin and up to 9 to 18 months for a complete response. The depigmentation with MEH leads to chalk-white coloration of the skin like that of vitiligo macules.[13] The health care provider can monitor this treatment regimen if it is prescribed by the specialist. Patients are generally pleased with the outcome of this treatment.

COMPLICATIONS

Treatment with steroids may involve atrophy and striae formation, which increases the risk for easy bruising and infection. Steroid-induced glaucoma and cataracts are complications of steroid application around the eyes. Complications of PUVA treatment include a phototoxic reaction and ocular damage if appropriate UV-protective sunglasses are not used. Consultation with the specialist is necessary if evidence of skin atrophy, adrenal axis suppression, or steroid-induced glaucoma is seen.

INDICATIONS FOR REFERRAL

After coexistent autoimmune disorders have been excluded, patients with vitiligo are referred to a dermatologist for treatment options. Health care providers can assist with monitoring of therapy, with a dermatology consultation for treatment questions. The involvement of eye pigment mandates a referral to an ophthalmologist for evaluation. A referral for mental health counseling may be indicated because this disorder can be psychologically stressful. In progressive forms of the disease, the patient should be referred to a specialist for depigmentation therapy. Laser therapy is an option for those trained in the use of this technique.

PATIENT AND FAMILY EDUCATION

Education includes teaching patients about the nature of the pigmentary changes and the lack of scientific knowledge concerning the true cause of the disease. Patients should be taught that the treatment response includes repigmentation that occurs first in areas with residual melanocytes. Vitiligo with late-life onset or long-standing lesions is less likely to respond to treatment. Risk factors associated with topical steroids include easy bruising, infection, and decreased vision. Patients are taught to observe the skin closely for the development of skin lesions suggestive of melanoma. The rule of fingertip units should be adhered to in prescribing topical steroids and monitoring patients. One fingertip unit weighs 0.5 g and is the amount expressed from a tube applied to the fingertip. One half of a fingertip unit will cover the dorsum of the hand, and 2.5 fingertip units will cover the face. For lesions affecting the face, a 30-g tube should last for 10 days.[13] Patients should avoid using more steroid cream than directed and should avoid applying steroids around the eyes and moist genital areas, where thin skin enhances systemic absorption. Patients should avoid sunlight for 48 hours after each PUVA treatment.

Assessment of the patient's psychological response to vitiligo includes body image adjustment, use of cosmetic coverings, and knowledge concerning the noncontagious nature of vitiligo. Family members should be included in the office visit for support and explanation concerning the benign nature of the disorder and the expected response to treatment. Instruction concerning the use of sunscreens to protect depigmented areas is critical.

CHAPTER 61

PRURITUS

Daniel W. O'Neill • Lauren E. Curtis

DEFINITION AND EPIDEMIOLOGY

Pruritus is a sensation that leads to a desire to scratch. It is a common symptom that can be found with many dermatologic and systemic illnesses and often leads to a high burden and impaired quality of life. A population-based cross-sectional study in 19,000 adults showed that about 8% to 9% of the general population experienced acute pruritus, and this was dominant across all age groups.[1]

PATHOPHYSIOLOGY

Pruritus is characterized by the activation of a network of distinct free nerve endings situated at the dermoepidermal junction by local mediators such as histamine and numerous other peptides and proteases as well as elevated levels of various substances associated with certain systemic diseases of renal, hepatic, endocrine, or hematologic origin.[2] These impulses are carried by unmyelinated C fibers to the central nervous system, where the impulses are modulated by opioid peptides. Prostaglandins in the skin lower the threshold for itching. The exact pathophysiologic mechanisms leading to itching in systemic disease are not well defined. Scratching leads to symptomatic relief by temporarily destroying the nerve endings or stimulating pain fibers. However, this often leads to the release of more mediators and the scratch-itch cycle, in which one scratch is too many and a million are not enough.

CLINICAL PRESENTATION AND PHYSICAL EXAMINATION

Dermatologic disorders can manifest with characteristic primary skin lesions; therefore after obtaining a basic history of the present illness the health care provider should perform a total skin examination to first identify or to exclude dermatologic disorders.[2] Secondary skin lesions, such as excoriations (scratches), secondary infections (e.g., impetigo), hyperkeratotic skin changes, and lichenification (thickening, which indicates chronicity), often obscure the primary lesion. If a specific diagnosis is not evident on initial examination, the history should be readdressed with particular attention to any diurnal rhythms, characteristics of associated symptoms, any variations in symptom severity, evolution of current lesion distribution, exacerbating and alleviating factors, and previous treatments. The history should also include medication use, alcohol use, past medical and psychiatric history, exposures (e.g., to people who are scratching, pets, soaps, detergents, dry air, chemicals), and complete review of systems. A complete physical examination with emphasis on evaluation for organomegaly and adenopathy is then performed. Pruritus of the scalp and face is the most common manifestation of psychogenic pruritus.[3]

DIAGNOSTICS

If the symptoms persist and no dermatologic cause is discovered, screening laboratory examinations include a complete blood count (CBC) with differential, serum glucose, aspartate and alanine transaminases, alkaline phosphatase, bilirubin, blood urea nitrogen (BUN), creatinine, thyroid panel, urinalysis, and chest radiograph. If indicated, a skin biopsy specimen can be sent for pathologic examination for mycosis fungoides, immunofluorescence (pemphigoid and dermatitis herpetiformis), or special staining (mastocytosis). Additional studies that may be indicated include serum ferritin level, protein electrophoresis, immunoelectrophoresis, and stool culture for ova and parasites.

On occasion, it is necessary to perform repeated evaluations in follow-up visits or to refer the patient for dermatologic or psychiatric evaluation.

DIFFERENTIAL DIAGNOSIS

Dermatologic disorders with pruritus as a predominant symptom are common. Some of these disorders are covered in detail in other chapters, and each has its own etiology, clinical presentation, and treatment considerations. Pruritus without diagnostic skin lesions that persists longer than 2 weeks and is undiagnosed after 2 weeks of evaluation is called *pruritus of undetermined origin* and may indicate a systemic disorder.[4] It has been reported that 10% to 50% of patients with pruritus but no rash have an underlying systemic disease and up to 70% have a psychiatric one.[3] Medications are also a significant cause of pruritus.

MANAGEMENT

Treatment of pruritus depends on successful identification of the underlying dermatologic or systemic cause. In addition to appropriate treatment of the cause, pruritus requires interventions to alleviate this annoying symptom, although often not completely.[5]

General measures include the following:

- Medications that cause pruritus should be stopped.
- Taking steps to avoid irritants (e.g., wool or misguided topical therapy), reducing stress, and keeping the nails trimmed should be pursued.
- Cooling of the skin by the use of light clothing, air conditioning, or frequent application of cool wet compresses and cooling lotions such as calamine or aqueous creams is useful.
- A tepid bath before retiring can alleviate pruritus long enough for the patient to fall asleep. Decreased bathing frequency and emollients are effective for any condition in which dry skin (xerosis) is present.
- Disruption of the scratch-itch cycle by alleviating pruritus is a mainstay of therapy for dermatitis.
- Pramoxine hydrochloride (often combined with other topical agents) and 5% doxepin cream, a topical tricyclic antidepressant, have proved effective in several trials.[6]
- Topical and oral corticosteroids should be reserved for cases of cutaneous inflammation.
- Topical antihistamines and anesthetics are sensitizers and therefore should be discouraged.
- A topical 1% naltrexone cream has been shown to reduce itch symptoms by 50% in 46 minutes after application and is especially useful for patients with long-lasting pruritus.[6]
- Capsaicin works for localized pruritus.

Ultraviolet B (UVB) phototherapy is effective for uremic pruritus (i.e., in those receiving dialysis). Psoralen plus UVA therapy, intralesional corticosteroid therapy, or other methods may be used. Other approaches to relieve pruritus include the use of

DIFFERENTIAL DIAGNOSIS

Pruritus

PRURITIC DERMATOLOGIC DISORDERS

Inflammatory Disorders
- Xerosis (asteatotic eczema)
- Atopic dermatitis (eczema, the "itch that rashes")
- Nummular eczema
- Dyshidrotic eczema
- Lichen simplex chronicus
- Contact dermatitis (chemical or allergic)
- Urticaria and dermatographism
- Lichen planus
- Psoriasis
- Aquagenic pruritus
- Rhus dermatitis (poison ivy and poison oak)
- Miliaria
- Neuropathic pruritus (nodular prurigo, brachioradial pruritus, or notalgia paresthetica)
- Bullous and prebullous pemphigoid
- Dermatitis herpetiformis
- Pruritic urticarial papules and plaques of pregnancy
- Polymorphic light eruption (and other photosensitive reactions)

Infectious Disorders
- Viral exanthem (e.g., varicella)
- Dermatophytes
- Folliculitis (e.g., hot tub)
- Impetigo

Infestations
- Scabies
- Pediculosis
- Sea bather's eruption (jellyfish larvae)
- Insect bites (e.g., fleas, mites, bedbugs)
- Parasitic infections (e.g., onchocerciasis, echinococcosis, schistosomiasis)

Neoplastic Disorders
- Mycosis fungoides
- Mastocytosis

Environmental Disorders
- Sunburn
- Fiberglass dermatitis
- Pernio (chilblains)
- Winter itch (dry ambient environment, excessive bathing)
- Other (wool, hairs, fabric softeners, brighteners, other chemicals)
- Aquagenic pruritus (histamine mediated; lasts 1 hour after exposure to water)

SYSTEMIC DISORDERS COMMONLY ASSOCIATED WITH PRURITUS

Metabolic and Endocrine Disorders
- Diabetes mellitus (anogenital pruritus is more common)
- Postmenopausal estrogen withdrawal (anogenital and generalized)
- Adrenal insufficiency
- Carcinoid syndrome
- Hypothyroidism (secondary to dry skin in myxedema)
- Hyperthyroidism (secondary to elevated skin temperature)

Hematologic Disorders
- Polycythemia vera (typically water induced, or "bath itch")
- Iron-deficiency anemia
- Paraproteinemia
- Waldenström macroglobulinemia

Malignant Neoplasms
- Lymphoma (Hodgkin) and leukemia
- Abdominal visceral carcinoma
- Central nervous system tumors
- Multiple myeloma
- Mycosis fungoides

Hepatobiliary Disorders
- Primary biliary cirrhosis (from bile salts and associated substances)
- Biliary obstruction (cholestasis)
- Cholestasis of pregnancy

Renal Disorders
- Chronic renal failure (80% of patients on hemodialysis; can be from secondary hyperparathyroidism)

Parasitic Infestations
- Hookworm, onchocerciasis, ascariasis, trichinosis

Infections
- HIV (pruritus is sometimes the primary presentation)
- Hepatitis

Psychological States
- Delusions of parasitosis
- Neurotic excoriations (can be extensive)
- Psychogenic pruritus (anxiety induced)

MEDICATIONS THAT CAUSE PRURITUS
- Opiates and derivatives
- Aspirin
- Quinidine
- Phenothiazines*
- Tolbutamide*
- Erythromycin estolate*
- Hormones* (e.g., anabolic steroids, estrogens, progestins, testosterone)
- Vitamin B complex
- Psoralen plus ultraviolet A light
- Antimalarials
- Subclinical sensitivity to any drug

*By cholestasis.
HIV, human immunodeficiency virus.

acupuncture, transcutaneous electrical nerve stimulation, and mechanical vibratory stimulation.

Systemic Therapy

- Systemic therapy consists of H_1 antagonists. Second-generation antihistamines such as cetirizine, levocetirizine, loratadine, desloratadine, ebastine, fexofenadine, and rupatadine have minimal activity on nonhistaminic receptors, little sedative effect, and a longer duration of action compared with the first-generation antihistamines such as diphenhydramine.[7] Diphenhydramine, 25 to 50 mg every 6 hours, or hydroxyzine, 25 to 50 mg every 6 hours, can be beneficial, especially at bedtime. Sedative side effects are common, which may explain their therapeutic benefit.

- The oral tricyclic antidepressant doxepin (Sinequan), 25 mg every night up to 150 mg daily (in divided doses), is a potent H_1 and H_2 receptor blocker that has anxiolytic effects. Mirtazapine (Remeron), 15 to 45 mg nightly, and paroxetine (Paxil), 10 to 20 mg nightly, have been useful in case reports.[1] Sertraline was also shown to be effective in resolving cholestatic pruritus.[8]
- Opiate antagonists such as naltrexone (ReVia), 50 to 150 mg daily, have been used for various causes of pruritus with success, although the effectiveness for uremic pruritus is questionable.[9]
- Oral activated charcoal is a safe, effective therapy for uremic pruritus.
- Cholestyramine (Questran), 4 g once to three times daily, is effective for pruritus caused by cholestasis, but it can have untoward gastrointestinal side effects and should be taken with vitamin K and multivitamin supplements. Colestipol (Colestid) works similarly but is better tolerated. In refractory cases of cholestatic pruritus, ursodiol, phenobarbital, and rifampin have been used with good results.
- Gabapentin (Neurontin), 200 to 300 mg nightly, is effective for dialysis patients and those with neurogenic pruritus.
- Patients with liver disease should have diets high in polyunsaturated fatty acids. Thalidomide (Thalomid), 50 to 200 mg daily, is used in some circumstances, but monitoring for neuropathy and thrombosis is necessary.
- Danazol (Danocrine) is effective therapy for myeloproliferative disorders and other systemic disorders.
- Aspirin and cyproheptadine (Periactin), 4 mg three times daily, have both been shown to help patients with pruritus from polycythemia vera.
- UVB, sunlight, and topical clobetasol are efficacious in pruritus associated with human immunodeficiency virus (HIV) disease.[8]
- Psychotherapy and psychotropic medication have been shown to be beneficial in some patients.[10]

LIFE SPAN CONSIDERATIONS

A study of cutaneous complaints in older adults identified pruritus as the most frequent, accounting for 29% of all complaints. Patients older than 85 years showed the highest prevalence of pruritus, and it was reported more frequently in winter months.[11] The exact pathophysiologic mechanism of chronic pruritus among elders is unknown.[1]

COMPLICATIONS

Secondary skin lesions from scratching (e.g., lichenification) and secondary infections are common. Other complications include an undiagnosed underlying systemic illness and untoward side effects from drug therapy.

INDICATIONS FOR REFERRAL OR HOSPITALIZATION

Consultation with a dermatologist should be considered for intractable cases of pruritus or when the cause remains unknown after the preliminary evaluation and follow-up. Some patients require a referral to a pain relief clinic. Psychotherapeutic interventions have been shown to be beneficial in some patients.[10] If a systemic disorder is discovered, referral to an endocrinologist, hematologist, oncologist, gastroenterologist, nephrologist, psychiatrist, or other subspecialist may be in order.

PATIENT AND FAMILY EDUCATION AND HEALTH PROMOTION

Lifestyle interventions to alleviate pruritus require a concerted effort at patient education to identify factors that provoke or worsen itching. Avoidance of dry skin through the use of humidifiers, limited bathing, mild soaps, and emollients is critical. Elimination of wool and other clothing irritants, stress reduction measures, and instructions on medication side effects are also helpful in the management of pruritus.

CHAPTER 62

PSORIASIS

Richard M. Prior

DEFINITION AND EPIDEMIOLOGY

Psoriasis is an inflammatory papulosquamous eruption characterized by well-circumscribed erythematous macular and papular lesions with loosely adherent silvery white scale. It is a chronic, unpredictable disorder that is characterized by remissions and exacerbations throughout the life span. From 1% to 3% of the population is affected by psoriasis, or around 7.4 million Americans, with 25% to 45% of cases beginning after the age of 10 years. First episodes often appear in young adulthood, but they can appear later in life as well. Stress, anxiety, and illness often precede flares. Time lost from school and work as well as the emotional and financial constraints on families mandate effective and convenient treatments. Symptoms can be treated; however, as yet there is no cure. Remissions are common and can last for short periods or years, with progression to arthritis in about 30% of cases. A genetic component appears to exist in this disorder; thus a familial tendency can increase risk.[1,2]

Patients with psoriasis score poorly on quality-of-life (QOL) measures. Patients are troubled by the appearance of the lesions and pruritus associated with the disease. Those with psoriatic arthritis often have disability and pain. Over 80% of those with the disorder report that psoriasis often affects their emotional state and decreases their satisfaction with life. Psoriasis and psoriatic arthritis can have negative economic effects on those with the disorder; more than 92% of unemployed patients attribute their lack of a job solely to their disease.[3]

Psoriasis should be viewed as a systemic disorder that causes additional morbidity in those affected. Patients with psoriasis are more prone to inflammatory bowel disease and cardiovascular disease. They are likely to be overweight, hypertensive, diabetic, and dyslipidemic when psoriasis symptoms are present. In addition, these patients are more likely to experience alcohol dependence and depression.[4]

PATHOPHYSIOLOGY

Psoriasis is a chronic, inflammatory, autoimmune disorder characterized by dermal hyperproliferation that develops in response to T-cell infiltration into the skin and overexpression of multiple cytokines, including interferon, tumor necrosis factor (TNF), and interleukin-23 (IL-23). T cells are activated and

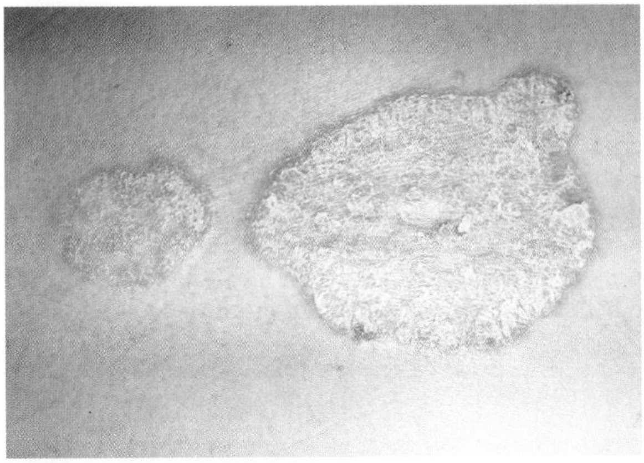

FIGURE 62-1 Psoriasis. Thick, red plaques have a sharply defined border and adherent silvery scale. (From Ignatavicius DD, Workman ML, *Medical-Surgical Nursing: Patient Centered Collaborative Care*, ed 8, St. Louis, 2016, Mosby.)

produce an inflammatory response that results in the hyperproliferation of keratinocytes. Psoriasis lesions often contain 30 times the number of keratinocytes as normal skin.[1]

Psoriasis is known to have strong genetic associations. Those who have first-degree family members with the disorder are often affected as well. There is an increased incidence of psoriasis in monozygotic twins.[1]

CLINICAL PRESENTATION AND PHYSICAL EXAMINATION

In psoriasis, scaly papules and plaques form and collect on skin surfaces in well-demarcated lesions (Fig. 62-1). The lesions have an erythematous base with silvery white plaques that are adherent. The dermis is highly vascular, and tiny bleeding points are revealed if the scales are removed (Auspitz sign). Common sites for these lesions include the elbows, knees, scalp, genitals, and intergluteal cleft. In contrast to adult psoriasis, childhood psoriasis often involves the face. Many patients exhibit concomitant nail dystrophies, including pitting, yellowing of the distal portion (oil drop sign), separation of the nail plate (onycholysis), and thickening of the entire nail (hyperkeratosis).[5]

Cutaneous trauma can induce psoriasis 1 to 3 weeks after injury. This isomorphic response, also known as the Koebner phenomenon, occurs in a linear fashion along the lines of a scratch, abrasion, sunburn, or pressure.

Discrete, scaly, "raindrop" plaques that are smaller than 1 cm, begin on the trunk, and spread to the extremities, sparing the palms and soles, are indicative of guttate psoriasis. Guttate psoriasis is occasionally seen after a streptococcal infection and is most common in adolescents. These patients are likely to develop psoriasis vulgaris (common, plaquelike psoriasis) later in life.[5]

Erythroderma and pustular psoriasis are more serious forms of the disease. They are most common in patients older than 50 years and may be precipitated by infection, withdrawal of systemic steroids, emotional stress, or severe illness. Erythrodermic forms generally appear over a large portion of the body and can be precipitated by various treatments themselves.[5]

Although most psoriatic lesions are asymptomatic, itching is variable. However, picking and scratching of the lesions can produce the Koebner response, and the lesions worsen. Skinfold lesions tend to itch more than common plaquelike lesions. The axilla, intramammary folds, groin, buttocks, and genitals are common sites for intense itching, or inverse psoriasis. The bright red appearance of the lesions and affinity for dark, moist folds can make distinguishing inverse psoriasis from *Candida* infections difficult based on appearance alone.

Psoriatic arthritis is a seronegative spondyloarthropathy that affects approximately 10% to 15% of the population with psoriasis. It is characterized by monoarthritis, often causing joint effusions; pain at the insertion point of tendons to bone (enthesitis); swelling of the fingers and toes (dactylitis); and changes to the nails (including pitting and splitting). In a small percentage of patients, psoriatic arthritis precedes the appearance of skin symptoms.

DIAGNOSTICS

The presence of silvery scales on red, erythematous plaques is characteristic; therefore the diagnosis is usually based on presentation. However, biopsy is useful in pustular cases, and nail cultures differentiate fungal disease. Uric acid levels may be elevated in psoriasis as well as in gout.

Psoriatic arthritis is diagnosed clinically based on symptom scoring models, as there is no diagnostic laboratory test. As many as half of those with psoriatic arthritis may be HLA-B27 positive. Almost all patients with psoriatic arthritis are rheumatoid factor negative. Many patients who develop erosive arthritis have radiographic findings in advanced stages of the disease.

DIFFERENTIAL DIAGNOSIS

In children, the plaques of psoriasis are thinner and less scaly than in adults with psoriasis and are often confused with seborrhea, atopic dermatitis, and diaper dermatitis. Seborrhea on the scalp tends to be patchy, red, and a bit oilier in appearance. Psoriasis is more plaquelike, with thick scales. Psoriasis typically appears on extensor surfaces, whereas atopic dermatitis is found on most flexor surfaces. Lichen planus papules have more of a purple hue, and patients exhibit Wickham striae (lacy, reticular, crisscrossed whitish lines) on many lesions. Flat warts do not have scale on the surface. Guttate psoriasis is often confused with pityriasis rosea; however, it lacks the characteristic herald patch, and the scale is thicker and more diffuse in psoriasis. Changes in the nails are often confused with onychomycosis. Culture for the presence of fungus will help establish the diagnosis. Yellow discoloration is common in both fungal and psoriatic changes, as is nail separation. The nails in psoriasis are not well formed because debris collects underneath, again because of rapid shedding of the skin layers. This debris leads to failure in the integrity of the nail and onycholysis.

DIFFERENTIAL DIAGNOSIS

Psoriasis

- Lichen planus
- Lichen simplex chronicus
- Flat warts
- Pityriasis rosea
- Rheumatoid arthritis
- Reactive arthritis
- Seborrheic dermatitis
- Atopic dermatitis
- Fungal infections (in nails)
- Gout
- Pseudogout
- Syphilis
- Nummular eczema
- Squamous cell carcinoma

Additional diagnoses to be considered are gout, pseudogout, reactive arthritis, syphilis, squamous cell carcinoma, nummular eczema, and lichen simplex chronicus.

MANAGEMENT

Topical Therapy

The goal of treatment is the restoration and maintenance of the barrier function of the skin. Good control can be achieved; however, it requires meticulous and consistent home care. Present therapy is aimed at reducing epidermal proliferation and decreasing inflammation. Topical corticosteroids produce rapid resolution of mild to moderate plaques. High-potency topical glucocorticosteroids applied ideally twice (but at least once) per day produce maximum benefit in 2 to 3 weeks. Current research suggests that combination therapy of a potent steroid combined with a vitamin D analogue (either as a single product or applied separately) may be the most effective topical treatment for lesions on the skin.[6] Intertriginous psoriasis, however, should be treated with low-potency steroids.

Ointments are the preferred vehicle because of better medicine penetration and support of the skin moisture barrier; however, ointments are not easily tolerated by the patient, especially if large skin surface areas are involved. Creams can be prescribed for patients who cannot tolerate ointments. Newer foam-based delivery systems provide advantages for some skin surfaces, such as the scalp, but they are expensive and often nonformulary. Solutions are available that are good vehicles for delivery of medicine to the scalp. Tolerance to steroid preparations rarely develops with plaque psoriasis, which can tolerate chronic application of high doses of steroids, but atrophy can occur with use on thinner lesions, as with inverse psoriasis. Occlusion with clear plastic wrap can increase the efficacy of therapy on large or thick plaques.

For severe, recalcitrant cases, intralesional injections with a corticosteroid suspension produce satisfactory results after one or two injections; this treatment requires a dermatology referral. Limitations of this therapy include atrophy and obvious discomfort from injections.

Scalp psoriasis is often characterized by thick scale, which not only produces embarrassing dandruff but interferes with the steroid's ability to penetrate the dermis. Scalp lesions also respond best to topical high-potency steroids. Combination therapy using vitamin D analogues in conjunction with topical steroids may also be helpful in the treatment of scalp lesions.[6]

Research suggests that coal tar preparations may not be any more effective than placebo in treating scalp lesions.[6] Shampoos containing the exfoliant salicylic acid are available to reduce scale buildup and to improve medication penetration. Use of topically applied mineral oil or vegetable oil and a bathing cap at bedtime is sometimes very effective at loosening and removing scale.

Phototherapy

Phototherapy in the form of ultraviolet B (UVB) light therapy has been shown to be effective for the treatment of psoriasis. The most common delivery method for the therapy is via a laser at a dermatologist's office. Targeted therapy is well tolerated, with some side effects such as blistering and erythema. The use of phototherapy requires multiple office visits, making it impractical or too expensive for some patients. Devices for home use are available, but some dermatologists are reluctant to prescribe them owing to concerns of misuse or abuse.[7]

Systemic Medications

Oral retinoids are used occasionally for psoriasis—particularly for pustular and erythrodermic psoriasis. However, they have side effects similar to those of isotretinoin and should be used with caution in women of childbearing age because they are teratogenic. Retinoids are less effective than methotrexate and cyclosporine but are safe in patients who are immunocompromised. Retinoids are not effective in patients with psoriatic arthritis.

Methotrexate, a folic acid antagonist, is highly effective in treating severe, recalcitrant psoriasis involving a large body area, acute pustular psoriasis, and psoriatic arthritis. Cell division is reduced, and the drug may also affect the inflammation. It should not be used in patients with liver or kidney disease, pregnancy, anemia, colitis, or debility. It should be reserved for patients unresponsive to other therapies and for those with psoriatic arthritis. Patients who take methotrexate are at risk for pancytopenia and should be monitored frequently with complete blood counts. Methotrexate should be avoided in pregnancy and in those who wish to become pregnant. Methotrexate and retinoid therapy should be co-managed with a dermatologist.

Cyclosporine (Neoral) is efficacious; however, it is also limited in use because of its potential nephrotoxicity. Blood pressure and serum creatinine concentration should be monitored. Relapse is also common once therapy is stopped. A dermatologist should manage patients who require cyclosporine therapy.

Biologic Agents

Biologic agents target the immune-mediated inflammation that is responsible for the psoriasis presentation. Currently, three TNF antagonists (etanercept, infliximab, and adalimumab), one T-cell modulator (alefacept), and one monoclonal antibody that targets IL-12 and IL-3 (ustekinumab) have been approved for the treatment of moderate to severe psoriasis. Several other biologic agents are approved for use in patients with psoriatic arthritis. Their use is increasing owing to their high degree of efficacy, low side effect profile, and improvement in QOL measures. They are given as self-administered subcutaneous or intramuscular injections or as intravenous infusions. In part because of the expense of the agents, use is restricted to patients with moderate to severe disease. Insurance companies often require that other treatment modalities have been attempted and have failed before patients are approved for the biologics.[8]

Safety data are available from the use of biologics in other disease states, such as rheumatoid arthritis. Several agents come with a Food and Drug Administration–mandated "black box" warning for safety concerns relative to increased susceptibility to infection from fungi, viruses, bacteria, and mycobacteria and a possible connection to lymphoma, hematologic diseases such as aplastic anemia, melanoma, nonmelanoma skin cancers, and other solid organ cancers. Each medication has its own particular safety profile; thus it is good practice that patients be screened for tuberculosis and hepatitis B before initiation of therapy to avoid latent disease activation. This is also a good time to check titers and to update the patient's vaccination status because live vaccines are contraindicated during treatment. They can, however, be administered before treatment. Histories of multiple sclerosis or other demyelinating disease and congestive heart failure are relative contraindications. Monitoring parameters include psoriasis lesion and surface area reduction, QOL assessments, periodic liver function tests and complete blood counts, and assessment for evidence of infectious disease.[8,9]

Combination Therapy

Combination therapy using several different treatment modalities is common, especially with particularly difficult-to-treat cases or when the treatment is poorly tolerated. Even in patients maintained with topical treatments alone, it is useful to use multiple agents simultaneously for their synergistic effects. For smaller flares or chronicity, early treatment with combination therapies centered on topical treatments can manage the disease and minimize risk.

Selected Therapy Considerations

Guttate psoriasis should clue the provider to the need to screen for *Streptococcus*. Treatment is guided by the results of the culture.

Oral steroids should be used with caution because they can induce a pustular flare. They may be useful in controlling persistent erythroderma; however, they are not indicated in the treatment of psoriasis.

Many patients are interested in the question of whether or not diet can positively influence the severity of psoriasis. Research suggests that weight loss is a useful adjunct therapy to medication and that maintaining a normal body weight may help limit or prevent the disorder.[10] In addition, supplements containing omega-3 fatty acids may be helpful for patients with psoriasis.[11]

COMPLICATIONS

Complications are usually related to infection. Scratching can introduce bacteria from beneath fingernails into lesions. Guttate psoriasis, erythrodermic psoriasis, and pustular psoriasis are also potential complications. Both erythrodermic psoriasis and pustular psoriasis are rare; however, serious sequelae, including congestive heart failure and sepsis, are potential hazards. Additional complications include psoriatic arthritis and cardiovascular disease, atrophy of skin with corticosteroid use, risk of skin cancer and cataracts with phototherapy if the eyes are not protected, and risk of effects on the metabolic profile with use of strong antimetabolites or retinoids.

INDICATIONS FOR REFERRAL OR HOSPITALIZATION

A patient with recalcitrant or unresponsive psoriasis should be referred to a dermatologist for management with phototherapy, oral therapies, and biologics. If a dermatology referral is not possible, an internist may be appropriate for oral therapy.

Psoriatic arthritis often follows psoriasis by about 10 years. Early referral, close monitoring, and co-management with a rheumatologist or dermatologist can help identify appropriate patients to prevent the further debilitation to psoriatic arthritis in susceptible individuals.

PATIENT AND FAMILY EDUCATION AND HEALTH PROMOTION

It is crucial for the patient and family to understand the chronic nature of psoriasis as well as the genetic and environmental factors. Adherence to the prescribed regimen is necessary for effective treatment; however, this requires meticulous and consistent home care.

Patients should understand the use of moisturizers and lubricants to maintain control. They should avoid injury to skin (i.e., sunburn and other physical trauma), triggering the Koebner phenomenon. Certain medications (beta blockers, lithium, and antimalarials) that are known to worsen psoriasis should be avoided when possible. An important part of treatment is education about treatment modalities and emotional support for families as well as for patients. Patients may contact the National Psoriasis Foundation (www.psoriasis.org), a not-for-profit organization dedicated to research, education, and support. Research is ongoing in the study of psoriasis. Patients and providers need to stay abreast of studies and treatment modalities and encourage ongoing collaborative practice across disciplines to meet the needs of these patients.

CHAPTER 63

PURPURA

Joanne Sandberg-Cook

DEFINITION AND EPIDEMIOLOGY

Purpura is a hemorrhaging into the skin. The size of the bleeding vessel determines the size of the lesion, which in turn may provide clues to the cause. Petechiae are lesions less than 3 mm (1/10 inch) in diameter; these indicate capillary bleeding. Lesions ranging from 3 mm to 1 cm (1/10 to 4/10 inch) are often referred to as purpura. Lesions larger than 1 cm are referred to as ecchymoses. All show a predilection for the limbs. Purpura is divided into two groups: inflammatory (palpable) and noninflammatory. Noninflammatory purpura is further divided into hemostatic defects, nonpalpable purpura, and nonhemostatic defects (vascular purpura).[1]

PATHOPHYSIOLOGY

Purpura is characterized by an extravasation of red blood cells into the dermis from small cutaneous vessels. Hemosiderin or hematoidin may be present if the purpura is chronic; this causes a characteristic red or brown discoloration. Purpura may be oval or round or irregularly outlined; it may be flat or raised (palpable) as a result of edema or induration.[1]

Palpable purpura consists of raised, erythematous lesions that do not blanch when the skin is pressed with a glass slide. Dilated superficial capillaries, in which the blood remains confined within the vessels, do blanch when pressed, thereby distinguishing them from true purpura.

Extravasation of blood from the vessel depends on the integrity of the blood vessel, which in turn depends on the strength of the vessel, the transmural pressure gradient that drives blood out of the vessel, and the competence of the mechanism that combats the basal level of vascular trauma.[1]

CLINICAL PRESENTATION

Because purpura is a symptom of many systemic diseases, these lesions seldom are seen without other symptoms. A review of systems should include an inquiry into other bleeding sites, abnormally heavy menstrual bleeding, trauma, recent infection (including sexually transmitted diseases), exposure to ticks or a

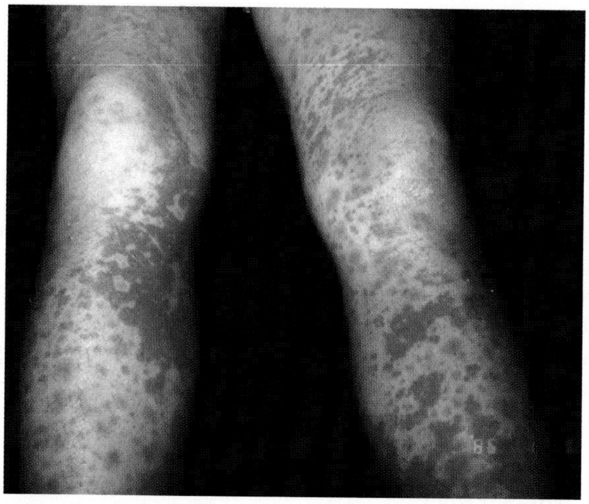

FIGURE 63-1 Palpable purpura (nonblanching red macules and papules) on the lower legs is typical of many types of cutaneous vasculitis. (From Goldman L, Schafer AI: *Goldman's Cecil medicine*, ed 24, Philadelphia, 2012, Elsevier.)

tick bite, and recent travel to areas where Rocky Mountain spotted fever, dengue fever, or Lyme disease is endemic or epidemic. A complete medication history (including over-the-counter medications and allergies) should be taken. Any history of autoimmune disease or other serious illnesses, such as leukemia or lymphoma, should be noted. Recent complaints of fever, chills, arthralgias, and myalgias should be noted.

PHYSICAL EXAMINATION

The skin is the focus of the physical examination. The size, location, and shape of the lesions should be documented. Bullae and ulcerations can develop within any lesion larger than petechiae.[2] Lesions should be palpated for swelling (palpable purpura) or flatness against the skin. Palpable purpura is usually associated with inflammation of the vessel (Fig. 63-1; see Chapter 220). A glass slide pressed against the lesion determines whether it is blanchable, thereby differentiating it from erythema or dilated superficial capillaries.[1] Excoriation may imply pruritus.

The remainder of the general examination includes an oral examination to look for lesions of the gums or tongue and a joint examination to look for swelling, inflammation, or deformities that would suggest connective tissue disease. Fever, nuchal rigidity, organomegaly, or a new heart murmur may imply serious systemic disease or infection.

Observations of weight, nutritional status, or skin turgor may suggest nutritional deficiencies. Evidence of trauma (healing bruises, fractures) may indicate ongoing trauma as a cause.

DIAGNOSTICS

Laboratory studies help differentiate between inflammatory and noninflammatory purpura. (Inflammatory purpura [vasculitis] is discussed in Chapter 220.) A complete blood count (CBC) with a platelet count (not an estimate) is most helpful. An erythrocyte sedimentation rate (ESR) or C-reactive protein (CRP) level can be beneficial in excluding an inflammatory cause. Bleeding time, platelet count, prothrombin time (PT), partial thromboplastin time (PTT), and international normalized ratio (INR) will determine the presence of coagulopathies. Blood urea nitrogen (BUN), creatinine, and liver function tests (LFTs) are necessary to exclude organ disease. Immune studies to exclude autoimmune diseases such as lupus, rheumatoid arthritis, cryoglobulinemias, or scleroderma may be indicated, depending on other physical findings and symptoms. Infectious disease screening would include screening for hepatitis B and C, human immunodeficiency virus (HIV) infection, and tuberculosis.[2]

DIAGNOSTICS

Purpura

LABORATORY	ESR
CBC and differential	Bleeding time
BUN	PT/PTT
Creatinine	INR
LFTs	Rheumatoid factor*
Hepatitis B and C virus antibodies	CRP
HIV screening	Antinuclear antibodies*
Platelet count	Antineutrophil cytoplasmic antibody*

*If indicated.

DIFFERENTIAL DIAGNOSIS

The differential diagnosis of purpura is extensive. Inflammatory and noninflammatory causes of purpura should be differentiated. Inflammatory purpura is most often palpable and is associated with the vasculitides. These syndromes can be life-threatening and require prompt treatment in conjunction with a specialist (see Chapter 220). Causes of noninflammatory purpura include serious infectious diseases, medication hypersensitivity, trauma, vascular disorders, and bleeding disorders.

Systemic infections such as HIV and acquired immunodeficiency syndrome (AIDS), cytomegalovirus, hepatitis B and C, herpes zoster, Lyme disease (see Chapter 234), Rocky Mountain spotted fever, meningitis, syphilis, and gonococcemia have been associated with purpura.[3-5] Subacute bacterial endocarditis manifests with fever, petechial rash, and a new heart murmur.

Noninfectious presentations are often related to medications, including the long-term use of oral steroids and fluorinated topical steroids. Drug-induced vasculitis, also known as hypersensitivity vasculitis or leukocytoclastic vasculitis, is the most common cause of palpable purpura and can occur at any time during the course of the medication. These allergic reactions to medication may be associated with fever, arthralgia, and urticaria. The most common causative agents are antibiotics (vancomycin), sulfonamides, trimethoprim, thiazide diuretics, phenytoin, and allopurinol. Nonsteroidal anti-inflammatory medications, including aspirin and ibuprofen, can also cause petechial rashes.[4] Heparin, low-molecular-weight heparin, and warfarin (Coumadin) can cause bleeding, which can result in purpura.

Trauma to blood vessels is initially seen as classic bruising, often involving the extremities, feet, hands (in the case of repetitive pounding), or face. The lesions associated with child abuse may involve bruising from pinching or grabbing or palpebral conjunctivae resulting from strangulation or smothering.[1] Senile purpura manifests as large ecchymoses on the extensor surfaces of the arms and hands of (usually) an older adult. Such lesions are a result of the skin thinning associated with age, sun damage, or prolonged steroid use in combination with minor trauma or shearing. Laboratory study results are normal, and the patient should be reassured that the lesions are benign. Use of a citrus bioflavonoid may be helpful in reducing the number of purpuras.[6]

A variety of syndromes associated with vascular diseases can cause purpura. Atheroemboli secondary to cholesterol can cause petechiae, purpura, nodules, ulceration, and occlusion leading to gangrene. Fat emboli that occur 2 or 3 days after severe trauma can be seen with petechiae of the upper extremity, thorax, and conjunctivae.[1] Disseminated intravascular coagulation (DIC) demonstrates both thrombotic and hemorrhagic features. Purpura fulminans is a rare complication of DIC and results in hemorrhagic necrosis of the skin.[4] Palpable purpura may, rarely, be the initial presentation of a paraneoplastic syndrome, especially lymphoproliferative disease.[7]

Immune thrombocytopenic purpura (ITP) is an acquired disorder of platelet aggregation in the microcirculation, not caused by a known condition, which can lead to bleeding. The bleeding associated with ITP can range from severe to only petechiae and easy bruising. Generally defined by a platelet count of less than 50,000/mm^3, this disorder can be seen in all age groups. Treatment is usually reserved for those with a platelet count of less than 50,000/mm^3 who are at risk of bleeding or those with active bleeding. High-dose steroids either by mouth or intravenously are the first-line treatment. Some patients require intravenous immunoglobulins.[8] WinRho (anti-D polyclonal antibody) can raise the platelet count in those severely affected. Rituximab and splenectomy are reserved as second-line therapy for those in whom medical treatment fails to raise platelet counts above 50,000/mm^3 and who remain at high risk of serious bleeding.[4,9]

Petechiae and ecchymoses are common concerns. Stasis dermatitis manifests with petechiae caused by capillary injury. This results from chronic venous stasis caused by valve incompetence. Later stages of chronic venous stasis are associated with an accumulation of hemosiderin, leading to the characteristic brown discoloration of the lower extremities.[4]

Miscellaneous causes of purpura include hemorrhagic gingivitis and stomatitis related to vitamin C deficiency (scurvy). Young girls occasionally tend to bruise easily because of hormonal changes. A tendency toward early stroke, multiple miscarriages, or thrombocytopenia may be associated with the presence of antiphospholipid antibodies, sometimes known as lupus anticoagulant. HIV/AIDS and cancers, including lymphomas and leukemias, can produce petechial or purpuric lesions.[3] Finally, defects in clotting factors or platelet abnormalities, including the quantity and quality of platelets, can lead to cutaneous bleeding (see Chapter 238).

DIFFERENTIAL DIAGNOSIS

Purpura

INFLAMMATORY (PALPABLE)

- Vasculitis
- Cryoglobulinemia

NONINFLAMMATORY

Hemostatic Defects

- Platelet abnormalities
- Coagulation abnormalities

Nonpalpable Purpura

- Increased pressure
  - Venous stasis
- Decreased vessel integrity
  - Senile purpura
  - Steroid excess
  - Vitamin C deficiency
  - Hormonal
- Trauma
  - Physical injury
  - Solar injury
- Infectious
  - Bacterial (meningococcemia)
  - Viral (dengue fever)
  - Rickettsial (Lyme disease, Rocky Mountain spotted fever)

Embolic

- Atheroembolic
  - Cholesterol

Neoplastic

- Leukemia
- Lymphoma

Allergic

- Medications
- Contact

Thrombotic

- DIC
- Purpura fulminans
- Antiphospholipid syndrome
- Idiopathic thrombocytopenic purpura

MANAGEMENT

Treatment of purpura is directed toward the cause. Patients with disorders of platelet count or function should be referred to a hematologist for possible bone marrow biopsy. Patients with palpable purpura should be advised that an extensive evaluation, including a skin biopsy, may be indicated. A referral to appropriate specialists, usually hematologists or rheumatologists, is indicated.

Patients with stasis dermatitis may benefit from the application of a moderate-potency topical steroid ointment to help with the associated pruritus and to reduce the risk for cellulitis from scratching. A reassurance that the lesions are benign is needed for young women who bruise easily because of hormonal changes and for older patients with senile purpura.

LIFE SPAN CONSIDERATIONS

Purpura associated with hormonal change is most often seen in young women. Senile purpura is primarily a disease of older adults but can result from chronic steroid use. Antiphospholipid antibodies are most commonly found in women of childbearing age, but men and older women can also be affected. The vasculitides are most often seen in middle-aged patients, with several notable exceptions (see Chapter 220).

COMPLICATIONS

Complications of the skin lesions themselves include the formation of bullae, skin breakdown, and ulcer formation. Ulcers are slow to heal and can involve a large area. Necrosis of the skin, especially the fingertips, can be a complication of vascular lesions.

INDICATIONS FOR REFERRAL OR HOSPITALIZATION

Any patient with fever and a petechial rash and serious bleeding should be hospitalized to exclude or to evaluate life-threatening infection, systemic vasculitis, or neoplasm. This is especially necessary if the patient has a known connective tissue disease such as lupus or rheumatoid arthritis, has a malignant neoplasm, or has been exposed to meningitis. Patients with acute bleeding disorders may require hospitalization to control bleeding and for transfusion (see Chapter 238). All patients with palpable purpura should be referred to a hematologist or rheumatologist for evaluation and treatment recommendations. Referral to a dermatologist is appropriate when a skin biopsy is needed for accurate diagnosis.

PATIENT EDUCATION AND HEALTH PROMOTION

Medications that may contribute to bleeding should be avoided unless the patient is advised to continue them as part of a treatment plan. Patients with stasis should be advised to avoid tight-fitting garments and prolonged sitting or standing. Sun protection remains important throughout life. Steroid creams or ointments should be used judiciously to prevent skin thinning and increased susceptibility to minor trauma.

CHAPTER 64

SCABIES

JoAnn Lepke

DEFINITION AND EPIDEMIOLOGY

Scabies is an infection caused by infestation of the *Sarcoptes scabiei* mite, sometimes referred to as the *human itch mite.* It can affect people of all ages and is more common in crowded living conditions and institutional facilities such as nursing homes, prisons, long-term care facilities, and day care centers. Worldwide cases number an estimated 130 million at any time, especially affecting the young and elderly in resource-poor countries. It is more prevalent in hot and humid environments and in poor, overcrowded areas.[1] Scabies is usually transmitted by direct, prolonged skin-to-skin contact with an infested person, commonly through sexual contact with an infected individual.[2]

Animals do not spread scabies.

PATHOPHYSIOLOGY

The scabies mite is not visible to the unaided eye. The female mite is responsible for the infestations. The mite is oval and has four pairs of legs (Fig. 64-1). It burrows no deeper than the stratum corneum and lays two to three eggs per day for 1 to 2 months before dying. The eggs and mites reach maturity in 28 to 30 days, starting a new cycle.[1] The intense pruritus experienced with scabies infestation is a hypersensitivity reaction to the mites. It usually begins 2 to 4 weeks after infection in a person who was not previously sensitized. Pruritus may begin within a day of reinfestation in a previously sensitized person. Scabies is usually acquired through close personal contact, although the mite can survive off the human host for up to 3 days.

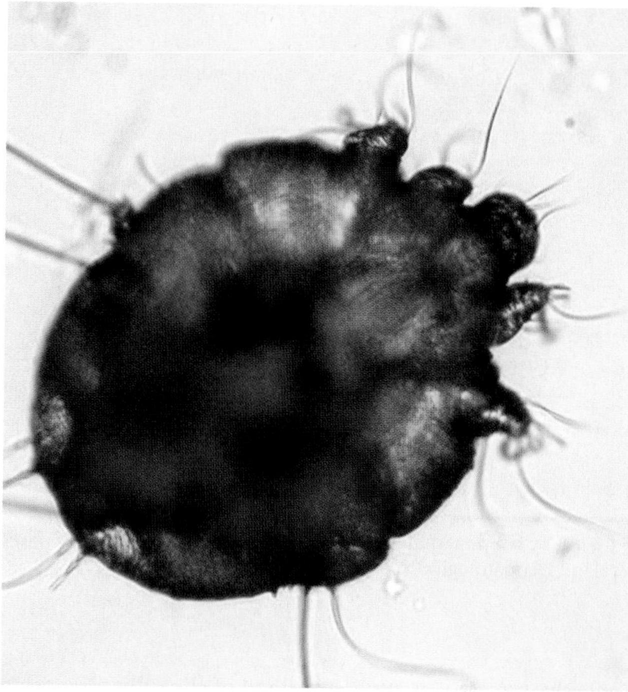

FIGURE 64-1 Scabies mite, highly magnified. (Courtesy New Zealand Dermatological Society Incorporated.)

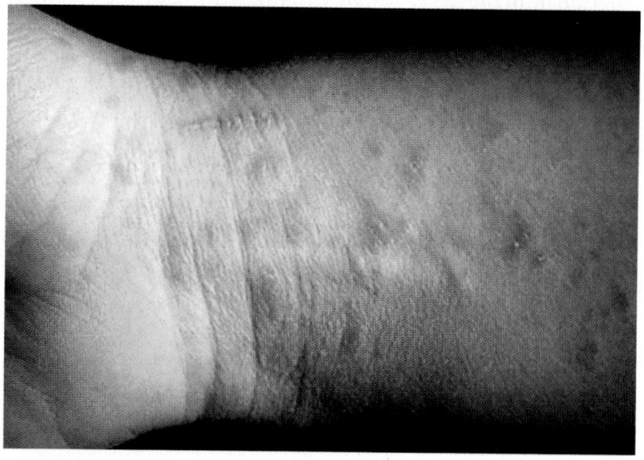

FIGURE 64-2 Scabies on the wrist. (Courtesy New Zealand Dermatological Society Incorporated.)

CLINICAL PRESENTATION AND PHYSICAL EXAMINATION

The clinical presentation of scabies is variable. Most commonly, there are minimal findings in the setting of intractable pruritus, especially at night. The skin lesions of scabies can be classified into two categories: lesions at the site of infestation and lesions secondary to hypersensitivity to the mite. Intraepidermal burrows are linear or serpiginous ridges that are produced by the infesting female mite. Common burrow sites are the interdigital spaces of the hands, flexures of the wrists and arms, genitals, feet, buttocks, and axillae (Fig. 64-2). A hypersensitivity reaction to the mites can manifest as urticaria, eczematous dermatitis, and scabetic nodules. Excoriations, lichen simplex chronicus, and secondary infection may result from scratching. Crusted scabies (Norwegian or hyperkeratotic) is found in immunocompromised or debilitated patients, and itching may be only mild.[2]

DIAGNOSTICS

The classic burrow, a straight or S-shaped ridge 2 to 10 mm long, is not always present and is less likely to be seen in warm, humid climates.[3] However, diagnosis is typically made with clinical findings. Dermoscopy may be of value in diagnosis, making burrows more visible, and the ability to see a "jet-plane" appearance of a mite at one end of a burrow (Fig. 64-3).[4] The

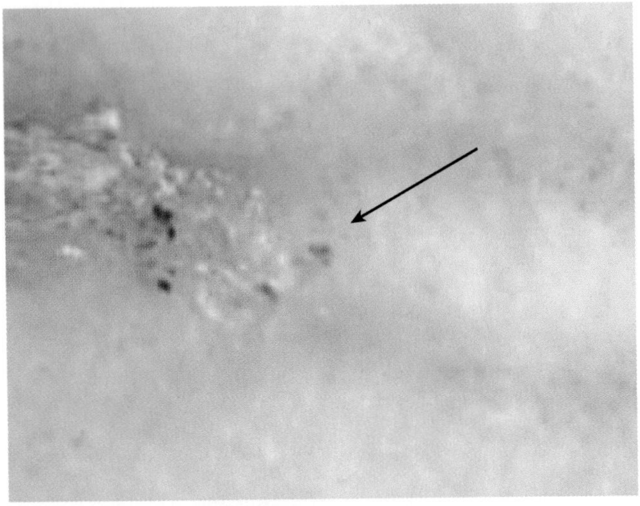

FIGURE 64-3 Scabies seen with dermatoscope. (Courtesy New Zealand Dermatological Society Incorporated.)

"adhesive tape test" is another method of clinically diagnosing scabies. Adhesive tape is adhered to the affected area, then rapidly removed. The tape is then applied to a slide and examined under a microscope.[5]

Definitive confirmation is made with a "scabies prep." A drop of mineral oil is placed on a burrow, and the lesion is scraped or shaved. The sample is viewed under a microscope and examined for mites, eggs, fragments, or feces. The lack of positive findings on a scraping does not rule out the diagnosis of scabies, as the total number of mites present on any host may be fewer than 10 to 15.[2]

DIAGNOSTICS

Scabies

LABORATORY

Microscopic examination for mites or eggs
Biopsy to rule out other conditions (if necessary)
Screening for sexually transmitted diseases

DIFFERENTIAL DIAGNOSIS

Scabies may easily be mistaken for other skin disorders. See the differential diagnosis box.[6]

DIFFERENTIAL DIAGNOSIS

Scabies

- Atopic dermatitis
- Insect bites
- Pediculosis
- Pityriasis rosea
- Animal scabies
- Seborrheic dermatitis
- Syphilis
- Contact dermatitis
- Psoriasis
- Drug reactions
- Viral exanthem
- Bullous pemphigoid
- Folliculitis
- Dyshidrotic eczema
- Id reaction
- Seabather's eruption
- Chickenpox
- Dermatitis herpetiformis

MANAGEMENT

Treatment is initiated with topical application of 5% permethrin cream (Elimite), applied from the neck down, giving attention to the interdigital webs, axillae, umbilicus, gluteal cleft, genitals, areas under the nails, and soles of the feet. The medication should be left on for 8 to 12 hours and then washed off. The treatment should be repeated in 1 to 2 weeks. Because scabies can infest the hairline of older adults, massage the permethrin cream into the skin from head to toe in these patients. Crotamiton cream is not first-line topical treatment; this product has been associated with resistance issues.[6] Sulfur ointment or lotion is an older treatment; however, sulfur preparations are not popular with patients owing to the strong odor and messiness associated with application.[6]

Oral ivermectin is used off label to treat crusted scabies or if topical treatments are not effective. The dose of ivermectin is 200 µg/kg, taken once only, but the dose may be repeated in 14 days.[6,7]

Lindane (Kwell) is no longer recommended as a first-line treatment of scabies because of toxicity concerns and side effects. However, it is considered an alternate regimen by the Centers for Disease Control and Prevention (CDC) to be used if other treatments are unavailable or have failed. One ounce of lotion (or 30 g of cream) is applied sparingly from the neck down and washed off in 8 hours.[7]

Pregnant and lactating women may be treated with permethrin or sulfur preparations. Ivermectin and lindane are pregnancy risk factor C; neither is recommended in breastfeeding women.

Infected patients' clothing and bedding should be machine washed and dried in a very hot dryer, or dry-cleaned. Personal or household contacts from the past 30 days should be evaluated and treated. Lubrication and topical corticosteroids are used to treat persistent pruritic papules and eczematous dermatitis resulting from infestation and treatment. Antihistamines may be used to treat pruritus.

COMPLICATIONS

Superinfection is a potential complication. A secondary infection may result from scratching. Pustules, impetigo, and ecthyma should be treated with appropriate antibiotics.

Acute glomerulonephritis has been associated with streptococcal superinfection.

INDICATIONS FOR REFERRAL OR HOSPITALIZATION

Deaths have been associated with the use of ivermectin for scabies in older adults; thus it should be used with caution. Dermatology referral is indicated with treatment failure. Recalcitrant infestation or persistent pruritus requires physician consultation.

PATIENT AND FAMILY EDUCATION

All household contacts should be identified and treated. All clothing and bedding must be washed in hot water and dried on the hot cycle, and stuffed sofas and chairs should be vacumed. Materials that cannot be washed should be placed in a plastic bag for 1 week. Patients should be given written and verbal instructions about how to use medication and how to eliminate mites in bedding and on furniture. Patients should be warned that symptoms may continue to be present for 2 weeks after treatment.

CHAPTER 65

SEBORRHEIC DERMATITIS

Theresa A. Bedford

DEFINITION AND EPIDEMIOLOGY

Seborrheic dermatitis is a chronic, common dermatosis that occurs across the life span. It is characterized by greasy, slightly erythematous scaling that occurs in areas with the highest concentration of sweat glands or sebaceous glands, including the scalp, face, and postauricular and intertriginous areas.[1,2] The disorder affects 1% to 5% of immunocompetent adults. Men tend to be affected more than women. Although the association is unclear, this disorder occurs in disproportionate numbers in patients with neurologic disorders (e.g., Parkinson disease, epilepsy, central nervous system disease or trauma) and may worsen with stress and fatigue.[2]

PATHOPHYSIOLOGY

The cause of seborrheic dermatitis is unknown. Sebaceous gland secretion, the presence of Malassezia yeast, and the host immune response are thought to contribute to the condition.[2]

CLINICAL PRESENTATION AND PHYSICAL EXAMINATION

Seborrheic dermatitis is seen in both young and old patients. In infants, the most common presentation is yellow or brown scaling lesions on the scalp, which are called cradle cap. In adolescents and adults, another common presentation is dry, flaky scales on the scalp. This disorder is known as dandruff.[3,4]

On the face and auricular area, seborrheic dermatitis is seen as greasy, erythematous, sharply marginated plaques. Polycyclic plaques are commonly seen on the sternal area. In the axillae and groin, the eruption manifests as more confluent plaques with fine scales and less well-defined borders. Lesions are usually asymptomatic, although pruritus is may be present.

DIAGNOSTICS AND DIFFERENTIAL DIAGNOSIS

There are many differential diagnoses. More common diseases that can resemble seborrheic dermatitis include eczema, psoriasis, impetigo, dermatophytosis, tinea versicolor, intertriginous candidiasis, otitis externa, blepharitis, and systemic lupus erythematosus. Psoriasis is often described with more circumscribed, thicker plaques with a bright silvery hue. Seborrheic dermatitis can often overlap with psoriasis in a condition known as *sebopsoriasis*. Pityriasis versicolor is often less inflamed with more extension and flatter lesions. Atopic or contact dermatitis generally is accompanied by pruritus; patch testing may be needed. If the diagnosis is uncertain, a skin biopsy and immunofluorescence studies should be completed.

DIAGNOSTICS

Seborrheic Dermatitis

INITIAL
KOH wet preparation

OTHER
ANA*
Skin biopsy*

*If indicated.
ANA, antinuclear antibody test; KOH, potassium hydroxide.

DIFFERENTIAL DIAGNOSIS

Seborrheic Dermatitis

- Dandruff
- Scabies
- Tinea capitis, versicolor, cruris, corporis
- Asteatotic eczema
- Allergic and irritant dermatitis
- Drug eruptions, drug-induced photosensitivity
- Psoriasis
- Extramammary Paget disease
- Impetigo
- Nummular dermatitis
- Dermatophytosis
- Acute lupus erythematosus
- Candidal infection
- Intertrigo infection
- Langerhans cell histiocytosis
- Pityriasis rosea
- Acrodermatitis enteropathica
- Pemphigus, pemphigus foliaceus
- Glucagonoma syndrome

Less common diseases that can resemble seborrheic dermatitis include Langerhans cell histiocytosis, acrodermatitis enteropathica, pemphigus foliaceus, and glucagonoma syndrome. If these disorders are considered, there should be consultation with a dermatologist.

MANAGEMENT

In general, when patients have symptoms suggestive of seborrheic dermatitis on the face or eyebrows, the scalp should be carefully examined because this is usually a "top-down" disorder, requiring treatment in that order as well. There is no cure. Treatment is targeted at controlling acute flares and maintaining remission. First-line therapy is topical antifungals or topical corticosteroids. Topical antifungals reduce *Malassezia* proliferation, thereby reducing the inflammatory response; topical corticosteroids serve to reduce inflammation. Topical antifungals are safe for all skin types.

Antiseborrheic shampoos (e.g., ketoconazole 2%, selenium sulfide 2.5%, ciclopirox 1%) used one to two times a week for 4 weeks may be used to treat flare-ups and prevent relapses. Some patients may require a topical steroid in the form of a lotion, solution, or foam applied once a day after washing with an antiseborrheic shampoo.[2] Ortonne and colleagues (2011) found that twice-weekly clobetasol propionate shampoo 0.05% alternating with twice-weekly ketoconazole shampoo 2% for 4 weeks was more effective for severe seborrheic dermatitis than ketoconazole shampoo alone.[5] Topical steroids should be used only for the short term. Derma-Smoothe/FS is effective for scalp plaques.[6]

There are several options for therapy on the face, trunk, and intertriginous regions. Tacrolimus 0.1% ointment, ketoconazole 2% cream, ciclopirox olamine 1% cream, sertaconazole nitrate 2% cream, and metronidazole 0.75% gel have been shown to be effective at clearing symptoms. If this intervention does not help, a mild topical steroid such as 1% or 2.5% hydrocortisone can be used daily until the eruption clears.[2] Shemer and colleagues (2008) found itraconazole (Sporanox), an anti-inflammatory and antimycotic, to be effective for moderate to severe symptoms; it is an alternative for those who do not respond to or do not wish to use topical treatment during exacerbations.[7] Pimecrolimus 1% (Protopic), a macrolactam immunomodulator, works by inhibiting T-cell activation and proinflammatory cytokine production and has shown effectiveness in the treatment of seborrheic dermatitis. Pimecrolimus may cause burning on initiation of treatment; however, this typically resolves within 72 hours and is not problematic for the majority of patients.[8] Steroid treatment may induce skin atrophy and early relapse. Secondary bacterial or candidal infections should be treated with antibiotic or antifungal agents.

COMPLICATIONS

Secondary candidal and bacterial infections may occur, especially around the eyes and in intertriginous areas. These should be treated with appropriate antifungal or antibiotic medications. Secondary changes such as flexural intertrigo, lichenification, otitis externa, and widespread disease may occur.[2] Periorificial dermatitis is a papular eruption that can occur around the eyes, nose, and mouth as a result of topical steroid overuse on the face. If this eruption occurs, topical steroids should be tapered off.[9]

LIFE SPAN CONSIDERATIONS

Older adult patients present a unique disease management challenge because of their individual physical and mental abilities. Their ability to comply with the treatment plan should be considered and simple topical therapies used to increase efficacy and compliance.

INDICATIONS FOR REFERRAL OR HOSPITALIZATION

Patients with unresponsive seborrheic dermatitis or secondary changes with therapy should be referred to a dermatologist for further workup. As indicated previously, several dermatoses can resemble seborrheic dermatitis but will not respond to standard therapies.[3]

PATIENT AND FAMILY EDUCATION

Seborrheic dermatitis is chronic and recurrent. Proper use of antiseborrheic preparations and monitoring for early flares will usually control the disorder.

CHAPTER 66

STASIS DERMATITIS

Ashley M. Taylor

DEFINITION AND EPIDEMIOLOGY

Stasis dermatitis is an eczematous eruption, inflammation, or chronic dermatitis of the lower extremities, the result of chronic venous insufficiency.[1] Recurrent swelling may cause pruritus, excoriation, hyperpigmentation, papules, and scaling and crusting of the skin on the lower extremities, with a predilection for the medial ankle.[1] Stasis dermatitis can lead to skin ulceration in approximately 30% of chronic venous insufficiency cases.[1] The condition is most often seen in persons older than 50 years and is more common in women because there is a higher incidence of comorbidities that affect the venous circulation, such as deep venous thrombosis (DVT), pregnancy, use of oral contraceptives, obesity, smoking, and immobility.[1,2]

PATHOPHYSIOLOGY

Stasis dermatitis is a recalcitrant condition resulting from ambulatory venous hypertension, which is caused by calf muscle pump dysfunction, valvular incompetence, or any abnormalities of the venous system that cause a reflux of blood.[2] Distention of the adjacent capillary beds ensues, creating stasis in these beds. Over time, ulcerations may result from the damage to the vessels themselves, surrounding skin, or supporting structures in the subcutaneous and dermal layers. There are two explanations for this damage. Stasis fosters the development of fibrous perivascular cuffs around the capillaries, which reduces blood flow to surrounding tissues, damaging these structures; alternatively, stasis produces endothelial damage, releasing damaging proteolytic enzymes and free radicals into surrounding areas.[3]

CLINICAL PRESENTATION AND PHYSICAL EXAMINATION

The hallmark sign of stasis dermatitis is bronzing (hemosiderin staining) of the affected skin. The eruption can be unilateral, usually as a result of trauma or surgery, or bilaterally symmetric and is initially localized to the ankle (Fig. 66-1). Edema, a common manifestation, progresses from distal to proximal, and varicose veins are often present. The condition is often insidious; full manifestation of the signs and symptoms may take months. Patients may be initially seen with mild pruritus, xerosis, a scaly and erythematous rash, cutaneous atrophy, and bulla formation. The skin may be cyanotic when the extremity is in a dependent position. Secondary bacterial infection (usually staphylococcal) ensues, and painful ulceration eventually occurs.

DIAGNOSTICS

Doppler ultrasound examination and venography are used to diagnose venous insufficiency or DVT. The D-dimer blood test, if the result is normal, can exclude DVT if it is suspected in conjunction with venous stasis dermatitis. Any nonhealing skin ulcerations should be cultured for bacterial infection.

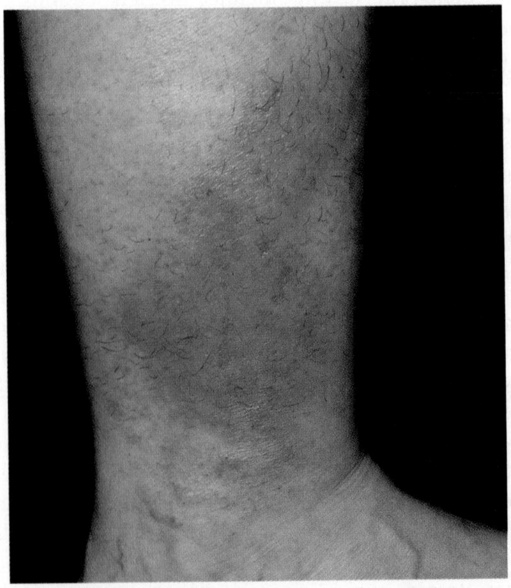

FIGURE 66-1 Stasis dermatitis in early stage with erythema and erosions. (From Habif TP, Campbell JL, Chapman MS, et al: Skin disease: diagnosis and treatment, ed 2, St Louis, 2004, Mosby.)

DIAGNOSTICS

Stasis Dermatitis

LABORATORY
Wound culture*
D-dimer test for suspected DVT*

IMAGING
Doppler ultrasound study or venography for suspected DVT*

*If indicated.

DIFFERENTIAL DIAGNOSIS

Differential diagnoses include diseases that cause the chronic skin changes associated with stasis dermatitis and those that result in lower extremity ulceration.

DIFFERENTIAL DIAGNOSIS

Stasis Dermatitis

CARDIOVASCULAR
- Arterial insufficiency
- Sickle cell anemia

DERMATOLOGIC
- Atopic dermatitis
- Carcinoma
- Cellulitis
- Contact dermatitis
- Necrobiosis lipoidica
- Nummular dermatitis
- Pigmented purpuric dermatitis
- Pyoderma gangrenosum
- Tinea pedis

MANAGEMENT

Specialist consultation is indicated for ulcerations recalcitrant to therapy or those that penetrate past the dermal layer.

Immediate emergency department referral is indicated for patients who have infections that require intravenous antibiotics.

Treatment of stasis dermatitis is based on the restoration of healthy circulation, healing of the eczematous skin response, and healing of any ulcerations that may have developed as a result of the disease process.

Compression therapy is considered the gold standard of care. The patient should be fitted for graduated compression hose and should be encouraged to elevate the extremities above the heart several times a day to decrease the edema and promote wound healing.[4] For patients at risk for comorbid arterial disease, adequate perfusion should be determined by ankle-brachial index before the application of compression therapy.[2,5]

Topical emollients should be applied daily. The use of plain petrolatum as a moisturizer avoids the potential risk of allergic contact dermatitis. Maintenance of optimum skin integrity entails avoidance of trauma, including hot water in showers or baths and irritants such as lanolin, wool, and alcohol. Use of mild soaps (e.g., Dove, Neutrogena) should be encouraged.

Systemic antibiotics are necessary for any cellulitis or wound infection. Topical corticosteroids are indicated for pruritic, nonulcerated areas. A midpotency steroid can be used for a short time, with gradual reduction to a low-potency steroid cream. However, steroids should not be used if there are any signs of infection.

Ulcerations should be treated with moist wound healing and compression therapy.[6] Compression can be applied as an Unna paste boot or a multilayer compression wrap. Intermittent pneumatic devices can be used for patients who cannot tolerate sustained compression.[4] Topical wound treatment may include alginates, antimicrobial hydrofibers, hydrocolloids, foams, or gels depending on the level of exudate the wound produces.[7] These dressings are considered "interactive" because they provide moisture required for debridement and an ideal environment for new tissue growth. "Active" dressings, such as topically applied growth factor, encourage formation of granulation tissue or enhance epidermal cell function. Platelet-derived growth factor and epidermal growth factor are two examples of growth factor for which supplementation has dramatically reduced ulcer size and promoted healing.[7]

Surgery to treat varicose veins now includes the newer minimally invasive endovascular technique, which results in more rapid recovery and fewer complications. Stasis pigmentation usually does not resolve even with proper treatment of venous hypertension, but intense pulsed light treatment has been shown by some authors to be beneficial.[3]

COMPLICATIONS

Many older adults have venous incompetence and stasis. As a result, stasis ulceration is responsible for substantial immobility and prolonged hospitalization of many otherwise healthy elders.[8] In addition, ulceration or cellulitis can progress to osteomyelitis or sepsis, which can cause significant morbidity and may even be fatal in compromised hosts.

Lipodermatosclerosis, progressive skin thickening with skin contraction, occurs in patients who, for unknown reasons, are more susceptible to fibrosis. Lipodermatosclerosis produces the classic "bowling pin" appearance in lower extremities.[5]

INDICATIONS FOR REFERRAL OR HOSPITALIZATION

Ulcerations that are recalcitrant to therapy or that penetrate past the dermal layer require referral to a wound care specialist. A consultation with a general surgeon or plastic surgeon for partial-thickness grafting may be necessary. Hospitalization is indicated for patients who require surgical intervention or have infections that require intravenous antibiotics.

EDUCATION AND HEALTH PROMOTION

Patients and caregivers need to receive instruction in and often closely monitored assistance with the application of compression hose, topical medications, or dressings. Compression therapy using hose, adjustable garments, or wraps is essential for the maintenance of a healthy venous system and reduce the rate of leg ulcer recurrence.[2] Success is directly correlated with patient adherence.[9] Measures to improve adherence include appropriate measuring and fitting by trained personnel, as well as proper education on home maintenance and application aides. The appropriate use, side effects, interactions, and contraindications of antibiotics should be carefully explained. Patients with chronic stasis dermatitis need to understand the importance of keeping the legs elevated as much as possible when seated, but home exercise and ambulation should also be encouraged. The need for good nutrition, supplemental vitamins when indicated, and weight reduction should be discussed.

CHAPTER 67

URTICARIA

Cené L. Gibson

DEFINITION AND EPIDEMIOLOGY

Urticaria, also referred to as hives, is caused by a vascular reaction that occurs in the upper dermis of the skin. It is characterized by the development of wheals on the body surface (Fig. 67-1). Acute urticaria is defined as episodes of hives lasting less than 6 weeks, whereas chronic urticaria is defined as hives persisting for more than 6 weeks.

Chronic urticaria can be categorized as idiopathic or autoimmune. On the continuum of urticaria, deeper release of vasoactive mediators into lower dermal and subcutaneous layers of the skin causes angioedema, and severe symptoms can result.[1,2]

Physical urticaria, which accounts for 15% to 25% of chronic cases,[3] is a distinct form of urticaria caused by exposure to physical triggers, such as mechanical or thermal triggers, water, or cold. The hives associated with physical urticaria typically fade within an hour, except in the case of pressure urticaria, in which case the hives take longer to develop and subsequently take longer to fade. In some cases, there is an association between thyroid autoimmunity and urticaria.[1] There may be an autoimmune component in some patients with chronic urticaria. An association between *Helicobacter pylori* and urticaria also has been identified, and recommendations include screening for and/or providing treatment for *H. pylori* colonization in patients without gastrointestinal complaints.[1]

Urticaria is a common disorder, affecting an estimated 20% of the population at some time during their lives.[3,4] In most cases, it is relatively mild in presentation, albeit frustrating for the patient. In other cases, however, it represents part of a continuum that includes anaphylaxis and can be life-threatening. Acute urticaria is more common in young adults, children, and atopic individuals, affecting 15% to 20% of the general population at some point in their lives.[3] This form of urticaria is often attributed to exposure to food allergens, food additives, medications, or radiocontrast media, with rare identification of a specific trigger. Chronic urticaria is slightly more common in middle-aged women and does not show the same predilection for individuals with atopy; 60% of all cases are idiopathic.[3,4]

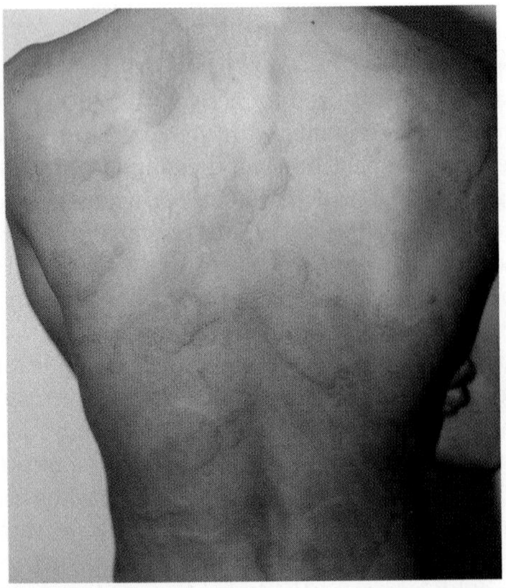

FIGURE 67-1 Urticaria. (Bolognia JL, Schaffer JV, Duncan KO, Ko CJ, *Dermatology Essentials*, ed 1, St Louis, 2015, Saunders.)

Immediate emergency department referral or physician consultation is indicated for urticaria patients with angioedema, respiratory failure, or hemodynamic compromise.

PATHOPHYSIOLOGY

Urticaria is an immediate hypersensitivity reaction that occurs after exposure to an allergen or antigen. Mast cells located in the loose connective tissue of the skin release histamine in response to the exposure. Histamine binds to H_1 receptors, leading to dilation of capillaries and vascular permeability. Arteriolar dilation leads to flaring around the lesions, and extravasation of fluid from the leaky capillaries leads to wheals, which are superficial itchy swellings in the skin. The histamine that is released causes the pruritus.[1,4] Deeper swellings of the skin and alimentary tract can occur in some cases; these swellings tend to be more painful than pruritic and are consistent with angioedema. Histamine also activates H_2 receptors, increasing gastric acid secretions.[1,4]

Mast cells can also be activated by immunoglobulin E (IgE) antibodies stimulated by foods, drugs, insect stings, latex, or animals. Alternatively, activation can occur directly from drugs, including opiates, nonsteroidal anti-inflammatory drugs, and radiocontrast media. Other cell mediators, such as complement and neuropeptides (substance P), may be involved.

Recent laboratory research has implicated the complement system in chronic urticaria, particularly C5a, found on cutaneous cells but not on pulmonary cells. This may explain the lack of pulmonary symptoms in chronic urticaria. Certain human leukocyte antigen (HLA) class II associations are also being investigated as possible links to chronic autoimmune urticaria (CAU), and evidence has recently emerged that an underlying autoimmune disease may manifest as CAU.[1,4]

CLINICAL PRESENTATION

Patients with urticaria initially note pruritus followed by the development of hives. Lesions appear in crops that last 2 to 3 hours and then disappear, only to flare up elsewhere later. They generally fade in less than 24 hours, leaving no trace. Episodes can occur as often as daily and in chronic urticaria can last up to 2 years.

Important history can be simplified into the six *I*s: infections, ingestants (food), injectants (drugs), insect stings, inhalants (pollen), and internal disease. Latex allergy is an increasingly common cause of urticaria. Other historical factors to be elicited are exposure to heat or cold, fever, exercise, change in menses, and emotional stress. In more severe cases of urticaria, the patient may experience angioedema and may report difficulty breathing.

PHYSICAL EXAMINATION

Physical examination reveals edematous pink or red wheals surrounded by a bright red flare. The center of the lesions may be clear or, rarely, may develop bullae. Lesions typically appear on the torso but may occur anywhere on the body. The patient with physical urticaria caused by exposure to some physical stimulus may show what is referred to as dermatographism on examination. Dermatographism is the development of a wheal-and-flare reaction when the skin is stroked with a pen or other physical stimulus. In severe cases of urticaria with angioedema, there may be swelling of the face or oropharynx and deeper swelling in the dermis.

DIAGNOSTICS

In general, laboratory tests are of little value unless the history or examination suggests that they are needed. In fact, most cases of urticaria require no laboratory investigation, especially if mild disease is responding to therapy. Tests may be helpful in cases of chronic urticaria in which physical causative agents have been excluded. Typical laboratory workup would include a complete blood count (CBC), white blood cell differential, and erythrocyte sedimentation rate (ESR). Urinalysis, hepatitis panel, thyroid panel, thyroid antimicrosomal antibody, antinuclear antibody, rheumatoid factor, *H. pylori* testing, serum complement C3 and C4, cryoglobulin, serum IgE and IgM, chest radiograph, and sinus series are less likely to be needed but may be ordered when indicated by history, physical examination, or consultation with a specialist. A skin biopsy may be done to assess for vasculitis if the sedimentation rate is increased or if hives are accompanied by arthralgia or burning sensation in the skin. Specific allergy or provocative tests may prove useful in certain patients (e.g., atopic individuals with severe urticaria) to establish sensitivity to certain foods that should be avoided.

DIAGNOSTICS

Urticaria

LABORATORY
CBC and differential
ESR
Urinalysis
Liver function tests (LFTs)
Thyroid-stimulating hormone (TSH)
Thyroid antimicrosomal antibodies
Antinuclear antibodies
Rheumatoid factor
Serum levels of complement C3 and C4
Cryoglobulin
Serum level of IgE
Serum level of IgM
Hepatitis
H. pylori

IMAGING
Chest x-ray examination

*If indicated and no physical causes are present.

DIFFERENTIAL DIAGNOSIS

There are many conditions that can be confused with urticaria. The following should be considered in the differential diagnosis: anaphylaxis,[1,5] insect bites, vasculitis, pityriasis rosea, syphilis, bullous pemphigoid, systemic lupus erythematosus, urticaria pigmentosa, drug eruptions, and erythema multiforme.

MANAGEMENT

Identification of the responsible trigger and elimination would be ideal.[2] However, most cases of urticaria are idiopathic, and providers often must turn to pharmacologic therapy. Evidence exists for the benefit of treatment of acute and chronic urticaria with H_1 receptor antagonists as first-line medication, augmented with H_2 receptor antagonists, tricyclic antidepressants, and, in some cases, leukotriene receptor antagonists and steroids for resistant episodes (Table 67-1).

TABLE 67-1 Medications Used in Management of Urticaria and Angioedema

Medication	Dose
H_1 RECEPTOR ANTAGONISTS	
Cetirizine HCl (Zyrtec)	Adults: 10-20 mg/day (tablet)
Loratadine (Claritin)	Adults: 10 mg/day (tablet)
Fexofenadine (Allegra)	Adults: 120 mg/day (capsules, tablets)
Desloratadine (Clarinex)	Adults: 5 mg/day (tablets, liquid)
H_2 RECEPTOR ANTAGONISTS	
Cimetidine (Tagamet)	300 mg qid (tablet, liquid)
Ranitidine HCl (Zantac)	150 mg PO bid (tablet, capsule, liquid)
Famotidine (Pepcid)	20 mg PO bid (tablet)
TRICYCLIC ANTIDEPRESSANTS	
Amitriptyline HCl (Elavil)	10-100 mg PO qd (tablet)
Doxepin (Sinequan)	25 mg PO qd (capsule, oral concentrate)
LEUKOTRIENE RECEPTOR ANTAGONISTS	
Montelukast sodium (Singulair)	Adults: 10 mg/day (tablet)
Zafirlukast (Accolate)	Adults: 20 mg PO bid (tablet)

Although older antihistamines such as diphenhydramine (Benadryl) and hydroxyzine (Atarax) were used commonly in the past, they have largely been replaced by newer, nonsedating H_1 blockers such as loratadine (Claritin), cetirizine (Zyrtec), fexofenadine (Allegra), and desloratadine (Clarinex). There is evidence for clinical benefit when these medications are used at higher doses.[2,5] Their efficacy combined with reduced sedation and anticholinergic side effects have made them first-line therapy for urticaria. Because treatment of the symptoms of urticaria often requires higher doses of the H_1 blockers—doses that in most individuals would lead to significant sedation with the older H_1 blockers—the newer nonsedating H_1 blockers have found favor.[2,5] However, the addition of a sedating antihistamine (e.g., chlorpheniramine, 4 to 12 mg, or hydroxyzine, 10 to 50 mg) at bedtime to the regimen of a patient already taking a nonsedating H_1 blocker may help the patient sleep better.[5] There is little evidence, however, that such an addition adds much to H_1 receptor blockade.

In the case of urticaria that is refractory to H_1 blockade, evidence exists for clinical benefit when an H_2 blocker is added, such as cimetidine (Tagamet), 300 mg orally four times a day; ranitidine (Zantac), 150 mg orally twice a day; or famotidine (Pepcid), 20 mg twice a day.[1] An H_2 blocker should be used only in conjunction with an H_1 blocker because the evidence pertains to the benefit of H_2 blockers in cases of chronic urticaria that is refractory to treatment with H_1 blockers alone.[1,5] Evidence also exists for the benefit of treatment of refractory chronic urticaria with tricyclic antidepressants.[2,4] Doxepin is the most potent H_1 blocker in the class; when it is used, it should be started at 25 mg orally at bedtime and titrated to effect with a maximum dose of 100 mg. Alternatively, amitriptyline (Elavil) may be used at the same dosage interval of 10 to 100 mg orally at bedtime. Either may help with depression and anxiety related to chronic urticaria.

Evidence also suggests that the leukotriene inhibitors may be useful in some patients with chronic refractory urticaria, but clinical trials remained inconclusive as to effectivenss.[1,6] Evidence exists for benefit of treatment of acute urticaria with oral corticosteroids, such as prednisolone at a dosage of 0.5 mg to 1 mg/kg/day tapered over 3 to 7 days.[2] Long-term oral corticosteroids should not typically be used in chronic urticaria but may be used in select refractory cases with specialty consultation.[1,6]

Remember that cases of acute urticaria typically last no more than 5 to 7 days. Chronic urticaria is different. Individuals affected by chronic urticaria must try to modify their lifestyle to avoid the irritant that triggers the symptoms. Patients with a history of severe urticaria or angioedema should carry an epinephrine auto-injector for emergency use. Epinephrine 1:1000, 0.3 mL subcutaneously, may be used in addition to the H_1 blocker if the patient exhibits any signs of angioedema or if urticaria is severe. A short course of oral corticosteroids may also be considered in the case of angioedema that affects the mouth.[6]

DIFFERENTIAL DIAGNOSIS

Urticaria

- Insect bites
- Vasculitis
- Pityriasis rosea
- Syphilis
- Bullous pemphigoid
- Systemic lupus erythematosus
- Urticaria pigmentosa
- Drug eruptions
- Erythema multiforme

COMPLICATIONS

Pruritus may lead to scratching, excoriation, and secondary infection. The most severe complication is angioedema or anaphylaxis accompanying the urticaria, which can lead to airway obstruction or cardiopulmonary arrest.

Immediate emergency department referral or physician consultation is indicated for patients with angioedema, respiratory failure, or hemodynamic compromise. Patients should be hospitalized if they require intubation or are at risk for airway compromise, severe anaphylaxis, or shock.

INDICATIONS FOR REFERRAL OR HOSPITALIZATION

Patients should be referred to a physician or specialist for further evaluation when the diagnosis is in question, when an underlying systemic disease is suspected or found, and when routine medical therapy is not effective.

PATIENT AND FAMILY EDUCATION AND HEALTH PROMOTION

Patients should be educated on the natural course and history of the disease, including the fact that the specific trigger may remain elusive. Quality of life is markedly reduced with chronic urticaria, and the index of suspicion for depression and anxiety should be high.[1,2] Surveillance should still be conducted in the form of diet or activity diaries. Patients and their families should be educated about the signs and symptoms of anaphylaxis and angioedema and should understand the importance of avoiding known precipitants because urticaria can plague them throughout their lives. Patients predisposed to severe urticaria, anaphylaxis, or angioedema should be educated in crisis management, including the use of subcutaneous epinephrine to avoid unnecessary morbidity or mortality. If patients have a history of anaphylaxis or angioedema, they should be provided with an injectable epinephrine preparation such as an EpiPen for emergency use. Both the patient and family members should be educated in its use.

CHAPTER 68

WARTS

Glen Blair

DEFINITION AND EPIDEMIOLOGY

Verruca, or warts, are benign epidermal neoplasms caused by various types of the human papillomavirus (HPV), a group of double-stranded DNA viruses of the family Papillomaviridae.

More than 200 subtypes of HPV have been identified.[1] Roughly 40 of these types affect mucosal surfaces, such as the vulva, vagina, penis, anus, and oral cavity; of these, 16 have been identified as high-risk oncogenic viruses implicated in the development of numerous cervical and anogenital cancers. The other virus phenotypes are apt to affect the nonmucosal cutaneous surfaces, such as the face, hands and feet.

Transmission is through direct skin contact, although contact with viral particles on inanimate objects has been known to cause infection. Genital infection is usually acquired through sexual contact. Wart subtypes with an affinity for the hands and feet typically do not affect the genitalia. Individuals with decreased cellular immunity are at risk for more recalcitrant HPV infection. In these patients, warts can be larger and involve a greater surface area.

Environmental and occupational factors increase the risk for development of warts. Periungual warts, for example, are much more common in butchers and in patients whose hands are exposed to chronic wet conditions. Recurrence is common for warts of all types.

Anogenital HPV infection is believed to be the most common sexually transmitted disease in the United States. Studies have shown that 76% of human immunodeficiency virus (HIV)–seropositive women and 42% of seronegative women are at high risk for anogenital HPV infection, and the rates for HIV-seropositive men who have receptive anal intercourse approach 100%.[2] Low-risk types 6 and 11 account for 90% of anogenital warts. The high-risk genotypes are responsible for 99% of the cases of cervical cancer and are emerging as the leading causes of oropharyngeal, vulvar, vaginal, and penile cancers, as well.[2] Of these, type 16 is the most common, and type 18 accounts for 70% of all cervical cancers. HPV types 31, 33, 45, 52, and 58 are believed to be responsible for an additional 19% of invasive cervical cancers.

There are currently three HPV vaccines available in the United States[3]:

- Cervarix, a bivalent vaccine targeting HPV types 16 and 18
- Gardasil 4, a quadrivalent vaccine targeting HPV types 6, 11, 16, and 18

- Gardasil 9, a nonavalent vaccine targeting HPV types 6, 11, 16, 18, 31, 33, 45, 52, and 58

Each of these vaccines has been shown to induce a significant antibody response. Although there is no national consensus on which vaccine to provide to which patients, the U.S. Advisory Committee on Immunization Practices (ACIP) advocates for the provision of the nonavalent vaccine as the most promising vaccine available to reduce the incidence of HPV-related cancers of all types, because the bivalent and quadrivalent vaccines fail to protect against 25% to 30% of cervical cancers. Vaccination for males and females can begin as early as age 9 but typically begins at age 11 or 12 and up to age 26 in high-risk individuals such as those infected by HIV.[3]

PATHOPHYSIOLOGY

Infection occurs when the virus comes in contact with skin that is broken or has been traumatized. The virus enters the host's epidermal epithelial cells and begins to use the host's resources to replicate. Infection remains contained within the epidermis, although the wart can become hypertrophic and behave as if it were a deep lesion, as it commonly does on the plantar surface.

Warts can occur singly or in groups and can coalesce to form plaques called mosaic warts. Autoinoculation can occur with cutaneous trauma, such as from shaving or scratching.

Vertical transmission of the virus from infected mother to the fetus during passage through the birth canal can cause anogenital warts and recurrent respiratory papillomatosis in the infant.

Infection by the wart virus depends on the number of viral particles, the extent of contact, and the host's cellular immunity. The virus spreads laterally for a considerable distance beyond the line that demarcates the wart from the normal skin. HPV may be actively replicating or may lie in a dormant, latent state. Spontaneous remission may occur in as many as two of three patients within 2 years. Lesions recur when the host's cell-mediated immunity can no longer hold the virus in check. Incubation periods range from 1 to 8 months.

CLINICAL PRESENTATION AND PHYSICAL EXAMINATION

HPV infection is often asymptomatic. When it becomes apparent, it manifests in several different morphologic characteristics. Verruca vulgaris, the common wart, is a skin-colored, hyperkeratotic papule that may occur on the backs of the hands, in periungual areas, and on the knees. Filiform warts are a variant of common warts that are distinguished by their fine, finger-like projections, They typically occur on the face and may be tender. Verruca plana, the flat wart, is commonly seen on the face and extremities in crops of 1- to 2-mm papules that are smooth, flat, and skin colored to brown. Verruca plantaris, the plantar wart, is a skin-colored papule or plaque on the weight-bearing plantar surfaces of the foot and digits; it is often studded with black pinpoint-sized areas that represent thrombosed capillaries. These warts may be extremely tender and interfere with weight bearing. The thickness of plantar warts makes them particularly resistant to multiple treatment modalities. Condylomata acuminata, or anogenital warts, are sexually transmitted and range from unobtrusive, small, skin-colored papules to large, cauliflower-like growths (Fig. 68-1). Warts have also been described on the oral and nasal mucous membranes, conjunctivae, and larynx.

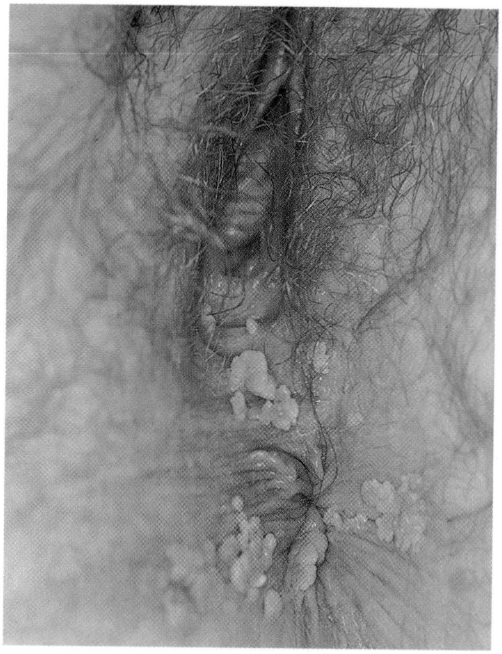

FIGURE **68-1** Multiple condylomata in the perineum and perianal area. (From Fisher BK, Margesson LJ: *Genital skin disorders: diagnosis and treatment*, St Louis, 1998, Mosby.)

The physical examination is generally by careful visual inspection. When warts are discovered on the perineum or perianal area, there is an indication to perform a vaginal examination, digital rectal examination, or anoscopy.

DIAGNOSTICS AND DIFFERENTIAL DIAGNOSIS

Diagnosis of most warts can be confirmed clinically. Debridement of the thickened hypertrophic epidermis with a scalpel or curet will reveal pinpoint capillaries that may bleed. On the foot, this can help differentiate it from a callus (or clavus), a different type of lesion that is commonly mistaken for a wart. When it is pared, the callus will have a punctate depression and no thrombosed capillaries. The absence of skin lines within the lesion is also considered a reliable diagnostic indicator for a wart.

The American College of Obstetricians and Gynecologists and the American Cancer Society recommend yearly or biennial Pap tests for women younger than 30 years and, with three consecutive normal Pap test results, every 2 to 3 years thereafter. Vaccination does not obviate the need for regular Pap tests.[2] Although there are no consensus recommendations for the screening for anal cancer yet, there is a growing body of evidence supporting the regular use of cytology-based (Pap) testing of the anus for patients at high risk, including men who have sex with men, HIV-infected patients, immunocompromised patients, and women who participate in receptive anal intercourse.[4]

Warts can appear in varied forms that mimic other common dermatologic lesions. The differential diagnosis of warts includes seborrheic keratosis, callus, lichen planus, squamous cell carcinoma, molluscum contagiosum, amelanotic melanoma, and foreign body.

DIFFERENTIAL DIAGNOSIS

Warts

- Seborrheic keratosis
- Callus
- Lichen planus
- Squamous cell carcinoma
- Molluscum contagiosum
- Amelanotic melanoma
- Foreign body

MANAGEMENT

Most warts are benign and asymptomatic. In general, they will regress spontaneously over time. There is, however, no cure for warts. Treatment decisions are influenced by a number of factors, including the degree of discomfort or disfigurement, the motivation of the patient to undergo treatment that may be painful and protracted, and the commitment to continuing treatment at home. Patients with anogenital infection need to be evaluated for anogenital cancer and screened appropriately.

Therapies are directed toward physical and chemical destruction of the lesions and the recruitment of the host's innate defenses.[2] Topical treatments need to extend at least 2 mm outside the visible confines of the wart to ensure that all infected cells are treated. Chemical destruction is done with a liquid agent or transdermal patches. Liquid preparations of salicylic acid and dichloroacetic or trichloroacetic acid are used on common, flat, periungual, and plantar warts. Application once or twice a day along with paring or filing of the lesion has resulted in cure rates that can exceed 60%.[5] Petrolatum ointment can be applied on the surrounding skin to protect it from chemical burn. Treatment may take up to 12 weeks or more.

Imiquimod (Aldara) is a topically applied immunomodulator approved for the treatment of anogenital warts but is commonly used for nongenital warts as well. It is useful in areas where scarring is of concern, such as the face, and for recalcitrant lesions in combination with regular lesion debridement.[5,6]

Cantharidin is an extract of a beetle that produces blistering of the skin hours after contact. It has the advantage of painless application but can be very painful hours later. It is not currently approved by the Food and Drug Administration, but its use is permitted when it is compounded, as with podophyllin or salicylic acid. It is still sometimes available, but its use is waning.[7] Other medications include topically applied 5-fluorouracil and tretinoin and oral cimetidine.

Injections of skin test antigens, such as mumps, *Candida*, and *Trichophyton* antigens, have shown significant success in nonblinded studies; controlled studies are lacking. Their use is suggested for facial lesions when scarring and pigmentation are of concern and for warts that have been resistant to treatment.[8]

Cryotherapy with liquid nitrogen (LN_2) is commonly used alone or in conjunction with other modalities to treat warts. For genital warts, flat warts, and filiform warts, a single freeze-thaw application with minimal involvement of surrounding skin is usually sufficient for each wart. For warts on the palmar or plantar surfaces, individual lesions and their bases are treated for two or three freeze-thaw cycles. The procedure can be painful. Tissue destruction can cause local redness, swelling, and blistering and may take up to 2 weeks to heal. People with dark skin are at risk of hyperpigmentation and hypopigmentation from LN_2 and are good candidates for trials of the topically applied medications before LN_2 is used. All patients are at risk for scarring. Treatment may be required every 2 to 4 weeks for months at a time.

Treatment of periungual warts can result in damage to the nail matrix and subsequent nail deformity. Nerve damage can occur if treatment is too vigorous in areas where the nerves are superficial, such as the lateral phalanges. Cryotherapy should be performed cautiously or not at all in patients with Raynaud phenomenon. Laser ablation therapy is an option for very resistant cases, but cure rates are not reported to be higher than with less painful and less expensive alternatives.

COMPLICATIONS

In general, treatment of warts can be painful. Blistering and hemorrhagic bullae can develop from typical doses of cryotherapy on frail skin.

Plantar warts can be particularly painful and if left untreated may result in altered activity, abnormal gait, or foot deformities. Bacterial infections are rare. Autoinoculation from one area to another is possible.

Genital warts (condylomata acuminata) are particularly contagious and increase the risk for anogenital carcinomas in both men and women. Genital warts can be transmitted from mother to infant during childbirth.

INDICATIONS FOR REFERRAL

- Dermatology referral is advised for large warts, warts on cosmetically sensitive areas, and treatment failures or when the diagnosis is in question.[9]
- Podiatry referral may be appropriate for resistant plantar warts.
- Obstetric-gynecologic evaluation is appropriate for women with intravaginal lesions or abnormal Pap test results.
- Urology referrals may be appropriate for lesions that are affecting normal urination or sexual performance.
- Gastroenterology for sigmoidoscopy may be indicated for patients with abnormal anal cytology or clinical findings suggesting rectal HPV infection.[4]

PATIENT AND FAMILY EDUCATION

For common warts, patients and families should understand that most warts are benign, viral lesions that can spread from person to person in places such as showers or locker rooms and often resolve spontaneously, although that may be only after many years. Education should include self-treatment options and the side effects of medications.

Patients should be instructed to pare hyperkeratotic warts regularly, especially those on the feet, with an instrument that is not used on any other skin surface. Soaking the area in warm water makes physical debridement easier, as does the use of an exfoliating cream or lotion, such as ammonium lactate or urea.

Some warts, however, have been linked to the development of cervical, genital, and mucosal carcinomas, and there are now multiple vaccines available to protect against cancers and warts related to HPV infection. Patients, parents, teens, and young adults need to be educated about the health implications of HPV infection, offered the appropriate screening, and advised of the availability of the vaccine. This is especially important information to be shared before a patient becomes sexually active and during routine health maintenance visits.

Routine Pap tests are still recommended regularly for sexually active women. Rectal Pap smears should become routine care for select patient populations.

CHAPTER 69

WOUND MANAGEMENT

Ashley M. Taylor

DEFINITION AND EPIDEMIOLOGY

Tissue trauma accounts for significant morbidity and financial concern. Treatment of chronic wounds conservatively costs the U.S. health care system $50 billion annually.[1] The incidence and prevalence of acute and chronic wounds vary with populations, geographic and demographic status, and general medical conditions. Acute wounds consist of lacerations, abrasions, avulsions, crush injuries, puncture wounds, insect or mammalian bites, traumatic or surgical wounds, burns, and skin tears. Chronic wounds consist of pressure ulcers, venous and arterial ulcers, diabetic foot ulcers, and nonhealing surgical or traumatic wounds.

Pressure and Venous Ulcers

An estimated 2.5 million pressure ulcers are treated each year in U.S. acute care facilities alone, and the cost of treating them ranges from $11 billion to $17.2 billion per year.[2] Development of a pressure ulcer increases the length of stay for hospitalized patients, and increases the mortality rate significantly.[2]

Venous ulcers account for 80% to 90% of ulcers found on the lower leg.[3] Approximately 26% to 28% of healed ulcers will recur within 1 year.[3] The annual cost of treating venous stasis ulcers to the U.S. health care system is $1.9 billion to $3.5 billion.[3] Arterial ulcers occur in a large percentage of patients with peripheral arterial disease. These ulcers are particularly difficult to heal as a result of poor perfusion, and revascularization is often needed to promote reperfusion and the hope of healing the ulcer.

Diabetic Foot Ulcers

There are more than 20 million people in the United States with diabetes, of whom 10% to 15% are at risk for ulceration.[2] Of all nontraumatic lower limb amputations in the United States, 50% to 75% are diabetes related.[2] Amputation and foot ulceration are the most common consequences of diabetic neuropathy and major causes of morbidity and disability in people with diabetes. People with diabetes are at higher risk for development of peripheral artery disease, which significantly increases the risk of amputation. The risk of ulcers or amputations also increases in people who have had diabetes for more than 10 years, are male, or have poor glucose control; risk is also increased with cardiovascular, retinal, or renal complications (Boxes 69-1 and 69-2).[4]

Surgical Wounds

Surgical wounds are often treated in the outpatient setting secondary to the rising costs of acute care management and reimbursement concerns. Wound dehiscence or infection can affect healing by secondary intention and may require tertiary healing, with the health care provider and home health nurse managing the care of these difficult-to-heal wounds.[5,6] A broad understanding of wound healing physiology and general management principles will assist the provider in facilitating maximum wound repair.

BOX 69-1

Foot Care Recommendations for Patients with Diabetes

- For all patients with diabetes, perform an annual comprehensive foot examination to identify risk factors predictive of ulcers and amputations. The foot examination should include inspection, assessment of foot pulses, and testing for loss of protective sensation (LOPS) (10-g monofilament plus testing any one of: vibration using 128-Hz tuning fork, pinprick sensation, ankle reflexes, or vibration perception threshold).
- Provide general foot self-care education to all patients with diabetes.
- A multidisciplinary approach is recommended for individuals with foot ulcers and high-risk feet, especially those with a history of prior ulcer or amputation.
- Refer patients who smoke, have LOPS and structural abnormalities, or have history of prior lower extremity complications to foot care specialists for ongoing preventive care and life-long surveillance.
- Initial screening for peripheral arterial disease (PAD) should include a history for claudication and an assessment of the pedal pulses. Consider obtaining an ankle-brachial index (ABI), because many patients with PAD are asymptomatic.
- Refer patients with significant claudication or a positive ABI for further vascular assessment, and consider exercise, medications, and surgical options.

From American Diabetes Association: Standards of medical care in diabetes—2010, *Diabetes Care* 33(Suppl 1):S11-S61, 2010.

BOX 69-2

Foot-Related Risk Conditions Associated with Increased Risk of Amputation

The risk of ulcers or amputations is increased in people who have the following risk factors:

- Previous amputation
- Past foot ulcer history
- Peripheral neuropathy
- Foot deformity
- Peripheral vascular disease
- Visual impairment
- Diabetic nephropathy (especially patients on dialysis)
- Poor glycemic control
- Cigarette smoking

From American Diabetes Association: Standards of medical care in diabetes—2010, *Diabetes Care* 33(Suppl 1):S11-S61, 2010.

CLASSIFICATION OF WOUNDS

Classification of wounds is unique to wound type, and reference to established classification systems is recommended.

Wounds involving only the epidermal layer are classified as superficial or partial thickness. Examples include simple lacerations, skin tears, first-degree burns, abrasions, and shallow ulcerations. These wounds usually heal quickly and require the least intervention. Full-thickness wounds involve the epidermis and dermis and may extend through subcutaneous tissue into muscle and bone. Examples include deep lacerations, second- and third-degree burns, various types of ulcers, and surgical or traumatic wounds.

BOX 69-3

Pressure Ulcer Staging (NPUAP/EPUAP Guidelines)

DEFINITION

A pressure ulcer is localized injury to the skin and/or underlying tissue, usually over a bony prominence, as a result of pressure, or pressure in combination with shear and/or friction. A number of contributing or confounding factors are also associated with pressure ulcers; the significance of these factors is yet to be elucidated.

STAGES

Suspected Deep Tissue Injury

Purple or maroon localized area of discolored intact skin or blood-filled blister caused by damage of underlying soft tissue from pressure and/or shear. The area may be preceded by tissue that is painful, firm, mushy, boggy, warmer or cooler as compared with adjacent tissue.

Further description: Deep tissue injury may be difficult to detect in individuals with dark skin tones. Evolution may include a thin blister over a dark wound bed. The wound may further evolve and become covered by thin eschar. Evolution may be rapid, exposing additional layers of tissue even with optimal treatment.

Stage I

Intact skin with nonblanchable redness of a localized area, usually over a bony prominence. Darkly pigmented skin may not have visible blanching; its color may differ from the surrounding area.

Further description: The area may be painful, firm, soft, warmer or cooler as compared with adjacent tissue. Stage I wounds may be difficult to detect in individuals with dark skin tones. May indicate "at-risk" persons (a heralding sign of risk).

Stage II

Partial-thickness loss of dermis manifesting as a shallow open ulcer with a red or pink wound bed, without slough. May also manifest as an intact or open or ruptured serum-filled blister.

Further description: Shiny or dry shallow ulcer without slough or bruising.* This stage should not be used to describe skin tears, tape burns, perineal dermatitis, maceration, or excoriation.

Stage III

Full-thickness tissue loss. Subcutaneous fat may be visible, but bone, tendon, or muscle is not exposed. Slough may be present but does not obscure the depth of tissue loss. May include undermining and tunneling.

Further description: The depth of a stage III pressure ulcer varies by anatomic location. The bridge of the nose, ear, occiput, and malleolus do not have subcutaneous tissue, and stage III ulcers can be shallow. In contrast, areas of significant adiposity can develop extremely deep stage III pressure ulcers. Bone or tendon is not visible or directly palpable.

Stage IV

Full-thickness tissue loss with exposed bone, tendon, or muscle. Slough or eschar may be present on some parts of the wound bed. Often includes undermining and tunneling.

Further description: The depth of a stage IV pressure ulcer varies by anatomic location. The bridge of the nose, ear, occiput, and malleolus do not have subcutaneous tissue, and these ulcers can be shallow. Stage IV ulcers can extend into muscle and/or supporting structures (e.g., fascia, tendon, or joint capsule), making osteomyelitis possible. Exposed bone or tendon is visible or directly palpable.

Unstageable

Full-thickness tissue loss in which the base of the ulcer is covered by slough (yellow, tan, gray, green, or brown) and/or eschar (tan, brown, or black) in the wound bed.

Further description: Until enough slough and/or eschar is removed to expose the base of the wound, the true depth, and therefore stage, cannot be determined. Stable (dry, adherent, intact without erythema or fluctuance) eschar on the heels serves as "the body's natural (biologic) cover" and should not be removed.

*Bruising indicates suspected deep tissue injury.

From National Pressure Ulcer Advisory Panel (NPUAP) and European Pressure Ulcer Advisory Panel (EPUAP): *Pressure ulcer prevention and treatment: clinical practice guideline*, Washington, DC, 2009, National Pressure Ulcer Advisory Panel.

A pressure ulcer is a localized injury to the skin or underlying tissue and is staged in accordance with the National Pressure Ulcer Advisory Panel's staging definitions. Pressure ulcer staging includes deep tissue injury, stages I to IV, and unstageable (Box 69-3). Burns are classified as first, second, or third degree (Box 69-4) and require a unique approach that often requires referral to a burn specialist (Box 69-5).

Skin tears are common in frail older adults, often occurring during routine daily activities such as washing and dressing. The shearing and friction forces against frail skin cause the tear, separating the epidermis from the dermis (partial thickness) or the dermis from underlying structures (full thickness).

Arterial and venous ulcers are classified as partial or full thickness; the diabetic foot ulcer is typically graded by one of two classification systems, the Wagner and the University of Texas classifications. The Wagner system uses grades 0 to 5 to assess wound depth (Table 69-1). The University of Texas system uses a matrix of grades and scales to assess the wound's depth and presence of infection or ischemia (Table 69-2).[7,8]

TABLE 69-1 **Wagner Classification System**

Grade	Lesion
0	No open lesions: may have deformity or cellulitis
1	Superficial ulcer
2	Deep ulcer to tendon or joint capsule
3	Deep ulcer with abscess, osteomyelitis, or joint sepsis
4	Local gangrene—forefoot or heel
5	Gangrene of entire foot

Modified from Wagner FW: The dysvascular foot: a system for diagnosis and treatment, *Foot Ankle* 2:64-122, 1981.

BOX 69-4

Burn Classification

FIRST-DEGREE (SUPERFICIAL OR EPIDERMAL) BURNS

These burns involve only the epidermis. They do not blister, but are red and quite painful. Over 2 to 3 days the erythema and the pain subside. By about day 4, the injured epithelium peels away from the newly healed epidermis underneath, a process that is commonly seen after sunburn.

SECOND-DEGREE (PARTIAL-THICKNESS) BURNS

Partial-thickness burns involve the epidermis and portions of the dermis and can be clinically categorized as either *superficial* partial-thickness or *deep* partial-thickness burns. Superficial partial-thickness burns characteristically form blisters between the epidermis and dermis. Because blistering may not occur for some hours after injury, burns that initially appear to be only epidermal in depth (first degree) may be determined to be partial-thickness burns 12 to 24 hours later. Most superficial partial-thickness burns heal spontaneously in less than 3 weeks, and do so typically without functional impairment or hypertrophic scarring. Second-degree burns often accumulate a layer of fibrinous exudate and necrotic debris on the surface, which may predispose the wound to heavy bacterial colonization and delayed wound healing, in addition to making more difficult the determination of wound depth by visual inspection.

Deep partial-thickness burns extend into the lower layers of the dermis. They possess characteristics that are distinctly different from superficial or mid-dermal partial-thickness burns. If infection is prevented and spontaneous healing is allowed to progress, these burns will heal in 3 to 9 weeks. However, they invariably cause considerable scar formation. Even with active physical therapy throughout the healing process, hypertrophic scarring is common and joint function is usually impaired. These burns are best treated by excision and grafting. For the patient, a partial-thickness burn that fails to heal within 3 weeks is functionally and cosmetically equivalent to a full-thickness injury.

THIRD-DEGREE (FULL-THICKNESS) BURNS

Full-thickness burns involve all layers of the dermis and often injure underlying subcutaneous adipose tissue as well. Burn eschar is structurally intact but dead and denatured dermis. Over days and weeks, if left in situ, eschar separates from the underlying viable tissue, leaving an open, unhealed bed of granulation tissue. Without surgery, these burns can heal only by wound contracture with epithelialization from the wound margins. Some full-thickness burns involve not only all layers of the skin, but also deeper structures such as muscle, tendon, ligament, and bone, and are classified as deep full-thickness or fourth-degree burns. Grafting may use autologous skin grafts or biologic dressings and skin substitutes or both. (Excision and grafting using biologic dressings or skin substitutes permits closure of extensive burns in stages, with autografting done at a later date; see detailed discussion elsewhere in this chapter.) Deep full-thickness burns may require amputation or closure with alternative techniques (such as adjacent tissue transfer or microvascular procedures).

From Kagan RJ, Peck MD, Ahrenholz DH, et al: Surgical management of the burn wound and use of skin substitutes: an expert panel white paper. *J Burn Care Res* 34(2):e60-e79, 2013.

BOX 69-5

Burn Center Referral Criteria

A burn center may treat adults, children, or both. Burn injuries that should be referred to a burn center include the following:

1. Partial-thickness burns of greater than 10% of the total body surface area.
2. Burns that involve the face, hands, feet, genitalia, perineum, or major joints.
3. Third-degree burns in any age group.
4. Electrical burns, including lightning injury.
5. Chemical burns.
6. Inhalation injury.
7. Burn injury in patients with preexisting medical disorders that could complicate management, prolong recovery, or affect mortality.
8. Any patients with burns and concomitant trauma (such as fractures) in which the burn injury poses the greatest risk of morbidity or mortality. In such cases, if the trauma poses the greater immediate risk, the patient's condition may be stabilized initially in a trauma center before transfer to a burn center. Physician judgment will be necessary in such situations and should be in concert with the regional medical control plan and triage protocols.
9. Burned children in hospitals without qualified personnel or equipment for the care of children.
10. Burn injury in patients who will require special social, emotional, or rehabilitative intervention.

From American College of Surgeons, Committee on Trauma: Guidelines for the operation of burn centers. In *Resources for optimal care of the injured patient,* Chicago, Ill, 2006, American College of Surgeons.

PATHOPHYSIOLOGY

Wound healing begins at the time of injury and often proceeds over a period of several months through the stages of inflammation, proliferation, and remodeling. Inflammation, which begins at the time of injury, is an essential first step in wound healing to provide local vasospasm and initiation of the clotting process. Neutrophils, oxygen, and nutrients are transported to the wound site, and proliferation begins. In this phase, epithelial cells migrate over the surface of the wound, collagen synthesis begins, and the wound begins to contract. Remodeling occurs during the next several months, with organized layering of type I collagen providing improved tensile strength.[2,7,9]

Wound healing is affected by many internal and external factors. Internal factors include age, preexisting comorbidities (e.g., diabetes mellitus, cardiovascular disease, autoimmune disorders), perfusion, oxygenation, nutrition, hydration, and some medications (especially steroids, immunosuppressants, and chemotherapeutic drugs). External factors include pressure, friction, shear, contamination (with bacteria, debris, or necrotic tissue), and wound environment (pH, moisture).[2,7]

Stages of wound healing may be interrupted by changes in the internal and external wound healing factors. Two common examples are the occurrence of anemia during wound healing, which slows the healing response as a result of decreased oxygenation, and pressure exerted over the site, which decreases perfusion and prolongs or delays wound healing.[7]

Surgical wounds heal by primary, secondary, or tertiary intention. Primary intention implies that the wound edges are

TABLE 69-2 **Diabetic Foot Ulcer Grades (University of Texas Classification System)**

		Wound Depth			
		0	1	2	3
Presence of infection or ischemia	A	Preulcerative or postulcerative lesion completely epithelialized	Superficial; not involving tendon, joint capsule, or bone	Penetrating to tendon or joint capsule	Penetrating to bone or joint capsule
	B	With infection	With infection	With infection	With infection
	C	With ischemia	With ischemia	With ischemia	With ischemia
	D	With infection and ischemia	With infection and ischemia	With infection and ischemia	With infection and ischemia

Modified from Lavery LA, Armstrong DG, Harkless LB: Classification of diabetic foot wounds, *J Foot Ankle Surg* 35:528-531, 1996.

approximated and sutured, stapled, taped, or glued. Secondary intention implies that the wound edges are not approximated, usually because of failed primary intention (dehiscence) or infection. Secondary intention healing is prolonged and results in significant scarring. Delayed primary intention, or tertiary intention, refers to wounds that were not initially closed (usually because of infection, contamination, or wound stress) and are closed after some secondary intention healing has occurred.

CLINICAL PRESENTATION

Any break in skin integrity in the immunocompromised or diabetic patient warrants timely and complete evaluation. Early evaluation and intervention in this population of patients may prevent complications of healing, including infection.

Acute wounds are most often caused by accidental injury and include lacerations, abrasions, burns, bites, and puncture wounds. Patients with comorbidities, especially diabetes mellitus and peripheral vascular disease, may be seen with lower extremity ulcers related to neuropathy and poor perfusion. Patients with decreased functioning resulting from brain injury, neurologic disease, or spinal cord injury often see their providers with complaints of pressure ulcers. Prevention, early identification, and appropriate management are of primary importance to avoid costly and irreversible tissue damage, especially in the medically compromised patient.

The patient's medication history is important to evaluate and guides management decisions. Immunosuppressive drugs, including chemotherapeutics and steroids, adversely affect wound healing by interrupting the inflammatory process, an important first step in mounting of a healing response. Critical factors to be elicited include the patient's age, allergies, occupation, nutritional status, drug or alcohol use, smoking history, and immune status, including the last tetanus booster. Moreover, the provider must identify conditions that adversely affect wound healing, including diabetes mellitus, autoimmune disorders, malnutrition, positive smoking history, chronic respiratory disease, and peripheral vascular disease; these affect management plans.[2,7,10,11]

PHYSICAL EXAMINATION

Assessment of the wound must follow a thorough history. The nature and age of the wound along with the patient's medical history determine management strategies. Wound location, type, depth, previous treatments, and surrounding tissue assessment guide treatment decisions.

In addition to a thorough wound evaluation (including observation for tunneling, the presence and odor of exudate, and the appearance of all tissue in and around the wound bed), a focused physical examination is important. In lower extremity wounds, perfusion is determined by pulse assessment and noninvasive diagnostic testing, if necessary. It is essential to determine the absence or presence of peripheral perfusion and associated changes of edema, tissue color and warmth, and neurovascular status.[3]

Wounds that are healing or have the potential to heal will demonstrate pink or red tissue and the absence of excessive exudate, infection, and debris. The size of the wound, measured weekly, should slowly decrease. Healing wounds are pink to red, robust, and bumpy (granulation tissue), with pink healing edges that demonstrate migration by contact with the wound bed. Tissue is not healing if it is pale or smooth, and it may have raised hard edges.

DIAGNOSTICS

X-ray studies may be necessary in acute injuries to identify bone or tendon involvement.[12] They are also helpful in evaluating infection, foreign bodies, and deformity in the diabetic foot, although they may lag behind the clinical presentation of osteomyelitis by as long as 2 weeks.[13] Separation, fracture, or dislocation usually requires referral to a specialist. Compound fractures, especially in hand injuries, require diligent management and antibiotic administration.

Noninvasive vascular studies such as ankle-brachial index or transcutaneous partial oxygen pressure are useful to determine arterial flow in patients with lower extremity ulceration.[14] Magnetic resonance imaging (MRI) is the most specific and sensitive noninvasive test for evaluation of osteomyelitis. For patients with a pacemaker, the Ceretec or indium white blood cell

DIAGNOSTICS

Wound Management

LABORATORY
CBC and differential*
Hemoglobin A_{1c} *
Albumin level*
Wound culture*

IMAGING
X-ray examination*
Bone scan*
MRI*
Noninvasive vascular studies*

OTHER DIAGNOSTICS
Biopsy*

*If indicated.

(WBC) can may be considered.[8] The complete blood count (CBC) is useful in detecting anemia, which can slow wound healing progression by decreasing perfusion and oxygenation. A slightly elevated WBC count may indicate the inflammatory response, whereas a WBC count that continues to rise may indicate an infection. Immunosuppressive disorders delay wound healing and may be first detected on CBC. A total lymphocyte count of less than 1500 cells/mm^3 coupled with an albumin level of less than 3.5 g/dL is indicative of malnutrition, which delays wound healing. Patients with diabetes who have a hemoglobin A_{1c} level of greater than 8% are at increased risk of failed wound healing as a result of hyperglycemia.[4]

DIFFERENTIAL DIAGNOSIS

The nature of the injury and the location of the wound determine diagnosis as well as treatment. Diagnosis and treatment of chronic wounds are determined by history of the patient, presence of medical conditions, and location and appearance of the wound.

Ulcers: Venous and Arterial

Ulcers are chronic wounds that can be caused by several different underlying medical conditions. The diagnosis of the underlying cause is essential because treatment of this condition affects ulcer recurrence rates. Most pressure ulcers occur over bony prominences, including the sacrum, greater trochanter, ischial tuberosity, heel, and lateral malleolus.

Venous ulcers are typically located on the medial lower leg, above the medial malleolus. The wound is often large with irregular wound edges; the wound bed usually has granulation tissue or fibrinous material over the surface, with moderate to heavy exudate and minimal pain. Associated skin changes include a hemosiderin pigmentation, edema, and lipodermatosclerosis.

Arterial ulcers occur most often on the lower extremity distal to the area of impaired perfusion. They are painful and dry, have well-demarcated edges, and can be very deep with exposed support structures. The limb is traditionally thin, cool, pale or hyperemic, hairless, and shiny as a result of decreased perfusion. Diabetic foot ulcers appear most commonly on the plantar surface of the foot, often over the head of the metatarsal joint bearing the greatest pressure. They are often painless secondary to neuropathy. The borders are often punched out with surrounding callus; the ulcer base varies on the basis of arterial perfusion. With good perfusion, they have red granulation; poorly perfused ulcers are often drier, with flattened pale granulation or black eschar, warranting further vascular evaluation.

Thermal Wounds

Thermal wounds are the most common type of burn. Many patients initially are seen in the outpatient setting but may require the attention of a burn specialist. Burn center referral is based on the criteria of the American Burn Association and the American College of Surgeons (see Box 69-5).[15]

MANAGEMENT

Immediate referral to a specialist is indicated for deep lacerations, especially when a fracture or tendon injury is suspected.

Immediate referral to a hand specialist is indicated for hand injuries.[12]

Consideration for referral to a plastic surgeon is indicated for facial and hand wounds because of the high priority for minimizing scarring and ensuring a return to normal motor function.[12]

Specialist referral is indicated for deep puncture wounds of the foot, hand, chest, abdomen, and head.

Specialist referral is indicated for wounds requiring significant debridement and wounds with continuous bleeding.

General Principles

The use of universal precautions is essential in wound assessment and treatment. Establishing the type and nature of injury guides wound management decisions. Documentation must include the nature of the injury; wound type, location, and size in centimeters (length, width, depth); integrity of supporting structures (bone, wound, vasculature); appearance of the periwound; and characteristics of the exudate (Box 69-7). Normal saline 0.9% is the cleansing and irrigating product of choice in most wounds because it is isotonic, readily available, and inexpensive. Gentle surfactants, or dermal wound cleansers, may also be used and often come in a delivery system to provide adequate pressure per square inch needed for irrigation. The use of cytotoxic products, including undiluted povidone-iodine (Betadine) and hydrogen peroxide, previously thought to be beneficial, is not currently recommended. Dakin solution (a diluted sodium hypochlorite solution) has been shown to be safe at concentrations less than 0.5% but should be considered a short-term treatment.[2] Regardless of wound type, the principles of moist wound healing guide management. However, chronic wounds require specific intervention based on cause. It is imperative to ensure wound bed moisture, nutrition, perfusion, pH balance, freedom from infection and debris, and protection. Antibiotic creams and ointments, including silver sulfadiazine (SSD), can be appropriate for short periods in infected wounds and are prescribed for only 14 to 21 days. Management of comorbid conditions and reduction of risk factors, including careful blood glucose monitoring and control, smoking cessation, correction of malnutrition, and enhancement of perfusion, are important strategies. Ensuring intake of adequate protein and essential vitamins and minerals such as vitamin C, zinc, copper, magnesium, and arginine may also enhance wound healing.[16,17]

Debridement. Debridement of necrotic tissue can be accomplished by surgical, mechanical, autolytic, biologic (larval), or chemical methods. Surgical debridement is used to remove hyperkeratotic or necrotic tissue and should cause only minimum healthy tissue trauma and bleeding. Mechanical debridement involves the use of high-pressure water sprays. Whirlpool treatments are not recommended by some sources because these treatments have a risk for skin burning and maceration in a population of patients in whom there are impaired healing mechanisms (the diabetic population).[2] In the office setting, a 30-mL syringe with an 18-gauge needle can be used for mechanical debridement. Standard wet-to-dry dressings are considered a form of mechanical debridement but should be avoided because of the nonselectivity and potential damage to healthy tissue.[18] Autolytic debridement with film, hydrocolloid, or hydrogel dressings allows leukocytes on the ulcer surface to degrade and release lysosomal enzymes that break down protein and mucopolysaccharide components of ulcer eschar; however, dressings that retain moisture are contraindicated in the presence of infection.[2,19] Biologic debridement occurs by application of sterilized medicinal maggots topically to the wound. Maggots have a unique capability of digesting bacteria and produce enzymes that break down necrotic tissue. Maggot therapy is not widely used in the United States because of psychological factors but is gaining more favor in Europe.[7] Chemical debridement can be achieved by the use of collagenase, a metalloproteinase made from the bacterium *Clostridium histolyticum*, which has been shown to expedite debridement by the degradation of denatured collagen and is more effective than hydrogel.[20,21] Dakin solution, used at 0.5% concentration, has also been proven to debride wounds by the degradation of collagen as well, but is less selective than collagenase. When used for a debriding agent, it should be applied by moist gauze packing twice a day and should be used short term.[2]

Dressings. A dressing is applied after wound exploration, irrigation, cleansing, debridement (when appropriate), and closure (when appropriate). Dressings serve the purposes of protection, drainage absorption, insulation, maintenance of moisture and cleanliness, and facilitation of gaseous exchange. They should be easily removed without traumatizing tissue and are often multilayered. No single dressing may afford all these properties; several hundred wound care products are available to choose from.[22]

Selection of dressing is based on function, availability, cost, and comfort. Topical wound treatment may include alginates, antimicrobial hydrofibers, hydrocolloids, foams, or gels, depending on the level of exudate the wound produces. The wound care product selection algorithm (Fig. 69-1) can guide the selection of a dressing based on the appearance of the wound.

Dressings may be secured with tape, roll gauze, stockinet, binders, or straps. Being mindful of minimizing tissue trauma can guide the choice of dressing security. For example, wounds that are large and highly exudative and require frequent changes should be secured with a nonadhesive bandage when possible. This will decrease skin tearing and trauma from frequent tape removal. Dressing change intervals vary and depend on the patient and wound characteristics along with specific manufacturer guidelines.[12,22]

Acute Wounds

Lacerations, Abrasions, Avulsions, Crush Injuries, Bites, Puncture Wounds, and Other Traumatic or Surgical Wounds. The primary management goals for all acute wounds are to control major hemorrhage, to protect the patient and the wound, and to promote comfort by providing appropriate pain medication.[12,23]

It is essential to assess vascular, neurologic, and musculoskeletal (i.e., muscle, tendon, joint) function and potential injury to supportive tissues and structures.[23,24] After examining the wound, the health care provider must clean and debride it to remove dirt, debris, and foreign bodies.[24]

Contaminated wounds should be irrigated with normal saline solution (0.9%) or tap water. A 19-gauge needle or plastic cannula and a 35-mL syringe held 2 inches from the wound is used for high-pressure irrigation. A low-pressure bulb syringe alone does not create enough pressure for adequate irrigation.[25] Hydrogen peroxide and concentrated povidone-iodine should be avoided because of cytotoxicity to healthy tissue.[24]

Decisions about wound closure depend on the wound type, location, and depth and tension of the wound edges. A wound with smooth edges that is not grossly contaminated (e.g., a laceration from a knife or razor) may be closed by approximation of the wound edges and application of wound adhesive or Steri-Strips or suturing with appropriate material. Staples are an efficient closure medium but are usually used when closure must be quick and the wound is not located in an area where scarring is of concern. Wounds easily closed include small lacerations not over a joint; wounds with clean, even edges approximated without inversion or eversion; and lacerations in areas with no redundant tissue.[12] Suturing guidelines are reviewed in Table 69-3. Abrasions, avulsions, crush injuries, bites, and puncture wounds are not usually closed.

Tissue adhesive, or glue, can be an excellent substitute for stitches or staples to close simple cuts; glue causes less pain, is quicker, and needs no follow-up removal. Glue should not be used for lacerations longer than 4 cm or wounds under tension, such as over joints.[24]

Tissue approximation, when appropriate, and the application of a sterile nonadherent dressing are standard practice. Follow-up care involves observing for signs and symptoms of infection and applying a dressing to keep the wound moist, clean, and free from physical trauma.[12,24]

Tetanus immunization should be reviewed for all patients after any type of tissue trauma. Tetanus and diphtheria toxoid and tetanus immune globulin should be administered if immunization status is unknown or if the patient has received fewer than three lifetime doses. All age groups are currently recommended to receive one dose of Tdap booster immunization (tetanus, diphtheria toxoids combined with acellular pertussis vaccine). Once an adult has received one dose of Tdap, immunization with tetanus diphtheria (Td) toxoid is recommended for all patients with tetanus-prone wounds (including all contaminated wounds) if the previous immunization was more than 5 years ago[24] (Table 69-4 and Box 69-6).

Skin Tears. Skin tears should be gently cleansed with normal saline or a gentle surfactant, and the skin flap should be as closely approximated as possible.[26] The flap should not be removed unless it is necrotic.[26]

An appropriate dressing should be selected based on moist wound healing principles. Dressings considered may include hydrogels, silicone foams, alginate, or nonadherent gauze mesh.[26]

Burns (see Chapter 46). Burns are described according to depth (see Box 69-4 for burn classification). Immediate action should be taken to stop the burning process by removal of the patient from the burn source, and the burn should be emergently treated with rapid and copious irrigation with cool (not ice) water.[27] Before dressing, burn wounds should be cleansed with normal saline or a gentle surfactant, necrotic tissue should be sharply debrided, and an appropriate dressing should be applied. SSD has been the standard of care for topical treatment of burns, but recent studies have shown that longer wear, sustained-release silver dressings may provide better outcomes and are more cost-effective.[27] Topical antimicrobials such as SSD, mupirocin, and bacitracin may used but necessitate frequent dressing changes.[27]

Chronic Wounds

Pressure Ulcers. Pressure ulcers are treated by removing pressure and avoiding friction, shear, and moisture.[7,11]

Pressure can be reduced by the use of specialty mattresses such as gel or foam overlays, alternating air pads, or low–air loss mattresses. For wheelchair-bound patients, the use of pressure-reducing chair cushions is beneficial.[7,11] Topical treatment is based on wound size, depth, exudate, presence of necrosis, and bacterial contamination.[7,11]

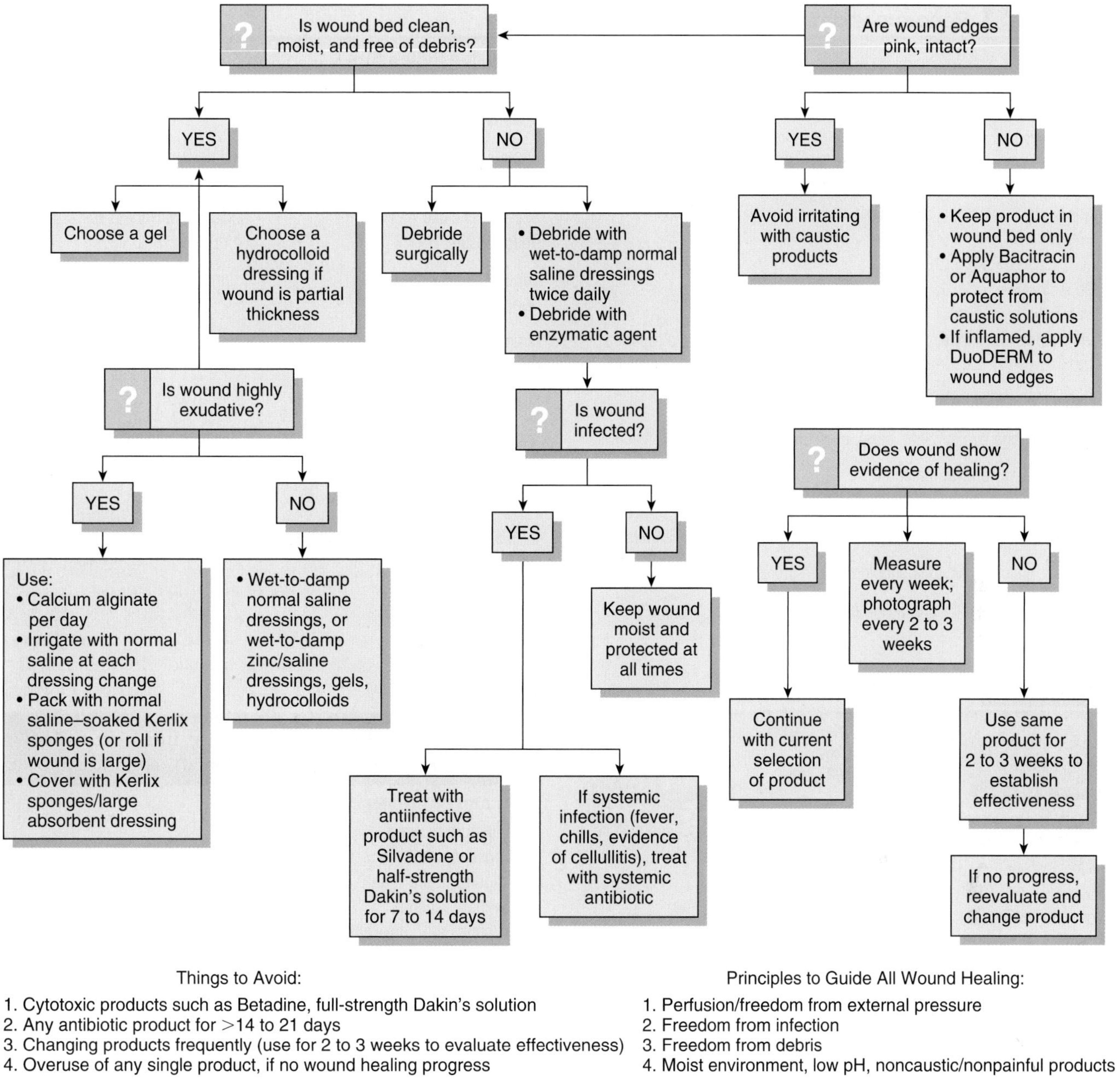

FIGURE 69-1 Algorithm for wound care product selection.

Ulcers are cleaned after each incontinent episode or bowel movement.[28] Stage I and stage II pressure ulcers with light or no exudate can be managed with a transparent film. Hydrogel can be used on stages II, III, and IV deep wounds and with necrosis or slough. Stage III and stage IV ulcers with heavy exudates can be managed by calcium alginate or biologic products. Foam dressings can be used for a primary dressing or as a secondary dressing for wounds that require packing and stage II or stage IV ulcers with drainage.[29]

Venous Ulcers. Treatment of venous ulcers involves reducing edema with leg elevation and graded compression.

Ulcerations should be treated with moist wound healing along with compression therapy.[30]

Compression can be applied as an Unna paste boot or a multilayer compression wrap. Intermittent pneumatic devices can be used for patients who cannot tolerate sustained compression.[31] Some patients may have arterial insufficiency along with venous disease. Measurement of the ankle-brachial pressure index to exclude the presence of peripheral vascular disease before the application of compression is necessary.[28,32] Adjunctive therapies to accelerate healing include skin grafting and grafting of living human skin equivalents.[29]

Arterial Ulcers. Management of arterial ulcers involves improving perfusion. Perfusion can be improved surgically and by the use of pharmacologic agents, lifestyle changes, and adjunctive therapies (such as hyperbaric oxygen therapy and arterial flow augmentation with intermittent pneumatic compression devices). The intervention selected would depend on the severity of the patient's ischemia.[2] Providing warmth to the lower extremities with cotton stockings and protecting from injury with well-fitting shoes can aid in prevention.

Topical therapy depends on the vascular supply. If there is adequate blood supply to support healing or if the patient has been successfully revascularized, debridement and a moist

TABLE 69-3 **Recommendations for Suturing**

Location	Suggested Suture Size	Suggested Suture Removal
Scalp	Superficial closure: 4 or 5 Deep closure: 4	6-7 days
Trunk	Superficial closure: 4 or 5 Deep closure: 3 or 4	6-8 days
Arms	Superficial closure: 4 or 5 Deep closure: 3 or 4	Extensor surfaces: 10-14 days All others: 7-10 days
Legs	Superficial closure: 4 or 5 Deep closure: 3 or 4	Same as for arms
Hands: referral indicated, although simple lacerations may be repaired	Superficial closure: 5 or 6 Deep closure: 4	Palms: 7-10 days Extensor surfaces: 10-14 days
Feet (soles): referral indicated for tendon or nerve injury	Superficial or deep closure: 3 or 4	7-14 days
Facial (including eyelids, lips, ears): pressure dressing; referral indicated		3-5 days
Penis, scrotum: referral indicated		
Dog bites: bites more than 6 hours old and puncture wounds should not be sutured; consultation suggested for wounds less than 6 hours old		
Cat bites: puncture wounds should not be sutured		
Human bites: wounds should not be sutured		

TABLE 69-4 **Tetanus Immunization***

Wound Type	Unknown Primary Immunization or Fewer than Three Doses	Three or More Doses
Tetanus-prone wounds	Tetanus and diphtheria toxoid (Td) and tetanus immune globulin (TIG)	Td if >5 years since booster
Non–tetanus-prone wounds	Td	Td if >10 years since booster

Adult patients should receive 1 dose of Tdap (tetanus and diphtheria toxoids combined with acellular pertussis vaccine) as a replacement for Td (diphtheria and tetanus toxoids).

*Doses (for age 7 years or older): Td, 0.5 mL IM; TIG, 250 units IM.

From Novak RT: *Tetanus.* Centers for Disease Control and Prevention. Available at www.nc.cdc.gov/travel/yellowbook/2014/chapter-3-infectious-diseases-related-to-travel/tetanus. Accessed September 2, 2014.

BOX 69-6

Tetanus-Prone Versus Non–Tetanus-Prone Wounds

TETANUS-PRONE WOUNDS

- Puncture wounds
- Crush injuries
- Wounds more than 6 hr old
- Stellate wounds
- Wounds with devitalized tissue
- Obviously contaminated wounds

NON–TETANUS-PRONE WOUNDS

- Wounds less than 6 hr old
- Wounds with clean margins
- Wounds without devitalized tissue
- Wounds without organic contamination
- Wounds with clearly defined edges

wound healing environment are recommended.[17] Arterial ulcers characterized by dry stable eschar should be left intact and treated by painting with Betadine daily to prevent infection.[2]

Standard compression therapy such as an Unna boot is inappropriate in the care of arterial ulcers because it dries an already dry wound bed and provides compression in a poorly perfused limb. Modified compression can be used in patients with concomitant edema if the ankle-brachial index is above 0.6.[3]

Diabetic Foot Ulcers. Management of blood glucose concentration is an essential component for foot ulcer prevention and healing.[17] Off-loading areas of pressure at risk for ulceration with appropriate shoes can be effective in preventing initial or recurrent ulceration and can aide in healing of current ulcers.[14] Specific ulcer management techniques include debridement to a clean ulcer base, treatment of any infection in the ulcer, and use of modalities to promote wound healing. Once the ulcer is debrided, prevention of infection is imperative to reduce risk of amputation; however, detection of infection is often difficult secondary to neuropathy and decreased inflammatory response. Prolonged hyperglycemia may be the first indication of infection. Systemic antibiotics and assessment for osteomyelitis are essential to prevent amputation.[4,17] There is evidence showing benefit for other treatment modalities, such as bilayered living cell therapy, tissue factors, hyperbaric oxygen therapy, total contact casting, electrical stimulation, and infrared light therapy.[19,33] Once ulcers are healed, patients require close, continuous monitoring to minimize recurrences. Pressure-relieving modalities, including therapeutic footwear, should be used.[14,17]

BOX 69-7

Documentation of Wounds

Wound
- Location
- Width
- Depth
- Edges
- Exudate

Presence of foreign bodies

Accompanying injuries
- Fractures
- Dislocations
- Tendon or ligament injuries
- Neurologic and cardiovascular findings

Diagnostic findings, radiologic conclusions

Treatments

Follow-up

Nonhealing Surgical or Traumatic Wounds

Wounds healing by secondary intention often have significant amount of devitalized tissue and bacterial loads.[2] Wound packing with a hydrogel (not indicated for highly exudative wounds) or calcium alginate to absorb exudate is often effective. Both of these items are now formulated with silver for antimicrobial coverage.[22]

The use of new technologic advances to enhance healing, such as negative pressure wound therapy, has promoted wound healing in large, open wounds.[34] Adjunctive therapies are useful in chronic wounds; hyperbaric oxygen therapy is an evidence-based therapy being used to treat diabetic foot ulcers with success. Negative pressure wound therapy is useful to promote healing in chronic stage III or stage IV pressure ulcers as well as nonhealing surgical wounds and some lower extremity ulcers. Ultrasound, biologic therapy, growth factors, and electrical stimulation may also be beneficial in certain wounds.[34]

COMPLICATIONS

Complications of wound healing include infection, dehiscence, delayed wound healing, extensive scarring, and sepsis. Serious infection of the face or hands and cellulitis that has not responded to oral antibiotic treatment require intravenous antibiotics or hospitalization.

INDICATIONS FOR REFERRAL OR HOSPITALIZATION

Referral decisions are guided by the location and nature of the wound; injury to bone, tendon, or vasculature; and the experience of the health care provider. Referral to a specialist is required for fractures, deep tissue injury, vascular or organ damage, facial and hand injuries, or severely contaminated wounds. Large, open wounds or deep puncture wounds most likely require referral for a surgical intervention. Chronic wounds, such as ulcers, are best managed by referral to a wound care specialist who is part of an interdisciplinary team. Facial or hand wounds that are infected may require hospitalization and intravenous antibiotics.

LIFE SPAN CONSIDERATIONS

Elderly patients tend to heal more slowly, and their wounds tend to lose tensile strength, which correlates with reduced collagen.[9] Impaired skin integrity is common in older adults as a result of age-related skin changes, immobility, malnutrition, incontinence, immunocompromised status, polypharmacy, sensory deficits, and comorbidities. Thinning of the epidermis, dermis, and subcutaneous tissue coupled with decreased tensile strength and elasticity and poor epidermal-dermal adhesion contributes to easy skin tears, pressure ulcers, and lower extremity ulcers.[9]

In addition, wound healing time is prolonged in older adults because of decreased oxygenation and perfusion and a decreased inflammatory response. Although the same principles of wound management apply in all populations, special diligence is recommended in caring for older adults. Consideration of the diminished ability to provide self-care and to travel easily to and from medical facilities should prompt the provider to select appropriate dressings and to consider a referral to home health agencies for wound evaluation and care in the patient's setting. The risk of delayed wound healing contributes to infection, pain, and a decreased quality of life in patients who may already be compromised.[9]

EDUCATION AND HEALTH PROMOTION

Signs and symptoms of wound infection should be reviewed with the patient and family both verbally and in writing. Infection of the wound can greatly affect outcome and may impede wound healing and return of function. Demonstrating wound dressing techniques with the patient and family and observing a return demonstration when possible are helpful in ascertaining the patient's and family's understanding. A patient teaching pamphlet or video with specific directions for wound cleansing and care reinforces teaching, especially if available in the patient's primary language.

Reevaluation and follow-up evaluation for suture removal should be scheduled before discharge. Sutures are removed according to the location of the wound and the type of suture used. Referral for a home health nurse may be important for dressing changes, support in managing medications (especially antibiotics), and wound evaluation in the home. Follow-up monitoring of most wounds should occur within 7 to 10 days.

Prevention of lower extremity ulcers and diligent foot care in patients with diabetes mellitus and peripheral vascular disease will prevent amputations, decrease the cost of multiple hospitalizations, and prolong and improve the overall quality of life. Pressure-relieving interventions such as callus removal, padded hosiery to reduce callous buildup, extra-depth shoes, and insoles to redistribute foot pressure have demonstrated some benefit in ulcer prevention. Emollient moisturizers can help prevent fissures and breaks in the skin of those with diabetes and venous insufficiency. Patients at risk for pressure ulcers should be instructed in proper positioning and pressure reduction techniques.

Promotion of healthy behaviors is an essential intervention in the prevention of traumatic wounds. Health care providers should encourage home safety and reinforce child safety practices including automobile safety, helmet use, gun safety, and safe behavior around animals.

REFERENCES

For a full list of references, scan the QR code or visit http://booksite.elsevier.com/9780323355018

PART 6

Evaluation and Management of Eye Disorders

CHAPTER 70

EVALUATION OF THE EYES

Daniel S. Churgin • James T. Banta

A complete ophthalmic examination is vital not only for routine patient care but for the diagnosis of critical local and systemic abnormalities. Whereas some problems may require a formal evaluation by an ophthalmologist, the primary care provider should be well versed in the basics of the eye examination. By achieving a better understanding of the eye examination, a primary care provider can assist patients with common complaints and refer them to a specialist when it is indicated. This chapter discusses basic eye anatomy, the components of a complete ocular evaluation, and the differential diagnosis of common presenting ophthalmic complaints.

SCREENING RECOMMENDATIONS

Because of the significant public health implications and vision's impact on quality of life, regular eye examinations are recommended at various intervals, depending on a patient's age and risk factors. Even in an otherwise healthy adult, the risk of visual impairment increases with age. Vision of 20/50 or less has been demonstrated in 9% of adults older than 60 years.

The American Academy of Ophthalmology (AAO) recommends that patients 65 years of age and older without risk factors for eye disease should have a comprehensive eye examination every 1 to 2 years. Several other academies, including the American Congress of Obstetricians and Gynecologists and the American Academy of Family Physicians, suggest similar recommendations for screening of older patients.[1,2]

In addition to more general screening guidelines, certain disease entities carry specific screening guidelines that are highly applicable to primary care providers. The AAO recommends that patients with diabetes receive eye screening—type 1 diabetics 3 to 5 years after the diagnosis, and type 2 diabetics at the time of diagnosis—to assess for diabetic retinopathy. In addition, these patients should continue to undergo screening on an annual basis. With regard to pregnancy, patients with diabetes should receive a screening examination before conception and early in the first trimester.[3] The U.S. Preventive Services Task Force (USPSTF) has also looked at screening for primary open-angle glaucoma (POAG) in adults but thus far has found insufficient evidence to justify routine screening.[4] However, the AAO has noted that screening for POAG may be more useful when it is targeted at populations at high risk for glaucoma, such as older adults, those with a family history of glaucoma, and African Americans and Hispanics.[5]

HISTORY

The basis of a good eye examination is a thorough history. As with any medical examination, details about the history of the present illness can help hone the physical examination and give clues about an aberrant process. For patients with a new eye complaint, such as pain or vision loss, it is important to determine the quality and nature of the presenting problem. The onset of the complaint is of particular importance in ophthalmology. For instance, although a patient with a gradual worsening of vision may simply need glasses or evaluation for cataracts, a complaint of acute vision loss should be referred for immediate evaluation by an ophthalmologist. Other details should be explored, such as the location (left eye, right eye, or both), duration, character, associated factors (pain, redness, discharge, headache, nausea, or neurologic changes), aggravating and alleviating factors (pain with eye movements or with bright lights), radiation, temporal association (worse in morning or night), and severity. In addition to acute vision loss, any patient with painful vision loss or trauma should be referred to an ophthalmologist. Similarly, a patient with acute vision loss associated with neurologic signs should be emergently evaluated to rule out a cerebrovascular accident or other central nervous system processes.

A patient's past medical and ocular history can also give insight into a new problem. Information should be gathered about any previous eye disease, trauma, and surgery (both medically necessary and cosmetic or refractive). In addition, many systemic medical problems have associated ophthalmic manifestations, as discussed in more detail later in this chapter. Medication reconciliation is equally important because systemic and topical medications can be associated with both systemic effects and changes in the eye. For instance, medications commonly prescribed for erectile dysfunction (e.g., sildenafil) are sometimes associated with cyanopsia, or blue-tinted vision. The beta blocker timolol is frequently prescribed for glaucoma and can exacerbate bradycardia and asthma in susceptible patients.

A thorough family history that includes ocular disease should be obtained because several ocular conditions are associated with a familial pattern of inheritance and can represent a threat to a patient's vision or life. Patients with a family history of glaucoma, color blindness, cataracts, macular degeneration, retinal degeneration, corneal dystrophy, and retinoblastoma have increased risks for these processes, which should be considered in the taking of the general family history. These patients should be referred to an ophthalmologist if care has not already been established.

Social and occupational factors are elucidated to better identify behaviors that increase risk for eye-related trauma or disease. Leisure or occupational activities associated with trauma to the eyes, such as construction work (particularly hammering or grinding), chemical work, and high-impact sports, should direct the physician to ask about the use of eye protection. Similarly, injection drug use or high-risk sexual behavior generates a higher risk for human immunodeficiency virus (HIV) and acquired immunodeficiency syndrome (AIDS) and can be important in correct identification of ocular diseases specific to immunocompromised states.

PHYSICAL EXAMINATION

An evaluation of the structure and function of the eyes should be approached systematically and incorporate a sound understanding of ocular and periocular anatomy. The primary measurements to determine the basic health and function of the eyes are visual acuity, pupil responses, intraocular pressure, visual fields, and extraocular movements. These metrics are analogous to vital signs for a systemic examination and are integral to every ophthalmic examination. After the assessment of these ocular vital signs, an evaluation of ocular structures should proceed from external and anterior segment structures inward to the posterior segment.

Visual Acuity

Visual acuity refers to the spatial resolving power of the eye. As the primary functional measure of the eye, it is important to measure vision accurately. Vision is typically measured at the beginning of the examination before any other test or intervention has been performed. Spurious results can otherwise be found as a result of dilating drops or corneal irritation from intraocular pressure measurements. Vision should be tested in each eye with use of the patient's refractive aids (e.g., glasses, contact lenses) or a pinhole (a technique of looking through a hole in a card to diminish refractive error). In patients with refractive error—especially high myopia—failing to test vision with the use of refractive aids or a pinhole can lead a provider to incorrectly suspect acute pathology, causing undue concern to the patient and provider.

There are many valid means of measuring vision, such as the Snellen chart, tumbling *E*s, and other instruments used for pediatric populations. Of these, the most commonly used and referenced is the Snellen chart. This chart consists of 11 lines of precisely sized block letters, or optotypes. By convention in the United States, the patient is directed to stand 20 feet away from the wall chart. With each eye, the chart is read down until the patient is unable to make out the letters. The patient's vision is recorded as a fractional value, such as 20/80, based on the last line that was successfully seen. This value indicates the equivalent distance that a person with normal vision could stand away from the chart and still read the indicated letters. In this example, a patient with normal vision could be 80 feet away from the chart and still read the letters that the patient in question can read at 20 feet. The tumbling *E* chart uses variously sized letter *E*s in different orientations for patients who have difficulty identifying letters or are illiterate.

If a patient is unable to read any letters on the Snellen chart (visual acuity <20/400), the vision can be tested by other means. The first alternative means of testing vision is to use a card of a 20/200 Snellen E. This card can be held starting directly in front of the patient's eye and slowly moved back until the patient is no longer able to identify it. This value is recorded as the number of feet the patient is able to see the letter over 200; for example, if a patient can read the card at 6 feet, the vision is recorded as 6/200. If this proves unsuccessful, finger counting can be employed. Similar to testing vision with the 20/200 card, any number of fingers are held at gradually increasing distances from the patient's eye. Vision is recorded as the maximum distance a patient can count fingers (e.g., CF at 6 feet). If a patient cannot count fingers, the patient is asked to identify the examiner's hand waving slowly in front of the eyes; a patient able to see the movement of a hand has vision recorded as HM for hand motions. If the patient fails the aforementioned tests, the final check of visual acuity is the patient's ability to perceive light. For this test, a light is shined into a patient's eye in a darkened room, and the patient is asked if any light can be seen. Care must be taken to fully cover the eye that is not being tested, as light may enter the unintended eye and lead to a false-positive result. A positive response is recorded as LP (light perception); a negative response is recorded as NLP (no light perception).

Near vision can be tested separately, as some pathologic processes yield good near vision with poor far vision and vice versa. Near vision can be tested with a Rosenbaum near card held at 14 inches. Again, each eye is tested independently, and the patient is asked to read the smallest line possible. Unlike distance vision, near vision is recorded on the Jaeger scale. This scale ranges from J16 (approximately 20/200) to J1+, which equates to 20/20 on the Snellen chart. On this scale, standard newspaper font is J5. All adults will begin to exhibit difficulties with near vision around the age of 42 or 43 years. This is because of a decrease in the flexibility of the human lens, a natural aging process known as *presbyopia*. Although this condition can cause significant patient distress, a trial of over-the-counter reading glasses generally produces a satisfactory improvement in the patient's near vision and therefore in the quality of life.

Pupil Response

Impaired pupil responses can give vital information about the function of a patient's visual system. Under standard fluorescent lighting conditions, the average adult pupil ranges from 2.6 to 5.0 mm and is round and symmetric.[6] Any variance in the size of the pupils between the eyes is defined as anisocoria. This finding can be benign, as physiologic anisocoria exists in 20% of the population[7] and demonstrates a difference of no more than 1 mm between two normally functioning pupils. However, anisocoria can also suggest a neurologic, pharmacologic, or anatomic abnormality. In addition, previous episodes of trauma or intraocular surgery can result in an anatomically abnormal pupil; thus a detailed history is vital.

Pupil function can be assessed with a standard penlight. On initial inspection, the examiner should test each pupil independently, shining the light from a slightly oblique angle to avoid a false response from accommodation. The pupil should respond briskly to the light and hold in its constricted position. A normal pupil should not redilate in direct light, but it might demonstrate a slight fluctuation in diameter. This phenomenon is referred to as *hippus* and is of no pathologic significance. When the examiner has established the independent functioning of each pupil, he or she must next verify symmetric pupil responses with the swinging flashlight test. To perform this technique, the patient is first asked to focus straight ahead on a distant object. It is important that the patient's fixation is at distance to prevent accommodation from causing pupillary constriction and confounding the swinging flashing test. A flashlight is then directed at one eye until the pupil constricts. The flashlight is then swung quickly to the opposite eye, and the response is observed. In a normally functioning eye, equal signal is received from each eye and transmitted across synaptic pathways to achieve consensual constriction. If the pathway or the input is damaged—usually through a defect in the optic nerve—the signal is disrupted and the eyes will respond asymmetrically. For instance, if a significant injury has occurred to the left optic nerve, a flashlight shined into the right eye will produce a normal constriction in both eyes from appropriate consensual response. However, when the flashlight is swung to the left, the pupils will paradoxically dilate because of the disruption of the afferent signal from the damaged nerve. This phenomenon is known as a *relative afferent pupillary defect* (RAPD) or *Marcus-Gunn pupil.* It is important to use the swinging flashlight test to identify this condition because both pupils may respond to light, and therefore it is the relative response that is essential. An RAPD indicates significant ocular dysfunction, and if it is present for an unknown reason, the patient should be referred for further evaluation by an ophthalmologist.

Intraocular Pressure

Normal intraocular pressure is generally considered to range from 10 to 20 mm Hg. Many methods exist to measure intraocular pressure. These include the air-puff tonometer, Tono-Pen, and Goldmann applanation tonometry. Of these options, the Tono-Pen is most accessible to nonophthalmologic offices. It consists of a penlike device that is tapped against the center of the patient's cornea after instillation of an ocular anesthetic such as proparacaine. The Tono-Pen provides an easy-to-use, quick estimation of intraocular pressure. Unfortunately, at higher pressures the Tono-Pen is not as accurate as other methods. The gold standard of measurement is Goldmann applanation tonometry, which requires the use of a slit lamp and is something that is not typically available in nonophthalmologic offices.

Although accurate measurement of intraocular pressure is essential to a complete eye examination, not all primary care settings have access to a measurement tool. In these cases, the physician can gather a rough estimation of the intraocular pressure by gently palpating the globes through closed lids. Under normal circumstances, the eyes should feel of a consistency similar to a grape and should be roughly symmetric. Any eye that feels rock-hard is abnormal and should be further evaluated. In addition, a firm, painful eye that is inflamed and associated with a cloudy cornea is indicative of an acute rise in intraocular pressure. This represents an ophthalmic emergency with a strong potential for irreversible vision loss; emergent referral is indicated.

Ocular Alignment and Extraocular Movements

Ocular movements are controlled by six extraocular muscles: the four rectus muscles (superior, inferior, medial, and lateral) as well as the two oblique muscles (superior and inferior). These muscles are controlled by cranial nerves III, IV, and VI. Under normal conditions, the eyes should be symmetric and aligned when the patient is looking forward and should move equally in all directions. Movements can be affected by a neurologic dysfunction (from trauma, compression of a cranial nerve, or ischemia), by a muscle dysfunction (such as a restrictive or inflammatory processes), or by congenital abnormalities.

The examination of ocular alignment consists of three general components: the Hirschberg test, the cover-uncover test, and the alternate-cover test. These maneuvers allow the examiner to determine the presence of strabismus, a condition that may influence visual prognosis in children or cause diplopia in adults. The Hirschberg test is performed with the patient looking in primary gaze, or directly at the observer. The examiner, standing in front of the patient, then shines a bright penlight directly at the patient's eyes. The light from the penlight is seen reflecting on the patient's corneas, prompting what is referred to as the *light reflex.* In a patient with normal alignment, these reflections should be symmetrically located within the pupils. If a reflection is deviated medially (nasally) or laterally (temporally), this indicates an exotropia or esotropia, respectively.

When a disorder of ocular alignment is suspected, the cover-uncover test and alternate-cover test can be used to further evaluate the nature of the disorder. The cover-uncover test involves having a patient fixate on a distant object. The examiner then places an occluder in front of one eye to disrupt binocular vision. The occluder is removed and the newly uncovered eye is observed. Movement of the newly uncovered eye suggests underlying strabismus. Similarly, in the alternate-cover test, the patient looks at a distant object and an occluder is passed from one eye to the other. Any resulting movement in the unobstructed eye is abnormal and represents a dysfunction of ocular motility. Ophthalmologists use prisms to quantify any noted deviations.

Once the ocular alignment has been evaluated, one must examine the patient's ocular motility. The examiner asks the patient to track an object such as a pen or the examiner's index finger without moving the head (The index finger should be moved slowly to avoid making the patient dizzy). Any gross deficit in motility should be noted. There are nine diagnostic positions of gaze: straight, right, upper right, up, upper left, left, lower left, down, and lower right. Of these gazes, six (right, upper right, upper left, left, lower left, and lower right) are considered the cardinal directions of gaze. With these six, one can localize a movement deficiency of one of the extraocular muscles. Dysfunctional extraocular movement with a paretic cause can often be identified by this examination technique.

Because the oculomotor nerve (cranial nerve III) innervates the majority of extraocular muscles as well as levator palpebrae and autonomic muscles, its injury or dysfunction can have diverse presentations. In a complete cranial nerve III palsy, the patient classically has a "down-and-out" position of the affected eye and is unable to adduct the eye or move it up or down. The eyelid may demonstrate complete or partial ptosis, and a third nerve palsy can also be associated with a nonresponsive pupil in the same eye. Multiple causes of third-nerve palsy are possible, ranging from the microvascular effects of hypertension and diabetes to compressive lesions such as tumors or aneurysms. Pupil function can give a clue to the cause of a third-nerve palsy and should be checked before the instillation of dilating drops. If a nonresponsive pupil is present, this is suggestive of a compressive lesion (often an aneurysm) and necessitates referral for emergent neuroimaging and evaluation.

A trochlear nerve (cranial nerve IV) palsy can be difficult to detect; the motility examination findings can appear grossly normal. However, some patients will exhibit a decreased ability to look down in the adducted position. A head tilt away from the affected side is often present and diminishes diplopia. A patient with an abducens nerve (cranial nerve VI) abnormality will be unable to abduct the involved eye. A head turn away from the affected side will diminish diplopia. Both cranial nerve IV and VI palsies are often ischemic or traumatic in nature.

Another important examination when evaluating the motility and position of the eyes is to check for protuberance of one or both eyes (exophthalmos or proptosis). This is especially important in a patient who reports pain or double vision or is suspected of having thyroid disease. The best way to check for proptosis is to have the patient lift up his or her chin while the provider looks at the prominence of the eyes from below. If proptosis is suspected, a referral to an ophthalmologist is recommended and should be done urgently if the patient is experiencing other ocular symptoms such as pain, headache, or double vision. Lastly, if the patient has noticed that one eye is becoming progressively proptotic, this is an indication for an urgent referral and potentially facial and head imaging.

Visual Fields

Visual field defects can result from any abnormality that affects the eye, optic nerve, optic radiations, or visual cortex. Several methods exist to precisely determine a patient's field of vision, but only confrontation visual field testing is used routinely during a standard ophthalmic examination. Confrontation field testing is performed with the examiner approximately 1 meter away from the patient. The patient has one eye covered at a time, and the patient is instructed to look at the examiner's nose. The physician then presents fingers (usually one, two, or five fingers, because they are easily distinguishable and yield more accurate results) to the patient in each quadrant of vision. It is important for the provider to ensure that the patient has not changed his or her focus from the provider's nose to another area, which can dramatically alter results. If the patient is unable to count fingers, a stronger stimulus such as hand motions or light can be presented in the deficient areas. In patients capable of good cooperation, the physician can present different numbers of fingers at once in multiple quadrants. The patient is then asked for the total sum of the fingers shown. This method can confirm a suspected visual field deficit. If a field defect with an unknown cause is identified on confrontational examination, the patient should be referred to an ophthalmologist for a formal visual field test. If a visual field abnormality is present with other symptoms of concern for cerebrovascular accident or transient ischemic attack, the patient should be referred immediately to the nearest emergency room.

External Structures

The periorbital structures are composed of the eyelids, eyelashes, and lacrimal system. The eyelids are vital to maintaining ocular lubrication and are tightly opposed to the globe under normal circumstances. Both the upper and lower eyelids contain oil-secreting glands necessary for maintaining the tear film. The eyelid margin contains a continuous row of lashes that serve to protect the eye from debris. Lash loss is most frequently a sign of chronic inflammation but can be associated with a neoplastic process. Whitening (poliosis) or loss (madarosis) of lashes should be evaluated by an ophthalmologist. The medial aspect of the eyelid contains the punctum, the opening of the canalicular drainage system. During the blink cycle, the lids work as a pump to move tears from the ocular surface into the lacrimal sac. Lid abnormalities can result in pathologic changes ranging from dryness and exposure to excessive tearing. Accordingly, the lids must be examined carefully for signs of irregularity, improper positioning (e.g., ectropion or entropion), punctal patency, inflammation, and swelling. The eyelids should completely cover the ocular surface when they are closed. Any lack of closure, or lagophthalmos, suggests an underlying anatomic or functional abnormality and should be investigated.

Anterior Segment

The sclera is the firm outer wall of the globe and is composed of dense connective tissue. Typically, it has a white appearance on examination, but several local and systemic conditions can cause color variations. For instance, in conditions of hepatic dysfunction associated with jaundice, the sclera assumes a yellowish hue known as *icterus*. Similarly, in the genetic condition osteogenesis imperfecta or after local inflammation of the sclera, the sclera can be thinned and appear blue.

The conjunctiva is composed of two parts: the bulbar portion, which overlies the sclera, and the palpebral portion lining the eyelids. The bulbar conjunctiva is a moist, shiny tissue that is typically devoid of large or significant blood vessels. For the conjunctiva to be appropriately assessed, the patient is instructed to look in all directions as the lids are retracted for full exposure. The presence of prominent vessels with redness, known as *injection*, is indicative of inflammation. Although injection is commonly seen in infectious, allergic, or chemical conjunctivitis, injection is also noted with many other inflammatory conditions. The presence of a mucopurulent or watery discharge would suggest bacterial or viral conjunctivitis, respectively. In cases of conjunctival injection, the palpebral conjunctiva should be examined with a penlight. Under normal circumstances, the palpebral conjunctiva should appear pink and smooth. In the setting of conjunctivitis, it assumes a rough appearance (e.g., conjunctival papillae or follicles). Conjunctival injection associated with severe photophobia or layered inflammatory debris in the anterior chamber (hypopyon) suggests intraocular inflammation or infection.

After trauma or Valsalva maneuvers (e.g., lifting, sneezing), conjunctival vessels can become compromised and bleed. Blood becomes trapped between the sclera and conjunctiva and results in a deep confluent red appearance that can be focal or diffuse (Fig. 70-1). This is known as a *subconjunctival hemorrhage*. Despite an often impressive appearance, it causes no ophthalmic problems and resolves without treatment, usually within 2 weeks.

A clear balloon-like swelling of the conjunctiva is known as *chemosis*. Chemosis can be associated with allergies, mechanical ventilators, trauma, and local inflammation. It is important to identify the source of chemosis. Severe chemosis can prevent proper closure of the eyelids. When it is present, aggressive lubrication with ophthalmic lubricating drops and ointments is required to prevent ocular exposure.

The cornea is a curved structure composed of collagen fibers precisely arranged to achieve optical clarity. It is composed grossly of an epithelial surface, stroma, and endothelium. Damage or irritation of the epithelium can produce significant pain and irritation. The corneal epithelium is best evaluated with fluorescein dye. Under a cobalt blue light, any abrasions or irregularities in the epithelium will glow bright green. Pain associated with epithelial abnormalities will resolve completely after the use of topical anesthetic. Under no circumstances should a patient be given a bottle of topical ophthalmic anesthetic for personal use because prolonged use can result in a

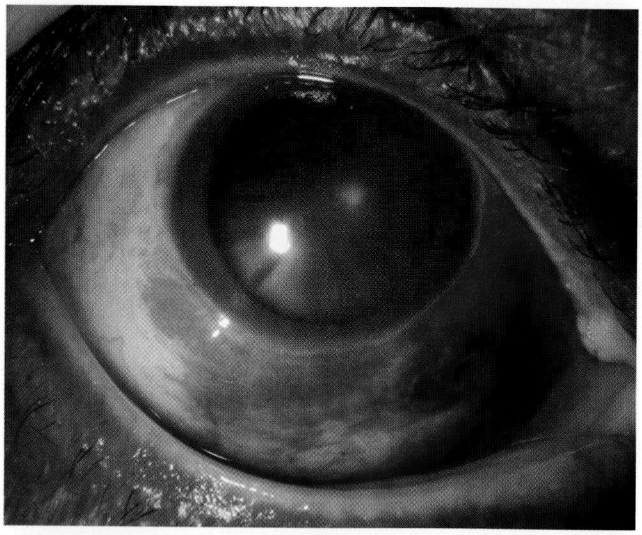

FIGURE 70-1 Despite the dramatic appearance, isolated subconjunctival hemorrhage is a benign condition that does not require treatment.

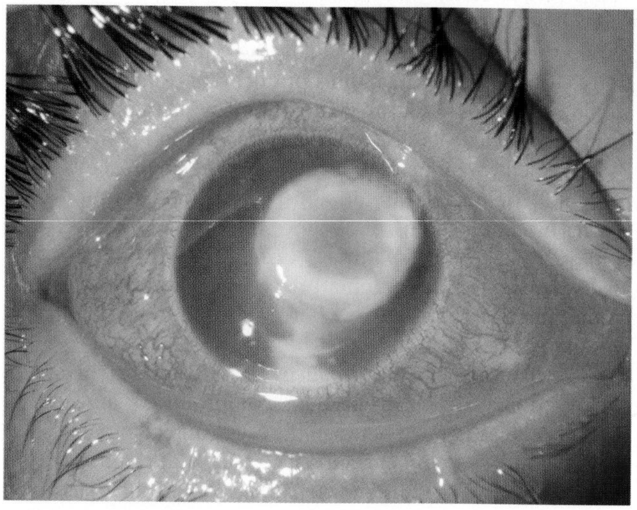

FIGURE 70-2 Inappropriate contact lens use is frequently associated with severe bacterial keratitis, as illustrated in this photograph. Note the hypopyon collecting in the inferior aspect of the anterior chamber.

corneal perforation. Abuse of topical anesthetics is often seen among health care workers, given their relatively easy access to the drops.

It is important to note any irregularities in the clarity of the cornea, which can signify infection (typically a focal white plaque) or edema (from decomposition of corneal function or elevated intraocular pressure). The evaluation of a corneal opacity is especially important in patients who wear contact lenses and have eye pain or redness. These patients must be carefully examined for suppurative, feathery, or ring-shaped white infiltrates on the cornea (Fig. 70-2). Contact lens–related ulcers are common in patients who exhibit poor contact lens hygiene (e.g., sleeping or swimming in contact lenses, prolonged use, and poor handwashing) and can evolve rapidly. Untreated, corneal ulcers may result in permanent and severe visual loss. Any patient with an acute change in corneal clarity should be referred to an ophthalmologist for further evaluation.

The anterior chamber is defined as the space between the iris and the cornea. Aqueous humor fills the anterior chamber and is produced by the ciliary body and drains through the trabecular meshwork. This space should be deep and clear. In the setting of trauma, a shallow anterior chamber can signify a violation of the globe (open globe injury). An open globe injury is sometimes associated with expulsion of intraocular tissue or a peaked pupil. An open globe is an ophthalmic emergency and must be emergently referred. In the case of a suspected open globe, it is important to place a hard shield over the eye to protect it from further serious damage, and to allow the ophthalmology team to evaluate and treat from that point. Typically, an open globe injury will require emergent surgery, so the patient should be restricted from eating and drinking in preparation for the operating room as soon as the diagnosis is suspected. This topic is addressed in greater detail in Chapter 79.

Numerous other severe conditions can lead to blood or inflammatory debris in the anterior chamber. Layering of blood (hyphema) or inflammatory debris (hypopyon) in the anterior chamber should prompt an immediate ophthalmic referral. In these cases, placing a hard shield over the eye is again advisable until an ophthalmologist can evaluate the eye.

The iris is the pigmented structure that forms the posterior aspect of the anterior chamber and acts as a shutter for the eye by controlling the amount of light through the pupil. The sphincter and dilator pupillae muscles produce constriction and dilation of the pupil in response to exogenous and endogenous stimuli. The iris is easily examined with a penlight with the aid of magnifying glass, if one is available. The color of the iris can vary greatly, but it should be of a uniform color and bilaterally symmetric. Inconsistencies in the color of an iris can represent nevi, neoplasms (melanoma), hamartomas (Lisch nodules), genetic abnormalities (Waardenburg syndrome), or inflammatory nodules (sarcoidosis). Blood vessels are typically not seen on the surface of the iris. The presence of abnormal blood vessels (iris neovascularization) suggests ocular ischemia, a condition most commonly seen in association with proliferative diabetic retinopathy or central retinal vein occlusion. Patients with iris neovascularization often develop severe, recalcitrant glaucoma and require urgent ophthalmologic consultation.

The crystalline lens is a transparent, biconcave structure aligned at the center of the pupil. The lens refracts light to achieve fine focus on the retina at various distances. A penlight can be used to assess the lens, although this is difficult through a nondilated pupil. Cataracts can appear as focal opacities or a more diffuse yellow to brown discoloration. Cataractous changes are most easily assessed in the primary care setting by use of a direct ophthalmoscope to observe irregularities in a patient's red reflex. Cataracts occur naturally with age, but they can also be a sign of trauma or certain systemic conditions (e.g., diabetes, myotonic dystrophy, Fabry disease, corticosteroid exposure). Although cataracts almost never represent an ophthalmic emergency, they can cause significant visual impairment and can be removed surgically to improve a patient's quality of life.

Posterior Segment

The posterior segment is composed of vital eye structures including the vitreous, retina, and optic nerve. Examination of the posterior segment requires the assistance of an ophthalmoscope. A complete assessment of the posterior segment requires a formal evaluation by an ophthalmologist; however, the primary care provider can use a direct ophthalmoscope to identify some important, visually significant abnormalities. The direct ophthalmoscope produces a highly magnified image of the retina and optic nerve (approximately 15×). The examination should be performed in a dark room with the examiner at approximately the same height as the patient. While the examiner is standing several feet from the patient, the light from the direct ophthalmoscope is used to assess the red reflex. Any asymmetry or opacity suggests ocular disease, which should be further investigated. The examiner then takes the ophthalmoscope, held to the same eye that is being evaluated, and approaches the pupil slowly. The ophthalmoscope should be aimed slightly nasally to identify the optic disk. As the retina becomes visible, the Rekoss disk (the dial on the side of the ophthalmoscope) is turned to correct for the combined refractive errors of the examiner and patient to bring the retinal features into focus.

The vitreous humor is the gelatinous material that fills the posterior segment and attaches to the retina at several points. Under normal circumstances, it should be optically clear, allowing a crisp view of the retinal structures. With normal aging, the vitreous undergoes degenerative changes and eventually detaches from the retina (posterior vitreous detachment), causing dark floating spots (floaters). Multiple pathologic conditions can cause an abrupt increase in floaters, including vitreous hemorrhage (e.g., trauma, diabetes, retinal tears), inflammatory conditions (e.g., uveitis, endophthalmitis), and retinal detachments. Floaters associated with flashing lights, a black curtain covering part of the visual field, or decreased vision could represent serious disease and should be urgently evaluated by an ophthalmologist.

The optic disk is the coalescence of the retinal nerve fiber layer as it leaves the globe to form the optic nerve. In the normal eye, it can be seen as a slightly oval pink-yellow disk with a small white depression at its center (optic cup). The cup normally encompasses 10% to 30% of the area of the optic nerve. A larger cup often represents a normal physiologic change but can be worrisome for glaucoma-related damage. With use of a direct ophthalmoscope, the optic disk should appear flat with distinct margins. A blurring of the margins suggests optic disk elevation, which can be seen with a multitude of conditions, including ocular inflammatory disorders or increased intracranial pressure. A flat, pale disk suggests optic atrophy associated with chronic ocular or neurologic disease.

The central retinal vein and artery travel along the center of the optic nerve and enter the globe through the optic disk. The vessels separate to form two main branches temporally, known as the *arcades,* and two smaller branches nasally. At the disk margin, the vessels can be identified by their size. Veins are approximately 1.5 times the size of arteries. In addition, the vessels should follow a smooth course with no significant tortuosity. The examiner should note the crossing of the arteries and veins. In a hypertensive patient, arteriovenous nicking is sometimes visible. The area between the temporal arcades is the macula. The fovea—responsible for central high-acuity vision—is located at the center of the macula. This region should be flat and regular and devoid of hemorrhages or exudates.

The peripheral retina, or the regions beyond the arcades, is difficult to evaluate with a direct ophthalmoscope. However, by having a well-dilated patient look in various cardinal directions, it is possible to view some extramacular retinal detail. If the decision is made to dilate the patient's pupils, the provider should always ensure that the anterior chamber appears grossly deep and ask the patient if there has ever been a negative reaction to dilation. If a pupil is dilated in a shallow chamber, there is a risk of causing acute angle-closure glaucoma—one of the most feared complications of dilating drops. Also, if the provider believes the patient requires urgent ophthalmic examination, it is best to leave the pupils undilated so that the ophthalmologist can make a formal assessment of the pupils. If the pupils are dilated, the peripheral retina should appear uniformly pink-orange. As with the macula, any elevation, hemorrhage, or exudates are abnormal and should be evaluated further by an ophthalmologist.

SIGNS AND SYMPTOMS OF OCULAR DISEASE

Red Eye

Red eye is one of the most common ocular concerns in the primary care setting. Often the underlying disorder is self-limited with minimum visual consequences, but it is important to recognize serious, vision-threatening conditions. The term *red eye* denotes hyperemia of the conjunctiva or sclera. It is also sometimes used to denote redness of the adnexal structures or periocular area.

The most common cause of red eye is conjunctivitis, which may be allergic, bacterial, or viral. Conjunctivitis is covered in great detail in Chapter 73. Patients may also be seen with a red eye from episcleritis or scleritis. These are inflammatory conditions, although scleritis may rarely have a microbial cause. Episcleritis is almost always self-limited and rarely requires topical anti-inflammatory therapy. This condition typically manifests with sectoral inflammation and is associated with foreign body sensation. Scleritis is a more serious condition that can be vision threatening and is often related to an underlying autoimmune disorder. Scleritis produces an exquisitely painful, boring eye pain, and the eye is very tender to palpation. Patients with possible scleritis should be promptly referred to an ophthalmologist.

The uveal tract of the eye consists of the iris, ciliary body, and choroid. Any or all of these structures may become inflamed, causing red eye. Uveitis is an inflammation of any of these layers, including the posterior uveal structures. Iritis is an inflammation of the anterior uveal structure, the iris. These inflammatory conditions are often associated with systemic disorders, many with an autoimmune component. Patients with uveitis should be referred to an ophthalmologist. Table 70-1 presents these and other ocular disorders that must be considered in the differential diagnosis of a patient with red eye.

Accurate diagnosis is critical in determining the appropriate therapy for red eye. For example, treatment of bacterial conjunctivitis with steroids may exacerbate the infection, and steroid use with a corneal abrasion or ulcer may lead to corneal melting and serious visual consequences. Similarly, treatment of herpetic keratitis with an antibacterial may delay appropriate therapy and lead to potentially serious consequences. Many ocular disorders can be difficult to diagnose accurately without a slit lamp. The health care provider should not hesitate to refer patients to an ophthalmologist when treatment does not produce the expected result or when the diagnosis remains obscure.

Vision Loss and Other Visual Disturbances

Visual disturbances can include decreased central or peripheral vision, metamorphopsia (distorted images), photopsia (light flashes), or vitreous opacities (floaters). Visual loss may

TABLE 70-1 Red Eye: Differential Diagnosis and Management Guidelines

Disorder	Signs and Symptoms	Pain	Management
DISORDERS ASSOCIATED WITH OCULAR ADNEXA REDNESS			
Blepharitis	Ocular burning; eyelid margins red with scaling or crusting	Yes	Warm compresses; daily lid scrubs; erythromycin or bacitracin ophthalmic ointment for anterior blepharitis; see Chapter 72
Cellulitis			
Orbital	Vision frequently affected; localized tenderness, erythema, edema; fever; proptosis	Yes	Referral to ophthalmologist for hospitalization, intravenous antibiotics; see Chapter 77
Preseptal	Vision usually not affected; localized tenderness, erythema, edema; fever sometimes present	Yes	Systemic, broad-spectrum antibiotics; office follow-up visit in 12-24 hr; see Chapter 77
Dacryocystitis	Chronic tearing; eyelash crusting; localized tenderness; circumscribed erythema, edema in the inferior medial canthal area; may be able to express purulent material from the nasolacrimal duct	Yes	Warm compresses; gentle massage; topical and/or systemic antibiotics; see Chapter 76
Eyelid lesions			
Chalazion	Nontender in chronic lesions; localized erythema, edema of eyelids	No	Warm compresses; daily lid scrubs; lid massage; see Chapter 72
Hordeolum	Localized tenderness, erythema, edema of eyelids; internal lesions pointing to external or internal eyelid surface; external lesions pointing to eyelid margin	Yes	Warm compresses; lid scrubs for recurrent lesions; see Chapter 72
Soft tissue hemorrhage	Localized tenderness sometimes present; erythema, ecchymosis, edema of affected area	±	Cold compresses; if orbital floor fracture suspected, computed tomography scan
DISORDERS ASSOCIATED WITH OCULAR SURFACE REDNESS			
Angle-closure glaucoma	Severe pain; nausea, vomiting; halos around lights; photophobia; cornea cloudy with variable decrease in vision; conjunctival hyperemia; pupil mid-dilated and fixed; firm globe; shallow anterior chamber	Yes	Emergent referral to ophthalmologist; with physician consultation, consider acetazolamide, 500 mg IV or PO, topical beta blocker
Chemical exposure	Pain; conjunctival hyperemia, chemosis; corneal haze; decreased visual acuity	Yes	Immediate copious irrigation essential; emergent referral to ophthalmologist; see Chapter 79
Conjunctivitis			
Allergic	Pruritus; conjunctival hyperemia, chemosis; watery or stringy discharge	No	Avoidance of allergens; cold compresses; topical and/or systemic medication; see Chapter 73
Bacterial	Photophobia with blepharospasm; mucopurulent discharge with eyelash mattering; edema, hyperemia; preauricular adenopathy only with hyperacute disorder	±	Topical antibiotic drops; systemic antibiotics necessary for gonococcal or chlamydial cause; see Chapter 73
Viral	Acute onset often associated with systemic illness; photophobia or foreign body sensation; preauricular adenopathy; hyperemia; chemosis; watery discharge; classic dendritic corneal lesion present with herpes simplex; periocular lesions present with herpes zoster ophthalmicus	±	Supportive treatment, including cool compresses, topical artificial tears; referral to ophthalmologist for herpetic conjunctivitis; see Chapter 73
Corneal foreign body, abrasion, or ulcer	Foreign body sensation with intense pain; photophobia; conjunctival hyperemia; may have decreased visual acuity; ulcers usually seen as white or opaque corneal lesion; immediate prior history of trauma common with abrasion but not erosion	Yes	Topical antibiotics (for prophylaxis) and systemic pain relievers in abrasions and after foreign body removal; no patching generally, never with ulcers or contact lens–related problems; urgent referral to ophthalmologist for erosions, emergent referral for ulcers; see Chapter 74
Dry eye	Sandy, gritty, foreign body sensation; burning; pruritus; conjunctival hyperemia; decreased visual acuity	±	Topical artificial tears; lubricating ointments at night; warm compresses; gentle eyelid massage; evaluation for systemic disorders; see Chapter 75

TABLE 70-1 Red Eye: Differential Diagnosis and Management Guidelines—cont'd

Disorder	Signs and Symptoms	Pain	Management
Episcleritis or scleritis	Mild to severe pain; circumscribed erythema of affected sclera; vision unaffected	Yes	Episcleritis usually self-limited; with possible scleritis, referral to ophthalmologist
Hyphema	Microscopic or visible blood layering in anterior chamber usually after blunt trauma; often associated with other ocular symptoms	Yes	Urgent referral to ophthalmologist
Iritis or uveitis	Pain; photophobia; conjunctival hyperemia; pupil constriction; may have epiphora but no mucopurulent discharge	Yes	Urgent referral to ophthalmologist
Keratitis	Pain, photophobia; conjunctival hyperemia; corneal cloudiness with stromal involvement	Yes	Urgent referral to ophthalmologist
Pinguecula and pterygium	Ocular irritation or pain when inflamed; dry eye symptoms; fleshy lesion medial on conjunctiva; with pterygium, lesion extending onto cornea	Yes	Ocular lubricants; topical NSAIDs; with pterygium, routine referral to ophthalmologist; see Chapter 78
Subconjunctival hemorrhage	No subjective symptoms; bright red spot of blood visible under overlying conjunctiva; remainder of conjunctiva white	No	Reassurance; no treatment necessary

NSAIDs, nonsteroidal anti-inflammatory drugs.

be unilateral or bilateral, may be transient or permanent, may occur suddenly or gradually, and may involve central or peripheral vision. Complaints of decreased peripheral vision are not common in the primary care setting because patients usually perceive only significant scotomas. "Sudden" vision loss must be distinguished from "suddenly noticed." A gradual vision loss in one eye may be suddenly noticed when the better eye is inadvertently occluded by a hand or some other object. The differential diagnosis box lists common causes of sudden and gradual vision loss. Table 70-2 presents the signs, symptoms, and management of sudden vision loss.

Amaurosis fugax is a transient, unilateral episode of vision loss. This condition is typically caused by small embolic plaques that transiently occlude retinal circulation. Patients typically notice a total loss of vision that lasts seconds to minutes. An embolic workup and cardiovascular evaluation are typically warranted.

Transient visual loss, photopsia, floaters, photophobia, metamorphopsia, or scintillating scotomas may accompany migraine headaches. Ocular symptoms common in migraines can occur without an associated headache. Unless the patient has a clear past history of ocular migraine, these patients should be referred to an ophthalmologist to rule out other potential problems, such as retinal or vitreous detachment.

Metamorphopsia (warped or distorted central vision) is commonly seen with macular degeneration as well as a host of other ocular conditions. Any patient reporting new-onset visual distortion or a change in previously noted metamorphopsia should be referred to an ophthalmologist. Effective treatments are available for certain types of age-related macular degeneration.

Photopsia (flashes or flickers of light) may result from a retinal problem or cortical stimulation. Photopsia may be an indication of a retinal tear or a posterior vitreous detachment with retinal traction. Cortically induced photopsia may indicate migraine headache or occipital epilepsy. Retinal detachment may also produce a persistent symptom described as a curtain, shadow, or veil falling over part of the visual field.

The vitreous degenerates and liquefies with aging. When this occurs, aggregates form vitreous floaters, which are perceived by the patient as gray or black shapes floating within the visual

DIFFERENTIAL DIAGNOSIS

Vision Loss

SUDDEN
- Acute angle-closure glaucoma
- Central retinal vessel occlusion
- Hyphema or other trauma
- Endophthalmitis
- Iritis or uveitis
- Migraine
- Optic neuritis
- Retinal hemorrhage (macular area)
- Stroke
- Vitreous hemorrhage
- Corneal ulcer
- Giant cell arteritis (temporal arteritis)

GRADUAL
- Amblyopia
- Cataracts
- Corneal opacities
- Primary open-angle glaucoma
- Iritis or uveitis*
- Macular degeneration*
- Pituitary tumor*
- Retinal detachment*
- Vitreous opacities

*May manifest with sudden-onset vision loss depending severity of disease or complications.

TABLE 70-2 Sudden Vision Loss: Management Guidelines

Disorder	Signs and Symptoms	Management
Acute angle-closure glaucoma	See Table 70-1	See Table 70-1
Central retinal vessel occlusion	Arterial occlusion: vision loss typically more profound; cherry red macula seen against paleness of surrounding retina Venous occlusion: metamorphopsia; flame hemorrhages and dilated tortuous veins in ocular fundus	Urgent referral to ophthalmologist; with arterial occlusion, permanent vision loss possible in <2 hr; physician consultation to determine underlying cause
Hyphema or other trauma	See Table 70-1	See Table 70-1
Endophthalmitis	May or may not be associated with pain; lid edema; conjunctival injection; retinal hemorrhage	Emergent referral to ophthalmologist; visual prognosis dependent on immediate treatment
Iritis or uveitis	See Table 70-1	See Table 70-1
Meningitis	Systemic presentation of meningitis; see Chapter 196	See Chapter 196
Migraine	Scintillating scotomas; photopsia; headache; photophobia; phonophobia; see Chapter 195	See Chapter 195
Optic neuritis	Variable vision loss; papilledema (present in 1/3 of patients); pain on eye movement; sore globe	Referral to ophthalmologist within 24-48 hr
Retinal hemorrhage (macular area)	Central vision loss with no associated pain	Ophthalmologist or physician consultation; management dependent on cause
Stroke	Visual field defects; amaurosis fugax; hemianopia; see Chapter 190	Immediate emergency department referral for all patients with suspected cerebrovascular accident
Vitreous hemorrhage	Ocular fundus possibly obscured in severe cases; if retina visible, examination may reveal signs of the underlying causative disorder (diabetic retinopathy, retinopathy of prematurity, retinal tear or detachment, vitreous detachment, trauma)	Ophthalmologist or physician consultation; management dependent on cause

field. Depending on the size and number, floaters may be simply annoying or may cause visual disability. If floaters occur suddenly or increase in frequency or quantity, urgent referral to an ophthalmologist is necessary. These symptoms may indicate the presence of a posterior vitreous detachment, primary vitreous hemorrhage, retinal tear, or retinal detachment.

Ocular and Periocular Pain

Ocular or periocular pain can include any discomfort in or around the eye and may be described as burning, aching, throbbing, boring, stabbing, or irritating, as with a foreign body sensation. Any condition that stimulates the numerous pain receptors in the eyelids, cornea, conjunctiva, and uveal tract will cause ocular or periocular pain. Any inflammatory disorder of the conjunctiva, superficial layers of the cornea, or uveal tract can cause ocular irritation, burning, discomfort, or frank pain. Symptoms may be related to exposure to environmental irritants such as tobacco smoke or chemical fumes. Pain may also be referred from adjacent structures innervated by the ophthalmic division of cranial nerve V (trigeminal nerve). Noninflammatory conditions affecting the optic nerve, retina, or vitreous do not usually result in pain.

Pain may occur coincidentally with other ocular symptoms, including decreased visual acuity, photophobia, ocular discharge, eyelid edema or erythema, ptosis, proptosis, or corneal cloudiness. Important history includes decrease in visual acuity, suddenness of onset, associated symptoms (including systemic symptoms such as nausea or vomiting), contact lens use, exposure to ultraviolet light (such as during outdoor activities or arc welding), neurologic or systemic disorders, and trauma.

A complete ocular assessment should be performed in any patient with ocular pain. It is also important to examine the structures of the head and neck in any patient with a history of trauma. However, the eye should never be manipulated if there is any possibility of laceration or rupture of the ocular tissues. A shallow anterior chamber or abnormally shaped pupil may indicate a loss of aqueous humor secondary to a penetrating injury. Acute glaucoma should be excluded by measuring the intraocular pressure with a Tono-Pen or similar device or by palpating the globes and comparing the affected eye with the unaffected eye. Patients with a painful eye from acute glaucoma usually have associated redness, nausea, and vomiting. The cornea and conjunctiva may be assessed to identify abrasions or ulcers by applying fluorescein dye and examining the external eye under fluorescent light. Application of a topical anesthetic such as proparacaine hydrochloride 0.5% (Ophthaine) or tetracaine hydrochloride 0.5% (Pontocaine) will help differentiate the superficial pain caused by corneal surface disorders from pain resulting from problems with the deeper structures.[8]

TABLE 70-3 Symptoms Associated with Ocular Pain and Possible Causes

Associated Symptom	Possible Causes
Photophobia	Acute glaucoma, migraine, corneal trauma, keratoconjunctivitis, iritis, uveitis, scleritis
Nausea and vomiting	Acute glaucoma, endophthalmitis
Itching	Chemical injury, severe dry eye, allergy
Pain on eye movement	Orbital pseudotumor, myositis, posterior scleritis, optic neuritis, trauma, orbital cellulitis
Foreign body sensation	Corneal ulcer or abrasion, conjunctivitis, overexposure to ultraviolet light, entropion, trichiasis, conjunctival or eyelid lesion (rule out actual corneal or conjunctival foreign body)

It may be useful to approach the differential diagnosis of ocular pain by grouping possible causes according to accompanying symptoms. This approach is summarized in Table 70-3.

Other Ocular Signs and Symptoms

Epiphora is excessive tearing. Causes include obstruction of the normal tear drainage system and excessive production of tears as a result of irritation or inflammation. Although persistent tearing of one or both eyes in an infant is a cardinal sign of congenital glaucoma, this is a rare condition. Tearing in infants is most often caused by congenital nasolacrimal duct obstruction. The patient should be referred to an ophthalmologist when no underlying cause is apparent or if the epiphora worsens.

Ocular discharge may be clear, watery, purulent or mucopurulent, stringy, or ropy. The differential diagnosis of an ocular disorder may be aided by observing the nature of abnormal ocular secretions. Pus in the conjunctival sac causes the eyelashes to stick together and is most common in mucopurulent conjunctivitis. A profuse watery discharge with a burning or gritty sensation and pain may be present in viral conjunctivitis. Pruritus associated with a discharge varying from watery to a stringy, mucus-like consistency may indicate allergic conjunctivitis.

Photophobia may occur for no known reason. However, almost any condition resulting in ocular irritation or inflammation may cause photophobia. Conditions to consider include uveitis, conjunctivitis, conjunctival or corneal foreign bodies, corneal abrasion, keratitis, congenital glaucoma in infants, and acute glaucoma in adults. Photophobia may also result from toxic exposures, as seen in arc welders, swimmers, or skiers who do not use lenses for protection from excessive direct or reflected ultraviolet light exposure.

Pruritus is the most common complaint in allergic conditions, including allergic conjunctivitis. The symptom is usually bilateral and may be seasonal with associated hay fever symptoms. Unilateral pruritus associated with erythema and chemosis may be iatrogenic or caused by an allergic reaction to topical ophthalmic preparations or, commonly, the preservative in the preparation. Patients with severe dry eye or a chemical injury may also experience pruritus.

CHAPTER 71

CATARACTS

Jack Stringham • James T. Banta

DEFINITION AND EPIDEMIOLOGY

Ancient physicians thought that a crystalloid structure (lens) rested in the center of the eye and was responsible for vision. People lost vision when an abnormal humor developed and flowed in front of the lens. They called this a *cataract* (Latin for waterfall).[1] Today, the term *cataract* refers to the opacification of the crystalline lens of the eye. The most recent World Health Organization estimate lists cataract as the leading cause of blindness worldwide, accounting for 48% of world blindness or affecting 18 million people. Cataract causes some degree of visual impairment in nearly 20.5 million Americans or one in six Americans aged 40 years and older.[2]

The most common form of cataract is associated with increasing age and progressive oxidative damage to the crystalline lens. Every person who lives long enough will develop some degree of cataract. As life expectancy increases and the population ages, visual loss from cataract will have an even greater medical and economic impact. In the United States, prevalence estimates of visually significant cataract increase with age for both men and women, from 4% and 10% for men and women aged 55 to 64 years to 39% and 46% for those older than 75 years.[2]

PATHOPHYSIOLOGY

The anatomic function of the crystalline lens is to focus incident light on the retina. Opacification of this lens, a cataract, prevents light from focusing on the retina, causing loss of vision. The natural aging process of the crystalline lens involves an increase in mass, thickness, and the development of a yellow hue with an associated loss of accommodative capacity. Initially these changes cause minimal visual impairment, but with time the lens becomes more opaque, leading to a significant decrease in vision and forming an age-related cataract. Cataracts develop in everyone who lives long enough, but their formation is hastened by trauma, exposure to certain medications (e.g. corticosteroids), metabolic disorders such as diabetes, and oxidative stress from smoking or ultraviolet light. Congenital cataracts can also form; these can be idiopathic in nature or can be caused by an underlying infection or metabolic disease.[2]

CLINICAL PRESENTATION

The classic presentation of age-related cataract is with nonpainful, progressive loss of visual acuity. Patients often describe blurred or hazy vision and haloes or significant glare with bright lights; a common complaint is difficulty driving at night. Another common presentation is frequent changes in a patient's eyeglass prescription. The majority of refractive changes (typically an increase in myopia) in older adults are the result of cataract progression.

Nuclear sclerotic cataracts tend to affect distance vision more than reading vision, whereas cortical cataracts result in more symptoms of glare in dim illumination. Posterior subcapsular cataracts tend to progress more rapidly and occur in younger patients than do nuclear sclerotic and cortical cataracts.

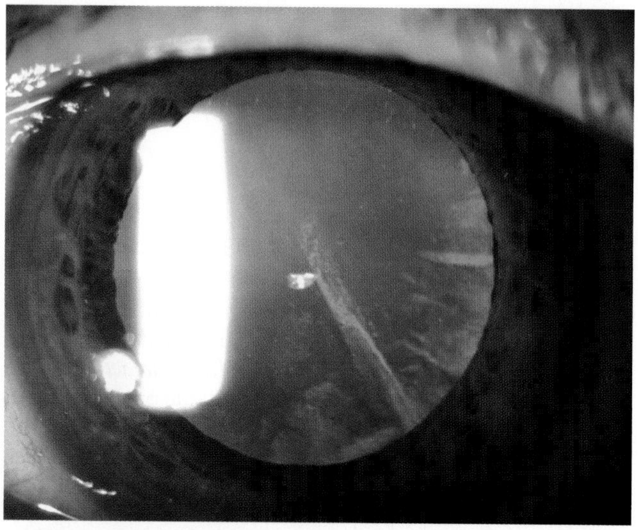

FIGURE 71-1 Retroillumination photo demonstrating cortical "spokes," a finding frequently seen in people with diabetes.

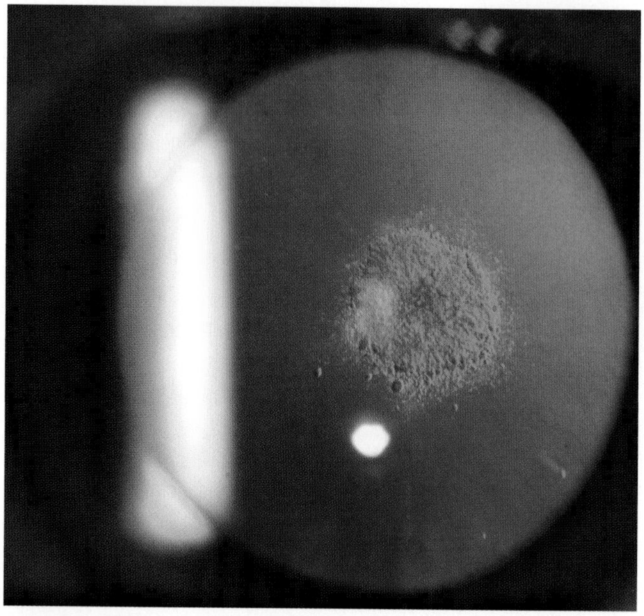

FIGURE 71-2 Retroillumination photo demonstrating a small paracentral posterior subcapsular cataract.

Posterior subcapsular cataracts can cause glare symptoms and difficulty reading in bright illumination.[2] Cataracts may progress during the course of months to years. Patients may occasionally report a sudden decrease in vision. In these patients the cataract has progressed slowly but just recently reached the point at which it noticeably inhibited the patient's ability to perform some activity. Nontraumatic cataracts are usually bilateral but may be asymmetric.[2]

PHYSICAL EXAMINATION

Cataracts are often an isolated finding, but a full ophthalmic examination is indicated to determine if other causes of visual loss may be present. A cataract will not cause injection of the conjunctiva, corneal opacification, or pain—except in rare instances of traumatic or hypermature cataracts. The pupils should constrict normally to light. Direct ophthalmoscopy may reveal hazy visualization of the optic nerve and retina as a result of the lens opacity. Cataractous lens changes are best appreciated with use of a direct ophthalmoscope with a dilated pupil, focusing on the red reflex. Nuclear sclerotic changes may cause the reflex to appear dull or asymmetric. Cortical lens changes may cause focal, segmental, or spokelike dark areas in the reflex (Fig. 71-1); posterior subcapsular changes typically appear as a central, dark plaque (Fig. 71-2).

DIAGNOSTICS

No diagnostic tests are recommended.

DIFFERENTIAL DIAGNOSIS

Many conditions can cause progressive loss of vision, such as age-related macular degeneration and diabetic retinopathy. A full ophthalmologic examination may be necessary to distinguish these entities in some patients.

MANAGEMENT

Early lens changes can usually be handled conservatively. A change in eyeglass prescription may improve the patient's visual acuity. Cessation of certain tasks made difficult by the cataract, such as driving at night, may be necessary. Magnifiers, increased font size, and other visual aids may temporarily ameliorate the visual acuity loss. No medical treatments are available to reverse lens opacification. Surgical cataract extraction is highly successful and safe, and it should be considered when a cataract has reduced visual function to the point at which activities of daily living are adversely affected.[2]

DIFFERENTIAL DIAGNOSIS

Cataracts

VASCULAR
- Vitreous hemorrhage
- Hypertensive retinopathy

NEOPLASTIC
- Retinoblastoma (pediatric)

TRAUMATIC
- Traumatic cataract
- Corneal scar
- Retinal detachment

METABOLIC
- Diabetic macular edema

AGE RELATED
- Macular degeneration
- Cataract

INFECTIOUS
- Toxocariasis

COMPLICATIONS

Complications of a cataract are very rare, but a hypermature cataract can cause intraocular inflammation and glaucoma, both of which are cured with surgical removal of the cataract.[2] To prevent surgical complications, it is vital for the patient to provide the ophthalmologist with a current medication list; of particular importance is the use of any systemic alpha$_1$-adrenergic antagonists, such as tamsulosin (Flomax). The current or prior use of such medications can cause intraoperative floppy iris syndrome (IFIS), which can complicate cataract surgery and result in longer postoperative recovery and poorer outcomes.[3] IFIS is most frequently associated with the selective alpha$_{1A}$ antagonist tamsulosin, but it has also been reported with other nonselective alpha$_1$ antagonists, such a terazosin

(Hytrin) and doxazosin (Cardura). IFIS has been reported to occur several years after the discontinuation of tamsulosin. Studies have shown that when the surgeon is forewarned about the use of tamsulosin, the risks associated with IFIS are greatly reduced.[3]

INDICATIONS FOR REFERRAL OR HOSPITALIZATION

Referral for surgical treatment of cataracts is indicated when the cataract has caused visual decline to the point at which the patient's vision no longer meets his or her needs. This level will vary from patient to patient according to the patient's daily activities and warrants a discussion with the ophthalmologist on the risks and benefits of surgery.

LIFE SPAN CONSIDERATIONS

In older individuals, cataracts have been associated with decreased quality of life by causing functional loss and decreased independence. Impaired vision has been shown to cause cognitive impairment that is improved by cataract surgery.[4] Impaired vision is also a safety risk. Drivers with cataracts are more likely to be involved in an at-fault automobile accident compared with those without cataracts.[5] Surgical treatment of cataract was also found to reduce the risk of falls and hip fracture.[6] Improved cataract surgical techniques, such as topical anesthesia and sutureless, clear corneal incisions, allow patients with significant medical comorbidities to be considered for cataract extraction.[7]

EDUCATION AND HEALTH PROMOTION

Patients should be educated that all crystalline lenses will eventually opacify; the rate varies from person to person. Medical management, visual aids, and alterations of activities may ameliorate the effect of early cataract formation. Patients should be counseled, however, that cataract progression will continue and surgery may eventually be required. It is up to the patient to determine when the cataract has become visually significant to the point that it affects activities of daily living.

Cigarette smoking, ultraviolet light, and glycemic control in diabetics are modifiable risk factors of cataract formation.[2] Patients at risk for contusive or penetrating ocular trauma and chemical exposure should be encouraged to use appropriate eye protection.

CHAPTER 72

BLEPHARITIS, HORDEOLUM, AND CHALAZION

Rebecca Shields • James T. Banta

DEFINITION AND EPIDEMIOLOGY

Inflammation of the eyelids, also known as *blepharitis,* is one of the most frequently encountered ocular diseases. Blepharitis may be of infectious or inflammatory etiology. The disease can be divided into two basic categories anatomically: anterior and posterior blepharitis.[1,2] Anterior blepharitis involves the anterior lid margin surrounding the eyelashes and is usually associated with staphylococcal infection or seborrhea. Staphylococcal blepharitis is a disorder that predominantly affects young to middle-aged women, with exacerbations and remissions of disease. Seborrheic blepharitis is seen in a somewhat older age group, with an equal incidence in men and women.[3] Posterior blepharitis involves the posterior lid margin and is characterized by meibomian gland dysfunction, sometimes associated with rosacea. Meibomian glands are enlarged sebaceous glands aligned in a row posterior to the eyelashes. They produce a clear lipid secretion that makes up the outer layer of the tear film. All forms of blepharitis may result in a disruption of the ocular surface, exacerbate dry eye syndrome, and result in the development of hordeola or chalazia. A chalazion is a chronic, sterile, lipogranulomatous inflammatory lesion of the meibomian gland, whereas a hordeolum is an acute infection of one of the glands in the eyelid. The most commonly associated organism is *Staphylococcus aureus.*

PATHOPHYSIOLOGY

Anterior staphylococcal blepharitis is thought to be caused by an abnormal cell-mediated response to *S. aureus,* ultimately resulting in lid margin inflammation. Anterior seborrheic blepharitis is associated with generalized seborrhea that may involve the scalp, nasolabial folds, skin behind the ears, and sternum. Posterior blepharitis is caused by meibomian gland dysfunction and alterations in meibomian gland secretions. Bacterial lipases may result in formation of free fatty acids, increasing the melting point of the meibum and preventing its expression from the glands, possibly enabling growth of *S. aureus* and the development of a hordeolum.[4] Certain persons may be predisposed to this condition, and hormones may play a role in creating an environment that promotes lipase-producing bacteria that alter glandular secretion.[5]

Once the meibomian gland is obstructed from excessive meibomian oil secretions or solidification of the meibum, a chalazion or hordeolum may develop (commonly referred to as a *stye*).

CLINICAL PRESENTATION

Symptoms of blepharitis are often caused by ocular tear film instability and dry eye. Patients complain of burning, foreign body sensation, tearing, photophobia, itching, redness, discharge, and swollen erythematous eyelids, often worse in the morning.[6] Remissions and exacerbations are characteristic. A hordeolum or chalazion may occur at any age as a gradually enlarging localized nodule (Fig. 72-1). A hordeolum is usually painful, whereas a chalazion does not normally cause pain. Both may cause cosmetic disfigurement and mechanical ptosis. If large, the lesion may mechanically press on the corneal surface to induce astigmatism and blurred vision.[7]

PHYSICAL EXAMINATION

The patient's face, ocular adnexa, and eye should be carefully inspected. Patients with staphylococcal blepharitis may have lid margin erythema with fine ulceration at the base of the lashes and collarettes of fibrin along the lash. Lashes may be absent, broken, or misdirected. Patients with seborrheic blepharitis may have greasy scales along the lid margin and lashes with excess oily meibomian secretion and foamy tears. These patients may also have diffuse seborrhea with dandruff of the scalp and scaling of the brows, behind the ears, and at the base of the nose. Patients with posterior blepharitis may have hyperemia and

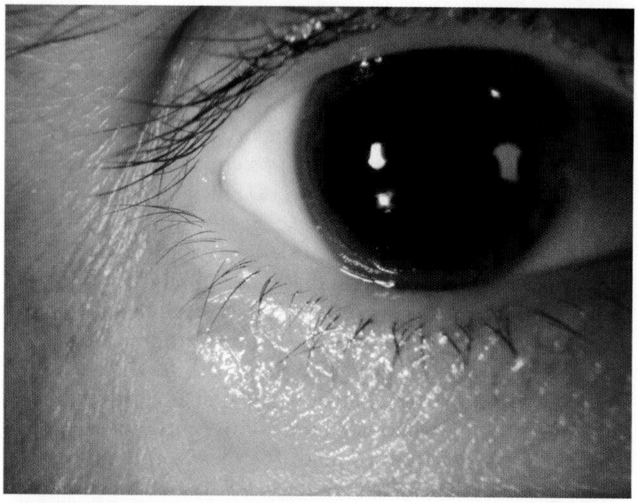

FIGURE 72-1 Unlike a hordeolum, a chalazion typically is a lid nodule with minimal erythema or pain, as illustrated in this photograph.

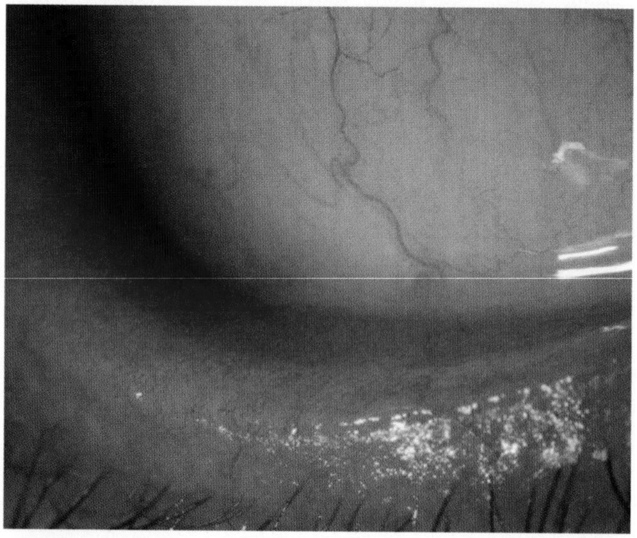

FIGURE 72-2 Lid margin telangiectasis and erythema, as demonstrated in this photograph, often accompany meibomian gland dysfunction in posterior forms of blepharitis.

telangiectasis of the lid margin (Fig. 72-2) and an oily and frothy tear film. Pressure on the lid margin results in expression of thick inspissated secretions. Rosacea is commonly associated with meibomian gland dysfunction, so these patients should be inspected for erythema with telangiectasis over the cheeks and nose, a pustular skin eruption, and sebaceous gland hypertrophy typified by rhinophyma.[3] All types of blepharitis may also cause conjunctival injection, corneal infiltrates, excess tearing, lid crusting, discharge, and inflammation of the lid margin (see Fig. 72-2).

When a patient with a hordeolum or chalazion is examined, the lid should be palpated for swelling and masses, and the eyelid should be everted. Hordeola and chalazia are often clinically indistinguishable. However, a hordeolum is often acute, tender, warm, and erythematous, whereas a chalazion is more chronic and nontender.

DIAGNOSTICS

No diagnostic tests are indicated.

DIFFERENTIAL DIAGNOSIS

DIFFERENTIAL DIAGNOSIS

Eyelid Disorders

- Hordeolum
- Blepharitis
- Benign or malignant tumors
- Chalazion
- Dry eye syndrome
- Conjunctivitis
- Herpes simplex infection
- Ocular rosacea
- Cellulitis
- Trauma
- Dermatitis
- Abscess
- Dacryocystitis

Chronic lid swelling and ulceration may rarely be caused by sebaceous carcinoma, which is a potentially life-threatening disease.[8] Any patient with chronic lid swelling, erythema, notching of the lid margin, or an atypical lid lesion associated with loss of lashes should be sent to the ophthalmologist for biopsy to rule out sebaceous carcinoma, basal cell carcinoma, squamous cell carcinoma, and other malignant or benign tumors. The differential diagnosis of blepharitis also includes dry eye syndrome, conjunctivitis (viral, bacterial, or allergic), contact dermatitis, atopic keratoconjunctivitis, herpes simplex infection, preseptal cellulitis, acute dacryocystitis, and ocular rosacea.

MANAGEMENT

Lid hygiene is the mainstay of all blepharitis treatment. Warm compresses, over both eyelid margins for 5 to 10 minutes, loosen lid margin debris and remove secretions. After use of the compresses, patients may use commercially available lid scrub kits or warm water with diluted baby shampoo on a cotton tip applicator at the lid margin to decrease bacterial colonization. After scrubs, a thin strip of antibiotic ointment, such as erythromycin or bacitracin, may be applied to the eyelid margins. Artificial tears may also be beneficial. Patients with a prominent conjunctivitis component can be treated with an antibiotic solution four times a day. An antimicrobial agent effective against the majority of staphylococci, such as tobramycin 0.3% (Tobrex ophthalmic solution), is a good choice for initial therapy. In severe cases, patients may benefit from tetracycline, 250 mg by mouth four times daily, or doxycycline, 50 mg by mouth twice daily.[9,10] Treatments for both anterior and posterior blepharitis often need to be maintained for months to years and occasionally indefinitely, given the chronic nature of the condition.

Hordeola are usually self-limited, spontaneously improving in 1 to 2 weeks with conservative treatment alone. Lesions may be treated with frequent application of warm, moist compresses with light massage over the lesion. Daily lid hygiene with lid scrubs is also beneficial. Topical antibiotics are generally not effective or indicated unless an accompanying infectious blepharoconjunctivitis is present. Systemic antibiotics are generally indicated only in rare cases of secondary eyelid cellulitis. Any patient for whom conservative treatment fails or who develops a secondary infection, such as conjunctivitis or cellulitis, should be referred to an ophthalmologist. Large persistent lesions may require incision and drainage by an ophthalmologist. Cultures are not indicated for isolated, uncomplicated cases of hordeolum.

TABLE 72-1 Management of Lid Disorders

Disorder	Compresses	Antibiotic	Steroid	Other
HORDEOLUM				
Internal: Zeis or Moll gland infection *External*: meibomian gland infection	Frequent warm, moist compresses to hasten drainage	Not indicated	None	Lid scrubs, especially if lesions recur
CHALAZION				
Meibomian gland inflammation	Frequent warm compresses to liquefy glandular secretions	Not indicated	Intralesional corticosteroid injection is often effective	Lid scrubs with gentle massage to help express impacted secretions
BLEPHARITIS				
Anterior staphylococcal	Daily warm compresses to loosen crusts	Topical ophthalmic erythromycin or bacitracin ointment	None	Daily lid scrubs to reduce sebaceous secretions
Anterior seborrheic	Daily warm compresses to loosen crusts	None	Occasional topical steroid if inflammation prominent	Daily lid scrubs to help remove oily secretions
Posterior	Daily warm, moist compresses	Oral doxycycline in severe cases	None	Daily lid scrubs and lid massage

Chalazia may be self-limited in 25% to 50% of cases and can be cured or improved with conservative treatment within 1 to 3 months.[11] Chronic chalazia may require steroid injection.[12] If this is not effective, lesions can be surgically incised and removed by an ophthalmologist. Table 72-1 summarizes the specific management of hordeola, chalazia, and the different forms of blepharitis.

LIFE SPAN CONSIDERATIONS

Hordeola can affect individuals of all ages but are more common in children and adolescents. Chalazia can affect individuals of all ages but are more common in adults. Anterior staphylococcal blepharitis is more common in younger patients, and posterior blepharitis is more common in older patients.[13]

COMPLICATIONS

In rare cases a hordeolum may progress to preseptal cellulitis or abscess and require systemic antibiotics. Large lesions can induce corneal astigmatism and mechanical ptosis and may restrict the superior visual field. Chronic blepharitis may result in scarring and the loss of protective eyelashes.

INDICATIONS FOR REFERRAL OR HOSPITALIZATION

Any patient for whom conservative treatment fails or who develops a secondary infection, such as conjunctivitis, eyelid cellulitis, or preseptal cellulitis, should be managed by an ophthalmologist. Patients with recurrent, atypical lesions or unexplained vision loss should also be referred to an ophthalmologist. Large persistent eyelid lesions may require incision and drainage by an ophthalmologist.

PATIENT AND FAMILY EDUCATION

Patient education should emphasize daily eyelid hygiene and lid scrubs. Patients should be instructed to apply lid scrubs at the base of the lashes with a moistened cotton-tipped applicator or a small, soft face cloth moistened with a dilute concentration of baby shampoo. After the scrub, the patient should thoroughly rinse the area and pat it dry. Alternatively, patients may prefer to perform lid scrubs with dilute baby shampoo while in the shower using a cotton-tipped applicator or the tip of the finger. Patients who wear mascara and eye makeup should replace their products on a regular basis to reduce the likelihood of reinoculating their lids with contaminated cosmetics.[14]

HEALTH PROMOTION

Daily eyelid hygiene helps reduce bacterial colonization and accumulation of sebaceous secretions, thereby modulating the symptoms of chronic blepharitis and preventing the formation of chalazia and hordeola.

CHAPTER 73

CONJUNCTIVITIS

Sarah P. Read • James T. Banta

DEFINITION

Conjunctivitis is inflammation of the bulbar or palpebral conjunctiva, the transparent mucosal tissue that lines the eye and inner surface of the eyelids.[1] Approximately 70% of patients with acute conjunctivitis visit a primary care provider for diagnosis and management.[1,2] Commonly referred to as *pink eye*, conjunctivitis actually consists of many different disorders. Infectious causes include viruses and bacteria. Noninfectious conjunctivitis can commonly be caused by allergy, atopy, or exposure to toxins.[2]

EPIDEMIOLOGY

Up to 70% of all infectious conjunctivitis is viral.[1] The most common causative organism is adenovirus, the same virus implicated in the common cold.[3] Bacterial conjunctivitis is the second most common cause of infectious conjunctivitis and the most common cause in the pediatric population.[4] Other infectious causes include virus infections such as herpes and molluscum contagiosum.

The most common cause of noninfectious conjunctivitis is allergic conjunctivitis, a condition seen most frequently in the spring and summer.[5] Approximately 15% of all eye-related complaints to a primary care provider are secondary to allergic conjunctivitis.[6] Other noninfectious causes include primary ocular diseases such as toxic or cicatricial conjunctivitis and systemic diseases such as graft-versus-host disease, systemic inflammatory disorders, or neoplastic processes.[7]

PATHOPHYSIOLOGY

Viral conjunctivitis is spread by direct contact or by proximity to an infected patient.[8] Because of its highly contagious nature, viral conjunctivitis is often seen in areas of overcrowding, such as schools, nursing homes, and summer camps.[1,9] Similarly, bacterial overgrowth in the conjunctiva occurs directly from hand-eye contact with an infected individual or from the transfer of organisms in one's own nasal and sinus mucosa.[1]

Commonly known as *hay fever*, seasonal allergic conjunctivitis is typically secondary to environmental allergens, with ragweed being the most common (75%).[6,10] Perennial allergic conjunctivitis is caused by common household allergens such as household chemicals or pet dander. In both conditions, an inflammatory response occurs once the airborne allergen comes into contact with the ocular surface.[9] Acute allergic conjunctivitis is characterized by an immunoglobulin E mast cell–mediated hypersensitivity.[6]

Vernal conjunctivitis and atopic conjunctivitis are chronic, mast cell–and lymphocyte-mediated immune processes. Both are considered to be more severe and chronic forms of allergic conjunctivitis.[10] Environmental allergens can trigger exacerbations.[7,10]

Conjunctivitis from a medication typically occurs with long-term use (>1 month) of an eye drop.[9] Any eye drop can be causative, but conjunctivitis is most commonly encountered with eye drops containing the preservative benzalkonium chloride (listed as an inactive ingredient). It can also be seen as a response to excessive use of a vasoconstrictor (e.g., naphazoline, tetrahydrozoline). Vasoconstrictors are excellent at removal of redness acutely, but if they are used for longer than 3 to 5 days, rebound vasodilation is frequently encountered. This may take as long as 4 weeks to resolve fully.[9] The use of vasoconstrictors should be uniformly discouraged except for infrequent, intermittent use. Other common causes of medication toxicity include topical antibiotics, especially aminoglycosides, and glaucoma medications.[9]

CLINICAL PRESENTATION AND PHYSICAL EXAMINATION

Viral Conjunctivitis

Evaluation of a patient with conjunctivitis should first start with a careful history. A recent upper respiratory infection or exposure to sick individuals can point to a diagnosis of adenoviral conjunctivitis.[1,11] Ocular symptoms include acute onset of a red eye with excessive watery discharge.[2] Classically, it begins in one eye and then involves the fellow eye within days due to the phenomenon of autoinnoculation.[11] Approximately half of patients will have bilateral involvement at the time of presentation.[11]

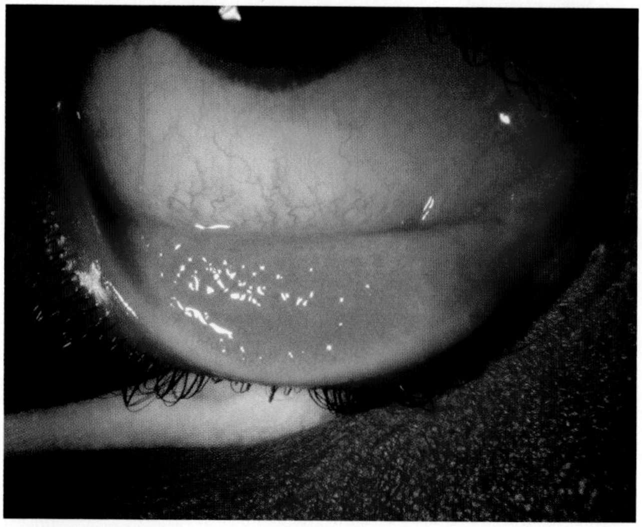

FIGURE 73-1 Follicles are typical of viral conjunctivitis and can frequently be appreciated without magnification.

Adenoviral conjunctivitis can occur in three different forms.[2,9] On examination, the lower eyelid should be pulled down and the palpebral conjunctiva evaluated. Follicles are clear bumps, ranging in size from pinpoint to 2 mm, with overlying conjunctival vessels (Fig. 73-1).[7,9] The second form is pharyngoconjunctival fever. The ocular examination is similar. However, the patient will have systemic disease: fever, headache, and sore throat.[2] Epidemic keratoconjunctivitis is clinically striking with significant, bilateral conjunctival hyperemia and chemosis. Petechial and larger subconjunctival hemorrhages may be present in this form.[1,9] Up to one third of patients with epidemic keratoconjunctivitis have corneal involvement, and it is appropriate to refer these patients to an ophthalmologist.[12]

When a patient with suspected adenoviral conjunctivitis is examined, it is important to palpate the anterior cervical chain of lymph nodes. At least 50% of patients have a tender preauricular lymph node.[2] The preauricular node is located just inferior and medial to the tragus. Of note, certain types of bacterial conjunctivitis can also manifest with lymphadenopathy (specifically, *Neisseria*- and methicillin-resistant *Staphylococcus aureus* [MRSA]–associated bacterial conjunctivitis).[1]

Herpes simplex virus (HSV) infection accounts for 1.3% to 4.8% of acute conjunctivitis.[2] It can be spread by direct contact but is more commonly spread by asymptomatic shedding of viral particles. Children with primary HSV infection will often have an antecedent respiratory infection. The disease is almost always unilateral and can cause concurrent vesicular skin lesions.[2] Recurrent HSV infection can manifest similarly but often involves other ocular structures. Therefore in patients with a history of prior cold sores and with presumed herpetic eye disease, referral to an ophthalmologist is recommended.[1,9]

Molluscum contagiosum is spread by direct contact. Because it typically occurs in children, human immunodeficiency virus (HIV) infection should be considered if it is seen in adults.[1,9] Patients have a chronic follicular reaction. On examination of

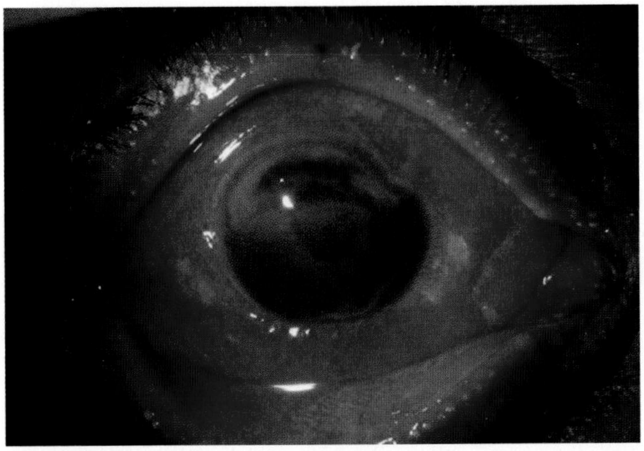

FIGURE 73-2 Gonococcal conjunctivitis can progress to severe corneal thinning and even corneal perforation if it is left untreated. Severe corneal thinning can be seen superiorly and inferonasally in this photograph.

the eyelid margin, an umbilicated nodule is characteristic. Referral to an ophthalmologist should be made for evaluation and potential excision.[9]

Bacterial Conjunctivitis

Bacterial conjunctivitis is typically accompanied by thick, purulent discharge.[11] On history, patients will often report that both eyes are sticky or glued shut. These symptoms persist throughout the day but are worse in the morning.[13] Bacterial conjunctivitis can result from the overproliferation of native ocular flora or from direct spread from an infected individual.[2]

Acute conjunctivitis is the most common form of bacterial conjunctivitis. Symptoms manifest over days. In children, the causative agents include *Haemophilus influenzae* and *Streptococcus pneumoniae*. *S. aureus* is more commonly seen in adults.[8,13] Symptoms typically last for 7 to 10 days.[2]

Hyperacute onset (12 to 24 hours) with severe purulent discharge is highly consistent with *Neisseria gonorrhoeae*.[9,13] Gonococcal conjunctivitis is typically seen in sexually active adults but can also occur in neonates via maternal-neonate transmission.[9,13] If it is seen in a child, child abuse should be suspected. Rapid progression is the hallmark of this disease. The cornea can become involved in less than 2 days and lead to permanent vision loss (Fig. 73-2).[9]

Chronic bacterial conjunctivitis is used to describe symptoms lasting longer than 4 weeks.[2] Chlamydial conjunctivitis should be suspected in sexually active adults with a nonresponsive conjunctivitis.[8] Patients typically have a concurrent genital infection.[2] Mild symptoms may be present for weeks to months, with exacerbations and remissions.[9]

Acute Allergic Conjunctivitis

Allergic conjunctivitis affects up to 40% of the U.S. population.[5] Seventy-five percent of patients with allergic rhinitis will have associated conjunctivitis. Patients often will have an associated headache and fatigue. Often patients will also have a positive family history of hay fever or atopy.[6] Unlike conjunctivitis from infectious causes, allergic conjunctivitis typically occurs simultaneously in both eyes. Its predominant feature is itching.[5,6] If discharge is present, it will be clear or stringy and white. The conjunctiva has a boggy appearance. Examination of the periocular skin shows lid discoloration, thickening, and erythema.[6] In addition, periorbital venous congestion can manifest as dark circles under the eyes (i.e., allergic shiners).[9]

Vernal and Atopic Conjunctivitis

Vernal conjunctivitis occurs in childhood, typically in the spring. It primarily affects males and resolves by the third decade.[1,9] Atopic conjunctivitis occurs in adults (>50 years) with a history of asthma, allergic rhinitis, and atopic dermatitis.[9] Twenty-five percent of elderly patients with eczema will develop atopic conjunctivitis.[1] Compared with acute allergic conjunctivitis, atopic conjunctivitis and vernal conjunctivitis have more severe symptoms of severe itching, burning, and tearing. Other symptoms include blepharospasm and photophobia. Discharge is often white, thick, and ropy.[7,9] Ninety-eight percent of cases are bilateral.[14]

Giant papillary conjunctivitis is a hallmark of vernal conjunctivitis. Eversion of the upper lid will reveal a cobblestone pattern of large (>1 mm), geometric bumps.[9,14] These giant papillae can cause a droopy eyelid. In addition, corneal involvement is more common than in acute allergic conjunctivitis. Patients with vernal disease will often have a shield ulcer (an oval corneal epithelial defect of the superior cornea) in addition to the conjunctivitis.[14] This can be identified by a decrease in vision or by fluorescein staining. If it is present, the patient needs close monitoring by an ophthalmologist.[11,12]

Medication Toxicity

A variety of topical medications can induce an allergic response in the conjunctiva.[2] In addition to conjunctivitis, a contact dermatitis of the lower lids with thickening and scaling of the skin is sometimes seen.[7] Discontinuation of the offending medication leads to resolution of symptoms.[7]

DIAGNOSTICS

For bacterial conjunctivitis, rapidity of onset, severity, and age at presentation often suggest the causative organism. Gram-stained smears and cultures are necessary in the immunocompromised (including neonates) as well as in severe or unresponsive cases.[9] For confirmation of a diagnosis of chlamydial conjunctivitis, polymerase chain reaction testing of the conjunctiva is frequently used.[9]

MANAGEMENT

Viral Conjunctivitis

Viral conjunctivitis is self-limited and typically lasts 5 to 14 days. Treatment is supportive with artificial tears and cool compresses. Patients should be advised that they are contagious as long as they are still tearing (i.e., shedding viral particles) or for at least 1 week.[11] Prior practice patterns recommended treatment of viral conjunctivitis with an antibiotic to prevent a bacterial superinfection. However, the occurrence of this is rare, and it is not recommended to prescribe topical antibiotics unnecessarily. In addition, topical corticosteroids should be avoided because they can prolong viral shedding and increase infectivity.[1,8]

The majority of patients with viral conjunctivitis do not have long-term sequelae. Two potentially sight-threatening consequences are corneal involvement, which can cause decreased vision, and conjunctival pseudomembranes, which can lead to scarring and chronic dry eye. Thus it is important to follow up in 1 to 4 weeks if symptoms have not fully resolved.[1,9,11]

Bacterial Conjunctivitis

Topical treatment with antibiotics is not always necessary. Evidence shows that outcomes with topical antibiotics are equivalent to placebo at 1 week.[15] To minimize cost and antibiotic resistance, some advocate a delayed treatment plan. Patients should be educated on the self-limited nature of their disease and start antibiotics only if there is no improvement in symptoms.[8] Others advocate use of topical antibiotics in all cases to reduce infectivity rates.[7]

High-risk patients with suspected bacterial conjunctivitis should always be prescribed topical antibiotics. These patients include immunocompromised patients, patients with uncontrolled diabetes, health care workers, and patients with any history of glaucoma surgery.[7,15,16] Reasonable initial choices for a topical antibiotic include trimethoprim–polymyxin B or fluoroquinolone drops, four times a day for 1 week. Corticosteroids are rarely indicated and should not be used without the supervision of an ophthalmologist.[11]

The following types of bacterial conjunctivitis require systemic treatment:

- *H. influenzae:* treat with oral amoxicillin-clavulanate (if not allergic) because of the potential for extraocular involvement (otitis media, pneumonia, and meningitis).[17]
- Gonococcal: ceftriaxone, 1 g intramuscularly, one dose (or ciprofloxacin, 500 mg orally if the patient has a penicillin allergy,) and one dose of azithromycin, 1g orally—requires same-day referral to an ophthalmologist.[17,18]
- Chlamydial: azithromycin, 1 g orally, one dose (or doxycycline, 100 mg twice daily for 7 days).[12,18]

One third of patients with gonococcal disease have concurrent chlamydial infection, and treatment for both diseases is recommended.[11] Remember to treat the sexual partners of patients with gonococcal or chlamydial conjunctivitis to prevent reinfection.[9]

Acute Allergic Conjunctivitis

A stepwise approach should be used. First, any allergens should be identified and eliminated. Typically, symptoms resolve quickly once the inciting allergen is removed.[6] Because allergic conjunctivitis is typically associated with systemic allergies, an oral antihistamine can be helpful in controlling ocular symptoms. Agents to consider include fexofenadine and loratadine.[17]

Treatment should start topically with supportive care: preservative-free artificial tears, cool compresses, and removal of contact lenses. If symptoms persist, an antihistamine-vasoconstrictor (e.g., naphazoline-pheniramine) can be added with caution.[5] With use for longer than 3 to 7 days, rebound vasodilation can occur, resulting in a medication-induced conjunctivitis. Mast cell stabilizers can be used as prophylaxis for recurrent or persistent allergic conjunctivitis. The patient should keep in mind that results take several weeks with a mast cell stabilizer. If the patient has any systemic allergies, an oral antihistamine can also be helpful in controlling ocular symptoms. Topical nonsteroidal anti-inflammatory drugs and steroids may be beneficial but should be used only under the supervision of an ophthalmologist.[5,7,17]

Vernal and Atopic Conjunctivitis

The treatment approach is similar to that for allergic conjunctivitis. However, because agents are nonspecific, simple avoidance of triggers is a difficult remedy. The provider should initiate mast cell stabilizers (e.g., cromolyn sodium, lodoxamide tromethamine) 2 weeks before the usual time of presentation for relief in vernal conjunctivitis.[9] Symptoms tend to be more refractory and severe. Ophthalmology referral is indicated in all cases.

Medication Toxicity

Treatment is twofold. First, the toxic medication must be eliminated. Second, symptomatic relief with preservative-free artificial tears should be provided.[7] A short course of topical steroids is sometimes used to reduce the duration of symptoms, particularly in more severe cases.[9,17]

DIFFERENTIAL DIAGNOSIS

Not all patients with a red eye have conjunctivitis.[3,11] Conjunctival inflammation can result from other ocular diseases. Effective treatment of the red eye depends on appropriate targeting of the underlying disease.[7] Multiple causes of red eye ranging from benign to potentially sight-threatening are listed in the differential diagnosis box.

DIFFERENTIAL DIAGNOSIS

Conjunctivitis

- Subconjunctival hemorrhage
- Blepharitis
- Dry eye
- Pterygium, pinguecula
- Episcleritis
- Eyelid malposition (e.g., ectropion, entropion, floppy eyelid)
- Canaliculitis, dacryocystitis
- Foreign body
- Corneal abrasion
- Corneal ulcer
- Glaucoma
- Lagophthalmos after Bell palsy or stroke
- Uveitis
- Scleritis
- Endophthalmitis

INDICATIONS FOR REFERRAL

On initial evaluation, if there is any concern for a sight-threatening disease, the patient should be immediately referred to an ophthalmologist. History can provide important clues. For example, patients with recent trauma, ocular surgery, or use of contact lenses need to be referred. In addition, physical examination is important. A decrease in vision or severe ocular pain is not consistent with conjunctivitis and warrants an ophthalmic consultation. Nonocular symptoms and signs, such as nausea and vomiting, should raise concern for acute glaucoma and prompt referral.[8,11,13]

Conjunctivitis in immunocompromised patients requires immediate attention by an ophthalmologist.[7]

In addition, in patients with conjunctivitis, if any of the following occur, the patient needs an evaluation by an ophthalmologist[7]:

- Vision loss
- Pain
- Severe, purulent discharge

- Corneal involvement
- No response or worsening symptoms despite treatment
- Recurrent episodes

Suspected herpetic infection (either by history of prior HSV infections or by presentation with a vesicular rash in the V1 dermatome) also warrants ophthalmic evaluation.[7,8]

EDUCATION AND HEALTH PROMOTION

Education is a key component of treatment. For example, patients with noninfectious conjunctivitis need to understand the underlying cause of their disease and the chronic nature of their condition. In patients with infectious conjunctivitis, the health care provider has a valuable role in interrupting the cycle of transmission. Patients should avoid touching their eyes, shaking hands with others, sharing towels or bedclothes, and swimming in public pools.[8,11,17] Teach patients and their families recommended hand washing techniques. The health care provider also must take care to wash hands with antimicrobial soap after examination of a patient with conjunctivitis. Infectious outbreaks have been linked to health care facilities. In addition, all exposed surfaces in the examination room should be decontaminated with sodium hypochlorite (a 1:10 dilution of household bleach) or other disinfectants.[7]

CHAPTER 74

CORNEAL SURFACE DEFECTS AND OCULAR SURFACE FOREIGN BODIES

Neda Nikpor • James T. Banta

DEFINITION AND EPIDEMIOLOGY

A corneal surface defect occurs when the corneal epithelium is interrupted. Direct trauma from foreign objects (e.g., fingers, tree branches, makeup applicators) typically causes these injuries. Airbags from motor vehicle accidents are another common source of injury. Contact lens wearers are particularly susceptible to corneal problems because prolonged use of lenses can result in injury and corneal epithelial breaks.[1] In most cases, the patient can recall a specific moment when trauma occurred.

Corneal surface foreign bodies are particularly common in workers who spend time around small particles or dust or who grind metal, such as construction workers, mechanics and landscapers (Fig. 74-1).[2] Chemicals, either splashed or inadvertently placed in the eye, can also cause surface defects. These injuries are almost universally preventable with the appropriate type of eye protection.

Corneal surface defects must be distinguished from other serious conditions, most notably corneal inflammatory conditions, lacerations, and infections. Full-thickness lacerations can occur with ocular trauma and sometimes appear clinically similar to epithelial defects. Infectious keratitis, or corneal ulcers, are common in contact lens users. An ulcer is an epithelial defect with an infiltrate, or white area in the cornea. Other common conditions with similar presentations include herpetic keratitis, staphylococcal marginal disease, and phlyctenulosis, the last two frequently manifesting as peripheral corneal opacities with associated epithelial defects.

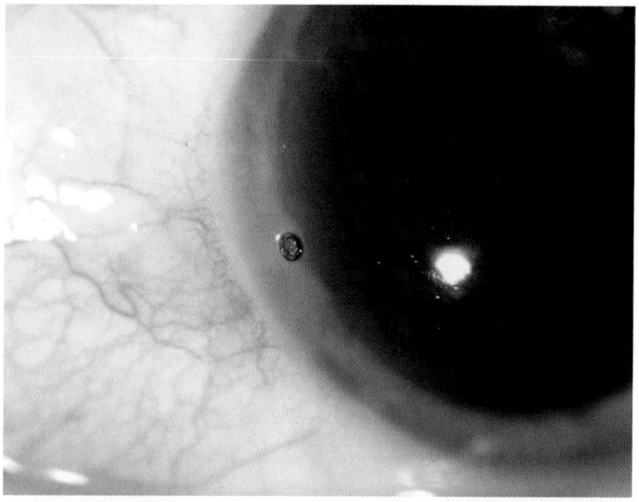

FIGURE 74-1 A metallic corneal foreign body is a common presentation in young male workers, often occurring while grinding or hammering metal on metal.

PATHOPHYSIOLOGY

An abrasion of the corneal epithelium may be caused by chemical or mechanical debridement resulting from trauma, chemicals, or ultraviolet radiation exposure. Corneal erosions occur if an abrasion disrupts Bowman's layer. Decreased evaporation during sleep results in the formation of a fluid layer above the incompletely healed Bowman's layer and below the epithelium. This can lead to repeated sloughing of the overlying epithelium when the patient awakens and opens the lid, given the relative lack of epithelial adherence. Epithelial defects, whether abrasions or erosions, may allow bacterial, viral, or fungal organisms to invade the corneal stroma, resulting in an ulcer. Sterile corneal ulcers may also occur.

CLINICAL PRESENTATION

The most common symptom of a corneal abrasion or foreign body is sudden onset of severe eye pain in the affected eye. This pain typically resolves after application of a topical anesthetic eye drop.[3] Some patients may report a foreign body sensation instead of severe pain. Other symptoms include blurred vision, redness, tearing, light sensitivity, eyelid swelling, and blepharospasm.[4]

PHYSICAL EXAMINATION

On examination, vision may be limited if the epithelial defect or foreign body falls within the visual axis. The pupils should react normally to light, and eye pressure is typically not affected. The eyelids may appear swollen in the affected eye, and the conjunctiva is typically injected. The cornea may have some mild haze but should not be focally opacified. If there is a significant corneal opacity, an alternative diagnosis such as infectious keratitis should be considered. A foreign body may be visible on the corneal or conjunctival surface. The anterior chamber should have normal depth, and the iris should have a normal, round appearance. Presence of a hypopyon (inflammatory debris layering in the inferior portion of the anterior

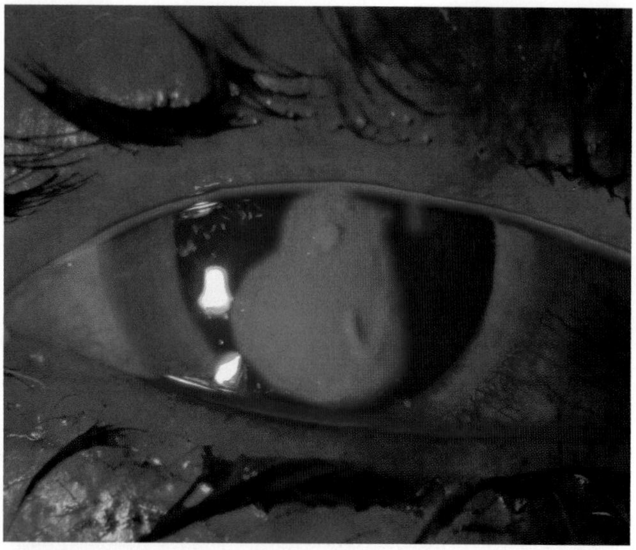

FIGURE 74-2 Corneal abrasion stained with fluorescein under a cobalt blue light. The patient was inadvertently poked in the eye and complained of severe pain, decreased vision, and lid swelling.

chamber) suggests a more serious diagnosis, and immediate referral should be made to an ophthalmologist. If the anterior chamber appears flattened or the pupil is peaked or irregular, this suggests a penetrating injury, and immediate referral should be made to an ophthalmologist.

DIAGNOSTICS

Use of topical fluorescein dye can assist in the diagnosis of a corneal surface defect. One drop of fluorescein can be applied and viewed under a cobalt blue light or Wood lamp. A corneal abrasion should appear as a bright green area, often polygonal (Fig. 74-2). Linear, vertically oriented epithelial defects are typically caused by subtarsal (trapped under the upper eyelid) foreign bodies and should prompt eversion of the upper eyelids to check for foreign material. Fluorescein staining of true surface defects should not change with the patient's blinking. If the defect appears to have a branching or dendritic pattern, a herpetic cause should be entertained. An irregular iris and a shallow anterior chamber associated with an area of fluorescein staining raise the specter of a full-thickness corneal laceration and should prompt emergent ophthalmology referral.

DIAGNOSTICS

Corneal Surface Defects and Foreign Bodies

INITIAL (CORNEAL ABRASION OR ULCER)
Fluorescein stain

LABORATORY (CORNEAL ULCER)
Culture and sensitivity (if immediate ophthalmology consultation is not available)

INITIAL (FOREIGN BODY)
Fluorescein stain
Evert eyelids and examine fornices if appropriate

DIFFERENTIAL DIAGNOSIS

The differential diagnosis of a corneal surface defect or corneal foreign body includes corneal ulcer, herpetic keratitis, dry eye syndrome, episcleritis, iritis, acute angle closure glaucoma, conjunctivitis, full-thickness corneal laceration, staphylococcal marginal disease, phlyctenulosis, and contact lens overuse, among others.

DIFFERENTIAL DIAGNOSIS

Corneal Surface Defects and Foreign Bodies

- Corneal lacerations
- Conjunctivitis
- Keratitis
- Contact lens intolerance
- Blepharitis
- Episcleritis
- Inflamed pinguecula or pterygium
- Hordeolum (early)
- Chalazion (early)

MANAGEMENT

Most patients with corneal abrasions or surface defects can be managed with supportive care. An ophthalmic antibiotic ointment, such as erythromycin or polymyxin B–bacitracin (Polysporin), may help with pain control by providing a physical barrier between the cornea and eyelid,[1] and it is often prescribed in lieu of antibiotic eye drops. Ophthalmic ointment can be applied on the ocular surface by pulling the lower lid away from the eye while having the patient look up. Ointment is then applied into the pocket that is opened. Pressure patching, although helpful in relieving pain, may encourage infection and should be avoided.[5] Oral analgesics are the first-line agents for pain control, but patients should be encouraged to use ointment and artificial tears frequently because this often provides more relief than oral analgesics. Steroids are contraindicated because they inhibit healing and may encourage infection. Topical anesthetics such as proparacaine should *never* be used or prescribed for pain control; their prolonged use may lead to corneal melting. Care should be taken to inform patients of this risk, and providers should avoid leaving patients in examination rooms with topical anesthetics within reach. Cycloplegic drops are occasionally used for pain control in severe cases, particularly if the injury is severe enough to produce intraocular inflammation as is sometimes seen with trauma. However, care should be taken to avoid cycloplegic drops (owing to their vasoconstrictive effect) in severe chemical burns.

A healthy corneal epithelium will repopulate rapidly, from just a few hours for a small, uncomplicated defect to 3 to 5 days with larger defects. Symptoms typically abate once the epithelium is reestablished. Patients should be informed of the typical time course and should be reassured that their pain should improve gradually over a few days. They should be advised to seek urgent ophthalmology evaluation if they develop sudden worsening of symptoms including redness, sensitivity to light, vision changes, or pain. The mnemonic *RSVP* can be given to help patients remember these precautions.

If a visible foreign body is present on the cornea, it must be removed. If it is not easily removed with a cotton-tipped applicator, an ophthalmology referral should be made so that the foreign body can be visualized with a slit lamp for removal. Even when a metallic foreign body is dislodged, a rust ring may

BOX 74-1

Irrigation After Chemical Injuries

- Position patient comfortably at an angle.
- Place basin to collect excess fluid.
- Apply 1 drop of topical anesthetic.
- Retract lids with lid retractor.
- Deliver 1 L of normal saline through standard intravenous tubing to affected eyes.
- Flush entire area for 1 hr, including fornices (areas between globe and eyelids).
- Test pH. If result is not 7.0 to 7.5, repeat irrigation.

BOX 74-2

Indications for Immediate Ophthalmology Referral

- Nonhealing epithelial defects
- Metallic foreign bodies
- Chemical injuries (after prompt irrigation)
- Infectious keratitis
- Hypopyon (evidence of a fluid line in anterior chamber near the bottom caused by inflammatory cells)
- Full-thickness corneal laceration
- Elevated eye pressure (>30) on tonometry

persist on the cornea and cause further inflammation if it is not completely removed.

If chemical injury is suspected, *immediate* irrigation of the affected eye should be performed (before referral). A full history, including the type of chemical, should be obtained; alkali injuries in particular can lead to rapid damage. Irrigation should be performed as described in Box 74-1.[6] After irrigation, pH should measure 7.0 to 7.5.[2] If the pH is not in this range after irrigation, further irrigation should be performed. After irrigation, immediately refer the patient to an ophthalmologist.

Chemical injuries can be broadly categorized into acid or alkali. Identification of the causative chemical agent is important, and referred patients should be provided a bottle of the chemical or at the very least specific information about the offending agent. Acid injuries tend to be less harmful; these materials cause corneal surface proteins to coagulate and create a barrier that prevents deeper penetration. On the other hand, alkaline materials (e.g., ammonia, bleach) lead to rapid damage because of saponification of fats and denaturation of collagen. Within *minutes,* alkaline materials can penetrate the anterior chamber and cause damage to intraocular structures.

COMPLICATIONS

The most concerning complication of a corneal epithelial defect or corneal foreign body is infection. Although rare, infection is often preventable with appropriate therapy and use of topical antibiotics. Trauma with vegetable matter (e.g. tree branch) should increase suspicion and concern for infection (often by atypical organisms, frequently fungus). Misdiagnosis of a corneal ulcer as a corneal epithelial defect can lead to scarring of the cornea and worsening of infection, leading to further vision loss. Corneal foreign bodies may leave behind rust that can cause future inflammation or vision loss. Patients who have previously sustained surface defects may occasionally develop recurrent corneal erosion syndrome, in which spontaneous erosion occurs at the site of a previous injury weeks to months after the initial injury. If a chemical injury is not promptly treated or irrigated, severe visual impairment and ocular damage may occur.

INDICATIONS FOR REFERRAL

After initial management of symptoms, patients with corneal surface defects, history of metallic foreign body removal, and persistent foreign bodies should be referred to an ophthalmologist. Chemical injuries should be irrigated before referral because of the risk of rapid progression. See Box 74-2 for additional situations requiring immediate referral.

PREVENTION

Many workplace injuries are caused by foreign bodies, chemicals, or direct trauma and can be easily prevented with appropriate eyewear. The Occupational Safety and Health Administration (OSHA) recommends use of safety glasses with side protection in situations such as hammering and metal grinding.[2] Safety glasses may be insufficient for workers who are performing tasks with high-velocity particles that can potentially reach the eye around the glasses. Polycarbonate safety goggles that fit snugly to the face are more appropriate in these settings. Welders can also develop painful corneal injuries and should wear appropriate safety equipment. Standards for eye protection are set in the American National Standards Institute (ANSI) guidelines Z78.1 and Z49.1.[7]

Chemical injuries require prompt therapy. Work environments with hazardous chemicals should have easily accessible eyewash stations for rapid treatment.[8] ANSI standard Z358.1 provides requirements for water temperature, flow rate, distance, and functioning of eyewash stations.

Nearly all eye injuries in the workplace are preventable. Further education and awareness can reduce the financial burden of these injuries as well as potentially sight-threatening accidents.

CHAPTER 75

DRY EYE SYNDROME

Scott D. Walter • James T. Banta

DEFINITION AND EPIDEMIOLOGY

Dry eye is a multifactorial disorder characterized by abnormalities in the tear film that result in symptoms of discomfort, visual disturbance, and tear film instability with potential damage to the ocular surface.[1] The disorder is known by many names including *dry eye syndrome, ocular surface disease, keratoconjunctivitis sicca, aqueous tear film deficiency,* and *dysfunctional tear syndrome.*

Dry eye is one of the most common reasons that adults consult an eye care professional. It is also treated frequently by primary care physicians, and, perhaps most commonly, by patients themselves. Prevalence estimates for dry eye have varied widely, ranging from as low as 0.6% to as high as 57% based on the population studied and the stringency of the definition of the disease.[2] Several large cross-sectional studies have estimated that 5 million Americans have moderate to severe dry eye disease, and up to 20% of the population report occasional dry eye symptoms.[3]

PATHOPHYSIOLOGY

Dry eye is a surprisingly complex condition. The tear film is responsible for nourishing and lubricating the ocular surface, as well as providing its immune protection. In addition, the tear film functions as the anterior refracting surface of the eye and, as such, plays a pivotal role in maintaining optical clarity.

A healthy tear film is created by complex interactions of the lacrimal glands and ducts, cornea and conjunctiva, eyelids, and meibomian glands and is maintained by autonomic and reflexive functions of the peripheral somatosensory and motor nervous system.[1] The tear film itself is formed with each blink and is composed of three layers: an inner mucin layer, an intermediate aqueous layer, and an outer lipid layer. The outer lipid layer, produced largely by secretions of the meibomian glands in the upper and lower eyelids, limits evaporative loss of the underlying aqueous layer between blinks.

A deficiency in any layer of the tear film or in any component of the lacrimal functional unit can lead to dry eye. Broadly speaking, dry eye can be classified into two mechanistic categories: *aqueous-deficient* and *evaporative* dry eye. Aqueous-deficient dry eye typically localizes to the lacrimal gland, and lacrimal gland insufficiency may be caused by Sjögren disease (a primary or secondary autoimmune infiltration of the lacrimal and salivary glands leading to dry eye and dry mouth), other infiltrative diseases of the lacrimal gland, or primary hyposecretion. Evaporative dry eye similarly has many causes, although the most common is meibomian gland dysfunction, in which the lipid-producing meibomian glands in the eyelids are obstructed at their openings (Fig. 75-1). Other causes of evaporative dry eye include poor eyelid closure (lagophthalmos), inadequate blinking, and ocular rosacea.

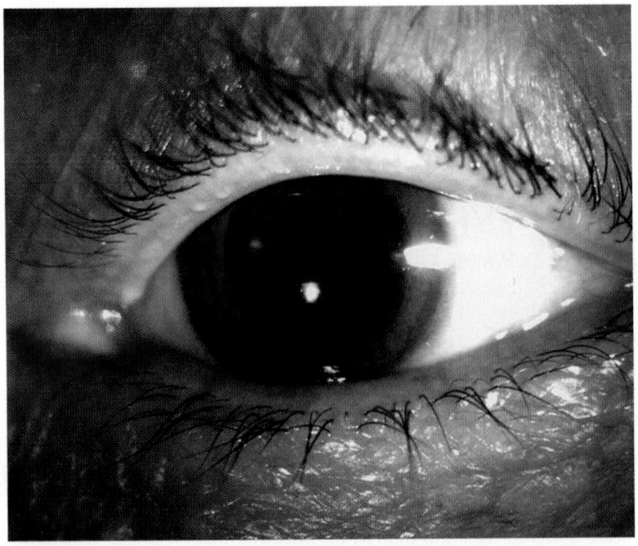

FIGURE 75-1 Meibomian gland dysfunction. Meibomian glands are situated in the upper and lower eyelids, posterior to the eyelashes, and secrete the outer lipid layer of the tear film. Clogged meibomian glands are visible along the nasal portion of the upper lid in the photograph. Blockage of the meibomian glands leads to decreased tear film lipids, increased evaporation of the underlying aqueous layer, and tear film instability.

Despite the apparent simplicity of this classification scheme, most patients with dry eye will have components of both mechanisms contributing to their disease. Regardless of the cause, inflammation plays a central role in exacerbating and perpetuating dry eye disease. Inflammatory cytokines affect tear film osmolarity, leading to increased tear film instability and evaporative loss, which in turn leads to further inflammation.[4] Breaking this inflammatory cycle is critical in the management of dry eye disease.[5]

As the disease becomes more chronic, dry eye may evolve into a corneal pain disorder. There is increasing evidence that a significant number of patients with chronic dry eye describe features of neuropathic pain.[6] Dysfunctional adaptation of the corneal pain apparatus, including changes in corneal nerve morphology and neurotransmission,[7,8] may also contribute to the development of a more persistently symptomatic disease phenotype.[9]

CLINICAL PRESENTATION

The symptoms of dry eye may be vague and nonspecific, and the clinician must carefully distinguish dry eye from other conditions that affect the ocular surface. Patients with dry eye most often have a chief concern of dryness, foreign body sensation (a scratchy or gritty feeling in the eyes), burning or stinging pain, itching, or ocular fatigue. They may also secondarily complain of redness or light sensitivity or note transient blurred vision that is relieved by blinking. Often their symptoms are worsened by activities that require visual concentration (e.g., reading or computer use) or by low-humidity environments (e.g., airplane travel). Paradoxically, some patients may demonstrate excessive tearing, a reflexive hypersecretion of tears caused by corneal irritation. Many contact lens users report increasing intolerance to their lenses.

A careful medical history, including current medications and a complete review of systems, should be obtained, because many systemic diseases and treatments can cause or exacerbate the symptoms of dry eyes. For example, many commonly prescribed anticholinergic drugs (including antihistamines and tricyclic antidepressants), alpha blockers (e.g., tamsulosin), antihypertensives (including diuretics and beta blockers), oral corticosteroids, and even vitamins have been associated with dry eye symptoms.[10] Autoimmune diseases including lupus and rheumatoid arthritis can cause a secondary Sjögren syndrome leading to aqueous-deficient dry eye. Similarly, infiltrative processes affecting the lacrimal gland, such as lymphoma, sarcoidosis, and graft-versus-host disease, can cause lacrimal gland insufficiency. Thyrotoxicosis and thyroid eye disease can cause exophthalmos, eyelid retraction, and incomplete eyelid closure.[11] Cranial nerve VII (e.g., Bell) palsies causing partial or complete paralysis of the orbicularis oculi muscle may also lead to eyelid malposition, poor eyelid closure, and exposure of the ocular surface. Reactivation of varicella zoster virus (shingles) within the ophthalmic division of the trigeminal nerve may lead to diminished corneal sensation, an impaired blink reflex, and exposure of the ocular surface.[12] Decreased corneal sensitivity and lower rates of spontaneous blinking are also seen in patients with Parkinson disease.[13]

PHYSICAL EXAMINATION

Physical examination by the primary care physician should include measurement of visual acuity (in each eye separately) as well as an external inspection of the ocular adnexa, including the skin, eyelids, conjunctiva, and cornea. If available, fluorescein dye can be used in conjunction with a cobalt blue–filtered light source to highlight pathology on the corneal surface. Attention should be given to eyelid and cranial nerve (especially V and VII) function, because incomplete eyelid closure (lagophthalmos) can cause corneal exposure and evaporative dry eye. The primary care physician should evaluate for eyelid retraction and proptosis (hallmarks of thyroid eye disease) and consider screening for thyroid dysfunction. In addition, a complete physical examination—with close attention to the skin and joints—should be completed to screen for an associated autoimmune condition.

Although examination of the ocular surface by an ophthalmologist can help establish a diagnosis of dry eye syndrome, there is often a poor correlation between signs and symptoms in dry eye syndrome.[16] Some patients will report severe symptoms with little objective evidence of ocular surface disease; others will note only mild symptoms despite dramatic findings clinically. This discrepancy between signs and symptoms can complicate the diagnosis and management of patients with dry eye.

DIAGNOSTICS

The diagnosis of dry eye is based primarily on symptoms subjectively reported by the patient. The Ocular Surface Disease Index (OSDI) is a simple, reliable, and reproducible way to assess dry eye severity and to monitor patients' response to treatment.[14]

Two basic tests help to distinguish aqueous-deficient from evaporative dry eye.

- A Schirmer test can be performed to assess aqueous production (Fig. 75-2). A narrow piece of filter paper is placed in the inferior cul-de-sac, and tear production is measured by the amount the paper is wet after 5 minutes. The test can be performed with topical anesthesia (to measure basal tearing) or without anesthesia (to measure basal plus reflex tearing). A cutoff of less than 5 mm (with anesthesia) or less than 10 mm (without anesthesia) is considered abnormal.[15] An abnormal Schirmer test result suggests aqueous-deficient dry eye.
  - For patients with aqueous-deficient dry eye suspected of having Sjögren syndrome, a serologic evaluation including SS-A (anti-Ro), SS-B (anti-La), rheumatoid factor, and antinuclear antibodies should be obtained.[15]

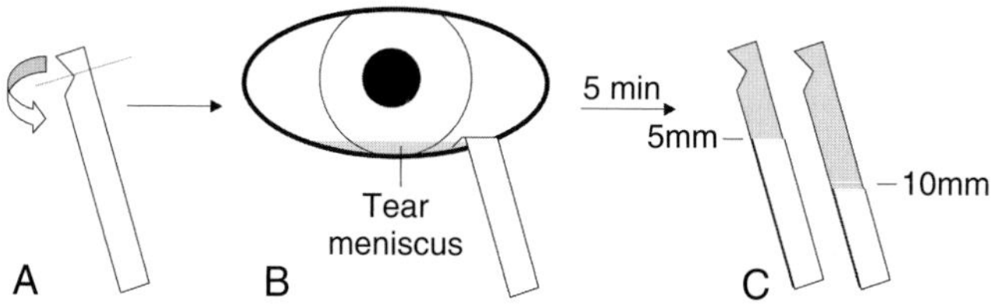

FIGURE 75-2 Schirmer test. A narrow strip of filter paper is used to measure the production of tears. The Schirmer strip is folded at the notch **(A)** and placed over the lower eyelid margin with the short end resting in the tear meniscus of the inferior fornix **(B)**. The strips are removed after 5 minutes, and the amount of moisture is measured **(C)**. If the test is performed with topical anesthesia, then only basal tear secretion is measured, and less than 5 mm of wetting is considered diagnostic of aqueous tear deficiency. If the test is performed without topical anesthesia, then basal plus reflex tear secretion is measured, and less than 10 mm of wetting is considered diagnostic of aqueous tear deficiency.

- Tear breakup time can be recorded with the aid of a slit-lamp biomicroscope. Fluorescein dye is instilled and the tear film is visualized with a cobalt blue filter. The amount of time between the last blink and the first discontinuity in the tear film is recorded as the tear breakup time, and less than 10 seconds is considered abnormal.[15] An abnormal tear breakup time suggests evaporative dry eye.

A number of more advanced diagnostic modalities (listed in the diagnostics box) are available to help stratify patients and predict their responses to different treatment options.

DIAGNOSTICS

Dry Eye

INITIAL

Ocular Surface Disease Index (OSDI) questionnaire
Schirmer test
Tear breakup time

ADVANCED

Tear osmolarity
Contact and noncontact meibography
Biomarker assays (e.g., lactoferrin, immunoglobulin E, matrix metalloproteinase 9)

DIFFERENTIAL DIAGNOSIS

Making a diagnosis of dry eye syndrome requires the exclusion of other, more serious diseases of the ocular surface. There is a broad range of possible causes of ocular surface irritation, with the most common and important disorders listed in the differential diagnosis box. It is important to localize the problem and distinguish among these conditions because each is managed differently.

DIFFERENTIAL DIAGNOSIS

Ocular Surface Irritation

EYELID DISORDERS

- Trichiasis (misdirected eyelashes that contact the ocular surface)
- Facial nerve paralysis (e.g., Bell palsy)
- Floppy eyelid syndrome

CONJUNCTIVAL DISORDERS

- Viral conjunctivitis
- Allergic conjunctivitis
- Topical medication toxicity (especially from glaucoma drops)
- Cicatrizing conjunctivitis (graft-versus-host disease, Stevens-Johnson syndrome, ocular cicatricial pemphigoid, trachoma)

CORNEAL DISORDERS

- Corneal abrasion
- Corneal foreign body
- Contact lens intolerance
- Thermal or chemical burns
- Herpes simplex or varicella zoster keratitis
- Pterygium (a benign, wing-shaped growth of tissue over the cornea)
- Decreased corneal sensation (neurotrophic keratopathy, Parkinson disease)
- Photokeratitis (typically seen after welding or tanning without ultraviolet light protection)

DRY EYE SYNDROMES (TEAR FILM DISORDERS)

- Aqueous-deficient dry eye
- Evaporative dry eye

MANAGEMENT

Specialist consultation with an ophthalmologist is warranted whenever patients complain of dry eye symptoms that are refractory to conservative management with behavioral changes, eyelid hygiene, and artificial tears.

Emergency department referral is rarely warranted. Patients should be referred promptly to the ophthalmologist on call for visual loss, severe pain, or corneal ulceration.[15]

Management of dry eye should be approached in a stepwise fashion. Most patients will require a systematic escalation of treatment combining several different behavioral, pharmacologic, and nonpharmacologic approaches. Lifestyle or workplace modifications can help alleviate the symptoms of dry eye, and patients should be advised to avoid windy, smoky, or low-humidity environments. Patients should be counseled to avoid direct exposure to the drying effects of air conditioning and fans and to limit the uninterrupted time spent reading or working on the computer without a break.

Eyelid inflammation (blepharitis) and meibomian gland dysfunction (see Fig. 75-1) can often be treated with lid hygiene measures. These measures include frequent warm compresses and gentle lid scrubs with nontearing baby shampoo.

The primary care provider can help to alleviate symptoms of dry eye by reviewing the patient's systemic medications and making dietary recommendations. Exacerbating medications, including anticholinergics, beta blockers, and diuretics, should be avoided (or substituted with medications in other drug classes) whenever possible. Many of the dietary modifications and supplements that primary care providers routinely recommend for cardiovascular health (e.g., Mediterranean diet, fish oil, omega-6 fatty acids, vitamin D) may have a beneficial effect on patients' dry eye symptoms.[17,18]

Artificial tears are usually the first line of treatment of dry eye disease and can be used by the patient as needed. A wide variety of artificial tear drops are available over the counter. Patients should be encouraged to try a variety of commercially available drops to find the artificial tear formulation(s) that work best for them. High-viscosity gels and ointments provide better tear retention time and protection of the ocular surface but tend to cause visual blurring; therefore they are recommended for nighttime use or in patients with more severe dry eye. The preservatives in topical eye drops can also irritate the ocular surface, so preservative-free formulations are often beneficial for patients requiring drops more than four to six times per day (including their other topical ophthalmic drops, such as those for the treatment of glaucoma).

As a general rule, use of eye drops that contain vasoconstrictive agents such as tetrahydrozoline (e.g., Visine) should be discouraged, because these drops can produce a rebound vasodilation and worsening conjunctival injection without addressing the underlying causes. Occasionally patients may report the illicit use of topical anesthetic drops obtained from a doctor's office. These should be confiscated from the patient because their abuse may lead to severe complications including corneal opacities, ulceration, and even perforation. When ocular lubricants and behavioral changes fail to alleviate the symptoms of dry eye, it is important to consult an ophthalmologist for consideration of pharmacologic treatment options.

Ophthalmologists may prescribe a short course of topical corticosteroids, which can help to quiet the inflammatory component of dry eye disease. However, this therapy should not be used chronically or without close follow-up, given the increased risk of glaucoma, cataract formation, and infection. Treatment with cyclosporine ophthalmic emulsion 0.05% (Restasis) can be recommended by an ophthalmologist. Restasis is the only option approved by the Food and Drug Administration for the long-term treatment of dry eye. Low-dose oral doxycycline is also gaining popularity in the management of aqueous-deficient dry eye secondary to meibomian gland dysfunction and/or ocular rosacea.[19] The ophthalmologist may also consider punctal occlusion, moisture goggles, or therapeutic contact lenses to improve tear retention. In extreme cases refractory to conventional therapies, some experts recommend autologous serum tears to lubricate the eyes and to reduce inflammation, although robust efficacy data from clinical trials are lacking.[20]

COMPLICATIONS

Failure to treat dry eye early in the course of disease can lead to chronic changes in corneal nerve morphology and neurotransmission[7,8] and neuropathic ocular pain,[9] making the disease more difficult to treat later. Severe dry eye can cause conjunctival adhesions, death of limbal stem cells leading to scarring and neovascularization of the cornea, or exposure of the ocular surface leading to corneal thinning, ulceration, and infection.

INDICATIONS FOR REFERRAL OR HOSPITALIZATION

Straightforward cases of dry eye with mild, intermittent symptoms can be self-managed by the patient—with lifestyle modifications, artificial tears, and eyelid hygiene—under the guidance of a primary care provider.

Patients should be referred to an ophthalmologist for dry eye symptoms that are moderate to severe, symptoms that are persistent or poorly controlled, despite use of artificial tears four to six times daily, or are associated with any known or suspected ocular or systemic disease.

Patients should be referred to an ophthalmologist before initiating any pharmacologic therapy for dry eye. A non–eye specialist provider should never initiate the use of ocular corticosteroids because of the risk of glaucoma, cataract formation, and infection.[5]

Hospitalization is rarely required, except in the case of patients with severe sight-threatening complications (e.g., corneal ulceration) who are unable to provide adequate care for themselves on an outpatient basis.

LIFE SPAN CONSIDERATIONS

Dry eye is a chronic condition that frequently requires long-term therapy. It is more common in older adults and particularly common in postmenopausal women.[21]

EDUCATION AND HEALTH PROMOTION

Patients should be advised that dry eye is a chronic condition that usually requires long-term management and treatment. The most effective treatment plan involves the patient, the ophthalmologist, and the primary care provider in a collaborative, ongoing, and stepwise approach to management. Many behavioral, nonpharmacologic, and pharmacologic treatment options are available to patients, and most report good control of their symptoms with appropriate therapy.

Patients with dry eye symptoms should avoid low-humidity, smoky, or windy environments. They should take frequent breaks during activities that require close visual attention, such as reading and computer work. They should also make a habit of performing eyelid hygiene, including frequent warm compresses and gentle lid scrubs with baby shampoo. Over-the-counter artificial tears are readily available as a first-line therapy for dry eye, although eye drops with preservatives should be limited to four to six times per day. Severe disease can be managed with more powerful anti-inflammatory topical medications, but only under the supervision of a trained eye care professional.

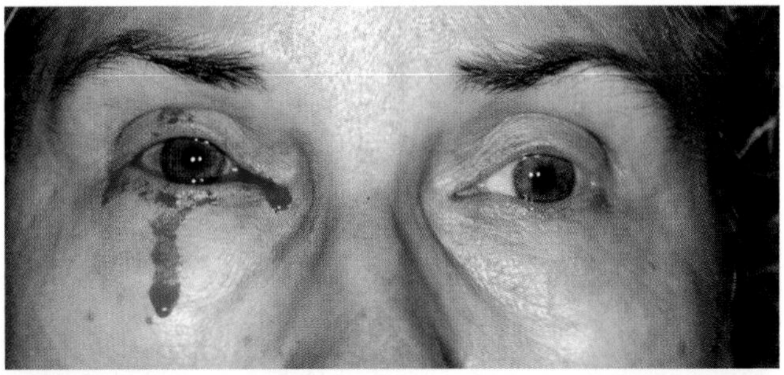

FIGURE 76-1 After the application of fluorescein in both eyes, normal clearance of the tears is seen on the left side. Pooling of tears and frank tearing are seen on the right side, indicative of nasolacrimal duct obstruction.

CHAPTER 76

NASOLACRIMAL DUCT OBSTRUCTION AND DACRYOCYSTITIS

Audrey C. Ko • James T. Banta

DEFINITION AND EPIDEMIOLOGY

The nasolacrimal duct, commonly known as the *tear duct,* is a tubular structure that drains excess tears from the eyes into the nose. A complete or partial obstruction at any point along this structure is called a *nasolacrimal duct obstruction* (NLDO).[1] There are two types of acquired NLDO: primary and secondary. Primary acquired NLDO is the most common clinical syndrome of acquired NLDO in adults and is typically caused by inflammation or fibrosis without any precipitating cause.[2] Secondary acquired NLDO is caused by myriad precipitating factors, including infection, inflammation, neoplasm, and trauma. Patients affected by NLDO have disruption of normal tear drainage, causing problems that range from the annoyance of constant tearing to the more serious dacryocystitis, an inflammation of the lacrimal sac.

PATHOPHYSIOLOGY

The lacrimal drainage system consists of the superior and inferior canaliculus, the lacrimal sac, and the nasolacrimal duct. Tear drainage begins with contraction of the palpebral orbicularis oculi muscle, which acts to pump fluid through the lacrimal ducts into the lacrimal sac. The tears then enter the nasal cavity through an opening under the inferior meatus.[3] In normal development, the nasolacrimal duct becomes patent to the inferior meatus of the nose during the first few weeks of life and before the onset of tear production. In 5% of newborns, the impatency persists beyond this period, and the parents may notice the clinical symptoms of congenital NLDO.[4,5]

Acquired inflammation originating at the eye, lacrimal system, nose, or sinuses can induce swelling of the lacrimal system's mucous membranes, resulting in acquired NLDO. Congenital or acquired forms of NLDO can lead to stasis of tear flow and the development of secondary infections, dacryocystitis, and abscess formation. Obstruction that is not congenital may result from involutional stenosis, trauma, neoplasia, or anatomic obstructions (e.g., a deviated septum, polyps, or hypertrophied inferior turbinates).

CLINICAL PRESENTATION

Adults with partial or complete obstruction of the nasolacrimal duct often have chronic tearing, ocular discharge, and eyelash crusting.[1] More serious cases may also cause painful swelling below the medial canthus and a mucopurulent discharge from the punctum. The clinical history is used to differentiate an excess accumulation of tears caused by drainage obstruction from excess tear production. Epiphora, the accumulation of tears in the palpebral fissure with eventual overflow down the cheeks, denotes evidence of excess tearing caused by lacrimal outflow deficiency (Fig. 76-1); hyperlacrimation denotes an excess production of tears. A history of chronic allergies, sinusitis, previous nasal or sinus surgery, prior midfacial fractures, or radiation therapy may predispose patients to NLDO.[6] Systemic inflammatory diseases such as Granulomatosis with polyangiitis, sarcoidosis, Crohn disease, and ulcerative colitis are other known associations.[7-9]

PHYSICAL EXAMINATION

The ocular adnexa and surface structures should be carefully examined for signs of inflammation such as the presence of telangiectasias or erythema. Gross examination findings may include overflow of tears, mucoid or purulent discharge, conjunctival infection, and erythema over the lacrimal sac. Pressure over the lacrimal sac may produce a mucoid reflux from the punctum, indicative of lower system obstruction. Close attention should be given to the medial canthal region for focal swelling, fluctuance, erythema, or tenderness overlying the nasolacrimal sac, suggestive of dacryocystitis (Fig. 76-2). Fever and leukocytosis may also be present in acute dacryocystitis. Finally, a nasal speculum may be used to examine the nares for any mucosal swelling, tumors, or other anatomic abnormality that could narrow the distal opening of the nasolacrimal duct in the vicinity of the inferior turbinate.

DIAGNOSTICS

Diagnostic tests are usually unnecessary. In some cases, the ophthalmologist will test the lacrimal drainage system by directly cannulating the canaliculus and injecting sterile water or saline to check for patency of the system. In select cases of suspected trauma, tumors, or anatomic abnormalities, computed tomography or magnetic resonance imaging of the lacrimal system can

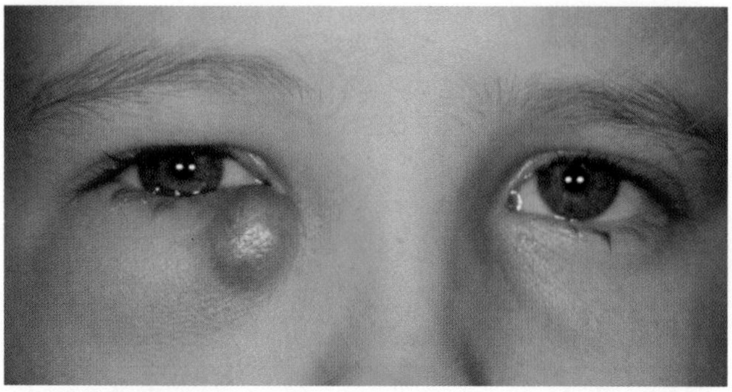

FIGURE 76-2 Dacryocystitis commonly manifests as erythematous, fluctuant swelling just inferior to the medial canthus.

be useful in the evaluation of patients with excess tearing. In cases of dacryocystitis or purulent discharge, culture and sensitivity testing may help guide antibiotic therapy. If fever is present, a complete blood count (CBC) may be considered to evaluate for leukocytosis.

DIAGNOSTICS

Nasolacrimal Duct Obstruction and Dacryocystitis

LABORATORY
Culture and sensitivity (if purulent discharge is present)
CBC and differential (if fever is present)

DIFFERENTIAL DIAGNOSIS

Chronic tearing and ocular irritation in an adult may also indicate dry eye syndrome, blepharitis, meibomian gland disease, conjunctivitis, punctal stenosis, eyelid malpositions, corneal foreign body, or Bell palsy. In patients with blood-tinged tears or if a mechanical obstruction is suspected, a neoplastic process must be ruled out. Preseptal or orbital cellulitis must also be considered in patients with severe swelling, mucopurulent discharge, and pain.[10]

DIFFERENTIAL DIAGNOSIS

Nasolacrimal Duct Obstruction and Dacryocystitis

- Conjunctivitis
- Blepharitis
- Meibomian gland disease
- Congenital glaucoma
- Dry eye syndrome
- Corneal abrasion
- Corneal foreign body
- Tumor
- Foreign body
- Eyelid malposition
- Punctal stenosis
- Bell palsy
- Preseptal cellulitis
- Orbital abscess
- Orbital cellulitis

MANAGEMENT

Acquired NLDO does not benefit from nasolacrimal duct probing, and definitive treatment usually requires surgery. Temporizing conservative management consists of warm compresses and topical antibiotics if infection is suspected. In cases of dacryocystitis, the initial treatment for adults includes warm compresses, topical broad-spectrum antibiotic eye drops, and oral penicillinase-resistant antibiotics. Antibiotic choice is further guided by Gram stain and cultures. Topical antibiotics include trimethoprim sulfate and polymyxin B sulfate (Polytrim), tobramycin (AKTob, Tobrex), ciprofloxacin 0.3% (Ciloxan), and ofloxacin 0.3% (Ocuflox),[11] one drop every 1 to 6 hours. Systemic therapy may include cephalexin (Keflex), amoxicillin and clavulanate (Augmentin), or erythromycin (Erythrocin).[6] In the absence of mucopurulent drainage, prolonged use of topical antibiotics is not necessary.

As a general rule, acute dacryocystitis is managed medically. However, if a painful lacrimal sac abscess is pointing to a head, incision and drainage of the abscess may be beneficial. Once the episode of acute dacryocystitis has resolved, definitive treatment is lacrimal bypass surgery with dacryocystorhinostomy.

COMPLICATIONS

Acquired NLDO may progress to secondary infection, dacryocystitis, mucocele, pyocele, chronic conjunctivitis, preseptal and orbital cellulitis, or abscess formation. Systemic antibiotics are necessary in cases of abscess formation, ineffective topical antibiotic therapy, orbital cellulitis, or recurrent dacryocystitis.

INDICATIONS FOR REFERRAL OR HOSPITALIZATION

Adults with acquired NLDO should be referred to an oculoplastic surgeon for further evaluation and possible lacrimal bypass surgery (dacryocystorhinostomy), a procedure that is successful in up to 95% of cases. If acute dacryocystitis develops, patients should be referred to an ophthalmologist after antibiotic therapy is initiated. After the infection has resolved, definitive treatment is lacrimal bypass surgery. Older adults or frail patients may develop sepsis as a result of acute dacryocystitis. The presence of dacryocystitis or abscess with systemic signs of fever, malaise, or leukocytosis may require hospitalization for intravenous antibiotic therapy in seriously ill patients.

PATIENT AND FAMILY EDUCATION

Adult patients should be informed about the signs and symptoms of dacryocystitis in the setting of NLDO, including mucopurulent discharge, pain, redness, and fever. Patients should also understand that the definitive treatment of NLDO and dacryocystitis is surgery and that antibiotics are used to treat the infection but will not resolve the obstruction.

CHAPTER 77

PRESEPTAL AND ORBITAL CELLULITIS

Nathan Blessing • James T. Banta

DEFINITION AND EPIDEMIOLOGY

Periorbital infections are classically divided anatomically into whether the findings are isolated anterior to the orbital septum (preseptal cellulitis) or involve structures posterior to the orbital septum (orbital cellulitis). The distinction is critical because infection of the orbit with extension to the orbital apex and beyond can lead to rapid blindness and have potentially fatal consequences. Both disease entities are more common in children, with preseptal infection occurring much more frequently than orbital infection, but individuals of all ages can be affected.[1,2] Males are disproportionately affected compared with females at a ratio of 2:1, and the mean age is 7 years in both boys and girls.[3]

PATHOPHYSIOLOGY

Infection arises from three principle sources: local spread from adjacent structures such as the sinuses and lacrimal system, inoculation after local trauma such as skin lacerations or bug bites, and bacteremic spread from remote foci including the upper respiratory system, middle ear, and heart. As previously mentioned, cellulitis may exist anterior to the orbital septum, with the septum acting as a natural barrier to the passage of microorganisms; however, an initial preseptal cellulitis may spread to involve the orbit as well. There are several anatomic factors that predispose the orbit to infection. Veins in the midface are valveless, permitting the direct posterior spread of infectious organisms into structures such as sinus cavities. The paranasal sinuses surround the orbit inferiorly, medially, and superiorly, and the ethmoid sinus is separated from the orbit by the lamina papyracea, meaning "of paper" because the bone is paper-thin. Unsurprisingly, local spread from ethmoid sinusitis is the most common cause of orbital cellulitis in all age groups, and more than 90% of all cases of orbital cellulitis occur as a secondary extension of acute or chronic bacterial sinusitis.[1,4] Causative organisms are usually *Streptococcus* species or *Staphylococcus aureus* (including methicillin-resistant *S. aureus* [MRSA]), but *Haemophilus influenzae* (less common because of vaccination against *H. influenzae* type b), *Moraxella catarrhalis*, and the anaerobic bacteria of the upper respiratory tract may also be implicated.[5] In children, the majority of culture results are typically positive for staphylococci or streptococci, with the remainder being polymicrobial. Patients over the age of 15 are more likely to have polymicrobial infections. In immunocompromised or diabetic patients, a fungal cause, such as *Aspergillus* or *Mucor*, should be considered.[1]

CLINICAL PRESENTATION AND PHYSICAL EXAMINATION

Careful physical examination will elucidate key information regarding whether an infection is located anterior or posterior to the orbital septum and the severity of the infection. Preseptal cellulitis typically manifests with eyelid edema, warmth, and erythema that may be severe (Fig. 77-1). The eye is typically spared, without conjunctival injection or chemosis. In contrast, orbital cellulitis causes axial proptosis, lid swelling, conjunctival chemosis and injection, elevated intraocular pressure, and pain or restriction with eye movement (Fig. 77-2).[4] The patient may report decreased visual acuity and diplopia. Decreased visual acuity and an afferent pupillary defect (see Chapter 70) are suggestive of optic nerve compromise, one of the most feared complications of orbital cellulitis. Patients with both preseptal and postseptal infections may be febrile, but systemic malaise is typically associated with postseptal disease. A history of sinusitis, local cutaneous infection, trauma, or dental infection is common. The condition is typically unilateral. A history of neck stiffness or mental status change is worrisome for underlying meningitis. If trauma is implicated, the patient usually is seen 48 to 72 hours after the inciting event. However, in the presence of a retained foreign body, the clinical presentation of cellulitis can occur weeks to months after the injury.[5]

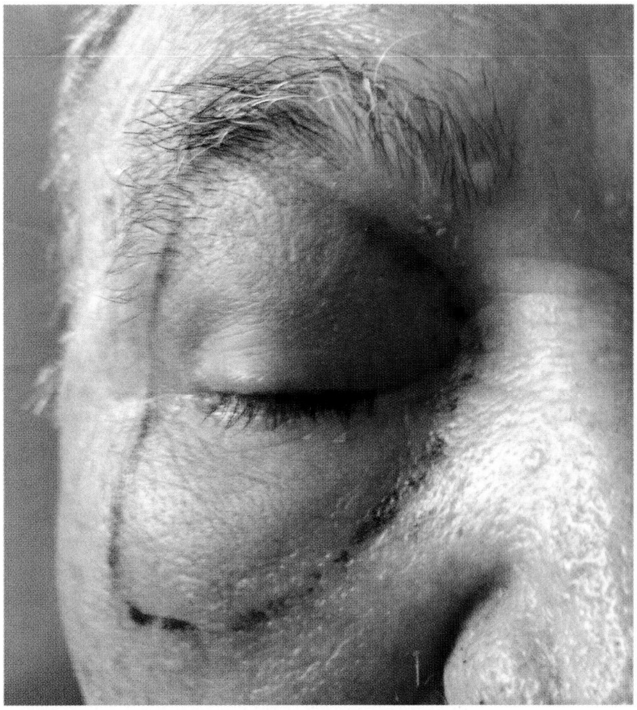

FIGURE 77-1 Warm, erythematous skin with sparing of the eye is typical of preseptal cellulitis. A skin marker can be used to outline the area of erythema and monitor the response to treatment.

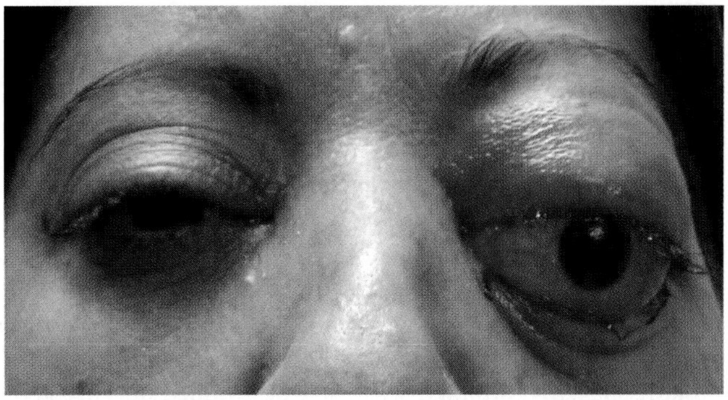

FIGURE 77-2 Orbital cellulitis often presents with a dramatic appearance of axial proptosis, chemosis, and restricted ocular motility. This is an emergency and requires immediate ophthalmic care.

A thorough examination should include an evaluation of the patient's vital signs, mental status, neck flexibility, visual acuity (including color vision), pupillary response, and extraocular muscle function (cranial nerves III, IV, XI) as well as any pain elicited with extraocular movements. If possible, intraocular pressure should be measured because venous congestion from orbital inflammation may lead to elevated pressures. The globe and ocular adnexa should be inspected for swelling, redness, focal tenderness, hypoesthesia, and fluctuance or drainage. Close inspection should be undertaken to rule out trauma, foreign bodies, or a focal source of infection such as dacryocystitis or eyelid abscess. In diabetic or immunocompromised patients a black eschar located in the nasal cavity or hard palate may herald underlying fungal infection.

DIAGNOSTICS

An accurate history and physical examination will provide most of the information required to reach a diagnosis. All patients with suspected orbital cellulitis should undergo a computed tomography (CT) scan of the orbits and paranasal sinuses (with contrast if possible) to confirm the diagnosis. Pertinent CT scan findings include signs of sinusitis (mucosal wall thickening, opacification, air-fluid levels), a foreign body, orbital fat stranding, and signs of periosteal abscess (a heterogeneous or homogeneous collection in the subperiosteal space surrounded by an enhancing border suggestive of pus or fluid). CT may also show displacement of extraconal fat or muscle as well as diffuse enhancement of the orbit.[6] Given that approximately 75% of patients with orbital cellulitis develop leukocytosis, a complete blood count (CBC) with differential is indicated. Blood cultures may be helpful when bacteremia is suspected, and culture specimens should be taken from any drainage or abscess that is directly accessible. However, imaging should not be delayed to perform any of the aforementioned ancillary tests.

DIAGNOSTICS

Preseptal and Orbital Cellulitis

LABORATORY

CBC with differential
Specimen samples for Gram stain, culture with sensitivity
Blood cultures

IMAGING

CT scan of the orbits and sinuses (with contrast if possible)

DIFFERENTIAL DIAGNOSIS

Preseptal and Orbital Cellulitis

INFLAMMATORY

- Thyroid eye disease
- Idiopathic orbital inflammatory syndrome (orbital pseudotumor)
- Sarcoidosis
- Granulomatosis with polyangiitis (formerly Wegener granulomatosis)
- Severe allergies
- Chalazion
- Pyogenic granuloma

INFECTIOUS

- Viral conjunctivitis
- Varicella zoster
- Dacryocystitis
- Dacryoadenitis
- Mucormycosis
- Cavernous sinus thrombosis

NEOPLASTIC

- Metastasis
- Rhabdomyosarcoma
- Lymphoma
- Cavernous hemangioma
- Optic nerve glioma

TRAUMATIC

- Orbital fracture
- Retrobulbar hemorrhage
- Foreign body
- Insect bites

MALFORMATIONS

- Cavernous hemangioma
- Lymphangioma
- Varix
- Buphthalmos and nanophthalmos

DIFFERENTIAL DIAGNOSIS

Both infectious and noninfectious orbital disease may cause eyelid swelling, bulging of one or both eyes, and double vision. Broadly speaking, orbital disease may be grouped into five general categories including inflammatory, infectious, neoplastic (both benign and malignant), traumatic, and related to malformation (e.g., congenital or vascular).

MANAGEMENT

Urgent hospitalization, imaging, and intravenous antibiotics are indicated for any patient suspected of having orbital cellulitis.

Referral to an ophthalmologist is indicated for preseptal cellulitis that fails to respond to initial therapy within 24 hours.

Appropriate oral therapy for preseptal cellulitis includes broad-spectrum antibiotics such as a third-generation cephalosporin or amoxicillin-clavulanate. In suspected MRSA infections, drugs such as clindamycin, doxycycline, and double-strength trimethoprim-sulfamethoxazole are effective. A follow-up evaluation should be scheduled within 12 to 24 hours to monitor for signs of progression or lack of response to antibiotic therapy. Regardless of age, patients with significant systemic symptoms, cellulitis that fails to respond to oral antibiotics, or possible orbital cellulitis should be referred to an ophthalmologist or otolaryngologist for hospitalization, urgent imaging, and intravenous antibiotic therapy. Patients are monitored closely during the first 24 to 48 hours of hospitalization for any clinical deterioration, which could suggest abscess formation or intracranial extension that may necessitate surgical intervention.[1,7]

Given the likelihood of the primary care provider to care for patients who are diabetic (or, less commonly, immunocompromised), it is imperative to identify a possible fungal cause. The most feared complication, rhino-orbital mucormycosis, can progress rapidly; the earliest signs include apical boring pain, increased cellulitis, proptosis, and abrupt visual failure. Early tissue biopsy and radical excision with both local antifungal irrigation and systemic antifungal administration may be both sight saving and lifesaving, underscoring the importance of aggressive treatment and prompt referral to an ophthalmologist.[8]

LIFE SPAN CONSIDERATIONS

Older adults and immunocompromised individuals may not demonstrate the same degree of inflammatory signs and may not be febrile in spite of a severe underlying infection; a heightened degree of suspicion is necessary to appropriately manage these individuals.[1]

COMPLICATIONS

Orbital cellulitis is a potentially fatal condition and blindness may occur in up to 11% of patients, necessitating prompt clinical identification of this disorder. Other complications include cavernous sinus thrombosis; central retinal artery or vein thrombosis; subperiosteal, orbital, epidural, subdural, or brain abscess; and optic neuropathy.[1,2,4]

INDICATIONS FOR REFERRAL OR HOSPITALIZATION

Patients with decreased visual acuity, proptosis, diplopia, restricted ocular movement, globe involvement, systemic symptoms, or neurologic signs should be referred to an ophthalmologist emergently or hospitalized for emergent imaging. Patients with preseptal cellulitis treated with oral antibiotics that does not improve within 24 hours should also be referred to an ophthalmologist. Patients with documented orbital cellulitis require hospitalization for initiation of intravenous antibiotics, imaging, and other supportive therapy as indicated.

PATIENT AND FAMILY EDUCATION

When oral antibiotic therapy is prescribed, patients should be instructed to return before their scheduled follow-up visit (in 12 to 24 hours) if their symptoms increase in severity. They should also be reminded to complete the full course of antibiotic therapy and to return before the end of therapy if signs and symptoms do not continue to improve or if there is any worsening of the condition. Patients and families should be informed that fever, lethargy, and irritability are signs of possible sepsis or meningitis.

EDUCATION AND HEALTH PROMOTION

Risk factors for frequent sinus infections, such as smoking and untreated allergic rhinitis, should be addressed. Diabetes is a risk factor for the development of more serious fungal infections and should be controlled.

CHAPTER 78

PINGUECULA AND PTERYGIUM

Eric D. Hansen • James T. Banta

DEFINITION AND EPIDEMIOLOGY

Pinguecula and pterygium are two of the most common ocular surface abnormalities with which patients visit primary care providers. Pingueculae are benign, elevated lesions of the bulbar conjunctiva, often located adjacent to the cornea. Pterygia are similarly benign and originate in the conjunctiva but have grown onto the surface of the cornea. The word *pterygium* derives its origin from the Greek word *pterygion* meaning "small wing"—an apt name because of the winglike shape the growth displays on the cornea. Both pingueculae and pterygia usually grow slowly and commonly manifest in patients 20 to 50 years of age. They are more common in lower latitudes with greater sun exposure.

PATHOPHYSIOLOGY

Pingueculae and pterygia have both degenerative and proliferative components. Pathologic analysis reveals fibrovascular proliferation and disruption of the basement membrane of the conjunctival epithelium along with basophilic and elastotic degeneration of the substantia propria. Corneal involvement in pterygia includes infiltration of the Bowman layer, a strong layer of collagen directly beneath the corneal epithelium. Disruption of this layer can lead to scarring and focal opacification of cornea.

Although the pathogenesis of these entities is multifactorial and incompletely understood, exposure to ultraviolet (UV) light, particularly UVB, has been associated with development of pterygia.[1,2] Heredity and chronic conjunctival inflammation also may contribute.[3,4] Pingueculae and pterygia have no common systemic associations, although they may occur more frequently in conditions that confer a proclivity for skin neoplasms, such as xeroderma pigmentosum. However, despite this association and the link to UV light exposure, pterygia and pingueculae carry no significant malignant potential. In addition, because they are degenerative processes, development before the age of 20 years is very unusual.

CLINICAL PRESENTATION

Both pingueculae and pterygia arise and grow slowly over the course of years. Common complaints on the part of the patient include dryness, irritation, redness, foreign body sensation, and itching, as well as the cosmetic appearance of the lesion itself. Severe dryness from tear film irregularity induced by the lesion may cause intermittent blurry vision. In more advanced stages of disease, pterygia may cause decreased vision by two other mechanisms: astigmatism, which is irregularity of the corneal shape as a result of the physical presence of the pterygium; and obstruction of the visual axis by extension of the lesion into the central cornea.

PHYSICAL EXAMINATION

The diagnosis of pinguecula and pterygium is often made clinically. Most lesions are detectable with the naked eye. The overwhelming majority of lesions appear in the horizontal meridian at either the 3-o'clock or 9-o'clock position, more frequently nasally than temporally. A single eye may have a pinguecula or a pterygium at both positions or a combination of a pinguecula at one and a pterygium at the other.

Pingueculae appear as elevated, yellowish-white lesions immediately adjacent to but not encroaching on the cornea. They do not typically have abnormal vasculature or large feeder vessels and do not bleed spontaneously. Pingueculitis, or inflammation of a pinguecula, may occur, in which case the lesion may be pinkish with dilated blood vessels over and surrounding it (Fig. 78-1). Patients typically report increased redness and irritation in the area.

Pterygia arise from preexisting pingueculae. They have a base in the conjunctiva with an extension of tissue onto the cornea (Fig. 78-2). Pterygia commonly extend only a millimeter or two onto the cornea; however, in advanced states they can involve a large portion of the cornea including the central visual axis. Mild elevation is typically seen. The corneal aspect of a pterygium ranges in coloration from white to clear and may be visible only by the change in corneal contour and the blood vessels that track from the conjunctival base. Similar to a pinguecula, an inflamed

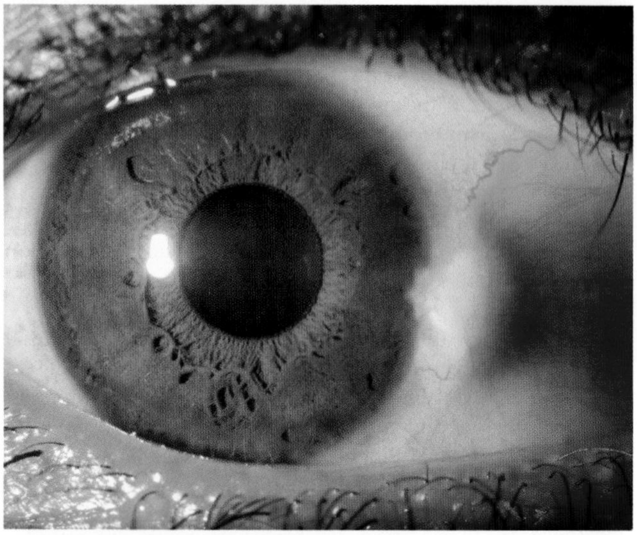

FIGURE 78-1 An elevated, inflamed pinguecula can cause foreign body sensation and chronic redness.

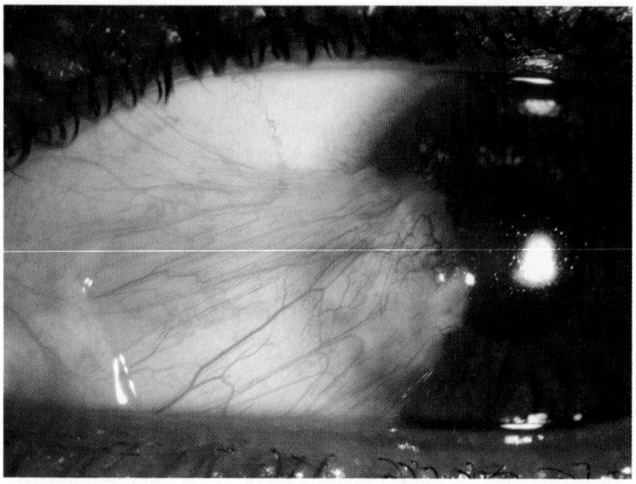

FIGURE 78-2 Typical appearance of a medium-sized pterygium.

pterygium will have overlying dilated blood vessels and a pink or reddish hue.

DIAGNOSTICS

Slit-lamp examination provides the best view of the ocular surface, but if it is unavailable, careful examination with the naked eye under adequate lighting is usually sufficient. Orienting the lighting obliquely may reveal subtle differences in elevation and coloration.

In differentiating pingueculae and pterygia from other ocular surface abnormalities, examination of the cornea under a cobalt blue light after fluorescein staining can be helpful. Fluorescein staining allows identification of epithelial defects on both the cornea and conjunctiva, and because neither pingueculae nor pterygia involve epithelial breakdown, they do not stain strongly with fluorescein. In addition, corneal epithelial defects often cause more acute pain and photophobia.

DIAGNOSTICS

Pinguecula and Pterygium

Initial examination
Fluorescein stain*

*If indicated.

DIFFERENTIAL DIAGNOSIS

It is important to keep in mind that pterygia and pingueculae may coexist with other, more urgent ocular lesions. Any evaluation of acute red eye or eye pain should include an assessment for corneal ulcers, epithelial defects, scleritis, and foreign bodies. As mentioned earlier, fluorescein staining will aid in differentiating between conditions. Pterygia and pingueculae grow very slowly and do not cause acute symptoms other than local irritation and redness. They do not cause fever, lymphadenopathy, severe pain, purulence, or rapid vision loss.

Other ocular surface lesions can resemble pterygia or pingueculae, such as squamous neoplasms, dermoids, and even lymphomas; however, the rarity of these lesions should be kept in mind. A lesion typical for a pterygium or pinguecula in its appearance, location, and time course is highly unlikely to be anything else.

DIFFERENTIAL DIAGNOSIS

Pinguecula and Pterygium

- Corneal ulcer
- Scleritis
- Episcleritis
- Conjunctivitis
- Epithelial defect
- Foreign body
- Limbal stem cell deficiency
- Conjunctival dermoid
- Squamous neoplasm
- Lymphoma

MANAGEMENT

Treatment should initially be directed toward improvement of symptoms and prevention. Dry eye, foreign body sensation, itchiness, and redness typically respond well to artificial tear drops, which may be purchased over the counter and are very well tolerated. They may be used as frequently as needed and do not interfere with other medications. UV protection in the form of wide-brimmed hats and sunglasses with UVB protection should be advised. Other over-the-counter eye drops, such as tetrahydrozoline (Visine) and naphazoline (Clear Eyes), induce vasoconstriction in the conjunctiva and should be avoided because their chronic use can cause rebound inflammation and worsening redness.

Inflamed pterygia or pingueculae respond well to a short course of topical steroid drops, such as loteprednol (Lotemax) or fluorometholone (FML). These particular topical steroids are preferred because of lower risk of complications such as elevation of intraocular pressure as compared with other steroid formulations. Corneal ulcers and epithelial defects should be definitively ruled out before anti-inflammatory treatment is started, and the treatment should not extend beyond 4 to 7 days without ophthalmic consultation. A general dosage guideline for these topical medications is four times daily for 4 to 7 days.

INDICATIONS FOR REFERRAL

An inflamed eye that has not responded within a few days should prompt a nonurgent ophthalmic examination. On occasion, pterygia require excisional surgery. The primary indications for surgery are (1) chronic pain and redness refractory to conservative therapy and (2) visual compromise as a result of induced astigmatism or obscuration of the visual axis. Recurrence and excessive scarring are the most common complications of excision.[5] The recurrence rate is reduced by placement of a conjunctival autograft (typically harvested from the superior conjunctiva of the same eye) or topical application of an antimetabolite intraoperatively (e.g., mitomycin C). Novel adjuvant management strategies targeting inflammation and angiogenesis are being developed and incorporated in efforts to reduce recurrence—a frustrating and not infrequent complication for both patients and providers.[4]

PATIENT EDUCATION AND HEALTH PROMOTION

Patients who spend a lot of time outdoors or those with preexisting pterygia and pingueculae should be encouraged to wear sunglasses with UV filters and wide-brimmed hats to reduce exposure to UV light.

CHAPTER 79

TRAUMATIC OCULAR DISORDERS

Ryan C. Young • James T. Banta

DEFINITION

Ocular trauma encompasses a number of physical injuries, both mechanical and chemical, sustained by the eye (globe) and ocular adnexa. These tissues can sustain myriad different injuries, some of which are listed in Box 79-1. For nonophthalmologists, these injuries may seem complex and foreign. To facilitate classification and communication among health care professionals, a terminology system was devised to allow a standardized description and classification of ocular trauma.[1,2] Table 79-1 lists the standard definitions that are used to describe traumatic ocular injuries.[3]

The most vital distinction is between open and closed globe injuries. This information is crucial because it determines the clinical management of the patient and provides important prognostic information.[4] If the patient has not sustained a full-thickness injury, then the patient has a *closed* globe trauma. If there is a full-thickness wound, it is an *open* globe trauma. Closed globe trauma is further divided into contusions and lamellar lacerations. Contusions are the most common form of ocular injury and occur when the eye is impacted but the wall of the eye remains intact. The sequelae of an ocular contusion are vast and include corneal abrasion, hyphema, and iridodialysis. A *lamellar laceration* refers to a partial-thickness wound of the eye wall, but the integrity of the globe is maintained.

Full-thickness injuries are often inappropriately described and lead to confusion between a referring provider and the ophthalmologist. Too often, both primary care providers and ophthalmologists describe a patient who has sustained a full-thickness injury to the globe as having a "ruptured globe." This is correct only if the person has sustained an ocular contusion (typically with a blunt object) resulting in a *rupture* of the eye wall. Common mechanisms for a ruptured globe include high-velocity projectiles (e.g., racquetball, bungee cord) and assault (e.g., fist, bat, paintball). These injuries are highly destructive to intraocular contents and have a guarded prognosis in all instances. By contrast, if a sharp object creates a full-thickness eye wall injury, it is classified as a laceration. Common mechanisms of lacerations include work-related activities (e.g., cutting tile, landscaping) and accidents (e.g., children playing with scissors). Lacerations can be further divided into penetrating injuries, perforating injuries, and intraocular foreign bodies. *Penetrating* injuries penetrate through the eye wall without an exit wound, whereas *perforating* injuries have both an entry and an exit wound. An *intraocular foreign body* is present when a portion of the insulting object enters and remains in the eye.

BOX 79-1

Manifestations of Ocular Trauma

ADNEXA AND ORBIT

- Eyelid laceration
- Orbital fracture
- Retrobulbar hemorrhage
- Traumatic optic neuropathy
- Orbital foreign body

CORNEA AND ANTERIOR SEGMENT

- Chemical burn
- Corneal abrasion
- Corneal or conjunctival foreign body
- Conjunctival laceration
- Subconjunctival hemorrhage
- Corneal laceration
- Traumatic iritis
- Hyphema
- Iridodialysis and cyclodialysis
- Traumatic glaucoma

POSTERIOR SEGMENT

- Vitreous hemorrhage
- Commotio retinae
- Traumatic choroidal rupture
- Chorioretinitis sclopetaria
- Purtscher retinopathy
- Shaken baby syndrome

COMBINED OR MIXED

- Globe laceration or rupture
- Intraocular foreign body

EPIDEMIOLOGY

The annual number of eye injuries treated by medical personnel was estimated at nearly 2 million by a large national survey.[5] The Baltimore Eye Survey reported a cumulative lifetime prevalence of eye injury of 14.4% in the general population of an urban area.[6] McGwin and colleagues estimated the rate of injury to be 6.98 injuries per 1000 persons. Of those injuries, 50.7% were treated in emergency departments, 38.7% in private offices of physicians, 8.1% in outpatient facilities, and 2.5% within inpatient facilities. Not surprisingly, most injuries were sustained by men younger than 30 years.[5,7] The most commonly encountered injuries were superficial injuries of the eye and adnexa and foreign bodies on the ocular surface.[5]

TABLE 79-1 Birmingham Eye Trauma Terminology

Term	Definition	Explanation
Eye wall	Sclera and cornea	Although the eye wall technically has three coats posterior to the limbus, for clinical and practical purposes, violation of only the most external structure is taken into consideration.
Closed globe injury	No full-thickness wound of the eye wall	
Open globe injury	Full-thickness wound of the eye wall	
Contusion	No (full-thickness) wound of the eye wall	The injury results from direct energy delivery by the object or from the changes in the shape of the globe.
Lamellar laceration	Partial-thickness wound of the eye wall	The wound of the eye wall is not "through" but "into."
Rupture	Full-thickness wound of the eye wall caused by a blunt object	Because the eye is filled with incompressible liquid, the impact results in momentary increase of the intraocular pressure. The eye wall yields at its weakest point (at the impact site or elsewhere; e.g., an old cataract wound dehisces even though the impact occurred elsewhere). The actual wound is caused by an inside-out mechanism.
Laceration	Full-thickness wound of the eye wall caused by a sharp object	The wound occurs at the impact site by an outside-in mechanism.
Penetrating injury	Entrance wound	If more than one wound is present, each must have been caused by a different agent.
Intraocular foreign body	Retained foreign object(s)	This is technically a penetrating injury but grouped separately because of different clinical implications.
Perforating injury	Entrance and exit wounds	Both wounds are caused by the same agent.

Modified from Kuhn F, Morris R, Witherspoon CD: Birmingham Eye Trauma Terminology (BETT): terminology and classification of mechanical eye injuries, *Ophthalmol Clin North Am* 15:139-143, 2002.

An interesting aspect of ocular trauma is its recurrent nature. In the Beaver Dam Eye Study, Wong and coworkers noted that an initial episode of ocular trauma increased the likelihood of recurrent trauma in the next 5 years by a factor of 3.27.[8] The rates of injury were also higher among blue collar and farm workers compared with white collar workers, with odds ratios of 1.58 and 1.32, respectively. Epidemiologic studies such as these assist in identifying at-risk populations and creating appropriate prevention strategies. For example, Dannenberg and associates found in their study of penetrating ocular trauma in the workplace that only 6% of the injured were wearing protective eyewear at the time of their injury,[9] clearly highlighting the need for protective eyewear in high-risk settings.

Children are not immune to ocular trauma. Open globe injuries are among the most serious of ocular injuries, and one study has shown that up to 43% of these injuries are sustained in patients younger than 18 years.[10] A large study of pediatric globe injuries in Los Angeles demonstrated that sharp objects cause the majority of injuries (67%) and that most injuries occur at home (72%).[11]

PATHOPHYSIOLOGY

Mechanical Injuries

When mechanical energy is imparted to the eye, the manner in which it is delivered and the amount imparted to the eye largely determine the type and degree of injury.[12] Minor trauma may cause only limited injuries, such as subconjunctival hemorrhage, superficial abrasions of the periocular skin, painful abrasions of the cornea, or lacerations of the conjunctiva.

Ocular trauma associated with a higher level of mechanical energy is often mitigated by the size of the object. Large objects will often not fit in the confines of the orbital rim within which the globe rests. Thus a large blunt object with high mechanical energy may create a blowout fracture of the thin orbital walls as a result of the pressure on the orbital rim and contents. The thin orbital bones act as a "crumple zone," allowing most of the energy to be absorbed by the orbit while sparing the eye. However, a similar amount of energy imparted by a smaller blunt object that fits in the confines of the orbital rim can cause more severe injuries, such as hyphema (caused by shearing of iris blood vessels), iridodialysis (disinsertion of the iris root), or even devastating rupture of the globe.

A globe rupture results when the eye is bluntly impacted and cannot sustain the forces imparted. Because the eye contains incompressible fluids, the sudden increase in pressure from a mechanical trauma can cause an enormous transfer of energy to the eye wall. The eye wall may rupture if the pressure is high enough at weak points, such as previous surgical sites, the insertions of the extraocular muscles, or the limbus (junction of the cornea and sclera). Ruptures often cause devastating visual loss secondary to retinal detachments, massive hemorrhage, loss of intraocular contents, intraocular infections, and a number of other complications.

Mechanical energy imparted from sharp objects typically results in lacerations of the eye wall. In contrast to ruptures, these injuries are sustained at the site of impact and mechanically disrupt the eye wall at that location. These injuries can be equally devastating but often have a better prognosis, especially if the injury is confined to the anterior segment of the eye.

Chemical Injuries

Chemical injuries to the eye depend on the nature of the chemical, the duration of exposure, and the degree of ocular penetration. Acids can be quite destructive to the ocular surface because the dissociated anions of the acid lead to denaturation and coagulation of the ocular proteins. Although destructive, the eye proteins act as an acid buffer to limit ocular penetration. By contrast, alkaline substances release hydroxyl ions that saponify cell membranes and cations that interact with the structural proteins of the eye wall. Both allow deeper ocular penetration of the agents and more extensive intraocular injuries. The initial treatment of any chemical exposure is immediate, copious irrigation with normal saline.

CLINICAL PRESENTATION

The clinical presentation of eye trauma is highly variable. Given this variability, patients may have multiple presenting symptoms including pain, redness, decreased vision, diplopia, and photophobia. The most commonly encountered traumatic injuries are superficial injury of the adnexa and external eye (e.g., corneal abrasion, subconjunctival hemorrhage) and a foreign body on the ocular surface.[5] These patients typically have an abrupt onset of redness, foreign body sensation, tearing, and photophobia. A complaint of pain with blinking is typical of a corneal or conjunctival foreign body.

Contusive trauma may affect the orbit or the globe itself. Patients who sustain orbital fractures may acutely report diplopia, pain with eye movement, hypesthesia of the cheek and upper lip, and subcutaneous or conjunctival emphysema. A hyphema is a layered collection of blood in the anterior chamber of the eye (Fig. 79-1) and is a common manifestation of contusive ocular injury. In general, patients report blurred vision and pain. Elevated intraocular pressure is the most feared complication and can lead to permanent loss of vision.

Open globe trauma usually is associated with a history of projectile injury or severe contusion of the eye (see Fig. 79-2). Not surprisingly, the clinical presentation of an open globe can be subtle or exceedingly obvious. A very high index of suspicion should be maintained, particularly in patients with a high-risk profile (e.g., construction, landscaping, mechanic).

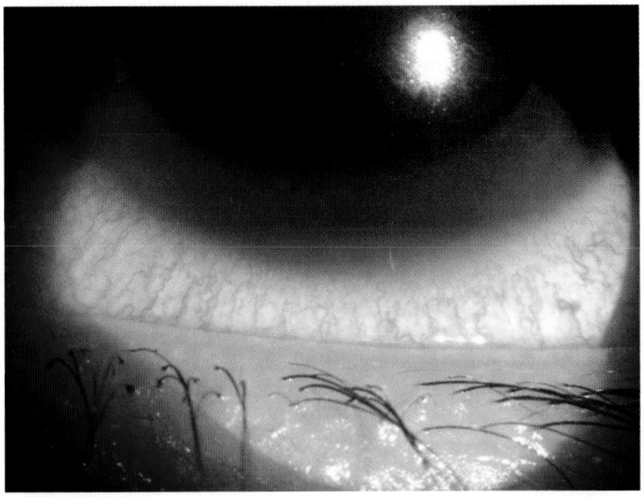

FIGURE 79-1 A small layered hyphema after an ocular contusion.

In any situation in which there is suspected or potential globe rupture, it is imperative not to touch or to manipulate the eye. If potential globe rupture is suspected, place a protective shield over the eye and refer the patient to an ophthalmologist immediately.

PHYSICAL EXAMINATION

Important elements of the examination are detailed in Chapter 70. Whereas intraocular pressure measurement and slit-lamp microscopy may not always be available, the other elements of the examination should be available in most clinic or emergency departments, and the information gathered will be invaluable to the accepting physician should the patient require referral. Measurement of the intraocular pressure is contraindicated if there is a possibility of an open globe injury.

With use of a bright light source (e.g., flashlight, penlight), the ocular surface and anterior chamber should be visualized to check the integrity of anterior segment structures. Frequent findings with severe trauma include subconjunctival hemorrhage, iris defects, hyphema, lens dislocation, and conjunctival chemosis. Periorbital lacerations should be explored to rule out foreign bodies or potential penetration sites. Prolapsed uveal contents, a shallow anterior chamber, or a more subtle finding such as an eccentric pupil often indicates a full-thickness injury to the globe. If a laceration or rupture is suspected, a protective eye shield rather than a patch should be placed over the eye. The goal is to eliminate any undue pressure on the injured globe.

DIAGNOSTICS

Once an adequate examination has been performed (see chapter 70), there are several diagnostic tools that can aid in establishing a diagnosis. If a laceration of the cornea is suspected, a Seidel test can be performed. A moistened fluorescein strip is liberally applied to the ocular surface. When it is viewed with a cobalt blue light source, a laceration is confirmed if a stream of aqueous disrupts the thick layer of fluorescein. Imaging studies are often very helpful and should be considered in eye injuries

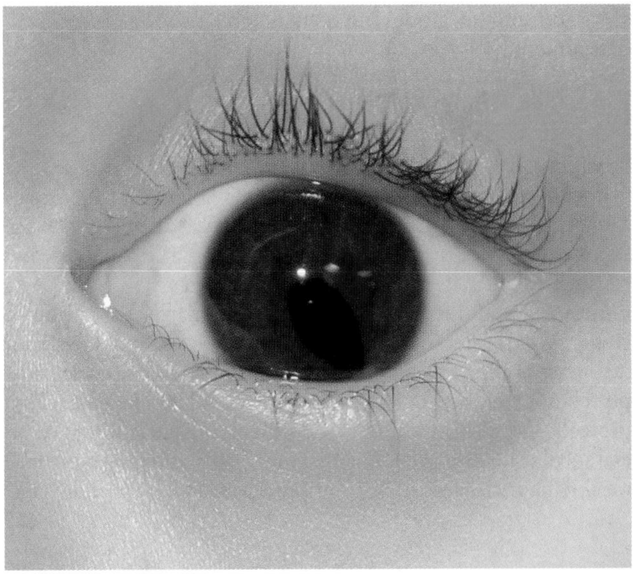

FIGURE 79-2 Peaking of the pupil after ocular trauma is indicative of an open globe injury and should lead to immediate referral to an ophthalmologist.

DIAGNOSTICS

Ocular Trauma

Seidel test
Ultrasound
CT scan
MRI

that have the potential for an intraocular foreign body. Computed tomography (CT) scan is the gold standard for eye injuries. In one study, CT was shown to be 73% sensitive and 95% specific for detection of open globe injuries.[13] The CT scan should include thin coronal and axial cuts (1 to 2 mm) of both orbits. This is especially important when an intraocular foreign body is suspected. CT is also vital in assessing the integrity of the bony orbit when orbital fractures are suspected. Magnetic resonance imaging (MRI) is less useful in the acute management of ocular trauma because it is less helpful in defining orbital bone trauma and is contraindicated if a metallic foreign body is suspected.

DIFFERENTIAL DIAGNOSIS

DIFFERENTIAL DIAGNOSIS

Ocular Trauma

- Foreign body
- Corneal abrasion
- Orbital fracture
- Globe rupture
- Hyphema
- Detached retina
- Thermal burns
- Radiation keratitis
- Chemical injury
- Subconjunctival hemorrhage

The manifestations of ocular trauma are numerous and varied. They range from mildly uncomfortable, self-limited lesions to potentially blinding and even systemically threatening conditions. Many of these lesions are listed in Box 79-1. One of the key elements to formation of a differential diagnosis is an attempt to determine which structures in the eye have been traumatized. Injuries restricted to the lids, conjunctiva, and superficial cornea have a very different differential diagnosis including more benign pathologic processes, such as corneal abrasion and subconjunctival hemorrhage. In contrast, more severe injuries open the differential diagnosis to more serious pathologic processes, such as ruptured globe, intraocular foreign body, and retinal detachment.

MANAGEMENT AND INDICATIONS FOR REFERRAL

Small corneal abrasions and subconjunctival hemorrhages are generally self-limited and do not require referral if further injury can be ruled out. Patients with corneal foreign bodies should be referred, even if the foreign body is partially removed, because residual material (e.g., rust ring) needs to be completely removed. Conditions that require an immediate intervention or emergency transfer of care to an ophthalmologist include chemical injury (after copious irrigation of the ocular surface), suspected open globe injury (after CT imaging and placement of a protective shield), orbital fractures involving entrapment of an extraocular muscle (after CT imaging), retrobulbar hemorrhage producing increased intraocular pressure, vitreous hemorrhage, large complex corneal abrasions, eyelid lacerations, hyphema, and unexplained visual loss after trauma.

COMPLICATIONS

Infections can sometimes complicate chemical injuries, lacerations of the periocular adnexa, and partial-thickness or full-thickness lacerations of the globe. A particularly hazardous complication is the development of post-traumatic endophthalmitis (intraocular infection) after open globe injury. Several large studies have shown that endophthalmitis can complicate open globe injuries with an incidence ranging from 6.8% to 11.9%.[14,15] Another serious complication is the development of retinal detachment in open and closed globe injuries. Serious chemical injuries are often complicated by the destruction of the normal ocular surface and intraocular structures, leading to corneal opacification and severe glaucoma. Hyphema can be complicated by glaucoma and corneal blood staining.

LIFE SPAN CONSIDERATIONS

Ocular trauma can have a debilitating effect on those who sustain it. It is estimated by the U.S. Eye Injury Registry that 500,000 years of eyesight are lost annually as a result of ocular trauma.[16] In addition, a total of approximately 4 billion dollars annually in direct costs has been attributed to workplace eye injuries alone.[16] The lifetime prevalence of sustaining an eye injury regardless of severity is approximately 20%.[6,8] This number of injuries highlights the importance of instituting preventive measures.

EDUCATION AND HEALTH PROMOTION

Extensive collection of epidemiologic data by researchers and organizations such as the U.S. Eye Injury Registry and Prevent Blindness has led to a better understanding of when and where eye injuries occur. It now behooves clinicians and employers to educate their patients and workers to implement the consistent use of protective devices. Protective eyewear has been shown to be an effective deterrent to ocular injury on the battlefield, in the workplace, in the sports arena, and at numerous other locations.[17,18] At a minimum, 2-mm polycarbonate safety glasses with side shields should be used for all high-risk activities (e.g., landscaping, construction, impact sports). For even higher-risk activities, such as hammering metal on metal or grinding, polycarbonate goggles should be used because foreign bodies can still reach the eye around spectacle lenses. Eyewash stations should be available in all workplaces in which splash injuries or chemical exposures are possible.

REFERENCES

For a full list of references, scan the QR code or visit http://booksite.elsevier.com/9780323355018

PART 7

Evaluation and Management of Ear Disorders

CHAPTER 80

AURICULAR DISORDERS

Terry Mahan Buttaro

DEFINITION AND EPIDEMIOLOGY

Auricular disorders are conditions that affect the external ear. The incidence and prevalence of the individual conditions vary. The auricular disorder may be a secondary issue or may be discovered during the physical examination. Auricular disorders may be benign conditions associated with other disease processes, may be related to cultural practices such as body piercing, or may be a symptom of a serious illness that requires immediate referral and treatment.

Certain disease processes are associated with specific abnormalities of the auricle. Patients with Addison disease may have calcification of the cartilage. The nodules of Hansen disease may appear on the earlobe and may initially be noticed as multiple nodules on the ear and face. Patients with chronic arthritis may have hard nodules develop in the auricle. These rheumatoid nodules are usually accompanied by similar nodules on the hands, elbows, knees, or heels. Auricular pain, erythema, and edema can be associated with relapsing polychondritis, a rheumatologic disorder that affects the cartilage of the ears, nose, and laryngobronchial system.[1,2] Relapsing polychondritis is often related to other disorders (e.g., systemic vasculitis or systemic lupus erythematosus) but can be related to nonrheumatologic disorders also (e.g., primary biliary cirrhosis, Hashimoto thyroiditis, or myelodysplasia).[2] Hearing loss, cardiac abnormalities, and glomerulonephritis are associated with relapsing polychondritis, which, although not common, can affect people of all ages.[2]

A more common auricular disorder is tophi: painless, hard or gritty, and irregular uric acid crystal deposits in the auricle. They form in relation to high uric acid levels. Pressure exerted on tophi may result in the expulsion of a white crystalline substance.

Injuries and infections are the more common auricular disorders seen in primary care offices. A hematoma of the auricle occurs in response to blood disorders or trauma. A bluish-tinged hematoma can develop in the pinna after an injury. This type of lesion may be accompanied by laceration and require incision and drainage by an ear, nose, and throat surgeon. If the lesion is not drained, the resultant deformity is commonly referred to as cauliflower ear.[3]

Other common auricular problems include infections and tears related to earlobe and helix piercing. Keloids, hypertrophic scar tissue that is not cosmetically acceptable but is otherwise benign, can also occur at the pierced site.[4] Keloids occur more often in dark-skinned people.[4] Multiple helix piercing can cause a perforation-like appearance.

Chondrodermatitis nodularis helicis is a benign, chronically inflamed lesion, usually found on the helix or antihelix.[5] The lesion most often affects elders, men more often than women, and is painful and possibly crusting. A shave biopsy is necessary to distinguish the lesion from carcinoma.[5] Photodynamic therapy (PDT), cryotherapy, intralesional steroid injection, electrodessication, and nodular excision are potentially successful treatment modalities.[5]

Malignant otitis externa is a severe form of otitis externa. It results in a severely edematous, erythematous, and tender auricle. It can quickly dissect through fascial planes and lead to a life-threatening infection of the head and face. It is most likely to occur in patients with diabetes and in those who have compromised immune systems. The causative organism is usually *Pseudomonas aeruginosa*, especially in people with diabetes.[6]

Skin cancer is probably the most common significant auricular disorder seen in primary care. Basal cell carcinoma (BCC) is the most common form of skin cancer found on the auricle and the least likely to be malignant. It is a slowly growing cancer often found in sun-exposed areas, such as the top of the auricle.[7] BCC is found more often in older persons, in fair-skinned patients, and in patients who have a history of sun exposure. A shiny, irregular, painless lesion, this form of cancer rarely metastasizes, but in some cases BCC can be invasive and thus concerning.[7] Squamous cell carcinoma (SCC) is also commonly found on the auricle, usually in fair-skinned patients and in patients with a history of sun exposure. The typical lesion has a raised, crusted border around a center ulcer. SCC is a more serious form of skin cancer, although still relatively benign compared with melanoma. SCC can potentially metastasize to regional lymph nodes and cause death.[7]

PATHOPHYSIOLOGY

The auricle is the external ear structure that is composed chiefly of cartilage covered by skin. It is firm and elastic. It is divided into three parts: the top portion is the helix, the midsection is the antihelix, and the lower portion is the lobe. The function of the outer ear is to aid in receiving sound waves from the environment.

CLINICAL PRESENTATION

The presentation of auricular disorders is myriad and depends on the underlying cause of the disorder. Often, the patient is being seen for a general examination or follow-up. The complaint related to an auricular disorder is usually a minor issue, but the parameters of the disorder should be noted and include the onset, duration, and intensity of any symptoms. Any medications, treatments, or remedies that have been used on the auricle or systemically should also be documented, as should all related symptoms and past history of treatments and outcomes. For tears and infection, the patient may be seen after a specific episode of trauma or with an erythematous, tender earlobe. Malignant otitis externa may manifest as a sequela to an infection or a respiratory illness and most often occurs in immunosuppressed or diabetic patients.[6] A detailed history and physical examination aid the diagnosis.

PHYSICAL EXAMINATION

A complete inspection and palpation of the auricle form the basis for evaluation. The top of the auricle crosses a line drawn from the occiput to the corner of the eye. The ears of neonates are usually flat; however, in older infants, this may indicate persistent side lying. Protruding ears should be examined to exclude edema from insect bites or infection. Normal earlobes are similar in size and placement and should move freely and painlessly. Infected pierced earlobes will be warm, tender, and erythematous and may have exudates. The lobes of older patients may be more prominent or pendulous. Dry or scaly skin of the external ear may indicate psoriasis, seborrhea, or eczema, which can occur on and be limited to the ear. The external ear may also have skin breakdowns or erosions from prolonged pressure from eyeglasses or oxygen tubing. Cancerous or precancerous lesions are most often found on the top of the auricle. They may appear as shiny, irregular, painless lesions (BCC) or as raised, crusted lesions around a center ulcer (SCC).[7] Painless lesions can sometimes be better palpated than observed.

DIAGNOSTICS

DIAGNOSTICS

Auricular Disorders

LABORATORY

Culture and sensitivity*
Uric acid*
Rheumatoid factor*
Endocrine studies*

OTHER DIAGNOSTICS

Biopsy*

*If indicated.

The diagnostic tests depend on the underlying disease process. A biopsy should be performed on any small, crusted, ulcerated, or indurated lesion that does not heal properly. If the biopsy findings are positive, a complete cancer screening should be ordered. Rheumatoid arthritis profiles should be obtained in patients with rheumatoid nodules. If tophi are present, a uric acid chemistry profile is indicated. Calcification nodules indicate the need for endocrine studies and further assessment for Addison disease.

DIFFERENTIAL DIAGNOSIS

The differential diagnosis includes all the diagnoses mentioned earlier.

DIFFERENTIAL DIAGNOSIS

Auricular Disorders

- Cancer
- Rheumatoid arthritis
- Gout
- Addison disease
- Infection
- Relapsing polychondritis

MANAGEMENT

Infections of the earlobe or pinna that are a result of piercing can be treated with topical alcohol and antibiotic ointment. Mild infections can be treated with oral cephalexin or dicloxacillin.[8] Patients with severe infections require hospitalization and usually treatment with intravenous cefazolin or nafcillin.[8]

Patients with perichondritis, malignant otitis externa, or signs of mastoiditis require immediate referral to a physician or an otolaryngologist, admission to a hospital, and aggressive antimicrobial therapy usually aimed against *Pseudomonas* and/or *Staphylococcus aureus*.[8] Patients with very early malignant otitis externa disease may be treated with an oral fluoroquinolone, with frequent follow-up.[8] A biopsy should be performed on any chronically inflamed lesion to determine if it is malignant.

LIFE SPAN CONSIDERATIONS

Life span considerations are related to the specific disease disorder. Complications from piercing are more likely in the young. Skin cancers are most likely to occur in middle-aged and older patients.

COMPLICATIONS

Complications are unusual but do occur. Trauma, if untreated, may result in painful nodules or a distorted cauliflower ear. Painless pinnal nodules may be a complication of Addison disease, and any painless nodule may represent a carcinoma. Infections, if untreated, may spread systemically. Recurring pinnal infections should prompt concern for relapsing polychondritis, a degenerative cartilage disease that can cause tinnitus or deafness.[2]

INDICATIONS FOR REFERRAL OR HOSPITALIZATION

Patients with torn earlobes are usually referred to a reconstructive plastic surgeon for repair. In addition, a trend that can lead to damage of the cartilage and subsequent deformity is high ear piercing in the pinna. If deformity and instability of the pinna are observed, a referral to a reconstructive surgeon is also recommended. A biopsy should be performed on any cancerous or suspicious lesion. Malignant otitis externa requires immediate referral to a physician or hospital admission.

PATIENT AND FAMILY EDUCATION

Understanding of the importance of sunscreen protection for the ears is essential. In addition, the signs of skin cancer—asymmetry, borders (irregular, ragged, notched, or blurred), color (irregular), and diameter (a lesion that is 6 mm [¼ inch] or growing)—should be carefully explained. The provider should stress the importance and correct way of cleaning and caring for the external ear canal and auricle. When selecting ear-piercing facilities, patients should look for facilities that employ licensed personnel and are inspected or approved by public health authorities. In addition, caution is advised if wearing heavy or dangling earrings because the earring might be torn from the ear.

HEALTH PROMOTION

Health promotion is primarily related to the specific disease. Sunscreens and protective clothing are the best choices for the prevention of skin cancer.

CHAPTER 81

CERUMEN IMPACTION

Diane Wink

DEFINITION AND EPIDEMIOLOGY

Cerumen impaction occurs when increased amounts of hard cerumen either partially or completely occlude the external ear canal. Cerumen is a natural substance that can become dry and immobile and occlude the canal. Although cerumen is an important defense against infection, many think a buildup of earwax is a sign of uncleanliness and make efforts to remove the wax. This can compromise the integrity of the ear's defenses against infection and actually contribute to cerumen impaction. Ear plugs, hearing aides, ear buds used to listen to music and talk on the phone, and probes such as cotton-tipped swabs used to clean the ear can cause cerumen impaction. The presence of cerumen can also decrease efficacy of hearing aides.[1]

Clinicians should diagnose cerumen impaction only when an accumulation of cerumen is associated with either or both of the following conditions: patient symptoms and prevention of needed assessment of the ear. An exception is when the patient is elderly or a young child or is cognitively impaired and not able to express symptoms. These individuals are at higher risk for cerumen impaction because they are often unaware of or unable to express any symptoms associated with it. Hearing loss associated with cerumen impaction may further impair cognitive function.[1]

PATHOPHYSIOLOGY

Cerumen is a soft, yellow, waxy protective substance that is secreted by glands in the external ear canal. It is part of the mechanism that protects the ear canal and tympanic membrane (TM) from dirt and debris. When cerumen is formed relatively close to the TM, it is soft and fluid, colorless, and odorless. As the cerumen moves toward the distal part of the ear canal through the process of mandibular movement, it becomes drier and darker and develops its characteristic odor. If an individual uses a swab to clean the ear canal or another item that obstructs normal movement of the cerumen, the harder cerumen that is not removed or allowed to naturally progress to the outer ear is pushed against the TM. Cotton-tipped swabs can leave fibers from the swab, which then hold the cerumen in a mass. Excessive cerumen production, a narrow ear canal, or obstruction may also predispose a patient to impaction.[2]

CLINICAL PRESENTATION

Patients with cerumen impaction typically complain of unilateral or bilateral fullness or hearing loss; otalgia, itching, discomfort, tinnitus, cough, vertigo, and dizziness are also common complaints. Because hearing changes thought to be from cerumen impaction can also be from other causes (e.g., TM rupture) an expanded history to identify such problems should be obtained.[1-3]

PHYSICAL EXAMINATION

The outer ear should be inspected for size, shape, color, and placement; the lobe, helix, and preauricular and postauricular lymph nodes should be bilaterally palpated. The body temperature and lymph nodes are usually normal. The ear should be inspected by having the patient tip his or her head toward the opposite shoulder. In adults, the pinna is pulled gently up and backward; for young children and infants, the ear is pulled downward. The largest speculum that fits into the ear canal is gently inserted. Cerumen impaction may prevent the speculum from being fully inserted.

An impaction appears as a light yellow to dark brown mass that prevents or partially blocks visualization of the TM. Blood in the external ear canal appears as bright red to black and may be liquid or a solid mass. Sanguineous drainage often appears as honey-colored fluid. Whenever a cerumen impaction is noted in one ear, the other ear should be examined as well.

DIAGNOSTICS

No diagnostics are indicated.

DIFFERENTIAL DIAGNOSIS

The primary differential diagnosis is a foreign body in the external ear canal. Perforation of the TM, otitis, middle ear disease, and dysfunction of the eustachian tube can also cause symptoms similar to cerumen impaction.

DIFFERENTIAL DIAGNOSIS

Cerumen Impaction

- Foreign body

MANAGEMENT

When cerumen removal is needed, first verify if patients have a history of a ruptured TM, tympanostomy tubes, or recent ear surgery. When such history is present, some modes of cerumen removal are contraindicated. Foreign objects such as beans or other vegetable matter tend to swell with the irrigating solution, complicating removal.[1,3]

- If there is a contraindication to instilling fluid into the ear canal, removal with a cerumen spoon or curette is appropriate. If direct visualization is possible, the cerumen is in the lateral third of the external ear canal, and the patient is able to remain still during removal.
- If there is no contraindication to instilling fluid into the ear canal, a commercial ceruminolytic agent (e.g., any brand of carbamide peroxide) or two or three drops of baby oil or mineral oil, liquid docusate sodium, or hydrogen peroxide can be inserted in the affected ear daily for 3 to 5 days. This may resolve the impaction.
    - If a patient is known to have dry skin in the ear canal, ceruminolytics containing hydrogen peroxide should be avoided because the peroxide can further dry the skin.[4]
    - Although any ceruminolytic agent seems to be better than no treatment at all, there is no evidence that any one particular ceruminolytic is superior to any other.[1,5] However, only carbamide peroxide has been approved by the U.S. Food and Drug Administration (FDA) for this use.[2]
- If the ceruminolytic agent does not cause resolution of the impaction, removal with a cerumen spoon or curette can be performed.
- If the cerumen is deeper in the canal or is not cleared with the ceruminolytic agent and/or curette, irrigation with water or normal saline at body temperature using an ear syringe, a device specifically designed for ear irrigation, or a regular syringe with a flexible catheter can be performed.

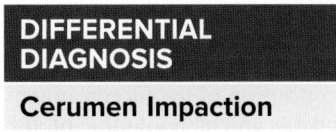

- If not already used, a ceruminolytic agent may be instilled in the canal for 15 to 20 minutes before the irrigation to soften the cerumen and aid in its removal.
- The auricle should be straightened as much as possible and the irrigant directed upward in the canal to minimize the pressure against the TM.
- The canal should be irrigated until clear unless the patient experiences pain or dizziness.
- If the patient is immunocompromised, a sterile solution should be used.[1,2]

- Pain, injury to the skin of the ear canal with hemorrhage, and acute otitis externa are possible complications after cerumen removal. Patients on anticoagulants are at higher risk for bleeding.[1]
- The clinical indication for use of antibiotics and topical steroids after removal of a cerumen impaction is determined by the amount of excoriation and other conditions, such as diabetes or an immunocompromised status.
    - When warranted, hydrocortisone–neomycin sulfate–polymyxin B sulfate (Cortisporin otic solution) or a mixture of white vinegar and rubbing alcohol in the canal every day for 2 or 3 days after the procedure can reduce the risk of otitis externa.[1]
- Reassess the patient at the conclusion of in-office treatment for cerumen impaction and document resolution of the impaction.[1]
- If the impaction is not resolved, additional treatment should be prescribed.
- If full or partial symptoms persist despite resolution of impaction, clinicians should consider alternative diagnoses and referral to an otolaryngology specialist.[1]

LIFE SPAN CONSIDERATIONS

In older adults, the glands that produce cerumen may become less productive, which can result in cerumen that is drier and more likely to collect in the canal and to become impacted. Those with cognitive or communication deficits may also be unable to express symptoms of cerumen impaction.

Adults who work in noisy industries and are required to wear hearing protection may have an increased risk of cerumen impaction. Individuals requiring use of hearing aids, earplugs, or swim molds and those who insert foreign bodies into the external auditory canal can increase the incidence of impaction by pushing the cerumen into the canal. Clinical practice guidelines recommend examination of such patients for cerumen impaction during health care encounters, although no more frequently than every 3 months.[1]

COMPLICATIONS

Cerumen accumulation can decrease auditory acuity and cause pressure on and perforation of the TM. Removal of cerumen that has adhered to the wall of the external ear canal may leave an abraded or irritated area that can develop into otitis externa. Hearing loss and injury to the TM are other potential complications. In addition, if the impaction is not completely removed, water retention behind the impaction can occur, predisposing the patient to infection.

INDICATIONS FOR REFERRAL OR HOSPITALIZATION

Patients with suspected perforation, chronic cerumen impaction, tympanostomy tubes, recent ear surgery, or pus or necrotic tissue in the ear canal should be referred to an otolaryngologist, as should patients who experience acute pain, dizziness, hearing loss, or damage to the external ear canal or TM during the ear lavage.

EDUCATION AND HEALTH PROMOTION

Patients should be educated that cerumen (earwax) is normal and that the external ear canal does not require cleaning. Gentle cleaning of the outer ear and canal with a cloth is all that is usually needed to remove wax and any dirt extruded from the canal. Avoidance of use of ear swabs and inserting other items into the ear will both prevent cerumen impaction and help prevent injury to the ear canal and TM. The American Academy of Otolaryngology–Head and Neck Surgery has a useful patient handout on earwax and care. This can be found at www.entnet.org/content/earwax-and-care.

Because patients who wear hearing aids or other ear-occluding items are more at risk for the development of cerumen impaction, they should try to decrease or to eliminate wearing of these items when not needed and while sleeping.

If not contraindicated, one or two drops of commercial ceruminolytic (carbamide peroxide) once or twice a week will help prevent cerumen from becoming hard and embedded. Ear syringes can also be used to gently direct clean warm water to the roof of the ear canal. Patients should be cautioned about the need to follow directions related to use and cleaning of ear syringes. Patients should be advised not to use any other home removal technique or device for cerumen removal. Although mentioned as an option for providers in the otolaryngology clinical practice guideline on cerumen impaction, oral irrigation tools should not be used by patients because they may rupture the TM even at low pressures.[1,2]

Patients should also be cautioned not to use cotton-tipped swabs or other implements to clean the ear canal. These items can push the cerumen farther into the ear and cause perforation of the TM. Soft cloths and soap and water should be used to clean the auricle. Patients must understand the importance of a medical evaluation if pain or discharge is noted.[1,6]

Patients should be cautioned to never use ear candling (also called *ear coning* or *thermal-auricular therapy*) for cerumen removal. This has no observable positive effects and is associated with considerable risks of burns to the tissues within the ear canal, perforation of the TM, external otitis, and temporary hearing loss. The FDA concluded that there is no validated scientific evidence to support the efficacy of ear candles and warns against their use.[1,2,6]

CHAPTER 82

CHOLESTEATOMA

Terry Mahan Buttaro

DEFINITION

A cholesteatoma (sometimes referred to as a keratoma) is an abnormal accumulation of squamous epithelial cells typically found within the middle ear, mastoid air spaces, or epitympanum.[1] Cholesteatomas can be acquired or congenital, but most often are acquired.

PATHOPHYSIOLOGY

The pathogenesis of congenital cholesteatoma is the presence of embryonic squamous epithelial cells in an ear without a history of tympanic membrane (TM) perforation or ear infection.[1] Congenital cholesteatomas arise in fetal development, but the exact cause is unclear. Primary acquired cholesteatomas are also the result of an unknown pathology but are related to retraction of the TM, usually in the pars flaccida.[1] The cause may be related to abnormal function of the eustachian tube or a chronic inflammatory cascade of events initiated by a middle ear infection.[2] The result is an accumulation of squamous epithelium, progressive erosion of the associated structures, and destruction of the delicate bones of the ossicular chain. Secondary acquired cholesteatomas develop as squamous epithelial cells enter the middle ear either after a surgical procedure (e.g., tympanoplasty) or as a direct consequence of epithelial cell shifting from the TM.[1] Advanced cholesteatomas can become secondarily infected. Typical organisms causing infected cholesteatomas include *Pseudomonas aeruginosa, Proteus* species, *Enterobacter, Staphylococcus, Streptococcus,* and anaerobes.[1] Over time, cholesteatomas can spread into intratemporal structures, causing tinnitus, otorrhea, hearing loss, twitching of the facial nerve, or paralysis of the facial nerve from infection or compression. Even with treatment, recurrence is possible.[3]

CLINICAL PRESENTATION

Congenital cholesteatomas may slowly enlarge for years and be asymptomatic. Otorrhea or hearing loss is often the presenting complaint. Acquired lesions are associated with recurrent or persistent purulent ear infections and tinnitus. Impaired hearing may be the first sign of middle ear destruction from a cholesteatoma.[4] Rarely the inflammatory process in the middle ear can result in vertigo, or the dizziness can occur from erosion of the labyrinth by the cholesteatoma.

PHYSICAL EXAMINATION

For a thorough otoscopic examination to be performed, several things should be taken into consideration. The light source on the otoscope must have adequate brightness to provide sufficient illumination of the inner ear. The entire TM should be inspected, particularly the posterosuperior quadrant and the anterosuperior quadrant, which are the most common locations of acquired and congenital cholesteatomas, respectively. Removal of cerumen or debris from infection may be necessary for adequate exposure of the entire TM.[4] On otoscopic examination, congenital cholesteatomas are typically identified as a pale whitish discoloration or spherical white cyst behind an intact TM. In primary acquired cholesteatoma, findings include retraction of the pars flaccida and, although less commonly, the pars tensa. Retraction pockets are identified by careful inspection of the TM and can be shallow or deep. Shallow pockets may be seen with otoscopy; deep pockets can contain debris and not be visible. Other common findings include a whitish keratin mass, purulent otorrhea, polyps, granulation tissue on the surface of the TM, and ossicular erosion. In secondary acquired cholesteatoma, the findings depend on the cause. The physical examination should include the entire ear, and the function of the facial nerve (cranial nerve VII) should be evaluated. Routine examination techniques for nystagmus and balance function may be warranted for patients with vestibular dysfunction.

DIAGNOSTICS AND DIFFERENTIAL DIAGNOSIS

An audiogram can reveal conductive hearing loss and is an important diagnostic tool,[1] though hearing can be unaffected if there is no damage to the ossicular chain. A computed tomography (CT) scan can aid in diagnosis and determination of the nature and extent of tumor involvement and complications[1] but does not differentiate between fluid and the dense tissue of a cholesteatoma. Tympanostomy tube placement may improve the quality of the CT scan. Magnetic resonance imaging (MRI) is useful if findings suggest a neoplasm or an encephalocele, but MRI technology is unable to determine tissue characteristics because of the small diameter of the ear and mastoid and the common presence of an inflammatory process.[1]

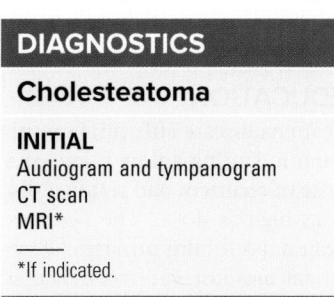

DIAGNOSTICS

Cholesteatoma

INITIAL

Audiogram and tympanogram
CT scan
MRI*

---
*If indicated.

The differential diagnoses include other white lesions of the TM such as tympanosclerosis, white foreign bodies, exostoses, prosthetic and grafted material in surgically repaired ears, and inclusion cysts of the TM. For patients with persistent or recurrent otorrhea, diagnoses to consider include chronic otitis media without cholesteatoma, otitis externa, malignant external otitis, neoplasms (such as squamous cell carcinoma of the ear) or other uncommonly occurring tumors (such as adenomas), adenocarcinoma, adenoid cystic carcinoma, and cerebrospinal fluid otorrhea (such as from an encephalocele).[2] In both children and adults with conductive hearing loss and a TM that appears intact or even normal, ossicular dysfunction resulting from either previous inflammatory disease of the ear or trauma should be considered. In children, congenital malformation of the ossicular chain is also a diagnosis that should be entertained, as is otosclerosis in adult patients.[1]

DIFFERENTIAL DIAGNOSIS

Cholesteatoma

- Tympanosclerosis
- White foreign bodies
- Exostoses
- Inclusion cysts of the TM
- Chronic otitis media
- Otitis externa
- Neoplasms
- Adenocarcinoma
- Adenoid cystic carcinoma
- Cerebrospinal fluid otorrhea
- Otosclerosis

MANAGEMENT

Removal of debris from the ear canal, avoidance of water entering the canal, and treatment with bacterial agents that cover the common bacterial organisms are included in the common management plan to reduce the inflammation and bacterial infection in the involved ear. If the TM is not intact, ototoxic agents such as aminoglycosides should not be prescribed. In many cases, the infection does not completely subside. Surgery is the definitive treatment for cholesteatoma.[4]

INDICATIONS FOR REFERRAL OR HOSPITALIZATION

All patients with a cholesteatoma should be referred to an otolaryngologist to confirm the diagnosis. Early detection and treatment of cholesteatomas reduce the likelihood of complications. Cholesteatomas that are not surgically removed continue to enlarge, which can lead to serious complications.[1]

PATIENT AND FAMILY EDUCATION

Recurrent and residual cholesteatoma disease after primary surgical intervention is fairly common. During a time frame of 5 years or more, the combined rate of recurrent and residual disease has been reported to be as high as 40%.[1] The pediatric population appears to be at greatest risk for this problem.[1] Postoperatively, regular follow-up to monitor for recurrence is recommended.[1]

CHAPTER 83

IMPAIRED HEARING

Michael L. Norris

DEFINITION AND EPIDEMIOLOGY

Impaired hearing is a defect in the detection and/or processing of sound waves. Impaired hearing affects both communication ability and personal safety and can be a socially isolating experience. Hearing loss occurs at all ages, although its prevalence increases with advancing age. A complaint of hearing loss can reflect a wide variety of abnormalities and requires different considerations in children than in adults.

Immediate specialist referral to an otolaryngologist or neurologist is indicated for patients with sudden hearing loss.

PATHOPHYSIOLOGY

The ear is the peripheral mechanism that converts sound waves into electrical impulses that are processed by the central auditory pathways. It is divided into three segments: the outer ear, middle ear, and inner ear. Each section must function properly for hearing to occur normally. The outer ear includes the auricle and ear canal. Its function is to collect sound waves and funnel them to the middle ear. The middle ear includes the tympanic membrane (TM) and the ossicles and the middle ear space that contains them. It transfers the sound waves to the inner ear, amplifying these vibrations as it does. Finally, the inner ear consists of the cochlea, the organ of hearing, and the semicircular canals, which function as a primary balance system. The cochlea converts the vibratory energy into electrical impulses that are then processed by the auditory nerve pathways in the brainstem, midbrain, and cerebrum.

Hearing losses are classified into three types. The first is conductive loss, which results from sound waves being attenuated at the external auditory canal or the middle ear. The second type is sensorineural loss, resulting from malfunction in the cochlea or central auditory pathways. Sensorineural losses can be subdivided into a peripheral (cochlear) loss or a central (nerve) loss. Finally, a mixed hearing loss has both conductive and sensorineural components. The vast majority of hearing losses are peripheral, and differential diagnosis is generally focused on the peripheral mechanism. It should never be forgotten, however, that the central auditory pathways are crucial to hearing and central losses will be encountered occasionally. A number of abnormalities may lead to hearing loss of each type.

In conductive hearing loss, any component of the anatomic structures of the outer or middle ear can be involved. In the outer ear, impacted cerumen, bacterial or fungal infection (swimmer's ear), overgrowth of the bony wall (exostoses), tumors, congenital atresia, and fibrotic stenosis from recurrent infection may attenuate the sound reaching the middle ear and cochlea. In the middle ear, perforation of the TM, scar tissue, negative pressure from eustachian tube dysfunction, barotraumas, cholesteatoma, glomus tumor, otosclerosis, or any other condition that impairs the mobility of the TM or ossicles can reduce hearing sensitivity. Causes of conductive loss from middle ear disease include acute otitis media, serous otitis media, and chronic serous otitis. While otitis media is primarily associated with early childhood, it may occur at any age. Otosclerosis, which is fusion of the stapes over the oval window, is a common cause of hearing loss in adults, usually appearing between the ages of 20 and 40.[1] Other conditions that interfere with the mechanical transmission of sound in the middle ear are trauma that damages the ossicles and congenital malformations.

Sensorineural hearing loss usually occurs from disorders of the cochlea. Less prevalent are disorders of the central auditory nervous system (CANS)—that is, cranial nerve VIII (acoustic), the internal auditory canal, or the brain. Congenital sensorineural hearing loss may result from noninherited factors such as maternal infections (toxoplasmosis, other, rubella, CMV, HSV [TORCH complex]) or medications or from inherited autosomal abnormalities. Adventitious sensorineural hearing loss can result from such factors as infections of the inner ear, Meniere disease, inner ear barotraumas, trauma, and tumors.

Presbycusis is a gradual degeneration within the cochlea that accompanies aging. Multiple factors may be at play in any given individual, including hair cell loss, metabolic changes, and circulatory insufficiency. Multiple factors influence the rate at which hearing loss occurs: genetics, medications, infections, and exposure to noise. High blood pressure, smoking, and diabetes may hasten presbycusis. There may also be degeneration of the mechanical structures and the central auditory connections.[2]

Noise trauma is a common cause of cochlear damage and may be a factor in presbycusis.[2] Persistent or repeated exposure to excessive noise causes stress and mechanical damage to the delicate hair cells of the inner ear. High frequencies are affected initially, and over time the loss spreads to middle and lower frequencies. A loud, explosive noise may cause severe or profound damage to these structures and result in immediate hearing loss. In the United States the Occupational Safety and Health Administration (OSHA) has set standards and guidelines for noise exposure to protect workers. The OSHA standards limit the noise level exposure and require that hearing protection be worn at certain levels and that the hearing of those working in noise be monitored annually.[3]

Sensorineural hearing loss can also be caused by diseases that involve the endocrine or metabolic systems, autoimmune disorders, and neurogenic disorders. Ototoxic medications can also cause sensorineural hearing loss. The prime suspects in ototoxicity include antineoplastics, salicylates, aminoglycosides, furosemide, and quinine-related drugs. Audiologic evaluation before inception of treatment and regular monitoring of hearing during treatment is recommended for patients receiving a course of antineoplastics or aminoglycosides.

Central sensorineural hearing losses may be caused by acoustic tumors (vestibular schwannomas), stroke, and meningiomas.

Mixed hearing loss is a combination of both conductive and sensorineural loss. Usually, the presence of a mixed hearing loss is the result of two unrelated disease processes. Occasionally, however, injury to the ear, infection, and congenital disorders may affect the outer and/or middle ear and the inner ear.

CLINICAL PRESENTATION AND PHYSICAL EXAMINATION

Hearing loss may be sudden, progressive, or fluctuating in nature. It is important to determine whether the problem is unilateral or bilateral. Associated symptoms of otalgia, ear fullness, vertigo, tinnitus, or cranial neuropathies should be documented. The medical history should incorporate current and past treatments with oral and intravenous medications or nonprescription drugs, particularly aminoglycosides, diuretics, antineoplastics, or large doses of aspirin. Chronic illnesses, hospitalizations, head injuries, and surgeries should be included in the history. A family history of hearing loss, neoplasms, renal disease, and balance disorders should be investigated. Finally, exposures to trauma and noise should also be noted.

A complete examination of the head, neck, and throat and an evaluation of cranial nerves and the auditory and vestibular system are essential. The pinna and external auditory canal should be inspected for malformations, lesions, exudates, and obstruction. Examination of the TM should assess for mobility (via pneumoscopy) and determine whether effusion, infection, perforation, or cholesteatoma is present.

DIAGNOSTICS

- Weber and Rinne tests, performed in conjunction, are used to differentiate conductive and sensorineural hearing loss.
  - The Weber test is performed by placing a vibrating tuning fork at the midline of the forehead. With normal hearing or symmetric sensorineural hearing loss, the sound is heard equally in both ears. With asymmetric sensorineural loss, the sound is heard in the better ear. With an asymmetric conductive loss, the sound is heard in the poorer (greater conductive loss) ear.
  - The Rinne test compares air conduction (AC) and bone conduction (BC). A vibrating tuning fork is held next to the ear and the patient reports when he or she can no longer hear the sound. The still-vibrating fork is then placed on the mastoid process behind the ear. In normal hearing, AC is better than BC (AC > BC)—that is, the patient does not hear the tuning fork when it is placed on the mastoid. With a conductive hearing loss, BC is better than AC—that is, the patient hears the tuning fork when it is placed on the mastoid. In the presence of a sensorineural hearing loss, AC remains better than BC but the patient does not hear it at as soft a level as a normal hearing person.[4]
- A screening audiogram is optimal.
  - A recent noise exposure history should be taken before administering a hearing test for more accurate results. Exposure to loud noises over the weekend, for example, may decrease hearing if tested on a Monday morning. If the individual works in a noisy environment, a test in the morning, before the patient has been to work, is preferred.
- Tympanometric screening is used to determine middle ear function.
- A formal audiogram, performed by an audiologist in a sound-treated environment, is recommended if hearing is impaired on clinical examination. Formal testing should include the following:
  - Pure tone tests by AC—to determine hearing thresholds for selected frequencies through earphones, and hence for the entire auditory system.
  - Pure tone tests by BC—to establish the thresholds for the same frequencies with a bone oscillator placed on the mastoid. This bypasses the outer and middle ear and determines the sensorineural component of the loss. Analogous to the Rinne tuning fork test, better response on this test than on the AC test indicates a conductive component to the loss.
  - Speech reception test under phones—to determine the softest level at which the patient can identify two-syllable words chosen from a closed set and to provide confirming evidence that the pure tone AC results are accurate.
  - Speech recognition testing—to evaluate the patient's ability to understand single-syllable words at a given presentation level.
  - Impedance audiometry—to evaluate middle ear function. The tympanogram determines whether the TM is intact, how well it moves, and what the air pressure is in the middle ear. Acoustic reflexes evaluate the movement of the stapedius muscle and are particularly sensitive to the presence of otosclerosis.
  - Additional specialized tests—to evaluate outer hair cell function (otoacoustic emissions [OAEs]) in the inner ear and integrity of the auditory nerve and brainstem auditory pathways (auditory brainstem response [ABR]). The tests are done when indicated by the results of conventional audiometry.
- Pediatric audiologists can evaluate hearing at any age. Behavioral tests provide good estimates of hearing thresholds, and objective tests such as OAEs and threshold ABR can provide reliable information about hearing in those patients too young to respond reliably to behavioral testing.
- Laboratory tests should also be done to evaluate the patient for systemic or metabolic causes for the hearing loss. For example, CBC/differential if anemia or infection is suspected; VDRL or RPR to exclude syphilis; ESR, antinuclear antibodies, rheumatoid factor, if autoimmune disorder is a consideration; TSH to exclude thyroid disorder.
- Magnetic resonance imaging (MRI) or computed tomography (CT) scans are useful in ruling out tumors; gauging the extent of chronic inflammatory middle ear disease and cholesteatomas; evaluating otosclerosis, erosion, or displacement of the ossicles; and identifying cochlear atresias or enlarged vestibular aqueducts,[5] which may cause sensorineural hearing loss.[6]

DIFFERENTIAL DIAGNOSIS

Once the site of lesion (outer, middle, or inner ear) is established, the differential diagnosis of hearing loss focuses on the nature of the presenting complaint: whether the loss was sudden, gradual, fluctuating, or progressive.

Causes of sudden hearing loss in adults can include sudden idiopathic sensorineural hearing loss, infections, perilymphatic fistula, ischemia of the inner ear or retrocochlear structures, multiple sclerosis, autoimmune diseases, trauma, chronic renal failure, and sickle cell anemia. Gradual hearing loss can be related to presbycusis, noise exposure, familial factors, retrocochlear neoplasm, chronic otitis media, cholesteatoma, otosclerosis, hypothyroidism, diabetes, and chronic renal failure. Differential diagnosis for fluctuating hearing loss includes otitis media, perilymphatic fistula, Meniere disease, multiple sclerosis, migraine headache, syphilis, autoimmune disorders, and sarcoidosis. Hearing loss that is rapidly progressive may result from causes such as autoimmune inner ear disease, meningeal carcinoma, vasculitis, Lyme disease, and ototoxic exposures.

DIFFERENTIAL DIAGNOSIS

Impaired Hearing

SUDDEN HEARING LOSS

- Sudden idiopathic sensorineural hearing loss
- Infection
- Ischemia of the inner ear or retrocochlear structures
- Multiple sclerosis
- Autoimmune diseases
- Trauma
- Chronic renal failure
- Sickle cell anemia

GRADUAL HEARING LOSS

- Presbycusis
- Noise exposure
- Familial factors, hypothyroidism, diabetes, and chronic renal failure
- Retrocochlear neoplasm
- Chronic otitis media
- Cholesteatoma
- Otosclerosis
- Hypothyroidism
- Diabetes
- Chronic renal failure

FLUCTUATING HEARING LOSS

- Otitis media perilymphatic fistula
- Meniere disease
- Multiple sclerosis
- Migraine headache
- Syphilis
- Autoimmune disorders
- Sarcoidosis

MANAGEMENT AND INTERDISCIPLINARY MANAGEMENT

Conductive hearing loss associated with cerumen impaction usually resolves with removal of the impaction. Conductive loss caused by infection usually responds to resolution of the infection, although improvement in hearing loss typically lags behind clinical improvement of the infection. Otolaryngology referral is indicated for patients with hearing deficit associated with trauma, congenital hearing loss, tumors, obstructions of the external auditory canal, nonhealing TM rupture, and otosclerosis. Treatment for otosclerosis may be stapedectomy or sound amplification. TM perforation may heal spontaneously or require a surgical patch or graft. Presbycusis and some other hearing impairments can be treated with hearing aids. Parents of children with congenital or progressive hearing loss or possible syndromic loss should be referred for genetic counseling.

LIFE SPAN CONSIDERATIONS

Hearing loss is most often associated with aging, but hearing loss may occur at any age. Hearing loss in infancy, either congenital or adventitious, can cause delays in speech, language, and cognitive development. Early identification and intervention can prevent speech and language delays and the consequent negative effects on cognitive development and educational attainment. In recent years there has been a movement to institute universal neonatal screening of hearing, and 44 states have requirements for universal screening.[7] The negative effects of hearing loss are not restricted to deafness or severe impairment. Even mild losses and unilateral losses have been shown to be educationally significant.[8]

COMPLICATIONS

Hearing impairment can result in frustration and anger at difficulties understanding speech and avoidance of situations in which communication is difficult. The resulting social isolation can lead to depressive symptoms. Frequent misunderstanding of speech at home can cause increased strain in marriage or other intimate relationships. Failure to hear warning signals can lead to accidents. In middle age hearing loss can cause restricted economic opportunities. Early hearing loss resulting in reduced educational attainment can result in lifelong reduction in earning ability.

Some missed diagnoses may result in significant health consequences. Untreated ear infection or cholesteatoma may result in erosion of the lamina between the middle ear space and the brain resulting in meningitis. Untreated acoustic neuroma can result in facial paralysis as the tumor impinges on other cranial nerves and ultimately death as the brainstem is displaced laterally. A number of syndromic hearing losses, such as branchio-oto-renal (BOR) syndrome and velocardiofacial (Shprintzen) syndrome, are associated with significant, even life-threatening dysfunction of the heart, kidneys, and neurologic and other systems.[9]

INDICATIONS FOR REFERRAL OR HOSPITALIZATION

Referral to an otolaryngologist is appropriate when the diagnosis is unclear, when preliminary assessment indicates a serious condition, or when surgical intervention is an option. Referral to an audiologist is always appropriate for definitive testing and rehabilitative intervention. Sudden hearing loss or unilateral symptoms indicate the need for immediate referral to an appropriate specialist, usually an otolaryngologist or a neurologist.

PATIENT AND FAMILY EDUCATION

Patients should be aware that a sudden hearing loss, difficulty understanding what other people are saying, or a constant ringing in the ear requires further evaluation. They should receive a careful explanation about their particular type of hearing loss, as well as how medications, such as aspirin, nonsteroidal anti-inflammatory drugs (NSAIDs), antibiotics, and diuretics, can cause hearing loss. Information about referral resources and options for management should also be presented to patients and their families. For patients considering hearing aids, establishing realistic expectations for amplification is paramount. It should be made clear that hearing cannot be completely restored and that the patient will have to relearn to use auditory information that they have not been hearing. Family members who live with a hearing-impaired person should understand the importance of decreasing background noise, facing the person when speaking so that the face and mouth are visible, and involving the hearing-impaired person in conversations.

HEALTH PROMOTION

Employees at risk for hearing loss from trauma or prolonged and elevated noise exposure are mandated by OSHA to limit their exposure and to wear protective equipment. Earplugs or protective equipment to reduce home, occupational, and recreational noise exposure should be encouraged to prevent hearing loss. Parents and children need to be informed of the risks of prolonged exposure to loud music from listening to mp3 players with ear buds.

Preschoolers should be monitored for recurrent otitis media, and periodic hearing screening of school-aged children should be encouraged.

Ototoxic medications should be monitored or, if possible, eliminated. Adults should be questioned periodically about hearing impairment. Questions should focus on specific areas of possible difficulty, such as difficulty hearing in noisy environments, difficulty hearing on the telephone, and difficulty understanding when the speaker's face is not visible. Ears should also be checked for ceruminosis and excess cerumen removed, if indicated.

CHAPTER 84

INNER EAR DISTURBANCES

Magen M. Lorenzi

Nearly 3% of all emergency department visits are a result of dizziness.[1] This complaint, as well as that of hearing loss or tinnitus, may indicate an inner ear disturbance. Vestibular neuritis, Meniere disease, and tinnitus are three of the most common inner ear disturbances.

VESTIBULAR NEURITIS

DEFINITION AND EPIDEMIOLOGY

Vestibular neuritis is an acute unilateral labyrinthine dysfunction, also called acute peripheral vestibulopathy or labyrinthitis. The condition is characterized by brief severe vertigo, nausea, vomiting, and disequilibrium lasting a few days followed by vertigo and disequilibrium with rapid head movement that may last for weeks to months.[2]

PATHOPHYSIOLOGY

Vestibular neuritis is most commonly caused by viral inflammation of the vestibular nerve, but otitis media is another possible cause. Increasing evidence suggests an association with latent herpes simplex virus type 1 (HSV-1) infection of the vestibular ganglia.[3] Inflammation of the eighth cranial nerve causes the sensation of vertigo. Acute suppurative labyrinthitis, an uncommon bacterial infection of the inner ear, is more serious and may be a complication of otitis media or meningitis.[4] Vestibular neuritis may also be caused by irritation from chemical products associated with acute or chronic otitis media.

CLINICAL PRESENTATION

Patients with vestibular neuritis complain of severe vertigo, nausea, and vomiting aggravated by head movement. Tinnitus may be present, but hearing remains intact.[3] The most severe symptoms of vertigo usually subside within 48 to 72 hours, but they can last 4 or 5 days. Although most episodes resolve spontaneously, up to half of patients will continue to experience dizziness and disequilibrium for many months.[2] Albeit not life-threatening, these symptoms can cause significant emotional and social stress for patients.

The history should include current medication use; history of head trauma; and duration, episodic nature, and severity of the vertigo. Past medical history and recent infection, particularly in the respiratory tract, should be elicited. Precipitating or aggravating factors, including cough, sneeze, or change in head position, and associated symptoms should be ascertained to help determine the cause of the vertigo.

PHYSICAL EXAMINATION

A thorough ear, nose, and throat examination and a careful neurologic evaluation, including balance testing (Romberg test), are recommended. A hearing screen reveals normal hearing.[3] Spontaneous nystagmus, horizontal or rotary, is often present with fast phases directed away from the affected ear. The nystagmus may need to be evaluated by use of Frenzel lenses for greater magnification.[3] Any abnormal finding on neurologic examination suggests a central cause and should be referred for immediate neurologic evaluation.[4]

DIAGNOSTICS

DIAGNOSTICS

Vestibular Neuritis

LABORATORY
CBC and differential*

IMAGING
MRI or CT scan*

*If indicated.

More definitive examinations to test hearing and to assess vertigo may be warranted. If a bacterial cause is suspected, a complete blood count (CBC) with differential may be helpful. If a tumor is suspected, magnetic resonance imaging (MRI) or a computed tomography (CT) scan is indicated.

DIFFERENTIAL DIAGNOSIS

Additional causes of peripheral vertigo and central vertigo must be considered. Benign paroxysmal positional vertigo (BPPV) (see Chapter 194) is associated with changes in head position, especially when the patient is recumbent. Meniere disease is associated with recurrent episodic vertigo, fluctuating hearing loss, and tinnitus.[3] Migrainous vertigo may occur in patients with a history of migraines.[5] Ramsay Hunt syndrome, caused by herpes zoster, includes hearing loss, facial palsy, and vertigo.[6] Central causes of vertigo, such as cerebellar disorders, are less common but potentially life-threatening.[4] Multiple sclerosis, head trauma, barotrauma, and toxins such as drugs and alcohol can also cause similar symptoms. Additional information about vertigo can be found in Chapter 194.

DIFFERENTIAL DIAGNOSIS

Vestibular Neuritis

- BPPV
- Meniere disease
- Migrainous vertigo
- Vascular disorders
- Trauma (head trauma, barotrauma)
- Toxins (medications, alcohol)
- Demyelinating disease (multiple sclerosis)
- Ramsay Hunt syndrome
- Cerebellar disorder
- Tumors

MANAGEMENT

Treatment focuses on three goals: (1) alleviating vertigo, nausea, and vomiting, (2) treating the cause of infection, and (3) improving ventral compensation through vestibular exercises.[3] Symptomatic relief can be achieved with anticholinergics, antihistamines, long-acting benzodiazepines, or antiemetics. Anticholinergics and antihistamines are first-line agents; benzodiazepines are reserved for patients who cannot take drugs with anticholinergic effects. Meclizine, 25 to 50 mg every 6 hours, is commonly used and acceptable in pregnancy. Antiemetics may be added during an acute episode to relieve vomiting.[7] These medications should be stopped after 3 days because continuing them may hamper vestibular recovery.[7] The use of antivirals as monotherapy has not proven effective and is typically not recommended.[3] Some studies report improvement of symptoms with corticosteroids; however, more recent studies have shown little benefit. Despite conflicting evidence, it is reasonable to begin steroid therapy during the acute phase of vertigo.[3] Methylprednisolone can be given once daily for 22 days beginning with diagnosis, beginning with a 100-mg dose and gradually tapering down every 3 days. Once the severe symptoms have passed, patients may benefit from vestibular enhancement exercises, which can be obtained through physical therapy services.[3,7]

LIFE SPAN CONSIDERATIONS

Medications for symptomatic relief of vestibular neuritis can cause drowsiness and sedation. In older adults, lower doses of medications (e.g., 12.5 mg of meclizine or less) should be considered for control of sedation.

COMPLICATIONS

Sensorineural hearing loss can occur after resolution of inner ear inflammation. In older adults especially, vertigo may increase the risk of falls.

INDICATIONS FOR REFERRAL OR HOSPITALIZATION

Consultation with an otolaryngologist is indicated if the diagnosis is unclear, the bacterial infection is severe, or symptoms do not resolve within 4 to 6 weeks. Associated suppurative otitis media or meningitis also necessitates referral. Severe dehydration indicates a need for intravenous rehydration and possible hospitalization.

PATIENT AND FAMILY EDUCATION

The provision of information about the disorder and reassurances will be helpful to patients and families. The importance of slowly changing positions should be discussed. In addition, adequate hydration and safety should be stressed. Patients, particularly older adults, may require assistance with activities of daily living or a walker or cane during the acute phase of the illness. Patients should avoid driving and operating heavy equipment while taking sedatives or antihistamines.

Because the disorder usually resolves within 4 to 6 weeks, patients should understand the importance of notifying the health care provider if the symptoms continue or increase in severity. Follow-up evaluation should be scheduled to reassess the patient and to ensure that the vertigo is resolving.

MENIERE DISEASE

DEFINITION AND EPIDEMIOLOGY

Meniere disease is a chronic condition of the inner ear characterized by recurrent vertigo and hearing loss. It is a complex of four symptoms that may or may not occur simultaneously: dizziness described as spinning vertigo, low-frequency sensorineural hearing loss, tinnitus, and a feeling of fullness in the affected ear. Studies estimate a prevalence of 40 to 50 cases per 100,000 people, with an annual incidence of three to four cases per 100,000.[8] Women are one to three times more likely to be affected than men, and the majority of patients acquire the disease in the fourth and fifth decades of life.[8]

PATHOPHYSIOLOGY

Meniere disease involves excess fluid and pressure in the labyrinth of the inner ear that episodically distends the structures of the labyrinth and damages the vestibular and cochlear hair cells. The exact cause remains unknown; however, the majority of cases are likely caused by viral infections or immune system–mediated mechanisms.[8] Up to one third of all cases seem to originate from an autoimmune process. Less common potential causes include tumors and trauma.

CLINICAL PRESENTATION

Along with eliciting a careful symptom analysis, the health care provider should ask patients about a history of recurrent symptoms. Early in the disease process, patients have intermittent attacks of vertigo that last from minutes to hours, often associated with nausea and vomiting. These episodes are commonly accompanied by pressure in the ear, low-pitched tinnitus fluctuating in intensity, and unilateral hearing loss. There can be long periods of remission. During later stages, the attacks of vertigo may occur frequently, and the hearing loss is constant.

PHYSICAL EXAMINATION

Diagnosis of Meniere disease is based on clinical criteria and/or response to treatment; however, it is important to differentiate Meniere disease from other causes of vertigo and hearing loss.[8] A thorough head and neck examination to exclude acute otitis media or another infectious process and a comprehensive neurologic examination are important. On physical examination, sound will lateralize to the unaffected ear in the Weber test; in the Rinne test, air conduction will be greater than bone conduction. Spontaneous nystagmus occurs during attacks and may not be present between attacks.

DIAGNOSTICS

Diagnostic criteria for Meniere disease include two episodes of spontaneous vertigo lasting at least 20 minutes each, audiometrically documented hearing loss, tinnitus or aural fullness, and the exclusion of other causes.[9] Basic testing for Meniere disease includes an audiogram, and MRI to rule out central nervous system (CNS) lesions. Laboratory testing should include thyroid-stimulating hormone (TSH), rapid plasma reagin (RPR) testing for syphilis, serum glucose, and Lyme serologies. Additional testing, done by an otolaryngologist, may include vestibular testing; glycerol urea, or sorbitol "stress" tests; electrocochleography; electronystagmography; and auditory brainstem testing.[9]

DIAGNOSTICS

Meniere Disease

INITIAL
Audiogram

LABORATORY
TSH
Serum glucose
RPR
Lyme serologies

IMAGING
MRI (to rule out neuroma)

DIFFERENTIAL DIAGNOSIS

Meniere disease is in large part diagnosed by excluding other disorders and is classified as idiopathic. Meniere disease can be seen with only hearing loss or vertigo, symptoms seen in many disorders. Conditions that must be considered and excluded in the workup for Meniere disease include acoustic neuroma, cerebellar tumors, diabetes, thyroid disease, and tertiary syphilis. Other differential diagnoses include BPPV, vestibular neuritis, head trauma, vertebrobasilar insufficiency, multiple sclerosis, transient ischemic attack, migraine headache, anemia, and Cogan syndrome.[9]

DIFFERENTIAL DIAGNOSIS

Meniere Disease

- Paroxysmal positional vertigo
- Vestibular neuritis
- Vertebrobasilar insufficiency
- Acoustic neuroma
- Migraine headache
- Head trauma
- Thyroid dysfunction
- Anemia
- Diabetes
- Multiple sclerosis
- Cerebellar tumor
- Transient ischemic attacks
- Cogan syndrome

MANAGEMENT AND INTERDISCIPLINARY MANAGEMENT

If Meniere disease is suspected, patients should be referred to an otolaryngologist for testing and management. There is no cure for the disease, and treatment can be difficult. The goals of therapy include managing the episodes of vertigo and arresting the disease process. The antiviral approach has almost eliminated the need for surgical intervention.[8,10] If an autoimmune process is suspected, diagnosis is typically confirmed after a positive response to steroid therapy.[8] Prompt treatment with steroids may even reverse inner ear damage.[8]

For symptomatic relief, meclizine and antiemetics such as promethazine (Phenergan) may be beneficial for some patients. Betahistine hydrochloride, a histamine H_1 agonist, and diuretic therapy may reduce the severity of the attacks if they are not controlled by diet, but evidence of benefit is unclear.[11] Studies suggest that betahistine may be effective for alleviating vertigo symptoms; however, it is unlikely to alleviate tinnitus in patients with Meniere disease.[12] In the United States, oral betahistine is not available, although it may be possible to obtain it by prescription from a compounding pharmacist. The Meniett device is a benign, noninvasive treatment that has been helpful in Meniere disease; it generates low-pressure pulses that may displace inner ear fluids, thereby relieving symptoms.[13]

Approximately 6% of patients with Meniere disease will go on to develop drop attacks, a potentially life-threatening condition, typically requiring surgical removal of the labyrinth of the affected ear.[14] Fortunately, intratympanic gentamicin has recently proven to be a long-lasting and effective treatment against drop attacks.[14]

LIFE SPAN CONSIDERATIONS

Although Meniere disease is more commonly diagnosed in middle-aged adults, older adults and children can also be affected.[8] The disorder can be particularly difficult to treat in pregnancy because medications are toxic to the fetus.

COMPLICATIONS

Hearing loss may be permanent. If the patient develops drop attacks, injury from falls is a possible complication, and proper safety education and evaluation should be performed.

INDICATIONS FOR REFERRAL OR HOSPITALIZATION

Referral to an otolaryngologist or a neuro-otologist is indicated for diagnostic evaluation and management. Hospitalization is rarely indicated unless the patient becomes dehydrated or injured as a result of a fall. Hospitalization is necessary for surgical intervention.

PATIENT AND FAMILY EDUCATION

Patient education should include information about the disease, expected course, and treatment choices. Reassurance will help allay anxiety. Patient safety during acute episodes of vertigo and the sedative side effects of prescribed medications should be emphasized.

TINNITUS

DEFINITION AND EPIDEMIOLOGY

Tinnitus is defined as the perception of a sound when there is no sound in the environment.[15] I It is usually a chronic, benign, but annoying ringing, buzzing, hissing, high-pitched screeching, whistling, or other noise in one or both ears that can be constant or intermittent. It can, however, herald a more serious disorder. It is estimated that 10% to 25% of the general population are affected. Prevalence increases with age (12% of those older than 60 years versus 5% of those aged 20 to 30 years).[15]

PATHOPHYSIOLOGY

The pathophysiology of tinnitus is not well understood but includes activity within the nervous system without any corresponding mechanical or vibratory activity within the cochlea.[15] Vestibular schwannoma, somatic sounds, otosclerosis, presbycusis, toxins, noise trauma, barotrauma, eustachian tube dysfunction, acoustic neuroma, vascular abnormalities, and neuromuscular conditions can all be potential causes of tinnitus.

CLINICAL PRESENTATION

Patients with tinnitus have varying degrees of symptoms and levels of debilitation, depending on the type and level of perceived sound. The history should include onset, duration, frequency, characteristics, and location of the sound as well as past ear disease or injury, allergy history, noise exposure, hearing status, and all medications. A description of the tinnitus can be helpful. High-pitched, continuous sounds are usually associated with sensorineural loss, and low-pitched sounds with idiopathic tinnitus or Meniere disease. Tinnitus described as pulsing or rushing is usually vascular in origin. Sounds similar to the ocean may result from eustachian tube dysfunction. Clicking sounds are usually somatic and may be caused by temporomandibular joint (TMJ) dysfunction or spasms of the muscular or middle ear structures. The spasms of ear structures may be symptomatic of an underlying neurologic disorder and warrant a thorough neurologic history, complete physical examination, and consultation. If the tinnitus is associated with hearing loss, any dizziness, vertigo, ear pressure, pain, or discharge should be noted. Tinnitus can either accompany or cause insomnia and depression, so it is important to inquire about both of these conditions.[15]

PHYSICAL EXAMINATION

The physical examination should include a complete ear, nose, throat, head, neck, and TMJ examination. If vascular tinnitus is suspected, the health care provider should include bilateral auscultation of preauricular areas, temples, orbits, mastoids, and jugular veins in various positions. Hearing tests and a complete neurologic examination (including cranial nerves) are also indicated.

DIAGNOSTICS

Questionnaires are available to determine the degree of tinnitus severity (e.g., the Tinnitus Handicap Questionnaire). All patients with tinnitus thought to originate in the auditory system should receive a complete audiologic evaluation performed by an audiologist. Tests may include pure tone audiogram, tympanometry, auditory reflex testing, determination of speech discrimination abilities, and otoacoustic emissions testing. An otolaryngologist or neurologist should evaluate any patient in whom vascular tinnitus is a concern.

There is little evidence to support routine laboratory testing for the evaluation of tinnitus, and therefore diagnosis must be guided by clinical impression.[16] Patients with unilateral sensorineural hearing loss and tinnitus should be tested for syphilis and Lyme disease.[16] Alternative laboratory testing may include a CBC and differential to rule out anemia and infection, erythrocyte sedimentation rate (ESR) to rule out autoimmune disease, serum glucose concentration, and thyroid function. If indicated, additional diagnostics include MRI and CT scan to exclude a CNS lesion.[16]

DIAGNOSTICS

Tinnitus

INITIAL
Audiology evaluation

LABORATORY
Lyme serologies
RPR
CBC and differential
ESR
Serum glucose
TSH

IMAGING
MRI or CT scan*

*If indicated.

DIFFERENTIAL DIAGNOSIS

The differential diagnosis should include those conditions that distinguish benign tinnitus from tinnitus caused by serious pathologic conditions. Excessive noise exposure and presbycusis are common causes of hearing loss and tinnitus. Medications such as aspirin can cause permanent or reversible tinnitus. Tinnitus of short duration is often caused by an acute process such as otitis, labyrinthitis, or noise exposure. Vascular disorders can cause pulsatile tinnitus and require in-depth evaluation by an otolaryngologist or neurologist. Spasm in the muscles of the ear or palate can be heard as an intermittent tapping sound. Eustachian tube dysfunction causes a sound like the ocean. Vestibular schwannoma, a benign tumor of the acoustic nerve, is usually associated with unilateral tinnitus.[16] Meniere disease is characterized by fluctuating tinnitus, hearing loss, aural fullness, or vertigo.

DIFFERENTIAL DIAGNOSIS

Tinnitus

- Noise exposure
- Medication
- Presbycusis
- Labyrinthitis
- Otitis
- Somatic sounds, eustachian tube dysfunction
- Vascular disorders
- Meniere disease
- CNS disorders (multiple sclerosis)
- Acoustic neuroma

MANAGEMENT

Intermittent tinnitus is not usually considered serious, but unilateral tinnitus has been associated with vestibular schwannoma; therefore MRI or CT scanning is often warranted.[16] Pulsatile tinnitus is also considered a serious symptom and necessitates evaluation by an otolaryngologist or neurologist. All ototoxic medications and excessive noise exposure need to be eliminated. Obvious local pathologic conditions should be treated (e.g., TMJ treatment or administration of antibiotics for infection).

Most patients with mild to moderate tinnitus adjust to the condition; although it is annoying, they do not find it debilitating. Patient education and reassurance are often all that can be offered. Other patients, with more severe tinnitus, find the condition disabling and should be referred to an otolaryngologist. If a sensorineural hearing loss is associated, referral for the application of other treatment modalities, such as hearing aids, sound masking, and cognitive behavioral therapy, may be indicated.[16] If no hearing loss is present, sound maskers alone, such as electronic noise-generating devices, mood tapes, and radio static, may diminish the intrusiveness of tinnitus.

The evidence of benefit is unclear for alternative therapies, including vitamins, herbal remedies, biofeedback, acupuncture, and electrical stimulation, but they may help individual patients. Various antidepressants have been used to treat both tinnitus and the depressive symptoms associated with tinnitus, but no one medication has as yet shown significant efficacy.

Because some patients also experience insomnia, a sleeping medication may be helpful. However, all sleeping medications should be used judiciously in older adults.[15]

COMPLICATIONS

No complications are associated with chronic, benign tinnitus. Missed diagnosis of tinnitus that is caused by a serious underlying pathologic condition may lead to untreated disease and major complications.

INDICATIONS FOR REFERRAL OR HOSPITALIZATION

Consultation with the primary care physician is necessary when referral to an otolaryngologist or a neurologist is indicated. If there is a suspicion that the tinnitus is not benign or if pulsatile or unilateral tinnitus is present, the patient should be seen by the appropriate specialist.

PATIENT AND FAMILY EDUCATION

Information on the causes of tinnitus and hearing loss increases understanding for most patients. A discussion of treatment options and resources for treatment is beneficial. Reassurance about the benign and common experiences of tinnitus is also helpful. Resources about tinnitus can be obtained from the American Tinnitus Association (www.ata.org).

CHAPTER 85

OTITIS EXTERNA

Jacqueline Rosenjack Burchum

DEFINITION AND EPIDEMIOLOGY

Otitis externa is a cellulitis of the external auditory canal that may extend to the auricle (pinna).[1] The condition is often referred to as *swimmer's ear,* although the causes are varied. Approximately 1 in 125 people develop acute otitis externa annually, with occurrence primarily in the warmer months and in regions with high humidity.[2] Chronic otitis externa affects 3% to 5% of the U.S. population.[2] A smaller percentage of patients with otitis externa will progress to malignant (necrotizing) otitis externa, which is a complication that is most often seen in people who are immunocompromised or who have comorbid conditions such as diabetes mellitus.[1,3]

PATHOPHYSIOLOGY

Risk factors for development of external otitis are typically those that compromise the integrity of the inherent defense mechanism against infection. These include removal of protective cerumen with damage to fragile skin that results from vigorous cleaning of the canal; maceration of skin that results from accumulation of moisture within the canal from swimming; and alterations to the tissues that result from wearing of devices such as headphones and ear plugs.[1,3] In the United States, over 90% of cases have a bacterial cause. The most common causative organisms are *Pseudomonas aeruginosa* and *Staphylococcus aureus.*[1,3] Fungi such as *Candida* and *Aspergillus* organisms are uncommon causes of acute otitis externa but may be present in chronic otitis externa or after antibiotic treatment of acute otitis externa.[1] Patients with recurrent otitis externa should be evaluated to determine whether the episode represents a fungal infection, treatment failure, or recurrence.

CLINICAL PRESENTATION

The usual presentation of acute otitis externa is pain of the affected ear and auricle developing over 48 hours or less. The pain is often accompanied by a feeling of fullness or itching. Other signs and symptoms that may be present include drainage from the affected ear and hearing loss.[2,4] Presentation of chronic otitis externa is primarily one of intense pruritus.[3]

PHYSICAL EXAMINATION

The classic finding in acute otitis externa is pain and tenderness on palpation of the tragus and on repositioning of the auricle to allow inspection of the canal.[1,3-5] The canal may be erythematous and edematous. Often the canal is filled with debris and sloughed tissue. The tympanic membrane may be erythematous; alternately, it may be poorly visualized because of edema or cerumen and exudate in the canal. Advanced cases of acute otitis externa are often accompanied by complete obstruction of the canal. The cellulitis may extend to the external ear with enlargement of periauricular lymph nodes.[1,4] Hearing deficits may occur in advanced cases.[1]

Chronic otitis externa has a very different presentation. The canal is often dry, and cerumen may be absent. Excoriations may be present secondary to use of objects inserted to relieve the itching that accompanies this condition. Discharge may be present. The canal may be narrowed, but this is secondary to thickened canal walls that occur over time rather than to the edema that is responsible for narrowed canals in acute otitis externa.[5]

DIAGNOSTICS

Diagnostic testing is usually unnecessary.

- A culture of canal drainage with antibiotic sensitivities is indicated if there is no improvement after 14 days of antibiotic therapy.[3]
- Microscopic analysis of drainage using potassium hydroxide (KOH) can identify a fungal cause.

DIAGNOSTICS

Otitis Externa

LABORATORY
Culture and sensitivity*
KOH preparation of drainage

*If indicated.

DIFFERENTIAL DIAGNOSIS

It is important to distinguish otitis externa from other conditions that cause ear pain, drainage, inflammation, or hearing loss. Patients with recurrent otitis externa should be evaluated to determine whether the episode represents a treatment failure rather than a recurrence.

DIFFERENTIAL DIAGNOSIS

Otitis Externa

- Acute otitis media
- Cerumen impaction
- Cholesteatoma
- Dermatoses
- Foreign body
- Furunculosis
- Malignant otitis externa
- Otitis media with effusion
- Referred dental pain
- Fungal infection

MANAGEMENT

Management of otitis externa focuses on clearing debris from the canal, managing the pain, and treating the infection and inflammation.

- Clearing debris from the canal
  - Because debris in the canal can interfere with healing and prevent penetration by topical medications, it should be gently removed.[1]
  - If the tympanic membrane is intact, aural lavage with hydrogen peroxide, saline, or even water may be helpful. These should be warmed to room temperature.[1]
  - Cleansing may also be accomplished by gently suctioning or using cotton-tipped swabs under direct observation via otoscope.[1]

Referral to an otolaryngologist may be indicated if the tympanic membrane is ruptured.

- Managing the pain
  - For mild to moderate pain, nonsteroidal anti-inflammatory drugs (NSAIDs) offer the benefit of both analgesia and control of inflammation; however, acetaminophen may be substituted if NSAIDs are not well tolerated.[1,3,5]
  - Opioids may need to be given during the initial 48 to 72 hours if the pain is severe.[1,3,5]
  - Topical anesthetics such as benzocaine otic solution may be helpful, but because they can mask evolution of underlying conditions, it will be important to recheck the patient within a couple of days if these are prescribed.[1] Topical anesthetics should not be used unless an intact tympanic membrane is verified.
- Treating the infection and inflammation
  - Systemic antibiotic therapy is indicated only if acute otitis externa has extended beyond the canal or if the patient has diabetes or is immunocompromised.[1,5]
  - Topical antibiotics are indicated for uncomplicated conditions in which inflammation is confined to the ear canal.[1] If the ear canal is severely swollen, insertion of a wick into the affected ear may be necessary to allow the medication to access the deeper recesses of the canal.
  - In the absence of culture and sensitivity results, it is important to choose medications that are effective against both *P. aeruginosa* and *S. aureus.*
  - Fluoroquinolone antibiotics are effective against *P. aeruginosa* and *S. aureus.*[1,3,5,6] Examples include ofloxacin (Floxin otic) and ciprofloxacin (Cetraxal, Ciloxan). These are also available as antibiotic-corticosteroid combinations such as ciprofloxacin with hydrocortisone (Cipro HC) to promote resolution of both infection and inflammation. Fluoroquinolones are safe to use in patients with nonintact tympanic membranes or tympanostomy tubes.[1,3]
  - Aminoglycoside antibiotics such as neomycin are another option for treating acute otitis externa.[1,3,5,6] Neomycin is effective against *S. aureus* but not *P. aeruginosa,* so it is commonly combined with polymyxin B for *P. aeruginosa* coverage in products such as Cortisporin otic. Aminoglycosides carry a risk for ototoxicity and should not be used in patients unless the tympanic membrane is verified to be intact.[1]
  - For fungal infections such as those that commonly cause chronic otitis externa, acidification with 5% acetic acid (white vinegar) or a 1:1[1] or 1:2[6] solution of vinegar and alcohol is often effective, though it may sting. Antifungal solutions such as clotrimazole otic are effective against common causative fungi. Fungal infections may also be treated with fluconazole (Diflucan).[6]

LIFE SPAN CONSIDERATIONS

Otitis externa is most common in young people.[1,2,4] Malignant otitis externa primarily affects older patients.[2-4]

COMPLICATIONS

Malignant otitis externa is an invasive osteomyelitis of the ear that occurs when the bacterial infection extends into cartilage and bone.[1,3,4] This condition is usually caused by *P. aeruginosa* and is most commonly seen in patients who are older, who have diabetes, or who are immunocompromised.[1,4] It is associated with severe pain, necrotic ulcerations, and fever. Facial paralysis and other cranial nerve abnormalities may also occur.[2,4]

INDICATIONS FOR REFERRAL OR HOSPITALIZATION

Because malignant otitis externa can become life-threatening, patients with suspected malignant otitis externa require immediate referral to an otolaryngologist for possible hospitalization for aggressive antimicrobial therapy.[1,3] Patients with otitis externa who are at high risk for development of malignant otitis externa, such as those who have diabetes or are immunocompromised, may also require a referral for specialized care.

Immediate physician or otolaryngologist consultation is indicated for patients with malignant otitis externa (Fig. 85-1).

EDUCATION AND HEALTH PROMOTION

Patients with otitis externa need to be educated about causes, management, and prevention of their condition. Many patients will not know how to administer topical otic medications so it will be important to review medication administration in addition to teaching about medication schedules and potential adverse effects.

Patients need to know that improvement should occur within 48 to 72 hours. If the condition should worsen rather than improve, they should be promptly reevaluated for complications. Resolution typically occurs in 7 to 10 days. If symptoms continue beyond this time, patients should be evaluated for treatment failure.

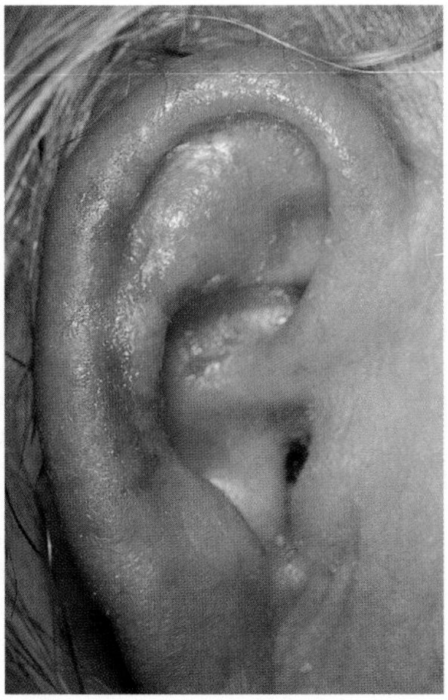

FIGURE 85-1 Malignant otitis externa. (From Habif TP, Campbell JL, Chapman MS, et al: *Skin disease: diagnosis and treatment*, ed 3, St Louis, 2011, Saunders.)

Prevention should center on avoidance of conditions that contribute to the development of otitis externa. Because cerumen provides a lubricant as well as a protective barrier against water and bacteria, patients should be instructed to avoid use of cotton-tipped swabs and similar objects to clean the ears. Because swimming allows prolonged exposure of the canal to water, it will be helpful to use a blow dryer to dry out the ear after swimming.[1,3] A 1:1 or 1:2 mixture of white vinegar and rubbing alcohol drops in each ear after swimming will restore an acidic environment and promote drying.[1,3,5] Ear plugs may also be used when swimming; however, these have also been identified as a risk factor for otitis externa.[1]

CHAPTER 86

OTITIS MEDIA

Margaret Thorman Hartig

DEFINITION AND EPIDEMIOLOGY

Otitis media, characterized by fluid in the middle ear, is a group of inflammatory or infective processes that may be bacterial, fungal, or viral in origin and is most often associated with upper respiratory tract infections or allergies. Otitis media is the most frequent childhood infectious illness, with the peak incidence at 6 to 15 months of age.[1] It accounts for a significant number of all antimicrobial prescriptions in primary care.[1,2] Severity and presentation vary. Symptoms and findings often are part of a continuum, despite the common practice of identifying discrete diagnoses. This continuum and its subtypes complicate diagnosis, as one condition often evolves into another.

Acute otitis media (AOM), with bacterial or viral infection of the middle ear fluid, has a rapid onset and short duration. Otitis media with effusion (OME) describes accumulation of serous fluid in the middle ear without acute inflammation. OME can precede or follow AOM, but barotrauma or allergy also can precipitate an occurrence. Middle ear effusion (MEE) signifies an accumulation of serous fluid in the middle ear and can be associated with AOM, often persisting for weeks or months after an episode of AOM.

Chronic effusion (known also as serous otitis media or glue ear) may persist for several months, with or without signs of infection.[2] Children aged 3 to 7 years old are most commonly affected. Recurrent otitis media is defined as three or more distinct episodes in 6 months or four or more episodes in the preceding 12 months with at least one episode in the past 6 months.[2]

PATHOPHYSIOLOGY

Otitis media is a dysfunction of the middle ear and middle ear mucosa.[1] The actual cause is multifactorial, related to anatomy, pathophysiology, and cell biology.[1] Antecedent events may be viral, bacterial, or allergic. Viral upper respiratory tract infections or allergies often precede otitis and result in edema of the eustachian tube and nasopharynx.[1] Narrow eustachian tubes, common in infants and young children, may predispose patients to episodes of otitis media. Exposure to cigarette smoke acts in several ways to increase the individual's risk for otitis media. Smokers are at higher risk for upper respiratory tract infections, plus the smoke may decrease the mucociliary functioning in the eustachian tube. When middle ear secretions accumulate in the eustachian tube, the opportunity for pathogen growth also increases. Causative pathogens are bacterial and viral. The most common bacterial causative agents are *Streptococcus pneumoniae* and *Haemophilus influenzae*. Group A β-hemolytic *Streptococcus, Staphylococcus aureus,* and *Moraxella catarrhalis* cause infection on a less frequent basis.[1]

Bacteria are the most frequent cause of otitis infections; however, in one study, two thirds of the infections were caused by a combination of bacteria and viruses.[1] This combination complicates recovery because viruses may increase inflammation, decrease neutrophil function, and interfere with antibiotic penetration.

CLINICAL PRESENTATION AND PHYSICAL EXAMINATION

Thorough otoscopic examination is key to accurate diagnosis of otitis. Clinical findings and severity of symptoms (otalgia and fever) experienced are aligned with criteria for categorizing the types of AOM, distinguishing it from OME and determining treatment. Three 2013 clinical practice guidelines presented by the American Academy of Pediatrics (AAP) consider age, severity of symptoms, otorrhea, and laterality in diagnosing and treating AOM.[2] These criteria require thoroughness in the physical examination that may not be well received by the child in pain.

Presence of rapid-onset otalgia, worse in a prone position, remains the common initial complaint of patients with AOM. Infants and younger children often have nonspecific symptoms, such as ear rubbing, rhinorrhea, vomiting, diarrhea, and fever. Specific symptoms and signs are linked with causative bacteria. Patients with OME or serous otitis may be asymptomatic or have mild pain with no symptoms of acute infection. Conductive hearing loss is most common. Other symptoms found in this condition include imbalance or vertigo, mild stuffiness, and a fullness or popping sensation in the ear.

History should include incidents (especially recent) of ear infections, upper respiratory tract infections, allergies, smoke exposure, and any treatments and their effectiveness. Examiners also should note development of the current illness, including the onset and duration of symptoms, ear pain or drainage, fever, irritability, hearing loss, tinnitus, and dizziness. Associated symptoms, including headache, eye drainage, nasal congestion, sore throat, and mouth pain, require investigation. Knowledge of activities that involve barometric pressure changes, such as scuba diving and flying, is helpful because these may affect equilibrium and cause discomfort from air in the middle ear. As with any infectious process, the patient's immune status must be considered.

Body temperature and other vital signs may be within normal range, or the temperature may be elevated. The findings on examination of the mouth, eyes, and nose may also be normal, or the patient may show signs and symptoms of upper respiratory tract infection. The frontal and maxillary sinuses often are tender on palpation and do not transilluminate. Mild to significant lymphadenopathy may be present with warm, tender, and enlarged posterior auricular and cervical lymph nodes.

Diagnosis of AOM requires thorough assessment with pneumatic otoscopy and adherence to defined diagnostic criteria. AAP guidelines[2] address and discourage the not uncommon practice of deferring aggressive visualization of the tympanic membrane (TM) and relying on symptomatology. The presence or absence of TM bulging is considered critical to accurate diagnosis and discrimination between AOM and OME.[2,3]

Cerumen removal may be necessary to obtain a clear view of the TM. The operating head of an otoscope provides direct visualization of the canal and access to remove the cerumen with a small plastic disposable ear curette.[3] Irrigation may be used in the absence of TM perforation. Hard or flaky cerumen can be softened with a variety of products at room temperature (e.g., sodium docusate solution, hydrogen peroxide, mineral oil) before removal with a curette removal, irrigation with soft bulb syringe, or use of a low-pressure water stream (Waterpik is a common choice).

Ideally, the otoscope uses a bright light source and airtight seal, usually achieved with the proper-size speculum. Nondisposable speculums are recommended for best seal and light conduction, as well as less painful examinations.[2,4] The importance and challenge of differentiating AOM from OME with and without effusion is commonly acknowledged. Web-based resources are available to improve examiner skills.[4] The interactive online learning site Enhancing Proficiency in Otitis Media (ePROM) is found at http://pedsed.pitt.edu/34_viewPage.asp?pageID=527326406.[4] Other findings include fluid behind the TM, which often affects the color, and fluid levels may be visible behind the membrane. Discharge in the canal without acute otitis externa suggests perforation. Purulent discharge in the ear canal may be sampled for culture and used as a basis for antibiotic selection. Bullae between the TM layers are most often associated with *Mycoplasma pneumoniae.*

Diagnosis of AOM requires bulging of the TM with obscured landmarks *or* new onset of otorrhea not caused by acute otitis externa.[2] Findings of moderate to severe bulging without other signs *or* mild bulging *and* recent (less than 48 hours) onset of ear pain *or* intense erythema of TM also quality for AOM diagnosis. Presence of MEE also is necessary for diagnosis of AOM. Fluid levels or air bubbles may be seen behind the TM, indicating accompanying effusion, though definitive diagnosis relies on pneumatic otoscopy and/or tympanometry.[2]

Pain assessment is necessary for both determining the presence of AOM and the need for pain relief. AOM usually is characterized by a throbbing, painful earache with impaired hearing. The Acute Otitis Media Severity of Symptom Scale (AOM-SOS) provides a seven-item, parent-reported symptom score.[5] Symptoms evaluated are ear-tugging, rubbing, and holding; excessive crying; irritability; difficulty sleeping; decreased activity, decreased appetite; and fever. The validated scale correlates with both the diagnosis and symptoms over time. Fever is often present, and the patient may have nausea or dizziness. The disease usually is accompanied by cold or influenza symptoms.[1,4]

In OME, fluid is present in the middle ear without signs or symptoms of acute infection. The TM often is dull gray, although it may appear injected.[1,2,6] Ear pain may still be present in infants, although it tends to be milder and often intermittent. Older children may report ear fullness and/or an ear popping sensation. Balance problems or hearing loss also may be noted. School performance may be affected. In chronic serous otitis, the TM may appear retracted and amber or bluish in color with a diffuse light reflex. TMs usually have limited movement, and bubbles or a fluid line is seen behind the membrane.

DIAGNOSTICS

Determine TM position or contour, color, translucency, and mobility.[2-4] Positions other than the usual neutral include retracted, full, and bulging. Moderate to severe bulging is the most important characteristic for the diagnosis of AOM.[2] Otorrhea may indicate MEE, especially if accompanied by abrupt relief of pain. Retraction is a common finding in OME.

Color options vary widely. The color of the TM may range from gray to red. Erythema of the TM often occurs in AOM, though it may be related to crying or fever. A very white TM may be the result of scarring from previous infections or purulence behind the TM. Translucency may be obscured and cloudy or opaque with illness. Decreased or absent mobility, determined by pneumatic otoscopy, indicates the presence of MEE and is one of the necessary criteria for accurate diagnosis of AOM.[2,4]

Cerumen removal may be necessary for adequate visualization of the TM. Tympanometry may help with diagnosis if otoscopic examination cannot determine whether there is fluid in the middle ear.[4] Acoustic reflectometry, the use of sound waves to determine TM mobility, may also be helpful for diagnosis, although it is rarely used.

Examination of the ear canal for otorrhea in the absence of external otitis media is necessary for classification of AOM. Temperature should be checked for presence of fever (above or below 39° C or 102.2° F).

Pain level (severe versus mild) may be determined by parental report in young children. The AOM-SOS is a sensitive option for evaluation.[5]

Weber and Rinne tests may be indicated to determine whether conduction and sensorineural hearing have been affected.

Laboratory or further diagnostic testing is not indicated for most patients with otitis media. There are special considerations for some patients, however.[3]

- A sinus x-ray study or a computed tomography (CT) scan of the sinuses may be indicated for patients who have recurrent or chronic otitis media, especially if intratemporal or intracranial complications are suspected. A contrast-enhanced CT scan of the temporal bones is the imaging study of choice.

- Allergy testing should be considered in patients who have recurrent or chronic otitis symptoms and a history of allergies or allergic rhinitis. Immune status should be considered in patients with atypical otitis media or those who do not respond to therapy.

DIAGNOSTICS

Otitis Media

INITIAL ASSESSMENT

Pneumatic otoscopy (position, color, translucency, mobility)
Tympanometry*
Acoustic reflectometry*
Weber test*
Rinne test*

IMAGING

Sinus x-ray study or CT scan of sinuses*
Contrast-enhanced CT scan of the temporal bone*

LABORATORY

CBC and differential*
Immune status*

OTHER DIAGNOSTICS

Allergy tests*
Tympanocentesis*
Culture and sensitivity*

*If indicated.

- A complete blood count (CBC) with differential should be ordered in immunocompromised patients.
- Tympanocentesis may be indicated for recurrent otitis media to identify causative organisms.

DIFFERENTIAL DIAGNOSIS

The primary challenge with differential diagnosis is distinguishing AOM from OME. The type of AOM also influences the management course.

MANAGEMENT

Specialist referral is recommended for children younger than 6 months for a possible sepsis workup or for those children with underlying conditions, such as tympanostomy tubes, anatomic or craniofacial abnormalities, or cochlear implants.[2]

Specialist referral may be necessary for any child who appears more toxic or lethargic than signs and symptoms would suggest.[3]

AAP guidelines define each of the AOM types and recommended treatments.[2] Antibiotic recommendations are found in Table 86-1.[7]

1. The type of AOM determines the most appropriate treatment for individual patients. The need for antibiotic therapy is determined on an individual basis based on history and presentation.
2. Increased incidence of antibiotic resistance, awareness of overprescribing for noninfectious OME, and recognition of antibiotic side effects are not without consequence. Current recommendations are for "watchful waiting" with close follow-up within 24 hours for nonsevere AOM.[2,3] Parental or caregiver preference is to be considered in these decisions.

TABLE 86-1 Recommended Antibiotics for (Initial or Delayed) Treatment for Children and for Pediatric Patients in Whom Initial Antibiotic Treatment Has Failed

Initial Antibiotic Treatment at AOM Diagnosis or After Observation		Antibiotic Treatment After 48-72 Hours of Initial Antibiotic Treatment Failure	
Recommended First-Line Treatment	**Alternative Treatment**	**Recommended First-Line Treatment**	**Alternative Treatment**
Amoxicillin (80-90 mg/kg per day)	Cefdinir (14 mg/kg/day in 1 or 2 doses)	Amoxicillin-clavulanate (90 mg of amoxicillin per kilogram per day, with 6.4 mg of clavulanate per kilogram per day)	Ceftriaxone, 50 mg/kg day, or clindamycin (30-40 mg/kg/ day in 3 divided doses), with or without second- or third-generation cephalosporin
OR	Cefuroxime (30 mg/kg per day in 2 divided doses)	OR	
Amoxicillin–clavulanate* (90 mg of amoxicillin per kilogram per day, with 6.4 mg of clavulanate per kilogram per day)	Cefpodoxime (10 mg/kg/day in 2 divided doses)	Ceftriaxone (50 mg/kg/day IM or IV for 3 days)	Clindamycin plus second- or third-generation cephalosporin
	Ceftriaxone (50 mg/kg per day IM or IV for 1 to 3 days)		Tympanocentesis† Consult specialist†

*May be considered in patients who have received amoxicillin in the previous 30 days or who have otitis-conjunctivitis syndrome.
†Perform tympanocentesis or drainage if skilled in the procedure or seek a consultation with an otolaryngologist for tympanocentesis or drainage. If the tympanocentesis reveals multidrug-resistant bacteria, then seek an infectious disease specialist consultation.
From Erratum. Lieberthal AS, Carroll AE, Chonmaitree T, et al: Clinical guideline: the diagnosis and management of acute otitis media. *Pediatrics* 131(3): e964-e999, 2013. In *Pediatrics* 133(2):346-347, 2014.

3. AOM with otorrhea in children 6 months or older: antibiotic therapy is recommended.
4. Severe AOM (bilateral or unilateral) in children 6 months or older with moderate to severe otalgia *or* fever of 39° C or higher: antibiotic therapy is recommended.
5. Nonsevere AOM, bilateral AOM in children younger than 24 months with mild otalgia for less than 48 hours and fever less than 39° C: antibiotic therapy is recommended.
6. Nonsevere AOM, unilateral in children aged 6 to 23 months with mild otalgia and fever below 39° C: may receive either antibiotics or observation with close follow-up.[2]
7. Nonsevere AOM (bilateral or unilateral) in children 24 months or older with mild otalgia for less than 48 hours and fever below 39° C may receive either antibiotics or observation with close follow-up.[2,3]
8. Initial observation includes a plan for treatment of associated symptoms, especially pain management, and planned provider contact within 24 hours for follow-up assessment.
9. Studies support the potential benefit of waiting 48 to 72 hours to administer antibiotics with minimal risk.[2,3]
10. Some providers find it effective to give parents a written prescription at the time of appointment with the proviso they will wait up to 72 hours to determine the need for antibiotic therapy.[2]
11. Amoxicillin is the recommended first-line antibiotic for children who are not allergic and have not received it in the last 30 days *or* do not have purulent conjunctivitis.[2]
12. Amoxicillin with β-lactamase is preferred for children not allergic *and* who have received amoxicillin in the last 30 days *or* have purulent conjunctivitis.[2]
13. Length of antibiotic treatment varies by AOM severity and child age.[2]
    a. Severe AOM in children younger than 2 is treated for 10 days.
    b. Mild or moderate AOM in children 2 to 5 years of age is treated for 7 days.
    c. Mild to moderate symptoms of AOM in children 6 years or older are treated adequately at 5 to 7 days.
14. Pain treatment should be provided for otalgia, whether or not antibiotics are prescribed.
    a. Acetaminophen or ibuprofen, with dose calculated according to weight, is effective for mild to moderate pain.
    b. Narcotic analgesia with codeine is effective for moderate to severe pain. However, there are continued concerns about the potential for significant side effects and even death for children who are prescribed codeine. The risks of prescribing codeine for children necessitate serious consideration and physician consultation.
    c. Topical agents may provide brief relief, but evidence is limited as to extended benefits.[2]
15. Antihistamines, decongestants, and steroids are not beneficial for treatment of AOM or OME.[2,3,7]

DIFFERENTIAL DIAGNOSIS

Otitis Media

- Otitis externa
- Transient MEE
- Mastoiditis
- Temporomandibular joint disorder
- Mumps
- Dental disorder
- Tonsillitis
- Foreign body
- Head or ear trauma

16. Treatment decisions should be reconsidered if symptoms worsen or fail to respond to initial antibiotic treatment within 48 to 72 hours.[2,3]
17. OME should be evaluated monthly for superimposed AOM (refer to ear, nose, and throat [ENT] specialist).[3]
18. Prophylactic antibiotic use for the treatment and prevention of chronic or recurrent otitis media in children is no longer recommended unless unusual circumstances exist.[2]

COMPLICATIONS

The most common short-term consequence is decreased conductive hearing loss. MEE and chronic OME may last for months and can be a barrier to learning and language development in young children.[1-3] Eardrum perforation is a common sequela of both AOM and OME. Hearing loss, perforation of the eardrum, cholesteatoma, acute mastoiditis, meningitis, and epidermal abscess are less common complications of otitis media, especially in developed countries. Of additional concern is the consequence of antibiotic resistance. Antibiotic treatment of OME in the absence of bacterial infection is linked with growing drug resistance.[2,3,6]

INDICATIONS FOR REFERRAL OR HOSPITALIZATION

The patient with AOM who does not respond to therapy in 48 to 72 hours should be switched to an alternative therapy.

Specialist referral is indicated for tympanocentesis for culture to determine antibiotic sensitivity for AOM that fails to resolve within 3 days of treatment with a second-line agent.[3]

Speech and audiology evaluation for speech delay is indicated in younger children at 3 months for OME that fails to resolve and the potential need for ventilating tubes with or without adenoidectomy.[3]

ENT referral for tympanostomy tubes is indicated for recurrent AOM (three episodes in 6 months or four or more episodes in 1 year with one episode in preceding 6 months).[2]

LIFE SPAN CONSIDERATIONS

AOM is primarily a disease of young children. The incidence decreases quickly after age 7 years, when the Eustachian tube matures. In adults, AOM most often occurs in smokers and in adults who are exposed to second-hand smoke.[1]

EDUCATION AND HEALTH PROMOTION

Education regarding otitis media risk reduction and treatment is focused most appropriately toward parents and caregivers when patients are younger. Treatment decisions should include the preferences of parents and caregivers regarding the prescription of antibiotics. Parental comfort with delaying antibiotic administration may be increased with provision of a written antibiotic prescription to be held while the child is under initial observation. Follow-up consultation initiated by the provider is critical to the decision to observe before antibiotic use. In addition, caregivers often require careful explanation about symptomatic treatment of OME and MEE, rather than antibiotic treatment in the absence of AOM.

Parents also need to understand that antibiotic treatment alone does not necessarily relieve pain and sleeplessness. Pain relief measures are necessary whether or not the provider is waiting to initiate antibiotics.

Otitis media, including AOM and OME, is not contagious, allowing children to return to day care or school once acute symptoms have resolved. All caregivers need to understand proper administration of antibiotics and management of pain and other symptoms. Teachers need to be aware of impaired hearing, which may continue for weeks or months after the acute infection stage.

Breastfeeding for 3 months or more is associated with reduced incidence of AOM during the first year of life. Recurrent AOM in infants may increase with pacifier use after 6 months of age.

The risk of otitis media can be decreased by not smoking and by minimizing exposure to smoke. Smoking cessation should be encouraged.

In children, recent research indicates that the pneumococcal conjugate vaccine (PCV7) and influenza vaccine may have a protective effect.[1-3]

CHAPTER 87

TYMPANIC MEMBRANE PERFORATION

Vincent Pair

DEFINITION AND EPIDEMIOLOGY

Tympanic membrane (TM) perforation is an opening in the otherwise intact membrane that, as a mechanical component of hearing, separates the external ear from the middle ear. TM perforation results from a variety of conditions and is a cause of conductive hearing loss. Most perforations heal spontaneously without incident; however, some TM perforations may necessitate referral to a specialist.

PATHOPHYSIOLOGY

Perforation can be caused by a variety of traumatic, infectious, and neoplastic processes. The TM can be lacerated or perforated by foreign objects in the external canal. Barotrauma, physical trauma, blast injury, or a fracture of the temporal skull can tear or perforate the TM. On occasion, the TM perforates with the pressure and inflammation of acute otitis media. Perforations often precede the development of a cholesteatoma.[1-4]

CLINICAL PRESENTATION AND PHYSICAL EXAMINATION

A thorough history will support the cause of the TM perforation.[1,4] TM perforations are often discovered at the time of trauma or during the evaluation for middle ear infection. Perforation may also be observed in association with a cholesteatoma. Most patients with traumatic perforation experience pain and some degree of hearing loss.[5] A thorough ear examination and an evaluation of hearing status should be included in the initial assessment.

DIAGNOSTICS AND DIFFERENTIAL DIAGNOSIS

After the perforation has healed, an audiogram is helpful in evaluating the presence or extent of hearing impairment. The differential diagnosis includes all causes of perforation, including trauma, infection, and neoplasm.

DIAGNOSTICS

Tympanic Membrane Perforation

Audiogram

DIFFERENTIAL DIAGNOSIS

Tympanic Membrane Perforation

- Barotrauma
- Trauma
- Blast injury
- Infection
- Neoplasm

MANAGEMENT

Most TM perforations heal spontaneously unless they become secondarily infected or are very large. Some TM perforations will require surgical repair with a patch or graft. Patients should keep water out of the ear until the perforation has healed. Antibiotic drops or systemic antibiotics are often necessary when infection is evident.[1] Special consideration must be given to the individual with known or suspected perforation of the TM or history of tubes, because antibiotics placed into the middle ear can cross the round window membrane and reach the inner ear. Ototoxic antibiotics delivered into the middle ear space of experimental animals, including primates, consistently cause severe hearing loss and ototoxic injury to the organ of Corti. Although clinical experience suggests that hearing loss does not occur after a single short course of therapy in humans, prolonged or repetitive administration of topical drops has resulted in severe hearing loss.[3]

COMPLICATIONS AND INDICATIONS FOR REFERRAL OR HOSPITALIZATION

A middle ear infection, cholesteatoma, and impaired hearing are potential complications of a TM perforation. A referral to an otolaryngologist is appropriate for large perforations or for those that do not show evidence of timely healing. Also, patients with TM perforations resulting from blast injury or major trauma should be referred to a specialist.[1,4] Blast injuries have been shown to cause inner ear trauma as well as the obvious TM perforation, which can lead to profound hearing loss.[6] Likewise, skull fractures can damage the inner ear structures, causing permanent damage.

PATIENT AND FAMILY EDUCATION

Patient education should include measures to protect the TM while it heals. Patients should not permit water to enter the ear until healing has occurred, and they should be encouraged to return for follow-up evaluation. The cause of the perforation should be determined so that repeated perforations can be avoided.[7] Special emphasis on the importance of not inserting objects (e.g., cotton-tipped applicators) into the external ear canal is also necessary.[1,2]

REFERENCES

For a full list of references, scan the QR code or visit http://booksite.elsevier.com/9780323355018

PART 8

Evaluation and Management of Nose Disorders

CHAPTER 88

CHRONIC NASAL CONGESTION AND DISCHARGE

Catherine M. Franklin • Patricia A. Reidy • Daniel E. Kane • Emily Karwacki Sheff • Elissa Ladd • Margaret Ann Mahoney • Patrice K. Nicholas

DEFINITION AND EPIDEMIOLOGY

Chronic rhinosinusitis (CRS) is a clinical syndrome characterized by persistent inflammation of the nasal and paranasal sinus mucosa with symptoms for longer than 12 weeks' duration.[1] It is estimated that 16% of the population experiences CRS,[2,3] ranking it second in prevalence among all chronic conditions.[3] CRS affects all major racial and ethnic groups,[4] is more common in men,[5] has a significant effect on quality of life,[6,7] and accounts for 11.5 million missed workdays with an estimated cost approaching $2449.00 per patient per year.[8]

CRS is classified into two main subtypes: CRS without nasal polyps (CRSsNPs) and CRS with nasal polyps (CRSwNPs).[1] This differentiation can be made only in a specialist's office; for purposes of primary care, both are considered under the same category of CRS.[9]

PATHOPHYSIOLOGY

Nasal congestion is primarily the result of vascular changes and chronic inflammation in the nasal mucosa induced by a combination of immunologic, infectious, and environmental factors.[9] Predisposing and associated factors include dysfunctional cilia as seen in smokers and those with cystic fibrosis, allergy, asthma, aspirin sensitivity, genetic factors, and pregnancy.[1,9-11]

CLINICAL PRESENTATION

The clinical presentation of CRS includes nasal blockage, nasal discharge (anterior or posterior nasal drip), facial pain or pressure, and reduction in or loss of smell for 12 weeks or longer[1] and is distinguished from symptoms of acute onset and allergic rhinitis. See Table 88-1 for distinction in symptoms.

A detailed history is critical to the diagnosis. It is important to ask the patient about the onset and timing of symptoms, location of congestion on one side or both, and associated symptoms such as rhinorrhea, sneezing, eye symptoms, itchiness, change in smell, fever, purulent discharge, facial pressure, and snoring. Ask about triggers such as pollutants, allergens, and occupational chemicals. Ask the patient if there is a history of allergies, asthma, aspirin sensitivity, acute sinusitis, nasal trauma, nasal surgery, nasal polyps, or a family history of seasonal or environmental allergies. A detailed medication history and a history of smoking, exposure to passive smoke, and recreational drug use should also be elicited.[9]

PHYSICAL EXAMINATION

The patient is observed for any asymmetry or deformity of the nasal structure. The patient should be asked to press on each nostril individually and breathe in to test for obstruction. Inspect each nostril with an otoscope with a wide speculum. Apply gentle pressure to the tip of the nose with the examiner's thumb to widen the nostrils, and then insert the lighted otoscope. The nasal mucous membranes are inspected for erythema, pallor, atrophy, edema, crusting, and discharge. The mucosa of the turbinates is often more erythematous in patients with chronic nasal congestion compared with the pale bluish hue or pallor seen in patients with allergic rhinitis. Any abnormalities, such as polyps, erosions, and septal deviations or perforations, should also be noted. Finally, the frontal and maxillary sinuses are palpated.[11]

DIAGNOSTICS

Selection of laboratory studies depends on the differential diagnoses and any suspected disease process. Skin and in vitro

TABLE 88-1 Comparison of Clinical Presentations of Chronic Rhinosinusitis and Allergic Rhinitis[1,9,12]

Variable	Chronic Rhinosinusitis	Allergic Rhinitis
Symptoms	Persistent nasal blockage May alternate sides Postnasal drip Facial pain Anosmia	Intermittent nasal blockage or rhinorrhea Usually bilateral Sneezing Itching or watery eyes Frequently associated atopic dermatitis
Onset	≥12 weeks	Acute or intermittent
Allergens	May be associated and identifiable	Associated and identifiable
Timing	Perennial May be exacerbated by weather	Typically seasonal Can also be perennial
Family history of seasonal or environmental allergies	Infrequent or absent	Typically present
Asthma	Less frequent	More frequent

tests for allergen-specific immunoglobulin E may be helpful in determining whether the symptoms are related to allergic or nonallergic disease. Plain x-ray studies and computed tomography (CT) are not recommended in primary care. The diagnosis of CRS is a diagnosis of exclusion in primary care, based on criteria and symptoms alone.[1,9]

DIFFERENTIAL DIAGNOSIS

Allergic Rhinitis

Allergic rhinitis is diagnosed based on symptoms and with allergy testing. Refer to Chapter 91 for more information.

Sinusitis

Sinusitis may manifest as an acute or chronic infection of the sinus cavities. Refer to Chapter 92 for more information on this topic.

Rhinitis Medicamentosa

Rhinitis medicamentosa occurs when nasal decongestants (e.g., oxymetazoline, phenylpropanolamine, pseudoephedrine) are overused, leading to a worsening of symptoms.[12] After more than 3 days of continuous use, response to these agents becomes blunted (tachyphylaxis). Once the response to these medications has changed, the patient is likely to increase the number of times that the medication is used to obtain a therapeutic response. Cessation of the medication at this point may result in rebound nasal congestion. The congestion is believed to be a result of reflex vasodilation. The nasal mucosa appears erythematous.

Cocaine Use

Cocaine abuse is becoming a more common cause of nasal congestion seen in the primary care setting. Nasal snorting of cocaine results in nasal congestion and discharge. Cocaine is a potent sympathomimetic, and the reaction of the nasal passages is similar to that of nasal decongestant abuse. Recurrent nasal use of cocaine causes the nasal septal mucosa to become ischemic. This leads to tissue atrophy and telltale septal perforation.[13]

Pregnancy Rhinitis

Pregnancy rhinitis manifests as nasal congestion without allergy or infection in 18% to 30% of pregnant women.[10] The rise in estrogen in the second and third trimesters leads to an increase in hyaluronic acid in the nasal mucosa, resulting in increased nasal edema and congestion. In addition, during pregnancy there is an increase in the number of mucous glands and a decrease in nasal cilia, both of which contribute to diminished clearance of mucus.[14]

Mechanical Obstruction

Congestion, discharge, and recurrent episodes of sinusitis that are unilateral are the classic signs of mechanical obstruction. The obstruction can be caused by a tumor, polyp, deviated septum, or foreign body in the nose. Neoplasms are rare, and polyps generally occur in association with allergic and idiopathic rhinitis, chronic sinusitis, aspirin-induced asthma, cystic fibrosis, and drug abuse.

Autoimmune Vasculitides

Autoimmune vasculitides such as Wegener granulomatosis or sarcoidosis affect the upper and lower respiratory tracts and kidneys, involving both small arteries and veins. A common presentation is paranasal sinus pain and nasal discharge.[1] (See Chapters 94 and 220.)

DIFFERENTIAL DIAGNOSIS

Chronic Rhinosinusitis

- Allergic rhinitis
- Rhinosinusitis
- Rhinitis medicamentosa
- Cocaine use
- Pregnancy rhinitis
- Mechanical obstruction
- Autoimmune vasculitides

MANAGEMENT

Patients with warning signs of complications and severe illness should be referred urgently to an otolaryngology specialist. These warning signs include periorbital edema, diplopia, displaced globe, reduced visual acuity, proptosis, and severe headache.[1,9]

The goal of management for CRS is symptom control of inflammation and reduction of infectious exacerbations. These patients typically are less responsive to oral pharmacotherapy.

1. Intranasal corticosteroids are the mainstay of treatment to minimize and control inflammation and are considered safe for long-term use.[1,3,9] Initial treatment should include the addition of saline lavage of the sinus cavities.[9]
2. Oral decongestants, such as pseudoephedrine and phenylephrine hydrochloride, should be used sparingly and only on days when symptoms are especially intolerable. Oral decongestants should not be recommended for patients with hypertension. Referral to an otolaryngologist of patients with severe congestion refractory to treatment is appropriate because surgery may be helpful for some patients.
3. Use of antibiotics may be considered if an exacerbation of CRS leads to bacterial sinusitis (see Chapter 92).
4. When topical decongestants have been abused, the rebound nasal congestion will resolve 2 to 3 weeks after the medication is stopped. If cocaine has been abused, the septum will slowly heal once the drug is stopped.
5. Nasal congestion associated with pregnancy will resolve after delivery. Use of saline lavage for symptomatic relief is recommended. There are no human data on the safety of intranasal corticosteroid in pregnancy.

COMPLICATIONS

Complications depend on the cause: ulcerations, infection, and septal perforation may occur if the underlying disorder is undetected.

INDICATIONS FOR REFERRAL OR HOSPITALIZATION

In most cases, CRS can be managed successfully in the primary care setting. Referral to an otolaryngologist specialist for further evaluation may be considered in the following instances:

- Patients with severe congestion refractory to treatment after 4 weeks of intranasal corticosteroids and saline lavage.
- Circumstances in which the health care provider is unable to easily remove a foreign body or if nasal polyp or tumor is suspected.

LIFE SPAN CONSIDERATIONS

CRS is a common condition in children and a diagnosis often overlooked in primary care practice. Symptoms may lead to chronic cough, malodorous breath, poor appetite, and interrupted sleep. Symptoms may be associated with asthma, allergic rhinitis, tonsillar hypertrophy, and recurrent otitis media.[15]

CRS is also a common condition in the older adult. Symptomatology is the same as in a younger population, and the management is the same.[1]

Patients with pregnancy rhinosinusitis should be counseled in symptom management and offered reassurance that the condition will most likely resolve after delivery.

PATIENT AND FAMILY EDUCATION AND HEALTH PROMOTION

All patients should be educated about the risks associated with decongestant abuse, cocaine, and chronic exposure to irritants and allergens. Patients should be instructed in the proper use of saline irrigations and nasal sprays. All patients should be advised that the effect of nasal corticosteroids may not be noticed for several days to weeks. Patients should be counseled that this may be a lifelong condition that will require chronic management.

CHAPTER 89

EPISTAXIS

Patricia A. Reidy • Emily Karwacki Sheff • Catherine M. Franklin • Daniel E. Kane • Elissa Ladd • Margaret Ann Mahoney • Patrice K. Nicholas

DEFINITION AND EPIDEMIOLOGY

Epistaxis (nosebleed) is a common problem experienced by most individuals at some time in their lives. Epistaxis occurs in 60% of the population and is the second most common reason for emergency admission to otolaryngology services.[1] The incidence is highest in individuals younger than 10 years and in individuals 70 to 79 years.[2] Most nosebleeds are idiopathic. Some individuals are more prone to nosebleeds because of fragile mucous membranes. Local predisposing factors include nasal trauma, rhinitis, drying of the nasal mucosa from low humidity, nasal septum deviation, alcohol use, and chemical irritants (e.g., cocaine). Systemic conditions from either genetic or acquired coagulation disorders, hematologic cancers, and anticoagulation medication can cause epistaxis.[2] Herbal supplements can inhibit platelet aggregation, causing adverse effects with other prescribed medications.[3]

PATHOPHYSIOLOGY

Bleeding can occur from the anterior or posterior nares. Ninety percent to 95% of nosebleeds occur within the Kiesselbach plexus, a vascular plexus on the anterior nasal septum, and are associated with irritated mucous membranes or trauma.[2,4] This plexus is particularly vulnerable and easily injured. Posterior nosebleeds occur within the posterior branches of the sphenopalatine artery and account for 5% of cases. In general, these nosebleeds are idiopathic or associated with vascular disease and can be difficult to control.[3] Studies have not found an association between hypertension and epistaxis, although there may be an elevated risk caused by vascular changes.[3]

CLINICAL PRESENTATION

Patients with epistaxis initially are seen with scant to copious amounts of blood emerging from the nares. Anterior nosebleeds are usually unilateral with continuous moderate bleeding. Depending on the amount of bleeding, small clots may also emerge. Patients may report that the bleeding began spontaneously or that nasal trauma preceded the bleeding. Posterior nosebleeds can occur bilaterally, are associated with severe bleeding, and are difficult to treat. Bleeding into the pharynx is indicative of a posterior epistaxis. If the patient's condition is stable, the provider should obtain a thorough health history regarding frequency, duration, trauma, nasal obstruction, and prior treatments. It is important to inquire about other systemic conditions, prescribed and complementary alternative medications, intranasal substances, and clotting disorders to establish the causative factors and initiate care.[1,3]

PHYSICAL EXAMINATION

Vital signs and airway safety should first be determined, and the patient should be instructed to sit up straight, tilt the head forward, and apply firm, continuous pressure for 15 minutes to the anterior aspect of the affected nostril.[2] The provider should assess for blood loss and risk for hemodynamic instability. If the epistaxis is the result of trauma, the nose should be checked for fractures. An internal examination may be deferred until the blood flow has subsided; but if the bleeding does not readily subside or nasal compression causes postnasal bleeding, the nose should be examined with a nasal speculum. The blood is cleared with suction or nose blowing to identify the site of bleeding. Topical vasoconstrictive agents such as 1:1000 epinephrine or 4% cocaine, applied either as a spray or on a cotton pledget, serves as both an anesthetic and a vasoconstricting agent. If this preparation is not available, a topical decongestant (e.g., oxymetazoline) can be used in conjunction with a topical anesthetic (e.g., lidocaine) to examine the nose.[2,3] The nose should be inspected to identify the bleeding site before further treatment is initiated. If the site cannot be identified, the posterior pharynx is inspected for any bleeding. Rinsing the oropharynx first with water will clear the area to permit identification of any new bleeding.[2]

DIAGNOSTICS

It is important to consider any underlying condition that may have caused the epistaxis. Laboratory assessment of bleeding parameters may be necessary to exclude underlying disease,

DIAGNOSTICS

Epistaxis

LABORATORY

CBC and differential (if infection or extensive blood loss is present)
Coagulation studies*
Type and screen/crossmatch (with extensive blood loss)*
Basic metabolic panel (if hemodynamically unstable)

*If indicated.

especially if the bleeding recurs without a clinical explanation. A complete blood count (CBC) with a type and screen/crossmatch should be obtained if severe bleeding has occurred. A prothrombin time (PT) and international normalized ratio (INR) should be obtained if the patient is taking an anticoagulant. Additional laboratory studies should be performed if the patient is hemodynamically unstable.[2,3]

DIFFERENTIAL DIAGNOSIS

Sudden epistaxis demands conscientious consideration. Although nasal trauma is the most common cause of nasal bleeding, it is critical to recognize other conditions that may result in bleeding from the nose. Other causes of recurrent epistaxis, such as systemic factors (e.g., hemophilia, von Willebrand disease, hereditary hemorrhagic telangiectasia [Osler-Weber-Rendu disease], thrombocytopenia, or tumor), chemical irritants, or warfarin toxicity should be considered.[3]

DIFFERENTIAL DIAGNOSIS[1-3]

Epistaxis

EAR, NOSE, AND THROAT
- Allergic rhinitis
- Nasal trauma
- Foreign body
- Septal perforation

GENETIC CAUSES
- Coagulation defect
- Hereditary hemorrhagic telangiectasia (HHT)
- von Willebrand disease
- Hemophilia

CARDIOVASCULAR CAUSES
- Hypertension
- Congestive heart failure

MEDICATIONS
- Aspirin, warfarin
- Nasal steroids
- Cocaine

OTHER CAUSES
- Neoplasm

MANAGEMENT

Anterior Epistaxis

Most cases of epistaxis can be successfully treated with the application of direct pressure to the anterior portion of the nose for 15 minutes. This technique is often successful because the most common source of epistaxis is the anterior part of the septum, where the Kiesselbach plexus is located. The patient should also be encouraged to sit upright because venous pressure is reduced in this position. The patient should also lean forward to decrease the swallowing of blood. Depending on the amount of bleeding, short-acting topical nasal decongestants (e.g., phenylephrine 0.125% to 1% solution, one or two sprays), which act as vasoconstrictors, may help stop the blood flow. One retrospective study reported that 65% of patients seen in the emergency department with epistaxis were successfully treated with oxymetazoline and nasal pressure.[3] Once the bleeding site has been identified, the area can be treated with chemical cautery (silver nitrate) or electrocautery.[2,3] After the bleeding has stopped, a small amount of petroleum is applied in the nares and the patient is observed for 30 minutes.

If the bleeding continues, nasal packing may be used. It is important to insert the packing properly in the nares to reduce bleeding. Two types of packing are commonly used. Merocel is a nasal polyhydroxylated polyvinyl tampon that expands when moistened. RapidRhino uses a coated inflatable balloon to increase the pressure and is effective as a platelet aggregator.[4,5] There should be minimal packing visible at the nares if placed appropriately. The packing strings or balloon should be taped to the face to avoid displacement.[4] Once it is in place, the pack is not removed for 24 to 48 hours.[3] If the bleeding continues, the opposite nostril should be packed in a similar fashion to increase nasal pressure. After insertion of the nasal pack, the patient must be observed for 30 minutes to determine that there is no posterior bleeding. Once there is evidence of no bleeding, the patient may be discharged home. Prophylactic antibiotics such as cephalexin (250 mg) four times daily or amoxicillin-clavulanate (875 mg/125 mg every 12 hours) are prescribed while the packing is in place to prevent infection.[3]

Posterior Epistaxis

Continued bleeding suggests that there is a posterior bleed and requires specialist consultation and possible hospitalization. Posterior packs with a balloon catheter (Epistat) provides bidirectional pressure to control the bleeding until the patient can be brought to surgery.[5] Nasal endoscopy is performed to visualize the bleeding site.[5] Surgical techniques such as arterial ligation or vascular embolization may be considered by an otolaryngologist. This technique is certainly necessary when the bleeding becomes life-threatening and other treatments have failed.

Epistaxis management is variable, but one study found that chemical cautery was most effective for initial treatment whereas direct vascular control (e.g., ligation, embolization) managed recurrent epistaxis.[6] Epistaxis management is variable.

COMPLICATIONS

Complications are rare because most nosebleeds are easily controlled. However, respiratory function can be compromised, and patients may become hypotensive if bleeding is severe. Other complications are usually related to treatment and include necrosis, abscess formation, septal perforation, and sinus infection.[1] Toxic shock syndrome has also been reported as a complication of nasal packing; thus, appropriate antibiotic therapy is necessary while the packing is in place.[1,5] Posterior packing can cause a vagal response resulting in hypotension and bradycardia.[1] One study showed that patients who undergo embolization are at higher risk for a stroke compared with a nasal packing procedure.[7] This may be related to comorbid conditions rather than to complications from the procedure.

INDICATIONS FOR REFERRAL OR HOSPITALIZATION

Patients should be referred to a specialist in a critical care setting if there is extensive bleeding or posterior epistaxis. Depending on the ability to access the site or control the bleeding, extensive packing may be required. Not all office settings are equipped to manage acute epistasis. If the bleeding cannot be managed within 15 minutes, patients should be transferred to an emergency department. The packing should be done in an operating room or specialist's office because of discomfort and risk of hypoxia. Nasal obstruction may require endoscopy or imaging studies by an otolaryngologist. Surgical intervention may be necessary if medical measures are not sufficient to eliminate epistaxis.

LIFE SPAN CONSIDERATIONS

The incidence of epistaxis is bimodal, occurring in ages below 10 years and above 70 years.[1] Posterior nosebleeds are more frequently seen in the older population and are a frequent cause of emergency department visits.[1]

PATIENT AND FAMILY EDUCATION AND HEALTH PROMOTION

Once the bleeding has stopped, the patient is advised to avoid vigorous exercise and aspirin-containing medications for several days or weeks. The patient and family should also understand the importance of calling the health care provider if the bleeding recurs (particularly while packing is in place) and recognize the necessity of follow-up evaluation within 48 to 72 hours to ensure healing of the lesion.

Avoidance of tobacco and hot, spicy foods is also advisable because they may cause vasodilation. Avoidance of nasal trauma, including digital self-trauma, is an obvious necessity. Lubrication of the mucous membranes with petroleum jelly, nasal saline, or bacitracin ointment may relieve nasal discomfort and reduce the need to manipulate the nasal passages.[3] Home humidification may also prevent the nasal irritation that results from a dry environment. Patients should also understand how to treat nosebleeds at home by applying firm pressure to the nostrils for 10 to 30 minutes.

CHAPTER 90

NASAL TRAUMA

Jason R. Lucey • Daniel E. Kane • Catherine M. Franklin • Patricia A. Reidy • Emily Karwacki Sheff • Kerry A. Decker • Margaret Ann Mahoney • Patrice K. Nicholas

DEFINITION AND EPIDEMIOLOGY

Nasal injuries are important not only because they may be associated with critical life-threatening complications but also because of the potential for long-term cosmetic disfigurement, which can lead to poor social and psychological outcomes for patients.[1] Nasal trauma occurs with high frequency owing to the prominence of the nose on the face and the relative fragility of the nasal bones compared with other facial bone structures.[2] The nasal bones are fractured more often than other facial bones, and these injuries occur more than twice as often in men as in women.[2]

PATHOPHYSIOLOGY

Nasal trauma is the result of a severe blow to the face. In adults, most facial blows are related to automobile accidents, sports injuries, or altercations.[2] Falls and abuse are also associated with nasal and orbital trauma. Because facial anatomy is complex, injuries to the nose and face can involve damage to skin, mucous membranes, muscle, nerve, bone, cartilage and vascular structures.[1]

CLINICAL PRESENTATION

Immediate emergency department referral is indicated for nasal trauma associated with airway compromise, evidence of intracranial injury, leaking cerebrospinal fluid, or suspicion for cervical spine injury.

If immediate emergent transfer is deemed to be unnecessary, a more focused history of the injury should be obtained. The mechanism of injury and the patient's past medical history, allergies, and current medications should be discerned. Distinguishing between an isolated nasal injury and one that is associated with other conditions such as concussion, facial or orbital injury, or cervical spine injury is of utmost importance. Questions about loss of consciousness, headache, nausea and vomiting, diplopia, visual changes, facial numbness, and malocclusion or other dental injury should be asked.[1,2] Interviewing a witness to the injury other than the patient may be helpful to describe the patient's behavior and appearance immediately after the injury occurred. Specific history questions related to nasal injuries might include the following: Can you breathe through both of your nostrils? Did you have any bleeding from the nostrils (one or both), and how long did it last? Have you ever had a broken nose or nasal surgery before?[1]

PHYSICAL EXAMINATION

During inspection, the health care provider should determine the presence of periorbital ecchymosis, edema, abrasions or lacerations, epistaxis, or cerebrospinal fluid leakage (clear or blood-tinged liquid); trauma to the teeth, neck, or chest; and obvious deformity. Inspection from multiple perspectives (e.g., frontal, worm's eye, and bird's eye views) can help identify subtle abnormalities.[1,2] Respiratory and cervical spine stability and vital signs should be assessed. Assessing patency of airflow through the nostrils can help determine the presence of potential obstruction caused by deviation of a fractured septum, soft tissue edema, or a potential septal hematoma.

The dorsum (bridge) of the nose should be gently palpated for deformity, instability, crepitus, and point tenderness. It is also important to assess for a palpable step-off of the infraorbital rim; this indicates a zygomatic complex fracture.[3] If orbital involvement is suspected, a detailed examination should include assessment of extraocular muscle function looking for diplopia caused by entrapment of the inferior rectus muscle as well as investigation for facial anesthesia secondary to infraorbital nerve injury.[1] Stability of the teeth and palate should also be evaluated. Intranasal examination with adequate lighting and use of a nasal speculum (if available) is conducted to visualize the internal nasal structures including the mucosa, septum, and turbinates. Septal fracture, displacement or deviation, hematoma, or laceration should be noted.[4] Epistaxis may be present when there has been trauma, and although bleeding is often a sign that the nose has been fractured, one third of patients with a fracture may not have any epistaxis.[4] If bleeding is active, internal examination of the nose may be deferred until it is controlled with a combination of direct pressure, topical vasoconstrictors, or nasal packing as needed. Exclude a septal hematoma, which appears as a rounded bluish or purplish mass against the nasal septum and requires urgent drainage to prevent cosmetic long-term complications (see the Complications section, later).[1]

DIAGNOSTICS

Choice of imaging techniques for a nasal injury is influenced by the associated findings and mechanism of injury. For injuries in which there is suspicion of intracranial involvement or facial skull fracture (e.g., cerebrospinal fluid rhinorrhea; orbital or facial or sinus step-off; extraocular muscle [EOM] palsy; or high-speed mechanism), computed tomography (CT) scan is the preferred modality.[1] For isolated nasal bone injuries, plain x-ray examination may confirm the findings from the physical examination; however, x-ray studies of the nasal bones seldom provide additional information and are not recommended unless there is suspicion of extensive trauma that extends beyond a simple nasal fracture.[1,2] Deferring initial x-ray examination of nasal bones is appropriate and will not influence the plan of care if tenderness and swelling are isolated to the nasal bridge; both nares are patent; there is no significant deformity or angulation seen; and no septal hematoma is present.[1] Another less widely available imaging option for nasal and facial injuries is high-resolution ultrasonography, which has been shown to be sensitive and specific in identifying nasal fractures.[5]

DIAGNOSTICS

Nasal Trauma

IMAGING
X-ray study
High-resolution ultrasound
CT scan*

*If indicated.

DIFFERENTIAL DIAGNOSIS

The differential diagnosis of nasal trauma is based on the force of the trauma, with higher-speed mechanisms being more concerning for potentially life-threatening or disfiguring injury. Frontal sinus fractures result from trauma to the forehead and, because of the location, may initially be seen as a nasal fracture. Brisk hemorrhage from the nasal cavity accompanies these fractures. Fractures of the posterior wall of the frontal sinus may cause dural tears and leakage of cerebrospinal fluid into the nasal cavity. Other injuries that should be included in the differential diagnosis include concussion, septal hematomas, zygomatic arch fractures, maxillary sinus fractures, and orbital fractures.

DIFFERENTIAL DIAGNOSIS

Nasal Trauma

- Nasal fracture
- Frontal sinus fracture
- Zygomatic or maxillary fractures
- Orbital fracture
- Septal hematoma
- Concussion

MANAGEMENT

Initial treatment consists of cool, local pressure to the affected areas to decrease edema and bleeding. A nasal fracture without deformity or septal hematoma may be treated with ice, head elevation, and analgesia (e.g., acetaminophen), with close otolaryngology follow-up in 3 to 5 days for reevaluation once swelling has subsided.[1] Ideally, a displaced fracture would be manually reduced under general or local anesthesia in the initial postinjury hours by a trained provider or otolaryngologist, but many specialists prefer to allow initial swelling to subside in the first 3 to 5 days after injury before manipulation.[1,2] Nasal fracture reduction in children is typically performed with the patient under general anesthesia.[2]

Antibiotics are typically prescribed for open fractures, injuries with grossly contaminated wounds, wounds involving nasal cartilage, or injuries in which nasal packing is used (e.g., incision and drainage of septal hematoma).[1] Assessment of tetanus vaccination status and appropriate prophylaxis are indicated for any nasal injury with a wound.[1]

COMPLICATIONS

Nasal trauma may result in a nasal septal hematoma that separates the septal cartilage from the adherent mucoperichondrium, which supplies the septum with nutrition.[6] A hematoma that remains untreated can result in the loss of nasal cartilage because the mucoperichondrium cannot reattach to the septum. Therefore the blood supply is lost and the septum becomes necrotic. The loss of nasal cartilage results in a saddle nose deformity. Treatment of a septal hematoma requires urgent surgical incision, drainage, and packing by a trained provider (emergency department or otolaryngologist).[1,2]

Deviations of the nasal septum are often a complication of nasal trauma. The deviation may cause varying degrees of nasal obstruction and predispose the patient to sinusitis and epistaxis. This is a result of the loss of natural defenses, such as the nasal cilia. Septal ulcers and perforations may occur after repeated trauma and even constant nose picking. In addition, nasal foreign bodies may mimic nasal trauma or fracture; this may occur as a result of trauma to the face in adults or introduction of a foreign body in the nasal cavity in the pediatric population.[7]

INDICATIONS FOR REFERRAL OR HOSPITALIZATION

Immediate emergency department referral is required for nasal trauma associated with airway compromise, evidence of intracranial injury, leaking cerebrospinal fluid, or suspicion for cervical spine injury.

In primary care practice, nasal injuries are frequently referred to otolaryngology for follow-up within the first week of the injury. After swelling has subsided (usually after 3 to 5 days), a more detailed examination for airflow obstruction deformity can be performed, and, if necessary, reduction and manipulation of the fracture can be done with the appropriate anesthesia. Again, any suspicion of leaking cerebrospinal fluid or a dural tear or other more complex skull or facial fractures mandates more immediate referral to the emergency department or specialist.

LIFE SPAN CONSIDERATIONS

Pediatric

Fractures of the nasal bones in infants and very young children are not as common as in older children and adolescents. Nasal skeletal structure in early childhood is mostly composed of cartilage and, in general, infants and younger children are engaged in activities with lower risk of high-impact trauma compared with older children and teens.[2] As with any injury in pediatric patients, the clinician should include abuse in the differential diagnosis and involve social services or legal authorities as mandated by reporting laws if the situation warrants it.[2]

Geriatric

Falls and associated trauma are a significant, common, and potentially life-threatening problem in geriatrics.[8] The nurse practitioner should include a general assessment of fall risk in the evaluation of any elderly patient with nasal trauma. The cause of a fall should be investigated and other comorbid conditions leading to fall should be considered. Risk factors for falls include but are not limited to neurologic diseases, syncope, polypharmacy, and alcohol use.[8]

Severe complications of head trauma (even with fairly minor mechanisms such as a fall from a standing position) in elderly patients, such as intracranial bleeding, may occur without overt neurologic deficits on initial examination.[9] The clinician should have a low threshold for referring elderly patients who have fallen for emergency department care and appropriate imaging and access to specialty care.[9]

PATIENT AND FAMILY EDUCATION

The patient should understand the signs and symptoms of complications and whom to call if problems develop. In particular, the patient should return for evaluation if the pain becomes intense, if bleeding is profuse, and if nasal discharge becomes purulent with a foul odor. Signs and symptoms of worsening intracranial injury (e.g., headache, confusion, vomiting, vision changes) should be reviewed, and the patient instructed to seek emergency care if they develop. If nasal packing (for epistaxis or septal hematoma drainage) has been placed, the patient should understand the importance of prompt scheduled follow-up for its removal. Routine risks and benefits of any analgesics or antibiotics should be reviewed. Ice application and elevation of the head of the bed for sleeping may provide comfort and control soft-tissue swelling.[1] The patient should avoid any nose touching or picking, increase the degree of humidified air at home, and increase fluid intake. The dressings should not get wet, and swimming is not allowed until dressings are removed and wounds adequately healed. Antihistamine use and smoking are discouraged during the recovery period. Lastly, prevention of sports-related nasal injuries should be encouraged through counseling on the use of protective headgear including face-shields available for many sports.[2]

CHAPTER 91

RHINITIS

Alexandra Wilder

ALLERGIC RHINITIS

DEFINITION AND EPIDEMIOLOGY

Allergic rhinitis is a condition characterized by sneezing, rhinorrhea, and nasal and pharyngeal itching in relation to an allergen exposure. In more severe cases, systemic symptoms of fatigue, headache, and cognitive impairment may be present. This disorder is caused by an immunoglobulin E (IgE)–mediated hypersensitivity response to foreign allergens and can affect individuals in any age group. The hallmark of this condition is the temporal correlation of symptoms with exposure to allergens, most commonly pollens, weeds, trees, grass, animal dander, dust mites, foods, insect stings, cockroach droppings, mold spores, and medications.

The prevalence of allergic rhinitis varies by location and depends on the type and quantity of airborne allergens. Recent estimates state that up to 14% of Americans experience allergic rhinitis, although that number may in fact be higher.[1]

PATHOPHYSIOLOGY

The nose contains a large surface area where inhaled particles are trapped before they can flow into the lower respiratory structures. Most allergens are large and become trapped in the mucous membranes of the nasal tissue. In the mucous membranes, there is an initial reaction between the allergen and intraepithelial mast cells, which proceeds deeper to the perivenular mast cells, both of which are sensitized with specific IgE. In addition to IgE, the mucosal surface in the nose also contains IgA. The IgE attaches to the mucosal and submucosal mast cells, and the intensity of the symptoms is directly related to the allergen dose. When an allergen is inhaled, the IgE attached to the mast cells within the mucosa and submucosa stimulates the release of histamine and leukotrienes, causing local tissue edema and increased drainage.

CLINICAL PRESENTATION

Allergic rhinitis should be suspected with seasonal or recurrent sneezing, disturbances of taste or smell, nasal congestion, dry mouth, postnasal discharge, and fatigue. Nasal discharge is thin and clear, and the patient may have nasal obstruction and facial discomfort. Watery, itchy, and puffy eyes commonly occur, but fever and chills are unusual. Typically the patient has a personal or family history of asthma, eczema, or other atopic disease.

A detailed environmental exposure history is essential. Dust mites, animal dander, and indoor allergens should be suspected when winter symptoms predominate because heating systems disseminate dust particles and aggravate symptoms during the winter months. Patients with seasonal symptoms are typically allergic to outdoor allergens such as pollen and ragweed. Symptoms that occur during late spring and early summer are generally triggered by grass pollens, whereas symptoms during late summer and early fall tend to be linked to weed pollens. Tree pollens tend to be associated with symptoms in late winter or early spring. These generalizations vary with geographic changes and daily fluctuations in allergen counts.

Because symptoms related to allergic rhinitis cause itching in the nose and throughout the upper respiratory tract, the pattern of symptoms is important. When is the patient asymptomatic? What medications has the patient been using? Where and when do symptoms occur? Is there associated itching, and if so, where?

The exact anatomic location of congestion should also be determined. Anatomic obstructions tend to cause unilateral nostril blockage, whereas nasal polyps generally cause bilateral obstruction.

PHYSICAL EXAMINATION

The physical examination can be performed with either a nasal speculum or an otoscope with an attached speculum. The nasal mucosa is typically pale (in contrast to viral or bacterial disease) because of chronic venous engorgement from the histamine and leukotrienes. The upper airway examination will also reveal swollen nasal turbinates with bleeding, mucus, crusting, and other signs of inflammation. Other common findings can include enlarged tonsils, postnasal drip, the well-recognized "allergic salute" (a crease across the nose from manipulating the tip of the nose), and conjunctival irritation.[2]

DIAGNOSTICS

Diagnosis of allergic rhinitis is primarily clinically based; patients report the hallmark symptoms of sneezing, rhinorrhea, and nasal and pharyngeal itching in the absence of infection. If there is a question about the cause of the symptoms, nasal cytologic studies (Wright stain) can demonstrate neutrophils or eosinophils and determine whether the symptoms are related to allergic rhinitis or infection. If further diagnostic tests are desired, the patient should be referred to an allergist for testing. Additional tests can include scratch or patch tests, which are used to test for skin response to suspected allergens. Radioallergosorbent tests (RASTs) determine serum levels of allergen-specific IgE titers, but skin testing is more sensitive and is the preferred diagnostic. However, RASTs are helpful in diagnosis of food-related allergies and can be used in patients with dermatographism or equivocal skin test results or in patients who cannot discontinue antihistamines.

DIAGNOSTICS

Allergic Rhinitis

LABORATORY	OTHER
Nasal cytology–Wright stain	Allergic scratch tests
RASTs	

DIFFERENTIAL DIAGNOSIS

Providers should exclude structural abnormalities within the nasopharynx, irritant exposure, pregnancy, hypothyroidism, idiopathic rhinitis, rhinitis medicamentosa, or prolonged use of topical alpha-adrenergic agents before making a diagnosis of allergic rhinitis. Many oral medications are also associated with rhinitis, including reserpine, methyldopa, nonsteroidal anti-inflammatory drugs (NSAIDs), and beta blockers.[3] Infectious rhinitis tends to be associated with fever, purulent sinus drainage, and other signs of infectious sinusitis.

DIFFERENTIAL DIAGNOSIS

Allergic Rhinitis

ALLERGIC
- Seasonal
- Perennial

INFECTIOUS
- Viral
- Bacterial

ANATOMIC
- Nasal polyps
- Deviated septum
- Neoplasm
- Adenoidal hypertrophy

IMMUNOLOGIC
- Acquired immunodeficiency syndrome (AIDS)
- Primary ciliary dyskinesia
- Cystic fibrosis
- Humoral deficiencies

ENDOCRINE
- Hypothyroidism
- Pregnancy

IATROGENIC
- Rhinitis medicamentosa
- Hydralazine
- Angiotensin-converting enzyme (ACE) inhibitors
- Aspirin
- NSAIDs
- Alpha-adrenoreceptor antagonists
- Guanethidine
- Psychotropic agents
- Chlorpromazine
- Methyldopa
- Estrogen and progesterone
- Reserpine
- Oral contraceptives
- Beta blockers
- Phosphodiesterase-5 inhibitors

OTHER CAUSES
- Idiopathic

MANAGEMENT

Environmental Control

The most important way to control allergic rhinitis is through environmental control. Because the patient is typically allergic to several allergens, control of the indoor and outdoor environment is crucial.[3] Nonspecific irritants (e.g., smoke) and indirect contact (e.g., secondary contact with animal dander) can cause symptoms that are indistinguishable from those of allergies.[4] Although techniques to control environmental allergens are arduous, time-consuming, and sometimes expensive, they are often essential for symptom control. In general, it tends to be the time commitment involved, not the cost, that makes environmental control difficult for patients.

If the allergen is outdoors, minimizing both direct and indirect exposure is recommended. Long-sleeved clothing and a mask may also be necessary to minimize direct contact. However, it is often the indirect contact—when the allergen is brought into the house—that proves to be most bothersome. Keeping the windows closed and bathing and changing clothes immediately after entering the home should minimize exposure.

An indoor allergen is often the cause of complaints. House dust contains the waste products of dust mites that live in furniture, carpets, bedding, and mattresses. Stuffed animals are a significant problem for some patients. Pets, particularly cats and dogs, are also a major cause of allergic symptoms. Removal of the pet is not an effective means of environmental control because many people are not willing to give up their animal. Effective strategies include keeping the pet out of the bedroom at all times; keeping the pet outdoors as much as possible; washing the pet and pet bedding weekly; ventilating the home frequently to promote air exchange; having a friend or family member who is not allergic clean regularly with a high-efficiency particulate air (HEPA) or double-bag vacuum; and minimizing carpeting, drapes, and upholstered furniture. Attempts to eliminate cockroach proteins include storing foods in tightly sealed containers and having the pest eliminated.[3] When possible, carpets should be eliminated, but if that is not an option, carpeting should be made of synthetic and short-napped fibers. Rugs should be washable; all loose or old rugs should be removed. Curtains (which should be cotton and, preferably, washable) and furniture should be cleaned and wiped regularly; dust-catching blinds should be avoided.

Other recommendations include keeping closet doors shut; covering machine-washable polyester pillows, mattresses, and comforters with allergy-free and zippered plastic covers; wet dusting; washing stuffed animals, sheets, and comforters in hot water (>54° C [130° F]) at least weekly; removing house plants and books; trimming bushes from the house; cleaning central heating and air-conditioning units; cleaning walls; using mold inhibitors when painting; reducing mold growth and humidity; and using a frost-free refrigerator. Although the efficacy of HEPA filters is unclear, HEPA furnace filters and room cleaners may also decrease allergen exposure.

Controlling environmental exposures is important in controlling symptoms, but the provider-patient relationship is also crucial. Environmental recommendations should be reasonable and made with compassion and clarity.

Medications

Pharmacologic interventions are appropriate if strict environmental control has not worked sufficiently, but they should be used only when allergies significantly affect quality of life. Because pharmacologic agents may be used for extended periods, the safety, side effect profile, and cost-effectiveness of each agent must be considered carefully. Pharmacologic therapy often combines several different medications to provide patients with optimum symptom relief.

Treatment of allergic rhinitis is multifaceted and includes a combination of medical therapies and behavior modifications. Intranasal steroids should be first-line treatment for allergic rhinitis[5] because systemic treatments do not target the nasal mucosa as effectively.[6] The benefit of intranasal steroids is that they provide a targeted dose of steroids, allowing maximal efficacy and sparing systemic steroid doses and side effects. Steroids exert their effects by reducing the inflammatory response and inhibiting cytokine release[5,6]; they begin working as soon as 6 to 8 hours after the dose. However, patients often need 2 to 4 weeks of continued use to see maximum benefit.[5,6] Several intranasal steroids are available for use, and there is no demonstrable difference among the different steroids, so patients may start with any of the available preparations.[5] If treating pregnant patients, the only intranasal steroid to receive a Category B rating from the U.S. Food and Drug Administration (FDA) is budesonide.[5]

Intranasal steroids have a good safety profile with few systemic side effects.[5] No studies have shown any effects on the hypothalamic-pituitary axis.[5] Most common side effects reported are nasal burning, stinging, and dryness.[5] Patients may also report headaches, epistaxis, and pharyngitis.[5]

Oral antihistamines are another mainstay of treatment in allergic rhinitis because histamine is the primary mediator of the nasal allergic reaction and increases nasal secretion; blocking of the histamine can potentially interrupt the damaging chemical mediator cascade, producing symptoms from both the allergic and viral pathologic processes.[5] Oral antihistamines can be effective in reducing sneezing, pruritus, and rhinorrhea, but overall are less effective than intranasal steroids in reducing the congestion associated with the allergic response.[5] The second-generation antihistamines are preferable because they have far fewer central nervous system side effects, require only once-daily administration, and offer quick relief with a 1- to 2-hour onset of action.[7] The second-generation antihistamines are effective throughout the allergic cycle. With the exception of cetirizine, the second-generation antihistamines do not produce significant sedation and should therefore be considered a first-line treatment of allergic rhinitis before use of first-generation antihistamines and for those who cannot tolerate inhaled nasal steroids or those with narrow-angle glaucoma or benign prostatic hyperplasia.[5,8] Initially more expensive than the first-generation agents, second-generation antihistamines, such as loratadine, cetirizine, and fexofenadine, are now available in generic formulations and can provide improved quality of life and work performance.

Although the second-generation antihistamines are very effective, they tend not to alleviate nasal congestion. Therefore, combination formulations with decongestants, such as fexofenadine and pseudoephedrine (Allegra-D) or loratadine and pseudoephedrine (Claritin-D), are useful. Unfortunately, the decongestant component can cause sleeplessness, tachycardia, tremors, and other side effects. Antihistamines and decongestants are contraindicated for patients with hypertension, prostate enlargement, or narrow-angle glaucoma.

First-generation antihistamines can also be considered as a treatment option for allergic rhinitis, but they are much more sedating than their newer counterparts. In addition to their sedating side effects, the first-generation antihistamines have poor selectivity for the H_1 receptors, and often have an effect on the muscarinic receptors as well, causing constipation, blurred vision, and urinary retention.[1] Several options are available over the counter, including diphenhydramine and chlorpheniramine, and there are also prescription agents including hydroxyzine or promethazine. Compliance with the first-generation antihistamines can be low, because they often need to be administered several times per day. Some studies have shown patients occasionally develop a tolerance to the sedating properties of these medications, but more study is needed.[1] Generally speaking, the first-generation antihistamines should be reserved for nighttime symptoms when patients may desire the sedating side effects of these medications.

Other intranasal agents that can be helpful in controlling allergic rhinitis include azelastine, cromolyn, and ipratropium bromide. Azelastine is an antihistamine spray, but it is expensive and can cause an unpleasant taste if it is not used correctly. One study has suggested that intranasal azelastine was superior to several second-generation antihistamines at relieving nasal symptoms.[1] Intranasal cromolyn affects the inhibition of mast cell degranulation; thus it affects local cytokine release. If it is taken regularly, cromolyn can prevent early- and late-phase allergic responses.[1] The major problem is the administration regimen, which is four times daily. Nevertheless, its safety profile makes it an appealing choice for some patients, and it is available over the counter.

Intranasal ipratropium bromide, an anticholinergic agent, is most effective for rhinorrhea and sneezing but is less useful for nasal congestion.[1] It is the treatment of choice for gustatory and vasomotor rhinitis and is often used to treat symptoms of the common cold.[1] It is generally safe and well tolerated. The most common drug-related problems are dryness and epistaxis.

Special consideration for patients who are pregnant includes use of chlorpheniramine and nasal cromolyn to alleviate symptoms. Intranasal beclomethasone may be used for intractable symptoms in place of oral therapy. Oral decongestants should be avoided during the first trimester and in breastfeeding mothers. As always, patients should inform their obstetrician/gynecologist of any medications they may be considering for treatment.

One nonpharmacologic intervention that has shown efficacy in allergic rhinitis is nasal saline irrigation. Patients can use a variety of devices, including a neti pot or plastic bottle to rinse the nares and potentially sinus cavities with isotonic saline. Few studies have examined the benefit of nasal saline irrigation, but one study has suggested that it is beneficial in pregnant women with allergic rhinitis.[1]

Co-Management with Specialists

Immunotherapy is a long-term treatment of allergic rhinitis that has not responded to traditional treatments even at maximal doses.[9] It may be effective if exposures cannot be avoided and is generally considered if symptoms are present for more than 6 months, if symptoms are not relieved by environmental control and pharmacologic agents, and if the cost of immunotherapy is less than that of pharmacologic therapy. Subcutaneous injections are given every week in progressively increasing doses until a maintenance dose has been achieved; after that, injections are given monthly. Sublingual preparations are also available and involve the patient taking a tablet under the tongue and allowing it to absorb for up to 2 minutes before swallowing. It is not yet clear if subcutaneous or sublingual forms have equal efficacy.[9]

There is a risk of immediate and delayed reactions with immunotherapy. Generalized reactions tend to occur within 20 to 30 minutes, but more systemic reactions can be delayed. Although the risk of a severe reaction is small, the response can be fatal. Therefore, patients should wait in the office for 30 minutes after the injection and carry an EpiPen if appropriate. The proper resuscitative equipment should be accessible if immunotherapy is offered, and a physician should be readily available.

COMPLICATIONS

Complications of allergic rhinitis are rare but potentially serious. Increased asthma and other pulmonary disease exacerbations are related to rhinitis, and sleep apnea can be a problem in untreated rhinitis.[10] Thus, treatment with medications and strict environmental control can be beneficial.

INDICATIONS FOR REFERRAL OR HOSPITALIZATION

Older adults with new-onset rhinitis may need a physician evaluation to exclude anatomic obstruction.

However, most patients with new-onset rhinitis have been recently exposed to a new and offending agent and can be managed effectively without a referral. Some patients require a referral to an otolaryngologist. Any patient who sees a health care provider because of new nasal congestion should undergo a nasal examination for assessment of anatomic problems. Although nasopharyngeal neoplasms are rare, nasal polyps are common and often require surgical intervention. These patients can also have aspirin sensitivity and allergic asthma. A deviated septum can also produce symptoms that mimic classic rhinitis.

A second careful review of the patient's history, medication use, exposure to cigarette smoke and perfumes, and occupational exposures is indicated before any referral is made. In addition, a home visit and review of inhaler technique are invaluable. Medications and medical problems that may be contributing to the symptoms should be investigated. T-cell deficiencies (e.g., with acquired immunodeficiency syndrome [AIDS]), cystic fibrosis, hypothyroidism, and humoral deficiencies should be considered. A referral to an allergist is indicated if the signs and symptoms continue and anatomic problems have been excluded.

Allergic rhinitis rarely requires hospitalization. Rare circumstances include anaphylaxis, a life-threatening hypersensitivity immune response, or the need for a surgical procedure (e.g., nasal polypectomy). Hospitalization is typically required for treatment and continued observation.

PATIENT AND FAMILY EDUCATION

Once the environmental allergens have been identified, recommendations can be made and a therapeutic regimen agreed on. Education is crucial in the management of allergic rhinitis. A dramatic improvement in symptoms is often noted when patients become experts on the triggers that activate symptoms. An allergy diary is therefore often useful. Reducing exposure to dust mites, animal dander, molds, cockroaches, pollens, smoke, and other irritants is essential. Patients should also understand how to use nasal inhalers correctly and the importance of using inhalers regularly to promote their effectiveness. The side effect profile of these medications and of over-the-counter and prescription antihistamines and decongestants should also be discussed.

IDIOPATHIC, OR VASOMOTOR, RHINITIS

DEFINITION AND EPIDEMIOLOGY

Vasomotor rhinitis, which is now known as *idiopathic* or *nonallergic* rhinitis, is an important, often overlooked, nonallergic, noninfectious cause of perennial nasal congestion and rhinorrhea. Idiopathic rhinitis is not associated with itchiness of the eyes and nose or sneezing. It occurs in response to environmental triggers, such as cold air, strong smells, irritants, changes in weather, some medications (angiotensin-converting enzyme [ACE] inhibitors, beta blockers), stress, exercise, and certain foods.[1] In contrast to the symptoms of allergic rhinitis, which tend to be seasonal and periodic, nonallergic symptoms tend to occur year-round and to be chronic.

PATHOPHYSIOLOGY

Symptoms of nonallergic rhinitis are provoked by environmental stimuli. It is distinguished from other types of rhinitis by its lack of purulent discharge. It has been postulated that the cause of nonallergic rhinitis is neurogenic, involving an abnormal balance that favors parasympathetic control over sympathetic control of the nasal mucosa,[1] leading to intermittent vascular engorgement of the nasal mucous membranes. The underlying cause of this imbalance is unknown.

CLINICAL PRESENTATION

With nonallergic rhinitis, patients often report perennial nasal congestion but little discharge. Any discharge is generally described as watery. There are few if any symptoms on arising, but nasal congestion can begin shortly after getting out of bed. Exposure to cold bedrooms or bathrooms, stress, odors, spicy foods, sunlight, and other environmental factors are often cited as causes. These irritants appear to be nonspecific triggers for exaggerated physiologic responses.

One characteristic that distinguishes idiopathic rhinitis from allergic rhinitis is that itching, sneezing, and other irritative symptoms tend to occur with allergic rhinitis, whereas obstructive symptoms and rhinorrhea tend to occur with nonallergic rhinitis.[1] Tearing and itching of the eyes and sneezing are common in allergic rhinitis but uncommon with nonallergic rhinitis. Sneezing can occur at times with idiopathic rhinitis, usually in response to temperature changes.

PHYSICAL EXAMINATION

The physical appearance of the nasal mucosa often differs in allergic rhinitis and nonallergic rhinitis. The nasal mucosa is typically pale in allergic rhinitis, but it is often erythematous in idiopathic rhinitis.

DIAGNOSTICS AND DIFFERENTIAL DIAGNOSIS

Idiopathic rhinitis can be difficult to distinguish from allergic rhinitis. Although there is no definitive test, certain diagnostic procedures can be useful. Skin testing results are often positive in allergic rhinitis but not in idiopathic rhinitis.[11] Patients with idiopathic rhinitis demonstrate little correlation between positive skin test results and exposure history.[11] A positive skin test response to a seasonal allergen in a patient with perennial symptoms is not clinically significant. Medication side effects, hypothyroidism, pregnancy, rhinitis medicamentosa, allergic rhinitis, aspirin sensitivity, infections, and nasal obstructions should also be considered in patients with symptoms of idiopathic rhinitis.

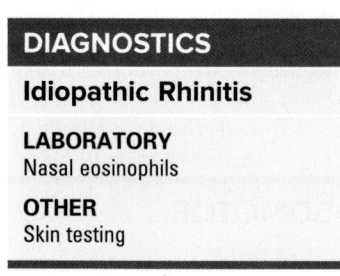

> **DIAGNOSTICS**
>
> **Idiopathic Rhinitis**
>
> **LABORATORY**
> Nasal eosinophils
>
> **OTHER**
> Skin testing

> **DIFFERENTIAL DIAGNOSIS**
>
> **Idiopathic Rhinitis**
>
> - Allergic rhinitis
> - Medication side effects
> - Hypothyroidism
> - Pregnancy
> - Rhinitis medicamentosa
> - Aspirin sensitivity
> - Infections
> - Nasal obstruction

MANAGEMENT

Unlike allergic rhinitis, idiopathic rhinitis does not usually respond to antihistamines.[11] Oral decongestants are often effective and are best used around the clock.[1] Intranasal steroids can also be effective. As with allergic rhinitis, environmental avoidance is the best treatment; immunotherapy is often not effective. Idiopathic rhinitis is chronic, and avoidance of stimuli is important. Smoking, use of perfumes or colognes, and eating of spicy foods should be discouraged.

COMPLICATIONS

Although little information is available on the long-term complications of idiopathic rhinitis, chronic problems can occur. Patients can experience sleep deprivation and a poor quality of life.

INDICATIONS FOR REFERRAL OR HOSPITALIZATION

Most patients can be managed effectively. A referral may be indicated if the diagnosis remains elusive, if treatments have not been effective, or if anatomic causes are being considered.

PATIENT AND FAMILY EDUCATION

It is important for the patient to understand that idiopathic rhinitis is a chronic condition and that the effectiveness of symptomatic treatment is limited. A detailed environmental history with minimization of potential exposures is most beneficial. Many of the measures that are effective for patients with allergic rhinitis will be effective for patients with idiopathic rhinitis. Regular use of topical decongestants should be avoided because of the potential for development of a tolerance to these agents.

OTHER CAUSES OF RHINITIS

INFECTIOUS

Upper respiratory tract infections typically are associated with rhinitis. A coexistent infection is present, and relatively prompt relief of symptoms occurs with resolution of the infection. Purulent discharge is common but not always present. Viral rhinitis is usually caused by a rhinovirus or coronavirus and has a specific incubation period and duration. Rhinoviruses are responsible for the majority of viral rhinitis (or the "common cold," as most patients term the illness).[10] Infection with the rhinovirus occurs through direct contact with infected secretions, usually hand-to-hand contact with an infected patient.[10] Once the virus has been passed, infection proceeds as the virus attaches to a variety of cellular receptors; the exact receptors are not well understood because there is little research regarding the pathogenesis of rhinovirus infections in humans.[10] The rhinovirus prefers to live at temperatures slightly lower than those in the lower respiratory tract, which explains the localized symptoms.[10] The virus then replicates and causes an infiltration of neutrophils, lymphocytes, and other inflammatory cells, which cause the mucus-secreting glands within the submucosa to become hyperactive.[10] The turbinates become engorged, and several mediators, including prostaglandins, histamine, interleukins, and tumor necrosis factor, are released and are responsible for the rhinorrhea patients experience during acute viral rhinitis.[10] Coronaviruses are similar, but they specifically infect the ciliated epithelial cells in the nasopharynx through either aminopeptidase N receptors or sialic acid receptors and damage the ciliated cells when the virus replicates, releasing the same cascade of mediators.[11] Coronaviruses are a less common cause of the common cold but tend to be more prevalent during late fall, winter, and early spring.[10]

Bacterial rhinitis, or infectious rhinitis, often originates from allergic or viral swelling of the nasal mucosa, affecting the drainage from the sinuses and trapping microorganisms within the warm, dark, moist environments of the sinuses. Signs and symptoms of a primary bacterial or primary viral rhinitis are indistinguishable, and a bacterial cause is recognized only after a secondary infection, such as sinusitis, develops.

ANATOMIC

Anatomic causes of rhinitis include a deviated nasal septum, nasal polyps, and nasal tumors.

In particular, neoplasms should be suspected in older adults. The most common cause of anatomic problems is nasal polyps, which can cause impressive obstructive symptoms. These are often found incidentally in patients with asthma who also have aspirin sensitivity. Symptoms can be perennial and difficult to differentiate from allergic rhinitis or idiopathic rhinitis. Treatment options include intranasal steroids and surgery.

RHINITIS MEDICAMENTOSA

Symptoms of nasal congestion may result from the chronic administration of sympatholytic drugs, NSAIDs, or topical decongestants. This most commonly develops with tolerance to topical decongestants. After the patient uses topical decongestants for approximately 1 or 2 weeks, the nasal mucosa develops rebound engorgement through increased blood flow. Although these symptoms tend to continue for days or weeks, discontinuation of the offending drug is curative. A 1- to 2-week course of nasal steroids or, rarely, systemic steroids can be helpful during the withdrawal period.

PHARMACOLOGIC

Various medications, including beta blockers, ACE inhibitors, chlorpromazine, estrogen, and oral contraceptives, can cause symptoms that mimic those of allergic rhinitis. Treatment involves discontinuation of the medication.

FOOD- OR DRINK-RELATED RHINITIS

Symptoms of rhinitis may occur after ingestion of food or alcohol. The exact cause is unknown, but it may be a cholinergic reaction or other mechanism.[1] If the rhinitis is caused by a food allergy, gastrointestinal, dermatologic, or systemic manifestations are usually present. Treatment involves avoidance of the trigger food or drink.

OTHER MEDICAL CAUSES

Pregnancy and hypothyroidism are other common causes of rhinitis. Other causes also include cocaine use and atrophic changes. Treatment is directed at the underlying medical problem.

CHAPTER 92

SINUSITIS

Melissa A. Hall

DEFINITION AND EPIDEMIOLOGY

Sinusitis is an inflammation of the mucosal surface of the paranasal sinuses. This common disorder develops in 20 million Americans per year, resulting in $5.8 billion in health care costs and 61.2 million work days lost annually.[1] Sinusitis has numerous subclassifications, but the most useful definitions include acute, subacute, and chronic sinusitis. Acute sinusitis resolves with treatment within 2 to 3 weeks; subacute sinusitis resolves within 4 to 12 weeks; and chronic sinusitis continues for 12 weeks or longer. This is an important distinction because treatment of chronic sinusitis is more complicated than treatment of acute sinusitis.[1]

Acute sinusitis is an inflammatory process in the paranasal sinuses caused by viral, bacterial, and fungal infections or allergic reactions. The most common cause of acute sinusitis is a bacterial infection caused by *Streptococcus pneumoniae, Haemophilus influenzae,* or *Moraxella catarrhalis; S. pneumoniae* is the most common pathogen in all age groups. Sinusitis is usually precipitated by an acute viral respiratory tract infection. Less common pathogens are *Chlamydia pneumoniae, Streptococcus pyogenes,* viruses, and fungi.[2]

The symptoms of acute sinusitis are often confused with those of an upper respiratory tract infection. The presenting signs and symptoms include nasal congestion, purulent nasal discharge, and a headache that becomes more intense when the patient bends forward. Fever, fatigue, and other constitutional symptoms are common. The onset is abrupt, with infection in one or more paranasal sinuses.[3] The benefits versus risks of antibiotic therapy in decreasing the symptoms and duration of illness have been documented.[4]

There is an association between sinusitis and asthma. The incidence of sinusitis in patients with asthma ranges from 40% to 75%. Treatment of the sinus infection results in improvement of asthma symptoms.[5]

Chronic sinusitis occurs with episodes of prolonged sinus infection (more than 12 weeks) that resist treatment or with recurrent acute infections that are inadequately treated and never resolve. The presentation of this disease is the frequent exacerbations of sinus infections that are caused by gram-negative or anaerobic microorganisms. Approximately 10% to 12% of cases of chronic maxillary sinusitis are secondary to dental infection.[6] Identification of an anaerobic infection that can result in an anaerobic brain abscess is vital to prevent hematogenous spread from the sinuses. Gram-negative bacilli may cause sinusitis in patients who are intubated through the nares or who have a nasogastric tube placed in the nares. The trauma and obstruction caused by these invasive devices can lead to a sinus infection.[7]

Physician consultation is recommended when there is evidence of visual changes, periorbital cellulitis, mental status changes, high fever, or acute focal pain.

PATHOPHYSIOLOGY

Most sinus disease involves the maxillary and anterior ethmoidal sinuses. The maxillary sinus is the largest of the paranasal sinuses, and its ostium into the nose is superiorly placed, thereby failing to take advantage of gravity. These anatomic characteristics cause it to be the most commonly infected sinus. In community-acquired sinusitis, the sinus may fill with fluid during a viral infection, such as influenza or the common cold; because the fluid is unable to drain, it becomes a good medium for bacterial growth. Bacterial sinusitis is most often a complication of viral rhinosinusitis but is also associated with allergies, dental infection, or fluid introduced into the sinuses by diving and swimming. Sinusitis may also develop when fluid is trapped in the sinuses by anatomic abnormalities, such as a deviated septum, adenoidal hypertrophy, neoplasms, or a foreign body. Patients with cystic fibrosis have thick mucus that is not easily expelled by the normal mucociliary clearance mechanism and are at increased risk for sinusitis.[8]

As the infection develops, the sinuses become inflamed; sensations of pain and pressure become intense and are the common symptoms of a sinus infection. Pain may be referred to the upper incisor and canine teeth through the branches of the trigeminal nerve, which traverse the floor of the sinus.[6]

Chronic sinusitis is thought to result from an acute sinus infection that has not completely resolved with antibiotic treatment because the sinuses have not drained completely. Patients with chronic sinusitis may have an anatomic abnormality that inhibits normal mucus clearance and thus may not be able to completely recover from a sinus infection.[9]

CLINICAL PRESENTATION

Acute sinusitis is characterized by nasal congestion, facial or dental pain, postnasal drip, headache, fever, and yellow or green nasal discharge. Sensations of pain in the teeth and forehead are worse in the morning and when the patient bends forward from the waist. Acute frontal sinusitis usually causes pain and tenderness of the forehead. This pain can be elicited by palpation of the orbital roof just below the medial end of the eyebrow. Palpation here is more accurate than percussion of the supraorbital area.[1] An infection in the frontal sinuses produces pain and tenderness in the lower portion of the forehead and purulent drainage from the middle meatus of the nasal turbinates. Maxillary sinus infections produce pain and tenderness over the cheek area and may also cause erythema over the upper, lateral aspect of the cheek. The anterior ethmoid cells drain through the middle meatus, and the posterior cells drain through the superior meatus. Sphenoid sinusitis is rare but may cause pain behind the eyes or at the vertex as well as facial pain. These sinuses drain through the superior meatus.

The common cold and allergic and idiopathic rhinitis are common antecedents to an acute sinus infection. A sore throat is common and may develop from the postnasal drip that is present with sinus infections. Postnasal drainage may cause the sensation of material in the back of the pharynx, a need to swallow frequently to clear the throat, and a persistent cough when the patient is in a prone position. Gastrointestinal symptoms result from the swallowing of mucus.[1]

Symptoms of chronic sinusitis may vary but typically involve one or more symptoms of acute sinusitis. Nasal congestion, discharge, and a cough that lasts for more than 30 days are common. Severe pain and headache are not usually present in chronic sinusitis. The pain that is present is usually a dull ache or pressure across the forehead or midface. Nasal drainage may be thick and green or yellow. A constant postnasal drip and chronic cough are present. Chronic sinusitis is thought to be one of the primary causes of reactive airway disease. Worsening of asthma is not unusual and may be a result of the sinobronchial reflex, mouth breathing, and postnasal drip containing inflammatory chemicals from the sinuses.[5] The patient with chronic sinusitis may also experience an increase in allergic symptoms, including nocturnal asthma, allergic rhinitis, and eczema.[5] When a patient is in a prone position, sinusitis symptoms worsen, especially at night.

PHYSICAL EXAMINATION

The presence of fever and vital signs should be determined, along with associated symptoms that are concerning to the patient. General inspection for facial asymmetry, periorbital edema, or cellulitis should be performed while the patient's history is obtained. Evaluation of the nasal tract for nasal turbinate edema and erythema as well as for discharge in the nasal cavity and in the area of the turbinates is necessary. The patency of both nares should be evaluated, and the nose should be inspected for septal deviation and polyps; however, examination of the nose with a nasal speculum is often inadequate in evaluating sinusitis. Transillumination of the sinuses can in some instances provide helpful information, although transillumination does not differentiate between a viral and a bacterial cause of the sinus inflammation. If the sinuses can be transilluminated, they are not likely to contain fluid; inability to transilluminate the sinuses suggests the presence of fluid in the sinuses. However, this test must be done with care because improper technique can result in a false reading.[10] Examination of the eyes, noting periorbital swelling, "allergic shiners" (dark circles under the eyes), and erythema, should precede palpation and percussion of the frontal and maxillary sinuses for tenderness—all of which indicate that a sinus infection is present. The pharynx should be examined for postnasal drip, erythema, and lymphoid hypertrophy. Because otitis media commonly occurs with sinusitis, otic examination is extremely important. The sinuses drain into the nasopharynx, and bacteria found in this discharge are easily transported to the eustachian tube, where they ascend to the middle ear, creating a middle ear infection. Because sinusitis is associated with fever and headaches, assessment and documentation for meningeal irritation (absence of Kernig and Brudzinski signs) are important for both children and adults.[11]

The teeth should be examined for caries, and the gingivae should be examined for inflammation. Approximately 10% to 12% of patients with maxillary sinus infections have dental root infection; therefore the maxillary teeth should be tapped to determine if the teeth are infected.[6]

DIAGNOSTICS

Acute sinusitis can be diagnosed empirically from the history and physical examination. However, computed tomography (CT) scanning without contrast enhancement may be indicated for children with recalcitrant symptoms that have not responded to two or more courses of antibiotic therapy.[12,13] CT scanning is also recommended for adults who have orbital complications, who have neurologic defects associated with the sinusitis, who are immunodeficient, or who are potential sinus surgical candidates. The CT image has the advantage of demonstrating both soft tissue and bone changes, compared with plain radiographs. Magnetic resonance imaging (MRI) with and without contrast enhancement may be necessary if a mass lesion is suspected.[12,13]

DIAGNOSTICS

Sinusitis

Clinical findings are usually sufficient.

LABORATORY

CBC and differential*

IMAGING

CT scan or MRI (for recalcitrant infections based on criteria recommended by the American College of Radiology)*

*If indicated.
CBC, complete blood count.

DIFFERENTIAL DIAGNOSIS

Other possible explanations for facial pain include dental abscess, trigeminal neuralgia, optic neuritis, viral rhinosinusitis,

DIFFERENTIAL DIAGNOSIS

Sinusitis

- Cold
- Dental abscess
- Trigeminal neuralgia
- Optic neuritis
- Atrophic, allergic, or idiopathic rhinitis
- Migraine or cluster headache
- Foreign body
- Tumor
- Nasal polyps
- Syphilis
- Rhinosporidiosis
- Leishmaniasis
- Blastomycosis
- Histoplasmosis
- Maxillary cysts
- Dentigerous cyst

and migraine headache. Chronic rhinitis may occur in syphilis, rhinosporidiosis, leishmaniasis, blastomycosis, and histoplasmosis. These are all conditions characterized by granuloma formation and destruction of soft tissue, cartilage, and bone. Mechanical obstruction and atrophic rhinitis can also manifest with the same symptoms as chronic sinusitis and should be included in the differential diagnosis.[3]

Dental Abscess

A dental abscess is an infection beside a tooth, usually near the root. The symptoms are localized or may radiate to the sinuses. An abscess is a collection of purulent material and is evidenced by inflammation, with fluctuation and pointing. Constitutional symptoms may be present. Fever, with chills and sweating, may progress to septicemia. If the abscess has been present for a long time, anemia may be present.[6]

Trigeminal Neuralgia

Trigeminal neuralgia is degeneration of or pressure on the trigeminal nerve, resulting in severe unilateral facial pain in and around the fifth cranial nerve. The pain is stabbing and radiates from the angle of the jaw along the branches of the nerve. Pain in the first branch is felt as lightning-like sensations along the eye and back over the forehead; it resembles the pain of a sinus infection.[1]

Optic Neuritis

Optic neuritis is an inflammation that causes hyperesthesia, paresthesia, dysesthesia, or paralysis. The pain that results from optic neuritis can resemble the pain of sinusitis.[1]

Viral Rhinosinusitis

The common cold often involves the paranasal sinuses. The common cold is an acute, afebrile infection of the respiratory tract, with inflammation of the upper airway, including the nose, parasinuses, throat, larynx, and often both bronchi.[3]

Migraine Headache

A paroxysmal disorder characterized by recurrent attacks of headache, migraine can occur with or without associated visual and gastrointestinal disorders. The mechanism is thought to be related to episodic reductions in systemic serotonin concentrations, which in turn lead to the observed vasomotor changes. There may or may not be an aura. The pain begins after the aura subsides and may be unilateral or generalized. Migraines often resemble the headaches that are present with a sinus infection.[14]

MANAGEMENT

Symptomatic treatment of the rhinorrhea, sneezing, and coughing associated with viral rhinosinusitis consists of a first-generation antihistamine, a nonsteroidal anti-inflammatory drug (NSAID), and a decongestant or cough suppressant.[4] The benefits of over-the-counter symptom relief products are not currently supported by evidence.[4]

Antibiotics are not recommended for viral rhinosinusitis in healthy adults.[4] If symptoms continue for more than 10 days or are accompanied by unilateral facial pain, purulent nasal secretions, cough, or postnasal discharge, antibiotic therapy and decongestants are recommended.[4] Few studies document treatment efficacy for acute or chronic bacterial sinusitis. If the patient has unresolved symptoms of acute bacterial rhinosinusitis, an antibiotic to combat the most common pathogens (*S. pneumoniae*, *M. catarrhalis*, and *H. influenzae*) may be considered. The choice of antibiotic in adults should be individualized and focused on geographic regional resistance patterns: amoxicillin-clavulanate, 500 mg/125 mg orally three times daily for 5 to 7 days or amoxicillin-clavulanate 875 mg/125 mg orally twice a day for 5 to 7 days. Doxycycline is an alternative in penicillin-allergic patients. Azithromycin could be considered a choice in pregnancy but should not be considered in adults otherwise because of resistance patterns.[4]

There is no evidence to support topical therapy in reducing obstruction and mucosal inflammation,[4] nor is there evidence to support the usefulness of saline solutions in liquefying secretions, although these products may provide relief for some patients.[4]

Decongestants such as oxymetazoline (Neo-Synephrine) may decrease nasal congestion and edema, promoting drainage, but the potential harm of these products without evidence to support their efficacy should alert the provider to recommend them with caution. Topical decongestants should not be used for more than 3 to 5 days, to prevent rebound congestion.

Nasal steroid preparations such as flunisolide (Nasalide), two puffs in each nostril twice daily, have weak evidence to support their benefits in decreasing nasal congestion.[4] Intranasal steroids in acute sinusitis could be considered, especially in patients with allergic rhinitis.

Oral decongestants, topical decongestants, mucolytics, and oral antihistamines have little support in efficacy and are not recommended in the treatment of acute viral rhinosinusitis. The benefits of these products do not outweigh their side effect profiles.[4]

COMPLICATIONS

In the antibiotic era, it is uncommon for sinusitis to become life-threatening. However, a chronic infection may interfere with quality of life because chronic sinusitis can continue for extended periods, possibly years. The cost in time, pain, expense, and emotional stress is significant.

Osteomyelitis of the frontal bone is a potential complication of sinusitis that has been increasing in the pediatric population.[15] If osteomyelitis develops, fever, pain, and edema over the involved bone will be present. The edema is called Pott puffy tumor.[16]

An orbital infection is another possible complication of sinus infection because the orbit is surrounded on three sides by the paranasal sinuses. This complication occurs more often when the ethmoid sinuses are infected and the bacteria can extend through the lamina papyracea. The orbital infection may cause so much edema that the patient has difficulty with vision. Visual loss can also result from pressure on the optic nerve, which can cause a permanent loss of vision. In addition, if the optic nerve becomes infected, the infection can spread to the intracranial vault. Intracranial suppuration can develop, creating a brain abscess or meningitis. Patients with this condition are usually acutely ill and have an elevated temperature, severe headache, and symptoms of increased intracranial pressure.[17]

Invasive fungal sinusitis is a rare but potentially fatal complication of chronic sinusitis in patients with a comorbid immunologic disorder, such as malignant neoplasm, human immunodeficiency virus (HIV) infection, diabetes, or drug-induced neutropenia. Prompt recognition of the serious signs and symptoms (fever, facial pain, epistaxis, and cognitive or visual changes in an immunocompromised patient) associated with invasive fungal sinusitis is essential to prevent proliferation of the infection.[18] Invasive fungal sinusitis should not be confused with allergic fungal sinusitis, a benign but unremitting sinus infection more common in young people with asthma.[18]

INDICATIONS FOR REFERRAL OR HOSPITALIZATION

The patient who is not symptom free after the second treatment with antibiotics should be referred to an otolaryngologist or allergist. If the patient with chronic recurrent sinusitis has allergies, immunotherapy as indicated by skin testing may be necessary. Surgery may be indicated if the symptoms of sinusitis do not respond to medical therapy, chronic pain is present, or recurrent reactive airway disease develops. Endoscopic transnasal surgery has become more common and involves irrigation and suctioning of the sinuses. External approaches, such as the Caldwell-Luc operation, provide better visualization but can have severe complications, such as optic nerve damage and blindness. Bone perforation is also a rare complication, and meningitis may result.[1]

Immediate specialist referral is indicated for immunocompromised patients with suspected fungal sinusitis and for patients with suspected acute bacterial sinusitis associated with visual changes, mental status changes, or periorbital edema.[18] Hospitalization for intravenous therapy and surgical consultation for biopsy or debridement are imperative.[18]

Scuba divers with chronic sinusitis can experience sinus barotraumas. This condition is not usually serious, but these patients can be at risk for neurologic compromise. For this reason, scuba divers with chronic sinusitis should be evaluated by an otolaryngologist.[19]

PATIENT AND FAMILY EDUCATION AND HEALTH PROMOTION

Patients should be aware that although the symptoms of an upper respiratory tract infection and sinusitis are similar, antibiotic therapy is not beneficial in viral rhinosinusitis.[4] However, upper respiratory tract infections that increase in severity, do not resolve after 10 to 14 days, and are accompanied by symptoms suggestive of bacterial sinusitis may require treatment. The patient treated for sinusitis should be instructed to return for further evaluation if the symptoms have not improved in 48 to 72 hours. In addition, the patient must be able to recognize complications such as periorbital swelling and know to contact the health care provider immediately.

Patients with upper respiratory tract infections should understand the importance of blowing the nose gently to prevent the introduction of nasal fluid into the sinuses.[20] Patients should also know the signs and symptoms of viral respiratory infections and be warned against the side effects of first-generation antihistamines, NSAIDs, decongestants, and cough suppressants.[4]

If allergic rhinitis is a precursor to sinusitis, environmental control should be stressed. Humidified air and increased fluid intake are important to relieve nasal discomfort and to liquefy secretions. Warm, moist air in the form of steam inhalation or warm compresses may relieve the feeling of pressure and headache, and any activity that might introduce fluid into the sinuses, such as swimming or diving, should be avoided. Smoking cessation and frequent handwashing are also strongly encouraged.

CHAPTER 93

SMELL AND TASTE DISTURBANCES

Margaret Mahoney • Catherine M. Franklin • Patricia A. Reidy • Emily Kawacki Sheff • Daniel E. Kane • Elissa Ladd • Patrice K. Nicholas • Jason R. Lucey

DEFINITION AND EPIDEMIOLOGY

Disorders of smell and taste can be seriously debilitating to patients and are often diagnostic dilemmas for health care providers. Olfactory dysfunction can be described as loss of the sense of smell (anosmia), smell distortion (parosmia), or diminished sense of smell (hyposmia).[1,2] These dysfunctions can result from aging, tobacco, toxins, medications, malignant neoplasms, nasal inflammation, infection, malnutrition, head or facial trauma, Parkinson disease, Alzheimer disease, multiple sclerosis, diabetes, or inflammatory autoimmune conditions.[1-10]

Taste disorders include diminished taste (hypogeusia), unpleasant taste (aliageusia), and any persistent taste (dysgeusia). Ageusia, or absent taste, does occur but is less common.[1] Taste disorders are often caused by conditions similar to those causing smell disorders but can also be associated with endocrinologic dysfunction, anesthesia, malignant neoplasms, head and neck irradiation, surgical procedures, iatrogenic causes, kidney or gastric dysfunction, metabolic or hepatic disorders, environmental exposure, substance abuse, or psychiatric disorders.[8,10-12]

PATHOPHYSIOLOGY

During the process of smelling, odorant molecules are taken in through the nose; these molecules must pass through the nasal cavity to reach the cribriform area and become soluble in the mucus that lies over the dendrites of the olfactory receptor cells.[13,14] The inability of odorant molecules to reach the receptor cells of the olfactory nerve (cranial nerve [CN] I) is the most common cause of olfactory dysfunction. Therefore, anosmia or hyposmia can be caused by any disease process that prevents the odorant molecules from reaching these receptor cells. The dysfunction may occur in reception or transmission. Barriers to reception may include physical barriers—polyps, septal deformities, rhinitis, and nasal tumors—or epithelial cell changes that occur with aging, trauma, and chemical or iatrogenic exposure.[3] Transmission may be affected by neurodegenerative diseases.[2,6,8]

Similar to the impact on smell of damaged nasal mucosa receptors, damaged taste receptors (buds) can impair taste. This is especially prevalent with aging, which results in the loss of taste buds.[1,10] Other conditions that can impair taste include heavy smoking, viruses, chemical exposure, environmental exposure, iatrogenic exposure, and radiotherapy of the head and neck.[1,15] Ageusia also may result from disease of the chorda tympani or the gustatory fibers but is rare. Lesions involving sensory pathways to the taste centers of the brain, or diseases of the taste centers of the brain itself, can also interfere with the sense of taste.[8,11,14]

CLINICAL PRESENTATION

Problems with taste and smell may or may not be associated with symptoms related to disorders that cause ageusia and anosmia. Most often, the presenting complaint is loss of taste or smell after an upper respiratory tract infection. In young adults, the loss of smell often results from head trauma. If a patient has lost or experienced a decreased sense of smell, a thorough evaluation for intranasal and intracranial disease is required. A complete medical, social (including substance abuse and occupation), and medication history is essential to diagnosis. Onset of symptoms (gradual versus acute) and associated symptoms should also be determined.[5]

PHYSICAL EXAMINATION

The examination should confirm the patient's subjective complaint. Assessment for the loss of taste and smell focuses on the CNs that provide information about taste and smell. The olfactory nerve (CN I) is a sensory nerve. Testing of this nerve begins with asking the patient to identify odors that are nonirritating and aromatic, such as coffee, isopropyl alcohol, and toothpaste. After testing of CN I, the provider should inspect the nasopharynx for abnormalities (e.g., polyps), crusting, amount of mucus present, and any signs of upper respiratory tract problems. The pharyngeal examination should determine the presence of lesions, inflammation, or exudate.[5]

The glossopharyngeal nerve (CN IX) is a mixed sensory-motor nerve. The sensory portion controls the taste sensation for the posterior third of the tongue. CN IX is tested along with the facial nerve (CN VII), which is also a mixed sensory-motor nerve. The sensory part of CN VII controls taste sensation for the anterior two thirds of the tongue. Each side of the tongue should be tested with sweet, salty, sour, and bitter flavors. The patient should protrude the tongue while identifying the taste and rinse the mouth before testing the other side. This process should be repeated with the posterior portion of the tongue.[8,12,15]

After determining whether the complaint is related to olfactory or taste dysfunction, the provider should perform a more comprehensive examination, including weight, vital signs, and a conscientious ear, nose, throat, and neurologic evaluation.

DIAGNOSTICS

Assessment of odor and taste identification is an essential component of diagnostic testing for the loss of taste and smell. Two tests that are appropriate for the primary care office are the University of Pennsylvania Smell Identification Test and the Sniffin' Sticks.[5,16] If these tests are unavailable, the patient should be referred to a specialist for specific assessment of smell and taste dysfunction. Laboratory testing should include a complete blood count (CBC), electrolytes, blood urea nitrogen (BUN), creatinine, liver function tests (LFTs), thyroid-stimulating hormone (TSH), antinuclear antibodies, and erythrocyte sedimentation rate (ESR). If Sjögren syndrome is suspected, antibodies to Ro/SSA and La/SSB should be assessed. Levels of vitamin and metal concentrations may be indicated, depending on social history. Magnetic resonance imaging (MRI) is used to evaluate soft tissues and mucosal edema; computed tomography (CT) is useful to assess the skull base and sinuses.[5] Further testing should be based on clinical presentation and physical findings.

DIAGNOSTICS

Smell and Taste Disturbances

LABORATORY
CBC and differential
Electrolytes
Creatinine
LFTs
TSH
Antinuclear antibodies
ESR
Anti-Ro/SSA and anti-La/SSB*
Lead*
Arsenic*
Vitamin B_{12}*

IMAGING
CT scan
MRI

*If indicated.

DIFFERENTIAL DIAGNOSIS

The differential diagnosis for the loss of taste or smell includes disease processes that can affect the upper respiratory tract. The most common conditions are allergic and bacterial rhinitis, viral infections, head trauma, sinusitis, nasal polyps, and benign neoplasms. Anosmia can also be congenital or related to a meningioma, glioma, dementia, or aneurysm. Depression can be a cause of dysosmia.[1,2,5,7,17] Aging, olfactory dysfunction, infection, radiotherapy, medications, malnutrition, Sjögren syndrome, gastroesophageal reflux, endocrine disorders, trauma, cancer, and cancer therapy should be considered in the differential diagnosis of taste disorders.[8,10-12,15,18]

DIFFERENTIAL DIAGNOSIS

Smell and Taste Disturbances

- Viral infection
- Allergic or bacterial sinusitis
- Nasal polyps
- Sinusitis
- Gastroesophageal reflux disease (GERD)
- Trauma
- Occupational or environmental exposure to chemicals and metals
- Cancer
- Benign neoplasms or tumors
- Sjögren syndrome
- Endocrine disturbances
  - Diabetes mellitus type 2
  - Hypothyroidism
  - Turner syndrome
- Irradiation
- Degenerative disorders
  - Parkinson disease
  - Alzheimer disease
  - Huntington disease
  - Multiple sclerosis
- Malnutrition
- Medications
- Depression

MANAGEMENT

Treatment will vary according to the cause of a disrupted sense of taste or smell. It is particularly important to distinguish between olfactory and taste disturbance. Treatment of rhinitis, sinusitis, infection, gastroesophageal reflux disease (GERD), or anemia may restore the lost function.[5,18] If possible, medications that may be associated with this disorder should be discontinued or changed.

If the cause of the change in smell sensation seems to stem from blockage of sinuses, oral or intranasal glucocorticoid steroid treatment is effective in most cases. Other adjunct treatments may include antihistamines and leukotriene inhibitors. Referral to a specialist may be indicated if these interventions are ineffective, in which case surgery is often performed with variable effects on restoration of smell and taste.[5]

Dysgeusia, in conditions other than aging, is treated with elimination of the offending agent. The diet should be reviewed and the overuse of condiments eliminated. Treatment of GERD with a proton pump inhibitor or H_2 receptor antagonist is often effective. Tricyclic antidepressants (TCAs), because of their analgesic proprieties, may be helpful for complaints of burning mouth.[19]

If these measures are unsuccessful, the patient should be referred to an otolaryngologist for a comprehensive nose and throat examination. Patients with suspected central nervous system disorders or conditions that cause destruction of the neuroepithelium or its central pathway require referral to a neurologist. Patients whose symptoms are related to allergies may benefit from consultation with an allergist, whereas those with dental disorders require referral to a dentist.

COMPLICATIONS

Complications of smell and taste disorders include a permanent loss of smell or taste. The loss of taste and smell can indicate a serious problem, such as a brain tumor or degenerative nerve disease. The loss of these senses profoundly affects quality of life, and depression is a potential problem.[2,17,20] Patients may lose their appetite and lose weight. Olfactory and taste dysfunction can also compromise safety, with decreased sensitivity to avoid harmful substances.[1,6,9,10]

INDICATIONS FOR REFERRAL OR HOSPITALIZATION

- Emergent referral for brain imaging (CT and/or MRI) and/or immediate neurologist evaluation—for patients whose symptoms are suspicious for an acute life-threatening intracranial process (e.g., intracranial hemorrhage related to significant head trauma or stroke, suspicion of malignancy based on history and examination findings).
- Otolaryngology referral—for suspected nasal pathway obstruction (e.g., polyps or deviated septum) and symptoms not abated with first-line primary care treatments (e.g., inhaled nasal corticosteroid). Also for persistent dysgeusia after controlling for GERD or persistent burning mouth syndrome despite first-line TCA therapy or elimination of potential medication cause.
- Neurology referral—for patients whose symptoms are suspicious for systemic central nervous system disorders (e.g., multiple sclerosis, Parkinson disease, Alzheimer disease, other neurodegenerative processes).
- Allergy referral—for poorly controlled allergic rhinitis or sinusitis despite first-line primary care interventions.
- Dental referral—for suspected dental disorder cause (if indicated by examination findings).
- Rheumatology referral—for suspected Sjögren disease (if indicated by initial laboratory test results).
- Endocrinology referral—for suspected endocrine disorders (if indicated by initial laboratory test results).
- Referral to smell and taste specialist—for any patient whose quality of life is significantly impaired or who has no easily treatable cause.[21]

LIFE SPAN CONSIDERATIONS

Pediatrics

- Because sinonasal disorders (allergic rhinitis, rhinosinusitis, nasal polyps, upper respiratory infections) account for the most common reasons for smell and taste disturbances, special attention to the ear, nose, and throat history and examination is called for with younger patients.[21]
- Head trauma history (e.g., sports injuries, use of helmets for recreational activities) and concussion history may help elucidate cause in pediatric patients.

Geriatrics

- Loss of taste in geriatric patients is largely related to decreased olfaction, which declines significantly with age.
- Decreased smell and taste sensation may lead to potentially dangerous situations (e.g., inability to detect smell of spoiled food or gas stove that is left on; decreased appetite and food intake, malnutrition).[21]
- Smell and taste disturbances may be early signs of neurodegenerative diseases such as Alzheimer disease or Parkinson disease.[21]
- Medications and polypharmacy should be considered in older patients as a potential cause.
- Nutritional deficiencies (e.g., zinc, copper, vitamin B_{12} or B_3) may play a role.[21]

PATIENT AND FAMILY EDUCATION AND HEALTH PROMOTION

If the sensory loss is permanent, the patient should be instructed to take extra care in avoiding harmful substances, both in environmental chemicals and in food. Patients who have lost the sense of smell should be counseled to install smoke detectors and to use electrical rather than gas appliances. Food in the refrigerator may need to be dated or handled with extra care. Personal hygiene should be based on routine and physical inspection.[3,6]

CHAPTER 94

TUMORS AND POLYPS OF THE NOSE

Emily Karwacki Sheff • Jason Lucey • Patricia A. Reidy • Catherine M. Franklinh • Daniel E. Kane • Kerry A. Decker • Margaret Ann Mahoney • Patrice K. Nicholas

NASAL TUMORS AND POLYPS

DEFINITION AND EPIDEMIOLOGY

Primary sites for malignant tumors can occur in the nose, nasopharynx, and paranasal sinuses. The broad spectrum of malignant lesions that occur in the nose and paranasal sinuses includes carcinomas, lymphomas, sarcomas, and melanomas. The most common, however, is squamous cell carcinoma.

The most common type of benign tumor is an inverted papilloma, which arises from the common wall between the nose and maxillary sinuses. A highly vascular benign tumor, the juvenile angiofibroma, is common in adolescent boys, bleeds easily, and can cause nasal obstruction. These tumors are nonmalignant, but they can cause considerable problems as they spread through the nasopharynx.[1]

Nasal polyps represent an inflammatory disorder of the nose and paranasal sinuses that can result in chronic nasal obstruction and a diminished sense of smell. The cause of these pale, edematous masses is unknown, but the lesions are commonly seen in patients with allergic rhinitis, which predisposes them to polyp formation, and in patients with acute or chronic infections.[2] Nasal polyps occur in up to one third of patients and children with cystic fibrosis, and a majority of cystic fibrosis patients have some form of sinus disease.[3]

PATHOPHYSIOLOGY

The pathophysiology of benign and malignant tumors of the nasopharynx is varied and makes diagnosis difficult. However, a basic understanding of the different pathologic conditions can assist in diagnosis. Squamous cell carcinomas arise from the keratinocytes of the epithelium. This cancer develops in normal skin, in preexisting actinic keratosis, or in a patch of leukoplakia. The incidence is higher in men and can be associated with smoking, alcohol consumption, and sunlight exposure.[4] The inverted cell papillomas develop from the squamous cells in which the epithelium is invaginated into the vascular connective tissue stroma. They are invasive and behave in a locally malignant manner. Potentially serious complications involve invasion of the orbit or cranial vault.[4] Juvenile or nasopharyngeal angiofibromas are vascular and may actually hemorrhage. These tumors may be associated with familial adenomatous polyps and almost exclusively occur in adolescent males who often have red hair and fair skin.[4] They also act in a locally malignant manner. They spread from the nasopharynx to the nasal cavity, the sphenoid, and the parasinuses and may extend extradurally.

Nasal polyps originate mostly from the mucous membrane linings of the maxillary sinuses and prolapse into the nasal cavity. Polyps may be classified into four types: *antrochoanal* (non-eosinophilic, unilateral masses), *idiopathic* (unilateral or bilateral eosinophilic without lower airway involvement), *eosinophilic* (associated with asthma or aspirin sensitivity), and *polyps with underlying systemic disease* (e.g., cystic fibrosis, Churg-Strauss syndrome, Kartagener syndrome).[2]

CLINICAL PRESENTATION

Malignant tumors can occur in the nose, nasopharynx, and paranasal sinuses. In general, these malignant neoplasms remain asymptomatic until late in their course. Early symptoms are nonspecific, mimicking those of rhinitis or sinusitis. Unilateral nasal obstruction and discharge accompanied by pain, recurrent hemorrhage, headache, or visual or olfactory changes suggest the presence of cancer. For this reason, any patient with unilateral or persistent nasal symptoms requires thorough evaluation.

Benign nasal tumors are associated with nasal obstruction, discharge, or facial swelling. These tumors can bleed easily and cause recurrent epistaxis. The tumor is usually easily visualized because of its growth and spread.

Symptoms of nasal polyps include nasal obstruction, hyposmia or anosmia, recurrent sinusitis, headache, and postnasal drip. In some patients, nasal polyps are accompanied by intrinsic asthma and intolerance to acetylsalicylic acid.[1] A developing polyp is teardrop shaped; when mature, it resembles a peeled seedless grape.

PHYSICAL EXAMINATION

A complete examination of the head and nasopharynx is essential. The vestibules should be inspected with a penlight while the patient's head is tipped back. The use of a nasal speculum and/or a topical vasoconstrictor spray such as phenylephrine (if available) can improve visualization of intranasal structures.[5] Each naris should be inspected for erythema, edema, discharge, bleeding, or tumor. Further examination includes pharyngeal inspection, sinus palpation, and determination of lymph node involvement.

DIAGNOSTICS

DIAGNOSTICS

Nasal Tumors and Polyps

LABORATORY
CBC and differential

IMAGING
Sinus x-ray studies
CT scan or MRI*

OTHER
Biopsy*

*If indicated.
CBC, complete blood count.

Diagnostic testing for benign tumors and nasal polyps can include sinus x-ray studies for information about fluid levels and bone involvement, but computed tomography (CT) scan or magnetic resonance imaging (MRI) is usually indicated if tumor is suspected. Endoscopic evaluation and biopsy are the gold standard for definitive diagnosis and treatment of suspected tumors.[5] Complete blood studies are necessary to determine the presence of anemia or other hematologic disease.

DIFFERENTIAL DIAGNOSIS

The differential diagnosis for tumors and polyps includes mucoceles; granulomas without systemic involvement; and granulomatosis with polyangiitis (GPA) (Wegener granulomatosis), a systemic vasculitis of unknown cause associated with granulomatous changes. GPA is associated with glomerulonephritis and granulomatous lesions in the upper and lower respiratory tract. Other organ systems can also be affected.

DIFFERENTIAL DIAGNOSIS

Nasal Tumors and Polyps

- Benign or malignant polyps
- Granulomatosis with polyangiitis (Wegener granulomatosis)

MANAGEMENT

The successful treatment of small polyps involves the use of nasal topical steroids. A short course of oral corticosteroid (e.g., prednisone, 6-day course of 21 5-mg tablets, with 30 mg on the first day and tapering by 5 mg each day) may also be therapeutic in the short term. When medical management is unsuccessful, evaluation by an otorhinolaryngologist is necessary. Polyps often require surgical removal. Benign and malignant tumors should be surgically excised and therefore necessitate referral to a specialist; benign tumors can be removed endoscopically, but malignant tumors require a large surgical excision.[6] If the tumor is malignant, chemotherapy or radiotherapy may be indicated. Patients with suspected GPA require specialist referral (usually rheumatology, but possibly also nephrology or pulmonology input may be required).

COMPLICATIONS

Complications of benign tumors and polyps include chronic nasal obstruction and olfactory dysfunction. Patients may have frequent recurrence of the tumors or polyps, necessitating frequent surgical procedures.[6] A cancerous tumor may carry a terminal prognosis despite extensive therapy.

INDICATIONS FOR REFERRAL OR HOSPITALIZATION

- Physical examination findings suggestive of airway compromise or acute neurologic changes caused by a facial mass necessitate urgent emergency department referral.
- All suspected tumors (benign or malignant) require ear, nose, and throat (ENT) and/or maxillofacial surgical evaluation.
- Nasal polyps/obstructive symptoms unrelieved by first-line primary care measures (i.e., nasal corticosteroids) merit ENT consultation.
- Patients with suspected Wegener granulomatosis should be referred to rheumatology and/or nephrology and pulmonology as indicated.

LIFE SPAN CONSIDERATIONS

Pediatric

- Juvenile angiofibroma should be considered in the differential diagnosis of obstructive nasal symptoms, especially in adolescent males (in particular those with fair complexion and red hair).[7]
- Cystic fibrosis patients (often children) frequently have nasal polyps or other sinus obstructive symptoms.[3]

Geriatric

Age is a risk factor for malignancy in general, and epidemiologic surveys have found that most malignant nasal cavity tumors are diagnosed when a patient is older than 60 years.[8]

PATIENT AND FAMILY EDUCATION

Patients with benign or malignant tumors need to understand the importance of therapy. The patient should be aware of the signs and symptoms of complications or disease recurrence and the importance of continued follow-up monitoring.

GRANULOMATOSIS WITH POLYANGIITIS (WEGENER GRANULOMATOSIS)

DEFINITION AND EPIDEMIOLOGY

In 2011, the American College of Rheumatology recommended that the name *Wegener granulomatosis* be changed to *granulomatosis with polyangiitis* with the support of several other worldwide organizations. GPA is a vasculitis characterized by glomerulonephritis plus granulomas of the nose and lung.[9] The most destructive lesions of bone, cartilage, and soft tissue of the nose and paranasal sinuses are ultimately found on biopsy to be malignant neoplasms, such as lymphomas or carcinomas. The cause of this rare disorder is unknown. Without treatment, GPA is invariably fatal; most patients survive less than a year after diagnosis.[10] However, the prognosis is good if the disease is diagnosed and treated early. The disease usually occurs in those older than 40 years, with equal frequency in men and women. It can also affect the skin, eyes, heart, gastrointestinal system, nervous system, and musculoskeletal system.[9]

PATHOPHYSIOLOGY

A necrotizing vasculitis associated with autoimmunity, GPA is one of the many autoimmune diseases that occur when the immune system reacts against self-antigens and destroys host tissue. The body has a hypersensitive response; inflammation results and causes the destruction of healthy tissue. In this disease, the probable self-antigen is unknown. The hypersensitivity results in chronic inflammation and causes the formation of a granuloma, a dense infiltration of lymphocytes and macrophages. If the macrophages cannot protect the body against tissue damage, the body attempts to wall off the infected site, and a granuloma is formed.[11] In the vasculitis of GPA, immune complex is deposited in the blood vessel walls. Complement is activated, resulting in direct cellular injury and a decrease in the circulating levels of the complement components. Once the process begins, the disorder usually develops during 4 to 12 months.[9]

CLINICAL PRESENTATION

Most patients with this condition initially complain of respiratory tract symptoms, such as nasal congestion, nasal ulcerations, rhinitis, sinusitis, otitis media, otorrhea, hearing loss, gingival hypertrophy, cough, dyspnea, or hemoptysis.[10] Fever, weakness, malaise, weight loss, conjunctivitis, rashes or skin lesions, and polyarthralgias are other common complaints. The lungs are affected in 40% of newly diagnosed patients.[10] As the disease progresses, the percentage of lung involvement progresses, eventually reaching 80%, but patients with pulmonary involvement can be asymptomatic.[10] Renal disease is rarely apparent on initial presentation, although hematuria, red blood cell casts, and impaired renal function suggest renal involvement.[7]

PHYSICAL EXAMINATION

Physical findings may be absent initially despite numerous subjective complaints. If physical signs are present, they are usually associated with the upper respiratory tract and include nasal congestion and crusting, rhinorrhea, ulceration of the nasal septum, and epistaxis. The destruction of the nasal septum that results in saddle nose deformity, a characteristic sign of GPA, occurs late in the disease process. Infrequently, there may be erosions through the skin that cover the nose and sinuses.[10] If there is pulmonary involvement, localized rales, rhonchi, and wheezing can be heard during auscultation. Other physical findings include unilateral proptosis, red eye, otitis media, symmetric polyarticular arthritis, and purpura.

DIAGNOSTICS

Routine laboratory studies add little to the diagnosis of GPA. Most patients have normocytic normochromic anemia, leukocytosis, thrombocytosis, and elevated erythrocyte sedimentation rate (ESR). A urinalysis, plus blood urea nitrogen (BUN) and creatinine, should be obtained to assess renal involvement.

A chest x-ray study is necessary to determine the presence of infiltrates, nodules, masses, and cavities as well as sarcoidosis, tumor, or infection. Sinus x-ray studies may also be indicated to determine whether sinusitis or sinus destruction is present.

Most patients with GPA test positive for circulating antineutrophil cytoplasmic antibodies (cANCAs), which are commonly found in this disorder.[10] Although a positive cANCA result suggests GPA, tissue biopsy of a suspicious lesion confirms diagnosis. Lung biopsy is preferred, although other sites can be used. The biopsy site depends on the severity of the illness, the risks of the surgical procedure, and the organ system involved.

DIAGNOSTICS

Granulomatosis with Polyangiitis (Wegener Granulomatosis)

LABORATORY
Urinalysis
cANCA
CBC and differential*
ESR

DIAGNOSTICS
BUN
Creatinine

IMAGING
Chest x-ray studies
Sinus x-ray studies*

OTHER DIAGNOSTICS
Biopsy*

*If indicated.

DIFFERENTIAL DIAGNOSIS

The differential diagnosis for GPA includes other pulmonary-renal syndromes such as Goodpasture syndrome, Churg-Strauss vasculitis, and systemic lupus erythematosus. Other vasculitides and rheumatic disorders should also be considered.

DIFFERENTIAL DIAGNOSIS

Granulomatosis with Polyangiitis (Wegener Granulomatosis)

- Goodpasture syndrome
- Churg-Strauss vasculitis
- Systemic lupus erythematosus
- Vasculitic disorders
- Rheumatic disorders

MANAGEMENT AND INDICATIONS FOR REFERRAL OR HOSPITALIZATION

A patient suspected of having GPA should be referred to a specialist as soon as the disease is suspected. In general, most patients will be hospitalized for diagnosis and the initiation of treatment: Initially, it is recommended that GPA be treated with immunosuppressive cytotoxic drugs such as cyclophosphamide (Cytoxan).[7] In patients with preserved renal function, therapy is started at a dose of 1 to 2 mg/kg/day orally as a single dose. A response to this drug occurs within 2 weeks, and remission can be induced in up to 75% of patients[10]; however, most patients have relapses of the disease. In most patients, therapy is started at a dose of 1 to 2 mg/kg/day orally as a single dose (not to exceed 80 mg/day). After 2 or 3 weeks, the steroids are slowly reduced to a maintenance dose; in some cases they may be discontinued after 4 months.[7] The cyclophosphamide is given for at least 1 full year and then is reduced by 25 mg every 2 to 3 months.[7] Treatment may differ for patients who have more critical pulmonary or kidney involvement, and other drug regimens (e.g., methotrexate, azathioprine, rituximab) may be indicated in some instances.[7,12]

The most serious side effect of cyclophosphamide is leukopenia; therefore the blood count needs to be checked on a routine basis. It is recommended that patients with GPA who are being treated with cyclophosphamide drink 1 to 2 quarts of liquid per day and empty the bladder frequently because of the risk of bladder cancer from the medication.

COMPLICATIONS

The complication for this disease is the inability to create a remission. If the patient does not receive early treatment, the disease is typically fatal. Once proteinuria or hematuria develops, progression to renal failure can be rapid.[10] Morbidity may result from the disease or be related to toxicity from the treatment.

Pneumocystis carinii pneumonia related to immunosuppression is a potential treatment complication necessitating prophylactic therapy with trimethoprim-sulfamethoxazole.[4,12]

PATIENT AND FAMILY EDUCATION

Patients need to understand the necessity of adherence to therapy and frequent follow-up evaluation. Medication and side effects must be explained and understood. These patients should also be able to recognize the signs of renal, pulmonary, and other complications. In particular, they should be alert for the recurrence of nasal discharge, sinusitis, fever, and pulmonary changes.

REFERENCES

For a full list of references, scan the QR code or visit http://booksite.elsevier.com/9780323355018

PART 9

Evaluation and Management of Oropharyynx Disorders

CHAPTER 95

DENTAL ABSCESS

Erin A. Lyden

DEFINITION AND EPIDEMIOLOGY

The term *dental abscess* is used to describe any abscess found in the tissues around the tooth. The most common type of dental abscess is an acute infection of the apical tissue.[1] These infections are often encountered in the general population among those who have untreated dental caries.[2] This type of dental abscess along with toothaches comprise more than half of all nontraumatic dental emergencies.[1] Proper evaluation and treatment of these infections are important in the prevention of life-threatening complications.[2]

PATHOPHYSIOLOGY

Poor dental hygiene resulting in dental caries, trauma, or an unsuccessful root canal can all lead to acute dental abscesses.[3] Dental abscesses arise as a result of infection by normal oral flora in a carious tooth or as a result of traumatized gingival mucosa.[1] Dental or apical abscesses begin with necrosis of the tooth pulp, leading to bacterial invasion of the pulp chamber and deeper tissues (root canals). Necrosis of these areas can occur with or without pain. However, once the bacteria are able to enter the root canal, bacteria with their toxic materials enter into the periodical space, creating an inflammatory response and pus formation. This response causes acute inflammation, which initiates a cascade of signs and symptoms. The abscess in the periapical tissue, if not handled appropriately, can enter deeper fascial spaces, leading to severe infections and mortality.[1,3]

Multiple organisms are common in acute dental abscesses.[1,3] These infections are usually a blend of both facultative anaerobes and strict anaerobes. Most of the facultative anaerobes found are *Streptococcus anginosus* or viridans streptococci. The strict anaerobes most frequently identified are species including *Prevotella and Fusobacterium.*[1,3]

CLINICAL PRESENTATION

Abscesses usually occur in the setting of carious teeth or poor dental hygiene and cause localized pain, edema, erythema, and purulent discharge from the affected site.[1,3,4] The site may be heat sensitive and friable. The tooth may be partially elevated out of the socket. The pain responds poorly to analgesic agents. If the abscess is minor, systemic signs may not be evident. More advanced infections may be associated with fever and lymphadenitis.[3] Althoughpain is a common sign with this type of infection, take special note in patients who have been on glucocorticoids, have diabetes mellitus, and are of an advanced age, because they may deny pain or report only mild pain.[5]

PHYSICAL EXAMINATION

A detailed history of the pain, symptoms, and previous dental care should be taken, followed by a thorough oral examination. Inspection of the gingiva surrounding the area of pain will reveal edema and erythema of the soft tissues and possibly a purulent discharge from a draining sinus tract.[2] The tooth may be mobile and painful to manipulation. The abscess should be visualized and palpated by the practitioner.[2] If the infection has progressed beyond the local area, orbital cellulitis, retropharyngeal space invasion, fascial plane invasion, or cavernous sinus thrombosis can occur. Signs of severe infection include trismus, airway compromise, and dysphagia. A patient unable to handle his or her own secretions or with involvement of the fascial spaces of the head and neck needs emergent care. Any patient whose outpatient therapy fails should receive inpatient treatment.[2,4,6]

DIAGNOSTICS

Physical examination remains the standard of diagnosis for an acute dental abscess. Routine radiologic screening is not recommended because thickening of the periodontal membrane is the only finding visible before abscess formation, and abscesses develop rapidly. Chronic abscesses may reveal a radiolucent area at the tooth apex.[1] A complete blood count (CBC) may be indicated if cellulitis is suspected. Other diagnostics depend on complications.

> **DIAGNOSTICS**
>
> **Dental Abscess**
>
> **LABORATORY**
> CBC and differential*
>
> **IMAGING**
> X-ray examination*
>
> *If indicated.

DIFFERENTIAL DIAGNOSIS

All oral lesions must be evaluated for potential malignancy. If there is doubt about the lesion, a biopsy is necessary to exclude malignant disease, especially in populations predisposed to oral cavity cancer. Individuals at high risk for oral cancers include those with a history of heavy tobacco and/or heavy alcohol use and individuals infected with human papillomavirus (HPV). Of all cancers diagnosed annually, oral cavity and pharyngeal cancer comprise approximately 3%, but a missed diagnosis significantly affects morbidity.[7]

MANAGEMENT

Management of a periapical abscess is primarily by incision and drainage (I&D).[1,2,3,6] However, definitive treatment may involve dental extraction, allowing the release of pressure and drainage of the abscess, or root canal of the involved tooth or teeth.[2]

Antibiotic coverage is controversial with uncomplicated abscess and not necessarily indicated, although commonly prescribed, despite increasing concerns about antibiotic resistance.[8] If there are signs of infection in adjacent tissues, antibiotics should be used without any delay to prevent further complications. With oral antibiotic therapy, penicillin or clindamycin are first-line recommendations. Macrolide antibiotics are acceptable alternatives. If there is a known resistance in the geographic area, then amoxicillin-clavulanate should be used.[1-3] Culture of the purulent discharge can result in a more specific bacterial diagnosis, and appropriate therapy can then be implemented. Analgesic therapy is instituted as an adjunct to antibiotic and surgical treatment. Hydration of the patient is necessary to ensure appropriate delivery of the antibiotic therapy chosen. Emergent surgery is indicated if there is a question of airway compromise or when the patient decompensates.[6]

Patients should be given follow-up instructions for dental consultation within 2 to 3 days of I&D.[2]

DIFFERENTIAL DIAGNOSIS

Acute Dental Abscess

- Gingivostomatitis
- Oral cancer

COMPLICATIONS

Complications arising from dental abscesses can range from minor to life-threatening. Minor complications include the need for antibiotic therapy, dental extraction, or endodontic work (i.e., root canal). Major complications can include orbital cellulitis, fascial plane infections, osteomyelitis, dentocutaneous fistula, cavernous sinus thrombosis, and bacteremia with sepsis.[1,9] Up to 57% of deep neck space infections may be caused by dental abscesses.[3] In addition, the life-threatening complication of Ludwig's angina is a possibility. This infection of the deep mandibular space is manifested with trismus, drooling, induration of the tongue and submandibular area, tachypnea, and dyspnea. Airway compromise can occur. Ludwig's angina is rare in children.[1,5]

INDICATIONS FOR REFERRAL OR HOSPITALIZATION

Dental abscesses are co-managed with dentists or endodontists to ensure adequate resolution of the initial infection, to prevent complications, and to institute preventive treatment. When signs and symptoms of periodontal abscess, periodontitis, bacteremia, orbital cellulitis, cavernous sinus thrombosis, or fascial plane involvement are present, prompt hospitalization and team management with a dentist or endodontist and an infectious disease consultant are indicated.[10] Other indications for hospitalization include edema and erythema of the eyelids, exophthalmos, and conjunctival edema. Deep neck space infection is also an indication for hospitalization.[1]

PATIENT AND FAMILY EDUCATION AND HEALTH PROMOTION

Early and proper dental care prevents most dental infections. Ninety-one percent of adult Americans have dental caries. It is important that primary care providers stress the importance of regular care and proper dental checkups.[11] Twice-daily brushing, flossing, and appropriate dental hygiene should be stressed. Early care of carious teeth can prevent future dental infections. Fluoride treatment of the local water supply and dietary fluoride supplements are excellent preventive measures.[11,12]

CHAPTER 96

DISEASES OF THE SALIVARY GLAND

Lisa M. O'Neal

DEFINITION AND EPIDEMIOLOGY

The salivary glands include the paired parotid glands, the submandibular and sublingual glands, and numerous minor salivary glands found in the upper aerodigestive tract; these glands produce saliva to aid in the breakdown of food. Diseases that affect the salivary glands are divided into neoplastic and non-neoplastic categories. The non-neoplastic category is further divided into infectious and noninfectious origins; neoplastic diseases are either benign or malignant. Acute suppurative sialadenitis (bacterial parotitis) is covered in Chapter 99.[1]

Salivary gland infections are found in all age groups and populations. However, malfunction of the salivary gland is most common in adults and typically involves a decrease in the production of saliva.[1] Malignant neoplasms involving the salivary glands account for less than 5% of all head and neck tumors, not including skin cancers.[2] The distribution of salivary tumors is more common among men than women.[3] Salivary tumors can occur at any age, and the risk of developing a salivary gland cancer increases with age. The average age at time of diagnosis is 64 years.[3]

Salivary tumors in older adults most commonly affect the parotid glands. Radiation treatment to the head and neck and workplace exposure to certain radioactive substances increase one's risk of developing a salivary gland cancer.[3] Several studies have identified an increased incidence of breast cancer in patients who have had mucoepidermoid carcinoma (MEC) of the salivary glands, and an increase in minor salivary gland adenocarcinoma has been associated with occupational exposure to woodworking and to furniture, boot, and shoe manufacturing.[3] There does not appear to be any increased incidence of salivary gland cancer from inheritance or in individuals with a history of family members with salivary gland cancer.[3] Recent studies have shown that a diet low in vegetables and high in animal fat may increase one's risk for developing salivary gland cancer.[3] Cell phone usage was shown in a singular study to increase the risk of developing benign parotid gland tumors. However, other studies have shown no relation; research is still ongoing.[3]

PATHOPHYSIOLOGY

Recurrent parotitis, sialolithiasis (salivary gland stones), branchial cleft anomalies, Sjögren syndrome, xerostomia, ptyalism (hypersalivation), sialosis, and benign lymphoepithelial lesion of Godwin are classified as noninfectious salivary gland disorders. Sialectasis (dilation of a salivary duct, either acquired or congenital) can lead to recurrent parotitis. Dilation of the duct and gland can be produced by either stone formation or strictures. Sialolithiasis, which mainly affects the submandibular glands, refers to the formation of stones or calculi in the glands. The stones are predominantly hydroxyapatite, and there may be more than one.[4] The higher mucin content of the saliva produced in the submandibular glands, combined with an antigravity flow of saliva, contributes to stone formation.[5] The stagnant saliva in the gland also leads to the formation of stones. Elevated serum levels of calcium and phosphorus are not associated with stone formation.[5] First branchial cleft anomalies affect the salivary glands, primarily the paired parotid glands. Infected cysts and sinus tracks associated with these anomalies usually are initially seen in the preauricular area and can affect the facial nerve.[4]

Sjögren syndrome is an autoimmune disorder that affects the salivary glands. On pathologic evaluation, a lymphocytic infiltrate with acinar atrophy, ductal epithelial hyperplasia, and metaplasia can be found. Benign lymphoepithelial lesion of Godwin is an inflammatory condition often found in association with human immunodeficiency virus (HIV) infection. It can be confused pathologically with malignant lymphoma, metastatic carcinoma, sarcoidosis, or chronic sialadenitis.[6]

Xerostomia means dry mouth. Several diseases as well as radiotherapy and drug therapy cause these symptoms. The production of excess saliva is called ptyalism; drug treatments (atropine) and other medical conditions are usually the underlying causes.[1] Sialosis refers to bilaterally recurring salivary gland edema. Acinar cell hypertrophy, interstitial edema, and striated duct atrophy may be present on pathologic examination. Alcoholism, metabolic disorders such as diabetes and various vitamin deficiencies, obesity, and malnutrition also initiate enlargement of the salivary glands. Certain drugs, including the phenothiazines, heavy metals, thiourea, and iodide-containing substances, cause salivary gland enlargement as a result of their cholinergic effects.[1]

Infectious diseases that affect the salivary glands include mumps parotitis and other viral infections, syphilis, HIV infection, and granulomatous diseases. Granulomatous diseases affecting the salivary glands include tuberculosis, sarcoidosis, cat-scratch disease, uveoparotid fever (Heerfordt syndrome), and actinomycosis.[4]

Neoplastic changes also affect the salivary glands. Studies have shown that 2% to 4% of all head and neck neoplasms are salivary gland tumors.[4] The majority (70%) of salivary gland tumors involve the paired parotid glands,[7] whereas, 8% of salivary gland tumors are found in the submandibular glands and 22% in the minor glands.[4]

Benign tumors that involve the salivary glands have been classified by the World Health Organization (WHO) into 13 subtypes (Table 96-1). Because of the epithelial and myoepithelial tissue components of the salivary glands, the tumors are defined by their dominant tissue type.[4] Of the benign tumors, pleomorphic adenoma (PA) is the most common and is most frequently found in the parotid gland. Warthin tumor, also known as adenolymphoma, is the second most common benign neoplasm of the salivary glands; this tumor is cystic and is found solely in the parotid glands.[4] Recent studies have questioned whether or not Warthin tumors are truly parotid neoplasms, but rather a disease of the parotid lymph nodes.[4]

The remaining subtypes of benign epithelial tumors make up approximately 15% of all tumors.[4] Diagnosis is dependent on definitive histology of the benign neoplasm.[4]

Malignant tumors of the salivary glands have been classified by WHO into 24 subtypes (see Table 96-1). The parotid gland is the most common site for metastatic disease. The majority (60% to 70%) of patients will have MEC, adenoid cystic carcinoma, acinic cell carcinoma, or polymorphous low-grade adenocarcinoma.[4]

MECs are the most common cancers of the major and minor salivary glands and are most commonly seen in the parotid gland. Furthermore, MEC has been found to have a strong

TABLE 96-1 WHO Classification of Epithelial Salivary Gland Neoplasms

Benign Epithelial Neoplasms	Malignant Epithelial Neoplasms
Pleomorphic adenoma Warthin tumor Myoepithelioma Basal cell adenoma	Acinic cell carcinoma Mucoepidermoid carcinoma Adenoid cystic carcinoma Polymorphous low-grade adenocarcinoma Epithelial-myoepithelial carcinoma Clear cell carcinoma not otherwise specified Basal cell adenocarcinoma Sebaceous carcinoma Sebaceous lymphadenocarcinoma Cystadenocarcinoma Low-grade cribriform cystadenocarcinoma Mucinous adenocarcinoma Oncocytic carcinoma Salivary duct carcinoma
Oncocytoma Canalicular adenoma	Adenocarcinoma, not otherwise specified Myoepithelial carcinoma Carcinoma ex pleomorphic adenoma Carcinosarcoma Metastasizing pleomorphic adenoma Squamous cell carcinoma Small cell carcinoma Large cell carcinoma Lymphoepithelial carcinoma Sialoblastoma
Sebaceous adenoma Lymphadenoma Sebaceous Nonsebaceous Ductal papillomas Inverted papillomas Intraductal papilloma Sialadenoma papilliferum Cystadenoma	

Data from Bradley P, O'Hara J: Diseases of the salivary glands. *Surgery* 30(11):611-616, 2012.

predilection for the lower lip.[8] The majority of MECs are low or intermediate grade and can be surgically treated. However, if the MEC is high grade, there is greater potential for metastasis.[4]

Adenoid cystic carcinoma accounts for approximately 10% of the malignant salivary gland tumors overall, but 30% of the minor salivary gland tumors.[4] These types of tumors often manifest with a nerve palsy because of their predilection for perineural spread. Prognosis after 10 to 15 years is poor (mortality 80% to 90%) because of metastases to other organs.[4]

Acinic cell carcinomas are found predominately (80%) in the parotid gland and are slow growing. They can occur in both parotids and can metastasize to the cervical lymph nodes.[4]

CLINICAL PRESENTATION

The noninfectious entities that cause enlargement of the salivary gland usually manifest with painless swelling of the salivary gland. One exception is sialolithiasis, evidenced by painful edema of the affected gland and increased symptoms with meals, "meal-time syndrome."[4] Sjögren's syndrome, commonly seen in woman aged 40 to 60 years, is associated with connective tissue diseases such as rheumatoid arthritis, polyarteritis nodosa, and systemic lupus erythematosus. Sjögren syndrome symptoms manifest with the classic xerostomia, abnormal taste, keratoconjunctivitis sicca, dry tongue, and intermittent unilateral or bilateral swelling of the salivary gland.[4] Bilateral salivary gland cysts characterize the benign lymphoepithelial lesion of Godwin, whereas a lack of saliva is associated with xerostomia; excess saliva production results in ptyalism. Other conditions associated with ptyalism include epilepsy, cerebral palsy, rabies, and stomatitis.

Infectious diseases of the salivary glands usually cause a rapid onset of colicky pain with meals, edema, induration of the affected gland, malaise, and chills.[6] With HIV infection, generalized parotid gland enlargement and xerostomia can be presenting features.[4]

Benign and malignant processes of the salivary gland are seen initially as painless, unilateral masses. These may be cystic, as in Warthin tumor. A prior history of radiation therapy may be elicited. A small number of patients complain of pain, and a few have facial nerve paralysis or palsy.[4] Squamous cell carcinoma and malignant mixed tumors have a history of rapid growth and may manifest with facial pain and fixation of underlying structures. The salivary glands may also be the sites of metastatic spread of other malignant neoplasms of the head and neck, most commonly squamous cell carcinoma and malignant melanoma; the primary sites are found above the clavicles.[5] Primary malignant lymphomas have been reported but are rare.

PHYSICAL EXAMINATION

The superficial location of the salivary glands allows the practitioner to thoroughly inspect and palpate the glands during physical examination. Inspection includes visual observation of the head, mouth, and neck. Both the major and minor salivary gland regions are inspected for enlargement.[4] Salivary gland swelling is more discrete, larger, and smoother than swelling of lymphatic origin. Any facial nerve paralysis is noted, because this type of paralysis can be indicative of a malignant parotid neoplasm.[4] Intraoral inspection includes visualization of the duct orifices to identify obstruction.[4]

Non-neoplastic, noninfectious diseases of the salivary glands manifest as unilateral or bilateral swelling of the affected gland. In the case of sialolithiasis, a stone may be palpated in the submandibular duct, or parotid stones may be noted at the orifice of the Sensen duct.[5] With Sjögren syndrome, xerostomia and keratoconjunctivitis accompany unilateral or bilateral swelling of the salivary gland. Dry papillae on the tongue may be present. Bilateral cystic masses may be palpated with a benign lymphoepithelial lesion of Godwin. Sialosis manifests as a bilateral, recurrent swelling of the affected glands.

Infectious diseases of the salivary gland result in inflammation, edema, and bilateral or unilateral involvement of the gland. Purulent discharge is present in acute bacterial infections. With a localized parotid abscess, pitting edema may be found. In viral infections such as mumps parotitis, a bilaterally and painfully enlarged gland and difficulty in opening the jaws (trismus) may be encountered.[5]

Neoplastic diseases are usually distinguished by painless, firm masses that may be fast or slow growing. Patients seen late in the course of their disease may exhibit paralysis of the facial nerve, fixation of underlying structures, and possible skin involvement.[4]

DIAGNOSTICS

Evaluation of salivary gland disease relies heavily on the patient's history and physical examination. It is important for the practitioner to determine chronicity and whether there is a history of chronic inflammatory disorders.[4] Patients often have vague complaints of pain and/or swelling with few or no other symptoms; therefore diagnosis can be difficult. Radiographic diagnostic studies (i.e., sialography, plain-film radiography, computed tomography [CT], and magnetic resonance imaging [MRI]) are extremely useful in clarifying the cause of vague symptoms.[9] In patients with known salivary gland disease, radiographic diagnostic studies can aid in planning and treatment of the disease.[4] Recent studies have shown that ultrasound combined with fine-needle aspiration cytology (FNAC) or core biopsy examination is useful, economical, and accurate in the diagnosis of major salivary gland disease and differentiation of malignant from benign disease in 90% of cases.[9] Ultrasound with FNAC is able to distinguish between salivary stones and cystic and noncystic disease.[9] Diagnostic examination of the deep parotid salivary gland lobes with ultrasound and FNAC is limited owing to location of these lobes near the mandible.[4]

Fine-needle aspiration is indicated for patients with chronic parotid lesions to exclude tuberculous parotitis, an uncommon disorder.[6]

A culture of purulent discharge from the affected ducts is performed if one suspects infectious entities. Anaerobic cultures diagnose actinomycosis. Systemic evaluation of blood serum establishes a diagnosis of HIV infection, mycobacterial disease, toxoplasmosis, and tularemia.[6] Identification of acid-fact bacilli on microscopy and culture, via drainage of pus or aspiration, gives a definitive diagnosis of *Mycobacterium tuberculosis*.[4] Cat-scratch disease is indicated with the presence of serum immunoglobulin G (IgG) and IgM.[4]

Viral titers are requested if viral infectious agents such as mumps paramyxovirus are suspected. Antibodies to the S and V antigen at levels greater than 1:192 are expected with mumps. Mumps virus can be isolated in urine samples. CT scans or ultrasonographic evaluations of the glands are used to exclude neoplastic disease. Sialography in conjunction with conventional radiographic films is used to diagnose sialolithiasis.[4] Conventional radiography is used to diagnose submandibular gland stones because 65% of these are radiopaque. Sjögren syndrome is diagnosed by minor salivary gland biopsy, usually performed on the mucosal surface of the lip, and by

DIAGNOSTICS

Diseases of the Salivary Glands

LABORATORY
Culture of discharge*
Viral titers*

IMAGING
CT scan*
Ultrasound of salivary gland*

OTHER
Fine-needle aspiration biopsy with cytology*
Oral mucosa biopsy (lip)*
Sialography*
Skin testing*

*If indicated.

measurement of salivary flow and autoantibodies (anti-Ro and anti-La).[4] Lidocaine with epinephrine is not used for this biopsy procedure because the epinephrine interferes with the pathologic diagnosis. Rheumatoid factors and antinuclear factor levels should be measured, serum protein electrophoresis performed, autoantibodies SSA and SSB assessed, and other autoimmune study results obtained, if indicated by the history and examination.

DIFFERENTIAL DIAGNOSIS

The differential diagnosis of noninfectious, non-neoplastic salivary gland disease includes drug therapy, sialolithiasis, branchial cleft anomalies, Sjögren syndrome, xerostomia, ptyalism, and metabolic disorders such as diabetes. Infectious conditions that can affect the salivary gland are numerous and include HIV infection; viral infections caused by mumps paramyxovirus, cytomegalovirus, and Epstein-Barr virus; bacterial infections, including *Staphylococcus aureus* and streptococci, tuberculosis, tularemia, actinomycosis, and cat-scratch disease; and parasitic diseases such as toxoplasmosis.[6]

Neoplastic involvement of the salivary glands includes both benign and malignant disease. Included in the differential diagnosis for benign lesions are PA, Warthin tumor, monomorphic adenoma, and oncocytoma. Malignant tumors affecting the salivary glands include MEC, acinic cell carcinoma, adenocarcinoma, adenoid cystic carcinoma, malignant mixed tumors, and squamous cell carcinoma.[4] The salivary glands can also be the site of metastatic disease to the head and neck. Included in these metastatic tumors are malignant melanoma, squamous cell carcinoma, and lymphoma. Primary malignant lymphoma of the salivary glands has been reported but is rare.[4]

DIFFERENTIAL DIAGNOSIS

Diseases of the Salivary Glands

- Infections (bacterial, viral, granulomatous, parasitic)
- Drug therapy
- Branchial cleft anomalies
- Sjögren syndrome
- Benign or malignant tumors
- Sialolithiasis
- Xerostomia
- Ptyalism
- Metabolic disorders (diabetes)

MANAGEMENT

Management of many noninfectious diseases of the salivary glands is conservative. This includes pain management and hydration. Many noninfectious, nonmalignant salivary gland problems are caused by lack of adequate hydration. Recurrent parotitis may be treated with surgical removal of the affected gland if the patient remains symptomatic. Sialolithiasis is managed with warm compresses, analgesics, and sialagogues. Sialagogues are agents that stimulate the production and flow of saliva, such as lemon balls and chewing gum. Fluid and electrolyte replacement should be addressed. Surgical removal of the offending stone may be required. Branchial cleft anomalies are treated with surgical excision. Sjögren syndrome is treated symptomatically with local and systemic therapy to address the xerostomia and xerophthalmia. Ptyalism may require surgical intervention, intraparotid injections of botulinum toxin A, or neodymium:yttrium-aluminum-garnet (Nd:YAG) laser treatment.[9]

Management of infectious diseases of the salivary glands depends on the cause of the disease. Management of acute suppurative parotitis is discussed in Chapter 99. Viral infection of the salivary glands, most commonly caused by the mumps paramyxovirus, requires conservative therapy that consists of adequate hydration, rest, and possibly diet modification. Hospitalization and consultation with infectious disease specialists is necessary if infection progresses to involve other organs or structures.[4] Infections that are suspected to be HIV infection should be evaluated by an HIV specialist. Granulomatous infection of the salivary glands should be treated with the appropriate agents. Tubercular infections and nontubercular mycobacterial infections may require surgical removal because these infections may not respond to traditional therapies. Actinomycosis is treated with intravenous penicillin, followed by the oral form for several months. Clindamycin or erythromycin can be substituted if the patient is allergic to penicillin.[10] Surgical removal may be required. Cat-scratch disease can be treated symptomatically without antibiotic therapy. Toxoplasmosis can be treated with combination therapy that consists of pyrimethamine and trisulfapyrimidines, although in most cases this regimen is reserved for those who have systemic disease, are immunocompromised, or are pregnant.[6] Parenteral antibiotics, such as the aminoglycosides streptomycin and gentamicin, can be used for tularemia. Tetracycline has also been used for tularemia, but with mixed results.

Suspected benign or malignant salivary gland masses are managed surgically. With surgery involving the parotid gland, preservation of the facial nerve is critical unless the nerve is already nonfunctional or has tumor involvement. A superficial parotidectomy is the surgical procedure of choice. Some surgeons propose that both the deep and superficial lobes of the parotid gland be treated with a total parotidectomy. Tumors of the minor salivary glands are treated with surgical excision. The extent of the procedure is dictated by the tumor site and the disease.[4] Radiotherapy as a primary treatment modality is no longer recommended, although postoperative radiotherapy may be necessary for certain tissue types.[9] Neck dissection performed at the time of the surgical procedure may be indicated for tumors larger than 4 cm (1⅗ inches), cancers that originate in the submandibular gland, and primary squamous cell carcinoma. If there is undifferentiated carcinoma or high-grade MEC, a neck dissection is performed at the time of the initial surgery.[4]

LIFE SPAN CONSIDERATIONS

Mumps paramyxovirus infection is decreasing in incidence in the pediatric population because of routine immunization (measles, mumps, and rubella [MMR]). Unimmunized children and adults are at risk for complications, including orchitis, encephalitis, meningitis, and cochleitis. Adults exposed to mumps paramyxovirus are more likely to develop serious complications such as mumps orchitis, pancreatitis, and nephritis. Adults who have not had mumps are encouraged to have the MMR immunization.

Older adults are at high risk for all types of salivary gland tumors. Sjögren syndrome has a higher incidence in postmenopausal women because of the increased incidence of connective tissue disorders in this population.

PAs are more common in people who have received prior radiation therapy. Smokers have an increased rate of Warthin tumors.[4]

COMPLICATIONS

Complications of diseases of the salivary glands include recurrent bouts of salivary gland swelling, pain, and stone formation, which may necessitate surgical intervention. Xerostomia produces serious dental caries because of the lack of saliva. Saliva has properties that aid in the prevention of caries. Dry mouth seriously affects the patient's quality of life, necessitating dietary changes and frequent sips of water. Infectious causes of salivary gland disease have a potential for sepsis. Encephalitis, orchitis, meningitis, and cochleitis are serious consequences of mumps paramyxovirus infection. On occasion, development of islet cell antibodies leading to acute onset of type 1 diabetes can occur. Bacterial infections and granulomatous diseases can be serious in patients who are immunocompromised. Patients diagnosed with Sjögren syndrome have a significantly increased risk of developing mucosa-associated lymphoid tissue lymphoma (MALT).[4]

Benign tumors of the salivary gland rarely cause complications unless they are neglected and invade the facial nerve, underlying structures, or overlying skin. The recurrence rate is low for tumors excised appropriately and properly. However, malignant tumors of the salivary glands can be difficult to treat. Tumors such as adenoid cystic carcinoma, squamous cell carcinoma, and adenocarcinoma may metastasize to other local and regional sites. To ensure a good outcome, it is important to initiate appropriate surgical consultation if a tumor is suspected.[4]

INDICATIONS FOR REFERRAL OR HOSPITALIZATION

Health care providers may manage many infectious and noninfectious diseases that affect the salivary glands. A team of qualified practitioners should manage acute suppurative parotitis (sialadenitis). Patients with suspected benign and malignant masses should be referred to an appropriate head and neck surgeon for proper diagnosis and treatment. Sialolithiasis requires consultation with an otolaryngologist. Hospitalization may be required to manage the underlying condition causing salivary enlargement or to manage complications. Sjögren syndrome may need to be managed by a specialist in autoimmune diseases.[3]

PATIENT AND FAMILY EDUCATION

Patients should be encouraged to examine themselves for signs of salivary gland disease. Painful or painless swelling of the salivary glands, xerostomia, ptyalism, and purulent discharge from salivary gland ducts are important conditions to investigate. Patients undergoing prolonged surgical procedures, especially gastrointestinal procedures, should maintain adequate hydration to avoid acute suppurative sialadenitis.

HEALTH PROMOTION

Important topics for health promotion include adequate hydration, attention to oral hygiene, and immunizations. In addition, it is important that the patient be instructed to avoid risk factors such as radiation exposure, tobacco smoking, and exposure to animals that may be vectors of disease.

CHAPTER 97

EPIGLOTTITIS

Lisa M. O'Neal

Immediate emergency department referral or physician consultation is indicated for patients with suspected epiglottitis.

DEFINITION AND EPIDEMIOLOGY

Epiglottitis (supraglottitis) is an acute inflammation of the supraglottic region of the oropharynx. Epiglottitis is characterized by inflammation and edema of the epiglottis, vallecular, arytenoids, and aryepiglottic folds.[1] Owing to the high vascularity and loose mucosa of the epiglottic region, sudden airway obstruction and possible death can result.[1] Epiglottitis is typically caused by a bacterial infection and less commonly results from a viral illness or caustic and thermal injury to the epiglottis. Thermal epiglottitis is a rare and potentially life-threatening disease caused by direct thermal injury or inhalation of steam or aspiration of heated liquids.[2,3] Crack cocaine use has been associated with thermal injury to the hypopharynx in teens and young adults.[4]

Epiglottitis is a rare but serious life-threatening condition because of the potential for laryngospasm and irrevocable loss of the airway.[5] From the 1950s to the early 1990s, epiglottitis typically occurred more often in children than in adults. The most common bacterial pathogen responsible for epiglottitis in children was *Haemophilus influenzae* type B (Hib). More recently, however, the incidence of epiglottitis in adults has shown a steady increase and is approximately 2.5 times greater than that in children.[5] In the United States, epiglottitis in adults is estimated to be 1.9 in 100,000 per year.[5] The dramatic decline in childhood epiglottitis is due to the advent of the vaccination for *Haemophilus* organisms. Overall, the incidence is now decreasing in all age groups, possibly as a result of a general decrease of Hib disease in the general population. It should be noted however, that a recent case report found *H. influenzae* type A as the responsible pathogen for severe invasive disease in countries with an Hib vaccination program.[6] Other pathogens associated with epiglottitis include groups A, B, and C streptococci; *Streptococcus pneumoniae; Klebsiella pneumoniae; Candida albicans; Staphylococcus aureus; Haemophilus parainfluenzae; Neisseria meningitidis;* varicella-zoster virus; and various other viral pathogens.[7]

Male predominance is reported with epiglottitis; however, male/female ratios have varied. The mean age of adults with epiglottitis is 44.94 years.[8] There is no seasonal predilection for epiglottitis; however, two studies have shown an increase in cases during the summer months.[5]

Epiglottitis among adults may follow an unpredictable clinical course, ranging from relatively benign disease to rapidly progressive disease with acute airway obstruction and possibly death. The mortality rate for children is less than 1%, but the mortality rate for the adult population is in the range of 6% to 7%.[9]

PATHOPHYSIOLOGY

Epiglottitis can be caused by a variety of microorganisms. In the postvaccine era, for children younger than age 5, Hib continues to be an important cause of epiglottitis.[6] In patients with underlying disease, *Aspergillus*, *Klebsiella*, and *Candida* organisms have been identified. A viral cause has been postulated for some cases of adult epiglottitis, especially the milder cases, although it is traditionally associated with infectious organisms. Investigators have identified noninfectious causes of epiglottitis, which can include inflammation in association with thermal injury (crack cocaine and marijuana smoking), ingestion of caustic substances (automatic dishwashing detergent), systemic disease (diabetes mellitus, hypertension, obstructive pulmonary disease, seizure disorder, alcohol and drug abuse, tobacco smoking), chemotherapy for head and neck cancer, trauma by foreign objects, and burns associated with bottle-fed infant formula.[5,8,10]

CLINICAL PRESENTATION

Patients with epiglottitis are initially seen with an acute occurrence of severe odynophagia, dysphagia, fever, and shortness of breath with sitting up and leaning forward in an effort to enhance air flow.[10] Other complaints include the inability to swallow their own secretions, neck tenderness, lymphadenopathy, cough, drooling, stridor, respiratory distress, and hoarseness. The patient may adopt the tripod position (leaning forward with hands braced on the knees), using accessory muscles for respiration.[5] Dyspnea and stridor are common signs of epiglottitis in children, whereas odynophagia, dysphagia, and voice change are common presenting symptoms in adults.[10] The onset and duration of symptoms before the patient's initial contact with the health care provider vary. Depending on the severity of symptoms, patients may seek treatment after having symptoms for less than 8 hours, or they may have had them for more than 4 days.

PHYSICAL EXAMINATION

Patients with epiglottitis may or may not have fever and a toxic appearance, depending on the severity of the infection or the cause of the inflammation. Generalized toxemia is a result of acute epiglottitis.[10] If assessment of the adult patient reveals the presence of anterior neck tenderness with severe sore throat, epiglottitis should be suspected.[5] Patients experiencing respiratory distress, posturing in the upright "sniff" or tripod position, dysphagia, and refusal to swallow are all reliable signs of epiglottitis.[5] Indirect laryngoscopy may reveal an erythematous, edematous epiglottis with a narrow glottic opening. Substernal and supraclavicular retractions, tachycardia, tachypnea, and inspiratory stridor are common. With severe respiratory distress, changes in mental status, anxiety, pallor, cyanosis, and other signs of hypoxia may be present.

Precautions during the physical examination are required. If epiglottitis is suspected, the pharynx should not be examined with a tongue depressor, because this may precipitate an airway emergency. Any inspection of the oral cavity requires that emergency airway management equipment be immediately available in case of laryngospasm; laryngospasm can cause sudden airway occlusion.

DIAGNOSTICS

The gold standard for a definitive diagnosis of epiglottitis is made by direct visualization via laryngoscopy with a flexible fiberoptic scope or a laryngeal mirror.[11] It provides accurate visualization of the epiglottis and it shows the extent of epiglottic swelling.[5] Indirect laryngoscopy is considered a safe diagnostic tool in the adult population but not in children.[12] A recent study showed that sonography is an accurate, noninvasive, and rapid diagnostic tool for epiglottitis in the emergency setting.[9] A positive diagnosis of epiglottitis is achieved by evaluating the diameter of the anteroposterior diameter of the epiglottis.[9]

A lateral neck film can be useful but is not always diagnostic in the adult population.[11] Findings on the lateral neck film suggestive of epiglottitis include a swollen epiglottis manifesting as a "thumbprint" sign (Fig. 97-1).[13] Because they have a low sensitivity rate (true positives), lateral neck films are not a true

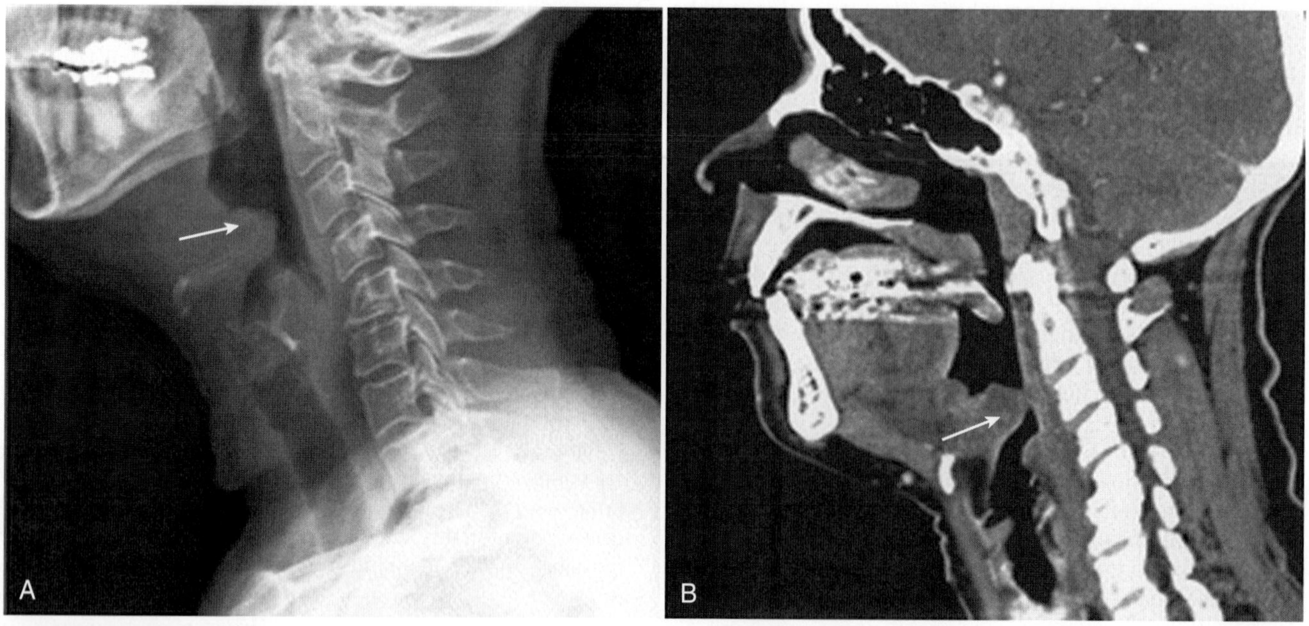

FIGURE 97-1 Epiglottitis in an adult. Lateral soft tissue radiography of the neck showed the "thumbprint sign" **(A)**, indicating a swollen epiglottis, suggestive of epiglottitis. Computed tomography of the neck revealed substantial swelling and edema of the epiglottis **(B)**, the base of the tongue, and the lingual tonsil. (From Angirekula V, Multani A: Images in clinical medicine. Epiglottitis in an adult. *N Engl J Med* 372[5]:e20, 2015.)

diagnostic tool and are being replaced with direct visualization of the epiglottis with fiberoptic nasopharyngoscopy.[11] It should be noted that if the thumbprint sign is present, it is a significant predictor for imminent airway compromise and rapid clinical deterioration.[10] Prophylactic airway management is not indicated for an adult with epiglottitis; however, securing the airway should take precedence over the performance of laboratory examinations or radiologic studies.[3] Computed tomography (CT) and magnetic resonance imaging (MRI) are not commonly used for the diagnosis of epiglottitis; however, they are useful in the evaluation of complications (infection and abscess formation) of epiglottitis.[5]

A complete blood count (CBC) often reveals leukocytosis with a shift to the left and bandemia.[12] Blood cultures may be obtained to guide antibiotic therapy and exclude septicemia. Recent literature indicates that microbiologic studies are not very helpful, because no definite organism is identified in the majority of cases of epiglottitis in adults.[5] The low percentage of positive pharyngeal and blood cultures is presumed to be related to anaerobic bacterial causes or cases of partially treated disease.[5] Analysis of arterial blood gases (ABGs) may also be indicated.

DIAGNOSTICS

Epiglottitis

INITIAL
Airway stabilization mandatory before further diagnostic evaluation
Pulse oximetry

LABORATORY
CBC and differential
Blood cultures
Culture and sensitivity
ABGs

IMAGING
Sonography (Ultrasound)
Lateral neck x-ray examination, chest x-ray examination

OTHER DIAGNOSTICS
Fiberoptic nasopharyngoscopy in the emergency room or surgical suite*

*Primary recommended imaging diagnostic.

DIFFERENTIAL DIAGNOSIS

Multiple conditions have a similar presentation. Conditions in the differential diagnosis of epiglottitis include Ludwig angina, retropharyngeal and peritonsillar infections, tumor, caustic ingestions, allergic drug reactions, laryngeal trauma, uvulitis, bacterial tracheitis, angioedema, foreign body aspiration, and thermal injury.

Signs and symptoms of Ludwig angina, retropharyngeal abscess, and peritonsillar cellulitis or abscess are similar to those of epiglottitis because all are seen with an infectious process. Ludwig angina is a severe diffuse form of cellulitis with an acute onset affecting the submental, sublingual, or submandibular spaces. Clinical presentation of Ludwig angina includes clinical signs of fever, dysphagia, inability to swallow, and stridor.[14] Ludwig angina typically results from a dental infection and can be easily diagnosed by CT scan.[14] Retropharyngeal abscess can also be identified by CT scan and can be excluded by negative findings on physical examination.[15] Peritonsillar cellulitis or abscess can be excluded by negative physical examination findings.

A tumor, gastroesophageal reflux disease, trauma to the larynx, allergic drug reaction, or angioedema may manifest with signs similar to those of epiglottitis. A tumor or trauma to the larynx may cause sore throat, hoarseness, dysphagia, and respiratory distress; however, infectious findings are negative. Allergic drug reaction or angioedema typically manifests with respiratory distress and dermatologic findings.[5] A history of illicit drug use or thermal injury or trauma to the neck should be elicited. Crack cocaine vaporizes at high temperatures, and the extreme heat of the inhaled vapors may incite acute inflammation of the epiglottis.[3]

DIFFERENTIAL DIAGNOSIS

Epiglottitis

- Ludwig angina
- Retropharyngeal and peritonsillar infections
- Tumor
- Trauma
- Allergic reaction
- Angioedema
- Gastroesophageal reflux disease
- Illicit drug use
- Thermal injury

MANAGEMENT

Patients should be allowed to sit upright in a quiet environment with humidified oxygen. Treatment of epiglottitis consists of close observation for airway management, antibiotics if indicated, and, in some cases, steroids. The patient should be hospitalized in the intensive care unit for aggressive airway monitoring. Sedation, racemic epinephrine, and inhaled medications should be avoided. The patient is considered to have an unstable airway, and equipment should be at the bedside to perform cricothyrotomy or emergent intubation if necessary.

Immediate consultation with otolaryngology is essential. Isolation is sometimes recommended for the first 24 hours after the initiation of antibiotic therapy. Patients with an increased risk of airway obstruction (those with respiratory distress, tachycardia, tachypnea, or increased white blood cell count) may require an artificial airway by intubation or tracheotomy; an anesthesia provider should be immediately available. Intubation is preferred, if indicated, over tracheostomy because of ease of removal of the endotracheal tube a couple of days after edema has subsided, the absence of surgical complications, and lower or equal mortality and complication rates.[12] Continuous oxygen therapy and monitoring of oxygen saturation are necessary.[10]

Intravenous broad-spectrum antibiotics should be initiated as soon as possible.[5] In the past, the usual treatment for epiglottitis was ampicillin and chloramphenicol; however, because of ampicillin-resistant *H. influenzae*, this regimen is no longer recommended. Chloramphenicol is not often used because of the increased risk of aplastic anemia. Until culture and sensitivity results are available, second- and third-generation cephalosporins (e.g., ceftriaxone given intravenously; cefotaxime), ampicillin-sulbactam, clindamycin, or levofloxacin is the recommended treatment.[5] Adult doses are as follows: ceftriaxone 2 g/day, cefotaxime 2 g every 4 to 8 hours, or ampicillin-sulbactam 1.5 to 3 g every 6 hours.[12] Antibiotic treatment is for 10 to 14 days.[12] Vancomycin is a consideration if methicillin-resistant *Staphylococcus aureus* (MRSA) or sepsis is a concern. Although many experts advocate the use of steroids, it is not a universal standard of treatment.[5] However, in the absence of any specific contraindications, a short course of steroids can be used to possibly decrease airway inflammatory edema and potentially negate the need for intubation and prolonged hospitalization. Randomized controlled trials proving benefit from steroid use are not available.[5]

If anaerobic bacteria are suspected, metronidazole may be added to the course of therapy.[5] Epiglottitis should resolve within 36 to 48 hours after initiation of treatment; this can be confirmed via flexible laryngoscopy. If not, other diagnoses should be considered.[5]

LIFE SPAN CONSIDERATIONS

With the changes in the ages of those affected by Hib infection, careful evaluation of all age groups is suggested. A suspicion of epiglottitis should prompt an immediate referral to an emergency department capable of airway support. A careful history, including illicit drug use, should be documented.[6]

COMPLICATIONS

Epiglottitis is a serious and potentially fatal condition. Death from airway obstruction may result. Rapid and careful intervention is required in an effort to avoid life-threatening complications. Other potentially fatal complications include septicemia and meningitis, resulting from the spread of infection. Other complications, such as pulmonary edema, epiglottic abscess, vocal cord granuloma, and pneumomediastinum, have been reported.

INDICATIONS FOR REFERRAL OR HOSPITALIZATION

All cases of epiglottitis or suspected epiglottitis require immediate referral. Hospitalization is necessary for close observation of the airway and initiation of appropriate antibiotic therapy.

PATIENT AND FAMILY EDUCATION

Explanation of all procedures is necessary to allay patient and family anxiety. The importance of the medical regimen should be stressed to enhance adherence. If steroids are prescribed, information on steroids and tapering of doses must be reviewed. If illicit drug use is documented, education and referral for counseling should be attempted. The causes of thermal epiglottitis should be discussed with patients who are at risk for the injury (parents of children, illicit drug users).[2]

HEALTH PROMOTION

Health promotion should include an age-appropriate immunization status review. Cases of thermal inhalation injuries resulting in epiglottitis have been documented in crack cocaine users. Caustic ingestions, foreign bodies, and other thermal inhalations have also resulted in signs and symptoms of epiglottitis.[2]

CHAPTER 98

ORAL INFECTIONS

Erin A. Lyden • Lisa O'Neal

DEFINITION AND EPIDEMIOLOGY

The American Academy of Periodontology has emphasized the direct connection between oral health and general health; accordingly, it is imperative for providers to treat oral infections and to promote oral hygiene.[1] The most common oral infectious lesions are candidiasis, herpes labialis, and recurrent aphthous stomatitis.[2,3] Other common oral lesions are also discussed in this chapter because their recognition is important in the differential diagnosis of systemic disease or oral cavity cancer.

Viral infections of the mouth include those caused by the common herpes simplex virus types 1 and 2 (HSV-1 and HSV-2). HSV-1 is the type most associated with oral lesions, believed to infect up to 90% of the population. Human papillomavirus (HPV) is also found in the oral cavity, manifesting with papillomatous soft tissue lesions. HPV can be transmitted by direct contact, including sexual contact. HPV-associated cancers are estimated to make up 30% of cancers in the United States.[3]

Bacterial infections of the mouth frequently cause periodontitis or gingivitis. Oral bacterial infections are under intense investigation because they have been linked to systemic diseases, such as cardiovascular disease and diabetes.[1]

Candida albicans is the most common fungus to infect the oral cavity. Fungal infections of the mouth are encountered across the spectrum of patient age. Thrush, or candidal infection of the oral mucosa, is caused by the overgrowth of *C. albicans*, fungi that are normally found in the flora of the gastrointestinal tract. Reports state that as many as 50% of adults may have *Candida* as part of their normal oral flora. Immunocompromised hosts and patients who wear dentures are susceptible to these oral mucosal lesions, as are patients with diabetes, ulcerative colitis, Crohn disease, gluten sensitivity, or poor oral hygiene and others with poor general health. These lesions may occur from infancy through maturity and can be a recurrent source of irritation. Inhaled steroids are also a risk factor for candidiasis.[3]

Aphthous ulcers (recurrent aphthous ulceration, canker sores) are defined as shallow, painful, and often recurrent lesions of the oral mucosa. These are the most common oral mucosal lesions in North America.[3,4] Prevalence is estimated at 5% to 50%.[4] Aphthous ulcers typically affect adolescents and young adults, with more females than males affected. Incidence has been noted to be 20% to 40% in the general population.[3] Patients with known ulcerative colitis, Crohn disease, or gluten-sensitive enteropathy may have aphthous ulcers as a feature of these conditions.[3,4]

Stomatitis is a general term that refers to the inflammation of the soft tissues of the oral cavity. Chemical or heat injuries can initiate stomatitis; aspirin can cause an ulcerative lesion when it is used as a topical anesthetic on the oral mucosa. Burns sustained from hot food or liquids can also cause mucosal irritations. Certain food substances, chewing gum, oral mouth rinses, and dental products can induce painful lesions.[3]

Aphthous ulcers and stomatitis are often encountered in primary care practice. Other entities are associated with oral lesions and may include mechanical irritation, drug reactions, local trauma (broken teeth, cheek gnawing), nutritional deficiencies, and stress. These forces irritate and inflame the sensitive oral mucosa. Conditions may be localized to the oral mucosa or associated with systemic disease; therefore it is important to accurately diagnose and appropriately care for oral lesions.[3,4]

PATHOPHYSIOLOGY

Herpes labialis occurs when HSV-1 is introduced to the oral mucosa through the oral secretions. After the initial outbreak, the virus typically remains in the trigeminal ganglion (HSV-1) and is commonly reactivated at a later time.[3,5] HPV invades the mucosal epithelium and the basal layer, where the viral DNA infects the host DNA. Over 150 HPV types have been identified, of which only nine are known to cause cancer (and another six are being investigated). HPV type 16 is most associated with oral cavity malignancy.[6]

Gingivitis is most commonly associated with bacterial overgrowth in persons with poor oral hygiene. As few as 4 or 5 days without oral care can initiate the infectious process, and continued inattention to dental health can eventually lead to tooth and bone loss.[7] There is much interest in investigating the role that oral health and gingivitis have in the development of coronary heart disease, atherosclerosis, and stroke.[8]

The most common fungal infection in the oral cavity is candidiasis. Overgrowth of *C. albicans* (thrush) occurs when the normal oral flora is out of balance or when the host immunity is somehow compromised.[9]

Aphthous ulcers are a common presenting problem for all age groups. Although the exact cause of these ulcers is unknown, it is thought to be autoimmune in nature.[2] Other proposed etiologic factors include physical or emotional stress; trauma associated with physical, chemical, or local agents; deficiencies of vitamin B_{12}, folic acid, or iron; familial or genetic predisposition; microbial agents; and hypersensitivity states such as gluten-sensitive enteropathy.[4] Generalized stomatitis may be caused by poor oral hygiene, ill-fitting dentures, and nicotine abuse. Mechanical trauma, chemical trauma from caustic substances, or hot foods may also traumatize the mucosa.[3] Thrush more typically occurs with underlying diabetes or with immunocompromised states. Parenteral antibiotic and steroid use have been implicated as precursors to oral candidiasis.[2,3]

CLINICAL PRESENTATION

Patients with herpes simplex typically report a prodromal set of symptoms that include localized pain, tingling, and burning with erythema.[2,3] These symptoms are followed by the eruption of vesicles that evolve into painful ulcerative lesions.[3] The patient may experience an incubation period of 4 to 7 days after exposure.[2]

HPV infections manifest as white, verrucous lesions individually or in clusters. The lesions can be found on the lips, hard palate, or gingiva. They are painless but may become ulcerative in response to local trauma.[6]

Thrush usually appears as white, cottage cheese–like lesions that are easily removed with a swab. The underlying tissue may bleed after manipulation. Children with thrush may have a white coating in the mouth, and they often have difficulty feeding.[2,3]

Gingivitis manifests as an inflammation of the gingiva, possibly with areas of ulceration with or without purulent discharge from the affected areas.[10] Patients typically report bleeding with eating (hard food such as chips and crusty breads) or tooth care. Chronic gingivitis may cause only minimal findings.[1,3]

Aphthous ulcers are painful, shallow ulcerations of the nonkeratinized oral mucosa and occur as solitary or multiple lesions. A prodrome of burning or pricking of the oral mucosa has been reported.[4] The lesions may be recurrent but are not typically found on the anterior hard palate or gingiva.[3] Ranging in size from 2 mm to several centimeters, aphthous ulcers may have a gray-yellow, pseudomembranous base surrounded by erythema. The disease itself is self-limited, usually lasting 10 to 14 days.[4]

There are three categories of aphthous ulcers. Minor aphthous ulcers are the most common and range in size from 2 to 10 mm (0.08 to 0.4 inch); healing occurs during 7 to 14 days. Many people attribute these minor ulcers to stress, trauma, or even menses. Major aphthous ulcers may be seen as painful lesions that are larger than 1 cm in diameter and are often in a state of cyclic eruption. Scarring is associated with these lesions. The third category is the herpetiform ulceration, which often is mistaken for lesions of HSV. These lesions are small (2 to 3 mm [0.08 to 0.12 inch]), are widely scattered or closely grouped, and may be recurrent. Cultures of these lesions are negative for virus.[2,3]

PHYSICAL EXAMINATION

The lesions of HSV are vesicular with an erythematous base. The vesicles may coalesce and ulcerate before healing. Recurrent lesions may be triggered by fever, stress, and exposure to sunlight.[3]

Examination of the patient with oral HPV reveals single or multiple verrucous, white, sessile growths.[3] The Pap smear is currently the screening tool for genital HPV, but there is currently no screening examination for oral HPV.[5]

Candidal infection manifests as white, curdlike lesions on the oral mucosa or tongue. Patients with xerostomia may have thrush more often, because saliva is an oral protectant against overgrowth of this yeast.[2,3]

Gingivitis may cause few physical findings. Minor manipulation of the gingiva may cause local bleeding.[9]

Aphthous ulceration can occur as a solitary lesion or multiple lesions. The usual presentation is a 2- to 10-mm (0.01- to 0.4-inch), ulcerative mucosal lesion that has a white-yellow central fibrinous pseudomembrane.[2,3]

DIAGNOSTICS

Herpes simplex infection can be diagnosed by clinical presentation. However several laboratory methods exist to verify diagnosis, including Tzanck smear, viral culture of specimens taken from an active lesion, and serum antibody titers.[2,3]

HPV lesions may be tentatively diagnosed by physical examination; excisional biopsy and pathologic evaluation provide definitive diagnosis. Specific typing of the virus is accomplished with immunohistochemical evaluation.[3]

Candidal infections can also be diagnosed from the physical examination and presentation, but a microscopic examination of oral scrapings will reveal the classic findings of hyphae. Cultures on a mycologic medium (Sabouraud dextrose agar, Pagano-Levin) may be obtained for confirmation.[2,3]

> **DIAGNOSTICS**
>
> **Oral Infections**
>
> **INITIAL**
> KOH preparation or Tzanck test*
>
> **LABORATORY**
> CBC and differential*
> Serum glucose*
> Vitamin B_{12}, folate*
>
> *If indicated.

Gingivitis is diagnosed by physical examination; no diagnostic studies are required. If a specific cause is suspected (systemic disease, medication), the appropriate laboratory test may be requested.[1,3,8]

Aphthous ulcerations as well as lesions of nicotinic and traumatic stomatitis are diagnosed by clinical presentation and physical examination.[2-4]

Laboratory examination may be performed to assess the patient's state of health or confirm diagnosis. This may include complete blood count (CBC); erythrocyte sedimentation rate; serum iron, folate, and vitamin B_{12} levels; potassium hydroxide (KOH) examination; and Tzanck smear.[2-4]

DIFFERENTIAL DIAGNOSIS

Carcinoma of the oral cavity should be suspected with oral erosive lesions that are slow to heal (longer than 2 weeks without resolution) or with thickened white patches that adhere to the oral mucosa.[6] Although similar in appearance to aphthous ulcers, herpetic lesions originate from vesicles and are usually found only on the oral mucosa attached to bone structures. Additional causes of mucosal ulceration that are indicative of systemic disease include bullous pemphigoid,[2] Behçet syndrome, Crohn disease, ulcerative colitis, immune dysfunction, and hand-foot-and-mouth disease.[3,4]

Bullous pemphigoid is a cutaneous disorder in which lesions commence as fixed urticarial plaques followed by clear bullae that appear on both normal and urticarial areas. This chronic eruption primarily affects flexor surfaces but may be generalized. The lesions occur in crops and transiently affect the oral mucosa.[2]

Behçet syndrome produces ulcerative lesions on oral and genital areas, with associated symptoms of uveitis and arthritis. Involvement of the central nervous system is less common; the ocular effects of Behçet syndrome include retinal vasculitis and necrosis. Loss of vision can occur, even with aggressive treatment.[3,4]

The lesions of Crohn disease affect the mucosal surfaces of the gastrointestinal tract, including the oral cavity. Extensive or recurrent oral lesions necessitate careful evaluation for gastrointestinal symptoms, investigation of immune status, and screening for diabetes or other systemic disorders.[2-4]

Hand-foot-and-mouth disease less commonly affects the buttocks and proximal extremities. This viral disease produces a mild, self-limited illness. Inquiry concerning the sudden onset of gastrointestinal symptoms is helpful when clear vesicular lesions that ulcerate are found in the mouth and on the hands and feet.[2,3]

DIFFERENTIAL DIAGNOSIS

Oral Infections

- Aphthous ulcers
- Mechanical, chemical, thermal injury
- Drug reactions
- Nutritional deficiencies
- Infectious causes (bacterial, viral, fungal)
- Carcinoma
- Systemic disease (diabetes, Crohn disease, Behçet syndrome, hand-foot-and-mouth disease)
- Immune dysfunction

MANAGEMENT

Management of localized oral manifestations of HSV infection in immunocompetent patients may include the topical or oral medications acyclovir and valacyclovir. These agents may be most effective if they are taken when the patient is in the prodromal phase.[2] Symptomatic treatment of acute and recurrent herpes labialis should always include hydration, analgesia, antipyretics, and nutritional support. Recurrent episodes of herpes labialis may benefit from oral suppressive therapy with antiviral agents.[2,3]

Oral papillomas are currently treated by surgical excision. There are HPV vaccines currently targeting genital HPV; these vaccines are not approved for prevention of oral papillomas.

Candidal infections may be treated in several ways because antifungal agents are now supplied in many forms. A nystatin oral suspension and troches are commonly prescribed. For patients with dentures, nystatin powder is applied to the dentures three or four times daily. Oral clotrimazole troches are also widely prescribed. Antifungal creams may be applied under dental appliances. Some infections may respond only to systemic therapy with fluconazole, 100 mg/day for 14 days (reduce dose for creatinine clearance <50 mL/min). In patients with diabetes, maintenance of proper glucose levels is an important therapeutic component.[2,3]

Gingivitis is commonly treated with attention to oral hygiene. Brushing twice daily and flossing at least once daily is also recommended.[1]

Aphthous stomatitis can be a vexing problem because recurrence is common. Treatment is directed at symptomatic relief. Methods of symptomatic relief with unclear benefit include the application of topical steroids (e.g., triamcinolone in Orabase, a dental paste) or a steroid mouth rinse with betamethasone syrup.[11] Dexamethasone elixir, 0.5 mg/mL, 5-mL swish and spit four times daily, has been used in adults for severe or recurrent episodes. Current treatments that are likely to reduce the severity and duration of episodes but are not likely to affect recurrence rates include (1) carbamide peroxide (Gly-Oxide) rinse, or bismuth subsalicylate (Kaopectate) and diphenhydramine (Benadryl) mixed in equal measures and applied to the irritated surfaces as a mouth rinse six times a day, and (2) avoidance of irritating, acidic, hot, or spicy foods. Other treatments with likely benefit are varied mouth rinse preparations. Viscous lidocaine is also used as a rinse, but careful observation is needed because this treatment may affect the swallowing and gag reflexes. Amlexanox oral paste, ¼ inch of paste four times daily after oral care, is also indicated.[11] Several preparations or "mouthwash" recipes have been developed to assist in the relief of patients with aphthous stomatitis. One such compounded suspension consists of 30 mL of diphenhydramine elixir and 60 mL of Mylanta (aluminum and magnesium hydroxide), taken as a 5-mL swish and swallow three times daily and at bedtime.[11] Another compound is 60 mL of Maalox and 4 g of sucralfate used in the same manner.[11] Other treatments include the combination of diphenhydramine liquid, dexamethasone, nystatin suspension, and tetracycline (from capsules), swished and swallowed, 1 tsp six times a day (after and between meals and at bedtime).[11] Advice from a pharmacist should be obtained concerning this formulation. Acemannan oral gel or rinse, as needed, can be used to soothe irritated tissue. For children and those in whom tetracycline is prohibited, amoxicillin-clavulanate can be substituted for the tetracycline.[11] However, severe eruptions may respond only to systemic steroids.

COMPLICATIONS

Complications associated with HSV oral infections are uncommon in immunocompetent individuals. In immunosuppressed patients, these infections may lead to widespread systemic infections.[2,3,5]

Candidal infections of the oral cavity can be managed without complication in most instances. However, care should be taken to identify patients who may be immunocompromised or nutritionally at risk so that their needs can be adequately assessed.[2]

Gingivitis is not considered to cause acute complications, but long-term inattention to oral hygiene can lead to painful and costly periodontitis and tooth loss. Investigators are researching the role of periodontal disease in the development of heart disease.[1,7,8]

Aphthous stomatitis is usually a short-lived entity with few if any complications. In patients with major aphthous ulcers, oral intake should be monitored.[2]

Oral HPV infection is often a silent disorder until the patient becomes symptomatic or an oral lesion is identified by a health care provider. HPV has been implicated in some oropharyngeal cancers, particularly cancer of the tonsils.[12]

INDICATIONS FOR REFERRAL OR HOSPITALIZATION

Aphthous stomatitis, dental and nicotinic stomatitis, and routine candidal infections rarely require referral. Severe cases of aphthous ulcers may need referral for assessment of the patient's immune status and need for systemic therapy.[2] A physician or subspecialist in infectious diseases should be consulted if questions arise concerning possible carcinoma or if the patient is immunocompromised. Patients with routine eruptions are not candidates for hospitalization, but severely immunocompromised patients or patients with diabetes may need hospitalization for treatment of the underlying disease.[2,3] Alcohol or tobacco use and HPV infection increase the risk for oral cancers, and patients with ulcers or nonhealing lesions present for more than 2 weeks without resolution or improvement should be referred for evaluation.[6]

PATIENT EDUCATION AND HEALTH PROMOTION

HSV infections are spread by contact with the virus, and this can include sharing of lip balms or other materials with a viral carrier. Kissing and sharing of drinking utensils should be avoided to prevent the spread of the virus. Asymptomatic viral shedding occurs frequently, and avoidance of contact only when lesions are present does not offer protection.[2,3,5] These same precautions should be offered to individuals with manifestations of HPV infection. Orogenital contact is a common method of transmission of HPV, and this information should be shared with the individual and his or her partner. Education about the risk of HPV-related oral cancer is essential.[3,6]

Candidal infections can be anticipated in patients who are taking long courses of steroids and antibiotics; treatment of these patients should be started as soon as symptoms occur. Patients who are known to be immunocompromised should be monitored regularly for the signs and symptoms of developing candidal infections and treated accordingly. Patients with diabetes should be instructed in proper glycemic control measures and routine surveillance of skin and mucosal surfaces.[2]

Careful, daily attention to dental hygiene is the key to prevention of gingivitis and periodontitis. A routine daily brushing and flossing regimen is recommended by dental health care providers.[1,3]

Aphthous stomatitis is usually a recurrent eruption. Treatment of the underlying causes, if known, may alleviate future outbreaks. Crohn disease, ulcerative colitis, stresses, deficiencies of vitamin B_{12} and folic acid, iron deficiency, and estrogen sensitivity have been implicated in outbreaks. Avoidance of irritating food, beverages, and chemicals may alleviate some of the symptoms and decrease the number of recurrences.[4]

CHAPTER 99

PAROTITIS

Lisa O'Neal

DEFINITION AND EPIDEMIOLOGY

The parotid gland is the largest of the three major salivary glands in the body. An inflammatory reaction of the parotid gland is defined as parotitis. This is not to be confused with sialadenitis, which is defined as the inflammation or infection of a salivary gland.[1] Parotitis may be caused by bacterial, viral, fungal, or mycobacterial invasion. The parotid gland is most commonly affected by an inflammatory process, and infections can range from acute to severe. Assessment of the disease process should differentiate between local primary infections of the parotid gland, such as bacterial sialadenitis, and systemic infection, in which the gland is inflamed from a generalized inflammatory process caused by a virus. Viruses most commonly associated with parotitis are the paramyxovirus (cause of mumps) and the human immunodeficiency virus (HIV).[2]

Inflammatory conditions of the parotid gland include acute viral inflammation, commonly caused by mumps, and acute suppurative sialadenitis, often caused by *Staphylococcus aureas.* Chronic inflammatory conditions of the parotid are caused by infection with *Mycobacterium tuberculosis* (tuberculosis [TB]) and HIV.[3] Noninfective causes of parotitis can be related to Sjögren syndrome (SS) and sarcoidosis.[3]

Acute suppurative parotitis is more likely to be encountered in the sixth to seventh decade of life, with a higher incidence in men and with the right side involved more frequently than the left.[2] Older adults are at a higher risk of development of acute suppurative parotitis because of a medication-induced (e.g., anticholinergics and antihistamines) decrease in salivary flow.[2] Other factors are associated with acute suppurative parotitis. These include chronic illness (e.g., diabetes mellitus, hypothyroidism, renal failure, rheumatoid arthritis), an immunocompromised host, poor oral hygiene, salivary duct obstruction, autoimmune disease (SS), recent surgical procedure, radiotherapy, and hypovolemia.[2] Acute suppurative parotitis has been identified as a common postoperative occurrence in patients undergoing major abdominal and hip repair surgery.[2] This has been attributed to postoperative dehydration and is usually identified within the first 2 weeks after surgery.[2] Acute suppurative parotitis is rarer now because antibiotic use in the perioperative setting is more common and there is increased attention to perioperative hydration, nutrition, and oral hygiene.[1]

PATHOPHYSIOLOGY

The parotid gland is most susceptible to infection because it secretes serous saliva versus mucinous saliva.[2] Serous saliva lacks lysosomes, immunoglobulin A antibodies, and sialic acid, all with bacteriostatic properties, thus predisposing the parotid gland to a greater risk of infection compared with its counterparts.[2] Multiple factors contribute to the development of parotitis. Most commonly, the infection begins with retrograde migration of oral cavity flora through the Stensen duct. Stasis of saliva, ductal obstruction, decreased stimulation of saliva, decreased mastication, and poor oral hygiene contribute to retrograde migration.[2,4] Ill patients, recent surgical patients, and those with acute or chronic hypovolemia can develop stasis and retrograde migration. Although most of these infections occur in adults, they can occur in children also. Presentation of parotitis in the pediatric population is usually an isolated occurrence and associated with a viral or bacterial infection.[5] Parotitis is also the classic symptom of infection with paramyxovirus (mumps).[6]

CLINICAL PRESENTATION

Usually the onset of parotitis is rapid and associated with localized pain, edema, and induration of the infected gland.[4] Systemic symptoms include fever, chills, anorexia, and malaise.[4] Viral inflammatory reactions most often are seen with edema (usually bilateral) and pain, which is exacerbated by mastication.[4] Parotitis associated with a bacterial infection (acute suppurative sialadenitis) often occurs in a hypovolemic elder and consists of unilateral parotid enlargement and cellulitis.[3] Intraorally, pus can be visualized with manual pressure on the parotid duct orifice.[4] Chronic inflammatory conditions of the parotid caused by the infective agent *M. tuberculosis* appear much like a malignant neoplasm, with enlargement of and pain in the affected gland.[3] The mass is usually unilateral and associated with matted lymph nodes.[3] Infection with HIV may produce bilaterally enlarged, painless parotid glands that gradually produce smaller amounts of saliva, resulting in complaints of xerostomia.[3]

PHYSICAL EXAMINATION

Bimanual palpation of the gland with attention to the Stensen duct should be performed. In bacterial parotitis, palpation of the gland elicits a suppurative discharge from the Stensen duct.[2] Bilateral edema is suggestive of viral infection, and a clear discharge is found on palpation of the duct. Suppurative discharge should be cultured. If the process has been present for several days, fluctuance of suppurative sialadenitis may not be palpable because of the anatomic septations in the parotid.

DIAGNOSTICS

DIAGNOSTICS
Parotitis

LABORATORY
CBC and differential
Culture and sensitivity

IMAGING
X-ray studies*
CT scan with contrast*
Ultrasound*
MRI*

*If indicated.

The diagnosis of parotitis is based on the clinical presentation and physical examination. A complete blood count (CBC) with differential may reveal leukocytosis with neutrophilia in suppurative cases.[1] Appropriate cultures and sensitivities should be performed and fungal and mycobacterial studies requested when indicated. Caution should be taken when evaluating cultured pus from the Stensen duct, because it is often contaminated by the normal oral flora.[1]

Radiographs or oblique soft tissue films of the mouth and jaw should be obtained if obstruction caused by a sialolith (calculus) is suspected.[1] Computed tomography (CT) scan with contrast medium is an excellent study because it may delineate ductal stones or a suppurative process.[1] Ultrasonography is the most cost-effective and safest diagnostic tool for identifying sialoliths and diagnosing inflammatory parotid disease.[1]

Magnetic resonance imaging (MRI) is most useful in identifying parenchymal changes of the parotid gland and possibly identifying atrophy, which is commonly associated with SS,[1] or if neoplasms or abscesses are suspected.[2] If a neoplasm is suspected, a biopsy is indicated.[7]

DIFFERENTIAL DIAGNOSIS

The differential diagnosis of parotitis should include bacterial, viral, mycobacterial, and fungal infections. In addition to paramyxovirus, identified agents of infection include cytomegalovirus, Coxsackie A virus, Epstein-Barr virus, influenza A, parainfluenza virus type 3, lymphocytic choriomeningitis, human herpesvirus type 6, echovirus, and HIV.[1] Mechanical or extrinsic factors, such as radiotherapy or drug-induced parotitis, should also be included in the differential diagnosis. In addition, anticholinergic medications can initiate parotitis. Such medications include antiparkinsonian agents, atropine, dicyclomine hydrochloride, glycopyrrolate, scopolamine, and hyoscyamine sulfate. Many psychotropic medications have an atropine-like effect and can cause parotid swelling.[2]

Painless enlargement of the parotid gland requires further investigation to exclude a malignant process. Fine-needle biopsy or surgical excision is indicated.

DIFFERENTIAL DIAGNOSIS
Parotitis

- Infection
  - Bacterial
  - Viral
  - HIV
  - Fungal
  - Mycobacterial
- Medications
- Mechanical obstruction

MANAGEMENT

Nonsurgical treatments include parenteral antibiotics and possibly hospitalization for parenteral antibiotic therapy. Culture and sensitivity testing is important because multidrug-resistant organisms are common.[8] Recommended antibiotic therapy is initially empirical and includes amoxicillin with clavulanate, dicloxacillin, clindamycin, or a cephalosporin in addition to metronidazole.[6,8] Results will further direct antimicrobial therapy and identify if methicillin-resistant *S. aureus* is present, thus requiring vancomycin or linezolid.[2] Response to antimicrobial therapy should be identified within 48 to 72 hours of initiation of therapy and should be continued for 1 week after symptoms have ceased.[2] Fluid and electrolyte replacement is necessary.[2] Attention to proper oral hygiene and the use of sialagogues (agents that stimulate the production and flow of saliva, such as sugar-free hard candy and chewing gum) are also recommended.[6] There is a questionable role for the use of steroids. Analgesics and local heat for relief of pain are beneficial. External bimanual massage (from distal to proximal) of the duct is

BOX 99-1

Severe Complications of Parotitis

Sepsis with or without shock
Soft tissue infection extending into the neck, face, mediastinum
Osteomyelitis of the mandible
Lemierre syndrome
Airway obstruction
Invasion of the external auditory canal
Facial nerve palsy (common with parotid malignancy)

also recommended.[2] Surgical drainage is appropriate if the infection is refractory for more than 3 or 4 days.[3] A CT scan or ultrasound examination of the parotid and neck is indicated if abscess formation has occurred after 3 or 4 days while the patient is taking aggressive parenteral antibiotics. Because of the usually debilitated states of patients predisposed to parotitis, a poor prognosis is associated with postoperative patients who develop parotitis. A 20% mortality rate is associated with the development of this infection.[2]

COMPLICATIONS

Complications include abscess formation and the need for surgical drainage.[2,5,6] The discomfort associated with this disorder may prevent the patient from eating and drinking, increasing the risk of hypovolemia and further compromising the patient. Suppurative parotitis is a rare occurrence postoperatively because of the routine use of preoperative and intraoperative antibiotic therapy. However, if it is left untreated, severe complications can arise (Box 99-1).[1] Chronic parotitis may develop as a result of an acute episode of suppurative parotitis.[4] Complications of viral parotitis include orchitis, pancreatitis, meningoencephalitis, and deafness.[3]

INDICATIONS FOR REFERRAL OR HOSPITALIZATION

Consultation with an otolaryngologist, a head and neck surgeon, is highly recommended. Patients who develop parotitis often require hospitalization for fluid replacement, careful monitoring, and intravenous antibiotics.

PATIENT AND FAMILY EDUCATION AND HEALTH PROMOTION

Preoperative attention to hydration and overall health status should be addressed if the patient is not a candidate for emergent surgery. After diagnosis, attention to hydration, parenteral antibiotics, oral hygiene, and sialagogue use should be addressed. Patients should be instructed in proper oral hygiene, which includes brushing and flossing the teeth and proper care of dentures and dental appliances. The side effects of medications should be discussed with the patient to determine whether medication is causing decreased salivary secretions.[1]

CHAPTER 100

PERITONSILLAR ABSCESS

Erin A. Lyden

DEFINITION AND EPIDEMIOLOGY

A peritonsillar abscess (PTA) is an accumulation of pus within the peritonsillar tissues, between the tonsil and the pharyngeal constrictor muscle.[1-3] PTA is a common deep infection of the head and neck.[1] The abscess frequently occurs in patients with a history of recurrent, chronic, or improperly treated tonsillitis.[1]

Peritonsillar cellulitis and abscess formation are common occurrences in the middle teenage years through age 40.[2,4] The incidence rate for PTA varies internationally; one source lists 1 in 6500 in the United States and 1 in 10,000 in Northern Ireland.[4] The incidence of PTAs reported is on the rise worldwide.[2] The recurrence of PTA is reported to be variable, from 9% to 22%.[5] The risk of recurrence is higher if the patient is younger than 30 years and for patients who smoke.[4]

Specialist referral is recommended for PTA.

PATHOPHYSIOLOGY

PTAs were previously believed to be a direct result of inadequately treated tonsillitis. The tonsillitis progresses to cellulitis, and eventually pus formation occurs in the peritonsillar tissue.[2,6] However, now there are two theories regarding the pathogenesis of PTAs.[2,6] One study found that 79% of patients reported symptoms of a sore throat before PTA, whereas another reported that 68% of the patients studied denied such symptoms before PTA diagnosis.[2] In addition to the theory that PTA is a complication of acute tonsillitis is the theory of blocked Weber glands.[2,6] These are salivary glands located on the upper soft palate.[6] It has been suggested that infection secondary to poor oral hygiene or other sources (e.g., infections and smoking) could cause scarring that leads to an eventual blockage of the ducts of the Weber glands.[2] These glands are reported to assist in the removal of debris in the tonsil area. If these glands are obstructed by debris, inflammation, or pus, their function is impaired, contributing to the development of PTA.[2,6] PTA has been found to have both aerobic and anaerobic bacteria.[1]

CLINICAL PRESENTATION

The presentation typically consists of fever, chills, fatigue, malaise, foul breath, dysphagia, severe sore throat, and otalgia.[6,7] One small Canadian study noted that only 24% of patients had fever over 38° C.[7] The patient may appear acutely ill and often reports pain radiating to the ear of the affected side. Trismus (spasms of the masticator muscles) is often noted. Drooling is typically present because of the inability to handle secretions. A "hot potato" (hoarse) voice is commonly noted.[6]

PHYSICAL EXAMINATION

With PTA, there is marked edema and erythema of the peritonsillar tissue and soft palate; this tissue is often fluctuant and covered with exudate.[6] The findings are almost always unilateral, with the tonsil typically displaced downward and medially. The uvula is often edematous and displaced to the opposite side.[7] Other findings include trismus, tender cervical adenopathy, tachycardia, pooling of saliva or drooling, and signs of dehydration.[6] In a small study published in 2013, the patient's physical examination revealed the "classic symptoms" of uvular deviation, trismus, and muffled voice in more than 90% of patients.[7]

DIAGNOSTICS

PTAs are easily diagnosed on the basis of physical findings. A computed tomography (CT) scan with contrast will confirm abscess formation and the presence of gas. Ultrasonography, either oral or cutaneous, in a cooperative, nonemergent patient can also be a useful diagnostic tool.[1]

A complete blood count (CBC) often reveals leukocytosis.[6,7] A Monospot heterophile antibody test may be performed to exclude infectious mononucleosis.[6] Culture and sensitivity testing of aspirate from the abscess typically reveals both aerobic and anaerobic bacteria.[1,6,7] Serum electrolytes may be ordered if the patient reports decreased oral intake. As with any other suspected infectious process, Gram stain and culture and sensitivity should be performed on any aspirated purulent material.[1]

DIAGNOSTICS

Peritonsillar Abscess

LABORATORY	IMAGING
CBC and differential	CT*
comprehensive metabolic panel (CMP)*	Ultrasonography, oral or cutaneous
Monospot test*	
Culture and sensitivity of abscess aspirate (by otolaryngologist)	

*If indicated.

DIFFERENTIAL DIAGNOSIS

When considering a diagnosis of PTA, the health care provider must exclude other conditions that manifest with similar signs and symptoms. These conditions include infectious mononucleosis; tumors; peritonsillar cellulitis; epiglottitis; retromolar or retropharyngeal abscesses; and lymphoma.[6,8,9]

Infectious mononucleosis can be excluded on the basis of clinical presentation, physical examination, and serologic findings. With mononucleosis, headache, malaise, fatigue, and anorexia are typically present before the sore throat. A tumor in the peritonsillar region is eliminated from diagnostic consideration by a lack of the physical findings usually present in an infectious process. A CT scan and, possibly, a biopsy are indicated if a tumor is suspected.

The signs and symptoms of PTAs are similar to those of epiglottitis, which is a potentially fatal condition if not diagnosed. Epiglottitis is less likely when there is peritonsillar swelling with preserved ability to swallow and no stridor auscultated over the larynx on physical examination. Indirect visualization of the epiglottis is a reliable method in the adult and may be necessary to exclude epiglottitis as a cause of symptoms.[10]

Retropharyngeal abscesses may be similar in their presentation. Both conditions reveal an ill or toxic patient, with signs of infection and neck pain. A retropharyngeal abscess can be identified with a CT scan.[6,8]

DIFFERENTIAL DIAGNOSIS

Peritonsillar Abscess

- Peritonsillar cellulitis
- Infectious mononucleosis
- Tumors
- Epiglottitis
- Retromolar or retropharyngeal abscess
- Lymphoma

MANAGEMENT

Oral antibiotic therapy is not sufficient for effective treatment of a PTA. Surgical intervention is required with needle aspiration, incision and drainage, or tonsillectomy. The majority of PTAs can be treated effectively with needle aspiration, antibiotics, pain medication, and maintenance of hydration.[6,9] A tonsillectomy may be indicated in certain situations, such as recurrent tonsillitis or history of PTA.[9,11] Careful attention to analgesia is required, along with adequate hydration. Optimum hydration of the patient must be maintained, either orally or intravenously. The use of intravenous antibiotics plus a single high dose of intravenous steroids versus intravenous antibiotics alone in PTA patients has been shown to be superior.[5,6,10] The steroid dose was determined to aid in relief of fever, pain, trismus, and dysphagia.[10]

As an adjunct to surgical intervention, the antibiotic regimen appears to vary based on otolaryngologist preference and geographic location. One review stated that the use of combined penicillin and metronidazole was effective in at least 98% of cases.[5] Clindamycin is another widely used antibiotic for PTA; in some cases it is preferred by the provider, and in others it is used if the patient has a known penicillin allergy.[7,10]

LIFE SPAN CONSIDERATIONS

Although PTA is usually seen in people from teenage to 40 years of age, a high index of suspicion must be maintained in all age groups.[2,5] Early detection and treatment can prevent a life-threatening complication.[10]

COMPLICATIONS

Serious and potentially fatal complications may result from a PTA. The abscess can result in airway obstruction from spread of the infection. Rupture of the abscess with aspiration of the infected material can cause severe and serious sequelae. If untreated, the infection may spread to involve the superior constrictor muscle, other deep spaces of the neck, and the mediastinum. Necrosis of the muscle may result. Internal jugular vein thrombosis with septic pulmonary embolism can also occur.[10]

Other complications of PTA include thrombophlebitis, chronic PTA, glottic edema, epiglottitis, septicemia, endocarditis, myocarditis, and hemorrhage. Poststreptococcal complications such as rheumatic fever and glomerulonephritis may result if the infected material consists of group A β-hemolytic streptococci. Thrombosis of the internal jugular vein (Lemierre syndrome) is a rare sequela, usually the result of infection with *Fusobacterium necrophorum*. Intravenous antibiotic therapy and surgical treatment of the abscess are required. Ligation or excision of the internal jugular vein is mandatory if septic emboli are noted. Extension of the abscess into the carotid artery sheath is a complication of extending infection.[6,9,10]

INDICATIONS FOR REFERRAL OR HOSPITALIZATION

After diagnosis of a PTA has been made, patients should be referred immediately to an otolaryngologist for an evaluation concerning surgical intervention and antibiotic therapy. Hospitalization may not be necessary, although the patient is usually hospitalized after aspiration and started on intravenous antibiotics. Patients may be discharged in 24 hours or less if symptoms subside and the abscess does not reappear. Follow-up should occur 24 to 36 hours. Referral to an otolaryngologist is necessary if tonsillectomy is indicated.[2,5,6]

PATIENT AND FAMILY EDUCATION

Education concerning PTA as a complication of tonsillitis is important. PTA can recur, and therefore the signs and symptoms should be described to the patient and family. These include fever, chills, malaise, odynophagia, ear pain, inability to open the mouth, dysphagia, drooling, and a "hot potato" voice.[5,6] The provider should also discuss the possible side effects of antibiotic therapy. These side effects may include nausea, vomiting, diarrhea, abdominal pain, lethargy, vaginitis, or a secondary yeast infection. Signs and symptoms of an allergic reaction, including urticaria, shortness of breath, wheezing, or tightness in the chest, indicate the necessity for immediate emergency treatment.

HEALTH PROMOTION

Patients with histories of recurrent tonsillitis, chronic tonsillitis, and inadequately treated tonsillitis should be monitored closely for signs of PTA. Consultation with an otolaryngologist is a must for these patients.[5,6,9] PTA is increased in individuals with poor oral hygiene and in smokers. For this reason the importance of good oral health and smoking cessation should be discussed with patients.[2,3]

CHAPTER 101

PHARYNGITIS AND TONSILLITIS

Erin A. Lyden

Immediate emergency department referral or physician consultation is indicated for pharyngeal abscess.

DEFINITION AND EPIDEMIOLOGY

Pharyngitis is a condition that encompasses inflammation of the pharynx from either infection or irritation.[1] An illness affecting both children and adults, pharyngitis is a common reason for people to seek health care and accounts for around 6% of visits to health care providers.[2] Pharyngitis can manifest as an acute illness or a chronic condition. The causes are numerous and include both infectious and noninfectious agents.[1]

Noninfectious causes of pharyngitis include referred pain, allergies, trauma from foreign bodies or burns, cancer, and irritation. Irritation of the pharynx may result from dust, smoke, dryness, or toxins, either inhaled or swallowed.[1,2]

Infectious agents responsible for pharyngitis include viruses, bacteria, and, uncommonly, fungi or parasites. Viral infection is the most common cause of pharyngitis in all age groups and can occur during any season.[1-3] Viruses are responsible for 30% to 60% of cases in adults. In those cases the most common cause is the rhinovirus.[1] Other responsible agents include Epstein-Barr virus (which causes mononucleosis), herpes simplex virus, influenza virus, parainfluenza virus, and coronavirus.[1,4]

Bacterial pharyngitis is more common in children (30% to 40%), peaking at ages 5 to 15, than in adults (5% to 10%).[1,2] *Streptococcus pyogenes* is the etiologic agent for an estimated 15% to 30% of acute pharyngitis cases.[5] *S. pyogenes* includes groups A, C, and G β-hemolytic streptococci. Group A β-hemolytic *Streptococcus* (GAS) is the most important to identify because it is responsible for acute rheumatic fever (ARF) and poststreptococcal glomerulonephritis. Infection with GAS typically peaks in the late winter and early spring, but it can be seen year-round.[1,2,6] Group C disease is more common among college students and adolescents. Community-wide and foodborne causes of pharyngitis have been connected to group G organisms.[1] Other offending agents include mycoplasmas, *Arcanobacterium haemolyticum,* chlamydiae, *Neisseria gonorrhoeae,* corynebacteria, and anaerobic bacteria.[1]

Tonsillitis and pharyngitis are similar in clinical presentation, physical findings, diagnosis, and management (Fig. 101-1). Tonsillitis is an acute or chronic inflammation of the tonsils and usually results from GAS infection, although it may be caused by other bacteria or viruses. Tonsillitis may not be a concern unless the patient is symptomatic.

PATHOPHYSIOLOGY

The normal flora of the oral pharynx region consists of various and numerous microorganisms. These microorganisms are not harmful unless the immune system is weakened, resulting in increased susceptibility to illness. Pharyngitis or tonsillitis develops from exposure to a viral or bacterial agent, although some people can harbor or be colonized with pathogenic bacteria and remain free of infection.[1]

CLINICAL PRESENTATION

The clinical presentation of pharyngitis or tonsillitis varies according to the offending agent. Noninfectious pharyngitis has an initial appearance somewhat different from that of infectious

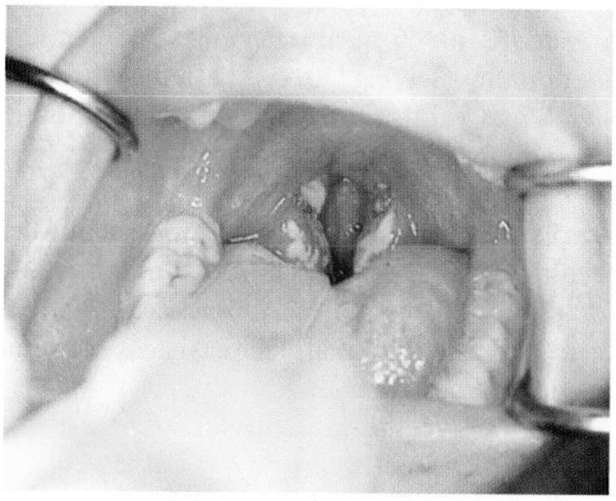

FIGURE 101-1 Pharyngitis and tonsillitis. (From Barkauskas VH, Stoltenberg-Allen K, Baumann LC, Darling-Fisher C: *Health and physical assessment,* ed 2, St Louis, 1998, Mosby.)

pharyngitis. Typically, with noninfectious pharyngitis the patient reports a sore throat and dryness; if environmental allergens are the cause, symptoms often include rhinorrhea, watery eyes, and postnasal drip. Patients receiving radiation therapy or chemotherapy may report pain, dryness, and dysphagia. Oropharyngeal candidiasis (thrush) may be present in these patients secondary to the immunosuppression.

The infectious causes of pharyngitis or tonsillitis are bacterial and viral. The presentation of symptoms can be similar. Viral causes are more common, and patients typically report the sudden onset of a sore throat, fever, malaise, cough, headache, myalgias, and fatigue. Patients may also report rhinitis, conjunctivitis (adenovirus), congestion, and a cough with sputum production.[7]

One of the most common causes of bacterial pharyngitis or tonsillitis is GAS. In the winter months, it is estimated that 15% to 25% of pharyngitis cases in children are caused by GAS.[5,7] This disease is most prevalent in children younger than 15 years. The transmission of GAS is by direct contact with respiratory secretions or large droplets, and the incubation period can be 2 to 5 days. It is often spread in the classroom setting.[5,7]

Patients may report a sudden onset of sore throat, painful swallowing, fever (temperature higher than 38.5° C [101.3° F]), chills, headache, nausea, vomiting, and abdominal pain.[1,5,7] With bacterial pharyngitis, rhinitis, cough, conjunctivitis, and myalgias are not typically present.[6,7]

Other bacterial causes should be investigated if indicated because *N. gonorrhoeae* and *Chlamydia* organisms can cause pharyngitis. Other bacteria, such as group C and G streptococci, *Mycoplasma pneumoniae,* and *A. haemolyticum,* can be involved.[7] These patients often report mild throat discomfort in addition to urethritis or vaginitis.

PHYSICAL EXAMINATION

In viral pharyngitis, findings include fever, cough, nasal symptoms, and mild erythema with little or no pharyngeal exudate, although the pharynx may appear swollen, boggy, or pale. Painful or tender lymphadenopathy is not typically present. Infectious mononucleosis typically produces headache, fatigue, high fever, pharyngeal erythema, tonsillar hypertrophy, white to gray-green exudate, petechiae at the junction of the hard and soft palate, and posterior cervical adenopathy. Hepatomegaly and splenomegaly may be identified in less than 50% of patients. Jaundice may be present, but that is unusual.[1,4,6]

In GAS infection, the physical examination reveals marked erythema of the throat and tonsils; patchy, discrete, white or yellowish exudate; pharyngeal petechiae; and tender anterior cervical adenopathy (see Fig. 101-1). Patients with previous exposure to GAS may exhibit the typical diffuse exanthem of scarlet fever, a sandpaper-type rash, and erythematous (strawberry) tongue.[1,6]

Pressure on the tonsillar pillars may produce purulent drainage. The uvula may also be edematous, and temperature higher than 38.3° C (101° F) is typical. On occasion, GAS infection may be seen with an erythematous, persistent sore throat with little fever and no exudate.[1,6]

DIAGNOSTICS

Although it is sometimes difficult to differentiate between viral and bacterial pharyngitis and tonsillitis, clinical presentation may indicate the diagnosis. No specific diagnostic test exists for viral pharyngitis.[1]

Diagnostic studies used to detect GAS infection include a throat culture, a rapid antigen detection test (RADT), and sometimes an antistreptolysin O (ASO) titer. The ASO titer is not used during initial diagnostic screening but is obtained to identify or to confirm a diagnosis of GAS infection weeks to months later. The RADT is often used because it is rapid and convenient. However, the RADT is less sensitive (true positives) than a throat culture. If the diagnosis of GAS infection is suspected and the RADT result is negative, a throat culture is performed for confirmation. A complete blood count (CBC) often reveals leukocytosis with GAS infection.

Many studies have evaluated the efficacy of a clinical scoring system in the diagnosis of GAS pharyngitis. Many medical societies have recommended various clinical indicators in an attempt to standardize diagnosis. The Centor criteria—tonsillar exudates, swollen and tender anterior cervical lymph nodes, lack of cough, and history of fever—have proved to be predictive of a positive diagnosis in adult patients.[5] To calculate a Centor score for an individual patient, 1 point is added for each of the following findings: absence of cough, tonsils with exudates or swelling, tender and swollen anterior cervical nodes, and temperature higher than 38° C (100.4° F); thus the score can range from 1 to 4.[8] Some sources use age to modify the score, subtracting 1 point if the patient is over 45.[3,5]

There remains disagreement concerning the precise use of the Centor score to guide diagnosis and testing. The differences in recommendations arise from concern about potential sequelae of rheumatic fever.[3] Some U.S. guidelines (Infectious Diseases Society of America, American Heart Association [AHA], American Academy of Pediatrics, and Institute for Clinical System Improvement) recommend culture and RADT testing based on presence of history of exposure to streptococci, previous history of rheumatic fever or poststreptococcal glomerulonephritis, or clinical signs and symptoms suggestive of streptococcal infection.[3] In addition, the AHA guidelines recommend throat culture, even if the RADT is negative.[3] The American College of Physicians–American Society of Internal Medicine (ACP-ASIM) guidelines use a Centor score of 2 to 3 to recommend testing with RADT with throat culture. In the ACP-ASIM guidelines, a Centor score of 4 indicates a presumptive diagnosis of GAS and confirmatory testing is not necessary.[3]

An investigation conducted in a large retail health system found that use of local biosurveillance data on the recent local proportion positive (RLPP) streptococci results on throat culture or DNA probe test to modify the Centor score improved the score's ability to predict GAS infection.[9] American College of Physician guidelines do not recommend testing adults with Centor scores of 0 or 1; the retail health system study found that in times of high RLPP, those patients with a Centor score of 0 typically have only a 15% risk for GAS, yet those with a Centor score of 1 when there is high RLPP should be tested because their risk is increased.[9]

DIAGNOSTICS

Pharyngitis and Tonsillitis

LABORATORY

Throat culture or RADT
CBC and differential*

*If indicated.

DIFFERENTIAL DIAGNOSIS

The presence of an inflamed pharynx requires further investigation. The differential diagnosis should include infectious mononucleosis, allergies, thrush, peritonsillar cellulitis or abscess, pharyngeal abscess, epiglottitis, leukoplakia, and upper respiratory tract infection (URI).

Infectious mononucleosis differs from pharyngitis or tonsillitis in clinical presentation, physical examination, and serologic findings. This diagnosis is seen more commonly in adolescents and young adults.[7] These patients usually are seen with headache, malaise, fatigue, and anorexia before the sore throat occurs. Hepatosplenomegaly may be noted during the physical examination. A CBC often reveals leukocytosis with atypical lymphocytes. A positive Monospot test result reveals heterophil antibodies.[1,6] The Monospot test is highly specific and sensitive, but it may take 2 to 3 weeks to produce a positive result. Therefore an initial false-negative finding may occur. Associated symptoms of teary eyes and watery discharge from the eyes, pruritus, rhinitis, postnasal drip, pale and boggy nasal mucosa, and erythematous pharynx with mucus are commonly seen with seasonal allergies. Thrush, a white, thick, cheeselike material that can be scraped off, is identified with a positive potassium hydroxide test result. Peritonsillar cellulitis differs from pharyngitis by the physical examination findings and the absence of pus on aspiration. Peritonsillar abscess can be diagnosed by presenting signs and symptoms and the aspiration of pus. Tonsillitis may be present with pharyngitis.[1]

Although presenting signs and symptoms of a URI are similar to those of viral pharyngitis, a URI usually has associated symptoms such as cough, congestion, rhinitis, sneezing, injected conjunctiva, erythematous and edematous nasal mucosa, and erythematous pharynx.[1,2,4,6] Epiglottitis must be excluded by radiographic imaging or direct laryngoscopy once it is suspected; typically, however, patients with epiglottitis cannot effectively swallow even their own saliva.[1]

Severe exudative pharyngitis or tonsillitis is usually present in mononucleosis. A thick, gray membrane over the tonsils and pharynx is indicative of diphtheria. Leukoplakia, a white patch, is a premalignant change that may arise anywhere on the oral mucosa (Fig. 101-2). If it is suspected, a thorough history is warranted. If the lesion remains for more than 2 weeks, a biopsy is indicated.

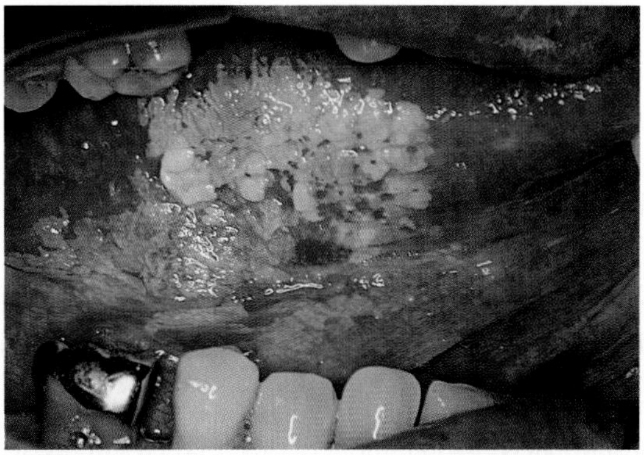

FIGURE **101-2** Leukoplakia on the ventral aspect of the tongue. (From Eisen D, Lynch DP: *The mouth: diagnosis and treatment,* St Louis, 1998, Mosby.)

DIFFERENTIAL DIAGNOSIS

Pharyngitis and Tonsillitis

- Infectious mononucleosis
- Viral, bacterial, or fungal infection
- Allergies
- Peritonsillar cellulitis or abscess
- Epiglottitis
- URI
- Diphtheria
- Trauma
- Cancer
- Chemotherapy
- Radiation therapy
- Irritation
- Thrush

MANAGEMENT

Treatment of viral pharyngitis includes rest, fluids, humidification, voice rest, and warm saline gargles to ease discomfort.[7] Acetaminophen or ibuprofen should be used for fever and general discomfort. Topical anesthetic sprays and throat lozenges are of benefit; however, they may produce further irritation in a small number of individuals.

In addition to the measures employed with viral pharyngitis, antibiotic therapy (penicillin V, 500 mg two or three times daily for 10 days) is indicated in GAS pharyngitis primarily to prevent complications, such as suppurative tonsillitis, glomerulonephritis, and rheumatic fever.[3] A one-time dose of benzathine penicillin, 1.2 million units intramuscularly, has also proved effective. Penicillin is often prescribed because of the low cost, safety, and efficacy. Amoxicillin, 250 mg three times daily to four times daily or 500 mg twice daily for 10 days, is also appropriate. Clarithromycin, 250 mg twice daily for 10 days, is indicated for patients with penicillin allergy.[3] Azithromycin, 12 mg/kg with a maximum dose of 500 mg daily for 5 days, and clindamycin, 20 mg/kg/day divided into three doses, maximum of 1.8 g/day for 10 days, can also be used in these patients.[3] Guidelines continue to recommend a 10-day course with penicillins.[3,6]

A first- or second-generation cephalosporin is effective initially or for recurrent disease and may have greater efficacy; however, it is not considered a first-line choice because of the cost and concern with building antibiotic resistance. There is a small chance of cephalosporin allergy if the patient is allergic to penicillin. The recent United Kingdom guidelines recommend treatment for Centor scores of 3 or above without confirmatory testing. The ACP-ASIM guidelines use a Centor score of 4 to initiate treatment without testing.[3]

Treatment of non–group A streptococcal infection is given for symptomatic relief because the organisms are not linked to serious sequelae and do not produce a major antibody response.[2] Penicillin or erythromycin is effective. Management of chronic pharyngitis or tonsillitis with GAS infection may require tonsillectomy, although tonsillectomy is not performed as often as in the past. Current recommendations suggest six or seven documented episodes of GAS pharyngitis or tonsillitis within 1 year, five episodes a year for 2 consecutive years, or three episodes a year for 3 years before tonsillectomy is warranted.

LIFE SPAN CONSIDERATIONS

More than 11 million visits occur annually for pharyngitis in the United States. Pharyngitis is an entity that affects all age groups and populations. A comprehensive head and neck examination and history are required for accurate assessment of the situation and for appropriate treatment to be prescribed. Pharyngitis that lasts more than 2 weeks in an adult smoker should be considered a cancer unless proven otherwise. Prompt and proper diagnosis of patients who truly have *S. pyogenes* infections can have a significant effect on the morbidity of the disease.[5]

COMPLICATIONS

Complications from chronic tonsillitis include upper airway obstruction, sleep apnea, and sleep disturbances. Complications from acute streptococcal infections can be divided into suppurative and nonsuppurative entities. Suppurative complications include streptococcal pharyngitis, otitis media, sinusitis, impetigo, pneumonia, and necrotizing fasciitis. Nonsuppurative complications associated with GAS infection include ARF and poststreptococcal glomerulonephritis.[1,6]

Unfortunately, glomerulonephritis may result even with proper treatment. ARF can be prevented by prompt antibiotic therapy for the prescribed time. Because diagnosis of GAS pharyngitis is difficult on the basis of clinical findings alone, the practitioner should use recommended guidelines in the assessment of the patient thought to have GAS pharyngitis.[6]

INDICATIONS FOR REFERRAL OR HOSPITALIZATION

An evaluation by an otolaryngologist should be sought for recurrent GAS infections or for complications that may result from pharyngitis. In addition, potential airway obstruction from pharyngitis or abscess requires immediate referral to an otolaryngologist and hospitalization. Peritonsillar abscess and retropharyngeal abscess require hospitalization for observation and intravenous antibiotics. Abscesses usually require incision and drainage. Patients with ARF and poststreptococcal glomerulonephritis may require hospitalization, depending on symptoms. Patients diagnosed with ARF require antibiotic prophylaxis, although debate exists about the duration of prophylaxis.[1]

PATIENT AND FAMILY EDUCATION

Education is extremely important, and adherence to antibiotic therapy must be stressed. Patients should understand that they are infectious until 24 hours after the start of antibiotic therapy and that a full course of antibiotics is required to prevent reinfection or complications.[10]

Education stresses adherence to prescribed therapy to ensure eradication of organisms. Possible side effects of antibiotic therapy, including allergic reaction, nausea, vomiting, diarrhea, abdominal pain, lethargy, vaginitis, and secondary yeast infection, should be explained. Signs and symptoms of an allergic reaction, such as urticaria (hives), shortness of breath, wheezing, or tightness in the chest, mandate immediate medical attention. Although the evidence is unclear concerning the effectiveness of oral contraceptives and concurrent antibiotic therapy, additional contraception is recommended for the entire pill cycle in which the antibiotics are used. All patients with GAS infection should be instructed to call the health care provider if symptoms escalate or if respiratory distress or difficulty swallowing develops. In general, patients should start to feel better 24 to 48 hours after the start of antibiotic therapy. Patients should be encouraged to use a new toothbrush 48 hours after antibiotic therapy is started to decrease the possibility of a recurrent infection. The old toothbrush should be discarded.

Education for the patient with viral pharyngitis is important. Supportive measures should be encouraged. Patients can expect symptom resolution of the pharyngitis during a 1- to 3-week period.[1] Antibiotics are inappropriate in viral infections, but patients and families may require considerable teaching to understand the importance of avoiding antibiotic therapy when appropriate.[1,2,10]

HEALTH PROMOTION

Health promotion involving pharyngitis covers many areas. Proper oral hygiene should be addressed with all age groups at all visits. Education regarding the misuse of antibiotic therapy for viral entities should also be stressed.[2,10] Of importance is teaching patients, families, and health care workers the need for appropriate handwashing technique. Limiting exposure to individuals with pharyngitis must also be included in patient teaching.[10]

REFERENCES

For a full list of references, scan the QR code or visit http://booksite.elsevier.com/9780323355018

PART 10

Evaluation and Management of Pulmonary Disorders

CHAPTER 102

ACUTE BRONCHITIS

Patricia Polgar-Bailey

DEFINITION AND EPIDEMIOLOGY

Acute bronchitis is an acute and self-limited inflammation of the trachea and major bronchi, generally characterized by cough lasting 1 to 3 weeks and without evidence of bronchial consolidation (as seen in pneumonia) or underlying cardiopulmonary disease.[1] Clinically, it is diagnosed on the basis of acute cough, with or without phlegm, and occasionally dyspnea and wheezing. It is typically viral in origin[2] and is considered part of the spectrum of upper respiratory infections (URIs), which also include acute otitis, pharyngitis, tonsillitis, and acute sinusitis; but by definition bronchitis is an inflammation of the lower respiratory tract.[3]

Cough is the most frequent reason for visits to primary care physicians, accounting for approximately 8% of all visits.[4] The most common causes of acute cough are URIs and acute bronchitis, which together account for approximately 60% of diagnosed cases.[3] In the United States, acute bronchitis affects approximately 5% of the population annually and is the most common cause of acute cough.[5] Symptom relief is the primary reason for seeking medical attention, and of those who seek care, most do so within the first week of illness.[6] Each episode of acute bronchitis results in approximately 2 to 3 missed work days.[7] A higher incidence of acute bronchitis has been noted during the autumn and winter months, when other URIs occur with frequency.[4] Environmental factors such as living in substandard housing also predispose individuals, particularly children, to higher rates of acute bronchitis.[8]

Viruses account for an estimated 85% to 95% of cases of acute bronchitis and include most commonly influenza A and B viruses, parainfluenza virus, and respiratory syncytial virus (RSV), and less commonly coronavirus, adenovirus, rhinovirus, and metapneumovirus.[4,6] Influenza occurs in distinct outbreaks and can result in significant morbidity because of its rapid spread.[6] The incidence of RSV is high in households with small children and in areas where the elderly predominate, such as geriatric wards, senior day care settings, and nursing homes, and it can be a significant cause of morbidity in older adults.[6] Severe acute respiratory syndrome (SARS), first defined by the World Health Organization in 2003, is caused by a novel coronavirus.[6]

Less than 10% of cases of acute bronchitis are bacterial in origin, and these are more common in patients with chronic health problems.[5] These less common nonviral causes of acute bronchitis include atypical bacteria that also cause community-acquired pneumonia (CAP), such as *Bordetella pertussis, Mycoplasma pneumoniae, Moraxella catarrhalis,* and *Chlamydia pneumoniae* (as distinguished from *Chlamydia trachomatis,* which causes pneumonia in neonates). Common upper respiratory flora such as *Haemophilus influenzae* and *Streptococcus pneumoniae* are often found in sputum samples of patients with acute bronchitis, but it is unclear if their presence contributes to disease development.[3]

PATHOPHYSIOLOGY

The causative pathogen for acute bronchitis is rarely identified; however, the cause of cough in uncomplicated acute bronchitis is multifactorial.[9] It is the result of edematous changes in the mucous membrane of the tracheobronchial tree, epithelial cell damage, the release of proinflammatory mediators, and an increase in secretions.[4] Destruction of the bronchial epithelium and loss of ciliary function are usually minimal with the common cold viruses but may be more extensive with *M. pneumoniae* and influenza viruses. Transient airflow obstruction and bronchial hyperresponsiveness occur in approximately 40% of previously healthy adults without concomitant conditions and usually resolve within 6 weeks.[6]

Acute bronchitis may be associated with a variety of symptoms, depending on anatomic distribution of the pathogen involved. For example, rhinovirus, a pathogen generally presumed to cause URI, has been found in a significant percentage of bronchoalveolar lavage specimens. Viral infection of lower airways may help explain the association between viral infection, such as that caused by rhinovirus, and asthma exacerbations.[4] Cigarette smoking and chemical irritants may increase the severity of the infection. Undiagnosed asthma may be a factor, but this can be difficult to establish because of the transient bronchial hyperresponsiveness and abnormal spirometry results that often accompany acute bronchitis.

CLINICAL PRESENTATION AND PHYSICAL EXAMINATION

A cough with or without sputum production is the most common symptom reported with acute bronchitis. Characteristics of the cough may vary. It is often described as dry and nonproductive, but it commonly progresses to a productive cough as the illness evolves. The sputum may be clear at the onset of the infection and become mucoid. Approximately 50% of patients with acute bronchitis report a cough productive of purulent sputum.[3] A common but inaccurate belief is that a productive cough or purulent sputum is indicative of a bacterial infection and requires antibiotic therapy. In fact, in otherwise healthy individuals, the production of purulent sputum is the often the result of sloughing of the tracheal bronchial epithelium and inflammatory cells.[3] The cough may also produce a burning substernal pain with inspiration. Nasal and pharyngeal symptoms subside after 3 or 4 days, but the cough usually remains prominent and progressive, typically lasting for 10 to 20 days, but it may occasionally persist for up to 5 to 6 weeks.[4] A low-grade fever, wheezes, rhonchi, and coarse rales may be present. However, substantial abnormalities in vital signs are infrequent, especially in older adults, even when symptoms have been present for a week or more.[4] Approximately 40% to 60% of patients may have significant reductions (a value below 80% of predicted) in forced expiratory volume in 1 second (FEV_1), with gradual improvement during the ensuing 5 to 6 weeks.[4,7] Individuals with *M. pneumoniae* or *C. pneumoniae* infections often have lower FEV_1 values and demonstrate a greater degree of reversibility than do those with viral causes.[6]

DIAGNOSTICS

Diagnostic tests are generally not necessary in the diagnosis of acute bronchitis. Cough and normal vital signs, in the absence of tachypnea, tachycardia, rales, and egophony, are strongly suggestive of acute bronchitis and minimize the likelihood of pneumonia. Routine sputum cultures are not helpful because they are often contaminated by bacterial flora that normally colonize the nasopharyngeal area. Viral cultures and serologic assays should not be routinely performed because they are rarely helpful in identifying the causative agent and as a result are not useful in guiding treatment.[3,6] Rapid diagnostic tests exist for several of the pathogens that cause acute bronchitis. However, not all of these tests are widely available, and routine use in outpatient settings is not cost-effective. Their use is indicated when there is suspicion of a treatable organism, an infectious outbreak in the community, and a patient with specific signs and symptoms that are identifiable—for example, testing of patients with cough and fever for influenza during influenza season.[4] Multiplex polymerase chain reaction testing of nasopharyngeal swabs or aspirates is being developed for diagnosis of infections resulting from *B. pertussis, M. pneumoniae,* or *C. pneumoniae*.[4]

A chest radiograph may be useful if the history and physical examination suggest the possibility of CAP. A heightened suspicion of CAP is reasonable in elders because they may be seen initially with more subtle symptoms of lower respiratory tract infections or cough without any other distinctive signs and symptoms. Data suggest that only one third of individuals 75 years of age and older who had CAP had temperatures higher than 38° C and heart rates above 100 beats per minute.[4] According to the American College of Chest Physicians (ACCP) 2006 clinical practice guidelines, the absence of the following findings reduces the likelihood of pneumonia sufficiently to eliminate the need for a chest radiograph: heart rate above 100 beats per minute; respiratory rate above 24 breaths per minute; oral body temperature higher than 38° C; and chest examination findings of focal consolidation, egophony, or fremitus.[6]

DIAGNOSTICS

Acute Bronchitis

LABORATORY
Complete blood count and differential*
Nasopharyngeal culture (for *B. pertussis* or influenza)

IMAGING
Chest x-ray studies (posterior or lateral)*

*If indicated.

DIFFERENTIAL DIAGNOSIS

Distinguishing between acute bronchitis and a simple URI within the first several days of illness is difficult, but a cough that persists for longer than 7 days is suggestive of acute bronchitis.[5] Because acute bronchitis is a clinical diagnosis, how providers assign the diagnosis varies. For example, some providers diagnose acute bronchitis only if a productive cough is present, whereas others make the determination based on the presence of purulent sputum. Discolored sputum is commonly but mistakenly interpreted by both patients and health care providers as clinical evidence of bacterial infection. There has been no evidence to indicate correlation between discolored sputum and a bacterial cause of acute bronchitis.[10] A cough that lasts for longer than 3 weeks should prompt consideration of another diagnosis.

Other causes of cough, with or without phlegm production, include the common cold, reflux esophagitis, acute asthma, chronic obstructive pulmonary disease (COPD), and pneumonia. The symptoms of the common cold or URI, such as nasal stuffiness, discharge, sneezing, sore throat, and cough, can also be present in acute and chronic bronchitis.[5] Acute sinusitis in the context of a cold may stimulate cough receptors.[5]

Because pneumonia is the third most common cause of cough (following asthma), usually not self-limited, often bacterial in origin, and associated with considerable morbidity and mortality when it is not treated with antimicrobial therapy, distinguishing between acute bronchitis and pneumonia is of primary importance. This is particularly true in elders, because older adults are less likely to have respiratory or nonrespiratory symptoms.[6]

CAP should be suspected if the patient's history includes dyspnea, high fever, tachycardia, evidence of consolidation on examination, or presence of symptoms for 2 weeks or more.[11]

Acute bronchitis is an inflammation of the trachea and bronchi and should be differentiated from asthma and bronchiolitis, which are acute inflammations of the small airway and generally characterized by wheezing, tachypnea, respiratory distress, and hypoxemia. Acute bronchitis should also be distinguished from bronchiectasis, which is associated with bronchial dilation and chronic cough.[4]

DIFFERENTIAL DIAGNOSIS

Acute Bronchitis

- Allergic rhinitis
- Asthma
- Chronic lung disease
- COPD exacerbation
- Common cold
- Foreign body aspiration
- Gastroesophageal reflux disease (GERD)
- Influenza and parainfluenza viruses
- Malignancy
- Pertussis
- Pneumonia
- Postinfectious cough
- Postnasal drip
- Rhinitis
- SARS
- Sinusitis
- Tuberculosis

Infection with *B. pertussis* should also be considered in adults who have a paroxysmal cough lasting longer than 2 weeks, especially in the context of a community outbreak. Fever is less common with pertussis infection than with viral bronchitis.[4] Although infection with *B. pertussis* is rarely life-threatening in adults, its diagnosis is important because of the complications it can cause in older adults or in infants who have not been vaccinated against the disease.

Epidemiologic data may be helpful in the diagnosis of acute bronchitis. For example, contact with a confirmed case of pertussis and paroxysmal cough or post-tussive vomiting strongly suggest *B. pertussis* infection. Outbreaks in specific populations, such as military personnel or college students, may suggest *M. pneumoniae* or *C. pneumoniae* infection.[6] Nursing homes and long-term care facilities tend to harbor a wide range of viral and bacterial pathogens, including influenza and parainfluenza viruses, RSV, and coronaviruses, some of which are difficult to detect with standard viral cultures.[12] Residents of these facilities are at increased risk for the nosocomial spread of respiratory viruses.

The diagnosis of chronic bronchitis should be considered only for those patients who have had cough and sputum production on most days of the month for at least 3 months of the year during 2 consecutive years. During influenza outbreaks, the presence of both cough and fever is highly predictive of influenza.[4] Other differential diagnoses include rhinitis, sinusitis, foreign body aspiration, tuberculosis, tumors, and other chronic lung diseases.

There is considerable clinical overlap in the symptoms of acute bronchitis, other respiratory symptoms, and asthma. Data suggest that many patients are misdiagnosed with acute bronchitis and their cough is more likely caused by asthma, an acute exacerbation of chronic bronchitis, or a mild URI such as the common cold.[4]

MANAGEMENT

The mainstay of treatment in acute bronchitis is directed toward symptom reduction. Data suggest that 85% of patients diagnosed with acute bronchitis will improve without specific treatment.[7] Despite evidence that only 5% to 10% of acute bronchitis cases have a bacterial cause, data indicate that antibiotics continue to be prescribed for approximately two thirds (approximately 71% to 73%) of patients in the United States.[13,14] Despite current Agency for Healthcare Research and Quality guidelines[15] that discourage the routine use of antibiotics for acute bronchitis, the percentage of patients receiving antibiotics for acute bronchitis has increased, and patient expectations for antibiotic therapy are largely responsible for this trend.[1] More than half of the antibiotic prescriptions are for extended-spectrum antibiotics.[6] Certain populations are more likely to receive unnecessary antibiotics, including elders and cigarette smokers. There is no evidence that cigarette smokers with acute bronchitis, in the absence of underlying COPD, are in need of antibiotics any more than nonsmokers are.[6] Studies of uncomplicated acute bronchitis in the general population demonstrate little benefit from antibiotic use when a treatable pathogen is not identified, even with smokers. Any benefit demonstrated has been of questionable clinical significance (i.e., decrease in symptoms by only a fraction of a day with the use of the three most commonly prescribed antibiotics[15]), which is offset by the risks of antibiotic use, including serious adverse effects (e.g., *Clostridium difficile* diarrhea, anaphylaxis), drug-drug interactions, financial burden, and the possibility of future antibiotic resistance.[6] In addition, antibiotic therapy for acute bronchitis has not been shown to have any impact on activity limitations.[16] The problem of antimicrobial resistance has become a serious public health threat, and rates of resistance to penicillin and macrolide antibiotics are particularly high. Decreasing the inappropriate use of antibiotics is the first step in decreasing antibiotic resistance.

Antitussive therapy is commonly prescribed, but the evidence for its effectiveness is weak.[6,7] According to the ACCP 2006 evidence-based guidelines for the diagnosis and management of acute bronchitis, antitussive agents are occasionally useful and can be offered for short-term symptomatic relief of coughing.[6] A dextromethorphan cough preparation (30 mg/5 mL, 1 to 2 teaspoons orally every 4 hours as needed; maximum of four doses per day) or benzonatate may help alleviate the cough. Codeine or hydrocodone may be useful at bedtime if the cough is severe. Antipyretics, bed rest, and increased fluid consumption to thin the secretions are also beneficial treatments. In trials involving the use of beta-adrenergic bronchodilators for uncomplicated acute bronchitis in adults, there was no demonstrated reduction in symptoms, including cough. Subgroups of patients with airflow obstruction and wheezing at the onset of illness did experience some benefit from the bronchodilators.[6] Based on these studies, the ACCP guidelines state that beta-adrenergic bronchodilators should not be routinely used to alleviate cough; but in those patients with acute bronchitis and wheezing associated with the cough, bronchodilators may be useful.[6] According to the ACCP guidelines, there is no consistent favorable evidence for the use of mucokinetic agents for cough, and they are not recommended.[6]

Antibiotic therapy is recommended if pertussis is suspected. Pertussis is an acute bacterial infection of the respiratory tract caused by *B. pertussis*, a gram-negative bacterium. *B. pertussis* is transmitted primarily through aerosolized droplets of respiratory secretions or by direct contact with an infected person.[17] Studies indicate that pertussis may be present in 10% to 20% of patients with cough lasting longer than 2 weeks. Unfortunately, distinguishing pertussis from other sources of acute cough is difficult because pertussis in adults with previous immunity does not lead to the classic features of whooping cough that are seen in children. Suspicion of pertussis should be limited to individuals with a high probability of exposure, such as in community outbreaks. Patients with confirmed and probable pertussis should receive antimicrobial antibiotic therapy and be isolated for 5 days from the start of treatment.[6] Early treatment of pertussis is very important. If treatment is started early in the course of illness, during the first 2 weeks before coughing paroxysms occur, symptoms may be reduced. Treatment before receipt of confirmatory test results should be considered if clinical history is strongly suggestive of pertussis or if the patient is at risk for severe or complicated disease.[17] If diagnosis is late and antimicrobial therapy is not started within the first 5 to 7 days of symptom onset, therapy is less likely to alter the course of the illness. However, antimicrobial therapy may still decrease shedding of the bacteria and in that way limit spread of the disease.[17] Persons with pertussis are infectious from the beginning of the catarrhal stage (runny nose, low-grade fever, common cold symptoms) through the third week after the onset of paroxysmal cough or until 5 days after the onset of antibiotic therapy.[17]

Macrolides are used as first-line therapy. Options include azithromycin at a dosage of 500 mg on day 1 and 250 mg on days 2 to 5 for a total of 5 days of therapy; erythromycin, 500 mg four times a day for 14 days; and clarithromycin, 500 mg twice daily for 7 days. Second-line therapy is trimethoprim-sulfamethoxazole, 160-800 mg (1 double strength tablet) orally every 12 hours for 14 days. Erythromycin has been the antimicrobial agent of choice for the treatment of postexposure prophylaxis of pertussis and is usually prescribed at 2 g/day in four divided doses for 14 days. Other macrolide antibiotics, including clarithromycin (1 g/day in two divided doses for 7 days) and azithromycin (500 mg on day 1, followed by 250 mg on days 2 to 5), can also be used.[17]

On March 12, 2013, the Food and Drug Administration (FDA) issued a warning that azithromycin can cause abnormal changes in the electrical activity of the heart that may lead to a potentially fatal irregular heart rhythm in some patients. An alternative to azithromycin should be considered in persons with known cardiovascular disease, including (1) those with known prolongation of the QT interval, a history of torsades de pointes, congenital long QT syndrome, bradyarrhythmias, or uncompensated heart failure; (2) those on drugs known to prolong the QT interval; and (3) those with ongoing proarrhythmic conditions such as uncorrected hypokalemia or hypomagnesemia or clinically significant bradycardia and patients receiving class IA (quinidine, procainamide) or class III (dofetilide, amiodarone, sotalol) antiarrhythmic agents.[17]

The most common pathogen isolated in acute bronchitis is influenza; therefore, anti-influenza agents, such as oseltamivir (75 mg twice daily for 5 days) or zanamivir (2 puffs [5 mg/puff] twice daily for 5 days), may be effective if influenza is diagnosed and treatment initiated within 48 hours after onset of symptoms (see Chapter 231).[4] Because pneumonia is the third most common cause of cough illness, the presence of pneumonia should be excluded.

Even though older adults may not always manifest the typical features of pneumonia, such as fever and other vital sign abnormalities, the predictive value of these simple clinical tools remains high and should not be neglected. For atypical manifestations of pneumonia in older adults, such as diminished appetite, increased falls, and altered mental status, see Chapter 111.

Studies suggest that several factors contribute to and influence the decision to prescribe an antibiotic, including patient beliefs, desires, and expectations and provider perceptions about what is indicated clinically and what is necessary to ensure patient satisfaction.[18] Patients frequently expect to receive antibiotics for acute bronchitis, perhaps because they received antibiotics for similar symptoms in the past. In one study, less than 50% of the general public accurately identified antibiotics as being effective against bacterial infections and not against viral infections.[4] Nonetheless, patient expectations are among the strongest predictors of a provider's decision to prescribe an antibiotic, even though providers' perceptions of patient expectations are unclear or inaccurate up to 50% of the time.[18] Some providers also erroneously believe that if they do not prescribe antibiotics, the patient is more likely to return for another visit and take up more time. A study by Li and colleagues found that patients who received antibiotics during the index visit did not have a decreased rate of return visits.[18] In fact, the results suggested that patients who received antibiotics may have had higher expectations for a rapid resolution of their symptoms compared with those who, in lieu of obtaining an antibiotic prescription, received more education and counseling about the natural history of viral infections.[18] Providers also perceive that visits in which an antibiotic prescription is given take significantly less time and result in higher patient satisfaction than do visits in which no antibiotic prescription is given. Neither of these perceptions has been supported by research. Patient satisfaction with an office visit for acute bronchitis does not depend on receiving antimicrobial therapy but rather is centered on the nature of the provider-patient relationship as experienced during that visit. Even though acute bronchitis is a common diagnosis that resolves on its own, patients' satisfaction is primarily related to how much time was spent explaining the illness and answering their questions.

COMPLICATIONS

Although acute bronchitis is often viral and self-limited, complications do occur. The development of a chronic cough, usually the result of postbronchitis reactive airway disease, can cause discomfort and sleep loss. Pneumonia results from bacterial superinfection and can cause dyspnea, chest pain, and anxiety in addition to other symptoms. If the cough lasts 3 weeks or longer, a chest x-ray study is indicated in the absence of other known causes. Acute respiratory failure, although uncommon, is a potential sequela. Individuals with chronic bronchitis are more susceptible to superinfection and can develop exercise intolerance and hypoxia.

INDICATIONS FOR REFERRAL OR HOSPITALIZATION

Acute bronchitis that does not respond to symptomatic treatment and lingers longer than 2 weeks may require physician referral. Patients with progressive dyspnea, oxygen saturation less than 90%, and signs of sepsis require hospitalization for intravenous therapy, enhanced pulmonary therapy, and intravenous antibiotics.

PATIENT AND FAMILY EDUCATION

Reassurance and education are probably the most important modalities for treatment of acute bronchitis. Education should include a realistic expectation of the duration of the cough (generally 10 to 14 days) and the general ineffectiveness of antibiotic therapy for this diagnosis. Rest, increased fluids, and breathing of moist air from a clean humidifier or warm shower should be encouraged. Patients should be counseled about smoking cessation and the need to avoid air pollution and irritants. An appropriate face mask can be helpful if work involves chemicals, dust, or other irritants. Patients should be encouraged to call their health care provider if the symptoms continue or increase in severity.

The Centers for Disease Control and Prevention (CDC) recommends that providers refer to acute bronchitis as a "chest cold" to minimize expectations that antibiotics are appropriate therapy. In addition, the CDC offers the following suggestions to decrease antibiotic prescribing and use:

- Explain that antibiotic use increases the risk of antibiotic-resistant infections, and provide educational materials on antibiotic resistance.
- Identify and validate patient concerns.
- Recommend specific symptomatic therapy.
- Spend time answering questions, and offer an alternative plan if symptoms worsen.[17]

Additional patient education information can be obtained from the American Lung Association, 61 Broadway, 6th floor, New York, NY 10006; 800-586-4872; www.lungusa.org.

CHAPTER 103

ASTHMA

Patricia Polgar-Bailey

DEFINITION AND EPIDEMIOLOGY

Asthma is a chronic inflammatory disorder of the airways characterized by increased responsiveness of the tracheobronchial tree to various stimuli, resulting in episodic reversible narrowing and inflammation of the airways.[1,2] In susceptible individuals, this bronchial inflammation causes recurrent episodes of wheezing, shortness of breath, chest tightness, and cough. These episodes are usually associated with widespread but variable airflow obstruction that is often reversible, either spontaneously or with treatment. The inflammation also causes an associated increase in the existing bronchial hyperresponsiveness to a variety of stimuli.[1,2]

Asthma attacks can vary from mild to life-threatening and can be triggered by many factors, including allergens, infections, exercise, abrupt changes in weather, and exposure to airway irritants such as tobacco smoke.[2] The concept of asthma as a chronic and inflammatory process represented a significant change in the previous understanding of the disease. During the past decade there have been substantial advances in the understanding of the genetics, pathogenesis, and natural course of the disease, which have had important implications for its management, particularly the development of new, targeted therapies, especially for severe asthma.[1]

Asthma is the most common chronic respiratory disorder among all age groups and affects 5% to 16% of people worldwide.[3] Although the global prevalence of asthma increased markedly during the latter half of the of the 20th century, it appears to have plateaued since then, especially in countries with the highest asthma rates such as the United Kingdom.[1] An exception to this is the United States, where the prevalence of asthma increased from 7.3% (20.3 million persons) in 2001 to 8.2% (24.6 million persons) in 2009, a 12.3% increase. Prevalence among children (persons aged <18 years) was 9.6% and was highest among poor children (13.5%) and among non-Hispanic black children (17.0%). Prevalence among adults was 7.7% and was greatest in women (9.7%) and in adults who were poor (10.6%). Looking at subgroups, a rising trend in asthma prevalence was observed for non-Hispanic black children (11.4% to 17.0%), non-Hispanic white women (8.9% to 10.1%), and non-Hispanic black men (4.7% to 6.4%).[4] In 2009, asthma prevalence was greater among children than adults (9.6% versus 7.7%) and was especially high among boys (11.3%) and non-Hispanic black children (17.0%). Prevalence among adults was greatest for women (9.7%) and adults who were poor (10.6%).[4] These statistics, as striking as they are, may still underestimate the actual prevalence of asthma, especially in communities where access to care, including emergency care, is limited.[5] Among racial groups, persons of multiple race had the highest asthma prevalence (14.1%), whereas Asian persons had the lowest rates (5.2%). Persons of black (11.2%) and American Indian or Alaska Native (9.4%) races had higher asthma prevalence compared with white persons (7.7%). Among Hispanic groups, asthma prevalence was higher among persons of Puerto Rican (16.1%) than Mexican (5.4%) descent.[6]

Asthma attack prevalence refers to the number of people who had at least one asthma attack during the previous year; it is a crude indicator of how many people have uncontrolled asthma or are at risk for a poor outcome, such as hospitalization.[6] In 2008, at least half (52.6%) of those diagnosed with asthma reported having an asthma attack within the past year.[7] Asthma attack prevalence decreases with age; a greater proportion of children than adults (57.2% versus 50.7%) were reported to have had an asthma attack within the preceding 12 months. Women have a 35% higher asthma attack prevalence than men, but this pattern is reversed among children, in whom the attack prevalence for boys was 45% higher than the rate for girls.[6] A greater proportion of persons who had an asthma attack reported being in fair or poor health (24.8%) than of those who did not have an asthma attack (17.9%).[7]

Asthma interferes with daily activities, including attending school and going to work. In 2008, on average, children missed 4 days of school and adults missed 5 days of work because of asthma, 26% reported emergency department (ED) or urgent care center visits, and 7% reported having been admitted to a hospital.[7,8] Occupational asthma is currently the most common occupational ailment. Widespread exposure in the workplace environment to airborne dusts, gases, vapors, or fumes contributes to both the development of asthma and the worsening of asthma for those already affected. An estimated 1.9 million cases of asthma among adults were work related, accounting for 15.7% of current adult asthma cases. Work-related asthma significantly differs by age; the incidence is highest among persons aged 45 to 64 years (20.7%).[8] Asthma accounts for 10.1 million lost work days annually and a total annual economic cost of $19.7 billion—$14.7 billion in direct costs, and another $5 billion in lost productivity.[8]

Asthma is one of the most common reasons for visits in ambulatory settings; in 2010 there were 14.2 million office visits with asthma as the primary diagnosis.[9] Asthma is still responsible for a disproportionate and increasing number of ED visits (1.8 million) and hospitalizations (0.5 million).[7] The type of medical setting in which persons receive health care for asthma differs for those with private health insurance and those without health insurance. From 2001 to 2009, health care visits for asthma per 100 persons with asthma declined in primary care settings, whereas asthma ED visit and hospitalization rates were stable. For the period of 2007 to 2009, black persons had higher rates for asthma ED visits and hospitalizations per 100 persons with asthma than white persons, and a higher asthma death rate per 1000 persons with asthma. Compared with adults, children had higher rates for asthma primary care and ED visits, similar hospitalization rates, and lower death rates. Asthma is a condition that can be treated effectively in primary care, resulting in fewer ED visits, improved continuity of care, and decreased health care costs based on Centers for Disease Control and Prevention (CDC) 2012 health statistics for U.S. adults.[9]

Although the asthma prevalence is higher among children, asthma deaths in children are relatively rare.[10] Women have an asthma death rate higher than that of men.[6] High mortality rates are associated with high rates of hospitalization in impoverished urban areas. Most of those hospitalized or seen in the ED had been there before, reflecting the fact that inadequate health care results in increased costs.[10,11]

Asthma hospitalization rates have been highest among African Americans, women, and children; likewise, death rates have consistently been disproportionately higher among African Americans, especially those aged 15 to 24 years.[6] Although prevalence is higher among racial and ethnic minorities, a more valid relationship may exist between socioeconomic status and increased asthma prevalence, morbidity, and mortality than between race and asthma prevalence. Asthma mortality has also been associated with poverty, urban living conditions, exposure to oxidant pollutants, and passive smoking.[7] Allergic asthmatic children exposed to high levels of indoor allergens, such as those associated with cockroaches, rodents, and mold, have more severe and more frequent episodes of asthma.[11]

The financial impact of asthma is considerable. At least 1% of all U.S. health care costs are spent on asthma—an estimated $3300 per person with asthma annually.[8] Direct and indirect asthma-related costs are estimated to be $56 billion per year, with ED visits and hospitalizations responsible for the majority of the cost.

Worldwide, an estimated 300 million people are affected by asthma, and the prevalence of asthma ranges from 1% to 18% of the population, depending on the country.[2] It is estimated that the number of people with asthma will grow by more than 100 million by 2025.[8] Workplace conditions, such as exposure to fumes, gases, or dust, are responsible for 11% of asthma cases worldwide. Prevalence rates vary widely depending on the country, which reflects a true difference in prevalence as well as different diagnostic standards. The prevalence has been increasing in low- and middle-income countries and plateauing in high-income countries.. Deaths from asthma worldwide have been estimated at 250,000 per year, but mortality does not appear to correlate well with prevalence.[12,13] Although the cost to control asthma on a global scale is high, the cost of not treating asthma is even higher.

Specialist referral is indicated for patients with Sa_{O_2} less than 90% on room air, peak flow less than 70%, and failure to improve with three nebulizer treatments or three epinephrine injections.

PATHOPHYSIOLOGY

It is now believed that the primary event in asthma is airway inflammation and that airway hyperresponsiveness and airflow obstruction are secondary and symptomatic features of the disease. Underlying airway inflammation (which involves cellular infiltration, edema, nerve irritation, and vasodilation) results in constriction of airway smooth muscle, increased production of mucus, and airway hyperresponsiveness. The airflow limitation associated with asthma is caused by a variety of changes in the airway, all of which are influenced by airway inflammation. These changes include bronchoconstriction (bronchial smooth muscle contraction that quickly narrows the airways in response to a variety of stimuli, including allergens and irritants), airway hyperresponsiveness (an exaggerated bronchoconstrictor response to stimuli), and airway edema (hypersecretion of mucus and mucous plugs as the disease becomes more persistent, which further limit flow).[12] With time, remodeling of airways may occur, and reversibility of airway obstruction may be incomplete in some persons. Possible changes in airway structure include sub-basement fibrosis, hypersecretion of mucus, epithelial cell injury, smooth muscle hypertrophy, and angiogenesis (the growth of new blood vessels from existing blood vessels).[12]

The development of asthma appears to involve an interplay among host factors, particularly genetics, and environmental factors that occur at a crucial time in the development of the immune system, although a definitive cause of the inflammatory process has not been established.[12]

Different immune responses influence the development of asthma, including the Th1-type and Th2-type cytokine responses. Numerous factors affect the balance between these responses early in life and increase the likelihood that the Th1 immune response—which fights infection—will be downregulated and that the Th2 immune response—which contributes to the development of allergic diseases and asthma—will dominate. This is known as the hygiene hypothesis, which postulates that early in life, exposure to other children (e.g., presence of older siblings and early enrollment in childcare, which increase the likelihood of exposure to respiratory infection), less frequent use of antibiotics, and "country living" are associated with a Th1 response and a lower incidence of asthma, whereas the absence of these factors is associated with a persistent Th2 response and higher rates of asthma.[12]

Asthma also has an inheritable component, but the genetic factors involved remain complex.[12] One factor involved is atopy, which is the genetic tendency for development of immunoglobulin E (IgE)–mediated hypersensitivity reactions in response to environmental antigens and allergens; it is considered one of the strongest predisposing factors for the development of asthma. Certain stimuli induce asthma by causing or increasing airway inflammation, whereas other stimuli provoke bronchoconstriction in individuals who already have asthma or airway hyperresponsiveness. Inducers, stimuli that are known to increase inflammation, include inhaled allergens, low-molecular-weight sensitizers, viral or mycoplasmal respiratory infections, and high concentrations of noxious gases. Stimuli that trigger or cause bronchoconstriction include exercise, cold air, laughter, emotional upset, and inhaled irritants. Triggers of sudden severe bronchoconstriction include acetylsalicylic acid or nonsteroidal anti-inflammatory drugs (NSAIDs), beta-adrenergic blockers, food allergens, certain food additives, stings, bites, injections (e.g., allergy shots), and inhaled allergens.

These stimuli set the stage for a cascade of cellular activation, which includes subsequent cytokine release and neurologic excitation. The antigenic response is limited by certain cellular processes such as mast cell activation through cytokines and infiltration by inflammatory cells, including neutrophils, eosinophils, and lymphocytes. The inflammatory cells are also the source of mediators that induce bronchoconstriction, excess production of mucus, airway edema, and further influx of inflammatory cells, all of which lead to bronchial obstruction. The late-phase reaction, which generally occurs 3 to 8 hours after antigen exposure, is the result of new cellular infiltration and activation. Nocturnal and early morning bronchospasm, which occurs with relative frequency in persons with asthma, may be related to circadian variations in cortisol and epinephrine levels, vagal tone, and inflammatory mediators.

One common, often overlooked, exacerbating factor of asthma is esophageal reflux of gastric contents. The incidence of gastroesophageal reflux in adults with asthma has been reported to range from 15% to 82% by pH monitoring.[13] Gastroesophageal reflux resulting in distal esophageal stimulation with acid may cause bronchoconstriction or may increase bronchial reactivity through vagal mechanisms. Although the potential mechanism exists for gastroesophageal reflux disease (GERD) to cause asthma symptoms, and it is fairly well accepted that GERD may be an exacerbating factor, particularly in difficult-to-control asthma, it remains unclear whether there is a true causal relationship between reflux episodes and asthma symptoms. A study involving the largest group of patients with difficult-to-control asthma to date found that the identification and treatment of GERD failed to improve asthma outcome in the group as a whole. However, this study did not exclude the possibility that antireflux therapy does contribute to asthma control in persons with well-controlled asthma.[13]

In addition to the aforementioned factors, environmental factors appear to play a role in the development of asthma, although the nature of specific environmental contributions is not clearly defined. Exposure in utero to tobacco smoke is associated with an increased risk of wheezing, but it is not clear whether this is linked to subsequent development of asthma.[12] Air pollution (ozone and particular matter) and diet (obesity or low intake of omega-3 fatty acids) have been associated with asthma, although the contribution of these factors to the development of asthma has not been clearly defined.

As mentioned, asthma has a strong genetic component. However, for this to manifest, interaction with environmental factors must occur. At least some of the difference in asthma prevalence between white and minority populations may be a result of differences in genetic susceptibility. Most of the evidence to date suggests that the explanation for these differences is most likely the disparity in socioeconomic, environmental, behavioral, and cultural factors and in access to routine health care.[14]

Asthma is a disease that varies within and among individuals, but inflammation of the airways is a persistent feature, even in persons with mild asthma. Although asthma is considered to be a disease of reversible airflow obstruction, chronic airway inflammation can lead to progressive airway remodeling and airflow obstruction, eventually resulting in an irreversible deterioration of airway function.[1] At present, asthma has no cure, but effective management can reduce its impact on quality of life and morbidity.

CLINICAL PRESENTATION

The clinical hallmarks of asthma include episodic wheezing associated with dyspnea, cough, and sputum production. Between episodes, symptoms may improve or completely resolve. Symptoms vary from mild to severe, with varying effects on activity. An increased index of suspicion for asthma is essential when respiratory symptoms, including cough, wheeze, shortness of breath, chest tightness, and soreness, persist or recur often.

Although wheezing is probably the symptom most typically associated with asthma, the most common symptom of asthma and often the most troublesome is cough. However, cough is also the third most common presenting symptom in the ambulatory setting, with a corresponding long list of potential causes. Coughing is the only asthma symptom 7% to 57% of the time; this type of asthma is referred to as cough-variant asthma. Cough can be the principal or only manifestation of asthma, especially in young children.[12] Cough is often treated symptomatically, which can easily result in a delayed or missed diagnosis of asthma. Asthma should be considered in the differential diagnosis of all patients with a cough because it is such a common cause. Most persons with a cough do not have associated variable airflow obstruction; if obstruction is present and reversible with bronchodilator medication, the diagnosis of asthma is confirmed.[15]

In addition to chronic cough, asthma has several common clinical presentations. An acute asthmatic episode is characterized by airway obstruction, manifesting with symptoms of breathlessness and anxiety and often accompanied by wheezing and sometimes coughing. These symptoms may resolve within several hours if treatment is given or within 1 to 3 days even without specific intervention, or they may progress to more severe airway obstruction and respiratory compromise if no therapy is provided. Between acute asthmatic episodes, airflow is normal and symptoms are absent. Several specific conditions are associated with acute asthma exacerbations.

Exercise-induced asthma refers to the development of airway obstruction in an individual after the cessation of exercise, even after brief periods of exercise. Symptoms usually begin 5 to 10 minutes after the completion of exercise and resolve within 1 to 4 hours. Certain forms of exercise, including skiing, ice hockey, and running in the cold, more commonly precipitate airway obstruction; other forms of exercise, such as swimming, less commonly precipitate airway obstruction, probably because of the warmer and more humid air being inspired. Cold or dry air often predisposes an asthmatic individual to airway obstruction, such as occurs when a person enters a dry, air-conditioned environment (such as an indoor mall) from the warmer, more humid outside air.

Common allergens that precipitate asthma include cat allergen (dander), house dust mite allergen, cockroach allergen, and tree and grass pollen. Viral illnesses can also induce airway obstruction in asthmatic individuals; symptoms may persist for weeks to months if therapy is not initiated. Occupational exposures are common asthma triggers. Early responses may occur within several hours; however, late responses may not occur for 8 to 12 hours after exposure. Often, occupation-induced asthma symptoms may persist long after the individual has left the workplace, an important consideration in the differential diagnosis.

Approximately 1% to 10% of individuals with moderate to severe asthma have aspirin exacerbated respiratory disease (AERD) (aspirin-induced asthma), which is characterized by symptoms of moderately severe airway obstruction, rhinorrhea, sneezing, tearing, dermal changes, and in some cases gastrointestinal symptoms (nausea, vomiting, cramping) on exposure to aspirin or other prostaglandin (H synthase type 1) inhibitors. The onset of AERD occurs most often when patients are in their 20s and 30s.[16] The diagnosis of aspirin-induced asthma is important for two reasons: aspirin-containing drugs should be avoided because these drugs may induce life-threatening asthma attacks, and effective treatment is available specifically for this type of asthma. In trials in which patients with AERD were challenged with selective NSAIDs, there was a small risk of respiratory symptoms with selective NSAIDs. However, cyclooxygenase 2 (COX-2) inhibitors with etoricoxib did not appear to exacerbate airway inflammatory or obstruction in persons with AERD.[16]

Acute severe asthma, although it is not pathologically distinct from acute asthma, represents a more severe and prolonged form of the illness. Acute severe asthma is often characterized by unremitting asthma symptoms (including shortness of breath, diminished exercise tolerance, and wheezing) for weeks with less-than-optimum response to therapy. Often, asthmatic individuals develop prolonged severe asthma by inappropriately self-medicating with beta$_2$-adrenergic agonist inhalers for weeks before seeking medical attention, at which point the risk of respiratory collapse and asphyxia may be great.[15]

Chronic stable asthma refers to asthma that is characterized by episodes of airway obstruction and airway symptoms. Although multiple asthma episodes may occur during a period of several months, most are of moderate severity and respond promptly to therapy. The two most important aspects of asthma therapy are pharmacologic therapy and environmental control. For severe asthma, treatment of comorbidities is also essential to achieve control, but may complicate asthma management.[1,2]

The National Asthma Education and Prevention Program (NAEPP) of the National Institutes of Health (NIH) developed sample questions for the diagnosis and initial assessment of asthma (Box 103-1).[12] In addition to an assessment of symptoms, an individual's family history is helpful when a diagnosis of asthma is being considered. Persons with asthma often have a family history of asthma or atopy. Also, family members are often able to identify specific exposures or circumstances that precipitate the patient's symptoms. Sample questions for the follow-up assessment of patients with previously diagnosed asthma are listed in Box 103-2.

Asthma can be classified according to the frequency and severity of symptoms and the pattern of airflow limitation or according to the treatment steps necessary to decrease symptoms, to improve lung function, and to prevent exacerbations to allow normal daily activities (Table 103-1). Asthma can have a variable course, and the degree of asthma control and the severity of asthma within an individual can change over time. Providers need to be aware of the difference between asthma control and severity. For example, severe asthma can be well controlled, that is, few exacerbations with intensive pharmacotherapy and good self-management. On the other hand, an individual with mild asthma and little need of intensive treatment may still have periods of poor control. Persons with well-controlled asthma are still vulnerable to acute exacerbations, especially if they are exposed to factors that precipitate their asthma symptoms.

There is increasing evidence that persons affected by problems of socioeconomic deprivation and psychosocial issues such as anxiety, depression, and stress are at increased risk for asthma exacerbations.[17] A study by Sandberg and colleagues[18] demonstrated that even in children with asthma, psychosocial stress can worsen asthma control and increase the risk of an acute exacerbation.

PHYSICAL EXAMINATION

The physical examination of the patient with asthma or suspected asthma can be divided into four objectives: (1) diagnosis and differential diagnosis, (2) assessment of asthma severity, (3) identification of adverse effects of medications, and (4) identification of concomitant medical problems. A complete physical examination is necessary if assessment of respiratory exertion or compromise is needed, coexisting medical conditions must be identified or evaluated, or the presentation is complex.

The diagnosis of asthma is based on the history, physical examination, and certain diagnostic tests, particularly spirometry. The physical examination, although an essential part of the evaluation, may correlate poorly with objective measures of airway obstruction, such as pulmonary function tests (PFTs). In the asymptomatic patient, the physical examination findings may be entirely normal. Nonetheless, assessment of the severity of asthma and airway obstruction is the most important objective in evaluating a person with asthma. Wheezing may be

BOX **103-1**

Initial Assessment of Asthma

KEY INDICATORS FOR CONSIDERING A DIAGNOSIS OF ASTHMA

The presence of multiple key indicators increases the probability of a diagnosis of asthma, but spirometry is needed to establish a diagnosis.

1. Wheezing—high-pitched whistling sounds when breathing out, especially in children. A lack of wheezing and normal chest examination findings do not exclude asthma.
2. History of any one of the following:
   - Cough (worse particularly at night)
   - Recurrent wheeze
   - Recurrent difficulty in breathing
   - Recurrent chest tightness
3. Symptoms occur or worsen in the presence of the following:
   - Exercise
   - Viral infection
   - Inhalant allergens (animals with fur or hair, house dust mites, mold, pollen)
   - Irritants (tobacco or wood smoke, airborne chemicals)
   - Changes in weather
   - Strong emotional expression (laughing or crying hard)
   - Menstrual cycles
4. Symptoms occur or worsen at night, awakening the patient.

SUGGESTED ITEMS FOR MEDICAL HISTORY*

A detailed history of the new patient who is known or thought to have asthma should address the following items.

1. Symptoms
   - Cough
   - Wheezing
   - Shortness of breath
   - Chest tightness
   - Sputum production
2. Pattern of symptoms
   - Perennial, seasonal, or both
   - Continual, episodic, or both
   - Onset, duration, frequency (number of days or nights, per week or month)
   - Diurnal variations, especially nocturnal and on awakening in early morning
3. Precipitating or aggravating factors
   - Viral respiratory infections
   - Environmental allergens, indoor (e.g., mold, house dust mite, cockroach, animal dander, or secretory products) and outdoor (e.g., pollen)
   - Characteristics of home, including age, location, cooling and heating system, wood-burning stove, humidifier, carpeting over

BOX 103-1

Initial Assessment of Asthma—cont'd

concrete, presence of molds or mildew, presence of pets with fur or hair, characteristics of rooms where patient spends time (e.g., bedding, floor covering, stuffed furniture)
- Exercise
- Occupational chemicals or allergens
- Environmental change (e.g., moving to new home; going on vacation; or alterations in workplace, work processes, or materials used)
- Irritants (e.g., tobacco smoke, strong odors, air pollutants, occupational chemicals, dusts and particulates, vapors, gases, and aerosols)
- Emotional expressions (e.g., fear, anger, frustration, hard crying or laughing)
- Stress (e.g., fear, anger, frustration)
- Drugs (e.g., aspirin, NSAIDs, beta blockers including eye drops, others)
- Food, food additives, and preservatives (e.g., sulfites)
- Changes in weather, exposure to cold air
- Endocrine factors (e.g., menses, pregnancy, thyroid disease)
- Comorbid conditions (e.g., sinusitis, rhinitis, GERD)

4. Development of disease and treatment
   - Age at onset and diagnosis
   - History of early-life injury to airways (e.g., bronchopulmonary dysplasia, pneumonia, parental smoking)
   - Progress of disease (better or worse)
   - Present management and response, including plans for managing exacerbations
   - Frequency of using short-acting $beta_2$ agonist
   - Need for oral corticosteroids and frequency of use
5. Family history
   - History of asthma, allergy, sinusitis, rhinitis, or nasal polyps in close relatives
6. Social history
   - Daycare, workplace, and school characteristics that may interfere with adherence
   - Smoking (patient and others in home or daycare)
   - Social factors that interfere with adherence, such as substance abuse
   - Social supports and social networks
   - Level of education completed
   - Employment (if employed, characteristics of work environment)
7. History of exacerbations
   - Usual prodromal signs and symptoms
   - Rapidity of onset
   - Duration
   - Frequency
   - Severity (need for urgent care, hospitalization, intensive care unit [ICU] admission)
   - Life-threatening exacerbations (e.g., intubation, ICU admission)
   - Number and severity of exacerbations in the past year
   - Usual patterns and management (what works?)
8. Impact of asthma on patient and family
   - Episodes of unscheduled care (ED, urgent care, hospitalizations)
   - Number of days missed from school or work
   - Limitation of activity, especially sports and strenuous work
   - History of nocturnal awakening
   - Effect on growth, development, behavior, school or work performance, and lifestyle
   - Impact on family routines, activities or dynamics
   - Economic impact
9. Assessment of patient's and family's perceptions of disease
   - Patient's, parents', and spouse's or partner's knowledge of asthma and belief in the chronicity of asthma and in the efficacy of treatment
   - Patient's perception and beliefs regarding use and long-term effects of medications
   - Ability of patient and parents, spouse, or partners to cope with disease
   - Level of family support and patient's and parents', spouse's, or partner's capacity to recognize severity of an exacerbation
   - Economic resources
   - Sociocultural beliefs

SAMPLE AND INITIAL ASSESSMENT OF ASTHMA

A yes answer to any questions suggests that an asthma diagnosis is likely.†

In the past 12 months …
- Have you had a sudden severe episode or recurrent episodes of coughing, wheezing (high-pitched whistling sounds when breathing out), or shortness of breath?
- Have you had colds that "go to the chest" or take more than 10 days to get over?
- Have you had coughing, wheezing, or shortness of breath during a particular season or time of the year?
- Have you had coughing, wheezing, or shortness of breath in certain places or when exposed to certain things (e.g., animals, tobacco smoke, perfumes)?
- Have you used any medications that help you breathe better? How often?
- Are your symptoms relieved when the medications are used?

In the past 4 weeks, have you had coughing, wheezing, or shortness of breath …
- At night that has awakened you?
- In the early morning?
- After running, moderate exercise, or other physical activity?

*This list does not represent a standardized assessment or diagnostic instrument. The validity and reliability of this list have not been assessed.

†These questions are examples and do not represent a standardized assessment or diagnostic instrument. The validity and reliability of these questions have not been assessed.

Modified from National Asthma Education and Prevention Program (NAEPP): *Expert panel report 3: guidelines for the diagnosis and management of asthma,* National Institutes of Health (NIH) Publication No. 08-5846, Bethesda, Md, 2007, U.S. Department of Health and Human Services, NIH, National Heart, Lung, and Blood Institute (NHLBI). Available at www.nhlbi.nih.gov/guidelines/asthma/asthsumm.pdf.

BOX 103-2

Components of Practitioner's Follow-Up Assessment: Sample Routine Clinical Assessment Questions*

MONITORING SIGNS AND SYMPTOMS

(Global assessment) Has your asthma been better or worse since your last visit?

Has your asthma worsened during specific seasons or events?

(Recent assessment) In the past 2 weeks, how many days have you:

- Had problems with coughing, wheezing, shortness of breath, or chest tightness during the day?
- Awakened at night from sleep because of coughing or other asthma symptoms?
- Awakened in the morning with asthma symptoms that did not improve within 15 minutes of inhaling a short-acting beta$_2$ agonist?
- Had symptoms while exercising or playing?
- Been unable to perform a usual activity, including exercise, because of asthma?

MONITORING PULMONARY FUNCTION

Lung Function

What is the highest and lowest your peak flow rate has been since your last visit?

Has your peak flow rate dropped below ____ L/min (80% of personal best) since your last visit?

What did you do when this occurred?

Peak Flow Monitoring Technique

Please show me how you measure your peak flow rate.

When do you usually measure your peak flow rate?

MONITORING QUALITY OF LIFE AND FUNCTIONAL STATUS

Since your last visit, how many days has your asthma caused you to:

- Miss work or school?
- Reduce your activities?
- *(For caregivers)* Change your activity because of your child's asthma?

Since your last visit, have you had any unscheduled or ED visits or hospital stays?

MONITORING EXACERBATION HISTORY

Since your last visit, have you had any episodes or times when your asthma symptoms were a lot worse than usual?

- If yes, what do you think caused the symptoms to get worse?
- If yes, what did you do to control the symptoms?

Have there been any changes in your home or work environment (e.g., new smokers or pets)?

MONITORING PHARMACOTHERAPY

Medications

What medications are you taking?

How do you feel about taking medication?

How often do you take each medication?

How much do you take each time?

Have you missed or stopped taking any regular doses of your medications for any reason?

Have you had trouble filling your prescriptions (e.g., for financial reasons, not on formulary)?

How many puffs of your inhaled short-acting beta$_2$ agonist (quick-relief medicine) do you use per day?

How many __________ (name short-acting inhaled beta$_2$ agonist) inhalers (or pumps) have you been through in the past month?

Have you tried any other medicines or remedies?

Side Effects

Has your asthma medicine caused you any problems?

- Shakiness, nervousness, bad taste, sore throat, cough, upset stomach, hoarseness, skin changes (e.g., bruising)

Inhaler Technique

Please show me how you use your inhaler.

MONITORING PATIENT-PROVIDER COMMUNICATION AND PATIENT SATISFACTION

What questions have you had about your asthma daily self-management plan and action plan?

What problems have you had following your daily self-management plan? Your action plan?

Has anything prevented you from getting the treatment you need for your asthma from me or anyone else?

Have the costs of your asthma treatment interfered with your ability to get asthma care?

How satisfied are you with your asthma care?

How can we improve your asthma care?

Let's review some important information:

- When should you increase your medications? Which medication(s)?
- When should you call me (health care provider)? Do you know the after-hours phone number?
- If you can't reach me, what ED would you go to?

*These questions are examples and do not represent a standardized assessment instrument. The validity and reliability of these questions have not been assessed.
From National Asthma Education and Prevention Program (NAEPP): *Expert panel report 3: guidelines for the diagnosis and management of asthma,* National Institutes of Health (NIH) Publication No. 08-5846, Bethesda, Md, 2007, U.S. Department of Health and Human Services, NIH, National Heart, Lung, and Blood Institute (NHLBI).

detectable or elicited during forced expiration. In general, mild bronchospasm is associated with expiratory wheezing. As obstruction becomes more significant, wheezing is heard during both the inspiratory and expiratory phases, with a prolongation of the latter. With profound obstruction, wheezing may be heard only during the inspiratory phase or may be entirely absent. With severe obstruction, the intensity of the breath sounds diminishes. As obstruction increases, accessory muscles of respiration are used; with significant obstruction, there may be evidence of hyperinflation with a low diaphragm and an increased anteroposterior diameter.

Severe asthma exacerbations are characterized by labored respirations, diaphoresis, anxiety, and breathlessness (inability to finish a complete sentence). A respiratory rate of 30 breaths

TABLE 103-1 Severity of Asthma Exacerbations

Parameter*	Mild	Moderate	Severe	Respiratory Arrest Imminent
Breathless	Walking Can lie down	Talking Infant: softer, shorter cry; difficulty feeding Prefer sitting	At rest Infant stops feeding Hunched forward	
Talks in ...	Sentences	Phrases	Words	
Alertness	May be agitated	Usually agitated	Usually agitated	Drowsy or confused
Respiratory rate	Increased	Increased	Often >30/min	Paradoxical
Normal Rates of Breathing in Awake Children				
	Age		**Normal Rate (Breaths per Minute)**	
	<2 mo 2-12 mo 1-5 yr 6-8 yr		<60 <50 <40 <30	
Accessory muscles and suprasternal retractions	Usually not	Usually	Usually	Paradoxical thoracoabdominal movement
Wheeze	Moderate, often only end-expiratory	Loud	Usually loud	Absence of wheeze
Pulse (beats per minute)	<100	100-120	>120	Bradycardia
Guide to Limits of Normal Pulse Rate in Children				
	Age		**Normal Rate (Beats per Minute)**	
	Infants, 2-12 mo Preschool, 1-2 yr School age, 2-8 yr		<160 <120 <110	
Pulsus paradoxus	Absent <10 mm Hg	May be present 10-25 mm Hg	Often present <25 mm Hg (adult) 20-40 mm Hg (child)	Absence suggests respiratory muscle fatigue
PEF after initial bronchodilator (% predicted or % personal best)	>80%	Approximately 60%-80%	<60% predicted or personal best (100 L/min adults) or response lasts <2 hr	
PaO_2 (on air)†	Normal (test not usually necessary)	>60 mm Hg	<60 mm Hg; possible cyanosis	
and/or				
$PaCO_2$†	<45 mm Hg	<45 mm Hg	>45 mm Hg; possible respiratory failure	
SaO_2% (on air)†	>95%	91%-95%	<90%	

Hypercapnia (hypoventilation) develops more readily in young children than in adults and adolescents.
*The presence of several parameters, but not necessarily all, indicates the general classification of the attack.
†Kilopascals are also used internationally; conversion would be appropriate in this regard.
PEF, peak expiratory flow.
From Global Initiative for Asthma (GINA): *Pocket guide for asthma management and prevention: a pocket guide for physicians and nurses*, updated 2011. Available at www.ginasthma.org.

per minute or more and a heart rate of 120 beats per minute or more suggest severe bronchospasm. Other signs and symptoms that often herald impending respiratory failure include agitation, confusion, somnolence, and cyanosis. Unilateral loss of breath sounds may reflect mucous plugging and secondary atelectasis, but pneumothorax must also be considered in this situation. However, even a careful physical examination provides only a crude estimate of airway obstruction, and significant airway obstruction is possible even when the physical examination findings are entirely normal. Assessment of respiratory status is best accomplished through measurement of lung function with spirometry or peak flow meters. The Global Initiative for Asthma (GINA) system of classifying the severity of asthma exacerbations is presented in Table 103-1. The physical examination is also important in identifying adverse effects of asthma medications. Side effects of $beta_2$-adrenergic medications and theophylline include tachycardia and tremors. Inhaled corticosteroids (ICSs) can cause oral thrush and dysphonia. Adverse effects of oral (systemic) corticosteroids include central adiposity, hypertension, ecchymoses, cataracts, kyphosis, muscle weakness, and alterations in mental status.

Coexisting medical problems can be conceptualized in two ways. Certain comorbid conditions, such as nasal polyps, allergic rhinitis, sinusitis, and eczema, are commonly associated with asthma. In addition, some coexisting medical problems may be unrelated to asthma, but their identification and management have important implications for asthma therapy and control. Such possible comorbidities include glaucoma, hypertension, gastroesophageal reflux, diabetes mellitus, arthritis, and current malignant neoplasms.

DIAGNOSTICS

A diagnosis of asthma is based on three components: (1) demonstration of episodic symptoms of airflow obstruction (e.g., wheeze, cough, shortness of breath), (2) evidence that airflow obstruction is at least partially reversible, and (3) exclusion of other conditions from the differential diagnosis.[12] A thorough history and physical examination are essential to making the diagnosis of asthma. Physical findings can be helpful in identifying significant obstruction as it occurs but at best provide only a crude estimate of the degree of obstruction. However, significant obstruction may not manifest as an abnormal physical finding; in addition, findings are likely to be completely normal between episodes. In fact, reduced expiratory flow rates (forced expiratory volume at 1 second [FEV_1]) and increased airway resistance may not be recognized as dyspnea until a 30% to 40% decline in FEV_1 has occurred.[19] Thus, objective measures of pulmonary function, such as spirometry and peak flow meters, are essential in establishing the diagnosis of asthma and assessing its severity. Spirometry is now recommended at the time of initial assessment to confirm the diagnosis of asthma, after treatment is initiated and symptoms and peak expiratory flow (PEF) have been stabilized, and at least every 1 to 2 years.[12]

Although spirometry provides many measures, the most useful for evaluation of asthma are the peak expiratory flow rate (PEFR), FEV_1, maximum mid-expiratory flow rate (MMEFR), and forced vital capacity (FVC). Results are compared with expected values, derived from a population of healthy, nonsmoking adults, and are expressed as a percentage of the expected value.

The most common pulmonary function abnormality in mild asthma is the decreased rate of airflow throughout the vital capacity as reflected by abnormalities in the PEFR, FEV_1, and MMEFR (forced expiratory flow [FEF_{25-75}]). During bronchospasm, spirometry reveals obstruction with decreases in FEV_1 and MMEFR. The FEV_1/FVC ratio is also reduced. As obstruction increases, an increased residual volume and functional residual are noted. One of the diagnostic hallmarks of asthma is reversal of obstruction after the administration of a bronchodilator, which corresponds with both clinical improvement and improved spirometric values. In addition to helping establish the diagnosis of asthma, spirometry helps assess the adequacy of therapy, the need for further therapy and evaluation during emergencies, and the need for hospital admission. The severity of asthma attacks must be assessed by accurate and reproducible measures of airflow. Health care providers tend to underestimate the degree of airway obstruction in individuals with acute asthma, and knowledge of a person's pulmonary function has potentially important implications for treatment. For this reason, the NAEPP guidelines recommend the use of PFTs as part of the assessment and monitoring during the treatment of acute asthma. During a severe asthma attack, recording of the entire spirogram may be difficult, but the FEV_1 can still be measured. As the asthma attack resolves, both the PEFR and the FEV_1 increase, whereas the MMEFR usually remains significantly diminished.

Most patients with controlled asthma will not exhibit reversibility in FEV_1 at each visit, particularly those who are being treated for asthma, and therefore the test lacks sensitivity. Repeated testing at different visits may be helpful.[2]

PEF measurements with use of a peak flow meter may also be helpful in the diagnosis and management of asthma, but measurements of PEF are not interchangeable with other measurements of lung function such as FEV_1 because values obtained with different peak flow meters vary and the range of predicted values is too wide.[2] In addition, PEF measurements are effort dependent and may not be an accurate reflection of a person's pulmonary function. PEF measurements done in the office should always be compared with the patient's previous "personal best" using his or her own peak flow meter.

The terms *reversibility* and *variability* refer to changes in symptoms accompanied by changes in airflow limitation that occur spontaneously or in response to treatment. Reversibility refers to rapid improvements in FEV_1 or PEF minutes after use of a quick-relief medication such as a bronchodilator or sustained improvement during days or weeks after the introduction of a long-term control medication such as an ICS.[2] In contrast, variability refers to the change (improvement or deterioration) in asthma symptoms and lung function occurring during a longer time.[12] Variability may be experienced in the course of a day (diurnal variability), from day to day, from month to month, or seasonally. Obtaining a history of variability is an integral aspect of asthma diagnosis and management.

Other laboratory tests that may be used to diagnose asthma or be included as part of the evaluation are airway responsiveness testing, arterial blood and other serum analysis, radiography, electrocardiography (ECG), and sputum cultures. Airway responsiveness testing measures the bronchoconstrictor response elicited by a standard stimulus. The FEV_1 is measured after inhalation of an aerosol containing graded amounts of a bronchoconstrictor agonist. The most commonly used bronchoconstrictor is methacholine, but histamine, exercise, eucapnic voluntary hyperventilation or inhaled mannitol can also be used for bronchial provocation. These tests are moderately sensitive for a diagnosis of asthma, but have limited sensitivity. For example, airway hyperresponsiveness to inhaled methacholine can also occur in patients with allergic rhinitis.[2] Individuals with asthma often have atopy, which is often reflected in blood eosinophilia. Total serum IgE levels are elevated in persons with asthma and associated with disease severity, but IgE levels cannot predict response to treatment.[20] The data from studies in pediatric populations unambiguously suggest a positive relationship between atopy and asthma severity, but studies in adults show an inconsistent relationship between the two.[21]

In general, the chest radiographs of individuals with asthma are normal. Therefore, chest radiography is not indicated in the routine evaluation of patients with asthma unless physical examination findings are suggestive of infectious illness or respiratory complications such as pneumomediastinum or pneumothorax. If an asthma exacerbation is severe enough to warrant hospital admission, a chest x-ray film should be taken. The x-ray film may show hyperinflation (indicated by diaphragmatic depression) and abnormally translucent lung fields.

Between asthma attacks, in the absence of respiratory infection, the sputum is usually clear. During an asthma attack, even in the absence of infection, the sputum may be yellow to green. This does not necessarily indicate infection; the color change may be from eosinophil peroxidase. Sputum culture specimens are generally not obtained unless there is suspicion of an acute contagious respiratory infection.

ECG is not part of the routine evaluation of a patient with asthma. If it is performed during an asthma exacerbation, ECG in the absence of cardiac disease is usually significant only for sinus tachycardia. In severe attacks, right-axis deviation, right bundle branch block, cor pulmonale, or even ST-T wave abnormalities may occur. If these abnormalities resolve as the asthma attack abates, no further cardiac evaluation is necessary. Electrocardiographic findings should be monitored during asthma attacks for patients with significant cardiac disease to monitor for myocardial infarction, which can result from attack-induced stress.

DIAGNOSTICS

Asthma

INITIAL
Peak flow meter
Pulse oximetry

LABORATORY
Complete blood count and differential
IgE*

IMAGING
Chest x-ray examination*

OTHER DIAGNOSTICS
PFTs, airway responsiveness testing
Arterial blood gases (ABGs)*
ECG*

*If indicated.

DIFFERENTIAL DIAGNOSIS

The medical conditions most likely to be confused with asthma involve the upper respiratory system (e.g., croup, vocal cord dysfunction [VCD]) and lower respiratory system (e.g., pneumonia, chronic obstructive pulmonary disease [COPD]), the cardiovascular system (e.g., valvular disease and cardiomyopathy), and the gastrointestinal system (e.g., GERD).

Not all wheezing is caused by asthma, and other causes should be excluded before a diagnosis of asthma is made. Spirometry can be used to help differentiate asthma from other possible conditions in the differential diagnosis. An FEV_1 of 80% of predicted or less with a reduced FEV_1/FVC ratio that normalizes or significantly improves with bronchodilator therapy raises the suspicion of asthma. Other causes of wheezing and upper airway obstruction include tracheomalacia, tracheal or bronchial masses, and laryngeal (vocal cord) dysfunction. The presence of stridor or focal wheezing on physical examination and with flow limitation on a flow-volume loop is characteristic of tracheomalacia and tracheobronchial masses. VCD can mimic asthma and may coexist with asthma, but it is a distinct disorder. VCD is caused by abnormal apposition of the vocal cords during the respiratory cycle and can generally be treated effectively by speech therapy. Laryngoscopy is needed to confirm VCD. VCD is often initially misdiagnosed as asthma and often inappropriately and ineffectively treated with high-dose systemic steroids. VCD should be considered in atypical asthma patients who do not respond well to asthma medications and in athletes who have exercise-related breathlessness unresponsive to asthma medication. COPD is characterized by airflow limitation that is not fully reversible, is usually progressive, and is associated with an abnormal inflammatory response of the lungs to noxious substances. Persons with COPD, including emphysema and chronic bronchitis, may have acute episodes of airway obstruction and wheezing, especially during exacerbations of their disease. COPD is often accompanied by a history of smoking, reduced response to bronchodilator therapy, and irreversible PFT changes over time. In addition, COPD may be distinguished from asthma by signs of hyperinflation, such as diminished breath sounds, decreased heart sounds, and a flattened diaphragm. Chest wall deformities are suggestive of restrictive lung diseases. Dullness to percussion may indicate pneumonia or a pleural effusion. Foreign body aspiration should be considered if lateralizing wheezes are heard. Although asthma can usually be distinguished from COPD, in some individuals who develop chronic respiratory symptoms, it may be difficult to differentiate between the two. It may be helpful for primary care providers to use symptom-based questionnaires to assist in differentiating COPD from asthma.

α_1-Antitrypsin (AAT) deficiency is an inherited disorder caused by an inborn error in the liver's production of AAT, which is the dominant protease in the lung and protects alveoli from the destructive effects of serine proteases. AAT deficiency causes a syndrome of abnormalities, including neonatal jaundice, airflow obstruction, premature emphysema, and cirrhosis of the liver. The primary respiratory effect of AAT deficiency is degradation of the protein elastin, a protein that is essential for the elastic recoil required for pulmonary expiratory function. As a result, chronic persistent airflow obstruction develops. AAT deficiency is a well-established cause of panacinar emphysema, but its role in the pathophysiologic process of asthma is less well understood. The prevalence of AAT deficiency is about 0.01% to 0.02% in those with emphysema; the prevalence of AAT deficiency among patients with asthma is not known.[22] Individuals with AAT deficiency often have symptoms similar to those of bronchial asthma; pulmonary function may be normal, especially among those who do not smoke. Hence, a diagnosis of AAT deficiency is often missed or delayed. However,

DIFFERENTIAL DIAGNOSIS

Asthma

- AAT deficiency
- Acute bronchiolitis (infectious, chemical)
- Airway obstruction by masses
- Bronchiolitis obliterans organizing pneumonia
- Bronchial stenosis
- Carcinoid syndrome
- Cardiac failure
- Central thoracic tumors
- COPD (chronic bronchitis or emphysema)
- Cystic fibrosis
- Endobronchial sarcoid
- Eosinophilic pneumonia
- Foreign body aspiration
- Interstitial fibrosis
- Metastatic cancer
- Pleural effusion
- Primary lung tumors
- Pulmonary emboli
- Substernal thyroid tumors
- Systemic mastocytosis
- Systemic vasculitis (polyarteritis nodosa)
- Tracheomalacia
- VCD

bronchopulmonary infections are common in persons with AAT deficiency, and their family history almost always includes lung disease. Asthmatic patients with AAT deficiency usually have more severe disease and often respond less to bronchodilators than do those without the disorder. Health care providers should have a high level of suspicion for AAT deficiency in young persons whose symptoms do not respond to appropriate asthma therapy, especially in the absence of smoking. Diagnosis of AAT deficiency is based on AAT serum levels but may also involve other diagnostic measurements, including PFTs, chest radiography, serum electrophoresis, and genotyping. Although management of AAT deficiency has some similarities to that of asthma, it also has important differences; diagnosis of AAT deficiency has critical implications for an individual's prognosis and quality of life.

MANAGEMENT

Although the role of inflammation in the pathogenesis of asthma was recognized in the 1991 National Heart, Lung, and Blood Institute (NHLBI) guidelines on asthma management, asthma was not defined as a chronic inflammatory disorder of the airways until later.[2] This new understanding of asthma pathology also suggests that much of asthma care will be provided by individuals and their families outside of and away from health care institutions and practitioners. In addition, inflammation is now understood to be one of the preeminent problems in asthma, which has shifted the focus of treatment from symptomatic to preventive therapy, including the need for anti-inflammatory medications, environmental controls, and patient education. GINA was created to increase awareness among health professionals, public health authorities, and the general public to improve the prevention and management of asthma through a concerted worldwide effort. GINA offers a framework for asthma management that can be adapted to local health care systems and resources.[2] Both the NAEPP of the NHLBI (NIH) and GINA have identified six goals of asthma treatment, which differ only with regard to GINA's emphasis on preventing the possible sequelae of asthma, including irreversible airflow limitation and asthma-related death.[2,6] GINA's goals for successful asthma management are listed in Box 103-3.

The NHLBI Expert Panel for the Diagnosis and Management of Asthma and GINA use the same classification system of asthma severity, which is based on the frequency and severity of symptoms. Characteristics of each of these categories are presented in Figures 103-1 and 103-2. According to the guidelines, individuals should be assigned to the most severe asthma category in which any characteristic occurs. The major change from previous classification systems is the division of asthmatic patients into those with and those without mild persistent symptoms. This distinction has important clinical implications because, in general, the only persons not requiring anti-inflammatory medications are those with intermittent symptoms.

Asthma pharmacotherapy is determined by the severity of the disease, and a summary of disease classification can also be found in Figures 103-1 and 103-2. The most effective medications for long-term control of asthma continue to be those with anti-inflammatory effects, including the ICSs, mast cell stabilizers such as cromolyn, long-acting $beta_2$-adrenergic agonists (LABAs), and leukotriene modifiers. These medications are referred to in the Expert Panel Report (EPR)[12] as long-term control medications and in GINA[2] as controller medications to emphasize their role in achieving and maintaining control of persistent asthma (Table 103-2). Relief of exacerbations and control of acute symptoms are achieved through the use of quick-relief medications (EPR) or reliever medication (GINA), chief among them being the short-acting $beta_2$-adrenergic agonists (SABAs) but also including anticholinergics and systemic glucocorticoids (Table 103-3). The new EPR guidelines also emphasize a stepwise management approach in which therapies should be initiated at higher levels (steps, not doses) to establish control as quickly as possible (see Figs. 103-1 and 103-2). After control has been achieved, therapy should be tapered for long-term management.[12]

Classification of asthma by severity of symptoms is helpful in guiding disease management at the initial assessment of a patient. However, as emphasized by GINA, it is important to recognize that asthma severity involves both the severity of the underlying disease process and its responsiveness to treatment.[2] Severity should not be considered an invariable or static feature of a person's asthma; rather, it is a factor that may change over time.

Despite the fact that the approach to asthma therapy has been recommended by the NHLBI since 1991, studies indicate that asthma control, as defined by the asthma management guidelines, is not being achieved in the majority of patients.[9,10] There remains an overreliance on short-acting bronchodilators and underuse of anti-inflammatory medications on the part of both practitioners and persons with asthma. This suggests that the underlying pathophysiologic mechanism of asthma and its implications for therapy are still not widely understood. As emphasized in the EPR stepwise approach, all patients except those with mild, intermittent asthma benefit from maintenance anti-inflammatory medication. The use of anti-inflammatory medications for maintenance (long-term control) of mild to moderate asthma results in fewer asthma exacerbations, fewer ED visits, decreased cost of care, fewer school or work days missed, and improved quality of life.[12] Despite the guidelines, research suggests that asthma is often undertreated because of inappropriate prescribing or underprescribing by physicians and poor adherence of patients to therapy.[23,24]

Adherence to the asthma management guidelines has been shown to lead to a reduction in health care use; the greatest gains were for those with moderate to severe disease.[25] Specifically, among both severe and less severe asthma groups, high use of inhaled short-acting beta agonists in the absence of ICS use (inconsistent with the guidelines) has been associated with as much as a fourfold increase in hospitalization. The risk of hospitalization was progressively reduced with both low and

BOX 103-3

Goals for Successful Asthma Management

- Achieve and maintain control of symptoms
- Maintain normal activity levels, including exercise
- Maintain pulmonary function as close to normal as possible
- Prevent asthma exacerbations
- Avoid adverse effects from asthma medications
- Prevent asthma mortality

Global Initiative for Asthma (GINA): Pocket guide for asthma management and prevention: a pocket guide for physicians and nurses, updated 2015. Available at www.ginasthma.org.

Youths ≥12 Years of Age and Adults

Assessing severity and initiating therapy in children who are not currently taking long-term control medication

Components of Severity		Classification of Asthma Severity: Intermittent	Persistent: Mild	Persistent: Moderate	Persistent: Severe
Impairment Normal FEV_1/FVC: 08 to 19 yr 85% 20 to 39 yr 80% 40 to 59 yr 75% 60 to 80 yr 70%	Symptoms	≤2 days/week	>2 days/week but not daily	Daily	Throughout the day
	Nighttime awakenings	≤2x/month	3 to 4x/month	>1x/week but not nightly	Often 7x/week
	Short-acting $beta_2$-agonist use for symptom control (not prevention of EIB)	≤2 days/week	>2 days/week but not daily, and not more than 1x on any day	Daily	Several times per day
	Interference with normal activity	None	Minor limitation	Some limitation	Extremely limited
	Lung function	• Normal FEV_1 between exacerbations • FEV_1 >80% predicted • FEV_1/FVC normal	• FEV_1 >80% predicted • FEV_1/FVC normal	• FEV_1 >60 but <80% predicted • FEV_1/FVC reduced 5%	• FEV_1 < 60% predicted • FEV_1/FVC reduced >5%
Risk	Exacerbations requiring oral systemic corticosteroids	0 to 1/year (see note)	≥2/year (see note) →		
		← Consider severity and interval since last exacerbation. → Frequency and severity may fluctuate over time for patients in any severity category.			
		Relative annual risk of exacerbations may be related to FEV_1.			
Recommended Step for Initiating Therapy (See Fig. 103-2 for treatment steps.)		Step 1	Step 2	Step 3 and consider short course of oral systemic corticosteroids	Step 4 or 5 and consider short course of oral systemic corticosteroids
		In 2 to 6 weeks, evaluate level of asthma control that is achieved and adjust therapy accordingly.			

Notes

- The stepwise approach is meant to assist, not replace, the clinical decision making required to meet individual patient needs.
- Level of severity is determined by both impairment and risk. Assess impairment domain by patient's/caregiver's recall of previous 2 to 4 weeks and spirometry. Assign severity to the most severe category in which any feature occurs.
- At present, there are inadequate data to correspond frequencies of exacerbations with different levels of asthma severity. In general, more frequent and intense exacerbations (e.g., requiring urgent, unscheduled care, hospitalization, or ICU admission) indicate greater underlying disease severity. For treatment purposes, patients who had ≥2 exacerbations requiring oral systemic corticosteroids in the past year may be considered the same as patients who have persistent asthma, even in the absence of impairment levels consistent with persistent asthma.

Key: *FEV_1*, forced expiratory volume in 1 second; *FVC*, forced vital capacity; *ICU*, intensive care unit; *x*, times; *yr*, years.

FIGURE **103-1** Classifying asthma severity and initiating treatment in youths 12 years of age or older and adults. (From National Asthma Education and Prevention Program [NAEPP]: *Expert panel report 3: guidelines for the diagnosis and management of asthma,* National Institutes of Health [NIH] Publication No. 08-5846, Bethesda, Md, 2007, U.S. Department of Health and Human Services, NIH, National Heart, Lung, and Blood Institute [NHLBI]. Available at www.nhlbi.nih.gov/guidelines/asthma/asthsumm.pdf.)

high use of ICSs. The protective effect of ICS on hospitalization has been reported in several studies, with the reduction rate ranging from 30% to 60%.[26]

In addition to long-term daily therapy to control symptoms and to prevent exacerbations, asthma management guidelines also include strategies for classifying and managing exacerbations. Early introduction of oral corticosteroids and frequent use of short-acting beta agonists should be initiated as symptoms worsen. Table 103-1 includes parameters for assessing the severity of asthma attacks. Home and hospital treatments of asthma exacerbations are found in Box 103-4 and Figure 103-3.

An integral component of asthma management is the treatment of coexisting diseases, including rhinitis, sinusitis, and GERD. Evidence from clinical trials suggests no benefit from antibiotic therapy for asthma exacerbations, whether it is administered routinely or when the suspicion of bacterial infection is low. The NAEPP EPR recommendation is that antibiotics not be used in the treatment of acute asthma exacerbation except for the treatment of certain comorbid conditions, such as fever and purulent sputum, evidence of pneumonia, and bacterial sinusitis.[12] Intranasal glucocorticoids may be helpful in the management of chronic rhinitis, whereas antibiotics are indicated for bacterial sinus infections.[12] Annual influenza vaccination is recommended for all persons with persistent asthma. For persons with GERD, acid-suppressive therapy may decrease asthma symptoms. Individuals with GERD often do not describe symptoms suggestive of GERD; approximately 25% to 30% of patients with asthma have clinically silent reflux.[27,28]

Given the known role of environmental triggers in the pathophysiologic process of asthma, it is essential that environmental interventions be implemented along with clinical approaches in the management of asthma. Interventions at the household level must include efforts to eliminate cockroaches, rodents, and mold. Individual efforts to sustain pest-free environments, especially in apartment complexes, will be effective only if efforts at the building, neighborhood, and city level are in place to bolster those efforts. Common asthma risk factors and actions to reduce exposure to them are listed in Table 103-4.[12]

MEDICATIONS

Long-Term Control Medications

Corticosteroids. Corticosteroids are the most potent and effective anti-inflammatory medications available for the treatment of moderate to severe asthma. Although the mechanism of action is not completely understood, they have been shown to reduce the synthesis of inflammatory mediators and to inhibit late responses to allergen (those occurring several hours after allergen exposure). Their ability to inhibit a wide variety

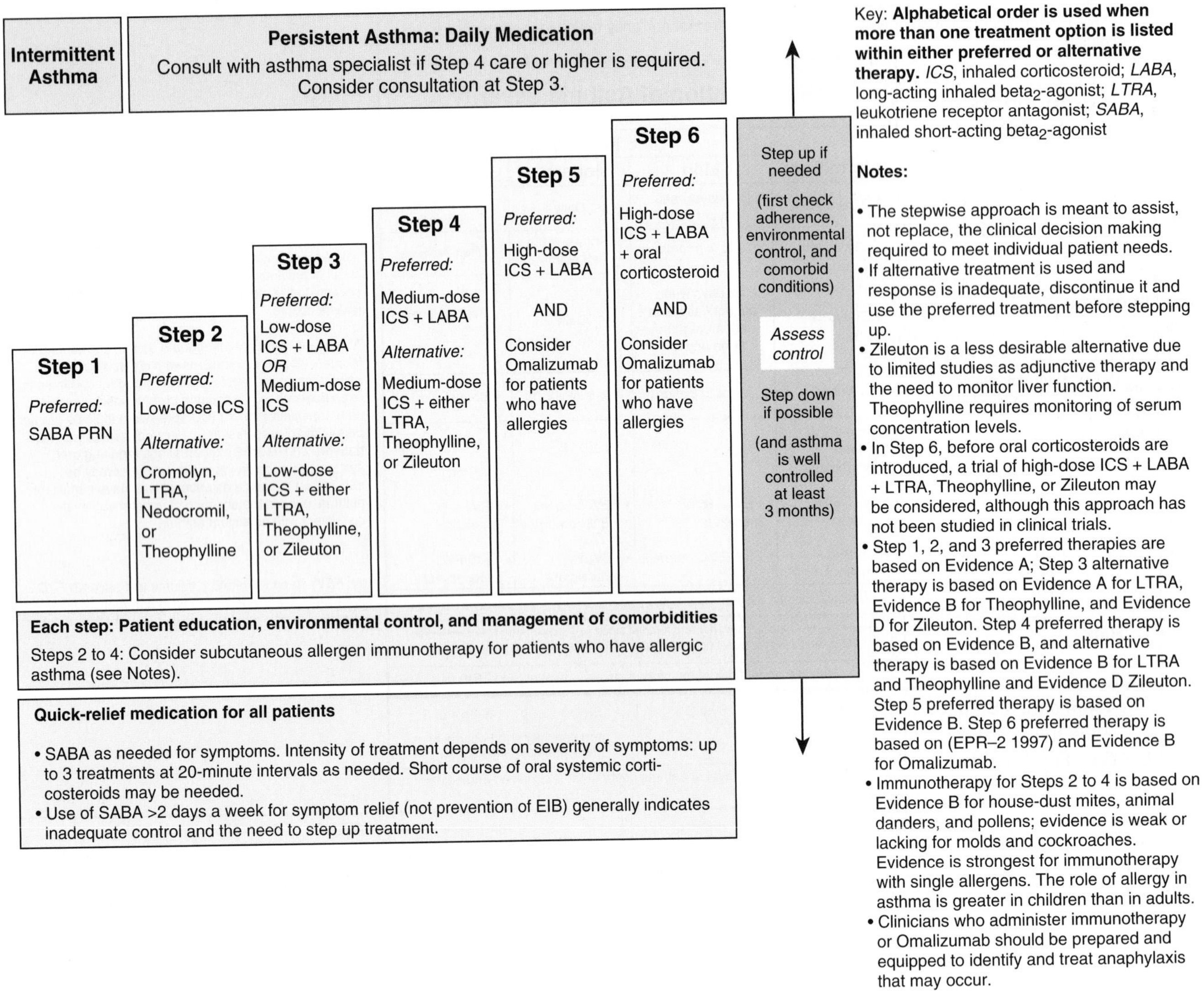
Intermittent Asthma
Persistent Asthma: Daily Medication
Consult with asthma specialist if Step 4 care or higher is required. Consider consultation at Step 3.
Step 1
Preferred: SABA PRN
Step 2
Preferred: Low-dose ICS
Alternative: Cromolyn, LTRA, Nedocromil, or Theophylline
Step 3
Preferred: Low-dose ICS + LABA OR Medium-dose ICS
Alternative: Low-dose ICS + either LTRA, Theophylline, or Zileuton
Step 4
Preferred: Medium-dose ICS + LABA
Alternative: Medium-dose ICS + either LTRA, Theophylline, or Zileuton
Step 5
Preferred: High-dose ICS + LABA
AND
Consider Omalizumab for patients who have allergies
Step 6
Preferred: High-dose ICS + LABA + oral corticosteroid
AND
Consider Omalizumab for patients who have allergies
Step up if needed
(first check adherence, environmental control, and comorbid conditions)
Assess control
Step down if possible
(and asthma is well controlled at least 3 months)
Each step: Patient education, environmental control, and management of comorbidities
Steps 2 to 4: Consider subcutaneous allergen immunotherapy for patients who have allergic asthma (see Notes).
Quick-relief medication for all patients
• SABA as needed for symptoms. Intensity of treatment depends on severity of symptoms: up to 3 treatments at 20-minute intervals as needed. Short course of oral systemic corticosteroids may be needed.
• Use of SABA >2 days a week for symptom relief (not prevention of EIB) generally indicates inadequate control and the need to step up treatment.
Key: Alphabetical order is used when more than one treatment option is listed within either preferred or alternative therapy. ICS, inhaled corticosteroid; LABA, long-acting inhaled beta2-agonist; LTRA, leukotriene receptor antagonist; SABA, inhaled short-acting beta2-agonist
Notes:
• The stepwise approach is meant to assist, not replace, the clinical decision making required to meet individual patient needs.
• If alternative treatment is used and response is inadequate, discontinue it and use the preferred treatment before stepping up.
• Zileuton is a less desirable alternative due to limited studies as adjunctive therapy and the need to monitor liver function. Theophylline requires monitoring of serum concentration levels.
• In Step 6, before oral corticosteroids are introduced, a trial of high-dose ICS + LABA + LTRA, Theophylline, or Zileuton may be considered, although this approach has not been studied in clinical trials.
• Step 1, 2, and 3 preferred therapies are based on Evidence A; Step 3 alternative therapy is based on Evidence A for LTRA, Evidence B for Theophylline, and Evidence D for Zileuton. Step 4 preferred therapy is based on Evidence B, and alternative therapy is based on Evidence B for LTRA and Theophylline and Evidence D Zileuton. Step 5 preferred therapy is based on Evidence B. Step 6 preferred therapy is based on (EPR–2 1997) and Evidence B for Omalizumab.
• Immunotherapy for Steps 2 to 4 is based on Evidence B for house-dust mites, animal danders, and pollens; evidence is weak or lacking for molds and cockroaches. Evidence is strongest for immunotherapy with single allergens. The role of allergy in asthma is greater in children than in adults.
• Clinicians who administer immunotherapy or Omalizumab should be prepared and equipped to identify and treat anaphylaxis that may occur.

FIGURE 103-2 Stepwise approach for managing asthma in youths 12 years of age or older and adults. (From National Asthma Education and Prevention Program [NAEPP]: *Expert panel report 3: guidelines for the diagnosis and management of asthma,* National Institutes of Health [NIH] Publication No. 08-5846, Bethesda, Md, 2007, U.S. Department of Health and Human Services, NIH, National Heart, Lung, and Blood Institute [NHLBI]. Available at www.nhlbi.nih.gov/guidelines/asthma/asthsumm.pdf.)

of inflammatory responses probably accounts for their effectiveness in many types of asthma. ICSs are the most effective long-term therapy for persistent asthma and are recommended for every individual with persistent asthma symptoms. ICSs are generally well tolerated in low to moderate doses and have fewer side effects for a given level of therapeutic effect than medications administered orally. There is no consensus on the specific type or dose of inhaled steroid to be used. In general, administration begins with 2 to 4 puffs or inhalations per day, and the dose is increased on the basis of the individual's response. Each of the inhaled steroids has its own maximum number of doses per day as summarized in Table 103-5 (EPR).

The usual estimated comparative daily doses for inhaled glucocorticoids and ICSs can be found in Table 103-5.

Combined medications (inhaled corticosteroids and long-acting beta$_2$ agonists) include fluticasone/salmeterol, budesonide/formoterol, and mometasone/formoterol. Daily doses can be found in Table 103-5.

The major side effect of inhaled steroids is oral thrush, which can be prevented by good oral hygiene and the use of aerosol spacers during delivery. The safety of long-term therapy with high-dose inhaled steroids has not been well established, and their use may be associated with untoward side effects, including adrenal suppression, bone loss, skin bruising, glaucoma, behavioral abnormalities, and the possibility of inhibited growth in children. It is still unknown whether the use of high-potency steroids increases the risk of adrenal suppression and other systemic side effects.[2]

Systemic corticosteroids are used in the management of asthma symptoms not responding to standard treatment. In general, a steroid "pulse" with initial doses of prednisone of 40 to 60 mg/day tapering to 0 mg in the ensuing 1 to 2 weeks is prescribed. If symptoms worsen during this period, the dose is increased and the taper restarted. For persons not responding to a prednisone taper or with life-threatening symptoms,

Continued on page 437

TABLE 103-2 Usual Doses for Long-Term Control Medications*

Medication	≥12 Years of Age and Adults	Potential Adverse Effects	Comments (Not All-Inclusive)
INHALED CORTICOSTEROIDS			
See Table 103-5			
ORAL SYSTEMIC CORTICOSTEROIDS			
Methylprednisolone 2-, 4-, 8-, 16-, 32-mg tablets Prednisolone 5-mg tablets, 5 mg/5 mL, 15 mg/5 mL Prednisone 1-, 2.5-, 5-, 10-, 20-, 50-mg tablets; 5 mg/mL, 5 mg/5 mL	7.5-60 mg daily in a single dose in AM or every other day as needed for control Short-course "burst": to achieve control, 40-60 mg/day as single or 2 divided doses for 3-10 days	Short-term use: reversible abnormalities in glucose metabolism, increased appetite, fluid retention, weight gain, mood alteration, hypertension, peptic ulcer, and rarely aseptic necrosis. Long-term use: adrenal axis suppression, growth suppression, dermal thinning, hypertension, diabetes, Cushing syndrome, cataracts, muscle weakness, and—in rare instances—impaired immune function. Consideration should be given to coexisting conditions that could be worsened by systemic corticosteroids, such as herpes virus infections, varicella, tuberculosis, hypertension, peptic ulcer, diabetes mellitus, osteoporosis, and *Strongyloides* infection.	For long-term treatment of severe persistent asthma, administer single dose in AM either daily or on alternate days (alternate-day therapy may produce less adrenal suppression). Short courses or bursts are effective for establishing control when initiating therapy or during a period of gradual deterioration. There is no evidence that tapering the dose after improvement in symptom control and pulmonary function prevents relapse. For patients unable to tolerate the liquid preparations, dexamethasone syrup at 0.4 mg/kg/day may be an alternative. Studies are limited, however, and the longer duration of activity increases the risk of adrenal suppression.
INHALED LONG-ACTING BETA$_2$ AGONISTS			
Salmeterol DPI: 50 μg/blister Formoterol DPI: 12 μg/single-use capsule	1 blister every 12 hr 1 capsule every 12 hr	Tachycardia, skeletal muscle tremor, hypokalemia, prolongation of QTc interval in overdose. A diminished bronchoprotective effect may occur within 1 week of chronic therapy. Clinical significance has not been established. Potential risk of uncommon, severe, life-threatening or fatal exacerbation; see text for additional discussion regarding safety of LABAs.	Should not be used for acute symptom relief or exacerbations. Use only with ICS. Decreased duration of protection against EIB may occur with regular use. Do not blow into inhaler after dose is activated. Each capsule is for single use only; additional doses should not be administered for at least 12 hours. Capsules should be used only with the inhaler and should not be taken orally.
COMBINED MEDICATIONS ICS/LABA			
Fluticasone/salmeterol DPI: 100 μg/50 μg, 250 μg/50 μg, or 500 μg/50 μg HFA: 45 μg/21 μg, 115 μg/21 μg, 230 μg/21 μg Advair	1 inhalation twice daily; dose depends on level of severity or control	See notes for ICSs and LABAs.	Do not blow into inhaler after dose is activated. 100/50 DPI or 45/21 HFA for patients who have asthma not controlled on low- to medium-dose ICS. 250/50 DPI or 115/21 HFA for patients who have asthma not controlled on medium- to high-dose ICS.
Budesonide/formoterol HFA MDI: 80 μg/4.5 μg, 160 μg/4.5 μg Symbicort	2 puffs twice daily; dose depends on level of severity or control	See notes for ICSs and LABAs.	There have been no clinical trials in children <4 years of age. Currently approved for use in youths ≥12 years of age. Dose for children 5-12 years of age based on clinical trials using DPI with slightly different delivery characteristics. 80/4.5 for patients who have asthma not controlled on low- to medium-dose ICS 160/4.5 for patients who have asthma not controlled on medium- to high-dose ICS

Continued

TABLE 103-2 **Usual Doses for Long-Term Control Medications*—cont'd**

Medication	≥12 Years of Age and Adults	Potential Adverse Effects	Comments (Not All-Inclusive)
CROMOLYN/NEDOCROMIL			
Cromolyn MDI: 0.8 mg/puff Nebulizer: 20 mg/ampule Nedocromil MDI: 1.75 mg/puff	2 puffs 4 times a day 1 ampule 4 times a day 2 puffs 4 times a day	Cough and irritation; 15%-20% of patients complain of an unpleasant taste from nedocromil.	One dose of cromolyn before exercise or allergen exposure provides effective prophylaxis for 1-2 hours. Not as effective for EIB as SABAs. 4- to 6-week trial of cromolyn or nedocromil may be needed to determine maximum benefit. Dose by MDI may be inadequate to affect hyperresponsiveness. Once control is achieved, the frequency of administration may be reduced. Safety is the primary advantage of these agents.
IMMUNOMODULATORS			
Omalizumab (anti-IgE) Subcutaneous injection, 150 mg/1.2 mL following reconstitution with 1.4 mL sterile water for injection	150-375 mg SC every 2-4 wk, depending on body weight and pretreatment serum IgE level	Pain and bruising of injection sites in 5%-20% of patients. Anaphylaxis has been reported in 0.2% of treated patients. Malignant neoplasms were reported in 0.5% of patients compared with 0.2% receiving placebo; relationship to drug is unclear.	Do not administer more than 150 mg per injection site. Monitor patients after injections; be prepared and equipped to identify and treat anaphylaxis that may occur. Whether patients will develop significant antibody titers to the drug with long-term administration is unknown.
LEUKOTRIENE MODIFIERS			
Leukotriene Receptor Antagonists			
Montelukast 4-mg or 5-mg chewable tablet 4-mg granule packets 10-mg tablet	10 mg every bedtime	No specific adverse effects have been identified. Rare cases of Churg-Strauss have occurred, but the association is unclear.	Montelukast exhibits a flat dose-response curve. Doses >10 mg will not produce a greater response in adults. No more efficacious than placebo in infants ages 6-24 months. As long-term therapy may attenuate exercise-induced bronchospasm in some patients, but less effective than ICS therapy.
Zafirlukast 10-mg tablet 20-mg tablet	40 mg daily (20-mg tablet twice daily)	Postmarketing surveillance has reported cases of reversible hepatitis and, rarely, irreversible hepatic failure resulting in death and liver transplantation.	For zafirlukast, administration with meals decreases bioavailability; take at least 1 hour before or 2 hours after meals. Zafirlukast is a microsomal P-450 enzyme inhibitor that can inhibit the metabolism of warfarin. INRs should be monitored during coadministration. Monitor hepatic enzymes (ALT). Warn patients to discontinue use if they experience signs and symptoms of liver dysfunction.
5-Lipoxygenase Inhibitor			
Zileuton 600-mg tablet	2400 mg daily (give tablets 4 times a day)	Elevation of liver enzymes has been reported. Limited case reports of reversible hepatitis and hyperbilirubinemia.	For zileuton, monitor hepatic enzymes (ALT). Zileuton is a microsomal P-450 enzyme inhibitor that can inhibit the metabolism of warfarin and theophylline. Doses of these drugs should be monitored accordingly.

TABLE 103-2 Usual Doses for Long-Term Control Medications*—cont'd

Medication	≥12 Years of Age and Adults	Potential Adverse Effects	Comments (Not All-Inclusive)
METHYLXANTHINES			
Theophylline Liquids, sustained-release tablets, and capsules	Starting dose: 10 mg/kg/day up to 300 mg maximum; usual maximum: 800 mg/day	Dose-related acute toxicities include tachycardia, nausea and vomiting, tachyarrhythmias (supraventricular tachycardia [SVT]), central nervous system stimulation, headache, seizures, hematemesis, hyperglycemia, and hypokalemia. Adverse effects at usual therapeutic doses include insomnia, gastric upset, aggravation of ulcer or reflux, increase in hyperactivity in some children, difficulty in urination in elderly men who have prostatism.	Adjust dosage to achieve serum concentration of 5-15 μg/mL at steady state (at least 48 hours on same dosage). Because of wide interpatient variability in theophylline metabolic clearance, routine serum theophylline level monitoring is essential. Patients should be told to discontinue if they experience toxicity. Various factors (diet, food, febrile illness, age, smoking, and other medications) can affect serum concentrations.

*Dosages are provided for those products that have been approved by the U.S. Food and Drug Administration or have sufficient clinical trial safety and efficacy data in the appropriate age ranges to support their use.

ALT, alanine transaminase; DPI, dry powder inhaler; EIB, exercise-induced bronchospasm; HFA, hydrofluoroalkane; INR, international normalized ratio; LABA, long-acting beta$_2$ agonist; MDI, metered dose inhaler; SABA, short-acting beta$_2$ agonist.

Modified from National Asthma Education and Prevention Program [NAEPP]: *Expert panel report 3: guidelines for the diagnosis and management of asthma,* National Institutes of Health (NIH) Publication No. 08-5846, Bethesda, Md, 2007, U.S. Department of Health and Human Services, NIH, National Heart, Lung, and Blood Institute (NHLBI). Available at www.nhlbi.nih.gov/guidelines/asthma/asthsumm.pdf.

TABLE 103-3 Usual Doses for Quick-Relief Medications*

Medication	≥12 Years of Age and Adults	Potential Adverse Effects	Comments (Not All-Inclusive)
INHALED SHORT-ACTING BETA$_2$ AGONISTS			
Albuterol CFC MDI: 90 μg/puff, 200 puffs/canister Albuterol HFA MDI: 90 μg/puff, 200 puffs/canister Levalbuterol HFA MDI: 45 μg/puff, 200 puffs/canister Pirbuterol CFC MDI Autohaler: 200 μg/puff, 400 puffs/canister	*Doses apply to all four SABAs.* 2 puffs 5 min before exercise 2 puffs every 4-6 hr, as needed for symptoms	Tachycardia, skeletal muscle tremor, hypokalemia, increased lactic acid, headache, hyperglycemia. Inhaled route, in general, causes few systemic adverse effects. Patients with preexisting cardiovascular disease, especially the elderly, may have adverse cardiovascular reactions with inhaled therapy.	*Comments apply to all four SABAs.* Drugs of choice for acute bronchospasm. Differences in potencies exist, but all products are essentially comparable on a per-puff basis. An increasing use or lack of expected effect indicates diminished control of asthma. Not recommended for long-term daily treatment. Regular use exceeding 2 days/wk for symptom control (not prevention of EIB) indicates the need for additional long-term control therapy. May double usual dose for mild exacerbations. For levalbuterol, prime the inhaler by releasing 4 actuations before use. For HFA: periodically clean HFA actuator, because drug may plug orifice. Nonselective agents (i.e., epinephrine, isoproterenol, metaproterenol) are not recommended because of their potential for excessive cardiac stimulation, especially at high doses.

Continued

TABLE 103-3 Usual Doses for Quick-Relief Medications*—cont'd

Medication	≥12 Years of Age and Adults	Potential Adverse Effects	Comments (Not All-Inclusive)
Albuterol Nebulizer solution: 0.63 mg/3 mL, 1.25 mg/3 mL, 2.5 mg/3 mL, 5 mg/mL (0.5%)	1.25-5 mg in 3 mL of saline every 4-8 hr, as needed	Same as with MDI.	May mix with cromolyn solution, budesonide inhalant suspension, or ipratropium solution for nebulization. May double dose for severe exacerbations.
Levalbuterol (R-albuterol) Nebulizer solution: 0.31 mg/3 mL, 0.63 mg/3 mL, 1.25 mg/0.5 mL, 1.25 mg/3 mL	0.63-1.25 mg every 8 hr, as needed for symptoms	Same as with MDI.	Compatible with budesonide inhalant suspension. The product is a sterile-filled preservative-free unit-dose vial.
ANTICHOLINERGICS			
Ipratropium HFA MDI: 17 µg/puff, 200 puffs/canister Nebulizer solution: 0.25 mg/mL (0.025%) Ipratropium with albuterol MDI: 18 µg/puff of ipratropium bromide and 90 µg/puff of albuterol, 200 puffs/canister Nebulizer solution: 0.5 mg/3 mL ipratropium bromide and 2.5 mg/3 mL albuterol	2-3 puffs every 6 hr 0.25 mg every 6 hr 2-3 puffs every 6 hr 3 mL every 4-6 hr	Drying of mouth and respiratory secretions, increased wheezing in some individuals, blurred vision if sprayed in eyes. If used in the ED, produces less cardiac stimulation than SABAs.	Multiple doses in the ED (not hospital) setting provide additive benefit to SABA. Treatment of choice for bronchospasm caused by beta blocker medication. Does not block EIB. Reverses only cholinergically mediated bronchospasm; does not modify reaction to antigen. May be an alternative for patients who do not tolerate SABAs. Has not proven to be efficacious as long-term control therapy for asthma. Ipratropium with albuterol nebulizer solution contains EDTA to prevent discoloration of the solution. This additive does not induce bronchospasm.
SYSTEMIC CORTICOSTEROIDS			
Methylprednisolone 2-, 4-, 6-, 8-, 16-, 32-mg tablets Prednisolone 5-mg tablets, 5 mg/5 mL, 15 mg/5 mL Prednisone 1-, 2.5-, 5-, 10-, 20-, 50-mg tablets; 5 mg/mL, 5 mg/5 mL	Short course "burst": 40-60 mg/day as single or 2 divided doses for 3-10 days	Short-term use: reversible abnormalities in glucose metabolism, increased appetite, fluid retention, weight gain, facial flushing, mood alteration, hypertension, peptic ulcer, and rarely aseptic necrosis. Consideration should be given to coexisting conditions that could be worsened by systemic corticosteroids, such as herpes virus infections, varicella, tuberculosis, hypertension, peptic ulcer, diabetes mellitus, osteoporosis, and *Strongyloides* infection.	Short courses or bursts are effective for establishing control when initiating therapy or during a period of gradual deterioration. Action may begin within an hour. The burst should be continued until patient achieves 80% PEF personal best or symptoms resolve. This usually requires 3-10 days but may require longer. There is no evidence that tapering the dose after improvement prevents relapse in asthma exacerbations. Other systemic corticosteroids such as hydrocortisone and dexamethasone given in equipotent daily doses are likely to be as effective as prednisolone.
Methylprednisolone acetate Repository injection: 40 mg/mL, 80 mg/mL	240 mg IM once		May be used in place of a short burst of oral steroids in patients who are vomiting or if adherence is a problem.

*Doses are provided for those products that have been approved by the U.S. Food and Drug Administration or have sufficient clinical trial safety and efficacy data in the appropriate age ranges to support their use.

CFC, chlorofluorocarbon; EDTA, ethylenediaminetetraacetic acid; EIB, exercise-induced bronchospasm; HFA, hydrofluoroalkane; MDI, metered dose inhaler; SABA, short-acting $beta_2$ agonist.

Modified from National Asthma Education and Prevention Program (NAEPP): *Expert panel report 3: guidelines for the diagnosis and management of asthma,* National Institutes of Health (NIH) Publication No. 08-5846, Bethesda, Md, 2007, U.S. Department of Health and Human Services, NIH, National Heart, Lung, and Blood Institute (NHLBI). Available at www.nhlbi.nih.gov/guidelines/asthma/asthsumm.pdf. Medications and dosages updated in September 2011.

BOX 103-4

Management of an Asthma Attack: Home Treatment

ASSESS SEVERITY

- Patients at high risk for a fatal attack require immediate medical attention after initial treatment.
- Symptoms and signs suggestive of a more serious exacerbation such as marked breathlessness, inability to speak more than short phrases, use of accessory muscles, or drowsiness should result in initial treatment while immediately consulting with a clinician.
- Less severe signs and symptoms can be treated initially with assessment of response to therapy and further steps as listed below.
- If available, measure PEF; values of 50%-79% predicted or personal best indicate the need for quick-relief medication. Depending on the response to treatment, contact with a clinician may also be indicated. Values below 50% indicate the need for immediate medical care.

INITIAL TREATMENT

- Inhaled SABA: up to 2 treatments 20 min apart of 2-6 puffs by MDI or nebulizer treatments.
- Exacerbations of lesser severity may need fewer puffs than suggested above.

RESPONSE TO INITIAL TREATMENT

Good Response	Incomplete Response	Poor Response
No wheezing or dyspnea (assess tachypnea in young children).	Persistent wheezing and dyspnea (tachypnea).	Marked wheezing and dyspnea.
PEF is ≥80% predicted or personal best.	PEF is 50%-79% predicted or personal best.	PEF is <50% predicted or personal best.
Actions	**Actions**	**Actions**
Contact clinician for follow-up instructions and further management.	Add oral systemic corticosteroid.	Add oral systemic corticosteroid.
May continue inhaled SABA every 3-4 hr for 24-48 hr.	Continue inhaled SABA.	Repeat inhaled SABA immediately.
Consider short course of oral systemic corticosteroids.	Consult clinician urgently (this day) for further instruction.	If distress is severe and nonresponsive to initial treatment: • Call your doctor **and** • **Proceed to ED** • Consider calling 911

MDI, metered dose inhaler; SABA, short-acting $beta_2$ agonist (quick-relief inhaler).
From National Asthma Education and Prevention Program (NAEPP): *Expert panel report 3: guidelines for the diagnosis and management of asthma,* National Institutes of Health (NIH) Publication No. 08-4051, Bethesda, Md, 2007, U.S. Department of Health and Human Services, NIH, National Heart, Lung, and Blood Institute (NHLBI). Available at www.nhlbi.nih.gov/guidelines/asthma/asthgdln.htm.

TABLE 103-4 **Risk Factors and Actions to Reduce Exposures**

Risk Factor	Actions
Domestic dust mite allergens (so small they are not visible to the naked eye)	Wash bed linens and blankets weekly in hot water and dry in a hot dryer or the sun. Encase pillows and mattresses in air-tight covers. Replace carpets with linoleum or wood flooring, especially in sleeping rooms. Use vinyl, leather, or plain wooden furniture instead of fabric-upholstered furniture. If possible, use vacuum cleaner with filters.
Tobacco smoke (whether the patient smokes or breathes in the smoke from others)	Stay away from tobacco smoke. Patients and parents should not smoke.
Allergens from animals with fur	Remove animals from the home, or at least from the sleeping area.
Cockroach allergen	Clean the home thoroughly and often. Use pesticide spray—but make sure the patient is not at home when spraying occurs.
Outdoor pollens and mold	Close windows and doors and remain indoors when pollen and mold counts are highest.
Indoor mold	Reduce dampness in the home; clean any damp areas frequently.
Physical activity	Do not avoid physical activity. Symptoms can be prevented by taking a rapid-acting inhaled $beta_2$ agonist, a chromone, or a leukotriene modifier before strenuous exercise.
Drugs	Do not take beta blockers or aspirin or NSAIDs if these medicines cause asthma symptoms.

Modified from Global Initiative for Asthma (GINA): *Pocket guide for asthma management and prevention: a pocket guide for physicians and nurses,* updated 2015. Available at www.ginasthma.org.

in-hospital treatment is necessary and intravenous methylprednisolone is often used.[2] Untoward side effects of systemic corticosteroids include hypothalamic-adrenal axis suppression, electrolyte imbalances, myopathy, osteoporosis, peptic ulcer, dermal atrophy, carbohydrate intolerance, increased intracranial pressure, and psychiatric disturbances. They have less of a therapeutic index in asthma as compared with ICSs and are therefore used primarily for management of exacerbations.[29]

Cromolyn. Cromolyn sodium (Intal) is an anti-inflammatory agent whose specific mechanism of action is not yet well understood. It is used in the prophylaxis of mild to moderate asthma rather than for the treatment of acute

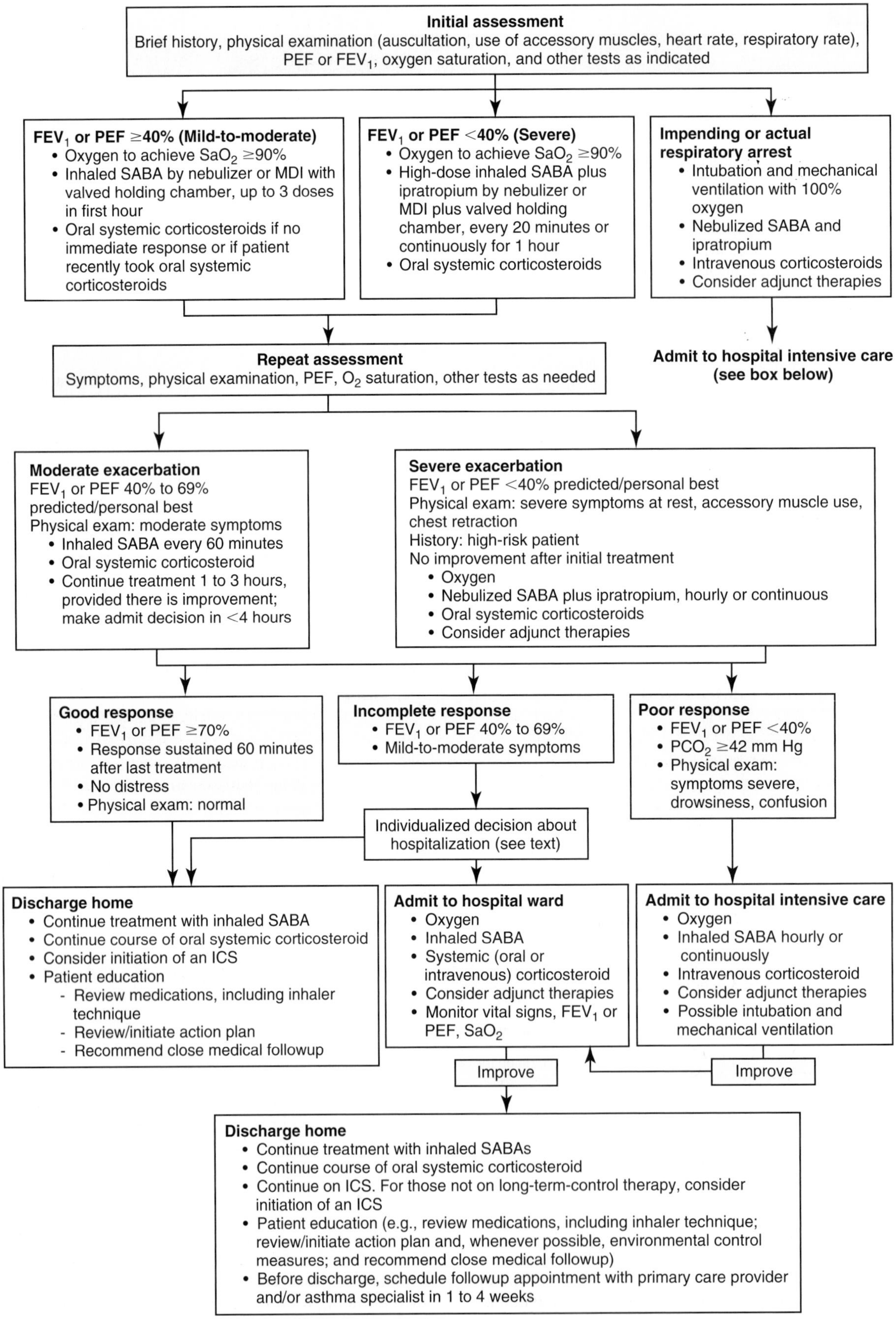

FIGURE **103-3** Management of asthma attacks: hospital-based care. (Modified from Global Initiative for Asthma [GINA]: *Pocket guide for asthma management and prevention: a pocket guide for physicians and nurses,* updated 2015. Available at www.ginasthma.org.)

TABLE 103-5 Estimated Comparative Daily Doses for Inhaled Corticosteroids

Drug	Low Daily Dose ≥12 Years of Age and Adults	Medium Daily Dose ≥12 Years of Age and Adults	High Daily Dose ≥12 Years of Age and Adults
Beclomethasone HFA 40 or 80 μg/puff	80-240 μg	>240-480 μg	>480 μg
Budesonide DPI 90, 180, or 200 μg/inhalation	180-600 μg	>600-1200 μg	>1200 μg
Flunisolide 250 μg/puff	500-1000 μg	>1000-2000 μg	>2000 μg
Flunisolide HFA 80 μg/puff	320 μg	>320–640 μg	>640 μg
Fluticasone HFA/MDI 44, 110, or 220 μg/puff	88-264 μg	>264-440 μg	>440 μg
Fluticasone DPI 50, 100, or 250 μg/inhalation	100-300 μg	>300-500 μg	>500 μg
Mometasone DPI 200 μg/inhalation	200 μg	400 μg	>400 μg
Triamcinolone acetonide 100 μg/puff	300-750 μg	>750-1500 μg	>1500 μg

DPI, dry powder inhaler; HFA, hydrofluoroalkane; MDI, metered dose inhaler.
Data from National Asthma Education and Prevention Program (NAEPP): *Expert panel report 3: guidelines for the diagnosis and management of asthma*, updated 2011. National Institutes of Health (NIH) Publication No. 08-5846, Bethesda, Md, 2007, U.S. Department of Health and Human Services, NIH, National Heart, Lung, and Blood Institute (NHLBI). Available at www.nhlbi.nih.gov/guidelines/asthma/asthsumm.pdf.

symptoms. It is more more useful when exposure to an identifiable factor (such as exercise, cold air, or animal dander) triggers symptoms and may be useful prophylactically when a known asthma trigger cannot be avoided. In such situations, cromolyn may be a good alternative to inhaled steroids because it has a better safety and side effect profile.[12]

Xanthine Derivatives. Xanthine derivatives, such as theophylline, are used for long-term asthma management and sustained relief of symptoms. Theophylline and aminophylline have a long history of use in asthma and have been traditionally considered to be bronchodilators of moderate potency. These drugs also have an inotropic effect on the diaphragm and anti-inflammatory activity, which may be beneficial in asthma. One of the major difficulties with use of theophylline is its relatively narrow therapeutic index and the potentially significant variations in plasma levels, both in a single individual and within a population over time. A number of drugs affect the metabolism of theophylline, and careful monitoring of serum levels during treatment is recommended (Table 103-6). Acceptable therapeutic plasma levels are between 10 and 20 μg/mL, although clinical improvement has been noted at subtherapeutic levels. Higher plasma levels are associated with gastrointestinal, cardiac, and central nervous system toxicity, including such symptoms as headache, nausea, vomiting, diarrhea, cardiac arrhythmias, and seizures.

The use of theophylline in asthma management has declined with the availability of other maintenance medications that have fewer side effects and do not require monitoring of serum levels. Nonetheless, theophylline may be useful in certain situations (e.g., as an additional agent to ICSs when better long-term control is still needed).

Leukotriene Modifiers. Four antileukotriene agents are currently on the market: montelukast, pranlukast, zafirlukast, and zileuton. These anti-inflammatory agents target a single group of inflammatory mediators; they interfere with the effects of leukotrienes by either blocking the leukotriene receptor or reducing the activity of enzymes required for leukotriene synthesis. As inflammatory mediators, leukotrienes increase endothelial permeability, which increases airway edema and secretion of mucus, further increasing airway obstruction. In addition, the leukotrienes directly potentiate bronchoconstriction mediated by leukotriene receptors on bronchial smooth muscle.[27] In persons with persistent asthma, the leukotriene modifiers have been shown to increase persistent bronchodilation, to reduce asthma symptoms (including nocturnal asthma symptoms), to reduce medication use, and to decrease the need for prednisone quick-relief therapy. All leukotriene modifiers can increase prothrombin times in persons receiving anticoagulant therapy; prothrombin times should be monitored more closely in these cases.

Zafirlukast, montelukast, and pranlukast are oral leukotriene receptor antagonists that prevent the binding of leukotrienes at receptor sites. Zafirlukast has a relatively rapid onset of action, and its effects are additive with beta-adrenergic bronchodilators. It has been shown to be helpful in reducing cold air–, exercise-, and allergen-induced bronchoconstriction and nocturnal asthma symptoms. Zafirlukast should be taken on an empty stomach. The leukotriene receptor antagonist montelukast is also rapidly absorbed after oral administration, with peak plasma levels achieved in 2.5 to 4 hours, depending on the dose. Montelukast is used in conjunction with other asthma therapies for the prophylaxis and chronic treatment of asthma. It should not be used as monotherapy for the treatment and management of exercise-induced bronchospasm and also should not be used for the treatment of acute asthma attacks. In clinical trials, the most common adverse side effects were similar to those

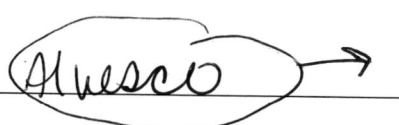

TABLE 103-6 Factors Affecting Serum Theophylline Concentrations*

Factor	Decreases Theophylline Concentrations	Increases Theophylline Concentrations	Recommended Action
Food	↓ or delays absorption of some sustained-release theophylline (SRT) products	↑ Rate of absorption (fatty foods)	Select theophylline preparation that is not affected by food.
Diet	↑ Metabolism (high protein)	↓ Metabolism (high carbohydrate)	Inform patients that major changes in diet are not recommended while taking theophylline.
Systemic, febrile viral illness (e.g., influenza)		↓ Metabolism	Decrease theophylline dose according to serum concentration level. Decrease dose by 50% if serum concentration measurement is not available.
Hypoxia, cor pulmonale, decompensated congestive heart failure, cirrhosis		↓ Metabolism	Decrease dose according to serum concentration level.
Age	↑ Metabolism (1- 9 years)	↓ Metabolism (<6 months, older adults)	Adjust dose according to serum concentration level.
Phenobarbital, phenytoin, carbamazepine	↑ Metabolism		Increase dose according to serum concentration level.
Cimetidine		↓ Metabolism	Use alternative H_2 blocker (e.g., famotidine or ranitidine).
Macrolides: erythromycin, clarithromycin, troleandomycin		↓ Metabolism	Use alternative macrolide antibiotic, azithromycin, or alternative antibiotic or adjust theophylline dose.
Quinolones: ciprofloxacin, enoxacin, pefloxacin		↓ Metabolism	Use alternative antibiotic or adjust theophylline dose. Circumvent with ofloxacin if quinolone therapy is required.
Rifampin	↑ Metabolism		Increase dose according to serum concentration level.
Ticlopidine		↓ Metabolism	Decrease dose according to serum concentration level.
Smoking	↑ Metabolism		Advise patient to stop smoking; increase dose according to serum concentration level.

*This list is not all-inclusive; for discussion of other factors, see package inserts.
From National Asthma Education and Prevention Program (NAEPP): *Expert panel report 3: guidelines for the diagnosis and management of asthma,* National Institutes of Health (NIH) Publication No. 08-5846, Bethesda, Md, 2007, U.S. Department of Health and Human Services, NIH, National Heart, Lung, and Blood Institute (NHLBI). Available at www.nhlbi.nih.gov/guidelines/asthma/asthsumm.pdf.

associated with zafirlukast. In addition, in rare cases, montelukast therapy has been associated with systemic eosinophilia, although a causal relationship has not been established.

Zileuton is an oral leukotriene synthesis inhibitor with similar effects in clinical trials to those of the leukotriene receptor antagonists. Zileuton can be taken without regard to meals. In clinical trials, zileuton therapy was associated with elevated liver enzyme levels in some subjects. For this reason, it is recommended that liver enzyme levels be obtained at baseline and monitored at regular intervals throughout the first year and periodically thereafter for persons receiving zileuton therapy. Its use is contraindicated in persons with active liver disease or with abnormal liver function test results. Zileuton also increases serum levels of theophylline, and in persons receiving concurrent theophylline therapy, the dose generally needs to be reduced by approximately 50%.[5] Several other antileukotriene agents are currently in clinical trials and are likely to receive U.S. Food and Drug Administration approval in the near future.

Because antileukotriene agents have only recently been approved for use in asthma management and because they are less potent than corticosteroids, specific guidelines for their use in asthma therapy have not yet been developed. Their use is recommended for the treatment of chronic persistent asthma. They may be helpful in reducing the quantity of inhaled or oral corticosteroids needed to control symptoms, which would be especially helpful for persons who experience troubling corticosteroid side effects. In addition, they may be effective alternatives to long-acting bronchodilators, such as salmeterol (Serevent) and theophylline. They may also be helpful for persons with aspirin-induced asthma because they offer some protection against a variety of environmental substances that often produce cross-reactions in persons with aspirin sensitivities.

Immunomodulators. Omalizumab (anti-IgE) is a monoclonal antibody that prevents binding of IgE to the high-affinity receptors on basophils and mast cells.[1] Omalizumab is used as adjunctive therapy for patients 12 years of age and older who have moderate to severe persistent asthma caused by hypersensitivity to environmental allergens (e.g., dust mites, cockroaches, cats, or dogs). Omalizumab is administered by subcutaneous injection (150 to 375 mg) every 2 to 4 weeks; the dose and frequency of injections are based on body weight and pretreatment IgE level.[12] The cost of omalizumab is high ($10,000 to $30,000 per year) compared with other drugs for asthma, and therefore its use is reserved for persons with severe, persistent asthma that is not controlled with high-dose corticosteroids. Like other protein and antibody drugs, omalizumab causes anaphylaxis in approximately one or two patients per 1000, and clinicians who administer it should be prepared and equipped to identify and to treat anaphylaxis that may occur.

Long-Acting $Beta_2$-Adrenergic Agonists. Salmeterol and formoterol are long-acting bronchodilators. Both have a much slower onset of action (1 to 2 hours after administration) and a much longer duration (at least 12 hours). Because of their slower onset of action, salmeterol and formoterol should never be used as quick-relief medications for short-term relief of acute symptoms or exacerbations or as monotherapy for long-term control of asthma.[1] LABAs are used in conjunction with ICSs for long-term control and prevention of symptoms in moderate or severe persistent asthma. Of the adjunctive therapies available, a LABA is the preferred therapy to combine with ICS in youths 12 years of age or older and adults. A LABA may be used before exercise to prevent exercise-induced bronchospasm, but the duration of action does not exceed 5 hours with chronic, regular use. Frequent or chronic use before exercise is discouraged because this may mask poorly controlled persistent asthma.[12]

Quick-Relief Medications

Short-Acting $Beta_2$-Adrenergic Agonists. SABAs act as bronchodilators by relaxing airway smooth muscle that has become constricted as a result of stimuli in the environment (see Table 103-3). Short-acting bronchodilators may also provide effective prophylaxis against anticipated asthma triggers, including exercise, cold air, and certain allergens. SABAs usually provide rapid relief of symptoms, but they do not affect the underlying inflammation associated with asthma. SABAs are not approved as maintenance medications because their use does not improve long-term asthma control. An increase in the use of bronchodilator therapy indicates worsening asthma; in fact, the need for more than 2 puffs of bronchodilator (quick-relief) medication once or twice daily or the use of more than one canister per month is generally an indication that a person's asthma is inadequately controlled. In such cases, the asthma management plan should be reviewed, and anti-inflammatory medication should probably be added to the therapy or, if it is already being used, prescribed at an increased dose. All $beta_2$-adrenergic agonists used routinely for asthma therapy have an onset of action of 10 to 15 minutes and a duration of effect of 4 to 6 hours. Side effects of the short-acting bronchodilators include tachycardia, hypertension, tremors, nervousness, headache, dizziness, hyperactivity, insomnia, nausea, and muscle cramps.

Because these medications are generally administered by metered dose inhaler, it is important that inhaler technique be reviewed on a regular basis. When bronchodilators do not promptly and completely resolve symptoms of bronchoconstriction, systemic glucocorticoid therapy is indicated for suppression and reversal of underlying airway inflammation.[12]

Anticholinergic Agents. Anticholinergic agents inhibit muscarinic cholinergic receptors, reduce intrinsic vagal tone of the airway, and are sometimes useful in reversing bronchoconstriction. Bronchial smooth muscle receptors, innervated by the vagus nerve, respond to acetylcholine, which induces bronchoconstriction. Anticholinergic agents (ipratropium bromide) have been shown to have a bronchodilator effect in persons with mild to moderate asthma, but the effect is generally not as significant as that of the short-acting $beta_2$-adrenergic agents. They may be used as alternatives for symptomatic relief for those who have difficulty tolerating the side effects of the $beta_2$-adrenergic bronchodilators.[12]

Monitoring Therapy and Asthma Severity

Asthma management guidelines stress the importance of assessment of pulmonary function with use of PEFR meters rather than basing assessment on the individual's perception of dyspnea (POD). Studies have shown that in 60% of individual, there is no correlation between POD and simultaneous peak flow measurements and that the majority of individuals have a blunted POD (i.e., an underestimation of respiratory compromise), resulting in undertreatment of asthma, a delay in treatment changes, and perhaps even a predisposition to fatal asthma attacks.[28] Therefore it is recommended that all individuals with moderate to severe asthma learn how to monitor PEF and have a flow meter at home. PEF monitoring during exacerbations should be encouraged for all those with moderate to severe, persistent asthma, and PEF should guide management. In addition, long-term daily peak flow monitoring is recommended for individuals with moderate to severe asthma to help maintain control of symptoms; however, if long-term monitoring is not done, periodic short-term monitoring is recommended for evaluating responses to therapy or assessing the effect of environmental exposures. All individuals with asthma who experience periodic severe asthma exacerbations may benefit from peak flow monitoring.[12]

Peak flow monitoring helps individuals follow the course of their disease, predict exacerbations, identify triggers, and assess their response to treatment. PEF values, specifically the individual's personal best PEF, should be used as the basis for an action plan. An individual's personal best PEF can be estimated after a 2- to 3-week period during which the PEF is recorded at least once a day in the early afternoon. Additional measurements should be made after $beta_2$-adrenergic inhalers are used for symptomatic relief. The personal best is usually achieved in the early afternoon after maximum effect of any therapy has stabilized or resolved the symptoms. The personal best should be reassessed periodically to account for progression of disease. A PEF value that is significantly higher than all the other measurements should be interpreted with caution; rather than reflecting a personal best, an outlying value may occur because of spitting or coughing into the peak flow meter.[12]

A zone system similar to a traffic light has been successfully used to help patients interpret their symptoms and PEFR results. The use of this system is particularly helpful for asthmatic patients who are unable to recognize the severity of their asthma on the basis of symptoms, which is estimated to be the case for more than 50% of patients. In addition, many studies have shown that asthma symptoms correlate poorly with the level of airway obstruction as determined by spirometry (FEV_1 and PEF). After treatment, subjective improvement in asthma symptoms may occur without a corresponding improvement in the degree of airway obstruction. For this reason, current guidelines recommend that airway obstruction be measured objectively in assessing patients with chronic asthma.[12]

The zone system consists of green, yellow, and red zones (or lights if the traffic light analogy is used). The green zone (or light) corresponds to a PEF measurement that is at least 80% of an individual's personal best or optimum control. For patients with irritable airways who decompensate quickly, the cutoff may be adjusted to 90%. A measurement in the green zone reflects good asthma control and that it is safe to proceed. The yellow zone means caution and refers to a PEF measurement that is within 50% to 80% of the individual's personal best or optimum control. Some guidelines use a range of 60% to 80% for the yellow zone; the more conservative value of 60% promotes earlier intervention as the patient's condition begins to deteriorate. Symptoms that interfere with daily activities may be present; typical symptoms include cough, wheeze, chest tightness, shortness of breath, and nocturnal awakening. A measurement in the yellow zone indicates the need for a temporary increase in medication dose or frequency. The specific medication change is tailored to each individual and may include increased bronchodilator therapy, increased or added corticosteroid therapy, and a short course of oral corticosteroids.

In many ways, the yellow zone is the key to the entire asthma action plan (AAP) because a measurement in this zone reflects worsening airway obstruction, which will usually continue to worsen if action is not taken. The written AAP should identify at what point the provider should be contacted; in general, patients should be instructed to contact their health care provider for mild to moderate symptoms that do not respond to treatment or for PEFs that remain within the yellow zone (50% to 80% of personal best). The presence of a PEF value or symptoms in the red zone means danger and indicates the need for emergency treatment. A reduction in the PEF of 50% (or 40%) and dyspnea are the general criteria for the red zone. Other associated symptoms may include inability to blow into the peak flow meter, accessory respiratory muscle use, difficulty walking or talking because of asthma, and cyanosis. Immediately using inhaled rescue bronchodilator therapy and initiating or increasing oral corticosteroid therapy are necessary. If the PEFR does not improve after emergency treatment, the individual should be instructed to call 911 (or an emergency number) or to proceed to the ED (or to his or her health care provider). The AAP should clearly state in the red zone portion when patients need to seek emergency care.

The NAEPP has developed a self-management program for asthma exacerbations that is based on the zone system (see Figs. 103-1 and 103-2). These asthma management guidelines emphasize the importance of teaching asthma self-management and prevention techniques to patients. This includes the provision of an individualized AAP, accompanied by regular medical visits and reviews by a health care provider.[12]

It has been well established that improving asthma adherence can lead to better control. Despite growing awareness of the importance of asthma education, however, adherence to asthma treatment, including medications, the use of peak flow meters, and avoidance of environmental irritants, is still poor. The provider-patient relationship is central to improving adherence; all specific strategies aimed at improving adherence (such as simplifying medication regimens or using AAPs) must be developed in a therapeutic, trusting provider-patient relationship to be effective. Studies have shown that asthma therapy based on influencing behavior and self-management of acute exacerbations results in improved control and decreased asthma morbidity.[27,28]

Current practice guidelines recommend follow-up visits at 1- to 6-month intervals, depending on the severity of asthma and the degree of control. Persons with mild asthma who, for example, experience occasional exacerbations only after exercise may need only an annual visit for asthma or have it addressed as part of an annual examination. On the other hand, persons with moderate to severe asthma with frequent exacerbations may need monthly visits to review PEFR readings and to assess the effectiveness of medications and self-management.

A wide range of risk factors contribute to poor asthma control, and these may be related to genetics, patient characteristics, variability of disease pathogenesis and severity, medication use, and environmental factors. Comorbidities such as GERD, sleep apnea, rhinitis, or rhinosinusitis may complicate disease management.[29] In addition, the association between obesity and asthma has become increasingly recognized during the past decade. A positive correlation between the risk of developing asthma and increased body mass index (in a dose-response manner) has been demonstrated.[30] There is an increased risk of morbidity from asthma among those who are morbidly obese. Treatment of obesity and other comorbidities can improve asthma control and enhance efficacy of medications.

Interdisciplinary Management

The current NIH guidelines state that all patients who have had an asthma-related hospitalization (and thus, by definition, have chronic severe asthma) be evaluated by an asthma specialist. In addition, general reasons for consultation with a specialist include poorly controlled asthma, asthma that is unresponsive to appropriate therapy, the desire to obtain a second opinion, and periodic patient evaluation. Specific reasons for specialist consultation may include classification of asthma type and severity, interpretation of PFT results, assessment of possible occupational asthma, allergy skin testing, and advice about pharmacotherapy. Evidence of poorly controlled asthma, including frequent missed days of work or school, dissatisfaction with the quality of life, and frequent ED visits and hospitalizations, may reflect lack of recognition of the disease severity by the patient or health care provider or treatment plans that are too simplistic. In such cases, referral to an asthma specialist is warranted and will likely improve control and the quality of life and decrease asthma-related morbidity and mortality.

LIFE SPAN CONSIDERATIONS

The preparation for pregnancy in women with asthma should, if possible, begin well in advance to achieve good asthma control before and during the pregnancy. In about equal proportions of women, the control of asthma will improve, worsen, or remain unchanged during pregnancy. Just as with any individual, unmanaged asthma in a pregnant woman may result in ED visits, hospitalizations, respiratory failure, and even death. In addition, poorly managed asthma has been associated with certain complications of pregnancy, including an increased incidence of preeclampsia, eclampsia, low birth weight, premature delivery, and infant death.[31] Given the potential for and possible consequences of asthma complications during pregnancy, it is vitally important that pulmonary function (minimally peak flow monitoring) be monitored throughout pregnancy. Because a 20% drop in peak flow often precedes the onset of symptoms, pregnant women need to be able to recognize when they fall below 80% of their baseline. In addition, an appreciation of ability to improve or lack of improvement is essential so that appropriate prompt treatment can be initiated.

The basic management of asthma during pregnancy is similar to that in nonpregnant individuals. To minimize the need for medications, environmental and lifestyle controls assume an even more important role. No asthma therapy has been proved to be absolutely safe during pregnancy. For women who require only beta$_2$-adrenergic agonists, metaproterenol is usually the drug of choice. For women requiring anti-inflammatory medication, the use of beclomethasone or cromolyn is considered relatively safe. During more severe exacerbations of asthma, tapered regimens of oral prednisone are used because the risks of anoxia to the fetus outweigh the possible risks of oral corticosteroid therapy.[1]

Asthma tends to be less well recognized among older adults because symptoms are often attributed to other respiratory ailments, such as COPD, congestive heart failure, pulmonary aspiration, pulmonary embolism, and bronchogenic carcinoma.[16] However, the tools usually used to diagnose asthma are still helpful in ruling out the differential diagnoses in this population.

If the clinical picture is indistinguishable from either COPD or asthma, it is often useful to consider age at onset; asthmatics have generally experienced symptoms at an earlier age and had a clearer history during their younger years.[32]

In addition, subjective awareness and perception of symptoms tend to be poorer among older adults. For these reasons, asthma remains underdiagnosed and suboptimally treated in this population. In older adults, chronic bronchitis may coexist with asthma, which may affect management. Asthma medications may aggravate coexisting medical conditions, such as cardiac disease and osteoporosis; adjustments in the pharmacotherapy may need to be made. Certain drugs commonly used in older people, including aspirin and beta blockers, may adversely affect asthma. Finally, older adults may have particular difficulty with inhaler administration; their technique should be carefully reviewed, and devices such as spacers may be especially helpful in improving drug delivery in this population. Overall, asthma in older adults tends to be associated with poor overall health and reduced mobility, despite adjustment for living conditions, depression, cognition, visual or auditory impairment, and joint pain.[23,24]

Nonetheless, appropriate care in older individuals is achievable. Most adverse reactions to asthma drugs may require dose adjustment but are typically not significant enough to warrant discontinuation of the drug. The use of a large-volume spacer improves the inhalation technique, and most older individuals prefer this device to the metered dose inhaler alone.

COMPLICATIONS

Complications of asthma include status asthmaticus and fatal asthma. Status asthmaticus is present when symptoms do not improve or remit with initial treatment of an acute exacerbation. During status asthmaticus, despite maximum therapy, respiratory failure may develop. Signs and symptoms of respiratory failure include paradoxical thoracoabdominal movement, absence of wheeze, bradycardia, and deterioration in mental status. If an exacerbation is severe enough that respiratory failure seems possible, intubation should be performed sooner rather than later.

The increasing rates of asthma morbidity and mortality are disturbing. The reasons for these increasing rates are unclear; however, certain risk factors for fatal asthma have been identified. Comorbidity (such as from cardiovascular disease or COPD) and serious psychiatric disease or psychosocial problems increase the risk of fatal or near-fatal asthma. Difficulty perceiving airflow obstruction or its severity and a history of sudden severe exacerbations also increase the risk of fatal asthma. However, a period of 2 to 7 days of worsening asthma symptoms rather than a sudden deterioration often precedes hospitalizations, providing a window of opportunity to implement more aggressive therapy in an effort to prevent fatal or near-fatal events. Additional risk factors include hospitalization or emergency care for asthma within the past month, prior asthma-related intensive care unit admission, three or more ED visits or two or more hospitalizations for asthma during the past year, and prior intubation for asthma. Other risk factors include current use or withdrawal from systemic glucocorticoids and the use of three or more canisters of inhaled SABAs per month. Urban residence, low socioeconomic status, and illicit drug use also increase the risk for fatal asthma.[12] These risk factors affirm the need for interventions designed to prevent and to control asthma as well as therapy that includes the self-management of asthma symptoms during periods of exacerbation, especially for those at high risk.

Research has demonstrated that in comparison with other patient groups, adults with asthma who have lower socioeconomic status and less education are likely to receive care that has less continuity and is less intensive after hospital or ED discharge. In addition, a minority of these patients tend to have AAPs or adequate communication with their health care providers during the acute stages of the exacerbation. In addition, those most at risk for fatal asthma are more likely to depend primarily on the ED for management of exacerbations. In other words, those individuals who are at highest risk for complications of asthma are likely to receive the type of care that increases rather than mitigates the risk of future complications.

INDICATIONS FOR REFERRAL OR HOSPITALIZATION

Referral to an asthma specialist for consultation or comanagement is recommended if there are any difficulties achieving or maintaining control of asthma or if step 3 or step 4 care is required. Hospitalization should be considered for all patients whose symptoms do not improve or remit with initial aggressive treatment of the acute exacerbation. The NHLBI's guidelines for the management of asthma exacerbations in the ED and hospital are included in Figure 103-3.

PATIENT EDUCATION

Patient education is both one of the most important and one of the most challenging aspects of asthma management. Asthma is a chronic disease and, like other chronic diseases, requires ongoing maintenance and prevention. Asthma that is treated only episodically when exacerbations occur will result in symptomatic relief at best. To achieve the other goals of asthma treatment (such as preventing symptoms, maintaining near-normal pulmonary function, minimizing the adverse effects of pharmacotherapy, and minimizing the need for ED visits and hospitalizations), patients and their families need to be well educated about the disease, its basis, and their role in monitoring symptoms and preventing exacerbations. Table 103-7

TABLE 103-7 Delivery of Asthma Education by Clinicians during Patient Care Visits

Assessment Questions	Information	Skills
RECOMMENDATIONS FOR INITIAL VISIT		
Focus on: Expectations of visit Asthma control Patient's goals for treatment Medications Quality of life *Ask relevant questions:* What worries you most about your asthma? What do you want to accomplish at this visit? What do you want to be able to do that you can't do now because of your asthma? What do you expect from treatment? What medicines have you tried? What other questions do you have for me today? Are there things in your environment that make your asthma worse?	*Teach in simple language:* What is asthma? Asthma is a chronic lung disease. The airways are very sensitive. They become inflamed and narrow; breathing becomes difficult. The definition of asthma control: few daytime symptoms, no nighttime awakenings because of asthma, able to engage in normal activities, normal lung function. Asthma treatments: two types of medicines are needed: Long-term control: medications that prevent symptoms, often by reducing inflammation Quick relief: short-acting bronchodilator relaxes muscles around airways Bring all medications to every appointment. When to seek medical advice. Provide appropriate telephone number.	*Teach or review and demonstrate:* Inhaler and spacer or valved holding chamber (VHC) use. Check performance. Self-monitoring skills that are tied to an action plan: Recognize intensity and frequency of asthma symptoms. Review the signs of deterioration and the need to reevaluate therapy: Waking at night with asthma Increased medication use Decreased activity tolerance Use of a written AAP that includes instructions for daily management and for recognizing and handling worsening asthma.
RECOMMENDATIONS FOR FIRST FOLLOW-UP VISIT (2-4 WEEKS OR SOONER AS NEEDED)		
Focus on: Expectations of visit Asthma control Patient's goals for treatment Medications Quality of life *Ask relevant questions from previous visit and also ask:* What medications are you taking? How and when are you taking them? What problems have you had using your medications? Please show me how you use your inhaled medications.	*Teach in simple language:* Use of two types of medications. Remind patient to bring all medications and the peak flow meter, if using, to every appointment for review. Self-assessment of asthma control using symptoms and/or peak flow as a guide.	*Teach or review and demonstrate:* Use of a written AAP. Review and adjust as needed. Peak flow monitoring if indicated. Correct inhaler and spacer or VHC technique.
RECOMMENDATIONS FOR SECOND FOLLOW-UP VISIT		
Focus on: Expectations of visit Asthma control Patient's goals for treatment Medications Quality of life *Ask relevant questions from previous visits and also ask:* Have you noticed anything in your home, work, or school that makes your asthma worse? Describe for me how you know when to call your doctor or go to the hospital for asthma care. What questions do you have about the AAP? Can we make it easier? Are your medications causing you any problems? Have you noticed anything in your environment that makes your asthma worse? Have you missed any of your medications?	*Teach in simple language:* Self-assessment of asthma control, using symptoms and/or peak flow as a guide. Relevant environmental control and avoidance strategies: How to identify home, work, or school exposures that can cause or worsen asthma How to control house-dust mites, animal exposures if applicable How to avoid cigarette smoke (active and passive) Review all medications.	*Teach or review and demonstrate:* Inhaler/spacer or VHC technique. Peak flow monitoring technique. Use of written AAP. Review and adjust as needed. Confirm that patient knows what to do if asthma gets worse.
RECOMMENDATIONS FOR SUBSEQUENT VISITS		
Focus on: Expectations of visit Asthma control Patients' goals of treatment Medications Quality of life Ask relevant questions from previous visits and also ask: How have you tried to control things that make your asthma worse? Please show me how you use your inhaled medication.	*Teach in simple language:* Review and reinforce all: Educational messages Environmental control strategies at home, work, or school Medications Self-assessment of asthma control, using symptoms and/or peak flow as a guide	*Teach or review and demonstrate:* Inhaler/spacer or VHC technique. Peak flow monitoring technique, if appropriate. Use of written asthma action plan. Review and adjust as needed. Confirm that patient knows what to do if asthma gets worse.

From National Asthma Education and Prevention Program (NAEPP): *Expert panel report 3: guidelines for the diagnosis and management of asthma,* National Institutes of Health (NIH) Publication No. 08-5846, Bethesda, Md, 2007, U.S. Department of Health and Human Services, NIH, National Heart, Lung, and Blood Institute (NHLBI). Available at www.nhlbi.nih.gov/guidelines/asthma/asthsumm.pdf.

BOX 103-5

Peak Flow Meters: Uses and Technique

Lung function measurements assess airflow limitation and help diagnose and monitor the course of asthma.

To assess the level of airflow limitation, two methods are used. Peak flow meters measure PEF, and spirometers measure FEV_1 and its accompanying FVC. The accuracy of all lung function measurements depends on patient effort and correct technique.

Several kinds of peak flow meters and spirometers are available, and the technique for use is similar for all. It is important to use a "low-flow" peak flow meter for younger children. Appropriate ages for use are usually indicated by the manufacturer. To use a peak flow meter:

- Stand up and hold the peak flow meter without restricting movement of the marker. Make sure the marker is at the bottom of the scale.
- Take a deep breath, put the peak flow meter in your mouth, seal your lips around the mouthpiece, and breathe out as hard and fast as possible. Do not put your tongue inside the mouthpiece.
- Record the result. Return the marker to zero.
- Repeat twice more. Choose the highest of the three readings.

Daily PEF monitoring for 2 to 3 weeks is useful, when it is available, for establishing a diagnosis and treatment. If during 2 to 3 weeks a child cannot achieve 80% of predicted PEF (predicted values are provided with all peak flow meters), it may be necessary to determine the child's personal best value (e.g., by a course of oral glucocorticosteroid).

Long-term PEF monitoring is useful, along with review of symptoms, for evaluating a child's response to therapy. PEF monitoring can also help detect early signs of worsening before symptoms occur.

Note: Examples of available peak flow meters and instructions for use of inhalers and spacers can be found at www.ginasthma.org.

Data from Global Initiative for Asthma (GINA): *Pocket guide for asthma management and prevention in children,* updated 2005. Available at www.ginasthma.org.

summarizes asthma education to be included as part of patient care visits.

Every patient with asthma should participate with his or her health care provider in setting up an individualized written asthma management plan, or AAP, that includes his or her own asthma triggers, detailed description of relevant environmental control measures, instructions on the role and use of medications and delivery devices (e.g., spacers, nebulizers), monitoring techniques (e.g., PEFR meters), and instructions on how to tailor therapy to deal with changing symptoms. The use of peak flow meters and proper inhaler technique are described in Boxes 103-5 and 103-6, respectively. Patients should be taught how to recognize symptom patterns, to interpret PEFR results, and to increase treatment during exacerbations of asthma. An AAP based on signs and symptoms or PEFR should be developed for each individual, with instructions on how and when to change pharmacotherapy and when to contact the health care provider. Emphasis should be placed on the long-term control medications (anti-inflammatory medications) used to achieve and to maintain control of persistent asthma and quick-relief medications (bronchodilators) used to treat acute symptoms and exacerbations.[12] In addition to allowing the early recognition of symptoms and earlier initiation of treatment, which can minimize the severity of exacerbations, AAPs also increase confidence, security, and ability for self-control in individuals with asthma and their families.

BOX 103-6

Proper Metered Dose Inhaler Technique with and Without a Spacer

1. Remove cap, hold inhaler upright, and shake inhaler well.
2. Tilting your head back slightly, exhale slowly and fully.
3. Place mouthpiece between lips, or open mouth widely and hold inhaler 1 to 2 inches from mouth.
4. Press down on inhaler once as you start to inhale slowly and deeply.
5. Continue to inhale slowly and deeply as long as you can.
6. Hold breath for 10 seconds (at least 4 seconds).
7. Exhale slowly through nose or pursed lips.
8. Repeat puffs as prescribed, waiting at least 1 minute between puffs.

Patients with asthma should have a copy of their AAP at home, work, and school, with all medications available at each location. In addition, they should be reminded and encouraged to plan ahead for vacations—to have an AAP with them and to know ED locations and phone numbers.

Persons with asthma and other household members need to be educated about the role of environmental triggers of asthma and efforts that they can take to reduce environmental hazards in the home and surrounding areas. Cleaning crews often require specialized training and equipment to decrease allergen levels in the environments they are servicing.

CHAPTER 104

CHEST PAIN (NONCARDIAC)

David Patrick Murphy • William A. Boller

DEFINITION AND EPIDEMIOLOGY

Noncardiac chest pain is a recurrent substernal chest pressure or other chest discomfort believed to be unrelated to the heart after a reasonable cardiac evaluation. Because heart disease is the leading cause of death in the United States and because patients are commonly initially seen with chest pain in the primary care setting, it is important to be able to distinguish cardiac from noncardiac causes of chest pain.[1] Research indicates that it is possible to accurately differentiate between the two in most cases. In a study of all patients initially diagnosed with noncardiac chest pain, 93.6% had no evidence of adverse cardiac events, 3.5% had possible evidence of adverse cardiac events, and only 2.8% had a definite cardiac event.[2]

Nevertheless, symptoms of chest pain are frightening to patients, but reassuringly, most episodes seen in the primary care setting are not of cardiac origin. According to one report, 67% of chest pain diagnoses were a result of musculoskeletal, gastrointestinal, psychiatric, or pulmonary disorders. Only 16% were secondary to cardiac causes of all types, and another 16% were idiopathic.[3] Table 104-1 summarizes the data from that study.

Interestingly, even when patients have risk factors or indications for invasive diagnostic workups, data consistently show that a large percentage of these patients' pain still does not have

TABLE 104-1 Causes of Chest Pain in the Primary Care Setting

Final Diagnosis	Percent of Episodes
Musculoskeletal conditions and chest wall pain	36.2
Gastrointestinal conditions	18.9
Nonspecific chest pain	16.1
Stable angina	10.5
Psychogenic pain	7.5
Respiratory condition	5.1
Nonischemic cardiac condition	3.8
Acute cardiac ischemia	1.5

Study included 399 patients in 12 family practice clinics in Michigan.[3]

BOX 104-1

Sample Questions for Patients with Chest Pain

- Where is the pain?
- How long have you had the pain?
- Do you have recurrent episodes of pain?
- How long does each episode last?
- What makes the pain better? worse? (breathing? lying flat? moving your arms, neck?)
- How would you describe the pain? (burning? crushing? throbbing? stabbing? knifelike?)
- When does the pain occur? (with exertion? after eating? when moving your arms?)
- Is the pain associated with shortness of breath? (cough? palpitations? nausea and vomiting? fever? leg pain? coughing up blood?)

Modified from Swartz MB, editor: The heart. In *Textbook of physical diagnosis: history and examination,* ed 5, Philadelphia, 2006, Elsevier.

a cardiac cause. For example, when patients undergo cardiac catheterization, approximately 20% to 30% are found to have normal or insignificantly diseased coronary arteries.[4] In another study, 81% of moderate-risk women with chest pain syndrome were prospectively demonstrated to be experiencing noncardiac discomfort. Of the remainder, only 2.5% of women actually experienced cardiac events.[5]

The correct diagnosis for chest pain is most often obtained with a detailed history, supporting physical examination findings, and an electrocardiogram (ECG) or chest radiograph if indicated. Ruling out cardiac causes of chest pain or other noncardiac life-threatening conditions is an essential first step. The evaluation of cardiac chest pain is discussed separately in Chapter 120.

Immediate emergency department referral or specialist referral is indicated for hemodynamic instability or suspected pulmonary embolism, pneumothorax, esophageal rupture, or aortic dissection.

PATHOPHYSIOLOGY

The sympathetic chain, vagus, and phrenic nerves are responsible for carrying pain impulses in the thoracic cage. All the structures in the chest, including the chest wall, esophagus, lungs, heart, and diaphragm, have overlapping innervation. Thus, pain from different organs, including those in the abdomen that abut the diaphragm (liver, spleen, stomach), may have similar referral patterns. In addition, patients may have a difficult time localizing pain from deep structures, whereas diseases involving more superficial structures, such as the chest wall and pleura, are more easily localized. Because there is no sensory innervation in the lung parenchyma, disease involving the alveoli or interstitium does not cause chest pain unless the pulmonary vasculature, bronchi, or pleura is involved.[6]

CLINICAL PRESENTATION

The history is crucial in determining the differential diagnosis and appropriate management in individuals complaining of chest pain. Careful questioning usually clarifies the cause. Some examples of questions are listed in Box 104-1. The following descriptions should be pursued when the patient is questioned[7]:

Quality: "Can you describe your pain?" Myocardial ischemia typically manifests as a tightness or viselike, constricting, or heavy pressure sensation. On the other hand, pleuritic pain or pain that is positional, sharp, or reproducible with palpation is often not cardiac.

Location: "Where is your pain?" Pain that localizes to a small area of the chest suggests pleural or chest wall involvement. Ischemic pain, however, is often difficult to localize. In fact, in an observational study in patients admitted with chest pain, patients who vocalized larger areas of discomfort were more likely be experiencing a cardiac event than patients who complained of smaller areas.[8]

Intensity: "How severe is your pain?" Pain from an aortic dissection, pneumothorax, or pulmonary embolism all tend to have an abrupt start with the greatest intensity at the beginning. Ischemic chest pain is more gradual, and psychogenic causes of chest pain have a vaguer onset.

Duration: "How long does your pain last?" If the chest pain lasts only seconds or has been constant for weeks, it is unlikely cardiac. Ischemic cardiac pain typically lasts for a few minutes.

Aggravation: "What provokes your pain or makes it worse?" Symptoms related to eating, such as dysphagia, odynophagia, and heartburn, are more suggestive of an upper gastrointestinal cause, whereas chest pain that worsens with physical exertion is usually more reflective of cardiac ischemia. Aggravation of the pain with position changes, deep breathing, or cough is often indicative of a musculoskeletal or pleural disorder.

Alleviation: "What makes your pain better?" Repeated palliation with antacids or food suggests a gastrointestinal source. Esophageal and cardiac causes are generally attenuated with sublingual nitroglycerin. Pain that lessens with rest and cessation of physical activity strongly suggests an ischemic cause.

The patient's description of his or her symptoms should be viewed in the context of any history of cardiac, pulmonary, psychiatric, or musculoskeletal diseases. It is important to determine whether the patient has a history of similar symptoms or other illness, such as heart disease, pulmonary disease, and diabetes, or a family history of heart disease. Other information to be elicited includes whether the patient has engaged in any recent unusual or strenuous physical activity; whether the patient has experienced any heartburn, difficult or painful swallowing, or water brash; and whether the patient tends to eat before bedtime. The patient should be questioned about whether there has been any blood in the stool or symptoms consistent with anemia. The presence of any recent emotional or psychological stress should also be assessed. Daily caffeine intake and any street or illicit drug use should be discussed as well. Lastly, a thorough review of current medications, both over-the-counter and illicit, should be obtained. All this information may contribute to the decision-making process.[4]

Diagnosis of chest pain in the clinical setting has classically been based on some of the factors listed earlier, including location, description, and precipitants of the pain. This has led to a widely accepted classic angina syndrome, which has been shown to correlate well with underlying coronary artery disease (CAD) in both men and women. However, research indicates that women, elderly individuals, and patients with diabetes with CAD often experience less-typical symptoms, which can result in a missed diagnosis and improper treatment.[5]

PHYSICAL EXAMINATION

Examination of a patient with chest pain starts with an assessment of his or her general appearance and vital signs. The evaluation must begin with an exclusion of cardiac disease. The general appearance suggests the severity and possibly the seriousness of the symptoms. Abnormalities in vital signs suggest an infectious, pulmonary, cardiac, or malignant process. Hemodynamic instability should prompt immediate referral to the emergency department. The majority of patients with noncardiac chest pain should have normal vital signs. The neck examination should focus on the presence of lymphadenopathy in the cervical chains or supraclavicular fossa. Elevation of the neck veins indicates volume overload and possible heart failure. Tracheal deviation points to a possible pneumothorax.

A general inspection of the chest may reveal a rash, such as the unilateral rash of herpes zoster in a thoracic dermatome. Evidence of trauma may confirm a history of domestic violence or indicate its existence, even if the patient did not discuss it.

Palpation of the chest and range of motion of the upper body may cause chest pain in the presence of costochondritis, musculoskeletal disease, fibromyalgia, rib fracture, or trauma. Dullness to percussion over a portion of the posterior chest indicates either a pleural effusion or a consolidative pulmonary process such as pneumonia.

Auscultation of the lungs may elicit asymmetric breath sounds, pleural friction rub, wheezing, crackles, or absent or decreased breath sounds, all of which should prompt additional investigation with a chest radiograph. The cardiac examination should evaluate for the presence of murmurs, extra heart sounds (S_3 or S_4), or friction rubs.

Examination of the abdomen may reveal tenderness in the epigastric area or right or left upper quadrants, causing irritation of the diaphragm and resultant referred chest pain. Finally, many patients with noncardiac chest pain will actually have completely normal physical examination findings.

DIAGNOSTICS

The diagnostic testing options for chest pain are often limited in the primary care setting. If the patient's chest pain seems cardiac in origin, a 12-lead ECG may demonstrate characteristic abnormalities. Although a normal ECG reduces the likelihood of an acute coronary syndrome by 70% to 90%, it does not completely rule it out. An ECG should always be interpreted in the context of the patient's history and risk factors for heart disease.[9]

In individuals younger than 40 years, a normal ECG may be sufficient to rule out cardiac disease. However, in older patients or in those with risk factors (e.g., smoking, obesity, diabetes, hyperlipidemia, stress), cardiac enzymes, stress testing, or coronary angiography may also be necessary.[2] Noninvasive electrocardiographic stress testing is less reliable in women than in men; in women, it is associated with an increased frequency of false-positive results and frequent failure to achieve target heart rates. For these reasons, image-based stress testing has a strong predictive value and may be more diagnostically helpful in women than other noninvasive stress test modalities.[5]

Empirical response to a proton pump inhibitor (PPI) has been shown in studies to be a reasonable first-line means to diagnose gastroesophageal reflux disease (GERD) as a source of chest pain, equal to or better than invasive and expensive testing, such as esophageal pH monitoring, manometry, and upper endoscopy, with sensitivity of 80% and specificity of 74%.[10,11] A short course of a high-dose PPI twice daily for 1 to 2 months demonstrating good clinical response is sufficient for diagnosis. After this, the dose should be tailored to the lowest once-daily regimen that provides symptom control.[12]

The chest x-ray study is a useful diagnostic tool for detecting cardiac and pulmonary abnormalities. Pulse oximeters should be available to determine the oxygen saturation. On occasion, other studies may be needed, such as an arterial blood gas (ABG) analysis or a complete blood count (CBC) with differential. In most cases, however, a detailed history, physical examination, and possibly an ECG or chest radiograph should give enough information for a hypothesis to be formed regarding the cause of the symptoms.

DIAGNOSTICS

Chest Pain (Noncardiac)

INITIAL
ECG
Pulse oximetry

LABORATORY
CBC and differential*
ABGs*
Serum cardiac biomarkers*

IMAGING
Chest x-ray studies (posteroanterior and lateral)
Echocardiography*

OTHER DIAGNOSTICS
Electrocardiographic stress testing (exercise or pharmacologic)*
Coronary angiography*

*If indicated.

DIFFERENTIAL DIAGNOSIS

The most common causes of noncardiac chest pain in the primary care setting are gastrointestinal, musculoskeletal, pulmonary, and psychiatric disorders.[3] In one study, gastroesophageal disease accounted for approximately 42% of all cases of chest pain and was the most common cause in persons for whom myocardial infarction (MI) was ruled out.[1] The gastroesophageal causes of chest pain include GERD, esophageal rupture or perforation (Boerhaave syndrome), esophageal spasm, pill-induced esophagitis, peptic ulcer, pancreatitis, and cholecystitis. Symptoms highly suggestive of an esophageal disorder, especially reflux disease, include dysphagia, odynophagia, regurgitation, heartburn, and cough.[1,13] Clinical history alone cannot reliably differentiate between cardiac and esophageal chest pain. For example, chest pain associated with GERD may also be triggered by exertion or have other characteristics similar to angina, such as relief with nitroglycerin.[14] However, pain related to an esophageal disorder is more likely to last for hours, to occur retrosternally without radiation, to interrupt sleep, and to be related to meals more often than cardiac chest pain. It is also more often related to other esophageal symptoms, such as dysphagia and heartburn. One important point to consider is that cardiac and gastrointestinal diagnoses can coexist, and the management of one should not eliminate consideration of therapy for the other. In fact, one publication interestingly revealed that over 30% of patients sent to cardiology had concurrent gastrointestinal disease and that patients with true CAD might still benefit from PPI therapy, because of decreased chest pain and fewer emergency department visits with the addition of gastroesophageal medical management.[15]

With regard to esophageal perforation, this is usually caused by instrument-induced damage, foreign body impaction, forceful straining or vomiting, and diseases of the esophagus, such as esophagitis or neoplasm. The classic history for esophageal perforation is profound, sudden, severe, and constant pain from the neck to the epigastrium that is worsened by swallowing. Pain may occur after severe retching and vomiting.

Recent use of prescriptions such as doxycycline, nonsteroidal anti-inflammatory drugs (NSAIDs), or alendronate may suggest pill-induced esophagitis. Although any pill, if it is not swallowed properly and with enough fluid, may cause esophagitis, alendronate has received much attention for this side effect, earning specific recommendations to swallow the pill with at least 6 to 8 ounces of water and to remain upright for at least 30 minutes after swallowing. In one study, 65.8% of cases of pill esophagitis were related to use of antibiotics, especially in the tetracycline group.[16] Accidental ingestion of caustic substances can also cause chemical esophagitis.

Musculoskeletal conditions are indeed a common cause of chest pain and in one study accounted for up to 28% of chest pain in patients for whom MI was ruled out.[1] Chest pain related to musculoskeletal conditions is often nagging and persistent, lasting anywhere from hours to weeks. Patients usually complain of superficial chest pain localized in a small area. The symptoms are aggravated by position, deep breathing, turning, or arm movement. Causes of musculoskeletal chest wall pain include costochondritis, routine muscle strains, rheumatologic diseases such as rheumatoid arthritis, ankylosing spondylitis, fibromyalgia, and other nonrheumatologic diseases such as neoplasms and fractures.

Fibromyalgia is a complex widespread pain syndrome, often with visceral and somatic pain components. It is often part of a larger spectrum of central sensitization that includes depression, chronic headaches, post-traumatic stress disorder, functional gastrointestinal disorders, and chronic fatigue. Complaints such as fatigue, nonrestorative sleep, chronic headache or gastrointestinal complaints, or cognitive disturbance may indicate fibromyalgia as the cause of chest pain. Specific tender points on the second rib lateral to the costochondral junction and the midpoint of the upper border of the trapezius, although not specific, are of importance in making the diagnosis.[17]

Herpes zoster can cause acute chest pain that is usually described as a burning sensation, usually in a unilateral dermatomic distribution. Pain often occurs before the onset of vesicular lesions, so physical examination findings may not be present at the time of the initial complaint, making diagnosis difficult.[1] A history of zoster or varicella may be helpful in making this diagnosis.

Finally, the cause of chest pain may be pulmonary if the vasculature, parenchyma, or pleural tissue is affected; the associated pain is frequently described as pleuritic in nature, such as pain worsened with breathing, coughing, chest movement, sneezing, or talking. Pleuritic pain may also be described as stabbing or shooting chest pain or, if mild pain, as "a stitch in the side." Pulmonary embolism is a common and often missed diagnosis and is suggested by the onset of dyspnea, pleuritic chest pain, severe hypoxia, and the presence of risk factors such as recent surgery, underlying malignant disease, and a sedentary lifestyle.[1] These symptoms are obviously nonspecific and require a high degree of clinical suspicion with special attention to known risk factors of pulmonary embolism, such as immobilization, history of previous venous thromboembolism, recent surgery, pregnancy, or malignant disease.

Another diagnosis that should be considered in patients with the sudden onset of sharp, stabbing chest pain is pneumothorax. Patients with primary spontaneous pneumothorax are typically young, tall, thin men who smoke and have no history of lung disease.[6] Secondary spontaneous pneumothoraces occur in patients with cystic fibrosis, chronic obstructive pulmonary disease, and human immunodeficiency virus (HIV) and *Pneumocystis* pneumonia. Patients who have pneumonia as the underlying cause of their chest pain are usually easily diagnosed on the basis of the cough, fever, sputum production, and findings on physical examination and chest x-ray study.

Psychiatric diseases may underlie symptoms of chest pain in some primary care patients. In one study, patients with noncardiac chest pain and no abnormalities on upper endoscopy or other explanation for their symptoms had a higher prevalence of panic disorder, obsessive-compulsive disorder, and major depressive episodes.[13] These patients tend to be younger and female and have atypical symptoms and other diagnosed psychiatric illnesses. In patients, especially older women, with acute life stressors and symptoms of a panic attack, Takotsubo stress cardiomyopathy should be considered whether or not the patient's ECG shows changes, especially if there are vital sign changes present such as bradycardia or hypotension.[18,19]

Finally, the cause of chest pain may be attributed to vascular or non-MI cardiac source. Important items to explore in a patient history are family history of sickle cell anemia, which would prompt evaluation of sickle crisis, or acute chest syndrome. Mitral valve prolapse may also cause chest discomfort without ECG changes, and patients may have a family history, an associated connective tissue disorder, and the characteristic mid-systolic click on examination. Patients with less than 50% stenosis on cardiac catheterization but with a change on their cardiac stress test result may still warrant follow-up appointments with cardiology, given the high percentage of patients, 20% to 30% in one study, with characteristic chest pain who may fall under the diagnosis of cardiac syndrome X.[20] These cardiac causes are discussed more in depth in other portions of this textbook.

DIFFERENTIAL DIAGNOSIS

Cardiac and Noncardiac Causes of Chest Pain

CARDIAC

Ischemic
- Angina
- Myocardial infarction
- Aortic stenosis
- Hypertrophic cardiomyopathy
- Coronary vasospasm

Nonischemic
- Pericarditis
- Aortic dissection
- Mitral valve prolapse

PULMONARY
- Bronchitis
- Malignant disease
- Pleurisy
- Pneumonia
- Pneumothorax
- Pulmonary embolism

MUSCULOSKELETAL
- Arthritis
- Costochondritis
- Compression radiculopathy
- Rib fractures
- Fibromyalgia

GASTROINTESTINAL
- Esophageal hyperalgesia
- Gastritis
- Reflux esophagitis
- Referred gallbladder, pancreatic, hepatic, or splenic pain
- Esophageal spasm
- Esophageal perforation

DERMATOLOGIC
- Herpes zoster

PSYCHIATRIC
- Major depression
- Panic disorder
- Generalized anxiety disorder
- Takotsubo stress cardiomyopathy

AGE CONSIDERATIONS

After cardiac and life-threatening noncardiac conditions have been excluded, the patient's age is often an important factor in determining the diagnosis. In general, younger patients' chest pain is caused by more benign underlying conditions, whereas older patients with more risk factors and comorbid conditions are more likely to have serious causes of their chest pain. Regardless of the patient's age, cardiac and life-threatening noncardiac conditions should be ruled out first.

MANAGEMENT

Management of patients with chest pain depends on the cause of the disease process (Fig. 104-1). As noted earlier, exclusion of CAD and life-threatening noncardiac causes of chest pain is an essential first step.

When the clinical picture suggests an esophageal source, the goals of therapy are to heal the esophagus, to control symptoms, and to prevent recurrence and complications. Mild to moderate GERD can be initially treated with once-daily administration of any of the H_2 receptor antagonists or PPIs. If symptoms remain, a trial of a PPI for 8 weeks with twice-daily administration is usually recommended. For persisting symptoms, the patient should then be referred to a gastroenterologist for formal pH testing or endoscopy, continuing his or her medical therapy until evaluated by the specialist.[21]

Musculoskeletal chest pain therapy includes the use of NSAIDs, rest, heat, or ice. Physical therapy may likewise be appropriate for some causes of musculoskeletal chest pain. Scheduled acetaminophen or ibuprofen may also be helpful in these patients, although careful discussion of kidney function and any history of GI ulcers should be considered before initiation of scheduled therapy.

If a pulmonary disorder is suspected and confirmed by a chest radiograph, treatment will be self-evident. In the case of pneumonia, first-line treatment with antibiotics is indicated (see Chapter 111). A follow-up chest x-ray study should be done 6 to 8 weeks after treatment in all patients older than 50 years to document resolution of the infiltrate and to assess for an underlying cause of the process, such as a malignant neoplasm or another structural defect. Patients with a pneumothorax or suspected pulmonary embolism should be referred to the emergency department. An intraparenchymal or pleura-based mass causing chest pain deserves additional workup with chest computed tomography (CT), pain management with analgesics, and a referral to a pulmonologist.

Psychiatric disease as a cause of noncardiac chest pain is common; however, it should always be a diagnosis of exclusion. If a diagnosis of panic disorder, depression, or generalized anxiety disorder is suspected, selective serotonin reuptake inhibitors are effective.

One study even demonstrated a benefit of reducing daily noncardiac chest pain by 50% in those patients who did not meet *Diagnostic and Statistical Manual of Mental Disorders,* Fourth Edition (DSM-IV) criteria for panic disorder, major depressive disorder, or generalized anxiety disorder but who did not otherwise have an explanation for their symptoms.[22] In addition, patients with these diagnoses have been shown to benefit from cognitive behavioral therapy.[23]

COMPLICATIONS

Pulmonary embolism can be life-threatening if diagnosis and treatment are delayed. Thus, clinical suspicion of pulmonary embolism is important in all patients who are seen with respiratory or cardiac complaints. A pneumothorax can develop into a tension pneumothorax if it is not treated appropriately. With a tension pneumothorax, there is a mediastinal and tracheal shift to the contralateral side, hypotension, and an increase in respiratory distress. This condition can be rapidly fatal if it is not diagnosed and treated. Pneumonia can proceed to respiratory failure even in young and otherwise healthy patients. Esophageal perforation leads to mediastinitis. Finally, acute aortic dissection can lead to cardiac valvular insufficiency, rapid hemodynamic collapse, and death if it is not addressed promptly.

INDICATIONS FOR REFERRAL OR HOSPITALIZATION

In patients with suspected reflux causing chest pain, a lack of response to high-dose PPI therapy should prompt a referral to a gastroenterologist.

A pulmonologist should be consulted for any mass on chest x-ray film and for patients with recurring or nonresolving pneumonia; these conditions may indicate an underlying malignant neoplasm or immune deficiency.

Patients with suspected pulmonary embolism who are stable require diagnostic testing (D-dimer and pulmonary CT scan).

Unstable patients with suspected pulmonary embolism require emergency care and transfer to the nearest emergency center.

Emergency department referral or specialist referral is necessary when a cardiac origin of chest pain or a life-threatening noncardiac cause cannot be excluded. See Box 104-2 for a list of common red flags that warrant escalation of care. A practitioner's clinical judgment is the ultimate reason to refer—this list is by no means all-inclusive.

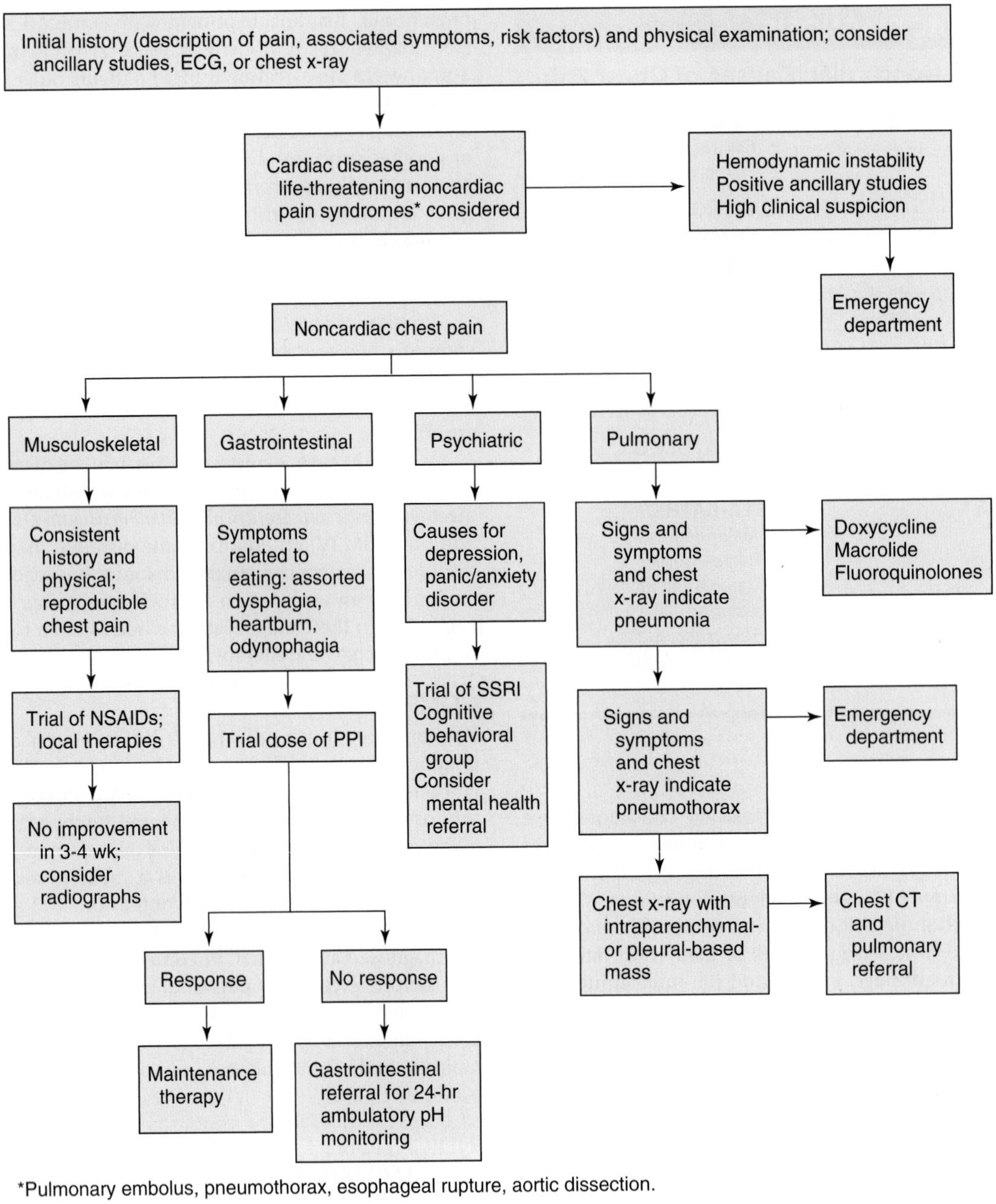

FIGURE 104-1 Approach to the patient with noncardiac chest pain. CT, computed tomography; PPI, proton pump inhibitor; SSRI, selective serotonin reuptake inhibitor. (Modified from Fang J, Bjorkman D: A critical approach to non-cardiac chest pain: pathophysiology, diagnosis, and treatment, *Am J Gastroenterol* 96:958-968, 2001.)

BOX 104-2

Clinical Signs Warranting Immediate Transfer to Higher Level of Care

- Respiratory distress (breathlessness, tachypnea, hypoxia, hypoxemia)
- Significant hypotension or hypertension
- Signs of abnormal perfusion—cyanosis, altered mental status
- Asymmetric breath sounds
- New heart murmurs, rubs, or gallops
- Pulsus paradoxus >10 mm Hg
- Abnormal ECG findings or cardiac enzymes if done in clinic
- Widened mediastinum on chest x-ray examination
- Significant hematemesis
- Pleuritic chest pain
- Sharp chest pain radiating through to the back
- Subcutaneous crepitus

PATIENT AND FAMILY EDUCATION AND HEALTH PROMOTION

Noncardiac chest pain can be a diagnosis with significant morbidity, depending on the cause. Ensuring that patients are well informed about their diagnosis, its natural history, and possible complications improves the probability of a positive outcome. Patient education should emphasize how to recognize cardiac, pulmonary, or musculoskeletal chest pain and what to do when it occurs, including when to call 911 (or universal emergency number). If the patient smokes, he or she should receive counseling on the importance of tobacco cessation at every visit. If any medications are prescribed, instructions should incorporate the correct administration of the drugs and their possible side effects.

CHAPTER 105

CHRONIC COUGH

Patricia Polgar-Bailey

DEFINITION AND EPIDEMIOLOGY

Cough is a common symptom in persons with a wide range of respiratory and nonrespiratory diseases, as well as individuals who are not ill.[1] Cough, an important reflex action and respiratory defense mechanism, is designed to prevent the aspiration of foreign material into the lower respiratory tract and to clear excessive secretions, mucus, fluids, foreign matter, and infectious organisms from the larynx, trachea, and large bronchi.[2] Cough has a protective role that is illustrated by the possible complications resulting from cough suppression, such as infections. However, cough can also transmit disease through airborne droplets and the contamination of objects, and it can be associated with complications, particularly when it is chronic. Excessive and chronic cough can result in numerous complications, including headache, anorexia, vomiting, throat pain, subconjunctival hemorrhages, fatigue, insomnia, myalgia, dysphonia, perspiration, urinary incontinence, syncope, rib pain and rib fractures, inguinal or abdominal wall herniations, diaphragmatic rupture, anxiety, and depression.[2,3] Chronic cough can have a profound psychological and emotional impact.[3] Many adults with chronic cough report feeling self-conscious about their cough and can become socially isolated owing to the associated complications, such as incontinence. In addition, older adults with chronic cough often feel anxious that "something's wrong"; in studies, a significant percentage have expressed a specific fear of cancer.[3] Chronic cough may be a symptom of underlying disease. For these reasons, a persistent chronic cough is a cause for concern for both the patient and the health care provider.

Coughs may be classified as acute (lasting less than 3 weeks), subacute (lasting 3 to 8 weeks), and chronic (persisting beyond 8 weeks).[3] Most coughs are acute and self-limited; 90% are caused by viral upper respiratory tract infections, two thirds of which clear within 2 weeks.[2] Nonviral causes of acute cough include exacerbations of asthma and exposure to environmental pollutants.[2]

A cough that persists for more than 3 weeks and for which initial treatment has failed should be investigated. Subacute cough is generally caused by bacterial sinusitis or asthma, but it can also be caused by upper respiratory infections. The cough that follows a viral or virus-like infection (e.g., *Mycoplasma pneumoniae* or *Bordetella pertussis*) is sometimes referred to as a postinfectious cough. A postinfectious cough, by definition, lasts no longer than 8 weeks; chest radiograph findings are normal, and the cough eventually resolves, generally without intervention.[4] Thus, subacute postinfectious cough can be distinguished from chronic cough by the duration of symptoms; the chronic cough lasts for 8 weeks or more and usually much longer.[3] The American College of Chest Physicians (ACCP) has developed evidence-based clinical practice guidelines for the management of postinfectious cough, which can be found at chestjournal.chestpubs.org.

Cough is reportedly the most frequent reason for visits to primary care providers and accounts for approximately 8% of all encounters.[5] In the United States and Europe, cough is estimated to affect 9% to 33% of the population, and its prevalence may be increasing as a result of worsening environmental pollution.[1,2] Chronic cough is often related to cigarette smoking, and the prevalence of chronic cough is three times higher in smokers than in nonsmokers or ex-smokers.[2] Chronic bronchitis (primarily from cigarette smoking) is another common cause of chronic cough. Exposure to secondhand smoke and other irritants also increases the risk for development of a chronic cough.

Chronic cough can have many causes in addition to exposure to cigarette smoke, but only a few diseases account for most cases. In adults, the three most common causes of chronic cough with normal chest radiography include the corticosteroid-responsive eosinophilic airway diseases (asthma, cough variant asthma, and eosinophilic bronchitis), upper airway cough syndrome (previously referred to as postnasal drip syndrome), and gastroesophageal reflux disease (GERD).[1] These have been referred to as the pathogenic triad of chronic cough, accounting for almost all cases of cough in immunocompetent, nonsmoking adults who have normal chest radiographs and are not taking angiotensin-converting enzyme (ACE) inhibitors. The incidence of ACE inhibitor–induced cough has been estimated at 10%, but there is geographic variation and in certain countries, such as China, the prevalence is estimated to be as high as 44%.[3]

An understanding of the anatomic, physiologic, and pathophysiologic aspects of cough is important for diagnosis and appropriate treatment. The systematic, diagnostic protocol uses the anatomic characteristics of the cough reflex and innervation as a guide to finding the cause of the cough (Box 105-1).

PATHOPHYSIOLOGY

When a neural receptor along the respiratory tree is stimulated, an afferent signal is transmitted to the "cough center" of the

BOX 105-1

Characteristics of Chronic Cough

- When did the cough start?
- Is it severe at night or during the day?
- Is it productive or dry?
- What characteristic does the sputum have?

brain, which is located in the medulla. From this center, through a complex reflex arc, the impulse is passed down the efferent pathway to the expiratory musculature.

The receptors of the afferent limb can be found anywhere along the respiratory tree. These include the vagus from the ears, larynx, trachea, bronchi, pleurae, and gastrointestinal tract; the trigeminal from the nose and the sinuses; the glossopharyngeal from the pharynx; and the phrenic from the diaphragm.

The efferent limb consists primarily of the phrenic and spinal nerves. After the stimulus reaches the cough center, the cough begins with a deep inspiration to approximately 50% of the vital capacity. This allows maximum expiratory flow by increasing the lung elastic recoil and by decreasing airway frictional resistance. During this phase, the glottis opens widely to allow rapid entry of large amounts of air into the lung. The glottis rapidly closes and the abdominal and intercostal muscles contract, increasing the intrapleural pressures to 100 to 200 mm Hg. In a fraction of a second, the glottis reopens, causing an explosive release of air. During this phase, the tracheobronchial tree narrows, resulting in forces sufficient to strip mucus off the walls, creating sputum.

CLINICAL PRESENTATION

A careful and detailed history will provide the diagnosis in the majority of cases of cough. Careful consideration of the various characteristics of cough may aid diagnosis (Fig. 105-1). A cough that lasts for 3 consecutive months for more than 2 consecutive years is indicative of chronic bronchitis. A sudden onset of cough in the supine position with an associated sour taste in the mouth suggests esophageal reflux. A cough associated with constant throat clearing and thick mucus production, especially on rising from bed, is consistent with upper airway cough and sinusitis. A cough associated with rhinorrhea or sneezing may be a viral syndrome or the common cold. If it recurs annually at the same time of year, allergic rhinitis is possible. Intermittent productive cough associated with wheezing is most probably asthma. A loud hacking cough during the daytime that is nonproductive, leads to exhaustion, and is associated with emotional stress may suggest psychogenic cough. In addition, some authors have attributed certain sputum characteristics to a particular disease process (Box 105-2). Evaluation of these attributes may also aid in diagnosis.

ACE inhibitors can cause a nonproductive cough more commonly in women, nonsmokers, and persons of Chinese ethnicity.[3] The onset of cough may occur within hours of the first dose or can be delayed for weeks to months after the initiation of ACE inhibitor therapy. The cough is not dose related and usually resolves within 1 to 4 weeks after cessation of therapy; however, in a small percentage of patients, the cough may linger for up to 3 months after termination of therapy.[3]

BOX **105-2**

Sputum Characteristics of Various Pulmonary Disorders

- Hemoptysis: bronchogenic cancer, pulmonary embolus, tuberculosis
- Yellow-green, purulent: bronchitis
- Pink frothy: pulmonary edema
- Fetid purulent: anaerobic infections
- Rust colored: pneumococcal pneumonia
- Foam, serous, mucopurulent layers: bronchiectasis

PHYSICAL EXAMINATION

The history and physical examination can help establish the cause of cough in the majority of cases. Obvious physical examination findings include the following:

- Pharyngeal erythema with or without cobblestoning of the mucosa and purulent secretions, as seen in sinusitis, upper airway cough, or allergic disease
- Diffuse inspiratory crackles characteristic of pulmonary edema or fibrosis
- Expiratory wheezes as in asthma or chronic obstructive pulmonary disease (COPD)
- Occasional hair rubbing against the eardrum or cerumen impaction in the canal resulting in the irritation of the auricular branch of the vagus nerve and triggering of cough[2]

If the cause of the cough remains elusive after a thorough history and physical examination, a chest radiograph should be obtained, even though radiographic findings are diagnostic in only a minority of cases. A normal chest radiograph usually excludes malignant disease, bronchiectasis, persistent pneumonia, sarcoidosis, and tuberculosis. The next step is to reconsider the most likely remaining causes of chronic cough, keeping in mind that chronic cough may fail to resolve because of inaccurate diagnosis or incorrect or insufficient therapy.

DIAGNOSTICS

A chest radiograph will reveal the presence of a lung mass or parenchymal abnormalities, such as sarcoidosis, fibrosis, emphysema, and congestive heart failure. If chest films reveal abnormalities, further diagnostic studies may be indicated, possibly including bronchoscopy, pulmonary function tests (PFTs), computed tomography (CT) scanning of the chest, barium esophagography, and cardiac studies. Bronchoscopy should be planned only for a specific diagnosis, keeping in mind that bronchoscopy has been shown to be of little diagnostic benefit when chest radiograph or CT findings are normal or nonlocalizing.[5] If the diagnosis is still not found, routine PFTs are indicated, and if these results are negative, a methacholine challenge test is necessary.

At this point, more than 50% of coughs will have been diagnosed. If the cause is still undetermined, a gastrointestinal evaluation with a barium swallow study and 24-hour pH esophageal monitoring should be considered. Further diagnostic tests include a CT scan of the sinuses and otolaryngologic evaluation. The majority of patients should now have a definitive diagnosis. Undiagnosed cases of cough may include psychogenic cough. There is a select group of patients who have a syndrome referred to as chronic idiopathic cough, for which the cause remains elusive. In some cases the precipitating cause of the cough may have disappeared, but its effect on the cough reflex may be more prolonged.[1] An example of this might be a transient upper respiratory tract viral infection or an exposure to respiratory toxins, which can cause inflammatory neuropathic changes in the sensory nerves, thereby inducing more prolonged damage to the respiratory mucosa.[1] Approximately 25% to 50% of patients have multiple causes of cough.[6]

Individuals with a compromised immune system require additional diagnostic testing as part of the initial workup. If a patient is immunocompromised, especially because of human immunodeficiency virus (HIV) infection, a chest radiograph and oxygen saturation level should be obtained earlier in the assessment. Chronic comorbid conditions and acute critical

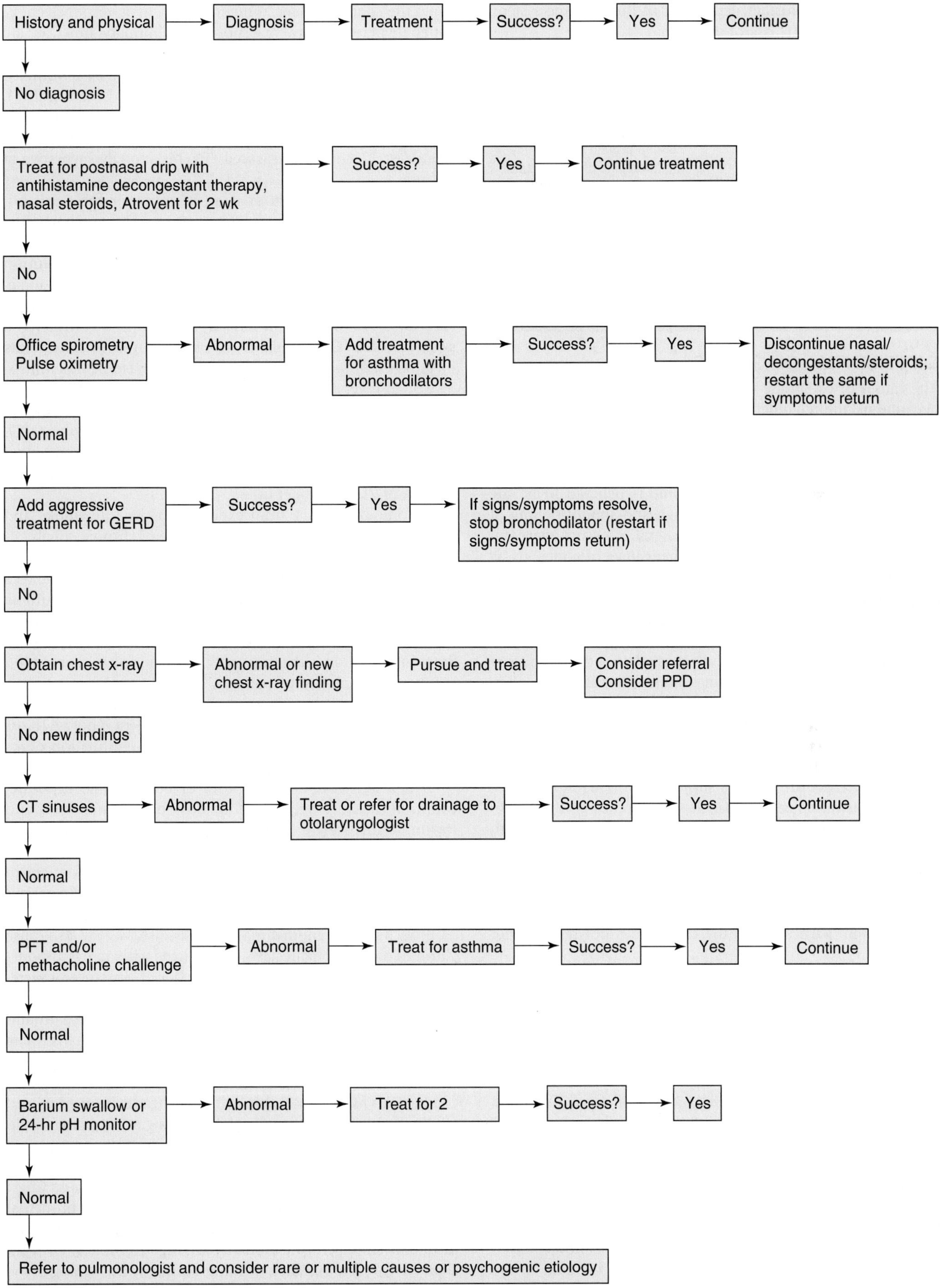

FIGURE 105-1 Diagnostic chronic cough protocol. CT, computed tomography; GERD, gastroesophageal reflux disease; PPD, purified protein derivative; PFT, pulmonary function tests.

illnesses can cause further depression of the immune system, thereby increasing the risk of infection.

DIAGNOSTICS

Chronic Cough

IMAGING
Chest x-ray examination*
Barium swallow*
Sinus CT*

OTHER DIAGNOSTICS
Bronchoscopy*
PFTs*
Purified protein derivative*
Methacholine challenge test*
24-Hour esophageal pH monitoring*
Oxygen saturation level*

*if indicated.

DIFFERENTIAL DIAGNOSIS

The causes of cough are plentiful and diverse. In adults of all ages and in children older than 1 year, corticosteroid-responsive eosinophilic airway diseases (asthma and eosinophilic bronchitis), upper airway cough syndrome (postnasal drip syndrome), and GERD are the three most common causes of chronic cough.[1] Upper airway cough syndrome is believed to be the most common cause of chronic cough and should be one of the first conditions considered. In general, it occurs after viral upper respiratory tract infections. Other causes of upper airway cough syndrome include perennial rhinitis (e.g., rhinitis caused by seasonal allergens), irritants, drugs, vasomotor responses, and chronic sinusitis. There are no signs and symptoms specific to the cough caused by upper airway cough syndrome; therefore it can be difficult to make the diagnosis based on the history and physical examination findings alone. Postnasal drip, often associated with rhinorrhea and nasal congestion, is characterized by a sensation of nasal secretions or a "drip" at the back of the throat, often accompanied by the need to clear the throat.[1] Throat clearing and a cobblestone appearance on the posterior pharynx are features suggestive of but not definitive for upper airway cough because they can occur in other conditions and these signs and symptoms often correlate poorly with cough.[3] The diagnosis of upper airway cough syndrome is often based on response to a trial of therapy. Upper airway cough syndrome may occur in association with some other chronic condition, so it is important to consider other possible causes of the cough, particularly if the cough does not resolve after therapy.

Early asthma and other related eosinophilic conditions may manifested as chronic cough. Bronchial asthma is the second most common cause of chronic cough in immunocompetent adults. Cough can be one of the first signs of worsening asthma (cough-variant asthma) as well as the symptom most reported by patients with chronic asthma, irrespective of having achieved good asthma control with inhaled bronchodilators.[2] The cough may precede audible wheezes, dyspnea, or airflow obstruction. A subset of asthmatics will have cough-variant asthma, in which cough is the only symptom with an otherwise normal physical examination.[3] In particular, older persons with asthma may have a history of chronic cough with no wheezing. Cough-variant asthma is often characterized by a dry, nocturnal cough and associated with a drop in early morning peak flows.[2] Given the high and increasing prevalence of asthma, it should always be considered a possible cause of chronic cough, especially when persistent cough is exacerbated by cold or exercise or when the cough worsens at night. Airway hyperresponsiveness, cough hypersensitivity, and normal pulmonary function are also suggestive of cough-variant asthma.[2] The degree and reversibility of obstruction are most accurately assessed by spirometry, which measures forced expiratory volume in 1 second (FEV_1). An FEV_1 of less than 80% predicted value that is strongly responsive to inhaled $beta_2$ agonist bronchodilators (an increase of at least 12% in the measured FEV_1) is strongly suggestive of asthma.

If the PFT results are normal, an attempt to induce bronchospasm with use of a bronchoconstrictor such as methacholine should be tried. This is known as the methacholine challenge test and is diagnostic in 25% of patients.[7] A nebulized solution of methacholine is administered in a stepwise fashion, incrementally increasing the dose and repeating the spirometry after each dose. A 20% drop in FEV_1 from baseline is considered a positive result. Other substances used as bronchoconstrictors include histamine, cold air exposure, and ultrasonic water mists.

Cough is reported by 70% of patients with COPD; 46% report daily cough.[2] Cigarette smoking is the most important risk factor for cough and sputum production in patients with COPD. Patients with COPD cough very frequently while awake, with a frequency of coughs ranging from 10 to 59 coughs per hour and a mean of 21 coughs per hour.[2]

Chronic bronchitis, from exposure to cigarette smoke and other irritants, is another common cause of chronic cough, although it accounts for a much smaller percentage of those who seek treatment, probably because many persons with "smoker's cough" do not seek medical care. Spirometry reveals an airflow obstruction that does not respond significantly to inhaled bronchodilators (or improvement in FEV_1 of more than 12%). Smoking cessation is the most effective therapeutic intervention because the majority of patients will have resolution or improvement of cough within 8 weeks. Unfortunately, the cough of persistent smokers is usually resistant to most if not all forms of therapeutic interventions, other than the elimination of tobacco smoke or other environmental irritants.

Cough is a common symptom of occupational exposure; common causative agents include dust, organic materials, and low-molecular-weight irritants, such as hydrochloric acid and organic oils.[2] The relationship between occupational exposures and cough should be suspected if there is an improvement in symptoms over the weekend or at other times when the patient is not at work.

Bronchiectasis, another major airway disease, may also cause chronic cough. Bronchiectasis is associated with an overproduction of secretions, combined with a reduced clearance of secretions, resulting in excessive airway secretions. As much as 30 mL of mucoid or mucopurulent sputum may be produced daily and may be accompanied by fever, hemoptysis, and weight loss.[2] The cough is functional; it helps clear secretions. Bronchiectasis may be associated with some of the other common causes of chronic cough, such as postnasal drip, asthma, chronic bronchitis, and GERD. Purulent sputum, when left standing in a cup, may separate into three layers—frothy top, serous middle, and purulent bottom—and cultures are often positive for *Haemophilus influenzae, Staphylococcus aureus,* and *Pseudomonas aeruginosa.* Chest radiography can show increased thickening of the bronchial wall, particularly in the lower lobes in advanced disease.[2] The most efficient diagnostic modality is a high-resolution CT scan; characteristic findings include intrapulmonary thickening of the airway wall, enlargement and distortion of the peripheral airways, mucous plugging, and evidence of bronchiolitis.[2]

Gastroesophageal reflux has been estimated to be a causative factor in up to 73% of chronic coughs and one of the three most common causes of cough in nonsmoking, immunocompetent adults who have normal chest x-ray films.[3] This cough can occur at any age, although it occurs most often in the middle to late 60s, and occurs slightly more often in women. Gastric reflux to the larynx can cause reflux laryngitis with associated thickening, redness, and edema of the posterior larynx.[2] Patients may report abdominal complaints, such as dyspepsia or heartburn, but may also have throat clearing, persistent cough, and hoarseness. It is also not unusual for patients to have no symptoms at all. The reflux material does not necessarily need to be aspirated or even to reach the glottis to cause cough or bronchospasm. Studies commonly used for diagnosis include barium swallow, esophagoscopy, manometry, and pH probe monitoring. Although the most sensitive and specific test for GERD is 24-hour esophageal pH monitoring, it is generally not recommended in the routine evaluation of GERD because of the inconvenience of this test. An alternative approach is to treat patients diagnosed with GERD empirically with antireflux medications such as proton pump inhibitors or H_2 histamines. If individuals do not respond well to medical therapy, additional diagnostic testing or surgery may be indicated. Patients with GERD may continue to cough despite the use of antireflux medications, supporting the evidence that other substances such as bile, pepsin, and other gastric enzymes may be causing the cough.[2]

Infectious causes such as pertussis and tuberculosis are becoming more prevalent and need to be considered as important differentials of chronic cough. The cough that follows a viral or virus-like infection has been referred to as a postinfectious cough and is a relatively common complaint in the primary care setting. An upper respiratory infection may result in a subacute postinfectious cough, lasting less than 8 weeks, or it may result in a cough lasting much longer.[4] The pathogenesis of postinfectious cough is not clearly understood, but it is thought to result from widespread disruption of the epithelial integrity and inflammation of the upper or lower airways, with or without airway transient hyperresponsiveness.[4] Persistent inflammation of the upper airways, especially the nose and paranasal sinuses, can cause or contribute to postinfectious cough. Despite the presence of bronchial hyperresponsiveness and transient inflammation of the lower airways, eosinophilic inflammation, typical of asthma, is absent.[4]

Ear canal irritation is a cause of cough in approximately 3% of healthy people.[2] Cerumen, foreign bodies, or any irritation of the auditory meatus can irritate the auricular branch of the vagus nerve and trigger a cough.

Chronic cough is a result of more than one cause in up to 20% of patients.[8] Cardiac disease (particularly left ventricular failure), interstitial lung disease, bronchogenic carcinoma, sarcoidosis, foreign body aspiration, postradiation pneumonitis, and metastatic lung carcinoma may have a cough as the sole presenting symptom. (Although many health care providers are concerned about missing lung carcinoma, isolated chronic cough is a rare presentation of lung cancer.) Other rare causes of cough include esophageal diverticulitis, stomach ulcer, and pericardial effusion.

The literature suggests that psychogenic cough is generally a loud, barking cough that is associated with high stress and typically does not occur at night. However, a cough that is not psychogenic can also be barking or honking, and most persons with chronic cough usually do not wake up during the night once they have fallen asleep. In addition to not coughing at night, patients with psychogenic cough are not awakened by cough and generally do not cough during enjoyable distractions. Because a psychogenic cough has no distinguishing features or diagnostic tests, it should remain a diagnosis of exclusion after all other possibilities have been eliminated. In a small percentage of cases, the cause will be undetermined.

DIFFERENTIAL DIAGNOSIS

Chronic Cough

MOST COMMON

- Upper airway cough syndrome (formerly postnasal drip)
- Asthma
- GERD
- Chronic bronchitis caused by cigarette smoking
- Nonasthmatic eosinophilic bronchitis
- Smoking and other irritants
- ACE inhibitors

LESS COMMON

- Bronchiectasis
- Medications
- Cardiac disease
- Postinfectious cough syndrome (pertussis, mycoplasma)
- Postradiation pneumonitis
- Gastrointestinal disturbances
- Obstructive sleep apnea
- Primary lung cancer
- Tuberculosis
- Heart failure
- Interstitial lung disease

UNCOMMON

- Tracheobronchial collapse
- Sarcoidosis
- Occupational or environmental exposures (e.g., pneumoconiosis from asbestosis)
- Foreign body or recurrent aspiration
- Chronic tonsillar enlargement
- Chronic irritation to auditory canal (cerumen or foreign body)
- Hyperthyroidism
- Retrosternal goiter
- Idiopathic pulmonary fibrosis
- Retained suture
- Hodgkin disease
- Zenker diverticulum
- Habit or tic cough
- Pulmonary abscess
- Endemic fungi
- Paragonimiasis
- Peritoneal dialysis
- Cystic fibrosis
- Tracheomalacia
- Aberrant innominate artery
- Irritable larynx
- Persistent pneumonia
- Psychogenic cough

Modified from Terasaki G, Paauw: Evaluation and treatment of chronic cough. *Med Clin North Am* 98:391-403, 2014

MANAGEMENT

Therapy is either antitussive (to prevent, control, or eliminate cough) or protussive (to make cough more effective and productive). Antitussive treatment is indicated when the cough serves no useful purpose, such as clearing the airway, and it can be specific or nonspecific. Specific treatment is directed at the aggravating factors or mechanism directly responsible, such as smoking cessation. Nonspecific therapy is directed at the symptom and is meant to control the cough when specific therapy has failed or is not possible (e.g., inoperable lung cancer). Protussive treatment is indicated for patients for whom coughing serves a useful function, as with cystic fibrosis.

Exposure to cigarette smoke and ACE inhibitor therapy are the most important potential aggravating factors of cough.[8] Removal of either of these factors often results in a substantial improvement in the cough. Persistence of cough after discontinuation of the ACE inhibitor is suggestive of another cause of cough. Treatment with ACE inhibitors may sensitize the cough reflex, which can exacerbate other causes of cough such as asthma, the onset of which has been associated with the use of ACE inhibitors.[8] In general, there is a temporal association between the onset of ACE inhibitor therapy and cough, but lack of such an association does not exclude ACE inhibitor therapy as a cause of the cough. According to the ACCP evidence-based clinical practice guidelines for ACE inhibitor–induced cough, therapy with ACE inhibitors should be discontinued "regardless of the temporal relationship between the onset of cough and the initiation of ACE inhibitor therapy."[9] If the ACE inhibitor is the causative agent, the cough usually resolves within 1 to 4 weeks after the cessation of therapy; however, in some patients, resolution of the cough may be delayed for up to 3 months after discontinuation of therapy. According to the ACCP guidelines, in patients for whom cough resolves after cessation of ACE inhibitor therapy and for whom there is a compelling reason to treat with this class of drugs, a repeated trial of ACE inhibitor therapy may be attempted. If cessation of ACE inhibitor therapy is not an option, pharmacologic therapy (including sodium cromoglycate, theophylline, sulindac, indomethacin, amlodipine, nifedipine, ferrous sulfate, and picotamide) should be attempted. The ACCP guidelines recommend that in patients with persistent or intolerable ACE inhibitor–induced cough, the patient's therapy be changed to an angiotensin receptor blocker, which does not appear to cause cough in patients with a history of ACE inhibitor–induced cough.[9] The ACCP guidelines can be found at chestjournal.chestpubs.org.

Specific therapy is encouraged for the causative agent if a definitive diagnosis is found. Empirical therapy is appropriate when there is a reasonable suspicion of a specific diagnosis. Asthmatic patients should be treated with inhaled $beta_2$ agonists, inhaled corticosteroids, or inhaled nonsteroidal anti-inflammatory medications (such as cromolyn sodium or nedocromil sodium) and occasionally oral steroids.

Upper airway cough caused by sinusitis is treated with oral decongestants, nasal steroids, and possibly but not necessarily antibiotics. When upper airway cough is related to allergic or nonallergic rhinitis, an H_1 antihistamine is an appropriate alternative to antibiotic therapy. Antibiotics are indicated when there is purulent nasal drainage and sinus tenderness.

Chronic bronchitis is best treated with smoking cessation, an ipratropium bromide inhaler, and a $beta_2$ agonist inhaler. When purulent sputum is present, a 7- to 10-day course of antibiotics is indicated.

Management of GERD involves a trial of antireflux therapy. A trial of acid suppression therapy, such as with a proton pump inhibitor, is reasonable if GERD is thought to be a contributing factor, even in the absence of specific gastrointestinal symptoms.[8] However, it may take several months before the full benefit of therapy is realized. In addition, preventive lifestyle changes, such as losing weight, stopping smoking, eating a diet low in acidic foods, and raising the head of the bed, may help reduce the tone of the lower esophageal sphincter, thus mitigating symptoms.

Demulcents are agents high in sugar content and are believed to coat the sensory receptors in the upper airways. They also promote swallowing, which may help suppress the cough reflex. Expectorants, such as guaifenesin, are believed to change the consistency of the sputum, thus making it easier to expectorate.

Opiates increase the latency threshold of the cough center. Codeine, oxycodone, and nonopiate dextromethorphan are standard therapy for severe nonproductive coughs. All are central nervous system depressants and, except for dextromethorphan, are addicting. Local anesthetics such as nebulized lidocaine are extremely effective and directly suppress the sensory nerve; however, these agents are difficult to administer.

COMPLICATIONS

Patients often develop costochondritis or hemoptysis as a result of strenuous coughing. Although usually not serious, these developments can be frightening for patients and families. Another recognized complication of cough is rib fracture, which occurs more commonly with chronic cough than with acute cough. Cough-induced rib fractures occur most often in ribs five through nine and along the lateral aspect of the rib cage (similar to the anatomic distribution of rib fractures seen in rowers), likely related to the repetitive mechanical stress to the ribs caused by coughing. Reduced bone density is a risk factor for cough-related rib fractures, although such fractures also occur in individuals with normal bone density. Chest radiography has a relatively low sensitivity for detecting cough-induced rib fractures. Other complications of chronic cough include ruptures, emphysematous blebs, syncope, wheezing, dyspnea, and sleep interruption.

INDICATIONS FOR REFERRAL OR HOSPITALIZATION

All patients with coughs that do not respond to or resolve with treatment require physician consultation. Patients with coughs related to cardiac disease, carcinoma, foreign body aspiration, or other suspected pathologic conditions require referral to the appropriate specialist with documentation of diagnostic evaluation, treatment, and treatment evaluation. Hospitalization may be indicated for wheezing and hypoxia as well as for bronchoscopy or other therapeutic interventions (Box 105-3).

BOX 105-3

Indications for Referral

POTENTIALLY SERIOUS CAUSES OF CHRONIC COUGH

Condition	Suggestive History of Clinical Features
Asthma	Wheezing, triggers such as exercise, cold air
Tuberculosis	Fever, weight loss, night sweats, hemoptysis, from an endemic area
Carcinoma (primary or metastatic)	Weight loss, hemoptysis, smoking history, older age, history of cancer
Chronic aspiration	History of cerebrovascular accident
Heart failure	History of cardiac disease, dyspnea, orthopnea, dependent edema
COPD	Smoking history, chronic sputum production
Interstitial lung disease	Dyspnea, possible environmental exposures, inspiratory crackles

ABNORMALITIES REQUIRING SPECIALIST INTERVENTION

- GERD requiring 24-hour pH monitoring
- Any suspicion of allergy requiring bronchoprovocation testing
- Occupational exposure requiring legal intervention
- Suspicion of sarcoid, carcinoma, bronchiectasis, carcinoid, Zenker diverticulum requiring bronchoscopy
- Retrosternal goiter requiring surgery
- COPD patients requiring home oxygen supplementation
- Chest x-ray film suggestive of empyema

PATIENT AND FAMILY EDUCATION

Cough is a major concern for patients that usually requires medical attention. Diagnostic studies are rarely needed, and a systematic and logical approach affords relief for most patients. Patients and families need to understand, however, that many coughs are viral in origin and that coughs may last 4 to 8 weeks. The health care provider should carefully explain the prescribed therapy, the need to use antibiotics only when indicated, and the signs and symptoms of serious cough-related illness.

CHAPTER 106

CHRONIC OBSTRUCTIVE PULMONARY DISEASE

Maureen Bell Boardman

DEFINITION AND EPIDEMIOLOGY

Chronic obstructive pulmonary disease (COPD) is a preventable and treatable disease characterized by airflow limitation; it is usually progressive, not fully reversible, and associated with an abnormal inflammatory response of the lungs. The chronic airflow limitations of COPD are caused by a combination of both small airway disease and parenchymal destruction.[1] *Chronic obstructive pulmonary disease* is a term used to describe two related lung diseases: chronic bronchitis and emphysema.[2]

Chronic bronchitis is defined clinically as a chronic, persistent cough or sputum production for 3 consecutive months each year for 2 consecutive years, with periodic acute exacerbations during which the symptoms worsen.[3] The pathologic features include inflammation of the cells lining the bronchial wall, hyperplasia of the mucous glands, and narrowing of the small airways.[4]

Emphysema is the permanent and abnormal enlargement of any part of the air spaces distal to the terminal bronchioles. Emphysema also involves destruction of the alveolar walls without fibrosis.[4]

COPD does not include other obstructive lung diseases such as asthma, even though asthma shares the same pathophysiologic common denominator as chronic bronchitis and emphysema, which is a slowing of the expiratory flow rate.[2] Asthma involves inflammation of the small airways. Although it is generally reversible, asthma can result in progressive airflow obstruction that over time becomes less and less reversible and resembles the obstruction seen with chronic bronchitis and emphysema. Persons with COPD can have a mix of emphysema, chronic bronchitis, and asthma that ranges from a "pure" emphysematous picture to a mixture of all three.

COPD is the third leading cause of death in the United States and the fourth leading cause of death worldwide.[1] Centers for Disease Control and Prevention statistics show that COPD has advanced from being the fourth to being the third leading cause of death between 1999 and 2010.[5] According to Social Security disability statistics, it is second only to coronary heart disease in causing disability. This shows a marked increase in the numbers of COPD cases worldwide since 1990, when it was ranked sixth. In the United States, where mortality from multiple chronic conditions declined from 1970 to 2002, COPD mortality rates increased.[1] Approximately 12.7 million adults in the United States have been diagnosed with COPD. However, almost 24 million U.S. adults have evidence of impaired lung function, indicating that the true prevalence of COPD is likely to be greatly underdiagnosed.[6]

COPD is predominantly a smoker's disease that clusters in families and worsens with age. Approximately 80% to 90% of COPD deaths are caused by smoking.[6] A hereditary pattern caused by α_1-antitrypsin deficiency contributes to the pure emphysematous form of this disease.

The risks for COPD include genetic, behavioral, socioeconomic, and environmental factors (Box 106-1). Cigarette smoke and an occupation that involves regular exposure to a dusty environment are the two major external factors. Because smoking cessation slows the decline in the expiratory airflow, it is clear that smoking is a powerful factor in determining outcome. When the disease is advanced, however, degeneration of lung function will probably continue even with smoking cessation. COPD is more common among individuals who are poor or undereducated. Cigarette smoking is also more common in these groups, but indigent populations still have worse lung function even with adjustment for smoking status. Other contributing factors include crowded living conditions with exposure to frequent viral infections, poorly ventilated homes, inadequate nutrition, exposure to passive cigarette smoke, and suboptimum care for childhood respiratory infections. Air pollution from the burning of wood and other biomass fuels has also been identified as a risk factor for COPD.[1]

Morbidity and mortality rates from COPD are higher in Caucasians than in African Americans or any other racial group in the United States.[7] Mortality has always been higher in men than in women. However, data from the past three decades have demonstrated a gender shift in the number of smoking-related COPD cases being diagnosed each year.[6] Some studies have suggested that women are more susceptible to the effects of smoking then men[1]; 2014 marked the eleventh consecutive year in which more women than men died as a result of COPD.[6]

Physician consultation is recommended for the initial diagnosis and management of patients with a significant change in condition or a failure to improve with prescribed therapies.

BOX 106-1

Risk Factors for Development of Chronic Obstructive Pulmonary Disease

- Cigarette smoking
- Airway hyperreactivity
- Childhood respiratory infections
- Occupational exposures
- Age
- Air pollution
- Passive exposure to smoke
- Poor nutrition
- Low socioeconomic status
- Crowded living conditions
- Family members with COPD
- α_1-Antitrypsin deficiency

PATHOPHYSIOLOGY

The cause of chronic bronchitis is not well understood, but chronic infection and airway hyperreactivity play important roles. The inflammatory process continues unabated even after withdrawal of prolonged exposure to bronchial irritants such as smoke, dust, and fumes. Airway edema, airway wall thickening, excess production of mucus, and loss of ciliary function result. Airflow is obstructed during both inspiration and expiration. Widespread bronchial narrowing with mucous plugging produces hypoxemia because of the mismatching of ventilation and perfusion. Hypercapnia results from the lack of ventilation. Chronic hypoxia and hypercapnia increase pulmonary arterial resistance and may lead to the development of pulmonary hypertension and, eventually, cor pulmonale. A sudden worsening of symptoms in severe chronic bronchitis can precipitate acute right-sided heart failure. Chronic bronchitis causes much less parenchymal damage than emphysema does; therefore, diffusing capacity, lung volumes, and compliance of lung tissue are not greatly altered.[4]

Enlargement of air spaces in emphysema is the result of alveolar wall destruction. This process is not completely understood but probably results from increased numbers of activated neutrophils that produce elastases, enzymes that destroy the elastin elements in the alveolar walls. Neutrophil-derived elastase is one of a group of destructive proteases contained in alveolar tissue. Usually, a small amount of neutrophil elastase is inactivated by antielastases (also known as antiproteases), which are found in the serum and lung lining layer. The prime antielastase, which is present in the largest quantities, is α_1-antitrypsin.

Even though they account for less than 3% of cases, patients with a hereditary deficiency of α_1-antitrypsin have less inhibition of elastase and a much higher risk for development of emphysema.[4] The primary role of α_1-antitrypsin is to inhibit the function of several proteases, most notably human neutrophil elastase. Human neutrophil elastase degrades the protein elastin, which is key to the elastic recoil mechanism necessary for the lung's expiratory function. The lack of α_1-antitrypsin can lead to panacinar emphysema. Because the alveoli have lost their recoil mechanism, the driving force during respiration decreases and causes a chronic persistent airflow obstruction. In addition to inhibiting proteases, α_1-antitrypsin inhibits the function of lymphocytes, macrophages, and neutrophils.[8] Patients with a hereditary deficiency of α_1-antitrypsin have less inhibition of elastase and a much higher risk for development of emphysema.

Cigarette smoking also increases elastase activity by causing an influx of elastase-rich neutrophils into the alveoli and by causing the oxidative inactivation of antitrypsin. These processes result in a 30-fold increase in the risk for COPD.

Regardless of the mechanism, the end result of COPD is the destruction of alveolar architecture and the capillary bed lying within the alveolar wall. Initially, the reduction in size of the vascular bed parallels the fall in alveolar surface area. Ventilation still roughly matches perfusion, and significant hypoxemia does not ensue. As the disease progresses, the elastic recoil of the airways is lost, and the poorly supported noncartilaginous airways collapse during expiration. Expiratory flow rates fall as a result, causing decreased airflow. Because this airflow obstruction is not uniform throughout the lung, there is uneven distribution of ventilation and blood perfusion. This uneven distribution causes arterial hypoxemia (decreased PaO_2); decreased ventilation causes hypercapnia (increased $PaCO_2$).

CLINICAL PRESENTATION

Diagnosis of COPD requires a thorough patient history, physical examination, and diagnostic testing. The most common presenting complaint is dyspnea on exertion. This symptom develops late in the course of this disease, when irreversible changes may have already occurred.

COPD must be considered as a diagnosis in every patient who smokes, even in the absence of respiratory symptoms. Discussing smoking habits at every visit is an important strategy in the prevention of irreversible disease. Documentation should include onset of smoking, the average number of packs per day, and whether the patient has made any successful cessation attempts. Information about other respiratory symptoms, such as cough, sputum production, and exertional dyspnea, should be elicited and quantified.

The important medical history includes any recurrent or prolonged respiratory tract infections that have required antibiotic treatment. A childhood history of frequent respiratory tract infections and bronchitis and any history of asthma, recurrent sinus infections, or nasal polyps should be documented because such conditions are common in patients with COPD.

The family history, including allergies, tuberculosis, cystic fibrosis, COPD, and other chronic lung conditions, should be elicited. A detailed occupational history with special attention to exposure to noxious inhalants such as fumes and mineral and biologic dust is essential.[1]

PHYSICAL EXAMINATION

Early in the disease process, the physical examination findings are often normal. Even without the findings of advanced COPD, it is impossible to exclude the diagnosis in the person at risk. However, if COPD is suspected based on the history and examination, it can be confirmed physiologically with simple spirometry.[1] In the late stages of COPD, the general physical findings include those resulting from hyperinflation. Inspection of the skin may show tobacco stains on the fingers and, occasionally, clubbing of the fingernails (convex nail plates). Chest inspection reveals an increase in the anteroposterior diameter, an increase in the intercostal spaces, and, in severe cases, abnormal retraction of the interspaces during inspiration. With inspiration, there is diminished movement of the rib cage and increased movement of the abdominal wall. Abdominal and sternocleidomastoid muscles may be well developed but accompanied by diminished muscle mass in the thighs and legs. A forward-sitting posture with both hands on the knees to fix the shoulders, thereby permitting more effective use of the accessory cervical muscles, may be noted. Pursed-lip breathing with prolonged expirations is also characteristic of COPD.[1]

There is increased resonance on chest percussion. The diaphragm seems low and moves poorly with deep inspiration and expiration. Diminished transmission of breath sounds on auscultation is the most reliable finding; this indicates chronic airflow limitation. Early inspiratory crackles are commonly found. Wheezing may be elicited with forced expiration, but it is a nonspecific symptom and is more characteristic of asthma.[1]

Lung disease causes hypertrophy of the right ventricle of the heart, resulting in cor pulmonale. Therefore, chronic cor pulmonale may be present in the advanced stage of COPD. The physical examination may reveal neck vein distention, peripheral edema, and hepatomegaly from an elevated right atrial pressure. Pulmonary hypertension and distention of the right ventricle cause a pronounced cardiac impulse in the epigastrium.

DIAGNOSTICS

Early detection of COPD is important for decreasing the associated morbidity and mortality. Symptoms of COPD do not usually occur until a significant amount of lung damage has occurred. A clinical diagnosis of COPD should be considered in any patient who has dyspnea, chronic cough, sputum production, and a history of exposure to risk factors for the disease, such as smoking or occupational exposures to dust and chemicals.[1] A simple office maneuver called forced expiratory time may help determine if further testing is needed. The patient is asked to take a deep breath in and then to breathe out as quickly and completely as possible with the mouth open. The practitioner auscultates the trachea with the diaphragm of the stethoscope and times the audible expiration. A forced expiratory time of 6 seconds or more suggests obstructive pulmonary disease.[9] The diagnosis should be confirmed by spirometry. Spirometry is considered the gold standard of diagnosis and assessment of COPD because it is the most reproducible, standardized, and objective way of measuring airflow limitation. Forced vital capacity (FVC), forced expiratory volume in 1 second (FEV_1), and the ratio of the two (FEV_1/FVC) are the primary spirometric measurements used for diagnosis. The presence of a postbronchodilator FEV_1/FVC of less than 0.70 and FEV_1 of less than 80% predicted confirms airflow limitation that is not fully reversible.[1] COPD is usually a progressive disease; the general patterns of symptom development are well established, and lung function usually worsens over time despite medical intervention (Box 106-2).

The concept of staging COPD based on FEV_1 alone is now thought to be inadequate. Newer research indicates the management of stable COPD should be based on a combination of factors including a symptomatic assessment, spirometric classification, and future risk of disease progression, with the focus on exacerbations.[1]

The COPD Assessment Test (CAT) is a short but comprehensive eight-item measure of health status impairment in patients with COPD.[1] It has been validated and can be easily used in a routine practice setting. It is scored from 0 to 40, with scores greater then 10 indicating more severe symptoms.

There is a large body of accumulated data in patients classified according to the Global Initiative for Chronic Obstructive Lung Disease (GOLD) spirometry grading system. The data show an increased risk of exacerbations, hospitalization, and death with worsening airflow limitations. The assessment of exacerbation risk is seen as a risk of poor outcomes overall[1] (Box 106-3).

A posteroanterior and lateral chest x-ray study is rarely diagnostic in COPD unless significant bullous disease is present. However, x-ray examination is useful in detection of COPD complications, such as pneumonia, pulmonary hypertension, and pneumothorax, as well as in establishing the presence of comorbidities, such as cardiac failure. Radiographic changes in COPD include flattening of the diaphragm and blunting of the costophrenic angle on the posteroanterior view, enlargement of the retrosternal space on the lateral view, flattening or concavity of the diaphragmatic contour on the lateral view, and irregularity of lung field lucency.[1]

BOX 106-2

Classification of COPD by Severity

STAGE I: MILD COPD

Mild airflow limitation (FEV_1/FVC < 70%; FEV_1 ≥ 80% predicted) and usually, but not always, chronic cough and sputum production. At this stage, the individual may not be aware that his or her lung function is abnormal.

STAGE II: MODERATE COPD

Worsening airflow limitation (50% ≤ FEV_1 < 80% predicted) and usually a progression of symptoms, with shortness of breath developing with exertion.

STAGE III: SEVERE COPD

Further worsening of airflow limitation (30% ≤ FEV_1 < 50% predicted), increased shortness of breath, and repeated exacerbations. Exacerbations that have an impact on a patient's quality of life and prognosis are seen in patients with FEV_1 < 50% predicted.

STAGE IV: VERY SEVERE COPD

Severe airflow limitation (FEV_1 < 30% predicted) or FEV_1 < 50% predicted plus chronic respiratory failure. At this stage, quality of life is very impaired and exacerbations may be life-threatening.

Modified from Global Initiative for Chronic Obstructive Lung Disease: *Global strategies for the diagnosis, management, and prevention of chronic obstructive pulmonary disease,* NHLBI/WHO Workshop Report, Washington, DC, 2009, U.S. Government Printing Office.

BOX 106-3

Combined COPD Assessment

PATIENT GROUP A—LOW RISK, FEWER SYMPTOMS

Typically GOLD 1 or GOLD 2 and/or no or one exacerbation per year and no hospitalization for exacerbation; and CAT score below 10.

PATIENT GROUP B—LOW RISK, MORE SYMPTOMS

Typically GOLD 1 or GOLD 2 and/or no or one exacerbation per year and no hospitalizations for exacerbation; and CAT score above 10.

PATIENT GROUP C—HIGH RISK, FEWER SYMPTOMS

Typically GOLD 3 or GOLD 4 and/or more than two exacerbations per year or more than one with hospitalization for exacerbation; and a CAT score below 10.

PATIENT GROUP D—HIGH RISK, MORE SYMPTOMS

Typically GOLD 3 or GOLD 4 and/or more than two exacerbations per year or more than one with hospitalization for exacerbation; and CAT score above 10.

Modified from Global Initiative for Chronic Obstructive Lung Disease: *Global strategies for the diagnosis, management, and prevention of chronic obstructive pulmonary disease,* NHLBI/WHO Workshop Report, Washington, DC, 2014, U.S. Government Printing Office.

Pulse oximetry to estimate oxygen saturation can be helpful, but blood gas measurements are necessary to assess and to manage patients during exacerbations and when oxygen therapy is indicated. Elevations of hematocrit and hemoglobin provide a measure of the severity of hypoxemia. Phlebotomy may become necessary if the elevation is severe. An electrocardiogram can indicate the severity of the lung disease and the presence of cor pulmonale. Significant findings include sinus tachycardia, multifocal atrial tachycardia, signs of right atrial enlargement (peaked P waves in leads II, III, and aVF), signs of right ventricular hypertrophy (a tall R wave in lead V_1 and a deep S wave in lead V_6), and right-axis deviation.[8]

Sputum is not routinely examined, but its inspection can help differentiate between a pulmonary infection and an exacerbation of reactive airways. The detection of neutrophils or eosinophils in the sputum will guide treatment between antibiotics and corticosteroids. Measurement of α_1-antitrypsin level is indicated in white patients who develop COPD before the age of 45 years or who have a strong family history of premature emphysema or α_1-antitrypsin deficiency.[1]

DIAGNOSTICS

Chronic Obstructive Pulmonary Disease

INITIAL
Spirometry (FVC and FEV_1)
Pulse oximetry

LABORATORY
CBC and differential*
ABGs*
α_1-Antitrypsin

IMAGING
Chest x-ray study (posteroanterior and lateral views)*

*If indicated
ABGs, arterial blood gases; CBC, complete blood count.

DIFFERENTIAL DIAGNOSIS

Distinguishing COPD from other causes of chronic cough or dyspnea is important for initial diagnosis and in acute exacerbations. A chronic cough may be secondary to chronic sinusitis or chronic rhinitis from allergies or postinfectious states. Gastroesophageal reflux, neoplasms, tuberculosis, interstitial lung diseases, and heart diseases (e.g., mitral stenosis or those causing chronic pulmonary edema) may also cause chronic cough. Chronic cough may be a side effect of certain drugs, including angiotensin-converting enzyme inhibitors, beta blockers, and amiodarone.

Diseases that cause chronic dyspnea include COPD, chronic bronchitis, emphysema, cystic fibrosis, and asthma. Less common entities include diffuse interstitial lung disease, pulmonary vascular disease (including recurrent pulmonary emboli, pulmonary hypertension, and arteriovenous malformation), and malignant neoplasms (including bronchogenic carcinoma and pulmonary metastatic disease). Phrenic nerve dysfunction or neuromuscular diseases can cause respiratory muscle weakness. Chest wall abnormalities, especially kyphoscoliosis, will cause chronic dyspnea. There are also nonpulmonary causes of dyspnea, including anemia, obesity, ascites, metabolic acidosis, hyperthyroidism, congenital heart disease, and abnormal hemoglobinopathies.

Certain features may help distinguish COPD from some of the most common pulmonary diseases that share similar signs and symptoms. The onset of COPD is more likely to be in midlife, with a long history of smoking and slowly progressing symptoms.[1] The onset of asthma is usually earlier in life, with varying symptoms occurring during the night and early morning. The patient often has a family history of asthma and may also have allergies, rhinitis, or eczema. The airflow limitations associated with asthma are largely reversible. Features suggestive of congestive heart failure include fine basilar crackles on auscultation and volume restriction versus airflow limitation on pulmonary function tests. A dilated heart and pulmonary edema may be noted on chest radiography. Bronchiectasis is associated with large volumes of purulent sputum and is commonly associated with bacterial infection. Coarse crackles may be noted on auscultation, and bronchial dilation and bronchial wall thickening may be seen on chest radiography or computed tomography. Tuberculosis can occur at any age. Lung infiltrates are usually noted on chest radiography with microbiologic confirmation. This occurs most often when there is a high local prevalence of tuberculosis.[1]

MANAGEMENT

Certain therapeutic interventions for symptomatic COPD improve survival, and some improve symptoms. In the presence of hypoxemia, smoking cessation and oxygen therapy improve survival. Interventions that improve symptoms include pharmacotherapy, education, exercise, psychological support, nutrition, and surgery.

The goals of treatment are to reverse or reduce airflow obstruction; to control cough and secretions; to prevent and eliminate infection; and to control complications, including polycythemia, hypoxemia, and right-sided heart failure. It is important to relieve underlying depression and anxiety, to maximize exercise tolerance, and to educate patients about avoidance of aggravating factors such as bronchial irritants.[1]

Smoking cessation is the single most important intervention to reduce the rapid decline of lung function in patients who smoke.[1] Treatment of tobacco use and dependence should be regarded as a primary and specific intervention. Smoking should be part of the routine evaluation of every health care visit, and every patient should be offered smoking cessation programs that involve multiple interventions that address the multifactorial causes of tobacco use.[1] In addition, providers should always express strong interest in helping their patients quit. Patients may be more inclined to stop smoking if they know their providers care that they stop smoking and if they understand that their smoking cessation is critical to prevention of premature loss of lung function. The most comprehensive smoking cessation guidelines are available at www.surgeongeneral.gov/tobacco.

Home oxygen is used in later stages of COPD because unlike some pharmacotherapeutics, it improves survival in hypoxemic COPD. The long-term administration of oxygen for more than 15 hours per day has been shown to increase survival in patients with chronic respiratory failure.[1] Other benefits of long-term oxygen include reduced polycythemia, reduced pulmonary artery pressures, reduced dyspnea, and improvement in neuropsychiatric test results. Another benefit may be the reduction of nocturnal arrhythmias, but it is unclear whether this translates into reduced mortality.

The Medicare criteria for 24-hour supplemental oxygen are PaO_2 of 55 mm Hg or less and an oxygen saturation of 88% or less while breathing room air (Box 106-4). Patients with cor pulmonale or erythrocytosis (hematocrit >55%) and a PaO_2 of 56 to 59 mm Hg also qualify.[1] Patients with exercise-induced desaturation below 88% should use oxygen during exercise to reduce dyspnea and to prevent hypoxemia. A number of studies have shown that use of oxygen during exercise can increase the

BOX 106-4

Criteria for 24-Hour Supplemental Oxygen

- PaO_2 of 55 mm Hg or less, or an oxygen saturation of 88% or less while breathing room air
- PaO_2 of 56 to 59 mm Hg or an oxygen saturation of 89% or less with evidence of pulmonary hypertension, cor pulmonale, or erythrocytosis

DIFFERENTIAL DIAGNOSIS

Chronic Obstructive Pulmonary Disease

CHRONIC COUGH
- Chronic sinusitis
- Chronic rhinitis
- Gastroesophageal reflux
- Neoplasm
- Asthma
- Tuberculosis
- Interstitial lung disease
- Congenital heart disease
- Cardiac disease (mitral stenosis, congestive heart failure)
- Medications (angiotensin-converting enzyme inhibitors, beta blockers, amiodarone)

DYSPNEA
- Asthma
- Cystic fibrosis
- Interstitial lung disease
- Pulmonary embolism
- Pulmonary hypertension
- Arteriovenous malformation
- Other pulmonary vascular diseases
- Phrenic nerve dysfunction
- Neuromuscular disease
- Kyphoscoliosis or chest wall abnormalities
- Malignant disease
- Anemia
- Obesity
- Ascites
- Metabolic acidosis
- Hyperthyroidism
- Congenital heart disease
- Abnormal hemoglobinopathies
- Hereditary emphysema (α_1-antitrypsin)

duration of exercise and reduce the severity of end-exercise breathlessness.[1] In the presence of daytime hypoxemia (PaO_2 <55 mm Hg), a hematocrit greater than 50% to 55%, morning headaches, daytime sleepiness, and poor exercise tolerance are indications of oxygen desaturation during sleep.[10] Monitoring of oxygen saturation during the night may be indicated for these patients because sleep can cause hypoventilation and nocturnal hypoxemia. Oxygen therapy at night will reduce the incidence of nocturnal hypoxemia.[10]

The need for long-term oxygen therapy should be reassessed 30 to 90 days after an acute exacerbation if that was the situation for which oxygen was prescribed. Oxygen therapy may be discontinued if the patient no longer meets the blood gas criteria. The development of simpler and more portable oxygen tanks and devices has helped improve the quality of life and increase mobility for persons requiring long-term oxygen therapy.

Pharmacotherapy

There is currently no pharmacologic treatment that mitigates the rate of decline of lung function or reduces or abolishes symptoms, but pharmacotherapy can improve exercise tolerance, reduce the number and severity of exacerbations, and improve lung function (Table 106-1). Pharmacotherapy should be based on the severity of disease and the patient's tolerance for certain drugs. In addition, a stepwise approach may be helpful.

Inhaled bronchodilators relieve bronchospasm; methylxanthine therapy further enhances bronchodilation, albeit within a narrow therapeutic range; and corticosteroids reduce inflammation. Antibiotics will not treat exacerbations of COPD unless these exacerbations are precipitated by infections. Even though few patients with COPD actually have α_1-antitrypsin deficiency and the long-term efficacy of replacement therapy is unclear, its identification and treatment are important. Diuretics may also be useful in patients with cor pulmonale.

Bronchodilators. Bronchodilators can alleviate the symptoms of COPD, improve exercise tolerance, decrease the frequency of exacerbations, and improve the quality of life. With most bronchodilators, the preferred route is inhalation of long-acting agents.

Some older patients may have difficulty effectively using a metered dose inhaler (MDI), and the use of a spacer may facilitate inhalation.

Bronchodilators include beta$_2$-adrenergic agonists and anticholinergics. Anticholinergics are a more effective first choice in patients with nonasthmatic COPD but are less effective than beta$_2$-adrenergic agonists in patients with asthmatic COPD. The American Thoracic Society recommends anticholinergics as the first line of maintenance therapy for patients with daily COPD symptoms. In patients who have intermittent symptoms, a short-acting beta$_2$-adrenergic agonist should be the first choice.[11]

Anticholinergic Therapy. Anticholinergics are effective first-line therapy for patients with COPD. Stimulation of the cholinergic nerves to the bronchial smooth muscle causes bronchoconstriction. Decreased cholinergic stimulation lessens bronchoconstriction. The cholinergic receptors are plentiful in the proximal airways, and these are the ones that influence COPD. Adrenergic receptors are more plentiful in the distal airways, which play a larger role in asthma.

The effects of anticholinergics are slower in onset but are more prolonged and intense, making them more useful for patients with sustained symptoms. There are now three anticholinergics on the market in the United States. Ipratropium bromide (Atrovent) in general has relatively few systemic side effects because of its poor systemic absorption. The usual dose is 2 six times daily, with a recommended maximum of 12 inhalations daily. This medication should be used on a regular basis, not as needed. There have been reports of an unexpected small increase in cardiovascular events in COPD patients treated regularly with ipratropium bromide, which requires further investigation.[1] Tiotropium (Spiriva) and aclidinium (Tudorza Pressair) are long-acting anticholinergics. Tiotropium is available in dry powder inhalers (Spiriva Handi-Haler, 18 µg, once a day; Spiriva Respimat, 5 µg, 2 inhalations once a day) that have a duration of action of 24 hours. Treatment with this long-acting anticholinergic drug improves the effectiveness of pulmonary rehabilitation.[1] Aclidinium (Tudorza Pressair), 400 µg, is a once daily oral inhalation. Caution is advised for patients with a severe milk protein allergy.

TABLE 106-1 **Pharmacologic Agents for COPD Therapy**

Agent	Recommended Dose Range	Notes
ANTICHOLINERGICS		
Short Acting		
Ipratropium bromide		
MDI, 20, 40 μg/inhalation	2-4 puffs 4-6 times per day	Poorly absorbed systemically; few side effects; should be used regularly (not prn)
Solution for nebulization, 500 μg/2.5 mL	3-4 times per day, separate doses by 6-8 hr	Precautions with narrow-angle glaucoma
Long Acting		
Aclidinium bromide, DPI, 400 μg/inhalation	1 inhalation twice a day	Same as ipratropium bromide
Tiotropium DPI, 18 μg/inhalation	1 inhalation daily	Same as ipratropium bromide
BETA$_2$-ADRENERGIC AGONISTS		
Short Acting		
Albuterol sulfate		
MDI, 90 μg/inhalation	1-2 puffs every 4-6 hr	Use on prn basis preferable to a fixed-use schedule
Solution for nebulization, 0.5 mL of 0.5% solution	3-4 times per day	No more than 12 inhalations daily Relatively short-acting drug; avoid excessive use Caution with cardiac disease, hyperthyroidism, diabetes, seizure disorders
Bitolterol mesylate		
MDI, 370 μg/inhalation	2 puffs at 1- to 3-min intervals every 8 hr followed by a third puff if needed Maximum dose: 3 puffs every 6 hr	Same as albuterol
Solution for nebulization, 2 mg/mL; dilute to 2-4 mL	2-4 times per day	
Levalbuterol		
MDI, 45 μg/inhalation	2 puffs every 4-6 hr	Same as albuterol
Solution for nebulization		
0.31 mg/3 mL of NS	3-4 times per day	
0.63 mg/3 mL of NS	3-4 times per day	
1.25 mg/3 mL of NS	3-4 times per day	
Metaproterenol sulfate		
MDI, 650 μg/inhalation	2-3 puffs every 3-4 hr	Same as albuterol
Solution for nebulization, 5.0% solution	0.2-0.3 mL of 5.0% solution in 2.5 mL of normal saline, 3-4 times per day	
Pirbuterol acetate, MDI, 200 μg/inhalation	2 puffs every 4-6 hr	Same as albuterol
Terbutaline sulfate, MDI, 200 μg/inhalation	2 puffs every 4-6 hr	Same as albuterol
Long Acting		
Salmeterol xinafoate		
DPI, 50 μg	1 puff every 12 hr	
MDI, 21 μg/inhalation	Maximum 2 doses/day	Not for treatment of acute attacks May be helpful for nocturnal symptoms in COPD because it is a long-acting preparation
Formoterol		
MDI, DPI, 4.5 μg, 12 μg	Maximum 2 doses/day	Same as salmeterol
Indacaterol		
MDI, 75 μg	1 inhalation daily	Same as salmeterol
Arformoterol		
Solution for nebulizer, 15 μg/2 mL	Maximum 2 treatments a day	Same as salmeterol

TABLE 106-1 Pharmacologic Agents for COPD Therapy—cont'd

Agent	Recommended Dose Range	Notes
METHYLXANTHINE		
Theophylline		
Immediate-release tablets	10 mg/kg/day in 4 divided doses	Follow serum levels to regulate dose between 8 and 13 mg/day; reduce dose in patients with liver disease, cardiac disease, or seizures
Sustained-release tablets	10 mg/kg/day in 1-3 doses	Check for drug-drug interactions
ORAL CORTICOSTEROIDS		
Methylprednisolone	40-48 mg/day in divided doses for 3-4 days	Used to treat acute exacerbations
Prednisone	3- to 4-week tapering course: begin with 40-60 mg; taper by 10 mg every 4-5 days, ending with 4 or 5 days of 5 mg/day 2- to 3-wk trial of steroids: 20-40 mg/day	Used to treat acute exacerbations Used for patients not responding to optimum doses of other drugs Steroid therapy associated with many side effects: osteoporosis, cataracts, hypertension, diabetes, peptic ulcers, psychic disorders, aseptic necrosis of hip, masking of infections, increased appetite, weight gain, and cushingoid effects Replace this form of steroid with inhaled form as soon as possible
INHALED CORTICOSTEROIDS		
Beclomethasone dipropionate, MDI, 40 μg/inhalation, 80 μg/inhalation	2 puffs 2 times a day	Teach patients that inhaled corticosteroids are not bronchodilators; must be used regularly to be effective; mouth should be rinsed after use Side effects: hoarseness, dry mouth, oral fungal infections
Budesonide, DPI, 90 μg/inhalation, 180 μg/inhalation	1-2 inhalations bid	Same as beclomethasone dipropionate
Ciclesonide, MDI, 80 μg/inhalation, 160 μg/inhalation	1-2 inhalations bid	Same as beclomethasone dipropionate
Mometasone furoate, MDI, 110 μg/inhalation, 220 μg/inhalation	1-2 inhalations daily to bid	Same as beclomethasone dipropionate
Fluticasone propionate, MDI, 44, 110, or 220 μg/puff	2-4 puffs bid; initial 88 μg bid; maximum 440 μg bid	Same as beclomethasone dipropionate
COMBINATION LONG-ACTING BETA$_2$ AGONIST PLUS GLUCOCORTICOSTEROID IN ONE INHALER		
Formoterol/budesonide, MDI, 80/4.5, 160/4.5 μg/inhalation	2 inhalations bid	Same as beclomethasone dipropionate
Fluticasone furoate, DPI, 100/25 μg/inhalation	1 inhalation daily	Same as beclomethasone dipropionate
Mometasone/formoterol, MDI, 100 μg/inhalation, 200 μg/inhalation	2 inhalations bid	Same as beclomethasone dipropionate
Salmeterol/fluticasone		Same as beclomethasone dipropionate
DPI 50/100, 50/250, 50/500 μg/inhalation	1 inhalation bid	
MDI 45/21, 115/21, 230/21 μg/inhalation	2 inhalations bid	
ANTICHOLINERGIC PLUS BETA$_2$ AGONIST		
Ipratropium bromide/albuterol, MDI, 20/100 μg 0.5 mg/2.5 mg/3 mL	1 inhalation qid 1 vial nebulizer 4-6 times a day	Same as ipratropium bromide and albuterol
ANTICHOLINERGIC PLUS LONG-ACTING BETA$_2$ AGONIST		
Umeclidinium/vilanterol, 62.5/25 μg/inhalation	1 inhalation daily	Severe hypersensitivity to milk proteins
PHOSPHODIESTERASE-4 INHIBITOR		
Roflumilast, 500 μg	1 tablet daily	Contraindicated in moderate to severe liver disease

DPI, dry powder inhaler; MDI, metered dose inhaler; NS, normal saline.

Beta$_2$-Adrenergic Agonist Therapy. Beta$_2$-adrenergic agonists (bronchodilators) cause bronchial smooth muscle dilation and can also improve mucociliary clearance. The major side effects include tachycardia and tremor from stimulation of beta$_1$ receptors in muscle. Unfortunately, recommended doses of these agents have been based on studies of patients with moderate, stable asthma. These doses may not be appropriate for patients with COPD. As the severity of bronchospasm increases, the efficacy of beta$_2$-adrenergic agonists decreases.

Most agents in this class have a 4- to 6-hour duration. The dose should not exceed 4 to 12 inhalations per day for the shorter-acting preparations (albuterol, pirbuterol acetate, metaproterenol sulfate, isoetharine, and terbutaline) or twice daily for the longer acting preparations (salmeterol xinafoate, formoterol fumarate). The longer-acting inhaled preparations or the oral form of these medications may be more helpful in patients with nocturnal symptoms.

Toxicity and drug-drug interactions must be avoided in older adults, especially those with coexisting heart disease.

Combination Therapy. The pairing of an anticholinergic and a short-acting beta$_2$ agonist in one MDI containing both ipratropium and albuterol has been shown in multiple studies to be superior in the treatment of COPD than either drug alone. The combination has also been shown to reduce exacerbations, to lower cost, and to improve lung function and quality of life.[1]

Anoro Ellipta is a combination long-acting anticholinergic agent (umeclidinium, 62.5 μg) and long-acting beta$_2$ agonist (vilanterol, 25 μg) that is now also available for COPD treatment. The dose is 1 inhalation daily, but this preparation is also contraindicated for patients with severe milk protein hypersensitivity.

Methylxanthine Therapy. Theophylline is considered a third-line agent because its bronchodilatory effect is limited and its therapeutic range is narrow. Theophylline is effective in COPD; low-dose theophylline reduces exacerbations in patients with COPD but does not increase postbronchodilator lung function, and because of the significant risk for toxicity, inhaled bronchodilators are preferred.[1] Newer slow-release preparations have improved the problems related to its narrow therapeutic index and complex pharmacokinetics, leading to more stable plasma levels. If levels rise, the risk of toxicity increases with little therapeutic gain. Theophylline is not recommended for patients receiving H_2 receptor blockers and fluoroquinolone or macrolide antibiotics because it is metabolized by cytochrome P-450 mixed function oxidases, and there is a likelihood of reduced theophylline clearance and an increased risk of toxicity.

Corticosteroids. Although oral corticosteroids improve airflow and gas exchange with acute exacerbations of COPD, their use in the management of COPD is discouraged secondary to an unfavorable risk/benefit ratio.[1] Complications, especially in older adults, make long-term therapy with oral corticosteroids problematic. These complications include skin damage, cataracts, diabetes, obesity, peptic ulcer disease, osteoporosis, and secondary infection. Oral steroids can be used to treat acute exacerbations. A 3- to 4-week tapering course of prednisone may be helpful. A dose of 40 to 60 mg of prednisone should be initiated and tapered by 10 mg every 4 or 5 days, ending with 4 or 5 days of 5 mg/day until discontinuation. Rebound bronchospasm can occur with faster tapers.

For patients who do not respond to optimum doses of other drugs, it is reasonable to try prednisone in doses of 20 to 40 mg/day. This trial of steroids should last 2 to 3 weeks. A 20% to 30% increase in FEV$_1$ must be demonstrated to justify continued use of oral steroids. Twice the lowest daily dose that maintains improvement should be prescribed on an every-other-day regimen to minimize side effects. If patients are taking corticosteroids long term, other measures to improve symptoms of COPD should be considered. Lung volume reduction surgery (LVRS) and lung transplantation are two possible options.

The World Health Organization's GOLD guidelines suggest that inhaled corticosteroid use is appropriate and reduces exacerbations for symptomatic COPD patients (i.e., stage III and stage IV COPD) with an FEV$_1$ of less than 60% predicted and repeated exacerbations. However, the GOLD guidelines also reveal that for most patients with COPD, inhaled glucocorticosteroids do not modify FEV$_1$ decline.[1]

There is a place for inhaled corticosteroids in the stepwise approach to the treatment of symptomatic COPD. The FEV$_1$ should be rechecked after 3 to 4 months of therapy with inhaled corticosteroids. If the FEV$_1$ improves or stays the same, the same dose should be continued. If the FEV$_1$ declines, discontinuation of the inhaled steroid should be considered. The side effects of inhaled corticosteroids are minimal. Oral candidiasis can be minimized by rinsing the mouth with water or mouthwash after every use or by using a spacer.

Combination Inhaled Glucocorticosteroid and Bronchodilator Therapy. The combination of an inhaled glucocorticosteroid with a long-acting beta$_2$ agonist is more effective than the individual components in improving lung function and health status and in reducing exacerbations. In patients with an FEV$_1$ of less than 60%, the combination therapy decreased the decline of lung function. However, combination therapy increased the likelihood of pneumonia and failed to demonstrate statistically significant effects on mortality in a large clinical trial.[1]

Phosphodiesterase-4 Inhibitors. Roflumilast (Daliresp), a phosphodiesterase-4 enzyme inhibitor, was approved for the treatment of patients with bronchitis-associated COPD.[1] Roflumilast breaks down intracellular cyclic adenosine monophosphate (cAMP) and reduces inflammation.[1] A once-a-day oral medication, roflumilast can be used with glucocorticoid therapy, salmeterol, or tiotropium, but cannot be used as monotherapy for patients with COPD. It is contraindicated in patients with moderate or severe liver dysfunction.[1]

Mucoactive Agents. Some patients with COPD form increased quantities of abnormal mucus. The value of mucoactive agents that decrease sputum viscosity and adhesiveness, which facilitates expectoration, has not been established in patients with COPD, although a few patients with viscous sputum may benefit from mucoactive agents. Increasing hydration by the intravenous route, aerosolized route, or oral route does not decrease the thickness of secretions. Oral iodinated glycerol, 60 mg four times daily, may help. Another option for patients who have trouble coughing up thick, tenacious sputum is supersaturated potassium iodide solution, although patients may need to take this medication for 7 to 10 days before a therapeutic effect occurs.

Antibiotics. The infectious agents in COPD exacerbations can be viral or bacterial. Several randomized placebo-controlled studies of antibiotic treatment in COPD exacerbations have demonstrated a small beneficial effect of antibiotics on lung function. The patients who showed significant beneficial effects were the ones with an increase in all three of the following cardinal symptoms: dyspnea, sputum volume, and sputum purulence. There was also some benefit in those patients with an increase in two of these cardinal symptoms if increased purulence of sputum was one of the two. Another study in patients with severe exacerbations that required mechanical ventilation indicated that not giving antibiotics was associated with increased mortality and an increased incidence of nosocomial pneumonia.[1] In bacterial infection, the most common pathogens include *Streptococcus pneumoniae, Haemophilus influenzae, Chlamydia pneumoniae,* and *Moraxella catarrhalis.*[1]

The antibiotic choice depends on several factors, including local resistance patterns and the cost of treatment. The mainstay antibiotics are broad-spectrum oral agents that the patient can keep at home to use at the first sign of an acute exacerbation. Typical choices are amoxicillin, ampicillin, cefaclor, doxycycline, and trimethoprim-sulfamethoxazole. Newer, more expensive antibiotics that extend the spectrum of coverage can be used for second-line therapy and include cefpodoxime, azithromycin, clarithromycin, levofloxacin, ciprofloxacin, and moxifloxacin. If the patient is moderately ill or needs to be hospitalized, the antibiotic choice needs to be supported by sputum culture and sensitivity testing.[1]

Pulmonary Rehabilitation

The principal goals of pulmonary rehabilitation are to reduce symptoms, to improve quality of life, and to increase physical and emotional participation in everyday activities.[1] The benefits of pulmonary rehabilitation are well documented in a large number of clinical trials. Pulmonary rehabilitation is a multidisciplinary team approach to care. It is designed to be highly individualized to meet the needs of each patient. The team makeup may vary from program to program but usually consists of a physician, respiratory therapist, exercise therapist or physical therapist, occupational therapist, psychosocial staff, and dietitian-nutritionist. Instruction on nutrition, exercise, upper body weight training, and breathing techniques and guidance for maximizing energy reserves are critical components of any rehabilitation program. Pulmonary rehabilitation programs are also an excellent source of support for both patients and family members.

Exercise Training

Patients at all stages of COPD appear to benefit from exercise programs, which have improved both patients' exercise tolerance and symptoms of dyspnea and fatigue.[1] Programs emphasize lower extremity training, upper extremity training, and strength training. Most pulmonary rehabilitation exercise programs consist of 10- to 45-minute sessions, daily to weekly, for 4 to 10 weeks, depending on resources.[1] Participants are also taught breathing strategies such as pursed-lip breathing and controlled coughing to improve their ability to perform activities of daily living.

Immunizations

There is evidence that persons with COPD benefit from immunization against respiratory pathogens. A yearly immunization with the influenza vaccine is essential to decrease morbidity and mortality from influenza epidemics and has been shown to reduce serious illness and death in COPD patients by about 50%.

Updated recommendations for the pneumococcal vaccine recommend not only that all patients with a diagnosis of COPD receive a pneumococcal vaccine regardless of age, but also that all smokers receive a pneumococcal vaccine. Patients 65 or older when they receive the pneumococcal vaccine should receive only a single dose. Patients aged 19 to 64 who have COPD or are smokers should receive another dose of the vaccine at age 65 or if at least 5 years have passed since their previous dose. Current guidelines do not recommend multiple revaccinations secondary to uncertainty regarding clinical benefit and safety.[12] All adults 65 years or older are advised to receive Prevnar 13 once, and Prevnar 13 is recommended for patients with COPD.[13] A patient who has already received Pneumovax must wait 1 year before receiving Prevnar 13, however.

Psychological Support

Patients with COPD may feel anxious, depressed, and fatigued. Counseling is recommended for those patients exhibiting signs and symptoms of major depression. COPD and associated dyspnea often result in immobility, which contributes to social isolation and depression. Pulmonary rehabilitation programs can be helpful in interrupting this vicious circle. In addition, antidepressants can be beneficial in COPD patients with depression. Depression and anxiety often improve when airflow obstruction is improved.

Nutrition

COPD often precipitates weight loss because the increased work of breathing can double resting energy expenditures. This, along with decreased physical activity, tends to diminish fat and muscle stores. Weight loss is also aggravated by disease exacerbations or anorexia from medications or emotional issues. Severe dyspnea, coughing, and sputum production can interfere with eating. A reduction in body mass index is an independent risk factor for mortality in COPD patients.[1] Patients should be encouraged to eat frequent, small meals instead of a large meal; large meals cause abdominal distention, which impairs diaphragmatic function. Vitamin supplementation and commercially prepared drinks are convenient, easily digested, and high in protein, calories, and vitamins. Nutritional counseling is a recommended component of pulmonary rehabilitation programs.

Surgery

Two types of surgery may be beneficial for some patients with COPD: LVRS and lung transplantation. The proposed benefit of LVRS is improved elastic recoil and diaphragmatic function, which is accomplished by reducing the volume of the lung and thereby decreasing hyperinflation. In addition, LVRS increases the elastic recoil pressure of the lung and thereby improves expiratory flow rates.[1] A large multicenter study of 1200 patients (National Emphysema Treatment Trial) compared LVRS with medical treatment in patients with upper lobe emphysema and low exercise capacity. In this small subset of patients, LVRS resulted in significant improvement. However, in patients who had other emphysema distribution or high exercise capacity before treatment, the advantage of surgery over medical treatment was less significant. Despite its beneficial results in a select group of patients, it is an expensive surgical procedure and therefore should be recommended only in the small number of patients who meet the criteria.[1]

Lung transplantation in appropriately selected patients with advanced COPD has been shown to improve both quality of life and functional capacity. However, lung transplantation is limited by the shortage of donor organs and its cost. Costs remain elevated for years after the surgery because of the high cost of both complications and the immunosuppressive regimens that must be used long term. Lung transplantation has also failed to show a survival benefit in patients with end-stage emphysema after 2 years.[1]

PALLIATIVE CARE AND HOSPICE

COPD is a chronic disease that consists of a gradual decline in health and increasing symptoms as well as episodes of acute exacerbation. Therefore, palliative care should be an essential component in the treatment of all patients with advanced COPD. Palliative care offers COPD patients a focus on quality of life, optimized function, and assistance with decision-making about end-of-life care, as well as providing emotional and spiritual support to both patients and their families. Unfortunately, patients with COPD are less likely to receive these services then patients with lung cancer.[1]

The National Hospice and Palliative Care Organization provides guidance for referring patients with noncancer diseases such as COPD for services.[14] These guidelines recognize the appropriateness of providing hospice services for patients with advanced COPD.

COMPLICATIONS

Complications may be caused not only by the condition of COPD but also by the treatment. Drug effects should always be considered if there is a change in clinical condition. Long-term corticosteroids increase the risk for compression fractures because of accelerated osteoporosis. Some of these complications can be prevented by keeping the corticosteroid dose as low as possible, encouraging calcium supplementation, and prescribing bisphosphonate therapy for patients who are unable to reduce their prednisone dose to less than 20 mg every other day.[8]

Theophylline toxicity should be considered in the presence of gastrointestinal symptoms, tremors, headache, or tachycardia. Other medications may affect the metabolism of theophylline. Corticosteroid or diuretic therapy may be responsible for hyperglycemia, hypokalemia, or azotemia.

Depression or marked anxiety often accompanies COPD. Patients with stable COPD tolerate antidepressant therapy, but depression most often improves when airflow obstruction improves.

Anti-inflammatory therapy needs to be maximized during acute infections. Atypical mycobacterial disease should always be considered if chest radiographs show cavitary apical disease. Placement of an intermediate-strength purified protein derivative (PPD) skin test and a sputum examination for acid-fast bacilli are indicated.[14]

Fungal infections are important in the differential diagnosis of certain infiltrates in patients with COPD. Histoplasmosis is endemic in the Ohio and Mississippi river valleys. In the southwestern United States, coccidioidomycosis is endemic and can be seen in epidemic proportions after a dust storm. *Aspergillus* organisms are fungi that can be particularly dangerous in patients with COPD. Consultation is recommended before specific antifungal therapy is initiated.[14]

Three other complications occur as a result of the COPD disease process: sleep disorders, acute respiratory failure, and cor pulmonale. Although it is not always recognized, nocturnal oxygen desaturation in patients with COPD is fairly common. It is not usually caused by sleep apnea but by ventilation/perfusion abnormalities and short-term hypoventilation during rapid eye movement sleep. Patients who are not obese rarely develop coexisting upper airway obstruction. However, in some individuals who are obese, there is an added obstructive component to the usual mechanisms of transient hypoxemia. Sleep-related hypoxemia is suggested by an increased hematocrit in a patient with morning headaches and daytime somnolence. Often, the patient's sleep partner reports intense snoring. Overnight home monitoring with pulse oximetry establishes the diagnosis. It is appropriate to prescribe home oxygen for nocturnal use if home monitoring with a pulse oximeter identifies an oxygen saturation of less than 88% and if symptoms of headache, fatigue, and poor exercise tolerance are present. Continuous positive airway pressure (CPAP) through a well-fitting nasal mask is helpful for patients with an obstructive component. If nocturnal oxygen desaturation is suspected, a referral should be made to a pulmonologist or sleep disorder specialist.[15]

Acute respiratory failure is the most severe complication of COPD. Acute worsening of arterial blood gases necessitates consultation and possible hospitalization.

Cor pulmonale is a severe complication of COPD and is an indication for consultation. Its pathologic definition is right ventricular enlargement, hypertrophy, or dilation secondary to lung disease.[15] Peripheral edema, elevation of the neck veins, and a congested liver reflect right-sided heart failure. In the presence of a significant degree of COPD and an elevated hematocrit with hypoxemia, the diagnosis of cor pulmonale as a complication of COPD can be made without further expensive tests other than electrocardiography. Standard therapy for cor pulmonale is to treat the underlying airflow obstruction and improve oxygenation. Restriction of salt intake to 2 g/day and a 24-hour diuretic can benefit those with mild heart failure. If decompensation continues, the addition of supplemental oxygen is indicated to achieve arterial oxygen saturation in the 90% to 95% range 24 hours a day. Hematocrit or hemoglobin levels should be monitored at 4- to 8-week intervals. If the patient is adequately oxygenated, the elevated hematocrit will resolve within that period. Persistent erythrocytosis reflects insufficient oxygen administration or the presence of desaturation during sleep despite the oxygen. A sleep study at this point may help determine whether additional therapy, such as CPAP, is needed during the night.

INDICATIONS FOR REFERRAL OR HOSPITALIZATION

Consultation is appropriate when the disease progresses and the need for oral corticosteroids is evident, when presentation includes escalation of symptoms and fever, when hospitalization is indicated, when continuous or nocturnal oxygen is required, and when there is evidence of right-sided heart failure and cor pulmonale is present. Petty[15] outlined 12 indications for consultation with a pulmonary specialist:

1. Particularly severe disease, including persistent dyspnea with activities of daily living despite therapy and frequent recurrent exacerbations
2. Evaluation for and maintenance of oxygen therapy, including consideration of nocturnal oxygen therapy or transtracheal oxygen therapy

3. Inability to successfully taper the patient from systemic corticosteroids
4. Preoperative assessment for thoracic surgery or other surgery, which places the patient at high risk for pulmonary complications
5. Failure to respond after two courses of antibiotics for an acute exacerbation
6. Consideration of long-term intermittent or continuous antibiotic therapy
7. Persistent pulmonary infiltrates on chest radiograph with no response to a course of antibiotics
8. Evaluation of sleep disturbances, including obstructive sleep apnea
9. Management of severe acute respiratory failure, especially if mechanical ventilation is a consideration
10. Cor pulmonale with clinical right-sided heart failure that is unresponsive to usual therapy
11. Consideration of new techniques in LVRS
12. Consideration of α_1-antitrypsin augmentation therapy

Hospitalization is based on the severity of the underlying respiratory dysfunction, the progression of symptoms, new or worsening cor pulmonale, or the existence of other comorbidities. Hypoxemia and hypercapnia are probably increasing if a patient does not respond adequately to treatment or is confused or unable to walk, eat, or sleep without aid. Hospitalization is warranted in these cases.

Some patients require admission to a specialized respiratory care unit. Issues that require admission include severe dyspnea that does not respond to initial emergency therapy; changes in mental status including confusion, lethargy, and coma; persistent or worsening hypoxemia or severe respiratory acidosis despite supplemental oxygen; the need for invasive mechanical ventilation; and hemodynamic instability and the need for vasopressors.[1]

PATIENT AND FAMILY EDUCATION

Education has always been considered a cornerstone of pulmonary rehabilitation. However, until recently, few studies unequivocally demonstrated the effectiveness of patient education, including behavior modification. A structured education program, specifically designed for patients with COPD, demonstrated that self-management and behavior modification can be achieved, resulting in a substantial decrease in morbidity.[16] Patients can better recognize and treat the symptoms of COPD if they understand the nature of the disease and the implications of treatment. The importance of medication, oxygen therapy, smoking cessation, nutrition, exercise, breathing techniques to minimize dyspnea, and health promotion should be stressed. Patients and families need to understand that acute exacerbations of COPD may produce respiratory failure, a possible need for ventilatory support, and the possibility of death. Providers should help patients and their family members make decisions about advance planning and their preferences for end-of-life care during stable periods of health. These discussions can help prepare patients with advanced COPD for a life-threatening exacerbation of the disease.

CHAPTER 107

DYSPNEA

David Patrick Murphy

DEFINITION AND EPIDEMIOLOGY

Dyspnea encompasses a broad array of discrete unpleasant sensations, such as air hunger, increased work of breathing, chest tightness, feelings of suffocation, and respiratory fatigue.[1] Although breathlessness is expected after vigorous exercise, dyspnea is a cardinal manifestation of cardiopulmonary disease that warrants appropriate evaluation and treatment. It is also a common and disabling symptom of chronic lung disease, and measures of dyspnea are commonly used in evaluating outcomes in these diseases.[2] Dyspnea is a very common complaint in the United States and accounts for 3 to 4 million emergency department visits annually. It was noted to be among the top three reasons for adults aged 65 and older to visit the emergency department. Its overall prevalence is about 9%, and this figure increases significantly with increasing age to about 17% of patients older than age 65.[3,4]

PATHOPHYSIOLOGY

The mechanisms that trigger dyspnea are complex and vary by disease. This is further complicated by a respiratory system that is unique in that respiratory motor drive has both autonomic (brainstem) and voluntary (cortical) sources of command. It has been suggested that dyspnea occurs whenever sensory input from receptors in the airways, lungs, and chest wall does not match up with respiratory drive.[5] These sensory receptors may respond to chemicals, stretch, irritation, or passive distention. For example, there appears to be a dissociation between sensory input and motor output in conditions that impose a mechanical load on the respiratory system by decreasing compliance of either the lung (e.g., pneumonia, pulmonary edema, fibrosis) or the chest wall (e.g., kyphoscoliosis, rib fractures, circumferential thorax burns) or by inhibiting airflow (e.g., asthma, chronic bronchitis, emphysema).[6] In addition, neuromuscular weakness or fatigue may cause dyspnea symptoms because of the inability of weakened muscles to generate an expected level of ventilation. Hypoxemia and hypercapnia stimulate chemoreceptors that may cause dyspnea through increased respiratory motor drive. Surprisingly, there is a poor correlation between dyspnea and blood gas abnormalities. Dyspneic patients are often perplexed to learn that they have adequate oxygen saturation or that supplemental oxygen administration does not relieve symptoms. Blood gases are of value in monitoring severity of illness, but many clinicians overestimate their value as measures of dyspnea.[1] Increased carbon dioxide production, lower pH, and, to a lesser degree, hypoxemia stimulate the efferent motor drive for ventilation; however, their importance physiologically in monitoring the adequacy of ventilatory response is less clear. What the physiologic mechanisms of dyspnea have in common is that some combination of stimuli triggers an awareness of a threat to the ability to breathe or a threat to self.[7]

CLINICAL PRESENTATION

Dyspnea is a common complaint, and the following dimensions are useful in elucidating the disease process that causes dyspnea: quality, timing, intensity, associated symptoms, and environmental exposures. These factors provide indications as to what the mechanism of the cause may be. A good history of the complaint is essential because dyspnea, like pain, is primarily dependent on a patient's perception and self-report of the symptom.

Quality

Dyspnea is typically described as the unpleasant sensation of tightness, increased work or effort, and air hunger or unsatisfied inspiration. The descriptors patients use for dyspnea sensations may be diagnostically useful.[8-10] For example, patients with obstructive lung disease such as asthma or chronic obstructive lung disease (COPD) tend to complain of "chest tightness" or "constriction." Diseases associated with an increased mechanical load (resulting from decreased compliance or increased airway resistance) such as interstitial lung disease or cystic fibrosis are often associated with feelings of excessive "work" or "effort." Patients with an increased drive to breathe (e.g., resulting from hypoxemia or hypercapnia) experience air hunger and may complain that they "can't get enough air in." This can also be related to decreased oxygen carrying capacity—for example, in severe anemia or carbon monoxide poisoning. It is important to note that causes of dyspnea probably activate multiple dyspnea mechanisms, leading to a composite of sensations that defy easy classification. For example, asthma that is mild may manifest as chest tightness only, whereas common later signs of more acute or severe disease include increased work of breathing or severe air hunger (Table 107-1).

Timing

Although it is often impossible to pinpoint the precise onset of dyspnea, it is important to distinguish between acute and chronic symptoms. Sudden onset of dyspnea often heralds serious cardiopulmonary disease that requires immediate evaluation and treatment (e.g., pulmonary embolism, pneumothorax, myocardial infarction). Relative stability, intermittent exacerbations, or progressive debilitating symptoms may characterize chronic dyspnea. Patients who experience increasing symptoms or intermittent exacerbations should be carefully reevaluated for worsening disease or a new problem.

Intensity

Dyspnea severity is difficult to quantify and there are many different proposed methods of trying to quantify it. This is an area of study that is still under development.[11] Activity limitation is commonly used as a surrogate marker because it is a more objective form of measure. Dyspnea is almost always first noticed with physical exertion and may progress to symptoms at rest. The degree of activity necessary to elicit symptoms may be quantified by asking questions such as "How many flights of stairs can you climb?" or "How far can you walk on level ground?" One commonly used scale for classifying the severity of dyspnea was proposed and published by the Medical Research Council (Table 107-2). Other measures that have been proposed include the Baseline Dyspnea Index. These measures may be repeated on subsequent visits to assess patient improvement with treatment. Another method for measuring intensity is use of quality-of-life measures such as the Chronic Respiratory Disease Questionnaire. There is no single broadly accepted form of measurement; the most important thing is to find the one that fits best in one's individual practice and use it consistently. Practitioners should be cautious, however, and not rely too heavily on a patient's grading of symptoms or ignore other clinical signs and symptoms.[12,13]

Associated Symptoms

In addition to dyspnea, cardinal symptoms of pulmonary disease are chest pain, cough, hemoptysis, and wheezing. Chest pain is one manifestation of ischemic heart disease but may also result from pneumothorax, pulmonary embolism, or rib trauma. A patient reporting leg or hip pain preceding or concurrent with onset of dyspnea should raise suspicion for pulmonary embolism. Hemoptysis is a distressing symptom that may accompany dyspnea. Expectorated blood can originate from the nose, airways, or lung parenchyma. Cough is a common symptom of acute and chronic pulmonary disease. Persistent cough is most often caused by upper airway cough syndrome (previously referred as postnasal drip syndrome), gastroesophageal reflux, or asthma. Wheezing signifies airway diseases, such as asthma and chronic obstructive pulmonary disease (COPD), or focal obstruction by a tumor, such as a carcinoid lesion, or aspirated foreign body. Patients who are initially seen with fever, chills, or night sweats should be evaluated for acute or chronic

TABLE 107-1 Respiratory Descriptions and Causes

Quality or Description	Common Causes
Tightness, constriction	Asthma, COPD, bronchiectasis, foreign body, bronchitis
Increased work or effort	Severe kyphoscoliosis, obesity, pleural effusion, myasthenia gravis, Guillain-Barré syndrome, spinal cord injury, myopathy
Air hunger, unsatisfied inspiration	Pulmonary embolism, pneumonia, CHF, altitude, metabolic acidosis, anemia, interstitial lung disease, cystic fibrosis

TABLE 107-2 Dyspnea Scale

Grade	Degree	Defining Clinical Characteristics
0	None	Not troubled with breathlessness except with strenuous exercise
1	Slight	Troubled by shortness of breath when hurrying on level ground or walking up a slight hill
2	Moderate	Walks more slowly than people of the same age when on level ground because of breathlessness or has to stop for breath when walking at own pace on level ground
3	Severe	Stops for breath after walking about 100 yards or after a few minutes on level ground
4	Very severe	Too breathless to leave the house or breathless when dressing or undressing

From Long-term domiciliary oxygen therapy in chronic hypoxic cor pulmonale complicating chronic bronchitis and emphysema. Report of the Medical Research Council Working Party, *Lancet* 1:681-686, 1981.

TABLE 107-3 Assessment of Dyspnea: Dos and Don'ts

Do	Don't
Ask about the qualitative experience of dyspnea (such as chest tightness, work of breathing).	Rely on blood gases for assessing the severity of dyspnea.
Ask about associated affective states (anxiety, panic, depression).	Rely on orders such as "Call physician for O_2 sat <90%" as a trigger for the reevaluation of dyspnea. Consider an order such as "Assess dyspnea intensity q shift. Call physician for dyspnea >6 (0-10 scale)."
Try to quantify the intensity of dyspnea and associated suffering (e.g., use a 0-10 scale).	
Ask how dyspnea is affecting the patient's life (e.g., reduced activity, sleep disorder).	
Ask about concerns for the future (fear of suffocation, greater disability).	

From Hallenbeck J: Pathophysiology and treatment of dyspnea, *Pulmonary, Critical Care, Sleep Update.* Available at www.chestnet.org/accp/pccsu/pathophysiology-and-treatment-dyspnea?page=0,3. Accessed January 24, 2012.

lung infections, including pneumonia, tuberculosis, and chronic bronchiectasis.

Dyspnea is often accompanied by fear and anxiety. A dyspnea-panic cycle has been described in which the sensation of breathlessness leads to anxiety, which creates muscle tension, which in turn leads to increased dyspnea and panic. Thus the anxiety associated with dyspnea can become a vicious circle leading to future attacks of dyspnea.[14,15]

Exposures

The lungs are uniquely susceptible to various environmental hazards, including air pollution, dust, smoke, carbon monoxide, and an array of occupational exposures (silica, asbestos, chemical exposure). A careful history of current and past tobacco use is essential in the evaluation of tobacco-related diseases such as asthma, chronic bronchitis, emphysema, spontaneous pneumothorax secondary to bullous disease, ischemic heart disease, respiratory bronchiolitis, and eosinophilic granuloma. In addition, many medications and therapeutic radiation are known to damage the lungs. Table 107-3 lists the steps to take in the assessment of dyspnea.[7]

PHYSICAL EXAMINATION

The physical examination begins with careful assessment of the patient's vital signs. Normal respiratory rate in adults ranges from 12 to 20 breaths per minute, and a rapid or labored breathing pattern is often but not always evident in dyspneic patients. Many practitioners consider pulse oximetry a "vital sign" because it usually provides a reliable measure of arterial oxygen saturation. A normal oxygen saturation level, however, does not rule out carbon dioxide retention and ventilatory insufficiency; carbon dioxide levels must be directly measured with an arterial blood gas sample. Expiratory peak flow measurement may also be included in the initial assessment of patients with known airway disease or wheezing.

Breathing pattern and body position provide important clues to disease severity. The acutely dyspneic patient often sits upright and leans forward to optimize breathing mechanics. The inability to speak in full sentences and accessory respiratory muscle use indicate increased work of breathing. Patients with COPD often adopt a characteristic "pursed-lip" appearance. Shallow, rapid breathing or panting is characteristic of interstitial lung disease in patients with poor or decreased lung compliance. The skin may be diaphoretic, and the patient may appear anxious. Bluish discoloration of the skin and mucous membranes (cyanosis) results from increased amounts of deoxygenated hemoglobin. Central cyanosis, detected in the tongue and mucous membranes, is a more reliable indicator of oxygenation than peripheral cyanosis, which can also result from intense vasoconstriction of vessels in the extremities. Mental status may be depressed by either severe hypoxemia or hypercapnia. Digital or finger clubbing is an important finding often attributed to various lung diseases, but it is also seen in other disorders, such as inflammatory bowel disease and congenital heart disease.

The lung examination includes careful inspection of the thorax and abdomen. Chest wall deformities may limit lung expansion and contribute to dyspnea. During inspiration, normally the chest rises and the abdomen moves outward because of the contraction of the diaphragm (which moves downward). During inspiration in a patient with inspiratory muscle fatigue, the chest rises (because of accessory muscle contraction) and the abdomen moves inward (because of upward movement of the diaphragm); this pattern of breathing is said to be paradoxical and indicates diaphragmatic weakness or fatigue. Palpation of the chest wall is useful in assessing tracheal position, symmetry of chest movement, areas of tenderness, and crepitus (subcutaneous air from pneumothorax or pneumomediastinum). Airless lung transmits sounds more efficiently than air-filled lung and is the basis for auscultatory consolidative findings, including bronchial breath sounds, egophony (E to A changes), and whispered pectoriloquy. The classic example of a disease that causes lung consolidation is pneumonia, although any process that fills (pus, water, blood, protein, cells) or collapses alveoli yields these findings. Abnormal, or adventitious, lung sounds are distinguished by whether they are continuous (high-pitched sounds are wheezing, low-pitched sounds are rhonchi) or discontinuous (crackles). Wheezing signifies bronchoconstriction or airway obstruction from secretions, tumor, or foreign body. Crackles are heard in a number of disease processes, including congestive heart failure (CHF) and interstitial lung disease. Pleural friction rubs are grating sounds that may occur on inspiration or expiration as inflamed pleural surfaces rub against each other.

A detailed discussion of the cardiac examination is beyond the scope of this chapter, but it is an important component of the evaluation of dyspneic patients. The pulse should be carefully analyzed for rate and rhythm. Atrial fibrillation is a common arrhythmia that can usually be diagnosed at the bedside by its "irregularly irregular" character. Left ventricular dysfunction and valvular heart disease also lend themselves to bedside diagnosis through palpation and auscultation. The extremities should also be assessed for pulse and edema.[16,17]

In summary, the physical examination is an essential part of the workup of dyspneic patients and should be used to help direct the diagnostic evaluation. The absence of specific physical examination findings can be of greater diagnostic usefulness than positive findings in patients with chronic dyspnea. For example, interstitial lung disease and CHF are unlikely causes of dyspnea in a patient without crackles on lung examination.

DIFFERENTIAL DIAGNOSIS

Dyspnea is most commonly caused by cardiopulmonary disease, although anemia, neuromuscular weakness, gastroesophageal reflux, deconditioning, and psychogenic causes must be considered. The most common causes of acute dyspnea are asthma, bronchitis, pneumothorax, pneumonia, pulmonary embolism, chest trauma with rib fractures or pulmonary contusions, ischemic heart failure, psychogenic causes, and acute blood loss. The majority of patients with long-standing dyspnea have one of four causes: asthma, COPD, interstitial lung disease, or cardiomyopathy.

DIFFERENTIAL DIAGNOSIS

Dyspnea

ACUTE

- Acute blood loss
- Airway obstruction
- Asthma
- Bronchitis
- Carbon monoxide poisoning
- CHF or pulmonary edema
- Foreign body aspiration
- Ischemic heart disease
- Neuromuscular weakness
- Pleural effusion
- Pneumonia
- Pneumothorax
- Psychogenic causes
- Pulmonary contusions
- Pulmonary emboli
- Trauma (rib fractures or pulmonary contusions)

CHRONIC

- Anemia
- Asthma
- Cardiomyopathy
- CHF
- COPD
- Cystic fibrosis
- Gastroesophageal reflux disease
- Interstitial pulmonary fibrosis
- Ischemic heart disease
- Obesity
- Pectus excavatum
- Pleural effusion
- Pulmonary hypertension
- Sarcoidosis
- Severe kyphoscoliosis
- Spondylitis

DIAGNOSTICS

After a thorough history and physical examination are completed, further diagnostic studies may be necessary. Diagnostic workup is often guided by history and physical examination findings and is affected by whether dyspnea is acute or chronic. A plain chest radiograph is helpful in elucidating many causes of dyspnea. Radiographic findings of hyperinflation, flattened hemidiaphragms, increased anterior clear space, and bullae support a diagnosis of COPD. Parenchymal infiltrates occur in many different disease processes but in the context of an acute infectious syndrome imply pneumonia. CHF is recognized by cephalization of vessels, Kerley B lines, and enlarged cardiac silhouette. Frank pulmonary edema manifests with bilateral perihilar air space filling (batwing appearance) and pleural effusions. Pneumothorax and pleural effusion are usually easily detected on a plain chest radiograph, although small effusions may require decubitus views for confirmation. The chest radiograph is usually normal or reveals only subtle abnormalities in asthma and pulmonary embolism.

Spirometry is essential to the diagnosis and management of asthma and COPD. A decrease in the ratio of forced expiratory volume in 1 second to forced vital capacity (FEV_1/FVC) is the spirometric hallmark of obstruction. Bronchoprovocation testing with either methacholine or exercise may be necessary to diagnose asthma in patients with normal baseline spirometry. Proportionately reduced FEV and FVC suggest restriction (a useful pneumonic for restrictive lung processes is *PAINT*: pleural disease, alveolar filling process, interstitial lung disease, neuromuscular disease, or thoracic cage abnormalities), which should be confirmed with lung volume measurements. Diaphragmatic and respiratory muscle weakness may be detected with maximum inspiratory pressure and maximum expiratory pressure maneuvers, although these tests are neither sensitive nor specific.

The workup for pulmonary thromboembolic disease can be complicated and is often driven by the availability and expertise of local medical resources. An appropriate evaluation may initially include a ventilation/perfusion ($\dot{V}/\dot{Q}$) scan or computed tomographic angiography. Symptomatic lower extremity clots (the source of most pulmonary emboli) are usually detected by ultrasound. Pulmonary angiography remains the definitive test for the diagnosis of pulmonary embolism.

Cardiac rhythm disturbances and hypertrophy may be noted on routine electrocardiography (ECG), although intermittent arrhythmias may be detected only by long-term monitoring (e.g., telemetry, Holter, or event monitoring). Echocardiography is extremely useful in assessing left ventricular function, cardiac valve status, pericardial effusions, and, in some cases, pulmonary hypertension.

Other routine studies with usefulness in the evaluation of patients with dyspnea include hemoglobin level to exclude anemia, thyroid function tests to exclude hyperthyroidism, and B-type natriuretic peptide (BNP) or its N-terminal prohormone precursor (NTproBNP) if heart failure is a consideration. BNP/NTproBNP testing has substantially higher sensitivity than specificity. This is why it is much better suited for ruling out heart failure in patients with a low to intermediate pretest probability of CHF. More sophisticated testing, such as formal cardiopulmonary exercise testing and cardiac catheterization, obviously requires referral to specialists.[17]

DIAGNOSTICS

Dyspnea

INITIAL

Peak flow
Pulse oximetry

LABORATORY

Complete blood count and differential*
Thyroid-stimulating hormone*
BNP*

IMAGING

Chest x-ray studies (posteroanterior and lateral)*
Computed tomography scan*

OTHER DIAGNOSTICS

Arterial blood gases*
ECG*
Echocardiography*
Exercise stress testing*
Pulmonary function tests
$\dot{V}/\dot{Q}$ scan or pulmonary angiography*
Holter or event monitor*

*If indicated.

MANAGEMENT

The treatment of dyspnea entails treatment of the underlying disease process and symptomatic relief. Supplemental oxygen should be administered initially to all acutely dyspneic patients and to chronically dyspneic patients who are hypoxemic. The standard Medicare criteria for supplemental oxygen are as follows: $Pa{O_2}$ at rest of less than 55 mm Hg or oxygen saturation of 88% or less. Patients with a $Pa{O_2}$ of 56 to 59 mm HG or an oxygen saturation of 89% or less warrant supplemental oxygen if they have underlying CHF or pulmonary hypertension. These criteria are based on two large studies that demonstrated improved survival in hypoxemic COPD patients treated with supplemental oxygen.[18-22] Patients who undergo desaturation during sleep or exercise also qualify for supplemental oxygen, although the data supporting these indications are not as strong. Administration of supplemental oxygen may worsen carbon dioxide retention in some patients with COPD. These patients require an arterial blood gas assessment to ensure adequate carbon dioxide elimination. Energy conservation strategies (e.g., walking slowly; periodically using resting positions, such as leaning forward while sitting in a chair; avoiding fatigue; and spacing chores at times of feeling well) and specific breathing techniques are often effective in patients with obstructive lung disease. Patients with difficulty mobilizing secretions (e.g., those with chronic bronchitis, bronchiectasis, cystic fibrosis) benefit from chest physiotherapy and airway clearance adjuncts, such as the flutter device or vest airway clearance system. Anxiolytics and narcotics are sometimes effective in relieving dyspnea but must be used cautiously because of inherent respiratory depressant properties. Opioid medications are among the most studied medications for the relief of dyspnea, and there can be significant relief of dyspneic symptoms; however, no improvement in oxygenation occurs. Typically these medications are used in palliative medicine at the smallest effective dose that does not cause significant side effects.

Formal pulmonary rehabilitation programs effectively incorporate dyspnea management for patients with long-term disease such as COPD. Therapies include exercise training, education, nutrition intervention, and psychosocial support. These programs have been shown to improve quality of life as well as reduce health care utilization and psychosocial issues.[23-26]

COMPLICATIONS

Dyspnea limits a patient's activities of daily living. The consequences of uncontrolled dyspnea symptoms may include anxiety, depression, loss of job, and social isolation. Physical deconditioning results from decreased exercise and leads to a downward spiral of ever-decreasing activity.

INDICATIONS FOR REFERRAL OR HOSPITALIZATION

Patients with chronic dyspnea should be referred to a pulmonary specialist when the cause is not obvious from the history, physical examination, and screening studies, including complete blood count (CBC), chest radiography, and spirometry. Echocardiography and treadmill stress testing may help differentiate between cardiac and pulmonary disease before the consultation.

The decision to hospitalize a patient depends initially on identifying the likely cause of respiratory distress. Conditions that need to be readily identified and mandate hospital admission include pulmonary embolism and myocardial infarction. Criteria for hospitalization of patients with other conditions such as pneumothorax, asthma, and COPD depend on the severity of the illness, response to treatment, and presence of comorbid conditions.

PATIENT AND FAMILY EDUCATION AND HEALTH PROMOTION

Patients with chronic dyspnea need to be taught techniques that control symptoms and warning signs of the need for medical assistance. Pulmonary rehabilitation programs provide intense education for patients with severe pulmonary disease but are expensive and not always available. All patients who use inhaled bronchodilators and corticosteroids should be regularly instructed in proper inhaler techniques, including the use of spacer devices. Asthmatic patients may benefit from home peak flow monitoring to detect worsening airflow obstruction, which offers an opportunity for early intervention. Smoking cessation is critical in the management of any cardiopulmonary disease, and providers play a pivotal role in educating their patients about the adverse effects of tobacco use and strategies to stop smoking.

CHAPTER 108

HEMOPTYSIS

Natalie Nicole Carrier

DEFINITION AND EPIDEMIOLOGY

Hemoptysis refers to the expectoration of blood from the lung parenchyma or airways. It can range from a small amount of blood-streaked sputum, which is commonly seen in bronchitis, to a massive hemorrhage, which is a medical emergency because it rapidly causes death by asphyxiation. The classifications—nonmassive and massive—are based on the volume of blood loss; however, there are no uniform definitions for these categories. Hemoptysis is generally classified as nonmassive if the blood loss is less than 100 to 200 mL/day, whereas massive hemoptysis refers to more than this amount in 24 hours.[1] Massive hemoptysis is uncommon, occurring in less than 5% of patients with hemoptysis. However, the associated mortality rate ranges from 7% to 30% to as high as 58%, which demonstrates the need for urgent evaluation and management.[1,2] Even slight bleeding may signify a serious condition, such as bronchogenic carcinoma, tuberculosis, or erosion of the thoracic aneurysm. Therefore, blood loss volume is more helpful in directing management than in making a diagnosis.

The most common causes of hemoptysis in the United States are, in descending order, acute and chronic bronchitis, lung cancer, pneumonia, and tuberculosis. Similarly, these are the most common causes of hemoptysis seen in the primary care setting. However, tuberculosis is a leading cause of hemoptysis in developing countries and should be high on the list of differential diagnoses for patients who are from countries with a high prevalence of the disease or who have traveled to countries where tuberculosis is endemic.[1] Less common causes of hemoptysis include influenza viruses, malignant carcinomas, and pulmonary barotrauma secondary to diving.[3,4] Hemoptysis can also be a sign of an underlying hereditary disorder, such as Osler-Weber-Rendu syndrome, also known as hereditary hemorrhagic telangiectasia (HHT). HHT is an autosomal dominant disorder that is typically characterized by a triad of telangiectasia (including pulmonary), recurrent epistaxis, and a family history of the disorder.[5]

PATHOPHYSIOLOGY

For hemoptysis to occur, there must be some communication between the airways and the blood vessels of the lungs. The lungs receive blood from two relatively independent circulations: pulmonary and bronchial. The pulmonary circulation is characterized by lower pressures and higher volumes and is supplied with mixed venous blood through the pulmonary arteries. In contrast, the bronchial circulation supplies oxygenated blood in a high-pressure, low-volume circuit.

The bronchial arteries can become enlarged and more numerous in association with a variety of inflammatory or neoplastic diseases. Chronic inflammation, often associated with infectious processes, can lead to destruction of the connective tissue of blood vessels or result in erosion through the vessel wall. Angiographic studies have revealed that hemoptysis typically originates from disruptions of the branches of the bronchial arterial tree. This is presumably related to the connection of these arteries to the proliferative nests of small vessels often found in areas of inflammation and tumors.

CLINICAL PRESENTATION

It is common for patients to confuse hemoptysis with hematemesis or epistaxis. Patient history, including factors such as age, nutritional status, occupational and environmental exposures, and comorbid conditions, can be useful in differentiating among the three conditions and can help narrow the differential diagnosis. Taking a thorough travel history is important because tuberculosis and bronchiectasis appear to be decreasing as causes of hemoptysis in the United States, whereas they are still frequent causes of hemoptysis in other parts of the world. Recent travel may have also increased the risk of parasitic infections, which can cause hemoptysis.

In addition, a description of the blood and accompanying symptoms can be helpful in differentiating between hemoptysis and hematemesis. Blood from the airways is usually bright red or pink, liquid or clotted in appearance, and frothy because of the presence of surfactant. The pH is alkaline, and it tends to be mixed with macrophages and neutrophils. Blood originating in the gastrointestinal tract is usually dark red, brown, or black; it has a coffee-ground appearance and is rarely frothy. It is acidic and may be intermixed with food particles. Absence of nausea and vomiting and a history of lung disease raise the suspicion of hemoptysis, whereas the presence of nausea and vomiting and coexisting gastric or hepatic disease suggest hematemesis.[1]

It is important to carefully determine the chronology and volume of hemoptysis. Quantifying blood loss may be difficult, even in patients who are clinically stable, because they are often anxious and, as a result, usually overestimate the amount of blood loss. However, every effort should be made to determine the rate and volume of blood loss, which can include observing as the patient coughs and using a graduated container. Urgent evaluation and possible hospitalization are indicated if more than 50 mL of blood has been expectorated in the previous 24 hours. For smaller amounts of blood loss, a thorough diagnostic evaluation can be initiated in the primary care setting.

Mild hemoptysis, recurring sporadically over a few years, is common in smokers, who may have chronic bronchitis with intermittent flares of acute bronchitis. However, abrupt hemoptysis associated with cigarette smoking can also be seen with bronchogenic carcinoma. A long history of small-volume, recurrent hemoptysis with little or no sputum production is suggestive of processes such as bronchogenic carcinoma, bronchial adenoma, and vascular malformation. A history of chronic sputum production suggests an infectious cause, such as bronchitis, bronchiectasis, lung abscess, or tuberculosis. Hemoptysis associated with bacterial pneumonia is suggested by an acute onset of fever, sputum production, and, commonly, pleuritic chest pain. Hemoptysis is commonly a late symptom of bronchogenic carcinoma and is preceded by a chronic cough, fatigue, and constitutional symptoms. Environmental exposure to asbestos, arsenic, chromium, nickel, and certain ethers can increase the risk for hemoptysis.[1] Occupational history may be helpful in elucidating the cause of hemoptysis. For example, after repetitive deep dives, breath-hold divers are often affected by a common syndrome characterized by typical symptoms such as cough, sensation of chest constriction, blood-striated expectorate (hemoptysis), and, rarely, an overt acute pulmonary edema syndrome, often together with various degrees of dyspnea. Similar clinical features had been previously observed in scuba divers, swimmers, and athletes engaged in strenuous efforts during terrestrial sport activities.[4] A travel history may be helpful. Tuberculosis is endemic in many parts of the world, and parasitic causes should be considered.[1]

PHYSICAL EXAMINATION

The presence of a fever suggests infection. A thorough examination of the ears, nose, and throat can detect upper airway sources of bleeding, such as laryngeal carcinoma lesions. Cervical, supraclavicular, or axillary adenopathy raises the suspicion of an intrathoracic malignant neoplasm. The presence of stridor or findings suggestive of chronic obstructive pulmonary disease, congestive heart failure, or pneumonia can be determined by auscultation of the chest.

Localized wheezing may indicate a local obstruction, foreign body, or bronchogenic carcinoma. A pleural friction rub may be the only sign of pulmonary infarction associated with a pulmonary embolism. Isolated crackles are nonspecific for the location of the primary disease because they may represent an inflammatory reaction to blood aspirated from another site.

Digital clubbing is suggestive of chronic lung disease, such as bronchiectasis or malignant neoplasm. Cardiac examination may help determine the presence of mitral stenosis. Localized adenopathy, especially a supraclavicular node, may be indicative of a lung malignant neoplasm. A bleeding disorder is suggested by the presence of petechiae or ecchymoses.

DIAGNOSTICS

- Chest radiography should be performed as part of an initial evaluation.
  - For all patients with hemoptysis; may help localize bleeding and identify cause; provides images for later comparison to evaluate resolution of disease
  - Important diagnostic findings include an air-fluid level of a lung abscess, the "crescent sign" of a mycetoma, a

nodule that suggests a neoplasm, evidence of volume loss, or consolidation distal to an airway obstruction.
- Computed tomography (CT) is suggested for initial evaluation of patients at high risk of malignancy who have suspicious findings on chest radiography.
  CT should be considered in patients with risk factors (e.g., 40 years or older, smoking history of at least 30 pack-years) who demonstrate negative or nonlocalizing findings.
- CT and fiberoptic bronchoscopy have complementary roles in the evaluation of patients with hemoptysis, and the combination of these two tests has been shown to give a higher yield of specific diagnoses than either test alone.
- Fiberoptic bronchoscopy allows direct visualization of the airways and localization of the bleeding source.
  - Biopsy specimens and lavage samples from the airways and alveolar spaces can be sent for cytologic and microbial studies.
  - This procedure is relatively safe, is well tolerated, and can be performed on an outpatient basis.
  - The proper timing for fiberoptic bronchoscopy is somewhat controversial. Most thoracic specialists prefer to perform bronchoscopy early in the course of hemoptysis. However, some believe that bronchoscopy is indicated primarily if hemoptysis has been present for longer than 1 week or if the likelihood of cancer is greater because of systemic symptoms or risk factors.
- Blood typing and crossmatch may be obtained for patients with hemodynamic instability from blood loss or those in whom a complete blood count (CBC) reveals anemia that warrants transfusion.
- Coagulation studies may be reasonable to obtain in patients with a history of coagulopathy or current anticoagulant use.
- A complete blood count is reasonable to obtain in all patients with hemoptysis to rule out thrombocytopenia and to evaluate for anemia and/or microcytosis indicative of chronic blood loss or malignancy.
- Renal function tests should be performed before imaging with contrast media and in patients with suspected vasculitis.
- Sputum testing (Gram stain, acid-fast bacilli smear, fungal cultures, cytology) should be obtained if massive hemoptysis or an infectious cause is suspected.

DIAGNOSTICS

Hemoptysis

LABORATORY
CBC and differential*
Coagulation studies*
Sputum for acid-fast bacilli, Gram stain, culture and sensitivity
Sputum for cytology*
Urinalysis*

IMAGING
Chest x-ray examination
CT scan*
Ventilation/perfusion scan*

OTHER DIAGNOSTICS
Fiberoptic bronchoscopy*
Transthoracic needle aspiration*
Bronchoscopy or open punch biopsy*

*If indicated.

- If a pulmonary embolus is suspected, especially if there are risk factors for deep venous thrombosis and pulmonary thromboembolism, a ventilation/perfusion lung scan should be obtained.

DIFFERENTIAL DIAGNOSIS

Minor hemoptysis is generally not life-threatening. Despite a thorough evaluation, many patients who are seen with hemoptysis do not receive a specific diagnosis, at least not initially. The goals of further evaluation are to determine the cause, to provide specific treatment (if available), and to rule out underlying disease. The differential diagnosis is extensive and includes airway diseases, neoplasms, pulmonary vascular diseases, cardiovascular disease, and miscellaneous causes such as the use of anticoagulants or fibrinolytics. The most common cause of acute mild hemoptysis is bronchitis or infections such as pneumonia. Other common causes include lung cancer and lung abscesses, tuberculosis, bronchiectasis, and pulmonary thromboembolism. A history of recurrent pneumonia or hemoptysis with onset during adolescence suggests possible intralobular pulmonary sequestration or hereditary syndromes such as HHT, although the presentation may be mistaken for other causes such as bronchiectasis or lung abscess.[5,6] Pulmonary embolism is an important diagnosis to consider when the presentation includes hemoptysis and pleuritic chest pain or when the patient's history is significant for malignant disease, especially adenocarcinoma, which can contribute to hypercoagulation, thus increasing the risk for a pulmonary embolism.[1,7]

DIFFERENTIAL DIAGNOSIS

Hemoptysis

PULMONARY
- Bronchial adenoma
- Bronchiectasis*
- Bronchitis*
- Bronchogenic carcinoma
- Bronchopulmonary sequestration
- Cystic fibrosis
- Foreign body
- Fungal infections
- Lung abscess*
- Lung cancer*
- Metastatic tumor
- Mycetoma (aspergilloma or fungus ball)
- Noninvasive aspergillosis or mucormycosis
- Nontubercular mycobacteria
- Parasitic infection
- Pneumonia*
- Pulmonary contusion or trauma
- Pulmonary embolism*
- Pulmonary-renal syndromes (Goodpasture syndrome, systemic lupus erythematosus, Wegener granulomatosis)
- Tuberculosis*

CARDIOVASCULAR
- Arteriovenous malformation
- Bleeding diathesis
- Congestive heart failure*
- Mitral valve prolapse and mitral stenosis

MISCELLANEOUS
- Medications (anticoagulants, fibrinolytics, amiodarone)
- Pulmonary artery rupture caused by pulmonary arterial (Swan-Ganz) catheterization*

*Common causes.

MANAGEMENT

Immediate emergency department referral is indicated when the rate of bleeding qualifies as massive hemoptysis (a rate of more than 200 mL/day).

The overall goals of management include bleeding cessation, aspiration prevention, and treatment of the underlying cause.

1. The most common presentation in primary care is acute mild hemoptysis caused by bronchitis.
2. Low-risk patients with normal chest films can be treated on an outpatient basis with close monitoring and appropriate oral antibiotics, if clinically warranted.
3. Outpatient evaluation by a pulmonologist should be considered if hemoptysis persists or if the cause remains unclear.
4. An abnormal mass on a chest radiograph necessitates outpatient bronchoscopy.
5. For patients with a normal chest radiograph and risk factors for lung cancer or recurrent hemoptysis, outpatient fiberoptic bronchoscopy is indicated to evaluate for neoplasm.
6. High-resolution CT scan is indicated when clinical suspicion for malignancy exists, when sputum and bronchoscopy do not offer a cause, or when chest radiography demonstrates peripheral or other parenchymal disease.
7. Patients with negative findings on chest radiography, CT, and bronchoscopy have a low risk of malignancy and can be observed for 3 years. No specific recommendations can be made regarding chest CT or radiography during that interval, but imaging should be based on risk factors. If hemoptysis recurs, multidimensional CT angiography should be considered. Bronchoscopy may also complement imaging during the observation period.
8. Patients with massive hemoptysis require rapid and decisive care; diagnosis and treatment must occur simultaneously.
9. Patients with massive hemoptysis require intensive care and early consultation with a pulmonologist.
10. As with any potentially serious condition, evaluation of airway, breathing, and circulation is the initial step in treatment, because asphyxiation is the primary cause of death.
11. Supplemental oxygen and fluid resuscitation are crucial.
12. Assistance from a cardiothoracic surgeon should be considered because emergency surgical intervention may be necessary.[1]
13. Emergency lung resection is feasible in appropriately selected patients with radiologically localized disease and massive hemoptysis.[8]
14. Bronchial artery embolization is an effective immediate treatment for massive hemoptysis. Because the bleeding recurrence rate is high in patients with lung cancer or idiopathic bronchiectasis, surgery should be considered in these patients after initial stabilization by bronchial artery embolization.[9]
15. Bronchial artery embolization may be best used as a temporizing measure in patients unsuitable for emergency lung resection.[8]
16. Other treatments modalities for massive hemoptysis include cold saline lavage, epinephrine, and endobronchial stent tamponade.[10]

COMPLICATIONS

Patients with hemoptysis resulting from noninfectious causes are at risk for frequent recurrences. Massive hemoptysis often recurs, both suddenly and without warning, and may be fatal. The most obvious complication is asphyxiation, which accounts for the majority of deaths from hemoptysis.

INDICATIONS FOR REFERRAL OR HOSPITALIZATION

- Cause with high risk of bleeding (e.g., lesions with pulmonary artery involvement or aspergillosis)
- Abnormal gas exchange (respiratory rate >30 breaths per minute, oxygen saturation <88% in room air, or need for high-flow oxygen [>8 L/min] or mechanical ventilation)
- Hemodynamic instability (hemoglobin <8 g/dL [80 g/L] and/or a decrease of more than 2 g/dL [20 g/L] from patient's baseline, consumptive coagulopathy, or hypotension requiring fluid bolus or vasopressors)
- Massive hemoptysis (>200 mL/48 hr or >50 mL per episode in patients with chronic pulmonary disease)
- Respiratory comorbidities (e.g., chronic obstructive pulmonary disease, previous pneumonectomy, cystic fibrosis
- Other comorbidities (e.g., need for anticoagulation, ischemic heart disease).[1]

PATIENT AND FAMILY EDUCATION

Hemoptysis is frightening for patients and their families and may be a symptom of serious underlying disease. Education should include information about the diagnostic evaluation, that management is tailored to the underlying cause, and the importance of adhering to the prescribed treatment. The rate of recurrence in patients who smoke is likely to be high because common causes, such as bronchitis and bronchogenic carcinoma, are often related to smoking. Therefore it is imperative that patients be encouraged to stop smoking. Because hemoptysis can be particularly disconcerting, emotional support for the patient and family is especially important.

CHAPTER 109

LUNG CANCER

Alexander Fuld

DEFINITION AND EPIDEMIOLOGY

Lung cancer, also referred to as *bronchogenic carcinoma*, encompasses multiple malignancies involving the lung or airways. The vast majority of lung cancers are categorized as non–small cell lung cancer (NSCLC) or small cell lung cancer (SCLC) based on the histologic characteristics.

Although lung cancer was notably uncommon near the turn of the 20th century, increased exposure to tobacco smoke has caused a global epidemic of lung cancer.[1] In 2015 there were projected to be an estimated 221,200 new cases of lung cancer and 158,040 deaths in the United States.[2] Although recently there has been a slight decline in the incidence of lung cancer within the United States, lung cancer remains the leading cause of cancer death among both males and females in this country. The 5-year survival rate for lung cancer as a whole is less than 20%.[1] The primary risk factor for lung cancer is smoking tobacco which accounts for 80% to 90% of cases.[3] Other risk factors include secondhand smoke, air pollution, radon, ionizing radiation, a family history of lung cancer, and occupational exposures such as asbestos, tar, and soot.[4]

PATHOPHYSIOLOGY

NSCLC represents approximately 85% of lung malignancies. The primary subtypes of NSCLC are adenocarcinoma (50%) and squamous cell carcinoma (25%), with the remainder consisting of large cell carcinomas and other less common variants.[5] Historically, these histologic subtypes have been grouped together as NSCLC and managed in a similar fashion, although there are some treatment considerations based on histology. SCLC comprises approximately 13% of lung cancers. Although smoking is linked with all forms of lung cancer, it is most strongly associated with SCLC and squamous cell carcinoma. Adenocarcinoma is the most common type of lung cancer in nonsmokers.

The precise path that causes the malignant transformation of bronchoepithelial cells is not fully understood. Smoking tobacco is the primary cause in the vast majority of lung cancers. Yet, only approximately 10% of smokers will develop lung cancer, which points to significant host factors that may control an individual's susceptibility to cancer.[6] Carcinogens such as tobacco smoke, radon, and asbestos fibers induce tissue injury with resultant genetic and epigenetic changes. Over time these changes cause various pathways that control cellular proliferation to become dysregulated, which ultimately leads to tumor formation, invasion, and metastasis.[7] Individuals have varying inherent genetic susceptibility to these carcinogens, and epidemiologic studies suggest there can be a familial predisposition to lung cancer independent of tobacco smoke exposure.[1] More recently, specific acquired genetic abnormalities in non–small cell lung tumors have been identified that have significant clinical implications. The two most important of these acquired abnormalities are the epidermal growth factor receptor *(EGFR)* gene mutations and the anaplastic lymphoma kinase *(ALK)* gene rearrangements. *EGFR* mutations are present in approximately 15% of adenocarcinomas in the United States and are more commonly seen in nonsmokers, females, and individuals of Asian descent. *EGFR* mutations are found in 35% of lung cancers in Asia. *ALK* rearrangements are identified in approximately 4% of adenocarcinomas in the United States, most frequently in nonsmokers and younger patients. As discussed later, specific therapies targeting these molecular defects have been developed with encouraging results.[1] Tumor specimens are now routinely being tested for these abnormalities. Other so-called driver mutations have also been identified in lung cancer (e.g., *ROS1*, *BRAF*), and efforts to develop additional targeted treatment agents are under way. Although SCLC cells also have characteristic mutations (e.g., loss of function of the tumor-suppressor retinoblastoma gene *RB1*, or p53 mutations), these have not yet resulted in targeted therapies.[8]

CLINICAL PRESENTATION AND PHYSICAL EXAMINATION

The typical lung cancer patient will be a current or former smoker in the seventh or eighth decade of life. At diagnosis, only approximately 15% of lung cancers are confined to the lung. Twenty-two percent have spread to regional lymph nodes, and nearly 60% have already metastasized. The majority of patients with lung cancer are symptomatic at presentation. Cough (up to 75% of cases), weight loss (up to 68%), and dyspnea (up to 60%) are the most common presenting signs and symptoms.[9] Cough is particularly seen with squamous cell carcinomas and small cell carcinomas owing to their tendency to involve central airways, whereas adenocarcinomas are more often peripherally located. Although cough is common in a smoking population in general, changes in a chronic cough should prompt consideration of malignancy. Other frequent presentations involve chest pain or discomfort and hemoptysis. Recurrent pneumonias in a similar anatomic area may indicate a neoplasm causing postobstructive changes, and further investigation is warranted. In addition, as with other malignancies, lung cancer is a hypercoagulable state, and patients may have deep vein thrombosis on presentation.

Although lung cancer can spread to any organ, the most common sites of metastasis are the liver, bones, adrenal glands, and brain. About a third of patients will have symptoms caused by distant metastasis at presentation. Weight loss of more than 10 pounds, focal skeletal pain (from bone metastases), or neurologic complaints such as headache or extremity weakness (from brain metastases) are the symptoms that most commonly indicate the presence of metastatic disease.[9] Patients with lung cancer often have abnormal blood counts with anemia, leukocytosis, and thrombocytosis. A hematocrit of less than 40% in males and 35% in females or an elevated calcium or γ-glutamyl transpeptidase (GGT) level also increases the likelihood of metastatic disease. On physical examination, the signs that most commonly indicate metastatic disease are palpable lymphadenopathy greater than 1 cm, bone tenderness, hepatomegaly, focal neurologic findings, or a soft tissue mass.[9]

Many of the signs and symptoms of SCLC and NSCLC are similar, but SCLC symptoms tend to progress more rapidly, typically over 8 to 12 weeks. NSCLC has a slower tempo, with tumor growth typically seen over many months. SCLC is also more frequently associated with paraneoplastic syndromes, with the most common entity, the syndrome of inappropriate antidiuretic hormone secretion (SIADH), seen in 15% to 40% of SCLC patients. Signs, symptoms, and associated syndromes of lung cancer are summarized in Table 109-1.

DIAGNOSTICS

When lung cancer is suspected based on history and physical examination findings, laboratory evaluation and imaging are indicated as summarized in the Diagnostics box. If there is a high degree of suspicion (e.g., an abnormal chest radiograph) a contrast-enhanced computed tomography (CT) scan of the thorax should be performed that includes the liver and the adrenal glands. Imaging should also include evaluation of any sites of suspected metastatic disease. As part of the staging evaluation, most patients will also eventually undergo a positron emission tomography (PET) scan to assess for spread to lymph nodes or distant sites. For patients with neurologic signs or symptoms or seemingly more advanced disease, brain imaging with magnetic resonance imaging (MRI) or CT scan is indicated. In general, the goal of this initial evaluation is to confirm the diagnosis and to establish the stage (i.e., the extent of disease). Staging considerations can be complex, and referral to a thoracic oncology program or a pulmonologist is indicated if the initial evaluation suggests likely lung cancer.

Staging for NSCLC is based on the TNM (tumor, nodes, metastases) system and is described in detail in the American Joint Committee on Cancer (AJCC) cancer staging manual.[10] The tumor stage (T1 to T4) is based on the size, location, and involvement of adjacent structures. The nodal stage (N1 to N3) is

TABLE 109-1 **Signs, Symptoms, and Syndromes of Lung Cancer**

Extent of Disease	Associated Signs, Symptoms, and Syndromes
Primary tumor in the lung	Cough, dyspnea, hemoptysis, chest pain or discomfort.
Tumor spread to regional nodes or intrathoracic structures	Dyspnea from airway compression as a result of bulky adenopathy. Pain and dyspnea from pleural or chest wall involvement. Hoarseness caused by recurrent laryngeal nerve palsy (particularly with left-sided tumors). Pancoast tumor: A superior sulcus tumor that causes shoulder and arm pain as a result of brachial plexus involvement. Horner syndrome (unilateral ptosis, meiosis, and lack of facial sweating): caused by ipsilateral invasion of the sympathetic chain. Superior vena cava (SVC) syndrome: Tumors obstructing the SVC will cause neck and facial swelling, dilated neck veins and dyspnea.
Metastatic disease	Weight loss and generalized fatigue are more common in metastatic disease. Bone metastases may cause bone pain or pathologic fractures. Lesions are usually osteolytic. Adrenal metastases may rarely cause adrenal insufficiency. Brain metastases can cause headache, weakness, nausea and vomiting, seizures, although they may be asymptomatic as well. Liver metastases can cause pain and hepatomegaly. Liver function tests will frequently be normal until very advanced. Pleural or pericardial effusions may cause pain or dyspnea.
Paraneoplastic syndromes	Hypercalcemia results from bony metastases or tumor secretion of parathyroid hormone–related peptide. This may cause altered mental status, constipation, nausea, polyuria, and dehydration. Syndrome of inappropriate antidiuretic hormone secretion (SIADH) causes hyponatremia and is more commonly seen with SCLC. Paraneoplastic neurologic syndromes are most commonly associated with SCLC. These include Lambert-Eaton myasthenic syndrome, cerebellar ataxia, and limbic encephalitis.

Data from Ost DE, Yeung SC, Tanoue LT, Gould MK: Clinical and organizational factors in the initial evaluation of patients with lung cancer. In Diagnosis and management of lung cancer, 3rd ed: American College of Chest Physicians evidence-based clinical practice guidelines. *Chest* 2013;143(5):E121–41.

DIAGNOSTICS

Lung Cancer

LABORATORY
Complete blood count
Comprehensive metabolic panel with liver function tests
Sputum or pleural fluid cytology

IMAGING
Chest x-ray study
Contrast-enhanced CT scan of the thorax (including the liver and adrenals)
PET scan or PET/CT scan
MRI or CT of the brain
Additional Diagnostic and Staging Evaluation
Conventional bronchoscopy
Endobronchial ultrasound with transbronchial needle aspirate (EBUS-TBNA)
Transthoracic needle biopsy with CT guidance
Surgical staging procedures (e.g., mediastinoscopy)
Thoracentesis

CT, computed tomography; MRI, magnetic resonance imaging; PET, positron emission tomography.

divided into three categories: N1 (ipsilateral peribronchial or hilar lymph nodes), N2 (ipsilateral mediastinal nodes), and N3 (contralateral or supraclavicular nodes). Metastatic (M) spread is present or absent. A simplified schema of staging and treatment is presented in Table 109-2. Staging will help identify patients who are candidates for curative therapies (surgery or definitive chemoradiation) as opposed to palliative therapies (chemotherapy and/or radiation therapy). SCLC uses a more simplified staging scheme wherein disease is determined to be either limited stage or extensive stage.

A diagnosis and stage should be determined in the least invasive manner possible. For example, if a patient with a new cough is found on imaging to have a lung mass, bulky mediastinal adenopathy, and bone lesions, a single biopsy of the bone lesion could confirm the diagnosis of lung cancer, identify the histology, and determine the stage to be stage IV (i.e., metastatic). Modalities for obtaining a cytologic or histologic diagnosis include sputum cytology, CT-guided needle biopsy, bronchoscopy including endobronchial ultrasound, thoracentesis with cytologic examination of pleural fluid, and surgical approaches including mediastinoscopy. In addition to determining the histology, a biopsy specimen can also be sent for molecular analysis (e.g., EGFR mutation testing), which may affect treatment.

In addition, if a tumor appears amenable to surgical resection, patients will be evaluated for surgical candidacy with pulmonary function testing to ensure that they have adequate pulmonary reserve to tolerate removal of part or all of a lung.

TABLE 109-2 Simplified Schema for Staging and Treatment of Lung Cancer

Stage	Simplified Staging Description	Typical Treatment Strategies
NON–SMALL CELL LUNG CANCER		
I	Small tumors without any lymph node involvement	Surgical resection Stereotactic body radiation therapy (SBRT) for nonsurgical candidates
II	Medium sized tumors that may invade adjacent structures (i.e., chest wall or diaphragm) OR Smaller tumors that have also spread to nonmediastinal (e.g., hilar) lymph nodes on the same side	Surgical resection with consideration of adjuvant chemotherapy Definitive chemotherapy or radiation for nonsurgical candidates
IIIA	All but the largest tumors that have also spread to the mediastinal lymph nodes on the same side OR The largest tumors (i.e., those that invade structures such as the heart, great vessels, trachea, vertebral body) but have not yet spread to the mediastinal lymph nodes	An area of ongoing debate May involve preoperative chemotherapy with or without radiation followed by surgery *or* definitive chemotherapy or radiation therapy
IIIB	Any size tumor that has also spread to the mediastinal lymph nodes on the opposite side or to any supraclavicular lymph nodes OR The largest tumors (as earlier) that have also spread to mediastinal lymph nodes on the same side	Not considered resectable Definitive chemotherapy or radiation therapy
IV	Tumors that have spread to distant sites (e.g., bone, brain, adrenals, or contralateral lung) or that cause malignant pericardial or pleural effusions	Not curable Palliative treatment involving chemotherapy or targeted therapy
SMALL CELL LUNG CANCER		
Limited	Disease that can be encompassed within one radiation port and that generally corresponds to one hemithorax with the associated lymph nodes	Chemotherapy and radiation
Extensive	Disease that has spread beyond the hemithorax or to distant sites	Palliative chemotherapy

Lung cancer staging and treatment are an evolving and complex science, and this table does not represent all the nuances of current staging or treatment. It is meant to give a general practitioner a working knowledge of the basic categories. For a more accurate and in-depth depiction of current staging, please refer to Goldstraw P, Crowley J, Chansky K, et al: The IASLC Lung Cancer Staging Project: proposals for the revision of the TNM stage groupings in the forthcoming (seventh) edition of the TNM classification of malignant tumours. *J Thorac Oncol* 2(8):706-714, 2007.

DIFFERENTIAL DIAGNOSIS

The differential diagnosis of lung cancer depends on the presenting signs and symptoms. Imaging may identify a pulmonary nodule (<3 cm in size) or a mass (>3 cm in size). Pulmonary nodules can be from benign (e.g., infections, granulomas) or malignant causes. NSCLC more commonly manifests with a solitary pulmonary nodule than with SCLC. The larger the nodule or mass, the more likely it is to be malignant. Metastases from another cancer (e.g., melanoma, renal cell carcinoma, breast cancer, or colorectal cancer) may sometimes manifest as a solitary lesion, although typically metastases have multiple foci on presentation.

MANAGEMENT

In general, the management of lung cancer involves one or a combination of treatment modalities including surgery, radiation therapy, chemotherapy or targeted therapy, or best supportive care. As discussed later, the treatment strategy is determined by the type of lung cancer (NSCLC versus SCLC), stage, performance status, pulmonary status, comorbidities, and patient preferences. Performance status (usually assessed by either the Karnofsky or ECOG [Eastern Cooperative Oncology Group] scales) is a particularly important consideration because patients with poor functional status may derive less or no benefit from certain treatments, and a supportive approach with palliative care may be the optimal course.

Stage I and II Non–Small Cell Lung Cancer

Surgery is the primary curative therapy for early-stage lung cancer (stages I and II). Overall survival rates at 5 years for pathologically staged stage I NSCLC are approximately 58% to 73%, and 36% to 45% for stage II.[11] Unfortunately, only 25% of patients in the United States will be at these early stages on presentation.[12] Surgical resection typically involves lobectomy (removal of one lung lobe) or pneumonectomy (removal of the entire lung). At the time of the surgery, the surgeon will also perform mediastinal lymph node sampling to allow for complete pathologic staging of the tumor. For patients who have stage I NSCLC according to the final pathologic assessment, there is typically no additional therapy after surgery. For patients with resected stage II NSCLC, adjuvant chemotherapy improves survival and is generally recommended.

To undergo a surgery, a patient must have adequate pulmonary function and anticipated reserve. Although formal testing should be performed with pulmonary function tests, a quick sense of pulmonary reserve adequacy can be assessed by whether or not a patient can climb a flight of stairs without stopping. Patients unable to do this task will likely have increased risk of perioperative complications and may not be good surgical candidates.

Some patients do not wish to undergo surgery or are not candidates because of comorbidities or poor pulmonary reserve. For patients who have stage I tumors (i.e., small tumors without apparent spread to the lymph nodes), an increasingly used treatment is stereotactic body radiation therapy (SBRT). In general, radiation therapy delivers energy to kill malignant cells in a region that is targeted via imaging by a radiation oncologist. With conventional radiation therapy, a specific amount of energy called a *fraction* is delivered daily to a specific target, and treatment may last for weeks. More recently, the technique of SBRT has allowed radiation oncologists to deliver the entire amount of energy in a single fraction or over just a few fractions to a very exact, though relatively small, targeted area. For nonsurgical candidates with stage II disease (i.e., larger tumors or those that have spread to hilar lymph nodes), a combination of chemotherapy and conventional radiation therapy is usually employed.

Stage III Non–Small Cell Lung Cancer

Most patients with stage III disease are treated with curative intent, although the 5-year overall survival is under 20%.[13] Treatment of stage III tumors is an area of controversy in lung cancer management, particularly for stage IIIA, wherein the precise role and timing of surgery remains unclear. Some patients with stage IIIA tumors will receive preoperative chemotherapy or chemoradiation therapy followed by surgical resection, others may receive definitive chemoradiation therapy without surgery, and some may have surgery followed by chemotherapy or radiation therapy. Stage IIIB tumors are considered unresectable, and the primary treatment is definitive chemoradiation therapy.[13]

Stage IV Non–Small Cell Lung Cancer

Stage IV or metastatic NSCLC is not considered curable. Treatment is palliative with the goals of reducing symptoms, improving quality of life, and prolonging survival. In good performance status patients, chemotherapy (usually two-drug combinations such as carboplatin and paclitaxel) has improved 1-year survival rates to 30% to 40% from 10%, and 2-year survival rates are now approximately 10% to 15%. The median overall survival for metastatic NSCLC is 8 to 10 months.[4]

Patients who do not have good performance status (i.e., those who spend 50% or more of their time in bed) typically do not benefit from chemotherapy.

An important advance in the last 10 years is the development of targeted therapies directed at the specific molecular defects that have been found in lung cancer cells such as the *EGFR* mutation and the *ALK* gene rearrangements. In patients with the *EGFR* mutations, the tyrosine kinase inhibitor erlotinib (Tarceva) can result in significant tumor response with fewer side effects and treatment-related deaths compared with conventional chemotherapy. Similarly, in patients with tumors that have *ALK* rearrangements, crizotinib (Xalkori) can induce significant tumor shrinkage. Unfortunately, despite the often dramatic initial responses to treatment, these agents are not curative and eventually the tumors will progress. Nonetheless, these targeted agents are a key breakthrough and may herald an era in which cancer treatment becomes "personalized" and tailored to an individual tumor's specific molecular composition.

In addition to systemic therapy for metastatic disease, radiation therapy is frequently employed to palliate specific symptomatic areas such as painful bone metastases, lesions that are obstructing airways, or brain metastases causing cerebral edema. Unfortunately, virtually all patients with stage IV NSCLC will die of their disease, and therefore addressing the palliative care needs of these patients is crucial. A recent randomized trial suggested that for patients with advanced lung cancer, the early initiation of palliative care as an integrated part of routine oncologic care improves quality of life and survival.[14]

Small Cell Lung Cancer

SCLC grows extremely rapidly, and therefore the majority of patients have metastatic disease at diagnosis. Even in patients who do not have apparent metastatic sites, the assumption is generally that they have "occult" micrometastases. Therefore, surgery does not play a significant role in the management of SCLC. The specific treatment for SCLC is based on the determination of whether the disease is limited stage or extensive stage. For limited-stage SCLC, treatment involves combined chemotherapy and radiation therapy, resulting in a 20% to 40% 2-year survival rate. Although SCLC often responds very well initially to chemotherapy, the majority of patients will relapse and the 5-year survival rates are approximately 10%.[1] For extensive-stage SCLC, treatment is palliative, using chemotherapy alone with a median survival of 8 to 13 months, and only 5% of patients are alive at 2 years.[8,15]

COMPLICATIONS

With lung cancer there can be many complications associated with both the underlying malignancy and the treatments. Patients may require urgent evaluation and treatment for myriad related conditions including epidural spinal cord compression, superior vena cava syndrome, hypercalcemia, pain crises, venous thrombosis, and chemotherapy-induced neutropenic fever (see later). Chemotherapy also has many potential side effects. It is important to note that because of improvements over the past two decades in antiemetics, notably the development of 5-hydroxytryptamine$_3$ (5-HT$_3$) receptor antagonists such as ondansetron, the burden of chemotherapy nausea and vomiting for the regimens typically used in the lung cancer treatment has been significantly reduced.[16]

INDICATIONS FOR REFERRAL OR HOSPITALIZATION

- As discussed earlier, when lung cancer is suspected, basic imaging and laboratory tests should be performed. When the suspicion remains high or is confirmed, referral is indicated, ideally to a full-service, multidisciplinary thoracic oncology program that has pulmonologists, thoracic surgeons, thoracic radiologists, and medical and radiation oncologists. If such a thoracic oncology program is not readily available, a pulmonologist can guide the initial staging and biopsy evaluation.

- Although there is no clearly identified optimal time frame for the staging and diagnosis evaluation, a reasonable expectation would be that a prompt and efficient diagnostic evaluation take place over 4 to 6 weeks and that treatment be initiated within 1 to 2 months after diagnosis. This time frame may need to be adjusted based on patient-specific factors such as the tempo of disease, patient anxiety, and patient comorbidities.[9]
- Of note, surgical outcomes in lung cancer are better when surgery is performed by board-certified thoracic surgeons with a focus on lung cancer, and thus national guidelines recommend lung cancer surgery be performed in highly experienced settings.[4,14]
- There are several presentations (potential oncologic emergencies) in patients with known or suspected lung cancer that require more urgent or emergent evaluation:
  - Severe back pain, particularly if associated with neurologic deficits (weakness, bowel or bladder changes, saddle anesthesia) may indicate spinal cord compression or cauda equina syndrome.
  - Dyspnea with plethora and dilated neck veins can be seen with superior vena cava syndrome.
  - Rapidly progressive or severe respiratory compromise may be the result of a large effusion, a lesion causing airway obstruction, or a pulmonary embolism.
  - Seizures, focal neurologic deficits, or altered mental status may indicate brain metastases.
  - Altered mental status, lethargy, and evidence of dehydration can be seen with severe hypercalcemia.
  - Unilateral lower extremity edema and pain may indicate venous thrombosis.
  - Severe pain from a metastatic lesion, particularly a bone metastasis, that cannot be easily controlled with oral analgesics may require parenteral narcotics.
  - Fever in a patient receiving chemotherapy requires urgent evaluation and treatment, especially in the context of neutropenia.

LIFE SPAN CONSIDERATIONS

Lung cancer is a highly lethal disease. Even when identified at an early stage (stage I or II) and treated with curative intent, a large percentage of patients (25% or more, depending on the exact stage) will develop relapse and ultimately die of their disease. With stage III cancer, 80% or more patients will die of their disease within 5 years. For patients with metastatic NSCLC, only 10% to 15% will live 2 years.

When making treatment decisions, age should always be considered in the context of comorbidities and performance status. The "functional age" of a patient is more important than the chronologic age. Older patients who are fit and have good performance status can be considered for similar treatment options as younger patients. However, a more individualized, case-by-case approach is likely better for patients with borderline performance status (i.e., symptomatic but out of bed more than 50% of the day) and/or who are very elderly. For patients with metastatic NSCLC who have poor performance status (i.e., in bed more than 50% of the day), treatment is unlikely to improve quality of life or survival, except in rare instances when the tumor possesses an *EGFR* mutation or *ALK* rearrangement and targeted agents can be used. For all other patients with poor performance status, best supportive care is the most appropriate treatment option.

EDUCATION AND HEALTH PROMOTION

The most pressing issue in lung cancer remains preventing exposure to tobacco smoke to stop new cases from developing. A smoker has 20 times the risk of developing lung cancer compared with a person who has never smoked. For individuals who do stop smoking, the risk of lung cancer diminishes significantly over time, although in the long term it still remains at least twice that of an individual who never smoked.[1] It is never too late to stop smoking. Even patients who have already been diagnosed with lung cancer will benefit from smoking cessation. Patients who continue to smoke after their diagnosis double their risk of dying of lung cancer.[17]

Given the high prevalence and lethality of lung cancer, many of studies have focused on early detection and screening. For years, studies using periodic imaging or sputum cytology analysis did not demonstrate a reduction in lung cancer-related mortality. More recently, however, the National Lung Screening Trial (NSLT), a large, randomized controlled trial involving more than 50,000 participants, showed a 20% decrease in lung cancer mortality in heavy smokers who were screened with annual low-dose CT scans for 3 years.[18] Based on these results, multiple medical societies including the U.S. Preventive Services Task Force (USPSTF) and the American Cancer Society now recommend lung cancer screening for high-risk individuals. For example, the USPSTF currently recommends annual screening for lung cancer with low-dose CT scans in high-risk individuals—namely, adults aged 55 to 80 who have a 30 pack-year smoking history and currently smoke or have quit with in the past 15 years.[19] Although this is a promising development, most likely smoking prevention and smoking cessation efforts will have a greater ability to reduce lung cancer–associated morbidity and mortality.

For those who have been treated with curative intent for lung cancer, issues of survivorship and surveillance may fall into the domain of the primary care provider. Specific guidelines vary, but it is generally recommended that patients have follow-up appointments and surveillance CT scans of the chest every 6 months for 2 years and then annually thereafter to detect recurrences or new primaries. Smoking cessation interventions are critical, and smoking status should be assessed at each visit. In addition, patients should be encouraged to maintain a healthy weight and an active lifestyle. Alcohol consumption should be limited. Routine blood work or PET scans are not considered beneficial and are not recommended.[4,20]

CHAPTER 110

PLEURAL EFFUSIONS AND PLEURISY

Patricia Polgar-Bailey

PLEURAL EFFUSIONS

DEFINITION AND EPIDEMIOLOGY

A pleural effusion is an abnormal amount of fluid within the pleural space. The pleura, a serous, semitransparent, elastic membrane, covers the lung parenchyma, mediastinum, diaphragm, and rib cage and is divided into the parietal and visceral pleurae. The parietal pleura lines the chest cavity, covering the chest wall, diaphragm, and mediastinum. It contains sensory nerves, and its blood supply comes from the systemic circulation and hence has hydrostatic pressure. The visceral pleura covers the entire surface of both lungs, including the interlobular fissures, and contains no pain fibers. Its blood flow is supplied by branches of the pulmonary circulation. The parietal and visceral pleurae are continuous at the hilum, where they are penetrated by both the pulmonary and bronchial vessels. The pleural space is an area approximately 10 to 20 mm in width, situated between the mesothelium of the parietal and visceral pleurae.[1] Pleural fluid is normally produced in quantities just sufficient to lubricate the parietal and visceral surfaces. This small amount of fluid is constantly replenished and reabsorbed; absorption is principally through the lymphatic system.

Approximately 0.16 to 0.36 mL of fluid per kilogram is normally contained within the pleural space, with a total volume of less than 20 mL and total fluid flow of 100 to 200 mL, unless some disease process or trauma has caused fluid or solid tissue to collect there. Pleural effusions are a common manifestation of many pulmonary and systemic diseases, most notably congestive heart failure (CHF), because of the elevation of pulmonary venous pressure. In addition, pleural effusions can result from a multitude of other diseases, including pulmonary tuberculosis, pulmonary embolus, and other lung diseases; chest injury or trauma; abdominal infections or pancreatitis; cancers, including lung, breast, and lymphoma; and connective tissue diseases, such as rheumatoid arthritis and lupus. Pregnancy and certain types of surgery (e.g., heart, lung, abdominal, and organ transplantation) also increase the risk for development of pleural effusions. Medical therapeutics, including radiotherapy and some medications (e.g., nitrofurantoin and amiodarone), can also increase the likelihood of developing a pleural effusion.[1,2] More than 90% of all pleural effusions in developed countries are caused by CHF, malignancy, pneumonia, and pulmonary embolism. Tuberculosis is a common cause of pleural effusions in tuberculosis endemic areas.[3] Viral infections are a common cause of pleural inflammation, which often manifests as pleural effusions. Some of the most common viruses implicated in the development of pleural effusions include influenza, coxsackievirus, respiratory syncytial virus (RSV), cytomegalovirus (CMV), adenovirus, human herpesvirus-8 (HHV-8), dengue virus, human T-lymphotropic virus 1 (HTLV-1), simian virus 40 (SV40), parvovirus B19, varicella, herpes simplex virus (HSV), and Epstein-Barr virus (EBV).[4] Although a malignant cause is always a concern with pleural effusions, at least 60 benign causes of pleural effusions have been identified and benign causes are at least twice as likely as malignant causes in most epidemiologic series.[3]

PATHOPHYSIOLOGY

An increased amount of fluid (an effusion) accumulates in the pleural space whenever the rate of fluid formation exceeds the rate of fluid absorption. Numerous conditions may lead to pleural effusions, including viral and bacterial infections, neoplasms, thromboemboli, cardiovascular dysfunction, and immunologic dysfunction (Box 110-1). Mechanisms that contribute to increased pleural fluid accumulation include an increase in microvascular pressure (e.g., CHF), a decrease in plasma

BOX 110-1

Potential Causes of Pleural Effusions

- Amyloidosis
- Atelectasis
- Benign asbestos-related effusions
- CHF (most common cause)
- Cirrhosis
- Drug-induced effusions
- Endocrine dysfunction
- Esophageal perforation
- Hemothorax
- Hepatic and splenic abscesses
- Immune conditions
  - Rheumatoid arthritis
  - Systemic lupus erythematosus
  - Sjögren syndrome
  - Wegner granulomatosis
  - Ankylosing spondylitis
  - Churg-Strauss syndrome
  - Sarcoidosis
- Infectious conditions (most common causes of exudative effusions)
  - Bacterial
  - Tuberculosis
  - Fungal
  - Viral (respiratory, cardiac, hepatic)
  - Parasitic
- Intra-abdominal abscesses
- Malignant disease
  - Primary lung cancer
  - Metastatic disease to pleura (most commonly in lung and breast carcinomas)
  - Mesothelioma
- Medications
  - Amiodarone
  - Bromocriptine
  - Dantrolene
  - Metronidazole
  - Nitrofurantoin
  - Procarbazine
- Nephrotic syndrome
- Pancreatic disease
- Peritoneal dialysis
- Peritonitis
- Pneumonia
- Postoperative
  - Postcardiac surgery
  - Lung transplantation
  - Abdominal surgery
- Pulmonary embolism
- Radiotherapy
- Viral illness, including human immunodeficiency virus (HIV) and acquired immunodeficiency syndrome (AIDS)

Modified from Quinn T, Alam N, Aminazad A, et al: Decision making and algorithm for the management of pleural effusions. *Thorac Surg Clin* 23:11-16, 2013.

osmotic pressure (e.g., hypoalbuminemia), an increase in the permeability of microcirculation (e.g., pneumonia), a decrease in pleural pressure (e.g., atelectasis), an impaired lymphatic drainage from pleural spaces (e.g., malignant effusions), and the movement of fluid across the diaphragm from the peritoneal cavity (e.g., inflammation from acute pancreatitis). Parapneumonic effusions are the most common type of effusion and are associated with bacterial infections such as pneumonia, lung abscesses, and bronchiectasis.[5] Malignant pleural effusions are a common problem encountered in persons with advanced cancer. Lung cancer in men and breast cancer in women are the most common causes of malignant pleural effusions.[6] Other common causes of malignant pleural effusions include lymphomas and genitourinary tract and gastrointestinal tract tumors.[6]

Pleural effusions are often categorized as transudates and exudates on the basis of the amount of protein detected in the pleural fluid. Exudative pleural effusions result primarily from pleural and lung inflammation (e.g., pneumonia) or impaired lymphatic drainage of the pleural space (e.g., malignant disease). In fact, a variety of disease mechanisms, including pneumonia and other infections, malignant carcinomas, immunologic and lymphatic abnormalities, and iatrogenic factors, can cause exudates. Transudative effusions develop when systemic factors alter the formation or absorption of pleural fluid, rather than from pleuritic disease. They are produced by imbalances in hydrostatic and osmotic pressures across the pleural membrane and are usually bilateral. Transudates have a lower specific gravity and lower concentrations of protein and lactate dehydrogenase compared with exudative effusions.[1] CHF is probably the most common cause of transudative pleural effusions, but other disease processes that cause movement of fluid from the peritoneal space or retroperitoneal space, such as cirrhosis, nephrosis, and glomerulonephritis, can cause transudates.[2]

Age-related changes affecting the respiratory system play an important role in the development of pleural effusions. In addition to the expected changes related to aging, years of exposure to particulate matter, dust, occupational toxins, and episodic respiratory infections increase the risk for development of a pleural effusion.[2]

CLINICAL PRESENTATION

Persons with pleural effusions often are asymptomatic when they are seen initially. When symptoms do occur, the most common presenting complaints include dyspnea, nonproductive cough, pleuritic chest pain, and activity intolerance. Dyspnea is the most common complaint and often increases with recumbent positions.[2] Cough tends to worsen as the size of the effusion increases. Pleuritic pain is associated with inflammation of the parietal pleura and is caused by irritation of its sensory fibers. This pain is often sharp, unilateral, and localized to the affected area, although it may also be experienced in the lower chest and ipsilateral shoulder or referred to the abdomen. Exacerbating factors include deep inspiration, cough, and other movement of the upper body. Constrictive pericarditis is a relatively common cause of pleural effusions, and chest pain and dyspnea are common associated symptoms.[7]

Malignant tumors involving the parietal pleura generally cause steady, dull pain compared with the sharp, intermittent pain associated with an acute inflammatory process. Pleural effusions cause compression of adjacent lung tissue and reduce the amount of possible lung expansion, which may result in varying degrees of dyspnea, depending on the size and functional status of the underlying lung and the rate of fluid accumulation. However, dyspnea does not necessarily correlate with blood oxygen levels or the size of the pleural effusion but rather seems to be related to the increased thoracic cage size, which affects respiratory muscle function. Dyspnea is a common presenting symptom associated with malignant pleural effusions and is occasionally accompanied by chest pain and cough. Chest pain is usually related to involvement of the parietal pleura, ribs and intercostal muscles, and other structures. The nonproductive cough is most likely a result of lung compression and bronchial irritation.[2] Associated constitutional symptoms include weight loss, malaise, and anorexia.

A thorough history is important and can be helpful in discriminating between the symptoms associated with the effusion and those of the primary underlying pathophysiologic process. Information about the presence of fever, cough, sputum production, dyspnea, or abdominal pain should be elicited. Past medical history, including systemic and chronic illnesses, previous surgeries, prior exposures (such as to tuberculosis and asbestos), and previous alcohol abuse, is important.

PHYSICAL EXAMINATION

Several findings on physical examination are suggestive of a pleural effusion; however, the clinical manifestations of the effusion may be overshadowed by the underlying disease process.[8] Common physical examination findings include decreased or absent breath sounds over the effusion, decreased respiratory excursion, dullness to percussion, reduced or absent tactile fremitus, and decreased or absent bronchial breath sounds, sometimes with egophony (E-to-A change) at the upper fluid borders. Pleural inflammation is often accompanied by a friction rub that is transitory and that generally disappears as fluid accumulates in the pleural space. Small effusions (<500 mL) may be associated with minimum or no findings. In situations in which effusions are greater (>1500 mL) or pulmonary compromise is more substantial, the use of accessory muscles of respiration, inspiratory lag, cyanosis, bulging intercostal margins, mediastinal shift, and jugular vein distention may be evident. In addition to assessing the respiratory status, the provider needs to perform a complete physical examination to identify signs that may be manifestations of systemic or acute illness and suggest the cause of the effusion. For example, nonthoracic signs such as jugular vein distention and an S_3 gallop are suggestive of CHF. A right ventricular heave or thrombophlebitis suggests pulmonary embolus. Lymphadenopathy or hepatosplenomegaly may be associated with hepatic disease, and ascites may be indicative of a hepatic cause.

DIAGNOSTICS

Once a pleural effusion is suspected, a chest radiograph should be obtained to confirm its presence and to look for other abnormalities that might help determine its cause. Normal amounts of fluid are not visible on chest radiographs; effusions of greater than 75 mL are usually visible.[6] Effusions that are detected appear as blunting and medial displacement of the sharp costophrenic angle, pleura-based densities, infiltrates, hilar adenopathy, or signs of CHF. A subpulmonary effusion is suspected if the diaphragm is elevated. Chest radiographs are limited in their ability to diagnosis pleural effusions and do not attain 100% sensitivity until pleural effusions are more than 500 mL.[6,9] However, they can provide other diagnostic clues to the cause of the effusion. For example, large unilateral effusions usually shift the mediastinum to the contralateral hemithorax, and lack of such a shift with a large effusion may indicate a bronchial obstruction, lung tumor, mesothelioma, or fixed mediastinum from tumor or fibrosis.[8]

Although most pleural effusions are seen on chest films, several conditions other than pleural effusions may produce similar findings. Chest ultrasound and computed tomography (CT) are more reliable for detection and localization of small pleural effusions.[6] Smaller effusions should be confirmed by ultrasonography, which will detect effusions of 5 to 50 mL and is 100% sensitive for effusions of more than 100 mL.[2] In addition to their use in detecting smaller effusions, ultrasound examinations are used to guide diagnostic thoracentesis, resulting in improved yield and decreased complication rates.[8] One of the benefits of chest CT is that it allows imaging of the underlying lung parenchyma or mediastinum and thereby permits identification of possible causes of the pleural effusion, such as pulmonary, bronchial, or pleural malignancy. In addition, chest CT can characterize the effusion in terms of its size and location and the presence of loculations.[6] Positron emission tomography (PET) scans are helpful in the evaluation of malignant pleural effusions.[6]

Once a pleural effusion has been discovered, identification of the disease process, procedure, or drug that caused the effusion is essential. Diagnostic evaluation relies heavily on examination of pleural fluid obtained by thoracentesis. In experienced hands, thoracentesis can be performed safely at the bedside. If there is any concern about damaging intradiaphragmatic or adjacent structures, such as in the setting of cardiomyopathy, the procedure should be done under the guidance of ultrasound.[6] The pleural fluid should always be sampled unless the underlying cause of the effusion has already been established. Although a definitive diagnosis, such as the finding of malignant cells, can be established in only 25% of cases, relevant information (from fluid analyses, including cellular counts, chemistry profiles, cultures, and stains) that is useful for clinical decision-making and for exclusion of certain causes of a pleural effusion is obtained in an additional 15% to 20% of cases.[2] In certain situations, when the clinical diagnosis and cause of the effusion are relatively secure and the clinical course is uncomplicated (e.g., uncomplicated CHF, small effusions after thoracic or abdominal surgery, postpartum effusion), therapy may be initiated and a thoracentesis performed only if the response to therapy is inadequate. However, whenever the cause of a pleural effusion is unclear, a diagnostic thoracentesis is generally warranted.[7]

Thoracentesis has no absolute contraindications. However, relative contraindications include bleeding diathesis or systemic anticoagulation, small volume of pleural fluid, mechanical ventilation, patient's inability to cooperate, and cutaneous disease such as herpes zoster infection at the needle entry site.[8] Preprocedure laboratory studies should include a complete blood count (CBC), prothrombin time, and partial thromboplastin time. Coagulation therapy should be considered if the platelet count is below 50,000/μL or if the clotting time is prolonged.[6] The complication rate of thoracentesis is approximately 20% and includes pain at the puncture site, cutaneous and internal bleeding, pneumothorax, cough, empyema, and spleen or liver puncture; therefore it is essential to obtain informed consent before the procedure is initiated.[2] The most common complications are vagal reactions and pneumothoraces.[6]

Other tests needed to establish a definitive diagnosis may include a CT scan of the chest, thoracoscopy, fiberoptic bronchoscopy, and pleural biopsy. A thoracotomy should be performed only if other diagnostic tests have not been helpful.[6] A chest CT scan is not obtained initially to confirm the presence of a pleural effusion; it is most useful after thoracentesis for further evaluation of suspected parenchymal or pleural abnormalities. Cytologic examination of the pleural fluid is an efficient and minimally invasive method to establish a diagnosis of cancer.[2] Fiberoptic bronchoscopy can be useful if an endobronchial malignancy is suspected, especially if symptoms include hemoptysis and stridor, because biopsy specimens can be taken at the time of the procedure.[6] Thoracoscopy allows for direct visualization of the visceral and parietal pleura, and biopsy of the pleura can be done simultaneously. Thoracoscopy is usually performed with the patient under general anesthesia, but it can also be done using local anesthesia or sedation.[6] Open pleural biopsy is required when other procedures have failed to provide a diagnosis.[7] It can be done using local anesthesia. Multiple biopsy specimens (at least four) should be taken at one site. Pleural biopsy can help establish a diagnosis of tuberculosis (sensitivity >85%), malignancy (sensitivity 45% to 60%) and amyloidosis.[6] Contraindications include thrombocytopenia (platelet count <50,000 μ/L), skin infections at the site of incision, small effusions (because of risk of injury to infradiaphragmatic viscera), and severe respiratory disease (because of risk of pneumothorax). Potential complications of pleural biopsy include hemothorax, pneumothorax, superficial and pleural infection, and injury to the liver or spleen.[6] In 15% of pleural effusions, the cause is not identified, despite repeated cytology and pleural biopsy.[6]

DIAGNOSTICS

Pleural Effusions

LABORATORY

Pleural fluid analysis (protein, lactate dehydrogenase, pH, cholesterol [including in exudative effusion], white blood cells, red blood cells, cultures, cytology, acid-fast bacilli)

IMAGING

Chest x-ray examination
Ultrasound*
CT scan*
Thoracoscopy*

OTHER DIAGNOSTICS

Thoracentesis*
Fiberoptic bronchoscopy*
Pleural biopsy*

*If indicated.

DIFFERENTIAL DIAGNOSIS

A number of diseases, including pneumothorax, pulmonary embolism, CHF, neoplasms, trauma, and tuberculosis, can cause symptoms similar to those characteristic of pleural effusions. Once a pleural effusion has been established, the differential diagnosis is based on the presence of transudative or exudative effusions, although a number of conditions can cause both. A transudative pleural effusion is generally associated with a systemic condition rather than with a pleural disease. An exudate usually suggests a pathologic condition that specifically involves the pleural space. Pleural fluid characterized by high erythrocyte counts ($>100,000/mm^3$) is most often seen in cases of trauma, malignant disease, and pulmonary embolism. Other laboratory evaluations, such as a pleural fluid eosinophil count, glucose concentration, and pH, can be used to help distinguish among the potential causes of the effusion. A predominance of neutrophils in the pleural fluid suggests that an acute process, such as pancreatitis, may be affecting the pleura.[9] A pleural fluid eosinophilia of greater than 10% is most often caused by blood or air in the pleural space and is uncommon in patients with cancer or tuberculosis, unless there is a history of repeated thoracenteses.[9] Pleural effusions with a low glucose concentration (<60 mg/dL) suggest a complicated parapneumonia or malignant effusion. Lactate dehydrogenase correlates positively with the degree of pleural inflammation. If the lactate dehydrogenase level increases with repeated thoracenteses, it suggests that the degree of inflammation is increasing, and it is important to aggressively pursue a diagnosis.[9]

DIFFERENTIAL DIAGNOSIS

Pleural Effusions

- Pneumothorax
- Pulmonary embolism
- CHF
- Neoplasms
- Trauma
- Tuberculosis

MANAGEMENT

Management is based on treatment of the cause of the effusion, and a number of specialists may be needed, depending on the cause. In addition, symptomatic treatment is aimed at making the patient more comfortable, beginning when the evaluation is initiated and while the underlying cause is being treated. When an effusion is large, the removal of only 300 to 500 mL through thoracentesis may result in a marked decrease in dyspnea. Indomethacin is often used successfully to treat pleuritic pain and does not suppress respirations, as do narcotics. Malignant pleural effusions, especially in the face of advanced disease, are generally difficult to treat, and management often focuses on providing comfort measures. Some effusions are caused by viral infections and most often resolve without medical intervention.

COMPLICATIONS

Complications depend on the cause and extent of the effusion, accompanying respiratory or systemic compromise, comorbid conditions, and treatment modalities available. Malignant pleural effusions are a major cause of morbidity in cancer patients with advanced disease. Treatment is usually palliative, although treatment of the primary malignant neoplasm and temporizing symptomatic relief (e.g., repeated thoracentesis for recurrent effusions) may be helpful.

INDICATIONS FOR REFERRAL OR HOSPITALIZATION

The evaluation and treatment of a pleural effusion depend on the underlying disease process, degree of respiratory distress, and other contributory factors such as coexisting health problems. Persons without evidence of respiratory compromise can often be assessed and treated on an outpatient basis. Those with substantial respiratory compromise should be admitted to the hospital for further evaluation and treatment. Referral to a specialist is necessary to establish a definitive diagnosis and management plan.

PATIENT AND FAMILY EDUCATION

Education varies, depending on the cause of the pleural effusion. In all cases, teaching must include an explanation of the diagnostic tests, such as thoracentesis, and the potential for chest tube placement and any additional surgical procedures. In addition, education should focus on relieving uncomfortable symptoms, such as dyspnea and pain, and helping patients deal with activity intolerance. Because multiple specialists are often involved in the evaluation of a pleural effusion, the health care provider's role in coordinating care and keeping the patient well informed and at the focus of decision-making is essential.

PLEURISY

DEFINITION AND EPIDEMIOLOGY

Pleurisy, also known as pleuritis, is an inflammation of the pleura. The chest pain of pleurisy is caused when the pleural layers rub together and pain fibers in the parietal pleura are stimulated. Pleurisy is not a diagnosis but rather a possible symptom of numerous localized and systemic disease processes.[10] Pleuritic pain is usually described as sharp or stabbing; it is generally exacerbated by deep breathing, coughing, or sneezing, and it is usually experienced over the lower portion of the chest.

PATHOPHYSIOLOGY

Pleurisy is caused by pleuritis, which is an inflammation of the pleural lining, with or without pleural effusion. The pleural layers are highly permeable and in close contact with microcirculation, which makes them responsive to local or systemic immunologic or inflammatory processes. Pleurisy has a variety of causes; it sometimes develops with excess fluid in the pleural cavity (wet pleurisy) and sometimes without (dry pleurisy). Secondary pleurisy is the result of some other chest disease, such as pneumonia, tuberculosis, or lung abscess, in which germs reach the pleura as well as the lungs and cause inflammation.

The most common causes of pleuritis include viral and bacterial infections as well as tuberculosis in areas of high tuberculosis prevalence.[11] Other common causes of pleuritis include pulmonary infarction and connective tissue diseases such as lupus erythematosus. Trauma to the chest wall is a less common cause of pleurisy, as is coronary bypass or valve replacement surgery (postpericardiotomy syndrome).[12]

Pleurisy is rarely caused by malignant processes; malignant tumors that involve the pleura generally cause a steady, dull pain compared with the sharp, stabbing, intermittent pain associated with pleural inflammation. Certain drugs, including nitrofurantoin, methotrexate, and procarbazine, have been associated with pleurisy.[12]

CLINICAL PRESENTATION

A thorough history is instrumental in determining the differential diagnosis for any type of chest pain. Pain on breathing (which may be mild to severe, depending on the degree of inflammation) and a stabbing or shooting chest pain are characteristics of pleurisy. Pain is usually localized, but sometimes the pain may be felt in the shoulder. Milder pleurisy may be described as a "stitch in the side." Pleuritic pain is generally made worse by breathing, deep inspiration or chest movement, or forced breathing movements such as coughing, sneezing, or talking. Patients will often adopt a position that limits movement of the affected area. The most comfortable position for the patient is often lying on the affected side, which limits expansion of the chest wall.[13]

PHYSICAL EXAMINATION

Pleuritic pain is usually located directly over the site of inflammation, and tenderness is increased with deep palpation. Rapid and shallow breathing may be associated symptoms, with limited chest wall expansion on the affected side. Percussion over the affected area may be dull if there is underlying consolidation or pleural effusion. Increased or diminished fremitus may also denote the presence or absence of consolidation. A pleural friction rub, which varies in intensity from a faint scratching sound to a loud creak, confirms the diagnosis of pleurisy. However, the absence of a pleural friction rub does not negate the presence of pleurisy because the presence of pleural fluid may mitigate or even nullify the rub.

A pleural friction rub may be heard during both phases of respiration but is often most pronounced at or near the end of inspiration. It disappears when patients hold their breath. A pleural friction rub may be localized or heard over a wider area and is generally most audible over the lateral and posterior regions of the inferior thorax. It is rarely heard over the upper thorax and lung apexes because of the limited movement of the lung in these areas compared with the lung bases. In general, a rub is heard only if the person takes a deep breath; a rub, even if it is present, is not audible during splinting or shallow breathing. Crackles can sometimes sound similar to a rub, but a cough usually diminishes crackles and has no effect on a rub. A sound similar to a pleural friction rub can be produced by sliding a stethoscope over the skin; firm pressure of the stethoscope on the skin should eliminate this "false rub" and intensify the sound of a real friction rub if it is present.

Pleuritic inflammation can sometimes lead to pleural effusions. Pleural effusions often ease the pain temporarily by providing a cushion between the inflamed membranes and, as a result, give a false sense of improvement when the situation is really getting worse. Large collections of pleural fluid can compress the lungs and further compromise respiration.

Some common symptoms associated with pleurisy may also suggest the underlying disease process giving rise to the pleurisy. A cough productive of purulent sputum may indicate an underlying lung disease, such as pneumothorax, pneumonia, tuberculosis, or pulmonary embolism.[10] Fever and chills suggest an underlying infectious process. Rigors can sometimes occur with bacterial pneumonia. Joint pain or rashes raise the suspicion of an underlying connective tissue disorder.

DIAGNOSTICS

Several laboratory tests, although not diagnostic of pleurisy, may help elucidate the underlying cause. An elevated leukocyte count with a shift to the left suggests a bacterial infection such as pneumonia, an esophageal rupture, or an abscess. Leukopenia may reflect a viral process or lupus erythematosus. A chest x-ray examination may help diagnose bacterial pneumonia, pneumothorax, esophageal rupture, or problems below the diaphragm, such as a subphrenic abscess or effusion. Thoracentesis and pleural fluid analysis can help identify the underlying cause once the existence of a pleural effusion has been established. If the cause of the pleurisy is still unclear, other studies, including CT scan of the chest, ventilation/perfusion scan, pleural biopsy, and esophageal contrast studies, may be indicated.

DIAGNOSTICS

Pleural Effusions

LABORATORY
CBC
Pleural fluid analysis*

IMAGING
Chest x-ray examination
CT scan*
Ventilation/perfusion scan*

OTHER DIAGNOSTICS
Thoracentesis*
Pleural biopsy*

*If indicated.

DIFFERENTIAL DIAGNOSIS

Problems that originate in other chest wall structures can produce pain similar to that of pleurisy; these conditions include pneumothorax, rib fractures, costochondritis, vertebral fractures, and nerve root pain from herpes zoster infection. The presence of a pleural friction rub confirms the pleuritis, but a patient history, physical examination, and pertinent diagnostic tests are still necessary to determine the most likely differential diagnosis.

Pleural effusion is a finding commonly associated with pleurisy and may be helpful in determining the diagnosis. Viral infections, rheumatic disease, and sarcoidosis often cause pleurisy in the absence of a pleural effusion. In contrast, pneumonia, *Mycobacterium tuberculosis* infection, lupus pleuritis, and postcardiac injury syndrome are typically associated with pleural effusions.[13]

The patient's history may be helpful in narrowing the differential diagnosis. For example, a recent leg fracture with casting raises the possibility of a pulmonary embolism. Occupational asbestos exposure might suggest asbestos pleurisy. A history of lupus erythematosus or sarcoidosis increases the suspicion of systemic connective tissue disease as the underlying cause of the pleurisy.[14]

Many types of pain experienced in the chest area are not pleuritic. Cardiac chest pain is often central and diffuse and is described as a pressing or squeezing rather than a sharp and intermittent pain. Cardiac pain (angina, acute myocardial infarction, dissecting aortic aneurysm) often radiates to the neck, jaw, or arms and worsens with exertion, which is not characteristic of pleurisy. Pericardial pain can be similar in character to pleuritic pain but is usually felt on the anterior side of the chest

DIFFERENTIAL DIAGNOSIS

Pleurisy

- Pneumothorax
- Rib fracture
- Costochondritis
- Vertebral fracture
- Nerve root pain from herpes zoster
- Cardiac condition (e.g., angina, acute myocardial infarction, dissecting aortic aneurysm, pericarditis)

and back and is exacerbated by lying down. Chronic chest pain is not usually a result of parenchymal lung disease because the lung and visceral pleura are not innervated by pain fibers.

MANAGEMENT

The management of pleurisy is based on treatment of the underlying disease. Co-management with a specialist is necessary for all except the most benign causes of pleural inflammation. Drainage of the pleural space may be indicated if a pleural effusion is present. Certain systemic causes of inflammation, such as lupus erythematosus, respond well to corticosteroids. Nonsteroidal anti-inflammatory drugs are used to provide symptomatic pain relief. Malignant diseases rarely cause pleurisy, and pleurisy usually resolves with appropriate and prompt treatment.[13]

COMPLICATIONS

The extent and complications of pleural inflammation depend on the underlying disease process. Some causes are self-limited and have no chronic sequelae or complications. If the inflammation is chronic or pleural repair processes cause fibrosis, an inelastic membrane (pleural peel) may form around the lung. This membrane causes lung entrapment and impairs respiratory function.[12]

INDICATIONS FOR REFERRAL OR HOSPITALIZATION

A referral is often necessary to determine or to treat the underlying cause of the pleurisy. The requisite evaluation and management depend on the cause of the inflammation. Patients without evidence of respiratory compromise or acute illness can often be evaluated and treated on an outpatient basis. Patients with more significant respiratory compromise or highly contagious disease (e.g., active pulmonary tuberculosis) may need to be hospitalized for further evaluation and treatment.

PATIENT AND FAMILY EDUCATION

Patient education varies according to the cause of the pleurisy. Teaching must include an explanation of and rationale for all diagnostic tests. Education should also focus on symptomatic relief. As in all cases in which multiple practitioners may be involved, the role of the health care provider is important in coordinating care and in keeping the patient well informed and at the focus of decision-making.

CHAPTER 111

PNEUMONIA

Geri C. Reeves

DEFINITION AND EPIDEMIOLOGY

Pneumonia remains one of the leading causes of morbidity and mortality in the United States, especially in older adults and in those with underlying chronic disease. In 2010, pneumonia and influenza combined were ranked as the ninth leading cause of death in the United States, with the majority of deaths attributable to pneumonia.[1] Worldwide, in children younger than 5 years, pneumonia remains the primary cause of death.[2] In 2011 in the United States, pneumonia was the primary cause of hospitalization death in adults, with costs exceeding 10 billion dollars.[3] Pneumonia and influenza together represented a cost to the U.S. economy in 2005 of approximately 40.2 billion dollars.[4]

The Infectious Diseases Society of America (IDSA) defines community-acquired pneumonia (CAP) as an acute infection of the pulmonary parenchyma that is frequently associated with at least two symptoms of active infection, occurring in individuals who have not been hospitalized or resided in a long-term care facility for 14 days before the onset of symptoms.[5] Hospital-acquired pneumonia (HAP; nosocomial pneumonia) is defined as pneumonia that occurs 48 hours or more after admission that did not appear to be incubating at the time of admission. Ventilator-associated pneumonia (VAP) is defined as a type of HAP that develops more than 48 hours after endotracheal intubation. Health care–associated pneumonia (HCAP), a relatively new clinical entity, is defined as pneumonia that occurs in a nonhospitalized patient with extensive health care contact, as defined by one or more of the following: intravenous therapy, wound care, or intravenous chemotherapy during the prior 30 days; residence in a nursing home or other long-term care facility; hospitalization in an acute care hospital for 2 or more days during the prior 90 days; or attendance at a hospital or hemodialysis clinic during the prior 30 days.[6]

PATHOPHYSIOLOGY

The lungs are usually a sterile environment maintained by a host of natural defenses. The airways act as a filtration and humidification system for inspired air. Epithelial cells line the entire respiratory tract and contain cilia that constantly beat upward toward the pharynx. This action is a physical means of elimination of foreign material. Also, an intact gag reflex prevents the entry of particles, mucus, and food debris. Finally, the immune system is responsible for defense mechanisms, such as the action of phagocytes, macrophages, neutrophils, complement, and immunoglobulins, which retard advancement of pathogenic organisms that do gain access to this normally sterile environment.

In the healthy adult, these host mechanisms prevent disease much of the time. However, a number of mechanisms allow pathogens to gain entry into the lungs; these mechanisms include an altered level of consciousness from stroke, seizure, anesthesia, alcohol abuse, intoxication, and the sleep state. Epiglottic closure may be compromised in these situations and allow normal oral flora to gain entry. Certain other conditions may predispose an individual to recurrent pneumonia. These include compromised immune function, cystic fibrosis, esophageal abnormalities, bronchial obstruction, and bronchiectasis.

Pneumonia can be classified as typical and atypical, although the clinical presentation is often similar.[7] Typical pneumonia is caused by organisms such as *Streptococcus pneumoniae,* which accounts for 60% to 70% of all bacterial CAP cases. Atypical pneumonia, so called because the organisms are not detectable on Gram stain or cultivatable on standard bacteriologic media, is caused by *Mycoplasma pneumoniae, Chlamydophila pneumoniae, Legionella* species, and respiratory viruses.[5] In addition, patients are more likely to be exposed to certain types of pneumonia according to the setting. The most common causes of CAP in outpatients include *S. pneumoniae, M. pneumoniae, Haemophilus influenzae, C. pneumoniae,* and respiratory viruses.[5] Common pathogens in inpatient, non–intensive care unit (ICU) settings include *S. pneumoniae, M. pneumoniae, C. pneumoniae, H. influenzae, Legionella* species, and respiratory viruses. Common causes in inpatient ICU settings include *S. pneumoniae, Staphylococcus aureus, Legionella* species, gram-negative bacilli, and *H. influenzae.*

Comorbidities also influence susceptibility to different types of pneumonia. *Moraxella catarrhalis* and *Klebsiella pneumoniae* infections are more commonly diagnosed when there is coexistent alcoholism. *S. aureus* and *H. influenzae* infections often occur after a primary influenza infection. *M. catarrhalis,* a gram-negative organism not thought to be pathogenic, is most commonly found in those with chronic lung conditions such as chronic obstructive pulmonary disease (COPD). It is also found in patients with other underlying chronic lung conditions such as malignant disease, with steroid use, and with diabetes.[8]

Another organism responsible for pneumonia is *Legionella pneumophila.* This organism was first implicated in 1976 after 182 people became ill in Philadelphia while attending an American Legion convention. The organism is a gram-negative bacillus that survives in water and soil. Contamination with the organism is acquired through inhalation of aerosolized droplets, thus making air-conditioning ventilating systems an obvious reservoir.

Clues to the specific cause of the pneumonia can be found in the patient's history. The CAPs include the organisms found in Table 111-1.

The incidence of some causes of pneumonia is linked to the season of the year and the geographic area. Influenza illness in the winter increases the prevalence of secondary *S. pneumoniae, S. aureus,* and *H. influenzae* pneumonias. *H. influenzae* is known to have a short incubation period and moves through communities quickly. Mycoplasmal infection usually moves through communities slowly because of a longer incubation period and lower communicability. *Legionella* organisms have been known to infect a large number of people simultaneously by infecting many within a group from a single reservoir.

CLINICAL PRESENTATION AND PHYSICAL EXAMINATION

In most cases of CAP, diagnosis is made by history and physical examination; identification of the causative agent is usually not

TABLE 111-1 Epidemiologic Characteristics Related to Specific Pathogens in CAP

Condition	Commonly Encountered Pathogens
Alcoholism	*Streptococcus pneumoniae,* oral anaerobes, *Klebsiella pneumoniae, Acinetobacter* species, *Mycobacterium tuberculosis*
COPD or smoking	*Haemophilus influenzae, Pseudomonas aeruginosa, Legionella* species, *S. pneumoniae, Moraxella catarrhalis, Chlamydophila pneumoniae*
Aspiration	Gram-negative enteric pathogens, oral anaerobes
Lung abscess	CA-MRSA, oral anaerobes, endemic fungal pneumonia, *M. tuberculosis,* atypical mycobacteria
Exposure to bat or bird droppings	*Histoplasma capsulatum*
Exposure to birds	*Chlamydophila psittaci* (if poultry: avian influenza)
Exposure to rabbits	*Francisella tularensis*
Exposure to farm animals or parturient cats	*Coxiella burnetii* (Q fever)
HIV infection (early)	*S. pneumoniae, H. influenzae, M. tuberculosis*
HIV infection (late)	The pathogens listed for early infection plus *Pneumocystis jiroveci, Cryptococcus, Histoplasma, Aspergillus,* atypical mycobacteria (especially *Mycobacterium kansasii*), *P. aeruginosa*
Hotel or cruise ship stay in previous 2 weeks	*Legionella* species
Travel to or residence in southwestern United States	*Coccidioides* species, hantavirus
Travel to or residence in Southeast and East Asia	*Burkholderia pseudomallei,* avian influenza, SARS
Influenza active in community	Influenza, *S. pneumoniae, Staphylococcus aureus, H. influenzae*
Cough 12 weeks with whoop or post-tussive vomiting	*Bordetella pertussis*
Structural lung disease (e.g., bronchiectasis)	*P. aeruginosa, Burkholderia cepacia, S. aureus*
Injection drug use	*S. aureus,* anaerobes, *M. tuberculosis, S. pneumoniae*
Endobronchial obstruction	Anaerobes, *S. pneumoniae, H. influenzae, S. aureus*
In context of bioterrorism	*Bacillus anthracis* (anthrax), *Yersinia pestis* (plague), *Francisella tularensis* (tularemia)

CA-MRSA, community-associated methicillin-resistant *Staphylococcus aureus;* HIV, human immunodeficiency virus; SARS, severe acute respiratory syndrome.
From Mandell LA, Wunderink R, Anzueto A et al: Infectious Diseases Society of America/American Thoracic Society consensus guidelines on the management of community-acquired pneumonia in adults, *Clin Infect Dis* 44(Suppl 2):S27-S72, 2007.

necessary. Although the list of organisms causing CAP is long and increasing, relatively few organisms are responsible for most cases of pneumonia. In primary care practice, two of the most important issues related to pneumonia are awareness of the most common infectious pathogens and their treatment and decisions about the appropriateness of outpatient treatment. The clinical presentation of pneumonia includes a history of fever, chills or rigors, malaise, and cough with or without sputum production.[9] The patient may also report hemoptysis, dyspnea, and pleuritic chest symptoms. The provider should focus on symptoms of bacterial, viral, and atypical pneumonia syndromes. Chest auscultation may reveal rales that do not clear with a cough, which may be found in both bacterial and atypical pneumonia. Consolidation, including dullness to percussion, bronchial breath sounds, and egophony (E-to-A changes), is found more commonly in the bacterial pneumonia syndromes. Chest radiographs are highly variable and may be normal in the early course of the disease. In addition, chest radiographs of patients with viral and mycoplasmal pneumonia may show large infiltrates with minimum outward symptoms. A prodrome of headache and sore throat is often associated with atypical pneumonia. Patients aged 18 to 44 years are almost twice as likely as those older than 75 years to complain of pleuritic chest pain and to have fever.

Some patients (e.g., older adults) may show none of the classic signs of pneumonia but may have atypical complaints such as fatigue, lethargy, decreased appetite, increased falls, and mental status changes (such as confusion, stupor, or coma). In addition, older adults are more likely to be seen initially with tachypnea but less likely to have a cough or fever.

Bacterial Pneumonia Syndromes

Gram-Positive Bacteria. *S. pneumoniae* is the leading cause of pneumonia in any adult age group with or without comorbid conditions.[7,8] Those at risk for *S. pneumoniae* infection characteristically have some chronic condition, such as diabetes, COPD, asplenia, advanced age, cigarette smoking, congestive heart failure, dementia, alcoholism, or immunosuppression. From 20% to 60% of all hospitalized patients are infected with pneumococci.[7]

The history may include an abrupt onset of high fever with shaking chills, productive cough with purulent sputum, and possibly pleuritic-type chest pains. Physical examination may reveal signs of consolidation (egophony, increased fremitus, dullness to percussion, rales, and rhonchi), and chest films reveal single or multiple lobar consolidation. Sputum analysis by Gram stain indicates gram-positive diplococci in pairs and short chains and large numbers of polymorphonuclear leukocytes.

S. aureus, although rarely a cause of CAP, must be considered, especially after a primary influenza infection, in older adults and in those with diabetes. Suppurative conditions, including empyema, lung abscess, and pneumothorax, are common complications. Seeding to distant sites, such as bones, joints, liver, endocardium, and the meninges, may also occur.

Group A streptococci rarely cause CAP but have been found in epidemics among close groups that live together, such as military units. Symptoms may be similar to those of *S. pneumoniae* infection, and Gram stain reveals clumped spherical cocci, similar in appearance to a bunch of grapes.

Gram-Negative Bacteria. *H. influenzae,* another causative agent of CAP, is a small, gram-negative rod with a polysaccharide capsule. There are six serotypes, of which type B is the most severe and invasive (causing meningitis and sepsis). Some strains of *H. influenzae* are nonencapsulated and therefore cannot be typed. These are also capable of causing disease, but the disease is usually noninvasive and therefore less severe. These nontypable strains of *H. influenzae* are usually found in acute bronchitis. Pneumonia caused by *H. influenzae* is usually caused by an encapsulated strain. Older adults and those with underlying chronic lung conditions are most susceptible to this bacterium. The history usually includes an abrupt onset of fever, shaking chills, and cough with purulent sputum. The patient may describe pleuritic chest pain, and physical examination reveals signs of consolidation. A bronchopneumonia pattern is seen on the chest radiograph.

Aerobic gram-negative bacilli rarely colonize the upper airway in healthy individuals but are often found in people with an underlying disease such as alcoholism and in those who reside in health care facilities or nursing homes. Aspiration of the organisms is thought to be the mode of infection. *Pseudomonas* organisms, *K. pneumoniae,* and *Escherichia coli* may also become pulmonary pathogens. The mortality rate associated with gram-negative pneumonia is relatively high compared with other types of pneumonia. Therefore, a history of recent hospitalization or nursing home residency should heighten suspicion for a gram-negative pathogenesis. Polymicrobial infection is seen more often in older adults, and increased colonization of gram-negative bacilli of the upper airway is related to recent antimicrobial use, decreased activity, diabetes, and alcohol use.

M. catarrhalis is a β-lactamase–producing gram-negative aerobic diplococcus that was recently identified as a common pathogen found in individuals with COPD.[7,8] In patients with COPD, it is often the only organism isolated from the lower respiratory tract. Other chronic conditions, such as alcoholism, steroid use, diabetes, and malignant disease, increase the risk for *M. catarrhalis* infection. The highest incidence of this infection tends to be in the winter months.

Atypical Pneumonia Syndromes

Atypical pneumonia syndromes largely refer to pneumonias caused by nonbacterial organisms and by bacterial organisms that do not share the expected characteristics of most bacteria. *M. pneumoniae* is one of the most common causes of atypical pneumonia in the United States and other parts of the world. Mycoplasma infection can occur at any age, but infection rates are highest among school-aged children, military recruits, and college students.[10] This atypical pneumonia syndrome is characterized by a prodrome of fever, headache, myalgias, and dry cough. These individuals usually appear less ill than those with bacterial pneumonia. Symptoms may last up to 6 weeks and include a dry, hacking cough that may require a narcotic cough suppressant. Because of the long incubation period, mycoplasmal infection may spread slowly among family members. It should be viewed as a systemic disease with a pulmonary component.

The physical examination usually reveals fine rales with no signs of lung consolidation. A cutaneous manifestation may be present in the form of maculopapular eruptions. Rarely, examination of the tympanic membranes shows evidence of bullous myringitis, which can be very painful. Chest radiographs reveal patchy alveolar densities or nonhomogeneous segmental infiltrates. The white blood cell count may be normal or only slightly elevated. Full recovery is expected with no residual effects in a previously healthy individual. However, the disease can be severe in those with sickle cell anemia, in older adults, and in those with immunosuppression.

C. pneumoniae (TWAR strain) has a higher incidence in older adults. Transmission of the organism is thought to be person to person and has been implicated in outbreaks of pneumonia in residents of long-term care facilities, in a prison, and among military recruits.[11-13]

Symptoms are similar to those of mycoplasmal infection. Clinical presentation may include laryngitis, a hoarse voice, and nonexudative pharyngitis in addition to the symptoms described for mycoplasmal infection. Laryngitis is not present in any other atypical pneumonia syndrome. Chest radiographs may show patchy consolidation, interstitial infiltrates, or funnel-shaped lesions. The white blood cell count is usually normal.

Multiple viruses, including adenoviruses, respiratory syncytial virus (RSV), and parainfluenza virus, may also cause pneumonia. Predilection for infection in children is most common. Cytomegalovirus and *Pneumocystis* may be the cause of pneumonia in the immunocompromised host. For years, *Pneumocystis* was referred to as *Pneumocystis carinii* pneumonia (PCP) and was known to be the most common serious acquired immunodeficiency syndrome (AIDS)–defining opportunistic infection in the United States. DNA analysis demonstrated extensive diversity within the genus *Pneumocystis*, with different host species having different DNA sequences. In recognition of its genetic and functional distinctness, the organism that causes human PCP is now named *Pneumocystis jiroveci*. Infection with hantavirus organisms was initially recognized in the southwestern United States. Caused by exposure to infected rodents (e.g., a rodent bite, breathing air contaminated with rodent excretion, or touching rodent droppings), hantavirus pulmonary syndrome (HPS) has now been identified in 34 states and in countries outside the U.S. A viral-like illness, HPS causes fever, myalgias, nausea, vomiting, dizziness, and thrombocytopenia.[14] HPS resembles acute respiratory distress syndrome and quickly can cause pulmonary failure.[7]

Causative agents associated with CAP include the coronavirus (CoV) responsible for severe acute respiratory syndrome (SARS), human metapneumovirus (hMPV), and community-acquired methicillin-resistant *Staphylococcus aureus* (CA-MRSA). Although SARS-CoV was not documented in humans until 2002, it has been hypothesized that a previously unknown animal CoV may have mutated and infected humans. SARS-CoV is highly contagious, so aggressive infection control measures are necessary to prevent spread of the disease. Middle East respiratory syndrome (MERS)–CoV is a more recently identified severe CoV that causes respiratory distress and death in 27% of cases.[15] MERS-CoV initially seemed to be associated with travel to the Arabian peninsula but has been identified in other countries as well.[15] Person-to-person contact is likely, but the actual cause is not yet known.[15]

Another pathogen associated with CAP is hMPV, a paramyxovirus first isolated in 2001 in children hospitalized with acute infections. Since then, hMPV has been reported in all age groups, with varying stages of disease, from those who are asymptomatic to those with severe bronchitis and pneumonia. There is no specific treatment for hMPV.[16]

CA-MRSA, a combination of well-known health care–associated strains and newer isolates with distinctive genotypes, is a virulent and resistant pathogen and causes outbreaks of serious infections, including skin and soft tissue infections and necrotizing pneumonia.[16]

RSV is an important cause of pneumonia in older adults, particularly those living in long-term care facilities. Treatment is supportive.[17]

L. pneumophila is the pulmonary pathogen responsible for legionnaires' disease. Symptoms of infection include dry cough, fever with a temperature of 38.3° C to 38.8° C (101° F to 102° F), altered mental status, relative bradycardia, headache, and gastrointestinal symptoms including diarrhea.

DIAGNOSTICS

Chest Radiography

Chest radiography is most valuable when the results are considered in the context of the history and physical examination. According to the IDSA and American Thoracic Society (ATS) guidelines, a chest radiograph is required for the routine evaluation of patients who are likely to have pneumonia, to establish the diagnosis and to aid in differentiating CAP from other common causes of cough and fever.[5] Posteroanterior and lateral chest radiographs confirm pneumonia when new infiltrates are found on the films. In addition, chest radiography may provide clues to the type of pneumonia. Bacterial patterns on the chest radiograph include lobar consolidation, cavitation, and large pleural effusions. Lobar consolidation is more common in typical pneumonia, and bilateral, diffuse infiltrates are seen more commonly in atypical pneumonia.[7] A chest radiograph that is normal does not exclude the diagnosis of pneumonia. Chest radiographs early in the course of the disease (i.e., first 24 hours) may be normal.[18] In addition, immunosuppression, dehydration, and neutropenia may result in false-negative findings. Comparison of the current chest radiograph with old radiographs is important to assess for changes. Computed tomography (CT) scan of the pulmonary system is a diagnostic consideration.[18]

Pulse Oximetry

All patients should be screened by pulse oximetry, which may suggest both the presence of pneumonia in patients without obvious signs of pneumonia and unsuspected hypoxemia in patients with diagnosed pneumonia.

Sputum Analysis

Analysis of sputum can be helpful in identifying a causative agent in pneumonia; however, ATS guidelines do not recommend this diagnostic test for outpatients diagnosed with CAP.[5] Culture and Gram stain are excellent methods of identifying the pathologic agent when needed. A good sputum sample comes from the bronchial tree; it is not the same as saliva from the mouth. Although it is not usually available during the clinic visit, sputum produced on awakening in the morning is typically a good sample because of the strong reflex to cough on rising to an upright position. Sputum that contains less than 10 squamous epithelial cells and more than 25 neutrophils is considered an adequate sample. The patient is encouraged to rinse the mouth with water several times before trying to produce a sample. Inhalation of a warmed 3% to 10% saline solution may help the patient provide an adequate sample.

Other Tests

ATS diagnostic recommendations for CAP patients requiring hospital admission include assessment of gas exchange by either telemetry or arterial sampling, complete blood count (CBC) with differential, blood chemistry, liver function tests, and two sets of blood cultures. Evidence for benefit of routine bronchoscopy does not exist.[5]

DIAGNOSTICS

Pneumonia

LABORATORY
Sputum analysis-culture and Gram stain*
CBC and differential*
Blood chemistries*
Blood cultures*
Complement fixation*
ABGs*
Viral culture*

IMAGING
Chest x-ray examination
CT scan*

OTHER DIAGNOSTICS
Bronchoscopy*

*If indicated.
ABGs, arterial blood gases.

DIFFERENTIAL DIAGNOSIS

Multiple organisms must be considered in the differential diagnosis of pneumonia. *S. pneumoniae* is the most common cause, followed by *H. influenzae,* influenza virus, and *Legionella.* Noninfectious diseases that can mimic symptoms of pneumonia should also be considered. These include bronchial asthma, hypersensitivity pneumonitis, pulmonary emboli, heart failure, pulmonary tumors, and some inflammatory lung diseases.

DIFFERENTIAL DIAGNOSIS

Pneumonia

- *S. pneumoniae*
- *M. pneumoniae*
- Respiratory viruses (including cytomegalovirus, hantavirus, RSV)
- *C. pneumoniae* (TWAR strain)
- *H. influenzae*
- *L. pneumophila*
- *S. aureus*
- SARS–CoV
- hMPV
- CA-MRSA
- *Mycobacterium tuberculosis*
- Endemic fungi
- Aerobic gram-negative bacilli (e.g., *Pseudomonas aeruginosa*)
- Anaerobic infections
- Polymicrobial infections
- Pulmonary embolus
- Congestive heart failure
- Pulmonary tumors
- Inflammatory lung diseases
- Acute and chronic bronchitis

MANAGEMENT

The treatment of pneumonia, both CAP and nosocomial, has been standardized to some degree by the publication of consensus guidelines by the IDSA and ATS. The initial management decision after diagnosis is to determine if the patient can be treated on an outpatient basis. The decision to admit the patient is the most costly issue in the management of CAP. Patients at low risk for death and who are treated appropriately in the outpatient setting do not require hospitalization. Severity assessment tools (e.g., the pneumonia severity index [PSI], CURB-65, A-DROP, SCAP) can assist in determining patients who require hospitalization. Successful treatment of pneumonia depends on the correct empirical antibiotic selection and knowledge of its proven effectiveness in vivo. A working knowledge of the organisms that most commonly infect different age groups and the habits or characteristics that put an individual at risk for specific causative agents is essential.

Resistance patterns to all antibiotics are an increasing problem—now more evident and widespread than at any other time in medical history. Careful, prudent use of antibiotics is absolutely necessary to curb this growing problem. The routine practice of trying to cover for all pathogens, especially gram-negative organisms, should be avoided to decrease increased resistance. Initiation of antibiotic treatment in patients with CAP is empirically determined because the history and physical examination will not determine a specific cause of the disease. Despite the use of sputum culture, Gram stain, and chest radiographs, providers cannot always accurately identify the causative organism. The patient's age, competency of the host immune system, underlying chronic conditions, patterns of resistance in the community, and knowledge of the most likely pathogens must be considered to accurately determine empirical antimicrobial therapy.

The recommendations for treatment of CAP are taken from the most recent guidelines and recommendations published by the ATS and IDSA in 2007.[5] Since the first publication of recommendations in 1993, there has been a shift in focus from age groups and comorbid conditions as the basis for drug selection to the most likely pathogens combined with modifying factors and coexisting cardiopulmonary disease. Empirical antibiotic therapy is based on whether the patient is being treated in an outpatient or inpatient non-ICU or ICU setting. In outpatient settings, for previously healthy individuals with no use of antimicrobial therapy within the previous 3 months, a macrolide antibiotic is recommended. Doxycycline is a secondary recommendation. For individuals with comorbidities, such as heart disease, lung disease, liver disease, renal disease, diabetes mellitus, alcoholism, malignant disease, asplenia, and immunosuppressive conditions or use of immunosuppressive drugs, a respiratory fluoroquinolone or β-lactam plus a macrolide is recommended.[5] For inpatients in non-ICU settings, a respiratory fluoroquinolone or a β-lactam antibiotic is recommended. For inpatients in ICU settings, a β-lactam (cefotaxime, ceftriaxone, or ampicillin-sulbactam) plus either azithromycin or a respiratory fluoroquinolone is recommended. For penicillin-allergic patients, a respiratory fluoroquinolone and aztreonam are recommended. Special concerns related to the selection of empirical antibiotic therapy include the possibility of *Pseudomonas* infection. In such situations, an antipneumococcal, antipseudomonal β-lactam (piperacillin-tazobactam, cefepime, imipenem, or meropenem) plus either ciprofloxacin or levofloxacin is recommended. Additional recommendations, particularly those based on Level III evidence, can be found in the IDSA/ATS consensus guidelines.

In addition, new antibiotics are now available for treatment of CAP. Recommendations for treatment of CA-MRSA include vancomycin and linezolid.[5] Linezolid is the first of a new class of antibiotics called the oxazolidinones. It is active against many gram-positive pathogens, including CA-MRSA, anaerobes, vancomycin-resistant enterococci, and penicillin-resistant *S. pneumoniae.* The main concern with CA-MRSA is the necrotizing aspect of the infection. Many of the treatment options mentioned before have not yet been shown to decrease toxin production. Therefore in some situations linezolid may be the best choice. Risk factors for other uncommon causes of CAP are included in Table 111-1.

Early treatment with oseltamivir or zanamivir is recommended for influenza A.[5] Use of oseltamivir and zanamivir is not recommended in patients with uncomplicated influenza with symptoms of more than 48 hours' duration, but these drugs may be used to decrease the risk of viral shedding in hospitalized patients or for influenza pneumonia. Patients with an illness comparable to influenza and with known exposure to poultry in areas with previous H1N1 infection should be tested for H1N1 and droplet precautions, and routine infection control measures should be observed. Patients with suspected H1N1 infection should be treated with oseltamivir and antibacterial agents targeting *S. pneumoniae* and *S. aureus,* the most common causes of secondary bacterial infection in patients with influenza.[5]

Older adults and those with coexisting illness are at increased risk for development of more virulent pneumonia, have longer healing times, need more supportive treatment, and require closer follow-up monitoring, especially with delayed resolution of pneumonia.

Younger individuals without comorbid disease who are infected with pneumonia usually respond more quickly and have fewer complications. According to the IDSA/ATS guidelines, patients admitted through the emergency department (ED) should receive their first dose of antibiotic while still in the ED. It is recommended that patients be switched from intravenous to oral antibiotics once they are hemodynamically stable and improving clinically, have a functioning gastrointestinal tract, and are able to tolerate oral medications.[5]

The choice of antibiotic therapy depends on careful consideration of the consequences of failure to respond to initial outpatient treatment, the need for hospitalization, and the likelihood of adherence to the treatment regimen. Other considerations include the existence of a supportive home environment, access to ED care if needed, the presence of an involved individual to identify significant changes in this illness should they occur, and the opportunity for follow-up in 24 to 48 hours. In addition, reducing health care costs while maintaining optimal care is a growing concern. Strategies for reducing the cost of antibiotic therapy include choosing monotherapy (if adequate) instead of combination therapy and using agents with longer half-lives to allow once-daily administration, which leads to improved compliance and decreased costs.[7] Transitioning patients to oral therapy as soon as it is clinically appropriate can significantly decrease the length of an inpatient stay, decreasing costs. Other strategies to reduce cost include avoiding agents with serious or costly side effects and avoiding agents with known resistance. In addition, avoiding agents that require therapeutic monitoring or laboratory tests or antibiotics with poor tissue penetration can reduce the costs associated with antibiotics.[7]

LIFE SPAN CONSIDERATIONS

Older adults have the highest rates of CAP in the United States. Advanced age is associated with a variety of age-related declines in immune-system function (immune senescence) and prevalent comorbidities. As a result, elders constitute the largest immunocompromised population in the United States, putting them at risk for new infectious agents. Pathogens that are not typical causative agents of pneumonia must be considered possible causative agents in elders. Both clinical features and physical examination findings may be lacking or altered in elderly patients.[5] Furthermore, older adults are more likely to have CAP caused by a resistant organism or tuberculosis and to require hospital admission.[19] Supportive treatment and closer follow-up monitoring are especially important in the elderly patient with pneumonia.

Symptoms and signs of pneumonia in children may be subtle. The combination of fever and cough is suggestive of pneumonia. Other respiratory findings, such as tachypnea or increased work of breathing, may precede cough. The longer fever, cough, and respiratory findings are present, the greater the likelihood of pneumonia.[20] Older children may complain of pleuritic chest pain, but this is an inconsistent finding. Occasionally, the predominant manifestation may be abdominal pain, caused by referred pain from the lower lobes.

COMPLICATIONS

With minimum diagnostic testing and empirical antibiotic treatment, most patients will improve and show resolution of pneumonia. In most cases, improvement is seen within 48 to 72 hours after initiation of antibiotics. Pneumonia that fails to resolve shows little clinical improvement after 4 weeks of therapy. Fever, cough, sputum production, and shortness of breath may still be present. Chest radiographs also do not show improvement within this time frame.

When there is poor response to therapy, possibly the initial antibiotic choice was not correct, there was poor adherence to the oral antibiotic therapy, or the diagnosis of pneumonia was not accurate. Considerations should include the possibility of opportunistic fungal infections, *P. jiroveci,* tuberculosis, bronchogenic carcinoma, Wegener granulomatosis, bronchiolitis obliterans with organizing pneumonia, and heart failure. Diagnostic bronchoscopy, CT scan, and transthoracic needle aspiration and biopsy may be warranted to exclude these. If the diagnosis is still undetermined and there is no resolution, an open lung biopsy may be considered, and consultation with a pulmonologist is clearly warranted. Other complications of pneumonia include abscess, empyema, pulmonary vascular congestion, and pulmonary embolism.

INDICATIONS FOR REFERRAL OR HOSPITALIZATION

Physician consultation is recommended for patients with oxygen saturation of less than 90% on room air, rigors, change in mental status, extremely abnormal vital signs, or comorbid disease (e.g., diabetes, human immunodeficiency virus [HIV], cancer, or COPD).

In addition, delayed resolution of pneumonia and inpatient treatment generally require consultation. Severity-of-illness scores, such as the CURB-65 criteria (*c*onfusion, *u*remia [blood *u*rea nitrogen >20 mg/dL], *r*espiratory rate >30 breaths per minute, low *b*lood pressure [<90 mm Hg systolic or 60 mm Hg diastolic], age 65 years or older), or prognostic models, such as the PSI, can be used to identify patients with CAP who may be candidates for outpatient treatment.[21,22] For patients with CURB-65 scores of 2 or higher, more intensive treatment through hospitalization or intensive in-home health services is usually warranted.[5] For the PSI, patients without a history of any of the following five co-existing conditions, neoplastic disease, heart failure, cerebrovascular disease, renal disease, liver disease, or vital sign abnormalities are assigned to class I (low risk for death within 30 days). If one or more risk factors are present, the evaluation of illness proceeds to step 2. This second step stratifies the remaining patients into risk classes II, III, IV, or V, based on the total number of points assigned to each risk factor.

The use of objective admission criteria can decrease the number of patients unnecessarily hospitalized with CAP. However, it is important to keep in mind that objective criteria do not replace the health care provider's clinical judgment. Determination of subjective factors, including the patient's ability to safely and reliably take oral medication and the availability of outpatient support resources should also be considered.[5] Certain clinical criteria observed in the patient warrant hospitalization. However, the health care provider's clinical judgment always supersedes written recommendations.

PATIENT AND FAMILY EDUCATION

Once the diagnosis of pneumonia has been made, patient education should include directions for use of the antibiotic and information on potential untoward effects of the drug. Follow-up instructions, depending on the clinical situation, may include 24-hour telephone contact or follow-up in the office after 24 to 48 hours. This will improve adherence to the prescribed therapy, provide an opportunity to address side effects of drug therapy, and allow progress to be monitored. The need for hospitalization should be assessed throughout the course of the illness. Education should include instructions to drink adequate fluids and to use an antipyretic to control fever and myalgias when needed. Use of cough medicines should be avoided because the cough reflex and sputum expectoration enhance removal of thick secretions. However, in the event of a constant, nonproductive cough, as found especially with mycoplasmal infection, a narcotic such as codeine at night allows more restorative sleep.

HEALTH PROMOTION

Patients at risk for pneumonia should receive the pneumonia vaccination and should also be encouraged to receive influenza vaccination (the flu shot) each year. Avoiding smoke and contact with persons who have a respiratory infection also decreases the risk of pneumonia. In an effort to reduce the spread of respiratory infections, respiratory hygiene measures, including the use of hand hygiene and masks or tissues for patients with cough, should be used in outpatient settings and EDs. Daily exercise and a diet of healthy foods high in vitamins, nutrients, and fiber should also be encouraged.

CHAPTER 112

PNEUMOTHORAX

Nena Tucker

DEFINITION AND EPIDEMIOLOGY

Pneumothorax is defined as the presence of air in the pleural space leading to a loss of negative intrathoracic pressure.[1] Processes leading to a pneumothorax may be spontaneous, traumatic, or iatrogenic. A spontaneous pneumothorax occurs in the absence of thoracic trauma and can be categorized into primary or secondary. A primary spontaneous pneumothorax (PSP) develops in the otherwise healthy patient without underlying lung disease or trauma.[2] A secondary spontaneous pneumothorax occurs in the presence of underlying lung disease but in the absence of trauma. A traumatic pneumothorax may result from penetrating or blunt force trauma to the chest wall.[3] An iatrogenic pneumothorax occurs secondary to a medical procedure such as a pleural biopsy, central venous line placement, or positive-pressure mechanical ventilation.[2] Any pneumothorax, regardless of type, may evolve into a tension pneumothorax in which there is increasing positive pressure in the pleural space caused by air being able to enter but not escape.

PSP occurs most frequently in young adults aged 20 to 30.[2] Additional risk factors include smoking, cannabis smoking, male gender, underlying lung disease, tall stature, and thin body habitus.[1,4] There is also evidence to suggest that pregnancy and family history may also be risk factors.

There is notable variance in the occurrence of primary pneumothorax between genders. This is evidenced by an incidence in men of 7.4 to 18 per 100,000 per year in the United States compared with 1.2 to 6 per 100,000 women per year in the United States.[2]

A pneumothorax can be potentially life-threatening. Astute assessment skills and prompt intervention are essential in the diagnosis and management of pneumothorax.

PATHOPHYSIOLOGY

The exact pathophysiology of PSP is unknown but is thought to be associated with subclinical or undiagnosed lung disease. The most common cause of PSP is spontaneous rupture of pleural apical blebs, lying in or just under the visceral pleura.[5] The cause of these blebs in otherwise healthy individuals is unclear, although smoking has been shown to play a clear role by increasing the lifetime risk for development of a pneumothorax.[4]

A secondary pneumothorax can result from underlying pulmonary diseases such as chronic obstructive pulmonary disease, tuberculosis, lung cancer, asthma, endometriosis, and cystic fibrosis.[4,5] Both penetrating and blunt force trauma can cause a traumatic pneumothorax irrespective of age, sex, or underlying lung disease. An iatrogenic pneumothorax is the complication resulting from a medical procedure, including invasive procedures such as the insertion of central lines and barotrauma related to surgery or mechanical ventilation.[2] There does not appear to be any relationship between physical activity and pneumothorax; most episodes of PSP occur at rest. Although many distinct factors may contribute to a pneumothorax, it is the loss of negative pressure when air enters the pleural space that causes the lung or a portion of it to collapse.

Immediate emergency department referral or physician consultation is indicated for patients with respiratory compromise. Tension pneumothorax is a medical emergency requiring immediate intervention. The diagnosis is clinical and should not await radiologic confirmation.[2]

CLINICAL PRESENTATION

The clinical history and physical examination findings associated with a pneumothorax vary and are primarily dependent on the size of the pneumothorax (volume of air in the pleural space).[6] The pertinent history would include history of previous pneumothorax, trauma, or smoking; current medications; allergies; history of strenuous exercise; recent medical procedures and other medical conditions.

Although some patients with pneumothorax may be asymptomatic, the most common complaints are an acute onset of breathlessness and unilateral pleuritic chest pain.[4,6] In general, the symptoms associated with a secondary pneumothorax are more severe than those associated with a primary pneumothorax.

PHYSICAL EXAMINATION

The physical findings reflect the size and nature of the pneumothorax. A tension or large pneumothorax is a medical emergency. Acute respiratory distress, diaphoresis, tachycardia, hypoxemia, tachypnea, tracheal deviation, and cyanosis are unmistakable and associated with a large or tension pneumothorax.[4,6] A smaller pneumothorax may cause mild dyspnea and chest discomfort, or the patient may be asymptomatic.

DIAGNOSTICS

The diagnosis of pneumothorax has historically been established by plain chest radiography, including upright posteroanterior (PA), anteroposterior (AP), and/or lateral views,[3] and portable chest radiography remains part of the standard workup for a suspected traumatic pneumothorax. However, chest radiography alone is inadequate for detection of pneumothoraces; sensitivities approximate 50%.[7] Ultrasound has emerged as a reliable method of detecting pneumothorax. Lung sonography is especially useful in detecting small occult pneumothoraces and traumatic pneumothoraces. A computed tomography (CT) scan is the gold standard for the identification of pneumothorax because of its ability to differentiate between a pneumothorax and underlying bullous lung disease, such as complex cystic lung disease, or when accurate size measurements are required. Chest CT is not widely used owing to delayed diagnosis and risk for hemodynamic compromise associated with transportation out of the clinical area. Pulse oximetry and arterial blood gases (ABGs) can be used to determine level of hypoxia.

DIAGNOSTICS

Pneumothorax

INITIAL	IMAGING
Pulse oximetry	Chest x-ray examination, PA and lateral views
LABORATORY	Ultrasound
ABGs*	CT scan*

*If indicated.

DIFFERENTIAL DIAGNOSIS

Dyspnea and chest pain are identified with a large number of clinical problems. It is important to ascertain whether there has been a history of lung disease (e.g., emphysema, cancer, or chronic obstructive pulmonary disease). Many pneumothoraces occur as a result of trauma, and therefore rib fractures, contusions, costochondral separation, and muscle strains need to be excluded. Other differential diagnoses to consider include pulmonary embolism, myocardial infarction, dissecting aortic aneurysm, pleurisy, pericarditis, and costochondritis. It is useful to remember that half of all patients with PSP have at least one recurrence, making a history of pneumothorax significant.[5] The final diagnosis of pneumothorax is made once the presence of air in the pleural space, seen as a visceral pleural line that parallels the chest wall without peripheral lung markings, is identified.[7]

Diagnosis should also include the size of the pneumothorax. Size can be expressed as the percentage of lung volume lost or measurement of distance from the outer edge of the pleural space to the most apical portion of the lung margin, or conversion tools such as the Rhea method and Collins method can be used.[1]

DIFFERENTIAL DIAGNOSIS

Pneumothorax

- Lung disease (acute or chronic)
- Trauma, blunt (contusion) or penetrating (fractured ribs)
- Pulmonary embolism
- Myocardial infarction
- Pericarditis
- Pleurisy
- Muscle strain, costochondritis
- Dissecting aortic aneurysm

MANAGEMENT

Controversy exists regarding the management of a pneumothorax.[8] Variation is based on pneumothorax type, size, and contributing factors. Treatment of pneumothorax can involve the following options: observation, needle aspiration, small-bore catheter, chest tube, chest tube plus pleurodesis, chest tube plus thoracotomy, and very rarely chest tube plus sternotomy.[1,4] Treatment strategies may also include methods to prevent recurrence, especially in PSP.

Traditionally, no treatment is needed if the pneumothorax is small (less than 2 to 3 cm between the lung and chest wall) and the patient is clinically stable.[2] Observation alone is appropriate for mildly symptomatic patients with small, closed pneumothoraces as well.[1] The risks associated with observation include expansion of pneumothorax and worsening of symptoms. The need to return for care in the event of worsening symptoms must be stressed to the patient and family before discharge.

Signs of cardiopulmonary compromise and/or worsening symptoms require intervention. Simple (needle) aspiration is considered first-line treatment for all primary pneumothoraces requiring intervention.[1] Research suggests that needle aspiration is at least as safe and effective as tube thoracostomy for management. Simple aspiration is not routinely recommended for secondary spontaneous pneumothorax because underlying lung disease is a relative contraindication. Placement of a small-bore catheter is another less invasive option. With the catheter-over-wire or catheter-over-needle technique, a small catheter is placed into the pleural space to allow release of the accumulated air. The catheter can also be attached to a one-way valve such as a Heimlich valve. This method is recommended for PSP as well as secondary spontaneous and recurrent pneumothorax. It is not contraindicated in the patient with underlying lung disease. Small-bore catheters are not indicated in the case of a traumatic pneumothorax. The final treatment option is placement of a tube thoracostomy, commonly known as a chest tube. Tube thoracostomy involves placing a hollow plastic tube into the pleural space; the tube is left in place until the lung re-expands and the leak seals. Tube thoracostomy is indicated for traumatic pneumothorax because of its ability to drain larger volumes of air in addition to blood and other fluids. Ventilatory support may be indicated in some cases. Options to decrease the likelihood of recurrences include the instillation of chemical sclerosing agents (such as talc, doxycycline, tetracycline, or minocycline) through a chest tube or thoracoscope, laser therapy, pleural abrasion, and thoracotomy.[2,4,5]

Secondary spontaneous pneumothorax usually requires more aggressive management because of the decreased reserve in patients with underlying disease. These patients should almost always be hospitalized for definitive treatment and prevention.[5]

A tension pneumothorax requires immediate intervention.[2] The diagnosis of tension pneumothorax can be made based on the clinical presentation. The clinician should not wait for radiographic confirmation to begin treatment. Treatment should be implemented immediately to prevent cardiopulmonary compromise and/or death. A large-bore angiocatheter is inserted into the pleural space at the second anterior intercostal space on the affected side. Air is released immediately, but the angiocatheter must be left in place until a chest tube can be inserted.[5]

In cases in which there is a persistent air leak or failure of the lung to re-expand, a respiratory specialist or thoracic surgeon should be consulted. In patients with human immunodeficiency virus (HIV) infection and underlying lung disease, such as cystic fibrosis, early and aggressive intervention and specialist referral are recommended.

LIFE SPAN CONSIDERATIONS

Efforts should be made to minimize and to treat all possible exacerbating and complicating factors. Patients who required no intervention should refrain from air travel until resolution of the pneumothorax is confirmed by chest radiography.[4] Diving should be permanently avoided after a pneumothorax unless the patient had bilateral surgical pleurectomy.

COMPLICATIONS

Complications resulting from a large pneumothorax may include cardiac and ventilatory compromise, which can be fatal. Chest tube placement can lead to numerous complications, including pulmonary edema, lung infarction, infection, trauma, bleeding, and subcutaneous emphysema.

INDICATIONS FOR REFERRAL OR HOSPITALIZATION

Outpatient treatment is reserved for those without evidence of pulmonary and cardiovascular compromise.[4] Traditionally, a patient with a large pneumothorax requires hospitalization for chest tube placement and close monitoring.[5] Patients with secondary spontaneous pneumothorax almost always require hospitalization, as do patients with respiratory compromise.[2,5] Patients with PSP, regardless of size, should be referred to a pulmonologist because of the large incidence of recurrence and the possibility of subclinical lung disease. All patients with pneumothorax (other than simple traumatic) warrant evaluation by a pulmonologist both to rule out underlying lung disease and to define clinical management. Because of the variation in treatment recommendations, the attending physician and/or pulmonologist should be consulted regarding the patient's plan of care.

PATIENT AND FAMILY EDUCATION

Patient education should center on information about the cause, prevention, and treatment of a pneumothorax. Recurrence is more likely to occur in those with preexisting lung disease.[4]

Smoking cessation is an important educational issue with any lung problem and is an issue for patients with a pneumothorax, regardless of the cause. It remains the only modifiable risk factor for PSP recurrence.[4] Patients need to be cautioned against air travel before confirmed resolution of the pneumothorax, as well as scuba diving. Health promotion is aimed primarily at the elimination of smoking and the prevention of trauma.

CHAPTER 113

PULMONARY EMBOLISM

Nena Tucker

DEFINITION AND EPIDEMIOLOGY

Pulmonary embolism (PE) is the blockage of one or more of the pulmonary arteries or their branches by a thrombus or other embolic material that dislodges and enters the pulmonary circulation.[1,2] Emboli may be caused by thrombi, fat, or other foreign material such as parasites. The most common cause of PE is a thrombus or blood clot that has formed in the pelvis or legs.[1] The focus of this chapter is pulmonary emboli caused by thrombi.

The true incidence of PE is unknown; more than half of all PEs go undiagnosed.[3] Estimates of PE incidence range from 300,000 to 600,000 people affected each year. It is the third most common cause of cardiovascular death, with approximately 100,000 to 200,000 deaths in the United States each year.[4] Of patients with acute PE, 8% to 10% die within the first hour.[1] Many occurrences go undiagnosed and are not identified until autopsy. It is estimated that as many as one in three cases are not identified.[2] A review of clinical studies from 1939 to 2000 found the prevalence of PE diagnosed at the time of autopsy to range from 9% to 55%.[3]

PATHOPHYSIOLOGY

PE is not a disease, but a complication of an underlying issue. Most frequently, the PE is the result of a thrombus that has entered pulmonary circulation.[1] Several factors contribute to susceptibility to thrombus formation, including stasis, vascular damage, and hypercoagulability.[3] Deep venous thrombosis (DVT) poses the greatest risk for PE; the thrombus develops most commonly in the lower extremities and pelvis.[1] The deep vein thrombus dislodges from the originating vessel, travels through the venous system, enters the lung via the right ventricle, and partially or completely occludes one or more of the pulmonary arteries or its branches or one or more of the pulmonary arteries or its branches.[1] The resulting hemodynamic response is dependent on the size of the embolism, cardiopulmonary reserve, and other neurohumoral effects.[2] It is estimated that 10% of emboli will cause pulmonary infarction.[1]

Immediate emergency department referral or physician consultation is indicated for all patients with suspected PE. A through, timely evaluation is warranted; the patient's condition may deteriorate rapidly, and long-term consequences may develop.

CLINICAL PRESENTATION

The clinical presentation is nonspecific and varies greatly, making the diagnosis of PE difficult. A key piece of the clinical picture is the patient's history. Those with a recent history of surgery, trauma, long bone fracture, travel, period of immobility, malignancy, stroke, paralysis, heart failure, smoking, central venous instrumentation, pregnancy or postpartum status, estrogen therapy, or a history of previous PE are at risk for PE.[2] The clinical assessment, inclusive of history, is not diagnostic but instead should prompt the provider to include PE in the differential diagnosis.

The classic presentation includes dyspnea, tachypnea, pleuritic chest pain, and calf or thigh pain and swelling.[3] Studies suggest that tachypnea is the most sensitive clinical sign.[2] Other symptoms include hemoptysis, orthopnea, tachycardia, jugular venous distention, and abnormal lung sounds.[3] Complaints of calf or thigh leg pain and swelling are not indicative of PE, but suggestive of DVT. Atypical presentations may include complaints of nonspecific malaise, weakness, dizziness, syncope, and extremity discomfort.[2]

PHYSICAL EXAMINATION

The physical findings vary greatly and reflect the nature of the PE.[2] The occult PE may be fatal because it is not routinely suspected or diagnosed; however, it may be benign because healthy lung tissue can filter out small emboli. An embolus of any size can produce cardiopulmonary signs depending on the effected area, including acute respiratory distress, tachycardia, hypotension, abnormal heart sounds, jugular vein distention, hypoxemia, tachypnea, cyanosis, and abnormal lung sounds.[1,5] A thorough, accurate physical examination is important because abnormal physical examination findings are subsequently used as part of clinical prediction tools.[1]

DIAGNOSTICS

An appropriate diagnostic workup varies and is patient and symptom specific. The combination of patient presentation, history, and physical examination findings should be used to guide diagnostic testing. A PE clinical prediction model can also be used to determine the risk of PE and suggest diagnostic tests. The Wells score, revised Geneva score, and pulmonary embolism rule-out criteria (PERC) score are three clinical decision rules that have been validated and can be used to determine the need for imaging.[3]

Laboratory tests are nonspecific to PE and are used primarily to detect the cardiopulmonary effects of PE as well as to exclude other differential diagnoses.[1,2,5] Arterial blood gases (ABGs) are used to evaluate oxygenation and the need for supplemental oxygenation or advanced ventilation.[3] Elevated troponin and brain natriuretic peptide (BNP) levels result in microinfarction and myocardial stretch. They are predictive of PE complications and mortality.[6] D-dimer is the product of the degradation of cross-linked fibrin.[7] This is an important measurement in the patient whose PE is caused by a thrombus, wherein the concentration increases in the presence of acute DVT.[5] Serum D-dimer assays have good negative predictive value and sensitivity but have poor positive predictive value and specificity, making them a useful tool for excluding but not confirming the diagnosis of PE.[8] D-dimer is not useful in the postoperative, trauma, hospitalized, or critically ill patient because of the coagulation and fibrolysis that occur as a result of the disease process.[4]

The electrocardiogram (ECG) is an integral part of PE evaluation. A ECG cannot diagnose PE but may demonstrate myocardial infarction, atrial fibrillation, and right ventricular dysfunction.[3] It is important to remember the ECG is neither sensitive nor specific and does not identify the cause of the ECG abnormality.

Abnormalities seen on the chest x-ray film may include pleural effusion, diaphragmatic elevation, Hampton hump, Westermark sign, or atelectasis but are not specific to PE.[2,3] The most widely used imaging modality for PE diagnosis has been the ventilation/perfusion ($\dot{V}/\dot{Q}$) scan.[5,6] A $\dot{V}/\dot{Q}$ scan measures both the ability of air to enter the lungs and the perfusion to the lungs. A defect in perfusion coupled with abnormal ventilation can suggest a low, intermediate, or high probability of PE. CT angiography has largely replaced the $\dot{V}/\dot{Q}$ scan and is the gold standard for PE diagnosis because of its rapid result and ability to directly visualize PE.[4] CT angiography is more invasive, expensive, and contraindicated in clinical scenarios in which contrast cannot be used.[3] Spiral chest computed tomography (CT) with intravenous (IV) contrast is commonly used because of its availability and noninvasive nature. Owing to the high levels of radiation and contrast that may be involved in PE imaging, clinical decision tools were designed to provide providers with a diagnostic strategy and mitigate patient exposure and risk.

DIAGNOSTICS

Pulmonary Embolism

INITIAL
Pulse oximetry
ECG

LABORATORY
ABGs*
Troponin
BNP*
D-dimer

IMAGING
Chest x-ray examination, posteroanterior and lateral views
$\dot{V}/\dot{Q}$ scan
Spiral CT scan of the chest with IV contrast
CT angiography

*If indicated.

DIAGNOSIS

Diagnosis is made based on the likelihood of PE combined with the presence of an alteration in ventilation. Patients can be categorized as low risk, intermediate or moderate risk, or high risk.[2] Risk factors can be classified into one of three

DIFFERENTIAL DIAGNOSIS

Pulmonary Embolism

- Lung disease (acute or chronic)
- Pneumothorax
- Myocardial infarction
- Pneumonia
- Acute respiratory distress syndrome
- Pericarditis
- Pleurisy
- Heart failure
- Dissecting aortic aneurysm

categories: venous stasis, endothelial or vessel wall injury, and hypercoagulability—the Virchow triad.[1] The PERC rule and Wells criteria can also be used to assign risk.[2] There is no diagnostic test capable of definitively diagnosing PE. Acute PE should be classified as massive or submassive; the term *massive* refers to a PE that causes hemodynamic instability or shock.[5] The presence of hypotension has a high correlation with acute right ventricular failure and subsequent death.

MANAGEMENT

Initial management is aimed at stabilization and ensuring adequate oxygenation.[3] Supplemental oxygen should be administered if hypoxemia is present. Pulse oximetry should be monitored with a goal of at least 92%. Bilevel positive airway pressure ventilation or intubation with mechanical ventilation is indicated with severe hypoxemia or hemodynamic compromise. Administration of IV fluid is indicated for the initial management of hypotension. IV fluids should be cautiously administered to prevent fluid overload with right-sided heart failure. Norepinephrine, dopamine, and epinephrine can be used when there has been a lack of response to IV fluids or if signs of shock are present.

Anticoagulation is the mainstay of PE management because it stops clot progression and allows endogenous fibrolysis to occur.[2] Unfractionated heparin, low-molecular-weight heparin, fondaparinux, warfarin, and rivaroxaban are anticoagulation treatment options. The American College of Chest Physicians suggests low-molecular-weight heparin as the first-line anticoagulant.[3] The recommended dose is 1 mg/kg given subcutaneously every 12 hours for enoxaparin, 200 U/kg once daily for dalteparin, and 175 U/kg once daily for tinzaparin.[2] Fondaparinux is given subcutaneously as a once-a-day injection at a dose based on weight categories. The advantages of low-molecular-weight heparins include standardized dosage without the need for regular monitoring and subcutaneous administration.[5] Low-molecular-weight heparins are frequently used to bridge the transition to an oral vitamin K antagonist.[2] Unfractionated heparan is administered intravenously at a bolus dose of 80 U/kg followed by an infusion starting at 18 U/kg/hr, titrated based on activated partial thromboplastin time (aPTT).[3] It is the treatment of choice for patients with renal impairment. Warfarin is the most commonly prescribed oral vitamin K antagonist. The dose should be adjusted until the patient has adequate anticoagulation, exhibited by an international normalized ratio (INR) of 2.0 to 3.0 with a goal of 2.5.[2] The duration of oral anticoagulant therapy is dependent on embolism characteristics and patient risk factors.[3] The average length of treatment is 3 months. Long-term treatment—longer than 3 months—is indicated for high-risk patients.

Surgical management may include removal of the embolism (embolectomy) and the insertion of an inferior vena cava (IVC) filter (IVCF). An IVCF prevents future pulmonary emboli in the patient with lower extremity DVT.[4] IVCFs are indicated in patients with recurrent PE, contraindications to anticoagulation, or significant risk for PE recurrence.[6]

Fibrinolytics may rapidly reverse right-sided heart failure and can lower the rate of death and PE recuurence.[6] Guidelines suggest fibrinolytic therapy for patients with massive PE who exhibit hypotension and have a low risk for bleeding.[3] The preferred regimen is 100 mg of recombinant tissue plasminogen activator (tPA) given intravenously over 2 hours.[6]

LIFE SPAN CONSIDERATIONS

Many patients who are diagnosed with acute PE will experience a recurrence.[5] The patient should be monitored for resolution of acute PE and associated complications. Daily use of vascular compression stockings is recommended to improve lower extremity venous blood return and to decrease the risk of deep vein thrombus formation. Indefinite anticoagulation may be indicated for high-risk patients who require lifestyle modifications because of bleeding precautions. Weight loss, smoking cessation, and control of chronic health conditions are suggested to limit the risk of recurrence.[5] In addition, avoiding extended periods of immobility and using prophylactic anticoagulation before surgical procedures should be encouraged.

COMPLICATIONS

Immediate complications resulting from PE include significant cardiopulmonary compromise leading to death. The acute PE usually resolves with few or no residual effects. For some, infarction occurs at the level of injury or the PE does not resolve and chronic thromboembolic pulmonary hypertension or post-thrombotic syndrome may develop.[5] In the case of chronic thromboembolic pulmonary hypertension, the patient will exhibit a mean pulmonary artery pressure that is greater than 25 mm Hg that persists for at least 6 months after the diagnosis of PE. Post-thrombotic syndrome is defined as chronic calf swelling, brownish discoloration of the lateral medial malleolus, and venous ulceration in severe cases.

INDICATIONS FOR REFERRAL OR HOSPITALIZATION

Because of the increased mortality rate, all suspected cases of PE should receive an immediate evaluation.[6] The initial management of PE traditionally takes place in the hospital setting with transition to outpatient management once the patient has been properly anticoagulated. Low-risk patients with adequate support and the ability to participate in care can be managed as outpatients if they are hemodynamically stable. Patients with chronic PE and infarction should be referred to a pulmonologist for long-term monitoring.

PATIENT AND FAMILY EDUCATION

Patients should be educated regarding management of risk factors associated with PE development because of the increased incidence of recurrent PE.[6] Avoidance of smoking and immobility should be discussed. The patient should also inform the provider of his or her history of PE when surgical intervention or venous catheterization is necessary or if the patient is pregnant. Women of childbearing age should not take combined oral contraceptive pills.

Those being treated with anticoagulant therapy should be instructed on bleeding precautions, including the use of a soft-bristled toothbrush, waxed floss, and an electric razor to reduce bleeding risk. Contact sports and other activities that can result in blunt trauma should be avoided. The prescribed anticoagulant should be taken exactly as prescribed, with routine monitoring by the outpatient provider.

CHAPTER 114

PULMONARY HYPERTENSION

Thuy D. Nguyen • Anthony S. Gemignani

DEFINITION AND EPIDEMIOLOGY

Development of pulmonary hypertension (PH) is the common end point for a number of disease processes whereby increased pulmonary vascular resistance results in impaired right-sided heart function. The hemodynamic definition for this condition consists of a mean pulmonary artery pressure (mPAP) greater than or equal to 25 mm Hg at rest or 30 mm Hg with exercise.[1] The World Health Organization (WHO) developed the model for characterizing the disease, dividing it into five distinct groups based on pathophysiology.[2] Proper identification of the specific type of PH is important because management strategies focus on reversal of the respective underlying pathology.

According to the modified WHO criteria from the 4th World Symposium on Pulmonary Hypertension, group 1 disease (also called pulmonary arterial hypertension [PAH]) is primarily caused by remodeling of the small arteries within the pulmonary circulation. Causes may be idiopathic, familial, or associated with a number of conditions that increase vascular resistance. These conditions include congenital heart disease, connective tissue disorders, portal hypertension, human immunodeficiency virus (HIV) infection, drugs and toxins, schistosomiasis, and chronic hemolytic anemia.[2] PAH is generally considered a diagnosis of exclusion, made only after PH groups 2 through 5 have been ruled out. The definition of PAH includes mPAP greater than or equal to 25 mm Hg, as well as pulmonary capillary wedge pressure (PCWP) less than 15 mm Hg and/or pulmonary vascular resistance greater than 3 Wood units.[3]

Group 2 represents PH associated with increased left-sided heart pressure. This can be caused by systolic heart failure, diastolic heart failure, or valvular heart disease (such as severe mitral or aortic stenosis). Patients with group 2 disease have an elevated PCWP and a modest transpulmonary gradient (usually less than 10 mm Hg difference between mPAP and PCWP).[1]

Group 3 is associated with chronic lung disease, with sleep apnea the most common cause of this type of PH. The presence of hypoxia is thought to play a key role in its development, although other mechanisms also appear to play a part.

Group 4 (also called chronic thromboembolic pulmonary hypertension [CTEPH]) is caused by multiple pulmonary emboli. This results in increased obstruction to arterial blood flow leading to elevated pulmonary arterial (PA) pressures.

Group 5 represents PH resulting from a heterogeneous collection of systemic disease processes including hematologic, inflammatory, and metabolic disorders. This final group also encompasses rare processes such as tumor obstruction, fibrosing mediastinitis, and chronic renal failure on dialysis.[2]

The overall prevalence of PH in the world and the United States is not known.[4] More data are available for group 1 specifically. A multicenter registry has estimated that the prevalence of group 1 disease in the United States is 10.6 cases per million adults, with an incidence of 2.0 cases per million adults per year. This type shows a female-to-male predominance of 3.9, with a mean age at time of diagnosis of 50 years. The median interval from symptom onset to diagnosis is 1.1 years.[5] The prognosis of PAH is poor, with an estimated median survival of 2.8 years and 1-, 3-, and 5-year survival rates of 68%, 48%, and 34%, respectively.[3] Prognosis is influenced by the severity of the underlying disease. Risk factors for poor prognosis include advanced functional class (New York Heart Association [NYHA] class III or IV), poor exercise capacity, high right arterial pressure, significant right ventricular dysfunction, evidence of right ventricular failure, and the presence of underlying connective tissue diseases (e.g., systemic sclerosis).[2,3,6] The median survival is 6 years for patients with functional class I and II symptoms, compared with 2.5 years for patients with functional class III symptoms and just 6 months for patients with functional class IV symptoms.[3]

PATHOPHYSIOLOGY

PH develops from restricted blood flow through the PA circulation as a result of increased resistance to flow through the pulmonary vascular tree, ultimately resulting in right-sided heart failure. This condition may be present at rest but is exacerbated with exercise. During exercise, cardiac output increases threefold to fivefold, and the increased flow in the pulmonary vasculature results in an associated rise in PA pressure. In healthy individuals, the pulmonary arteries are relatively compliant and accommodate the increased flow through distention of the vessels with relatively little increase in arterial pressures. In the disease states associated with PH, a number of different pathologic processes result in the common end point of increased resistance to flow through the pulmonary circulation.[7] In PAH (group 1 PH) the primary pathologic feature is vascular remodeling at the level of the small arteries, resulting in smaller-caliber vessels with increased stiffness. Several factors play a role in this process, including genetic predisposition, endothelial dysfunction, and abnormal vasomotor control.[2]

The pathologic state in group 2 PH is related to increased pulmonary venous pressure associated with elevated left-sided heart pressures. This results in impaired blood flow through the lungs and elevation in PA pressures. As for group 3 PH, which is associated with lung disease, increased pulmonary vascular resistance is most commonly caused by hypoxia-mediated vasoconstriction. However, thickening of the vascular media (vascular remodeling) and polycythemia also play a role.[8] Group 4 PH is a condition in which multiple, usually small, pulmonary emboli progressively obstruct the PA circulation,[9] resulting in increased pulmonary because of unknown or multifactorial mechanisms (Box 114-1).

Although increased pulmonary vascular resistance is the primary driver of PH, it is important to know that a number of other pathologic states can contribute to increased pulmonary pressures. These include increased blood viscosity, increased baseline pulmonary blood flow (i.e., left-to-right intracardiac shunting), and more rare conditions such as extrinsic compression of the pulmonary vasculature by chest masses. Although an increase in PA pressures is the distinctive characteristic of PAH, it is the ability of the right ventricle to cope with the progressive increase in PA pressures (rather than the pressure itself) that determines functional capacity and survival.[10]

CLINICAL PRESENTATION

Patients with PH are generally asymptomatic until the condition becomes severe. Sixty percent of patients initially have dyspnea. Other associated symptoms include fatigue, angina, syncope, cough, edema, and decreased exercise tolerance.

BOX 114-1

Updated Clinical Classification of Pulmonary Hypertension

1. Pulmonary arterial hypertension (PAH)
    1.1. Idiopathic PAH
    1.2. Heritable
        1.2.1 *BMPR2*
        1.2.2 ALK1, endoglin (with or without hereditary hemorrhagic telangiectasia)
        1.2.3 Unknown
    1.3. Drug- and toxin-induced
    1.4. Associated with
        1.4.1 Connective tissue diseases
        1.4.2 HIV infection
        1.4.3 Portal hypertension
        1.4.4 Congenital heart diseases
        1.4.5 Schistosomiasis
        1.4.6 Chronic hemolytic anemia
    1.5. Persistent pulmonary hypertension of the newborn
2. Pulmonary veno-occlusive disease (PVOD) and/or pulmonary capillary hemangiomatosis (PCH)
3. Pulmonary hypertension caused by left heart disease
    3.1. Systolic dysfunction
    3.2. Diastolic dysfunction
    3.3. Valvular disease
4. Pulmonary hypertension caused by lung diseases and/or hypoxia
    4.1. Chronic obstructive pulmonary disease
    4.2. Interstitial lung disease
    4.3. Other pulmonary diseases with mixed restrictive and obstructive pattern
    4.4. Sleep-disordered breathing
    4.5. Alveolar hypoventilation disorders
    4.6. Chronic exposure to high altitude
    4.7. Developmental abnormalities
5. Chronic thromboembolic pulmonary hypertension (CTEPH)
6. Pulmonary hypertension with unclear multifactorial mechanisms
    6.1. Hematologic disorders: myeloproliferative disorders, splenectomy
    6.2. Systemic disorders: sarcoidosis, pulmonary Langerhans cell histiocytosis, lymphangioleiomyomatosis, neurofibromatosis, vasculitis
    6.3. Metabolic disorders: glycogen storage disease, Gaucher disease, thyroid disorders
    6.4. Others: tumoral obstruction, fibrosing mediastinitis, chronic renal failure on dialysis

ALK1, activin receptor-like kinase type 1; BMPR2, bone morphogenetic protein receptor type 2; HIV, human immunodeficiency virus.

Modified from Simonneau G, Robbins IM, Beghetti M, et al. Updated clinical classification of pulmonary hypertension, *J Am Coll Cardiol* 54:S43, 2009.

Symptoms are insidious, and the average time from the onset of symptoms to diagnosis is more than a year.[6] It is important to take a careful history when PH is suspected, because clues to the underlying cause of the disease may be elicited through careful questioning. The corollary is also true. In diagnosing a condition commonly associated with PH (e.g., obstructive sleep apnea, mitral stenosis, or an autoimmune disease), it is important to assess the patient for signs of PH because early diagnosis may result in more effective treatment.

PHYSICAL EXAMINATION

Physical findings of PH may initially be subtle. Findings suggestive of PH include a loud second heart sound (specifically resulting from an enhanced pulmonic component), murmurs of tricuspid and/or pulmonic regurgitation, evidence of right ventricular dilation (lifts or heaves, loud S_3 on inspiration, or "right-sided" S_3), and decreased carotid pulse. As right ventricular dysfunction develops, patients may manifest jugular vein distention, increased liver size, ascites, and edema (all signs of volume overload associated with advanced disease). In general, lung fields are clear to auscultation. Patients with PH can also experience tachyarrhythmia, most commonly atrial flutter.[2,3,9]

DIAGNOSTICS

When PH is suspected, the initial workup should include electrocardiogram (ECG), chest radiography, and pulmonary function tests (PFTs), because these studies may identify other causes for a patient's dyspnea. In patients with PH, the ECG may show evidence of right-sided heart strain (e.g., S wave in lead I, Q wave in lead III, and an inverted T wave in lead III). Chronic right ventricular pressure overload may result in right-axis deviation and an R wave–to–S wave ratio of more than 1 in lead V_1.[6] Chest x-ray examination often reveals prominent pulmonary arteries and cardiomegaly, and PFTs may show evidence of a reduction in gas transfer.[11] Normal ECG, chest x-ray studies, and PFT results do not exclude the diagnosis of PH.

Imaging modalities to evaluate for PH include echocardiography or cardiac magnetic resonance imaging (cMRI). Echocardiography using Doppler techniques can be a useful screening tool for the presence of PH because it is capable of providing an estimate of pulmonary artery systolic pressure. In addition, other findings such as the presence of septal flattening, right ventricular hypertrophy, and right-sided chamber dilation may provide additional clues to disease severity. A recent meta-analysis of Doppler echocardiography for the assessment of PH found a sensitivity and specificity of 88% and 56%, respectively.[12] This modality, although generally useful, is subject to technical limitations. Additional studies, such as right-sided heart catheterization (RHC), may be indicated if other findings suggest more severe PH than is estimated by Doppler.

cMRI is becoming an increasingly popular tool when an accurate assessment of right ventricular size and function is necessary. The study provides information about stroke volume, cardiac output, PA distensibility and stiffness, and alterations in right ventricular morphology.[13-15] In addition, cMRI may be useful in serial assessments to follow therapeutic response in PH because of its high accuracy and low interobserver variability.[16]

Additional workup may include arterial blood gases (ABGs) to demonstrate hypoxia and respiratory alkalosis, chest computed tomography (CT) or ventilation/perfusion ($\dot{V}/\dot{Q}$) scan to exclude pulmonary embolism, serologic studies to screen for connective tissue diseases, and brain natriuretic peptide (BNP) for patients with known PAH to aid in monitoring progress.[17] In rare cases, a lung biopsy may be necessary to exclude interstitial lung disease.[3,6]

Although the aforementioned studies may help evaluate for PH, RHC is the standard for hemodynamic assessment and definitive diagnosis of PH. The purpose of RHC is to assess for elevated left-sided pressures and pulmonary venous hypertension (via assessment of wedge pressure), determine severity and prognosis (via evaluation of mPAP, right atrial pressure, and cardiac index), evaluate for pulmonary vasoreactivity, and tailor therapeutic interventions.[16]

DIAGNOSTICS

Pulmonary Hypertension

IMAGING	OTHER DIAGNOSTICS
Chest x-ray examination	Cardiac catheterization
Doppler studies	PFTs
Echocardiography	ABGs
CT scan or magnetic resonance imaging*	BNP*
$\dot{V}/\dot{Q}$ scan*	Biopsy*

*If indicated.

DIFFERENTIAL DIAGNOSIS

Although definitive diagnosis of PH is made by measurement of PA pressure, elucidating the cause can be quite challenging because of the myriad diseases that lead to PH. The differential diagnosis of the underlying causes resulting in PH includes lung disease (restrictive, obstructive, and granulomatous), chronic liver disease, heart disease (congenital, valvular, and myocardial), PA stenosis, pulmonary venous hypertension, thromboembolic disease, connective tissue disease (especially systemic sclerosis), sarcoidosis, and sickle cell disease. Other causes to consider include parasitic infection and intravenous drug use. Although it is rare in the United States, schistosomiasis is the leading cause of PH worldwide.[18]

MANAGEMENT

The ultimate treatment goals for patients with PH are slowing disease progression and improving survival. Surrogate markers for this include reduction of PA pressures with normalization of cardiac output, improvement in symptoms (most commonly dyspnea), and enhancement of functional capacity (as measured by exercise endurance, usually a 6-minute walk test). Management is directed by the causative factor; therefore, thorough diagnostic workup is of the utmost importance. Treatment of group 1 PH is primarily accomplished with vasodilators (calcium channel blockers, prostanoids, endothelin receptor antagonists, or phosphodiesterase inhibitors). Although less than 10% of patients demonstrate pulmonary vasoreactivity (reduction in mPAP greater than or equal to 10 mm Hg to an absolute mPAP less than 35 to 40 mm Hg with either no change or an increase in cardiac output after the administration of short-acting vasodilators), this subset of patients has been shown to derive significant long-term benefit from calcium channel blockers.[3] Calcium channel blockers have been shown to reduce mPAP and pulmonary vascular resistance as well as improve quality of life and survival in those who exhibit pulmonary vasoreactivity. Treatment doses of calcium channel blockers for PAH are higher than those used for treatment of systemic hypertension.[16] (See Table 114-1.)

Prostacyclin synthase is reduced in patients with PAH, resulting in inadequate production of prostacyclin I_2, a vasodilator with antiproliferative effects.[3] Prostanoids induce vasodilation and prevent platelet aggregation and inflammation through activation of cyclic adenosine monophosphate. The three U.S. Food and Drug Administration (FDA)–approved prostanoids are epoprostenol, treprostinil, and iloprost. Epoprostenol, administered by continuous intravenous infusion, is the first-line treatment for functional class IV patients and also serves as a rescue therapy for patients in whom other drugs have failed. Epoprostenol improves functional class, exercise tolerance, hemodynamics, and survival of patients with idiopathic PAH. However, drawbacks to epoprostenol include its short half-life of approximately 6 minutes, instability at room temperature, and risk of infection with intravenous administration. Treprostinil (available for intravenous infusion or subcutaneous injection) has a longer half-life, minimizing the risk of cardiovascular collapse with inadvertent infusion cessation. Newer inhaled prostanoids (e.g., iloprost) were developed with the thought that intrapulmonary selectivity would decrease right-to-left shunt blood flow and minimize systemic side effects. However, because of the short half-life of iloprost, it requires inhalation six to nine times daily.[16]

Patients with PAH are found to have increased levels of circulating plasma endothelin-1, a potent vasoconstrictor that promotes pulmonary artery smooth muscle cell proliferation.[16] Bosentan and ambrisentan are endothelin receptor antagonists that combat vasoconstriction and improve exercise capacity. Bosentan is associated with reversible hepatotoxicity in 5% to 10% of patients; therefore serial monitoring of a patient's hepatic function is necessary.[19] Ambrisentan is often prescribed to those who cannot tolerate bosentan, given its lower risk of hepatotoxicity.

Naturally occurring nitric oxide works to increase pulmonary vascular relaxation and reduce cellular proliferation through cyclic guanosine monophosphate. Phosphodiesterase type 5 degrades nitric oxide. Two phosphodiesterase inhibitors, sildenafil and tadalafil, have been shown to improve functional capacity and reduce mPAP by inhibiting degradation of nitric oxide.[11,16]

A number of adjuvant therapies for PAH also exist. Diuretics can be used for symptomatic relief in those with tricuspid regurgitation, right ventricular volume overload with systemic venous congestion, and increased right ventricular wall stress.[16] Digoxin has been shown in animal studies to offer some benefit in preserving right ventricular contractility, reducing circulating norepinephrine levels, and increasing resting cardiac output.[20] Anticoagulation is recommended to counteract thrombin deposition that occurs in the pulmonary circulation.[17,18]

Group 2 PH may be treated with medicine or surgery to correct the underlying heart disease. Treatment strategies for group 3 PH may include curtailing nicotine addition (if present) and using supplemental oxygen, continuous positive airway pressure (to treat obstructive sleep apnea), and vasodilators. Group 4 PH is primarily caused by emboli, and treatment can include elimination of acute clots (e.g., with tissue plasminogen activator) and long-term prevention of future emboli with anticoagulation therapy. Treatment of group 5 PH is aimed at treatment of the causative disease in addition to therapy for PH, including vasodilator therapy.[21,22]

General treatment recommendations include regular physical activity, maintenance of ideal body weight, prevention of infection, avoidance of pregnancy, maintenance of adequate hemoglobin, oral anticoagulation, oxygenation, digoxin, diuretic with avoidance of orthostasis, and psychological assistance. Graded balloon dilation atrial septostomy may be indicated for patients with idiopathic PAH that is unresponsive to vasodilator therapies.[23]

TABLE 114-1 Therapies for Pulmonary Arterial Hypertension

Medications	Year FDA Approved	Indications	Dose	Side Effects
CALCIUM CHANNEL BLOCKERS				
Amlodipine	1995	Responsive to vasodilator testing	2.5-20 mg PO daily	Peripheral edema, pulmonary edema, palpitations, flushing, fatigue, dizziness
Diltiazem	1995	Responsive to vasodilator testing	60-240 mg PO daily to tid	Edema, headache, AV block, bradycardia, hypotension, vasodilation, dizziness
Nifedipine	1995	Responsive to vasodilator testing	30-240 mg PO bid	Flushing, peripheral edema, dizziness, headache, nausea, heartburn
PROSTANOIDS				
Epoprostenol	1995	NYHA III-IV	2-40 ng/kg/min IV	Tachycardia, flushing, hypotension, dizziness, headache, anxiety, nausea, vomiting
Treprostinil	2002 (subcutaneous) 2004 (intravenous) 2009 (inhalation)	NYHA II-IV	0.625-40 ng/kg/min IV or SC 18-54 μg inhaled qid	Flushing, headache, rash, diarrhea, nausea
Iloprost	2004	NYHA III-IV	2.5-5 μg inhaled at maximum 9 doses/day	Flushing, hypotension, headache, nausea, flulike syndrome, cough, jaw pain
ENDOTHELIN RECEPTOR ANTAGONISTS				
Bosentan	2001	NYHA II-IV	62.5-125 mg PO bid	Edema, headache, hepatotoxicity, inhibition of spermatogenesis, respiratory tract infection
Ambrisentan	2007	NYHA II-IV	5-10 mg PO daily	Peripheral edema, headache, flushing, palpitations, decrease in hemoglobin, nasal congestion
PHOSPHODIESTERASE INHIBITORS				
Sildenafil	2005	NYHA II-IV	2.5 mg or 10 mg IV daily 5 mg or 20 mg PO tid (taken 4-6 hr apart)	Flushing, headache, dyspepsia, visual disturbances, epistaxis
Tadalafil	2009	NYHA II-IV	40 mg PO daily	Flushing, headache, dyspepsia, myalgia, respiratory tract infection

AV, atrioventricular; FDA, U.S. Food and Drug Administration.

The American College of Cardiology Foundation and the American Heart Association, in collaboration with the American College of Chest Physicians, the American Thoracic Society, and the Pulmonary Hypertension Association developed consensus guidelines for the diagnosis and management of PH. The guidelines, with updated information and services, can be obtained online at journal.publications.chestnet.org/article.aspx?articleid=1881654.

COMPLICATIONS

Complications of PH include the development of right ventricular hypertrophy, dilation, and eventual failure with associated symptoms of volume overload. Cardiac arrhythmias, both atrial and ventricular in origin, are also possible. PH is a common manifestation of cor pulmonale, which is defined as right ventricular enlargement caused by pulmonary or cardiac disease.[17] Other complications include acute pulmonary embolism, pulmonary hemorrhage, and pneumonia. In addition to physical symptoms associated with PH, other factors, such as anxiety, depression, adverse effects of therapy, functional limitations, and social isolation, may lead to impaired quality of life.[10] Hospitalization may be necessary for medication adjustment, monitoring, and imaging. The most common cause of death in patients with clinically severe PH is usually right ventricular failure.[18]

INDICATIONS FOR REFERRAL OR HOSPITALIZATION

Because accurate diagnosis is crucial, referral to an appropriate specialist is recommended. Imaging, cardiac catheterization, pulmonary function testing, medication recommendations, and lung transplantation all require specialist referral. Both cardiologists and pulmonologists have expertise in the workup and management of PH.

PATIENT AND FAMILY EDUCATION

Patients with PH often require a tremendous amount of support from health care providers. Careful explanation of the disease process and the need for moderation during activity is important because exercise may increase pulmonary vascular resistance and hypoxia. The side effects and adverse reactions of all medications should be carefully explained and understood by both patients and families. The importance of a low-salt diet and the avoidance of over-the-counter medications (unless approved by the health care provider) should be stressed.[18,24]

For patients with end-stage PH, lung transplantation (or heart-lung transplantation if heart damage is extensive) may be an option, although the waiting list for organ transplants is often long. Transplantation criteria include the patient's age, medical history, and overall condition at the time of transplantation. The risk management and complications of transplantation should be thoroughly explained.

Familial PH accounts for 6% to 10% of patients with PAH.[3] Most cases occur in individuals with no known family history.[22,24] Families need education and support if a genetic workup is chosen.

HEALTH PROMOTION

Group 1 PH is a relatively rare disease process, and the exact mechanisms of the disease are still being investigated. Overall prognosis has been poor, and patients had little hope for remission of this progressive disease until recently. Because PH occurs in association with other disorders, such as chronic obstructive pulmonary disease, sleep apnea, sickle cell crisis, connective tissue diseases, cardiac diseases, and thromboembolism, these disease processes must be monitored for the onset of complications. Lung diseases are the most common causes of PH; therefore raising awareness of lung disease prevention is crucial.[23] One of the most important preventive measures for elimination of lung disease is smoking cessation.

CHAPTER 115

SARCOIDOSIS

Joanne Sandberg-Cook

DEFINITION AND EPIDEMIOLOGY

Sarcoidosis is a multisystem, inflammatory, granulomatous disease of unknown origin that commonly affects young and middle-aged adults. It involves the lungs and intrathoracic lymph nodes in more than 90% of affected patients, but it may essentially affect any organ (Table 115-1). More than 80% of patients are 20 to 45 years of age; the disease is rare in children and older adults. The incidence may vary with geographic location. In Europe, the United Kingdom, Japan, and North America, incidence rates of 5 to 40 per 100,000 population have been cited. The incidence of sarcoidosis in the United States is higher in African Americans than in whites, with greater morbidity reported. Reports of sarcoidosis appear to be rare in Africa, India, and Central and South America, probably because of the absence of mass screening programs and the presence of more common granulomatous diseases such as tuberculosis.[1] No clear genetic basis has been established for sarcoidosis, but genetic factors may modulate its evolution and expression. Sarcoidosis is commonly seen in families; the likelihood for development of the disease ranges from 26% to 73% in individuals with an affected first-degree relative.[2]

Physician consultation is indicated for all suspected cases of sarcoidosis.

TABLE 115-1 **Clinical Features of Sarcoidosis**

Organ System	Symptoms or Presentation
Pulmonary	Dyspnea, cough, wheezing, chest pain
Upper airway	Dyspnea, nasal congestion, hoarseness, stridor, polyps
Dermatologic	Nodules, papules, plaques
Ocular	Photophobia, tearing, pain, decreased visual acuity, lacrimal gland enlargement, uveitis, glaucoma, blindness
Rheumatologic	Polyarthropathy, monoarthropathy, myopathy
Neurologic	Headache, hearing loss, paresthesias, seizures, cranial nerve palsy
Cardiologic	Syncope, dyspnea, arrhythmias, congestive heart failure, cardiac tamponade
Gastrointestinal	Dysphagia, abdominal pain, jaundice, hepatomegaly
Hematologic	Lymph node enlargement, hypersplenism
Renal	Kidney failure, calculi

PATHOPHYSIOLOGY

The characteristic pathologic feature of sarcoidosis is the noncaseating granuloma. The collection of macrophages and T cells that compose the granuloma releases various chemokines and cytokines, including tumor necrosis factor-α.[2]

The granuloma is likely to be preceded by an alveolitis that involves the interstitium more than the alveolar spaces. Although the initial antigen is unknown, the alveolitis begins an accumulation of helper T lymphocyte (CD4) cells and macrophages. It is believed that activated macrophages may be responsible for the eventual development of fibrosis in some patients with sarcoidosis.

In the lung, granulomatous inflammation and fibrosis result in ventilation/perfusion imbalance and widening of the alveolar-arterial oxygen gradient. In the early stages, Pao_2 may be within the normal range at rest but decreases with exertion.

CLINICAL PRESENTATION AND PHYSICAL EXAMINATION

Sarcoidosis may affect almost any organ system; however, 90% of affected individuals have pulmonary involvement.[3] Sarcoidosis can occur in acute, subacute, or chronic form and is initially discovered asymptomatically with an abnormal chest radiograph in approximately 50% of patients.[2] Patients who are symptomatic with this disorder often have nonspecific pulmonary symptoms—dry cough, dyspnea, chest pain, fever, fatigue, anorexia, weight loss, and, occasionally, chills and night sweats. The nonspecificity of these symptoms can delay diagnosis.[1] The symptoms and related organ involvement consistent with sarcoidosis are listed in Table 115-1. Involvement of the upper airways and posterior pharynx may result in upper airway obstruction with worsening symptoms of dyspnea. Hoarseness and nasal obstruction may occur as a result of vocal cord and nasal mucosa granulomas (polyps). Hemoptysis is rarely seen; when present, it suggests mycetoma.[4]

It is unusual for adventitious lung sounds to be detected on auscultation. Wheezing is occasionally audible in patients with advanced disease. Digital clubbing is rare. Dyspnea, dry cough, and chest pain occur commonly. Chest pain can be severe and difficult to distinguish from cardiac chest pain.[3]

Rheumatologic symptoms occur in 4% to 38% of patients with sarcoidosis.[5] These can manifest as an acute arthritis commonly involving the ankle, chronic polyarthritis, or myopathy.

Ocular lesions are seen in 20% of patients; anterior uveitis is seen most commonly. Symptoms may include redness, photophobia, and decreased visual acuity.[1] Other ocular lesions seen include posterior uveitis, retinal vasculitis, keratoconjunctivitis, and conjunctival follicles.[2]

Skin lesions are seen in 20% to 30% of patients. A maculopapular rash over the face and hairline is the most common subacute lesion.[3] Erythema nodosum is seen more commonly in women; when it occurs in combination with hilar adenopathy, polyarthralgias, and fever, it is referred to as Löfgren syndrome.[3]

Clinical involvement of the central nervous system is unusual, but cranial nerve involvement can be seen. Asymptomatic granulomas can occur in any part of the female reproductive system, including the breast.

DIAGNOSTICS

Chest radiographs are abnormal in more than 90% of patients. In general, one of the following patterns is demonstrated: (1) bilateral hilar lymphadenopathy (BHL; 50% to 80% of cases); (2) parenchymal interstitial infiltrates (25% to 50%), with a predilection for upper and mid lung field distribution; or (3) both lymphadenopathy and interstitial disease. BHL is often the lesion that suggests the diagnosis of sarcoidosis.

Unless lymphadenopathy is present, the appearance of the chest radiograph may be indistinguishable from that of other interstitial lung disorders. Typically, radiographic lesions are bilateral and are distributed relatively symmetrically; asymmetric involvement is occasionally seen.

Staging systems based on the appearance of the chest radiograph have been in widespread use since 1957. The consensus now favors the following classification[2]:

Stage 0: Normal chest radiograph
Stage 1: BHL
Stage 2: BHL with pulmonary infiltrates
Stage 3: Pulmonary infiltrates without BHL
Stage 4: Pulmonary fibrosis

Computed tomography (CT) and high-resolution computed tomography (HRCT) of the chest are superior to conventional chest radiography in defining the extent of parenchymal abnormalities in sarcoidosis. HRCT can help differentiate between reversible (mostly inflammatory) changes and irreversible (presumably fibrotic) alterations.

Hypergammaglobulinemia is seen in 30% to 80% of cases of sarcoidosis. Rheumatoid factor can be positive. The serum level of angiotensin-converting enzyme (ACE) is elevated in approximately 60% to 75% of patients with sarcoidosis; this level may be useful in following the course of the disease. Anemia occurs in 4% to 20% of patients.[4] Leukopenia, eosinophilia, and thrombocytopenia can be seen, although not commonly. The erythrocyte sedimentation rate (ESR) is often elevated, but this can be a nonspecific finding. Hypercalcemia and hypercalciuria occasionally occur secondary to increased gastrointestinal absorption, abnormal vitamin D metabolism, and increased calcitriol production by sarcoid granulomas. Skin testing often reveals cutaneous anergy.

Pulmonary function test (PFT) results may be normal or may reveal a restrictive pattern. This may be of most value in monitoring the course of the disease in individual cases. Radionuclide scanning reveals high uptake of gallium 67 (^{67}Ga) in pulmonary lesions of sarcoidosis. However, ^{67}Ga is also taken up by the lungs in patients with a large number of other diseases; therefore a high level of ^{67}Ga is not specific for sarcoidosis, and determination of the level is not recommended as part of the routine evaluation.[2]

It is often reassuring to have a tissue diagnosis, and there are many techniques for this. The most specific location for biopsy is the lung. Bronchoscopy with transbronchial biopsy specimens is positive in 50% to 60% of patients who do not have radiographic evidence of parenchymal disease. This positivity increases to 85% to 90% when there are radiographic abnormalities. Bronchoalveolar lavage performed at the time of fiberoptic bronchoscopy retrieves inflammatory and immune effector cells from the lower respiratory tract that can also be diagnostic. Open lung biopsy through mediastinoscopy may yield tissue diagnosis when bronchoscopy has failed.[6] Biopsy specimens can also be taken from other organ systems suspected to have sarcoid involvement (conjunctivae, skin, lymph nodes).

DIAGNOSTICS

Sarcoidosis

LABORATORY
- CBC and differential
- Electrolytes
- Glucose
- BUN
- Creatinine
- Calcium
- Phosphorus
- LFTs
- ESR
- Serum level of gamma globulin
- Serum level of ACE

IMAGING
- Chest radiography
- CT scan

OTHER DIAGNOSTICS
- PFTs
- Bronchoscopy
- Purified protein derivative

BUN, blood urea nitrogen; CBC, complete blood count; LFTs, liver function tests; PFTs, pulmonary function tests.

DIFFERENTIAL DIAGNOSIS

Many conditions can be seen with dyspnea, diffuse pulmonary infiltration, and granulomas. Hypersensitivity pneumonitis, asbestosis, silicosis, drug effects, bacterial or fungal infections, and

DIFFERENTIAL DIAGNOSIS

Sarcoidosis

- Hypersensitivity pneumonitis
- Asbestosis
- Silicosis
- Infection, including tuberculosis, histoplasmosis, atypical mycobacterial infections, actinomycosis
- Malignant disease: lymphoma
- Drug effects
- Vasculitis: Wegener granulomatosis

malignant neoplasms should all be considered. It is most important to differentiate sarcoidosis from tuberculosis, another granulomatous disease with public health implications. Tuberculin skin testing should be included as part of the evaluation.

MANAGEMENT

The indications for treatment are not standardized, and there is no U.S. Food and Drug Administration–approved therapeutic agent. Response to therapy is variable, and a large number of patients undergo a natural remission or follow a benign course.[2] No treatment is recommended for asymptomatic patients with stage 1 or stage 2 disease. Patients with fever, erythema nodosum, or joint pains often respond to nonsteroidal anti-inflammatory drugs (NSAIDs). Low-dose prednisone (Deltasone), 15 to 20 mg/day, may occasionally be needed to control symptoms that do not respond to NSAIDs. If there are symptoms of dyspnea or if a cough develops, airway obstruction may be present and corticosteroid therapy is advisable. Oral corticosteroids are used cautiously with great respect for potential toxicity. In some cases, inhaled corticosteroids may be effective.[2]

Patients with stage 2 disease who are symptomatic are treated with corticosteroids. Only observation is suggested for patients who are asymptomatic and have only mild impairment of lung function; treatment is needed for individuals who have progressive impairment of lung function. Patients with stage 3 or stage 4 sarcoidosis almost always require treatment with corticosteroids or another type of immunosuppressive treatment, but this is often unsatisfying. Sarcoidosis is very sensitive to corticosteroids. Typical regimens consist of a single daily dose of 20 to 40 mg of prednisone, which is gradually tapered during 6 months.[7] Some patients require a maintenance dosage of prednisone of approximately 10 to 15 mg/day, whereas others remain off prednisone indefinitely or for extended periods.

Alternatives to steroids are used for patients who develop severe side effects, do not respond to prednisone, or prefer not to take oral corticosteroids. Disease progression despite adequate corticosteroid therapy for longer than 1 year is also an indication for treatment with these agents.[7,8] Methotrexate (Trexall), cyclophosphamide (Cytoxan), and azathioprine (Imuran) have been used most extensively both as treatment and as steroid-sparing agents. All have shown modest efficacy in reducing symptoms. Thalidomide (Thalomid) and chloroquine (Aralen) have also been used with modest effect.[8] The use of these agents is clearly valuable for selected patients, but there are no controlled studies of indications for use or efficacy. These agents, along with antimalarial agents such as chloroquine and hydroxychloroquine (Plaquenil), are also often used as the initial drug of choice in the treatment of chronic skin lesions from sarcoidosis. Studies have been conducted using infliximab (Remicade), a tumor necrosis factor inhibitor, for patients who did not improve after first- or second-line therapies. In one study, 90% of patients treated with infliximab (N = 10) reported symptomatic improvement.[8] More and larger studies are required before these drugs can be recommended as part of the routine therapy for sarcoidosis.

LIFE SPAN CONSIDERATIONS

Sarcoidosis does not affect pregnancy but may flare after delivery. Sarcoidosis in children younger than 15 years showed the same organ distribution as in adults. The prognosis for children seems better than that for adults.[3] Patients older than 70 years are more likely to be seen with systemic symptoms[2] and have a higher likelihood of adverse reactions to treatment, particularly corticosteroids.

BOX 115-1

Complications of Sarcoidosis

Lung scarring. Untreated pulmonary sarcoidosis can lead to irreversible interstitial scarring (fibrosis) and pulmonary hypertension.

Skin involvement. Skin involvement is common with hyperpigmented papules and erythema nodosum.

Eye disease. Inflammation can affect almost any part of the eye and usually causes watering, redness, and pain. In a few cases, sarcoidosis can lead to blindness or serious eye diseases, such as cataracts and glaucoma.

Nervous system problems. Cranial neuropathies are the most common manifestations. A small percentage of people with sarcoidosis develop problems related to the central nervous system when granulomas form in the brain and spinal cord. Inflammation in the facial nerves can cause facial paralysis.

Fertility problems. In men, sarcoidosis can affect the testes and possibly cause infertility. Severe sarcoidosis may make it difficult for some women to become pregnant, but many women with the disease give birth to healthy children.

Heart and liver problems. Arrhythmias or cardiomyopathy can be seen in the most severe cases. Granulomas that form in the liver can affect its ability to function.

Muscle and joint problems. Muscle and joint problems, including acute and chronic arthritis and myopathy, can occur.

Data from Mayo Clinic: *Sarcoidosis: complications.* Available at www.mayoclinic.com/health/sarcoidosis/DS00251/DSECTION=complications. Accessed May 31, 2015.

COMPLICATIONS

Many complications of sarcoidosis (Box 115-1), including osteoporosis, hypertension, hyperglycemia, and gastric ulcers, occur as a result of corticosteroid therapy. Relapses are common and are determined by the reappearance of clinical signs and symptoms, chest radiograph abnormalities, and an elevated ACE level. In this situation, a return to a previously high maintenance dose is sufficient to control recurrence.

Patients with sarcoidosis have demonstrated high levels of depression and stress as measured by health-related quality-of-life (HRQOL) assessments. This is likely because young people in the prime of their professional lives are most commonly affected by the disease or side effects of the medications. In one study, those taking corticosteroids had lower HRQOL scores, reflecting worse HRQOL, compared with unmatched historical controls not treated with corticosteroids.[9] Possible reasons for the association between corticosteroid use and poorer HRQOL include increased disease severity, medication side effects, and concomitant mental health issues, such as depression and stress. This relationship needs to be further investigated.

In a few cases, sarcoidosis can be fatal. Death is usually a result of progressive scarring of the lungs and respiratory failure or the result of an arrhythmia, which may lead to sudden death.[10]

INDICATIONS FOR REFERRAL OR HOSPITALIZATION

Sarcoidosis is a serious multisystem disease that requires physician consultation. Lung biopsies are usually necessary for diagnosis and require referral to a pulmonary specialist. If other biopsies are indicated, the appropriate specialist should be consulted. Therapy during the acute and chronic phases should be directed by the physician or specialist to ensure proper treatment. Hospitalization may be necessary for patients with severe dyspnea and hypoxia or severe cardiac dysfunction.

PATIENT AND FAMILY EDUCATION

The nature of the disease, including its varied presentation, must be carefully explained to patients. Medications, if indicated, and their side effects need to be discussed. It is important that patients understand the risk for worsening lung impairment or other organ damage if compliance with therapy is poor. It is important that patients be familiar with the clinical signs suggestive of recurrence of sarcoidosis.

REFERENCES

For a full list of references, scan the QR code or visit http://booksite.elsevier.com/9780323355018

PART 11

Evaluation and Management of Cardiovascular Disorders

CHAPTER 116

CARDIAC DIAGNOSTIC TESTING: NONINVASIVE ASSESSMENT OF CORONARY ARTERY DISEASE

Susan Sanner

Since the advent of coronary artery disease (CAD) as a diagnosis, numerous ways for the proper assessment of this illness noninvasively have flourished. Although each test has its advantages, each also has limitations (Table 116-1). The optimum assessment of CAD is a thorough history and physical examination that includes prior medical history of myocardial infarction or CAD and the patient's present complaint (e.g., angina, radiating pain, tingling, or numbness) in conjunction with ascertaining the family history of CAD. In addition, immediate electrocardiographic (ECG) and laboratory biomarker testing should be considered to ensure a proper diagnosis and an adequate interventional plan.[1] (Cardiac catheterization is indicated if ECG findings and biomarkers indicate an acute myocardial infarction.) This chapter addresses the evaluation of suspected CAD in the absence of acute infarction.

Once all the results of the initial laboratory and ECG testing are reviewed, a pretest probability of disease can be generated and additional tests can be ordered.[2] The probability of CAD can be calculated by considering the chosen noninvasive test's sensitivity and specificity.[2] Selection of the proper cardiac test (see Table 116-1) for an individual depends on the person's risk stratification, age, and tolerable level of activity. The most common and least invasive test for diagnosis of CAD is the stress test, also called the exercise tolerance test (ETT) or treadmill exercise.

PATHOPHYSIOLOGY OF CORONARY ARTERY DISEASE

CAD exists when coronary arteries are narrowed by atherosclerotic plaque formation, plaque rupture, or spasm. This narrowing impedes coronary blood flow, resulting in hypoperfusion of the myocardium. The hypoperfusion produces first diastolic, and then systolic dysfunction, with characteristic signs and symptoms, including chest pain. Typical ECG changes of ischemia result, although the ST-segment and T-wave changes that are central to demonstration of ischemia occur relatively late in the ischemic cascade.

Role of Inflammation and Atherogenesis

Inflammation has been implicated as one of the major processes that mediate the acceleration and progression of CAD and its complications. Inflammatory pathways have been very closely linked with the early development of atherosclerotic disease with plaque formation in coronary arteries, producing CAD. Inflammation and plaque composition both have an impact on the occurrence of acute plaque rupture, a cause of acute myocardial infarction.

Relation to Cardiac Stress Testing

Unlike most other circulatory beds in the body, the coronary circulation allows maximum oxygen extraction from the blood when the body is at rest. In a stress test or ETT, patients are asked to perform incremental exercises that result in positive chronotropic (rate) and inotropic (strength of contraction) stimulation of the cardiovascular system, which in turn increases myocardial oxygen demand. Increases in oxygen demand obligate an increase in myocardial blood flow. The healthy coronary circulation can increase flow approximately five times above the baseline level. The fundamental pathophysiologic change in CAD is a limitation of the ability of the coronary arterial circulation to vasodilate appropriately. As a result, the ability to increase coronary blood flow in the face of increased myocardial oxygen demand is limited, leading to an imbalance between oxygen supply and demand and resulting in myocardial ischemia.

OVERVIEW OF CARDIAC DIAGNOSTIC TESTING

Noninvasive Tests and Biomarkers for Coronary Artery Disease

There is accumulating evidence that supports the use of noninvasive markers for the diagnosis of subclinical CAD. C-reactive protein, interleukin-6, and monocyte-macrophage colony-stimulating factor are markers that have shown promising results with their predictive value for future adverse cardiovascular events. A growing number of research studies have consistently suggested that either injury or insult to the vascular endothelium is a precursor for the process of atherogenesis to begin.[3] These investigations have led to tests such as carotid intima-media thickness, augmentation index, flow-mediated dilation of the brachial artery, and pulse wave velocity; however, which of these noninvasive markers have a role in risk stratification for primary and secondary CAD prevention is under investigation.

Recent American College of Cardiology (ACC) guidelines give some guidance about noninvasive testing and markers for asymptomatic CAD based on an individual patient's risk for CAD. ACC guidelines have as a Class 1 recommendation (suggested) based on Level B evidence (limited populations studied)

TABLE 116-1 **Exercise Testing Comparisons**

Test	Benefits and Indications	Limitations
Treadmill exercise	Assesses ischemia, functional capacity, prognosis Equipment widely available Accuracy established in different populations	Lower sensitivity than other tests listed Poor specificity with women, resting ECG ST-T abnormalities, LVH does not indicate site or extent of infarct
Exercise myocardial perfusion imaging	Reproducible results Improved sensitivity and specificity higher diagnostic accuracy	Increases costs over treadmill testing Requires longer than treadmill exercise alone Modest radiation exposure Artifacts from soft tissue (breast) or in obese patients attenuate signal, decrease specificity
Cardiac magnetic resonance imaging (MRI)	High resolution of cardiac structure, function, and morphology No radiation exposure Stress perfusion MRI an option Can be used with most cardiac stents	Use in claustrophobic patients can be difficult because of patient ability to stay in MRI machine contraindicated in patients with implantable ferromagnetic objects (debrillators)
Exercise radionuclide angiography	Well validated to identify patients with severe disease Risk stratification after MI Good images with obese patients or those with COPD Accurate information about ejection fractions	Limited availability and high expense Uses bicycle, not treadmill exercise Inaccurate when heart rate is irregular Reduced specificity with women, abnormal resting left ventricular function
Exercise echocardiography	Shorter test time, lower cost than nuclear imaging Assesses multiple parameters: global and regional ventricular function, chamber size, wall thickness, valve function Used with resting ECG abnormalities, LBBB Detects reversible ischemia (wall motion abnormalities develop with stress)	Images limited with obesity or obstructive lung disease Does not detect non–blood flow limiting blockages Reduced accuracy with resting wall motion abnormalities (prior MI, paced rhythm, certain types of cardiac surgeries)
Pharmacologic stress with dipyridamole or adenosine	Accurate assessments in patients unable to complete exercise protocol Useful assessment in patients with claudication or musculoskeletal limitations Side effects rapidly reversible by ending infusion or administering aminophylline	Cannot assess functional capacity Contraindicated with hypotension, sick sinus syndrome, high-grade heart block, hyperreactive airways, caffeine or theophylline dependence, oral dipyridamole therapy Chest pain during test not indicative of CAD
Dobutamine echocardiography	Improves CAD assessments in patients unable to exercise Side effects rapidly reversible by terminating infusion or administering a beta blocker) Perfusion defects represent true myocardial ischemia	Cannot assess functional capacity Contraindicated with recent MI (<1 week), unstable angina, high-grade heart block, BBB, severe aortic stenosis, hypertrophic obstructive cardiomyopathy, supraventricular dysrhythmias, ventricular tachycardia (history or current), uncontrolled hypertension, large aneurysm, severe pulmonary hypertension, beta blocker dependence

BBB, bundle branch block; COPD, chronic obstructive pulmonary disease; ECG, electrocardiographic; LBBB, left bundle branch block; LVH, left ventricular hypertrophy; MI, myocardial infarction.

Data from McCaffery JT, Geraci SA: Cardiac stress testing in women, *J Nurse Pract* 5(10):760-766, 2009; Merz NB, Bonow RO, Sopko G, et al: AHA/NHLBI conference proceedings: women's ischemic syndrome evaluation: current status and future research directions: report of the National Heart, Lung, and Blood Institute workshop, October 2-4, 2002: executive summary, *Circulation* 109: 805-807, 2004; American Heart Association (AHA): *AHA summary: cardiac stress testing: selecting the right stress test,* 2010. Available at www.cardiacscience.com/blog/2010/12/cardiac-stress-testing-selecting-the-right-stress-test. Accessed September 17, 2015.

that health care providers ascertain risk for cardiovascular disease in asymptomatic individuals by use of a global assessment such as the Framingham score.[4] The ACC guidelines use the level of risk determined by these scores to evaluate the evidence and to classify recommendations for the use of various testing modalities in the investigation and determination of subclinical cardiovascular disease. For example, the ACC guidelines suggest that C-reactive protein can be used in asymptomatic men older than 50 years and women older than 60 years with low-density lipoprotein cholesterol below 160 mg/dL to determine if statin therapy is indicated and in asymptomatic intermediate-risk men older than 50 years and women older than 60 years to assess risk of cardiovascular disease.[4] Ankle-brachial index assessment is acceptable for intermediate-risk individuals to determine their risk for subclinical cardiovascular disease.[4]

Recent evidence suggests that the Coronary Artery Calcium Score (CACS) may be beneficial for identifying CAD and is most likely to be useful in approaches for improving risk assessment in individuals who are at intermediate risk, although its role is not completely clear. The CACS is directly related to the plaque burden where zero constitutes a normal CACS; less than 10 is a low score and greater than 400 is a high score.[5,6] Even with a designated score, evidence does not support targeted treatment of patients with high-risk CACS to improve outcomes.[7] According to the American College of Cardiology Foundation (AACF)/American Heart Association (AHA) 2013 guidelines for assessment of cardiovascular risk, CACS may also be beneficial in asymptomatic adults with cardiovascular disease. Its primary advantage is that no patient preparation is required. However, owing to the issue of cost for a CACS determination, the exposure to radiation, and the unclear role of calcium scoring in low- to intermediate-risk patients with acute coronary syndrome, the ACC/AHA guidelines recommend CACS for individuals for whom, after having undergone a quantitative risk assessment, the treatment decision is unclear. CACS, in this case, may be able to help inform treatment.[8]

Overall, adequate risk assessment is the most challenging for individuals who are considered at low or intermediate risk for a cardiac event. Therefore the usefulness of inflammatory markers to predict a future cardiac event remains unclear and warrants further research.[9,10]

Exercise Tolerance Test

The standard first-line approach to initial testing for CAD is the ETT, during which the patient (attached to a 12-lead electrocardiogram) is continuously monitored during graded exercise. Multiple protocols are available for the ETT. The bicycle and treadmill are the two most often used. The primary goal of the ETT is to increase workload incrementally to induce ischemia or until a predetermined workload is reached. Multiple studies are available that have validated the efficacy and safety of ETT in patients with low risk of chest pain. Studies have also reported on the safety and efficacy of immediate exercise testing in low-risk patients who have normal ECG findings and biomarker levels and are not serially evaluated before stress testing.[11] The ETT also provides data on the patient's functional capacity, which has been shown to be a significant predictor of future cardiac events.[11] In an ETT, patients are asked to perform incremental exercises based on standardized protocols. These result in positive chronotropic (rate) and inotropic (strength of contraction) response of the cardiovascular system, increasing myocardial oxygen demand. The normal hemodynamic response to these stimuli is an increase in absolute coronary blood flow. However, this ability is reduced in the presence of CAD, which leads to an imbalance between oxygen supply and demand, resulting in myocardial ischemia and ischemic changes in the electrocardiogram.

The ECG response of normal hearts is maintenance of an "isoelectric" ST segment during exercise and recovery. By standard criteria, a positive test result for CAD is defined by the development of horizontal or downsloping ST-segment depression of 1 mm measured 80 msec after the J point of the QRS complex (the junction between the QRS complex and the ST segment). ECG changes such as upsloping ST segment (elevation) or isolated T-wave downsloping (depression) have not demonstrated significant predictive value.

Because the interpretation of the test is based primarily on the development of characteristic ischemic ST-segment and T-wave changes, it is not surprising that resting ECG abnormalities can lead to a reduction in test sensitivity and specificity. The specificity of the routine ETT is reduced if the patient has had a prior myocardial infarction or if the patient has a resting bundle branch block conduction abnormality, paced rhythm, preexcitation syndromes, or inability to exercise because this produces persistent ST-segment and T-wave abnormalities.[12]

A number of other factors can interfere with the sensitivity of the exercise test in detecting CAD. Because an increase in coronary blood flow is related to an increasing heart rate and systolic blood pressure, clearly the sensitivity of the test is effort dependent. The standard is the peak heart rate achieved during exercise. Specifically, a test result is considered negative for CAD only if the patient exercises to at least 85% of the age-predicted maximum heart rate without evidence of inducible ischemia (maximum heart rate = [220 − age]). If the patient fails to achieve this "target" heart rate, the test should be considered nondiagnostic or insufficient to exclude ischemia. On the other hand, if there is evidence of ischemia (typical angina, ischemic ST changes) before the patient's target heart rate is reached, the test is considered strongly predictive of significant CAD. A second important predictor of more advanced CAD is exercise-induced hypotension (i.e., a fall in systolic blood pressure of at least 20 mm Hg at any point during exercise). It is helpful to correlate the ischemic leads on exercise electrocardiography to the underlying coronary anatomy to roughly identify the culprit artery or arteries.

Medications such as beta blockers, digoxin, certain calcium channel blockers, and other antihypertensives can attenuate the heart rate, making the rest of the exercise test less diagnostic.[13] The decision to discontinue beta blockers 1 or 2 days before testing is influenced by the purpose of the exercise test. For ETTs ordered to detect angina, it is recommended that the cardiologist be consulted about withholding the medication before the test is performed. ETTs performed to assess effectiveness of pharmacologic therapy require normal daily medication regimens. Imaging studies such as nuclear cardiac scanning may be useful in patients who undergo a stress test during beta blocker therapy.[2]

Another potential contributor to the ETT's lack of sensitivity is derived from the limitations of the surface electrocardiogram related to the spatial distribution of the electrical abnormalities that occur in ischemia. This concept may be better understood if the electrocardiogram is considered an imaging tool that examines the electric forces of cardiac depolarization and repolarization. To detect ischemia, the repolarization phase of the cardiac cycle—the ST segment and T wave—is examined for abnormalities. ST-segment and T-wave changes in the surface electrocardiogram are related to both the extent and the severity of myocardial ischemia. As might be expected, the ETT is more sensitive for the detection of severe disease. Ischemia that is confined to the posterior or lateral segments of the left ventricle can be more difficult to detect.

When considering ETT, health care providers should be aware of its relative contraindications. For these patients, consultation with a cardiologist is recommended. Some pertinent contraindications to ETT include acute myocardial infarction, supraventricular ectopy, sustained ventricular arrhythmias, high-grade heart block, Wellens syndrome (highly correlated with CAD), hemodynamically significant aortic stenosis, severe hypertension, acute venous thromboembolic disease (deep venous thrombosis, pulmonary embolism), pericarditis, myocarditis, endocarditis, symptomatic congestive heart failure, and serious coexisting illness (such as diabetic ketoacidosis, pneumonia, or renal disease).[13]

Imaging Adjuncts to the Exercise Tolerance Test

In the evaluation of patients with stable chest pain syndromes and normal surface ECG recordings, the conventional ETT

BOX 116-1

Indications for Coupling of Nuclear or Ultrasound Imaging to Standard Exercise Tolerance Test

- Left ventricular hypertrophy with ST-segment and T-wave abnormalities on resting electrocardiography
- Baseline ST-segment and T-wave abnormalities on resting electrocardiography for any reason
- Recent myocardial infarction, particularly with persistent rest ST-segment abnormalities
- Clinical use of digoxin
- Wolff-Parkinson-White syndrome
- Bundle branch block
- Ventricular pacemaker

typically provides adequate clinical information for diagnostic purposes. Similarly, in patients with known CAD and stable coronary syndromes, the ETT is typically adequate as a means of observing disease progression for purposes of prognostication and timing of revascularization procedures. However, with respect to the delineation of damaged myocardial regions and residual myocardial viability in zones of prior injury, it has become clear that adjunctive radiopharmaceutical or cardiac ultrasound imaging substantially improves test sensitivity and specificity (Box 116-1).

The various imaging modalities that can be used as adjuncts to the graded exercise test can be viewed in the context of the ischemic cascade. Myocardial perfusion imaging (MPI) is designed to detect the spatial distribution of myocardial blood flow (i.e., to define the regional heterogeneity of flow that characterizes regional ischemia). Cardiac ultrasound imaging (two-dimensional echocardiography [2DE]) is designed to detect the abnormalities in regional wall motion that develop as a consequence of regional myocardial ischemia.

Examining the limitations of routine exercise testing from a historical perspective yields interesting information. The limitations detailed previously were clinically acceptable when the exercise study was performed principally as a binary diagnostic test (to determine whether CAD was present or absent) in patients with chest pain. The limited sensitivity of this test in a subgroup of patients with minimum CAD did not produce significant consequences. However, even for patients with minimum CAD, the ETT did not yield significant answers about CAD status, primarily because these patients have a cardiovascular event rate of only 1% to 2% per year.

With the advent of effective coronary revascularization surgery, the ETT has assumed additional predictive clinical relevance. It is clear that powerful predictors of outcomes reside in clinical data and in ETT results independent of the ST-segment response, such as the hemodynamic response and the aerobic work capacity as reflected by exercise duration.

In contrast, the more recent expansion of interventional therapies for coronary revascularization has resulted in an important shift in the data that practitioners seek from provocative testing. For example, in patients with stable coronary syndromes, the judicious application of percutaneous coronary intervention requires that both the presence and territorial distribution of ischemia be defined. Furthermore, in patients who have sustained prior myocardial injury, decisions about revascularization require a definition of ischemia both within and remote from the site of injury as well as tissue viability within the zone of infarction.

The usefulness of these adjunctive imaging modalities depends in part on the prevalence of disease in the population of patients being studied. In general, these adjunctive modalities are most useful in populations with an intermediate pretest clinical probability of disease.[14]

Myocardial Perfusion Imaging. MPI offers a method of visualizing blood flow to the heart by injection of a radioactive cardiac-specific tracer. This improves the diagnostic accuracy of a stress test because it gives another method of detecting perfusion defects aside from measuring ST depression on the electrocardiogram. MPI also offers the additional advantage of estimating left ventricular function. The technique is also used independently of a stress test in the evaluation of patients with acute active chest pain.[13]

At present, thallium chloride Tl-201 and technetium Tc 99m sestamibi are the radiopharmaceutical agents used for the detection of CAD in MPI. They appear comparable for CAD detection in patients with stable coronary syndromes. A number of sources have documented the clinical efficacy of sestamibi and thallium.

Thallium 201 was the first agent used in clinical practice. It is a cation that acts similarly to potassium and is taken into viable cardiac myocytes. It distributes in cardiac tissue roughly in proportion to regional blood flow. It has a half-life of 73 hours. Clinically, it is injected while the patient is at peak exercising or shortly after the pharmacologic stress test agent is administered. Images are taken immediately and then again in 3 to 4 hours. On the initial image, the defects may represent either regional ischemia or nonviable myocardium.[13]

The second agent that is commonly used is ^{99m}Tc sestamibi. It acts as a calcium analogue when it is taken up by the myocytes. It has a shorter half-life of about 6 hours. Once it is taken up by the myocytes, its distribution is quite different from that of thallium, and it is well suited to the imaging of patients with acute coronary syndromes. When a sestamibi scan is performed, a second injection is given at the time of the delayed image. Interpretation of the scan is very similar to that of thallium imaging.[13]

Unlike thallium-based perfusion imaging, sestamibi image acquisition can be performed up to several hours after tracer injection. This allows appropriate treatment and triage of patients with acute myocardial infarction and unstable angina; the image acquired after such treatment will represent the status of myocardial perfusion at the time of tracer injection. Tracer injection can be repeated at a later time to assess myocardial salvage—residual viability in infarct patients—or to define the presence, extent, and territorial distribution of ischemia in patients with unstable angina. Sestamibi imaging provides the capacity to "simultaneously" define left ventricular systolic function and myocardial perfusion. This offers a means to assess the impact of reperfusion therapies in patients with acute coronary syndromes.

Researchers have found that sestamibi imaging in the emergency department may be useful in identifying low- versus high-risk patients with suspected myocardial ischemia.[15] Furthermore, although MPI with ^{201}Tl is typically coupled with exercise or pharmacologic stress, rest-redistribution imaging may provide valuable information in patients with unstable coronary syndromes who are not suitable candidates for stress studies.

Because the diagnosis of perfusion defects requires the detection of decreased flow in one region relative to another, there will be occasional instances of false-negative scans in patients with severe three-vessel or left main CAD. These "balanced" flow disturbances (i.e., a decrease in coronary flow in more than two geographic territories) should be suspected in patients in whom clinical suspicion of severe CAD is high but whose MPI reveals uniform tracer uptake.

Because MPI increases diagnostic accuracy of stress testing, the ACC/AHA guidelines recommend its use in several patient subsets. It should be used if there is any baseline ECG abnormality that would interfere with measurement of stress-induced ST-segment changes, such as left ventricular hypertrophy, bundle branch blocks, and digoxin use. MPI is also a useful tool for use with high-risk diabetic patients.[11]

Exercise Echocardiography. The practice of exercise echocardiography has expanded dramatically in recent years. Current data suggest that adjunctive echocardiographic imaging enhances the sensitivity and specificity of CAD detection to an extent comparable to that provided by nuclear techniques.[1] The 2DE evidence for ischemia includes an abnormal left ventricular ejection fraction (LVEF) response to exercise or the development of regional wall motion abnormalities. The exercise is performed with a bicycle or treadmill, and dobutamine is the most common pharmacologic agent used simultaneously with the echocardiography imaging. The image quality may be enhanced by the injection of echogenic microbubbles.

As previously demonstrated in thallium imaging, the sensitivity of the 2DE technique for CAD detection is enhanced in patient subsets with multivessel CAD or prior myocardial infarction. In addition, the sensitivity of exercise echocardiography is decreased in patients with resting wall motion abnormalities. In practical terms, patients in whom adequate ultrasound imaging views cannot be obtained (often including obese patients and those with severe emphysematous lung disease or tachycardia) should be considered for alternative imaging modalities.

A positive exercise echocardiogram is defined by stress-induced decrease in regional wall motion, decreased wall thickening, or regional compensatory hyperkinesis. Some of the advantages of this test are that it is faster to perform than a nuclear stress test because the delayed images are obtained much sooner, there is no associated radiation exposure, it is less costly, and it can be more readily performed in an office setting. A limitation of the test is that it is dependent on the operator's experience. Test results can also be altered by obesity, lung disease, and tachycardia.

Comparison of Myocardial Perfusion Imaging with Two-Dimensional Echocardiography. Exercise 2DE with Doppler flow study is comparable to MPI for the detection of CAD. There is a greater accumulation of literature for MPI with respect to prognostication in patients with CAD. In addition, it appears that MPI may be preferable to 2DE for the recognition of incremental ischemia in myocardial regions characterized by abnormalities of resting wall motion. Furthermore, quantification of myocardial perfusion data has been more extensively validated than comparable quantification of cardiac ultrasound data; cardiac ultrasound imaging has been limited by the technical difficulties in the endocardial border recognition. The majority of studies with exercise 2DE have been limited to qualitative visual assessment. It is also clear that the early 2DE data were acquired in patient groups with a relatively high incidence of significant CAD. Finally, MPI (e.g., rest-redistribution ^{201}Tl scintigraphy and rest-injected ^{99m}Tc- sestamibi) is more amenable to the detection of ischemia in patients with unstable coronary syndromes, in whom exercise is contraindicated. Serial rest 2DE images acquired in patients with unstable coronary syndromes may occasionally be useful if new or more extensive wall motion abnormalities can be detected during recurrent ischemia.

In contrast, 2DE offers access to the incremental information about left ventricular contractile performance that is analogous to that provided by exercise radionuclide ventriculography. LVEF response to exercise provides important prognostic information in patients with CAD; such information is available only inferentially by myocardial perfusion scintigraphy (i.e., pulmonary thallium uptake). Finally, with respect to viability assessment, the detection of preserved contractile function in myocardial segments supplied by diseased coronary arteries is essential.

Three-Dimensional and Doppler Flow Echocardiography. Three-dimensional (3D) echocardiographic techniques are currently available that use magnetic resonance imaging (MRI) and computer-assisted 3D acquisition systems for 2DE. Three-dimensional technology has recently become available and provides a unique view of structure and function within the heart. Current evidence-based guideline evaluations, however, center on 2DE with Doppler flow study.[2] Doppler flow studies are used to localize and to quantify obstructions in the cardiovascular system. Primarily, the addition of a Doppler flow study to echocardiography enhances the ability to evaluate prosthetic valve function, to detect and to evaluate the blood shunting from a septal defect, and to gauge the severity of valvular stenosis or regurgitation.[2]

Cardiac Magnetic Resonance Imaging and Ultrafast Computed Tomography Cardiac Scans. Historically, it has been difficult to image the moving structures of the heart, and MRI has served as a less than reliable diagnostic tool. However, technology is rapidly advancing so that the MRI techniques can present precise and detailed reflections of cardiac blood flow and tissue viability to assist with diagnosis of CAD or the degree of damage from a heart attack. MRI has also been found to be useful in evaluating patients with a dissecting aortic aneurysm before surgery to determine the precise location and extent of dissection. Cardiac MRI is, with further technologic refinement, anticipated to provide accurate data to distinguish between stable and unstable plaque and to assist with quantifying CAD, replacing the diagnostic cardiac catheterization.[12]

Current investigations of 3D technology also involve ultrafast electron beam computed tomography (EBCT). This emerging 3D technology performs a heart scan at a rapid rate, thus "freezing" cardiac motion. Coronary artery calcification is analyzed, and a total calcium score for a patient's coronary arteries is calculated on the basis of the areas of calcification and the maximum CT calcium density. Calcium generally does not appear in normal coronary arteries, so calcium deposits are determined to be a strong marker of atherosclerosis. However, EBCT does not define the location and extent of cardiac disease, and it does not image soft noncalcified plaque. A negative calcium score does not imply the absence of plaque. With significant CAD (50% stenosis), only 2.5% of coronary segments have no detectable calcium on EBCT.[2] However, coronary calcium scoring has recently been proved to be accurate in predicting cardiovascular disease risk in apparently healthy middle-aged men in several studies.[8] EBCT scanning has also been found to be beneficial in motivating patients to adopt lifestyle changes and to implement aggressive cardiovascular risk reduction strategies. Recent ACC guidelines suggest calcium scoring for intermediate-risk individuals (class IIa, benefit outweighs cost); in individuals at low to intermediate risk, calcium scoring is considered class IIb (beneficial only in selected patients).[4]

Pharmacologic Stress Testing

The clinical usefulness of adjunctive imaging modalities has been expanded by coupling such techniques to "pharmacologic" stress, an important advantage in patients who are unable to perform conventional treadmill or ergometer exercises. Pharmacologic agents currently in use are coronary vasodilators (e.g., dipyridamole [Persantine] and adenosine) and inotropic-chronotropic drugs (e.g., dobutamine).

The vasodilator drugs are applied to assess the effective coronary flow reserve (i.e., the ratio of maximum flow to basal flow). Because the extraction of tracer is proportional to blood flow, the coupling of vasodilators with MPI allows the detection of regional flow disturbances. These regional perfusion abnormalities can be characterized as reversible (normal uptake at baseline, with decreased uptake after vasodilator) or fixed (indicative of prior infarction). The fact that vasodilators do not induce ischemia but simply unmask regional variations in flow reserve means that the ECG portion of the test will rarely demonstrate ischemic changes. However, on rare occasions, ECG changes may be observed, and up to 20% of patients may experience angina. Ischemia may be caused by "coronary steal." The effects of dipyridamole can be reversed by intravenous administration of aminophylline, and the effects of adenosine and dobutamine can be reversed by discontinuation of the infusion.

Another approach is to induce cardiac ischemia by use of a beta agonist such as dobutamine, which is administered in gradually increased doses until the goal heart rate is achieved (the provocation of ischemic chest pain or ST-segment changes may also lead to termination of the test). Dobutamine increases cardiac work, initially by an inotropic effect; a normal cardiac response to dobutamine is an increase in global left ventricular contractility. The chronotropic effects of this agent become apparent at higher infusion rates (20 to 50 mg/kg/min). Most commonly, inducible ischemia occurs at these higher infusion rates. Dobutamine is useful in patients who cannot tolerate the bronchoconstriction associated with adenosine administration.

As previously described, the development of regional wall motion abnormalities is often an early manifestation of ischemia. For this reason, dobutamine is most commonly coupled with 2DE (which is performed after each increase in dose) to determine regional abnormalities in left ventricular function or decreases in LVEF. The onset of new regional hypokinesis in a previously normally contracting segment is highly predictive of CAD in the artery supplying the dysfunctional segment. Alternatively, MPI can be coupled with dobutamine in patients with poor echocardiographic windows. The accuracies of dobutamine echocardiography and dobutamine MPI are comparable.

In a study by Sawada and colleagues,[16] dobutamine echocardiography was shown to have comparable usefulness in patients with baseline normal wall motion (89% sensitivity and 85% specificity); however, the sensitivity was somewhat lower in patients with abnormal resting wall motion (81% sensitivity and 86% specificity). In another study, adenosine had similar sensitivity (86%) to dipyridamole when coupled with nuclear imaging but lower specificity (specificity 71% and accuracy 80%).[17] The poor performance of adenosine echocardiography (sensitivity 58%, specificity 87%, and accuracy 69%) underscores the importance of coupling vasodilators with perfusion imaging rather than with cardiac ultrasound, which requires the induction of ischemia to produce regional contractile dysfunction.

Another study found the sensitivity of dobutamine stress 2DE to be comparable to that of dobutamine single-photon emission CT (85% versus 80%, respectively). The specificity of the two techniques was also comparable (82% versus 74%, respectively), as were the predictive values.[17]

In summary, on the basis of these data, the following conclusions can be drawn:

- Vasodilator stress echocardiography is less sensitive than similar stress tests coupled with perfusion scintigraphy for the detection of CAD.
- Vasodilator stress echocardiography is less sensitive than exercise or dobutamine 2DE for disease detection.
- Vasodilator perfusion scintigraphy compares favorably with exercise-dobutamine scintigraphy or exercise-dobutamine 2DE with respect to CAD detection.

DIAGNOSTIC TESTING FOR CARDIOVASCULAR DISEASE IN WOMEN

Cardiovascular disease is the leading cause of death for women in the United States, but a considerable body of research has demonstrated that women have different patterns of CAD and different responses to cardiac testing than their male counterparts do.[13,14] Although cardiovascular disease is the leading cause of death in women, this disorder often is not diagnosed expeditiously. Unfortunately, studies investigating women and cardiovascular disease are limited. Women are more likely to have nonobstructive or single-vessel disease compared with men, which decreases the diagnostic accuracy of stress testing.[7,18]

Single-photon emission CT imaging is technically limited in women because of breast tissue and smaller coronary artery size.[6,18] Recent evidence, particularly from the Women's Ischemia Syndrome Evaluation study, a multicenter study sponsored by the National Heart, Lung, and Blood Institute, has demonstrated that many women without obstructive CAD continue to have symptoms and a poor quality of life.[19] Many of these women have evidence of stress-induced ischemia, which is likely to be related to endothelial dysfunction of the microvasculature.[18]

As a result, there is limited evidence to suggest the most appropriate cardiovascular diagnostic testing for women. To address this issue, the AHA reviewed existing studies and developed guidelines to aid primary care providers in choosing suitable diagnostic tests for women with suspected cardiovascular disease.[19]

All patients, even if asymptomatic, require risk stratification according to the Framingham risk score (low, intermediate, or high) to identify CAD risk equivalents.[19] At present, the ACC/AHA guidelines do not recommend stress tests for asymptomatic patients, unless the patient (men 45 years or older, women 55 years or older) is sedentary and wishes to begin exercising aggressively.[19] The exception is asymptomatic women with diabetes and peripheral arterial disease. These women are classified as high risk; diabetes and peripheral arterial disease are CAD risk equivalents. The recommendation for asymptomatic women with diabetes, peripheral vascular disease, and possible kidney disease is for secondary prevention strategies to prevent future cardiac events.[19]

For women who are symptomatic but who have a normal resting ECG recording, good exercise tolerance, and no coronary risk factors, an exercise stress test is appropriate; diagnostic imaging is not recommended for low-risk women who are asymptomatic.[19] For women who are symptomatic and have known CAD, an abnormal resting ECG recording, questionable exercise tolerance, or coronary risk factors (e.g., diabetes, peripheral arterial disease), stress test imaging is recommended.[19]

SUMMARY

Cardiologists are generally aware of the test limitations inherent in exercise testing. The use of additional testing to better diagnose CAD noninvasively has evolved in the development of numerous testing modalities that are yielding more sensitive results. Tests that provide diagnostic information of the left ventricle specifically along with status reports of the regional myocardial perfusion gradient have obviously gained widespread use as adjunct modalities to arrive at a more comprehensive cardiac diagnosis with improved treatments and outcomes.

Cardiac ultrasound and MPI are of comparable usefulness in detecting CAD. The data with respect to prognostication are most extensive for MPI techniques, but ultrasound-based data are accumulating.

Both functional studies and perfusion imaging have demonstrated clear usefulness in addressing the complex question of myocardial viability. These testing modalities are used to assess the presence of functional heart muscle in patients with ischemic heart disease and regional contractile dysfunction.

MPI techniques and ultrasound-derived techniques are competitive. It is clear that these modalities may in fact be complementary in the evaluation of selected patients with CAD. The ACC/AHA Task Force on Practice Guidelines suggested that exercise MPI or exercise echocardiography may be used as the initial test for diagnosis in patients with chronic stable angina who are able to tolerate exercise.[20] The ACC/AHA Committee on Clinical Application of Echocardiography recognizes that exercise or pharmacologic stress echocardiography can be used to evaluate the presence or extent of ischemia, even when there is an underlying ECG abnormality that affects interpretation of the ECG recording, such as prior ischemia, left bundle branch block, or Wolff-Parkinson-White syndrome.[2] There is conflicting evidence on whether echocardiographic techniques are preferable when there are no resting ECG abnormalities.[2] For asymptomatic patients at risk for CAD, it is unclear whether exercise testing is beneficial because there have been no clinical trials investigating exercise testing in this population.[21]

In addition, multiple studies have documented gender-related differences associated with cardiovascular disease. In women, cardiovascular disease is less frequently diagnosed, which in turn helps contribute to making it the leading cause of death in women. Women are more likely to have single-vessel or nonobstructive cardiac disease compared with men, which makes it less likely for an accurate diagnosis by use of stress exercise.

CHAPTER 117

ABDOMINAL AORTIC ANEURYSM

Patricia Jordano

DEFINITION AND EPIDEMIOLOGY

An abdominal aortic aneurysm (AAA) is a progressive, permanent, localized dilation of the abdominal aorta with aortic diameter of 3.0 cm or more, or a 50% increase in diameter compared with the adjacent normal segment.[1-3]

The aorta is a conduit that carries blood to the body. The aorta is divided by the diaphragm into the thoracic and abdominal aorta. It is composed of three layers: the tunica intima, tunica media, and tunica adventitia. In adults, the normal diameter of the abdominal aorta varies with age, height, gender, and body habitus, but the average infrarenal aortic diameter in an adult is approximately 2.0 cm and typically less than 3.0 cm. The prevalence of an AAA located in the infrarenal section of the aorta is at least three times greater than a thoracic aortic aneurysm.[4]

Aneurysms are described by their shape, which help identify a true aneurysm. A true aneurysm involves all three layers of the aorta. The more common, fusiform aneurysm is a symmetric weakness of the entire circumference of the aorta that produces a bulge. A saccular aneurysm is an asymmetric weakness or bleb on the side of the aorta; these defects result from trauma or an internal wall defect caused by an ulcer. A pseudoaneurysm, or false aneurysm, is an enlargement of only the outer layer of the blood vessel wall. AAAs are also described by size (a small aneurysm has a diameter <4.0 cm, a medium aneurysm has a diameter of 4.0 to 5.4 cm, a large aneurysm has a diameter ≥5.5 cm, and a very large aneurysm has a diameter ≥6.0 cm), as well as involvement of the renal or visceral vessels.

AAA is an important clinical diagnosis because it is associated with considerable risk of rupture and death as the aneurysm enlarges to a diameter of more than 5.0 cm (1.96 inches).[2,5] In the United States, 15,000 deaths per year are attributed to AAAs, and it is the 10th leading cause of death in men older than 55 years.[6-8] Treatment is usually recommended when an AAA grows to larger than 5.5 cm in diameter. Most patients who have a ruptured AAA will die before reaching the hospital, and of those who make it to the hospital and have surgery, the outcome is dependent on their presenting clinical condition, but typically the mortality rate has been stated as anywhere from 50% to 80%. The high mortality rate has not changed over the past 20 years despite improvement in operative technique and preoperative management.[2,5,8]

Aortic aneurysms are a complex disease with genetic and environmental risk factors. Major risk factors for AAA include advancing age (>65), male gender, family history of an AAA, and cigarette smoking (current or past). Additional risk factors include atherosclerotic vascular disease, hypertension, hyperlipidemia, and other vascular aneurysms (e.g., iliac, femoral, popliteal aneurysms).[2,3,5,9-11] The association between chronic obstructive pulmonary disease (COPD) and AAA remains elusive. The high prevalence of AAA in patients with COPD may be related to medications (oral steroids) and coexisting disease

TABLE 117-1 Risk Factors for Aneurysm Development, Expansion, and Rupture

Symptom	Risk Factors
AAA development	Tobacco use Hypercholesterolemia Hypertension Male gender Family history (male predominance)
AAA expansion	Advanced age Severe cardiac disease Previous stroke Tobacco use Cardiac or renal transplant
AAA rupture	Female gender Low FEV_1 Larger initial AAA diameter Higher mean blood pressure Current tobacco use Cardiac or renal transplant Critical wall stress–wall strength relationship

From Chaikof EL, Brewster DC, Dalman RL, et al: The care of patients with an abdominal aortic aneurysm: the Society for Vascular Surgery practice guidelines, *J Vasc Surg* 50(4 Suppl):S2-S49, 2009.

rather than to a common pathway of pathogenesis involving plasma elastase or α_1-antitrypsin deficiency.[10-12] Those treated with corticosteroids have a more rapid rate of AAA expansion. Individuals younger than age 60 are not as affected by AAA. Males are affected more than females at a 6:1 ratio.[2,5,9-11] Smoking is the greatest environmental risk factor for AAA development. An AAA is over seven times more likely to develop in a smoker than a nonsmoker, with duration of smoking being a key variable.[5] First degree male relatives of patients with AAA have two to four times the normal risk for AAA. Female first-degree relatives appear to have similar risk, but the data are less certain.[2,11] Those with a decreased risk of AAA development include women, non-Caucasians, and diabetics.[1,2,5,9,11] Factors associated with an increased risk of rupture include female gender, large initial aneurysm diameter, low forced expiratory volume in 1 second (FEV_1), current smoking, and elevated blood pressure.[2,5,11] Risk factors for aneurysm development, expansion, and rupture are listed in Table 117-1.

PATHOPHYSIOLOGY

AAA is a disease of the medial wall layer of the aorta. It is characterized by degeneration of the extracellular matrix proteins and the presence of an inflammatory cell infiltrate composed predominantly of T cells. Degradation of the cell wall proteins in the medial layer occurs as a result of complex interactions among genetic factors, inflammatory cytokines, matrix metalloproteinases (MMPs), tissue inhibitors of MMPs, and others. The consequences include dissolution and fragmentation of collagen and elastin, leading to expansion of the vessel wall.[2-5,9] When the aortic wall tension exceeds the tensile strength of the wall collagen and the wall can no longer withstand the repetitive force of systolic contraction, the aneurysm ruptures.

CLINICAL PRESENTATION

Although an AAA may cause symptoms as a result of the pressure on surrounding structures, about 75% are asymptomatic at initial diagnosis.[13,14] Asymptomatic AAAs are generally detected during an incidental radiologic or surgical procedure. Alternatively, in thin patients, a supine abdominal examination may readily show a pulsatile abdominal mass.

Thromboembolic phenomena may herald the presence of an AAA. Microembolic infarcts in the lower extremity of a patient may suggest either abdominal or popliteal aneurysm. Embolization of mural thrombus from an abdominal aneurysm may be seen with acute limb ischemia caused by femoral or popliteal occlusion.[13]

The classic diagnostic triad of ruptured AAA is hypotension, pulsatile abdominal mass, and abdominal pain or back pain. The triad is encountered in less than 50% of patients with a ruptured AAA.[14] Symptoms of AAA may include a sensation of abdominal discomfort, back pain, pulsation of abdomen, or flank pain.[5,14] Less frequently, individuals may complain of pain in the legs, chest, or groin area. They may also report anorexia, nausea, vomiting, or dyspnea. In a patient with a history of aneurysm or pulsatile mass, abdominal pain must be considered to represent a rapidly expanding or ruptured aneurysm and must be treated accordingly.

PHYSICAL EXAMINATION

Palpation of the abdomen for AAA is one of the few physical examination maneuvers that is an evidence-based recommendation in the periodic health examination of older men.[15] For detection of AAA on physical examination, the patient is positioned supine with knees flexed to relax the abdominal wall. The examiner places the palm over the epigastrium to detect a transmitted pulsation. The examiner then places both hands on the abdomen with palms down and an index finger on either side of the pulsating area to measure the aortic width. An aneurysm expands laterally with each systole. An AAA is suspected when the aorta is judged to be at least 3.0 cm (1⅕ inches) in maximum diameter. Auscultation may reveal a bruit over the mass, but abdominal bruits are not specific for AAA formation.

Unfortunately, only 30% to 40% of aneurysms are noted on physical examination, with detection dependent on the skill of the examiner and the size of the aneurysm. The sensitivity of abdominal palpation increases with AAA diameter, from 29% for AAAs of 3.0 to 3.9 cm to 76% for AAAs of more than 5.0 cm. The sensitivity of abdominal palpation also increases (91%) when the abdominal girth is less than 100 cm (40-inch waistline) compared with 53% when abdominal girth is 100 cm or greater. Overall, when the girth is less than 100 cm and the AAA is more than 5.0 cm, abdominal palpation is highly sensitive (100%) for detection of AAA.[14,15] If on examination one finds a pulsatile mass in the groin or popliteal fossa, this raises suspicion for an AAA, because multiple aneurysms often coexist.[5,14]

DIAGNOSTICS

Given the high mortality associated with emergent AAA repair, early detection and repair before rupture are the mainstay of AAA management. The American College of Cardiology (ACC) and American Heart Association (AHA) practice guidelines for management of peripheral arterial disease recommend that "Men 60 years of age or older who are either a sibling or offspring of patients with AAAs should undergo physical examination and ultrasound screening for detection aortic aneurysms." And "men who are 65-75 years of age who have ever smoked should undergo a physical examination and a 1-time ultrasound screening for detection of AAAs."[11] The U.S. Preventive Services Task Force (USPSTF) recommendation statement recommends "1-time screening for AAA with ultrasonography in men aged 65-75 years who have ever smoked."[16] The USPSTF recommends that clinicians selectively offer screening for AAA in men aged 65 to 75 who have never smoked rather than routinely screening all men in this group. The Screening Abdominal Aortic Aneurysms Very Efficiently (SAAAVE) Act was approved by the United States Congress in January 2007. The SAAAVE Act permits a single screening aortic ultrasound examination as part of the "Welcome to Medicare" package for patients with defined risk factors for AAA. Males aged 65 to 75 years who have smoked more than 100 cigarettes in their lifetime or patients of any age or either sex with a strong family history are eligible for this screening examination.[2,17,18]

Ultrasonography is the imaging study ordered most often for screening and initial confirmation of an aneurysm. It can measure anteroposterior, transverse, and longitudinal dimensions of an AAA. Ultrasonography can provide a reasonably accurate measurement of initial size and can be used for serial follow-up evaluation.[5,14,19] This modality is widely available, is painless, does not expose the patient to ionizing radiation, and is inexpensive. It can also visualize important anatomic markers such as relation of major arterial branches and adjacent organs. Duplex ultrasound can provide additional information on aortic flow.

Computed tomography angiography (CTA), often with three-dimensional imaging, is the preferred and most widely used imaging modality before aortic aneurysm repair. It accurately demonstrates dilation of the aorta and the relationship to major branch vessels, both proximally and distally. It will show the degree of calcification, presence of mural thrombus, inflammatory aneurysms, aneurysmal leakage, penetrating aortic ulcer, length of the aneurysm neck, iliac artery, and whether other organs have become displaced.[14,19] It is noninvasive but does expose the patient to ionizing radiation and contrast medium, which can be harmful, especially in patients with kidney disease.

Standard contrast aortography is infrequently used but may be indicated in select individuals, including those with suspected suprarenal extension, suspected visceral or renal artery disease, iliofemoral occlusive disease, horseshoe kidney, prior aortic or colonic surgery, and unusual aneurysms (e.g., mycotic, aortocaval fistula).[19] The procedure uses ionizing radiation and contrast. Most institutions, however, are using CTA or magnetic resonance imaging (MRI) or magnetic resonance angiography (MRA) for the preoperative evaluation of AAA.

MRI and MRA may also be used to diagnose aortic disease and for preoperative planning. MRI and MRA have limitations, including inability to be used for patients with pacemakers or other metallic hardware that would affect the magnetic field. In addition, for certain patients, claustrophobia or unstable medical conditions would preclude their being in the tube during the necessary acquisition time. The advantage of MRI or MRA is its absence of iodinated contrast material and radiation exposure. The use of gadolinium is contraindicated in patients with renal failure. With pre–endovascular aneurysm repair (EVAR) planning, contrast-enhanced MRA is comparable to CTA.

DIAGNOSTICS

Abdominal Aortic Aneurysm

IMAGING

Abdominal ultrasound
CTA*
MRI or MRA*

*If indicated.

DIFFERENTIAL DIAGNOSIS

The differential diagnoses for AAA include conditions associated with abdominal pain or back pain. These conditions are listed in the differential diagnosis box. CT is the most readily available method to rule out alternative causes of abdominal pain.

DIFFERENTIAL DIAGNOSIS

Abdominal Aortic Aneurysm

- Nephrolithiasis
- Myocardial infarction
- Esophageal rupture
- Perforated gastric ulcer
- Pancreatitis
- Bowel obstruction
- Cholelithiasis
- Diverticulitis
- Gastrointestinal bleed
- Appendicitis
- Pyelonephritis
- Ischemic bowel
- Back strain
- Arthritis
- Neoplasm

MANAGEMENT

Once an AAA has been identified, it can be managed with traditional open surgical repair, minimally invasive abdominal EVAR, or continued surveillance. The goal of AAA management is to prevent aneurysmal rupture while minimizing surgical risk. Thus the size of the aneurysm, the shape of the aneurysm, and the patient's medical status, life expectancy, and preference are critical factors in deciding the timing of elective AAA repair.[5] AAA size is the best predictor of rupture risk.[2,5,11] A fair amount of controversy persists about the best timing for and method of AAA repair (operative or endoluminal) when preoperative risk factors and postoperative complications are considered (Box 117-1).[11]

The majority of aneurysms expand slowly at a rate of 0.2 to 0.3 cm per year, or 10% of the diameter. However, the risk of rupture increases significantly when an AAA exceeds 5.0 cm

BOX 117-1

Factors Affecting the Risk for AAA Rupture

- Size (>6.0 cm [2.36 inches])
- Rapid expansion*
- Female gender
- Smoking
- COPD
- Family history of AAA
- Asymmetric AAA

*It is difficult to predict the average expansion of an AAA because intervention is planned in all but high-risk patients and those who refuse treatment.

in diameter. The ACC/AHA 2005 practice guidelines for management of patients with peripheral arterial disease note that "data suggest the eventual risk for rupture is approximately 20% for aneurysms larger than 5.0 cm in diameter, 40% for those at least 6.0 cm in diameter, and greater than 50% for aneurysm that exceed 7.0 cm in diameter."[11] A 2011 focused update of these practice guidelines did not address or update these statistics.[20] An older population-based study also demonstrated increased risk of rupture as AAA size increases.[21] In the United Kingdom Small Aneurysm Trial (UKSAT), the relative risk of rupture was increased in women, those with AAAs of increased diameter, smokers, and patients with COPD.[22] Another factor found to be important in rupture risk was asymmetry in the aneurysm.[21,22]

Data from the UKSAT[22] and the Veterans Affairs Aneurysm Detection and Management (ADAM) trial[21] help guide decision-making about the timing of surgical repair of small AAAs (4.0 to 5.0 cm) versus surveillance with serial ultrasound examinations or CT. These studies concluded that unless the aneurysm exceeds 5.5 cm, there is no long-term survival advantage of early surgery over serial ultrasonographic surveillance at 6-month intervals. Elective repair is appropriately indicated for healthy patients with AAAs measuring 5.0 to 6.0 cm.[5] During the 9-year follow-up of the UKSAT, 74% of the surveillance group needed interventions, indicating that intervention is almost always necessary.[22]

PREOPERATIVE CARDIAC RISK STRATIFICATION

Several older, large surveys have demonstrated that coronary artery disease is the most important underlying medical illness contributing to morbidity and mortality among individuals who undergo major vascular surgery, regardless of the type of peripheral vascular surgery, particularly when they are 70 years of age or older.[23-26] The ACC/AHA developed guidelines to aid in cardiac risk stratification before noncardiac surgery. According to the ACC/AHA guidelines,[11] aortic and other vascular procedures are considered high risk. Patients with an active cardiac condition such as unstable coronary syndrome, decompensated heart failure, significant arrhythmia, or severe valvular disease may require cancellation or delay of surgery until further testing, which may include coronary angiography or even cardiac bypass surgery, and/or implementation of medical management is done. Patients should proceed to surgery without further cardiac evaluation only when they have no clinical predictors or minor clinical predictors (minor clinical predictors include advanced age older than 70, electrocardiogram [ECG] with left ventricular hypertrophy, left bundle branch block, nonspecific ST-T abnormalities, cardiac rhythm other than sinus, uncontrolled hypertension) with moderate to excellent functional capacity (≥4 metabolic equivalents [METs]).[5,11,25,26] Four to 7 METs include activities such as climbing a flight of stairs or walking up a hill, running a short distance, doing heavy housework such as scrubbing floors, or moving furniture. Poor functional capacity (1 to 3 METs) includes activities such as doing light housework (washing dishes), eating, walking at 2 to 3 miles per hour, and getting dressed.[5,11,25,26]

Preoperative noninvasive testing, such as a resting 12-lead ECG, is recommended for all within 30 days of the planned procedure. Pharmacologic stress testing is indicated when patients are undergoing high-risk vascular surgery and they have two or more intermediate predictors of clinical risk (mild angina pectoris, prior myocardial infarction, compensated or prior congestive heart failure, diabetes mellitus, renal insufficiency) and unknown or poor functional capacity (≤4 METs). Preoperative echocardiography is recommended for patients with dyspnea or heart failure. Results of noninvasive testing are then used to plan further perioperative management. This may include intensified medical therapy and/ or further cardiac testing, and perhaps cancellation or delay of surgery.[5]

Other medical conditions may increase the mortality rate of aneurysm repair by twofold or threefold. They include chronic renal failure (serum creatinine level >3 mg/dL or hemodialysis), COPD (FEV/FEV_1 <0.70), and liver cirrhosis with portal hypertension. These conditions increase the mortality rate from between 3% and 5% to between 8% and 10%.[5] In a Canadian North American study, the most significant predictors of mortality were electrocardiographic changes indicative of ischemia, COPD, and increased creatinine concentration.

Open Surgical Repair

Open surgical repair of an AAA is usually approached through a midline or a left flank retroperitoneal incision. Overall, these two approaches are generally interchangeable in the treatment of infrarenal aneurysm, although specific indications for the transperitoneal approach include right renal graft, right iliac artery aneurysm, prior left colectomy, and aneurysmal neck that turns to the right. Indications for the retroperitoneal approach include multiple prior laparotomies or abdominal surgeries, selected abdominal stoma, horseshoe kidney, inflammatory aneurysms, obesity, and juxtarenal and suprarenal aortic aneurysms.

During open surgical repair of an AAA, the aneurysm is exposed and normal segments of the proximal and distal aorta are cross-clamped. The aneurysm is incised. Lumbar arteries, which back-bleed into the aneurysm, are oversewn. A prosthetic graft is positioned in the aorta, extending from a segment of normal aorta above the aneurysm to a segment of normal aorta below the aneurysm. If the aneurysm extends to the iliac arteries, a bifurcated prosthetic graft is used. The distal ends of the bifurcated limbs extend into the iliac or femoral arteries. The wall of the aneurysm is closed over the newly placed graft. The posterior peritoneum and then the abdomen are closed in the standard manner.

Today, most patients undergoing surgical repair of an AAA have their preoperative workups done on an outpatient basis and are admitted for same-day surgery. Hospital discharge ranges from 5 to 7 days postoperatively, and recovery ranges from 6 weeks up to 3 months depending on health status and the patient's overall medical condition. CTA should be performed within 5 years after open repair of AAA to detect aneurysmal degeneration.

Endovascular Stent Grafts

Endovascular AAA repair (EVAR) was first performed in 1991. A number of studies have documented the efficacy and generally satisfactory results of a variety of transluminally placed endovascular grafts.[27,28] Endoluminal AAA repair is associated with reduced length of hospital stay, decreased recovery time, a smaller incision, and fewer complications, which accounts for its appeal to patients and physicians as well as an upsurge of enthusiasm for the development and use of such devices.[27,29] In 2006, 21,725 EVAR procedures were performed in the United States, exceeding for the first time the number of open surgical

AAA repairs. At present, more than 80% of AAA repairs in the United States are performed by EVAR.[30,31]

EVAR requires accurate preoperative imaging evaluation for appropriate patient selection based on aneurysm morphology and access vessel size and patency. The proximal aortic neck and iliofemoral arteries are important areas of imaging. Endoluminal repair of AAA is achieved through exclusion of the aneurysm from the circulation by means of a prosthetic graft that is inserted from a remote site to the desired intraluminal location, under radiologic guidance, and then secured by an expandable stent attachment system. The devices may be commercially manufactured or custom made. They include a bifurcated graft or a tube graft with a single limb (aorto–uni-iliac), uncovered, branched, and fenestrated devices. New devices have allowed EVAR to be offered to a greater number of patients.[29] The development of the superspecialty of vascular therapy and the dissemination of skills have increased the rate of endoluminal use.

The initial successful deployment of a stent graft has been reported in 95% to 97% of cases.[32] The procedure time is usually less than 2 hours. Most procedures are performed with the patient under epidural anesthesia combined with conscious sedation. Only infrequently does an endovascular patient require an intensive care unit stay. Patients are sent home after computed tomography (CT) confirmation of graft placement and the absence of a leak at the attachment sites for the graft, with more than 85% of patients discharged on their first or second postoperative day.[27] Patients report a return to a sense of preoperative health status 11 days after endoluminal repair versus 47 days after open surgical repair.[27]

The first routine follow-up visit with the vascular surgeon occurs 1 month after hospital discharge, at which time another CT scan is obtained to reaffirm the position of the graft, presence or absence of any leak, and evidence of sac shrinkage. It appears that smaller AAAs have fewer endoleaks than larger ones.[33,34] Thereafter, CT scans are obtained at prescribed intervals, usually again at 6 months, then 12 months and yearly thereafter, depending on stability of the aneurysm and prosthesis. Aortic remodeling after EVAR is a slow process that continues for several years.[29]

Ruptured AAAs present a unique challenge to endovascular repair. Because the first indication of their presence is often the back pain and hypotension associated with acute enlargement and rupture, the primary goal is stabilization of the patient. This is accomplished by gaining control of the rupture and preventing further hemorrhage. Once the patient is stabilized, repair of the aorta can be accomplished. With increasing surgical experience, improvement in technology, and the availability of a range of graft sizes, this less invasive method of repair has been applied with success.[35-39]

Multiple guidelines recommend lifelong annual imaging after EVAR to identify complications such as endoleaks or residual aortic sac enlargement, and to prevent death from aneurysm rupture after EVAR.[29-31,40,41] Compliance with follow-up imaging is strongly recommended, and patients need to be educated about this before the procedure. Those having an EVAR AAA repair emergently appear to be at a higher risk of loss to follow-up imaging.

LIFE SPAN CONSIDERATIONS

In general, AAA is considered a disease of older white men (≥65 years), but younger individuals with certain risk factors may be affected and need to undergo repair. Aneurysms are more commonly symptomatic in younger patients. Perioperative mortality and morbidity rates are not significantly different for young patients compared with older patients (≥65 years) with degenerative (atherosclerotic) AAAs. Technique (open versus endovascular) is determined not by age but by the assessed risk to the patient and the size of the AAA.

COMPLICATIONS

Complications vary for surgical repair and endoluminal repair of AAAs. Mortality rates and short- and long-term graft complications are comparable for the two techniques.

In most large series, the 30-day mortality rate for surgical repair is 3% to 5%. If electrocardiographic changes of ischemia, COPD, and elevated creatinine concentration are present, the mortality rate at 30 days is 50%. By comparison, patients with none of these factors have a perioperative mortality of less than 2%. Early surgical complications of arterial thrombosis, anastomotic rupture or bleeding, peripheral emboli, and limb loss are rare (1% to 3%) at centers with experience. In a 36-year population-based study of late graft complications, the 1-, 3-, and 5-year rates of survival free of graft complications were 97%, 95%, and 93%, respectively.[36] The primary cause of death was myocardial infarction. The rate of open conversion during endovascular repair is less than 5%. Furthermore, the incidence of long-term complications is very low but includes anastomotic pseudoaneurysm, graft thrombosis, aortoenteric fistula, graft infection, anastomotic hemorrhage, colonic ischemia, and atheroembolism.

The 30-day mortality rates for stent graft repairs are similar (3%) to those for standard surgical repair. However, for patients at high risk, mortality rates have been as high as 10% to 13%. The most common early complications include groin hematoma, arterial thrombosis, iliac artery rupture, and thromboemboli.

The most common long-term problem is endoleak.[42-44] An endoleak involves persistent filling of the aneurysm from either an anastomotic site or collateral blood vessels, most commonly caused by persistent bleeding from lumbar or inferior mesenteric artery branches in the AAA sac. Endoleaks occur in about one third of cases. Appropriate classification is crucial for subsequent management. Endoleaks close spontaneously in more than 50% of cases by 6 to 12 months after the procedure. Secondary catheter-based reinterventions are required to close an additional 10%. Surgical intervention has been required to treat 2% to 3% of long-term leaks. Even after successful EVAR, aneurysm expansion may occur, leading to eventual rupture. This occurs in 1% of patients within 1 to 2 years. Other common late complications include severe graft kinking, graft migration, graft thrombosis, and renal dysfunction.

INDICATIONS FOR REFERRAL OR HOSPITALIZATION

Patients with an AAA of 4.0 cm or larger should be referred to a vascular physician. Recent evidence suggests that outcomes for open repair of intact AAAs are better at large, urban institutions.[5] Therefore, referral to a center with a vascular service experienced in treating AAAs is indicated with elective repairs. Using ultrasound examination, the vascular physician will obtain an ultrasound 6 months after the initial ultrasound to look for rapid expansion, and thereafter monitors for expansion by ultrasound or CT scan every 6 to 12 months for AAAs measuring 4.0 to 5.4 cm.[45] Although elective repair is usually considered when the AAA enlarges into the range of 5.0 to 6.0 cm, smaller aneurysms may be repaired if the patient cannot commit to the surveillance program. Rapid expansion beyond 10% of the diameter per year is also an indication for surgical repair. Finally, repair may be delayed until the diameter is 6 cm or larger in poor-risk patients.[5] If the aneurysm enlarges and is being considered for repair, the vascular physician will order a CT scan for evaluation for stent graft placement.

PATIENT EDUCATION

During the period of surveillance of small aneurysms, patient education addresses modification of risk factors such as hypertension and smoking to slow AAA expansion, and management of diabetes and hyperlipidemia.[5]

Physical activity is encouraged, such as walking, bike riding, or other aerobic exercise, but patients should avoid activities that include heavy lifting or exercises that involve undue strain. Also addressed are protocols for surveillance, indications for emergent evaluation, and surveillance of first-degree relatives.

During the periprocedural phase, patient education focuses on the trajectory of care, including hospital stay and postdischarge recovery. Reinforcement of the vascular surgeon's instructions including care of the incision or catheterization site, resumption of activities of daily living, and protocols for long-term monitoring are also discussed.

Hypertension and cigarette smoking are critical risk factors for expansion of AAA. Although beta blockade has not demonstrated a significant difference in the rate of expansion of small AAAs or the need for surgery, treatment with beta blockers continues because of its effect on reducing coronary events.[5,21,26,46] Smoking cessation needs to be addressed and encouraged at every visit, along with referral to a smoking cessation councilor. However, smoking cessation does not preclude the development of AAA, nor will smoking cessation prevent expansion of AAA.[3,5]

The frequency of surveillance depends on the size of the aneurysm at the most recent ultrasonographic study. Patients must commit to serial ultrasonographic examinations or consider early repair of a small aneurysm with the inherent risks and benefits of open surgical or endovascular repair.

At the initial visit with the vascular physician, the patient will be educated about both the standard open surgical procedure and the endovascular stent graft procedure. The explanation should include early and late results of both types of procedures to inform the patient and to assist in decision-making.

After the detection of an AAA, patients should be counseled to report new-onset symptoms of aneurysmal enlargement, such as abdominal or back pain, to the vascular physician. Symptoms of impending rupture requiring immediate emergency care include severe abdominal pain, flank pain, or back pain unrelieved by position change. The abdominal pain may be characterized as deep, boring, or tearing. Low back pain may be dull, radiating to the legs, similar to musculoskeletal pain. The flank pain may radiate to the groin and be associated with hematuria.

HEALTH PROMOTION

There is strong evidence to suggest a genetic predisposition to AAA.[2,4,5,11] First-degree male relatives of patients with AAA have two to four times the normal risk for AAA,[11] suggesting the importance of periodic ultrasonographic screening after the age of 50 years in these family members.[11]

There is also strong evidence suggesting the relationship between smoking and the development of AAA in men.[2,5] For this reason, the USPSTF recommends screening with ultrasonography for men older than 65 years with a past or current history of smoking.[16]

CHAPTER 118

CARDIAC ARRHYTHMIAS

Andrea Efre

Cardiac arrhythmias are electrical abnormalities of the cardiac conduction system that can vary in severity from trivial to life-threatening. These may occur in the presence or absence of structural heart defects or cardiac disease. Arrhythmias may be divided into categories by rate or location. Rate classifies the arrhythmia by the speed of the heart rate: tachyarrhythmia (>100 beats per minute) and bradyarrhythmia (<60 beats per minute). Location identifies where the arrhythmia originates: ventricular (originates from the ventricles) and supraventricular (originates from above the ventricles). Arrhythmias may arise from conductive tissue anywhere within the atria, atrioventricular (AV) junction, or the ventricles. However, symptoms are more closely related to the ventricular rate and to the severity of underlying heart disease than to the origin of the arrhythmia. Cardiac arrhythmias may cause minor symptoms such as palpitations or dizziness but may also predispose to the development of lethal conditions such as stroke, embolism, or sudden cardiac death.[1]

DEFINITION AND EPIDEMIOLOGY

Tachyarrhythmias

More than half of all cardiac arrhythmias arise from or involve the atria. Atrial fibrillation (AF), atrial flutter, and other supraventricular tachyarrhythmias occur frequently in patients with ST-elevation myocardial infarction (STEMI). They are triggered by excessive sympathetic stimulation, atrial stretch caused by ventricular overload, atrial infarction, pericarditis, electrolyte abnormalities, hypoxia, or underlying lung disease.[2] By far the most common supraventricular arrhythmia is AF (estimated 2.3 million Americans), which is often associated with structural heart disease or other co-occurring chronic conditions. It is slightly more common in men, and there is an increased prevalence with age (older than 60 years of age).[3,4] AF occurs in 8% to 22% of patients with STEMI, and new-onset AF is associated with shock, heart failure (HF), stroke, and 90-day mortality.[2]

Ventricular tachyarrhythmias, especially in the presence of serious underlying organic cardiac disease, may predispose the patient to sudden cardiac death and increased mortality rates. Sudden cardiac death claims 300,000 to 400,000 lives annually in the United States, with the majority being older adults; approximately 80% of these deaths are caused by ventricular fibrillation (VF) in the context of ischemic heart disease. Structural cardiovascular anomalies and congenital rhythm abnormalities (such as long QT syndrome or Brugada syndrome) are thought to be the cause of unexplained deaths in the younger population.[1]

Ventricular arrhythmias such as sustained ventricular tachycardia (VT) and VF are common early after the onset of STEMI and are also the most common cause of out-of-hospital cardiac arrest with STEMI. There are multiple factors in the possible cause of these arrhythmias, which include ongoing ischemia, hemodynamic instability, electrolyte abnormalities, enhanced automaticity, and reentry mechanisms.[2] Ventricular arrhythmias such as accelerated idioventricular rhythm may follow myocardial insult and are known as reperfusion arrhythmias; they are related to the restoration of normal myocardial blood flow and may occur after myocardial infarction (MI) or revascularization procedures such as percutaneous coronary intervention.

Bradyarrhythmias

Bradyarrhythmias may result from abnormalities in conduction between the sinoatrial (SA) node and atrium, within the AV node, or in the intraventricular conduction pathways. The rhythm of sinus bradycardia may be noted as an incidental finding and considered normal in highly trained athletes. The presence of symptoms with sinus bradycardia should lead to further investigation and a possible treatment plan.

Bradyarrhythmia may result from intrinsic disease of the sinus node or AV conduction system, but the cause of intermittent bradyarrhythmia can be difficult to determine.[5] Idiopathic fibrosis is a major cause of AV block, particularly in older adults.[4] Other causes may include hypothyroidism, advanced liver disease, hypothermia, or severe hypoxia or medications such as calcium channel blockers or beta blockers. Other causes of disruption in normal conduction may include coronary spasm, myocarditis, rheumatic fever, mononucleosis, Lyme disease, sarcoidosis, amyloidosis, and neoplasms.

Bundle branch block (BBB) may be intermittent or chronic, and symptomatic or asymptomatic. Possible causes include structural heart disease, congenital conditions, cardiac disease, and coronary artery disease. Right bundle branch block (RBBB) is associated with right ventricular hypertrophy, ischemic heart disease, pulmonary embolus, atrial septal defect, rheumatic heart disease, myocarditis, cardiomyopathy, and Brugada syndrome. Left bundle branch block (LBBB) is associated with ischemia, MI, aortic stenosis or regurgitation, dilated cardiomyopathy, and Lyme disease. The rhythm disturbances of BBB do not always require treatment, but it is imperative to determine and manage the underlying cause as well as to treat any associated symptoms.

PATHOPHYSIOLOGY

The functional components of the cardiac conduction system subdivide into (1) impulse-generating tissue (SA and AV nodes) and (2) impulse-propagating tissue (e.g., His-Purkinje system). The SA node is the impulse-generating node with the highest intrinsic firing rate. It has complex dimensional tissue composed of ion channel and gap junction expression profiles, which have different action potential characteristics and conduction properties.[6] Rhythmic release of calcium contributes to the SA nodal diastolic depolarization. The local intracellular calcium elevations drive the sodium-calcium exchange current to substitute intracellular calcium for extracellular sodium, producing positive-charge results in membrane depolarization.[6]

The SA node is the natural pacemaker of the normal heart; if stimulated, suppressed, or blocked, it will induce tachyarrhythmias or bradyarrhythmias. The pacemaker function may then be assumed by "escape" foci in the atrial tissue, the AV node, the bundle of His, the Purkinje fibers, or the ventricular myocardium. The intrinsic rates of each part of the conductive system may be influenced (increased, decreased, or blocked) by factors such as cardiac disease, ischemia, medications, electrolytes, or changes in the endocrine system. Impaired conduction through the cardiac conduction system may be related to altered action potential (usually a result of ion channel defects) or defective coupling between cardiomyocytes (e.g., AV nodal block or BBB).[6]

Cardiac arrhythmias are a result of abnormal impulse formation or conduction and can be categorized into one or more of three mechanisms: (1) abnormal automaticity, (2) triggered activity, or (3) reentry.

- *Abnormal automaticity (enhanced or suppressed):* Automaticity is a natural property of all myocytes, which may be suppressed or enhanced by factors such as electrolyte imbalance, medications, hypoxia, ischemic heart disease, scarring, or increased age, and can result in atrial or ventricular tachyarrhythmias.[7] Abnormal or enhanced automaticity is a deficit in the ability of the cardiac cells to depolarize spontaneously. Enhanced automaticity results in increased conduction of impulses and results in tachycardia (e.g., sinus tachycardia). Abnormal automaticity may lead to irregularity of the impulse conduction, causing erratic or ectopic rhythms of the atria or ventricles. Suppressed automaticity decreases conduction of the SA node and can result in sinus node dysfunction or sick sinus syndrome.
- *Triggered activity:* Triggered activity usually occurs after an early or delayed depolarization that precipitates multiple depolarizations and causes ventricular arrhythmias. They may be induced by electrolyte imbalances or medications, as in antiarrhythmic or digoxin toxicity.[7] An example of a triggered arrhythmia is torsades de pointes.
- *Reentry:* Reentry arrhythmias require a circular movement of the impulse across the myocardium. Most tachyarrhythmias are thought to be caused by a reentry mechanism and include bidirectional conduction and unidirectional block.[7] They may start and terminate suddenly and are often paroxysmal. If a large area is involved, it is known as a macro-reentry arrhythmia and occurs through concealed accessory pathways; the best example is Wolff-Parkinson-White (WPW) syndrome, but macro-reentry arrhythmias can also cause AF and atrial flutter. Micro-reentry arrhythmias affect a small area; examples include VT or VF after MI. An example of a reentry arrhythmia is AV nodal reentry tachyarrhythmia.

The pathophysiology of arrhythmias is additionally defined in the differential diagnosis section to include the expected electrocardiographic changes.

CLINICAL PRESENTATION

Tachyarrhythmias

Tachyarrhythmias may be entirely asymptomatic or may cause symptoms that affect the patient's activities of daily living. When symptoms occur they are in large part related to the ventricular rate, extent of underlying heart disease, ventricular function, and associated precipitating factors. Palpitations are the most common symptom caused by tachyarrhythmias. In patients with paroxysmal attacks, palpitations start and terminate abruptly and are usually rapid but regular. In patients with AF the palpitations are typically irregular and tend to be more sustained. Extrasystoles may also cause palpitations or an awareness of isolated extra beats; and the pause that follows may be symptomatic. Other causes of palpitations include thyrotoxicosis, hypovolemia, regurgitant valvular disease, anemia, hypoglycemia, pheochromocytoma, fever, anxiety, symptoms of menopause, stimulants such as caffeine, street drugs, and medications. Any history of underlying heart disease or previous rhythm disturbance and its treatment is relevant, as are the family history and evaluation of coronary risk factors. Pertinent history also includes inquiring about the use of alcohol, tobacco, caffeine, sympathomimetics (commonly found in over-the-counter cold medicines or diet aids), and prescription medication use (e.g., theophylline or thyroid supplements). When interviewing the patient with tachyarrhythmias and/or palpitations, it is prudent to ask about the use of street drugs, especially those known to be stimulants, such as cocaine, methamphetamines, synthetic cannabinoids, and synthetic cathinones (bath salts).

Tachyarrhythmias tend to shorten diastole, and ventricular filling may become compromised, causing a drop in blood pressure, cardiac output, and coronary perfusion. Irregularity in the ventricular rate control, loss of coordinated atrial contraction (e.g., AF), or beat-to-beat variability in ventricular filling causes symptoms that may include lightheadedness, dizziness, syncope, dyspnea, or fatigue, with fatigue being the most common presenting symptom of AF.[3] A serious tachyarrhythmia may result in hemodynamic decompensation, causing hypotension, chest pain, HF, change in level of consciousness, or even sudden cardiac death. It is important to assess both the arrhythmia and its tolerance by the patient to determine the degree of urgency and the appropriate setting for intervention.

Bradyarrhythmias

Bradycardia may cause symptoms or may be asymptomatic (especially in healthy individuals), discovered as an incidental finding on routine electrocardiography. In such cases it is most likely that the needs of the body are being met despite the slow heart rate. Symptoms accompanying bradycardia are largely dependent on the ventricular rate relative to metabolic demand and on the presence of underlying cardiac disease. Those with limited cardiac reserve are less tolerant of a slow rate than those with normal hearts. The American Heart Association recognizes two types of bradycardia: absolute and relative. Absolute bradycardia refers to any heart rate below 60 beats per minute. Relative bradycardia refers to a heart rate that is too slow to maintain normal blood pressure or cardiac output even if the rate is greater than 60 beats per minute.[8]

Symptomatic bradycardia is thought to be directly responsible for the development of frank syncope or near-syncope, transient dizziness, lightheadedness, or confusion resulting from decreased cerebral blood flow attributable to the slow ventricular rate.[5,8] Subtle symptoms of irritability, lassitude, inability to concentrate, apathy, or forgetfulness are common symptoms of bradyarrhythmia, and palpitations may be the presenting complaint when the bradyarrhythmia is a manifestation of sick sinus syndrome. Other symptoms may occur at rest or with exertion in persistent bradyarrhythmias, and include fatigue, reduced exercise capacity, or symptoms of HF.[5,8] In addition, lethargy; weight gain; changes to the skin, hair, or nails; constipation; or eyelid edema may be subjective findings of hypothyroidism, which may be the cause of a bradyarrhythmia.

Relevant aspects of the history include a careful review of all medications and the identification of any underlying cardiac disease. It is important to discern whether the symptoms occur at rest or with exertion and if there are outstanding, aggravating, or alleviating factors. A vagal mechanism for bradycardia may be implicated—for instance, if the symptoms occur only with straining, such as with vomiting or moving the bowels.

PHYSICAL EXAMINATION

The initial examination should include evaluation of blood pressure, pulse, temperature, mental status, evidence of diaphoresis, respiratory effort, and manifestations of anxiety. Alterations in rate and pulse volume and irregularity may accompany ventricular ectopic beats, depending on the timing and force of ventricular contractions, which may be observed by labile blood pressure. Orthostatic vital signs are helpful to exclude orthostatic hypotension as a cause of syncope, dehydration, or hypovolemia, which could be the cause of reflex tachycardia (requiring prompt intervention). The patient's hydration status also includes examination of skin turgor and status of mucous membranes.

Assessment of the neck should include inspection, observing the neck veins for jugular venous distention (a sign of HF), and for the presence of a goiter (suggesting thyroid disorder). Assessment of the neck veins may provide information about atrial activity. The *a wave* (atrial contraction) reflects atrial pressure and occurs just before S_1 and the carotid pulse. The *v wave* (venous filling) occurs just before or coincides with S_2.[9] Absence of the a wave suggests AF as atrial systole is lost. A more prominent a wave than v wave may be observed with 2:1 AV block. Cannon a waves, or forceful, irregular expansions in the jugular pulse, may occur with AV dissociation as the atria contract against closed AV valves, causing a reflux of blood to the jugular veins.[10]

The carotid pulses are palpated for amplitude, contour, timing, and presence of thrills. Auscultation of the carotid arteries should be performed initially with the diaphragm of the stethoscope to detect the higher frequency of the arterial bruits, then with the bell to detect the low-pitched sounds of higher-grade stenosis.[9] The presence of a bruit would suggest atherosclerosis and contraindicates carotid massage as a diagnostic or treatment option.

The chest is inspected and palpated for parasternal lifts, heaves, and thrills. Palpation of the point of maximum impulse (PMI) and percussion of the left side of the chest will establish the size and location of the heart. Enlargement of the cardiac silhouette may suggest ventricular hypertrophy or cardiomyopathies, which are triggers for some arrhythmias. Auscultation of the heart sounds for regularity, rate, murmurs, clicks, or the presence of extra heart sounds is essential. An accentuated S_1 may be heard in some tachyarrhythmias, and a diminished S_1 may be found in AV nodal blocks. A varying S_1 may be a sign of complete heart block or AF as the mitral valve is in varying positions before ventricular contraction. The splitting of S_2 may be heard in patients with premature ventricular contractions (PVCs) or RBBB; and paradoxical splitting of S_2 may be related to LBBB.[9] An S_3 is a significant finding of increased ventricular filling and can be caused by fluid overload, HF, or decreased myocardial contractility, which may be end points of an arrhythmia. Note that S_3 may be a normal finding in a child, young adult, or pregnant female, who may also have the presence of a cardiac arrhythmia. The presence of an S_4 is pathologic and is caused by resistance in ventricular filling. It may be associated with AV nodal conduction delays.

The presence of an S_3 and/or S_4 in an athlete should be investigated because it may be a sign of athletic heart syndrome.

Electrocardiographic findings may include sinus bradycardia, AV nodal block, or RBBB, and there may be lateral displacement of the PMI owing to the increased heart size. These patients should be referred to a cardiologist for further evaluation because the differentiation of benign findings from the ominous possibility of sudden cardiac death can be difficult to determine.

A heart murmur is most often associated with underlying valve disorders; however, a benign systolic ejection murmur may accompany a tachycardia with or without valvular disease. Absence of a murmur is not necessarily a significant finding because rapid rates can often make accurate auscultation difficult. The patient should always be reexamined after the heart rate is controlled. An S_3 sound is a significant finding, as are jugular venous distention (JVD) and peripheral edema—signs of fluid overload—and may warn of impending HF or be an indication that the rhythm is poorly tolerated by the patient.

As part of the complete assessment, the examiner auscultates the lungs for rales, wheezes, or rhonchi. Other important findings include exophthalmos, an enlarged or nodular thyroid gland, or skin, nail, and hair changes commonly associated with hyperthyroidism or hypothyroidism. When the presenting complaint is syncope, near-syncope, dizziness, confusion, or altered level of consciousness, a neurologic examination should be performed to explore the possibility of noncardiac causes.

If there is a positive history, or suspected use, of street drugs, physical manifestations will depend on the type of drug and route used. The examiner should be observant for signs of use: needle markings (e.g., intravenous use), burns to the mouth or fingers (e.g., from pipe use), sores to the nasal area, epistaxis or increased rhinorrhea (e.g., insufflation), or skin or gum abscesses or rotten teeth noted from chemically manufactured drugs or methamphetamine.

INITIAL DIAGNOSTICS

12-Lead Electrocardiogram

The 12-lead electrocardiogram (ECG) is indicated for initial evaluation of a suspected arrhythmia. This diagnostic tool has the notable limitation of providing only a 12-second view of the heart's electrical activity. Although sustained rhythms may easily be captured, paroxysmal rhythms may be elusive. However, even when the rate and rhythm are normal, the resting ECG may yield valuable information about the cause of the arrhythmia. The first priority is to identify ST- or T-wave changes that indicate MI or myocardial ischemia. Other significant findings are ventricular hypertrophy, effects of medication toxicity, and electrolyte imbalance, such as peaked T waves noted in hyperkalemia.

Indications of conduction abnormalities may also be present and include the widened QRS complex of intraventricular conduction delay, the shortened PR interval that accompanies preexcitation syndromes such as WPW syndrome, and the prolonged QT interval that may accompany idiopathic long QT syndrome or drug effects.[4,10] When abnormal rhythms are captured on the 12-lead ECG, it is prudent to record a rhythm strip by allowing the tracing to continue for several minutes to fully evaluate the rhythm. With tachyarrhythmias, minor depressions of the ST segment and inversion of the T wave could be rate related rather than indications of coronary disease.[10] However, these changes should be reevaluated once the rate is controlled. Arrhythmias can be a sign of underlying acute coronary syndrome (ACS), and the 12-lead ECG should be interpreted carefully.

Laboratory (Serum Testing)

Based on presenting symptoms, history, and clinical findings, laboratory testing may assist in determining the underlying cause of the arrhythmia. These tests might include a complete blood count (CBC) to determine the presence of anemia or infection; and serum electrolyte values including potassium, calcium, and magnesium to evaluate disturbances such as hypokalemia, hyperkalemia, hypocalcemia, hypercalcemia, or hypomagnesemia. A blood glucose measurement is helpful if hypoglycemia is suspected, and blood urea nitrogen (BUN) and creatinine levels are beneficial in determining fluid volume status. A thyroid-stimulating hormone (TSH) level should be drawn if hyperthyroidism or hypothyroidism is suspected. Measuring a toxicity level may be useful for patients being treated with medications that might cause arrhythmia (e.g., digoxin). Toxicology screening for stimulants such as cocaine or amphetamines may beneficial. Cardiac biomarkers should be measured if ACS or coronary ischemia is suspected as the cause of the arrhythmia (evaluate coronary risk factors for questionable ACS).

Echocardiography

Two-dimensional transthoracic echocardiography with Doppler should be performed during the initial workup of all arrhythmia patients to determine left atrial and left ventricular size, systolic function, and underlying structural heart disease. This is useful in guiding decisions for antiarrhythmic and antithrombotic therapy, particularly with regard to the patient with AF.

Radiologic Imaging

Chest radiography is useful to identify structural disease or the presence of HF or pneumonia.

Stress Testing

Stress tests are an example of provocative testing and can be performed by exercise (usually on a treadmill) or pharmacologically. Causes of exercise-induced arrhythmias may include ischemia, increased sympathetic activity, congenital conduction disturbances, and medications. It is important to verify the absence of coronary ischemia before initiating antiarrhythmic agents. Nuclear images of the myocardium at baseline and after exercise show disruption of myocardial blood flow from ischemia. When the history suggests symptoms such as palpitations, exercise stress testing can be used to provoke electrocardiographic changes or arrhythmias, which may remain unidentified at rest. This is especially useful if the symptoms occur or are worsened with activity. Exercise testing can also be useful to evaluate the adequacy of rate control in AF.[3]

OTHER DIAGNOSTICS

Holter Monitor

Continuous ambulatory electrocardiographic rhythm monitoring such as with a Holter monitor is a useful option for evaluation of a suspected arrhythmia, especially when symptoms are inconsistent or paroxysmal in nature. Ambulatory monitoring may also be useful in the definitive correlation of bradyarrhythmias when evaluating the need for a pacemaker. Use of this portable device allows continuous recording of the heart's activity during a 24- to 48-hour period. The patient keeps a diary of activities and symptoms that can later be correlated with the tracing. This is worn while patients go about their usual activities. Ventricular arrhythmias such as PVCs, ventricular couplets, and nonsustained VT may have no similarity among the days, making it unlikely that a single Holter recording for 24 hours may capture this phenomenon, suggesting that additional recordings may be necessary.[11]

Event Monitor and Loop Recorder

For the patient with infrequent symptoms, intermittent ambulatory electrocardiography (event recording) may be more appropriate because these devices can be worn for a long time. There are two types of these recorders. One type is worn externally; this recorder remains dormant until it is activated by the user at the onset of symptoms.[4] Patient-activated electrocardiographic event recorders can help assess the relation to symptoms, whereas auto-triggered event recorders may detect asymptomatic episodes. These technologies may also provide valuable information to guide drug dosage for rate control or rhythm management.[3]

The second type is an implantable loop recorder for long-term monitoring, used for diagnosis in patients with recurrent unexplained episodes of palpitations or syncope. The implanted device records the ECG during activity or symptoms or can record when it is activated by the patient. The device has an automatic recording triggered by arrhythmia and has an additional feature that allows the patient to activate the recording. New devices may offer remote transmission of the data back to the cardiologist. Implantable loop recorder monitoring is useful in detecting arrhythmias and guiding treatment plans,. It may be used to evaluate for lethal bradycardias and sudden cardiac death in hemodialysis patients.[12] The implantable loop recorder may stay in place for months or several years; battery life tends to last 24 months or more. It can provide additional diagnostic value in patients with syncope or nonsyncopal, real or apparent, transient loss of consciousness.[13,14]

Tilt-Table Test

Provocative testing in the form of a tilt-table test is used to evaluate syncope. The patient is observed as the table is angled in varying degrees. Symptoms and hemodynamic status are monitored to see if syncope is related to a vasodepressor or a cardiac or neurologic reason. Arrhythmias, usually bradyarrhythmias, may be elicited with position change and induce syncopal symptoms. An example is malignant vasovagal syndrome, which is evidenced by exaggerated vagal response to emotional or painful stimuli. Tilt-table tests are performed in a monitored setting by a specialist, usually a cardiologist or an electrophysiology (EP) cardiologist, or a neurologist if syncope is suspected to be non-cardiac.

Electrophysiologic Studies

Rhythms that put the patient at high risk for adverse events warrant referral to a specialist for electrophysiologic studies to properly identify and treat the problematic rhythm. The arrhythmias are often tachycardic in nature and may include very rapid supraventricular tachycardia (SVT), WPW syndrome, complex ventricular ectopy, and VT. EP studies may also be indicated for investigation of palpitations and syncope when noninvasive techniques have failed to definitively identify the problem.[4] If congenital heart defects are suspected to be the source of an arrhythmia, electrophysiologic studies may be useful in evaluating if the arrhythmia is related to extra electrical pathways (known as accessory pathways). The procedure will evaluate the origin and specific location of extra pathways and (if reachable and appropriate) may lead to ablation of the offending source cells.

Transesophageal Echocardiography

Transesophageal echocardiography (TEE) is performed by a specialist physician and is used to determine the presence or absence of left atrial thrombus before consideration of cardioversion.[4] For patients with asymptomatic WPW syndrome, the TEE procedure can be very helpful in determining their risk for sudden cardiac death.[15]

Carotid Sinus Massage and Valsalva Maneuvers

Valsalva maneuvers and carotid sinus massage may be used as a diagnostic test to induce bradycardia. Transient AV block results in the slowing of the ventricular response, enabling identification of the underlying rhythm. These techniques may terminate rhythms for which the AV node is part of the reentry circuit, such as in atrioventricular nodal reentry tachycardia (AVNRT), and are therefore used as therapeutic treatments. The provider should evaluate atherosclerotic risk factors, assess for carotid bruits, and ensure correct technique is used before performing carotid massage. Carotid sinus massage during simultaneous recording of the ECG is useful to provoke symptomatic bradycardia in carotid sinus syndrome, a disorder in which bradycardia occurs in response to carotid sinus hypersensitivity. Carotid sinus massage is usually performed by a physician specialist in a monitored setting (e.g., emergency provider, cardiologist or EP cardiologist).

DIAGNOSTICS

Arrhythmias

INITIAL DIAGNOSTICS

12-Lead ECG
Vital signs

LABORATORY (SERUM TESTING)

CBC
Serum electrolytes including calcium and magnesium, BUN, creatinine, and glucose
TSH
Digoxin level or other medication levels*
Toxicology, especially cocaine and amphetamines*
Cardiac biomarkers*

IMAGING

Echocardiography (to evaluate underlying structural heart disease)
Chest x-ray examination (to identify structural disease)
Stress test

OTHER DIAGNOSTICS

Holter monitor
Event monitor
Implantable loop recorder
Tilt-table test
Electrophysiologic studies
TEE
Valsalva maneuver and/or carotid sinus massage*

*If indicated.

DIFFERENTIAL DIAGNOSIS OF TACHYARRHYTHMIAS

Narrow Complex Tachycardia

Narrow complex tachycardia includes rhythms with a rate over 100 beats per minute and QRS duration of 0.12 second or less. The rhythms in the following paragraphs are included in this group and are described as they appear on the ECG.

Sinus Tachycardia. In sinus tachycardia, there is a P wave preceding each QRS complex in a consistent 1:1 relationship. The rhythm is regular, the P waves are identical, the QRS complexes are normal and narrow, and the PR and QRS intervals are within normal ranges. The rate is above 100 beats per minute (Fig. 118-1).

Multifocal Atrial Tachycardia. In multifocal atrial tachycardia, the heart rate is usually 100 to 130 beats per minute and the rhythm is irregular. The P waves have three or more different morphologic appearances. The P-P interval and the PR interval will be variable. This rhythm is usually seen in patients with pulmonary, cardiovascular, or metabolic disturbances.

Paroxysmal Supraventricular Tachycardia. Paroxysmal supraventricular tachycardia (PSVT) is a rapid (rate of 140 to 240 beats per minute), generally regular rhythm that is typically initiated by a single beat and starts and stops abruptly. P waves may differ slightly in morphologic appearance compared with the sinus rhythm. The QRS complex is most typically narrow. P and QRS waves may exist in a 1:1 relationship, or variable AV block may alter this relationship. If the rate is very fast, P waves may be buried in the previous beat. Paroxysmal atrial tachycardia (PAT), particularly PAT with block, is often associated with digoxin toxicity.[16]

Atrioventricular Nodal Reentry Tachycardia. The reentry tachyarrhythmia of AVNRT is the most common mechanism for SVT. There are dual pathways within the AV node that are responsible for the reentrant circuit conduction. P waves, when they are visible, exist in a 1:1 relationship with the QRS complex. In very fast rhythms they are buried within the QRS complex and may not be visible or may be seen as a distortion at the end of the QRS complex. This distortion appears as a pseudo-S wave in leads II, III, and aVF or a pseudo-R wave in lead V_1.[16] The rate is usually 140 to 180 beats per minute and regular. The QRS complex is narrow and morphologically similar to that of the sinus rhythm. It is typically paroxysmal in nature and will terminate with the Valsalva maneuver or carotid sinus massage.

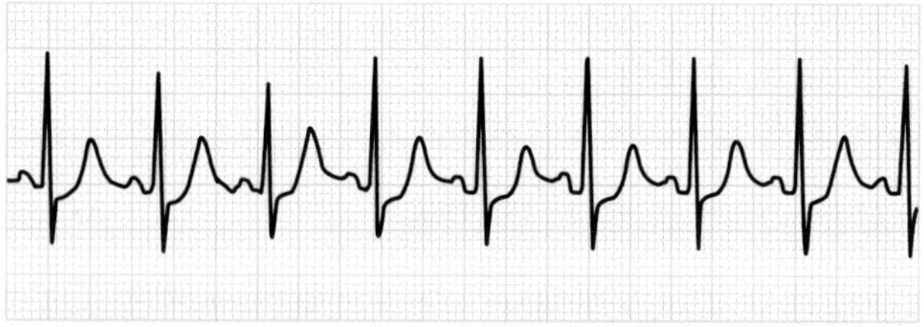

FIGURE 118-1 Sinus tachycardia. (From Goldman L, Schafer AI, editors: *Goldman's Cecil medicine*, ed 24, Philadelphia, 2011, Elsevier.)

Atrioventricular Reentry Tachycardia. With atrioventricular reentry tachycardia (AVRT), the reentry is the result of an accessory pathway between the atria and ventricles that bypasses the AV node. This mechanism is responsible for preexcitation syndromes, the most common being WPW syndrome.

Wolff-Parkinson-White Pattern. In WPW syndrome an AV bypass tract connects the atria and the ventricles, circumventing the AV junction and causing preexcitation of the ventricles. The physiologic lag through the AV junction may result in a shortened PR interval of less than 0.12 second, but a normal PR interval remains possible. The delta wave is the key identifier on the ECG and is observed by an upstroke slurring of the QRS complex.[16]

Atrial Flutter. In atrial flutter, the atrial rate ranges from 250 to 350 beats per minute, producing a sawtooth appearance of the P waves. The atrial rate of 300 beats per minute usually has a 2:1 conduction to the ventricle, producing a QRS rate of 150 beats per minute.

Atrial Fibrillation. In AF the normal P wave is replaced by fibrillatory F waves, producing a wavy baseline. The atrial rate is estimated to be between 350 and 650 beats per minute. There is an irregularly irregular ventricular response because the AV node will allow only a fraction of the atrial impulses to reach the ventricle (Fig. 118-2).

Wide-Complex Tachycardia

Wide-complex tachycardia involves rhythms with a rate over 100 beats per minute and QRS duration of 0.12 second or greater. The rhythms in the following paragraphs are included in this group and are described as they appear on the ECG.

Supraventricular Tachycardia with Aberrancy. In SVT with aberrancy the QRS duration is longer than 0.12 second but typically not more than 0.14 second. Often, a triphasic RSR right bundle branch pattern is seen in lead V_1. Because of the

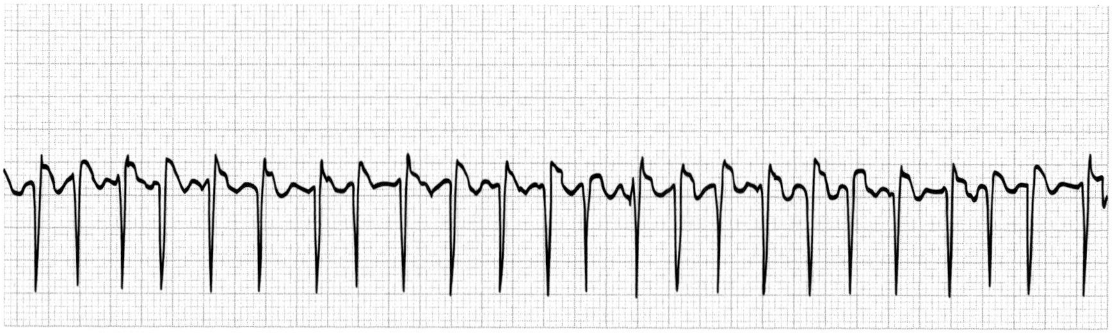

FIGURE 118-2 Atrial fibrillation with rapid ventricular response. (From Marx JA, Hockberger RS, Walls RM, et al, editors: *Rosen's emergency medicine*, ed 7, Philadelphia, 2009, Elsevier.)

fast ventricular rate, the P wave may be buried in the previous beat or may present as a peaked or notched T wave in the previous beat. Carotid sinus massage may slow or even terminate the tachycardia. Differentiation between SVT with aberrant conduction ventricular tachycardia may be challenging but is critical because treatment approaches differ significantly according to the origin of the arrhythmia. A combination of leads is superior to one lead in making this differentiation.[17]

Ventricular Tachycardia. VT is defined as three or more consecutive ventricular ectopic beats. The rhythm may be sustained (>30 seconds) or nonsustained (<30 seconds). The QRS width is usually greater than 0.14 second, with a rate between 100 and 300 beats per minute. VT may be monomorphic in nature (QRS complexes appear the same) or polymorphic (the QRS shape changes from beat to beat).

Differentiation of VT from SVT with aberrancy is not always possible. Usually SVT with aberrancy would have a BBB morphology, so the absence of BBB on the ECG suggests it may be VT. Another criterion is AV dissociation; P waves are independent and unrelated to the QRS complex. Other indicators that favor a diagnosis of VT are extreme right-axis deviation (northwest) between 180 and −90 degrees; concordance of the QRS pattern in all precordial leads (e.g., all have negative deflections); and a wide QRS pattern inconsistent with typical right or left bundle branch patterns.[17] Using carotid sinus massage may assist in the differentiation of VT and SVT with aberrancy; it may slow down the rate of SVT long enough to offer an improved view of the rhythm, but VT will not respond (Fig. 118-3).

Ventricular Outflow Tract Tachycardia. One of the most common causes of idiopathic VT is right ventricular outflow tract (RVOT) tachycardia, which is monomorphic and originates from the outflow tract of the right ventricle. It is usually triggered by sympathetic stimulation (anxiety, excitement, exercise, and stimulants) and typically seen in younger patients (20 to 30 years) without underlying structural heart disease. Typical ECG findings for this type of VT have an appearance of LBBB, usually with an onset of positive R wave in V_4 and positive deflections in the inferior leads. Precordial leads that show a transition of the R wave in V_3 are more likely to be septal in the origin of the right outflow tract. These ECG changes rarely occur during rest, so exercise stress testing is beneficial to provoke the arrhythmia so that a more definitive diagnosis may be made. It is possible that the VT is originating from the left ventricular outflow tract and manifests in a similar fashion on the ECG. This makes diagnosis challenging and should be referred to EP cardiology.

Torsades De Pointes. The most common polymorphic VT is torsades de pointes, which is characterized by polymorphic QRS complexes that change in amplitude and cycle length. It is associated with QT prolongation, which may be congenital or idiopathic or a result of electrolyte imbalances (particularly hypokalemia or hypomagnesemia). The arrhythmia may also be induced by long QT intervals produced by medications, such as quinidine, antiarrhythmic agents, and some antibiotics used routinely in primary care (including azithromycin and moxifloxacin). Patient outcome will be improved if differentiation of this arrhythmia is made early, because the treatment for torsades de pointes differs markedly from standard VT treatments.

Other types of polymorphic VT may be congenital or acquired. Congenital causes include long QT syndrome (corrected QT interval >0.40 second); Brugada syndrome (ECG exhibits RBBB pattern and ST-segment elevation in the precordial leads); and the more unusual diagnosis of catecholamine-induced polymorphic VT. Acquired polymorphic VT is usually induced by drug toxicity or electrolyte abnormalities. Differential diagnosis of these types of VT can be difficult and should be referred to a cardiology specialist.

Ventricular Fibrillation. VF is a rapid, disorganized electrical activity within the ventricles with no discrete QRS complexes. The heart is unable to contract, and therefore no systole (pulse) is possible. Recognizing this arrhythmia is vital to the patient's chances of survival because defibrillation is required immediately.

Additional Complexes

Premature Atrial Contractions. Premature atrial contractions (PACs) are irregularities rather than a tachyarrhythmia but are important to identify because they may initiate a tachyarrhythmia in the susceptible heart.[10] Also, if they are numerous, they may cause the patient to complain of palpitations or a skipped or extra beat. They are typically identified on the ECG within a prevailing sinus rhythm, which would be completely regular were it not for the premature beats. The PAC is a normal-looking beat in every way except that it occurs prematurely. The PR interval may differ slightly from that of the prevailing rhythm, although it remains within the normal range. Because the beat depolarizes the sinus node, there is typically a partially compensatory pause before the next sinus beat (Fig. 118-4).

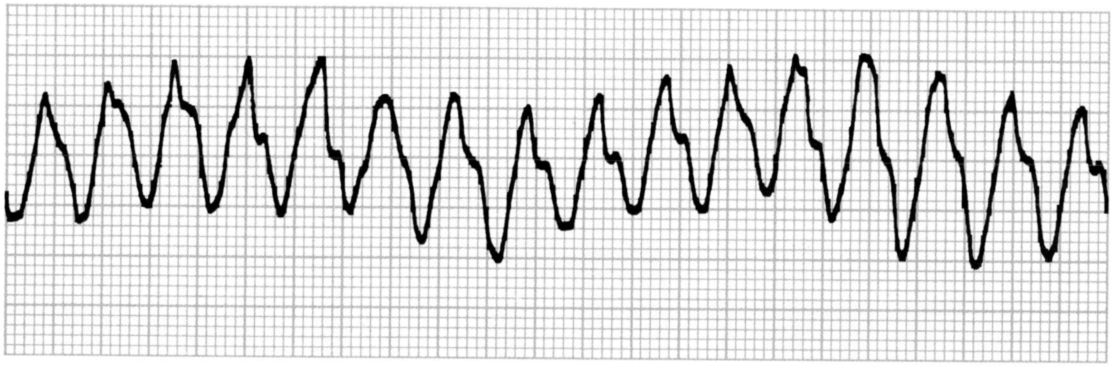

FIGURE 118-3 Ventricular tachycardia. (From Marx JA, Hockberger RS, Walls RM, et al, editors: *Rosen's emergency medicine*, ed 7, Philadelphia, 2009, Elsevier.)

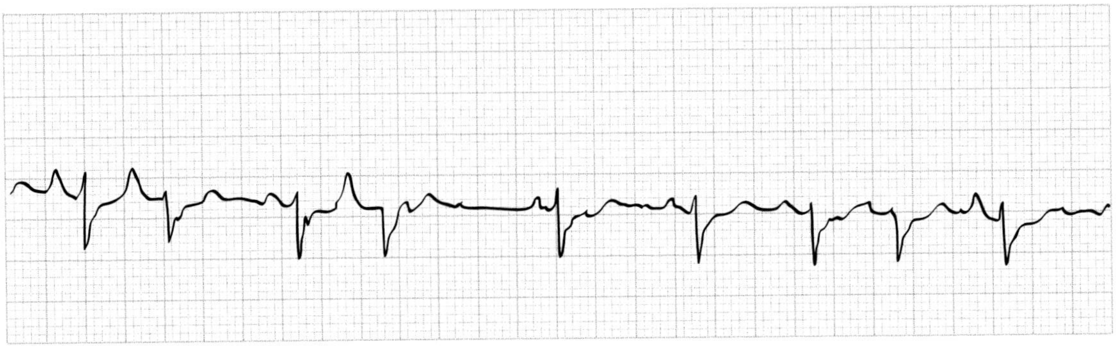

FIGURE 118-4 Premature atrial contractions. (From Goldberger AL: *Clinical electrocardiography: a simplified approach*, ed 7, Philadelphia, 2006, Elsevier.)

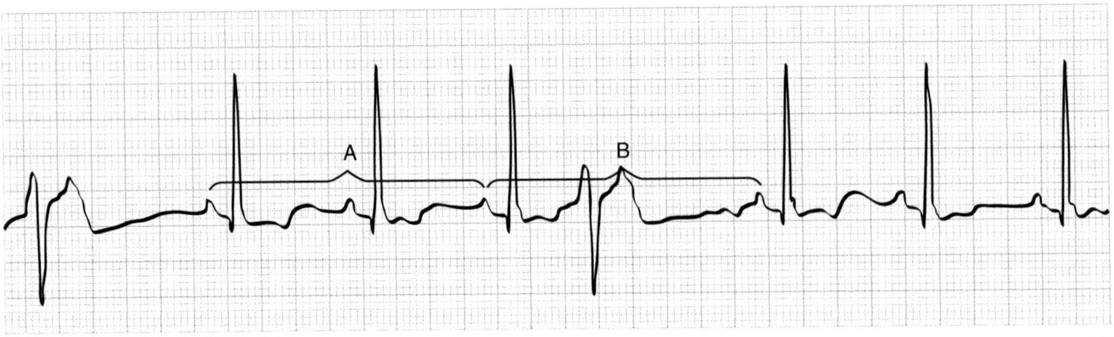

FIGURE 118-5 Premature ventricular contractions with compensatory pause. (From Marx JA, Hockberger RS, Walls RM, et al, editors: *Rosen's emergency medicine*, ed 7, Philadelphia, 2009, Elsevier.)

Premature Junctional Contractions. Premature junctional contractions (PJCs) originate in the AV node and are another cause of irregularity in the heart rhythm. The impulse is carried to the ventricles along normal pathways; the resultant QRS complex is narrow and appears similar to the QRS complexes of the sinus rhythm. There may be retrograde conduction to the atria, yielding a P wave that can occur before, during, or after the QRS complex. If the P wave occurs before the QRS complex, the PR interval is less than 0.12 second. When a P wave is visible, it is typically negative in leads II, III, and aVF.[16]

Premature Ventricular Contractions. PVCs are extra premature beats that originate in the ventricle. They are characterized by wide, bizarre QRS complexes (>0.12 second) that interrupt the prevailing rhythm. They may be unifocal (originating from one focus) or multifocal (originating from multiple points of focus). The P wave is typically absent, and the beat is most often followed by a full compensatory pause (the distance from the QRS preceding the PVC to the QRS that follows it is equal to twice the R-R interval of the prevailing sinus rhythm). Typically the T-wave deflection is in opposition to that of the QRS complex.[17] The description of PVCs is included here because of their association with ventricular tachyarrhythmias (Fig. 118-5).

DIFFERENTIAL DIAGNOSIS OF BRADYARRHYTHMIAS

Sinus Bradycardia

In sinus bradycardia, the SA node fires at a rate of less than 60 beats per minute with a 1:1 relationship between each P wave and QRS complex. The time that is taken for each electrical conduction is normal, PR intervals are 0.20 second or less, and QRS intervals are 0.12 second or less.

Sinoatrial Exit Block

SA exit block is the sudden cessation of sinus rhythm that results in long pauses. These pauses usually occur in a fixed pattern.

Atrioventricular Nodal Blocks

When conduction through the AV node is delayed or blocked completely, it is categorized as an AV nodal block rhythm. These types of block are separated in to three groups: first-degree AV block, second-degree AV block, and third-degree AV block. The AV block may be transient, intermittent, or permanent and may be differentiated further by measuring the length of the PR interval and identifying the presence of a QRS complex.

First-Degree Block. In first-degree AV block the PR intervals are equal and longer than 0.20 second, but every P wave is conducted to the ventricle, resulting in a related QRS complex.

Second Degree Block. There are many types of second-degree AV block, but two are specifically identified in primary care: type I (sometimes referred to as Mobitz type I) and type II (Mobitz type II). The differentiating factor for second-degree AV block when compared with other blocks is the consistent absence of a QRS complex that is missed or "skipped" in a timed fashion (e.g., three complete complexes followed by a P wave where a QRS is missing. The atrium-ventricle conduction ratio is usually 3:2 or 4:3, and a typical pattern of complexes occurs.

Second Degree, Type I. In second-degree AV block Mobitz type I, there is progressive prolongation of the PR interval until

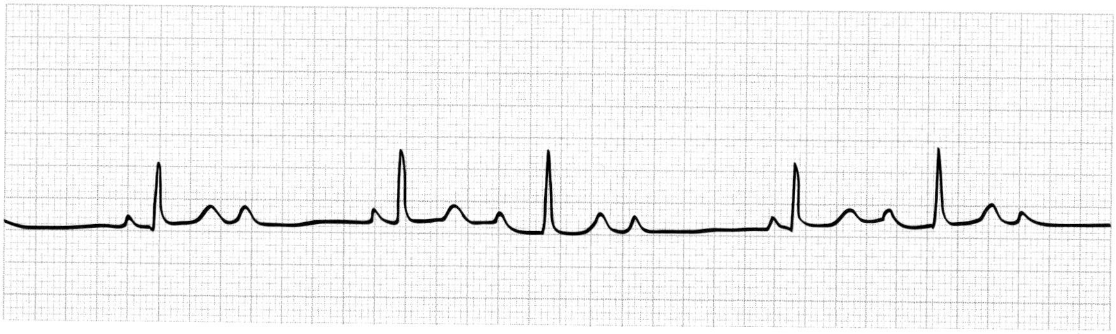

FIGURE 118-6 Second-degree atrioventricular block, Mobitz type I. Note the prolongation of the PR interval between the second and third beats followed by a nonconducted atrial impulse. (From Marx JA, Hockberger RS, Walls RM, et al, editors: *Rosen's emergency medicine,* ed 7, Philadelphia, 2009, Elsevier.)

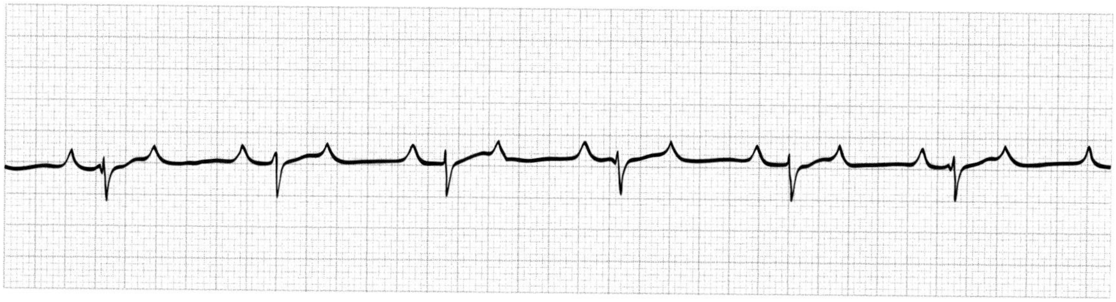

FIGURE 118-7 Second-degree atrioventricular block, Mobitz type II. (From Goldberger AL, Goldberger E: *Clinical electrocardiography,* ed 2, St Louis, 1981, Elsevier.)

a P wave is not conducted to the ventricle. This rhythm is also called Wenckebach block (Fig. 118-6).

Second Degree, Type II. In second-degree AV block Mobitz type II there is a constant PR interval until a P wave does not conduct to the ventricle and the QRS complex is skipped (missing). This type of second-degree AV block is less common and a little more severe than Mobitz type I and has a higher propensity to progress to complete heart block (Fig. 118-7).

Third-Degree AV Block. In third-degree AV block none of the atrial impulses are conducted to the ventricle. This rhythm is often referred to as complete heart block or AV disassociation. The P waves have no relationship to the QRS complexes (they are dissociated). Typically, the pacemaker function is picked up by an escape focus, resulting in either a junctional or ventricular escape rhythm. A junctional escape rhythm is characterized by a slow rate (40 to 60 beats per minute) with QRS complexes of normal width that are not related to P waves. A ventricular escape rhythm typically produces a bradycardia of less than 40 beats per minute and is characterized by wide QRS complexes (>0.12 second) that are also not connected to, or associated with, P waves.

Bundle Branch Blocks

As conduction of the impulse passes across the AV node, conduction continues rapidly to all sections of the ventricular muscle by way of the right and left bundle branches. In BBB the conduction is disrupted as it journeys down the bundle branches. The impulse is stopped at the blocked bundle and is forced to travel across the myocardium to depolarize the opposite ventricle. This depolarization across the ventricle takes longer than the normal bundle conduction, which causes a time lapse that

DIFFERENTIAL DIAGNOSIS

Cardiac Arrhythmias

TACHYARRHYTHMIAS

Narrow Complex
- Sinus tachycardia
- Multifocal atrial tachycardia
- PAT
- AVNRT (WPW)
- AV reciprocating tachycardia
- Atrial flutter
- AF

Wide Complex
- SVT with aberrancy
- VT
  - Ventricular outflow tract tachycardia
  - Torsades de pointes
- VF

Additional Complexes
- PACs
- PJCs
- PVCs

BRADYARRHYTHMIAS
- Sinus bradycardia
- SA exit block

Atrioventricular Nodal Blocks
- First-degree AV block
- Second-degree AV block
  - Second-degree AV block Mobitz type I
  - Second-degree AV block Mobitz type II
- Third-degree AV block (complete heart block)

Bundle Branch Block
- RBBB
- LBBB
- Hemiblock (left anterior fascicle and left posterior fascicle)

increases the QRS duration. A QRS duration of 0.10 to 0.11 second results from incomplete BBB, whereas a QRS duration of 0.12 second or longer results from complete BBB.

Right Bundle Branch Block. The ECG shows a small R wave followed by an S wave and then a final R in lead V_1, whereas V_6 will show a deep, slurred S wave after initially normal Q and R waves.

Left Bundle Branch Block. The ECG shows a broad, slurred S wave in lead V_1 and an R in lead V_6.

Hemiblocks. The left bundle branch is further divided into the left anterior fascicle and the left posterior fascicle. When conduction is impaired in only one of the fascicles, a hemiblock occurs (which is usually related to loss of blood supply, and mostly found after MI). In addition to the LBBB, a right-axis deviation will be noticed on the ECG with left posterior hemiblock, and a left-axis deviation will occur with left anterior hemiblock.

MANAGEMENT

Immediate emergency medical transportation to the closest emergency department is essential for patients with life-threatening arrhythmias such as VT or VF and for patients with an arrhythmia who are hemodynamically compromised or when indications of ischemia are present on the ECG. Emergency department referral is also required for patients with an arrhythmia in the presence of chest pain and coronary risk factors. It is important to consider that ischemia may be the cause of the arrhythmia and must be further evaluated. Best morbidity and mortality rates occur if a reperfusion procedure is achieved within 60 minutes of diagnosis.

Emergency department referral is additionally indicated if further testing is required that cannot be achieved on an outpatient basis or if the specialist requires the emergency department setting for testing. For example, the provider may determine that the patient needs an urgent stress test for evaluation of ischemia as a cause of arrhythmia. Hospitalization with inpatient monitoring is required if the arrhythmia has the potential to become unstable or for the initiation of medications that require monitoring (see section on indications for hospitalization).

Referral to a cardiologist or EP cardiologist is indicated when additional evaluation of arrhythmia is required for new-onset rhythm disturbances, symptomatic arrhythmias, or treatment failure. Most electrophysiologists require a referral from a cardiologist before being involved in the management of the patient.

Managing the patient with an arrhythmia starts with establishing the stability of the patient's condition by assessing hemodynamic status. When an arrhythmia causes a patient's condition to be unstable, immediate intervention is indicated. "Symptomatic" implies that an arrhythmia is causing the symptoms but that the patient is not in imminent danger[8]—sometimes referred to as stable arrhythmias. The basic premise for treating unstable arrhythmias is the introduction of an electrical intervention. Tachycardic unstable rhythms are evaluated for synchronized cardioversion, and the bradycardic rhythms will be assessed for pacemaker intervention. These interventions require hospitalization and are most often used by the emergency department.

When managing a stable patient with an arrhythmia, the provider carefully evaluates symptoms to assist in the treatment plan. If the symptoms affect activities of daily living, suppression of the symptom is the goal. For many arrhythmias (especially tachycardia), converting back to normal sinus rhythm may be achieved by synchronized cardioversion or use of pharmacologic agents. If restoration of sinus rhythm is not achieved or not appropriate, controlling the heart rate will assist in symptom reduction, which may also be achieved with medications.

For the purposes of managing arrhythmias in this chapter, the treatment is broken down into tachyarrhythmias and bradyarrhythmias. This information will focus on the medical management of the arrhythmia; discussion of emergency treatment and procedures and inpatient management will be brief and further emphasized in the section on indications for referral or hospitalization.

Management of Tachyarrhythmias

Although many of the symptoms caused by arrhythmias are the result of the heart rate and the hemodynamic response, the individual patient response is variable between episodes. The effect of an arrhythmia on hemodynamics is largely dependent on the rate rather than its cause. This may be a result of shortened ventricular filling time, the severity of underlying heart disease, the presence of AV synchrony, the ventricular activation sequence, and the autonomic balance. For patients with atrial tachyarrhythmias who are hemodynamically unstable, immediate synchronized cardioversion is be recommended.[3,4] For stable patients, medications may be more appropriate

The decision to initiate antiarrhythmic therapy depends on the severity and frequency of the arrhythmia and the hemodynamic consequences versus the risks associated with the therapy itself. The need for long-term therapy must be individualized to each patient's needs because the severity of symptoms is highly variable, based on the clinical situation and the presence or absence of underlying coronary artery disease.[4,18] Multiple clinical trials have radically altered antiarrhythmic therapy as the results identified the concept of proarrhythmia—that is, antiarrhythmic agents inducing the very arrhythmia they are used to suppress.[3,4]

The two general conditions for which antiarrhythmic therapy is appropriate are a potentially life-threatening arrhythmia and an arrhythmia that is hemodynamically significant or symptomatic, which mostly involve ventricular arrhythmias and AF. The Vaughn-Williams classification separates antiarrhythmic medications into four classes based on their mechanism of action and target cell (excluding digoxin and adenosine).[4,19]

- Class I: sodium channel blockade drugs; further divided into three subgroups as follows:
  - Class Ia—quinidine, procainamide, and disopyramide
  - Class Ib—lidocaine, mexiletine, and tocainide
  - Class Ic—flecainide, propafenone, and moricizine
- Class II: beta blockers
  - Selective agents such as atenolol, bisoprolol, and metoprolol
  - Nonselective agents such as nadolol and propranolol
  - Nonselective and alpha receptor blockers such as carvedilol and labetalol
- Class III: potassium channel blocking and include sotalol, dofetilide, ibutilide, amiodarone and bretylium.
- Class IV: calcium channel blockers
  - Dihydropyridines such as amlodipine, felodipine, nicardipine, nifedipine

- Nondihydropyridines—SA and AV node depressants such as diltiazem and verapamil

Sinus Tachycardia

Sinus tachycardia is typically treated by treatment or elimination of the underlying cause (e.g., fever, hypovolemia, hyperthyroidism, anxiety). Elimination of tobacco, alcohol, caffeine, stimulants, or sympathomimetics (such as those found in over-the-counter cold medications, nasal sprays, and diet supplements) may result in a return to normal heart rate.

If the tachycardia is unresolved by removal of the underlying cause, a diagnosis of syndrome of inappropriate sinus tachycardia (IST) may be considered. It is defined as a sinus-initiated heart rate higher than 100 beats per minute at rest for longer than 24 hours (mean >90 in 24 hours), usually associated with palpitations. Before managing this diagnosis, the provider should ensure that all possible underlying causes have been investigated and should eliminate possible stimulants with lifestyle modifications. Pending approval for IST in the United States, ivabradine (Corlanor) holds considerable promise for treatment, with 70% of patients reporting reduction of symptoms and increased exercise performance.[20] Beta blockers are not the primary therapy but may be useful when combined with ivabradine.[20]

Multifocal Atrial Tachycardia

Multifocal atrial tachycardia occurs primarily in older patients with comorbid disease. Sixty percent of these patients have significant pulmonary disease.[17] The diagnosis often occurs in the setting of congestive HF, exacerbation of the underlying pulmonary condition, or electrolyte imbalance. As with sinus tachycardia, therapy is directed at correction of the precipitating factor (e.g., improving oxygenation, correcting electrolyte imbalance).[17]

Paroxysmal Supraventricular Tachycardia

The use of vagal maneuvers or carotid massage may be useful in slowing the ventricular rate. A trial of adenosine is a reasonable treatment option in narrow-complex tachycardia and may be attempted before cardioversion. It may also be used in wide-complex tachycardia if the rhythm is regular and monomorphic.[8] Adenosine is contraindicated in patients with asthma because it may precipitate AF. Narrow-complex PSVT may also be treated pharmacologically by slowing of AV conduction with digoxin, calcium channel blockers, or beta blockers or by suppression of atrial automaticity with class IA, IC, or III antiarrhythmic agents.[17]

Caution is necessary when managing wide-complex PSVT; careful monitoring is required during medication administration. Pharmacologic agents that increase the refractoriness of the AV node (digoxin, calcium channel blockers, and beta blockers), when used alone, may decrease the refractoriness of the accessory pathway and have the potential to cause a faster ventricular rate. Class IA, IC, and III agents are preferred because they increase the refractoriness of the bypass tract.[17]

Most cases of PSVT are reentrant and amenable to radiofrequency ablation when symptoms are significant and recurrent. Ablation is most often preferable to antiarrhythmic agents because of safety and tolerability concerns. Wide-complex PSVT should be managed with caution in conjunction with a cardiologist and usually necessitates hospitalization.

Atrial Fibrillation or Atrial Flutter

Management of the patient with AF or atrial flutter may be challenging because the best approach is often not clear and treatment must be highly individualized. Although AF is not considered a lethal arrhythmia, it carries a significant risk of stroke and embolism and increased risk of HF. Initially an attempt at restoration of normal sinus rhythm may be made with synchronized cardioversion and/or a pharmacologic converting agent, such as amiodarone. However, evaluation of thromboembolism risk should be made before restoration of atrial contraction.

Therapeutic goals of long-term treatment are rate control and prevention of thromboembolism. The risks and benefits of each treatment are patient specific, and consideration of the patient's lifestyle and socioeconomic situation will help in choosing options that encourage treatment compliance. Reasons to opt for restoration of sinus rhythm include symptom relief, prevention of embolism, and reduction in the risk of cardiomyopathy or HF. However, prolonged duration of the AF and left atrial enlargement can reduce the ability to be successful in maintaining normal sinus rhythm.[17,18]

When initially diagnosing AF for the first time, management starts with a search for the cause, as some are reversible. Common causes include MI, pericarditis, myocarditis, cardiomyopathy, rheumatic heart disease, mitral valve disease, hyperthyroidism, electrocution, cardiothoracic and noncardiac surgery, acute alcohol intoxication or withdrawal, stimulant ingestion, pneumonia, or pulmonary embolism.[3,4]

In deciding to use a pharmacologic cardioverting agent, consider the side effects and proarrhythmia of antiarrhythmics. Flecainide, ibutilide, propafenone, amiodarone, and dronedarone are the drugs of choice. Although there are risks inherent with each of these medications, several precautions are necessary with dronedarone. Dronedarone should not be used for ventricular rate control in permanent AF, HF, or left ventricular systolic dysfunction because it increases the risk of stroke, MI, systemic embolism, and cardiovascular death.[3] Administration of other antiarrhythmics with dronedarone should be avoided; there can be interactions with calcium channel blockers, antiseizure medications, and other medications metabolized by the CYP3A or CYP2D6 hepatic pathways.

Amiodarone is the most effective antiarrhythmic drug for maintenance of sinus rhythm in patients with paroxysmal or persistent AF and is more effective than dronedarone, sotalol, or propafenone.[3] Amiodarone should be initiated in the hospital with a loading dose (intravenous bolus, followed by a maintenance therapy). Proarrhythmias are a serious side effect, and lethal arrhythmias are possible with both intravenous and oral medication. Amiodarone has a very long half-life (40 to 50 days) and accumulates in the skin, liver, and cornea. Before initiation of amiodarone, baseline monitoring parameters should be attained, including liver and thyroid function tests and pulmonary function tests. Routinely observe for hepatic and pulmonary toxicity, and refer to optometry or ophthalmology specialists for corneal monitoring.

Rate control is easier to achieve then conversion of the rhythm and is an acceptable goal in hemodynamically stable patients. Beta blockers and nondihydropyridine calcium channel blockers are the drugs of choice for rate control alone (of the calcium channel blockers, only verapamil and diltiazem control rate). Digoxin can be added to assist in rate control, and its inotropic properties can be useful. A recent study, indicated that patients with AF have increased mortality when digoxin is used.[3a] Periodic serum levels should be measured to establish a therapeutic level (0.8 to 2 ng/mL for AF, and toxicity level >2 ng/mL).

One major consideration in determining treatment is the patient's tolerance of the lost atrial contraction that accompanies AF. Loss of AV synchrony and the irregularity of the ventricular rhythm both contribute to a decline in cardiac output that has been estimated to be about 15%.[4] The presence of mitral stenosis, restrictive or hypertrophic cardiomyopathy, pericardial disease, or ventricular hypertrophy increases the likelihood of hemodynamic deterioration. Decisions in AF management are sometimes less obvious when the patient is hemodynamically stable, and the loss of atrial contraction is not as critical. Neither conversion, rate control, nor maintenance of sinus rhythm is clearly superior.[4] The duration of AF is an important determinant of success: the longer a patient experiences AF, the lower the odds of maintaining sinus rhythm.

Finally, those with problematic or refractory AF may be candidates for nonpharmacologic approaches. These include electrical synchronous cardioversion, AV nodal ablation or modification, and/or pacemaker implantation. The surgical maze procedure has been shown to be useful in controlling the tachyarrhythmia that occurs with AF.[4]

Electrical and pharmacologic cardioversion carry the risk of thromboembolism. When the rhythm has been sustained for longer than 48 hours, anticoagulation therapy should be uninterrupted for 4 weeks before and for at least 4 weeks after elective cardioversion. TEE may be used to evaluate or exclude the presence of left atrial thrombus before cardioversion. If an atrial thrombus is present, cardioversion is postponed for more adequate anticoagulation (usually 3 to 4 weeks) and TEE can be repeated.[3]

Prevention of Thromboembolism in Atrial Fibrillation

Thromboembolism is a major complication of recurrent or persistent AF. Stroke risk is measured using the CHA_2DS_2-VASc score. For patients with nonvalvular AF with prior stroke, transient ischemic attack, or a CHA_2DS_2-VASc score of 2 or higher, oral anticoagulants are recommended.[3]

Anticoagulation may be accomplished with warfarin, a vitamin K antagonist. It is effective at multiple sites of action in the coagulation cascade, which is why it has been the mainstay oral anticoagulant treatment in the prevention of stroke for patients with AF for decades.[3] However, it is not without its drawbacks. The constant monitoring and the risk of bleeding make it a medication requiring thoughtful consideration. Warfarin dose should be titrated to maintain the international normalized ratio (INR) between 2 and 3. The INR is measured at least weekly during initiation of therapy, and monthly when stable.[3]

Use of a direct thrombin or factor Xa inhibitor is an alternative to warfarin and does not require serum monitoring. Currently there are four medications available in this category: dabigatran (Pradaxa), a direct thrombin, and the factor Xa inhibitors rivaroxaban (Xarelto), edoxaban (Savaysa), and apixaban (Eliquis). They are substrates for the efflux transporter P-glycoprotein and indicated for use in nonvalvular AF to prevent thromboembolism.[3] Dabigatran (factor IIa inhibitor) is a prodrug with the advantage that it is not metabolized by the cytochrome P-450 system; rivaroxaban, edoxaban, and apixaban are direct inhibitors of factor Xa and are partially metabolized by cytochrome P-450 enzymes, and therefore are contraindicated with drugs that are strong P-450 3A4 (CYP3A4) inducers or combined with P-glycoprotein.[3]

Severe bleeding is a side effect of both warfarin and the factor Xa inhibitors; the risks of bleeding versus the benefits of stroke prevention must be considered. Interaction with other medications may increase or decrease the potency and effectiveness of the drugs. P-glycoprotein inhibitors (ketoconazole, verapamil, amiodarone, dronedarone quinidine, and clarithromycin) may increase plasma concentrations. In addition, P-glycoprotein inducers (phenytoin, carbamazepine, rifampin, and St. John's wort) can decrease levels to subtherapeutic levels. These medications should not be used for patients with AF and mechanical heart valves and are not recommended in patients with AF and end-stage chronic kidney disease (or dialysis) because of a lack of clinical trial evidence establishing safety and efficacy.[3] Before initiation of therapy with one of these medications, renal status should be established with serum creatinine and then periodically during use of the medication. Edoxaban is contraindicated for patients with nonvalvular AF if the creatinine clearance is greater than 95 mL/min. No antidote is currently available to reverse the effects of these medications, but the limited half-life lessens the need for a reversal agent. Research continues with this group of medications to establish better understanding of clinical variables such as the patient's age, dose and administration interval, and renal function.

For those who cannot take anticoagulants, aspirin, 325 mg/day, may be used as an alternative. However, it is ineffective in preventing severe strokes or strokes in patients older than 75 years and has not been studied in a population at low risk of AF.[3,4] Clopidogrel plus aspirin is superior to aspirin alone in stroke prevention but is still significantly less effective than warfarin. Anticoagulation in low-risk patients (those younger than 60 years without heart disease) may be accomplished with this combination. Although the risk of stroke is decreased with the combination therapy, there is a risk of bleeding complications.[3,4]

Older adults potentially have multiple comorbidities and a higher risk factor for stroke. (CHA_2DS_2-VASc identifies 65 to 74 years as a minor risk factor and 75 years or older as major risk factor.) Symptoms may be minimal and somewhat atypical with increased age. The risks and comorbidities must be factored into management decisions.[3]

Premature Atrial and Junctional Contractions

In general, PACs and PJCs do not usually require treatment, but the cause should be investigated. In a nondiseased heart of normal structure these irregularities of the rhythm may be a result of increased stimulation as discussed in the section on sinus tachycardia. Their occurrence may diminish or disappear when these stimuli are withdrawn. More concerning causes include ischemia, hypokalemia and hypomagnesemia, hypoxia, and myocardial stretch in early congestive HF. If possible, correct the underlying cause. Symptom management may be necessary, based on individual patient situations, and possibly achieved with beta blockers.

Premature Ventricular Contractions

PVCs occur in both normal and diseased hearts and are of no prognostic significance in the structurally normal heart. As with PACs and PJCs, management follows identifying and treating the underlying cause; beta blockers are the drugs of choice. Complex ventricular ectopy (defined as more than 10 PVCs per minute during 24 hours or nonsustained VT) is rare in the normal heart and should provoke an evaluation for underlying cardiac disease.

Ventricular Tachycardia

Clinical management of nonsustained VT first includes identification and management of any underlying cause (e.g., digoxin toxicity, electrolyte imbalance, hypoxia, ischemia). Patients with previous MI, structural heart disease, or low ejection fractions who have nonsustained VT are at particularly high risk for adverse events, including sudden death. Beta blockers reduce these risks, but referral for electrophysiologic testing should be considered for this group as well as for those with severe symptoms.[17]

Right ventricular outflow tract (RVOT) is the most common form monomorphic nonsustained VT. It is usually initially treated by a cardiologist or electrophysiologist by radiofrequency ablation or beta blockers for symptom relief. However, it is common for the primary care nurse practitioner to continue managing the long-term beta blocker therapy. Nadolol is the nonselective beta blocker of choice. It is long acting and is taken daily, which increases compliance for long-term use. The dose of nadolol for ventricular tachyarrhythmias is often much higher than the dose used for the control of hypertension, and may be titrated up or down for symptom relief.

The patient with cardiac disease and complex ectopy is at increased risk for sudden death. However, antiarrhythmic therapy has not been shown to decrease mortality even though it may reduce the ectopy. In some clinical trials, it was actually shown to increase the risk of sudden cardiac death.[4]

Sustained VT requires emergency treatment and will not be managed in primary care, but the management of the arrhythmia is worth mentioning. Pulseless VT is treated in the same way as VF and requires immediate defibrillation and cardiopulmonary resuscitation. Sustained VT with a pulse requires treatment at an acute care facility, and hemodynamic status is evaluated. Synchronized cardioversion with 100 to 360 joules is recommended for VT with hemodynamic compromise.[8] Therapy to prevent recurrent sustained VT may include pharmacologic management, implantable cardioverter-defibrillator (ICD) implantation, or a combination of the two.

Antiarrhythmic therapy for VT has remained unchanged for the past decade and continues to be limited by the potential for toxicity and proarrhythmia side effects. Amiodarone and sotalol remain the principal agents used in the chronic treatment of VT.[19] Sotalol has a significant adverse effect of torsades de pointes and therefore is initiated in an inpatient setting with continuous ECG monitoring. Beta blockers remain the first-line therapy for patients with systolic HF and after acute MI.

The treatment of polymorphic VT requires consultation with a cardiologist. Beta blockers may be useful in the management of congenital VT, such as long QT syndrome and catecholaminergic polymorphic ventricualr tachycardia (CPVT).[19] Long QT syndrome and Brugada syndrome usually require implantation of an internal defibrillating device in patients with syncope and complex ventricular arrhythmias. Torsades de points is an emergency ventricular arrhythmia that requires immediate intervention and defibrillation. Intravenous magnesium sulfate can facilitate termination of torsades de pointes, but only when the VT is associated with a prolonged QT interval. Magnesium sulfate is not likely to be effective in terminating irregular or polymorphic VT in patients with a normal QT interval.[8]

Electrophysiologic studies with radiofrequency ablation are appropriate for some patients with reentrant VT, and the electrophysiologist will evaluate ventricular function before treatment. Patients may be best managed with ICD implantation. Biventricular pacing can be incorporated into a combination device with an ICD. The use of an ICD is the gold standard therapy in patients with structural heart defects who are at risk of ventricular arrhythmias.[19]

MANAGEMENT OF BRADYARRHYTHMIAS

The initial management of bradyarrhythmias begins with evaluating the hemodynamic stability of the patient and investigating an underlying cause (as with tachyarrhythmias). If the patient is hemodynamically compromised, emergent treatment and referral to the closest hospital are needed. Initial management depends on the underlying cause of the bradycardia. Hemodynamically compromised patients will need a temporary pacemaker, which can be achieved rapidly through transcutaneous electrodes or the insertion of a transvenous pacer wire.

The initial medication used for bradyarrhythmias is atropine, which reverses cholinergic-mediated reductions in heart rate and increases the atrial rate. If the bradyarrhythmia is symptomatic or becoming unstable, atropine is used as a temporary measure while awaiting the placement of a temporary pacemaker. Atropine must be used with great caution if ACS is suspected, because increases in the heart rate may worsen ischemia and cause MI. Atropine may not be effective in patients who have undergone cardiac transplantation because of vagal innervation.[8] The decision to administer atropine to increase heart rate also depends on the underlying rhythm (see section on management of heart blocks). Although they are not first-line agents, intravenous dopamine and epinephrine are alternatives when atropine is ineffective or not appropriate for the patient.[8] These medications require emergency or inpatient monitoring.

In the primary care setting, management of the patient with a bradyarrhythmia who is hemodynamically stable is dependent on finding a reversible cause. Medications routinely prescribed for chronic disease processes should be reviewed. These include beta blockers, calcium channel blockers, digoxin, clonidine, and opiates. Withdrawal of the offending drug may be all that is required for restoration of adequate ventricular rate. Correction of electrolyte imbalances, in particular hyperkalemia, may also resolve the problem. Underlying conditions of hypothyroidism or Lyme disease could also be the causative factor of bradyarrhythmias and are mostly reversible with appropriate treatment of the disease. In general, patients with symptomatic bradycardia should be referred to a cardiologist unless a reversible cause can be identified and corrected, which effectively restores sinus rhythm. Patients with asymptomatic bradycardia may or may not require further intervention; this is largely determined by the type of rhythm and described in the following paragraphs.

Sinus Bradycardia

Sinus bradycardia is treated only if the patient is symptomatic (e.g., lightheadedness or syncope associated with decreased heart rate). Withdrawal of drugs that produce an increase in vagal tone (e.g., edrophonium chloride or digitalis) or that decrease sympathetic tone (e.g., beta blockers, calcium channel blockers, amiodarone, or reserpine) may result in an increase in sinus node activity. A drug such as atropine, which blocks vagal tone, will increase the heart rate. A permanent pacemaker may be necessary for patients with chronic, symptomatic bradycardia.

Sinoatrial Exit Block

SA exit block is managed by removal of the offending cause. Medications, ischemia, or excessive vagal tone may induce this arrhythmia. In the absence of a reversible cause, the rhythm is managed as a sinus bradycardia.

Heart Blocks

Heart block is treated first by correction of any underlying causes. The initial priority for any type of new heart block is to identify coronary risk factors and investigate for coronary ischemia with a 12-lead ECG. Immediate transfer to an emergency facility with interventional cardiology would be the goal for this type of patient in order to rapidly address reperfusion.

If the heart is free from disease and is structurally normal, the causes of heart block are usually acquired. These causes may include hyperkalemia, hypothyroidism, overactive vagus nerve, or sensitivity reaction to medications or toxicity. Pharmacologic agents such as digitalis, beta blockers, calcium channel blockers, or class III agents (sotalol, amiodarone) could be responsible for the arrhythmia. Removal of the offending agent or treatment of the underlying cause should assist in the cessation of most heart blocks.

Atropine reverses cholinergic-mediated reductions in AV nodal conduction and heart rate and may be useful in treating first-degree AV block. However, it is not likely to be as effective in second- or third-degree AV block. Hemodynamic instability is more likely in third-degree AV block and may require intervention with a temporary pacemaker while the underlying cause is treated. Virtually all patients with third-degree AV block will require a permanent pacemaker unless the block is likely to be resolved after the underlying condition is treated. An example is a chronic kidney disease patient with third-degree AV block, hyperkalemia, and digitalis toxicity. The patient may require hemodialysis to address the underlying cause of the heart block but will most likely also require stabilization with a temporary pacemaker until serum potassium and digoxin levels resolve. Discussion regarding a permanent pacemaker would then be warranted based on the unstable nature of renal failure with chronic hemodialysis.

The sudden development of a BBB requires evaluation for coronary disease, structural defects, or medication that could have initiated a new-onset rhythm. Management focuses on treatment of the underlying cause and treatment of any specific symptoms. Once a BBB becomes chronic it is periodically monitored and usually remains asymptomatic. A temporary pacemaker may be necessary in the initial management while the underlying cause is treated.

Use of a temporary pacemaker (transcutaneous or intravenous) may be necessary in the emergency treatment of heart blocks. As soon as the need for continuous pacing is determined, referral to a cardiologist or EP cardiologist will be necessary for the implantation of a permanent pacemaker. Patient follow-up and periodic checks of the pacemaker's function will be managed by the cardiologist.

COMPLICATIONS

An important determinant of mortality from an arrhythmia is the degree and nature of left ventricular dysfunction. Sudden cardiac death is a real and present danger with complex ventricular arrhythmias, particularly in the setting of underlying cardiac disease. Exacerbation of cardiac ischemia or infarction or HF may also occur with tachyarrhythmias or bradyarrhythmias. Reduction in cardiac output will result in decreased perfusion to other vital organs (e.g., brain, kidney). The risk of thromboembolism and stroke with AF has been previously discussed, as have the proarrhythmic effects of many of the antiarrhythmic agents. Lethal proarrhythmias are a serious adverse reaction that must be considered and monitored for in patients receiving antiarrhythmic therapy.[8,17,19]

INDICATIONS FOR REFERRAL OR HOSPITALIZATION

Hospital

Immediate emergency department referral was discussed under management of the arrhythmia, and hospitalization is required for any arrhythmia that produces hemodynamic decompensation such as hypotension, syncope, or chest pain. A loss of pulse requires initiation of cardiopulmonary resuscitation.

Cardiologist

The treatment of serious, recurrent, or potentially life-threatening arrhythmias requires referral to a cardiologist. Therapies may be initiated on an inpatient basis and managed on an outpatient basis. Patients requiring treatment of severe bradycardias and AV blocks will also be referred to a cardiologist; treatment usually requires a single- or dual-chambered permanent pacemaker.

Electrophysiology Cardiologist

Referral to an electrophysiologist is required if treatment of the arrhythmia warrants electrophysiologic studies or procedures such as a pacemaker, catheter radiofrequency ablation, or ICD implantation. Radiofrequency ablation is an option provided by electrophysiologists to locate the source of an arrhythmia and manipulate or eradicate it. Electrophysiologic studies are also required for guided pharmacologic therapy in the treatment of complex, potentially life-threatening arrhythmias, if the patient is refractory to standard drug therapy, or if the drug therapy itself produces life-threatening proarrhythmia.

LIFE SPAN CONSIDERATIONS

Older patients have the highest incidence of arrhythmias as well as other comorbid conditions. Renal, hepatic, and cardiovascular disease will greatly affect left ventricular function, tolerance of the arrhythmia, and ability for clearance of antiarrhythmic agents. Interactions with other agents must also be considered in treating an older patient for arrhythmias. Prescribing an agent such as amiodarone to a patient who is already taking warfarin or digoxin will, for example, increase the plasma levels of these drugs.

PATIENT AND FAMILY EDUCATION

First, the nature of any particular arrhythmia should be explained to the patient. When the arrhythmia is benign or harmless, this information may serve to alleviate unnecessary fears. When a potentially serious arrhythmia does exist, a frank discussion of the problem and treatment options may serve to enhance understanding and guide the decision-making process.

Lifestyle modifications may be needed to eliminate the source of the arrhythmia, particularly in tachyarrhythmias induced by stimulants or stressors. Therefore, discussion regarding the avoidance of any potential stimuli is important (e.g., alcohol, caffeine, decongestant medications, cocaine, cigarettes). Recommendations concerning steps to follow when the arrhythmia occurs should include a plan that addresses where and when to seek treatment. Careful medication teaching, including proper scheduling of doses, potential side effects, and interactions with over-the-counter medications, is essential.

Information should be provided about the relative efficacy and potential side effects of antiarrhythmic agents and antiarrhythmic devices. Risks and benefits of all appropriate interventions will need to be discussed with the patient and family before initiation, and better results are achieved when the patient has input into the decision-making process. When implantation of a device is the most appropriate option (such as permanent pacemaker or automatic ICD), a review of special precautions should be presented. The manufacturer is often able to provide excellent educational materials specific to any particular device.

Finally, the importance of involving family and significant others in teaching cannot be overemphasized. Depending on the nature of an arrhythmia, an individual may be rendered incapable of intervening on his or her behalf during an acute event. Family or others who are able to act in a timely and appropriate fashion may influence the outcome and survival of the affected individual. The families of patients with arrhythmias should learn cardiopulmonary resuscitation and develop an emergency plan.

CHAPTER 119

CAROTID ARTERY DISEASE

Virginia Curtin Capasso • Alicia Wierenga

Stroke is now the fourth leading cause of death, behind heart disease, cancer, and chronic lower respiratory disease (CLRD), when considered separately from other cardiovascular diseases (CVDs).[1] Stroke remains the leading cause of serious long-term disability in the United States.[2] Each year, more than 795,000 people have a stroke, over 75% of which are new attacks.[1] In the United States, in 2011, stroke accounted for approximately 1 in 20 deaths.[1] The age-adjusted death rate for stroke as an underlying cause of death was 37.9 per 100,000.[1] Because of the larger number of elderly women, more women than men die of stroke each year, with women accounting for 60% of the U.S. stroke deaths.[1] Between 2001 and 2011, the stroke death rate decreased 35.1% and the actual number of stroke deaths decreased 21.2%—a finding associated with a greater decline for persons aged 60 years or older than younger individuals, and whites as compared with most racial and ethnic minority groups except Hispanics, who have lower mortality rates for ischemic stroke and intracerebral hemorrhage (ICH).[3] Factors contributing the most substantial influence on declining stroke mortality include control of hypertension and control of diabetes mellitus (DM) and high cholesterol, especially in combination with treatment of hypertension.[1]

The vast majority of strokes (80% to 90%) are ischemic strokes.[4] Approximately 20% of ischemic strokes result from carotid artery disease,[5] which is defined as atherosclerotic narrowing of the extracranial arteries (60% to 99%),[4] most often at the bifurcation of the carotid artery with involvement of the proximal internal carotid artery (ICA). Carotid stenosis (CS) increases from the fifth decade of life onward. The overall estimated prevalence of CS (defined as 70% or 75% to 99% stenosis) is 0.5% to 1%.[6]

CS may be symptomatic or asymptomatic. Symptomatic CS manifests with its sequelae: transient ischemic attack (TIA), ischemic stroke, or a range of more subtle but enduring neurologic deficits.[7] TIA is defined as a syndrome of acute neurologic dysfunction referable to the distribution of a single brain artery and characterized by symptoms that last for less than 24 hours without acute infarction.[8,9] Ischemic stroke involves neurologic deficit that persists longer than 24 hours.[8] Even in the presence of high-grade CS, patients may truly be asymptomatic or may exhibit nonspecific symptoms, which do not qualify as symptomatic ischemic events.[7]

The age-, sex-, and race-adjusted incidence of TIA is 0.83 per 10,000.[10] The prevalence increases with age and varies by sex and race or ethnicity. Men, blacks, and Mexican Americans have higher rates of TIA than women and non-Hispanic whites.[11-13] A TIA is an important predictor that precedes approximately 15% of strokes. The risk of stroke is highest during the first week after the initial event, 17.3% in the first 30 days, as high as 20.1% in the first 90 days, and up to 30% within 5 years.[14] Data from the Framingham Heart Study (FHS) of the National Heart, Lung, and Blood Institute (NHLBI) during three timeframes (1950 to 1977, 1978 to 1989, and 1990 to 2004) showed a progressively decreasing age-adjusted incidence of first stroke per 1000 person-years of 7.6, 6.2, and 5.3 in men and 6.2, 5.8, and 5.1 in women, respectively. Lifetime risk of stroke at 65 years of age decreased significantly, from 19.5% to 14.5% in men and from 18.0% to 16.1% in women. Age-adjusted stroke severity did not vary across periods; however, 30-day mortality rate decreased significantly in men (from 23% to 14%) but not in women (from 21% to 20%).[15]

In a study of a European general population,[15] the prevalence of moderate asymptomatic carotid artery stenosis (ACAS) (≥50% stenosis measured by Doppler ultrasonography) increased with age and was higher for men. The prevalence of severe stenosis was higher among individuals aged 60 years or older who had a history of vascular disease. For men, the prevalence of moderate ACAS increased from 0.2% (95% confidence interval [CI] 0.0%-0.4%) to 7.5% (95% CI 5.2%-10.5%) and the prevalence of severe ACAS (≥70% stenosis) increased from 0.1% (95% CI 0.0%-0.3%) to 3.1% (95% CI 1.7%-5.3%). Among women, the prevalence of moderate ACAS increased from 0% (95% CI 0.0%-0.2%) to 5.0% (95% CI 3.1%-7.5%); for severe ACAS, the prevalence increased from 0% (95% CI 0.0%-0.2%) to 0.9% (95% CI 0.3%-2.4%).

PATHOPHYSIOLOGY

Atherosclerotic CS originates near the bifurcation of the common carotid artery (CCA) in the region of the bulb.[8,16] Conditions near the bulb, including low shear stress, flow separation, and nonlaminar flow, increase the contact time between blood-borne particles, such as lipids, and the vessel wall. A fatty streak, consisting of monocytes that differentiate into lipid-laden macrophages, or foam cells, eventually develops into an atherosclerotic plaque. As the plaque enlarges, blood flow to the brain can be reduced or interrupted by severe narrowing or occlusion of the ICA. In addition, turbulence may actually damage the atherosclerotic plaque, resulting in loss of intimal continuity or ulceration. Platelets and fibrin aggregate on the roughened intimal surface, and there is subsequent thrombosis. Fragments of a fractured plaque or thrombus may embolize to smaller distal arteries. Interruption of cerebral blood flow and cerebral infarction are the potential life-threatening sequelae.

CLINICAL PRESENTATION

As noted earlier, CS may be symptomatic or asymptomatic. Patients with severe CS may be asymptomatic if the circle of Willis is competent and adequately perfuses the territory of the middle cerebral artery.

The presentation of symptomatic CS may consist of transient or permanent focal neurologic symptoms related to the ipsilateral retina or cerebral hemisphere, including retinal ischemia manifesting with a brief, fleeting attack of monocular blindness (amaurosis fugax), weakness or numbness of the contralateral arm, leg, and/or side of the face, visual field defect, dysarthria, and, in the case of involvement of the dominant hemisphere (usually left), aphasia. Asymptomatic CS may be detected on a routine physical examination or during a workup for ill-defined symptoms, such as dizziness, generalized weakness, syncope or near-syncopal episodes, blurred vision, or transient visual phenomena such as "floaters" or "stars."

In the history of individuals with CS, there are important nonmodifiable and modifiable risk factors. The nonmodifiable risk factors include age, gender, race, and ethnic background. The modifiable risk factors include high blood pressure, cigarette smoking, hyperlipidemia, DM, hyperhomocysteinemia, obesity, nutrition, physical inactivity, and chronic kidney disease (CKD). Other modifiable risk factors may include heavy alcohol consumption, sleep apnea,[17] and depression.[2,17-19]

Numerous studies have demonstrated that CS is present and, without medical therapy, worsens with advancing age.

On average, women who sustain a stroke are approximately 4 years older than their male counterparts (75 years versus 71 years).[20] Women aged 45 to 54 years are twice as likely to have had a stroke as age-matched male peers. Furthermore, women aged 45 to 54 years are four times more likely than women aged 35 to 44 years to have had a stroke. Women with atrial fibrillation are at significantly higher risk of stroke than men.[21] Migraine with aura is associated with ischemic stroke in younger women, particularly if they smoke or use oral contraceptives.[22] In generally healthy postmenopausal women, hormonal treatment with combination estrogen and progestin and conjugate equine estrogen alone increases stroke risk by 44% and 55%, respectively. The proportion of antenatal and postpartum hospitalizations for stroke increased between the mid-1990s and the first decade of 2000, specifically attributable to hypertensive disorders during the postpartum period.[23] Menopause before age 42 years is associated with twice the risk of stroke experienced by postmenopausal women in other age groups.[19]

Blood pressure is a powerful determinant of CS, ischemic stroke, and ICH.[1,19] In the FHS, there was a twofold greater risk of CS of more than 25% for each 2-mm Hg increase in systolic blood pressure.[24] In the Systolic Hypertension in the Elderly Program (SHEP), systolic blood pressure of 160 mm Hg or higher was the strongest independent predictor of CS.[25] For each 10-mm Hg increase in blood pressure, the risk of stroke increases by 8% in whites. In contrast, a threefold increase in stroke risk, at 24%, is noted in African Americans.[1]

Cigarette smoking also is a strong independent risk factor for ischemic stroke. Current smokers are at a risk of stroke that is two to four times higher than nonsmokers or those who have quit for more than 10 years.[26,27] Smoking increases the relative risk (RR) of ischemic stroke by 25% to 50%.[8] Cigarette smoking is associated with extracranial carotid artery intima-media thickness (IMT) and the severity of CS. Furthermore, the severity of CS has been shown to be greater among current smokers than nonsmokers and is significantly related to pack-years of smoking.[28]

Epidemiologic studies consistently have shown an association between cholesterol and carotid IMT, although only a modest or weak association between elevated total cholesterol or low-density lipoprotein cholesterol (LDL-C) and increased risk of ischemic stroke.[8,18] Conversely, in the Women's Health Study, total cholesterol and LDL-C levels were strongly associated with increased risk of ischemic stroke.[29] The literature also supports an inverse association between high-density lipoprotein cholesterol (HDL-C) and stroke or carotid atherosclerosis.[30]

DM is associated with a twofold to fivefold increase in ischemic stroke.[11] Patients with DM who sustain an ischemic stroke typically are younger, more likely to be black, and more likely to have hypertension, myocardial infarction (MI), and high cholesterol than counterparts without diabetes.[31] Although the absolute number of hospitalizations for acute ischemic stroke decreased 17% between 1997 and 2006, the number of hospitalizations for acute ischemic stroke with comorbid DM rose by 27% during the same time period.[32]

Numerous studies have demonstrated an association between diabetes and progression of carotid IMT. In the Epidemiology of Diabetes Interventions and Complications (EDIC) study, progression of IMT was greater among patients with diabetes than those without diabetes, although it was less among patients with diabetes who were treated with intensive insulin therapy.[33] In several studies, intensive therapy to reduce blood glucose has not reduced the risk of stroke in patients with type 2 DM. In contrast, long-term follow-up of patients in the Diabetes Control and Complications Trial (DCCT) who had type 1 diabetes treated with intensive insulin therapy has shown a 57% reduction in the rate of nonfatal MI, stroke, and death, although the absolute risk reduction was small at less than 1% over 17 years of follow-up.[34]

Hyperhomocysteinemia increases the risk of stroke. Among elderly patients with elevated homocysteine levels, there is a twofold risk of development of CS of more than 25%. In the Atherosclerosis Risk in Communities (ARIC) study,[35] increased carotid IMT was three times more likely among patients with the highest quantile versus lowest quantile of homocysteine. Intake of grain products enriched with folic acid has been associated with decreased stroke rates and plasma concentrations of homocysteine. However, studies of patients with vascular disease have not confirmed a benefit of homocysteine lowering by B-complex vitamin therapy on cardiovascular outcomes, including stroke.

Obesity, defined as body mass index above 30 kg/m^2, has been established as an independent risk factor for coronary heart disease (CHD) and premature mortality. The relationship of obesity to stroke has been studied mostly in relationship to primary prevention. In studies of components of the metabolic syndrome (i.e., blood glucose, hypertension, dyslipidemia, body mass index, waist/hip ratio, and urinary albumin excretion), a strong relationship exists between obesity and carotid atherosclerosis, behind hypertension and hypercholesterolemia.[11]

Several studies have demonstrated the effect of nutrition on risk of stroke. In a randomized clinical trial in Spain, a Mediterranean-style diet that is rich in nuts and olive oil was associated with a reduced risk stroke (hazard ratio [HR] 0.54; 95% CI 0.35-0.84).[36] The Nurses' Health Study showed that each one-serving increase in sugar-sweetened soda was associated with a 13% increase in risk of ischemic stroke. However, each one-serving increase in low-sugar soda was associated with a 7% increase in ischemic stroke as well as a 27% increase in hemorrhagic stroke.[37] In Sweden, individuals without hypertension who consumed seven or more servings of fruits and vegetables each day had a 19% lower risk of stroke than those who ate only one serving per day.[38]

Physical inactivity is a well-documented, modifiable risk factor for stroke. Individuals who exercised four or more times per week had a 20% lower risk of stroke than persons who exercised fewer than four times per week. The effect is largely caused by reduction of other risk factors such as DM and obesity.[39]

CKD is an independent risk factor for CVD. In a study of 1003 patients aged 50 years or older who underwent carotid ultrasonography and evaluation of kidney function by estimated glomerular filtration rate (eGFR) and presence of proteinuria, eGFR was significantly correlated with mean maximal carotid IMT but not carotid calcification.[40] Furthermore, in multiple regression analysis, reduced eGFR, proteinuria, age, male sex, CVD, hypertension, DM, and smoking were independently associated with mean max-IMT. In a secondary analysis of the outcomes of patients with and without CKD among those enrolled in the North American Symptomatic Carotid Endarterectomy Trial (NASCET), individuals who had a glomerular filtration rate (GFR) below 30 mL/min/1.73 m^2 with symptomatic high-grade CS (≥70%) and who were treated medically had much higher rates of stroke, MI, or death than counterparts with normal GFR.[41]

PHYSICAL EXAMINATION

The physical examination should include a complete cardiovascular and neurologic examination. Important components of the cardiovascular examination include palpation of all bilateral peripheral pulses and auscultation for bruits, as well as blood pressures in bilateral upper extremities in the lying and sitting positions. The neurologic examination should include an examination of mental status, cranial nerves (including funduscopic examination), and motor and sensory function.

Carotid auscultation for bruit is a marker for generalized atherosclerosis and may be used to screen asymptomatic patients with vascular risk factors. However, because bruits are produced by turbulent flow, they may be pronounced with mild stenosis and less audible or undetectable with severe or critical stenosis. Thus, carotid bruits have relatively low sensitivity for detection of moderate to severe CS[8,42] and auscultation of the neck for carotid bruits is of limited value in evaluating patients with symptoms of TIA or stroke. Symptomatic patients must undergo imaging studies.

DIAGNOSTICS

Catheter-based angiography is the criterion standard for defining the degree of stenosis and morphologic characteristics of offending plaque in CS, although it has inherent cost and risks including risk of stroke in about 1% of patients and death in 0.1%.[43] Thus, duplex ultrasound, which measures blood flow velocity as an indicator of severity of stenosis, is now the primary diagnostic tool for CS. Indications for carotid duplex ultrasound include the following[8]:

- Cervical bruit in an asymptomatic patient
- Serial surveillance of known stenosis (>20%) in asymptomatic individuals
- Vascular assessment in a patient with multiple risk factors for atherosclerosis
- Stroke risk assessment in patient with CAD or peripheral arterial disease (PAD)
- Amaurosis fugax
- Hemispheric TIA
- Stroke in a candidate for carotid revascularization
- Serial surveillance after carotid revascularization procedure
- Intraoperative assessment during carotid endarterectomy (CEA)

A meta-analysis of studies of color duplex ultrasound demonstrated that when the peak systolic velocity is 130 cm/sec or greater, the sensitivity and specificity are very high—98% and 88%, respectively—in detecting stenotic ICA lesions of 50% or greater. In the setting of a peak systolic velocity of 130 cm/sec or greater, the sensitivity and specificity of duplex ultrasound are 90% and 94%, respectively, in the detection of stenotic lesions of 70% or greater.[44] For recognizing carotid occlusion, duplex ultrasound has been shown to have a sensitivity of 96% and specificity of 100%.[45] There is also high agreement between duplex ultrasound and arteriography in the detection of more than 45% stenosis in the carotid artery.[44,46]

Magnetic resonance angiography (MRA) and computed tomography angiography (CTA) may be indicated as alternatives or adjuncts to duplex ultrasound in the following scenarios: (1) when duplex ultrasound cannot be obtained, (2) when results of duplex ultrasound are inconclusive, (3) when further evaluation of the severity of stenosis and identification of intrathoracic or intracranial vascular lesions is needed before intervention for severe CS. CTA may be preferred for patients who are not suitable candidates for MRA because of claustrophobia, implanted pacemakers, or other incompatible devices. CTA can provide imaging from the aortic arch to the circle of Willis, defining bone and soft tissue structures surrounding the diseased carotid arteries, tracing the course of a vessel that is tortuous or has a high bifurcation, and directly imaging the vessel lumen and allowing evaluation of stenosis. However, CTA may underestimate CS as compared with rotational angiography. Catheter-based angiography may still be necessary to detect and characterize extracranial cerebrovascular disease when noninvasive imaging is inconclusive or not feasible because of technical limitations or when noninvasive imaging studies yield discordant results.[8]

DIFFERENTIAL DIAGNOSIS

The differential diagnosis of symptomatic CS includes intracranial arterial stenosis, atheromatous disease of the aortic arch, partial seizure, radiculopathy, neuropathy, microvascular cerebral or spinal pathology, and lacunar stroke. Causes of intracranial arterial stenosis include atherosclerosis, intimal fibroplasia, vasculitis, adventitial cysts, or vascular tumors. Intracranial arterial occlusion may occur as a result of thrombosis or embolism arising from the aortic arch, cardiac chambers, heart valves, or a defect in the septum of the heart allowing a right-to-left shunt. Symptoms and signs of ischemia or infarction in the vertebrobasilar system may include ataxia, cranial nerve deficits, visual field loss, dizziness, imbalance, and incoordination.[8] Partial seizure may be associated with brief, stereotyped, repetitive behaviors, and electroencephalography is required to confirm the diagnosis. Causes that account for purely sensory symptoms (i.e., numbness, pain, or paresthesia) include radiculopathy, neuropathy, microvascular cerebral or spinal pathology, and lacunar stroke.

MANAGEMENT

Current options for management of CS include medical therapy alone and carotid revascularization (i.e., CEA or carotid angioplasty and stenting [Carotid Angioplasty and Stenting]) *plus* medical management. To date, there have been no reported studies involving head-to-head comparison of the three treatment approaches. Thus, according to the 2011 collaborative guidelines from the American Heart Association (AHA), the effectiveness of revascularization by CEA or CS versus medical therapy alone has not been well established, especially in asymptomatic CS.[8] To address this gap, the Carotid Revascularization and Medical Management for Asymptomatic Carotid Stenosis Trial (CREST-2), a clinical trial funded by the National Institute of Neurological Disorders and Stroke (NINDS) of the National Institutes of Health (NIH), began enrolling patients in December 2014.[47] The study involves two parallel, randomized trials. In one trial, patients with at least 70% stenosis of the cervical ICA are randomized to either the combination of CEA and intensive medical management or intensive medical management alone. In the second trial, patients with at least 70% stenosis of the cervical ICA are randomized to either the combination of CS and intensive medical management or intensive medical management alone.[48] The primary end point is any stroke or death during the periprocedural period and ipsilateral stroke thereafter, out to 4 years of follow-up.

Of note, carotid revascularization is not recommended in the setting of the following three conditions: (1) narrowing of the ipsilateral ICA by less than 50%, (2) chronic total occlusion of the affected carotid artery, and (3) severe disability consequent to cerebral infarction that precludes preservation of useful function.

Medical Therapy

Analysis of data from several studies published in the early 1990s, which included either an arm of medical therapy alone or initial therapy with only medical therapy, revealed that the stroke rate has decreased since the mid-1980s. In NASCET, symptomatic patients treated for 18 months with medical therapy alone without revascularization had stroke rates of 19% for individuals with 70% to 79% initial stenosis, 28% with 80% to 89% stenosis, 33% with 90% to 99% stenosis, and diminished risk near occlusion.[49] Among asymptomatic individuals managed with medical therapy alone in the ACAS trial, the rate of ipsilateral stroke or death during a 5-year period was 11%.[50] In the Asymptomatic Carotid Surgery Trial (ACST), the risk of ipsilateral stroke or death during a 5-year period in patients with 70% or greater stenosis randomized to initial medical therapy was 4.7%.[51]

From 1999 to 2003, the Warfarin-Aspirin Symptomatic Intracranial Disease (WASID) trial was conducted involving 567 patients with symptomatic high-grade intracranial atherosclerotic stenosis who were randomized to treatment with aspirin or warfarin and standard approaches to risk factor management that were prevalent during that time period.[52] The 30-day rate of stroke or death of 10.7% and a 1-year rate of the primary end point (ischemic stroke, brain hemorrhage, or death from vascular causes other than stroke) was 25.7%. In a subsequent study, the Stenting and Aggressive Medical Management for Preventing Recurrent Stroke in Intracranial Stenosis (SAMMPRIS) study, 451 similar patients were randomized to intracranial stenting or medical therapy from 2008 to 2011.[52] In the SAMMPRIS study, medical therapy was much more aggressive, guideline driven, and more intensely monitored than in the WASID trial. In the SAMMPRIS study the stroke and death outcome (5.8%) and the stroke, MI, and death composite primary outcome (12.2%) for medical therapy were 5.8% and 12.2%, respectively—about half of rate achieved in WASID.

Carotid Endarterectomy

The effectiveness of CEA plus medical management versus medical management alone on event rates has been studied in symptomatic patients and asymptomatic patients. Studies of the effectiveness of CEA in symptomatic patients (i.e., history of TIA or mild stroke and 30% to 99% ipsilateral CS) include two large randomized trials: NASCET[49] and the European Carotid Surgery Trial (ECST).[34] In these studies, randomization was stratified by severity of stenosis, although the trials differed on method of measurement of CS and definitions of outcome events. Three studies compared the effectiveness of CEA plus medical therapy versus medical therapy alone in asymptomatic patients, including ACAS,[50] ACST,[51] and the Veterans Affairs Cooperative Study (VACS).[32]

Carotid Endarterectomy for Symptomatic Patients. In NASCET, high-grade stenosis was defined as 70% to 99% reduction of the diameter of the vessel lumen at the point of greatest stenosis. Lower grade stenosis was defined as 30% to 69% reduction in luminal diameter. After 18 months of follow-up, NASCET stopped enrolling patients in the high-grade stenosis group (70% to 99%) because the benefit of CEA over medical therapy alone was clear. At 2 years, the cumulative risk of stroke was significantly lower for the CEA group (9%) than for the medical management group (26%). NASCET also demonstrated a benefit of CEA for patients with 50% to 69% CS. The 30-day rate of death or stroke was 6.7%. At 5-years, the rate of ipsilateral stroke was 15.7% for the CEA group versus 22% for the medical management group. No benefit was found for CEA among individuals with less than 50% CS.

In the ECST, randomization also was stratified according to severity of stenosis, which was defined as mild (10% to 29%), moderate (30% to 69%), and severe (70% to 99%).[53] ECST also showed highly significant benefit of CEA for patients with severe stenosis but no benefit for patients with lower grade stenosis. After adjustment for primary end points and duration of follow-up, the benefit of CEA for symptomatic patients with high-grade CS was similar for men and women in NASCET and ECST.

The Very Urgent Carotid Endarterectomy Confers Increased Procedural Risk Study found that patients who sustained a neurologic event and were treated with CEA were at higher risk for mortality and stroke if the procedure was done at day 0 to 2 after event (11.5%) versus day 3 to 7 (3.6%).[54]

Carotid Endarterectomy for Asymptomatic Patients. Several studies have examined the effect of CEA in asymptomatic patients (i.e., atherosclerotic narrowing of the proximal ICA exceeding 50% to 60% in the absence of previous referable symptoms of TIA or stroke[49]), although the end points of the studies varied. VACS[52] compared the rates of TIA, stroke, and death among individuals treated with surgery plus aspirin and risk factor modification versus with medical management alone. At 30 days, the death rate was 1.9%, stroke rate was 2.4%, and combined event rate was 4.3% for patients who underwent surgery. At 5 years, the rate of adverse events was significantly lower for patients undergoing CEA (10%) versus medical therapy (20%).

In ACAS, TIA was not included as an end point.[50] The trial was stopped early, when an advantage of CEA was apparent among patients with greater than 60% CS. The 30-day death rate was 2.3%. After mean follow-up of 2.7 years, the projected 5-year rates of ipsilateral stroke, perioperative stroke, and death for patients treated surgically and medically were 5.1% and 11%, respectively.

In ACST, asymptomatic patients with hemodynamically significant CS were randomized to two groups: (1) immediate surgery, and (2) delayed surgery.[51] At 30 days the risk of stroke and death was 3.1% in both groups. The 5-year adverse event rate demonstrated an important advantage for the early surgery group (6.4%) over the delayed surgery group (11.4%).

In summary, the AHA 2011 collaborative guidelines[8] recommend CEA within 6 months for patients with symptomatic CS. Criteria for CEA include (1) average to low surgical risk; (2) reduction of the diameter of the lumen of the ipsilateral ICA by more than 70% as measured by noninvasive imaging, or more than 50% as measured by catheter angiography; and (3) an anticipated rate of perioperative stroke or mortality of less than 6%. When compared with CS, CEA may be preferred when arterial anatomy is unfavorable for endovascular intervention.

Periprocedural Care. Before CEA, cardiac risk assessment is conducted. Blood pressure is controlled with beta blockers and angiotensin inhibitors. Antithrombotic therapy begins with aspirin 81 mg to 325 mg daily, clopidogrel (75 mg daily), or a combination of low-dose aspirin (25 mg daily) plus extended-release dipyridamole (200 mg daily), for 1 week before CEA. If not previously prescribed, statin medications also are administered for 1 week before CEA.

CEA may be performed using general anesthesia or local anesthesia. The procedure begins with an incision along the anterior border of the sternocleidomastoid muscle, repositioning and protecting the internal jugular vein and vagus nerve to expose the common, internal, and external carotid arteries.[55] After the patient is heparinized, the common and external carotid arteries are clamped sequentially. A longitudinal incision is made in the CCA, extending distally through the bifurcation to the ICA beyond the offending plaque. The plaque is everted from the external carotid artery (ECA) then the ICA. The arteriotomy is closed using a patch of autogenous vein, Dacron, or bovine pericardium, although no single material has been shown to be superior. Flow is restored to the ECA then the ICA. Completion angiogram or duplex ultrasound may be done to evaluate residual stenosis, which occurs in less than 1% of cases.

Patients who have undergone CEA initially stay in the postanesthesia care unit (PACU) for about 4 hours, then are transferred to the acute care unit for neurologic, cardiac, and vascular monitoring. In our institution, stable patients usually are discharged to home on the first postoperative day (POD). Skilled nursing visits for blood pressure checks are scheduled for POD 2 or 3 and POD 7 or 8.

Medical management includes control of blood pressure with beta blockers and angiotensin inhibitors and antithrombotic therapy with aspirin (75 mg to 325 mg daily indefinitely after surgery), clopidogrel (75 mg daily), or a combination of low-dose aspirin (25 mg daily) plus extended-release dipyridamole (200 mg daily), and statin medications.

Surveillance of the extracranial carotid arteries by noninvasive imaging, to detect new ipsilateral or contralateral lesions, is recommended at 1 month, 6 months, 1 year, and annually after CEA.[8] Surveillance may be discontinued when the patient is no longer a candidate for intervention.

Complications of Carotid Endarterectomy. Possible complications of CEA include hypertension (20%), hypotension (5%), hemorrhage, acute arterial occlusion, stroke, MI (1%), venous thromboembolism (0.1%), cranial nerve palsy, infection, arterial restenosis, and death. The risk of stroke or death is higher among symptomatic patients (3.2%) than asymptomatic patients (1.4%), patients with hemispheric symptoms versus retinal symptoms, urgent operation versus nonurgent operation, reoperation versus primary surgery, and those with renal insufficiency.[56] ICH may occur as a consequence of hyperperfusion syndrome, although the rate is less than 1% among patients whose blood pressure is stable preoperatively and well controlled perioperatively.

Cranial nerve injuries occur in 5% to 7% of cases, which, in decreasing order of frequency and with most common clinical presentation, usually involve the hypoglossal nerve (atrophy of tongue musculature), marginal mandibular nerve (asymmetric smile), recurrent laryngeal nerve (hoarseness), spinal accessory nerves (weakness of trapezius muscle), and Horner syndrome. Cranial nerve dysfunction is linked to a duration of surgical procedure longer than 2 hours. Approximately 25% of cranial nerve injuries resolve before discharge from the hospital.

Wound complications include infection (≤1%) and hematoma (≤5%). Factors contributing to wound complications include perioperative antiplatelet therapy, duration of surgery, and perioperative heparin and protamine therapy.

Arterial restenosis occurs at two predictable timeframes: within 18 months (but usually within 6 months after CEA), and at 5 years or more after surgery. The earlier restenosis is a result of intimal hyperplasia. The later restenosis is caused by progressive atherosclerotic disease. When outcomes of CEA were compared with those of CS, rates of early restenosis (>70%) were lower in the CEA group than the CS group in the Carotid and Vertebral Artery Transluminal Angioplasty Study (CAVATAS)[57] (4% versus 14%, respectively) and Stent-Protected Angioplasty Versus Carotid Endarterectomy (SPACE) trial[58] (4.6 versus 10.7%, respectively), although the rate of restenosis at 1 year was higher in the CEA group (4.2%) versus the CS group (0.8%) in the Stenting and Angioplasty with Protection in Patients at High Risk for Endarterectomy (SAPPHIRE) study.[59] Two years after the SPACE trial, there was no difference in the rate of restenosis between the CS and CEA groups at 9.5% and 8.8%, respectively.[60] The collaborative AHA guidelines[8] recommend repeat CEA or CS for symptomatic patients with greater than

50% recurrent stenosis or asymptomatic patients with greater than 80% recurrent CS and risk of periprocedural risk of stroke or death below 6%. Revascularization by CEA or CS is not recommended in symptomatic patients with less than 70% CS that has remained stable over time.

Carotid Angioplasty and Stenting

Numerous studies have compared the outcomes of CEA and CS. These studies include the Carotid Revascularization Using Endarterectomy or Stenting Systems (CaRESS) study and the SAPPHIRE Study.

CaRESS was a nonrandomized study that compared symptomatic patients with greater than 50% CS and asymptomatic patients with greater than 75% CS who underwent CEA and CS.[61,62] Study results revealed no significant differences in event rates (i.e., MI, stroke, and death at 30 days and 1 year and restenosis and revascularization at 1 year) for patients undergoing the two types of revascularization procedures.

SAPPHIRE is the only study that has compared the outcomes of high-risk patients (i.e., age >80 years, New York Heart Association Class III or IV heart failure, chronic obstructive pulmonary disease, >50% contralateral CS, prior CEA or CS, or prior coronary artery bypass graft [CABG] surgery) undergoing CEA and CS. Rates of periprocedural MI, stroke, and death were twice as high for CEA as for CS at 30 days and 1 year, possibly as a consequence of determining the rate of MI only on the basis of sensitive cardiac serum biomarker data. Among symptomatic patients, the periprocedural event rate was similar following CEA (16.5%) and CS (16.8%). Among asymptomatic patients, the rate of MI, stroke, and death after CEA (21.5%) was over twice the event rate after CS (9.9%).[63] At 1 year, CEA was associated with significantly higher rates of cranial nerve palsy (4.9% and 0%, respectively) and target-vessel revascularization (4% and 0.6%, respectively) than CS. At 3 years, the rates of stroke and target-vessel revascularization were similar for CEA and CS.[64]

Several other studies have compared the outcomes of conventional-risk patients who underwent CEA and CS. In CAVATAS, which compared endovascular and medical therapy, the rate of stroke or death at 30 days was 10% in both groups; at 1 year, the rates of cranial neuropathy, major hemorrhage, MI, and pulmonary embolism were lower and the rate of restenosis was higher among patients who underwent CS; at 3 years, the stroke and death rate was similar (14.2%) in both groups. In the SPACE trial, which randomized symptomatic patients with high-grade CS (>70% by ultrasound), TIA, or stroke, there was no significant difference between treatment groups on outcomes at 30 days. The Endarterectomy Versus Angioplasty in Patients with Symptomatic Severe Carotid Stenosis (EVA-3S) study was terminated early because of a significantly higher rate of stroke in the CS group (24%) versus the CEA group (9%) ($P = .01$).[65] In the International Carotid Stenting Study (ICSS), a European multicenter randomized controlled trial that compared the safety and effectiveness of CEA versus CS in symptomatic patients with greater than 50% stenosis, the 120-day composite adverse event rate for stroke, death, or MI was 5.2% in the CEA group versus 8.5% in the CS group ($P = .006$).[66]

The Carotid Revascularization Versus Endarterectomy Trial (CREST)[67] compared the periprocedural risk of stroke, death, and MI and ipsilateral risk of stroke up to 4 years after CEA and CS in conventional-risk, symptomatic patients with greater than 50% CS and asymptomatic patients with greater than 60% stenosis. After mean follow-up of 2.5 years, results revealed that there was no significant difference in the overall rate of primary events for CEA (6.8%) and CS (7.2%). However, significant differences existed between CEA and CS on the periprocedural rate of stroke (2.3% versus 4.1%, respectively) and MI (2.3% versus 1.1%, respectively). At 1 year, major and minor stroke was shown to have a greater impact on quality of life than MI. Furthermore, improved outcomes were observed with CEA for patients older than 70 years, whereas patients younger than 70 years had better outcomes with CS. Similar to the SAPPHIRE study, the rate of cranial nerve palsy in CREST was higher after CEA than CS.

The collaborative AHA guidelines[8] recommend CS only for symptomatic patients who meet the following criteria: (1) average or low risk of complications associated with endovascular intervention; (2) narrowing of the arterial lumen of more than 70% as shown by noninvasive imaging, or more than 50% as demonstrated by catheter angiography; and (3) risk of periprocedural stroke or death below 6%. CS may be preferred over CEA when the neck anatomy is unfavorable for arterial surgery (e.g., previous neck surgery or radiation injury).

Procedure. At least 2 days before the planned procedure, patients undergoing CS are started on aspirin, 81 to 325 mg by mouth once per day, and clopidogrel, 75 mg by mouth twice per day. CS is performed with minimal or no local sedation; patients may be asked to squeeze an audible toy with the contralateral hand to allow assessment of gross neurologic function during instrumentation of the carotid artery.[36] During the procedure, cardiac rate and rhythm, oxygen saturation, and blood pressure are monitored because instrumentation of the carotid bulb may be associated with bradycardia and hypotension.

Traditional Approach to Carotid Angioplasty and Stenting. The traditional approach to catheterization has been a retrograde femoral approach, although iliofemoral occlusive disease may necessitate brachial or radial access, and anomalies of the aortic arch may necessitate direct cannulation of the cervical CCA.

Once a decision has been made to proceed with CS, a loading dose of heparin, 100 IU/kg, is administered. Heparin dose is adjusted to maintain the activated clotting time (ACT) of 250 to 300 seconds throughout the procedure.

After insertion of a 5-F catheter over a 0.035-inch guidewire into the CCA, the wire is positioned in the ECA. A series of stents and catheters are deployed into the CCA within a few centimeters of the lesion, with care taken to avoid inadvertent arterial dissection. To prevent embolization and consequent neurologic complications, an embolic protection device (EPD) is positioned in the straight portion of the distal ICA. Over-the-wire exchanges are carefully executed to prevent ICA trauma, spasm, dissection, and thrombosis.

Once the EPD is deployed, atropine (0.5 mg to 1.0 mg intravenously) may be given to prevent a vasovagal response during angioplasty. Subsequently, angioplasty is performed with a 3- to 4-mm balloon to ensure safe passage of the stent and retrieval of the stent delivery system. A self-expanding stent is deployed to cover the entire lesion (usually 30 to 40 mm). Post-stenting angioplasty is performed using a balloon that is undersized by 20% to 40% of the ICA diameter and stent length to avoid dissection, atheroembolization, and vasovagal response. Stents may continue to expand, enlarging the vessel lumen over time. Thus, moderate residual stenosis may be tolerated after post-stenting angioplasty.

At the end of the procedure, the EPD is removed. Completion angiogram visualizing the extracranial and intracranial circulation in two or more views is performed. Anticoagulation is discontinued. If an arterial closure device is used, the need for normalization of the ACT is eliminated.

Innovative Approach to Carotid Angioplasty and Stenting. The findings of ICSS[66] demonstrated a higher adverse event rate that may be attributable to the use of EPDs, especially of the distal filter type.[68] As described by Schnaudigel, diffusion-weighted magnetic resonance imaging (DW-MRI) has shown a higher incidence of new ischemic brain lesions in the contralateral hemisphere in CS versus CEA patients (14.5% versus 0.1%, $P < .01$), suggesting embolization into the contralateral carotid artery from guidewire and catheter manipulation in the aortic arch.[69] A large number of ipsilateral ischemic brain lesions also are attributed to manipulation of the aortic arch and CCA during transfemoral access. These findings have prompted several iterations of innovation in neuroprotection devices and strategies, leading to (1) direct transcervical access to the CCA, thereby avoiding the embolic risk of traversing the aortic arch and supra-aortic vasculature, and (2) a low-resistance shunt between arterial and venous circulations with high and low flow rates, thereby eliminating the need for ECA occlusion and reducing or eliminating an active aspiration step.[68] There is inferential evidence from the Proximal Protection with the MO.MA Device During Carotid Stenting (ARMOUR)[70] and Embolic Protection with Reverse Flow (EMPiRE)[71] trials that flow reversal is a better protection strategy than distal filters. The Silk Road Trial, which completed enrollment in 2014, was a single-arm study that enrolled 400 high-risk symptomatic and asymptomatic patients and incorporated transcarotid access with a flow reversal system.[68] The Silk Road system (Silk Road Medical) has been associated with a very low overall stroke risk, in the 1% range, which is comparable to the rate achieved with CEA.[72]

Postprocedural Care. Patients who have undergone CS usually return to the cardiac catheterization laboratory or radiology recovery room or the acute care unit for management of the vascular access site and neurologic, cardiac, and vascular monitoring. If an arterial closure device is not used, the ACT must normalize (≤150) before the sheath can be removed. While the coagulation study results normalize, the patient is on bed rest with immobilization of the affected extremity to avoid bleeding and hematoma formation. After the sheath is removed, manual pressure is applied to the access site for an average of 20 minutes until hemostasis is achieved.

Medical management includes dual-antiplatelet therapy with aspirin (81 to 325 mg daily) and, for at least 4 weeks, clopidogrel (75 mg daily). For patients intolerant of clopidogrel, ticlopidine (250 mg daily) may be substituted. Medications for blood pressure control, hyperlipidemia, and diabetes also are resumed or initiated. The patient is usually discharged on postprocedural day 1 or 2. If the patient has persistent hypotension, hospitalization may be extended for hydration and oral adrenergic therapy using ephedrine (25 to 50 mg by mouth three or four times daily).

Long-term postprocedural management includes continued antithrombotic therapy with aspirin and serial surveillance for stent patency and areas of recurrent stenosis using noninvasive imaging techniques. Serial surveillance should occur at 1 month, 6 months, 1 year, then annually thereafter. Surveillance can be terminated when the patient is no longer a candidate for intervention.

Complications of Carotid Angioplasty and Stenting. Complications of CS are categorized as cardiovascular problems, neurologic issues, device malfunction, general medical issues, access-site complications, restenosis, and mortality.

Cardiovascular complications include baroreceptor reflexes, MI, arterial dissection or thrombosis, transient vasospasm, and recurrent stenosis. The rates of target-vessel perforation and MI are generally low, at 1%. Baroreflex responses (i.e., bradycardia, hypotension, and vasovagal reaction) occur in 5% to 10% of patients undergoing CS. Transient vasospasm occurs in 10% to 15% of procedures as a result of instrumentation with guidewires, catheters, and protection devices. Restenosis after CS, which ranges from 3% to 5%, can be minimized by avoiding multiple high-pressure balloon inflations, particularly in heavily calcified vessels.

In order of decreasing frequency, neurologic complications include stroke (as high as 5.5%), nondisabling stroke (2.9%), disabling stroke (1.5% to 2%), TIA (1% to 2%), intracranial hemorrhage and hyperperfusion syndrome related to hypertension and anticoagulation (<1%), and seizures related to hypoperfusion (<1%).

Device malfunction can involve deployment failure of the stent and EPD. In addition, the stent may be malformed or, rarely, migrate after deployment.

General risks include access-site injury (5%), although most of these injuries involve pain or hematoma and are self-limiting. Other risks include groin infection (<1%), pseudoaneurysm (1% to 2%), bleeding from the access site, retroperitoneal hematoma, and contrast-induced nephropathy.

LIFE SPAN CONSIDERATIONS

In review, in the absence of medical therapy, CS advances with age, increasing from the fifth decade and affecting about 10% of those older than 80 years.[73] The severity of CS is generally worse for men than women. The prevalence of TIA also increases with age, although the lifetime risk of stroke decreased significantly for both men and women between 1950 and 2004. Among women, the risk of stroke increases with age. Higher risk is associated with menopause before age 42 and postmenopausal hormonal therapy.

The CREST trial, which compared outcomes of symptomatic patients and asymptomatic patients treated with CEA and CS, revealed that for patients younger than 70 years, CS had more favorable outcomes whereas CEA yielded better outcomes for patients older than 70 years. Even octogenarians safely underwent CEA.

INDICATIONS FOR REFERRAL OR HOSPITALIZATION

All patients with amaurosis fugax, TIA, or stroke should undergo noninvasive imaging to determine the extent of CS. Noninvasive imaging is also indicated for patients with carotid bruit or other nonspecific symptoms, such as dizziness.

Symptomatic patients with CS greater than 70% on noninvasive imaging or greater than 50% on catheter angiography and with perioperative risk of stroke below 6% should be referred for carotid revascularization, by CEA or CS. CEA may be preferred for patients older than 70 years and those with arterial anatomy that precludes endovascular instrumentation. CEA also may be indicated for asymptomatic patients with CS greater than 60%. Patients who require CEA should be referred to vascular surgeons or neurosurgeons in centers in which more than

100 CEAs are performed each year.[8] CS may be preferred for patients younger than 70 years and those with unfavorable neck anatomy (e.g., previous ipsilateral neck surgery or radiation injury). Patients who require CS should be referred to a vascular surgeon, interventional cardiologist, or interventional radiologist.

PATIENT EDUCATION

Patient education focuses on the pathogenesis and consequences of CS, indications, approaches and complications of treatment approaches (i.e., CEA and CS), associated medical management, risk factor reduction to prevent recurrent CS, and the plan for ongoing follow-up.

During the periprocedural period, the patient must be able to recognize and report signs of complications of CEA or CS. For patients in both groups, the importance of adherence to the antihypertensive and statin regimen in preventing hyperfusion syndrome and stroke is emphasized, as is the need for the patient to report transient loss of consciousness, severe headache, and transient or persistent neurologic deficit. For patients who have undergone CEA, signs and symptoms of infection of the neck incision are stressed. Immediate treatment and reporting of bleeding, hematoma, and groin complications are emphasized with patients who have undergone CS. Secondary prevention of recurrent CS and ischemic stroke is directed at reducing cardiovascular risk factors.[24] The target for normal blood pressure is less than 120/80 mm Hg, which may require a regimen of antihypertensive medications. Additional lifestyle modifications include salt restriction (<1500 mg/day)[74]; weight loss, if necessary, to achieve a body mass index below 30 kg/m^2; consumption of a diet rich in fruits, vegetables, and low-fat dairy products; and moderate-intensity exercise for 30 minutes one to three times per week. Glycemic control and blood pressure control are important for patients with diabetes. Statin therapy may be titrated to achieve LDL-C below 75 mg/dL and reduce cholesterol, and niacin or gemfibrozil may be added to the medication regimen to increase HDL-C. Smoking cessation is a critical component of secondary prevention; counseling, nicotine products, and smoking cessation medications have been shown to be effective at promoting successful smoking cessation. Alcohol consumption should be limited to light to moderate levels (i.e., two drinks per day for men and one drink per day for women who are not pregnant.)

CHAPTER 120

CHEST PAIN AND CORONARY ARTERY DISEASE

Patricia Lowry

DEFINITION AND EPIDEMIOLOGY

Coronary heart disease (CHD) remains the primary cause of death for both men and women in the United States. CHD includes acute myocardial infarction (MI), angina pectoris, atherosclerotic cardiovascular disease (ASCVD), and all forms of chronic ischemic heart disease. In 2011, 375,295 Americans died of CHD. Each year, an estimated 525,000, Americans have a new coronary attack (defined as first hospitalized MI or CHD death), and approximately 210,000 have a recurrent attack.[1] It is estimated that an additional 155,000 silent first MIs occur each year. Approximately every 34 seconds one American has a coronary event, and approximately every 84 seconds an American will die of CHD.[1] Disparities in the treatment of racial and ethnic minorities appear to be improving over time. In an assessment of a statewide program for treatment of ST-elevation myocardial infarction (STEMI), institution of a coordinated regional approach to triage and management was associated with significant improvements in treatment times that were similar for whites and blacks and for women and men.

At least 68% of people older than 65 years with diabetes die of some form of heart disease. Heart disease death rates among adults with diabetes are two to four times higher than the rates for adults without diabetes. Diabetes mellitus is associated with higher short- and long-term mortality after STEMI, and in patients with diabetes mellitus both hyperglycemia and hypoglycemia are associated with worse outcomes. Myocardial tissue perfusion after restoration of epicardial coronary flow is more impaired in patients with diabetes mellitus.

Patient-Related Delays and Initial Treatment

Early reperfusion for patients with an acute MI improves left ventricular (LV) systolic function and survival; therefore every effort must be made to minimize hospital delay. Although time is critical in the treatment of MI, it is patient delay, not transport or system inadequacy, that has proved to be the biggest obstacle to timely medical treatment. Half of patients experiencing STEMI do not seek medical care for approximately 1.5 to 2 hours after symptom onset, and one quarter delay seeking care for up to 6 hours. Little has changed in this time interval for the past 10 years, despite community-wide educational efforts to increase patient awareness of symptoms. Patient delay times are often longer in women, blacks, older adults, and Medicaid-only recipients and are shorter for Medicare recipients (compared with privately insured patients) and patients who are taken directly to the hospital by emergency medical services (EMS) transport. Patients may delay seeking care because their symptoms differ from their preexisting belief that a heart attack should manifest dramatically with severe, crushing chest pain. Approximately one third of patients with MI experience symptoms other than chest pain.

Other reasons for delay in seeking treatment include (1) inappropriate reasoning that symptoms will be self-limited or are not serious; (2) attribution of symptoms to other preexisting conditions; (3) fear of embarrassment should symptoms turn out to be a "false alarm"; (4) reluctance to trouble others unless "really sick"; (5) preconceived stereotypes of who is at risk for a heart attack, an especially common trait among women; (6) lack of knowledge of the importance of rapid action, the benefits of calling EMS or 911, and the availability of reperfusion therapies; and (7) attempted self-treatment with prescription and/or nonprescription medications.[2] To avoid such delays, health care providers should assist patients when possible in making anticipatory plans for timely recognition and response to an acute event.[3] Family members, close friends, or advocates also should be enlisted as reinforcement for rapid action when the patient experiences symptoms of possible STEMI. Discussions should include a review of instructions for taking aspirin and nitroglycerin in response to chest pain.

Immediate emergency department referral or physician consultation is indicated for patients with suspected MI.

Risk Factors for Coronary Artery Disease

It is currently believed that it is the composition, morphology, and stability of the coronary artery plaque rather than the degree of plaque stenosis that determines the risk of cardiovascular events. Modification of controllable cardiac risk factors has been shown to decrease the frequency of cardiovascular morbidity and mortality.

Historically, risk factors have been subdivided into factors that are nonmodifiable, such as gender, age, and family history, and factors that are modifiable, such as smoking cessation, dyslipidemia, diabetes mellitus, increased waist-to-hip ratio, physical inactivity, poor diet, psychosocial stress, and hypertension. There are specific recommendations to modify risk factors for patients who already have coronary artery disease (CAD) (Table 120-1). Studies suggest that 90% of the variability of acute MI can be attributed to modifiable risk factors. It is now known that some cardiac risk factors are more predictive of coronary artery events than others are.

LIPID GUIDELINES

Lifestyle modifications, including adherence to a heart-healthy diet, regular exercise habits, avoidance of tobacco products, and maintenance of a healthy weight, remain an important component of health promotion and ASCVD risk reduction. Lipid lowering with the use of statins has also been supported for the primary prevention of ASCVD in many higher-risk individuals and for secondary prevention in all individuals. In 2013 the American College of Cardiology (ACC) and American Heart Association (AHA) released new guidelines on the treatment of blood cholesterol.[4] Four statin benefit groups have now been identified and include individuals in need of primary or secondary prevention. The first group includes those in need of secondary prevention who have demonstrated clinical ASCVD. This is defined by an acute coronary syndrome (ACS), history of MI,

TABLE 120-1 AHA/ACC Secondary Prevention for Patients with Coronary Artery Disease and Other Atherosclerotic Vascular Disease*

Risk Factor	Goal
Smoking	Complete cessation
Blood pressure control	<140/90 mm Hg <130/80 mm Hg if patient has heart failure or renal insufficiency
Lipids	Initial evaluation before statin initiation Fasting lipid panel Check ALT and CK level Age <75 years without contraindications, conditions, or drug-drug interactions influencing statin therapy—begin on high-intensity statin therapy Age >75 years or with conditions or drug-drug interaction or a history of statin intolerance—initiate moderate-intensity statin therapy Educate on healthy lifestyle habits Reduce saturated fats to <7% calories Triglycerides <200 mg/dL If triglycerides are ≥200 mg/dL, non-HDL-C should be <130 mg/dL Non-HDL-C = Total cholesterol − HDL-C
Physical activity	30 minutes, 7 days per week (minimum 5 days per week)
Weight management	Body mass index of 18.5-24.9 kg/m^2 Waist circumference: men <40 inches, women <35 inches
Diabetes mellitus	Hemoglobin A_{1c} <7% is advised
MEDICATIONS	
ASA	75-162 mg PO daily; if ASA is contraindicated, use clopidogrel or warfarin. ASA is used alone or in combination with antiplatelet medications, depending on clinical situation.
Beta blockers	All patients who have had myocardial infarction, acute coronary syndrome, or left ventricular dysfunction with or without heart failure symptoms, unless contraindicated
ACE inhibitors	All patients with left ventricular ejection fraction ≤40% and those with hypertension, diabetes, or chronic kidney disease, unless contraindicated
Influenza vaccination	All patients

*Includes peripheral arterial disease, atherosclerotic aortic disease, and carotid artery disease.
ACC, American College of Cardiology; ACE, angiotensin-converting enzyme; AHA, American Heart Association; ALT, alanine aminotransferase; ASA, acetylsalicylic acid; CK, creatine kinase; HDL-C, high-density lipoprotein cholesterol.
From Smith SC Jr, Benjamin EJ, Bonow RO, et al: AHA/ACCF secondary prevention and risk reduction therapy for patients with coronary and other atherosclerotic vascular disease: update. *J Am Coll Cardiol.* 2011;58(23):2432-2446.

TABLE 120-2 High-, Moderate-, and Low-Intensity Statin Therapy

High-Intensity Statin Therapy	Moderate-Intensity Statin Therapy	Low-Intensity Statin Therapy
Daily dose lowers LDL-C on average by approximately >50%	Daily dose lowers LDL-C on average by approximately 30% to <50%	Daily dose lowers LDL-C on average by 30%
Atorvastatin 40-80 mg Rosuvastatin 20-40 mg	Atorvastatin 10-20 mg Rosuvastatin 5-10 mg Simvastatin 20-40 mg Pravastatin 40-80 mg Lovastatin 40 mg Fluvastatin 40 mg bid	Simvastatin 10 mg Pravastatin 10-20 mg Lovastatin 20 mg

From Stone N, Robinson, J, Lichtenstein A et al: ACC/AHA guideline on the treatment of blood cholesterol to reduce atherosclerotic cardiovascular risk in adults: a report of the American College of Cardiology/American Heart Association Task Force on Practice Guidelines. *J Am Coll Cardiol.* 2014 Jul 1;63(25 Pt B):2889-2934.

stable or unstable angina, coronary or other arterial revascularization, stroke, transient ischemic attack (TIA), or peripheral vascular disease (PVD). The other three categories involve patients in need of primary prevention. The first of these categories involves those with elevations of low-density lipoprotein cholesterol (LDL-C) above 190 mg/dL without a secondary cause such as high saturated fats or causative drugs. The next category involves those primary prevention patients with diabetes aged 40 to 75 years with LDL-C of 70 to 189 mg/dL. The last category involves those without diabetes aged 40 to 75 years with LDL-C of 70 to 189 mg/dL and an estimated 10-year ASCVD risk score[5] higher than 7.5%. The new guidelines base the intensity of statin therapy to reduce ASCVD risk according to those most likely to benefit (Table 120-2). There are therefore no more low-density lipoprotein (LDL) treatment targets. For those individuals unable to tolerate high-intensity statin therapy, moderate-intensity statin therapy is recommended. Nonstatin therapies (e.g., niacin, fibrates, ezetimibe), whether alone or in addition to statins, were not found to provide acceptable ASCVD risk reduction benefits and should be avoided.[6]

PATHOPHYSIOLOGY

Chronic Stable Angina

Chronic stable angina is precipitated by exertion and relieved by rest. A reduction in myocardial oxygen supply or increases in myocardial oxygen demand are the determinants of coronary ischemia. Although the pathologic process for unstable angina and the pathologic process for chronic stable angina both result from atherosclerotic lesions in the coronary arteries, the pathophysiologic mechanism of each varies.

Under normal circumstances, an increase in myocardial oxygen demand is balanced by an increase in myocardial oxygen supply. The three most important factors that determine myocardial oxygen demand are heart rate, systemic blood pressure (peripheral vascular resistance), and LV wall tension. The heart rate and the systolic blood pressure exert independent influence on myocardial oxygen requirements because both determine myocardial workload (heart rate × systolic blood pressure = myocardial workload). Therefore, activities (e.g., exercise, hurrying, lifting) and increased metabolic demands (e.g., with fever, anemia, thyrotoxicosis) that increase the workload of the heart in the presence of a fixed and limited oxygen supply will increase myocardial oxygen requirements and thus precipitate ischemia and angina.

The coronary arteries exhibit changes in vascular tone (vasomotion). These changes play a significant role in the development of coronary ischemia. Under normal circumstances, the endothelial or innermost lining of the coronary artery responds to vasoactive stimuli, such as mental stress, cold, and catecholamines, by releasing endothelium-derived relaxing factor (EDRF) to maintain vasodilation. In the presence of atherosclerosis, however, the endothelial function is impaired; hence, the vasoconstrictive response is unopposed, leading to constriction at the site of atherosclerosis and adjacent areas. This results in a decrease in myocardial blood flow and induces coronary ischemia.

Silent Myocardial Ischemia (Asymptomatic Coronary Heart Disease)

It has been recognized that asymptomatic occurrences of ischemia are more common than symptomatic episodes in patients with exertional angina symptoms. Silent myocardial ischemia occurs when there is objective evidence of ischemia in the absence of symptoms. Since the advent of continuous ambulatory electrocardiographic monitoring, many patients with typical stable angina have been found to have frequent episodes of asymptomatic ischemia.[7]

The full clinical implications of silent ischemia are not well understood, but there is increased incidence of ischemia, MI, and sudden death in asymptomatic patients with positive exercise stress test results. In addition, patients with asymptomatic ischemia who have had an MI are at greater risk for a second coronary event. Ischemia can occur with or without evidence of increased myocardial oxygen demand (increased product of heart rate and blood pressure). Diabetic patients are at a twofold to fourfold greater risk of cardiovascular mortality compared with those without diabetes, and silent myocardial ischemia on stress testing occurs more often in patients with diabetes than in patients without diabetes.

The pathogenesis of silent myocardial ischemia is not well understood, although several hypotheses exist. It has been suggested that some individuals have a higher endorphin level than others do, which may play a role in the perception of pain. In addition, some patients have a higher ischemic pain threshold and greater tolerance of cold-induced ischemia. Finally, autonomic dysfunction, particularly in patients with diabetes, is thought to contribute to silent ischemia.

Microvascular Angina (Syndrome X)

The cause of microvascular angina is still not fully understood, although studies have demonstrated that some patients with this syndrome have an abnormal vasodilating response of their small or resistance vessels (diminished coronary reserve). Still other patients may have a low pain threshold or other noncardiac causes of pain. Most patients with microvascular angina have cardiac risk factors such as family history of heart disease, hypertension, tobacco abuse, diabetes, hyperlipidemia, and abdominal obesity. Women seem to be more prone to this than men, especially those with decreased estrogen levels. The diagnosis of microvascular angina (syndrome X) is suspected when there is a convincing history of anginal chest pain with or without documented reversible ischemic electrocardiographic changes, angiography fails to demonstrate obstruction or spasm of a major coronary artery, and other conditions have been excluded from the differential diagnosis.

Variant Angina (Coronary Artery Spasm, Prinzmetal Angina)

In variant angina, coronary artery spasm should be suspected on the basis of the patient's history. Spasm can occur in any coronary artery; however, the right coronary artery and, to a lesser extent, the left anterior descending artery are more commonly affected. The spasm tends to be focal and reproducible at the same location. However, diffuse single-vessel coronary artery spasm may occur. Multivessel spasm is extremely rare; when it occurs, it is associated with intractable ventricular tachycardia. The cause of coronary artery spasm is abnormal endothelial cell function. This is especially true when injury to the endothelium results in decreased concentration of EDRF.

Unstable Angina and Non–ST-Segment Elevation Myocardial Infarction

The pathophysiologic mechanism of acute MI has been controversial since Hippocrates first postulated that heart disease could cause sudden death. The causes of MI can be divided into those that decrease myocardial oxygen supply and those that increase myocardial oxygen demand. Atherosclerotic plaque results in a reduction of coronary blood flow, thereby reducing oxygen supply. These plaques reduce the cross-sectional area of the coronary artery lumen, thus reducing coronary perfusion pressure. When a critical stenosis develops, coronary blood flow is adequate at rest but cannot increase to meet metabolic demands during exertion.

The development of a vulnerable coronary artery lesion is multifactorial and depends on the biochemical and physical properties of that lesion. Unstable angina can be divided into those that decrease myocardial oxygen supply and those that increase myocardial oxygen demand by a nonocclusive thrombus that has developed from a ruptured atherosclerotic plaque. Plaque rupture initiates an inflammatory response, which stimulates chemotactic factors for circulating monocytes. Monocytes enter the vessel wall, transform into tissue macrophages, and ingest oxidized LDLs. Over time, lipid-filled macrophages (foam cells) die, creating an extracellular lipid pool with eventual formation of a fibrous cap. Proteolytic enzymes produced by activated macrophages erode the fibrous cap, producing areas that are fragile and prone to rupture. Increases in shear stress and vasomotor changes placed on this vulnerable lesion make it highly likely to rupture. Plaque rupture causes vessel damage and initiates platelet activity. Platelet aggregation and activation develop a platelet-rich "white clot" over the endothelial damage, causing partial obstruction of flow in the artery and thus unstable angina and non–ST-segment elevation myocardial infarction (NSTEMI). Therefore the role of the inflammatory response as a trigger for plaque rupture cannot be overemphasized. Bacterial and viral infections make plaques more vulnerable and unstable with a predisposition to rupture and thrombose. A number of studies have shown the benefit of evaluating high-sensitivity C-reactive protein to determine cardiovascular risk.[8]

When plaque rupture occurs, the size of the resultant thrombus, whether it is a small mural thrombus or an occlusive thrombus, depends on several factors, including the amount of thrombogenic substrate that is exposed, the amount of local blood flow disturbance, and the actual thrombotic propensity of the vessel.

Therefore, lesion disruption is a dynamic process that may lead to transient vessel occlusion and ischemia by a labile thrombus, resulting in unstable angina. These thrombotic occlusions often resolve spontaneously; however, they can recur within hours or days. In other cases, formation of a fixed thrombus and a more chronic occlusion may occur, resulting in acute MI.

Coronary artery narrowing of less than 80% typically does not induce development of collateral vessels. For this reason, smaller plaques that rupture are more likely to cause a significant clinical event during thrombotic occlusion of the vessel as a result of the absence of protective collateral flow.

Acute ST-Segment Elevation Myocardial Infarction

In most cases, MI occurs when an atherosclerotic plaque ruptures, which serves as a nidus for thrombus formation with resultant coronary artery occlusion. The atherosclerotic plaque most likely to rupture is the nonocclusive plaque, which may rupture several times before MI is produced. With each rupture, blood, fibrin, and platelet aggregates accumulate in the plaque, forming intraintimal or intraplaque thrombus and resulting in increases in plaque size, intraplaque pressure, and obstruction of the coronary lumen. When such a plaque ruptures, fissures, or ulcerates, MI or sudden death may occur. Plaque rupture with resulting thrombus formation is the common physiologic mechanism underlying unstable angina, MI, and sudden death. The amount of myocardial injury sustained is directly related to several factors, including the amount of thrombus present, the ability of the intrinsic lytic system to promote lysis, the impact of local vasoconstrictor substances on impeding blood flow, whether the vessel affected is partially or totally occluded, the presence or absence of collateral vessels and the quantity of blood they supply to the affected area, and the amount of myocardium supplied by the affected vessel.

The platelet is not only the smallest cell but also the most active in thrombus formation. The platelet consists of membranes, tubules, granules, and receptors. During activation, the resting platelet undergoes a dramatic change that induces platelet-platelet interaction or aggregates. Such platelet aggregates play an important role in ACS and MI. Patients who died of unstable angina, MI, and sudden cardiac death have platelet aggregation, fibrin, and microthrombi as common findings. Because platelets are important in the pathophysiologic process of acute ischemic syndrome and MI, inhibition of platelet activation should be beneficial in reducing and preventing ACS.

MINOCA: Suspected Myocardial Infarction with Nonobstructed Coronary Arteries

Myocardial infarction with nonobstructed coronary arteries (MINOCA) is an emerging syndrome. Cardiac registries' prevalence measurements indicate that 10% of patients with diagnosed MI do not have obstructions in their coronary arteries.[9] In 2015, researchers used PubMed and Embase to conduct a meta-analysis of studies mentioning nonobstructed coronary arteries in the setting of MI. For this review, these researchers defined MINOCA as documented presence of MI with angiographic findings of less than 50% stenosis in any epicardial artery. Findings from this meta-analysis indicate that MINOCA is a finding in 6% of MI patients, confers a better 12-month mortality prognosis than in documented CAD (prognosis for patients with MINOCA is still guarded), and has structural dysfunction, coronary spasm, and thrombotic disorders found in association.[9] Current recommendations are to consider MINOCA as a working diagnosis while evaluating these patients for treatable underlying causes with magnetic resonance imaging (MRI), provocative testing, and evaluation for thrombophilia.[9]

CLINICAL PRESENTATION

Chronic Stable Angina

The patient with chronic stable angina demonstrates characteristic symptoms that occur with predictable frequency, severity, duration, and provocation. These symptoms occur with exertion, are relieved by rest or no more than one nitroglycerin tablet, and in general last for only 1 to 3 minutes. Chronic stable angina remains constant unless an acceleration of the disease process intervenes. The clinical presentation can best be evaluated by a detailed history of angina quality, location, radiation, severity, duration, and precipitating and relieving factors. Associative factors such as dyspnea, diaphoresis, nausea, vomiting, eructations, diarrhea, and fatigue should also be evaluated (Box 120-1).

William Heberden first defined the peculiar discomfort of myocardial ischemia as angina pectoris, which translated means "strangling in the chest." The majority of patients do not refer to their angina symptoms as pain; thus, questioning related to "chest pain" may prove misleading, and the diagnosis of angina pectoris may be missed. Discomfort originating in the chest may arise from many structures, including the skin, subcutaneous tissue, bone, muscle, vascular structures, nerves, pleura, lungs, pericardium, heart, esophagus, and gastrointestinal viscera.

Adjectives used to describe the quality of angina can be variable; it is often conveyed as a pressure, heaviness, aching, constriction, tightness, squeezing, numbness, or burning sensation. Patients may demonstrate a clenched fist over the sternal area (Levine sign) to further elucidate this feeling. The location of discomfort is predominantly behind the midsternum (retrosternal) or just to the left of the sternum, in an area approximately the size of a clenched fist. If the patient is able to localize the area of discomfort as being no larger than a fingertip, the sensation is seldom related to myocardial ischemia, and other causes should be considered. Myocardial ischemia can also encompass the territory between the epigastrium and the lower jaw, lower teeth, and hard palate, with sensations of tightness or constriction in the throat area. Atypical symptoms are more common in women, the elderly, and diabetic patients.

Radiation symptoms are not uncommon and are related to involvement of the C8 to T4 spinal ganglia. These ganglia receive impulses from the heart and from peripheral dermatomes that are transmitted to the spinal cord through afferent nerve fibers. When myocardial ischemia occurs, the sharing of these ganglia can produce discomfort to the other dermatomal areas. Thus, stimulation of the dermatomes affecting the brachial plexus can result in discomfort or numbness anywhere along the medial surface of the left arm, including the fourth and fifth digits. Isolated wrist discomfort has also been reported. The right arm and lateral surfaces can be affected, although with less frequency.

Stimulation of the cervical plexus can result in suprascapular and intrascapular discomfort. Precipitating factors, including increased exertion, coitus, and emotion, tend to induce myocardial ischemia by increasing circulating catecholamine levels. This increases the metabolic oxygen needs of the heart in the setting of a limited oxygen supply, thereby producing angina symptoms. Eating of a large meal may precipitate discomfort, as can the increased metabolic demands from fever, chills, thyrotoxicosis, anemia, hypoglycemia, exposure to cold air, and the nicotine from cigarette smoking.

Relief of stable angina symptoms generally occurs within 1 to 3 minutes after the discontinuation of activity or with rest. When angina is related to emotional upheaval, it may take longer for catecholamine levels to decrease, and angina symptoms may persist for a longer period. Nitroglycerin administration will usually provide relief within 5 minutes and is a useful diagnostic tool. When symptoms persist for longer than 20 minutes, the patient should no longer be considered to be having chronic stable angina and should be instructed to seek prompt medical attention.

Although cessation of activity generally produces relief of pain, it has been noted that some patients who develop angina with walking are able to continue walking, with eventual alleviation of the angina. These patients are able to "walk through" the angina event. There are several proposed hypotheses for the relief of angina during exercise. These include dilation of functioning collateral blood vessels during exercise; relief of coronary arterial spasm; and vasodilation of systemic blood vessels with a corresponding decline in systemic arterial blood pressure and heart rate, which in turn reduces myocardial oxygen demand.

The Canadian Cardiovascular Society classification (CCSC) is a useful tool to determine the exercise tolerance of patients with stable angina pectoris and to determine the degree of disability that angina symptoms are imposing on the patient (Box 120-2). This simple instrument can be used to risk stratify and to manage patients with angina.[10]

BOX 120-1

History Questions for the Patient with Angina

Chest pain information
- Precipitating factors (exertion, meals, stress, cold)
- Quality (pressure, squeezing, burning, stabbing)
- Radiation (shoulders, arm, wrist, neck, jaw, back)
- Relief measures (rest, nitroglycerin [hallmark], food)
- Severity (1-10 scale)
- Timing (activity, bedtime, meals, history of occurrence, duration)

Associative factors
- Dyspnea
- Provoked by activity (chest pain first or dyspnea)
- Orthopnea (how many pillows)
- Paroxysmal nocturnal dyspnea (how soon after retiring to bed)
- Diaphoresis
- Gastrointestinal complaints (nausea, vomiting, diarrhea)
- Fatigue

Cardiac risk factors

Current medication profile

Anginal Equivalents

Myocardial ischemia can be experienced as dyspnea, indigestion, nausea, numbness in the upper extremities, and fatigue rather than actual chest pressure; this is particularly true in women.[11]

Symptoms of dyspnea are generally noted to be stable when they occur with moderate exertion and unstable when they occur with minimum exertion or with rest or when they begin to awaken the patient during the night. The cause of stable

BOX 120-2

Canadian Cardiovascular Society Classification

Class I: Prolonged exertion evokes angina, without limits to normal activity.
Class II: Walking more than 2 blocks evokes angina, with slight limits to normal activity.
Class III: Walking less than 2 blocks evokes angina, with marked limits to normal activity.
Class IV: Minimal activity or rest evokes angina, with severe restrictions to activity.

symptoms is related to increased myocardial demand, and the cause of unstable symptoms is related to decreased myocardial supply. The dyspnea produced is caused by myocardial ischemia resulting in diastolic dysfunction, which produces increased left-sided filling pressures. Fatigue often follows an activity and resolves within several minutes. The cause is related to LV dysfunction resulting in decreased cardiac output.

Microvascular Angina

The clinical presentation for microvascular angina is chest pain, which is often unpredictable and may occur with rest, routine physical activity, or stressful events. Unlike chest pain from stable angina, chest discomfort from microvascular disease is generally more intense, lasts for longer periods of time, and does not go away with rest. Discomfort is generally not responsive to nitroglycerin. Although there is no apparent gender difference in the perception of angina, the syndrome of microvascular angina is found predominantly in women.

Variant Angina

The sine qua non of variant angina pectoris is a history of spontaneous or unprovoked episodes of typical angina. Discomfort occurs predominantly at rest and is usually not provoked by exertion. Patients sometimes note that beta blockers exacerbate symptoms. The differential diagnosis on presentation should be unstable angina until it is proven otherwise.

Unstable Angina and Non–ST-Segment Elevation Myocardial Infarction

Diagnosis of unstable angina and NSTEMI depends predominantly on a detailed patient history. The most important factors from the initial history that enhance the likelihood of the patient's experiencing an episode of ischemia are the nature of symptoms, prior history of CAD, age older than 65 years, and number of risk factors present for CAD. The Thrombolysis in Myocardial Infarction (TIMI) risk score is one of several valued tools for use in the emergency department for risk stratification and therapeutic decision-making (Table 120-3).[12] The risk score encompasses these factors and adds electrocardiographic findings and cardiac marker data as well as aspirin use in the previous 7 days. The use of aspirin and concomitant angina was found to be a powerful predictor of unstable angina or NSTEMI. In addition, several factors may suggest an acceleration of the patient's chronic angina symptoms to unstable angina or NSTEMI. These factors may include occurrence of the angina event with less provocation or at rest, prolongation of the angina symptoms, increase in the severity of symptoms, and newly associated findings with the chest discomfort. Physical examination findings of pulmonary edema, new or worsening mitral regurgitation murmur, S_3 heart sound, hypotension, bradycardia, or tachycardia suggest that the patient is at high risk. According to guidelines, a 12-lead electrocardiogram (ECG), preferably with and without chest pain, should also be obtained. It is particularly important to assess the duration of

TABLE 120-3 **TIMI Risk Score for Patients with Unstable Angina and NSTEMI: Predictor Variables**

Predictor Variable	Point Value of Variable	Definition
Age ≥65 years	1	
≥3 risk factors for CAD	1	Risk factors: Family history of CAD Hypertension Hypercholesterolemia Diabetes Current smoker
Aspirin use in last 7 days	1	
Recent, severe symptoms of angina	1	≥2 anginal events in last 24 hr
Elevated cardiac markers	1	CK-MB or cardiac-specific troponin level
ST deviation ≥0.5 mm	1	ST depression >0.5 mm is significant; transient ST elevation ≥0.5 mm for <20 min is treated as ST-segment depression and is high risk; ST elevation ≥1 mm for more than 20 minutes places these patients in the STEMI treatment category
Prior coronary artery stenosis ≥50%	1	Risk predictor remains valid even if this information is unknown
CALCULATED TIMI RISK SCORE	**RISK OF ≥1 PRIMARY END POINT* IN ≤14 DAYS**	**RISK STATUS**
0 or 1	5%	Low
2	8%	Low
3	13%	Intermediate
4	20%	Intermediate
5	26%	High

*Primary end points: death, new or recurrent MI, or need for urgent revascularization.
CK-MB, creatine kinase muscle-brain fraction.
From O'Connor RE, Brady W, Brooks SC, et al: 2010 American Heart Association guidelines for cardiopulmonary resuscitation and emergency cardiovascular care: part 10: acute coronary syndromes, *Circulation* 122:S787-S817, 2010.

angina events and whether rest pain has been present to determine the patient's short-term risk of complications. Patients who develop NSTEMI have a 70% higher risk of death and an 8.5% higher potential for reinfarction than do those with unstable angina alone.[13]

Acute ST-Segment Elevation Myocardial Infarction

Classically, acute MI is diagnosed as a constellation of symptoms. Chest pain described as pressure, heaviness, squeezing, crushing, and aching is often associated with nausea, vomiting, diaphoresis, or dyspnea. In general, the pain involves the sternum or epigastrium; in many cases, it may radiate to the arm, elbow, jaw, or neck. Any combination of these symptoms may occur in an individual patient. Epigastrium pain secondary to acute MI may be misdiagnosed as indigestion, and referred pain to the shoulder on deep inspiration may be misdiagnosed as being splenic in nature. In the older patient, MI may manifest as a sudden onset of dyspnea, weakness, loss of consciousness, or confusion. Although chest discomfort may be the most common presenting symptom, it may be atypical or absent in some patients with ACS (silent acute MI).

PHYSICAL EXAMINATION

Inspection of the chest may reveal the point of maximum impulse (PMI) to be downward or laterally displaced, suggestive of cardiomegaly, perhaps from hypertension. The PMI may also have a rocking quality, perhaps related to a LV aneurysm from a previous MI. The thorax should be inspected to determine the presence of any rashes or vesicles, which may suggest a herpetic cause of the discomfort. Inspection of the neck veins should be performed to assess the jugular venous pulse for any elevation. The contour of the internal jugular waveforms should also be noted. A funduscopic examination may reflect hypertension or diabetic retinopathy. Xanthomas or an early arcus senilis may be indicative of elevated cholesterol levels. The peripheral circulation should be assessed for any vascular lesions suggestive of arterial or venous disease.

Palpation during cardiac assessment is confined to assessment of the upstroke of the carotid artery pulse and the PMI of the cardiac apex. The carotid upstroke should be of normal volume and intensity. A prolonged carotid upstroke may indicate aortic stenosis because ventricular emptying becomes delayed when it is ejected across a significantly stenotic valve. Conversely, a brisk carotid upstroke may indicate aortic regurgitation or hypertrophic cardiomyopathy.

The PMI should be confined to the fifth intercostal space at the midclavicular line. With any downward or lateral displacement of the PMI, cardiomegaly should be considered. In a follow-up inspection, palpation of the PMI should confirm any aneurysm formation.

Auscultation of the chest may reveal a ventricular gallop (S_3) produced just after the second heart sound, which may be either physiologic or pathologic in nature. A physiologic S_3 may be heard in children and adults up to 35 to 40 years old. It may also be noted in women during their third trimester of pregnancy. A pathologic S_3 may be related to decreased myocardial contractility and is suggestive of heart failure caused by volume overload of the ventricles. This may be related to either mitral or tricuspid regurgitation.

An atrial gallop (S_4) may be noted just before the first heart sound and is produced by an increased resistance to ventricular filling caused by ventricular stiffness after atrial contraction. LV causes of an S_4 include cardiomyopathy, hypertension, MI, and aortic stenosis. Right ventricular (RV) causes include pulmonary hypertension and pulmonary stenosis. An S_4 may also be noted in trained athletes.

A pansystolic murmur audible at the apex during an episode of chest pain is most likely consistent with mitral regurgitation. It is often secondary to papillary muscle dysfunction as a result of LV ischemia. A ventricular septal defect after MI should also be considered and further evaluated with echocardiography.

Inflammation around the pericardium may produce a pericardial friction rub, which generally has one systolic and two diastolic components. The systolic component is produced when the ventricles contract in systole, whereas the diastolic components are produced in early and late diastole. The early diastolic component is a result of rapid, passive ventricular filling, whereas the late diastolic component occurs with atrial contraction. The sound produced is very high and of a scratching or grating quality.

Adventitious breath sounds suggest heart failure. Their occurrence and the presence of any vascular bruits, indicating further vascular disease, should prompt further evaluation.

The physical examination findings are usually normal when the patient is not having episodes of variant angina; however, during episodes, the patient may develop hypertension and tachycardia in response to the pain. In addition, the patient may have associated diaphoresis, nausea, and radiation of pain to the arm. Auscultation of the chest during an episode may reveal a gallop or transient systolic murmur originating from the mitral valve.

Approximately 90% of the diagnosis of an acute coronary event is made from the patient's history, ECGs and laboratory data. The physical examination findings will support this diagnosis and help determine whether the patient is in heart failure or is manifesting evidence of a cardiac arrhythmia. The patient will understandably be anxious and on occasion will be diaphoretic. The pulse rate and blood pressure may be normal; however, with an extensive area of MI, the patient may have a compensatory tachycardia and be hypotensive (Box 120-3).

DIAGNOSTICS

Chronic Stable Angina

Electrocardiography. In chronic stable angina, the ECG can be useful for detection of cardiac ischemia during actual episodes of angina. During this period, ST-segment depressions with symmetric T-wave inversions in the affected leads may be noted. During pain-free intervals, however, the ECG will revert to normal limits. Other possible changes include evidence of a prior MI, LV hypertrophy, and repolarization abnormalities.

Exercise Tolerance Testing (Stress Testing). Because of the nondiagnostic potential of the ECG in patients with intermittent episodes of chest pain, for those patients in whom the diagnosis of coronary ischemia remains unclear, an exercise tolerance test within 72 hours of presentation of symptoms should be obtained. Stress testing, which may be pharmacologic or exercise based, is performed for diagnostic, prognostic, and management purposes. With an overall sensitivity of 50% and specificity of 90%, exercise stress testing can be a cost-effective strategy for evaluation of CAD.

Stress testing for patients with a history of chest pain or angina-type symptoms should always be implemented with imaging. Imaging with either thallium or sestamibi should be added for those patients with uninterpretable resting ECGs

BOX 120-3

Cardiac Physical Assessment

INSPECTION

PMI: displaced downward and laterally, aneurysmal
Skin and extremities: color, edema, xanthomas, lesions
Neck veins: elevated jugular venous distention, contour of internal jugular pulse
Thorax: rashes, zoster
Funduscopic examination: evaluation for risk factors—diabetes mellitus, elevated cholesterol

PALPATION

Carotid upstroke: may be prolonged with aortic stenosis
PMI: may be diffuse with cardiac enlargement

AUSCULTATION

Ventricular gallop (S_3): heart failure
Atrial gallop (S_4): hypertension, myocardial infarction; caused by resistance of ventricular filling
Systolic mitral regurgitation murmur consistent with an ischemic papillary muscle
Pericardial friction rub: inflammation around the pericardial sac; may have one systolic and two diastolic components
Adventitious breath sounds
Carotid bruits: other vascular location

BOX 120-4

Dukes Treadmill Score

$$\text{DTS} = \text{Exercise time (minutes)} - (5 \times \text{ST deviation in mm}) - (4 \times \text{angina index})$$

Patients are categorized as low, intermediate, or high risk.

- Low risk (score >5) indicates a 5-year survival of 97%.
- Intermediate risk (score between 4 and −11) indicates 5-year survival of 90%.
- High risk (score < −11) indicates 5-year survival of 65%.

In high-risk patients, 74% had three-vessel or left main occlusive coronary disease on angiography.

Mark DB, Hlatky MA, Harrell FE, et al: Exercise treadmill score for predicting prognosis in coronary artery disease. *Ann Intern Med* 106:793-800, 1987.

resulting from the following conditions: preexisting 1-mm ST-segment depressions, LV hypertrophy with strain, left bundle branch block (LBBB), digoxin therapy, ventricular pacing, or Wolff-Parkinson-White syndrome.

The most commonly used definition for a positive result of exercise tolerance testing is the development of electrocardiographic changes consistent with ischemia. The standard criteria for test positivity include horizontal or down-sloping ST depression of 1 mm (0.1 mV) or more at 60 to 80 msec after the J point. When modest resting ST depression is present on the upright control ECG before exercise, only additional ST depression during exercise is measured for analysis. Markedly depressed up-sloping ST-depression responses to exercise (2.0 mm at 80 msec after the J point) could identify under lying CAD and future adverse events in highly symptomatic patients with angina.

The ST-segment changes on a stress test are indicative of viable cardiac muscle being supplied by a narrowed coronary artery. The time frame in which symptoms or electrocardiographic changes appear should be noted, as should the hemodynamic response. Stress testing should not be performed in individuals with exacerbation of heart failure, uncontrolled cardiac arrhythmias, severe hypertension, unstable angina, acute evolving MI, or critical aortic stenosis.

The Duke's Treadmill Score (DTS) was developed in 1987 and continues to be used to this day. It is a pint system to predict 5-year mortality utilizing a treadmill stress test with a standard Bruce protocol. The scoring system itself is based on the duration of exercise, ST-segment deviation (depression or elevation) and the presence and severity of angina during the exercise.

$$\text{DTS} = \text{Exercise time (minutes)} - (5 \times \text{ST deviation in mm}) - (4 \times \text{angina index})$$

See Box 120-4.[14]

CT Angiography. Since 1999, newer imaging techniques in noninvasive coronary arteriography with multidetector computed tomography (MDCT) or multislice computed tomography (MSCT) scanners have permitted imaging of the beating heart with no or little motion artifact. The presence and extent of coronary artery calcification serve as a marker of the extent of coronary atherosclerosis rather than the actual severity of coronary artery vessel stenosis. Coronary artery calcifications can be seen without a dye load; however, for the provider to visualize the coronary artery anatomy for stenosis, intravenous iodine containing contrast needs to be administered. With this in mind, one absolute contraindication to this type of testing is pregnancy. Relative contraindications to this testing include a contrast allergy, hyperthyroidism, and renal insufficiency. It is important to note that coronary computed tomography angiography (CTA) is highly sensitive, with a detection rate over 90%, but is not very specific. This means that a negative result will essentially rule out CAD with 90% accuracy, but if the test result is positive, this result is less conclusive and further imaging studies such as with an invasive cardiac catheterization procedure will need to be considered.

The Dilemma

Once the decision has been made that a noninvasive imaging study is needed to further evaluate the patient with chest pressure, the decision then becomes whether to perform a nuclear stress test or cardiac CTA. It may be helpful to understand the benefits and concerns with each study. One fact that may not be well appreciated is the amount of radiation exposure for each test. Historically, radiation exposure had been a major concern for CTA, with some centers exposing a patient to 25 to 30 mSv (millisieverts) of radiation. However, advances in technology can now allow CTA with 1 to 3 mSv or less. (Think of a chest radiograph as exposing a patient to 0.1 mSv of radiation.) Nuclear stress testing, on the other hand, exposes the patient to approximately 13 mSv of radiation. Given the enhanced degree of temporal resolution, newer scanners can image the heart with improved accuracy without the need to slow the heart rate (hence there is not always a need to administer beta blockers). Further CTA can often provide information about noncardiac findings, including pulmonary embolism, aortic dissection, and lung masses, which nuclear testing does not provide. Thus, given the low radiation exposure, higher amount of diagnostic accuracy, and additional noncardiac information that is obtained, many would argue that CTA is indeed the gold standard.

However, morbidly obese patients may have decreased penetration, which can result in poor image quality, making it difficult to visualize the mid to distal coronary arteries, although newer scanners have made improvements in this area. Reimbursement continues to be a major issue, and many insurance companies will approve a CTA only based on their "appropriateness criteria," and then only after a stress test has been performed and has yielded equivocal results. Some centers are concerned with the coronary calcium score, which is obtained first, and will not proceed to coronary artery CT scan if the value is greater than 800. Artifact from the calcium reduces the accuracy of testing; however, newer technology is able to subtract the calcium interference, so at centers with newer scanners this is no longer an issue. For patients who have had coronary artery bypass graft surgery, CTA can be effective in evaluating the potency of the bypass grafts. Unfortunately for patients with coronary artery stents, it is challenging to image the inside of the stent to determine any evidence of in-stent restenosis, and therefore CT scanning has generally not proven helpful for this patient population.

Microvascular Angina

Diagnosing microvascular disease has been challenging, because standard testing used to diagnose CAD in the larger vessels has not proven helpful in these smaller vessels. This type of angina usually does not result in any wall motion abnormality on a cardiac echo. Stress testing may produce ST changes similar to those of CAD, but perfusion imaging will be abnormal only 30% of the time. Anemia, thought to slow the growth of cells needed to repair damaged blood vessels, should be ruled out.

Variant Angina

Electrocardiography. Transient ST-segment elevation on a 12-lead ECG during an episode of variant angina is essential to make the diagnosis. Electrocardiographic changes are usually observed in the leads related to the ventricular areas supplied by the affected vessels. On occasion, electrocardiographic changes may be dramatic but resolve readily with the use of sublingual nitroglycerin or nifedipine.

Echocardiography. An echocardiogram obtained during a period of variant angina may reveal segmental wall motion abnormality, depending on the severity of the spasm and duration of the episode.

Exercise Tolerance Testing. An exercise tolerance test should be performed to exclude atherosclerotic disease. Most patients with noncritical CAD who have variant angina have a negative exercise tolerance test result.

Coronary Angiography. Patients with unprovoked chest discomfort at rest that is typical of angina may have variant angina. An exercise tolerance test should be the initial testing modality. On occasion, the result of this test may be negative for ischemia, even though the patient is still experiencing chest discomfort. At that time, patients may undergo coronary arteriography to evaluate further for CAD. If variant angina is indeed suspected, all vasoactive medications should be discontinued at least 24 hours before coronary arteriography or any other provocative testing. Provocation of spasm with acetylcholine has been used to induce endothelial cell vasoreactivity. However, this practice has fallen out of vogue because of the potential to induce global spasm and hence lethal cardiac arrhythmias. Therefore, diagnosis of variant angina is typically made from a patient history revealing nonexertional events that often are nocturnal.

Unstable Angina and Non–ST-Segment Elevation Myocardial Infarction

Electrocardiography. In patients with chest pain or other symptoms suggestive of an ACS, a 12-lead ECG should be obtained and evaluated for ischemic changes within 10 minutes of the patient's arrival at an emergency facility. Serial electrocardiography should be performed for the next 15 to 30 minutes if chest pressure persists despite the lack of initial ECG changes coupled with continuous telemetry monitoring. During an episode of angina the electrocardiographic findings depend on several factors, including location of the involved vessel, amount of myocardium involved, duration of ischemia, and transient nature of the pathophysiologic process. During an episode of ischemia, the electrical properties of the myocardial cells within and surrounding the area of ischemia are altered, producing changes on the surface ECG. ST-segment depression, along with symmetrically inverted T waves, is generally present within minutes during an acute ischemic event. According to guidelines of the Agency for Healthcare Research and Quality, ST depressions of more than 1 mm indicate a high likelihood of an unstable angina event, whereas ST depressions of 0.5 to 1 mm indicate an intermediate likelihood. These changes generally return to baseline once the ischemic event has resolved. As a rule, Q waves do not develop, and there is no distinct change in the R wave. Persistence of ST-segment depression for longer than 48 hours usually differentiates an unstable angina event from NSTEMI. An absence of ST-segment or T-wave changes does not exclude the possibility of myocardial ischemia. In particular, ischemia affecting the left circumflex territory is not always demonstrated on the ECG.

In addition, ST-segment and T-wave changes may be seen in a variety of disease processes, including infiltrative myocardial disease (neoplasm, sarcoidosis, amyloidosis, hemochromatosis), chest deformities; muscular dystrophy; electrolyte abnormalities; cerebrovascular accidents; pharmacologic treatments (digoxin, tricyclics); hyperventilation; and anxiety.

Exercise Tolerance Testing. An exercise stress test is not performed in those individuals experiencing MI.

Laboratory Data. Laboratory blood work for the patient with a potential unstable angina pattern should consist of hemoglobin and hematocrit levels to exclude anemia as a precipitating factor. Measurements of sodium, potassium, chloride, carbon dioxide, blood urea nitrogen, and creatinine should be obtained. A fasting blood glucose level and fasting cholesterol profile should be obtained to identify potential coronary risk factors. Thyroid functions should be considered to exclude hyperthyroidism or hypothyroidism. Magnesium levels should be considered for repletion purposes. Serial cardiac troponin I or T levels (when a contemporary assay is used) should be obtained at presentation and 3 to 6 hours after symptom onset (Table 120-4). Samples for C-reactive protein analysis may also be drawn to determine the presence of an inflammatory response. Measurement of B-type natriuretic peptide f N-terminal pro-B type natriuretic peptide may be considered to assess risk for heart failure.

Echocardiography. The echocardiogram is helpful during an acute ischemic event in several ways. Most important, it assists in detecting the location and extent of regional or global

LV dysfunction. Second, it assists in risk stratification before discharge. Finally, it is helpful for future evaluation of the remodeling. Echocardiography detects ischemia by evaluating the motion and thickening of the LV walls. This becomes particularly helpful when the patient has chest pressure and nondiagnostic electrocardiographic findings.

Although there are many techniques to assess ventricular wall motion, the method most commonly used is two-dimensional echocardiography with M-mode echocardiography. In acute coronary ischemia, two-dimensional and M-mode echocardiography may demonstrate abnormal wall motion of the ischemic section, which occurs almost immediately. Wall motion abnormalities, however, can be influenced by any abnormalities in the adjacent muscle to which the ischemic area is attached. Perhaps a more specific finding for ischemic cardiac muscle would be the inability of the affected myocardial muscle to thicken during systolic contraction. The nonischemic, or normal, region reveals normal motion and thickening toward the LV cavity during systole. The M-mode echocardiogram is ideal for measuring wall thickness and chamber dimensions, whereas the color Doppler study is used in conjunction with M-mode echocardiography to assess a regurgitant lesion.

ST-Elevation Acute Myocardial Infarction

STEMI is a clinical syndrome defined by characteristic symptoms of myocardial ischemia in association with persistent ST elevation in the absence of LV hypertrophy or LBBB coupled with the release of cardiac biomarkers. MI is defined as new ST elevation at the J point in at least two contiguous leads of 2 mm (0.2 mV) or more in men or 1.5 mm (0.15 mV) or more in women in leads V_2 to V_3 and/or of 1 mm (0.1 mV) or more in other contiguous chest leads or the limb leads. The majority of patients will evolve ECG evidence of Q-wave infarction. New or presumably new LBBB has been considered a STEMI equivalent but should not be considered diagnostic of acute MI in isolation. Baseline ECG abnormalities other than LBBB (e.g., paced rhythm, LV hypertrophy, Brugada syndrome) may obscure ECG interpretation. In addition, ST depression ≥ to 2 mm in the precordial leads (V_1 to V_4) may indicate transmural posterior injury; multilead ST depression with coexistent ST elevation in lead aVR has been described in patients with left main or proximal left anterior descending artery occlusion. Rarely, hyperacute T-wave changes may be observed in the very early phase of STEMI, before the development of ST elevation. Although the 12-lead ECG is useful in localizing the region of myocardial ischemia, it is limited in both the sensitivity and the specificity needed to distinguish the culprit coronary artery (Table 120-5 and Figures 120-1 to 120-3).

It is important to note that other disease states can demonstrate ST-segment elevations, such as hypertrophic cardiomyopathy, Prinzmetal angina, pericarditis, hyperkalemia, and early LV repolarization. Early depolarization changes can be differentiated from the ST-segment elevation of an acute MI by the

TABLE 120-4 Cardiac Markers

Cardiac Marker	Rises	Peaks	Normalizes
CK-MB isoforms	3-12 hr	24 hr	48-72 hr
Myoglobin	1-3 hr	6 hr	24 hr
Troponins T and I	3-12 hr	3-4 hr	14 days

CK-MB, creatine kinase muscle-brain fraction.

TABLE 120-5 Twelve-Lead ECG and Myocardial Infarction Territory

Lead	Territory
II, III, aVF	Inferior wall
II, III, aVF, V_5, V_6	Inferoapical wall
I, aVL, V_5, V_6	Inferolateral wall
V_1-V_4	Anterior wall
I, aVL, V_1-V_6	Anterolateral wall
V_1-V_3	Anteroseptal wall (ST-segment elevations)
V_5-V_6	Apical wall
I, aVL, V_5-V_6	Lateral wall
V_1-V_3	Posterior wall (ST-segment depressions; tall, upright R wave)
V_1-V_2	Septal wall (ST-segment elevations)

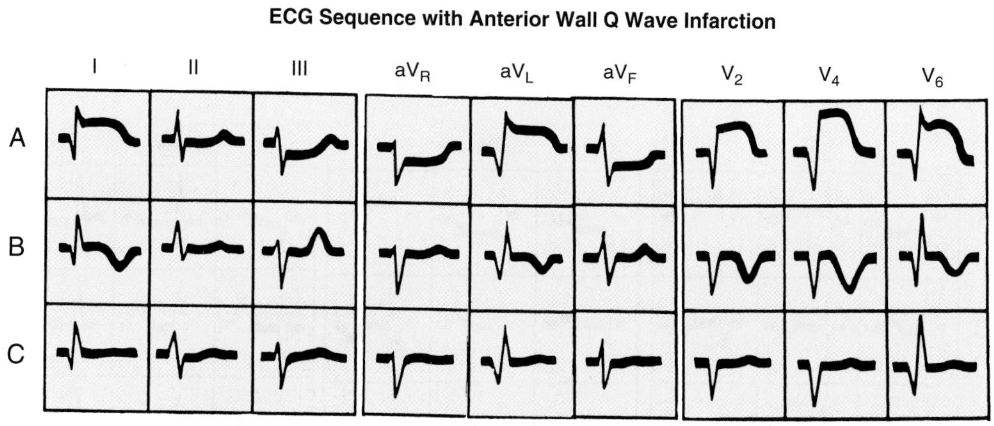

FIGURE 120-1 **A,** Acute phase of an anterior wall infarction: ST elevations and new Q waves. **B,** Evolving phase: deep T-wave inversions. **C,** Resolving phase: partial or complete regression of ST-T changes (and sometimes of Q waves). In **A** and **B**, note the reciprocal ST-T changes in the inferior leads (II, III, and aVF). (From Goldberger AL: Goldberger clinical electrocardiography: a simplified approach, ed 8, Philadelphia, 2012, Elsevier.)

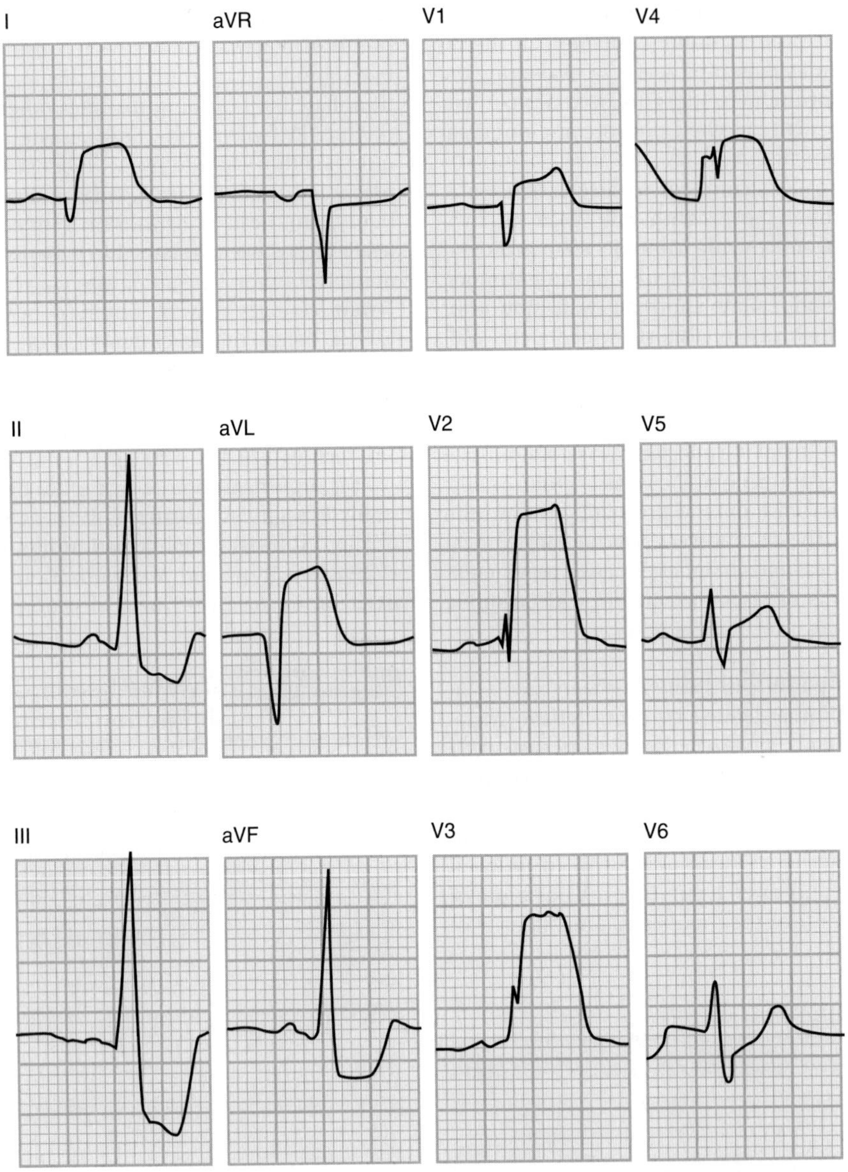

FIGURE 120-2 Large anterior (or anterolateral) myocardial infarction. There is marked ST-segment elevation in leads V1 through V5 and in leads I and aVL. This infarction, caused by occlusion of the proximal left anterior descending artery, therefore covers the anterior, septal (V1 through V3/V4), and lateral (V4 to V5 and I/aVL) portions of the left ventricle. In addition, reciprocal ST-segment depression is seen in the inferior leads (II, III, aVF). A Q wave is present in aVL. (From Sidebotham D, McKee A, Gillham M, et al: *Cardiothoracic critical care,* Philadelphia, 2007, Butterworth Heinemann.)

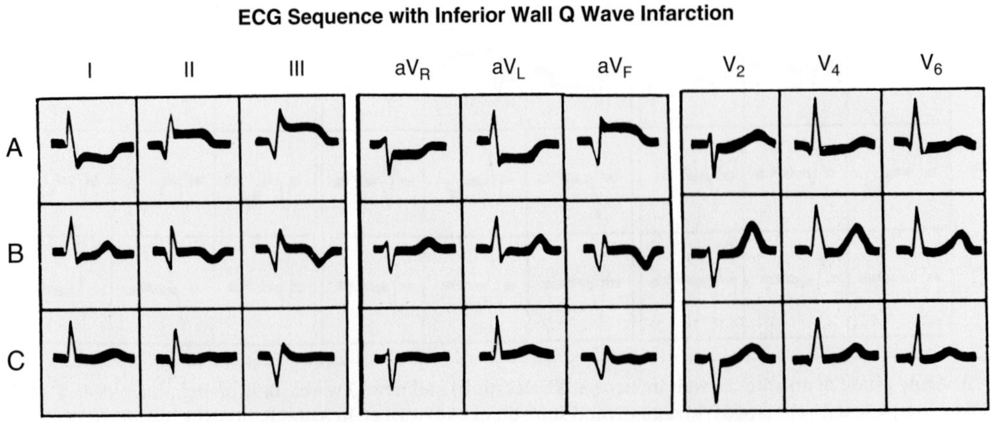

FIGURE 120-3 **A,** Acute phase of an inferior wall myocardial infarction: ST elevations and new Q waves. **B,** Evolving phase: deep T-wave inversions. **C,** Resolving phase: partial or complete regression of ST-T changes (and sometimes of Q waves). In **A** and **B,** notice the reciprocal ST-T changes in the anterior leads (I, aV_L, and V_2). (From Goldberger AL: *Clinical electrocardiography: a simplified approach,* ed 7, Philadelphia, 2006, Mosby.)

following: an upward concavity of the ST segment, an elevated takeoff of the ST segment at the J point (the junction of the end of the QRS complex and the beginning of the ST segment), and a distinct notching or slurring on the downstroke of the R wave. Therefore the history and presenting symptoms remain the important factors in the diagnosis of an acute or chronic coronary syndrome.

Echocardiography may provide evidence of focal wall motion abnormalities and facilitate triage in patients with ECG findings that are difficult to interpret. If doubt persists, immediate referral for invasive angiography may be necessary to guide therapy in the appropriate clinical context.

Laboratory Data

For almost 30 years, the creatine kinase (CK) and creatine kinase muscle-brain (CK-MB) levels were used to detect myocardial cell injury. They were found to be moderately sensitive and specific. The ACC has recommended the use of troponin I and troponin T as the new definitive diagnostic markers because of their high sensitivity and specificity. Like CK-MB levels, cardiac troponin levels become elevated within 3 to 4 hours. Troponins continue to be released for up to 11 days (7- to 14-day range) after a cardiac event. Thus, troponin is a more useful diagnostic test than CK-MB in predicting an acute coronary event and serving as a late cardiac marker. Myoglobin is found exclusively in both cardiac and skeletal striated muscle. It is released within 1 to 3 hours after a myocyte cell injury, which currently makes it the earliest marker of cell injury. Unfortunately, myoglobin lacks the cardiac specificity of the troponins. This can lead to false-positive results because of skeletal, renal, or other cardiac issues. In addition, a mild leukocytosis of approximately $15,000/mm^3$ may persist for up to 1 week.

Stress Testing. Stress testing is not performed during an ST-elevation myocardial event. Based the ACC/AHA guidelines and each patient or risk/benefit profile, stress testing is, however, often performed after an MI to determine the risk of future ischemic events and to provide an exercise prescription for cardiac rehabilitation.

Echocardiography. Two-dimensional echocardiography can be of value in identifying wall motion abnormalities; estimating left ventricular ejection fraction (LVEF); assessing for pericardial effusion, ventricular aneurysm, and LV thrombus; and corroborating clinical and physical diagnosis of RV infarction. Doppler echocardiography is useful in the detection of valvular regurgitant lesions as well as ventricular and atrial septal defects. Echocardiography performed early in the course of an evolving MI is helpful in diagnosis and can aid in the decision-making process. In addition, the echocardiogram can provide prognostic information about LV function and identify patients who may be at risk for development of complications. Therefore, serial echocardiograms are beneficial for future comparison.

DIFFERENTIAL DIAGNOSIS

The primary focus in the ambulatory care setting is to differentiate cardiac from noncardiac chest pain. Four chest pain syndromes have a particularly high mortality rate and therefore need to be expediently detected, diagnosed, and managed. These conditions are aortic dissection, MI, pulmonary embolus, and spontaneous pneumothorax. Conditions in the differential diagnosis that have a lower mortality rate include gastrointestinal, pulmonary, valvular, inflammatory, integumentary, and psychological disturbances (Table 120-6).

MANAGEMENT

Chronic Stable Angina

Treatment of chronic stable angina involves many modalities. Because this is a chronic disease, it is important to have a good provider-patient relationship and a means of objectively evaluating specific therapeutic interventions. Such an objective measure of evaluation and classification is the previously noted classification of the CCSC.

The majority of patients should initially undergo noninvasive stress testing for diagnosis and risk stratification. Coronary angiography is appropriate only when the information derived from the procedure will significantly influence patent management, and the patient is agreeable to, and a candidate for, a percutaneous or surgical revascularization. As an alternative to invasive angiography many clinicians proceed to CTA, which may be a more appropriate and safer approach than routine invasive angiography. The medication regimen should include acetylsalicylic acid, beta blockers, lipid-lowering agents, and nitrates as needed. Nitrate tolerance is a major limitation to continuous nitrate therapy. To avoid tolerance, it is recommended that a daily nitrate-free interval of a minimum of 8 hours be provided. This interval is usually scheduled during the night when angina is less likely to occur. Calcium channel blockers are reasonable options for symptom relief if beta blockers are contraindicated or poorly tolerated or as an additional agent for symptom relief. Renin-angiotensin-aldosterone system blockers such as angiotensin-converting enzyme (ACE) inhibitors or angiotensin blockers should be implemented in patients with LVEF less than 40% and patients with diabetes, hypertension, or chronic kidney disease. Ranolazine is recommended to be used as a substitute for beta blocker therapy or in addition to beta blockers and/or calcium channel blockers for the treatment of chronic angina. Ranolazine is thought to inhibit the late inward sodium current during systole, which leads to reductions in intracellular calcium accumulation, LV wall tension, and oxygen consumption. It does not affect heart rate, blood pressure, contractility, or coronary blood flow. One of the major concerns is that ranolazine may cause QT prolongation and is contraindicated with concurrent QT-prolonging drugs or with a preexisting prolonged QT interval. It should also be avoided with the use of CYP3A4 inhibitors and in patients with hepatic impairment.

From an education perspective, patients should be cautioned about specific angina triggers. Lifting of a heavy load or performing arm exercise (isometric exercise) may precipitate angina symptoms because of an increase in myocardial oxygen demand. Walking in cold air may induce coronary vasoconstriction. It is advisable, therefore, to educate patients to cover the nose and mouth with a scarf when walking in cold weather. Finally, patients should be encouraged to exercise to a level below their anginal threshold to avoid the potential complications resulting from inactivity.

Silent Myocardial Ischemia

Myocardial ischemia can occur without symptoms. It has been observed that asymptomatic ST segment depression during ambulatory ECG monitoring occurs more often than symptomatic

TABLE 120-6 Differential Diagnosis: Chest Pain

Diagnosis	Symptoms	Physical Examination Findings
INTEGUMENTARY		
Herpes zoster	Prodromal symptoms of chest pressure Tingling, tenderness, and pain along involved dermatomes	Grouped vesicles along erythematous base
CHEST WALL DISCOMFORT		
Costochondritis	Anterior chest pain, sharply localized	Reproducible by pressure on costochondral junction
LUNGS		
Pneumonia	Pain when inflammatory process extends to pleura, resulting in chest pain that worsens with inspiration Fever, chills, cough, sputum production, dyspnea	Crackles, rales, or decreased breath sounds over affected area Bronchial breath sounds with dense consolidation, increased fremitus, and egophony (E-to-A changes) Dullness to percussion
Pneumothorax	Sudden-onset, severe unilateral chest pain, generally pleuritic in nature Dyspnea	Diminished breath sounds on affected side Mediastinal emphysema may be present
Pneumothorax, tension	Same as pneumothorax, yet with substernal chest pressure with throat tightness	Same as pneumothorax, but hypotension may be present Tracheal and mediastinal shift
Pulmonary embolus	Dyspnea Chest pain secondary to pulmonary infarction or inflammatory response (pleuritic)	Decreased breath sounds in affected area Hypotension with massive pulmonary embolus as a result of low cardiac output Hemoptysis, tachycardia, and hypoxia
Pulmonary hypertension	Mimics symptoms of ischemic chest pain Dyspnea	Prominent parasternal lift at lower left sternal border or xiphoid Pulmonic, tricuspid, or mitral regurgitation murmur S_4 may be audible
HEART		
Aortic stenosis	Easy fatigability, dyspnea on exertion, syncope or near-syncope, anterior chest pressure	Systolic murmur best heard over right base Delayed carotid upstrokes
Aortic dissections	Sudden onset of severe tearing, stabbing pain over anterior chest (proximal dissection) or interscapular-abdominal region (distal dissection) Diaphoresis, nausea, vomiting, near-syncope	Hypertension in 50% of patients Pulses diminished or absent Neurologic symptoms (decreased cerebral–spinal cord perfusion) Aortic regurgitation murmur may be present as a result of aortic root dissection
Mitral valve prolapse	Sharp left anterior chest pain, generally occurring in response to stress or emotional events Chest discomfort lasting seconds to days Palpitations and dyspnea	Mitral valve click may be noted in systole at left lower sternal border
Pericarditis Takotsubo cardiomyopathy	Anterior chest pain that may radiate to shoulder area if diaphragmatic surface of pericardium is involved Sharp chest pain that increases with inspiration or supine positioning (pleuritic) and lessens with forward positioning Chest pain, dyspnea	Fever with bacterial or viral cause Friction rub may or may not be present Possible hypotension, tachypnea, tachycardia, S_3 gallop, systolic ejection murmur (SEM) or holosystolic murmur, jugular venous distention (JVD), and/or bibasilar rales Clinical signs may be absent
GASTROINTESTINAL SYMPTOMS		
Reflux (gastroesophageal reflux disease) Acute cholecystitis	Substernal burning that may radiate to neck; occurs 30 to 60 minutes after eating Nausea, vomiting, and anorexia	Right upper quadrant pain, epigastric pain Right upper quadrant tenderness plus Murphy sign Fever may be present
PAIN DISORDERS		
	Intense anxiety that may last for several days Avoidance behavior because of inability to seek a safe refuge during an attack period Chest pain that is atypical Hypertension may be noted	

ST-segment depression in patients with CAD. The Asymptomatic Cardiac Ischemia Pilot Study (ACIP) enrolled patients in the 1990s and found that revascularization was better than medical therapy in reducing silent ischemic episodes and possibly cardiovascular events.

Management of patients with asymptomatic myocardial ischemia must be individualized. Exercise stress testing should be considered for evaluation of ischemia in asymptomatic male patients older than 45 years with one or more of the following risk factors: hypercholesteremia, hypertension, history of tobacco use, diabetes, or family history of early CAD. Diabetic patients with only one of the following risk factors should undergo exercise stress testing: age older than 35 years, type 2 diabetes for longer than 10 years or type 1 diabetes for longer than 15 years, any additional atherosclerotic risk factors for CAD, PVD, or presence of microvascular disease. Asymptomatic patients with silent ischemia and significant left main CAD or three-vessel CAD and impaired LV function are appropriate candidates for coronary artery bypass graft (CABG) surgery. Among patients with recent MI, silent ischemia verified by exercise stress test imaging and followed by percutaneous coronary intervention (PCI) reduced long-term risk of major cardiac events.

Microvascular Angina (Syndrome X)

The treatment of microvascular disease is aimed to relieve pain. Beta blockers are regarded as first-line therapy. They work by lowering adrenergic tone and reducing myocardial oxygen demand, as well as enhancing endothelium-dependent vasodilation. Calcium-channel blockers (nifedipine and diltiazem) may be used in combination with beta blockers; however, their efficacy has not yet been proven. Sublingual nitrates may benefit symptomatic episodes, but long-acting nitrates have proven disappointing. Xanthine derivatives such as aminophylline have been shown to improve the time to exercise-induced angina, time to ST depression, and magnitude of ST depression. They could be used when chronic airway disease and microvascular angina coexist. Some studies have found imipramine may be beneficial in pain modulation. Metformin has also been suggested, even in women without diabetes, because it may improve vascular function and decrease myocardial ischemia; however, further trials are required.[15] Lifestyle changes to incorporate risk factor modifications and the initiation of physical activity should also be implemented. Many patients will have resolution of symptoms but may have periods of exacerbations. It is important to note that there does not appear to be a risk for MI or sudden cardiac death despite the presence of symptoms, and therefore reassurance of the patient is an important part of therapy.

Variant Angina

Acute treatment of the chest pain episode is usually sublingual nitroglycerin. Calcium channel and beta blockers are the long-term treatments of choice for this condition. Continuous nitrate therapy is not recommended because of problems with tolerance, but targeted nitrates may be helpful in patients with a predictable pattern of pain.

The natural history of spasm is one of periods of symptomatic exacerbation followed by periods of relative quiescence. Once a patient who is receiving therapy has been without symptoms for 6 to 12 months, medication withdrawal can be attempted. Patients with spasm without significant fixed coronary stenosis are not candidates for mechanical intervention.

Unstable Angina and Non-ST Segment Elevation Myocardial Infarction

Early risk stratification should be performed to determine the likelihood of an acute cardiac ischemic event from NSTEMI. The immediate management of this population of patients consists of a detailed patient history, physical examination, and 12-lead ECG within 10 minutes of arrival at an emergency facility. Cardiac specific troponin (troponin I or T) levels should be measured at presentation and at 3 to 6 hours after symptom onset. From this information, the health care provider can usually assign the patient with chest pain to one of four categories: a noncardiac cause, a stable angina cause, a possible acute coronary artery syndrome, or a definite coronary artery syndrome. All patients with unstable angina or NSTEMI should be referred to a cardiologist for further management.

Low-risk patients should be immediately started on aspirin therapy, 160 to 325 mg, unless contraindicated, daily beta blocker therapy provided there are no contraindications, and sublingual nitroglycerin as needed. Identifiable precipitating clinical circumstances should be uncovered, as should any secondary causes (e.g., fever, anemia, hypotension, cardiomyopathy, aortic stenosis, thyrotoxicosis, or recent stressful events). Symptoms of unstable angina may resolve once the precipitating event has been treated. Low-risk patients should be seen for follow-up evaluation within a 72-hour period, at which time symptoms should be reevaluated for any further instability. Early exercise tolerance testing should also be performed. Patients should be educated about cardiac risk factors and aggressive plans for risk factor modification.

Patients in the intermediate or high-risk category should be hospitalized for careful monitoring, risk stratification, and management. If the symptoms of ACS are identified in the office setting, immediate referral to an emergency department should be undertaken. The patient should be given sublingual nitroglycerin and chewable aspirin immediately. If chewable aspirin is not available, a regular aspirin tablet should be crushed and given to the patient. Once the patient is in the emergency department setting, beta blocker therapy should be initiated within 24 hours if the presenting hemodynamic profile permits, with the dose titrated to a heart rate of 50 to 60 beats per minute. Contraindications to beta blocker therapy include (1) signs of heart failure; (2) evidence of a low-output state; (3) increased risk for cardiogenic shock; or (4) PR interval greater than 0.24 seconds, second- or third-degree heart block without a cardiac pacemaker, active asthma, or reactive airway disease.

ACE inhibitors and angiotensin II receptor blockers have improved survival rates in patients with acute MI and are most beneficial to patients experiencing anterior wall infarction, pulmonary congestion, or LVEF less than 40%, according to AHA guidelines.

Heparin should be considered with a bolus of 80 units/kg of body weight and then infused at 14 units/kg/hr. The dose is then titrated to achieve an activated partial thromboplastin time of 1.5 to 2.0 times the control value. Low-molecular-weight heparin may also be considered in lieu of intravenous heparin therapy. Guidelines indicate that initiation of statins within 24 hours of acute MI or ACS has reduced major cardiac events.

High-intensity statin therapy should be initiated or continued in all patients who have no contraindications to its use. A P2Y12 inhibitor (e.g., clopidogrel or ticagrelor) in addition to aspirin should be administered for up to 12 months in all patients who undergo PCI. For some patients, longer dual-agent therapy may be a consideration.[16] An urgent immediate invasive strategy is indicated in patients who have refractory angina or hemodynamic or electrical instability.

Acute ST-Segment Elevation Myocardial Infarction

Treatment goals for the patient with an acute MI are to restore blood supply to cardiac muscle, relieve pain, and decrease the incidence of complications (such as heart failure, myocardial rupture, valvular dysfunction, and fatal and nonfatal arrhythmias). With these goals in mind, patients with an acute evolving STEMI should be transferred to a hospital with a dedicated chest pain center and interventional cardiac program within 90 minutes. Primary PCI is the recommended method of reperfusion when it can be performed in a timely fashion by experienced operators. At non–PCI capable hospitals, when the anticipated time of transfer would exceed 120 minutes, fibrinolytic therapy should be administered within 30 minutes of the time of first medical contact to patients with an evolving STEMI in the absence of contraindications. Reperfusion therapy should be administered to all eligible patients who experienced the onset of symptom within the previous 12 hours because benefit can still be achieved when therapy is instituted 3 to 6 hours after the onset of infarction, and some benefit is possible when therapy is given up to 12 hours after the onset of infarction if chest pain is ongoing and ST-segment elevation is apparent in electrocardiographic leads that do not demonstrate new Q waves. Delays in reperfusion have been shown to increase mortality rates. General contraindications to lytic therapy include recent surgery or head trauma, active internal bleeding, suspected aortic dissection, pregnancy, diabetic hemorrhagic retinopathy, severe hypertension, and history of cerebrovascular accident or allergic reaction to the thrombolytic agent. Hemorrhagic stroke is the most common complication. The rate increases with advancing age. Patients older than 70 years have strokes at twice the rate of younger patients; however, older patients may benefit from lytic therapy. Decisions about thrombolytic therapy must be made on a case-by-case basis in these patients.

Adjunctive antithrombotic therapy at the time of primary PCI would include aspirin in doses of 162 to 325 mg before PCI, and after PCI should be continued indefinitely. Heparin is usually administered by weight adjustment to keep the partial thromboplastin time at 1.5 to 2 times normal. Unless contraindicated, a loading dose of a P2Y12 receptor inhibitor (clopidogrel, prasugrel, or ticagrelor) should be given as early as possible or at the time of primary PCI to patients with evolving STEMI and should be continued for at least 1 year in patients with drug-eluting stents (DESs). Most recently, the Dual Antiplatelet Therapy (DAPT) Study showed that continuation of a P2Y12 receptor inhibitor and aspirin therapy for up to 30 months, when compared with the continuation of aspirin alone, in patients with a DES resulted in a significantly reduced rate of stent thrombosis.[16]

Oral beta blocker therapy should be initiated in the first 24 hours in patients with STEMI who do not have any symptoms of heart failure, a low output state, or cardiogenic shock. Other concerns related to beta blocker therapy would include a PR interval greater than 0.24 seconds, second- or third-degree heart block, active asthma, or reactive airway disease. Patients with initial contraindications should be reevaluated to determine if the prior contraindications have resolved.

The use of ACE inhibitors has improved the mortality rate and the prevention of heart failure and recurrent MI in patients with LVEF of 40% or less. If possible, ACE inhibitors should be started once the patient is hemodynamically stable. Renal issues should also be considered when ACE inhibitor therapy is started; renal artery stenosis is a contraindication to this therapy. Among lower-risk patients with normal LVEFs, ACE inhibitor therapy initiated early in the course of hospitalization has improved survival rates for patients with acute MI.

Calcium channel blockers have been shown to be effective in acute and chronic stable angina, to lower blood pressure and to control heart rate with atrial fibrillation in patients who are intolerant of beta blockers. They have not been shown to have any beneficial effect on infarct size or the rate of reinfarction. They should not be given to patients with LV systolic dysfunction. The use of immediate-release nifedipine is contraindicated in patients with STEMI because of hypotension and reflex sympathetic activation with tachycardia.

Nitrates can assist with relief of symptoms by decreasing LV preload and to some extent increasing coronary blood flow. Nitrates are further useful to treat hypertension or heart failure. Nitrates should not be given to STEMI patients with hypotension, marked bradycardia, RV infarction, or phosphodiesterase type 5 inhibitor use within the previous 24 to 48 hours.

Pharmacologic Therapy for Coronary Artery Disease

Aspirin. Aspirin is effective in the treatment of CAD because of its effects on platelets and vascular endothelial cells. In platelets, aspirin irreversibly inhibits the synthesis of cyclooxygenase, preventing the formation of thromboxane A_2, which is responsible for platelet aggregation. In vascular endothelial cells, aspirin temporarily inhibits the synthesis of cyclooxygenase, which inhibits prostacyclin production and platelet aggregation. The clinical benefits of aspirin have been demonstrated at doses of 75 to 325 mg/day.

Aspirin reaches appreciable plasma levels within 20 minutes and results in platelet inhibition within 60 minutes. The antiplatelet effect of aspirin lasts for the 10-day life of the platelet; however, 10% of circulating platelets are replaced on a daily basis. Normal hemostasis can be achieved with only 20% of aspirin-free platelets. This becomes an important consideration in the timing of aspirin withdrawal for elective surgical procedures.

Aspirin therapy has proved to benefit patients in the acute phase of an evolving MI and should be routinely administered orally with an initial loading dose of 325 mg unless an anaphylactic aspirin allergy is known. Enteric-coated tablets should be chewed or crushed for more rapid absorption. The U.S. Preventive Services Task Force recommends aspirin use in men ages 45 to 79 years when the potential benefit resulting from a reduction in MIs outweighs the potential harm resulting from an increase in gastrointestinal hemorrhage. Aspirin is recommended for women ages 55 to 79 years when the potential benefit to reduce ischemic stroke outweighs the potential harm of an increase in gastrointestinal hemorrhage. The American Diabetes Association and AHA jointly recommend 75 to 162 mg a day of aspirin as primary prevention of heart disease for persons with diabetes who are older than 40 years and who also have additional risk factors for cardiovascular disease and no contraindications to aspirin therapy.

Beta Blockers. Beta blockers have become the mainstay of therapy for patients with CAD. Beta blockers decrease myocardial oxygen consumption by decreasing the heart rate at rest and with exercise, by lowering the blood pressure, and by reducing myocardial contractility, thereby eliciting a negative inotropic effect. In contrast, these agents are not useful for vasospastic angina and may worsen the condition. Beta blockers have been shown to reduce total mortality, rate of nonfatal infarction, infarct size, cardiovascular mortality, and sudden cardiac death.

Beta blockers can be classified according to their relative cardioselectivity and lipid solubility. Beta blockers may be nonselective (have an affinity for both $beta_1$ and $beta_2$ receptors) or selective (have an affinity for $beta_1$ receptors). $Beta_1$ receptors are located in the myocardium, with small amounts of $beta_2$ receptors in the atrium. $Beta_2$ receptors are primarily located in the bronchioles, peripheral vascular smooth muscles, and other specialized sites, such as pancreatic islet cells. Thus, blockade of $beta_2$ receptors may lead to bronchoconstriction or bronchospasm and peripheral vascular constriction, resulting in claudication. In addition, the mechanism whereby insulin-induced hypoglycemia is countered by stimulation of the liver to mobilize liver glycogen is $beta_2$ receptor dependent. Thus, blockade of $beta_2$ receptors in a patient with diabetes may lead to an inappropriate response to hypoglycemia. This is important because patients with CAD and asthma, COPD, diabetes, or intermittent claudication may benefit from a low dose of $beta_1$-selective agents administered with caution. However, as the dose of such agents is increased, selectivity is lost, and both types of receptors become blocked (Box 120-5).

Side effects of beta blockers include fatigue, impotence, cold extremities, bronchospasm, worsening claudication, bradycardia, and cardiac conduction disturbances. Central nervous system side effects are based on the agent's lipid solubility property. Agents that are lipid soluble readily cross the blood-brain barrier and are more likely to cause insomnia, depression and nightmares; this may be seen in any patient but is commonly observed in older adults. Patients should be cautioned that sudden discontinuation of beta blocker therapy may precipitate angina symptoms or lead to MI as a result of rebound tachycardia. Although much has been written about the beta blocker withdrawal syndrome, the incidence is low. However, in discontinuing the drug, one should be prudent and taper the drug during several days. Some beta blockers have the capacity to stimulate either one or both $beta_1$ and $beta_2$ receptors—hence the term *intrinsic sympathomimetic activity,* as seen with pindolol. This property limits the efficacy of treating patients with angina because at higher doses the heart rate is not decreased and may even be increased. These agents may be beneficial in patients who have symptomatic sinus bradycardia when they are treated with other beta blockers. The major effect of beta blockers with sympathomimetic activity is lowering of blood pressure. Labetalol possesses both beta- and alpha-blocking actions. This drug can be used to treat patients with angina as well as patients with significant hypertension.

BOX 120-5

Beta Blocker Agents

NONSELECTIVE $BETA_1$ AND $BETA_2$ BLOCKERS
Propranolol (Inderal)
Timolol (Blocadren)
Nadolol (Corgard)
Sotalol (Betapace)
Penbutolol (Levatol)

NONSELECTIVE, VASODILATORY
Labetalol (Trandate, Normodyne)
Pindolol

CARDIOSELECTIVE, $BETA_1$ RECEPTORS ONLY
Acebutolol (Sectral)
Atenolol (Tenormin)
Metoprolol (Lopressor, Toprol-XL)
Esmolol (Brevibloc)
Bisoprolol (Zebeta)
Nebivolol (Bystolic)

COMBINATION $ALPHA_1$ AND NONCARDIOSELECTIVE BETA BLOCKER
Carvedilol (Coreg)

Nitrates. Nitrates are recommended for the treatment of stable and unstable angina and the management of an acute MI. The clinical effectiveness of nitrates is in their ability to promote vascular smooth muscle relaxation, resulting in arteriolar and venous dilation. In smaller doses, nitrates dilate the venous system, which causes peripheral pooling and decreased venous return to the heart (preload). This reduction in preload decreases the LV size, ventricular filling pressures, and myocardial wall tension. In larger doses, nitrates dilate the arterial vasculature, lowering systemic blood pressure (afterload) and thereby decreasing the resistance to ventricular ejection, making it easier for the heart to contract. This overall reduction in LV workload decreases myocardial oxygen consumption. The arteriolar dilating effect, however, may produce a reflex tachycardia, thereby increasing myocardial oxygen consumption. This effect may be attenuated by concurrent use of beta blockade. In addition, the combination of nitrates with calcium channel blockers should be undertaken cautiously because postural hypotension may be a problem.

Coronary vasodilation is induced through the exogenous production of nitric oxide from nitrate metabolism, which is now known to be EDRF. In the coronary circulation, damage to the endothelial layer from atherosclerosis results in decreased availability of EDRF and hence a decreased vasodilatory response. Nitrates are endothelium-independent vasodilators and therefore do not require a functioning endothelium to deliver a vasodilating response. Nitrate administration results in the endogenous production of nitric oxide, which replaces the vasodilating effects of EDRF and promotes coronary vessel vasodilation.

Three nitrate preparations are currently available for use in the United States (Table 120-7): nitroglycerin, isosorbide dinitrate (ISDN), and isosorbide mononitrate (ISMN). Sublingual nitroglycerin tablets in doses of 0.4 mg are most useful for acute angina events because of the rapid course of action of sublingual nitroglycerin. Sublingual nitroglycerin is also recommended for prophylactic use before the patient engages in a physical activity or a stressful event that has historically precipitated an angina event. Sublingual nitroglycerin works within 3 to 5 minutes; however, anti-ischemic effects last for less than 30 minutes. Because of its short duration of action, sublingual nitroglycerin should be combined with oral nitrates for sustained effectiveness. According to the ACC/AHA 2007 guidelines for the

TABLE 120-7 **Nitrate Preparations***

Preparation	Starting Dose	Maximum Dose	Onset of Action	Duration of Action
Nitroglycerin (Nitrostat)	0.4 mg (1 tablet)	3 tablets in 15 min	1 min	<30 min
Nitroglycerin (Nitrolingual)	0.4 mg (metered spray)	3 sprays in 15 min	1 min	<30 min
ISDN (Isordil, Sorbitrate)	20 mg every 4-6 hr	240 mg/day	60-90 min	4-6 hr
ISDN-SR (Dilatrate-SR)	40 mg every 8-12 hr			
ISMN (Ismo, Monoket)	20 mg in AM and 20 mg 7 hr later			
ISMN-SR (Imdur)	30-60 mg/day	120-240 mg/day		
Nitroglycerin ointment (2%) (Nitro-Bid, Nitrol)	½ inch every 4-6 hr	4-5 inches every 3-4 hr	30-60 min	3-6 hr
Nitroglycerin patch (Transderm-Nitro, Nitro-Dur, Nitrodisc, Deponit)	5 mg/24 hr (0.1 to 0.4 mg/hr)	2-3 patches of 15 mg in 24 hr	30 min	24 hr

*Regimen for nitrate preparations should include a dose-free interval each day to prevent refractory tolerance.

management of patients with unstable angina or NSTEMI, "Health care providers should instruct patients with suspected ACS for whom nitroglycerin [NTG] has been prescribed previously to take not more than 1 dose of NTG sublingually in response to chest discomfort/pain. If chest discomfort/pain is unimproved or is worsening 5 min after 1 NTG dose has been taken, it is recommended that the patient or family member/friend/caregiver call 911 immediately to access EMS before taking additional NTG. In patients with chronic stable angina, if symptoms are significantly improved by 1 dose of NTG, it is appropriate to instruct the patient or family member/friend/caregiver to repeat NTG every 5 min for a maximum of 3 doses and call 911 if symptoms have not resolved completely."

Nitroglycerin tablets retain their potency for up to 6 months after the bottle has been opened. Patients should be encouraged to keep nitroglycerin tablets in their amber-colored glass bottle, protected from moisture and extremes of temperature and light.

Nitroglycerin spray is particularly useful for patients with visual or neurologic impairments, who may have difficulty handling a small tablet. The spray is delivered at a metered dose of 0.4 mg and should be applied to the surface of the tongue. Patients should be reminded not to inhale the spray. Each canister contains approximately 200 doses, and the canister will maintain its potency for up to 3 years.

Oral nitroglycerin is the nitrate of choice in the ambulatory population and can be taken as either ISDN or ISMN. ISDN is extensively metabolized in the liver, where more than half of it is converted to ISMN. Because of this bypass effect, ISDN is not effective for treatment of angina or enhancement of exercise capacity in doses of less than 20 mg every 4 hours. In 1991, the U.S. Food and Drug Administration approved ISMN, which does not undergo hepatic degradation, so that 100% of it is available after oral administration. The main advantage of the ISMNs is that they can be administered once or twice daily, whereas ISDNs must be administered three or four times per day. The main disadvantage is the cost. ISMN preparations cost several times more than the generic ISDN, and this needs to be considered in prescribing practices. Aside from these two factors, there is no distinct advantage in use of one of these preparations over the other.

Topical nitroglycerin is absorbed through the skin and can be administered either as a 2% ointment or by premeasured skin patches in doses of 5, 10, 15, or 20 mg/day. The advantage of nitroglycerin ointment over other methods of administration is that the ointment can be removed promptly if any side effects develop. However, its disadvantages seem to outweigh its advantages in the ambulatory population. The ointment is messy to apply, can soil clothing, is seldom dosed consistently each time, and may produce a localized rash. The nitroglycerin patch produces a more controlled dose and is generally favored over the ointment. Although topical nitroglycerin is initially effective, long-term use can lead to nitrate tolerance and thus a decreased therapeutic effect. It is therefore recommended that topical nitroglycerin be removed from the skin for 8 to 12 hours daily.

Nitrate tolerance results from plasma nitrate levels sustained from continued nitrate administration. It is important to identify nitrate tolerance because it leads to a reduction in anti-ischemic benefits. The cause of nitrate tolerance is a complex, multifactorial phenomenon, and the mechanism remains elusive. However, the theory that is commonly associated with nitrate tolerance involves vascular depletion of sulfhydryl groups. The metabolism of nitrates requires the use of sulfhydryl to form intracellular nitric oxide from nitrates. This is the active molecule that stimulates guanylate cyclase to produce vasodilation. Continuous use of nitrates produces excess nitric oxide formation, thus depleting sulfhydryl groups. A sulfhydryl donor such as acetylcysteine has been used in experiments to counteract nitrate tolerance.

To avoid the effects of nitrate tolerance, intervals free of nitrates must occur. For oral ISDN administration, an administration schedule of three times per day (8 AM, 1 PM, and 6 PM) rather than four times per day should be prescribed. With sustained-release ISDN administration, administration at 8 AM and 2 PM would support nitrate-free intervals in the evening. Topical nitrates should be removed for 8 to 12 hours daily. This schedule provides periods during the evening hours when the patient is without anti-ischemic therapy. For this reason and because of the reflex tachycardia often seen with vasodilation in response to nitrate therapy, combination therapy with beta blockers or calcium channel blockers is recommended.

Calcium Channel Blockers. Calcium channel blockers are used in the treatment of hypertension and angina pectoris. They selectively inhibit the influx of calcium into the calcium

BOX 120-6

Calcium Channel Blockers

DIHYDROPYRIDINES

Amlodipine (Norvasc)
Isradipine (DynaCirc)
Felodipine (Plendil)
Nicardipine (Cardene)
Nifedipine (Procardia, Adalat)
Nisoldipine (Sular)

NONDIHYDROPYRIDINES

Diphenylalkylamine derivative: verapamil (Calan, Covera-HS, Isoptin, Verelan)
Benzothiazepine derivative: diltiazem (Cardizem, Dilacor, Tiazac)

L-channel in both smooth muscle and myocardial cells. All have a peripheral arteriolar and coronary vasodilating effect and a negative inotropic effect, although the latter is modest in the case of nifedipine. Two distinct classes of calcium channel antagonists have emerged on the basis of molecular structure (Box 120-6): the dihydropyridines (DHPs), with a chemical structure similar to nifedipine; and the non-DHPs, such as verapamil (papaverine derivative) and diltiazem (benzothiazepine derivative).

The DHPs are more vascular selective; thus their dominant effect is peripheral and coronary vasodilation. They have minimum or no effect on the sinus and atrioventricular nodes. The rapid vasodilatory effects of these agents may lead to reflex tachycardia, exacerbation of heart failure, and stimulation of the renin-angiotensin system. These undesirable effects are more common among the short-acting DHPs, which should be avoided in the patient with an acute MI. Extended-release non-DHPs may be considered in patients with unstable angina or NSTEMI instead of beta blockers or as adjuncts to beta blocker therapy in the presence of ongoing ischemia or hypertension.

Angiotensin-Converting Enzyme Inhibitors and Angiotensin II Receptor Blockers. The conical shape of the heart is designed for optimum efficiency in performance and energy use. MI induces alteration in the contour of the heart, leading to decreased LV performance and increased energy requirement for a given workload. Preservation of the contour of the heart after MI is essential for effective LV performance and prevention of the development of left-sided heart failure. Studies have shown significant survival benefits for older patients with heart failure who are compliant with ACE inhibitor therapy.

It is clear that stimulation of the renin-angiotensin-aldosterone system plays an important pathophysiologic role in the development of heart failure and poor LV performance. ACE inhibitors can therefore inhibit or counteract the adverse hemodynamic and neurohumoral effects (increased preload, afterload, heart rate, sympathetic tone, catecholamines, and renin-angiotensin system activity) contributed by the system.

Heart failure guidelines have shown that administration of ACE inhibitors shortly after acute MI, once the patient is hemodynamically stable, has prevented the development of heart failure in patients with LV dysfunction but without clinical heart failure. In addition, ACE inhibitors reduced long-term mortality in patients with and without clinical evidence of heart failure through the ability of the inhibitors to reverse the major hemodynamic and neurohumoral abnormalities associated with poor LV performance. Angiotensin receptor blockers should be used in patients who are intolerant of ACE inhibitors and have heart failure or have had an MI with LVEF of less than 40%.

Anticoagulation. The use of anticoagulation with aspirin and heparin has significantly reduced the short-term risk of thromboembolic complications during an acute MI. With the use of heparin infusion, therapeutic levels may be difficult to maintain. An alternative to unfractionated heparin is the use of low-molecular-weight heparin. Enoxaparin and fondaparinux have been shown to reduce mortality and reinfarction but can be administered only to patients with normal renal function.

A significant percentage of patients with ACS experience major vascular events either during or within the first few months after their hospital stay. Another recommended adjunctive therapy for ACS is clopidogrel, which irreversibly binds to the adenosine diphosphate receptors on platelets, causing a decrease in platelet aggregation. Clopidogrel has been shown to reduce cardiovascular morbidity and mortality when it is administered to patients with NSTEMI. In patients up to 75 years of age experiencing a STEMI, there is a reduction in major cardiac event mortality.

Cases in which there is a mural thrombus represent another circumstance for anticoagulation. Ventricular mural thrombi are more common in patients with a large rather than a small area of MI. Thrombi are often observed in the left ventricle, particularly in the apex, where aneurysm and pseudoaneurysm commonly form. On rare occasions, with extensive infarction, thrombus may be observed in the RV apex. Warfarin (Coumadin) therapy is indicated in patients with a mural thrombus, especially in cases in which the thrombus is mobile, has an irregular surface, and is protruding. Warfarin therapy is generally initiated for 3 to 6 months, after which time echocardiographic evaluation to assess the presence or absence of mural thrombus is performed. If the thrombus persists after warfarin therapy, it does not necessarily indicate continued embolic potential unless there is evidence of mobility. In addition, warfarin therapy is indicated in patients with severe LV dysfunction and an LVEF of less than 20%.

LIFE SPAN CONSIDERATIONS: WOMEN AND HEART DISEASE

Approximately 6.6 million women alive today have CHD. Of these, 2.6 million have a history of MI. Each year new and recurrent MI and fatal CHD will affect an estimated 385,000 women. Of women age 45 and older who have an initial recognized MI (heart attack), 26% die within a year compared with 19% of men. This is in part because women have heart attacks at older ages than men do, they're more likely to die from the heart attack within a few weeks.

It has been observed that 64% of women who died suddenly of CHD had no previous symptoms. In 2010, 518,000 women diagnosed with CHD were discharged from short-stay hospitals.

The gender differences between men and women with respect to coronary anatomy, clinical presentation, and treatment modalities have recently been under investigation. The clinical presentation of women often is not the typical midsternal chest tightness with shoulder and arm radiation that men often experience. Instead, women may be seen initially with indigestion as their only symptom. Because the mortality rate from STEMI is higher in women than in men, it is important that gender bias be eliminated from the clinical decision-making and that the nuances of CAD in women be acknowledged. Current data continue to show disparity in diagnosis and management of ACS and acute MI in women.

The diagnosis of CAD in women has also proved difficult because of false-positive results of exercise tolerance testing in women. The electrocardiographic response to such testing in women has been shown to be an abnormal ischemic response in up to 67% of those tested, despite normal coronary arteries. Speculation in this area suggests women's lower hematocrit levels and higher circulating estrogen levels as plausible culprits. Radionuclide testing may be performed to provide greater test sensitivity and specificity. Despite the increased accuracy of this testing, a significant number of false-positive results still occur, mainly as a result of breast attenuation artifact, which may produce septal and anterior wall defects. Stress echocardiography may prove a more accurate method of noninvasive CAD testing in women.

COMPLICATIONS

The complications of ischemic heart disease and MI are potentially life-threatening. Recurrent ischemia and reinfarction can increase the area of nonfunctioning myocardial tissue, creating mechanical complications such as papillary muscle rupture, ventricular aneurysm, and ventricular septal defect. Rhythm and conduction disturbances may arise without premonitory signs. Chest pain and anxiety associated with cardiac disease can produce hypertension, increasing afterload and oxygen demand. Heart failure, hypotension, and shock impair systemic perfusion and cardiac function.

INDICATIONS FOR REFERRAL OR HOSPITALIZATION

The patient whose condition is complicated by multiple comorbid diseases (e.g., diabetes mellitus, hypertension, heart failure, hyperlipidemia, and PVD) should be referred to a cardiologist. Patients with chronic stable angina who develop a change in angina pattern should also be referred to a specialist. In addition, all patients with a documented history of coronary ischemic syndrome should be co-managed with a cardiologist. The patient's symptoms and comorbid diseases should determine the frequency of visits to the specialist.

Ischemic CAD represents a spectrum of coronary insufficiency ranging from chronic stable angina, unstable angina, or non Q wave MI (subendomyocardial infarction) to transmural MI. Hospitalization is based on specific criteria.

Patients who have unstable angina pectoris, defined as new-onset angina (angina occurring within 1 month), angina occurring at rest and with minimum exertion, or crescendo angina, should be admitted to the hospital. All patients who are thought to be having or are having an acute MI should be immediately brought to the nearest emergency department.

PATIENT AND FAMILY EDUCATION

Considerations for patients with CAD include careful management of comorbid illnesses along with a thorough understanding of their disease process and prescribed medical regimen. Women who are candidates for hormone replacement therapy should be offered information about the risks and benefits of estrogen or hormone replacement therapy after menopause.

Patients need to be educated about CAD and heart attack warning signs. Angina symptoms are often present days to weeks before the onset of an acute MI. Therefore, education to assist patients in recognizing cardiac symptoms and the formation of an early action plan should be undertaken. The National Institutes of Health educational materials emphasize recognition of heart attack warning signs and the importance of activation of EMS immediately. Risk factor identification and the ability to plan ahead in case of a heart attack are also educational goals for the community.

It is well established that deaths from acute MI occur within the first hour of onset. Therefore, the importance of education regarding symptoms of an MI and rapid transport and early admission to a hospital cannot be overemphasized.

Both patients and families should understand the importance of calling 911 or an ambulance if the symptoms of a heart attack occur. These symptoms include chest pressure or discomfort; pain radiating to the arm, neck, or jaw; diaphoresis; nausea or vomiting; shortness of breath; dizziness; rapid or irregular pulse; and loss of consciousness. All families who have a family member with CAD should be encouraged to learn cardiopulmonary resuscitation.

HEALTH PROMOTION

Adherence to the guidelines for ideal cardiovascular health (see earlier) is paramount. Despite growing evidence from clinical trials establishing that risk factor modification can decrease coronary artery morbidity and mortality, the majority of patients still are not being treated. The AHA has developed the Get with the Guidelines program to ensure that patients are being discharged with prescription of appropriate medications and with risk factor counseling. These guidelines focus on smoking cessation, lipid lowering, ACE inhibitor use, beta blocker therapy, hypertension management, weight and exercise management, diabetes management, atrial fibrillation management, aspirin or other antithrombotic medication, and alcohol and drug abuse management.

CHAPTER 121

HEART FAILURE

Virginia L. Beggs

DEFINITION AND EPIDEMIOLOGY

Heart failure (HF) is a complex syndrome characterized by the inability of the heart to meet the body's metabolic demands; it is a clinical diagnosis. It results from any structural or functional cardiac disorder that impairs the ventricle's ability to fill or to eject blood properly. HF is not the same as cardiomyopathy or left ventricular dysfunction (Table 121-1). HF has been divided into two main types:

1. HFrEF: heart failure with reduced ejection fraction of 40% or lower, notable for a reduction in the contractility of the left ventricle. Left ventricular systolic dysfunction is often associated with clinical symptoms when the left ventricular ejection fraction (LVEF) falls below 40%, resulting in pump failure. HFrEF has historically been associated with symptomatic HF, and is also known as systolic HF.

TABLE 121-1 HFrEF Versus HFpEF in Heart Failure: Differences in History, Physical Examination Findings, and Diagnostic Test Results*

Parameter	HFrEF	HFpEF
HISTORY		
Coronary artery disease	+++	++
Hypertension	++	++++
Diabetes	++	++
Valvular heart disease	++++	+
Paroxysmal dyspnea	++	+++
PHYSICAL EXAMINATION		
Cardiomegaly	+++	+
Soft heart sounds	++++	+
S_3 gallop	+++	+
S_4 gallop	+	+++
Hypertension	++	++++
Mitral regurgitation murmur	+++	+
Rales	++	+
Edema	+++	+
Jugular venous distention	+++	+
CHEST X-RAY EXAMINATION		
Cardiomegaly	+++	+
Pulmonary congestion	+++	+++
ELECTROCARDIOGRAPHY		
Low voltage	+++	–
Left ventricular hypertrophy	++	++++
Q waves	++	+
ECHOCARDIOGRAPHY		
Left atrial enlargement	++	++
Low ejection fraction	++++	–
Left ventricular dilation	++	–
Left ventricular hypertrophy	++	++++

*Plus signs indicate "suggestive" (the number reflects relative weight). Minus signs indicate "not very suggestive."
Modified from Young JB: Assessment of heart failure. In Colucci WS, editor: *Atlas of heart failure: cardiac function and dysfunction,* ed 3, Philadelphia, 2002, Current Medicine.

2. HFpEF: heart failure with preserved ejection fraction of 50% or higher, associated with impairment of ventricular filling and relaxation, wherein the left ventricular filling pressures are often high, resulting in a reduced stroke volume with exertion, causing HF symptoms. HFpEF now accounts for approximately 50% of all patients with HF.[1]

Although coronary artery disease is the most common cause of HFrEF, hypertension, atrial fibrillation, and diabetes are common antecedents of HFpEF. It has been hypothesized that HFpEF may be more than just one problem. The Organized Program to Initiate Lifesaving Treatment in Hospitalized Patients with Heart Failure (OPTIMIZE-HF) registry shows a similar postdischarge mortality risk and rehospitalization rate for both HFpEF and HFrEF patients. Clinical presentation of HF is wide ranging, from mild, exertionally related dyspnea resulting from fluid retention to cardiogenic shock and lethal arrhythmias. Cardinal symptoms of HF are dyspnea and fatigue, often but not always associated with volume overload.[2-4]

Etiology

The etiology of HF can be divided into the following three broad categories:

1. Anatomic or functional abnormalities of the coronary vessels, myocardium, or cardiac valves, of either sudden or gradual onset
2. Neurohormonal overexpression that causes activation of the adrenergic nervous system and renin-angiotensin system
3. Extracardiac factors that cause excessive demand on the cardiovascular system[1]

The most common diseases associated with HF are coronary artery disease, hypertension, and dilated cardiomyopathies (Box 121-1). Most forms of heart disease predispose the patient to HF over time; viral, metabolic, and toxic insults to the myocardium can cause acute symptomatic HF that may become chronic if left untreated. Common antecedents of HFpEF include hypertension, diabetes, and atrial fibrillation. Early diagnosis and treatment can improve quality of life and life expectancy for people who have HF.

The 30-day, 1-year, and 5-year case fatality rates after a hospitalization for HF are 10.4%, 22%, and 42.3%, respectively. The OPTIMIZE-HF registry shows a similar postdischarge mortality risk and rehospitalization rate for both HFpEF and HFrEF.[4]

Physician consultation is indicated for new onset of HF in a patient with no previous history of cardiac disease.

Physician consultation is recommended for patients with deterioration of previously stable HF.

Cardiomyopathy. Cardiomyopathy, the most common cause of HF, is a disease process of the myocardium that affects the heart's pumping ability. Classification of heart muscle disease is complex; an expert panel defined cardiomyopathies as "a heterogeneous group of diseases of the myocardium associated with mechanical and/or electrical dysfunction that usually (but not invariably) exhibit inappropriate ventricular hypertrophy or dilatation and are due to a variety of causes that frequently are genetic. Cardiomyopathies either are confined to the heart or are part of generalized systemic disorders, often leading to cardiovascular death or progressive heart failure–related disability."[5]

Cardiomyopathies have been divided into two major groups:

1. Primary (including genetic, nongenetic, and acquired cardiomyopathies)—confined to the heart muscle
2. Secondary—heart muscle involvement as part of a general or systemic disease or disorder

An example of a primary cardiomyopathy would be the genetic disorder hypertrophic cardiomyopathy; an example of an acquired cardiomyopathy would be myocarditis or an inflammatory cardiomyopathy. Stress cardiomyopathy (Takotsubo), infiltrative cardiomyopathy such as amyloidosis, and

BOX 121-1

Causes of Heart Failure

ANATOMIC OR FUNCTIONAL ABNORMALITIES OF THE CORONARY VESSELS, MYOCARDIUM, OR CARDIAC VALVES

Ischemic heart disease
Valvular heart disease
Pericardial disease
Congenital defects
Chronic tachycardia
Idiopathic cardiomyopathies
- Dilated
- Hypertrophic
- Restricted

EXTRACARDIAC FACTORS THAT CAUSE EXCESSIVE DEMAND ON THE CARDIOVASCULAR SYSTEM

Toxic cardiomyopathy (e.g., alcohol, chemotherapeutic agents)
Hypertension
Endocrine or metabolic disorders (contractility not usually impaired; rather, metabolic demands are in excess of normal cardiac output; volume overload of the left ventricle)

NONCARDIAC DISEASE

Viral illness (parvovirus, cytomegalovirus, Epstein-Barr virus, hepatitis, Lyme disease, varicella, and others)
Thyrotoxicosis
Anemia
Iron overload disease
Pregnancy
Fever, systemic infection
Arteriovenous fistulas
Vitamin B_1 deficiency (beriberi)
Amyloidosis, sarcoidosis

CONNECTIVE TISSUE DISEASES

Systemic lupus erythematosus
Polymyositis
Progressive systemic sclerosis (scleroderma)

PULMONARY DISEASES

Cor pulmonale secondary to chronic obstructive pulmonary disease
Pulmonary hypertension

Data from Funk M, Winkler CG: Epidemiology of heart failure. In Moser DK, Riegel B, editors: *Cardiac nursing: a companion to Braunwald's heart disease,* St Louis, 2008, Elsevier.

peripartum cardiomyopathy are other examples of secondary cardiomyopathy.[5]

Incidence, Prevalence, and Epidemiology

HF is a societal epidemic in our country because of its incidence, prevalence, and high cost. HF is a leading cause of morbidity and mortality; 670,000 new cases are identified each year. The lifetime risk of HF for both men and women at 40 years of age is 1 in 5. Worldwide, 1% to 2% of the population has HF in developed countries; the prevalence approaches 10% in those older than 70 years. In the United States, the estimated direct and indirect cost of HF by 2030 is estimated to be $70 billion. This total includes the cost of health care services, medications, and lost productivity.[4]

Risk Factors. Many individuals with HF have antecedent hypertension or myocardial infarction (MI). Other risk factors include coronary artery disease, diabetes, renal disease, obesity, smoking, and increasing age. African Americans have a higher prevalence of HF than other ethnicities and a greater 5-year mortality than whites. Hypertension is believed to account for some of the risk difference; socioeconomic factors that affect access to health care may be another important factor after control for conventional risk factors.[4]

PATHOPHYSIOLOGY

HF is a clinical syndrome characterized by signs and symptoms of volume excess. Whereas there can be several causes of the HF, common pathophysiologic mechanisms characterize this important condition. Understanding these mechanisms is critical to selection of successful therapeutic interventions.

Systolic Dysfunction: Heart Failure with Reduced Ejection Fraction

Systolic dysfunction, which accounts for about half of all HF cases, is a decrease in both ejection fraction (40% or less) and cardiac output. In systolic dysfunction, when looking at a hemodynamic model, the three determinants of ventricular function—preload, contractility, and afterload—are usually altered. Preload is the degree of myocardial fiber stretch at the end of ventricular filling. When the heart ejects subnormally, there is an increased volume of blood left in the ventricular chambers (increased left ventricular end-systolic volume). This excess volume leads to distention of the ventricles and increased interventricular pressure at the onset of diastole. Filling must then occur at higher pressures during diastole. At small increases of volume and pressure, nonfailing myocardial fibers have the intrinsic property of increasing their force of contraction in an attempt to "revert" the subsequent volume and pressure conditions of both heart ejection and filling back to normal. This intrinsic property also enables the heart to maintain cardiac output during states of pressure or volume overload. However, in the failing heart, the failing myocardial fibers are both excessively overloaded and stretched beyond lengths commensurate with the normal reflex-increased force of contraction. This results in left ventricular remodeling, with dilation and impaired contractility, and activation of the sympathetic and renin-angiotensin-aldosterone systems. The ventricular dysfunction in HFrEF is accompanied by a decrease in myocardial contractility, a reduction in ejection fraction, and often a reduction in stroke volume and cardiac output. If HF is left untreated, symptoms develop and worsen, with declining functional capacity, recurrent acute decompensated events, life-threatening arrhythmias, and pump failure. Effective treatment of HF, primarily pharmacotherapy, depends on the interruption of left ventricular remodeling and the pathophysiologic processes that accompany it.

Afterload is the amount of left ventricular wall tension that develops during systole; it is determined by both the size of the ventricular chamber and the dynamic vascular resistance against which the heart contracts. According to Laplace's law, an increase in the radius of the ventricle results in an increase in wall tension. Because systolic blood pressure closely approximates afterload, it is a clinically important indicator of myocardial load or afterload. The LVEF is a function of afterload and an afterload-dependent measure of contractility. Chronic elevation of cardiac afterload can lead to ventricular enlargement, reduction in ejection fraction, and reduction in stroke volume and cardiac output. Several systemic mechanisms exist for the body to compensate for the reduction in cardiac output. Early on, these compensatory mechanisms serve to increase cardiac output and tissue perfusion. In the long run, however, they lead to further cardiac injury and further decompensation.[1]

Heart Failure with Preserved Ejection Fraction

The prevalence of HFpEF has increased dramatically. Controversy surrounds the true cause(s) of HFpEF. One mechanism believed responsible is increased ventricular stiffness and reduced compliance of the left ventricle, which produces a rise in cardiac filling pressures during diastole. Left ventricular distensibility is reduced during part or all of diastole, and filling pressures must increase to maintain a constant ventricular volume. Whereas filling pressures in the left ventricle are increased during both rest and exercise, the failure of a normal rise in cardiac output during exertion results in characteristic symptoms of HF, particularly dyspnea. The heart attempts to initially compensate for this impaired distensibility through the "booster" effect of augmented left atrial contraction, resulting over time in left atrial dilation.

The incidence of HFpEF increases with age and is more prevalent in older adult women. Recent studies have examined the role of inflammation contributing to diastolic abnormalities. The most common factors associated with HFpEF are hypertension, ischemia resulting from coronary artery disease, aortic stenosis, and infiltrative or restrictive myocardial diseases.[2]

Compensatory Mechanisms

Several interrelated compensatory mechanisms attempt to maintain normal ventricular contractility, ventricular pressures, cardiac output, and blood pressure. The three primary compensatory mechanisms are increased sympathetic adrenergic activity with a resultant increase in circulating neurohormones, neuroendocrine activation of the renin-angiotensin-aldosterone system, and ventricular remodeling. In addition, as HF progresses, neurohormonal alterations in peripheral vasculature and renal function occur. Sodium and water retention through the renal tubules results in decreased renal perfusion and rising blood urea nitrogen and creatinine concentrations, broadly called cardiorenal syndrome, which can be chronic or acute. The same compensatory mechanisms in early and acute stages gradually fail as HF progresses, and they are responsible for the eventual deterioration in cardiac function.[1]

Sympathetic Adrenergic Activity. Baroreceptors and chemoreceptors in the heart and vascular system, sensitive to stretch, pH and CO_2, help regulate blood pressure. Cardiac reflexes regulate heart rate. Abnormalities in both baroreceptor and cardiac reflexes have been documented in HF.[1] In a healthy heart, stimulation of the baroreceptor reflex results in activation of the parasympathetic nervous system and inhibition of the sympathetic nervous system. Heart rate and systemic vascular resistance are reduced, and normal blood pressure and cardiac output are maintained.

In HF, however, a decrease in cardiac output leads to activation of the sympathetic nervous system and blunting of the baroreceptor reflex. The result is an elevation in heart rate, compensating for low cardiac output in an attempt to maintain perfusion to vital organs. As HF progresses, further depression of the baroreceptor function leads to greater sympathetic overactivity despite intense vasoconstriction and volume retention.

Increasing activation of the sympathetic nervous system stimulates release of catecholamines from cardiac adrenergic nerves and the adrenal medulla; this in turn causes vasoconstriction in less metabolically active organs (e.g., skin, kidneys). It results in venoconstriction, which increases preload by increasing venous return. Catecholamines also affect the cardiac cells, producing an increased myocardial oxygen demand, myocyte hypertrophy, and tissue necrosis. Progressive HF occurs as cardiac cells progressively enlarge and die. As a result of sympathetic activation, plasma norepinephrine levels are elevated. The degree of plasma norepinephrine elevation correlates with the severity of HF and may be predictive of mortality, especially in patients with markedly elevated norepinephrine levels.[6,7]

Neuroendocrine Activation. Two additional vasoconstrictor systems act as compensatory mechanisms and therefore are affected by HF: the renin-angiotensin-aldosterone system and arginine vasopressin. The renin-angiotensin-aldosterone system is activated by a decline in blood pressure in the renal juxtaglomerular cells, which causes an increase in the release of the enzyme renin. The release of these hormones causes maladaptive remodeling of the ventricles; blockade of these hormones has been found to be beneficial in HF treatment.[1]

Ventricular Remodeling. Cardiac remodeling is an alteration in both the structure and function of the heart as a response to cardiac injury or hemodynamic strain in association with neurohormonal activation. Remodeling can be physiologic (adaptive; as in the case of pregnant women and trained athletes) or pathologic (maladaptive; in disease states). Both myocardial hypertrophy and dilation occur in varying degrees as a progressive process, even in the absence of further myocardial injury, infection, or ischemic events.[8] Dilation is an increase in the ventricular end-diastolic volume and represents an early compensatory response in volume overload in an attempt to increase contractility and to maintain cardiac output. In dilation, each individual myocyte lays down additional sarcomeres in series. Dilation preserves stroke volume and maintains cardiac output, but it also significantly increases wall stress, which increases myocardial oxygen demand, a deleterious condition if significant coronary artery disease is present. Also, excessive wall stress may lead to myocyte loss and fibrosis of cardiac tissue.

The condition of ventricular hypertrophy is a direct result of attempts to compensate for the increase in wall stress. Ventricular hypertrophy is an increase in the number of sarcomeres within each myocyte of ventricular heart muscle; these abnormal, large cells cannot contract as efficiently. Initially, myocardial hypertrophy distributes the greater degree of wall stress to a greater myocardial mass and thus "normalizes" the increased load per myocyte. Hypertrophy also increases the force of the ventricular contraction. Ultimately, however, ventricular remodeling in HF progresses to the point that it can no longer offer any compensatory advantage, especially when loading conditions remain abnormal or when myocardial disease causes myocyte loss.[9]

Recurrent Acute Decompensated Heart Failure. At the onset of HF, compensatory mechanisms described are beneficial; however, over time, compensatory mechanisms may themselves exacerbate HF. The fluid retention intended to enhance contractile force can cause pulmonary and systemic congestion. Arterial vasoconstriction can cause impaired tissue perfusion and increased afterload. Myocardial hypertrophy and the sympathetic activity can increase myocardial oxygen consumption. The result of all these responses is an increase in myocardial burden and an escalation in frequency and severity of HF exacerbations.

CLINICAL PRESENTATION AND PHYSICAL EXAMINATION

HF is a constellation of symptoms occurring as a result of heart muscle damage and the body's physiologic response mechanisms. A careful history and review of symptoms are extremely important because they yield clues to the cause of HF; HF should never be the only diagnosis (Box 121-2).

The cardinal symptoms of dyspnea and fatigue and the typical signs of HF, such as lower extremity edema and jugular venous distention, are nonspecific and must be evaluated along with a patient's history, review of symptoms, and physical examination findings, corroborated by further cardiac investigations. Patients may describe symptoms of paroxysmal nocturnal dyspnea and orthopnea as well as shortness of breath with exertion or at rest. Some people experience abdominal fullness or bloating along with lack of appetite (Table 121-2). Certain signs, such as jugular venous distention, cardiac enlargement, and a third heart sound (S_3), are specific for HF (70% to 90%), as is lower extremity edema, but these signs are only 11% to 55% sensitive (Table 121-3).[10]

BOX 121-2

Critical Components of a Patient's History That Assist with Diagnosis and Management of Heart Failure

- History of HF (American Heart Association [AHA]/American college of Cardiology [ACC] stage C)
- Known coronary artery disease
- History of high blood pressure
- History of or current arrhythmias
- History of hypertension
- Family history of cardiomyopathy, sudden cardiac death, coronary artery disease
- Recent viral illness, fevers
- Travel outside of the United States (particularly Mexico or South American countries)
- Any history of Lyme disease, tuberculosis, human immunodeficiency virus (HIV) infection, hepatitis; recent rashes
- History of substance abuse (e.g., heavy alcohol use, diet pills, cocaine, cigarettes)
- Any medications that could exacerbate volume status, such as nonsteroidal anti-inflammatory drugs (NSAIDs), prednisone
- History of any chemotherapy or any radiation therapy to the chest
- Recent pregnancy
- History of autoimmune disease (sarcoid, amyloid, thyroid disease)
- Recent extreme stress

REVIEW OF SYSTEMS

- Presence of fatigue
- Lightheadedness or dizziness
- Syncope or presyncope
- Dyspnea on exertion
- Dyspnea at rest
- Orthopnea
- Paroxysmal nocturnal dyspnea
- Cough
- Chest pain, heaviness, or tightness
- Palpitations
- Abdominal bloating or fullness
- Loss of appetite
- Weight gain (or loss)
- Edema or swelling

CLASSIFICATION OF HEART FAILURE

Symptoms and activity limitations have been quantified to assist in classifying a patient's status. The American College of Cardiology (ACC) and the American Heart Association (AHA) have devised a classification system that grades HF by stage (Table 121-4) to include patients at risk for the development of HF (stage A) and those with end-stage, advanced disease (stage D). Complementary to the ACC/AHA staging system is the New York Heart Association (NYHA) classification, which illuminates the patient's reported functional status and symptom burden. As an example, a patient with a prior history of HF who experiences shortness of breath while making the bed may be assigned to ACC/AHA stage C and NYHA class III HF.[11]

DIAGNOSTICS

Signs and symptoms of HF, such as fatigue, dyspnea, and peripheral edema, are often nonspecific. Fortunately, routine cardiac investigations can provide useful information to confirm a diagnosis. However, there is no single diagnostic test for HF, largely because it is a clinical spectrum that is based on a careful history and examination. The diagnostic evaluation should be aimed at those studies necessary to determine the type and degree of ventricular dysfunction (primarily systolic or diastolic), to uncover correctable causes of cardiomyopathy, to determine prognosis, and to guide treatment.

When HF is suspected, the diagnostic evaluation is preceded by a history and physical examination, followed by an assessment of cardiac structure and function. Patients should be evaluated for coronary disease and ischemia. In addition, important aspects in the diagnostic evaluation of each patient with HF are establishment of the risk of arrhythmia, identification of exacerbating factors (e.g., anemia, ischemia, or infection) for HF, and diagnosis of any comorbidities. Echocardiography, chest radiography, electrocardiography, cardiac catheterization, cardiac magnetic resonance imaging (MRI), positron emission tomography–computed tomography (PET/CT), blood hematology, serum laboratory testing, and, in selected cases, exercise tolerance testing are common diagnostic tests used in the evaluation of patients with HF.

The 2013 HF guidelines suggest the usefulness of a multivariate risk score to estimate subsequent risk of mortality in both ambulatory and hospitalized patients with HF.[11]

Echocardiography

The value of echocardiography cannot be overestimated in the diagnostic evaluation of suspected HF. It represents the single most effective tool in widespread clinical use for the assessment of HF.

Approximately 50% of patients with HF have left ventricular systolic dysfunction, defined as a LVEF of less than 40%. Transthoracic Doppler echocardiography is rapid and safe and

TABLE 121-2 Symptoms of Heart Failure

Symptoms	Why It Happens	What Patients with Heart Failure May Describe
Shortness of breath (dyspnea)	Pressure is increased in the pulmonary veins because the heart cannot keep up with the supply. This can cause pulmonary congestion or pulmonary edema (interstitial and alveolar congestion), which leads to left ventricular overload and worsening symptoms of failure.	Breathlessness during activity, at rest, or while sleeping (called paroxysmal nocturnal dyspnea); these symptoms worsen with severity of HF. Difficulty breathing while lying flat (orthopnea) or complaints of waking up tired or feeling anxious and restless.
Persistent coughing, bronchospasm, or wheezing	Persistent pulmonary interstitial or alveolar edema (sometimes called cardiac asthma), worsen when recumbent.	Coughing that produces white or pink blood-tinged mucus may not always be present.
Edema	As blood flow out of the heart is impeded, blood returning to the heart through the veins backs up, causing fluid to build up in the tissues. The kidneys are less able to dispose of sodium and water, also causing fluid retention. This is evidence of right-sided HF.	Swelling in the feet, ankles, legs, or abdomen or weight gain. Patients may find that their pants or shoes feel tight.
Tiredness, fatigue	The heart cannot pump enough blood to meet the needs of body tissues, resulting in decreased oxygen saturation. The body's normal vascular response to exercise is altered; blood is diverted away from less vital organs, particularly muscles in the limbs, and sent to the heart and brain. Muscle deconditioning plays a role here as well. Loss of potassium induced by increased aldosterone also leads to muscle fatigue.	Tired feeling all the time and difficulty with everyday activities, such as shopping, climbing stairs, carrying groceries, or walking.
Lack of appetite, nausea	The digestive system receives less blood, causing problems with digestion. Medications, particularly diuretics, may be poorly absorbed. Hepatic congestion may often lead to discomfort.	Feeling of being full or nauseated, or loss of appetite.
Confusion, impaired thinking, lightheadedness	Changing levels of certain substances in the blood, such as sodium, can cause confusion. Poor cardiac output with decreased perfusion to the brain may also cause these symptoms.	Memory loss and feelings of disorientation; a caregiver or relative may notice this first.
Increased heart rate	Compensatory mechanism for the loss in stroke volume; the heart beats faster.	Heart palpitations, described by patients as a sensation that the heart is racing or throbbing.
Nocturia	Nocturnal diuresis lessens the degree of fluid retention. Nocturnal diuresis results from fluid reabsorption and redistribution in the supine position as well as a reduction in renal vasoconstriction that occurs at rest.	Patient reported; diuretics confound the picture.

provides information about biventricular systolic performance, wall thickness, and chamber dimensions as well as segmental or regional wall motion abnormalities and valvular function. Evaluation of the mitral, tricuspid, and aortic valves with regurgitation grading is important, as is a determination of estimated pulmonary artery pressures from secondary tricuspid regurgitation. LVEF is determined. Diastolic function can often be detected as well; Doppler echocardiography allows the characterization of abnormal left ventricular filling in diastole. The ACC and AHA guidelines recognize echocardiography as the preferred diagnostic tool for evaluation of the cause of HF.[11]

Evaluation for myocardial ischemia should be considered in most patients who have developed new left ventricular systolic dysfunction by echocardiography. Referral to a cardiologist is recommended. The evaluation modality ultimately chosen depends on pretest probability of disease and whether the patient is a candidate for an intervention.

Electrocardiography

An electrocardiogram should be obtained as part of the assessment of patients with possible HF. It may be a useful diagnostic test in the workup of patients thought to have HF to assist in evaluation of heart rhythm, presence of wide QRS (left ventricular bundle branch block) or left ventricular hypertrophy, and evidence of MI or ongoing ischemia.

Chest Radiography (Chest X-Ray Examination)

In patients with a new diagnosis of HF, a chest radiograph (posteroanterior and lateral) is recommended.[11] The size and shape of the cardiac silhouette and the presence of interstitial and

TABLE 121-3 Signs of Heart Failure

Sign	Indicates	Physical Examination
Jugular venous distention	An index of right atrial pressure; when elevated, it is an indicator of volume overload. (Tricuspid regurgitation may alter the examination findings.) With normal pressure, the upper level of visible jugular vein is approximately 4 cm above the sternal notch.	With the patient at a 45-degree angle, note the upper limit of visible pulse in the internal jugular. In some patients, this pressure may be normal at rest, but it rises to abnormal levels with compression of the right upper quadrant. This sign is known as the hepatojugular or abdominal jugular reflex. The internal or external jugular vein is compressed in the supraclavicular fossa, and as the examiner's finger strips the vein cephalad, blood rises in the more proximal portion of the vein; the height of this blood volume above the patient's clavicles reflects the central venous pressure. The height of the venous column normally falls during inspiration as a result of the accompanying decrease in intrathoracic pressure.
Crackles, frothy or pink sputum, pleural effusions	Pulmonary fluid transudate moves to interstitial spaces and alveoli, usually in lung bases because of gravity. Pulmonary edema. Occur with volume overload—transudative.	Lung examination. Dull or absent breath sounds.
Third heart sound	Early diastolic rapid ventricular filling associated with left ventricular systolic dysfunction.	S_3 is best heard with patient in left lateral position.
Fourth heart sound	Overdistention of ventricles during late diastole as the stiff ventricles expand further to accommodate final diastolic filling by atrial contraction (atrial "kick").	Best heard with patient in left lateral position; absence of S_3 suggests early failure or the presence of diastolic dysfunction.
Aortic stenosis	Small volume, high velocity.	Harsh murmur, usually loud.
Mitral regurgitation	Large volume, low turbulent flow.	Soft holosystolic murmur.
Tricuspid regurgitation	Large volume in right ventricle.	Hepatic congestion, edema, ascites.
Hepatomegaly, right upper quadrant tenderness	Liver enlargement or stretching of the hepatic capsule.	Right upper quadrant tenderness indicates enlarged or tender liver.
Ascites, anasarca, or edema	Caused by volume overload.	Edema of subcutaneous tissue may be found in abdomen, chest, buttocks. Ascites may be suggested by protuberant abdomen, but the examination is not reliable. Pitting or firm edema of lower extremities is common in HF.
Altered hemodynamics	Changes in cardiac output by stroke volume and heart rate.	May appear with symptoms and signs of low output, such as lightheadedness, impaired cognition, tachycardia, cool extremities, hypotension.
Tachycardia	Changes in heart rate caused by arrhythmia or activation of baroreceptors, which in turn activate sympathetic nervous system. These compensatory mechanisms along with the renin-angiotensin-aldosterone and vasopressin release help modulate heart rate early on with a drop in pressure. Ultimately tachycardia will ensue, unless it is masked by medication (such as beta blockers, digoxin, calcium channel blockers).	Heart rate measurement; evaluation of rhythm is important.
Displaced point of maximal impulse	Displacement of the palpable apical impulse away from the midclavicular line toward the anterior axillary line indicates left ventricular enlargement.	The palpable apical impulse should be a quick tap, narrow in distribution, not more than 1 to 2 cm (⅖ to ⅘ inch) in diameter. An impulse that is palpable with the palm of the hand, lasts longer, or is forceful indicates increased cardiac output or ventricular hypertrophy. Palpable impulse may be elicited with the palm placed on the sternum. This finding is a right ventricular tap or heave, indicating right ventricular enlargement and volume overload.
Hypotension, cool extremities	Caused by low cardiac output; sometimes medication related.	Blood pressure measurement.

TABLE 121-4 Classification of Heart Failure

NEW YORK HEART ASSOCIATION FUNCTIONAL CLASSIFICATION	
Class I	No limitations. Ordinary physical activity does not cause undue fatigue, dyspnea, or palpitations.
Class II	Slight limitation of physical activity. Such patients are comfortable at rest. Ordinary physical activity results in fatigue, palpitations, dyspnea, or angina.
Class III	Marked limitation of physical activity. Although patients are comfortable at rest, less than ordinary activity will lead to symptoms.
Class IV	Inability to carry on any physical activity without discomfort. Symptoms are present even at rest. With any physical activity, discomfort is experienced or increased.
ACC/AHA HEART FAILURE STAGES	
Stage A	At high risk for HF with no identified structural or functional abnormality; no signs or symptoms.
Stage B	With structural heart disease that is strongly associated with the development of HF but without signs or symptoms.
Stage C	Symptomatic HF associated with underlying structural abnormalities.
Stage D	Advanced structural cardiac disease and marked symptoms of HF at rest with maximal medical therapy or requiring advanced therapies.

Data from Yancy CW, Jessup M, Bozkurt B, et al: 2013 ACCF/AHA guideline for the management of heart failure: a report of the American College of Cardiology Foundation/American Heart Association Task Force on Practice Guidelines. *J Am Coll Cardiol* 62(13):1497-1532, 2013; and the Criteria Committee of the New York Heart Association: *Diseases of the heart and blood vessels: nomenclature and criteria for diagnosis*, ed 6, Boston, 1964, Little, Brown.

alveolar edema comprise the radiologic evidence of HF. A common chest radiographic finding in HF is cardiomegaly, with a cardiothoracic ratio (the ratio of the diameter of the heart at its widest point to the maximum width of the thoracic cavity; the normal ratio is less than 1:2) that is increased more than 50%. This ratio is nonspecific, and widespread use of echocardiography has rendered chest radiography less important and insensitive for the diagnosis of HF.

Cardiac Catheterization

Clinical information gleaned from cardiac catheterization and measurement of hemodynamics is invaluable in patients with HF who have advanced symptoms or suboptimum response to medical therapy. Hemodynamic evaluation or right-sided heart catheterization provides hemodynamic measurements and assessments along with a measurement of cardiac output, which can guide medical therapy and provide data to identify the timing of valvular surgery. It is useful when patients have respiratory distress and impaired perfusion and when determination of volume status is uncertain based on clinical assessment. Left-sided heart catheterization (coronary artery angiography) is reasonable to diagnose the presence, extent, and severity of coronary artery disease when ischemia may be contributing to HF.[11]

Endomyocardial Biopsy

The role of right ventricular endomyocardial biopsy in the diagnostic evaluation is controversial. The AHA/ACC 2013 guidelines suggest performing it if it might be deemed useful; otherwise it is not routinely recommended.[12]

Cardiac Magnetic Resonance Imaging

Cardiac MRI is becoming an important imaging technique for the diagnosis of myocardial infiltrative processes and scar burden. Cardiac MRI allows a reproducible and accurate evaluation of myocardial morphology, function, perfusion, and tissue damage in a noninvasive way. If there is suspicion of an infiltrative disease process or uncertainty about scar burden, MRI may be useful. Currently, use of MRI is not widespread, and it is recommended only if other imaging techniques are not diagnostically satisfactory.

Positron Emission Tomography–Computed Tomography

PET/CT is currently an accepted standard in noninvasive imaging of coronary perfusion in patients with suspected or known coronary artery disease. PET/CT allows accurate noninvasive clinical decision-making about coronary artery disease. Because of its high negative predictive value, PET/CT is playing an important role in noninvasive selection of coronary artery disease patients for revascularization. It is not mentioned in the AHA/ACC guidelines specifically.

Laboratory

The initial evaluation of the patient with symptoms of HF includes the hematology and serum laboratory tests listed in Table 121-5 B-type (brain) natriuretic peptide (BNP), combined with history, physical examination findings, other values such as echocardiographic indices, and cardiovascular risk factors, augments the assessment of patients with suspected HF and is recommended as a screening test in all patients with suspected HF.[11]

Brain Natriuretic Peptide. BNP is a peptide synthesized and secreted almost exclusively by ventricular myocardial cells in response to elevations in end-diastolic pressure and volume. The Vasodilator Heart Failure Trial (V-HeFT) confirmed this test as the strongest predictor of outcome in HF compared with other neurohormones and clinical markers. BNP is helpful in differentiating cardiac from pulmonary causes because values less than 100 have 100% sensitivity and 97.1% specificity, making this extremely useful in ruling out CHF. A BNP value of 400 has a high positive predictive value for determination of CHF; additional research shows values of 1000 to 4000 to be associated with CHF and values above 4000 to be directly related to CHF. BNP can be elevated in both diastolic and systolic dysfunction and therefore cannot be used to distinguish between these two types of HF. In addition, serial BNP levels can be measured over time and compared with steady-state levels to allow detection of trends that lead toward decompensation.[13]

Although it has a longer half-life, the sensitivity to detect early-stage left ventricular dysfunction is similar for NT-proBNP and BNP. The NT-proBNP value is approximately 7.9 times higher than the BNP value.[14]

TABLE 121-5 Laboratory Evaluation

Laboratory Test	Comments
Complete blood count	Anemia, iron deficiency, or iron overload can exacerbate HF.
Serum electrolytes, including calcium and magnesium	Hyponatremia can be associated with volume overload and diuretic use. Potassium aberrations should be detected and corrected. Helpful before initiation of aldosterone antagonist. Abnormalities in calcium or magnesium may aggravate or induce arrhythmias.
Blood urea nitrogen and serum creatinine	Before initiation of ACE inhibitors. Renal function may be altered in HF because of poor renal perfusion, medications, age, or diabetes.
Lipid profile	Risk factor modification.
Fasting blood glucose concentration or glycohemoglobin level	Diabetes.
Urinalysis	Evaluate for proteinuria, evidence of kidney disease.
Liver function tests	Hepatic congestion may cause abnormalities.
Serum albumin	Low albumin level may cause edema.
Thyroid-stimulating hormone	Hypothyroidism or hyperthyroidism can lead to HF.
Brain natriuretic peptide (BNP) or pro-BNP	See Diagnostics.

Exercise or Stress Testing for Heart Failure

The exercise test, or stress test, for functional capacity is not currently recommended as part of the routine evaluation for HF. It is sometimes done as part of a pre–cardiac transplantation workup to evaluate symptoms that are disparate from what other objective indicators would suggest or to distinguish between cardiac and pulmonary causes of symptoms. It is sometimes used in disability determinations.

Differential Diagnosis

Dyspnea is a common presenting symptom in primary care. Initial evaluation of the patient with dyspnea is to determine the severity of the dyspnea; acute symptoms require immediate evaluation. Dyspnea is most commonly caused by underlying respiratory or cardiac disease but can also be associated with other conditions, such as metabolic diseases, psychogenic disorders, mechanical obstruction, and neuromuscular diseases. Therefore, systematic evaluation of dyspnea is critical for proper diagnosis of the underlying disease. Differential diagnoses that should be considered when there are signs and symptoms consistent with HF are shown in the differential diagnosis box.

Cardiac Conditions

Dyspnea is a known anginal equivalent in many patients who have coronary artery disease but who lack classic anginal symptoms. Women and diabetics, in particular, frequently do not have classic anginal symptoms of chest pain but will have dyspnea or dyspnea on exertion. These patients should be thoroughly evaluated for coronary artery disease. In addition, valvular disorders, pericardial disease, and cardiac arrhythmias can also cause dyspnea. A careful history and negative physical examination findings suggestive of HF (e.g., elevated jugular venous pressure, edema, S_3) can lead the clinician to further focused diagnostic testing or cardiology consultation for more extensive evaluation.

DIFFERENTIAL DIAGNOSIS

Heart Failure

- Myocardial ischemia
- Pulmonary disease (pneumonia, asthma, chronic obstructive pulmonary disease, pulmonary embolus, primary pulmonary hypertension)
- Symptoms of embolic events
- Symptoms of arrhythmia
- Symptoms of possible cerebral hypoperfusion (syncope, presyncope, lightheadedness)
- Sleep-disordered breathing
- Obesity
- Deconditioning
- Malnutrition
- Anemia
- Hepatic failure
- Chronic kidney disease
- Hypoalbuminemia
- Venous stasis
- Anxiety and hyperventilation syndromes
- Hyperthyroidism or hypothyroidism

Data from Lindenfeld J, Albert NM, Boehmer JP, et al: HFSA 2010 comprehensive heart failure practice guideline, *J Card Fail* 16:e1-e194, 2010.

Chronic Pulmonary Conditions

The dyspnea of HF might be confused with chronic pulmonary conditions. The most common obstructive disorders are chronic obstructive pulmonary disease (COPD), chronic bronchitis, and asthma; restrictive disorders include underlying pulmonary diseases (e.g., interstitial fibrosis) and extrapulmonary causes (e.g., obesity and thoracospinal abnormalities). COPD represents a spectrum of disease severity and pathophysiologic changes and is a common comorbidity in patients with HF.

Mortality and morbidity rates in patients with coexistent HF and COPD are high, and these patients present unique diagnostic and management issues.[14]

Orthopnea and paroxysmal nocturnal dyspnea may result from either COPD or HF or a combination of both. These entities may be difficult to identify on the basis of symptom analysis; past medical history, risk for HF, and physical examination findings (sudden weight gain, S_3, S_4, jugular venous distention, peripheral edema) in combination with other symptoms, such as increased fatigue, may help elucidate the cause as HF.

Asthma and Upper Respiratory Tract Infection

In clinical practice, new-onset HF is often mistaken for asthma or an upper respiratory tract infection because dyspnea is the predominant symptom. However, the duration of the dyspnea can be a clue to distinguish new-onset HF from asthma or upper respiratory tract infection. The asthmatic patient is usually free of chronic dyspnea but experiences episodic dyspnea. Other asthmatic symptoms can include prominent inspiratory and expiratory wheezing, cough, and chest tightness; not all asthmatic patients will experience all symptoms. Because pulmonary edema can trigger bronchospasm and wheezing, also called cardiac asthma, an acute asthma attack may mimic acute pulmonary edema, but airflow limitation and wheezing are usually more marked in acute asthma; in addition, other signs and symptoms of HF, such as an S_3 gallop or edema, are absent in acute asthma.

Pleural Effusions

A pleural effusion is an abnormal collection of fluid in the pleural space, which lies between the lung and the chest cavity. Fluid accumulation may result from excess fluid production or decreased absorption and is indicative of underlying disease from pulmonary or nonpulmonary causes. Approximately 1.5 million cases of pleural effusion occur annually in the United States. Common causes include HF, infections, malignant disease, and pulmonary embolus.

Dyspnea associated with pleural effusions is usually more chronic in nature. Symptoms may worsen with exertion, and hypoxia may occur in some patients. Pleural effusions produce dyspnea through compression of underlying lung parenchyma and reduction in ventilated lung volume. Diminished breath sounds, dullness to percussion, and diminished tactile fremitus are noted on physical examination.

Pleural effusions are primarily transudative or exudative, which can help distinguish among the causes. Differentiation between transudative and exudative is based on the protein content and lactate dehydrogenase levels in the pleural fluid compared with those levels in the serum. Transudative effusions have similar protein and lactate dehydrogenase levels to levels found in serum. A large majority of transudative effusions are caused by HF because of abnormally high pleural capillary pressures. Transudative effusions can also result from liver failure, chronic renal failure, or hypoalbuminemia.[15]

Pulmonary Embolism

Pulmonary embolism is a common and potentially deadly medical condition that may mimic the acute dyspnea of pulmonary edema. However, the symptoms of pulmonary embolism may be subtle and range from none to mild dyspnea with pleuritic chest pain to cardiac arrest. The most common cause of a pulmonary embolus is lower extremity deep venous thrombosis, which can cause unilateral leg pain and swelling that can suggest embolus as a cause of chest pain and dyspnea. Patients at risk for pulmonary embolus include those with previous thrombosis or hereditary factors (hypercoagulable states); those with acquired factors, such as prolonged immobility, cardiac disorders (atrial fibrillation, prosthetic cardiac valve), obesity, hormonal therapy, and malignant neoplasms; and postoperative patients. In pulmonary embolus, arterial blood gas analysis may show hypoxemia, but this is nondiagnostic. Diagnostic tools that can be used in the evaluation of suspected pulmonary embolus include a moderately sensitive D-dimer assay, which has a high negative predictive value in low probability patients; a ventilation/perfusion scan, which exhibits ventilation/perfusion mismatch in a pulmonary embolus; and a helical CT scan of the chest.

Neuromuscular Disorders

Neuromuscular disorders, such as myasthenia gravis, amyotrophic lateral sclerosis, and Guillain-Barré syndrome, may cause dyspnea by weakness of the respiratory muscles. A careful history and significant neurologic physical examination findings can differentiate dyspnea caused by HF from neuromuscular disorders.

Anxiety

Anxiety as the sole cause of dyspnea is uncommon and is always a diagnosis of exclusion. Health care providers must remember that anxiety is common with dyspnea of any cause, adds to the perceived severity, and prolongs the duration of the dyspnea.

Additional Causes

Many other medical conditions can cause dyspnea and should be included in the differential diagnosis in the evaluation of a patient who has symptoms at rest or with exertion. Anemia, obesity or deconditioning, kyphoscoliosis, and hypersensitivity reactions (allergens, medications) are a few common conditions that should be considered.

MANAGEMENT

Chronic or acute HF requires sufficient diagnostic testing for determination of the specific cause. Coronary artery disease, valvular heart disease, and pericardial disease may be treatable either percutaneously or surgically, mandating appropriate diagnostic studies. Once a specific diagnosis has been made, the first strategy in the treatment of HF is to relieve congestion; next, specific reversible causes are treated. Once reversible causes have been treated, management of the residual HF can be initiated. HF caused by diastolic dysfunction must be differentiated from that caused by systolic dysfunction because treatment options differ; currently, there are evidence-based guidelines for HFrEF but only recommendations for the treatment of HFpEF.

In general, the primary objectives in treatment of HF are fourfold: relief of symptoms and signs, prevention of further myocardial injury, prevention of recurrence of clinical failure (congestive or low output), and improvement in prognosis.[1] Correct selection and application of pharmacologic therapy require a careful history and physical examination as well as an understanding of the physiologic process of HF.

Use of ACC/AHA Classifications to Guide Therapy

The ACC/AHA classification stages represent a framework for management of left-sided HF (see Table 121-3). In patients assigned to stage A (at high risk, no structural abnormality), clear benefit exists for control of systolic and diastolic hypertension. Studies support treatment of lipid disorders, angiotensin-converting enzyme (ACE) inhibitor or angiotensin receptor blocker (ARB) use in patients with diabetes and other cardiovascular risk factors, and control of arrhythmias and tachycardic ventricular rates. According to expert consensus opinion, these patients should be screened periodically for signs and symptoms of HF, and primary prevention issues should be addressed: smoking cessation, dietary salt reduction, avoidance of illicit drug use, limitation of alcohol consumption, regular exercise. The use of nutritional supplements for prevention of HF is not recommended.[11]

For patients assigned to stage B (those with structural heart disease, previous MI, left ventricular systolic dysfunction, and asymptomatic valvular disease, but without symptoms of failure), clear evidence exists for the use of ACE inhibitors, or ARBs if the patient is intolerant of ACE inhibitors, and beta blockers, irrespective of the ejection fraction. Valvular repair or replacement for hemodynamically significant stenosis or regurgitation is recommended according to contemporary guidelines outlined by the ACCF/AHA. The use of digoxin for patients with systolic dysfunction in sinus rhythm, in the absence of HF symptoms, is not recommended, nor is the use of calcium channel blockers or nutritional supplements. Patients with ischemic or nonischemic cardiomyopathy who have LVEF of less than 35% and are receiving maximally tolerated medical therapy should be considered for a prophylactic implantable cardioverter-defibrillator (ICD).[11]

Management of patients assigned to stage C (with known structural heart disease and with prior or current symptoms of failure) includes the health promotion measures previously mentioned in conjunction with daily weights, dietary sodium restriction, reduced exercise during periods of acute decompensation, and close monitoring for decompensation. In these patients, nonadherence to prescribed medication and dietary regimens can precipitate rapid deterioration.

Identification and treatment of sleep-disordered breathing and sleep apnea can be beneficial and improve functional status. Cardiac rehabilitation and exercise training may improve overall clinical status in clinically stable patients and may improve functional status, quality of life, and even perhaps mortality.[11]

Avoidance of medications that can adversely affect these patients, such as nonsteroidal anti-inflammatory drugs (NSAIDs) and calcium channel blockers, should be stressed. Pharmacologic therapy in stage C typically involves four classes of medications: a diuretic, an ACE inhibitor or ARB, a beta blocker, and an aldosterone antagonist.[11]

In stage C, additional interventions have demonstrated value in selected patients. These include the use of digoxin for symptom control, hydralazine and nitrates, and biventricular pacemakers and ICDs in appropriate patients. Patients assigned to stage D with refractory HF require meticulous control of fluid balance. Clear evidence exists for benefit of ACE inhibitors or ARBs and beta blockers. However, the increased role of neurohormonal factors in compensation of severe HF can place stage D patients at risk for hypotension and renal insufficiency with ACE inhibition, as well as at greater risk for increasing failure with beta blockade. Thus, these agents should be used with caution in these patients, and dose reductions may be needed. Selected stage D patients may be candidates for specialized interventions, such as circulatory support measures, cardiac transplantation, and left ventricular assist devices (LVADs); these patients need to undergo rigorous evaluation for appropriateness of these advanced therapies. In addition, palliative care measures may include inotropic support and morphine to relieve breathlessness. End-of-life care issues should be addressed early and compassionately, because symptom management becomes a main focus of care in these patients.

Pharmacologic Therapy Overview

Pharmacotherapy for the treatment of HF can be subdivided by the pathophysiologic process (HFrEF versus HFpEF) and by the level of symptomatic presentation defined by the NYHA classification system. Whereas evidence-based therapies for the treatment of systolic dysfunction and HF are clearly defined, the treatment of HFpEF remains less clear. In patients with HF in the setting of either reduced LV function or preserved LV function as well as signs and symptoms of volume overload, initial therapy focuses on the relief of symptoms by treatment of volume excess with diuretics. In all patients with HFrEF (ejection fraction ≤40%), with or without evidence of volume overload, ACE inhibitor therapy is recommended. For patients who are intolerant of ACE inhibitors because of cough or other side effects, an ARB should be considered. Beta blocker therapy is beneficial in all patients with current or prior symptoms of HFrEF. Currently only three beta blockers—carvedilol, metoprolol, and bisoprolol—are proven to reduce mortality in patients with HF. In patients who have signs of fluid overload, such as elevated jugular venous pressure, weight gain, or pulmonary crackles, initial therapy should be a diuretic to reduce volume excess and an ACE inhibitor (or ARB). Beta blocker therapy should not be considered until the patient is decongested and has stabilized. Digoxin is an appropriate therapy for symptom control and has been shown to reduce hospitalizations. Additional drug therapy includes the use of aldosterone antagonists, such as spironolactone for patients who are NYHA functional class II to IV.[11] Although not currently endorsed in the HF management guidelines, there are data to support benefit in patients with NYHA functional class I symptoms.[16] Hydralazine-isosorbide combination therapy is beneficial in the African-American population and in patients intolerant of ACE inhibitors or ARBs. Renal function, potassium level, and other comorbid conditions may affect decisions for therapy.[11]

The 2013 American College of Cardiology Foundation (ACCF)/AHA guideline for the management of heart failure recommends blood pressure control (i.e., both systolic and diastolic) according to the currently published practice guidelines in patients with HFpEF. Ventricular rate control in patients with atrial fibrillation is recommended. Diuretic therapy in the setting of volume excess such as pulmonary congestion, peripheral edema, and abdominal bloating is recommended for relief of symptoms.[11]

ACE Inhibitors. The role of the ACE inhibitor emerged from the recognition that neurohormonal activation contributes to the pathogenesis of HF. By suppressing the production of angiotensin II, a potent vasoconstrictor, ACE inhibitors decrease systemic and pulmonary vascular resistance by preventing the release of aldosterone and norepinephrine while elevating the levels of the vasodilator hormone bradykinin. Multiple large randomized trials have shown that ACE inhibitor therapy improves mortality in symptomatic and asymptomatic patients with HFrEF, decreases HF symptoms, and improves overall clinical status. Therefore, ACE inhibitor therapy remains the cornerstone of chronic medical management in patients with HFrEF and should be considered a priority in all symptomatic or asymptomatic patients, unless there is an absolute contraindication. ACE inhibitors should be used with caution in patients with prior allergy including anaphylaxis, hyperkalemia, baseline hypotension, bilateral renal artery stenosis, or serum creatinine level greater than 3 mg/dL.[11] There is no creatinine level that absolutely limits the use of ACE inhibitors, although in patients with chronic kidney disease, renal function should be monitored closely. Creatinine increases typically occur quickly and are less than 10% to 20% of baseline levels. If creatinine increases exceed 20% of baseline levels, the drug should be withheld and additional evaluation of renal function explored. Often patients can be rechallenged with ACE inhibitors if renal function recovers and other contributors are treated.[17] Absolute contraindications include angioedema associated with ACE inhibitors and pregnancy. Cough can occur as a side effect of ACE inhibitors in close to 20% of treated patients. Although not dangerous, this can be annoying, and alternate therapy with ARBs is often considered.[11] Patients who begin ACE inhibitors should have their blood pressure, renal function, and serum potassium level monitored within 7 to 10 days. Target doses should be attempted in all patients.

Angiotensin Receptor Blockers. ARBs act directly on the angiotensin-renin-aldosterone system. These agents modify the effects of angiotensin II, the substance that promotes vasoconstriction, abnormal cell growth, and the release of aldosterone, but do not interfere with kinins, resulting in fewer adverse drug reactions.[11] ACE inhibitors remain the first-line choice for inhibition of the renin-angiotensin system, but as a result of multiple trials, ARBs have been endorsed as an effective option for those who are ACE inhibitor intolerant.[18-20] Cautions, contraindications, and monitoring parameters are similar to those outlined for ACE inhibitors.

Hydralazine and Oral Nitrates. The 2013 ACCF/AHA Guidelines for the Management of Heart failure state that hydralazine combined with oral nitrate is an appropriate alternative for patients who are unable to tolerate ACE inhibitors.[10] In addition, there are data to support the use of this combination in addition to standard HF treatment in the African-American population. Studies have shown a reduction in mortality and hospitalizations in this population of patients.[21,22]

Hydralazine is a direct arteriolar vasodilator, and isosorbide dinitrate is a venodilator. The combination of these agents results in an increase in cardiac output secondary to decreased impedance to ventricular ejection and decreased preload. Side effects include headache, palpitations, gastrointestinal (GI) issues, and nasal congestion. Compliance with this regimen has been problematic because of these side effects and the three-times-daily administration, with large number of tablets required with uptitration. Initiation of both drugs is at low doses with weekly uptitration as tolerated.[11]

Aldosterone Antagonists. Aldosterone contributes to the detrimental neurohormonal activation that is associated with ACE and the renin-angiotensin system. Interrupting this effect leads to improved endothelial function and reduced left ventricular remodeling as well as positive effects on heart rate variability and ventricular arrhythmias. The Randomized Aldactone Evaluation Study (RALES) suggested a benefit from the addition of spironolactone in patients with symptoms of dyspnea at rest currently or within the past 6 months or "severe" or NYHA class IV HF. This potassium-sparing diuretic and aldosterone antagonist has been shown to decrease both mortality and hospitalization rates in these patients through reverse ventricular remodeling.[23] Further data support the use of spironolactone and eplerenone in patients with NYHA functional class II symptoms and in post-MI patients with LVEF of 40% or less.[24,25] Although not endorsed in any of the currently accepted HF treatment guidelines, there are data to support benefit in patients with NYHA class I symptoms as well.[16] Use of these agents promotes hyperkalemia and requires careful patient selection, initiation, and monitoring. Concomitant potassium supplementation should be avoided. Interruption in therapy or discontinuation may be necessary for worsening renal function or acute kidney injury. Renal function and potassium concentration should be measured at 1 and 4 weeks after initiation or uptitration of therapy and periodically thereafter. Gynecomastia or breast tenderness occurs in approximately 10% of patients using spironolactone. This is less frequent with eplerenone.[11]

Diuretics. Diuretics are used to relieve symptoms of systemic and pulmonary congestion caused by volume overload in both systolic and diastolic HF. Many factors contribute to the sodium and water retention that causes volume overload in HF. Diuretics promote sodium and fluid excretion, thus relieving both the symptoms and the accompanying signs of volume overload.

Initial therapy with a thiazide diuretic or low-dose loop diuretic may be appropriate in mild HF. A loop diuretic, which is more potent, should be used for more symptomatic HF, renal insufficiency, or persistent edema. Persistent congestion despite a thiazide diuretic trial necessitates changing to a loop diuretic. Symptoms of severe HF or significant renal dysfunction will require a loop diuretic agent, either orally or intravenously. Patients may become resistant to oral diuretic therapy in increasing doses from a single class. Response may improve with oral diuretics in combination from two different classes (i.e., loop diuretic and metolazone) or intravenous diuretic therapy. Patients unresponsive to intravenous diuretics or with anasarca from excessive volume overload may benefit from advanced therapies, such as ultrafiltration. Diuretic dosage is summarized in Table 121-6. The standing dose of a diuretic depends on the patient's body size, age, estimated glomerular filtration rate, renal function, amount of edema, and compliance with a low-sodium and fluid-restricted diet.[11]

Use of high- dose diuretic therapy can cause electrolyte abnormalities, such as hypokalemia and hypomagnesemia, that require close monitoring and cautious repletion. An aldosterone antagonist, such as spironolactone, may minimize potassium wasting in patients with hypokalemia and can be used in these patients with close monitoring of electrolyte and renal function. With disease progression, the use of intermittent intravenous diuretics to overcome the neurohormonal responses that are antecedent to the increase in sodium and fluid retention may be necessary. Eventual diuretic resistance is common in advanced HF or in long-term diuretic therapy. Metolazone, a potent oral thiazide-like agent, can be added with caution to loop diuretic therapy to enhance the effect. Metolazone may be effective in patients with reduced renal function, but it should in general not be prescribed on a daily basis.[11]

Digoxin. The cardiac glycosides, such as digoxin, have been used to treat HF for more than 200 years. Digoxin improves symptoms and reduces hospitalization rates, but it does not

TABLE 121-6 Diuretics Used in Treatment of Chronic Heart Failure

Drug	Initial Dose	Recommended Maximum Dose	Potential Adverse Reactions
THIAZIDE DIURETICS			
Hydrochlorothiazide	12.5-25 mg/day	200 mg/day	Postural hypotension, hypokalemia, hyperuricemia
Chlorthalidone	25 mg/day	100 mg/day	
LOOP DIURETICS			
Furosemide	20-40 mg/day to twice daily	600 mg/day	Same as with thiazide diuretics
Bumetanide	0.5-1 mg/day	10 mg/day	
Torsemide	10-20 mg/day		
POTASSIUM-SPARING DIURETICS			
Spironolactone	12.5-25 mg/day	50 mg/day for HF	Hyperkalemia (especially if given with ACE inhibitors), gynecomastia, rash
Eplerenone	25 mg/day	50 mg/day	Less gynecomastia than with spironolactone
THIAZIDE-RELATED DIURETIC			
Metolazone (Zaroxolyn)	2.5 mg as single dose initially	5-10 mg/day	Same as with thiazide diuretics

Modified from Yancy CW, Jessup M, Bozkurt B, et al: 2013 ACCF/AHA guideline for the management of heart failure: a report of the American College of Cardiology Foundation/American Heart Association Task Force on Practice Guidelines. *Circulation* 128:e240-e327, 2013.

improve mortality in patients with systolic dysfunction.[26] Digoxin may be used to slow ventricular rates in patients with HF and atrial fibrillation. In addition, digoxin may be used as an add-on therapy in patients who are tolerating other standard HF medical therapy.[11]

Digoxin acts as a positive inotropic agent by increasing intracellular calcium concentration in myocytes by altering calcium-sodium exchange. In addition, digoxin may resensitize baroreceptors that have been suppressed by increased neurohormonal sympathetic activity. Digoxin is not indicated in patients with primary diastolic dysfunction and preserved systolic function.[27]

Loading doses of digoxin are not necessary in HF. In the presence of normal renal function, a daily dose of 0.125 to 0.25 mg is adequate. In patients with abnormal renal function, conduction defects, and small body size as well as in older patients, digoxin should be started at 0.0625 to 0.125 mg/day. There are numerous interactions between digoxin and other drugs, particularly amiodarone, quinidine, procainamide, diltiazem, verapamil, antibiotics, and anticholinergic agents. There are no data to support regular measurement of serum digoxin levels. Electrolyte abnormalities can exacerbate digoxin toxicity.

Beta Blockers. One of the most important mechanisms responsible for progression of HF is activation of the sympathetic nervous system. This observation led to the hypothesis that drugs that interfere with the actions of the sympathetic nervous system (e.g., beta blockers) can be beneficial in HF. Beta blockers reduce heart rate and thereby reduce myocardial oxygen consumption, inhibit the release of renin, and decrease the activation of the renin-angiotensin system.[11]

In numerous trials, beta blockers in selected patients with HF have been shown to improve ventricular function, hemodynamics, functional status, and exercise tolerance, reduce HF exacerbations, and improve mortality. However, this is not a beta blocker class effect. Only carvedilol, metoprolol, and bisoprolol have been shown to reduce mortality by at least 34% in patients with HF.[28,29] Trials using nebivolol and bucindolol have not led to the same mortality benefit.[30]

Beta blockers are currently recommended for all patients with LVEF of 40% or less. Beta blockade should be used with caution in those with HF who have bradycardia, high-degree heart block, or severe COPD. The benefits are especially well described for patients with a history of MI and most patients with left ventricular dysfunction. In addition, a study showed that continuation of beta blocker therapy in patients with acutely decompensated systolic HF did not delay improvement in these patients.[31] Initiation of therapy is recommended at low doses and only when patients are hemodynamically stable. Suppression of compensatory tachycardia with beta blockade can result in hypotension and cardiogenic shock.[10]

Ivabradine. Ivabradine is the first new medication approved for use in HFrEF in over 10 years. It is a hyperpolarization-activated cyclic nucleotide-gated channel blocker that inhibits sinus node activity without affecting ventricular repolarization or myocardial contractility. It has been shown to reduce HF hospitalization and death from worsening HF in patients with LVEF of 35% or less and heart rate of 70 beats per minute or more who are being treated with standard HF medical therapy. It is not indicated for patients in atrial fibrillation because its action is directed at the sinus node. Common adverse reactions include bradycardia, hypertension, atrial fibrillation, and visual brightness.[32] Because of its recent U.S. Food and Drug Administration (FDA) approval, it is not in the current ACCF/AHA guidelines. Ivabradine is mentioned in the 2012 European Society of Cardiology ESC guidelines as a treatment that may be valuable in patients with systolic HF.[33] European approval occurred in 2012.

Aspirin. The use of aspirin in patients with HF remains controversial. Aspirin provides cardioprotective benefit in patients with concomitant coronary artery or vascular disease, but studies have suggested an increase in HF hospitalizations in patients taking aspirin.[34]

Anticoagulants. There are no data to support routine use of anticoagulation in patients with HFrEF. However, HF patients with other indications for thromboembolic prophylaxis including atrial fibrillation, hypercoagulable states, or a previous thromboembolic event should follow current guidelines for concomitant comorbid conditions.[11,35]

Device Therapy

Implantable Cardioverter-Defibrillators and Cardiac Resynchronization Therapy. In patients with reduced ejection fraction, with or without prior MI, who are receiving standard HF medications, ICDs prevent sudden cardiac death. Numerous studies have shown that ICDs detect and terminate malignant ventricular arrhythmias, therefore reducing mortality. ICDs are appropriate for both primary and secondary prevention of sudden cardiac death in patients with LVEF of 35% or lower.[36-38] Patients with LVEF of 35% or lower who are on optimal HF medical therapy; are at least 40 days post-MI; or are 90 days from index diagnosis if the cause is nonischemic, have NYHA class II to III symptoms, and have life expectancy of at least 1 year may be candidates for prophylactic ICD implantation.[11]

ICD implantation is a prophylactic therapy for patients with HFrEF. Cardiac resynchronization therapy (CRT) or biventricular pacing is a therapeutic intervention indicated in patients with ventricular dyssynchrony evidenced by left bundle branch block (LBBB), QRS duration of 150 msec or less, and LVEF of 35% or less who have NYHA class II or III symptoms. This therapy has been shown to modify the disease process by improving LVEF and reducing LV size and functional mitral regurgitation as well as reversing ventricular remodeling. Only about 35% of qualifying patients show benefit from this therapy, and benefit is usually evident by 3 months after implantation, although some patients show late improvement. Although benefits can be significant, permanently implanted device therapy is not without drawbacks including device malfunction, lead integrity issues, infection, and inappropriate shocks, which can all decrease quality of life.[11,39,40] Cardiac electrophysiologists are the experts in this subspecialty and can counsel patients regarding the risks and benefits of device therapy as well as guide device selection.

Revascularization

Some HF patients may benefit from revascularization. Most patients with newly diagnosed systolic dysfunction should be evaluated for cardiac ischemia by either stress testing or coronary angiography. Certain patients with reduced ejection fraction and coronary artery disease may benefit from revascularization, such as percutaneous coronary intervention or coronary artery bypass grafting, because this may improve survival as well as reduce symptoms. Decision criteria related to revascularization are beyond the scope of this chapter.

Advanced Heart Failure Therapies

Inotropic Agents. Positive inotropic agents, which are given by intravenous infusion, increase the force of myocardial contraction. Long-term parenteral administration of positive inotropic agents such as phosphodiesterase inhibitors (milrinone) and beta-adrenergic agonists (dobutamine) has resulted in improved symptoms but increased rates of sudden cardiac death because of their potential proarrhythmic effect. The continuous or intermittent parenteral administration of positive inotropic agents remains largely palliative in patients with stage D HF. Inotrope infusion can be a bridge to recovery, a bridge to decisions regarding further advanced HF therapy, or a bridge to cardiac transplantation. These agents can be helpful as short-term infusions for patients with refractory volume overload or threatened end-organ dysfunction. The temporary institution of an intravenous inotropic agent can transiently improve systolic function, palliate low-output states, and improve end-organ dysfunction.[11]

Mechanical Circulatory Support. Mechanical circulatory support (MCS) can be considered for short-term management in the acutely ill hospitalized patient or for longer-term therapy. Short-term devices are placed percutaneously and used in the critical care areas of specialized centers. These devices are a bridge to recovery or a bridge to decisions regarding a longer-term therapy. LVADs are the most commonly used longer-term MCS device. LVADs have emerged as a destination or bridge to transplant therapy in patients with stage D HF. These devices are implanted and managed in specialty centers. They are designed to augment cardiac output and improve survival, functional capacity, and quality of life in selected stage D patients.[41]

Cardiac Transplantation. Cardiac transplant is the gold standard of advanced HF therapies. It is the most effective therapy for stage D HF. Five-year post-transplant survival is approximately 70%. Patients who may be be considered should be referred to an advanced HF program or cardiac transplant center. Unfortunately, cardiac transplantation is an option for relatively few patients because of the limited supply of donor hearts. Life expectancy of patients who qualify for transplant is typically less than 1 year. Because of recent advances in LVAD technology, this therapy has emerged as a more viable option for patients waiting for transplant.[11]

Nonpharmacologic Therapy

Education. Patient education regarding self-care principles has been shown to improve medication adherence and understanding of disease process and reduce hospitalizations. The current ACCF/AHA HF treatment guidelines include self-care education as a Class 1 recommendation for patients with HFpEF and HFrEF. Self-care principles, such as smoking cessation, medication compliance, immunization updates, fluid restriction, and daily weight monitoring, should be discussed with all HF patients and reinforced frequently. Patients with sleep apnea should be treated.[11,42]

Diet. Reduced-sodium diets have been recommended for the management of HF, although no clinical studies have as yet evaluated a specific sodium restriction. Dietary sodium restriction of 2 to 3 g is advised for HF patients, including those with preserved systolic function and patients with reduced ejection fractions. More rigid dietary sodium restriction (<2 g) may be more appropriate for patients with moderate to severe HF.[31] Most patients with HF can benefit from specific dietary instructions and guidelines on how to read the labels on all food packages. A licensed dietitian with specialized training in HF can be an invaluable asset to the HF patient and family. Involvement of family members who prepare the foods cannot be underestimated; they should be included in all dietary education.

Sudden increases in sodium intake in patients with well-compensated but relatively severe HF can lead to acute decompensation. Holidays and seasonal festivities are particularly a problem because of the alteration in food preparation, increase in daily activity levels, and increase in emotional stressors during these times. Patients with alcohol-induced cardiomyopathy should completely abstain from alcohol. Alcohol is a cardiac toxin; therefore patients with HFrEF should be advised to limit or avoid alcohol completely.[43]

Exercise. The benefits of a regular exercise program have been well documented for patients with HFpEF and HFrEF. The HF-ACTION trial (Heart Failure: A Controlled Trial Investigating Outcomes of Exercise Training), a large randomized trial of stable class III and class IV systolic HF patients who underwent a structured exercise program, demonstrated a modest reduction in all-cause mortality, cardiovascular mortality, and hospitalization rates. Patients demonstrated improved exercise tolerance and reported improved health-related quality of life.[10,44] It has been suggested that this benefit is a result of improved endothelial function, blunted catecholamine response, and improved peripheral oxygen uptake.

All major societies with HF treatment guidelines include an exercise training recommendation, although a program is not clearly outlined. A consensus paper from the ESC and Heart Failure Association is an effort to provide clearer recommendations for exercise training in this group of patients.[10,33,45] In 2014, Medicare expanded its coverage to include cardiac rehabilitation programs in patients with LVEF of 35% or lower and NYHA class II to IV symptoms who are on optimal medical therapy for at least 6 weeks.

INDICATIONS FOR REFERRAL OR HOSPITALIZATION

Patients with HF may benefit from cardiology consultation when symptoms appear to be refractory to the standard therapies of diuretics, ACE inhibitors, aldosterone antagonists, and beta blockers. The onset of arrhythmias, coronary ischemia, or MI should prompt consultation. In addition, consideration of input from a cardiologist should be entertained in all young patients with either ischemic or nonischemic dilated cardiomyopathy, hypertrophic cardiomyopathy, worsening ejection fraction over time, NYHA class III or class IV symptoms, need for device therapy (ICD), or HF advanced therapies evaluation.

Even with pharmacologic advances in HF management, the 30-day hospital readmission rate among older patients remains above 20%, with the lowest rates of readmission occurring among patients who are seen by a care provider within 1 week after hospital discharge. This high readmission rate is multifactorial, possibly involving inadequate diuresis during hospitalization, inadequate symptom management by the patient, nonadherence to complex and expensive pharmacologic schedules and dietary regimens, social isolation, and the natural illness trajectory. Early post-hospital follow-up with a health care provider supports a lower rate of readmission.[46]

With the rapidly increasing prevalence of HF worldwide and the financial burden this is placing on the health care system, disease-management programs and strategies to manage HF patients are important interventions for reducing hospital readmission rates. Several types of disease-management programs have been studied, including HF clinics, home health advanced practice nurses, community-based case managers, patient telemanagement, cardiac rehabilitation, emergency department observation units, and HF subacute care. Recently hospitalized HF patients as well as those at high risk for hospital admission (renal insufficiency, multiple comorbid illnesses) should be considered for referral to a disease-management program.[11]

HF clinics have provided a mechanism for patients to be seen in a clinic for physical assessment, medication instruction and frequent diuretic titration, dietary education, and exercise training. Some nurses run clinics that focus on patient education and resource finding; advanced practice registered nurses who run HF clinics are instrumental in frequent diuretic titration, uptitration of medical therapy, and referral for appropriate advanced therapies. For patients with HF who are unable to attend clinic sessions, the home health advanced practice nurse may be an appropriate referral. The advanced practice nurse with expertise in HF can see the patient in his or her home for assessment of weight, vital signs, heart and lung sounds, and other physical examination findings to assess for HF. During the home visit, the advanced practice nurse can continue patient teaching about medications, diet, and activity and develop a plan with the patient and family for emergency care and when to call the health care provider.

The use of telemedicine technology as a tool in disease management is expanding rapidly to meet the needs of patients in integrated health care delivery systems. A number of innovative attempts at telemedicine with patients with HF are under way and may be potential alternatives for management of these patients at home. Specifically, patients with HF are using telephone and computer technology to transmit data on vital signs, symptoms, and weight to a central repository where the health care providers can review trends. The data are currently variable regarding the effectiveness of this intervention in reducing HF hospitalizations.[47]

Indications for hospitalization include new-onset HF with symptoms of congestion for treatment and diagnostic evaluation, clinical or electrocardiographic evidence of acute myocardial ischemia (acute coronary syndrome), pulmonary edema or acute decompensated HF, oxygen saturation below 90%, severe medical complications (e.g., pneumonia, renal failure), anasarca, symptomatic hypotension or syncope, hemodynamically significant cardiac arrhythmias, HF refractory to maximal outpatient oral treatment program, and need to evaluate home support for safe management in the community. In addition, hospitalization may be necessary for intravenous administration of intravenous diuretics or for more advanced therapies, such as inotropic support for low-output states or initiation of antiarrhythmic medications.[11]

LIFE SPAN CONSIDERATIONS

HF with preserved systolic function is more prevalent with increasing age. All comorbidities should be treated in these patients with HF, particularly anemia, thyroid abnormalities, diabetes, and sleep apnea. Recommendations include management of systolic hypertension with diuretics, ACE inhibitors, and beta blockers and use of beta blockers and nitrates to treat myocardial ischemia. NSAIDs should be avoided in older adult patients at risk for HF because of the propensity of these agents to promote fluid retention and to affect renal function.[11]

HF is a progressive and deadly disorder; less than 50% of patients are alive at 5 years after diagnosis, and less than 25% are alive at 10 years. Consideration should be given to early involvement of HF patients in a palliative care program. Palliative care specialists provide decision support surrounding advanced therapies and assistance with symptom management and facilitate discussions about end-of-life decisions. The trajectory of this disease process is variable, and prognosis statistics are simply predictions. Early involvement of the palliative care team is critical for emotional support of patients and families as they negotiate their way through a progressive, chronic disease process.[11,33,43]

EMERGING EVIDENCE

Our knowledge about the origins, mechanisms, and treatments of HF is continually evolving. Health care providers are advised to monitor specialty organizations, journals, and other guideline sources for timely information to make the best treatment decisions for their HF patients. Early referral to a cardiologist or HF disease management program should be considered for their expertise in evaluating and treating HF patients. Epidemiologic studies have shown the importance of primary care intervention long before HF develops to treat and to assist patients in modifying health risks that have been shown to lead to the development of HF.[48]

Cardio-oncology is a rapidly growing area; both oncologists and cardiologists recognize the increasing prevalence of HF in cancer patients and screen patients more aggressively both before and after potentially cardiotoxic chemotherapy or radiation therapy or during stem cell transplant evaluation. Primary care clinicians should be aware of the potential for chemotherapy-induced cardiomyopathy and HF in patients, even years after they have completed chemotherapy, and refer appropriately.

Newer medical therapies include neprilysin inhibition. The PARADIGM-HF trial (Prospective Comparison of ARNI with ACEI to Determine Impact on Global Mortality and Morbidity in Heart Failure) was stopped early because of the significant improvement in survival in patients with LVEF of 40% or below with class II to IV symptoms who were treated with ARB-neprilysin inhibition compared with enalapril.[48] There are guideline-driven therapies for systolic HF patients; however, patients with preserved systolic function (diastolic failure) continue to present a clinical challenge because treatment remains empirical. Ongoing research into the underlying pathophysiologic mechanism of and treatment approaches for diastolic HF will lead to improved therapies and outcomes for these patients. These are exciting developments in the understanding and management of HF. Further investigations and consultations with cardiac specialists will guide use of these in individual patients with HF.

PATIENT AND FAMILY EDUCATION

Many of the important concepts for management of HF are discussed in previous sections of this chapter. Patients and their families can take an active role in management of their disease process if they understand the condition and its treatments. Support for weight reduction and smoking cessation, if applicable, may be helpful. Reinforcement of the self-care principles is a valuable intervention.

Increasing weight is an early sign of decompensation. Therefore, all patients should know their target weight and be counseled regarding importance of daily weights. A phone call to their health care provider (primary or specialty) regarding weight gain of more than 2 pounds in a day or 5 pounds in a week can prompt diuretic uptitration and reduce need for hospitalizations.

HEALTH PROMOTION

Prevention of HF is linked to prevention of ischemic heart disease as well as to control of hypertension in the primary care setting. Accordingly, all patients should be screened for heart disease risk and encouraged to reduce their risk by adopting a healthy lifestyle, including maintenance of normal weight, low-fat diet, tobacco avoidance, and exercise. Interventions to screen for heart disease risk include a family history, blood pressure measurement, lipid screen, and blood glucose concentration or hemoglobin A_{1c} level to screen for diabetes. Patients should be encouraged to seek medical attention promptly for any heart attack signs or symptoms, unexplained fatigue, or dyspnea. In addition, patients should be screened for familial cardiac conditions, such as hypertrophic cardiomyopathy and sudden cardiac death, and referred to a cardiologist if family history is positive. Other cardiovascular diseases need close monitoring with timely intervention for any condition change.

CHAPTER 122

HYPERTENSION

Maryjane Giacalone • Randall M. Zusman

DEFINITION AND EPIDEMIOLOGY

Blood pressure is the force in arterial structures created by interplay of flow, volume, and constriction. High blood pressure, or hypertension, has been defined by determining the levels of blood pressure that cause target organ damage, morbidity, and mortality as arterial flow is delivered. It is known that 95% of all hypertension is primary, or essential, hypertension and has no known cause. The remaining 5% is termed secondary hypertension and is directly attributable to structural, circulatory, or chemical abnormalities.

In 1972, the National Heart, Lung, and Blood Institute initiated a campaign to improve public awareness of the need for treatment of hypertension. The campaign has been successful in improving awareness and increasing treatment, but control of hypertension in the general population has progressed slowly, reaching 51% in 2009 to 2012.[1]

Approximately one third of adult Americans have hypertension. Hypertension is a risk factor for coronary artery disease (CAD), heart failure, stroke, peripheral arterial disease, kidney disease, and retinopathy and therefore represents a significant public health threat.

In 2011, hypertension was directly responsible for 65,123 deaths and indirectly responsible for 377,258 deaths.[2] Research has shown that small gains in the control of hypertension can result in health improvements. Data extrapolated from the Intersalt study have shown that an overall drop of 2 mm Hg in the distribution of blood pressure would result in a 6% annual reduction in stroke, a 4% reduction in CAD, and a 3% reduction in all-cause mortality.[3] The most recent data available reveal that although 82% of Americans with high blood pressure are aware of it, 74.7% are undergoing treatment, with 68.9% having adequate blood pressure control.[1]

As knowledge evolves, guidelines change after reevaluation of past studies and incorporation of findings from new studies to account for different risk levels and treatment regimens. The most recent guidelines from the Eighth Joint National Committee (JNC 8)[4] and from the American Society of Hypertension (ASH) and the International Society of Hypertension (ISH)[5] have established blood pressure parameters based on these criteria.

INCIDENCE AND PREVALENCE

Both systolic and diastolic blood pressures rise throughout childhood and early and middle adulthood; each is an independent predictor of cardiovascular and cerebrovascular disease, occurring alone or concurrently, in individuals younger than 50 years. The rate of rise in diastolic blood pressure tends to level off or to drop slightly in approximately the fifth decade of life. Systolic blood pressure continues to rise with advancing age, making isolated systolic hypertension more prevalent in the older adult. There is a higher prevalence of hypertension among men until they reach the mid-50s. From 55 to 64, the prevalence of hypertension among men and women is relatively equal. From age 65 to 74, 68% of women have hypertension versus approximately 62% of men, and after 74 years of age, the prevalence increases to 76.4% of men and 79.9% of women.[1]

In general, people of lower socioeconomic means have a higher prevalence of hypertension. In these groups, poor diet, stress, and poor or less frequent access to health care may play a role in the development of high blood pressure.[1]

Black adults have higher rates of hypertension than do white or Hispanic adults through age 75. African Americans have a higher incidence of cardiovascular, stroke, and renal complications and have a higher mortality rate related to hypertension than do people of other ethnic backgrounds.[2] Enhanced renal sodium reabsorption occurs in 57% of African Americans compared with 27% in other groups. This salt sensitivity contributes to the problem of high blood pressure among African Americans.

Risk Factors

Obesity, metabolic syndrome, high dietary intake of fat and lower intake of potassium, excessive amount of dietary sodium, physical inactivity, obstructive sleep apnea, excessive alcohol intake, smoking, and stress are associated with the development of hypertension.[2] In general, the risk for hypertension is significant for both systolic and diastolic measurements. Prevention, detection, and treatment of hypertension should be public health priorities. The development of hypertension is likely multifactorial and therefore necessitates a coordinated, thoughtful, and individualized approach to diagnosis and treatment.

PATHOPHYSIOLOGY

Blood pressure is the product of cardiac output (heart rate, myocardial contractility, and circulating volume and its impact on myocardial stretch) and peripheral resistance (vascular constriction and compliance). Anything that affects any part of this equation can affect blood pressure. In a properly functioning system, feedback loops maintain homeostasis.

Primary Hypertension

Primary or essential hypertension is affected by the sympathetic nervous system, either through response to perceived hypovolemia (baroreceptor response) or physical or psychological stressors. Hyperkinetic myocardial muscle, related to neurohormonal stimulation, may cause mild hypertension, primarily in young adults. Hypertension also leads to ventricular hypertrophy.

The primary effect of sodium on blood pressure is probably related to excess circulating volume, but sodium may also directly affect hypertrophy, contractility, and vascular resistance. Hypertension associated with salt sensitivity has been postulated to be caused by (1) inability to normally excrete sodium through the kidneys; (2) resetting of the pressure-natriuresis curve, requiring higher blood pressures to maintain normal sodium and water balance; (3) abnormal electrolyte transport, resulting in disturbances in the cytosolic sodium and calcium balance and increased vasoconstriction; or (4) low renin levels, reduced numbers of nephrons, and modified sympathetic nervous system activity.[6]

Epidemiologic studies generally support a link between higher salt intakes and the prevalence of hypertension.[6,7] Age, African-American heritage, diabetes, low renin levels, and nonmodulating hypertension often predict salt sensitivity.

Renin is released by the juxtaglomerular apparatus of the kidney in response to a low-flow state (reduced renal perfusion pressure or low circulating intravascular volume), sympathetic nervous system stimulation or catecholamine release, and hypokalemia. Once released, renin acts on angiotensinogen to create angiotensin I. In the pulmonary circulation, angiotensin-converting enzymes (ACEs) change angiotensin I to angiotensin II, a potent vasoconstrictor that over time and with prolonged production causes arterial stiffening and hypertrophy. Vascular hypertrophy results in increased peripheral resistance, depression of angiogenesis, or vessel regression. Angiotensin II also causes aldosterone stimulation, which enhances sodium and water reabsorption from the renal tubules and effectively increases circulating volume. The resulting higher blood pressure should provide feedback to maintain homeostatic responses; however, feedback loops may not work properly in some individuals, allowing higher circulating levels of renin and thus higher blood pressure.

There may also be a correlation among obesity, insulin resistance, and hypertension, resulting in impaired salt excretion and enhanced sodium reabsorption, increased sympathetic nervous system activation, and increased angiotensin II and aldosterone production, all of which are associated with higher blood pressure readings.[8]

The Dietary Approaches to Stop Hypertension (DASH) study showed a relationship between lower potassium intake and hypertension. In this study, it was found that blood pressure also decreased in response to a universally recommended diet that contains generous servings of fruits, vegetables, and low-fat dairy products with reduced sodium and saturated and total fat and increased potassium.[7,9]

Excessive alcohol consumption (more than two drinks per day) has been associated with hypertension and other cardiovascular risks and should be suspected in individuals who have been resistant to treatment. Alcohol may raise blood pressure by causing increases in sympathetic nervous system activity, activation of the renin-angiotensin system, or decreases in peripheral vascular tone and impairment of baroreceptor effectiveness. Marked increases in blood pressure may occur with acute alcohol withdrawal but are unrelated to mechanisms of chronic hypertension. Overall reduction of alcohol intake results in a lowered blood pressure and overall cardiovascular risks in hypertensive heavy drinkers.[10]

Blood pressure rises with acute exercise and is most dramatic and serious in those with uncontrolled hypertension. However, regular exercise can be beneficial if the person can adhere to an established exercise routine. The Centers for Disease Control and Prevention recommend regular exercise as an aid in lowering blood pressure. Regular isometric exercise has been shown to prevent the development of hypertension.[6] Regular aerobic exercise has been shown to reduce the incidence of cardiovascular events.

Secondary Hypertension

Secondary hypertension can be ascribed to renal artery stenosis (RAS), pheochromocytoma, hyperaldosteronism, coarctation of the aorta, Cushing syndrome, sleep apnea, and thyroid disease; alcohol and the use of steroids, oral contraceptives (hormone replacement therapy is an infrequent cause), or nonsteroidal anti-inflammatory drugs (NSAIDs) are exogenous causes (Table 122-1).[11] Although secondary causes account for approximately 5% to 10% of all hypertension cases, it is important to keep in mind that 5% translates to more than 3 million cases.

Renal Artery Stenosis. RAS results in hypertension when there is a 70% to 80% blockage of a renal artery, often activating the renin-angiotensin system. Two different mechanisms have been shown to cause RAS. In individuals younger than 30 years, fibrodysplasia or fibromuscular dysplasia causes tight fibrous bands that alternate with normal or thin tissue along the renal artery, usually the medial portion. Fibrodysplasia affects more women than men. After the age of 50 years, atherosclerosis is the more likely cause of RAS and usually manifests in the proximal artery, extending from aortic plaque. Hypertension from RAS can coexist with essential hypertension; in elderly persons, RAS is likely to be a frequent contributor to hypertension. Angioplasty with or without stenting is the preferred treatment of fibromuscular dysplastic RAS. Atherosclerotic RAS may also be treated with angioplasty, often with stenting if there is elastic recoil in the vessel; an ostial lesion is more difficult to resolve percutaneously. Surgical bypass of the renal artery is another option as long as the individual is healthy enough to undergo surgery.[11]

Pheochromocytoma. Pheochromocytoma is a catecholamine-producing tumor of the adrenal glands and is a fairly rare cause of hypertension (see Chapter 205). A small percentage of these tumors are malignant. Hypertension seen with pheochromocytoma is constant in 50% of cases and labile in the other 50%. Approximately 50% of cases involve the five *Hs*: hypertension, headache, hyperhidrosis, hypermetabolic state, and hyperglycemia. Bilateral headache, hyperhidrosis, and palpitations occur in 95% of the cases.[11]

Primary Hyperaldosteronism. Primary hyperaldosteronism is seen in less than 0.5% of all cases of hypertension and is more common in women. Adrenal adenoma accounts for 70% of all cases of primary hyperaldosteronism and is correctable by surgery. The other 30% results from bilateral adrenal hyperplasia, which must be managed medically. Primary hyperaldosteronism is suspected in patients with unprovoked hypokalemia.[11]

Coarctation of the Aorta. Coarctation of the aorta (a localized stricture of the aorta) is usually found in youth. It is typified by hypertension in the presence of claudication, delayed femoral pulses, decreased blood pressure in the lower extremities, and notching of ribs on chest x-ray films.[12] Treatment usually involves surgical repair, with angioplasty and stenting a less frequent option.

Cushing Syndrome. Eighty percent of individuals with Cushing syndrome have hypertension (see Chapter 205).[12] Cushing syndrome is caused by hypersecretion of glucocorticoids by the adrenal cortex. This hypersecretion results from an adrenal tumor or overstimulation by the anterior pituitary.

Use of Certain Medications. The use of oral corticosteroids and anabolic steroids may also result in hypertension. All NSAIDs have been associated with hypertension.[13]

Obstructive Sleep Apnea. Obstructive sleep apnea, which affects up to 5% of the Western population, is associated with hypertension and is thought to result from a hypoxia-driven sympathetic nervous system discharge. It is more common in individuals with elevated body mass index and appears to plateau at 65 years of age. There is a possible association with leptin, which may be associated with the development of obesity, obstructive sleep apnea, and hypertension.[8,11] Use of continuous positive airway pressure (CPAP) resulted in improvement in resistant hypertension over a 12-week study.[14]

Renal Parenchymal Disease. Renal parenchymal disease is associated with the development of hypertension and is also considered a result of hypertension.[11] Renal insufficiency is apparent when creatinine levels rise higher than 1.5 mg/dL and the glomerular filtration rate falls to less than 50 mL/min. Renal parenchymal disease encompasses glomerular diseases (e.g., chronic renal failure, systemic lupus erythematosus, nephritis, diabetic nephropathy, glomerulonephritis, renal vasculitis) and interstitial diseases (e.g., polycystic kidney disease, chronic interstitial nephritis).

The pathophysiologic mechanism of renal parenchymal disease and hypertension probably involves factors that impair sodium excretion and lead to increased circulating volume.

Genetics. Some studies have found a genetic link to some secondary causes of hypertension, such as hyperaldosteronism. No single significant association has been found for a genetic basis of essential hypertension.

CLINICAL PRESENTATION

Because most patients with hypertension are asymptomatic, the importance of screening cannot be overemphasized. Symptoms of high blood pressure usually occur only after the physical consequences of end organ damage arise. Stroke, CAD or heart failure symptoms, renal dysfunction, retinopathy, and aortic dissection are potential presenting conditions that result from long-standing undiagnosed hypertension. Secondary causes of hypertension are more likely to manifest with early symptoms reflective of the underlying cause, such as diabetic nephropathy and Cushing syndrome. Blood pressure should be measured at each patient visit.

The medical history, physical examination, and laboratory data obtained from a patient with high blood pressure should focus on eliciting the presence of cardiovascular risk factors, dysfunction of target organs, and evidence of possible secondary causes of hypertension.[5]

Cardiac risk factors are assessed in the medical history. The health risks associated with hypertension are compounded by tobacco use, hyperlipidemia, left ventricular hypertrophy,

TABLE 122-1 Secondary Hypertension

	Clues			
	History and Physical	**Screening**	**Diagnostic Testing**	**Treatment**
CONDITION: ENDOGENOUS				
Renovascular condition (RAS)	Age <30 yr (fibromuscular) or >50 yr (atherosclerotic) History of atherosclerosis or risk factors Family history of RAS Abdominal bruits	Urinalysis Creatinine	Captopril flow scan Renal magnetic resonance arteriography Renal arteriography	Control hypertension: beta blockers Avoid ACE inhibitors Angioplasty Bypass surgery
Pheochromocytoma	Five *H*s (hypertension, headache, hyperhidrosis, hypermetabolic state, hyperglycemia) Hypertension after anesthetics, tricyclics Family history of endocrine disorders Hypertension after abdominal palpation Labile hypertension	Spot urine VMA 24-Hr urine VMA and metanephrines	Spot urine VMA 24-Hr urine VMA and metanephrines Plasma catecholamines (clonidine suppression test) CT scan of abdomen and pelvis Scintigraphy/MIBG imaging	Control hypertension: alpha blocker followed by beta blocker, or alpha-beta blocker Surgery (to check for extrarenal and malignant masses)
Hyperaldosteronism	Weakness Headache Fatigue Hypertension Hypokalemia	Unprovoked hypokalemia	Aldosterone levels before and after saline challenge Renin levels 24-Hr urinary aldosterone 17-Hydroxycorticosteroids CT scan of abdomen and pelvis Adrenal scintigraphy (if CT scan is normal) Adrenal vein catheterization (if CT scan and scintigraphy are normal)	If adrenal tumor: surgery If bilateral hyperplasia: potassium-sparing diuretics
Coarctation of the aorta	Young age Arm blood pressure > leg blood pressure Possible claudication Fatigue Late systolic murmur Apical heave	Chest x-ray study	Echocardiography Chest CT scan Aortography	Surgery Angioplasty Stent
Thyroid disorder	Weight change Fatigue Metabolic change Temperature intolerance Edema Change in bowel habits Thyromegaly	Thyroid-stimulating hormone Weakness Muscle spasms Unprovoked hypokalemia	Triiodothyronine Thyroxine Thyroid-binding hormone	Treatment of underlying disorder Control hypertension in interim
Renal parenchymal disease: Polycystic kidney disease Glomerulonephritis Diabetic nephropathy Chronic renal failure Obstruction Creatinine	Edema Nocturia Diabetes History of UTIs Pruritus Family history of polycystic kidney disease 24-Hr urine: protein, creatinine, creatinine clearance	Urinalysis	Renal ultrasound Intravenous pyelography Diabetes testing	Depends on specific cause; control of volume intake, diuretics, and additional medical therapy; ACE inhibitor if diabetic (otherwise use with caution), control of glycemia, relief of obstruction

TABLE 122-1 Secondary Hypertension—cont'd

	Clues			
	History and Physical	**Screening**	**Diagnostic Testing**	**Treatment**
Cushing syndrome	Hirsutism Edema Buffalo hump Moon facies Truncal obesity Red-purple striae	24-Hr urine: free cortisol	Dexamethasone suppression test Pituitary MRI CT scan of thorax, abdomen	Surgery Control hypertension
Other: Anxiety Pregnancy Sleep apnea				
CONDITION: EXOGENOUS				
Alcohol	History of use			
Cocaine				Cessation of substance
NSAIDs	History of arthritis			Alternative treatment if necessary
Steroids	History of steroid-dependent conditions			
Sympathomimetics (over-the-counter cold remedies)	History of recent URI			
Weight control remedies				
Erythropoietin				
MAOIs				

CT, computed tomography; MAOIs, monoamine oxidase inhibitors; MIBG, metaiodobenzylguanidine; MRI, magnetic resonance imaging; URI, upper respiratory tract infection; UTI, urinary tract infection; VMA, vanillylmandelic acid.

glucose intolerance, and positive family history. In addition, a complete cardiovascular, cerebrovascular, renovascular, endocrine, and family history is documented.

Any recent surgical, psychological, social, environmental, or traumatic stress should be elicited. Such events may precipitate a temporary elevation in blood pressure or suggest a secondary cause of hypertension. For example, pheochromocytoma can adversely affect hemodynamic stability during surgery.

All over-the-counter and prescribed medications (both currently and formerly used by the patient) should be listed, including nicotine, herbal treatments, steroids, oral contraceptives, NSAIDs, sedatives, sympathomimetics, amphetamines, cyclosporine, erythropoietin, tricyclic antidepressants, monoamine oxidase inhibitors, and alpha- and beta-adrenergic agonists.[5] The dosage, frequency, and duration of medications should be documented. A dietary assessment of sodium, cholesterol, fat, and alcohol intake must also be obtained.

The provider should elicit clues for potential secondary causes of hypertension, such as sleep apnea (loud snoring, erratic sleep, daytime somnolence), pheochromocytoma (severe headaches, diaphoresis, palpitations), aldosteronism (muscle cramps, weakness, polyuria, polydipsia, nocturia, rhabdomyolysis, paresthesias), mineralocorticoid alteration (licorice intake, chewing tobacco, oral steroid use), and renovascular conditions (hypokalemia).

Symptoms indicative of target organ damage must be sought. These symptoms can be neurovascular (transient weakness or blindness, loss of visual acuity, severe headache, confusion, lethargy, seizures), vascular (coarctation, impotence, claudication), cardiovascular (chest pain, dyspnea, palpitations, syncope), and renal (oliguria, hematuria, dysuria).

PHYSICAL EXAMINATION

Accurate assessment of blood pressure is crucial. A blood pressure cuff of the appropriate size (with the bladder of the cuff encompassing at least 80% of arm circumference) is applied 1 cm (⅖ inch) above the antecubital fossa. The patient's arm is positioned with support level with the heart; the sphygmomanometer must be at the provider's eye level. The systolic value is the level at which the first Korotkoff sound appears; the diastolic value is the level at which sound disappears. An average of at least two measurements is recommended. Blood pressure and heart rate are measured in each arm while the patient is seated with feet on the floor; when it is warranted by concerns for orthostasis, these measurements are repeated after the patient has been standing for at least 2 minutes.

Height and weight are recorded and guide weight management decisions. Other components of the physical examination gather evidence of end-organ impairment and secondary causes for hypertension.

Sustained hypertension produces a vascular effect. Retinal changes include arteriolar narrowing, arteriovenous nicking, exudates, hemorrhages, and, in severe cases, papilledema. The carotid arteries and aorta may have bruits, and impaired cerebral circulation may manifest as deficits on neurologic testing. Evidence of cardiac dysfunction (e.g., adventitious lung sounds, cardiac gallops, or displaced apical pulse) or left ventricular enlargement indicates complications of hypertension and affects treatment decisions. Pulse changes (diminished or absent) and skin changes (thinning, loss of extremity hair) point to peripheral circulatory impairment.

Hypertension may be produced as a result of other processes that affect multiple organ systems. It is important to note striae, neurofibroma, and pruritic areas. Radial-femoral pulse delays and differences in blood pressure between arms or between arms and legs require further evaluation. Renal artery bruits or enlarged kidneys are evidence of kidney involvement. Thyroid findings of enlargement, bruits, or nodules necessitate additional testing.

DIAGNOSTICS

Because multiple factors may transiently increase or decrease blood pressure values, a diagnosis of hypertension is usually based on measurements obtained during at least two office visits.[5] Anxiety, oral contraceptives, nicotine, caffeine, and appetite suppressants are some of the more common causes of increased blood pressure. Fluid loss and bed rest can decrease blood pressure. Classification and treatment of hypertension are guided by age, ethnicity, and comorbidities. Per the JNC 8 panel, blood pressure of 140/90 or higher is classified as hypertension in individuals younger than 60 and blood pressure of 150/90 or higher is hypertension for those 60 years of age or older. The ASH/ISH guidelines differ slightly, with blood pressure of 140/90 or higher classified as hypertension in individuals younger than 80 and blood pressure of 150/90 or higher as hypertension in those 80 years of age or older.[4,5] Blood pressures in the 120 to 139/80 to 89 range can be considered prehypertension.[5] The recommendations of the JNC 8 have been controversial in that some providers, including specialists, feel that the traditional target of lowering the blood pressure to below 140/90 is applicable in general. Each patient should be evaluated individually, and target blood pressure values established based on the patient's unique characteristics, comorbidities, and tolerance to medication.

Routine evaluation of hypertension includes urinalysis and complete blood count (CBC) and determination of serum potassium, blood urea nitrogen (BUN), serum creatinine, fasting blood glucose, plasma lipoprotein, serum uric acid, and calcium concentrations. Electrocardiography (ECG) is performed to assess evidence of ischemic heart disease or left ventricular hypertrophy. Left ventricular hypertrophy manifests on ECG with a large S wave in V_1 and a large R wave in V_5. These two deflections add up to more than 35 mm.

DIAGNOSTICS

Hypertension

LABORATORY
Urinalysis
CBC and differential
Serum glucose
Serum electrolytes
BUN
Creatinine
Fasting lipid profile
Calcium
Phosphorus
Uric acid
Thyroid-stimulating hormone (TSH)*
24-Hour urine cortisol (if Cushing syndrome is suspected)
24-Hour creatinine, catecholamines, and metanephrines (if pheochromocytoma is suspected)

IMAGING
Chest x-ray examination*
Abdominal ultrasound*
Renal angiography*

OTHER DIAGNOSTICS
ECG
Echocardiography*

*If indicated.

DIFFERENTIAL DIAGNOSIS

The initial evaluation of a patient with hypertension should exclude the possibility of secondary hypertension. Diagnosis and treatment of an underlying secondary cause may ultimately resolve the hypertension. The more commonly noted secondary causes of hypertension are noted later; their symptoms and diagnostic testing can be found in Table 122-1.

Among the differential diagnoses is white coat hypertension, which is an elevated blood pressure related to the anticipation or anxiety associated with visiting a health care provider. When white coat hypertension is suspected, home or ambulatory blood pressure monitoring may be beneficial. If home monitoring is recommended, the patient's sphygmomanometer should be evaluated for comparative efficacy in the office and the patient should be instructed or supervised in proper technique. If ambulatory blood pressure monitoring is considered, coverage by insurance should be confirmed. Some cases of white coat hypertension are thought to be predictive of high blood pressure; in such cases, patients may benefit from nonpharmacologic primary prevention techniques.

DIFFERENTIAL DIAGNOSIS

Hypertension

- White coat hypertension
- Hypertension, primary
- Secondary hypertension (see Table 122-1)

CARDIOVASCULAR
- Renal vascular disease
- Coarctation of the aorta

RENAL
- Renal parenchymal disease

ENDOCRINE
- Primary aldosteronism
- Cushing syndrome
- Hypercalcemia caused by hyperparathyroidism
- Hypothyroidism
- Pheochromocytoma
- Acromegaly

SLEEP DISORDERS
- Central sleep apnea
- Obstructive sleep apnea

EXOGENOUS
- Alcohol
- Pregnancy
- Medications, drugs

INDICATIONS FOR REFERRAL OR HOSPITALIZATION

Hospitalization is recommended for those with a blood pressure of 180/120 mm Hg and evidence of target organ dysfunction. Retinopathy may be the first presenting sign; grade 3 or grade 4 retinopathy with exudates and hemorrhage is a significant physical finding.[4] Target organ symptoms should be rapidly assessed. Neurologic symptoms include altered mental status, dizziness, blurred vision or loss of vision, focal neurologic deficits, and gastrointestinal symptoms. Cardiac symptoms include chest pain (or an anginal equivalent) or dyspnea accompanied by electrocardiographic changes, rales, and an S_3 on physical examination and possibly heart failure on chest x-ray study. Vascular symptoms may include tearing or burning chest pain and interscapular pain, with a variation in bilateral arm or leg blood pressure measurements, decreased pulses in lower extremities, or widened mediastinum on the chest x-ray film. Renal signs may include oliguria, hematuria, proteinuria, and red cell casts by urinalysis. If evidence of acute end organ damage is not present, blood pressure control can be managed on an outpatient basis.

A physician consultation is necessary when hypertension is resistant to therapy (failure of three full-dose, or maximally tolerated, antihypertensive drugs, including a diuretic) and when secondary causes attributable to lifestyle considerations or habits have been excluded. Most secondary causes may be best diagnosed and managed collaboratively.

A patient who has known secondary hypertension caused by RAS should be referred to a vascular interventionalist or surgeon.

Primary aldosteronism may require specialized input from an endocrinologist. Pheochromocytoma will require collaboration with medical physician and surgeon. Patients with autonomic failure who have orthostatic hypotension but hypertension while supine are challenging and would benefit from a consultation with a specialist in autonomic dysfunction or hypertension.[15]

GENERAL TREATMENT FOR PRIMARY HYPERTENSION IN ADULTS

Nonpharmacologic Treatment

Lifestyle modifications, which include regular exercise, the maintenance of a healthy weight, tobacco cessation, a reduction of daily dietary sodium to below 2300 mg, and moderation of alcohol intake are essential first steps. These nonpharmacologic recommendations apply to those with hypertension, as well as to those who fit into the category of prehypertension. Specific exercise recommendations and guidelines for alcohol use are found in Chapter 16 and under Education and Health Promotion. Strategies for smoking cessation are found in Chapter 16. Other options such as relaxation and meditation exercises can also be considered.

Pharmacologic Treatment

Medical regimens are based on age, ethnicity, and comorbidities, as well as patient preferences. Antihypertensives come in many different categories. Thiazide-like diuretics, ACE inhibitors, angiotensin receptor blockers (ARBs), and calcium channel blockers (CCBs) are the primary categories; these and others are listed in Table 122-2.

As noted previously, the JNC 8 panel recommends treating to a goal blood pressure of less than 140/90 for adults ages 18 to 59 and to less than 150/90 for those 60 and older unless the patient's blood pressure is less than 140/90 on medication and he or she is tolerating that regimen. For ASH/ISH, the recommendation is target blood pressure below 140/90 for individuals aged 18 to 79, and below 150/90 for individuals 80 years old and older. The clinician will need to use judgment regarding the patient's safety and stability in determining the best plan with the patient.

In the setting of chronic kidney disease and/or diabetes, regardless of age or ethnicity, the target blood pressure is below 140/90. Medical treatment should include an ACE inhibitor or an ARB either as initial treatment or as a second agent.

For nonblack individuals with or without diabetes, treatment is started with a thiazide-like diuretic, a CCB, an ACE inhibitor, or an ARB.

For black individuals with or without diabetes, treatment is started with a thiazide-like diuretic or a CCB. Although the JNC 8 panel did not suggest an ACE inhibitor or ARB for black individuals, these medications are still considered a mainstay of treatment in the presence of diabetes regardless of race.

Beta blockers are not recommended as baseline hypertension therapy but are indicated in settings of known CAD or heart failure with reduced ejection fraction (HFrEF). Nondihydropyridine CCBs (e.g., diltiazem, verapamil) are contraindicated in patients with HFrEF, but dihydropyridines (e.g., amlodipine) are acceptable to use for blood pressure control. Also in patients with HFrEF, loop diuretics, such as furosemide or torsemide, along with spironolactone may be used for volume management as well as blood pressure management.

The majority of people require two medications for adequate blood pressure control.[5] For nonorthostatic patients whose blood pressures are at or below 160 mm Hg systolic or 100 mm Hg diastolic, two-drug therapy is suggested as initial pharmacologic treatment.[5] Drugs that combine two medications may improve adherence, provided the insurance copay is affordable for the patient.[16]

Follow-up should be performed in 1 to 4 weeks to assess blood pressure results. If blood pressure is not at target, either the dose of the initial drug can be increased or a second drug can be added. The provider should continue to follow blood pressures until at target and to uptitrate and/or add a third drug as needed.

A patient has resistant hypertension when blood pressure readings are not at target despite maximal dose of three drugs, including a thiazide-like diuretic.

Potassium and renal function must be monitored after initiation of diuretics, ACE inhibitors, or ARBs.

Other Considerations

Clinical trials are ongoing to study renal denervation in individuals with resistant hypertension. Renal denervation is done percutaneously by inserting catheters into the renal arteries and performing radiofrequency ablation of renal artery tissue where nerves exist, to target and disable an area of renal sympathetic hyperactivity.[17]

LIFE SPAN CONSIDERATIONS

In general, systolic blood pressure rises with age, whereas diastolic blood pressure reaches a peak at around 50 to 60 years of age and then may begin to decrease mildly. Isolated systolic hypertension is especially a problem for patients older than 60 years and is thought to result from aging, stiffening, and lack of compliance of the arteries. Isolated systolic hypertension responds well to most antihypertensive medications and especially to diuretics and CCBs. Advancing age does not preclude pharmacologic therapy. In this population, pharmacologic therapy may require gentle initiation and advancement to prevent excessive drops in blood pressure or orthostatic hypotension, which can result in falls. Blood pressure target goals are slightly

Text continued on p. 583

TABLE 122-2 **Hypertension Medications**

			Effect on Coexisting Conditions		Efficacy		Side Effects		
Medication	**Dose**	**Compelling Indications**	**Favorable**	**Unfavorable**	**Increase**	**Decrease**	**Caution with**	**Short-Term Use**	**Possible**
DIURETICS		Hypertension, heart failure	Type 2 diabetes (low dose); osteoporosis (thiazides)	Type 1 and 2 diabetes (high dose); gout; renal insufficiency	Combination diuretics with different sites of action	Steroids; NSAIDs; resin-binding drugs	Lithium (increased levels); potassium-sparing diuretics and ACE inhibitors may cause hyperkalemia	Increases cholesterol, blood glucose	Hyponatremia, hypokalemia (except potassium-sparing diuretics), hypomagnesemia, hyperuricemia, hypercalcemia, hyperglycemia, orthostatic hypotension, renal dysfunction, sexual dysfunction
Thiazide and Thiazide-like									
Chlorthalidone: recommended as initial thiazide	12.5-50 mg/day								
Hydrochlorothiazide	12.5-50 mg/day								
Indapamide	1.25-5 mg/day								
Metolazone	2.5-10 mg/day								
Loop									
Bumetanide	0.5-4 mg divided 2-3 times a day; up to 10 mg/day (requires intermittent use and monitoring)								
Ethacrynic acid	25-100 mg divided 2-3 times a day								
Furosemide	40-240 mg divided 2-3 times a day								
Torsemide	2.5-10 mg/day								

Potassium Sparing									
Amiloride	5-10 mg/day								
Eplerenone	25 mg/day to 50 mg twice a day								
Spironolactone	25-100 mg/day								
Triamterene	25-100 mg/day								
ALPHA BLOCKERS		Hyperlipidemia; benign prostatic hypertrophy							Decreased clearance of verapamil with prazosin
Doxazosin	1-16 mg/day								
Prazosin	2-40 mg/day divided two/three times a day								
Terazosin	1-20 mg/day								
BETA BLOCKERS		MI (nonintrinsic sympathomimetic activity)	Angina; atrial tachycardia and atrial fibrillation; essential tremor; migraine (noncardioselective); hyperthyroidism; preoperative hypertension	Bronchospasm; depression; diabetes type 1 and 2; hyperlipidemia; AV heart block; peripheral vascular disease	Concomitant use of hepatically metabolized beta blockers; cimetidine; quinidine; food	NSAIDs; rifampin; phenobarbital; inducers of hepatic metabolism	Severe heart failure; asthma, bronchospastic COPD; diabetes (decreased hypoglycemic awareness); heart block; hypertriglyceridemia (associated with nonintrinsic sympathomimetic activity)		Bradycardia; fatigue; impaired circulation in extremities; sexual dysfunction; depression
Acebutolol	200-800 mg/day								
Atenolol	25-100 mg/day divided twice a day								
Betaxolol	5-20 mg/day								
Metoprolol	50-125 mg/day divided twice a day								

Continued

TABLE 122-2 Hypertension Medications—cont'd

Medication	Dose	Compelling Indications	Effect on Coexisting Conditions		Efficacy		Side Effects		
			Favorable	Unfavorable	Increase	Decrease	Caution with	Short-Term Use	Possible
Metoprolol extended release (Toprol XL)	50-100 mg/day								
Nadolol	40-320 mg/day								
Pindolol	10-60 mg/day								
Propranolol	40-480 mg/day divided								
Timolol maleate	20-60 mg/day divided twice a day								
ALPHA-BETA BLOCKERS									
Carvedilol	12.5-50 mg twice a day		Heart failure						Postural hypotension; bronchospasm
Labetalol	200-1200 mg twice a day			Liver disease					
CALCIUM CHANNEL BLOCKERS (CCBS)									
	Isolated systolic hypertension (long-acting dihydropyridine)	Angina; cyclosporine-induced hypertension; diabetes type 1 and 2 Nondihydropyridine: atrial tachycardia, atrial fibrillation, and migraine headache	Heart failure (except amlodipine) and second- and third-degree AV block (nondihydropyridine)	Cimetidine or ranitidine with CCBs hepatically metabolized	Rifampin; phenobarbital; inducers of metabolism				Dihydropyridines only: lower extremity edema, flushing, headache L-channel nondihydropyridines only: conduction defects, heart failure, lower lithium levels (with verapamil); increased levels of quinidine, digoxin, sulfonylureas, and theophylline (competitive hepatic metabolism) with nondihydropyridines Do not use diltiazem or verapamil with rivaroxaban or apixiban

Dihydropyridines						
Amlodipine	2.5-10 mg/day					
Felodipine	2.5-10 mg/day					
Isradipine	5-20 mg/day					Bradycardia; fatigue; impaired circulation in extremities; sexual dysfunction; depression
Nicardipine	30-60 mg twice a day (long-acting only)					
Nifedipine (long-acting only)	30-120 mg/day					
Nondihydropyridines (Long-Acting Only)			Atrial arrhythmias	HFrEF		
Diltiazem	120-360 mg*					
Verapamil	90-480 mg*					
ANGIOTENSIN-CONVERTING ENZYME (ACE) INHIBITORS						
	Heart failure; diabetes type 1; MI with systolic dysfunction	Diabetes type 1; renal insufficiency (with creatinine <3 mg/dL)		Kidneys in RAS; pregnancy	NSAIDS, antacids, food may decrease some absorption	Angioedema, anaphylaxis, hyperkalemia, cough, cholestatic jaundice. Monitor renal function carefully especially in older adults (consider lowest dose ACE or discuss dc with MD in elders with 20% increase in creatinine). Increased risk renal insufficiency if used in combination with diuretic therapy. Do not use with aliskiren

Continued

TABLE 122-2 Hypertension Medications—cont'd

			Effect on Coexisting Conditions		Efficacy		Side Effects		
Medication	Dose	Compelling Indications	Favorable	Unfavorable	Increase	Decrease	Caution with	Short-Term Use	Possible
Captopril	25-100 mg divided 2-4 times a day								
Enalapril	5-40 mg/day								
Fosinopril	10-40 mg/day*								
Lisinopril	5-40 mg/day								
Moexipril	7.5-30 mg/day								
Perindopril	4-8 mg/day								
Quinapril	10-80 mg/day								
Ramipril	2.5-20 mg/day								
Trandolapril	1-4 mg/day								

ANGIOTENSIN II BLOCKERS				
Candesartan	8-32 mg/day divided daily to twice a day			Side effects of angiotensin blockers: cough, hypotension, diabetic nephropathy, muscle weakness, anaphylaxis, facial edema. Do not use with aliskiren
Eprosartan	400-800 mg/day to twice a day			
Irbesartan	150-300 mg/day			
Losartan	25-100 mg/day			
Olmesartan	20-40 mg/day			
Telmisartan	20-80 mg/day			
Valsartan	80-320 mg/day			
ANGIOTENSIN II BLOCKERS		Heart failure	RAS	
Candesartan	8-32 mg/day divided daily to twice a day			
Eprosartan	400-800 mg/day to twice a day			
Irbesartan	150-300 mg/day			
Losartan	25-100 mg/day			
Olmesartan	20-40 mg/day			
Telmisartan	20-80 mg/day			
Valsartan	80-320 mg/day			
Azilsartan (Edarbi)	40-80 mg/day			

Continued

TABLE 122-2 Hypertension Medications—cont'd

Medication	Dose	Compelling Indications	Effect on Coexisting Conditions		Efficacy		Caution with	Side Effects	
			Favorable	Unfavorable	Increase	Decrease		Short-Term Use	Possible
VASODILATORS			Heart failure (with hydralazine along with the nitrates when ACE inhibitors cannot be prescribed)						
Hydralazine	10-50 mg/day four times a day, up to 300 mg a day total								Edema, orthostatic, hypotensiontachycardia, drug induced lupus-like syndrome
Minoxidil	5-100 mg/day								Angina, edema, heart failure, pericarditis or pericardial effusion
DIRECT RENIN INHIBITOR			Hypertension						
Aliskiren	150-300 mg/day								Hyperkalemia, renal dysfunction is possible in patients CrCl< 30 mL/min. Do not use with ACE or ARB

Beta blockers are now not recommended for initial hypertensive control, but may be indicated in patients with coronary artery disease
$Alpha_1$ blockers are also not recommended antihypertensive therapy but may be indicated in specific circumstances
*Frequency depends on formulation.
AV, atrioventricular; HFrEF, heart failure with reduced ejection fraction; MI, myocardial infarction.
Modified from National Heart, Lung, and Blood Institute: *The seventh report of the Joint National Committee on Prevention, Detection, Evaluation, and Treatment of High Blood Pressure,* NIH Publication No. 03-5233, Bethesda, Md, December 2003, U.S. Department of Health and Human Services and the Joint National Commission (JNC 8) Guidelines.

higher with older persons except in the setting of chronic kidney disease. Progress toward those goals has been associated with improved or preserved cognitive function.[18,19]

Secondary hypertension should be considered when hypertension develops before the age of 30 years (e.g., coarctation of the aorta or fibromuscular RAS) or after the age of 65 years (e.g., atherosclerotic RAS). Hypertension during pregnancy (preeclampsia) is outside the scope of this discussion.

COMPLICATIONS

Long-term complications of hypertension include left ventricular hypertrophy, heart failure, CAD, myocardial infarction, sudden death, aortic dissection, cerebrovascular disease, proteinuria, renal insufficiency, atherosclerotic conditions, retinopathy, and hypertensive urgencies and emergencies. Complications can be caused by long-term uncontrolled hypertension that assails target organs over time or by sudden surges of acute hypertension that result, for example, from acute glomerulonephritis or cocaine ingestion. A decline in cognitive functioning and a higher incidence of dementia and Alzheimer disease have been associated with hypertension in older individuals.[19]

Hypertensive Crises

Hypertensive emergencies are relatively rare events. Earlier and more pervasive diagnosis and treatment have reduced the incidence of malignant hypertension from untreated high blood pressure and have reduced mortality rates. A hypertensive crisis is present when blood pressure is high enough to threaten target organs acutely. JNC 7 differentiated between hypertensive emergencies and hypertensive urgencies as shown in Box 122-1.[20]

The initial assessment of hypertensive crises should be aimed at two primary goals: (1) determining a threat to the most commonly affected target organs (fundi, brain, heart, and kidneys) and (2) finding a cause. Various diagnostic options may be contaminated by drugs; therefore blood and urine samples should be collected quickly before treatment but without delaying it (Box 122-2).

Parenteral antihypertensive therapy is often indicated for hypertensive urgencies, but oral therapy may be appropriate. Newer very-short-acting agents such as clevidipine may be indicated urgently when organ damage is ongoing.[21] It may be advisable to coordinate the treatment of the cause (e.g., relief of pain in a postoperative patient) with the adjustment or initiation of medication. Observation of the patient for several hours after treatment to determine safety and efficacy is recommended.

BOX 122-1

Hypertensive Crises

Hypertensive Emergency Characteristics	Hypertensive Urgency Characteristics
Hypertensive encephalopathy	Upper levels of stage 2 hypertension
Intracranial hemorrhage	Hypertension with optic disc edema
Unstable angina pectoris	Progressive target organ complications
Acute myocardial infarction	Severe perioperative hypertension
Pulmonary edema	
Eclampsia	

National Heart, Lung, and Blood Institute. *The seventh report of the Joint National Committee on Prevention, Detection, Evaluation, and Treatment of High Blood Pressure.* NIH Publication No. 04–5230. Bethesda, Md: U.S. Department of Health and Human Services; 2004.

Hypertensive emergencies require admission to an intensive care unit and may require parenteral treatment (Table 122-3). The goal of treatment should be to reduce blood pressure slowly over a few hours because rapid lowering of blood pressure can produce a shock effect in target organs. The brain maintains cerebral perfusion pressure by autoregulation, which balances perfusion by cerebral vasoconstriction or vasodilation in response to rises and falls in blood pressure. Normal autoregulation is easily maintained with blood pressure ranges of 70/40 to 190/130 mm Hg (allowing for some individual variation). However, the autoregulation curve skews to the right and upward in patients with chronic hypertension. If blood pressure exceeds the limits of autoregulation or if blood pressure drops precipitously, signs of cerebral hypoperfusion may be present.

Initially, patients with severe hypertension may appear with headache, dizziness, altered consciousness (lethargy, slowed mentation, confusion, agitation), and nausea. Other target organs may produce profound symptoms in response to severe hypertension; pulmonary edema may occur in the setting of diastolic heart failure from excessively high afterload (peripheral resistance); retinal hemorrhage may occur. The physical

BOX 122-2

Diagnostic Tests Affected by Drugs Used to Treat Hypertensive Crises

Drug	Interferes With
Labetalol	Catecholamine assays (alpha blocker)
Diuretics, potassium	Primary aldosteronism evaluation
Renin-suppressing drugs	Renovascular evaluation

TABLE 122-3 Parenteral Medications for Severe Hypertension

Drug (Type)	Duration	Cautions and Comments
Nitroprusside (vasodilator)	1-10 min	Most rapid; use arterial monitoring; raises intracranial pressure
Nitroglycerin (vasodilator)	Minutes	Good for heart failure, CAD; tolerance may develop
Labetalol (alpha-beta blocker)	3-6 hr	Avoid in asthma; caution in heart failure
Esmolol (beta blocker)	<30 min	Avoid in heart failure and asthma
Nicardipine (CCB)	3-6 hr	Prevents cerebral vasospasm; may cause ischemia
Furosemide (diuretic)	4 hr	Use with vasodilators
Hydralazine (diuretic)	>1 hr	Indicated for eclampsia; avoid in CAD, dissection
Fenoldopam (peripheral vasodilator and diuretic)	15 min	Contraindicated in glaucoma; may cause reflex tachycardia
Clevidipine (CCB)	5-15 min	Contraindicated in patients allergic to eggs or soy

examination, especially the retinal examination, should focus on target organ damage. Groups 3 and 4 Keith-Wagener-Barker funduscopic changes may be the only or the initial sign of rapid deterioration with severe hypertension. Other possible changes may include blood pressure variation between the arms resulting from coarctation or aortic dissection, electrocardiographic changes and chest pain consistent with unstable angina or myocardial infarction, and hematuria resulting from renal decompensation.

JNC 7 recommends initial reduction of blood pressure gradually in the first 2 hours as dictated by comorbid conditions.[20] The rate of decrease should be tightly controlled. Effort should be made to control the pressure and to avoid precipitous drops that could result in neurologic symptoms related to too rapid a decrease in autoregulation of pressure within the brain. For this reason, the prior practice of using sublingual, short-acting nifedipine is contraindicated.[20] Particular caution should be exercised with older adults, patients with chronic hypertension, patients who might have hypovolemia (diuretic use, recent loss of appetite, vomiting, or diarrhea), and patients who are taking vasoactive medications. In patients of all ages, overly aggressive therapy has been associated with adverse outcomes such as blindness, coma, and death. The necessity of preventing permanent cerebral damage must be carefully achieved while lowering blood pressure enough to protect vital organs in circumstances such as acute heart failure, threatened myocardial infarction, or acute aortic dissection.

EDUCATION AND HEALTH PROMOTION

Topics that must be addressed include dietary instructions, exercise recommendations, other risk factor modification, lifestyle issues, and side effects associated with the medication prescribed. Patient comprehension is increased when handouts are given as references after the office visit.

Salt intake should be restricted to a maximum of 2.3 g/day and potentially less if possible. The DASH study showed that the lower the salt intake, the lower the blood pressure.[9] As noted previously, adherence may be difficult for many patients at extremely low income levels. Measures that help with salt restriction include avoiding the addition of salt to food, cooking with herbs, using fresh fruits and vegetables instead of canned, choosing fresh meats instead of deli or processed meats (e.g., bacon, sausage), and avoiding obviously salty foods (e.g., potato chips, pretzels, salted nuts). Products with food labels showing sodium free (5 mg/serving), very low sodium (<36 mg/serving), or low sodium (<141 mg/serving) should be selected.

Exercise recommendations are geared to provision of a specific exercise prescription (see Chapter 16), with consideration of screening for CAD by physician consultation or stress testing in men older than 40 years and women older than 50 years.

The goal should be an established routine of exercise that is enjoyable and maintains interest with consistent progression of activity. Factors that need emphasis include adequate hydration, stretching, and warm-up and cool-down periods with more strenuous exercise.

Self-monitoring of blood pressure is a reasonable goal. If the patient agrees, family members should be provided with information concerning therapeutic recommendations. Individual knowledge concerning the optimum level of blood pressure, the factors affecting blood pressure, the necessity of treatment for control rather than cure of high blood pressure, and the dangers of quick weight loss programs is crucial. When a patient is prescribed medication, the dose, the medication's mechanism of action, the monitoring required, and the side effects are important topics to discuss to ensure patient understanding. Involvement of patients in the decision-making process, exploration of feelings concerning treatment regimens, exit interviews, and regular follow-up visits help the patient achieve therapeutic goals.

CHAPTER 123

INFECTIVE ENDOCARDITIS

Jean P. Hartin Del Castillo • Isabella Rosa-Cunha

DEFINITION AND EPIDEMIOLOGY

Infective endocarditis (IE) refers to a microbial infection within the endothelium of the heart. Vegetations form and adhere to the endothelial structures. The heart valves are most often involved, but the disease may also occur within a septal defect, on the chordae tendineae, or on the mural endocardium. The majority of IE cases are the result of bacterial infections. However, increasing numbers of cases of IE caused by fungal, chlamydial, and rickettsial organisms have been reported; hence the change in name from *bacterial endocarditis* to *infective endocarditis.*[1-5] Despite diagnostic and therapeutic advancements, IE remains a life-threatening disease associated with serious complications and carries a high mortality.

Historically, IE has been classified as acute or subacute according to its clinical course. Acute IE is a fulminant process; death can occur within days to less than 6 weeks. The usual culprit organisms are *Staphylococcus aureus, Streptococcus pyogenes, Streptococcus pneumoniae,* and *Neisseria gonorrhoeae.* Subacute IE (death occurring within 6 weeks to 3 months) and chronic IE (death occurring later than 3 months) are usually classified together. These two forms of IE have a more subtle, indolent course; the usual causative organisms are the viridans streptococci. Although classifications based on acuity are helpful, a more descriptive system has been introduced and is of greater therapeutic and prognostic value. IE may be classified according to the evolution of the disease, the infectious pathogen, and the presence of a preexisting disease or risk factor (e.g., acute native valve endocarditis [NVE] involving viridans streptococci).[3,6,7]

Currently more than half of patients diagnosed with IE are older than 50 years; the ratio of male to female patients is greater than 2:1.[4] Although the overall incidence of IE is relatively low, certain populations are at higher risk, including but not limited to users of injectable drugs; individuals with structural cardiac abnormalities, implantable devices, or cardiac and vascular prostheses; immunosuppressed patients; and individuals with a history of IE.[2,3] In the United States alone, approximately 10,000 to 15,000 new IE cases annually as well as an alarming 20% to 30% mortality rate have been reported.[2] *S. aureus* is the most common cause of IE in the industrialized world, mainly because of development of risk associated with health care contact.[2,3,4,7] Successful management of IE requires a multidisciplinary collaborative effort in this extremely challenging population of patients.[1-4,7]

Native Valve Endocarditis

NVE is the most common type of IE and affects the mitral valve (28% to 45%), the aortic valve (5% to 36%), and both mitral and aortic valves (35%); the tricuspid valve is rarely affected (0% to 6%).[3,7,8]

Native Valve Endocarditis Risk Factors. Predisposition to NVE seems to be greatest when structural heart disease has created a defect, resulting in turbulent blood flow.[3,4] Any structural heart disease (e.g., rheumatic heart disease, mitral valve prolapse, congenital heart disease) or degenerative cardiac lesion (e.g., calcification of the mitral annulus, calcified nodular lesions secondary to atherosclerotic disease, post–myocardial infarction thrombus) may predispose a patient to IE.

In many countries rheumatic heart disease is still a common cause of IE; it has been implicated in 37% to 76% of infections.[3] IE has been associated with mitral valve prolapse, especially in the setting of mitral valve regurgitation. Mitral valve prolapse without mitral insufficiency is a more common abnormality and is associated with a small risk of endocarditis. Previous endocarditis is a risk factor for IE owing to the valvular damage that results from the infection.[3,8]

Congenital heart disease anomalies including bicuspid aortic valve, patent ductus arteriosus, ventricular septal defect, coarctation of the aorta, bicuspid aortic valve, tetralogy of Fallot, and pulmonic stenosis account for 10% to 20% of the cases.[2] Advances in the management of structural abnormalities and surgical correction of congenital abnormalities have significantly reduced the number of individuals at risk for IE.[2,3,6,8]

IE can occur on valves that are morphologically normal; in recent years, an increasing number of patients have no detectable predisposing cardiac lesion. Other predisposing factors for NVE are advanced age, diabetes, injection drug use, long-term hemodialysis, and immunosuppression, including human immunodeficiency virus (HIV) infection.[4,9]

Native Valve Endocarditis Infectious Organisms. Streptococcal and staphylococcal species account for 80% of NVE in non–injection drug users.[2,3] Higher mortality is seen in patients with *S. aureus* infection, diabetes, advanced age, and IE complications (stroke, congestive heart failure [CHF], paravalvular abscess). *S. aureus* is the culprit organism in most cases of acute IE; it causes systemic toxicity, often with metastatic infection, and carries a 40% mortality.[3,5]

Viridans streptococci are normal inhabitants of the oropharynx and account for approximately 30% to 40% of all streptococcal IE.[2,3] *Streptococcus bovis,* a group D *Streptococcus* species, is the causative organism in a small percentage of cases and is strongly associated with malignant or premalignant gastrointestinal lesions; therefore evaluation for colon cancer should be conducted in patients with *S. bovis* IE.[2]

Group B streptococci are normal flora of the gastrointestinal tract, oropharynx, vagina, and urethra in 5% to 12% of the population. Group B streptococci account for less than 5% of cases, yet these organisms are capable of affecting normal valves, leading to rapid destruction of the valve and embolization of vegetative matter. Mortality rates can approach 50%.[2,3] Enterococci are indigenous to the gastrointestinal tract and urethra; the number of IE cases caused by enterococci appears to be increasing. IE caused by enterococci is usually seen in both older men and younger women who have a recent history of genitourinary surgery, trauma, or malignant disease. Albeit rarely, it may also occur in women who have undergone an obstetric procedure.[2,3]

Other potential pathogens in NVE include fastidious gram-negative organisms grouped by the acronym of *HACEK* (*Haemophilus aphrophilus* [subsequently called *Aggregatibacter aphrophilus* and *Aggregatibacter paraphrophilus*]; *Actinobacillus actinomycetemcomitans* [subsequently called *Aggregatibacter actinomycetemcomitans*]; *Cardiobacterium hominis; Eikenella corrodens;* and *Kingella kingae*). These organisms are components of the flora of the oropharynx and upper respiratory tract and account for approximately 3% to 10% of cases of IE in patients who do not use injection drugs.[2] Although the clinical course is typically subacute, these organisms are capable of producing large friable vegetations with high risk of embolization, causing CHF and often necessitating valve replacement. Although it was previously difficult to identify the HACEK organisms, they are now reliably isolated with automated blood culture systems.[2,3,5]

NVE caused by other gram-negative organisms including *Pseudomonas* species and *Escherichia coli* is rare and usually associated with central venous catheters and implantable endovascular devices. Recent health care contact is common in these patients.[3]

Fungal IE represents less than 5% of NVE cases. *Candida* and *Aspergillus* species account for the majority of fungal endocarditis, usually in patients with predisposing conditions including but not limited to central venous catheters, dialysis catheters, prosthetic valves, immunosuppression, and implanted cardiac devices. Large vegetations often develop, extension into surrounding tissue and apparatus is seen, and surgical intervention frequently is required. The prognosis remains poor, despite aggressive combined medical and surgical interventions.[2,5]

Culture-negative endocarditis occurs in 5% to 15% of cases of IE. It is usually associated with previous exposure to antibiotics or infection with extremely fastidious organisms or intracellular bacteria that cannot be routinely cultured in blood with the standard blood culture techniques, including *Bartonella* species and *Coxiella burnetii.* Close work with the microbiology and pathology laboratories can help to identify organisms that may require longer incubation periods, enhanced culture mediums, special serology testing, and tissue biopsy [2,3,7]

Prosthetic Valve Endocarditis

Prosthetic valve endocarditis (PVE) comprises 10% to 20% of all IE cases and occurs with similar frequency in both the aortic and mitral valves. The first 12 months after valve replacement surgery represent the highest risk of infection; bioprosthetic and mechanical prostheses are infected with similar frequency.[2,3,9-11] Risk factors associated include prior NVE, long cardiopulmonary bypass time during valve replacement, and male sex.

PVE is categorized as early when symptoms occur within 60 to 365 days after surgery, or late when symptoms occur more than 1 year after surgery; the time frame usually relates to the varying virulence of the organisms. Early PVE is usually nosocomial, and the result of perioperative or immediate postoperative infection; it occurs either intraoperatively through direct contamination of the surgical field or postoperatively through contamination of central lines, pacemaker wires, or other indwelling sources. Despite prophylactic antibiotic therapy, the majority of early infections are the result of *S. aureus,* coagulase-negative staphylococci, or fungi.[3,7,10] The organisms involved in

PVE are similar to those seen in NVE. Infections associated with early PVE usually result in rapid valvular dysfunction and destruction of the integrity of the suture line, thus heralding an acute and rapidly deteriorating course with a high morbidity and mortality rate. *Streptococcus* species, enterococci, gram-negative bacilli, and diphtheroids are often involved within the first year after surgery.[3,7,10]

Because late PVE is often caused by less virulent organisms, it usually has a subacute course;, however, if the offending organism is virulent, late PVE may also manifest as an acute, fulminant infection. Common presentations in PVE include but are not limited to CHF, conduction system abnormalities, valve dehiscence, and regurgitant murmurs.[7] Late fungal endocarditis accounts for 10% to 15% of cases and carries a higher mortality.[2,3,9] Staphylococci, streptococci, and enterococci are the organisms mainly responsible for community-acquired late PVE.[3,7] PVE usually requires a combination of medical and surgical approaches.[2,5]

Endocarditis in Injection Drug Users

Those who develop endocarditis associated with injection drug use tend to be 20 to 40 years of age (80%) and are most often male (4:1).[3,5] The actual risk of infection among injection drug users is variable, depending on the drugs injected, the method of preparation, and the frequency of use. In this population, infection involving the tricuspid valve or in combination with another valve is most common (50% to 60%). Up to 75% of these patients may develop septic pulmonary emboli.[2,3] Right-sided endocarditis is otherwise rare; therefore injection drug use should be suspected. Involvement of the mitral valve alone is seen in 10.8% of cases, and in the aortic valve, 18.5% of cases. Involvement of both the aortic and mitral valves is seen in 12.5% of patients. The majority of individuals (66% to 75%) who develop IE have structurally normal valves before the infection; a minority have an underlying cardiac lesion from congenital heart disease or previous endocardial infection. Use of injection drugs predisposes the patients to recurrent and polymicrobial IE.[2,3]

Skin flora is the most common source of pathogenic microorganisms in users of injection drugs; contaminated drugs and drug paraphernalia are also bacterial sources. *S. aureus* is the most common offending organism; it is isolated in 50% to 60% of total cases and tends to be less virulent in IE originating from the right side. *Streptococcus* species, *Pseudomonas aeruginosa*, polymicrobial infections, and diphtheroids have also been implicated as causative pathogens.[2,3,5]

Right-sided endocarditis is associated with pneumonia and septic pulmonary emboli as a result of direct embolization in approximately 75% to 85% of patients. These patients appear ill, with high fevers and shaking chills. Patients with a clinical syndrome consistent with tricuspid valve endocarditis should also be evaluated for a potential extracardiac source of the endovascular infection, such as septic thrombophlebitis. The overall mortality rate for right-sided endocarditis is approximately 2% to 6%, whereas left-sided involvement is associated with a much higher mortality.[2,5]

Health Care–Associated Endocarditis

Health care–associated endocarditis refers to IE in patients with history of out-of-hospital health care system contact (e.g., wound care, care in a dialysis center or specialty nursing home, or chemotherapy within the last 30 days; or hospitalization for 2 or more days within the last 90 days). Community-acquired IE is defined as diagnosis within 48 hours of admission, without extensive health care contact. Non-nosocomial IE is defined as the occurrence of symptoms within 48 hours of hospital admission, with extensive health care contact. Nosocomial IE is defined as IE that is diagnosed more than 48 hours after hospital admission.[3,7] Data suggest that most cases of nosocomial and non-nosocomial IE are caused by *S. aureus*, and at higher rates than previously reported; *Enterococcus* species were second in frequency.[3,9] Most patients with health care–associated IE had indwelling central catheters, were on hemodialysis, had undergone recent surgical procedures, or were immunosuppressed. A study of hospitalized patients on hemodialysis through a central venous catheter indicated a 28% IE rate (mainly isolated was *S. aureus*); the overall death rate was 55.6%, and death occurred in all with methicillin-resistant *S. aureus*.[12]

CARDIAC IMPLANTABLE ELECTRONIC DEVICE ENDOCARDITIS

Permanent pacemakers and implantable cardioverter-defibrillators are examples of cardiovascular implantable electronic devices (CIEDs). Advances in cardiovascular device technology have had a positive impact on patient outcomes with respect to quality and quantity of life. According to the American Heart Association, implantation rates for permanent pacemakers and implantable cardioverter-defibrillators increased dramatically over the study period from 1993 to 2008.[13] With the population living longer and greater numbers of devices being implanted, rates of infection have markedly increased to 0.13% to 0.19%; infection may occur in the device pocket or leads as well as in valvular or nonvalvular endocardium.[2,13] Elevated risk of infection also appears correlated to the following: advanced age; comorbid conditions (diabetes, CHF, malignancy, renal failure); device revision; absence of preprocedure antibiotic prophylaxis; hematoma formation; inexperienced operators, and low-volume implantation centers.[13,14] Early infections, within 6 months of implantation, are generally caused by skin flora organisms, mainly *Staphylococcus* species. Those organisms demonstrate the ability to form biofilm. Biofilm is an accumulation of bacteria on bacteria, adherent to the surface of the device and encased in extracellular slime; this dense formation of bacteria is more resistant to antibiotics as well as to host defenses.[13,15]

PATHOPHYSIOLOGY

The development of endocarditis depends on the invasion of the bloodstream by a pathogen capable of attaching to an endothelial surface. The normal endothelium is not conducive to bacterial deposition. A high-velocity jet stream, a narrow valvular orifice, and a flow from a high- to a low-pressure chamber are hemodynamic features that predispose the patient to endocarditis. The forceful flow denudes the endothelium and allows platelet and fibrin deposition. The layering of platelets and fibrin creates nonbacterial sterile vegetation (nonbacterial thrombotic endocarditis [NBTE]), which in turn provides an ideal medium for bacterial adherence and growth.[3,16] Virulent microorganisms, especially the staphylococcal species, are capable of attaching to even normal endothelium.[3,4]

Microorganisms typically attach just distal to the narrowed orifice of a turbulent jet, such as on the atrial surface of the mitral leaflets in mitral regurgitation or on the ventricular surface of the aortic cusps in the setting of aortic insufficiency. After colonization of the endothelial surface, bacteria begin the replication process. Further platelet and fibrin deposition over the bacteria provides insulation from phagocytic cellular defenses, which allows the microorganisms to thrive and to form vegetations. Proliferation of the microorganism leads to local valvular destruction, tissue invasion, and possible embolization of the vegetative material.[2-4]

Morphologic characteristics of the vegetations depend on the offending organism and the duration of the infection. Lesions range from small, flat, or granular deposits to large, pedunculated, and friable formations. During the course of effective antimicrobial therapy, leukocytes and fibroblasts penetrate vegetations. This healing process results in fibrosis, occasionally with calcification, and eventual re-endothelialization of the valvular surface.[3]

Embolization of vegetative matter is not uncommon and most often involves the renal, splenic, coronary, or cerebral circulation. Myocardial infarction can be the result of embolization of the vegetative material to the coronary arteries. Pulmonary embolism is a complication associated with right-sided endocarditis in injection drug users, or in individuals with fungal infections. Embolization of septic material can lead to abscess formation. Mycotic aneurysms occur as a direct result of septic invasion into the arterial wall or septic embolization, which weakens the vessel wall and predisposes it to rupture.[3]

Persistent bacteremia triggers an immune complex response of both the humoral and cell-mediated immune systems. As seen in many chronic infections, a generalized hypergammaglobulinemia develops. Immune complexes containing immunoglobulins G, M, and A along with complement are deposited along the glomerular basement membrane of the kidney, precipitating glomerulonephritis. Peripheral manifestations of arthritic discomforts and cutaneous vasculitis may also be attributed to deposition of immune complexes in the joints and mucocutaneous vessels.[3,7]

CLINICAL PRESENTATION AND PHYSICAL EXAMINATION

The onset of symptoms usually occurs within days to weeks of the introduction of the microorganisms, but the symptoms may initially be nonspecific. Early symptoms of infection include generalized fatigue, malaise, night sweats, chills, weight loss, weakness, nausea and vomiting, and anorexia. A highly pathogenic organism such as *S. aureus* may manifest with an abrupt onset that prompts the patient to seek early medical attention. The virulence of the invading microorganism, underlying health of the patient, duration of infection, valvular structures involved, and presence or absence of CHF dictate the pace and severity of the disease course.[1-3]

Fever

Fever is present in the majority of patients but may be absent in older adults, immunocompromised hosts, patients with CHF or renal failure, or patients previously treated with antibiotics.[2-4] The degree of fever depends on the causative microorganism; high-grade fevers are primarily associated with virulent organisms and acute infections. Most patients defervesce with 3 to 7 days of appropriate antimicrobial therapy; however, fever may be protracted in some patients, usually resolving within 2 weeks of treatment. Persistent fever may suggest drug failure, secondary infection, an ineffective antimicrobial regimen, or intracardiac or extracardiac abscess formation.[2,3,7]

Neurologic Findings

Evidence of cerebral emboli may be seen in approximately 20% to 30% of patients with IE, and is the most common clinical neurologic finding. In recent studies, there is indication of a higher rate of cerebral emboli, varying from 65-82%; the formerly lower rate is due to silent presentations of IE. Even with appropriate therapy, stroke is seen in 4.82 cases per 1000 patient-days in the first week but improves by nearly two thirds in the second week.[3] Staphylococcal IE may manifest with neurologic phenomena as the first sign. The middle cerebral artery is the most commonly involved territory.

Mycotic aneurysms are potentially life-threatening complications that occur in a small percentage of patients. They typically occur early in the course of the disease but can occur months or even years after a bacteriologic cure has been achieved. A severe unrelenting headache, transient neurologic changes, or signs of cranial nerve involvement suggest the possibility of an intracranial mycotic aneurysm. Brain abscesses, seizures, purulent meningitis, arteritis, cerebral emboli, intracerebral bleeding, subarachnoid hemorrhage, and encephalopathy have also been reported.[2,3,5,7]

Ophthalmologic Findings

A complete funduscopic examination in those diagnosed with or suspected to have IE is recommended. Roth spots are exudative, edematous hemorrhagic lesions of the retina. They may cause changes in visual acuity. Endogenous endophthalmitis can be one of the consequences of IE; usual symptoms are decreased vision and/or eye pain. It can cause severe vision impairment and vision loss.[3]

Cardiac Findings

The signs and symptoms of IE vary according to the causative organism and the degree of systemic involvement. Valvular infection can result in the disruption of valvular integrity, including perforation of a valve leaflet, rupture of chordae tendineae or papillary muscles, and leaflet prolapse. Penetration of bacteria into the adjacent myocardium can result in myocardial or perivalvular abscesses, which may contribute to development of conduction system disturbances, heart block, and pericarditis.[7] Further penetration of infection may produce fistulas between cardiac chambers. Large vegetations associated with fungal or *Haemophilus* infections can cause obstruction of the valvular orifice. Even after a bacterial cure has been achieved, fibrosis of the valve leaflets can result in hemodynamically significant valvular stenosis or regurgitation.[3]

Heart murmurs are detectable in the majority of patients but may be absent early in the course of the illness, in patients with right-sided endocarditis, or in older adults. A new murmur of regurgitation or change in an existing murmur suggests an acute, virulent process and often heralds the development of CHF. The diagnosis of IE must be entertained in any patient with a new heart murmur or a change in an existing heart murmur and fever of unknown origin.[2-4,7]

CHF, regardless of acuity, predicts a grave prognosis; poor surgical outcome is also demonstrated. Nevertheless, substantially reduced mortality rates are seen in the individual who undergoes valve surgery, if necessary. CHF may be secondary to valvular destruction, rupture of one of the chordae, obstruction of the valve by bulky vegetations, coronary embolization resulting in myocardial infarction, myocarditis, myocardial abscess formation, or prosthetic dehiscence.[2,3,5]

Pulmonary Findings

Pulmonary embolism is most often associated with tricuspid valve endocarditis in injection drug users. It may also occur in patients with indwelling central venous catheters or in patients with left-sided endocarditis who have left-to-right shunting from a septal defect.[2,5] Patients may have clinical pulmonary signs and symptoms; abnormal chest x-ray findings, pleural effusion, infiltrates or pneumonia, pleuritic chest pain, and cough with or without blood-streaked sputum. Pneumothorax may also be a complication of septic pulmonary emboli.[3]

Splenic and Dermatologic Findings

Splenomegaly has declined significantly, with rates reported at 11%, possibly because of increasing acute IE and/or shorter time to diagnosis. Splenic septic emboli, although common, are usually asymptomatic. Prolonged fever or localized symptoms should prompt CT scan to rule out splenic abscess.

Petechiae may be noted on the conjunctivae, palate, buccal mucosa, and extremities; they are present in 20% to 40% of patients and usually only for the first few days. Splinter hemorrhages are linear, subungual hemorrhages appearing in the proximal nail bed; common in subacute IE, they are also found in patients of advanced age or in the setting of occupational trauma.[2,3] Janeway lesions and Osler nodes are cutaneous lesions associated with endocarditis. Janeway lesions are nontender, hemorrhagic macules (1 to 4 mm) on the palms and soles and are the result of septic embolization. Osler nodes are painful nodules on the finger and toe pads that last hours to days. They have also been noted on the forearms, ears, and dorsa of the feet and are associated with immune complex deposition. The resulting inflammatory response leads to swelling, redness, and pain that characterize these lesions. Osler nodes are rare in acute IE but are present in 10% to 25% of subacute cases; they are not specific to IE. Clubbing may be seen in 10% to 20% of patients with subacute IE or more prolonged cases, and may improve with therapy.[2,3]

Renal Findings

Renal failure is associated with severe and/or prolonged IE and is usually reversible with treatment of the infection. Uremia is often the result of glomerulonephritis secondary to immune complex deposition on the glomerular basement membrane.[3,7] It may also occur secondary to septic embolization leading to renal infarction or abscess formation (uncommon), or in the setting of severe sepsis and/ or cardiogenic shock. The urinalysis may reveal microhematuria with or without proteinuria.[7]

Musculoskeletal Findings

Musculoskeletal manifestations may be seen early in the course of IE;d these findings number approximately 44%. Complaints of arthralgias and myalgias are common. Arthralgias tend to involve the proximal joints and lower extremities and may be monoarticular. Myalgias, often localized to the thigh or calf, are commonly unilateral and have no radicular pattern. These discomforts are often described at the time of presentation and may in part be a manifestation of elevated circulating immune complexes.[3,7]

Findings with Cardiovascular Implantable Electronic Devices

IE in patients with CIEDs can manifest as an acute or subacute process. Infection may be indolent and ongoing for weeks, or acute and associated with symptoms such as sepsis, high fever, rigors, and organ dysfunction. Local inflammatory changes at the pocket site are often seen. Examples are exposure of the leads or device, pain, discomfort, erythema, and drainage. Malaise, anorexia, presence or absence of fever, and decreased functional capacity are also possible complaints.[3,13]

DIAGNOSTICS

For establishment of the diagnosis of IE, every effort should be made to isolate the pathogenic microorganisms from the blood. Three sets (two bottles to each set) of blood cultures should be obtained from different venipuncture sites before antimicrobial therapy is initiated. Additional blood cultures may be useful in patients who have been recently exposed to antibiotics. Culture specimens can be obtained at any time; a febrile state at the time of culture is not critical.[2,3,5,7] Negative blood cultures may be present in 10% of patients. The laboratory should be notified when the presence of culture-negative bacteria or fungi or a fastidious pathogen is suspected.[2,4,10]

Normochromic normocytic anemia is present in 70% to 90% of cases of IE and worsens with the duration of illness. The white cell count is usually within normal limits in less virulent infections, perhaps with a slight shift to the left. A marked leukocytosis with a shift to the left is a common finding in endocarditis caused by a virulent microorganism. The erythrocyte sedimentation rate (ESR) is elevated except in patients with cardiac or renal failure. Rheumatoid factor can be detected in half of the patients who have an infection lasting longer than 3 to 6 weeks. Circulating immune complexes are present in most patients; these levels decline as the infection is effectively treated. The serum complement level is usually decreased, especially in patients with glomerulonephritis. The urinalysis result is most often abnormal with proteinuria, microscopic hematuria, or pyuria. Serum creatinine concentration may be elevated and reflects the degree of renal involvement secondary to glomerulonephritis or renovascular embolization. Although these laboratory findings are common, they are of limited diagnostic value in IE.[2,3,7]

Echocardiography plays an important role in the evaluation of highly suspected or documented endocarditis. Vegetations appear as abnormal sessile or pedunculated echogenic masses attached to valve leaflets. Unfortunately, vegetations smaller than 2 mm can be difficult to identify with transthoracic echocardiography (TTE); body habitus and emphysema limit the sensitivity of this study (46% to 65%).[7,10] With its greater resolution, transesophageal echocardiography (TEE) has been shown to be more sensitive in detection of abscesses (87%) and vegetations (95%).[2,3,5]

Identification of vegetations in the presence of a prosthetic valve is more difficult because the prosthesis causes acoustic shadowing of parts of the ultrasound image; in this setting, the sensitivity of TTE falls to approximately 36%.[2] TEE is capable of imaging prosthetic valves reliably; its sensitivity for vegetations in this setting is 82% to 95%. Consequently, TEE is preferred for evaluation of suspected endocarditis in patients with valve prostheses.[2,3,7,8]

In addition to documenting the presence of vegetations in patients with endocarditis, echocardiography provides additional data of prognostic importance. First, the size, location, and mobility of vegetations as determined with echocardiography may be useful predictors of subsequent embolism. Second, echocardiography reliably identifies leaflet damage or associated valvular regurgitation that arises as a consequence of endocarditis. Finally, echocardiography can detect evidence of local invasion by an aggressive infection, such as an abscess or a fistula formation, that may be an indication for surgical repair.[8,9]

DIFFERENTIAL DIAGNOSIS

The diagnosis of IE is based on careful history and physical examination, blood cultures and laboratory results, electrocardiography, chest radiography, and echocardiography. Several sets of criteria for IE have been described. The most widely accepted are the Duke criteria (Box 123-1). This diagnosis must be considered in any patient with a cardiac murmur, changes in an existing murmur, and/or a fever of unknown origin. IE should also be entertained in any febrile injection drug user, patient with a prosthetic valve and evidence of valvular dysfunction, or patient with a cerebrovascular accident.[3] Last, IE should be suspected in any patient with an implantable device (i.e., permanent pacemaker or implantable cardioverter-defibrillator) even if there is not fever, erythema at the pocket site, cutaneous erosion of the device itself or drainage from the pocket.[12,13] The definitive diagnosis of IE requires the isolation of a pathogenic organism from the blood or embolic material or the demonstration of endocardial vegetations on echocardiography or at the time of surgery or autopsy.[2,4,12] For patients with suspected device endocarditis, additional cultures of the device pocket and hardware should be obtained on explantation.[12,13]

Other conditions can mimic the signs and symptoms of IE, which makes a definitive diagnosis difficult at the time of initial presentation. A comprehensive diagnostic evaluation will usually yield an accurate diagnosis in a timely manner. Disease processes such as acute rheumatic fever, atrial myxoma, lymphoma, systemic lupus erythematosus, tuberculosis, thrombotic thrombocytopenic purpura, connective tissue disorders, sickle cell disease, and nonbacterial thrombotic endocarditis can produce a similar constellation of symptoms. Diagnosis of IE

BOX 123-1

Duke Criteria for Diagnosis of Infective Endocarditis

MAJOR CRITERIA

1. Positive blood cultures: one of the following:
   a. Typical organisms consistent with infective endocarditis from two separate cultures (viridans streptococci, *Streptococcus bovis,* HACEK group, *Staphylococcus aureus,* or community-acquired enterococci in the absence of a primary focus)
   b. Microorganisms consistent with infective endocarditis from persistently positive blood cultures (two positive cultures >12 hours apart; or all of three or a majority of four or more separate cultures with the first and last sample at least 1 hour apart)
   c. Single positive blood culture for *Coxiella burnetii* or anti–phase I immunoglobulin G antibody titer >1:800
2. Evidence of endocardial involvement: echocardiogram demonstrating vegetation, abscess, new prosthetic valve dehiscence, or new valvular regurgitation (worsening or changing of preexisting murmur not sufficient). (Transesophageal echocardiography is recommended for prosthetic valves rated at least "possible infective endocarditis" by clinical criteria or complicated infective endocarditis, such as paravalvular abscess. Transthoracic echocardiography is the first approach in other patients.)

MINOR CRITERIA

1. Predisposition: preexisting heart conditions or injection drug use
2. Fever: temperature of 38° C (100.4° F) or higher
3. Vascular phenomena: arterial emboli, septic pulmonary emboli or infarcts, mycotic aneurysms, intracranial hemorrhage, conjunctival hemorrhage, Janeway lesions
4. Immune phenomena: nephritis, Osler nodes, Roth spots, rheumatoid factor
5. Microbiologic evidence: positive blood cultures that do not meet major criteria or serologic evidence of active infection with a microorganism consistent with endocarditis

DEFINITION OF INFECTIVE ENDOCARDITIS ACCORDING TO THE DUKE CRITERIA

Definite Infective Endocarditis

Pathologic criteria
- Microorganisms: documented by culture or histologic examination of vegetation, embolic material, or intracardiac abscess; or
- Pathologic lesions: presence of vegetation or intracardiac abscess, histologic confirmation of active endocarditis

Clinical criteria
- Two major criteria; or
- One major criterion and three minor criteria; or
- Five minor criteria

Possible Infective Endocarditis

Presentation and findings that are consistent with diagnosis but fall short of definite criteria (but not "rejected"—one major criterion and one minor criterion or three minor criteria)

Infective Endocarditis Rejected

Firm alternative diagnosis established; or
Resolution of symptoms after 4 days or fewer of antibiotic therapy; or
No pathologic evidence at surgery or autopsy after 4 days or fewer of antibiotic therapy

Modified from Baddour LM, Wilson WR, Bayer AS et al: Infective endocarditis: diagnosis, antimicrobial therapy, and management of complications: a statement for healthcare professionals from the Committee on Rheumatic Fever, Endocarditis, and Kawasaki Disease, Council on Cardiovascular Disease in the Young, and the Councils on Clinical Cardiology, Stroke, and Cardiovascular Surgery and Anesthesia, American Heart Association: endorsed by the Infectious Diseases Society of America, *Circulation* 111:e394-e434, 2005 [erratum in *Circulation* 112(15):2373, 2005]; and Li JS, Sexton DJ, Mick N et al: Proposed modifications to the Duke criteria for the diagnosis of infective endocarditis, *Clin Infect Dis* 30:633-638, 2000.

requires a high degree of suspicion given its complexity; the Duke criteria remain the most sensitive and specific diagnostic tool available.[2,3,5,7]

Blood cultures are essential in the diagnosis and management of IE and should not be delayed more than 2 or 3 hours in the toxic patient. In recent reports, 2.1% to % of patients may have negative blood cultures with IE already established.[2] Negative culture data should prompt further investigation into other possible causes of the fever and symptoms. If there is high clinical suspicion of IE in a patient with negative blood cultures, intensive efforts should be undertaken to identify fastidious microorganisms; these include prolonged incubation periods, culturing on special media, and serologic assessment. Microorganisms including *C. burnetii* (Q fever), *Chlamydia*, *Tropheryma whipplei*, and *Bartonella* organisms are difficult to isolate. Pathogens may potentially be isolated from embolized material or excised valve tissue.[2,11]

DIFFERENTIAL DIAGNOSIS

Infective Endocarditis

- Acute rheumatic fever
- Atrial myxoma
- Systemic lupus erythematosus
- Thrombotic thrombocytopenic purpura
- Connective tissue disorders
- Sickle cell disease
- Nonbacterial thrombotic endocarditis

MANAGEMENT

Specialist consultation and immediate referral to the emergency department are both indicated for the patient with fever who is suspected to have IE.

The identification of the infecting organism and the institution of high-dose bactericidal therapy are the cornerstones of treatment. Parenteral administration of antibiotics is preferred to ensure predictably high serum levels. Throughout the prolonged course of treatment, ongoing assessment of the patient's response to therapy and vigilance for the development of potential complications are crucial. Clinical improvement with reduction of fever is usually seen within 1 week of appropriate antimicrobial therapy. Blood cultures should be rechecked and should become negative after effective antimicrobial treatment. Persistent fevers and/or bacteremia should raise the suspicion of an intracardiac abscess, metastatic foci of infection, or inadequate antimicrobial therapy.[2,3,7]

The selection of antimicrobial agents and the duration of therapy vary by microorganism isolated and the duration of infection. IE caused by highly penicillin-sensitive viridans streptococci can often be cured within 2 weeks with a dual regimen of penicillin G or ceftriaxone and an aminoglycoside. Intracardiac prostheses or infections of longer duration (which produce large vegetations) require a prolonged antibiotic course for a successful cure to be achieved.[5]

Multiple organisms are the infectious agents in NVE. The prominent infectious agents are streptococci, enterococci, staphylococci, HACEK organisms, and fungal organisms. Viridans streptococci usually infect abnormal valves and are typically highly sensitive to penicillin, although some strains are exhibiting variable penicillin resistance.[4] Other organisms in this group include *Streptococcus sanguis*, *Streptococcus salivarius*, *Streptococcus mutans*, *Streptococcus mitis*, and *S. bovis*. *S. bovis* is a virulent microorganism associated with significant valvular damage and resultant hemodynamic compromise as well as a high risk of embolism. Surgical intervention may be necessary in cases of valvular destruction and persistent large vegetations. Treatment options are guided by the degree of penicillin sensitivity; concurrent use of aminoglycosides may be required.[2,4]

Group B streptococci may not be eradicated by penicillin alone, and aminoglycoside adjuvant antibiotic therapy may be necessary.[3,5] Enterococci may be resistant to penicillin; the treatment of these organisms has become further complicated by β-lactamase–producing and aminoglycoside-resistant strains. Overall, enterococcal IE therapy will need to be tailored according to the antibiotic susceptibilities.[2,3,5,7]

Staphylococcal species are highly resistant to penicillin because of their ability to produce β-lactamase. Either oxacillin or vancomycin is the preferable therapy, depending on the methicillin sensitivity profile of the organism.[3,5,7] Increasing resistance to these antibiotics has complicated the treatment in recent years.[5]

Valve infection with fungal organisms represents a challenge. Historically, therapy is a combination of parenteral antifungal therapy and valve replacement surgery. The availability of new antifungal agents presents the opportunity for reevaluation of therapy principles.[3,4,6]

Suspicion of CIED endocarditis warrants TEE to rule out involvement of the valves.[13,15] Complete removal of all hardware including the leads and generator, regardless of location, is recommended when CIED infection has been identified.[13,15] Local or superficial infection may not warrant complete removal of all hardware. Antimicrobial therapy should be directed toward oxacillin-resistant staphylococcal species; vancomycin should be administered until the source of infection is known.[13]

Early recognition of cardiac decompensation and intensive intervention are critical. Failure of antimicrobial therapy and/or the development of refractory CHF is an indication for surgical intervention. A recent study showed decreased 1-year mortality rates for patients with IE and heart failure who underwent valve surgery rather than medical treatment alone.[16,17] Other intracardiac complications requiring surgical intervention include valvular dehiscence, ruptured chordae tendineae, perforation of valve leaflets, and formation of an aneurysm or abscess. In these situations, surgical intervention may be lifesaving; therefore the presence of an active infection is not considered a surgical contraindication.[4] Surgical intervention is usually indicated in the following conditions: infection with brucellae, fungi, or resistant bacteria; left-sided IE caused by gram-negative bacteria; and recurrent emboli, early PVE, or late PVE secondary to *S. aureus*.[5,9]

Table 123-1 summarizes the current treatment recommendations formulated by a consensus group of the American Heart Association. Although these recommendations do not include all subgroups or potential pathogens, they do provide treatment regimens for the most commonly encountered causes of IE and incorporate recommendations for antibiotic resistance.

Co-Management with Specialists

IE is a potentially life-threatening infection and should be managed collaboratively with a cardiologist, infectious disease specialist, cardiac surgeon, and pathologist.[1-3,5]

Text continued on p. 595

TABLE 123-1 Some Suggested Antibiotic Regimens

Antibiotic*	Dose†	Duration of Treatment	Comments
NATIVE VALVE ENDOCARDITIS CAUSED BY PENICILLIN-SENSITIVE VIRIDANS STREPTOCOCCI AND *STREPTOCOCCUS BOVIS*			
Penicillin G (evidence exists for benefit)	12-18 million units/24 hr IV, continuously	4 wk	Preferred in most patients older than 65 years and in patients with impaired renal or cranial nerve VIII function.
Or			
Ceftriaxone (evidence exists for benefit)	2 g/24 hr IV or IM in 1 dose	4 wk	
Alternative treatments: Penicillin G	12-18 million units/24 hr IV, either continuously or in 6 equal doses	2 wk	
Or			
Ceftriaxone‡	2 g/24 hr IV or IM in one dose	2 wk	
Plus			
Gentamicin (evidence exists for benefit)	3 mg/kg/24 hr IV or IM in a single dose	2 wk	Gentamicin dosage is based on ideal body weight, not actual body weight.
Vancomycin (evidence exists for benefit)	30 mg/kg/24 hr IV in 2 divided doses, levels monitored not to exceed 2 g/24 hr unless serum levels monitored	4 wk	Recommended for patients allergic to penicillin or ceftriaxone. Follow recommended peak-trough levels.
PROSTHETIC VALVE OR OTHER PROSTHETIC MATERIAL ENDOCARDITIS CAUSED BY VIRIDANS STREPTOCOCCI AND *STREPTOCOCCUS BOVIS*			
Penicillin-Susceptible Strains			
Penicillin G (evidence exists for benefit)	24 million units/24 hr IV, either continuously or in 4-6 doses	6 wk	
Or			
Ceftriaxone‡ (evidence exists for benefit) with or without:	2 g/24 hr IV or IM in 1 dose	6 wk	
Gentamicin†	3 mg/kg/24 hr IV or IM in 1 dose	2 wk	The addition of gentamicin has not demonstrated higher cure rates compared with monotherapy. Not recommended with creatinine clearance <30 mL/min.
Vancomycin‡ (evidence exists for benefit)	30 mg/kg/24 hr IV in 2 divided doses, not to exceed 2 g/24 hr	6 wk	Recommended only for patients allergic to penicillin or ceftriaxone.
Penicillin-Resistant Strains			
Penicillin G (evidence exists for benefit)	24 million units/24 hr IV, either continuously or in 4-6 doses	6 wk	For relatively or fully resistant strains with MIC >0.12 µg/mL.
Or			
Ceftriaxone (evidence exists for benefit)	2 g/24 hr IV or IM in 1 dose	6 wk	
Plus			
Gentamicin (evidence exists for benefit)	3 mg/kg/24 hr IV or IM in 1 dose	6 wk	See above for gentamicin recommendations.
Vancomycin (evidence exists for benefit)	30 mg/kg/24 hr IV in 2 divided doses, not to exceed 2 g/24 hr	6 wk	Recommended only for patients allergic to penicillin or ceftriaxone.

Continued

TABLE 123-1 Some Suggested Antibiotic Regimens—cont'd

Antibiotic*	Dose†	Duration of Treatment	Comments
NATIVE VALVE ENDOCARDITIS CAUSED BY STRAINS OF VIRIDANS STREPTOCOCCI AND *STREPTOCOCCUS BOVIS* RELATIVELY RESISTANT TO PENICILLIN G			
Penicillin G	24 million units/24 hr IV, either continuously or in 4-6 equal doses	4 wk	Patients with penicillin-resistant strains (MIC >0.5 μg/mL) should be treated with the regimen recommended for enterococcal endocarditis (see below).
Or			
Ceftriaxone‡	2 g/24 hr IV or IM in a single dose		
Plus			
Gentamicin (evidence exists for benefit)	3 mg/kg/24 hr IM or IV in a single dose	2 wk	Dose should be adjusted to achieve a peak concentration of 3-4 μg/mL.
Vancomycin (evidence exists for benefit)	30 mg/kg/24 hr IV in 2 equal doses, not to exceed 2 g/24 hr unless serum levels monitored	4 wk	Vancomycin is recommended for patients allergic to penicillin or ceftriaxone.
ENTEROCOCCAL ENDOCARDITIS§			
Ampicillin (evidence exists for benefit)	12 g/24 hr IV in 6 doses	4-6 wk	4 wk if native valve and symptoms ≤3 mo in duration; 6 wk if symptoms >3 mo.
Or			
Penicillin G	18-30 million units/24 hr IV, either continuously or in 6 equal doses	4-6 wk	A minimum of 6 wk for prosthetic valve or prosthetic cardiac material.
Plus			
Gentamicin (evidence exists for benefit)	1 mg/kg IV or IM every 8 hr	4-6 wk	
Vancomycin	30 mg/kg/24 hr IV in 2 equal doses, not to exceed 2 g/24 hr unless serum levels monitored	6 wk	Vancomycin is recommended for patients allergic to penicillin.
Plus			
Gentamicin‖ (evidence exists for benefit)	1 mg/kg IM or IV every 8 hr	6 wk	
ENTEROCOCCAL ENDOCARDITIS§ (FOR STRAINS SUSCEPTIBLE TO PENICILLIN, STREPTOMYCIN, AND VANCOMYCIN BUT RESISTANT TO GENTAMICIN)			
Ampicillin (evidence exists for benefit)	12 g/24 hr IV in 6 doses	4-6 wk	4 wk if native valve and symptoms ≤3 mo in duration; 6 wk if symptoms >3 mo.
Or			
Penicillin G	24 million units/24 hr IV, either continuously or in 6 equal doses	4-6 wk	Minimum of 6 wk for prosthetic valve or prosthetic cardiac material.
Plus			
Streptomycin (evidence exists for benefit)	15 mg/kg/24 hr IV or IM in 2 doses	4-6 wk (a minimum of 6 wk for prosthetic valve or prosthetic cardiac material)	
Vancomycin	30 mg/kg/24 hr IV in 2 equal doses, not to exceed 2 g/24 hr unless serum levels monitored	6 wk	Vancomycin is recommended for patients allergic to penicillin.
Plus			
Streptomycin (evidence exists for benefit)	15 mg/kg/24 hr IV or IM in 2 doses		

TABLE 123-1 Some Suggested Antibiotic Regimens—cont'd

Antibiotic*	Dose†	Duration of Treatment	Comments
ENTEROCOCCAL ENDOCARDITIS§ (FOR STRAINS RESISTANT TO PENICILLIN BUT SUSCEPTIBLE TO AMINOGLYCOSIDE AND VANCOMYCIN)			
β-Lactamase–Producing Strain			
Ampicillin-sulbactam	12 g/24 hr IV in 4 doses	6 wk	Unlikely that organism is susceptible to gentamicin; if strain is gentamicin resistant, >6 wk of ampicillin-sulbactam is required.
Plus			
Gentamicin (limited evidence exists for benefit)	1 mg/kg IM or IV every 8 hr	6 wk	
Vancomycin	30 mg/kg/24 hr IV in 2 equal doses, not to exceed 2 g/24 hr unless serum levels monitored	6 wk	Vancomycin is recommended for patients allergic to penicillin.
Plus			
Gentamicin‖ (limited evidence exists for benefit)	1 mg/kg IM or IV every 8 hr		
With Intrinsic Penicillin Resistance			
Vancomycin	30 mg/kg/24 hr IV in 2 equal doses, not to exceed 2 g/24 hr unless serum levels monitored	6 wk	Infectious disease consultation is recommended.
Plus			
Gentamicin‖ (limited evidence exists for benefit)	1 mg/kg IM or IV every 8 hr		
ENTEROCOCCAL ENDOCARDITIS§ (FOR STRAINS RESISTANT TO PENICILLIN, AMINOGLYCOSIDE, AND VANCOMYCIN)			
Enterococcus Faecium			
Linezolid	1200 mg/24 hr IV or PO in 2 doses	≥8 wk	Use with infectious disease consultation. Rate of bacteriologic cure with antimicrobial therapy is <50%. Reversible thrombocytopenia is a risk with linezolid after 2 wk of therapy.
Or			
Quinupristin-dalfopristin (limited evidence exists for benefit)	22.5 mg/kg/24 hr IV in 3 doses	≥8 wk	Use with infectious disease consultation.
Enterococcus Faecalis			
Imipenem-cilastatin	2 g/24 hr IV in 4 doses	≥8 wk	
Plus			
Ampicillin (limited evidence exists for benefit)	12 g/24 hr IV in 6 doses		
Or			
Ceftriaxone‡	4 g/24 hr IV or IM in 2 equally divided doses	≥8 wk	
Plus			
Ampicillin (limited evidence exists for benefit)	12 g/24 hr IV in 6 doses		

Continued

TABLE 123-1 Some Suggested Antibiotic Regimens—cont'd

Antibiotic*	Dose†	Duration of Treatment	Comments
STAPHYLOCOCCAL ENDOCARDITIS IN THE ABSENCE OF PROSTHETIC MATERIAL			
Oxacillin-Susceptible Strains			
Nafcillin or oxacillin (evidence exists for benefit)	12 g/24 hr IV in 4-6 doses	6 wk	For uncomplicated right-sided infective endocarditis, 2 wk.
With optional			
Gentamicin‖	3 mg/kg/24 hr IV or IM in 2-3 doses	3-5 days	Benefit of additional aminoglycoside is unclear.
In Patients Who Are Penicillin Allergic (Nonanaphylactoid Type)			
Cefazolin‡ (evidence exists for benefit)	6 g/24 hr IV in 3 doses	6 wk	Avoid cephalosporins in patients with anaphylactoid-type reactions to penicillin.
With optional			
Gentamicin‖	3 mg/kg/24 hr IV or IM in 2-3 doses	3-5 days	Benefit of additional aminoglycoside is unclear.
Oxacillin-Resistant Strains			
Vancomycin (evidence exists for benefit)	30 mg/kg/24 hr IV in 2 doses	6 wk	Adjust dose to achieve peak serum concentration of 30-45 μg/mL and trough levels of 10-15 μg/mL.
STAPHYLOCOCCAL ENDOCARDITIS IN THE PRESENCE OF PROSTHETIC MATERIAL			
Oxacillin-Susceptible Strains			
Nafcillin or oxacillin	12 g/24 hr IV in 6 doses	≥6 wk	Vancomycin should be used in patients with anaphylactoid reactions to penicillin.
Plus			
Rifampin	900 mg/24 hr IV or PO in 3 doses	≥6 wk	
Plus			
Gentamicin‖ (evidence exists for benefit)	3 mg/kg/24 hr in 2-3 doses	2 wk	
Oxacillin-Resistant Strains			
Vancomycin	30 mg/kg/24 hr in 2 doses	≤6 wk	
Plus			
Rifampin	900 mg/24 hr IV or PO in 3 doses	≤6 wk	
Plus			
Gentamicin‖ (evidence exists for benefit)	3 mg/kg/24 hr IV or IM in 2-3 doses	2 wk	
ENDOCARDITIS CAUSED BY HACEK MICROORGANISMS¶			
Ceftriaxone‡ (evidence exists for benefit)	2 g/24 hr IV or IM in a single dose	4 wk	Cefotaxime or other third- or fourth-generation cephalosporin may be substituted.
Or			
Ampicillin-sulbactam (limited evidence exists for benefit)	12 g/24 hr IV in 4 doses	4 wk	

TABLE 123-1 Some Suggested Antibiotic Regimens—cont'd

Antibiotic*	Dose†	Duration of Treatment	Comments
Or			
Ciprofloxacin (limited evidence exists for benefit)	1000 mg/24 hr PO or 800 mg/24 hr IV in 2 doses	4 wk	Recommended only for patients unable to tolerate cephalosporin or ampicillin therapy. In patients with prosthetic valves, treatment is recommended for 6 wk.

*Desirable peak serum gentamicin level (1 hr after infusion) is approximately 3-4 μg/mL. Desirable peak serum vancomycin level (1 hr after infusion) is 30-45 μg/mL for twice-daily administration.
†Doses recommended are for adults with normal renal function.
‡Cephalosporins should not be used in patients with immediate-type sensitivity reactions to penicillins (urticaria, angioedema, anaphylaxis).
§All enterococcal endocarditis must be tested for antimicrobial susceptibility.
‖Gentamicin should be given close to nafcillin, oxacillin, or vancomycin doses.
¶HACEK microorganisms include *Haemophilus parainfluenzae, Haemophilus aphrophilus, Haemophilus paraphrophilus, Actinobacillus actinomycetemcomitans, Cardiobacterium hominis, Eikenella corrodens,* and *Kingella kingae.*
MIC, minimal inhibitory concentration.
Modified from Baddour LM, Wilson WR, Bayer AS et al: Infective endocarditis: diagnosis, antimicrobial therapy, and management of complications: a statement for healthcare professionals from the Committee on Rheumatic Fever, Endocarditis, and Kawasaki Disease, Council on Cardiovascular Disease in the Young, and the Councils on Clinical Cardiology, Stroke, and Cardiovascular Surgery and Anesthesia, American Heart Association: endorsed by the Infectious Diseases Society of America [erratum in *Circulation* 112(15):2373, 2005], *Circulation* 111:e394-e434, 2005.

BOX 123-2

Cardiac Conditions Associated with High Risk of Adverse Outcome from Infectious Endocarditis

ENDOCARDITIS PROPHYLAXIS RECOMMENDED (HIGH RISK)*

Prosthetic valves—mechanical, bioprosthetic, and homograft valves
Prosthetic material used for valvular repair
Prior episode of infective endocarditis
Unrepaired cyanotic congenital heart disease (CHD)
Repaired CHD with prosthetic material or device (surgical or catheter intervention within 6 months)
Repaired CHD with residual defects at or adjacent to repair site
Cardiac transplant recipients with development of valvulopathy

*In 2008 the American College of Cardiology and American Heart Association issued a focused update to their guidelines for the prophylaxis of infective endocarditis in patients with valvular heart disease, and it is recognized that "some clinicians and some patients may still feel more comfortable continuing with prophylaxis for infective endocarditis, particularly for those with bicuspid aortic valve or coarctation of the aorta, severe mitral valve prolapse, or hypertrophic obstructive cardiomyopathy. In those settings, the clinician should determine that the risks associated with antibiotics are low before continuing a prophylaxis regimen."[16]
Modified from Nishimura RA, Carabello BA, Faxon DP et al: ACC/AHA 2008 guideline update on valvular heart disease: focused update on infective endocarditis, *J Am Coll Cardiol* 52(8):676-685, 2008; and Wilson W, Taubert KA, Gewitz M et al: Prevention of infective endocarditis: guidelines from the American Heart Association: a guideline from the American Heart Association Rheumatic Fever, Endocarditis, and Kawasaki Disease Committee, Council on Cardiovascular Disease in the Young, and the Council on Clinical Cardiology, Council on Cardiovascular Surgery and Anesthesia, and the Quality of Care and Outcomes Research Interdisciplinary Working Group, *Circulation* 116:1736-1754, 2007.

BOX 123-3

High-Risk Procedures and Endocarditis Prophylaxis*

ENDOCARDITIS PROPHYLAXIS RECOMMENDED

Dental Procedures

Perforation of oral mucosa
Manipulation of gingival tissue (most dental procedures, such as cleanings, extractions, implant placements, periodontal procedures)
Exposure or manipulation of periapical region of tooth

Respiratory Tract Procedures

Procedures involving incision or biopsy of respiratory mucosa
- Tonsillectomy, adenoidectomy
- Bronchoscopy (only with incision of respiratory mucosa)

Infected Skin, Skin Structure, or Musculoskeletal Tissue Procedures

Surgical procedures involving infected skin or musculoskeletal structures

*For patients with underlying risk factors listed in Box 123-2.
Modified from Nishimura RA, Carabello BA, Faxon DP, et al: ACC/AHA 2008 guideline update on valvular heart disease: focused update on infective endocarditis, *J Am Coll Cardiol* 52(8):676-685, 2008; and Wilson W, Taubert KA, Gewitz M et al: Prevention of infective endocarditis: guidelines from the American Heart Association: a guideline from the American Heart Association Rheumatic Fever, Endocarditis, and Kawasaki Disease Committee, Council on Cardiovascular Disease in the Young, and the Council on Clinical Cardiology, Council on Cardiovascular Surgery and Anesthesia, and the Quality of Care and Outcomes Research Interdisciplinary Working Group, *Circulation* 116:1736-1754, 2007.

Primary Prevention

Because IE is associated with significant morbidity and mortality, primary prevention for patients at risk needs to be considered. The cardiac conditions believed to predispose patients to IE are listed in Box 123-2. Identification and education of patients at risk are essential and are the responsibility of all providers. The American Heart Association's current recommendations for endocarditis prophylaxis, with prophylaxis being reserved for those at high risk, are summarized in Box 123-3 and Table 123-2. The 2008 American College of Cardiology focused update recognized that these recommendations are inconsistent with practices common for decades and suggested that "some clinicians and some patients may still feel more comfortable continuing with prophylaxis for infective endocarditis,

TABLE 123-2 Antibiotic Prophylaxis for Dental, Oral, or Respiratory Tract Procedures

Patient Situation	Antibiotic	Route	Adult Dose	Pediatric Dose
Standard prophylaxis*	Amoxicillin	Oral	2 g	50 mg/kg
Inability to take standard oral medication*	Ampicillin	IM or IV	2 g	50 mg/kg
	or			
	Cefazolin	IM or IV	1 g	50 mg/kg
	or			
	Ceftriaxone	IM or IV	1 g	50 mg/kg
Allergy to penicillin or ampicillin*	Cephalexin†‡	Oral	2 g	50 mg/kg
	or			
	Clindamycin	Oral	600 mg	20 mg/kg
	or			
	Azithromycin	Oral	500 mg	15 mg/kg
	or			
	Clarithromycin	Oral	500 mg	15/mg/kg
Allergy to penicillin or ampicillin and inability to take oral medications*	Cefazolin†	IM or IV	1 g	50 mg/kg
	or			
	Ceftriaxone†	IM or IV	1 g	50 mg/kg
	or			
	Clindamycin	IM or IV	600 mg	20 mg/kg

*All regimens: to be given in a single dose, 30 to 60 min before the procedure.
†Cephalosporins should not be used in patients with hypersensitivity reaction to penicillins.
‡Other first- or second-generation oral cephalosporins may be used in equivalent adult dose.
Modified from Nishimura RA, Carabello BA, Faxon DP et al: ACC/AHA 2008 guideline update on valvular heart disease: focused update on infective endocarditis, *J Am Coll Cardiol* 52(8):676-685, 2008.

particularly for those with bicuspid aortic valve or coarctation of the aorta, severe mitral valve prolapse, or hypertrophic obstructive cardiomyopathy. In those settings, the clinician should determine that the risks associated with antibiotics are low before continuing a prophylaxis regimen. Over time, and with continuing education, the committee anticipates increasing acceptance of the new guidelines among both provider and patient communities."[16] Patients at high risk for IE should receive antibiotics with gastrointestinal and genitourinary procedures if they have infections, as prevention for wound infection, or to sterilize infected urine before genitourinary manipulation.[16]

Special consideration is required in addition for patients with rheumatic heart disease who are receiving long-term penicillin therapy for the prevention of recurrent episodes of rheumatic fever. In this setting, oropharyngeal organisms may have become resistant to penicillin. Consequently, before the procedure, these patients should receive prophylaxis with another appropriate antibiotic, such as clindamycin. One exception is rheumatic prophylaxis with monthly injections of benzathine penicillin. This regimen does not usually result in penicillin resistance, and therefore penicillin prophylaxis may be used safely.[18]

COMPLICATIONS

The acute complications associated with IE are numerous, may involve all major organ systems, and are potentially life-threatening. Cardiac complications are often the result of direct pathogen invasion, whereas metastatic complications result from septic embolization or immune complex deposition.

Another concern is the possibility of a relapse. After completion of the antibiotic course, the following should be completed: new baseline TTE, referrals for drug rehabilitation services (if necessary) and dental evaluations, prompt removal of intravenous catheter, and ongoing patient education about IE. Short-term follow-up should include physical examination, evaluation for antibiotic toxicity, and at least three sets of blood cultures for any febrile illness.[5] Patients with a relapse in NVE often respond to further antimicrobial treatment, but surgical intervention should be considered, especially in patients with prosthetic valves.[2,5]

On occasion, it is impossible to completely eradicate the microorganism with antimicrobial therapy, and surgery may not be an option because of the high operative risk associated with comorbid conditions. In this case, chronic suppressive therapy may be considered in an attempt to prevent the manifestations and complications of endocarditis.

INDICATIONS FOR REFERRAL OR HOSPITALIZATION

Immediate consultation and hospitalization are warranted if the history, symptoms, and clinical findings raise a suspicion for IE. Diagnostic evaluation, including blood cultures and echocardiography, must be performed. After blood culture specimens are obtained, the early initiation of an intravenous antibiotic regimen is vital in minimizing risks of valvular destruction and metastatic complications associated with pathogenic invasion.

Outpatient parenteral antibiotic therapy (OPAT) makes home therapy an option after adequate treatment in the hospital has been accomplished and the patient is stable for discharge home. OPAT requires scheduled home health care visits by the registered nurse and regular follow-up with the patient's primary experienced clinician.

LIFE SPAN CONSIDERATIONS

Aging is associated with an increased morbidity and mortality in this already potentially deadly infection. Compromised physical functions are in danger of decompensation in this fragile population. Nutritional fitness is usually compromised at baseline, and reserve is low. Prompt evaluation by the medical team should be initiated if endocarditis is in the differential diagnosis.

PATIENT EDUCATION AND HEALTH PROMOTION

Education of patients and family members is crucial. The etiology and treatment of IE as well as the diagnostic tests should be carefully explained. Patients should understand the importance of preventive therapy and current prophylaxis recommendations. Emphasis on oral health and improved access to dental care should be a primary focus, especially for those with highest risk of predisposition and adverse outcome from IE.[18] Patients should understand the risk of relapse, the early recognition of signs and symptoms, and the importance of obtaining follow-up diagnostics; health care provider evaluations should be emphasized. Every effort should be made to actively engage the patient with prescribed treatment because lack of patient adherence to regimens may adversely affect treatment outcomes.[16]

CHAPTER 124

MYOCARDITIS

John R. Butterly

DEFINITION AND EPIDEMIOLOGY

Myocarditis is the term used to include any pathologic process in which inflammation involving the myocardium is identified. The basic definition given by the World Health Organization (WHO) is "an inflammatory disease of the myocardium diagnosed by established histological, immunological and immunochemical criteria."[1] There are multiple potential causes and therefore varying degrees of clinical presentations and outcomes. In addition, the presently accepted gold standard diagnostic test, endomyocardial biopsy (EMB), is infrequently used, so the criteria of this very specific definition will likely not apply to the majority of patients ultimately diagnosed with this condition. To further confuse this issue, the Dallas criteria,[2] defined as histologic evidence of inflammatory infiltrates within the myocardium associated with myocyte degeneration and necrosis of nonischemic origin, have been criticized as too insensitive, nonspecific, and inadequate to predict response to therapy in view of newer modalities of immunologic and molecular testing.[3] Because of the aforementioned factors and the infrequent use of EMB, the actual incidence of myocarditis is not actually known, and there is a wide variation of reported incidences. For example, in autopsy studies of sudden cardiac death in adolescents and young adults, the prevalence of microscopic evidence of myocarditis has been variably reported to be 2% to 42%[4,5]; biopsy-proven myocarditis has been reported at 9% and 16% in adults diagnosed with nonischemic, dilated cardiomyopathy[6,7] and in 46% of children with an identified cause of dilated cardiomyopathy.[8]

It is important to note the distinction between cardiomyopathy and myocarditis. Cardiomyopathy refers to any situation in which myocardial systolic or diastolic function is impaired and is generally categorized in three separate types; dilated, hypertrophic, or restrictive. There are multiple causes of systolic myocardial dysfunction, the most common in developed nations being ischemic in origin as a result of the presence of coronary artery disease. The most common cause of dilated cardiomyopathy is idiopathic (unexplained), whereas myocarditis is only one cause of dilated cardiomyopathy and accounts for less than 10% of all cases.[9]

PATHOPHYSIOLOGY

Myocarditis is a heterogeneous condition and can be caused by a multitude of insults to the myocardium. The causative agent may be infectious, such as viral (including human immunodeficiency virus [HIV]), bacterial, protozoal (Chagas disease, a major cause of dilated cardiomyopathy in Latin America), spirochetal (Lyme disease), rickettsial, or fungal. A number of toxins can cause severe myocarditis; ethanol and certain chemotherapeutic agents belonging to the anthracycline family are among the most common. Myocarditis may also be the result of drug-induced allergies (including penicillin allergy) or autoimmune diseases such as systemic lupus erythematosus. Histologic diagnosis is made by examination of tissue obtained by EMB and depends on analysis of the type of inflammation present (lymphocytic, polymorphic, eosinophilic) as well as correlation with other systemic and physical findings. Frequently the cause remains undetermined, although new molecular techniques have shown that viruses seem to be the most important cause in North America and Europe. Viruses that have been identified include enteroviruses, adenoviruses, influenza, herpesvirus, Epstein-Barr virus, cytomegalovirus, hepatitis C, and HIV.[10]

The myocardium is damaged by direct viral cytopathic effects as well as by damage by autoantibodies that are triggered by the ongoing inflammatory process. Families with a genetic predisposition for developing viral-induced autoantibodies and subsequent dilated cardiomyopathy have been identified.[11]

CLINICAL MANIFESTATIONS

Initial presentation can be varied and ranges from mild symptoms of fever, atypical chest pain, fatigue, and palpitations with possible transient electrocardiographic changes to potentially fatal cardiogenic shock and/or arrhythmias and sudden death. Should myocarditis progress to significant systolic dysfunction, the symptoms would be the same as seen in any cause of left ventricular dysfunction (dyspnea on exertion, fatigue, orthopnea, paroxysmal nocturnal dyspnea). In cases involving the right ventricle, either through direct involvement or because of the underlying left-sided failure, the patient may report ankle swelling, bloating, or loss of appetite as a result of the development of bowel edema. Chest pain, usually of the pleuritic kind, may be a prominent finding if there is pericardial involvement.

Myocarditis is more frequent in younger age groups, although it can occur at any age. The presentation may well be subtle, so the diagnosis should be considered in any patient with symptoms suggestive of a cardiac cause, with the understanding that other cardiac diagnoses such as coronary artery disease, endocarditis, or a noncardiac inflammatory process should always be ruled out. It must also be recognized that patients with established cardiac diagnoses, such as coronary disease or valvular heart disease, may also develop acute myocarditis, which should especially be considered if the signs and symptoms do not correlate well with the known existing condition. When this is suspected, the gold standard for diagnosis remains EMB.

PHYSICAL EXAMINATION

Resting tachycardia with an exaggerated chronotropic response to any exertion would be an expected finding on physical examination. Mild cases of myocarditis may include normal physical examination findings or just a low-grade fever and tachycardia. In cases that progress to significant systolic dysfunction, the physical findings would be the same as seen in any cause of left ventricular dysfunction (pulmonary rales, third or fourth heart sounds, or occasionally a murmur of mitral regurgitation [MR] caused by the functional MR seen in moderate to severe left ventricular dilation). There may be a pericardial friction rub in cases involving the pericardium. In cases in which right ventricular dysfunction is a prominent finding, one would see an elevation of the jugular venous pressure, evidence for hepatic congestion in the form of hepatic enlargement and possible right upper quadrant tenderness, and pedal edema, with development of ascites and anasarca in extreme cases. The astute clinician will be aware of the fact that patients with chronic heart failure may be symptomatic but have few if any obvious physical findings.

DIAGNOSTICS

There are no accepted, specific criteria for making a diagnosis of myocarditis short of EMB. The diagnosis is most frequently made by a combination of clinical presentation coupled with the results of noninvasive testing, most frequently echocardiography. Documentation of decreased left (and sometimes right) ventricular function in a more global distribution, and lack of regional wall motion abnormalities (RWMAs) that would be more suggestive of an ischemic cause, in the right clinical setting (e.g., fever, recent flulike illness) is suggestive of a diagnosis of acute myocarditis. In facilities experienced in cardiac magnetic resonance imaging (MRI) a more sensitive finding, in addition to the lack of RWMAs, would be evidence of patchy, focal edema and the presence of subepicardial foci of late gadolinium enhancement (LGE), a finding that is typical of acute myocarditis. Because of the lack of specific criteria in making this diagnosis, it is presently recommended that patients with a suspected diagnosis be referred to a tertiary center with expertise in cardiac MRI or EMB if deemed necessary.[10]

As is true with all patients suspected of having a cardiac diagnosis, an electrocardiogram (ECG) should be obtained initially. This is most often abnormal in patients with acute myocarditis, although there are no findings that would be specific for this diagnosis. The ECG might demonstrate all degrees of atrioventricular (AV) block, right or left bundle branch block, nonspecific ST-T wave changes or T-wave abnormalities, atrial fibrillation, or, more ominously, ventricular tachycardia. Of some possible help, the ST elevations that can be seen in acute myocarditis are more frequently concave upward, as they are in pericarditis, and more likely to be diffuse—that is, not restricted to any one specific vascular distribution.

All patients with suspected myocarditis should have an initial echocardiogram to evaluate degree of left and right ventricular dysfunction, chamber size, and wall thickness and to rule out other potential diagnoses such as valvular or ischemic disease. Although global ventricular dysfunction is the most common finding, one might see RWMAs, although not in the expected distribution of any one vascular territory. In addition, the echocardiogram may demonstrate significant wall thickening and depression of systolic function consistent with the acute edema seen in marked inflammatory conditions. Sequential echocardiograms are very useful in following possible progression or response to therapy. At present, echocardiography is preferable to nuclear studies owing to a lack of sensitivity and specificity of the latter with present techniques. As mentioned earlier, cardiac MRI, where available, can be very helpful and may be the imaging modality of choice in a facility with that expertise. Stress testing is not recommended in cases of suspected myocarditis owing to the risk of precipitating an arrhythmia in this setting (unless there is a need to rule out an ischemic cause for symptoms).

Biomarkers are helpful and confirmatory in making the diagnosis of acute myocarditis. The markers of acute inflammation, such as erythrocyte sedimentation rate (ESR) and C-reactive protein (CRP) will frequently be elevated, but of course are nonspecific as to cause. Specific cardiac biomarkers are more explicit, with troponins being more sensitive than creatine phosphokinase (CPK). These tests will not necessarily, however, help differentiate myocarditis from other cardiac conditions, and the results may be normal at the time of testing. This is also true of brain natriuretic peptide (BNP).

Testing for specific viral antibodies can be unreliable because infection with these agents is frequent in most populations without causing acute myocarditis. Proof of progression from immunoglobulin M (IgM) to IgG antibodies might be helpful, as might testing for HIV when suspected or Lyme disease in areas where it is known to be endemic. Testing for cardiac autoantibodies may be useful, although these tests are not routinely available.

DIAGNOSTICS

Myocarditis

LABORATORY	IMAGING
Complete blood count and differential	ECG
ESR	Echocardiogram
CRP	Cardiac MRI (if available)
Troponins	
IgM to IgG progression	

DIFFERENTIAL DIAGNOSIS

The differential diagnosis in patients with symptoms and signs consistent with a diagnosis of myocarditis includes those conditions associated with similar symptoms of dyspnea, fatigue, fever, chest discomfort, palpitations, and presyncope or syncope. Because acute myocarditis is a potentially dangerous condition that can rapidly progress to a life-threatening situation or fatal outcome, rapid diagnostic testing, very close follow-up, and, in general, immediate hospitalization are warranted in all cases of suspected myocarditis.

Other important diagnoses to consider and exclude are those that are more common and potentially dangerous. These include atypical presentations of acute coronary syndromes or myocardial infarction, pulmonary embolism, or other, potentially reversible cause of dilated cardiomyopathy. Other considerations would include underlying valvular disease, cardiomyopathy, endocarditis, pneumonia, or other causes of systemic inflammation not necessarily involving the heart.

DIFFERENTIAL DIAGNOSIS

Myocarditis

- Atypical presentation acute coronary syndromes (myocardial infarction)
- Cardiomyopathies
- Pulmonary embolism
- Endocarditis
- Pneumonia
- Sepsis
- Deteriorating valvular heart disease

MANAGEMENT

Immediate specialist referral is indicated for all cases of suspected myocarditis.

Immediate emergency department referral is indicated for all cases in which immediate specialist referral is not available or there are clear symptoms or signs of congestive heart failure or persistent arrhythmia.

Hospitalization is indicated when acute myocarditis is strongly suspected or is diagnosed based on clinical findings with evidence for ventricular dysfunction. Patients who are asymptomatic or mildly symptomatic also require hospitalization for monitoring, because myocardial damage and the attendant risks of progressive heart failure and arrhythmias are unpredictable and can advance rapidly.

The fundamental principles of clinical management include bed rest and avoidance of stimulants such as alcohol, caffeine, and nicotine. Exercise is to be avoided, especially in athletes. Strenuous exercise should not be resumed for 6 months from the date of symptom onset.[12,13] Medical therapy should be instituted in co-management with a physician (preferably a cardiologist if available) or directly by a consulting cardiologist, and consists of the same regimen one would use in any cause of heart failure; angiotensin-converting enzyme (ACE) inhibitors or angiotensin receptor blockers (ARBs), loop diuretics (furosemide or torsemide), and beta blockers as tolerated. Caution is advised in the use of beta blockers in patients with severe left ventricular dysfunction, and they may be held until congestive heart failure comes under control. Arrhythmias are treated as in any other situation: temporary pacing for symptomatic bradyarrhythmias or high-grade AV block, rate control or consideration of cardioversion for atrial fibrillation, and antiarrhythmic therapy as indicated for ventricular arrhythmias. Anticoagulation with heparin or warfarin may be indicated in cases of persistent atrial fibrillation or severe left ventricular dysfunction.

Antiviral therapy may be helpful in specific cases depending on the viral agent. Involvement of an infectious disease specialist is recommended if antiviral therapy is being considered. High-dose intravenous immune globulin (IVIG) may be helpful in cases refractory to conventional therapy in either virally mediated or autoantibody-mediated cases, as might immunoadsorption, although neither has proven efficacy.[14] Immunosuppressive therapy has not been shown to be effective except possibly in autoimmune forms. In patients with hypereosinophilia, consideration should be given to the possibility of drug-induced hypersensitivity. The offending agent must be discontinued and should not be reintroduced.

PROGNOSIS AND LIFE SPAN CONSIDERATIONS

The eventual outcome and prognosis of myocarditis depend on the cause, clinical status at presentation, and severity of disease. In about 50% of cases, acute myocarditis resolves in 2 to 4 weeks. Twenty-five percent of patients will progress to chronic cardiac dysfunction, and 12% to 25% can acutely deteriorate and die or progress to end-stage congestive heart failure requiring consideration of transplantation. Biventricular dysfunction at the initial presentation is a main predictor of death or eventual need for transplantation.[1,14,15]

Close follow-up at appropriate intervals—depending on degree of left ventricular function, physical functionality of the patient, and response to therapy for residual heart failure (or lack thereof)—is important both to track recovery as well as to monitor for possible relapse.

PATIENT AND FAMILY EDUCATION

Any visit to a caregiver is likely to be associated with some degree of trepidation or anxiety. This can be especially true in any person who is not feeling well, and any existing anxiety can be magnified when the diagnosis in question involves cardiac issues. Because myocarditis is a potentially life-threatening or disabling disease, it is important to clearly and compassionately explain the process, its effects on cardiac function, and the possible complications that might ensue. This should be explained in the context of the overall good prognosis in many patients and the fact that there are advanced therapies for myocarditis, its potential complications, and heart failure. Most important, it should be made clear that the provider, as caregiver, will be there to see the patient and family through this potentially complex, intimidating, and frightening experience.

CHAPTER 125

PERIPHERAL ARTERIAL AND VENOUS INSUFFICIENCY

Ann Guttendorf

PERIPHERAL ARTERIAL INSUFFICIENCY

Peripheral arterial insufficiency is the condition that results when there is insufficient blood flow to the extremities. It is much more likely to occur in the lower extremities, although the use of catheter interventions has made the incidence of upper extremity problems more common. In the United States it is estimated that 8 to 10 million people have arterial occlusive disease, and the incidence is more prevalent in those 50 years of age and older.[1] The incidence in this population is estimated to be 1 in every 20 individuals.[1] When defining peripheral artery disease disease (PAD), if the symptoms have been present for weeks or months, the condition is defined as chronic. If the symptoms develop during hours or days, it is referred to as acute.

Immediate physician or vascular surgeon referral is indicated for suspected arterial occlusion or dissecting aneurysm.

CHRONIC ARTERIAL INSUFFICIENCY

DEFINITION AND EPIDEMIOLOGY

Chronic arterial insufficiency is a disease that has increasing prevalence as the population ages. Because the major cause of PAD is atherosclerosis, the risk factors are the same as those for coronary artery disease. Diabetes, hypertension, hyperlipidemia, hyperhomocysteinemia, and tobacco use are all independent risk factors. Smokers are twice as likely to develop claudication.[2] Vascular disease is one of the most common complications of diabetes. Genetic factors have also long been recognized as playing a role in the development of PAD, and an increased level of homocysteine has been shown to be associated with atherosclerosis.[2] Even in younger patients, premature atherosclerosis is the most common cause of chronic arterial insufficiency, although rare causes also include entrapment syndromes and adventitial cystic disease of the popliteal artery.

Numerous studies have confirmed that most patients with clinically obstructive arterial disease have underlying coronary artery disease or diabetes. These patients have a 40% increased risk of stroke and a 20% to 60% risk of myocardial infarction (MI), with a twofold to sixfold increase in the risk for cardiac death.[2]

In cases of severe obstructive disease and acute limb ischemia, the risk for amputation is determined by disease severity, sudden appearance of limb ischemia, and the timeliness and ability to restore limb circulation, not by the mere appearance of claudication.[2] The occurrence of acute limb ischemia carries with it a 30-day amputation rate of 10% to 30% regardless of whether thrombolysis has been used.[3]

PATHOPHYSIOLOGY

Chronic arterial insufficiency results from diverse systemic conditions that can affect the arteries in various parts of the circulatory system, even in the absence of clinical symptoms in more than one arterial system.[2] The disease entities that result in arterial insufficiency include degenerative diseases (collagen abnormalities found in Marfan or Ehlers-Danlos syndrome), dysplastic disorders (e.g., fibromuscular dysplasia), and vascular inflammatory processes (e.g., arteritis). Arterial insufficiency can also be a result of thrombosis, thrombotic embolism, radiation-induced arteritis, autoimmune conditions, and, the most common cause, arteriosclerosis.[2]

In patients without atherosclerosis, the pathophysiology of chronic arterial insufficiency involves loss of structural integrity of the artery wall. This loss of structural integrity produces arterial dilation and favors aneurysm formation with its associated risk of rupture or occlusion as a result of aneurysmal dissection.[2] This loss of structural integrity can affect arteries in the carotid, renal, and iliac circulation most commonly, but is not restricted to those circulatory beds.[2]

In patients with underlying arteriosclerosis, the atherosclerotic plaque causing leg ischemia is identical to that seen in coronary artery disease and carotid disease. The plaque is an intimal lesion that may affect any of these vessels. The blockage may build up slowly, allowing collateral vessels to develop and thereby minimizing symptom progression until such time as the flow is inadequate to support the metabolic needs. Alternatively, intraplaque hemorrhage and thrombosis may lead to sudden expansion and acute symptoms.[2]

The infrarenal aorta and iliac arteries are classified as the inflow arteries, whereas the femoral, popliteal, and tibial vessels are classified as the outflow vessels. Obstruction of the aortoiliac and femoral arteries is often seen in smokers, whereas disease in the smaller vessels such as that seen in tibial artery disease is much more common in patients with diabetes. There is evidence that the presence of reduced ankle-brachial index (ABI) and diabetes are associated with the development of rest pain and ulcerations from inadequate perfusion.

CLINICAL PRESENTATION

Certain groups of patients are at risk for PAD. This includes patients who are older than 65 years (21% had asymptomatic or symptomatic PAD in one study),[2a] patients who are older than 50 with a history of diabetes or smoking, and patients younger than 50 who have diabetes and another risk factor for atherosclerosis (e.g., smoking, dyslipidemia, hypertension, hyperhomocysteinemia). It also includes patients with exertional leg symptoms suggestive of claudication or with ischemic rest pain, patients with abnormalities of lower extremity pulses, and patients with known atherosclerotic coronary, carotid, or renal artery disease. All of these patients should undergo a comprehensive vascular review of symptoms (Box 125-1).[2]

It is imperative to recognize that each patient with PAD is unique; the reported discomfort associated with PAD includes "tiredness," "giving way," "soreness," or "pain."[4] Although the classic or "textbook" symptom of peripheral arterial insufficiency is claudication, patients report two or more symptoms in two or more locations.[4] Primary care providers must take a careful history of each symptom, including the impact of each symptom on work, activities of daily living, and recreational activities; the symptoms should be interpreted in the context of patient comorbidities and the presence of previously discussed PAD risk factors.[3] When present, claudication is a tightening or cramping pain that is precipitated by exercise and is relieved by rest. These symptoms most frequently occur in the calf muscles but also can occur in the thighs or buttocks depending on the location of the stenosis. Claudication occurs with exercise because of an increased demand for blood that cannot be met by the stenotic vessels. Subsequently, lactic acid and other metabolites build up in the muscle, causing discomfort. Claudication

BOX 125-1

Components of a Vascular Review of Symptoms (Includes Family History)

Assess for presence of:

- Exertional leg symptoms (fatigue, aching, numbness, or pain; record location of symptoms such as buttock, thigh, calf, or foot)
- Poor wound healing in legs or feet
- Pain at rest in lower leg or feet; note whether occurs when patient is recumbent or upright
- Abdominal pain that occurs after eating and is associated with weight loss
- First-degree relative with abdominal aortic aneurysm

From Wennberg PW: Peripheral arterial disease, *Circulation* 128:2241-2250, 2013.

is assessed by how far a patient can walk before pain ensues. Although the distance may be reduced by an incline, cold weather, or a recent meal, it tends to be fairly consistent. Pain is always relieved immediately by stopping the activity and never occurs when the patient is at rest. The thigh or buttock muscles are sometimes affected first. This is indicative of iliac artery obstruction (Leriche syndrome).

As the obstruction becomes more severe, the patient may develop pain at rest because circulation to the feet is impaired. Characteristically, the patient will go to bed and be awakened after a couple of hours by pain in the toes that is relieved only by gravity to enhance peripheral blood flow (e.g., getting out of bed or hanging the feet over the side of the bed). The patient may resort to sleeping in a chair to avoid the pain. Ischemic rest pain tends to be consistent; it occurs every night, unlike the intermittent leg cramps seen so often in older adults, which are not related to arterial insufficiency.

PHYSICAL EXAMINATION

For effective, collaborative care of the patient with suspected vascular insufficiency, there must be a standard set of measurements. The American College of Cardiology (ACC) and American Heart Association (AHA) guidelines recommend components of the vascular physical examination supplemented by vascular testing (see the section on diagnostics, later). Components of the vascular physical examination include measurement of blood pressure; palpation for pulse, quality, and amplitude; abdominal aortic pulsation assessment; auscultation for bruits; estimation of pulse intensity; and full foot examination and lower extremity skin assessment (Box 125-2).[2]

On physical examination, inspection of the limbs may reveal muscle wasting and loss of hair. With more severe disease, there is not enough blood to sustain viability, and tissue loss ensues, usually beginning in the toes or heels. Tissue loss may manifest as ulceration, dry gangrene, or wet gangrene. Reduced temperature in an affected limb may be noted. Careful pulse examination is important. Absent femoral pulses suggest inflow disease, whereas the absence of popliteal pulses implies isolated tibial disease.

One physical sign that can be helpful in the diagnosis of peripheral vascular disease is dependent rubor. If the ischemic leg is elevated for 30 seconds, it becomes pale because blood is unable to travel uphill. This renders the tissue ischemic, and the capillaries vasodilate. If the leg is then made dependent, blood travels down to those dilated capillaries, and a deep red color ensues. The longer the rubor takes to develop, the worse the ischemia. A careful history and physical examination will allow a good assessment of the functional severity of the obstruction and the likely location.

The severity of the patient's peripheral arterial insufficiency can be graded based on the vascular history and physical examination findings. Fontaine's stages or Rutherford's categories are the most widely used tools to provide a standardized system of classifying the severity of peripheral disease, based on symptoms, gangrene, or ulcerations.[3] The distances that define mild, moderate, and severe claudication is part of the Fontaine classification and is based on a distance of 200 meters (650 feet). It is not specified in the Rutherford classification of symptoms. In addition, there is a separate Rutherford scale for acute limb ischemia.[5,6] Any patient with intermittent claudication, leg pain at rest, or nonhealing wounds in the lower extremity that persist for 4 weeks or more warrants an evaluation for PAD.

BOX 125-2

Components of the Vascular Physical Examination

- Measure blood pressure in both arms; record findings and note any discrepancy.
- Auscultate carotid arteries bilaterally for bruits; record findings.
- Palpate carotid pulses bilaterally; record upstroke and pulse amplitude.
- Auscultate abdomen and flank for bruits; record findings.
- Palpate abdomen; measure and record width of aortic pulsation.
- Palpate, estimate, and record the intensity of the following pulses bilaterally: brachial, radial, ulnar, femoral, popliteal, dorsalis pedis, and posterior tibial.
- Use the following scale for pulse intensity documentation: 0 = absent, 1 = diminished, 2 = normal, 3 = bounding.
- If upper extremity insufficiency suspected, perform Allen test and record results.
- Auscultate femoral arteries for bruits; record findings.
- Assess lower extremities for indications of more severe peripheral artery disease such as distal hair loss, trophic skin changes, or hypertrophic nails; record findings.
- Remove shoes and socks; assess feet for color, temperature, skin integrity, ulcerations;
- examine intertriginous areas for lesions or ulcerations; record findings.
- Measure and record ankle-brachial index (ABI).

From Hirsch AT, Haskal ZJ, Hertzer NR, et al: ACC/AHA 2005 practice guidelines for the management of patients with peripheral artery disease (lower extremity, renal, mesenteric, abdominal aortic). *Circulation* 113:e463-e654, 2006.

DIAGNOSTICS

There is a role for noninvasive testing to supplement the history and physical examination depending on the clinical scenario and the urgency of the patient's condition. The level of testing should be limited initially to those studies that confirm the presence of arterial disease and those that will alter the course of treatment. The main reason for physiologic testing is to verify a vascular origin for the patient's complaints and to localize the level of the lesion. In addition, it can be used to assess the adequacy of tissue perfusion and wound healing potential.

Lower extremity PAD is diagnosed by the resting ABI in patients with one or more of the following: exertional leg symptoms, nonhealing lower extremity wounds, history consistent with PAD in patients 65 years and older, or symptoms in patients 50 years and older with a smoking history or diabetes.[3] The most useful tools in assessing peripheral arterial insufficiency in the office are a portable Doppler instrument and a sphygmomanometer cuff. With these tools, it is possible to compare the systolic pressure at the brachial artery with that in the dorsalis pedis and posterior tibial arteries. This measurement is expressed as the ABI and should be lower in the affected extremity than in the normal one. An ABI of 0.9 or less is indicative of PAD. An ABI of 0.75 to 0.5 is consistent with claudication, and an ABI below 0.5 is consistent with rest pain and/or tissue loss. An ABI of higher than 1.4 is also considered abnormal and can indicate the potential for noncompressible calcified vessels. Along with low ABI, high ABI is also associated with higher cardiovascular risk.[3,7-9]

Patients with mild claudication may have palpable pulses at rest but lose them with exercise. This is best demonstrated in the vascular laboratory with an exercise noninvasive study.

During this test, the patient is placed on a treadmill and ABIs are measured at rest, while exercising, and on recovery.

Related medical conditions, such as obesity and peripheral edema, sometimes make it impossible to assess the pulse status. In these situations, the pocket Doppler instrument may be invaluable. A normal pulse is triphasic but becomes increasingly monophasic with proximal obstruction. With practice, it is relatively simple to distinguish these pulses. If Doppler ultrasonography reveals good triphasic pulses in the feet, there is not likely to be significant ischemia in that extremity.

A variety of tests are now available to accurately assess vascular status. Patients should be referred to the vascular laboratory for formal evaluation if there is concern for arterial insufficiency or to ascertain the location and severity of occlusive lesions. Once arterial disease is confirmed, the level of the disease and the extent of the severity can be further assessed with segmental limb pressures. This testing is also done with specialized equipment in the vascular lab and can be performed on both the upper and lower extremities. Vascular laboratory evaluation will provide the ABIs, the level at which the pulse becomes monophasic, the pulse volume recording (a plethysmographic test that records the volume of the pulse in the extremity with each heartbeat) and other important measurements (see Diagnostics box). The forefoot tracing is helpful for the vascular surgeon to determine whether there is enough circulation to heal a foot lesion. This is particularly important in patients with diabetes, in whom ABIs are often inaccurate.[10]

Other tests are available but are used less often except in research protocols. Chief among these is the measurement of transcutaneous oxygen ($TcPO_2$), which reflects the metabolic state of the target tissues. Unfortunately, variants such as ambient temperature make this test impractical as a routine part of the evaluation. The level at which $TcPO_2$ indicates tissue healing remains controversial and will vary in the setting of diabetes and tissue edema It also can be affected by skin temperature and emotional state.[11] An analysis from pooled data from the women in the Nurses' Health Study (1990 to 2010) and from men enrolled in the Health Professionals Follow-Up Study (1994 to 2008) found that elevated levels of β-macroglobulin are associated with increased risk for symptomatic PAD and are indicative of the presence of atherosclerosis promoting kidney disease.[12]

DIAGNOSTICS

Chronic Arterial Insufficiency

INITIAL
- Doppler ankle, arm indexes
- Laboratory
- Serum glucose, lipid profile, high-sensitivity C-reactive protein, and homocysteine

IMAGING
- Digital subtraction angiography
- Color-assisted duplex ultrasonography
- Magnetic resonance angiography
- Computed tomography angiography

OTHER DIAGNOSTICS
- Segmental limb pressure measurement
- Pulse volume recording
- Toe-brachial index assessment
- Velocity waveform analysis
- Treadmill testing
- Plethysmography

Instead of a treadmill test, it is possible to use reactive hyperemia as a marker of disease severity. This is obtained after inflation of a pressure cuff to a suprasystolic pressure to produce vasodilation; however, this is somewhat uncomfortable and is not currently used routinely.

DIFFERENTIAL DIAGNOSIS

Diabetic Peripheral Neuropathy

The presence of peripheral neuropathy in diabetes makes the diagnosis of peripheral insufficiency difficult. Damage to the peripheral nerves may mask the symptoms of arterial insufficiency. Thus, if patients have no feeling in their legs, they may simply complain that their legs get tired of walking. Without sensation, there may be no rest pain, and patients may be initially seen with nonhealing ulcers and possibly painless gangrene. Other conditions that should be considered include cauda equina syndrome, Buerger disease, leg cramps, and musculoskeletal disorders.

Cauda Equina Syndrome

Spinal stenosis causing pressure on the nerve roots may result in symptoms of claudication from the hip downward, which can easily be confused with Leriche syndrome. This is becoming increasingly common as the population ages and progressive degenerative joint disease becomes more prevalent. Patients with spinal stenosis will often not have relief until they sit down, and usually they have to wait longer for relief than patients who have claudication. The correct diagnosis can be made by ordering noninvasive exercise studies. In cauda equina syndrome, there will be no pressure drop when the patient exercises on a treadmill. Magnetic resonance imaging of the lumbar spine will reveal the arthritic changes.

Buerger Disease

Buerger disease is an inflammatory occlusive disease involving primarily the medium and smaller arteries of both the upper and lower extremities. Although it is less common in the United States, it is seen more often in the Middle East and Asia and appears to be directly related to the effects of smoking. Patients manifest the signs and symptoms of chronic arterial insufficiency but apart from smoking have no other risk factors for atherosclerosis. Bypass surgery is rarely indicated because disease is more distal, but patients will experience remission if exposure to nicotine is avoided.

Upper Extremity Arterial Disease

It is important not to forget about the upper extremities in evaluating patients with known or suspected arterial disease. Patients with compromised flow to the upper extremities can have typical ischemic pain of one or more muscle groups but also may have atypical pain or no symptoms at all. The presentation may be only a difference in the systolic blood pressure between one arm and the other.

In other cases, patients may report dizziness during arm exertion that can be indicative of disease in the subclavian artery. Subclavian steal syndrome implies the presence of significant symptoms caused by arterial insufficiency in the brain (vertebrobasilar insufficiency) or the upper extremity, which is also supplied by the affected subclavian artery.[13]

A review of symptoms and upper extremity vascular examination need to be performed in all patients at risk for or with documented PAD. Further testing would be determined based on examination findings and on patient symptoms. This may include duplex ultrasound, transcranial Doppler studies, magnetic resonance angiography, or computed tomography (CT) angiography.[14-16]

DIFFERENTIAL DIAGNOSIS

Chronic Arterial Insufficiency

- Acute peripheral arterial occlusion
- Peripheral neuropathy
- Cauda equina syndrome
- Buerger disease
- Musculoskeletal condition
- Leg cramps

MANAGEMENT

Management of chronic arterial insufficiency depends on the severity of the symptoms. If the patient has stable claudication and is managing without much difficulty, it is reasonable to treat the patient conservatively. Patients with mild, recent-onset claudication are likely to improve with conservative measures alone. These include lifestyle modifications as indicated, particularly tobacco cessation. Hypertension, hyperlipidemia, and diabetes must be treated aggressively to reduce long-term risk. Compression stockings may be used in selected PAD patients to treat leg swelling and reduce deep venous thrombosis (DVT) risk, providing the ABI is 0.8 or higher and the use of the compression stockings does not compromise circulation to the extremity or increase claudication symptoms.[17]

Studies comparing exercise with angioplasty have shown that a daily exercise program involving walking to the point of pain as often as possible is as effective as angioplasty in providing relief of symptoms.[18] Components of a structured exercise program to relieve claudication include (1) an initial session of treadmill or track walking of 30 minutes, with an increase of subsequent sessions to reach 1 hour per session, three times a week; (2) in each session, walking at a speed and grade that produce moderate claudication pain within 3 to 5 minutes; (3) resting until claudication resolves; and (4) repeating the exercise and rest cycles until the session duration is achieved.[3] Because the ABI does not change, it is believed that this beneficial effect is produced by training the muscles rather than by increasing flow to the foot.

These patients are at high risk for coronary artery disease, so it is prudent to start them on a daily aspirin dose as well. The literature on the role of aspirin, dipyridamole, and ticlopidine in peripheral vascular disease is extensive and confusing.[3,19] There is much disagreement as to whether aspirin confers benefit either preoperatively or postoperatively in patients with peripheral vascular disease. There is agreement, however, that low-dose aspirin (325 mg/day) reduces the incidence and mortality of subsequent MI in patients older than 50 years.

There has never been a study demonstrating a benefit of adding dipyridamole to that regimen. Ticlopidine, another antiplatelet agent, is at least as effective as aspirin, but it is expensive and has significant side effects. Clopidogrel can be used as an alternative to aspirin or in combination with aspirin (reserved for high-risk patients not at risk for bleeding).[3] Any antiplatelet regimen needs to be based on an individual patient's clinical characteristics (risk of PAD, risk of bleeding) and tolerance for the medications in conjunction with cost and future guidance from regulatory bodies.[3]

It has been shown that statin therapy helps stabilize plaque and lowers the low-density lipoprotein (LDL) level, and studies have suggested that bypasses are more durable if the patient is taking a statin.[20,21]

Pentoxifylline (Trental) has been shown to increase the distance that 30% of patients with claudication can walk, although the effect has been small. Trials of cilostazol (Pletal), a phosphodiesterase type 3 inhibitor, have demonstrated significant improvement over both placebo and pentoxifylline in distance walked without symptoms for patients with claudication.[21] The main contraindication for using cilostazol is a history of congestive heart failure.

COMPLICATIONS OF PERIPHERAL ARTERIAL DISEASE

Lower extremity ulcers may result from neuropathy, arterial insufficiency, infection, or a combination of these. Infection such as cellulitis, or ulcers with extensive involvement may result in osteomyelitis. The presence of infection can also disturb blood glucose control, complicating diabetes management.

Peripheral neuropathy is associated with the development of calcification of the arteries. This is not directly related to the atherosclerotic lesion, which is an intimal lesion, but it does render the vessels relatively incompressible. This means that the ABI may be artificially elevated and less helpful in assessing the degree of ischemia. In these cases, the pulse volume recording can be particularly helpful.

Thirty percent of patients with neuropathy also have an autonomic neuropathy, which is sometimes called an autosympathectomy. This condition results in diversion of blood from the nutrient vessels to the skin, making the skin unnaturally warm. Thus it is possible to see a diabetic patient with a minor skin lesion but with no symptoms and a warm foot that is critically ischemic. Failure to recognize this may result in further loss of tissue.

Diabetic Foot Ulcer

Diabetic neuropathy is a polyneuropathy and has a motor component. The paralysis of the intrinsic muscles results in clawing of the foot, and the patient tends to develop traumatic lesions over the metatarsal heads and on the tops of the toes. Healing may be impaired by relative arterial insufficiency.

Infection

Any infection requires treatment with appropriate debridement and antibiotics. Bed rest is indicated to minimize damage that may go undetected if neuropathy is present. If the ulcer is superficial, it can be treated on an outpatient basis, with non–weight bearing, dressing care, and a first-generation cephalosporin. If the ulcer is deep or has significant cellulitis, hospitalization is advised, and broad-spectrum antibiotics are instituted. Failure to heal with treatment suggests arterial insufficiency and merits referral to a vascular surgeon or vascular medicine specialist for possible arteriography.

INDICATIONS FOR REFERRAL OR HOSPITALIZATION

If patients have severe claudication, rest pain, or gangrene, they should be referred promptly for further evaluation. Once the extent of the severe ischemia has been identified, arteriography is indicated to demonstrate the extent and location of the obstruction. Treatment may involve angioplasty (with or without stent placement) or surgery. Magnetic resonance arteriography was a popular alternative to arteriography, but the risk of gadolinium-induced complications has limited its use in patients with renal failure. CT angiography has become more popular, particularly in patients with aortoiliac disease, because it is less invasive. In general, neither arteriography nor CT should be ordered without consultation with a vascular medicine specialist or a vascular surgeon.

The vascular specialist can perform arteriography and decide at that time whether to proceed with an angioplasty or stent or to refer the patient for surgery. Patients are often treated with a hybrid procedure in which an inflow stent is placed at the same time as an outflow surgical procedure is performed.[22]

Diabetic patients with neuropathy or arterial insufficiency require regular podiatry consultation. The podiatrist will determine the frequency of visits based on callus development. With appropriate shoes and care of calluses and nails, many patients with ischemia can avoid problems for long periods. Regular podiatric visits enable early recognition of potential problems and ensure expeditious referral and treatment.

Patients with superficial ulcers who do not improve with bed rest and treatment require referral to a vascular specialist. More extensive ulcers require immediate vascular consultation.

LIFE SPAN CONSIDERATIONS

The AHA published a scientific statement highlighting the underdiagnosis of women with PAD. Women, particularly postmenopausal women, exhibit complications associated with PAD at a higher rate than men, yet risk assessment, risk modification, and early detection and intervention do not occur at the same rate as in male patients.[23] Complicating the picture is the nonspecific symptoms that women with PAD exhibit—extremity fatigue and rest discomfort.[23] Primary care providers are well advised to consider the holistic nature of atherosclerotic disease, whether found in the coronary, peripheral, renal, or cerebral arteries, and incorporate PAD risk screening and risk reduction for patients with CAD risk factors such as hypertension, diabetes, and hyperlipidemia.[23]

EDUCATION AND HEALTH PROMOTION

All patients should be advised to follow a low-carbohydrate, low-fat diet; to exercise regularly; and to avoid all tobacco products. Patients should understand the importance of lifestyle modification to reduce the risk of cardiovascular disease and diabetes.

Patients with diabetes, particularly if neuropathy is present, should be instructed to visually inspect their feet daily and to seek professional help for any foot lesion. Many patients with diabetes are terrified of amputation and should be reassured that with good podiatric care and immediate attention to any problem, amputation can possibly be avoided. All patients with arterial insufficiency should have their toenails cut by a podiatrist. In addition, patients should be given instructions about general foot protection measures, including the importance of properly fitting shoes, avoiding synthetic materials in shoes that causes them not to "breathe," and always wearing shoes or slippers to protect their feet. Direct contact with very hot or very cold substances or surfaces must be avoided. It is imperative to seek immediate medical evaluation for prolonged pain, sudden color changes, or a numb feeling in the extremities.

ACUTE ARTERIAL INSUFFICIENCY

DEFINITION AND EPIDEMIOLOGY

Acute arterial insufficiency is the sudden onset of the symptoms of ischemia. The incidence of acute arterial occlusion seems to be increasing,[24] partly as a result of better diagnosis and recognition, but also because patients with advanced heart disease are living longer and undergoing more invasive procedures. It is critical to make the diagnosis expeditiously to avoid loss of limb or life.

PATHOPHYSIOLOGY

Acute ischemia may result from an embolus (from another source) that occludes or obstructs flow to a distal vessel. The most common source of an embolus is the heart. This may be a clot that forms on the ventricular wall after an MI or a clot from the atrium in patients with atrial fibrillation. Rarely, a tumor in the heart, such as atrial myxoma, may break off and travel to the peripheral vessels.

Acute thrombosis of preexisting atherosclerotic lesions is the other major cause of acute ischemia. This type may be less severe than acute ischemia secondary to embolization because collateral circulation has had time to develop. Aneurysms of the abdominal aorta or popliteal artery may cause acute ischemia secondary to acute thrombosis of the aneurysm. Once the embolus becomes lodged, the arteries and veins distal to the occlusion go into spasm. After a few hours, vasodilation occurs, and the thrombus begins to organize. At this point, the ischemia becomes irreversible. It is generally accepted that if acute occlusion of the limb occurs and there is no collateral circulation, necrosis will begin after 6 hours unless the ischemia is relieved.

CLINICAL PRESENTATION

Classically, the patient reports a sudden onset of pain in an extremity. A history of recent MI or atrial fibrillation and the presence of normal circulation in the other limb suggest an embolus as the source of acute limb ischemia. A previous history of peripheral vascular disease would suggest acute thrombosis as the cause.

PHYSICAL EXAMINATION

On examination, the limb is usually pale and pulseless with absent or diminished capillary refill. If there is loss of sensation or immobility of the foot, tissue loss is imminent. These signs and symptoms are often referred to as the five *P*s: pain, pallor, pulselessness, paresthesias, and paralysis.

If left untreated, the limb becomes edematous, mottled, and eventually gangrenous. The sudden onset of pain with signs of acute ischemia and mottling from the waist down suggests acute aortic occlusion and demands immediate diagnosis and treatment if the patient is to survive.

DIAGNOSTICS

Diagnosis of acute limb ischemia is generally based on the clinical presentation and physical examination. Doppler studies may be necessary to confirm the presence or absence

DIAGNOSTICS

Acute Arterial Insufficiency

INITIAL	IMAGING
Doppler studies	Arteriography*

*If indicated.

of arterial pulses. Arteriography may be indicated in some circumstances.

DIFFERENTIAL DIAGNOSIS

The patient history usually suggests whether the ischemia is related to an embolus or thrombus. The most common error is misdiagnosis of acute ischemia as an acute neurologic event. The consequent delay in treatment can result in limb loss or, in the case of acute aortic occlusion, death. Careful pulse examination at the time of presentation will avoid this problem. Other causes of acute arterial insufficiency or arterial occlusion include blue toe syndrome and aneurysms.

Blue Toe Syndrome

Bluish discoloration or localized gangrene of the feet without evidence of ischemia, infection, or peripheral neuropathy is known as blue toe syndrome. Blue toe syndrome results from microemboli from the heart, aorta, or peripheral arteries that are small enough to lodge in the capillaries. These emboli may be small thrombi from the heart or from an aortic or popliteal aneurysm. They may also be cholesterol emboli or atheroemboli from atherosclerotic plaques in the aorta, iliac arteries, or femoral arteries.

When blue toe syndrome is suspected, careful physical examination for the presence of an abdominal or popliteal aneurysm is mandatory. If there is no evidence of ischemia, infection, or peripheral neuropathy, cardiac echocardiography and an abdominal ultrasound study should be obtained. If these tests are negative for a clot or abdominal aneurysm, antiplatelet therapy is initiated and the patient closely monitored. Consultation with a vascular specialist is necessary. The lesion will usually improve during the next few weeks, but if it does not or if emboli recur, transesophageal echocardiography and aortography of the thoracic aorta to the femoral arteries are indicated. If a localized lesion is discovered, it can be addressed, although diffuse atherosclerosis of the suprarenal aorta is often the source. In these cases, recurrent embolization often leads to renal failure and distal gangrene. Ligation of the iliac arteries with axillobifemoral bypass and preparation for dialysis are the some of the available therapies.

Aneurysm

An aneurysm is a localized enlargement of an artery that causes symptoms by expansion, rupture, or thrombosis. A true aneurysm is said to be present when the wall of the aneurysm is an arterial wall. If the wall is compressed connective tissue, however, the rupture is a contained rupture, or false aneurysm.

Infrarenal aortic aneurysms are a common cause of death secondary to rupture. They are often asymptomatic, although they may cause an acute onset of back or abdominal pain. If a pulsatile abdominal mass is discovered on physical examination, further evaluation with either an abdominal ultrasound study or a CT scan is indicated. If the presence of an aneurysm is confirmed, referral to a vascular surgeon is indicated.

Femoral or popliteal aneurysms are less common but may be detected on physical examination and usually cause symptoms by expansion and thrombosis. They are often associated with aortic aneurysms, and an abdominal ultrasound study should also be obtained if either of these is detected.

Patients with aneurysms should be advised that this condition is often congenital and that any blood relatives older than 50 years should consult their primary care provider about when they should have an abdominal ultrasound examination to screen for an aortic aneurysm.

DIFFERENTIAL DIAGNOSIS

Acute Arterial Insufficiency

- Ruptured aneurysm
- Thrombotic event
- Embolic event
- Neurologic event

MANAGEMENT

As soon as the diagnosis of acute arterial occlusion is made, a bolus of intravenous heparin (5000 units) should be given to prevent a clot from forming distal to the occlusion. Hospitalization and prompt referral to a vascular specialist for evaluation with treatment are essential.

Treatment of the occlusion includes surgical or percutaneous embolectomy, percutaneous arterial thrombolytic delivery, or intravenous thrombolytic therapy. No matter the options available, treatment should be instituted within 6 hours of the occlusion to prevent permanent injury.

COMPLICATIONS

Complications are dependent more on the effect of the acute occlusion than on the cause. Thus, patients with an embolus at the time of a massive MI will do poorly in comparison with those whose clot is from atrial fibrillation. Studies show a mortality rate with arterial occlusion of 22% to 39% and an amputation rate of 11% to 17%.[25]

INDICATIONS FOR REFERRAL OR HOSPITALIZATION

Once arterial occlusion is identified, immediate evaluation by a vascular specialist is imperative. Acute arterial occlusion is an emergency in which treatment delay can impair limb viability or threaten life.

EDUCATION AND HEALTH PROMOTION

It is important to review the signs and symptoms of acute arterial occlusion with the patient and family members at regular intervals. For other educational points for review, see the Education and Health Promotion section under Chronic Arterial Insufficiency.

PERIPHERAL VENOUS INSUFFICIENCY

Peripheral venous insufficiency occurs whenever there is obstruction to venous return in the superficial or deep veins of the upper or lower extremities. Important clinical syndromes related to venous insufficiency include DVT, venous stasis, varicose veins, stasis dermatitis, and leg ulceration.

Physician consultation is indicated for all patients with DVT as documented by Doppler ultrasound study.

DEEP VENOUS THROMBOSIS OF THE LOWER EXTREMITY

DEFINITION AND EPIDEMIOLOGY

DVT is the development of a blood clot in the deep veins of the lower or occasionally the upper extremity. A DVT may also involve the iliac veins and the vena cava. DVT is characterized by a relatively loose thrombotic attachment to the vein wall until the healing process starts. This loose attachment puts the patient at risk for mobilization of the clot until it stabilizes.

Although the term *phlebitis* is often used to describe DVT, it should in fact be reserved for superficial phlebitis. Superficial phlebitis is an inflammation of the affected superficial veins as a result of local trauma, venous stasis, or infection; chemical injury may result from an intravenous injection. Because the clot is part of an inflammatory process that involves the vessel wall, there is no risk of pulmonary embolism unless the process extends to involve the deep system.

PATHOPHYSIOLOGY

The deep veins of the lower extremity are the main conduit by which the legs are emptied of blood. Blood travels back to the heart as a result of compression of the deep veins by leg muscles. Valves in the vein prevent reflux back down the vein because of gravity. Blood runs from the superficial system to the deep veins through perforator veins, which are also protected from reflux by the presence of valves. Any condition that produces stasis or hypercoagulability is likely to result in the formation of clots in the deep veins.[25] A major risk factor is surgery, particularly gynecologic operations and orthopedic procedures on the hip and knee. Bed rest produces stasis and may result in DVT. Long airplane or car rides are also risk factors.[26]

Patients who have a tendency for hypercoagulation, particularly patients with malignant disease, may also be seen with DVT. A lesser but definite risk factor for DVT is use of estrogen preparations (e.g., contraceptives or hormone replacement therapy), and this should be considered in patients with other risk factors.[26]

A clot may form in any part of the deep venous system and may either propagate or remain localized. It may cause symptoms in two ways. First, there is a local effect in obstruction of blood flow, which rarely is so significant that it results in venous gangrene. Second, the clot may become detached and migrate to the lungs, forming an embolus. This is a common cause of death in at-risk patients.

CLINICAL PRESENTATION AND PHYSICAL EXAMINATION

A history of previous DVT, prolonged inactivity, estrogen use, or recent surgery or trauma should be obtained from the patient. The classic signs of DVT are leg edema and calf tenderness. Calf pain on dorsiflexion of the foot is known as Homans sign. All these signs are relatively nonspecific; up to 50% of patients with DVT have no symptoms at all. Together, extensive thrombosis and extreme leg swelling have in the past been known as phlegmasia alba dolens.

The history and examination for superficial phlebitis differ from those for DVT. The patient may have a localized area of edema, erythema, and tenderness over a superficial vein, with increased temperature in the surrounding skin.

DIAGNOSTICS

The diagnosis of superficial phlebitis is based on the clinical findings; diagnostic tests are not usually needed. However, every patient with superficial phlebitis should undergo a duplex ultrasound examination to make sure that he or she does not have a DVT as well. If a DVT is suspected on the basis of clinical signs or risk factors, the diagnosis can be made simply by duplex ultrasound examination of the legs.[27] Test results should document clot visualization, normal blood flow, compressibility of the veins, augmentation of flow with respiration, or reflux in the deep and superficial systems.

The D-dimer level is a global marker of coagulation activation and fibrinolysis. Plasma D-dimer levels have been found to be an aid to the diagnosis of DVT in selected patient populations with medical diagnoses; a negative D-dimer level has been used to rule out DVT.[28] Surgical patients present a challenge to the use of this assay, because surgical patients will exhibit D-dimer elevations postoperatively as a result of the coagulation response. One study conducted on patients who had undergone total hip and knee replacement surgery found that D-dimer levels were higher for a week postoperatively and that levels in these patients did not significantly differ from levels in patients with known DVT.[28] Investigations have suggested that there is variability in the sensitivity of the various D-dimer assays; in addition, the assays are less sensitive when patients have distal DVT and more sensitive when they are combined with assessment of pretest probability of DVT.[29,30]

The most common sites for DVT are the femoral veins; in this situation, the duplex ultrasound examination is as accurate as venography. Isolated tibial or iliac vein thrombosis may be more difficult to diagnose; venography or magnetic resonance venography may be indicated if there is a high index of suspicion. Appropriate testing for anatomic abnormality, malignant disease, connective tissue disorders, or inherited coagulation deficiencies may be necessary. The need for further investigation is guided by the clinical presentation, past medical history, and family history.

DIAGNOSTICS

Peripheral Venous Insufficiency

DEEP VENOUS THROMBOSIS	**CHRONIC VENOUS STASIS**
Imaging	None indicated
Duplex ultrasound*	Varicose veins
Venography, magnetic resonance venography*	*Imaging*
	Duplex scan
Laboratory	
D-dimer, protein C, protein S	**VENOUS STASIS ULCERATION**
Antithrombin III	*Initial*
Antiphospholipid antibodies	Doppler ultrasound
Factor V Leiden	

*If indicated.

DIFFERENTIAL DIAGNOSIS

It is not possible to diagnose DVT accurately on the basis of clinical presentation or physical examination alone. Other differential diagnoses that should be considered are superficial phlebitis, cellulitis, ruptured Baker cyst, strained muscle, and a malignant neoplasm that is compromising the veins.

The possibility of an underlying malignant neoplasm or the existence of a connective tissue disorder must also be considered. Inherited deficiencies of protein C, protein S, or antithrombin III are important (albeit less common) causes, particularly in recurrent cases or in patients with a family history of DVT.

DIFFERENTIAL DIAGNOSIS

Peripheral Venous Insufficiency

DEEP VENOUS THROMBOSIS
- Superficial phlebitis
- Cellulitis
- Ruptured Baker cyst
- Strained muscle
- Malignant neoplasm

CHRONIC VENOUS STASIS
- Heart failure
- Malnutrition
- Lymphatic obstruction

VARICOSE VEINS
- Venous-arterial insufficiency
- Peripheral neuritis
- Arthritis

VENOUS STASIS ULCERATION
- Ischemic ulceration
- Neuropathic ulceration

MANAGEMENT

Management of superficial vein phlebitis consists of nonsteroidal anti-inflammatory agents, leg elevation, and compression with an elastic bandage; because of the risk of deep vein thromboembolism, low-molecular-weight heparin (LMWH) (e.g., enoxaparin) or a factor Xa inhibitor (e.g., fondaparinux) for 6 weeks is recommended.[31] Antibiotics are indicated if there is evidence of an infection.

Management of DVT requires that heparin be initiated immediately to prevent a pulmonary embolism. Traditionally, this has meant admission to the hospital for systemic heparinization. Typically, a bolus of 5000 units is given, followed by a continuous infusion at 800 to 1400 units/hr (80 units/kg heparin bolus followed by an infusion of 18 units/kg/hr) to maintain a partial thromboplastin time (PTT) that is twice the normal rate. The PTT should be checked after 6 hours. The heparin infusion should be continued until the PTT has been in the therapeutic range for a minimum of 2 consecutive days. Warfarin (Coumadin) is started within the first 24 hours, and the patient is discharged once the international normalized ratio (INR) is between 2 and 3 for 72 hours.[32] Fondaparinux, a direct selective inhibitor of factor Xa, or LMWH (e.g., enoxaparin) is increasingly used in the management of DVT and patients being bridged to warfarin until the PT/INR is 2 to 3 for 3 consecutive days, at which time the LMWH can be discontinued.

The regimen of oral anticoagulation is usually continued, based on into which of three patient groups the patient with DVT falls. Group 1 consists of patients with a first episode of DVT associated with a reversible risk factor (surgery or trauma); these patients can typically have anticoagulation stopped after 3 months. Group 2 consists of patients with recurrent DVT, unexplained DVT, or a coagulopathy. These patients are considered for treatment for an indefinite period, with periodic reassessment of risk and the benefit of continuing anticoagulation. Group 3 consists of DVT patients with cancer. These patients are treated for at least 3 to 6 months, or as long as the patient is undergoing chemotherapy and/or has an active cancer diagnosis.[33]

Rivaroxaban and apixaban (factor Xa inhibitors) and dabigatran (a direct thrombin inhibitor) have been studied in patients requiring dual-antiplatelet therapy after cardiac stenting and an anticoagulant to prevent or treat thromboembolic events.[33] Because these medications have no required laboratory monitoring, and fewer medication and food interactions than warfarin, they are replacing standard warfarin therapy in select patient populations.[34] However, it is important to remember that the novel anticoagulants (e.g., dabigatran, rivaroxaban, apixaban) currently have no known readily available reversal agents to use in case of hemorrhage.

Providers are reminded that before use of any of these medications, a comprehensive review of their indications for use and their contraindications as well as dosage regimens and monitoring intervals needs to be performed. All patients receiving heparin should have the platelet count checked every 6 to 8 hours until stable and then daily or per hospital protocol. A sudden drop in the platelet count may be indicative of heparin-induced thrombocytopenia requiring immediate cessation of the heparin infusion and discussion with the physician. If precipitous thrombocytopenia occurs or if the patient has a known allergy to heparin, treatment with a direct thrombin inhibitor is a consideration in consultation with hematology. LMWH (e.g., enoxaparin) given by subcutaneous injection has been shown in studies to be safe for at-home treatment of uncomplicated DVT.[35] These studies show the same or a lower incidence of complications compared with standard heparin. Because enoxaparin has a long half-life, it can be given twice a day subcutaneously; its predictable anticoagulant response obviates the need for PTT monitoring. This has become the standard treatment in uncomplicated cases of DVT. The use of LMWH is contraindicated in patients with renal failure, and adjustments in dose and frequency are indicated in those patients with decreased creatinine clearance.

In patients with massive swelling of one limb (phlegmasia), there is increasing enthusiasm for thrombectomy and lytic therapy, although the long-term effectiveness of this in reducing long-term swelling is not yet clear.

LIFE SPAN CONSIDERATIONS

DVT that is diagnosed during pregnancy should be managed on an individual basis after consultation with a vascular specialist and the patient's obstetrician.[36] Heparin is generally safe during pregnancy and can be given to pregnant women for treatment of DVT. The use of warfarin is contraindicated during pregnancy. Any woman of childbearing age who is taking this medication should be advised of the risks of pregnancy. The introduction of enoxaparin has made the management of these patients much simpler.

A number of measures have been shown to be effective for DVT prophylaxis in patients undergoing surgery. Cuffs that provide intermittent leg pressure to reduce stasis are combined with subcutaneous heparin or LMWH until the patient is mobile. LMWH has been approved for DVT prevention in very-high-risk procedures (e.g., hip replacement) and is now being used. Once or twice daily LMWH (depending on DVT risk) may be used for medical patients who have been prescribed bed rest.

COMPLICATIONS

Pulmonary embolism is one of the major causes of postoperative morbidity and mortality.[37] In high-risk patients, the key to prevention is appropriate surveillance for DVT with the duplex scan. Pulmonary embolism usually occurs within 2 weeks of DVT. After this time, the clot is sufficiently organized to make detachment unlikely. Signs and symptoms of a pulmonary embolus may include pleuritic chest pain, shortness of breath, cough, tachypnea, tachycardia, and/or syncope. The patient may be hypoxic; however, signs and symptoms differ, so it is essential to be aware of the risk factors associated with pulmonary embolism and have a high clinical suspicion if a patient complains of chest pain or shortness of breath. A D-dimer, if within normal limits, is helpful to exclude pulmonary embolism. A chest x-ray film can appear normal, although there are changes suggestive of pulmonary embolism. Evidence of a clot in the leg by duplex scan raises the likelihood of a pulmonary embolism, but the diagnosis is easily verified with CT pulmonary angiography with contrast enhancement.

Postthrombotic syndrome (PTS), postphlebitic syndrome, or secondary venous stasis syndrome is a range of symptoms and physical examination findings consistent with chronic venous insufficiency in a limb affected by DVT; the occurrence of PTS is 20% to 50% of patients over 12 months to as long as 20 years after DVT.[38] Signs and symptoms include leg swelling, chronic severe limb pain, persistent limb edema, and venous stasis ulcers.[33]

Prophylactic placement of an inferior vena cava filter to trap the thrombus and thus prevent pulmonary embolism should be considered if other medical conditions prevent the use of anticoagulation therapy.[39]

INDICATIONS FOR REFERRAL OR HOSPITALIZATION

A documented DVT in any patient requires a physician consultation, during which the need for hospitalization and intravenous administration of heparin versus outpatient treatment with LMWH can be determined. Vascular consultation is necessary for patients who may require placement of a vena cava filter.[40] If the inflammatory process continues despite treatment, excision may occasionally be indicated; in such cases, a vascular consultation should be sought.

PATIENT AND FAMILY EDUCATION

Anticoagulant therapy should be carefully explained to patients and families, and the importance of routine laboratory testing to monitor warfarin therapy should be stressed. Patients should understand the necessity of contacting the health care provider if any abnormal bleeding occurs. In addition, patients should be familiar with the signs and symptoms of pulmonary embolism (e.g., chest pain, dyspnea) as indications for emergency care. A list of foods high in vitamin K and a careful explanation of how excess ingestion of these foods may decrease the action of warfarin are also necessary.

HEALTH PROMOTION

Other options for birth control should be discussed with female patients, particularly those who smoke. High-risk patients should understand the risks associated with long plane and automobile journeys. They should also be advised to wear support stockings and to take low-dose aspirin (81 to 325 mg) while traveling. Adequate fluid intake, frequent rest breaks to stretch and exercise the legs, and passive intermittent contraction of the calf muscles enhance blood flow to the lower extremities during prolonged, confined travel conditions.

CHRONIC VENOUS STASIS

DEFINITION AND EPIDEMIOLOGY

Chronic venous stasis results from increased pressure in the deep veins. This condition produces edema, varicose veins, chronic skin changes, and ulceration.

PATHOPHYSIOLOGY

Human beings are relatively poorly adapted to walking on two legs for extended periods. The distribution of blood to the feet is accomplished by the heart in concert with gravity, but it is only the muscle pump and fragile venous valves that return the blood to the heart. Prolonged standing and a tall stature increase hydrostatic pressure on the valves. During pregnancy, the hormone relaxin, which allows the pelvis to stretch, also causes the veins to distend and the valves to become incompetent. Resolution of this condition after pregnancy is often incomplete, resulting in increased venous stasis. Obesity and age-associated loss of tissue turgor are also factors that produce venous stasis.

Increased pressure may also result from proximal venous obstruction secondary to an old DVT or more commonly from reflux secondary to valvular incompetence. Valvular incompetence may result from recanalization after a DVT, or it may be primary in nature.

Even if the valves of the perforator and saphenous veins remain competent, deep venous hypertension affects the foot and ankle. The foot tends to swell, particularly if the patient stands much of the day. The point of maximum pressure is the ankle, and the skin becomes thickened and may react to the pressure with an eczematous reaction known as stasis eczema. Consequently, blood cells in the tiny venules break down under high pressure; hemosiderin is deposited under the skin to produce a characteristic brown staining that progresses with time.

CLINICAL PRESENTATION AND PHYSICAL EXAMINATION

The clinical appearance of chronic venous stasis varies according to whether the superficial or deeper veins are affected. Chronic edema and skin discoloration on the legs and ankles may be present. Varicose veins, ulceration, and even cellulitis may result.

DIAGNOSTICS AND DIFFERENTIAL DIAGNOSIS

Diagnostic tests are unnecessary because the diagnosis is based on the clinical history and physical findings. The physical findings also guide the diagnosis. However, the peripheral edema associated with chronic venous stasis may also be caused by other disease entities. Medications, congestive heart failure, lymphatic obstruction, and malnutrition may all be associated with lower extremity edema (see the Diagnostics and Differential Diagnosis boxes for peripheral venous insufficiency).

MANAGEMENT

Compression stockings or elastic bandages (e.g., Profore) and periodic leg elevation are the most important methods for controlling chronic venous insufficiency and preventing skin ulcers. Careful monitoring is important when venous ulcers occur. Normal saline wet-to-dry dressings or topical antibiotic therapies are indicated. Ulcer infections should be treated with the appropriate antibiotic.

COMPLICATIONS

Venous ulcers are the most common complication of chronic venous stasis. A superimposed infection and cellulitis are additional concerns. Severe edema may result in decreased mobility and an increased risk for falls or DVT.

INDICATIONS FOR REFERRAL OR HOSPITALIZATION

Venous ulcers or peripheral edema that does not respond to conventional therapies may require a referral to the appropriate specialist. Severe ulcers with extensive tissue loss may require evaluation by a plastic surgeon for possible grafting. Most patients can be successfully managed with careful outpatient follow-up visits. However, hospitalization may be indicated for severe edema, infection, or surgical valvuloplasty.

PATIENT AND FAMILY EDUCATION

The most effective treatment of leg swelling and stasis dermatitis is the use of support stockings.[41] Severe stasis eczema may require the use of 0.5% hydrocortisone cream in combination with compression. The hydrocortisone cream should be discontinued once the condition has resolved.

VARICOSE VEINS

PATHOPHYSIOLOGY

Varicose veins are caused by pathologic distention and proliferation of the superficial veins. Varicose veins include primary and secondary varicose veins as well as spider veins.

Primary varicose veins are usually familial. There is no previous history of DVT, and the varicosities are usually exacerbated by pregnancy. Progressive dilation of the superficial veins may be local or more extensive. Primary varicose veins result from incompetent perforators, which produce local varicosities, or from incompetence of the saphenous vein valves, which produces more generalized varicosities. Secondary varicose veins result from a previous DVT. Most commonly, these are caused by incompetent valves after recanalization. When the deep venous system is totally occluded, these varicose veins may represent the main venous drainage from the leg; in this instance, removal of the veins would be harmful. Telangiectasia or spider veins may result from increased pressure in the superficial veins. It is not clear why this condition is more predominant in some patients.

CLINICAL PRESENTATION AND PHYSICAL EXAMINATION

The pooling of blood in large varicose veins tends to produce symptoms of heaviness and discomfort in the legs while standing. Large varicose veins are unsightly and may produce severe anxiety and cause major lifestyle changes. Trauma to varicose veins may result in severe bleeding, particularly in older adults because their skin may be atrophic and thereby provides less protection.

DIAGNOSTICS AND DIFFERENTIAL DIAGNOSIS

Diagnosis is based on inspection of the lower extremities when the patient is standing. The important diagnostic for varicose veins is the duplex scan to determine whether the deep system is patent and whether there is saphenofemoral reflux. Individual incompetent perforators in the leg may also be identified. If varicosities are not present, venous and arterial insufficiency, peripheral neuritis, and arthritis should be considered (see the Diagnostics and Differential Diagnosis boxes for peripheral venous insufficiency).

MANAGEMENT

Asymptomatic varicose veins do not require treatment. There is no effective way to reduce venous pressure in the lower legs except with support stockings.

COMPLICATIONS

A superficial varicosity will occasionally rupture, and significant bleeding may be noted. Topical compression and elevation of the extremity usually control the bleeding. Skin ulcerations are an additional complication of varicose veins.

INDICATIONS FOR REFERRAL OR HOSPITALIZATION

Referral to a vascular specialist is indicated if support stockings are not effective in controlling symptoms or are poorly tolerated by the patient.

Treatment by a specialist may involve removal of the varicose veins or, alternatively, injection or laser treatment. Large veins are more appropriately removed in outpatient surgery, whereas smaller veins can be injected. Spider veins can be treated by either injection or laser treatment. Increasingly, obliteration of the long saphenous vein with use of a catheter and a radiofrequency generator or a laser has reduced the morbidity of saphenectomy; this can be done with the patient under local anesthesia in the office.[42]

PATIENT AND FAMILY EDUCATION

It is important to inform patients that none of the treatments for varicose veins eradicate the problem of high venous pressure. Therefore recurrence is the rule rather than the exception. This knowledge may affect a patient's decision to proceed with surgery. Patients should also understand that compression stockings and periodic leg elevation are beneficial.

VENOUS STASIS ULCERATION

DEFINITION AND EPIDEMIOLOGY

Venous stasis ulceration is the most severe complication of PTS and rarely occurs without a history of DVT. With the introduction of heparin and the prompt diagnosis and treatment of DVT, venous stasis ulceration is now less common.

PATHOPHYSIOLOGY

A number of factors contribute to venous ulceration. At first, peripheral edema increases as a result of incompetent valves in the venous system. This edema leads to capillary distention and the leakage of fluid and other substances into the surrounding tissue. If there is trauma to the skin of the affected extremity, oxygen and essential nutrients for healing are prevented from reaching the injured area. As a result, a superficial, irregularly shaped ulceration occurs. These ulcers can continue to erode, and cellulitis and superimposed infection can occur.

CLINICAL PRESENTATION AND PHYSICAL EXAMINATION

The patient with venous stasis ulceration typically is seen with an ulcer above the medial malleolus, and other signs of venous stasis are usually present. The ulcers have a distinctive presentation that permits differentiation from ischemic or diabetic ulcers (Box 125-3). At the time of presentation, the wound may be secondarily infected. Pulses may not be palpable because of local swelling or coexistent ischemia.

BOX 125-3

Characteristics of Leg Ulcers by Cause*

VENOUS STASIS
Occur around ankle, particularly medial side
History of phlebitis
Signs of venous stasis
Painful when secondarily infected
Improved by elevation

ISCHEMIC
Occur at tips of extremities or heel
History of claudication common
Very painful, but much worse on elevation
Absent pulses on physical examination
Secondary infection likely to spread very quickly

NEUROPATHIC (DIABETIC)
Occur at pressure points
Painless, but coexistent neuritic pain possibly confusing
Often present after secondary infection

*More than one cause may be involved.

DIAGNOSTICS AND DIFFERENTIAL DIAGNOSIS

Diagnostic tests are usually unnecessary. A portable Doppler instrument can be used to assess pulses if they are not readily palpable. The differential diagnosis should encompass all peripheral ulcers (see the Diagnostics and Differential Diagnosis boxes for peripheral venous insufficiency).

MANAGEMENT

Management of venous stasis ulceration consists of wound debridement by an experienced practitioner and an appropriate dressing that will manage the wound exudate without causing further skin irritation or damage.[43] Antibiotics are appropriate if the wound is infected or cellulitis is present.[43] A nonstick dressing may be less painful once the ulcer is clean.

COMPLICATIONS

Superimposed infection and cellulitis are potential concerns with venous stasis ulceration. Osteomyelitis is an additional complication of infected ulcers.

INDICATIONS FOR REFERRAL OR HOSPITALIZATION

A surgical or wound clinic referral is indicated if the ulcer is not responding to treatment. If the ulcer is clearly deteriorating, hospitalization may be required.

PATIENT AND FAMILY EDUCATION

Patient education is important in preventing reoccurring venous stasis ulcers. Patients need to understand the importance of appropriately fitted compression stockings worn daily. If severe edema is present, an external pneumatic compression stocking may be necessary to control end-of-day lower extremity edema.

Many patients fail to wear their prescribed support stockings because the wrong stockings are provided. In general, knee-high stockings are much better tolerated than any tight support that crosses the knee. The main exceptions are for pregnant women and women with varicose veins in the thigh, who may find support pantyhose comfortable. In ordering of stockings, the key factor is pressure (Table 125-1). The thick or fine-knit quality of the stockings affects only durability and patient acceptance.

TABLE 125-1 **Recommendations for Support Stockings***

Pressure (mm Hg)	Recommendations
0-10	Normal socks
10-20	Over-the-counter support stockings Recommended for individuals who are on their feet all day and for prophylaxis for DVT when traveling
20-30	Lowest pressure therapeutic stocking Good for individuals who are looking for more pressure than over-the-counter stockings or who cannot tolerate the higher pressures
30-40	Standard pressure for therapeutic stockings Instruct patients to shower in the evening so that these stockings can be put on before getting out of bed; otherwise, they will be difficult for many patients, particularly older adults, to put on
40-50	Should be prescribed only for patients who do not have enough compression with 30-40 mm Hg Almost impossible to get on!

*Consult vascular specialist for use in patients with PAD.

CHAPTER 126

VALVULAR HEART DISEASE AND CARDIAC MURMURS

Cathleen Crowley-Koschnitzki

When a murmur is heard for the first time, it is important to determine whether it is from a pathologic condition and what type of condition it may represent. The cause of a murmur, whether benign or malignant, is difficult to determine by auscultation alone. What distinguishes benign from pathologic murmurs is often the characteristics of the murmur, associated physical findings, or symptoms (Table 126-1). Some patients require referral for diagnostic testing, whereas the clinical assessment of others suggests that diagnostic testing is unnecessary.

DEFINITION

A murmur is the relatively lengthy series of sounds produced by the turbulent flow of blood. Under normal conditions, blood flow is uniform or laminar within the vessel or chamber and is therefore free of audible vibration. When flow velocity is excessively high or when normal flow occurs across an obstruction, turbulence and its resultant audible vibration occur. In a classic article on auscultation of the heart, Leatham[1] noted that all murmurs are related to one of three factors: (1) high rates of flow through a normal or abnormal valve; (2) forward flow through a constricted or irregular valve or into a dilated vessel; or (3) backward flow through a regurgitant valve, septal defect, or patent ductus arteriosus.

EVALUATION OF MURMURS

Murmurs may be characterized by a number of factors: location, intensity, pitch, radiation, and timing. Of these, timing is the most important factor. Timing delineates the critical division between systolic and diastolic murmurs as well as the relationship to the heart sounds (S_1 and S_2; e.g., ending well before, right at, or continuing through S_2). As the heart rate increases, diastole shortens, and systole and diastole approach similar intervals. When this occurs, differentiation between S_1 (beginning of systole) and S_2 (beginning of diastole) on the basis of cadence alone becomes difficult. Palpation of the carotid pulse while simultaneously auscultating the heart at the base will easily permit the listener to focus and time S_1 (the onset of systole), which will occur slightly before the onset of the carotid pulse rise. The two components of S_2 (aortic, or A_2, and pulmonic, or P_2) are almost superimposed at end-expiration, with inspiration P_2 splits later, creating an easily audible gap. This will be best appreciated over the upper left sternal border. A systolic murmur that ends at or before A_2 will be a left-sided murmur (e.g., aortic stenosis [AS] or mitral regurgitation [MR]), whereas one that extends beyond A_2 will be emanating from the right side of the heart (i.e., pulmonic stenosis or tricuspid regurgitation).

Intensity, or loudness, which is related to the velocity of blood flow, describes how audible the murmur is. However, loudness does not equate with the severity of the underlying problem. Some of the loudest murmurs are caused by a small muscular ventricular septal defect (VSD) in an adolescent that is destined to close spontaneously. Murmurs are graded 1 (barely audible), 2 (faint but clearly heard), 3 (easily heard but without being able to palpate the vibrations on the chest wall), 4 (heard with a palpable thrill), 5 (heard with the stethoscope only partially in contact with the chest wall with a palpable thrill), or 6 (heard without a stethoscope with a palpable thrill). The location where a murmur is best heard is also generally noted (e.g., at the upper right sternal border [second intercostal space], upper left sternal border, lower left sternal border, or apical areas of the chest wall). These terms have largely superseded the earlier descriptors of aortic, pulmonic, tricuspid, and mitral locations because of the variable radiation or transmission of the sounds.

SYSTOLIC MURMURS

Systolic murmurs are classified into two general types: ejection type (midsystolic) and regurgitant type (pansystolic). In the ejection type, the murmur is grade 1 or 2, and there is a period between S_1 (closure of the mitral and tricuspid valves) and the onset of the murmur. During this time, the ventricle is generating pressure (isovolumetric contraction) to overcome the pressure in the great vessels (aorta and pulmonary artery) and to open the aortic and pulmonic valves. The murmur builds in intensity as velocity increases, followed by a decrease in intensity, which occurs well before S_2 (closure of the aortic and pulmonic valves). Thus, the murmur is diamond shaped, or crescendo-decrescendo. This murmur occurs with left ventricular outflow obstruction whether the obstruction is from rheumatic or calcific AS, idiopathic hypertrophic subaortic stenosis (IHSS, also known as hypertrophic obstructive cardiomyopathy), or pneumonic stenosis. Most murmurs are of this type.

In contrast are the murmurs resulting from flow from a high-pressure chamber to a low-pressure chamber, which occurs in incompetent valves (mitral or tricuspid regurgitation) or with a VSD. As soon as pressure starts to develop, flow occurs throughout systole (pansystolic flow). The pressure gradient and therefore the intensity of the murmur are largely unchanged throughout systole. Such murmurs are described as plateau shaped. The murmur of chronic tricuspid regurgitation or MR is the epitome of the pansystolic murmur. However, when a significant gradient or differential of pressure does not exist between chambers, the murmurs will be truncated. Thus, the murmur of severe acute MR may occur only during early systole because of rapid equalization of left atrial pressure with left ventricular pressure. Similarly, the classic murmur of a VSD, which may ordinarily be indistinguishable from that of chronic MR, may be truncated or even totally absent in the face of pulmonary hypertension (Eisenmenger complex). The murmur of mitral valve prolapse (MVP) is classically late systolic, often after a midsystolic click. Variation in intensity of the murmur with respiration is strongly associated with right-sided (pulmonic or tricuspid valve) abnormalities.[2]

DIASTOLIC MURMURS

Diastolic murmurs are related to regurgitation across either the aortic or the pulmonic valve or to filling rumbles caused by flow across a normal (in exaggerated flow states) or obstructed mitral or tricuspid valve. Listening for the high-pitched diastolic murmur of aortic or pulmonic insufficiency (regurgitation) is difficult and may require proper positioning of the patient. These murmurs are loudest early in diastole, when there is a large

TABLE 126-1 Murmurs

Diagnosis	Characteristic	Location, Radiation	Physical Examination Findings	Effect of Valsalva Maneuver	Electrocardiographic Findings	Chest X-Ray Findings
COMMON SYSTOLIC MURMURS						
Aortic stenosis	Harsh, crescendo-decrescendo	Right sternal border; radiation to neck	Delayed carotid upstroke; narrowed pulse pressure; systolic thrill at second right intercostal space	Decreased murmur	Left atrial enlargement; left axis deviation; atrioventricular conduction delay; left ventricular hypertrophy	Aortic valve calcification; left ventricular hypertrophy
Mitral regurgitation	Pansystolic blowing	Apex; radiation to axilla	Laterally displaced, hyperdynamic apical impulse; brisk carotid upstroke	No change	Left ventricular hypertrophy	Left ventricular enlargement
Mitral valve prolapse	Midsystolic to late systolic; occasionally honking; may have midsystolic click; click and murmur can be intermittent	Lower left sternal border	May have scoliosis or pectus excavatum in connective tissue disorder	Murmur or click may move to later systole or disappear	Usually within normal limits; occasionally flat or inverted T in leads II, III, aVF	Skeletal abnormalities, if present
Tricuspid regurgitation	Early systolic, midsystolic, late systolic, or pansystolic	Lower left sternal border; radiation to right sternal border	Sustained precordial lift	Decreased murmur	Right atrial hypertrophy; right axis deviation	Usually normal
Hypertrophic cardiomyopathy	Peaks midsystole	Left sternal border	Murmur decreased with change from standing to squatting; S_4 gallop may be present	Increased murmur	Left atrial enlargement; increased voltage; may have left ventricular hypertrophy	May have slight cardiac enlargement
Benign or innocent*	Early systolic; crescendo-decrescendo; changes intensity with rate	Variant	No underlying systemic findings; no findings of cardiac enlargement or failure; murmur disappears with breath holding	Murmur disappearing	Normal recording	Normal findings
Ventricular septal defect	Pansystolic; louder in midsystole	Left sternal border; radiation to right sternal border	May have systolic thrill at lower left sternal border	Increased murmur	May have left atrial and ventricular enlargement	
COMMON DIASTOLIC MURMURS						
Aortic regurgitation	Loud, blowing, high pitched	Lower left sternal border	Widened pulse pressure; abrupt rise and fall in carotid upstroke	Increased murmur	Left ventricular hypertrophy; sinus tachycardia	Left ventricular hypertrophy; aortic valve calcification; ascending aortic dilation
Mitral stenosis	Low-pitched, diastolic rumble (mid)	Apex, left lateral position	Opening snap	No change or increased murmur	Left atrial enlargement; right axis deviation	Left atrial enlargement; calcified mitral valve
Tricuspid stenosis	Decrescendo, low pitched	Fourth or fifth left intercostal space	Absent right ventricular impulse; diastolic thrill; lower left intercostal border may have opening snap at fourth left intercostal space	Decreased murmur	Height of P wave in lead II >2.5 mm; PR shortened; right atrial hypertrophy	Right atrial and vena cava shadows

*Whether a murmur is benign or innocent cannot be determined with 100% accuracy.

pressure gradient between the aorta and the left ventricle; they then fall in intensity as the pressure gradient falls, producing a decrescendo pattern of sound. They are best heard with the patient sitting, leaning forward, and exhaling, all of which minimize the distance from the stethoscope to the heart. The diaphragm of the stethoscope should be used because of the high-frequency response of the murmur.

The cause of the murmur cannot be discerned by the character of the murmur; however, it is generally acknowledged that aortic insufficiency murmurs heard best at the upper right sternal border are more likely to be related to dilation of the aortic root, in contrast to murmurs caused by damage to the aortic valve. If the aortic insufficiency is acute and severe, the duration of the murmur may be truncated as a result of the rapid and premature equalization of pressures between the left ventricle and the aorta. Pulmonic insufficiency is usually found in the setting of pulmonary hypertension with dilation of the pulmonic artery and produces a Graham Steell murmur, which by clinical examination is almost indistinguishable from the murmur of aortic insufficiency. Low-pitched rumbles in diastole are caused by forward flow across a stenotic mitral or tricuspid valve. Such low-pitched murmurs are best appreciated by use of the bell of the stethoscope at the apical area with the patient lying slightly on the left side. Because the filling of the ventricles occurs primarily in early diastole (the rapid filling phase) and at the end of diastole (from atrial contraction), the murmur is loudest during these times. Therefore patients with atrial fibrillation will lack the presystolic accentuation of their diastolic rumbles because they have no atrial contraction.

The duration, not the intensity, of the murmur correlates with the severity of the obstruction. Less-severe stenosis will result in a shorter gradient across the stenotic valve and a shorter murmur; more severe stenosis will result in a longer gradient across the stenotic valve and a longer murmur (to the end of diastole). Hyperdynamic states, such as anemia and fever, or the presence of atrial septal defects or VSDs producing shunting of blood from one chamber to the other during diastole may produce murmurs in mid-diastole. Left atrial myxomas may obstruct flow across the mitral valve during diastole, producing a similar rumble but one that is associated with a "tumor plop" instead of an opening snap.

CONTINUOUS MURMURS

Continuous murmurs begin in systole and extend at least partway into diastole. Continuous murmur causes include rapid blood flow, high to low pressure shunts, or localized stenosis.[3] The classic continuous murmur is exemplified by the murmur associated with a patent ductus arteriosus. Intracardiac shunting between a high-pressure system (aorta) and a low-pressure system (pulmonary artery) exists throughout the cardiac cycle and may be heard in the region just beneath the left clavicle. Fistulas or localized arterial obstructions may also produce continuous murmurs. In addition, continuous murmurs are often associated with benign high-flow states. A continuous murmur known as a venous hum and heard in the neck is commonly noted in children and adolescents. It may be abolished by compression of the jugular vein. Similarly, women in the late stages of pregnancy or lactating women shortly postpartum may develop a continuous "mammary shuffle" over the breast that may be obliterated with firm pressure.

FLOW MURMURS (BENIGN AND PATHOLOGIC)

Murmurs that are not caused by any pathologic obstruction to flow are termed innocent, benign, or functional. As noted previously, the acoustic-mechanical phenomena that create benign or innocent murmurs are the same as those that create pathologic conditions. The differentiation is based on the lack of other findings (e.g., abnormal carotid or peripheral pulses, associated symptoms). Several clues may help distinguish innocent murmurs from pathologic ones.[3] Murmurs that are caused by an increased cardiac output (e.g., as a result of fever, thyrotoxicosis, anemia) may be termed functional because they are caused by excess flow across the outflow tract. Many older adults have decreased mobility of the aortic valves as a result of fibrosis and calcification (aortic sclerosis), which distorts the flow without producing a significant gradient across the valve. Other older patients may have outflow murmurs that are caused by ejection of blood into a kinked, tortuous aorta.

2014 American College of Cardiology/American Heart Association Guidelines

The 2014 American College of Cardiology (ACC) and American Heart Association (AHA) guidelines for the management of patients with valvular heart disease (VHD) updated the recommendations for evaluation and management of adult patients. General recommendations include a through history and complete physical examination on all patients with suspected or known heart disease. The presence or absence of symptoms guides progression staging and treatment (Table 126-2). Recommendations for initial diagnostics of VHD include transthoracic echocardiogram (TTE) with two-dimensional (2D) imaging and Doppler studies, which provides necessary anatomic and hemodynamic measurements. Transthoracic echocardiography is the standard diagnostic test for the initial evaluation of patients with suspected or known VHD. Classification of the severity of valve disease is determined from physical examination findings and TTE results.[4] Monitoring of asymptomatic VHD patient status by periodic TTE varies based on lesion, severity level, and valvular function. For patients with known VHD, a change in symptoms or the physical examination findings warrants a repeat TTE. Cardiac catheterization is recommended for symptomatic patients with inconclusive TTE results or when there is

TABLE 126-2 Stages of Progressive Valvular Heart Disease (VHD)

Type	Description
A (At risk)	Risk factors for development of VHD
B (Progressing)	Asymptomatic patients with mild to moderate severity of VHD
C (Severe but asymptomatic)	Asymptomatic patients who meet criteria for severe VHD: C1: Asymptomatic patients with severe VHD with compensated left or right ventricle C2: Asymptomatic patients with severe VHD with left or right ventricle decompensation
D (Severe and symptomatic)	Symptomatic VHD patients

a discrepancy between physical examination findings and noninvasive testing results (see Table 126-2).[4]

AORTIC STENOSIS

DEFINITION AND EPIDEMIOLOGY

AS is a disorder associated with advancing age. Purely based on clinical findings, it is more difficult to assess the degree of severity of AS than it is to assess any other valvular abnormality. Valvular AS may be caused by rheumatic damage, congenital abnormality (bicuspid aortic valve), or degeneration by the aging process (calcific AS of older adults).[5] During the past three decades, with the successful treatment of streptococcal pharyngitis, the etiology has shifted away from rheumatic to calcific. A history of 20 to 30 years of repetitive mechanical trauma of the blood against the valve results in inflammation, fibrosis, calcification, and eventually stenosis. This progression of calcification within the valve cusps is usually seen during the latter decades of life. An inflammatory process similar to that causing the development of atherosclerotic plaques in coronaries may be a possible cause of the progression of AS.[5] AS is staged based on symptomatology, valve anatomy, and hemodynamics.

PATHOPHYSIOLOGY

Any reduction of the normal aortic valve orifice of approximately 3 cm^2 (1⅕ square inches) will cause obstruction to the flow of blood from the left ventricle into the aorta during ventricular systole. A systolic pressure gradient develops between the left ventricle and the aorta. Left ventricular pressure rises, increasing systolic wall stress. The left ventricle hypertrophies as a compensatory mechanism to maintain adequate cardiac output. Valvular stenosis is generally considered to be significant when the valve area is reduced to 25% of normal. Therefore, hemodynamically significant AS would be an aortic valve area of less than 0.75 cm^2 ($\frac{3}{10}$ square inch) in an adult, which is associated with a gradient of more than 50 mm Hg. A large pressure gradient across the aortic valve may be sustained for many years without a reduction in contractile function, with left ventricular dilation generally a very late manifestation. Persistent pressure overload to the left ventricle may eventually lead to left ventricular dilation, left atrial enlargement, and pulmonary hypertension.

CLINICAL PRESENTATION

Chest pain, syncope, exercise intolerance, and dyspnea are the classic symptoms associated with severe AS. With chronic AS, there generally is a long latent period before the development of symptoms. By the time clinical symptoms are present, AS can be advanced.[5] Angina and syncope manifest whereas the left ventricular function remains preserved; dyspnea indicates congestive heart failure (CHF) and left ventricular dysfunction. Angina pectoris is a frequent symptom among patients with AS. Anginal symptoms in AS may be caused by an increased myocardial oxygen demand related to increased wall tension combined with a reduction in coronary blood supply.[5] This may occur even in the presence of normal coronary arteries. [4] Heart failure is a late clinical sign and is associated with poor prognosis.[5]

Although it is uncommon, patients with severe AS are at a higher risk of sudden death when anginal symptoms are present. Dizziness or frank syncope occurs in patients and has been attributed to an abrupt fall in systemic vascular resistance in the presence of a fixed cardiac output, abrupt failure of the overloaded left ventricle during effort, or arrhythmia.[5] Left ventricular failure eventually occurs with symptoms of fatigue, cough, progressive dyspnea on exertion, orthopnea, and paroxysmal nocturnal dyspnea.[5]

PHYSICAL EXAMINATION

No physical finding can reliably assess the severity of AS obstruction. Classically, the carotid pulse has a slow rise with delayed peak and small volume (pulsus parvus and pulsus tardus). A notch or shudder in the upstroke (anacrotic notch) may be appreciated. Auscultation reveals a harsh (grade 3/6 or greater) crescendo-decrescendo systolic ejection murmur that begins after the first heart sound. The murmur of AS is loudest at the second right sternal edge and radiates to the left lateral sternal border and carotids. A thrill is often present. The murmur may become softer or even inaudible in patients with end-stage AS. Paradoxical splitting of the second heart sound (S_2) occurs as a result of delay in closure of the aortic valve. In severe stenosis, the A_2 is often inaudible; therefore, no splitting of S_2 is appreciated. An additional early systolic ejection sound or click may be heard, more commonly in younger patients with congenital or bicuspid AS. Left ventricular hypertrophy (LVH) produces a sustained thrust or heave of the apical impulse. Displacement of the apical impulse downward and to the left occurs after left ventricular failure develops and the ventricle dilates.

DIAGNOSTICS

Recommendations for initial diagnostics include electrocardiography (ECG), chest x-ray examination, and TTE with 2D imaging and Doppler studies. TTE is the standard diagnostic test for the initial evaluation of patients with suspected or known VHD.[4] In patients with AS, normal findings (e.g., lack of LVH or normal chest x-ray findings) do not exclude severe disease. ECG demonstrates normal sinus rhythm with signs of LVH. Atrial fibrillation usually represents either end-stage disease with left ventricular decompensation or other associated disease. Conduction abnormalities, such as first-degree atrioventricular block, bundle branch block, and intraventricular conduction disturbances, are fairly common. The chest x-ray film may demonstrate rounding or prominence of the left ventricle as a result of concentric hypertrophy of the left ventricle, poststenotic dilation of the aorta, and calcification of the valve cusps, or the chest x-ray findings may be completely normal.

In contrast, a technically satisfactory, well-performed 2D echocardiogram has the ability to exclude significant obstruction of the aortic valve. The Doppler portion of the examination is able to provide an assessment of the outflow gradient that closely approximates that obtained by cardiac catheterization. By combining Doppler ultrasonography and echocardiography, the examiner may make a reasonable calculation of the aortic valve area. Thickened, calcified, and immobile leaflets are readily noted by transthoracic 2D echocardiography. The echocardiogram also demonstrates poststenotic dilation of the aorta and left ventricular wall thickening. Dilation of the left ventricle or reduced contractility (ejection fraction) occurs with myocardial failure. Equally important, additional valvular abnormalities (e.g., MR or mitral stenosis [MS]) are apparent, as are the findings of IHSS.

Cardiac catheterization can determine the severity of obstruction by recording the gradient across the valve and by calculating the valve area. Additional functional assessment of the left ventricle is possible. In the current era, these findings often confirm those obtained by Doppler echocardiography. In adults, the major indication for cardiac catheterization is to delineate the coronary anatomy. Even in patients without angina, approximately 50% will have significant coronary obstructions.[6]

DIAGNOSTICS*

Murmurs

INITIAL TESTING	OTHER DIAGNOSTICS
ECG	Stress ECG*
Chest x-ray examination	Cardiac magnetic resonance imaging (cMRI)*
TTE (echocardiography including 2D and Doppler studies)	Cardiac catheterization*

*If indicated.

DIFFERENTIAL DIAGNOSIS

The major condition in the differential diagnosis for a systolic ejection murmur without valvular disease is the functional or innocent murmur (i.e., flow murmur without disease). The absence of symptoms or other physical abnormalities will generally lead to this diagnosis. In adults, the major pathologic state that must be differentiated is IHSS, or hypertrophic obstructive cardiomyopathy. These patients may have similar symptoms; however, the carotid upstroke is very brisk, with at times two distinct humps (pulsus bisferiens). The primary distinguishing characteristic is the murmur's response to maneuvers that increase or decrease the dynamic obstruction. Thus, standing or the strain phase of the Valsalva maneuver decreases venous return, resulting in a smaller left ventricular outflow tract and an increase in the murmur intensity.

DIFFERENTIAL DIAGNOSIS

Systolic Murmurs

EJECTION MURMURS
- AS
- IHSS
- Pulmonary stenosis

REGURGITANT MURMURS
- Mitral regurgitation or insufficiency
- Tricuspid regurgitation or insufficiency
- VSD

LATE SYSTOLIC MURMURS
- Mitral valve prolapse

CONTINUOUS MURMURS
- Patent ductus arteriosus
- Benign (innocent) murmur
- Mammary shuffle

MANAGEMENT

Patients with asymptomatic AS require periodic monitoring for symptom development and disease progression. With severe AS, once symptoms manifest, however mild, valve obstruction must be relieved to prevent poor outcome. Recommendations for aortic valve replacement (AVR) are usually reserved for patients in stages C and D; consideration for AVR should be given to those patients who are in stage B with aortic velocity 3.0 to 3.9 m/sec for whom other cardiac surgery is contemplated.[4] Management of the patient with symptomatic AS is almost entirely surgical. Two options—surgical replacement and transcatheter aortic valve replacement (TAVR)—are available. TAVR is a minimally invasive procedure for patients who are too high risk for traditional valve replacement. In the TAVR procedure, a valve is inserted into the place of the old valve, but the old valve is not removed. When the replacement valve is expanded, the old valve is pushed out of the way and the new valve begins to function. Medical therapy for the asymptomatic patient with AS is no longer a recommended by the AHA unless the patient has associated high-risk medical conditions that would warrant treatment.[4] Recommendations for medical therapy in AS are management of hypertension.[4] Statin therapy is not recommended for prevention in patients with mild to moderate calcific AS (stages B to D).[4] See Box 126-1 and Chapter 123 for current recommendations for infective endocarditis. Patients with moderate or severe AS should not engage in competitive sports that require high dynamic and static muscular activity.[4]

Interdisciplinary Management

Interdisciplinary management is reasonable for patients with AS. Patients with significant obstruction and modest symptoms or those who are asymptomatic yet have severe obstruction may require more frequent evaluation. The AHA/ACC guidelines have specific recommendations for TTE based on the patient's stage of VHD. Any significant changes in status such as murmur changes or onset of symptoms necessitates TTE.

COMPLICATIONS

The initial symptoms associated with AS are angina and syncope or presyncope as well as dyspnea and frank CHF, which in the patient with just AS are manifestations of a failing left ventricle. Atrial fibrillation occurs in less than 10% of patients with AS, and its occurrence should raise the possibility of concomitant mitral valve disease. If it occurs, prompt cardioversion is often required because loss of atrial contraction may significantly impair left ventricular performance as a result of the markedly noncompliant left ventricle.

LIFE SPAN CONSIDERATIONS

AS is a condition most often seen in the aging population. However, if a women of childbearing age is diagnosed with AS and is planning a pregnancy, she should be referred to a cardiologist for evaluation, testing, and guidance.

INDICATIONS FOR REFERRAL OR HOSPITALIZATION AND PATIENT AND FAMILY EDUCATION

See Indications for Referral or Hospitalization and Patient and Family Education under Mitral Stenosis.

AORTIC REGURGITATION

DEFINITION AND EPIDEMIOLOGY

Aortic regurgitation (AR) occurs when the aortic valve fails to close completely, allowing blood to flow back into the left ventricle during ventricular diastole. This process may be either chronic or acute. It may occur as a result of involvement of the

BOX 126-1

Summary of Current Recommendations for Prevention of Infective Endocarditis*

CARDIAC CONDITIONS ASSOCIATED WITH HIGH RISK OF ADVERSE OUTCOME FROM INFECTIOUS ENDOCARDITIS (ENDOCARDITIS PROPHYLAXIS RECOMMENDED [HIGH RISK][†])

Prosthetic valves—mechanical, bioprosthetic, and homograft valves
Prosthetic material used for valvular repair
Prior episode of infective endocarditis
Unrepaired cyanotic congenital heart disease (CHD)
Repaired CHD with prosthetic material or device (surgical or catheter intervention within 6 months)
Repaired CHD with residual defects at or adjacent to repair site
Cardiac transplant recipients with development of valvulopathy

HIGH-RISK PROCEDURES AND ENDOCARDITIS PROPHYLAXIS* (ENDOCARDITIS PROPHYLAXIS RECOMMENDED)

Dental Procedures

Perforation of oral mucosa
Manipulation of gingival tissue (most dental procedures, such as cleanings, extractions, implant placements, periodontal procedures)
Exposure and manipulation of periapical region of tooth

Respiratory Tract Procedures (Involving Incision and Biopsy of Respiratory Mucosa)

Tonsillectomy, adenoidectomy
Bronchoscopy (only with incision of respiratory mucosa)

Infected Skin, Skin Structure, or Musculoskeletal Tissue Procedures

Surgical procedures involving infected skin or musculoskeletal structures

*Please refer to Chapter 123 for more information on infective endocarditis.
[†]In 2008 the ACC/AHA issued a focused update to the guidelines for the prophylaxis of infective endocarditis in patients with VHD, which recognized that "some clinicians and some patients may still feel more comfortable continuing with prophylaxis for infective endocarditis, particularly for those with bicuspid aortic valve or coarctation of the aorta, severe mitral valve prolapse, or hypertrophic obstructive cardiomyopathy. In those settings, the clinician should determine that the risks associated with antibiotics are low before continuing a prophylaxis regimen."[12]

leaflets themselves or as a result of distortion of the aortic root. Pathologic processes affecting the aortic valve that lead to chronic AR are inflammation (e.g., resulting from rheumatic fever, syphilis, rheumatoid arthritis), structural processes (e.g., unicuspid, bicuspid, aneurysm), disruptive processes (e.g., trauma, infective endocarditis, dissection), congenital conditions, and stress from hypertension; acute AR most commonly is a result of infective endocarditis, with dissecting aortic aneurysm and acute chest trauma being less-common causes.

PATHOPHYSIOLOGY

AR produces a volume overload to the left ventricle during diastole. In chronic AR, the slow disease progression results in increased left ventricular volume. The left ventricle adapts to the increased volume, which over time causes LVH.[4] In acute AR there is no time for this adaptation to occur. The left ventricle volume overload leads to severe pulmonary congestion and decreased cardiac output.

CLINICAL PRESENTATION AND PHYSICAL EXAMINATION

Patients with chronic AR may be asymptomatic for decades. When symptoms do occur, the patient usually reports symptoms of CHF, especially dyspnea and fatigue. Patients may also have angina in the absence of significant coronary artery disease (CAD). Patients with acute AR may have symptoms of severe left-sided heart failure (dyspnea at rest, orthopnea, paroxysmal nocturnal dyspnea, fatigue, exhaustion) that have occurred suddenly. Symptoms of low forward cardiac output (fatigue and exhaustion) are overshadowed by symptoms of pulmonary congestion in patients with acute AR.

A number of physical findings differ between acute and chronic AR. In chronic AR, the rate of rise of the peripheral pulse is rapid with quick collapse (Corrigan or water-hammer pulse) as a result of the forceful ejection of blood in early systole and regurgitation during early diastole. The carotid pulse is often bisferious. Arterial blood pressure usually demonstrates a low diastolic pressure (Korotkoff sounds may even be zero) with a normal systolic blood pressure, thus causing a widened pulse pressure in a patient with moderate or severe chronic AR. Patients with acute AI usually demonstrate a carotid arterial pulse with a sharp rise to a single, rapidly collapsing peak without a widened pulse pressure. Pulsus alternans may be present in severe acute AR, but it is unusual in patients with chronic AR. With chronic AR, the apical impulse is displaced to the left and downward and is hyperdynamic.

In patients with mild or moderate AR, a diastolic regurgitant murmur is not always auscultated.[4] The diastolic murmur of chronic regurgitation is usually high pitched and blowing, with the duration correlating best with the severity of the insufficiency. In acute AR, the murmur may be very short or even absent. A rumbling mid-diastolic or late diastolic murmur, the Austin Flint murmur, may be heard at the apex in the presence of at least moderate insufficiency. This represents functional stenosis of the mitral valve from the torrential regurgitant flow produced by the impingement of AR on the anterior mitral valve leaflet. A loud systolic ejection murmur is common in both acute and chronic AR, even in the absence of valvular stenosis. In chronic AR, hepatomegaly and ascites may be present in patients with associated heart failure.

DIAGNOSTICS

Recommendations for initial diagnostics include ECG, chest x-ray examination, and TTE with 2D imaging and Doppler studies. TTE is the standard diagnostic test for the initial evaluation of patients with suspected or known VHD.[4] The characteristic finding on ECG for a patient with chronic AR is LVH, especially in the precordial leads. Conduction disturbances may occur with AR secondary to inflammatory processes. In severe acute AR, the electrocardiographic recording is usually normal except for sinus tachycardia, without evidence of LVH.

As the severity of chronic AR increases, the left ventricular contour enlarges, producing a boot-shaped heart silhouette on the chest x-ray film. The aortic knob and ascending aorta become prominent with moderate to severe chronic AR. Patients with acute AR do not demonstrate cardiac enlargement but will exhibit increased venous redistribution to the upper lobes because of pulmonary venous and capillary hypertension secondary to an increased left ventricular end-diastolic pressure and left atrial pressure.

TTE with 2D imaging and Doppler studies provides the necessary anatomic and hemodynamic measurements for staging of AR. TTE (echocardiography combined with color Doppler imaging) confirms the presence, severity, and cause of AR.[4] Evidence of mild AR may be detected on TTE long before it is audible on auscultation. TTE may help identify possible causes of the regurgitation by documenting flail or prolapsing leaflets, a dilated aortic root, or evidence of vegetation. The greatest impact, however, is the ability of Doppler echocardiography to assess the severity of the regurgitation and assist in determining the optimum time for valve replacement, especially in the asymptomatic patient. Color Doppler imaging provides an assessment of the amount of regurgitation, which depends not only on the "size of the hole" but also on both the upstream and downstream pressures. Echocardiography is able to quantify the ventricular dimensions and ventricular function (ejection fraction). Evidence of reduction in systolic function or marked or progressive ventricular dilation is an indication for surgery.

Routine follow-up TTE is used to monitor for disease progression toward surgical intervention. Any new onset of symptoms in patients diagnosed with mild to moderate AR, such as angina or dyspnea, may indicate progression and warrants further diagnostic testing.

DIFFERENTIAL DIAGNOSIS

The murmur of AR is an early diastolic murmur that must be differentiated from other early diastolic murmurs (pulmonary regurgitation and VSD). Most early diastolic murmurs are related to either pulmonary regurgitation or AR. However, an early diastolic flow murmur can also sometimes be heard in patients with a VSD and a large left-to-right shunt.

MANAGEMENT

Appropriate management of AR requires accurate diagnosis of the cause and staging of the disease process. Clinical staging of chronic AR is determined by symptomatic status, regurgitation severity, left ventricular volume, and systolic function. Chronic AR patients who are hypertensive should be treated with calcium channel blockers, angiotensin-converting enzyme (ACE) inhibitors, or angiotensin receptor blockers (ARBs). Vasodilators are not recommended for asymptomatic patients with normal blood pressures and preserved ventricular function.[4] Medical therapy is also appropriate for symptomatic patients considered at high risk for surgery. Patient status is monitored by TTE. The frequency of monitoring is based on AR staging. It is currently recommended that symptomatic AR patients at stage C or higher undergo evaluation for surgical treatment.[4] See Box 126-1 and Chapter 123 for current recommendations for infective endocarditis.

The primary therapy for an incompetent valve is valve replacement. The critical issue is the timing of surgery. Surgery is advocated for patients based on staging and is determined by the patient's symptoms and hemodynamic function. AVR is recommended for patients in stage D (with symptoms); patients without symptoms (stage C) who have left ventricular ejection fraction (LVEF) less than 50%; and patients in stage C or D who have other cardiac surgery planned.[4] AVR should be considered in patients in moderate AR (stage B) and other cardiac surgery and in patients with AR and normal LVEF who have enlarged left ventricular size (left ventricular end-systolic dimension [LVESD] >50 mm) or progressing left ventricular enlargement (left ventricular end-diastolic dimension [LVEDD] >65 mm).[4]

DIFFERENTIAL DIAGNOSIS

Diastolic Murmurs

EARLY DIASTOLE
- Aortic insufficiency
- Pulmonary insufficiency
- VSD

MID-DIASTOLE TO LATE DIASTOLE
- Mitral stenosis
- Tricuspid stenosis
- Austin Flint murmur

Interdisciplinary Management

Interdisciplinary management is considered when the patient with AR becomes symptomatic. Management is based on staging. Patients may live for years or decades with AR before the development of symptoms. However, as with AS, once symptoms develop, progressive deterioration will occur during the next few years unless surgical intervention occurs.

COMPLICATIONS

Progressive deterioration of ventricular function is a complication. The onset of dyspnea and angina is a complication and is an indication for immediate evaluation by TTE; diagnostic results will guide the need for treatment and referral.[4]

INDICATIONS FOR REFERRAL OR HOSPITALIZATION AND PATIENT AND FAMILY EDUCATION

See Indications for Referral or Hospitalization and Patient and Family Education under Mitral Stenosis.

MITRAL REGURGITATION

DEFINITION AND EPIDEMIOLOGY

Mitral insufficiency (or MR) may result from a disturbance of any of the functional components of the mitral valve or its supporting structures, which include the valve leaflets, papillary muscle, mitral valve annulus, chordae tendineae, and left ventricle itself. Rheumatic heart disease was generally the most common cause of chronic MR. However, with the reduction in the incidence of rheumatic fever, other causes have become more prevalent, such as ischemic heart disease and MVP. Additional causes of MR, either acute or chronic, include congenital abnormalities, isolated rupture of the chordae tendineae, papillary muscle dysfunction, CAD, collagen vascular disease, and infective endocarditis.[4] Dilation of the left ventricle from any cause is likely to cause the mitral leaflets to fail to coapt. Acute regurgitation may be a result of spontaneous rupture of the chordae tendineae, blunt chest trauma, or necrotic disruption of a papillary muscle as a sequela of a myocardial infarction, most often an inferior infarct.

PATHOPHYSIOLOGY

Chronic MR is usually classified as either primary or secondary (functional). Primary refers to an abnormality of the valve or valve components (leaflets, chordae tendineae, papillary muscles, or annulus), usually seen with infectious endocarditis, connective tissue disorders, radiation cardiac disease, rheumatic heart disease, or progressive MVP.[4] Functional MR is usually caused by a damaged left ventricle (common causes are CAD, myocardial infarction), which causes deformation of a normal valve.[4] The burden placed on the heart as a result of MR is dependent on the amount of reflux and the ventricular and atrial ability to compensate. During systole, the left ventricle simultaneously ejects blood forward through the aortic valve and backward across an incompetent valve into the left atrium. The volume of mitral regurgitant flow in either chronic or acute MR therefore depends on the size of the regurgitant orifice and on the pressure gradient between the left ventricle and the left atrium, which is affected by the balance between the ease of regurgitation into the "low-pressure sump" of the left atrium and the flow out to the aorta. Regurgitant flow is decreased by any agent that decreases left ventricular size (such as diuretics) or shifts the balance toward forward output (such as afterload-reducing vasodilators). In contrast, regurgitation is increased by any factor that enlarges the left ventricle, depresses myocardial function, or increases resistance to forward flow (such as hypertension or AS). With chronic MR, the increased volume of blood ejected back into the left atrium causes stretching and thinning of the atrial wall. The large, thin-walled atrium accommodates the large volume of blood ejected into it during ventricular systole. Although the pressure in the left atrium and pulmonary capillaries and veins is elevated during systole, the left atrial pressure decreases to nearly normal during ventricular diastole. The left ventricle dilates and becomes hypertrophied in response to the increased volume from the left atrium, so that sufficient cardiac output is maintained. Initially, the additional volume to be ejected by the ventricle (increased preload) results in enhanced emptying. Therefore the ejection fraction is increased. "Normal" ejection fraction or other measures of cardiac systolic performance actually are likely to represent significantly abnormal ventricular function. Pulmonary hypertension rarely develops in the patient who has developed MR gradually over time. However, in functional MR there is long-standing left ventricular dysfunction increasing the atrial pressures, leading to increased pulmonary pressures and eventually to failure.[4]

In contrast, patients with acute MR develop a rapid increase in left atrial pressure as a result of the sudden volume overload into a normal, nondilated left atrium and ventricle. This results in suddenly increased left ventricular end-diastolic, left atrial, and pulmonary venous pressures, producing interstitial edema that leads to pulmonary congestion. Pulmonary hypertension may develop.

CLINICAL PRESENTATION AND PHYSICAL EXAMINATION

Patients with MR may have murmur. Severe MR may not cause murmur because of the equalization of left ventricular and left atrial pressures. The patient with MR may remain asymptomatic for decades. Patients typically report fatigue and, later in the course of the disease, dyspnea on exertion. The fatigue is a result of reduced forward cardiac output, whereas the dyspnea occurs with the onset of left ventricular dysfunction. The severity of symptoms and clinical outcome of chronic MR depend not only on the degree of regurgitation but also on associated additional valvular abnormalities, underlying ventricular dysfunction, and concomitant CAD. Palpitations are often noted, even in the patient without evidence of atrial fibrillation. Symptoms of CHF appear late in the course of chronic MR as a result of the gradual increase in volume overload. By the time symptoms appear, the degree of ventricular dysfunction may have progressed to such an extent as to be irreversible.

Those who develop acute MR have an abrupt onset of symptoms resulting from the sudden overload of the left atrium. A patient with rupture of a few chordae from subacute bacterial endocarditis or trauma usually reports easy fatigue, dyspnea, pedal edema, and occasionally intermittent chest pain. A patient with a complete rupture of a papillary muscle usually has severe hypotension and florid pulmonary edema. With MR, palpation of the carotid pulse typically demonstrates a rapidly rising pulse. The apical impulse is hyperkinetic and displaces downward and to the left. Auscultation of the patient with chronic MR reveals a soft S_1. A loud P_2 or an accentuated pulmonic component of S_2 suggests the presence of pulmonary hypertension. An audible S_3 is present when there is hemodynamically significant MR; in combined MS and regurgitation, S_3 is indicative of predominant regurgitation. The hallmark murmur of MR is the pansystolic, blowing murmur best heard at the apex and radiating to the axilla or back. The murmur may radiate to other locations such as the back or sternum if papillary muscle dysfunction or partial rupture of supporting structures is present. Maneuvers that decrease left ventricular volume by decreasing impedance to left ventricular outflow or venous return (such as sudden standing or inhalation of amyl nitrite) will result in a decreased murmur, as will more chronically decreasing ventricular volume with diuresis. Increasing the impedance to left ventricular ejection (asking the patient to squeeze both fists in a handgrip) will increase regurgitation and thereby the intensity of the murmur.

DIAGNOSTICS

Recommendations for initial diagnostics include ECG, chest x-ray examination, and TTE with 2D imaging and Doppler studies. TTE is the standard diagnostic test for the initial evaluation of patients with suspected or known VHD.[4] ECG in chronic MR usually demonstrates normal sinus rhythm with left atrial hypertrophy in the early stage and atrial fibrillation later. If the MR is secondary to underlying ventricular dysfunction and dilation, evidence of LVH is usually noted on ECG. The chest x-ray film demonstrates an increase in both left ventricular and left atrial size.

TTE detects the high-velocity jet of regurgitant flow back into the left atrium. It permits sensitive detection of regurgitation of even a mild degree. Although the ability to quantify the degree of the regurgitation remains imprecise, the technique permits the more important prediction of clinical outcomes. The severity can be roughly estimated by the distance the jet goes into the atrium. Chronic MR usually produces a volume overload pattern and a large left atrium. Echocardiography can detect structural abnormalities such as flail leaflets, endocarditic vegetation, and thickened, rheumatic chordae.

For patients with acute MR, accurate diagnosis and urgent intervention can be lifesaving. TTE will confirm diagnosis by visualization of the MR. In cases where TTE is not diagnostic, cardiac magnetic resonance imaging can be useful.[4]

DIFFERENTIAL DIAGNOSIS

The murmur of MR or mitral insufficiency is a pansystolic murmur. Other pansystolic murmurs include the murmurs of tricuspid regurgitation and VSD. On rare occasions, the murmur of patent ductus arteriosus can be pansystolic also. Often, if the patient is tachycardic, these murmurs are difficult to distinguish from long systolic ejection murmurs. Because pansystolic murmurs are pathologic murmurs, differentiation is essential.

MANAGEMENT

MR is a progressive disease. The management of chronic primary MR is determined by severity and the presence or absence of negative prognostic features, which include symptoms, left ventricular dysfunction and size increase, and pulmonary hypertension. Patients with MR should be referred for co-management with cardiologist at a Heart Valve Center of Excellence to establish an individualized monitoring plan.

Medical management includes beta-adrenergic blockade, ACE inhibitors or ARBs, and possibly aldosterone antagonists. These therapies aid in reducing the severity of MR in a failing heart. Vasodilator therapy is not indicated for normotensive asymptomatic patients with chronic primary MR.[4]

Asymptomatic patients with MR and normal sinus rhythm, and without atrial or left ventricular enlargement, can participate in exercise without any restrictions.[4] Patients with MR associated with pulmonary hypertension, left ventricular enlargement, or evidence of heart failure cannot engage in competitive athletic exercise.[4] See Box 126-1 and Chapter 123 for recommendations regarding infective endocarditis.

Interdisciplinary Management

Progression of MR varies with each patient, and prognosis worsens with delayed MR correction. Referral to a Heart Valve Center of Excellence for early repair or very careful surveillance is required.[4] Interdisciplinary management should be considered for patients with acute MR or once the patient with chronic MR becomes symptomatic and surgery is considered. Surgical therapy is aimed at improving symptoms, relieving severe pulmonary hypertension, and decreasing left ventricular volume and mass. The goal of treatment is to correct MR before onset of left ventricular systolic dysfunction to prevent adverse effect on patient outcomes. Mitral valve surgery should be performed when the patient's left ventricle nears but does not exceed the parameters of systolic dysfunction (LVEF ≤60% or LVESD ≥40 mm).[4]

Patients with marked left ventricular dysfunction may remain symptomatic even after surgical treatment. Such patients may show a decrease in ejection fraction and an increase in end-systolic volume immediately after surgery as the abolition of MR removes their low-pressure sump, essentially increasing the afterload that the ventricle faces. These patients may require vasodilator treatment in the immediate postoperative period and in fact may be difficult to wean off bypass. Such patients may benefit from only partial repair of the valve, leaving some regurgitation.

Surgical repair of MR is very successful for resolution of MR. Surgical techniques used to treat MR are valve repair or reconstruction and valve replacement. Valve repair, the preferred treatment, repairs the disrupted functional component of the valve. Mitral valve repair retains the tethering effect of chordal attachments, which may prevent postoperative dilation of the left ventricle and decreases the chance of left ventricular dysfunction that occurs after mitral valve replacement. Surgery recommendations are based on MR stages.[4]

LIFE SPAN CONSIDERATIONS

Life span considerations for patients with MR depend on the degree of symptoms and the status of the left ventricular function. All female patients planning a pregnancy should be referred to a cardiologist for evaluation, testing, and guidance. Patients with MR may remain asymptomatic for decades, with only a small percentage progressing to more severe MR requiring surgery.[4] Patients commonly may tolerate even significant MR for decades without development of symptoms.

COMPLICATIONS

Atrial fibrillation affects approximately 75% of patients with MR and is related to the size of the left atrium. Other complications include systemic embolization (generally in the presence of atrial fibrillation) and bacterial endocarditis.

INDICATIONS FOR REFERRAL OR HOSPITALIZATION AND PATIENT AND FAMILY EDUCATION

See Indications for Referral or Hospitalization and Patient and Family Education under Mitral Stenosis.

MITRAL VALVE PROLAPSE

DEFINITION AND EPIDEMIOLOGY

A unique subset of patients with MR, affecting 2% to 4% of the general population, consists of those with MVP.[8] Although the regurgitation is usually mild and often free of associated papillary muscle dysfunction, MVP appears to occur more often in patients with small ventricles resulting from thoracic deformities, such as the straight back syndrome or pectus excavatum. The syndrome seems to be more prevalent in women, although it has been detected in males of all ages, with men older than 45 years at increased risk for development of complications of severe MR and endocarditis.[9] Women are diagnosed earlier and more frequently than are men. Physiologically, women tend to have more valve thickening (myxomatous degeneration) and less MR. On the other hand, men tend more often to have flail leaflets and have a higher incidence of MR.[10]

PATHOPHYSIOLOGY

MVP is typically described as the posterior displacement or prolapse of one or both (more commonly the posterior) leaflets of the mitral valve into the left atrium during systole. This billowing back of the leaflet places stress on the chordae tendineae and papillary muscles, which may be the cause of the nonischemic chest discomfort. The myxomatous degeneration may, over time, result in thickened and redundant valves. As the valvular dysfunction progresses, insufficient coaptation will result in MR. The connective tissue changes may extend into the mitral anulus, enhancing the tendency for MR, and into the chordae tendineae, potentially resulting in sudden chordal rupture.

CLINICAL PRESENTATION AND PHYSICAL EXAMINATION

Most persons with MVP are asymptomatic. When symptoms do occur, the patient usually reports chest discomfort, palpitations, mild dyspnea, fatigue, and anxiety. These symptoms are similar to those reported in the panic disorder syndrome. Both disorders may be a result of autonomic dysfunction.[9] The chest symptoms, along with the tremendous frequency of this disorder in the general population, mandate familiarity with its presentation. Before the 1980s, as many as 38% of healthy teenage girls may have been misdiagnosed with MVP after auscultatory findings suggestive of this syndrome were identified on physical examination. A more valid estimate relying on newly established echocardiographic criteria developed in the 1980s would place the frequency at 2% to 3% with equal distribution among both sexes.[9] MVP should probably be thought of as a continuum from the exaggeration of the normal, slight billowing of the mitral valve into the left atrium during systole, to a fully "floppy" valve, and finally to variable degrees of MR when the floppy, redundant leaflets no longer are able to coapt. At times, the regurgitation may become severe, often as a result of the rupture of the chordae tendineae. Most commonly, the disorder exists by itself, generally in association with a characteristic pathologic myxomatous degeneration of the mitral valve. There appears to be a strong hereditary predisposition to the condition, although it may be associated with other conditions, some rare (e.g., Ehlers-Danlos syndrome) and others common (e.g., atrial septal defect). MVP has been noted in patients with CAD. The ischemic discomfort is usually described as brief attacks of severe, piercing pain localized to the apex. Palpitations are common and may result from a variety of arrhythmias.

Most cases of MVP are diagnosed on routine physical examination. Auscultation of the patient with MVP reveals a midsystolic click. This is a snapping extra heart sound heard best at the lower left sternal border or at the apex, and it may be only intermittently appreciated. The presence of an apical systolic murmur varies with the degree of MR. This systolic murmur is usually a late systolic crescendo type that can be loud and musical. Maneuvers that decrease the left ventricular volume, such as standing, will both move the click earlier in systole and make the murmur longer. Pansystolic murmurs are usually an indication of pronounced MVP resulting in a more severe form of MR.

DIAGNOSTICS

Recommendations for initial diagnostics include ECG, chest x-ray examination, and TTE with 2D imaging and Doppler studies. TTE is the standard diagnostic test for the initial evaluation of patients with suspected or known VHD.[4] Patients with MVP, most commonly those who are symptomatic, may demonstrate inverted T waves and nonspecific ST-segment changes in the inferior and left precordial leads of the electrocardiogram. These changes may be a manifestation of the ischemia to the papillary muscles resulting from the strain placed on these muscles by the prolapsed valve leaflets. Stress ECG and thallium Tl-201 or sestamibi exercise scans should be used when there is a need to differentiate MVP from CAD. This is especially important when the patient with suspected MVP complains of chest discomfort.

Supraventricular tachycardia is not uncommon in MVP. Other ventricular and supraventricular arrhythmias and conduction disturbances may also occur. There seems to be a slightly increased incidence of sudden death, presumably as a result of ventricular fibrillation, although this finding has not been firmly established.

TTE shows the posterior mitral valve leaflet or both leaflets bowing or bulging back into the left atrium during systole. Such displacement, noted solely on the four-chamber view, is now recognized as a normal finding. Patients with thickened mitral leaflet of more than 5 mm and redundant mitral valves form a higher-risk subgroup for subsequent complications.[9] Other echocardiographic findings include MR and flail leaflets in patients with ruptured chordae.

DIFFERENTIAL DIAGNOSIS

The murmur of MVP is a late systolic murmur and is characterized by a midsystolic click. This click heralds the onset of the murmur. Because it is a murmur of mitral insufficiency, it should be differentiated from the pansystolic murmur of mitral insufficiency.

MANAGEMENT

Most persons with MVP are asymptomatic and require no intervention other than periodic clinical and echocardiographic follow-up evaluation every 3 to 5 years. Asymptomatic patients need reassurance that the condition is benign and usually uncomplicated and that the prognosis is good. If a systolic murmur is present, however, the patient with MVP, even if asymptomatic, requires more frequent monitoring. Those with pansystolic murmurs are more likely to have more MR and require the same approach as noted for MR. However, even in the face of severe MR, many patients with normal ventricular ejection fraction continue to do well.[9] See Box 126-1 and Chapter 123 for recommendations regarding infective endocarditis.

Patients with a history of palpitations or prolonged QT intervals should have 24-hour ambulatory monitoring. Beta blocker therapy is often useful for palpitations or nonischemic chest pain. Patients with syncope or near-syncope should be referred for more complete arrhythmia evaluation.

Interdisciplinary Management

Interdisciplinary management and life span considerations for MVP are related to the severity of the MR and are the same as previously described for MR. Surgical treatment of MVP is necessary when the MR has been progressive and severe. Mitral reconstruction with ring annuloplasty has been successful.

COMPLICATIONS

In addition to chordal rupture and progressive MR, infective endocarditis, atrial fibrillation, and sudden death have been associated with this disorder[9]; however, their incidence remains uncertain. Most reviews have concluded that endocarditis and sudden death are rare. All of the complications are more common in men older than 50 years and those with MVP and leaflets 5 mm or greater in thickness.[4,9]

INDICATIONS FOR REFERRAL OR HOSPITALIZATION AND PATIENT AND FAMILY EDUCATION

See Indications for Referral or Hospitalization and Patient and Family Education under Mitral Stenosis.

MITRAL STENOSIS

DEFINITION AND EPIDEMIOLOGY

MS is almost always caused by rheumatic heart disease. Thus, with the marked reduction of rheumatic carditis during the past four decades, the occurrence of MS has lessened. Less-common causes of obstruction across the mitral valve that prevents normal emptying of the left atrium into the left ventricle during diastole include congenital stenoses, masses such as vegetation and clots or benign tumors (atrial myxomas), and profound calcification of the mitral anulus. Damage to the mitral valve from rheumatic fever will cause the commissures of the leaflets themselves to fuse, the leaflets to thicken and fibrose, and the chordae to thicken and shorten, resulting in a thickened, scarred valve that is funnel shaped with a "fish mouth" appearance.

PATHOPHYSIOLOGY

The central pathophysiologic feature of MS is obstruction across the mitral valve during diastole. This results in a pressure gradient between the left atrium and the left ventricle. The increased left atrial pressure is transmitted to the pulmonary veins and capillaries and eventually to the pulmonary arteries and right side of the heart. The normal mitral valve area (MVA) is 4 to 5 cm^2.[11] There is usually no detectable pressure gradient across the normal mitral valve, even when flow is increased with exercise. As the valve area is reduced, the gradient across the valve increases. When the valve area is reduced to 2.5 cm^2, hemodynamically significant stenosis is present.[11] MS usually becomes symptomatic when the mitral valve opening is reduced to 1.5 cm^2 or less.[11] With this degree of obstruction, the mean gradient, even at rest, is likely to be more than 20 mm Hg throughout diastole. With a further rise to 25 to 30 mm Hg, the left atrial pressure will exceed plasma oncotic pressure, and episodes of orthopnea or paroxysmal nocturnal dyspnea will develop. Chronic elevation of left atrial pressure produces a passive pressure load on the pulmonary vessel and causes hypertrophy and hyperplasia. In addition, there is a reactive vasoconstrictive aspect. Pulmonary hypertension may develop, which over time may produce right ventricular hypertrophy.

CLINICAL PRESENTATION AND PHYSICAL EXAMINATION

The principal symptom of MS is dyspnea, which is graded according to the New York Heart Association (NYHA) classification. Patients with asymptomatic MS are assigned to functional class I. Patients with dyspnea that occurs with greater than ordinary exertion are assigned to class II; patients with dyspnea that occurs with only mild exertion (less than ordinary activity) are assigned to class III; and those with dyspnea on minimum exertion, with episodes of orthopnea, paroxysmal nocturnal dyspnea, or pulmonary edema, are assigned to class IV.

Fatigue is also common with MS and in some cases may be more severe than the dyspnea. If atrial fibrillation develops, patients may also complain of palpitations. Hemoptysis may occur as a result of pulmonary hypertension and in rare instances may be massive.[11] Hoarseness (Ortner syndrome) may develop from compression of the left recurrent laryngeal nerve by a dilated left atrium. A small number of patients report angina-like chest pain, which may be caused by concomitant CAD, pulmonary embolus, or pulmonary hypertension. Thromboembolism may be the presenting symptom in some patients.

Auscultation will typically reveal a loud S_1, an accentuated pulmonic component of S_2 (P_2) if pulmonary hypertension is present, and an opening snap heard with the diaphragm of the stethoscope. This snap is the snapping of the thickened mitral valve as it reaches the end of its maximum excursion during early diastole. This must be distinguished from an S_3 gallop sound, which is lower in pitch and occurs later in diastole (typically 0.12 second after S_2) than the opening snap, which occurs 0.04 to 0.10 second after S_2. The classic diastolic rumble of MS is heard with the bell of the stethoscope near the apex. It begins shortly after the opening snap and may have a presystolic accentuation in patients who are still in normal sinus rhythm. The murmur may be difficult to appreciate in the early stages of MS and can be better appreciated by listening with the patient in the left lateral decubitus position or by increasing the flow by having the patient perform mild exercise. As the severity of MS increases and valve leaflets become markedly calcified, the S_1 sound will decrease in intensity while the diagnostic rumble progresses to a pandiastolic murmur.

DIAGNOSTICS

Recommendations for initial diagnostics include ECG, chest x-ray examination, and TTE with 2D imaging and Doppler studies. TTE is the standard diagnostic test for the initial evaluation of patients with suspected or known VHD.[4] The characteristic findings on ECG are evidence of left atrial enlargement (widened, notched P wave in lead II with pronounced terminal negativity in V_1) in patients still in normal sinus rhythm and evidence of right axis deviation of the QRS or right ventricular hypertrophy. Atrial fibrillation is common. Chest x-ray examination may reveal a straightening of the left-sided heart border or "double density" in the midportion of the cardiac silhouette, both of which are manifestations of left atrial enlargement. With chronic pulmonary hypertension, the pulmonary vessels become prominent, and flow redistributes fluid in the upper lobes. Chronic accumulation of transudated fluid in the interstitial spaces of the lungs and lymphatic engorgement result in linear shadows perpendicular to the pleura, which are known as Kerley B lines.

TTE quantifies the magnitude of the gradient and valve area, determining the presence of additional valvular lesions, and assessing ventricular function. M-mode echocardiography is able to demonstrate the characteristic motion of the mitral valve, which resembles a square wave. In MS, the anterior and posterior leaflets demonstrate concordant movement (both leaflets moving in concert anteriorly during diastole) as opposed to the normal discordant movement (leaflets moving in opposite directions). Two-dimensional echocardiography demonstrates the reduced excursion of the valve, with "doming" of the valve during diastole, and permits accurate assessment of the valve area by planimetry of the valve on the cross-sectional, or short-axis, view. Two-dimensional echocardiography will also assess the size of the left atrium and identify other causes of mitral obstruction, such as atrial myxoma. Doppler study not only documents the presence of regurgitation but also permits another accurate method for estimating valve area by means of either the pressure half-time technique or the continuity equation. In the presence of tricuspid regurgitation, some degree of which is almost always present, pulmonary pressure can be estimated. Coronary arteriography still may be required in adults to exclude CAD in patients with conflicting TTE and transesophageal echocardiogram (TEE) results. Exercise testing can provide information for patents whose TTE does not correspond with symptom presentation.

DIFFERENTIAL DIAGNOSIS

The murmur of MS is classified as a mid-diastolic to late diastolic murmur. Other mid-diastolic to late diastolic murmurs that should be considered in the differential diagnosis include an atrial presystolic murmur, the Austin Flint murmur, and the murmur of tricuspid stenosis.

MANAGEMENT

Medical management of MS is determined by identification of the cause and accurate staging of disease. Stages are determined by patient symptoms, valve anatomy, hemodynamics, and the effect of valve obstruction on the left atrial and pulmonary circulation. Stage A (risk of MS) has normal left atrial size and normal flow velocities with only doming of the valve during diastole.[4] Stage B (progressive) is characterized by rheumatic valve changes with commissural fusion, diastolic valve doming, MVA greater than 1.5 cm^2, and diastolic pressure half-time below 150 msec.[4] Stage C is severe, asymptomatic MS; valve changes are accompanied by MVA equal to or less than 1.5 cm^2 and diastolic pressure half-time exceeding 150 msec; with stage C and above, left atrial enlargement and elevated pulmonary artery pressures are present.[4] Stage D is termed severe symptomatic MS; the valve anatomy, hemodynamics, and valve obstruction sequelae are accompanied by decreased exercise tolerance and exertional dyspnea. Treatment of the underlying obstructive lesion of MS is an operative procedure—percutaneous mitral balloon valve commissurotomy. The disorder has multiple characteristics; shape of valve, presence of symptoms, MVA, size of left atrium, presence of left atrial thrombus, new onset of atrial fibrillation, and whether other cardiac surgery is planned are all considered when making the decision about surgical intervention to correct MS and the type of procedure that is used. Medical therapy aims include treatment of atrial fibrillation and prevention of recurrent episodes of rheumatic fever and systemic embolism. Patients who have had one episode of rheumatic fever are at risk for a second episode. Recurrent episodes of rheumatic fever are dramatically reduced with secondary prophylaxis against streptococcal infections. Anemia and infections should be promptly treated because they increase the heart rate and therefore the gradient. Similarly, occupations that demand strenuous physical exertion should be avoided by patients with more than mild MS. Patients who are symptomatic should be treated with oral diuretics and sodium restriction. See Box 126-1 and Chapter 123 for recommendations regarding infective endocarditis.

Patients with MS who have atrial fibrillation associated with ventricular dysfunction can be treated with digoxin. Other patients with MS and atrial fibrillation or who have symptoms with exercise can be treated with beta blockers or calcium channel blockers to slow the ventricular rate.[4,11]

Patients with MS in chronic atrial fibrillation are at a much higher risk of embolic events if they are not receiving anticoagulant therapy. This risk more than doubles if there has been a previous embolic episode.[10] Furthermore, it may be reasonable to consider anticoagulation for those patients found to have moderate MS by echocardiography or those with symptoms because systemic embolization is well recognized in these patients. No benefit of anticoagulation has been shown for patients in normal sinus rhythm without a prior history of embolism.

There are three procedures that have been found to be effective in the treatment of MS. These are balloon mitral valvulotomy (BMV), open commissurotomy, and valve replacement. BMV is an interventional procedure in which a large balloon is inflated across the mitral valve and the leaflets are dilated. This allows better excursion of the leaflets and a larger valve area. Degree of calcification and regurgitation, valve morphology, and presence of thrombi in the atrium are considerations in determining the type of surgical intervention needed.[4] Open commissurotomy is attempted to repair the valve. If the valve cannot be repaired, a valve replacement is performed. Because atrial fibrillation is so common in patients with MS, a surgical ablation can be performed during surgery, thus eliminating possible thrombotic complications.[4]

Interdisciplinary Management and Life Span Considerations

Interdisciplinary management is necessary. Consultation with or referral to a Heart Valve Center of Excellence is recommended to discuss treatment options for asymptomatic patients with severe VHD and patients who may benefit from valve repair or replacement.[4] Consultation should occur when the diagnosis is unclear or when cardioversion, surgery, or balloon valvuloplasty is being considered.

COMPLICATIONS

Patients with MS are at risk for thromboembolization. An additional complication is severe pulmonary hypertension. This, in turn, could lead to tricuspid regurgitation because of atrial dilation. The possibility of having to repair or replace both valves should be considered if MS surgery is contemplated.

INDICATIONS FOR REFERRAL OR HOSPITALIZATION

Any patient with VHD requires cardiology referral. Consultation with or referral to a Heart Valve Center of Excellence is recommended to discuss treatment options for asymptomatic patients with severe VHD and patients who may benefit from valve repair or replacement.[4] Hospitalization for cardiac catheterization, balloon angioplasty, or surgical intervention may be necessary. Patients with acute bacterial endocarditis require intravenous antibiotics. Hospitalization may also be required for the management of complications, such as heart failure or pulmonary edema.

PATIENT AND FAMILY EDUCATION

Patients with valvular disorders, whether from a stenotic valve or regurgitant valve, require basic knowledge of their condition to prevent complications. Patients are told to immediately report the development of or any change in their symptoms, such as fatigue, dyspnea, weight gain, rapid heart beat, or chest discomfort, because a change in or onset of symptoms can signify disease progression. All female patients with MS planning a pregnancy should be evaluated by a cardiologist to determine needed testing and management guidelines. The patient's medication regimen should be explained and its importance reinforced at every visit. The indications for antibiotic prophylaxis have changed; new indications for antibiotic prophylaxis before instrumentation procedures should be discussed with patients and a mutually satisfactory decision made in this challenging area.

REFERENCES

For a full list of references, scan the QR code or visit http://booksite.elsevier.com/9780323355018

PART 12

Evaluation and Management of Gastrointestinal Disorders

CHAPTER 127

ABDOMINAL PAIN AND INFECTIONS

Terry Mahan Buttaro

DEFINITION AND EPIDEMIOLOGY

Abdominal pain is a common reason patients seek care in primary care offices, urgent care centers, and emergency rooms. Gastrointestinal discomfort is also a challenging condition to diagnose because the pain can be related to abdominal gas or a more serious condition requiring emergency care.[1] There are many causes of abdominal pain, and the patient's description of the discomfort may be vague, but for any patient reporting abdominal discomfort, the health care provider's first priority is to determine whether the patient's pain is the result of an acute abdomen, indicating an emergency referral.[1]

PATHOPHYSIOLOGY AND CLINICAL PRESENTATION

There are several major mechanisms of abdominal pain, including pain from obstruction of a hollow viscus, capsular distention, peritoneal irritation, mucosal ulceration, vascular insufficiency, altered body motility, nerve injury, abdominal wall injury, and pain referred from an extra-abdominal site. Determination of the specific type of pain gives a provider valuable information about the possible cause of the pain. Abdominal wall pain is often described as a constant achy feeling. Visceral pain, the pain arising from a hollow viscus, is usually the result of distention or spasm of a hollow organ, as in early intestinal obstruction; it is commonly described as dull and crampy and is poorly localized. Parietal pain is a sharp, well-localized pain arising from irritation of the parietal peritoneum, such as the pain of acute appendicitis with inflammation spread to the peritoneum. Referred pain is an aching type of pain experienced away from the disease process and is perceived to be near the surface of the body. The pain referral phenomenon is a result of the shared central pathways for afferent neurons from different locations (e.g., pain from an inflamed gallbladder may be felt in the right scapula[1]).

Location of the abdominal pain is another factor that can aid in identifying the cause of the patient's discomfort. Pain localized to the right upper abdominal quadrant generally emanates from the chest cavity, liver, gallbladder, stomach, bowel, or right kidney or ureter. Left upper quadrant pain is usually associated with the heart or chest cavity, spleen, stomach, pancreas (especially acute pancreatitis), or left kidney or ureter. The source of left lower abdominal pain can include the bowel, left ureter, or pelvis and is most commonly associated with diverticulitis, particularly when the pain is protracted and severe.[2] Right lower quadrant pain is associated with the appendix, bowel, right ureter, or pelvis, with the most common diagnosis being appendicitis. Cholecystitis or peptic ulcer perforation also must be considered. Pain that migrates across several quadrants is typically associated with the bowel, whereas abdominal wall pain from trauma or inflammation can occur in any quadrant.

In some patients, abdominal pain can be subtle and the diagnosis obscure. This is particularly true in older adults, who are less likely than younger ones to have a fever or pain and more likely to be hypotensive, lethargic, or confused.[3]

Lower abdominal or pelvic discomfort in females can suggest a gynecologic problem (e.g., an ovarian cyst). In women of childbearing age, even those with a history of tubal ligation, abdominal pain, or abnormal vaginal bleeding, it is imperative to perform a pregnancy test to exclude the possibility of ectopic pregnancy.[4]

An accurate diagnosis in patients complaining of acute abdominal pain is highly dependent on history, physical examination, and appropriate laboratory and radiologic procedures. Previous abdominal surgery, medication history (including over-the-counter drugs, vitamins, and supplements), allergies, social and sexual history, last menstrual period, dietary history, last food or fluid ingested, and family history of abdominal pain are important considerations that should be elicited. Causes of acute abdominal pain include appendicitis, cholecystitis, diverticulitis, small bowel obstruction, perforated peptic ulcer, peritonitis, ruptured ectopic pregnancy, pelvic inflammatory disease, ruptured abdominal aortic aneurysm (AAA), hypercalcemia, superior mesenteric artery syndrome, and acute intermittent porphyria.[5-7] In female patients, it is important to obtain a sexual history and to consider pelvic inflammatory disease. It is also essential to remember that acute diseases of the chest, including myocardial infarction, congestive heart failure, pulmonary infarction, and pneumonia, may mimic primary diseases of the abdomen.

Specialist referral is indicated for suspected gastrointestinal bleeding, bowel obstruction, orthostatic vital sign changes, abnormal findings, jaundice, positive pregnancy test result, severe localized or unilateral lower abdominal pain, or a history of trauma and any indication of peritoneal irritation.

APPENDICITIS

DEFINITION AND EPIDEMIOLOGY

Acute appendicitis is an inflammatory disease of the wall of the appendix that may result in perforation with subsequent peritonitis. In the United States, appendicitis affects about 300,000 people yearly, often resulting in emergency surgery.[8]

PATHOPHYSIOLOGY

Appendicitis is primarily thought to be caused by the blockage of the appendiceal lumen, leading to distention of the appendix as a result of accumulated intramural fluid with secondary bacterial infection. Acute appendicitis is described as simple, gangrenous, or perforated on the basis of operative findings. In simple appendicitis, the appendix is viable and intact. Gangrenous appendicitis is characterized by necrosis of the appendiceal wall. Perforated appendicitis refers to disruption of the appendix. Acute appendicitis is thought to be secondary to obstruction of its orifice, with secondary bacterial infection.[9]

When the appendiceal lumen becomes obstructed, the mucosa continues to secrete fluid until the intraluminal pressure exceeds venous pressure. At this point, the appendix becomes hypoxic, the mucosa ulcerates, and bacteria invade the wall. Infection causes additional swelling and ischemia as a result of thrombosis of small intramural vessels.[9] Gangrene and perforation usually develop in 24 to 36 hours. Perforation leads to a release of the luminal contents into the peritoneal cavity.

CLINICAL PRESENTATION

The most reliable historical feature in the diagnosis of acute appendicitis is the sequence of symptoms. The three signs and symptoms most predictive of acute appendicitis include pain that starts in the epigastrium or periumbilical area, migration of the pain to the right lower quadrant, and abdominal rigidity.[6,9] The pain can be diffuse or occur at other sites in the abdomen, including the left lower quadrant.[6] Another predictor is the duration of the pain; patients with appendicitis have been shown to have pain of a shorter duration than that of patients with other disorders.[10]

Anorexia, nausea or vomiting, constipation, or rarely diarrhea accompanied by low-grade fever follows the onset of pain. Not all patients will have every symptom; however, when the symptoms occur in any other order, the diagnosis of appendicitis should be questioned.[6,10]

PHYSICAL EXAMINATION

The diagnosis of acute appendicitis requires a careful history and a thorough physical examination (including a pelvic examination for female patients). Often the symptoms are subacute and nonspecific; crampy abdominal discomfort that comes and goes, some malaise, and possibly a change in bowel habits occur initially.[1] Anorexia and nausea are quite common, with the latter occurring after the pain onset; vomiting is possible.[1] A fever is usually present. In some patients diarrhea and urinary symptoms are possible.[1] Abdominal tenderness is elicited by asking the patient to cough. Localized tenderness is a valuable physical finding, and the patient can often specify the painful spot with one finger. By systematically performing a thorough abdominal examination starting in the upper abdomen in an area without pain and ending in the area of pain, localized tenderness can be determined, usually in the right lower quadrant between the umbilicus and the anterosuperior iliac spine (McBurney point). The Rovsing sign (right lower quadrant pain) is elicited by palpating the left lower quadrant.[1] There may be signs of peritoneal irritation, including guarding, rebound tenderness, and obturator sign (elicited by passive rotation of the right leg with the patient supine and the right hip and knee flexed) and psoas sign (the supine patient raises the straightened right leg against resistance by the practitioner). A rectal examination is necessary and may reveal tenderness or a mass.

DIAGNOSTICS

Acute appendicitis is suggested by the history and physical examination findings. An elevated white blood cell count is present in 70% to 90% of patients with acute appendicitis. The health care provider should immediately refer a patient with suspected appendicitis for surgical consultation. Elevated white blood cell count is present in 70% of patients with acute appendicitis; a left shift is present 95% of the time.[1] A serum beta-human chorionic gonadotropin (β-hCG) level should be obtained in women of childbearing age because appendicitis is common in pregnancy and it is necessary to exclude a ruptured ectopic pregnancy. Serum amylase and lipase levels are necessary. Sickle cell disease should be excluded in patients of African, Indian, Mediterranean, or Spanish descent.[1] A C-reactive protein level is also necessary, as is a urinalysis.

Imaging studies are not required in most cases of suspected appendicitis. However, imaging modalities may be necessary if the presentation is atypical or in patients at the extremes of age. Plain abdominal radiographs show nonspecific signs and are not recommended. Ultrasonographic evidence of appendicitis includes appendiceal wall thickening, luminal distention, and lack of compressibility. Ultrasound is useful in children and in pregnant women and if the cause of the discomfort seems gynecologic, although, in general, ultrasound can be limited by operator skill and interpretation. A computed tomography (CT) scan is most useful for diagnosis if the cause of the abdominal pain is unclear.[1]

DIAGNOSTICS

Appendicitis

LABORATORY	IMAGING
CBC and differential	Ultrasound*
C-reactive protein	CT scan*
Serum β-hCG*	
Sickeldex test*	**OTHER**
Urinalysis	Laparoscopy or laparotomy*

*If indicated.

DIFFERENTIAL DIAGNOSIS

Conditions that mimic acute appendicitis include gastroenteritis, mesenteric lymphadenitis, acute salpingitis, mittelschmerz, ruptured ectopic pregnancy, ruptured corpus luteum cyst, ureteral colic, Meckel diverticulitis, sigmoid diverticulitis, perforated peptic ulcer, cholecystitis, intestinal obstruction, cecal diverticulitis, intestinal ischemia, and perforated colonic carcinoma. Basilar pneumonia may also be confused with appendicitis.

MANAGEMENT

Abdominal discomfort in older patients should always be evaluated and appropriate treatment initiated. Treatment of appendicitis is usually a prompt appendectomy, preferably within 24 hours of symptom onset to prevent perforation and peritonitis. In patients with uncomplicated appendicitis, antibiotic therapy is a possible option, though controversial because appendicitis can recur.[11]

DIFFERENTIAL DIAGNOSIS

Appendicitis

- Gastroenteritis
- Mesenteric lymphadenitis
- Acute salpingitis
- Mittelschmerz
- Ruptured ectopic pregnancy
- Ruptured corpus luteum
- Ureteral colic
- Meckel diverticulitis
- Sigmoid diverticulitis
- Perforated peptic ulcer
- Cholecystitis
- Intestinal obstruction
- Cecal diverticulitis
- Perforated colonic carcinoma
- Basilar pneumonia
- Pyelonephritis
- Intestinal obstruction
- Ureteral calculus
- Salpingitis, pelvic inflammatory disease
- Ruptured corpus luteum cyst
- Endometriosis
- Regional enteritis (Crohn disease)

If surgery is required, patients should have nothing by mouth and intravenous fluid and electrolyte repletion initiated as necessary. Perioperative systemic antibiotics, such as metronidazole and ceftizoxime, have been shown to prevent wound infection in simple appendicitis. If the appendix is perforated, antibiotic therapy to cover anaerobic as well as aerobic pathogens is initially indicated until culture results are available. Antibiotics are also indicated for patients with suspected septicemia and patients scheduled for laparoscopic surgery. Surgery for an appendiceal abscess may spread a localized infection to other parts of the peritoneal cavity; therefore, percutaneous CT-guided drainage of an abscess is used to allow the acute inflammation to resolve before elective appendectomy is performed.[12]

COMPLICATIONS

Complications of appendicitis include gangrene, perforation with peritonitis, and abscess formation. Pylephlebitis, which is septic thrombophlebitis of the portal venous system, should be suspected in any patient with appendicitis who has shaking chills. Septicemia, urinary retention and infection, small bowel obstruction, and mesenteric thrombophlebitis may also occur. Common complications associated with appendectomy include wound infection, pneumonia, intraperitoneal abscesses, enterocutaneous fistulas, wound or inguinal hernias, and possibly minor bleeding.

INDICATIONS FOR REFERRAL OR HOSPITALIZATION

Immediate surgical referral or a transfer to the emergency department is indicated for suspected appendicitis or other acute abdominal pain. Hospitalization is indicated for monitoring and surgical care, if necessary.

PATIENT AND FAMILY EDUCATION

Patients must understand that abdominal pain may be a sign of serious illness or may be related to a chronic disorder. Localized abdominal pain or pain that increases in severity warrants discussion with the health care provider. Patients must also understand that abdominal pain accompanied by fever, chills, severe vomiting or diarrhea, significant rectal bleeding, black and tarry stools, weakness, or dizziness requires a visit to the health care provider.

Families of older patients should understand that pain perception may be diminished; the associated delay in presentation results in more than 30% of older adults with appendicitis having perforation at presentation.[13] In older adults, any of the previously listed symptoms, even if unaccompanied by abdominal pain, should be evaluated by a medical professional.[14]

SMALL BOWEL OBSTRUCTION

DEFINITION AND EPIDEMIOLOGY

Small bowel obstruction, a common cause of acute diffuse abdominal pain, refers to either a partial or complete obstruction of the bowel lumen or paralysis (ileus) of the intestinal musculature. As a result, fluid and gas accumulate proximal to the obstruction, causing nausea, vomiting, abdominal distention, and pain. It is essential to recognize bowel obstruction because it can cause vascular compromise, bowel ischemia, and peritonitis. Adhesions, hernias, and tumors are the most common causes of small bowel obstruction, although other conditions, such as fecal impaction, ischemia, abscesses, inflammatory bowel disease, volvulus, intussusception, strictures, and radiation enteritis, can also be responsible.[15] Ileus is associated with abdominal surgery; abdominal and other infectious processes (e.g., pneumonia, sepsis); electrolyte disorders; and medications (e.g., anticholinergics, calcium channel blockers, narcotics, tricyclics, and other drugs).[16]

PATHOPHYSIOLOGY

In a bowel obstruction, distention results in decreased absorption and increased secretions that cause further distention and fluid and electrolyte imbalances. Bacterial proliferation may occur as a result of stasis. Distention increases the risk of bowel perforation and diffuse peritonitis. Mechanical obstruction of the bowel lumen may occur from lesions (e.g., adhesions; congenital, inflammatory, or neoplastic lesions), femoral or indirect inguinal hernia, polypoid tumors, intussusception, volvulus, gallstone ileus, impacted feces, or bezoar formation.[17] Intussusception, often recognized as an abdominal mass on examination with a history of acute symptom onset, occurs when a bowel segment telescopes into the adjacent bowel, resulting in symptoms of intermittent bowel obstruction. Volvulus results from abnormal twisting of a bowel segment along its mesenteric axis.

CLINICAL PRESENTATION

Bowel obstruction manifests with intermittent and crampy abdominal pain, vomiting, obstipation, abdominal distention, hyperactive bowel sound, and fever. The pain is usually relieved by vomiting, intestinal tube decompression, or the passage of intestinal contents through a partial obstruction. Pain that progresses in severity, localizes, or becomes constant demonstrates progression to a strangulated obstruction; this condition requires urgent surgery. The presentation of a patient with ileus differs slightly in that bowel sounds are more frequently decreased or absent.[16]

A careful history of the chronicle of the illness, the patient's medication history, the last bowel movement, and the presence of flatus is necessary. A prior history of bowel obstructions, abdominal irradiation, abdominal inflammation or cancer, or abdominal or pelvic operations should be identified because these conditions are all associated with bowel obstructions.

PHYSICAL EXAMINATION

For any patient with an intestinal obstruction, the provider must pay attention to the patient's general appearance and vital signs. A fever suggests an infectious process, whereas hypovolemia is associated with tachycardia and orthostatic hypotension. The physical examination should determine whether the patient's symptoms are related to a nonabdominal cause (e.g., pneumonia, myocardial infarction) or an abdominal process. A distended, tympanic abdomen accompanied by peristaltic rushes and high-pitched tinkling sounds may be present initially, but bowel sounds may be absent as the disorder progresses. Diffuse midabdominal tenderness is common; localized tenderness, abdominal guarding, rebound tenderness, and rigidity are concerning signs. The rectal examination may reveal stool, masses, tenderness, or occult blood. Particular attention needs to be placed on examination of potential hernial orifices, especially the area of the femoral ring because of its small opening and potential for bowel strangulation.[5]

DIAGNOSTICS

A small bowel obstruction can be diagnosed with plain radiography or ultrasound, although an abdominal CT is often used and is indicated if an abdominal infection or mechanical obstruction is suspected and to determine the underlying cause of the obstruction.[16] If x-rays are appropriate, upright and supine views of the abdomen and an upright view of the chest are necessary. The upright abdominal film identifies a distended bowel proximal to the obstruction in addition to air-fluid levels. It may show free air if perforation has occurred. The supine radiograph may distinguish between ileus and obstruction. If an ileus is present, the radiograph will show distended loops in both the large and small bowel; with an obstruction, the segment proximal to the obstruction is distended, and the distal bowel loops are decreased in caliber. Diagnostic evaluation should determine the presence of intraperitoneal masses, ascites, gallstones, renal calculi, foreign bodies, and gas within the bowel wall, portal venous system, or biliary tree and may require magnetic resonance imaging (MRI).[18]

Laboratory data usually reflect a progressively increasing white blood cell count and electrolyte abnormalities. Other diagnostics include a urinalysis and, if indicated, a lactate dehydrogenase test and liver panel.[17] Serum β-hCG should be measured to exclude pregnancy in women of childbearing age.

DIAGNOSTICS

Small Bowel Obstruction

LABORATORY	IMAGING
CBC and differential	Abdominal x-ray studies (upright and supine) *
Serum electrolytes, blood urea nitrogen (BUN), creatinine	Chest x-ray studies*
Liver panel*	CT scan*
Lactate dehydrogenase*	MRI*
Serum β-hCG (in women of childbearing age)	Transabdominal ultrasound*

*If indicated.

DIFFERENTIAL DIAGNOSIS

The differential diagnosis of small bowel obstruction includes appendicitis, constipation, gastroenteritis, pancreatitis, paralytic ileus, intestinal perforation, ischemic colitis, inflammatory bowel disease, mesenteric thrombosis, and retroperitoneal hemorrhage. Addison disease, poisoning, diabetes mellitus, ovarian torsion, and tertiary syphilis (e.g., tabetic crisis) may also mimic small bowel obstruction.[19]

DIFFERENTIAL DIAGNOSIS

Small Bowel Obstruction

- Gastroenteritis
- Paralytic ileus
- Intestinal perforation
- Ischemic colitis
- Idiopathic inflammatory bowel disease
- Mesenteric thrombosis
- Retroperitoneal hemorrhage
- Addison disease
- Poisoning
- Diabetes mellitus
- Tertiary syphilis

MANAGEMENT

Suspected small bowel obstruction requires immediate hospitalization and consultation with a surgeon. Initial management of bowel obstruction includes restriction of all oral intakes, intravenous fluid therapy, electrolyte and acid-base correction, and optimization of cardiopulmonary and renal function; an antiemetic can be administered for systemic relief. Nasogastric tube for decompression may be necessary in some situations.[15] Urgent laparotomy is required if the patient does not respond to supportive care or has advanced illness, ischemia, or perforation. Otherwise, patients can be observed with serial physical examinations and radiographs. Antibiotic therapy is usually not indicated. However, broad-spectrum intravenous antibiotics are indicated in cases of strangulated bowel or as an adjunct to surgery.[15]

COMPLICATIONS

A bowel obstruction may progress to bowel ischemia. Physical and diagnostic signs of ischemic bowel include fever, severe and continuous pain, hematemesis, peritoneal signs, hypotension, gas in the bowel wall or portal vein, abdominal free air, and acidosis.

INDICATIONS FOR REFERRAL OR HOSPITALIZATION AND PATIENT AND FAMILY EDUCATION

See Indications for Referral or Hospitalization and Patient and Family Education under Appendicitis.

PERFORATED PEPTIC ULCER

DEFINITION AND EPIDEMIOLOGY

The prevalence of peptic ulcer disease (PUD) in the United States is decreasing, largely because of proton pump inhibitor therapy and treatment of *Helicobacter pylori* infection. However, peptic ulcer perforation still occurs and is a life-threatening complication that occurs more commonly with duodenal ulcers than with gastric ulcers.[20] Perforation may lead to a free perforation into the peritoneal cavity or perforation of an adjacent organ such as the pancreas, with resulting peritonitis or pancreatitis. Factors that predispose a patient to peptic ulcers are *H. pylori* infections, medications (e.g., aspirin, bisphosphonates, nonsteroidal anti-inflammatory drugs, potassium chloride), gastric malignancy, tobacco abuse, and hypersecretory states such as Zollinger-Ellison syndrome.

PATHOPHYSIOLOGY

Peptic ulcer perforations can be classified as (1) those in which the luminal contents freely escape into the peritoneal cavity and (2) those in which the penetration is sealed by surrounding structures of peritoneum.[21] Because the anterior walls of the stomach and duodenum are not defended by contiguous tissue, ulcers in these locations are more likely to be complicated by free perforation, which leads to generalized peritonitis and the accumulation of air in the abdominal cavity.[21] Posterior gastric ulcers perforate into the lesser peritoneal sac, where the inflammatory reaction may be contained and form an intra-abdominal abscess. Ulcers may also penetrate into the pancreas, liver, or greater omentum and cause intractable symptoms.

CLINICAL PRESENTATION

The most common presentation of a perforated peptic ulcer is the abrupt onset of severe abdominal pain followed rapidly by peritoneal signs.[6] Pain begins in the epigastrium and spreads rapidly throughout the abdomen with frequent early radiation of pain to the scapular areas. Vomiting of coffee-ground emesis, hematemesis, or melena or hematochezia occurs in some patients. The abruptness, severity, and rapid progression of symptoms lead the patient to seek prompt medical attention. Clinically, patients often demonstrate signs of improvement, such as decreased pain and vomiting, 6 to 12 hours after perforation. However, peritoneal signs remain and the clinical improvement does not last long, and the patient can then become obviously ill within several hours.

PHYSICAL EXAMINATION

In some patients, especially older adults, the pain may be absent or slight. The patient may have a history of abdominal discomfort and at presentation usually complains of severe upper abdominal tenderness, especially in the epigastric region. The pain of peptic ulcer perforation is accompanied by boardlike rigidity of the abdomen.[20] Tachycardia is common, as is orthostasis if vomiting or bleeding occurs.[20] Continued spilling of gastric and intestinal contents into the peritoneum causes chemical peritonitis and subsequent hypovolemia with the development of progressive hypotension and fever.[22]

DIAGNOSTICS

Perforation is suggested by the history and physical examination. The suspected diagnosis is confirmed by the detection of pneumoperitoneum on upright abdominal or chest x-ray films. A left lateral decubitus radiograph usually demonstrates air over the liver. Perforation is also confirmed with upper gastrointestinal contrast with water-soluble contrast medium; extravasation of contrast material is evidence of perforation.[22] When the diagnosis is suspected and the x-ray studies are normal, the diagnosis may be confirmed by endoscopy. Laboratory tests include a complete blood count (CBC) with differential; serum electrolyte values; blood urea nitrogen (BUN), creatinine, and serum amylase levels; *H. pylori* testing and urea breath test; and stool specimen for occult blood. A serum β-hCG measurement is necessary for women of childbearing age.

DIAGNOSTICS

Perforated Peptic Ulcer

LABORATORY
- CBC and differential
- Serum electrolytes, BUN, creatinine
- Serum amylase
- Stool for occult blood
- *H. pylori*
- Serum β-hCG (in women of childbearing age)

IMAGING
- Abdominal x-ray studies (upright, left lateral decubitus)

OTHER DIAGNOSTICS
- Endoscopy
- Urea breath test

DIFFERENTIAL DIAGNOSIS

The differential diagnosis of a perforated peptic ulcer includes acute pancreatitis, acute cholecystitis, perforated acute appendicitis, colonic diverticulitis, intestinal obstruction, ruptured ectopic pregnancy, and postemetic esophageal rupture. Myocardial infarction may also mimic a perforated peptic ulcer.

DIFFERENTIAL DIAGNOSIS

Perforated Peptic Ulcer

- Acute pancreatitis
- Acute cholecystitis
- Perforated appendix
- Colonic diverticulitis
- Myocardial infarction
- Intestinal obstruction
- Perforated colon

MANAGEMENT

Immediate hospitalization and consultation with a gastroenterologist and, if indicated, surgeon are essential. Endoscopy is effective in some situations,[23] but surgery may be necessary for patients in whom the bleeding is not controlled and who are hemodynamically unstable, show signs of peritonitis, or have free extravasation of contrast material on upper gastrointestinal studies.[24] Management includes intravenous fluid resuscitation, correction of electrolyte abnormalities, and continuous nasogastric suction for decompression. Intravenous proton pump inhibitors and broad-spectrum antibiotics are also required. Blood transfusions may be necessary in the presence of hemorrhage. Early suspicion, recognition, and endoscopic or surgical repair are the keys to survival and decreased morbidity.[23,24]

COMPLICATIONS

Despite the widespread use of H_2 blockers and proton pump inhibitors, the mortality rate of patients with perforated peptic ulcers continues to be significant, especially in older patients.[8] Vitamin deficiencies and dumping syndrome are possible surgical complications.[21]

INDICATIONS FOR REFERRAL OR HOSPITALIZATION AND PATIENT AND FAMILY EDUCATION

See Indications for Referral or Hospitalization and Patient and Family Education under Appendicitis.

PERITONITIS

DEFINITION AND EPIDEMIOLOGY

Spontaneous bacterial peritonitis refers to an ascetic fluid infection in the absence of a clear precipitating factor, such as a perforated viscus. The most common cause of primary spontaneous bacterial peritonitis in adults is cirrhosis complicated by variceal hemorrhage and ascites.[25] Secondary peritonitis refers to spillage of gastrointestinal or genitourinary microorganisms into the peritoneal space and is most often the result of peritoneal dialysis or a perforated viscus (e.g., acute pancreatitis, appendicitis, diverticulitis, cholecystitis, perforated gastric or duodenal ulcer) or penetrating wounds of the bowel.[25] In these instances, a secondary infection may occur as either generalized peritonitis or a localized abscess.

PATHOPHYSIOLOGY

Primary peritonitis is thought to result from a hematogenous and lymphogenous spread of bacteria through an intact gut wall from the intestinal lumen. The gut wall is thought to be more permeable to bacterial translocation because of wall edema from portal hypertension. In patients with cirrhosis, microorganisms removed from circulation by the liver may not be properly phagocytosed by impaired liver macrophages and thus contaminate hepatic lymph and pass into the ascitic fluid. Portosystemic shunting also diminishes hepatic clearance of microorganisms, which perpetuates bacteremia and increases the potential for ascitic fluid infection.[21] Enteric microorganisms account for the majority of pathogens in patients with cirrhosis. *Escherichia coli* is the most commonly identified pathogen, but viridans streptococci, *Staphylococcus aureus, Klebsiella,* and enterococci have also been identified.[25] Primary bacterial peritonitis is almost exclusively monomicrobial; if multiple organisms are identified, the diagnosis should be questioned and other sources of infection sought, such as perforated viscus.[26]

CLINICAL PRESENTATION

Many patients have a high fever and acute abdominal pain that can be diffuse, localized, or referred. Patients with cirrhosis may not complain of pain; a temperature higher than 37.7° C (100° F) may be the only manifestation of peritoneal infection.[27] Additional complaints include diffuse abdominal pain, tenderness, nausea, vomiting, and diarrhea or constipation.

PHYSICAL EXAMINATION

Abdominal distention, rigidity, decreased bowel sounds, diffuse abdominal tenderness, rebound tenderness, and guarding are prominent physical examination findings. Fever, tachycardia, tachypnea, and hypotension may also be present. Rectal examination may reveal tenderness if abscesses occur near this area.

DIAGNOSTICS

The diagnosis of peritonitis should be suspected on the basis of fever, abdominal pain and tenderness, and leukocytosis. Initially, a chest and abdominal x-ray study, CBC and differential, and serum electrolyte values with BUN and creatinine levels may be obtained in the primary care setting. Suspected peritonitis, especially that accompanied by decreasing bowel sounds, increasing tenderness, and rebound tenderness, warrants a laparotomy for confirmation of the diagnosis. Hospitalization and consultation with an internist, gastroenterologist, and surgeon are therefore required.

Patients with cirrhosis and spontaneous bacterial peritonitis should be diagnosed on the basis of the clinical appearance, presence of ascites, and ascitic fluid analysis, not by laparotomy.[28] Patients with ascites require a paracentesis in the hospital setting with peritoneal fluid analysis for cell count, differential, protein concentration, and Gram stain and culture.[19] The diagnosis of primary bacterial peritonitis requires more than 250 to 500 white blood cells/mm^3 in the ascitic fluid, with more than 50% of them being polymorphonuclear neutrophils.[29] More than 500 white blood cells/mm^3 indicates a possible perforated viscus.[30] The ascitic fluid analysis will typically show a neutrophil count greater than 250/mL, low protein concentration, pH of less than 7.35, and a lactate concentration of more than 25 mg/dL.[26,29] In primary bacterial peritonitis, 30% to 50% of ascites fluid cultures are negative.[30] When a suspected intra-abdominal abscess is present, CT- or ultrasound-guided aspiration is indicated.[26]

DIAGNOSTICS

Peritonitis

LABORATORY	OTHER DIAGNOSTICS
CBC and differential	Chest x-ray studies
Serum electrolytes	Kidney, ureter, and bladder (KUB) studies
BUN, creatinine	CT scan
Ascitic fluid analysis*	Laparotomy or endoscopy*
Serum β-hCG (in women of childbearing age)	Ultrasound-guided aspiration, if indicated

*If indicated.

DIFFERENTIAL DIAGNOSIS

Diseases that may mimic peritonitis include pancreatitis, appendicitis, diverticulitis, gastroenteritis, salpingitis, ischemic colitis, or other abdominal infection. Pneumonia and secondary causes of peritonitis should also be considered, including perforated duodenal or gastric ulcer, small bowel infarction or perforation, large bowel perforation, and cholecystitis with or without perforation or pericholecystic abscess.

DIFFERENTIAL DIAGNOSIS

Peritonitis

- Pancreatitis
- Appendicitis
- Diverticulitis
- Gastroenteritis
- Salpingitis
- Ischemic colitis
- Perforated duodenal ulcer
- Perforated gastric ulcer
- Small or large bowel perforation
- Cholecystitis
- Ruptured ectopic pregnancy
- Pneumonia
- Acute granulomatous peritonitis
- Chylous ascites
- Mesenteric lipodystrophy

MANAGEMENT

With primary bacterial peritonitis, the peritoneal fluid Gram stain is often negative; therefore, antibiotic therapy is usually empirical and is based on the most likely pathogens.[27,29] Current empirical therapy recommendations for primary bacterial peritonitis include a third- or fourth-generation cephalosporin or a quinolone until culture results are available.[29] Antimicrobial therapy should be continued for those patients in whom peritoneal cultures are sterile but there is a strong suspicion of primary bacterial peritonitis.[29] Clinical improvement and a decline in the ascitic fluid leukocyte count (<250/mm^3) should occur after 24 to 48 hours of antimicrobial therapy; a failure to respond to therapy should prompt investigation for other pathologic conditions. Fluid resuscitation and careful monitoring of vital signs and fluid balance are critical. A nasogastric tube may be necessary. Patients with secondary bacterial peritonitis may require surgical management and will require metronidazole in addition to ertapenem or another carbapenem.[29] A β-lactam/β-lactamase combination can be substituted for the carbapenem in the treatment of secondary bacterial peritonitis.[29]

Preventive treatment in patients with cirrhotic ascites is recommended to reduce the incidence of spontaneous bacterial peritonitis. Prophylaxis may not change the mortality rate for cirrhotic patients, which is related to their underlying hepatic dysfunction.[26]

COMPLICATIONS

Primary peritonitis is an ominous sign in the cirrhotic patient. Renal failure, recurrent gastrointestinal bleeding, and liver failure are potential concerns that increase morbidity and mortality.

INDICATIONS FOR REFERRAL OR HOSPITALIZATION AND PATIENT AND FAMILY EDUCATION

See Indications for Referral or Hospitalization and Patient and Family Education under Appendicitis.

RUPTURED AORTIC ANEURYSM

DEFINITION AND EPIDEMIOLOGY

An AAA is an abnormal dilation of the abdominal aorta that may rupture and cause exsanguination into the peritoneum.[6] Most aneurysms are diagnosed on routine examination and do not rupture[5]; when they do rupture, the mortality rate is high. In 2009, almost 11,000 people (mostly men) died from a ruptured aortic aneurysm.[31] Fortunately, screening and risk management recommendations have decreased the prevalence of this potentially fatal disorder.[32]

Most AAAs are atherosclerotic in origin. Risk factors for AAA include atherosclerosis, hypertension, peripheral vascular disease, smoking (90% of patients with aortic aneurysm have used tobacco), male gender, advancing age, Marfan syndrome, and Ehlers-Danlos syndrome.[31]

PATHOPHYSIOLOGY

The pathogenesis of most dissecting AAAs is atherosclerosis; the common underlying defect is vessel wall weakness secondary to continued stress on wall of the aorta and a lack of infiltrative vasa vasorum in the media layer.[32] The focal loss of elastic and muscle fibers in the media leads to cystic spaces filled with a metachromatic myxoid material. Weakening and replacement of elastin and collagen over time lead to increased aneurysm diameter and length. The initial event triggering the medial dissection is controversial, but the resultant rupture typically causes significant hemorrhage and profound hemodynamic instability.

CLINICAL PRESENTATION

Although AAA is a leading cause of sudden death, patients may be asymptomatic before rupture. In some cases, rupture may be preceded by abdominal, flank, or back pain. Patients with a contained rupture can be seen several days after the rupture with abdominal, flank, or back pain.[33,34] In many cases, rupture of an AAA is accompanied by the sudden onset of severe abdominal pain that may be confined to the flank, low back, or groin with radiation to the back that brings the patients in urgently. Faintness and syncope may occur as a result of blood loss and gradually worsen until shock finally supervenes.[33] The patient might also have urinary retention and renal colic.[33]

PHYSICAL EXAMINATION

During dissection, a pulsatile, painful mass can be palpated in the abdomen between the xiphoid process and the umbilicus. In AAAs, the pulsations are felt directly over the mass and displace the examining fingers laterally. An aortic bruit may be present. Peripheral pulses may be unequal or absent but can be normal. Profound shock may rapidly ensue as a result of intraperitoneal leakage of blood. Abdominal examination findings might include abdominal distention and abdominal, flank, or back tenderness.[33,34]

DIAGNOSTICS

Additional diagnostic tests are not required if a ruptured AAA is suspected. The patient should be hospitalized immediately, with resuscitation and therapy in the operating room. If the diagnosis of rupture is in doubt and time allows, a CT scan is the standard for evaluation of an AAA because it can determine the extent of the aneurysmal process. Angiography is used preoperatively in elective repairs to demonstrate aortic and vascular anatomy and renal vessel involvement. An ultrasound examination can be a helpful screening tool in the early stages of the disease process or in the questionable emergency department patient. Abdominal plain x-ray films may show a soft tissue mass in the region of the abdominal aorta. A chest radiograph should also be obtained to evaluate the thoracic aorta. Laboratory tests should include a CBC, type and crossmatch, electrolytes, and renal function tests.[33,34]

DIAGNOSTICS

Ruptured Aortic Aneurysm

LABORATORY
- CBC and differential
- Serum electrolytes
- BUN
- Creatinine
- Serum β-hCG (in women of childbearing age)
- Type and crossmatch

IMAGING
- Chest x-ray studies
- CT scan or MRI
- Transthoracic echocardiography
- Angiography
- Ultrasound
- Abdominal x-ray studies

OTHER DIAGNOSTICS
- Electrocardiography

DIFFERENTIAL DIAGNOSIS

The most common misdiagnosis of ruptured AAA is myocardial infarction. Other diseases or conditions that may mimic AAA include a perforated peptic ulcer, diverticulitis, appendicitis, peritonitis, acute pancreatitis, pyelonephritis, renal colic, renal infarct, and mesenteric ischemia.[33] Consideration of a ruptured AAA is essential in the differential diagnosis for all these disorders.

DIFFERENTIAL DIAGNOSIS

Ruptured Aortic Aneurysm

- Myocardial infarction
- Perforated peptic ulcer
- Diverticulitis
- Appendicitis
- Peritonitis
- Acute pancreatitis
- Pyelonephritis
- Renal colic or infarct
- Mesenteric ischemia

MANAGEMENT

A patient with abdominal pain and shock should immediately have a surgical consultation to determine whether the patient should be taken directly to surgery. When a rupture is strongly suspected, resuscitation procedures should happen as testing is being done. After rupture confirmation with imaging, the decision should be made to take the patient directly to the operating room because emergency surgery is the only chance the patient has for survival.[33,34] The surgeon can do either endovascular or open repair.

COMPLICATIONS

Postoperative complications of ruptured AAA repair include colon infarction, sepsis, congestive heart failure, myocardial infarction, arrhythmias, liver dysfunction, renal failure, respiratory failure, pneumonia, and lower extremity ischemia.

INDICATIONS FOR REFERRAL OR HOSPITALIZATION AND PATIENT AND FAMILY EDUCATION

See Indications for Referral or Hospitalization and Patient and Family Education under Appendicitis.

CHAPTER 128

ANORECTAL COMPLAINTS

Pamela Slaven-Lee

Benign anorectal disorders of structure and/or function include defecatory disorders, fecal incontinence, anal fissure, pruritus ani, proctalgia syndromes, and anorectal abscess and fistula.[1] However, other anorectal conditions, such as polyps, condylomata acuminata, malignant neoplasm, and dermatologic disorders, should be considered, because all of these disorders may cause similar symptoms. The correct diagnosis and treatment of any of these disorders require a careful patient history and thorough physical examination. Dietary history should also be obtained because inadequate fiber intake, suboptimal fluid intake, and foods known to alter bowel habits may be revealed as contributory to hemorrhoidal symptoms.[2]

HEMORRHOIDS

DEFINITION AND EPIDEMIOLOGY

Hemorrhoids are masses of vascular tissue that, along with connective and muscular tissue, form a cushion in the submucosal layer of the anal canal. One of their functions is to help maintain anal closure and continence. They are part of normal human anatomy, and therefore symptomatic hemorrhoids can potentially develop in all adults. External hemorrhoids lie below the dentate line and are covered by squamous epithelium. Internal hemorrhoids are located above the dentate line and are covered by columnar epithelium. Although they are normal anatomic structures, they are infrequently referred to until symptomatic issues arise. Symptomatic hemorrhoidal disease will develop in 50% of the population at some point in their lives, with a peak incidence between the ages of 45 and 65 years. Development of hemorrhoids before the age of 20 is rare,[3-5] and pregnancy is associated with a higher risk of symptomatic hemorrhoidal disease.[6]

PATHOPHYSIOLOGY

The exact cause of hemorrhoids is not completely understood. The development of hemorrhoidal disease is most likely multifactorial and influenced by diet, toileting habits, and genetics.[2] However, it is thought that submucosal vascular cushions enlarge or prolapse as a result of increased pressure applied to the pelvic floor, causing external or internal hemorrhoids to develop.[1,2] Potential causes include pregnancy, straining, lifting, prolonged standing, and irregular bowel habits that contribute to the downward sliding of the vascular cushions in the submucosal layer of the anal canal.[2]

CLINICAL PRESENTATION

The most common presenting symptoms of hemorrhoids are bleeding, pruritus, protrusion, and pain. Internal hemorrhoids, which are usually painless, are associated with intermittent, painless, bright red rectal bleeding and intermittent, reducible protrusion that occurs after defecation. The blood may be seen on the toilet paper, in the toilet water, or sometimes on the outside of the stool. Blood mixed in with the stool or dark-colored blood often indicates more proximal disease, whereas bright red blood on the outside of the stool may be suggestive of anorectal pathology.

Internal hemorrhoids can be divided into four categories classified by the degree of prolapse. First-degree hemorrhoids cause bright red, painless bleeding and may bulge but do not prolapse through the anal orifice. Second-degree hemorrhoids prolapse during defecation but reduce spontaneously; patients with second-degree hemorrhoids report bleeding and perineal itching from chronic moisture secreted by the anal canal mucosa. Third-degree hemorrhoids prolapse with defecation and require manual reduction; patients with third-degree hemorrhoids have pain secondary to local ischemia and mucoid drainage.[7] Fourth-degree hemorrhoids are permanently prolapsed and are not reducible. It is important to note that the degree of prolapse does not imply incarceration, but nor does prolapse dictate the need for intervention. Hemorrhoidal symptomology and effect on quality of life should guide therapy.[1,2] However, incarcerated fourth-degree hemorrhoids require urgent surgical intervention.[7] External hemorrhoids are less likely to bleed and are often asymptomatic unless thrombosis develops. The patient can also be seen with anal irritation, pruritus, or a palpable nodule. Symptoms of a thrombosed external hemorrhoid include edema and moderate to severe pain.[1]

PHYSICAL EXAMINATION

The entire perineum and perianal area should be inspected with the patient in a comfortable position (knee-chest, lithotomy, or left lateral prone position) while the patient is both at rest and straining.[1] External hemorrhoids can be visualized around the anal orifice as the patient bears down, whereas internal hemorrhoids are best visualized with use of an anoscope as the patient bears down. A careful rectal examination is also necessary. An internal hemorrhoid is not palpable on rectal examination unless the hemorrhoid is thrombosed. Inflamed external hemorrhoids are erythematous and sensitive, whereas a thrombosed external hemorrhoid is tender and has a dark, bluish nodular appearance on the anal verge.

Severe rectal pain is unusual but if present suggests a gangrenous or thrombosed hemorrhoid. Gangrenous hemorrhoids are fourth-degree internal hemorrhoids and require immediate surgical evaluation.

DIAGNOSTICS

If the history reveals heavy, prolonged bleeding, a complete blood count (CBC) should be obtained to exclude anemia. To screen for bleeding from a more proximal site in the colon, the adult patient should be given stool cards for serial fecal occult blood testing once all hemorrhoidal bleeding has resolved. Any patient who complains of rectal bleeding should undergo endoscopic evaluation to exclude malignant disease. In patients older than age 50 or with a family history of colorectal cancer, the entire colon should be visualized via colonoscopy.[1]

DIAGNOSTICS

Hemorrhoids

LABORATORY	OTHER
Serial fecal occult blood testing	Endoscopic evaluation
CBC and differential*	

*If indicated.

DIFFERENTIAL DIAGNOSIS

The differential diagnosis includes other anorectal conditions that can cause pain, bleeding, or protrusion. Examples are rectal prolapse, anal skin tags, hypertrophied anal papillae, rectal polyps or cancer, anal fissure, anal papillitis, proctitis, inflammatory bowel disease, and condyloma or other sexually transmitted disease.

DIFFERENTIAL DIAGNOSIS

Hemorrhoids

- Rectal prolapsed
- Anal skin tags
- Anal fissure
- Anal fistula
- Anorectal abscess
- Hypertrophied anal papillae
- Rectal polyps
- Anal papillitis
- Inflammatory bowel disease
- Condyloma acuminatum
- Intraepithelial neoplasms
- Cancer of colorectum and/or anus

MANAGEMENT

Guidelines for the treatment of benign anorectal disorders such as hemorrhoids were published by the American Gastroenterological Association in 2014.[1] The treatment of hemorrhoids is usually based on the degree of the patient's symptoms and may be categorized as medical management, in-office procedures, and surgical intervention.[2] Most hemorrhoids are managed conservatively, and some patients require little or no treatment. A high-fiber diet and increased fluid intake are almost always recommended for the treatment of symptomatic hemorrhoids; according to a Cochrane review, fiber is an effective treatment for symptomatic hemorrhoids, with reduction in hemorrhoidal prolapse and bleeding. Fiber (20 to 30 g/day) absorbs water and helps soften the stool, thus preventing constipation and straining. Bulk-forming agents and stool softeners are sometimes used in addition to diet therapy to keep stools soft. Topical analgesics or hydrocortisone creams and suppositories or foams (Table 128-1), frequent warm water sitz baths, and oral analgesics can help reduce inflammation and promote patient comfort. Laxatives have a limited role in the initial management of hemorrhoids, because the variability in stool consistency associated with chronic laxative use makes hemorrhoid management more difficult.[2] Patients with first- to third-degree hemorrhoids that remain symptomatic after diet modification should be referred for in-office procedures such as banding, sclerotherapy, and infrared coagulation.

If a thrombosed external hemorrhoid is identified within 3 days of onset, it can be evacuated by first infiltrating a local anesthetic into the base of the hemorrhoid. An elliptical incision is then made into the thrombus, and the clot is expressed. Relief is immediate. This procedure can usually be carried out in the clinic setting by an experienced health care provider but is not indicated in children or in patients who have bleeding disorders, are immunocompromised, or are pregnant. Postoperative care includes a gauze pad applied to the site for 12 hours, followed by a sitz bath to remove the bandage and cleanse the area. Continued daily sitz baths and a minipad to protect clothing are recommended for several more days. If a thrombosed external hemorrhoid has been present for more than 3 days or is not too painful, conservative measures, including mild analgesics, sitz baths, and topical anesthetic ointments, can be used.[1,4,7]

Researchers continue to investigate newer anesthetic, analgesic, anti-inflammatory, and vasoconstrictive preparations to relieve the discomfort associated with hemorrhoids. In a small study, Rectogesic (glyceryl trinitrate 0.2%) ointment relieved pain, high anal canal resting pressures, and rectal bleeding.[8] Phlebotonics, most often composed of natural plant compounds, have proven effective in the management of first- and second-degree hemorrhoids by decreasing vascular endothelial inflammation and normalizing capillary permeability.[9]

LIFE SPAN CONSIDERATIONS

Symptomatic hemorrhoids are a common disease entity. Although they can occur at any age in both sexes, they are more common in adults between 45 and 65 years of age. The

TABLE 128-1 Topical Anorectal Anti-inflammatory Preparations*

Preparation	Actions	How Supplied	Usual Dosage and Administration
ProctoCream-HC 2.5% (hydrocortisone acetate)	Anti-inflammatory and antipruritic	Cream	Apply to affected area 2-4 times per day, depending on severity of condition.
Anusol-HC 2.5% (hydrocortisone)	Anti-inflammatory and antipruritic	Cream	Apply to affected area 2-4 times per day, depending on severity of condition.
Analpram-HC 1% and 2.5% (hydrocortisone acetate and pramoxine)	Anti-inflammatory and antipruritic, topical anesthetic	Cream	Apply to affected area 2-4 times per day, depending on severity of condition.
Anusol-HC suppositories (hydrocortisone acetate)	Anti-inflammatory and antipruritic	Suppositories	Place 1 suppository in rectum in morning and 1 at night for 2 weeks.
ProctoFoam-HC (hydrocortisone acetate and pramoxine)	Anti-inflammatory and antipruritic, topical anesthetic	Aerosol container and anal applicator	Apply to affected area nightly for 2 weeks; may be used up to 3-4 times a day.

*Topical anal preparations containing hydrocortisone should not be used continuously for more than 2 weeks to avoid skin atrophy.

prevalence in the United States has been estimated to be as high as 75% of adults older than 50 years.[10]

COMPLICATIONS

Fourth-degree hemorrhoids are at risk for strangulation because they are irreducible. Strangulated hemorrhoids can become gangrenous, requiring immediate surgical intervention.[7]

Rubber band ligation has been associated with increased pain, infection, and sepsis. Hemorrhoidectomy has been associated with urinary tract infections, urinary retention, fecal impaction, delayed hemorrhage, and, rarely, infection. Stapled hemorrhoidectomy has been associated with a higher recurrence of hemorrhoids and complications.[1,11]

INDICATIONS FOR REFERRAL OR HOSPITALIZATION

Referral for rubber band ligation, sclerotherapy, or infrared coagulation is indicated for patients with symptomatic third degree hemorrhoids.[1] If necessary, hemorrhoidectomy may alleviate symptoms. Patients who are unable to tolerate in-office procedures, who have large, associated external anal skin tags, or who have third- or fourth-degree hemorrhoids should be referred for surgical intervention. This includes traditional hemorrhoidectomy, stapled hemorrhoidopexy, and Doppler-assisted hemorrhoidal artery ligation.[1] In general, increased complications are associated with hemorrhoidectomies, and this procedure is recommended for only a small number of patients.

PATIENT AND FAMILY EDUCATION

Patients should be instructed in how to increase dietary fiber and in the correct use of topical anti-inflammatory agents; topical corticosteroids should be used judiciously to avoid thinning of the perianal skin with risk for maceration secondary to excess wiping.[2] Patients should also be taught preventive measures, including increasing fluid intake, keeping the stool soft, avoiding straining during bowel movements, exercising regularly to help promote regular bowel movements, and keeping the anal area clean and dry. The patient should understand the importance of follow-up care, particularly if symptoms do not resolve with conservative measures.

ANAL FISSURE

DEFINITION AND EPIDEMIOLOGY

Anal fissures, painful linear cracks or tears in the lining of the anal canal distal to the anatomic dentate line, are a frequent cause of rectal bleeding and are common in children and middle-aged adults. A fissure present for less than 6 weeks is considered acute, whereas fissures present for longer than 6 weeks are designated chronic.

PATHOPHYSIOLOGY

Anal fissures are sometimes seen in patients with inflammatory bowel disease, cancer, Crohn disease, tuberculosis, human immunodeficiency virus (HIV) infection, syphilis, or leukemia.[12,13] Most anal fissures are caused by trauma to the anal canal from passage of a large, hard stool. Pathophysiology is associated with high resting sphincter tone coupled with relative ischemia in the posterior midline of the internal anal sphinter.[13] Other causes include frequent diarrhea, which can result in a chemical burn from severe alkalinity, and anal stenosis, which may predispose the patient to fissure formation. An acute fissure often resolves without intervention. However, a chronic ulcer surrounded by scar tissue may develop if the underlying sphincter goes into involuntary spasm, leading to diminished blood flow to the area.

CLINICAL PRESENTATION

Many patients seek treatment with the thought that they have hemorrhoids. Classic symptoms of an anal fissure are severe rectal pain during and after bowel movements and small amounts of bright red rectal bleeding seen on the toilet paper. Some patients avoid having a bowel movement because of the pain and thus produce even harder stools, which exacerbates the problem.[12] Acute anal fissure appears to be a laceration, whereas a chronic anal fissure is associated with an indurated, fibrotic appearance and an anal skin tag or polyp.[13]

PHYSICAL EXAMINATION

Because of the severe pain associated with an anal fissure, the physical examination should be done gently and with reassurance. The patient should be placed in the left lateral decubitus position and a topical anesthetic applied to enable adequate visualization of the rectum and anus. The fissure is most easily visualized by spreading the buttocks to expose the anus. Ninety percent of fissures are located at the posterior midline, and the remainder are situated in the anterior midline.[10] A fissure located in a more lateral position usually indicates a sexually transmitted disease, tuberculosis, HIV infection, ulcerative colitis, Crohn disease, malignant neoplasm, or other underlying disorder and necessitates referral to a subspecialist.[13] If the fissure is extremely painful, digital rectal and anoscopic examination may be deferred. If the fissure is touched with a cotton-tipped applicator, the symptoms will often be reproduced, helping to confirm the diagnosis.

DIAGNOSTICS

There are no routine laboratory abnormalities.

DIFFERENTIAL DIAGNOSIS

Sharp, burning pain during bowel movements is indicative of anal fissure. Chronic anal fissures are often misdiagnosed as hemorrhoids because of the presence of a sentinel tag. Sometimes a large hypertrophied anal papilla can be mistaken for a polyp on digital rectal examination. Inflammatory bowel disease, carcinoma of the anus, leukemia, lymphoma, tuberculosis, syphilis, and other sexually transmitted diseases are also included in the differential diagnosis.

DIFFERENTIAL DIAGNOSIS

Anal Fissures

- Hemorrhoids
- Polyps
- Inflammatory bowel disease
- Carcinoma
- Syphilis
- Proctalgia fugax

MANAGEMENT

Increased fiber, stool softeners, and sitz baths are proven effective treatment for acute anal fissures and should be considered first-line treatment.[1] Suppositories or foam-containing anti-inflammatory agents may also be used (see Table 128-1). Topical anesthetic gel (lidocaine [Xylocaine] 2% jelly) applied before bowel movements can be helpful in reducing pain and spasm. Chronic anal fissures may be treated with topical or oral calcium channel blockers or topical nitrates. Topical 2% diltiazem applied twice daily for 6 to 8 weeks has proven effective in the healing of chronic anal fissures without the vasodilatory side effects associated with topical nitrates.[14] Patients with chronic anal fissures that fail to respond to topical treatment strategies should be referred for local botulism toxin injection. Surgical internal anal sphincterotomy is recommended for patients in whom botulism toxin injections fail.[1]

LIFE SPAN CONSIDERATIONS

Anal fissures are commonly seen in young and middle-aged adults but can occur at any age. Both sexes seem to be equally affected. Although they are common, the exact incidence of this disease is unknown.[15]

COMPLICATIONS AND INDICATIONS FOR REFERRAL OR HOSPITALIZATION

Patients with chronic or recurrent fissures that do not respond to conservative therapy should be referred for surgery. Subcutaneous internal anal sphincterotomy reduces internal sphincter tone, allowing the fissure to heal. Complications of this procedure can include poor wound healing and rectal incontinence but are usually avoided.[15]

PATIENT AND FAMILY EDUCATION

Patients need to be informed that healing can take up to 6 weeks with conservative measures. They should be advised to return for follow-up if symptoms do not resolve or if they recur. Prevention includes keeping the stools soft with a high-fiber diet and adequate fluid intake and avoiding straining during bowel movements.

If topical nitrates or calcium channel blockers are prescribed, patients should understand how to use these preparation and be able to recognize associated side effects. Nitrates are contraindicated in patients using sildenafil citrate.

PRURITUS ANI

DEFINITION AND EPIDEMIOLOGY

Pruritus ani, or itching of the anus and perianal skin, is a fairly common condition affecting up to 5% of the population.[15] Although the true prevalence of this disorder is unknown, men are affected four times more often than women are.[10,15]

PATHOPHYSIOLOGY

There are many different causes of pruritus ani. In many patients, the condition has no identified cause. Most causes are idiopathic and are classified as primary pruritus.[15] Secondary causes can be related to cancer, dermatologic conditions, anal disorders, hyperhidrosis, infections or infestations (e.g., scabies, pediculosis, fungus, or pinworms), medications, malignant neoplasms, and common systemic illnesses (e.g., renal insufficiency, liver disease, or diabetes).[10,15] Pruritus ani may also be related to improper hygiene or to the ingestion of certain foods or beverages that may affect the function of the internal anal sphincter.

CLINICAL PRESENTATION

The patient often reports an uncontrollable urge to scratch the anus. The symptoms tend to be worse at night or after a bowel movement. Sometimes the itching will involve the perianal area, buttocks, and vulva or scrotum. Scratching provides only transient relief and can lead to an itch-scratch cycle that exacerbates the condition.[16]

PHYSICAL EXAMINATION

Diagnosis is made by a careful history and physical examination. The anus should be thoroughly inspected for obvious anorectal, infectious, or dermatologic disease. A digital rectal examination is also indicated. If the pruritus is chronic, the perianal skin may appear moist, excoriated, and macerated.

DIAGNOSTICS

Some cases of pruritus ani are related to an infectious process (e.g., β-hemolytic streptococci, *Staphylococcus aureus,* and *Corynebacterium minutissimum*).[15] Thus cultures may be useful. If the pruritus is primarily nocturnal, cellophane tape can be applied to the perianal skin in the early morning. The tape is then placed on a glass slide and examined under a microscope for pinworm eggs. For patients with intractable pruritus or a suspected dermatologic disease or malignant neoplasm, a biopsy sample obtained by a dermatologist can help confirm the diagnosis. Suspected sexually transmitted disease requires the appropriate workup to exclude chlamydia, gonorrhea, syphilis, and other diseases.

DIAGNOSTICS

Pruritus Ani

LABORATORY	OTHER
Cultures*	Biopsy*
Microscopic examination for pinworm eggs*	

*If indicated.

DIFFERENTIAL DIAGNOSIS

Anorectal disorders, diarrhea, and constipation are common causes of pruritus ani.[15] The *ITCH* acronym is helpful in the initial evaluation and exploration of differential diagnoses associated with pruritus ani:

*I*nfections—Infections such as *Candida albicans,* herpes, HIV, pinworms, and other bacterial infections should be considered.

*T*opical irritants—Soaps, detergents, and restrictive clothing are all topical irritants that should be considered.

*C*utaneous causes—Cutaneous causes such as cancer should be considered.

*H*ypersensitivities—Hypersensitivities to foods and medication should be determined.[16]

DIFFERENTIAL DIAGNOSIS

Pruritus Ani

ANORECTAL DISEASES
- Diarrhea
- Fissures
- Fistulas
- Hemorrhoids
- Incontinence
- Skin tags
- Squamous cell cancer

DERMATOLOGIC DISEASES
- Atopic dermatitis
- Contact dermatitis
- Hidradenitis suppurativa
- Lichen planus
- Neurodermatitis
- Psoriasis
- Seborrheic dermatitis

INFECTIONS OR INFESTATIONS
- Bacterial infection
- Candidal infection
- Condyloma acuminatum
- Gonorrhea
- Herpes simplex
- Pinworms
- Scabies
- Pediculosis
- Sexually transmitted infections
- Syphilis

MALIGNANT NEOPLASMS
- Bowen disease
- Paget disease

OTHER CAUSES
- Dietary
- Medication
- Idiopathic cause
- Overzealous hygiene
- Poor hygiene
- Psychogenic cause
- Warmth and moisture

MANAGEMENT

Any identified infectious or dermatologic disease should be treated. Once other pathologic causes of pruritus ani have been excluded, patient education should be aimed at perianal hygiene and breaking the itch-scratch cycle that leads to the chronicity of the condition.[16]

The anal area should be kept clean and dry, and overly vigorous wiping or scratching should be avoided. According to Markell and Billingham, a hair dryer on the cool setting can help dry the anal area more thoroughly.[15] Perfumed toilet paper, soaps, and hygiene products should not be used, but cornstarch applied sparingly can be helpful.[15] Tight-fitting clothing should also be avoided, and constipation prevented.[15] A 1% hydrocortisone cream can be used initially but should be discontinued after 2 weeks to avoid skin atrophy.[15] Patients should be encouraged to wear clean cotton underwear and to avoid tight-fitting clothing.

Dietary restrictions of possible offending foods should be tried. A psyllium product can be used to bulk the stool in an attempt to prevent fecal soilage if loose stools are a problem. Medications and foods that cause loose stools should be avoided if at all possible. If severe nocturnal itching is a problem, an antihistamine with antipruritic properties, such as hydroxyzine (Atarax), can help the patient sleep and assist in breaking the itch-scratch cycle.[15] Relief of symptoms usually occurs in 4 to 6 weeks.[15] For patients who do not respond to these therapies, intradermal methylene blue injections have relieved the disorder for some patients.[15]

LIFE SPAN CONSIDERATIONS

Pruritus ani is most common in the fourth, fifth, and sixth decades. However, this disorder can occur at any age.[15]

COMPLICATIONS

Scratching associated with pruritus ani can cause excoriations and dermatologic changes. These can become infected and require antibiotic therapy. Vaginal infections are also potential complications. Pruritus ani related to pinworm infestation can be easily spread to others, and reinfection is common.

INDICATIONS FOR REFERRAL OR HOSPITALIZATION

Patients with persistent symptoms after 2 weeks of appropriate therapy should be referred to dermatology for further evaluation.[16] Suspicious lesions require biopsy, and any signs or symptoms suggesting bowel pathologic conditions require colonoscopy to exclude malignant disease. If medical treatment has failed, referral to a gastroenterologist is indicated.

PATIENT AND FAMILY EDUCATION

The patient should be educated about the possible cause of this condition. To help identify offending foods, the patient can be taught an elimination diet. The patient should be instructed about proper anal hygiene habits and to avoid scratching the area.

ANORECTAL ABSCESS OR FISTULA

DEFINITION AND EPIDEMIOLOGY

An anorectal abscess is an infection that occurs from obstruction of the duct of a perianal gland in the intersphincteric space. An anorectal fistula is the drainage of an abscess through an abnormal communication to the perianal skin. An abscess is the acute manifestation of an infection, and a fistula is the chronic manifestation. The incidence is two times higher in men than in women,[17] with the most common ages being the third and fourth decades of life.[10] Up to 35% of patients with

Crohn disease are affected by at least once instance of perianal fistula formation.[18]

PATHOPHYSIOLOGY

The most common cause of anorectal abscesses and fistulas is bacterial infection of the anal crypt glands. These glands may become infected if obstruction with resulting stasis occurs from trauma, hard stools, foreign bodies, or diarrhea. Other possible causes of anorectal abscesses or fistulas include neoplasms, ruptured diverticula, and inflammatory bowel disorders (e.g., Crohn disease).[19] Abnormal communication between the anorectal canal and the perianal skin results in fistula formation with resultant drainage of purulent material.

CLINICAL PRESENTATION

Symptoms of an abscess include acute pain and swelling. The pain increases with movement, sitting, or bowel movements. Malaise and fever may also be present. The most common complaint of patients with an anorectal fistula is a persistent purulent drainage with a history of abscess that has either been drained surgically or spontaneously. A careful history is necessary to determine whether the patient has a history of immunocompetence, diabetes, Crohn disease, or anorectal abscess or fistula.

PHYSICAL EXAMINATION

Inspection of the perineum may reveal erythema, heat, swelling, and tenderness. If the abscess is located higher in the anorectum, the perineum may be unrevealing and the abscess may manifest as localized tenderness on rectal examination. On anoscopy, pus may be seen exuding from the fistula tract into the anal canal. A fistula may be seen with purulent drainage oozing from a sinus or opening in the perineal skin. Inguinal lymph nodes may be enlarged.

DIAGNOSTICS

A CBC may reveal leukocytosis. Ultrasound, computed tomography (CT), or magnetic resonance imaging (MRI) is indicated in cases of recurrent and complex cases such as those involving inflammatory bowel disease.[17]

DIAGNOSTICS

Anorectal Abscess

LABORATORY	OTHER
CBC and differential*	Colonoscopy* Small bowel examination*

*If indicated.

DIFFERENTIAL DIAGNOSIS

With recurrent fistulas, Crohn disease should be considered. Also included in the differential diagnosis are pilonidal sinus, hidradenitis suppurativa, anorectal malignant neoplasm, actinomycosis, sexually transmitted diseases, and lymphoma.

DIFFERENTIAL DIAGNOSIS

Anorectal Abscess

- Crohn disease
- Pilonidal sinus
- Hidradenitis suppurativa
- Carcinoma
- Actinomycosis
- Sexually transmitted diseases

MANAGEMENT, COMPLICATIONS, AND INDICATIONS FOR REFERRAL OR HOSPITALIZATION

Use of incision and drainage is indicted for acute anorectal abscess. The severity and location of the abscess dictates the treatment setting. Perianal and ischiorectal abscesses may be treated in an outpatient setting, whereas more complex abscess presentations require management in the operating room.[17]

Management of anal fistulas can include treatment with metronidazole; however, medical management alone is rarely recommended. Consultation regarding appropriate re-treatment should be obtained; it is dictated by patient comorbidities and path of the fistula tract. Surgical options for the management of chronic anal fistulas include fistulotomy, fistulectomy, debridement with seton placement, fibrin glue, fistula plug, ligation of the intersphincteric fistula tract (LIFT), and sphincter-sparing advancement flaps.[17]

PATIENT AND FAMILY EDUCATION

After surgery, the patient should be instructed to keep the stools soft with bulk-forming agents, a high-fiber diet, and stool softeners. Warm sitz baths can help with hygiene, promote healing, and provide comfort until healing is complete. The importance of follow-up visits to effectively manage conditions contributing to anorectal abscess and subsequent fistula formation should be emphasized.

CHAPTER 129

CHOLELITHIASIS AND CHOLECYSTITIS

Meghan Glynn

DEFINITION AND EPIDEMIOLOGY

Cholelithiasis and cholecystitis are worldwide disorders that result from inflammatory, infectious, neoplastic, metabolic, and congenital conditions. Gallbladder disease affects all cultures and is prevalent in most Western countries.[1] The highest incidence of acute cholecystitis occurs in adults of middle age and older. Although gallbladder disease also occurs in adolescents, it is seen at increased rates after the age of 40 years. Acalculous cholecystitis is less common but is associated with more severe morbidity. Risk factors for gallbladder disease include ethnicity, with Native Americans having an increased incidence in North America. Moreover, gallbladder disease is more common in females and during pregnancy. Other risk factors include family history, diet, medications (e.g., estrogen, oral contraceptives, thiazide diuretics), obesity, rapid weight loss, history of gastric bypass surgery, and hyperalimentation, as well as comorbid disorders such as diabetes, Crohn disease, alcoholic and biliary cirrhosis, and hyperparathyroidism (Box 129-1).

Physician consultation is indicated for acute cholecystitis.

BOX 129-1

Risk Factors for Gallstone Formation

*A*ge: Increasing age*
*B*ody habitus: Obesity, rapid weight loss
*C*hildbearing: Pregnancy
*D*rugs: Fibric acid derivatives (or fibrates), contraceptive steroids, postmenopausal estrogens, progesterone, octreotide (Sandostatin), ceftriaxone (Rocephin)
*E*thnicity: Pima Indians, Scandinavians
*F*amily: Maternal family history of gallstones
*G*ender: Females
*H*yperalimentation: Total parenteral nutrition,† fasting†
*I*leal and other metabolic diseases: Ileal disease (Crohn disease), resection or bypass,* high triglycerides, diabetes mellitus, chronic hemolysis,* alcoholic cirrhosis,* biliary infection,* primary biliary cirrhosis, duodenal diverticula,* truncal vagotomy, hyperparathyroidism, low level of high-density lipoprotein cholesterol

*Risk factors for pigment gallstone formation.
†Risk factor for cholesterol and pigment gallstone formation.
From Ahmed A, Cheung RC, Keefe EB: Management of gallstones and their complications, *Am Fam Physician* 61(6):1673-1680, 1687-1688, 2000.

BOX 129-2

Risk Factors Associated with Acute Acalculous Cholecystitis

Coronary artery disease
Previous myocardial infarction
Diabetes
Peripheral or cerebral vascular disease
Polyarteritis nodosa
Prolonged labor
Prolonged fasting
Immediate postoperative period
Hyperalimentation
Dehydration
Fibrosis of the gallbladder
Obstruction of the biliary or pancreatic ducts
Thrombosis of the cystic artery
Critical illnesses (e.g., bone marrow transplantation)
Severe illnesses
- Trauma
- Burns
- Sepsis

Major diseases
- AIDS
- Leptospirosis

AIDS, acquired immunodeficiency syndrome.

PATHOPHYSIOLOGY

Gallstones are formed from bile constituent crystals and are divided into three primary types of stones: cholesterol, pigmented, and mixed. Small gallstones pass uneventfully through the common bile duct and do not cause distress. Larger stones may obstruct the cystic or common bile duct, causing increased pressure to the ductal system that results in pain, nausea, and vomiting as a result of the contractile spasms of the smooth muscle. Because of the blockage, bile is prevented from entering the duodenum, reducing the body's ability to digest fat. The undigested fat passes from the small intestine into the large intestine, where bacteria convert the excess undigested fat into fatty acid derivatives. The fatty acid derivatives alter water absorption from the colon, which results in diarrhea and excess fluid loss. The obstruction prevents bile secretion into the small intestine, causing jaundice.

The gallbladder becomes inflamed as a result of various processes, including continued blockage of the cystic or common bile duct. This inflammation causes the release of prostaglandins and other chemicals that further inflame gallbladder tissue. In the majority of cases, bacterial infections contribute to the inflammatory response in acute cholecystitis.[2] Human immunodeficiency virus (HIV) disease may lead to opportunistic infections of the biliary tract. The most common bacteria involved in biliary tract infections are *Escherichia coli*, *Klebsiella* organisms, *Enterobacter*, and enterococci.[3] Gangrene of the gallbladder and possible perforation can result if the process is not stopped.

Cholecystitis can also occur in the absence of stones; this condition is labeled *acute* or *chronic acalculous cholecystitis*. Acalculous cholecystitis is classified as acute if the duration of symptoms is less than 1 month and as chronic if the symptoms have been present longer than 3 months. The pathophysiology of this condition is poorly understood. The inflammatory process is similar to that of cholecystitis except that gallstones are not present. A common cause of chronic acalculous cholecystitis is biliary dyskinesia. Risk factors associated with acute acalculous cholecystitis are outlined in Box 129-2.

CLINICAL PRESENTATION

Most patients with gallstones are asymptomatic.[4] Classically, symptomatic cholelithiasis manifests as biliary colic with intermittent or steady, right upper quadrant abdominal pain that radiates to the right posterior shoulder within an hour of eating any type of large meal, specifically a meal with a high fat content. The pain may be constant or intermittent and tapering, sometimes without complete relief. It is described as mild to severe and lasts 1 to 6 hours. The biliary colic is accompanied by nausea and vomiting. There can be a history of these episodes, which increase in frequency.

Acute cholecystitis develops in a manner similar to symptomatic cholelithiasis, but biliary colic lasts longer than 4 to 6 hours. There usually is a history of intermittent colic consistent with chronic cholecystitis, and the patient may have anorexia, fever, and chills with the nausea and vomiting observed in symptomatic cholelithiasis. As the gallbladder becomes progressively inflamed, the pain in the right upper quadrant becomes sharp. The Charcot triad of right upper quadrant abdominal pain, fever, and jaundice can be observed if a stone is lodged in the common bile duct.

Patients with chronic cholecystitis often describe a recurrent, mild to moderate, right upper quadrant and epigastric abdominal pain accompanied by nausea and vomiting. The pain may radiate to the region of the posterior right shoulder and scapula and is often associated with the eating of fatty foods.

Traditionally, patients with acute acalculous cholecystitis are critically ill and require hospitalization. Presentation includes generalized complaints, fever, nausea, vomiting, and loss of appetite. The patient often has no significant medical history, although surgery, trauma, burns, and other disorders have been associated with acalculous cholecystitis. This condition should be considered in all patients who are seen with right upper quadrant pain in the absence of gallstones.

PHYSICAL EXAMINATION

Depending on the severity of the condition, the physical examination in symptomatic cholelithiasis and chronic cholecystitis may be unremarkable. Right upper quadrant abdominal pain may be accompanied by tenderness. The diagnosis is based on the history, the exclusion of other disorders, and the results of the gallbladder ultrasound examination.

With acute cholecystitis, patients may have moderate distress from systemic toxicity, including tachycardia and fever. The right upper quadrant abdominal pain is associated with tenderness and muscle guarding or rigidity. The gallbladder is not commonly palpable, but a distended tender gallbladder confirms the diagnosis. Hypoactive bowel sounds and presence of Murphy sign (an inability to take a deep breath because of the discomfort during palpation beneath the right costal margin) may be noted. Dehydration is not uncommon. Jaundice is present in some patients and is the result of biliary obstruction or chronic hemolysis.

The physical findings in acalculous cholecystitis are similar to those of symptomatic gallstones: right upper quadrant pain, vomiting, fever, jaundice, and presence of Murphy sign.

DIAGNOSTICS

Laboratory testing should be individualized, but a complete blood count (CBC) with differential, urinalysis, liver function tests (LFTs), and serum pancreatic enzymes are usually indicated (Table 129-1). Serum electrolyte values and blood urea nitrogen (BUN) and creatinine concentrations are necessary to determine fluid and electrolyte status as well as renal function. Blood cultures are indicated if sepsis is suspected. A test for human chorionic gonadotropin (hCG) is essential in women of childbearing age if potentially teratogenic clinical imaging studies are considered. Electrocardiography is necessary if cardiac risk factors are present or if cardiac involvement is suspected.

DIAGNOSTICS

Cholelithiasis and Cholecystitis

LABORATORY

CBC and differential
LFTs (bilirubin, alkaline phosphatase)
Serum electrolytes, BUN, and creatinine*
Serum pregnancy test, hCG*

IMAGING

Ultrasound
Biliary scintigraphy
Endoscopic retrograde cholangiopancreatography*

*If indicated.

Although history and physical examination findings help to support diagnosis of cholecystitis, an ultrasound is ordered to help confirm diagnosis. Ultrasound is the most practical imaging study for evaluation of the gallbladder and is not contraindicated in pregnancy. In addition to detecting the gallstones, ultrasound may show gallbladder thickening and "sonographic Murphy sign"; the examination is similar to the physical examination techniques, except that when performed during the ultrasound examination, there is confirmation that the gallbladder is being pressed when the patient responds. Follow-up diagnostics are based on ultrasound findings and include computed tomography (CT), preferably with contrast; cholescintigraphy (hepatobiliary iminodiacetic acid [HIDA] scan); or magnetic resonance imaging (MRI).[4,5]

Plain abdominal radiographs will demonstrate biliary air, marked hepatomegaly, and, in some cases, gallstones. A chest x-ray study will exclude right lower lobe pneumonia. An abdominal CT scan may be indicated in some instances if other imaging tests are not conclusive.

DIFFERENTIAL DIAGNOSIS

Cholecystitis has an extensive number of differential diagnoses. See the differential diagnosis box for a list of the more common ones.

TABLE 129-1 Expected Laboratory Values in Biliary Tract Disease

	Serum Laboratory Tests						
	White Blood Cell Count	Bilirubin	Alkaline Phosphatase	Aspartate Aminotransferase	Alanine Aminotransferase	Amylase	Lipase
Chronic cholecystitis	Normal	Normal	Normal	Normal	Normal	Normal	Normal
Symptomatic cholelithiasis	Normal	Normal or slight rise	Normal or slight rise	Normal	Normal	†	†
Acute cholecystitis	Normal or rise	Rise in 45% of patients	Rise in 23% of patients	Rise in 40% of patients	Normal	Rise in 13% of patients†	Normal
Acute acalculous cholecystitis	Rise	Slight rise	Slight rise	Slight rise	Slight rise	Normal	Normal
Chronic acalculous cholecystitis	Normal	Normal	Normal	Normal	Normal	Normal	Normal
Choledocholith	Rise	Rise	Rise	Rise*	Rise*	Rise†	Rise†

*A rise in the transaminases is associated with prolonged obstruction leading to hepatocellular destruction.
†A rise in the serum amylase and lipase is associated with pancreatitis secondary to ampulla of Vater stone obstruction.

DIFFERENTIAL DIAGNOSIS

Cholelithiasis and Cholecystitis

- Bowel obstruction
- Chronic cholecystitis
- Diverticulitis
- Gastritis
- Gastroenteritis
- Herpes zoster
- Hepatitis or hepatic abscess
- Irritable bowel syndrome
- Myocardial ischemia or infarction
- Neoplasm
- Pancreatitis
- Peptic ulcer disease
- Pelvic inflammatory disease
- Pleuritis
- Pneumonia (right lower lobe)
- Pyelonephritis
- Renal colic
- Appendicitis
- Fitz-Hugh–Curtis syndrome

MANAGEMENT

In general, asymptomatic gallstones do not require surgical intervention. However, there is a chance that the patient will become symptomatic. Thus, it is possible that gastroenterologists and surgeons would consider the benefit of a prophylactic cholecystectomy in some instances.[6]

The initial management of symptomatic gallbladder disease begins with isotonic intravenous rehydration and correction of electrolyte abnormalities. Oral hydration is contraindicated during this time. Antispasmodic and antiemetic medications are used for uncomplicated cholelithiasis. In addition to an antiemetic, a nasogastric tube should be used for protracted vomiting to decompress the stomach. Although meperidine was frequently used in the past to manage pain, an injectable nonsteroidal anti-inflammatory prostaglandin inhibitor (e.g., ketorolac tromethamine) is also an effective pain reliever in nonbacterial gallbladder distention.[6]

With uncomplicated symptomatic cholelithiasis, discharge is appropriate once the condition has stabilized and oral hydration is maintained. Surgical consultation before discharge is advised because many patients will have recurrent symptoms.

Acute cholecystitis should be suspected if the symptoms do not resolve within 4 to 6 hours; in this case, timely surgical referral for laparoscopic cholecystectomy is essential.[7] Prophylactic antibiotics may be indicated for patients with acute complicated cholecystitis.[8]

Co-Management with Specialists

Medical dissolution, biliary lithotripsy, or surgical intervention requires further consultation to ensure optimum health care. Patients who have diabetes or asymptomatic disease or who are not candidates for surgery should have a consultation with a gastroenterologist or surgeon to determine whether further management is required.

After initial stabilization of the patient, treatment options for uncomplicated symptomatic cholelithiasis include medical dissolution therapy (oral or direct gallbladder irrigation), biliary lithotripsy, cholecystostomy (as an alternative surgical procedure), and open or laparoscopic cholecystectomy.

Ursodeoxycholic acid alone or in combination with chenodeoxycholic acid can decrease the pain associated with biliary disease and aid in gallstone dissolution.[9, 11] This treatment is an option for patients with mild symptoms, stone size less than 0.5 to 1 cm, and normal gallbladder function. However, side effects such as diarrhea can make this treatment intolerable for patients. Moreover, the addition of a 3-hydroxy-3-methylglutaryl-coenzyme A (HMG-CoA) inhibitor may help to reduce the cholesterol saturation index. Studies disagree as to whether or not the addition of statin will assist with the dissolution and prevention of gallstones. Ezetimibe has also been considered because it inhibits cholesterol absorption; however, its ability to prevent or dissolve gallstones needs further studying.[10] These treatments take time, but they may be appropriate for patients who are not surgical candidates.

Although becoming less common, biliary lithotripsy can be considered in some patients with gallstones. The relatively painless shock waves fracture the stones into smaller pieces that are then passed into the small intestine. The criteria for biliary lithotripsy are specific; eligibility may include stone size or calcification and gallbladder function.

Cholecystostomy is an alternative surgical procedure to open or laparoscopic cholecystectomy and is used if the patient has too much inflammation or is too ill for cholecystectomy. Either operatively or percutaneously, stones and bile are removed through the gallbladder fundus, and a tube is placed as an external drain.

In some instances, an open cholecystectomy may be indicated. The open surgical approach is necessary when the laparoscopic method is contraindicated. Contraindications include coagulopathy, cirrhosis, portal hypertension, pregnancy, peritonitis, severe cardiopulmonary disease, and prior surgical adhesions. Cholecystostomy is the treatment of choice with severe disease or extensive inflammation.[11]

Because of its safety, convenience, reduced postoperative pain, and shorter hospitalization (outpatient surgery at some facilities) leading to reduced costs, laparoscopic cholecystectomy is the standard treatment of symptomatic gallbladder disease. Surgical drainage or removal of the gallbladder is indicated with laparoscopic cholecystectomy or ultrasound-guided percutaneous cholecystotomy. Choledocholithiasis, or stones in the common bile duct, can also be managed through the laparoscopic approach, although this will be too difficult in some instances to manage safely. Some laparoscopic approaches require a conversion to the open cholecystectomy procedure.

In addition to the initial treatment of gallstone disease, antibiotics may be indicated. Bacteria associated with acute cholecystitis include *E. coli*, *Klebsiella pneumoniae*, *Clostridium welchii*, *Clostridium perfringens*, and *Streptococcus faecalis*. Therapeutic antibiotics are used for preoperative prophylaxis, acute cholecystitis, and cholangitis. In acalculous cholecystitis, broad-spectrum antibiotics with gram-negative coverage (e.g., piperacillin) are necessary.[4,11]

COMPLICATIONS

Potential organ damage depends on the location of the gallstone obstruction in the biliary system. The most common complication is choledocholithiasis. In general, symptomatic gallstones require surgical intervention. If it is left untreated, the disease has potential complications, including a pus-filled gallbladder, which can lead to perforation. Local perforation can occur within 1 week after the onset of acute cholecystitis and can lead to the formation of a pericholecystic abscess and potential mortality. Should a large gallstone pass into the intestinal lumen, a small bowel obstruction (also known as a *gallstone ileus*) can occur. Gas-forming bacteria (*Clostridium* and coliform organisms) can lead to an emphysematous cholecystitis that also can result in gallbladder perforation. The gallbladder may become gangrenous if extensive inflammation occurs and causes necrosis and thrombosis of the cystic artery. Gangrenous cholecystitis is more common in older patients who have co-morbidities or who delay treatment. These patients not only will have the symptoms of cholecystitis, but they also will have sepsis.[4] Stones lodged in the ampulla of Vater can cause gallstone pancreatitis. The porcelain gallbladder, an uncommon condition associated with cancer, is observed on plain radiographs. The porcelain appearance of the gallbladder rim is caused by calcification of the gallbladder.

The complication rate of gallstone disease varies and depends on the procedure chosen to manage the disease, the size of the gallstone, the patient's age, and comorbid issues.

INDICATIONS FOR REFERRAL OR HOSPITALIZATION

Asymptomatic cholelithiasis does not require referral for surgical management except as previously discussed. Symptomatic gallstones or evidence of acalculous disease supported by ultrasound examination or oral cholecystography requires further medical or surgical consultation for management and maintenance.

Acute cholecystitis requires hospitalization for intravenous antibiotics and fluid therapy. The length of the course of antibiotic prophylaxis is dependent on the severity of the presentation as well as the patient's risk factors. Patients diagnosed with acalculous cholecystitis are admitted to the hospital and are also given antibiotic prophylaxis as well as fluid therapy.[8] If percutaneous catheter placement is used to drain the gallbladder, the catheter may be in place for 6 to 8 weeks; if no stones are present at postdrainage cholangiography, cholecystectomy may be unnecessary.

The postoperative course after cholecystectomy is variable. Laparoscopic cholecystectomy patients have a shorter hospitalization and usually return to work sooner.[4] If a patient has an open cholecystectomy, the recovery is longer.

PATIENT AND FAMILY EDUCATION

Patients who are obese should be counseled about the increased risk of gallstone formation and understand the importance of lifestyle and dietary changes.[1] Some risk factors have been implicated in but not clearly demonstrated for cholelithiasis; still, physical exercise and weight control are beneficial for all patients.

If gallstones are incidentally noted on x-ray, ultrasound, or other clinical imaging studies of the abdomen, reassurance that asymptomatic stones do not require surgery is needed. Patients with symptomatic gallbladder disease need an explanation of laboratory and imaging tests, referral, and management.

Many patients who are anticipating laparoscopic cholecystectomies underrate or have unrealistic expectations about postoperative pain and activity. Preparatory guidance in this area may be efficacious to ensure a more realistic understanding of the postoperative course. Older patients can expect to spend additional time in the hospital or in rehabilitation after cholecystectomy.

CHAPTER 130

CIRRHOSIS

Donna Glynn

DEFINITION AND EPIDEMIOLOGY

Cirrhosis is the end-stage consequence of progressive hepatic fibrosis affecting normal liver function. It is a serious, irreversible disease—the result of exposure to persistent toxins and resulting in liver failure and death.

The most common causes of cirrhosis in the United States are alcoholic liver disease, hepatitis C, non alcoholic fatty liver disease (NAFLD) and nonalcoholic steatohepatitis (NASH).[1] Various pharmacotherapeutics including acetaminophen, amiodarone, methotrexate, isoniazid, varied antibiotics, and carbon tetrachloride are also associated with cirrhosis. The cause can be inherited or idiopathic, but primary and secondary biliary cirrhosis, infections, viruses, hemochromatosis, polycystic liver disease, right-sided heart failure, autoimmune hepatitis, and other disorders play a key role in the development of cirrhosis (Box 130-1).

Fibrosis, the replacement of normally functioning liver tissue by injured scar tissue, results in varied-size nodules that impair function. In advanced stages, the impaired hepatic vasculature results in a shunting of the portal and arterial blood supply, causing portal hypertension, obstructive biliary channels, destruction of liver cells, hepatocellular carcinoma, and eventual liver failure.[2]

Liver biopsy is necessary in the diagnosis of cirrhosis to stage the severity of the fibrosis and to establish a plan of care. Cirrhosis is typically classified as micronodular, macronodular, or mixed.[3] Micronodular cirrhosis, often associated with alcoholic liver disease, occurs when the repeated presence of an offending agent prevents the regeneration of normal tissue. As a result, the regenerating tissue produces small nodules that have limited functional abilities. As the disease progresses, the liver becomes

BOX 130-1

Diseases That Cause Cirrhosis

Metabolic disease (diabetes mellitus)
Wilson disease
Hemochromatosis
α_1-Antitrypsin deficiency
Cardiac failure (congestive heart failure, myocardial infarction, valvular heart disease)
Cystic fibrosis
Primary sclerosing cholangitis
Biliary tract obstruction
- Primary obstruction (calculi)
- Secondary obstruction (tumor)

Veno-occlusive disease (Budd-Chiari syndrome)
Autoimmune disease (lupus erythematosus)
Autoimmune hepatitis
Chronic viral hepatitis B or C
Non alcoholic fatty liver disease

smaller in size and the nodules become larger with diffuse fat accumulation. Macronodular cirrhosis is seen in chronic viral hepatitis and hepatocellular carcinoma and is distinguished by larger nodules (2 to 3 cm [⅘ to 1⅕ inches] in diameter) that may contain their own blood supply. The larger nodules resemble scar tissue and also have limited functional abilities. Mixed-form cirrhosis, a combination of both macronodules and micronodules, has mixed characteristics, and liver functions are also varied.[3]

Data regarding the prevalence and progression of cirrhosis are limited and variable, likely because of undiagnosed cirrhosis in the adult population. In the United States, 36,427 deaths were attributed to cirrhosis in 2013.[4] The Model for End-Stage Liver Disease (MELD) is a prognostic tool for cirrhosis. Based on the underlying cause of the cirrhosis and the serum creatinine, bilirubin, and international normalized ratio (INR), the MELD tool is used as a prediction tool for patients with cirrhosis and for prioritizing candidates for liver transplantation (www.mdcalc.com/meld-score-model-for-end-stage-liver-disease-12-and-older).[2,5,6]

The prognosis of cirrhosis depends on the cause and classification of the disease. If the cirrhosis is related to alcohol or hepatotoxic drugs, the major factor that determines survival is the patient's ability to stop drinking alcohol or taking hepatotoxic drugs.

PATHOPHYSIOLOGY

Primary biliary cirrhosis (PBC) is the autoimmune destruction of the intrahepatic bile ducts and eventual development of cirrhosis and liver failure. Hepatocellular injury occurs when the liver is continually exposed to toxins (e.g., alcohol, elevated triglycerides) or diseases (e.g., hepatitis) that produce toxemia, inflammation, ischemia, and necrosis of the hepatic tissue. The persistent inflammation and necrosis stimulate hepatocellular regeneration, causing the development of fibrous (scar) tissue such as collagen by fibroblasts. As the regeneration process progresses, rigid nodules form, distorting the normal surrounding hepatic tissue. This deformation produces increased resistance to normal blood circulation, decreased blood flow, and even obstruction of normal portal venous flow, resulting in decreased liver functional abilities.[2,6]

Portal hypertension develops when increased hydrostatic pressure within the portal venous circulation occurs, the result of inflammation and obstruction of blood flow. As cirrhosis progresses, the rising pressure in the portal circulation will increase resistance to portal venous flow. Collateral circulation develops new vascular channels and shunts that bypass areas of obstruction to maintain adequate blood flow.[2,6] The collateral path to portal circulation occurs most commonly in the peritoneum, retroperitoneum, and thoracic cavities, but also in the rectum, esophagus, and gastric areas. The complications of the collateral circulation include ascites, splenomegaly, and esophageal varices. These collateral vessels contain varicosities susceptible to spontaneous rupture, hemorrhage, and subsequent death.

CLINICAL PRESENTATION

The onset of symptoms can be insidious, and patients with cirrhosis can be asymptomatic. In PBC, the earliest reported symptoms include pruritus, weight loss, and fatigue.[5] Other concerns associated with cirrhosis are nonspecific and include weakness, malaise, dark urine, or pale stools. As the patient's condition worsens, anorexia is present and is often associated with nausea and vomiting. Hematemesis can also be a common presenting concern. Abdominal pain, if present, is related to ascites and the stretching of the muscles around the enlarged liver. Chest pain caused by cardiomegaly has also been reported. Menstrual abnormalities, impotence, and sterility are other concerns. Neuropsychiatric symptoms such as difficulty concentrating, irritability, and confusion are associated with liver function failure. Jaundice is a late-stage presenting symptom. The initial clinical presentation of patients with advanced cirrhosis is common.

A careful history, particularly a personal history of alcohol, toxic drug, or substance use and a specific review of the patient's social and work history, can identify high-risk behaviors such as intravenous drug use. Additional information necessary includes a thorough review of all medications, including herbal and over-the-counter products; allergies; past medical history; and family history. A history of recent blood transfusion or residence in an area of high hepatitis virus incidence also can suggest the diagnosis of cirrhosis.

PHYSICAL EXAMINATION

Jaundice, spider angiomata, gynecomastia, ascites, splenomegaly, palmar erythema, digital clubbing, and asterixis may be the presenting signs of cirrhosis. Low-grade fever, anorexia, and right upper quadrant pain can be present. The liver may be nodular, firm, enlarged, or shrunken (seen in late stages of cirrhosis), and the spleen may be enlarged. A fluid wave and increased abdominal girth will be evident if ascites is present. The presence of high pressures in the portal circulation often leads to the development of a venous hum (best heard over the epigastrium) and rectal and esophageal varices. As a result of the fluid shifts, peripheral edema is found in the feet, legs, and hands. Delirium, lethargy, and coma occur in the later stages of cirrhosis.[5]

Other physical signs associated with cirrhosis include weight loss; tremors; cheilosis or glossitis; spider angiomata on the face, chest, and abdomen; palmar erythema; Dupuytren contracture; horizontal white bands on nail beds (Muehrcke nails); whitening of the proximal two thirds of the nails and reddening of the remainder (Terry nails); digital clubbing; gynecomastia and testicular atrophy in men; and changes in body hair distribution in women. A sweet breath odor may be discernable in patients, referred to as *fetor hepaticus*. Asterixis, or liver flap, can be elicited with severe cases of liver failure.[3]

In patients with portal hypertension, a Cruveilhier-Baumgarten murmur may be heard. This murmur is described as a venous hum and is best auscultated over the epigastrium, and may be augmented by the Valsalva maneuver.[5]

DIAGNOSTICS

In the early stages of cirrhosis, there are often no significant diagnostic findings. It is with the presence of laboratory abnormalities that the potential for liver dysfunction is questioned. No single diagnostic biochemical marker is available regarding cirrhosis. Although not found in all patients, hypoalbuminemia, elevated serum protein, hyperbilirubinemia, and elevated liver enzymes (aspartate transaminase [AST] and alanine aminotransferase [ALT]) all indicate hepatocellular inflammation or injury. ALT is used to evaluate acute versus chronic liver injury. The alkaline phosphatase and γ-glutamyl transpeptidase levels are also often elevated. The evaluation of liver function test results and the decision to proceed with further testing and possible biopsy are based on the history and physical examination findings.[3]

Prothrombin time (PT), partial thromboplastin time (PPT), and serum albumin should be evaluated to determine hepatic synthesis and clotting function[2]; such measurements are a useful tool in the MELD score. Albumin synthesis is directly correlated to liver function, and levels of albumin will decrease as the cirrhosis advances. In addition, decreased levels of platelets are common in patients with chronic liver disease, placing the patient at increased risk for bleeding.[2,7]

The Lok index is an online calculator that uses blood chemistries to determine the likelihood of cirrhosis in patients with hepatitis C virus. The index uses the platelet count, AST, ALT, and INR to assess that probability.[8]

Additional diagnostics depend on the patient presentation, but it is important to determine the exact cause of the cirrhosis in newly diagnosed patients. Initial serologic workups may include a screen for antimitochondrial antibodies (a marker of PBC that distinguishes PBC from secondary biliary cirrhosis), antinuclear antibodies, anti–smooth muscle antibodies, antibodies to hepatitis C, hepatitis B surface antigen, and antibodies to hepatitis B core antigen and surface antigen. Fasting serum ferritin, transferrin saturation, and total iron-binding capacity should be obtained to exclude hereditary hemochromatosis.[2] If the transferrin saturation is significantly elevated (>45%), genetic testing for hereditary hemochromatosis (C282Y and H63D) is indicated. FibroTest (FT) is a serum marker that combines the quantitative results of five serum markers (α_2-macroglobulin, haptoglobin, γ-glutamyl transpeptidase, total bilirubin, and apolipoprotein A-I) with the patient age and gender and provides a measure of the degree of fibrosis in the liver.[9]

Other abnormalities in laboratory results are common. Pancytopenia, anemia (frequently macrocytic), thrombocytopenia, abnormal clotting mechanisms, and prolongation of PT all contribute to an increased potential for gastrointestinal bleeding.[7] Hyponatremia can indicate advanced illness, but other electrolyte abnormalities and renal insufficiency are also common. Ultrasound is used to assess liver size, portal circulation, and the presence of occult ascites or tumor. The imaging will also detect portal hypertension, ascites, and portal vein thrombosis.

Computed tomography (CT) is not used to diagnosis cirrhosis, and the benefits of magnetic resonance imaging (MRI) in the diagnosis and management of cirrhosis are still unclear.

Non invasive serum and radiologic markers for staging and diagnosis of fibrosis and cirrhosis are being studied. [9] However, at this time, liver biopsy, unless contraindicated, is still necessary for the diagnosis of cirrhosis and staging of fibrosis.[9] A biopsy specimen may be obtained by a radiographically guided percutaneous procedure or via the transjugular or laparoscopic route. Bleeding is a concern because of the risk of platelet abnormalities. However, in patients with a history of heavy alcohol use and ascites, liver biopsy is not necessary if the clinical, laboratory, and ultrasound results strongly support the diagnosis of cirrhosis.

Magnetic resonance elastography (MRE) estimates liver stiffness resulting from fibrosis. MRE is a safe, effective method of evaluating fibrosis in patients with chronic hepatitis C.[10]

DIFFERENTIAL DIAGNOSIS

Hepatocellular injury has varied causes, but it can be idiopathic. PBC is a chronic, progressive cholestatic disease of unknown cause. Nonsuppurative, granulomatous inflammatory destruction of the small interlobular bile ducts occurs within the liver and results in the development of cholestasis, liver failure, and cirrhosis.

Secondary biliary cirrhosis occurs when the disease is related to extrahepatic disease, as seen with cardiac failure, hemochromatosis, or Wilson disease. Patients with neuropsychiatric symptoms should be evaluated for Wilson disease. Uremia, nephrotic syndrome, metabolic disorders, pericarditis, various blood dyscrasias, biliary disease, and hepatitis are conditions that impair liver function and mimic cirrhosis. Thrombosis that is the result of cardiac or hematologic manifestations can obstruct blood flow and alter liver function. The presence of a tumor (hepatocellular carcinoma or metastatic tumors) can be detected by imaging and is suspected if the serum alpha-fetoprotein concentration is elevated. The presence of diabetes and endocrine disturbances in an older patient may suggest hemochromatosis. NASH, primary sclerosing cholangitis, or a parasitic infection such as *Schistosoma mansoni* should also be considered as a possible cause of hepatocellular injury.

DIAGNOSTICS

Cirrhosis

LABORATORY
CBC and differential
Serum electrolytes
Serum glucose
BUN
Creatinine
Serum protein
Albumin
Globulin
LFTs
Bilirubin
Alpha fetoprotein*
Hepatitis screen
Fasting serum ferritin
Transferrin saturation
Total iron-binding capacity
Serum protein electrophoresis*
Serum ceruloplasmin*

IMAGING
Ultrasound
MRI
Doppler studies
Hepatic elasticity measurement

OTHER DIAGNOSTICS
Liver biopsy
Esophagogastroscopy

*If indicated.
BUN, blood urea nitrogen; CBC, complete blood count; LFTs, liver function tests.

DIFFERENTIAL DIAGNOSIS

Cirrhosis

- Primary biliary cirrhosis (PBC)
- Secondary biliary cirrhosis
- Cardiac failure
- Hemochromatosis
- Wilson disease
- Uremia
- Nephrotic syndrome
- Metabolic disorders
- Pericarditis
- Blood dyscrasias
- Biliary disease
- Hepatitis
- Thrombosis
- Tumor
- α_1-Antitrypsin deficiency
- Nonalcoholic steatohepatitis (NASH)
- Primary sclerosing cholangitis
- Parasitic infection
- Pancreatitis
- Common bile duct obstruction

MANAGEMENT

Cirrhosis is considered an irreversible disease process, but recent advances provide hope that early identification and future

BOX 130-2

Hepatotoxic Drugs and Substances

ENVIRONMENTAL TOXINS
- Arsenic
- Fluorine
- Trichloroethylene
- Copper
- Vinyl chloride
- Toluene

DRUGS
- Isoniazid
- Folic acid analogues
- Sodium valproate
- Quinolone antibiotics
- Acetaminophen
- L-Asparaginase
- Purine antimetabolites
- Heavy metal chemotherapeutics
- Phenothiazines
- Ketoconazole
- Cytidine analogs
- Anthracenediones
- Megadose vitamin E
- NSAIDs
- Iron salts
- Gold sodium thiomalate
- Tetracycline
- Testosterone and derivatives
- Thioxanthenes
- Aspirin (high dose: >2 g/day)
- Nitrofurantoin
- Interleukins
- Inhaled anesthetics
- Retinoic acid and derivatives
- Estrogen antagonist and agonists
- Alkylating agents
- Hetastarch
- Flutamide, goserelin
- Griseofulvin
- Clozapine
- Butyrophenones
- Methyldopa
- Dantrolene

therapies will permit reversibility. Currently, progression is dependent on the cause, treatment, and patient adherence to treatment recommendations. The main focus of treatment involves the prevention of further liver dysfunction and the treatment of complications. The MELD classification tool can also be used for 3-month predication of survival with cirrhosis regardless of cause.

Primary care providers must focus on the elimination of causative factors and the promotion of a healthy lifestyle to delay the long-term consequences of cirrhosis. Patients should be immunized with polyvalent pneumococcal vaccine, yearly influenza vaccine, and, unless already immune, both hepatitis A and B vaccines.[3] Reversible causes of cirrhosis such as alcohol or hepatotoxic medications such as nonsteroidal anti-inflammatory drugs (NSAIDs) must be eliminated (Box 130-2) because continued use will result in a limited life expectancy. Patients who have ongoing viral hepatitis B or C infection can have increased life expectancy with antiviral therapy.[11] Polymerase inhibitors and protease inhibitors used in the treatment of hepatitis C have been shown to be effective in eradication and therefore prevention of cirrhosis.[12]

Esophageal varices and the risk of bleeding is a serious complication of decompensated cirrhosis. Management is directed to both control and prevent bleeding (Box 130-3). The use of nonselective beta blocker therapy has been proven to reduce the risk of bleeds by 40%. Patients should undergo esophagogastroduodenoscopy routinely to evaluate for varicies.[13] When beta blocker therapy is contraindicated or the patient is unable to tolerate it, endoscopic variceal ligation is considered. The combination of beta blocker therapy and endoscopic variceal ligation has been proven effective in recurrent variceal bleeding.[13]

To identify the cause of ascites and develop an effective treatment plan (Box 130-4), diagnostic paracentesis is necessary.

BOX 130-3

Management of Ascites

DIETARY MANAGEMENT
- Restrict sodium to 2 g/day.
- Obtain dietary consultation.
- Encourage protein intake 1.2 to 1.5 g/kg/day.

FLUID MANAGEMENT
- Restrict fluid to 1500 mL when there is marked hyponatremia.
- Consider referral for large-volume paracentesis (5-6 L); admit for procedure.

PHARMACOLOGIC MANAGEMENT
- When sodium levels remain high, begin spironolactone 100 mg/day.
- Check sodium levels in 1 week, and if natriuresis and diuresis do not occur, increase daily dose by 100 mg every 4-5 days to a maximum of 400 mg/day. Monitor carefully for hyperkalemia.
- Adjust diuretic doses so that no more than 0.5 kg (1 pound) of fluid is lost per day. Consider furosemide in combination with spironolactone to promote diuresis.
- If patient has ascites and peripheral edema, no more than 1 kg of fluid loss is acceptable.
- Decrease dose of diuretics by 50% if patient has signs and symptoms of hypovolemia.

LABORATORY TESTS
- Monitor weight, serum electrolytes, BUN, and creatinine every week or more often if patient's condition warrants it.

BOX 130-4

Prevention of Gastrointestinal Bleeding

- Administer a beta blocker (propranolol) for prophylaxis in patients at increased risk for bleeding (because of ascites, encephalopathy, or confirmed presence of varices).
- Consider consultation with a gastroenterologist for patients to undergo sclerotherapy and shunt procedures for prevention of recurrent variceal bleeding.
- Monitor PT and platelet count. Although patients can have severe alterations in PT and PTT, bleeding may not occur, and treatment is not indicated. To be certain that a vitamin K deficiency is not contributing to the alterations in PT/PTT, consider administering vitamin K, 5-10 mg PO or 10 mg SQ, or IV, if major bleeding. May repeat in 12 hours if indicated.

Management of ascites includes dietary sodium restriction to 1 to 2 g/day. Spironolactone is also a consideration to improve fluid diuresis; furosemide may be added to augment diuresis and prevent hyperkalemia. Monitoring of electrolytes, blood urea nitrogen (BUN), and creatinine is required. If ascites is refractory to diet and pharmacologic intervention, placement of peritoneovenous shunts or repeated large-volume paracentesis may be required.

Spontaneous bacterial peritonitis (SBP) is an infection of the ascitic fluid in patients with cirrhosis, necessitating careful monitoring for patients at risk. The presentation includes abdominal pain, fever, and altered mental status. Hospitalization is required, and patients are treated with cephalosporin or fluoroquinolone therapy.[13] For patients with recurrent bacterial peritonitis, antibiotic prophylaxis is required.[13]

Hepatorenal syndrome (HRS) results from renal vasoconstriction and progressive renal failure. Treatment is difficult because diuretic therapy needs to be discontinued and dehydration needs to be corrected. Fluid overload is a common complication, and hemodialysis is a necessary consideration.[13]

Hepatic encephalopathy is associated with severe liver disease. Symptoms of hepatic encephalopathy include changes in cognition, mood disturbance, and disorientation. Numerous factors, including infections, medications, gastrointestinal bleeding, and constipation, are associated with the development of hepatic encephalopathy requiring careful management (Box 130-5). The serum ammonia level may or may not be elevated. Lactulose 30 to 45 mL by mouth three times per day (tid) or four times per day (qid) to produce two or three daily soft stools helps treat and prevent hepatic encephalopathy, but the underlying cause should also be corrected. If the patient develops diarrhea, the dose should be decreased to prevent fluid and electrolyte imbalance. Rifaximin is used in addition to lactulose to treat hepatic encephalopathy. Neomycin is also used to treat hepatic encephalopathy. Because the nutritional state of the patient is compromised, close oversight of all systems is necessary to ensure management of iron deficiency, fluid and electrolyte balance, and protein-calorie malnutrition. The health care provider and nutritionist can design a patient-centered plan that will focus on consumption of a low-sodium diet, combined with protein 1.2 to 1.5 g/kg/day and adequate fiber (25to 45 grams daily), with foods that meet the patient's physical, emotional, and cultural needs. Multivitamin supplementation each day is also advised. Patients with Wernicke encephalopathy also require thiamine supplementation.[13]

Co-Management with Specialists

Management of the patient with cirrhosis is complex and requires coordinated effort with a gastroenterologist and other specialists.[14] For patients with drug or alcohol abuse, the initial priority is to assist in eliminating the offending agent from use. Drug and alcohol treatment programs can help both the patient and the family. Collaboration with mental health specialists provides information about the patient's progress with alcohol or drug abuse and determines safe medication choices for patients if pharmacologic support for detoxification is needed.

The availability of social services is helpful in acquiring financial, physical, or psychologic assistance; attaining therapeutic home aides and home health nursing care; recommending support groups; or arranging transportation. If long-term care is needed, the social worker can provide information about available facilities that will meet the patient's and family's needs.

COMPLICATIONS

The complications that occur in cirrhosis are discussed in the management of the disease and the disease process. Individuals with a diagnosis of cirrhosis will undergo many complications during the course of the disease, and early identification and treatment are critical to improve their quality of life.

INDICATIONS FOR REFERRAL OR HOSPITALIZATION

Health care providers manage most patients with cirrhosis and monitor for complications. Prompt consultation and hospitalization are indicated for gastrointestinal bleeding, encephalopathy, increasing azotemia, peritoneal irritation, or unexplained fever. A hepatologist should be consulted once decompensation is apparent. Consultation with a gastroenterologist is indicated for ascites unresponsive to fluid and sodium restriction, diuresis, large-volume paracentesis (5 to 6 L), or gastrointestinal bleeding from varices. Patients with intractable ascites, variceal bleeding, progressive encephalopathy, Wilson disease, end-stage liver disease, or hemochromatosis and candidates for liver transplantation are managed by a hepatologist. Consultation with a nephrologist is indicated for patients with oliguria, anuria, or azotemia.

PATIENT AND FAMILY EDUCATION

The patient and family should understand the benefits of the treatment plan. Dietary discipline, avoidance of hepatotoxic drugs (including NSAIDs), and support group activities are ways to achieve a successful outcome (Box 130-6).[15] The importance of reducing the risk of gastrointestinal bleeding, recognizing the signs of variceal bleeding, and taking the appropriate course of action if bleeding occurs should be discussed.

Patients with cirrhosis may be depressed. However, the use of antidepressant drugs is not usually indicated because of the high risk of oversedation and toxicity. Consultation with a

BOX 130-5

Hepatic Failure Management

1. Determine underlying cause of encephalopathy (e.g., infection, dehydration, gastrointestinal bleeding, medication or other cause of mental status change).
2. Consult dietitian to ensure patient's intake of amino acids is adequate.
3. Monitor mental status; check asterixis by using a five-point star or signature testing.
4. Monitor ammonia levels.
5. Consider oral lactulose 15-30 mL q4-6h, with subsequent adjustments in dose to allow two or three soft stools per day. Consider adding rifaximin 550 milligrams orally twice a day or neomycin, 250 milligrams g bidto q-i-d, or metronidazole , if lactulose does not decrease ammonia levels.

BOX 130-6

Patient and Family Education

1. Eliminate use of alcohol and any hepatotoxic drugs.
2. Maintain strict dietary discipline.
   - Sodium restriction to 2 g/day.
   - Consult dietitian when in doubt about any phase of the diet.
3. Follow exercise plan.
   - Consult with physical therapist to determine plan for patient.
4. Participate in support group activities.
   - Alcoholics Anonymous
   - Al-Anon
5. Watch for signs of peripheral edema; call office for weight gain greater than 0.9 kg (2 lb) per day.
6. Instruct patient's family to report any changes in patient's sensorium, posture, or gait.

psychopharmacologist can assist in designing a treatment regimen that could help the patient through this depression. Signs and complications of depression, as well as indications for immediate intervention, should be reviewed with the patient and family.

RESOURCES

www.mdcalc.com/meld-score-model-for-end-stage-liver-disease-12-and-older
medcalc3000.com/LokIndex.htm

CHAPTER 131

CONSTIPATION

Courtney L. Betts

DEFINITION AND EPIDEMIOLOGY

Constipation, one of the most common gastrointestinal complaints in the United States, results in almost 8 million primary care visits each year, with an estimated 230 million dollars spent annually in medical costs and more than 820 million dollars spent on laxatives.[1,2] This chronic disorder disproportionally affects women, children, older adults, people of low socioeconomic status, obese patients, and non-white individuals.[3] Whereas older adults are more affected and may be predisposed to constipation, there are no significant studies showing that the colonic musculature atrophies with age.[4] Rather, the increased incidence in older adults is most likely secondary to diminished vitality, decreased fluid intake, diets high in fat and protein and low in fiber, decreased activity, and the consequences of many illnesses and medications (Box 131-1).[4] Although it is not usually considered life-threatening, constipation can be disconcerting and disabling and can cause a decrease in quality of life, especially for older women.[5] It can also be associated with hemorrhoids, anal fissures, rectal prolapse, impaction, and ileus.[6]

Constipation is usually defined by practitioners as a decrease in the frequency of bowel movements to fewer than three per week.[7] However, for the Rome III criteria for constipation to be fulfilled, two or more of the following must have been present for at least 3 months with onset 6 months before diagnosis: fewer than three bowel movements per week, the passage of hard or lumpy stools, a sensation of straining, a feeling of incomplete evacuation or anorectal obstruction, and use of manual maneuvers to aid defecation in more than 25% of defecations.[8] In addition, soft, easily passed stools are not present without the use of medication such as laxatives, and the patient does not meet criteria for irritable bowel syndrome.[8] A true clinical diagnosis is the finding of a large amount of feces in the rectal ampulla on digital examination or excessive feces in the colon, rectum, or both on the abdominal radiograph.

BOX 131-1

Medications Associated with Constipation

- 5-HT_3 receptor antagonists (Ondansetron)
- Antacids
- Anticholinergics
- Antidepressants (selective serotonin reuptake inhibitors and tricyclic antidepressants)
- Antihistamines
- Anticonvulsants
- Calcium channel blockers
- Clonidine (Catapres)
- Calcium supplements
- Diuretics
- Iron supplements
- Levodopa (Larodopa)
- Narcotics
- Nonsteroidal anti-inflammatory drugs
- Psychotropics
- Sympathomimetics

Data from Bharucha AE, Pemberton JH, Locke GR: American Gastroenterological Association technical review on constipation. *Gastroenterology* 144:218-238, 2013.

PATHOPHYSIOLOGY

The primary function of the large intestine is to store and to concentrate fecal material before defecation. If the fecal contents remain in the large intestine for long periods, almost all water is absorbed, resulting in hard stools. Normal colonic motility depends on the integrity of the central nervous system, autonomic nervous system, gut wall innervation and receptors, circular smooth muscle, gastrointestinal neurotransmitters, and hormones. Healthy adults have normal gut transit time; total gut transit time is prolonged in patients with constipation.

Causes of constipation can be classified as either primary or secondary. Primary causes are disordered colonic transit (normal or slow transit) and defecatory disorders (a failure to adequately empty the rectal contents).[2] Secondary causes are related to medical and psychogenic conditions, medications, structural abnormalities, and lifestyle.[1,2] These include ignoring the urge to defecate; inadequate fiber or fluid intake; medications; pregnancy; Hirschsprung disease; hypothyroidism; hypoparathyroidism; diabetes; hypokalemia; hypercalcemia; motility disorders; psychological disturbances; and neurologic disorders, such as Parkinson disease, multiple sclerosis, and disorders of the peripheral or central nervous system.[1,2,9] Fistulas, hemorrhoids, rectoceles, abscesses, neoplasms, and other functional abnormalities are also associated with constipation, but the cause can be idiopathic or even related to irritable bowel syndrome. Parasitic infections, such as with *Ascaris lumbricoides* (an intestinal roundworm), have been identified with intestinal obstruction and should be considered in patients who travel to or live in endemic areas.[10]

CLINICAL PRESENTATION AND PHYSICAL EXAMINATION

Constipation is a subjective complaint and varies from one individual to another. Patients may have daily bowel movements but still feel constipated.[7] Patients may complain of constipation and describe a feeling of nausea, bloating, straining, and cramping and difficulty passing stools. The patient history should include when the change in bowel pattern occurred; the number of stools per day and week; the last bowel movement; the need to strain during defecation; the sensation of incomplete evacuation; the need to self-disimpact; and any episodes of fecal incontinence, diarrhea, abdominal pain, or blood or pain with defecation.[7,11] Patients who indicate that their main concerns are incomplete evacuation, feeling of obstruction, and manual disimpaction may have a defecatory disorder.[9] Possible systemic, neurologic, or other related symptoms should be elicited in addition to a past history of associated illnesses, a 24-hour dietary and fluid review, and a complete medication review (including laxative and over-the-counter medication use). Alarm symptoms and factors include sudden change in bowel habits, weight loss of 10 pounds or more, blood in the stool, anemia, family history of colon cancer or inflammatory bowel disease, constipation resistant to treatment, and age older than 50.[1,11]

Although it is not uncommon to have normal findings, the physical examination is performed to exclude or to verify the symptoms of constipation. Orthostatic hypotension or tachycardia implies dehydration; weight loss suggests anorexia or carcinoma. The oral examination may suggest poor dentition, ill-fitting dentures, lesions, or dehydration. Abdominal scars indicate a surgical history. Peristalsis and bowel sounds may be increased or decreased, suggesting a threatened obstruction or ileus. There may be increased dullness over areas of stool, and masses may be palpated. Rebound tenderness suggests a peritoneal inflammation. A gynecologic examination may demonstrate a rectocele. A digital rectal examination should determine anal abnormalities, sphincter tone and function, pain, lesions, rectal prolapse, impaction, hemorrhoids, or fissures. The neurologic examination may elicit autonomic dysfunction or neuropathy. Perineal descent is assessed by having the patient bear down while lying in the left lateral position (normal perineal descent while straining is 1 to 4 cm [2⁄5 to 1 3⁄5 inches]).

DIAGNOSTICS

- If abdominal discomfort, nausea, or vomiting is present, abdominal x-ray studies or abdominal computed tomography (CT) scan and complete blood count (CBC) with differential are necessary to exclude obstruction, ileus, megacolon, and volvulus.[12]
- Alarm symptoms mandate an evaluation for an obstructing neoplasm with colonoscopy.[2]
- CBC and thyroid-stimulating hormone (TSH) and chemistry profile, including calcium and blood glucose concentrations, are indicated in chronic constipation.[13]
  - However, the American Gastroenterological Association recommends only a CBC unless other signs and symptoms warrant further investigation.[7]
- Urinalysis and culture may reveal chronic cystitis, which is often related to constipation.
- Stool culture is indicated if the parasite *Ascaris* is suspected.[10]
- Further testing for chronic constipation after pharmacologic interventions have failed includes the following:
  - Balloon expulsion testing, barium enema, colonic transport, anorectal manometry, dynamic pelvic magnetic resonance imaging, colonoscopy, defecography[1,13]

DIAGNOSTICS

Constipation

LABORATORY	IMAGING
CBC with differential	Abdominal radiography (KUB, flat plate and upright)*
Urinalysis*	Abdominal ultrasound*
Stool for occult blood	**OTHER DIAGNOSTICS**
TSH	Barium enema*
Chemistry profile (including creatinine, calcium, potassium, serum glucose)	Colonoscopy*
Stool culture*	Anorectal manometry*
	Balloon expulsion*
	Defecography*
	Colonic transport studies*

*If indicated.
KUB, kidney, ureter, and bladder.

DIFFERENTIAL DIAGNOSIS

It is critical to recognize the pathologic conditions that first manifest as constipation. Acute-onset constipation requires emergent evaluation to identify ileus, intra-abdominal infection (e.g., appendicitis, diverticulitis), toxic megacolon, or an obstructing lesion.[12,14] Causes of chronic constipation that must be considered include anxiety or other psychogenic disorder, colorectal carcinoma, colonic obstruction, ovarian cancer, hypothyroidism, hypopituitary disorder, hypokalemia, hypercalcemia, parasitic infection, motility disorder, rectal fissure, and irritable bowel syndrome with alternating constipation and diarrhea.[1,2,9,10]

DIFFERENTIAL DIAGNOSIS

Constipation

ACUTE CONSTIPATION
- Intra-abdominal infection
- Ileus
- Toxic megacolon
- Obstructing lesion

CHRONIC CONSTIPATION
- Colon cancer
- Ovarian cancer
- Obstruction
- Endocrine disorder
- Electrolyte disorder
- Parasitic infection
- Motility disorders
- Neurologic disorders
- Psychological disorder
- Rectal fissure
- Irritable bowel syndrome

MANAGEMENT

Immediate emergency department referral is indicated for volvulus and obstruction, because the patient will need emergent surgical evaluation. Ileus and pseudo-obstruction can be medically managed with nasogastric suction and intravenous fluid.

The initial approach should include management of secondary causes, dietary measures, periodic exercise, and bowel training.[11]

- Manage secondary causes such as medical and psychogenic conditions, medications, structural abnormalities, and lifestyle.[1,2] See Box 131-1 for a list of medications.
- Advise patient to keep a stool diary.
  - Patients should be encouraged to keep a stool diary (note frequency of stooling and associated symptoms), both to substantiate the constipation and to aid in determining the effectiveness of interventions.[4]
- Have patient increase fiber.
  - Fiber should be increased to 25 to 30 g/day over a period of weeks.[2]
    - It is important to increase fiber slowly because it can cause bloating, gas, and abdominal discomfort.
    - Five prunes per day are often adequate.

- Fiber supplements such as psyllium (Metamucil) or polycarbophil (FiberCon) combined with increased fluids are recommended if a patient is unable to consume the required diet.
- Soluble fiber (psyllium) is more effective than insoluble fiber (bran).[1,15]

- Patient should initiate physical activity.
  - Initiation of a mild exercise program increases gas clearance and decreases bloating.[1]
  - Physical inactivity may lead to prolonged colonic transit.[11]
- Patient should develop regular bowel habits.
  - Instruct patients to allow enough time for satisfactory bowel elimination and to attempt to defecate during a specific time period each day.
  - Encourage the patient to toilet 30 minutes after eating a meal because eating stimulates the gastrocolic response.
- Fluids may be increased to 1.5 to 2 L daily.
  - However, there is no evidence supporting increase in fluids unless a patient is dehydrated.[1,16]

Pharmacologic treatment is appropriate if there is no response to conservative measures.

- Recommend use of bulking agents (psyllium, methylcellulose, polycarbophil).
  - Fiber, as mentioned earlier, should be trialed first either through diet or with fiber supplements (bulking agents).
  - Fiber increases the stool's water absorbency, which in turn increases bulk and weight of the stool, making it easier to pass.[4]
  - It should be noted that fiber can worsen constipation in patients with slow transit constipation or outlet dysfunction.[2] In addition, fiber will likely not help constipation caused by medications.[1]
- Stool softeners or emollients (docusate sodium, mineral oil) may be considered.
  - Docusate sodium may be added to soften the stool if bulk-forming agents are ineffective; however, there is little evidence suggesting the use and effectiveness of stool softeners for treatment of chronic constipation.[4]
  - Mineral oil, an emollient, will soften stool, but it has been associated with aspiration and lipoid pneumonia, prevents absorption of fat-soluble vitamins, and can cause fecal incontinence; it is not generally recommeneded.[2,6]
- Use of probiotics may be considered.
  - Probiotics may help increase stool frequency, but currently there are insufficient data for recommendation.[17]
- Prescribe osmotic laxatives (magnesium hydroxide, polyethylene glycol (PEG), lactulose, sorbitol).
  - Osmotic laxatives are hypertonic medications that cause secretion of water through osmosis into the intestinal wall, resulting in diarrhea.[1]
  - Osmotic laxatives, such as polyethylene glycol (PEG), are first-line treatment compared with stimulant laxatives, because there is more research showing efficacy of PEG.[1] PEG is also more effective than lactulose.[11]
  - Lactulose should be used cautiously in patients with diabetes.
  - PEG or milk of magnesia should be used judiciously in patients with a history of congestive heart failure or renal insufficiency to avoid fluid and electrolyte abnormalities.[1,11]
- Recommend use of stimulant laxatives (senna, bisacodyl).
  - Stimulant laxatives increase intestinal motility by stimulating colonic mucosa and decreasing water absorption.[4]
  - The chronic use of senna or bisacodyl was previously contraindicated, but new studies show no evidence of injury to the enteric nervous system with long-term use.[1]
- Have patient use suppository, Fleet enema, or tap water enema.
  - Enemas are useful when there are mobility issues and fecal impaction is a concern.[6]
- 5-Hydroxytryptamine receptor 4 (serotonin) agonists (tegaserod maleate, prucalopride) have either been taken off the U.S. market or have restricted use because adverse cardiovascular events reported in some users.[2,11]
- Prescribe intestinal secretagogues (lubiprostone and linaclotide).
  - Lubiprostone and linaclotide are both newer drugs that activate chloride channels, which then increases chloride secretion into the lumen, allowing passive diffusion of sodium and then water to enter the stool.[1,2,4]
  - Lubiprostone, a chloride channel activator, does not cause electrolyte imbalances; nausea is a common side effect.[2]
    - Women who may potentially be pregnant should have a negative pregnancy test before starting lubiprostone and should use contraceptives while taking lubiprostone.[1]
  - Linaclotide, a guanylate cyclase-C receptor agonist, is generally safe and effective; a common side effect is diarrhea.[17]
  - There are no current research studies comparing lubiprostone or linaclotide with standard therapy (such as PEG or lactulose), but only with placebo.[17]
- Use methylnaltrexone bromide and alvimopan.
  - These are peripherally active opioid antagonists approved for use in opioid-induced constipation.[11]

Other treatments include the following:

- Biofeedback training
  - Patients with constipation related to pelvic floor dysfunction or neurologic injury may benefit from biofeedback training.[7]
- Surgery
  - Surgical evaluation is necessary for patients with rectal prolapse and for those who require surgical intervention.
- Sacral nerve stimulation
  - Sacral nerve stimulation is used for some patients with intractable constipation.[9]

The phases of constipation management are listed in Box 131-2.

LIFE SPAN CONSIDERATIONS

Older adults are more prone to constipation. Common causes include medications, disease, diet, and lack of physical activity.[4] Older women with constipation are particularly at risk for depression and a diminished quality of life, and in addition have higher mortality rates than women who do not have constipation.[5]

COMPLICATIONS

Complications of constipation include the development of ileus, ischemic bowel, megacolon, hernia, hemorrhoids, fecal impaction, or rectal or uterine prolapse.

BOX 131-2

Constipation Management

PHASE 1

Make lifestyle changes.

- Exercise regularly.
- Develop regular bowel habits.

Make dietary changes.

- Increase dietary fiber to 25-30 g/day (prunes, bananas, bran, beans, broccoli, spinach, carrots, corn, potato, apple, and pears with skin).
- Decrease fats, particularly cheese.
- Increase fluids to 1.5-2 L/day.

PHASE 2

Use bulk-forming laxatives.

- Psyllium (Metamucil) 10-15 g daily in divided doses
- Methylcellulose (Citrucel) 6-9 g daily in divided doses
- Calcium polycarbophil (FiberCon), 2 tablets with 8 oz of water 1-3 times daily, followed by a second glass of water

PHASE 3

Use stool softeners.

- Docusate sodium: 100 mg PO twice daily followed by 8 oz of water

PHASE 4

Use osmotic laxatives.

- MiraLax: 17 g in 8 oz of water prn daily*
- Milk of magnesia: 30 mL PO prn at bedtime
- Lactulose: 15-30 mL PO daily to twice a day, up to 60 mL/day in divided doses*

PHASE 5

Use stimulant laxatives.

- Bisacodyl: 5-15 mg PO daily prn
- Senna (Senokot): 2 tablets PO prn at bedtime
- Bisacodyl (Dulcolax) suppository: 1 per rectum every 3 days prn

PHASE 6

Use intestinal secretagogues.

- Lubiprostone 24 μg twice a day* for chronic constipation
- Linaclotide 145 μg daily* for chronic constipation

PHASE 7

Severely constipated patients may require both oral laxatives and enemas or a suppository to alleviate constipation.

*These products may be expensive.

Data from Bharucha AE, Dorn SD, Lembo A, Pressman A: American Gastroenterological Association medical position statement on constipation. *Gastroenterology* 144:211-217, 2013; Costilla VC, Foxx-Orenstein AE: Constipation: understanding mechanisms and management. *Clin Geriatr Med* 30(1):107-115, 2014; and Greenberger N: *Constipation.* Available at www.merckmanuals.com/professional/gastrointestinal_disorders/symptoms_of_gi_disorders/constipation.html?qt=constipation&alt=sh. Accessed August 12, 2014.

INDICATIONS FOR REFERRAL OR HOSPITALIZATION

Nausea, vomiting, fever, and abdominal pain may indicate an ileus or ischemia and must be managed accordingly. Treatment is usually supportive and requires physician consultation when hospitalization is necessary to provide parenteral fluids and pain management. Referral to a gastroenterologist is indicated if a pathologic condition is suspected or if therapies are unsuccessful.

PATIENT AND FAMILY EDUCATION

It is imperative that lifestyle changes be reinforced to establish consistent bowel habits. Patients should not delay in responding to the call to defecate and should be encouraged to sit on the toilet, with feet placed on a stool, at the same time each day for approximately 10 minutes; this should occur preferably after meals or the ingestion of a warm liquid to stimulate the gastrocolic reflex. The promotion of a low-fat, high-fiber diet and 2 L of fluid per day are recommended. However, dietary fiber should be gradually introduced to avoid severe cramping and bloating. It is important that patients receive a careful explanation of medication side effects and understand the importance of avoiding laxatives during pregnancy or unless necessary. Patients should also contact the health care provider for any change in bowel habits or if the constipation is associated with fever, bleeding, weight loss, and abdominal pain.

CHAPTER 132

DIARRHEA, NONINFECTIOUS

Michelle Freshman

DEFINITION AND EPIDEMIOLOGY

Diarrhea is generally appreciated as an increase in stool frequency of more than three stools per day, typically appearing loose or liquid, consistent with a stool weight greater than 200 g daily. Diarrhea can range from a mild, self-limited episode to a severe, life-threatening illness. Acute diarrhea, lasting less than 2 weeks, whether it is infectious or noninfectious, usually improves without intervention. Persistent diarrhea over 2 to 4 weeks might be associated with a protozoal or other endemic infection and is more commonly described by pediatric gastroenterologists.[1] When diarrhea continues for a month without improvement, it is considered chronic. Hyperdefecation, an increase in stool frequency without a concomitant change in stool consistency, and fecal incontinence, involuntary loss of stool, are distinct.

Among industrialized country inhabitants with adequate sanitation, chronic diarrhea may account for 3% to 5% of cases annually,[1,2] whereas an individual might experience acute diarrhea once every 18 months.[3] Community-dwelling and hospitalized elderly patients are at increased risk.

Approximately 10% of acute diarrhea is noninfectious, caused by trauma, medications, toxins, transient ischemia, diverticulitis, or flares of irritable bowel syndrome (IBS) or inflammatory bowel disease (IBD). Chronic diarrhea is usually noninfectious and related to a host of malabsorptive, autoimmune, endocrine, malignant, and surgical conditions. Chronic diarrhea can be intermittent or continuous and can be manifested with extraintestinal processes or complications.

Prompt medical evaluation is indicated if diarrhea is associated with fever, abdominal pain, dehydration, or bloody stool.

PATHOPHYSIOLOGY

Approximately 10 L of fluid daily enters the jejunum, yet only a fraction leaves the body within stool. In 95% of individuals, 200 mL of fluid or less is excreted—more with higher dietary fiber.[3] The colon is able to recover up to four times its usual volume but is dependent on a tempered flow rate, allowing enough time for the maximum reabsorption of 800 mL to occur. Between the small and large intestines, this volume accounts for 99% of the excess water reabsorption; a decrease of as little as 1% may result in significant diarrhea.[3] A key mechanism in balancing colonic electrolyte and water flow is sodium (and chloride) regulation by cholinergic, adrenergic, and serotonergic mediators, among others.

Multiple mechanisms create the conditions for diarrhea. Although some focus on three categories—watery (osmotic and secretory diarrhea), inflammatory, and fatty diarrhea—noting many overlapping presentations, others separately account for secretory, osmotic, fatty, motility, inflammatory (including noninvasive infections), and functional disorders.

Secretory diarrhea is the most common type. The circumstances typically involve chemical, mechanical, or functional disruptions that produce an excess of electrolyte, nutrient, and water content in the colon. Secretory diarrhea is defined as an imbalance in fluid and electrolytes that cannot be adequately reabsorbed when water enters the bowel after a high solute or high anion load. Caused by proximal hypersecretion of the gut and a breakdown in the normal reabsorption of electrolytes and water from the colon, the result can be large-volume isotonic or hypertonic fluid in the colon, which affects patients even during fasting. For example, loss of intrinsic factor from surgery or damaged ileum will result in unconjugated bile salts that spill into the colon, pulling additional water into the lumen. Nonosmotic medications, endocrine disorders, and cancers are examples. By contrast, osmotic diarrhea includes malabsorptive disorders and results from solute-rich molecules (e.g., laxatives with magnesium, phosphate, or sulfate-containing ingredients)[3] leaving the vascular space and entering the colon, which in turn draws more water and salt into the intestinal lumen or may prevent water from entering the vascular space (Fig. 132-1). This can result in excretion up to 1 L/day.[2] Diarrhea starts postprandially and typically ends with fasting or discontinuation of the identified ingredient. Short-chain fatty acids produced as a result of bacterial metabolism of the undigested small carbohydrates result in the retention of fluid distally as well as a lower fecal pH.

Steatorrhea, another secretory diarrhea known as *fatty diarrhea*, is usually associated with malabsorption or maldigestion involving mucosal changes, ileal disease or surgery, bile acid deficiency, or pancreatic exocrine insufficiency. Type 1 bile acid diarrhea is associated with ileal disease. Cases involving 100 cm of ileum or less produce diarrhea typically; more than 100 cm of resected or diseased ileum causes steatorrhea.[4] Type 2 is diarrhea that responds to bile acid binders in the absence of structural change, a group that includes a significant number of patients with chronic diarrhea, IBS with diarrhea (IBS-D), and microscopic colitis.[4] Pale, sticky, floating, foul-smelling stool can also be the result of celiac disease caused by malabsorption of gluten. Malabsorption of bile acids resulting from use of biguanides in diabetics may cause vitamin B_{12} malabsorption with diarrhea and may play a role in acquired immunodeficiency syndrome (AIDS) diarrhea.[4] Likewise, small intestinal

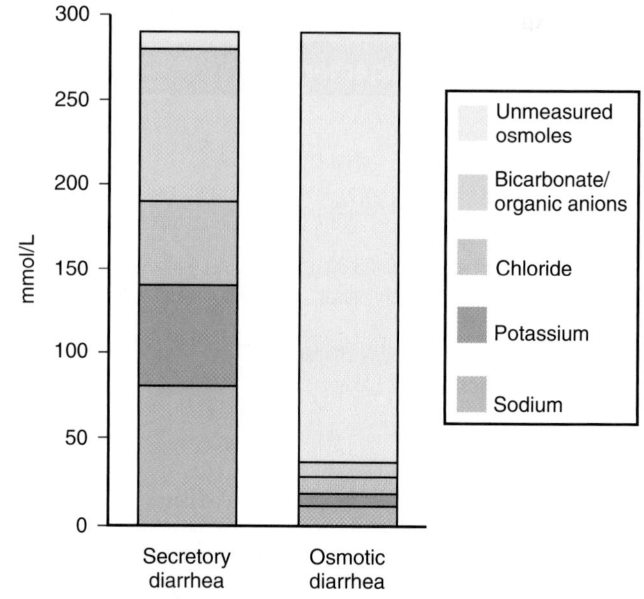

FIGURE 132-1 Fecal electrolyte composition in osmotic and secretory diarrhea. (From Schiller LR: Definitions, pathophysiology, and evaluation of chronic diarrhea. *Best Pract Res Clin Gastroenterol*. 26:677-687, 2012.)

bacterial overgrowth syndrome (e.g., after cholecystectomy) is associated with malabsorption. Maldigestion results from decreased bile salts as a result of congestion (e.g., cirrhosis, bile duct obstruction) and pancreatic dysfunction (e.g., chronic pancreatitis, cystic fibrosis).[1]

Secretory and osmotic mechanisms rather than exudative conditions are more likely to result in a very watery stool. Exudative or inflammatory conditions resulting in febrile illness or blood and pus in stool are typically associated with pain. Diverticulitis, ischemic colitis, IBD (if not pseudomembranous colitis from *Clostridium difficile* invasion after antibiotic exposure), and a range of other viral, bacterial, and parasitic infections represent the inflammatory causes.

Cancer treatment–induced diarrhea may be considered a subcategory of the exudative or even secretory type, inclusive of radiation enteritis. Nonulcerative, microscopic colitis (usually without blood, pus, or pain) may be as common as IBD.[5] Colon cancer, mastocytosis, invasive or inflammatory infections (*C. difficile*, cytomegalovirus, *Entamoeba histolytica*, tuberculosis, or ischemia is indicative[1]; rarely, Aeromonas and *Yersinia* are included in this category).[3]

Motility or regulation dysfunctions drive gastrointestinal contents along the tract more quickly, resulting in inadequate absorption of fluid from the colon. These transit dysfunctions may also be considered secretory-type diarrheal disorders but include such a variety of conditions as to warrant separate mention. Postsurgical complications may result in diarrhea. Surgeries with a high likelihood of this adverse effect include cholecystectomy, Whipple procedure (pancreaticoduodenectomy), Billroth II (gastrojejunostomy), gastric bypass (Roux-en-Y), ileocolonic resection, and ileocecal valve removal or compromise. Bile salt malabsorption features largely in significantly resected or diseased ileum, causing an overflow into the colon and an osmotic gradient (with secretory and osmotic features in the barrier crossing). Rapid transit may result from limited exposure to mucosal surface or from changes in the mechanical stretch receptors or neural stimuli.[6]

Motility disorders also include diarrhea-predominant IBS. Defined by commonly accepted Rome III diagnostic criteria for functional gastrointestinal disorders, IBS is thought to result from altered central nervous system pathways involving the limbic and paralimbic connectors, which communicate stress and receive pain signals,[6] sometimes referred to as *visceral hypersensitivity.* Serotonin reuptake transporter has a critical effect on the increase or decrease in gastrointestinal motility through the 5-HT_3 and 5-HT_4 receptors.[6] Although the mechanism is not yet known, these activators are thought to be involved[6] and have been harnessed in medical therapy directed against diarrhea-predominant IBS. In older adults, there may be significant enteric neuron loss over time, especially in the cholinergic neurons, causing motility changes as well as a blunting of cellular and humoral immunity, autoantigen recognition, and disturbed gut flora.[3]

Finally, a range of functional disorders are included. A subset of patients with functional bowel disease have significant psychological disorders that are more likely to respond to psychiatric co-management. A smaller group of patients perpetuate symptoms for secondary gain or out of emotional distress.[7]

CLINICAL PRESENTATION

The initial history should include the patient's normal stool pattern compared with the new-onset diarrhea. Charting of when the diarrhea began—whether the onset was abrupt or gradual, the course's duration, and daily stool frequency (discrete or continuous) as well as when diarrhea occurs with respect to meals and sleep—will help frame the clinical picture. Any improvement or worsening of the condition or associated symptoms should be elicited as part of the history.

Attention should be given to new-onset urgency; lower abdominal spasms, whether across the abdomen or localized to one side; relief of spasms after a movement; rectal discomfort; a sense of incomplete evacuation; or fecal incontinence. Bloody or mucopurulent exudates in the stool might reveal an inflammatory source. Greasy, bulky, rancid-smelling stool is suggestive of fat or carbohydrate malabsorption related to small bowel or pancreatic dysfunction. Whether the stool is mostly watery or unformed is also helpful in sorting out a potential secretory. Alternating patterns of diarrhea and constipation, diarrhea that awakens the patient from sleep, and any history of hemorrhoids will help determine the diagnosis. A previous history of manual disimpaction and chronic constipation or recent narcotic use might suggest overflow diarrhea in the setting of fecal impaction.

It is important to ascertain symptom relief achieved in relation to diet and over-the-counter or prescription medication. Associated signs and symptoms (e.g., nausea, vomiting, dehydration, abdominal cramping, pain, fever, chills, and rash) must also be explored. Recent history of illness may point to postinfectious IBS. Foreign travel may contribute. Other pertinent information includes increased thirst, dark or concentrated urine, oliguria, dizziness, and urinary tenesmus in consideration of renal insufficiency or undiagnosed diabetes.

Determination of whether unintentional weight loss (gradual or acute) has occurred is critical; this may prompt a diagnosis of Addison disease, hyperthyroidism, or malignant disease in the absence of other findings, especially in older adults. Growth retardation or delayed onset of puberty can suggest celiac disease, juvenile-onset diabetes, or cystic fibrosis.

Medications are also commonly associated with diarrhea as much as 4% of the time, particularly magnesium; antihypertensives; nonsteroidal anti-inflammatory drugs (NSAIDs), associated to some extent with microscopic colitis[5]; antibiotics; theophyllines; and chemotherapy agents.[2] Drugs highly associated with diarrhea include α-glucosidase inhibitors (acarbose), biguanides (metformin), cholinergic drugs, colchicine, digoxin, gold salts, highly active antiretroviral agents, metoclopramide, osmotic laxatives, prostaglandins, tyrosine kinase inhibitors, selective serotonin reuptake inhibitors, some immunosuppressive agents, and ticlopidine.[7] Chronic prednisone use can result in hypercortisolism with symptomatic diarrhea. Finally, over-the-counter and complementary products warrant further investigation for possible adverse effect or toxicity.

Allergic reactions to prescription medications and environmental exposures as well as food-related reactions are important. A dietary history should include any nutritional or dietary supplements or diet aids, especially sugar-free products that contain xylitol, sorbitol, or mannitol, which are poorly absorbed. Patients whose food sources lack vitamin B_3 or niacin (from tryptophans) or who have chronic vitamin deficiency secondary to alcoholism or food deprivation may develop pellagra, which is associated with diarrhea, dementia, and dermatitis.

The history should elicit previous medical conditions, in particular Addison disease, Behçet disease, common variable immunodeficiency disease, cystic fibrosis, celiac disease with signs of dermatitis herpetiformis or osteoporosis, diabetes mellitus type 1 or acquired diabetes mellitus, human immunodeficiency virus (HIV) infection or AIDS, hyperthyroidism or potentially overmedicated hypothyroidism, ischemia or renal blood flow difficulties, pancreatic insufficiency or other pancreatic conditions, protein-losing enteropathies, short bowel syndrome, and Zollinger-Ellison syndrome, a pancreatic neuroendocrine tumor in which 90% of patients have peptic ulcer disease.[8] Personal history of intestinal lymphoma, carcinoid, or other gastrointestinal tumors or prior radiation therapy is important because radiation enteritis can result in diarrhea many years later. Gastric bypass, Billroth II, or a Whipple procedure and associated complications, such as fistulas, blind loops, and strictures, may contribute to bacterial overgrowth and chronic mucosal surface changes, leading to diarrhea. Obstetric injury to the anal sphincter may be especially pertinent if there is fecal incontinence, which is perceived as diarrhea. A family medical history of the same or other chronic gastrointestinal conditions or cancers would be clinically relevant.

A social history of tobacco product use, alcohol abuse, or illicit drug or recently unsupervised narcotic use may contribute to diarrhea. Smoking has been shown to increase the risk and earlier presentation of lymphocytic and collagenous colitis.[5] Diarrhea can be associated with weight loss medications, in particular amphetamines and caffeinated products, such as stimulating energy drinks and tea preparations. Finally, laxative abuse and other disturbed eating, such as bulimia, might raise concern for self-injurious behavior. Munchausen syndrome, factitious diarrhea for secondary gain, malingering, and hypochondriasis are also seen. Situational stress, heightened anxiety, and panic attacks, which can be seen in association with depression, might contribute to a change in bowel pattern.

PHYSICAL EXAMINATION

The physical examination includes temperature and orthostatic vital signs (blood pressure and heart rate [lying, sitting, and standing]) to assess volume depletion. The patient's mental status should be noted along with other signs or symptoms of wasting, including weight loss.

Dry mucous membranes, decreased skin turgor, and absent jugular venous pulsation would suggest significant dehydration. A close assessment should be done for skin pallor or hair thinning in patients with anemia, rashes, flushing, and warmth; adrenocorticotropic hormone (ACTH)–related darkening of palmar creases and other sites, as in Addison disease; dermatographia (mast cell disease); icteric conjunctiva in advanced liver disease; evidence of exophthalmos and eyebrow thinning (hyperthyroidism); eye redness and pain of uveitis (Whipple disease, episcleritis or dry eyes associated with IBD); subcutaneous bleeding resulting from lack of vitamin K or prolonged prothrombin time (cirrhosis); and erythema nodosum (ulcerative colitis). The head and neck should be assessed for evidence of immunocompromise, such as lymphadenopathy or oral leukoplakia in those undergoing cancer treatment or AIDS patients, macroglossia (in rare cases of amyloidosis), or mouth ulcers in IBD, as well as thyromegaly. Carotid bruits may indicate arterial flow disease. Flushing might relate to carcinoid syndrome or mastocytosis.

A cardiovascular examination is indicated to exclude the cardiac complications associated with some illnesses, such as tachycardia in hyperthyroidism. Chest findings would be unusual except in suggesting systemic or metastasized diseases. Wheezing might signify a carcinoid tumor. During the abdominal examination, particular care should be taken in noting abdominal scars, visible distention, and audible activity of the bowel including a succussion splash, which may provide evidence of delayed gastric emptying. In addition, an indication of impaired arterial flow would be seen in bounding abdominal pulses, heard as bruits. For completion of the examination, palpation should be performed for tenderness, rigidity, rebound, guarding, masses, organomegaly, or ascites. Gauging anorectal sphincter tone as well as performing a digital rectal examination for masses, fecal impaction, or bleeding would be included. In the female patient with lower abdominal symptoms, a pelvic examination is imperative.

Tremor may be a sign of hyperthyroidism. Joint pains might point to IBD, reactive arthritis after enteritis such as Reiter syndrome, or a vitamin D and calcium deficiency resulting from malabsorption. Distal extremity edema suggests interstitial fluid shift, possibly from extravascular fluid leak or protein malabsorption as a result of chronic malnutrition or protein-losing enteropathy.

DIAGNOSTICS

Acute Diarrhea

For the patient who has mild, afebrile, acute diarrhea, diagnostic evaluation is not usually indicated. These brief episodes are typically viral or food-borne illnesses, are self-resolving, and require little or no intervention (Box 132-1). If an infectious source is suspected, stool for fecal leukocytes, ova, and parasites; a stool culture; and sensitivity testing are necessary.

In the absence of an infectious cause, plain abdominal x-ray examination of the kidneys, ureters, and bladder (KUB), flat and upright, is necessary if a small bowel obstruction or stool impaction with overflow incontinence is suspected. Emergent indications for upper endoscopy with small bowel follow-through include small bowel torsion causing partial or full obstruction, possibly resulting from colitis-related strictures, bowel perforation, toxic megacolon, or ileus.

If diarrhea continues after 2 weeks and the suspected cause is noninfectious, then colitis, diverticulitis, pancreatitis, irritable bowel, and IBD would lead the list of differential diagnoses. The patient's weight is a key indicator, especially in persistent or chronic cases.

A complete blood count (CBC) with differential revealing an elevated white blood cell count may indicate general inflammation or infection; low hematocrit and hemoglobin would indicate anemia, potentially as a result of acute blood loss, which may corroborate a positive stool guaiac test result over time. A complete metabolic panel including liver function would reveal electrolyte or enzyme abnormalities. A compromise in kidney function would suggest dehydration or concomitant illness is a factor.

In patients with a temperature above 38.8° C (102° F), bloody diarrhea, abdominal pain, more than six unformed stools in a 24-hour period, profuse watery diarrhea, and dehydration or in patients who are frail or older, immunocompromised, or toxic appearing, a stool sample should be sent for *C. difficile* toxin A or B analysis, with secondary consideration of IBD.

DIAGNOSTICS

Acute Diarrhea

LABORATORY
- CBC with differential*
- Serum electrolytes
- Serum glucose
- BUN
- Creatinine*
- Stool for fat, osmolality, laxative screen*
- Stool for occult blood and fecal leukocytes (infectious transmission or inflammatory disease)*
- Stool for ova and parasites, culture for *C. difficile* (infectious transmission)*

IMAGING
- KUB*
- CT of abdomen*
- Sigmoidoscopy or colonoscopy*
- Upper endoscopy with small bowel follow-through and biopsy*

*If indicated.
BUN, blood urea nitrogen; CT, computed tomography.

Chronic Diarrhea

The cornerstone of diagnosis in chronic diarrhea is stool analysis (see Box 132-1). A case of persistent, now chronic diarrhea in the setting of blood in stool and pus should prompt a Wright stain for white blood cells in cases of bacterial bowel disease or IBD. Also, HIV infection, recent chemotherapy, transplantation, and antibiotic or antiretroviral use would suggest an infectious cause (see Chapter 230).

A 24-hour stool pH, electrolyte panel, osmotic gap, weight, elastase, and qualitative and quantitative fecal fat along with a stool screen for laxatives if indicated (which have an alkalinizing effect on feces; stool will likely be phenolphthalein positive) should help in the diagnosis of malabsorption, maldigestion, or laxative abuse. A small osmotic gap (<50 mOsm/kg) points to a low electrolyte concentration and secretory diarrhea; a large gap (>125 mOsm/kg) points to more electrolyte polarity,

BOX 132-1

Evaluation of Acute and Chronic Diarrhea

EVALUATION OF ACUTE DIARRHEA

Symptomatic therapy
- Hydration (PO or IV)
- Diet modification

Symptoms persist: order fecal leukocytes
- Hypovolemia
- Bloody stools
- Fever
- >6 liquid stools per day
- >48 hr
- Severe abdominal pain
- Older adults (>70 years)
- Immunocompromised

EVALUATION OF CHRONIC DIARRHEA

Osmotic diarrhea
- Stool osmolarity (osmolar gap >50 mOsm/kg, often ≥125 mOsm/kg)
- Stool analysis (low pH → carbohydrate malabsorption)
- Breath H_2 test, D-xylose test for lactose intolerance or lactate assay
- Magnesium level (inadvertent ingestion or laxative abuse)

Secretory diarrhea
- Exclude persistent infectious pathogens (*Aeromonas*, microsporidia, epidemic cholera)
- Stool osmolarity (osmolar gap <50 mOsm/kg)
- Serum gastrin, secretin stimulation test, if necessary (Zollinger-Ellison syndrome)
- Thyroid-stimulating hormone, T_4 (hyperthyroidism)
- Calcitonin, prostaglandins, or 5-hydroxyindoleacetic acid (medullary carcinoma of the thyroid)
- Histamine and tryptase levels (mastocytosis)
- ACTH stimulation (Addison's disease)
- Tissue transglutaminase and antiendomysial antibodies if normal IgA level (celiac disease)
- 72-Hour fecal α_1-antitrypsin level with α_1-antitrypsin plasma clearance (intestinal protein loss)
- Immunoglobulins, serum protein electrophoresis (multiple myelomas, common variable immunodeficiency)
- Antienterocyte or antigoblet antibodies, may be detected (autoimmune enteropathy)
- Metanephrines
- Small bowel series, endoscopic ultrasonography, upper endoscopy with small bowel follow-through and biopsy with aspirate for quantitative culture, CT of abdomen and pelvis, CT and magnetic resonance enterography, sigmoidoscopy or colonoscopy with biopsy, positron emission tomography combined with CT or MRI for small bowel lymphomas, radioligand scintigraphy (e.g., OctreoScan) for certain neuroendocrine tumors, device-assisted enteroscopy with balloon or spiral overtubes, possibly capsule endoscopy

Inflammatory diarrhea
- Fecal leukocytes or lactoferrin (limited usefulness)
- Small bowel series, upper endoscopy with small bowel follow-through and biopsy, CT of abdomen and pelvis, CT and magnetic resonance enterography, sigmoidoscopy or colonoscopy with biopsy; in graft-versus-host disease, sigmoidoscopy and biopsy of distal colon instead of duodenum to mitigate risk

Fatty diarrhea
- Stool fat test (72-hour collection)
- Small bowel series, upper endoscopy with small bowel follow-through and biopsy with aspirate for quantitative culture, CT of abdomen and pelvis, CT enterography
- Exclude pancreatic insufficiency (amylase, lipase, stool chymotrypsin of fecal elastase, secretin stimulation test, trial of pancreatic supplements)

Modified from Schiller LR: Definitions, pathophysiology, and evaluation of chronic diarrhoea. *Best Pract Res Clin Gastroenterol* 26:677-68, 2012; and ASGE Standards of Practice Committee, Shen B, Khan K, et al: The role of endoscopy in the management of patients with diarrhea. *Gastrointest Endosc* 71(6):887-892, 2010.

creating a hypertonic gradient. This concentration gap is characteristic of an osmotic mechanism wherein the ingested ions are poorly absorbed, such as in carbohydrate malabsorption.

Although stool weight can be used as a guide to excess output, a more precise indicator is fecal liquidity, which in cases of diarrhea refers to the marked inability of the stool to absorb excess water. A fecal elastase below 200 µg/g points to chronic pancreatitis with exocrine insufficiency.[8] Serum trypsin levels below 20 ng/mL point to advanced chronic pancreatitis or tumor obstruction.[8] A steatocrit determines pancreatic exocrine function.[8] In some cases, a 72-hour screen for osmolality, stool fat, and laxative use may also be indicated. Qualitative fecal fat or Sudan III stain will be misleading if the condition results from ingestion of Olestra or use of the diabetic medication acarbose. Clinicians may prefer the quantitative 72-hour collection screening, which is performed after the patient's intake of a high-fat regimen (>100 g/day). Steatorrhea often points to small bowel disturbances. Small bowel bacterial overgrowth syndrome might also show up as a significantly elevated folate level in the setting of gastrointestinal bloating, flatulence, and diarrhea.

Serum eosinophilia may reflect eosinophilic gastroenteritis, eosinophilic colitis (rare, but suggestive based on place of birth, travel, or immunocompromise)[5] or mastocytosis, which could be confirmed by a serum tryptase level, especially if there is a significant association with the use of various medications (penicillin, NSAIDs, or narcotics), or by mast cells on skin biopsy.

In cases of watery diarrhea, poorly absorbed carbohydrates or magnesium overload should be considered. A hydrogen breath test using lactose, D-xylose (if available), or similar sugar molecules may help make the diagnosis of lactose intolerance, small bowel bacterial overgrowth syndrome, or carbohydrate malabsorption such as in sucrase or fructase enzyme deficiencies, especially if fecal pH is acidic. A separate stool magnesium level in excess of 45 µmol/L (90 mEq/L) might raise suspicion of factitious tampering through laxative overuse.

A wider investigation of secretory diarrheal causes might include a cosyntropin stimulation test for Addison disease if fatigue, weight loss, and malaise persist in the absence of other signs, even absent electrolyte shifts. Low albumin and abnormal liver function test results might point to cirrhosis or chronic illness states. In patients with a low albumin level but normal kidney and liver function, a protein-losing enteropathy can be gauged by calculation of α_1-antitrypsin clearance during 24 hours, which combines a 72-hour fecal α_1-antitrypsin collection with a serum α_1-antitrypsin level.[3]

A serum blood glucose or hemoglobin A_{1c} (HbA_{1c}) level would help establish diabetes mellitus, as would physical signs of neuropathy and acanthosis nigricans in patients with insulin resistance if not associated with Cushing disease or polycystic ovary syndrome. An abnormally low thyroid-stimulating hormone concentration obtained as a result of tachycardia and weight loss should prompt consideration of hyperthyroidism.

Other laboratory tests may include immunoglobulin A (IgA) with anti–tissue transglutaminase, which may be used alone given its high positive predictive value, and antiendomysial antibodies for celiac disease in the absence of IgA deficiency. IgA or IgM deficiency in the setting of an already low IgG level may lead to the diagnosis of common variable immunodeficiency (CVID) or common variable hypogammaglobulinemia, with its constellation of infectious, pulmonary, gastrointestinal, and potentially malignant manifestations.

Various pancreatic conditions might lead to secretory diarrhea. Plain abdominal radiography and computed tomography (CT) scan will help differentiate pancreatitis from pancreatic mass. Magnetic resonance imaging (MRI) is the best structural test in cases of suspected pancreatic insufficiency if anatomic landmarks can be seen. A secretin stimulation test, which would follow a positive stool chymotrypsin level, may be performed when a pancreatic exocrine disorder or a tumor is suspected. In practice, pancreatic enzyme replacement often precedes if not replaces this test as a more cost-sensitive approach. Other rare neuroendocrine disorders might be implicated in situations of low potassium concentration or fatigue. Urine excretion of 5-hydroxyindoleacetic acid in the setting of facial flushing or wheezing might lead to a diagnosis of carcinoid, gastrin in consideration of Zollinger-Ellison syndrome, calcitonin for medullary thyroid adenocarcinoma or bone metastases, and vasoactive intestinal polypeptide (VIP) for VIPoma, but these tests area usually low yield, given a high false-positive rate in the absence of leading clinical indicators.

Fecal leukocytes on Wright stain with microscopy or a fecal calprotectin or lactoferrin level can lead the investigation for bacterial infection or IBD, although it is limited by variable sensitivity. The fecal marker tests are thought to be better than C-reactive protein levels in determining an organic versus a functional cause; a normal erythrocyte sedimentation rate is also thought to be more likely to point to functional bowel disease, although the role of these fecal and inflammatory marker tests is controversial. Thiopurine methyltransferase (TPMT) and the metabolite panel is sometimes ordered if there is clinical suspicion.

Further diagnostic tools include magnetic resonance angiography for ischemic colitis, sigmoidoscopy, colonoscopy, and abdominal and pelvic CT scan. For IBD or those conditions known to disrupt intestinal mucosa or to shed white or red blood cells in stool but that are not deemed infectious, the diagnosis is made histologically. This category tends to overlap with secretory diarrheal causes in cases in which inflammation does not produce detectable fecal leukocytosis or blood and thus must be ascertained on biopsy. Another consideration is that an infection may overlie preexisting colitis.

IBD is best appreciated on upper endoscopy with small bowel follow-through as well as on colonoscopy with microscopic analysis of the gastrointestinal mucosa. Ulcers, fistulas, and strictures may lead the clinician to a diagnosis of IBD. Both sigmoidoscopy (for left-sided symptoms) and colonoscopy with biopsy are useful to diagnose chronic laxative use, colonic carcinoma, collagenous and lymphocytic colitis, and IBD.

A small bowel biopsy will distinguish amyloidosis, bacterial overgrowth, Behçet disease (a vasculitis more prominent in the Middle East), celiac disease, Crohn disease or ulcerative colitis, eosinophilic gastroenteritis, jejunal diverticulitis, intestinal lymphangiectasia (congenital as well), lymphoma, mastocytosis, and small bowel carcinoma. Wireless capsule endoscopy, increasingly preferred over small bowel follow-through, might be necessary for an enhanced three-dimensional visualization and biopsy of the distal ileum if the lesions are very small. A ^{75}SeHCAT (radiation) retention study (available in Europe) provides evidence of bile salt malabsorption, although a trial of bile salt resin replacement is typically prescribed in the United States before further testing would be ordered. It may be the that fibroblast growth factor 19 (FGF-19) ileal hormone, arising from a failure of the liver to make it, may serve as a marker for bile acid diarrhea (BAD).[4]

Gastroenterologist consultation is warranted if the initial workup does not suggest a cause. Further endoscopic visualization and biopsy as well as serum testing for rare endocrine tumors are likely to be necessary.

DIAGNOSTICS

Chronic Diarrhea

LABORATORY
- CBC and differential
- Serum glucose
- BUN
- Creatinine
- Liver biochemical tests
- Calcium
- Phosphorus
- Albumin
- Glycosylated hemoglobin (Hb_{A1c})
- Thyroid-stimulating hormone
- Prothrombin time
- Serum immunoglobulins (particularly IgG and IgA)
- Tissue transglutaminase and antiendomysial antibodies
- Serum vasoactive intestinal peptide†
- Serum calcitonin†
- Serum gastrin*
- Serum glucagon†
- Urine 5-hydroxyindoleacetic acid†
- Urine vanillylmandelic acid†
- Urine metanephrine†
- Serum tryptase†

IMAGING
- KUB
- CT of abdomen
- Barium study
- Sigmoidoscopy
- Colonoscopy with biopsy*
- Upper endoscopy with small bowel follow-through and biopsy*
- MRI*
- CT-PET scan for evaluation of cancer metastasis

*If indicated.
†Very rare, low-yield test in the absence of compelling diagnostic features.
BUN, blood urea nitrogen; PET, positron emission tomography.

DIFFERENTIAL DIAGNOSIS

Acute Noninfectious Diarrhea

Once the commonly occurring infectious causes are no longer under consideration, medications rise to the top of the differential list. Magnesium-containing antacids and laxatives lead the list in contributing to acute noninfectious diarrhea. Antibiotics are commonly implicated as well. In fact, over 700 medications have been associated with diarrhea after initiation.[7] Toxins such as organophosphate insecticides (typically found in migrant farm workers), unpasteurized milk, mushrooms, lead, mercury, arsenic, food additives such as monosodium glutamate (MSG), and ciguatera and scombroid (environmental toxins found in fish) also cause diarrhea. Abrupt-onset, large-volume diarrhea with bleeding, pain, or fever may result from mesenteric vascular insufficiency or intestinal angina (an emergency that may lead to bowel necrosis and death without revascularization or stenting), ischemic colitis involving low flow to the inferior mesenteric artery of the left lower quadrant, diverticulitis, or obstruction.

Chronic Noninfectious Diarrhea

Toxins from bacterial processes are the most likely cause of chronic diarrhea; however, many noninfectious causes are possible (e.g., HIV-associated noninfectious diarrhea or tube feedings and pseudomembranous colitis associated with *C. difficile*). There is also a graft-versus-host disease phenomenon that results in chronic diarrhea.

Chronic noninfectious diarrheas represent a multitude of disease entities, some with overlapping features. Celiac disease, which produces secretory diarrhea, involves mucosal changes of the duodenojejunal brush border, malabsorption of gluten, and fatty stool. Diabetes, an endocrine disorder with pancreatic effects, is a secretory cause of diarrhea featuring a glucose malabsorption component, which can eventually lead to protein-losing enteropathy and dysmotility. Therefore, categorical delineations may not be as well circumscribed as suggested.

Excess magnesium, sulfate, and phosphate ingestion, most often associated with antacids and laxatives, can cause osmotic diarrhea. Cathartics or saline purgatives likewise draw water into the gut. Other highly osmotic molecules include sugar alcohols such as sorbitol and mannitol found in sugar-free (diabetic) candy or chewing gum and undigested lactulose. Sucrase-isomaltase malabsorption can be controlled through avoidance diets. Other carbohydrate malabsorption (maltose, glucose-galactose, fructose) may result from disaccharide insufficiency, although excess fructose can cause diarrhea in healthy individuals.

Cow's milk or soy milk protein intolerance as well as lactose intolerance may be discovered early in life. Whereas the majority of individuals have lactase enzyme activity until they are weaned in early childhood, a minority of those of northern European descent appear to have lactase enzyme activity continuing into adulthood, which is considered the result of a genetic mutation. Typically, no diagnostics are indicated other than a trial of abstinence from foods or liquids that contain lactose.[1] However, if the lactose-free diet trial fails to resolve the symptoms, a further workup including a lactose hydrogen breath test may be advised. A retrial of lactose-containing foods in smaller quantities throughout the day, after a hiatus, will sometimes allow some tolerance, particularly if calcium supplementation cannot be achieved any other way.

Watery diarrhea that persists despite efforts to eliminate potential sources can result from a secretory disorder. There is usually no blood or white blood cell debris or constitutional symptoms. Causes of secretory diarrhea include primary gastrointestinal disorders, nongastrointestinal inflammatory diseases, and endocrine disorders such as unusual neuroendocrine tumors. Although celiac disease might be considered a gluten malabsorption or mucosal disorder, it is treated as a secretory one. Alcoholism-associated malnutrition, low vitamin B_{12} intake, and resulting pernicious anemia can also lead to secretory diarrhea.

Chronic diarrhea can also be inflammatory and accompanied by pain, fever, and pus and bleeding. Examples include lymphogenous or collagenous colitis, Crohn disease and ulcerative colitis (including ulcerative jejunoileitis), ischemic colitis, diverticulitis, Behçet syndrome, pseudomembranous colitis, primary or secondary immunodeficiency, eosinophilic gastroenteritis, diarrhea after cancer treatment, and radiation colitis. Malabsorption disorders that cause protein-losing enteropathy and gluten malabsorption are similar.

When changes in the intestinal mucosa occur, whether or not they are caused by an autoimmune disease or inflammation, muscle innervation and in turn peristalsis can be affected. This causes malabsorption of fluid and nutrients and rapid transit in a state of overactive motility or inflammatory bowel diseases, such as ulcerative colitis and Crohn disease. Crohn disease may strike anywhere along the whole gut (mouth to anus) and affects the full thickness of the bowel wall. Ulcerative colitis usually affects the mucosal layer in the distal sigmoid but has been known to arise occultly in the left side of the colon or distal ileocecal valve, causing high-volume stool with pus and bloody exudates, significant cramps, and even fever in severe cases. Mucosal changes associated with inflammation as a result of IBD, collagenous and lymphocytic colitis, diverticulitis, or Behçet disease cause secretory diarrhea. Small intestinal ischemic colitis is often associated with poor vascular flow. Other than infectious and neoplastic sources, further inflammation of the intestinal wall and ulceration of the mucosa can result from diverticulitis and radiation enteritis.

Another cause of chronic secretory diarrhea is disruption of fat absorption. Pancreatic insufficiency can produce a malabsorption of fats, causing fatty stool, bloating, and malodorous gas. Small bowel surface loss as a result of bacterial overgrowth can cause malabsorption, as is the case in cystic fibrosis. An example of small intestinal malabsorption is gluten-sensitive enteropathy, or celiac disease, which causes an inflammatory reaction with loss of mucosal surface area resulting in steatorrhea and malnutrition. Gluten-sensitive enteropathy is a complex disorder composed of impaired absorption, increased intestinal permeability, and, in 10% of patients, pancreatic insufficiency. Chronic pancreatitis is the most common, but develops into permanent scarring and progressive dysfunction. BAD may be more closely linked to IBS-D, microscopic colitis, and perhaps functional diarrhea, accounting for one third of the 1% of people in Western countries experiencing chronic diarrhea.[4] Diarrhea resulting from motility dysfunction is highly prevalent, whether it is caused by use of stimulant laxatives or NSAIDs, diabetic enteropathy, hyperthyroidism, scleroderma, strictures or adhesions from surgery, radiation enteritis, or prokinetic agents.

Although functional disorders are typically grouped separately, stress and anxiety may also come into play in both IBS and the more generally defined functional disorders, which ultimately affect transit time. The Rome III consensus statement defines IBS as recurrent abdominal pain or discomfort, 3 days per month in the last 3 months, associated with at least two of the following: improvement with defecation, onset noted by a change in stool frequency or form (appearance) of stool, with symptom onset at least 6 months before diagnosis[9]; functional diarrhea, in contrast, is loose (mushy) or watery stool without

DIFFERENTIAL DIAGNOSIS

Noninfectious Diarrhea

ACUTE NONINFECTIOUS DIARRHEA

- Bowel trauma
- Diverticulitis
- Irritable bowel syndrome flare
- IBD flare (Crohn disease, ulcerative or collagenous colitis)
- Ischemic colitis
- Medication or toxin exposure (<4 wk of diarrhea)
- Mesenteric vascular insufficiency

CHRONIC NONINFECTIOUS DIARRHEA

Medications and Supplements (Secretory or Osmotic Dysfunction)

- Antacids (magnesium, sulfate, or phosphate containing)
- α-Glucosidase inhibitors (acarbose)
- Antiarrhythmic (quinidine)
- Antibiotics (especially ampicillin)
- Antidepressants
- Antihypertensives
- Biguanides (metformin)
- Chemotherapeutics
- Cholinergics
- Colchicine
- Diuretics
- Gold salts
- Highly-active antiretroviral agents
- Lactulose
- Laxatives (magnesium containing or lactulose)
- Metformin
- Metoclopramide
- Narcotic withdrawal
- NSAIDs
- Polyethylene glycol
- Prostaglandins
- Selective immunosuppressive agents
- Selective serotonin reuptake inhibitors
- Sugar substitutes (maltitol, mannitol, sorbitol, xylitol)
- Theophylline
- Ticlopidine
- Tyrosine kinase inhibitors
- Vitamins
  - Niacin deficiency
  - Excess fish oil ingestion (omega-3 fatty acids)
  - Excess vitamin A, C, D, or E ingestion

Toxins, Environmental or Food Related

- Heavy metals (lead, mercury, arsenic)
- Insecticides
- Monosodium glutamate
- Mushrooms
- Organophosphates
- Sulfites

Osmotic Disorders of the Intestine

- Enzyme deficiency
  - Cow's milk protein intolerance
  - Fructose or carbohydrate malabsorption
  - Lactose intolerance
  - Soy milk protein intolerance
  - Sucrase-isomaltase deficiency
- Osmotic laxatives
- Poorly absorbable ions (excess magnesium, sulfate, phosphate, bicarbonate, or chloride)

Secretory Disorders of the Intestine

- Autoimmune disorders
  - Amyloidosis
  - Autoimmune enteropathy*
  - Common variable immune disorder (multiple gastrointestinal manifestations)*
  - Mastocytosis (mast cell disease)*
  - Scleroderma
  - Vasculitis (e.g., Behçet disease)*
- Endocrine disorders
  - Addison disease
  - Carcinoid syndrome*
  - Diabetes mellitus (diabetic diarrhea—20% of diabetics)
  - Gastrinoma (Zollinger-Ellison syndrome, small intestine, or metastases to liver)*
  - Hyperparathyroidism
  - Hyperthyroidism or hypothyroidism
  - Medullary carcinoma of the thyroid*
  - Somatostatinoma*
  - VIPoma*
- Malabsorption (damage affecting or loss of absorption)
  - Bile salt malabsorption (see detail on following page)
  - Celiac disease (gluten-sensitive enteropathy)
  - Chronic mesenteric ischemia
  - Eosinophilic gastroenteritis
  - Malnutrition (many causes, including alcoholism)
  - Pernicious anemia
  - Small intestinal bacterial overgrowth
  - Whipple disease (long-term *Tropheryma whipplei* infection)
- Inflammatory or exudative disorders of the intestines
  - Collagenous colitis
  - Crohn colitis
  - Diversion colitis
  - Diverticulitis (segmental colitis)
  - Ischemic colitis
  - Lymphocytic colitis
  - Radiation enteritis or colitis
  - Ulcerative colitis (including ulcerative jejunoileitis)
- Malignant neoplasms
  - Colonic tumor, especially villous adenoma
  - Esophageal tumor
  - Gastric tumor
  - Lymphoma
  - Neuroendocrine tumors*
  - Pancreatic tumor
  - Small intestinal tumor
- Invasive or inflammatory infections
  - Bacterial—*Aeromonas, C. difficile,* cholera, cytomegalovirus, *Yersinia, Mycobacterium tuberculosis*; parasitic—*Cryptosporidium, E. histolytica, Giardia;* viral—cytomegalovirus, herpes simplex virus, HIV/AIDS
  - Diverticulitis
  - Inflammatory bowel disease (Crohn disease and ulcerative colitis)
  - Ischemia
  - Mastocytosis

Motility or Structural Disorders of the Intestine (Secretory or Osmotic Dysfunction)

- Congenital chloridorrhea*
- Diabetic enteropathy, autonomic neuropathy

DIFFERENTIAL DIAGNOSIS—cont'd

Noninfectious Diarrhea

- Eosinophilic gastroenteritis
- Fistulas, diverticula, strictures, blind loops
- Gastrojejunostomy
- Ileocecal valve removal or compromise
- Impaction with leak around as a result anorectal dysfunction
- Intestinal lymphangiectasia (protein-losing gastroenteropathy; can be congenital)
- NSAIDs (protein-losing enteropathy)
- Postcholecystectomy
- Postgastrectomy (gastric bypass, Billroth II, or Whipple procedure)
- Postvagotomy
- Prokinetic agents (metoclopramide, erythromycin)
- Pseudo-obstruction
- Radiation enteritis
- Short bowel or short gut syndrome
- Small bowel intestinal overgrowth

Steatorrhea Resulting from Pancreatic Disorders

- Bile salt malabsorption
  - Bacterial overgrowth syndrome
  - Stimulant laxatives (senna, castor oil, cascara, bisacodyl)
  - Terminal ileal disease (>100 cm of ileum is removed or compromised)
- Pancreatic insufficiency syndromes from maldigestion
  - Alcohol-related pancreatitis or cirrhosis
  - Carcinoma of pancreas
  - Chronic pancreatitis or pancreatic exocrine insufficiency
  - Cystic fibrosis
  - Diabetic steatorrhea usually with pancreatic exocrine insufficiency
  - Zollinger-Ellison syndrome (typical primary site)

Functional Disorders

- Factitious
- Irritable bowel disease, diarrhea predominant (or alternating with constipation)
- Laxative abuse
- Malingering
- Munchausen syndrome (or Munchausen by proxy)

Other Disorders

- Heightened physical demands (e.g., intensive running)
- Idiopathic diarrhea

*Very rare.

pain occurring at least 75% of the time during the past 3 months, for at least 6 months (see Chapter 139).

Stress or psychiatric disease may play a role in functional bowel disease. Self-neglect or substance abuse (e.g., alcoholism) may result in malabsorption, a cofactor or prevailing cause of diarrhea. Unsupervised narcotic withdrawal causes rapid transit in the gut. Other severe malnutrition states as a result of socioeconomic or behavioral neglect may set the stage for further illness or infectious complications. Last, factitious diarrhea includes those cases caused by deception or self-injury. The motivation is often secondary gain, such as for sympathy, treatment with controlled medications, or relief of responsibilities. Factitious causes may account for up to 15% of otherwise unexplained cases, made more difficult on occasion by patient tampering with samples. In some cases of severe psychological illness, the behavior may perpetuate without insight.

MANAGEMENT

Fluid and electrolyte replacement is essential in the treatment of acute diarrhea. Oral fluid replacement should be initiated at home or in the office to manage a mild, uncomplicated episode of diarrhea. A hyperosmolar solution containing glucose and electrolytes is advised to prevent future intestinal intraluminal fluid overload. If the patient's condition fails to respond to oral rehydration or worsens or if the patient has persistent symptoms, intravenous hydration may be indicated. Solid food products should be reintroduced as symptoms resolve and stools become more formed.

Medications can be used for symptomatic relief of nausea and vomiting, abdominal cramping, and diarrhea. If nausea is the main complaint, treatment with promethazine (Phenergan) or prochlorperazine maleate (Compazine), which have anticholinergic effects, or ondansetron, a serotonin 5-HT_3 antagonist, can be effective. Absorbents such as attapulgite (Kaopectate), 30 mL by mouth every 30 minutes as needed to a maximum of eight doses a day, and bismuth subsalicylate (Pepto-Bismol), 30 mL by mouth every 30 minutes if needed to a maximum of eight doses per day, typically serve to control diarrhea (as do activated charcoal, kaolin-pectin, attapulgite, and smectite).[2] The tablet form of bismuth subsalicylate, 1 or 2 tablets every 4 to 6 hours to maximum 8 tablets in 24 hours, and antispasmodic-anticholinergic sedatives such as atropine-scopolamine-hyoscyamine-phenobarbital (Donnatal, immediate release), 1 or 2 tablets up to three times a day, are used to decrease abdominal cramping. Because these products may cause aspirin intoxication, they should be used cautiously. Patients taking warfarin should be warned as well, because anticoagulation will be affected. Also, Pepto-Bismol should not be used with HIV-positive or immunocompromised patients, who are at risk for encephalopathy. Secretory diarrhea related to neuroendocrine tumors (VIPomas, carcinoids) is treated with octreotide, 50 to 250 μg subcutaneously three times a day. This agent is a somatostatin analogue that stimulates intestinal fluid and electrolyte absorption and stops intestinal fluid secretions. Octreotide is also used to treat AIDS-related chronic noninfectious diarrhea.

Depending on the cause of chronic diarrhea, treatment may be curative, suppressive, or empirical. If the cause of the diarrhea is not known but is not thought to be worrisome, treatment may include an opiate such codeine, 15 to 60 mg up to four times daily (maximum daily dose 320 milligrams), or deodorized tincture of opium, 2 or 3 drops four times daily. These intestinal transit inhibitors aid in slowing motility, decreasing secretions, increasing fluid absorption, and increasing blood flow. Because narcotic agents are potentially habit-forming, they should be reserved for patients with chronic, intractable diarrhea, prescribed in consultation with the physician and pharmacist. Clonidine is an $alpha_2$-adrenergic agonist that inhibits intestinal electrolyte secretion. Octreotide, as mentioned (natural somatostatin or its analogues), provides further antisecretory support.[2]

For IBS-D in women, one agent, alosetron hydrochloride, is available under strict supervision and requires prescription by a gastroenterologist enrolled in the Prescribing Program for Lotronex (see Chapter 139). One popularly adopted, evidence-based approach to symptom management is adhering to a low FODMAP diet (consisting of low levels of fermentable oligo-di-monosaccharides and polyols).[7,10] Celiac disease is managed by a gluten-free diet (i.e., strictly avoiding wheat, buckwheat, oat, rye, barley, and malt). A mere one third of an average-sized piece of bread is enough to lead to symptoms. Church wafers or inert ingredients in medications have been known to be unexpected culprits. Because there is some correlation with celiac disease and microscopic colitis, strict gluten avoidance may also help in these conditions. For collagenous colitis and lymphocytic colitis, budesonide has been shown to be effective. Alternatively, bismuth subsalicylate (2 tablets four times a day for 8 weeks), colesevelam (1875 mg daily up to twice daily), or cholestyramine (4 g daily up to four times a day) can be helpful.

Acute insult to the bowel, such as through trauma or ischemic attack, necessitates hospitalization because significant complications may arise. Diverticular disease also may necessitate hospitalization and treatment if unresponsive to past outpatient therapy (see Chapter 133).

For some patients, postoperative diarrhea can persist for years. In patients who have dumping syndrome after vagotomy or gastric surgery affecting transit, concentrated carbohydrates can be a trigger. Avoidance of liquids with meals and lying down afterward can help relieve a common postprandial sweating, dizziness, and flushing reaction. Some gastrointestinal surgeries will lead to motility disorders stemming from stagnation in the small intestine. Empirical treatment with antibiotics should be considered in cases of small intestinal bacterial overgrowth syndrome if it is likely that excessive dyspepsia with flatulence and watery diarrhea might be associated with an elevated folate level. Rifaximin, 400 mg three times daily for a week, is currently recommended; an alternative is metronidazole, 250 mg three times daily, or ciprofloxacin, 500 mg twice daily for a week, with the caveat that its use may cause tendon injury. Ideally, any antibiotic used for this purpose would be alternated with a second, if there are likely to be repeated courses, to prevent antibiotic resistance. Probiotics that stimulate the bowel to colonize increased levels of *Lactobacillus* GG, although controversial, may be used as an adjunct.

If *C. difficile* colitis is diagnosed, metronidazole, 500 mg three times a day for 10 to 14 days, or vancomycin, 125 mg orally four times a day for 10 to 14 days, may be used. Unfortunately, some resistant strains have arisen, and a small subset of patients can have a difficult time surmounting this secondary infection. Rifaximin, 200 to 400 mg twice a day to three times a day, is another treatment option, as is, in limited use, fecal transplant.[11] Inflammatory diarrhea from infectious causes would also respond to systemic antibacterial, antifungal, antiviral, antiprotozoal, or anthelmintic therapy.

For diarrhea caused by bile salt malabsorption as a result of intestinal resection or terminal ileal disease, colesevelam hydrochloride (Welchol), 1875 g twice daily, although not approved by the Food and Drug Administration for this indication, is a preferred agent in practice, despite the fact that cholestyramine (Questran), 4 g one to two times a day, is typically recommended. Antimotility agents should not be used with IBD. Finally, some clinicians will resort to a trial of codeine, which has been used in variable immunodeficiency disease but may lead to tolerance, heightened nausea, and sedation. Following a low-fat diet is no longer recommended because fat-soluble vitamins must be absorbed; weight should also be maintained if therapy is successful.[11]

Anti-inflammatory treatments are appropriate for inflammatory causes such as Crohn disease and ulcerative colitis. Depending on severity of presentation, location, and history of the course of IBD, sulfasalazine or mesalamine would be advised in addition to a steroid course or ongoing treatment. In more severe cases, azathioprine or 6-mercaptopurine, with or without mesalamine suppositories or enemas, with ongoing steroid suppression or weaning, might lead to a remission. Some patients cannot tolerate 6-mercaptopurine or azathioprine treatment if their TPMT enzyme level is too low (see Chapter 138). Monoclonal antibodies are now in common use for moderate to severe cases of Crohn and ulcerative colitis disease: infliximab, adalimumab, certolizumab, natalizumab, and vedolizumab.

For overflow incontinence, manual disimpaction and subsequent low-volume tap water or solute-filled enemas, along with the side-lying position and turning back and forth, may help move the bowel contents along. For fecal incontinence unresponsive to bulking agents or loperamide, if there is documented anorectal dysfunction captured though defecography, anorectal manometry, and MRI, then biofeedback administered by a specialized physical therapist is highly useful.

COMPLICATIONS

Complications from diarrhea are usually a result of dehydration. Regardless of the cause, attention should be directed toward fluid and electrolyte replacement. Electrolyte disorders, particularly hypocalcemia, hypomagnesemia, and hypokalemia, are common in persistent diarrhea. Continuous diarrhea can necessitate hospitalization for fluid and electrolyte replacement if the patient is unable to maintain hydration with oral fluid replacement. Sepsis and cardiovascular collapse are potential complications, and infants, older adults, and immunosuppressed patients are more susceptible to these complications. Refractory diarrhea is usually a symptom of a more serious illness and requires diagnostic evaluation and immediate physician consultation.

Relapses of *C. difficile* colitis are common in older adults and are more likely in cases of extended fever, stool incontinence, and use of H_2 receptor antagonist acid suppression therapy, for which probiotic and immunogenic therapy is under investigation.[3] Nosocomial diarrhea, arising after 2 days in hospital, can stem from noninfectious sources such as medications (particularly antibiotics). Enteral feedings or comorbidities may further complicate the condition, particularly in those who are immunocompromised.

In celiac disease, patients may first notice a persistent erythematous rash specifically associated with it, called *dermatitis herpetiformis*. In addition to the abdominal bloating and steatorrhea coupled with foul-smelling stool, there is a potential for weight loss caused by anorexia and resulting stunted growth. Untreated or recalcitrant celiac disease can lead to other endocrine, hematologic, neurologic, and oncologic conditions as well anemia, osteopenia, or osteoporosis, and sometimes infertility.

Untreated IBD can lead to bowel perforation, stricture or blockage, obstruction, and sepsis. For those diagnosed with IBS, there is a phenomenon in which the entity is associated with interstitial cystitis and endometriosis, which may mean that a patient seeks specialty management from three specialists instead of one. Complications of CVID can lead to significant dehydration, bowel blockage, and anemia. The effects of a surgically shortened ileum can range from anemia resulting from lack of intrinsic factor to dumping syndrome. Gastric bypass surgery has a host of complications necessitating adequate vitamin and electrolyte replacement and nutrient supplementation.

Amyloidosis is a multiorgan syndrome in which damage may manifest in the heart and elsewhere. Recalcitrant, high-volume diarrhea may lead to dangerous levels of potassium loss, and hypokalemia has cardiac implications. Laxative abuse may lead to metabolic acidosis if there is a severe decrease in sodium bicarbonate, which may affect the heart.

INDICATIONS FOR REFERRAL OR HOSPITALIZATION

In patients with severe dehydration or protracted vomiting, intravenous fluids should be initiated in a medical setting. If the illness persists beyond 3 weeks despite treatment measures, chronic lactose intolerance, malignant neoplasms, and disease states such as diabetes, thyrotoxicosis, lupus, HIV infection, and IBD should be further considered.

IBD can manifest as a bowel obstruction or severe anorectal fistula. Surgery, potentially colectomy, in severe, protracted cases might be a primary consideration. Renal and cardiac comorbidity would be a factor in ischemic colitis, considered a gastrointestinal emergency.

Older adults are more likely to be hospitalized with diarrheal illness and have higher mortality. Urgent physician or hospital-based consultation with surgical staff is imperative in these cases.

LIFE SPAN CONSIDERATIONS

In young adults, IBS may occur as a postviral complication. In general, IBS has a bimodal distribution, appearing in young adults or older adults for the first time, with a female and constipation predominance. Crohn disease and ulcerative disease are split roughly equally by sex and disease type and are considered to have a bimodal distribution by age at onset, although these groupings are clustered closely in time. These two peaks in symptom onset occur between the ages of 15 and 40 years and the ages of 50 and 80 years, and both entities have a genetic and ethnically Jewish predisposition, although new-onset diarrhea late in the seventh decade (median age at onset) is more likely to be microscopic colitis. Microscopic colitis typically affects women in the fifth to seventh decades of life. Detection of celiac disease is on the rise because of more sensitive and specific testing assays; it can first manifest in children, sometimes in pregnancy, or as late as the sixth decade as diarrhea. A history of small birth size, childhood illnesses, Irish or Scottish descent, and concomitant diabetes are risk factors. Diabetic complications, such as diabetic enteropathy, are more likely to affect patients with long-standing disease.

Older adults are more likely to have a worse case of *C. difficile* colitis, with a higher risk of relapses and a higher risk of death. Medications have a multitude of side effects. The majority of patients older than 65 years have diverticula. Tube feeding in elders can be a cause of iatrogenic diarrhea, causing a dumping syndrome from the high solute content when it is infused directly into the small bowel. In the geriatric patient, fecal impaction must be ruled out.

PATIENT EDUCATION AND HEALTH PROMOTION

Diseases of malabsorption or complications of intestinal surgery that have led to malabsorption offer an opportunity to promote healthful choices in nutrient and vitamin supplementation, with periodic laboratory surveillance. For those with celiac disease, multiple societies provide online resources to find food alternatives, medical information, and support. Regular exercise programs in many instances are thought to be of benefit to the patient with chronic, noninfectious diarrhea.

If infectious, toxin- or medication-related, autoimmune, endocrine, surgical, and other gastroenterologic causes have been excluded, the clinician is left with a host of functional diseases for which symptom management is key. Functional bowel disease, including IBS-D as well as mixed IBS (involving alternating diarrhea and constipation predominance at baseline), is thought to be influenced by diet and stress, with further insults from caffeine, nicotine, and alcohol. Therapeutic support or referral for psychological counseling is paramount for those with a significant psychological component to their illness.

CHAPTER 133

DIVERTICULAR DISEASE

Mellisa A. Hall

Diverticular disease is a common disorder of the colon occurring more often as life expectancy increases and as dietary practices include more refined foods. The disease manifests in a variety of clinical spectrums and in three different clinical patterns: (1) diverticulosis, or uncomplicated diverticular disease, the asymptomatic or symptomatic presence of noninflamed multiple colonic diverticula; (2) diverticulitis, or complicated diverticular disease associated with inflammation in one or more of the diverticula, with possible resultant perforation leading to abscess or fistula formation; and (3) hemorrhage, another complication of diverticular disease, often associated with a right-sided diverticulum or diverticula.[1]

DIVERTICULOSIS

DEFINITION AND EPIDEMIOLOGY

Diverticulosis derives its name from the basic unit of diverticular disease, the diverticulum, which is an outpouching of mucosa through the colon wall. The occurrence of a single diverticulum is uncommon; hence, the term *diverticulosis* is used to describe the condition of numerous diverticula in the colon.

This term is an anatomic descriptor. Clinically, diverticulosis is an uncomplicated, asymptomatic or symptomatic disease without inflammation or bleeding.

The prevalence of colonic diverticulosis varies greatly in different geographic areas of the world. It is most common in the Western Hemisphere and is rare in Africa, Asia, and many parts of South America. This disease is considered an acquired disease of 20th-century Western civilization. Its emergence parallels a change in dietary habits that occurred during the Industrial Revolution of the 1850s, including the mechanical milling of crude cereal grain and wheat flour and the resultant loss of the nonabsorbable fiber content. At this time, there was also an increased consumption of white flour, refined sugar, conserves, and meat.[2]

Studies from less industrialized regions (e.g., Africa and Asia) document prevalence rates of diverticulosis of less than 0.2%.[3] Incidence of diverticulitis in Africa and Asia commonly involve the right colon compared with left colon involvement in Western countries.[4] The worldwide prevalence of diverticular disease is not truly known; but in the United States and other developed countries, its prevalence approaches a third of the population older than 45 years and two thirds older than 85 years. In advancing age, women are affected more than men.[3] Diverticulosis also affects a significant proportion of younger adults, with increasing prevalence of diverticular disease in all age groups. Patients younger than 40 years are more commonly male.[3] A familial pattern is noted from twin studies.[5]

PATHOPHYSIOLOGY

Colonic diverticula are defects of the large colon, especially the sigmoid, that develop with advancing age. They are saclike herniations of the mucosa through the muscularis propria and are actually pseudodiverticular because they do not contain the muscle layer.

The pathophysiologic changes common to all cases of diverticulosis of the colon are not entirely clear. Herniation of the muscle layer of the colon is the result of two factors: (1) an increased pressure gradient between the colonic lumen and the serosa and (2) areas of relative weakness in the colonic wall.[1]

One commonly accepted hypothesis of diverticula formation is that low-fiber diets decrease the amount of intraluminal bulk in the colon, causing muscle hypertrophy as the colon tries to move the fecal matter along.[1] Lack of fecal bulk is thought to produce uncoordinated and irregular colonic peristalsis, which creates sacculations in the colon wall. There is increased pressure within these sacs, which results in diverticular outpouchings. These sacs occur at weak points, or natural breaks, in the muscle layer of the colon where the nutrient vessels, the vasa recta, pass through the muscularis propria into the submucosa. In addition, the colon wall, which is covered by connective tissue, loses its flexibility and tensile strength with age. A weakened bowel wall develops and may predispose an individual to formation of diverticula.

Increasing dietary fiber intake will reduce the incidence of diverticular disease; accordingly, vegetarians have a reduced risk for diverticular disease.[1] Additional risk factors for diverticular disease include consumption of red or processed meats, obesity, and smoking.[3]

In terms of size and distribution, diverticula range from 1 or 2 mm to giant diverticula. In Western societies, diverticula occur predominantly in the sigmoid colon. In Asians, right-sided diverticula are more common.[4]

CLINICAL PRESENTATION

Patients with uncomplicated colonic diverticula, or diverticulosis, are often asymptomatic and rarely seek medical attention; approximately 75% of these individuals are never seen with a clinical problem.[1,6] Of the 25% of patients with acute diverticulitis who are seen, 15% will develop significant complications including fistulas, abscesses, and perforations.[3] Symptomless diverticula are often noted when the colon is studied for another reason with a barium enema, colonoscopy, computed tomography (CT) scan, or ultrasound examination.

Symptomatic patients may complain of irregular defecation, intermittent abdominal pain, bloating, or excessive flatulence. In general, there is a change in stool caliber, with descriptors that can range from flattened or ribbon-like to hard pellets. Associated complaints include urinary dysfunction, anorexia, nausea, vomiting, and heartburn. Older individuals often relate recurrent bouts of steady or crampy pain (mostly in the left lower quadrant) in combination with constipation or alternating periods of diarrhea and constipation. They may also have abdominal distention that is relieved by the passage of flatus or stool. These symptoms can often mimic irritable bowel syndrome except that they are experienced at an older age. Patients with right-sided pain tend to be younger, and their pain is easily mistaken for appendicitis. Immunocompromised patients may be asymptomatic longer because of ineffective inflammatory response, making them at higher risk for complications.[1]

PHYSICAL EXAMINATION

For patients with uncomplicated symptoms, the findings of the physical examination (including both pelvic and rectal examinations) are usually normal. Fever is possible but may not be present. The other vital signs are often normal except in the presence of a massive diverticular bleed; tachycardia and hypotension are not uncommon. Most often, physical findings reveal mild, left lower quadrant tenderness with a thickened palpable sigmoid and descending colon. Isolated right lower quadrant tenderness also may be related to diverticulitis. Tenderness throughout the abdomen suggests perforation and peritonitis.[7] Rectal bleeding is infrequent, but painless bright red bleeding or maroon-colored stools suggest a diverticular bleed.[7]

DIAGNOSTICS

A complete blood count (CBC) and urinalysis should be obtained. Screening laboratory values should be normal in uncomplicated diverticulosis; leukocytosis may be present in diverticulitis. A stool specimen for occult blood is necessary because uncomplicated diverticulosis is not known to cause occult rectal bleeding. Plain abdominal x-ray films will be normal and are unnecessary, although they are sometimes ordered to exclude the presence of free air in the abdomen. Rigid sigmoidoscopy usually cannot be performed beyond the rectosigmoid junction and for this reason is not particularly useful. The diagnosis of diverticulosis is most often established with a barium enema examination; this method is the best for determination of the extent and severity of the disease. Barium enemas should be avoided in acute diverticulitis because of the risk of extravasation of barium into the peritoneal cavity, causing chemical peritonitis. Chemical peritonitis increases the risk of mortality. A substitution for barium enema would be a water-soluble enema. Although it is often used as a diagnostic tool, colonoscopy is best used to assess the large bowel for a coexisting pathologic

DIAGNOSTICS

Diverticulosis

LABORATORY	IMAGING
CBC and differential	Barium enema
ESR*	KUB*
Urinalysis	CT scan*
Stool for occult blood	**OTHER DIAGNOSTICS**
	Colonoscopy*

*If indicated.
ESR, erythrocyte sedimentation rate; KUB, kidney, ureter, and bladder study.

condition rather than for an actual diagnosis of diverticular disease.[1]

A CT scan of the abdomen and pelvis with contrast enhancement is the preferred imaging study if acute diverticulitis is suspected. However, CT scan is not indicated for all patients but should be considered if peritonitis, a diverticular abscess, or other complication is suspected. Unless pregnancy is ruled out, the recommended imaging modality for women of childbearing age with acute abdominal pain is sonography.[8,9]

DIFFERENTIAL DIAGNOSIS

The hallmark of symptomatic diverticulosis is colicky abdominal pain in the absence of an inflammatory process. The cause of this pain is not fully understood but possibly is related to spasms in the sigmoid colon or an element of obstruction related to the spasms. This clinical entity must be differentiated from diverticulitis and any disease that causes abnormal intestinal motility.

The challenge is not so much in making the diagnosis as it is in distinguishing patients who have symptomatic diverticular disease from those who have diverticula plus other lesions that may be responsible for the symptoms. Irritable bowel syndrome and colorectal cancer should be considered in the differential diagnosis. In patients with localized right-sided abdominal pain, appendicitis must be considered.[1]

DIFFERENTIAL DIAGNOSIS

Diverticulosis

- Diverticulitis
- Irritable bowel syndrome
- Cancer
- Cystitis
- Appendicitis
- Inflammatory bowel disease
- Crohn disease
- Peritonitis
- Chronic ulcerative colitis
- Ischemic colitis
- Infectious colitis
- Radiation-induced colitis
- Gynecologic inflammatory or neoplastic diseases
- Vascular ectasia
- Ectopic pregnancy
- Anorectal disease
- Small or large bowel obstruction
- Gastroparesis
- Chronic constipation

MANAGEMENT

Fiber is essential to reduce the risk of constipation. In the United States, adults consume approximately 11 to 23 g of fiber per day, half of the 27 to 40 g of daily fiber recommended by the World Health Organization and less than the 20 to 35 g proposed by the American Dietetic Association.[2] Increased fiber intake can be achieved through the consumption of whole grains and cereals, fruits, vegetables, and legumes. These foods should be introduced gradually during a period of weeks to months to avoid excessive bloating and flatulence. Bran, a concentrated form of fiber, can be used as an adjunct to fiber consumption but should not be a replacement for other high-fiber foods. Some patients may need 2 g of bran three times a day to provide the bulk; it should be soaked or mixed in media such as hot cereal, applesauce, juice, or milk.[2] Fiber can also be given through commercially available high-fiber supplements or bulk formers such as psyllium hydrophilic mucilloid, methylcellulose, and calcium polycarbophil. These products work similarly to bran and must be taken with several glasses of fluid to be effective. They produce a softer, more frequent stool.[10]

Current literature does not support the elimination of certain dietary foodstuffs in the management of diverticulosis. Diets high in dietary fiber and low in saturated fat, along with the avoidance of red meat, have minimal evidence in reducing the risk of diverticulosis. They do have promising support in clinical trials to lower the risks of colon cancer.[11,12]

Anticholinergic and antispasmodic agents have been used without substantiated evidence of their effectiveness. They may be used to relieve spasms. Care should be taken to avoid constipation.

Surgical resection for pain relief, in the absence of documented inflammatory complications, is associated with a high rate of symptom recurrence and is therefore not recommended.[1]

LIFE SPAN CONSIDERATIONS

Diverticular disease is usually observed in adults older than 40 years, and incidence increases with age. Younger adults, however, can develop diverticular disease and associated complications such as diverticulitis and diverticular bleeding.[1]

COMPLICATIONS

The most common complication of diverticular disease is acute diverticulitis. Hemorrhage from diverticula is also a common complication, occurring in 5% to 15% of patients; 3% to 5% of cases are severe. Hemorrhage is more common from the right colon. Other complications that are less common include abscess, bowel perforation, peritonitis, strictures, fistulas, and small bowel obstructions.[3]

INDICATIONS FOR REFERRAL OR HOSPITALIZATION

Uncomplicated diverticular disease can be managed in the primary care setting. Questionable radiographic findings on any barium studies necessitate referral to a gastroenterologist for further evaluation. Patients with suspected diverticular abscess or rectal bleeding need further evaluation, and a referral or consultation is indicated for lower endoscopy.

Although the health care provider assumes responsibility for patient education, a referral to a dietitian may be beneficial for patients with recurrent, painful disease.

PATIENT AND FAMILY EDUCATION AND HEALTH PROMOTION

The patient's diet and symptoms should be reviewed at every session for prevention and health promotion. All patients need to be instructed about a nutritionally well-balanced diet that includes whole-grain breads and cereals and fresh fruits and vegetables to attain the benefits of both types of fiber. The goal of 30 to 35 g of fiber per day requires the consumption of five fruits and vegetables (15 g), four high-fiber starches (8 g), and one high-fiber cereal (7 g).

It is important that patients be advised to increase their fiber intake gradually to prevent flatulence and abdominal discomfort. Patients can often tolerate 5- to 10-g increments every few weeks on the basis of symptoms. Bloating or flatulence resulting from bran intake usually resolves with continued use. If patients are taking pharmaceutical fiber supplements, it is especially important that they increase their fluid intake to at least eight 8-ounce glasses of fluid per day. Maintenance of ideal body weight, daily exercise, reduced consumption of red and processed meats, and avoidance of tobacco and alcohol and the routine use of nonsteroidal anti-inflammatory drugs also reduce the risks of development of diverticula.[13-15]

DIVERTICULITIS

DEFINITION AND EPIDEMIOLOGY

Diverticulitis, or complicated diverticular disease, is the most common complication of diverticulosis. An inflammatory condition that involves one or more colonic diverticula, diverticulitis is almost always symptomatic. Diverticulosis must be present before there can be an attack of diverticulitis.[1,3] Complicated diverticulitis occurs in up to 25% of cases, and the majority of the patients have no prior knowledge of the disease. Patients may have perforation as the first symptom; perforation is the most significant cause of morbidity and mortality.[1]

PATHOPHYSIOLOGY

The inflammation associated with diverticulitis is thought to result from the stagnation of fecal material in a single diverticulum. This produces a fecalith that leads to pressure necrosis of the mucosa and subsequent inflammation. This inflammatory process progresses, and either a microperforation or a macroperforation ensues. A small perforation is easily contained by the pericolic tissues and becomes a localized phlegmon. A larger perforation may result in a walled-off pericolic abscess whose erosion may produce fistulas into adjacent structures, such as the urinary bladder, vagina, small bowel, and anterior abdominal wall. If there is free perforation in the abdominal cavity, fecal peritonitis may occur.[16]

CLINICAL PRESENTATION

The diagnosis of diverticulitis is often clinical, especially in a patient with known diverticula. Most patients with infection or localized inflammation have mild to moderate, colicky to steady, aching abdominal pain usually present in the left lower quadrant (93% to 100%) accompanied by fever (57% to 100%) and leukocytosis (69% to 83%).[1] Constipation or loose stools may or may not be present. There may be nausea and vomiting. Hematochezia is uncommon in diverticulitis and is more suggestive of other diagnoses. In some instances, the patient is initially seen with complications of diverticulitis, such as recurrent urinary tract infections or feculent vaginal discharge resulting from fistulization. In other cases, a patient may exhibit few or no symptoms and therefore does not seek medical attention for several days. Older patients or patients who are immunocompromised may have minimum abdominal pain, no fever, and relatively benign findings on physical examination but still have sepsis.[1]

PHYSICAL EXAMINATION

The physical examination of patients with diverticulitis may reveal mild distention. Bowel sounds are hyperactive if there is obstruction but are otherwise normal. In general, there is tenderness in the suprapubic region or over the involved colonic segment (often in the left lower quadrant). A mass may or may not be palpated. Pain in the right lower quadrant can be mistaken for acute appendicitis. There can be involuntary guarding and percussion tenderness localized in this area, indicating localized peritoneal inflammation. Patients who experience generalized abdominal pain and abdominal wall rigidity could have a perforated viscus. A rectal examination may reveal some tenderness in the pelvis, and a mass is occasionally palpated anteriorly. Stools are not usually positive for occult blood, but hematochezia is possible. In female patients, a pelvic examination is a necessary component of the physical examination. Fever may or may not be present, depending on the severity of the infection and the age and immune status of the patient.[1]

DIAGNOSTICS

Initial laboratory studies may not be useful in diagnosis of diverticulitis. Although a CBC is usually obtained, leukocytosis is not a requisite symptom of this condition. Urinalysis may reveal white blood cells if the inflammatory process is adjacent to the bladder or ureter. The presence of bacteria in the urine sample consistent with urinary tract infection is suggestive of a fistula. A pregnancy test is indicated for premenopausal and perimenopausal women.

Supine and upright plain x-ray films can be obtained to assess for ileus, a small or large bowel obstruction, or free abdominal air (which indicates perforation). A CT scan of the abdomen and pelvis has been used increasingly to evaluate patients with diverticulitis. It is the test of choice if diverticular complications are suspected because it gives a more accurate estimate of the degree of inflammation than other studies do.[9] Some authorities suggest that not all patients with acute diverticulitis require a CT scan for successful management but recommend that it be performed under the following conditions: with a questionable diagnosis; when an abscess or fistula is suspected; with inadequate clinical improvement with medical treatment; as a diagnostic for patients who are immunocompromised (e.g., steroid dependent), when clinical evaluation is not a reliable indicator of the patient's condition; and in an unusual clinical situation, such as right-sided diverticulitis. A barium enema is not recommended with acute diverticulitis because of the risk of barium peritonitis.[9]

Additional tests include ultrasonography, flexible sigmoidoscopy, and colonoscopy. Ultrasonography is used to reveal extracolic fluid collections and to guide percutaneous drainage of pelvic and paracolic abscesses; however, ultrasonography is more operator dependent than CT is.[9] Patients may not be able to tolerate the external pressure, and imaging is limited in an obese patient. Flexible sigmoidoscopy is often used during an episode of suspected diverticulitis. Its main usefulness arises in the event of colonic obstruction to differentiate an obstructing carcinoma from an obstructing diverticular mass. Colonoscopy is useful after the inflammatory process subsides.[16]

DIAGNOSTICS

Diverticulitis

LABORATORY
CBC and differential
ESR*
Stool for occult blood
Urinalysis
BUN, creatinine (before CT scan in elders or in patients with renal insufficiency)*

IMAGING
Angiography (if the patient is bleeding)
CT scan*
Ultrasound*
Water-soluble contrast enema*

OTHER DIAGNOSTICS
Colonoscopy*
Flexible sigmoidoscopy*

*If indicated.
BUN, blood urea nitrogen; ESR, erythrocyte sedimentation rate.

DIFFERENTIAL DIAGNOSIS

Diverticulosis is sometimes associated with marked local tenderness and a palpable sigmoid loop and therefore may be mistaken for diverticulitis; however, fever and leukocytosis are typically absent with diverticulosis.[1,16] Other differential diagnoses include acute appendicitis, peritonitis, cystitis, neoplasm, inflammatory bowel disease, ischemic colitis, radiation colitis, infectious colitis, small bowel obstruction, and gynecologic disorders (such as pelvic inflammatory disease, endometriosis, ovarian cysts, and ectopic pregnancy).[1]

DIFFERENTIAL DIAGNOSIS

Diverticulitis

- Diverticulosis
- Acute appendicitis
- Gastroenteritis
- Peritonitis
- Cystitis
- Neoplasm
- Inflammatory bowel disease
- Ischemic colitis
- Radiation colitis
- Infectious colitis, bacterial abscess
- Small bowel obstruction
- Pelvic inflammatory disease
- Endometriosis
- Ovarian cysts
- Ectopic pregnancy
- Testicular torsion

MANAGEMENT

The clinical spectrum of acute diverticulitis is diverse. Spontaneous resolution is common for many patients with low-grade fever, mild leukocytosis, and minimum abdominal tenderness. These patients do not require hospitalization. In general, treatment consists of taking clear liquids for 2 or 3 days, limiting physical activity, and taking oral antibiotics such as trimethoprim-sulfamethoxazole (Bactrim DS, 160 mg/800 mg twice daily) plus metronidazole (500 mg three times daily), amoxicillin–clavulanate potassium (Augmentin, 875 mg/125 mg), or ciprofloxacin (500 mg twice daily) plus metronidazole (500 mg three times daily) for 7 to 14 days.[1] Antibiotic selection is based on coverage of the usual gram-negative and anaerobic pathogens responsible for the infection.[1,16] As the patient begins to feel better, the diet is slowly advanced as tolerated. Conservative therapy of clear liquid diet, hydration, and oral antibiotics is effective in managing 85% of cases; unfortunately, one third of patients will have a recurrence. Anti-inflammatories including mesalamine and probiotics are newer therapies that have been used successfully for diverticulitis.[12] Additional clinical trials are needed to support their routine use in prevention.

If fever and leukocytosis are absent, the patient may have only painful diverticular disease and not diverticulitis; for this condition, antibiotics are withheld. The duration of treatment is determined by clinical response; treatment is usually discontinued when symptoms have resolved and the patient is afebrile. Pain medication is discouraged; symptomatic relief may be achieved with warm packs. Nonopiate analgesics may be used if necessary.[1]

Immediately after an attack of diverticulitis, a short-term, low-fiber diet that consists of 15 g or less of dietary fiber is prescribed to reduce the volume of fecal material in the lower bowel and to prevent irritation to the colon. When the patient is asymptomatic, a gradual modification to a diet high in fiber (and free of seeds) may help reduce pressure inside the colon, thus reducing the chances of future attacks.[17] A colonoscopy is recommended after symptoms resolve to exclude carcinoma.[1]

Patients can be acutely ill with systemic peritonitis, sepsis, and hypovolemia. Any patient with a temperature of 38.5° C (101.3° F) or higher and with marked tenderness, signs of localized peritonitis, intestinal obstruction, or suspected intra-abdominal or pelvic abscess must be admitted to the hospital. Hospitalization is also recommended for diabetic or immunosuppressed patients, older adults, and patients with chronic renal failure in whom diverticulitis is suspected in the absence of the previously listed criteria.[1] Older adults are especially prone to complications from diverticular disease, including risk of diverticular rupture and peritonitis.[18] Hospital management includes assessment of fluid status and intravenous replacement, nasogastric suction if there is an obstruction or ileus, blood cultures, and broad-spectrum intravenous antibiotics that cover gram-negative anaerobes and gram-negative aerobes. Treatment time depends on symptom resolution and is usually maintained for 7 to 10 days. Further evaluation and management depend on patient assessment and response to initial treatment. If fever, abdominal signs, and leukocytosis have mostly resolved and bowel function has returned with the passage of flatus, a liquid diet can be started and slowly advanced to a low-fiber diet. When the patient is asymptomatic, a high-fiber diet can be gradually introduced. The patient is discharged with a regimen of oral antibiotics, such as metronidazole, 500 mg three times daily for 7 to 10 days. Studies such as a barium enema or colonoscopy should be performed 4 to 6 weeks after hospital discharge. A CT scan with contrast enhancement is required if the patient's condition does not improve after 2 to 4 days of medical treatment; if the diagnosis is in doubt; or if a pelvic or abdominal abscess, fistula, or obstruction needs to be excluded.[1]

Most patients with uncomplicated diverticulitis recover with medical treatment and do not have recurrences of acute disease; thus, surgery is not routinely recommended. However, in patients who require hospitalization for treatment of diverticulitis, surgical management is necessary in 15% to 30% of patients. Younger patients and immunocompromised patients are managed surgically more often than other patients with diverticulitis.[16] Elective surgical intervention should be considered after the second episode of acute diverticulitis at any age because of the risk of perforation. Urgent surgical intervention is also sometimes necessary. Elective surgical management typically consists of a single-stage procedure to decrease morbidity and mortality. Factors that guide surgical management include the patient's age, comorbidities, frequency and severity of attacks, and CT-graded severity of attacks. A laparoscopic approach has been used for sigmoid resection. This approach decreases hospitalization time and shortens recovery.[16]

COMPLICATIONS

Complications of diverticulitis include free perforation with fecal peritonitis, suppurative peritonitis secondary to ruptured abscess, abdominal or pelvic abscess, fistula, and obstruction. It is estimated that 30% of patients will have recurrent diverticulitis; patients who experience a second episode have more than a 50% chance of having a third episode.[4] The chance of recurrence after the first episode is 90% within 5 years. Fiber can reduce the risk of recurrence in up to 70% of patients.[17]

Patients between 40 and 50 years old are at increased risk for development of complications.[1] Medical management may not be successful, recurrences with complications are common, and aggressive treatment with early surgery when the patient's condition is stabilized is sometimes recommended. Immunosuppressed patients are at especially high risk for complications because they may not experience a normal inflammatory response and subsequently can develop spontaneous colon perforation and perforated diverticula.[1] Aggressive management of these patients includes emergency surgical intervention.[1,6]

INDICATIONS FOR REFERRAL OR HOSPITALIZATION

The diagnosis of diverticulitis is, unfortunately, based on clinical findings that can be diagnostically nonspecific. The presentation, course of illness, and treatment plan can be challenging. Referral to a gastroenterologist is appropriate if the diagnosis is unclear, attacks are recurrent, or hospitalization is indicated. A surgical consultation is required for patients with suspected complications or those who are readmitted because of a second episode of diverticulitis.[18]

PATIENT AND FAMILY EDUCATION

During the convalescent period, patients require a low-fiber diet (<15 g/day) and careful diet instruction. Whole-grain breads and cereals, raw fruits and vegetables, nuts and seeds, and legumes should be avoided. Canned fruits and well-cooked vegetables are allowed in limited quantities. The diet can be liberalized as the patient's condition improves. Once stable and pain free, patients can reintroduce a high-fiber diet slowly, during several weeks, to avoid any abdominal distention or excessive flatulence. Symptoms often guide the treatment plan. A fiber preparation may be necessary for patients who are unable to follow a diet reasonably high in fiber. Regardless of fiber supplementation, many patients who have had surgical treatments will continue to experience symptoms.[1,6]

Patients should avoid laxatives, enemas, and any other form of bowel cleansing therapy because these substances increase colonic pressure.[16] It is important that patients establish a regular bowel movement pattern of once or twice a day to once every 2 or 3 days. With a high-fiber diet, the stools should be softer and thus easier to pass.

In addition, patients should be aware of the importance of reporting recurrent pain promptly, especially if the pain is associated with chills or fever. Urgent hospitalization may be necessary.

DIVERTICULAR BLEEDING

DEFINITION AND EPIDEMIOLOGY

Severe bleeding is not a frequent complication of diverticulosis; however, diverticular disease is the most common cause of massive lower gastrointestinal bleeding.[1] Hemorrhage from a colonic diverticulum generally begins without warning in an older individual with otherwise asymptomatic diverticulosis. Painless rectal bleeding is associated with diverticulosis in 3% to 15% of patients and is usually self-limited. Diverticular hemorrhage stops spontaneously in 70% to 90% of cases.[19]

PATHOPHYSIOLOGY

Bleeding arises from the rupture of one of the branches of the vasa recta adjacent to a diverticulum. The most common site for massive bleeding is the right colon, particularly in older adults.[1,18] Diverticular bleeding is neither chronic nor occult. Iron deficiency anemia associated with occult blood in the stool can never be attributed to diverticulosis without an appropriate diagnostic evaluation.

CLINICAL PRESENTATION

Diverticular bleeding usually occurs in an older patient with diverticulosis who has previously been asymptomatic or undiagnosed. The patient may or may not experience abdominal cramping and passes a large volume of bright red to dark maroon blood with or without signs of hypovolemia. The patient may have one or two more such movements and then no more, or the bleeding may continue for several days. Bleeding stops spontaneously in 70% to 90% of patients, with the rate of additional bleeding after one episode being 20% to 38%.[19] There are no distinctive features by which to distinguish diverticular bleeding from other causes of lower gastrointestinal bleeding.

PHYSICAL EXAMINATION

The physical examination findings are typically normal, although the digital rectal examination can reveal anorectal lesions as the source of bleeding. The upper alimentary canal should be examined as well, including the oropharynx, nasopharynx, abdomen, perineum, and anal canal, to exclude other sources of bleeding. If blood loss is excessive, signs of hypovolemia with postural vital signs or shock may be present.[1]

DIAGNOSTICS

A CBC will help determine not only the blood loss but also whether the bleeding has been ongoing. The initial assessment includes a rectal examination and a proctosigmoidoscopy, which may reveal bleeding from anorectal lesions, rectal cancer, or acute colitis. Upper gastrointestinal bleeding must be excluded by aspiration of gastric contents, and esophagogastroduodenoscopy is indicated in some instances.[20] A barium enema study should never be the initial test in patients with diverticular bleeding because angiography or colonoscopy is precluded until the contrast material has been evacuated. With slow bleeding, colonoscopy is the best approach, and a study suggests that colonoscopy is an effective diagnostic adjunct even in aggressive bleeding.[21] Scintigraphic or angiographic localization is necessary with brisk bleeding. Mesenteric angiography can be used as a diagnostic tool for localization of the bleeding site and as a therapeutic intervention in which vasoconstrictive

DIAGNOSTICS

Diverticular Bleeding

LABORATORY
CBC and differential and manual platelet count
Stool for occult blood
Coagulation studies, including liver function tests

IMAGING
Nuclear scintigraphy
Angiography
RBC nuclear bleeding scan

OTHER DIAGNOSTICS
Proctosigmoidoscopy
Esophagogastroduodenoscopy
Colonoscopy

RBC, red blood cell.

drugs or an artificial blood clot can be infused to control the hemorrhage.

DIFFERENTIAL DIAGNOSIS

Diverticular bleeding is a diagnosis of exclusion. Patients who come in to see the health care provider with a massive hemorrhage often have no prior history of diverticular complications. Bleeding is characteristically sudden and brisk and is usually self-limited. Any gastrointestinal lesion that has the potential for massive hemorrhage (e.g., a duodenal ulcer or Meckel diverticulum) can manifest in a manner similar to diverticular bleeding and must be excluded.[22] Gastric aspiration is a crucial part of the evaluation. Lower tract sources (vascular ectasias; inflammatory diseases; and anorectal lesions such as hemorrhoids, fissures, lacerations, polyps, ulcers, and neoplasms) must be considered.[22]

DIFFERENTIAL DIAGNOSIS

Diverticular Bleeding

- Colon or rectal cancer
- Colon polyp
- Ischemic colitis
- Duodenal ulcer
- Meckel diverticulum
- Vascular ectasia
- Anorectal lesion
- Inflammatory disease
- Angiodysplasia
- Hemorrhoids
- Foreign body

MANAGEMENT

Although massive gastrointestinal bleeding is a life-threatening condition, the prognosis for diverticular bleeding is generally favorable. Most bleeding stops spontaneously and does not recur. The exception for recurrence includes advanced age, documented diverticulitis, a history of peripheral vascular disease, or a history of chronic renal failure. Any of these factors increase the risk for a repeat bleed.[23] Treatment of diverticular bleeding should begin with conservative medical management. Most patients can be observed as inpatients without the need for urgent diagnostic or invasive therapeutic maneuvers. For those who do need intervention, the evaluation and treatment of diverticular bleeding are interrelated.

The primary interventions for diverticular bleeding are hemodynamic stabilization and resuscitation. Anal or rectal bleeding should first be excluded with a digital rectal examination and proctoscopy. Most cases of mild to moderate hemorrhage stop spontaneously with medical management that includes establishment of intravenous access and insertion of a nasogastric tube to exclude an upper gastrointestinal source of bleeding. Laboratory tests should include electrolytes, CBC, coagulation studies, and blood type with crossmatch.

Patients, especially older patients, who have massive, active bleeding require observation in an intensive care unit. As previously discussed, several diagnostic options are available, including radionuclide scanning, angiography, and endoscopy.

The patient with persistent diverticular bleeding also has several therapeutic options, including selective intra-arterial infusion of vasopressin, angiographic embolization, and surgical resection.[6]

Surgical intervention is required for massive and persistent bleeding that does not respond to medical treatment and interventional radiology. Surgery may also be recommended on an elective basis for patients with recurrent hemorrhages.[22]

COMPLICATIONS

The complications of diverticular hemorrhage are related to hypovolemia and circulatory collapse. Older patients tolerate the hemorrhage poorly because of the ischemic risk to major organs with each bleeding episode.

INDICATIONS FOR REFERRAL OR HOSPITALIZATION

Massive bleeding is an urgent situation and requires collaboration and referral to a gastroenterologist. Surgical intervention may also be necessary. In older patients with bleeding, transient hypovolemia can be a serious problem for major organs, and immediate hospitalization must be considered.

PATIENT AND FAMILY EDUCATION

Explicit patient education is essential because of the risk for recurrent bleeding after the first episode. It is important to advise patients to report symptoms immediately to avoid complications such as hypovolemia and circulatory collapse.

CHAPTER 134

DYSPHAGIA

Talli McCormick

DEFINITION AND EPIDEMIOLOGY

Oropharyngeal dysphagia is a swallowing disorder that involves dysfunction of one or more stages in the normal sequence of swallowing. This type of dysphagia differs from upper gastrointestinal disorders in that the dysfunction involves oral, pharyngeal, and laryngeal structures. The dysphagia may be mild or severe, resulting in malnutrition, dehydration, choking, aspiration, pneumonia, and even death. Estimates of incidence in the community vary, but a significant number of residents in nursing homes may have feeding difficulties. Patients with aspiration are thought to have a 1-year mortality rate of 45%.[1]

PATHOPHYSIOLOGY

Dysphagia may be either oropharyngeal or esophageal. The cause can be neurologic, neuromuscular, metabolic, pharmacologic, infectious, psychiatric, environmental, or structural. Identification of the causative agent or disease is paramount in the assessment and treatment of dysphagia. Structural causes are more common in esophageal dysphagia, and functional causes are more likely in oropharyngeal dysphagia (Box 134-1). Structural causes include trauma or surgery, tumor, webs, strictures or stenoses, diverticula, infection, and, in some cases, cervical osteophytes or cricopharyngeal bars.[1]

To more fully understand dysphagia, it is essential to appreciate the anatomy and physiology of normal swallowing. Swallowing has three commonly described phases: oral, pharyngeal, and esophageal. In addition to these three phases, there are preparatory phases to the act of eating. Most of us decide when we are hungry and what, and how much, we would like to eat. We prepare it or go to a restaurant. We decide with whom we will eat. These decisions involve autonomy, fairly intact cognition, and neuromuscular function. Nursing home residents and homebound older adults may have significant limitations or restrictions in this preparatory phase.[2]

During the oral phase, a multitude of sensory information is gathered about the food and the involved structures. Quantity, shape, consistency, and moisture content are determined, along with the temperature, taste, and location of the food. The touch and pressure exerted on the oral structures, especially the tongue and hard and soft palates, are transmitted to the brainstem for further action and distribution. This continuous assessment by the sensory system allows precise communication with the muscles of mastication.

Chewing (mastication) involves cranial nerves (CNs) V (trigeminal), VII (facial), IX (glossopharyngeal), and XII (hypoglossal) in addition to the muscles of the jaw, cheeks, tongue, and palate. The lips remain closed during chewing, while the tongue and teeth prepare the food into a bolus of the proper size and consistency. The soft palate descends to help hold the food within the mouth during chewing. The teeth close, the tongue places the bolus in its central groove, and the bolus is then rapidly pushed, or transferred, through the pillars (fauces) into the pharynx.

At this point, the bolus passes a ring of sensory receptors at the base of the tongue, pillars, soft palate, and posterior pharyngeal wall. The transmission of a sensory impulse indicating the presence of a bolus is sent by CN IX to the swallowing center

BOX 134-1

Potential Causes of Oropharyngeal Dysphagia

IATROGENIC
- Medication side effects (e.g., xerostomia, chemotherapy, neuroleptics)
- Postsurgical muscular or neurogenic disorders (e.g., head and neck cancers, stroke)
- Radiation therapy
- Corrosive (pill injury, intentional)

INFECTIOUS
- Diphtheria
- Botulism
- Lyme disease
- Syphilis
- Mucositis (e.g., herpes, cytomegalovirus, *Candida* organisms)

METABOLIC
- Amyloidosis
- Cushing syndrome
- Thyrotoxicosis
- Wilson disease

MYOPATHIC
- Connective tissue disease
- Myasthenia gravis
- Myotonic dystrophy
- Oculopharyngeal dystrophy
- Polymyositis
- Sarcoidosis
- Paraneoplastic syndromes

NEUROLOGIC
- Brainstem tumors
- Head trauma
- Stroke
- Cerebral palsy
- Guillain-Barré syndrome
- Huntington disease
- Multiple sclerosis
- Polio
- Postpolio syndrome
- Tardive dyskinesia
- Amyotrophic lateral sclerosis
- Parkinson disease
- Dementia

STRUCTURAL
- Cricopharyngeal bar
- Zenker diverticulum
- Cervical webs
- Oropharyngeal tumors
- Osteophytes and skeletal abnormalities
- Congenital disorders (cleft palate, diverticula, pouches)

PSYCHIATRIC
- Grief
- Depression
- Globus

ENVIRONMENTAL
- Poor positioning
- Eating or being fed too quickly
- Eating or being fed too large a bolus
- Inappropriate consistency
- Poor oral health or hygiene
- Distractibility

Modified from Cook IJ, Kahrilas PJ: AGA technical review on management of oropharyngeal dysphagia, *Gastroenterology* 116(2):455-478, 1999; and Blackington E, McCormick T, Willson B et al: Oropharyngeal dysphagia in the elderly, *Adv Nurse Pract* 9(7):45, 2001.

in the brainstem, which then initiates the involuntary phase of the swallow.[2] Sensory input is also crucial to the pharyngeal stage. As the tongue pushes the bolus to the posterior pharynx, the soft palate flattens upward and backward (CN V), sealing off the nasopharynx. Simultaneously, the hyoid and larynx begin to move upward and forward (CN X [vagus]), tipping back the epiglottis and widening the esophageal opening. The pillars lower, and the tongue presses against the posterior pharyngeal wall (CN IX) to block retrograde movement of the bolus into the oral cavity. Sensory fibers of CN X transmit information to the swallowing center in the brainstem. The impulse returns by the motor component of the vagus nerve and initiates peristalsis of the pharyngeal constrictors to propel the bolus toward the esophagus, passing the valleculae and piriform sinuses. The soft palate descends, the larynx continues to rise, and the epiglottis descends. As the epiglottis descends to block the laryngeal opening, the upper esophageal sphincter (UES) or cricopharyngeal sphincter opens to allow the bolus to pass into the esophagus.[2]

As the food bolus enters the esophagus, these processes begin in reverse. Once the food bolus is in the esophagus, the UES closes and peristalsis and gravity propel the bolus toward the stomach. The lower esophageal sphincter (LES) opens, and the bolus enters the stomach. Normal transit time depends on bolus consistency but is generally 2 to 4 seconds.[2] The cerebellum plays a significant role in the control and choreography of the swallowing process.[3]

CLINICAL PRESENTATION

Dysphagic patients can be initially seen with malnutrition, weight loss, dehydration, coughing or choking with eating, or pneumonia. Problems in the oral stage include poor bolus control, spillage either from the lips or into the pharynx, dry oral membranes, pocketing or oral residue, and difficulty with chewing. Pharyngeal dysphagia often results from weakness or poor coordination of the pharyngeal muscles. This can cause delayed swallow, failure of airway protection, nasal or oral regurgitation, or residue remaining in the pharynx after swallow, manifesting as coughing, choking, or gurgling.

Xerostomia (dry mouth), either intrinsic or extrinsic, can be a contributing factor in dysphagia. Globus, which is the sensation of a lump in the throat, can occur alone or coexist with esophageal dysphagia, particularly when it is accompanied by chest pain or heartburn.[4] Globus alone is merely a sensory experience; swallowing itself is unimpaired.

A detailed history is the most important step in differential diagnosis. Because dysphagia can be associated with neurologic disease, a thorough neuromuscular history is also important. Obtaining of an accurate history can be complicated by reduced alertness and cognitive and speech impairments, which can also affect the patient's ability to participate in examination, diagnostics, and treatment strategies. Assessment of the impact of dysphagia on patient function and quality of life is paramount. The Quality of Life in Swallowing Disorders (SWAL-QOL) instrument has been established as a reliable and valid tool for assessment of quality of life in patients with swallowing dysfunction.[5]

Onset, progression, location, duration, and food consistency aid in diagnosis. A short duration associated with weight loss can indicate malignant disease.[1] Abrupt onset associated with neurologic impairment suggests a cerebrovascular accident. Studies have estimated that one third to one half of new stroke patients will have dysphagia, and in 10% to 15% of these, the dysphagia will persist beyond 1 month. Swallowing of thin liquids is often a problem after a stroke. Gradual progressive onset is more likely to be associated with Parkinson disease, amyotrophic lateral sclerosis, sarcoidosis, myasthenia gravis, Alzheimer disease, or other chronic diseases. Parkinson disease is the most common movement disorder in older adults and leads to tongue rigidity and tremor, making bolus formation and transfer into the pharynx difficult. Difficulty in swallowing of only solids suggests a structural cause but not necessarily the location of the impairment. Ability to point to where the food "sticks" is useful for oropharyngeal obstructions and correlates well with radiographic studies.

Eating or being fed too rapidly may result in either oral or nasal regurgitation and choking. Coughing up food after meals can indicate a pharyngeal diverticulum.[1] Frequent swallowing can indicate oral or pharyngeal residue. Positioning of the patient, degree of distraction, companions or assistants, utensils used, food consistency, and likes and dislikes can all provide information useful not only in differential diagnosis but also in deciding on treatment strategies.

A complete review of all medications is necessary because some medications can cause or contribute to swallowing dysfunction; others, such as alendronate sodium (Fosamax), nonsteroidal anti-inflammatory drugs (NSAIDs), and potassium, can cause direct damage to the esophageal mucosa (Box 134-2). Xerostomia, altered esophageal sphincter pressure, and reduced alertness are other medication side effects that can affect swallowing.[2]

PHYSICAL EXAMINATION

A thorough physical examination aids in the differential diagnosis, establishes the existence of deficits and impairments, and determines whether malnutrition or pneumonia is present.[1] A complete oral examination will reveal oral health and hygiene, including dentition, oral sensation, tongue strength, mobility, coordination, and specific CN function. Altered speech or voice, particularly nasal speech or a gurgling voice, should be noted. Nasal speech can indicate soft palate dysfunction, whereas a gurgling or wet voice is more indicative of weak pharyngeal constrictors. The presence or absence of the gag reflex is not predictive of swallowing dysfunction or risk of aspiration because the gag reflex may be absent in 20% to 40% of healthy adults.[6] Trial sips of water or spoonfuls of applesauce or pudding can reveal specific deficits. Observation and palpation of laryngeal elevation can detect delayed swallowing. The pharyngeal swallow should occur within approximately 1 second.

The complete neuromuscular examination includes CN function (particularly V, VII, IX, X, and XII) and assessment of muscle strength or weakness, muscle atrophy, or altered coordination. Involuntary movements, tremor, or gait disturbance should also be determined. A mental status assessment with particular emphasis on level of alertness and ability to concentrate and cooperate is important. Deformities of or past operations on the head, neck, or trunk may affect dysphagia or the ability to participate in diagnostic studies. Despite skillful and comprehensive physical examination, the risk for aspiration may not be fully appreciated without the use of radiographic studies.[7]

DIAGNOSTICS

Videofluoroscopy (VFS), also called videofluoroscopic examination of swallowing (VFES) or modified barium swallow (MBS), is the most appropriate and commonly used imaging

BOX 134-2

Medication-Related Conditions That Cause Oropharyngeal Dysphagia

XEROSTOMIA
- Antidepressants
- Antispasmodics
- Antihypertensives
- Anticholinergics
- Antihistamines
- Bronchodilators
- Sedatives

CENTRAL NERVOUS SYSTEM DEPRESSION
- Anticonvulsants
- Antianxiety agents (alprazolam, diazepam, chlordiazepoxide)
- Antispasmodics (dantrolene, baclofen)
- Antidepressants (trazodone, amitriptyline, desipramine)
- Neuroleptics (haloperidol, chlorpromazine, thioridazine)
- Sedatives

IMMUNOSUPPRESSION
- Antibiotics
- Cytotoxic agents

INCREASED SALIVATION
- Anticholinesterase
- Clonazepam
- Clozapine

NEUROMUSCULAR JUNCTION BLOCKADE
- Aminoglycoside antibiotics
- Botulinum toxin (Botox)

MYOPATHY
- Corticosteroids
- Lipid-lowering agents
- Colchicine
- L-Tryptophan

MUCOSAL INJURY
- Alendronate (Fosamax)
- Tetracycline
- NSAIDs
- Potassium
- Ferrous sulfate

LOWER ESOPHAGEAL SPHINCTER PRESSURE
- Theophylline
- Nitrates
- Calcium channel blockers
- Beta blockers
- Hormone replacement therapy
- Anticholinergics

procedure. This is the only study that visualizes the actual swallow. The primary purpose of the MBS is to determine if and to what degree aspiration occurs. Patients must be able to sit upright, to hold still, and to follow commands during the examination. With the use of contrast material, this radiographic study is designed to assess functional impairment of swallowing in four categories: delay in swallowing initiation, nasopharyngeal regurgitation, aspiration, and pharyngeal residue. A variety of consistencies and bolus volumes are usually assessed during the MBS. This study not only aids in diagnosis but also helps determine the effectiveness of various positions, consistencies, or maneuvers used in treatment.

If a structural rather than functional cause is suspected, nasoendoscopy should be considered. Nasoendoscopy permits direct visualization of the oral cavity, nasopharynx, pharynx, and larynx. Lesion biopsy samples can be obtained during the procedure.

If muscle weakness or problems with sphincter relaxation are suspected, manometry can measure intraluminal pressures during the swallow. Manometry can be synchronized with VFS (manofluorography) to distinguish more subtle findings.

The fiberoptic endoscopic examination of swallowing (FEES), ultrasound examination, electromyography, and electroglottography are other diagnostic procedures that can be appropriate, although these tests are more limited. Computed tomography (CT) or magnetic resonance imaging (MRI) of the head and neck can aid in diagnosis but does not describe the actual swallow mechanism.

DIAGNOSTICS

Oropharyngeal Dysphagia

IMAGING	OTHER DIAGNOSTICS
MBS	Fiberoptic endoscopic examination of swallow
CT or MRI*	

*If indicated.

DIFFERENTIAL DIAGNOSIS

See the differential diagnosis box.

MANAGEMENT

Structural causes of dysphagia, such as tumors, strictures, webs, and diverticula, are usually treated with surgery or dilation. Chemotherapy or radiation therapy may be used for tumors. No randomized controlled trials have been conducted, but a number of case series indicate that webs and strictures are amenable to dilation. Cricopharyngeal myotomy is the most common surgical treatment for oropharyngeal dysphagia of structural origin, and consistent evidence of its benefit is available.[8]

Studies exploring the use of myotomy for dysphagia of neurogenic origin are very different. Data conflict and are often methodologically weak and sometimes qualitative. Nonetheless, myotomy may offer benefit to 50% of patients with neurogenic dysphagia.[1] It is suggested that patients who benefit may be those with a higher preoperative hypopharyngeal intrabolus pressure related to resistance of flow across the UES.[8] In patients with problems with coordination of the UES or cricopharyngeal muscle and the pharynx, some improvement in swallowing has been shown with botulinum toxin (Botox) injections into the UES[9] and with cricopharyngeal myotomy.[10] Other structural radiographic abnormalities exist, but their impact on swallowing is unclear.

The relationship of pharyngeal sensation, silent aspiration, and cough reflex has been explored in many Japanese studies. Ebihara and colleagues found that oral stimulation and awareness were key in addressing swallowing dysfunction. They

DIFFERENTIAL DIAGNOSIS

Oropharyngeal Dysphagia

MECHANICAL PROBLEMS

Acute inflammations
- Herpes simplex
- Tonsillitis, epiglottitis, pharyngitis, esophagitis
- Infectious and inflammatory bone and mucosal disorders

Chemical agents (aspirin, lozenges, gargles, alcohol)
Medications (see Box 134-2)
Skeletal anomalies
Muscle anomalies
Macroglossia
Pharyngoesophageal diverticulum
Carcinoma
Surgery
- Oral or palatal resections
- Glossectomy
- Supralaryngectomy; partial or total laryngectomy
- Tracheoesophageal puncture
- Chest surgery (coronary artery bypass graft)
- Endarterectomy
- Anterior cervical spine surgery

Irradiation
Cervical spine disease
Nasoenteric tubes
Tracheostomy tubes
Esophageal stenosis, webs, rings, stricture

NEUROGENIC PROBLEMS

Riley-Day syndrome
Acquired central nervous system disorders
- Stroke syndromes and vascular disorders
- Capsular infarct
- Pseudobulbar palsy
- Apraxias and agnosias
- Lacunar disease

Movement disorders
- Parkinson disease
- Dystonias and dyskinesias
- Huntington disease
- Palatal myoclonus

Poliomyelitis and other systemic infections
- Diphtheria
- Botulism
- Rabies
- Tetanus

Amyotrophic lateral sclerosis
Acquired peripheral nervous system disorders
Recurrent laryngeal neuropathies
CN neuropathies
- Guillain-Barré syndrome
- Diabetes
- Leukemia
- Lymphoma
- Carcinoma
- Other neuropathies

Neurodevelopmental disorders
- Cerebral palsy
- Abnormal oral and pharyngeal reflexes
- Abnormal salivation
- Others

MYOGENIC PROBLEMS

Myasthenia gravis
Neuromuscular esophageal disorders
- Scleroderma
- Achalasia
- Diffuse spasm
- Others

OTHER CONDITIONS

Dementias
Multiple sclerosis
Tuberculosis
Syphilis
Neoplasms
Degenerative disorders
Psychopathology
Feeding phobias
Atypical parent-child interactions
Sensory deficits

found that capsaicin stimulated warm receptors whereas menthol stimulated cold receptors, both of which improved delayed swallowing reflex. In addition, black pepper oil was effective in reducing latent time to swallow in patients with diminished consciousness.[11]

It has long been known that cough can be stimulated by angiotensin-converting enzyme (ACE) inhibitors, which has been of interest to researchers in dysphagia. Takahashi and colleagues used ACE inhibitors in older adult Japanese patients and found a decrease in aspiration pneumonia.[12]

Antipsychotics inhibit dopamine and thereby affect swallowing, and sedatives may reduce the level of consciousness, both of which may increase the risk of aspiration. Avoiding these medications in dysphagic patients may reduce risk of aspiration pneumonia.[13]

There is some support for the idea that the respiratory system may have a role in optimum swallowing. Gross and colleagues found that pharyngeal swallowing time was longer in subjects at residual lung volume than in persons at total lung capacity or functional residual capacity.[14] This implies a possible regulatory role of subglottic air pressure in optimum swallowing.

Intensive oral care and hygiene have been considered as a means of reducing pathogen load in aspirators, Sjögren and colleagues have suggested that 1 in 10 deaths from pneumonia among elderly nursing home patients may be prevented by improved oral hygene.[15]

Verin and others have discussed the use of electrical stimulation. Submental sensitive transcutaneous electrical stimulation (SSTES) of the submental muscles has been shown to improve swallowing coordination and reaction time by VFS and quality of life measures. The SSTES is more recognizable to the layperson as transcutaneous electrical nerve stimulation (TENS).[16]

Aspiration and Nonoral Feeding in Dysphagia of Functional Origin

Standard practice has been that patients found to have severe aspiration not treatable with dietary or positional modifications should receive nonoral feeding to prevent aspiration. It is clear that aspiration is evidence of severe swallowing dysfunction and that death is associated with aspiration pneumonia.[1] However, the relationship between aspiration and the risk for development of pneumonia is not as obvious. DiBardino and Wunderink found aspiration did not predict the risk of respiratory morbidity.[17] Similarly, Falsetti and coworkers discovered that 6 of 49 dysphagic patients had normal VFS findings.[18] A study by Terpenning and others suggested an increased risk of aspiration pneumonia in patients who have chronic obstructive pulmonary disease or diabetes mellitus or who require assistance with feeding.[19] Aspiration pneumonia was also more common in subjects with oral *Porphyromonas gingivalis,* decayed teeth, and visible dental plaque. Although these authors hypothesized that poor healing associated with diabetes and poor pulmonary clearance could contribute to the development of pneumonia, they did not find an association with stroke.[19] Harvey and colleagues proposed that patients with compromised functional capacity may be fed too quickly or with too large a bolus.[20] In summary, it appears that aspiration probably contributes to the risk of pneumonia but may not be the only important contributor; nonoral feeding may not reduce this risk in all patients, and it may increase this risk in some patients.

Swallowing Strategies and Therapies

Head positioning, swallowing maneuvers, and dietary textural modifications seem to demonstrate evidence of benefit in the treatment of functional dysphagia.[1] Newer interventional techniques also show promise, though studies regarding efficacy are small and some swallowing improvement may be related to normal recovery.[21] Table 134-1 provides data on swallowing therapy techniques, indications, and rationale. Many therapeutic measures require autonomy and fairly intact cognitive function for memory and learning. For patients with certain strokes, Alzheimer disease, and some other neurologic diseases, this requirement may limit the usefulness of these techniques. Dietary modifications may be the best choice for many of these patients.

TABLE 134-1 Swallowing Therapy Techniques, Rationales, and Indications

Technique	Execution (Rationale)	Indication
DIETARY MODIFICATION		
Thickened liquids	Reduced tendency to spill over tongue base	Disordered tongue function Preswallow spill or aspiration Impaired laryngeal closure
Thin liquids	Offers less resistance to flow	Weak pharyngeal contraction Reduced cricopharyngeal opening
MANEUVERS		
Supraglottic swallow	Breath hold, double swallow, forceful expiration (closes vocal folds before swallowing)	Aspiration: reduced or late vocal fold closures
Supersupraglottic swallow	Effortful breath hold (closes vocal folds before and during swallow) Increased anterior tilting of arytenoids	Aspiration (poor closure of laryngeal introitus)
Effortful swallow	Effortful tongue action (increases posterior motion of tongue base)	Poor posterior tongue base motion
Mendelsohn maneuver	Prolong hyoid excursion guided by manual palpation (prolongs UES opening)	Poor pharyngeal clearance and laryngeal movement
POSTURAL ADJUSTMENTS		
Head tilt	Tilt posteriorly at swallow initiation (gravity clears oral cavity) Tilt laterally to unaffected side (directs bolus down stronger side)	Poor tongue control Unilateral pharyngeal weakness
Chin tuck; positive improvement in swallowing scores	Chin down (widens valleculae, displaces tongue base and epiglottis posteriorly)	Aspiration, delayed pharyngeal response, reduced posterior tongue base motion
Head rotation	Rotate head to affected side (isolates damaged side from bolus path, reduces LES pressure) Rotate head to affected side with extrinsic pressure on thyroid cartilage (increases adduction)	Unilateral pharyngeal weakness Unilateral laryngeal dysfunction Unilateral pharyngeal dysfunction
Lying on side, elevation	Right or left lateral (bypass laryngeal introitus)	Aspiration, bilateral pharyngeal impairment, or reduced laryngeal elevation

TABLE 134-1 Swallowing Therapy Techniques, Rationales, and Indications—cont'd

Technique	Execution (Rationale)	Indication
FACILITATORY TECHNIQUES		
Strengthening exercises	Various	Nonprogressive disease
Biofeedback	Augment volitional component	Poor pharyngeal clearance
Thermal stimulation; reduces transition and swallow duration	Cold, tactile stimulation to anterior faucial pillar	Delayed or absent swallow response
Surface electrical stimulation; increases swallowing improvement	Electrical stimulation of pharyngeal and laryngeal musculature	
Gustatory stimulation	Sour bolus (facilitates swallow response)	Huntington chorea, stroke

From Cook IJ, Kahrilas PJ: AGA technical review on management of oropharyngeal dysphagia, *Gastroenterology* 116(2):470, 1999; and Speyer R1, Baijens L, Heijnen M, Zwijnenberg I: Effects of therapy in oropharyngeal therapy by speech and language therapists: a systematic review. *Dysphagia*, 25(1):40-65, 2010.

COMPLICATIONS

Complications associated with dysphagia include impaired quality of life, coughing, choking, aspiration, malnutrition, dehydration, pneumonia, and death. Gastrostomy tube placement may be necessary and appropriate for some patients.

INDICATIONS FOR REFERRAL OR HOSPITALIZATION

Dysphagic patients and their families should be offered dietary consultation. Other referrals will be dictated by the cause of the dysphagia. A gastroenterologist should be consulted for a suspected gastroesophageal problem. Structural abnormalities may require surgical intervention.

Moderate to severe cases of oropharyngeal dysphagia require referral to a speech therapist, particularly if therapeutic swallowing techniques are needed. Referral to a neurologist is warranted if the cause of the dysphagia is neurogenic. If oral health and hygiene are a concern, referral to a dentist for evaluation and treatment is indicated. Counseling or psychiatric consultation is necessary for patients experiencing grief or depression associated with the dysphagia.

Other comorbid illnesses or conditions may affect dysphagia or contribute to the development of pneumonia. Pulmonary rehabilitation may be indicated for patients with concurrent lung disease. Suspected pneumonia should usually be evaluated at the hospital, especially if gastric fluid is thought to be the aspirate. Malnutrition, dehydration, or acute dysphagia may require hospital admission.

PATIENT AND FAMILY EDUCATION

The most important aspects of education include patient feeding, positioning, maneuvers, and dietary textural modifications. Speech therapists can teach patients and families positioning and maneuvers to improve swallowing efficacy. The Silver Spoons program, a volunteer program, was designed to facilitate safe feeding and can also assist family members or institutional staff.[20] Paying careful attention to bolus size and consistency, allowing plenty of time for meals, and ensuring proper positioning of the patient for meals improve safety.

Discussion concerning the risks and benefits of feeding tubes in specific disease entities is important for patients, families, and, often, staff. Feeding tubes may not be appropriate for patients with severe dementia.[22] Cultural and religious preferences must be respected. Other concurrent illnesses may be important considerations. More research is needed, but for any given patient, the decision to place a feeding tube must remain individualized and be carefully considered.

HEALTH PROMOTION

Regular health screenings and recommendations for diet, exercise, and smoking cessation can prevent or delay the onset of disease, particularly in those with a strong family history of stroke. Once dysphagia is established, good oral hygiene, dental care, careful attention to positioning and swallowing techniques, and management of comorbid illnesses, particularly respiratory illnesses and diabetes, can help prevent pneumonia. Counseling can be beneficial for patients with a family history of hereditary neurologic or myopathic disorders associated with dysphagia. Support for families caring for dysphagic members may also help reduce caregiver stress.

CHAPTER 135

GASTROESOPHAGEAL REFLUX DISEASE

Michelle Freshman

DEFINITION AND EPIDEMIOLOGY

Gastroesophageal reflux refers to the retrograde movement of gastric contents from the stomach to the esophagus. This occurs in the general population approximately once per hour, followed by rapid clearance of refluxed material from the distal esophagus, without injury.[1] Swallowing initiates primary peristalsis; distention of the esophagus or acidification promotes secondary peristalsis. When the capacity of the esophageal mucosa to tolerate caustic refluxate is overwhelmed, this normal physiologic process can produce pathologic signs and symptoms in the oropharynx, larynx, esophagus, and respiratory tract. An individual is said to have *gastroesophageal reflux disease* (GERD) in the setting of chronic symptom distress with or without mucosal damage.

GERD is one of the most prevalent[1] clinical conditions of the gastrointestinal tract, affecting 10% to 20% of adults at least weekly in Western countries, although these accounts are subjective.[2] Prevalence among American (15% to 20%), British (10% to 15%), Swedish (5% to 10%), and Chinese citizens (0.1% to 5.0%) is variable,[3] and estimates of U.S. expenditure range from $9.3 billion to $12.3 billion per year.[4] Whereas body mass index (BMI) may be a factor, sex and older age appear to be less so.[3] Some 4% to 7% of patients with GERD experience progressive disease associated with aspiration (most often related to age, comorbidities, or large hiatal hernia).[2]

The most common symptoms of GERD are heartburn (retrosternal area pain, pyrosis) and acidic regurgitation. Although their sensitivity is high,[5] the sensitivity of either symptom is lower than originally thought.[6] Thoracic pain has been offered as a consideration in the definition.[2] Aside from typical symptoms, atypical and extraesophageal symptoms (EESs) are frequently reported.[5] Atypical symptoms include epigastric fullness, epigastric pressure, epigastric pain, dyspepsia, nausea, bloating, and belching, which may suggest GERD but actually represent microaspirations and overlap with other entities.[5] Symptomatic GERD affects quality of life, may contribute to tissue injury, and is associated with EESs such as dental erosions, sore throat, laryngitis, hoarseness, chronic cough, wheezing, asthma, and bronchospasm, to which some add burning of mouth and tongue, globus sensation, or shortness of breath.[3] As proposed with atypical symptoms of GERD, in cases of EESs, microaspirations or a vagally mediated response triggered by the distal esophagus has been theorized, although GERD may not be involved at all.[5]

Nevertheless, severity of symptoms is not a reliable indicator of mucosal damage or prognosis. There are three main types of GERD: nonerosive, erosive, and functional heartburn. Nonerosive, endoscopically negative GERD is the most prevalent type. In fact, 50% to 85% of patients have nonerosive reflex disease.[3] Although it is defined as heartburn in the absence of esophageal mucosal damage, a significant proportion of individuals with endoscopically negative GERD have been shown to have pH testing abnormalities on impedance testing. Esophageal damage is marked by erosions, ulcers, or strictures in the esophagus, exclusive of malignant disease. A small percentage of endoscopically negative, symptomatic GERD will progress to erosive GERD.[7] In patients with no findings on EDG or pH monitoring, functional GERD is suspected, which still may be responsive to standard GERD therapy.

Alarm symptoms include gastrointestinal bleeding, anemia, dysphagia, odynophagia, unintentional weight loss, early satiety, age older than 55 at presentation, and recurrent vomiting.[3,6]

PATHOPHYSIOLOGY

No single mechanism explains all cases of symptomatic GERD; however, multiple factors are thought to be involved in the pathogenesis of reflux[2]:

- Transient lower esophageal sphincter (LES) relaxations (TLESRs)
- Low resting LES pressure
- Poor esophageal acid clearance, with increased volume and causticity
- Defects in esophagogastric motility or peristalsis
- Impaired mucosal resistance and other protective defenses
- Altered hiatal and gastroesophageal anatomy (involving hiatal crura, phrenoesophageal ligament, esophageal shortening)
- Hypersensitivity to gastric acid

TLESRs, the first factor, have been shown to be the cause of most reflux events. Intervals of LES relaxation, which allow the gastric contents to reflux into the esophagus, result in esophageal damage. It is not necessarily the more frequent TLESRs but the higher percentage of relaxations that is associated with acid migration (often closer to a meal), leading to more discomfort and damage.[1] TLESRs account for over 90% of reflux events[8] and can occur when a patient lies flat or performs a Valsalva maneuver. Anatomic variations such as hiatal hernia, shortened abdominal length or obesity can contribute.[3]

The second factor, low resting pressure of the sphincter (normally 10 to 20 mm Hg), has been demonstrated in a minority of patients with reflux esophagitis.[1] A shorter LES (<2 to 5 cm) has been indicated as a potential contributor.[1] In addition, the absolute minimal pressure is 4 mm Hg (other cutoffs are <6 mm Hg)[1]; the normal range is 10 to 30 mm Hg higher than the gastric pressure. The pressure is lowest in the daytime and during the postprandial period and highest at night.[1] It remains unclear whether low LES pressure is a cause or consequence of esophagitis because chronic inflammation may also reduce the sphincter's ability to close.[1]

LES pressure is maintained or increased by acetylcholine; relaxation of the LES occurs in response to nitric oxide, as seen in response to swallowing, often augmented by the crural diaphragm and phrenoesophageal ligament[7] when intra-abdominal pressure increases.[1] Patients with chronic symptoms usually have a hiatal hernia, which reflects movement of the proximal stomach upward through the diaphragm into the chest, where the crural diaphragm becomes separated from the LES. This separation is highly correlated with severe esophagitis, especially in the setting of esophageal stricture or Barrett esophagus.[1] However, the presence of a hiatal hernia alone does not confirm the presence of reflux esophagitis because the majority of patients with hiatal hernias do not have any symptoms. Other conditions increase intra-abdominal pressure and cause retrograde movement of refluxate. In pregnancy there is an increased prevalence of reflux, especially in the final trimester, which results from the relaxant effects of circulating estrogen and progesterone on the LES.

A third factor is intensity of acid exposure. The proton pump ultimately drives the production of acid in the stomach.[1] This acidification pathway results from gastric parietal cells in response to histamine, acetylcholine, and gastrin,[3] using hydrogen-potassium adenosine triphosphate molecules in the secretory canaliculi to dislodge hydrogen ions, which in turn acidifies the stomach pH to 1.5 to 3.5.[1,3] Once acid reflux has occurred, impaired acid clearance prolongs exposure of the mucosa to the damaging effects of the reflux. Evidence suggests that the acid component of the refluxate is the primary cause of heartburn and subsequent erosion. Other factors include the duration of the acid reflux event on the esophageal mucosa and the extent and composition of refluxate. Secondary causes of GERD involving heightened acid exposure include rare hypersecretory disorders. The most common of these disorders, Zollinger-Ellison syndrome, is caused by gastrin-producing tumors of the duodenum, pancreas, or both. In this disease, an overproduction of gastrin-driven acid output refluxes upward, causing severe GERD pain or peptic stricture.

A fourth pathogenic factor is the inability of the esophagus to clear itself of reflux material, resulting in longer exposure to gastric contents. This is more common in patients with severe esophagitis.[1] Abnormalities in peristalsis increase the risk for esophagitis. This includes delayed gastric emptying when gastric contents wash back into the esophagus as a result of their increased time in the stomach. Connective tissue disorders, gastric outlet obstruction caused by ulceration and stricture, and delayed gastric emptying from a variety of causes (such as postviral infections, gastric stasis, neuromuscular disease, vagal nerve disorders, idiopathic gastroparesis, pyloric dysfunction, duodenal dysmotility, duodenogastroesophageal bile reflux, and functional disorders of the gut) may account for up to half of the inadequate refluxate clearance.[1] A decrease in esophageal peristalsis can be more pronounced in patients with scleroderma, diabetes mellitus, hypothyroidism, amyloidosis, and eating disorders.[1]

A fifth factor is the integrity of the protective barrier of the mucosal lining. The inability of the mucosa to resist breakdown in the face of excessive refluxed gastric acid, along with pepsin, bile, trypsin, and pancreatic enzymes of the small intestine, may lead to erosive esophagitis in the majority of patients and ulcers and strictures in the minority.[1] Saliva, along with alkaline secretion from the esophageal glands, serves as a potent buffer in neutralizing acid. Salivation decreases during sleep, which in turn prolongs acid clearance and may correlate with increased symptom severity at night. Reduced salivary secretion, such as in Sjögren disease or sicca syndrome, can lead to esophagitis. Eosinophilic esophagitis, both proton pump inhibitor (PPI) responsive and non–PPI responsive, is an allergy-mediated disease. Altered structural anatomy is also a factor in establishing an accurate diagnosis.

Finally, there is evidence to support the prevalence of GERD in individuals evaluated for excessive acid exposure despite normal findings on 24-hour pH monitoring studies. Of 128 patients in one study, 55% had confirmed normal acid exposure, but within 4 to 6 years 87% of these subjects continued to complain of GERD, leading to the suspicion that hypersensitivity plays a significant role.[3]

CLINICAL PRESENTATION

The most common symptom of GERD is heartburn, which is usually described as a burning, retrosternal discomfort. Other terms for heartburn include *indigestion, acid regurgitation, sour stomach,* and *bitter belching*. A hot sensation usually begins inferiorly and radiates up the entire retrosternal area to the neck, occasionally to the back, and rarely into the arms. The sensation may become so intense that it is described as pain. Heartburn is usually relieved with antacids, baking soda, or milk, but these remedies are often short-lived.

Heartburn is frequently precipitated by food intake and occurs within 1 hour of eating, particularly after a large fatty meal. Other foods that precipitate heartburn are foods high in fat or sugar, chocolate, coffee, and onions, because they lower pressure in the LES. Alcohol may also lower LES pressure. Tobacco smoking may have a dual role in causing harm: promoting bile movement from the intestine to the stomach while prolonging effective neutralization by delaying saliva secretion.[1] Other foods that commonly cause heartburn are citrus products, tomato-based foods, and spicy foods. These foods do not affect LES pressure but instead are direct mucosal irritants. Other direct irritants include aspirin, nonsteroidal anti-inflammatory drugs (NSAIDs), potassium, and even swallowing of large tablets. The prevalence of GERD is higher in patients on benzodiazepines, calcium antagonists, and aspirin, but GERD is less often seen in patients on oral contraceptives and hormone replacement therapy.[3] Patients may also report heartburn or acid regurgitation that increases after going to bed, especially after eating late in the evening. This pain usually occurs within 1 to 2 hours of bedtime and may awaken a patient from sleep. Several other maneuvers, including bending over, lifting, straining, and exercising, or even sleeping position[1] may also precipitate heartburn because of increased intra-abdominal pressure.

Other symptoms of GERD, outside of esophageal burning and regurgitation, are termed *extraesophageal symptoms*, involve the respiratory and oropharyngeal tracts, and may be associated with other entities as well. A subset, extraesophageal reflux (EER), involves the respiratory tract.[2] Another subset is laryngopharyngeal reflux (LPR).[4] Because these conditions may relate to GERD, they are included in the workup and treatment. Some variations of cough, sore throat, hoarseness, postnasal drainage, globus sensation, asthma, water brash, dysphagia, odynophagia, chest pain, sleep disturbance, nausea, and vomiting are described as EESs, but a consensus has not emerged.[2-4] The cost of investigating and treating this disparate group of patients is substantially higher than in PPI-controlled GERD.[4]

Acid regurgitation, bitter acidic fluid in the mouth, usually occurs at night or when bending over. Acid regurgitation may be associated with extraesophageal complications should the refluxate extend beyond the esophagus to the lungs, larynx, pharynx, or oral cavity. This symptom should be differentiated from vomiting. Water brash is the appearance of salty-tasting fluid in the mouth because of stimulated saliva secretion. If delayed gastric emptying is the cause of GERD, abdominal fullness, nausea, and early satiety may be present.

Dysphagia, which may affect up to 30% of patients with GERD,[1] and odynophagia are more predictive of severe disease and should be considered alarm symptoms. Dysphagia, an impairment of swallowing food into the stomach, is experienced immediately after swallowing. Patients may say that the food "sticks," "hangs up," or "stops." This may be stemming from the oropharynx in the upper esophageal area or lower in the esophagus and reflects peristaltic dysfunction, inflammation, peptic stricture, or a Schatzki ring.[1] Esophageal strictures are highly correlated with hiatal hernia.[9] Dysphagia and food impaction are hallmarks of eosinophilic esophagitis, which may be driven by reflux as a precursor and is thought to depend on the role of impaired esophageal mucosa and immune activation.[10] Alternatively, GERD may be associated with a globus sensation, which is considered a heightened perception of something stuck like a "lump" in the throat, despite the lack of a diagnosable artifact. A recent onset of severe dysphagia might reflect esophageal cancer[1] (see Chapter 143). Odynophagia is sharp pain on swallowing and usually occurs under the sternum. Odynophagia is more commonly associated with infectious esophagitis (fungal, viral, or bacterial) or pill ulceration[1] (see Chapter 134).

Chest pain can mimic angina, which may be explained by shared neural pathways. Esophageal disorders are considered the most common cause of noncardiac chest pain.[1] Symptoms that are more suggestive of esophageal problems include pain that continues for hours, interrupts sleep, or is retrosternal without lateral radiation and pain that is meal related or relieved with antacids. Some association of GERD symptoms with obstructive sleep apnea has been observed, but causal direction with respect to reflux and apnea has yet to be determined.

Obesity may be a confounder in both. Pain that is not exercise induced is also suggestive of an esophageal disorder.[1]

When GERD is overlooked as a factor, many of these atypical GERD symptoms can be refractory to treatment. As described earlier, some conditions, such as dyspepsia, may overlap with GERD; erosive esophagitis and nonerosive esophagitis are said to be present in 20% of patients with dyspepsia, the most common finding, followed by peptic ulcer.[7] However, symptom control in response to standard GERD treatment, including surgery, may serve to uncover reflux as a factor. Co-management, especially in respiratory illnesses such as asthma, pulmonary fibrosis, and aspiration pneumonia, increasingly is standard practice.

Medications may contribute to GERD by decreasing salivation, esophageal motility, LES tone, or a combination of these factors.[1] Decreased LES pressure results from the administration of nitrates, tricyclic antidepressants, benzodiazepines among other sedatives, anticholinergics, bronchodilators, and methylxanthine derivatives (such as caffeine, aminophylline, and theophylline) as well as a wide assortment of cardiac medications including alpha-adrenergic blockers, beta blockers, and calcium channel blockers.[1,3]

PHYSICAL EXAMINATION

A careful history is likely to be more important than the physical findings. Because there is an association between dental erosions and GERD, an oral examination may suggest GERD in a patient with extensive loss of enamel and exposed dentin. Halitosis might also be a sign. Cutaneous evidence of smoking can be associated with GERD, as well as scleroderma, evidenced as thickened, tight, shiny skin or sclerodactyly as well as facial telangiectasia. Weight loss is a concern, particularly in patients who have dysphagia; by contrast, obesity can lead to symptoms. Respiratory wheezes and cough may be seen if there is associated asthma. Epigastric tenderness or Hemoccult-positive stool may be the result of esophageal erosions, ulcerations, or even severe inflammation. Any abdominal mass would suggest malignant neoplasia.

DIAGNOSTICS

Further diagnostic testing should be considered in patients with a failed empirical trial suggesting an alternative diagnosis, with sudden onset of symptoms in a patient aged 50 years or older, with alarm symptoms suggesting complicated disease (anemia, dysphagia, bleeding, odynophagia), and with long-standing symptoms of sufficient duration to put patients at risk for Barrett esophagus. The purpose of evaluating patients with long-term symptoms is to exclude complications of GERD.

Although barium radiography will help characterize mechanical obstructions such as strictures, hiatal hernia, and esophageal shortening to inform surgical approach, it has poor sensitivity and specificity and should not be used as a screening test. However, it may be used in refractory GERD along with high-definition, high-resolution, flexible video esophagogastroduodenoscopy (EGD) and mucosal biopsy.[8,11]

EGD is appropriate for patients with long-standing or poorly controlled GERD or in the presence of alarm features. In fact, a rise in the prevalence of GERD and an older population correlate with a 40% rise in the number of screening EGDs among Medicare beneficiaries.[6] The American College of Physicians EGD Clinical Guidelines Committee members published best practices in 2012. Because EGD is notoriously problematic as a screening tool in those with reflux symptoms, it is better used (1) to examine patients who have breakthrough symptoms despite 4 to 8 weeks of twice-daily PPI therapy; (2) to monitor severe erosive esophagitis after 2 months of PPI therapy to assess healing or rule out Barrett esophagus; (3) to monitor patients with a history of esophageal stricture who have recurrent dysphagia; (4) to screen high-risk individuals with chronic GERD or to survey high-risk individuals with GERD and Barrett esophagus with or without dysplasia; and (5) to screen atypical or extraesophageal presentations as part of a presurgical evaluation or to perform stricture dilation.[3,9]

Because heartburn and regurgitation lead the clinician to GERD above other diagnoses, patients are commonly treated with PPI therapy without EGD. This risks missing a potential case of Barrett esophagus, eosinophilic esophagitis, and PPI-responsive eosinophilia, because they may overlap.[6,10] Barrett esophagus is an important diagnosis to be made; it represents a change in typically observed esophageal mucosa and may develop into esophageal adenocarcinoma within a rare, unfortunate group of patients with GERD. The Montreal consensus definition for classification of Barrett's esophagus includes all three types of columnar metaplasia (specialized intestinal, characterized by goblet cells; gastric junctional type, also known as cardiac type; and gastric fundic type), but the presence of metaplasia (goblet cells) in the columnar epithelial lining of the distal esophagus is the only type of esophageal columnar epithelium known to predispose to malignancy, so it is a preferred diagnosis.[2]

In cases of dysphagia, EGD is always indicated initially because dilation of a possible stricture can occur at the same time as the diagnostic procedure. Biopsy specimens of the gastric mucosa obtained during EGD may reveal gram-negative *Helicobacter pylori*, which affects 20% to 50% of the industrialized world's population and 80% of the developing world's.[12] Opinion is divided as to whether patients should be tested and treated for *H. pylori* before long-term PPI therapy. There is some association with the location of *H. pylori* and gastric and duodenal ulcers (in 1% to 10%), gastric carcinoma (0.1% to 3%, a sixfold increased risk), and gastric mucosa–associated lymphoid tissue lymphoma (rare); the majority will develop symptoms.[12] It is also linked to vitamin B_{12} and iron deficiency. In general, patients treated for *H. pylori* have a decrease in GERD symptoms.[3] Although *H. pylori* is associated with some protective effects with respect to developing GERD, esophageal carcinoma, pediatric allergies, and asthma, on the whole it is thought better eradicated in cases of peptic ulcer disease, carcinoma of the stomach, and functional dyspepsia, given that its cost-effectiveness is not established in broad testing and treatment.[12]

Gastric emptying scans are useful for early satiety, nausea, and vomiting symptoms. Dynamic barium videography is useful to examine swallowing irregularities and look for structural defects.

Ambulatory pH testing (24-hour catheter based or ≥48-hour wireless) and high-resolution esophageal manometry are of benefit to patients with refractory symptoms and before reflux surgery. Esophageal pH testing can be performed with or without PPI and H_2 receptor antagonist acid suppression therapy. Esophageal pH testing with a single- or dual-sensor pH probe positioned above the LES (and below the upper esophageal sphincter, if the second sensor is used) for 24 hours contributes to the composite DeMeester score.[8]

DIAGNOSTICS

Gastroesophageal Reflux Disease (GERD)

LABORATORY
CBC and differential*
Stool for occult blood × 3*
H. pylori fecal antigen*

OTHER DIAGNOSTICS
EGD with biopsy specimens*
24-hr ambulatory pH monitoring by transnasal catheter*
48-hr ambulatory pH monitoring by radiotelemetry capsule*
Multichannel intraluminal impedance testing*
High-resolution manometry*
EndoFLIP*
Gastric scintigraphy*
Barium esophagram (for complications of GERD)*
Gastric emptying scan*

*If indicated.
CBC, complete blood count.

Esophageal manometry measures LES sphincter compliance and is especially useful in fundoplication surgeries in clarifying presurgical cofactors; it is sometimes repeated postsurgically if there are significant, persistent symptoms that medication cannot relieve. Whereas these studies can be useful, the most common manometric finding in patients with GERD is a normal LES pressure with normal esophageal motility.

New advances in technology using a radiotelemetry capsule, such as the Bravo (Medtronic) capsule, allow remote-controlled testing without the discomfort of a nasogastric tube to capture esophageal pH during a 48-hour period. Also, in some settings, multichannel intraluminal impedance pH technology is used to look at acidic and nonacidic volume in the distal esophagus. Esophageal impedance detects retrograde bolus movement, pH, and location of reflux whether on or off of suppressive therapy. This test is especially important in identifying potential surgical candidates.

High-resolution manometry excludes motor disorders by closely measuring the esophagus during swallowing with reproducible pressure gradient measurements to mark severity of LES incompetence and to plan the surgical approach. There is work being done to add a cross-sectional view and volume estimation with a high-frequency intraluminal ultrasound probe.[8] The EndoFLIP looks at distensibility data in patients suspected of having large-volume reflux, by using a cylindric bag in the distal esophagus in patients for surgical planning should an anatomic correction be indicated.[8] In the face of atypical symptoms, proof of reflux is essential.[2]

DIFFERENTIAL DIAGNOSIS

The symptoms of GERD can be similar to those of cholelithiasis, peptic ulcer disease, gastritis, angina, esophageal motility disturbances, and gastrointestinal malignant neoplasms. These disorders can be distinguished from GERD through the use of ultrasonography, upper gastrointestinal x-ray studies, endoscopy, esophageal manometry, electrocardiography, or coronary angiography, depending on the degree of clinical suspicion, particularly if the patient has a poor response to empirical GERD treatment.

Because symptoms and tests do not offer satisfactory correlations, different phenotypes have emerged. There are patients who respond to PPI therapy who have evidence of abnormal acid exposure on ambulatory pH reflux testing and/or normal acid exposure with an acid hypersensitivity and a positive symptom reflux correlation, as well as patients who report a positive symptom reflux correlation without an abnormal distal esophageal acid exposure attributable to hypersensitivity. Both situations are thought more likely to respond to PPIs.[6] Patients with a third phenotype cannot stop their PPI treatment, and are proven to have improvement on some PPI treatment, but are no better with more aggressive PPI regimens, suggesting they have an additional factor. A fourth phenotype includes functional heartburn patients who do not need PPIs but alternative strategies for acid suppression and reflux mitigation.[6]

GERD may be the most common cause of esophagitis, but there are other causes, including cytomegalovirus, herpes, or *Candida* infections in patients who are immunocompromised. Medications such as tetracycline and potassium chloride, if dissolved in the esophagus, result in "pill esophagitis." In unexplained cases of chest pain, cough, hoarseness, or asthma, GERD should be considered.

Another consideration is eosinophilic esophagitis, which is seen more often in young men with a history of atopy in the setting of reflux, dysphagia, odynophagia, and even stricture. It is a uniquely managed entity that is captured on histology since diagnosis has become more standardized Prompt treatment is recommended with steroid inhaler solutions, such as fluticasone propionate, 220 μg, used twice daily. Leukotriene modifiers and other antihistamines or oral steroids may be used, depending on the severity.

There are many extraesophageal manifestations of GERD. These atypical symptoms of GERD may come to the attention of otolaryngologists, cardiologists, or pulmonologists initially

DIFFERENTIAL DIAGNOSIS

Gastroesophageal Reflux Disease

- Achalasia
- Angina
- Amyloidosis
- Apnea
- Aspiration pneumonia
- Barrett esophagus
- *Candida* infection in patients who are immunocompromised
- Cardiac disease
- Cytomegalovirus infection in patients who are immunocompromised
- Cholelithiasis
- Chronic bronchitis
- Chronic cough
- Diabetes mellitus
- Dental complications
- Eating disorders
- Gastritis
- Gastric obstructing tumor
- Gastroparesis
- Eosinophilic esophagitis
- Esophageal cancer
- Esophageal hypersensitivity (central and peripheral)
- Esophageal motility disturbances (esophageal spasm, "jackhammer esophagus")
- Esophagitis secondary to infection
- Functional disorders of the gut
- Functional dyspepsia (reflux-like dyspepsia)
- Herpesvirus infection in patients who are immunocompromised
- Idiopathic pulmonary fibrosis
- Medication-induced "pill esophagitis"
- Neuromuscular disease affecting the oropharynx and esophagus
- Otitis media
- Peptic ulcer disease
- Postviral infections
- Pyloric stenosis
- Scleroderma
- Sinusitis
- Sjögren's disease or sicca syndrome
- Vagal nerve disorders
- Zollinger-Ellison syndrome

and include odynophagia, tooth decay, gingivitis, sour or brackish water taste, halitosis, dysphagia or globus sensation, cough, hoarseness, laryngitis, earache, sinus pain, hiccups, noncardiac chest pain, asthma, bronchiectasis, aspiration pneumonia, idiopathic pulmonary fibrosis, and sleep disturbances, as discussed earlier. GERD is also associated with irritable bowel syndrome and peptic ulcer disease.[3] Moreover, newer entities proposed by the Montreal consensus meeting incorporate GERD in their classification: reflux cough syndrome, reflux laryngitis syndrome, reflux asthma syndrome, reflux dental erosion syndrome, and associated possibilities—pharyngitis, sinusitis, idiopathic pulmonary fibrosis, and otitis.[2]

Finally, in patients with persistent symptoms of reflux disease despite EGD-negative, biopsy-negative, pH-negative, manometry-negative results, the differential diagnosis includes a hypersensitivity syndrome, which parallels reflux events, or a functional syndrome, which does not.

MANAGEMENT

Goals of therapy are prompt and sustained symptom control; healing of the injured esophageal mucosa; and prevention of complications, including stricture formation, Barrett esophagus, and adenocarcinoma (Fig. 135-1).

Lifestyle Modifications

Lifestyle modifications may benefit patients with GERD, although these changes alone are unlikely to control symptoms (Box 135-1). Modifications include elevating the head of the bed, lowering fat intake, ceasing smoking, loosening restrictive clothing, and avoiding recumbency for 2 to 3 hours after a meal. The true efficacy of these changes is lacking in the literature, even in studies that support weight loss and head-of-bed elevation.[3] Avoidance of chocolate, alcohol, carbonated drinks, peppermint, coffee, citrus, onion, and garlic can guard against chemically reduced LES pressure.

BOX 135-1

Lifestyle Changes for Management of Gastroesophageal Reflux Disease

- Decreased meal size
- Raised head of bed
- Reduced alcohol consumption
- Reduced carbonated drinks
- Reduced dietary fat
- Smoking cessation
- Weight loss

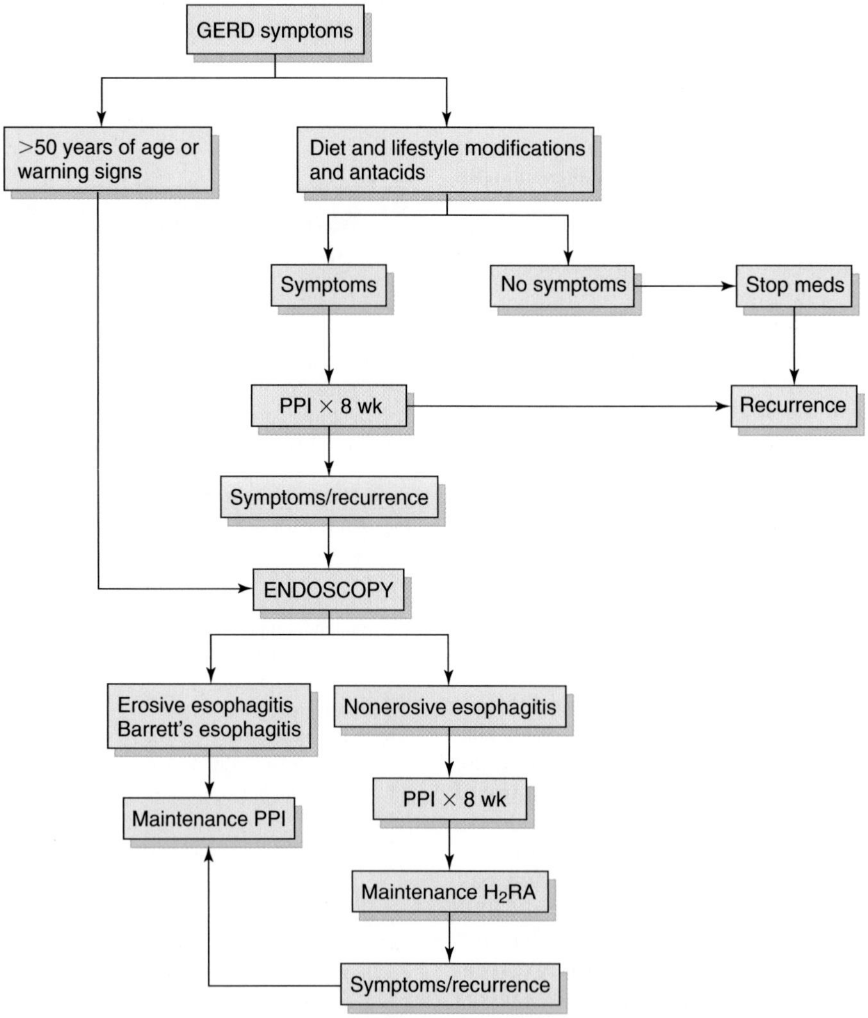

FIGURE 135-1 Gastroesophageal reflux disease (GERD) algorithm. H_2RA, H_2 receptor antagonist; PPI, proton pump inhibitor.

Acid Suppression Therapies

Many heartburn patients do not seek medical care but rather choose antacids and over-the-counter acid suppressants. Antacids are helpful but have a shorter duration. Alginate-based antacids provide effective relief but are less effective in non–acid reflux and regurgitation management.[2]

All four of the histamine$_2$ receptor antagonists (H_2RAs) approved for use in the United States are available over the counter and decrease gastric acid, particularly after a meal. They are often taken before an activity known to cause reflux symptoms. H_2RAs in divided doses may be effective in a patient with mild GERD and are considered equivalent in equipotent doses. Unfortunately, there is a risk of tolerance.[2] Over-the-counter PPIs have disclaimers that patients seek medical advice if treatment for more than 14 days is required. Prescription treatment for 2 months is sufficient to determine efficacy and to promote esophageal healing, as necessary (see Fig. 135-1).

The use of prescription-dose PPIs for acid suppression and maintenance therapy is well documented as the treatment of choice for GERD.[8] Because PPIs prevent acid production at the final juncture of the histamine, gastrin, and acetylcholine pathways, they tend to outperform H_2RAs. Because of interaction and reduced efficacy when taken together, PPIs and H_2RAs can be used together if administered at different times of day to offer an alternative to high-dose PPIs. Reduced dosages of PPIs, such as alternate-day or weekend therapy, have been shown to be ineffective long-term prescriptions.[8] Twice-daily administration is seen as more effective than a single higher dose initially.[8]

PPIs are superior to H_2RAs (even in high doses multiple times a day) in controlling symptoms, healing esophagitis, and improving quality of life. PPIs should ideally be given 1 hour before breakfast. Administration can be increased to twice daily. The first dose should be given 1 hour before breakfast, and the second dose should be given 1 hour before the evening meal. In the face of persistent symptoms, confirmation of correct timing of PPI administration and compliance with daily or twice-daily administration should be sought, along with lifestyle modifications, before considering the trial an inadequate response, because adherence to this regimen has been seen to hover around 50%.[6] Despite daily use of PPIs, 10% to 40% of patients still have GERD.[3] The thought is that some may have weakly acidic or weakly alkaline refluxate associated with regurgitation or atypical GERD symptoms, even bile salt exposure in nonacidic esophageal environment, but this is still not well established.[8] Sometimes a stepdown approach with successful PPI use can allow reduction in use (although up to half of patients may need H_2RAs instead),[5] or patients with nonerosive reflux disease (NERD) can use PPIs on demand.[5] With PPIs, a reduction in dose should happen slowly so as not to produce a rebound of GERD symptoms. Another concern has been increased risk of PPI-associated *Clostridium difficile* infection. This has been borne out by the U.S. Food and Drug Administration (FDA), which has led to the recommendation of testing for this pathogen in cases of unremitting diarrhea after recent start of PPI therapy.[3] This is more salient than the earlier concern for PPI-associated pneumonia.[3] Another consideration is the concern for reduced gastric acid associated with increased risk of gastric cancer, gastric carcinoids, or colorectal cancer; PPI use risk is associated with no greater contribution to these.[3] Fracture risk in men and women has not yet borne a clearly delineated association with PPIs; vitamin B_{12} and nonheme iron have yet to be evidenced by any association with PPIs. Iron malabsorption with PPIs is still controversial, as is the suspected negative impact of PPIs on magnesium absorption in the context of loop diuretic use. Finally, clopidogrel, a platelet aggregation inhibitor, is affected by omeprazole and esomeprazole and is associated with more cardiac events when taken together with these agents. PPIs may reduce the effect of bisphosphonates on bone modeling, although there has been no formal guidance on this.[3]

Another strategy in GERD management is to promote gastric emptying and to increase LES pressure. Promotility agents (e.g., metoclopramide, bethanechol, domperidone) may be used in selected patients as an adjunct to acid suppression, particularly if there is an element of delayed gastric emptying. The currently available agents are not ideal for monotherapy because they may produce undesirable side effects. Another consideration is the use of tricyclic antidepressants in significantly reduced doses for pain receptor modulation as well as trazadone or selective serotonin reuptake inhibitors.

TLSER reducers and pain modulators for weakly acidic refluxate might better address the perception of pain experienced by the patient. Medication strategies using γ-aminobutyric acid (GABA) type B ($GABA_B$) agonists such as baclofen (especially at nighttime) and cannabinoids have been useful; medications derived from the cholecystokinin CCK family are under investigation.

Endoscopic Therapies

Several endoscopic techniques for GERD have been developed. These techniques are less invasive than the standard surgical approach, laparoscopic fundoplication, but are considered experimental because they have not been subject to randomized, controlled trials or have been associated with complications.

A range of endoscopic techniques are available short of surgery. LINX involves placement in the distal esophagus of a small expandable ring of magnetic-linked beads that hold the LES closed unless it is overcome by swallowing, belching, or vomiting.

The Stretta system consists of a radiofrequency generator and a delivery catheter to remodel the esophageal junction and LES. The catheter is positioned, and needles are deployed into the muscles of the gastroesophageal junction. Energy is delivered to create a series of thermal lesions, which is thought to thicken the sphincter for more resistance. It may be used in a stepwise progression before antireflux surgery or in addition to other techniques.

Surgery

In patients responsive to PPI treatment, with documented reflux, LES incompetence with inadequate control and surgery can improve symptom control and quality of life.[2] Moreover, EER symptoms in patients with typical GERD symptoms and a pH below 4 more than 12% of the time over a 24-hour period were more significantly likely to resolve after Nissen fundoplication.[13] The laparoscopic approach to open Nissen fundoplication was developed in 1991 and is considered the standard of care, with fewer complications than the open approach.[8] Laparoscopic partial and total fundoplication are the best options for the patient with well-documented chronic, symptomatic GERD. The best predictors of surgical success for GERD include age younger than 50 years and typical reflux symptoms that completely resolve with medical therapy. Patients with atypical symptoms and EESs and those whose symptoms are refractory respond less effectively to surgery, although patients with respiratory symptoms, NERD, hypersensitive esophagus, or LPR may be candidates, depending on symptom correlation with acid or nonacid reflux.[2] Inappropriate patients include those with achalasia, diffuse esophageal spasm, nutcracker esophagus, eosinophilic esophagus, or scleroderma.[2]

Complications include a high rate of postoperative dysphagia, bloating, and flatulence. To address this, there are several variations on approach, particularly the anterior partial fundoplication, and reoperative procedures if necessary. The posterior partial fundoplication is indicated for qualifying normal-weight patients with GERD. In contrast, gastric bypass surgery would be a good choice for patients with BMI above 40. With all surgeries, repair of hiatal hernia is obligatory and correlated with improvement; still, there is an antireflux failure rate of 10% to 15%, wherein symptoms persist or new symptoms develop.[2]

Many studies support the role of surgery in decreasing acid exposure and increasing LES pressure, and therefore symptomatic Barrett esophagus is seen as an indication. However, this has not revealed an improvement in adenocarcinoma rates, even though metaplastic changes are seen to regress to a great degree. Nevertheless, there are symptomatic patients who choose to discontinue PPI therapy in favor of surgery.

The best candidates for surgery have a BMI between 25 and 35; do not have severe delayed gastric emptying suggested by symptoms of bloating, nausea, vomiting, or abdominal pain and fullness (documented on radionuclide testing as an excess of 150 minutes to move more than half of meal content from the stomach); do not have a debilitating psychiatric illness; and are psychologically prepared to accept a lack of improvement. The morbidly obese patient with GERD may achieve better results after a gastric bypass.

COMPLICATIONS

In one series, up to 30% of patients with nonerosive esophagitis progressed to having erosive esophagitis annually. In a different, smaller sample of patients with nonerosive GERD with abnormal pH testing results and normal EGD findings, 5% progressed; progression was associated with smoking and the absence of PPIs.[1] A relapse of reflux esophagitis (seen both endoscopically and clinically) as a result of the discontinuation of medication typically affects those with higher grades of symptomatic reflux.[1]

Complications of GERD include esophageal ulcers, peptic strictures, Barrett esophagus, hemorrhage, and perforation. Dental erosions, pharyngeal ulcerations, laryngeal damage, esophageal ulcerations, strictures, adenocarcinoma, and sleep derangements are complications.[3] Strictures, which form from mucosal scarring, may impede the progress of food from the mouth to the stomach. These inflamed bands develop over time and are characterized by dysphagia and a possible reduction in heartburn because the stricture may block some of the reflux. Dilation may be necessary if symptoms are persistent despite PPI therapy and may need to be repeated months to years later.

Barrett esophagus, an infrequent, premalignant condition, is associated with chronic (>5 years) esophageal injury resulting from reflux. It is estimated that 10% of patients with chronic GERD develop Barrett esophagus.[3] It is diagnosed histologically, when patches of normal gray-white, stratified squamous cell mucosa of the esophagus change into the light pink columnar epithelium. Biopsy specimens of the gastroesophageal junction are critical for accurate diagnosis and staging. The gastroesophageal junction shifts proximally in Barrett esophagus. The Montreal consensus definition for Barrett esophagus incorporates endoscopically suspected esophageal metaplasia of the proximal gastroesophageal junction, subcategorized histologically into gastric metaplasia–positive, specialized intestinal metaplasia–positive, and intestinal metaplasia–negative disease. Biopsy findings that are positive for intestinal metaplasia are further delineated: low-, high-, or indeterminate-grade dysplasia. Samples from suspected metaplastic areas less than 3 cm in length are thought to be less likely to develop into cancer; longer segments are considered more likely, although the emphasis of late is on inclusion of all suspected areas, including short-segment Barrett esophagus.

In half of Barrett esophagus cases, patients have undergone endoscopy in the absence of prior reflux symptoms. In fact, a history of erosive esophagitis has not been established as a clear risk factor for Barrett esophagus in patients with GERD symptoms. However, those with GERD and Barrett esophagus tend to develop symptoms at an earlier age and have more complications. Patients with Barrett esophagus with intestinal metaplasia require ongoing surveillance once it has been identified by histology, particularly those with high-grade dysplasia because this is a significant risk factor for esophageal adenocarcinoma.

The risk for esophageal adenocarcinoma (with a survival rate of 15% to 20% at 5 years) is 30 to 150 times higher in individuals with Barrett esophagus.[2] Risk factors include chronic (>5 years) of GERD as well as male sex, white race, age older than 50, tobacco use, hiatal hernia, nocturnal symptoms, and obesity.[9] *H. pylori* infection may be a protective factor. If Barrett esophagus is present, periodic EGDs with biopsies are recommended to assess and to grade the development of dysplasia or malignant transformation. Surveillance endoscopy every 3 to 5 years in patients without dysplasia, with four-quadrant mucosal biopsies of every 2 cm of involved mucosa, is generally recommended; in 6 months to confirm low-grade dysplasia and then annually; and every 3 months if high-grade dysplasia has been identified, with consideration of endoablative therapy for dysplasia.[9,11] Advanced imaging techniques, such as electronic or virtual chromoendoscopy, have been associated with increased yield of dysplasia detection[9]; probe-based confocal endomicroscopy is a newer technique, and volumetric laser endomicroscopy may be next.[9]

For those with complete eradication of intestinal metaplasia, whether by medication, an endoluminal procedure, or surgery (preferred in younger patients with hiatal hernia and LES incompetence),[2] surveillance should continue in accordance with baseline histology. Barrett esophagus may still progress despite PPI therapy; evidence supports antireflux surgery to forestall development of esophageal adenocarcinoma in patients with symptomatic Barrett esophagus.

As for other complications arising from antireflux surgery, a proportion of antireflux postoperative patients continue acid-blocking medication despite negative results of 24-hour pH monitoring.[4] Laparoscopic fundoplication complications represent 5%, often associated with dysphagia, flatulence, and the inability to belch, among other bowel complaints. Furthermore, the surgical wrap around the LES is also known to weaken over time.

INDICATIONS FOR REFERRAL OR HOSPITALIZATION

It is important to identify patients who might either benefit from maximum long-term medical therapy or experience complications. Patients who initially receive 2 months of empirical treatment without success or whose symptoms recur when medications are stopped should undergo EGD to determine whether esophagitis is present (see Fig. 135-1).

A gastroenterology referral is indicated if the patient is older than 50 years or has the warning signs of dysphagia (both solid and liquid), odynophagia, unexplained iron deficiency anemia, weight loss, fecal occult bleeding, new-onset motility disorder (which is more often seen in cases of respiratory complaints, such as obstructive symptoms of nausea, vomiting, and early satiety),[1] or anorexia.

Patients who have refractory symptoms will need further consultation and management, ideally within a multidisciplinary framework. When otolaryngologists, allergists, cardiologists, pulmonologists, surgeons, speech language pathologists, and nutritionists might be brought into the fold to make the diagnosis and propose a management strategy, the challenge is to continue to provide cross-disciplinary communication to optimize the patient's outcome.

LIFE SPAN CONSIDERATIONS

GERD can affect adults of any age, including infants. Both age and nutritional status affect esophageal mucosal resistance, which is less robust than that of the stomach.[1] Weight loss alone will probably not control symptoms but is recommended, especially in conjunction with other strategies.[1]

Patients with pregnancy-related reflux can use antacids, sucralfate,[1] and H_2RAs. As women enter perimenopause and postmenopause, the use of exogenous hormone replacement, including estrogen, progesterone, tamoxifen, selective estrogen receptor modulators, and over-the-counter hormone preparations, rises. Each of these medication classes has been shown to raise the risk of GERD in women.

With advanced age, arthritic pain as well as bone health in the prevention and management of osteopenia and osteoporosis may lead patients to the use of bisphosphonates and NSAIDs, which can exacerbate mild GERD symptoms. Although symptom severity in patients aged 60 years and older may be similar to that in younger patients, evidence suggests that the proportion of patients with heartburn alone may decrease in an older cohort, whereas incidence of erosive esophagitis and Barrett's esophagus may increase.[5] Older patients on H_2-receptor antagonists may experience drowsiness or falls, and there is a caveat in use in this population owing to increased risk of delirium or renal clearance concern.[3]

Long-term results of antireflux surgery appear to show a benefit in patients achieving their best control of symptoms with PPIs, whereas those refractory to intensive therapy have more variable responses postoperatively. If surgery is indicated for a patient older than 65 years, outcomes are thought to be comparable to those of younger patients, although postoperative stay is potentially longer because of comorbidities.

EDUCATION AND HEALTH PROMOTION

Education is essential for patients with GERD. Patients should avoid fatty foods, caffeinated and carbonated drinks, acidic and spicy foods, chocolate, peppermint, and excessive alcohol consumption. Foods that may elicit symptoms for one person may not necessarily produce symptoms in another; therefore, selective avoidance of foods that precipitate symptoms is necessary. Lifestyle modifications are numerous and were outlined earlier. Screening endoscopy is recommended in cases of chronic GERD or difficult-to-treat symptoms to determine if there is an erosive component or if complications are present.

CHAPTER 136

GASTROINTESTINAL HEMORRHAGE

Michael Huang • David H. Kerman

DEFINITION AND EPIDEMIOLOGY

Gastrointestinal (GI) bleeding is a common finding in the ambulatory care setting. Patients may report the symptoms as black tarry stools (melena), bright red stools (hematochezia), and even bright red vomitus (hematemesis).[1] GI hemorrhage can occur anywhere in the GI tract from the mouth to the anus and can be overt or occult[2] (Box 136-1). Overt GI bleeding is considered major when it is accompanied by hemodynamic instability and minor when it is not. Occult bleeding is nonvisible bleeding that can be detected by stool testing or indirectly suggested by iron deficiency anemia.[3]

GI bleeding may be related to ulceration, inflammation, erosion of a blood vessel, or neoplasm. Management of GI bleeding has remained constant for several decades. Hemodynamic stabilization of the patient, cessation of active bleeding, and prevention of recurrent bleeding have long remained the goals of medical management for this disorder, which occurs in approximately 100 individuals per 100,000 per year.[4] Many of these patients require emergency treatment, hospitalization, and intensive care monitoring.

Upper and lower GI tract bleeding are differentiated according to anatomic source. Patients with upper gastrointestinal tract bleeding (UGIB) from a source proximal to the ligament

BOX 136-1

Bleeding Definitions

Overt: Visible bright red or maroon blood in feces or emesis
Occult: No visible blood in feces or emesis
Obscure: Patient may be seen with iron deficiency anemia (IDA) or may have a positive fecal occult blood test (FOBT) result
Obscure/Occult: IDA recurrent or persistent; positive FOBT result; may or may not have visible bleeding; no bleeding source found at time of original endoscopy
Obscure/Overt
- IDA recurrent or persistent; positive FOBT result; no visible blood in feces; no source identified
- Blood visible in feces and emesis; bleeding recurrent or persistent; no source found at original endoscopy

Modified from Zuckerman GR, Prakash C, Askin MP, Lewis BS: AGA technical review on the evaluation and management of occult and obscure gastrointestinal bleeding. *Gastroenterology* 118(1):201-221, 2000.

of Treitz may be asymptomatic, have subtle signs of anemia and hypovolemia, or have a dramatic presentation with hematemesis, melena, or hematochezia.[5] Causes of UGIB are classified as variceal and nonvariceal bleeding. The most common cause of nonvariceal bleeding is peptic ulcer disease, with gastric ulcers occurring more frequently than duodenal ulcers.[5] Nonspecific mucosal abnormalities, such as erosions, are the second most common cause of nonvariceal bleeding.[6] Low-dose aspirin and other nonsteroidal anti-inflammatory drugs (NSAIDs) are frequently implicated in UGIB and are associated with morbidity and mortality.[5,7,8] Other causes of UGIB include anticoagulants, antiplatelets, esophagitis, and gastroesophageal varices. Lower gastrointestinal tract bleeding (LGIB) from a source distal to the ligament of Treitz can cause occult blood loss or massive hematochezia and shock. The most common cause of LGIB is diverticulosis (40%). Other sources include cancer, polyps, colitis, ulcers, angiodysplasia, and miscellaneous causes such as postpolypectomy bleeding, aortocolonic fistula, stercoral ulcer, anastomotic bleeding, anorectal hemorrhoids, fissures, and rectal ulcers.

PATHOPHYSIOLOGY

GI bleeding can be associated with esophagitis, peptic ulcer disease, gastritis, *Helicobacter pylori*, esophageal or gastric varices, diverticulosis, gastric and colonic cancers, gastric and colonic polyps, and angiodysplasia.[2,4] Peptic ulcers are defects in the mucosa of the duodenum or stomach caused by a breakdown in normal mucosal defenses and ulcer erosion into a blood vessel. Contributing factors include smoking, NSAIDs, excess stomach acid production, and *H. pylori*.

Bleeding caused by gastritis is related to diffuse superficial lesions in the gastric mucosa that are usually associated with local irritants or *H. pylori*. Gastritis can also be caused by major physiologic stressors, including burns, sepsis, trauma, and long-distance running, secondary to decreased splanchnic blood flow and the resultant decrease in mucus production, bicarbonate secretion, and prostaglandin synthesis, all leading to a breakdown in the normal mucosal defenses. NSAIDs inhibit cyclooxygenase, decreasing the synthesis of protective prostaglandins, and may have direct effects on the gastric mucosa, causing both irritation and superficial lesions. Alcohol ingestion causes gastric mucosa production of leukotrienes, which may be responsible for vascular stasis, engorgement, and increased vascular permeability, resulting in hemorrhage.[9,10]

H. pylori was first described in 1984. This gram-negative spiral bacterium has adaptive mechanisms to survive in the human stomach, including the conversion of urea, water, and acid to ammonia and bicarbonate. It is the secretions of toxins, disruption of the mucous layer, and direct adherence to the gastroduodenal surface epithelium that render the underlying mucosa vulnerable to peptic acid damage. Excluding NSAIDs, approximately 100% of cases of chronic superficial gastritis, 90% to 95% of duodenal ulcers, and 80% of gastric ulcers are believed to be caused by *H. pylori*. However, improved hygiene and eradication have caused the prevalence of *H. pylori* in peptic ulcer disease to markedly decrease.[11] Treatment of this organism has been shown to cure ulcer disease and to decrease the incidence of ulcer recurrence and rebleeding.[12,13,14]

Esophageal varices are dilated submucosal veins arising as a consequence of portal hypertension.[15] The most common cause of portal hypertension in the United States is cirrhosis from alcoholic and chronic active hepatitis; however, worldwide the most common cause is parasitic disease (particularly schistosomiasis).[12-16] Approximately one third of all patients with cirrhosis will bleed from varices; overall mortality is 30%.[17]

Diverticulosis is a common cause of acute LGIB.[4] Diverticula can occur at the penetration site of colonic arteries, which can rupture into the diverticular sac, resulting in LGIB.[10]

Angiodysplasias, small vascular tufts formed by capillaries, veins, and venules, representing an acquired arteriovenous malformation[14,15] are the most common vascular lesions found in the GI tract. A small percentage of these lesions are present at birth, but most angiodysplasias are detected in people older than 60 years.[14,18] Although massive bleeding is occasionally associated with these lesions, bleeding is more often slow, chronic, and occult.

CLINICAL PRESENTATION

Overt blood loss from the GI tract can manifest in numerous ways. Hematemesis is bloody vomitus that is either fresh and bright red or older and like coffee grounds in appearance. Melena is stool that is black, shiny, and foul smelling as a result of blood degradation. These clinical signs generally originate from an upper GI source. The presence or history of black or red hematemesis confirms an upper GI source after bleeding from the nose and oropharynx has been excluded. Melena represents an upper GI source 85% to 95% of the time, and hematochezia from a briskly bleeding upper GI source accounts for 15% of cases. Patients with UGIB with hematochezia have a worse prognosis in terms of morbidity and mortality than those with melena.[6] Hematochezia is the passage of bright red to mahogany-colored blood from the rectum as pure blood, blood mixed with stool, blood clots, or bloody diarrhea. These manifestations are more overt or obvious, but occult blood loss is often more subtle. In general, patients with a lower GI source of bleeding have hematochezia, a clear nasogastric (NG) aspirate, and a normal blood urea nitrogen (BUN)/creatinine ratio.[19] In addition, patients can have symptoms associated with blood loss, such as presyncope, dyspnea, angina, postural hypotension, and shock, with no overt bleeding source. Occult blood loss can manifest as iron deficiency anemia or as a positive result of a routine fecal occult blood test (FOBT) with use of a chemical reagent.[18]

Patient history should include the amount, duration, and source of any signs of bleeding along with any associated symptoms, including dizziness, abdominal pain, chest pain, shortness of breath, diaphoresis, and weakness. The patient should be questioned about prior episodes of bleeding and about other illnesses that can result in bleeding, such as cirrhosis, cancer, coagulopathies, and connective tissue disease. All significant past medical and surgical conditions as well as any allergies and medication use, including alendronate, potassium chloride, anticoagulants, and over-the-counter preparations (especially aspirin and NSAIDs), should be elicited and documented. A careful history of alcohol, tobacco, and illicit drug use is also necessary.

PHYSICAL EXAMINATION

The physical examination is brief and focused. The initial general appearance and mental status of the patient should be noted. Vital signs are the most important factor in considering initial triage and should be obtained early and frequently. The earliest sign of hypovolemia is tachycardia; hypotension does not occur until volume loss approaches 40%.[18] The skin should be examined for color, temperature, turgor, moisture, and capillary refill. Cutaneous lesions on upper extremities, lips, and oral mucosa may reveal hereditary hemorrhagic telangiectasia or blue rubber bleb nevus syndrome. These can be related to a family history of GI bleeding. Other cutaneous manifestations that should be noted on the physical examination include signs of cirrhosis such as spider nevi, palmar erythema, and scleral icterus.

The cardiovascular examination should focus on the heart rate and the character of the peripheral pulses. Postural change in blood pressure should be immediately noted. Orthostasis suggests a blood volume loss of 15% to 20%.[18] If the systolic blood pressure falls more than 20 mm Hg, the diastolic blood pressure decreases more than 10 mm Hg, or the heart rate increases by more than 20 beats per minute when an adult patient stands from a supine position, intravascular fluid loss is likely and hospital admission should be considered (level of evidence: moderate).[20]

The abdomen should be auscultated and palpated to identify a mass, tenderness, guarding, or rigidity. Abdominal pain, particularly cramping in the periumbilical area and abdominal distention, may indicate rapid intestinal transit of blood and a major bleed. A careful rectal examination can detect hemorrhoids, fissures, or rectal carcinoma. The stool should be examined for gross blood or melena, indicating acute bleeding that may require urgent intervention. Occult blood testing is usually reserved for colorectal cancer screening purposes, although it can be useful in the appropriate context.[21] One must be aware of the highly variable specificity and sensitivity rates of stool occult blood testing. After the patient is stabilized, a thorough physical examination should be performed in search of non-GI sources of bleeding, such as increased or irregular menstrual bleeding in the presence of iron deficiency anemia.[22]

DIAGNOSTICS

Laboratory evaluation of all patients with GI bleeding should include hemoglobin, hematocrit, and platelet count to assess baseline blood loss and platelet adequacy.[19] The patient's blood should be typed and crossmatched for 4 to 6 units of packed red blood cells. Laboratory studies include BUN, creatinine, and glucose concentration; liver function tests (LFTs); and prothrombin time (PT) and activated partial thromboplastin time (aPTT). An increased BUN level with normal creatinine concentration is suggestive of an upper GI source.[12] Arterial blood gases (ABGs) may be helpful in assessing oxygenation and clarifying the patient's acid-base status. Electrocardiography (ECG) should be performed for all patients older than 40 years with chest or abdominal pain or a history of cardiac or pulmonary disease. Radiographic studies may include an acute abdominal series if there is suggestion of a perforated viscus or intestinal obstruction accompanying bleeding.

NG tube lavage that reveals blood or coffee ground–like material confirms the diagnosis of UGIB and may suggest that the bleeding is caused by a high-risk lesion.[23] It is worth noting that 16% of patients with actively bleeding lesions at endoscopy may not demonstrate blood in the NG tube aspirate and therefore have a low sensitivity for UGIB.[21,22,24] The gastric lavage may not be positive for blood if the bleeding has ceased or if the bleeding is occurring beyond a closed pylorus in cases such as duodenal ulcers. Bilious fluid return on NG lavage indicates an open pylorus, thus increasing the sensitivity for detection of postpyloric bleeding. NG tube lavage has also been used to clear the stomach for improved visualization before endoscopic evaluation.

Further diagnostic studies, such as endoscopy, barium studies, bleeding scans, and angiography, should be performed at the discretion of the consulting gastroenterologist or surgeon.[19,21,22,25] Early consultation should be prompted if an acute bleed is suspected.

DIAGNOSTICS

Gastrointestinal Bleeding

LABORATORY
- Stool for occult bleeding
- CBC with differential
- Platelets
- BUN
- Creatinine
- Serum glucose
- Calcium
- LFTs
- Serum electrolytes
- Amylase level
- PT/aPTT
- ABGs
- *H. pylori*
- Type and crossmatch

IMAGING
- Abdominal x-ray studies
- Bleeding scans or angiography*
- Upright chest x-ray study (for severe abdominal pain)
- Computed tomography (CT) of abdomen and surgical consultation (if all other test results remain negative and the patient continues to have severe abdominal pain with intestinal bleeding)

OTHER DIAGNOSTICS
- Blood pressure tilts for orthostatic hypotension
- ECG (if >40 years or with cardiac history)
- Endoscopy*
- Barium studies*
- Air-contrast enema*
- Nuclear scintigraphy*†
- Selective mesenteric angiography*†
- Enteroscopy*
- Anoscopy†
- Sigmoidoscopy†
- Colonoscopy†

*If indicated.
†For evaluation of LGIB.

DIFFERENTIAL DIAGNOSIS

The sources of GI bleeding may be categorized as inflammatory, mechanical, vascular, neoplastic, systemic, or anomalous. Vomiting, coughing, retching, or blunt abdominal trauma before bleeding suggests a Mallory-Weiss tear, the majority of which occur in the upper stomach. Painful UGIB is suggestive of peptic ulcer disease, gastritis, esophagitis, or duodenitis; severe pain and peritoneal signs suggest a perforated viscus. The bleeding of esophageal varices is suggested by a history of cirrhosis and painless bleeding.[5]

Bleeding from colonic diverticula is the most common cause of acute LGIB. The bleeding is an arterial bleed at the neck or dome of the diverticulum but ceases spontaneously the majority of the time. Ischemic colitis, a common cause of LGIB, is usually associated with acute, temporary reduction in mesenteric blood flow in the "watershed" areas of the colon at the splenic flexure and the rectosigmoid junction. This transient ischemic event causes necrosis of the colonic mucosa and, as a result, diarrhea, abdominal pain, and bleeding. Postprandial abdominal pain or pain that is disproportionate to the physical findings is also suggestive of ischemic colitis. Other lower GI sources of bleeding associated with abdominal pain include inflammatory bowel disease and infectious colitis. Infectious diarrhea should not be overlooked in a patient with bloody

DIFFERENTIAL DIAGNOSIS

GI Bleeding

UGIB (ORIGINATING ABOVE THE LIGAMENT OF TREITZ)

- Oral or pharyngeal lesions: swallowed blood from nose or oropharynx
- Swallowed hemoptysis
- Esophageal: varices, ulceration, esophagitis, Mallory-Weiss tear, carcinoma, trauma
- Gastric: peptic ulcer (including Cushing and Curling ulcers), gastritis, angiodysplasia, gastric neoplasms, hiatal hernia, gastric diverticulum, pseudoxanthoma elasticum, hereditary hemorrhagic telangiectasia (Rendu-Osler-Weber syndrome)
- Duodenal: peptic ulcer, duodenitis, angiodysplasia, aortoduodenal fistula, duodenal diverticulum, duodenal tumors, carcinoma of ampulla of Vater, parasites (e.g., hookworm), Crohn disease
- Biliary: hematobilia (e.g., penetrating injury to liver, hepatobiliary malignant neoplasm, endoscopic papillotomy)

LGIB (ORIGINATING BELOW THE LIGAMENT OF TREITZ)

Small Intestine

- Ischemic bowel disease (mesenteric thrombosis, embolism, vasculitis, trauma)
- Small bowel neoplasm: leiomyomas, carcinoids
- Hereditary hemorrhagic telangiectasia
- Meckel diverticulum and other small intestine diverticula
- Aortoenteric fistula
- Intestinal hemangiomas: blue rubber bleb nevi, intestinal hemangiomas, cutaneous vascular nevi
- Hamartomatous polyps: Peutz-Jeghers syndrome (intestinal polyps, mucocutaneous pigmentation)
- Infections of small bowel: tuberculous enteritis, enteritis necroticans
- Volvulus
- Intussusception
- Lymphoma of small bowel, sarcoma, Kaposi sarcoma
- Irradiation ileitis
- Arteriovenous malformation of small intestine
- Inflammatory bowel disease
- Polyarteritis nodosa
- Other: pancreatoenteric fistulas, Henoch-Schönlein purpura, Ehlers-Danlos syndrome, systemic lupus erythematosus, amyloidosis, metastatic melanoma

Colon

- Carcinoma (particularly left colon)
- Diverticular disease
- Inflammatory bowel disease
- Ischemic colitis
- Colonic polyps
- Vascular abnormalities: angiodysplasia, vascular ectasia
- Radiation colitis
- Infectious colitis
- Uremic colitis
- Aortoenteric fistula
- Lymphoma of large bowel
- Hemorrhoids
- Anal fissure
- Trauma, foreign body
- Solitary rectal or cecal ulcers

diarrhea. Enterohemorrhagic *Escherichia coli* (especially *E. coli* O157:H7) is responsible for numerous infections worldwide[26] and is commonly associated with the ingestion of undercooked ground meat, contaminated water, or unpasteurized milk.

Painless bleeding may be related to diverticulosis, angiodysplasia, or hemorrhoids. Rectal pain may be associated with bleeding from anal fissures or anal or rectal carcinoma. Constipation may suggest malignant disease or hemorrhoids.

MANAGEMENT

The most important concept in the management of acute GI bleeding is that resuscitation and stabilization must precede diagnostic and therapeutic interventions. The initial priorities are the establishment of an adequate airway, ensuring oxygenation and ventilation, followed by restoration of the circulatory status to normal. All patients with hemodynamic instability (shock, orthostatic hypotension, decrease in hematocrit of at least 6%, or active bleeding) should be admitted to the intensive care unit (ICU) for resuscitation and close monitoring.

Any patient thought to have significant bleeding should immediately have two large-bore intravenous lines or a central line placed. Fluid resuscitation should be vigorous and should consist of crystalloid infusions of either normal saline or lactated Ringer's solution at rates as rapid as the patient's cardiopulmonary system will allow to correct the volume deficit. Consideration of a central venous pressure line or a Swan-Ganz catheter should be given for patients with underlying cardiac, pulmonary, renal, or hepatic disease to prevent fluid overload. A Foley catheter should be placed to assist with determination of volume status, with a minimum urinary output of 30 to 50 mL/hr in the adult.

The blood product of choice initially is packed red blood cells for patients continuing to bleed, patients in shock, patients with very low hematocrit values, or patients who have symptoms related to poor tissue oxygenation (e.g., angina).[21] High-risk patients, such as older adults and those with severe comorbid conditions such as coronary artery disease, should maintain hemoglobin above 7 g/dL.[20,27] Indications for transfusions have become more restrictive, with recent data suggesting more judicious use of blood products. Animal studies suggest that overtransfusion in cirrhotic patients may actually increase bleeding related to portal hypertension.[28] Randomized trials with cirrhotic patients have shown that transfusions should be used to maintain a hemoglobin at or above 7 g/dL. Furthermore, this threshold has been shown to improve outcomes for noncirrhotic patients with UGIB as well.[29] For patients with massive blood loss, whole blood may be used. Close monitoring of coagulation parameters and serum calcium concentration must accompany transfusion. Fresh-frozen plasma may be used to correct coagulopathy (international normalized ratio [INR] >1.5).[30] Patients with platelet counts of less than 50,0000 should be transfused with platelets.

Many patients, especially elderly patients, will often be taking medications that may exacerbate bleeding. Aspirin or other antiplatelet medications such as Plavix are frequently used in patients with prior history of coronary artery disease or stroke. Coumadin, low-molecular-weight heparin, and new antithrombin inhibitors such as dabigatran or rivaroxaban may be used in patients with a history of atrial fibrillation, pulmonary embolism, deep vein thrombus, or mechanical valves. Some of the anticoagulation can be reversed with medication. Vitamin K and FFP can reverse the coagulopathy from Coumadin.[31] Antiplatelet agents in general bind irreversibly, and transfusion of platelets may be necessary to counter the antiplatelet effects. The newer antithrombin inhibitors may not have reversal agents. The risks and benefits of the anticoagulation should be weighed and individualized with every patient before reversal of the anticoagulation.[31]

In most cases of suspected acute UGIB, acid suppressive therapy with proton pump inhibitors (PPIs) can be started empirically because the majority of upper GI lesions are acid responsive. Meta-analysis of randomized controlled trials in patients with UGIB suggests that PPI therapy is associated with reduced rebleeding and reduced need for surgery.[32] In addition, high-dose bolus and continuous infusion intravenous PPI (80 mg intravenous push followed by 8 mg/hr) has been shown to reduce the proportion of UGIB patients with bleeding sources that need to be treated with specific endoscopic therapy.[33] Given the broad efficacy of PPI in UGIB, patients with symptoms of UGIB should be started empirically on PPI therapy.[30] H_2 receptor antagonists (e.g., ranitidine, famotidine) should not be routinely used for patients with acute ulcer bleeding.[30]

Pre-endoscopy risk in UGIB can be assessed several different ways. Two models, the Glasgow Blatchford score and its modified version, are validated systems used to calculate a given patient's risk for requiring endoscopic intervention.[34,35] The modified Glasgow Blatchford score is simplified with use of fewer clinical parameters.[34]

The diagnostic test of choice in UGIB is endoscopy.[2,21] Endoscopy has the advantage of identifying patients with continued bleeding or high-risk lesions who will benefit from endoscopic therapy. Therapeutic endoscopy can achieve hemostasis once a bleeding lesion has been identified. High-risk endoscopic findings include arterial bleeding, adherent clot, visible vessels, and varices. Endoscopy is also helpful in stratifying those patients found to have lesions with low risk of rebleeding to early discharge. Those at risk for rebleeding, resulting in increased morbidity and mortality, are patients older than 60 years, those with coagulopathies and other concurrent illnesses, and anyone hospitalized at the time of bleeding.[21]

All patients who are diagnosed with gastric or duodenal ulcers should be screened for *H. pylori* infection by biopsy or noninvasive methods, including urea breath tests and serum serologies, and treated appropriately.[36] In addition, treatment with PPIs is recommended for patients with peptic ulcer disease. Intravenous PPI drip should be reserved for patients with high risk of rebleeding or those who are unable to tolerate oral intake.

Esophageal varices are related to increased portal hypertension causing variceal rupture and bleeding. Octreotide, a long-acting analogue of somatostatin, has become the vasoactive agent of choice for a patient experiencing acute GI bleeding. Octreotide decreases splanchnic and hepatic blood flow along with decreasing transhepatic and variceal pressures, thus reducing portal pressures. Octreotide is given as a 100-μg intravenous bolus followed by a continuous infusion of 50 μg/hr.[21] In patients with GI bleeding and cirrhosis, prophylactic broad-spectrum antibiotics (typically third-generation cephalosporins) should also be given for 7 days from the time of bleeding presentation to prevent the risk of infectious complications.[37,38]

The most common definitive therapy for gastroesophageal varices is endoscopic sclerotherapy or band ligation. According to Sarin and colleagues,[39] endoscopic variceal ligation is as effective as propranolol for the prophylactic treatment of high-risk varices. Endoscopic sclerotherapy involves intravariceal injection of a sclerosing agent. It has proven to be as effective as somatostatin alone for actively bleeding varices. However, a combination of medical and endoscopic therapy is superior to either treatment alone. For patients who rebleed despite endoscopic therapies, alternative therapies include balloon tamponade, surgical operations, and transjugular intrahepatic portosystemic shunt (TIPS). Balloon tamponade with a Sengstaken-Blakemore tube has a success rate of 70% to 80% but may cause severe complications, including aspiration, ulceration, and perforation if it is used improperly.[4] Surgical operations include shunt procedures to decompress the portovenous system, esophageal transection, and devascularization of the gastroesophageal junction. A TIPS procedure is performed by interventional radiologists and involves creation of a shunt between the portal and hepatic vein to decompress the portal system and to achieve hemostasis. An additional benefit of a TIPS procedure as salvage therapy is that in certain high-risk patients it has been shown to significantly decrease overall mortality if used early.[40]

Diagnostic modalities available for the evaluation of overt LGIB include sigmoidoscopy, colonoscopy, nuclear scintigraphy, selective mesenteric angiography (with vasopressin infusion or selective embolization), enteroscopy, and operative therapy.[17] The evaluation of the patient with LGIB depends on the severity of the bleeding.[14] Vigorous fluid resuscitation should precede any diagnostic evaluation. Patients who are hemodynamically stable should first undergo colonoscopy. Colonoscopy in this setting is the diagnostic procedure of choice because of its accuracy and therapeutic capability.[17,26] In addition, urgent colonoscopy has been associated with a decreased hospital length of stay.[41] Preparation facilitates endoscopic evaluation and increases safety and visualization and diagnostic yield.[42]

Radionuclide evaluation or a bleeding scan (red blood cell scan) is capable of detecting a hemorrhage as slow as 0.1 mL/min.[43] Technetium 99m–labeled red cells are injected, and scans are taken shortly thereafter to look for extravasation. Because technetium has a short half-life in the intravascular space, detection of abnormality requires the patient to be actively bleeding at the time of the evaluation. Unfortunately, red blood cell scans have a low diagnostic yield but may have a role in localizing an active bleed before more invasive imaging. Mesenteric angiography is useful in patients with continuous active bleeding who have had a normal finding on endoscopic evaluation or a positive nuclear medicine scan or who are too unstable for conventional endoscopic evaluation. Angiography also offers therapeutic interventions for bleeding cessation, including vasopressin infusion and targeted embolization.

Approximately 5% of patients with evidence of overt bleeding will have normal endoscopic evaluation findings and are classified as having overt, obscure GI hemorrhage. Evaluation should then focus on looking for small bowel sources of bleeding through either wireless capsule endoscopy (WCE) or enteroscopy. WCE involves ingestion of a capsule that records images throughout the intestine, which are transmitted to a recorder given to the patient. The images are then reviewed by a gastroenterologist; if small bowel bleeding is seen, further action can be taken with small bowel enteroscopy. Enteroscopy involves the passage of either a colonoscope or special enteroscopes beyond the ligament of Treitz to directly examine the small bowel. Methods of enteroscopy include push, intraoperative, spiral, and balloon enteroscopy, all of which differ in their ability to examine the distal small bowel. Causes of small bowel bleeding that can be detected by enteroscopy or WCE include angioectasias, small bowel tumors, and ulcerations from inflammatory bowel disease or NSAID enteropathy.[3] WCE should be performed first because it has been shown to have a higher diagnostic yield than push enteroscopy, but it does have the disadvantage of not having any therapeutic capabilities. In patients who have clinical evidence of small bowel obstruction, WCE should be used with caution.

Indications for surgical management of LGIB include transfusion of 4 units or more in 24 hours or more than 10 units overall and significant rebleeding that occurs within 1 week of initial cessation and in the presence of comorbid disease.[4] Emergency surgery can be lifesaving but associated with high morbidity and mortality if the location of the lesion is not identified before the surgical procedure. Surgical resection can be associated with rebleeding in up to 30% of cases.[2]

Interdisciplinary Management

Asymptomatic patients in whom GI bleeding is suggested during routine screening or hemodynamically stable patients with minor bleeding may be appropriately evaluated on an outpatient basis with specialty referral for endoscopy or radiologic studies.[21] For cases of chronic GI loss, management should be based on whether the patient has anemia. A patient with a positive FOBT result should undergo colonoscopy to exclude malignancy. If the study findings are negative or there are upper GI symptoms or concomitant anemia, evaluation with upper endoscopy should be considered as well, given that up to 40% of patients with a positive FOBT result can have peptic ulcer disease or esophagitis.[44]

For intermittent scant hematochezia, examination of the full colon versus a focused examination with sigmoidoscopy and anoscopy can be tailored based on the age of the patient. Healthy patients younger than 40 years most likely have a distal lesion such as hemorrhoids and fissures and may not need to undergo full colonoscopic evaluation. Anyone older than age 50 or having worrisome symptoms such as weight loss or change in bowel habits should undergo a full colonoscopic evaluation.[42]

LIFE SPAN CONSIDERATIONS

Mortality associated with GI bleeding is higher in older adults, primarily a result of comorbid disease. Variceal bleeding occurs in more than 40% of patients with chronic liver disease; 30% to 50% of patients die of a variceal bleeding episode. The patient with LGIB tends to be older than the patient with UGIB and hence has more comorbid illness. The incidence of LGIB is unclear. Overall mortality for hospitalization for LGIB has been reported to be approximately 3.5%; positive predictors of mortality include intestinal ischemia, comorbid illness, male gender, and age older than 70 years.[45] This increase in age may be related to the increased incidence of diverticulosis, angiodysplasia, and neoplasms in older adults.[4]

COMPLICATIONS

Many of the complications of GI bleeding are associated with the diagnostic or therapeutic modalities used in its treatment. Serious complications of angiography include bowel ischemia and infarction, dye allergy, and potential renal failure.[9] Complications of upper or lower endoscopy include perforation, bleeding, aspiration, and adverse reactions to conscious sedation.

INDICATIONS FOR REFERRAL OR HOSPITALIZATION

All patients with acute UGIB require urgent consultation with a gastroenterologist.[5,43] Patients with hematochezia or signs of ongoing bleeding should also be immediately referred. A surgical consultation should be obtained for any patient who is hemodynamically unstable, has an abdominal aortic aneurysm or graft, has high risk of rebleeding despite endoscopic therapy, or has a suspected perforation.[5,43]

Admission to the ICU is recommended for all high-risk patients with hemodynamically unstable GI bleeding or rebleeding and for patients who have red hematemesis or grossly bloody gastric aspirate, an abdominal aortic aneurysm or a graft, any bleeding with severe anemia, a large drop in hematocrit, or unstable comorbid disease.[5,43]

Hospitalization is recommended for patients with melena who are hemodynamically unstable or who have had recent bleeding with significant but stable comorbid disease.[5] A select group of patients may be discharged home after urgent endoscopy, provided they are hemodynamically stable, have no comorbid disease, and have no high-risk endoscopic findings.[5]

PATIENT AND FAMILY EDUCATION

Patients should understand that NSAIDs, alcohol, tobacco, and stress can affect peptic ulcer disease. NSAIDs and aspirin products need to be avoided in newly diagnosed ulcer disease to promote healing. If these medications cannot be stopped, concurrent use of a PPI is paramount to prevent recurrence; however, the risk of rebleed can be significant. In addition, older adults may be particularly susceptible to GI bleeding and should understand the risks associated with aspirin and NSAIDs and the importance of taking these medications with food.

Substance abuse should be identified and patients actively encouraged to participate in alcohol or tobacco cessation programs. Stress management classes can be indicated for those patients whose lifestyles indicate that behavioral change in this area could be beneficial. All patients should have thorough education and demonstrate an understanding of all medication use, interactions, and possible side effects.

HEALTH PROMOTION

Screening colonoscopy is recommended for all men and women of average risk to begin at age 50 years. For those with a strong family history of colon cancer in a first-degree relative diagnosed before the age of 60 years, screening should begin at the age of 40 years or 10 years before the age at diagnosis of the youngest affected relative.[46] Esophagogastroduodenoscopy for variceal screening is recommended for all newly diagnosed patients with cirrhosis.[40]

CHAPTER 137

HEPATITIS

Wendy L. Biddle

DEFINITION AND EPIDEMIOLOGY

Hepatitis is a general term meaning inflammation in the liver. Hepatitis has numerous causes, which can include viruses, alcohol, medications, autoimmune disease, and metabolic defects. Inflammation that continues for 6 months is considered chronic liver disease (CLD) and can eventually result in cirrhosis, characterized by scarring and death of hepatocytes or liver cells and hepatocellular carcinoma (HCC). CLDs are major causes of morbidity and mortality. Liver failure and the need for transplantation can occur if the cirrhosis progresses. An evaluation of data from 1988 to 2008 demonstrated that the prevalence rates for most of the major causes of CLD have remained stable except for nonalcoholic fatty liver disease (NAFLD) which has been increasing.[1] From 2005 to 2008 the prevalence of CLD was 14.78%. In 2007 2.6 million people were diagnosed with CLD.[2] In 2013 there were more than 15,000 people older than age 18 on the waiting list for liver transplantation, with the largest group being ages 50 to 64 years. The most common diagnoses for liver transplantation are chronic hepatitis C virus (HCV) infection, followed by NAFLD and alcoholic cirrhosis.[3]

Physician specialist consultation and referral are indicated for patients with newly diagnosed hepatitis.

Viral Hepatitis

Most viral hepatitis is attributed to five main groups of viruses that attack the liver: hepatitis A virus (HAV), hepatitis B virus (HBV), hepatitis C virus (HCV), hepatitis D virus (HDV; also known ~~as hepatitis delta virus~~ and occurring only as a coinfection with HBV), and hepatitis E virus (HEV). The features of the viruses are described in Table 137-1. Other viruses may cause a secondary hepatitis that never becomes chronic and resolves with the viral infection. Acute viral hepatitis can range in severity from a clinically asymptomatic infection to fulminant hepatic failure and death (rare). Chronic viral hepatitis is considered to be the presence of virus at least 6 months after initial exposure and can range in severity from mild disease with minimum inflammation to cirrhosis, liver failure, and need for transplantation.

The prevalences of chronic hepatitis B and C have been stable for the past 20 years.[1] There are many risk factors, including intravenous drug use, high-risk sexual behavior, and tattoos. Viral hepatitis is common among inmates of correctional

TABLE 137-1 Features of Viral Hepatitis

	Hepatitis A	Hepatitis B	Hepatitis C	Hepatitis D	Hepatitis E
Incubation period	2-6 wk	2-6 mo	2-22 wk	4-8 wk	2-9 wk
Onset	Usually acute	Usually insidious	Usually insidious	Usually acute	Usually acute
Symptoms					
Nausea and vomiting	Common	Common	Common	Common	Common
Fever	Common	Uncommon	Uncommon	Uncommon	Uncommon
Jaundice	50%	33%	25%	?	10%-20%
Arthralgias	Rare	Common	Rare	Rare	Rare
Diagnosis	IgM anti-HAV	HBsAg	Anti-HCV	IgM anti-HDV	Anti-HEV
Transmission					
Fecal-oral	Usual	Rare	No	?	Usual
Parenteral	Rare	Usual	Usual	Usual	No
Sexual	Yes	Yes	Yes	?	?
Perinatal	No	Yes	Yes	?	No
Sequelae					
Chronic carrier	No	5%-10%	Up to 75%	? Most	No
Chronic active hepatitis	No	Approximately 5%	75%	Up to 70%	No
Fulminant hepatitis	Approximately 0.1%	0.2%-1.0%	No	Up to 17%	2%-10%*
Recovery	99%	85%-90%	—	?	90%-98%*
Epidemiology					
Epidemics	Food-borne or water-borne	Contaminated blood products	Injection drug abuse and contaminated blood products	Contaminated blood products	Food-borne or water-borne
Post-transfusion	Extremely rare	<5% of cases	85%-95% of cases	Possible	No
Prevention	ISG	HBIG vaccine	? ISG	Hepatitis B vaccine	? ISG from endemic areas

*15% to 20% fatalities in pregnant women.
HBIG, hepatitis B immune globulin; HBsAg, hepatitis B surface antigen; ISG, immune serum globulin (human immune globulin).
Modified from Stein JH, Klippel JH, Reynolds HW: *Internal medicine*, ed 5, St Louis, 1998, Elsevier.

facilities. There are multiple prison-based programs in place that include HAV and HBV vaccinations, needle exchanges, risk reduction, and management strategies aimed at decreasing transmission among inmates. The Centers for Disease Control and Prevention (CDC) has published recommendations for prevention and control of viral hepatitis in incarcerated people in the United States.[4]

HAV, HBV, and HCV all cause inflammation by affecting the hepatocytes, which causes acute disease with similar symptoms but differing levels of pathogenicity.[5] HAV, an RNA virus identified over 20 years ago, is a common cause of acute viral hepatitis in the United States. In 2010, there were 1670 new cases in the United States, and worldwide it is responsible for approximately 1.5 million cases each year.[6] The highest incidence occurs in areas of low socioeconomic status, poor sanitation, and poor access to clean drinking water, including Africa, Asia, and Central America. In developing countries, HAV accounts for up to one third of all cases of viral hepatitis. There have been intermittent outbreaks in the United States, most recently in 2014. HAV is transmitted by the fecal-oral route, through person-to-person contact, through the ingestion of contaminated food or water, and through blood. The virus can survive for months in fresh and salt water. Ingestion of shellfish from polluted water is another means of transmission. HAV can be found in liver cells, bile, stool, and blood and has an incubation period of 2 to 6 weeks. The incidence of hepatitis A has decreased in the United States because of vaccination recommendation and use.[7,8] All strains of this virus belong to the same serotype; as a result, HAV immune globulin provides worldwide protection. The vaccination involves an injection followed by a booster, which can provide immunity for 20 years. The virus can be inactivated by boiling for 1 minute or by exposure to formaldehyde, chlorine, or ultraviolet radiation.

Patients are most infectious in the late incubation period because the virus excretes a large amount of virus 11 days before the antibodies appear in the blood. Clinical symptoms appear approximately 4 weeks after exposure, but more than 75% of adults and 70% of children younger than 6 years are asymptomatic when they are infected. This contributes to the easy spread of the virus.[8] The virus can be found in the stool 2 to 3 weeks before and up to 1 week after the development of clinical jaundice. Despite the presence of HAV in the liver, viral shedding in feces, viremia, and infectivity rapidly decrease once jaundice appears. Therefore, most patients are contagious when they are asymptomatic and are no longer contagious by the time they become diagnosed with jaundice. An important exception involves neonates, who can be infectious for up to 6 months after clinical jaundice develops. It is an acute disease, and, rarely, relapses can occur 30 to 90 days after the primary illness. There are rare cases when extrahepatic manifestations, including vasculitis, nephritis, myocarditis, encephalitis, and others, occur. HAV infection never progresses to chronic hepatitis.[8]

Hepatitis B is endemic worldwide, especially in Asia, where the carrier rate is estimated to be 1 in 4. In the United States, 1 in 10 Asian Americans have chronic hepatitis B, and of those, 1 in 4 will die of liver failure or liver cancer. Worldwide it is estimated that 400 million people have chronic HBV, with the highest rate in China.[9] It is less prevalent in the United States, and new infections are decreasing, but it was estimated that there were between 700,000 and 1.4 million people infected with chronic HBV in 2014.[10] Five percent to 10% of those infected are expected to develop chronic HBV.[5] The migration of Asians to the United States is contributing to the public health burden because it is estimated that up to 14% are carriers of chronic HBV.[9] There were 3050 reported new cases of HBV in the United States in 2010 for an incidence of reported acute HBV of 0.9 per 100,000.[6] However, because HBV can be asymptomatic, the estimated rate of new cases is 10 times higher, or 19,764 newly infected persons in 2013.[10]

BOX 137-1

High-Risk Groups for Hepatitis Screening

Born in areas of high-prevalence HBV
- Asia and Pacific Islands
- Middle East
- Mediterranean: Italy, Greece, Malta, Portugal, Spain
- Indigenous to the Arctic region
- South America
- Eastern Europe
- Caribbean

Other risk factors
- Household or sexual contact
- Injection drug use
- Multiple sexual partners, male same-sex partners
- Inmates of correctional facilities
- Chronically elevated alanine aminotransferase (ALT) or aspartate aminotransferase (AST)
- Human immunodeficiency virus (HIV) or HCV infection
- Hemodialysis
- Pregnancy

Modified from Keefe EB, Dieterich DT, Han SH, et al: A treatment algorithm for the management of chronic hepatitis B virus infection in the United States: 2008 update, *Clin Gastroenterol Hepatol* 6:1314-1340, 2008.

In Asia and Africa, HBV infection is seen mostly among newborns and young children and is spread by vertical transmission from mother to child. People with chronic HBV have an increased lifetime risk of cirrhosis and HCC.[11] It is recommended that individuals in high-risk groups (Box 137-1), including all who were born in Asia or have direct family members born in Asia, be screened for hepatitis B surface antigen (HBsAg) for HBV. In North America and Europe, hepatitis B is more common among adolescents and young adults and is spread by sexual contact and percutaneous exposure. Other risk factors are listed in Box 137-1. It is estimated that up to 40% of those infected with HBV will develop significant complications including cirrhosis, liver failure, and liver cancer. Almost 5000 people die of HBV-related cirrhosis or HCC annually. The number of new cases of hepatitis B reported has declined each year since 1985. A safe and effective vaccine against HBV was introduced in 1982.[12]

Recommendations to prevent transmission of HBV include universal vaccination of infants beginning at birth, screening of all pregnant women to prevent perinatal infection, and immunoprophylaxis of infants born to HBsAg-positive women, which indicates infection. All children and adolescents not vaccinated need to be immunized, as do unvaccinated adults at risk of infection.[11]

Hepatitis B can present a clinical picture similar to that of the other subtypes, with a severity that can range from asymptomatic to fulminant and fatal liver failure; it can progress to CLD and possibly cirrhosis and HCC. HBV can be found in blood, tears, cerebrospinal fluid, breast milk, saliva, vaginal secretions, and seminal fluid. HBV is transmitted parenterally, by sexual contact, and perinatally. Heterosexual contact with a person infected with HBV is the most common mode of transmission, followed by injection drug use, homosexual activity, and vertical transmission from mother to child at the time of birth. Transmission from blood transfusions is rare in the United States because of extensive blood transfusion screening processes. HBV is not transmitted through the fecal-oral route or by arthropod vectors. Compared with the general population, health care workers, especially surgeons, phlebotomists, and dialysis nurses, and the spouses of infected persons are at an increased risk for contracting hepatitis B.[13]

Hepatitis C, the number one cause of cirrhosis, HCC, and liver transplantation, has reached epidemic proportions in the United States; an estimated 4 million people are infected and anti-HCV seropositive (prevalence of 1.68%), and 2.7 to 3.9 million are chronically infected.[1] These estimates are likely to be low because the homeless, incarcerated, and hospitalized are not taken into account. Chronic HCV affects 12% to 31% of incarcerated persons, which results in substantial morbidity and risk of premature death. Worldwide, this disorder has also reached epidemic proportions, with an estimate of 200 million people infected.[14] Of those in the United States with chronic HCV, over 130,000 are children under the age of 19 years.[15] Approximately 75% of people with HCV are "baby boomers," born between 1945 and 1965. They are five times more likely to be infected with HCV than the rest of the population. Fortunately, new infections with HCV in the United States are uncommon; the primary cause of the approximately 850 new acute clinical cases that occurred in 2010 was likely injection drug use.[6] Estimates predict that 25% of people with chronic HCV will develop cirrhosis approximately 30 years after initial infection. Hispanics and African Americans have higher rates of HCV infection than whites. There appears to be greater disease and fibrosis progression, and the mortality rate is almost doubled.[16]

HCV, first identified in 1989, is a single-stranded RNA genome with a high rate of replication (10^{12} virions/day) and mutation. These characteristics lead to chronic infection, making it difficult to treat. At least six strains and multiple subtypes of the virus have been identified. Genotypes 2 and 3 respond better to treatment than does genotype 1, but 70% of people in the United States have genotype 1.[17]

Once a person is infected with HCV, the body initiates humoral and cellular mechanisms. The Third National Health and Nutrition Examination Survey found that approximately 75% of patients with HCV develop chronic infection. It is rare to see fulminant hepatic failure with acute HCV. The 25% who cleared the virus may have had a strong cellular immune response to HCV. Ineffective cellular immune responses lead to inflammation and damage in the liver. Extrahepatic manifestations of chronic HCV occur when humoral immune responses are continually stimulated. These can involve the skin, kidney, and nerves. Factors associated with rapid disease progression and cirrhosis include older age at time of infection, alcohol abuse, male gender, and coinfection with human immunodeficiency virus (HIV).[18]

HCV has been transmitted through blood transfusions given before July 1992, receipt of clotting factor concentrates produced before 1987, chronic hemodialysis, any injection of illegal drugs, and intranasal drug use (sharing needles or straws). There is no evidence that arthropod vectors transmit HCV. Other possible risk factors include tattoos, manicures or pedicures, and body piercings. These practices are not regulated and should be considered possible risk factors, especially if there have been multiple exposures or the work is done in questionable environments. Data from other countries have shown an association with some of these factors and HCV infection, but studies in the United States have not shown an association. Health care workers and emergency medical personnel are at risk from needle sticks, sharps, or mucosal exposure to HCV-positive blood, although the rate of transmission is low. Sexual transmission may be responsible for up to 20% of new cases, but the overall rate is believed to be less than 5%. Those with multiple partners have a two- to five-times higher risk of acquiring HCV through sexual contact. Long-term partners of a person with chronic HCV should be tested every 5 years. The rate of vertical transmission from mother to child during delivery is approximately 5%. Certain subgroups are believed to have an especially high rate—for instance, 20% of those on hemodialysis, and even higher rates in prisoners. Coinfection of HCV and HIV is becoming more prevalent, creating unique challenges in management. The prevalence of hepatitis C among HIV-infected people is estimated at 15% to 30%.[18]

HDV is a defective RNA virus that requires coinfection with HBV for replication and is considered to be the most severe form of viral hepatitis. Of the 350 million people worldwide with chronic HBV, 5 % are coinfected with HDV.[19] Several genotypes are known. It can be transmitted with HBV or may superinfect an individual who is already infected with HBV. It is transmitted parenterally through injection drug use and, rarely, through sexual contact. Perinatal transmission is rare and can be prevented through HBV prophylaxis. When it is seen in the Mediterranean region, HDV is endemic with HBV. In nonendemic areas such as the United States, HDV is associated with percutaneous exposure and blood transfusions. HDV is not transmitted through the fecal-oral route or by casual contact. During the past two decades, HDV circulation has decreased because of the use of HBV vaccine; however, the challenge of migration of infected persons from endemic areas continues to be a major problem.[19,20]

HEV is another RNA virus with four known human genotypes that has been responsible for large outbreaks in developing countries. It is often considered an important cause of acute hepatitis in Africa and Asia. This virus has a short incubation period of 15 to 60 days and usually results in a self-limited disease in an immune-competent host. There are groups that are at risk for severe disease and possible chronicity. Similar to HAV, HEV is enterically spread, most commonly by the ingestion of contaminated water. Areas endemic for HEV infection are Asia, northeast Africa, the Middle East, and Mexico, with up to 70% prevalence. In the United States, up to 20% of blood donors are seropositive for HEV. Prevalence is highest in states that have large producers of swine. Infection during pregnancy can lead to liver failure and death, especially during the third trimester, with mortality rates as high as 15% to 20%.[21]

Alcoholic Hepatitis

Alcoholic hepatitis is a common and life-threatening cause of liver failure. This is a type of toxic liver injury associated with excessive alcoholic consumption on a chronic basis, usually 10 years or longer. In the United States, alcoholism is the one of the most common cause of cirrhosis. It is estimated that 10%

to 35% of heavy drinkers develop alcoholic hepatitis. Studies suggest that an increased risk of cirrhosis occurs with ingestion of 10 to 20 g of alcohol a day in women and 20 to 40 g a day in men. Additional factors that increase the risk of alcoholic hepatitis include a genetic predisposition, environment, age when person started consuming alcohol, and body mass index higher than 25 in women and 27 in men. One drink of 10 g of alcohol is equal to 10 ounces of beer (5% ethanol), 3 to 4 ounces of wine (12% ethanol), or 1 ounce of hard liquor (40% ethanol, 80 proof).[22] Recent evidence suggests that the drinking pattern may play a role and that daily drinking increases the risk compared with drinking less frequently. It was suggested that recent alcohol intake and not lifetime consumption could be a strong predictor of alcoholic cirrhosis.[23] The excessive alcohol might lead to fat and inflammation of the liver, which can lead to cirrhosis.

Nonalcoholic Fatty Liver Disease

NAFLD and nonalcoholic steatohepatitis (NASH), a spectrum of chronic disorders associated with the metabolic syndrome, is the most common CLD in the United States. The prevalence of NAFLD steadily increased from 5% in 1988 to 11% in 2008. It now accounts for 75% of CLDs in the United States. These increases correspond with increases in obesity (33%), visceral obesity (51%), type 2 diabetes (9%), insulin resistance (35%), and hypertension (34%). In addition, obesity is an independent predictor of NAFLD.[1] There is a 10% to 20% incidence of NASH in those who have NAFLD. NASH is more serious because it is characterized by the development of inflammation (steatohepatitis) and scarring of the liver that can progress to cirrhosis, end-stage liver disease, and failure. NASH is now the third most common cause of cirrhosis and is expected to be the most common reason for liver transplantation by 2020.[24]

NASH may be a part of the metabolic syndrome. Abdominal obesity, hyperlipidemia, and diabetes are associated with increased liver fat content, and insulin resistance is proposed to be the cause of the liver's storing too much fat.[25] A strong predictor of fatty liver and progression to NASH is obesity, especially central obesity. In addition, certain races have a higher risk of NAFLD; these include, in decreasing order of risk, East Asian Indians, Hispanics, and Asians. Caucasians and African Americans have less of a risk.[24]

Drug-Induced Liver Injury

Drug-induced liver injury (DILI) is a rare reaction associated with common medications, including nonsteroidal anti-inflammatory drugs (NSAIDs) and antimicrobial agents. Half of all cases of acute liver failure are caused by drug hepatotoxicity, and it is thought that there is a genetic predisposition to DILI. Some drugs produce a predictable, dose-related injury, such as with acetaminophen, but most reactions are unpredictable. These reactions usually occur in one of two patterns: (1) an allergic reaction that occurs within 6 weeks of initiation of the drug, such as with phenytoin (Dilantin); or (2) a metabolic reaction that occurs with up to 1 year of continuous use, such as with isoniazid.[26] More than 800 therapeutic agents, including prescription drugs, over-the-counter medications, nutritional supplements, and herbal remedies, have been implicated in DILI. The National Institute of Diabetes and Digestive and Kidney Diseases has created the Drug-Induced Liver Injury Network. Since its inception in May 2004, more than 889 cases have been documented. The top offending drugs were amoxicillin–clavulanic acid, isoniazid, nitrofurantoin, sulfamethoxazole-trimethoprim, and minocycline.[27] A thorough drug history should include information about recent and past exposure to therapeutic agents, supplements, and herbal products. Details about the patient's occupation and work environment as well as the use of herbal preparations and "traditional" medications should be obtained.[26]

Autoimmune Hepatitis

Autoimmune hepatitis is a rare condition that can occur in anyone and is seen throughout the world. The peak age at onset is 50 to 60 years, but it has been documented in individuals aged 10 to 80 years and occurs in women three times as often as in men. There are no clear racial differences. The incidence is estimated at 1.9 in 100,000. Autoimmune hepatitis is associated with other autoimmune diseases in the patient or the family. The clinical spectrum varies from asymptomatic or mild symptoms to severe symptoms with acute or fulminant liver failure; the course can fluctuate. One third of newly diagnosed patients have already developed cirrhosis. Treatment is with corticosteroids; fulminant disease may require liver transplantation.[28]

PATHOPHYSIOLOGY

Process of Inflammation and Development of Cirrhosis

The process of inflammation and development of scarring and cirrhosis is similar for all causes of hepatitis. The pathologic process of hepatitis involves inflammation and damage to the hepatocytes. Fibrosis and scarring with isolated hepatocyte injury and focal necrosis can develop. Mononuclear infiltration, which consists mostly of lymphocytes, invades the tissue, particularly around the portal triads. Cellular edema and death can occur. There may be a minor degree of periportal necrosis of hepatocytes around these triads, which gives the liver an appearance of piecemeal necrosis on microscopic examination. After the hepatocyte degenerates, its cytoplasm shrinks and condenses to form an acidophil body. The available space is then temporarily filled by monocytes. Although characteristic of acute viral hepatitis, these cytologic changes are not specific to this disease and can also be found with drug-induced injuries and other disease processes.[29]

The inflammatory and scarring processes can lead to "bridging" fibrosis between portal triads. This level of fibrosis and moderate inflammation is a sign that cirrhosis will develop if the damage continues. Increased numbers of liver cells begin to die, which may lead to more collapse and condensation of the liver stroma. This may occur during months in a severe acute injury but is more commonly seen in chronic infection, taking 10 years or more to develop.[29] Bridging necrosis and confluent necrosis can resolve, enabling complete regeneration and histologic recovery in acute hepatitis. Chronic hepatitis, however, can remain mild, with little or no scarring ever developing. If scarring does develop, it is unlikely to improve without treatment. Over time, cirrhosis can lead to liver failure or HCC and death. Approximately 20% of people with cirrhosis from chronic hepatitis will develop a carcinoma.

Pathogenesis of Hepatitis

HAV is in the family of viruses that includes polio, which causes a self-limiting acute disease. The replication cycle is slow and has not been shown to cause chronic infection. The virus is thought to be transported across the intestinal epithelium after oral inoculation and is taken up by hepatocytes. It is shed in the feces, which continues the fecal-oral transmission.[8] Viral loads peak at 2 weeks postexposure and are undetectable by 6 to 8 weeks. It is suggested that CD4 T cells may play a role in immune clearance of HAV. Symptoms usually develop at week 4 at the same time as the beginning of the humoral response to the viral proteins.[5] HEV is also transmitted by the fecal-oral route. It does not cause CLD, but it is associated with mortality in pregnancy (15% to 20%) and in patients with cirrhosis. After oral ingestion, it is taken up in the portal circulation and produces viremia. It is excreted in the feces, and it is not known if it replicates in the small bowel.[21]

HBV is a DNA virus in the Hepadnaviridae family. The virus enters the hepatocyte nucleus and begins replication. The viral load peaks at 7 to 8 weeks after exposure. HBV initiates a type I interferon (IFN) response, and it is thought that viral clearance occurs in part with CD4 and CD8 T cells.[5] The infection has separate phases: immune tolerance (minimal activity in the liver), immune clearance (active with chronic inflammation in the liver), inactive carrier of HBsAg (minimal fibrosis), resolution (scant fibrosis), and reactivation (active, moderate fibrosis). Progressive fibrosis leads to cirrhosis. Each phase has serologic markers that help determine the phase. Ongoing viral replication leads to cirrhosis, hepatocellular cancer, or both.[13]

HDV is spread through parenteral exposure. It occurs only when a person is infected with HBV and HBsAg positive; this is required for transmission. It is associated with a severe course of hepatitis, fibrosis, decompensation, and cancer. It is an immune-mediated disease process, but the level of viremia is not directly associated with the stage of liver disease. The degree of control of infection may be associated with cellular immune responses.[20]

HCV is an RNA virus from the Flaviviridae family and has a remarkable ability to persist within a host by evading the adaptive and innate components of the immune system. More than 60% of people infected will develop chronic HCV. The life cycle and survival mechanisms of HCV are increasing. HCV enters the host cell, uncoats the viral genome, translates viral proteins, replicates the genome, and assembles and releases virions. The HCV infection impairs all parts of the adaptive immune system with multiple viral factors that allow it to evade detection and elimination.[30]

HCV is unique compared with HAV and HBV. The virus cycle has rapid turnover and elicits a strong type I IFN response. Multiple factors affect the course of the infection, including age, sex, presence of symptoms, antiviral T-cell response, and immunogenetic polymorphisms.[31]

Although the exact mechanism of alcohol damage to the liver is not known, there are several hypotheses. Ethanol is oxidized in the mitochondria, producing toxins that have harmful effects on lipid and carbohydrate metabolism. Acetaldehyde is increased, causing hypoxia at the terminal veins in the liver, and oxygen-derived free radicals may cause damage of the liver cells. Proinflammatory cytokines are expressed, stimulating cells to produce collagen, which leads to fibrosis.[22]

Liver damage from hepatotoxins, such as chlorpromazine, rifampin, and estrogens, is variable, depending on the drug, dose, and individual hypersensitivity. Damage can appear quickly or may take weeks to months after the medication is begun. Proposed mechanisms include alteration of the membranes, interference with the hepatic uptake process, and free radicals causing lipid peroxidation.[26]

CLINICAL PRESENTATION

Most people are not aware when they develop acute hepatitis because the symptoms are similar to those of any other mild viral illness. Symptoms can include anorexia, fatigue, myalgias, nausea, fever, headaches, arthralgias, vomiting, and abdominal pain. Jaundice can occur, especially with HBV, but it is rare in other viral hepatitis illnesses. Acute viral hepatitis occurs after an incubation period of varying lengths based on the specific virus. HBV and HDV are clinically indistinguishable from one another. Suspicion of HEV should be increased in patients with clinical symptoms of hepatitis and a recent travel history to an underdeveloped country.[21] The signs and symptoms of hepatitis are presented in Box 137-2.

People with alcoholic hepatitis can have a widely variable presentation and can be asymptomatic. Severe cases can give the appearance of sepsis or biliary obstruction. It is important to obtain a thorough alcohol intake history. Patients can have nonspecific symptoms, such as nausea, vomiting, abdominal discomfort, or diarrhea. Those with advanced liver disease appear ill and malnourished and can be feverish. There may be signs of cirrhosis such as jaundice, ascites, encephalopathy, and upper gastrointestinal bleeding.[22]

BOX 137-2

Signs and Symptoms of Hepatitis

HEPATITIS A

- May be asymptomatic
- Fever, jaundice, anorexia, nausea, malaise, myalgia
- Infectious 2 weeks before symptoms and 1 week after
- No carrier state or chronic illness
- Multiple extrahepatic manifestations can occur in rare cases

HEPATITIS B

- May be asymptomatic
- Anorexia, nausea, myalgia, malaise, jaundice to fatal hepatitis
- Infectious 4 to 6 weeks before symptoms and for unpredictable time after symptoms
- Carrier state and chronic illness

HEPATITIS C

- Patients may be asymptomatic
- Anorexia, nausea, malaise, rarely jaundice, myalgia
- Infectious 4 to 6 weeks before symptoms and unpredictable after symptoms
- 75% progress to chronic hepatitis

HEPATITIS D

- May be asymptomatic
- Anorexia, nausea, malaise, jaundice, myalgia
- Infectious 4 to 6 weeks before symptoms and unpredictable after symptoms
- Occurs only with HBV as coinfection or as superinfection in chronic HBV infection

HEPATITIS E

- May be asymptomatic
- Fever, jaundice, anorexia, nausea, malaise, myalgia
- Infectious 2 weeks before symptoms and 1 week after symptoms
- No carrier or chronic state

The presentation of drug-induced liver disease can be a nonspecific febrile or viral-like illness. The diagnosis of chronic hepatitis can be challenging because patients often are not symptomatic until liver damage has progressed. Risk factors for the development of chronic hepatitis include a young age and immunosuppression. Autoimmune hepatitis may manifest with fatigue, pain in the right upper quadrant of the abdomen, polymyalgia, and arthralgia of small joints. NAFLD usually has no symptoms. People can have right upper quadrant pain, especially if there is a large amount of fat in the liver and the liver is slightly enlarged.

PHYSICAL EXAMINATION

A low-grade fever with acute hepatitis is far more common with HAV and HEV, although patients with HBV can develop a serum sickness–like syndrome that can include fever, arthralgias, and rash. Dark-colored urine and clay-colored stools may precede the onset of clinical jaundice by 1 to 5 days. With the onset of jaundice, these constitutional symptoms usually diminish.

On examination, patients with jaundice often have both hepatomegaly and splenomegaly. The onset of jaundice or the icteric phase can be observed when the serum bilirubin concentration is higher than 4 mg/dL and is most easily observed in the sclera or under the tongue. Symptomatic hepatitis is difficult to miss, but half the patients with acute hepatitis do not develop jaundice. In alcoholic hepatitis, the physical findings may be consistent with cholestasis. Fever, jaundice, and leukocytosis may be present. Rashes are common, and patients can have tender hepatomegaly, ascites, or encephalopathy (ranging from asterixis to coma), but splenomegaly is uncommon. There may be findings of malnutrition, and there may be a hepatic bruit. Physical signs of alcoholic and nonalcoholic cirrhosis are similar, but spider telangiectasia (especially on the trunk and upper extremities), parotid enlargement, gynecomastia, palmar erythema, and hepatomegaly may be more common with alcoholic cirrhosis.[22]

The presence of extrahepatic manifestations can suggest drug-induced hepatitis. Fever, rash, and eosinophilia suggest drug hypersensitivity but are relatively nonspecific findings. Presenting signs may include pseudomononucleosis syndrome (phenytoin), systemic vasculitis (allopurinol and sulfonamides), and bone marrow suppression (NSAIDs).

DIAGNOSTICS

Initial testing should include a complete blood count (CBC) and liver function tests (LFTs). The first sign of hepatitis may be the elevation of the serum aminotransferases aspartate aminotransferase (AST) and alanine transaminase (ALT). These enzymes increase proportionately during the prodromal phase of hepatitis and can reach 20 times normal (in acute hepatitis). The levels in chronic hepatitis can be normal but may be mildly elevated or two or three times normal.

The total bilirubin level can be elevated with acute hepatitis, and it can continue to increase as the aminotransferases decline and may reach 20 mg/dL. There are equal proportions of direct and indirect bilirubin in patients with hepatitis, and bilirubin will also be present in urine. The prothrombin time (PT) is usually normal in patients with acute hepatitis but may become prolonged in patients with severe hepatitis; thus PT can be used as a marker of prognosis. If the PT is more than three times normal (international normalized ratio [INR], 1.5), the patient should be evaluated for fulminant hepatic failure. The white blood cell count and hemoglobin level and hematocrit are usually within normal limits. The platelet count may be normal or may be decreased in fulminant hepatic failure.

Other laboratory tests that may indicate advancing liver damage are platelet and albumin levels, which will be lower than normal with the progression to cirrhosis. Anemia may be present. Alkaline phosphatase levels are usually normal or mildly elevated. Alkaline phosphatase is not specific to the liver. An elevated alkaline phosphatase level can indicate a fatty liver or obstruction or disease in the bile ducts. If an elevated alkaline phosphatase level is documented, it is useful to determine how much of it is from the liver. Fractionation will show the percentages from the liver, bone, and intestines.

The elevation of aminotransferase levels does not seem to correlate with the histologic severity of the disease. HAV should be suspected if hepatitis infection occurs after the ingestion of contaminated food or shellfish, after natural disasters, in institutionalized adults or children, in patients returning from travel to an endemic area, or in children or families of children in day care facilities. Diagnosis can be confirmed by the presence of immunoglobulin M (IgM) anti-HAV during the acute illness. Eventually, the IgM anti-HAV decreases during several months, and IgG anti-HAV rises and persists indefinitely.

Initial testing for hepatitis B and C can be done with a hepatitis panel, which usually includes HBsAg, hepatitis B surface antibody (HBsAb), hepatitis B core antibody (HBcAb IgM and IgG), and HCV antibody. Patients positive for HBsAg and HBcAb should be referred for more detailed testing because interpretation can be difficult. Positive HBsAb indicates immunity from vaccination or resolved infection. There are several published tables that explain the various combinations of results for HBV. If HCV antibody is present, the viral load should be tested by polymerase chain reaction (HCV RNA). The level of virus load detected ranges from a few to more than several million international units per milliliter. If the viral load is detectable, the patient is considered to have chronic HCV. The testing of the genotype for HCV can help with decisions about treatment.

HDV infection should be considered in patients with acute HBV infection who develop fulminant hepatic failure or in patients with chronic HBV infection who show evidence of deterioration. Anti-HDV can be detected to confirm the diagnosis of HDV infection. HEV infection should be considered in patients returning from travel to endemic areas. Diagnosis can be made by testing IgM antibody to HEV, but the results can be variable. Viral load testing is not available in the United States, but testing can be done by contacting the CDC.[21]

Alcoholic hepatitis typically manifests as a cholestasis type of liver disease, with abnormalities seen as elevations in bilirubin and alkaline phosphatase levels. The ratio of AST to ALT is often greater than 2.0, which is considered diagnostic of this disease. Anemia is present in more than 90% of patients with alcoholic hepatitis, and leukocytosis is seen in 41% of patients. In more severe disease, PT may be prolonged, and the albumin concentration is often low. These two tests are measures of the capacity of the liver to synthesize proteins.

Laboratory testing in the diagnosis of suspected drug-induced liver disease is helpful in excluding other causes of liver disease. Liver biopsy is indicated when the diagnosis remains unclear. Diagnosis depends on the history of exposure; consistent clinical, laboratory, and liver biopsy findings in select cases; and the resolution of liver injury after the presumed toxin has been removed.

The most accurate test that can determine the amount of inflammation and scarring in the liver is a biopsy. Liver biopsy is also done when diagnosis is uncertain or certain conditions, such as autoimmune hepatitis, are suspected. Scoring mechanisms can be used to provide a fairly standardized measure of the severity of liver disease. Ultrasonography and computed tomography (CT) scan are equally useful in documenting tumors, fatty tissue, and size of the liver. The ultrasound examination is more cost-effective, providing screening information. There are noninvasive liver fibrosis tests, a reasonable alternative to liver biopsy, that are currently implemented. The tests can provide an estimate of the severity of steatosis, fibrosis, and inflammation. The tests are specific for NASH and hepatitis C. The tests are improving and can be used as an adjunct to the management of these conditions.[32]

DIAGNOSTICS

Hepatitis

LABORATORY

ALT, AST, alkaline phosphatase, bilirubin total and direct, protein, globulins, albumin

CBC and differential, platelets

PT/INR, partial thromboplastin time

Hepatitis serologic tests (HAV antibodies, HBsAg, HBsAb, HBcAb, HCV antibodies; if hepatitis B is positive, hepatitis B e antibody [HBeAb], hepatitis B e antigen [HBeAg])

Antimitochondrial antibodies, antinuclear antibodies, smooth muscle antibodies

Lipid panel

Thyroid-stimulating hormone

FibroSpect testing for fibrosis and inflammation

OTHER DIAGNOSTICS

Abdominal ultrasound or CT scan

Liver biopsy (ultrasound or CT guided)*

*If Indicated.

DIFFERENTIAL DIAGNOSIS

It is always important that patients be evaluated for other causes of liver disease. For instance, chronically elevated results of liver function tests (LFTs) may be caused by alcoholic liver disease, drug- or toxin-induced hepatitis, hepatic steatosis, cholestatic conditions, metabolic diseases, granulomatous hepatitis, pericholangitis associated with inflammatory bowel disease, celiac sprue, or biliary or pancreatic disease. The most common cause of chronically elevated results of LFTs is NAFLD, affecting up to 20% of the general population.

The most common drugs known to cause hepatitis are acetaminophen (especially with concomitant alcohol), isoniazid, methotrexate, amoxicillin–clavulanic acid, minocycline, methyldopa, nitrofurantoin, rifampin, and the cholesterol-lowering statins. Regular monitoring of LFTs is necessary because elevations can indicate the presence of liver inflammation. A secondary hepatitis can be caused by other viruses, such as Epstein-Barr virus, cytomegalovirus, HIV, herpes simplex virus, varicella-zoster virus, adenovirus, and coxsackievirus. Secondary hepatitis resolves along with the viral illness, in general.

Hemochromatosis, iron overload, is the most common inherited disorder in the United States. Testing of iron saturation and ferritin is used for screening. If elevated levels of iron are found, a genetic test for hemochromatosis is available. Autoimmune hepatitis, seen primarily in young women, can be screened for with antinuclear and smooth muscle antibody. Wilson disease, an autosomal recessive condition that results in toxic copper accumulation in the liver and other organs, must also be considered. Low levels of serum ceruloplasmin, elevated levels of urinary copper, and Kayser-Fleischer rings in the eyes can establish a diagnosis of Wilson disease. Sarcoidosis can affect the liver and is seen primarily in African Americans. Obtaining an angiotensin-converting enzyme level may be used to screen for sarcoid.

Celiac sprue has been known to elevate LFTs, which may be the only clinical sign of the disease. A celiac antibody panel and, if positive, a small bowel (duodenal) biopsy by endoscopy can confirm the diagnosis.

DIFFERENTIAL DIAGNOSIS

Hepatitis

- Alcoholic liver disease
- α_1-Antitrypsin deficiency
- Autoimmune hepatitis
- Celiac sprue (gluten intolerance)
- Cholestatic conditions (primary sclerosing cholangitis, primary biliary cirrhosis)
- Granulomatous hepatitis (sarcoidosis)
- Hemochromatosis
- Medication- or toxin-induced hepatitis
- Metabolic diseases
- NAFLD, NASH
- Wilson disease

MANAGEMENT

The management of acute HAV and HBV consists primarily of treating the acute symptoms and providing supportive care. Most patients do well and experience no chronic sequelae. More than 99% of patients with HAV and up to 90% of patients with HBV recover without incident. HAV infection does not develop chronicity, whereas 6% to 10% of patients infected with HBV in the United States develop chronic HBV. In the acute, uncomplicated course, the majority of patients do not require hospitalization, and only symptomatic care is needed. LFTs should be monitored every 2 weeks until normalization.

Pegylated IFN, entecavir, lamivudine, and tenofovir are some of the approved treatments for chronic HBV. With the onset of the antiviral age associated with the new anti-HIV drugs, many new chronic hepatitis drugs are currently under investigation.

Treatment of chronic hepatitis B is recommended when the person is hepatitis B e antigen (HBeAg) positive and has an HBV DNA viral level of at least 20,000 IU/mL. For levels below 20,000 IU/mL, only monitoring every 6 to 12 months is recommended unless there is evidence of histologic disease by biopsy. Entecavir or tenofovir (both preferred for high levels of DNA) are considered safe and effective treatment and are recommended. Treatment should be continued for 12 months after HBsAg seroconversion to negative and HBV DNA is undetectable. Long-term treatment may be needed if there is not seroconversion. Resistance can be an issue, and medications can be added or changed as needed.[13]

Treatment for chronic HCV has greatly improved. Pegylated IFN is improved with pegylation, which decreases clearance and breakdown of the drug, allowing the IFN to stay in the system longer. Treatment is usually 6 to 12 months, depending on early response (by 12 weeks of treatment), genotype, and other factors. Increased efficacy of treatment is seen with extension of treatment to 72 weeks if there is a late response that occurs between 13 and 24 weeks. A sustained virologic response is the goal of treatment, meaning an undetectable viral load that continues for 6 months after treatment is complete. Currently, the overall response is up to 88% with genotypes 2 and 3 but only 39% to 46% for genotype 1. Some patients relapse after an initial response; others do not respond at all. There are multiple factors that affect the response rate, and those with cirrhosis do not respond as well.[16]

Factors that predict a response in patients with cirrhosis (similar factors for those without cirrhosis) include non–genotype 1, overall dose and treatment adherence of 80% or greater, serum γ-glutamyl transferase below 76 IU/mL, baseline viral load below 6×10^{12}, and absence of ultrasound evidence of portal hypertension. After 4 weeks of treatment, a drop in the viral load of at least 1×10^{10} predicts a sustained viral response. The association between HCV and primary liver cancer is strong, and prevention of cirrhosis with eradication of the virus supports early antiviral treatment.[33] Protease inhibitors (telaprevir, boceprevir), when used in combination with IFN and ribavirin, have increased response rates in nonresponders.[14,34]

The most recent treatments includes imeprevir with pegylated IFN and ribavirin; sofosbuvir with ribavirin for HCV genotypes 2 and 3; and ledipasvir-sofosbuvir for genotype 1. Response rates are 95% or better with some treatments, and these therapies are also effective in patients with and without cirrhosis.

Side effects are more intense with pegylated IFN than with regular IFN. Many of the side effects, which include anemia, neutropenia, thrombocytopenia, depression, and fatigue, can be adequately managed, although some patients cannot tolerate them enough to complete treatment.[17] Adherence to therapy is very important, and research shows that missing doses, decreasing doses, and poor compliance affect treatment response. Improved response rates are associated with at least 80% compliance, taking at least 80% of the IFN and 80% of ribavirin at least 80% of the time.[35]

The mainstay of therapy for alcoholic hepatitis is alcohol abstinence. Involvement of family, friends, counseling, and support groups may be helpful. Patients should be hospitalized with an acute episode because it can be life-threatening. Discharge is considered when the patient is stable and the bilirubin level decreases. Malnutrition is a strong contributor to the morbidity and mortality associated with alcoholic hepatitis, and therefore assessment by a dietitian, adequate diet therapy, and vitamin replacement for deficiencies are essential. Parenteral administration of vitamin B is preferred to oral therapy for better absorption in alcoholic patients. Multivitamin preparations that include folic acid, thiamine, vitamins A and D, and essential minerals are also important. In the absence of hepatic encephalopathy, a high-protein diet is recommended. Corticosteroid therapy in the treatment of alcoholic liver disease has been equivocal and has significant risk. Pentoxifylline has recently been shown to have efficacy with severe alcoholic hepatitis and may help prevent hepatorenal syndrome, a complication that is a major cause of mortality. It is safe to be given for months. Transplantation is considered in patients with proven long-term abstinence, but recidivism is a concern. For successful treatment a focus on reducing recidivism rates with early and frequent outpatient visits is important. Baclofen started in the last few days of hospitalization has been shown to decrease alcohol cravings and to lengthen time to relapse. Carbohydrate-deficient transferrin may be used for identification of heavy alcohol use and is not detectable after 2 weeks of abstinence. It may be useful for monitoring on an outpatient basis.[22]

The most important principle in the management of drug-induced liver disease is removal of the suspected drug or offending agent. Supportive care of patients with acute hepatitis and liver failure is provided as necessary. In the case of severe, drug-induced liver failure, urgent liver transplantation can be lifesaving. Currently, the only specific treatment available is the administration of *N*-acetylcysteine for acetaminophen overdose. In general, corticosteroids have no value in the treatment of drug-induced liver disease.

Rifaximin is indicated for the treatment of hepatic encephalopathy, along with lactulose. Encephalopathy occurs with the development of cirrhosis and accumulation of ammonia in the brain. Hepatic encephalopathy can lead to coma and death. Rifaximin is a poorly absorbed antibiotic that has its effect in the intestinal tract and has a wide antibacterial spectrum. It helps reduce blood ammonia and has been effective in treating hepatic encephalopathy.[36] It is recommended to use rifaximin in combination with lactulose, which requires a large enough dose to produce three loose stools a day. Compliance can be an issue.

NAFLD is on the path to be the number one CLD. It can be considered a new pandemic for the 21st century. As a consequence of metabolic dysregulation, NAFLD also affects the continued dysregulation and increases the risk of type 2 diabetes and cardiovascular disease. Diagnosis and monitoring are important. Treatment consists of weight loss with diet and exercise (3% to 5% for NAFLD and 7% to 10% for NASH). Treatment of hyperlipidemia with diet and medication is important, because this plays a role in the development of NAFLD. Patients with diabetes should be on a low-carbohydrate diet and medication as appropriate for control of blood glucose levels. Low saturated fats and 25% polyunsaturated fats in the diet should be a goal. There is no effective pharmacologic treatment at this time.[24]

LIFE SPAN CONSIDERATIONS

The liver is a remarkable organ that is capable of regeneration. The treatment of hepatitis has been shown to halt progression and to improve liver histology, if the causative agent is removed. If hepatitis is treated and cirrhosis does not develop, patients can lead normal lives and their life span will be unaffected. If cirrhosis develops, the life span can be greatly reduced because cirrhosis is a leading cause of death.

Hepatitis is often insidious, and liver damage can be ongoing without the patient's knowledge. Signs or symptoms often do not appear for many years. Lifestyle becomes an important factor, but it is not the sole issue in deteriorating liver disease. Some patients have aggressive disease, and treatment is difficult. Thus, it is imperative that health care providers screen for risk factors and routinely monitor LFT results. Abnormal LFT results should never be ignored. The sooner identification and treatment can begin, the better the prognosis.

COMPLICATIONS

The most significant complications of hepatitis are cirrhosis, liver failure, and cancer. The greatest risk with chronic HBV is the development of hepatocellular cancer, which can be seen without development of cirrhosis. All patients with chronic HBV need HCC surveillance with imaging and laboratory tests every 3 to 6 months. Fulminant hepatic failure does occur in a small percentage of patients (<1%) with acute hepatitis A and hepatitis B. Rapid elevation of PT (more than three times normal), hyperbilirubinemia, and hepatic encephalopathy indicate fulminant hepatic failure. Hospitalization with rapid organ transplantation is the only treatment option; without transplantation, the mortality rate is very high.

Some people with chronic HCV may do well, without complications developing. Treatments have greatly improved and cure rate is very high (greater than 90% chance). The barrier to treatment is the cost, which can be exorbitant. Access and insurance coverage can be significant factors in the decision to treat HCV. An important factor in the progression of liver damage is alcohol intake. Those who drink regularly can increase their risk for development of cirrhosis to 50% in 5 years and their risk of cancer to 25% (develops in the presence of cirrhosis). HCC surveillance should be undertaken with anyone with cirrhosis. Alcoholic hepatitis has a significant risk of cirrhosis, liver failure, or cancer if the patient continues to drink alcohol. Physical and psychosocial problems and malnutrition are other complications associated with alcoholism.

NAFLD has become a significant issue with the rise of obesity and the metabolic syndrome. It is becoming a leading cause of cirrhosis and liver transplantation and is the only CLD on the rise. People will not be aware that they have NAFLD unless their liver enzymes begin to rise. Screening for NAFLD is important and should be done in patients who are obese, diabetics, those with metabolic syndrome, and patients with any transaminase elevations. Once diagnosed, patients need regular monitoring of their liver function at least every 6 months.

The prognosis of drug-induced liver disease is highly variable and depends on the clinical circumstances and the causative agent involved. The overall fatality rate is approximately 5%. There is a much poorer prognosis with some agents because they induce acute hepatic necrosis or cause progressive CLD and cirrhosis.

INDICATIONS FOR REFERRAL OR HOSPITALIZATION

Patients should be referred when abnormal LFT results are found (AST or ALT > 40 units/L or elevated alkaline phosphatase) on two separate testing dates. Interpretation of testing, need for liver biopsy, and management require specialist input. Even patients with mild acute hepatitis should be referred because there can be many complicating factors and long-term issues, management needs, and follow-up care. Patients with chronic HCV or HBV infection should be referred after initial testing. Any patients with signs of increasing liver failure or decompensation of cirrhosis should be emergently admitted to the hospital and gastroenterology and hepatology consultation obtained.

PATIENT AND FAMILY EDUCATION

The diagnosis of HCV has a profound effect on patients and families and their quality of life. A study examined illness intrusiveness and demonstrated an impact on all areas of daily life including work, recreation, finance, health, and intimacy.[37] Patients with all forms of hepatitis require careful education about the infection, prevention, transmission, treatment options, and complications. The benefit of rest, diet, avoidance of hepatotoxic substances (especially alcohol), and medications should be emphasized.

HAV can be prevented. Contact with obviously contaminated food or water should be avoided, and infected individuals should not handle or prepare food. In addition, personal objects should not be shared, and hands should be washed thoroughly after patient contact. Health care workers should wear gloves when handling blood or body fluids. Travelers to underdeveloped countries should avoid eating uncooked shellfish, fruits, or vegetables or drinking water that could be contaminated.

Currently, the CDC recommends immune globulin for all travelers to developing countries where HAV is endemic. Hepatitis A immune globulin should be considered for travel that is going to be longer than 6 months. Prophylaxis against hepatitis A should be given as soon as possible after exposure (0.02 mL/kg intramuscularly), although it is of no benefit if it is not given within 2 weeks of exposure. Immunization with immune globulin lasts for 6 months. A hepatitis A vaccine is now currently available.

Prevention of hepatitis B involves routine screening of pregnant women, prophylaxis of infants born to infected women, and routine infant immunization. The hepatitis B vaccine should also be offered to persons at risk. The vaccine is given in a series of three injections; the first two doses are given 1 month apart, and the third dose is given 6 months after the second dose. Antibodies to HBV develop in approximately 90% to 95% of vaccinated individuals but may be as low as 50% to 70% among individuals who are immunocompromised. A positive HBsAb indicates immunity. To prevent transmission, therapy should be initiated immediately after exposure to HBV. The recommendations for prophylaxis after sexual exposure to HBV include hepatitis B immune globulin (0.06 mL/kg intramuscularly) within 14 days of exposure and simultaneous hepatitis B vaccination, with the second and third injections at 1 and 6 months, respectively. HBV and HCV are transmitted by blood; therefore patients need to understand the importance of not sharing razor blades, toothbrushes, or nail clippers. Partners of infected patients need to be tested because sexual transmission is possible. Barrier protection should be used, and partners should be told about the patient's hepatitis infection. Long-term monogamous partners can use their discretion if the partner is hepatitis negative, but all partners should be tested every few years to detect any seroconversion. Household contacts have an extremely low risk of infection. Patients with chronic hepatitis should clean up their blood spills with bleach and bag any blood-stained material before placing it in the trash.

All patients with liver disease should understand the significant risk for development of cirrhosis, liver failure, and cancer with alcohol ingestion. Patients should be counseled and resources provided to help them stop drinking. Referral to psychotherapy, substance abuse counselors, Alcoholics Anonymous, and support groups can be helpful. Family members and significant others need to be included in counseling and therapy.

Patients with chronic hepatitis should be vaccinated for both HAV and HBV as appropriate. Education regarding their disease, possible complications, importance of adherence to the treatment regimen, and contributing factors to the disease needs to be addressed. Patient education can be a valuable tool that can improve patient adherence.[38]

HEALTH PROMOTION

Prevention of hepatitis is possible with healthy lifestyles and avoidance of situations that increase risk. A healthy lifestyle includes alcohol and substance abuse avoidance, safe sexual practices, vaccinations, and regular checkups that include monitoring of LFT results.

Once hepatitis has been diagnosed, complications and disease progression can be deterred by abstaining from alcohol and substance abuse, obtaining vaccinations, becoming knowledgeable about the disease, and maintaining regular follow-up with the health care provider.

CHAPTER 138

INFLAMMATORY BOWEL DISEASE

Wendy L. Biddle

DEFINITION AND EPIDEMIOLOGY

Ulcerative colitis (UC) and Crohn disease (CD) are chronic inflammatory bowel diseases (IBDs) that are on the rise. Both are thought to be heterogeneous groups of intestinal inflammatory disorders.[1] A third category known as IBD–unclassified can account for up to 10% of all patients with IBD. The unclassified disease involves the colon but the distinction between UC and CD cannot be made. A diagnosis may be later determined as UC or CD as symptoms and features manifest. The diagnosis of indeterminate colitis should be used only after colectomy and histopathology of the colon could not distinguish between UC and CD. IBD typically has periods of remission and exacerbation. There is no known drug cure, and often there is significant morbidity over years. Although UC and CD have many similarities, there are significant differences.[1,2]

UC is a chronic inflammation of the lining of the colonic mucosa and to some extent, the submucosal layer. Beginning in the rectum, the inflammation is diffuse and continuous and may involve the entire colon (pancolitis) or only part of the colon. The worst of the disease is seen in the rectum and may be indicative of the disease above, but it is not usually found worse higher in the colon compared with the rectal involvement. The disease can involve only the rectum (proctitis) or the rectosigmoid colon, accounting for approximately 40% to 50% of the cases of UC. An additional 30% to 40% of patients have disease extending proximally to the splenic flexure (left-sided UC). Many patients experience a major impact on their quality of life, and approximately 50% do not experience a stable period of remission for any significant amount of time.[2-5]

CD also involves chronic inflammation, but all layers of the intestinal tract wall (transmural inflammation) and any portion of the intestinal tract from the mouth to the anus can be affected. CD is heterogeneous, with a variable presentation and a variable response to treatment. The presentation is affected by site involvement and whether the disease is only inflammatory or also complicated with fibrostenosis or penetration of the bowel wall creating fistulous tracts. Approximately 40% to 50% of patients with CD have disease only in the small intestine (ileitis or regional enteritis), 30% to 40% in the small and large intestines (ileocolitis), and 10% to 30% only in the colon (Crohn colitis, not to be confused with UC). CD occurs in the mouth, stomach, and duodenum in a very small percentage of patients.[6]

The transmural involvement in CD is responsible for many of the complications that occur. Research has shown that many patients with CD will have a worsening course over time. A study of Olmsted County, Minnesota found 18.6% of patients developed either a stricture or a penetrating complication within the first 90 days of diagnosis and that 50% had developed complications by 20 years after diagnosis.[7] Although the inflammation can be patchy (unlike UC, which is nearly always continuous), the involvement of all layers of the bowel wall creates many problems. Fibrostenosis occurs from the inflammation and can partially or completely obstruct the lumen of the intestinal wall (stricturing). Weakening of the intestinal wall from inflammation results in sinus tracks or fistulas (penetrating disease), abscesses, and perforation. Fistulas can develop from bowel to bowel (enteroenteric), bowel to skin (enterocutaneous), bowel to bladder (enterovesical), or bowel to vagina (enterovaginal). The fistulas frequently occur perianally, and other complications include abscesses, large tender skin tags, and the need for surgically placed drains and repair.[3] For a comparison of UC and CD, see Table 138-1.

There are approximately 1.5 million persons with IBD in the United States. The annual incidences of UC and CD are similar in both age at onset and worldwide distribution. The highest incidence of IBD is in colder climates and industrial-urbanized societies with a Westernized lifestyle, which includes North America, Europe, and Australia, but the incidence is rising in developing countries and in Asia, and IBD is seen as an emerging global disease. The annual incidence per 100,000 persons in the United States is 7 to 8 each for UC and CD, but in Canada the rate is 19 to 20 for each.[2] The prevalence in North America is estimated to be 249 cases per 100,000 persons for UC and 319 per 100,000 population for CD.[2] IBD affects men and women equally, but there may be some regional differences. The peak age at onset is the second and third decade, but 25% of IBD patients are younger than age 20 years at presentation. The incidence in the pediatric population is increasing, especially for CD.[1] However, IBD can appear at any age from infancy to older adulthood, and new onset of CD has been seen in the eighth decade. The rates in the elderly are increasing as well, and 4% to 12% are diagnosed after 60 years of age.[8]

The cause of IBD is unknown, although there have been many advances in the understanding of the pathogenesis. The most recent research has focused on the microbiome. There appears to be an abnormal immune response to intestinal microbial flora, shifting the composition of the flora in the affected individual. Altered interactions between the intestinal flora and the immune system in the mucosa of the intestines may be contributing to the inflammatory response. Although genetics plays a role, twin monozygotic studies show a low concordance with IBD. Multiple environmental factors also play a role. These include long-term dietary patterns and age, both of which affect the gut microbiota.[9]

Genetics are also proposed to be significant in the cause of IBD and may be a link with the microbiome as well. Several genes have been identified to increase the susceptibility of the

TABLE 138-1 Crohn Disease (CD) Versus Ulcerative Colitis (UC)

Factor	Crohn Disease	Ulcerative Colitis
Section of gastrointestinal tract involved	Potentially any area from mouth to anus: 30% small bowel 30%-50% colon 10%-30% small bowel and colon	Colon: partial to entire length
Mucosal appearance of inflammation	Patchy, may have a cobblestone appearance if colon involved	Continuous, beginning at rectum
Inflammatory involvement	Transmural, affecting all layers of bowel wall	Mucosal and submucosal layers only
Corticosteroid use	15% with mild disease and up to 50% of those with CD will not need corticosteroids Used to treat moderate to severe disease 30% severe disease, no maintenance dose	15% severe disease, indicated for induction, not maintenance
Response to mesalamine	May be effective for mild disease Minimal effect for moderate to severe disease	Good to excellent first-line therapy
Complications	Arthritis, skin lesions, eye, mouth, liver 10% present with stricturing or penetrating disease: fistulas, stenosis, obstruction, perianal disease, malabsorption	Arthritis, skin lesions, eye, spine, mouth, liver, perianal disease
Surgical risk	75% will have surgery during lifetime Up to 65% will need a second surgery	10%-20% will need total colectomy, may be curative
Effect of cigarette smoking	Risk for active disease; 2.5-fold risk of reoperation, especially for women	Risk for disease onset after quitting May be protective for active disease
Family history	20% have family member with IBD	5% have family member with IBD
Remission maintenance	May have long periods of remission but likely will need lifelong treatment	80% will relapse without treatment

individual to IBD, with different genetic patterns for UC and CD. Mutations of these genes have an impact on the microbiome, which increases the inflammatory response.[9] In these individuals, the immune system is dysregulated, triggered by an environmental factor. These factors may include luminal bacteria, infection, or tobacco. For some persons with IBD, there seems to be a familial tendency in that these individuals have a first-degree relative with IBD. This is more commonly found in children with IBD than in adults.[1] In these families, most have the same form of IBD, although both UC and CD can occur in the same family. Persons of Jewish ethnicity originating in Europe (Ashkenazi Jews) have been shown to have a higher risk (up to fivefold to eightfold) for development of IBD.[2]

Cigarette smoking has been shown to be one of the strongest environmental factors affecting IBD. Many studies have documented a higher risk of UC in former smokers. Smoking may also affect the course of UC, demonstrating a protective role. The opposite relationship is evident with CD. Current smoking is a strong, independent risk factor for early development of structuring and fistulizing CD, postoperative recurrence of ileal CD, and disease requiring maintenance therapy, especially biologics. A higher level of tobacco pack-years will increase the risk. Researchers have documented that smokers are twice as likely to develop CD. Continued smoking after surgery increases the risk of needing further surgery. Smokers are also more likely to need immunosuppressives and have a poorer quality of life. Smoking cessation can improve the disease course, and individuals who quit can do better than those who continue to smoke.[10]

PATHOPHYSIOLOGY

It is thought that several factors are responsible for IBD. A proposed mechanism of inflammation is an infection or other toxin that releases cell wall products that upregulate macrophages and granulocytes. Macrophages and granulocytes activate circulating cells that migrate into the mucosa, releasing a variety of inflammatory factors, such as cytokines, proteases, and oxygen-derived free radicals. These factors all promote inflammation, and the patient has no means of downregulating the system to inhibit the inflammation. Either the tissue responds by resolving with scarring or other secondary immune reactions continue to create irreversible damage.[11]

Advances in pathophysiology over the past decade have included the role of the microbiome, and the impact from genetic profiles and environmental factors link together to help explain the development of IBD. It is known that *NOD2* (CD susceptibility gene) mutations are associated with an altered gut microbiota structure.[9] Anti–*Saccharomyces cerevisiae* antibodies (ASCAs) are associated with CD, and antineutrophil cytoplasmic antibodies (ANCAs) are associated with UC. More than 70 genes have been identified that are associated with IBD—UC, CD, or both.[12] Further studies have examined associations among genotype, phenotype, disease course, and response to treatment. This knowledge is contributing to the further understanding of the clinical manifestations of IBD, such as disease location, behavior, natural history, and response to and side effects of medications.[13]

CLINICAL PRESENTATION

UC and CD can have similar presentations and can be difficult to distinguish. Approximately 10% of people will have IBD–unclassified, colitis that cannot be distinguished as UC or CD.[1] People may complain of symptoms for varying lengths of time, and it is not unusual to have someone report abdominal pain or diarrhea intermittently for years before other symptoms develop. Abdominal pain may be the only presenting complaint. The symptoms of abdominal pain and diarrhea are present in most persons with both diseases. The abdominal pain may be diffuse (generalized lower pain) or localized to the right or left lower quadrants. The pain is usually a cramping sensation and can be intermittent or constant.[14]

Tenesmus, spasms in the rectum, urgency, and fecal incontinence may be reported with active rectal inflammation. Stools are often loose or watery and may have blood if the colon is involved. Rectal bleeding is usually present with colitis, either UC or Crohn colitis (if the lower colon is involved). Patients may report blood seen only on the toilet paper after wiping, blood in the stool, clots, or large amounts of blood.[15] With proctitis, rectal bleeding may be the only complaint, or constipation may be reported rather than diarrhea.

Other complaints may include fatigue, weight loss, anorexia, fever, chills, nausea, vomiting, joint pains, and mouth sores. CD may manifest with only vague complaints of fatigue and abdominal cramping, but it can also cause intestinal obstruction and symptoms of vomiting, bloating, and no stool as well as perianal disease of anal fissures, perirectal abscess, or fistula. Some patients, especially in late adolescence and early adulthood, have obstruction, abscesses, or fistula and are diagnosed at surgery.[16]

Pertinent history includes recent antibiotic use or travel, the health of other household members, family history of IBD, previous history of abdominal pain or diarrhea, and a thorough medication review.

PHYSICAL EXAMINATION

The presentation can vary from minimal or no distress to severe illness. Fever and accompanying tachycardia can be present but often are not. All weight ranges are seen, from underweight to obese. People, especially the young and the elderly, can demonstrate significant weight loss and failure to thrive. Conjunctival inflammation or oral aphthous ulcers may be present. Abdominal examination usually reveals a tender lower abdomen, which may be more prominent on one side or the other, although the abdomen can be diffusely tender. Hyperactive bowel sounds and palpation of loops of bowel may be noted as "fullness" in the lower abdomen. A mass, especially in the lower right quadrant, can signify ileocecal inflammation. Rectal examination for occult blood may be positive, with frank blood and tenderness. Perianal lesions, such as skin tags, anal fissure, and perianal fistula, are more suggestive of CD but can be seen in UC. Anal stenosis, abscess, or purulent drainage from a fistulous tract may be seen on rectal examination. Perianal disease is suggestive of IBD but can also be seen in healthy people. Joints do not usually appear red or edematous. Skin lesions (e.g., erythema nodosum, pyoderma gangrenosum, papulonecrotic skin lesions or rashes) may also be noted.

DIAGNOSTICS

Blood Tests

A complete blood count (CBC) is useful to determine the presence of anemia. The platelet count will often be elevated in the presence of active inflammation or infection. C-reactive protein (CRP) and erythrocyte sedimentation rate (ESR) can be elevated but are nonspecific markers of inflammation. CRP can be useful as a monitor of disease activity if it is elevated with active disease, but 20% of the population does not have a CRP response to active inflammation. None of these tests are useful for diagnosis, although they may have value in following a patient's progress. In addition, CD may result in malabsorption, especially after a small bowel resection. Monitoring of electrolyte values, liver function test (LFT) results, and glucose, blood urea nitrogen, creatinine, vitamin D, vitamin B_{12}, and folate levels should be done to determine status.

Anemia is the most frequently seen extraintestinal complication in IBD; iron deficiency is the most common cause. Indices that should be monitored include iron saturation, ferritin, and reticulocyte count. Depending on small bowel involvement of IBD and adverse gastrointestinal effects of oral iron supplements, patients may need iron supplementation parenterally. A hematology consultation would be appropriate for iron deficiency refractory to oral supplementation. There are also some data to suggest that oral iron may cause disease exacerbation.[16]

Genetic testing has continued to advance and may be helpful in identifying IBD, distinguishing CD from UC, and demonstrating the likelihood of more aggressive CD (prognostic test). The serogenetic markers include ANCAs and perinuclear antineutrophil cytoplasmic antibodies (pANCAs); ASCA immunoglobulin A (IgA) and IgG; outer membrane protein C (anti-OmpC) IgA; and flagellin (anti-Fla2, anti-FlaX, and anti-CBir1).[17] Other markers can be tested in an IBD panel. *NOD2/CARD15* genetic testing is prognostic for CD and can provide the likelihood of more aggressive disease over time.

A recent study reported sensitivity and specificity of biomarker testing in patients younger than 18 years of age (sensitivity for IBD 86%, CD 91%, UC 82%; specificity for IBD 86%, CD 76%, UC 91%).[18] A positive test result can be helpful for diagnosis, but it does not obviate the need for other diagnostic testing. False-negative test results can happen with approximately one third of patients and clinical judgement would override the test results. For this reason testing may be useful on a limited basis. The additional markers that are continually being refined may help to distinguish subtypes of disease.[19]

Stool Tests

Initial presentation of diarrhea as well as subsequent flares should be evaluated for infection. Stool testing for ova and parasites should be performed three times to eliminate the most common pathogens. Testing for *Clostridium difficile* is important during flares, especially if the patient recently used antibiotics, and has become a significant factor in IBD. Special cultures for other organisms can be requested. Fecal leukocytes can be tested in the stool specimen and are present with inflammation. Fecal calprotectin has become a frequently used test to demonstrate inflammation in the bowels.[20]

Radiography

Enterography by computed tomography (CT) or magnetic resonance imaging (MRI) is a diagnostic and monitoring tool that has become important in the management of CD. It is a more accurate test for small bowel disease. CT scans can detect bowel wall inflammation, perforation, and abscess and are used selectively when appropriate. There is growing concern about exposure to excessive radiation that occurs especially with CT scans. Responsible practitioners need to carefully weigh the benefits of the scan versus the increasing radiation risk. This is especially important in IBD as a chronic, lifelong illness that potentially will require multiple radiologic tests. MR enterography is safer because there is no radiation and is an alternative to view the small bowel.

Small bowel series are used infrequently to determine small bowel involvement and can demonstrate an abnormal terminal ileum and fistulas, but they are not as sensitive as other testing. The barium enema is of limited use in diagnosis of IBD and is most useful in detecting colonic distention, obstruction, fistulas, strictures, or tumors. There are moderate false-positive and false-negative rates with barium studies, which needs to be considered. A barium enema should not be used in patients with moderate to severe colitis because there is perforation risk when the colon is weakened from inflammation. MRI may be helpful in detecting fistulas and abscesses in patients with perianal CD. A laxative should be taken by the patients after barium studies because they can become extremely constipated and the barium can remain for weeks in the intestines.

Endoscopy

Flexible sigmoidoscopy examines the lower 76 cm (30 inches) of the colon and is useful to determine the source of bright red rectal bleeding. Colonoscopy can be useful in differentiating UC and CD. Bowel cleansing is necessary for colonoscopy, and there are several preparations available. The most effective method to cleanse the bowel is splitting the dose, half taken the night before and the rest taken the morning of the procedure. Hydration is extremely important and must be emphasized to the patient. Caution must be exercised for patients with a history of congestive heart failure or decreased kidney function (serum creatinine >1.5).

Both UC and CD may have distinguishing features endoscopically that, if found, may help differentiate one from the other. On endoscopy, UC mucosal inflammation will be continuous with disease in the rectum, up to the point that the inflammation stops. CD can have "skip areas," patchy sections of normal mucosa intermixed with inflamed mucosa. This skipping gives a cobblestone appearance to the mucosa. However, these distinguishing features may not be present, making the diagnosis difficult. Another useful endoscopic finding is an inflamed or abnormal terminal ileum that is more indicative of CD. Capsule endoscopy involves swallowing a capsule with a camera inside that takes pictures of the small intestine and transmits them to a box worn by the patient. It has excellent resolution and demonstrates many lesions and abnormalities missed by small bowel radiology. It is covered by insurance but requires specific indications and other testing to be completed first. It can be valuable in diagnosis and monitoring of CD, but caution should be exercised to ensure that there is no stricture or narrowing of the small bowel because the capsule may become lodged. Small bowel enteroscopy is evolving, and a detailed explanation of new and promising techniques can be found in a recent review.[21]

Mucosal biopsy samples, usually 3 to 4 mm, are especially helpful in diagnosis and monitoring of IBD. On microscopic examination, acute and chronic inflammation can be seen. It may be difficult to distinguish UC from CD; in these patients, the disease may be labeled indeterminate colitis until a clear diagnosis can be made. UC can have cryptitis and crypt abscesses, whereas CD can show aphthous ulcers and granulomas.

Virtual colonoscopy is an alternative to screening colonoscopy for colon cancer. This is done with a CT scan and requires the patient to be inflated with a large amount of air, after cleansing of the bowel. The test can be uncomfortable and costly (variable with insurance coverage); it does not examine the rectum and has a varying miss rate for polyps, especially small or flat polyps. It is not recommended as yet and has no role in diagnosis or management of IBD.

DIAGNOSTICS

Inflammatory Bowel Disease

LABORATORY

CBC and differential
Platelet count
CRP
ESR
Complete metabolic panel, including LFTs, creatinine, glucose
Vitamin B_{12} and folate
Celiac antibody panel
Genetic testing—minimal usefulness, reserve for specialist testing
Stool tests*

- Culture and sensitivity: *C. difficile, Escherichia coli, Campylobacter, Bacillus, Salmonella, Vibrio cholerae, Shigella*
- *Giardia lamblia, Entamoeba histolytica* organisms
- Ova and parasites
- Fecal leukocytes
- Fecal calprotectin

IMAGING AND ENDOSCOPY*

MRI of abdomen/enterography
CT scan of abdomen/enterography
Small bowel series
Upper endoscopy (esophagogastroduodenoscopy [EGD])
PillCam (small bowel capsule endoscopy)
Flexible sigmoidoscopy
Colonoscopy with biopsy
Barium enema

*if indicated.

DIFFERENTIAL DIAGNOSIS

When a patient is seen with the common symptoms of IBD, several diagnoses should be excluded: abdominal pain, rectal bleeding, and diarrhea. Rectal bleeding should never be ignored or assumed to be benign and should always be further evaluated. Bleeding may be hemorrhoids, ischemia, diverticular disease, a fissure, drug induced (e.g., by aspirin, nonsteroidal anti-inflammatory drugs [NSAIDs], anticoagulation), infection, or a colonic polyp or cancer. Abdominal pain can be diverticulitis and, in women, endometriosis or pelvic inflammatory disease. Abdominal pain and diarrhea without bleeding may signify irritable bowel syndrome, diarrhea predominant (IBS-D) or appendicitis. IBS is a chronic, benign functional disorder with no organic disease present. The classic symptoms of IBS-D are altered loose bowel habits, bloating, and abdominal pain relieved by defecation.

Infectious causes of diarrhea (with or without bleeding) need to be excluded. The most common pathogenic organisms to consider are *Giardia* organisms, *Campylobacter jejuni, C. difficile* (especially with a history of recent antibiotic use), *Escherichia coli, Salmonella,* and *Shigella.* Other causes include viral infection, celiac disease, lactase deficiency, bacterial overgrowth, bile acids (after cholecystectomy), hyperthyroidism, and diabetes (enteropathy). If a host is immunocompromised, infections with such organisms as cytomegalovirus, *Cryptosporidium,* and *Mycobacterium avium-intracellulare* should be excluded.

Noninfectious causes include acute self-limited colitis, ischemic colitis (especially in patients older than 60 years), radiation enteritis or colitis (history of radiation to abdomen or pelvis; may be a late sequela), Behçet syndrome, lymphoma, and systemic vasculitis. A rare cause of diarrhea (usually with excessive watery stools and flushing) is neuroendocrine tumors and carcinoid syndrome.

Over-the-counter medications that can be a source of diarrhea include antacids with magnesium, mints with sorbitol, and laxatives. Other medications that can cause diarrhea include metformin and proton pump inhibitors. Medications associated with microscopic (lymphocytic, collagenous) colitis include antibiotics, chemotherapeutic agents, NSAIDs, and gold.

DIFFERENTIAL DIAGNOSIS

Inflammatory Bowel Disease*

- IBS
- Infection
- Lactase deficiency, nonabsorbed or poorly absorbed sugars and other dietary factors
- Postcholecystectomy bile salt induced
- Pelvic inflammatory disease and other gynecologic disorders
- Appendicitis
- Diverticulitis
- Microscopic, collagenous, or lymphocytic colitis
- Ischemic colitis
- Radiation enteritis or proctitis
- Lymphoma, adenocarcinoma, carcinoid tumor, neuroendocrine tumors, metastatic cancer
- Systemic vasculitis and other vasculitides
- Medications causing diarrhea, such as antibiotics, magnesium-containing antacids, metformin, proton pump inhibitors, colchicine, and misoprostol
- Bleeding from hemorrhoids, anal fissures, colon polyps, anticoagulation, NSAID-induced ulceration

*Not inclusive.

MANAGEMENT

Pharmacotherapy

5-Aminosalicylic Acid. First-line treatments of UC are the 5-aminosalicylic acid (5-ASA, mesalamine) products. Sulfasalazine is a sulfapyridine and a 5-ASA product connected by a bond. The 5-ASA has been shown to be the active ingredient, and the sulfapyridine is responsible for most of the side effects. Several 5-ASA products have become available during the years (Table 138-2). Studies have shown that 4 g/day in divided doses is effective in establishing remission in colitis. 5-ASA suppositories are effective for proctitis. The rectal suspension of mesalamine is effective at inducing and maintaining remission in UC, especially left-sided UC. The combination of rectal and oral therapy can be effective for pancolitis.[5] Rarely, a patient may be allergic to 5-ASA; if so, the drug should be stopped. Patients will have a worsening of their colitis symptoms, which improves with discontinuation of the medication. 5-ASA medications are most useful for UC and disease in the colon. They are indicated for mild to moderately active disease and maintenance of remission of UC. There is some suggestion that 5-ASA may help prevent colon cancer. Its role in CD is very limited because it is a topical agent, affecting only the mucosal lining, and CD involves transmural inflammation.

Corticosteroids. Oral and parenteral steroids can be useful for moderate to severe disease but are avoided (or limited) if possible because of potential long-term side effects, including diabetes, osteoporosis, and cataracts. Steroids are currently used for moderate to severe UC that is not responding to

TABLE 138-2 Comparison of Mesalamine Medications

Brand Name	How Supplied	Daily Dose for Active Disease	Daily Dose for Maintenance of Remission	Common Side Effects
Azulfidine (sulfasalazine)	500-mg tablets	4 g in divided doses	2 g in divided doses	Headache, nausea, allergy to sulfa
Asacol HD	800-mg delayed release tablets	2.4 g in divided doses	1.6 g in divided doses	Dyspepsia, abdominal pain
Pentasa	500-mg capsules	4 g in divided doses	1.5 g in divided doses	Gastrointestinal upset, headache
Colazal (balsalazide)	750-mg capsules	2.4 g in 24 hours in divided doses	N/A	Gastrointestinal upset, headache
Lialda	1.2 g	4 tablets every morning	2-4 tablets every morning	Headache, gastrointestinal upset
Apriso	0.375 g	4 capsules every morning	2-4 capsules every morning	Headache, diarrhea, upper abdominal pain, nausea
SF Rowasa (sulfite free)	4 g/60 mL	4 g (1 bottle) per rectum	1 bottle every other night or less often per rectum	Hemorrhoids, rectal pain
Canasa	1000-mg suppositories	1 twice a day per rectum	1 every night or less often per rectum	Rectal irritation

mesalamine. Steroids have been shown to induce remission in mild to moderately active CD. Budesonide is a synthetic steroid that is enteric coated and subject to high first-pass metabolism, potentially decreasing the risk of side effects. It has similar (or slightly less) efficacy to corticosteroids and releases more in the distal ileum and right colon (useful for CD), but there is an oral preparation (Uceris) that is designed to release throughout the colon and is indicated for UC. It may be stopped without taper.[22] Once remission is achieved, corticosteroids are tapered off as soon as possible, although long, slow tapers (over 2 to 3 months) may be necessary to prevent a flare.

Rectal steroids in the form of a retention enema or foam can provide relief of urgency and spasm in the rectum, in addition to healing the inflamed mucosa. Rectal steroids are used for a few weeks, usually until there is an improvement of rectal symptoms. There is some absorption of the steroid systemically; thus, long-term use (more than a few months) is not routinely recommended.

Immunomodulators. There is a trend to use immunomodulators earlier in the course of disease than they have been used in the past. Azathioprine and 6-mercaptopurine (6-MP) may allow the patient to avoid steroids and are useful for prevention of steroid dependency.[23] These medications must be taken for 4 to 5 months before the full effect is seen. The initial dose of 6-MP is 50 mg. Phenotype and metabolite testing of 6-MP can determine those in whom the drug is likely to become toxic and who should not take it. The recommendation is to monitor CBC, LFT results, and amylase and lipase levels at baseline, weekly for 4 weeks, monthly for 3 months, and then every 3 months.

The development of leukopenia, thrombocytopenia, or pancreatitis warrants immediate discontinuation of the drug. If an elevated liver enzyme level is found, the test should be repeated in 1 to 2 weeks. If the levels remain elevated or continue to rise, the drug should be discontinued and the patient referred to the gastroenterologist for further evaluation. Levels that are twice normal or higher are especially concerning and should prompt immediate referral to a gastroenterologist. Parenteral methotrexate has been shown to be effective in CD, although few long-term data are available. It is infrequently used, especially since the approval of biologic therapy.[23]

Biologics. Biologics, as a class of medications, are a significant breakthrough in treatment of IBD, especially with CD (Table 138-3). Infliximab, an anti–tumor necrosis factor (anti-TNF) monoclonal antibody, is indicated for induction and maintenance of remission in CD. It is effective in treating fistulas, allowing patients to avoid or taper off steroids (steroid sparing), and is also indicated for UC. It is administered intravenously every 2 months, but 50% of patients need the interval shortened to every 6 weeks for efficacy. The standard treatment regimen is to give a dose at 0, 2, and 6 weeks and then every 8 weeks thereafter. Infusion reactions and a serum sickness–like reaction can occur because of the development of autoantibodies with infliximab, which is 25% mouse antibody and 75% human. Given alone or in combination with other immunomodulators, infliximab has induced remission in 25% to 35% and improvement in 45% to 54% of patients with refractory CD. Infusion reactions may be avoided by not extending the interval beyond 2 to 3 months and pretreating with corticosteroids and antihistamines.[4]

Adalimumab (fully human anti-TNF monoclonal antibody) was approved for CD in 2007 but had been tested on humans since 1997. It is indicated for induction and maintenance of remission in moderate to severe CD that has not responded to conventional therapy. It is a subcutaneous injection given every 2 weeks after an induction dose. Research studies showed a 56% response and 36% remission rate in 4 weeks. Certolizumab is a pegylated monoclonal antibody (10% mouse antibody, 90% human) that is given by subcutaneous injection every 4 weeks. It was approved in 2008. The response rates and remission rates are similar for all three medications for CD.[4]

Newer biologics are available for UC, and others are available for CD. The class continues to expand as other proinflammatory mediators beyond TNF are targeted.[4]

TABLE 138-3 Biologics Approved for Moderate to Severe IBD

Brand Name (Generic)	Indication	Induction of Remission Dose	Maintenance of Remission Dose	Cytokine Target Antibody Formulation
Remicade (infliximab)	CD and UC induction and maintenance of remission	IV infusion at wk 0, 2, and 6 5 mg/kg, increase to 10 mg/kg if no response	Every 8 wk 5 mg/kg, increase to 10 mg/kg if response is lost	TNF antagonist (75% human, 25% mouse)
Humira (adalimumab)	CD induction and maintenance of remission	160 mg, 4 SC injections in wk 0 80 mg, 2 injections in wk 2	40 mg, 1 SC injection every 15 days	TNF antagonist (100% human)
Cimzia (certolizumab pegol)	CD induction and maintenance of remission	400 mg, administered as 2 SC injections in wk 0, 2, and 4	400 mg, 1 injection every 4 wk	TNF antagonist, pegylated (90% human, 10% mouse)
Entyvio (vedolizumab)	UC induction and maintenance of remission	300 mg administered as IV infusion wk 0, 2, 6	300 mg every 8 wk	Integrin receptor antagonist
Simponi (golimumab)	UC induction and maintenance of remission	200 mg administered as IV infusion wk 0, 2	100 mg every 4 wk	Integrin receptor antagonist
Tysabri (natalizumab)	CD induction and maintenance of remission	300 mg administered as IV infusion wk 0	300 mg every 4 wk Limited prescription rights	Integrin receptor antagonist

TNF, tumor necrosis factor.

There are multiple serious risks with the class of biologics; these include life-threatening and serious infections, lymphoma and malignant neoplasms, activation of tuberculosis and other viruses, worsening or development of congestive heart failure, cytopenia, and a lupus-like syndrome. The risks are serious but small (<5%). All patients must have a negative tuberculin test response (purified protein derivative [PPD]) before beginning therapy and repeat the PPD test yearly as long as they are receiving a biologic. It is recommended that patients be tested for hepatitis B and C, and testing of other viruses that may be dormant should be considered. They should be up-to-date on vaccines including tetanus, Pneumovax, and influenza. Vaccination history is important, and guidelines have been developed for IBD patients.[24] Patients need to report any sign of infection or new symptom, and the biologic must be stopped until the infection is treated.

Research shows that patients with moderate to severe CD who begin biologics have a better course of disease if treatment is initiated as close to diagnosis as possible. The trend is to start a biologic earlier in the course and to taper off other medications for IBD. Immunomodulators are not recommended as concurrent therapy unless absolutely necessary. There is an increased risk of lymphoma with the combination.

Patients receiving biologics need regular follow-up and laboratory studies at least every 3 to 6 months. Compliance is important for the greatest efficacy to be maintained. At this time, patients are continued on a biologic indefinitely if they are doing well. Newer therapies are being developed, and extensive research is ongoing.

Antibiotics. Metronidazole can be effective in treating perianal disease and in healing fistulas associated with CD, but treatment with biologics is superior. Antibiotics mainly are used for possible infection because *C. difficile* is common with IBD. Probiotics have some limited use.

Surgery

Approximately 20% of patients with UC and 60% to 75% of patients with CD require surgery for refractory disease. Patients with intractable disease are generally not responding to high doses of medications and may be systemically sick, with weight loss, anemia, nausea, and vomiting. Surgery is also indicated when dysplasia or cancer is found on biopsy. In UC, a total colectomy is usually necessary. After surgery, patients no longer have the colonic disease, and all IBD medications can be discontinued. Complications such as liver disease and ankylosing spondylitis may still be present, and treatment of these and other complications needs to be continued. Options for surgical treatment include an ileostomy and an ileal pouch–anal anastomosis (IPAA). With an IPAA, the colon is removed except for some rectal tissue, the small intestine is anastomosed to the rectum, and an internal pouch is created to store stool. Patients have no external bag but have several loose stools a day and can develop complications, including pouchitis.[14]

In CD, the average time from diagnosis to surgery is about 3 years. Surgery is indicated for medical therapy that failed, small bowel obstruction, fistulas, and abscesses. Up to 10% to 15% of patients are diagnosed with CD by surgery. A small bowel or colonic resection is the most common surgical procedure, although colectomy may be necessary in some patients. Many patients do well after surgery, but recurrence can develop in up to 80% of patients within 6 months.[23] Approximately one third of patients who had a resection will require a second procedure, and a smaller number of patients will require additional surgical procedures.

Many novel surgical techniques are being tried at various centers, which are constantly seeking better ways to help patients. Variations on ileoanal pouch procedures, strictureplasties, and a multitude of other procedures continue to be advanced with the goals of preserving continence and repairing fistulas. Laparoscopic surgery can be done for CD of the small bowel or terminal ileum and total colectomy for UC or CD. There is also an increase in the level of sophistication with robotic surgery.

COMPLICATIONS

Studies have demonstrated an increased risk of colorectal cancer in patients with IBD. The risk is related to the extent of colonic involvement in both UC and Crohn colitis. Patients with proctitis have no increased risk over that of the general population. The risk in UC begins to increase after 8 years of disease and continually rises. A cumulative risk of colorectal cancer in a patient with UC has been 2% at 10 years of disease, rising to 18% at 30 years, but more recent data suggest that the risk is lower, only 7.6% at 30 years. Initial colorectal cancer screening for those with pancolitis or left-sided colitis should begin at 8 years after disease onset and then be performed every 1 to 3 years.[10]

A number of extraintestinal manifestations can occur with IBD. These primarily involve the eyes, mouth, peripheral joints, skin, and blood vessels. Some are related to the inflammatory activity of the bowel and can occur with active inflammation, improving when the IBD improves. These manifestations include aphthous stomatitis, iritis, uveitis, episcleritis, arthritis, and skin lesions (i.e., pyoderma gangrenosum, erythema nodosum).

Peripheral arthritis occurs in 10% to 12% of patients with UC and in up to 22% of patients with CD. Knees, ankles, and shoulders are most often affected. From 1% to 26% of patients with UC and 3% to 16% of patients with CD develop ankylosing spondylitis. Treatment of the underlying IBD is the best management approach for the arthritis, although symptomatic treatment can be used. Caution should be used in treating with NSAIDs because they can trigger a flare of IBD.

Other complications include liver disease (primary sclerosing cholangitis), gallstones, malabsorption (CD of the small bowel), and adrenal stones. Both men and women with IBD are at risk for osteoporosis, independent of steroid use. All patients need a bone density scan at baseline and every 2 years.[10]

INDICATIONS FOR REFERRAL OR HOSPITALIZATION

The diagnosis of IBD can be difficult and requires physician consultation. Referral for diagnostic and follow-up endoscopy procedures as well as for management is the best approach. Once a patient has a treatment regimen, health care providers may be able to co-manage the IBD. Continual, close consultation with a gastroenterologist is necessary for optimum management and various treatment options.

Hospitalization is necessary at times for bowel rest, hydration, and parenteral medications. Patients who develop systemic symptoms, such as weight loss, nausea, vomiting, severe abdominal pain, significant blood loss, and malnutrition, should be evaluated and referred immediately.

LIFE SPAN CONSIDERATIONS

IBD does not decrease the life span unless complications develop or the patient is not managed properly. Issues of malnutrition, malignant disease, and infection are factors that could have an impact. Compliance with treatment regimens, surveillance for colorectal cancer, and attention to complications will maximize the health of the patients.

PATIENT AND FAMILY EDUCATION

IBD has a significant impact on the quality of life of patients and their families.[15] The stigma of a chronic bowel disease creates a unique set of problems. Patients may be afraid or unwilling to discuss their disease with loved ones, friends, and coworkers. Embarrassment about the symptoms and the need to be near a bathroom can prevent patients from participating in activities and outings. Fear of pain and diarrhea may keep them from eating, and they may become malnourished. Frequent visits and embarrassing, uncomfortable procedures may prevent them from seeking medical care when it is needed. There is a tendency for patients to accept their symptoms and not expect to be in remission; they need to be reminded that the goal is remission, not just improvement. Patients receiving a biologic or immunomodulator need to seek medical attention for any signs of infection or new symptom.[25]

There is a great need for patient education for better disease management. Understanding of the disease process, potential complications, medication side effects, and risks (such as cancer) is imperative. The need for regular health care visits and the importance of treatments and scheduled procedures should be emphasized. The patient should be educated about the need for a well-balanced diet and informed that there is no specific diet to follow for IBD. Written materials, videos, and educational meetings are available. The Crohn's and Colitis Foundation of America is a national patient organization that can provide information and support. Many local support groups also can provide a forum for learning and support for patients and their families.

When teaching patients with IBD, the provider should remember that they will be overwhelmed. Repetition is necessary to ensure that patients understand. Many visual aids are available that can help patients understand the disease and the procedures and tests that are necessary. In addition, because patients can obtain a great deal of misinformation from the media and well-meaning friends, relatives, and others, correction of misinformation and misconceptions will help. Above all, establishing a trusting, comfortable relationship and listening carefully to patients are vital to the long-term management of IBD.

HEALTH PROMOTION

IBD is a disease of remission and exacerbation. Family history plays a limited role; up to 20% of patients have a family member with IBD. Cigarette smoking exacerbates CD, and the effect can be as strong as taking a medication. Patients should be encouraged to stop smoking because the risks of smoking far outweigh any benefit.

IBD is a chronic disease with no known cause or cure. Patients should be encouraged to maintain a healthy lifestyle, which should include a well-balanced diet and stress management. Compliance with the prescribed treatment regimen and regular follow-up are the two most important strategies a patient can implement to maximize health. Maintenance of remission can be achieved with medications, with the right dose. People with IBD are at higher risk for colon cancer and need regular colon cancer surveillance. Maintaining regular follow-up with their health care providers and contacting their providers with early signs of a flare-up will minimize problems. Patients need to understand their medication regimen, the importance of not self-adjusting doses, and what monitoring is necessary. Family members need to be a part of the health care team as well. Health care providers can play a significant role in keeping the patient on track with appointments, medications, and testing, ensuring that the patient will obtain the highest level of wellness possible.

RESOURCES

American College of Gastroenterology: www.acg.gi.org
Centers for Disease Control and Prevention: www.cdc.gov/ibd
Crohn's and Colitis Foundation of America: www.ccfa.org; info@ccfa.org; 800-932-2423
National Diabetes, Digestive Diseases and Kidney Diseases (NIDDK) Information Clearinghouse: www.niddk.nih.gov/health-information/health-topics/digestive-diseases; 301-496-3583
www.CrohnsAndColitis.com
www.Mayoclinic.org/ibd
www.nlm.nih.gov

CHAPTER 139

IRRITABLE BOWEL SYNDROME

Deborah Allen

DEFINITION AND EPIDEMIOLOGY

Irritable bowel syndrome (IBS) is the most common gastrointestinal (GI) complaint seen in primary care offices and is the most common diagnosis for gastroenterologists.[1] It is classified as a "functional" GI disorder because there are problems with normal gut function; however, no identifiable organic or structural causes explain its development.[1-3] A correlation appears to exist among abnormalities in GI tract motility, alterations in autonomic regulation, sensitivity in abdominal viscera, brain-gut interaction abnormalities, and changes within the GI flora.[4-7] IBS is characterized by abdominal bloating, flatulence, abdominal pain, and bowel dysfunction.[6]

IBS has been defined by the American College of Gastroenterology as abdominal discomfort associated with altered bowel habits and symptoms of constipation, including infrequent stools, straining, passage of hard stools, and feelings of incomplete or difficult evacuation.[7] The 1998 Rome II diagnostic criteria for IBS were updated in 2006 to Rome III, and these criteria are currently still being used for the diagnosis of IBS (Box 139-1).[2,7,8] Additional features that support the diagnosis of IBS include abnormal stool passage (i.e., straining, urgency, or feeling of incomplete evacuation), changes in the form of feces, effort needed to defecate, passage of mucus, and bloating or sensation of abdominal distention.[1,9] It is recommended that health care professionals also consider IBS if a patient reports abdominal pain or discomfort, bloating, or a change in bowel habit consistently for 6 months.[1] In the past, IBS was described as spastic

BOX 139-1

2006 Rome III Diagnostic Criteria for Irritable Bowel Syndrome

For diagnosis, criteria must be met at least once per week for at least 2 months before diagnosis.

Both of the following must be included:

1. Abdominal discomfort or pain at least 3 days per month in the last 3 months, with two or more of the following features:
   - Improvement with defecation
   - Onset associated with change in frequency of stool (fewer than three bowel movements per week or more than three bowel movements per day)
   - Onset associated with change in appearance of stool (lumpy and hard or loose and watery)
2. No evidence of an inflammatory, anatomic, metabolic, or neoplastic process that can explain symptoms

From Rome Foundation: Rome III diagnostic criteria for functional gastrointestinal disorders. Available at www.romecriteria.org/criteria/. Accessed July 14, 2014.

colon, mucous colitis, nervous bowel, spastic colitis, and functional bowel.[5,10] Functional disorders are often characterized by intestine movement or intestine sensitivity because no known structural disorder is identified. Therefore the diagnosis is based on patient symptoms and the diagnostic criteria for each disorder.[11]

The lack of sensitive diagnostic criteria, a reluctance to seek care for fluctuating symptoms, faulty perceptions, ambiguities in defining the condition, absence of specific and reproducible examinations and markers, and potentially demeaning connotations of IBS sometimes cause health care providers, patients, and others to feel ill at ease with the diagnosis of IBS. These influences make accurate estimates of worldwide IBS prevalence difficult.[1,2,9,12-14] Reports of prevalence vary widely from 2.5% to 37% worldwide,[2,6,9,12-15] yet only 5% to 7% percent are diagnosed with the condition.[5,10] Most epidemiologic studies demonstrate that IBS is up to 50% more common in females than in males, appears to be familial, and is estimated to affect 10% to 30% of the adult population in Western countries.[1,5,9,10,16,17] Some studies show that the prevalence of IBS appears to be similar among racial groups.[18] Other studies show an increase in whites and African Americans, but a lesser prevalence among Asians.[17] The influence of socioeconomic status is also controversial. Zhu and colleagues found no difference in socioeconomic classes[2]; others reported low socioeconomic class as a risk factor for IBS.[18,19] Although IBS symptoms can been seen in childhood, symptoms typically have their onset in late adolescence to early adulthood; peak prevalence occurs in the third and fourth decades of life, and the condition is usually diagnosed before age 50. However, IBS symptoms often persist into the seventh and eight decades of life.[1,2,18,19] Annually, IBS accounts for approximately 3.5 million physician visits in the United States, affecting 10% to 15% of Western populations, and is the most common condition referred by primary care providers to gastroenterology specialists.[1,3,9,13] The number of office visits for patients with IBS has been estimated to comprise 25% to 28% of all gastroenterology consultation office visits.[9,15] Persons with IBS miss three times as many work days as do healthy individuals, see health care providers more often for GI and non-GI complaints, and consume 50% more health care resources than similar groups. The costs associated with IBS are an estimated $20 billion in direct and indirect expenses in the United States.[9,15,19] Impairments to quality of life are often higher in patients with IBS, which affects personal and social relationships and overall well-being.[2,14,15,17,18,20]

The goals of clinical management are twofold: (1) to exclude the presence of underlying organic disease while considering the risk and expense of a thorough diagnostic evaluation; and (2) to provide support, education, and reassurance to optimize the quality of life of those for whom IBS has become a chronic condition.

PATHOPHYSIOLOGY

Research during the past decade has dramatically improved our understanding of the etiology of IBS as a complex, multifactorial disorder involving a number of physiologic processes including altered GI motility, microscopic inflammation, bacterial overgrowth, increased gut sensitivity, mental health problems, and brain-gut signal problems, with suspected genetic linkage; however, no specific physiologic reason has been identified.[1,3-5,18] Studies have demonstrated that patients with IBS process sensory information from the gut differently than do persons without IBS.[14] The signs and symptoms of IBS appear to be predominantly related to changes in central nervous system processing of sensory information; exaggerated normal intestinal motility patterns; or sensory abnormalities in the colon, rectum, or small intestine.[6,9,10] A number of theories of the mechanisms for altered intestinal motility and sensitivity have recently evolved.

Altered Motility

Although altered motility is often mentioned as a cause of IBS, controversy remains about the exact electrical and contractile activity of the colon in IBS. Normal bowel motility predominantly consists of segmenting contractions that function to inhibit the transit of bowel contents. Any increase in segmenting contractions with decreased transit time results in constipation, whereas a decrease in contractions with increased transit time results in more frequent stools.[10] In patients who have IBS, the colon delays the movement of feces, allowing an increase in absorption of the feces.[5,9] This altered motility leads to changes in stool consistency. The increase in intestinal peristalsis and motility that usually follows the ingestion of a meal is thought to be increased in patients with IBS.[3,19] More consistently demonstrated in IBS is an exaggeration of normal colonic motility in response to external and enteric stimuli, such as psychological stress, anxiety, anger, various drugs, acute intestinal infection, and (more recently discovered) small bowel bacterial overgrowth.[1,2,5,6,10,13] Postinfectious IBS has been the topic of recent research; a few studies have demonstrated that as many as 10% to 30% of post–acute gastroenteritis patients with previously normal bowel function develop long-term symptoms suggestive of IBS.[5,10,18] The exact cause of postinfectious IBS is unknown but could involve injury to the enteric nervous system, immune hypersensitivity, or chronic mucosal inflammation that results in an alteration of gut motility.[1,5] Proponents of the postinfectious theory speculated that IBS patients are postinfectious and that efforts should be directed toward measures to prevent and treat severe cases of acute gastroenteritis.[5,10,18] Research has also shown that the the use of antibiotics in acute gastroenteritis for the purpose of preventing IBS may reduce symptoms.[3,5,9,10] Another factor possibly affecting the development of IBS is the role of small bowel bacterial overgrowth.[3] Intestinal flora provides nutrition to the host, keeps the mucosal immune system in check, and regulates epithelial growth and function. However, it has been reported that a large portion of patients with IBS have small bowel bacterial overgrowth.[3] Therefore treatment of IBS symptoms may be improved with the use of probiotics.[3-5,9,10]

Enhanced Visceral Sensation

Balloon distention studies used to determine the pathogenesis of IBS in the sigmoid, ileum, and colorectum demonstrate that painful symptoms at significantly lower pressures and higher pain frequency and severity are often seen in persons with IBS compared with healthy individuals. This concept, known as *hyperalgesia,* suggests that altered visceral sensation plays a role in the pathogenesis of IBS.[6,16] Other diagnostic tests include endoscopy, radiology, stool samples (fecal calprotectin measurements, fecal ova and parasites, fecal occult blood), thyroid function tests, flexible sigmoidoscopy, and colonoscopy.[5,10,15] However, there are no biochemical, histopathologic diagnostic tests that can determine all causes of IBS.[1]

Research suggests that with IBS there is increased sensitivity to mechanical stimulation in the small bowel and colon, increased or unusual somatic referral of visceral pain, and increased sensitivity to normal intestinal functions. Several possible mechanisms of visceral afferent dysfunction have been suggested to explain the increased visceral sensitivity in IBS. These mechanisms include altered receptor sensitivity at the viscus, increased excitability neurons of the spinal cord, and altered central modulation of sensation.[3,9,16,18]

Role of Enteric Neurotransmitters

Evidence suggests that abnormalities in extrinsic autonomic innervation of the viscera occur with functional bowel disorders and that neuroimmune interactions may mediate stress-induced GI responses.[16,18] Research has focused on the role of enteric nervous system neurotransmitters, such as serotonin, in controlling intestinal motility and visceral afferent (sensory) responses to normal stimuli (gas, sugars, bile acids, fatty acids) and noxious stimuli (allergens, infectious agents, balloon distention).[18] Eighty percent of the body's serotonin is located in the gut, manufactured and released from enterochromaffin cells located in the mucosa. Increases in intraluminal pressures result in the release of serotonin.[9] These neurotransmitters stimulate afferent fibers in the mucosa and initiate a peristaltic reflex, enhancing GI motility and mediating visceral pain.[18] A preliminary study demonstrated increased plasma levels of postprandial serotonin in women with IBS compared with healthy controls.[3] Serotonin, along with corticotropin-releasing hormone (CRH), may also play a role in mediating psychological, stress-induced GI responses through the brain-gut axis.[13,16] Although defecating often relieves pain, stress and food increase it.[5,19]

Psychosocial Factors

Studies of the relationship between psychosocial factors and IBS suggest that although emotional responses to stress affect GI function and produce symptoms in all persons, these symptoms are believed to play a role in the development and pathogenesis of IBS symptoms to a greater extent in persons with IBS.[1] Several studies have reported that persons with IBS have a greater incidence of psychosocial stressors and abuse than healthy individuals. It has also been shown that patients with IBS have increased incidences of psychiatric illnesses such as depression, anxiety, or other abnormal illness behaviors.[1,10,13,16] In addition, patients diagnosed with IBS seek more professional medical advice, have increased absences from work, and request to be seen by a gastroenterologist more frequently than controls.[3,9,19,20] People with IBS often believe that stress triggers their symptoms[5]; however, many physicians are reluctant to refer patients for psychological treatment.[20]

CLINICAL PRESENTATION

Abdominal pain must be present for an IBS diagnosis.[1,6,8,13,18] The pain associated with IBS is often described as nonradiating, intermittent, and crampy; pain can occur anywhere but is usually located in the left lower abdominal quadrant.[10,15,19,20] Symptoms frequently occur after food or alcohol consumption.[10] Because IBS is a functional chronic disorder in which symptoms fluctuate over time, it is critical to establish the absence of nocturnal symptoms to diagnosis IBS.[16,19]

Diarrhea, constipation, or a pattern of alternating diarrhea and constipation may be reported in conjunction with abdominal pain.[4,6,8,18] It is necessary to clarify what is meant by these complaints because normal patterns of defecation can range from three bowel movements per week to three bowel movements per day, so this needs to be defined by the individual patient's norm. Mucus in the stool is sometimes reported. Complaints of abdominal distention, bloating, nausea, lethargy, and backache are common[1,10,18,19] and most likely reflect increased sensitivity to normal amounts of intestinal gas rather than an actual increase in gas.

The likelihood of organic disease is indicated by an acute onset of GI symptoms or an onset of symptoms in patients older than 50 years. Nocturnal symptoms, bloody or greasy stool, weight loss, malnutrition, evidence of GI bleeding, anemia, recurrent nausea, vomiting, and fever are incompatible with a diagnosis of IBS and require immediate diagnostic evaluation or referral.[10,18,19] Although bleeding is not associated with IBS, it may occur secondary to an anal fissure or hemorrhoids aggravated by an alteration in bowel habits associated with IBS. However, careful diagnostic evaluation is required before rectal bleeding can be ascribed to distal benign causes.

A complete health history should be elicited in the presence of abdominal pain with an alteration in bowel habits.[10] The history should include a thorough investigation of the presenting symptoms, the associated symptoms, and the presence of nocturnal symptoms. The patient should be questioned about previous diagnostic evaluations for similar symptoms. A past medical history and family history of GI problems, such as colon cancer, inflammatory bowel disease, and celiac disease, should be obtained. These are often associated with other disease processes and need further evaluation. The patient should be asked about recent travel, GI infections, and the use of any prescription or over-the-counter medications that could cause diarrhea or constipation. A thorough review of diet, with particular emphasis on any food allergies or sensitivities such as lactose or fructose intolerance, should be undertaken.[19] The review of symptoms should focus on the differential diagnoses for abdominal pain with an alteration in bowel habits. A menstrual history and gynecologic review of symptoms are essential in women to exclude urogenital sources of abdominal pain, such as pelvic inflammatory disease (PID), ovarian cysts, uterine fibroids, or endometriosis. A sensitive psychosocial history should be elicited to determine sources of stress, coping mechanisms, support systems, reactions to stress in the past, and the use of psychological counseling services to cope with past stressors. A history of physical or sexual abuse as a child or an adult should also be explored at some point.

Comorbidities

Patients with IBS often have symptoms consistent with other disease processes. Most patients with IBS have comorbidities including other functional gastrointestinal disorders (FGIDs); gastroesophageal reflux disease (GERD); psychiatric disorders such as depression, anxiety, and obsessive-compulsive disorders; chronic fatigue syndrome; fibromyalgia; gynecologic disorders; and asthma.[1,16,18]

PHYSICAL EXAMINATION

A thorough physical examination should be performed to exclude organic disease and to reassure the patient.[10] With IBS, the physical examination findings are often unremarkable. An abdominal, pelvic, and rectal examination should be performed. Increased tympany to percussion, a palpable and tender cordlike sigmoid colon, and tenderness on rectal examination have been reported. Significant abdominal tenderness or rectal tenderness, masses, or blood in the stool warrants further investigation.

DIAGNOSTICS

The diagnostic goals for patients with suspected IBS are to establish an early diagnosis, exclude the presence of alternative or coexisting diagnoses, and avoid unnecessary diagnostic testing.[10] When planning a diagnostic strategy for the patient with an alteration in bowel habits, the provider should consider several factors, including the duration and severity of symptoms, current medications, the demographic features, any family history of colon cancer, the nature and extent of psychosocial issues, and previous diagnostic evaluations for similar symptoms.[1,3,5,19] An initial approach should be based on the Rome III criteria, a thorough history and physical examination, and a limited diagnostic screen to exclude organic disease.[1,3,5,11,18,19] Few, if any, diagnostic tests are required in young healthy patients who meet the symptom-based criteria for IBS and do not have "red flags" suggestive of organic disease.[1,2,5,10,18,19,21] A diagnosis of IBS with adequate initial evaluation is rarely associated with a need for additional diagnostics in the future.[5,10]

Although the diagnosis of IBS is based on patient symptoms, a limited screen for organic disease should be completed at the first visit, including a complete blood count (CBC) with differential; erythrocyte sedimentation rate (ESR); electrolyte values; albumin, blood urea nitrogen (BUN), creatinine, and glucose concentrations; thyroid-stimulating hormone (TSH) level; and stool specimen for occult blood and fecal leukocytes. If fecal leukocytes are present, stool culture specimens for enteric pathogens, ova and parasites, and *Clostridium difficile* should be obtained. If the result for occult blood is positive, the patient should be referred to a gastroenterologist for evaluation. A colonoscopy is typically recommended for young (<40 years), healthy patients with an acute change in bowel habits or rectal discomfort. A colonoscopy should also be performed for patients older than 50 years or patients with weight loss, anemia, occult blood, or risk factors for colorectal cancer.[5]

Many patients with IBS are also lactose intolerant.[5] Any patient with bloating, gas, distention, and diarrhea who cannot be diagnosed as having IBS on symptoms alone should undergo a 2-week trial of a lactose-free diet or a hydrogen breath test to exclude lactase deficiency; otherwise, no testing is required. An alternative is to have patients drink a quart of milk. If the patient does not experience symptoms, lactose intolerance is unlikely.

Liver function tests (LFTs) and an abdominal ultrasound to exclude gallstones may be required, depending on the constellation of symptoms. Patients with persistent pain, diarrhea, and weight loss should undergo serologic testing for celiac disease.[19] Complaints of excess gas and bloating should be evaluated with a kidney, ureter, and bladder (KUB) scan of the abdomen. Patients with suspected urogenital causes of abdominal pain require further diagnostic testing or referral to a gynecologist.

DIAGNOSTICS

Irritable Bowel Syndrome

LABORATORY
CBC with differential
ESR
Serum electrolytes, BUN, creatinine, glucose
TSH
Stool for occult blood and fecal leukocytes (if fecal leukocytes are present, test for enteric pathogens, ova and parasites, and *C. difficile*)
LFTs*
Serum IgA tissue transglutaminase antibody (if celiac disease is a consideration)*
Hydrogen breath test*

IMAGING
KUB study (flat plate and upright)*
Barium enema*
Abdominal ultrasound*

OTHER DIAGNOSTICS
Flexible sigmoidoscopy or colonoscopy*

*If indicated.
IgA, immunoglobulin A.

If the initial diagnostic screen is negative, treatment of symptoms should be initiated and reevaluated in 3 to 6 weeks. This diagnostic strategy allows a more conservative and cost-effective evaluation. If the initial treatment fails, additional diagnostic studies or a referral to a gastroenterologist may be considered. IBS patients older than 50 years with new or changed symptoms require repeated evaluation.

DIFFERENTIAL DIAGNOSIS

A number of organic diseases have presentations similar to those of IBS. It is essential that they be considered in the diagnostic reasoning process. Colon cancer, inflammatory bowel disease, cholecystitis, pancreatic insufficiency, intestinal ischemia, intestinal parasites, lactase deficiency, fructose intolerance, malabsorption syndromes such as celiac disease, and viral gastroenteritis can cause abdominal pain or a change in bowel habits. Medications can cause constipation or diarrhea. Hypothyroidism can cause constipation, whereas hyperthyroidism and diabetes can cause diarrhea. Psychiatric conditions, including anxiety disorders, depression, and somatization, should be considered in the evaluation of the patient with a change in bowel habits.[1,10,19] Urogenital causes, such as PID, endometriosis, ovarian cyst, and uterine fibroid, should be considered in women with lower abdominal pain and gynecologic symptoms.

DIFFERENTIAL DIAGNOSIS

Irritable Bowel Syndrome

Endocrine disorders
- Thyroid disease
- Diabetes-related diarrhea

Gastrointestinal disorders
- Cholecystitis
- Fructose intolerance
- Intestinal ischemia
- Intestinal parasites
- Malabsorption syndromes (celiac disease)
- Pancreatic insufficiency
- Viral gastroenteritis

Medication effects

Psychiatric disorders
- Anxiety
- Depression
- Somatization

Urogenital causes
- PID, endometriosis, ovarian cysts, uterine fibroid

MANAGEMENT

The focus of IBS treatment is symptomatic and includes dietary modifications, medications, supportive and behavioral therapy, education, and reassurance. At times, patients will require medications.[1,3,5,16] One important factor in the successful management of IBS appears to be the establishment of a therapeutic relationship. A nonjudgmental, attentive approach is essential to assist patients in shifting their focus from finding the cause of their symptoms to finding a way to cope with them. Health care providers must make the correct diagnosis as early as possible, initiate appropriate treatment, and avoid expensive or unnecessary tests.

Because both physiologic and psychosocial factors appear to play a role in the severity of symptoms and the expression of illness, both must be considered in the development of a management plan.[1,3,5,10,22] Diagnosis and treatment of any underlying psychological disorder, such as anxiety and depression, are essential.[1,3,5,10] Most patients (75%) with IBS have mild symptoms and can be managed in a primary care setting. They usually respond to education, reassurance, and dietary and lifestyle modifications. A smaller number have moderate symptoms that can be intermittent and disabling. Patients may have psychological distress from their symptoms, but their symptoms correlate with gut physiology.[14,15,18] Cognitive behavioral therapy can be effective for patients with IBS, depression, and anxiety. In some cases, psychological counseling may be indicated (quality of evidence: low).[22,23] A small number of patients have severe and refractory symptoms associated with psychosocial difficulties and require antidepressant medication, mental health referral, and possibly a pain management evaluation.[5] These patients require a team approach that includes comanagement with a gastroenterologist.

Dietary Modification

Although true food allergies are uncommon, many patients with IBS report food intolerances.[10,13,19] Some studies suggest a correlation between various ingested allergens and the symptoms of IBS.[13] In some cases, it is not what the patient eats but rather the act of eating that precipitates symptoms; large meals can cause cramping and diarrhea.[5,10] Gas, bloating, distention, and a change in bowel habits are often attributed to the intake of certain foods (Box 139-2). Dairy products and gas-forming foods are the most common offenders. Other foods and beverages that may cause or aggravate symptoms include items artificially sweetened with fructose or sorbitol, carbonated beverages, caffeine, and alcohol.[5,10,13,24]

BOX 139-2

Common Gas-Forming Foods

- Beans, lentils, and other legumes
- Beer
- Broccoli
- Brussels sprouts
- Cabbage
- Carbonated beverages
- Cauliflower
- Coffee
- Grapes
- Plums
- Raisins
- Raw onions
- Red wine

Although care should be taken to avoid unnecessary dietary restrictions because evidence of benefit is unclear,[25] the initial recommendations should focus on elimination of foods suspected of causing or aggravating individual symptoms.[1] Use of a diary to record food intake and symptoms can help identify offending foods.[5] Some patients may benefit from referral to a nutritionist. Lactose intolerance should be excluded in all patients who initially are seen with symptoms of IBS.[1] Consideration should be given to hydrogen breath testing or recommendation of a 2- to 3-week trial of a lactose-free diet. Although there is no evidence that food allergy testing and food elimination diets are effective, many patients recognize these triggers and may choose to avoid these foods.[9,19] Instructions should also include a recommendation to avoid medications that could aggravate symptoms, such as stimulant laxatives and antacids with laxative effects in patients with cramping or diarrhea-predominant IBS. Stimulant laxatives usually do not improve abdominal pain. Soluble fiber therapy in IBS is now recommended (quality of evidence: moderate).[5,23] Fiber is likely to decrease constipation, but its role in relieving abdominal pain and diarrhea is less clear. Fiber is a safe and inexpensive way to treat IBS. Insoluble fiber, such as that found in wheat bran and corn, often increases symptoms of bloating and abdominal pain because of colonic distention and should therefore be provided in incremental steps of 2 to 3 g each day.[5] Clinical experience has demonstrated that many patients benefit from fiber after an initial period of bloating and abdominal discomfort. A trial of a minimum of 20 g of fiber per day, which should be gradually added, seems reasonable for the treatment of IBS.[5,19]

Synthetic fiber supplements are more soluble than natural fiber and may be better tolerated.[5] Slow introduction of the fiber load helps reduce gas and bloating. A number of commercial products are available as over-the-counter formulations. No one brand seems to have an advantage over another, although individual responses vary. Providers should instruct patients to try a different brand if one seems ineffective or produces side effects. Use of psyllium (Metamucil), calcium polycarbophil (FiberCon), or methylcellulose (Citrucel) taken daily with food or 8 ounces of liquid is a pharmacologic consideration (quality of evidence: moderate).[23] An alternative to synthetic fiber is a diet high in whole grains and natural fiber, a daily fluid intake of 64 ounces, and a set time each day to use the bathroom. Exercise has been shown to improve many health problems[5]; however, no data provide support for routine exercise and the improvement of symptoms.

Pharmacotherapy

Antispasmodics. Despite a lack of clinical evidence to support benefit, antispasmodics seem to slow bowel contractions, decreasing symptoms of diarrhea and discomfort (quality of evidence: low).[23] Anticholinergics act to reduce sigmoid motility in response to a fatty meal. Medications such as dicyclomine (Bentyl), 10 to 40 mg four times daily as needed, may be tried by patients who experience postprandial abdominal pain, gas, and bloating. For maximum effectiveness to be achieved, the medication should be taken 30 to 60 minutes before meals. Hyoscyamine sulfate, the active ingredient in Levsin and Donnatal, is also an effective antispasmodic but has several side effects, including urinary retention, tachycardia, and dry mouth. Clidinium, the active ingredient in Librax and Clindex, has fatigue as a common side effect. Dicyclomine acts more selectively on the smooth muscle of the GI tract and may produce fewer side effects than the nonselective anticholinergics. Analgesic medications, particularly narcotics, should be avoided if at all possible.

Antidiarrheal Agents. Loperamide (Imodium), 2 to 4 mg four times daily as needed, decreases intestinal transit time, enhances intestinal water absorption, and strengthens rectal sphincter tone, thereby improving the diarrhea, urgency, and fecal soiling in IBS patients with diarrhea (quality of evidence: low).[23] Patients may take a maximum of 16 mg per day as needed to control symptoms. Polycarbophil can be added to help increase stool bulk. Pepto-Bismol, Kaopectate, and bile acid–sequestering agents, such as cholestyramine (Questran, Prevalite), should also be considered in the treatment of diarrhea-predominant IBS. Rifaximin (Xifaxan), a miscellaneous antibiotic, has also been used successfully in the treatment of diarrhea-associated IBS (quality of evidence: moderate).[23] Alosetron (Lotronex), a 5-HT_3 receptor antagonist, is used for the treatment of abdominal pain, diarrhea, and bloating in women with severe, chronic diarrhea associated IBS who have not responded to other therapies (quality of evidence: moderate).[23] However, alosetron should be prescribed only by physicians participating in a prescribing program for this medication.

Anticonstipation Agents. Synthetic fiber is beneficial in treating constipation associated with IBS. In addition to fiber therapy, increase in fluids, and regular exercise, patients with constipation may benefit from stool softeners and osmotic laxatives such as lactulose and polyethylene glycol (MiraLax), though evidence is lacking to support its use (quality of evidence: very low).[23] Stimulant laxatives should be avoided whenever possible. Lubiprostone (Amitiza) was approved by the U.S. Food and Drug Administration (FDA) for chronic constipation and IBS associated with constipation (quality of evidence: moderate).[23] The newest anticonstipation agent to be approved is linaclotide (Linzess). Linaclotide works on the guanylate cyclase-C receptor to decrease the absorption of sodium ions, which allows the secretion of water to assist in defecation; the drug is also approved for IBS associated with constipation (quality of evidence: high).[23,25]

Psychotropic Agents. Antidepressants, including tricyclic agents and selective serotonin reuptake inhibitors (SSRIs), are often used to treat IBS, particularly in patients with severe or refractory pain and symptoms, impaired daily function, and associated depression or panic attacks (quality of evidence: high).[1,5,10,23,25] The anticholinergic properties of the tricyclic antidepressants (amitriptyline, nortriptyline, desipramine) are believed to contribute to their effectiveness in treating the pain, gas, bloating, and frequent stools associated with IBS. Small clinical trials have shown benefit in alleviating abdominal pain. Because of their tendency to decrease transit times, which in turn causes constipation, the use of tricyclic agents should be avoided in IBS patients with constipation.[1]

Because of the lower side effect profile of SSRIs, these should be considered in patients with constipation instead of tricyclic agents.[1,5,10] These medications reduce depression, anxiety, and somatization rather than relieving abdominal pain per se. A common side effect of SSRIs is diarrhea; therefore these drugs may prove most beneficial in treating IBS patients with constipation. There is no clinical research to support the use of benzodiazepines in IBS; their use should be avoided because of their addictive potential.

Alternative Therapies

Several alternative therapies have been studied in IBS, including cognitive behavioral therapy, hypnosis, guided imagery, relaxation techniques, and stress management.[5] Acupuncture decreased symptoms in some studies, but not all.[3,25] Alternative therapies seem to have some value in reducing GI symptoms, anxiety, and other psychological symptoms.[3] Patients with underlying psychological issues may benefit from a referral to a psychologist, mental health clinical nurse specialist, or psychiatric nurse practitioner. Patients with severe, refractory pain should be referred to a pain management program.[3,5]

Probiotics are live microorganisms similar to the normal bacterial flora of the GI tract. Some studies have shown a stimulation of the immune response that improved IBS symptoms.[1,5] Probiotics reduce inflammation or alter gut flora, and seem to decrease flatulence and relieve bloating; however, the use of probiotics remains controversial (quality of evidence: low).[3,5,10,23]

Peppermint oil is a natural spasmodic. Its GI effects are similar to those of calcium channel blockers, causing smooth muscle relaxation and aiding postprandial pain and bloating (quality of evidence: moderate).[23]

LIFE SPAN CONSIDERATIONS

IBS is a chronic recurrent disorder that frequently develops in late adolescence to early adulthood and continues throughout the life span. Exacerbations are common and often correlate with life stressors. Once thought to be a disease of young women, IBS is increasingly being recognized in men and older adults. An IBS diagnosis in an older person must be made cautiously and in consultation with a gastroenterologist to avoid missing a more serious diagnosis.

COMPLICATIONS

It is important to recognize that IBS is a chronic recurrent GI disorder in the majority of cases; serious complications from IBS are extremely rare. In some patients, the chronic nature of symptoms leads to a reduced quality of life and clinical depression. Chronic constipation may also result in hemorrhoids, anal fissures, fecal impaction, and, rarely, intestinal obstruction.

INDICATIONS FOR REFERRAL OR HOSPITALIZATION

Nocturnal symptoms, bloody stools, fever, and weight loss are incompatible with a diagnosis of IBS and require immediate further diagnostic evaluation or referral (Box 139-3). Physician consultation and referral to a gastroenterologist are indicated if initial treatment of IBS fails, if organic disease is suspected or found, or if the patient is older than 50 years or has an established diagnosis of IBS and is reporting a change in the usual

BOX 139-3

Emergency "Red Flag" Criteria

Symptoms that are incompatible with irritable bowel syndrome and require immediate diagnostic evaluation or referral include the following:

- Nocturnal symptoms
- Rectal bleeding
- Bloody stools
- Fever
- Unintentional weight loss
- Anemia
- Recurrent nausea or vomiting
- First-degree relative with gastrointestinal malignant disease, IBS, or ovarian cancer
- Abnormal physical examination findings
- Signs of anemia
- Abdominal mass
- Elevated CA 125
- Rectal mass

BOX 139-4

Indications for Referral

- Initial treatment failure
- Suspicion of organic disease
- Change in bowel habits in a patient older than 50 years
- Change in usual IBS symptom pattern

pattern of symptoms (Box 139-4). Gastroenterology specialists are also helpful in the co-management of a patient with complex IBS.

PATIENT AND FAMILY EDUCATION

Dietary and lifestyle modifications, such as avoiding foods that trigger symptoms, increasing fluids and fiber, getting regular exercise, and using alternative therapies, should be discussed with patients.[1,10] Information about what constitutes "normal" bowel habits should be provided. Bowel retraining should be encouraged by recommending sitting on the toilet (without straining) for 15 to 20 minutes each morning after breakfast. Medications for symptom control should be reviewed, including a conversation about laxative abuse.

Patients should be informed that the symptoms of IBS are very real and are caused by increased sensitivity and reactivity of the gut to stimuli, resulting in pain or abnormal motility. They should be reassured that IBS is a chronic condition characterized by periods of remission and exacerbation that often correlate with physical and psychological stressors but that IBS usually does not lead to cancer or inflammatory bowel disease.[3,5,10,19] Patients need to understand that although there is no cure, there is help, and most patients learn to cope with their symptoms and lead productive lives.[3,10]

HEALTH PROMOTION

The chronic nature of IBS symptoms may cause a patient with IBS to ignore a change in bowel habits resulting from an organic condition. Patients need to be instructed that although IBS does not increase their risk for colorectal cancer, a change in bowel habits that is atypical for their usual pattern of symptoms should be reported to the health care provider. In addition, screening for colorectal cancer per current guidelines is important for all patients.

CHAPTER 140

JAUNDICE

Melissa A. Hall

DEFINITION AND EPIDEMIOLOGY

Jaundice, or icterus, is a yellow or greenish discoloration of the skin, sclerae, and mucous membranes caused by bile pigments of conjugated or unconjugated bilirubin.[1] There are multiple causes of jaundice, necessitating determination of the underlying disorder.

Jaundice can be divided into three categories: prehepatic, hepatic, and posthepatic. Prehepatic jaundice is caused by conditions that produce excessive bilirubin. Examples include any condition that causes hemolysis. Hepatic jaundice is a result of hepatic injury, including infections, toxins, autoimmune disorders, and tumors. Posthepatic jaundice, also called *obstructive jaundice,* is a result of complete or partial obstruction of the bile ducts. Pancreatic tumors and gallstones are the most common causes of posthepatic jaundice.[2]

The causes of jaundice are categorized according to (1) symptoms (acute or chronic), (2) evidence of bile duct dilation, and (3) jaundice of the conjugated or unconjugated varieties.[1] Jaundice is common in newborns and occurs in 60% to 80% of term infants 4 to 14 days after birth.[2] In older children and young adults, common causes include viral hepatitis (accounts for 75% of jaundice in patients younger than 30 years), Gilbert syndrome, drug-induced hepatitis, pregnancy, cirrhosis, and alcoholic hepatitis. In older patients, the most common causes are cirrhosis (accounts for 30% of jaundice in the 30- to 60-year-old age group), pancreatic cancer, metastatic cancer to the liver, sepsis, common bile duct stone, and medication-induced hepatitis.[3] Alcoholic liver disease, associated with loneliness and depression, is a common cause in older adults.[3] Common causes of jaundice are presented in Box 140-1.

Physician consultation is indicated for patients with new-onset jaundice.

PATHOPHYSIOLOGY

The liver plays a major role in the metabolism of bile pigments. This process is divided into three distinct phases: (1) hepatic uptake, (2) conjugation, and (3) excretion.[1] A byproduct of hemolysis is bilirubin, which is produced through the breakdown of hemoglobin in red blood cells (RBCs). There are two forms of bilirubin: indirect, or unconjugated, bilirubin (which is protein bound) and direct, or conjugated, bilirubin. The direct form circulates freely in the blood until it reaches the liver, where it is conjugated with glucuronide transferase and excreted into the bile.[1] An increase in unconjugated bilirubin is often

BOX 140-1

Classification and Causes of Jaundice

UNCONJUGATED HYPERBILIRUBINEMIA (PREDOMINANTLY INDIRECT-ACTING BILIRUBIN)

- Increased bilirubin production
- Hemolytic anemias (thalassemias, sideroblastic anemias, some pernicious anemias), hematoma, infarction
- Decreased hepatic uptake
- Posthepatitis, drug reactions, sepsis, prolonged fasting
- Decreased bilirubin conjugation (decreased hepatic glucuronosyltransferase)
- Hereditary transferase deficiency (Gilbert syndrome, Crigler-Najjar syndrome)
- Acquired transferase deficiency: drug inhibition (e.g., chloramphenicol), breast milk, hepatocellular disease
- Neonatal jaundice
- Ineffective erythropoiesis (megaloblastic anemias)
- Hematomas
- Pulmonary emboli
- Chronic hepatitis

CONJUGATED HYPERBILIRUBINEMIA (PREDOMINANTLY DIRECT-ACTING BILIRUBIN)

- Impaired excretion: intrahepatic defects
- Familial defects (Dubin-Johnson syndrome, Rotor syndrome), recurrent intrahepatic cholestasis, cholestatic jaundice of pregnancy
- Acquired disorders: viral or drug-induced hepatitis, cirrhosis, sepsis, postoperative complications, androgens, chlorpromazine, acetaminophen, sulfonamides, NSAIDs, aspirin, industrial poisons
- Impaired excretion: extrahepatic defects
- Gallstones, biliary malformation or strictures, infection, biliary or pancreatic tumors, chronic pancreatitis, pancreatic pseudocyst, metastasis to the hepatic hilum, primary bile duct lymphoma

NSAIDs, non-steroidal anti-inflammatory drugs.

associated with an increase in the destruction of RBCs. An increase in conjugated bilirubin is more likely seen with liver dysfunction or obstruction.[1] Disturbance in the passage of conjugated bilirubin from the liver to the intestine accounts for 60% of jaundice in patients older than 60 years. With bile duct obstruction, bilirubin is conjugated by the hepatocytes but cannot flow into the duodenum.[1] Therefore bilirubin accumulates in the liver and enters the bloodstream, causing hyperbilirubinemia.

Extrahepatic obstructive jaundice develops if the common bile duct is occluded by gallstones or tumors, especially pancreatic carcinoma or strictures.[1,2] Because conjugated bilirubin is water soluble, it is excreted in the urine. This produces the characteristic orange urine with elevated conjugated bilirubin produced by inflammation.

Intrahepatic obstructive jaundice involves disturbances in hepatocyte function or obstruction of bile canaliculi. The uptake, conjugation, and excretion of bilirubin are affected, resulting in increased levels of conjugated and unconjugated bilirubin.[1]

Failure of liver cells to conjugate bilirubin causes hepatocellular damage, resulting in increased plasma concentrations of unconjugated bilirubin. In addition, bilirubin cannot pass from the liver to the intestine.[1] The causes of hepatocellular damage include infections, medications, toxins, and genetic defects causing decreased enzyme production.

Hemolytic jaundice is caused by excessive hemolysis of RBCs. An increased amount of unconjugated bilirubin is formed through metabolism of the heme component of destroyed RBCs and exceeds the conjugation ability of the liver.[1,4] This causes the blood levels of unconjugated bilirubin to rise. Hemolysis can occur with blood transfusion reactions, after cardiopulmonary bypass, with sickle cell anemia, and with marrow or splenic destruction of RBCs. In sickle cell anemia, abnormal hemoglobin and a fragile cell membrane lead to hemolysis and an increase in the amount of free, unconjugated bilirubin.[1] Bone marrow development problems and defective erythropoiesis are conditions in which poorly manufactured erythrocytes are fragile and have a short life span. The result is an excess of unconjugated bilirubin that reaches the liver for conjugation.[1] The most common causes of jaundice are hepatocellular destruction and mechanical obstruction of the biliary tracts.[1,2]

CLINICAL PRESENTATION

Jaundice is most commonly observed in the face, trunk, and sclera. Bilirubin is distributed uniformly in the sclera and is differentiated from the normal occurrence of the yellow subscleral fat that collects in the periphery.[5] In African Americans, the hard palate or ventral surface of the tongue helps clinical jaundice to be observed.[5] Jaundice caused by carotene does not stain the sclera but rather is seen in the forehead, around the alae nasi, and in the palms and soles. The patient with jaundice may have pruritus, which often accompanies obstructive jaundice. The pruritus is caused by nerve injury in the skin by the bile pigments.[5] Cutaneous xanthomas may be seen in patients with jaundice from chronic cholestasis and suggest hypercholesterolemia. The presence of spider angiomas, palmar erythema, and ascites combined with malaise, anorexia, and right upper quadrant discomfort suggests chronic hepatocellular disease or cirrhosis. Colicky right upper quadrant pain, weight loss, and light-colored stools may be present in obstructive jaundice. Intermittent, colicky right upper quadrant pain before the onset of jaundice suggests choledocholithiasis.[5] Fever and chills may accompany biliary obstruction and virus- or drug-induced hepatitis. Occult blood in the stools suggests cancer as a cause of jaundice.[6]

Appropriate history includes determining whether the jaundice is acute or chronic and ascertaining associated symptoms (e.g., fever, weight loss, anorexia, rash, pruritus, abdominal pain, or musculoskeletal aches and pains). In acute jaundice, inquiry focuses on hepatitis risks: recent travel; transfusions; tattoos; intravenous drug use; alcohol intake; medications (prescription drugs, herbals, or over-the-counter preparations); food, toxin, animal, or infected person exposures; unsafe sexual practices; and symptoms of biliary tract disease.[2] Chronic jaundice may suggest hepatitis (B, C, D, or autoimmune), biliary tract disease, pancreatitis, or chronic alcohol intake. Weight loss, anorexia, malaise, and other symptoms of cancer are noted. In addition, a list of medications (including over-the-counter medications) and a complete family history, including cancer, Wilson disease, Gilbert syndrome, hemochromatosis, and hereditary hemolytic anemias, provide vital information for an appropriate diagnosis. Exposure to toxins, including use of herbal products, and a surgical history should also be elicited.[2,7]

PHYSICAL EXAMINATION

Acute jaundice requires a complete examination for the cause of the illness to be determined. Essential components are determination of vital signs (including temperature); evaluation of the skin (including the palms and soles), sclera, and mucous membranes; assessment of the cardiovascular system for congestive heart failure; and evaluation of the abdomen for ascites, organomegaly, guarding, and tenderness.[1,3] Fever and right upper quadrant tenderness are most often associated with choledocholithiasis, cholangitis, or cholecystitis. An enlarged, tender liver suggests acute hepatic inflammation or a rapidly growing hepatic tumor.[2] Splenomegaly suggests portal hypertension from acute or active chronic hepatitis as well as cirrhosis.[5]

Chronic jaundice mandates evaluation for chronic liver disease. Gynecomastia, testicular atrophy, and splenomegaly are strongly associated with cirrhosis.[5] In addition, palmar erythema, facial telangiectasia, and Dupuytren contractures are associated with cirrhosis from chronic ethanol ingestion.[8] Lymphadenopathy suggests malignant disease and can be related to a pancreatic tumor obstructing the splenic vein or to a metastatic lymphoma. When malignant disease is suspected, the investigation should concentrate on determining the location of the primary tumor as indicated by heme-positive stool, abdominal masses, breast masses, thyroid nodules, or supraclavicular lymphadenopathy.[6] Physical findings associated with specific liver diseases include distended neck veins and hepatojugular reflux (right-sided heart failure), xanthomas (primary biliary cirrhosis), and Kayser-Fleischer rings (Wilson disease).[5]

DIAGNOSTICS

Liver function tests (LFTs)—including albumin, aspartate aminotransferase (AST), and alanine aminotransferase (ALT); total and direct serum bilirubin; serum alkaline phosphatase; stool guaiac; and urine bilirubin—are performed in addition to a complete blood count (CBC) with platelet count and a prothrombin time (PT). Elevated ALT and AST levels result from hepatocellular necrosis or inflammation.[1] An AST level that is more than twice the ALT level is typical with alcoholic liver injury. Elevated alkaline phosphatase levels suggest cholestasis, primary biliary cirrhosis, or infiltrative liver disease (e.g., tumor, abscess, granulomas).[7] In obstructive liver disease, the alkaline phosphatase may be more than three times the normal level.[8]

When the jaundice is not related to a biliary disorder or hepatic injury, the liver enzymes will be normal. A normal serum albumin concentration suggests a more acute disease process than the chronic disease associated with low serum albumin levels.[9]

Unconjugated (indirect) hyperbilirubinemia suggests a hemolytic disorder, such as an autoimmune or microangiopathic hemolytic anemia. The most common cause of mild elevations of unconjugated bilirubin is Gilbert syndrome, which affects up to 7% of the population with a male predominance.[1]

Direct hyperbilirubinemia results from hepatocellular inflammation, cholestatic liver disease, or extrahepatic biliary obstruction. The presence of direct hyperbilirubinemia without liver enzyme abnormalities is uncommon but is seen in pregnancy, in sepsis, or after recent surgery.[10,11] Patients with elevated conjugated bilirubin should be evaluated for evidence of viral hepatitis, drug toxicity, or hepatic congestion. Serologic studies are used to diagnose hepatitis A, B, C, and D.[2] Common causes of toxic hepatitis include acetaminophen, allopurinol, androgenic steroids, aspirin and other salicylates, nitrofurantoin, azathioprine, contraceptive steroids, chlorpromazine, erythromycin, glucocorticoids, mercaptopurine, methotrexate, plicamycin, nonsteroidal anti-inflammatory drugs (NSAIDs), and sulfonamides.[12]

In patients with chronic liver disease lacking a defined cause, serum iron, transferrin saturation, and ferritin should be measured to screen for hemochromatosis. In hemochromatosis, the serum ferritin concentration is substantially elevated. Plasma iron levels may exceed 200 μg/dL, and transferrin saturation exceeds 70%.[13] In patients younger than 30 years with abnormal LFT results or in patients with hepatitis who test negative for viruses A, B, C, and D and neurologic dysfunction, measurements of serum ceruloplasmin and urine copper levels are recommended to screen for Wilson disease.[2] Other laboratory diagnostics to consider include antimitochondrial antibodies (for primary biliary cirrhosis), antinuclear anti–smooth muscle and liver-kidney microsomal antibodies (for autoimmune hepatitis), and α_1-antitrypsin activity (for α_1-antitrypsin deficiency).[2]

Hepatobiliary imaging is recommended if the liver chemistry profile suggests cholestasis or extrahepatic obstruction. Ultrasonography is more than 90% specific and close to 90% sensitive in detecting obstruction. A computed tomography (CT) scan with and without the administration of contrast material is indicated in cases in which ultrasound examination is unsatisfactory.[14] However, ultrasonography is an effective means of detecting stones in the gallbladder and is somewhat more sensitive than a CT scan.[14] Endoscopic retrograde cholangiopancreatography (ERCP) or percutaneous transhepatic cholangiography is indicated if extrahepatic obstruction is strongly suspected.[14] ERCP may relieve the obstruction in the majority of cases. Newer imaging techniques to evaluate biliary obstruction and suspected malignant neoplasms include magnetic resonance cholangiopancreatography and endoscopic ultrasonography.[14]

DIAGNOSTICS

Jaundice

LABORATORY
- LFTs
- CBC and differential, platelets
- PT/PTT
- Hepatitis profile*
- Serum electrolytes, BUN, and creatinine
- Serum iron, transferrin saturation, ferritin
- Serum ceruloplasmin
- Antimitochondrial antibodies
- Antinuclear anti–smooth muscle and liver-kidney microsomal antibodies
- α_1-Antitrypsin activity
- Urine copper
- Urine bilirubin
- HIV

IMAGING
- Ultrasonography
- Helical CT scan

OTHER DIAGNOSTICS
- ERCP or percutaneous transhepatic cholangiography*
- Magnetic resonance cholangiopancreatography and endoscopic ultrasonography
- Percutaneous transhepatic cholangiography
- Liver biopsy

*If indicated.
BUN, blood urea nitrogen; HIV, human immunodeficiency virus; PTT, partial thromboplastin time.

Percutaneous liver biopsy is the definitive study for determination of the cause and extent of hepatocellular dysfunction or infiltrative liver disease, particularly if metastatic disease or a hepatic mass is suspected.[2]

DIFFERENTIAL DIAGNOSIS

The etiology of jaundice is multifactorial; consequently, the presence of coexisting disease is an important aspect of the evaluation. The finding of unconjugated hyperbilirubinemia can be related to increased bilirubin production (hemolytic anemia) or impaired bilirubin uptake and storage (hepatitis sequelae, posthepatitis conditions, Gilbert syndrome, drug reactions). Hereditary syndromes such as Crigler-Najjar and Gilbert syndromes (resulting from impaired glucuronosyltransferase activity) and Dubin-Johnson and Rotor syndromes (resulting from faulty excretion of bilirubin) are examples of causes of unconjugated bilirubin.[1] Conjugated hyperbilirubinemia can be caused by hepatitis, cirrhosis, cholestasis, postoperative jaundice, spirochetal infections, infectious mononucleosis, sarcoidosis, lymphomas, and industrial toxins. Fever and chills suggest cholangitis. Causes of biliary obstructions include tumors, choledochal cysts, choledocholithiasis, pancreatitis, pancreatic neoplasms, and cholestatic jaundice of pregnancy. Jaundice during pregnancy is most commonly related to viral hepatitis.[10]

DIFFERENTIAL DIAGNOSIS

Jaundice

- Hepatitis, infective
- Hepatitis, autoimmune
- Gilbert syndrome
- Drug reaction, including over-the-counter and herbal products
- Hemolytic anemia
- Hereditary syndromes
- Cirrhosis
- Cholestasis
- Postoperative jaundice
- Cholestatic jaundice of pregnancy
- Spirochete infection
- Infectious mononucleosis
- Sarcoidosis
- Lymphoma
- Toxins
- Cholangitis
- Tumor
- Choledochal cysts
- Choledocholithiasis
- Pancreatitis
- Hepatobiliary tuberculosis

MANAGEMENT

The treatment of jaundice relates to the underlying disease process. Most patients with viral hepatitis can be treated symptomatically on an outpatient basis (see Chapter 137). When liver enzymes fail to return to normal levels within 6 months, liver biopsy is indicated.[2] Cholangitis requires antibiotic therapy and surgical consultation. For patients with cholangitis, nonoperative biliary drainage can be performed through ERCP with transhepatically placed stents.[15] Surgical therapy is usually required for extrahepatic biliary obstruction. Gilbert disease, Dubin-Johnson syndrome, and Rotor syndrome beyond the neonatal period rarely require treatment to lower the bilirubin level. However, treatment of the primary disease process may require corticosteroids if the presentation of these diseases is complicated by hemolytic anemia.

The treatment of uncomplicated cirrhosis consists of voluntary restriction of activity if the patient has weakness and fatigue. The diet should be high in protein but low in sodium, and alcohol should be avoided. This regimen almost invariably results in improvement of hepatocellular function in patients with alcohol-induced cirrhosis.[16] Multivitamins and folic acid (1 mg/day) may be given if the patient's diet is inadequate. Tranquilizers and sedatives should be avoided. When serum potassium concentration falls below 3.5 mEq/L, the deficit of body potassium is approximately 300 to 500 mEq. This can be replaced during a few days with oral solutions of 10% potassium chloride, which provide 40 mEq of potassium/30 mL.[17] Protein can be restricted in stable cirrhotic patients to 45 g/day as long as there is a minimum of 400 g of carbohydrates ingested each day. Vegetable protein contains smaller amounts of ammonia, methionine, and aromatic acids and is better tolerated by these patients.[18] Lactulose is a nonabsorbable synthetic disaccharide that reduces blood ammonia and improves encephalopathy in the majority of patients when it is administered in doses of 20 to 30 g three or four times daily.[17] Rifaximin, 550 mg twice daily, can be considered if encephalopathy is worsening with lactulose alone. It reduces encephalopathy risk by killing ammonia-producing bacteria in the gut.[17] Patients with decompensated cirrhosis who are not responding to therapy should be considered for liver transplantation.[2] A one-time dose of vitamin K, 5 to 25 mg orally or 10 mg subcutaneously or intramuscularly, may improve clotting times. The dose may be repeated in 12 hours if necessary. An intravenous infusion of vitamin K is not recommended because of the risk of anaphylaxis.[17]

Pruritus, which is commonly associated with jaundice, may be disabling to some patients, resulting in depression. Early treatment with agents such as cholestyramine three times per day and antihistamines three or four times daily is recommended.[19] Fragrance-free soaps, less frequent bathing, and use of emollients may also reduce the severity of pruritus.[19] Continued monitoring of LFT results, serologic values, and the results of hematologic studies of blood counts, platelets, and PT as indicated are recommended for all patients with jaundice for detection of complications.

COMPLICATIONS

The complications of jaundice are directly related to the underlying disease process. In cirrhosis, infection and gastrointestinal bleeding often precipitate decompensation. Potassium deficiency is common in cirrhosis and may contribute to hepatic encephalopathy.[2]

Patients with hepatitis may experience one or two relapses during their recovery period. Complications of other underlying diseases associated with jaundice range from anemia to gastrointestinal infection, hepatocellular damage, encephalopathy, and postsurgical complications. The most serious postsurgical complication of stenting is recurrent jaundice from stent occlusion and recurrent cholangitis.[15]

INDICATIONS FOR REFERRAL OR HOSPITALIZATION

The management of patients with jaundice is often a complex process because of the myriad underlying disease processes and the potential complications. The primary care physician is always consulted to determine the diagnosis and initial management plans. Consultation with a gastroenterologist, hepatologist, or surgeon is also often indicated. For patients with hepatitis B or C infection, referral to a gastroenterologist is necessary to ensure appropriate serologic testing and treatment.

PATIENT AND FAMILY EDUCATION

It is imperative that patients understand the underlying disease process and prevention regimens. The Centers for Disease Control and Prevention (CDC) now recommends that all high-risk individuals be screened for hepatitis B and hepatitis C and that all individuals born in the years 1945 to 1965 be offered hepatitis C screening once.[20] The CDC makes recommendations for immunization against hepatitis B and hepatitis C for all age groups.[21] The appropriate levels of activity and rest, the importance of medication adherence, the need for avoidance of over-the-counter medications that interfere with hepatic function, and the avoidance of any liver-toxic chemicals including alcohol should be emphasized. Appropriate dietary instruction is essential for patients with hepatic disease, and referral to a dietitian for instruction in specific diets is desirable.

CHAPTER 141

NAUSEA AND VOMITING

Brad E. Franklin

DEFINITION AND EPIDEMIOLOGY

Nausea and vomiting significantly affect quality of life and are common presenting complaints in primary care.[1] One study of primary practice reported that nausea and vomiting ranked second to upper respiratory infections as presenting problems in primary care.[2] Nausea and vomiting present a diagnostic challenge to health care providers because of the varied causes such as infection, chronic medical conditions, and even treatment modalities. The health care provider needs not only to control the symptoms and to prevent complications but also to successfully diagnose and treat the underlying disease.[2,3]

Nausea is defined as an unpleasant or queasy, but painless, sensation that one is about to vomit. Actual vomiting may or may not occur.[1,4] Nausea usually lasts longer than vomiting and is generally relieved by vomiting. Vomiting, the forceful expulsion of liquid or food from the stomach through the mouth, should be differentiated from other symptoms that are often described by patients as vomiting, such as retching (rhythmic contractions of the respiratory and abdominal muscles without expulsion of gastric contents) or regurgitation (an effortless backward flow of food and liquids from the stomach to the mouth).[4,5] Vomiting is a protective mechanism from harmful ingested substances, but it can result from underlying disease affecting the gastrointestinal tract or surrounding structures, metabolic or endocrine function, or the central nervous system, or it can be an adverse effect of disease interventions (e.g., chemotherapy).[1,2]

Emergency consultation is indicated if nausea and vomiting are accompanied by pain, severe dehydration, acute abdomen, fever, neurologic changes, or a metabolic imbalance.

PATHOPHYSIOLOGY

Vomiting is a reflex action controlled by two major central nervous system centers: the vomiting center (VC) and the chemoreceptor trigger zone (CTZ).[2,5,6] The VC, a collection of neurons within the medulla, is stimulated by input from multiple mechanisms including pharyngeal, vagal, and midbrain afferents and the limbic system. Mechanical irritation can stimulate the pharyngeal afferents, leading to retching and then vomiting. The presence of noxious substances in the stomach and duodenum and the mechanical distention and contraction can sensitize chemoreceptors, and mechanical receptors can stimulate the vagal afferent pathways, which in turn stimulate the VC, leading to vomiting.[5,7]

The CTZ, located on the floor of the fourth ventricle, is directly sensitive to chemical agents with known emetogenic potential. It is sensitive to stimulation from serotonin, dopamine, histamine, cholinergic, adrenergic, and opiate receptors. The pharmacologic basis of most antiemetics is to block these neurotransmitters. The CTZ identifies harmful substances and transmits the information to the VC, which then initiates the vomiting reflex. Neurotransmitters, vagal afferents, or noxious agents can stimulate the CTZ, resulting in the stimulation of the VC.[5,7]

THE VOMITING REFLEX

No matter the cause of the stimulation of the VC, once stimulated it initiates a sequence of events that end with vomiting. There are three phases of vomiting: pre-ejection, ejection, and postejection. During pre-ejection, there is an increase in salivation and swallowing and a decrease in gastric tone; tachycardia, pallor, and diaphoresis occur. Relaxation of the proximal stomach and contraction of the small intestine ensue, leading to regurgitation of contents into the stomach. Pre-ejection is mediated by acetylcholine and the vagus nerve. In the ejection phase, abdominal muscles and the diaphragm contract and the lower esophageal sphincter relaxes, allowing contents into the esophagus and then into the mouth. The palate is elevated, thereby preventing propulsion of contents through the nasopharynx. Postejection is the period after expulsion of the stomach contents, usually resulting in some relief of the nausea.[7]

CLINICAL PRESENTATION

Nausea and vomiting are common presenting symptoms in primary care and can be associated with a variety of clinical presentations. The vomiting act varies very little regardless of cause.[2] The symptoms can be mild and self-limited or severe and prolonged, which can result in anorexia, weight loss, dehydration, and malnutrition. Nausea and vomiting might dominate the presentation or may be only a part of a symptom complex.[2]

When obtaining history, the clinician must have a clear determination of the patient's symptoms because a detailed history can provide clues to the diagnosis. The presentation of nausea and vomiting can vary from the gradual onset of symptoms noted with medication side effects, gastric retention, or early pregnancy to the abrupt episodes caused by viral gastroenteritis, food poisoning, increased intracranial pressure, or acute abdominal emergency.[1,4] Associated symptoms can include pain, headache, dizziness, tinnitus, diarrhea, fever, mental status changes, anxiety, and other symptoms associated with pregnancy.[1,2]

HISTORY

A thorough history should include such details as the timing of the symptoms and their relation to meals, characteristics of the emesis, and any associated complaints. For example, early morning vomiting is associated with metabolic disturbances, alcoholic bingeing, and pregnancy. Vomiting that is triggered by meals is suggestive of pyloric channel ulcer, gastritis, or possibly a psychogenic problem. Learning the appearance of the vomitus is helpful (e.g., coffee-ground emesis suggests gastritis or ulcer disease, vomiting of gastric juice is suggestive of peptic ulcer disease and Zollinger-Ellison syndrome, and vomiting of feculent material is a sign of distal small bowel obstruction). Learning the onset, duration, and severity of symptoms is important.

The clinician should also ask about associated symptoms, past medical history, and psychosocial history. Inquiry should be made about the presence of abdominal pain, fever, jaundice, weight loss, dizziness, headache, visual disturbances, or abdominal surgery; a history of diabetes, cancer, irritable bowel syndrome, or heart disease is ascertained; and current medications and therapies including radiation therapy or chemotherapy are reviewed. Gentle questioning about eating habits (binge eating), self-image, and self-induced emesis should also be conducted. A woman of childbearing age needs to be asked about the last menstrual period and whether she is sexually active, with or without contraception. Essential epidemiologic data include a history of recent foreign travel,[2] any recent exposure to commonly contaminated foods, and any recent exposure to sick contacts. It is also necessary to determine the relationship of nausea and vomiting to food (Does it happen before, during, or after eating? Is it predictable?); the force of vomiting (projectile versus retching); and the quality of the emesis (bile, undigested food, coffee-ground emesis). Acute nausea and vomiting without warning signs can be indicative of infectious or iatrogenic causes. A 24-hour dietary review, with bowel symptoms (diarrhea versus constipation) and the time of the last void, should also be determined.[1,2]

Acute episodes of nausea and vomiting may be caused by viruses, bacterial food poisoning, or medication overdose. Acute emergencies, such as pancreatitis, appendicitis, bowel obstruction, peritonitis, or cholecystitis, may be accompanied by fever or pain. These symptoms can also occur in acute episodes of Crohn disease, colitis, and diverticulitis. Chronic or recurrent nausea and vomiting may be psychogenic or the result of radiation therapy or chemotherapy, gastric disorders, migraine headaches, diabetic gastroparesis, or a metabolic or endocrine abnormality.[1,2]

PHYSICAL EXAMINATION

A thorough physical examination should be directed toward searching for complications of nausea and vomiting and identifying any signs that might point to the cause. Each area of the abdomen assessed should help narrow the possible differential diagnoses specific to that region.[8] The examination should focus on signs of dehydration, including evaluation of skin turgor, mucous membranes, and orthostatic vital signs (positional blood pressure, pulse). The general examination should include assessment of the skin for jaundice, moisture, rashes, or hyperpigmentation. Fingers should be assessed for calluses on dorsal surfaces suggesting self-induced vomiting. If self-induced vomiting is suspected, the clinician should examine the parotid gland for enlargement and check for the presence of lanugo hair and loss of tooth enamel; the patient should also be evaluated for signs of depression and anxiety. The head and neck should be assessed for evidence of dehydration, acute infection, lymphadenopathy, rigidity, or signs of thyrotoxicosis. A cardiovascular examination is necessary to determine the patient's response to the illness or other signs of infection. The abdomen should be observed for distention, visible peristalsis, abdominal or inguinal hernias, and surgical scars; auscultated for bowel sounds (presence or absence, increased or sluggish) and succussion; then palpated for rigidity, tenderness or masses, and flank tenderness. When palpating, the provider begins in areas where no discomfort is reported. Abdominal wall rigidity is indicative of an acute surgical abdomen. A rectal examination is used to assess for fecal impaction and bleeding, if indicated. A neurologic examination including mental status, gait, muscle weakness, asterixis, and cranial nerve function is also an essential component of the evaluation, if neurologic involvement is suspected.[1,2,4]

DIAGNOSTICS

There are currently no randomized controlled studies to guide the diagnostic evaluation; most recommendations are based on expert opinion.[1] The presentation of nausea and vomiting and the physical findings should guide diagnostic testing.[3] Even though there are no specific tests to determine the cause of nausea and vomiting, laboratory tests can be used to evaluate for the complications as well as to determine the underlying causes. The laboratory tests may include urinalysis for specific gravity; erythrocyte sedimentation rate; serum glucose concentration; electrolyte values; serum levels of ketones; blood urea nitrogen (BUN), creatinine, and amylase concentrations; liver function tests (LFTs); and drug levels (if indicated). A serum level of human chorionic gonadotropin should be obtained in women of childbearing age. Urinalysis with culture and sensitivity, complete blood count (CBC), thyroid-stimulating hormone, or further endocrine studies may be indicated in some cases.[1,4]

Abdominal upright and plain x-ray films are necessary if an obstruction is suspected. An ultrasound examination, barium swallow study, computed tomography (CT) scan, or endoscopic examination may be indicated for masses, dysphagia, or suspected gastrointestinal bleeding or ulceration. If a cerebral hemorrhage or mass is suspected, the patient should be urgently referred to the nearest hospital where a head CT scan can be performed. Severe indigestion, epigastric pain, and vomiting could indicate a myocardial infarction.[8] Electrocardiography is indicated if myocardial infarction suspected.

DIAGNOSTICS

Nausea and Vomiting

LABORATORY
Urinalysis*
Serum electrolytes*
Serum glucose*
BUN*
Creatinine*
Serum ketones*
Amylase*
LFTs*
Drug levels*
Human chorionic gonadotropin*
CBC and differential*

IMAGING
Abdominal x-ray studies*
Ultrasound*
Barium swallow*
Endoscopic examination*
Head CT scan*

OTHER DIAGNOSTICS
Electrocardiography*

*If indicated.

DIFFERENTIAL DIAGNOSIS

Nausea and vomiting may be caused by an acute or chronic process. Differentiation of the cause will assist in treatment of the underlying disease and in patient education efforts.

DIFFERENTIAL DIAGNOSIS

Nausea and Vomiting

ACUTE

- Cardiac
  - Myocardial infarction
- Gastrointestinal
  - Acute abdomen (appendicitis, ischemic bowel, peritonitis, abdominal aortic aneurysm, volvulus)
  - Cholecystitis
  - Constipation
  - Infection (viral, bacterial, or parasitic)
  - Intestinal obstruction
  - Medication (chemotherapy, toxic level of some medications, anesthesia, or side effect of medications)
  - Metabolic disturbances (diabetic ketoacidosis, adrenal crisis)
- Neurologic
  - Acute labyrinthitis, Meniere disease
  - Increased intracranial pressure
  - Migraine headache
  - Motion sickness
- Pain
- Pregnancy
- Renal conditions
- Uremia

CHRONIC

- Cancer
- Drug or alcohol use or withdrawal
- Gastrointestinal
  - Achalasia
  - Cirrhosis
  - Crohn disease
  - Diabetic gastroparesis
  - Diverticular disease
  - Hepatitis
  - Irritable bowel syndrome
  - Pancreatitis
  - Peptic ulcer disease
- Psychological
  - Anorexia nervosa or bulimia
  - Psychogenic

MANAGEMENT

Before initiating a treatment protocol, the clinician must identify the warning signs and consult with a specialist as warranted. In managing nausea and vomiting, priority should be given to recognition and correction of complications, followed by identification and treatment of underlying causes and finally, if necessary, treatment to suppress or to alleviate symptoms.[1,3,5,7] The possibility of intestinal obstruction or acute abdomen should be eliminated before other treatment options are initiated. How nausea and vomiting are managed should be individualized to patient-specific variables, including presence of comorbidities, current medications, success of previous therapies, severity of symptoms, and age of the patient.[1,4]

Uncomplicated viral gastroenteritis (without metabolic imbalance or dehydration) can be managed with nonpharmacologic interventions including increased fluid intake and diet restrictions. A clear liquid diet should be followed for 24 hours, followed by 24 hours of the BRAT (banana, rice, applesauce, and toast) diet. This regimen will provide the bowel with sufficient rest. A bland diet may be necessary the following week if the patient is still symptomatic.

Control of vomiting is important for the comfort of the patient and prevention of complications. The use of antiemetics may be indicated. Unfortunately, only a few high-quality studies have compared the efficacy of the different antiemetic drugs on the market.[9] Antiemetic medications should be selected on the basis of the patient's medical history and the suspected cause of the nausea and vomiting. In practice, the choice of antiemetic is also influenced by provider experience, safety, and cost.[10] Adequate fluid intake must be maintained to prevent dehydration, especially if the illness is prolonged or severe. Intake should exceed output by at least 500 mL in a 24-hour period. Assessment for hydration status should include postural vital signs along with the patient's ability to void every 2 to 3 hours. Oral hydration should be attempted in the office if the patient has postural hypotension and is able to tolerate fluid intake. If the patient is too nauseated or does not respond to oral fluid intake, intravenous hydration should be started. In general, 1 to 2 L of intravenous normal saline or lactated Ringer's solution over a few hours is well tolerated. Slower rates are recommended for older adults or patients with significant comorbidities. Emergency provider consultation is recommended if postural hypotension is not corrected or if metabolic alkalosis or severe dehydration is present.

Antiemetic medications are administered to treat or to prevent nausea and vomiting (Box 141-1). These medications can be given alone or in combination with other agents. Presently, the 5-hydroxytryptamine$_3$ (5-HT$_3$ [serotonin]) receptor antagonists are the cornerstone of antiemetic therapy and are used to treat postoperative emesis and chemotherapy-induced emesis. However, there are concerns about QT prolongation with ondansetron and dolasetron.

The phenothiazines were initially used to prevent chemotherapy-induced emesis. The 5-HT$_3$ receptor antagonists are also used for the prevention of nausea and vomiting associated with chemotherapy.[7] These agents used in combination with corticosteroids may offer the greatest antiemetic treatment.[7] For the refractory nausea and vomiting associated with chemotherapy, the cannabinoids may be useful.[6]

For the prevention of motion sickness, vertigo, and migraines, antihistamines and anticholinergics are excellent choices. These include diphenhydramine (Benadryl), meclizine (Antivert), dimenhydrinate (Dramamine), transdermal scopolamine, promethazine (Phenergan), and cyclizine (Marezine).[6]

COMPLICATIONS

The complications of nausea and vomiting must be identified and treated. The severity of complications is associated with the underlying condition. Untreated, nausea and vomiting can cause dehydration, hypokalemia, and metabolic acidosis. Although it is uncommon in alert patients, aspiration pneumonitis is a possibility in patients with decreased levels of consciousness.[5] Continual vomiting may result in malnutrition and dental erosion. Forceful vomiting has been the cause of Mallory-Weiss syndrome and esophageal ruptures.

INDICATIONS FOR REFERRAL OR HOSPITALIZATION

In the majority of patients with nausea and vomiting, the cause can be determined from a thorough history and physical examination without the need for additional testing.[1,11]

- An urgent referral for hospital admission and consultation with a specialist is indicated for patients when nausea and vomiting are accompanied by pain, severe dehydration, acute abdominal findings, neurologic changes, or a metabolic or electrolyte imbalance.

BOX 141-1

Antiemetic Medications

FOR GENERALIZED NAUSEA AND VOMITING

Bismuth Subsalicylate

For nausea with or without diarrhea

- Pepto-Bismol: 30 mL PO every 30-60 min; maximum 8 doses/24 hr; available over the counter

Benzamides

Metoclopramide Hydrochloride

For nausea related to diabetic gastroparesis: 10 mg PO 30 minutes before meals and at bedtime for 2-8 wk, depending on response

For gastroesophageal reflux: 10-15 mg PO 4 times daily prn 30 min before meals and at bedtime; do not use for more than 12 wk

For nausea and vomiting associated with chemotherapy: 1-2 mg/kg IV slowly during 1-2 min or infused over 15 min after diluting in 50 mL of D5W, D5½NS, normal saline, Ringer's solution, or lactated Ringer's solution; give first dose 30 min before chemotherapy, then every 2 hr prn; do not exceed 5 doses/day; may produce dystonic reaction when given IV; premedicate with diphenhydramine

Phenothiazines

Prochlorperazine (Compazine)

For severe nausea and vomiting: 5-10 mg PO 3 or 4 times daily, 5-10 mg IM every 3-4 hr prn (maximum 40 mg/day), or 25 mg rectal suppository every 12 hr prn; may give 2.5-10 mg IV at a rate not to exceed 5 mg/min; give IM injections in the upper outer quadrant of the gluteal muscle; use this drug when only a few doses are required for treatment

Promethazine Hydrochloride (Phenergan)

For nausea: 12.5-25 mg PO, IM, or rectally every 4-6 hr prn; use cautiously in ambulatory patients because of possible pronounced sedative effects

Trimethobenzamide Hydrochloride (Tigan)

For mild to moderate nausea and vomiting: 300 mg PO 3 or 4 times daily, 200 mg IM 3 or 4 times daily; give IM injections in the upper outer quadrant of the gluteal muscle; for short-term treatment

FOR NAUSEA AND VOMITING ASSOCIATED WITH CHEMOTHERAPY

5-HT (Serotonin) Receptor Antagonists (also used for postoperative emesis)

For prevention of postoperative and chemotherapy-induced emesis

- Granisetron (Kytril): 1 mg or 0.01 mg/kg once daily IV, or 2 mg once daily PO
- Ondansetron (Zofran): 4-8 mg or 0.15 mg/kg once daily IV, or 4-8 mg 3 times daily PO
- Palonosetron (Aloxi): 0.25 mg IV

Dopamine Receptor Antagonists

Phenothiazines

For prevention of chemotherapy-induced events

- Prochlorperazine (Compazine): 5-10 mg PO every 6-8 hr, 5-10 mg IM, 2.5-10 mg IV every 3-4 hr, or 25 mg suppository every 12 hr
- Chlorpromazine (Thorazine): 10-25 mg PO every 4-6 hr, 25 mg IV every 3-4 hr, or 100 mg suppository every 6-8 hr

Butyrophenones

For postoperative nausea

- Droperidol (Inapsine): 0.625-1.25 mg IV; 1.25-5 mg IM

Benzamides

For nausea caused by cytotoxic drugs

- Metoclopramide (Reglan): 0.5 mg/kg IV every 6-8 hr or 10-20 mg PO every 6-8 hr
- Trimethobenzamide (Tigan): 300 mg PO every 6-8 hr or 200 mg IM or suppository every 6-8 hr

Cannabinoids

For chemotherapy-induced nausea and vomiting

- Dronabinol (Marinol): 5 mg/m^2 PO 1-3 hours before chemotherapy; repeated every 2-4 hr prn to maximum 6 doses daily[6]

Substance P/Neurokinin$_1$ Antagonists

For acute and delayed nausea and vomiting associated with chemotherapy

- Aprepitant (Emend): 125 mg PO 1 hour before chemotherapy, then 80 mg/day for 2 days; may be given with other agents (e.g., steroids, Zofran)

Benzodiazepines

For adjunct therapy to decrease anxiety and anticipatory emesis

- Alprazolam (Xanax): 0.5-1 mg once daily PO up to 3-6 mg/day
- Lorazepam (Ativan): 0.5-2 mg PO or IV every 4-6 hr

Antihistamines and Anticholinergic Agents

For motion sickness, vertigo, and migraines

- Diphenhydramine (Benadryl): 25-50 mg PO every 6 hr or 10-50 mg IV or IM
- Dimenhydrinate (Dramamine): 50 mg PO every 4 hr
- Meclizine (Antivert): 12.5-50 mg PO every 24 hr
- Promethazine (Phenergan): 12.5 to 25 mg every 4 to 6 hours PO, IM, or IV
- Transdermal scopolamine (Transderm-Scop): 1 patch 4 hr before travel, remove after 72 hours; for surgery, apply 1 patch the evening before surgery, remove 24 hours after surgery

- Hospitalization may also be indicated if the patient is unable to maintain hydration status at home.
- Referral to an appropriate specialist may be necessary if the nausea or vomiting is not controlled by supportive measures such as hydration, diet change, and antiemetics; the patient's condition worsens or does not respond to treatment; a psychological component is present; the acuity of the patient's condition exceeds the experience and comfort level of the treating provider; or adequate resources are not readily available.

- Metabolic disturbances; pregnancy; and altered medication, drug, or alcohol levels should be managed in consultation with an interdisciplinary team.
- Consultation is required for emergencies such as acute myocardial infarction or for patients with neurologic changes.
- Prolonged or recurrent nausea or vomiting may indicate gastric paresis, irritable bowel, or pancreatitis and requires consultation with a gastroenterologist or appropriate specialist.

PATIENT AND FAMILY EDUCATION

Patients should be educated about adequate fluid intake, with special attention given to the types of fluid ingested. Oral rehydration solutions and broths are especially helpful in maintaining electrolyte balance. Dairy products and carbonated fluids should be avoided. A minimum of 96 to 120 ounces of fluid should be consumed each hour. An oral rehydration solution may be prepared by mixing 1 cup of orange juice, ¾ teaspoon of salt, 1 teaspoon of baking soda, 4 tablespoons of sugar, and 1 L of water.

Because dehydration can occur easily in the presence of persistent vomiting, patients should be instructed to notify the health care provider if the following occur:

- Vomiting persists despite antiemetic use.
- Vomiting is accompanied by fever, severe abdominal pain, severe headache, neck pain, or lethargy.
- Urinary output becomes dark, or the patient does not void at least every 2 hours during the day.
- Dizziness or lightheadedness occurs with or without position change.
- Patient is vomiting blood or fluid that has the appearance of coffee grounds.

HEALTH PROMOTION

Patients should be instructed in the proper handling and storage of food products to prevent contamination and possible food poisoning. Patients traveling abroad should receive the necessary vaccinations and treatments appropriate for the country visited. Guidelines are available from the Centers for Disease Control and Prevention or through local travel clinics.

CHAPTER 142

PANCREATITIS

Jodie A. Barkin • Henrique J. Fernandez • David H. Kerman

Gastroenterology consultation is indicated for patients with suspected acute pancreatitis.

ACUTE PANCREATITIS

DEFINITION AND EPIDEMIOLOGY

Acute pancreatitis is an inflammatory condition of the pancreas that may range in severity from mild to severe. The patient with acute pancreatitis typically has abdominal pain and an elevation of pancreatic enzymes. The clinical course can range from mild disease to life-threatening multiorgan failure, sepsis, and possibly death. The Atlanta symposium classified acute pancreatitis into mild (minimal organ dysfunction and self-limited) and severe (with organ failure or a local pancreatic complication, such as necrosis or pseudocyst formation).[1-3] Acute nonnecrotic pancreatitis has an associated mortality rate as low as 1%, with no or minimal necrosis present. Computed tomography (CT) primarily shows homogenous enhancement of the pancreas. Conversely, acute necrotizing pancreatitis shows areas of non-enhancement on CT with intravenous contrast, with necrosis in the pancreas, peripancreatic tissue, or a combination thereof, with the most common presentation being the combination. Furthermore, necrotizing pancreatitis is graded by CT as involvement of the gland of less than 30% or 30% or more, with the latter being more severe. Severe necrotizing pancreatitis may manifest with organ failure; when present, it has a mortality rate of 10% with aseptic necrosis and up to 30% with infected necrosis.[2,4]

The causes of pancreatitis are varied. A number of factors have been implicated as precipitants and can easily be identified using the ABCs of causes of acute pancreatitis (Boxes 142-1, 142-2, and 142-3). The most common cause of pancreatitis is gallstones, which are responsible for 45% of all cases of pancreatitis in the United States.[5] Toxins are another leading cause of acute pancreatitis, with ethyl alcohol as the precipitant in the majority of cases.[5] Standardized by gender, ethyl alcohol is the most common cause in males, with a worldwide incidence of 7.9 cases per 100,000 people per year. Gallstones are the most common cause in women, with a worldwide incidence of 4.8 per 100,000 people per year.[2,6] Other causes of pancreatitis include trauma from injury and surgery, which may disrupt the ductal system or damage the pancreas.[5] Endoscopic retrograde cholangiopancreatography (ERCP) is an important iatrogenic cause of pancreatitis and can occur in up to 5% of cases.[7] Conditions that cause hypercalcemia, such as hyperparathyroidism, are also implicated in the development of pancreatitis. However, the reasons for this are not clearly understood. Hyperlipidemia associated with triglyceride levels of more than 1000 mg/dL is known to increase the risk of pancreatitis.[5] Parasites and viral infections, such as human immunodeficiency virus (HIV) infection, have been implicated in the development of pancreatitis. Some medications are associated with pancreatitis such as thiazide diuretics and furosemide; the exact relationship is unknown but may be related to a hypersensitivity reaction that

BOX 142-1

The ABCs of Causes of Acute Pancreatitis

A: Alcohol, autoimmune disorders, arteritis
B: Biliary, blunt trauma
C: Congenital—pancreas divisum
D: Drugs or medications
E: ERCP, eosinophilia
F: Formations—primary and metastatic tumors
G: Genetic—*CFTR, SPINK*
H: Hyperlipidemia, hypercalcemia
I: Idiopathic, infectious—human immunodeficiency virus (HIV), inflammatory bowel disease

Courtesy Jamie S. Barkin, MD, University of Miami, Leonard M. Miller School of Medicine, Department of Medicine, Division of Gastroenterology. Miami, Florida.

BOX 142-2

Extended List of Factors Associated with Acute Pancreatitis

MOST FREQUENT CAUSES

- Gallstones
- Alcoholism
- Idiopathic (may be related to diverse causes)

FREQUENT CAUSES

- Toxins
- Ethyl alcohol
- Methyl alcohol
- Organophosphorus insecticides
- Scorpion venom
- Medications
  - Acetaminophen
  - Aminosalicylates
  - Angiotensin-converting enzyme inhibitors
  - Asparaginase (Elspar)
  - Azathioprine (Imuran) or 6-mercaptopurine
  - Chlorthalidone
  - Cimetidine
  - Corticosteroids
  - ddI (2′,3′-dideoxyinosine; associated with concurrent pentamidine treatment)
  - Erythromycin
  - Estrogens (identified with type IV or V hyperlipidemia)
  - Ethacrynic acid
  - Furosemide (rare)
  - Iatrogenic hypercalcemia
  - Intravenous lipids
  - L-Asparaginase
  - Methyldopa (rare)
  - Metronidazole (rare)
  - Nitrofurantoin
  - Nonsteroidals
  - Olsalazine, 5-ASA (rare)
  - Pentamidine (rare)
  - Phenformin (rare)
  - Ranitidine
  - Sulfonamides (rare)
  - Sulindac
  - Tetracycline (rare)
  - Thiazide diuretics
  - Valproic acid
- Blunt abdominal trauma
- Crohn disease of the duodenum
- End-stage renal disease with chronic dialysis
- Iatrogenic trauma: cardiopulmonary bypass, endoscopic retrograde cholangiopancreatography, endoscopic sphincterotomy, manometry of the sphincter of Oddi, organ transplantation, postoperative pancreatitis after abdominal or thoracic surgery
- Hyperparathyroidism associated with hypercalcemia
- Infection
  - Parasitic: *Ascaris* worms, clonorchiasis
  - Viral: coxsackievirus, cytomegalovirus, mumps, and fulminant viral hepatitis
  - Bacterial: *Campylobacter jejuni, Mycoplasma pneumoniae, Salmonella* organisms, microlithiasis
- Lipid abnormalities (hypertriglyceridemia)
- Metabolic abnormalities: hypercalcemia associated with excessive doses of vitamin D, parathyroid adenoma, familial hypocalciuric hypercalcemia, hypercalcemia associated with total parenteral nutrition
- Pancreatic divisum
- Pancreatic outflow obstruction: afferent loop obstruction, annular pancreatitis
- Penetrating peptic ulcer
- Pregnancy
- Surgery (endoscopic retrograde cholangiopancreatography)
- Trauma
- Tumor: primary and metastatic

LESS FREQUENT CAUSES

- Hereditary
- Pancreatic cancer
- Periampullary duodenal diverticulum
- Refeeding after fasting
- Rheumatologic disorders: systemic lupus erythematosus, mixed connective tissue disorders, scleroderma
- Thrombotic thrombocytopenic purpura
- Vasculitis

BOX 142-3

Factors Associated with Acute Pancreatitis in HIV-Positive Patients

INFECTION

- Cytomegalovirus
- *Cryptococcus*
- Cryptosporidia
- *Mycobacterium avium* and *Mycobacterium tuberculosis*
- *Toxoplasma gondii*

MEDICATIONS

- Didanosine
- Pentamidine
- Trimethoprim-sulfamethoxazole

results in pancreatic injury. Thiopurines, often used in autoimmune and chronic inflammatory disorders, carry up to a 3% risk of development of pancreatitis that is independent of dose.[8] Lesions that result in pancreatic ductal obstruction, such as tumors, also may cause pancreatitis.

PATHOPHYSIOLOGY

The exact mechanism of pancreatitis is not well understood, but the most common explanation is related to autodigestion of the pancreas. For reasons unknown, pancreatic enzymes become activated in the pancreas rather than in the intestine. Trypsinogen, an inactive enzyme produced by the pancreas, is normally released into the intestines through the pancreatic ducts and activated by trypsin. In pancreatitis, trypsin is present in the pancreas and not only digests the pancreas but also activates other enzymes, such as elastase and phospholipase A. Elastase and phospholipase A are also involved in the autodigestion of the pancreas. Elastase causes hemorrhage through breakdown of the elastic fibers of the blood vessels. Phospholipase A has been implicated in fat necrosis.[9]

Although most patients typically experience minimum organ dysfunction as a result of pancreatitis, approximately 10% to 20% develop systemic inflammatory response syndrome (SIRS). SIRS is defined by the presence of at least two of the following features: temperature below 36° C or above 38° C; heart rate above 90 beats per minute; respiratory rate above 20 breaths per minute or $PaCO_2$ below 32 torr; white blood cell count above 12,000 cells/mm^3, below 4000 cells/mm^3, or above 10% immature cells (bands).[10] SIRS appears to be caused by the activation of an inflammatory cascade mediated by cytokines, immunocytes, and the complement system. The inflammatory cytokines cause macrophages to migrate to the lungs, kidneys, and other tissues distant from the pancreas. SIRS leads to a fulminant course with pancreatic necrosis and multiorgan failure and is used to classify patients as having mild, moderate, or severe disease.[11]

CLINICAL PRESENTATION

The main presentation of acute pancreatitis is the sudden onset of constant, sharp, poorly localized abdominal pain that radiates to the back in about 50% of patients. The pancreas is in a retroperitoneal location, and signs of peritoneal irritation, such as rebound tenderness, are frequently absent.

PHYSICAL EXAMINATION

Early recognition of pancreatitis in clinical practice is of utmost importance. Given the nonspecific nature of symptomatology, acute pancreatitis may be misdiagnosed by physical examination alone. The most common presentation is intense abdominal pain so severe that the patient is reluctant to take a deep breath. This results in hypoventilation and contributes to the increased incidence of respiratory complications, such as atelectasis; therefore crackles may be present in lungs on examination. The pain is worse in the supine position and often increases in severity with time. Many patients are initially seen with symptoms of dehydration caused by nausea and vomiting, which may result in tachycardia, orthostatic hypotension, and shock. Abdominal distention caused by the leakage of fluid into the retroperitoneum is common and results in protrusion of abdominal contents forward. Direct and rebound tenderness secondary to peritonitis are late signs associated with severe acute pancreatitis, which is associated with a grave prognosis.[12] Upper abdominal palpation of a mass may suggest the presence of a pancreatic pseudocyst. Evidence of retroperitoneal hemorrhage, although rare, may be observed. Cullen sign (bruising of the periumbilicus) or Grey Turner sign (bruising of the flank) is consistent with the hemorrhagic findings in acute severe pancreatitis. The occurrence of Cullen and Grey Turner signs is rare and associated with increased mortality. Jaundice, an uncommon finding, also may occur and is related to compression of the common bile duct by edema or a mass of the head of the pancreas.

DIAGNOSTICS

Serum amylase and lipase are the most common laboratory tests used to diagnose acute pancreatitis. Rising 6 to 12 hours after the onset of symptoms, serum amylase levels usually return to normal within 3 to 5 days in uncomplicated cases. This elevation is not always seen in alcoholic pancreatitis, especially in patients with chronic alcoholic pancreatitis, or in hypertriglyceridemia-associated pancreatitis because of laboratory delineation. Serum amylase elevation is considered a nonspecific finding because serum amylase may be elevated in other conditions with an extrapancreatic cause, such as diseases of the salivary glands, which also produce amylase. A threefold elevation of serum lipase level is more diagnostic, especially in patients seen several days after the acute attack, and serum lipase is elevated in both alcoholic and nonalcoholic pancreatitis.[13] Trending of amylase and lipase levels in an acute episode is not indicated, and management should be driven only by symptomatology.

Hemoconcentration, hyperglycemia, and electrolyte abnormalities are commonly found as a result of intravascular volume depletion. Hyperbilirubinemia and transient hypocalcemia may also be present. Elevated bilirubin and alkaline phosphatase, with or without the presence of elevated aminotransferases, should raise the suspicion for biliary obstruction, a common presentation of biliary pancreatitis.

Abdominal radiographs are useful in the exclusion of other causes of abdominal pain, such as bowel obstruction or perforated bowel, but are not diagnostic for acute pancreatitis. Chest x-ray studies may show infiltration, left lower lobe atelectasis, or effusion. Although abdominal ultrasonography offers the most sensitive evaluation for cholelithiasis, ultrasonographic evaluation of the pancreas may be limited owing to overlying bowel gas. Additional imaging should be used only when the diagnosis is not conclusive from the history, physical examination, and laboratory findings or when the medical practitioner suspects a complicated course. Intravenous contrast-enhanced CT scanning is the most useful imaging technique, not only for diagnosis but also for detection of a pseudocyst (collection of fluid around or within the pancreas) and recognition of pancreatic necrosis. This should be delayed until the patient is rehydrated if there is uncertainty of diagnosis. If not, it can be used after 4 or more days to classify the level of necrosis. Magnetic resonance imaging (MRI) and magnetic resonance cholangiopancreatography (MRCP) are used in the diagnosis of acute pancreatitis. MRI is considered more useful in the effort to categorize acute fluid collections and assess main pancreatic duct anatomy and is more sensitive in diagnosis of milder forms of pancreatitis. MRCP is better able to delineate the pancreatic and bile ducts.

In 30% of patients diagnosed with pancreatitis, the cause is unknown. The majority of these patients will have no further episodes. Patients with recurrent acute pancreatitis may benefit from endoscopic ultrasound (EUS) for further evaluation of pancreatic parenchyma and ducts, or ERCP as a therapeutic modality to remove common bile duct stones or debris.[14] Patients with unexplained pancreatitis who are older than 40 years are at increased risk of pancreatic malignancy and should have further imaging with CT or EUS. ERCP should be used only as a therapeutic modality because it can exacerbate biliary pancreatitis with manipulation of the pancreatic duct.

One of the most important topics in diagnosis and staging of acute pancreatitis is the use of prognostic scoring systems. The most commonly used scoring systems currently are the Apache II criteria and the Bedside Index of Severity in Acute Pancreatitis (BISAP) (Box 142-4).[15,16] These scoring systems can be applied at admission and assess severity and prognosis of disease. Unfortunately, the Apache II score is cumbersome to

BOX 142-4

Bedside Index of Severity in Acute Pancreatitis

WITHIN FIRST 24 HOURS

Blood urea nitrogen >25 mg/dL
Impaired mental status
Presence of SIRS
Age >60 years
Presence of pleural effusion on imaging

A BISAP score of 3 or greater indicates increased risk of complications from acute pancreatitis.

Modified from Singh VK, Wu BU, Bollen TL, et al: A prospective evaluation of the bedside index for severity in acute pancreatitis score in assessing mortality and intermediate markers of severity in acute pancreatitis. *Am J Gastroenterol* 104(4):966-971, 2009.

calculate, which may limit its use. The BISAP score is easily calculated and can be recalculated daily to assess progression and prognosis. The BISAP criteria include five components assessed within 24 hours of presentation: blood urea nitrogen (BUN) above 25 mg/dL, impaired mental status, presence of SIRS, age older than 60, and pleural effusion on imaging. A BISAP score of 3 or greater is indicative of increased risk of complications from acute pancreatitis. Previously, the most widely used system was the Ranson criteria, but this has fallen out of favor more recently because of the requirement to wait until 48 hours after admission to calculate a score.[17] The first 48 hours after admission are the most critical, wherein medical therapy can make a tangible clinical difference in prognosis, and waiting to calculate a score may delay aggressive therapy.

DIAGNOSTICS

Acute Pancreatitis

LABORATORY
CHEM-12 (electrolytes, BUN, creatinine, hepatic function panel)
Fasting lipid profile*
CBC
TSH*
Serum hCG (in women of childbearing age)

IMAGING
KUB
Abdominal ultrasound
Chest x-ray study
MRI with or without MRCP
CT scan if no improvement after 72 hours only
HIDA scan*

OTHER DIAGNOSTICS
ECG
EUS*
ERCP*

*If indicated.
CBC, complete blood count; ECG, electrocardiogram; hCG, human chorionic gonadotropin; HIDA, hepatobiliary iminodiacetic acid; KUB, kidney, ureter, and bladder study; TSH, thyroid-stimulating hormone.

DIFFERENTIAL DIAGNOSIS

The patient who is seen with abdominal pain requires meticulous assessment, because many disease processes may have symptomatic overlap. A thorough history of the pain, including location, time of onset, severity, and quality, in addition to associated symptoms will assist in determining the diagnosis. Questions about gastrointestinal function, such as appetite, nausea, vomiting, and the presence of blood in the stool, will be useful. The possibility of gynecologic conditions also must be considered in women with abdominal pain.[18]

DIFFERENTIAL DIAGNOSIS

Acute Pancreatitis

- Myocardial infarction
- Bowel obstruction
- Acute cholecystitis
- Biliary or renal colic
- Peptic ulcer disease
- Ruptured aortic aneurysm or acute aortic dissection
- Gynecologic conditions
- Pneumonia
- Diverticulosis
- Pulmonary embolus
- Mesenteric ischemia or infarction

MANAGEMENT

Recognition of underlying abdominal emergencies and the need for quick surgical intervention for extrapancreatic processes is essential. Treatment of pancreatitis is generally aimed at decreasing pancreatic inflammation with rehydration and correcting any predisposing factors, such as removal of gallstones in gallstone pancreatitis. Hospitalization is generally indicated for analgesia and intravenous rehydration as well as for monitoring of vital signs, volume status, and electrolytes. Level of treatment should be based on severity criteria previously mentioned, and one should have a low threshold for intensive care unit monitoring. Patients should be treated as if they have a burn injury because third spacing of fluids is commonly seen. Monitoring of fluid status is critical; these patients require large amounts of fluids for correction of intravascular volume depletion. The foundation of therapy is early intravenous hydration. This should be administered with at least 1 L initially and then continued at 150 to 250 mL/hr during the initial 24 hours of hospitalization depending on the comorbidities of the patient. This has been shown to decrease morbidity and mortality of acute pancreatitis. Strict monitoring of intake and output should be used to follow overall fluid balance. BUN and hematocrit should be followed every 6 to 12 hours and should decrease with rehydration.[19] Oral intake of liquids, food, or medications should be limited until adequate pain control has been achieved.

Pain is typically treated with opioid analgesia. Meperidine is used cautiously because of the propensity of its metabolites to accumulate and to cause neuromuscular irritation and possibly seizures. Morphine has been shown in human studies to cause an increase in pressure of the sphincter of Oddi; however, there is no evidence that this has a negative effect on the condition of the pancreas. Fentanyl is sometimes used, but like all opioids, it can cause respiratory depression.

Antibiotic therapy for acute pancreatitis is not appropriate when the patient is admitted; it has not been shown to prevent pancreatic infection.[20] If the patient later in the course develops a secondary infection or suspected infected pancreatic necrosis, antibiotics can be used. Fluid aspiration via interventional radiology or EUS can be obtained for culture and sensitivities if there is no clinical response to antibiotics. Antibiotic prophylaxis is contraindicated because of the potential development of resistant bacterial or fungal pancreatitis and has not been associated with any statistically significant differences in subsequent morbidity or mortality. Probiotics have also been examined and have not been shown to have any benefit for preventing complications, and may lead to increased mortality.[21]

Pain cessation plus normalization of vital signs, radiographic studies, and laboratory values indicates resolving pancreatitis. Liquids can be resumed and small amounts of food gradually added once pain has subsided. The recurrence of pain indicates the need to again restrict oral intake and also to look for complications, such as fluid collections, necrosis, or development of pseudocysts. For patients with protracted attacks of pancreatitis and who are unable to meet caloric needs by day 7, enteral feedings should be used. Enteral feeding has been shown to be superior to parenteral nutrition for overall decreased morbidity and mortality.[22] Initiation of enteral feeding within 48 hours of onset of pancreatitis is associated with fewer complications and may decrease severity of the episode of pancreatitis. A jejunal feeding tube can be used to support enteral feeding if indicated.[23,24]

Intravenous contrast-enhanced CT scanning to determine the presence of necrosis or other complications is indicated for patients who do not respond to supportive measures. CT scanning should be performed no earlier than 72 hours after the start of the episode to enable appropriate estimation of the extent of pancreatic necrosis. ERCP with or without EUS may be necessary for management of common bile duct stones causing biliary pancreatitis. Pancreatic necrosis should be managed conservatively with a step-up approach focusing on supportive care measures, followed by catheter drainage if there are ongoing symptoms and need for drainage of infected necrosis. Intervention with EUS or a minimally invasive surgical approach should be considered for those patients with walled-off infected necrosis who are not clinically improving despite treatment with antibiotics.[25] Timing of the intervention is of utmost importance, and treatment should be delayed for at least 3 to 4 weeks after the initial episode of acute pancreatitis to allow for maturation of fluid collection walls and to enable delineation of tissue planes. Open necrosectomy should be reserved for severe refractory cases in which minimally invasive approaches fail; this procedure is associated with poor prognosis.[26]

COMPLICATIONS

Patients who have recovered from acute pancreatitis are at significant risk for recurrence if the initial cause has not been elucidated and corrected. Continued pain, malabsorption, or new-onset diabetes mellitus warrants immediate investigation. The majority of patients will recover with supportive therapy, although approximately 25% of patients will have complications. These complications include hypocalcemia and other metabolic abnormalities, blindness (Purtscher retinopathy), pseudocysts, necrosis, hemorrhage, and multisystem organ failure. The majority of deaths are caused by multiorgan system failure mediated by the SIRS.

INDICATIONS FOR REFERRAL OR HOSPITALIZATION

The treatment of acute pancreatitis is primarily supportive and requires physician consultation. Hospitalization is indicated for all patients for early large-volume intravenous fluid replacement, careful observation, frequent assessment of vital signs, laboratory analyses including electrolytes and glucose concentration, and parenteral analgesia. Nutritional, gastroenterologic, and surgical consultations are also recommended.

PATIENT AND FAMILY EDUCATION AND HEALTH PROMOTION

Patients should understand that severe abdominal pain with or without radiation, nausea, vomiting, or diaphoresis requires immediate evaluation. It is also important that patients understand the risk of repeated attacks of pancreatitis, the need to avoid possible precipitants, and the importance of adherence to prescribed therapy. Patient education about contributing factors, such as alcohol use, must be discussed. Because the mortality rate from alcoholic pancreatitis is high, alcohol should be avoided. A low-fat diet, weight loss, exercise, and normalization of triglyceride levels, with medications if needed, should be the goal for patients with pancreatitis associated with hypertriglyceridemia. Medications that may have caused the pancreatitis should also be avoided.

CHRONIC PANCREATITIS

DEFINITION AND EPIDEMIOLOGY

Chronic pancreatitis, an inflammatory condition of the pancreas, is characterized by morphologic and histologic changes in the pancreas that result in exocrine and endocrine insufficiency. Chronic pancreatitis differs from acute pancreatitis in that acute pancreatitis usually does not result in long-term pancreatic insufficiency, whereas the inflammatory changes in chronic pancreatitis permanently impair the exocrine and endocrine function of the gland. There are, however, reports of chronic pancreatic insufficiency in patients with acute pancreatitis with severe necrosis, especially in the head of the pancreas. The prevailing opinion regarding the parenchymal injury in acute pancreatitis, such as that induced by passage of a gallstone, is that it is both pathologically and morphologically different from the injury that occurs in chronic pancreatitis.

Chronic pancreatitis is a disease of multiple causes including chronic alcoholism, duct obstruction from tumors, strictures, hypercalcemia, hyperlipidemia, genetic mutations, congenital anatomic abnormalities such as pancreas divisum, and autoimmune and possibly dietary or environmental causes (Box 142-5). The TIGAR-O system can be used to identify major predisposing risk factors for chronic pancreatitis: (1) toxic-metabolic, (2) idiopathic, (3) genetic, (4) autoimmune, (5) recurrent and severe acute pancreatitis, (6) obstructive.[27] In a substantial number of cases (approximately 10% to 20%), no identifiable cause can be found.

Alcohol is a major factor in both acute and chronic pancreatitis. Alcohol abuse accounts for 50% to 70% of cases of chronic pancreatitis.[28] Although the exact pathogenesis is not clearly understood, the risk appears related to the duration and amount of alcohol consumed rather than to the type of alcohol or the pattern of consumption.[28] A small group of patients may have hereditary causes for chronic pancreatitis. Pancreatic duct obstruction from trauma, calcific stones, or tumors can result in chronic pancreatitis. Tropical pancreatitis is a common cause of pancreatitis in parts of India and the tropics. Systemic diseases, such as lupus erythematosus and cystic fibrosis, have been linked to chronic pancreatitis as well. Malnutrition or consumption of sorghum may play a role in the development of chronic pancreatitis in southern India, Indonesia, and central Africa and South Africa. Uncommon causes of chronic pancreatitis include

BOX 142-5

Causes of Chronic Pancreatitis

- Alcohol abuse
- Hereditary pancreatitis
- Ductal obstruction
- Congenital anatomic abnormalities
- Tropical pancreatitis
- Autoimmune disease
- Cystic fibrosis
- Hyperparathyroidism
- Hypertriglyceridemia
- Hereditary pancreatitis (mutation of trypsinogen gene)
- Idiopathic pancreatitis (associated with atherosclerotic disease)
- Nutritional deficiencies (of antioxidants, such as selenium or vitamin C or E)

Data from Freedman SD, Lewis MD: *Etiology and pathogenesis of chronic pancreatitis in adults*. Available at www.uptodate.com/contents/etiology-and-pathogenesis-of-chronic-pancreatitis-in-adults?source=search_result&search=chronic+pancreatitis&selectedTitle=3~93. Accessed February 22, 2012.

severe malnutrition, hemochromatosis, trauma, sicca syndrome, radiation injury, gastric surgery, and tuberculosis.

In patients older than 40 years, the finding of pancreatic exocrine dysfunction mandates an evaluation for pancreatic cancer. Pancreatic exocrine dysfunction in adults aged 20 to 40 years should trigger an investigation for cystic fibrosis because 85% of patients with cystic fibrosis have some pancreatic insufficiency and may have a delayed presentation of their underlying cystic fibrosis. Fifty percent of patients with chronic pancreatitis die within 25 years of diagnosis; up to 49% of those deaths are related to complications including pancreatic cancer. The remainder die of disease associated with chronic alcohol abuse.[29]

The most widely used classification for chronic pancreatitis is the Marseilles-Rome classification system modified by Sarles. It divides the condition into categories based on morphology, epidemiology, and molecular biology.[2,30]

PATHOPHYSIOLOGY

The pathophysiologic mechanism of chronic pancreatitis is multifactorial and not completely understood. It is postulated that increased pancreatic secretion causes proteinaceous plugs to form within the interlobular and intralobular ducts, with obstruction of the ducts and subsequent scarring and damage because of inflammatory changes, resulting from autodigestion.[31]

CLINICAL PRESENTATION

Chronic pancreatitis most commonly manifests with abdominal pain, and signs and symptoms related to pancreatic exocrine or endocrine insufficiency. Abdominal pain may be severe, recurrent, or constant and is typically epigastric, with potential referral to the upper back, anterior chest, or flank. Nausea and vomiting may accompany the pain. Usually the discomfort is not relieved by food or antacids and intensifies with alcohol or fatty food. Pain often occurs 15 to 20 minutes after eating. Weight loss, diarrhea, and steatorrhea with oily stools may be reported as a result of fat malabsorption. When the destruction of pancreatic function results in diabetes, the typical symptoms of polyuria, polydipsia, and polyphagia may be observed. Glucose intolerance occurs frequently, typically requiring insulin administration as the disease progresses. Patients with severe pancreatic dysfunction have difficulty digesting complex foods or absorbing products of digestion. Significant protein and fat deficiencies occur when more than 90% of pancreatic function is lost.[31,32]

PHYSICAL EXAMINATION

Even in the presence of severe pain, physical examination may reveal few overt findings. Weight loss or abdominal tenderness may be present. Jaundice, signifying common bile duct obstruction, is less common. If pancreatic dysfunction results in severe malabsorption, signs of malnutrition will be evident.[32]

DIAGNOSTICS

Laboratory data are useful to exclude other causes of abdominal pain and to determine whether pancreatic insufficiency exists. In contrast to acute pancreatitis, elevated serum amylase and lipase levels are not typically present. There is a minimal if any increase in pancreatic enzymes in the blood because of significant fibrosis, which results in decreased concentration of these enzymes within the pancreas. Complete blood count (CBC) and liver chemistry results are typically normal. Increased bilirubin and alkaline phosphatase levels can indicate compression of bile ducts and should prompt investigation for fibrosis, edema, or tumor. The presence of pancreatic insufficiency is indicated by elevated blood glucose concentration or steatorrhea. Steatorrhea can be diagnosed with Sudan stain of the feces and examination for fecal fat. The patient should eat a minimum of 100 g of fat daily, and stool is collected during a 72-hour period. A fecal fat level of more than 7 g is diagnostic of malassimilation.[32]

When the diagnosis is not clear clinically, the next step is pancreatic imaging. Imaging studies visualizing structure and pancreatic function tests complement one another. Abdominal radiography, EUS, CT scan, MRI, ERCP, and MRCP are diagnostic imaging studies that are useful in chronic pancreatitis. In one third of patients, abdominal radiographs (kidney, ureter, bladder [KUB]) may demonstrate pancreatic calcifications, thereby supporting the diagnosis. Abdominal ultrasonography may expedite early diagnosis because pancreatic enlargement and calcifications can be seen earlier than on abdominal radiography. The sensitivity of CT and MRI approaches 90% for diagnosis of advanced chronic pancreatitis. Evidence of ductal dilation with focal enlargement, fluid collections, or calcifications on CT or MRI indicates chronic pancreatitis. EUS is an increasingly common diagnostic and therapeutic modality in the management of chronic pancreatitis. It is now the gold standard because one can visualize the pancreatic parenchyma and comment on characteristics of the ductal system with much less risk for complications compared with ERCP. Stone formation seen on EUS is the most predictive feature of chronic pancreatitis. Other EUS findings include visible side branches, cysts, lobularity, irregularity or dilation of a main duct, hyperechoic foci, hyperechoic strands, and a main duct with hyperechoic margins. The severity of chronic pancreatitis correlates with the number of EUS findings observed. The Rosemont classification system has been proposed as a means to diagnose chronic pancreatitis using EUS, and takes into account a hyperechoic or echogenic appearance of the pancreas as well as measurements and appearance of the pancreatic ducts, side branches, and presence of strictures.[33,34] MRCP is useful in assessing the pancreatic ducts as a noninvasive method. ERCP should not be used as a primary diagnostic modality for chronic pancreatitis, and should be used only for therapeutic interventions.

The secretin stimulation test is considered the definitive test in assessing pancreatic function. This diagnostic test involves measurement of the bicarbonate concentration originating from the pancreas in the duodenal fluid after the administration of secretin. Secretin causes the secretion of bicarbonate-rich fluid from the pancreas. A peak bicarbonate concentration of less than 80 mEq/L is consistent with chronic pancreatitis. Laboratory tests may be used to diagnose autoimmune chronic pancreatitis, including erythrocyte sedimentation rate, immunoglobulin G4, rheumatoid factor, antinuclear antibodies, and anti–smooth muscle antibody.[32]

DIAGNOSTICS

Chronic Pancreatitis

LABORATORY	IMAGING
CBC and differential	KUB, abdominal ultrasound
Serum amylase	CT scan, MRI, MRCP
Serum lipase	**OTHER DIAGNOSTICS**
Serum bilirubin	EUS*
Serum glucose	ERCP*
Serum alkaline phosphatase	Secretin stimulation test*
Stool for steatorrhea (fecal fat)	

*If indicated.

DIFFERENTIAL DIAGNOSIS

A strong history of alcoholism suggests the diagnosis of chronic pancreatitis in the patient with abdominal pain. However, pancreatic cancer, peptic ulcer disease, cholelithiasis, biliary tract obstruction, irritable bowel syndrome, and pancreatic stones should be excluded when the diagnosis of chronic pancreatitis is being considered.

In addition, because pancreatic cancer may manifest with signs and symptoms similar to those of chronic pancreatitis, patients may require MRCP or EUS for diagnosis. Pancreatic cancer should be suspected as a cause of chronic pancreatitis when a patient is older than 50 years or has any of the following: (1) new-onset diabetes mellitus; (2) change in bowel habits; (3) negative history of alcohol use; (4) recent weight loss; (5) a short duration of symptoms and/or the presence of other constitutional signs and symptoms (e.g., fatigue, insomnia, anorexia). These symptoms can originate from pancreatic cancer and should be considered a "red flag," prompting additional workup with EUS and tumor markers, given a high suspicion for malignancy. Tumor markers (carcinoembryonic antigen, CA 19-9) may be normal with early pancreatic cancer.[32]

Further imaging with ultrasound or angiography can be used to exclude mesenteric vascular disease as the origin of chronic abdominal pain. Finally, the health care provider must recognize that chronic pancreatitis can occur in the setting of autoimmune diseases such as Sjögren syndrome, systemic lupus erythematosus, and primary biliary cirrhosis, and use appropriate testing to exclude associated conditions as warranted by the patient's history and presentation.

MANAGEMENT

The treatment of pancreatic exocrine and endocrine dysfunction, pain control, and correction of symptomatic pancreatic structural abnormalities are the goals of chronic pancreatitis treatment. These management modalities require medical and possibly surgical intervention.

Pain Control

The strong relationship between alcohol consumption and pancreatitis underscores the importance of alcohol abstinence to prevent further damage and to reduce pain. The intense pain of chronic pancreatitis coupled with inconsistent pain relief is a risk factor for narcotic addiction. A short course of opiates with low-dose amitriptyline and nonsteroidal medication may break the pain cycle. Nerve blocks have not been found to provide long-term pain relief in the treatment of chronic pancreatitis. Studies have found that the celiac nerve block provides relief of pain for 2 to 4 months, if at all, and poses a risk for irreversible nerve damage.[32] Early involvement of a pain management team may provide additional benefit to patients and potentially minimize addiction sequelae. Uncoated pancreatic enzymes combined with acid suppression to allow for maximal absorption are thought to be useful for pain control to suppress the production of pancreatic enzymes.

Nutritional Interventions

In chronic pancreatitis, patients experience nutritional deficiencies and chronic pain. Nutritional deficiencies result from malassimilation of ingested food from exocrine pancreatic insufficiency, and endocrine insufficiency resulting in diabetes mellitus with loss of calories. Steatorrhea and diarrhea are produced by exocrine dysfunction. Malassimilation is managed by pancreatic enzyme replacement. The starting dose of pancreatic enzyme replacement in patients with severe chronic pancreatitis may be as high as 90,000 United States Pharmacopeia (USP) units of lipase with each meal and 45,000 USP units with snacks.[35,36] Pancreatic enzyme function may be increased by intake of acid-suppressing medications. Enzyme supplementation is recommended for all patients with chronic pancreatitis and may have a role to decrease pain that has not responded to other conservative measures. Pancreatic enzyme replacement therapy comes in coated and uncoated forms; the uncoated form requires acid suppression, because an acidic environment will neutralize the pancreatic enzymes. The coated form of enzymes is usually used to correct pancreatic exocrine insufficiency. Additional nutritional support with supplementation of fat-soluble vitamins may be necessary.

Surgical Interventions

When a patient has pain nonresponsive to medical therapies, surgical interventions may be necessary. Extracorporeal shock wave lithotripsy of calcified pancreatic stones can be helpful in relieving the obstruction of pancreatic ducts, blocking secretions in the 22% to 60% of patients with chronic pancreatitis who have pancreatic duct stones. Endoscopic therapy may provide pain relief in some patients by decompressing an obstructed pancreatic duct with placement of a stent or pancreatic duct sphincterotomy and stone extraction. However, studies have shown that the presence or absence of stones does not correlate with the existence of pain.[32] A randomized controlled trial examining patients with chronic pancreatitis and a dilated duct showed that surgical drainage resulted in better pain scores than for those patients undergoing endoscopic drainage.[37]

Surgical options for chronic pancreatitis include denervation procedures, which involve interruption of the nerve fibers passing through the celiac ganglion and splanchnic nerves from the pancreas. Another surgical intervention for patients with a dilated duct involves decompression and drainage of the pancreatic duct. Gastric and biliary drainage may be necessary as well because of obstruction or strictures of the bile duct or duodenum. Resection of a portion of the pancreas may be an option for those patients with ongoing pain who are not considered candidates for drainage procedures. Resection of the pancreatic head may provide pain relief in up to 85% of patients. Patients who have undergone pancreatectomy may have exocrine and endocrine dysfunction. Pancreatic insufficiency can result with extensive resection, and severe diabetes can ensue. Autologous islet cell transplantation after entire gland resection is a topic under current exploration. Total pancreatectomy is a last resort in patients who have not responded to all other treatments. Despite the availability of these techniques, the criteria for surgical intervention are controversial. Consultation with a gastroenterologist is advised for diagnostic verification and collaborative management. Invasive studies may be indicated as the patient's condition changes or as complications follow.[31]

LIFE SPAN CONSIDERATIONS

Steatorrhea, diabetes, and pancreatic calcifications are complications commonly experienced by older adults with longstanding chronic pancreatitis. Also, idiopathic senile chronic pancreatitis may occur in adults older than 60 years. Two variants of senile chronic pancreatitis have been identified. In the first type, patients exhibit the typical symptoms of steatorrhea, weight loss, or diabetes; there is no pain. Primary inflammatory pancreatitis, the second and less common version, occurs primarily in women and manifests with weight loss, steatorrhea, atypical or absent pain, fever, hypergammaglobulinemia, or chronic hepatitis. Other causes of malabsorption in older adults should be considered. Celiac disease, small bowel bacterial overgrowth, and pancreatic cancer must be excluded.

COMPLICATIONS

Chronic pancreatitis can be associated with a variety of complications. The most common complications are pseudocyst formation and mechanical obstruction of the duodenum and common bile duct.[38] Diabetes, exocrine insufficiency, malnutrition, pancreatic ascites, pleural effusion, splenic vein thrombosis, gastric varices, and pain are other complications associated with chronic pancreatitis.[38] The most feared complication of chronic pancreatitis is development of pancreatic cancer. The development of extrahepatic biliary obstruction is signified by serum alkaline phosphatase levels that are twice the normal level for longer than 2 months. Portal hypertension may occur as a result of thrombosis in the splenic or portal veins, pancreatic abscess, common bile duct obstruction, peptic ulcer, pseudoaneurysm of adjacent arteries, gastrointestinal bleeding, ascites from a leaking pseudocyst or damaged duct, and pancreatic cancer.

INDICATIONS FOR REFERRAL OR HOSPITALIZATION

The primary care or collaborating physician is consulted for the initial diagnosis and management. Subsequent deterioration or complications in the patient's status warrant continued physician guidance. Initial testing for stable, uncomplicated patients can be accomplished in the outpatient setting. Patients with chronic pancreatitis may have superimposed episodes of acute pancreatitis, which should be appropriately managed as described in the acute pancreatitis section. Hospitalization is required for the management of serious complications and for surgical drainage or resection procedures. Given the complications and risk of progression to pancreatic cancer, patients with chronic pancreatitis should be referred to a gastroenterologist to tailor long-term management plans and ensure close follow-up. Incidentally found suspicious lesions or changes in imaging of the pancreas in a patient with known chronic pancreatitis should also prompt immediate referral to a gastroenterologist for further evaluation.

PATIENT AND FAMILY EDUCATION

It is vital that patients and families understand the recurrent, chronic character of the disease. Careful explanation of each individual's etiologic factors and the need for alcohol abstinence is necessary. Patients with pancreatic endocrine insufficiency should receive diabetic education, because they are susceptible to macrovascular and microvascular complications. Patients with pancreatic exocrine insufficiency must understand the origin of steatorrhea, the purpose and dosage of dietary supplements and pancreatic enzyme replacement when appropriate, and supplementation with fat-soluble vitamins and calcium. It is important to clarify and to update guidelines for follow-up care, pain management, and symptoms requiring immediate attention.

PANCREATIC PSEUDOCYST

DEFINITION AND EPIDEMIOLOGY

Pseudocysts develop in approximately 10% of patients with chronic pancreatitis. They are the result of an encapsulation by fibrous tissue of an acute fluid collection. Pancreatic pseudocysts can contain blood, tissue, fluid, pancreatic digestive enzymes, and cellular debris accumulated in a cystlike mass. The prefix *pseudo-* is used because this localized collection of material does not have an epithelial lining, a hallmark of a true cyst.

Pseudocysts form as sequelae of acute pancreatitis or in association with chronic pancreatitis. Other, less common causes include gallbladder disease causing pancreatitis, and surgery or trauma to the pancreas. Pseudocysts, occurring singularly or as multiple lesions, develop primarily in the body or tail of the pancreas but are found outside the pancreas.

PATHOPHYSIOLOGY

Pseudocysts develop as a result of ductal disruptions and contain a large concentration of pancreatic enzymes. Pseudocysts may be single or multiple, small or large, and located in or outside of the pancreas. An absence of epithelial tissue distinguishes pseudocysts from pancreatic cysts.

CLINICAL PRESENTATION

Most pancreatic pseudocysts are asymptomatic. When symptoms occur, the presenting symptoms are typically related to the location and extent of the fluid collection, or its complications—that is, leakage, infection, or erosion into adjacent organs such as the splenic vein. Abdominal pain may be a presenting symptom related to expansion of the pseudocyst. Other symptoms associated with pseudocyst formation include low-grade fever, jaundice, diaphragm inflammation, pleural effusion, and ascites. Pseudocyst expansion may also contribute to duodenal or biliary obstruction, vascular occlusion, and fistula formation into adjacent viscera. Gastrointestinal bleeding can result when a pseudoaneurysm forms from adjacent vessel necrosis and bleeds into a pancreatic duct.[39] Secondary infection of pseudocysts is uncommon compared with walled-off necrosis.

DIAGNOSTICS

Diagnostics include pancreatic imaging by CT, MRI, or ultrasonography. If pleural effusion or ascites is present along with the pseudocyst, the thoracentesis or paracentesis fluid has amylase levels above 1000 international units (IU)/L when the origin is pancreatic.[39] Biopsy and carcinoembryonic antigen levels of cystic fluid from suspicious cystic lesions exclude premalignant growths and malignant neoplasms.[40,41] This is accomplished by CT-guided percutaneous needle aspiration or via EUS with fine-needle aspiration. MRCP, EUS, or ERCP before surgery is indicated to determine ductal and pseudocyst anatomy. Serologic analysis includes amylase, glucose, alkaline phosphatase, and bilirubin concentrations. Elevations of blood glucose and amylase levels are common. Increased serum alkaline phosphatase or bilirubin levels indicate compression of the common bile duct as it passes through the pancreas from extrahepatic biliary obstruction.

DIAGNOSTICS

Pancreatic Pseudocyst

LABORATORY	IMAGING
CBC and differential	CT scan, MRI, or ultrasound
Serum amylase	**OTHER DIAGNOSTICS**
Serum glucose	ERCP, biopsy
Alkaline phosphatase	
Bilirubin	

DIFFERENTIAL DIAGNOSIS

The presence of pancreatic fluid masses requires investigation. Pseudocysts can be confused with and should be distinguished from pancreatic cystic tumors including cystadenomas, cystadenocarcinomas, intraductal papillary mucinous neoplasms (IPMNs), and other pancreatic cysts including retention cysts, and congenital conditions. Concerns that a fluid collection is not a pseudocyst are prompted by a patient's history of no prior episodes of acute pancreatitis, signs or symptoms of chronic pancreatitis, or pancreatic trauma, and by the absence of inflammatory changes on CT scan. The cyst on imaging may have features that suggest it is not a pseudocyst—for example, thick walls or septations.[39] EUS with fine-needle aspiration is used to exclude malignancy in cystic lesions because pancreatic neoplasms may be cystic.

DIFFERENTIAL DIAGNOSIS

Pancreatic Pseudocyst

- Congenital cysts
- Retention cysts
- Non-neoplastic—serous cystadenomas
- Neoplastic—mucinous cystadenomas
- Cystadenocarcinomas
- IPMNs

MANAGEMENT

The decision process for pseudocyst management contains several steps. First, alternative diagnoses, particularly the possibility that the cyst may represent a neoplasm, must be excluded. Next, the provider considers whether a complication of pseudocyst (e.g., biliary or duodenal obstruction) is present. If the pseudocyst is increasing rapidly in size and/or the hemoglobin is decreasing, consideration should be given to a pseudoaneurysm, which occurs in approximately 10% of patients with a pancreatic pseudocyst.[39] Complication rates rise dramatically after the presence of the pseudocyst for longer than 13 weeks. In patients without discomfort, neoplasm, or complications, conservative management may be possible and the pancreatic pseudocyst safely monitored.[39] Currently, there are several drainage options for pseudocysts that are based on the cyst's location and the patient's symptoms. These options are multiple internal drainage procedures that can be performed endoscopically and percutaneously guided by CT. Indications for drainage include rapid enlargement, compression of surrounding structures, pain, and signs of infection. One should allow maturation of the pseudocyst wall for at least 6 weeks before arranging for drainage.

Interdisciplinary Management

Initial evaluation, laboratory tests, and imaging studies can be performed in the primary care setting. Complications, invasive diagnostics, and evaluation for surgery require collaboration with specialists in radiology, surgery, and gastroenterology.

COMPLICATIONS

Infected pseudocysts may cause severe pain, high fever, chills, and leukocytosis. If infection is clinically suspected, guided needle aspiration is indicated. If infection is confirmed, then CT or EUS guided drainage is indicated. Furthermore, pseudocysts may erode and perforate structures, resulting in rupture into the peritoneal cavity or gastrointestinal tract. Stomach perforation can manifest with few symptoms and require no treatment; acute peritoneal perforation necessitates surgical intervention and can be fatal, as opposed to gradual leakage, which results in pancreatic ascites. Colon perforation is seen with abdominal pain and self-limited bloody diarrhea. Pseudocysts can also erode blood vessels, creating a pseudoaneurysm and producing hemorrhage and shock. Three clinical findings are associated with pseudoaneurysm formation: gastrointestinal bleeding, sudden pseudocyst enlargement, and unexplained decrease in hematocrit.[40] Elevated serum amylase levels and ascitic fluid containing amylase and protein suggest a leaking pseudocyst.

INDICATIONS FOR REFERRAL OR HOSPITALIZATION

If a pseudocyst or another complication is suspected, the collaborating physician is consulted during the initial visit.

Long-term management requires careful and continued collaboration with the primary care physician.

PATIENT AND FAMILY EDUCATION

Patients at risk for pseudocyst formation should be educated about the symptoms of a pseudocyst and the necessity to contact their health care provider for increased or persistent pain. Patients with known pseudocysts should receive instruction concerning the cause of their condition, complications, symptoms, and indications to seek medical attention.

ACKNOWLEDGMENTS

The authors wish to extend their thanks to Jamie S. Barkin, MD, for reviewing this chapter.

CHAPTER 143

TUMORS OF THE GASTROINTESTINAL TRACT

Lindsey Law

Tumors of the gastrointestinal tract may be benign or malignant. It is essential that malignant tumors be identified as early as possible and treated appropriately. This chapter focuses on the common malignant neoplasms of the esophagus, stomach, small intestine, and colon; common benign tumors of the gastrointestinal tract are also discussed.

TUMORS OF THE ESOPHAGUS

DEFINITION AND EPIDEMIOLOGY

Esophageal carcinoma is a malignant neoplasm of the esophagus. The two most common types of malignant neoplasms are adenocarcinoma and squamous cell carcinoma. Squamous cell carcinoma accounts for 95% of esophageal cancers worldwide, and adenocarcinoma accounts for 50% to 80% of esophageal cancers in the United States.[1] Squamous cell carcinomas develop from cells in the proximal portion of the esophagus, and adenocarcinomas develop from glandular cells in the distal portion of the esophagus. Squamous cell carcinoma is more common in African Americans, whereas adenocarcinoma is more common in whites. Men are three times as likely as women to develop esophageal cancer. In the United States, the rates of squamous cell carcinoma have decreased among African-American men, whereas the rates of adenocarcinoma in white men have increased.[1] The incidence of esophageal cancer increases with age. The majority of persons affected by esophageal cancer are aged 50 to 70 years, and approximately 40% of older adults with Barrett esophagus will develop adenocarcinoma of the esophagus. The prevalence of esophageal cancer is higher in northern China, South Africa, France, Iran, and parts of Asia.[2] Survival rates are poor for persons with esophageal cancer. The overall survival rate is approximately 14%.[3]

Older age, male gender, drinking, smoking, and cancer of the head and neck are risk factors for the development of esophageal cancer. Nutritional deficiencies of vitamins and trace elements have also been implicated.[4] The major risk factors for squamous cell esophageal carcinoma are chronic smoking and alcohol consumption, achalasia, and tylosis.[5] The single most important risk factor for the development of adenocarcinoma of the esophagus is esophageal reflux leading to the premalignant condition of Barrett esophagus.[5] Obesity is emerging as a significant risk factor for esophageal cancer, although a causal relationship has not been established.[5]

PATHOPHYSIOLOGY

Esophageal cancers are usually related to squamous cell carcinoma or adenocarcinoma.[6] The majority of esophageal tumors are located in the lower third of the esophagus (55%), but one tenth are found in the upper esophagus and these are usually squamous cell carcinomas.[6] Esophageal adenocarcinomas arise in Barrett esophagus, a metaplasia of the distal esophagus occurring in association with long-term gastroesophageal reflux.[6] The extensive lymphatic system of the esophagus allows cancers of the esophagus to spread locally and into adjacent mediastinal structures regardless of tumor type.[7]

CLINICAL PRESENTATION

Dysphagia is the classic presenting symptom of esophageal carcinoma. This symptom indicates that the esophageal lumen has been reduced by at least half of its normal diameter.[8] Other symptoms include anorexia, weight loss, and odynophagia with radiation to the back. Hoarseness results from tumor involvement of the recurrent laryngeal nerve, and a tracheoesophageal fistula may produce a chronic cough.[8] The clinical features of esophageal adenocarcinoma are similar to those of squamous cell carcinoma, but it may also produce early satiety, nausea, vomiting, and bloating because of tumor encroachment into the stomach.

PHYSICAL EXAMINATION

Fixed supraclavicular, cervical, and axillary lymphadenopathies are signs of advanced disease. Both hepatomegaly secondary to metastatic disease and superior vena cava syndrome indicate a poor prognosis.[7,8]

DIAGNOSTICS

New-onset dysphagia should prompt an evaluation for an esophageal tumor. Diagnostic evaluation of the patient with a suspected esophageal carcinoma is a two-step procedure that begins with barium esophagography and is followed by upper gastrointestinal endoscopy with biopsy and cytologic tests.[5] Barium esophagography and endoscopy are used in evaluating the primary tumor. Endoscopic ultrasound examination will

DIAGNOSTICS

Esophageal Tumors

IMAGING	OTHER DIAGNOSTICS
Contrast radiography	Barium esophagography
Chest x-ray examination*	Bronchoscopy*
CT scan*	Upper gastrointestinal endoscopy with biopsy and cytologic tests
PET/CT scan	
Radionuclide bone scans*	
Ultrasound*	

*If indicated.

help determine the extent of disease locally.[5] A clinical examination, biochemical assay, chest x-ray examination, computed tomography (CT) scan, positron emission tomography–computed tomography (PET/CT) scan, radionuclide bone scan, ultrasonography, and guided fine-needle aspiration biopsy of lymph nodes may be useful in the evaluation of metastasis.[5]

DIFFERENTIAL DIAGNOSIS

In the adult patient with a new onset of progressive, solid dysphagia, the differential diagnosis includes esophageal squamous cell carcinoma, esophageal adenocarcinoma, adenocarcinoma of the gastric cardia, benign peptic stricture, corrosive stricture, and esophageal motor disorders such as achalasia and scleroderma. Symptoms of dysphagia, especially in a patient older than 45 years, mandate a complete evaluation to exclude esophageal carcinoma.

DIFFERENTIAL DIAGNOSIS

Esophageal Tumors

- Benign esophageal leiomyoma
- Esophageal carcinoma
- Esophageal adenocarcinoma
- Adenocarcinoma of the gastric cardia
- Benign peptic stricture
- Corrosive stricture
- Esophageal motor disorders
- Achalasia

MANAGEMENT

Gastroenterologic, oncologic, and surgical consultations are critical for the evaluation of esophageal tumors. Surgical resection is the primary treatment of early-stage esophageal cancer. Chemotherapy with cisplatin and 5-fluorouracil plus radiation therapy with or without surgery may provide the best potential for cure in locally advanced disease.[7] However, palliation for dysphagia may be the only realistic goal because most patients have incurable disease at the time of diagnosis. Palliation can be accomplished by peroral stenting through the stenosis and transendoscopic ablation of obstructing tumors by laser photocoagulation.

For advanced disease, esophagectomy provides superb palliation.[9] Radiotherapy may provide palliation for patients who are not candidates for surgery.[9]

Systemic chemotherapy is a preferred method of palliation for metastatic disease. There are many chemotherapy agents available; however, there is not one particular regimen that is standard of care in the first-line setting.

Postoperative elevation of serum carcinoembryonic antigen (CEA) levels may be the first objective sign of recurrent disease and should prompt additional therapy, such as surgery or chemotherapy.[10]

COMPLICATIONS

Because of the distensibility of the esophagus, esophageal carcinoma tends to be silent until late in its course. Complications are usually related to mediastinal extension or esophageal narrowing and may include obstruction, hemorrhage, perforation, and fistula formation. Because the esophagus lacks a true serosa, cancer is often not contained at the time of diagnosis. The lungs and liver are the most common sites of hematogenous metastasis. Complications of esophageal resection include torsion or gangrene of the gastric, colonic, or jejunal pull-up; anastomotic leak; anastomotic stricture; subphrenic abscess; chylothorax; hemorrhage; wound infection and dehiscence; sepsis; dumping syndrome; vocal chord paralysis, and reflux esophagitis.

PATIENT AND FAMILY EDUCATION

Dietary instructions should be consistent with the degree of dysphagia experienced. Patients who have responded to therapy but continue to use alcohol and tobacco products during treatment demonstrate a poor response to treatment and an increased rate of local recurrence.[9] Therefore, patients should be encouraged to discontinue the use of these products and should be provided with therapeutic interventions for alcohol and tobacco cessation.[9,11]

HEALTH PROMOTION

Patients should be regularly questioned about the presence of heartburn or other signs of gastroesophageal reflux so that appropriate diagnostics and treatment can be initiated. Primary prevention of esophageal cancer includes avoidance of all tobacco products and of heavy alcohol consumption. It is also important to consume a diet that is rich in fruits and vegetables and to maintain a normal weight. With obesity, there can be increased acid reflux, thus multiplying the risk for adenocarcinoma of the lower esophagus and stomach.[9,11]

TUMORS OF THE STOMACH

DEFINITION AND EPIDEMIOLOGY

Gastric cancer is the second most common cause of cancer-related deaths worldwide. The prevalence of gastric cancer remains very high (70 per 100,000) in Japan, eastern Asia, eastern Europe, Chile, Colombia, and Central America.[5] The incidence of gastric cancer in the United States has declined dramatically during the past 70 years.[5] In this country, approximately 22,000 persons are diagnosed with gastric cancer each year, and about 11,000 people die of gastric cancer yearly.[5] The decline in gastric cancer has been attributed to improved refrigeration and the reduced consumption of preserved foods.[5] Gastric carcinoma occurs more often in African Americans, Hispanics, and Native Americans.[5] Common benign tumors of the stomach include leiomyomas and epithelial polyps.

Helicobacter pylori is noted as the primary risk factor for gastric cancer.[12] Other risk factors for gastric adenocarcinoma include chronic atrophic gastritis, pernicious anemia, and gastric polyps.[4] Dietary risk factors include a decreased consumption of fruits and vegetables and an increased intake of salt, nitrates and nitrites, and smoked and poorly preserved foods.[4] Genetic factors linked to gastric carcinoma include hereditary nonpolyposis colorectal cancer, familial polyposis, and first-degree relatives of patients with gastric cancer. A partial gastrectomy for peptic ulcer disease is also associated with an increased risk of gastric carcinoma.

PATHOPHYSIOLOGY

Gastric cancer is divided into two histologic types, intestinal and diffuse.[5] The intestinal type of gastric adenocarcinoma is characterized by distinct, large glands lined by columnar cells; it resembles intestinal cancer and is more common than the diffuse type.[5] The diffuse type of gastric cancer is poorly differentiated, lacks a glandular structure, and is more aggressive.[5] Gastric carcinomas spread by direct extension, lymphatic spread, hematogenous metastasis, and peritoneal seeding.

CLINICAL PRESENTATION

Unexplained weight loss, upper abdominal pain, anorexia, nausea, and vomiting are the most common symptoms of advanced gastric carcinoma.[4] The abdominal pain begins as insidious upper abdominal discomfort that ranges in intensity from a vague sense of postprandial fullness to a severe, steady pain. Other symptoms include change in bowel habits, dysphagia, melena, anemic symptoms, and hemorrhage.[4]

PHYSICAL EXAMINATION

Patients with advanced gastric cancer may be initially seen with cachexia, small bowel obstruction, epigastric mass, ascites, hepatomegaly, or lower extremity edema. Metastases may also manifest as an enlarged left supraclavicular lymph node (Virchow node) or an enlarged left anterior axillary lymph node, an enlarged periumbilical lymph node (Sister Mary Joseph node), an enlarged ovary (Krukenberg tumor), or a mass on the Blumer shelf on rectal examination.[5]

DIAGNOSTICS

Blood studies may reveal hypochromic, microcytic anemia secondary to iron deficiency. The stool is often positive for occult blood. Upper gastrointestinal endoscopy is the imaging modality of choice for stomach tumors because it allows direct visualization and biopsy of the tumor.[5] Once the diagnosis of gastric cancer is confirmed, abdominal and chest CT scans along with endoscopic ultrasound examination are indicated to establish the invasiveness of the primary tumor and the extent of metastasis.[5]

DIFFERENTIAL DIAGNOSIS

The differential diagnosis for tumors of the stomach includes gastric lymphoma; leiomyosarcoma; carcinoid tumors; and gastric metastasis from the lung, breast, and melanoma. Kaposi's sarcoma of the stomach, which may be present in patients with acquired immunodeficiency syndrome (AIDS), and hypertrophic gastropathy (Meniere disease) are also included in the differential diagnosis.

MANAGEMENT

Gastroenterologic, surgical, and oncologic consultations are essential for a patient with gastric cancer. Complete resection of the gastric carcinoma and adjacent lymph nodes offers the only chance for cure. A palliative resection should be considered for patients with advanced lesions who are initially seen with obstruction or bleeding.

In patients with locally advanced tumors or in those who are not surgical candidates secondary to comorbidities, combination chemotherapy plus radiation can be definitive. Pathologic complete response can be obtained in up to 30% of patients. Systemic chemotherapy is a preferred method of palliation for metastatic disease. There are many chemotherapy agents available; however, there is not one particular regimen that is standard of care in the first-line setting.

Obstruction and bleeding from large carcinomas of the gastric cardia can be managed by stent therapy, endoscopic laser therapy, or angiographic embolization.[5]

COMPLICATIONS

Gastric carcinomas are detected at an advanced stage, and the prognosis of this neoplasm remains poor. Intraperitoneal dissemination of the tumor may occur with involvement of the omentum, peritoneum, and serosa of the intestine. Other complications include gastric outlet obstruction, gastrointestinal bleeding, linitis plastica, malnutrition, and ascites.

DIAGNOSTICS

Stomach Tumors

LABORATORY
LFTs
CBC and differential
Stool for occult blood
Tumor markers (CEA, CA-125)

IMAGING
Contrast radiography
CT scan of abdomen

OTHER DIAGNOSTICS
Upper gastrointestinal endoscopy and biopsy
Endoscopic ultrasound
Barium upper gastrointestinal series (if endoscopy is not available)
Diagnostic laparoscopy

CBC, complete blood count; LFTs, liver function tests.

DIFFERENTIAL DIAGNOSIS

Stomach Tumors

- Gastric lymphoma
- Leiomyosarcoma
- Carcinoid tumors
- Gastric metastasis
- Kaposi sarcoma of the stomach
- Hypertrophic gastropathy

PATIENT AND FAMILY EDUCATION

Although gastric tumors and small colon tumors may be associated with aging, cancer can affect younger patients. Weight loss, anorexia, difficulty swallowing, abdominal pain, change in bowel habits, and blood in the stool are signs of gastrointestinal cancers. Patients should be reminded to notify their health care provider if any of these symptoms occurs. In addition, patients should routinely be asked about a family history of gastrointestinal or other cancers.

HEALTH PROMOTION

A well-balanced diet rich in fruits and vegetables is important for overall good health. Such a diet will provide sufficient vitamins and antioxidants to maintain health. Consumption of smoked and highly salted, nitrated food should be avoided or severely limited. Only food that is refrigerated and kept under safe conditions should be consumed. Avoidance of all tobacco products is strongly recommended.[11] Because infectious agents have been associated with gastric cancer, it is important to practice good hygiene. Diagnosis of *H. pylori* infection and subsequent treatment also contribute to a reduction in the incidence of gastric cancer. Exposure to glycol ethers, hydraulic fluids, and leaded gasoline should also be limited. Education of the public along with increasing protection and surveillance in the workplace will limit or eliminate exposure to these products.

TUMORS OF THE SMALL INTESTINE

DEFINITION AND EPIDEMIOLOGY

Cancer of the small bowel is not as common as other gastrointestinal cancers, although small bowel cancers may be more difficult to diagnose.[13] Adenocarcinomas of the small intestine account for 50% of malignant neoplasms of the small bowel.[6,7,13] After resection of small bowel adenocarcinomas, there is a 5-year survival rate of 30%.[5] The peak incidence of symptomatic tumors is in the sixth decade of life.[5] The highest rate of small bowel adenocarcinoma occurs in African-American men.[14] Other malignant neoplasms of the small intestine include carcinoid tumors, lymphomas, and leiomyosarcomas.[6] All carcinoid tumors should be considered malignant. Metastasis occurs in the majority of patients with carcinoid tumors larger than 2 cm (⅘ inch).[5] More than 50% of all gastrointestinal carcinoids occur in the appendix, rectum, and small intestine.[5]

The three most common benign tumors of the small intestine are adenomas, leiomyomas, and lipomas.[6,14] Multiple adenomas may occur in the small intestine in Peutz-Jeghers syndrome and are considered benign; however, in some instances, adenocarcinoma may develop.[6]

Risk factors for adenocarcinoma of the small bowel include Crohn disease, celiac sprue, ileostomy stomas, ileal pouches and conduits, familial adenomatous polyposis, hereditary nonpolyposis colorectal cancer, cystic fibrosis, and Peutz-Jeghers syndrome.[15] Patients with Crohn disease have an increased risk for development of carcinoma of the small bowel, and adenocarcinoma develops years earlier than expected for this malignant neoplasm.

PATHOPHYSIOLOGY

Adenocarcinomas of the small intestine may be polypoid, ulcerative, or annular and stenosing. The tumors infiltrate through the bowel wall and invade adjacent organs. Venous invasion of the lymph nodes occurs by either metastasis or direct extension of the tumor. Carcinoid tumors are well-differentiated endocrine tumors that arise from the enterochromaffin cells at the base of the crypts of Lieberkühn. These cells give the tumor its most clinically distinctive feature—its ability to secrete tumor products that induce the carcinoid syndrome.[6,14] Serotonin is believed to be the humoral mediator responsible for the diarrhea that occurs with carcinoid syndrome.[16] Other carcinoid features include asthma-type wheezing, skin lesions, and cardiac manifestations.[16] The cardiac effects of carcinoid include endocardial fibrotic plaques on the tricuspid and pulmonic valves, the endocardium of the right cardiac chambers, and the pulmonary artery.[16]

CLINICAL PRESENTATION

Abdominal pain is the most common symptom expressed by patients with either benign or malignant small bowel tumors. Other symptoms include nausea, vomiting, cramping, abdominal distention aggravated by eating, and weight loss. Unless patients manifest the carcinoid syndrome—characterized by flushing, diarrhea, wheezing, and sweating—no specific signs or symptoms suggest cancer of the small bowel.[5]

PHYSICAL EXAMINATION

A palpable abdominal mass may be present in up to 40% of patients with a small bowel malignant neoplasm.[15] Duodenal adenocarcinomas that involve the Vater ampulla may cause obstructive jaundice or pancreatitis.[6,14] Hepatomegaly, ascites, and jaundice may indicate advanced metastatic disease. Pulmonic stenosis may cause a systolic murmur in patients with carcinoid syndrome.

DIAGNOSTICS

In the evaluation of small bowel tumors, the stool should be tested for occult blood. However, the diagnostic modality of choice is a small bowel follow-through (SBFT), an extension of the conventional barium meal in which the barium is ingested orally.[15] Enteroclysis, synonymous with a small bowel enema, may be performed by infusing approximately 1 L of barium until bowel distention occurs and the barium reaches the terminal ileum.[15] Enteroclysis is superior to SBFT in the diagnosis of small bowel disease, except for lesions of the terminal ileum.

DIAGNOSTICS

Small Intestine Tumors

LABORATORY	Endoscopy*
CBC and differential	Capsule endoscopy*
Stool for occult blood	Arteriography*
Serotonin and metabolites	Scintigraphy*
Urinary 5-HIAA*	CT scan*
IMAGING	**OTHER DIAGNOSTICS**
SBFT	Laparotomy*
Enteroclysis	

*If indicated.
CBC, complete blood count.

Additional studies after barium radiology may be indicated and include CT scanning, arteriography, serotonin and metabolite levels, scintigraphy, endoscopy, and possibly capsule endoscopy.[16,17] Endoscopy is indicated for duodenal lesions that are accessible with gastroduodenoscopy and for terminal ileal lesions accessible with colonoscopy. A CT scan is indicated to determine metastasis, including hepatic involvement, by possible malignant tumors. Arteriography is indicated in cases of obscure gastrointestinal bleeding. Measurement of serotonin and metabolites (5-HIAA) as well as scintigraphy may be necessary for suspected carcinoid tumors.[15] A laparotomy may be necessary when the diagnostic modalities are insufficient.

DIFFERENTIAL DIAGNOSIS

Small bowel tumors may be considered one of the less common causes of intestinal obstruction, occult gastrointestinal blood loss, weight loss, and unexplained abdominal pain. The diagnosis of a small bowel tumor often is not made before laparotomy. Therefore the differential diagnosis includes adhesions, hernias, intussusception, volvulus, intra-abdominal abscesses and hematomas, endometriosis, pelvic inflammatory disease, Crohn disease, ischemia, hematoma associated with oral anticoagulant therapy, radiation enteritis, amyloidosis, ingested foreign bodies, gallstones, bezoars, and worms.

MANAGEMENT

Gastroenterologic, oncologic, and surgical consultations are essential to provide optimum care for patients with small bowel tumors. These cancers are managed surgically, which offers the

DIFFERENTIAL DIAGNOSIS

Small Intestine Tumors

- Adhesions
- Hernias
- Intussusception
- Volvulus
- Intra-abdominal abscess or hematoma
- Endometriosis
- Pelvic inflammatory disease
- Crohn disease
- Ischemia
- Hematoma associated with oral anticoagulant therapy
- Radiation enteritis
- Amyloidosis
- Foreign body, bezoars, worms
- Gallstones
- Malignant tumors (including lymphoma)
- Benign tumors

only hope for cure. Because adenocarcinomas metastasize early to regional lymph nodes, a wide resection is undertaken.[15] If the lesions cannot be resected for cure, a palliative resection of the main lesion is recommended. Chemotherapy and radiotherapy are adjuvant therapies. Because carcinoid tumors larger than 1 cm (⅖ inch) in diameter are capable of metastasizing, a wide resection should be undertaken. Nonresectable intestinal and hepatic metastatic carcinoids should have aggressive debulking to alleviate symptoms of the carcinoid syndrome and possibly to prolong survival.[5,15]

Carcinoid syndrome may be treated with injections of octreotide (a synthetic somatostatin analogue that is a serotonin antagonist) to provide symptomatic relief until surgical management of the hepatic metastasis can be performed.[5,15] Hepatic artery occlusion and chemotherapy may control symptoms associated with hepatic metastasis.[5]

INDICATIONS FOR REFERRAL OR HOSPITALIZATION

Large lesions of the small intestine may produce partial or intermittent obstruction, bleeding, intussusception, and volvulus. Carcinoid tumors spread locally to regional lymph nodes, the liver, other intra-abdominal organs, and the lung. Small carcinoid tumors normally do not invade or obstruct the bowel lumen but can penetrate the muscle layer and lead to adhesions, bowel kinking, angulation, and obstruction. Massive fibrosis of the mesenteries, omentum, and peritoneum may result from the leakage of serotonin and other vasoactive substances. High serum levels of 5-HIAA may cause endocardial fibrotic plaques that stiffen and fix the tricuspid and pulmonic valves, which may lead to right-sided heart failure.

PATIENT AND FAMILY EDUCATION

Patient and family education for tumors of the small intestine is the same as for tumors of the stomach.

HEALTH PROMOTION

See the Health Promotion section under Tumors of the Colon.

TUMORS OF THE COLON

DEFINITION AND EPIDEMIOLOGY

Colorectal cancer is the third most common cancer in the United States and is the second leading cause of cancer deaths.[18] Adenocarcinomas account for the majority of all malignant tumors of the large bowel.[5] Risk factors for the development of colorectal cancer include greater than age 50, prior colorectal cancer, ulcerative colitis, hereditary and genetic factors, familial polyposis syndromes, history of breast or female genital cancer, long-term cigarette smoking, and a high-fat high-caloric diet.[6] Benign tumors of the colon include polyps and polyposis syndromes.

PATHOPHYSIOLOGY

Genetic and environmental factors contribute to the development of colorectal cancer. Colon cancer develops from mucosal polyps. Adenomatous and hyperplastic are the most common types. The majority of colon cancers arise from adenomas. Colorectal adenocarcinomas may be polypoid, ulcerating, or infiltrative. Adenocarcinomas arise from a varied progression of events that can be genetic in origin and involve a series of mutations that result in a malignant neoplasm. Colorectal adenocarcinoma can spread intraluminally or by direct extension, hematogenous spread, lymphatic dissemination, or transperitoneal seeding. More than 80% of colorectal cancers are a result of malfunction of tumor suppressor genes *p53*, *APC*, and *DCC*.[5]

CLINICAL PRESENTATION

The symptoms of colon adenocarcinoma depend on the location of the tumor. Cancers of the proximal colon usually attain a larger size before becoming symptomatic compared with cancers of the left side of the colon and rectum. Fatigue, shortness of breath, angina caused by hypochromic microcytic anemia, and melenic liquid stool may be the principal means of presentation of right-sided colonic masses. Abdominal discomfort may be present as the tumor increases in size. Obstruction is uncommon because of the large diameters of the cecum and ascending colon. The left side of the colon has a smaller lumen than the proximal colon, and therefore obstructive symptoms may occur. Left-sided symptoms include cramps, gas pain, and decrease in the caliber of the stool. Adenocarcinomas of the descending and sigmoid colon are often circumferential and may also cause obstruction.

Patients with colon adenocarcinoma may experience colicky abdominal pain, especially after meals, and a change in bowel habits. Constipation may alternate with an increased frequency of defecation. Hematochezia may be present with distal rather than proximal lesions, and bright red blood passed through the rectum may be seen with cancers that involve the left side of the colon and rectum. Approximately half of patients with colon cancer experience anorexia and weight loss.

PHYSICAL EXAMINATION

Patients may initially be seen with a palpable abdominal mass and signs of distention or intestinal obstruction. Inguinal nodes may be enlarged with left-sided cancer, and the liver may be enlarged because of metastasis.

DIAGNOSTICS

Visual inspection and digital examination of the anus and distal rectum are important in the evaluation of colorectal tumors to permit palpation of a possible tumor and to obtain stool to test for occult blood. A complete blood count (CBC) should also be obtained. The air-contrast barium enema can diagnose many colon cancers but does not permit biopsy. Colonoscopy as well as flexible sigmoidoscopy allows direct visualization and biopsy of the colon, but colonoscopy provides more thorough colon visualization. Virtual colonoscopy, a high-resolution CT scan, is also used in some instances to detect colon tumors. However, there are continued concerns that virtual colonoscopy may not detect small tumors, and there is no evidence that virtual colonoscopy is superior to colonoscopy.[6] CEA is not useful for screening but may be a valuable marker for recurring cancer.[5] The metastatic evaluation includes a CT scan, a chest x-ray study, CEA, and liver function tests (LFTs).[5]

DIAGNOSTICS

Colon Tumors

LABORATORY
CBC and differential
Stool for occult blood
LFTs
CEA

IMAGING
CT scan*
Chest x-ray studies
Barium enema x-ray studies

OTHER DIAGNOSTICS
Colonoscopy

*If indicated.

DIFFERENTIAL DIAGNOSIS

The differential diagnosis of colon carcinoma includes benign tumors, diverticulitis, ulcerative colitis, Crohn disease, tuberculosis, amebiasis, fungal masses, schistosomiasis, viral lesions such as cytomegalovirus, feces, lymphoid polyps and lymphoma, carcinoid tumors, metastatic lesions, and Kaposi sarcoma. Obstructing lesions may include strictures from inflammation, radiation and ischemic colitis, and volvulus. In addition, extrinsic compression may occur from endometriosis and pancreatitis.

DIFFERENTIAL DIAGNOSIS

Colon Tumors

- Benign tumors
- Diverticulitis
- Ulcerative colitis
- Crohn disease
- Tuberculosis
- Amebiasis
- Fungal masses
- Schistosomiasis
- Viral or metastatic lesions
- Feces
- Lymphoid polyps, lymphoma
- Carcinoid tumors
- Kaposi sarcoma
- Inflammatory bowel disease
- Strictures
- Extrinsic compression from endometriosis or pancreatitis

MANAGEMENT

Gastroenterologic, oncologic, and surgical consultations are necessary to provide optimum care for patients with colorectal tumors. The primary treatment of colorectal cancer is surgical resection of the primary colon or rectal tumor and removal of at least 12 regional lymph nodes.[5] The CEA sample should be drawn before removal of a primary tumor[6] because not all cancers produce this glycoprotein. If the preoperative value is not elevated, the test is not informative in the postoperative period. If the CEA value is elevated before surgery, the measurement should be repeated every 3 months after surgery for tumor recurrence.[6] Adjuvant chemotherapy for colon cancer has been used in an attempt to reduce the recurrence rate of metastatic disease.[5,6] Adjuvant therapy with 5-fluorouracil and oxaliplatin has been shown to decrease the recurrence rate and distant metastasis in stage II and III disease.[5]

The use of chemoradiotherapy for rectal cancer is usually recommended as an adjunctive treatment but is not beneficial for colon cancers outside of the rectum.[6]

COMPLICATIONS

Colorectal cancer may cause large bowel obstruction or perforation in cancers that reach an advanced stage. Rate of recurrence within the abdominal cavity, including liver metastasis, is high. Distant metastases, which are thought to be disseminated by hematogenous spread, may occur to the lungs, adrenal glands, bones, and brain. Weight loss, fatigue, rectal bleeding, abdominal and pelvic pain, coughing, change in bowel habits, and bone pain may signal recurrent disease.

PATIENT AND FAMILY EDUCATION

Individuals 50 years of age and older should be screened for colorectal cancer.[5] Also recommended is sigmoidoscopy at the age of 45 years, or 10 years younger than the youngest family member with colon cancer, and then every 3 to 5 years thereafter. In patients with familial polyposis of the colon, colorectal cancer is inevitable 10 to 15 years after the onset of polyposis, and elective complete colectomy is required. Other family members must be screened for the dominant inheritance pattern. The American Cancer Society recommends that routine screening for colon cancer begin at 50 years of age with annual fecal occult blood testing, sigmoidoscopy every 5 years, and colonoscopy every 10 years.[5] If polyps are present, repeated flexible sigmoidoscopy is indicated in 3 to 5 years. However, the guidelines may differ for older patients. Annual digital rectal examinations are also recommended for all patients older than 40.[6]

Individuals at high risk for the development of colon carcinoma, such as those with familial polyposis syndrome, prior adenomatous colonic polyps or cancer, or long-standing ulcerative colitis involving the entire colon, may require screening before 40 years of age and more frequent periodic screening tests (including examination of the entire colon) (see Chapter 19).[5]

Healthy diets with increased fiber and decreased fat intake may help prevent colon cancer. Therefore, these diets should be explained and encouraged routinely. Patients should be evaluated every 3 months for 3 to 5 years with history, CEA level, and physical examination to detect the postoperative recurrence of colorectal carcinoma.[5] A screening colonoscopy should also be performed 1 year after surgery and, if findings are normal, then every 3 to 5 years.[5]

HEALTH PROMOTION

Promotion of a healthy lifestyle is essential in the prevention of colorectal cancer. Patients should be encouraged to exercise on a regular basis, 30 minutes at least three times weekly. More vigorous exercise may provide more benefit. It is important to limit the fat intake to 25% to 30% of the total calorie intake. Increasing the amount of fiber to 20 to 30 g/day in a diet that provides five servings of fruits and vegetables daily may be beneficial, but this is not yet proven.[6] However, these recommendations will help maintain a normal body weight. Avoidance of tobacco products and heavy alcohol consumption is also important.[11]

CHAPTER 144

PEPTIC ULCER DISEASE

Donna M. Glynn

DEFINITION AND EPIDEMIOLOGY

Peptic ulcer disease (PUD) is a pathologic, destructive, chronic disorder characterized by ulceration of the gastric and duodenal mucosa. The two common causes of peptic ulcers in the United States are *Helicobacter* infections *(Helicobacter pylori)* and the use of nonsteroidal anti-inflammatory drugs (NSAIDs). During the last decades of the 20th century, the incidence of PUD declined dramatically. This decline is attributed to the discovery and effective use of acid suppressants and the treatment of *H. pylori* infections. However, gastric and duodenal ulcers continue to have a serious impact on the economics of health care and society because of recurrence rates, increased office visits, medication costs, diagnostic costs, and patient quality-of-life concerns. Therefore it is essential to obtain a thorough health history, to identify potential risk factors, and to provide a cost-effective diagnosis and treatment plan.

PUD may be defined as a full-thickness defect in the mucosa of the stomach or duodenum caused by an imbalance both in the amount of acid and pepsin production and in the ability of the gastric and duodenal lining to protect itself. It is estimated that approximately 4.5 million people in the United States are affected annually, and the hospitalization rate for PUD is approximately 30 patients per 100,000 cases. Lifetime prevalence is estimated at 11% to 14% in males and 8% to 11% in females.[1] *H. pylori*, a spiral, flagellated, gram-negative, rod-shaped bacterium, was first identified and linked to gastritis in the 1980s and is a major causative organism in the development of ulcer disease. With the discovery of the bacterium, the treatment of PUD has changed from acid suppression to eradication of the bacterium. Excluding individuals who are using NSAID therapy, 61% of duodenal ulcers and 63% of gastric ulcers have been found to test positive for *H. pylori.*[1]

The second most common cause of PUD is the use of NSAIDs and low-dose aspirin. NSAIDs are commonly prescribed medications and available over the counter. As many as 30% of individuals taking NSAIDs will have adverse gastrointestinal (GI) events. Increasing the risk of an adverse event in individuals using NSAID therapy are a previous history of PUD, advanced age, long-term NSAID use, comorbidities, and concurrent use of anticoagulants.[1] Because of advancing age and the increased prevalence of osteoarthritis, the risk of PUD is significant in older patient populations. The discovery of cyclooxygenase 1 (COX-1) and COX -2 led to the development of COX-2–selective NSAIDs as an alternative therapy. COX-2 inhibitors are generally considered safer for the GI tract; however, this class of medication, which is commonly prescribed for arthritis pain, can also cause gastric or duodenal ulcer formation and has been linked to adverse cardiovascular events.[2]

Other risk factors for the development of PUD include family history, cigarette smoking, chronic obstructive pulmonary disease, major trauma, oral steroids, bisphosphonate therapy, caffeine ingestion, alcohol, cirrhosis, and physiologic stress. Certain conditions and genetic factors have also been identified as risk factors for the development of PUD. Zollinger-Ellison syndrome, antral G cell hyperplasia, cystic fibrosis, short bowel syndrome, hyperparathyroidism, and noncompliance with an *H. pylori* treatment regimen are documented in the development of PUD.[1]

PATHOPHYSIOLOGY

The function of the GI tract is the digestion of food and absorption of nutrients. This process is achieved by high concentrations of acid and pepsin that are secreted from the parietal cells of the stomach. The surface of the mucosa secretes alkaline mucus that protects the mucosa from self-digestion. Under normal conditions, a balance is present between gastric acid secretion and gastroduodenal mucosal defense. However, when this system is interrupted, the protective tissue is damaged, and erosion or ulcer formation occurs. A peptic ulcer can affect one or all layers of the gastric lining or duodenum. Gastric ulcers are commonly found distal to the junction between the antrum and the acid secretory mucosa. Duodenal ulcers are primarily located in the duodenal bulb or at the pyloric duodenal junction. Most patients with duodenal ulcers have impaired bicarbonate secretion, which is associated with *H. pylori.*[3] Reduction of the production of acid and pepsin is key to the promotion of healing and prevention of recurrence. Spontaneous remissions and exacerbations are commonly associated with PUD.

H. pylori, a spiral, flagellated organism, is acquired through the orofecal route. Once it is ingested, *H. pylori* attaches to the gastric mucosa, colonizes the entire gastric epithelium, and produces local tissue injury that results in the release of cytotoxins and proteases. NSAID therapy has been shown to damage the gastric mucosa by suppression of gastric prostaglandin synthesis. Acid suppression continues to be the key component in the management of NSAID-associated PUD.

CLINICAL PRESENTATION

Although some patients are asymptomatic, the most common presenting chief complaint is epigastric pain or dyspepsia. Upper abdominal pain or discomfort is the most common presentation, with pain centered in the epigastrium. This discomfort is often described as a sharp, burning, aching, gnawing pain occurring 2 to 5 hours after meals or in the middle of the night. The patient will report that the pain is usually relieved with the ingestion of food or antacids; however, the symptoms are recurrent, with episodes lasting from hours to days to months. Peptic ulcers may be associated with food provoking symptoms. Patients may report pain with eating, postprandial belching, fullness, fatty food intolerance, nausea, and vomiting. Changes in the intensity, duration, or location of the pain may indicate penetration or perforation of an ulcer.[4]

PHYSICAL EXAMINATION

Inspection, auscultation, and percussion generally yield negative findings. In rare presentations, auscultation may reveal a succussion splash 4 hours or longer after meals, which would indicate a duodenal or pyloric channel ulcer, causing gastric outlet obstruction. Palpation may produce epigastric tenderness midline between the umbilicus and xiphoid process. If a perforation has occurred, the patient will have a rigid abdomen and generalized rebound tenderness. Rectal examination should be included with testing for melena.

DIAGNOSTICS

There is no reliable blood testing that can accurately confirm PUD. A complete blood count (CBC) will exclude anemia.

Blood chemistries will assess liver function and calcium levels. Serum culture for *H. pylori* is also indicated initially because of cost and availability. Breath test and stool antigen testing for *H. pylori* are available noninvasive testing methods. However, endoscopy is the standard diagnostic method.[5]

Endoscopy will provide the most accurate diagnosis of PUD and allows for multiple biopsies to exclude malignancy and confirm *H. pylori*. Barium radiography is still performed, but only in patients who are not eligible or who are unwilling to undergo endoscopy.[5]

DIAGNOSTICS

Endoscopy

LABORATORY
- CBC and differential
- *H. pylori* testing (serum, breath, fecal)
- Serum chemistries
- Stool for occult blood

DIAGNOSTICS
- Barium radiography

DIFFERENTIAL DIAGNOSIS

Differential diagnosis for PUD is based on the symptoms reported and the location of the pain. Cholecystitis causes right upper quadrant abdominal discomfort. Vague abdominal pain with reports of diarrhea or constipation may be associated with diverticulosis, irritable bowel syndrome, or nonulcer dyspepsia. Gastroesophageal reflux disease (GERD), pancreatitis, and malignant disease should also be considered. Zollinger-Ellison syndrome is a condition of excessive acid production. This should be considered if the individual does not respond to the traditional diet, smoking cessation, and pharmacologic therapy.

DIFFERENTIAL DIAGNOSIS

Ulcer Disease

- Cholecystitis
- Diverticulosis
- Irritable bowel syndrome
- Nonulcer dyspepsia
- GERD
- Pancreatitis
- Malignant disease
- Zollinger-Ellison syndrome

MANAGEMENT

First-line treatment of PUD is antisecretory therapy. If NSAID or COX-2 inhibitor use is documented, the medications should be discontinued. If objective findings include anemia, GI bleeding, rigid abdomen, weight loss, or new-onset dyspepsia in an individual older than 50 years, an immediate physician consultation is indicated. If symptoms persist after a limited course of antisecretory therapy, referral to a gastroenterologist for endoscopy is appropriate.

Treatment options for PUD include histamine$_2$ receptor antagonists (H_2RAs), proton pump inhibitors (PPIs), and prostaglandin therapy. The H_2RAs include cimetidine, famotidine, nizatidine, and ranitidine. These preparations inhibit gastric acid secretion by blocking the H_2 receptors of the parietal cells. H_2RA therapy is associated with 75% to 98% healing during a 4- to 6-week period in documented PUD. Therapy needs to be continued with maintenance administration at bedtime for 1 year to prevent recurrence. H_2RA therapy is available over the counter, which presents new challenges for the primary care providers. Again, an in-depth history that includes over-the-counter medication use is extremely important in contemplating treatment options.

PPIs are the most potent and most expensive treatment option for PUD. Omeprazole, lansoprazole, rabeprazole, and esomeprazole effectively block the production of acid secretion. Daily administration eliminates acid production and also improves patient compliance. Investigation of over-the-counter medication use is once again required because PPI therapy is available for purchase without prescription.

Prostaglandin therapy protects the gastric and duodenal mucosa and should be considered for individuals with documented PUD who are unable to discontinue NSAID use. Misoprostol is the only available agent for the prevention of NSAID-induced gastric ulcers; it inhibits acid production and prevents duodenal damage. The therapeutic dose has been shown to produce transient side effects of cramping and diarrhea, which can be eliminated with a lower dose. Sucralfate is also indicated for treatment of active duodenal ulcer and maintenance of healed duodenal ulcers.

Treatment options for *H. pylori* eradication continue to be closely evaluated for efficacy and compliance. Treatment for *H. pylori*–associated ulcer disease is achieved with a combination of acid-inhibiting therapy and antibiotics. Current studies support the use of two antibiotic preparations, which produces higher efficacy and coverage for resistant organisms. PPI therapy has documented improved efficacy over H_2RA therapy, but cost and adherence must be considered before therapy is initiated. In the United States, the recommended treatment for the eradication of *H. pylori* infection includes a PPI and clarithromycin for 14 days. An alternative approach includes a PPI or H_2RA, bismuth, metronidazole, and tetracycline for 10 to 14 days (Table 144-1).[6]

TABLE 144-1 Treatment of *Helicobacter pylori* Infection

Medication	Duration
OPTION 1	
Omeprazole, 40 mg PO daily Clarithromycin, 500 mg twice a day Then omeprazole, 20 mg daily for 14 days	14 days
OPTION 2	
Ranitidine bismuth citrate, 400 mg twice a day Clarithromycin, 500 mg 3 times daily Then ranitidine, 400 mg twice a day for 2 weeks	14 days
OPTION 3	
Bismuth subsalicylate, 525 mg 4 times per day Metronidazole, 250 mg 4 times a day Tetracycline, 500 mg 4 times a day Ranitidine, 150 mg twice a day for 4 weeks	14 days
OPTION 4	
Lansoprazole, 30 mg twice a day for 10 days Amoxicillin, 1 mg twice a day Clarithromycin, 500 mg 3 times daily	

Many concerns about successful eradication exist in the treatment of *H. pylori* infection. The most important predictors of treatment failure are antibiotic resistance and poor patient adherence to the prescribed regimen. Clinicians need to be aware of the local data regarding antibiotic resistance and educate the patients about medication side effects, duration of therapy, and consequences of treatment failure. In patients with persistent *H. pylori* infections, previously prescribed antibiotics need to be avoided. Gastroenterology consultation should be obtained for individuals with suspected resistance. Disadvantages of the bismuth-based quadruple therapy include the daily pill count, administration frequency, and side effects, which need to be discussed with the patient to improve adherence. Eradication rate of the U.S. Food and Drug Administration (FDA)–approved treatments range from 61% to 94%, and longer duration of treatment results in improved eradication rates.[6]

COMPLICATIONS

Perforation of gastric or duodenal ulcers is a life-threatening complication of chronic ulcer disease. This is most common in older patients and requires emergency care. Other complications include hemorrhage, gastric outlet obstruction, and ulcers refractory to treatment.

INDICATIONS FOR REFERRAL OR HOSPITALIZATION

Gastroenterology referral is indicated for endoscopy if bleeding is suspected or for examination of the mucosal lining. Surgical referral is indicated for emergency intervention and in cases of prolonged refractory ulcer disease.

PATIENT AND FAMILY EDUCATION

Patient education involves the identification and modification of risk factors, specifically cigarette smoking, alcohol abuse, stress, and NSAID and aspirin use. Once a diagnosis of ulcer disease has been established, education should also include the signs and symptoms of hemorrhage, perforation, GI bleeding, and anemia. In addition, the consequences of lack of adherence to the medication regimen related to the treatment of PUD and *H. pylori* infection should be carefully reviewed.

REFERENCES

For a full list of references, scan the QR code or visit http://booksite.elsevier.com/9780323355018

PART 13

Evaluation and Management of Genitourinary Disorders

CHAPTER 145

INCONTINENCE

Joanne Sandberg-Cook

DEFINITION AND EPIDEMIOLOGY

Urinary incontinence is the involuntary transient or persistent loss of urine (Box 145-1). It is experienced by 30% to 50% of women and 17% of men older than 60 years as well as up to 50% of elderly nursing home residents.[1] Incontinence is considered to be one of the major causes of institutionalization in the geriatric population, but incontinence is not limited to the elderly. Twenty percent to 30% of young community dwellers are also affected by this disorder.[1] Urinary incontinence should not be considered normal at any age and is not an expected outcome of aging. Impaired mobility, pelvic floor weakness, race and ethnicity, weight, other comorbidities (asthma, depression, heart disease, or a history of frequent urinary tract infection [UTI]), benign prostatic hyperplasia (BPH), medications, and bowel status may all contribute to incontinence.[2]

The annual cost of managing incontinence for all age groups in the United States was nearly $66 billion in 2007 with much of the cost associated with nursing home placement.[3] However, despite its financial impact on society, incontinence is rarely addressed by patients with their health care providers. Thus, it behooves health care providers to identify patients who could benefit from therapeutic regimens to minimize the overall impact of incontinence.

PATHOPHYSIOLOGY

Urinary incontinence is usually the symptom of an underlying bladder or sphincter condition, but it may also be related to an extrinsic problem that can be easily treated. There are five main types of urinary incontinence: stress incontinence, urge incontinence, mixed incontinence, overflow incontinence, and functional or transient incontinence.

BOX 145-1

Incontinence Definitions

Stress incontinence: Loss of urine associated with activities that increase intra-abdominal pressure
Urge incontinence: Involuntary loss of urine usually preceded by a strong, unexpected urge to void
Mixed incontinence: Urge and stress incontinence together
Overflow incontinence: An involuntary loss of urine associated with incomplete emptying

Stress Incontinence

Stress urinary incontinence (SUI) is leakage of urine with any maneuvers that increase intra-abdominal pressure (coughing, sneezing). The increase in intra-abdominal pressure is transmitted to the bladder, which then overcomes the sphincteric and urethral pressure, resulting in an open urethra and urinary leakage. Stress incontinence is seen in those who have either or both of the following issues.

Anatomic Stress Urinary Incontinence. Previously termed genuine stress incontinence, anatomic incontinence refers to hypermobility of the bladder neck (vesicourethral junction). In general, the sphincter is competent at rest, and an increase in abdominal pressure leads to increased closure pressure. When the bladder neck is mobile, a rise in intra-abdominal pressure results in rotation of the bladder neck and urethra below the pelvic floor muscles so that intra-abdominal pressure is no longer transmitted to the bladder neck and urethra. The sphincter is overcome by the increase in abdominal pressure, which is transmitted to the bladder, and leakage occurs.[4]

Intrinsic Sphincter Deficiency. Intrinsic sphincter deficiency (ISD) indicates an open bladder neck at rest. Even a mild increase in intra-abdominal pressure in individuals with ISD can result in leakage.[4] Although ISD can occur naturally, patients who have had radical pelvic surgery may also experience a compromise of their intrinsic sphincter, predisposing them to incontinence. Contemporary theories suggest that all patients with sphincteric incontinence have some degree of ISD.[4]

Urinary Urge Incontinence

Urge is the most common cause of incontinence in older adults and manifests as the sudden, often uncontrollable sensation to void.[5] This urge can then lead to urinary urge incontinence (UUI). However, in patients with severe urge, incontinence may not be realized until actual leakage occurs. Overactive bladder is a newer term used to describe the phenomenon of urgency and frequency with or without UUI.[5] Urge and urge incontinence occur because of a rise in detrusor pressure that may be a phasic contraction, detrusor overactivity (DO), or poor bladder compliance.

Detrusor Overactivity. DO is instability of the detrusor muscle during bladder filling as a result of idiopathic or neurogenic causes. In both idiopathic and neurogenic DO, bladder pressures surpass sphincter and urethral pressures, causing the bladder neck to open and incontinence to occur.

Idiopathic Causes. When no defined neurologic contributor can be identified, DO is idiopathic. Prominent theories for DO include increased stimulation of alpha$_1$ receptors in the bladder, disruption of somatic and autonomic nervous systems that help regulate voiding, disruption of afferent and efferent pathways, and increased activation of muscarinic (M_2/M_3) receptors in the bladder.[4]

Neurogenic Causes. Patients who have spinal cord injuries below T11-L1,2 or neurologic conditions, such as multiple sclerosis, diabetes mellitus, and spina bifida, can have a disruption in voluntary micturition control. Reflex micturition often results, leading to detrusor hyperactivity and urge incontinence.[4]

Poor Bladder Compliance. Normal bladder compliance allows large amounts of urine to be stored with minimum changes in bladder pressure.[6] With poor compliance, large bladder pressures are seen with small increases in volumes.[6] This can be a result of the loss of viscoelasticity in detrusor muscle or changes in neuroregulatory activity.

Mixed Incontinence

A combination of SUI and UUI is referred to as mixed incontinence.

Overflow Incontinence

Incomplete emptying of urine often results in passive loss of small amounts of urine when bladder pressures elevate, either episodically or continuously, as the bladder fills beyond capacity. The rise in bladder pressure may occur because of either transmitted abdominal pressure or an increase in detrusor pressure. Overflow incontinence is seen in patients with either bladder outlet obstruction or poor detrusor contractility. Bladder pressure surpasses sphincter and urethral pressure, which allows "overflow" of urine to occur. This is more commonly seen in men than in women, and causes include BPH, radical pelvic surgery, detrusor inactivity, neurologic issues, and certain medications.

Functional or Transient Incontinence

Pathologic conditions external to the urinary tract can also cause incontinence. Such factors are indicated in Resnick's DIAPPERS mnemonic (Box 145-2). Reversal of these conditions may improve the urinary incontinence.

CLINICAL PRESENTATION

The presentation of incontinence can vary depending on the cause. A careful history and physical examination should exclude causes of transient incontinence that can be easily treated. SUI, UUI, mixed incontinence, and overflow incontinence can manifest similarly, so careful history taking may help delineate the type of incontinence experienced. A history should include a detailed review of symptoms related to incontinence; bowel habits; medications; medical, surgical, and genitourinary histories; history of pelvic trauma; and neurologic issues.[5] Onset, precipitants, duration, characteristics (frequency, timing, and amount), alleviating factors, and treatments tried should all be documented. Alterations in bowel or bladder habits, number of pads used, and response to previous treatments should be noted as well.

BOX 145-2

Resnick's DIAPPERS Mnemonic

*D*elirium or confusional state
*I*nfection—urinary (only symptomatic)
*A*trophic urethritis, vaginitis
*P*harmaceuticals
*P*sychological, especially severe depression (rare)
*E*xcess urinary output (e.g., congestive heart failure, hyperglycemia)
*R*estricted mobility
*S*tool impaction

From Resnick NM: Urinary incontinence. In Cassel CK, Cohen HJ, Larson ER et al, editors: *Geriatric medicine,* ed 3, New York, 1997, Springer.

PHYSICAL EXAMINATION

The physical examination for incontinence includes abdominal, genitourinary, pelvic, and rectal components. A neurologic and functional assessment as well as an assessment of the extremities for edema should also be made. Medication history (especially that of diuretic use), mental status, mobility, and social evaluations should be performed, especially in older adults, because impairment in any of these realms may contribute to functional incontinence.

Examination findings in men including phimosis, balanitis or infection, rectal masses, prostate nodules or asymmetry, and fecal impaction suggest underlying causes of the incontinence. In women, an assessment of urethral mobility is performed by examining the bladder neck and urethra with the patient supine while she strains. A stress test is also performed by observing for urine loss when the patient performs a Valsalva maneuver or by having the patient cough. If incontinence is not seen when the patient is examined supine, the examination should be repeated with the patient standing.

Bladder neck hypermobility can also be determined with the Q-tip test. If the Q-tip moves more than 30 degrees from a horizontal plane when it is inserted superficially into the urethra, lack of urethral support is delineated.[7] Furthermore, pelvic organ prolapse and effectiveness of the patient's ability to perform Kegel exercises (contraction of the pelvic floor) should be noted. General observation of pelvic anatomy should be made, and any abnormalities, including atrophy, should be documented. The relationship between estrogen and incontinence in perimenopausal and menopausal women has not been well defined. However, lack of estrogen and subsequent vaginal atrophy may contribute to symptoms of stress incontinence.[8]

UUI may not be detectable on physical examination. Subjective complaints may be most beneficial in detecting urge incontinence and UUI. However, examination of pelvic anatomy and pelvic floor strength may reveal contributors to bladder symptoms, such as constipation and vaginal atrophy. Mixed incontinence requires a physical examination to assess for SUI and UUI. This should be performed as previously discussed.

Finally, overflow incontinence can often be determined through abdominal and vaginal examinations. Bladder distention may be easily palpated abdominally or vaginally. Evaluation of general pelvic anatomy should also occur.

DIAGNOSTICS

A urinalysis is performed to exclude hematuria, pyuria, glucosuria, or proteinuria. Hematuria, defined as more than three red blood cells per high-power field on urinalysis with a negative urine culture,[9] warrants further workup with cytology, upper tract imaging, and bladder cystoscopy. Urine cytologic studies should also be performed in patients with gross or persistent microhematuria, risk factors for bladder cancer, or irritative symptoms.[9] A urine culture is necessary to exclude a UTI in patients with pyuria or irritative symptoms, including urge and urge incontinence.[5] Blood urea nitrogen (BUN) and creatinine levels should be obtained if compromised renal function is suspected, especially with overflow incontinence. If polyuria is suspected, serum glucose and calcium tests are also recommended.

A postvoid residual (PVR) is helpful to exclude incomplete emptying and can be obtained through either pelvic ultrasound or catheterization.[5] In general, a PVR of less than 50 mL is considered normal, whereas residuals of more than 100 mL are considered abnormal and require further evaluation.[10]

Additional testing is usually not needed for the basic evaluation of urinary incontinence unless onset is sudden, symptoms are severe, or suprapubic pain or hematuria is present. The patient should be referred to a urologist if further diagnostic testing (e.g., cystoscopy, urodynamics) is necessary or if the diagnosis is uncertain.[5] The health care provider should refer the patient if an effective care plan cannot be devised, if hematuria is present without infection, if surgical intervention is being considered, or if therapy has failed.

DIAGNOSTICS

Incontinence

LABORATORY
- Urinalysis
- Urine culture and sensitivity
- BUN
- Creatinine
- Serum glucose*
- Calcium*
- Urine for cytology*

OTHER DIAGNOSTICS
- PVR
- Urodynamic testing
- Cystoscopy*

*If indicated.

DIFFERENTIAL DIAGNOSIS

If incontinence is believed to be functional, the first step in treatment is to manage the underlying condition. This may be as simple as moving a commode to the bedside of a newly immobile patient recovering from orthopedic surgery. Medical conditions that may exacerbate incontinence should be treated, and conditions that contribute to incontinence should be minimized or discontinued, if possible. When all nonurologic causes of incontinence have been ruled out, the type of incontinence—based on history, physical examination, and diagnostic data—can be determined. Once it has been identified, a management plan for the type of incontinence can be initiated.

DIFFERENTIAL DIAGNOSIS

Incontinence

- Stress urinary incontinence
  - Anatomic SUI
  - ISD
- Urge incontinence
  - Detrusor overactivity (idiopathic or neurogenic)
  - Poor bladder compliance
- Mixed incontinence
- Overflow incontinence
- Functional or transient incontinence
- Increased urinary production
- Lower urinary tract conditions (bladder cancer, stricture, prolapse)
- Medication contribution

MANAGEMENT

The treatment of incontinence varies according to cause, but behavioral and pharmacologic therapies are generally first-line therapies in the treatment of urinary incontinence. Surgical therapies may be indicated in some individuals (Box 145-3).

BOX 145-3

Management of Incontinence

STRESS INCONTINENCE
- Behavioral therapies: timed or double voiding, smoking cessation, weight loss, pelvic muscle exercises with or without a physical therapist, pessary, bowel management
- Medical therapies: alpha-adrenergic agonists, tricyclic antidepressants, estrogen
- Surgical therapies: injectables, bladder neck suspensions, slings, artificial sphincters

URGE INCONTINENCE
- Behavioral therapies: as above with bladder training, scheduled voiding, bladder irritant minimization, and urge suppression
- Medical therapies: anticholinergic-antimuscarinics
- Surgical therapies: neurosacral modulation, bladder augmentation, botulinum toxin injections

MIXED INCONTINENCE
- Combination of therapies for stress and urge incontinence

OVERFLOW INCONTINENCE
- Behavioral therapies: timed or double voiding, clean intermittent catheterization, pessary
- Medical therapies: $alpha_1$ blockers, 5α-reductase inhibitors
- Surgery to relieve urethral obstruction or stricture or to reduce prolapse

FUNCTIONAL OR TRANSIENT INCONTINENCE
- Treatment of underlying cause

Stress Incontinence

Behavioral Therapies. Behavioral therapies for SUI include timed voiding, double voiding, smoking cessation, weight loss, pelvic muscle exercises, pessary placement, and bowel management.[11] Timed voiding—voiding every 2 hours during the day—allows adequate time for the patient's bladder to fill but not overdistend. This will minimize the amount of urine in the bladder to leak when a stress maneuver does occur.[11] Use of a bladder diary may be beneficial to map voiding occurrences so the patient and health care provider can identify problematic bladder habits.

Double voiding is used for patients who empty incompletely with urination. It consists of having the patient change positions on the toilet, get up and sit back down, or just allow a few extra minutes for the bladder to contract and fully empty. In a patient with stress incontinence and incomplete emptying, improved emptying may allow improved control.

Smoking cessation helps minimize events that increase intra-abdominal pressure; smokers are often more likely to cough because of respiratory side effects and infections. Tobacco is also a bladder irritant and can increase the sense of urgency.[5] Weight loss can help minimize SUI because increased abdominal girth may apply more pressure to the bladder when stress maneuvers occur.[12]

Pelvic muscle exercises, or Kegel exercises, strengthen the pelvic floor. These exercises are beneficial because when they are performed correctly, pelvic floor contraction can help minimize stress incontinence by preventing rotation and descent of the urethra and bladder neck during physical activities that may cause symptoms.[11] They may also improve resting pressure in the urethra and increase bulk around the urethra, which may prevent stress and urge incontinence. Kegel exercises are performed by tightening only the pelvic floor muscles as if controlling defecation or urination. Contraction of abdominal, thigh, and gluteal muscles should be avoided. Appropriate technique is best assessed by placing a finger in the vagina so the appropriate muscles can be isolated. Contractions should be held for up to 5 seconds followed by a period of relaxation. Exercises should be performed as three sets of 10, three times a day, for 6 months, even though benefit may not be seen for 4 to 8 weeks.[13]

Referral to a physical therapist (PT) is often beneficial for patients who are unable to appropriately isolate the pelvic floor muscles or are unsure if they are performing Kegel exercises correctly. The PT may use adjuncts such as biofeedback and electrical stimulation—for instance, with a transcutaneous electrical nerve stimulation (TENS) unit or similar device—to further improve the patient's ability to contract the pelvic floor. Biofeedback is used to increase awareness of pelvic floor function and help change responses in an attempt to improve urination.[14] One of the simplest forms of biofeedback is the use of vaginal weights.[14] Patients are instructed to insert a weight intravaginally and to retain it during ambulation by contraction of the pelvic floor muscles.[14] Exercises should start with light vaginal weights (20 g) and gradually increase to use of heavier weights. If electrical stimulation is used, training must be performed by a professional skilled in this procedure.[5]

Pessary placement may be helpful in patients with stress incontinence or bladder or pelvic organ prolapse. There are pessaries specifically designed for incontinence that work by elevating the bladder neck. Referral to a skilled pessary fitter for appropriate fitting and management is important because patients may need to try a variety of types and sizes before obtaining a good fit.

Bowel management is important in minimizing incontinence. Stool impaction can increase the likelihood of bladder irritability by an increase in external pressure on the bladder and from increased activity in the sacral nerves. Excessive straining with defecation may also contribute to denervation of the external anal sphincter and pelvic floor muscles.[15] This denervation is thought to result in bladder symptoms.[15] Ideally, the goal is moderation of the gastrointestinal tract so that one large, soft bowel movement per day or every other day is achieved.

Medical Therapies. Alpha-adrenergic agonists, such as pseudoephedrine (Sudafed), increase urethral pressure and outlet resistance to decrease incontinence. Although not curative or approved for this indication, alpha-adrenergics may improve symptoms without significant side effects.

Estrogen replacement may be helpful in treating postmenopausal stress incontinence in women who have signs of vaginal atrophy, although controversy still exists about whether oral estrogen therapy provides benefit because many studies have not found symptom improvement with estrogen use.[8] Local applications of estrogen cream can provide a measurable reduction in urinary incontinence and are generally safe for most women.[8] A trial of estrogen may be efficacious in women who have no contraindications to estrogen therapy with the understanding that if beneficial, all benefit will gradually disappear after discontinuation of oral estrogen.[8] Given the results of the Women's Health Initiative and other studies, women must be counseled about the risks versus benefits of hormone replacement therapy and therapy used for the shortest possible time.[8]

Conjugated estrogen may be given orally, and risks in relation to benefit should be thoroughly discussed before it is started. If oral estrogen is started in a woman with an intact uterus, oral progesterone should also be given. Periurethral estrogen creams have very low systemic levels and can be administered daily for 2 weeks, and then twice weekly thereafter with excellent results.

Imipramine or other tricyclic antidepressants may be recommended, especially in younger patients, if other therapies have proved ineffective. At doses of 10 to 25 mg orally one to three times daily, imipramine has both alpha-agonist and anticholinergic effects, which make it useful for patients with SUI or mixed incontinence.[16]

In general, these drugs should be used carefully in older adults because of potential adverse effects, mostly cardiac and anticholinergic. Orthostatic hypotension with an increased risk of falls may be more likely in the elderly.

Other possible anticholinergic side effects include dizziness, fatigue, dry mouth, and constipation. If a patient decides to stop the tricyclic antidepressant, a gradual taper should be used. Duloxetine, commonly used in Europe for stress incontinence and not approved for use in the United States, should be used with caution when it is prescribed, because worsening of depression may occur initially before benefit is seen.

Surgical Therapies. Surgery should be considered if treatment regimens are ineffective or if patients are not able to adhere to other treatment plans. Stress incontinence is the most common type of incontinence treated with surgery. Surgery is done either to lift or to provide support to the urethra or bladder neck. Choices include retropubic suspensions, a variety of sling procedures, urethral bulking agents, and artificial urinary sphincters. Referral to a urologist or urogynecologist is recommended if surgery is being considered. The type of surgery performed depends on patient anatomy, urodynamic findings, and patient expectations.

Urge Incontinence

Behavioral Therapies. Behavioral methods for treatment of UUI also include timed and double voiding, use of a voiding diary, pelvic floor exercises with or without the assistance of a PT, weight reduction, smoking cessation, and bowel management as indicated. However, bladder training, scheduled voiding, urge suppression techniques, and overall minimization of bladder irritants can also be recommended.

With UUI, a voiding diary documenting time and amount of each void and the time of any incontinent episode will help illustrate which treatments could be most beneficial. The patient with urge incontinence on the way to the toilet after waiting 4 to 5 hours to void may need to incorporate timed voiding every 2 hours into his or her daily routine.

Bladder training is of benefit to the patient who voids frequently (every 30 minutes to 1 hour) during the day but can sleep through the night and void 300 mL in the morning. Bladder training requires the patient to postpone voiding, to resist the sense of urgency, and to void on a predetermined schedule.

Intervals of 10 to 15 minutes should be added to the current voiding pattern and then gradually increased so the patient can reach a goal of voiding every 2 to 3 hours. The bladder should be emptied at the scheduled intervals, and voiding should be delayed if urge occurs. Four or five quick Kegel exercises ("quick flicks") may alleviate bladder spasms, allowing the patient to get to the bathroom without rushing or leaking.[13]

Scheduled or prompted voiding by a caregiver may be effective when a patient cannot use the toilet independently.[11] Assistance with toileting should be provided every 2 to 4 hours during the day and night to minimize incontinence. Habit training, another method for decreasing incontinence in dependent patients, occurs when a toileting schedule is developed in accordance with the patient's past voiding habits. Based on a record of incontinence, a schedule can be developed to minimize episodes of incontinence.

Regulation of bladder irritants can help decrease urgency and UUI. Spicy, acidic, and caffeinated foods tend to irritate the bladder and increase the sense of urgency.[16] Chocolate, tomatoes, citrus fruits or juices, most nuts, coffee, tea, dark sodas, alcohol, and tobacco can contribute to irritative symptoms. Furthermore, moderation of overall fluid intake to 48 to 64 ounces per day can help maintain hydration while mitigating the frequency of voiding. A voiding diary may be helpful in assessing this.

Medical Therapies. Medications are generally helpful in moderating urge incontinence. Anticholinergic-antimuscarinic agents are the cornerstone of medical therapy because they work to block impulses to muscarinic acetylcholine receptors (M_2/M_3) found in the bladder.[17] In turn, the number and strength of involuntary bladder contractions decrease, and urinary frequency is moderated. Anticholinergic agents can have side effects of dry mouth, confusion, constipation, dizziness, blurred vision, and tachycardia.

Tolterodine tartrate (Detrol) and oxybutynin chloride (Ditropan) are examples of antimuscarinic agents.[18] Oxybutynin has greater anticholinergic side effects than other anticholinergics and may be reserved for younger patients. Ditropan XL (an extended-release formulation of oxybutynin), Oxytrol (transdermal oxybutynin in a patch), and Gelnique (transdermal oxybutynin in a gel) have been shown to produce fewer anticholinergic side effects than regular oxybutynin.[18] Newer anticholinergics, such as fesoterodine (Toviaz), continue to be developed in an effort to increase efficacy while reducing side effects. Trospium (Sanctura) is a quaternary amine and, in theory, has less ability to cross the blood-brain barrier. Darifenacin (Enablex), solifenacin (VESIcare), and mirabegron (Myrbetriq) are selective for M_3 receptors, which may increase efficacy and decrease M_2-mediated side effects.[19] However, because all these drugs have the potential to cause side effects in the frail geriatric patient, they should be started at low doses and gradually titrated until either symptoms improve or nontolerability indicates further medication trials.

Tricyclics may be helpful for certain patients with UUI. Again, low doses of these drugs should be used in older adults because of the potential for adverse effects.

Surgical Therapies. Surgical therapies may be indicated in some patients with severe urge incontinence. Surgical therapies, done to counteract bladder contractions or to increase bladder capacity, include botulinum toxin injections, neurosacral modulation, and bladder augmentation. Botulinum injections are now licensed by the Food and Drug Administration for the treatment of overactive bladder and neurogenic DO and can be helpful for these conditions.[20] Referral to a urologist is indicated if botulinum injections or surgical therapy is being considered.

Mixed Incontinence

After careful diagnostic evaluation, the patient may be found to have mixed incontinence. Treatment with a combination of previously described behavioral or medical therapies is warranted.

Overflow Incontinence

Overflow incontinence can be managed with timed and double voiding but also with clean intermittent catheterization (CIC), a pessary, medical therapies, or surgical options. CIC is recommended for patients who have poor emptying secondary to poor detrusor function or for patients with urethral obstruction who are poor surgical candidates. This should be done often enough that CIC amounts, if the patient does not void volitionally, or total void plus CIC amounts remain less than 500 mL with each catheterization-void event.

A pessary may be helpful for prolapse that causes partial urethral obstruction. A pessary provides support to the vaginal canal so the bladder can empty more completely. However, when it is placed, stress incontinence may become more prevalent once the bladder is in proper anatomic position.

Medications are used to relieve overflow incontinence in relation to BPH. The $alpha_1$ blockers tamsulosin hydrochloride (Flomax) and terazosin (Hytrin) as well as the 5α-reductase inhibitors finasteride (Proscar) and dutasteride (Avodart) can be used. There is no role for these medications in women.

Surgery is often indicated to relieve urethral obstruction caused by BPH, stricture, or a nonreducible prolapse. Referral to a urologist should occur if surgery is being considered.

Functional Incontinence

Functional incontinence can be resolved through treatment of the underlying cause. Behavioral therapies may be beneficial as well.

LIFE SPAN CONSIDERATIONS

Incontinence can occur at any age but is more prevalent in the older adult. Changes in the urinary tract that occur with aging can contribute to the development of incontinence. Bladder capacity, contractility, and the ability to postpone voiding are thought to decline with age. Prostate size, urethral obstruction, involuntary bladder contractions, and PVRs, on the other hand, may increase.[21] These changes as well as increased chronic health conditions and medications that affect the urinary tract explain why incontinence is so prevalent in the geriatric population.

COMPLICATIONS

Incontinence can contribute to medical morbidities, including perineal candidal infections, pressure ulcers, UTIs, urosepsis, falls, and sleep interruption. At the same time, incontinence can contribute to poor self-esteem, social withdrawal, depression, and sexual dysfunction secondary to embarrassment. Because of this, patients in the home environment may try to limit fluid intake in an effort to control incontinence. By minimizing fluid intake, patients may put themselves at risk for dehydration and its sequelae.

CONSIDERATION FOR REFERRAL

Consultation with a urologic specialist is important when there is difficulty determining the type of incontinence or when traditional treatment regimens provide inadequate relief of symptoms. Incontinence that does not respond adequately to initial treatment may be managed more effectively in collaboration with a PT, continence nurse, urologist, urogynecologist, or specialized nurse practitioner.

Referral to a specialist is indicated with incontinence and an abnormal PVR, prostate examination that suggests prostate cancer, a neurologic condition, symptomatic pelvic prolapse, recurrent symptomatic UTIs, a history of radical pelvic or incontinence surgery, or persistent symptoms of difficult or incomplete bladder emptying. Further testing is warranted when the diagnosis is uncertain, when hematuria without infection is present, when surgical intervention is being considered, or when therapy of reasonable duration has failed.

PATIENT EDUCATION

Effectiveness of behavioral strategies in the treatment of incontinence depends on the education and adherence of patients, families, and caregivers to the treatment plan agreed on. Plans for behavioral interventions should be realistic and meet the needs of patients and caregivers. Regular follow-up visits will help reinforce therapeutic options, support efforts to obtain treatment goals, and allow care plan modification so optimum outcomes can be obtained.

CHAPTER 146

PROSTATE CANCER

Kenneth Peterson

DEFINITION AND EPIDEMIOLOGY

Other than skin cancer, cancer of the prostate is the most common malignant neoplasm in men in the United States and the second leading cause of cancer death in men of all races and Hispanic origin populations.[1] The National Cancer Institute estimated that in 2014 the United States had 233,000 new cases diagnosed and 29,480 deaths from prostate cancer.[2] One in seven men in the United States will be diagnosed with prostate cancer in his lifetime, and more than 2 million American men are living with prostate cancer.[3] Risk factors for prostate cancer include advancing age, African-American race, and a positive family history of prostate cancer. Geography is considered a risk factor; prostate cancer is more common in Caribbean men of African ancestry and men living in North America, northwestern Europe, and Australia. The majority of cases are diagnosed in men older than 65 years, with incidence rates higher in African-American men than in white men.[2] The mortality rate of African-American men is estimated to be twice that of white men.[2] As a result of early, effective screening and the aging of the U.S. population, the number of prostate cancer cases diagnosed has increased; however, deaths from prostate cancer have decreased significantly in recent years, and the majority of men diagnosed with prostate cancer do not die of the disease.[2,3]

PATHOPHYSIOLOGY

The most common type of prostate cancer is adenocarcinoma. It develops in the acinar glands located in the posterior peripheral zone of the prostate. Histologic grading is an important predictor of prognosis. The Gleason system incorporates clinical and physiologic parameters for grading of the malignant neoplasm.[4] Tumors can arise in one or both lobes of the prostate and can spread within the prostate, through the prostatic capsule, and through the seminal vesicles or the base of the bladder, with metastasis occurring through the lymphatic and circulatory systems.

CLINICAL PRESENTATION

Presenting symptoms of prostate cancer may include urinary hesitancy, urgency, nocturia, frequency, and hematuria, although the patient is usually asymptomatic in early stages of the disease. Symptoms tend to increase in intensity during a 1- to 2-month period, which is different from the slow, gradual progression in symptoms that occurs in benign prostatic hyperplasia (BPH). In more advanced disease, presenting symptoms may include back pain, impotence, and other bone pain that suggests metastasis. Other symptoms of metastasis include weight loss, constipation, malaise, hematuria, and rectal pain or symptoms related to nerve root compression, such as paresthesias or extremity weakness.

Rarely, prostate cancer can be non–prostate-specific antigen (PSA) producing, and tumor burden will not correlate with PSA values. These patients will have the same presentation as others, with symptoms of bone pain or obstruction, and will likely have abnormal digital rectal examination (DRE) findings but a low PSA level. Patients with signs and symptoms of prostate cancer should be referred to a urologist for evaluation, even in the presence of a normal PSA level.

PHYSICAL EXAMINATION

The DRE is used to detect initial physical abnormalities of the prostate gland. A firm nodule on rectal examination, induration, or a stony, asymmetric prostate is suggestive of prostate cancer. In early-disease stage, the findings on prostate examination will generally be normal.

DIAGNOSTICS AND DIFFERENTIAL DIAGNOSIS

Measurement of the PSA level combined with DRE if elevated is considered the most sensitive and specific screening method for prostate cancer. Some controversy exists regarding initial PSA screening and interval testing. The American Urological Association (AUA) recommends that men who are considering prostate screening should discuss the benefits and harms of testing with their health care providers. The American Cancer Society recommends that men have the opportunity to make an informed decision with their care provider about prostate cancer screening.[5] The U.S. Preventive Services Task Force continues to support the recommendation against PSA-based screening for prostate cancer. The recommendation applies to all men in the general U.S. population regardless of age.[6] (See Life Span Considerations for age-specific screening recommendations.)

PSA is a protease enzyme secreted by the prostate gland, and levels may be elevated in both benign and malignant conditions of the prostate. A prostate level below 4 ng/mL is considered normal, although a prostate tumor may be present with a PSA level below 4 ng/mL. Algorithms exist to adjust normal values for age and race. In addition, some medications (e.g., finasteride) can decrease PSA values, thus requiring adjustment. Values of 4 to 10 ng/mL may be seen in early prostate cancer and other benign conditions; values above 10 ng/mL suggest prostate cancer. The use of the free PSA test and determination of PSA velocity (rate of rise) may increase specificity for prostate cancer, especially if the PSA level is elevated. A rate of rise of more than 0.75 ng/mL per year is considered highly sensitive for prostate cancer.[7,8] Different age-specific reference ranges are sometimes considered, especially in African-American men, because cases in this population might be missed with use of the traditional reference ranges.

Similar to decisions about when PSA screening should occur, the decision regarding when to perform tissue biopsies for prostate cancer diagnosis confirmation remains controversial. In men older than 60 years, if the PSA level is higher than 4.0 ng/mL or findings on DRE are abnormal, transrectal ultrasound (TRUS) of the prostate with TRUS-guided biopsy is recommended. TRUS allows guided biopsy of suspicious hypoechoic areas. In younger men, biopsy is considered if the PSA level is above 2.6 ng/mL.

In cases with a positive finding on biopsy of the prostate and a PSA level above 10 μg/L, a radionuclide bone scan may be necessary to determine the presence of bone metastases. Magnetic resonance imaging (MRI) of the abdomen and pelvis is important to assess the regional lymph nodes and metastasis. A chest x-ray study can exclude metastasis to the lungs. An elevated alkaline phosphatase level suggests bone metastasis, and an elevated acid phosphatase level suggests prostatic metastasis.

The differential diagnosis includes BPH and prostatitis when there is an abnormal DRE finding and PSA test result. Other potential differential diagnoses include bladder cancer, urinary tract infection, and urethral stricture.

Based on data from the Prostate, Lung, Colorectal, and Ovarian (PLCO) Cancer Screening Trial, the rate of death from prostate cancer did not differ significantly by whether the prostate cancer screening test used was PSA or DRE.[9]

DIAGNOSTICS

Prostate Cancer

LABORATORY
- PSA
- Complete blood count and differential*

OTHER DIAGNOSTICS
- Needle biopsy

*If indicated.

DIFFERENTIAL DIAGNOSIS

Prostate Cancer

- Bladder outlet obstruction
- Urinary tract infection
- Prostate calculi
- BPH
- Prostatitis

MANAGEMENT

Treatment options are based on the stage or extent to which the cancer has spread. There are several different staging systems for prostate cancer, but the most widely used is the American Joint Committee on Cancer (AJCC) TNM system. The TNM system describes the following:
- Extent of the primary tumor (T category)
- Whether the cancer has spread to nearby lymph nodes (N category)
- Absence or presence of distant metastases (M category)

Localized disease (T1) has the most options: watchful waiting (monitoring with PSA and DRE), radiation therapy (brachytherapy or external beam radiation therapy), hormonal therapy (with the goal of suppression of testosterone), and surgery. Patients with disease that has gone beyond the prostatic capsule but without evidence of metastatic spread (T2) may be offered watchful waiting, radiation therapy, hormonal therapy, or a combination of radiation and hormonal therapy. Patients with either local or distant metastatic disease will generally be offered hormonal therapy or watchful waiting; however, palliative radiation therapy (beam therapy aimed at bone lesions) or palliative chemotherapy as well as salvage chemotherapy may be offered.

Treatment decisions are based on the stage at diagnosis; prognostic features of the tumor; and the patient's age, medical condition, and treatment preference. Decisions about therapy are complex and controversial. The current therapy with disease classified as stage A or stage B is radical prostatectomy or radiation therapy. Cryotherapy is being used more commonly in localized prostate cancer.

Hormonal therapy, androgen deprivation therapy (ADT), has been used for symptomatic patients with advanced disease or for patients who do not want surgery, but evidence is mixed as to whether androgen suppression improves long-term outcome.[10] Hormone treatments include oral estrogens, orchiectomy, luteinizing hormone–releasing hormone (LHRH) agonists, antiandrogens, and progestational agents. LHRH agonists act by initially stimulating pituitary gonadotropin production and later inhibiting it. Therapy to prevent osteoporosis may be necessary in men receiving hormonal therapy. The National Cancer Institute provides a very helpful treatment by stage section for patients on their prostate cancer treatment (PDQ) site.

Pain management is often an important treatment issue in more advanced disease. Palliative treatment with chemotherapy or radiation therapy and medication may help relieve the pain.

LIFE SPAN CONSIDERATIONS

The early detection of prostate cancer remains the key consideration in caring for male patients. In addressing this concern for men, primary care providers must demonstrate an evidence-based shared decision-making approach to care. Providers should be prepared to discuss screening recommendations and all related aspects of prostate health with adult males of all ages.

The AUA offers the following prostate cancer screening recommendation in its recent early detection of prostate cancer guideline.[11] PSA screening is not recommended for men younger than age 40 years. Routine screening is not recommended for men aged 40 to 54 years who have average risk. For patients younger than 55 years with higher risk, providers should individualize decisions for prostate screening. A shared decision-making approach to prostate cancer screening for men 55 to 69 years should be implemented. The greatest benefit of PSA screening is evidenced for men 55 to 69 years. For those men who have made the decision to screen, a screening interval of 2 years is preferred over annual screening. Evidence supporting the AUA guideline suggests that a two-year screening interval may reduce harm and improve benefits including a reduction in overdiagnosis and false positives.[11] PSA screening is not recommended for men older than 70 years or men with less than a 10- to 15-year life expectancy. The AUA guideline suggests that PSA screening may be of value to healthy males older than 70 years.[11]

COMPLICATIONS

The major complication of prostate cancer is metastatic disease. Risks of surgery include hemorrhage and injury to the obturator nerve, ureter, or rectum. Incontinence and impotence are also potential complications. Problems associated with radiation therapy include urinary problems, intestinal sequelae, impotence, and transient edema. Intestinal problems include diarrhea, fecal incontinence, rectal bleeding, intestinal obstruction, rectal strictures, mucous discharge, and tenesmus. Potential urologic problems include cystitis, hematuria, frequency, dysuria, and urethral stricture. The main complications of cryotherapy include urethral stricture, irritative symptoms, urinary incontinence, impotence, rectourethral fistula, bladder neck contracture, and urinary retention.

INDICATIONS FOR REFERRAL OR HOSPITALIZATION

A referral should be made to a urologist when an abnormality is found on DRE or the PSA level is elevated (after options and implications for treatment have been discussed with the patient; some patients may decline referral). After treatment, the health care provider can offer follow-up care that includes monitoring of the PSA levels. After radical prostatectomy, the PSA level should fall to less than 0.2 μg/L. PSA levels also fall after radiation therapy and continue to decrease for 12 months after completion of therapy. PSA levels should be tested at 6 and 12 months after treatment and annually thereafter. An increase in PSA should be evaluated with TRUS and biopsy. Hospitalization may also be necessary in the case of advanced metastatic disease.

PATIENT AND FAMILY EDUCATION

Prostate health education that incorporates shared decision-making approaches is more likely to produce successful outcomes that align with patient and family preferences and values. The use of shared decision-making in health care can improve care quality and reduce costs.[12] Providers should emphasize education that incorporates best evidence of prostate cancer screening and treatment recommendations. Patients should receive individualized, well-informed treatment options.[13] Primary providers should collaborate with urologic specialty providers and remain fully engaged and responsive to the patients' and families' needs.

HEALTH PROMOTION

As with most cancers, the exact cause of prostate cancer is not certain. Mutations in the genetic structure and a cadre of risk factors related to age, race, location, and diet are considered causes. Evidence to support significant benefits including reduction in morbidity and mortality related to prostate health is limited. There is limited evidence supporting specific nutritional recommendations to prevent prostate cancer. Despite these limitations, health promotion strategies to address modifiable lifestyle factors such as diet, stress management, and overall health are the current approaches considered. Primary care providers should promote health through lifestyle interventions that encourage overall health and wellness.

CHAPTER 147 PROSTATIC HYPERPLASIA (BENIGN)

Kenneth Peterson

BENIGN PROSTATIC HYPERPLASIA

DEFINITION AND EPIDEMIOLOGY

Benign prostatic hyperplasia (BPH), an almost ubiquitous phenomenon among older men, is a noncancerous enlargement of the prostate gland. Although the exact prevalence of BPH is unknown, by the eighth decade of life BPH is present in more than 90% of all men.[1]

PATHOPHYSIOLOGY

The prostate gland undergoes its first growth spurt during puberty and attains an average size of 20 g ($\frac{7}{10}$ ounce) by the age of 20 years. The gland then undergoes a second growth spurt during the fifth decade of life.

The development of the prostate gland depends on androgen secretion, and both the presence of testes and advancing age are necessary for the development of BPH. Dihydrotestosterone (DHT) is the main mediator of the growth and secretory function of the prostate and is the active metabolite that results from testosterone conversion.[2] BPH seems to be related to a complex interaction between androgen and estrogen secretion; abnormal serum elevations of androgen and estrogen stimulate prostatic growth. Other factors that contribute to prostatic enlargement appear to be related to the elaboration of certain growth factors, the formation and maintenance of DHT levels, and the functioning of androgen receptors.[2]

CLINICAL PRESENTATION

Men with BPH can also have bladder outlet obstruction (BOO), lower urinary tract symptoms (LUTS), or a combination of these problems.[3] Thus, the symptoms of BPH are either obstructive or irritative in character, depending on the particular BPH components involved. Obstructive symptoms include urinary hesitancy, decreased caliber and force of the stream, and postvoid dribbling. These symptoms are related to BOO. Irritative symptoms include frequency, urgency, and nocturia and occur as a result of decreased functional bladder capacity and instability or infection. In men, the term *LUTS* was originally used to describe the irritative symptoms primarily associated with BPH but has been expanded to include symptom related to bladder storage and/or voiding disturbances; the term used now is *male LUTS* or *MLUTS*.[3] On occasion, hematuria accompanies BPH.

Episodic symptoms may be present during many years with a gradual increase in the intensity of symptoms over time.

A thorough history is important and should include questions related to general health, history of type 2 diabetes, and sexual health. A family history of BPH or prostate cancer should be explored as well as any past history of urethral trauma, urethritis, or urethral instrumentation. Current over-the-counter and prescription medication use should be explored to determine the use of anticholinergics (including diphenhydramine and those in cold preparations), which can impair bladder contractility, or sympathomimetics such as pseudoephedrine, which increase outflow resistance. Diuretics, which can cause an increased output of urine, may lead to urinary retention, especially in the presence of a partially decompensated detrusor muscle. Frequency volume charts or voiding diaries can be used to evaluate nocturia.[3]

BPH symptoms may be quantified by a symptom index developed by the American Urological Association to aid in classifying symptom severity and in developing a treatment plan[4] (Table 147-1). Symptoms are rated according to frequency of occurrence.[4]

PHYSICAL EXAMINATION

A digital rectal examination (DRE) is done to evaluate the prostate gland for size, consistency, shape, symmetry, and abnormalities and to evaluate anal sphincter tone. Prostatic nodules or induration should be noted on rectal examination because these findings suggest prostate cancer. The normal prostate is heart shaped and measures approximately 4 × 3 × 2 cm (1⅗ × 1⅕ × ⅘ inches). With BPH, there may be uniform or focal enlargement of the prostate. The size of the prostate does not always correlate with symptom severity, however, and should not direct therapy. The median sulcus is often obliterated in BPH, and it is often difficult to palpate over the base of the prostate because of the gland's enlarged size in advanced stages. With BPH, the gland is nontender and should be rubbery and smooth in consistency. A focused neurologic examination is done to assess sacral nerve roots to identify neurologic problems that could be contributing to bladder symptoms. A lower abdominal examination is necessary to ascertain bladder distention from urinary retention.[3,5]

DIAGNOSTICS

A urinalysis should be performed to exclude a urinary tract infection or hematuria. Determination of the creatinine level may be prudent to assess renal function. Office-based bladder ultrasound examination to determine postvoid residual is helpful in the diagnosis and treatment of BPH.

According to American Urological Association guidelines, measurement of serum prostate-specific antigen (PSA) is appropriate for men with a life expectancy of more than 10 years in the presence of physical findings suggestive of prostate cancer (abnormal DRE findings) and if 5α-reductase inhibitor therapy is planned.[6]

TABLE 147-1 American Urological Association Symptom Index for Benign Prostatic Hyperplasia[4]

Questions to be Answered	Not at All	Less Than One Time in Five	Less Than Half the Time	About Half the Time	More Than Half the Time	Almost Always
Over the past month, how often have you had a sensation of not emptying your bladder completely after you finish urinating?	0	1	2	3	4	5
Over the past month, how often have you had to urinate again less than 2 hours after you finished urinating?	0	1	2	3	4	5
Over the past month, how often have you found you stopped and started again several times when you urinated?	0	1	2	3	4	5
Over the past month, how often have you found it difficult to postpone urination?	0	1	2	3	4	5
Over the past month, how often have you had a weak urinary stream?	0	1	2	3	4	5
Over the past month, how often have you had to push or strain to begin urination?	0	1	2	3	4	5
Over the past month, how many times did you most typically get up to urinate from the time you went to bed at night until the time you got up in the morning?	0 (None)	1 (1 time)	2 (2 times)	3 (3 times)	4 (4 times)	5 (5 times)

A score of 0 to 7 indicates mild symptoms; 8 to 19, moderate symptoms; and 20 to 35, severe symptoms.

From Holtgrewe HL, Mebust WK, Dowd JB, et al: The American Urological Association symptom index for benign prostatic hyperplasia (abstract 1042), *J Urol* 167(2):265, 2002.

Men with BPH should be advised that data from the Prostate Cancer Prevention Trial revealed that BPH is not a risk factor for prostate cancer.[7] Assessment of free PSA and PSA velocity (the rate of rise per year) may help increase specificity for prostate cancer. Noncancerous prostate growth rarely results in a PSA velocity of more than 0.75 ng/mL/yr.[8] The use of finasteride, a medication indicated for BPH, may increase the accuracy of PSA testing and even decrease the incidence of prostate cancer in select men at increased risk of prostate cancer.[9]

DIAGNOSTICS

Benign Prostatic Hyperplasia

LABORATORY	IMAGING
Urinalysis	Bladder scan for postvoid residual*
Creatinine	Other imaging at discretion of urologist
PSA*	

*If indicated.

DIFFERENTIAL DIAGNOSIS

Symptoms of BOO mandate evaluation for bladder calculi, urethral stricture, cancer of the prostate, and bladder neck contracture. Bladder cancer (as well as renal cancer) should be a consideration in a male patient with unexplained hematuria. Urinary tract infection must be excluded if there are complaints of irritative voiding symptoms. If abnormalities are found on neurologic examination and problems with urinary retention are present, neurologic disease must be considered. Prostate cancer should be considered when an asymmetric enlargement, nodule, or induration is palpated on rectal examination.

DIFFERENTIAL DIAGNOSIS

Benign Prostatic Hyperplasia

- Bladder calculi
- Urethral stricture
- Bladder neck contracture
- Cancer
- Urinary tract infection and prostatitis
- Neurologic disorder

MANAGEMENT

The traditional management goal for treatment of BPH has been relief of symptoms to improve quality of life. Treatment focuses on balancing the severity of the patient's symptoms with potential side effects of therapy. For men with BPH who have mild symptoms and no complications, behavioral modifications including limiting fluids before bedtime, limiting use of caffeine and alcohol, and double voiding can be helpful. Treatment options include watchful waiting and lifestyle modifications, $alpha_1$-adrenergic antagonist therapy, 5α-reductase enzyme inhibitor therapy or combination drug therapy, balloon dilation, and surgery.[6] The benefits and risks associated with each treatment should be explained. It is important to advise the patient that if he chooses watchful waiting, other treatment approaches can be considered at any time if symptoms increase.

Alpha-adrenergic antagonists have long been the main treatment of BPH. They work by relaxing smooth muscle in the bladder neck, prostate capsule, and prostatic urethra. Doses can be titrated up while monitoring for side effects. Terazosin and doxazosin need to be initiated at bedtime to reduce dizziness and postural effects. If patients cannot tolerate this class of medications, 5α-reductase inhibitor therapy (e.g., dutasteride and finasteride) can be initiated as monotherapy. These drugs work by shrinking prostatic glandular hyperplasia by decreasing tissue DHT levels, but it may take up to 6 to 12 months to see improvement in symptoms based on reduced prostate size. Phosphodiesterase-5 (PDE5) inhibitors such as sildenafil or tadalafil can be used for men with mild to moderate BPH symptoms and erectile dysfunction. Combination therapy with alpha-adrenergic antagonists and 5α-reductase inhibitors can also be used for men with large prostates and severe symptoms.[6]

Use of herbal preparations such as saw palmetto, Cernilton, and *Pygeum africanum* may be increasing, but there is limited evidence as to their safety and efficacy.[10-12] Saw palmetto may contribute to increased risk of bleeding, and patients need to notify their providers so that it can be stopped before invasive procedures. Balloon dilation reduces symptoms in the short term, but long-term follow-up after the procedure has not been adequately studied. Transurethral resection of the prostate (TURP), transurethral incision of the prostate, and open prostatectomy are surgical procedures that are effective for severe BPH. TURP has long been considered the gold standard treatment of BOO, but it is limited to prostates weighing less than 100 g and is associated with significant complications and mortality.[13]

COMPLICATIONS

Urinary tract infection and urinary retention are common sequelae of BPH. In addition, urinary retention can result in renal problems if it is not detected early.

INDICATIONS FOR REFERRAL OR HOSPITALIZATION

Referral to a urologist is necessary for patients with urinary retention; intractable symptoms related to obstruction; recurrent or persistent urinary tract infection; recurrent prostatic bleeding; significant postvoid residual; changes in the kidneys, ureters, or bladder caused by prostatic obstruction; abnormally low urinary flow rate; and bladder calculi. Filling cystometry, uroflowmetry, urethrocystoscopy, pressure-flow studies, and measurement of postvoid residuals may be helpful in individual situations, and their need can best be determined by a urologist. These tests are not recommended as standard tests for the evaluation of BPH.[6] Surgery may be indicated for patients who do not tolerate medical management.

Acute urinary retention with a distended bladder confirmed by ultrasound examination or catheterization increases the risk of infection and renal complications, and hospitalization may be indicated.

PATIENT AND FAMILY EDUCATION

Patients should understand the advantages and risks of each treatment option so that they can make informed decisions. Patients should be advised of the importance of monitoring symptom progression and reporting any abrupt change in symptom pattern, which may indicate a complication or another pathologic process.

PROSTATITIS

DEFINITION AND EPIDEMIOLOGY

Prostatitis, or inflammation of the prostate gland, is a common problem in the adult male population. There are four basic types of prostatitis: acute bacterial, chronic bacterial, nonbacterial, and prostatodynia. Accurate diagnosis to differentiate these urologic problems is a prerequisite for effective management.

The prostate gland is an organ located adjacent to and inferior to the bladder. The urethra passes through the prostate gland. Bacterial prostatitis (both acute and chronic) is caused by bacterial inflammation. However, nonbacterial prostatitis, for which there is no identifiable cause, is the most common cause of prostatic inflammation. Prostatodynia is characterized by symptoms of prostatic inflammation but without signs of inflammation on physical examination.

PATHOPHYSIOLOGY

The organisms responsible for acute and chronic prostatitis are usually gram-negative organisms, those responsible for most of the lower urologic tract infections. *Escherichia coli* or *Proteus* species and *Klebsiella, Enterobacter,* and *Serratia* are the most common causative bacteria. *Pseudomonas aeruginosa* is also implicated as an infective organism. Some gram-positive cocci are considered responsible for prostatitis including *Staphylococcus aureus,* streptococci, and enterococci. *Neisseria gonorrhoeae* and *Chlamydia trachomatis* are important organisms to consider in relation to infections in men at higher risk for sexually transmitted infection.

Acute bacterial prostatitis results from the ascent of organized, colonized bacteria from the lower urethra to the prostate. The urethral bacteria may be a result of infection or normal fecal flora. Increases in intraurethral pressure as a result of intercourse can result in bacterial deposition into the prostate. Challenges associated with bacterial eradication increase the risk of chronic infection. The use of instruments during urologic procedures is another common cause of acute bacterial prostatitis.

The cause of nonbacterial prostatitis is less clear. Causative factors contributing to the development of nonbacterial prostatitis include prior bacterial infection; bicycle riding; organisms such as *Ureaplasma urealyticum, Chlamydia, Gardnerella,* and *Mycoplasma;* irritation from urine flow problems, chemical irritants, lower urinary tract nerve disorders and pelvic muscle abnormalities; sexual abuse; and viruses.[14]

The cause of prostatodynia is also unknown. There is some evidence that it may be related to a neurologic disorder that results in voiding dysfunction and in dysfunction of the pelvic floor musculature.[14]

CLINICAL PRESENTATION

Fever, chills, malaise, myalgias, and arthralgias are common with acute bacterial prostatitis. Genitourinary symptoms include hesitancy, frequency, urgency, nocturia, dysuria, and a sensation of incomplete bladder emptying. Accompanying complaints may be low back pain, perineal pain, or suprapubic pain. PSA levels are often markedly elevated and should not be checked in the acute stages of prostatitis because they are not reliable indicators of either infection or cure.

The presentation of chronic prostatitis tends to be more varied than that of acute prostatitis and may include a history of recurrent urinary tract infection (usually with the same organism) and complaints of urinary frequency, urgency, and burning on urination. Perineal, inguinal, or suprapubic pain may be present.[14]

Nonbacterial prostatitis is characterized by prostatic pain or vague discomfort of the suprapubic, scrotal, inguinal, lower back, or perineal areas. Pain on ejaculation may also occur. Urinary symptoms, such as hesitancy, a decrease in the urinary stream, frequency, urgency, and burning on urination, may also be present.

Symptoms suggestive of prostatodynia include pain and discomfort in the pelvic area and problems related to urinary flow, such as hesitancy, interrupted flow, postvoid dribbling, and decreased flow. Frequency, urgency, and nocturia may be present. Penile and urethral pain as well as discomfort in the lower back, suprapubic area, testicles, groin, and perineum is often reported. The patient usually has no history of urinary tract infection but may have a lifetime history of voiding difficulty.

PHYSICAL EXAMINATION

Abdominal and rectal examinations are important components of the physical examination for symptoms related to the prostate. The abdominal examination should exclude bladder distention, and the prostate gland should be examined for size, consistency, and tenderness. Normally, the prostate is heart shaped and measures approximately $4 \times 3 \times 2$ cm ($1\frac{3}{5} \times 1\frac{1}{5} \times \frac{4}{5}$ inches). In acute bacterial prostatitis, the prostate is typically enlarged, with tenderness and induration. The prostate examination should be performed gently without excessive manipulation to avoid inducing bacteremia. Urinary retention and fever may be present.

The prostate examination in chronic bacterial prostatitis may be nonspecific or may reveal a tender or boggy prostate. In nonbacterial prostatitis, the prostate examination findings are usually normal, but a soft, boggy prostate with tenderness may occasionally be present. Physical examination in prostatodynia is unremarkable with the exception that increased anal sphincter tone and paraprostatic tenderness may be present.

DIAGNOSTICS

The history and physical examination are often adequate for diagnosis of prostatitis. Examination of expressed prostatic secretions (EPSs) and the premassage and postmassage test (PPMT) are two diagnostic tests for prostatitis. These tests are infrequently used in primary care. There is weak clinical evidence regarding benefits of their use. These tests are considered by some as helpful to the diagnosis and differentiation of types of prostatitis. These tests should not be done if acute prostatitis is suspected. Because gram-negative organisms almost always cause bacterial prostatitis, many clinicians choose to empirically treat suspected prostatitis based on history and physical examination findings.

If acute bacterial prostatitis is suspected, prostatic massage should be avoided to minimize risk of bacteremia. In acute bacterial prostatitis, the urinalysis results may reveal pyuria, bacteriuria, and varying degrees of hematuria; urine culture is necessary for organism identification. A complete blood count (CBC) is significant for increased numbers of leukocytes with a left shift. In chronic bacterial prostatitis, the urinalysis is usually normal unless there is coexistent cystitis.

Urine cultures are negative with nonbacterial prostatitis, but increased numbers of leukocytes are often seen in the specimen.

DIAGNOSTICS

Prostatitis

LABORATORY
Midstream urine specimens for culture and sensitivity
CBC and differential
Blood urea nitrogen
Creatinine

IMAGING
At discretion of urologist

In prostatodynia, the urine and EPS specimens are normal. Urodynamic testing may show signs of dysfunctional voiding.

DIFFERENTIAL DIAGNOSIS

The diagnosis of acute prostatitis is usually made on the basis of the clinical presentation and the markedly tender prostate on physical examination. It can be distinguished from acute pyelonephritis, acute epididymitis, and acute diverticulosis by a careful history, physical examination, and urinalysis. Prostatic enlargement from BPH or prostate cancer causing urinary retention can usually be distinguished from acute bacterial prostatitis on rectal examination.

Chronic bacterial prostatitis can be differentiated from chronic urethritis and cystitis with segmented urine cultures. Common causes of urinary outflow problems, such as BPH, urethral stricture, and prostate cancer, should be considered in the differential diagnosis. Bladder carcinoma, sphincter dyssynergia, and neurogenic bladder also can cause lower urinary tract irritative symptoms.[14] Rectal examination should help to exclude anal disease, such as tumors, which may manifest similarly to chronic prostatitis.

The primary condition to be considered in the differential diagnosis of nonbacterial prostatitis is chronic bacterial prostatitis. The absence of positive cultures and a negative history of urinary tract infection support the diagnosis of nonbacterial prostatitis.

A urinary cytologic examination and cystoscopy are indicated to exclude bladder cancer in the older man with irritative voiding symptoms and negative cultures.[15]

Interstitial cystitis and carcinoma in situ of the bladder may be seen with similar symptoms in the younger man.

DIFFERENTIAL DIAGNOSIS

Prostatitis

- Urinary tract infection, urethritis or cystitis
- Acute or chronic bacterial prostatitis
- Acute pyelonephritis
- Acute epididymitis
- Acute diverticulitis
- Prostatic cancer or bladder cancer
- Benign prostatic hyperplasia
- Urethral stricture
- Sphincter dyssynergy
- Neurogenic bladder
- Interstitial cystitis
- Obstructive calculus

MANAGEMENT

Many patients with acute prostatitis are severely ill and require broad-spectrum antibiotic therapy. Depending on the severity of the illness, hospitalization and intravenous antibiotic therapy may be indicated. Patients who are febrile should be considered for hospitalization. Intravenous fluoroquinolones such as levofloxacin or ciprofloxacin may be selected for treatment. Intravenous therapy is changed to oral therapy when the patient is afebrile for 24 to 48 hours and able to tolerate oral intake.

Those who are less acutely ill may be treated on an outpatient basis with oral antibiotics. Trimethoprim-sulfamethoxazole and fluoroquinolones are effective and usually considered first-line treatment choices.[16] Penicillins and cephalosporins do not penetrate the prostatic epithelium and are not considered desirable options for treatment.[16] The length of appropriate treatment ranges from 2 to 6 weeks. In general, acute bacterial prostatitis requires antibiotic therapy for a minimum of 3 weeks to prevent the development of chronic bacterial prostatitis. Six weeks of antibiotic therapy is recommended to ensure eradication of the bacteria.[16,17] Experts suggest obtaining urine cultures 7 days after initiation of antibiotic therapy.[18] This approach ensures correct antibiotic selection and predicts cure at completion of therapy. Overall cure of acute bacterial prostatitis can be established through urine culture analysis 14 days after treatment.[18] Local measures may be helpful in reducing discomfort. Sitz baths, three times per day, may reduce perineal pain. Analgesics, antipyretics, stool softeners, and bed rest may also be beneficial.

The treatment of chronic bacterial prostatitis is more complex because of the difficulty in attaining therapeutic intraprostatic antibiotic levels in a noninflamed prostate. The antibiotics that have demonstrated the highest effectiveness for penetration into prostatic tissue include fluoroquinolones, sulfonamides, tetracyclines, and macrolides. Fluoroquinolones are a good choice for men who have an initial occurrence of chronic bacterial prostatitis.[19] Ciprofloxacin, 500 mg orally every 12 hours, and levofloxacin, 500 mg daily, have shown cure rates of 60% to 70% after 6 months of follow-up.[20,21] Trimethoprim-sulfamethoxazole generally provides effective treatment but will need to be prescribed for a longer duration and a minimum of 6 weeks.[21] Treatment length is often 3 weeks to 4 months.[21] It is recommended that a urine culture be performed for all men being treated with antibiotics 4 weeks into treatment. If the urine is not sterile at that time, treatment change should be considered.

It may be difficult to cure chronic bacterial prostatitis. If a relapse occurs, a longer course of antibiotic therapy is necessary. If a cure is not achieved, a low dose of antibiotics may be prescribed to prevent symptomatic infection. Commonly used medications include trimethoprim-sulfamethoxazole DS (160 mg/800 mg, 1 tablet per day or every other day) and nitrofurantoin (50 to 100 mg/day). In older patients, drug dosages for any medication may require adjustment depending on creatinine clearance.

Supportive measures, such as warm water baths, may be helpful in the treatment of chronic bacterial prostatitis. Beverages that produce rapid bladder expansion, such as coffee, tea, and alcohol, should be avoided. The use of medications that impair bladder function (e.g., anticholinergics, sedatives, antidepressants) should be assessed.

The treatment of nonbacterial prostatitis or chronic pelvic pain syndrome is controversial because of the inability to isolate a causative organism. If *Ureaplasma* or *Chlamydia* organisms are suspected and prostatic discharge reveals leukocytes exceeding 1000/μL, treatment with doxycycline, erythromycin, trimethoprim-sulfamethoxazole DS, or a fluoroquinolone for 4 to 6 weeks is an option.[22] If the patient does not respond to treatment, antibiotic therapy should be discontinued and the emphasis shifted to symptomatic relief. Supportive measures as described previously may be helpful, including warm tub baths and the use of nonsteroidal anti-inflammatory drugs (NSAIDs). Normal sexual activity is not contraindicated. If patients complain of irritative voiding problems, a trial of anticholinergic medications, such as oxybutynin chloride, may be effective. If spicy foods, alcohol, and caffeine aggravate symptoms, they should be avoided.

The treatment of prostatodynia includes the use of alpha-adrenergic blocking agents that relax the muscles of the bladder neck. To minimize the risk of hypotension, therapy should be initiated with a low dose. The use of biofeedback, referral to a mental health professional for stress and emotional problems, and the use of sitz baths and NSAIDs may also be helpful in prostatodynia.

LIFE SPAN CONSIDERATIONS

In the older man, the possibility of coexistent BPH or prostate cancer, which can potentiate the signs and symptoms of prostatitis, should be considered.

COMPLICATIONS

A prostatic abscess rarely occurs as a complication of acute bacterial prostatitis except in immunocompromised patients. The symptoms are similar to those of acute bacterial prostatitis, but on rectal examination there is a fluctuance of the affected lobe. Diagnosis can be confirmed with transrectal ultrasonography (TRUS). The treatment usually includes surgical drainage and antibiotics. Other complications of acute bacterial prostatitis may include pyelonephritis, epididymitis, seminal vesiculitis, and bacteremia. Chronic prostatitis/chronic pain syndrome may occur and includes LUTS, sexual dysfunction, and reduced quality of life.[23] The syndrome is diagnosed on the basis of symptoms, particularly pain or discomfort in the pelvic region.

INDICATIONS FOR REFERRAL OR HOSPITALIZATION

Because of the severity of the illness associated with acute bacterial prostatitis and the potential chronicity of bacterial and nonbacterial prostatitis and prostatodynia, co-management with a urologist is often indicated. Urologic referral is indicated for severe cases of acute bacterial prostatitis, when comorbidity increases the risk of sequelae, or when signs of urinary retention are present. Refractory chronic prostatitis in the presence of prostatic stones also requires urologic referral. If symptoms do not resolve after the treatment of nonbacterial prostatitis or prostatodynia, a urologic referral is necessary to exclude cystitis[24] or bladder cancer and to confirm the original diagnosis.

Hospitalization is indicated for acute illness. If prostate enlargement results in urinary retention, urinary catheterization is contraindicated and a percutaneous suprapubic tube is necessary until the prostatic enlargement subsides.

PATIENT AND FAMILY EDUCATION

Education about the cause of the patient's symptoms and treatment is necessary. The long duration of antibiotic treatment in several of these conditions requires that patients understand the necessity of maintaining an adequate therapeutic level for the duration of therapy. The importance of follow-up care as well as the use of condoms to prevent the reintroduction of bacteria into the urethra with sexual intercourse should be stressed. Anal intercourse should be avoided with acute bacterial prostatitis.

CHAPTER 148

PROTEINURIA AND HEMATURIA

Joanne Sandberg-Cook

Proteinuria and hematuria are relatively common findings on routine urinalysis. However, these findings can also be signs of serious disease or neoplasm. For example, research demonstrates that there is a positive linear association between the magnitude of proteinuria and an increase in the risk of cardiovascular disease and end-stage renal disease (ESRD).[1] Hematuria is the most common sign of bladder cancer. Because of the potential seriousness of these findings, careful, systematic evaluation is essential.

PROTEINURIA

DEFINITION AND EPIDEMIOLOGY

Approximately 15 kg of protein is filtered through the adult kidney each day, with normally less than 150 mg excreted.[2] Proteinuria, generally defined as urinary protein excretion of more than 150 mg/day (10 to 20 mg/dL), is the hallmark of renal disease. Microalbuminuria is defined as the excretion of 30 to 150 mg of protein per day and is a sign of early renal disease, particularly in patients with diabetes.[3] Macroalbuminuria is occasionally used to describe rates of more than 300 mg/day.

Proteinuria can be classified as transient or persistent. Transient proteinuria is caused by a temporary change in glomerular hemodynamics, which causes the excess of protein. These conditions are usually of a benign or self-limited nature and include orthostatic (postural) proteinuria, dehydration, fever, exercise, and emotional stress. Congestive heart failure and seizures can also cause transient proteinuria.[4] Persistent proteinuria is defined as 1+ protein on a standard dipstick (which corresponds to approximately 30 mg/dL) two or more times during a 3-month period.[4] Persistent proteinuria indicates a pathologic process, and the etiology must be investigated. Some common causes of persistent proteinuria are listed in Box 148-1.

Although isolated proteinuria is not necessarily associated with excess morbidity and mortality, it can be a sign of serious systemic disease. Evidence suggests that changes in low levels of proteinuria are predictive of the annual decline in glomerular filtration rate and the development of ESRD in persons with nondiabetic kidney disease.[1] Even a slight increase in proteinuria has been shown to be an independent risk factor for ESRD. Therefore, asymptomatic proteinuria warrants further evaluation.

BOX 148-1

Common Causes of Proteinuria

DRUG INDUCED
- Lithium
- Cyclosporine
- Cisplatin
- Nonsteroidal anti-inflammatory drugs (NSAIDs)

HEREDITARY
- Polycystic kidney disease
- Medullary kidney disease

IMMUNE
- Drug allergies
- Collagen vascular disorders (lupus, vasculitis)
- Immunoglobulin A nephropathy (Berger disease)
- Sarcoidosis

INFECTIOUS
- Bacterial, fungal, or parasitic infection
- Tuberculosis

METABOLIC
- Hyperuricemia
- Hypercalcemia
- Amyloidosis

VASCULAR
- Diabetes mellitus
- Hypertension
- Sickle cell disease
- Radiation nephritis

INCREASED PRODUCTION
- Multiple causes

In the United States, diabetes is the leading cause of ESRD, and in both type 1 and type 2 diabetes, microalbuminuria is the first sign of deteriorating renal function (see Chapter 206). As kidney function declines, microalbuminuria becomes full-fledged proteinuria. Hypertension is the second leading cause of ESRD. ESRD has a high annual mortality worldwide, with millions having no access to treatment.

Urinary albumin excretion has also been shown to predict blood pressure progression in nondiabetic, nonhypertensive individuals and appears to precede progression to higher blood pressure stages.[5] Therefore, proteinuria may be a useful biomarker for identification of individuals who are at risk for development of hypertension. In addition, persistent proteinuria in excess of 1 g/day has been associated with increased cardiac morbidity and mortality, especially heart failure.[6]

Certain population groups, including African Americans, Native Americans, Hispanic Americans, and Pacific Islanders, are at increased risk for development of proteinuria. Aging and obesity are also risk factors for development of proteinuria.[7]

PATHOPHYSIOLOGY

Protein excretion is affected by three factors: (1) prevention of excretion by the glomerular capillary wall, (2) reabsorption and catabolism by the proximal tubule cells, and (3) production of low-molecular-weight proteins.[3] Therefore, proteinuria is classified as glomerular, tubular, or overflow in origin. Glomerular proteinuria is the most common type of persistent proteinuria, and albumin is the primary urinary protein.[3] Tubular proteinuria results when malfunctioning tubule cells no longer metabolize or reabsorb the protein that has been normally filtered. In this condition, low-molecular-weight proteins are the predominant type of protein, and the amount rarely exceeds 2 g/day. Overflow proteinuria occurs when low-molecular-weight proteins overwhelm the ability of the tubules to reabsorb filtered proteins.[2]

CLINICAL PRESENTATION

The clinical presentation of the patient with proteinuria can vary from healthy young adults with functional proteinuria related to prolonged exercise to seriously ill diabetic patients with nephrotic syndrome. All individuals should therefore be screened for proteinuria by routine dipstick testing. Especially important is the routine screening of pregnant women. Proteinuria before 24 weeks' gestation indicates a likely glomerulonephritis, whereas proteinuria after 24 weeks' gestation is usually a sign of preeclampsia.[8]

Persistent proteinuria in patients with diabetes is usually a result of diabetic nephropathy. However, uncontrolled diabetes mellitus may cause transient proteinuria, most likely as a result of hyperfiltration and decreased tubular reabsorption.[9]

PHYSICAL EXAMINATION

With proteinuria, a complete and thorough history is essential. Specific areas of focus should include recent acute or chronic illness, surgery, diagnostic procedures (especially those requiring contrast media), urinary frequency or symptoms suggesting infection, risk factors for human immunodeficiency virus (HIV) infection, medications taken (including over-the-counter medications), family history of renal disease or diabetes, and recent physical activity (especially exercise or cold weather activities). The physical examination should be comprehensive and thorough; in the case of coexistent diabetes, the severity of the diabetes should be assessed to determine whether it correlates with the severity of proteinuria. Diabetic retinopathy is often present in patients with diabetic renal disease.[10]

DIAGNOSTICS AND DIFFERENTIAL DIAGNOSIS

Proteinuria is usually detected on routine dipstick testing, and any value of 1 or greater on two or more occasions should be investigated. Limitations of dipstick testing include false-negative results caused by dilution, inability to detect microalbuminuria (although ultrasensitive dipstick tests are now available that can measure low rates of microalbuminuria), false-positive results caused by certain medications, and inability of dipstick reagents to detect light-chain proteins.[4]

Once proteinuria has been identified, unless the cause is readily apparent (e.g., preeclampsia or diabetes), the urine should be tested for Bence Jones proteins (the presence of which suggests multiple myeloma). In addition, a full blood chemistry panel with fasting blood glucose concentration, hemoglobin A_{1c} (HbA_{1c}), lipid profile, urine culture and sensitivity, and complete blood count (CBC) with differential are indicated. Further evaluation of persistent proteinuria usually includes determination of 24-hour urinary protein excretion or spot urinary protein/creatinine ratio, microscopic examination

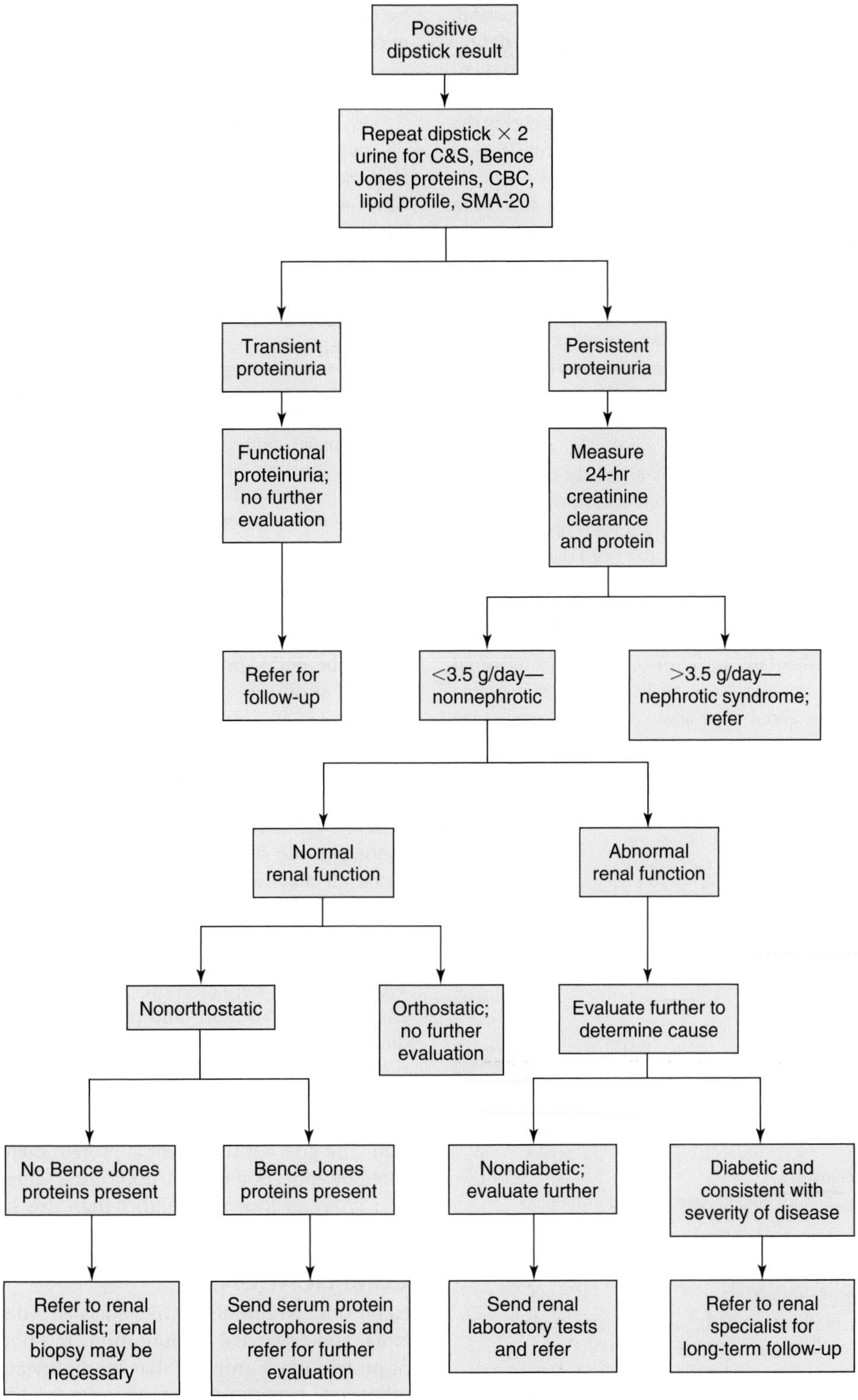

FIGURE **148-1** Algorithm for the evaluation of proteinuria.

of urinary sediment, urinary protein electrophoresis, and additional assessment of renal function.[4] A diagnostic flowchart for the evaluation of proteinuria is provided in Figure 148-1.

It is important to determine whether the proteinuria is persistent or transient. Transient proteinuria in an otherwise healthy patient that is secondary to an identifiable cause (e.g., exercise, fever, congestive heart failure) may be classified as functional proteinuria and does not require further diagnostic testing or evaluation.

Persistent proteinuria that cannot be classified as functional proteinuria requires further investigation. Investigation should begin with a 24-hour measurement of urine protein and creatinine clearance to determine the urinary protein excretion and the protein/creatinine ratio.[11] Although this has been the gold standard, it is complicated for patients and errors are common. If the excretion rate is 3.5 g/day or more, the patient by definition has nephrotic syndrome,[11] which is usually accompanied by hypoalbuminemia, hyperlipidemia, and edema. Nephrotic syndrome mandates a nephrologist's evaluation. Diabetes is the leading cause of nephrotic syndrome and accounts for 75% of all cases.[11]

If the 24-hour urinary protein excretion rate is less than 3.5 g/day, renal function should be classified as normal or abnormal. Proteinuria in the presence of normal renal function is defined as "isolated" proteinuria; in these patients, the next step is to determine whether the proteinuria is orthostatic or nonorthostatic.[11] Urinary protein excretion can increase after prolonged standing, and therefore three early morning voids should be checked for protein. If all the results are negative, a diagnosis of orthostatic proteinuria can be made, and no further diagnostic tests are necessary.[11] However, referral to a renal specialist is also appropriate because this is a poorly understood although generally benign and self-limited condition.

An alternative to 24-hour urine testing for total protein is the measurement of the urine protein/creatinine ratio using a single urine specimen and a single blood draw. The ratio is the same as the amount of grams excreted daily, so a ratio of 3.5 is equal to 3.5 g of protein per day excreted.

Patients with nonorthostatic proteinuria and normal renal function and without an elevation in Bence Jones proteins should be referred to a renal specialist. A renal biopsy may be needed to determine the cause of the proteinuria. The presence of Bence Jones proteins warrants serum protein electrophoresis and a referral for further evaluation to exclude multiple myeloma.

Other diagnostic tests depend on presentation and differential diagnosis. Collagen disease, glomerulonephritis, hepatitis-induced vasculitis, urate-related renal disease, diabetes, and other systemic disease or structural abnormalities should be considered in the evaluation of proteinuria.[11]

DIAGNOSTICS

Proteinuria

LABORATORY

- Urine dipstick
- Urine specimen for Bence Jones proteins
- CBC and differential
- Serum electrolytes
- Serum glucose/HbA_{1c}
- Blood urea nitrogen (BUN)
- Creatinine
- Serum albumin
- Calcium and phosphorus
- Lipid profile
- Urinalysis
- Urine culture and sensitivity*
- 24-hour urine collection for volume, protein, and creatinine clearance*
- Three early morning urine specimens for protein*
- Serum protein electrophoresis*
- Urine protein electrophoresis*
- Erythrocyte sedimentation rate (ESR), antinuclear antibodies, lupus profile (if lupus is suspected)*
- Antistreptolysin O titer, complement (C3, C4) if glomerulonephritis is suspected
- Hepatitis B surface antigen (if hepatitis vasculitis is suspected)

IMAGING

Intravenous urography
Renal ultrasound
Spiral computed tomography (CT)

OTHER DIAGNOSTICS

Renal biopsy*

*If indicated.

DIFFERENTIAL DIAGNOSIS

Proteinuria

- Transient proteinuria
- Persistent proteinuria
- Orthostatic proteinuria or nonorthostatic proteinuria
- Glomerulonephritis
- Diabetic nephropathy
- Nephrotic syndrome
- Vasculitis
- Medications

MANAGEMENT

Management of proteinuria depends on the underlying cause, but some general principles apply. A careful medication review should be performed, and any medications implicated in proteinuria should be discontinued. Both angiotensin-converting enzyme (ACE) inhibitors and angiotensin receptor blockers (ARBs) inhibit the renin-angiotensin system and reduce proteinuria by decreasing the systemic arterial pressure and the intraglomerular filtration pressure.[9] ACE inhibitors incompletely block the formation of angiotensin II, which is the main effector peptide of the renin-angiotensin system. ARBs do not block all angiotensin II type 1 receptors at clinically recommended doses. Diabetes and hyperlipidemia, if present, should be aggressively managed; blood pressure control is also important. Patients with chronic kidney disease should be managed aggressively to help prevent or delay the onset of ESRD (see Chapter 149). Sodium- and protein-restricted diets may be indicated for some patients. No matter what the cause, persistent proteinuria should be aggressively managed, both by controlling the underlying disease and by directing specific therapy (usually ACE inhibitors or ARBs) at reduction of protein excretion. The goal for treatment is protein excretion rates (as measured by collection of a 24-hour urine sample for total protein) of 1 g/day or less; rates higher than this have been shown to increase cardiovascular disease.

COMPLICATIONS

Nephrotic syndrome with associated edema, hypoalbuminemia, and extrarenal complications is a potential consequence of proteinuria. Cardiovascular morbidity and mortality, immobilization, hyperlipidemia, hypercoagulability, and electrolyte disturbances are additional complications.

INDICATIONS FOR REFERRAL OR HOSPITALIZATION

All patients with renal disease or abnormal renal function should be referred to a renal specialist for consultation and management guidance. Referrals for patients with isolated orthostatic proteinuria should be based on a thorough risk assessment and evaluation of their general health, life span considerations, and concerns for aggressive management.

Any patients seen with nephrotic syndrome, acute renal failure, renal failure of unknown origin, or unstable vital signs should be urgently referred for hospitalization. New-onset proteinuria in pregnant women should be considered a medical emergency, and urgent referral to exclude eclampsia is indicated.

PATIENT AND FAMILY EDUCATION

Patient education depends on the cause of proteinuria, but diet education, diabetic teaching for patients with diabetes, and education concerning blood pressure management are usually necessary. Especially critical is that the patient and family understand the importance of diagnostic testing and regular follow-up care.

HEMATURIA

DEFINITION AND EPIDEMIOLOGY

Hematuria is generally defined as three or more red blood cells (RBCs) per high-power field.[12] Transient hematuria is defined as hematuria that occurs on one occasion, whereas persistent hematuria is defined as hematuria that occurs on two or more consecutive occasions.[4,12] Exercise-induced hematuria in healthy young adults is not associated with any known morbidity or mortality, but both transient and persistent hematuria can be signs of serious disease. Common causes of hematuria are listed in Box 148-2.

The rates for asymptomatic microscopic hematuria in the general population range from 2.4% to 31% and vary with gender and age.[12] In older men, who are at higher risk for urologic disease, the prevalence of asymptomatic microscopic hematuria is high. Ten percent of men older than 50 years have asymptomatic hematuria on presentation. Gross hematuria in older men denotes a significant risk of malignant disease. Most bladder cancers are diagnosed because of hematuria.[13]

BOX 148-2

Common Causes of Hematuria

GLOMERULAR
- Glomerulonephritis
- Lupus nephritis
- Interstitial nephritis
- Pyelonephritis
- Vasculitis
- Alport syndrome
- Thin basement membrane disease

NONGLOMERULAR
- Infection
- Neoplasm of the bladder, ureter, prostate, or kidney
- Renal or bladder calculi
- Polycystic kidney disease
- Sickle cell (disease or trait)
- Trauma
- Increased bleeding time
- Hemorrhagic cystitis
- Schistosomiasis
- Nutcracker phenomenon

MISCELLANEOUS
- Drug induced
  - Warfarin, heparin
- Exercise induced
- Endometriosis

PSEUDOHEMATURIA
- Menstrual contamination
- Hemoglobinuria
- Myoglobinuria
- Porphyrins
- Red food dyes, red foods (e.g., beets)
- Drugs
  - Dilantin
  - Quinine
  - Phenothiazines
  - Rifampin
  - Pyridium
  - Sulfonamides
  - Cascara, Ex-Lax

PATHOPHYSIOLOGY

Normal urinary excretion of RBCs is 2 million/day, which results in two or three RBCs per high-power field.[4] Isolated hematuria (hematuria unaccompanied by any other abnormal urine components) can result from bleeding anywhere from the renal pelvis to the urethra but is rarely caused by systemic disease. Hematuria related to renal disease enters the tubular field along the nephron and produces RBC casts that are indicative of the renal origin.[3,4] Bacterial infections are a common cause of hematuria, and the presence of bacteria on urinalysis is suggestive of an infectious cause. Acute cystitis or urethritis can cause gross hematuria and is more common in women than in men. The presence of proteinuria and hematuria is suggestive of glomerular or interstitial nephritis.[3]

CLINICAL PRESENTATION

Hematuria is often accompanied by clinically significant symptoms or by abnormalities in the urinalysis that can aid in identifying the source of bleeding. The patient's age, gender, and level of physical activity should always be considered (long-distance runners have been documented to have rates of hematuria as high as 13%).[14] Hematuria associated with pyuria suggests an infectious process, whereas colicky flank pain suggests pain originating from a ureter. A prostatic or urethral source is likely when bleeding occurs only at the beginning or end of micturition. The presence of hemoptysis, acute renal failure, and hematuria is highly suggestive of Goodpasture syndrome. Postinfection glomerulonephritis is signified by hematuria and proteinuria accompanied by edema, hypertension, and a history of sore throat or skin infection, although patients often may not report any recent signs or symptoms of infection. This form of glomerulonephritis results in transient reduction of renal function in most cases.[15]

PHYSICAL EXAMINATION

A thorough patient history should be obtained, including urinary patterns, urine color, timing of hematuria (beginning, end, or throughout micturition; transient or persistent), flank pain, history of renal calculi, urinary tract infections (UTIs), hemoptysis or bloody nasal secretions, recent acute or chronic illness, medications (including over-the-counter and illicit drugs), history of sexually transmitted disease, risk behaviors for HIV infection, and history of travel to areas with endemic schistosomiasis, a common cause of hematuria in Asia and Africa. A complete family history specifically related to renal disease, sickle cell disease or traits, and congenital deafness (indicating Alport syndrome) is also necessary. A comprehensive physical examination, including a pelvic examination in women and a prostate examination in men, is warranted. In women, urethral and vaginal examinations are indicated to determine if there are any local causes of microscopic hematuria.[12] In uncircumcised men, the foreskin should be retracted to expose the glans penis. In both men and women, a catheterized urinary specimen is indicated if a clean-catch specimen cannot be reliably obtained.

DIAGNOSTICS AND DIFFERENTIAL DIAGNOSIS

Laboratory analysis of hematuria begins with a comprehensive examination of the urine and urinary sediment (Figure 148-2).[12] A urinalysis with RBC casts indicates hematuria originating from the renal parenchyma.[2] Further evidence of a renal source

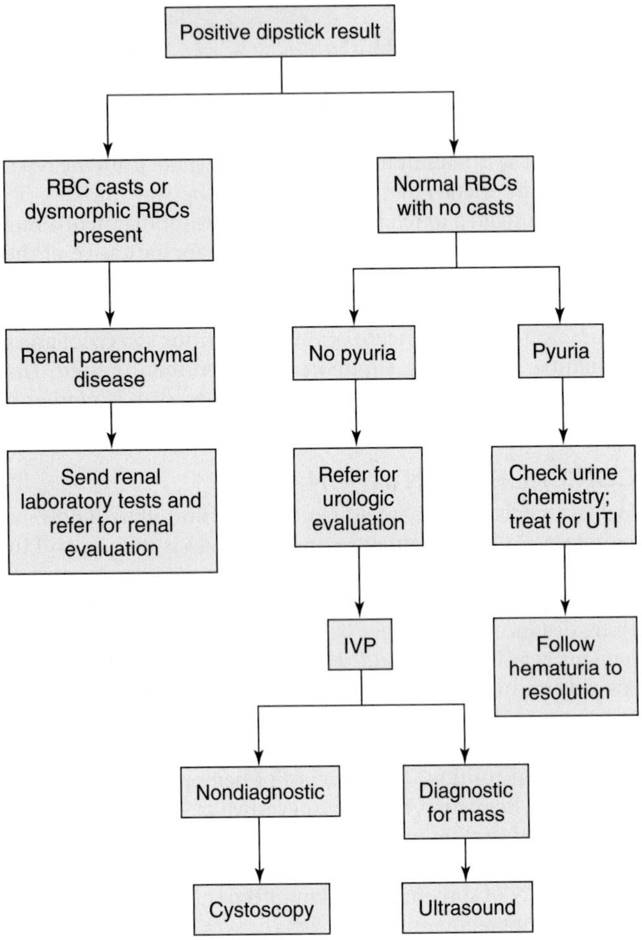

FIGURE 148-2 Algorithm for the evaluation of hematuria.

is significant proteinuria (>1 g/24 hr), dysmorphic RBCs, cola-colored urine, or renal insufficiency.[3,4] One major limitation of dipstick testing is that it detects the peroxidase activity of erythrocytes, not RBCs, in the urine. However, myoglobin and hemoglobin will also catalyze this reaction, so a positive test result may indicate hematuria, myoglobinuria, or hemoglobinuria. If the dipstick is positive for heme but no increased numbers of RBCs are seen on microscopic examination, the urine should be tested for myoglobinuria and hemoglobinuria.

Hematuria can be divided into glomerular, renal (i.e., nonglomerular), and urologic causes. Glomerular hematuria is typically associated with significant proteinuria, erythrocyte casts, and dysmorphic RBCs. However, 20% of patients with biopsy-proven glomerulonephritis are seen with hematuria alone. Berger disease (immunoglobulin A nephropathy), Alport syndrome, and thin basement membrane disease are three common causes of glomerular hematuria.[16] Nonglomerular or renal hematuria is caused by tubulointerstitial, renovascular, or metabolic disorders. As with glomerular hematuria, there is often coexisting proteinuria but no dysmorphic RBCs or erythrocyte casts. The evaluation of glomerular and nonglomerular hematuria requires an assessment of renal function and 24-hour urine or spot urinary protein/creatinine ratio. Urologic causes of nonglomerular hematuria include tumors, calculi, and infections. It is distinguished from other types of hematuria by the absence of proteinuria, dysmorphic RBCs, and erythrocyte casts. Up to 23% of patients with gross hematuria have a urinary tract malignant neoplasm, so a full workup, including cystoscopy and imaging of the upper urinary tract, needs to be done.[17]

When hematuria originates from the lower urinary tract, intact and uniform RBCs should be present.[17] The presence of intact RBCs, white blood cells, and bacteria suggests hematuria resulting from a UTI. The decision to obtain a urine culture and sensitivity should be guided by the patient's age and gender and the presence of resistant organisms in the local population. After treatment has been completed, repeated urinalysis is necessary to ensure that the hematuria has resolved. Failure to follow hematuria to resolution may result in failure to diagnose a serious condition (see Chapter 153).

If the hematuria resolves after treatment of the UTI, no further diagnostic testing is indicated, although repeated UTIs in low-risk populations such as young men should always be fully investigated. If hematuria fails to resolve despite resolution of the UTI, or if it is of renal origin, a referral for a urologic evaluation is required.

In the absence of RBC casts or bacteria and white blood cells, a urologic evaluation should be performed. There are limited data on the impact of intravenous urography (IVU), ultrasonography, computed tomography (CT), or magnetic resonance imaging (MRI) on the management of patients with microscopic hematuria. Although IVU has been the long-standing initial imaging study, CT scanning is now recommended.[12] The advantage of CT over IVU is that CT has the highest efficacy rate for the range of possible underlying pathologic processes, especially of the upper tract. If the CT scan shows a solid mass or is nondiagnostic, referral to a urologic surgeon for excision and pathologic testing is advised. The presence of renal or bladder calculi generally requires genitourinary referral for definitive treatment. If the CT scan is nondiagnostic, the next step in the evaluation is cystoscopy, which includes inspection, biopsy, and culture of the bladder tissue. Cystoscopy is highly diagnostic for uroepithelial neoplasms. If the cystoscopy is nondiagnostic, the urologist may request a renal biopsy (see Figure 148-2).

DIAGNOSTICS

Hematuria

LABORATORY

- Urinalysis
- Urine culture and sensitivity*
- Urine for cytology*
- CBC and differential*
- Serum glucose*
- Serum electrolytes*
- Blood urea nitrogen (BUN)*
- Creatinine*
- Prothrombin time/partial thromboplastin time (PT/PTT)*
- Antinuclear antibodies
- Immunoglobulins, cryoglobulins
- Cytoplasmic antineutrophil cytoplasmic antibodies*
- Anti–glomerular basement membrane antibodies*
- Antistreptolysin O titer*
- Serum protein electrophoresis*
- Venereal Disease Research Laboratory (VDRL) tests*
- 24-Hour urine collection for calcium, uric acid*

IMAGING

- Ultrasound of kidney, ureters, bladder*
- CT scan, MRI*

OTHER DIAGNOSTICS

- Cystoscopy*
- Renal biopsy*

*If indicated.

DIFFERENTIAL DIAGNOSIS

Hematuria

- UTI
- Sexually transmitted disease
- Tuberculosis
- Malignant disease
- Renal calculi
- Exercise, medication, or food induced
- Glomerular disease
- Bladder outlet obstruction

MANAGEMENT

Management of hematuria consists mainly of identification, diagnosis, and referral. Further management considerations are based on the underlying pathologic condition, not on the presence of the hematuria itself.

COMPLICATIONS

Complications of hematuria depend on the underlying pathologic condition. Urinary obstruction, renal failure, anemia, infections, and hydronephrosis are potential complications.

INDICATIONS FOR REFERRAL OR HOSPITALIZATION

Isolated, transient hematuria or hematuria related to a UTI does not require a urology consultation. Referral to a renal or urology specialist is indicated to evaluate other causes of hematuria, given the high incidence of malignancy associated with this sign. Patients with large amounts of frank hematuria, severe flank pain suggestive of renal calculi, unstable vital signs, signs of urologic obstruction, or acute renal failure should be referred for urgent evaluation and possible hospitalization.

PATIENT AND FAMILY EDUCATION

Patient education largely depends on the cause of the hematuria; advice and educational material specific to the underlying pathologic process are appropriate. Because smoking is a major risk factor for bladder cancer, smoking cessation assistance should be offered to all smokers. One of the major goals of education in asymptomatic hematuria is to reinforce the importance of the diagnostic evaluation. Other guidance should focus on the explanation of tests, medications, untoward effects, and the need for careful follow-up evaluation when indicated.

CHAPTER 149

RENAL FAILURE

Chris Winkelman • Evelyn Duffy

DEFINITION AND EPIDEMIOLOGY

Kidney damage causes loss of filtration and the retention of waste products in blood. Patients with kidney damage experience a complex and common health condition that demands the involvement of both the primary care provider and specialists. The loss of kidney filtration has two patterns of damage: chronic kidney disease (CKD) and acute kidney injury (AKI). These patterns of damage may result in impaired kidney function, although AKI is considered potentially reversible. However, both AKI and CKD can also progress to kidney failure or the absence of kidney function. Kidney failure is also known as end-stage renal disease (ESRD) and stage 5 CKD. CKD, AKI, and kidney failure or ESRD replace other terms that have been used, such as *renal insufficiency, acute renal failure,* and *acute-on-chronic kidney disease.*[1,2]

In 2002, the National Kidney Foundation (NKF) published a landmark clinical practice guideline for the evaluation, classification, and stratification of CKD.[3] This guideline provided a common language for classifying CKD based on glomerular filtration rate (GFR). This 2002 guideline also resulted in changes in how creatinine was measured and reported by laboratories, generated new codes for the International Statistical Classification of Diseases and Related Health Problems (ICD), improved estimation of GFR, and increased awareness on the part of providers of the importance of early identification of kidney damage. Over time, it became evident that the use of the guidelines needed refinement because some patients without kidney damage, particularly older adults, were diagnosed as having CKD based on GFR estimation. In 2012 an updated guideline was published.[1]

The Kidney Disease: Improving Global Outcomes (KDIGO) group refined the definition of CKD as "abnormalities in kidney structure or function for greater than 3 months with implications for health," and this definition now includes measures of kidney damage detailed in Table 149-1.[4] The 2012 guideline recommended that CKD be categorized based on the cause, GFR, and amount of albuminuria; these categories are illustrated in Tables 149-2 and 149-3.[4] This international guideline was reviewed for its usefulness in the United States and was accepted by the NKF.[4]

The Centers for Disease Control and Prevention estimates that over 20 million Americans, 10% of the population, have CKD and that the majority of those are undiagnosed.[5] Both providers and patients have demonstrated a lack of awareness of the diagnosis of kidney disease. Studies of provider and patient awareness of CKD have consistently found that the majority of cases are not recognized by providers and that patients themselves are unaware of their damaged kidneys.[6,7] Although CKD is more prevalent in adults aged 65 years and older, about one third of older adults do not experience progressive disease.[7,8]

TABLE 149-1 Guidelines: Diagnosing CKD

Markers of kidney damage (one or more)	Albuminuria (AER ≥30 mg/24 hr; ACR ≥30 mg/g [≥3 mg/mmol]) Urine sediment abnormalities Electrolyte and other abnormalities resulting from tubular disorders Abnormalities detected by histology Structure abnormalities detected by imaging History of kidney transplantation
Decreased GFR	GFR <60 mL/min/1.73 m^2 (GFR categories G3a-G5)

ACR, albumin/creatinine ratio; AER, albumin excretion rate.

From Kidney Disease: Improving Global Outcomes (KDIGO): KDIGO 2012 clinical practice guideline for the evaluation and management of chronic kidney disease. *Kidney Int Suppl* 3(1):1-150, 2013.

TABLE 149-2 Categories of CKD

GFR Category	GFR (mL/min/1.73 m^2)	Terms
G1	≥90	Normal or high
G2	60-89	Mildly decreased*
G3a	45-59	Mildly to moderately decreased
G3b	30-44	Moderately to severely decreased
G4	15-29	Severely decreased
G5	<15	Kidney failure

*Relative to young adult level.
From Kidney Disease: Improving Global Outcomes (KDIGO): KDIGO 2012 clinical practice guideline for the evaluation and management of chronic kidney disease. *Kidney Int Suppl* 3(1):1-150, 2013.

TABLE 149-3 Albuminuria Categories in CKD

ACR (Approximate Equivalent)				
Category	AER (mg/24 hr)	(mg/mmol)	(mg/g)	Terms
A1	<30	<3	<30	Normal to mildly increased
A2	30-300	3-30	30-300	Moderately increased*
A3	>300	>30	>300	Severely increased†

*Relative to young adult level.
†Including nephrotic syndrome (albumin excretion usually >2200 mg/24 hr [ACR >2220 mg/g; >220 mg/mmol]).
From Kidney Disease: Improving Global Outcomes (KDIGO): KDIGO 2012 clinical practice guideline for the evaluation and management of chronic kidney disease. *Kidney Int Suppl* 3(1):1-150, 2013.

Similar to CKD, AKI has undergone a succession of definitions and refinement of stages. The most recent international source is from the KDIGO Acute Kidney Injury Work Group (2012).[2] AKI is defined as an increase in serum creatinine of 0.3 mg/dL over 48 hours or an increase of serum creatinine to 1.5 times baseline over the prior seven days; or a urine volume output of less than 0.5 mL/kg/hr for 6 hours. According to this guideline, AKI severity is classed from 1 to 3, with 1 being the most severe as illustrated in Table 149-4.

AKI is an abrupt loss of kidney function that occurs over 48 hours, although progressive damage may occur over as long as 7 days.[2] AKI can progress to CKD when kidney damage persists for 3 months or longer. AKI occurs in as many as 30% of adults admitted to the intensive care unit and about 7% of all hospital admissions in the United States.[9] AKI is a significant contributor to mortality and morbidity during hospitalization and in the year after discharge from acute care.[10] Older adults, particularly those older than 75 years, are at increased risk for AKI and its complications.[11]

Both AKI and CKD can progress to kidney failure in a small but significant percentage of people.[12] Kidney failure (ESRD) is characterized by anuria and the need for renal replacement therapy or kidney transplant. The kidneys and the urinary tract

TABLE 149-4 Staging of AKI

Stage	Serum Creatinine	Urine Output
1	1.5-1.9 times baseline *or* >0.3 mg/dL (>26 µmol/L) increase	<0.5 mL/kg/hr for 6-12 hr
2	2.0-2.9 times baseline	<0.5 mL/kg/hr for >12 hr
3	3.0 times baseline *or* Increase in serum creatinine to >4.0 mg/dL (>353.6 µmol/L) *or* Initiation of renal replacement therapy *or* In patients <18 years, decrease in estimated GFR to <35 mL/min/1.73 m^2	<0.3 mL/kg/hr for >24 hr *or* Anuria for >12 hr

Data from Kidney Disease: Improving Global Outcomes (KDIGO) Work Group for Acute Kidney Injury: KDIGO clinical practice guideline for acute kidney injury. *Kidney Int Suppl* 2(Suppl):1-138, 2012.

system no longer filter blood, create filtrate, or excrete urine in amounts sufficient to clear waste and balance fluid intake with output. In addition to being a clinical diagnosis, ESRD has administrative implications because those patients who receive dialysis or a kidney transplant as a result of this diagnosis are eligible for health insurance through Medicare regardless of their age.

PATHOPHYSIOLOGY

The basic pathophysiologic process of kidney disease is loss of functioning nephrons. As filtration capacity falls to less than 50%, the remaining healthy nephrons exhibit hyperfiltration and hypertrophy. This process is hypothesized to contribute to increased glomerular capillary pressure, leading to secondary nephron damage and progressive disease.[13] The results are a decrease in GFR; an increase in circulating biomarkers of kidney disease, including creatinine and blood urea nitrogen (BUN); and albuminuria.

The pathophysiology of AKI is any process that interferes with perfusion, filtration, or excretion.[14] Disruption to perfusion is categorized as prerenal. Filtration abnormalities are intrinsic causes of AKI and refer to the pathology of vessels, glomeruli, or tubules and interstitium.[15] Postrenal causes of AKI include obstruction to the renal pelvis, ureters, bladder, or urethra. However, AKI can also result from combined pathologic processes. For example, poor perfusion and subsequent ischemic damage to the nephron comprise a combined prerenal and intrinsic cause of AKI. Consider the hospitalized patient with prolonged poor renal perfusion (i.e., prerenal) from a hypotensive shock state (e.g., cardiogenic, septic, or hemorrhagic shock) with concurrent acute tubular necrosis (related to endotoxin exposure or ischemic necrosis of the nephron tubules), an intrinsic cause of AKI. As a second example of combined pathology, consider the patient with untreated kidney stones

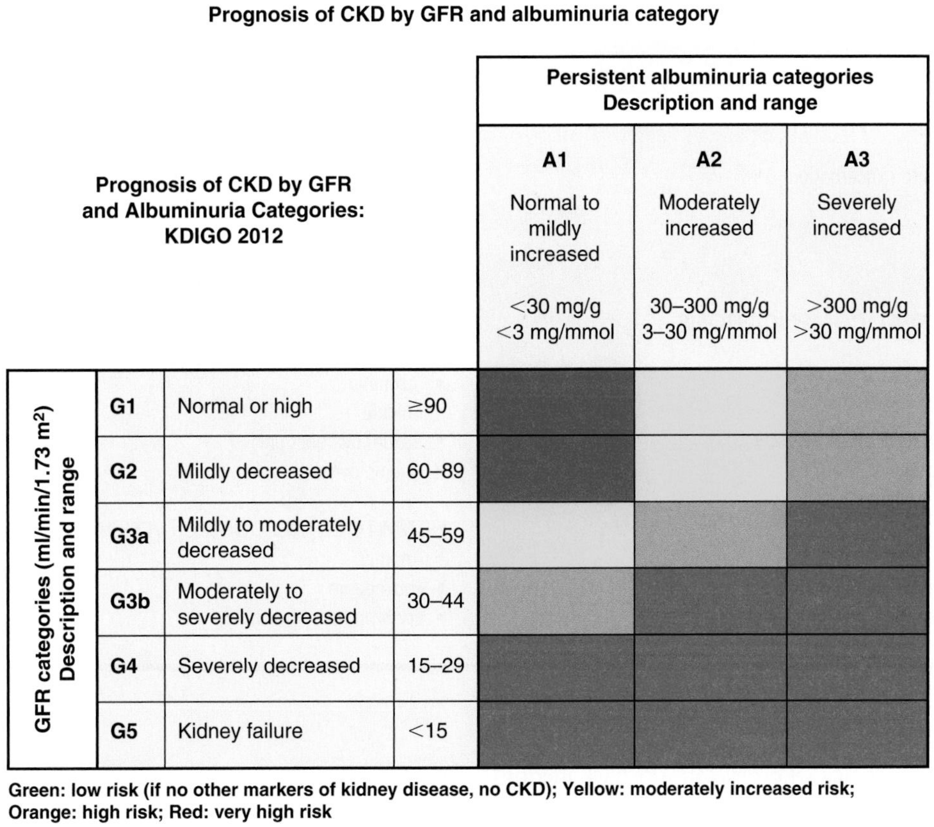
Prognosis of CKD by GFR and albuminuria category
Persistent albuminuria categories
Description and range
Prognosis of CKD by GFR and Albuminuria Categories: KDIGO 2012
A1
Normal to mildly increased
<30 mg/g
<3 mg/mmol
A2
Moderately increased
30–300 mg/g
3–30 mg/mmol
A3
Severely increased
>300 mg/g
>30 mg/mmol
GFR categories (ml/min/1.73 m²)
Description and range
G1 Normal or high ≥90
G2 Mildly decreased 60–89
G3a Mildly to moderately decreased 45–59
G3b Moderately to severely decreased 30–44
G4 Severely decreased 15–29
G5 Kidney failure <15
Green: low risk (if no other markers of kidney disease, no CKD); Yellow: moderately increased risk;
Orange: high risk; Red: very high risk

FIGURE 149-1 Risk for progression of kidney damage. (From Kidney Disease: Improving Global Outcomes [KDIGO]: KDIGO 2012 clinical practice guideline for the evaluation and management of chronic kidney disease. *Kidney Int Suppl* 3[1]:1-150, 2013.)

leading to urinary tract obstruction—postrenal AKI—leading to fibrosis and atrophy of the obstructed kidneys—an intrinsic pathology.

Risk factors of comorbidities, age, and drugs can also contribute to prerenal, intrinsic, and postrenal AKI. For example, comorbidities that affect blood flow to the kidneys such as chronic heart failure (HF) or cirrhosis increase the risk for AKI. Hypovolemic states from acute blood loss, diarrhea, or dehydration lead to prerenal injury. Contrast from imaging studies may contribute to AKI.[16] Small vessel vascular pathology from diabetes, clotting disorders, and hypertension contributes intrinsic structural changes leading to AKI.[17] Renal artery stenosis from atherosclerosis or dysplasia can cause ischemic intrinsic nephropathy.[16] Inflammatory conditions, sepsis, kidney infection, drug-induced nephritis, and malignancies damage tubules and the interstitium, leading to intrinsic causes of AKI.[18-20] Postrenal (obstructive) AKI may be caused by neoplasm, prostatic enlargement, neurogenic bladder, strictures, or nephrolithiasis.

An alternative approach to AKI suggests that it is the balance of injurious and repair processes that may drive the rapidity of decline in kidney function in AKI.[18] This molecular approach to the diagnosis and management of AKI has led to investigation of new biomarkers that detect glomerular or nephron injury earlier and provide guidance to early treatment, with a potential for improved patient outcomes.[21] For example, cystatin C is emerging as a potential marker for the early diagnosis of AKI and CKD and may be useful in determining if management is contributing to improvement such as return to baseline kidney function (i.e., reversal of AKI) or stability with cessation of progression of CKD.[1,2] Figure 149-1 illustrates the risk for progression of CKD.

CLINICAL PRESENTATION

CKD and AKI have few symptoms in the early stages. Ongoing progression of CKD and destruction of nephrons result in a variety of symptoms, complications, and a steady and predictable decline in functional health. ESRD and its management (dialysis or kidney transplantation) have significant complications that need to be co-managed with nephrologists and other experts.

The hallmark clinical signs of CKD and AKI are a decreased GFR, an increased serum creatinine, and albumin in the urine. The clinical symptoms are subtle and uncommon, with a GFR above 35 mL/min/1.73 m^2. Therefore, suspicion for kidney disease should be based on recognition of the risk for kidney damage, particularly in patients with diabetes mellitus and hypertension. Because diabetes and hypertension are highly associated with CKD, clinical guidelines for management of both diabetes and hypertension recommend regular urinalysis with a calculation of the urinary albumin/creatinine ratio (ACR) to allow for early detection of kidney damage.[13,19] Early detection of renal disease—for both CKD and AKI—is advocated to slow progression or kidney damage and decrease complications from uremia and disrupted metabolism.

The most common cause of AKI is hospitalization with concomitant reduced renal perfusion and exposure to

BOX 149-1

Major Complications of Stages 4 and 5 CKD

CARDIOVASCULAR COMPLICATIONS
- Atherosclerosis
- HF (chronic and acute exacerbation)
- Hypertension
- Pulmonary edema
- Pericarditis

GASTROINTESTINAL COMPLICATIONS
- Nausea, vomiting
- Anorexia

NEUROLOGIC COMPLICATIONS
- Peripheral neuropathy
- Muscle cramps or twitching
- Pruritus

METABOLIC COMPLICATIONS
- Electrolyte abnormalities
- Metabolic acidosis
- Alterations in vitamin D, calcium, and phosphorus metabolism and absorption
- Mineral and bone disorders (MBDs)
- Hyperparathyroidism
- Hyperlipidemia

PSYCHOSOCIAL COMPLICATIONS
- Depression
- Fatigue
- Insomnia
- Suicide
- Sexual dysfunction
- Unemployment

HEMATOLOGIC COMPLICATIONS
- Anemia
- Leukopenia
- Erythropoietin deficiency

nephrotoxins.[12] Most patients who develop AKI have identifiable risk factors, such as CKD, advanced age, liver disease, diabetes, or vascular disease. Therefore it is essential to identify those at high risk before AKI develops. It is equally important to follow up with monitoring after a diagnosis of AKI because patients with AKI are at risk for developing CKD in the future and may be discharged with early-stage CKD.[20]

Once the GFR falls below 35 mL/min/1.73 m^2, a variety of cardiovascular, gastrointestinal, neurologic, metabolic, hematologic, and psychosocial problems occur. These complications are listed in Box 149-1. Clinical presentation at this point depends on the particular complication and on the underlying cause of kidney failure. All individuals with CKD should undergo screening for the complications of kidney disease to prevent morbidity and to establish a credible baseline for the individual.

PHYSICAL EXAMINATION

The physical examination should include both a focused examination to identify primary diseases that contribute to kidney damage (e.g., diabetes mellitus or hypertension) and a broader examination that evaluates the effects of kidney disease. Staging or categorizing kidney damage (i.e., AKI stage 1 to 3; CKD category 1 to 5) can guide the primary care provider in determining the frequency of monitoring and providing anticipatory guidance about self-management. CKD may be asymptomatic until it is in the advanced stages. In older adults there may never be clear symptoms related to declining renal function.

The provider should assess for hypotension and hypertension by taking vital signs (including measurement of bilateral arm and orthostatic blood pressure); performing funduscopic evaluation for signs of arteriovenous nicking, diabetic retinopathy, and papilledema; and evaluating peripheral pulse characteristics. Volume status is determined with auscultation of lung sounds; evaluation of jugular vein distention; presence of edema; and evaluation of heart sounds. Pericarditis and pleural effusions can be a complication of CKD. A full abdominal examination includes auscultation for renal artery bruits, palpation of the kidneys, inspection for distention that may be caused by ascites, and percussion of the suprapubic area to determine bladder distention. The skin is examined for ecchymosis, rashes (especially those suggesting collagen vascular disorders), or uremic frost. The patient is asked about pruritus. A rectal examination is performed to evaluate the prostate (to exclude obstruction) in male patients. A thorough mental status examination is included to screen for depression, anxiety, substance use, and cognitive dysfunction associated with CKD.

DIAGNOSTICS

The most important diagnostic tool in monitoring both patients at risk for and those with diagnosed CKD is a serum creatinine test with an estimated GFR and a first morning or random urine sample to assess for the presence of albuminuria.[1,4]

Serum creatinine is a product of muscle metabolism. In patients with very high muscle mass, such as weight lifters, or very low muscle mass as a result of sarcopenia, the estimated GFR will be inaccurate. There is ongoing evaluation of the use of serum cystatin C in patients in whom more precise measurement of estimated GFR is necessary.[21] The estimated GFR may be limited as a screening and diagnostic tool among older adults, who may have lower muscle mass (leading to reduced creatinine production) or reduced kidney mass (leading to elevated creatinine but without concerning progression).

Most laboratories now report GFR along with serum creatinine, but if that is not available there are recommended GFR calculators. The preferred method is the CKD Epidemiology Collaboration (CKD-EPI) 2009 creatinine equation. Other methods include (in order of preference) the Modification of Diet in Renal Disease (MDRD) equation, the CKD-EPI 2012 creatinine equation, and the Crockhoff-Gault formula.[1] These calculators are available at www.kidney.org/professionals/KDOQI/gfr.

The preferred screening strategy for albuminuria is measurement of the urine ACR in an untimed urinary sample.[1,4] If the ACR is greater than 30 mg/g, a confirmatory test is done on the first morning urine.

In the absence of available ACR determination, the KDIGO guidelines recommend alternatives in the following order:

- Protein/creatinine ratio (PCR)
- Reagent strip analysis for total protein with automated reading
- Reagent strip analysis for total protein with manual reading

Another method for determining kidney damage is urinalysis. Examination of urine sediment or dipstick for red or white blood cells is recommended.[4,5]

If AKI or CKD is identified, a more comprehensive assessment of causative factors and possible complications is recommended. Not all patients require all of the evaluation; the primary care provider can individualize diagnostics based on history, established previous diagnoses or comorbidities, and an estimate of cost-effectiveness. The evaluation may include the following:

- A comprehensive serum metabolic panel including sodium, potassium, chloride, bicarbonate, BUN, creatinine, glucose, albumin, total protein, calcium, alkaline phosphatase, total protein, aspartate aminotransferase (AST), alanine aminotransferase (ALT), and bilirubin
- Glycosylated hemoglobin (HbA_{1c})
- Lipid profile
- Complete blood count (CBC) with differential
- Renal ultrasound

DIFFERENTIAL DIAGNOSIS

Differential diagnoses related to AKI and CKD include conditions that contribute to renal damage. Vigilance is necessary to determine any underlying correctable pathologic process that may be causing kidney damage. Identifying and reversing disorders that occur acutely can mitigate the severity or progression of kidney damage. In general, a mean arterial pressure of 65 mm Hg is recommended to avoid hypoperfusion to kidneys and subsequent damage.[2,18] Nephrotoxin exposure, including drugs, heavy metals, and byproducts of infection, should be avoided or eliminated.[18,22] Recognition and treatment of inflammatory conditions that contribute to AKI can mitigate intrinsic causes of AKI.

The most common type of AKI seen in primary care is prerenal AKI related to volume depletion or hypotension. Common drugs and toxins that contribute to intrinsic AKI include nonsteroidal anti-inflammatory drugs (NSAIDs) used chronically, renin-angiotensin-aldosterone system (RAAS) antagonists (i.e., angiotensin-converting enzyme [ACE] inhibitors and angiotensin receptor blockers [ARBs]), many antibiotics (including aminoglycosides, quinolones, cephalosporins active against β-lactamase, sulfonamides), illicit drugs (amphetamines, heroin), antineoplastic agents, immunosuppressants, the human immunodeficiency virus (HIV) drugs indinavir and ritonavir, heavy metals, industrial chemicals, organic solvents, pesticides, and bacterial exotoxins and endotoxins.[23] Radiation can also cause AKI. Contrast used in radiographic imaging has undergone signification reformulation in recent years with a reduced profile in terms of causing direct kidney damage, particularly when patients are well hydrated before testing.[24] Inflammatory conditions that contribute to AKI include systemic lupus erythematous, renal artery stenosis, Wegener granulomatosis, Alport syndrome, polycystic kidney disease, diabetic nephropathy, Goodpasture syndrome, multiple myeloma, nephrolithiasis, and rapidly progressive glomerulonephritis; these conditions need to be recognized.[15] In general, acute inflammatory conditions are co-treated with corticosteroids; early and appropriate administration is essential to good patient outcomes.[12,15]

Often, patients who experience AKI have preexisting conditions, such as advanced age, liver disease, diabetes, and cardiovascular disease.[12] It is not uncommon to see a patient with early-stage CKD experience AKI while hospitalized and then progress to a more serious stage of CKD; this is known as AKI on CKD. The astute primary care provider will assess the presurgical patient for CKD and risk for AKI. Recently hospitalized patients should be tested for renal function in the first 2 to 3 months after discharge to determine if kidney damage is present or if it is progressing during recovery.[27]

DIFFERENTIAL DIAGNOSIS

Renal Failure

- AKI resulting from one or more of the following:
  - Prerenal issues (hypoperfusion)
  - Intrarenal issues (glomerular and tubular inflammation, infection, and toxin exposure)
  - Postrenal issues (from obstruction of urine outflow)
- CKD

MANAGEMENT

Specialist referral: Primary care providers need to consider the timing of referral to a nephrologist. In one study it was noted that 64% of patients did not receive referral until the late stage of their disease.[28]

The 2012 KDIGO guidelines[1,4] provide suggestions for timely referral. These include:

- AKI or abrupt sustained fall in GFR
- GFR less than 30 or CKD stage 4 or 5
- Significant albuminuria (ACR greater than 300 mg/g)
- Progression of CKD defined as a decrease in any GFR category and a 25% or greater drop in GFR from baseline
- Urine red blood cells (RBCs) greater than 20 per high-power field (hpf)
- Hypertension refractory to treatment with four or more agents
- Persistent abnormalities of serum potassium or low serum albumin
- Recurrent or extensive nephrolithiasis
- Hereditary kidney disease

Urgent or emergent referrals: A diagnosis of stage 4 CKD requires an urgent referral to the nephrologist to establish patient preferences around renal replacement therapy (dialysis). Because it takes about 4 to 6 weeks for a fistula to mature sufficiently for intermittent hemodialysis, this surgical procedure, completed by a vascular surgeon, needs to be planned in advance of starting hemodialysis.

Kidney failure will require interdisciplinary management with a nephrologist. Complications for late-stage CKD or ESRD may also require an urgent referral for interdisciplinary management. For example, symptomatic hyperkalemia discovered in primary care may require an urgent request for dialysis, managed by the nephrologist. New onset or acute exacerbation of HF may require referral to a cardiologist. Box 149-1 details major complications from ESRD.

When a patient has a diagnosis of AKI, an emergent referral is made to a nephrologist for initiation of dialysis to manage the following life-threatening conditions: metabolic acidosis with a pH <7.1; refractory hyperkalemia >6.5 mEq/L; volume overload unresponsive to diuretic use (particularly when hypervolemia impairs perfusion or ventilation); uremic encephalopathy; and removal of toxins or drugs that can be removed with dialysis.[12,14] The goals of management of a patient with AKI are to reverse the causes of AKI and stop progression of kidney damage.[25]

An excellent resource for the most current recommendations for management of CKD as well as information for patients with CKD is the NKF website, www.kidney.org. The NKF publication *Making Sense of CKD: A Concise Guide for Managing Chronic Kidney Disease in the Primary Care Setting* is a summary of the most current recommendations as well as patient information sheets and guidelines for referral. The goal of management for a patient with CKD is to slow progression of disease. The following management steps reflect best practices in primary care.

Blood pressure is managed to a target of less than 140/90. Some experts suggest a lower systolic value.[26] Lifestyle modifications are essential to management and include sodium restriction and weight loss. The use of RAAS antagonists (ACE inhibitors or ARBs) is recommended for treatment of hypertension in any patient with CKD and albuminuria. These drugs should not be used concurrently, nor should they be used in patients with bilateral renal artery stenosis. Their use in CKD increases the risk of hyperkalemia. Serum potassium, BUN, and creatinine measurements are repeated 1 week after initiation of ACE inhibitor or ARB therapy. Serum potassium levels must be monitored to attain a goal of 5 mEq/L or lower. The addition of a thiazide diuretic may be useful for improved management of hypertension and to manage hyperkalemia. NSAIDs increase the risk of hyperkalemia, and patients should be advised to avoid these over-the-counter medications. If an ACE inhibitor or ARB is not tolerated, nondihydropyridine calcium channel blockers may be used an alternative.[27]

Reducing albuminuria may be accomplished by the use of RAAS antagonists; tobacco cessation may also be helpful.

Partnering with the patient who has diabetes is essential to manage both CKD and diabetes. The HbA_{1c} must be monitored; guidelines recommend maintaining a level below 7%, although this may need to be increased for older adults owing to the risk for harm from hypoglycemia.[19,28] Certain diabetic medications may need to be adjusted or eliminated in patients with CKD. Metformin, for example, is contraindicated in patients with a GFR below 60 or those older than 80.

Dietary management is essential to the overall management of CKD. Referral to a registered dietitian for medical nutritional therapy (MNT) is beneficial for optimum care, especially in patients with comorbidities of diabetes and those who are under or over ideal body weight. Medicare provides an MNT benefit for patients with CKD or diabetes at no cost and may be provided yearly. Although protein restriction is widely recommended at 0.6 to 0.8 g/kg/day, the issue of how much to restrict protein remains controversial.[1,4] To help prevent hyperkalemia, patients should be instructed to avoid potassium-containing salt substitutes. Diets low in phosphorus (0.8 to 1 g/day) have been shown to delay the progression of kidney failure, probably as a result of the prevention of deposition of phosphate and calcium in the interstitium of the kidney.[29]

Calcium-containing foods are recommended. Calcium supplements vary in amount of elemental calcium as well as in absorption. Calcium carbonate provides 40% elemental calcium but requires stomach acid for absorption. It must be taken with meals. Calcium citrate provides 21% elemental calcium and it may be taken without regard for food. Calcium acetate, recommended for patients with later stages of CKD, provides 25% elemental calcium and helps to remove phosphate. Use of aluminum or magnesium antacids as replacement for calcium should be avoided because these can cause aluminum or magnesium toxicity. It is important to monitor serum calcium levels. Serum calcium levels need to be corrected if the patient has a concomitant low serum albumin. Calcium is bound to protein, and when albumin is decreased for any reason the serum value will be lower than the actual calcium level. Tools are available to perform this calculation. If the corrected calcium level is high or low, an ionized calcium measurement should be ordered to confirm the result.

Vitamin D insufficiency is identified by measurement of 25-hydroxyvitamin D levels. Vitamin D replacement should be initiated when levels are below 30 ng/mL. Replacement can follow recommendations established for the general population; either ergocalciferol (D_2) or cholecalciferol (D_3) may be prescribed.[29]

Lipids must be controlled. Hyperlipidemia is both a complication of CKD and a potential factor in the progression of the disease.[1,19] Patency of vessels anywhere in the body is compromised by hyperlipidemia. Lowering of low-density lipoprotein (LDL) cholesterol in patients with coronary artery disease is recommended.[30] Many statins have limitations based on renal function, but atorvastatin and fluvastatin are two medications that do not require dosage based on renal function.

Anemia is a frequent complication of CKD but may have other causes. All potential causes of anemia should be explored to establish optimal treatment; iron deficiency, B_{12} or folate deficiency, and thalassemia screening tests should be completed before concluding that anemia is exclusively a result of CKD.[31] The CBC with differential is monitored at least annually in patients with stage 3 CKD without anemia and twice yearly in patients with stage 4 or 5 CKD. Additional tests for anemia evaluation conducted annually are an absolute reticulocyte count, serum ferritin level, serum transferrin saturation, and serum B_{12} and folate levels. Iron replacement therapy is often required in patients with anemia related to CKD. Replacement with iron should precede initiation of erythropoiesis-stimulating agents (ESAs) because RBC production is dependent on adequate iron and iron stores. Although treatment with ESAs may be necessary in patients with CKD, all correctable causes of anemia should be treated first. Treatment with ESAs should be considered only if hemoglobin concentrations fall below 10 g/dL and must be stopped before normal values are achieved. Judicious use of ESAs avoids RBC transfusion and improves quality of life. Decisions regarding the use of intravenous iron or ESAs should be made in conjunction with a nephrologist.[31]

Changes resulting from damage in the kidneys cause CKD-related mineral and bone disorders (CKD-MBDs), a syndrome previously called renal osteodystrophy.[29] These changes affect parathyroid hormone (PTH) and both activated and inactive forms of vitamin D. Beginning in CKD stage 3, excretion of phosphate is decreased, resulting in a need to decrease dietary phosphate. Hyperphosphatemia and hyperparathyroidism contribute to calcium removal from bones. The bone demineralization is associated with an increased incidence of atraumatic and traumatic fractures.

For a patient with ESRD, the goal is to maximize patient survival with the use of dialysis or through kidney transplantation. Optimizing function and a sense of well-being are also important goals shared by the primary care provider, and achieving these goals can occur even when the patient does not elect to manage kidney failure with dialysis or transplant.[32] Patients with ESRD are likely to be older adults who have multiple comorbid conditions.[33] The presence of a high symptom burden and the potential for early mortality among patients with ESRD suggests that primary care providers have a significant role in ensuring education about options for dialysis, establishing advance directives, and using structured shared communication with the nephrologist and other specialists to avoid or reduce complications that occur during ESRD and its treatment.[34,35] Co-management with an expert in symptom management (i.e., a specialist in palliative care) may increase quality of life and function among patients with ESRD.[32]

COMPLICATIONS

When CKD or AKI results in ESRD, complications are systemic and require significant intervention for maintenance of health. Understanding patient preferences and values can help the primary care provider communicate options for treatment, such as discussing the advantages of peritoneal dialysis or the strategies that promote adherence to a complicated medical regimen. Coaching for self-management and ongoing communication between the primary care and specialist provider (e.g., nephrologist, cardiologist, or vascular surgeon) are also valuable to achieving goals of care. The current mortality rate for U.S. patients with ESRD is more than 20% per year, and the primary care provider can lead a discussion about end-of-life care after a diagnosis of ESRD.

Cardiovascular Management and Complications

Cardiovascular complications are the leading cause of death among patients with kidney failure (ESRD), accounting for more than 50% of deaths in the first year of dialysis.[1] Prevention of cardiovascular complications is therefore of the utmost priority in primary care, and management or co-management of cardiovascular disease falls within the primary care provider's scope of practice. Hypertension and hyperlipidemia should be aggressively managed.[27] Unfortunately, 70% of patients who begin dialysis treatment already have left ventricular hypertrophy and 40% have chronic HF.[17] Pulmonary edema and acute exacerbation of HF are major concerns in ESRD. If the patient is unstable, hospitalization and urgent dialysis may be necessary. All episodes of HF and pulmonary edema should be reported to the renal specialist so that adjustments can be made in the dialysate fluid to compensate for fluid overload.

Dietary Management and Metabolic Complications

Dietary management should be aimed at balancing electrolytes (including calcium, phosphorus, and potassium), preventing malnutrition, and maintaining fluid volume balance.[23] Daily dietary requirements for patients with ESRD depend on the type of dialysis chosen (continuous ambulatory peritoneal dialysis [CAPD] versus hemodialysis). All patients with ESRD should be referred to a dietitian for optimization of nutritional status.

Hematologic Management and Complications

The anemia of CKD, if untreated, leads to significant functional decline, including cardiac damage and cognitive impairment. The options to treat CKD-related anemia are transfusion of RBCs, and ESAs. ESAs given subcutaneously are more effectively absorbed than ESAs given intravenously or into extracorporeal blood during hemodialysis. Bleeding risk increases with uremia from impaired platelet function. In the presence of concerning hemorrhage, administration of coagulation factors (e.g., cryoprecipitate) may help, and emergent dialysis will reduce uremia. Patients with CKD are at increased risk for infection, and careful attention should be paid to preventive measures, including vaccination with influenza, pneumococcal, and hepatitis B vaccines.

Psychosocial Management and Complications

The stress of dealing with severe chronic illness can be psychologically devastating. Patients with ESRD (especially patients on hemodialysis) are known to have high rates of depression, insomnia, and anxiety.[34] Often ignored, sexual dysfunction occurs at high rates in both male and female patients with ESRD. The treatment of these and other psychosocial complications should begin before the onset of ESRD.

INDICATIONS FOR REFERRAL OR HOSPITALIZATION

Potential problems associated with AKI, CKD, or ESRD that necessitate referral are innumerable. Referrals should be considered if the patient is experiencing cardiovascular, pulmonary, bone-mineral derangement, or psychiatric problems or complications that do not respond to first-line treatments. A referral to a palliative care specialist to manage distressing symptoms that affect function or quality of life may be considered.

Hospitalization should be considered for any acute, life-threatening disorder and new-onset encephalopathy. Patients with the following conditions should be considered for hospitalization:

- Symptomatic acute fluid and electrolyte derangements (see Chapters 208 to 210).
- Acute hypotensive or hypertensive emergency regardless of cause.
- Pulmonary edema or pleural effusion resulting a peripheral oxygenation (SpO_2) below 92% or, if chronically hypoxemic, below 88%, particularly if there is a decrease in consciousness or cognition that cannot be improved with the administration of oxygen at less than 5 L by nasal cannula.
- Acute exacerbation of HF or pericarditis that compromises mean arterial pressure, systolic blood pressure, or ventilation.
- Metabolic acidosis (or large anion gap on basic metabolic panel) that contributes to new-onset encephalopathy and requires emergent dialysis.
- Symptoms of systemic inflammatory response or sepsis.

LIFE SPAN CONSIDERATIONS

Age increases the risk for AKI and CKD. GFR declines by about 5% each decade after age 40 years. Note that a decline in GFR alone is not diagnostic of CKD without the presence of other markers, particularly in older adults. All individuals with CKD should undergo screening for the complications of renal disease to prevent morbidity and to establish a credible baseline for the individual.

PATIENT AND FAMILY EDUCATION

Patient education related to a diagnosis of AKI, CKD, or ESRD is highly complex. CKD and ESRD require carefully coordinated care. Numerous resources to support patient and family education along the trajectory of kidney disease are available at www.kidney.org or via phone at 1-855-NKF-CARES (1-855-653-2273). At this site, patients can access a food coach and receive help with insurance coverage and medication costs as well as information about clinical trials, transplant, and dialysis. There is a special link on the site for older adults with information specific to their unique needs. Guiding patients and family members to appropriate Internet and social media sites is part of essential patient and family education. By gradually introducing different educational materials and prompting self-management to help control the course of the kidney disease, the primary care provider can help restore a sense of independence and confidence in the patient.

CHAPTER 150

SEXUAL DYSFUNCTION (MALE)

Patricia Polgar-Bailey

DEFINITION AND EPIDEMIOLOGY

Sexuality is a fundamental aspect of human identity and an important determinant of one's quality of life. Sexual dysfunction can lead to sexual frustration, guilt, loss of self-esteem, and interpersonal problems. It often results in a change in partner relationships and dynamics, decreased sexual intimacy, and reduced quality of life. Despite the high prevalence of male sexual dysfunction worldwide, and an even higher incidence among certain populations—such as those with neurologic, endocrine, and other comorbidities; those with combat-related mental health disorders; and cancer survivors[1-4]—concerns about sexual health are often not elicited by providers owing to a lack of appreciation of the impact of sexual dysfunction or fear of patient embarrassment.

Men with sexual dysfunction are often embarrassed about discussing their problem openly with health care providers. In addition, many men associate declining sexual function with aging and do not appreciate that this is a problem for which there is treatment. In addition, men are generally less likely to seek medical care than women, and men's heath as a concept and discipline is not nearly as well developed as women's health. However, men are more inclined to see a provider for problems that specifically affect men most such as baldness, sports injuries, and erectile dysfunction (ED).[5] ED, the most common sexual problem in men, often causes serious distress and prompts men to seek care when they otherwise might not.[6] In addition, the aging population, the increase in available therapies, and the publicity regarding new pharmacologic agents for the treatment of ED have increased the awareness of the scope of this problem and resulted in an increased number of men seeking treatment. Incorporation of an understanding of male sexual health and available treatment options can have a tremendous impact on the sexual health and quality of life of men affected by sexual dysfunction.

Sexual dysfunction is broadly defined as the difficulty or inability to fully enjoy sexual intercourse and more specifically includes disorders that interfere with a full sexual response cycle. The human sexual response can be described as a cycle with four phases: desire, excitement, orgasm, and resolution. Sexual dysfunction affects one or more of the first three phases. Resolution is simply the relaxation and reduction in arousal after orgasm. Resolution to the preexcitement phase occurs more rapidly with age, although this is most noticeable in older men. The amount of time that must pass before a man is capable of another ejaculation increases as men age.

The desire phase of the cycle consists of an urge to have sex, sexual fantasies, and sexual attraction to others. Hypoactive sexual desire is a lack of interest in sex or sexual activity, although the actual sexual experience may be normal. The perception or stereotype of men in our culture is that they want sex as often as they can get it; however, hypoactive sexual desire affects as many as 16% of men, and the number of men seeking treatment for it has increased during the past decade.[7] There is an important distinction between people who have normal sexual desires but choose as part of their lifestyle not to engage in sexual relations and people with hypoactive sexual desire. Hypoactive sexual desire is also different from sexual aversion, which refers to people who find sex distinctly unpleasant or repulsive.

The excitement phase of the sexual response cycle is marked by physical changes of arousal: increases in heart rate, blood pressure, rate of breathing, and muscle tension. ED affects the excitement phase. ED is the persistent inability to achieve and to maintain an erection sufficient to permit satisfactory sexual performance. Since the National Institutes of Health Consensus Conference in 1988, the term *erectile dysfunction* has replaced the term *impotence*. ED is now recognized as a medical problem with potential psychological consequences that may interfere with a man's quality of life, self-esteem, and interpersonal relationships.

Based on data from the National Health and Social Life Survey (NHSLS), the prevalence of sexual dysfunction in males is approximately 31%. Some degree of ED, the most common male sexual problem,[8] was reported by 52% of respondents in the Massachusetts Male Aging Study (MMAS),[5,9] a large epidemiologic study by as many as 65.6% in a Brazilian study, and almost 60% in a Ghanian study.[1] It is estimated that globally more than 150 men are affected by ED, and this number will likely double by 2025. After adjustment for age, men with certain comorbidities, including diabetes, heart disease, and hypertension, have significantly higher probabilities for ED than men as a whole.

During the orgasmic phase of the sexual response cycle, an individual's sexual pleasure peaks, sexual tension is released, and the man's semen is ejaculated. Male sexual dysfunctions during this phase include premature ejaculation (PE) and male orgasmic disorder. In 2013 the International Society for Sexual Medicine (ISSM) developed the first evidence-based definition for PE: "a male sexual dysfunction characterized by: (1) ejaculation that always or nearly always occurs prior to or within about

1 minutes of vaginal penetration (lifelong PE) or a clinically significant and bothersome reduction in latency time, often to about 3 minutes or less (acquired PE); (2) the inability to delay ejaculation on all or nearly all vaginal penetrations; and (3) negative personal consequences, such as distress, bother, frustration, and/or avoidance of sexual intimacy."[10] Although previous definitions of PE included some of these dimensions, there was need for an evidence-based definition; a more accurate definition was necessary for diagnosis and treatment selection and to improve research design.[10] The previous lack of a standardized definition for PE has resulted in conflicting prevalence rates for PE. A study by Serefoglu and colleagues reported an overall PE prevalence of approximately 19.8%.[11] A study by Gao and colleagues reported a prevalence of 25.8% among Chinese men.[12] Data from both studies suggested that the prevalence of acquired PE in the community is approximately 4% among sexually active adults and that men with acquired PE are more likely to seek treatment than men with lifelong PE.[10] The reasons for this difference are unclear, but it has been hypothesized that men with lifelong PE may have accommodated to their rapid ejaculation, whereas those with acquired PE may be bothered to the point of seeking treatment.[10] It is estimated that approximately 30% to 50% of men with PE have concurrent ED, which typically results in early ejaculation with an incomplete erection.[13,14] Men with ED may required higher levels of stimulation to achieve an erection or may intentionally "rush" intercourse to prevent the early detumescence of a partial erection, resulting in PE.[10]

The cause of PE is not completely understood, but PE appears most commonly to result from performance anxiety, inexperience, hurried masturbation experiences, relationship factors, or psychological issues. Although less frequent, it may also be caused by prostatitis, hyperthyroidism, and withdrawal or detoxification from prescribed or recreational drugs.[10] Men with acquired PE have a higher incidence of concomitant ED and other comorbidities, including hypertension, diabetes mellitus, and chronic prostatitis, than men with lifelong PE.[10]

Men are often hesitant to discuss sexual problems with their providers and in general consult them for health-related problems less frequently than women do. In addition, the emphasis in health care visits, particularly for men, tends to be on cardiovascular diseases and other common chronic illnesses, such as hypertension and diabetes, whereas conditions that may be of a more sensitive nature are ignored, thereby reducing the opportunity for the recognition and treatment of problems that substantially affect the quality of life.[15] Research shows that health care providers do not regularly ask about sexual dysfunction with men who are at risk, citing as reasons a lack of time and the belief that the patient will initiate the discussion.[16] Reluctance to discuss ED on the part of both the patient and the health care provider results in underdiagnosis and lack of treatment. The partner in a relationship significantly influences a man's health-seeking behavior. Men who do not have a supportive partner or who feel particularly vulnerable or fearful or are in denial are less likely to seek help for issues related to sexual dysfunction.[15]

Although sexual dysfunction affects a sizable portion of the male population, a lack of discussion of the condition prevents a significant number of affected men from receiving treatment. Health care providers have become well versed in asking questions about patients' sexual practices in screening for sexually transmitted diseases (STDs) and human immunodeficiency virus (HIV) infection but are less experienced and more uncomfortable when it comes to investigating sexual satisfaction among patients and their partners.[16] It is important for health care providers to include sexual assessment as a component of routine health care surveillance and to become comfortable in eliciting the information that will help identify sexual dysfunction, give insight into its cause, and guide further intervention. It is also important to remember that ED is often a sentinel or early marker for concomitant cardiovascular disease, as well as a risk factor for metabolic comorbidities. Research indicates that men with ED are at significantly greater risk of having a cardiovascular event—angina, myocardial infarction (MI), or stroke—than those without ED.[5] In addition, the relationship between "incident ED" (the first report of ED of any grade) and cardiovascular disease is comparable to that associated with current smoking, family history of MI, and hyperlipidemia.[5] The meaning of this relationship appears to vary depending on age. When ED occurs in a younger man (age below 60) it is associated with a marked increase in future cardiovascular events, whereas in older men it appears to be less of a prognostic indicator.[5]

Eliciting information about sexual health is essential for a thorough assessment of health. In particular, ED can be viewed as a "barometer" of cardiovascular health, and its identification can provide an opportunity to identify and treat modifiable risk factors.[5] Health care providers are in a unique position to address sexual and relationship issues that exist between their patients and their partners. In addition to representing more holistic care, discussing and addressing sexual health concerns may uncover underlying comorbid conditions, improve quality of life and self-esteem, foster a better patient-provider relationship, and increase patient satisfaction.

PATHOPHYSIOLOGY

Disorders of Desire

The etiology of disorders of desire or reduced libido is multifactorial and involves a combination of biologic, psychological, and sociocultural factors. Several hormones combine to produce sexual desire, and lower levels of them can lower the sex drive. In men and women, sexual desire is linked to levels of androgen, testosterone, and dehydroepiandrosterone (DHEA). In men, testosterone levels peak at 19 years of age and demonstrate a linear decline of 1% per year thereafter.[17] DHEA levels begin to decline in the 30s and continue to decline steadily until a low is reached by the age of 60 years.[18] Because a decrease in male hormones begins early, it is suggested that screening for hypogonadism should begin at 50 years of age.[17] Chronic physical illness as well as stress, pain, or depression related to the illness directly affects the desire to have sex. The sex drive can also be lowered by some pain medications, certain psychotropic drugs, and a number of illegal drugs, such as cocaine, marijuana, and amphetamines. In addition, low levels of alcohol can enhance the sex drive by reducing inhibitions; but at high levels, alcohol can reduce sex drive. Circumstances and social pressures such as job stress, marital discord and divorce, death in the family, and infertility difficulties can affect one's desire to have sex.

Disorders of Excitement

Erectile function is a neurovascular event initiated by cognitive or tactile stimulation that is processed in the brain. Chemical mediators cause the essential relaxation of tissue and perfusion of the corpora cavernosa and corpus spongiosum. Nitric oxide and cyclic guanosine monophosphate (cGMP) are the primary noncholinergic and cholinergic mediators responsible for the neurogenic aspect of erection. Engorgement of the corpora cavernosa and corpus spongiosum, in turn, compresses the veins to prevent the venous outflow of blood. This is how the erection is maintained and accounts for the vascular component of erection. Any factor that interferes with this process may lead to ED.

The cause of ED may be clearly identified (e.g., a radical prostatectomy) or may be multifactorial, requiring comprehensive assessment. Although ED was believed in the past to be psychogenic, it is now understood to result from organic causes (e.g., vascular, neurogenic, hormonal, anatomic, or drug induced), psychological causes, or a combination of the two. A normal sexual erectile response is a complex interaction among neurotransmitter, biochemical, and vascular smooth muscle responses initiated by parasympathetic and sympathetic neuronal triggers that integrate physiologic stimuli and sexual desire.[6] Alterations in vascular supply, hormonal changes, neurologic dysfunction, or medications and associated systemic disease may contribute to or exacerbate ED. A list of common organic and psychological risk factors for ED can be found in Box 150-1.

BOX 150-1

Common Risk Factors for ED

NEUROLOGIC CONDITIONS
- Multiple sclerosis
- Peripheral neuropathy
- Radical prostatectomy
- Spinal cord injury
- Stroke
- Parkinson disease

CARDIOVASCULAR CONDITIONS
- Cardiovascular or peripheral vascular disease
- Congestive heart failure
- Hypertension
- Hyperlipidemia
- Cigarette smoking

TRAUMATIC INJURY OR PENILE ABNORMALITIES
- Trauma to perineum, pelvis, penis
- Peyronie disease (penile curvature)
- History of priapism
- History of penile fracture

RADIATION THERAPY
- Pelvic irradiation for malignant conditions

HORMONAL CAUSES
- Decreased testosterone
- Increased prolactin
- Increased luteinizing hormone
- Increased prostate-specific antigen

ENDOCRINE DISORDERS
- Diabetes mellitus
- Hypothyroidism
- Hyperthyroidism
- Pituitary adenoma
- Hypogonadism
- Obesity

PSYCHOGENIC FACTORS
- Performance anxiety
- Depression
- Psychological stress
- Relationship problems

MEDICAL CONDITIONS
- Chronic disease states
- Multiple sclerosis
- Renal failure
- Diabetes mellitus
- Sleep apnea

MEDICATIONS
- See Box 150-2

Psychogenic. Psychological factors that may be of etiologic significance include performance anxiety, guilt, and strict religious constraints. Life events, such as a business failure, loss of health, or deterioration in the partner relationship, may also contribute to ED because of their impact on mood, anxiety, self-esteem, and depression. Developmental vulnerabilities, such as a history of child abuse, may have a profound effect on sexual function. Psychological issues, when combined with physiologic problems, can result in significant erectile difficulties.

Hormonal Risk Factors. Testosterone deficiency may be caused by hypothalamic or pituitary tumors or treatment aimed at suppression of testosterone, such as hormonal therapy for prostate cancer. Although the primary effect of testosterone deficiency is decreased libido, ED may result as well. Other conditions that may precipitate decreased libido or ED because of their hormonal effects include hyperprolactinemia, hyperthyroidism, hypothyroidism, Cushing syndrome, and Addison disease.

Cardiovascular Risk Factors. Cardiovascular disorders that affect the penile vasculature can affect different stages of erection, including a failure to initiate erection, a failure to achieve erection, and a failure to sustain erection.

Pharmacologic Risk Factors. The major classes of drugs that affect erectile function include antihypertensives, antidepressants, and major tranquilizers. ED may result from pharmacologic effects on the central nervous system, vascular system, hormone levels, and libido (see Box 150-2). Other medications that have been associated with ED include hormonal agents (e.g., antiandrogens), protease inhibitors, antihistamines, benzodiazepines, selective serotonin reuptake inhibitors (SSRIs), and cytotoxic agents.[6]

Surgical Risk Factors. ED may occur after major surgery that potentially alters either the innervation of or the blood flow to the penis. These procedures may also affect a man's body image and self-perception of masculinity. Examples of such procedures are the radical prostatectomy, radical cystectomy, and abdominal-perineal resection. Nerve-sparing surgical techniques minimize this risk and may result in the preservation of erectile function.

Other Factors. Pelvic radiotherapy (e.g., to treat prostate cancer) may damage nerves and blood vessels, potentially resulting in ED.

Disorders of Orgasm

Male orgasmic disorders (i.e., problems with ejaculation) can be caused by low testosterone levels, certain neurologic diseases, and some head and spinal cord injuries. Certain drugs, including hypertensive medications, antidepressants, anxiolytics, antipsychotics, and alcohol, can slow down the sympathetic nervous system and can also affect ejaculation. An important psychological cause of male orgasmic disorder seems to be performance anxiety and the spectator role. If a man focuses on reaching orgasm, he stops being an aroused participant and instead has a tendency to be a self-critical and fearful observer.

CLINICAL PRESENTATION

Men may not readily offer information about sexual dysfunction, even though it may be the reason for the visit. Because men often avoid routine visits and are known to underuse primary care in general, the provider could suspect that a man with

BOX 150-2

Pharmacologic Agents Implicated in the Development of ED

CARDIOVASCULAR AGENTS

- Angiotensin-converting enzyme inhibitors
- Beta blockers
- Calcium antagonists
- Centrally acting agents
- Antiarrhythmics

PSYCHOGENIC AGENTS

- Anxiolytics
- Hypnotics
- Selective serotonin reuptake inhibitors (SSRIs)
- Serotonin-norepinephrine reuptake inhibitors (SNRIs)
- Tricyclic antidepressants
- Antipsychotics, mood stabilizers

NEUROLOGIC AGENTS

- Anticonvulsants (phenytoin [Dilantin], phenobarbital)
- Antiparkinson agents (bromocriptine [Parlodel], levodopa, trihexyphenidyl)

OTHER PHARMACOLOGIC AGENTS

- Analgesics (e.g., opiates)
- Anticholinergics
- Antihistamines (diphenhydramine [Benadryl], hydroxyzine [Vistaril], meclizine [Antivert], promethazine [Phenergan])
- Cytotoxic agents (methotrexate)
- Diuretics (spironolactone, thiazides)
- Immunomodulators (interferon alfa)
- Miscellaneous: clofibrate, dichlorphenamide, fenfluramine, ketoconazole, methadone, metoclopramide, methazolamide, norethindrone, thiabendazole
- Recreational and illicit drugs (amphetamines, cocaine, marijuana, heroin), alcohol, nicotine

vague somatic complaints might actually be in the office because of concerns about sexual dysfunction. The interactions between the provider and patient are vital in establishing rapport, and the patient's anticipation of the discussion or concern about bringing up the issue may be the source of considerable anxiety or stress. Thus, sensitively introducing the subject of sexual health may help create a more comfortable atmosphere and facilitate discussion.

Providers should obtain a broad history, which includes not only sexual concerns but also relationships and life events. Open-ended questions help elucidate the onset of concerns, course over time, and factors that may improve or worsen symptoms. It is helpful to start by asking general questions about sexual activity and interest and then relate this to healthy "masculine" intimacy, rather than by directly asking questions about sexual function. It is important to keep in mind the impact that physical, psychological, and relationship issues can have on sexual health. Compassionate and normalizing statements can be helpful, such as "It is common for men who have had prostate cancer to notice changes in their interest in sexual activity."

In obtaining a history from the patient or partner, the provider may find it useful to identify three types of factors that can contribute to sexual dysfunction: predisposing factors (e.g., restrictive upbringing, disturbed relationships, traumatic sexual experiences), which might make a man more susceptible to sexual dysfunction; precipitating factors (e.g., dysfunction in the partner, discord in the relationship, depression or anxiety, comorbid medical conditions), which may have triggered the onset of the problem; and maintaining factors (e.g., performance anxiety, relationship issues, impaired self-image, poor communication), which sustain the problem.

Specific inquiries about ED should include questions that address the onset of ED (gradual or abrupt), whether there is difficulty in achieving or maintaining an erection, and the presence and quality of nocturnal erections. In addition, the onset of ED, particularly if it is associated with a specific event (e.g., stress), should be determined. Additional information to elicit includes quality and timing of the orgasm, volume and appearance of the ejaculate, presence of sexually induced genital pain or penile curvature (Peyronie disease), and partner sexual function.[6] A brief urologic questionnaire, such as the five-item version of the International Index of Erectile Function Questionnaire is a validated survey instrument that can be used to assess the nature and severity of ED.[6,19] The clinical history should include current health problems, a review of systems, and current medications including nonprescription drugs and herbal formulations. Cardiovascular risk stratification is an essential component of the evaluation of ED because of the increased incidence of cardiovascular disease. Questions about exercise tolerance, history of cardiovascular disease, and past and current medication use are important. Men with risk factors for cardiovascular disease should undergo further evaluation and management before treatment of ED is initiated.[9]

In eliciting information about sexual health, the provider also must consider generational issues. The sexual behaviors and interests of aging "baby boomers" are now beginning to emerge through surveys, such as those conducted by AARP. For example, baby boomers appear to hold traditional values about extramarital relationships but are more willing than former generations to experiment with new activities, such as watching pornography with their partners and trying new sexual positions.[15] Another issue to consider is the growing population of divorced and single adults who engage in sexual relationships and may be at risk for STDs, including HIV infection.[15] Relationship issues are a major factor in the decline of sexual activity among older adults.

Relatively little research has been done on the needs and interests of sexual minority patients, but it is important to consider that homosexual men may be reluctant to disclose their sexual orientation or to discuss sexuality because of the negative associations with being gay. Transgender health and the use of cross-sex hormones (estrogens in male-bodied people and androgens in female-bodied people) is increasing around the world, and health care providers must educate themselves to adequately care for these individuals in the primary care setting. Maintaining a nonjudgmental and accepting attitude can increase the comfort level of a patient who finds it difficult to discuss issues related to sexual identity.

PHYSICAL EXAMINATION

The history will guide the physical examination, which, if indicated, also focuses on detecting signs of endocrine, vascular, or neurologic deficits and penile abnormality. Testicular atrophy, gynecomastia, or signs of hypothyroidism or hyperthyroidism may indicate hormonal abnormalities. Vascular assessment includes checking pulses in the lower extremities and observing for vascular skin changes in the lower extremities (e.g., hair loss). The presence of a femoral bruit may indicate possible pelvic blood occlusion. Neurologic assessment is focused on testing for genital reflexes (bulbocavernosus, cremasteric, scrotal, sphincter tone) and light touch discrimination. During the genital examination, it is important to palpate for penile plaques, which may indicate Peyronie disease. Plaques in the tunica albuginea limit penile distensibility, causing a bend in the penis with erection. This may interfere with sexual activity by making penetration difficult.

Although approximately 75% of patients with ED have an organic cause (resulting from vascular, neuronal, or endocrine factors), psychosocial, cognitive, and interpersonal variables, often related to illness or disease, play a role in exacerbating or maintaining ED. Assessment of these issues is essential in the evaluation of ED and other types of sexual dysfunction.

DIAGNOSTICS

The history and physical examination will determine which diagnostic and laboratory tests are indicated. Detection of underlying medical problems is essential in the evaluation of sexual dysfunction, and appropriate diagnostic testing is indicated. There is no preferred first-line diagnostic test for ED, and routine screening is not recommended. History and physical examination are sufficient to make an accurate diagnosis in most cases.[5,20]

The American Urological Association (AUA) and the World Health Organization (WHO) recommend limited diagnostic testing for men with ED.[5] Initially, nocturnal penile tumescence is evaluated to determine whether ED is attributable to a psychogenic or organic condition. The snap gauge, a Velcro band with three colored films arranged parallel to one another, is fitted around the penis. Each film ruptures to correspond with the intracavernosal pressures found in erection. Response is gauged by the number of films broken, with none or one indicating absent rigidity and two or three indicating rigid erection. The accuracy of snap gauge results is variable.

The RigiScan (Dacomed Corporation, Minneapolis) is a more sophisticated device that provides continuous tumescence monitoring and can distinguish functional from inadequate erections in the majority of cases.[1]

Studies to evaluate penile vasculature include the intracavernosal injection of a vasoactive drug, duplex Doppler study of the penis, dynamic infusion cavernosometry and cavernosography (DICC), and internal pudendal arteriography. These tests can evaluate for anatomic abnormalities such as Peyronie disease and measure both penile inflow and outflow.[1] Neurologic studies include bulbocavernous reflex latency and nerve conduction studies.

In the absence of a reliable test, the clinician must rely on the patient's history, physical examination, and laboratory testing to determine the cause of ED. Laboratory tests include thyroid-stimulating hormone (TSH) and luteinizing hormone concentrations; serum electrolyte values; serum glucose, blood urea nitrogen (BUN), creatinine, serum testosterone, and prolactin levels; and lipid panel. Serum testosterone to detect hypogonadism maybe useful, especially in older men because the disorder is common in this population.

DIAGNOSTICS

Erectile Dysfunction

LABORATORY

Complete blood count and differential
Fasting serum glucose or hemoglobin A_{1c} (HbA_{1c})
Serum electrolytes
BUN and creatinine
Lipid profile
TSH
Prostate-specific antigen
Prolactin
Morning total serum testosterone level
Luteinizing hormone

OTHER DIAGNOSTICS

As indicated (see Diagnostics section)

DIFFERENTIAL DIAGNOSIS

See differential diagnosis box.

DIFFERENTIAL DIAGNOSIS

Erectile Dysfunction

- Decreased libido
- Anorgasmia
- Ejaculatory dysfunction

MANAGEMENT

Research supports a multidisciplinary approach to the treatment of sexual dysfunction. Health care providers need to determine their own comfort level with discussions about sexuality and sexual dysfunction. In addition, health care providers need to determine whether the patient's major issues are psychogenic, relational, or organic (often all three are involved) and whether referral to a psychologist, marriage counselor, or sex therapist might be helpful. Relationship counseling (or referral) may be appropriate to help the patient and partner with any emotional and communication barriers to sexual success. Effective communication is essential, and the provider can recommend some excellent self-help books and videos.

Anxiety reduction techniques have been a prominent part of psychological approaches for sexual dysfunction. These techniques are based on the principle that by removal of the source of the anxiety (e.g., by forbidding intercourse and permitting only nondemand caressing), men can overcome performance anxiety and inhibitions. Providers can help alleviate the anxiety by encouraging sensuality, extended foreplay, and a focus on pleasure rather than arousal. It is important to remind the persons involved that treatment often takes time to be fully effective and to be comfortably integrated into their sex lives.[15]

Cognitive restructuring techniques can be used to overcome sexual ignorance and to challenge unrealistic expectations that couples may have about sexuality. Sexual dysfunction, such as ED, and associated anxiety can sometimes lead to the cessation of all sexual activity. In these situations, couples can be coached to give and to receive pleasure in other ways, such as manual or oral stimulation. Increased stimulation may also be necessary for the male partner to achieve an erection and thus can augment pharmacologic therapy.[15]

An important first step in management is to determine where in the sexual response cycle the problem lies. For example, loss of sexual desire can be the result of life stressors, which may begin or worsen at midlife and can subsequently result in feelings of failure and low self-esteem. Testosterone replacement therapy (TRT) has been shown to improve libido in older men with low testosterone levels; however, the role of testosterone in the physiology of erections is unclear. Thus, TRT for the treatment of ED and androgen deficiency is controversial. There is an FDA warning regarding the potential for cardiovascular or cerebrovascular events related to TRT.[22] TRT may increase prostate size and cause lower urinary tract symptoms, but a causal relationship between testosterone supplementation and prostate cancer has not been demonstrated.[20]

The primary goal in the management of ED is to determine its cause and treat it when possible, rather than treating the symptom alone. ED may be associated with modifiable and reversible risk factors, including lifestyle and drug-related issues. Addressing these factors can be done before or concurrently with other specific therapies.[1] As a rule, ED can be treated successfully with current treatment options but cannot be cured. The exceptions to this are psychogenic ED, post-traumatic arteriogenic ED in young men, and ED from hormonal causes, which may resolve with specific treatment.[1] Most ED therapy is not cause specific, but rather follows a structured treatment strategy that depends on a number of factors including efficacy, safety, invasiveness, cost, and patient preference.[1]

For ED with concomitant risk factors, lifestyle changes and risk factor modification should precede or accompany any pharmacologic therapy. The potential benefits of lifestyle modification are particularly apparent in men with specific comorbidities, such as cardiovascular or metabolic disorders (e.g., diabetes and hypertension). In such situations, lifestyle changes have the potential to improve not just ED and cardiovascular and metabolic health, but also overall health.[1]

Psychotherapy is the preferred treatment for psychogenic ED. Sexual counseling can enhance communication, ease some of the stress associated with ED, and dispel myths. For instance, men may not realize that they do not have to have an erection to have an orgasm and may believe intercourse to be their only means of sexual expression. In mixed psychogenic and organic ED, psychotherapy may relieve anxieties and increase the success of medical or surgical intervention.

Oral phosphodiesterase type 5 (PDE5) inhibitors are a class of medications that facilitate erection by enhancing the effects of nitric oxide and blocking the degradation of cGMP. Inhibition of PDE5 results in smooth muscle relaxation with associated increased arterial flow, which leads to compression of the subtunical venous plexus and penile erection.[1] These medications do not initiate an erection, and sexual stimulation is required for an erection to occur. They are the first-line pharmacotherapy for ED in patients with no contraindications to their use. Currently, four PDE5 inhibitors are available in the United States: sildenafil (Viagra), vardenafil (Levitra), tadalafil (Cialis), and avanafil (Stendra).[20,21] They are similar in their action and efficacy. Common to all four drugs is the need for sexual stimulation to effect the release of nitric oxide. Evidence has shown the PDE5 inhibitors to be effective in a wide range of patients with ED. They are not the preferred option for men with neurogenic ED and are absolutely contraindicated in patients who are taking nitrates secondary to increased vasodilation with concomitant use (Table 150-1).

Although PDE5 inhibitors have a similar mechanism of action, there are significant differences among the agents in terms of pharmacokinetics; the ones that most directly affect patient preference are onset and duration of action. Sildenafil, vardenafil, and avanafil have a rapid onset of action and remain effective for a short time. In addition, sildenafil and vardenafil are more effective if they are taken on an empty stomach; eating of a high-fat meal before either drug is taken reduces the peak plasma concentration. Avanafil is rapidly absorbed (within 30

TABLE 150-1 Phosphodiesterase Type 5 Inhibitors

Drug	Sildenafil (Viagra)	Vardenafil (Levitra)	Tadalafil (Cialis)	Avanafil (Stendra)
Dose	25-100 mg on an empty stomach Starting dose is 50 mg	5-20 mg	5-20 mg 2.5 or 5 mg for once-daily use	100-200 mg about 30 min before sexual intercourse
Peak time	1 hr	42-54 min	2 hr	30-45 min
Excretion	8-12 hr	8-12 hr	36 hr	5 hr
Contraindications	Nitrates Resting blood pressure <90/50 or >170/110 mm Hg Cardiac failure Unstable angina Retinitis pigmentosa (applies to all PDE5 inhibitors) Caution with alpha blockers	Nitrates Same as sildenafil Associated with minor QT interval prolongation Those taking class I or class II antiarrhythmics Caution with alpha blockers	Nitrates Same as sildenafil Caution with alpha blockers other than tamsulosin (Flomax)	Nitrates Same as sildenafil Caution with alpha blockers Caution with concomitant use of CYP3A4 inhibitors
Adverse side effects	Headache Flushing Nasal congestion Abnormal vision Dyspepsia Hearing loss	Headache Flushing Nasal congestion Abnormal vision Dyspepsia Hearing loss	Headache Flushing Nasal congestion Abnormal vision Dyspepsia Back pain Myalgias	Headache Flushing Nasal congestion Sore throat Abnormal vision Dyspepsia Back pain

to 45 minutes), and food does not appear to delay or decrease drug absorption.[9,21] Tadalafil has a longer median half-life than the other two drugs, resulting in a period of responsiveness of 24 to 36 hours. The Food and Drug Administration approved the use of once-daily tadalafil at doses of 2.5 to 5 mg for men who anticipate more frequent sexual activity.[20] In addition, neither the consumption of a high-fat meal nor the timing of administration (morning or evening) has an effect on changes in plasma concentration or time to maximum response.

By facilitating a sexual response, PDE5 inhibitors may help couples return to a more satisfying sexual lifestyle. However, even with these agents, other underlying or unresolved issues may require counseling or other types of psychological interventions.

Second-line therapies for the treatment of ED include intraurethral suppositories, intracavernous injections, and vacuum pump devices. Alprostadil (prostaglandin E_1) is indicated for the treatment of ED related to angiogenic, neurogenic, psychogenic, or mixed causes. Alprostadil is available as a urethral suppository (Muse) or as a solution for intracavernosal injection (Caverject, Edex).[1] The dose is highly individualized, which requires the patient to receive a test dose in the clinical setting. For this reason, patients wishing to pursue this option are usually referred to a urologist. Efficacy rates for intracavernous alprostadil in the treatment of ED overall appear to be greater than 70%, with similar rates in certain patient subgroups such as those with diabetes or cardiovascular disease.[1] Reported satisfaction rates appear to be quite high for both patients (87.5% to 93%) and partners (86% to 90%). Complications of intracavernous alprostadil include penile pain, prolonged erections (5%), priapism (1%), and fibrosis (2%). Pain is usually self-limited after prolonged use and can be alleviated by the addition of sodium bicarbonate or local anesthesia. Contraindications to its use include men with a hypersensitivity to alprostadil, those at risk for priapism, and those with a history of bleeding disorders.[1]

For men whose only difficulty is maintaining an erection, a constriction band (e.g., Actis venous flow controller) applied at the base of the penis after erection is achieved may be all that is needed. Vacuum devices are associated with an 80% to 90% success rate and are among the least invasive and least expensive of the current treatment options. They produce an erection by creating a vacuum around the penis that triggers passive blood flow into the corpora cavernosa. Erection is then maintained by a constriction band applied at the base of the penis. A certain amount of manual dexterity is required to use these devices, but once men become comfortable with their use, many men can create an erection sufficient for vaginal penetration and intercourse.

Sexual dysfunction is a common side effect of some antidepressant medications, particularly SSRIs and other antidepressants such as venlafaxine (Effexor), a serotonin-norepinephrine reuptake inhibitor (SNRI), and clomipramine (Anafranil), a tricyclic, and is a common reason for discontinuation.[23] In one study, patients taking bupropion sustained release (Wellbutrin SR) in addition to their existing SSRI antidepressant reported an increase in the desire to engage in sexual activity and the frequency of sexual activity compared with a group taking placebo.[24] Although the combination of bupropion and an SSRI resulted in a few adverse side effects, including irritability, dry mouth, and headache, the authors of the study concluded that "improvements in sexual function and residual depressive symptoms when bupropion SR is added to an SSRI may improve quality of life in patients with SSRI-induced sexual dysfunction."[3]

Hormonal imbalance, such as low levels of testosterone or high levels of prolactin, is a less common cause of ED. Testosterone replacement is available by injection or transdermal patch with the goal of keeping the serum testosterone level within normal limits.

Surgical management includes vascular surgery or implantation of a penile prosthesis. The goal of vascular surgery is to increase arterial inflow to the corpora cavernosa and to increase venous outflow resistance. Candidates are selected only after careful vascular examination, measurement of intracavernous pressures, and observation of the patient's response to certain pharmacologic agents. Younger men with discrete lesions, usually sustained from pelvic or perineal trauma, seem to be the best candidates for vascular surgery.

Placement of a penile prosthesis remains the third-line treatment of ED and is a therapeutic option for individuals in whom first- and second-line therapies have failed and those who cannot tolerate these therapies. Penile prostheses may be malleable, mechanical, or inflatable devices and provide girth and rigidity; they do not increase length. The decision to proceed with implant therapy often comes after treatment with the less-invasive options has been unsuccessful. Complications of penile implants are infection, erosion, and component failure, and patients must be counseled regarding the risks, benefits, expectations, and possible complications of these procedures. Because of improvements in design and more durable materials, the complication rate has significantly decreased during the past few years, and patient-partner satisfaction has increased.

Group or individual cognitive behavioral therapy, psychosexual therapy, and relationship or couples therapy may improve sexual dysfunction. Research suggests that men who have received psychosocial interventions in addition to pharmacotherapy may have had more successful intercourse compared with those receiving medications alone.[9] In addition, psychoeducation about the medical and psychosocial causes of ED in conjunction with reassurance and support may be adequate to restore normal sexual function.[6]

COMPLICATIONS

Unfulfilled or even destroyed relationships, lack of self-esteem, and depression are common complications of sexual dysfunction. Difficulties related to sexual health often cause the cessation of all sexual activity. This withdrawal of affection can lead to diminished sexual desire and can exacerbate whatever distance or conflict already exists in the relationship.

INDICATIONS FOR REFERRAL

Underlying or refractory medical problems should be referred to the appropriate specialist. Persistent sexual dysfunction requires consultation with a urologist who has a subspecialty in sexual dysfunction. Patients with hormonal abnormalities should be referred to an endocrinologist or urologist. Referral for sexual counseling or psychotherapy should be considered when appropriate. Modern sex therapy is short term and instructive, typically lasting 15 to 20 sessions. It centers on specific sexual problems and includes assessment and conceptualization of the problem, education about sexuality, recognition of mutual responsibility and attitude change if necessary, elimination of performance anxiety, and help with improving sexual and general communication skills to change destructive lifestyle or marital interactions. Sex therapy does not deal with broad personality issues, and if these are contributing factors, psychotherapy is indicated.

LIFE SPAN CONSIDERATIONS

Physical, social, and sexual maturation can be a source of satisfaction as well as confusion and anxiety for adolescents, who would like to talk with their health care provider about sexual issues, particularly those they are curious about. Masturbation is a normal and healthy activity at all ages and may serve as a substitute for partnered sexual behavior during adolescence. Creation of a trusting environment for discussion around issues of consensual or forced sexual experiences, sexual orientation, risk factors for unprotected intercourse (e.g., alcohol and drug use), and family planning will assist the adolescent in developing healthy sexual behaviors as an adult.

Reduction in sexual functioning in the later years may be associated with hormonal changes and concurrent physiologic illnesses, such as vascular and coronary artery disease, stroke, diabetes, hypertension, and hyperlipidemia. Complications from medical or surgical treatments (e.g., genitourinary and prostate surgeries) can also play a role in sexual dysfunction. Older adults are at higher risk for sexual dysfunction related to pharmacologic agent side effects and effects of prolonged cigarette smoking. The normal physical changes that accompany the aging process are inevitable, but health care providers can be helpful in preventing loss of sexual activity as a result of preventable conditions. Physical intimacy and sexual activity are integral to an individual's overall quality of life, and health care providers should assist patients of all ages in achieving and maintaining healthy sexual function.

PATIENT AND PARTNER EDUCATION

Patient education is essential to the success of treatment for sexual dysfunction. The health care provider must take the necessary time to counsel patients about the available options appropriate to their individual needs. It is important to remember that sexual dysfunction is a couple's problem and to include the partner whenever possible. The patient and partner should have realistic expectations of treatment and understand their role in its success.

Whether patients are using a vacuum device, taking an oral medication, using a urethral suppository, or undergoing penile injection therapy, it is important that they be instructed in its use. If the patient has elected injection therapy, it is important that the patient and partner feel comfortable with the injection process and be able to demonstrate accurate administration. Instructions should be provided in writing along with numbers to call should they have further questions or problems. Follow-up is important to determine whether further intervention is needed. Patients appreciate knowing that their providers are concerned about their sexual health and are open to discussing these issues with them.

HEALTH PROMOTION

Early detection and screening for patients at high risk for sexual dysfunction should be considered in the primary care setting. Such patients include those with a history of heavy cigarette use, obesity, sleep apnea, chronic medical problems (such as hypertension, diabetes, or cardiovascular disease), psychological issues, and unresolved life stressors. Sexual dysfunction may be the first indication of underlying cardiovascular disease or serious comorbidity. Health promotional behaviors, such as smoking cessation, daily exercise, low-fat diet, and stress reduction, can minimize risk for sexual dysfunction.

CHAPTER 151

TESTICULAR DISORDERS

Daniel A. Blaz

DEFINITION AND EPIDEMIOLOGY

Scrotal pain may be a symptom of an underlying pathologic condition of the scrotum or testis. The pain may be described as sharp, dull, aching, uncomfortable, or tender, and it is characterized as mild, moderate, or severe. The pain may be sudden in onset, remitting, or progressively escalating in severity. Scrotal pain may be the chief complaint or an incidental finding during the history and physical examination. It is necessary to determine the cause of the pain to evaluate the need for emergent referral or intervention and to exclude potentially life-threatening or fertility-threatening conditions.

Scrotal masses may be nodules or cystic changes on the skin of the scrotum; may involve intrascrotal contents, such as the testis, epididymis, spermatic cord, and tunica vaginalis; or may be the result of herniation of abdominal structures into the scrotal sac. Palpation may reveal single or multiple nodules of varying sizes with consistencies that range from soft to firm. The mass may be freely movable or fixed and may range from nontender to extremely painful to touch or manipulation. Masses may be found during testicular self-examination (TSE) or are discovered during examination and palpation of the scrotum by a health care provider. The mass may go undetected if it is small, if enlargement is gradual, or if discomfort is minimum or absent.

Scrotal swelling, or edema, may involve only one side of the scrotum (left or right hemiscrotal edema) or both sides (bilateral scrotal edema) and may indicate an underlying pathologic condition. Edema caused by a hydrocele may be benign, whereas swelling related to testicular torsion or a malignant tumor of the testis may be potentially life-threatening. The clinical presentation of testicular cysts and dysplasia is enlarged testes, and both are clinically interpreted as neoplasms until otherwise evaluated. Testicular malignancy has doubled over the past 40 years and accounts for approximately 1% of all malignant neoplasms in men in the United States.[1,2]

The epidemiology of scrotal pain, masses, and swelling depends on the cause of the disorders that manifest these symptoms. Specific disorders may occur more often in certain age groups. The causes of scrotal pain, masses, or swelling discussed in this chapter are limited to those most commonly encountered in primary care: varicocele, epididymitis, epididymo-orchitis, spermatocele, hydrocele, hematocele, testicular torsion and torsion of the appendix testis, trauma, scrotal hernia, and testicular tumors.

PATHOPHYSIOLOGY

A varicocele is an abnormal dilation of the pampiniform plexus and spermatic veins in the spermatic cord.[3-5] The cause of a varicocele has been determined to be a multifactorial process that involves anatomic variations (the left gonadal vein is longer than the right, and the left testicular vein inserts at an angle into the left renal vein) and incompetent valves within the pampiniform venous plexus, which results in a backflow of blood and venous pooling.[3,4] Varicoceles usually develop slowly, are often symptomatic, and can lead to testicular damage or dysfunction and male infertility.[5] They occur in less than 1% of boys younger than 10, but this gradually increases to 15% in the young adult male age range.[4,6] Varicoceles are commonly identified in men with primary infertility, with approximately 35% to 40% of infertile males being diagnosed with a left-sided varicocele.[3,5,6] In addition, the prevalence of varicocele increases as men age, with 42% of the geriatric population having an identified varicocele.[4] Although the majority of varicoceles are left sided, bilateral varicoceles occur in approximately 30% to 80% of males.[5] A right-sided varicocele is a rare occurrence and should raise concern for a secondary cause of the varicocele, specifically an abdominal, pelvic, or retroperitoneal mass.[4,5]

Epididymitis is an acute or chronic inflammation of the epididymis and is the most common cause of acute scrotal pain in men, with the majority of cases occurring at ages 14 to 35.[7] The cause may be bacterial, viral, parasitic, chemically induced, or related to trauma, and it is further categorized as a nonspecific or specific infection or traumatic injury. Nonspecific infections are caused by gram-negative rods, gram-positive cocci, or anaerobic bacteria associated with a group of diseases with similar symptoms. Inflammation of the epididymis is occasionally caused by trauma or urinary reflux from the urethra through the vas deferens.[7,8] The two most common causes, especially in younger men, are *Chlamydia trachomatis* and *Neisseria gonorrhoeae.*[7,9] Other causative agents include *Escherichia coli, Haemophilus influenzae,* tuberculosis, cryptococci, and *Brucella* organisms in men who engage in unprotected anal intercourse.[7,10] Epididymitis has several nonsexually transmitted causes, including Enterobacteriaceae and *Pseudomonas aeruginosa,* which are associated with urinary tract infections and prostatitis.[10] In men older than 35 years, epididymitis is most often associated with urinary tract pathogens, structural abnormalities, and urologic procedures or instrumentation, such as transurethral resection of the prostate and urethral catheterization.[10,11] Epididymitis can also spread to the entire testicle (epididymo-orchitis) as a result of many of the same pathogens (*C. trachomatis, N. gonorrhoeae,* and *E. coli*) that cause epididymitis or from reflux of urine from straining, although the exact cause is unclear.[12,13]

Orchitis is a systemic, blood-borne infection that results in an acute inflammation of one or both testicles. It may coexist with infections of the prostate and epididymis; be a consequence of systemic viral infections, such as mumps; or be a complication of syphilis, mycobacterial infections, or fungal infections.[9] Orchitis is commonly caused by *C. trachomatis* and *N. gonorrhoeae* in adolescents and urinary tract pathogens such as *E. coli* in men older than 35.[12,14] When orchitis is a complication of mumps, it is seen in 25% of postpubertal males and may be accompanied by a hydrocele and scrotal wall thickening.[12,14]

A spermatocele is a benign, painless sperm-filled cyst of the epididymis located between the head of the epididymis and the testes and arising from the tubules that connect the rete testis to the head of the epididymis.[15,16] Spermatoceles typically form from the obstruction of the efferent duct and contain a milky fluid that consist of spermatozoa, lymphocytes, and debris.[15,17,18] Spermatoceles have been reported to commonly occur after vasectomies and may be present in 30% of males.[16,18]

A hydrocele is an accumulation of fluid within the tunica vaginalis surrounding the testicle; it may also result from a patent processus vaginalis at birth and sometimes closes spontaneously within the first 1 to 2 years of life.[16,19] Hydroceles are the most common cause of painless scrotal swelling; in adults they are often the result of trauma, a hernia, testicular tumor, or torsion or a complication of epididymitis.[13,15,18]

Similar to a hydrocele, a hematocele is a collection of fluid in the tunica vaginalis of the testes and manifests as a mass.[18] However, a hematocele is a collection of blood (rather than serous fluid) and usually is precipitated by trauma and can be painful and tender on palpation.[13,18,20]

Testicular torsion is an obstruction of blood flow to the testes because of a twisting of the arteries and veins in the spermatic cord.[21-23] Testicular torsion has an overall incidence of 1 in 4000, with the majority of cases occurring from 12 to 18 years of age.[22] Testicular torsion is most often unilateral (commonly involving the left testis). There are two different types of torsion: extravaginal and intravaginal.[22] Extravaginal torsion occurs with the twisting of the spermatic cord, testis, and process vaginalis; intravaginal torsion is failure of the testis to adhere to the scrotal wall, creating a "bell clapper deformity."[14,22] Extravaginal torsion is rare and is more commonly seen in neonates; intravaginal torsion is mostly seen in adolescents.[14,22] An appendage (appendix testis) on the testicles that is vestigial tissue may twist, making it difficult to distinguish from a testicular torsion.[21] The appendix testis is located at the superior pole of the testicle and is the most common cause of acute scrotal pain in children.[14]

Trauma to the scrotum and testicles results in 4% to 8% of testicular torsions.[20] This condition results in congestion of venous blood flow and concomitant edema of the testis. Trauma to the scrotum can be caused by burns, blunt force, or penetrating injury or may be sports related; it can involve the testicle.[20] The majority of blunt force testicular trauma is isolated, but approximately half of such injuries occur during sporting activities.[20] Therefore, no matter what the mechanism is for testicular torsion, it should be included within the differential diagnosis for any scrotal trauma.[20]

A scrotal-inguinal hernia results when a segment of the bowel slips through the internal inguinal ring, where it may remain in the inguinal canal or pass into the scrotal sac. An inguinal hernia may occur as a result of a defect in the anterior abdominal wall or because of a patent process vaginalis.[8] Inguinal hernias predominantly affect men (9:1) and have the highest incidence in men aged 40 to 59.[24] A hernia may move freely between the abdomen and the scrotum or can be spontaneously reduced by digital manipulation.[8] When a hernia becomes strangulated or is unreducible, this compromises the blood supply and requires emergent surgical reduction.[8] Strangulation should be suspected when a tender mass is palpated in the scrotum in addition to redness, nausea, and vomiting.[24]

The origin of testicular tumors can be divided into two primary categories: germ cell and stromal tumors.[1] On the basis of the histologic and genetic origin of the tumor, neoplasms of germ cell origin may be further divided into seminomas and nonseminomas.[1]

Testicular malignant neoplasms are relatively uncommon in the general population and account for only 1% of all cancers in men in the United States.[2] Testicular cancer occurs most often at ages 20 to 39 years and is the most common form of cancer in men aged 15 to 34 years, although these tumors have also been reported in infants and in older men.[2,17,25] The risk for testicular cancer in Caucasian men is more than five times that of African-American men and more than double that of Asian men.[17] Although the exact cause of testicular tumors is unknown, tumors have been associated with scrotal trauma, atrophy, undescended testicles (cryptorchidism), exogenous estrogen exposure, and family history of testicular cancer.[2,17] Males that have an undescended testicle (cryptorchidism) have an approximately 17% higher incidence of developing testicular cancer than the general population.[2] Germ cell tumors (GCTs) are the most common type of testicular tumor and account for 90% to 95% of all primary malignant neoplasms.[1,17,25] Stromal tumors are rare and usually consist of Leydig and Sertoli cell tumor types.[17] GCTs are associated with serum tumor marker products alpha fetoprotein (AFP), human chorionic gonadotropin (hCG), and lactate dehydrogenase (LDH) and are critical to diagnosing, prognosing, staging, and monitoring treatment response of testicular cancer.[1,25] Metastasis from testicular tumors occurs primarily through the lymphatic system, usually to the retroperitoneal lymph nodes.[1,17]

Elephantiasis is caused by a filariasis (parasitic disease) that affects the scrotum, causing massive scrotal lymphedema.[26,27] Filariasis is caused by threadlike roundworms, called filariae, that are transmitted by various mosquitoes, flies, and biting midges and is most often caused by *Wuchereria bancrofti*.[27] Although this is a rare cause of testicular problems in the United States, it should be considered in the differential diagnosis in persons who have recently traveled to Africa or Asia or in health care workers involved in humanitarian missions in those areas.[27]

CLINICAL PRESENTATION

With testicular disorders, the history and presenting symptoms often suggest the underlying pathologic condition. Because some disorders may not cause significant discomfort, however, all male patients should be queried about changes in testicular size or the presence of nodules or masses, pain, or penile discharge. The following disorders may be identified by the presenting complaint.

Varicocele

There are usually no visible outward signs other than a blue color through light-colored scrotal skin. The patient may be asymptomatic or complain of a dull pain, ache, or heaviness in the affected hemiscrotum that worsens with activity or straining.[4,15] Male patients may report enlargement in a testicle that decreases in the supine position; however, the mass may not be seen or palpable on lying down.[5]

Epididymitis

The patient may have a low-grade fever, chills, and a heavy sensation.[22] The history includes a sudden onset of severe pain that may be partially relieved by elevating the scrotum (Prehn sign).[10,22] Additional signs and symptoms include blood in semen, penile discharge, lower abdominal discomfort, groin pain, lump in the testicle, and pain with intercourse or ejaculation. Symptoms may also include dysuria, flank pain, and testicular pain that is made worse by a bowel movement or straining.[17]

Orchitis

The patient may report a gradual onset of acute or moderate pain, testicular swelling, and fever; he may have a concomitant hydrocele and scrotal wall thickening.[14,22]

Spermatocele

A spermatocele typically is a painless, cystic mass that is separate from the testis and located superior or inferior to it.[16] It is in general movable, firm, and painless, with distinct borders and it is easily visible on transillumination.[15,16]

Hydrocele

Hydroceles are usually painless and may be present for long periods, partially resolve, and recur before the patient seeks medical attention.[15] Gradual enlargement of the scrotum occurs with marked edema, which may be uncomfortable because of the added weight. A hydrocele may occur secondary to a tumor when excess serous fluid accumulates in the scrotal sac.[15]

Hematocele

The patient may report a painful scrotum that is tender to palpation. The hematocele is not visible on transillumination. It may have begun after recent surgery, trauma, or a sports-related injury.[18,20]

Testicular Torsion

Testicular torsion, which involves twisting of the spermatic cord and resultant occlusion of the blood flow, is sudden in onset, is extremely painful, and may awaken the patient from sleep or be trauma induced.[20,23] In addition to testicular pain, the patient may experience abdominal pain, nausea, and vomiting; 25% of patients have a fever.[20] Two clinical signs that are suggestive of testicular torsion are a testicle that rides high in the scrotum and an absent cremasteric reflex on examination.[20]

Torsion of the Appendix Testis

The classic presentation is a gradual onset of unilateral testicular pain, edema, and tenderness over the head of the testicle.[8,21] The "blue dot sign" is often present, in which a blue discoloration is noted on transillumination, usually indicating an infarcted or ischemic appendage.[10,22]

Trauma

There may be a history of blunt or penetrating injury to the scrotum that may involve the scrotal contents, leading to severe pain, bruising, edema, nausea, vomiting, or syncope.[20] Depending on the type and extent of the injury, the patient may be in excruciating pain, have minimal pain, have a noted hematocele, or have loss of normal testicular shape because of testis rupture.

Scrotal-Inguinal Hernia

Scrotal swelling, mild to moderate pain on straining, scrotal heaviness, and the possible presence of a bulge are common complaints.[28] The edema is increased after standing in an erect position but decreases when the patient is recumbent.[29]

Testicular Tumor

The patient usually seeks medical care for evaluation of an abnormal mass found during self-examination or has symptoms similar to those of epididymitis, orchitis, or hydrocele.[25] The most common symptom or finding associated with a testicular tumor is a palpable mass that is often accompanied by edema or a sensation of fullness or heaviness in the scrotum.[2,25] Complaints, such as back or abdominal pain, nausea, anorexia, or bowel and bladder symptoms, may occur with retroperitoneal lymph node involvement and suggest metastatic disease.[1]

Elephantiasis

Elephantiasis leads to massive scrotal lymphedema, thickened scrotal skin, and in severe cases skin ulcerations.[27]

PHYSICAL EXAMINATION

Examination begins with inspection of the scrotum. Scrotal size can change with temperature variations because of the cremaster muscle response. Asymmetry is expected because the left hemiscrotum is normally positioned lower than the right.[30] The skin of each hemiscrotum should be inspected carefully, spreading the rugae between the fingers. Care should be taken to inspect both the anterior and posterior surfaces to detect any lesions. Each hemiscrotum should be palpated with the thumb and first two fingers of both hands. The scrotal contents should be easily movable in a sliding fashion. The testes should be smooth, equal, firm but rubbery, and the shape is round in the newborn transitioning to ovoid during puberty.[14] The size of a testicle after puberty is on average 4 to 5 cm in length, 2 to 4 cm in width, and 3 cm anteroposteriorly.[30] The normal epididymis is divided into the head, body, and tail and is located in the superior, posterior portion of the testis.[14,30] It is softer than the testis, nontender, and smooth. To palpate the spermatic cord, the provider should slide the fingers and thumb up from the epididymis. The cord should feel smooth and nontender. Documentation should include any tenderness or pain, discoloration, edema, or abnormal findings, such as those seen in the conditions discussed in the following sections.

BOX 151-1

Aspects of the Scrotal Examination

INSPECT

Ensure appropriate pubic hair distribution
Identify scrotal skin lesions
Look for bulging masses
Evaluate symmetry of left and right hemiscrotums

PALPATE

Ensure testes are firm but not hard
Assess epididymides
Identify vasa bilaterally
Examine vascular cord structures
Check for intact external ring on Valsalva maneuver

CHARACTERIZE MASSES

Assess the following:

- Location
- Size
- Texture (e.g., hard, cystic)
- Tenderness

Data from Montgomery JS, Bloom DA: The diagnosis and management of scrotal masses. *Med Clin North Am* 95(1):235-244, 2011.

Varicocele

Bluish color shows through the scrotal skin; when the patient stands, palpation of the soft mass reveals a "bag of worms" on the proximal spermatic cord, more frequently encountered on the left side.[4,5] Varicoceles become smaller when the patient is supine and are better seen when the patient is upright or performs a Valsalva maneuver.[4] If a right varicocele is identified, it is noted to be rare and may indicate venous obstruction, a retroperitoneal process, or abdominal or renal neoplasm.[5,31]

Epididymitis

The scrotum is red, enlarged, and extremely tender and may be difficult to distinguish from the testis.[10] The position of the testicle should be noted; it should be located in its normal anatomic position.[22] The examination should include evaluation for strong predictors of epididymitis, which include an intact cremasteric reflex, a positive Prehn sign (pain relief with the elevation of the affected testicle), and pain along the upper pole of the testicle.[10] Other elements that may be noted during the examination are fever, tachycardia, urinary tract infection symptoms (dysuria, urgency, frequency), and inflammation of the testis (orchitis).[13,22]

Orchitis

As with epididymitis, testicular edema may be so pronounced that it is difficult to distinguish the testes from the epididymis. Palpation may reveal swollen, very tense testes that are painful, and the patient may be febrile. Inflammation of the testis usually involves systemic viral infections (commonly mumps) and includes unilateral or bilateral erythema, edema, and scrotal tenderness, which occurs 4 to 7 days after initial fever.[9,11]

Spermatocele

The spermatocele is palpated as a small, nontender, freely movable mass above and behind the testis.[15,16] The mass may arise from the vasa efferentia (tubules that connect the rete testis to the epididymis), the epididymis, or cystic structures on the upper pole of the testis.[16] Transillumination of the mass in a darkened room may help visualize the mass.[15]

Hydrocele

Palpation reveals a painless mass that appears easily on transillumination.[15,17] The hydrocele may fluctuate in size and is identified by a smooth, tense scrotal mass.[15] A hydrocele that is noted in men older than 30 years can be secondary to a testicular tumor.[15,32]

Hematocele

Palpation reveals scrotal swelling that does not transilluminate and may be tender to palpation.[18,20]

Testicular Torsion

Torsion is more common in the left hemiscrotum. The scrotum may be edematous and erythematous, and the affected side may have a higher position as a result of rotation.[20,33] The spermatic cord is swollen and extremely tender, the epididymis may be felt anteriorly, and the majority of patients will have an absent cremasteric reflex.[20,33] In some instances a small area of cyanosis (blue dot sign) may be present on the scrotal skin and indicates torsion of the appendix testis.[20]

Torsion of the Appendix Testis

Torsion of the appendage testis commonly occurs in children and frequently is seen at ages 7 to 12 years.[14] On examination, the testicle will be tender along the superior pole of the testis, with scrotal edema and enlargement of the epididymis, and often the blue dot sign is identified.[14,21] Occasionally nausea and vomiting occur, but are less frequent than with a testicular torsion.[8]

Trauma

Bruising, bleeding, edema, and severe pain may be present and are highly suspicious for scrotal trauma.[18,20] Inspection should include careful comparison of coloration to determine the extent of bruising or expanding hematoma. A ruptured testis should be suspected if there is evidence of increasing hematoma or hematocele; edema; and pain.[20] Palpation should include external skin and scrotal contents. Documentation includes the time and date of injury, type of trauma, and any change in signs or symptoms since the time of injury.

Scrotal-Inguinal Hernia

Inspection reveals an enlarged hemiscrotum or a bulge in the groin area that may spontaneously reduce when the patient is supine or with manual reduction.[24] The provider will not be able to move the fingers above the mass, which should be soft and mushy but painless unless it is incarcerated and ischemic. Scrotal hernias do not transilluminate. Auscultation of bowel sounds over the mass is significant for the diagnosis of bowel in the scrotal sac.

Testicular Tumor

Inquiry should focus on previous trauma to the scrotum or perineal area and the history or presence of cryptorchidism, pain, swelling, or sensations in the scrotum. The physical examination should include inspection and palpation of the abdomen, perineal area, scrotal sac, testes, and surrounding lymph nodes. Palpation should be performed with both hands to assist in differentiating between a mass located on the body of the testicle and a mass located on or within the epididymis. The location, size, mobility, and degree of tenderness of normal structures as well as any abnormal findings should be noted.[17] Any solid, firm mass within the body of the testicle should be considered a tumor unless proven otherwise.[18] Additional examination of the abdomen and chest should be completed while also evaluating for gynecomastia (a sign of elevated β-hCG).[22] One in three patients is misdiagnosed with epididymitis, orchitis, or a hydrocele on initial presentation.[1] Evaluation of lymph nodes in the abdomen and groin should be performed, because bulky lymphadenopathy is noted in metastatic disease.[1] Scrotal transillumination performed in a darkened room may be used to visualize abnormalities and to detect solid versus fluid-filled masses.[7,22]

Elephantiasis

Obstruction of the lymphatic vessels leads to swelling in the torso, genitals, and lower extremities and is classically characterized by massive scrotal lymphedema.[27]

DIAGNOSTICS

Many testicular disorders are readily recognized at the time of presentation and do not require further evaluation. In general, clinical presentation and physical examination guide the choice of appropriate diagnostics.

Varicocele

Varicoceles have a grading system from 1 to 3. Grade 1 is considered small and palpable only with the patient standing while performing a Valsalva maneuver. Grade 2 is moderate and palpable with the patient standing and no Valsalva maneuver. Grade 3 is large and palpable with the patient standing and can been seen through the scrotal skin.[5]

- Semen analysis may reveal oligospermia or azoospermia, but findings can be normal.[5]
- Measurement of serum testosterone levels may be considered; varicoceles have been shown to have a negative impact on Leydig cell function.[5]
- Ultrasound examination will reveal a dilated pampiniform plexus vessel larger than 2 to 3 mm.[18]

Epididymitis

- Doppler ultrasound examination shows heterogeneous hypoechoic epididymis with hyperemia and increased intratesticular blood flow.[18,30]
- Urinalysis and complete blood count (CBC) may reveal white blood cells and bacteriuria.
- A nucleic acid amplification test (NAAT) will assist with diagnosing chlamydia and gonorrhea.[12]

Orchitis

- Doppler ultrasound examination shows heterogeneous hypoechoicity.[18]

Spermatocele

- A mass is located at the proximal aspect of the spermatic cord and can be transilluminated.[15]

Hydrocele

- A hydrocele will transilluminate and be anechoic on ultrasound examination.[18]

Hematocele

- Ultrasound examination is used to evaluate blood flow and will show echogenic debris.[18] Surgical exploration may be necessary to rule out cancer.

Testicular Torsion

- Ultrasound examination will demonstrate an enlarged testicle with diffuse hypoechogenicity, usually associated with a reactive hydrocele and edema of the epididymis and scrotum.[14] Absent blood flow seen on color flow Doppler ultrasound is both sensitive and specific for testicular torsion.[14]

Torsion of the Appendix Testis

- Transillumination may reveal a blue dot sign, and ultrasound examination of the appendage will demonstrate an oval nodule in the superior pole of the testis. If the appendage has infarcted, it can calcify and may later appear as a "scrotal pearl" during imaging.[14]

Trauma

- Ultrasound examination of the scrotum after trauma may reveal a hematocele or hematoma, which can become quite large.[14] If there is testicular rupture, a testicular fracture line may appear on ultrasound images and should be considered an emergency; prompt surgical repair should be considered.[14]

Scrotal-Inguinal Hernia

- A scrotal hernia does not transilluminate and is easily identified on ultrasound examination, showing the bowel mass within the scrotum.[18]

Testicular Tumor

- To assist practitioners in assessing the extent of testicular disease, the staging system commonly used is the American Joint Committee on Cancer staging system, which is based on surgical findings and histologic examination of retroperitoneal lymph nodes: stage I, tumor confined to testis; stage II, tumor spread to retroperitoneal nodal involvement; stage III, tumor spread beyond retroperitoneal nodes.[1]
- The diagnosis of testicular cancer is usually confirmed through direct surgical exploration of the testes and serum tumor markers (hCG, AFP, and LDH) along with chest, abdominal, and pelvic imaging.[1]
- Tumor markers are drawn before and after orchiectomy to obtain information on staging, prognosis, and treatment outcome.[1,25] A negative marker does not necessarily exclude disease, but an elevated marker is considered clinically significant.[1]
- High levels of hCG are seen in both seminomatous and nonseminomatous tumors, whereas AFP levels are elevated only in nonseminomas.[25]
- Ultrasonography is useful in evaluating testicular masses and in confirming the size and location of palpable tumors.[1]

Abdominopelvic and chest computed tomography (CT) along with other imaging studies may be necessary to determine the extent and location of metastases.[1]

Elephantiasis

- The only definitive way to make the diagnosis of lymphatic filariasis is by detecting the parasite itself, either the adult worms or the microfilariae.[27]
- The microfilariae can sometimes be detected by microscopic examination of a blood sample, but people with chronic infection often do not have the microfilariae in their blood. In such cases, the urine, hydrocele fluid, or other clinical tests are necessary.
- Blood samples should be obtained during the night, when microfilariae are more numerous in the bloodstream.
- A CBC and ultrasound examination are additional diagnostics that can be considered.[27]

DIAGNOSTICS

Testicular Disorders

VARICOCELE
Laboratory
Semen analysis
Testosterone

Imaging
Doppler ultrasound

EPIDIDYMITIS
Laboratory
Urinalysis and NAAT
CBC and differential
Human immunodeficiency virus (HIV) and syphilis (<35 years of age)

Imaging
Doppler ultrasound

ORCHITIS
Imaging
Doppler ultrasound

TESTICULAR TORSION
Imaging
Doppler ultrasound

TORSION OF THE APPENDIX TESTIS
Imaging
Doppler ultrasound

TRAUMA
Laboratory
Urinalysis

Imaging
Ultrasound

TESTICULAR TUMOR
Laboratory
Serum tumor markers: hCG, AFP, LDH
Clinical staging

Imaging
Ultrasound
CT scans and magnetic resonance imaging

DIFFERENTIAL DIAGNOSIS

The differential diagnosis for any testicular disorder or acute scrotal mass or pain should first exclude the possibility of a testicular tumor. The differential diagnosis for testicular tumors includes cysts, testicular torsion, epididymitis, and epididymo-orchitis.[7] A hydrocele, hernia, hematoma, or spermatocele may also mimic a testicular tumor.[32] The presence of a testicular mass is suggestive of a tumor and indicates the need for immediate referral. It is often difficult to differentiate between epididymitis and orchitis because the symptoms are similar and at times may coexist. A varicocele is more discernible than other scrotal masses because this mass classically resembles a bag of worms on palpation.[4] However, many other testicular conditions (specifically, testicular cancer in men older than 30) may have hydrocele development as a symptom.[15] A detailed history, a thorough physical examination, and key diagnostics (urinalysis, urine culture, ultrasound, CT, tumor markers) all aid in clarity for determining the precise diagnosis.

MANAGEMENT

Specialist or surgical consultation is indicated for testicular or scrotal trauma, complicated epididymitis, painless testicular mass, right varicocele, and varicocele in conjunction with infertility.

Immediate emergency department referral or surgical consultation is indicated for patients with sudden-onset unilateral scrotal pain, testicular torsion, incarcerated or strangulated hernia, testicular trauma with concern for rupture, and Fournier disease.

Management of testicular disorders depends on the specific type of disorder.

Varicocele

- A volume discrepancy of more than 20% along with an abnormal semen analysis usually prompts surgical intervention. Surgical treatment by ligation of the spermatic vein (varicocelectomy) is often the treatment of choice, and there are several different surgical approaches.[4] The microsurgical subinguinal technique appears to have the highest spontaneous pregnancy rate in previously infertile couples.[4]
- Alternative treatment options include vascular ablation or embolization, and percutaneous sclerotherapy.[4]

TABLE 151-1 Differential Diagnosis of Testicular Disorders

Diagnosis	Symptoms	Signs	Evaluation
Appendage torsion (appendix testis)	Typically a more indolent onset of symptoms compared with testicular torsion; less likely to present with nausea or vomiting	Tender nodule typically at head of testicle or epididymis; "blue dot sign" pathognomonic	Ultrasound examination may demonstrate infarcted appendage.
Epididymitis	Typically a more indolent onset of symptoms compared with testicular torsion; less likely to present with nausea or vomiting	*Early:* firmness and nodularity isolated to epididymis *Late:* with progression, inflammation may become contiguous with testicle (termed epididymo-orchitis	Ultrasound examination may reveal increased intratesticular blood flow, although this is a nonspecific finding.
Epididymo-orchitis	More likely to present with systemic findings, including nausea, vomiting, fever	Large, swollen scrotal mass typically with indistinct border between testicle and epididymis	Ultrasound examination may reveal increased intratesticular blood flow, although this is a nonspecific finding.
Fournier disease	Perineal swelling, redness; fever, vomiting, lethargy	May present with an absence of visible local findings on skin inspection in early stages (pain out of proportion to examination); ecchymosis, crepitus, necrotic eschar may be present in more advanced disease	Emergent surgical consultation for debridement, broad-spectrum antimicrobials.
Hematocele	Large, painful scrotal mass; often antecedent history of trauma	Ecchymosis of scrotal skin; testicular tenderness or firmness	Ultrasound examination may reveal fluid-filled tunica vaginalis.
Hernia	Unilateral inguinal or scrotal swelling and pain	Reducible, incarcerated and strangulated forms; incarcerated or strangulated hernia may be particularly tender on examination	Emergent surgical consultation when incarcerated or strangulated; outpatient surgical referral reasonable if readily reducible.
Hydrocele	Typically a gradual progression of swelling	Scrotal transillumination may be helpful	Ultrasound examination may reveal fluid-filled tunica vaginalis.
Idiopathic scrotal edema	Typically unilateral scrotal swelling and edema; primarily seen in boys younger than 10 years	Scrotal, perineal, inguinal erythema and edema; may be difficult to distinguish from an acute skin or soft tissue infection	Ultrasound examination.
Orchitis	Typically gradual onset of unilateral (or bilateral) testicular swelling and pain	Swelling and tenderness isolated to testis or testes, without epididymal involvement	Ultrasound examination; often seen in conjunction with other systemic diseases (viral, other); treatment is disease specific.
Scrotal skin infection	Variable depending on cause	Must distinguish between lesions localized to scrotal wall and those contiguous with deeper scrotal structures	Ultrasound or CT imaging may be helpful in determining the depth and extent of involvement if invasive process suspected.
Spermatocele or epididymal cyst	Typically a painless well-defined nodule Spermatocele is present on the head of the epididymis; epididymal cysts arise throughout the epididymis	Spermatocele will have proteinaceous fluid and spermatozoa. Epididymal cysts contain clear serous fluid	Ultrasound examination. Spermatoceles and epididymal cysts are indistinguishable.
Testicular torsion	Typically a sudden and severe onset of pain; more likely to be associated with nausea or emesis	Classic findings include an elevated testis with a transverse lie	Emergent surgery consultation in high probability cases.
Trauma	History of blunt or penetrating mechanism of injury	Variable depending on mechanism	Ultrasound examination; low threshold for surgical consultation in all but the most minor injuries.

Continued

TABLE 151-1 Differential Diagnosis of Testicular Disorders—cont'd

Diagnosis	Symptoms	Signs	Evaluation
Tumor	Typically a gradually progressive testicular mass; may be painless or painful	May palpate testicular mass, firmness, or induration	Ultrasound examination.
Varicocele	Typically a gradual onset of unilateral swelling, often painless	Abnormally enlarged spermatic cord (pampiniform) venous plexus (often described as a "bag of worms")	Ultrasound examination.
Vasculitis (e.g., Henoch-Schönlein purpura [HSP])	Testicular swelling and pain	Associated vasculitis findings (such as buttock or lower extremity purpura and renal involvement in HSP)	Ultrasound examination, other diagnostic testing guided by suspected cause (e.g., CBC, serum electrolytes with renal function in HSP).

Modified from Davis JE, Silverman M: Scrotal emergencies. *Emerg Med Clin North Am.* 29(3):469-484, 2011.

Epididymitis and Orchitis

- Anti-infective therapy is recommended, with guidance by local sensitivity reports. The following antibiotic regimens are effective against the most common causes of epididymitis: single-dose ceftriaxone given intramuscularly (IM), 250 to 500 mg, and doxycycline, 100 mg twice daily for 10 days for men younger than 35 years; in men older than 35 years, levofloxacin (given intravenously [IV] or orally [PO]), 500 to 750 mg/day, or ciprofloxacin, 500 mg (IV or PO), for 10 to 14 days.[11,12] In severe cases, it may be necessary to use intravenous antibiotics.
- Antipyretics should be used to reduce discomfort and fever, and an anti-inflammatory agent should be prescribed.[10] An antiemetic can also be prescribed for nausea and vomiting.
- Bed rest and scrotal elevation are also recommended for epididymitis.[10] Hot or cold compresses may be helpful for orchitis.

Spermatocele

- No treatment if asymptomatic or scrotal support.
- If significant discomfort is present or there is concern because of the increasing size of the mass, excision is recommended.[15]

Hydrocele

- Congenital hydroceles that occur in newborns usually resolve themselves within the first year of life; if not, surgical correction can be completed.[15,29]
- Treatment of asymptomatic hydroceles can consist of watchful waiting.[15]
- Symptomatic hydroceles can be treated with surgical aspiration, resection, or sclerotherapy.[15]

Testicular Torsion

- Treatment is prompt surgical consultation with surgical exploration with the intent to prevent ischemia and restore blood flow.[21] It is critical to restore vascularity as soon as possible because salvage rates are higher than 90% within 6 hours, higher than 50% within 12 hours, and lower than 10% in 24 hours.[21]

Torsion of the Appendix Testis

- Treatment of an appendix testis with torsion often is self-limiting, but management revolves around conservative measures of anti-inflammatories, rest, ice, and scrotal support.[10] If pain persists and conservative management does not provide relief, surgical referral is appropriate.

Trauma or Hematocele

- If all scrotal contents are intact, trauma injuries can be treated symptomatically with ice, elevation, scrotal support, and bed rest.[20] However, if there is concern that the testicle has been ruptured or penetrated, or if other contents are not palpated as intact, immediate surgical exploration and intervention should be undertaken.[8,20]

Scrotal-Inguinal Hernia

- If the herniated bowel is reducible, surgical referral for possible future repair is indicated. Difficulty in reducing a hernia is cause for urgent surgical intervention. However, pain may indicate incarceration of the bowel or complete inability to reduce the hernia, which is cause for immediate emergency department referral and surgical exploration.[29]

Testicular Tumor

- Prompt evaluation is essential. The mainstays of testicular cancer treatment are surgery, chemotherapy, and radiation.[2]
- Primary treatment for seminomas involves radical orchiectomy followed by irradiation of the retroperitoneal lymph for low-stage seminomas and chemotherapy for more advanced stage seminomas.[2,25]
- Nonseminomas are also treated with radical orchiectomy followed by retroperitoneal lymphadenectomy and chemotherapy, because they are more responsive to chemotherapy.[2]
- Additional management is monitoring of tumor markers hCG, AFP, and LDH.[25] Follow-up visits should include a thorough physical examination, chest imaging, and measurement of serum tumor markers monthly for the first year, every 2 months for the second year, and every 3 to 6 months for up to 5 years. Regardless of the disease stage, more than 90% of all newly diagnosed cases of testicular cancer will be cured.[25]

Elephantiasis

- The recommended treatment for *W. bancrofti* infection is diethylcarbamazine, but some research has shown response to doxycycline.[34] Diethylcarbamazine is no longer sold in the

United States or approved by the U.S. Food and Drug Administration (FDA), but it can be obtained from the Centers for Disease Control and Prevention (CDC) with positive laboratory confirmation.[34]

COMPLICATIONS

Varicoceles are associated with infertility and produce abnormal semen parameters, testicular atrophy, and Leydig cell dysfunction.[4] The condition can be reversed if the varicocele is surgically corrected, and this has been shown to improve spontaneous pregnancy rates by almost 40%.[4] Infertility is also the most serious complication of epididymitis, orchitis, and spermatocele.[9]

Testicular torsion is a medical emergency and should be surgically explored and relieved as quickly as possible to prevent the development of gangrene. A delay in treatment could result in testicular infarction and loss of the affected testicle. Manual detorsion can be attempted in certain situations with the standard medial-to-lateral rotation method (as in opening a book), but residual torsion may still remain.[8] Torsion of the appendix testis is frequently seen in adolescents and is a self-limiting condition that is treated with pain relief and limited activity.[8] In some instances, torsion of the appendix testis can recur.[8] In scrotal trauma, the most pressing concern is whether the testis has been ruptured or the blood supply compromised from trauma-induced torsion of the spermatic cord.[20] A referral to a urologist or surgical consultation is required to verify that the testis and other scrotal contents are intact.[20]

Scrotal-inguinal hernia repair can have complications associated with the procedure, the most common being hematomas, scrotal ecchymosis, seromas, and infection.[24] Testicular cancer is the most common malignancy in males aged 15 to 35 years.[2] The mainstays of testicular cancer treatment are surgery (inguinal orchiectomy), chemotherapy, and radiation therapy; with these treatments, complications may occur.[2] Potential complications that may occur as a result of testicular cancer treatment are infertility, recurrent or secondary malignancy (lymphoma and myeloid dysfunctions), cardiac disease, ventral hernia, and bowel obstruction.[2,7]

INDICATIONS FOR REFERRAL OR HOSPITALIZATION

- Patients suspected of having a testicular mass, testicular torsion, or an incarcerated scrotal hernia require immediate referral to a urologist or surgeon.
- Epididymitis and minor scrotal trauma can be managed by the health care provider unless complications are present or the testis is involved in a traumatic injury. Any suspicion of testicular rupture, torsion, epididymal injury, hematocele, or other testicular defect warrants evaluation by a surgeon.[20]
- Any patient with a hydrocele that is expanding, is causing pain, or potentially was caused by a scrotal tumor should be referred to a urologist.
- Patients with varicoceles that do not respond to conservative treatment (scrotal support and anti-inflammatory medications) should be referred to a urologist for more definitive treatment. Patients with an identified varicocele in addition to an abnormal semen analysis, known infertility, and testicular atrophy should be referred to a urologist.[5]
- Hospitalization should be considered for any unremitting testicular or scrotal pain, if a testicular mass is suspected, or if edema from testicular involvement cannot be excluded.

LIFE SPAN CONSIDERATIONS

Issues critical in the assessment and treatment of conditions involving the scrotum or testes are threat to life, immediate pain or discomfort, potential for infertility or impotence, and quality of life. Treatment success may depend on the patient's overall health, available treatment options, and age-related issues affecting treatment decisions. Although the patient's age may influence concerns about fertility, the potential loss of testicular function should not be disregarded in men of advanced age. Surgical intervention for testicular tumors may result in body image disturbances and altered sexuality in adolescence and later life. After an orchiectomy, counseling may be indicated to assist in coping with loss related to alterations in the genitals and reproductive system. For children, adolescents, or young men with a single testicle, it is recommended that protective equipment be used during athletic participation.[20]

EDUCATION AND HEALTH PROMOTION

Diagnosis, treatment options, potential outcomes, and the need for follow-up care should be carefully explained to patients. All patients should be encouraged to discuss their concerns or fears about the diagnosis and treatment or treatment options. These concerns and fears about potential complications and the severity of the condition should be addressed truthfully.

Patients with testicular masses require ongoing education and support from the time of diagnosis through all phases of treatment. Whenever possible, the spouse or significant other should be educated about the disease process, prognosis, treatment, and effects of treatment on relationships and sexuality. The patient and family should be encouraged to verbalize feelings and to support one another throughout the process.

Male patients, from adolescence to older age, should be instructed in the correct method of TSE and the importance of the examination for other men in their family (including teenagers, because this is the beginning of the age range for testicular cancer). The TSE should be performed monthly and is best performed after a warm bath or shower when the skin of the scrotum is relaxed.[2] Patients should see their health care providers if any abnormalities are detected in the scrotum or testes.

CHAPTER 152

URINARY CALCULI

Daniel A. Blaz

DEFINITION AND EPIDEMIOLOGY

Renal and urinary calculi are calcifications or "stones" that can form anywhere within the urinary tract, specifically the kidneys (nephrolithiasis), urinary system (urolithiasis), or ureters (ureterolithiasis), or they may migrate to the lower urinary tract (bladder or urethra).[1-3] The majority of stones are found within the kidney, but stone formation may also occur in the ureter, bladder, and urinary diversion structures (e.g., ileal conduit, orthotopic bladder).[1,4] Renal stone formation and disease revolve around a multifactorial process that involves environmental and genetic factors and a delicate balance of substances within the urine.[5,6] In the United States stone disease is associated with nearly $2 billion in health care costs and accounts for nearly 2 million outpatient care visits each year.[7] Understanding the epidemiology, particularly the etiology of stone formation and the interaction among different factors, may help elucidate and define approaches to reduce the risk of stone formation and mitigate the health care costs related to stone disease.[8]

The prevalence of kidney stones in American adults was most recently reported from the National Health and Nutrition Examination Survey (NHANES 2007 to 2010) at 8.8%, with men having a higher prevalence (10.6%) than women (7.1%).[9] Kidney stones are most common in men, specifically white males, and development of stones is most prevalent in individuals aged 20 to 50 years, with a peak incidence at age 30.[4,7] Males have a threefold greater lifetime incidence for stone development, but the gender gap has recently been closing.[7] This is thought to be related to the rise in obesity rates among individuals, specifically in women.[9] Women have a bimodal age distribution, with peaks at 35 and after age 60 believed to be related to the development of menopause and the decline of estrogen.[3] In children, stone disease is not very common, although 40% of children who develop stones have a positive family history, pointing to a probable genetic metabolic cause.[10] The lifetime risk for kidney stone disease in Americans is 9%. The recurrence rate for stone formation is approximately 15% in the first year, with a 50% chance of experiencing another stone within the next 5 to 10 years and a 75% chance within the next 20 years.[4,7,9,11] Fifty-five percent of those with recurrent stones have a family history of stones, which increases the risk for stone formation threefold.[7] The incidence of stone formation has several ethnic (age, gender, heredity) and geographic (geography, climate, season) implications that affect the development of renal stones; the highest frequency occurs in the Middle East regions of the world and the Southeast region of the United States.[12] Living in a hot tropical or desert climate has been shown to increase the risk of forming stones.[12]

The genetic predisposition to stone development is becoming clearer to health care providers when diagnosing hereditary stone disease.[10] Certain metabolic and genetic disorders have been shown to occur most frequently in inherited cases, with cystinuria (in adults) and primary hyperoxaluria (PH; in children) being the two most common.[10] A positive family history of kidney stones has been documented to occur in 15% to 20% of familial cases and is a risk factor for stone development.[10] In addition, certain lifestyle factors have shown increased stone risk such as chronic laxative use, excess antacid use, betel nut chewing, tropical holidays, strenuous exercise, and stress.[6,13] Other risk factors include insulin-resistant states, history of hypertension or gout, primary hyperparathyroidism, chronic metabolic acidosis, and surgical menopause.[5,9] Obesity is associated with insulin resistance and compensatory hyperinsulinemia, both of which can contribute to stone formation. In addition, body mass index and waist circumference have been positively associated with kidney stone formation in both men and women. Obese individuals who form stones excrete higher amounts of sodium, calcium, uric acid, and citrate, with uric acid stones found most commonly in this population.[14] Diet-related factors such as a diet that is high in salt and animal protein and excessive ingestion of substances that produce stones, such as purines (e.g., seafood, organ meats), oxalates (e.g., colas, chocolate), calcium (e.g., dairy products), and phosphate, increase the incidence of stone formation.[6] Other predisposing factors include occupation (e.g., chefs, taxi drivers), sedentary activity level, risk of dehydration, and medications (e.g., acetazolamide, antacids, ascorbic acid in doses of 2 g or more daily, hydrochlorothiazide, and indinavir [Crixivan]).[6] Environmental factors, such as exposure to drinking water high in minerals, may contribute to stone formation, but it has been widely accepted that the role of increased water intake can reduce risk of stone formation by up to 39%.[13] Other beverages (tea, grapefruit juice, apple juice, and cola) have been shown to contribute to the risk of stone development, and with the rise of energy and sport drink use these products could increase the risk of stone formation.[13]

PATHOPHYSIOLOGY

The formation of kidney stones is a multifaceted process that incorporates a delicate balance between elevated levels of stone-forming salts and inadequate inhibitory proteins.[3] Renal and urinary calculi are mineral deposits that develop from microscopic crystals in the loop of Henle, the distal tubule, or the collecting ducts, and they aggregate to form visible structures.[7] The cause of renal and urinary calculi formation has traditionally narrowed on two agreed-on theories. The first theory involves the process of the supersaturation of urine with calcium, oxalate, and uric acid, whereby microscopic crystals form on these substances and adhere to the urothelium, creating the nidus for stone formation.[7,11] The second theory primarily involves the formation of calcium oxalate stones whereby deposits (Randall plaques) of subepithelial interstitial calcium act as nuclei for the formation of a stone.[6,7] In addition, more recent theories centralize on the aspect of surface molecules that promote or inhibit the formation of crystals.[11] These molecules are further influenced by the urothelial injury and repair cycle after a stone has formed, which increases the expression of the molecules and promotes enhanced crystal adhesion.[6]

One of the most common risk factors for stone formation is reduced urinary flow, and any factor that reduces urinary flow or urinary volume (e.g., dehydration or inadequate fluid intake) allows stone constituents to supersaturate and increases the risk of kidney stones.[11] Other risk factors for the formation of urinary calculi include excess dietary intake of oxalate and sodium, which promotes hyperoxaluria and hypercalciuria, respectively; gout, which promotes hyperuricosuria; and primary hyperparathyroidism, which can result in persistent hypercalciuria.[11] Excess dietary animal protein (meat, poultry, and fish) creates an acidic urinary milieu, resulting in citrate depletion and hyperuricosuria.[11] Obesity may contribute to hypercalciuria and uric acid stone formation owing to an increase in refined sugars, low fluid intake, high calcium and oxalate, and excess dietary ingestion of meat.[14] Short bowel syndrome can contribute to low urine volume, acidic urine (which depletes available citrate), and hyperoxaluria.[11] Insulin resistance can result in an alteration in urinary pH, and gout increases the risk of hyperuricosuria, both of which increase the risk of stone formation.[6,14,15] The entire process of stone formation is influenced by multiple chemical, physical, physical-chemical, biochemical, and physiologic events.

Calculi can be broadly classified as calcareous (i.e., calcium containing) stones, which are visible on imaging, and noncalcareous stones, which are often radiolucent or poorly visible on plain film radiography.[3,16] Renal and urinary calculi can be more specifically classified into five types based on their composition:

calcium oxalate (75% to 80%), which are calcareous, and struvite (10% to 25), calcium phosphate (5% to 10%), uric acid (5% to 10%), and cystine (1% to 2%) stones, which are all noncalcareous.[3,4,11,14]

Calcium oxalate stones are the most common type of urinary calculi.[11] They are radiopaque and usually visible on plain radiography or unenhanced computed tomography (CT).[2,3] Hypercalciuria (>250 mg/24 hr) is the most common metabolic abnormality associated with calcium oxalate stones.[17] The next most common cause is hypocitraturia (<320 mg/24 hr), which involves a generally idiopathic deficiency of citrate (a naturally occurring stone inhibitor).[3,17,18] High acid loads, such as from excess intake of meat, and dehydration can contribute to or exacerbate hypocitraturia.[18] Urine levels of oxalate, normally a metabolic byproduct, may increase as a result of the ingestion of foods high in oxalate, such as rhubarb, nuts, cocoa, tea, beans, lime peel, and green leafy vegetables; this condition is termed hyperoxaluria.[18] The most common causes of hyperoxaluria are bowel resection and intestinal disease such as malabsorptive small bowel disorders, including Crohn disease, jejunoileal bypass, celiac sprue, chronic pancreatitis, and biliary obstruction.[18] More recently, an increasing cause of hyperoxaluria has been bariatric surgical procedures.[18] In addition, PH, which is a rare inherited autosomal recessive disorder of glyoxylate metabolism, should be highly considered in stone-forming children and adults with oppressive hyperoxaluria.[3,18]

Calculi that consist predominantly of calcium phosphate occur more often in women, specifically pregnant women, than in men.[3,19,20] They are most often associated with acidification disorders such as renal tubular acidosis (RTA) , which results in metabolic acidosis, defective urinary acidification, hypokalemia, and reduced urinary citrate concentrations.[11,19] Less common causes of defective urinary acidification include primary hyperparathyroidism, excessive alkalinization, and sarcoidosis.[19] Favorable conditions for calcium phosphate stone formation are high urine pH, reduced citrate excretion, and increased urinary concentration of calcium and phosphate.[19]

Uric acid stones account for approximately 5% to 10% of all stones and are more prevalent in patients with diabetes.[21] Uric acid is an end product of purine metabolism; increased uricosuria is often a result of dehydration and excessive purine intake.[2] Other risk factors include a consistently low urine pH, gout, myeloproliferative disorders, insulin-resistant states, cytotoxic drugs, end ileostomies, and conditions that predispose a patient to concentrated urine.[18,22] Uric acid stones are radiolucent and may be difficult to see on radiography; however, they are readily apparent on noncontrast CT.[2]

Struvite stones are composed of magnesium phosphate, ammonium phosphate, and calcium phosphate and are referred to as triple phosphate stones.[2] Struvite stones account for approximately 10% to 25% of all stones, are more prevalent in women, and are the leading cause of staghorn calculi.[2,14] Struvite stones grow rapidly, recur frequently, and occurs from urea splitting by urease, which results in high ammonium concentration and alkaline urine (pH range of 6.8 to 8.3).[3] This alkaline urine causes crystals to precipitate, creating the struvite stone. Struvite stones are an index of a urinary tract infection (UTI) usually from urea-splitting microorganisms.[22] Neurogenic bladders, foreign bodies in the urinary tract, and recurrent UTIs with urea-splitting microorganisms (e.g., *Proteus mirabilis, Ureaplasma urealyticum, Klebsiella pneumoniae*) increase the risk of struvite calculi.[3] Struvite calculi are radiopaque on radiography but may appear faint on imaging and therefore may not be immediately detected.[2]

Cystinuria is an autosomal recessive disorder in which there is excessive urinary excretion of the amino acids cystine, ornithine, lysine, and arginine.[2,11] The low solubility of cystine results in stone formation, accounting for approximately 1% to 2% of all stones.[2] Cystine stones tend to be yellow, round, and radiolucent or faintly radiopaque.[2,23] Cystine stones are more common in males than females, commonly appear in the second decade of life with the median onset at age 12, and ultimately can lead to kidney failure.[11,23]

Xanthinuria is caused by two conditions: an inherited deficiency of the enzyme xanthine oxidase, and an accelerated purine metabolism pathway (Lesh-Nyan syndrome), which results in stone formation and increased excretion of xanthine.[22] These stones are radiolucent and are often mistaken for uric acid stones.[2]

Lastly, stone formation is encouraged by anatomic abnormalities that reduce urine flow or cause stasis, including horseshoe kidney, genitourinary diverticula, obstructive disorders, and medullary sponge kidney.[2] Renal and urinary calculi can range from simple to complex in composition; identification of the cause of the stone can be challenging until a complete stone workup and formal stone analysis can be completed.

CLINICAL PRESENTATION

Symptoms vary and depend on the size and anatomic location of the stones. In general, symptoms include acute renal or ureteral colic, nausea and vomiting, hematuria (microscopic or occult blood in the urine), fever and chills, dysuria, increased urinary frequency, and vague abdominal, flank, or groin pain.[5,7,24] Individuals with calculi most commonly have hematuria and renal colic or severe flank pain that may migrate anteriorly and into the groin as the stone moves from the kidney toward the bladder.[7] Renal or ureteral colic is a result of obstruction of the urinary tract by the stone. This obstruction is usually in one or more of five locations: (1) the calyx; (2) the ureteropelvic junction; (3) at or near the pelvic brim, where the ureter begins to arch over the iliac vessels; (4) the posterior pelvis, where the ureter is crossed anteriorly by the pelvic blood vessels and the broad ligament; and (5) the ureterovesical junction, which is the most constricted area. Renal or ureteral colic is often associated with nausea and vomiting, gross hematuria, and dysuria. Fever and chills may be present if infection occurs with the stone. Patients are often extremely restless as they attempt to find a comfortable position. Less often, there may be persistent microhematuria or intermittent dull pain that lasts for weeks or months. Once a stone enters the bladder, dysuria, frequency, and urgency may be the only symptoms. Once the stone passes out of the bladder, symptoms resolve.

PHYSICAL EXAMINATION

A careful medical history should be obtained and should include personal stone history, medical problems and conditions (diabetes, gout, hyperparathyroidism, recurrent UTIs, immunosuppression, and solitary functioning kidney), surgical history (kidney transplant), medications (specifically ones that are associated with kidney stone formation: allopurinol, laxatives, topiramate, sulfonamides, quinolones, triamterene, sulfonylureas, and potassium channel blockers), family history (to include kidney stone disease), occupation, dietary habits and history, and fluid intake.[3,24] The physical examination includes assessment of systemic symptoms; meticulous abdominal examination to exclude other sources of pain, including intra-abdominal pathology (abdominal aortic aneurysm, diverticulitis, appendicitis, and gynecologic pathology), is essential.[25] Typical examination findings include fever; tachycardia; diaphoresis; pale, cool, and clammy skin; and costovertebral angle tenderness.[3]

DIAGNOSTICS

The cornerstones of diagnostics are a detailed history and physical examination, after which the appropriate urinalysis, laboratory studies, and imaging can be ordered. Urinalysis and culture and sensitivity are essential to determine pH and to identify the presence of bacteria, crystals, and red blood cells.[3,24] Hematuria may be microscopic or gross and may occur with or without infection. An increase in the urine pH and the presence of crystals may give clues as to the stone's composition and whether the stone is alkaline or acidic.[9] In addition, the urine should be strained, and if a stone is made available, stone analysis should be completed.[9] Urine pH above 7.0 suggests urea splitting microorganisms, and a urine culture should be obtained to evaluate for a UTI.[9] Urine pH below 5.4 associated with metabolic acidosis is seen in the presence of distal RTA, whereas the presence of hexagonal cystine crystals is diagnostic of cystinuria.[10,26] Further metabolic testing of the urine can be completed through the use of a 24-hour urine test. Currently there is conflicting opinion regarding whether a single 24-hour urine sample is adequate and reliable to identify abnormalities within the urine.[9] Therefore either one or two 24-hour urine samples with the patient on his or her usual diet should be obtained and measured for calcium, oxalate, citrate, magnesium, sodium, and sulfate, but two samples are preferred.[9] As part of the screening evaluation for patients with newly diagnosed renal or urinary calculi, serum chemistry should be performed. The serum chemistry will aid in evaluating underlying medical conditions (e.g., gout, hyperparathyroid) and should include sodium, potassium, chloride, bicarbonate, calcium, creatinine, and uric acid.[9] In the presence of elevated serum calcium, primary hyperparathyroidism should be suspected and parathyroid hormone (PTH) levels should be measured; vitamin D levels should be assessed because low vitamin D can mask primary or secondary hyperparathyroidism.[9] A complete blood count (CBC) may be obtained and will assist in ruling out an infectious cause.[7] Imaging is a key diagnostic tool to aid practitioners in the diagnosis and management of patients with renal and urinary calculi.[3] An abdominal x-ray study (plain film) of the kidneys, ureter, and bladder (KUB) is often the first imaging study used and will identify renal stones that are radiopaque.[3] Only about 60% of stones are found visible on plain film, but it is helpful in documenting the number, size, and location of the stones in the urinary tract.[3] A plain film is also helpful in identifying nephrocalcinosis, hyperparathyroidism, primary hyperparathyroidism, PH, RTA, or sarcoidosis.[9] The intravenous pyelogram (IVP) was previously the gold standard of imaging for kidney stones, with a detection rate near 90%, but newer, more precise imaging modalities have replaced it.[3,25] The IVP uses contrast to demonstrate the entire anatomy of the urinary tract but can detect only radiopaque stones.[3,25] Limitations of the IVP include radiation exposure, contrast reaction, lengthy study time, and a risk of nephrotoxicity.[25] Ultrasound is the imaging modality of choice for special populations such as pregnant women, children, and individuals in whom radiation is contraindicated.[3] A renal ultrasound examination will aid in diagnosis and can be used as a screening tool for hydronephrosis or stones within the ureters, kidney, or renal pelvis.[3] Renal ultrasonography can also determine the amount of renal parenchyma involved in an obstructed kidney.[25] Some recent studies have suggested that the use of ultrasonography along with a KUB study may improve the diagnostic accuracy for stones and is comparable to those observed with noncontrast CT.[25] The helical CT scan (spiral CT) is considered the gold standard radiographic tool for renal and urinary calculi, and it may be performed both with and without the administration of contrast material.[4,7,27] CT creates images of the urinary tract and shows delayed penetration of intravenous contrast material through the obstructed kidney, which is the hallmark of an acute urinary obstruction.[27] CT findings indicative of acute urinary obstruction because of a stone include renal enlargement, hydronephrosis, ureteral dilation, perinephric stranding, and periureteral edema.[25,27] In the event that a stone is not visualized with CT, secondary signs of a stone can be identified (nephromegaly, hydronephrosis, hydroureter) or an alternate diagnosis can be made from the CT findings.[25] Magnetic resonance (MR) urography can be considered, but currently there is no specific indication for its use in diagnosing and imaging kidney stones.[25]

DIAGNOSTICS

Renal and Urinary Calculi

Laboratory
Urinalysis with urine culture and sensitivity
CBC and differential*
Complete metabolic panel
PTH
Vitamin D*
24-Hour urine (for calcium oxalate, citrate, magnesium, sodium, and sulfate)*

IMAGING
Helical CT scan (gold standard)
Abdominal x-ray studies (plain film) of KUB*
Renal ultrasound (imaging of choice in children and pregnant women)
Cystoscopy*
Intravenous pyelography*
Retrograde pyelography*

OTHER DIAGNOSTICS
Urine strain for stone analysis

*If indicated.

DIFFERENTIAL DIAGNOSIS

Urolithiasis can mimic other causes of visceral pain. Therefore, in persons with abdominal symptoms, it is essential to consider other causes of abdominal and flank pain, such as appendicitis, cholecystitis, peptic ulcer, pancreatitis, ectopic pregnancy, and dissecting aortic aneurysm. Other diagnoses to consider are listed in the differential diagnosis box.

MANAGEMENT

The majority of acute renal and urinary calculi can be managed conservatively through oral hydration, pain management, and expectant stone passage.[24,25] Stone management guidelines depend on the size and location of the stone, the presence or absence of associated infection, the presence of one or two kidneys, and the severity of symptoms.[25] Most stones pass spontaneously without any residual damage.[3] Urinary calculi 1 mm or

DIFFERENTIAL DIAGNOSIS

Renal Colic Mimics

GYNECOLOGIC
- Hemorrhagic cyst
- Dermoid cyst
- Endometrioma
- Ovarian neoplasm
- Ovarian torsion
- Fibroid
- Ectopic pregnancy
- Pelvic inflammatory disease

GASTROINTESTINAL
- Appendicitis
- Diverticulitis
- Biliary disorders
- Pancreatitis
- Small bowel obstruction

UROLOGIC
- Pyelonephritis
- UTI

VASCULAR
- Abdominal aortic aneurysm with or without aortic dissection
- Renal artery thrombosis
- Renal infarction
- Mesenteric artery dissection or embolism
- Intraperitoneal or retroperitoneal hemorrhage

MUSCULOSKELETAL
- Mechanical low back pain
- Fractures

MISCELLANEOUS
- Herpes zoster infection (shingles)

Data from Rucker CM, Menias CO, Bhalia S: Mimics of renal colic: alternative diagnoses at unenhanced helical CT. *Radiographics* 24(Suppl 1):11-28, 2004.

less in diameter pass spontaneously in approximately 90% of patients. Stones 2 to 4 mm pass spontaneously in approximately 75% of patients; stones 5 to 7 mm pass spontaneously in approximately 60% of patients; stones 7 to 9 mm pass spontaneously in approximately 50%; and stones larger than 9 mm pass in only 25% of patients.[25] The shape of the kidney stone is just as important as the size; the width of the stone influences spontaneous passage.[25] Urinary calculi that have migrated to the distal ureter have a high incidence of spontaneous passage.[25] Patients with recurrent stones should undergo a stone analysis to assist in identifying the chemical composition and guide appropriate treatment.[4]

The acute management of renal colic symptoms and kidney stones should initially focus on pain relief through the use of narcotics or nonsteroidal anti-inflammatory drugs (NSAIDs).[4,25] As kidney stones pass into the ureter, pain intensifies owing to the increasing pressure on the collecting system, ureteral spasm, and renal capsular distention.[25] NSAIDs provide relief through prostaglandin inhibition, and recent literature has suggested that NSAIDs have similar efficacy as narcotics for renal colic pain.[25] Special issues need to be considered in prescribing NSAIDs, specifically in geriatric patients who have preexisting renal disease, severe dehydration, and other comorbidities that can lead to acute kidney injury.[25] Fluid therapy as part of acute stone management is something that has been used frequently. Recent literature is mixed on high-volume fluid therapy for stone management, and current evidence supports fluid volume replacement for those who are dehydrated or have increase creatinine levels.[3,25] For prevention of stone recurrence, increased water intake has been shown to reduce the supersaturation of the urine with stone-forming substances.[3] In conjunction with pain relief and adequate fluid hydration, several medical expulsion therapy medications are known to aid in the passage of kidney stones. The two most frequently used types of medications are calcium channel blockers and alpha blockers, which aid in relaxing smooth muscle and widen channels to allow stone passage.[4,25] Nifedipine and tamsulosin have been the best studied medical expulsion therapy medications and have produced stone passage rates of greater than 75%.[4] Lastly, two other medications have been used with uncertain results. Desmopressin is an antidiuretic hormone that is thought to decrease pressure from stone obstruction. However, the drug has a significant side effect profile that makes it not an ideal choice for the geriatric population or those with significant comorbidities.[25] Corticosteroids have also been used as part of the management of kidney stones, but there is no significant evidence that supports their efficacy and therefore routine use is not recommended.[25]

Larger stones were considered a major problem before the 1980s, and extensive surgical procedures were often needed. The morbidity associated with stone disease has been greatly reduced with the advent of extracorporeal techniques for stone treatment and with the refinement of endoscopic surgery. Kidney stones larger than 8 mm usually require surgical management because they will rarely pass spontaneously.[7] The three major endourologic procedures are extracorporeal shock wave lithotripsy (ESWL), percutaneous nephrolithotomy (PCNL), and ureteroscopy (URS).[4] ESWL is the least invasive treatment and is the treatment of choice for 75% to 85% of patients with retained stones.[7,25] It is indicated for stones that cannot be passed spontaneously, can be visualized on x-ray film, are located in the renal pelvis or upper ureter, and are smaller than 2 cm.[25,28] PCNL is the treatment of choice for complex renal and proximal ureteral calculi larger than 2 cm or when simple renal calculi do not respond to ESWL.[7,28] URS is used mainly in the ureter and involves the use of a fiberoptic scope through the urethra to relieve obstruction, allow basket extraction of stones, or use a laser or lithotripsy to break apart the stone.[4,28]

Calcium stones are the most complex of all stones in their causes and treatments. The accepted theory regarding their cause is an imbalance between urinary excretion of insoluble salts and water, which results in an environment of supersaturation.[11] Therefore, treatment is aimed at raising the urine flow rate and reducing excretion of stone-forming salts. Stone formation associated with idiopathic hypercalciuria can be decreased with a twice-daily dose of thiazides and a normal-calcium (1000 to 1200 mg/day), low-protein, low-sodium diet.[9] The use of thiazides (hydrochlorothiazide, 25 mg orally twice daily or 50 mg orally once daily; chlorthalidone, 25 mg orally once daily; indapamide, 2.5 mg orally once daily) has been shown to be beneficial in preventing renal stones because thiazide diuretics decrease urinary calcium excretion by augmenting tubular reabsorption of calcium, but do not decrease intestinal absorption in absorptive hypercalciuria.[9,29] Although the role of allopurinol is not well understood in the prevention of calcium stones, it has been shown to reduce the risk of recurrent calcium oxalate stones.[9] Calcium stones associated with hyperparathyroidism are best prevented by treatment of the underlying condition; referral to an endocrinologist is indicated (Fig. 152-1).[9]

The main cause of hyperoxaluria seems to be related to diet and is most easily regulated by omitting foods high in oxalate, such as colas, chocolate, and peanuts. Management of hyperoxaluria related to bowel disease and malabsorption syndromes is multifaceted and may include a low-fat diet, restrictive oxalate intake, and administration of calcium.[9] Pyridoxine (vitamin B_6)

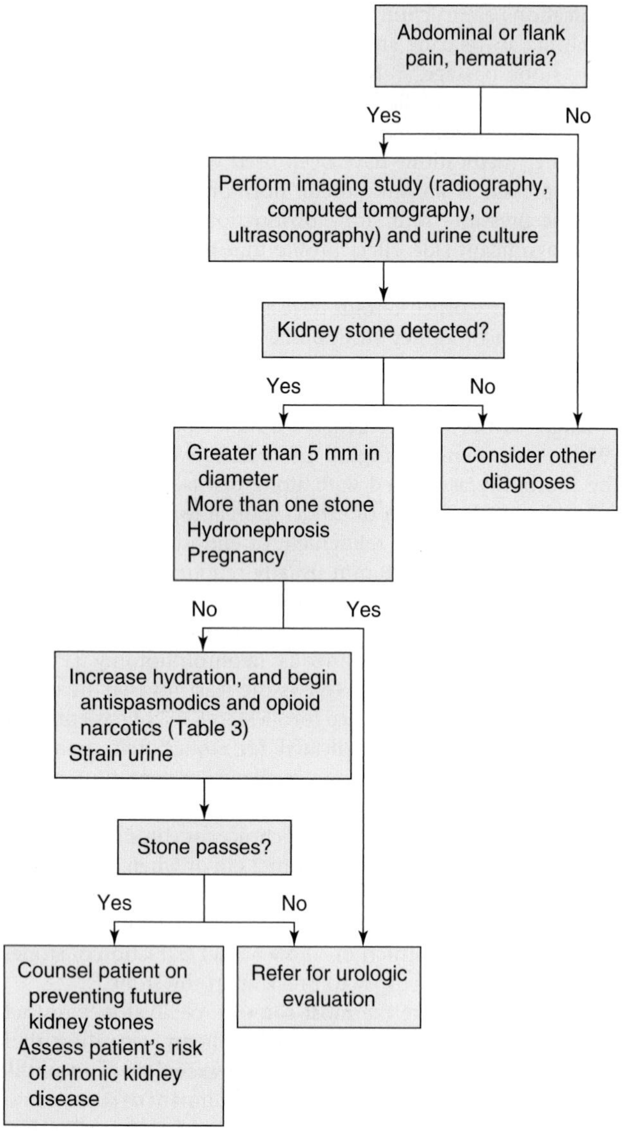

FIGURE **152-1** Diagnosis and management of acute kidney stones. (From Frassetto L, Kohlstadt I: Treatment and prevention of kidney stones: an update. *Am Fam Physician* 84[11]:1234-1242, 2011.)

may reduce the production of oxalate by reducing enzyme activity; in one epidemiologic study, high intake of vitamin B_6 (>40 mg/day) was inversely associated with oxalate stone formation in women.[29]

Hyperuricosuria, which is associated with calcium oxalate stones, is most simply managed by reducing the intake of foods that cause elevated uric acid excretion. Persistent stone formation may be treated with allopurinol to inhibit uric acid synthesis and to decrease urinary uric acid excretion.[29] Potassium citrate should also be given to increase urine pH because uric acid precipitates in acidic urine; potassium citrate has been shown to benefit calcium phosphate stone formers with hypocitraturia.[9]

Uric acid stones are managed most practically by maintaining a urinary output of more than 2.5 L/day and alkalinizing the urine.[21] Previously, allopurinol was offered as initial therapy for uric acid stones, but more recently first-line therapy is aimed at alkalinizing the urine with potassium citrate.[9] The initial dose of potassium citrate is 30 to 40 mEq/day with a maximum daily dose of 100 mEq/day.[21] A secondary choice of alkalinizing agent is sodium citrate or bicarbonate for those who do not tolerate potassium citrate.[21] Allopurinol, which inhibits the formation of uric acid, is reserved for use in uric acid stone treatment when diet control and alkalinizing agents fail to control the condition; the commonly used dose is 100 to 300 mg daily.

Management of magnesium ammonium phosphate (struvite) stones has centrally focused on eliminating urease-producing bacteria within the urine and stones that are colonized with bacteria.[29] Antimicrobial therapy to sterilize the urine is necessary to treat the infection, and, if needed, surgical intervention is required to remove the colonized stone.[29] Urease inhibitors may be used to prevent struvite formation or to slow the growth of existing calculi. The most commonly used urease inhibitor is acetohydroxamic acid (AHA).[29] It is an irreversible inhibitor of urease and can prevent the crystallization of struvite stones. However, because of its associated risk of deep venous thrombosis, it is generally reserved for patients who cannot tolerate surgical interventions.[9,29] Hydroxyurea, once thought to be a potent inhibitor, is no longer considered effective and also has demonstrated high toxicity rates. To adequately sterilize the urine, it is paramount that surgical intervention be performed to remove the offending stone.

Prevention of cystine stones includes reduced intake of protein-rich foods, low sodium intake (≤2300 mg daily), and high intake of fluids (4 L/day).[9] The mainstay of cystic stone treatment is the combination of urinary alkalinization and thiol binding medications.[29] D-Penicillamine and tiopronin (Thiola) have been shown in several studies to effectively decrease the number of recurrent stones in patients who are cystinuric stone formers.[29] Among the more common side effects of long-term D-penicillamine therapy is vitamin B_{12} deficiency. Tiopronin has fewer side effects but still poses some risk for hematologic changes, fever, proteinuria, and rash.[29] For patients who are taking these medications, specific laboratory testing should be completed at least twice a year (CBC, liver function tests, and urine protein/creatinine ratios).[29]

COMPLICATIONS

Renal calculi are associated with an increased risk of UTIs with the potential for progression to pyelonephritis, sepsis, or chronic kidney disease.[24] Hydronephrosis, which is associated with partial or complete obstruction of the renal pelvis or ureter, is another possible complication. Additional potential sequelae include renal tissue damage, scarring, and renal failure as a result of obstruction or stone movement and nephrocalcinosis as a result of deposition of calcium phosphate in the renal parenchyma.[15,25]

INDICATIONS FOR REFERRAL OR HOSPITALIZATION

Management of kidney or urinary tract stones often requires both medical and surgical interventions. Specific treatment depends on a number of factors, including stone type and location.

- The presence of infection, obstruction, urosepsis, acute renal failure, anuria, or retractable pain is an indication for emergent urologic referral or hospitalization.[25]

- Severe obstruction, infection, pain, and serious bleeding may necessitate hospitalization. Urgent urology referral follow-up within 1 to 2 days should be considered for patients in a nonacute condition with nonobstructing kidney stones who also have a UTI.[25]
- A patient with a kidney stone larger than 10 mm in whom conservative therapy fails and who does not pass the stone, who has a history of multiple stones, or who has uncontrolled pain should follow up with a urologist in 5 to 7 days.[25]
- Patients with persistent pain, gross hematuria, fever, or chills should be referred to a urologist.[25]

LIFE SPAN CONSIDERATIONS

Two special populations of individuals in whom kidney stones may develop are children and pregnant women. More children have been developing kidney stones; this is thought to be related to the rise in childhood obesity.[24] The development of kidney stones in children should raise a red flag because these stones are more likely the result of a genetic, anatomic, or metabolic abnormality.[24] Children who develop cystinuria or other forms of hereditary kidney stones at risk to develop impaired renal function.[24]

The development of kidney stones during pregnancy is increased owing to urinary stasis, elevated progesterone levels, and decreased bladder capacity.[25] Calcium phosphate stones occur more frequently in women than any other type of kidney stone, and stones occur more often in the second and third trimesters.[24] Ultrasound is the diagnostic imaging modality of choice for evaluating pregnant women with kidney stones.[24] The majority of kidney stones will pass spontaneously, but pregnant women have an increased risk of UTIs, and those who are symptomatic have double the risk for preterm labor.[24] If surgical intervention is indicated, ESWL is contraindicated, but ureteroscopic stone removal can be used and has similar safety outcomes as in nonpregnant women.[25]

EDUCATION AND HEALTH PROMOTION

Patients suspected of having stones should be instructed to increase fluid intake, to strain all urine, and to use analgesics as necessary. An emphasis on healthy lifestyle habits, such as regular exercise, generous fluid intake (2 to 4 L/day), and a balanced diet high in fiber, is integral to stone prevention.[11] Effective stone prevention depends on the stone type and identification of risk factors for stone formation. Therefore, specific patient education is based on individual risk factors, the type of stone produced by the patient, a prescribed medical regimen, and comorbidities. Research has demonstrated that obesity is a significant factor in stone formation owing to dietary choices such as low fluid intake, high-oxalate foods, protein-rich foods, and refined sugars and overall increases the risk for uric acid stones.[14] Therefore the importance of exercise and weight management must be emphasized as a recommendation to reduce stone risk, but also to improve renal function and insulin sensitivity.[14] Patients should be informed that the basic approach to stone management and prevention is a delicate balance among fluid hydration, a diet low in sodium and low in animal protein, and potential limitation of oxalate-rich and high-purine foods.

CHAPTER 153

URINARY TRACT INFECTIONS AND SEXUALLY TRANSMITTED INFECTIONS

Joann D. Lepke

URINARY TRACT INFECTIONS

DEFINITION AND EPIDEMIOLOGY

Urinary tract infection (UTI) is a broad term used to describe acute or chronic infection and/or inflammation of the bladder (cystitis), urethra, prostate, ureter, or kidney (pyelonephritis) with microbial colonization of the urine.[1] UTIs have six categories of classification: uncomplicated, complicated, isolated, unresolved, reinfection, and relapse.[2] UTIs are considered complicated if they include the presence of pyuria, positive urine culture, fever, or structural or functional abnormality of the urinary tract or if they occur in the presence of urinary catheterization. All UTIs in males are considered complicated.[3] Uncomplicated UTIs include those typically occurring in otherwise healthy, immunocompetent, nonpregnant women with no significant history of UTIs or structural abnormalities and are characterized by recent onset of mild to moderate symptoms.

Infection of the urinary tract is one of the most common diagnoses seen in primary care, and the most frequent urologic disorder encountered.[4] These infections are responsible for more than 7 million office visits yearly in the United States, with costs exceeding $1 billion per year.[5]

UTIs are a particular problem in certain patient groups, with young, sexually active women and elderly individuals being disproportionately affected.[4] Fifty percent of women have reported having at least one UTI by age 32. There are 1000 to 4000 cases of UTI per 100,000 females annually, and fewer than 100 cases per 100,000 men.[6] Most of these infections are sporadic, with about 25% being recurrent infections.[1] Over 33% of infections in long-term care facilities are attributed to UTIs, and UTI is one of the most common diagnoses in older adults.[7,8] The risk of having a UTI in childhood is 2% in boys and 8% in girls. Uncircumcised boys younger than 6 months are at a higher risk to have a UTI than circumcised boys in the same age group.[9] Overall, 3% to 8% of girls and 1% to 2% of boys will have a UTI.[4]

UTIs are unusual in men younger than 50 years with normal urologic structures but become more common with age. Common reasons for UTIs in men include prostatitis, epididymitis, orchitis, pyelonephritis, cystitis, and urethritis. Risk factors associated with UTI in men include previous UTI; enlarged prostate; history of instrumentation, catheterization, or surgery of the urinary tract; human immunodeficiency virus (HIV) infection; comorbidities; immunosuppression; abnormalities or family history of abnormalities in the urinary tract; and anal intercourse.[10] After the age of 65 years, the incidence of UTIs in men is about 10%, whereas the incidence is 20% in similarly aged women.[11] Asymptomatic bacteriuria refers to a colony count of at least 100,000/mL in the absence of symptoms. It is estimated that 8% of women have asymptomatic bacteriuria.[2] It is more common in women, increases in both sexes with advancing age, and is found in as many as 43% of older women and 21% of older men, especially those living in nursing homes. In addition to advancing age and nursing home residence, asymptomatic bacteriuria is also associated with pregnancy, history of indwelling catheterization, instrumentation, urinary incontinence, diabetes, multiple medical illnesses, obstructive uropathy, postmenopausal status, and impaired functional and mental status.[12]

PATHOPHYSIOLOGY

Most UTIs in women are secondary to ascending infection from the periurethral or perianal area. Bacteria from the colon, vagina, or skin are the usual organisms causing the infection.[13] Cystitis is more common in women than in men because of the short length of the urethra and the proximity of the urethral opening and vagina to the perianal area. Bacteria reach the bladder through the urethra and have the opportunity to ascend to the kidneys through the ureters.[14]

A relatively narrow spectrum of microorganisms cause the majority of UTIs. The most prominent pathogens are gram-negative organisms including *Escherichia coli, Klebsiella pneumoniae, Proteus mirabilis,* and *Pseudomonas aeruginosa. E. coli* represents 75% to 95% of infections in the bladder and ureters in normal genitourinary tracts. *Staphylococcus saprophyticus* is a species of gram-positive bacteria responsible for about 5% to 10% of uncomplicated bacterial UTIs.[10] Nosocomial infections are caused by *E. coli* about 50% of the time; 40% of occurrences are caused by *Klebsiella, Proteus, Enterobacter, Pseudomonas,* and *Serratia aeruginosa;* 10% are caused by *Enterococcus faecalis, S. saprophyticus,* and *Staphylococcus aureus. Pseudomonas* is responsible for most UTIs found in catheterized patients.[10,13] See Table 153-1 for a tabular representation of the causes of UTI.

Most UTIs in women are not associated with complicating conditions or serious problems. Common precipitants include sexual intercourse, use of spermicidal agents, impaired voiding, recent antibiotic use, and estrogen deficiency. UTIs frequently occur in individuals with diabetes, obesity, urinary tract calculi, sickle cell trait, and frequent or indwelling bladder catheterization.[6] In men, the reservoirs of microorganisms are not in close proximity to the urethral opening as in women; anatomic abnormalities of the urinary tract are more likely associated with UTIs in men. Risk factors associated with UTI in men include lack of circumcision, anal intercourse, HIV infection, and prostatic hypertrophy.[15]

Urethritis is characterized by an inflammation (mechanical, chemical, viral, or bacterial) of the urethra. Nongonococcal urethritis (NGU) is most common, with *Chlamydia* being the most frequent causative organism. Other urethral pathogens include *Ureaplasma urealyticum, Mycoplasma hominis,* herpes simplex virus (HSV), cytomegalovirus, and, in women, *Trichomonas vaginalis* and *Gardnerella vaginalis.* Noninfectious causes include Stevens-Johnson syndrome, Wegener granulomatosis, use of spermicides, and ingestion of some acidic foods.[12] Risk factors for urethritis include being a man aged 20 to 35, being a female of reproductive age, having multiple sexual partners, engaging in high-risk sexual behavior, and having a history of a sexually transmitted disease (STD).[15]

Children's bladders hold a small quantity of urine compared with an adult. Constipation is a greater risk factor for UTI in children, because hard stool may further reduce the capacity of the bladder and/or restrict the flow of urine. Bacteria have a better opportunity to grow in these conditions.[9]

Risk factors for UTIs are listed in Boxes 153-1 and 153-2.

CLINICAL PRESENTATION

UTIs can be subdivided into several distinct classifications: uncomplicated, complicated, isolated, unresolved, reinfection, and relapse. Different characteristics are associated with each of these categories.

Uncomplicated UTIs are characterized by signs and symptoms of bladder irritation: increased frequency, urgency, dysuria, suprapubic pain, odorous urine, and occasionally hematuria. The term *uncomplicated infection* implies that this is a relatively uncommon occurrence in the affected individual who is also otherwise healthy, that there are a small number of responsible pathogens susceptible to first-line narrow-spectrum antimicrobial agents, and that there are no underlying urologic or gynecologic abnormalities.

TABLE 153-1 Common Bacteria Responsible for Urinary Tract Infections

	Normal Genitourinary Tracts	Nosocomial Infections	Catheterized Patients	Diabetic Patients
GRAM-NEGATIVE BACTERIA				
Escherichia coli	75%-95%	50%		
Klebsiella pneumonia	0%-20%	40%		Frequent
Proteus mirabilis				
Pseudomonas aeruginosa			Most common	
Serratia				
GRAM-POSITIVE BACTERIA				
Enterococcus faecalis	5%-10%	10%		
Staphylococcus saprophyticus				
Staphylococcus aureus				
Group B *Streptococcus*				Frequent

Data from U.S. Department of Health and Human Services Food and Drug Administration, Center for Drug Evaluation and Research: *Guidance for industry complicated urinary tract infections: developing drugs for treatment;* draft guidance, clinical/antimicrobial revision 1. 2012, pp. 1-30; and Imam TH: Bacterial urinary tract infections. In *Merck manual for health care professionals.* Merck Sharp & Dohme Corp, November 2013. Available at: www.merckmanuals.com/professional/genitourinary_disorders/urinary_tract_infections_uti/bacterial_urinary_tract_infections.html. Accessed August 2, 2014.

A more acute presentation, including high fever, chills, flank pain, costovertebral angle (CVA) tenderness, nausea, and vomiting, is suggestive of complicated UTI (pyelonephritis or urosepsis). A sustained bladder infection increases the risk for a complicated infection. However, kidney infection may also manifest with only bladder irritation and the absence of any of the classic signs or symptoms. Pyuria in the presence of positive urine or blood culture is indicative of a complicated UTI. Risks associated with complicated UTI include presence of urinary catheter, residual urine of 100 mL or more after voiding, obstruction in the urinary tract, azotemia resulting from kidney disease, and urinary retention.[3]

UTI is considered isolated with the first occurrence or a repeat occurrence at least 6 months from the previous episode. About 25% to 40% of infections are considered isolated. Unresolved infections persist when prescribed medications are not effective because of drug resistance or the presence of more than one organism with different drug sensitivities.[2] UTIs are considered recurrent if they occur at least three times in 1 year or twice in 6 months.[4] There are two basic patterns of recurrence: relapse and reinfection. Relapse refers to infection caused by bacterial persistence—infection by the previously treated pathogen, which was not completely eradicated by the course of antimicrobial therapy. Reinfection refers to recurrence of infection by introduction of a new bacterial strain or regrowth of the same organism after complete eradication with treatment. Recurrent UTIs in women are usually are a result of reinfection rather than relapse, but it is difficult to determine reinfection versus relapse.[16] Groups often bothered by recurrent infections are listed in Table 153-2.[2]

In men, symptoms of urethritis are usually mild and gradual in onset and include dysuria and irritative symptoms, frequency, urethral discharge, and pruritus at the distal end of the penis. Women may experience vaginal discharge or bleeding from concomitant cervicitis and lower abdominal pain. Urinalysis often demonstrates pyuria and less commonly, hematuria. Urine cultures generally show a colony count of less than 100/mL in urethritis.

BOX 153-1

Risk Factors for Urinary Tract Infections

WOMEN
- Inherent anatomic risk (4-cm urethra in females versus 20-cm urethra in males)
- Fecal contamination
- History of recent urinary tract infection
- Decreased fluid intake
- Irregular bladder emptying
- Vaginal pH >4.5
- Sexual intercourse
- Failure to void within 10-15 minutes of coitus
- Spermicide use
- Symptomatic partner
- Pregnancy
- Menopause
- Hyperuricemia
- Neurogenic bladder
- Kidney disease
- Urologic abnormalities
- Instrumentation
- Immunosuppression
- Comorbidities (e.g., diabetes)

MEN
- Urologic abnormalities
- Neurogenic bladder
- Instrumentation
- Benign prostatic hyperplasia
- Anal intercourse
- Immunosuppression
- Comorbidities (e.g., diabetes)

CHILDREN
- Constipation
- Anatomic abnormalities
- Dysfunctional voiding
- Immunosuppression

PHYSICAL EXAMINATION

Important history to elicit from the woman with complaints of UTI symptoms includes urinary frequency, nocturia, dysuria,

BOX 153-2

Risks for Recurrent Urinary Tract Infections

WOMEN

Current Conditions
- Sexually active
- Immunosuppression
- Pregnancy
- Spermicide use
- New sexual partner
- Voiding problems

Past Medical History
- Post-coital UTI symptoms
- Pyelonephritis
- UTI in pregnancy

MEN
- Immunosuppression
- Voiding problems

Data from Al-Badr A, Al-Shaikh G: Recurrent urinary tract infections, management in women. A Review. *Sultan Qaboos Univ Med J* 13(3):359-367, 2013.

TABLE 153-2 **Outpatient Oral Antibiotic Treatment Regimens for Acute Bacterial Urinary Tract Infection in Nonpregnant Adults**

Antimicrobial Agent	Dose (Uncomplicated Infection)	Dose (Complicated Infection)*
Nitrofurantoin monohydrate, macrocrystals	100 mg twice daily for 5 days	
Trimethoprim-sulfamethoxazole (TMP-SMX)	1 double-strength tab 160 mg TMP/800 mg SMX twice daily for 3 days (avoid if used within last 3 months, or >20% resistance)	1 double-strength tab, 160 mg TMP/800 mg SMX twice daily for 14 days
Fosfomycin tromethamine	3 g, single dose	
Ciprofloxacin	250 mg twice daily for 3 days†	500 mg twice daily for 7 days
Levofloxacin	250 mg once daily for 3 days†	750 mg once daily for 5 days
Ofloxacin	200 mg twice daily for 3 days†	200 mg twice daily for 10 days

*Men should be treated for a minimum of 10-14 days, preferably with fluoroquinolones.
†Use in uncomplicated UTI only if nitrofurantoin, TMP-SMX. or fosfomycin is contraindicated.
From Gupta K, Hooton TM, Naber KG, et al: International clinical practice guidelines for the treatment of acute uncomplicated cystitis and pyelonephritis in women: a 2010 update by the Infectious Diseases Society of America and the European Society for Microbiology and Infectious Diseases. *Clin Infect Dis* 2011 52(5):e103-e120, 2011.

pruritus, fever or chills, hematuria, vaginal discomfort or discharge, pelvic discomfort, back or flank pain, date of last menstrual period, any prior history of UTIs, cervicitis, or pelvic inflammatory disease (PID). Patients should be queried about medical history, specifically immunocompromising disease or drugs, and recent instrumentation. A recent study has shown that women with a history of UTI correctly diagnose themselves (as confirmed by urine culture) as having a UTI 61% to 90% of the time.[17]

Vaginal symptoms, external irritation on urination, and dyspareunia are helpful in sorting out vaginal causes from those referable to the urinary tract. Male patients should be asked about urethral discharge, penile lesions, history of UTIs or sexually transmitted infections (STIs), and prior treatment. It is important to ask all patients about sexual history and risk factors for gonorrhea or chlamydia, including new or symptomatic sex partners.

The physical examination should include assessment of vital signs, signs and symptoms of acute illness, and dehydration. A careful abdominal examination including the assessment of CVA tenderness is an important aspect of the physical examination. A pelvic examination in females should be performed if there is any indication that infection is not solely associated with the urinary tract. The vulva, vagina, cervix, periurethral area, and perianal area should be assessed for discharge, excoriations, tenderness, and ulcerations. In male patients, the penis should be checked for discharge, lesions, ulcerations, and swelling. The prostate should be checked for tenderness, swelling, masses, or nodules. A rectal examination showing a tender prostate may be indicative of acute prostatitis, and a normal or enlarged prostate indicates chronic bacterial prostatitis.

The presence of cloudy urine, dysuria, and nocturia in women has shown a positive predictive value of greater than 80% for presence of UTI.[18] Approximately half of women with one UTI symptom actually have the infection.[4] Malodorous urine is not found to be indicative of infection.[18] The diagnosis of UTI is suggested by the history and physical examination findings and confirmed by examination of the urine.

DIAGNOSTICS

The urinalysis is the most important initial study, with a urine dipstick as a reasonable rapid diagnostic aid. A clean-voided specimen minimizes contamination from nearby sources. Leukocyte esterase reflects the presence of white blood cells (WBCs) in the urine, but not all UTIs are associated with WBCs in the urine. Evidence-based guidelines from the University of Michigan Quality Management Program report that the presence of pyuria has a sensitivity of 80% to 90% and a specificity of 50% in predicting UTI. The nitrite test is not as good at detecting UTI; not all bacteria produce nitrate reductase, and false-positive results may occur with intake of ascorbic acid.[5] However, in a more recent study of older women, these dipstick findings only resulted in 57% with a positive urine culture.[19] In addition to leukocyte esterase and urinary nitrite, the presence of blood on the dipstick is another variable that is useful in predicting the presence of a UTI. In a study on the sensitivity and specificity of dipstick variables, the presence of nitrites was most predictive, followed by leukocytes with blood.[20]

Urine may also be examined microscopically, which allows easier detection of red blood cells, WBCs, bacteria, and WBC casts. Correlation with subsequent culture is approximately 90%. This diagnostic is typically ordered by the provider and performed by a laboratory before culturing. Abnormalities of pH, protein, and blood are nonspecific with respect to UTIs. In the presence of symptoms but a negative dipstick result, direct demonstration by microscopy or culture should be done before the possibility of infection is excluded.

Urine culture is the definitive test; specimens should be obtained from all patients who are pregnant, are febrile, are seriously ill, have a history of frequent UTIs, live in a community with high rates of antibiotic resistance, or have recently been hospitalized, or in whom empirical treatment has failed.[21] Cultures should be obtained in young men because these infections are unusual and suggestive of underlying problems.

The presence of multiple bacterial species identified by culture usually suggests contamination of the specimen, except in the case of catheterization or other special circumstances. Small numbers of certain pathogens, including *Klebsiella* organisms and *E. coli*, should be regarded as suspicious. Large numbers of skin flora, such as *Staphylococcus epidermidis*, diphtheroids, and β-hemolytic streptococci, can usually be ignored. Anaerobic bacteria do not usually cause UTIs; their presence suggests communication from the bowel. *Candida* organisms usually suggest vaginal contamination.

Sterile pyuria is defined as a negative urine culture despite a positive urinalysis (e.g., positive leukocyte esterase). This condition requires further investigation because the absence of pathogens on culture does not imply the absence of infection. Renal tuberculosis, systemic illness, vaginal contamination, and kidney stones can also cause leukocytosis in the absence of a positive culture. Some infectious organisms, such as those causing NGU, do not grow on standard laboratory media. Cultures specific for these organisms should be considered if the history and physical examination findings suggest a chlamydial or nongonococcal cause. However, many patients with urethral syndrome do not have a demonstrable infectious agent even when special culture media are used. Test of cure urine cultures should be obtained in men and whenever there is suspicion that an infection may not have been eradicated. Routine test of cure cultures are not indicated unless a persistent UTI is suspected. The recurrence of a UTI within 2 weeks is suggestive of a persistent UTI.[22]

Renal ultrasound is useful to diagnose structural abnormalities, calculi, masses, and hydronephrosis. Persistent UTIs require more extensive urologic evaluation with referral to a urologist. Indications for ultrasound evaluation of patients with UTIs include frequent recurrent UTIs in females or failure to eradicate infection despite appropriate therapy; acute pyelonephritis in males; recurrent pyelonephritis in females; and palpable bladder or renal mass. Ultrasound is recommended for children younger than 2 years with their first febrile UTI, patients of any age with recurrent febrile UTIs, patients with a family history of kidney or urologic problems, and children with high blood pressure or retarded growth.[23]

DIFFERENTIAL DIAGNOSIS

The differential diagnosis of an acute uncomplicated UTI includes urethritis, vaginal infections, STIs that may lead to cervicitis or PID, and other STIs that may mimic symptoms of UTI but are considered distinct from UTIs. The diagnosis is usually made on the basis of the history, presenting signs and symptoms, and findings on urinalysis and culture. In the case of a negative urine dipstick result in the presence of urinary symptoms, microscopic evaluation or culture should be performed before it is decided that a UTI is not present. The combination of cervical discharge, cervical motion tenderness, and adnexal tenderness suggests cervicitis or PID. Atrophic vaginitis should be considered in a postmenopausal woman not using topical estrogen therapy. Chlamydial and gonorrheal cultures should be obtained in sexually active individuals.

Clinical syndromes in women that mimic UTIs include acute urethral syndrome (also referred to as symptomatic abacteriuria) and interstitial cystitis. Clinical presentation is characterized by bladder irritation, frequency, urgency, and dysuria. The urinalysis is often unimpressive, with few leukocytes, no bacteria, and occasionally hematuria. Urine cultures show no significant colony counts, and urethral cultures are often negative. Symptoms of interstitial cystitis also include suprapubic discomfort, especially with a full bladder, and symptoms are often relieved with voiding. No definitive therapy for interstitial cystitis has been developed.

The differential diagnoses for chronic or recurrent UTIs include structural abnormalities (such as obstructive uropathy, congenital anomalies, urinary tract fistulas), neurologic dysfunction, renal calculi and renal masses, intrarenal and perirenal abscesses, bladder tuberculosis, and prostate enlargement in men.

DIFFERENTIAL DIAGNOSIS

Urinary Tract Infections

ACUTE URINARY TRACT INFECTIONS

Genitourinary
- Urethritis
- Vaginitis
- Cervicitis
- PID
- Herpes simplex
- Acute urethral syndrome
- Interstitial cystitis
- Epididymitis
- Orchitis
- Prostatitis
- Pregnancy
- Urolithiasis
- Gonorrhea, chlamydia

Gastrointestinal
- Bowel dysfunction
- Appendicitis
- Pancreatitis

Neurologic
- Neurogenic bladder

CHRONIC URINARY TRACT INFECTIONS

Genitourinary
- Chronic pelvic pain syndrome and prostatodynia
- Benign prostate hyperplasia
- Sarcoidosis, tuberculosis, granulomatous diseases
- Urinary tract obstruction
- Vesicoureteral reflux
- Intrarenal or perirenal abscess
- Overactive bladder
- Genitourinary cancer
- Polycystic kidney disease

Gastrointestinal
- Bowel dysfunction

Neurologic
- Neurogenic bladder

MANAGEMENT

Specialist referral is indicated for complicated UTIs; consideration to hospitalize should be discussed.

Indications for urology referral include presence of macroscopic hematuria, suspected malignancy, recurrent UTIs or infections that do not respond to standard antimicrobial therapy, urinary tract anomalies or obstructions, acute scrotum, and all forms of prostatitis. Hospitalization is recommended for pregnant women with pyelonephritis.[24]

TABLE 153-3 Oral Antibiotic Treatment Options for Urinary Tract Infection During Pregnancy

Antibiotic	Pregnancy Category	Dose
Amoxicillin	B	500 mg, twice daily for 7 days
Amoxicillin-clavulanate	B	500/125 mg twice daily for 7 days
Fosfomycin tromethamine	B	3 g in single dose
Cefuroxime	B	250 mg twice daily for 7 days
Cephalexin	B	500 mg twice daily for 7 days
Nitrofurantoin monohydrate/macrocrystals	B (avoid during first trimester)[26] X (38-42 weeks' gestation)	100 mg twice daily for 7 days

1. Uncomplicated UTIs are typically managed on an outpatient basis with oral antibiotics. Recommended antimicrobials for treatment of UTI are shown in Table 153-2.[25]
2. UTI in males should be treated with fluoroquinolones for 10 to 14 days. Acute bacterial prostatitis requires 2 weeks of oral antibiotic treatment with trimethoprim-sulfamethoxazole (TMP-SMX) or fluoroquinolones. Chronic bacterial prostatitis may require 4 to 6 weeks of treatment.
3. UTI in pregnancy: see Table 153-3 for antimicrobial choices. TMP-SMX is no longer recommended for UTI in pregnancy because it is pregnancy risk factor D and may be associated with increased risk of congenital malformations.[26]
4. UTIs in children are commonly treated with the antimicrobials.
5. Phenazopyridine may be prescribed along with an antibiotic as a urinary analgesic. The adult dosage is 200 mg orally after meals for 2 to 3 days; the drug is pregnancy risk factor B. The children's dosage is 12 mg/kg/day in three divided doses for 2 to 3 days.
6. The effectiveness of specific nonpharmacologic therapies, especially cranberry juice, is still unclear, although the consensus of the lay public is that cranberry juice is helpful in treating and preventing UTIs. A recent literature review (2013) found insufficient evidence to recommend the use of cranberry juice for management of UTI.[27]
7. Recurrent cystitis can be managed by one of several strategies: continuous prophylaxis, postcoital prophylaxis, or therapy initiated by the patient. Prophylaxis should not be initiated until the existing UTI has been eradicated, confirmed with negative culture 1 to 2 weeks after treatment. Recommended antibiotics include TMP-SMX, nitrofurantoin, cephalexin, trimethoprim, or a quinolone.[28]
8. Postmenopausal women who experience recurrent UTIs may find symptomatic relief with topical estrogen cream.
9. Co-management with a urologist is recommended for patients with frequent recurrent or relapsing UTIs. In addition, those with underlying functional, metabolic, or structural

urologic abnormalities, which increase the risk of UTIs, should be managed in conjunction with a specialist.

Complications

The most common complication of UTI is pyelonephritis, a bacterial infection of the kidney resulting from ascending, untreated or inadequately treated lower UTI. Pyelonephritis can be treated effectively on an outpatient basis, and clinical response should occur within 48 to 72 hours of starting therapy. If no improvement is noted or if the patient's condition worsens, aggressive investigation for complications of renal infection or urinary obstruction should be undertaken, which generally requires hospitalization. Acute pyelonephritis is the most common serious medical complication of pregnancy, and 1% to 2% of pregnant women are admitted for this condition despite perinatal screening and treatment for bacteriuria.[29] Urosepsis is a potentially life-threatening systemic complication of UTI that requires hospitalization with high-dose parenteral antimicrobial therapy.

Acute urinary infections may be associated with severe complications and even death, particularly in patients with underlying comorbidities such as diabetes and in those with indwelling urologic devices or chronic disease. Individuals with diabetes are also more likely to develop rare complications, such as emphysematous cystitis and pyelonephritis, abscess formation, and renal papillary necrosis, compared with those who do not have diabetes mellitus.

Indications for Referral or Hospitalization

Any patient who appears acutely ill or with signs and symptoms of obstruction or urosepsis requires immediate hospitalization. Specific signs and symptoms requiring consideration for hospitalization or referral include rigors, high fever, flank pain, nausea, and vomiting.

Older adults and those with acute, severe symptoms are candidates for hospitalization and often require parenteral therapy. A history of diabetes mellitus, sickle cell anemia, nephrolithiasis, or excessive analgesic use increases the risk of renal papillary necrosis and subsequent obstruction and can be considered an indication for hospitalization.

LIFE SPAN CONSIDERATIONS

Asymptomatic UTIs are more prevalent in pregnant women. The U.S. Preventive Services Task Force recommends screening at the first prenatal visit or at 12 to 16 weeks' gestation with urine culture. Prompt treatment of infection is indicated in these women to decrease the risk of acute pyelonephritis, premature delivery, and low birth weight.[21]

UTIs are the most common cause of bacterial infection in older adults but are often not accompanied by the classic signs and symptoms. Symptoms are often subtle and may include a vague change in mental status, decreased appetite, lethargy, and increased falls (sustained during efforts to get to the bathroom). UTIs are also the most common cause of sepsis, the second most common cause of bacteremia in the geriatric population, and an important cause of morbidity and mortality in nursing facilities.[30]

PATIENT AND FAMILY EDUCATION

Nonpharmacologic measures have been demonstrated to prevent episodic or recurrent UTIs. Sexual intercourse and failure to void within 10 to 15 minutes after coitus are two factors most consistently associated with UTIs. In discussing the association between these two factors and UTIs with a patient, the provider must distinguish between UTIs and STIs. Drinking plenty of fluids (64 to 80 ounces daily), urinating frequently (at least every 4 hours), wiping from front to back, and using tampons during menstruation may also be helpful in preventing UTIs. Avoiding the following will help in the prevention of UTIs: using of sanitary napkins during menstruation, wiping more than once with the same tissue, extended soaking in a bathtub, wearing tight-fitting underwear made of nonbreathable fabric, and using spermicidal products. Women who have had previous UTIs should be encouraged to seek treatment as soon as symptoms are recognized.[31]

Women with recurrent UTIs should be educated about the possible benefits of antimicrobial suppression or postcoital prophylaxis, depending on the situation. Intravaginal estrogen cream may be helpful for postmenopausal women with recurrent UTIs. Patients should be informed that no reliable evidence is available showing that cranberry ingestion is associated with prevention of UTIs.[32]

SEXUALLY TRANSMITTED INFECTIONS

DEFINITION AND EPIDEMIOLOGY

The terms *sexually transmitted infection* and *sexually transmitted disease* are used interchangeably. They encompass more than 25 infectious organisms that are transmitted through sexual activity along with the dozens of clinical syndromes associated with these organisms. The most common STIs in the United States, from highest number of new occurrences to lowest, are human papillomavirus (HPV), chlamydia, trichomoniasis, gonorrhea, genital herpes, syphilis, HIV, and hepatitis B.[33,34] HPV, trichomoniasis, HIV, and hepatitis B are discussed elsewhere in this book.

STIs are spread by anal, oral, or vaginal sex with an infected individual. Symptoms are not always present, and knowing if sexual partners are infected can be challenging.[35] Pregnant women infected with an STI may infect infants in utero or during birth; women may also infect infants through breastfeeding.

There are approximately 20 million new cases of STIs annually in the United States, which cost the U.S. health care system $16 billion annually.[34] The latest data from the Centers for Disease Control and Prevention (CDC) surveillance report states that there has been an increase of 4.1% in gonorrhea and 0.7% in chlamydia cases reported in 2011 to 2012. Chlamydia is one of the most widespread STIs in the United States. Reported syphilis cases rose 11% in 2011 to 2012 after remaining stable in 2010 to 2011. The number of cases of congenital syphilis (transmitted from mother to infant) are at the lowest rate since 1988. The CDC's surveillance report includes data on only those STIs (syphilis, chlamydia, and gonorrhea) for which there is mandatory reporting, underestimating the true prevalence of STIs.[36]

STIs affect males and females of all racial, cultural, and socioeconomic groups, but wide disparities are present. The CDC's data show much higher rates of reported STIs among certain racial and ethnic groups, with blacks being disproportionally affected by chlamydia, gonorrhea, and primary and secondary syphilis. Figure 153-1 shows a graphical representation of the racial distribution of gonorrhea and chlamydia. Many factors contribute to this disparity, including poverty, lack of access to

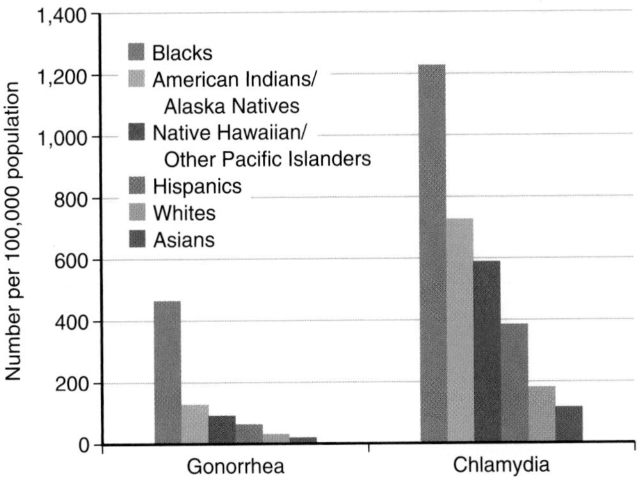

FIGURE 153-1 Sexually transmitted diseases by race. (Data from U.S. Department of Health and Human Services, Centers for Disease Control and Prevention (CDC): *A guide to taking a sexual history.* CDC Publication: 99-8445.)

health care, and a relatively high prevalence of STIs in the community.[36]

Adolescents and young adults are at the greatest risk of acquiring an STI, with 58% of gonorrhea and 69% of chlamydia reported in those aged 15 to 24.[37] The CDC estimates that one in four sexually active adolescent females have an STD. Behavior that includes multiple partners and inconsistent use of condoms contributes to the higher risk in this age group. Adolescents may also be faced with barriers to access for STD prevention resources. Women are more vulnerable to STIs because they are more biologically susceptible than men to certain STIs, may be reluctant to insist on condom use, and are dependent on the behavior of the male partner to practice safe sex.[36]

CLINICAL PRESENTATION

A significant number of persons with STIs have no apparent signs or symptoms. More than one site may be infected simultaneously (e.g., cervix plus urethra), and symptoms may overlap and involve more than one pathogen. Diseases are tentatively classified into syndromes to narrow the field of possible pathogens.

Because STIs do not always manifest with distinct clinical features, determination of which patients are at risk necessitates a thorough sexual history. Eliciting the history for an STI needs to be routine, standardized, and guided by the individual's age. An effective sexual history is critical for diagnosis and for counseling individuals with regard to risk reduction behaviors. The CDC suggests talking with patients about the five *Ps*: partners, practices, protection from STDs, past history of STDs, and prevention of pregnancy.[38] See Box 153-3 for sexual history questions and topics. With few exceptions, adolescents in the United States can be provided with confidential diagnosis and treatment of STIs without parental consent or knowledge.

PHYSICAL EXAMINATION

The physical examination for an STI incorporates the same principles as for the history. It is routine, standardized, and sensitive to the patient's age, individual needs, and cultural heritage.

BOX 153-3

Sexual History Questions

- Are you currently sexually active? (Are you having sex?)
  - If not, have you ever been sexually active?
- In the past 12 months, how many sex partners have you had?
- Are your sex partners men, women, or both? (If both, ask first two questions for each gender)
- What kind of sexual contact do you have or have you had? Anal, vaginal, or oral?
- Do you and your partner(s) use any protection against sexually transmitted diseases?
  - If not, tell me your thoughts about this.
  - If so, what kind of protection and how often do you use this protection?
  - If sometimes, in what situations or with whom do you use protection?
- Have you ever been diagnosed with an STD?
  - When?
  - How were you treated?
  - Have you had any recurring symptoms or diagnoses?
- Have you ever been tested for HIV or other STDs?
- Has your current or any former partner ever been diagnosed or treated for an STD(s)?
  - Were you tested for the same STD(s)?
  - If yes, when were you tested?
  - What was the diagnosis and how was it treated?
- Are you currently trying to conceive or father a child?
- Are you concerned about getting pregnant or getting your partner pregnant?
- Are you using contraception or practicing any form of birth control?

ADDITIONAL HISTORY

- Travel: location, date
- Dysuria, frequency, hematuria
- Adenopathy
- Fatigue, weight loss, night sweats, unexplained diarrhea, fever
- Rash, lesions, sores: location
- Pruritus: anogenital, oral, other
- Rectal bleeding, discharge, pain, constipation

ADDITIONAL HISTORY FOR WOMEN

- Vaginal discharge, bleeding, consistency, color
- Pain (abdominal, vaginal, vulvar, anal, headache, joints)
- Consistency of contraception use
- Last menstrual period, description, changes

ADDITIONAL HISTORY FOR MEN

- Penile discharge
- Pain (testes, joints, headache, anal)

Consistent examination of all areas reduces the chance of a missed diagnosis. Minimum physical examination procedures for women and men are listed in Box 153-4.

Every effort should be made to reduce anxiety. All steps of the examination should be explained before they are initiated. Female patients normally void before the examination; the necessity of obtaining a urine specimen to test for UTI, gonorrhea, or chlamydia should be kept in mind.

BOX 153-4

Minimum Physical Examination for Sexually Transmitted Infections

- Examination of the mouth
- Examination of the lymph nodes
- Examination of the skin on the thorax, abdomen, limbs, palms, soles
- Examination of the anogenital area
- Palpation for inguinal and femoral adenopathy

ADDITIONAL EXAMINATION FOR WOMEN

- Pelvic examination, including speculum examination and bimanual examination
- Assessment for cervical motion tenderness

ADDITIONAL EXAMINATION FOR MEN

- Examination of the external genitals and anus

DIAGNOSTICS

After completing the routine screening history and examination, the health care provider may be able to assign the patient to one of several clinical syndromes. This narrows the field of possible pathogens that cause the syndrome and guides treatment. If the patient is asymptomatic, therapy is determined by the laboratory results. Partners of persons with identified STIs are evaluated and treated on the basis of their last sexual encounter and the particular STI in question. Early, specific diagnosis and treatment of symptomatic and asymptomatic persons will prevent further transmission of disease to their partners. However, appropriate diagnosis of an STI often requires multiple diagnostic tests because of the variety of STIs. Culture, nucleic acid hybridization tests, and nucleic acid amplification tests (NAATs) are critical tools used to diagnose chlamydia and gonorrhea. In most cases, urine can be used to test for gonorrhea and chlamydia; first-voided urine is preferred.[39] Use of a urine sample for NAAT is the recommended testing method to detect gonorrhea and chlamydia.[39] Table 153-4 outlines various STIs and their associated pathogens and syndromes, appropriate diagnostics, and differential diagnoses.

MANAGEMENT

Specialist referral is recommended for newly diagnosed syphilis.

The management of STIs is often confounded by the inclusiveness of the term itself. A number of different organisms may be associated with different syndromes; for example, genital ulcers can result from herpes, chancroid, syphilis, or other infections. Because there is a broad spectrum of sources with STIs, treatment is individualized to the cause. Major curable syndromes in adults include genital ulcers, urethritis vaginitis, cervicitis, and PID. In the United States, treatments are frequently initiated against common pathogens causing these syndromes while laboratory results are pending; coinfection with more than one organism is common. Antimicrobial therapy is available for all bacterial STIs as well as for those caused by protozoa and ectoparasites. Drugs for viral STIs are largely limited to symptom alleviation because they cannot eradicate the organism.

1. The standards published by the CDC in 2010 and updated in 2012 use the regimens listed in Box 153-5.
2. For most STIs, the partners of patients should be examined.
   a. Expedited partner treatment (EPT) is considered permissible in 35 states, potentially allowable in 9 states and prohibited in 6 states.
   b. EPT is a treatment practice whereby a provider gives prescriptions or medications to the patient for treatment of an STD in his or her sexual partner.
   c. In many states, the local state or health department can assist in partner notification for selected STIs (e.g., HIV infection, syphilis, gonorrhea, hepatitis B, and chlamydia).

Interdisciplinary Management

All pregnant and HIV-positive patients should be co-managed with a specialist or collaborating physician. All treatment failures necessitate management with a specialist. Consultation or co-management with a specialist is necessary for all cases of syphilis. See Table 153-4 for further information.

LIFE SPAN CONSIDERATIONS

Prevalence rates for many STIs are highest among adolescents and young adults. Screening of asymptomatic high-risk patients, with sensitivity to age-related developmental and cultural characteristics, is required. STI prevention should be initiated before sexual activity begins, with education about healthy, safe, sexual practices and continual reinforcement throughout the life span. Additional life span considerations relate to the development of PID in women, with possible consequences of infertility, ectopic pregnancies, and chronic pelvic pain.

Prevention of viral STIs requires the adoption of lifelong healthy sexual behaviors to help avoid acquisition and spread of infection. The prevalence of herpes increases with age because once acquired, the disease stays within the body. Factors related to the spread and acquisition of STIs often include other high-risk behaviors, such as multiple partners, use of illicit drugs, excessive alcohol use, and unsafe sexual practices such as inconsistent or no use of condoms.

DISEASES CHARACTERIZED BY CERVICITIS AND URETHRITIS

Urethritis, or inflammation of the urethra, may be caused by an infection characterized by the discharge of mucoid or purulent material and by burning during urination. Among men, most urethral infections with *Neisseria gonorrhoeae* are symptomatic, causing the patients to seek treatment and to avoid serious sequelae, but this may occur after the STI has already been transmitted to others.[40] However, most presentations of chlamydia in both sexes are asymptomatic. Urethritis is classified as gonococcal if it is caused by *N. gonorrhoeae* (gonorrhea) or as NGU if *N. gonorrhoeae* is not detected. NGU in younger men is most commonly caused by *Chlamydia* but may be associated with other pathogens.

GONORRHEA

Definition and Epidemiology

Gonorrhea is an STI caused by the gram-negative diplococcus *N. gonorrhoeae*. In men, it is often characterized by a purulent urethral discharge, but it is asymptomatic in up to 80% of women.[41] Laboratory confirmation of the presence of *N. gonorrhoeae* is required for the establishment of the diagnosis.[42]

Text continued on p. 790

TABLE 153-4 Summary of Sexually Transmitted Infections

Pathogen, Differential Diagnosis	Clinical Presentation	Diagnosis	Consultation, Co-Management	Complications	Management
GONORRHEA *Neisseria gonorrhoeae* **Differential diagnosis:** NGU, PID, candidiasis, bacterial vaginosis, endometriosis, pregnancy, salpingitis, orchitis, trichomoniasis, UTI, epididymitis	Purulent urethral discharge Dysuria Pruritus Anorectal burning Skin lesions **Female:** Frequently asymptomatic; dysuria; leukorrhea; abnormal uterine bleeding; cervical motion tenderness; vaginal discharge; pharyngeal edema or erythema	NAATs: vaginal swab, first-catch urine Culture	Treatment failure Complications	Prostatitis Epididymitis Cystitis PID Gonococcal conjunctivitis	Treat presumptively for chlamydia. Specimen testing for gonorrhea should occur before other testing. Partners are evaluated and treated. Perform syphilis serology. Offer HIV counseling and testing.
CHLAMYDIA *Chlamydia trachomatis* **Differential diagnosis:** PID, gonorrhea, candidiasis, bacterial vaginosis, endometriosis, pregnancy, salpingitis, orchitis, epididymitis, trichomoniasis, UTI	Often asymptomatic May infect lungs and eyes **Female:** Abnormal vaginal discharge (yellow or green), vaginal bleeding, dysuria, cervical friability or edema **Male:** Dysuria, penile discharge, itching **Those having receptive anal intercourse:** Rectal pain, discharge, bleeding	NAATs: vaginal swab, first-catch urine, pharyngeal or rectal samples Culture	Treatment failure HIV-positive patients	Reactive arthritis Chronic conjunctivitis **Female:** PID, infertility, ectopic pregnancy, chronic pelvic pain **Male:** Epididymitis, orchitis, proctocolitis **Infant:** Conjunctivitis, pneumonia	Collect specimen. Treat presumptively in patients with PID, NGU, gonococcal infection, epididymitis in men <35 years old. Perform syphilis serology. Offer HIV counseling and testing.
NONGONOCOCCAL URETHRITIS *C. trachomatis* (23%-55% of cases) *Ureaplasma urealyticum* (20%-40% of cases) *Trichomonas vaginalis* (25% of cases) Herpes simplex virus **Differential diagnosis:** Same as for Chlamydia	Dysuria Mucoid or purulent discharge Pruritus Hematuria Frequency Urgency Endocervical exudate, friability	Gram stain Wet mount Tests for gonorrhea and chlamydia	Treatment failure Complications	Epididymitis Penile edema Reiter syndrome Tenosynovitis	If microscopic test results are not available, treat for both gonorrhea and chlamydia.

Continued

TABLE 153-4 Summary of Sexually Transmitted Infections—cont'd

Pathogen, Differential Diagnosis	Clinical Presentation	Diagnosis	Consultation, Co-Management	Complications	Management
PRIMARY SYPHILIS *Treponema pallidum* **Differential diagnosis:** Genital herpes; chancroid; lymphogranuloma venereum (LGV); balanitis, excoriation of nonulcerative lesions; squamous cell carcinoma	Painless, firm, round chancre(s) at site of inoculation, lasts 3-6 weeks Discrete, enlarged, painless regional lymph nodes Incubation: 10-90 days; average, 21 days	Darkfield microscopy Nontreponemal serology (RPR, VDRL) Confirm with treponemal serology (MHA-TP, FTA-ABS) Sequential serologic testing; use same testing method and laboratory	Positive diagnosis of disease All HIV-positive patients	Secondary syphilis Meningitis Cardiovascular or neurologic disease Facilitates HIV transmission Left untreated, can cause perinatal death or congenital syphilis in infants	Systemic disease: Chancre is unnoticed in 15%-39% of cases. Perform nontreponemal serology and clinical follow-up at 6 and 12 months. Note fourfold drop in titer; evaluate for HIV infection. Treatment failure: re-treatment and consultation with specialist are indicated; patients may need lumbar puncture.
SECONDARY SYPHILIS *T. pallidum* **Differential diagnosis:** All undiagnosed mucocutaneous skin eruptions (e.g., drug eruption, pityriasis rosea, scabies)	Nonpruritic rash: rough, red, red-brown spots, sometimes very faint; may occur on mucous membranes, vagina, anus, palms, soles, trunk Appears 2-8 weeks after chancre, may be present while chancre is resolving Generalized adenopathy Fever Sore throat Patchy alopecia Malaise, arthralgias, weight loss Oral mucous patches Condylomata lata Hepatosplenomegaly Increased incidence is associated with crack cocaine and illicit drug use.	As for primary syphilis	As for primary syphilis	As for primary syphilis	At 6- and 12-month follow-up, assess for fourfold drop in titer. A fourfold increase in titer at any time may represent treatment failure or reinfection.

LATENT SYPHILIS (EARLY LATENT, LATE LATENT)					
T. pallidum	Occur after primary and secondary symptoms resolve Difficulty coordinating muscle movements Paralysis Numbness Gradual blindness Dementia Positive serology without evidence of clinical disease	Reactive VDRL or RPR Reactive FTA-ABS or MHA-TP	All cases managed with specialist	Progression of disease	Latent syphilis is diagnosed as probable on the basis of documented seroconversion or a fourfold increase in titer of nontreponemal test. History of symptoms or exposure to partner during previous 12 months. Evaluate for aortitis, neurosyphilis iritis.
CHANCROID					
Haemophilus ducreyi **Differential diagnosis:** Genital herpes; primary syphilis; LGV; infected or traumatic lesions	One or more painful genital ulcers with tender inguinal adenopathy May have suppurative inguinal adenopathy and undermined ulcer borders	Isolation of H. ducreyi Most cases diagnosed on clinical grounds Painful ulcers 4-7 days after exposure Usually coronal sulcus in men Prepuce in women	Treatment failure	Successful treatment cures infection In extensive cases, scarring despite successful therapy	Topical cleansing with gentle soaks. Symptomatic treatment to reduce swelling. Antibiotic administration to patients with nonfluctuant buboes. No need to drain lesions. Reexamine patients at 3-7 days. Larger ulcers heal more slowly. No evidence of T. pallidum appears on darkfield examination or by serology. Culture is negative for herpes simplex virus. Partner contact: Examine and treat within 10 days. Perform syphilis serology. Offer HIV counseling.

Continued

TABLE 153-4 Summary of Sexually Transmitted Infections—cont'd

Pathogen, Differential Diagnosis	Clinical Presentation	Diagnosis	Consultation, Co-Management	Complications	Management
GENITAL HERPES (PRIMARY, RECURRENT)					
HSV-2 and HSV-1 **Differential diagnosis:** Primary syphilis; chancroid; candidiasis; hand-foot-and-mouth disease, herpes zoster; fixed drug eruption; folliculitis	**Primary:** Vesicular lesions on erythematous base **Male:** Penis shaft, glans, urethra, rectum **Female:** Vulva, vagina, anus, cervix Painful lesions Malaise Fever Painful adenopathy Lesions ulcerative to superficial ulcers **Recurrent:** Clinical prodrome—pain, itching, burning, tingling Constitutional symptoms rare Vesicles Superficial ulcers	History and physical examination with confirmation by viral culture Moist swab of unroofed or weeping vesicle from base of ulcer Tzanck smear of scrapings from lesion looking for multinucleated giant cells Testing for HSV routine in all atypical and all undiagnosed genital ulcers	Secondary infection Ocular infection Persistent constitutional symptoms Urinary retention Primary or recurrent infection during pregnancy HIV-positive patients	Secondary infection Ocular infection Neonatal infection Premature delivery Spontaneous abortion Intrauterine growth retardation Fetal infection	Treatment is symptomatic. Infection may recur. HSV may be transmitted to sex partners even when no lesions are present. Support groups are available. Many educational resources are available.
LYMPHOGRANULOMA VENEREUM (LGV)					
C. trachomatis **Differential diagnosis:** Chancroid Colitis Granuloma Inguinale Herpes simplex Syphilis	Small, nonpainful, ulcerative genital papule Painful inguinal or femoral lymph nodes follow 2-6 weeks later Proctocolitis in third stage				Drainage of infected buboes. Treat with antibiotics.
GRANULOMA INGUINALE					
Klebsiella granulomatis **Differential diagnosis:** Chancroid Herpes simplex LGV Syphilis		Difficult to culture			Difficult to culture.

FTA-ABS, fluorescent treponemal antibody absorption; HSV, herpes simplex virus; MHA-TP, microhemagglutination assay for antibody to *Treponema pallidum;* RPR, rapid plasma reagin; VDRL, Venereal Disease Research Laboratory.
From Reference 41-b.

BOX 153-5

Treatment of Sexually Transmitted Infections

UNCOMPLICATED GONOCOCCAL INFECTIONS

Recommended Regimens

Ceftriaxone 250 mg IM in a single dose
plus
Azithromycin 1 g PO in a single dose, *or*
Doxycycline 100 mg PO twice daily for 7 days *(azithromycin preferred)*

Alternative Regimens

If Ceftriaxone Not Available

Cefixime 400 mg PO in a single dose
plus
Azithromycin 1 g PO in a single dose, *or*
Doxycycline 100 mg PO twice daily for 7 days *(azithromycin preferred)*
plus
Test-of-cure in 1 week

If Patient Has Severe Cephalosporin Allergy

Azithromycin 2 g PO in a single dose
plus
Test-of-cure in 1 week

Uncomplicated Gonococcal Infections of the Pharynx

Ceftriaxone 250 mg IM in a single dose
plus
Azithromycin 1 g PO in a single dose, *or*
Doxycycline 100 mg PO twice daily for 7 days *(azithromycin preferred)*

Pregnant Women

Ceftriaxone 250 mg IM in a single dose
plus
Azithromycin 1 g PO in a single dose

Alternative Regimens for Pregnant Women

Azithromycin 2 g PO in a single dose

CHLAMYDIA

Recommended Regimens

Azithromycin 1 g PO in a single dose, *or*
Doxycycline 100 mg PO twice daily for 7 days

Alternative Regimens

Erythromycin base 500 mg PO 4 times daily for 7 days, *or*
Ofloxacin 300 mg PO twice daily for 7 days, *or*
Levofloxacin 500 mg PO once daily for 7 days

Pregnant Women

Azithromycin 1 g PO in a single dose, *or*
Amoxicillin 500 mg 3 times daily for 7 days

NONGONOCOCCAL URETHRITIS

Recommended Regimens

Azithromycin 1 g PO in a single dose, *or*
Doxycycline 100 mg PO twice daily for 7 days

Alternative Regimens

Erythromycin base 500 mg PO 4 times daily for 7 days, *or*
Erythromycin ethylsuccinate 800 mg PO 4 times daily for 7 days, *or*
Ofloxacin 300 mg PO twice daily for 7 days *or*
Levofloxacin 500 mg PO once daily for 7 days

TREATMENT OF DISEASES CHARACTERIZED BY GENITAL ULCERS

Primary, Secondary, or Latent Syphilis of Less Than 1 Year's Duration

Recommended Regimens

Benzathine penicillin G 2.4 million units IM in a single dose

If Allergic to Penicillin

Doxycycline 100 mg twice a day for 14 days *or*
Tetracycline 500 mg PO 4 times a day for 14 days

Early Latent Syphilis

Recommended Regimens

Benzathine penicillin G 2.4 million units IM in a single dose

Late Latent Syphilis of More Than 1 Year's Duration or Unknown Duration

Recommended Regimens

Benzathine penicillin G 7.2 million units total, administered as 3 doses of 2.4 million units IM each, at 1-week intervals

Genital Herpes: First Clinical Episode

Recommended Regimens

Acyclovir 400 mg PO 3 times daily for 7-10 days, *or*
Acyclovir 200 mg PO 5 times daily for 7-10 days *or*
Famciclovir 250 mg PO 3 times daily for 7-10 days, *or*
Valacyclovir 1 g PO twice daily for 7-10 days

Genital Herpes: Recurrent Episodes

Recommended Regimens

Acyclovir 400 mg PO 3 times daily for 5 days, *or*
Acyclovir 800 mg PO 3 times daily for 2 days, *or*
Acyclovir 800 mg PO twice daily for 5 days, *or*
Famciclovir 125 mg PO twice daily for 5 days, *or*
Famciclovir 1000 mg PO twice daily for 1 day, *or*
Famciclovir 500 mg PO once, followed by 250 mg PO twice daily × 2 days, *or*
Valacyclovir 500 mg PO twice daily for 3 days, *or*
Valacyclovir 1 g PO once daily for 5 days

Chancroid

Recommended Regimens

Azithromycin 1 g PO in a single dose, *or*
Ceftriaxone 250 mg IM in a single dose, *or*
Ciprofloxacin 500 mg PO twice daily for 3 days, *or*
Erythromycin base 500 mg PO 3 times daily for 7 days

LGV

Recommended Regimens

Doxycycline 100 mg PO twice daily for 21 days, *or*
Erythromycin base 500 mg PO 4 times daily for 21 days

Asymptomatic Partners

Doxycycline 100 mg PO twice daily for 7 days, *or*
Azythromycin 1 g PO in a single dose

Quinolones should not be used for infections in men who have sex with men or in those with a history of recent foreign travel or who have partners with a recent history of foreign travel, infections acquired in California or Hawaii, or infections acquired in other areas with increased quinoline-resistant *Neisseria gonorrhoeae* prevalence.

From Workowski KA, Berman S, Centers for Disease Control and Prevention (CDC): Sexually transmitted diseases treatment guidelines, 2010, *MMWR Recomm Rep* 59(RR-12): 1-112, 2010. Consult these guidelines for more detailed recommendations, including guidelines for treatment of pregnant patients, HIV-infected patients, allergic patients, and other specific groups.

Gonorrhea is the second most commonly reported infectious disease in the United States, with 334,826 infections reported in 2012.[37] The CDC has estimated that approximately 820,000 cases actually occur yearly in the United States, because not all cases are reported.[43] Populations at risk for gonorrhea include young, sexually active individuals; nonwhite urban poor; and other individuals who engage in high-risk behaviors, such as using illegal drugs or engaging in prostitution.[37] Drug resistance continues to be of concern in the treatment of gonorrhea, with 14.7% of isolates demonstrating resistance to ciprofloxacin. Cephalosporins are the only class of antimicrobials currently meeting the CDC efficacy standards; and oral cephalosporins are no longer recommended owing to resistance. Frequently persons with gonorrhea have a coexistent chlamydial infection. Current guidelines recommend dual treatment with ceftriaxone and azithromycin, to treat both chlamydia and gonorrhea.[44] Providers are urged to check the CDC and state health departments for the most current treatment recommendations.

Pathophysiology

N. gonorrhoeae infects mucus-secreting columnar and transitional epithelium in the mucocutaneous surfaces of the genitourinary tract, pharynx, conjunctiva, and anus. Transmission occurs by sexual contact with an infected individual, by autoinoculation to the eyes, or to the neonate during childbirth via the birth canal of a pregnant woman with gonorrhea. The incubation period is usually 1 to 14 days after exposure. If untreated, gonorrhea spreads from its initial sites upward into the genital tract, prostate, and epididymis in men and into the fallopian tubes in women. Menstruation increases the risk of intraluminal ascent from the cervix and predisposes the patient to gonococcal bacteremia.

Clinical Presentation

Many women and some men are asymptomatic. If symptoms develop, they usually manifest in women within 10 days of contact and in men within 2 to 5 days of infection.

Signs and symptoms of infection in females with *N. gonorrhoeae* include thin, purulent, and mildly odorous leukorrhea; dysuria; intermenstrual bleeding; dyspareunia or mild lower abdominal pain; or pharyngitis. Progression to PID may occur in 10% to 20% of females in whom symptoms are initially not present or are unrecognized. Symptoms of PID include lower abdominal pain, vaginal discharge, mucopurulent urethral discharge, dysuria, cervical motion tenderness, adnexal tenderness or mass, intermenstrual bleeding, fever, chills, nausea, and vomiting.[45]

Gonorrhea in men usually manifests as urethritis, burning on urination, and serous penile discharge. This progresses over the next few days to copious, purulent, and sometimes blood-tinged discharge.

Infections of the pharynx, rectum, and eye may occur in men or women. Pharyngeal infection usually occurs in association with orogenital contact. The majority of pharyngeal infections are asymptomatic, but they may cause symptoms of pharyngitis with cervical lymphadenopathy. Anorectal infection may manifest with anorectal burning, mucopurulent discharge, and painful bowel movements. Ocular infections occur via autoinoculation into the eye from another infection site, such as the genitalia. Typical presentation is unilateral and purulent conjunctivitis.[45]

Diagnostics

The CDC recommends testing for gonorrhea with U.S. Food and Drug Administration (FDA)–approved NAATs. Vaginal swabs are preferred for detection in women, and first-catch urine in men. However, urine collection is frequently performed in women and is a less invasive method of detection. Culture should be obtained in cases of suspected treatment failure or instances of child sexual assault in boys and extragenital infections in girls.[46]

Complications

Left untreated, infection can result in a range of complications from acute salpingitis in female patients, perihepatitis (Fitz-Hugh–Curtis syndrome), and disseminated gonococcal infections to ophthalmia neonatorum in newborns. Infections caused by gonorrhea are a major cause of PID, ectopic pregnancy, and chronic pelvic pain in the United States. In untreated men, gonorrhea can cause epididymitis, a painful condition of the testicles that can result in infertility. Untreated ocular gonorrhea may result in panophthalmitis and possibly loss of the eye if not treated immediately.[45]

CHLAMYDIA

Definition and Epidemiology

Chlamydia is an STI caused by an intracellular parasitic organism, *Chlamydia trachomatis,* and organisms of the genus *Chlamydophila.* Clinical syndromes associated with *C. trachomatis* include NGU, mucopurulent cervicitis, PID, lymphogranuloma venereum (LGV), acute urethral syndrome, ocular infections, proctocolitis, epididymitis, and reactive arthritis. *C. trachomatis* may be acquired by infants through an infected birth canal, causing pneumonia and conjunctivitis.

Chlamydia is the most commonly reported STI in the United States. More than 1.4 million cases were reported in 2012, a rate of 456.7 per 100,000 population. Rates of infection with chlamydia are highest in black men and women, about seven times the rate in whites. The number of reported cases in women exceeds the number reported in men by about 2.4 times. This likely reflects that the sex partners of women with chlamydia are either not reporting their infection or not being diagnosed.[36]

Pathophysiology

There are 18 strains of *C. trachomatis,* with variants affecting the eyes and genital tract. It is usually spread by sexual contact. In women, the organism infects the columnar epithelial cells, most commonly at the transition zone of the endocervix, resulting in an inflammatory cascade. Each sexual encounter with an infected male has about a 25% chance of infecting a female. Infected mothers spread the disease to their newborns about 50% to 60% of the time, usually resulting in conjunctivitis but possibly pneumonia. The incubation period is typically 1 to 2 weeks. Coinfection with gonorrhea is common; 20% to 40% of men and women with chlamydia are likely to also have gonorrhea.[47]

Clinical Presentation

Most chlamydial infections are asymptomatic. Symptoms may not appear for several weeks after contact with the organisms and include abnormal vaginal discharge, burning with urination, penile discharge, and discomfort and edema in testicle(s). The rectum may also show symptoms such as pain, discharge, and bleeding. Chlamydia should be suspected in female patients with cervicitis on the basis of mucopurulent discharge from the cervical os, easily induced bleeding, and edema in the area of ectopy.[48]

Diagnostics

NAATs are the preferred method of testing for chlamydia and are used for both endocervical swabs and urine-based evaluation. Testing for chlamydia can be coupled with liquid-based Pap smears during routine well-visit examinations, similar to testing for gonorrhea. *Chlamydia* organisms are found within urethral, cervical, and rectal epithelial cells but not in exudate or pus.

Complications

Chlamydia can cause damage to the reproductive system, including PID, perihepatitis, and reactive arthritis, regardless of the presence or absence of symptoms. Pregnant women with chlamydia are at risk for preterm delivery, chlamydial conjunctivitis, and pneumonia in the newborn.[48]

Education and Health Promotion

All sexually active women younger than 26 and all pregnant women should be screened for chlamydia. Routine screening is not currently recommended in men but should be encouraged in geographic areas with high prevalence. Men who have sex with men (MSM) who have receptive anal sex should be screened annually, and every 3 to 6 months for those who have multiple and/or anonymous partners.[48]

DISEASES CHARACTERIZED BY GENITAL ULCERS

In the United States, most young, sexually active patients who have genital ulcers are infected with genital herpes, syphilis, or chancroid. Other infectious causes of genital ulcers include LGV and HIV; noninfectious causes include trauma, Behçet syndrome, neoplasms, and fixed drug eruptions. More than one of these diseases may be present concurrently.

SYPHILIS

Definition and Epidemiology

Syphilis is a complex systemic STI caused by *Treponema pallidum*. In 2012 there were close to 50,000 reported cases in the United States (5 cases per 100,000 population), an increase of 8.4% from 2011. Increasing numbers of MSM represent newly diagnosed cases, accounting for 75% of primary and secondary syphilis. Blacks and Hispanics account for a majority of the remaining cases. It is interesting to note that the rate of congenital syphilis (passed from pregnant mother to infant) is about twice the rate of perinatal HIV transmission.[36,49]

Syphilis has been classified into a series of overlapping stages, which is used to guide treatment and follow-up (Box 153-6).[40] Patients may initially demonstrate signs and symptoms of primary infection (ulcer or chancre at the infection site; see Figure 153-2), secondary infection (rash, mucocutaneous lesions, and adenopathy), or tertiary infection (cardiac, neurologic, ophthalmic, auditory, or gummatous lesions). Primary and secondary syphilis are the most infectious states of the disease.

BOX 153-6

Stages of Syphilis

- Primary syphilis
- Secondary syphilis
- Latent syphilis
  - Early latent syphilis
  - Late latent syphilis
- Latent syphilis, unknown duration
- Neurosyphilis
- Tertiary (late) syphilis
- Syphilitic stillbirth

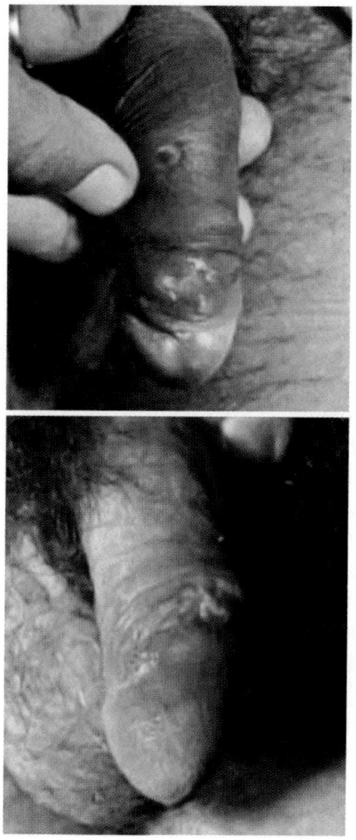

FIGURE 153-2 Chancre in primary syphilis. (From Wisdom A: *Color atlas of sexually transmitted diseases.* Year Book, 1989.)

Pathophysiology

Syphilis is usually spread through contact with infectious lesions called chancres; the infection usually enters the host during sexual activity through sites where the epithelium has been disrupted from minor trauma. Sexual contact with a partner who has early syphilis is associated with the highest risk for development of the disease. The mean time from exposure to the development of active infection (chancre formation) is 21 days (range, 10 to 60 days). Syphilis may also be transmitted from an infected pregnant woman to her developing child.[49]

Clinical Presentation

Chancres typically develop at the site of inoculation. Syphilitic lesions are painless and some patients may not be aware of them. Secondary syphilis causes more widespread findings, including macules and papules on the trunk, neck, palms, and soles. Condylomata lata, which are raised, flat, broad, grayish papular lesions, may occur in moist areas such as the anus, scrotum, and vulva. Mucous patches (small, asymptomatic, shallow ulcerations) may develop in the oral or genital mucosa or at the angles of the mouth.[49]

The signs of primary and secondary syphilis may resolve spontaneously even without treatment. The patient then enters the latent stage of the disease, in which there are generally no clinical signs or symptoms of infection and diagnosis is made on the basis of serology. A pregnant woman with latent disease can infect her fetus.

Tertiary syphilis (late-stage syphilis) manifests after a variable period of latency in approximately one third of patients who do not receive treatment. Late-stage syphilis may occur 10 to 20 years after initial infection. It may appear as gummatous disease (rubbery lumps or lesions found in subcutaneous tissue), cardiovascular disease, or neurosyphilis. Neurosyphilis can occur in all stages of syphilis, and the diagnosis is based on clinical findings and examination of the serum and cerebrospinal fluid.

Diagnostics

Darkfield examinations and direct fluorescent antibody tests of lesion exudate or tissue are the definitive methods for diagnosis of early syphilis. These are not typically performed in practice today owing to their complexity. Simple serologic testing with nontreponemal tests (e.g., Venereal Disease Research Laboratory [VDRL] and rapid plasma reagin [RPR]) are used for screening but are not specifically diagnostic for syphilis. These initial tests correlate with disease activity and are reported quantitatively. False positives may be associated with hepatitis, viral pneumonia, pregnancy, infectious mononucleosis, and other viral infections. Treponemal testing (e.g., fluorescent treponemal antibody absorption [FTA-ABS], *Treponema pallidum* particle agglutination [TP-PA], various enzyme immunoassays [EIAs], and chemoluminescence immunoassays) is done for diagnosis, and a positive result is usually present throughout the lifetime, regardless of treatment.[49] Chronic false-positive treponemal findings are associated with connective tissue diseases such as systemic lupus erythematosus.[50]

Complications

Untreated, syphilis may cause systemic disease involving neurologic and cardiovascular problems including stroke, meningitis, decreased hearing, changes in vision, and dementia.

GENITAL HERPES

Definition and Epidemiology

Genital infection with HSV infection is a condition characterized by primary involvement of the genital or anal area with visible, painful genital or anal lesions or grouped vesicles at the site of inoculation and regional lymphadenopathy. Recurrent HSV infections are characterized by a normal course of recurring outbreaks of vesicles at the same site. In the past, HSV-2 was the predominant serotype present in genital herpes. Now an increasing number of cases are represented by HSV-1, typically associated with orofacial infection.[51,52]

About 776,000 people in the United States get a new herpes infection every year. It is estimated that 16% of the U.S. population aged 14 to 49 is HSV-2 seropositive, and 50% to 80% is positive with HSV-1. It is estimated that more individuals are affected by genital herpes, because HSV-1 is also responsible for the infection. Of those infected, as many as 80% or more could be unaware of infection or be asymptomatic.[51,52]

More women than men have herpes. Racial and ethnic distribution is similar to that of other STIs, with blacks representing 39.2% of cases, more than triple the rate in whites.

Genital herpes is spread by direct contact with lesions, mucosal membranes, or genital or oral secretions. Transmission is higher from men to women than from women to men. Shedding occurs in asymptomatic individuals about 10% of days. Most transmissions occur from an infected person with no known sores who may not be aware of harboring the infection.[51] Most neonatal herpes is caused by HSV-2 infections transmitted during delivery. Infants of mothers who have been infected for the first time during their pregnancy, especially in the third trimester, are at high risk of serious complications. Delivery via cesarean section is recommended for all pregnant women with active lesions or early symptoms.[51]

Pathophysiology

After an inoculation, the virus undergoes primary replication, resulting in the production of the characteristic lesion (a thin-walled vesicle on an erythematous base). Incubation ranges from 2 to 12 days, averaging 4 days. With primary infection, HSV travels along sensory nerves and establishes latency within sensory nerve fibers for life.

Reactivation may be triggered by stimuli such as fever, trauma, stress, sunlight, and menstruation. Immunocompromised individuals are likely to experience more frequent and severe reactivation. Shedding occurs in both symptomatic and asymptomatic reactivations. Recurrences for genital HSV-2 are typically more frequent than those for HSV-1.[52]

Clinical Presentation

Many people are infected with herpes but have never been symptomatic. Those experiencing symptoms usually show an outbreak of vesicles on or around the genitals, rectum, or mouth. These vesicles erode and leave painful ulcerations that may linger for 2 to 4 weeks before healing.

An initial outbreak of herpes usually lasts longer than subsequent outbreaks, has a higher rate of viral shedding, and includes symptoms such as fever, body aches, lymphadenopathy, and headache. Subsequent outbreaks are common in the first year after initial episode, with later recurrences being shorter and milder. Recurrent outbreaks may produce prodromal symptoms several hours or days before lesions appear, including tingling and shooting pains in the lower extremities and buttocks.[53]

Diagnostics

Diagnosis of HSV infection is often a clinical decision based on the patient's history and the morphologic characteristics of the lesions. Isolation of HSV in cell culture is the preferred virologic test and requires a sample from an active lesion. Unfortunately, healing lesions affect the sensitivity of virologic testing. Several enzyme-linked immunosorbent assay (ELISA) serologic tests are available, and most are able to distinguish between HSV-1 and HSV-2. Serologic test results will not be positive at the time of the primary outbreak; seroconversion takes 2 to 12 weeks after infection. A positive serologic test result will be lifelong.[53]

Complications

Having herpes may increase the likelihood of contracting other STDs. Infants of mothers who have been infected for the first time during their pregnancy are at high risk of serious complications.

Indications for Referral or Hospitalization

Patients for whom any suspicion of HSV in the eyes is present should be promptly referred to an ophthalmologist.

Education and Health Promotion

The CDC does not currently recommend screening for HSV.[54]

CHANCROID

Definition and Epidemiology

Chancroid is an STI characterized by painful genital ulceration and inflammatory inguinal adenopathy. The disease is characterized by infection with *Haemophilus ducreyi*. In 2012, only 15 cases were reported to the CDC. It is more prevalent in poorer regions of Africa, Asia, and the Carribean.[36]

Pathophysiology

A destructive toxin is produced by *H. ducreyi*, which breaks down skin and mucus membrane barriers.

Clinical Presentation

Chancroid is a genital ulcer disease characterized by one or a few painful ulcers that develop after an incubation of 4 to 7 days. The most distinguishing feature is deep, raw, and painful ulcerations. Painful inguinal adenopathy, often unilateral, develops in 50% of patients 1 to 2 weeks after the primary lesion. Buboes occur and may drain spontaneously, leaving behind a nonhealing ulcer.[55]

Diagnostics

Diagnosis is often clinical. Confirmation is based on isolation via culture of *H. ducreyi* from a clinical specimen.

OTHER ULCERATIVE DISEASES

LGV and granuloma inguinale are two other causes of genital ulcers. These genital ulcers are rare in the United States but endemic to certain tropical areas.

Granuloma Inguinale

Definition and Epidemiology. Granuloma inguinale, also known as donovanosis, is caused by *Klebsiella granulomatis* and occurs occasionally in the United States (fewer than 100 cases per year), but is more common in tropical and developing areas. As with most STIs, blacks have a higher incidence than whites.[56]

Pathophysiology. Granuloma inguinale is primarily transmitted via sexual contact but may be spread fecally or to the neonate through an infected mother's birth canal. Incubation varies from 1 day to 1 year, but the median incubation is 50 days.[57]

Clinical Presentation. This infection is characterized by painless progressive ulcers and regional lymphadenopathy. The lesions bleed easily on contact. There are four types of skin lesions: nodular, ulcerovegetative, cicatricial, and hypertrophic/verrucous. Nodular lesions (pseudobubo) are soft and may be pruritic and erythematous. They eventually erode to ulcerations. Ulcerovegetative lesions are the most common, showing painless, large, beefy-red, pus-filled ulcers, with raised borders. They are frequently found in skin folds. Cicatricial lesions appear as dry ulcers resembling scars. Hypertrophic/verrucous ulcers appear similar to genital warts.[56]

Diagnostics. Granuloma inguinale is difficult to culture; however, it may be seen on a smear from the base of the lesion. Samples may be obtained via punch, curettage, or wedge resection and sent to pathology for review.

Lymphogranuloma Venereum

Definition and Epidemiology. LGV is a systemic STI caused by a variety of *C. trachomatis*. It rarely occurs in the United States. Providers in the United States should be aware of this infectious disease, especially if caring for MSM.[58]

Clinical Presentation. A primary lesion that is a small, nonpainful genital papule that ulcerates after an initial 3- to 30-day incubation period characterizes LGV. Painful inguinal or femoral lymph nodes follow 2 to 6 weeks later. Proctocolitis is present in the third stage of the presentation and is more common in women.[58]

INDICATIONS FOR REFERRAL OR HOSPITALIZATION

It is not common for patients with STIs to require hospitalization. Indications include signs and symptoms of systemic disease not appropriate for outpatient treatment; ineffective outpatient treatment; and complications related to an STI, such as PID. Referral to a specialist in infectious disease is indicated for all patients with LGV, syphilis, or granuloma inguinale as well as for all treatment failures.

PATIENT AND FAMILY EDUCATION

Patient education efforts need to focus on preventing the establishment of high-risk behaviors before sexual activity is initiated. The general public is largely unaware of the health consequences of STIs because many infections are asymptomatic. Major health consequences, such as infertility and chronic disease, can occur years after initial infections, and the stigma associated with STIs often inhibits frank and open discussion. Population-specific educational efforts and screening for specific STIs must be established to help curb this hidden epidemic.

HEALTH PROMOTION

Efforts to prevent STIs include promotion of healthy sexual practices and targeting of high-risk behaviors often associated with the acquisition of an STI. These behaviors include excessive alcohol intake, substance abuse, and high-risk sexual practices such as inconsistent or no condom use and multiple sex partners. Patients who are sexually active, regardless of age, should be educated on the risk of transmitting or acquiring the different STIs and on the various transmission modes. Sensitivity to the patient's age, culture, religion, and setting are integral to successful health promotion and disease prevention activities.

Adolescents are at higher risk for STIs. Efforts targeting this age group must include an awareness of peer pressures and self-esteem, which may affect the patient's health behavior patterns. Sex education can become a controversial issue for patients, families, and schools. This age group, with few exceptions, is able to consent to confidential diagnosis and treatment of STIs. This provides the opportunity for promotion of healthy sexual practices in a nonthreatening environment.

A great deal of information is available on the Internet, for both the health care provider and the patient, from numerous reputable and informative resources. The CDC Division of STD Prevention has the current treatment guidelines and STI fact sheets with valuable links to other sites. For more information, contact the following:

- CDC, Division of STD Prevention: www.cdc.gov/STD
- CDC National STD Hotline: 800-232-4636 (24 hours/day, 7 days/week)
- American Sexual Health Association (ASHA): www.ashasexualhealth.org

CHAPTER 154

UROPATHIES (OBSTRUCTIVE) AND TUMORS OF THE GENITOURINARY TRACT (KIDNEYS, URETERS, AND BLADDER)

Melisa A. Hall

DEFINITION AND EPIDEMIOLOGY

Obstructive uropathy refers to structural or functional changes in the urinary tract that impair urine flow. Left untreated, obstruction can result in progressive renal damage and potential renal failure.[1] The degree, duration, and location of obstruction determine the extent of functional and pathologic alterations in the kidney. Tumors of the genitourinary tract may be benign or malignant. Benign renal tumors include adenomas, oncocytomas, and angiomyolipomas and are often incidentally found on imaging studies. Adenomas are small tumors of the renal cortex and are most often asymptomatic. Oncocytomas are adenomas of the renal collecting tubule and represent 1% to 14% of renal tumors; although considered benign, they have on rare occasions demonstrated malignant potential. Angiomyolipomas, as the name implies, contain vascular tissue, smooth muscle cells, and fatty elements. Because of the potential for hemorrhage, they may become symptomatic, manifesting with pain, hematuria, or hypertension.[2]

Obstructive uropathy is common, can occur at any age, and can be seen anywhere in the urinary tract from the urethral meatus to the renal tubules.[1] It can be classified by cause (congenital or acquired), duration (acute or chronic), degree (partial or complete), and level (upper or lower urinary tract).[1] In children, congenital disorders are seen most commonly. For adults, acquired disorders are more prevalent. Urolithiasis is the most common disorder in young adults.[3] In individuals older than 60 years, men are affected more than women, and benign prostatic hyperplasia (BPH) and prostate carcinoma are the most prevalent culprits in this age group.[4]

Renal cell carcinoma (RCC) is the most common malignant renal tumor in adults and constitutes more than 90% of all adult renal cancers.[5] Known risk factors for RCC include abdominal imaging, smoking, obesity, long-term dialysis, and a family history.[6] Occupations such as leather tanning and shoe making and exposure to asbestos, gasoline, petroleum, tar, and pitch are considered risk factors, but more data are needed to determine the amount of risk.[6] Tobacco abuse is the strongest known risk factor for RCC. There is a higher prevalence of RCC in men than in women (2:1); black men have the highest incidence of all ethnic groups.[2]

Wilms tumor, the most common tumor of childhood, affects approximately 1 in 10,000 children younger than 15 years. The tumor is more common in blacks than in whites, and bilateral disease is more common in females.[7,8]

Cancer of the bladder is the second most common cancer of the genitourinary tract. The male/female ratio for bladder cancer is 3:1, and it is more common in whites than in blacks and peaks in the sixth to seventh decade of life.[9] Known risk factors for urothelial cancers of the bladder are aging, cigarette smoking, occupational chemical exposure including iron and aluminum processing, working with metals, industrial painting, gas and tar manufacturing, transport equipment operation, and mining. Genetic abnormalities, radiotherapy, and chronic bladder irritation also increase the risk for bladder cancers.[9,10] Current tobacco smokers have a threefold increased risk for bladder cancer, and ex-smokers have a twofold increased risk.[9,11]

PATHOPHYSIOLOGY

Urinary Tract Obstruction

Obstruction of urine flow can result from intrinsic or extrinsic mechanical blockage as well as from functional defects not associated with a fixed occlusion. Lesions causing mechanical obstruction can occur at any level of the upper or lower urinary tract.[12] When the lesion is above the level of the bladder, unilateral dilation of the ureter and kidney (hydronephrosis) can occur. When the lesion is below the level of the bladder, bilateral involvement of the kidneys occurs, unless there is a solitary kidney. Forms of mechanical obstructions are listed in the differential diagnosis box.

Obstruction of urine flow causes urinary retention and increased pressure proximal to the obstruction.[1] A significant or prolonged pressure increase can lead to considerable renal tissue damage with resultant renal insufficiency or failure.[1]

Functional impairment of urine flow can also result from disorders that involve both the ureter and bladder. Neurogenic bladder dysfunction can be caused by upper neuron damage or lower spinal cord injury. Upper neuron damage may produce involuntary micturition against a closed bladder neck or external sphincter, whereas lower spinal tract injury can cause the bladder to become atonic.[13] In many cases, a significant urinary residual volume may occur, resulting in increased bladder pressure and subsequent upper tract pressures.[1,13] This may or may not be accompanied by reflux of urine into the ureters. Ischemia of the upper tracts can occur when pressures are elevated, leading to substantial renal injury and even tissue death.[1,13]

Renal Cell Carcinoma

RCC is an adenocarcinoma of the kidney that most frequently originates from the proximal tubule.[2] Evidence of metastasis is present in one third of patients at the time of diagnosis. The most common site of metastasis is the lungs.[5] RCCs are often associated with paraneoplastic syndromes, which may produce the initial signs and symptoms (e.g., fever, anemia, cachexia, hypercalcemia, erythrocytosis, hypertension, hepatic dysfunction).[2]

RCC occurs with equal frequency in either kidney and may occur in the upper, middle, or lower poles. Tumor size at presentation varies from 1 to 10 cm or larger, and tumor size has been inversely correlated with survival.[2] Prognosis and treatment recommendations are based on the stage of disease. Two systems are commonly used for staging: the Robson staging system and the TNM (tumor, nodes, metastasis) classification of kidney cancer.[6]

Wilms Tumor

Wilms tumor is unilateral in 95% of cases and is associated with several congenital anomalies, including cryptorchidism, ureteral duplication, and hypospadias.[7] Acquired von Willebrand disease has been associated with Wilms tumor and should be considered in children with coagulation abnormalities or bleeding symptoms.[2]

Wilms tumor may be familial or sporadic in occurrence, and 15% to 20% of cases are associated with chromosomal abnormalities. The familial type is thought to be inherited by autosomal dominant transmission.[7]

Wilms tumors are usually large and multilobulated with focal areas of hemorrhage and necrosis. Metastasis (e.g., lungs, liver) is present in 10% to 15% of cases at the time of diagnosis.[7] Staging of Wilms tumor is based on the National Wilms' Tumor Study staging system and consists of five stages. The range is from stage I (tumor limited to kidney and completely excisable) to stage IV (hematogenous metastasis to lung, liver, bone, and brain) and stage V (bilateral renal involvement).[8]

Bladder Cancer

In 2014, 74,690 new cases of bladder cancer were anticipated to be diagnosed in the United States.[14] Bladder cancer develops within the urothelium, the lining of the urinary tract. The urothelium is composed of three to seven layers of transitional cells that cover the muscle layers of the bladder wall. Proliferative changes of the transitional cells may result in cancer, which may remain superficial or progress to invasive or metastatic disease.

Urothelial carcinoma (transitional cell carcinoma [TCC]) accounts for approximately 90% of all bladder cancers and may appear as papillary lesions or, less commonly, sessile or ulcerated lesions.[11] A papilloma or papillary tumor is a less aggressive transitional cell tumor. Non-TCCs include adenocarcinomas, squamous cell carcinomas, undifferentiated carcinomas, and mixed carcinomas. Squamous cell carcinomas account for 2% to 5% of bladder cancers and are more resistant to treatment.[11] They may be seen with high-grade urothelial carcinomas in which squamous differentiation has occurred or as a result of chronic infection, bladder stones, long-term indwelling urethral catheter use, or schistosomiasis.[6]

Carcinomas of the bladder are graded and staged in an effort to define the aggressiveness and extent of disease. Staging defines the depth of invasion within the bladder and progression of disease: stage 0 (mucosal changes) to stage D (lymph node involvement). The depth of invasion into muscle layers and perivesical fat increases the risk for metastasis.[11] Grading refers to the degree of cellular differentiation from normal urothelium. TCCs are graded on a numeric scale from 1 to 4, with the higher-grade tumors being more invasive and aggressive in behavior.

TCCs can progress to or initially appear as upper tract lesions. At least 90% of malignant neoplasms arising within the renal pelvis and ureter are TCCs. TCC of the upper tract is seen in nearly 5% of patients who have had bladder cancer. Conversely, at least 50% of patients first seen with upper tract urothelial carcinoma have or develop bladder cancer.[11]

CLINICAL PRESENTATION

Obstructive Uropathy

The presentation of obstructive uropathies can vary by cause. The health care provider should obtain a history with detailed review of symptoms, including onset, duration, location, aggravating and alleviating factors, characteristics of symptoms, changes in voiding or bowel patterns, and management therapies previously tried. Further inquiry should address current medications, medical and surgical histories, genitourinary history, family history (especially related to urologic issues), and history of pelvic trauma or neurologic issues.

In acute obstruction, pain is typically the most common presenting symptom.[1] Flank pain occurring in a crescendo-decrescendo pattern radiating to the lower abdomen, testes, or labia is common in acute obstruction. Flank pain that occurs only with urination is pathognomonic of vesicoureteral reflux, although reflux can also be asymptomatic.[1]

Chronic (slowly developing) obstructive lesions may be asymptomatic. Polyuria with resultant nocturia can be seen in chronic partial obstruction, whereas anuria and acute renal failure can be seen in total complete bilateral obstruction or obstruction of a solitary kidney. A pattern of oliguria or anuria alternating with polyuria or sudden onset of anuria suggests some type of obstructive uropathy.[1]

When it is incomplete, bladder outlet obstruction is often accompanied by other lower urinary tract symptoms, including frequency, nocturia, urgency, urge incontinence, hesitancy, poor stream, straining to initiate a urinary stream, postvoid dribbling, and overflow incontinence.[1,13] It is important to note changes in the pattern of urinary output, abrupt alterations versus gradual changes, and fluctuation in urinary symptoms. Recurrent urinary tract infections (UTIs) can also occur with chronic partial obstructions, so UTIs should be ruled out in patients with urologic symptoms.[1]

Clinical Presentation of Tumors

The classic triad of flank pain, hematuria, and renal mass occurs in less than 10% of patients, and consequently RCC is often not diagnosed until metastasis has occurred. Pain, hematuria, and flank mass therefore indicate advanced disease. A significant number of RCCs are found incidentally on imaging for other clinical problems.[2]

Wilms tumor affects children; the mean age at diagnosis is 3½ to 4 years. In Wilms tumor, the prevalent feature is an abdominal mass. Abdominal pain, which may suggest an acute abdomen, occurs in 30% to 40% of these patients.[7]

More than 70% of bladder cancer patients are first seen with intermittent painless gross hematuria that is often described as continuing throughout urination. Irritative voiding symptoms (e.g., urgency, frequency, dysuria) may or may not be present.[9] The presence of microhematuria also may herald a urothelial malignant neoplasm and requires further investigation.[15]

PHYSICAL EXAMINATION

A general physical examination should be performed on all patients. Blood pressure measurement is critical because both acute and chronic hydronephrosis can be accompanied by severe hypertension.[16] Signs of azotemia (pallor, skin changes, dizziness, and lethargy) should be monitored if kidney function is thought to be disrupted.[1] A fever may indicate infection. Palpation and percussion of the abdomen can often reveal bladder distention. An enlarged, tender kidney may be noted, especially in thin patients, and it may manifest as a flank mass or increased abdominal girth. Costovertebral angle or flank tenderness can be related to urolithiasis or infection.[1] The majority of genitourinary tract tumors are not associated with specific findings on physical examination. However, approximately 80% of children with Wilms tumor will have a large, smooth, firm flank mass that often extends across the midline.[7]

In men, a digital rectal examination will help determine the size of the prostate gland and the presence of nodules posteriorly. Prostate size does not directly correlate with intensity of lower urinary tract symptoms. However, symptoms are related to the degree of obstruction caused by the prostate.[4] The penis should be inspected for evidence of meatal stricture or phimosis.

A pelvic examination should be performed for women. Careful inspection of the external genitalia, vaginal and uterine cavities, and rectum may reveal contributors to urinary obstruction. It may also yield information about anatomy, such as prolapse, that might contribute to obstruction.

DIAGNOSTICS

Several diagnostic studies may be helpful in diagnosing urinary obstruction. A postvoid residual provides information about the residual urine in the bladder. Catheterization provides a sterile urine specimen for analysis, and a urine culture should be done to exclude infection. Urinalysis is necessary for all patients for whom obstructive uropathy is suspected. This can detect pyuria, microscopic hematuria, and abnormalities in urine pH that can occur with calculi or infection.[1] Gross hematuria is often seen in acute obstruction and is usually caused by calculi or bladder tumor but can be a result of infection as well.[1] Uric acid crystals in the urine sediment suggest uric acid nephropathy or calculi.

Routine blood studies are nonspecific. Complete blood count (CBC) and electrolyte values may be helpful in identifying anemia and alterations in fluid status. Blood urea nitrogen (BUN) and creatinine levels and glomerular filtration rate will be helpful in determining alterations in renal function if renal insufficiency is suspected.[1] Blood glucose concentration or hemoglobin A_{1c} level can help assess for diabetes. Further workup depends on results from these tests and the suspected cause of symptoms.

In patients with flank pain, renal calculus must be excluded (see Chapter 152). A stone protocol non–contrast-enhanced computed tomography (CT) scan is the best test to detect a stone and obstruction without use of contrast media.[17] If stones are not suspected, a diagnostic ultrasound evaluation is the preferred procedure for visualization of the renal pelvis and diagnosis of hydronephrosis.[1] Urodynamics may be helpful in diagnosis of lower tract obstruction such as bladder outlet obstruction. Other procedures useful in determining the site of obstruction include anterograde and retrograde pyelography.[1]

A hematuria workup should include cystoscopy and an imaging study of the upper tracts. Intravenous pyelography is being used less frequently in favor of the spiral CT scan (CT urography) for imaging of the kidneys, ureters, and bladder (KUB).[17]

DIAGNOSTICS

Obstructive Uropathy and Genitourinary Tumors

OBSTRUCTIVE UROPATHY

Initial
- Postvoid residual
- Urine dip for leukocytes, nitrites, blood

Laboratory
- CBC and differential
- Serum glucose, serum electrolytes, BUN, and creatinine
- Glomerular filtration rate
- Microalbumin
- Urinalysis
- Urine cultures*
- Blood cultures*

Imaging
- KUB
- Intravenous pyelography
- Ultrasound (duplex Doppler ultrasonography)
- CT scan
- Anterograde and retrograde pyelography
- Diffusion-weighted magnetic resonance imaging (MRI)

Other Diagnostics
- Cystoscopy
- Urodynamics
- Diuretic renography
- Perfusion pressure-flow study

RENAL CELL CARCINOMA

Laboratory
- Urinalysis
- Urine cytology*
- CBC and differential
- Serum glucose, electrolytes, BUN, and creatinine
- Liver function tests
- Calcium

Imaging
- Intravenous pyelography
- Ultrasound
- CT scans, MRI
- Renal angiography*
- Retrograde pyelography*

Other Diagnostics
- Cystoscopy

WILMS TUMOR

Laboratory
- Urinalysis
- CBC and differential
- BUN, creatinine
- Coagulation screening
- Imaging
- Ultrasound
- CT scan
- Chest x-ray studies*

BLADDER CANCER

Laboratory
- Urine for cytology
- Imaging
- Spiral CT (CT urography)
- Ultrasound
- Intravenous pyelography
- CT scan

OTHER DIAGNOSTICS
- Cystoscopy with biopsy

*If indicated.

DIFFERENTIAL DIAGNOSIS OF URINARY TRACT OBSTRUCTION AND RENAL TUMORS

See differential diagnosis box.

MANAGEMENT

Treatment to relieve partial obstruction is indicated when the patient has recurrent infections, significant symptoms, urinary retention, and impaired renal function. Urinary tract obstruction complicated by infection should be relieved as soon as possible to prevent development of sepsis, to preserve renal function, to normalize blood pressure, to correct fluid and electrolyte imbalances, and to treat pain. Acute treatment of lower tract obstruction is catheterization.[1]

Obstruction caused by BPH is not always progressive, and the patient need not be treated unless retention, recurrent infection, or unacceptable symptoms are present. Irritative symptoms often include frequency, nocturia, difficulty initiating a urinary stream, dribbling, and incontinence. Chronic urinary retention because of prostatic hypertrophy may respond

DIFFERENTIAL DIAGNOSIS

Obstructive Uropathy and Genitourinary Tumors

OBSTRUCTIVE UROPATHY

Intrinsic (Outflow Obstruction)

Intraluminal
- Stones
- Papilla
- Clots
- Fungal balls

Structural
- Stricture
- Tumors, polyps
- Infection: granuloma
- Anatomic defects
- Valve or sphincter abnormalities

Functional
- Vesicoureteral reflux
- Adynamic ureters
- Neurogenic bladder

Extrinsic (Outflow Obstruction)

Autoimmune
- Vascular, glomerular, or tubulointerstitial disease

Abdominal
- Ileum, left colon, duodenum, gallbladder disease
- Aneurysms (aortic or renal)
- Appendicitis

Pelvic
- Prostatic hypertrophy
- Cysts, tumors of the uterus, ovaries
- Endometriosis
- Pregnancy, ectopic pregnancy
- Phimosis, meatal stenosis

Retroperitoneal
- Fibrosis
- Tumor, lymphoma

GENITOURINARY TUMORS

Renal Cell Carcinoma

Simple cyst
Angiomyolipoma
Renal abscess
Arteriovenous malformations
Renal lymphoma
TCC of renal pelvis
Adrenal cancer
Oncocytoma

Wilms Tumor

Neuroblastoma
Hepatoblastoma
Germ cell or teratoma
Hydronephrosis
Mesoblastic nephroma
Fecal mass
Renal tumor, non-Wilms tumor

Bladder Cancer

UTIs
Interstitial cystitis
Hemorrhagic cystitis
Fibrous polyp
Endometriosis
Hematoma
Bladder calculi

to $alpha_1$ blockers such as terazosin (Hytrin) and doxazosin (Cardura).[18] There are at least three subtypes of $alpha_1$ receptors, with the 1A subtype being most predominant in the prostate. Alpha blockers specific for the 1A subtype include tamsulosin hydrochloride (Flomax) and alfuzosin (Uroxatral).[18]

5α-Reductase inhibitors—antitestosterone products such as finasteride (Proscar) and dutasteride (Avodart)—can be effective for relieving symptoms of BPH by reducing prostate size, thereby increasing urinary flow (see Chapter 147).[18,19]

The decision to undertake surgical or instrumental procedures for the relief of obstruction depends on the location of obstruction, presence of infection, and status of renal function. Relief of complete obstruction should occur as soon as possible after diagnosis. Infection in the face of an acute obstruction requires emergent treatment because relief of obstruction and antibiotics are both essential in treating the infection. Furthermore, antibiotics are given before any surgical intervention used to relieve obstruction. In cases of chronic incomplete obstruction, such as BPH, surgery is ideally done only when the urine is sterile.[1]

Renal Cell Carcinoma

The prognosis for RCC is poor unless it is diagnosed and treated before metastasis occurs. Surgical intervention for localized disease offers the only potential for cure.[2] Surgical options include a radical nephrectomy, which may be done as a laparoscopic procedure or as an open procedure. A nephron-sparing partial nephrectomy may be an option in select situations.[6]

Preoperative renal artery embolization may be used to minimize blood loss or to minimize pain or hematuria in the case of a nonresectable tumor.[2,6] For patients with disseminated disease, radiotherapy is used for palliation of metastatic lesions (e.g., to the brain, bone, or lungs). RCC has shown limited response to biologic response modifiers (e.g., interferons, interleukin).[2]

Targeted therapies for metastatic RCC have been employed for the treatment of advanced disease, with variable outcomes. Small-molecule therapy is another targeted treatment of metastatic RCC that may increase survival rates.[2]

Wilms Tumor

For the child with Wilms tumor, multimodality therapy has been successful, with cure rates currently greater than 90%.[7] Chemotherapy is recommended for bilateral disease before kidney resection. Radiation therapy is recommended in advanced cases.[8]

Bladder Cancer

Transurethral resection of the bladder tumor is usually the initial treatment of superficial bladder cancer. In cases of less aggressive cancer, follow-up surveillance may include interval urine cytologic studies and repeated cystoscopy with transurethral resection as necessary. Adjuvant intravesical therapy (e.g., bacillus Calmette-Guérin, mitomycin-C, thiotepa, doxorubicin) may be used for tumors with unfavorable prognostic features (e.g., frequent recurrence, multifocal tumors, carcinoma in situ). For muscle-invasive bladder tumors, a radical cystectomy with urinary diversion remains the standard therapy. Options for urinary diversion include ileal conduit, continent diversion, and orthotopic neobladder. Bladder conservation therapy, with combined modalities of radiation therapy and chemotherapy, may be an option for some patients.[9,11]

LIFE SPAN CONSIDERATIONS

Obstructive uropathy can occur at any age. Prenatal ultrasound has made it possible to diagnose obstruction in the fetus during pregnancy. In the young adult, acute obstruction is most likely a result of calculi. In women, pelvic cancer is an important cause of obstruction, and in men, BPH and prostate cancer are common causes.[1]

Because clinical evidence of RCC occurs late in the disease and discovery is usually accidental, survival rate at 5 years with stage IIIB is 18%. If the tumor is localized to the kidney, the average 5-year survival is 96%.[2,11] Even in muscle-invasive bladder cancer, survival rates can reach 70%. Lifetime follow-up is recommended to detect recurrences and to improve survival rates for bladder cancers.[20]

Wilms tumors boast the second highest cure rates of childhood cancers, with the survival rates at 5 years being greater than 90%.[7] Prognosis is poorer with diffuse anaplasia.

BOX 154-1

Complications of Obstructive Uropathy and Genitourinary Tumors

URINARY TRACT OBSTRUCTIONS
- Azotemia
- Life-threatening sepsis
- Chronic renal insufficiency or renal failure
- Surgical procedures: infection, sepsis, bleeding, voiding difficulty, pain from surgical intervention
- Postobstructive diuresis

GENITOURINARY TUMORS

Renal Cell Carcinoma
- Complications of metastasis
- Anemia
- Pain
- Hypercalcemia
- Erythrocytosis
- Hypertension
- Hepatic dysfunction

Wilms Tumor
- Treatment-related morbidity including surgical complications, chemotherapy, and scoliosis from partial vertebral irradiation
- Metastasis-related morbidity
- Complications of associated congenital anomalies

Bladder Cancer
- Bladder perforation
- Hematuria
- Clot retention
- Metastasis
- Treatment-related morbidity
- Obstruction

COMPLICATIONS

Complications of untreated urinary tract obstruction include azotemia, life-threatening sepsis, and obstructive nephropathy that can lead to chronic renal insufficiency or renal failure. Complications of surgical procedures include infection, sepsis, bleeding, voiding difficulty, and pain.

Profound and prolonged diuresis, known as postobstructive diuresis, can follow relief of complete obstruction.[1] This diuresis—characterized by marked losses of water and solutes such as sodium, potassium, and magnesium—is usually self-limited. However, loss of solutes can often result in hypovolemia, hyponatremia, hypokalemia, and hypomagnesemia. Careful fluid replacement and monitoring of weight and serum and urine electrolyte values should be performed in these patients.[1] Box 154-1 lists complications of both obstructive uropathy and genitourinary tumors.

INDICATIONS FOR REFERRAL OR HOSPITALIZATION

Renal calculi larger than 5 to 7 mm usually do not pass spontaneously and should be treated surgically.[3] These patients as well as those with other obstructive symptoms should be referred to a urologist for consultation and initiation of an appropriate care plan. In cases of anuria and acute renal failure, a nephrology referral should be made for appropriate management because hospitalization or dialysis may be needed. In patients with a history and clinical presentation suggestive of genitourinary tumors, specialist referral and consultation should be obtained as soon as possible. Hospitalization may be indicated for cases of acute illness or advanced disease.[21]

PATIENT EDUCATION

Patients with urinary tract obstruction are frequently uncomfortable and often frightened. Every effort should be made to alleviate discomfort and to provide information and reassurance. All patients with obstruction should be taught the signs and symptoms of infection and how to take their temperature. If obstruction is a result of calculi, patients need to understand that the likelihood of recurrence is high.[3] Patients with BPH taking nonselective alpha blockers need to be advised of the potential for postural hypotension and confusion, especially if they are elderly.[22] All patients need to know how to access the health care system in an emergency situation, whether they are at home or traveling.

Patient education for tumors of the genitourinary tract should include information about prevention, the disease process, diagnostic and staging procedures, treatment options, prognosis, and symptom management. The importance of lifelong surveillance and follow-up should be emphasized.

HEALTH PROMOTION

Adequate daily fluid intake may help prevent recurrence of urinary tract obstructions related to nephrolithiasis. Dietary modification, depending on the type of stone, may be indicated as well.

Unfortunately, there currently are no screening tests for cancers of the kidneys, ureters, or bladder. Urine cytologic testing may be done, but it is most sensitive and specific in high-grade urothelial cancers. Urine cytology may be falsely negative in as many of 50% to 75% of cases of low- to moderate-grade urothelial cancers.[23]

Cigarette smoking remains the greatest risk factor for bladder cancer. Health promotion that emphasizes no smoking or smoking cessation is a critical aspect of prevention.[9]

REFERENCES

For a full list of references, scan the QR code or visit http://booksite.elsevier.com/9780323355018

PART 14 Evaluation and Management of Gynecologic Concerns

CHAPTER 155

AMENORRHEA

Marie Elena Botte

DEFINITION AND EPIDEMIOLOGY

Amenorrhea is the absence or abnormal cessation of menstrual bleeding. *Primary amenorrhea* is defined as the absence of both spontaneous uterine bleeding and secondary sexual characteristics (delayed puberty) at the age of 14 years or by 2 years after sexual maturation or the absence of menarche at the age of 16 years regardless of the presence of secondary sexual characteristics. *Secondary amenorrhea* has been variously defined and refers to the absence of menstrual bleeding in a woman with prior menstruation.[1] Although the average age for menarche in the United States is 12.7 years[1] (12.8 years for white adolescents and slightly earlier, 12.6 years, for African American adolescents), there is a range of 9 to 16 years, and factors other than race, such as nutritional status, body fat, and maternal age at menarche, are also contributory.

Primary amenorrhea has an estimated prevalence of 0.1% to 0.3%. Secondary amenorrhea is much more common, affecting 1% to 3% of women of reproductive age in the general population. Higher prevalence has been noted in specific subgroups of women, such as college students, endurance athletes (particularly runners and elite athletes in sports and activities that emphasize thinness,[2] such as ballet), and women who are obese.

Up to 25% of female athletes experience exercise-induced amenorrhea. The female athlete triad involves the combination of amenorrhea, osteoporosis, and disordered eating; it affects female athletes in all sports and at all levels of training, as well as both professional and amateur dancers.[3] Approximately 2.5% of healthy adolescents will experience pubertal delay.

PATHOPHYSIOLOGY

Aside from physiologic amenorrhea resulting from constitutional delay, pregnancy, lactation, or menopause, the pathophysiologic mechanisms for amenorrhea generally involve disorders of the sex chromosomes, hypothalamic-pituitary-ovarian axis, and related hormone production; the responsiveness of the uterine endometrium to various hormones; and the patency of the outflow tract. Because normal ovarian development depends on the presence of at least two X chromosomes, abnormalities involving X and Y chromosomes can result in gonadal failure, agonadism, gonadal dysgenesis, and androgen resistance (testicular feminization). Problems with hypothalamic synthesis or release of gonadotropin-releasing hormone (GnRH) can result in hypogonadotropic hypogonadism. Müllerian agenesis, obstruction of the vaginal outflow tract (such as with an imperforate hymen), cervical stenosis, and transverse vaginal septa are structural causes of primary amenorrhea.

Disorders of the hypothalamic-pituitary-ovarian axis can cause primary or secondary amenorrhea. Leptin, a hormone secreted by adipocytes, signals energy availability in energy-deficient states and may have a major role in the regulation, synthesis, and secretion of sex steroids, gonadotropins, and GnRH. In the face of significant energy expenditure, the body may lack a compensatory response in terms of adequate calorie intake; decreased luteinizing hormone (LH) secretion and a subsequent lack of estrogen production may result. Other pituitary hormones (triiodothyronine, growth hormone, and insulin-like growth factor 1) may also be affected. Hypothalamic causes of dysfunction have been linked to weight loss, intensive exercise, starvation, eating disorders, and psychogenic stress in nonathletic, normal-weight women and can result in pubertal delay or secondary hormonal insufficiency. Persistent amenorrhea has also been correlated with a longer duration of eating disorders and the presence of a concomitant anxiety disorder. The majority of young women with amenorrhea are estrogen deficient; a minority have normal estrogen levels that are unopposed by progesterone secondary to anovulation. Neurotransmitter abnormalities (central dopaminergic and opioid activity) may modulate the response of LH to GnRH. Amenorrhea can also be seen in obese patients; reduction of body fat can bring about return of regular menstrual flow.

Prolactinemia associated with amenorrhea after normal puberty may be caused by breastfeeding, microadenomas or macroadenomas of the pituitary, renal failure, or the use of medications (e.g., psychoactive drugs such as haloperidol, amitriptyline, benzodiazepines, cocaine). Anovulation associated with hyperprolactinemic amenorrhea is primarily caused by both impaired gonadotropin pulsatility and derangement of the estrogen-positive feedback effect on LH in the face of a continued ovarian response to gonadotropin. In polycystic ovary syndrome (PCOS), a low ratio of progesterone to estrogen is associated with menstrual irregularity and amenorrhea. Drugs (chemotherapeutic agents, thalidomide, leuprolide, heroin, gabapentin) may affect menstruation. Autoimmune disorders (systemic lupus erythematosus, Addison disease, hypothyroidism, and toxic thyroiditis) have also been associated with amenorrhea. In thalassemic patients with secondary amenorrhea, severe and progressive damage to the hypothalamic-pituitary axis has been demonstrated by gonadotropin pulse abnormalities, marked reduction in GnRH-stimulated gonadotropin levels, and even apulsatility.

CLINICAL PRESENTATION

Relevant history in the evaluation of amenorrhea includes a thorough menstrual history (age at menarche; frequency, duration, and flow of menstrual periods; last menstrual period; history of missed menses). Obtaining a complete sexual history (number of partners; date of last intercourse; method of birth control and percentage of use; number of pregnancies, abortions, miscarriages, or ectopic pregnancies; and surgical history) as well as the age at menarche and menopause for family members and any family history of infertility is also necessary.

Probable signs of past ovulatory cycles include breast tenderness, cyclic abdominal pain or bloating, and changes in the cervical mucus. The past medical history should be examined specifically for autoimmune disorders, childhood onset of type 1 diabetes mellitus, previous irradiation or chemotherapy, frequent fractures or osteoporosis, and thyroid or adrenal dysfunction. A complete medication history regarding prescribed, over-the-counter, and illicit drug use should be obtained. Nutritional and exercise factors, including disordered eating behavior, recent weight loss or gain, and athletic training, are evaluated, along with endocrinologic markers of growth and development (growth charts and the presence or absence of secondary sexual characteristics, specifically breast development and pubic hair).

A review of systems may reveal indications of systemic illness, such as thyroid dysfunction, headaches or visual disturbances (possibly indicating a cranial mass in the area of the pituitary or hypothalamus), galactorrhea, and signs of hyperandrogenism (hirsutism, truncal obesity, deepening of the voice) or hypoestrogenism (hot flashes, vaginal dryness, headaches, depression, dyspareunia, decreasing breast size). A social history may indicate substance abuse or stressful life events (e.g., going away to college, entering religious life or the armed forces, sudden changes in the environment, death or divorce in the family), which have been linked with amenorrhea.

PHYSICAL EXAMINATION

In addition to an evaluation of general growth and development (the presence of congenital short stature together with neck webbing and a pigeon chest suggests Turner syndrome), the physical examination may reveal signs of androgen excess (hirsutism, acne, male pattern hair loss, truncal obesity, clitoromegaly >1 cm [⅖ inch]), androgen insensitivity (complete absence of axillary and pubic hair), hyperprolactinemia (galactorrhea on breast examination), decreased estrogen status (pale, dry vaginal mucosa; scant cervical mucus), or eating disorders (cachexia, hypothermia, lanugo hair, decreased blood pressure, bradycardia, dry skin, tooth decay, chipmunk cheeks, Chvostek sign). Assessment of visual acuity and a funduscopic examination are important because vision changes or retinal abnormalities may reflect an intracranial mass. The thyroid is palpated for masses or nodules. A pelvic examination assesses estrogen status by vaginal epithelium and cervical mucus; it may identify an imperforate hymen and also provides a gross evaluation of the cervix, uterus, and ovaries. Enlarged ovaries are palpable in 60% of women with PCOS and, in combination with acne, obesity, and acanthosis nigricans, suggest this diagnosis. Abdominal striae on nulliparous women may be indicative of hypercortisolism, and skin tags, fissures, and fecal occult blood may indicate inflammatory bowel disease.

DIAGNOSTICS

The possibility of pregnancy or lactation-induced amenorrhea must be excluded in all women of childbearing age before any other diagnostic evaluation is initiated. Next, follicle-stimulating hormone (FSH) and LH should be checked (anovulation); thyroid-stimulating hormone (TSH) concentration is determined to evaluate for hypothyroidism; and prolactin levels are obtained to check for hyperprolactinemia or possibly an early presentation of acromegaly, which produces excess prolactin and growth hormone. If prolactin levels are elevated, a magnetic resonance imaging (MRI) or computed tomography (CT) scan of the sella turcica to identify microadenomas and macroadenomas is necessary (MRI is more effective than CT in detecting empty sella syndrome). If these scans are normal, a progesterone challenge test, which classically consists of 10 mg of medroxyprogesterone administered daily for 5 to 7 days, can be used to further evaluate estrogen status. Any vaginal bleeding within 2 to 7 days after the cessation of progesterone signals a positive progesterone challenge, indicating both adequate estrogen stores and patency of the outflow tract. A negative progesterone challenge (i.e., no bleeding 2 to 7 days after cessation of progesterone) indicates either inadequate estrogen stores or an obstruction of the outflow tract. To further differentiate hypoestrogenism from obstruction, the test can be repeated after daily administration of 2.5 mg of estrogen for 21 days, followed by 10 mg of progesterone for the next 5 days. If there is still no withdrawal bleeding, investigation into structural or outflow reasons for the amenorrhea should ensue.

If amenorrhea is secondary to anovulation, potential causes include Cushing syndrome, adrenal or ovarian tumors, premature ovarian failure, and, more commonly, PCOS. An FSH level elevated beyond 20 IU/L after repeated measurements is indicative of ovarian failure. An elevated LH/FSH ratio (>0.2) is suggestive of PCOS; an FSH level greater than 30 IU/L indicates menopausal status.

To differentiate between pituitary and hypothalamic amenorrhea, an LH-releasing hormone test is typically performed in conjunction with imaging of the sellar region by CT or MRI. Long-term administration of pulsatile GnRH can indicate hypothalamic amenorrhea by an ovulatory response within two treatment cycles. In the absence of an ovulatory response, a pituitary cause of the amenorrhea should be suspected.

MRI has been shown to be an effective and accurate tool to evaluate the cause of primary amenorrhea and to plan for surgery, particularly when this involves congenital disorders of sexual differentiation and localization of the gonads. A hysterosalpingogram or sonohysterogram can be used to outline the uterine cavity if a bicornuate uterus or double cervix is suspected.

The clomiphene challenge test may provide information necessary for an early diagnosis to be made of waning ovarian function in hypergonadotropic amenorrhea. Increased serum dehydroepiandrosterone (DHEA; >700 mg/dL) indicates an adrenal origin for androgens in women with hirsutism, and elevated plasma testosterone levels (>90 ng/dL) suggest tumors of adrenal and ovarian origin or congenital adrenal hyperplasia; levels above 200 ng/dL are found in the rare Sertoli-Leydig cell tumors. The level of sex hormone–binding globulin, which binds potent androgens such as testosterone and thereby controls the level of active androgens in circulation, may also provide useful clinical information.

Chemistry profiles (including serum electrolyte values and serum glucose, blood urea nitrogen [BUN], and creatinine concentrations), urinary free cortisol, thyroid antibodies, erythrocyte sedimentation rate (ESR), and hemoglobin A_{1c} can help differentiate possible causes of autoimmune-related amenorrhea[4] (Addison disease, diabetes mellitus, thyroiditis, and hypoparathyroidism), which are responsible for 20% to 40% of cases of primary ovarian insufficiency. The diagnosis of premature ovarian failure in a young woman (in general, younger than 25 or 30 years) warrants karyotyping to exclude the presence of a Y chromosome.

DIAGNOSTICS

Amenorrhea

LABORATORY

Initial Diagnostics
- Serum human chorionic gonadotropin
- Thyroid profile
- LH
- FSH
- Prolactin

Additional Testing, if Indicated
- DHEA
- Serum electrolytes
- Thyroid antibodies
- Serum glucose
- BUN
- Creatinine
- ESR
- Urinary free cortisol
- Glucose tolerance test

IMAGING
- CT or MRI

OTHER DIAGNOSTICS
- Clomiphene challenge test

DIFFERENTIAL DIAGNOSIS

Primary Amenorrhea

Physiologic primary amenorrhea may be attributable to constitutional delay, although 97% to 99% of young women experience menarche by age 16 years and 95% by 14.5 years. Failure of the gonads to develop normally accounts for half of all cases of primary amenorrhea. Other possible causes include Turner syndrome (45,X) mosaicism; abnormal X chromosomes; the presence of an intact or fragmented Y chromosome; complex chromosomal rearrangement; chromosomal deletions; pure gonadal dysgenesis (may manifest with hyperandrogenism); steroidogenic factor 1 (SF-1) mutation; and the rare 17α-hydroxylase deficiency, which is seen with hypernatremia, hypokalemia, and hypocortisolism.

Additional causes of primary amenorrhea include structural abnormalities (imperforate hymen, transverse septum, congenital absence of the uterus or vagina), premature ovarian failure (may be idiopathic or secondary to radiation therapy or chemotherapeutics), malnutrition, systemic illness, tumors (ovarian, hypothalamic, parasellar, or adrenal), and any of the disturbances in the hypothalamic-pituitary-ovarian axis that also cause secondary amenorrhea. Rare causes of primary amenorrhea include mutations in the beta subunit of FSH, vaginal inversion and uterus acollis, multiple endocrine neoplasia, progesterone-producing adrenal adenoma, increased melatonin secretion from a cystic pineal lesion, and childhood trauma.

Secondary Amenorrhea

Pregnancy is the most common cause of secondary amenorrhea; lactation and early menopause are other physiologic possibilities. Transient amenorrhea may occur in the first two postmenarchal years, after discontinuation of oral contraceptives, and in the majority of women who receive medroxyprogesterone (Depo-Provera) for contraception. Aside from these causes, secondary amenorrhea is most often linked to disordered functioning somewhere along the hypothalamic-pituitary-ovarian axis.

Other causes of secondary amenorrhea include primary ovarian insufficiency (previously referred to as *premature ovarian failure*), which may be of an autoimmune cause,[4] and chronic anovulatory disorder (PCOS, obesity-related disorder, idiopathic disorder). Less common conditions include pituitary tumors, hyperprolactinemia, Sheehan syndrome (postpartum pituitary necrosis), hypogonadotropic hypogonadism, thyroid disease, tuberculosis, and late-onset 21-hydroxylase deficiency. For the majority of women, a clinical history, physical examination, and laboratory determination of TSH, LH, FSH, and prolactin levels are sufficient for diagnosis.

Categorization of amenorrhea by cause (hyperprolactinemic, hyperandrogenic, hypergonadotropic, and hypogonadotropic) provides a helpful framework for consideration of the differential diagnosis, evaluation, and management.

Hyperprolactinemic amenorrhea can be caused by drugs (including reserpine, phenothiazines, oral contraceptives, metoclopramide, and α-methyldopa), prolactin-secreting tumors of the pituitary, or systemic illness such as acromegaly or hypothyroidism. Physiologic causes of increased prolactin levels include lactation and nipple stimulation.

Hyperandrogenic amenorrhea is seen most commonly in women with PCOS (also called *hyperandrogenic chronic anovulation* or *Stein-Leventhal syndrome*) but may also be caused by obesity, Cushing syndrome, hyperprolactinemia, thyroid disease, adrenal disease (hyperplasia, adenoma, carcinoma), androgen-secreting ovarian tumors, or drug abuse.

DIFFERENTIAL DIAGNOSIS

Amenorrhea

PRIMARY AMENORRHEA
- Structural abnormalities
  - Vaginal inversion
  - Uterus acollis
  - Trauma
- Disturbances of the hypothalamic-pituitary-ovarian axis
  - Premature ovarian failure
  - Primary ovarian insufficiency
- Systemic illness
  - Malnutrition
  - Multiple endocrine neoplasia
- Genetic or chromosomal problems
  - Turner syndrome
  - 17α-Hydroxylase deficiency
  - Gonadal dysgenesis (chromosomal translocation)
- Tumors: ovarian, hypothalamic, parasellar, or adrenal

SECONDARY AMENORRHEA
- Physiologic causes
  - Pregnancy
  - Lactation
  - Menopause and perimenopause
- Medications (oral contraceptives, reserpine, metoclopramide, medroxyprogesterone)
- Disorders of the hypothalamic-pituitary-ovarian axis
  - Premature ovarian failure
  - Hypogonadotropic hypogonadism
  - Chronic anovulatory disorder (polycystic ovary syndrome, obesity-related disorder, idiopathic disorder)
  - Pituitary tumor
  - Hyperprolactinemia
- Other causes
  - Sheehan syndrome
  - Thyroid disease
  - Tuberculosis
  - Late-onset 21-hydroxylase deficiency

Hypergonadotropic amenorrhea affects about 1% of women younger than 40 years. The differential diagnosis for ovarian failure includes chromosomal (mosaicism and gonadal dysgenesis), autoimmune (Hashimoto thyroiditis, Addison disease, diabetes mellitus, hypoparathyroidism), metabolic (ovarian enzymatic defects), familial, infectious (mumps), idiopathic, and iatrogenic (irradiation, chemotherapy) causes as well as resistant ovary syndrome.

Hypogonadotropic amenorrhea, a clinical syndrome of gonadal failure caused by abnormal pituitary gonadotropin levels, can be a result of either congenital or acquired causes,[2] including functional and organic forms. Although relatively common in young women as a result of emotional or physical stress (including athletic training), depression, nutritional deficiency, weight loss, and eating disorders, it can also be caused by thyroid or adrenal dysfunction, isolated gonadotropin deficiency (Kallmann syndrome), or hypothalamic or pituitary lesions (craniopharyngiomas, germinomas, pituitary adenomas, endodermal sinus tumors, pituitary apoplexy, empty sella syndrome, postpartum ischemia, necrosis of the pituitary gland). Amenorrhea is one of the cardinal features of anorexia nervosa. Head injuries (especially head-on automobile collisions resulting in whiplash) and external irradiation can damage the hypothalamus; infections (tuberculosis, human immunodeficiency virus [HIV]) can disrupt pituitary function.

In addition to disorders of the hypothalamic-pituitary-ovarian axis, secondary amenorrhea can be caused by uterine pathologic conditions, including endometrial hyperplasia, postpartum uterine adhesions, and iatrogenic Asherman syndrome. Rare causes of secondary amenorrhea include hydrocephalus, Pendred syndrome, onchocerciasis, inhibin-secreting ovarian tumors, Sjögren syndrome, and neurosarcoidosis.

MANAGEMENT

Women with eating disorders, such as anorexia nervosa, are best managed in collaboration with psychiatric or other specialized eating disorder services. Evidence of anatomic or endocrinologic abnormalities mandates co-management with the appropriate specialist.

1. In amenorrhea caused by systemic illness or endocrinopathy, treatment of the underlying cause, such as diabetes mellitus or hypothyroidism, generally resolves the amenorrhea as a result of renewed ovarian function.
2. Spontaneous recovery of menses also occurs after diagnosis of premature ovarian failure, after prolonged irradiation-induced ovarian failure from treatment of Hodgkin disease, and in cases of chemotherapy-induced ovarian failure; there is evidence to suggest that taxane, as an adjuvant agent, may help prevent chemotherapy-related amenorrhea and that the use of oral contraceptives during chemotherapy may also decrease post-treatment amenorrhea. Gonadal function should be reassessed periodically in these women, and oral contraceptives are a good choice for hormone replacement in women not desiring pregnancy.
3. Menses generally return 6 to 14 months after a last injection of medroxyprogesterone and within 6 months after stopping of oral contraceptives in post–oral contraceptive amenorrhea. Eventual return of menstruation has been shown, after a variable interval, for less than half of women with medically refractory menorrhagia after endometrial ablation and uterine resection.
4. In perimenopausal women, amenorrheic intervals are common and do not require any treatment aside from adequate contraception when pregnancy is not desired; in these women, unplanned pregnancy is possible unless FSH levels have been consistently elevated (>30 IU/L) and the amenorrhea has been present for more than 1 year.
5. Complete recovery of gonadal function in hypothalamic amenorrhea depends on restoration of the hypothalamic-pituitary-adrenal and the hypothalamic-pituitary-thyroidal axes, and so psychological interventions[5] (such as cognitive behavioral therapy [CBT]) that focus on changing behaviors and attitudes and pharmacologic interventions that target the resultant hormonal dysfunction are often necessary; multidisciplinary approaches to treatment are generally encouraged.
6. Whereas women with anorexia or other eating disorders and endurance athletes have benefited from increased calorie intake and decreased exercise,[6] some overweight and hirsute women with hyperandrogenism may recover normal menses with control of excess body weight by calorie restriction. Menstrual return can often be predicted by a return to the weight at which previous function ceased.
7. Recombinant human leptin has been used in research settings in women with hypothalamic amenorrhea, resulting in normalization of levels of reproductive hormones, follicular development, and menstrual cyclicity.
8. Pulsatile GnRH has also been used to induce ovulation[7] in hypothalamic infertile women with PCOS. GnRH administration on alternate days has also been used to increase FSH levels, to reinstate LH pulsatility, and, in conjunction with clomiphene therapy, to induce ovulation in women with weight loss–associated amenorrhea.
9. Clomiphene has also been used alone, and naltrexone hydrochloride, an oral antiopioid, has also been studied as an agent in the management of amenorrhea resulting from hypogonadotropic syndromes.
10. Estrogen, the current standard of pharmacologic care, does not address the underlying infertility or neuroendocrine dysfunction associated with hypothalamic amenorrhea in anorexia nervosa, but early research does suggest a possible a role for the administration of a weak estrogen, estriol,[8] in the spontaneous and GnRH-induced LH secretion in women with functional hypothalamic amenorrhea.
11. One review of the available literature on the use of oral contraceptives or hormone replacement therapy by these women determined that available evidence was both of low quality and mixed,[9] in terms of improving lumbar spine and total body bone mineral density. Although supplemental estrogen and progesterone (as with oral contraceptives) have been recommended for the prevention of further bone loss and subsequent fracture development in women with decreased estrogen levels, normalization of body weight is the single most important factor in regaining bone density. Irreversible bone loss can occur after 3 years of amenorrhea. Although scant direct evidence supports the use of hormone replacement therapy in amenorrheic women, there is some evidence that taking long-term triphasic oral contraceptives can increase total lumbar spine bone mineral density in women with hypothalamic amenorrhea and osteopenia and can improve both endothelial function and dyslipidemia in amenorrheic athletes.

12. Adequate calcium and, if indicated, vitamin D intake or supplementation plus weight-bearing exercise should be encouraged in women who are amenorrheic for any reason to help maintain bone density.
13. Administration of estrogen and progesterone is also necessary after hysteroscopic adhesiolysis to reestablish a functional endometrium in women with Asherman syndrome.
14. No treatment is required if women maintain normal estradiol and prolactin levels in post–oral contraceptive amenorrhea.
15. Amenorrhea caused by heroin use has been reversed with methadone maintenance.
16. Bromocriptine has been widely studied with demonstrated effectiveness for promoting menstrual bleeding and ovulation and for years has been the drug of choice for hyperprolactinemic amenorrhea and the syndrome of galactorrhea-amenorrhea. In case of relapse, this treatment should be resumed and continued.
17. An alternative, cabergoline, may be more effective and better tolerated than bromocriptine, with fewer gastrointestinal symptoms; this drug may be a better first choice initial treatment[10] in many women. Subcutaneous pulsatile GnRH therapy combined with human chorionic gonadotropin has been proposed as a method of ovulation induction if these women should desire pregnancy.

LIFE SPAN CONSIDERATIONS

The prognosis for present or future fertility is a major concern of many women with amenorrhea and will guide the treatment plan in most instances. For women with hypothalamic amenorrhea resulting from stress, weight loss, or exercise, reassurance about the reversible nature of the problem after requisite lifestyle modification may be all that is necessary. For other women, such as those with primary ovarian insufficiency, cryopreservation of oocytes or ovarian tissue[11] (the only option for prepubertal girls) is becoming increasingly possible. For women with structural or chromosomal abnormalities incompatible with achieving a natural pregnancy, alternatives such as adoption, egg donation, or surrogacy may need to be considered.

COMPLICATIONS

Untreated amenorrhea is associated with significant long-term morbidity, especially when it occurs in younger women. Loss of body weight is adversely related to pituitary-ovarian function, and in 20% to 30% of women with weight loss–related amenorrhea, no restoration of function is attained despite recovery of body weight.

Hypoestrogenemic amenorrhea, which includes the female athlete triad, has been associated with an increased risk of decreased bone mineral density[12] that can manifest decades later as osteoporosis and fractures. The female athlete triad has also been linked to endothelial dysfunction,[13] with potential for cardiovascular consequences. Although some improvements in bone mineral density have been observed with appropriate treatment of amenorrhea, this recovery in bone mass has not been substantial, emphasizing the importance of early diagnosis and treatment.

The hypoestrogenemic state has also been associated with endothelial dysfunction, unfavorable lipid profiles, and a significantly increased risk of cardiovascular events. Anovulatory amenorrhea puts women at increased risk for endometrial hyperplasia and endometrial carcinoma. Women with PCOS and women with chronic hyperandrogenic anovulation have a high risk of metabolic syndrome and cardiovascular disease.[14]

INDICATIONS FOR REFERRAL OR HOSPITALIZATION

Suspected or confirmed genetic abnormalities that result in primary or secondary amenorrhea warrant referral to a specialist for more thorough evaluation. Young women with either Y chromosome fragments or an entire Y chromosome will need to have their gonads removed after pubertal development is complete because of the increased risk of malignant gonadoblastoma. Referral to an infertility specialist is indicated for women with ovarian reserve factors, anovulatory cycles, hyperprolactinemia, and genetic or structural factors.

Hospitalization may be necessary for women with anorexia nervosa who have lost more than 30% of their desired body weight and fail to gain weight, as well as for those with suicidal ideation. Inpatient surgical care may be indicated for women with tumors or adenomas associated with amenorrhea.

PATIENT AND FAMILY EDUCATION AND HEALTH PROMOTION

Women will have varying educational needs depending on the cause of their amenorrhea, but all women should receive basic nutritional counseling with an emphasis on obtaining sufficient calcium from either food sources or supplementation. Women should also be reminded that pregnancy can occur in the presence of amenorrhea; sexually active women not desiring pregnancy, especially adolescents, should receive appropriate contraceptive counseling. Women with genetic or congenital abnormalities may wonder about their ability to become pregnant and need to be apprised of their reproductive potential. The necessity for gonadectomy to prevent future malignant neoplasms should be discussed with women who have Y chromosome fragments or a Y chromosome.

The reversible nature of most cases of hypothalamic amenorrhea resulting from stress, weight changes, or exercise as well as the temporary (6 months or less) duration of post–oral contraceptive amenorrhea can be stressed when relevant. When counseling athletes, the health care provider should remind them, as well as trainers and coaches, that amenorrhea can be an indication of overtraining and can contribute to future performance deficits, especially in light of the long-term health consequences, such as fractures and osteoporosis. Like hypoestrogenemic women, women with androgen excess are at increased risk of lipid abnormalities and coronary artery disease. Counseling may be required in an effort to reduce other contributing risk factors, such as obesity.

CHAPTER 156

BARTHOLIN GLAND CYSTS AND ABSCESSES

Marie Elena Botte

DEFINITION AND EPIDEMIOLOGY

Bartholin glands, also known as the greater vestibular or vulvovaginal glands, were first discovered by the French anatomist

Joseph-Guichard du Verney in the late 17th century[1]; their physiology was described by the Danish anatomist Gaspard Bartholin in 1677.[2] These paired glands, homologous to the male bulbourethral glands in structure, placement, and function, have narrow ducts about 2.5 cm (1 inch) long that open into the vestibule just distal to the hymenal ring at the 5-o'clock and 7-o'clock positions. The glands become active at puberty and continuously secrete mucus through their narrow ducts. This mucus lubricates the vulva, and the glands are generally not palpable unless a cyst or abscess develops. Bartholin gland cysts are usually noninfectious enlargements of the gland related to ductal obstruction, which can occur as a result of inflammation, mucus, or congenitally even narrower ducts. Bartholin gland abscesses, also called bartholinitis or Bartholin adenitis, are the result of acute infection followed by obstruction.

Bartholin gland cysts occur most often during women's reproductive years, and an individual woman's lifetime risk of developing a Bartholin cyst or abscess is approximately about 2%.[3] A Korean study[4] found that the incidence increases until menopause and then declines. Another study designed to estimate the prevalence of Bartholin gland cysts in asymptomatic women serving as controls in research studies found that 3% of the participants had cysts of the gland that were visible on magnetic resonance imaging (MRI).[5] Half of these were on the right, nearly 43% were on the left, and the remaining 7% were bilateral. The cysts ranged in size from 0.5 to 2.7 cm, and on average the cysts were 1.3 × 1.2 × 1.3 cm. Clinicians are likely to encounter cysts of this gland approximately once per 46 pelvic examinations.[6]

PATHOPHYSIOLOGY

Cysts of the Bartholin gland are related to obstruction of the duct orifice. They are most commonly the result of trauma, parturition, or episiotomy and can be the result of inflammatory scarring, epithelial metaplasia, or inspissated secretions that accumulate. In the presence of an infectious process, inflammation of the gland's acinus may lead to abscess. Most cases are self-limited but can be severely discomforting.

Any opportunistic genital or genitourinary organism can be the cause of an acute inflammation, and infections can be the result of single organisms or polymicrobial in nature. Although it has long been generally held that most abscesses of the gland are caused by polymicrobial and sexually transmitted infections, one 6-year retrospective study found that *Escherichia coli* was the single most common (47%) pathogen identified on culture,[3] and less than 8% of all cases were polymicrobial. Nevertheless, studies have also demonstrated the presence of *Chlamydia trachomatis, Neisseria sicca,* "usual genital flora,[7]" methicillin-resistant *Staphylococcus aureus,*[7] and *Brucella melitensis; Bacteroides* species have been detected in cultures from abscess formations in human immunodeficiency virus (HIV) antibody–positive women. Capnophilic bacteria, gram-negative bacteria (*Proteus* organisms), *Neisseria gonorrhoeae,* and polymicrobial flora including gram-negative and gram-positive anaerobes have also been cultured. Anaerobic and facultative aerobic organisms have also been implicated in abscess formation.

CLINICAL PRESENTATION

Bartholin gland cysts are often asymptomatic, are generally unilateral, and range in size from 1 to 3 cm (⅖ to 1⅕ inches); they can be chronic or recurrent. Associated pain is usually a sign of an infectious process and development of an abscess, which can often grow large and rapidly during 2 to 4 days. Women may be seen with pain (especially while walking or standing), swelling, dyspareunia, or tenderness. Specific inquiry into recent history of an infectious process may yield clues to the cause. A recent vaginal delivery or history of localized trauma should be explored.

PHYSICAL EXAMINATION

Physical examination includes vital signs, visualization of the affected area, and assessment of accompanying inguinal node involvement. Patients usually exhibit a unilateral, erythematous, edematous mass located lateral to the vestibule that ranges from tender to extremely painful. The size may vary, and discharge is usually present. A speculum or bimanual examination may be too painful until the cyst or abscess has been treated.

DIAGNOSTICS

DIAGNOSTICS

Bartholin Gland Cysts and Abscesses

LABORATORY
Culture and sensitivity
CBC and differential

Culture of cystic contents and the cervix for sexually transmitted diseases is recommended to ensure adequate treatment of women and their sexual contacts. A complete blood count (CBC) can identify leukocytosis.

DIFFERENTIAL DIAGNOSIS

Cysts or abscesses of the Bartholin gland represent the majority of cysts in the vulvar region and are the most common diseases of the gland. Although solid benign tumors, adenocarcinomas, high-grade squamous intraepithelial neoplasias, carcinomas,[8] sarcomas,[9] mixed tumors, leiomyomas, adenofibromas, mucinous cystadenomas, myxoid leiomyosarcomas,[10] papillary tumors, mucocele-like changes, endometriosis,[11] and malacoplakia all can originate in (or, in the case of endometriosis, infiltrate) the Bartholin gland, these presentations are rare. Carcinoma of the Bartholin gland, which can be primary, accounts for less than 1% of all genital neoplasms in female patients. Tuberculosis of the Bartholin gland is also rare (vulval and vaginal infections account for less than 2% of genital tuberculosis) but should be considered if swelling does not resolve after excision. Primary neuroendocrine carcinoma (Merkel cell carcinoma) of the vulva can both originate in Bartholin gland and mimic Bartholin gland abscess.

DIFFERENTIAL DIAGNOSIS

Bartholin Gland Cysts

- Tumors
- Genital tuberculosis

MANAGEMENT

The goal of management is to preserve the gland and its function if possible. Many options are available, including antibiotics and office procedures, such as catheter placement for drainage.

Antibiotics

When it is initiated early, empirical antibiotic treatment can potentially prevent full-blown abscess formation and should focus on both aerobic and anaerobic organisms as potential sources of infection. Treatment is generally initiated with broad-spectrum antibiotics to decrease the chance of abscess formation or the need for surgical intervention. Metronidazole, 500 mg twice daily, and erythromycin, 250 mg four times daily for 10 days, are reasonable first-line therapies, followed by doxycycline, 100 mg twice daily for 10 days (not for pregnant women), or cephalexin, 250 mg four times daily for 10 days, for those who are allergic to or cannot tolerate erythromycin. Follow-up evaluation after antibiotic therapy is recommended at 7 to 10 days or sooner if there is fever or increased pain.

Surgical Treatments

A variety of surgical options to treat Bartholin gland cysts and abscesses have been cited in the literature, ranging from simple incision and drainage techniques (with or without the insertion of a catheter) to fistulization and marsupialization (the most commonly employed surgical techniques),[12] alcohol sclerotherapy, hydrodissection procedures, and the application of silver nitrate or carbon dioxide (CO_2) lasers. Adequate pain control is an important issue for all women who have surgical intervention for Bartholin gland cysts and abscesses.

Incision and Drainage. A commonly used management strategy for Bartholin gland cysts and abscesses and once the mainstay of treatment is incision and drainage followed by packing with gauze. The procedure requires minimal surgical skill but is not without disadvantages. Although the procedure is effective for temporary relief of symptoms, the recurrence rate is high. Weekly follow-up monitoring is recommended after placement of a drain.

Excision of Bartholin Gland. Removal of the entire gland, once standard procedure, is now recommended only when there is suspicion of malignancy or for recurrent abscess. Current surgical practices emphasize preservation of the gland's function.

Marsupialization and Window Operation. Both these treatments seek to create and to maintain a patent fistula for drainage of the cyst or abscess. The techniques differ significantly only in that the cyst is excised in the marsupialization procedure, whereas a "window" is cut into the cyst or abscess in the window procedure. In both marsupialization and window techniques, pudendal or local anesthesia is used, and the edges of the opened cyst cavity are sutured to the adjacent labial skin to make a permanent opening. The gland remains functional after both procedures, and the size of the fistulas created gradually decreases over time. Recurrence rates for marsupialization are 5% to 15%. Recommended follow-up care after marsupialization is 4 to 6 weeks.

Catheter or Drain Placement. The goal of catheter or drain placement is the creation of a fistula through which the gland can continue to drain. The drain can be placed after a simple stab wound or a marsupialization procedure and typically is left in place for 6 to 8 weeks to ensure fistula patency. The recurrence rate is about 24%. Both the Word catheter and the rubber Jacobi ring have been used effectively; the Jacobi ring may be better tolerated than the Word catheter.

Carbon Dioxide Laser Therapy. With the patient under local anesthesia, the CO_2 laser is used first to create a defect from the vulvar skin to the cystic cavity as near as possible to the original duct track and then to vaporize cyst contents. The neostoma that is created permits continued drainage after the procedure without the presence of sutures or mechanical devices such as catheters or drains and allows an epithelium-lined tract to form. Glandular function is maintained, sexual function is not impaired after a 2-week healing period, and the size of the created defect is substantially reduced with complete healing (shrinking from approximately 1.5 to 0.2 cm [$\frac{3}{5}$ to $\frac{2}{25}$ inch]). Healing typically occurs without scarring. A disadvantage of this approach is that the laser equipment is expensive to install and to maintain, but in one study the relapse-free rate exceeded 85%.[13,14]

Silver Nitrate. Insertion of silver nitrate into a scalpel-formed incision is a simple and inexpensive option for treatment; it is as effective as traditional excision techniques and has fewer complications and less scar formation[15] than marsupialization. However, chemical burning of the vulva has been observed. There is evidence to suggest that alcohol sclerotherapy to Bartholin gland cysts or abscesses is as effective as silver nitrate and is associated with fewer complications.[16]

LIFE SPAN CONSIDERATIONS

Bartholin gland cysts and abscesses are most common in women of reproductive age; yet, when adequately treated, women maintain function without reproductive or other sequelae such as dyspareunia.

COMPLICATIONS

Cyst recurrence often follows incision and drainage or aspiration alone,[17] and gland excision may be accompanied by hemorrhage, hematoma formation, trauma to surrounding tissues, rectovaginal fistula,[18] scarring, a long healing process, and subsequent dyspareunia from loss of vaginal lubrication. Toxic shock syndrome, a very rare complication, has been noted in the literature, both before and after corrective surgical procedures. True necrotizing fasciitis[19] has been noted after abscess.

INDICATIONS FOR REFERRAL OR HOSPITALIZATION

Health care providers not comfortable managing Bartholin gland cysts and abscesses are encouraged to refer these patients to experienced surgeons for appropriate therapy. In general, Bartholin gland cysts or abscesses are managed successfully on an outpatient basis, but systemic infection or other complications remain valid indications for hospitalization.

Women who have been treated by surgeons for Bartholin gland cysts or abscesses should have continued follow-up care with their health care providers. Providers can also check for possible sequelae to treatment, including dyspareunia, in the course of routine gynecologic or other primary care provision.

PATIENT AND FAMILY EDUCATION

Explaining to patients the basic physiology of the Bartholin gland and the pathophysiology involved in cyst or abscess may help demystify the condition and the treatment experience. Women may also benefit from an explanation of what to do and expect after a treatment strategy is used. After CO_2 therapy, for example, patients are instructed to refrain from sexual intercourse for 2 weeks; potential postoperative discomfort is managed with saltwater soaks. Women should be counseled to expect drainage of mucus for 2 or 3 days after certain procedures while the cyst or abscess resolves. Proper hygiene, sitz baths or soaks, and condom use are also helpful in the treatment and prevention of future Bartholin gland cysts and abscesses.

CHAPTER 157

BREAST DISORDERS

Elizabeth B. McCabe

Evaluation of breast complaints and screening for breast cancer account for a significant number of primary care visits. The most frequent breast complaints include breast pain, breast masses, and nipple discharge. Most breast masses and other breast complaints are a result of benign conditions, but some breast disease can impart actual risk for the development of breast cancer.[1] Studies have shown that women with certain kinds of benign breast disease have a relative risk for breast cancer of 1.35 to 1.6 compared with women in the general population.[2]

For these reasons, accurate evaluation of all breast complaints and appropriate follow-up are essential. In addition, failure to adequately reassure women about their breast symptoms after a benign diagnosis heightens the need for appropriate support for women with ongoing breast symptoms.[1] Research shows that even after a benign diagnosis, up to one third of women report that they are either unsure or not reassured about their breast symptoms. A significant percentage of women who undergo evaluation and receive a benign diagnosis for their breast symptoms remain anxious about the possibility of breast cancer or another form of breast disease.

The initial breast evaluation should be comprehensive and include a risk assessment to determine average to high-risk status, history of the present breast concern, workup to date including imaging and pathology reports of recent or past breast biopsies, past relevant medical and surgical history, and family history of both breast and ovarian cancer on both the maternal and paternal sides of the family. Education about breast health tailored to age and risk status, including screening recommendations and follow-up, should be clearly outlined for every patient regardless of the underlying breast condition.

RISK ASSESSMENT

Risk Factors

A thorough history and breast cancer risk assessment should be performed for every woman who sees her health care provider with a breast complaint. The absolute lifetime risk for development of breast cancer is approximately 12%.[3] Determination of level of risk is an important part of the risk assessment process. Several well-established risk factors associated with the development of breast cancer have been thoroughly studied and are defined by four major groups: family history or genetic factors, reproductive or hormonal factors, proliferative benign breast disease, and mammographic density.[4]

Individuals with a single first-degree relative with breast cancer have an estimated twofold risk. Individuals with two first-degree relatives have a threefold risk, and three or more impart a fourfold risk. A first-degree relative younger than 40 years at the time of diagnosis results in a threefold risk compared with a twofold risk for relatives 40 to 50 years old and a 1.5-fold risk for relatives 50 to 65 years old. Risks are also greater if relatives have bilateral breast cancer.[4] Other risks in this category include male breast cancer, ovarian cancer, and Ashkenazi Jewish ancestry.

In terms of reproductive factors, nulliparous women have the same risk as that of women who delivered their first child at the age of 30 years of age or older. Subsequent births and substantial periods of breastfeeding offer some degree of risk protection. Early menarche and late menopause result in increased duration of ovulation with the resultant hormonal effects. Women who are using hormone replacement therapy (HRT) have up to a 5% increased risk per year of use, which returns to baseline levels within a year of stopping hormone use.[4]

Certain types of benign breast disease impart significant risk for development of invasive breast cancer. Women with lobular carcinoma in situ have a 10-fold relative risk, and women with atypical ductal hyperplasia and atypical lobular hyperplasia carry a fourfold to fivefold relative risk. A doubling of risk is seen with proliferative lesions without atypia, such as intraductal papillomas. Nonproliferative lesions, such as fibroadenomas and cysts, do not increase risk.[4]

Mammographic density, estimated by the percentage of the mammogram covered by opaque tissue, has been determined to be the single most important risk factor in the population of women receiving mammograms. Description of density can be found on the final mammogram report and is described as extremely dense, heterogeneously dense, scattered density, or fatty replacement of the breast tissue. Fifty percent to 75% density on a mammogram imparts a twofold to threefold risk. Approximately 14% of the population falls into this category, compared with 5% whose density is greater than 75%. Mammographic density as a risk is not well understood.

It is also known that other risk factors are largely independent of one another. Efforts are ongoing at looking at all risk factors and using the information to provide individual risk status and prevention strategies.[4]

Risk Assessment Models

There are varied breast cancer risk assessment tools available (www.cancer.gov/bcrisktool). Two models that have been used to determine a woman's absolute risk for development of breast cancer are the Gail model and the Claus model. The Gail model is based on several risk factors: age, race, age at menarche, number of breast biopsies, number of biopsies with atypical hyperplasia, number of first-degree relatives with breast cancer, and age at first live birth. (ww5.komen.org/BreastCancer/GailAssessmentModel.html). A 5-year score of 1.67% or greater is considered high risk. The Gail model was not designed for women younger than 35 years, with a personal history of breast cancer or ductal or lobular carcinoma in situ, or whose history suggests a possible hereditary breast cancer.[5] The Claus model predicts the cumulative probability for development of breast cancer of a woman who has a family history with both first- and second-degree relatives. This model has been most useful in assessing risk in younger women (aged 29 to 35 years) with a family history of breast cancer. There have been more validation studies performed on the Gail model, and this model tends to be more frequently used in the clinical setting.[5]

Genetic Testing

Women with a strong family history of breast cancer may be candidates for genetic testing for *BRCA* mutations. The decision to undergo genetic testing raises many psychosocial and ethical issues and should be considered after a discussion with a genetics counselor. Strong consideration to involve family members is recommended. Women who are known *BRCA1* or *BRCA2* mutation carriers have a 40% to 70% lifetime risk for development of breast cancer.[6,7] These women are considered to be at extremely high risk and require education and counseling about screening and risk reduction strategies. Screening recommendations include clinical breast examination every 6 months, annual mammography, and breast magnetic resonance imaging (MRI).

Risk Reduction

The best nonsurgical risk reduction strategy for *BRCA* mutation carriers is adjuvant MRI. It has been shown to be successful in detecting twice as many invasive cancers as mammography, with the majority of cancers being at an early stage at diagnosis.[8] Surgical risk reduction strategies include prophylactic mastectomy and oophorectomy. Women who undergo mastectomy reduce their breast cancer risk by 90%, and premenopausal women who undergo prophylactic oophorectomy decrease their breast cancer risk by 75%.[6] Once a woman has been identified as a mutation carrier, choices for risk reduction are typically made on the basis of age and childbearing status.

SCREENING RECOMMENDATIONS

There is ongoing debate about the appropriate age at which to initiate screening mammography in the average-risk patient, defined as a woman whose relative risk for developing breast cancer is 1.5-fold or lower and whose 5-year Gail score is below 1.7%.[6] In addition to mammography, clinical breast examination and breast self-examination have historically been recommended as routine screening practices for women.

In 2015, the U.S. Preventive Services Task Force (USPSTF) issued a continued biennial recommendation for screening mammography for women aged 50 to 74 years of age and determined that the evidence to continue screening women after age 75 was inconclusive.[9] USPSTF screening recommendations for women aged 40 to 49 continue to be individualized based on the risks and benefits of biennial screening, although the American College of Radiology (ACR), Society of Breast Imaging (SBI), and American College of Obstetricians and Gynecologists (ACOG) recommend annual mammography for women ages 40 to 74.[9] For women aged 75 or older, the USPSTF found there was insufficient evidence to recommend for or against breast cancer screening, yet the American Cancer Society and American College of Obstetricians and Gynecologists continue to recommend annual mammography.[9] Teaching breast self-examination to patients is still not recommended by the USPSTF, although women should be encouraged to discuss breast changes with their primary care provider.[9,10]

There is strong evidence to suggest that mammography is most useful in women aged 50 to 65 years and that mammography remains the best method for breast cancer screening among average-risk patients.[9,10] Regular breast self-examination is a very individualized decision. For those women who are interested in learning proper techniques for performing self-examination and who are interested in promoting awareness of their breast health, time needs to be allotted for providing this information.

High-risk women are those with a 5-year Gail score higher than 1.7% and whose relative risk is 1.5- to 5-fold. Screening recommendations for this group include annual clinical breast examination and mammography, consideration for chemoprevention, and discontinuation of hormonal therapy if the patient has been receiving it for more than 2 years.[6]

Very-high-risk women include those with a personal history of invasive breast cancer, ductal carcinoma in situ, or lobular carcinoma in situ. This imparts a fourfold to fivefold risk for development of a new primary breast cancer. Other women who fall into this category are those with a prior breast biopsy showing atypical hyperplasia, known *BRCA* mutation carriers, and those with a history of mantle radiation of the chest wall for Hodgkin disease before the age of 30. Screening recommendations for this group include clinical breast examination every 6 months, annual mammography, consideration for chemoprevention, and genetic testing.[6] Screening for this population may begin as early as 25 years of age. Digital mammography and adjuvant MRI may be recommended for many of these women.[10]

Determination of average- or high-risk status for each patient is an integral step in the process of providing individualized care. Both average- and high-risk women require education about the screening tools available and how the use of these tools can be tailored to meet their individualized needs.

BREAST PAIN (MASTALGIA, MASTODYNIA)

DEFINITION AND EPIDEMIOLOGY

Breast pain, often referred to as mastalgia or mastodynia, is the most common breast problem encountered in primary care and surgical practices.[11] Although increased awareness and overestimation of breast cancer risk may prompt women to be more inclined to seek medical treatment for breast concerns, mastalgia is generally underreported.[12] Premenstrual, or cyclic, breast pain is the most common type of mastalgia and usually occurs during the late luteal phase of the menstrual cycle, in association with the premenstrual syndrome or independently, and resolves after menses.[13] Studies of healthy women in the United States have shown that 11% have moderate to severe cyclic breast pain and 58% have mild discomfort.[13]

Noncyclic mastalgia involves constant or intermittent pain that is unrelated to the menstrual cycle.[12,13] It is less common than cyclic mastalgia and occurs most frequently in women 40 to 50 years old. It accounts for about 31% of women being seen for mastalgia.[12] Noncyclic mastalgia may result from pregnancy, mastitis, thrombophlebitis, macrocysts, benign tumors, fibrocystic breast changes, or cancer; however, these conditions explain only a minority of noncyclic mastalgia cases. Most noncyclic mastalgia occurs for unknown reasons, but it is thought to be related more often to an anatomic cause than to a hormonal one. Noncyclic breast pain usually resolves spontaneously without treatment.[12]

PATHOPHYSIOLOGY

The actual pathophysiologic mechanism of breast pain is not well understood. Cyclic mastalgia occurs during the luteal phase of the menstrual cycle and resolves with the onset of menstruation.[14] This predictable pattern of pain is likely to be hormonally mediated, despite the failure of studies to show any difference in estrogen levels among women with or without pain. It has also been shown that progesterone levels may be lower in these women and that prolactin release may be increased as a response to thyrotropin-releasing hormone.[15]

Essential fatty acids such as dietary gamma-linolenic acid have been suggested as inhibitors of prostaglandins, which possibly cause breast pain. Low plasma levels of these essential fatty acids may result in a hypersensitivity of breast tissue to circulating hormones.[14]

There is little evidence to support a relationship between breast pain and histologic findings consistent with cysts, apocrine metaplasia, and ductal hyperplasia.[15]

CLINICAL PRESENTATION

Cyclic mastalgia usually starts in the luteal phase of the menstrual cycle, increases in intensity until menses begin, and then dissipates, although pain may be present during the entire cycle with increased intensity premenstrually.[12] Cyclic mastalgia usually begins in the third or fourth decade of life. It is usually bilateral and poorly localized, although it typically involves the upper outer breast area and radiates to the upper arm and axilla. Women will describe the pain as dull, heavy, or aching. Symptoms tend to persist with intermittent relapses, but remission can occur with hormonal events such as pregnancy and menopause. Only 14% of women with cyclic mastalgia experience spontaneous resolution of symptoms, whereas 42% experience resolution at menopause.[12] In contrast, noncyclic mastalgia is often unilateral, localized, and described as a sharp, burning pain. Mastalgia is rarely the sole presenting symptom of breast cancer.[11]

There may be an association between breast pain and anxiety, depression, emotional distress, somatization, and a history of emotional abuse. Women with breast pain may experience greater cyclic fluctuations in anxiety and depression, but it remains unclear whether there is any kind of causal or consequential relationship between breast pain and psychological distress.[12]

PHYSICAL EXAMINATION

A thorough history and breast examination must be performed for every woman who is seen with any breast problem and must be directed at identification and characterization of breast-related symptoms. The provider should elicit current symptoms, such as type of pain (cyclic, noncyclic, bilateral, or unilateral), presence or absence of nipple discharge with characteristics of the discharge (color, whether it is spontaneous or nonspontaneous, large or scant volume), presence of a breast mass, change in mass with the menstrual cycle, axillary masses, skin dimpling, ulceration, inflammation, and history of recent breast infections or trauma.

The history should include current medications, including hormone therapy. Prior history of any breast surgery for both cancerous and noncancerous reasons including cosmetic procedures should be obtained. In addition, age at menarche and menopause, pregnancy and lactation history, and relevant past medical and surgical history should be included. Breast cancer screening history should include the date and results of the last clinical breast examination and breast imaging. Family history of breast and ovarian cancer on both maternal and paternal sides should be obtained.

The breast examination must be methodical, and the breasts should be inspected for differences in size, skin changes, retraction or dimpling of the skin or nipple, prominent venous patterns, lesions, and signs of inflammation. The axillary, supraclavicular, and infraclavicular areas should be palpated with the woman in the sitting position. Inspection of the breasts should be performed with the woman both sitting and supine, with her hands behind her head or raised over her head. The examiner should use the flat surface of the fingertips to palpate all of the breast tissue against the chest wall. In women with a history of nipple discharge, the nipple-areola complex is compressed very gently in all directions. If this technique does not elicit discharge, firm equal pressure should be applied from the periphery toward the nipple. To distinguish discharge from multiple or single ducts, pressure must be distributed evenly over all of the ductal structures. Benign or physiologic nipple discharge is typically creamy, gray, or green. Watery, serous, or bloody fluid is considered abnormal.

Breast masses palpated on physical examination may be moveable or fixed and are typically discrete. Description of the size and location of the mass is important before obtaining any radiographic studies.

On examination of the patient with a complaint of breast pain, it is important to note if the pain is focal, regional, or diffuse. Some breast pain actually originates from the chest wall and can manifest as point tenderness.

Skin changes that may signify cancer include erythema, edema, retraction, dimpling, peau d'orange, and nipple excoriation or crustiness.

DIAGNOSTICS

Noncyclic breast pain is initially investigated with bilateral mammography in postmenopausal women, although the likelihood of an abnormal finding is low. A focused ultrasound examination is often performed to evaluate persistent, focal mastalgia in young women and in addition to mammography in older women.[12] Mammography is not indicated in young women with cyclic breast pain in the absence of focal pain, suspicious findings, or risk factors. However, mammography should be considered in women 30 to 35 years or older who have a family history of breast cancer or other risk factors for breast cancer.[12]

Laboratory studies are not useful in general, but a pregnancy test should be done for a woman of reproductive age if the history or physical examination findings suggest that pregnancy is possible. Other hormone levels, such as estrogen, progesterone, and prolactin, are usually within normal limits in women with breast pain and therefore are not indicated as part of the workup.[12]

DIAGNOSTICS

Breast Pain (Mastalgia, Mastodynia)

IMAGING
Mammography
Ultrasound*

OTHER
Biopsy

*If indicated.

DIFFERENTIAL DIAGNOSIS

The differential diagnosis of breast pain includes a normal physiologic event, recent or past trauma with or without hematoma or fat necrosis, microcysts or macrocysts, infection, and malignant or benign tumor.

Chest wall or nonbreast pain accounts for about 7% of women seen with complaints of mastalgia. Pain that is limited to a particular area and characterized by a burning or knifelike sensation may be chest wall pain. There are several distinct types of chest wall pain, including localized or diffuse pain, radicular pain from cervical arthritis or slipping and cracking ribs, and pain from Tietze syndrome (also known as costochondritis).[12]

The pain can be reproduced with pressure over the costal cartilage rather than in the more generalized pattern of mastalgia. Movement may also precipitate chest wall pain, and there is no relationship to the menstrual cycle.[13] Chest wall syndromes can occur even in the absence of a clear precipitating event, which sometimes heightens the woman's concern that the pain has a suspicious or malignant cause.[12]

DIFFERENTIAL DIAGNOSIS

Breast Pain (Mastalgia, Mastodynia)

NONBREAST CAUSES
- Achalasia
- Angina
- Cervical radiculopathy
- Cholecystitis
- Cholelithiasis
- Costochondritis (Tietze syndrome)
- Fractured rib
- Hiatal hernia
- Myalgia
- Neuralgia
- Peptic ulcer disease
- Pleurisy
- Systemic infections (including tuberculosis, syphilis, fungal infections)
- Trauma (nonbreast)

BREAST CAUSES
- Hormone therapy
- Macrocysts
- Fibrocystic breast changes
- Sclerosing adenoma
- Duct ectasia
- Mastitis
- Pregnancy
- Postpartum engorgement
- Trauma
- Thrombophlebitis
- Breast cancer
- Breast abscess
- Periductal mastitis

MANAGEMENT

After a thorough history, evaluation, and risk assessment, reassurance is all that is needed for 85% of women with cyclic mastalgia. For the 15% of the women not helped with reassurance alone, use of a pain chart for at least two cycles may elucidate any patterns of mastalgia. Patients can also be reassured that breast pain has a high spontaneous remission rate (60% to 80%).[4] Management of cyclic mastalgia should also include reevaluation of the breast pain at a different time during the menstrual cycle, preferably soon after the menses.

Proven benefits for the treatment of cyclic mastalgia are few. Because of the extreme variability in mastalgia, only treatments that have been tested in randomized controlled trials (RCTs) can be confidently considered. Danazol (Danocrine), an antigonadotropin, is the only drug labeled by the U.S. Food and Drug Administration for the treatment of mastalgia. RCTs have demonstrated a response rate of 50% to 75% in women with cyclic breast pain who received danazol, 100 to 400 mg/day orally in two divided doses. Approximately 75% of women with noncyclic pain responded to the drug.[11] Typically, the initial dose is 200 mg daily, eventually tapering to lower doses, with alternate-day or luteal-phase administration. However, initial dosages of 50 to 400 mg/day have been described. Unfortunately, side effects plague 30% of women, eventually resulting in discontinuation of the drug in approximately 15% of women, even when breast pain is improved. Adverse effects are primarily dose related and androgenic, including hirsutism, acne, hair loss, lowered voice pitch, weight gain, headache, nausea, rash, anxiety, and depression.[12] The severe side effect profile and teratogenic potential of danazol support referral or collaboration before initiation of treatment.

Other pharmacologic agents used to treat mastalgia include dopamine agonists, such as bromocriptine, because one of the hormonal abnormalities detected in women with mastalgia has been an increase in thyrotropin-induced prolactin secretion. Although clinical improvement occurs in 47% to 88% of symptomatic women, up to 29% of women in some studies have stopped taking the medication because of side effects.[12]

The selective estrogen receptor modulator tamoxifen is used to prevent and to treat breast cancer but has also been effective in reducing pain in 71% to 96% of women with cyclic mastalgia and 56% of women with noncyclic mastalgia. Tamoxifen has a serious potential side effect profile, including deep venous thrombosis and endometrial cancer, as well as the more benign side effects of hot flashes, nausea, menstrual irregularity, vaginal dryness, and weight gain. Tamoxifen compares favorably with danazol and bromocriptine with regard to efficacy and adverse effects. As with the other hormonal agents, use of tamoxifen for breast pain should be reserved for women with severe mastalgia that is not responding to other forms of therapy.[12]

Supportive bras and the use of nonsteroidal anti-inflammatory drugs (NSAIDs) can be helpful. Oral contraceptives may be discontinued or changed to an alternative agent with a lower estrogen and higher progesterone content. Caffeine avoidance has been a popular treatment measure in women with breast pain, although a therapeutic benefit for caffeine restriction has not been consistently demonstrated in controlled studies. Vitamin E supplementation has also been advocated for treatment of breast pain. However, two double-blind, placebo-controlled RCTs demonstrated no benefit to this approach.[11] Similar studies using evening primrose have been conducted and have shown minimal benefit in relieving breast pain.[16,17]

It may be difficult to quantify breast pain because it is often variable. However, assessment of pain with a pain-rating instrument or scale can be particularly useful in evaluating cyclic breast pain and response to treatment.

COMPLICATIONS

Mastalgia is infrequently associated with breast cancer. Despite this fact, any persistence in a patient's symptoms should prompt further evaluation. Failure to treat or a delay in diagnosis of an underlying problem may affect a woman's quality of life or long-term outcome.

INDICATIONS FOR REFERRAL OR HOSPITALIZATION

Treatment of cyclic mastalgia with antigonadotropic agents should be managed by or in consultation with a specialist because of the severity of the side effect profile and the teratogenicity of this class of drugs.

Women with mastalgia, without evidence of disease on physical examination and imaging, whose pain is refractory to basic interventions may be considered candidates for a chronic pain referral. If the pain is severe enough and interferes with a woman's quality of life, a general surgery referral can be considered to discuss mastectomy. The benefit of this extreme intervention is not well proven.

PATIENT EDUCATION

Many women are initially seen with mild forms of mastalgia, fearful that they have cancer. Women who experience breast pain should receive a thorough clinical breast examination and reassurance that pain is an uncommon presenting symptom of breast cancer.

For most patients, a thorough evaluation without clinical or radiographic findings should provide sufficient reassurance in addition to knowing that the pain they are experiencing is typically self-limited and improves over time. A follow-up breast examination on an interval basis may be offered.

MASTITIS

DEFINITION AND EPIDEMIOLOGY

Mastitis refers to inflammation of the breast tissue. It can occur in both men and women. The frequency of mastitis increases with lactation, but it can occur in the nonlactating or pregnant patient. Approximately one third of women who breastfeed develop mastitis. *Staphylococcus aureus* is the most common organism. *Haemophilus parainfluenzae, Streptococcus,* and *Escherichia coli* can be seen as well but are less common.[18]

Any clinical presentation of mastitis should be promptly treated. If resolution of symptoms does not occur after the initial treatment, inflammatory breast cancer should be considered and a referral should be made for biopsy. Inflammatory breast cancer represents 1% to 3% of all breast cancer diagnoses in the United States. Almost 50% of women with inflammatory breast cancer have metastatic disease at the time of diagnosis.[19]

PATHOPHYSIOLOGY

In lactational mastitis, organisms enter the ductal system from the infant's mouth through the nipple. Infection frequently occurs in a segment of the breast where milk drainage is poor. Breast milk provides a good culture medium for these microorganisms.

Because of the increase in incidence of methicillin-resistant *Staphylococcus aureus* (MRSA) soft tissue infections seen in the United States, providers who treat women with mastitis should consider MRSA as a causative organism if traditional treatment fails. MRSA mastitis in the postpartum period is more likely to result in a breast abscess.[18]

Nonpuerperal mastitis can manifest as periductal mastitis with or without periareolar abscess or whole-breast cellulitis. Periductal mastitis occurs secondary to blockage of the milk ducts by breast secretions and cellular debris.[19]

CLINICAL PRESENTATION

Puerperal mastitis is typically unilateral and may occur any time during lactation. Women with puerperal mastitis often are seen with breast engorgement and tenderness, fever, chills, anorexia, headache, and malaise. Erythema is usually confined to the area of a single breast lobule. A discrete mass is suggestive of abscess formation. The axillary lymph nodes may be tender and enlarged. Nonpuerperal mastitis is often seen in women who are immunocompromised (e.g., women with diabetes or who have undergone radiation treatment) and those with autoimmune disorders. Nonpuerperal mastitis may also be accompanied by nipple discharge. Periductal mastitis manifests with periareolar inflammation with or without an erythematous subareolar mass.[19] Mastitis is typically associated with pain, malaise, fever, and leukocytosis.

Persistent erythema involving the entire breast, accompanied by increased breast firmness and size, with or without pain, is suggestive of inflammatory breast carcinoma and necessitates immediate referral.[19]

Inflammatory breast cancer is a clinical diagnosis characterized by breast edema (peau d'orange) and erythema, with or without a palpable mass. Biopsy confirms the presence of invasive cancer.[20]

DIAGNOSTICS

Mammography, if it is tolerated, should be considered when a breast infection does not respond to appropriate antibiotic therapy within 3 to 7 days. A focused ultrasound examination is indicated in any patient with symptoms of mastitis with a mass or an area of focal fullness or fluctuance. Ultrasonography may detect abscess formation. Mammography is not indicated in pregnant or lactating women with an initial presentation of mastitis.

Diagnosis of inflammatory breast cancer should be considered in patients who do not respond to antibiotic therapy. The diagnosis cannot be made with radiographic examination alone; pathologic examination is required for confirmation. A skin biopsy reveals dermal lymphatics congested with cancer cells, and the core biopsy of breast tissue reveals invasive breast cancer.

DIFFERENTIAL DIAGNOSIS

In lactating women, the differential diagnosis for mastitis includes breast engorgement, which is usually bilateral. In nonlactating women, inflammatory breast cancer can mimic acute mastitis or cellulitis. Failure to respond to appropriate antibiotic therapy is a concerning sign of a malignant neoplasm. Other differential diagnoses include duct ectasia, breast abscess, granulomatous mastitis, and periductal mastitis.

MANAGEMENT

Methods to facilitate removal of milk from the breast include breastfeeding followed by pumping and the use of warm compresses, good support, massage of the painful areas while nursing, and analgesics.[18]

Traditional antibiotic therapy includes dicloxacillin and cephalexin. Clindamycin is recommended for penicillin-sensitive patients. MRSA should be considered when women do not respond to traditional therapy. It may be necessary to obtain a culture of the abscess fluid if it is present, breast milk, or nipple discharge to confirm the diagnosis. MRSA infections may respond to treatment with oral clindamycin, trimethoprim-sulfamethoxazole, linezolid, or intravenous administration of vancomycin.[18]

Continuation of breastfeeding during treatment is encouraged, provided the infant is healthy and full term.[18] If an abscess is present, incision and drainage of the infected fluid is required. In both puerperal and nonpuerperal mastitis, acetaminophen or NSAIDs and moist heat may be beneficial.

COMPLICATIONS

Concerns for an underlying abscess may be present in any patient with mastitis who does not respond to a standard course of antibiotics. A focused ultrasound examination should be performed to further evaluate any area of the breast that has a mass or an area of focal prominence.

INDICATIONS FOR REFERRAL

Any patient with an abscess or suspected abscess requires a surgical referral. Surgical intervention for incision and drainage is indicated when a fluctuant mass, suggestive of an underlying abscess, accompanies mastitis. Intravenous antibiotics may be required to treat acute mastitis unresponsive to oral agents. Surgical referral is also indicated when inflammatory breast cancer is suspected. The diagnosis is confirmed after a skin biopsy and core needle biopsy.

PATIENT EDUCATION

Lactating women should also be reassured that mastitis is a common complication of lactation, the nutrition of the breast milk is unaffected by the infection, and a history of mastitis is not associated with an increased risk of breast cancer.

Nonpuerperal mastitis typically resolves after a course of antibiotics. Women should be instructed to monitor their breast examination after resolution of their symptoms.

In the absence of clinical concerns, the timing of the next screening mammogram should be no earlier than 3 months from the resolution of symptoms.

NIPPLE DISCHARGE AND GALACTORRHEA

DEFINITION AND EPIDEMIOLOGY

Nipple discharge is commonly seen in approximately 20% to 25% of women with breast complaints.[15] It is classified as physiologic, pathologic, or galactorrhea. Nipple discharge causes significant anxiety and fear that there may be an underlying malignant neoplasm.[15]

Physiologic nipple discharge is common in premenopausal and pregnant women. It is typically bilateral and may be spontaneous or nonspontaneous. Pathologic nipple discharge is often spontaneous, bloody, serous, and involving one duct. Galactorrhea or milky discharge is associated with pituitary adenomas or hypothyroidism.[21]

PATHOPHYSIOLOGY

Most nipple discharge is physiologic in nature and is not symptomatic of any pathologic condition. It is seen in nonlactating and lactating breasts. Hormonal influences from estrogen, progesterone, and prolactin, as well as the presence of growth hormones, insulin, and adrenal hormones, may stimulate nipple discharge. When the physiologic fluid is secreted through the nipple, it is generally bilateral, arising from multiple ducts, and not spontaneous.

The most common cause of pathologic nipple discharge is intraductal papilloma, followed by duct ectasia. The presence of an associated palpable mass increases the likelihood of cancer.[11] The most common cause of bloody nipple discharge is intraductal papilloma. Approximately one third of bloody or serous discharges are the result of a malignant neoplasm.[21]

Galactorrhea is caused by hypothyroidism, hyperprolactinemia, and medications. Brain MRI is indicated when elevated prolactin levels are seen, to rule out prolactin-secreting pituitary tumors.[15]

CLINICAL PRESENTATION

The primary goal in evaluating nipple discharge is to determine whether it is physiologic, pathologic, or galactorrhea. Physiologic nipple discharge is characterized by discharge only with compression and by multiple duct involvement. These discharges are often bilateral, and the fluid may be clear, gray, yellow, white, or dark green.[11] Although it is not common, lactational secretions may persist for years after weaning if the breasts continue to be manually stimulated.

Nipple discharge requires further investigation if it is spontaneous, bloody, watery, large volume, or associated with a mass. Pathologic discharge is usually unilateral and involves a single duct.

Galactorrhea manifests as bilateral milky discharge and is seen with endocrine disorders such as hypothyroidism and hyperprolactinemia. Clinical signs and symptoms indicative of these complaints include lethargy, cold intolerance, constipation, dry skin, headache, amenorrhea, and defects in peripheral vision.[15]

PHYSICAL EXAMINATION

A thorough breast examination as previously described should be performed to assess for an underlying breast mass and should include gentle compression of the nipple-areola complex between the thumb and index finger. Milking of the ducts with equal pressure from various directions is required to determine the origin of the discharge from either a single duct or multiple ducts.

In the presence of galactorrhea, funduscopic examination to exclude papilledema as well as evaluation of visual acuity, visual fields by confrontation, and extraocular movements is indicated to detect a bitemporal field defect and asymmetry of field loss, which are common in parapituitary lesions. Neurologic and thyroid examinations should also be performed.

A complete medication and past medical history, including endocrine and reproductive histories, should be obtained at the time of the evaluation.

DIAGNOSTICS

Nipple discharge that is serous or watery should be tested for occult blood. Cytologic studies are not recommended because the absence of malignant cells does not exclude malignant disease or distinguish intraductal from invasive cancer.

Diagnostic mammography should be performed to assess for any nonpalpable masses or calcifications.[15] A focused periareolar ultrasound examination may be performed in an attempt to identify any intraductal masses or ductal abnormalities such as duct ectasia.

Pregnancy should be excluded by obtaining a human chorionic gonadotropin level in all premenopausal women experiencing amenorrhea and galactorrhea. The serum prolactin level is the single most important determination that can establish a lesion of pituitary or central nervous system (CNS) origin.

DIAGNOSTICS

Nipple Discharge and Galactorrhea

LABORATORY	IMAGING
Prolactin level, thyroid-stimulating hormone (TSH) (or thyroid profile)	Mammography
Serum human chorionic gonadotropin	Periareolar ultrasound
Hematest	Ductography*
	Brain MRI for hyperprolactinemia
	Breast MRI

*If indicated.

The serum prolactin level may be normal or only slightly elevated when galactorrhea is drug related. Thyroid profiles should also be obtained because primary hypothyroidism can cause elevation of serum prolactin level and galactorrhea.

MRI of the brain is indicated for the patient with symptoms suggestive of an intracranial mass, galactorrhea with amenorrhea, or elevated prolactin level.[15]

DIFFERENTIAL DIAGNOSIS

Duct ectasia, nonpuerperal mastitis, intraductal papilloma, and breast cancer must be considered in the presence of a nonmilky nipple discharge.

The differential diagnosis of galactorrhea includes pituitary adenomas, neurologic disorders, hypothyroidism, numerous medications, breast stimulation, chest wall irritation, and physiologic causes.[22]

MANAGEMENT

Treatment of the underlying infection, as previously described, is required if nipple discharge is related to acute mastitis. When a chemical origin for galactorrhea is suspected, discontinuation or substitution with a comparable pharmacologic agent may be attempted when possible. Restoration to the euthyroid state is indicated if hypothyroidism is present. Minimum intervention is required for galactorrhea of idiopathic, drug-related, or physiologic origin.

Mammary duct ectasia is not related to neoplasms. Treatment is not necessary unless there is associated periductal

DIFFERENTIAL DIAGNOSIS

Nipple Discharge and Galactorrhea

BREAST-RELATED CAUSES
- Breast cancer
- Duct ectasia
- Intraductal papilloma
- Nonpuerperal mastitis

CHEMICAL AGENTS
- Amphetamines
- Anesthetics
- Arginine
- Atypical antipsychotics (clozapine, loxapine, risperidone)
- Benzamides (metoclopramide, sulpiride*)
- Benzodiazepines
- Butyrophenones (haloperidol)
- Cimetidine
- Danazol
- Dronabinol
- Estrogen
- Flunarizine*
- Isoniazid
- Methyldopa
- Monoamine oxidase inhibitors
- Opiates
- Oral contraceptives
- Phenothiazines
- Progestins
- *Rauwolfia* alkaloids
- Reserpine
- Selective serotonin reuptake inhibitors
- Thioxanthenes
- Thyrotropin-releasing hormone
- Tricyclic antidepressants
- Verapamil

IDIOPATHIC CAUSES
- Conditions related to abnormal dopamine secretion

MEDICAL (NONMALIGNANT) CONDITIONS
- Addison disease
- Ahumada–del Castillo syndrome†
- Chiari-Frommel syndrome†
- Chronic renal failure
- Chest wall lesions
- CNS lesions (involving hypothalamus or pituitary)
- Cushing disease
- Endocrine anovulatory syndromes
- Forbes-Albright syndrome
- Hand-Schüller-Christian disease
- Head trauma
- Liver failure
- Multiple sclerosis
- Polycystic ovaries
- Postencephalitis
- Primary hypothyroidism
- Renal failure
- Sarcoidosis
- Thoracic herpes zoster

MEDICAL (MALIGNANT) CONDITIONS
- Adrenal carcinoma
- Breast carcinoma (rare)
- Bronchogenic carcinoma
- Chest wall lesions
- CNS lesions (involving hypothalamus or pituitary)
- Ovarian cystic teratoma
- Renal adenocarcinoma

PHYSIOLOGIC CONDITIONS
- Cyclic menstrual hormone variations
- Nipple stimulation
- Pregnancy (after first trimester)
- Postlactation (a few months to 5 years)
- Stress

SURGICAL PROCEDURES‡
- Implantation of breast prostheses
- Reduction mammoplasty
- Thoracic procedures

PSEUDODISCHARGES
- Atopic dermatitis
- Herpes simplex
- Infected Montgomery glands
- Inverted nipples
- Lactiferous sinuses
- Molluscum contagiosum
- Nipple trauma
- Paget disease
- Sebaceous cysts of the nipple

*Not available in the United States.
†May be associated with pituitary tumors.
‡Procedures that may result in irritation to the afferent arc.

mastitis. With recurrent infections, effective treatment is surgical excision of the involved ducts.

Spontaneous bloody or large-volume watery discharge with or without a palpable mass can be caused by intraductal papillomas. Surgical referral is recommended to determine the need for duct excision and to rule out malignant disease.

Co-Management with Specialists

Nipple discharge that is spontaneous, unilateral, bloody, serous, or watery and arising from a single duct may be pathologic in nature and requires further investigation with a mammogram and ultrasound examination. If imaging is normal, a referral to a breast surgeon is indicated.[23] Recurrent periductal mastitis necessitates a surgical referral as well.

Controversy exists about the frequency of follow-up care for pituitary microadenomas. Repeated MRI examinations are often recommended until the growth of the lesion is established, and these should be performed in conjunction with the consulting specialist. (See the section Indications for Referral or Hospitalization.)

LIFE SPAN CONSIDERATIONS

Most women are concerned about breast cancer, and nipple discharge usually heightens concerns about possible malignant disease. Although nipple discharge is not commonly associated with cancer, care must be taken to ensure that a complete workup is conducted. Galactorrhea is more common in premenopausal women, and duct ectasia is seen more often in perimenopausal and postmenopausal women. Periductal mastitis is often seen more frequently in smokers; therefore counseling for smoking cessation is indicated.

INDICATIONS FOR REFERRAL OR HOSPITALIZATION

All patients with spontaneous or unilateral nipple discharge, regardless of color, should be referred for surgical evaluation. Intraductal papillomas require surgical biopsy and excision.[11] Galactorrhea accompanied by decreased visual fields, deterioration in visual acuity, papilledema, progressive headache, and nausea or vomiting should be promptly discussed, and the patient referred to a neurologist, endocrinologist, or neuroendocrinologist. When idiopathic galactorrhea is suspected, referral to a specialist for confirmation of the diagnosis is also indicated.

PATIENT AND FAMILY EDUCATION

Patients should be reassured that most causes of breast discharge are nonmalignant. In the presence of a normal prolactin level and menses, women with galactorrhea should be informed of its normal physiologic association with nipple and breast stimulation. Patients with pituitary adenoma should be reassured of the generally favorable response to treatment. Accurate and clear information, support, and close follow-up will help minimize the anxiety that many women with nipple discharge have.

PAGET DISEASE OF THE NIPPLE

Paget disease of the nipple is a superficial manifestation of an underlying breast carcinoma, most often of ductal origin. Paget disease is believed to represent 1% to 3% of all breast cancers. It is rare in men but is associated with a poorer prognosis.[24]

PATHOPHYSIOLOGY

Controversy exists about the origin of the malignant cells seen in Paget disease. They may represent malignant breast ductal epithelial cells, which then migrate into the epidermis of the nipple.[24]

CLINICAL PRESENTATION

Paget disease manifests clinically as a unilateral, well-demarcated, erythematous, scaly plaque first appearing on the nipple and subsequently spreading to the areola. The surrounding skin is usually spared. Serous or sanguineous discharge, pain, crusting, pruritus, burning, epithelial thickening, erythema, ulceration, nipple retraction, and underlying breast mass (in up to 60% of patients) may be seen. A small vesicular lesion on the nipple, persistent soreness, pain, or pruritus of the nipple-areola complex in the absence of other clinical symptoms should be evaluated thoroughly because these may be early manifestations of Paget disease.[24]

PHYSICAL EXAMINATION

A thorough breast examination as described previously must be conducted. Paget disease may manifest as scaling of the nipple, but it may also be accompanied by erythematous and excoriated, retracted nipples. The erosion of the areolar tissue may produce copious clear or viscous yellow exudate. As the disease steadily progresses, the excoriated surface of the nipple may result in a bloody discharge and associated adenopathy. There may or may not be an associated periareolar mass.

DIAGNOSTICS

If Paget disease is suspected, punch biopsy of the nipple may be performed as an office procedure, or the patient may be referred to a dermatologist or a general surgeon. As with all breast abnormalities, mammography is indicated but should not delay referral to a specialist.

DIAGNOSTICS

Paget Disease of the Nipple

IMAGING	OTHER
Mammography	Biopsy*
MRI	
Ultrasound	

*If indicated.

DIFFERENTIAL DIAGNOSIS

For patients with lesions involving the nipple, Paget disease should be suspected until proven otherwise. This is true even for a lesion that has healed spontaneously, because patients have been identified with healed nipple lesions that were subsequently diagnosed as Paget disease. Paget disease is most commonly misdiagnosed as eczema (Table 157-1). Eczema involving the nipple (versus the areola) is rare and, when present, is usually bilateral. The differential diagnosis of Paget disease includes psoriasis, contact dermatitis, tinea, basal cell carcinoma, Bowen disease, and benign intraductal papilloma of the nipple. Direct spread of invasive carcinoma from the underlying breast may be considered after Paget disease has been excluded.[24]

TABLE 157-1 Eczema Versus Paget Disease of the Nipple

Eczema	Paget Disease of the Nipple
Usually bilateral	Unilateral
Intermittent history with rapid progression	Continuous history with slow progression
Moist initially	Moist or dry
Indistinct border	Irregular but distinct border
Areola involved, nipple may be spared	Nipple always involved and disappears in advanced cases
Itching common	Itching common

DIFFERENTIAL DIAGNOSIS

Paget Disease of the Nipple

- Eczema
- Psoriasis
- Contact dermatitis
- Lichen sclerosus
- Nevoid hyperkeratosis of areola
- Malignant melanoma
- Bowen disease
- Carcinoma
- Intraductal papilloma
- Herpes
- Tinea versicolor

MANAGEMENT

Paget disease is treated with mastectomy or breast conservation surgery, which may be followed with radiation treatments.[24]

INDICATION FOR REFERRAL

Because histologic diagnosis of Paget disease is required, surgical referral for skin biopsy or excisional biopsy of the underlying mass is indicated. Biopsy-proven Paget disease should be viewed as an invasive breast cancer, and the patient must be referred to an oncologist for management.[24]

PATIENT EDUCATION

Patients undergoing evaluation for Paget disease require the same accurate information, support, and well-coordinated care that all patients anticipating a possible diagnosis of cancer are provided.

BREAST MASSES

DEFINITION AND EPIDEMIOLOGY

Currently, one in eight women will develop breast cancer in her lifetime.[3] Up to 85% of women with newly diagnosed breast cancer do not have a family history of breast cancer.[21]

Most breast cancers are diagnosed after a biopsy of a mammographic abnormality has been performed.[25] Ninety percent of breast masses are caused by benign lesions such as cysts, fibroadenomas, and fibrocystic changes.[13] Breast masses are different entities in women who are younger than 30 years, 31 to 50 years of age, or older than 50 years. Nine of 10 new masses in premenopausal women are benign.[13]

The breast undergoes substantial morphologic changes between early adolescence and menopause, ranging from a predominance of ducts, lobules, and interlobular stroma to fibrous change and cyst formation, formerly referred to as fibrocystic disease of the breast. The term *fibrocystic changes* is now preferred because 50% to 60% of women without breast disease may have fibrocystic changes, such as breasts with nondiscrete nodules, which entail no increased risk of breast cancer and are distinguished from those that confer a small increase in relative risk.[13]

Simple cysts are the most common type of discrete mass and are characterized as a distinct entity consisting of a palpable, fluid-filled sac within the breast tissue. Although cysts may be found in younger women, they are most commonly found in women aged 35 to 50 years. Cysts are rare in postmenopausal women not receiving HRT and should be viewed as breast cancer until proven otherwise. Fibroadenomas are the most common benign solid lesion of the female breast. Characteristically, fibroadenomas are painless, well-circumscribed, freely movable masses with a rounded, lobulated, or discoid configuration. They usually have a rubbery feeling but may appear hard, especially if calcified. Fibroadenomas occur most often in women in their 20s and 30s but may occur anytime after puberty and even during menopause. They are hormonally responsive and may increase in size toward the end of the menstrual cycle.

Benign phyllodes tumors are solid tumors of the breast that can manifest as a rapidly enlarging breast mass.

Focal areas of firm tissue in the breast when biopsied are often described as stromal fibrosis and represent a benign finding.

Common malignant tumors of the breast may manifest as a breast mass; these include invasive ductal carcinoma and invasive lobular carcinoma. Malignant phyllodes tumors are less often seen but often manifest as a breast mass.

Ductal carcinoma in situ may manifest as a breast mass but is frequently diagnosed as a mammographic abnormality.

PATHOPHYSIOLOGY

Breast development begins at puberty under the influence of increased levels of estradiol and progesterone. These influences promote the growth of ductal structures and glandular or lobular units. During the luteal phase of the menstrual cycle, there is an increase in the rate of cell proliferation.[13]

Fibroadenomas are thought to develop in the lobules and stroma as a result of hormonal stimulation. This occurs more frequently between adolescence and the mid-20s. Women in their 30s and 40s develop adenosis or enhancement of the lobular tissue with hypertrophy, resulting in palpable fullness of the breast tissue. By their 40s and toward menopause, more patients may develop hypertrophy of the stroma.[13]

The incidence of cysts increases with late menopause, use of HRT, and low body fat.[13] Evidence suggests that the incidence of benign breast lesions increases in response to hormonal events. Many investigators believe that breast lesions progress in a linear fashion from usual ductal hyperplasia to atypical ductal hyperplasia to ductal carcinoma in situ and then to invasive cancer.[13]

CLINICAL PRESENTATION

Discrete masses can be solitary lesions or multiple lesions, unilateral or bilateral. Cysts, fibroadenomas, hematomas, and breast cancer can manifest as a discrete palpable mass. Cysts are fluid-filled lesions that may or may not be associated with pain.

Symptomatic cysts occur in conjunction with the menstrual cycle.[21] Oil cysts may form as a result of fat necrosis.

Fibroadenomas are seen more often in adolescents and young women. They vary in size and are bilateral in approximately 10% of patients.[21] During pregnancy, fibroadenomas may enlarge. Clinically, they are discrete with well-circumscribed smooth borders. They may feel rubbery or firm and may be tender. Giant or juvenile fibroadenomas may enlarge quickly.[26]

Phyllodes tumors can be seen in young adults but more frequently occur in women in their 40s. On pathologic examination, they are benign or malignant. Clinically, they can be well circumscribed and can become very large in a short time.[26]

A palpable mass in the face of recent breast injury is often a hematoma. A mass that develops months after a traumatic injury may be caused by fat necrosis. These masses may be tender.[26]

The clinical presentation of breast cancer may include a firm, discrete mass or an area of diffuse firmness of the breast tissue, with or without skin thickening.

PHYSICAL EXAMINATION

Physical examination should be performed as previously described. Key historical features in the evaluation of a breast lump are the length of time the mass has been present, pain, associated skin changes, presence of axillary adenopathy, change in size or texture over time, relationship to menstrual cycle, and nipple discharge.

The clinical breast examination of a woman with a complaint of a discrete breast mass should assess the mass, including the location, consistency or texture, mobility, size, and shape and the presence or absence of palpable lymph nodes. Nipple discharge should also be assessed if it is reported. The presence or absence of a corresponding finding in the contralateral breast should be included.

DIAGNOSTICS

Clinical breast examination is a method of detection, not an independent diagnostic test. Diagnostic mammography and ultrasonography are usually the initial tests for a palpable mass in women older than 35 years. Ultrasonography alone is typically done in average-risk women younger than 35 years. Use of mammography in women younger than 35 years is individualized on the basis of risk status, clinical presentation, and findings on ultrasound examination. Negative imaging should not deter follow-up evaluation because 15% to 18% of mammograms appear negative in the presence of a palpable cancer. Decision to perform biopsy is based on the outcome of the radiographic findings and the level of clinical suspicion. A discrete mass with normal imaging always requires surgical referral for consideration of biopsy.

DIAGNOSTICS

Breast Masses

IMAGING	OTHER
Mammography	Biopsy
Ultrasound	Aspiration
MRI	

DIFFERENTIAL DIAGNOSIS

The differential diagnosis of a dominant breast mass includes breast cancer, macrocyst (clinically evident cyst), fibroadenoma, and phyllodes tumors (malignant or benign). In addition, prominent areas of fibrocystic change, fibrosis or fat necrosis as a result of surgical or extraneous trauma, and a galactocele (a milk cyst in a lactating woman) may be seen as a breast mass.[11]

MANAGEMENT

Management of the patient with a breast mass is governed by the patient's age, clinical history, and clinical findings. The incidence of malignant palpable masses increases after the age of 40 years. Any discrete mass requires thorough evaluation to include imaging, aspiration, or biopsy.[15]

If a cyst is detected, aspiration can be performed for both diagnosis and relief of pain. Cysts require cytologic analysis of aspirate fluid and surgical biopsy only if the aspirated fluid is bloody or if the palpable abnormality does not resolve completely after the aspiration of fluid. This approach has been supported by large studies of benign-appearing cyst fluid aspirates.[11] No cancers were ultimately identified in 6782 aspirates of low-probability samples. It is recommended that patients with a solitary breast cyst be reexamined 4 to 6 weeks after cyst aspiration to determine whether the cyst has recurred.[11]

Noncystic masses in premenopausal women that are different from the surrounding breast tissue require tissue sampling by core, needle, or excisional biopsy. Observation for one or two menstrual cycles is appropriate only for vague asymmetry or nodularity when it is unclear that a dominant breast mass is present.[11]

Any discrete, solid mass requires a tissue diagnosis to rule out malignant change.[15] Solid masses with ultrasound features consistent with a fibroadenoma can be followed clinically with serial ultrasound examinations. Core biopsy to confirm the diagnosis can be performed if there is any doubt about the ultrasound or clinical finding. Surgical excision is recommended if the mass enlarges or if the patient requests surgical removal.[15]

DIFFERENTIAL DIAGNOSIS

Breast Masses

- Malignant neoplasm
- Cyst
- Fibroadenoma
- Fibrocystic breast disease
- Intraductal papilloma
- Galactocele
- Lipoma
- Fat necrosis

LIFE SPAN CONSIDERATIONS

Approximately 90% of women have some degree of fibrocystic breast changes. Hormonal status and menopause status are associated with these changes, which at times may manifest as a breast mass. Awareness of breast changes with a willingness to seek evaluation for any new finding is always recommended.

INDICATIONS FOR REFERRAL OR HOSPITALIZATION

A palpable solid mass in all women, regardless of age, necessitates both consultation with a radiologist and a breast specialist and referral for surgical evaluation. Women should be referred for mammography or ultrasound examination and a clinical breast examination. Even when fibrocystic changes are suspected, surgical evaluation of a persistent, palpable dominant mass or lump is required. Tissue diagnosis will provide a definitive diagnosis and determine the presence of high-risk lesions.

PATIENT AND FAMILY EDUCATION

Most women are worried about developing breast cancer. Women need reassurance about the benign nature of breast lesions that wax and wane with hormonal variation as well as the rationale behind conservative versus surgical management. Education must also focus on the need for prudent breast evaluation of all breast symptoms and lesions regardless of the improbability of malignant disease. Screening recommendations should be tailored based on whether the patient is at average or high risk.

GYNECOMASTIA

DEFINITION AND EPIDEMIOLOGY

Gynecomastia is a benign enlargement of the male breast. Unlike pseudogynecomastia or lipomastia, which refers to an excess of adipose tissue of the breast, gynecomastia is the result of proliferation of the ductular elements.[27] Gynecomastia is common in older men and during puberty. Palpable breast tissue is appreciated on physical examination in 30% to 65% of men, and 50% to 70% of boys experience breast enlargement during puberty.[27] Physiologic pubertal gynecomastia typically lasts for approximately 6 months before regressing.[28]

PATHOPHYSIOLOGY

Gynecomastia is caused by the effects of an imbalance between free estrogen and free androgens. During puberty, production of estrogen by the testes and the peripheral tissues exceeds production of testosterone, resulting in breast enlargement. As men age, the testes may secrete too little testosterone. Numerous pathways that produce androgens and estrogen can be altered. Gynecomastia is the result of an enhanced estrogen effect or a diminished androgen effect on breast tissue.[28]

Exposure to many medications and recreational drugs may cause gynecomastia. The mechanism of action for this is not well understood.[27] Gynecomastia is also associated with disease processes including Klinefelter syndrome, adrenal and testicular tumors, thyrotoxicosis, some forms of liver disease, large cell carcinoma of the lung, and some gastric and renal cell cancers.[28]

CLINICAL PRESENTATION

Gynecomastia is often an incidental finding on physical examination. Men are often asymptomatic and can describe stable enlargement of their breast tissue. Clinical findings may present unilaterally or bilaterally or as asymmetry. A thorough physical examination is required to distinguish among a benign finding, a breast cancer, and a finding indicative of a serious endocrine or systemic disease.[27]

PHYSICAL EXAMINATION

A family history to determine the presence of breast or ovarian cancer, male breast cancer, and *BRCA* mutation carriers is essential.

A detailed history should include onset and duration of symptoms, presence of pain, underlying systemic illness, medications, exposures to environmental estrogens, and recent weight gain or loss.[27]

On physical examination, the axilla should be evaluated for adenopathy. Both breasts are examined by comparing subareolar tissue with the adjacent subcutaneous fat. Tissue in gynecomastia can be soft, elastic, or firm but is not typically hard. A unilateral hard or asymmetric mass that is fixed to the skin is worrisome for a malignant neoplasm. Skin dimpling or nipple retraction may be seen with breast cancer.[28]

In addition to a breast examination, a testicular and general physical examination should be considered to evaluate for systemic illness.[27]

DIAGNOSTICS

When a clinical diagnosis cannot be differentiated between gynecomastia and breast cancer, the patient should undergo diagnostic mammography. Mammography is 90% sensitive and specific to distinguish malignant from benign breast tissue.[28]

For long-standing asymptomatic gynecomastia, laboratory tests may not be necessary. A decrease in morning testosterone and luteinizing levels reflects hypogonadism, often seen with advancing age.[28]

Suspicion of systemic illness as a causative factor should be worked up appropriately.[27]

DIFFERENTIAL DIAGNOSIS

Adolescents with persistent gynecomastia should be further evaluated for Klinefelter syndrome, testicular or adrenal tumors, hyperthyroidism, and other hormonal causes. Further history taking to determine ongoing use of anabolic steroids, alcohol, opioids, or marijuana as a causative factor may be helpful. Persistent gynecomastia in adults should be further evaluated with hormone levels to confirm hypogonadism. A unilateral mass should suggest breast cancer until proven otherwise.[28]

MANAGEMENT

If it is thought that the gynecomastia is related to a medication, the suspected agent should be discontinued and the breast reassessed for resolution of the gynecomastia. Mammography is indicated for any clinical presentation worrisome for a breast malignant neoplasm. There are currently no professional guidelines for management of gynecomastia.[28]

INDICATIONS FOR REFERRAL OR HOSPITALIZATION

Patients with gynecomastia should be referred when breast cancer is suspected or when concern exists for other serious disease processes, such as endocrine disorders, other malignant neoplasms, or liver disease.

Surgical referral is indicated when there is a discrete mass and/or a clinically abnormal nipple or nipple areolar complex, with or without a mammographic abnormality. Painful large masses or segments of breast tissue may be surgically excised.

PATIENT AND FAMILY EDUCATION

Patients and their families can be informed that asymptomatic gynecomastia is relatively common. In adolescents, gynecomastia resolves over time, and reassurance and clinical follow-up are all that is needed. Reassurance is indicated for adults whose gynecomastia is related to an adverse reaction to a medication. Any patient whose symptoms persist and who is concerned about cosmesis may be referred for surgical removal of the affected breast tissue.[28]

CHAPTER 158

CHRONIC PELVIC PAIN

Patricia Polgar-Bailey

DEFINITION AND EPIDEMIOLOGY

Chronic pelvic pain (CPP) is a continuous or episodic, nonmenstrual pain of at least 6 months' duration, which may be sudden or gradual in onset, occurs at or below the umbilicus, and is severe enough to interrupt normal activities of daily life.[1] CPP may involve gastroenterologic, urologic, gynecologic, oncologic, musculoskeletal, and psychosocial systems, and its cause is often multifactorial, making it challenging for patients and providers.[2] Ideally, the cause of CPP is elucidated; however, in up to 50% to 60% of patients no clear cause is established and the absence of pathology often exacerbates the challenge of CPP.[2,3] CPP affects both men and women. Chronic prostatitis/chronic pelvic pain (CP/CPP) is a well-established cause of pelvic pain in men[2]; however, this chapter refers to the assessment and management of CPP in women. Chronic cyclic pelvic pain (CCPP) is a subset of CPP and is generally used to describe a CPP syndrome that occurs in relation to the menstrual cycle.[1] However, CCPP may also be used to describe pelvic pain that occurs in a cyclic pattern that is unrelated to the menstrual cycle.[4]

CPP is one of the most common medical problems affecting women today. In the United States CPP is estimated to affect approximately 15% of the female population aged 18 to 50.[2] In other parts of the world the prevalence of CPP is estimated to be higher. Recent studies demonstrated prevalence rates of approximately 25% in the United Kingdom and New Zealand.[2] Data indicate that the prevalence of CPP (38 per 1000) is similar to that of migraine, back pain, and asthma.[5] CPP is considered the principal indication for 40% of gynecologic laparoscopies and 12 of all hysterectomies performed for benign disease annually in the United States.[6] Epidemiologic studies have found that women with CPP are more likely to have a history of spontaneous abortion, nongynecologic surgery, and nonpelvic complaints than women without CPP.[2] In addition, a positive correlation has been demonstrated between CPP and a history of multiple sexual partners and psychosocial trauma and abuse. Women with CPP are four times more likely to have a history of pelvic inflammatory disease (PID), as well as higher incidences of constipation, irritable bowel syndrome (IBS), depression, and anxiety than those not affected by CPP.

Potential visceral sources of CPP include the reproductive, genitourinary, and gastrointestinal tracts; potential somatic sources include the pelvic bones, ligaments, muscles, and fascia. CPP may result from psychological disorders or neurologic diseases, both central and peripheral.[7] It may be caused by one disorder, or it can be the end result of several diagnoses, with each contributing to the generation of pain and requiring management. Women with diagnoses that involve more than one organ system have greater pain than do women with only one system involved.[8] The distinction between acute and chronic pain is significant. In acute pain, the pain is often a symptom of underlying tissue damage, such as anal fissure, and the diagnosis can be precise, but with CPP, the pain itself becomes the disease; CPP is itself the diagnosis.[2,9]

Populations at Increased Risk of Chronic Pelvic Pain

Physical and Sexual Abuse. A significant association exists between physical and sexual abuse and CPP. If a history of abuse is obtained, it is important to ensure that the woman is not currently being abused or in danger.

Pelvic Inflammatory Disease. Approximately 18% to 35% of all women with acute PID develop CPP.[10] The mechanisms by which CPP results from PID are not known, but the extent of adhesive disease, tubal damage, and pelvic tenderness present 30 days after treatment correlates with the likelihood of development of CPP. Whether acute PID is treated with inpatient or outpatient regimens does not appear to alter the odds for development of subsequent CPP (34% with outpatient therapy versus 30% with inpatient therapy).[10]

Endometriosis. Endometriosis is the one of the leading causes of CPP in women and the most common diagnosis made at the time of gynecologic laparoscopy for the evaluation of CPP. Most often, women diagnosed with CPP in the setting of endometriosis are nulliparous, in their 20s to 30s, with symptoms associated with their menstrual cycle, including dysmenorrhea or pain.[2] Although endometriosis is diagnosed laparoscopically in approximately 33% of women with CPP, up to 40% of women with endometriosis and CPP will have no findings on laparoscopy.[2] There is often no correlation between severity of pain and pathologic findings.[2]

Interstitial Cystitis. Interstitial cystitis is a chronic inflammatory condition of the bladder. It is clinically characterized by bladder pain, urinary frequency or urgency, or nocturia in the absence of evidence of another disease that could cause the symptoms.[2] Pain is often present in the suprapubic area but may also occur in the lower back or buttock. As many as 50% of women complain of dyspareunia; fibromyalgia, vulvodynia, anxiety, and depression are often associated complaints.[2]

Irritable Bowel Syndrome. Approximately one third of women with CPP have IBS,[8] and an estimated 65% to 70% of person with IBS have CPP.[2] IBS is a functional gastrointestinal disorder characterized by intermittent or chronic abdominal pain that is associated with bowel symptoms such as bloating, urgency, diarrhea, and constipation. IBS is associated with certain gynecologic problems, such as endometriosis, dyspareunia, and dysmenorrhea.[11] Women with both CPP and IBS are more likely to have screening and diagnostic procedures done and are less likely to have improvement after laparoscopy compared with women with only CPP.[11]

Musculoskeletal Disorders. Faulty posture may contribute to weak and deconditioned muscles, which allow imbalances in the pelvis with formation of trigger points and hypertonicity and, as a result, pelvic pain. Other musculoskeletal disorders, such as trigger points, lumbar vertebral disorders, pelvic floor myalgia, and fibromyalgia, may cause or contribute to pelvic pain.

Postsurgical Pain. Chronic pain has been reported after several types of surgical procedures, including after cholecystectomy and groin hernia repair in less than 30% of patients and after cesarean section in 6% of patients. A study also found a

48.4% incidence of CPP in patients up to 5.6 years after surgery for pelvic fracture.[12]

PATHOPHYSIOLOGY

The pathogenesis of CPP remains poorly understood, and diagnostic studies, such as laparoscopy, reveal no obvious cause of the pain in up to 35% of cases.[2] In a U.S. population study, 61% of women with CPP did not have a clear cause of their pain.[5] Thus, chronic pain is thought to be a dynamic interaction of the combined influences of the mind and nervous system on the body. In addition to the organ system where the pain originated, other organ systems become involved and emotional changes occur with the long-term tension of CPP. For example, pain can cause muscle tension, which can in turn cause changes in the muscles of the pelvis, adjacent urinary tract (bladder, urethra), bowel, connective tissue, and even skin of the area. These secondary changes often become more significant than the original cause of the pain and also may overshadow the original disease process, making it more difficult to diagnose.

There are different theories about the development of chronic pain. According to an older theory of pain, called the cartesian theory, neurons carry pain signals from the damaged areas through the spinal cord directly to the cortex of the brain, where the pain is perceived. This theory is now thought to be an oversimplification of the development of chronic pain.

A newer theory, the gate control theory, posits that pain signals arise from the injured or adversely affected tissues and travel through specialized nerve cells to the spinal cord, where they can be intensified, reduced, and even blocked before they are transmitted to the brain. The spinal cord acts as a functional "gate" with respect to the pain signals. This gate is influenced by local factors such as nerve inputs in the spinal cord and by descending signals from higher brain centers. Thus, internal influences, other than the pain itself, and external environmental factors affect the nature of the pain's impulse transmission. If the gates are damaged by chronic pain, they may remain open even after the tissue damage has resolved or been controlled. In other words, the pain remains despite the fact that the original cause of the pain has been treated; this type of pain is referred to as neuropathic pain, a key factor in CPP.[9]

CLINICAL PRESENTATION

The evaluation of CPP can require many office visits and become a highly frustrating experience for both patient and provider. A complete and thorough history and physical examination are crucial in developing a rational approach to women with CPP. It is important that the patient understand early on that visits are not only for evaluation and treatment but also for the formation of a continued therapeutic relationship between patient and provider.

The history should include a description of the nature, intensity, distribution, radiation, location, and daily pattern of the pain, as well as the relationship of the pain to each organ system. Associated events, including complaints of fever, sweats, fatigue, anorexia, nausea, vomiting, and constipation, should be elicited. The relationship of the pain to posture, meals, bowel movements, voiding, menstruation, intercourse, and medications as well as any factors that aggravate or alleviate the pain should be determined. Past surgeries, pelvic infections, and a history of infertility are important diagnostic clues to the origin of the pain.

BOX 158-1

Chronic Pelvic Pain Questionnaire (Sample Questions)

- How and when did the pain begin?
- What actions or activities make it better or worse?
- Does it vary based on time of day, week, or menstrual cycle?
- Does it affect your sleep?
- Has it spread beyond where it first was noted?
- Is it associated with abnormal skin sensations, muscle or joint pain, or back pain?
- Do you have any urinary pain or problems, constipation, diarrhea, or other bowel complaints?
- Has it affected your daily routine at home and at work?
- Has it led to emotional changes such as anxiety or depression?
- What have you personally done to attempt to alleviate the pain?
- What has your physician done?
- Have these methods been successful to any degree?
- What medications are you currently using?
- What do you think is causing your pain?
- What concerns you most about your pain?

Modified from the International Pelvic Pain Society: *Chronic pelvic pain, a patient education booklet,* 1999. Available at www.pelvicpain.org/pdf/Patients/CPP_Pt_Ed_Booklet.pdf.

It is helpful to obtain an understanding from the woman of the past and present status of her pain, the chronology, and how it developed. It can be helpful to have the woman complete a detailed pain questionnaire before her first visit. Box 158-1 includes some questions that should be included on a CPP questionnaire.

PHYSICAL EXAMINATION

The physical examination should be thorough, complete, and guided by the history. It will differ from a standard gynecologic examination because it is designed to provide information beyond the condition of the female genitals. The initial part of the examination should begin with observation of the patient's general demeanor during the interview. The five major sources that contribute to pelvic pain should be completely evaluated: gynecologic, gastrointestinal, psychological, musculoskeletal, and urologic.

The abdomen should be examined to elicit a point or area of tenderness. It is important that the patient be allowed to indicate the location of the pain and the depth of palpation necessary to elicit the discomfort. If pain is experienced during palpation of the abdomen, a trigger point, hernia, endometriosis, or hematoma is likely. Costovertebral angle tenderness should also be elicited if there is tenderness with suprapubic palpation. The groin should be evaluated for inflamed lymph nodes and hernias.

The back should be examined for lordosis, scoliosis, and any tenderness over the paraspinal musculature, sacroiliac joints, or spine prominence. Range of motion should be evaluated. By having the patient lie in the lateral decubitus position, the examiner can accomplish passive thigh extension, which may reveal psoas muscle tenderness.

The pelvic examination should be performed in a gentle, stepwise manner. Attention should be given to any evidence of a vulvar pathologic condition. Pelvic relaxation should be evaluated by having the patient bear down while the practitioner separates the labia and observes for a significant cystocele, rectocele, enterocele, or cervical or uterine prolapse.

A single-digit transvaginal examination (monomanual) is necessary to elicit any tenderness or mass in the adnexa, in the cervix or posterior vagina, along the vaginal side walls, or near the base of the bladder or urethra. Special attention during palpation of the levator ani muscles, piriform muscles, and coccyx is important because all have been implicated as a cause of CPP and discomfort.

A careful speculum examination is performed to visualize the cervix and vagina and to inspect for neoplasms, prolapse, or infections. This examination may reveal vaginismus, with involuntary spasms of the vaginal musculature that make insertion of the speculum difficult.

The bimanual examination and rectovaginal examination complete the genitourinary evaluation. Particular attention should be given to areas of tenderness. Cervical motion tenderness has been associated with endometriosis, pelvic adhesive disease, inflammatory bowel disease (IBD), and ureteral colic. A fixed retroverted uterus or an enlarged boggy uterus, the hallmark of adenomyosis, may be noted. Uterine fibroids do not classically cause pain unless they are degenerating or infarcting, but their enlargement may cause a feeling of heaviness and pressure on nerve endings in the lower abdomen and pelvis. Finally, the rectovaginal examination may reveal nodularity in the cul-de-sac that is associated with endometriosis. The examination may also help identify any rectal masses, and the piriform muscle can be evaluated for spasms and tenderness.

DIAGNOSTICS

Laboratory studies should be based on the history and physical findings. The usual evaluation for CPP should include vaginal and cervical cultures, urinalysis, urine culture, complete blood count (CBC), pregnancy test, and erythrocyte sedimentation rate (ESR). A transvaginal ultrasound examination may be beneficial if the bimanual examination was difficult; if it revealed adnexal tenderness, a mass, or uterine enlargement; or if irregularity was noted.

Laparoscopy may be indicated, especially if the pelvic examination or imaging findings are abnormal. Commonly found abnormalities include endometriosis, adhesions, and chronic PID. Referral to a gynecologic surgeon should be made if abnormalities are noted.

DIAGNOSTICS

Chronic Pelvic Pain

LABORATORY
Cervical cultures*
CBC and differential
Serum human chorionic gonadotropin
ESR
Urinalysis*
Culture and sensitivity*
Pregnancy test

IMAGING
Transvaginal ultrasound
Renal ultrasound
Magnetic resonance imaging or computed tomography scan

OTHER DIAGNOSTICS
Laparoscopy*
Trigger point injection*

*If indicated.

DIFFERENTIAL DIAGNOSIS

The differential diagnosis for CPP is extensive. From a primary care perspective, a good history and physical examination aid in the differential diagnosis. Direct questioning of the patient's view of what is wrong or of concern may be very helpful in developing a differential diagnosis.[4] IBS is believed to account for 35% to 50% of all cases of CPP.[5,8] IBS is a chronic functional bowel disorder that is often accompanied by gynecologic complaints and labeled as CPP. IBS consists of a constellation of symptoms, including abdominal pain or discomfort that is relieved with defecation; it is usually associated with alternating constipation and diarrhea. The pain of IBS is usually worse around the time of menstruation and may be associated with dyspareunia.

CPP and IBS are both believed to be multifactorial in origin and share some of the same psychosocial factors, including a high prevalence of depression and a history of physical or sexual abuse A diagnosis of IBS should be included in any differential diagnosis of CPP, but CPP should also remain a diagnosis of exclusion.[2] As with any other gastrointestinal complaint, more serious disease entities need to be excluded, including IBD, diverticulitis, and malignant disease.

Urinary tract problems may manifest as CPP. Because the gynecologic and urinary systems share embryologic origins, differentiation of the source of pain can be difficult. A pathologic condition of the urinary tract can demonstrate a constellation of symptoms, including pelvic pain, dysuria, urgency, hesitancy, dyspareunia, postcoital voiding difficulties, and incontinence. Urethral syndrome, chronic urethritis, interstitial cystitis, urethral diverticulum, and bladder spasms should be considered in the differential diagnosis.

Musculoskeletal diseases are also associated with CPP. These conditions include postural problems, herniated disk disease, chronic pelvic tilt, degenerative joint disease, and myofascial trigger points. Levator ani muscle spasms and piriform muscle spasms are two conditions that are easy to evaluate on physical examination and may be a source of pain and discomfort.

Levator syndrome is generally attributed to muscle spasms of the pelvic floor musculature and and is associated with a wide range of musculoskeletal disorders, including piriformis and puborectalis syndromes.[2] Levator ani muscle spasms are more common in women, with an incidence of approximately 6%,[2] and are usually initially seen as sacral pain and overlooked as a possible cause of CPP. The pain is caused by contraction and spasm of the levator ani muscles. Palpation of this muscle group reveals tenderness and increasing pain with voluntary contraction. Teaching the patient to relax these muscles and the vaginal muscles will help alleviate the discomfort.

Piriform syndrome or spasms of the piriform muscle during external rotation of the leg can be reproduced by contraction of the externally rotated leg against resistance. Because the piriform muscle can be palpated transvaginally, tenderness along the muscle should be evaluated during bimanual examination. Physical therapy is usually indicated to help relieve the spasms.

An alteration in the processing of the stimuli by the spinal cord and brain in women with CPP has also been suggested as a possible cause.[5] This may be a component in other types of chronic pain, in which normal body sensations are perceived as painful.[5]

A gynecologic source of pain should always be considered. Although a pathologic condition is more likely with acute pain, certain entities are more commonly seen with CPP.

Endometriosis is one of the leading causes of CPP in women.[2] Endometriosis is caused by the development of implants outside the endometrium. Because these implants can be found anywhere and are responsive to the cyclic hormonal cycle, the point source of the pain can be elusive. On physical examination, either tenderness in the cul-de-sac or along the uterosacral ligaments (early finding) or nodularity in the same locations (late finding) may be noted. The diagnosis should be confirmed by laparoscopy. In spite of laparoscopic confirmation of endometriosis, definitive criteria to determine the actual cause of the pain of endometriosis are lacking.[2]

Adhesions are scar tissue that can form between any two abdominal organs, usually after surgery or intra-abdominal infections such as PID. The pain occurs because of the stretching of usually mobile structures that are now scarred. Patients usually complain of a substantial positional component to the pain. The diagnosis can be confirmed by laparoscopy.

Other gynecologic origins of CPP include pain with ovulation, dysmenorrhea, functional ovarian cysts, ovarian torsion, chronic PID, pelvic congestion of the reproductive organ venous system, adenomyosis, and leiomyomas.

If a patient admits to depression and attributes it to the pain, management in collaboration with a psychiatrist or psychologist may be helpful.[4] Disclosure of childhood physical or emotional abuse should elicit a referral to an appropriate mental health provider but will likely not affect immediate management of the pain.[4]

If no other pathologic entity or explanation can be found for the pain, a psychiatric component such as clinical depression or somatization disorder should be considered. Screening for depression and referral to a psychiatrist can assist in this area.

DIFFERENTIAL DIAGNOSIS

Chronic Pelvic Pain

MUSCULOSKELETAL
- Myofascial
- Coccygodynia, piriformis or levator ani syndrome
- Low back pain
- Scoliosis and other postural problems
- Spasm of the pelvic floor
- Fibromyalgia

GASTROINTESTINAL
- IBS
- Diverticulosis or diverticulitis
- IBD
- Celiac disease

UROLOGIC
- Interstitial cystitis
- Recurrent urinary tract infection
- Urethral diverticulum

GYNECOLOGIC
- Dysmenorrhea
- Pain with ovulation
- Chronic pelvic inflammatory disease
- Adhesions
- Endometriosis
- Adenomyosis
- Endometritis
- Uterine fibroids
- Ovarian mass

PSYCHOLOGICAL
- Depression
- Physical or sexual abuse
- Opiate dependency
- Somatization

MANAGEMENT

Information for evidence-based management of CPP is not widely available, and there is little specific evidence for the role of analgesic drugs in the treatment of CPP.[4] Success in treating women with CPP is greatly facilitated by winning their trust and confidence. In general, positive reinforcement and general psychological support are important in the early diagnostic phase of CPP. Women suffer for years, and many are told the problem is psychosomatic. Consideration of depression and sleep disorders is important because treatment of these conditions enhances management of the chronic pain syndrome. If a cause of the pain is identified, appropriate management should be undertaken with the assistance of the appropriate physician specialist.

During the diagnostic evaluation, the pain component should be treated effectively and promptly. First-line treatment is generally nonsteroidal anti-inflammatory drugs (NSAIDs) to decrease pain and inflammation.[2] Narcotics are not recommended owing to concerns for abuse and addiction potential, as well as risks of constipation or antimotility side effects, which could exacerbate the pain.

There are data to suggest that tricyclic antidepressants are effective for neuropathic pain and, for this reason, may be helpful in CPP.[4] There are limited data for the use of selective serotonin reuptake inhibitors for relief of pain in CPP and insufficient evidence for the use of any other antidepressant.

Anticonvulsants have been used for pain management for many years. Recently, gabapentin has begun to be used for chronic pain syndromes and is thought to have fewer side effects than other anticonvulsants.[4] There remains insufficient good-quality evidence for the efficacy of neuropathic medications in the context of CPP, but they may be helpful for some women.[2]

Neurostimulation has been used successfully for the treatment of neuropathic pain. It is believed that there may be a role for sacral neuromodulation in CPP syndromes.[4] Neuroablative techniques and chemical neuroablation have been used with some success in pain management. Botox has been used with some success for both pelvic floor muscle spasms and undifferentiated CPP.[2]

Laparoscopy has been used as both a diagnostic and a therapeutic tool in CPP. Adhesions are often thought to be a cause of CPP, and some women may experience improvement after laparoscopic adhesiolysis.[2] An estimated 10% of hysterectomies have been performed for CPP, but up to 40% of women will have recurrent pain after hysterectomy.[2]

Counseling and a supportive patient-provider relationship are very important, particularly because diagnostic procedures such as ultrasound and laparoscopy are used to exclude serious conditions and to provide reassurance.[5] Menstrual cycle suppression with oral, transdermal, transvaginal, or subcutaneous contraceptives (medroxyprogesterone [Depo-Provera]) may be helpful. The Mirena intrauterine device and a gonadotropin-releasing hormone agonist such as leuprolide (Lupron) may also be helpful in management of CPP.

Complementary and alternative medicine (CAM) options most commonly used for CPP include dietary supplements and herbs, acupuncture, and mind-body methods.[6] Some of these adjunctive therapies have shown promise, but more studies are necessary to demonstrate efficacy in the management of CPP.

Regardless of the treatment used, regular office visits are important for patients with CPP. These visits enable discussion of the progress of the diagnostic process and assessment of therapy, and they provide reassurance and support during the evaluation period.

LIFE SPAN CONSIDERATIONS

CPP usually occurs during a woman's late 20s and early 30s but can be seen across the reproductive life span, and the population group is varied. This can be a stressful period in a woman's life. She may be married, considering pregnancy or raising children, and involved in a career. CPP can profoundly affect a woman's personal and professional life. An open mind and the pursuit of appropriate diagnostics as well as support of the patient's fears, anxieties, and stresses can have a profound impact on the understanding of CPP and ultimate pain control.

COMPLICATIONS

Numerous pathologic conditions have been identified with CPP, and the potential for complications is incalculable. Many women suffer great frustration associated with the diagnosis and treatment of this disorder. In addition, there is often a psychogenic component to the disorder that is not easily addressed.

INDICATIONS FOR REFERRAL OR HOSPITALIZATION

The cause of CPP is often complex and multifaceted, and treatment may involve several specialists. A coordinated multidisciplinary approach has been advocated. Prompt referral to physical therapy, gastroenterology, urology, and pain management programs as indicated should be considered. Working with a consulting physician is essential to assess the need for surgical evaluation, in addition to consultation for diagnostic testing, appropriate referral to collaborating providers, and assistance with treatment planning as indicated.

PATIENT AND FAMILY EDUCATION

Reassurance that the causes of CPP, although real and concerning, tend to be less urgent than the causes of acute pelvic pain can be helpful. In addition, it is important that the patient understand that additional diagnostic testing may not be indicated. Education should include information about the possible sources of pain and an explanation that the alleviation of pain may be best achieved by a combination of therapies, including medical, psychological, and behavioral treatments.

HEALTH PROMOTION

Helping a woman understand her body and the sources of possible pain can assist her in coping. As always, a healthy diet, regular exercise, moderation of alcohol intake, and relaxation techniques can go a long way toward improving a woman's management of the stress and anxiety associated with CPP.

CHAPTER 159

DYSMENORRHEA

Elke Jones Zschaebitz

DEFINITION AND EPIDEMIOLOGY

The term *dysmenorrhea,* from the Greek word meaning "difficult monthly flow," refers to painful menstruation. Dysmenorrhea is classified as either a primary or a secondary gynecologic disorder. Primary dysmenorrhea is defined as painful menses despite normal pelvic anatomy and ovulation occurring within 6 to 12 months after menarche, when ovulatory cycles are established.[1,2] However, primary dysmenorrhea can begin as late as 1 to 3 years after menarche and is characterized by cramping pelvic pain just before or with the onset of menstrual flow and typically lasting 1 to 3 days,[3] with a peak in the second and third decades of life and subsequently decreasing with advancing age. Secondary dysmenorrhea usually appears later in life, after some years of painless menstruation, and is associated with underlying pathologic processes such as endometriosis, uterine fibroids, adenomyosis, pelvic inflammatory disease, infertility problems, ovarian cysts, polyps, intrauterine adhesions, cervical stenosis, other pelvic pathologic conditions, or an intrauterine contraceptive device (IUD).[2,4]

Dysmenorrhea prevalence rates around the world vary widely and range between 20% and 90%.[4] In the United States, dysmenorrhea is one of the most commonly encountered gynecologic disorders, estimated to affect 50% to 60% of reproductive age women overall and up to 90% of adolescents.[5] The peak incidence of dysmenorrhea is highest during adolescence, and approximately 15% of women who experience dysmenorrhea have discomfort that interferes with normal daily activity for 1 to 3 days each month, with 51% of women having missed work or school because of their symptoms.[1,5,7] It is difficult to estimate the economic burden of missed work from dysmenorrhea, but clearly it accounts for significant lost wages and diminished quality of life. Nevertheless, many women "suffer silently" and do not discuss dysmenorrhea with any health care provider. Adolescents, in particular, are unlikely to consult a health care provider about dysmenorrhea and have a tendency to self-medicate with over-the-counter medications.[1] Providers should be aware that the quality of a woman's life can be improved by reducing or relieving the discomfort of dysmenorrhea. In addition, the willingness to discuss this common but possibly sensitive issue may pave the way to a more satisfying patient-provider relationship.

PATHOPHYSIOLOGY

Primary dysmenorrhea has been attributed to ovulatory cycles, with the maturation of the hypothalamic-pituitary-gonadal axis.[2] Dysmenorrhea is caused by an excess or imbalance of prostaglandins, vasopressin, and chemical substances originating from phospholipids. These chemicals cause uterine contractions, cramping, nausea, vomiting, and diarrhea. Risk factors for dysmenorrhea include adolescence, anxiety, depression, stress, body mass index below 20 or above 30 kg/m^2, menorrhagia, metrorrhagia, nulliparity, and smoking. Contractions in the menstruating uterus and pain have been attributed to the production of prostaglandins, specifically $PGF_{2\alpha}$ and PGE_2.[2,3] The prostaglandins also cause the nausea and diarrhea associated with dysmenorrhea. Current evidence shows that the menstrual fluid of women with primary dysmenorrhea has higher-than-normal levels of these prostaglandins.[1,8,9] Anovulatory cycles are associated with lower levels of prostaglandins and as a result usually no dysmenorrhea.[3]

Despite the supporting evidence for a link between higher prostaglandin levels and dysmenorrhea, it is likely that the explanation for menstrual pain is not as simple as the cyclic production of one hormone. Women with dysmenorrhea may have complex alterations in hormonal patterns that exist throughout the cycle and affect a number of factors, including higher basal body temperature and disrupted sleep patterns.[2] Vasopressin may also play a role by increasing uterine contractility and causing ischemic pain as a result of vasoconstriction. Elevated vasopressin levels have been reported in women with primary dysmenorrhea.[1] In addition, women have differing perceptions of pain, and this may affect how they experience dysmenorrhea.[2] Research suggests that many factors are related to dysmenorrhea, including younger age, low body mass index, smoking, early menarche, pelvic infections, genetic influence, and history of pelvic assault.[4]

There is no convincing evidence that mechanical cervical obstruction or severe uterine flexion causing obstructed uterine flow is present in patients with primary dysmenorrhea, although heavy menstrual flow is associated with dysmenorrhea. Some studies have suggested that young age and nulliparity are associated with dysmenorrhea, but the correlation with age was not substantiated in other studies once parity and other factors were controlled for.[1] There is also no evidence to support an association between tubal sterilization and the prevalence of dysmenorrhea.[1,10]

Although dysmenorrhea is no longer considered a psychological disorder, risk factors for dysmenorrhea have been investigated, including the varied socioeconomic and behavioral variables in many studies. Factors such as smoking; higher body mass index, which can also include obesity; earlier age at menarche; nulliparity; longer and heavier menstrual flow; and family history of dysmenorrhea have been examined.[2] In addition, depression, stress, level of education attained, marital status, employment, alcohol consumption, and physical activity levels have also been investigated.

A systematic review of several studies has suggested a significant inverse relationship between age and the risk of dysmenorrhea. A concurrent family history of dysmenorrhea, perceived stress levels, and heavy or irregular menstrual cycles have also been linked to dysmenorrhea in many studies. Stress has been demonstrated to indirectly affect prostaglandin synthesis and concentrations through the release of corticotropin-releasing hormone. Prostaglandins affect uterine muscle and vascular tone, and an imbalance of prostaglandins has been linked to the occurrence of dysmenorrhea.[1,9,11] Stress inhibits the release of follicle-stimulating hormone and luteinizing hormones, leading to impaired follicular development. This pathway can alter progesterone synthesis and release, which can alter the activity of prostaglandin. Stress-related hormones also appear to influence prostaglandin synthesis and/or binding in the myometrium of the uterus.

Fruit and vegetable intake has been found to have some benefit in the treatment of dysmenorrhea. The protective effect of oral contraceptives or other hormonal contraceptive forms such as IUDs has been evident and consistent across different study types[2]; IUDs containing hormones were found to have a positive effect on dysmenorrhea pain. Interestingly, there was no significant association between tubal ligation and dysmenorrhea.

Conflicting results were found in studies examining sociodemographic factors such as employment, socioeconomic status, body mass index, and the effect of exercise on dysmenorrhea. No associations between alcohol consumption and dysmenorrhea were found, and the association with cigarette smoking yielded mixed results.[1,2] The lack of data and the conflicting data are attributed to the limited number of studies as well as the small study samples in examining variables and the biases noted in systematic reviews.

Cultural and family influences may have a profound effect on how a woman experiences dysmenorrhea. The attitudes a woman has toward menstruation are often formed early in life and may be influenced by factors that include culture, religion, family, friends, and sexual partners. Additional emotional influences may be related to perceptions of fertility, the ability to bear children, or the relationship with the sexual partner. Many women begin menstruating with little or no accurate information, and menstrual sensations and discomfort may be distressing, frightening, or viewed as punishment. A woman's beliefs about menstruation may directly affect the way she experiences it and her willingness to report any problems to her provider or to seek treatment. The variation rates examining the prevalence globally in studies are attributed to the lack of standard methods for assessing the severity of dysmenorrhea in various cultures.[1]

Secondary dysmenorrhea is associated with underlying pelvic pathology and needs to be investigated to determine the cause. Secondary dysmenorrhea is caused by a pathologic process that affects the uterus, fallopian tubes, ovaries, or pelvic peritoneum. These processes can cause pain by altering pressures in or around pelvic structures, changing or restricting blood flow, or irritating the pelvic peritoneum. They can occur with the normal physiology of menstruation or act completely independently, with symptoms appearing during specific points in the menstrual cycle. Extrauterine causes must also be considered in the differential diagnosis; associated pelvic, bladder, and abdominal structural problems as well as causes related to previous surgical history may exist with chronic pelvic pain syndromes that suggest dysmenorrhea.[5]

CLINICAL PRESENTATION

The diagnosis of primary dysmenorrhea is based on clinical features determined with a careful and detailed history of symptoms. The history should include age at menarche, menstrual history, last menstrual period, location and severity of discomfort, associated symptoms (headache, dizziness, nausea, vomiting, diarrhea, dyschezia), amount of school or work missed, medications, method of birth control, and whether the birth control is being used correctly. Abdominal and pelvic pain not related to the menstrual cycle should also be considered in the differential diagnosis.

Pain descriptions can vary significantly from individual to individual. Young women will generally report recurrent sharp, crampy pelvic pain, spasmodic lower abdominal pain, or pain over the suprapubic area.[4] The pain will often radiate to the back, sacrum, or inner thighs. The pain usually begins a few hours before or just after the onset of menstruation and lasts the first 1 to 3 days of menstruation; it can be associated with nausea, vomiting, diarrhea, low back pain, or headache. Some young women also have associated systemic symptoms, including nausea, vomiting, loose bowel movements, and dizziness. Consideration should be given to symptoms exacerbated by dysmenorrhea such as irritable bowel syndrome, interstitial cystitis, or migraines.[2,3]

Secondary dysmenorrhea is distinguished from primary dysmenorrhea by a history of pain that is inconsistent with the kind of low anterior pelvic pain described as beginning in adolescence and associated specifically with menstrual cycles. The signs and symptoms of secondary dysmenorrhea are related to an underlying pathologic process. The onset of secondary dysmenorrhea usually occurs in women 30 or 40 years of age rather than shortly after menarche. The pain is often not limited to the menses and is less related to the 48 to 72 hours of menstrual flow. There may be an array of associated symptoms in secondary dysmenorrhea including dyspareunia, infertility, and abnormal bleeding.

PHYSICAL EXAMINATION

Physical examination findings are normal in primary dysmenorrhea. The diagnosis is based on a careful history. It is appropriate to perform only an abdominal examination in young women with a typical history of low anterior pelvic pain beginning in adolescence and associated specifically with the menstrual cycle.

When the history or physical examination suggests secondary dysmenorrhea (i.e., an atypical history or physical findings of pelvic mass, abnormal vaginal or pelvic tenderness not limited to the menstrual cycle), the evaluation should follow accordingly and is based on the suspicion of an underlying pathologic condition. The physical examination for secondary dysmenorrhea must include a thorough abdominal, pelvic, and rectovaginal examination. Clues to diagnosis may be asymmetric enlargement of the uterus or adnexa (indicating myomas or other tumors), symmetric enlargement (indicating adenomyosis), painful nodules in the posterior cul-de-sac together with restricted motion of the uterus (indicating endometriosis), cervical stenosis (suggesting retrograde menstruation), or restricted motion of the uterus together with thickened adnexal structures (indicating pelvic scarring or adhesions).

DIAGNOSTICS

No diagnostic studies are needed for the diagnosis of primary dysmenorrhea. However, if the diagnosis of primary versus secondary dysmenorrhea is not clear or the pelvic examination suggests pelvic disease, additional diagnostic tests are indicated. Pelvic ultrasonography is often a helpful initial diagnostic test to rule out anatomic abnormalities, such as ovarian cysts and endometriomas.[1] Sonovaginography (i.e., transvaginal ultrasonography with saline infusion of the uterus) may be more helpful than transvaginal ultrasonography in diagnosis of endometriosis.[1] In some instances an abdominal or pelvic computed tomography (CT) scan may be indicated. Laboratory evaluation may include a complete blood count (CBC), erythrocyte sedimentation rate (ESR), and genital cultures for pathogens. If the final diagnosis is still unconfirmed, the patient may require a laparoscopy, hysteroscopy, or dilation and curettage.

DIAGNOSTICS

Secondary Dysmenorrhea

LABORATORY

CBC and differential
ESR
Serum human chorionic gonadotropin (hCG)
Urinalysis*
Gonococcal, chlamydial cultures
Pap test

IMAGING

Pelvic ultrasonography (transvaginal, vaginal)*

OTHER DIAGNOSTICS

Laparoscopy*
Hysterosalpingography*
Hysteroscopy*
Dilation and curettage*
Abdominal or pelvic CT*

*If indicated.

DIFFERENTIAL DIAGNOSIS

The diagnosis of primary dysmenorrhea is made by a careful history and clinical presentation. Secondary dysmenorrhea is more concerning because the cause can be pathologic, requiring treatment, and difficult to determine.[5] The causes can be broadly classified as intrauterine or extrauterine. Intrauterine causes include myomas, adenomyosis, polyps, an IUD, infection, cervical stenosis, and cervical lesions. Unilateral dysmenorrhea is relatively rare and may manifest as an acute abdomen, but it should also raise the suspicion of uterine malformation.[6] Extrauterine causes include endometriosis, tumors (myomas or malignant), inflammation, sexually transmitted infections, adhesions, psychogenic causes such as pelvic congestion syndrome, and nongynecologic causes (urologic, gastrointestinal, musculoskeletal, and psychiatric conditions). Pregnancy and especially ectopic pregnancy should always be a consideration in a female patient of childbearing age.

DIFFERENTIAL DIAGNOSIS

Dysmenorrhea

INTRAUTERINE CAUSES

- Myomas
- Adenomyosis
- Polyps
- IUD
- Infection
- Cervical stenosis
- Cervical lesions
- Uterine malformation
- Infection (pelvic inflammatory disease [PID] or sexually transmitted disease [STD])
- Adhesions
- Imperforate hymen
- Psychogenic causes
- Pelvic congestion syndrome

EXTRAUTERINE CAUSES

- Ectopic pregnancy
- Endometriosis
- Tumors
- Fibroids
- Inflammation

NONGYNECOLOGIC CAUSES

- Urologic conditions
- Gastrointestinal conditions
- Musculoskeletal conditions
- Psychiatric conditions

Chronic cyclic pelvic pain (CCPP) is a subset of chronic pelvic pain that occurs in relation to the menstrual cycle; however, CCPP also refers to cyclically occurring pelvic pain that may not be related to the menstrual cycle.[12] For example, pain associated with ovulation (mittelschmerz) or pain associated with intercourse may occur with a cyclic pattern but is not related to menstruation as is dysmenorrhea.

Dysmenorrhea (primary and secondary) is also a distinct and separate entity from premenstrual syndrome (PMS), and the two should not be confused. PMS describes a predictable set of physical and affective symptoms that occur cyclically during the luteal phase and resolve quickly on or near the onset of the menstrual cycle. The American College of Obstetricians and Gynecologists define this condition as at least one symptom associated with "economic or social dysfunction; that occurs during the 5 days prior to onset of menses and is present in at least three consecutive menstrual cycles." These symptoms may be concurrent with dysmenorrhea; however, their characteristics are distinct.[5] The cause of PMS is not known, but it is a relatively uncommon disorder during adolescence, in contrast to primary dysmenorrhea, which affects the majority of adolescent girls.[2]

MANAGEMENT

A variety of therapies have been used to treat dysmenorrhea, but the standard treatments have not been well examined over the past 30 years. The mainstays for treatment of primary dysmenorrhea are nonsteroidal anti-inflammatory drugs (NSAIDs), which are antiprostaglandins, and hormonal contraceptives. NSAIDs are the best established initial therapy for dysmenorrhea. They inhibit prostaglandin synthesis and thereby provide pain relief. In addition, they decrease the volume of menstrual flow, which may mitigate the dysmenorrhea.[8] Randomized controlled trials of NSAIDs suggest that all of the NSAIDs studied are more effective in treating dysmenorrhea than acetaminophen is, although no studies have clearly determined which NSAIDs are the most efficacious. Typical examples of NSAIDs that are approved by the U.S. Food and Drug Administration for treatment of primary dysmenorrhea are listed in Box 159-1. NSAIDs may be the most effective when therapy is started before the onset of menstrual pain and flow, and they need not be continued for the entire menstrual cycle.[1]

Small studies have shown that cyclooxygenase-2 (COX-2) inhibitors are as beneficial as NSAIDs in the treatment of dysmenorrhea.[1,2] The choice for any particular drug may be determined by a woman's preference based on individual experience, administration patterns, side effects, or cost.[2]

Treatment of dysmenorrhea is a well-recognized off-label use for oral contraceptive pills,[13] although more studies need to address the efficacy of oral contraceptives in the management of dysmenorrhea. Combined oral contraceptives, and in particular monophasic contraceptives, that are in continuous use without a placebo can be of benefit.[2,7] Oral contraceptives suppress ovulation and creation of a cyclic pattern of serum estrogen and progesterone, resulting in diminished endometrial thickening, decreased prostaglandin release during menstruation, and in turn pain reduction.[1,2,8] If the discomfort of primary dysmenorrhea is not controlled with NSAIDs or oral contraceptives, further diagnostic evaluation is indicated to exclude a pathologic pelvic condition.

There is some evidence that Mirena, the levonorgestrel-releasing IUD, may reduce dysmenorrhea because the progestin may act directly on the endometrium to reduce endometrial proliferation, menstrual flow, and pain. This IUD has been introduced in Europe for the management of primary and secondary dysmenorrhea but is not currently labeled for this use in the United States.[1,2] Another option that may be available in the near future is a vasopressin receptor antagonist.

BOX 159-1

Examples of NSAIDs for Treatment of Dysmenorrhea

- Ibuprofen, 400-800 mg PO every 6 hr for 3 days
- Naproxen, 500 mg as initial dose, and then 250 mg every 6-8 hr for 3 days
- Naproxen sodium, 550 mg as initial dose, and then 275 mg every 6-8 hr for 3 days
- Mefenamic acid, 500 mg as initial dose, and then 250 mg every 4-6 hr for 3 days
- Meclofenamate, 100 mg as initial dose, and then 50 to 100 mg every 6 hr (not to exceed 400 mg/day) for 3 days

Other approaches used in the management of dysmenorrhea, including calcium channel blockers (such as nifedipine or diltiazem), tocolytic agents (such as albuterol [Salbutamol]), progestogens, acupuncture, herbal remedies, exercise, a low-fat vegetarian diet, increased dietary fiber, castor oil packs to the abdomen, vitamin E (500 IU for 2 days before and 3 days after the onset of menses or 500 IU daily during the menstrual period), fish oil supplements, psychotherapy, and hypnosis, have proven beneficial in some studies.[1,14] A more recent meta-analysis found moxibustion and acupoint therapy effective in treating the pain associated with dysmenorrhea, although more studies are needed.[15] High-intensity transcutaneous electrical nerve stimulation (TENS) was also associated with pain improvement in dysmenorrhea in one small study (level of evidence: moderate).[16]

The role of nutrition (e.g., arachidonic acid as a precursor to prostaglandin formation) has led to an inquiry of a low-fat diet rich in fish (especially salmon, tuna, and halibut), beans, seeds (particularly pumpkin, sesame, and sunflower), whole grains, fruits, and vegetables to decrease arachidonic acid. Similarly, the impact of nutritional supplements on menstrual pain has been studied in small trials including vitamin B_1 (thiamine), vitamin B_3 (niacin), vitamin B_6 (pyridoxine), zinc, calcium, magnesium, and omega-3 fatty acids. Patients frequently ask about herbal therapies for dysmenorrhea. The Society of Obstetricians and Gynaecologists of Canada has noted that Toki-shakuyaku-san, an herbal preparation, may or may not be helpful for some patients with dysmenorrhea (Grade C, Level II: evidence is conflicting).

Narcotic analgesics should not be used for the typical level of discomfort associated with dysmenorrhea. Not only do narcotics raise issues related to prescription drug abuse, but the side effects of narcotics, such as sedation, and potential drug interactions may further affect a woman's ability to fully participate in daily life activities.[2]

Other interventions include behavioral interventions such as relaxation training, biofeedback, and mind-body awareness, as well as an examination of the impact of exercise, chiropractic and osteopathic treatment, acupuncture, and TENS. Heat therapy has been used for millennia (e.g., hot water bottles, hot baths, and heating pads). New modalities such as heat patches and wearable heating devices should not be dismissed as a treatment option.

Hysterectomy is considered a viable option for the treatment of severe, refractory dysmenorrhea.[1] Presacral neurectomy and uterosacral ligament division were used in the past to treat dysmenorrhea but are rarely performed today.[2] These treatments of primary dysmenorrhea may also assist in the treatment of secondary dysmenorrhea. However, successful treatment of secondary dysmenorrhea depends on an accurate diagnosis of the cause of the pelvic pain.[2] In the absence of a clear diagnosis, nonacute pain can be treated empirically for a short time with some of the interventions described.

COMPLICATIONS

Dysmenorrhea may be a difficult and frustrating condition to treat in some patients. If patients diagnosed with primary dysmenorrhea do not respond to conventional treatment, the diagnosis may need to be reassessed.

INDICATIONS FOR REFERRAL OR HOSPITALIZATION

Patients with recalcitrant primary dysmenorrhea and no apparent secondary causes found by physical examination and laboratory and radiologic studies need to be referred to a gynecologist for possible surgical diagnostic evaluation and treatment. Referral is also necessary if a secondary cause requiring surgical intervention is found. In difficult cases, psychological factors must be considered, and mental health referral may be warranted.

PATIENT AND FAMILY EDUCATION

Women with dysmenorrhea must be educated about the disorder and the rationale for certain treatments. Women receiving NSAID therapy should understand the potential gastrointestinal adverse effects associated with NSAIDs. Studies suggest that certain modifiable risk factors, such as smoking and pelvic infections, may contribute to dysmenorrhea. Thus, education directed toward reducing or eliminating these risk factors may be helpful. Given the possible association between stress and dysmenorrhea, stress reduction may be an effective preventive strategy for some and should be included in education about a healthy lifestyle.

Primary dysmenorrhea is a common condition throughout the world with a wide range of treatments available based on evidence and ongoing trials. The opportunity to recognize and support this condition, particularly for women who are incapacitated by their symptoms, is a need that the primary care provider can successfully fill while helping to counsel healthy lifestyle choices.

CHAPTER 160

DYSPAREUNIA

Marie Elena Botte

DEFINITION AND EPIDEMIOLOGY

Dyspareunia is defined as recurrent or persistent genital pain associated with sexual intercourse. The condition is not unique to women; men can have dyspareunia from a variety of causes, including dermatologic infections, structural abnormalities, exposure to alloplastic materials via partners who have had pelvic floor surgery,[1] and anodyspareunia in men who have receptive anal sex. However, it is much more commonly encountered in women and is therefore almost exclusively described as a women's health issue. Dyspareunia can develop secondary to other vulvar problems, such as localized provoked vulvodynia (LPV), vaginismus, or vulvodynia. LPV, formerly known as vulvar vestibulitis, refers to severe pain on vestibular contact or with attempted vaginal entry, tenderness to pressure within the vestibule, and vulvar erythema. Vaginismus is involuntary spasm of the muscles surrounding the outer third of the vagina brought on by real, imagined, or anticipated attempts at vaginal penetration. Vulvodynia refers to chronic vulvar discomfort that may involve complaints of rawness, burning, stinging, or irritation; it is not necessarily related to sexual activity.

Dyspareunia is a common gynecologic complaint, with a widely varying estimated prevalence of 4.7% to 39.5% of women,[2,3] and can be thought of as either superficial (pain around the vaginal opening) or deep (pain in the lower abdomen or pelvic organs). Factors influencing dyspareunia include spontaneous and postabortive pelvic inflammatory disease; early postpartum or perimenopausal status; generalized urogenital sensitivity[4]; history of sexual abuse or cervical cancer; and psychosocial factors, such as rigid religious upbringing, low physical and emotional satisfaction, decreased general happiness, or previous painful sexual experience. Dyspareunia has not been consistently associated with factors such as age, parity, marital status, race, income, or education, and there is no increase in prevalence among women seeking fertility treatment.[3] Hormonal and sexual history factors including oral contraception use[5] (especially before age 17 years) and first intercourse before age 15 years have been proposed as causes of LPV. Women with LPV have demonstrated lower pain threshold, higher magnitude estimation of pain, higher trait anxiety, increased somatization, poorer body image than controls, hypervigilance for coital pain, and selective attentional bias toward pain stimuli.

PATHOPHYSIOLOGY

Pain in the vulvar area can result from inflammatory or atrophic dermatologic conditions, assorted pelvic pathologies, neoplasm, neurologic dysfunction, trauma (horseback riding, sexual abuse, genital mutilation), chemotherapy, and genital manifestations of other systemic diseases such as discoid lupus erythematosus, nonalcoholic liver disease (by decreasing vaginal lubrication), Ehlers-Danlos syndrome,[6] and Charcot-Marie-Tooth disease.[7] Vulvar pain may be a sequela of iatrogenesis (pelvic radiation, chemotherapy, graft-versus-host reaction, pelvic surgery) or an acute or chronic infectious process (human semen carries the irritating toxin in ciguatera), or the result of psycho-social-sexual disturbance. Although the *Diagnostic and Statistical Manual of Mental Disorders* currently classifies dyspareunia as a sexual pain disorder, there is debate[5] as to whether dyspareunia reflects a predominant psychopathology, a condition of sexual dysfunction, or a physical pain syndrome. However it is classified academically, there is evidence of high levels of psychological distress in some women with dyspareunia,[8-10] particularly those with provoked vestibulodynia (PVD) and vulvodynia.

Dyspareunia is often a result of inadequate vaginal lubrication. This can be attributable to insufficient stimulation or arousal during sexual activity or can be related to decreased estrogen, a condition noted in postmenopausal women, women taking tamoxifen for chemoprevention of breast cancer, and breast cancer survivors. Superficial dyspareunia has been associated with lichen planus and lichen sclerosis,[11] factitious urticaria, vulvovaginal candidal infection and recurrent candidiasis,[12] bacterial vaginosis, herpes simplex virus (HSV) types 1 and 2 infection, human papillomavirus (HPV) infection, urinary tract infections,[13] urinary incontinence, occlusion of Bartholin gland duct, Bowen disease, and interstitial cystitis. Tiny mucosal tears have been implicated in focal vulvitis, and perivascular inflammation has been proposed as a mechanism causing dyspareunia in women with Sjögren syndrome. Dyspareunia after a normal pelvic examination has been linked with overexertion of the levator ani muscles and subsequent myalgia after the initiation of Kegel exercises. When the levator ani muscles are hypertonic, vaginismus can result.

In PVD, a conditioned, protective, muscle-guarding response has been proposed, leading to a pelvic floor pathologic condition. Vaginismus cannot easily be distinguished from vestibulitis or PVD by vaginal spasm and pain alone, but women with vaginismus demonstrate significantly greater vaginal and pelvic muscle tone and lower muscle strength, have a higher frequency of defensive and avoidant distress behaviors during pelvic examinations, and recall past attempts at intercourse with more affective distress.

By far the most common cause of deep dyspareunia in premenopausal women is endometriosis, especially when it involves the rectovaginal area.[14] One of the key factors recently proposed for the promotion of nerve fiber growth and for the onset and maintenance of pain in this condition is nerve growth factor (NGF).[15] Women with deep infiltrating endometriosis of the uterosacral ligament can have severe impairment of sexual function, and many have had deep dyspareunia for their entire sex lives. Structural abnormalities that can cause dyspareunia include glomus tumors; leiomyomas of the uterus and urethra; vaginal, urethral, and hymenal abnormalities; bladder stones; postobstetric or postoperative vulvar outlet stenosis; and stenosing lichen planus. Aortoiliac or atherosclerotic disease can diminish pelvic blood flow and lead to vaginal wall and clitoral smooth muscle fibrosis. Pelvic floor surgery can either ameliorate preexisting dyspareunia or cause it.[16,17] Episiotomies, particularly those involving the mediolateral technique and glycerol-impregnated chromic catgut, have been tied to significant increases in dyspareunia.[18] Obstetric instrumentation and perineal trauma during delivery contribute to postpartum dyspareunia.

CLINICAL PRESENTATION

Health care providers need to take an active role in inquiring specifically about discomfort during or after sexual intercourse and not simply assume that women will raise the issue if it is a problem. Women often will not voice this concern even if it is the main reason for their visit. Although some women will discuss dyspareunia with their partner, far fewer consult a health care provider for the problem.[2]

A thorough symptom analysis will guide the physical examination and should specifically include questioning about the onset of the discomfort and its relationship to particular partners, positions, times in the menstrual cycle, contraceptive devices and substances (such as latex condoms, spermicides, or lubricants), and products (such as douches, soaps, tampons, or detergents). Women may report pain with tampon use or pelvic examinations. Important information to gather includes number of pregnancies and type of delivery, surgical history, history of rape or sexual abuse, and menopausal signs and symptoms. Knowing whether the pain is on entry, postcoital, generalizable to the entire vulva, felt only with deep thrusting, or localized to a particular anatomic structure or area is helpful in determining the cause of the discomfort. Several symptom-related scales have been proposed, such as the Female Sexual Function Index, but are not widely used in clinical practice.

EXAMINATION

A thorough pelvic examination is necessary for all complaints of dyspareunia. The experience can be educational for the woman and more informative for the provider if the patient sits somewhat upright and holds a small hand mirror; this allows the woman to see what is happening and feel more in control. It is important to correlate the discomfort elicited during the pelvic examination with specific physical findings whenever possible. In addition, clarification should be sought for pain elicited to determine whether it is similar to what the woman has been experiencing during intercourse because many women find pelvic examinations generally uncomfortable.

The external genitals should be examined for erythema, pigment changes, lesions (including herpes and condyloma), and indications of trauma or abuse. Touching of the vestibule and the hymen with a moistened cotton swab (the Q-tip test) may elicit the pain of PVD, a condition in which there is exquisite tenderness to pressure at specific sites, often accompanied by erythema.

A finger inserted gently into the introitus and gradually pressed in a posterior direction may elicit the spasms of vaginismus; conscious control of the pelvic floor musculature can be evaluated by asking the woman to squeeze and relax the muscles around the examiner's finger. Bartholin glands, which are normally not palpable, may be tender and enlarged. A narrow, well-lubricated speculum should be used to evaluate the vagina. A bimanual examination can assess for uterine and ovarian size, fibroids, ovarian cysts, other pelvic masses, cervical motion tenderness (seen with pelvic inflammatory disease), and position of the uterus. Hemorrhoids or prolapse of the uterus, bladder, or rectum may be evident. A rectal or rectovaginal examination is generally not necessary.

DIAGNOSTICS

Wet mounts, potassium hydroxide (KOH) preparation and cultures of vaginal discharge, endocervical Papanicolaou test, and *Chlamydia trachomatis* and *Neisseria gonorrhoeae* cultures will help rule out infection as a cause of either superficial or deep dyspareunia. The Q-tip test (assessing for localized discomfort by means of touching a swab to the vulvar or vaginal epithelium) can identify local sites of allodynia. A complete blood count (CBC) and erythrocyte sedimentation rate (ESR) can help identify inflammation and infection; a urinalysis evaluates for urinary tract infection; and a human chorionic gonadotropin level can exclude ectopic pregnancy.

DIAGNOSTICS

Dyspareunia

LABORATORY

Initial Diagnostics
- Wet mount, KOH preparation
- Gonorrhea and chlamydia cultures
- ESR
- Urinalysis
- Serum level of human chorionic gonadotropin

Further Diagnostics if Indicated
- Pap test
- CBC and differential

IMAGING
- Pelvic ultrasound

DIFFERENTIAL DIAGNOSIS

Potential causes of dyspareunia include both psychological and pathophysiologic factors. Most cases are probably a combination of both. A problem that is initially physical often has a continued and escalating psychological impact. Potential causes of dyspareunia are listed in the differential diagnosis box and are arranged according to the phase of intercourse during which the symptom is experienced.

DIFFERENTIAL DIAGNOSIS

Dyspareunia

SURFACE (OCCURS WITH PENETRATION)
- Insufficient arousal
- Hypoestrogenic mucosa
- Vaginitis
- Vaginismus
- Hymenal abnormalities
- Dermatopathology
- Postherpetic neuralgia

FOCAL
- PVD or Vulvar vestibulitis
- Bartholin gland cyst or abscess
- Episiotomy scar
- Residual sutures
- Introital tear
- Herpetic lesions
- Urethral problems

DEEP (OCCURS WITH PENILE THRUSTING)
- Endometriosis
- Fibroids
- Pelvic inflammatory disease
- Hemorrhoids
- Inflammatory bowel disease
- Retroverted uterus
- Uterine prolapse
- Pelvic adhesions or masses

POSTCOITAL
- Urinary tract infection
- Vulvodynia

IRRITANTS
- Contraceptive devices
- Spermicides
- Douches
- Feminine hygiene products
- Soaps

PSYCHOSOCIAL FACTORS
- Anxiety
- Prior painful sexual experience
- Rigid upbringing

MANAGEMENT AND HEALTH PROMOTION

Women with dyspareunia related to severe psychological distress or anxiety may be best managed in collaboration with psychiatric or other counseling services.

Women with dyspareunia resulting from insufficient lubrication may benefit significantly from education about the physiology of female arousal and the importance of allowing adequate time before vaginal penetration for the vascular engorgement of genital tissues that results in glandular secretions. If the problem is estrogen-insufficient vaginal dryness, topical estrogen cream is the most effective way to build up the vascularity of the vaginal epithelium and thereby induce physiologic lubrication in moderate to severe vulvovaginal atrophy.[19] Ultra-low-dose vaginal tablets (10 mg estradiol) provide symptom relief with minimal absorption[20] and no risk of endometrial hyperplasia or carcinoma.

Women with mild symptoms may obtain relief from nonhormonal therapies, with or without a prescription. Alternative vaginal lubrication[21] (water-based products such as glycerin [Astroglide] for those women using condoms or diaphragms), olive oil,[22] ospemifene[23] (a selective estrogen receptor modulator), and topical aqueous lidocaine[24] have been used by women for whom supplemental estrogen is not wanted or is contraindicated, such as breast cancer survivors.

Alternative sexual positioning (female astride to control penetration) or position changes can alleviate the pain of dyspareunia for some women, as can nonsteroidal agents, botulinum toxin type A injections,[25] pelvic floor relaxation exercises or a warm bath before sex.

Potent topical steroids are indicated for lichen sclerosis.

Dyspareunia secondary to endometriosis has been treated successfully both hormonally and with surgical intervention[26-28]; a combination of both may be more effective than either alone[29] and results in the lowest incidence of recurrence. Some women have had a reduction in endometriosis-related dyspareunia on a gluten-free diet,[30] and others have had success with antioxidant (vitamins E and C) supplementation, suggesting a link with oxidative stress in the peritoneal cavity.[31]

Behavioral treatment is first-line therapy for PVD or vulvar vestibulitis syndrome. PVD has been treated successfully with a low-oxalate diet and calcium citrate supplementation to neutralize urinary oxalates and tricyclic agents, and topical amitriptyline cream (2% in sorbolene).[32] Other therapeutic strategies include pelvic floor surface electromyography biofeedback, the manual techniques of pelvic floor physical therapists, topical estrogen cream applied twice a day for 4 to 8 weeks, intralesional injections of interferon, and local application of capsaicin cream. Surgical intervention, such as a modified vestibulectomy[33] and vaginal apex repair, can be effective in cases refractory to more conservative approaches.

Treatment of vaginismus-related dyspareunia focuses on helping the woman regain voluntary control of the muscles of the pelvic floor,[34] and pelvic floor physical therapy is often quite helpful: therapeutic approaches most often involve pelvic floor contraction-relaxation exercises and use of fingers or dilators to progressively desensitize the woman to vaginal penetration. Surgical intervention is rarely required and may be detrimental to the resolution of vaginismus.

LIFE SPAN CONSIDERATIONS

Dyspareunia affects sexually active women of all ages but may become increasingly evident at times of major transition in a woman's life, including onset of sexual activity, childbirth, and menopause.[35]

COMPLICATIONS

Dyspareunia is known to have a detrimental effect on relationships[36] and can continue unacknowledged and unaided for years in the absence of clinician inquiry and therapeutic involvement. Although the morbidity associated with dyspareunia varies widely with its attendant cause, the impact on a woman's quality of life can be profound and should not be underestimated.

INDICATIONS FOR REFERRAL

For severe PVD and/or vulvar vestibulitis unresponsive to conservative behavior-based therapies, perineoplasty or posterior vestibulectomy can be performed as a last resort and involves a crescent-shaped posterior vestibular excision followed by vaginal advancement. Surgery is less successful if there is concomitant vaginismus (unless the vaginismus is treated first), in dyspareunia present since first intercourse, and in women with associated persistent vulvar pain. For some women in whom dyspareunia is related to prior hysterectomy, surgical excision of the vaginal apex has been a successful surgical procedure.

PATIENT AND FAMILY EDUCATION

Education is central in the management of dyspareunia, particularly when the cause of discomfort is attributable to insufficient sexual arousal time and lubrication, spasms of vaginismus, control of concomitant infections, or use of irritating or allergenic products. Taking the time to educate individuals about their bodies and the particular strategies necessary to attain or to resume sexual activity without discomfort is an important aspect of comprehensive, holistic primary care.

CHAPTER 161

ECTOPIC PREGNANCY

Marie Elena Botte

DEFINITION AND EPIDEMIOLOGY

Ectopic pregnancy (from the Greek *ektopos,* meaning "out of place") occurs when a fertilized ovum implants anywhere outside of the uterus. Ectopic pregnancy occurs in up to 2.6% of pregnancies[1] and in 6% to 16% of women who visit the emergency department with pain or bleeding (or both) in early pregnancy. The mortality rate related to ectopic pregnancy is still high,[3] even in developed countries; ectopic pregnancy is the second leading cause of maternal mortality and the leading cause of pregnancy-related death in the first trimester, representing approximately 6% to 9% of maternal deaths.[2,4] The rate of ectopic pregnancy in the United States has risen dramatically in the past few decades.[4] Prevalence has risen sixfold since 1970, peaking in the late 1980s, perhaps because of an attendant increase in sexually transmitted diseases, increased frequency of sterilization procedures, and delayed childbearing. The incidence plateaued around the turn of the 21st century and has since increased, perhaps in part related to worldwide increases in chlamydia infections.[5] The rate of ectopic pregnancy has been found to increase dramatically after the age of 30 years, especially beyond the age of 35 years.

Identified risk factors[6] for ectopic pregnancy are all maternal, and include tubal pathologic conditions and infections, prior tubal surgery including sterilization, particularly at younger (<28) age,[7] prior ectopic gestation,[8] in vitro fertilization (embryo transfer and assisted hatching), endometriosis,[9] irritable bowel syndrome,[10] and smoking. In one Danish historical prospective controlled cohort study, daughters of mothers who experienced ectopic pregnancy had a 50% higher risk of ectopic gestation.[11] Prior medical abortion is not associated with increased risk. Risk of rupture is increased with parity and previous ectopic gestation.

Risk factors for ectopic pregnancy should be elicited for any woman when pregnancy is suspected, although identifiable factors may be absent in many women with ectopic gestation. Risk factors that interfere with fallopian tube function include past or current history of sexually transmitted infections and pelvic inflammatory disease (PID) (including recurrent chlamydial infection), pregnancy occurring while taking oral contraceptives (because of the mechanism of action of the birth control pill on the ciliary movement of the fallopian tube), previous history of ectopic pregnancy, history of infertility, in utero diethylstilbestrol (DES) exposure, documented tubal pathologic condition, prior appendectomy or pelvic operation, cesarean section, prior tubal sterilization or operation (Essure[12]), history of in vitro fertilization, and congenital malformation of the fallopian tubes. Cigarette smoking, vaginal douching, multiple sexual partners, and early age at first intercourse have weaker evidence for association. Although intrauterine devices do not increase the risk for ectopic pregnancy, pregnancies that occur with these devices in place are more likely to be ectopic. Previous induced abortion has not been associated with subsequent ectopic pregnancy.

PATHOPHYSIOLOGY

Proposed pathophysiologic explanations for ectopic pregnancy include abnormal embryogenesis (with serious chromosomal aberration in one third of cases), ascending *Chlamydia trachomatis* infection that scars the fallopian tubes, and luteal phase defects. History of or current PID and in utero DES exposure may also result in ectopic gestation. Cases have been reported that involve clear cell hyperplasia of the fallopian tube development in a cesarean section scar and occurrence after ethinyl estradiol–levonorgestrel for emergency contraception. Although implantation can occur anywhere on the cervix, in the abdomen, or on the ovary, 95% of ectopic pregnancies implant in the distal portion of the fallopian tube, and on the ipsilateral side to the corpus luteal cyst.

Cervical pregnancy is the rarest form of ectopic pregnancy (accounting for less than 1% of all ectopic pregnancies), and has been associated with cervicouterine instrumentation. Ovarian pregnancy has been associated with ovulation induction, intrauterine insemination, and vaginal douching. Heterotopic pregnancy (simultaneous intrauterine and extrauterine gestations) is increasing in incidence, occurring in 0.3% to 0.8% of the general population and 1% to 3% of women whose pregnancies resulted from assisted reproductive technologies.[2] Persistent ectopic pregnancy involves residual trophoblastic activity and a beta-human chorionic gonadotropin (β-hCG) level that rises or plateaus, whereas chronic ectopic pregnancy contains no active trophoblastic tissue and results in an hCG level that is low or absent.

CLINICAL PRESENTATION

Symptoms of unruptured ectopic pregnancy can be vague and subacute. The most common symptom of ectopic pregnancy is abdominal pain, which may manifest in isolation or in combination with vaginal bleeding or spotting, dizziness, and shoulder pain (which suggests blood irritating the diaphragm); symptoms typically appear between 6 and 12 weeks of gestation. Amenorrhea for 1 to 2 months and the usual early signs of pregnancy (nausea, fatigue, breast heaviness) are often part of the initial presentation. Women can also be seen with generalized or unilateral pelvic or abdominal pain described as sharp, cramping, continuous, or intermittent. Less common presenting symptoms include acute urinary retention and abnormal dark, scant vaginal bleeding. Painless vaginal bleeding is the most common presentation for cervical pregnancy. Pain that radiates to the shoulder is more common in a ruptured ectopic pregnancy. Acute syncopal episodes and hypotension are possible secondary to rupture-induced peritoneal hemorrhage. Chronic ectopic pregnancy usually appears as a pelvic mass, with minimum symptoms such as intermittent pain and a low or absent hCG titer.

PHYSICAL EXAMINATION

Any suspicion of ectopic pregnancy warrants a thorough physical examination, although the history and physical examination, with a combined sensitivity of 50%, can neither exclude nor confirm an ectopic pregnancy. Postural vital signs and temperature are essential to indicate the presence of hypotension or infection. Speculum examination may reveal a bulging cul-de-sac (indicative of hemoperitoneum in rupture), a bluish coloration of the cervix (a normal finding in any pregnancy), and vaginal bleeding or spotting (the uterus is not able to maintain a stable endometrium at low hCG levels). Uterine enlargement occurs in roughly one fourth of women with ectopic pregnancy, but its size may be less than expected according to dates (generally smaller than expected size at 8 weeks). Approximately 75% of women with ectopic pregnancies have abdominal tenderness, but the abdominal examination findings may be normal if the ectopic pregnancy has not ruptured; cervical motion tenderness may also be present. An adnexal mass, involuntary guarding, and peritoneal signs, although uncommon, are highly predictive of ectopic gestation.

The pelvic examination may also reveal signs that suggest a cause other than ectopic pregnancy as the source of the bleeding, such as hemorrhoids, urethral irritation, cervical lesions, or condyloma. Although tissue at the os is a sign of spontaneous abortion and an open os and heavy vaginal bleeding are predictive of an abnormal intrauterine pregnancy, absence of these signs does not differentiate ectopic from intrauterine gestation.

DIAGNOSTICS

Pregnancy tests have become increasingly sensitive in recent years and are the first step in the diagnosis of any suspected ectopic pregnancy. The slope of a rising hCG titer has been found to be a useful determinant of early ectopic pregnancy below the ultrasonographic discriminatory zone. In normal pregnancy, this titer doubles every 1.4 to 3.5 days, with a minimum of 66% increase suggesting viable pregnancy in clinical practice; a titer that plateaus or falls suggests either ectopic pregnancy or miscarriage, although some ectopic pregnancies (and nonviable intrauterine pregnancies) do have abnormally rising hCG levels.

One prospective study that sought to distinguish viable pregnancy from ectopic pregnancy and spontaneous miscarriage at presentation (of women to the emergency department with abdominal pain and a positive pregnancy test) with single point biomarkers[13] found that a serum hCG level below 3736 mIU/mL was 100% sensitive, and 76% specific, for distinguishing ectopic from viable pregnancy, but that these measurements alone could not distinguish between ectopic gestation and spontaneous miscarriage. Serum CA-125 level below 41.98 U/mL, however, was 100% sensitive and 43% specific in distinguishing ectopic gestation from spontaneous miscarriage. The study suggested that the serial use of hCG and CA-125 cutoffs followed by ultrasound could detect 100% of ectopic pregnancies with 87% specificity for intrauterine gestation. Recent evidence suggests that declining hCG levels in spontaneous abortions can be distinguished from those in ectopic gestation; ectopic gestation (or retained trophoblastic tissue) has a rate of decline that is less than 21% at 2 days or 60% at 7 days. Because nearly all ectopic pregnancies have hCG titers less than 50,000 mIU/mL, a single value above this level can help rule out ectopic pregnancy.

Initial diagnostic tests also include a complete blood count (CBC) (because women with ectopic gestation are often anemic) and a blood type and Rh determination. Serum progesterone is a useful marker of viable pregnancy[14] (levels above 22 ng/mL); levels below 16 ng/mL are consistent with a failing pregnancy (whether ectopic or miscarriage), and levels below 5 ng/mL indicate nonviable pregnancies with nearly 100% sensitivity.

Ultrasonography, particularly transvaginal sonography, is the single best diagnostic tool for demonstration of viable intrauterine pregnancy, nonviable pregnancy, and ectopic gestation.[15] Ultrasound can reliably diagnose a failed pregnancy[16] in an embryo larger than 7 mm (crown rump length) in the absence of cardiac activity or the absence of an embryo when the mean sac diameter is in excess of 25 mm. Spontaneous heterotopic pregnancy was once so rare that detection of intrauterine pregnancy on ultrasound essentially ruled out ectopic gestation, but the incidence of these simultaneous intrauterine and extrauterine pregnancies has been increasing.

At low hCG levels, ultrasound is often nondiagnostic; but when hCG levels are greater than 1800 mIU/mL, sonography is helpful in establishing the location and viability of the pregnancy and is an essential investigation for all women requesting termination of pregnancy. At hCG levels of 1500 to 1800 mIU/mL, a gestational sac should be visible[4] on transvaginal ultrasound (in a singleton pregnancy); at more than 5000 mIU/mL, a yolk sac is visible. When hCG levels are 2000 mIU/mL or more and the mean sac diameter is 3 mm or more, the sensitivity for diagnosis of an intrauterine pregnancy is increased. The β-hCG discriminatory zone (the hCG level at which, if no intrauterine pregnancy is visualized on ultrasound, one can be reasonably confidant that a healthy singleton intrauterine pregnancy is not present[17]) is debated at somewhere between 1000 and 2500 mIU/mL[18,19] and is a surrogate marker for gestational age. Transvaginal ultrasound has been shown to be effective at diagnosis of ectopic gestation at even lower levels for some patients. Ultrasound can detect ectopic pregnancy in one third of women with β-hCG levels of less than 1000 mIU/mL. By 3 weeks after missed menses, virtually all viable intrauterine pregnancies, half of nonviable intrauterine and viable ectopic pregnancies, and one fourth of nonviable ectopic pregnancies can be detected with this method. A trilaminar pattern (specific but not sensitive in ectopic pregnancy) and the thickness of the endometrium (it is thinner in ectopic gestation) as well as something called the leash sign[12] have also been studied as ways to differentiate ectopic from viable uterine gestations on ultrasound examination.

There is broad agreement regarding the combined use of transvaginal sonography and β-hCG levels in evaluating possible ectopic gestation, because of an ability to detect earlier and smaller ectopic pregnancies without the attendant risks of a surgical procedure. When ultrasound findings are indeterminate, diagnostic laparoscopy is considered by many to be the definitive test for diagnosis of ectopic pregnancy. However, the advent of new strategies, particularly very sensitive pregnancy tests and ultrasonography, contributes to "nearly perfect" noninvasive diagnostic acumen and permits medical management of the condition in carefully selected instances.

DIAGNOSTICS

Ectopic Pregnancy

LABORATORY	IMAGING
Serum level of β-hCG	Pelvic ultrasound
CBC and differential	Pelvic computed tomography or magnetic resonance imaging*
Type and crossmatch*	
Rh titers*	

*If indicated.

DIFFERENTIAL DIAGNOSIS

Ectopic pregnancy must be considered a likely possibility in any woman of childbearing age with abdominal pain or bleeding (or both) until it is proved otherwise. Other possible differential diagnoses include appendicitis, salpingitis, cholecystitis, PID, intrauterine pregnancy with inaccurate dates, corpus luteum cyst, gestational trophoblastic neoplasm, incomplete or missed spontaneous abortion, endometriosis, pelvic mass, ureteral calculi, and adnexal torsion. A twisted cystic teratoma or a ruptured malignant ovarian tumor may appear similar to a ruptured ectopic pregnancy.

DIFFERENTIAL DIAGNOSIS

Ectopic Pregnancy

- Appendicitis
- Salpingitis
- Cholecystitis
- PID
- Intrauterine pregnancy
- Corpus luteum cyst
- Gestational trophoblastic neoplasm
- Incomplete abortion
- Endometriosis
- Pelvic mass
- Ureteral calculi
- Adnexal torsion
- Cystic teratoma
- Ruptured malignant ovarian tumor

MANAGEMENT

Immediate emergency department referral or physician consultation is indicated for female patients with a positive test result for serum hCG, abdominal pain, and vaginal bleeding. Ruptured ectopic pregnancy is a surgical emergency and requires immediate admission and attention.

The major factor in determining appropriate therapy in ectopic gestation (i.e., expectant, medical, or surgical) is what is referred to as the level of activity of the ectopic gestation.[3] Signs of a very active ectopic gestation (those that have already ruptured or that are at high risk of tubal rupture) include hemodynamic failure, hemoperitoneum, high hCG levels, pain, and syncope. These situations require immediate surgical intervention. Less active (medically treatable) gestations are generally agreed to have lower hCG levels (typically below 5000 IU/L, but there is considerable debate as to the cutoff[3]), and no fetal cardiac activity in an asymptomatic woman who is hemodynamically stable. In very inactive ectopic gestation (low and plateauing hCG <1500), expectant management may be the most appropriate strategy.

Expectant management for appropriately selected women[20] (hCG <1500, mild clinical symptoms, small nonviable tubal ectopic pregnancy, and no significant intra-abdominal bleeding on ultrasound in a woman who is able to adhere to close follow-up) involves an intensive follow-up of the woman until she has fully recovered and includes serial hCG measurements, initially every 2 days and then weekly, until the hCG drops below 2 IU/L. Success with expectant management is inversely related to hCG level at diagnosis of ectopic pregnancy.[21] Spontaneous resolution is not uncommon, occurring in up to 80% of cases that are less vascular and less advanced (1 to 3.5 cm [⅖ to 1⅖ inches]) and in which hCG levels are initially low[21] (<1000 mIU/mL) or declining.

During the course of resolution, associated β-hCG levels become undetectable in 3 to 45 days (mean, 15.8 days). An increase in serial CA-125 levels has been explored as an aid in the early diagnosis of tubal rupture in ectopic pregnancies being managed expectantly or with medical treatment.

Methotrexate therapy, with or without leucovorin rescue or accompanying mifepristone, has been widely used as a nonsurgical intervention for early unruptured ectopic pregnancies[22] smaller than 3.5 cm (1⅖ inches) and with β-hCG levels below 3000 mIU/mL.[23]

A folic acid antagonist that inhibits purine and pyrimidine synthesis, methotrexate interferes with DNA synthesis and cellular multiplication. Rapidly growing tissues such as fetal and trophoblastic cells are most susceptible. Various dosage strategies have been explored,[3] with decreased occurrence and severity of side effects observed in single, low-dose intramuscular injections and increased success rates with flexible protocols and "variable dose" regimens.

Methotrexate or potassium chloride has also been used in ultrasound-guided local injections, equally successfully, in unruptured live ectopic pregnancies. Methotrexate has been used successfully to decrease the incidence of persistent ectopic pregnancy after salpingostomy, in cervical pregnancy[24] when followed by curettage, and in women eligible for expectant management. Uterine embolization with methotrexate for selected cases of early interstitial gestation may decrease the risk of hemorrhage. Appropriate candidates for methotrexate therapy should be hemodynamically stable, have no active renal or hepatic disease, and have no evidence of thrombocytopenia or leukopenia. Initial hCG levels in this population should be low, the gestational sac should be small (<3.5 cm [1⅖ inches]) or absent, and there should be no discernible fetal cardiac activity on ultrasound examination.

Methotrexate therapy has a 94% success rate as long as the woman fits the appropriate criteria. Methotrexate (1 mg/kg or 50 mg/m^2) is given intramuscularly, followed by a repeated hCG titer and symptom assessment on day 4 and another hCG titer on day 7. For women whose hCG titers do not decline significantly (by 15%), a second injection of methotrexate is indicated; this is more likely to be necessary if a yolk sac was visualized on ultrasound examination. If a woman's hCG titer declines by the seventh day, she should be monitored weekly until it is undetectable.

Side effects of treatment with methotrexate include diarrhea, nausea, perioral irritation, and transient transaminase elevations. Similar tubal patency rates have been shown after both methotrexate treatment and expectant management; subsequent fertility[22] and ovarian reserve are not affected,[25] and subsequent risk of recurrent ectopic gestation is not increased with conservative methotrexate treatment.[26]

Surgical laparoscopy[27] or laparotomy remains the only treatment choice for ruptured ectopic pregnancy, and laparoscopy is the cornerstone of treatment in most cases of ectopic gestation. Although laparoscopy is the standard treatment of all ectopic pregnancies, attendant risks include perioperative and postoperative complications, such as uncontrollable hemorrhage, adhesion formation, subcutaneous emphysema and pneumothorax, and reduced subsequent fertility.

In women with a healthy contralateral fallopian tube, salpingotomy does not confer a significant increase in future fertility over salpingectomy.[18] Regardless of treatment modality, every woman with Rh-negative blood should receive anti-D immunoglobulin (RhoGAM).

LIFE SPAN CONSIDERATIONS

All sexually active women of reproductive age are theoretically at risk for ectopic pregnancy, especially if they have one or more of the risk factors mentioned earlier. Women in their 20s are more likely to have ectopic gestation, but adolescents and perimenopausal women are also at risk. Women, including those for whom infertility is an issue, may require the provider's support in expressing and grieving the loss of the pregnancy and the baby who was expected.[28]

COMPLICATIONS

Ruptured ectopic pregnancy can result in acute, massive bleeding and poses an immediate threat to life. Rupture is more likely at higher presenting levels of hCG and with multiple ovulation or ovulation induction. Misdiagnosis, which occurs in as many as 12% of cases, can result in sudden death secondary to internal hemorrhage and infection. Nonfatal sequelae of delayed diagnosis include infection and an increased rate of salpingectomy, potentially affecting future fertility. Missed or delayed diagnoses and subsequent ruptures occur more often in women previously treated with therapeutic abortions when ectopic pregnancies were not suspected. In addition, the risk of a missed or delayed diagnosis is higher in women considered to be less at risk for an ectopic pregnancy, including those with no history of ectopic pregnancy, those with at least one child, and those who have a history of tubal ligation.

Methotrexate has adverse effects, including mucositis, abdominal cramping, and malaise. Its administration has been associated with cases of anaphylaxis, alopecia, and life-threatening neutropenia; high doses can cause bone marrow depression, hepatotoxicity, stomatitis, pulmonary fibrosis, and photosensitivity. The risk of persistent ectopic pregnancy ranges from 3% to 20% after conservative surgical therapy and is 9.8% for treatment with methotrexate. Research has shown a significantly reduced fertility rate postoperatively for some women after ectopic pregnancy and a relationship among advancing age, prior ectopic pregnancy, and declining future pregnancy rates.

INDICATIONS FOR REFERRAL OR HOSPITALIZATION

Suggestive hCG levels (<1000 mIU/mL) and an indeterminate vaginal ultrasound examination necessitate further evaluation, preferably on an inpatient basis. Although transient abdominal pain is common in the second week after methotrexate administration and generally resolves within 24 hours, severe pain is an indication for hospital-based observation because it may indicate tubal rupture.

PATIENT AND FAMILY EDUCATION

All women should be apprised of their subsequent risk of reduced fertility and recurrent ectopic pregnancy. Condom use should be encouraged to reduce the likelihood of infection and PID because declining rates of chlamydial infection have been associated with declining rates of ectopic pregnancy. Women taking birth control pills should be reminded to take them as directed. Women at risk for ectopic pregnancy should alert their provider when they become pregnant. Women who have received methotrexate therapy for unruptured ectopic pregnancy need to refrain from sexual activity and consumption of alcohol or vitamins containing folic acid until after resolution of the ectopic pregnancy, preferably at least 3 months, because of the potential teratogenic effects of methotrexate. These women should also be alerted to the possibility that they may experience increased abdominal pain 5 to 10 days after therapy. Further clinical evaluation would be necessary at this point because severe pain may indicate tubal abortion and rupture. Good subsequent fertility rates have been demonstrated in women who received methotrexate for ectopic pregnancy (more than half conceive within 1 year of attempting pregnancy), which suggests that fertility in these cases depends more on prior medical history than on the treatment of the ectopic pregnancy.

CHAPTER 162

FERTILITY CONTROL

Richard M. Prior

DEFINITION AND EPIDEMIOLOGY

In the United States, 99% of sexually active women have used contraception at some time in their lives. From 2006 to 2010, 62% of women aged 15 to 44 years reported that they were currently using contraception. The most common types of contraception are oral contraception, female sterilization, and condoms. Unfortunately, 47% of the women who have used more than one method of contraception have chosen to change or stop owing to dissatisfaction.[1]

From 2006 to 2010, 37% of all births were unintended.[2] Given the high frequency of unplanned pregnancy, it is essential that health care providers educate and counsel women and their partners on the variety of feasible contraception options. It is imperative that the woman (and her partner, if desired) be involved in the care plan rather than be merely a recipient of the provider's expertise and advice. Discussion of contraceptive options should include information about the risks and benefits, potential side effects, rate of efficacy, and effects on future fertility.

When possible emotional and health care costs are factored in, all methods of contraception have been shown to be more cost-effective than unintended pregnancy.[3] Current methods of contraception are continuously improved and new contraceptives are constantly being developed, resulting in an ever-evolving variety of patient-centered, cost-effective choices.

HORMONAL CONTRACEPTION

Oral Contraceptives

The oral contraceptive pill (OCP) is a highly effective means of preventing pregnancy and has played an important role in contraception since its approval by the U.S. Food and Drug Administration (FDA) in 1960. The terms *birth control pill, combined oral contraceptive,* and *oral contraceptive* generally refer to pills containing both estrogen and progestin. In this chapter, these terms are not used to refer to progestin-only pills, also known as *minipills.*

Estrogen is one of the two major hormonal components in combined oral contraceptives. The role of estrogen in combined oral contraceptives is to promote bleeding regularity and to suppress the release of follicle-stimulating hormone.[4,5] The basic chemical structure of estrogen has been modified by pharmaceutical manufacturers to increase effectiveness, leading to the development of the two synthetic estrogens (ethinyl estradiol and less commonly mestranol) that are used in combined oral contraceptives today. The doses of ethinyl estradiol used in the first oral contraceptives were often in excess of 100 µg, resulting in side effects that decreased the safety profile of the medication. Subsequent research and experience have proved that doses of 50 µg or less are sufficient to aid in the suppression of ovulation while minimizing side effects.

These estrogen compounds are delivered with a synthetic progestin, the second active hormonal compound. The progestin component provides the majority of the contraceptive effect by suppressing follicle-stimulating hormone and luteinizing hormone. This altered hormonal environment prevents ovulation, thickens cervical mucus, and promotes a uterine atmosphere that is hostile to implantation.[4,5] Several different formulations of synthetic progestins are commonly used in combined oral contraceptives in the United States. Newer third- and fourth-generation progestins are less adrenergic, limiting such side effects as acne, hirsutism, and hyperlipidemia.[4]

Several different types of OCPs are available and vary according to the dose of hormones and the formulations within each cycle pack. Monophasic OCPs have a constant dose of estrogen and progestin in each of the active tablets of the cycle pack. Phasic OCPs have alternating doses of progestin and, in some cases, estrogen throughout the cycle. The aim of manufacturers in lowering the total monthly exogenous hormone dose while trying to simulate a woman's normal menstrual cycle is to reduce the metabolic side effects associated with OCP use.

The first oral contraceptive regimens provided 21 days of active hormone followed by 7 days of inert pills, resulting in a withdrawal bleed. The 21/7 regimen was initially adopted because the creators of the OCP believed that women would appreciate the reassurance of a monthly period. Alternating regimens offer additional benefits of decreasing unpleasant symptoms and inconvenience associated with withdrawal bleeding. The FDA has approved the use of several extended OCP regimens consisting of 84 days of active pills and 7 days of nonhormonal pills. Other preparations provide a regimen of 24 active days followed by 4 days of inert pills, resulting in decreased side effects caused by estrogen withdrawal, lighter menses, and decreased likelihood of ovulation.[6,7]

With perfect use, OCPs are 99.7% effective in preventing pregnancy. However, with typical use in the United States, the rate of efficacy drops to 91%.[8] At the time of prescription, the absence of pregnancy should be verified via standard laboratory tests. Traditionally, women have been instructed to begin the regimen of OCPs on either the first day of menses or on the first Sunday after menses begin, a method known as the *conventional start*. This approach ensures that the patient is not pregnant and in the case of a Sunday start aligns the days on the packaging with the actual day of the week. Another approach, known as the *quick start*, has the patient begin the regimen on the day of the visit, as the hormones in the contraceptive do not harm the fetus if the woman is pregnant at that time. Studies have shown that both methods have similar rates of effectiveness and side effects, leaving opportunity for provider and patient choice.[9]

Women should be encouraged to take OCPs at the same time every day and to associate pill taking with a certain daily habit or ritual if that facilitates compliance. Daily compliance is essential to ensuring efficacy. Women who miss one or two tablets should take two tablets for each of the missed days. Women who miss more than 2 days should continue taking the pills as prescribed but use an additional form of birth control for the remainder of the cycle. Women who often miss doses of OCPs should be encouraged to consider a form of fertility control that does not depend on daily compliance.

Secondary analysis of National Survey for Family Growth data suggests that 29% of women discontinued oral contraceptives because of dissatisfaction. Of those women, 64.6% discontinued because of side effects, and 13.1% of women discontinued OCPs because they were worried about side effects.[2] The extent and type of side effects differ slightly among individual OCPs because of variations in the amount and kind of estrogen and progestin contained within each product.

Nausea, breast tenderness, and mild fluid retention resulting from the estrogen component of OCPs are common side effects. Menstrual changes, including intermenstrual (breakthrough) spotting or bleeding, occur in 25% of women during the first 3 months of OCP use and decrease significantly during subsequent prolonged use. Other estrogen-related side effects include increased breast size (ductal and fatty tissue), cervical hyperplasia, benign hepatocellular adenomas, increased skin pigmentation, and cholelithiasis.[10]

Women with persistent intermenstrual bleeding after 3 months of OCP use should be evaluated for possible causes of bleeding unrelated to OCP use. Amenorrhea may also occur, especially in women who have been using OCPs for a prolonged period. Other possible side effects include a decreased libido (decreased interest in sex or the decreased ability to have an orgasm), fluid retention, leukorrhea, pruritus, and headaches.

Some of the "short-lived" side effects associated with OCPs tend to dissipate by the third or fourth cycle. Once the responsible hormonal component has been identified, the provider can determine whether the side effect is caused by an excess or deficiency and can present potential alternative contraceptive options that may lead to increased satisfaction.

Benefits of oral contraceptives extend beyond that of preventing pregnancy. There is a reduced risk of formation of ovarian cysts. Lighter menses may result in a decrease in the incidence or severity of iron deficiency anemia. Some women may notice a decrease in premenstrual mood symptoms and premenstrual cramping. OCPs are known to decrease the incidence of fibrocysts in the breasts. Most combined oral contraceptives—in particular some triphasic preparations—are known to help control acne. Other advantages may include increased bone density and decreases in the incidence of pelvic inflammatory disease (PID), endometrial and ovarian cancers, and rheumatoid arthritis.[11]

OCPs also have significant health risks and disadvantages, including a lack of protection against human immunodeficiency virus (HIV) infection, a greater threat to the health of many sexually active individuals than an unplanned pregnancy. To protect against HIV infection and other sexually transmitted infections, barrier methods (e.g., condoms) must be used in conjunction with OCPs.

The estrogen component in OCPs has been shown to cause mild increases in both systolic and diastolic blood pressure, which may be more pronounced in some patients. Blood pressure returns to baseline after the cessation of OCPs. There is a lack of data demonstrating a link between OCPs and myocardial infarction, although women who have hypertension and smoke may be at risk. Current practice recommendations are that women with a blood pressure lower than 140/90 mm Hg are good candidates for OCPs. Women with well-controlled hypertension who are younger than 35 years and do not smoke, have no comorbidities, and have no end-organ damage are also considered good candidates for combined oral contraceptives. All women should have their blood pressure monitored at each clinic visit.[5,12,13]

Potential for thromboembolism is another infrequent but serious adverse effect associated with combined oral contraceptives. Although the risk is quite low, thromboembolism occurs three times more frequently in women who take OCPs than in those who do not. The effect appears to be more pronounced in women who are obese; in women with a history of thromboembolism; and in women who have venous stasis, coagulopathies, and vascular injury.[12-14]

There is a questionable relationship between OCPs and stroke. The risk is most likely increased in women who have coagulopathies, women who smoke, and those older than 35 years of age. There may also be an increased risk of ischemic stroke with OCP use in women with a history of migraines with aura. Although the risk is low, morbidity associated with stroke is devastating enough that current recommendations suggest that migraine sufferers use a progestin-only contraceptive or nonhormonal form of contraception.[12-14]

The potential impact of OCP use on breast cancer is a concern for a great number of women interested in this form of fertility control. There continues to be debate as to the degree of effect of OCPs on the development of breast cancer. Many of the studies showing an association between OCP use and breast cancer are older and apply to preparations that included a much higher dose of estrogen than is used today. Women should be counseled that there may be a slightly increased risk of breast cancer with OCP use. Studies have not proved an increased risk in OCP users with a first-degree relative who has a history of breast cancer; therefore, current practice guidelines do not treat family history as a contraindication.[12,15,16]

The World Health Organization's medical eligibility criteria for contraceptive use, published in September 2010, provide comprehensive guidance for the safety of use of different contraceptive methods. OCPs should not be prescribed for the following women: those who are breastfeeding and are less than 6 weeks postpartum; smoke more than 15 cigarettes per day; have a systolic blood pressure of 160 mm Hg or higher or a diastolic blood pressure of 100 mm Hg or higher; have a current or past history of deep vein thrombosis or pulmonary embolus; are immobilized for extended periods of time after surgery; have a history of coronary artery disease or stroke; have a genetic disease that predisposes them to clotting; or have systemic lupus erythematosus, diabetes and end-organ damage, or severe liver diseases. Caution should be used in prescribing OCPs to the following women: those who have blood pressure higher than 140/90 mm Hg; have adequately controlled hypertension; are less than 3 weeks postpartum; are breastfeeding and are 6 weeks to 6 months postpartum; smoke fewer than 15 cigarettes per day; have diabetes mellitus; have hyperlipidemia; have migraines without aura and are older than 35 years; or are taking anticonvulsants.[14]

The warning signs to teach OCP users can be summarized with the acronym *ACHES*:

- Abdominal pain (severe)
- Chest pain (severe), cough, or shortness of breath
- Headaches (severe), dizziness, weakness, or numbness
- Eye problems (vision loss or blurring) or speech problems
- Severe leg pain (calf or thigh)

Women who experience any of these signs or symptoms or who develop depression, jaundice, or a breast lump should discontinue taking the pill and consult their providers. OCP users who smoke should be encouraged to quit smoking; if quitting is not possible, they should consider discontinuation of OCPs after the age of 35 years.

Progestin-Only Pills (Minipills). Progestin-only pills were developed in the early 1960s in response to the side effect profile associated with the estrogen component of OCPs. Several types of progestins have been used in oral contraception products and are often referred to by generation: first, second, third, and now fourth. Progestin-only pills prevent pregnancy mainly by thickening the cervical mucus to slow sperm motility and interfering with or preventing sperm penetration. Progestins may also work by inhibiting ovulation and creating an endometrial environment inhospitable to implantation.[4] Progestin-only pills are taken on a daily basis, with no pill-free days. Progestin-only pills have a failure rate equivalent to those of OCPs; however, they must be taken at the same time each day. Because of the lack of an estrogen component, minipills are preferred in women who are lactating; their efficacy rate for these women is close to 100%. Progestin-only pills are also useful for women who wish to use an OCP but have contraindications to combined pills.[4,12,17]

The structural similarity of the progestins to testosterone largely determines their androgenic activity. This androgenic activity is often associated with the side effects of progestins, which may include menstrual cycle disturbances, weight gain, breast tenderness, increase in functional ovarian cysts, ectopic pregnancy, interactions with anticonvulsants, and bone density decrease. Because of the lack of estrogen, minipills are not associated with some of the same potential side effects of combination oral contraceptives, such as thromboembolic disorders (e.g., myocardial infarction and cerebrovascular disease) and gallbladder disease. Minipills are associated with a higher incidence of ectopic pregnancy compared with other contraceptive measures.[4,10]

Newer Progestins. The spironolactone derivative drospirenone has been combined with ethinyl estradiol (30 μg) to form several newer monophasic oral contraceptives. Drospirenone is a fourth-generation progestin that is a spironolactone analogue with antimineralocorticoid and antiandrogenic properties. A dose of 3 mg/day displays antimineralocorticoid activity similar to that of 25 mg of spironolactone, which may be a good choice in women who experience significant sodium and water retention during their cycle. Drospirenone also is thought to be less likely to exacerbate acne and to mitigate premenstrual symptoms. Hyperkalemia is a potential adverse effect related to the potassium-sparing effects of drospirenone.[18]

Dienogest is a relatively new and very potent antiandrogenic progestin that also allows for good cycle control. Dienogest is available in both biphasic and quadriphasic preparations. Although similar to drospirenone, dienogest does not require the monitoring of potassium levels, because it lacks antimineralcorticoid activity.[18]

Injectable Contraception

The only available injectable form of contraception available in the United States is depot medroxyprogesterone acetate (DMPA;

Depo-Provera). DMPA prevents pregnancy by inhibiting ovulation. A 150-mg injection of DMPA suppresses ovulation for 14 weeks. A 104-mg subcutaneous preparation may be associated with fewer side effects because of the lower dose. With a prescribed dose given every 3 months, contraceptive efficacy is 99.8%.[8] Although DMPA has traditionally been started immediately before or during menses, new research suggests improved effectiveness if given at the time of the initial visit, as long as the provider is reasonably sure that the patient is not pregnant. DMPA injections should be administered every 12 weeks, which provides a 2-week "grace" period given the 14-week duration of action. The possibility of pregnancy should first be excluded for any woman who is more than 2 weeks late for her DMPA injection. Side effects include irregular menses, and reversible bone loss.[9,17,19]

Menstrual changes occur in almost all women who use DMPA and are the most common cause for dissatisfaction and discontinued use of this form of fertility control. Irregular bleeding usually resolves within the first month of use. Amenorrhea is the most common menstrual change with persistent use of DMPA. Women for whom menstrual irregularities are disconcerting should be counseled about alternative contraceptive choices. Other side effects of DMPA include headache, abdominal or breast bloating, fatigue, mood changes, decreased libido, and weight gain of 5 pounds or less.[19] DMPA is a reversible form of contraception, but a return to fertility is often delayed after discontinuation of DMPA. Average return to fertility occurs in 5 to 7 months after cessation of DMPA, but fertility may not be restored for as long as 18 months in some women. DMPA is associated with certain noncontraceptive benefits, such as a reduction in or elimination of premenstrual symptoms, a reduced risk of PID, a decreased risk of endometrial cancer, and hematologic improvement in women with sickle cell disease. DMPA-induced amenorrhea may make DMPA a good contraceptive choice for women with menorrhagia, dysmenorrhea, and iron deficiency anemia as well as for women with intellectual disabilities who have menstrual hygiene problems.

DMPA is linked with certain health risks. As is the case with OCPs, DMPA provides no protection from many sexually transmitted diseases (STDs), including HIV infection. Currently, no data suggest that either OCPs or DMPA are associated with an increased risk of breast, endometrial, ovarian, or cervical carcinoma. Decreased bone density has been noted among some DMPA users, but this was reversed with discontinuation of DMPA.[17,19] The only absolute contraindication to DMPA is active breast cancer.[14]

Women should be counseled to use an additional form of contraception for the first 2 weeks after the first DMPA injection. Women who are at risk for STDs should use a barrier method of contraception, preferably condoms. Women who become concerned about their menstrual irregularities while taking DMPA or who develop signs or symptoms of infection should consult their health care providers. Women need to be informed about the likely delay in fertility after discontinuation of DMPA. DMPA is not the best choice for women who wish to become pregnant within the next 1 to 2 years; these women should be counseled about alternative contraceptive options.

Contraceptive Implants

In 1990, the contraceptive levonorgestrel (Norplant) ushered in the era of implantable progestin rods. Although Norplant is no longer being manufactured, there is currently one contraceptive implant available in the United States. A single-rod implant (Implanon) was approved by the FDA in 2006 for use by women in the United States. Implanon is a thin, flexible plastic subdermal insert, approximately 4 cm long, that delivers ethylene vinyl acetate impregnated with 68 mg of etonogestrel. The rod delivers an average of 40 μg of etonogestrel every day, inhibiting ovulation and thickening cervical mucus.[6,17,18] The etonogestrel implant is reported to be 99.9% effective at preventing pregnancy.[8]

A provider trained in Implanon insertion can perform this procedure in the office. The implant prevents pregnancy for 3 years and does not interfere with fertility once the rod has been removed. Menstrual periods usually return to normal within a few months after removal of the rod.[17] The rod is typically inserted into the inside portion of the upper arm. If the rod is inserted within 5 days of the start of menses, a backup form of contraception is not needed during the remainder of the cycle. The most common side effect is irregular menstrual bleeding.[6,17,19]

Contraceptive Patch

Norelgestromin–ethinyl estradiol transdermal system (Ortho Evra) is the only contraceptive patch currently available in the United States. The 20-cm^2 patch delivers 20 μg of ethinyl estradiol and 150 μg of norelgestromin daily and is 99.7% effective with perfect use and 91% effective with typical use.[8,17] It inhibits ovulation in much the same way as OCPs do. Each cycle consists of a contraceptive patch applied to the lower abdomen, buttocks, upper outer arm, or upper torso (excluding the breasts) once a week for 3 weeks. After the third week, the patch is removed for a contraceptive-free week during which withdrawal bleeding occurs.[17,20]

Although questions have arisen about the effectiveness of the patch when prescribed to obese women, the most recent evidence suggests no link between a woman's body mass index (BMI) and patch efficacy.[20] Advantages of the contraceptive patch include ease of use, improved adherence, reversibility, and steady-state hormone levels. Spotting rates are comparable to those of OCP use. Additional side effects include breast discomfort, headache, nausea, dysmenorrhea, and skin irritation at the patch site.[17] In November 2005, the FDA issued a warning that the birth control patch could be associated with an increased risk of thromboembolism, although studies have not conclusively defined whether there is increased risk of thromboembolism compared with similarly dosed OCPs. The patch carries the same risks, warnings, and contraindications as OCPs. All patients starting on the contraceptive patch or hormonal birth control should understand the risks of thromboembolism and the importance of stopping the medication and calling their health care providers immediately if they develop a severe headache, chest pain or pressure, shortness of breath, abdominal pain, or leg pain.[17,20]

Postcoital Contraception

Postcoital contraception, also referred to as *emergency contraception* (EC) or the *morning-after pill,* is intended for women who have experienced a single episode of unprotected intercourse within a given menstrual cycle. Postcoital contraception can also be used in cases of sexual assault. In the United States, three types of EC are widely accepted for use: levonorgestrel, ulipristal acetate (UA), and the copper intrauterine device (IUD).[17,21]

The commercial formulation Plan B One-Step contains the progestin levonorgestrel as single dose 1.5 mg pill that should be taken as soon as possible within 3 days of unprotected sex. In April 2013, the FDA approved (with 3 year marketing exclusivity) Teva Pharmaceuticals Plan B One-Step for nonprescription use by women 15 years of age and older. Within 72 hours of intercourse, levonorgestrel can reduce the risk of pregnancy by 85%. From 72 to 120 hours after intercourse, there is a significant drop in efficacy. Studies have demonstrated that a single dose of 1.5 mg is as effective as the split dose, providing an additional option to providers. Common side effects include bleeding irregularities, nausea, headaches, vomiting, and abdominal pain.[17,21]

Another option includes the prescription-only selective progesterone receptor modulator UA, know by the brand name Ella. UA is prescribed as a single-dose 30-mg tablet that is taken within 120 hours of unprotected sexual intercourse. Studies indicate that UA is as effective as levonorgestrel up to 72 hours after intercourse and may be more effective from hours 72 to 120. Side effects are similar to those of levonorgestrel.[17,21]

Perhaps the most effective method is the copper IUD, which can be used as EC as long as there is no established pregnancy and the woman has no other contraindications to IUDs.[21] Providers who prescribe EC should engage the patient in a discussion about the benefits of a sustained contraception plan.

BARRIER METHODS

Barrier methods of fertility control are so named because they act as mechanical barriers and prevent pregnancy by blocking the passage of sperm through their surfaces. In addition, they prevent or reduce contact with genital lesions, discharges, or secretions.

Condoms

Most condoms made in the United States are manufactured from latex; approximately 3% are made from other materials. Contraception and disease prevention efficacy data are available only for latex condoms. Failure rates with condoms are as low as 2% with perfect use and as high as 18% with typical use.[8] Polyurethane female condoms have the benefit of affording women direct control of contraception and disease prevention. However, failure rates for the female condom are significantly higher (5% with perfect use, 21% with typical use) than for male condoms.[8] Condoms remain the only immediately reversible method of contraception for men.

Patient education about condom use should include information about how to put on and to remove a condom, the need to leave a receptacle at the tip of the condom to avoid breakage, what to do in case of condom slippage or damage, and the importance of avoiding oil-based products (e.g., petroleum jelly, cold cream) when extra lubrication is needed.

Diaphragms and Cervical Caps

Diaphragms and cervical caps are female barrier methods of contraception. Both must be individually fitted to be effective; even with correct use, failure rates are as high as 32% for nulliparous users and 16% for parous users during the first year of use.[22] Both the diaphragm and the cervical cap are used with spermicidal cream or jelly.

The diaphragm is a dome-shaped rubber cap that comes in a variety of sizes. It fits into the vagina, covering the cervix and the anterior vagina from the pubic symphysis to the posterior fornix. The diaphragm should remain in place for at least 6 hours after intercourse, but no more than 24 hours (to minimize the risk of toxic shock syndrome). Once it is in position, the diaphragm provides effective contraception for 6 hours, after which fresh spermicide must be applied if additional contraceptive protection is desired. The postpartum patient should not be fitted for a diaphragm for at least 6 weeks after childbirth.

The cervical cap is a deep, soft rubber cup that covers the surface and fits snugly around the base of the cervix. There are several sizes of cap that correspond to the woman's obstetric history. The cap provides continuous contraceptive protection during 24 hours regardless of how often intercourse occurs. Additional spermicide or jelly can be inserted vaginally without removal of the cap for repeated intercourse.[22]

Advantages of the female barrier methods include a lack of dependence on partners for contraception and none of the side effects of systemic hormones. With the exception of the female condom, all female vaginal barrier methods are used in conjunction with spermicides. Some protection against HIV infection is afforded if the spermicide contains nonoxynol-9. On the other hand, research has demonstrated that vaginal irritation caused by nonoxynol-9 may increase susceptibility to HIV infection. Reduction in the risk of other STDs, including gonorrhea and chlamydia, varies from 10% to 50%, depending on the study. Risks associated with the use of diaphragms and cervical caps include latex allergy, toxic shock syndrome, and recurrent urinary tract infections.[17,22]

Spermicides

A variety of over-the-counter spermicidal products are available in the United States and include foams, creams, gels, suppositories, and films. The active ingredient in all spermicides available in the United States is nonoxynol-9 or a similar agent that destroys the membrane of the sperm cell. Spermicides can be used alone but, as noted earlier, are also essential for the effective functioning of diaphragms and cervical caps.[17,22] Effectiveness varies with the type of use and compliance; failure rates vary from 29% with typical use to 18% with perfect use.[8]

One major advantage of spermicides is that they are available over the counter. Many women also appreciate that there is no partner involvement with this method. Side effects include allergic reactions to the active ingredient or to the particular spermicide base or vehicle, which generally manifests as vulvar pruritus or a rash. Women who are prone to yeast infections may notice an increased frequency of this problem when spermicides are used. Although women do not need to consult a health care provider to use spermicides, it is nonetheless important for this option to be discussed in any family planning session.

Cervical Sponge

The cervical sponge is available without a prescription. With perfect use, it is 91% effective for nulliparous women and 80% effective for parous women.[8] The sponge is moistened with water and inserted into the vagina. The sponge provides its contraceptive effect for up to 24 hours and must be left in place for 6 hours after intercourse, to a maximum 30-hour total. The Today Sponge available in the United States is impregnated with the spermicide nonoxynol-9.

Intrauterine Devices

Intrauterine contraceptive devices are one of the safest, most effective, and most cost-effective contraception options. Many negative perceptions of the IUD are based on the first-generation models, which were removed from the market because of side effects and morbidity. The current-generation IUDs are safer and are engineered to produce fewer side effects than their predecessors.

Two types of IUDs are currently available in the United States. The oldest is the copper T 380A (ParaGard), a T-shaped, polyethylene device with a stem and cross arms partly covered by copper wire and tubing; the device can remain in place for 10 years. In addition, there are two levonorgestrel-containing IUDs: the Mirena device, which releases 20 µg of levonorgestrel per day, and the newer Skyla device, which releases 13.5 µg/day. The 20-µg IUD can be left in place for 5 years, and the 13.5-µg IUD can be left in place for 3 years.[17,23]

Copper IUDs prevent fertilization primarily by creating a spermicidal environment. The IUD causes the endometrium to initiate a foreign body reaction, which results in sterile inflammation and inhibits sperm from reaching the fallopian tube. In addition, the copper ions permeate the cervical mucus and decrease sperm motility. Progesterone-releasing IUDs thicken the cervical mucus, cause atrophy of the endometrium, and perhaps inhibit ovulation. Both forms of IUD are more than 99% effective,[8] although the copper IUD causes heavier bleeding, particularly in the first 6 months.[17,23]

Far fewer complications are associated with the IUDs currently in use than with the early copper-containing IUDs (including the Dalkon Shield) of the 1980s. Copper-containing IUDs can increase bleeding and dysmenorrhea, whereas the levonorgestrel system lessens these symptoms. Historically, one of the concerns about IUDs had been that women are at a greater risk for developing PID. This was believed to be attributed to the multifilament strings in the Dalkon Shield, which provided a convenient route for bacteria to ascend to the pelvic organs. Current IUDs possess a monofilament string that is much less likely to harbor bacteria.

Current recommendations are that women should be warned of the very small risk of PID in the 20-day postinsertion period. Only women who are symptomatic or those who are at risk for having an STD should be tested before insertion. Women who develop PID can be treated with antibiotics with an IUD in place unless they fail to improve with 72 hours of therapy.[17,23]

Of the pregnancies that do occur with IUDs in place, 50% result in spontaneous abortion. In contrast to the older-generation IUDs, neither type of IUD increases the overall risk of ectopic pregnancy compared with the risk for noncontraceptive users.[17,23]

IUDs should not be prescribed for women with known pregnancy, an active sexually transmitted infection, or active PID; in the period immediately after a septic abortion; in the presence of unexplained vaginal bleeding or untreated cervical cancer; or for women with anatomic abnormalities of the uterus (such as fibroids that disrupt the uterine cavity). IUDs are generally not recommended in women less than 4 weeks postpartum. The levonorgestrel IUDs are not recommended in women who are breastfeeding, have an acute deep vein thrombosis or pulmonary embolus, have had breast cancer within the past 5 years, or have ovarian cancer or severe liver disease.[14]

IUDs have been demonstrated to be safe for both nulliparous and parous women, although in some circumstances an IUD may be inappropriate. The 13.5-mg Skyla was specifically tested on nulliparous women and does not include a recommendation against use in that population. Patient education should include information about checking for the IUD string as well as the signs and symptoms of possible complications, including pain, bleeding, odorous discharge, fever, and missed menses.

Vaginal Ring

The etonogestrel–ethinyl estradiol vaginal ring (NuvaRing) is a 54-mm-diameter vaginal contraceptive ring that delivers 15 µg of ethinyl estradiol and 120 µg of etonogestrel each day. The flexible, circular ring is inserted in the vagina by the woman and kept in for 3 weeks. Unlike the diaphragm, the ring does not have to be in a specific position because the hormones can be absorbed anywhere in the vagina. If for some reason the ring is out of the vagina for more than 3 hours, backup contraception should be used until the ring has been back in place for 7 days. After 3 weeks, the ring is removed for 1 week. Withdrawal bleeding usually begins within 2 or 3 days of the ring-free week. For prevention of pregnancy, a new ring must be inserted after the ring-free week (7 days). The ring is reported to be 91% effective with typical use and 99.7% effective with perfect use.[8] The vaginal ring provides contraception with use of lower hormonal doses than in other contraceptive methods, is readily reversible, and is easy for patients to use. Side effects include vaginal complaints and headaches. It has the same contraindications as the combined oral contraceptives.[17,24]

SURGICAL STERILIZATION

Methods of surgical sterilization include tubal sterilization and vasectomy. Sterilization is the most commonly reported method of fertility control; in the United States in 2006 to 2008, it was the method used by 33% of contraceptive users aged 15 to 44 years.[1] Advantages of both male and female sterilization include its permanence, high rate of efficacy (0.5% failure rate for women and 0.15% for men), cost-effectiveness, lack of significant long-term side effects, and lack of need for partner compliance.[8] Permanence is also a disadvantage of sterilization; the procedures can sometimes be reversed, but this is difficult and expensive. In addition, sterilization provides no protection against STDs, including HIV infection.

HYSTEROSCOPIC STERILIZATION

A newer type of nonsurgical permanent sterilization is gaining popularity as an alternative to tubal ligation. The Essure method involves placement of microinserts into the fallopian tubes through a hysteroscope. Over the course of 3 months, fibers in the inserts promote tissue growth and occlusion of the fallopian tubes, preventing conception. The procedure can be performed in the office setting with or without use of conscious sedation or local anesthesia. Occlusion is verified radiologically. Adverse effects are rare. This method has been shown to be slightly more effective than surgical sterilization but without the surgical risks.[25]

NATURAL FAMILY PLANNING

Natural family planning (NFP) includes any method of family planning that is based on observations of the signs of fertility rather than on interference with physiologic function. Although

NFP is infrequently used,[1] it is important for health care providers to suggest NFP to those who might otherwise be unaware of its benefits or have spiritual or religious beliefs that preclude the use of barrier and hormonal contraceptives. With perfect use, NFP methods can be as high as 97% effective.[8]

NFP began in the 1920s with the rhythm method, which taught couples to avoid intercourse on days on which the woman was likely to be ovulating. Typically, starting at day 1 for menses, women avoided intercourse on days 12 to 19 and then altered those days depending on menstrual cycle length. Another older method, basal body temperature, relied on spikes of 0.05° F to 1° F in morning temperatures as an indicator of ovulation. Newer, more accurate methods of NFP primarily rely on identification of more sensitive physiologic indicators of fertility.

There are several methods of cervical mucus testing as a means of measuring fertility. All involve testing the quality and character of the mucus before intercourse. Mucus produced during fertile periods is clear, moist, and slippery and stretches. In contrast, mucus produced during periods of infertility is dry, cloudy, and sticky and breaks when stretched. The couple cannot adequately evaluate cervical mucus the day after intercourse and must abstain. After developing and identifying patterns, the couple can learn to identify periods of fertility and infertility. The Billings Ovulation Method and Creighton Method are formalized programs that provide the couple with education and visual aids.[26]

Another method of family planning, the symptothermal method (STM), is similar to the ovulation method but uses two other fertility signs in addition to cervical mucus: basal body temperature and the position, shape, and consistency of the cervix. STM is the most widely used method of NFP in the United States. Advocates of this method place particular emphasis on the cooperation of man and woman in fertility regulation.[27]

With STM, the menstrual cycle is separated into three phases. The relatively infertile phase lasts from the beginning of menstruation to the onset of any mucus. The fertile phase lasts from the first sign of mucus until the beginning of the third phase. The third phase, known as the *postovulatory infertility phase* (or the *absolute infertility phase*), begins on the fourth day of a temperature elevation and the fifth day of the drying of the cervical mucus. A basal thermometer (useful for measuring subtle variations in body temperature between 35.5° C and 37.7° C [96° F and 100° F]) is used to record morning body temperatures. Typically, a biphasic curve is observed during the course of the menstrual cycle, with low temperatures recorded before ovulation and slightly higher temperatures recorded after ovulation. A typical postovulatory elevation ranges from 0.4° F to 1° F above the average of the last 6 ovulatory days. The temperature rise is caused by the presence of progesterone, which is released by the empty follicle after ovulation. At least 3 days of elevated temperatures must be recorded before the postovulatory infertile phase begins on the evening of that third day. Basal body temperature does not give any advance warning of ovulation but indicates when ovulation has passed.[27]

Palpation of the cervix is performed as an adjunct to the other signs of fertility. During the infertile period, the cervix is firm and low in the vagina, and the cervical os is closed. As ovulation approaches, the cervix softens and elevates until it is almost out of reach, and the cervical os opens. Some women find this to be a helpful sign; others do not. In some cycles, these signs provide information as to when the woman is capable of conceiving. Couples who wish to avoid pregnancy should wait to have intercourse until all signs indicate that the fertile time has passed.

REASONS FOR CONTRACEPTIVE NONUSE

In the United States, where contraception is generally widely available, it is surprising that almost 50% of pregnancies are still considered unintended. Unintended pregnancy may occur for many reasons, including nonuse of contraception, failure to use contraceptive methods consistently and correctly, and, far less frequently, method failure. Studies show that reasons for nonuse differ by event and by age at the time of the event. Common nonuse reasons include difficulty obtaining contraception, side effects, and displeasure with the current method.

Given the high rates of unintended pregnancy and the high rates of dissatisfaction with contraceptive methods, it is imperative that health care providers be skilled in prescribing contraception. This requires a well-informed, nonjudgmental approach in which the provider listens to the patient's concerns and desires, assesses risks, and sifts through that information to present a thoughtful list of contraceptive choices.

CHAPTER 163
GENITAL TRACT CANCERS

Patricia Polgar-Bailey

Gynecologic malignant neoplasms are cancers of the female genital tract; they include cancers of the endometrium, ovary, fallopian tube, vulva, vagina, and cervix. In the United States, endometrial cancer is the most commonly diagnosed gynecologic malignant neoplasm, and ovarian cancer accounts for the most deaths annually.[1] Although endometrial cancer is more common than ovarian cancer, it is easier to cure with surgery alone. Ovarian cancer is usually diagnosed at a later stage and therefore is difficult to cure. Fallopian tube cancers are rare and are managed like ovarian cancers.

Vulvar and vaginal cancers are rare and are less familiar to patients. Few women are aware that a cancer of the vulva or vagina can develop and therefore do not seek health care at the onset of symptoms, usually burning or itching. Most vulvar or vaginal cancers are detected during a careful gynecologic examination. Of the gynecologic cancers, cervical cancer is the only one with a standardized screening tool—the Papanicolaou (Pap) test.

As a primary care provider, it is important to have a clear understanding of these six types of gynecologic cancers.

ENDOMETRIAL CANCER

DEFINITION AND EPIDEMIOLOGY

The endometrium is the inner glandular lining of the myometrium (muscle) of the uterus. This layer proliferates to prepare for implantation of a fertilized egg and sloughs on a regular cycle during the reproductive years. Once a woman reaches menopause, the endometrium remains thin because estrogen is no longer secreted from the ovaries. The proliferative characteristic of this lining is what can lead to neoplasia.

Endometrial cancer is the most common female genital tract cancer, but it is rare in women younger than 45. Three out of four cases are found in women ages 55 and older. Only 20% to 25% of endometrial cancers are diagnosed before menopause.[2] In 2015, approximately 55,000 new cases of uterine cancer were projected to be diagnosed in the the United States, and approximately 10,000 of these women will die of the disease.[1] Up to 8% of uterine body cancers are sarcomas, so the actual number of endometrial cancers is actually slightly lower.[1] The 5-year relative survival rate is approximately 84%.[3] Whereas more white women are diagnosed with endometrial cancer, more African American women die of the disease; this occurs because of a variety of socioeconomic issues related to access to care and education.[4]

PATHOPHYSIOLOGY

Endometrial cancers are divided into two types, type I and type II. Type I is associated with excess estrogen that is unopposed by progesterone. It typically occurs in women who are overweight and have the following characteristics: hyperlipidemia, hyperestrogenism, anovulatory bleeding, infertility, low parity, and late menopause.[5] Type I is associated with a favorable prognosis and usually is at an early stage on presentation. The excess androgen in the obese patient is converted to estrogen. Type II is not associated with these risk factors; it is most often seen in normal-weight women and has a poor prognosis.[6]

Type I endometrial cancer is associated with exposure to abnormal estrogen levels. Estrogen that is not opposed by progesterone causes the endometrium to become thicker and hypervascular (hyperplasia). Without progesterone, the structural support needed to sustain vascularity of the thickened endometrium is not present, and spontaneous superficial random hemorrhages occur.[7]

This hyperplastic appearance is classified by pathologists into two categories: benign endometrial hyperplasia and endometrial intraepithelial neoplasia (EIN). This is a recent change in the classification system intended to stratify the patient's risk for development of malignant endometrial cells. Benign endometrial hyperplasia shows cysts, remodeled glands, vascular thrombi, and stromal microinfarcts; these are changes resulting from the duration and combination of hormonal exposures. In contrast, EIN is the premalignant state that is demonstrated microscopically as cells with altered cytologic features and crowded architecture. Patients with EIN have a 45-fold greater risk for development of an endometrial cancer, and hysterectomy is recommended.[8] According to a recently published paper by the Collaborative Group on Epidemiological Studies on Endometrial Cancer, medium- to long-term use of oral contraceptives (i.e., for 5 years or longer) results in substantially reduced risk of endometrial cancer.[9] The reduction in risk associated with ever having used oral contraceptives differed depending on the type of tumor, with the risk reduction being stronger for carcinomas than sarcomas. In high-income countries, use of oral contraceptives for 10 years was estimated to reduce the absolute risk of endometrial cancer arising before age 75 years from 2.3 to 1.3 per 100 women.[9]

Factors that influence the risk of endometrial cancer include things that affect hormone levels (e.g., estrogen after menopause, birth control pills, tamoxifen), the number of menstrual cycles (over a lifetime), pregnancy, obesity, certain ovarian tumors, polycystic ovarian syndrome, use of an intrauterine device, age, diet and exercise, diabetes, a history of breast or ovarian cancer, history of endometrial hyperplasia, and a history of radiation therapy to the pelvis to treat another type of cancer.[10]

The risk of endometrial cancer is increased among first-degree relatives of patients with endometrial cancer and those with a personal history of colon and breast cancers. Patients with Lynch II syndrome, or hereditary nonpolyposis colorectal cancer (HNPCC), have a 40% to 60% lifetime risk for development of endometrial cancer.[10,11] HNPCC is an autosomal dominant inherited cancer that is caused by a germline mutation in a DNA mismatch repair gene. These patients should be referred to an oncologist to ensure careful and frequent screening.

CLINICAL PRESENTATION AND PHYSICAL EXAMINATION

The most important sign or symptom of endometrial cancer in the postmenopausal patient is bleeding. Patients often have complaints of a single episode of postmenopausal bleeding or a fullness or pressure in the pelvis. For some women who may not bleed because of cervical stenosis, a transvaginal ultrasound examination is a helpful tool. In a postmenopausal woman, endometrial thickness (also called endometrial stripe) on transvaginal ultrasonography should not be more than 5 mm. An endometrial thickness of more than 5 mm should be assessed with either biopsy in the office or dilation and curettage in the operating room. These procedures are usually performed by gynecologists.[12]

The perimenopausal presentation is more challenging. These patients often have irregular menses that are heavier and more frequent than their cycle previously. This is an important sign because bleeding should become lighter and less frequent during perimenopause, not heavier and more frequent. Providers must be careful not to assume that changes in menses are related to the onset of menopause.[6]

A detailed history of menstruation, dyspareunia, pelvic pain, fever, trauma, and intrauterine contraceptive device use should be elicited, and risk factors for endometrial cancer reviewed.

Other complaints that either premenopausal or postmenopausal women might express to the primary care provider are painful urination, dyspareunia, pelvic pain, cramping, pelvic discomfort, and postcoital bleeding. These symptoms warrant further evaluation, and transvaginal ultrasound examination is a good place to start.

In addition to a thorough general physical examination, the patient should undergo bimanual pelvic examination (including rectovaginal examination) and transvaginal ultrasound examination. If endometrial cancer is considered as a differential diagnosis, the patient requires endometrial sampling, either in the office with a Pipelle (a small suction catheter that is passed into the uterus in the office) or in the operating room with dilation and curettage. Endometrial biopsy is accurate 90% of the time; if there is high suspicion for cancer and the biopsy finding is normal, dilation and curettage should also be performed. If abnormalities are palpated on general or pelvic examination, a computed tomography (CT) scan with contrast enhancement of the abdomen and pelvis should be obtained to assess for spread of disease to adjacent organs or lymph nodes. Most common spread of disease is to the pelvic and para-aortic lymph nodes.

Workup for endometrial cancer is most often performed by the gynecologist. On occasion, if the sampling is difficult or there is high suspicion for cancer, these patients should be referred directly to a gynecologic oncologist.

DIAGNOSTICS AND DIFFERENTIAL DIAGNOSIS

There are multiple benign causes of dysfunctional uterine bleeding; however, bleeding in the postmenopausal woman should be assumed to be cancer until proven otherwise. If a postmenopausal patient has vaginal bleeding, the priority should be tissue sampling; 20% of these patients will have a malignant neoplasm on biopsy.[6] If a perimenopausal patient has worsening vaginal bleeding, tissue sampling should be obtained to rule out malignant disease.

Once a malignant neoplasm has been ruled out, the provider can sift through the myriad benign causes to determine the correct one. Atrophic vaginitis is a common cause of postmenopausal bleeding.

DIAGNOSTICS

Endometrial Cancer

LABORATORY

- Serum human chorionic gonadotropin (if of reproductive age)
- Complete blood count (CBC) and differential, platelets
- Cultures
- Vaginal wet preparations and cultures
- Coagulation profile
- Blood urea nitrogen (BUN)
- Prothrombin time/partial thromboplastin time (PT/PTT)*
- Creatinine
- Hormone levels*

OTHER DIAGNOSTICS

- Biopsy (endometrial)
- Hysteroscopy or dilation and curettage
- Transvaginal ultrasound

*If indicated.

DIFFERENTIAL DIAGNOSIS

Endometrial Cancer

- Atrophic vaginitis
- Cervicitis
- Cervical polyp
- Ovarian cyst
- Inflammation
- Infection
- Endometriosis
- Systemic disease
- Uterine fibroids
- Uterine prolapse
- Uterine polyp
- Pelvic inflammatory disease
- Trauma
- Medications
- Pregnancy

MANAGEMENT AND INDICATIONS FOR REFERRAL OR HOSPITALIZATION

Surgery is the treatment of choice for endometrial cancer. In early-stage disease, surgery can be curative; approximately 75% of patients with endometrial cancer have stage I disease (confined to the uterus) on presentation for evaluation.[6] Ideally, even patients with disease that has spread outside the uterus will undergo hysterectomy to remove the bulk of the disease and the source of bleeding.

Endometrial cancer surgery includes removal of the uterus, fallopian tubes, ovaries, and lymph nodes. Recently, there is a trend toward minimally invasive staging surgeries that use laparoscopy or robotically assisted vaginal hysterectomy with lymph node sampling. The surgery should be performed in collaboration with a gynecologic oncologist who is trained to perform lymphadenectomy and lymph node sampling. Adjuvant treatment (in addition to surgery) includes radiation therapy, hormonal therapy, and chemotherapy. Treatment decisions are made after surgery is complete and the stage (where it is located) and grade (type and morphologic features) of the disease have been assigned.

LIFE SPAN CONSIDERATIONS

The average age at diagnosis of endometrial cancer is 60 years, and the incidence increases with advancing age. When endometrial cancer occurs before the age of 40 years, it is usually associated with chronic obesity or anovulation.[13]

PATIENT AND FAMILY EDUCATION

Patients should understand that the use of estrogen plus progesterone for postmenopausal hormone replacement therapy does not increase the risk of endometrial cancer. It is also necessary that women understand the importance of evaluation for any postmenopausal bleeding even if it occurs only once or is a small amount.

OVARIAN CANCER

DEFINITION AND EPIDEMIOLOGY

Among women, ovarian cancer represents the fifth leading cause of death from cancer.[1] In 2015, the American Cancer Society estimated that there were approximately 21,290 new cases diagnosed and 14,180 deaths from ovarian cancer. A woman's lifetime risk of getting ovarian cancer is about 1 in 75, and the lifetime chance of dying from ovarian cancer is about 1 in 100. This cancer develops mainly in older women, and approximately half of the women who are diagnosed with ovarian cancer are 63 years or older. It is more common in white women than African-American women.[1] The rate at which women are diagnosed with ovarian cancer has gradually decreased over the past 20 years.

Because of socioeconomic factors, there is a big difference in survival of white women versus black women. The 5-year relative survival is 45.4% for white women and 36.8% for black women.[14]

During the last decade, advances have been made in the treatment of ovarian cancer; however, little advance has been made in the development of tools for early diagnosis of ovarian cancer. This disease often progresses to advanced stages with only subtle signs and symptoms. It is important that the primary care provider be tuned in to the possible signs of early disease.

PATHOPHYSIOLOGY

Ovarian cancer develops in the ovary. Typically, it occurs in women 65 years and older. There are numerous histologic types of ovarian cancer: epithelial, germ cell, and mesenchymal (stromal and sex cord). The epithelial ovarian cancers are further subdivided: serous, mucinous, endometrioid, clear cell, transitional cell tumors (Brenner tumors), carcinosarcoma, mixed epithelial tumor, and undifferentiated carcinoma. Clear cell and endometrioid ovarian carcinomas are often associated with endometriosis. Serous carcinomas are often discovered at more advanced stages (III and IV); clear cell and endometrioid carcinomas are more often confined to the ovary and therefore are at an earlier stage at diagnosis. Although all of these types are labeled ovarian cancers, it is important for the provider to understand that each histologic type is slightly different from its counterparts, and therefore the oncologist might manage the disease for each type slightly differently.[15] Although the management of each type of ovarian cancer might differ, what does not differ is the need for all patients with suspected ovarian cancer or pelvic mass to undergo surgery.

The risk for development of ovarian cancer is influenced by genetic, hormonal, and environmental factors. Approximately 5% to 10% of women have a genetically acquired risk of ovarian cancer because of inherited mutations in the *BRCA1* and *BRCA2* tumor suppressor genes. The overall risk for development of ovarian cancer is 20% to 60% for those with *BRCA1* mutations and 10% to 35% for those with *BRCA2* mutations. Some data suggest that women with *BRCA* mutation–mediated ovarian cancer may have survival rates better than those of woman with sporadic ovarian cases. This may be a result of improved tumor response to platinum-based chemotherapy in those with *BRCA*-related cancer.[16]

Increased age and family history are risk factors; family history is the best predictor of risk. One second-degree relative with ovarian cancer increases the lifetime risk to 2.9%; one first-degree relative with ovarian cancer increases the lifetime risk to 4% to 5%; and two or more affected first-degree relatives increases the risk to 30% to 50%.[7] Whereas these hereditary syndromes are rare, if a patient with a family history of ovarian cancer reports pelvic pain, fullness, early satiety, or urinary frequency, the provider must carefully evaluate the patient and rule out malignant disease.

Other risk factors include late menopause, nulliparity, and early menarche. There is debate as to whether or not infertility drugs increase the risk for ovarian cancer; at this time, the data do not fully support either argument. In general, these theories are based on a theory of ovulation without stopping, in which the ovary itself is somehow disrupted and is sensitive to events of ovulation. Therefore, methods to suppress ovulation, such as oral contraceptive use, multiparity, late menarche, and early menopause, would potentially decrease a patient's risk. The use of oral contraceptives confers protection for up to 10 years after they are discontinued.[7]

CLINICAL PRESENTATION AND PHYSICAL EXAMINATION

In 2007, Goff and colleagues[17] developed a symptom index to improve early detection of ovarian cancer. These specific symptoms, if persistent, should be considered red flags for the provider: pelvic pain, abdominal pain, urinary urgency, urinary frequency, increased abdominal size, abdominal bloating, difficulty eating, and early satiety. The provider must consider all differential diagnoses for these symptoms and should not presume that they are related to menopause or stress. Ovarian cancer must be considered as a differential diagnosis in these cases. Goff's research was groundbreaking in that it brought new public attention to common symptoms that warrant suspicion of ovarian cancer.

A pelvic examination that includes a rectovaginal examination should be done but is not sensitive for detection of ovarian cancer. This examination should be done routinely on all women to adequately assess the entire pelvis for mass, fullness, or tenderness. Despite a careful examination, it is rare that an ovarian cancer is detected. DiSaia and Creasman[6] stated that it takes 10,000 routine pelvic examinations to detect one ovarian cancer.

DIAGNOSTICS AND DIFFERENTIAL DIAGNOSIS

Other conditions can manifest as a pelvic mass. These include sigmoid diverticulitis; pregnancy; a distended bladder; a low-lying distended cecum; stool in the sigmoid colon; a pelvic kidney; and a fallopian tube, uterine, or gastrointestinal tumor. Included in the differential diagnosis are fallopian tube carcinomas, which are rare and are managed and treated like ovarian cancers.

The differential diagnoses can be sorted out through the use of radiographic imaging. Transvaginal ultrasonography is the gold standard assessment of the pelvis. If the ultrasound study is inconclusive, pelvic CT scan and pelvic magnetic resonance imaging (MRI) are both useful. However, if a primary care provider suspects a pelvic mass or diagnoses a mass on ultrasound examination, the patient should be referred to a gynecologist for further workup.

If the provider suspects a pelvic mass, the first diagnostic test that should be ordered is a transvaginal pelvic ultrasound study. Once the diagnosis of a pelvic mass is established, a serum cancer antigen 125 (CA-125) test should be ordered. CA-125 is a serum protein that is produced by ovarian cancer cells. It is elevated in most epithelial ovarian cancers. CA-125 can be elevated in myriad conditions including many nonmalignant conditions (Box 163-1). Because it is also elevated in nonmalignant conditions, it is not an adequate screening tool. When the CA-125 test and transvaginal ultrasound examination are used in the general population, they are found to be inadequate screening tools, with false-positive rates that are greater than 75%. As a result, women undergo unnecessary surgery.

BOX 163-1

Causes of Elevation of CA-125

- Acute pelvic inflammatory disease
- Endometriosis
- Functional ovarian cyst
- Meigs syndrome
- Ovarian hyperstimulation
- Uterine myoma
- Acute infection: hepatitis, pancreatitis, colitis, pericarditis, pneumonia, congestive heart failure, polyarteritis nodosa
- Renal disease
- Chronic liver disease
- Mesothelioma
- Postoperative period
- Rodent exposure (human anti-mouse antibody [HAMA] response)
- Systemic lupus erythematosus
- Autoimmune disease
- Poorly controlled diabetes

Data from DiSaia PJ, Creasman WT: *Clinical gynecologic oncology*, ed 7, St Louis, 2007, Mosby.

However, if the patient has a pelvic mass and plans to undergo surgery, a CA-125 value that is above the laboratory's designated normal value (usually 35 U/mL) may guide the surgeon to plan a cancer staging operation rather than a simple removal of the mass.

In addition to the CA-125 test alone, new to the market is a test called OVA1. This is a serum test that combines the results of five immunoassays into a single numeric result. The five assays are prealbumin (transthyretin), apolipoprotein, β_2-microglobulin, transferrin, and CA-125. It is indicated for women who have a pelvic mass for which surgery is already planned. It is intended to aid in the assessment of the likelihood that the pelvic mass is malignant. It is particularly useful when the pelvic examination and radiographic imaging do not clearly indicate a malignant neoplasm. It is not a useful test for screening. The test result is divided into two categories, premenopausal and postmenopausal. When the probability of malignant disease is high, the test is designed to help the general gynecologist decide whether the patient's surgery should be performed by a gynecologic oncologist, who can perform a complete debulking and staging surgery.

In premenopausal women, there is low probability of malignant disease with an OVA1 result below 5.0 and high probability of malignant disease with an OVA1 result of 5.0 or higher. In postmenopausal women, there is low probability of malignant disease with an OVA1 result below 4.4 and a high probability of malignant disease with an OVA1 of 4.4 or higher.[18]

If an ovarian cancer is suspected, the patient should undergo CT scanning to further delineate the disease process. On CT, the provider is looking for lymphadenopathy, ascites, omental caking, diaphragmatic thickening, and pleural effusion. These are all signs of advanced-stage disease; these patients should be referred directly to a gynecologic oncologist for complete debulking surgery, which usually includes hysterectomy, bilateral salpingo-oophorectomy, omentectomy, and node sampling; diaphragmatic stripping, bowel resection, and splenectomy are sometimes performed as well.

DIAGNOSTICS

Ovarian Cancer

LABORATORY
CA-125
OVA1

IMAGING
Ultrasound (abdominal, vaginal)
CT scan (pelvic)*
MRI (pelvic)*

OTHER DIAGNOSTICS
Laparoscopy
Biopsy

*If indicated.

DIFFERENTIAL DIAGNOSIS

Ovarian Cancer

- Sigmoid diverticulitis
- Pregnancy
- Distended bladder
- Distended cecum
- Stool in sigmoid colon
- Pelvic kidney
- Fallopian tube, uterine, or gastrointestinal tumor

MANAGEMENT AND INDICATIONS FOR REFERRAL OR HOSPITALIZATION

All patients with suspected ovarian carcinoma should be referred for surgery with a gynecologic oncologist. The standard surgery is a laparotomy to facilitate careful evaluation of the upper abdomen for evidence of disease spread that might not have been detected on radiographic imaging preoperatively.

LIFE SPAN CONSIDERATIONS

Older women are more likely to develop ovarian cancer and have worse outcomes than younger women. This is likely because of comorbidities and tolerability of aggressive treatment with surgery and chemotherapy.

PATIENT AND FAMILY EDUCATION

Patients with a familial history of ovarian cancer or known genetic abnormality associated with *BRCA1* or *BRCA2* or HNPCC should be referred to a gynecologist and possibly a gynecologic oncologist for careful surveillance. These families will benefit from referral to genetic counseling. There are many emotional challenges related to screening the relatives of the patient with ovarian cancer. The decision to undergo screening should be done with the expertise of a genetic counselor.

Families and patients undergoing treatment of ovarian cancer should understand that although the disease is rare, it is generally sensitive to chemotherapy. There is an increasing number of drugs available to offer ovarian cancer patients; some of them are novel agents that do not have the same toxicities of traditional chemotherapies. These patients generally receive chemotherapy intermittently or targeted therapy for the rest of their lives.

VULVAR CANCER

DEFINITION AND EPIDEMIOLOGY

In the United States, vulvar cancer accounts for about 4% of cancers of the female reproductive organs and 0.6% of all cancers in women. In the United States, approximately 5150 cases of vulvar cancer were projected to be diagnosed in 2015 and approximately 1080 women will die of this disease. In the United States, women have a 1 in 333 chance of developing vulvar cancer at some point during their life.[19]

The median age at death from vulvar cancer is 79 years; the 5-year combined survival rate is 75.6%.[20]

PATHOPHYSIOLOGY

There are several types of vulvar cancers: squamous cell carcinoma, melanoma, basal cell carcinoma, Paget disease, and adenocarcinoma. Squamous cell carcinoma accounts for the large majority of invasive vulvar cancers; these arise from the skin of the vulva. Adenocarcinomas of the vulva arise from the glandular cells of the vulva, such as Bartholin gland.

It is not entirely clear what causes vulvar cancer. Fifty percent of squamous cell cancers of the vulva are caused by human papillomavirus (HPV). Prognosis of these lesions is related to size of the lesion and lymph node involvement.

Melanoma is a rare and aggressive form of vulvar skin cancer that is often without any symptoms of burning, itching, or pain. It is thought to arise from a lesion that contains a junctional or compound nevus.[6] It is the second most common cancer of the vulva. These lesions are usually pigmented, raised, and often ulcerated. Most of these lesions occur on the labia minora and clitoris. Prognosis is related to size of the lesion and depth of invasion.

Basal cell carcinoma is usually small and occurs on the labia majora; it often has a central ulceration. It usually progresses slowly and rarely involves the lymphatics. Usually, the patient reports a repeated pattern of mild itching, slight bleeding, and then healing.

Paget disease is a lesion of unknown cause that arises from the apocrine-bearing part of the vulvar skin. These lesions usually are present for years before the patient seeks medical attention. It occurs most often in women older than 70 years; however, it can occur earlier. Paget disease manifests with pruritus, tenderness, erythematous skin, and hyperkeratotic plaques and may be confused with candidiasis. The lesions are hyperemic, well-demarcated, thickened plaques with foci of excoriation and induration. The skin is usually smooth and thick, reminiscent of leukoplakia. The hyperemic areas are often associated with a superficial white coating that is described as "cake icing effect." This is a classic presentation and indicative of the disease. These patients have an increased risk for development of an associated adenocarcinoma and concurrent adenocarcinoma somewhere else in the body. Therefore, routine cancer screening with mammography, colonoscopy, and chest radiography is important. The primary treatment of Paget disease is surgical resection.[6]

Adenocarcinoma of the Bartholin gland is rare. It represents 1% of vulvar cancers. Peak incidence occurs in women in their 60s. This cancer usually presents with a mass in the deep vulvar tissues. Women often experience dyspareunia before they realize there is a problem. Although the Bartholin gland can form an abscess, enlargement of the Bartholin gland in a postmenopausal woman should be presumed to be carcinoma. Treatment involves radical pelvic surgery to extensively dissect the tissues around the gland.[6]

Risk factors for vulvar cancers include cigarette smoking (particularly with the vulvar cancers that are caused by HPV), human immunodeficiency virus (HIV) infection or other conditions that cause immunosuppression, low socioeconomic status, vulvar intraepithelial neoplasia, other genital cancers, and lichen sclerosus.[21]

CLINICAL PRESENTATION AND PHYSICAL EXAMINATION

Most patients have a history of vulvar irritation, burning or pain, pruritus, local discomfort, excoriation, fissuring, painful irritation, bleeding and discharge, or painful vulvar lump. The lesion may be white, raised, hyperkeratotic, or pigmented. Many tumors are diagnosed at advanced stages because women are generally unaware of the possibility of vulvar cancer or they are embarrassed about letting symptoms worsen and develop into a frank tumor. A long-term "lump" or mass and pruritus are present in more than 50% of women who are diagnosed with vulvar cancer. There is a reported delay of 2 to 16 months after symptoms begin before medical attention is sought.[6]

Early diagnosis of vulvar cancer is important. The initial lesion may appear as a small raised area or as an ulceration that will not heal, or it may be associated with a secondary infection. The entire vulva is composed of squamous cells, and therefore lesions can arise anywhere on the vulva; 70% are usually found on the labia.[6] The size of the tumor correlates with the risk of lymph node metastases. Careful examination of the inguinal lymph nodes is important because the cancer can metastasize easily along the inguinal lymph channels. The presence of palpable lymph nodes often represents malignant spread.[21]

DIAGNOSTICS AND DIFFERENTIAL DIAGNOSIS

Definitive diagnosis requires a biopsy and further evaluation, for which the patient should be referred to a gynecologist. Biopsy is usually done in the office with a punch biopsy procedure and local anesthetic.

Vulvar carcinoma can be mistaken for other conditions, including eczema or dermatitis, ulcerative lesions such as syphilis, and granuloma inguinale. These lesions are often cultured and treated for infection before a biopsy is done, which delays diagnosis. Crohn disease can manifest as an ulcerative area on the vulva, and a lesion, on rare occasion, could be a metastasis from a distant site.

DIAGNOSTICS

Vulvar Cancer

Biopsy

DIFFERENTIAL DIAGNOSIS

Vulvar Cancer

- Carcinoma
- Dermatitis
- Syphilis
- Granuloma inguinale
- Eczema
- Crohn disease

MANAGEMENT AND INDICATIONS FOR REFERRAL OR HOSPITALIZATION

Treatment of vulvar cancer is usually surgery consisting of wide local excision or vulvectomy with unilateral or bilateral inguinal lymph node dissection. On occasion, the urethra or the rectum may be involved, and the oncologist will opt to treat the patient with radiation therapy or chemotherapy before resection of the tumor. Postoperatively, these patients may develop lymphedema of the lower extremity. This is managed with lymph compression stockings or compression pumps.

LIFE SPAN CONSIDERATIONS

Invasive vulvar cancer occurs most often in patients aged 65 to 70 years. Seventy-five percent of vulvar cancers occur in women older than 50 years.[2]

PATIENT AND FAMILY EDUCATION

All patients should understand the necessity of screening to ensure early detection of vulvar cancer. In addition, primary care providers have an opportunity to educate patients and families on the possibility of development of a malignant neoplasm of the vulva and the importance of seeking care as soon as symptoms arise. Screening methods include an annual pelvic examination and Pap test, monthly genital self-examination, and prompt reporting of unusual symptoms.

VAGINAL CANCER

DEFINITION AND EPIDEMIOLOGY

Vaginal cancer is an uncommon tumor that accounts for 1% of genital tract cancers. In the United States, there are 2500 cases of vaginal cancer annually and fewer than 1000 deaths from vaginal cancer. More than 50% of vaginal cancers are diagnosed in women 70 years of age and older. Sixty-eight percent of vaginal cancers are squamous cell carcinoma; 17% are adenocarcinomas, 9% are melanomas, and the remaining cases are of other rare histologic types. The combined 5-year survival rate for squamous cell carcinomas and adenocarcinomas of the vagina is 50% to 60%. Eighty percent of vaginal cancers are secondary (originating from other sites, such as the gastrointestinal tract or the breast). When the cancer involves the vagina only, it is considered a primary vaginal cancer. The grade of the tumor, the stage, and the histologic type will all affect survival.[22]

PATHOPHYSIOLOGY

Squamous cell carcinoma and adenocarcinoma are the most common types of vaginal cancer. Squamous cell carcinomas arise from surface epithelial cells; adenocarcinomas arise from glandular cells; sarcomas arise from connective tissue; and melanomas arise from melanocytes. Non–clear cell adenocarcinoma is very rare, occurs predominantly in postmenopausal women, and has a worse prognosis than squamous cell carcinoma.[6] Clear cell adenocarcinoma is usually associated with diethylstilbestrol (DES) exposure in utero.

Risk factors that increase a woman's risk of vaginal cancer are young age at coitarche, greater number of lifetime sexual partners, smoking, in utero DES exposure, HPV infection, previous history of pelvic irradiation, and personal history of cervical cancer.[6] Fifty percent of vaginal cancers are caused by HPV infection.[23] Vaginal cancers metastasize by direct extension into the surrounding tissues. The pelvic bones, bladder, rectum, and soft tissues are commonly involved.

CLINICAL PRESENTATION AND PHYSICAL EXAMINATION

Five percent to 10% of vaginal carcinomas are asymptomatic and found on a routine pelvic examination. Three percent to 7% of vaginal intraepithelial neoplasias will progress to invasive carcinoma despite treatment of the precancerous lesions.[6] The most common symptom is painless vaginal discharge that is often bloody. The symptomatic patient may report vaginal pain, pelvic pain, dyspareunia, postcoital bleeding, dysuria, constipation, or vaginal discharge or mass. Tenesmus can be associated with posterior vaginal disease. The most common site for a primary tumor is the upper third of the vagina.[6]

DIAGNOSTICS AND DIFFERENTIAL DIAGNOSIS

If a gross lesion is noted on vaginal examination, the provider should obtain a smear by use of the Pap broom and refer the patient for further evaluation by a gynecologist; if a lesion is detected on routine Pap testing, the patient should also be referred to a gynecologist. In both cases, the patient will undergo colposcopy by the application of dilute acetic acid to improve visualization and directed biopsies of the abnormal tissue.

If the patient has a history of DES exposure in utero, she should be referred to a gynecologist for surveillance because of the increased incidence of clear cell adenocarcinoma in this population. These patients should undergo Pap test of the cervix and vaginal fornix to screen for vaginal adenosis and coexisting adenocarcinoma. Of note, adenosis rarely progresses to adenocarcinoma.[24]

Vaginal cancer is staged clinically, not surgically. Careful pelvic and rectovaginal examination is essential to determine the amount of direct extension of the disease into surrounding tissues. Metabolic imaging with positron emission tomography and CT scan is more sensitive than CT or MRI for the detection of metastatic disease. All patients diagnosed with a vaginal cancer should be assessed for metastatic disease.

DIAGNOSTICS

Vaginal Cancer

Pap test
Colposcopy
Biopsy

DIFFERENTIAL DIAGNOSIS

Vaginal Cancer

- Vaginal intraepithelial neoplasia
- Metastatic lesion
- Trophoblastic disease

MANAGEMENT AND INDICATIONS FOR REFERRAL OR HOSPITALIZATION

Patients with suspicious lesions require colposcopy and biopsy. The primary treatment involves surgery; wide excision or upper vaginectomy is the most common. Adjuvant treatment includes chemotherapy and radiation therapy. In rare cases, the gynecologic oncologist may perform a pelvic exenteration.

LIFE SPAN CONSIDERATIONS

Age is a risk factor for squamous cell cancer of the vagina. In the 1970s, more vaginal adenocarcinoma was seen in a younger population because of the use of DES during the first trimester in the 1950s. Because DES is no longer used, there are fewer cases of clear cell adenocarcinomas of the vagina.

PATIENT AND FAMILY EDUCATION

These patients and families should be educated about the importance of routine screening. This is especially true for women who have a history of cervical cancer or radiation therapy because vaginal cancers can be detected on routine examination with the Pap test and careful inspection.

CERVICAL CANCER

DEFINITION AND EPIDEMIOLOGY

Cervical cancer is a malignant neoplasm that develops in the squamous or glandular cells of the uterine cervix. In the United States, it is estimated that approximately 12,900 new cases of invasive cervical cancer will be diagnosed in 2015 and about 4100 women will die from this disease. Cervical precancers are diagnosed far more often than invasive cervical cancer.[25]

Cervical cancer used to be one of the most common causes of cancer death for American women, but over the last 30 years, the cervical cancer death rate has gone down by more than 50%. The main reason for this change was the increased use of the Pap test.

Cervical cancer generally occurs in midlife. Most cases are found in women younger than 50, and it rarely develops in women younger than 20. Many older women do not realize that the risk of developing cervical cancer is still present as they age. More than 15% of cases of cervical cancer are found in women older than 65. However, these cancers rarely occur in women who underwent regular tests to screen for cervical cancer before they were 65.[25]

In the United States, Hispanic women are most likely to get cervical cancer, followed by African Americans, Asians and Pacific Islanders, and whites. American Indians and Alaskan natives have the lowest risk of cervical cancer in this country.[25]

There are significant differences in racial and ethnic incidence of cervical cancer and related deaths in the United States. The incidence for African Americans is 1.5 times higher than for white women. The incidence for Hispanic women is also higher than for white women. The death rate for black women related to cervical cancer is twice that of white women.[26]

Each year, 50 million women undergo screening with the Pap test, which was invented by George Papanicolaou in the 1940s to obtain a cytologic sample of the cervix to screen for cancer or precancerous cells. It involves use of a brush or broom-like tool to sample the cells of the cervix and endocervix. The advent of the Pap test has reduced the incidence of cervical cancer in the United States by approximately 75%.[26]

Approximately 3.5 to 5.0 million of these Pap tests require some follow-up. Of these, 2 to 3 million will involve atypical cells of undetermined significance, 1.25 million will be low-grade squamous intraepithelial lesions, and 300,000 will be high-grade squamous intraepithelial lesions.[26]

PATHOPHYSIOLOGY

Approximately three quarters of all cervical cancers in the United States are squamous cell carcinomas; the remaining are adenocarcinomas. HPV is a precursor for the development of cervical cancer and precancer. An estimated 14 million persons in the United States are newly infected with HPV every year.[26] High-risk HPV types 16 and 18 account for approximately 70% of all cervical cancers; the remaining are caused by other high-risk strains of HPV (of which there are approximately 40).[27] Cervical cancers occur when high-risk HPV infection persists more than 2 years. Approximately 90% of HPV infection will become undetectable in the first 2 years after exposure to the virus. Therefore it is the remaining 10% that persists that causes cervical squamous cell and adenocarcinomas.

The transformation zone of the cervix (where the columnar cells of the endocervix are undergoing metaplasia to become squamous cells) is particularly sensitive to microtrauma and therefore to HPV infection. Ninety-nine percent of HPV-related cancers occur in this zone.[28] As women age, the transformation zone regresses into the endocervical canal. Adolescents, who have a large transformation zone on the cervix, are at an increased risk of HPV infection; this explains why early sexual debut and multiple sex partners would increase one's risk of HPV infection and in turn one's risk for development of cervical cancer if monitoring is not done on a regular basis with Pap testing.

Another important risk factor for cervical cancer is smoking. Women who smoke have a two to three times greater risk for development of cervical cancer.[29] Immunosuppression, other cervical infections such as herpes simplex virus and chlamydia, and multiparity are other risk factors.[30]

CLINICAL PRESENTATION AND PHYSICAL EXAMINATION

Early symptoms include abnormal uterine bleeding (postmenopausal, postcoital, after douching, or intermenstrual) and foul vaginal discharge. Vaginal discharge is often described as thin and watery. Bleeding usually begins as light and serosanguineous and becomes heavier and more persistent as the tumor enlarges. Late symptoms include pain, leg edema, and urinary and rectal symptoms.

A vaginal examination may reveal an enlarged cervix (described as a barrel cervix), friable tumor on the cervix, or ulcerative lesion that bleeds easily on contact. A Pap test will detect precancerous and cancerous lesions on the cervix or within the endocervix even if the cervix appears normal. The Pap test should include a scraping from the cervical os and a brushing from the endocervical canal. The specimen should be sent for interpretation by an experienced cytopathologist.

DIAGNOSTICS AND DIFFERENTIAL DIAGNOSIS

The Pap test is a screening test that uses a liquid-based medium (cytology) that is spun down and plated on a slide for the pathologist. It is only a screening test and has a high false-negative rate. However, it is an effective screening tool when it is used routinely. It does not render a diagnosis; this must be obtained by tissue sampling with colposcopy (the application of acetic acid to improve visualization of abnormal cells for directed biopsy). Both the Pap test and the histologic features are described by the terminology of the Bethesda System, which was last updated in 2006. Management of abnormal Pap tests is discussed in Chapter 165.

The Bethesda System scores cervical intraepithelial neoplasia (CIN) on a grading system (1 to 3). CIN 1 is well differentiated and involves the initial third of the epithelial layer. CIN 2 is less differentiated and involves one third to two thirds of the epithelial layer. CIN 3 is undifferentiated in two thirds and involves the full thickness (carcinoma in situ) up to the basal cell layer. Invasive cervical cancer involves cancerous cells that penetrate below the basal cell layer or the basement membrane.[30]

There are no differential diagnoses for cervical cancer. The use of the Pap test will aid in detection. If a cervix has an abnormal appearance on examination and the Pap test is normal, the primary care provider should refer the patient to a gynecologist. The liquid-based medium used for Pap tests allows the pathologist to distinguish between HPV-infected cells and inflammatory cells. In particular, this medium allows the pathologist to test the sample for the presence of HPV DNA.

Newly diagnosed cervical cancer patients should undergo careful pelvic examination, which includes a rectovaginal examination. Cervical cancer spreads by direct extension into the adjacent tissues (bladder, rectum, parametrium, bone). It is staged clinically, not surgically. Therefore the stage is assigned at initial examination by a gynecologic oncologist. Patients should be evaluated for invasion of the tumor into the bladder and the rectum. This is done during an examination under anesthesia by cystoscopy and proctoscopy. Urine cytology can be used to detect bladder wall invasion.[6]

DIAGNOSTICS

Cervical Cancer

Pap test
Biopsy
Colposcopy

MANAGEMENT AND INDICATIONS FOR REFERRAL OR HOSPITALIZATION

The patient should be referred to a gynecologic oncologist for evaluation and consideration of surgery versus chemotherapy combined with radiation therapy. This determination is based on the assigned stage of the disease.

In 2006, the first HPV vaccine, Gardasil, was approved by the U.S. Food and Drug Administration (FDA). Gardasil is a quadrivalent vaccine that contains four types of HPV (16, 18, 6, 11). This is the first vaccine developed to prevent cervical cancer, precancerous cervical lesions, vulvovaginal cancer, and genital warts caused by HPV. The vaccine is highly effective against four types of HPV, including types 16 and 18, which account for 70% of cervical cancer. The vaccine is currently available for girls and women 9 to 26 years of age and is recommended for girls 11 or 12 years old.

In 2009, a second vaccine, Cervarix, was approved by the FDA. Cervarix is a bivalent vaccine that contains HPV types 16 and 18. It is indicated to prevent cervical precancerous lesions and cervical cancer caused by HPV types 16 and 18. It is available for girls and women 10 to 26 years of age. It is also highly effective.

Both vaccines are given in a three-injection series during the course of 6 months. The side effect and adverse event profiles for both vaccines are favorable. They are both Pregnancy Category B.[31]

LIFE SPAN CONSIDERATIONS

Cervical cancer is unique in life span considerations. In most cases, women who are diagnosed with and die of cervical cancer have had HPV-related precancerous lesions for many years and have not been screened on a regular basis. In addition, this is the only cancer for which there is a preventive vaccine. By the vaccination of young girls, there is the possibility of dramatically reducing the incidence of cervical cancer in the United States 20 years from now. In addition, both vaccines significantly lower the rate of procedures to treat precancerous lesions by approximately 40%.[31]

PATIENT AND FAMILY EDUCATION

Patients and families, and the public, can be educated on the role of HPV in the genital health of women. Young girls who are naive to all types of HPV should be vaccinated to prevent precancerous lesions in the future as well as to prevent the spread of HPV to partners. Cervical cancer is a preventable disease that can be treated successfully if it is detected early. Routine Pap testing is the key to cervical cancer prevention.

CHAPTER 164

INFERTILITY

Marie Elena Botte

DEFINITION AND EPIDEMIOLOGY

Whereas a healthy couple has a 20% to 25% chance of conceiving in a given month (natural cycle fecundity), infertility is defined as a couple's inability to conceive after 1 year of regular, timed, unprotected intercourse or therapeutic donor insemination.[1] Impaired fecundity is defined as physical difficulty in getting pregnant or the inability to carry a pregnancy to live birth. Infertility affects one couple in six, and prevalence increases dramatically with paternal and maternal age. In this chapter, infertility is contrasted with sterility, a term that applies to those members of a population for whom there is no possibility of attaining a natural pregnancy. The most recent national U.S. data suggest that some form of infertility or subfertility was reported by 12% of men aged 25 to 44 and by 11% of women aged 15 to 44.[2] An estimated 15% of all couples experience infertility. The recent increase in the numbers of individuals who see health care professionals for help with infertility is most likely attributable to a combination of factors, including an increasing number of women delaying the birth of their first child and widespread media attention regarding new reproductive technologies. Even after targeted interventions, up to half of these couples remain unable to have a biologic child of their own.[3]

PATHOPHYSIOLOGY

Potential causes of infertility include genetic, anatomic, endocrine, and behavioral factors. Physiologic dysfunction in men accounts for approximately 20% to 50% of all cases of infertility; ovulatory dysfunction in women contributes to up to 40% of infertility cases[4]; and tubal factors (20%), endometriosis (5%), and unexplained causes (between 10% and 25%) are other factors. Male factors alone are the cause of infertility in 20% of infertile couples, and combined male and female factors occur in about 30% to 40%.[5] In 10% to 25% of cases, no specific factor can be identified. The odds of delivering a healthy infant drop 3.5% per year after the age of 30 years. For women younger than 25 years, the rate of impaired fertility is 11.7%; this rate rises to 42.1% for women older than 35 years.

Male factor infertility can in general be attributable to chromosomal or structural defects or to endocrine abnormalities of the hypothalamic-pituitary-testicular axis. Contributing hypothalamic-pituitary disorders include congenital gonadotropin-releasing hormone (GnRH) deficiency (Kallmann syndrome); hemochromatosis; pituitary and hypothalamic tumors; infiltrative disorders (tuberculosis, sarcoidosis); hormonal disturbance (androgen, cortisol, and estrogen excess; hyperprolactinemia); and systemic disorders, such as chronic illness, obesity, and nutritional deficiencies. Structural causes include cryptorchidism, aplasia or obstruction in the male genital tract, varicoceles (usually a problem only when accompanied by other factors, such as abnormal semen analysis), congenital bilateral absence of the vas deferens (which can indicate partial expression of a gene mutation for cystic fibrosis), impotence, and ejaculatory dysfunction. Factors influencing spermatogenesis or motility include inflammation or infection (postpubertal mumps, gonorrhea, chlamydial infection), direct injury or trauma (including postoperative), and use or abuse of substances (including alcohol, caffeine, cocaine, steroids, and marijuana).

Male factor infertility can involve a low sperm concentration (oligospermia), poor sperm motility (asthenospermia), abnormal sperm morphology (teratospermia), or, more commonly, a constellation of all three variables (oligoasthenoteratozoospermia). Poorer semen quality (reduced motility, increased DNA fragmentation, chromosomal aberrations) has been demonstrated in older men[6,7]; as men age, they produce fewer motile sperm, which are less able to travel in a straight line.[8]

Reproductive hazards for both men and women include environmental exposures,[9] possibly but not necessarily in an occupational setting, to solvents, pesticides, heavy metals, pharmaceuticals, anesthetic gases, ionizing radiation, and lead. Occupational exposures in male workers can affect the male reproductive system, leading to sperm abnormalities, hyperestrogenism, impotence, infertility, or increased spontaneous abortions in their partners. Even benzene levels at the U.S. Occupational Safety and Health Administration (OSHA)–permissible level of 1 ppm have been associated with sperm aneuploidy[10,11]; because stem cells are affected, such exposures may have persistent reproductive effects in previously exposed workers. The websites of the National Institute for Occupational Safety and Health (www.cdc.gov/niosh/homepage.html) and OSHA (www.osha.gov) provide information on reproductive hazards and their management. Cigarette smoking is associated with infertility in both women and men,[12-14] as is obesity.[6,15] In women, being underweight at age 20,[16] doing shift work, and having occupational exposure to chemotherapeutic drugs have also been associated with an increased subsequent risk of infertility.

In women, ovulatory dysfunctions range from congenital absence of the ovaries and premature ovarian failure to various disruptions in the hypothalamic-pituitary-ovarian axis and other metabolic or endocrine conditions, such as hypothyroidism and hyperthyroidism. Uterine and fallopian pathologic conditions include current or past pelvic inflammatory disease resulting in salpingitis, endometriosis, iatrogenic Asherman syndrome after overly vigorous curettage, fibroids, bicornuate uterus, and postinfectious or operative tubal scarring and adhesions. Tubal infertility has been associated with lower family income. Preembryonic developmental problems and implantation problems have been postulated as possible causes of idiopathic infertility.

The pathophysiology of infertility includes theories relating to energy deficits inhibiting GnRH and luteinizing hormone (LH) secretion, interference with circadian rhythms, and the temporal pattern of endocrine functions in shift work. In addition, endogenous opioid–mediated inhibition of the hypothalamic GnRH pulse generator has been implicated in hypothalamic ovarian failure. The link between infertility and various autoimmune disorders may be related to the fact that the segment of the major histocompatibility complex that contains genes affecting reproduction also contains genes associated with various autoimmune disorders. Diabetes mellitus has been linked at least in part to a functional deficit of hypothalamic noradrenergic neurons, and cystic fibrosis has been connected to congenital bilateral absence of the vas deferens.

CLINICAL PRESENTATION

Ideally, both members of the couple are present for the initial interview; this is invaluable not only for the comprehensiveness of the medical history but also for providing insight into the couple's communication and decision-making style, emotional status, ability to support each other, coping strategies, and current level of functioning. Subsequent interviews with either partner alone may reveal information (e.g., previous pregnancies, abortions, or infections) that the individual is not comfortable disclosing otherwise. Essential components of relevant history to be elicited include coital frequency and timing, duration of the couple's infertility, previous pregnancy or siring of children, and age, because these factors have been consistently demonstrated to affect the prognosis.

Other relevant historical information includes a thorough obstetric and gynecologic history (contraceptive use, prior pregnancy, therapeutic abortion, miscarriage, infection, pathologic conditions, or procedures). Particular attention is given to the menstrual history for cues related to ovulatory cycles, including midcycle discomfort, regular menses, premenstrual symptoms, and periods that occur every 27 to 30 days. The past medical history focuses on infections, surgeries, medications, and developmental, systemic, and autoimmune disorders. Family history is assessed for relatives with infertility or early menopause, autoimmune disorders such as lupus, and maternal diethylstilbestrol (DES) exposure. A review of systems may reveal weight changes; signs of estrogen deficiency or excess; signs of thyroid imbalance; hyperandrogenism or virilism; hyposmia (which may be related to Kallmann syndrome); or signs of galactorrhea, headaches, or visual disturbances (which are possibly suggestive of a pituitary pathologic condition).

Social history should include patterns of smoking, use of alcohol or other substances such as caffeine, exercise patterns, level of stress and coping strategies, potential eating disorders, and frequency of intercourse. Occupational history may reveal a host of potential reproductive threats, including the prolonged waiting time to pregnancy observed in female shift workers. Laboratory workers, health care workers (including anesthetists, dental assistants, and hospital personnel), farmers, painters, and construction workers may be exposed to reproductive toxins such as lead, nitrous oxide, waste anesthetic gases, and solvents. Domestic exposures include recent home renovation, contaminated air or ground water, and domestic pesticide use. Various population-based studies have failed to find a correlation between consanguinity (uncle-niece, first cousins, and first-degree cousins once removed) and primary sterility. Infertility has also been shown not to be related to prior cervical laser surgery.

PHYSICAL EXAMINATION

Examination of the male partner includes inspection of the genitals for abnormalities, including phimosis, varicocele (the most commonly identified genital abnormality in subfertile men), and hypospadias. The bilateral presence of the vas deferens is established, and the testes are palpated for maldescent, consistency, and size. Decreased testicular size is related to impaired spermatogenesis; the length of the testes (measured in a warm room, after the patient has been standing for several minutes) should be more than 4 cm (1⅗ inches) and the volume more than 20 mL by orchidometry.

Physical examination of the female partner includes palpation of the thyroid; breast examination to check for galactorrhea; and evaluation of signs of hypoestrogenic status (dry, pale vaginal mucosa), androgen excess (hirsutism, male pattern hair loss, acne, obesity), or virilization (changes in body fat distribution, a lowering of the voice, or clitoromegaly). A pelvic examination also provides a gross indication of the state of the reproductive organs and may detect enlarged ovaries or other masses such as uterine fibroids. Changes in visual acuity or visual fields may be indicative of a cranial (pituitary) mass.

DIAGNOSTICS

Considerable debate surrounds the selection and interpretation of diagnostic studies in the context of a basic fertility workup because of the difficulty in establishing cutoff points for "abnormal" findings of investigations such as semen analysis and the demonstrated inability of many analyses to differentiate between fertile and infertile individuals. Complicating the issue is the likelihood that many couples have a constellation of factors, such as varicoceles and low-normal sperm count; although each may be relatively insignificant in isolation, they combine synergistically to produce clinical infertility.

According to World Health Organization guidelines, semen analysis should be performed early in the evaluation, after 36 to 48 hours of abstinence. National guidelines from England and the U.S. Institute for Clinical Systems Improvement suggest repeated semen analysis after 4 months if the first test result was normal and there has been no intervening pregnancy. If semen analysis indicates oligospermia, follicle-stimulating hormone (FSH) and testosterone levels should be obtained before referral to a male infertility specialist; if the serum testosterone level is low or the patient has other symptoms of hypogonadism (decreased libido or potency), a prolactin level should also be obtained. Testicular volume assessment with an orchidometer combined with basal serum FSH level can also be used to estimate future fertility in individuals who are long-term survivors of malignant disease in childhood or adolescence. The postcoital test (PCT) has received mixed reviews in the literature and is generally not recommended. It can be useful to confirm that intercourse has taken place, but it has poor sensitivity, specificity, positive predictive value, and negative predictive value. Although tests for sperm DNA fragmentation are available, they are not yet recommended in best-practice guidelines from the American Society for Reproductive Medicine (ASRM) and the European Society of Human Reproduction and Embryology (ESHRE).[17]

Although the only definitive proof of ovulation in a particular cycle remains a subsequent pregnancy, ovulatory assessment has traditionally been done with menstrual calendars (a cycle normal in duration and frequency is suggestive of ovulation), and basal body temperature charting (biphasic curve demonstrating a consistently raised temperature in the latter half of the cycle is one of the simplest, most inexpensive, and most practical ways to assess ovulatory function, but the resultant curves can be difficult to interpret.). Urinary LH can identify the LH surge that precedes ovulation by 1 or 2 days, and kits are available for home use. Such home testing, especially when done with an afternoon or evening urine sample, correlates well with peak serum LH. A plasma midluteal progesterone concentration higher than 3 ng/mL on day 21, or about 1 week before the expected onset of the next menses, is presumptive of ovulation but cannot assess the quality of the luteal phase. All female patients merit a rubella titer (if indicated), cervical cytology (Papanicolaou test), and *Chlamydia* culture or serum antibody. Evaluation of tubal patency is most commonly done by hysterosalpingography and can even be therapeutic in that women have been known to conceive soon after this procedure. For women older than 35 years, a day-3 FSH level and an estradiol level are indicated to assess ovarian reserve (elevated day-3 FSH levels indicate a poorer outcome with assisted reproductive technologies [ARTs]). Additional laboratory assessment is indicated by the patient's history and physical examination findings and is not warranted for all women concerned about their fertility, especially those with regular menstrual cycles. These tests include prolactin and thyroid assays, testosterone, and dehydroepiandrosterone (DHEA) and 17-hydroxyprogesterone tests when indicated and clomiphene challenge or day-3 FSH to evaluate ovarian reserve. Anticardiolipin antibody, antiphospholipid antibody, and antinuclear antibody assessments can be performed to exclude lupus.

DIAGNOSTICS

Infertility

MEN

Laboratory

Semen analysis

Further Testing if Indicated

FSH
Testosterone level
Prolactin level
Hepatitis screen
Human immunodeficiency virus (HIV) infection
Testicular volume assessment

WOMEN

Laboratory

Chlamydia culture or serum antibody gonococcal culture

TO EVALUATE FOR AN ANOVULATORY DISORDER

FSH
LH
Prolactin
TSH
Estradiol

If Polycystic Ovary Syndrome or Nonclassic Congenital Adrenal Hyperplasia Is Suspected

Androgens (total testosterone, DHEA, 17-hydroxyprogesterone)

Other Testing if Indicated

Gonococcal culture
Pap test
Rubella titer
Purified protein derivative
Antiphospholipid antibody
Antinuclear antibody
Clomiphene stimulation test
DHEA
Erythrocyte sedimentation rate (ESR)
Hepatitis screen
HIV infection
Hysterosalpingography

DIFFERENTIAL DIAGNOSIS

A wide range of conditions can contribute to infertility and early pregnancy loss, including genetic, structural, and endocrine disorders; acquired infections (*Trichomonas, Chlamydia* organisms); treatment of other conditions with radiation therapy or chemotherapy; body mass index; personal behaviors such as alcohol consumption and maternal cigarette smoking; medications; sexual dysfunction; antisperm antibodies; previous genital or pelvic surgery; exposure to reproductive toxins; and other chronic medical diseases, such as thyroid dysfunction, celiac disease, inflammatory bowel disease, and hemochromatosis. Congenital causes include gonadal dysgenesis; chromosomal mosaicism; congenital bilateral absence of the vas deferens or the uterus; Klinefelter syndrome (small hard testes, gynecomastia); Turner syndrome (short stature, pigeon chest, webbed neck); deletions in the Y chromosome genes; and isolated corticotropin deficiency, which is rare but treatable. Male factors contributing to infertility are in general determined by semen analysis.

Ovulatory dysfunction can be attributable to hyperprolactinemia; hypogonadotropic hypogonadism (these women have

DIFFERENTIAL DIAGNOSIS

Infertility

- Genetic disorder
- Structural disorder
- Endocrine disorder
- Comorbid illness
- Infection
- Body mass index
- Exposures
  - Medications (including chemotherapy)
  - Alcohol
  - Smoking
  - Chemicals
  - Irrradiation
- Other
  - Antisperm antibody
  - Sexual dysfunction

decreased serum estradiol levels and no withdrawal bleeding after a progesterone challenge); hypergonadotropic hypogonadism (elevated FSH levels indicating premature ovarian failure and possible presence of Y chromosome in young women); and normogonadotropic anovulatory conditions, including polycystic ovary syndrome (PCOS; a hyperandrogenic condition often seen with acne, weight gain, hirsutism, or acanthosis nigricans when hyperinsulinemia is also contributing), luteal phase defects, and multifollicular ovaries.

The term *unexplained infertility* refers to a diagnosis of exclusion, one in which the findings of standard investigations (semen analysis, tests of ovulation, tubal patency) are normal; this accounts for roughly 30% to 40% of all infertile couples.[18,19]

MANAGEMENT

Although the provision of infertility services is beyond the scope of practice of most primary health care providers, they perform an important initial exploration of historical, physical examination, and selected diagnostic factors that can facilitate expedient referral to appropriate specialists when indicated. Individuals warranting an expedited workup and referral to a specialist include women without periods, with irregular periods, or with bleeding between periods as well as those who have pain with intercourse and a history of abdominal surgery, ruptured appendix, or upper genital tract infection. Men for whom similar expedited workup and referral are appropriate include those with difficulty sustaining an erection or an inability to ejaculate during intercourse and those with a history of testicular injury, infection, or maldescension.

1. Health care providers can intervene early in terms of improving modifiable lifestyle risk factors, improving coping mechanisms, providing basic preconception education and care such as updating immunization status,[20] and improving overall health for all patients who are attempting conception. General health-promoting interventions for the couple include normalizing weight, especially in overweight and obese individuals with PCOS[15]; improving nutritional status[21]; taking folate supplementation; reducing stress; and eliminating potential detrimental factors, such as cigarette smoking, caffeine, alcohol, nonsteroidal anti-inflammatory drugs,[22] illicit drugs, and exposure to potential reproductive toxins. These interventions, which may increase a couple's chances of attaining successful pregnancy, might also improve their psychological health.
2. Education regarding prognosis. Of all couples diagnosed as infertile in one prospective U.S. trial,[23] 28% of those untreated achieved pregnancy, and the rates were higher in all of the treatment modes—up to 85% in the first two cycles of medications, up to 71% in the first three intrauterine insemination (IUI) cycles, and 57% to 59% in the first two in vitro fertilization (IVF) cycles. For all of these cycle-based treatment modalities, there was a diminishing return of efficacy as treatments continued beyond this point. In a European longitudinal multicenter cohort study, most couples (81%) diagnosed with unexplained infertility achieved an ongoing pregnancy, and the majority of these pregnancies (nearly 74%) were spontaneous.[24] Prognosis is more encouraging for shorter duration of infertility (less than 3 years), for younger women, and for those who have previously conceived a child in the same relationship. Prognosis is worse for situations involving endometriosis, male factor infertility, and tubal pathologic conditions or multiple factors.
3. It is essential from the outset to reinforce with any couple seeking treatment that appropriately directed therapy, excluding advanced reproductive technologies, is unsuccessful up to 50% of the time. Expectant management for unexplained infertility (encouraging couples to have intercourse during the "fertile window," roughly 5 days before until the day of ovulation) can be an effective strategy, especially for younger women with a shorter duration of infertility.[15] More elaborate ARTs, such as IVF and the newer intracytoplasmic sperm injection along with donor gametes and surrogacy, may provide hope for pregnancy otherwise unattainable through more conventional means. However, these approaches can be expensive[25] (upwards of $10,000 for a single IVF cycle) and risky,[26] and their use often raises moral and ethical dilemmas.
4. Any treatment plan should follow a full discussion of all possible treatment options, including adoption, child-free living without intervention of any kind, and the possibility of stopping at any time in the treatment process. Discussion must address attendant benefits, risks, time required for participation, and costs along with reasonable estimations of probability for achieving pregnancy based on relevant infertility factors both with and without treatment.
5. Ongoing counseling for the couple should be offered and encouraged. Counseling may help the couple discontinue treatment when appropriate, solicit second opinions, participate in support groups, establish a (necessarily arbitrary) time limit for treatment, and take time off from treatment to give them a sense of control and balance in their lives.

Pharmacologic Therapy

1. When infertility is a result of hypothalamic-pituitary insufficiency in the male partner (as is the case in 1% to 2% of couples with male factor infertility), these men often respond well to gonadotropin or GnRH therapy.
2. Induction of ovulation according to a variety of protocols involving gonadotropins has been used for hypogonadotropic hypogonadism in women.
3. Chronic opiate agonist administration (naltrexone) can normalize ovarian function for women with hypothalamic ovarian failure.
4. Bromocriptine or other, newer dopamine agonists, such as cabergoline, are indicated in the treatment of hyperprolactinemia.
5. Metformin is a reasonable first-line intervention for nonobese women with anovulatory PCOS.[27,28]
6. Antiestrogens such as clomiphene citrate and tamoxifen are used for the induction of ovulation in women with POPS, and Chinese herbal medicine has shown some promise in increasing the efficacy of clomiphene citrate therapy.[29]
7. Estrogen replacement for women with hypergonadotropic hypogonadism is important to prevent osteoporosis; ovulation-inducing therapies are neither useful nor indicated for these women.
8. For women with chemotherapy-induced ovarian failure, ovarian function should be reassessed periodically because spontaneous recovery has been noted.
9. Pharmacologic management of unexplained infertility[15,24] is by definition empirical; clomiphene, human menopausal gonadotropin, and various ART procedures are often used in these cases.

10. ARTs include such technologies as gamete intrafallopian transfer (GIFT), IVF, direct intraperitoneal injection of sperm, intrafollicular injection of sperm, and preimplantation genetic diagnosis. The induction of superovulation is often followed by artificial insemination of some kind; success is highly influenced by the woman's age, with cycle fecundity dropping from an average of 0.23% to 0.05% after the age of 40 years.

Women or men being managed by specialists for infertility still require basic primary care services. This enables the health care provider to assess and to intervene on behalf of the couple's functional, emotional, and psychospiritual responses to continuing therapy. Somatization is a common manifestation of the psychological stress of infertility, as are sexual problems, depressive reactions, emotional instability, relationship difficulties, and reduced self-confidence and self-esteem as well as feelings of anger, guilt, grief, isolation, and anxiety.

LIFE SPAN CONSIDERATIONS

A cultural tendency to delay childbearing combined with decreased fecundability with increasing age[30] necessitates prompt investigation into infertility in certain cases. According to the ASRM, an infertility evaluation is warranted after 1 year of coital exposure for couples in which the woman is younger than 35 years and after 6 months when she is older than 35 years. Immediate referral is reasonable for women older than age 40 or for men with suspected male factor infertility. Future fertility preservation for young men faced with a diagnosis of cancer can be assisted with sperm banking procedures.[10]

COMPLICATIONS

In general, women with PCOS do not respond to ovulation induction as well as women with other ovulatory disorders do, and have an increased risk of ovarian hyperstimulation and spontaneous abortion when they do respond. Women with fibroids have a lower implantation rate with ART, women with endometriosis have a decreased pregnancy rate after ART procedures than do controls, and women 40 years of age or older have a higher risk for cesarean delivery after infertility treatment that is independent of other risk factors. Women who conceive with ART are more likely than their naturally conceiving counterparts to enter pregnancy with a chronic condition (such as diabetes or incompetent cervix) and to develop complications during pregnancy (pregnancy-induced hypertension, gestational diabetes mellitus, uterine bleeding), labor, and delivery.[11] Infants born after ART procedures are also at increased risk of adverse health outcomes (preterm delivery, very preterm delivery, low birth weight, infant not discharged home).[11] Other infertility treatment–related complications include a controversial association between fertility drugs and ovarian cancer and the protracted psychic anguish that can accompany successive failed treatment cycles.

The incidence and risks of multiple gestations associated with ARTs have been well documented in the literature; ART births are 18 times more likely to be twin, triplet, or higher-order births.[11] Twins that are the result of IVF also have an increased rate of preterm birth compared with spontaneously conceived twin controls.[12] (For all initial numbers of fetuses in an ART-induced multifetal pregnancy, including twins, reduction to a lower number decreases subsequent fetal loss, prematurity, and infant morbidity and mortality.[13]) Even resultant singleton pregnancies represent obstetric risks (given an increased incidence of pregnancy-induced hypertension, placenta previa, elective cesarean delivery, and preterm labor), an increased risk for major malformation, and a lower mean birth weight in ART pregnancies. Although the medical problems associated with ART-assisted multiple gestations have been widely emphasized in the medical literature, several studies note a desire among fertility patients for multiple births[14]; one study found that 67% to 90% of infertile couples expressed a desire for twins, and the majority of these couples rejected concerns about multiple gestations.[15] In another study, a significant proportion (41%) of fertility patients considered multiple birth an ideal treatment outcome.[16] This clearly indicates a need for additional education about the risks and complications associated with ARTs.

INDICATIONS FOR REFERRAL OR HOSPITALIZATION

Referral to a reproductive urologist is indicated for male factors identified on semen analysis. Referral to a reproductive endocrinologist or fertility specialist is indicated for an abnormal PCT result, for a basic infertility workup that does not disclose the source of the problem, or for any of the various ART procedures, should they be a couple's only hope for conception. Couples interested in exploring complementary therapeutic options may find some success with acupuncture.[17] Pathologic conditions, including adhesiolysis and various testicular, uterine, or tubal conditions, may require surgical repair. In addition, complications from therapy (moderate to severe ovarian hyperstimulation syndrome) may necessitate hospitalization.

PATIENT AND FAMILY EDUCATION

Infertility and its often unsuccessful medical treatment present a conglomerate of stresses and losses with which the couple must contend, including the loss of biologic children and the experiences of pregnancy and breastfeeding. Individuals endure the stresses of complicated, expensive, and invasive treatment interventions, which can be experienced as humiliating, embarrassing, frustrating, and disappointing for women and their partners. Adjusting to infertile status is easier for individuals with positive self-esteem, an internal locus of control, and higher socioeconomic status, whereas increased anxiety and distress have been associated with advancing age, undifferentiated sex role identity, and low self-esteem. In one study, pregnant women with a history of infertility were at increased risk for alcohol abuse and were more likely to experience psychiatric disorders (phobia, generalized anxiety, bulimia, major depression, and panic disorder).[17]

Motives for medical consultation by infertile couples, in addition to the desire to have a child, include a desire for education and understanding regarding the cause of the infertility. Health care providers should be aware of a potential disparity between the medical diagnosis and the perception of the diagnosis in infertile persons, along with a tendency for patients to blame themselves for the infertility. Basic education for infertile persons includes advising them to have intercourse about twice a week and to avoid lubricants that may be spermicidal, such as K-Y Jelly, petroleum jelly, and Surgilube. In contrast, raw egg white and vegetable oil do not seem to affect sperm motility. The provider should also encourage cessation of alcohol or illicit drug use, smoking cessation, proper nutrition, normalization of body mass index (especially for women), and strategies for stress reduction. Health care providers can also provide an initial infertility workup that focuses on explaining the various diagnostic procedures and addressing couples' concerns and questions as they arise. The ASRM website (www.asrm.org) is a good source of patient information.

It is particularly important to provide couples with an accurate estimation of the success rates that are expected for various procedures and the concordant risks, discomforts, and expenses. Unfortunately, there have been fewer randomized clinical trials in the area of infertility management than in other branches of medical science, and many studies have small sample sizes, inappropriate design, and pseudorandomization. For couples that are able to conceive with treatment, providers of primary care can stress the normalcy of the pregnancy and help the couple through the normative developmental processes of pregnancy and parenthood.

Because the length of time that a woman has been infertile is related to her future fecundability and because fertility decreases exponentially with increasing age, many infertile individuals confront the necessity of redefining their expectations and goals related to establishing a family. Providers play an important role in facilitating the grieving process for the many losses sustained throughout the experience of diagnosis and treatment. This process is important because it constitutes the experiential prerequisite to acceptance and is essential for the couple to move on with their lives. Many providers emphasize helping couples to determine their own end point and timeline for intervention attempts, because there always seems to be some promising or potential development around the corner. Clinician support can enforce an "unsuccessful" couple's eventual realization that they have been thorough and have tried sufficient therapeutic interventions and that cessation of such interventions is reasonable and advisable. Couples can then be supported in their efforts to plan their lives in ways that may include consideration of adoption or child-free living as valid alternatives to biologic parenthood.

CHAPTER 165

MENOPAUSE

Diane C. Seibert • Diane Pace

Like the onset of menstruation (menarche), menopause is a normal life event that every woman will experience if she lives past age 50. Unlike the onset of puberty, in many women the hormonal and physiologic changes associated with menopause are superimposed on disorders that manifest primarily in older adults, many of which can be traced to a complex mix of genetic predisposition, environmental exposures, health care access, and long-standing lifestyle choices. During midlife, many women experience significant psychological and social changes; adult children may begin families of their own, and aging parents may need help and support, all of which can adversely affect physical, emotional, social, and financial well-being. To optimize quality of life and health outcomes, providers need to consider all of these factors when developing an individualized care plan for women at or after midlife.

DEFINITION AND EPIDEMIOLOGY

Menopause is the final step in a series of reproductive stages in a woman's life that began decades earlier when she was a 4-week old embryo. At that time, several primordial germ cells (PGCs) split off from the female embryo and begin dividing as they migrated through the embryonic gut, eventually finding their way to the ovary at approximately 16 weeks' gestation. Unlike somatic cells, which form the rest of the human body, PGCs have the unique ability to divide by both mitosis (up to 5 million copies are made of the initial PGCs) and later by meiosis, wherein the cells are "frozen" in prophase 1 (dictyotene), entering a form of suspended animation that may last years or even decades, until ovulation.[1] At birth, a female infant will have approximately 2 million viable oocytes because 1 million will already have degraded. By the time she has her first menstrual period, the number of viable oocytes will have dropped to around 500,000, and she will enter menopause when the final oocyte degrades and disappears, typically at age 52.5. Atresia (cell death and degeneration) is responsible for the loss of almost all of the ova that disappear during a woman's life. Although the rate varies from woman to woman, the decline in the number as well as the quality of follicles is linear until approximately age 37, when atresia accelerates until menopause.[2]

As the number of functional ovarian follicles declines, levels of inhibin B fall and follicle-stimulating hormone (FSH) rises, which for a time sustains both follicular development and ovulatory function. The first clinically measurable sign of perimenopause therefore is a high FSH concentration (>10 IU/L) during the early follicular phase (days 2 to 5 of the menstrual cycle). Higher FSH levels may recruit relatively more follicles per cycle, possibly contributing to the acceleration of follicular atresia.[3] Overproduction of estradiol by this large cohort of recruited follicles may be responsible for many perimenopausal symptoms, including bloating, irritability, mastalgia, menorrhagia, uterine fibroid growth, vasomotor symptoms (VMSs), insomnia, migraines, and premenstrual syndrome (PMS) dysphoria.[4] Although rare, pregnancy is still possible late in the perimenopausal period and women are at risk for unplanned pregnancy until they have been amenorrheic for more than 1 year. Several terms associated with menopause are defined in Table 165-1.

The mean age at menarche in the United States has dropped steadily from the early 1800s and continues to decline in some populations,[5] but the age of onset of menopause has remained relatively stable for generations. The Study of Women's Health Across the Nation (SWAN) trial, which followed over 3000 women from multiple states and racial and ethnic groups, found that menopause occurred at age 52.54 years irrespective of racial or ethnic group, age of menarche, or number of lifetime pregnancies.[7] Some health and socioeconomic factors, such as self-rated health, higher body weight, lower physical activity levels, negative smoking history, prior oral contraceptive use, higher education level, and employment, were significantly associated with a later onset of menopause, suggesting that the onset of menopause is influenced by a number of factors, perhaps explaining some of the relationship between reduced morbidity and mortality in women who enter menopause later in life.[2]

Before 2001, there was no clear definition of menopause, nor was there a staging system to clearly communicate the physiologic changes occurring during the final 10 to 15 years of a

TABLE 165-1 Terms Related to Menopause

Term	Definition
Menopause	The permanent decline in gonadal hormone levels confirmed by 12 months of amenorrhea (12 months after final menstrual period [FMP]) in women with a uterus. The diagnosis can be established using other criteria including history of bilateral oophorectomy, symptoms, and/or serial measurement of endocrine markers.
Premenopause	The phase of life that precedes menopause.
Premenopausal	Relating to premenopause.
Postmenopause	The phase of life after menopause. The 2010 U.S. Census Bureau reported that nearly 40 million U.S. women were older than 55 years, past the age of natural menopause, which occurs at approximately ages 51-52 years years in the United States.
Postmenopausal	Relating to postmenopause.
Menopausal transition	Begins with the onset of intermenstrual cycle irregularities and/or other menopause-related symptoms and extends through menopause.
Perimenopause (sometimes called *climacteric*)	A clinically useful term that encompasses the most symptomatic years. Perimenopause begins with the onset of intermenstrual cycle irregularities and/or other menopause-related symptoms and extends beyond menopause to include the 12 months after menopause, thus lasting 1 year longer than the menopausal transition.
Early menopause, late menopause	Vague terms that have been used to describe menopause that occurs earlier or later than the normal range of menopause.
Premature menopause	Menopause that occurs before age 40. Approximately 1% of U.S. women experience premature natural menopause, so of the 49 million U.S. women who were projected to be age 15 to 44 years in 2015, approximately 490,000 would have experienced premature natural menopause.[6]
Primary ovarian insufficiency or failure	Hypergonadotropic hypogonadism in a woman younger than age 40 years.
Induced menopause	Cessation of menstruation after either surgical removal of both ovaries (the most common cause) or iatrogenic ablation of ovarian function (by chemotherapy or pelvic radiation therapy).
Premature ovarian failure	The North American Menopause Society as well as the American Congress of Obstetricians and Gynecologists recommend that this term no longer be used.

Modified from *Menopause practice: a clinician's guide,* ed 5, Mayfield, OH, 2014, North American Menopause Society.

woman's reproductive life. Since that time, the Stages of Reproductive Aging Workshop (STRAW) has met twice, once in 2001 and again in 2011 (STRAW +10), to develop a clear and simple set of definitions and descriptions to simplify the criteria for menopausal bleeding.[8] Consistent use of the STRAW +10 criteria holds the promise of improving clinical decision-making by clearly articulating where a woman is along the continuum, and supporting research efforts because it offers a structure within which to compare studies conducted on women in midlife (Fig. 165-1).

The STRAW +10 criteria divide the perimenopause, menopause, and postmenopause periods into seven phases, five of which occur before the final menstrual period (FMP) and two of which occur after the FMP. As with every other developmental phase in life, individual variability is the norm, with some women moving rapidly through one or more stages, some skipping stages altogether, and some shifting back and forth between stages. In general, the transition through these 7 phases is predictable, but chronologic age does not accurately predict reproductive ability, so menopause should be included in the differential diagnosis whenever a woman reports menopausal symptoms. Because most American women will spend nearly one third of their lives in the postmenopausal period, the implications for women, clinicians, and the health care system are huge.

PHYSIOLOGY

Reproduction is controlled by a highly complex series of interactions among a number of different hormones. A complete discussion of all of them is beyond the scope of this chapter, but the structure and function of a few key hormones (estrogen, progestogen, androgens) are discussed here to provide a frame of reference for the management section, later.

In the early 1970s, estrogen's effects were believed to be primarily reproductive, having little effect on tissues outside the uterus and mammary glands. Over the past 40 years, however, evidence has revealed that estrogen exerts its effects on many organs. At least two distinct estrogen receptors (ER-α and ER-β) have been identified, both of which are present in ovarian and central nervous system (CNS) tissues. In other body tissues, however, one form or the other predominates. For example, ER-α is found in hepatic, uterine, and breast tissue, whereas ER-β is found in bone, blood vessels, lungs, and urogenital tissues.[9] Further complicating the estrogen picture, there are three known forms of human estrogens: estrone (E1), estradiol (E2), and estriol (E3). E1, the least abundant, is derived from stored body fat and is the primary estrogen in postmenopausal women. E2, produced by the ovarian follicle during the reproductive years, is the most potent and abundant (10% to 29%). E3, the least potent, predominates during pregnancy. Serum estradiol

	Menarche					FMP (0)				
Stage	–5	–4	–3b	–3a	–2	–1	+1a	+1b	+1c	+2
Terminology	**REPRODUCTIVE**				**MENOPAUSAL TRANSITION**		**POSTMENOPAUSE**			
	Early	Peak	Late		Early	Late	Early			Late
					Perimenopause					
Duration	*variable*				*variable*	1–3 years	2 years (1 + 1)		3–6 years	*Remaining lifespan*
PRINCIPAL CRITERIA										
Menstrual Cycle	Variable to regular	Regular	Regular	Subtle changes in Flow/ Length	*Variable Length* Persistent ≥7-day difference in length of consecutive cycles	Interval of amenorrhea of ≥60 days				
SUPPORTIVE CRITERIA										
Endocrine										
FSH			Low	Variable	↑ Variable	↑ >25 IU/L**	↑ Variable		Stabilizes	
AMH			Low	Low	Low	Low	Low		Very Low	
Inhibin B				Low	Low	Low	Low		Very Low	
Antral Follicle Count			Low	Low	Low	Low	Very Low		Very Low	
DESCRIPTIVE CHARACTERISTICS										
Symptoms						Vasomotor symptoms *Likely*	Vasomotor symptoms *Most Likely*			*Increasing* symptoms of urogenital atrophy

*Blood draw on cycle days 2–5 ↑ = elevated

**Approximate expected level based on assays using current international pituitary standard[67–69]

FIGURE **165-1** STRAW +10. (Menopause © 2012 The North American Menopause Society.)

levels vary widely during the menstrual cycle—below 10 pg/mL early in the follicular phase, then rising above 800 pg/mL at midcycle, then dropping back down to 200 to 340 pg/mL during the luteal phase. More than 95% of the circulating E2 is produced by the dominant follicle, and less than 5% is derived from peripheral conversion of E1.[9]

Progesterone, secreted during the luteal phase of the menstrual cycle, first appears right after ovulation and rises steadily for about 10 days before dropping back down to baseline if no pregnancy occurs. Normal progesterone levels range from 2 to 20 ng/mL depending on the day the level is drawn.[10]

There are five clinically important androgens in women: testosterone, dihydrotestosterone (DHT), androstenedione, dehydroepiandrosterone (DHEA), and dehydroepiandrosterone sulfate (DHEAS). Although often referred to as androgens, androstenedione, DHEAS, and DHEA are actually prohormones that are converted to active androgens in body tissues. DHEA in particular plays an important role in the production of ovarian testosterone. In reproductive-age women, a slight but significant rise in serum testosterone is measurable immediately before ovulation. Evaluating serum androgen levels can be challenging for several reasons. First, only 1% to 2% of testosterone is free to circulate because two thirds is bound to sex hormone–binding globulin (SHBG) and the remainder is bound to albumin, so changes in SHBG production or albumin levels can affect the amount of testosterone available to tissues.[11] Second, serum androgen levels do not accurately reflect the amount of androgens available to androgen-dependent or androgen-sensitive tissues such as the skin, the clitoris, or the vulva, because the ratio of plasma DHT levels to serum testosterone levels is low (0.3:1) whereas the ratio is much higher (2:1) in tissues where conversion from DHT to testosterone is actively occurring.[12]

Antimüllerian hormone (AMH) produced by the follicular granulosa cells plays an important role in follicle recruitment and selection and has recently been found to be a useful marker of ovarian reserve. After rising in adolescence and early adulthood, AMH levels gradually decline, becoming undetectable approximately 5 years before the FMP.[13] To date, AMH levels have primarily been used in infertility settings, but serial AMH levels may soon be used to predict the age of menopause.

The first sign that a woman is entering perimenopause (stage −3a) might be (but is not always) menstrual cycle changes. In response to declining ovarian reserve, inhibin B levels drop, and FSH levels rise to more aggressively stimulate the remaining follicles, and although the luteal phase of the cycle remains 14 days, the follicular phase shortens by 2 to 4 days, causing the overall cycle to become shorter (i.e., 25 to 26 days rather than 28 days).[8] The STRAW +10 staging illustrates this because stages −2 and −1 are characterized by significant menstrual cycle irregularity, reflecting the increasingly wide swings in hormonal levels and the increasingly frequent anovulatory cycles.

Although the FMP marks the onset of menopause, it is difficult to tell clinically when that FMP has occurred. No serum marker sensitive enough to definitively mark this transition has yet been identified, and a single assessment of several hormone levels (FSH, luteinizing hormone [LH], and estradiol, for example) is unreliable when trying to determine when the FMP has occurred. Recent large studies such as SWAN have found that using a combination of factors such as comparing E2 levels with a level drawn earlier in the perimenopausal period, race or ethnicity, and timing of the serum collection (early follicular phase) is a better predictor of the probability of a woman having had her FMP.[14] It is important to remember that although the STRAW +10 criterion of one episode of more than 60 consecutive days of amenorrhea is enough to consider a women older than 45 years in late menopausal transition, it is unreliable in women younger than 40 years who have prolonged (>120 days) episodes of amenorrhea, even when their FSH levels are in the menopausal range. These women should be evaluated for other causes of amenorrhea because once treated, many will resume regular menstruation and have had successful spontaneous pregnancies.[8]

RESEARCH AND CLINICAL TRIALS

The Coronary Drug Project (1966 to 1975) was the first clinical trial to examine whether estrogen would reduce mortality in men with a history of myocardial infarction (MI).[15] A total of 8341 men ages 30 to 64 participated in the study. They were randomly assigned to one of six treatment arms: 2.5 mg of conjugated equine estrogen (CEE) per day, 5.0 mg of CEE per day, 1.8 g of clofibrate per day, 6.0 mg of dextrothyroxine sodium per day, 3.0 g of niacin per day, or 3.8 g of lactose placebo per day. It is important to note that the doses (2.5 and 5 mg) of CEE are extremely high compared with doses (0.325 to 0.625 mg) prescribed today, and that CEE contains several different estrogenic compounds. The primary estrogen in CEE (>50%) is estrone, but the drug also contains equilin (15% to 25%), sodium sulfate conjugates, 17α-dihydroequilin, 17α-estradiol, and 17β-dihydroequilin—all target ERs in different body tissues. The estrogen arm was stopped prematurely because men taking 5 mg CEE had an early excess of heart attacks, thromboembolic events, and estrogenic symptoms, and men taking 2.5 mg CEE were experiencing no benefits. The study concluded that high-dose estrogen is not good for men, but it did not advance our understanding of the effects of estrogen in women.[15]

The first randomized prospective controlled trial examining the effects of estrogen in postmenopausal women began in 1965 and continued for 22 years. In this study, Nachtigall and her team randomized 84 matched pairs of chronically hospitalized women to placebo or hormone therapy (HT), exploring a wide array of clinical end points (MI, cancer, thromboembolism, gallbladder disease). During the first 10 years, the women were randomized to placebo or CEE 2.5 mg and medroxyprogesterone acetate (MPA) 10 mg, but during the final 12 years of the trial, the CEE dose was decreased to 0.625 mg and the women were permitted to stop or to switch groups. Overall, Nachtigall and her colleagues found that women taking CEE had a higher incidence of gallbladder disease, but there were no differences in MI, endometrial cancer, or thrombophlebitis between groups. Women taking hormones were found to have a decreased incidence of breast cancer (no cases in the HT group versus six cases in the placebo group).[16]

Since those early days, many large studies have been conducted exploring the impact of postmenopausal hormones on a variety of clinical end points, particularly cardiovascular health, osteoporosis, breast cancer, and colorectal cancer (CRC). The majority of the earlier observational and randomized clinical trials and meta-analyses found that standard-dose estrogen-alone HT decreased coronary heart disease (CHD) and all-cause mortality in women who were younger than age 60 and recently (within 10 years) menopausal. The data on combined estrogen-progestogen HT were not as compelling, however. Most studies examining the effect of combined HT on a number of different health outcomes did not find a significant increase or decrease in CHD.[17] Two large randomized controlled trials, the Heart and Estrogen/Progestin Replacement Study (HERS) and the Women's Health Initiative (WHI), were launched in the late 1990s to find answers to important questions about the impact of HT on the cardiovascular system.

HERS, a two-phase, randomized, blinded, placebo-controlled trial of continuous-combined estrogen-progestogen (refers to either progesterone or progestin) therapy (EPT) in postmenopausal women, was designed to determine whether combined EPT (CEE plus MPA) altered the number of cardiovascular disease (CVD) events in postmenopausal women with established CHD. The study was almost terminated early because women in the treatment arm (receiving HT) experienced more cardiac events during the first year of hormone use than the placebo group did. After the first year, however, this difference in risk reversed and women receiving HT were found to have experienced slightly fewer CVD events overall. To see whether this trend toward fewer CVD events continued, the study was extended for 3 additional years (HERS II), but no continuing CVD benefit was found. The HERS study clearly demonstrated that HT does not provide CVD protection in women with established heart disease, and during the first year of HT use, women with existing heart disease were at increased risk for cardiac events. The authors postulated that the estrogen's prothrombotic, arrhythmic, and ischemic effects during the first year counteracted any improvement in lipids.[18]

The WHI was a large multicenter, multiyear trial consisting of three interrelated randomized, blinded, placebo-controlled hormone trials and an observational study designed to examine the risks and benefits of HT in healthy postmenopausal women aged 50 to 79. Women with a uterus were assigned to the EPT arm and women without a uterus were assigned to the estrogen therapy (ET)–only arm. Participants were then randomly assigned to receive either the appropriate HT or a placebo. Before the study began, researchers identified two major clinical outcomes (CVD and invasive breast cancer), six minor outcomes (stroke, pulmonary embolism, endometrial cancer, CRC, hip fracture, and death from other causes), and a global index (a number reflecting the balance of risks and benefits).[19] The EPT arm was terminated 3 years early, in July 2002, because the global index rose above a predetermined risk threshold. Although the absolute risk of harm was very small and there was no difference in the number of deaths between the EPT and placebo groups, the trend toward increasing risk could not be ignored. The ET group continued to the projected end point because the global index threshold was not crossed.

Overall, the WHI demonstrated that the health risks and benefits of HT vary depending on the type of hormones used (estrogen or EPT), the age of the woman, and how remote from menopause a woman is when she begins taking them. Systemic HT has been shown to reduce moderate to severe menopausal symptoms and decrease fracture risk. Although the absolute risk for harm was very low, the WHI clearly showed that both estrogen and EPT increased the risk for developing venous thromboemboli (and associated disorders such as stroke and CVD), although the risk of ischemic stroke was rare in the 50- to 59-year age group.[20] The risks and benefits for other health outcomes at different ages varied. After 5 years or more of continuous use of EPT, the study found an increased risk of breast cancer, which decreased after the HT was discontinued. This was not found in the estrogen-alone group even after 7 years of follow-up. Counseling women about the risks and benefits of HT is complex; the evidence shows that although HT is helpful and appropriate for managing menopausal symptoms in some women, HT should not be used for chronic disease prevention. For a detailed summary of the final WHI findings, see the article by Manson.[19]

CLINICAL PRESENTATION

The clinical presentation and symptoms of menopause may vary significantly from one woman to another depending on the woman's age and underlying health status. Some manifestations such as VMSs are clearly associated with menopause, but others such as sexual dysfunction are much more elusive. Management of symptoms in women at midlife must therefore be considered in the context of healthy aging, because age is a confounder for symptoms and diseases that may be associated with or directly affected by menopausal management. The primary driver for the physiologic changes associated with menopause is the dramatic decline in estrogen levels, causing a number of short- and long-term physical changes including cycle irregularity, VMSs (hot flashes), urogenital atrophy (vaginal dryness, urinary incontinence, pelvic floor dysfunction), mood changes, and poor sleep and sexual functioning.

Irregular Bleeding

Abnormal uterine bleeding (AUB) is the most frequently reported perimenopausal symptom, with nearly 90% of women reporting 4 to 8 years of menstrual cycle changes before experiencing their FMP. Although some women experience fewer cycles with lighter bleeding during the menopausal transition, many women seek medical assistance for prolonged or heavy menstrual bleeding (HMB), which can cause significant anemia, avoidance of activities, including sexual intercourse, and a diminished quality of life.[21] Early in the menopausal transition, cycle irregularities are caused by disruption of the communications among the hypothalamus, pituitary, and ovaries, but as the FMP approaches, anovulation becomes more common, increasing the risk for unopposed estrogen exposure, endometrial hyperplasia, and cancer. Although most perimenopausal women with heavy or irregular bleeding do not have anatomic pathology, common causes of HMB such as thyroid dysfunction, pituitary adenoma, cervical polyps, uterine fibroids, endometriosis, and endometrial hyperplasia or cancer should be ruled out before attributing the cycle changes to the menopausal transition.

Depending on the clinical presentation, a comprehensive AUB workup could include laboratory tests to rule out pregnancy and sexually transmitted infections, hematologic parameters (complete blood count, liver function, coagulation profile), and serum hormone levels (thyroid, prolactin, FSH, estradiol, progesterone, testosterone, and DHEAS). Depending on these results, additional procedures might include endometrial biopsy and/or dilation and curettage, transvaginal ultrasonography, hysteroscopy, or sonohysterography.

AUB can be managed medically, hormonally, and/or surgically, and treatment should be individualized based on the severity of the AUB, the impact of the bleeding on a woman's quality of life, her personal preferences and contraceptive needs, and her overall health status. Often the first therapy tried is medical management, which includes nonsteroidal anti-inflammatories, tranexamic acid, and desmopressin (for women with underlying bleeding disorders). Medical management is often combined with hormonal management, which includes gonadotropin-releasing hormone (GnRH) agonists, oral progestogens and contraceptive options such as low-dose oral contraceptive pills, depot MPA, and levonorgestrel-releasing intrauterine devices (IUDs). Referral for consideration of surgical options (endometrial ablation, polypectomy, myomectomy, and/or hysterectomy) is usually reserved for women who have anatomic pathology such as fibroids, endometrial hyperplasia, and cervical disorders such as dysplasia and polyps, and procedures are tailored to treat those specific conditions.[21]

Vasomotor Symptoms

VMSs, considered the hallmark of the female climacteric, are characterized by vasomotor instability, hot flashes, day sweats, and night sweats. As many as 75% of perimenopausal and postmenopausal women report experiencing VMSs for 6 months to 2 years, although some women will report having hot flashes for more than 10 years. The peak incidence of hot flashes is within 2 years of the FMP,[22] but the physiologic mechanisms are still not completely understood. The term *hot flash* is used to describe the sudden onset of head, neck, and chest flushing, accompanied by a feeling of intense body heat, profuse perspiration, and modest heart rate increases that lasts generally from 1 to 5 minutes. Often as skin temperatures return to normal, there are decreases in core body temperatures with significant heat loss resulting in chills for some women. According to the SWAN study, the prevalence of hot flashes differs across U.S. racial and ethnic groups. Within this study of over 15,000 women, black women reported VMSs most frequently, followed by Hispanic, white, Chinese, and Japanese women.[22] Other variables for increasing VMS include obesity, low socioeconomic status, and surgically induced menopause. Factors such as depression, history of depression, anxiety, perceived stress, and poor physical health have also been associated with a higher risk. Higher education levels appear to be somewhat protective, but other factors, such as age, current smoking, alcohol use, and employment status do not appear to be significantly associated with an increased risk for developing severe VMSs.[23] Conditions such as thyroid disease, infection, insulinoma, pheochromocytoma, autoimmune disorders, new-onset hypertension, diabetes, and autonomic dysfunction may also cause hot flashes and should be considered if appropriate in the differential diagnosis.[22]

Fluctuating hormone levels are associated with hot flashes. Although there have been numerous research studies and theories developed regarding the causes of hot flashes, specific mechanisms or brain areas involved in thermogenesis and heat perception are still being explored and more research is needed.[22]

Mild to moderate hot flashes can often be managed with lifestyle changes, such as getting regular exercise; wearing layers of light clothing; lowering the thermostat; avoiding spicy foods, caffeine, or alcohol; and engaging in relaxation exercises. If medical management is necessary, ET is both the primary indication and most effective treatment for VMSs, and every systemic ET and estrogen-progestogen therapy (EPT) product has received regulatory agency (U.S. Food and Drug Administration [FDA]) approval for vasomotor instability. Estrogen options include systemic estrogen; combination products including combined estrogen-progestogen or estrogen/bazedoxifene (BZA); a selective estrogen receptor modulator (SERM) combined with conjugated estrogen; or combined oral contraceptives (in women requiring contraception).[21] Other therapies available for women who either cannot or do not want to take HT include low-dose, 7.5-mg paroxetine (Brisdelle), which received FDA approval for treatment of vasomotor flushes. Some options that do not have FDA approval for this indication include clonidine; and gabapentin. In addition, some antidepressants (e.g., venlafaxine, escitalopram) have been shown to be helpful for VMSs.[21] Many herbal or alternative remedies including soy, isoflavone supplements, black cohosh, vitamin E, and omega-3 fatty acids are popular and generally low risk, but none has been proven to be significantly more effective than placebo, and some may be harmful.[21] Clinical trials on a new supplement, Relizen, available in Europe for more than 10 years and introduced in the United States for management of VMSs, suggest that it improves symptoms and is an effective nonestrogenic alternative to HT.[24] Refer to the North American Menopause Society (NAMS) resources for a list of products and complementary and alternative options.

Genitourinary Syndrome of Menopause

Vulvovaginal Atrophy. Vulvovaginal atrophy (VVA) refers to changes in the vagina and vulva that develop during the postmenopausal period as a result of declining estrogen levels in these tissues. VVA is a chronic, progressive disorder that often causes significant discomfort and worsens without treatment.[25] The vagina may be narrow and less elastic, with thin, pale, dry, or inflamed side walls with petechia. As a result of these changes, women with VVE often report dryness, burning, irritation, vaginal pain, and dyspareunia. These changes may be seen throughout the genitourinary tract. As many as half of midlife and older women may experience urinary symptoms such as frequency, urgency, dysuria, and recurrent urinary tract infections.[21]

Two large studies—Vaginal Health: Insights, Views and Attitudes (VIVA) and Real Women's View of Treatment Options for Menopausal Vaginal Changes (REVIVE)—examined the impact of VVA on women, and found that VVA negatively affects women's lives, lowers their quality of life, and has negative consequences on their sexual health.[26,27] The REVIVE survey also noted that women reported that few health care practitioners had had any conversations with them about VVA, prompting the need for clinicians to initiate this conversation with patients before the onset of symptoms, to assess for early clinical changes, and to discuss options for preventing and/or treating this disorder.

Not only did these surveys point out that clinicians are reluctant to initiate discussions about VVA, but medical societies and others have noted that the media and the general public are uncomfortable with using the term *vagina* in public discourse, and the term *atrophy* has a negative connotation for many women.[25] Given that the term *VVA* does not include the anatomic areas of the urinary tract that are also affected by estrogen deficiency of menopause, a panel was convened in 2012 to discuss the need for more acceptable terminology to replace VVA. Two large societies, NAMS and the International Society for the Study of Women's Sexual Health (ISSWSH), acknowledged that a new term was needed that would be more "scientifically accurate, descriptive, inclusive, and socially acceptable." The term *genitourinary syndrome of menopause* (GSM) was adopted by both organizations. It is anticipated that this term will be accepted by other professional societies, providers, researchers, educators, women, and the media and will improve communication, research, education, and the treatment in this area of women's health.[25]

GSM should be evaluated and interventions individualized for each woman as appropriate based on her symptoms and how these symptoms may be creating distress. Nonhormonal over-the-counter (OTC) lubricants and moisturizer products are often first-line therapies for symptoms of vaginal dryness and to reduce friction on atrophic tissue during sexual activity. Regular sexual activity or nonpenetrative sexual activity through use of oral stimulation or self-stimulation with massage promotes blood flow to the genital area and helps to maintain vaginal health. For symptoms requiring intervention for severe symptoms, including dyspareunia, minimally absorbed vaginal low-dose ET is the treatment of choice for women who have no medical contraindications to its use. Benefits of low-dose vaginal estrogen include restoration of vaginal blood flow, a decrease in vaginal pH, and improvement in the thickness and elasticity of the tissues. The FDA has also approved ospemifene, an oral SERM, for the treatment of moderate to severe dyspareunia associated with VVA.[22]

Central Nervous System Effects

Mood Changes. Mood disorders (particularly depression) are nearly twice as common in women as in men. Recent randomized, controlled trials have demonstrated that the hormone shifts associated with menopause can significantly increase the risk for new-onset and recurrent depression. It does not appear to be the estrogen alone, however, because a number of menopausal symptoms are independent risk factors for depression, including VMSs, insomnia, severe premenstrual or postpartum mood swings and depression, stressful life events, history of depression, high body mass index, low socioeconomic status, and hormone or antidepressant use. Estrogen helps modulate several neurotransmitter pathways, particularly serotonin and norepinephrine, helping to regulate mood. Studies have also shown that transdermal estrogen and serotonergic and noradrenergic antidepressants relieve both mood and VMSs.[28] If depressive symptoms appear when a woman begins taking HT, the provider should examine the type of HT being used. Progestogens have been shown to worsen mood in some women, particularly those with a history of PMS, premenstrual depressive disorder, or clinical depression.

Insomnia. Insomnia may occur in association with or independent of hot flashes, and HT has been shown to provide substantial relief for early morning waking, even in women without significant VMSs. The irritability that so often accompanies insomnia also responds positively to HT. Women receiving HT have been shown to have shorter sleep latency and more frequent and prolonged rapid eye movement sleep.

Sexual Functioning. Decline in sexual activity during the menopausal years is probably influenced more by culture and attitudes than by nature and physiology. Significant determinants of sexual activity for older women are the availability and health status of a sexual partner.[29] Data from the PRESIDE (Prevalence of Female Sexual Problems Associated with Distress and Determinants of Treatment Seeking) study point out, however, that sexual problems are reported by approximately 40% of U.S. women and peak in women at midlife.[30] Psychological, sociocultural, interpersonal, and biologic factors occurring at midlife also contribute to sexual issues at midlife.[22] Changes in mood and well-being and untreated anxiety or depression may have an effect on sexual disorders associated with menopause. Low estrogen levels at menopause often leading to GSM, also have been associated with a decline in sexual function. Although testosterone is an important factor in midlife sexual changes for women, playing a role in motivation, desire, and sexual sensation, an association between decreased androgen levels and impaired female sexual function is not clearly supported in the evidence.[22]

Taking a sexual history can facilitate a discussion on sexuality and sexual health, addressing the woman's concerns and identifying any potential issues such as intimate partner violence or risk for acquiring a sexually transmitted infection. The online handout *Talking to Patients About Sexuality and Sexual Health* published by the Association of Reproductive Health Professionals provides a good reference guide for clinicians.[31]

CHRONIC DISEASE

With rare exceptions, menopause occurs as women enter late midlife, when many of the disorders associated with the aging process emerge. Estrogen has been shown to improve quality of life and to reduce risk for some diseases associated with aging. More recently, estrogen has been shown to increase risk for adverse outcomes from some diseases in some women. The question for clinicians is how to best manage menopausal symptoms while maintaining optimal health in older women. To address these important questions, NAMS has published a series of position statements to help inform and guide clinicians in the management of midlife women.[32] In addition, in October 2014 NAMS published its most current guidelines, the North American Menopause Society Recommendations for Clinical Care of Midlife Women.[21] This 25-page publication is a wonderful resource for clinicians because it both identifies key points and provides clinical recommendations to assist in optimizing health for older women.

The disorders that are of most concern to clinicians working with menopausal women include CVD (venous thromboembolism [VTE], stroke, and CHD), osteoporosis, atrophic vaginitis, cognitive decline (Alzheimer dementia [AD]), and certain cancers (endometrial, breast, ovarian, lung, and colorectal), all of which are described here. A brief discussion of the disease is followed by what is known about the risks and benefits of HT for that particular condition.

Cardiovascular Disease

Cardiovascular disease is a broad term encompassing three distinct but related disorders: CHD, stroke, and VTE. According to the World Health Organization (WHO), in 2008 more than 7.3 million people died from CHD and another 6.2 million died from a stroke, making CVD responsible for more deaths worldwide than any other condition.[33] The classic description of MI (heart attack) often includes chest, left arm, or jaw pain or pressure, but many women are not aware that other, more atypical symptoms such as pain at rest, shortness of breath, nausea, and fatigue may be more common presenting manifestations in women. It is important, therefore, for health care providers to not dismiss a woman's reports of chest pain, fatigue, or shortness of breath as benign or noncardiac in nature.

Osteoporosis

Osteoporosis is a serious and disabling disease that has become a major public health problem as the American population has aged. A study by the National Osteoporosis Foundation (NOF) estimates that 10.2 million Americans currently have osteoporosis and another 43.4 million have osteopenia. Assuming that disease prevalence is unchanged. It is predicted that within 5 years, the number of Americans affected by this disease will increase from 54 million (nearly half of all adults) to 64.4 million, and that by 2030, 71.2 million people will be affected. Osteoporosis is a major risk factor for fracture, and the NOF estimated that in 2014 approximately 2 million fractures could have been attributed to the disease.[34] Osteoporosis is often site specific, affecting the femur, hip, spine, and forearm, but not necessarily uniformly in the same woman; one woman might have osteoporosis of the spine but normal bone density in the femoral neck, whereas another woman may have osteopenia in both areas. As the incidence of osteoporosis increases, so does the incidence of pathologic fracture. Interestingly, after adjusting for age and gender, the relative death rates after fractures sustained in severe trauma were lower than the death rates associated with pathologic fractures sustained after no more than moderate trauma. The estimated 10% overall increase in mortality was just as high regardless of fracture site (excluding hands and feet), and persisted for at least a decade after the initial pathologic fracture.[35]

The most important factors affecting risk for osteoporosis are gender, age, dietary calcium intake, hormone status, genetics, medication use, and certain disease states. Additional risk factors include low vitamin D levels, excess alcohol intake, sedentary lifestyle, low lean body mass, smoking, and early onset of menopause (Box 165-1). Risk factors specifically applicable to postmenopausal women are discussed here; a more in-depth discussion of osteoporosis risk factors can be found in Chapter 182.

Age plays a significant role in the development of osteoporosis. Bone matrix is the strongest in young adults, and nontraumatic (low-velocity) fractures are unusual in this population; with age, however, fracture risk steadily increases. Women are at increased risk for osteoporosis compared with men (2:1 ratio) because their bones are not as dense in young adulthood.

BOX 165-1

Risk Factors for Postmenopausal Osteoporosis

MEDICATIONS

- Corticosteroids (7.5 mg or more of prednisone per day, or equivalent, for ≥6 months)
- Long-term use of certain anticonvulsant medications (e.g., phenytoin)
- Anticoagulant agents (e.g., heparin, warfarin)
- Immunosuppressive drugs (e.g., cyclosporine)
- Levothyroxine
- Intramuscular medroxyprogesterone in premenopausal women
- Lithium
- Tamoxifen (premenopausal use)

MENSTRUAL STATUS

- Early menopause without ET or HT
- Premenopausal hypogonadism
- Previous amenorrhea (e.g., because of anorexia nervosa or exercise-induced amenorrhea)
- Hyperprolactinemia

DISEASE STATES

- Osteoporotic fracture as an adult
- Primary hyperparathyroidism
- Thyrotoxicosis
- Cushing syndrome
- Multiple myeloma
- Rheumatoid arthritis
- Malabsorption syndromes (e.g., celiac disease, Crohn disease)
- Chronic obstructive pulmonary disease
- Anorexia nervosa
- Chronic liver disease
- Chronic renal disease

Hormones, particularly estrogen, also play an important role in osteoporosis in determining the rate of bone resorption. Low estrogen levels cause bone to be resorbed more quickly while concurrently decreasing bone formation in weight-bearing bones. In early menopause, the abrupt decline of estrogen is associated with a striking loss of bone mass during the first 3 to 5 postmenopausal years.

Many genes are involved in the creation and maintenance of healthy bone, and both structural and regulatory genes have been implicated in the development of osteoporosis. Mutations in genes involved in the regulation of bone mass and/or turnover are estimated to account for 60% to 90% of difference in bone mineral density (BMD) among individuals. Other gene pathways are involved as well, including genes involved in vitamin D absorption and activity, ERr formation, and the *COLIA1* and *COLIA2* genes encoding for type I collagen. Because genes are passed down through generations of family members, osteoporosis screening should include a detailed three-generation family health history. Genetic variability also assorts by ethnic group. Caucasian and Asian Americans are most susceptible to osteoporosis. The lifetime risk for a pathologic fracture in a 50-year-old Caucasian-American woman is approximately 40%, double that of an African-American woman; the risk for Hispanic women falls somewhere in the middle.[36]

BMD testing can be done to obtain information about a woman's fracture risk. Dual-energy x-ray absorptiometry (DXA) is the technical standard for measurement of BMD at the spine and hip. Other tests can be used to evaluate BMD (single-energy x-ray absorptiometry, radiographic absorptiometry, quantitative computed tomography [CT], and ultrasound densitometry) but should be used only when DXA is not available. DXA is noninvasive, takes 10 to 15 minutes, and exposes patients to only a small amount of radiation. BMD testing should be offered to all postmenopausal women younger than 65 years who have one or more risk factors for osteoporotic fracture besides menopause, all women 65 years of age and older regardless of additional risk factors, postmenopausal women who have experienced a fracture (to confirm diagnosis and to determine severity), and women who are considering therapy for osteoporosis if BMD testing would facilitate the decision.

Most menopause-related bone loss occurs within 3 to 5 years after the onset of menopause, and significant bone loss may continue for up to 20 years in some women. Both oral and transdermal estrogens and oral BZA combined with conjugated estrogen (BZA/CE) are approved for osteoporosis prevention (decreasing bone loss, reducing fractures, and preventing height loss), and for women in whom alternative therapies cause side effects or are ineffective or when the benefits outweigh the risks. Estrogens are not FDA approved for primary treatment of osteoporosis. Studies have shown that if HT is started early, the incidence of osteoporotic fractures is reduced by 20% to 50%, and that if HT is used for at least 5 years, the protection against major osteoporotic fractures persists after HT is discontinued.[37] Overall, recent studies have suggested that if HT is prescribed to prevent bone loss, the drugs should be continued for 5 years or longer to reduce fracture risk after discontinuation of the hormones. It should be remembered that although estrogen is FDA approved to prevent postmenopausal osteoporosis, because of the estrogen-associated risks, alternative osteoporosis prevention and nonhormonal alternative therapies should be discussed with every woman (Boxes 165-2 and 165-3).

Cognitive Decline

Multiple factors occurring at midlife may affect the ability to concentrate at menopause, such as sleep disturbances, hot flashes, fatigue, mood changes, physical symptoms, and midlife stressors. Women participating in SWAN showed a trend toward worsening memory during menopausal transition; however, this returned to the same level after the transition.[22] However, cognitive performance declines gradually with age regardless of gender, and although this is frustrating, it is part of the normal aging process.

Dementia, however—a progressive and often rapid deterioration in cognitive function—is caused by brain damage or disease. More than 5 million Americans currently live with AD, the most common form of the disease, and the number of Americans with AD doubles every 5 years beyond age 65.[38] U.S. Census data estimating future AD prevalence rates indicate that unless new prevention strategies are developed, the number of older adults with AD will increase to 14 million by 2050, a nearly threefold increase over current rates.[39] Because women comprise an ever-increasing percentage of older adults, they are disproportionally affected by this disease.

The effect of estrogens on the brain varies based on the age of the woman at the time of treatment. Ovarian estradiol produced during the reproductive years and HT initiated early in

BOX 165-2

Prevention and Treatment Interventions for Osteoporosis

WEIGHT-BEARING EXERCISE

- Early in life, promotes higher peak bone mass
- Weight bearing and strength training (most beneficial for bone health)
- Increases muscle mass and strength
- Exercise programs for elderly to increase muscle strength and to reduce the risk of falls

SMOKING CESSATION

- Smoking leads to lower bone mass and fractures.

NUTRITION

- Calcium intake is stratified by age group.
  Children 1-3 years: 500 mg/day
  Children 4-8 years: 800 mg/day
  Adolescents: 1300 mg/day
  Women 19-50 years and men <71 years: 800 mg/day
  Women >50 years and men >71 years: 1000 mg/day
- Vitamin D recommendations*
  On average, most Americans should receive 400 IU/day.
  Men and women older than 71 years should receive up to 800 IU/day.

*Vitamin D is essential for intestinal absorption of calcium and therefore for bone health. Making population-wide recommendations for supplementation is complicated, however, because vitamin D is absorbed in the diet but is also synthesized in the skin through sunlight exposure. Dietary intake and sun exposure vary widely among individuals, and excess sun exposure increases the risk for skin cancer. The Institute of Medicine therefore assumed minimal sun exposure (as in home-bound individuals) when establishing vitamin D recommendations.

Data from Institute of Medicine (IOM): *Dietary reference intakes for calcium and vitamin D,* 2010. Available at www.iom.edu/Reports/2010/Dietary-Reference-Intakes-for-Calcium-and-Vitamin-D.aspx. Accessed September 20, 2011.

BOX 165-3

Nonhormonal Agents Approved for Postmenopausal Osteoporosis

BISPHOSPHONATES

- Alendronate (Fosamax): prevention and treatment
  Prevention: 5 mg/day or 35 mg/wk
  Treatment: 10 mg/day or 70 mg/wk
- Alendronate plus cholecalciferol (Fosamax Plus D): treatment
  70 mg plus 2800 IU/wk *or* 70 mg plus 5600 IU/wk
- Risedronate (Actonel): prevention and treatment
  5 mg/day, 35 mg/wk
  75 mg in 2 consecutive doses/mo
  150 mg/mo
- Risedronate plus calcium carbonate (Actonel with calcium): prevention
  35 mg/wk (day 1) plus 1250 mg calcium for no-risedronate days (2-7) of 7-day cycle
- Ibandronate (Boniva): prevention and treatment
  Prevention and treatment: 150 mg/mo (oral tablet)
  Treatment: 3 mg every 3 mo (intravenous injection)
- Zoledronic acid (Reclast): treatment
  5 mg/yr (intravenous infusion)

SERMS

- Raloxifene (Evista): prevention and treatment
  60 mg/day

CALCITONIN

- Calcitonin, salmon (Fortical, Miacalcin): treatment >5 years after menopause
  200 IU/daily (nasal spray)
  100 IU every other day (subcutaneous injection)

PARATHYROID HORMONE

- Teriparatide (recombinant human parathyroid hormone [PTH]1-34; Forteo): treatment for high fracture risk
  20 μg/day (subcutaneous injection)

Data from North American Menopause Society (NAMS): *Government-approved postmenopausal osteoporosis drugs in the United States and Canada,* July 2008. Available at www.menopause.org/edumaterials/otcharts.pdf. Accessed September 20, 2011.

the menopausal transition have been shown to be neuroprotective, but HT begun late in menopause (after age 65) has been associated with an increased risk for cognitive decline and dementia.[40] The neuroprotective effect of HT may be particularly important to discuss with women who undergo bilateral oophorectomy before the onset of menopause and with all women when they first enter menopause, but HT should not be prescribed to women already diagnosed with dementia or AD, and HT is not recommended for treatment of dementia.[40]

Cancers

Endometrial Cancer. It has long been known that most of the risk for developing endometrial cancer involves prolonged or unopposed exposure to estrogen. Risks include early menarche, late menopause, unopposed estrogen or tamoxifen use, chronic anovulation, estrogen-secreting ovarian tumors, obesity, and a history of breast or ovarian cancer. The magnitude of the risk varies depending on the dose and duration of exposure to estrogen. Women taking a standard dose of estrogen (0.625 mg of conjugated estrogens per day, or the equivalent) for more than 3 years incur up to a fivefold increased risk for endometrial cancer, and the risk increases to 10-fold if unopposed estrogen is taken for more than 10 years.[28] Interestingly, when taken as prescribed, HT can also reduce the risk for endometrial cancer in postmenopausal women. Women in the CEE plus MPA arm of the WHI trial had a lower risk (hazard ratio [HR] 0.83, confidence interval [CI] 0.49-1.40) for developing endometrial cancer than women in the placebo arm.[19] Endometrial cancer is a relatively common cancer among postmenopausal women. Because the presenting symptom is typically AUB, any bleeding must be promptly and thoroughly evaluated. Postmenopausal women with an intact uterus using systemic estrogen-only therapy are at risk of developing endometrial hyperplasia and cancer and should be treated with adequate progestogen or BZA to reduce the risk of endometrial cancer.[21]

Breast Cancer. After skin cancer, breast cancer is the most common cancer in women worldwide (American Cancer Society [ACS],[42] 2013 to 2014), and it is estimated that one in every eight American woman will develop the disease during her lifetime.[41] Approximately 75% of breast cancers cases are sporadic (not inherited), and approximately 79% of cases are diagnosed in postmenopausal women over the age of 50.[42] Older age, female gender, and high lifetime hormone exposure (early menarche, late menopause, lack of childbearing or breastfeeding, and obesity) are the greatest risk factors, although family history, race and ethnicity (white, black and Hispanic), and low economic status are also associated with increased risk. Although older women are the most likely to develop the disease, menopause itself does not appear to have an impact on breast cancer incidence.

A number of large randomized clinical trials have explored the relationship between HT and breast cancer. Most studies show an association, with greater risk with use of EPT versus ET alone.[22] In the WHI trial, breast cancer risk was increased in women using EPT beyond 3 to 5 years, but no increase in risk was seen in the ET users after 7 years compared with those on placebo. The risk for developing breast cancer decreases after HT is discontinued. There may also be differences in risk depending on the hormone formulations (CEE versus estradiol and MPA versus micronized progestin versus BZA/CE), and lower doses of HT have not been studied. Although hormones themselves do not appear to directly damage DNA, they do stimulate breast cell growth (including estrogen-responsive cancer cells) and influence other hormones that stimulate breast cell division.[17,19] In general, HT is contraindicated in women with breast cancer unless the decision to treat a survivor experiencing debilitating menopause-related symptoms without relief from nonhormonal alternatives follows an informed discussion and is managed with an oncology consultation.

A decline in deaths from breast cancer has been occurring over the past several decades as a result of increasing screening and the introduction of earlier interventions for disease management.[21]

Ovarian Cancer. Ovarian cancer is both rare (approximately 3% of cancer diagnoses) and deadly (fifth leading cause of cancer deaths in the United States), primarily because it often remains undetected until it has reached an advanced stage.[42] If the cancer is identified and treated early (stage I), the 10-year survival rate for epithelial ovarian cancer, the most common type of ovarian cancer, can be as high as 99%; but unfortunately, up to 75% of cases are detected at stage III or IV, and survival rates are much lower than when the cancer is still localized to the ovary.[43]

The relationship between hormone use and ovarian cancer is bimodal. During the reproductive years, combined hormonal contraception (birth control pills, vaginal contraceptive ring, contraceptive patch) and bilateral tubal ligation have both been shown to decrease ovarian cancer risk by 50%.[21] In the WHI, ovarian cancer incidence was slightly higher in the intervention (CEE plus MPA) group than it was in the control group. Although the difference was not statistically significant (HR 1.41), in their conclusion the authors stated, "Treatment with CEE plus MPA reduced the risk of endometrial cancer; however, both hormone therapy regimens may increase ovarian cancer risk."[21]

Lung Cancer. Lung cancer is the second most commonly diagnosed cancer (after nonmelanoma skin cancer), and more Americans die of the disease than of breast, prostate, and colon cancer combined. In 2014, 224,210 Americans were diagnosed with lung cancer and 159,000 persons died of the disease, 66% of whom were older than 65.[42] Men are at greater risk than women overall, and cigarette smokers are at higher risk in both groups; but, interestingly, among nonsmokers, women are more likely than men to develop lung cancer, which raises the question of whether hormones increase the risk.

Although menopause itself has not been shown to increase the risk for developing lung cancer, studies are limited and results are inconsistent. Large observational trials have shown that hormonal contraception and HT are protective, but secondary analyses of WHI data have found that CEE plus MPA was associated with an increased risk for dying from lung cancer (HR 1.10) after 8 years of use.[19,21] Combined, these data suggest that starting HT in older women who either are currently smoking or who have a history of tobacco use may promote the growth of existing lung cancers.

Colorectal Cancer. Although its overall incidence has been declining over the past two decades, CRC is still the third most commonly diagnosed cancer in the United States. The ACS estimated that in 2014 96,830 Americans would be diagnosed with colon cancer and 40,000 more would be diagnosed with rectal cancer.[42] CRC risk increases with advancing age, so menopausal women are at increased risk compared with younger women.

Although menopause itself has not been associated with an increased risk for the disease, the WHI showed that the type of HT used does influence CRC risk. Women taking *combined* HT (CEE plus MPA) were at significantly lower risk for developing CRC (HR 0.62; 95% CI 0.43-0.89), but if they did develop the disease, their cancer was diagnosed at a more advanced stage. CRC risk for women taking CEE alone was markedly different; they were at the same CRC risk as the placebo group (HR 1.15; 95% CI 0.81-1.64).[42] Screening for CRC has been found to detect early-stage disease and improve mortality rates. According to established guidelines, women should be screened for CRC at age 50 and in general should undergo repeat testing every 10 years until age 75.

PHYSICAL EXAMINATION

Regular physical and preventive health examinations are recommended for people of all ages, but the frequency and focus of the examination vary by the individual's age and gender and the presence of any comorbid conditions. Although no group recommends a routine "annual" visit, all older adults should be seen for preventive care on a regular basis. Several groups, including federal agencies, medical specialty societies, independent panels, and private advocacy groups, have published preventive services guidelines, but for the purposes of this chapter, screening recommendations published by NAMS will be highlighted (see Table 165-4).

MANAGEMENT

Lifestyle Changes

Because there is no single menopausal syndrome, it is important to collaborate and individualize a plan of care with each woman. For most women, menopause is a normal physiologic and developmental life event.[28] Many studies have found women have mostly positive or neutral attitudes toward the transition through menopause, but for some women, symptoms do affect their quality of life, and they may seek out interventions from their primary care provider. For all women, some modification of lifestyle can have a significant and positive impact on overall health regardless of age, and some lifestyle changes can improve menopausal symptoms as well.

Personal attitudes, culture, lifestyle, and even social and demographic factors may influence a woman's perception of menopause. Smoking cessation reduces the risk of lung cancer and may reduce VMSs. Weight-bearing exercise improves bone density. Eating a healthy diet, limiting alcohol intake, and maintaining a normal body weight can decrease cardiovascular and breast cancer risks. Reducing stress levels can improve mental health and emotional well-being. These are all important reasons for clinicians to begin any discussion with an assessment of lifestyle behaviors and discussion on health promotion and risk reduction.

Vitamins and Minerals

A balanced diet rich in fruits and vegetables is always preferable to taking supplements. However, a woman's daily diet may not contain all the nutrients required for optimal health, and a daily multivitamin and mineral supplement may be necessary. However, a systematic review published in 2013 for the U.S. Preventive Services Task Force (USPSTF) found a lack of evidence that supplements prevent either cancer or CVD.[44]

Vitamin D. Vitamin D is essential for the efficient intestinal absorption of calcium and for bone health and has been found to improve muscle strength and balance and to reduce the risk of falling. Although available in two forms—vitamin D_2 and vitamin D_3—D_3 (25-hydroxyvitamin D [25OHD]) is the naturally occurring form, is more potent, and is the one most commonly referred to when discussing this vitamin.[45] In 2011, the Institute of Medicine (IOM) published new guidelines for both vitamin D serum levels (20 to 50 ng/mL [50 to 125 nmol/L]) and Recommended Daily Allowances (RDAs) for vitamin D supplementation (women <70 years, 600 IU per day; >70 years, 800 IU per day; upper tolerable limit = 4000 IU regardless of age) in adults. Although the IOM stopped short of recommending universal vitamin D screening, it did recommend routine screening in vulnerable populations (e.g., older adults or institutionalized adults; people at increased risk for micronutrient deficiency, for instance, post–bariatric surgery patients; individuals at increased risk for osteoporosis; and those taking selected medications such as oral steroids).[46]

The NOF and NAMS recommend 800 IU to 1000 IU of vitamin D_3 per day for women aged 50 years and older.[22]

Calcium. The importance of an adequate calcium intake for skeletal health has been well established, although its requirements fluctuate throughout a woman's life. Although results from studies are conflicting, they have suggested nonskeletal benefits of calcium, such as reduction of CRC, hypertension, and obesity, but supplements may slightly increase the risk of nephrolithiasis. If adequate calcium cannot be obtained from the diet, a separate calcium supplement may be required to reach the recommended 1200 mg of calcium per day. Women should be encouraged to divide the doses throughout the day and to take calcium with food because absorption is better when it is taken with meals. However, there is no practical limit to the amount that can be taken at one time.[28]

Iron. Iron may be needed during the time of menopausal transition for the woman who is having AUB and may develop iron deficiency anemia. After the FMP of menopause, iron is no longer lost through menstrual bleeding. Women can be counseled that iron is readily available in food (e.g., organ meats, beef, turkey, clams, oysters, oatmeal, beans) and fortified foods (e.g., breakfast cereals). The daily requirement of elemental iron for menstruating women is 18 mg per day; after menopause, 8 mg per day is sufficient. Postmenopausal women choosing to take a multivitamin should be advised to use an appropriate formulation. Further supplementation is not necessary unless chronic illness leads to iron deficiency anemia.[28]

Further Intervention

The next phase for developing a collaborative plan is to discuss the woman's view of menopause and her desire for intervention for symptoms affecting her quality of life.

NONPHARMACOLOGICAL THERAPIES

Vasomotor Symptoms

1. Although randomized clinical trials have been few or inconsistent in validating effectiveness, some women have found the following lifestyle options to be effective in reducing VMSs:
   a. Dress in layers.
   b. Maintain healthy weight.
   c. Avoid smoking.
   d. Avoid triggers such as hot drinks, caffeine, spicy foods, alcohol.
   e. Pace respirations (deep, slow, abdominal breathing).
2. Women who choose not to use or have contraindications to pharmacologic interventions have found some of the following OTC devices or products to be helpful in moderating VMSs:
   a. Chillow Pillow
   b. Bed Fan
   c. Clothing and pajamas or gowns, bedsheets, and pillowcases made from wicking material
3. Herbal preparations. Many women purchase OTC supplements to alleviate minor menopausal symptoms. Because these products are not regulated by the FDA, there are significant concerns regarding the consistency, safety, and purity of the supplements, as well as the potential for adverse interactions with other drugs or herbal products. Women should also be aware that just because a product is labeled "natural" does not mean it is safe, and women should be counseled to discuss any new medication or OTC product with their health care provider before taking it. For more information, consult the National Center for Complementary and Alternative Medicine (NCCAM) at http://nccam.nih.gov.

   Several herbal products have been identified as options for managing VMSs:
   a. Black cohosh. Study results are inconsistent compared with placebo, but this herb has been found to be at least as effective as placebo for relieving VMSs in some women.[21] One OTC product, Remifemin, has been tested in randomized, controlled trials. Long-term safety of black cohosh has not been established because most studies for managing menopausal symptoms have been conducted for only 6 months or less.
   b. Relizen. Recently available in the United States, this supplement has been available in Europe for more than 10 years for the treatment of vasomotor flushes. It is a pollen extract that has been shown in several small randomized clinical trials to have no estrogenic effects. It does not have FDA approval and is considered an alternative product.[24]
4. Progesterone creams. In the United States, many brands of topical progesterone can be purchased without a prescription as lotion, gel, and cream preparations and have been used by women for treating VMSs. There have been limited,

small studies suggesting relief of symptoms with these products. However, because of absence of FDA oversight of these products, data regarding safety and efficacy are lacking. The effects of transdermal progesterone on endometrial protection with estrogen use are unknown, and this should not be recommended as an option for endometrial protection for women with a uterus who are taking an estrogen.[28]

5. Small limited studies have demonstrated reduction in VMSs through yoga, exercise, and acupuncture.

Genital and Sexual Symptoms

Vaginal Moisturizers and Lubricants. Menopausal women may experience symptoms of vaginal dryness, irritation, and dyspareunia, although these symptoms may not become problematic until late in the postmenopausal period. Although few clinical studies have been conducted on the efficacy of these products, first-line therapies include nonhormonal OTC vaginal lubricants and moisturizers. Products can be water based (e.g., Astroglide, Just Like Me, K-Y Jelly, Slippery Stuff), oil based (Elegance Women's Lubricants, olive oil), or silicone based (Astroglide X, ID Millennium, K-Y Millennium, Pink). Some products are pH balanced (Replens, RepHresh). Some OTC products, such as Luvena, have combination benefits such as a moisturizer and lubricant. Although no OTC vaginal product treats the underlying estrogen deficiency that is causing the dryness and irritation, these products often provide significant short-term symptom relief. Women should be encouraged to experiment with products to find ones that meet their personal needs, but should also be told that moisturizers may provide more relief if they are used regularly (several times a week), whereas lubricants are more helpful when used to minimize friction and irritation during sexual intercourse. Women should be discouraged from using products that contain perfumes, flavors, or warming ingredients that might cause irritation to the vaginal tissue, and douching disrupts the normal genital flora, increasing the risk for infection, and should be avoided by all women regardless of age.[28]

Stimulators or Vibrators. Regular sexual activity helps to maintain normal vaginal lubrication and blood flow to the vagina. When sexual activity is decreased or absent, use of clitoral stimulators or vibrators for self-stimulation or with partner assistance can be encouraged. Devices can be purchased OTC at drugstores (e.g., the Trojan Mini vibrator) or online (e.g., www.middlesexmd.com), and more information is available on the NAMS website (www.menopause.org).

PHARMACOLOGIC THERAPY

Deciding which pharmacologic intervention to recommend to a particular woman depends on several factors, including her underlying health status, her personal preference, the cost, and the potential adverse effects of a particular medication. Several prescription therapies have been approved by the FDA to manage menopausal symptoms, including estrogens and progestogens (available in oral, transdermal, and topical formulations), and two nonhormonal therapies. In addition, some FDA-approved pharmacologic options are also used off label to manage VMS symptoms. Because women may experience troublesome VMSs and vaginal symptoms before reaching menopause, women should be counseled regarding contraception options that can relieve perimenopausal symptoms while preventing an unintended pregnancy.

Contraceptive Therapy

Because there are no reliable laboratory tests to confirm definitive loss of fertility in a woman, both the American Congress of Obstetricians and Gynecologists (ACOG) and NAMS recommend that women continue contraceptive use until menopause or age 50 to 55 years.[47] Women of older reproductive age may also experience perimenopausal symptoms. Hormonal contraception offers a viable option for both symptomatic perimenopausal women and those who wish to avoid an unintended pregnancy. Low-dose combination estrogen/progestin contraceptives (pills, patch, ring) may be appropriate for healthy, lean, nonsmoking perimenopausal women but are contraindicated in women older than age 35 who smoke. Other potential contraindications include hypertension, diabetes, obesity, and other comorbidities. Progestin-only options offer potentially safer alternatives for women with these contraindications. Options for women who desire long-term contraception include long-acting reversible contraception (LARC) methods, such as the copper IUD, the two levonorgestrel-releasing intrauterine systems (LNG-IUSs), and the etonogestrel subdermal implant. The Centers for Disease Control and Prevention (CDC) has issued evidence-based guidelines, making contraceptive provision and clinical decision-making easier through publication of their "Selected Practice Recommendations" and "Medical Eligibility Criteria for Contraceptive Use." These guidelines can assist clinicians in recommending contraceptive methods according to age and medical conditions based on risks and advantages.[47]

Hormone Therapy

Consistent terminology is needed for discussion of pharmacologic choices for HT. In place of the old term *hormone replacement therapy* (HRT), the following terminology should be used:

1. HT—hormone therapy. The FDA uses this term to distinguish therapy that includes only combination estrogen-progestogen. NAMS uses this term to encompass both types of therapy, estrogen and estrogen-progestogen therapy.
2. ET—estrogen therapy alone.
3. EPT—combined estrogen-progestogen therapy.
4. Progestogen—encompassing both natural progesterone and synthetic progestins.

Estrogens are available in many prescription preparations, including as single agents in oral preparations; transdermal patch, gel, or topical emulsion preparations; and vaginal preparations for systemic or topical administration. Combination (EPT) preparations are also available in oral and transdermal preparations (see Tables 165-2 and 165-3.)

Individualization of the plan of care in collaboration with the clinician is important because no consensus has been established regarding the perfect risk/benefit ratio for initiating or continuing HT. A plan should be based on the woman's needs and desires after conducting a thorough history and physical examination and after a discussion with her regarding her risks and benefits for the interventions.

In October 2014, NAMS released a free app at the Apple App Store to help clinicians in prescribing HT. The Menopause Decision-Support Algorithm, discussed in an article published in Menopause: The Journal of the North American Menopause Society,[19] and the companion iPhone/iPad app, developed in collaboration with NAMS, are designed to help clinicians decide which patients are candidates for pharmacologic treatment of menopausal symptoms. The app provides clinicians with

TABLE 165-2 Pros and Cons of Hormone Therapy Routes of Administration

Type of Product	Pros	Cons
Oral estrogen products	Familiar, easy to use, usually low cost Beneficial effect on HDL-C, LDL-C, and total cholesterol Large amount of data	Risk of thrombosis, stroke Increase in triglycerides, C-reactive protein, other hepatic proteins Risk of reduced libido through SHBG effect
Transdermal and topical estrogens	Avoids first pass effect Compared to oral ET, lower incidence of the following: • Triglyceride increase • C-reactive protein increase • Reduced libido • GI side effects • Thrombosis risk (probably) Topical emulsion is moisturizing	Patch adhesive sensitivity and residue Patch less private Often higher cost Gels and creams can transfer hormone to others
Vaginal (local) estrogens	Vaginal benefit at lower dose Avoids systemic effects	Increased vaginal discharge May be less convenient to use Lack of long-term uterine safety data
Progestogens	Less adverse effect on endometrium Some reduce adverse effects of oral estrogen on triglycerides Nighttime administration can decrease insomnia, improving sleep	Some can increase risk for breast cancer Some can reduce estrogen's beneficial effect on HDL-C Some adverse effects such as bloating Dysphoria in some women

GI, gastrointestinal; LDL-C, low-density lipoprotein cholesterol.
Modified from *Menopause practice: a clinician's guide,* ed 5, Mayfield, OH, 2014, North American Menopause Society.

TABLE 165-3 Coping Strategies for Estrogen Therapy or Estrogen-Progestogen Therapy Adverse Events

Adverse Effect	Strategy
Fluid retention	Restrict salt; maintain adequate water intake; exercise; try a mild prescription diuretic.
Bloating	Switch to low-dose nonoral continuous estrogen; lower progestogen dose to a level that still protects the uterus; switch to another progestin or to micronized progesterone.
Breast tenderness	Lower estrogen dose; switch to another estrogen; restrict salt; switch to another progestin; cut down on caffeine and chocolate.
Headaches	Switch to nonoral continuous estrogen; lower dose of estrogen or progestogen or both; switch to a continuous-combined regimen; switch to progesterone or a 19-norpregnane derivative; ensure adequate water intake; restrict salt, caffeine, and alcohol.
Mood changes	Investigate preexisting depression or anxiety; lower progestogen dose; switch progestogen; switch from systemic progestin to the progestin intrauterine system; change to a continuous-combined EPT regimen; ensure adequate water intake; restrict salt, caffeine, and alcohol.
Nausea	Take oral estrogen tablets with meals or before bed; switch to another oral estrogen; switch to nonoral estrogen; lower estrogen or progestogen dose.

Modified from *Menopause practice: a clinician's guide,* ed 5, Mayfield, OH, 2014, North American Menopause Society.

treatment options based on the woman's risk factors and her individualized choices. Within the app are links to other resources such as the Gail model breast cancer screening tool, the FRAX (Fracture Risk Assessment Tool) osteoporosis screening tool, CV screening tools, and the NAMS HT tables. This new algorithm and mobile app for menopausal symptom management incorporate current evidence-based data and research to clarify the decision-making process for clinicians; the app also includes a component for patients to seek answers to their questions about HT. Future plans include a version of the app for Android systems.

For resources that provide evidence-based approaches to prescribing HT, see the NAMS website (www.menopause.org). The following resources on the NAMS website are helpful:

1. Shifren JL, Gass ML, NAMS Recommendations for Clinical Care of Midlife Women Working Group: The North American Menopause Society recommendations for clinical care of midlife women. *Menopause* 21(10):1038-1062, 2014.
2. Manson JE, Ames JM, Shapiro M, et al: Algorithm and mobile app for menopausal symptom management and hormonal/non-hormonal therapy decision making: a clinical decision-support tool from The North American Menopause Society. *Menopause* 22(3):247-253, 2015.
3. MenoPro. For Apple devices: free download app to help with prescribing HT.
4. North American Menopause Society: The 2012 hormone therapy position statement of The North American Menopause Society. *Menopause* 19(3):257-271, 2012.
5. de Villiers TJ, Gass ML, Haines CJ, et al: Global consensus statement on menopausal hormone therapy. *Climacteric* 16:203-204, 2013.

In reviewing these key resources the clinician can consider the following important points about prescribing HT:

1. Estrogen and progesterone agonists share common features and effects and have potentially different properties.

Although only two products were studied in the WHI, all HT products, including bioidentical and compounded hormones, are assumed to have similar risks until proven otherwise. Without randomized control trials, data for one agent should be generalized to all agents.

2. The option of HT is an individual decision in terms of quality of life and health priorities as well as personal factors such as age, time since menopause, and the risk of VTE, stroke, ischemic heart disease, and breast cancer. The dose and duration of HT should be consistent with treatment goals and safety issues and should be individualized.
3. HT is the most effective treatment for VMSs associated with menopause at any age, but benefits are more likely to outweigh risks for symptomatic women younger than 60 years or within 10 years after menopause. Absolute risks in healthy women ages 50 to 59 are low. Long-term use or HT initiation in older women, however, has greater risks.
4. HT should not be prescribed for the prevention of chronic illness, such as CVD.
5. Some oral and transdermal products are approved for prevention of postmenopausal osteoporosis, but not for treatment.
6. The risk of VTE and ischemic stroke increases with oral HT but the absolute risk is rare in patients younger than 60 years. Observational studies point to a lower risk with transdermal therapy.
7. ET alone is appropriate in women after hysterectomy. Additional progestogen or BZA is required if the woman has a uterus. Administration of unopposed estrogen in a woman with a uterus increases the risk of endometrial cancer. Research is insufficient to recommend one regimen over another.
8. Local low-dose ET is preferred for women whose symptoms are limited to only vaginal dryness or associated discomfort with intercourse. A progestogen is generally not indicated when ET is administered locally in a low dose for vaginal atrophy, although trials have been limited to only 1 year.
9. Vaginal ET may help decrease recurrent urinary tract infection in postmenopausal women. Local ET may benefit some women with overactive bladder. Systemic HT may worsen or provoke stress incontinence.
10. The risk of breast cancer in women older than 50 years associated with HT is a complex issue. The increased risk of breast cancer in the WHI was primarily associated with the addition of a progestogen to ET and related to the duration of use. Women with an intact uterus who choose to extend duration of EPT use beyond 5 years need to be candidly counseled regarding these concerns. No increase in risk of breast cancer with ET was seen in the WHI. Current safety data do not support the use of HT in breast cancer survivors.
11. Extending HT use is acceptable for women who are well aware of potential risks and benefits; at the lowest effective dose; for prevention of further osteoporosis-related fracture and bone loss when alternate therapies are inappropriate or the risk/benefit ratio is unknown; and/or with clinical supervision.
12. The decision to continue or discontinue HT must be individualized. There is a 50% chance of VMSs recurring when HT is discontinued. Symptom recurrence is similar whether the drug is tapered or abruptly discontinued.
13. There is insufficient evidence to support the use of HT for treating depression. Progestogens in EPT may worsen mood when there is a history of PMS, premenstrual depressive disorder, or clinical depression.
14. For postmenopausal women older than age 65, HT does not improve cognition. The Women's Health Initiative Memory Study (WHIMS) reported an increase in dementia incidence when HT was initiated at age 65 or older. HT is not recommended at any age for the sole or primary indication of preventing cognitive aging or dementia. There are inadequate data regarding whether HT started soon after menopause will increase or decrease later dementia risk.

Estrogen and progesterone both have unique side effects that must be reviewed with patients before beginning therapy with either drug. Estrogen side effects include breast tenderness, nausea, peripheral edema, and headaches (sometimes migraine). Scientific evidence has found no association between HT or menopause and weight gain. Common progestin side effects include the induction of menses in premenopausal women and withdrawal bleeding (often undesired in postmenopausal women) as well as bloating and mood changes.[28]

Contraindications to HT include undiagnosed vaginal bleeding; known, suspected, or a history of breast cancer; known or suspected estrogen-dependent neoplasia; acute liver disease; chronic severe hepatic dysfunction (aspartate aminotransferase level more than two times normal); and recent or active thrombophlebitis or thromboembolic disorders. HT is not contraindicated in women with controlled hypertension, diabetes mellitus, or elevated cholesterol levels but should be used cautiously in women with a history of endometriosis, uterine fibroids, atraumatic thrombophlebitis or thromboembolic events, gallbladder disease, seizure disorders, and migraine headaches.

Oral estrogen is the most widely used formulation. Because of the first-pass liver uptake, there is greater stimulation of certain proteins including a 25% increase in triglycerides,[28] so women with hypertriglyceridemia, or who are at increased risk based on family history, should consider transdermal administration. Oral ET also stimulates hepatic globulins, coagulation factors, and some inflammatory markers such as C-reactive protein, which have been associated with an increased risk of gallbladder disease.

Transdermal and topical estrogens are not subject to first-pass liver metabolism and therefore have both known and theoretical advantages as well as disadvantages compared with oral formulations. There is no effect on increasing triglycerides. For patients with metabolic syndrome or hypertriglyceridemia, transdermal estrogen would be a better option. However, with transdermal administration and the lack of the first liver pass, there is also no improvement in high-density lipoprotein cholesterol (HDL-C) as happens with oral administration. Although there have been no large randomized controlled trials, several observational studies have suggested that transdermal ET is associated with a decreased risk of VTE. However, in the 4-year randomized controlled Kronos Early Estrogen Prevention Study (KEEPS), involving 727 healthy women, there were no differences in stroke and VTE events among oral estrogen, transdermal estrogen, and placebo. (NAMS. KEEPS report).[28] Presented at NAMS 23rd Annual Meeting: October 3 to 6, 2012; Orlando, FL. www.menopauses.org/annual-meetings/2012-meeting/keeps-report).[28] Women using topical estrogen sprays and gels should be instructed to cover areas of drug placement until it has been absorbed to avoid exposing partners, children, and pets to the medication. The most common side effect of a transdermal patch is skin irritation at the patch application site. Rotating the patch to other areas such as the buttocks, maintaining a clean site, and applying talcum powder around the patch edge to prevent formation of dirt rings may help to reduce irritation.

Vaginal estrogen can be administered through creams, rings, and tablets. For symptomatic vaginal atrophy that does not respond to nonhormonal vaginal lubricants and moisturizers, low-dose vaginal ET is effective and well tolerated. Maintenance is achieved with either twice weekly application or insertion of 17β-estradiol cream, conjugated estrogen cream, or estradiol hemihydrate 10-μg tablets or insertion of a 17β-estradiol ring that releases hormone for 90 days. Regardless of the product used, systemic absorption is limited and progestogen therapy is usually not indicated for a woman with a uterus. However, clinical monitoring should be continued because endometrial safety data do not extend beyond 1 year. Low-dose, local ET can be continued for as long as distressing vaginal symptoms continue to occur.[28] Product labeling for vaginal estrogen products often includes the same warnings, contraindications, and listing of adverse effects as labeling for other systemic estrogen products, despite the fact that low-dose vaginal ET does not typically result in significant systemic estrogen levels. A number of menopause, clinical, and scientific experts have initiated conversations with the FDA regarding changing the "black box" labeling of topical vaginal estrogen products. One vaginal estrogen product, the estradiol acetate ring, releases estradiol at a higher dose, so although it has been FDA approved for managing VMS symptoms, a progestogen is also needed to protect the endometrium in women with a uterus. Instructions to the patient should include that if the ring falls out it can be rinsed off and reinserted, and that the ring does not usually interfere with sexual intercourse but it can be removed if it is uncomfortable for either partner.

Progestogen therapy can be an option to treat VMS. However, the primary role for this hormone in menopausal management is to reduce the risk of endometrial cancer associated with unopposed estrogen. Combined EPT products are available. All government-approved progestogen formulations will provide endometrial protection if the dose and duration are adequate. The progestogen product most structurally related to progesterone is an oral capsule containing micronized progesterone (Prometrium), which can be administered as an independent dose with an estrogen product. Prometrium is contraindicated for women who have an allergy to peanuts, and because of potential side effects of drowsiness and dizziness is recommended for administration at bedtime. A dose of 100 mg is usually effective for endometrial protection if administered in a continuous combined dosage schedule.[29]

EPT can be prescribed in many regimens. There is no consensus, and there is insufficient evidence to recommend any one regimen. Regimens are classified as continuous-cyclic sequential, continuous cyclic long-cycle, continuous-combined, and intermittent-combined. Each may have advantages and disadvantages, and clinicians using each regimen should be aware of any special monitoring of the endometrium that might be advised during clinical supervision of the patient. The continuous-combined regimen, which was developed to address withdrawal uterine bleeding, a major reason for discontinuation of EPT, has been the predominant regimen used in North America.[28] Breakthrough uterine bleeding has been observed in 40% of women on a continuous-combined regimen during the first 3 to 6 months, but most women will become amenorrheic within 12 months. Adjusting doses and evaluating for other causes of bleeding can be considered.

A tissue-selective estrogen complex (TSEC), which pairs BZA 20 mg, a novel SERM, with CEE 45 mg was approved by the FDA in October 2013 for the treatment of moderate to severe VMSs and for prevention of osteoporosis in postmenopausal women with a uterus. This gives women another option instead of pairing estrogen with a progestogen for endometrial safety.

Androgen therapy is receiving increasing attention for treatment of postmenopausal women with sexual dysfunction. New guidelines published in October 2014 by the Endocrine Society recommend a 3- to 6-month trial of testosterone therapy for women diagnosed with hypoactive sexual desire disorder (HSDD) but state that more evidence is needed to determine whether the benefits of testosterone outweigh the risks. The guidelines go on to say that because there are insufficient data to support its use, testosterone therapy is not recommended for managing infertility, sexual dysfunction, or osteoporosis, nor should it be used to treat women with androgen deficiency caused by other conditions such as hypopituitarism, adrenal insufficiency, or surgical menopause or pharmacologic glucocorticoid administration.[12]

Currently there are no government-approved androgen-containing prescription products for treating female sexual interest/arousal disorder, and androgen therapy for women remains controversial. The potential risks of androgen therapy for women are not well defined, and the risk of CVD or breast cancer is unknown.[28] There is, however, some evidence to support the use of testosterone therapy in postmenopausal women with female sexual interest/arousal disorder with no other cause identified for their sexual dysfunction.[22] When recommending such therapy, clinicians should fully inform women of potential risks and monitor for adverse events including acne, weight gain, excess facial and body hair, permanent lowering of the voice, clitoral enlargement, changes in emotion (e.g., increased anger), and adverse changes in lipids and liver function test results.

As with most medications, the clinical goal for HT management is to use the lowest effective dose for the shortest time consistent with treatment goals. NAMS recommends ongoing clinical monitoring of women using HT to include at least yearly return visits, during which time the woman and her clinician should review the decision to use HT, including a discussion of any new research findings. It is recognized that more frequent visits may be required, especially for women just starting HT or for those having bothersome side effects. Although clinical guidelines and societies may differ, NAMS recommends annual mammography for women who are prescribed HT. Endometrial surveillance is not required for women using systemic ET and adequate progestogen. Data are insufficient to recommend annual endometrial surveillance in asymptomatic women using low-dose vaginal ET for the treatment of vaginal atrophy. If a woman is at high risk for endometrial cancer, is using a higher dose of vaginal ET, or is having symptoms (spotting, breakthrough bleeding), closer surveillance may be required.[28]

Bioidentical Hormone Therapy Products. Many well-tested FDA-approved bioidentical brand-name products are available in the United States. However, the term bioidentical is typically used to mean custom-made HT formulations compounded for an individual according to a provider's prescription. Custom-compounded bioidentical hormone therapy (BHT) may provide doses, ingredients, and routes of administration not commercially available, but no formulation has been approved by any regulatory agency. Custom-compounded BHT agents are not tested for efficacy, safety, batch standardization, or purity and do not include package inserts like those required for FDA-approved HT products, explaining benefits and risks. Often, third-party payers do not reimburse prescription costs for these compounded drugs. Most of the large national organizations (NAMS, ACOG, Endocrine Society) do not support the use of custom-compounded BHT unless the patient must have the hormone prescription compounded because of an allergy to an ingredient in the commercial formulation. Clinicians are encouraged, if they decide to use a compounding pharmacy for whatever reason, to check whether the company supplying the drug is accredited by the Pharmacy Compounding Accreditation Board. Also, the clinician should educate the patient on the drug's risks, benefits, safety, administration, dosage.

FOOD AND DRUG ADMINISTRATION–APPROVED NONHORMONAL PHARMACOLOGIC OPTIONS

Nonhormonal pharmacologic options are available for management of VMSs. Two new drugs were approved by the FDA in 2013.

1. Paroxetine (Brisdelle) 7.5 mg is a nonhormone selective serotonin reuptake inhibitor (SSRI) that provides an alternative for women to manage VMSs, especially women who cannot or choose not to use HT. Higher doses of paroxetine were originally approved in 1992 for treatment of psychiatric conditions that currently include depression, anxiety disorder, social anxiety disorder, panic disorder, obsessive compulsive disorder, and generalized and post-traumatic stress disorder. Although study findings are contradictory, a potential exists for paroxetine to interact with tamoxifen owing to its potent cytochrome P-450 2D6 inhibitors.
2. Ospemifene (Osphena), a SERM, is an estrogen-like compound that acts as an estrogen agonist or antagonist. Ospemifene is an oral option for treating moderate to severe dyspareunia, a symptom of vulvar and vaginal atrophy resulting from menopause. It has not been shown to cause any increased risk of endometrial proliferation in trials up to 52 weeks. Although risks of thromboembolic stroke, hemorrhagic stroke, and VTE have been similar to those of placebo in healthy postmenopausal women studied for up to 52 weeks, concern remains about potential risk of VTE because of potential class effect.[28]

NON–FOOD AND DRUG ADMINISTRATION–APPROVED NONHORMONAL PHARMACOLOGIC OPTIONS

1. SSRIs and serotonin-norepinephrine reuptake inhibitor (SNRIs):
   a. Fluoxetine, 20 mg/day
   b. Paroxetine, 12.5 to 25 mg/day
   c. Citalopram, 10 to 20 mg/day
   d. Escitalopram, 10 to 20 mg/day
   e. Venlafaxine, 37.5 to 75 mg/day
   f. Desvenlafaxine, 100 mg/day
2. Clonidine: Initial oral dose for hot flash treatment is 0.05 mg twice daily, but some women may require at least 0.1 mg twice daily or the patch, 0.1 mg per day. The drug has a modest effect on symptoms. Adverse side effects include insomnia, dry mouth, constipation, and drowsiness. This may be a good choice for patients with hypertension.
3. Gabapentin may be initiated at a daily dose of 300 mg at bedtime; the dose can be increased to 300 mg twice daily and then to three times daily at 3- to 4-day intervals.

Estrogens are available in many prescription preparations, including as single agents in oral preparations; transdermal patch, gel, or topical emulsion preparations; vaginal preparations; and combination (EPT) preparations (Table 165-4).

TABLE 165-4 Approved Prescription Products for Menopausal Symptoms in the United States and Canada

Product	Product Name(s)	Doses (mg/day)
ORAL ESTROGEN PRODUCTS		
17β-estradiol	Estrace Various generics	0.5, 1.0, 2.0
CEE	Premarin	0.3, 0.45, 0.625, 0.9, 1.25
Synthetic conjugated estrogens, A	Cenestin	0.3. 0.45, 0.625, 0.9, 1.25
Synthetic conjugated estrogens, B	Enjuvia	0.3, 0.45, 0.625, 0.9, 1.25
Conjugated estrogens, CSD (synthetic)	CSD, PrC.E.S. Prpms-Conjugated estrogens	0.3, 0.625, 0.9, 1.25
Esterified estrogens	Menest Estragyn	0.3, 0.625, 1.25, 2.5 0.3, 0.625
Estropipate	Ogen Various generics	0.625 (0.75 estropipate) 1.25 (1.5), 2.5 (3.0) 0.625 (0.75), 1.5 (3.0), 5.0 (6.0)

Continued

TABLE 165-4 Approved Prescription Products for Menopausal Symptoms in the United States and Canada—cont'd

Product	Product Name(s)	Doses (mg/day)
TRANSDERMAL ESTROGEN PRODUCTS		
17β-estradiol		
Patch	Alora	0.025, 0.05, 0.075, 0.1 twice/wk
	Climara	0.025, 0.0375, 0.05, 0.075, 0.1 once/wk
	Estradot	0.025, 0.0375, 0.05, 0.075, 0.1 twice/wk 0.014 once/wk
	Estraderm	0.05, 0.1 twice/wk
	Menostar	0.0375, 0.05, 0.075, 0.1 twice/wk
	Minivelle	0.05, 0.1 twice/wk
	Oesclim	0.025, 0.0375, 0.05, 0.075, 0.1 twice/wk
	Vivelle	0.025, 0.0375, 0.05, 0.075, 0.1 twice/wk
	Vivelle-Dot	0.05, 0.06, 0.025, 0.0375, 0.75, 0.1 once or twice/wk
	Various generics	
Transdermal gel	Divigel EstroGel Elestrin	0.003, 0.009, 0.027 0.75 (use lowest effective) 0.0125, 0.0375 (use lowest effective)
Topical emulsion	Estrasorb	0.05 (2 packets) (use lowest effective)
Transdermal spray	Evamist	1.53 (1/day initially, adjust dose by response)
VAGINAL ESTROGEN PRODUCTS		
Creams		
17β-estradiol	Estrace *VVA*	Initial: 2-4 g/d for 1-2 wk Maintenance: 1 g 2-3 times/wk (0.1 mg active ingredient per gram)
Conjugated estrogens	Premarin Vaginal Cream *Atrophic vaginitis* *Kraurosis vulvae* *United States: Moderate to severe dyspareunia* *Canada: Dyspareunia*	*United States:* *Atrophic vaginitis and kraurosis vulvae:* 0.5-2 g/d (0.625 mg active ingredient per gram) for 21 days then off 7 days *Moderate to severe dyspareunia:* 0.5 g/d for 21 days then off 7 days, or twice/wk *Canada:* Low dose: 0.5 g intravaginal or topical twice/wk Maximum recommended dose: 0.5 g/day intravaginally or topically for 21 days then off 7 days Start with 0.5 g/day; dose adjustments (0.5 to 2 g) may be made based on individual response
Estrone	Estragyn Vaginal Cream *Senile vaginitis* *Pruritus vulvae* *Kraurosis vulvae*	2-4 g/day (1 mg active ingredient per gram) adjusted to the lowest amount that controls symptoms; administration should be cyclic (e.g., for 21 days then off 7 days)
Rings		
17β-estradiol	Estring *United States: Moderate to severe urogenital symptoms caused by postmenopausal atrophy of the vagina and/or the lower urinary tract* *Canada: Atrophic vaginitis, dyspareunia, dysuria, and urinary urgency*	2 mg (releases 7.5 μg/day) for 90 days
Estradiol acetate	Femring *VMSs* *Severe vulvar and vaginal atrophy*	Releases 50 or 100 μg of estradiol per day for 90 days; both doses release systemic levels and require consideration of a progestogen if the uterus is intact
Estradiol	Vagifem *Atrophic vaginitis*	Initial: 1 tablet/day for 2 wk Maintenance: 1 tablet twice/wk (tablet containing 10 μg of estradiol hemihydrates, equivalent to 10 μg estradiol)

TABLE 165-4 Approved Prescription Products for Menopausal Symptoms in the United States and Canada—cont'd

Product	Product Name(s)	Doses (mg/day)
COMBINATION ESTROGEN-PROGESTOGEN PRODUCTS		
Oral Continuous Cyclic		
Conjugated estrogens plus MPA	Premphase	0.625 mg estrogen + 5.0 mg progestogen 2 tablets: estrogen, and estrogen + progestogen Estrogen alone days 1-14, estrogen + progestogen days 15-28
Oral Continuous Combined		
Conjugated estrogens plus MPA	Prempro Premplus	0.3 or 0.45 mg estrogen + 1.5 mg progestogen, 0.625 mg estrogen + 2.5 or 5.0 mg progestogen
Ethinyl estradiol plus norethindrone acetate	femhrt, FemHRT Lo femhrt, FemHRT	2.5 μg estrogen + 0.5 mg progestogen 5 μg estrogen + 1 mg progestogen
17β-estradiol plus norethindrone acetate	Activella Activelle LD Activelle	0.5 mg estrogen + 0.1 mg progestogen, 1 mg estrogen + 0.5 mg progestogen 0.5 mg estrogen + 0.1 mg progestogen 1 mg estrogen + 0.5 mg progestogen
17β-estradiol + drospirenone	Angeliq	1 mg estrogen + 0.5 mg progestogen, 0.5 mg estrogen + 0.25 mg progestogen, 1 mg estrogen + 1 mg progestogen
Oral Intermittent-Combined		
17β-estradiol plus norgestimate	Prefest	1 mg estrogen and 1 mg estrogen + 0.09 mg progestogen Estrogen alone for 3 days, then estrogen + progestogen for 3 days Repeated continuously
Conjugated estrogens plus MPA	Premplus Cycle	0.625 mg estrogen + 10 mg progestogen 2 tablets: estrogen, and estrogen + progestogen Estrogen alone for 14 days, then estrogen + progestogen for 14 days
Transdermal Intermittent-Combined		
17β-estradiol plus norethindrone acetate	CombiPatch Estalis	0.05 mg estrogen + 0.14 mg progestogen 9 cm^2 patch, twice/wk 0.05 mg estrogen + 0.25 mg progestogen 16 cm^2 patch, twice/wk
17β-estradiol plus levonorgestrel	Climara Pro	0.045 mg estrogen + 0.015 mg progestogen 22 cm^2 patch, once/wk
PROGESTOGENS		
MPA	Provera Provera Pak Various generics	2.5, 5, 10
Micronized progesterone	Prometrium	100, 200
OTHER ORAL PRODUCTS		
Conjugated estrogens plus bazedoxifene	Duavee *Moderate to severe VMSs*	0.45 + 20 mg/day
Ospemifene	Osphena *Moderate to severe dyspareunia, a symptom of vulvar and vaginal atrophy, caused by menopause*	60 mg/day
Paroxetine	Brisdelle *Moderate to severe VMSs*	7.5 mg/day

Data from North American Menopause Society, 2015. www.menopause.org/docs/default-source/2014/nams-ht-tables.pdf 7-1-2014.

IMPLICATIONS FOR PRACTICE

The perimenopausal period offers a perfect opportunity to recommend healthy lifestyle choices and to address individual health risks as women transition into late midlife. Part of this discussion should include a conversation about the risks and benefits of HT, particularly if a women is experiencing premature or induced menopause.

In women using cyclic HT, endometrial sampling should be considered any time bleeding occurs at other than the expected time of withdrawal bleeding. Women using continuous-combined therapy should be evaluated if irregular bleeding persists more than 6 months after HT is started.

It is very important to remember that unexplained vaginal bleeding, particularly in a menopausal women, is cancer until proven otherwise. It is also important to recognize that although an endometrial biopsy may be the first diagnostic test conducted, it may not be the only test needed to evaluate the bleeding because the endometrium is not the only potential source of bleeding; bleeding and profuse watery discharge are also associated with fallopian tube carcinoma. Therefore, even if an endometrial sample is normal, if unexplained bleeding persists, additional tests and procedures, including hysteroscopy, laparoscopy, and possibly hysterectomy, may be required to diagnose the problem.

CHAPTER 166

PAP TEST ABNORMALITIES

Michelle Collins

DEFINITION AND EPIDEMIOLOGY

The Papanicolaou (Pap) test is a screening test for cervical cancer that involves collection of exfoliated cervical cells for cytologic staining and examination. Among the 30 million Pap tests performed annually in the United States, approximately 1.4 million (2.1%) reveal cytologic abnormalities requiring follow-up.[1] Cervical cancer affects approximately 12,000 U.S. women annually, with 4000 women dying from cervical cancer every year.[2] Cervical cancer mortality has decreased by 70% since the introduction of the Pap test 50 years ago; however, health disparity research has revealed that poor women, and particular ethnic minorities, have a higher incidence of cervical cancer mortality within the United States, with rates higher in African-American and Hispanic women than in white women.[3] Women immigrating to the United States from countries where cervical cytology screening is not routinely practiced are a group at particularly high risk.[4]

It is well known that particular strains of human papillomavirus (HPV) are involved in the etiology of cervical cancer. Papillomaviruses are small, double-stranded DNA viruses. Among the more than 100 types of HPV, 30 to 40 are genital subtypes; approximately 13 of those are high-risk types, particularly types 16 and 18, which are implicated as the cause of approximately 70% of all cervical cancers. HPV-16 accounts for approximately 50% of cervical cancers worldwide. Low-risk HPV subtypes, such as HPV-6 and HPV-11, are associated with genital warts and are not implicated in the etiology of malignant cervical disease.[5] HPV is the most common sexually transmitted infection in the United States, with at least 50% of sexually active persons becoming infected with at least one type of urogenital HPV during their lifetime; some estimates extend that to 80%. Although it is known that the presence of HPV is a necessary component for the development of cervical cancer, only a very small proportion of those women who are infected with HPV actually develop cervical cancer, which suggests that cervical cancer is a multifactorial phenomenon. It is the persistence of the HPV infection that is thought to be the impetus for precancerous and cancerous lesions.[6] Most HPV lesions resolve spontaneously, particularly in young women. This information, the result of research tracking women with HPV for several successive years, has led to the significant revision of screening and management guidelines for women younger than age 24.

PATHOPHYSIOLOGY

The development of cervical cancer is multifactorial. Some identified associated factors include older age, infection with particular high-risk HPV types, vaginal pH changes, hormonal changes, cellular trauma, long-term use of combined hormonal contraception, young age at coitarche, multiparity, history of sexually transmitted infections, having a sexual partner with a history of a sexually transmitted infection, having a higher number of lifetime sexual partners (defined as more than 5), younger age at first pregnancy, and cigarette smoking.[7]

HPV contains genes that encode proteins with particular functions in the life cycle of the virus. Among high-risk HPV types, the role of E5, E6, and E7 proteins is unique, allowing high-risk types of HPV to take control of an infected host cell for its own replication and survival. A normal host cell contains two important tumor suppressor genes (*p53* and *pRb*) that act as the guardians of the cell. Among high-risk HPV types, such as HPV-16, E6 and E7 proteins interfere with the *p53* and *pRb* host cell tumor suppressor genes, disrupting the normal cell life cycle. In a normal nonreplicating cell, *pRb* is bound to another protein, E2F, which is required for DNA replication. When HPV viral protein E7 displaces the connection between *pRb* and E2F, the usual control that *pRb* exerts over cell replication is disabled. Unbound E2F causes a normally nonreplicating cell to begin the complex sequence of cell replication necessary for the survival and reproduction of HPV. Usually, if *pRb* is dysfunctional, the other guardian of the cell, *p53*, recognizes this dysfunction and initiates a mechanism that suspends the cell cycle processes to repair the damage. Normally, when *p53* recognizes that the damage is not reparable, it triggers apoptosis (programmed cell death), preventing the damaged cell from future replication. However, HPV also disables *p53*, thereby allowing damaged cells to escape death and HPV to thrive. This aberrant replication process increases susceptibility to gene mutation. An unstable genome gives rise to carcinogenesis.[8,9]

HPV enters the body during vaginal, anal, or oral sexual contact, or by skin-to-skin transmission through intimate sexual contact. The virus passes through the cervical epithelium to the basal cell layer, where it enters the normally replicating basal cell and exploits the replicating machinery of the basal cell to establish itself and then begins to reproduce insidiously. It then accompanies the host cell through natural epithelial cell maturation until it is detectable in the normally nonreplicating suprabasal cells and surface epithelium.[10] After initial infection, HPV may exist as a latent infection for a period of months. Then it enters its productive phase, during which the virus produces a protective capsule that allows it to survive attached to superficial and exfoliated squamous cells. This protective capsule makes HPV highly infectious and sexually transmittable. Persistent HPV infection, combined with other cofactors, gives rise to cervical dysplasia, also described as cervical intraepithelial neoplasia (CIN). Low-grade lesions detected by Pap test and confirmed by cervical biopsy have a fairly high regression rate and frequently resolve spontaneously; the probability of regression of CIN 1 is approximately 70% to 80% in adult women, and greater than 90% in adolescents and young women.[11] However, high-grade lesions detected by Pap tests and confirmed by cervical biopsy are more likely than CIN 1 lesions to progress to cervical cancer than to regress, particularly for lesions that are CIN 3 as compared with those that are CIN 2.[12] In women who are immunocompromised, there is an even greater likelihood that cervical disease will ultimately progress.

CLINICAL PRESENTATION AND PHYSICAL EXAMINATION

Although frank cervical cancer may appear as a visible cervical lesion on the cervix, most cervical lesions detected as Pap test abnormalities are not visible by routine speculum and pelvic examination.

DIAGNOSTICS: CERVICAL CANCER SCREENING

Two techniques are currently available for Pap test specimen collection. The traditional Pap test involves collection of endocervical cells with a cytobrush or cotton swab, and collection of ectocervical cells with a wooden or plastic spatula. A slide is prepared, and fixative is applied immediately after specimen collection. A more recent technology for Pap test specimen collection and processing uses a liquid-based medium (SurePath, ThinPrep). The examiner uses either a plastic spatula and endocervical brush, or a cytobroom, for cell collection and then places the specimen in the liquid medium. The laboratory centrifuges the specimen, allowing the separation of cervical cells from blood, mucus, and cellular debris. When liquid-based cytology is used in the collection of a Pap test specimen, additional testing for gonorrhea, chlamydia, and HPV can be performed from the same specimen. Additional testing is not able to be done with the slide method of Pap testing.

HPV DNA testing has been approved by the U.S. Food and Drug Administration (FDA) as an adjunct to Pap testing when atypical squamous cells of undetermined significance (ASCUS) are detected. The FDA has also approved HPV DNA testing as a screening test for women older than 30 years as an adjunct to the Pap test. This age limitation is based on the concern that the high prevalence of inconsequential, transient HPV infections among women younger than 30 years would lead to an abundance of positive HPV results, resulting in unnecessary procedures and psychosocial concerns. HPV infection among women 18 to 25 years is more commonly transient and appears to frequently resolve spontaneously or to become undetectable within a period of 2 years.[13] Women older than 30 with a normal Pap test result and negative high-risk type HPV DNA test result can extend Pap test screening intervals to every 5 years rather than annually.[12]

The accuracy of Pap test screening depends, in large part, on proper specimen collection technique. Optimally, a Pap specimen should not be obtained during menses, or within 24 to 48 hours of having had intercourse or having used topical medications for vaginal infections. Health care providers should be aware that the Pap test sample should be obtained from the transformation zone of the cervix. The normal ectocervix (external surface of the cervix) is covered by stratified squamous epithelium. The endocervix (internal surface of the cervix) contains mucus-secreting columnar epithelium. The normal physiologic process of metaplasia transforms columnar epithelium into squamous epithelium, with the border between the columnar and squamous epithelium known as the squamocolumnar junction. The region of the cervix where columnar epithelium transforms into modified squamous epithelium is aptly named the transformation zone. The location of the squamocolumnar junction and the transformation zone varies according to a woman's age and hormonal influences. It may be located on the ectocervix, at the cervical os, or just inside the endocervix.[9,12]

MANAGEMENT

In 2012, existing consensus guidelines for the management of women with cytologic abnormalities, based on the Bethesda system of classification for the reporting of abnormal cervical cytologic findings, were revised (Box 166-1). ASCUS or low-grade squamous intraepithelial lesion (LSIL) is classified as low-grade lesions. High-grade squamous intraepithelial lesion (HSIL) and carcinoma in situ (CIS) are classified as high-grade lesions. The Pap result "atypical squamous cells, cannot rule out high grade" (ASC-H) is associated with high-grade lesions. High-grade lesions represent precursor lesions for the development of squamous cell carcinoma of the cervix. Atypical glandular cells, which are less frequently reported, may represent a precursor lesion for adenocarcinoma of the cervix.

The Pap test is the screening test for cervical cancer, whereas the biopsy is the definitive diagnostic test that guides treatment decisions. If there is no evidence of biopsy-proven cervical dysplasia, or CIN, then surveillance can include repeat cytology at particular intervals. If the biopsy reveals CIN 1, patients can be managed conservatively by repeating surveillance (which would be Pap, or Pap plus HPV, according to guidelines by age) at particular intervals. In some cases of persistent low-grade lesions, patients are given the option of surveillance versus treatment. If the biopsy reveals CIN 2, CIN 3, or more advanced abnormalities, treatment is indicated.[14] The 2012 Consensus Guidelines for the Management of Women with Abnormal Cervical Cancer Screening Tests guide the practitioner as to what is indicated after an abnormal Pap test result.

LIFE SPAN CONSIDERATIONS

According to the latest guidelines, Pap screening should begin no earlier than the age of 21 years, regardless of a woman's sexual history. Pap tests are then recommended every 3 years from the ages of 21 to 29 years. HPV testing (defined as testing for high risk HPV types only) for screening purposes is not appropriate for women in this age range. Between the ages of 30 and 65, HPV testing with the Pap test (also known as "co-testing") is the preferred method of cervical surveillance. Currently, screening by HPV alone, without a Pap test done simultaneously, is not recommended, though there may be a place for sole HPV DNA testing in the future according to very recent research. Cytology alone (i.e., Pap testing) every 3 years is an acceptable method of surveillance in the 30 to 65 age range, although Pap and HPV testing together is the preferred method. For women older than 65, no screening is recommended, given there has been adequate negative prior screening (defined as at least three consecutive normal Pap test results). Those women who have a history of CIN 2 or greater should continue screening past the age of 65 for a minimum of 20 years. Women who have had a hysterectomy and had their cervix removed should have screening discontinued unless they have a history of CIN 2 or greater in the past 20 years, or have ever had cervical cancer.[15] Immunosuppressed women, those infected with human immunodeficiency virus, women exposed to diethylstilbestrol in utero, and those previously treated for CIN 2 or 3 or cancer may require more frequent screening.[16]

INDICATIONS FOR REFERRAL

Clinicians' decisions for management should always be guided by the most recent screening and management guidelines.[14] Colposcopy is an office procedure conducted by a trained colposcopist in which the cervix and vagina are viewed directly under magnification, during which an ectocervical biopsy and endocervical sampling of cells may be obtained. According to most recent guidelines, patients with ASCUS lesions with a concurrent positive HPV DNA test result should be referred for colposcopy, unless they are younger than 24 years. Because HPV tends to clear the cells more impressively in younger women, those aged 21 to 24 with an ASCUS HPV-positive result no longer require colposcopy—only repeat cytology in 12 months. Although it is preferable to have a reflex HPV test run after the initial result of ASCUS is found, it is also acceptable to plan for repeat cytology in 12 months, without running a reflex HPV test. Women older than age 24 with an ASCUS HPV-positive result should be referred for colposcopy. For LSIL Pap results, as with ASCUS results, follow-up is age dependent. Women aged 21 to 24 with LSIL can be advised to follow up with cytology in 12 months. Women older than age 24 with LSIL should be referred for colposcopy as a next step, not repeat cytology. A reflex HPV DNA test is not indicated to be done after LSIL results because the vast majority of LSIL Pap results involve HPV. All patients with HSIL and ASC-H Pap results should be directed to undergo colposcopy. Women who have Pap results of "atypical glandular cells of undetermined significance" (AGUS or AGC) should have subsequent colposcopy with endocervical sampling, and women with this result who are 35 or older or who have risk for endometrial cancer should also undergo endometrial sampling. AGC Pap results can be indicative of either cervical or endometrial malignancies, or premalignant states.[14]

In addition, if a clinician notes a visible cervical lesion, particularly an erythematous, exophytic lesion, the patient should be directed to undergo colposcopy for further evaluation regardless of the Pap test result, because some frank cervical cancers may not be detected by Pap test.

PATIENT AND FAMILY EDUCATION

HPV infection should be discussed during disclosure of an abnormal Pap test result; patient education should include information about prevalence of HPV, course of infection, risk of cervical cancer, regression rates, cofactors influencing development of cancer, and health practices that may minimize progression of dysplasia. It is important for patients to understand that Pap testing remains the primary screening test for both persistent and recurrent cervical disease and that treatment decisions are based on both Pap (and HPV testing if indicated) (cytology) and biopsy (histology) results. Reassurance that cervical cancer may be preventable when precancerous lesions are detected and treated early in the course of dysplasia is appropriate.

BOX 166-1

The 2001 Bethesda System (Abridged)

SPECIMEN ADEQUACY

Satisfactory for evaluation
Unsatisfactory for evaluation
- Specimen rejected/not processed
- Specimen processed and examined, but unsatisfactory for evaluation of epithelial abnormality

GENERAL CATEGORIZATION

Negative for intraepithelial lesion or malignancy
Epithelial cell abnormality
Other

INTERPRETATION OF RESULT

Negative for intraepithelial lesions or malignancy
Organisms identified
- Trichomonas vaginalis
- Fungal organisms consistent with Candida species
- Shift in flora suggestive of bacterial vaginosis
- Bacteria consistent with Actinomyces species
- Cellular changes consistent with herpes simplex virus

Other non-neoplastic findings may include (optional to report; list not comprehensive):
- Reactive cellular changes associated with inflammation (includes typical repair), radiation, intrauterine contraceptive device
- Glandular cells status posthysterectomy
- Atrophy

Epithelial cell abnormalities
Squamous cell abnormalities
- Atypical squamous cells (ACS)
- Atypical squamous cells of undetermined significance (ASCUS)
- Atypical squamous cells, cannot exclude high-grade squamous intraepithelial lesion (ASC-H)
- Low-grade squamous intraepithelial lesion (LSIL) encompassing HPV, mild dysplasia, CIN 1
- High-grade squamous intraepithelial lesion (HSIL) encompassing moderate and severe dysplasia, CIN, CIN 2, CIN 3
- Squamous cell carcinoma

Glandular cell abnormalities
- Atypical glandular cells (AGC)
- Atypical glandular cells, favor neoplastic (AGC)
- Endocervical adenocarcinoma in situ (AIS)
- Adenocarcinoma

Other (list not comprehensive)
Endometrial cells in a woman ≥40 years of age

Modified from Solomon D, Davey D, Kurman R et al: The 2001 Bethesda system: terminology for reporting results of cervical cytology, *JAMA* 287(16):2114-2119, 2002.

In 2006, Gardasil, the first vaccine designed to prevent HPV infection, was approved by the FDA. Gardasil was developed to prevent cervical cancer, precancerous genital lesions, and genital warts caused by HPV. The vaccine is highly effective against four types of the HPV virus, including two (types 16 and 18) that cause 70% of cervical cancers. The vaccine is currently recommended for girls and women aged 11 to 26 years but can be given to girls as young as 9 years. Gardasil is licensed as a three-dose series given at 0, 2, and 6 months. The vaccine is given intramuscularly.[17]

In 2009 the FDA approved a second HPV vaccine, Cervarix, which provides protection against HPV types 16 and 18. It is approved for girls and women aged 10 to 25 years and is administered on a schedule similar to Gardasil, at 0, 1, and 6 months.[18] Ideally, the vaccines should be administered before the onset of sexual activity, but sexually active women should still be vaccinated. Women already infected with a type of HPV are also still candidates for the vaccination because they will be afforded protection from the types of HPV that they have not contracted.

In 2012 the American Academy of Pediatrics (AAP) recommended that the vaccine be given to both boys and girls at 11 or 12 years of age. Rationale for giving the vaccine at the prescribed ages is to vaccinate adolescents before the onset of sexual activity. If an individual is exposed to a strain of HPV included in the vaccine before immunization, there is no protection afforded. Another reason for the AAP age range recommendation is that children have the most efficacious antibody responses to vaccines when they are administered at ages 9 to 15.

In 2015 the Advisory Committee on Immunization Practices (ACIP) announced its recommendation for the 9-valent HPV vaccine (Gardasil). 9vHPV, approved by the FDA, contains HPV types 6, 11, 16, 18, 31, 33, 45, 52, and 58 virus-like particles (VLPs).[19] The FDA recommended 9vHPV for use in females aged 9 through 26 years and males aged 9 through 15 years.[19]

Of the three vaccines available in the United States, only Gardasil is approved for use in both boys and girls. Cervarix is approved only for use in girls.[20] Because the presence of HPV combined with the fear of potential cervical cancer often produces considerable psychological distress, it remains imperative to offer adequate counseling and information about the nature of HPV and abnormal Pap test results when giving women their results. Women may express concerns about future fertility, the stigma of harboring a sexually transmitted virus, and how to appropriately talk about HPV with their partners. They may be fearful of diagnostic and/or treatment procedures and may also have misconceptions about HPV. Women may also be confused by the medical jargon associated with HPV infection discussions, abnormal Pap results, colposcopies, biopsies, and treatment. All providers who perform Pap screening are responsible for being able to educate and to inform their patients about the abnormal Pap test result as well as further diagnosis and treatment. Excellent resources for patient education and support regarding abnormal Pap tests and HPV include the American Society for Colposcopy and Cervical Pathology (www.asccp.org), Association of Reproductive Health Professionals (www.arhp.org), American Social Health Association (www.ashastd.org), and National Women's Health Resource Center (www.healthywomen.org).

HEALTH PROMOTION

Women should be advised to have regular Pap screening according to the latest consensus screening guidelines. Although condom use does not completely prevent transmission of HPV, it appears to afford modest protection against cervical HPV infection as well as to possibly slow progression of viral spread and dysplasia development after HPV infection.

Recent work in the area of nutrition and HPV has found that the ingestion of certain foods, such as nuts, fish, fruits, and vegetables, may be a protective factor against HPV infection. Foods high in vitamin A and retinol, calcium, long-chain polyunsaturated fatty acids, and antioxidants (e.g., vitamins C and E, lutein, carotene, and lycopene) have been shown to reduce the risk of cervical cancer.[21] Healthy lifestyle habits, including adequate sleep, exercise, and avoidance of smoking, should be encouraged. There is evidence that certain practices that promote good health, including good nutrition, dietary supplementation of substances such as folic acid and beta-carotene, adequate sleep, and exercise, can help the body's cells fend off HPV's effects.[22]

In addition, one of the most important steps that health care providers can take toward decreasing the incidence of cervical dysplasia is to educate women on, and recommend, vaccination for HPV protection. Vaccination continues to be under-recommended and underused, according to the Centers for Disease Control and Prevention 2013 National Immunization Survey–Teen (NIS-Teen). Survey results noted that only 57% of adolescent girls and 35% of adolescent boys had received one or more doses of HPV vaccine.[23]

Health care providers must be vigilant in their efforts to screen patients of both sexes.

CHAPTER 167

PELVIC INFLAMMATORY DISEASE

Sheila Ann Medina

DEFINITION AND EPIDEMIOLOGY

Pelvic inflammatory disease (PID) refers to a spectrum of inflammatory disorders of the upper genital tract in women. It can include any combination of endometritis, salpingitis, tubo-ovarian abscess (TOA), and pelvic peritonitis.[1] There is a wide variation in the signs and symptoms associated with PID; although acute signs and symptoms are often moderately severe, many women have subtle or mild symptoms that go unrecognized. Nonetheless, the long-term sequelae resulting from fallopian tube damage and scarring can be serious and include ectopic pregnancy, recurrent episodes of PID, chronic pelvic pain, and infertility.[2,3]

It is estimated that each year in the United States, more than 750,000 women experience an episode of acute PID and 75,000 women are more likely to become infertile as a result of PID.[4-6] PID is the most common gynecologic reason for emergency department (ED) visits and hospitalizations in the United States. Women with PID make 2 million ED and office visits and incur health care costs exceeding $4 billion. PID affects more women of reproductive age, with a disproportionately higher incidence of African-American women.[7] Although the number of PID-related ED visits and hospitalizations remains high, more than three fourths of women treated for PID in the United States are now treated as outpatients, a trend that has been increasing during the past two decades.[2] Based on research looking at trends in PID from 2001 to 2013, cases of PID (based on hospitalizations and estimated ambulatory cases) have decreased significantly, but the annual estimate of acute and unspecified PID cases diagnosed in the United States for 2009 and

2010 was greater than had previously been published.[3] It is evident that PID remains an important public health concern for women and health care providers, especially those working in outpatient settings.

Direct costs for care of acute PID and its sequelae are estimated at $1.88 billion yearly, even though the majority of women receive care as outpatients.[4] The high financial and social costs related to PID are important to consider if the full impact of this disease is to be appreciated.

Risk factors for PID include being younger than 25 years, having multiple sexual partners, not currently or consistently using contraception, and living in an area with a high prevalence of sexually transmitted diseases (STDs). There is a strong correlation between the incidence of STDs and PID in any given population. Other risk factors for PID include penetration of the cervical mucus barrier during medical procedures, including the insertion of an intrauterine contraceptive device, vaginal douching, and cigarette smoking.[2] A woman's risk for PID is decreased if she uses barrier contraception, takes oral contraceptives, or has had a tubal sterilization.

The risk of PID in young women is significant; one in five cases of PID occur in women younger than 19, and one in eight adolescent girls will develop PID compared with one in 80 women older than 24 years.[1,8] From 2001 to 2013, 46.8% of all U.S. high school students had engaged in sexual intercourse, and 15% had had four or more partners, making STDs a major public health problem for adolescents.[9] Contact with multiple sexual partners, inconsistent use of contraception, and biologic vulnerability can account for the increased incidence of STDs in women younger than 25 years, although it does not fully account for the increased incidence of PID. Younger women with chlamydial infections of the cervix have a higher incidence of upper genital tract infection than do older women.[10]

Previous diagnosis of PID is a risk factor for subsequent episodes, with approximately 15% to 25% of all women with PID experiencing more than one episode.[10] These subsequent infections are generally new, primary attacks of PID, not flares of latent or chronic infection. Reinfection is often related to contact with untreated sexual partners. In addition, one third of women with PID will develop chronic pelvic pain.[8]

PATHOPHYSIOLOGY

PID is usually a polymicrobial infection caused by organisms that ascend from the vagina and cervix along the mucosa of the endometrium to infect the mucosa of the fallopian tubes. The most common organisms implicated in PID (one third to three quarters of cases) include *Neisseria gonorrhoeae* and *Chlamydia trachomatis;* however, microorganisms that can be part of the normal vaginal flora (e.g., anaerobes, *Gardnerella vaginalis, Haemophilus influenzae,* enteric gram-negative rods, and *Streptococcus agalactiae*) can also cause PID.[1,2] Newer data suggest that *Mycoplasma genitalium* may also play a role in PID and may be associated with milder symptoms.[1,11] *Mycoplasma hominis* and *Ureaplasma urealyticum* are also possible causative agents.[1] The mildest form of salpingitis involves tubal hyperemia, edema of the tubal wall, and exudate on the tubal surface and fimbriated ends.[12] If salpingitis is left untreated, further inflammatory changes of the pelvic organs occur, including tubal adhesions, pyosalpinx, and TOA.

The increased incidence of PID in young women may be explained by a larger cervical squamocolumnar junction, allowing easier colonization with *N. gonorrhoeae* or *C. trachomatis,* and by a decreased antibody response.[10] However, PID is uncommon in pregnancy because of the physiologic changes in the uterus.[11] The uterotubal junction is closed as early as the seventh week of gestation, and the chorioamnion covers the endocervix around the 12th to 15th week. An ascending infection before the 12th week often leads to endometritis and spontaneous abortion. After the 12th week, it results primarily in chorioamnionitis.

Rarely, PID can result from secondary extension of infection of adjacent organs, as in appendicitis or diverticulitis. It may also result from hematogenous dissemination of tuberculosis or as a rare complication of a tropical disease such as schistosomiasis. The following discussion refers only to ascending infections resulting in PID.

CLINICAL PRESENTATION

The clinical presentation of PID varies widely. Although some women are truly asymptomatic, others remain undiagnosed because of their mild or nonspecific signs and symptoms. These symptoms vary based on the pathogen responsible.[13] These can include fever or chills, cramping, dysuria, low back pain, nausea and vomiting, abnormal vaginal bleeding (postcoital or intermenstrual bleeding), dyspareunia, and vaginal discharge. The most common presenting symptom is lower abdominal and pelvic pain of less than 2 weeks' duration. The pain is typically described as dull and constant and is worsened by movement and sexual intercourse. The onset of symptoms occurs most commonly in the proliferative phase of the menstrual cycle. Complaints of fever or abnormal vaginal discharge may also be present.[13]

PID caused by gonococci is usually associated with a more intense inflammatory reaction in the tubal lumen than the reaction caused by chlamydial infection. Therefore the woman with a gonococcal PID may have a more acute presentation, often requiring hospitalization.[14]

Women with Fitz-Hugh–Curtis Syndrome (FHCS) are initially seen with right upper quadrant pain, pleuritic pain, and tenderness on liver palpation. These symptoms are often mistaken for hepatic disease, cholecystitis, or pneumonia.[15]

PHYSICAL EXAMINATION

The clinical diagnosis of acute PID is imprecise; lower abdominal pain may be mistakenly attributed to pregnancy (ectopic), ovarian cysts, or even appendicitis. No single history, physical, or laboratory finding is both sensitive and specific for the diagnosis of acute PID. According to the Centers for Disease Control and Prevention (CDC), empirical treatment of PID should be initiated in sexually active young women and other women at risk for STDs if they are experiencing pelvic or lower abdominal pain, if no cause of the illness other than PID (e.g., diverticulitis, ectopic pregnancy, or appendicitis) is identified, and if the pelvic examination is significant for one or more of the following criteria: cervical motion tenderness, uterine tenderness, or adnexal tenderness.[1] These criteria may not be sensitive enough to identify the more subtle cases of PID, and the following additional criteria enhance the specificity of the aforementioned minimum criteria and support a diagnosis of PID:

- Oral temperature above 38.3° C (101° F)
- Abnormal cervical or vaginal mucopurulent discharge
- Presence of white blood cells (WBCs) on saline microscopy of vaginal secretions
- Elevated erythrocyte sedimentation rate (ESR)

- Elevated C-reactive protein (CRP)
- Laboratory documentation of cervical infection with *N. gonorrhoeae* or *C. trachomatis*

Most women with PID have either mucopurulent cervical discharge or WBCs on microscopic evaluation of vaginal fluid. If the cervical discharge appears normal and no WBCs appear on the wet mount, the diagnosis of PID is unlikely and alternative causes of pain should be considered.[1]

DIAGNOSTICS

Acute PID is difficult to diagnose because of the wide variation in signs and symptoms. The clinical diagnosis of symptomatic PID has a positive predictive value for salpingitis of 65% to 90% compared with laparoscopy.[1] A pregnancy test should be performed immediately to assess for the possibility of ectopic pregnancy, although a negative result is not conclusive. Pelvic ultrasound evaluation is indicated when TOA is suspected. Additional studies to consider include the rapid plasma reagin (RPR) test for syphilis and serologic studies for human immunodeficiency virus (HIV) infection. PID can be diagnosed clinically, and empirical therapy initiated on the basis of some of the aforementioned findings. However, an evaluation that includes more extensive studies may be necessary if the diagnosis is unclear.

The most specific criteria for diagnosis of PID include endometrial biopsy with histopathologic evidence indicative of endometriosis; transvaginal ultrasonography, magnetic resonance imaging (MRI), or Doppler studies suggesting pelvic infection; and laparoscopic abnormalities consistent with PID.[16] However, these extensive procedures may not be warranted in all cases. Thus, an accurate diagnosis of PID is difficult, given the wide variation in symptoms on presentation. However, the potential damage to the reproductive health of women with even mild or atypical PID is well documented.[1] Diagnosis and management of other causes of lower abdominal pain are unlikely to be affected by the initiation of empirical therapy for PID.

DIAGNOSTICS

Pelvic Inflammatory Disease

LABORATORY

Serum level of human chorionic gonadotropin
Complete blood count and differential
ESR
CRP
Laboratory confirmation of cervical infection with *Neisseria gonorrhoeae* or *Chlamydia trachomatis*
RPR (to exclude concurrent syphilis infection)
HIV serology*

IMAGING

Pelvic ultrasound
Transvaginal sonography or MRI*
Endometrial biopsy with histopathologic evidence of endometritis*

OTHER

Laparoscopy

*If indicated.

DIFFERENTIAL DIAGNOSIS

The most important conditions in the differential diagnosis of PID are ectopic pregnancy, acute appendicitis, ovarian torsion, and ovarian cyst. Other conditions to consider include endometriosis, corpus luteum bleeding, pelvic adhesions, benign ovarian tumor, inflammatory bowel disease (IBD), irritable bowel syndrome (IBS), diverticulitis, pyelonephritis, nephrolithiasis, and cystitis.[2]

Gastrointestinal conditions and PID can give rise to lower abdominal pain, making it difficult to determine the cause of the symptoms. Thus, at-risk women with lower abdominal pain or pelvic pain and no other identified cause for their pain should be presumed to have PID.[5]

DIFFERENTIAL DIAGNOSIS

Pelvic Inflammatory Disease

- Ectopic pregnancy
- Acute appendicitis
- Ovarian or adnexal torsion
- Ovarian cyst
- Endometriosis
- Corpus luteum bleeding
- Pelvic adhesion
- Benign ovarian tumor
- IBS
- Diverticulitis
- Pyelonephritis
- Cystitis

MANAGEMENT

Treatment regimens for PID must provide empirical, broad-spectrum antimicrobial coverage, including anaerobic coverage. No single antibiotic agent is adequate; thus, combination therapy is necessary. In choosing therapy, the provider should consider availability, cost, patient acceptance, and antimicrobial susceptibility. The CDC provides periodic treatment recommendations for PID and other STDs.

Estimates for the percentage of cases of PID caused by infection with *C. trachomatis* or *N. gonorrhoeae* vary from 25% to 75%.[2] Nonetheless, most women are treated with antibiotics directed toward these bacteria.[17] However, in a study of women with clinically suspected PID, gram-negative and anaerobic gram-positive bacteria were also isolated and strongly associated with endometriosis.[17] For this reason, it has been recommended that all women with PID be treated with medication regimens that include metronidazole. This approach may reduce some of the frequency of potential PID sequelae, including recurrent PID, ectopic pregnancy, chronic pelvic pain, and infertility. Current guidelines from the CDC for treatment of PID include the addition of metronidazole for full coverage against anaerobes and bacterial vaginosis.[1]

Oral and parenteral therapy for PID is outlined in Box 167-1.[1] Patients receiving oral therapy should be reevaluated within 72 hours. Clinical improvement is indicated by defervescence; reduction in direct or rebound abdominal tenderness; and reduction in uterine, adnexal, and cervical motion tenderness. If significant clinical improvement is not seen within 72 hours after initiation of therapy, the patient should be reevaluated to confirm the diagnosis and to initiate parenteral therapy or surgical intervention. Patients should be tested for cure of infection with *C. trachomatis* and *N. gonorrhoeae* 4 to 6 weeks after the completion of therapy.

Patients receiving parenteral therapy should show substantial improvement within 72 hours after therapy is initiated. Those who do not receive parenteral therapy usually require further diagnostic evaluation or surgical intervention.

The trend has been toward outpatient treatment of PID, but concerns have been raised that outpatient treatment may be less effective than inpatient treatment at preventing some of the

BOX 167-1

Oral and Parenteral Therapy for PID

PARENTERAL TREATMENT

Parenteral Regimen A

Cefotetan (Cefotan) 2 g IV every 12 hr
Plus
Doxycycline (Vibramycin) 100 mg PO or IV every 12 hr
Or
Cefoxitin (Mefoxin) 2 g IV every 6 hr
Plus
Doxycycline (Vibramycin) 100 mg PO or IV every 12 hr

Note: Because of pain associated with infusion, doxycycline should be administered orally when possible, even when the patient is hospitalized. Both oral and intravenous administrations of doxycycline provide similar bioavailability.

Parenteral therapy may be discontinued 24 hours after a patient improves clinically, and oral therapy with doxycycline (100 mg twice a day) should continue to complete 14 days of therapy. When TOA is present, many health care providers use clindamycin or metronidazole with doxycycline for continued therapy rather than doxycycline alone because the combination provides more effective anaerobic coverage.

Parenteral Regimen B

Clindamycin 900 mg IV every 8 hr
Plus
Gentamicin loading dose IV or IM (2 mg/kg of body weight) followed by a maintenance dose (1.5 mg/kg) every 8 hr. Single daily administration (3-5 mg/kg) may be substituted.

Note: Parenteral therapy can be discontinued 24 hours after a patient improves clinically; continuing oral therapy should consist of doxycycline 100 mg PO twice a day or clindamycin 450 mg PO 4 times a day to complete a total of 14 days of therapy. When TOA is present, clindamycin may be preferable over doxycycline because clindamycin provides more anaerobic coverage.

Alternative Parenteral Regimens

Ampicillin-sulbactam 3 g IV every 6 hr
Plus
Doxycycline (Vibramycin) 100 mg PO or IV every 12 hr

Note: Ampicillin-sulbactam plus doxycycline has good coverage against *Chlamydia trachomatis, Neisseria gonorrhoeae,* and anaerobes and is effective for patients who have TOA.

ORAL TREATMENT

Recommended Intramuscular and Oral Regimens

Ceftriaxone (Rocephin) 250 mg IM in a single dose
Plus
Doxycycline (Vibramycin) 100 mg orally twice a day for 14 days
with or without
Metronidazole (Flagyl) 500 mg orally twice a day for 14 days
Or
Cefoxitin 2 g IM in a single dose and probenecid 1 g orally administered concurrently in a single dose
Plus
Doxycycline 100 mg orally twice a day for 14 days
with or without
Metronidazole 500 mg orally twice per day for 14 days
Or
Other parenteral third-generation cephalosporin (e.g., ceftizoxime or cefotaxime)
Plus
Doxycycline 100 mg orally twice per day for 14 days
with or without
Metronidazole 500 mg orally twice per day for 14 days

Note: The optimal choice of a cephalosporin is unclear; although cefoxitin has better anaerobic coverage, ceftriaxone has better coverage against *N. gonorrhoeae.* Clinical trials have demonstrated that a single dose of cefoxitin is effective in obtaining short-term clinical response in women who have PID; however, the theoretical limitations in its coverage of anaerobes may require the addition of metronidazole to the treatment regimen. Metronidazole also will effectively treat bacterial vaginosis, which is often associated with PID.

Alternative Oral Regimens

There are data to suggest that amoxicillin–clavulanic acid and doxycycline are effective when used together in obtaining short-term clinical response; however, gastrointestinal symptoms might limit compliance with this regimen. Azithromycin has demonstrated effectiveness in one randomized clinical trial; in another study, azithromycin (1 g orally once a week for 2 weeks) was effective when used in combination with ceftriaxone 250 mg IM single dose. When alternative regimens are used, the addition of metronidazole should be considered because of the presence of anaerobic organisms. In addition, metronidazole will also treat bacterial vaginosis.

As a result of the emergence of quinolone-resistant *N. gonorrhoeae,* regimens that include a quinolone are no longer recommended for the treatment of PID.

From Centers for Disease Control and Prevention (CDC): *2015 Sexually transmitted diseases treatment guidelines.* Available at www.cdc.gov/std/treatment/2015/pid.htm. Accessed August 11, 2015.

complications of PID, such as recurrent PID or infertility. However, studies comparing the inpatient and outpatient treatment regimens of the CDC have found no differences between inpatient and outpatient treatment groups in the rates of pregnancy, time to pregnancy, recurrence of PID, chronic pelvic pain, or ectopic pregnancy among women with mild to moderate PID.[11] In at least one subsequent study comparing the effectiveness of inpatient and outpatient treatments among women with suspected PID, ectopic pregnancy was found to occur rarely and more frequently in the outpatient group, but this difference was not significant.[8] Because of the high risk for maternal morbidity and preterm delivery, pregnant women with PID should be hospitalized and treated with parenteral antibiotics.[1] Aside from pregnancy, the CDC recommends hospitalization of women based on health care provider discretion and in certain situations (see Indications for Referral or Hospitalization).

Despite documented effective outpatient care for PID, studies have demonstrated that adolescents treated in outpatient settings have similar results to those treated in the inpatient setting. The absence of data to support any type of benefit from hospitalization for adolescent girls with PID led the CDC to not list adolescence among the criteria for hospitalizations and to suggest that a decision to hospitalize adolescents with PID should be based on the same criteria used for older women.[11]

Given the significant risk of future health problems associated with PID, efforts to adhere to recommended practice guidelines and to ensure patient adherence to care are critical in this high-risk population. Treatment of sexual partners of women with PID is imperative because of the risk for reinfection of the patient and the high incidence of urethral gonococcal or chlamydial infections in the male sexual partner. Partners who have had sexual contact with the patient during the 60 days preceding the onset of symptoms should be treated empirically with regimens effective against *C. trachomatis* and *N. gonorrhoeae*, regardless of the apparent cause of PID or pathogens isolated from the patient.[1] Sexual abstinence should be recommended until both partners have completed treatment.

COMPLICATIONS

Sequelae of PID include a significantly increased risk of tubal factor infertility, ectopic pregnancy, and chronic pelvic pain. A small number of deaths annually result from a ruptured TOA. Furthermore, the duration, severity, and number of episodes of PID are proportional to the prevalence of long-term sequelae.

FHCS involves perihepatic inflammation that is caused by the transperitoneal, lymphatic, or vascular spread of *N. gonorrhoeae* or *C. trachomatis*. There is inflammation of the liver capsule without parenchymal involvement.[12] FHCS develops in 5% to 10% of women with PID.[10] Chronic FHCS is characterized by adhesions between the anterior liver surface and the parietal peritoneum beneath the diaphragm. The treatment is the same as for PID.

INDICATIONS FOR REFERRAL OR HOSPITALIZATION

Referral for hospitalization of the patient with PID is indicated if:

- There is a surgical emergency, such as appendicitis or an ectopic pregnancy that cannot be excluded.
- The patient is pregnant.
- The patient has failed to respond clinically to outpatient therapy.
- The patient is unable to follow or unable to tolerate an outpatient regimen.
- The patient has severe illness, nausea and vomiting, or a high fever.
- The patient has a TOA.
- The patient is immunodeficient (e.g., HIV positive with a low CD4 count or receiving immunosuppressive therapy).

In early observational studies, HIV-infected women with PID were more likely to require surgical intervention.[1] A subsequent and more comprehensive study showed that despite a more severe clinical presentation, HIV-infected women with PID responded equally well to standard parenteral therapies.[1]

Gynecologic or surgical consultation is indicated when the diagnosis is unclear. Unilateral pelvic pain or a mass is a strong indication for laparoscopy.

PATIENT AND FAMILY EDUCATION

Patient education is an extremely important component in the treatment of the woman with PID. It must provide clear information about the diagnosis, including transmission and sequelae. The need for completion of therapy regardless of symptoms, timely follow-up, and partner treatment cannot be overemphasized. It is also helpful to encourage the patient in appropriate medical care–seeking behavior, including seeking care immediately when symptoms recur. The behaviors that increase the risk for PID also increase the risk for HIV infection. Rates of recurrent PID, chronic pelvic pain, and infertility have been shown to be highest among nonpersistent condom users.[1] Referral for HIV testing and counseling is recommended. Finally, information about prevention of future infections must be reviewed and repeated at all follow-up visits.

CHAPTER 168

SEXUAL DYSFUNCTION (FEMALE)

Sheila Ann Medina

DEFINITION AND EPIDEMIOLOGY

Sexual health plays an integral role in overall health, yet it is often overlooked and undertreated. Sexual dysfunction is an important aspect of sexual health that may affect a woman's self-esteem and quality of life. Several large-scale studies have confirmed that sexual satisfaction in women is strongly associated with life satisfaction and general well-being. Sexual health concerns should be taken seriously because they can lead to serious distress and interfere with relationships.[1] Sexual problems are highly prevalent, affecting between 40% to 45% of women in the United States in their lifetime.[2]

The *Diagnostic and Statistical Manual of Mental Disorders,* Fifth Edition (DSM-5) classifies female sexual dysfunction (FSD) into three major categories: (1) female sexual interest/arousal disorder; (2) female orgasmic disorder; and (3) genito-pelvic pain/penetration disorder.[3] FSD is further classified as to duration (lifelong versus acquired), as generalized versus situational, and by etiologic origin and/or treatment.

American Psychiatric Association guidelines specify that for the diagnosis of a female sexual disorder to be established, all of the sexual dysfunctions (except substance/medication induced sexual dysfunction) now require a minimum duration of approximately 6 months, and more precise severity criteria. The sexual problem must be recurrent or persistent, cause personal distress or interpersonal difficulty, and not be better accounted for by another mental disorder, drug-related cause, or medical condition.[3] The presence of distress is an essential criterion for the diagnosis; therefore a diagnosis of sexual disorder is not indicated unless the sexual dysfunction is associated with distress. Distress may be experienced because of a lack of sexual interest or arousal or as a result of significant interference with a woman's life and well-being.

Female sexual interest/arousal disorder is defined as diminished or absent sexual interest or arousal manifesting with at least three of six indicators for a minimum duration of approximately 6 months. Female sexual interest/arousal disorder is frequently associated with problems in experiencing orgasm, pain experienced during sexual activity, infrequent sexual activity, and couple-level discrepancies in desire.[3]

Five factors must be considered during the assessment and diagnosis of the patient, in addition to the subtypes "lifelong/acquired" and "generalized/situational." These factors may be relevant to the cause and/or treatment and include (1) partner factors (e.g., partner's sexual problems, partner's health status); (2) relationship factors (e.g., poor communication, discrepancies in desire for sexual activity); (3) individual vulnerability factors (e.g., poor body image, history of sexual or emotional abuse), psychiatric comorbidity (e.g., depression, anxiety), or stressors (e.g., job loss, bereavement); (4) cultural or religious factors (e.g., inhibitions related to prohibitions against sexual activity; attitudes toward sexuality); and (5) medical factors relevant to prognosis, course, or treatment.[3]

Female orgasmic disorder is defined as the persistent or recurrent inability of a woman to achieve orgasm, markedly diminished intensity of orgasmic sensations, or marked delay of orgasm during any kind of sexual stimulation despite self-reported high sexual satisfaction and arousal. The prevalence rates for female orgasmic disorders in women range from 10% to 42% and are varied based on multiple factors (e.g., age, culture, duration, and severity of symptoms).

Genito-pelvic pain/penetration disorder is defined as persistent or recurrent difficulties involving one (or more) of the following: (1) difficulty with intercourse, (2) genitopelvic pain, (3) fear of pain or vaginal penetration, and (4) tension of the pelvic floor muscles. This diagnosis is frequently associated with other sexual dysfunction, particularly sexual interest and arousal disorders. The five factors discussed under sexual dysfunction must also be considered during the assessment and diagnosis of genito-pelvic pain/penetration disorder because they may be relevant to the cause and/or treatment.[3]

Epidemiologic studies have yielded widely varied estimates of the prevalence of FSD, depending on the definition used as well as the population and specific dysfunction studied. The prevalence of female sexual interest/arousal disorder as defined in DSM-5 is unknown. Low sexual desire and problems with sexual arousal as defined by the the *Diagnostic and Statistical Manual of Mental Disorders,* Fourth Edition (DSM-IV) and International Classification of Diseases, Tenth Revision (ICD-10) may vary markedly in relation to age, cultural setting, duration of symptoms, and presence of distress. Low desire is a common sexual problem in women across all age groups worldwide; however, some older women report less distress about low sexual desire than younger women, although sexual desire may decrease with age.[3]

Studies reveal that the prevalence rate for dysfunction tends to increase as women become older, with approximately 40% to 45% of adult women revealing at least one sexual dysfunction.[4] Women also corroborate low levels of sexual interest, and report that with age sexual desire decreases. In general, arousal and lubrication problems are prevalent in 8% to 15%, although three studies have reported this at a higher level of 21% to 28% in sexually active women. In the United States, Australia, Canada, and Sweden, the prevalence of manifest orgasmic dysfunction is about 16% to 25% in 18- to 74-year-old women.[5] Estimates from multiple studies suggest that the prevalence of problems with women who experience difficulties with arousal or pain may range up to 28% for each.[5]

Prevalence rates are affected by a variety of factors including age, partner's age, duration of marriage, medical illness, menopause, family planning, and frequency of sexual intercourse had significant association with FSD. Studies have shown that prevalence of most sexual dysfunctions is higher in clinical than in community samples.[6]

PATHOPHYSIOLOGY

Female sexual response is a complex interaction of psychological, interpersonal, environmental, genetic, biologic, and physiologic factors that change throughout the life cycle. Thus, the pathophysiologic mechanism of a sexual complaint is typically multifactorial and complex, involving organic, functional, etiologic, and psychological factors. Vascular, neurogenic, hormonal, anatomic, medication-induced, and emotional factors have been implicated as major contributors to the development of FSD (Box 168-1).[3,7]

Any disease of the nervous system (e.g., multiple sclerosis, neuropathies, stroke) can result in neurogenic FSD with resultant impaired lubrication and orgasm. Any condition that affects blood flow, such as cardiovascular disease, hyperlipidemia, atherosclerosis, renal disease, and smoking, can affect sexual functioning. Vascular insufficiency with subsequent diminished genital blood flow may directly contribute to genital arousal disorder because of impairment of vaginal and clitoral engorgement. Decreased pelvic blood flow can lead to smooth muscle fibrosis of the clitoris and vagina, which may in turn cause symptoms of vaginal dryness and dyspareunia. Pelvic surgeries may injure autonomic pelvic nerves or interrupt blood flow, both of which may result in FSD.

Dysfunction of the hypothalamic-pituitary axis from natural menopause, surgical or medical castration, premature ovarian failure, or exogenous hormones can result in hormonally based FSD. The most common symptoms associated with estrogen deficiency are vaginal dryness, coital pain, and decreased desire. Diminished testosterone levels in women have been implicated as a cause of decreased arousal, libido, and orgasm.

The muscles of the pelvic floor contribute to sexual arousal and are responsible for the involuntary rhythmic contractions

BOX 168-1

Medical Conditions That May Affect Sexual Function

Cardiovascular: Hypertension, coronary artery disease, angina, myocardial infarction
Endocrine: Diabetes, thyroid disorders, adrenal insufficiency, congenital adrenal hyperplasia, hypopituitarism, hyperprolactinemia, metabolic syndrome, polycystic ovary syndrome
Neurologic: Parkinson disease, spinal cord injury, multiple sclerosis, neuropathies, stroke, seizure disorder, dementia
Rheumatologic: Arthritis, autoimmune diseases, fibromyalgia
Pulmonary: Chronic obstructive pulmonary disease, emphysema
Cancer-related: Breast and gynecologic cancers, ostomy surgery, chemotherapy, radiation therapy
Urologic: Urinary infections, interstitial cystitis, urinary incontinence, renal failure
Psychological: Depression, anxiety, premenstrual dysphoric disorder, history of sexual assault
Gynecologic: Vaginal atrophy, scarring, intact hymen or thick hymenal tags, vulvar vestibulitis, vulvodynia, vulvar dystrophy, vaginitis, vulvitis, endometriosis, pelvic masses, pelvic infection, pelvic floor dysfunction, prolapse

during orgasm. Increased tone of the levator ani muscle may cause dyspareunia and vaginismus, whereas hypotonia is associated with decreased vaginal sensation, coital anorgasmia, and urinary incontinence during sexual intercourse or orgasm. Anatomic causes such as uterine prolapse, pelvic tumors, and endometriosis are commonly associated with deep dyspareunia.

In addition, chronic illnesses, certain medications, substance abuse, and psychogenic issues, with or without organic disease, may contribute to the development of FSD. Self-esteem, body image, sociocultural factors, relationship issues, depression, and other mood disorders may significantly affect sexual response. Furthermore, many of the medications used to treat depression, especially the selective serotonin reuptake inhibitors (SSRIs), are associated with sexual side effects.

Most often, the cause of FSD is mixed, involving a combination of neurogenic, vascular, psychological, and hormonal causes. For example, women with diabetes may experience sexual dysfunction owing to disease-related neurovascular changes, medication side effects, and the psychological effects of coping with a chronic illness. In women, those who report excellent health compared with good, fair, or poor health are less likely to have sexual dysfunction. Sexual dysfunction is common in women with hypertension who use hypertensive drugs and seems to be associated with lubrication and orgasm dysfunction.[5]

CLINICAL PRESENTATION

It is important for clinicians to recognize that most women will not initiate a discussion of their sexual concerns. A recent study identified that 71% of symptomatic women never discussed their sexual concerns with their health care provider.[8] An open, understanding, nonjudgmental attitude is necessary to create a comfortable environment for patients to discuss this topic. Inclusion of sexual health questions in the history and review of systems legitimizes that sexual issues are appropriate to discuss. Asking open-ended questions (e.g., "Many women experience sexual changes after menopause. What changes have you noticed?") normalizes sexual concerns.

Basic screening for sexual dysfunction may begin merely with three key questions: (1) Are you currently sexually active? (2) If so, with men, women, or both? (3) Do you have any concerns or difficulties with sexual intercourse?[2] There are also several validated screening tools available for assessment of sexual problems. A self-administered sexual health questionnaire is the initial component of the evaluation. The abridged version of the Female Sexual Function Index (FSFI) questionnaire consists of six questions, each associated with a 5-point rating scale, and can be completed by patients very quickly in the office setting.[9,10]

A sexual history can be brief or extensive but should include the gynecologic history, sexual activity, number of partners, homosexual or heterosexual relationships, difficult or abusive sexual experiences, and satisfaction with sexual experiences. Problems with desire, arousal, lubrication, orgasm, pain, bleeding, or lesions should also be reviewed; sexually transmitted disease exposure and the need for contraception should be elicited. In addition, exploration of recent life events (e.g., divorce, separation, or recent losses) and cultural attitudes toward sexual activity should be considered.

A detailed psychosocial assessment is an important component of the evaluation of FSD. Given the interpersonal context of sexual problems, past and present partner relationships should be explored.[11] Because medications can affect all phases of the sexual response cycle, a drug review is also imperative.

PHYSICAL EXAMINATION

A complete history should be taken and a complete physical examination performed for every patient. In most cases, the physical examination will not identify the specific cause of sexual dysfunction but may be useful in uncovering relevant chronic diseases and identifying contributing anatomic, endocrine, vascular, or neurologic pathology. The presence of secondary sexual characteristics and hair distribution can be assessed during the general examination. A complete pelvic examination is required for evaluation of any sexual pain disorder and may be performed as indicated for evaluation of other FSDs.[12]

The external genitalia can be visually inspected for any lesions, anomalies, tenderness, erythema, edema, atrophy, thickening, prolapse, rectocele, or cystocele. Sensitivity to touch, pressure, vibration, and temperature may also be assessed. Presence of the bulbocavernosus and anocutaneous reflexes demonstrates integrity of the sacral nerves, which form the neurologic foundation of the sexual response cycle. Speculum examination may uncover lesions, inflammation, atrophy, or infection of the cervix or vagina. Bimanual palpation of the vagina, cervix, uterus, and adnexa may suggest the presence of pelvic tumor, infection, or endometriosis. Vaginal muscle tone can be evaluated by inserting two fingers in the vagina and having the patient squeeze them.

DIAGNOSTICS

FSD is complex and requires a multidisciplinary approach because currently there is no universally recommended battery of tests for its diagnosis. Diagnostic studies are guided by the history and physical examination findings. Laboratory tests may include wet mount, testing for gonorrhea and chlamydia, complete blood count (CBC), hormonal studies, fasting glucose concentration, lipid panel, renal panel, and liver function studies.[11-13] Pelvic ultrasound examination may be performed as indicated to rule out pelvic mass or anatomic anomaly. Screening for depression may also be indicated.

DIAGNOSTICS

Female Sexual Dysfunction

LABORATORY

- Luteinizing hormone (LH)*
- Follicle-stimulating hormone (FSH)*
- Dehydroepiandrosterone (DHEA)*
- CBC and differential*
- Thyroid profile*
- Liver enzymes*
- Prolactin*
- Testosterone*
- Serum estradiol*
- Hemoglobin A_{1c}*
- Fasting glucose*
- Blood urea nitrogen (BUN)*
- Creatinine*
- Wet mount*
- Testing for chlamydia and gonorrhea*

*If indicated.

DIFFERENTIAL DIAGNOSIS

Psychosocial difficulties, depression, post-traumatic stress disorder (PTSD), hormonal imbalance, thyroid disorders, adrenal disorders, liver disorders, kidney disorders, diabetes, infection, injury, substance abuse, arterial insufficiency, and neurologic

TABLE 168-1 Medications That May Affect Sexual Response

Category	Classification	Examples
Antihypertensives	Diuretics, angiotensin-converting enzyme inhibitors, alpha-adrenergic agents, beta blockers, calcium channel blockers, vasodilators	Clonidine, captopril, lisinopril, metoprolol, propranolol, methyldopa, spironolactone
Antidepressants	Monoamine oxidase inhibitors (MAOIs), tricyclic antidepressants (TCAs), SSRIs, serotonin-norepinephrine reuptake inhibitors (SNRIs)	Paroxetine, duloxetine, amitriptyline, venlafaxine, fluoxetine, sertraline, imipramine, trazodone
Antipsychotics	Phenothiazines, dopamine inhibitors	Chlorpromazine, olanzapine, risperidone, haloperidol, lithium, thiothixene
Anxiolytics	Benzodiazepines, barbiturates	Alprazolam, clonazepam, diazepam
Hormonal agents	Oral contraceptives, progestogens, aromatase inhibitors, gonadotropin-releasing hormone (GnRH) agonists	Medroxyprogesterone acetate, danazol, leuprolide (Lupron)
Anticonvulsants	γ-Aminobutyric acid (GABA) analogues, sulfamates	Gabapentin, topiramate
Miscellaneous	H_2 receptor antagonists, antihistamines, interferon alfa	Cimetidine, diphenhydramine, pravastatin (Pravachol), digoxin, niacin

disease or injury are important conditions that should be considered in the differential diagnosis. In addition, it is important to consider that many commonly used drugs, especially antihypertensives, psychotropics, and hormonal agents, may have negative effects on sexual function (Table 168-1).[10,13]

MANAGEMENT

Many sexual concerns can be addressed during a routine office visit by a primary care provider with accurate, unbiased information about female sexuality, referral to educational resources, suggestion for lifestyle changes, and referrals for individual or couples counseling.[14] The PLISSIT model of sex therapy is a graduated counseling system that provides a useful framework for addressing sexual concerns.[15] First proposed in 1976, the PLISSIT model remains useful in primary care practice today. The acronym stands for four levels of interventions: permission, limited information, specific suggestions, and intensive therapy. Examples of giving permission are letting patients know that sexual concerns are appropriate to discuss and reassuring them that their sexual anatomy or practices are normal. The second step involves providing limited information, such as dispelling myths or explaining the sexual response cycle. At the next level, specific suggestions, such as position changes, use of lubricants, or methods of self-exploration, may be offered. Finally, patients may be referred to a specialist if intensive therapy is indicated; however, the majority of sexual concerns may be adequately addressed within the context of a routine office visit employing the lower levels of this hierarchical model.

Psychological treatments include cognitive behavioral therapy, directed masturbation, sensate focus, and systematic desensitization.[16] Relationship issues and disparities in sexual desire between partners can be addressed in couples therapy. Women with focal muscular vaginal pain may be referred for pelvic floor physical therapy or trigger point injections. Pelvic floor muscle exercises are done to increase strength, to decrease incontinence, to improve blood flow, and to facilitate a orgasm. Symptoms related to vaginal dryness may be managed with use of supplemental lubricants.[16]

The Eros Clitoral Therapy Device (Eros-CTD) is a hand-held vacuum device that is available by prescription and approved by the U.S. Food and Drug Administration (FDA) for the treatment of female sexual arousal and orgasmic disorders. The device works by improving blood flow and stimulation to the clitoris and external genitalia. An implantable neurostimulation device is currently being evaluated for effectiveness in treating neurogenic FSD.

Local estrogen therapy, in the form of vaginal tablets, rings, creams, and pessaries, is highly effective for alleviating symptoms of urogenital atrophy. Because conjugated equine estrogen cream is well absorbed from the vagina, it should be paired with progestogen to prevent unopposed estrogen stimulation of the endometrium. Topical estradiol and estriol preparations have low systemic absorption and therefore do not require addition of progestogen for endometrial protection. Vaginally applied dehydroepiandrosterone (DHEA) and ospemifene, a selective estrogen receptor modulator, show promise as future therapies for treatment of vaginal atrophy.

In clinical trials, treatment with a testosterone patch resulted in significantly increased desire and arousal in postmenopausal women who were experiencing a decrease in sexual desire or interest; however, there are no data to support its use in premenopausal women.[17] Potential side effects of weight gain, acne, deepening of voice, clitoral enlargement, increased facial hair, hypercholesterolemia, and the risk of a cardiac event must be weighed against any potential benefits of treatment. Tibolone is a synthetic steroid sex hormone demonstrated to improve multiple dimensions of sexual function in clinical trials. Both the testosterone patch and tibolone have been approved for use in Europe; however, neither is FDA approved for the treatment of FSD in the United States.[16]

The selective phosphodiesterase type 5 inhibitors sildenafil, vardenafil, and tadalafil are approved for the treatment of erectile dysfunction in men but are not FDA approved for the treatment of sexual dysfunction in women. Although studies have shown that sildenafil may benefit women with sexual dysfunction related to SSRI use, spinal cord injury, or diabetes, results in other patient populations have shown no benefit.[17] Phentolamine is an alpha-adrenergic antagonist that causes vasodilation by relaxing smooth muscle and may improve lubrication and arousal in menopausal women with sexual arousal disorder but is not FDA approved for that indication.

Centrally acting agents show some promise for targeting low desire. Studies have demonstrated the effectiveness of the antidepressant bupropion in improving both arousal and orgasm in nondepressed women with decrease in sexual desire, interest, or arousal and in increasing desire in depressed women with SSRI-associated sexual side effects.[17] Flibanserin (Addyi), a 5-hydroxytryptamine agonist-antagonist, gained FDA approval in 2015 to treat hypoactive sexual desire disorder.

Herbal therapies, marketed as "natural" remedies for FSD, abound despite a lack of data on their efficacy and safety. A few very small randomized controlled trials of products containing yohimbine, ginseng, *Ginkgo biloba*, and damiana have shown promising results for improving sexual function and satisfaction. More research is needed to establish their role in the treatment of FSD.

COMPLICATIONS

Sexual dysfunctions can interfere with intimacy, adversely affect relationships, and have a negative impact on a woman's self-esteem, health, and sense of well-being. Failure to address a patient's sexual concerns may lead to eroded relationships, depression, self-medication with drugs and alcohol, and other psychosocial consequences. Primary care providers are in a unique position to uncover and to address sexual dysfunctions, thereby preventing these sequelae.

INDICATIONS FOR REFERRAL

The decision of whether to refer a patient with sexual dysfunction will depend on the provider's level of comfort and expertise as well as the complexity of the dysfunction. Many sexual concerns and dysfunctions can be treated with good anticipatory guidance and education about sexuality and sexual health. For some patients, the underlying medical condition is treated. For those who may require extensive general or sex therapy, referral to a reputable, certified sex therapist is warranted. The following professional organizations maintain listings of credentialed therapists on their websites:

- American Association of Sexuality Educators, Counselors, and Therapists (www.aasect.org)
- American Board of Sexology (www.americanboardofsexology.com)
- Society for Sex Therapy and Research (www.sstarnet.org)
- American Association for Marriage and Family Therapy (www.aamft.org)

Evaluation in a women's sexual health clinic, if it is available, may allow a better elucidation of the problem and a more comprehensive treatment approach.

LIFE SPAN CONSIDERATIONS

Providers should be aware of the range of sexual changes that occur across the life span. Each life stage may have unique physical and emotional influences to be considered. The transitional periods of adolescence, childbearing, menopause, and widowhood may profoundly influence sexual response.

EDUCATION AND HEALTH PROMOTION

Professional organization websites, such as the Association of Reproductive Health Professionals (www.arhp.org), the North American Menopause Society (www.menopause.org), and the American Congress of Obstetricians and Gynecologists (www.acog.org), are excellent sources of patient education materials pertaining to female sexual health. Condition-specific brochures are available from the American Cancer Society (www.cancer.org), the National Vulvodynia Association (www.nva.org), and many other medical organizations. Healthy Women (www.healthywomen.org and www.sexandahealthieryou.org) is an online organization dedicated to women's health issues and has developed a comprehensive series of publications addressing FSDs.

Education should be directed toward the understanding of normal sexual response, basic genital anatomy and physiology, and self-care measures. The importance of diet, exercise, and adequate sleep cannot be overstated because stress and fatigue are significant factors that affect sexual desire. Promotion of cholesterol reduction, tobacco cessation, and blood pressure and glycemic control may go a long way in the prevention of potential vasculogenic causes of FSD.

CHAPTER 169

UNPLANNED PREGNANCY

Cara Cohen

DEFINITION AND EPIDEMIOLOGY

The term *unplanned pregnancy* is defined as a pregnancy that is undesired at the time of conception or that is mistimed (occurs earlier than desired).[1,2] However, use of a single term to refer to unplanned pregnancies masks some of the differences between women with mistimed pregnancies and those with unwanted pregnancies. Women with unwanted or unintended pregnancies are more likely to have health risks that could negatively affect pregnancy outcomes. Unintended pregnancies are associated with greater unfavorable maternal behaviors and increased health risks for both mother and child than mistimed pregnancies are. Therefore, clarification of the difference between mistimed pregnancy and unintended pregnancy may help guide clinicians as they provide direct services to women and infants.[2]

Women with unintended pregnancies are less likely to receive the appropriate prenatal care, take prenatal vitamins and supplements, exercise during pregnancy, become vaccinated, eat a healthy diet, and gain the recommended amount of weight.[3] In addition, they are more likely to engage in high-risk sexual behaviors, smoke cigarettes, drink alcohol, and abuse drugs and have a higher risk for developing mental health issues.[3] Some but not all studies suggest that there is an increased risk of negative perinatal outcomes, such as low birth weight, preterm birth, and lower breastfeeding rates, associated with unintended pregnancies. Infants born to a mother with an unintended pregnancy are more likely to be readmitted to the hospital after discharge home. One study suggests that the emotions associated with having a child who was not planned for have long-term negative consequences for the parent-child relationship.[4] In addition, significant social and economic costs, at both the personal and community levels, are associated with unintended pregnancies.[5] In 2002, the medical costs associated with unplanned pregnancies in the United States totaled close to 5 billion dollars.[6]

The overall pregnancy rate for women 15 to 44 years of age in recent years is about 100 pregnancies per 1000 women; that is, approximately 10% of women of reproductive age become pregnant in any single year. Approximately 50% of those pregnancies are unintended. The rate of unintended pregnancies varies on the basis of several factors, including ethnicity, education, income, and marital status. Approximately 35 per 1000 white women have unintended pregnancies, compared with 78 per 1000 Hispanic women and 98 per 1000 black women. Unintended pregnancies occur in 26 per 1000 college graduates and in 76 per 1000 women who do not have a high school diploma.[7,8] One in 10 women aged 18 to 24 will have more than one unintended pregnancy.[9] This is twice the rate for all women of childbearing age.[9] Women whose income level is below 100% of the federal poverty level have an unintended pregnancy rate of 112 per 1000 women. Women whose income is twice the poverty level have an unintended pregnancy rate of 29 per 1000 women.[10] Adolescent women have the highest proportion of unintended pregnancies, with at least 75% of pregnancies in women younger than 19 years being unintended.[1] Approximately 750,000 adolescents in the United States become pregnant each year, and most of these pregnancies are unintended.[11] Thirty-five percent of these adolescents will have a rapid repeat pregnancy, which is a pregnancy within 2 years of a previous pregnancy. Of these rapid repeat pregnancies in adolescents, 35% are unplanned.[12] The United States has one of highest rates of adolescent pregnancies among developed countries.

Approximately 14% of unintended pregnancies end in miscarriage. There are no official statistics kept on the number of children adopted each year, but estimates range from 1% to 3% of unplanned pregnancies.[13] This number remains low despite changes to the adoption system over the past several decades that have resulted in an increase in support for birth parents.[14]

The high prevalence of unintended pregnancy is surprising, given that contraception is widely available in the United States. Although approximately 62% of women aged 15 to 44 years used contraception in 2006 to 2008, the proportions were significantly lower in four groups: teenagers 15 to 19 years of age (28%); never married, non-cohabitating women, some of whom are teens (39%); childless women (44%); and women who intend to have (more) children in the future (47%).[7] Reasons for contraceptive nonuse differ according to the age of the woman and the circumstances surrounding the event. For example, contraceptive nonuse at first intercourse and hence unintended pregnancy were most often related to concerns that parents would find out about sexual activity. Older women with a second or higher-order pregnancy were more likely to discontinue contraception because of its side effects and medical complications.[1] Interestingly, experts estimate that 48% of the unintended pregnancies in the United States occur in women who use contraception but are not using it correctly.[15]

Although three fourths of reproductive-age women see a health care provider annually, less than 50% receive contraceptive or family planning services.[13] Because women receive most of their preventive care from nongynecologic providers, primary care providers (PCPs) have a unique opportunity to provide contraceptive counseling to prevent unintended pregnancy.[16] Studies suggest that PCPs vary in their knowledge and perceived competence in providing contraceptive counseling. In addition, PCPs may inaccurately assess a woman's need for contraceptive counseling, misunderstand reasons for contraceptive nonuse, relegate the responsibility for contraceptive counseling to a subspecialist, or wait for the patient to initiate the discussion about contraception.[16] PCPs should ask women about their reproductive life plan. This includes an assessment of how many children they have, if they want more children, and when they want more children. The answers to these questions can help guide appropriate care for women of childbearing age.[17]

CLINICAL PRESENTATION

Patients may visit a provider because of signs and symptoms of possible pregnancy, without having taken a pregnancy test. These signs and symptoms may include a missed period, nausea and vomiting, breast pain, dizziness, and fatigue. Patients who feel especially vulnerable and are in denial about a pregnancy may not take a test at home and may want to take the test in a health care setting so that they have immediate guidance. Taking a test in a provider's office can prove to be beneficial for patients who have minimal support at home and those with mental health problems.

A positive result of a pregnancy test can generate a variety of responses. For some patients, the news brings joy and excitement; for others, the news can be a crisis of varying proportions. Given this, the provider should use neutral language when delivering the news of a positive pregnancy test result. Although many personal and socioeconomic factors may affect a woman's individual reaction, one common denominator is ensured: the woman's life is changed.

The health care provider is often the patient's first confidant in the first few minutes after delivery of the news of an unplanned pregnancy and is in a unique position to assist her in meeting her total health and wellness needs. For women for whom the pregnancy represents a crisis, several types of reactions can occur. With an unplanned pregnancy, the health care provider's response is critical in establishing and maintaining an environment that feels safe and supportive to the patient. The provider's initial role is to listen; both verbal and nonverbal communications provide information that is useful in developing the care plan. The patient needs to be allowed time to express her feelings. It is important that the provider not congratulate the patient or console her until the patient's feelings have been assessed.

Patients feel especially vulnerable and pressured to find a quick and easy solution. Many report feeling as though they are racing against the clock, and they look to the significant people in their life for support and advice. Support may be lacking, or advice from these sources may differ from what the patient desires. A study by Joyce and colleagues found that the parents' disagreement over the pregnancy was the most important predictor of instability in the mother's intention regarding the pregnancy.[18] In addition, a woman's intentions regarding the pregnancy are not fixed and may change, depending on where she is on the continuum from preconception to postpartum.

In many cases, the pregnancy is not the only issue that concerns the patient. In fact, the patient's reaction to the pregnancy may conceal her real concerns—finances, relationship problems, domestic violence, sexual abuse, or other issues. A woman's reaction to an unplanned pregnancy is in part based on her evaluation of the obstacles she faces in life. Nelson and O'Brien found that women who decide to continue with pregnancy and have trouble organizing and coping with their emotions are at risk for developing a pattern of negativity that will affect the quality of the parent-child relationship.[4] Assessment of these concerns is essential in the decision-making process for healthy outcomes.

MANAGEMENT AND COUNSELING

Counseling of a woman with an unplanned pregnancy can be challenging and emotionally difficult for both the health care provider and the woman involved. This challenge is accentuated by the personal feelings that each provider may have about unplanned pregnancy, the options available, and the fact that an unplanned pregnancy can be a crisis in a woman's life.[11] Health care providers need to understand and accept that a woman's perspective and her goals and way of achieving them may conflict with their own. Before a provider can put aside his or her own beliefs and biases about reproductive choices and options, he or she needs to thoughtfully reflect on what those beliefs might be and how they might influence the education and counseling provided to a woman with an unplanned pregnancy. It is virtually impossible for a provider to rid himself or herself of personal values and biases, but the provider must be committed to and vigilant about keeping those biases out of the interaction with the woman and other people involved in the situation. If a provider feels that he or she is unable to put personal beliefs and values aside, the patient should be referred to someone else for counseling and management.[14]

Every woman has the right to factual and unbiased information about reproductive choices to make an informed decision about the pregnancy. Based on this, it is important for the provider to keep in mind that the woman is responsible for defining how the unplanned pregnancy is a problem for her, and she is responsible for her own exploration, assessing her options, and ultimately making a decision and acting on it. The provider's role is to actively listen to the woman, to provide information and support, and to help the woman assess her options. A patient may ask the provider what she should do or what the provider would do if he or she were in the woman's situation. It is important for the provider to remind the patient that it is her decision and that the provider will support her through that decision, whatever it may be. Patients often ask health care providers what they would do, often deeming a provider's answer to be "the right answer." The solution to the unplanned pregnancy lies with the woman.[13]

After the patient has expressed herself, the health care provider can assist with prioritizing the patient's concerns and needs by focusing on one issue at a time. By exhibiting a willingness to listen and help, the provider helps build the patient's confidence. An exploration of the patient's feelings about pregnancy, the child, abortion, and abortion alternatives provides an opportunity to further process the situation. It is also helpful for the provider to know whether the patient has previously experienced an unplanned pregnancy or whether she knows anyone who has dealt with an unplanned pregnancy and the decision to have an abortion, to raise the child, or to surrender the child for adoption. A critical piece of information concerns the woman's support system and the role of the child's father in the woman's life and in the decisions about this pregnancy. Although patients seek a rapid solution to the crisis of an unplanned pregnancy, the provider should encourage the patient to take the time necessary to make an informed decision about this life-changing situation because even a decision to end the pregnancy can have long-term effects.

Patients may need time to process their emotions and to discuss the pregnancy with the significant people in their lives. A scheduled follow-up visit provides an opportunity to further discuss with the patient her reactions and their effect on decision-making as well as to provide information and available support services. These initial meetings play an important role in how patients react to their pregnancy and assist with the decision-making process.

The health care provider should inform the patient of the full range of available options. For someone experiencing an unplanned or a crisis pregnancy, abortion is often viewed as the only solution. However, other viable options do exist. Referrals to crisis pregnancy centers can provide patients with the expertise of trained staff and can broaden their options. If the patient does not want to go to a crisis pregnancy center or if one is not accessible to her, a referral to a professional counselor is appropriate. The provider should keep in mind that in some cultures abortion is illegal, so a patient may need be forthcoming about her true wishes.[19] The more informed the patient is, the less likely it is that she will regret the eventual decision. It is important to assure the patient that all information discussed will be kept confidential. Regardless of the decision, continued and unconditional acceptance of and compassion toward the patient will contribute to her overall wellness at this critical time.

Counseling a patient who is experiencing a crisis pregnancy can be very challenging. The following framework, which contains lists of questions for the health care provider to ask the patient, may help make this interaction fruitful for both patient and provider.

Focus on the patient. There is often a great deal of conversation about and concern for the infant. However, it is the woman who is experiencing the crisis, and it is she who ultimately makes the most adjustments.

Inquire about the patient's feelings. The health care provider should ask some of the following questions:

- How are you feeling about this pregnancy? *or* What does the pregnancy mean to you?
- Before finding out that you were pregnant, what were your feelings about abortion? Adoption? Parenting?
- Under what circumstances do you believe abortion (adoption, parenting) is okay? Not okay? Why?
- Under what circumstances would you like to become a parent?
- Who knows that you are pregnant?
- What is your relationship with the father of the baby? How involved is he in the decision-making? How supportive will he be of your decision?
- Who is your support system?
- Are you considering an abortion?
- Are you considering alternatives to abortion?

Make abortion real. If a patient is considering an abortion, it is important that she have as much accurate information as possible about the procedures involved, the risks, and the possible complications.

- Have you ever been pregnant before?
- Have you ever had an abortion?
- What does abortion mean to you?
- Do you know how abortions are performed?
- Do you know the physical risks of having an abortion?
- Do you know anyone who has had an abortion?
- What were your opinions about abortion before you learned you were pregnant?

Make the infant real. To make an informed decision, the patient needs to learn about the development of the fetus. Pictures of fetal development may be helpful for some patients. This should be done cautiously so the provider does not unintentionally sway a patient's decision. The health care provider should be prepared to discuss the different stages of fetal development.

- Do you know the present physical development of the fetus?

Focus on the woman and her future. The health care provider should ask the following:

- Under what circumstances would you like to become a parent?
- How would you feel if this was your only pregnancy?
- What are your goals for the next year? The next 5 years? How would each alternative help or hinder the achievement of these goals?
- What part of your circumstances is the most frightening or challenging?
- What is the worst thing you think might happen?
- How would you like for things to turn out for you ideally?

Remind the patient that she has time to make her decision. The provider should discuss the hormones of pregnancy and how they affect the decision-making process, especially during the first few months.

Use caution when adoption is mentioned as an option. The word *adoption* can generate negative or even painful feelings. In counseling patients, it is helpful to listen for any hints as a guide to the patient's feelings about this topic. Both the health care provider and the patient need to remember that adoption is an option. It is not a quick decision but rather a process to work through.

Develop a care plan. For patients who are committed to continuing the pregnancy, a care plan needs to be developed and should cover the following topics:

- Referral to an obstetrician for prenatal care
- Prenatal vitamins for the patient to take while awaiting her first prenatal visit
- Information on diet and healthy lifestyle
- Basic treatment for dealing with early pregnancy discomforts
- Financial resources
- Type of aid available to the patient, if needed, before and after birth
- Plans with regard to work or school
- Type of housing arrangements available during the pregnancy and after delivery
- The patient's relationship with the father of the baby
- Marriage
- Single-parenting issues
- Adoption (Even if the patient plans to keep her infant, she needs to consider the issues involved in adoption and the impact of adoption on herself and the infant.)
- Child support
- Day care
- Support from family and friends

For the patient who has decided to have an abortion, the complexities involved should be realistically reviewed. For example, a woman who is being pressured by the father of the child to have an abortion runs the same risk of being abandoned after the abortion as she would if she were to keep the child. A woman who has had repeated abortions needs to consider the possibility of future gynecologic, obstetric, and psychological complications. It is not uncommon for women who have had an abortion to experience a subsequent miscarriage, ectopic pregnancy, placenta previa, abruptio placentae, or premature birth. Psychological problems can include guilt, remorse, anger, eating disorders, addictions, and spiritual alienation. These manifestations are categorized under a condition called *postabortion stress syndrome* and may be similar to those of post-traumatic stress disorder.

The health care provider should provide factual information and be understanding as the patient makes plans and considers her options. The provider should avoid exerting pressure or being judgmental. The decision must be made by the patient; preparation is directed toward helping the patient make a decision that she can live with in the future.

If the patient plans to place the infant for adoption, assistance should be provided to establish future life goals. Professional counseling and support services are critical to prepare for the legal termination of parental rights and to assist the woman with some of the psychological aspects of releasing her infant. The patient should be encouraged not to view adoption as an indication of lack of love for her infant or as an indication that she is any less of a mother than a woman who keeps her infant. The choice of adoption can be viewed as providing both the patient and the infant with opportunities not otherwise possible.

Attempts should be made to thoroughly explore the possibilities of keeping the infant. Failure to go through this thinking and feeling process may contribute to future regrets concerning this decision.

LIFE SPAN CONSIDERATIONS

Research on unintended pregnancies indicates, as expected, that the age of the mother is strongly associated with intention. Studies show that more than 80% of mothers younger than 18 years indicated that they did not intend to become pregnant. In contrast, only 19% to 22% of women in their early 30s reported that they did not intend to become pregnant. Although a significant number of older women may not intend to become pregnant, the percentage is still considerably lower than in the group younger than 18 years.[8] Given this profile of unintended pregnancy, it is important for providers to ask all women of childbearing age about their plans for having children and to discuss the potential risks inherent in unplanned pregnancy and the benefits of planning. Several studies have documented a positive relationship between parent-adolescent communication and adolescent contraceptive use.[20] Thus, interventions designed to facilitate and to enhance parent-adolescent communication may help decrease the rate of unintended pregnancies in this high-risk age group.

COMPLICATIONS

Unplanned pregnancy has different associated risks, depending on whether the pregnancy was unwanted or untimed. According to a study comparing the mood states and parental attitudes of mothers with unplanned pregnancies, women with unplanned pregnancies demonstrate greater mood disturbances during their last month of pregnancy and during the first year postpartum than do women with planned pregnancies. In particular, during the last month of pregnancy, women with unintended pregnancies had greater levels of anxiety, depression, irritability, weariness, and confusion than women with planned pregnancies.[21]

INDICATIONS FOR REFERRAL

Referrals are based on a woman's decision about her pregnancy. Providers need to be aware of resources in the community to support a woman's choices. There may be situations in which a patient with an unplanned pregnancy must see a specialist immediately. These situations include the following:

- A patient who verbalizes thoughts of hurting herself or the fetus
- A patient who is in immediate danger because of domestic violence
- A patient who is experiencing bleeding and/or severe abdominal pain

PATIENT EDUCATION

Health care providers are in a unique position to provide counseling regarding pregnancy options for women experiencing the crisis of an unplanned pregnancy. This type of counseling is based on a commitment to respect the patient's autonomy, to provide accurate information, and to support women in their choices. It is helpful to give the patient written information to refer to as she goes through the decision-making process.

CHAPTER 170

VULVAR AND VAGINAL DISORDERS

Heidi Collins Fantasia

VULVAR DISORDERS

DEFINITION AND EPIDEMIOLOGY

Benign vulvar disorders, which encompass a broad range of dermatologic conditions, account for significant patient concern. Women may delay seeking treatment owing to fear, embarrassment, or confusion over which health care provider would best understand their condition. Therefore, symptoms may be present for some time before women seek care. Signs and symptoms of benign vulvar disorders can include pruritus, pain, burning, irritation, and a mass and/or growth. Women have often tried nonprescription remedies before coming to a provider.[1]

Pruritus is often the chief patient complaint for most vulvar disorders, and skin breakdown is common from scratching. Vulvar pruritus is a nonspecific vulvar symptom that may be unrelated to vaginitis, sexually transmitted infections (STIs), Bartholin duct cysts, or neoplasms. Proper treatment of vulvar pruritus depends on an accurate diagnosis. Women with vulvar pruritus often receive multiple treatments in the absence of a correct diagnosis; women are commonly prescribed therapy over the phone without ever having been examined, even if symptoms have been recurrent.[2]

In examining women with vulvar pruritus, the provider is advised to ask about and to inspect other areas of the body; many conditions affecting other organ systems, including tuberculosis, Crohn disease, and endometriosis, can have vulvar manifestations. For example, vulvar psoriasis may have an unusual presentation, but more typical psoriatic lesions are often seen simultaneously elsewhere on the body and may provide a diagnostic clue. Even with an experienced clinician, several visits may be needed to diagnose and to improve certain vulvovaginal conditions.

The visual inspection is essential in identifying vulvar changes. A hand-held microscope, or in some cases a colposcope, may allow more detailed inspection. Vaginitis, cervicitis, and other STIs should be excluded. Some of the common vulvar conditions causing pruritus are presented in this chapter.

LICHEN SCLEROSUS

Pathophysiology

Lichen sclerosus (LS) is a chronic condition with an unclear cause. Multiple factors are most likely involved in the development of this disorder. LS can have an autoimmune component, and women with LS may also develop other autoimmune diseases such as thyroid disorders, anemia, vitiligo, and alopecia areata. It has also been postulated that LS may be triggered by an infectious process, a genetic predisposition, and decreased estrogen levels.[3]

LS is primarily seen in perimenopausal and postmenopausal women, and the incidence increases with age. Although LS can occur in females of all ages, postmenopausal women are affected more frequently than women of other age groups. Approximately 1 in 30 older women has LS, and it is especially common in women with psoriasis.[4] It also affects males but at rates much lower than in females. LS is primarily found in the anogenital region, but it can be seen elsewhere on the body, such as the neck and shoulders.

Clinical Presentation and Physical Examination

Although it is sometimes asymptomatic, LS often results in severe vulvar pruritus and/or dyspareunia. Affected areas include the labia minora, vulvar vestibule, perineum, and clitoris; the vagina is usually spared. Early LS can be particularly difficult to diagnose. Early in the disease process, women may report vague vulvar burning and generalized irritation or itching that is difficult for them to localize and quantify. On examination, white papules can be seen, and the epithelium may appear normal or thin, resembling parchment.[5] Typically, tissue elasticity is decreased and edema may be present, depending on the disease stage. Fissures and secondary infections may develop, especially with sexual activity or scratching, which may make diagnosis especially difficult. With disease progression, papules develop into large, hypopigmented, symmetric plaques, often hourglass or keyhole shaped, on the labia minora, vulva, and anal area, which can resemble hyperplasia.[6] If these are not treated, there is eventual loss of vulvar architecture such that the labia minora are no longer seen, and introital stenosis may develop, resulting in dyspareunia, ecchymosis, fissures, and telangiectasis.

Diagnostics

- Thorough history is obtained to assess timing, onset, location, and duration of symptoms and any factors that may alleviate or aggravate the condition.
  - Fungal infections such as external yeast have a more rapid onset and are associated with erythema.
- Physical examination is performed to visualize any skin changes.
  - May be performed with hand-held magnifying glass or colposcope to improve visualization of the skin.

- Punch biopsy of the affected area will confirm diagnosis if examination findings are inconclusive. Biopsy is also important to exclude atypia or mixed diagnoses. Findings on histologic examination include hyperkeratosis, epithelial thinning, cytoplasmic vacuolation of the basal layer of cells, follicular plugging, homogenization of the subepithelial layer, and inflammatory cell infiltration consisting of lymphocytes with few plasma cells.
- Other diagnostics to consider include the following:
  - Complete blood count (CBC) if infection is suspected from scratching or skin breakdown.
  - Autoimmune laboratory tests including thyroid function tests, antinuclear antibodies, vitamin B_{12}. Autoimmune testing is not routinely done because the link between an autoimmune process and LS is not strong enough to justify the expense of the laboratory work.

DIAGNOSTICS

Lichen Sclerosus

LABORATORY

Consider autoimmune laboratory testing if autoimmune process strongly suspected

CBC with differential if clinical signs of skin infection

OTHER DIAGNOSTICS

Punch biopsy

Differential Diagnosis

It is important to establish the correct diagnosis of LS. This condition requires long-term treatment. Women should be prepared for the chronicity of the disorder and expected length of time to symptom improvement.

DIFFERENTIAL DIAGNOSIS

Lichen Sclerosus

- Lichen planus
- Vitiligo
- Contact or allergic dermatitis
- Atrophic vaginitis with atrophy
- Fungal infections

Management

Specialist referral is indicated for biopsy results that indicate hyperplasia or atypia. Surgical consultation is warranted if there is evidence of severe architectural changes or scarring. Women with LS have a slightly increased risk of developing squamous cell carcinoma. If there is evidence of severe architectural changes and/or vaginal, urethral, or anal stenosis, a surgical consultation is warranted.

The primary goals of treatment are symptom relief and prevention of disease progression.

1. Superpotent corticosteroids currently provide the best outcomes. However, treatment with ultropotent steroids is recommended for only 4 to 6 weeks.[7]
2. Clobetasol, halobetasol, or betamethasone dipropionate augmented 0.05% in an ointment base is recommended.
3. A typical regimen is a thin layer of steroid applied to the affected area once or twice daily for 2 to 4 weeks, then tapered to three times per week for maintenance therapy.[8] Long-term sequelae of potent topical corticosteroids (atrophy and thinning of skin and subcutaneous tissues) have not been clinically significant in this disorder because the vulvar skin is steroid resistant and can tolerate long-term application of superpotent steroids.[9] Contact dermatitis is a rare but reported side effect of this medication.
4. Subsequent LS recurrences are managed by reinstating the corticosteroid therapy.[9] It may be appropriate to switch to a milder corticosteroid such as betamethasone valerate 1% (high potency) or triamcinolone ointment 0.1% or fluocinolone acetonide ointment 0.025% (moderate potency) for long-term management.[10]
5. Topical antibiotic ointment can use used to treat signs of mild infection caused by scratching and excoriation.
6. Prescription (e.g., hydroxyzine, 25 to 50 mg) and over-the-counter (OTC) (e.g., diphenhydramine, 25 to 50 mg) antihistamines given at bedtime may also help relieve pruritus associated with LS.
7. Topical tacrolimus or systemic acitretin or etretinate may be beneficial
8. Application of topical estrogen cream can improve symptoms if LS exists in the presence of menopausal vulvovaginal atrophy.
9. Other relief measures to consider include the application of cool compresses and cool soaks and wearing loose-fitting clothing.

Life Span Considerations

LS is more common among menopausal women and may exist in the presence of atrophy related to estrogen deficiency. In addition, skin changes associated with aging predispose skin to trauma owing to thinning and decreased elasticity.

Complications

Thin, nonelastic tissue associated with LS can cause stenosis of the vaginal opening and result in painful intercourse (dyspareunia). This can often be corrected with topical steroids and/or estrogen therapy. A more serious complication is permanent scarring; surgery may be required to lyse adhesions and restore vulvovaginal functioning.

Indications for Referral or Hospitalization

If there is indication of atypia, hyperplasia, or a mixed diagnosis on biopsy, a gynecologic referral is indicated, especially in older women.

LS is often seen in combination with hyperplasia and requires closer follow-up monitoring.[5] Women with LS have a slightly increased risk of developing squamous cell carcinoma.

If there is evidence of severe architectural changes and/or vaginal, urethral, or anal stenosis, a surgical consultation is warranted. The role of surgery is defined in LS and should be limited to repair of introital stenosis or confirmed malignant disease.[11]

Patients who do not respond to a course of topical, high-potency steroids or who report ongoing pain should be referred to a gynecologic dermatology specialist. Other treatment modalities can include oral tricyclic antidepressants (amitriptyline, desipramine, and nortriptyline) and steroid injections.

Patient and Family Education

LS requires a long-term treatment plan that will span the lifetime. Women should be educated that this condition is chronic

BOX 170-1

Patient Education and Resources

1. Wear loose, soft clothing as much as possible, such as skirts without underwear while at home. Avoid spandex and stockings, or try thigh-high or shorter stockings.
2. Wear all-white, all-cotton underwear always (not just cotton crotch panel).
3. Use only white, unscented toilet paper.
4. Use mild laundry detergent and rinse underwear a second time in hot water.
5. When bathing, use mild soap and carefully rinse vulvar area with plain water. Ensure that all soaps and shampoos are completely rinsed from the area.
6. Avoid deodorant tampons and pads; instead of panty liners on light days, wear old underwear that can get stained. Another option is reusable cotton menstrual pads, available from GladRags (www.gladrags.com).
7. Avoid douches and deodorant sprays or powders in the groin area.
8. Use pure vegetable oil or mineral oil for lubrication with sex; avoid other commercial lubricants and spermicides.
9. Maintain as much nonpenetrating sexual activity as possible.
10. Rinse vulva after voiding with plain water spray bottle.
11. Keep detailed symptom diary that includes at least the following: characteristics of symptoms, their severity and duration, and triggering event if identified.
12. Contact national resources for local support groups, additional information, and newsletters:
    VP (Vulvar Pain) Foundation: www.vulvarpainfoundation.org
    National Vulvodynia Association: www.nva.org

and episodes of symptom control will be interwoven with disease exacerbations. Each woman will respond differently to steroid treatment and it may take some time and different dosing regimens to discover the best treatment plan. Women who are sexually active will need guidance on methods to reduce dyspareunia. Because women with LS have a slightly higher risk of squamous cell carcinoma, the importance of yearly skin checks should be stressed. General patient education information for all women with vaginal and vulvar complaints is listed in Box 170-1.

LICHEN PLANUS

Pathophysiology

Lichen planus (LP) is an acute or chronic inflammatory dermatosis affecting the skin, scalp, and the mucous membranes of the mouth, vulva, and vagina. The frequency of LP varies according to the population studied, but there is an estimated prevalence of 1% to 2% in the United States.[12] LP affects middle-aged people most often, although childhood LP has been described in the literature. Women are affected as often as men.[12] The cause is uncertain, but evidence suggests that it may have an autoimmune component, and inflammation precedes the appearance of lesions. Other possible triggers for LP can include infection with the hepatitis C virus and exposure to certain metals and chemicals.

Clinical Presentation and Physical Examination

In the genital area, there are two presentations of LP: classic or erosive. The appearance of classic LP includes well-defined delicate, white, reticulated papules. Erosive LP involves the presence of erythematous, erosive lesions and a desquamating process. Large denuded areas may lead to profuse leukorrhea or can become adherent, causing stenosis of the vaginal introitus.

Physical examination findings can vary with vulvar LP. Erythema is possible, as well as erosions and a lacy appearance on the skin. As with LS, the examination may reveal architectural changes that include loss of genital features, scarring of the vulva and anus, and urethral and vaginal stenosis. Women with LP often complain of a variety of vulvar symptoms, including pain, pruritus, burning, dyspareunia, and dysuria.

Diagnostics

- Diagnosis is established based on a thorough history and clinical examination findings.
  - Erosive LP may also have clinical features of herpes simplex virus (HSV) and Bechet disease.
- Physical examination is performed to visualize any skin changes.
  - May be performed with hand-held magnifying glass or colposcope to improve visualization of the skin.
- Biopsy of the affected area will confirm diagnosis if examination findings are inconclusive. Findings on histologic examination include chronic inflammation, presence of lymphocytes with few plasma cells, colloid bodies, and acanthosis and thinning of the epithelium.
- Other diagnostics to consider include the following:
  - Viral culture for HSV if erosive presentation
  - Hepatitis C antibodies
  - Autoimmune or allergy testing

DIAGNOSTICS

Lichen Planus

LABORATORY	OTHER DIAGNOSTICS
Consider hepatitis C antibody testing Consider autoimmune or allergy tests	Punch biopsy

Differential Diagnosis

Because LP may have two different clinical presentations, establishing a correct diagnosis can be challenging. As with LS, this is a chronic condition that requires long-term treatment. Symptoms with vary depending on presentation (classic versus erosive), and women should be prepared for the chronicity of the disorder and expected length of time to symptom improvement.

DIFFERENTIAL DIAGNOSIS

Lichen Planus

- Lichen sclerosus
- Ulcerative STIs: HSV, syphilis, chancroid
- Bechet disease
- Contact or allergic dermatitis
- Atrophic vaginitis with atrophy
- Fungal infections

Management

Specialist referral is indicated for biopsy results that indicate hyperplasia or atypia. Surgical consultation is warranted if there is evidence of severe architectural changes or scarring.

The primary goals of treatment are symptom relief and prevention of disease progression. LP requires lifelong management and treatment that is similar to that for LS.

1. Superpotent corticosteroids are the first-line treatment.
2. Clobetasol, halobetasol, or betamethasone dipropionate augmented 0.05% in an ointment base is recommended. A typical regimen is a thin layer of steroid applied to the affected area once or twice daily for 2 to 4 weeks, then tapered to three times per week for maintenance therapy.[8] Long-term sequelae of potent topical corticosteroids (atrophy and thinning of skin and subcutaneous tissues) have not been clinically significant in this disorder because the vulvar skin is steroid resistant and can tolerate long-term application of superpotent steroids.[9] Contact dermatitis is a rare but reported side effect of this medication.
3. The frequency of maintenance applications of topical steroids will vary depending on individual response and extent of the disease. Lifelong management is necessary to decrease pain and scarring.
4. Topical antibiotic ointment can be used to treat signs of mild infection caused by scratching and excoriation.
5. Prescription (e.g., hydroxyzine, 25 to 50 mg) and OTC (e.g., diphenhydramine, 25 to 50 mg) antihistamines given at bedtime may also help relieve pruritus associated with LP.
6. Application of topical estrogen cream can improve symptoms if LP exists in the presence of menopausal vulvovaginal atrophy.
7. Petrolatum ointment may be applied as a barrier for sensitive skin.
8. Other relief measures to consider include the application of cool compresses, cool soaks, and use of loose-fitting clothing.

Life Span Considerations

LP often manifests at midlife. For women this often coincides with the perimenopausal and postmenopausal years. LP may exist in the presence of atrophy related to estrogen deficiency, which can further increase discomfort. In addition, skin changes associated with aging predispose skin to trauma as a result of thinning, decreased elasticity, and a decreased ability to act as a first-line protection against injury.

Complications

Severe LP can cause significant pain, decreased quality of life, and interference with daily activities. Thin, nonelastic tissue associated with classic LP can cause stenosis of the vaginal opening and result in painful intercourse. This can often be corrected with topical steroids and/or estrogen therapy. A more serious complication is permanent scarring; surgery may be required to lyse adhesions and restore vulvovaginal functioning. Erosive LP can cause chronic pain, sexual dysfunction, and dysuria.

Indications for Referral or Hospitalization

If there is indication of atypia, hyperplasia, or a mixed diagnosis on biopsy, a gynecologic referral is indicated, especially in older women.

- If there is evidence of severe architectural changes and/or vaginal, urethral, or anal stenosis, a surgical consultation is warranted. The role of surgery is limited; surgery is used only to repair introital stenosis or confirmed malignant disease.[11]
- Patients who do not respond to a course of topical, high-potency steroids or who report ongoing pain should be referred to a gynecologic dermatology specialist and possibly a pain management specialist. Other treatment modalities can include topical application of an immunomodulating medication (tacrolimus)[13] and intramuscular injection of triamcinolone acetate.[14]

Patient and Family Education

Similar to LS, LP is a chronic condition that requires treatment over the life span. Symptoms and subsequent treatment will vary depending on whether the woman has classic or erosive LP. Pain is common with LP and can significantly affect a woman's quality of life and sexual functioning. Symptom management may involve a multidisciplinary approach that includes gynecologists, dermatologists, pain specialists, and pelvic floor physical therapy. The use of vaginal dilators may be necessary to prevent scarring and stenosis of the vaginal introitus. Women with LP should receive education on general vulvar care, including loose-fitting clothing; mild soaps; gentle patting of the vulvar area to dry; mild laundry detergent; cotton underwear; and sleeping without underwear or pajama bottoms. See Box 170-1.

LICHEN SIMPLEX CHRONICUS

Pathophysiology

Lichen simplex chronicus (LSC), or squamous cell hyperplasia, is the result of repetitive surface trauma from irritants that cause scratching or rubbing—a perpetual itch-scratch cycle. LSC is characterized histologically by epithelial thickening, lichenification, hyperkeratosis, and eczematous inflammation. It manifests, as do most of the non-neoplastic epithelial disorders, as pruritus, which may be secondary to degeneration and inflammation of terminal nerve fibers. The cause is not completely known, but atopic dermatitis is a common finding in women affected by LSC.

Clinical Presentation and Physical Examination

Intense itching (vulvar pruritus) is often the chief complaint. The pruritus may be aggravated by friction, heat, perspiration, or tight clothing. The affected woman may complain of a history of chronic scratching, which causes further pruritus. The pruritus often occurs at night and therefore sleep disturbances and fatigue are common. Painful erosions and fissures can result from the chronic scratching.

LSC may affect the labia majora, outer aspect of the labia minora, and anal area. On examination, the skin may exhibit thickening, and fissures are possible. Often, LSC initially manifests with small red papules. Reddened plaques develop from the papules, or if the condition has been ongoing without treatment, the skin may be more deeply colored, rough, and furrowed. Areas of excoriation are common.[10]

Diagnostics

- The condition is difficult to differentiate from other pruritic vulvar conditions. Diagnosis is made by history of chronic pruritus with scratching and examination findings that

support LSC. The underlying cause of the pruritus is often not immediately apparent.
- Physical examination is performed to visualize any skin changes. Magnification is often not needed.
- Punch biopsy of the affected area will confirm diagnosis if examination findings are inconclusive. Biopsy is also important to exclude other pruritic vulvar conditions such as LS, LP, and eczema and also to exclude atypia. The most important areas from which biopsy specimens should be taken are those of fissuring, ulceration, induration, and thick plaques. Findings on histologic examination include lichenification, hyperkeratosis, and chronic inflammation.

DIAGNOSTICS

Lichen Simplex Chronicus

LABORATORY	OTHER DIAGNOSTICS
None	Punch biopsy

Differential Diagnosis

Because LSC has a presentation and symptoms similar to those of many other pruritic vulvar conditions, it is important to establish a correct diagnosis. Treatment for LSC focuses on interrupting the itch-scratch cycle.

DIFFERENTIAL DIAGNOSIS

Lichen Simplex Chronicus

- Lichen sclerosus
- Lichen planus
- Psoriasis
- Eczema or allergic dermatitis
- Fungal infections

Management

Specialist referral is indicated for biopsy results that indicate atypia.

Treatment is aimed at relief of the itch-scratch cycle.

1. Topical steroids applied twice daily will reduce inflammation. Choice of strength will depend on the patient's subjective report of severity and examination findings.
2. Superpotent steroids (clobetasol, halobetasol) can be initiated if symptoms are severe. Moderate-potency (betamethasone valerate) or low-potency (hydrocortisone 2.5%) steroids can also be used for milder cases.
3. Removing any potential skin irritants is imperative.
4. Thickened plaques can be soaked in warm water or 5% Burow solution.[1] After thorough drying, an emollient such as petrolatum can be applied as a skin barrier.
5. Systemic antihistamines such as diphenhydramine, doxepin, or hydroxyzine taken at bedtime will reduce nighttime pruritus and scratching.
6. Tricyclic antidepressants such as amitriptyline taken at bedtime will also help control pruritus.
7. Screen for secondary fungal and bacterial skin infections.
8. Women should be reevaluated 4 to 8 weeks after beginning treatment.

Life Span Considerations

Although LSC can occur in children, it most often occurs after age 30 and can coincide with the menopausal transition. This is a chronic condition that women will need to manage throughout the midlife and older adult years. Aging skin is more susceptible to trauma from scratching, and advising patients to wear soft cotton gloves to bed may help reduce skin breakdown from scratching. As women age, urinary incontinence is more common, and wet skin from exposure to urine increases the risk of excoriation and infection. LSC in the presence of atrophy from estrogen deficiency of menopause may need to be treated with topical estrogen therapy.

Complications

LSC can cause skin changes such as hypopigmentation or hyperpigmentation that may be permanent. The severe pruritus that is a hallmark symptom of LSC can cause sleep disturbances, fatigue, and decreased quality of life. Skin breakdown places patients at risk for superimposed bacterial and fungal infections that can be painful. Decreased sexual function from pruritus and pain is possible.

Indications for Referral or Hospitalization

If there is indication of atypia, hyperplasia, or a mixed diagnosis on biopsy, a gynecologic referral is indicated, especially in older women.

- Women with LSC very rarely need hospitalization for this condition.
- Women who do not respond to a course of steroids, who report ongoing pain, or who have a superimposed skin infection that has not responded to antibiotics should be referred to a gynecologic dermatology physician.
- If an underlying allergic component is suspected, consultation with an allergist is important to identify allergens.
- LSC can have a psychological component to the chronic pruritus and scratching. Mental health evaluation and treatment may be appropriate for some women.

Patient and Family Education

Similar to LS and LP, LSC is a chronic condition that requires treatment over the life span. Tricyclic antidepressants at bedtime are often prescribed to help control itching and scratching symptoms and not to control depressive symptoms. Women need education regarding their treatment plan and the multifaceted approach to the management of this disorder.

CONTACT DERMATITIS

Pathophysiology

Contact dermatitis of the vulvovaginal area results when the area comes in contact with an allergen or irritant. This causes localized inflammation and edema. Pruritus is common. Contact dermatitis occurs when there is an immediate irritation of the area after exposure to an offending substance. Allergic responses, on the other hand, develop several days after exposure.[10]

Clinical Presentation and Physical Examination

Women with vulvar contact dermatitis often report a recent onset of vulvar irritation, pruritus, burning, soreness, or discomfort. These symptoms often worsen with friction or if skin is wet. Dysuria may result when acidic urine passes over inflamed or excoriated skin. On examination, erythema is typically present, and excoriation can result from scratching. Skin may be thickened if contact with the irritant or allergen has occurred over an extended period of time. Vaginal discharge is not common.

Diagnostics

- Diagnosis is established through history and physical examination.
- Physical examination findings include erythema or edema.
- A thorough history is crucial to a correct diagnosis.
- No specific laboratory tests are indicated.
- A punch biopsy may be considered if LS, LP, or LSP is suspected in addition to the contact dermatitis.

DIAGNOSTICS

Contact Dermatitis

LABORATORY
None

OTHER DIAGNOSTICS
Punch biopsy only if other dermatoses are suspected

Differential Diagnosis

Vulvar pruritus, irritation, burning, and pain are associated with a variety of vulvar conditions. Although erythema and edema are hallmark symptoms of contact dermatitis, other vulvar conditions must be considered.

DIFFERENTIAL DIAGNOSIS

Contact Dermatitis

- Lichen sclerosus
- Lichen planus
- Lichen simplex chronicus
- Psoriasis
- Eczema
- HSV
- Fungal infections

Management

- The goal of management is identifying the triggering substance and eliminating it.
- The list of possible irritants is extensive (Box 170-2). Women should be asked about treatments to the vulva (either prescribed or OTC medications) and use of feminine hygiene products (such as douches, sprays, and deodorants), tampons or pads, condoms, spermicides, lubricants, laundry detergents, soaps, and shampoos.
- Burow compresses, sitz baths, or emollients may improve symptoms.
- Antihistamines may help control pruritus.
- The use of a low potency topical steroid (triamcinolone 0.1% or hydrocortisone 2.5%) can be useful to bring acute symptoms under control.
- Allergic dermatitis usually takes a long time to resolve after exposure is terminated; resolution may be facilitated by a short course of topical steroids.

Life Span Considerations

Contact dermatitis can occur at any point in the life span. Some women report a lifelong history of sensitive skin that is easily irritated. Women with vulvar contact dermatitis should introduce any new treatments slowly to avoid possible increased irritation from the treatment. Aging skin is more susceptible to trauma, and women with contact dermatitis should be instructed on gentle vulvar care that will not increase symptoms or excoriation.

BOX 170-2

Potential Vulvar Irritants

1. Tight clothing, spandex clothing, synthetic underwear, latex and elastic in clothing
2. Laundry detergent, fabric softener, dryer sheets, bleach
3. Rough, scented or colored toilet paper; personal wipes
4. Menstrual hygiene and incontinence products, including pads, panty liners, and tampons (especially if scented)
5. Personal hygiene products, including soap, shampoo, conditioner, bubble bath, and shower gel
6. Perfumes, body sprays, deodorants, douches, powders, lotions, creams, hair removal products (wax, razors, shaving cream, depilatories)
7. Urine, feces (especially if incontinent), seminal fluid, sweat
8. Commercial vaginal lubricants, condoms, spermicide

Complications

Serious complications from contact dermatitis are rare. Pruritus can lead to scratching and possible skin breakdown and superimposed bacterial and fungal infections. Decreased sexual function from pruritus and discomfort is possible.

Indications for Referral or Hospitalization

If systemic symptoms occur in conjunction with a localized reaction, women should be instructed to seek immediate health care for angioedema or respiratory involvement.

- Localized dermatitis does not require hospitalization.
- Referral is indicated for women who do not respond to standard treatment or appear to worsen.
- If an allergic component is suspected, then a referral to an allergist is appropriate.

Patient and Family Education

Contact dermatitis of the vulva can be a very frustrating condition for women. The list of potential irritants and allergens is extensive, and it may take some time to uncover the causative agent. Trial and error are involved while specific agents are eliminated, and this involves patience and time.

ECZEMA AND PSORIASIS

Pathophysiology

Like eczema elsewhere on the body, vulvar eczema is typically a result of persistent scratching or aggravation of an area after an allergic trigger. It can be an acute or chronic condition. The diagnosis is made by the symptom history, vulvar examination, and presence of eczema on other parts of the body; biopsies are not beneficial. Psoriasis and seborrhea are often confused with eczema, and any diagnosis will be hampered if the area has been scratched. The provider should be alert to the possibility of secondary infection with continued dermal irritation.[5]

Often seen on the knees or elbows, psoriasis is an inherited chronic condition in which new skin cells are produced too rapidly, leading to pruritic, red and scaly, or thick white patches with clear-cut borders. It is often exacerbated by stress and occurs simultaneously on various parts of the body. In addition, new psoriatic lesions may develop at an injury site (referred to as Koebner phenomenon). Psoriasis usually affects the labia and is not typically present in mucous membranes or the urethra.

Clinical Presentation and Physical Examination

The typical presentation of eczema includes severe pruritus lasting several weeks or more. A red rash or erythema without distinct borders is usually observed on examination and, if left untreated, can progress to the thickened scaly plaques seen in squamous cell hyperplasia.[5] On the vulva, crusts are less likely, but the cycle of vulvar itching and scratching can lead to LSC.[4] Psoriasis of the vulva often initially manifests as a nonscaly area of smooth erythema. Pruritus is common and repeated scratching can result in excoriation, skin thickening, and a continued cycle of itching and scratching. Often eczema and psoriasis cause similar symptoms and can be difficult to differentiate. Other areas of the body should be examined for eczema and psoriasis because the vulva is usually not the only location for these conditions.

Diagnostics

Often eczema and psoriasis cause similar symptoms and can be difficult to differentiate.

DIAGNOSTICS

Eczema and Psoriasis

LABORATORY
None

OTHER DIAGNOSTICS
Punch biopsy only if other dermatoses are suspected

Differential Diagnosis

As with many vulvar conditions, initial symptoms often overlap and many differential diagnoses are possible.

DIFFERENTIAL DIAGNOSIS

Eczema and Psoriasis

- Lichen sclerosus
- Lichen planus
- Lichen simplex chronicus
- Contact dermatitis
- Fungal infections

Management

- For both eczema and psoriasis, biopsies are rarely useful unless there is suspicion that either condition exists concurrently with other dermatoses such as LS, LP, or LSC.[5] Psoriasis treatment is aimed at symptom relief.
- In severe cases of eczema, a potent topical corticosteroid ointment, such as clobetasol, can be used twice a day for 2 to 4 weeks and then gradually reduced in frequency until the symptoms are gone.[4] Low-potency corticosteroid creams can be used when appropriate.
- The pruritus can also be treated with cold compresses, Burow solution, and antihistamines.
- Triamcinolone acetonide injections can be used for recalcitrant eczema.
- Calcipotriene ointment (Dovonex), a topical vitamin D_3 preparation, is effective without the risk of skin atrophy.[1]
- Ultraviolet treatments are used to treat psoriasis; efficacy for vulvar lesions may be limited, and the dose of ultraviolet light needs to be reduced to avoid burning the genital skin.

Life Span Considerations

Eczema and psoriasis can occur across the life span. Although acute exacerbations are possible, both conditions are often chronic and management will change depending on stage of life. Women who are pregnant or breastfeeding should seek consultation before treatment because certain medications to control the symptoms of eczema and psoriasis should not be taken while pregnant or nursing. Aging skin is more susceptible to trauma, and women with these conditions in the presence of atrophy from estrogen deficiency of menopause may need to be treated with topical estrogen therapy to improve bothersome symptoms.

Complications

Serious complications from eczema and psoriasis are rare. Pruritus can lead to scratching and possible skin breakdown and superimposed bacterial and fungal infections. Decreased sexual function from pruritus and discomfort is possible.

Indications for Referral or Hospitalization

- Women with eczema or psoriasis do not require hospitalization.
- Referral is indicated for women who do not respond to standard treatment.

Patient and Family Education

Eczema and psoriasis are chronic conditions that require treatment over the life span. Symptoms often go through periods of remission and exacerbation that can frustrating. Pruritus is common and can affect a woman's quality of life and sexual functioning. Gentle care of vulvar skin, loose clothing, and avoidance of harsh cleansers and irritants need to be lifelong habits.

VULVAR PAIN

Definition and Epidemiology

Vulvodynia is an umbrella term for chronic vulvar pain or discomfort characterized by burning, stinging, irritation, and rawness of the vulva or exquisite sensitivity to touch on the vulvar area or on attempted vaginal entry.[15] The cause of vulvodynia is uncertain. It is estimated to affect up to 16% of women in the general population.[16]

Although burning vulvar symptoms can be attributed to conditions such as vaginitis, human papillomavirus (HPV) infection, or dermatoses such as those described in this chapter, the term is generally reserved for conditions such as vulvar vestibulitis syndrome (VVS) and essential vulvodynia (EV), which have no known cause.

VULVAR VESTIBULITIS SYNDROME AND ESSENTIAL VULVODYNIA

Pathophysiology

VVS is a chronic inflammatory condition of the vulvar vestibule that is characterized by burning pain on touch, which can persist for several days after the touch is removed. In 1987, Friedrich defined the condition and included three criteria for diagnosis: (1) severe pain on vestibular touch or attempted vaginal entry, (2) tenderness to pressure localized within the vulvar vestibule, and (3) physical findings confined to vestibular erythema of various degrees.[17] Although VVS is now better understood, the cause and most appropriate treatment of this condition remain unknown. Vulvar vestibulitis is found almost exclusively in women of reproductive age who are or have been sexually active. The true prevalence is unknown. The majority of affected women are white (97%) and nulliparous (75%).[18] Many women report having a relative who experienced similar symptoms or at least difficulty with tampon insertion.[19,20] Primary (no identifiable initial trigger or time of onset) and secondary (such as after HPV infection or vaginitis treatment or postpartum) categories of VVS have been suggested.

EV is characterized by spontaneous and unprovoked vulvar burning not limited to the vestibule. This condition may represent a neuropathic process such as a reflex sympathetic dystrophy or pudendal neuralgia.[21] Other than more widespread symptom distribution, physical findings on examination are similarly unremarkable, as with VVS. It is described more often in older women who have burning that extends beyond the vaginal introitus to involve the labia majora and sometimes the inner thighs and anus.[22,23] Studies have failed to demonstrate an association between vulvodynia and physical and sexual abuse. Some studies have suggested that patients with vulvodynia have more depressive and somatic complaints, but these studies do not demonstrate cause and effect.[22]

Causes of VVS and EV, including HPV and a *Candida*-triggered autoimmune response, have been suggested but not supported in the literature. In fact, treatments of HPV infection, such as topical acid or laser therapy, can lead to secondary VVS. A causal association between VVS and *Candida* organisms has not been established, but as more women treat themselves repeatedly with OTC vaginal fungicides, sensitivity to ingredients in these preparations may develop, increasing the risk for development of VVS. Other theories include an association between VVS or EV and interstitial cystitis, both of which are inflammatory conditions of tissues that share embryologic origins. Many of these women have overlapping urinary and vulvar symptoms. VVS may also be associated with a sympathetically maintained pain feedback loop that is perpetuated by an underlying pelvic floor muscle instability or hypertonicity that is initially triggered by a superficial tissue insult.[22-24]

The association between VVS and oral contraceptives remains controversial. It has been suggested that oral contraceptives downregulate receptors enough to cause epithelial thinning, but research has not demonstrated a clear association between oral contraceptives and the incidence of VVS. Although reports include exacerbation of symptoms related to the menstrual cycle or pregnancy, no mechanism has been identified.[20] In addition, various hormonal creams have been shown to be generally ineffective in treatment of VVS.

Given the lack of obvious clinical findings, VVS and EV were long thought to be a result of sexual dysfunction, childhood trauma, or some other psychological disorder, theories now recognized as fallacious. A chronic pain syndrome that heavily affects sexual relationships and daily activities is likely, not surprisingly, to be accompanied by anxiety or depression. These issues should be addressed, but to assume a causal link with VVS and EV is inappropriate.

Clinical Presentation and Physical Examination

A thorough history is essential to management of VVS and EV. Presentation of VVS commonly includes complaints of severe, burning vulvar pain during introital penetration with sexual intercourse or tampon use, during bicycle or horseback riding, or when wearing tight or bulky clothing. Pain may last a few minutes or as long as a few days after the trigger has been removed. Symptoms have often been present for months or years, resulting in a long history of frequent consultations. The history should include information about the initial onset of symptoms (if an initial onset can be identified), along with symptom characteristics, duration, and frequency. The impact of symptoms on sexual function should be determined, including how often intercourse is attempted and how often it is stopped because of pain. Assessment should also be made as to the impact of symptoms on daily activities and how often thoughts are distracted by symptoms during the course of a day. The presence of back pain, muscle soreness, and bowel and urinary patterns may be helpful in identifying related disorders. Previous ineffective treatment should be documented. Prior management has often included repeated treatment for yeast or bacterial infections; determination of whether treatment was empirical or culture based is essential. A review of previous medical records can be helpful. Women should also be asked if they have developed any techniques of their own to ease discomfort.

The vulvar burning of EV occurs with no demonstrable skin abnormalities. There is also a lack of focal tenderness typically seen in VVS. In EV, pain is not confined to coital attempts or other known triggers. Complaints of concomitant urethral, rectal, or back pain are more common than with VVS.[23]

Visual examination of the vulva and introitus is generally unremarkable, although with VVS erythema near the vestibular glands may be present. The most revealing test is the use of a water- or saline-moistened cotton-tipped applicator to test for sensitivity to touch. This is done by simply touching with the applicator in multiple locations around the labia minora, vestibule, clitoris, and urethra to determine any areas of tenderness, to elicit burning, and to rate the degree of discomfort. With VVS, tenderness or burning is usually triggered near the Bartholin glands, near the posterior fourchette, and to either side of the urethral opening. Use of the smallest speculum possible and a gentle, unhurried examination with extra lubrication will be better tolerated. Colposcopic evaluation of the involved areas, although advocated by some, is not appropriate in general unless physical findings suggest HPV infection or vulvar intraepithelial neoplasia. Vulvar biopsies typically show inflammation and should be performed only if a pathologic condition is suggested by the physical examination.

Diagnostics

- Careful visual inspection of the entire vulva to look for obvious causes of pain, including infections and lesions
- Use of a cotton-tipped swab to gently touch areas on the vulva to identify local areas of pain
- Wet prep examination of vaginal fluid
- Cultures for gonorrhea and chlamydia, HSV if lesions are present
- Cultures for *Ureaplasma* and β-hemolytic streptococci
- Urinalysis, culture and sensitivity if dysuria is present

DIAGNOSTICS

Vulvar Vestibulitis Syndrome and Essential Vulvodynia

INITIAL
Cotton-tipped applicator sensitivity test

LABORATORY
Gonorrhea and chlamydia cultures, HSV culture if indicated
Ureaplasma cultures
β-Hemolytic streptococci cultures
Potassium hydroxide (KOH) wet preparation for yeast and bacterial vaginosis (BV)

OTHER DIAGNOSTICS
Biopsies*
Colposcopy*

*Only if indicated.

Differential Diagnosis

STIs should be excluded and cultures performed for β-hemolytic streptococci and *Candida* and *Ureaplasma* organisms. The diagnosis of VVS is made on the basis of the history, positive physical examination findings, and negative cultures.[17]

DIFFERENTIAL DIAGNOSIS

Vulvar Vestibulitis Syndrome

- Sexually transmitted diseases
- Infection with *Candida* or *Ureaplasma* organisms
- Infection with β-hemolytic streptococci

Management

1. Although spontaneous resolution of symptoms is possible, treatment of VVS or EV is often a matter of trial and error and requires a solid provider-patient relationship. Goals of treatment include pain control and improved quality of life.
2. Reassurance that this condition is real and that the concerns are legitimate is important.
3. Women should be informed that partial symptom relief is likely, but that it will take time for adequate treatment trials. Realistic goals and time frames should be established and extra time planned for appointments.
4. Each woman should be involved as much as possible and should keep a daily symptom log, noting any possible pain triggers and rating the severity and duration of symptoms. Decisions to seek alternative forms of treatment, such as acupuncture, should be supported and incorporated into the overall management plan.
5. Treatment of VVS is dictated by the woman's history.
6. If recurrent candidiasis is suspected, the provider could institute a trial of fluconazole, 150 mg weekly, for 2 months, then biweekly for another 2 months, followed by one dose monthly. Careful evaluation for possible drug interactions (e.g., oral hypoglycemics, anticoagulants) is required.[18] Topical antifungal creams such as terconazole, miconazole, and clotrimazole may further irritate the vestibule.
7. Any positive cultures should be followed by appropriate treatment.
8. Other oral treatments aimed at interfering with the pain feedback loop include antidepressant medications (tricyclic antidepressants and SSRIs). Low-dose antidepressants are used to manage pain, and it should be carefully explained that this is the indication for which the antidepressant is being prescribed.
9. Another noninvasive approach involves education about calcium oxalate restriction and calcium citrate supplementation. Many common foods, such as peanut butter, are high in calcium oxalates, and although restriction of intake may be difficult, some have found it helpful. Symptom reduction has been achieved with calcium citrate and a low-oxalate diet.[25]
10. Application of topical xylocaine can temporarily relieve pain during sexual intercourse.
11. In women who are postmenopausal, application of topical estrogen cream may decrease pain.
12. Standard pain medications, including opiates, do not control the pain of VVS or EV and should not be prescribed.
13. Pelvic floor physical therapy may help reduce tension and improve pelvic floor tone, thus decreasing pain.[23,26]
14. Alternative forms of chronic pain management, such as guided imagery and acupuncture, may be useful as well.
15. Surgery to remove the affected area has produced mixed results, including worsening of symptoms, and should be discussed only after every other treatment option has been exhausted.[27]
16. Local application of a topical anesthetic before intercourse can be helpful in some cases.

Life Span Considerations

Women of all ages can experience vulvodynia. Women with VSS or EV can experience so much pain that intercourse is impossible and achieving a pregnancy is difficult. If women with one of these vulvar pain syndromes becomes pregnant, there is often concern over pain relief during delivery and how the delivery might affect the mother's pain in the postpartum period. Regardless of age, these syndromes can negatively affect sexual functioning throughout the life span. Pain may also increase as a result of estrogen deficiency during menopause.

Complications

Patients with vulvar pain may be reticent to discuss physical and sexual concerns and reluctant to have pelvic examinations. The disorder may be embarrassing and frustrating and may prohibit some patients from enjoying life or an intimate sexual relationship. These patients require considerable support and understanding and often will benefit from psychological counseling.

Indications for Referral or Hospitalization

- Consultation with a physical therapist is helpful to evaluate for pelvic asymmetry and problems with the pelvic floor musculature, which typically shows instability and increased resting tone in patients with VVS.[22,24] Trigger point physical therapy for myofascial release may be therapeutic, especially for patients with back pain or persistent muscle soreness.[26]
- Continued pelvic floor muscle dysfunction may perpetuate the sympathetically maintained pain feedback loop.
- Twice-daily biofeedback exercises may help reestablish muscle stability during the course of many months and may provide significant if not complete symptom relief.[22]
- If the response to any of the aforementioned interventions has been inadequate, referral should be made to a

gynecologist knowledgeable about medical, surgical, and behavioral treatment options.[27]

- In VVS, surgical excision of varying amounts of vestibular tissue (vestibulectomy) is the intervention with the highest reported success rate, but studies are often weakened by methodologic flaws, and the benefits of medical and behavioral management may be underreported.
- Conservative treatment has been recommended by the American College of Obstetricians and Gynecologists.[27]

Patient and Family Education

The impact of VVS on intimate relationships is significant, and the woman's partner should be included in discussions when possible and appropriate. Counseling referrals should be offered with the understanding that the health care provider does not believe symptoms are psychogenic in nature but rather that there are real emotional challenges to living with a chronic pain syndrome; the provider should also acknowledge that hope often gives way to disappointment before symptom relief is experienced.

When discussing treatment options, providers should first counsel women to avoid vulvar irritants and to implement the self-care measures described in Box 170-1. Many topical treatment options can be trialed, including estrogen and progesterone creams and topical anesthetics such as lidocaine 2% jelly. Although some women may respond to these therapies, others will experience an exacerbation of symptoms with any topical medication.[28,29]

VAGINITIS AND VAGINOSIS

DEFINITION AND EPIDEMIOLOGY

Vaginitis and vaginosis are disorders of the vagina that are characterized by vaginal discharge, odor, or vulvovaginal irritation. Vaginitis involves inflammation, whereas vaginosis does not. Both have historically been grouped under the term *vaginitis*. They result from an imbalance in the vaginal ecosystem, which may be caused by infection (bacterial, fungal, protozoan, or viral),[30] hypoestrogenic states, foreign bodies, contact dermatitis, or allergy. Many times the cause of the imbalance is not immediately clear. Recurrent vaginitis is defined as four or more episodes within a year.

Affecting women of all ages, vaginitis is the most common gynecologic problem encountered by health care providers. Bacterial vaginosis (BV) is the most common cause of vaginitis, with an incidence of 15% to 65%, depending on the location of practice.[30] Approximately 50% of the women meeting the diagnostic criteria for BV are asymptomatic.[30] Another common cause of vaginitis is vulvovaginal candidiasis (VVC), and an estimated 75% of all women will experience at least one episode of VVC in their lifetime.[30]

BACTERIAL VAGINOSIS

Pathophysiology

BV is characterized by the replacement of the normal, hydrogen peroxide–producing *Lactobacillus* organisms in the vagina with high concentrations of anaerobic bacteria, *Gardnerella vaginalis, Mycoplasma hominis,* and *Bacteroides* and *Mobiluncus* organisms.[30] Among women seeking care, BV is the most common cause of vaginal discharge or malodor, although data suggest that many women with BV are asymptomatic.[30]

In the presence of BV infection, protective hydrogen peroxide–producing lactobacilli are significantly reduced. This change is accompanied by an elevated pH. This alkaline environment facilitates the growth of the pathogenic organisms and their adherence to vaginal epithelia, seen as clue cells on a saline wet mount. The anaerobes facilitate the release of amines, which produce the characteristic "fishy" odor, especially on alkalization of the vaginal discharge. The cause of microbial alterations in BV is not fully understood. It is not classified as an STI but is considered to be sexually associated. It is more common among women who have multiple sexual partners or a new sex partner and women who do not use condoms.[30] However, women who have never been sexually active also get BV. Women with BV are at an increased risk for acquiring some STIs, such as infection with HIV, *Neisseria gonorrhoeae, Chlamydia trachomatis,* and HSV type 2. Treatment of male sex partners has not been beneficial in preventing the recurrence of BV and is not recommended.[31]

Clinical Presentation and Physical Examination

Symptoms of BV most often include an increased quantity of malodorous vaginal discharge, most noticeable after intercourse and during menses because of the alkaline nature of semen and blood. Some patients experience mild to moderate vulvovaginal irritation.

The physical examination should include inspection of the vulva and vagina. Assessment is important: skin turgor and elasticity; normal or sparse pubic hair; and whether the labia are full, atrophic, or dry will help identify if the symptoms are associated with estrogen deficiency. Any vulvovaginal erythema, lesions, discharge, or prolapse should be noted. A speculum examination is necessary to determine the color, consistency, viscosity, and odor of any vaginal or cervical discharge. The characteristic vaginal discharge of BV is often thin, homogeneous, and adherent to the vaginal walls and cervix. The fishy amine odor may be present, and rarely there is vaginal inflammation.[30] A bimanual examination will reveal any cervical motion tenderness, pelvic pain, or masses.

Diagnostics

- Wet prep examination of vaginal discharge and assessment of vaginal pH are point-of-care tests that can establish a diagnosis of BV.
- The diagnosis of BV can be made by clinical criteria. Clinical criteria require the presence of three of the following[30]:
  1. Homogeneous, white, noninflammatory discharge that adheres to the vaginal walls
  2. The presence of clue cells on microscopic examination
  3. pH of vaginal fluid above 4.5
  4. Vaginal discharge with a fishy odor before or after the addition of 10% potassium hydroxide (KOH)—positive whiff test result
- If wet prep evaluation is inconclusive or not available, a vaginal culture can be obtained.

DIAGNOSTICS

Bacterial Vaginosis

LABORATORY
pH of vaginal fluid
Wet mount with normal saline and 10% KOH
KOH whiff test
Vaginal culture (if wet prep inconclusive or unavailable)

Differential Diagnosis

Increased vaginal discharge can be caused by many different factors. Thorough history, examination, and microscopy evaluation will assist in establishing a correct diagnosis.

DIFFERENTIAL DIAGNOSIS

Bacterial Vaginosis

- Trichomoniasis
- Candidiasis
- Gonorrhea
- Chlamydia
- Atrophic vaginitis
- Foreign body
- Cervicitis
- Contact dermatitis or hypersensitivity reaction
- Physiologic discharge

Management

The goals of treatment are elimination of symptoms and relief from any vaginal irritation. Pharmacologic measures are the first-line treatment. Options include the following:

1. Recommended regimen for nonpregnant women[30]:
   - Metronidazole, 500 mg PO twice a day for 7 days, *or*
   - Metronidazole gel 0.75%, 1 full applicator (5 g) intravaginally once daily for 5 days, *or*
   - Clindamycin cream 2%, 1 full applicator (5 g) intravaginally at bedtime for 7 days, *or*
2. Alternate regimen for nonpregnant women[30]:
   - Clindamycin, 300 mg PO twice a day for 7 days, *or*
   - Clindamycin ovules, 100 g intravaginally every night at bedtime for 3 days, *or*
   - Tinidazole, 2 g orally once daily for 2 days, *or*
   - Tinidazole, 1 g orally once daily for 5 days
3. For pregnant women[30]:
   - Metronidazole, 500 mg PO twice a day for 7 days, *or*
   - Metronidazole, 250 mg PO twice a day for 7 days, *or*
   - Clindamycin, 300 mg PO twice a day for 7 days
4. Treatment of BV in pregnancy is of particular importance because of its association with adverse pregnancy outcomes, including preterm and low-birth-weight deliveries, intra-amniotic infection, postpartum endometriosis, and postcesarean wound infection.[32]
5. For pregnant women, treatment should include one of the oral therapies listed above to penetrate the chorion, amnion, and decidua.[32]
6. Although metronidazole was previously contraindicated in the first trimester, multiple studies and meta-analyses have not demonstrated an association between metronidazole use during pregnancy and teratogenic or mutagenic effects in newborns.[30]
7. Intravaginal clindamycin is not recommended in pregnancy because of an increased risk of preterm delivery.[30]
8. Screening of the asymptomatic pregnant woman for BV remains controversial, even in women at high risk for preterm delivery.[30]
9. For recurrent BV infections, options include the use of alternative first-line agents and prophylactic use of intravaginal metronidazole, twice a week for 4 to 6 months.[30,33]

Life Span Considerations

BV can occur at any point in a woman's reproductive life and more commonly affects women who are sexually active. The symptoms of increased vaginal discharge and odor can mimic symptoms of STIs and sexually active adolescents may be uncomfortable discussing their symptoms with parents, especially if their parents are unaware they are sexually active.

During the perimenopausal and postmenopausal years, BV can occur in the presence of atrophic vaginitis as a result of the alteration in vaginal lactobacilli and a more alkaline vaginal environment. Treatment with a topical estrogen preparation may help reduce recurrences in postmenopausal women.

Complications

Once considered benign, BV is now associated with gynecologic and obstetric complications. Perhaps of greatest concern is the possible link between BV and infection with human immunodeficiency virus (HIV). The shift in vaginal pH from acidity to alkalinity associated with the presence of semen may favor male-to-female transmission of HIV, and HIV infection is consistently associated with reduced levels of vaginal lactobacilli.[34]

The bacterial flora of BV have been implicated in pelvic inflammatory disease (PID) and have also been associated with endometritis, PID, and vaginal cuff cellulitis after invasive procedures. Evidence supports screening for and treatment of BV before therapeutic abortion,[30] but the evidence is less clear about the benefit of screening patients at high risk for preterm labor.

Indications for Referral or Hospitalization

BV rarely requires hospitalization and can often be treated without referral or consultation.

- BV very rarely requires hospitalization.
- The bacterial flora of BV have been implicated in PID and have also been associated with endometritis after invasive procedures or pelvic surgery. Physician referral is indicated if a pelvic infection is suspected.
- Referral is indicated in cases of multiple recurrent episodes of BV despite adequate treatment.

Patient and Family Education

BV recurs within 1 to 2 months for many women. Persistence of pathogens, an unidentified host factor, failure of lactobacilli to recolonize the vagina, and reinfection from a male partner are possible explanations. Recurrent episodes can be frustrating for women. The importance of completing the full course of treatment is essential to reduce regrowth of bacteria. Women should also be educated on general vaginal hygiene measures such as no douching, avoiding perfumed or scented vaginal cleansers or sprays, and wearing loose-fitting clothes. Safer sexual practices such as using condoms and reducing sexual partners are also helpful in reducing recurrent BV. Because BV has been linked to preterm labor and birth, pregnant women with BV should be educated on the subtle signs and symptoms of preterm labor, including increased watery vaginal discharge, spotting, lower abdominal pain, and low back pain.

The most common side effect of oral metronidazole is gastrointestinal upset. Women taking metronidazole should be advised to avoid the use of alcohol during treatment and for 24 hours thereafter to avoid a disulfiram-like reaction (severe nausea and vomiting). Oral clindamycin has been shown to be as effective as oral metronidazole, but it is more expensive and may cause diarrhea. Clindamycin cream is oil based and may weaken latex condoms and diaphragms for 5 days after use.[30] The results of clinical trials indicate that a woman's response to therapy and the likelihood of relapse or recurrence are not affected by treatment of a woman's sex partner. Therefore, routine treatment of sexual partners is not recommended.

VULVOVAGINAL CANDIDIASIS

Pathophysiology

VVC is caused by growth of the fungus *Candida* in the vagina. Most infections involve *Candida albicans,* although up to 17% may be caused by non–*C. albicans* species.[30,35] The most common non–*C. albicans* species involved in VVC are *Torulopsis glabrata* and *Candida tropicalis,* which may manifest atypically and may be more resistant to standard therapies. Women with HIV infection or recurrent VVC are twice as likely to have non–*C. albicans* VVC.[30,35] An estimated 75% of women will have at least one episode of VVC, and approximately 35% will have more than one.[36]

Several factors may trigger the change from colonization to proliferation, which results in the development of symptomatic VVC. These include changes in the vaginal ecosystem and possible phenotypic changes in the *Candida* organism. Symptomatic VVC involves candidal tissue invasion, causing inflammation, mucosal swelling, erythema, and exfoliation of epithelia. Factors that cause an increased susceptibility to VVC include antibiotic therapy, pregnancy, uncontrolled diabetes mellitus, use of oral contraceptives (especially high-dose formulations), immunosuppression, and occlusive synthetic clothing.[31]

Recurrent VVC is defined as four or more documented episodes of VVC in 1 year. The pathophysiologic mechanism of recurrent or chronic VVC remains controversial. It affects less than 5% of women annually, and the majority have no predisposing condition, such as diabetes or immunosuppression. Earlier theories on the cause of recurrent VVC have included reinfection from an intestinal reservoir; sexual transmission; and the vaginal relapse theory, which proposes that incomplete eradication of *Candida* organisms occurs after treatment and that the small numbers of *Candida* organisms present then multiply and result in recurrence. More recent theories propose deficiencies in the normal protective vaginal flora; a deficiency in antigen-specific, cell-mediated immunity to *Candida* organisms; and a possible local hypersensitivity to *Candida* organisms, predisposing the patient to recurrences.

Clinical Presentation and Physical Examination

Typical symptoms of VVC include pruritus and vaginal discharge. Other symptoms may include vulvar burning, dyspareunia, vulvar dysuria, and vaginal irritation. Vaginal discharge is not always present, and there may be only a small amount. The thick whitish gray discharge is typically described as cottage cheese–like, although it can vary from thin to thick.[30,35] On physical examination, the vulva and vagina may be hyperemic and edematous. Vulvar excoriation may be present from scratching, and irritated skin may have fissures. The vaginal discharge is usually whitish, curdlike, and adherent to the vaginal walls. Variations in the vaginal discharge are possible, although care must be taken to exclude concurrent infections.

Diagnostics

- Wet prep examination of vaginal discharge and assessment of vaginal pH are point-of-care tests that can establish a diagnosis of VVC.
- *Candida* vaginitis is associated with a vaginal pH below 4.5. A normal pH will help rule out a differential diagnosis of BV or trichomoniasis.
- Vaginal culture (if wet prep is inconclusive or unavailable).
- The diagnosis of VVC can be made on demonstration of pseudohyphae or yeast buds on a 10% KOH wet mount or by culture.
- Use of KOH on microscopy improves visualization by disrupting cellular material, which may obscure the yeast forms.
- Identification of yeast in the absence of symptoms is not an indication for treatment.

DIAGNOSTICS

Vulvovaginal Candidiasis

INITIAL	Wet mount with normal saline and 10% KOH
LABORATORY pH of vaginal discharge (to rule out BV or trichomoniasis)	Vaginal culture if wet prep inconclusive or unavailable

Differential Diagnosis

Vaginal pruritus, often the main symptom of VVC, can be difficult to diagnose. Many different differential diagnoses exist.

DIFFERENTIAL DIAGNOSIS

Vulvovaginal Candidiasis

- Atrophic vaginitis
- Trichomoniasis
- BV
- Chlamydia
- Gonorrhea
- Foreign body
- LS, LP, LSC
- Contact dermatitis or hypersensitivity reaction

Management

The goals of treatment are normalization of vaginal flora, elimination of symptoms, and restoration of skin integrity. Pharmacologic measures are the first-line treatment. For options for nonpregnant women, see the following:

1. OTC vaginal agents[30]:
   - Butoconazole 2% cream, 5 g given intravaginally for 3 days, *or*
   - Clotrimazole 1% cream, 5 g intravaginally for 7 to 14 days, *or*
   - Miconazole 2% cream, 5 g intravaginally for 7 days, *or*
   - Miconazole 4% cream, 5 g intravaginally for 3 days, *or*
   - Miconazole 100-mg vaginal suppository, 1 suppository for 7 days, *or*
   - Miconazole 200-mg vaginal suppository, 1 suppository for 3 days, *or*
   - Miconazole 1200-mg vaginal suppository, 1 suppository for 1 day, *or*
   - Tioconazole 6.5% ointment, 5 g intravaginally in a single application
2. Prescription vaginal agents[30]:
   - Butoconazole 2% cream, 5 g sustained release, single intravaginal application, *or*

- Nystatin 100,000-unit vaginal tablet, 1 tablet for 14 days, *or*
- Terconazole 0.4% cream, 5 g intravaginally for 7 days, *or*
- Terconazole 0.8% cream, 5 g intravaginally for 3 days, *or*
- Terconazole 80-mg vaginal suppository, 1 suppository for 3 days

3. Prescription oral agents[30]:
   - Fluconazole 150-mg oral tablet, 1 tablet in a single dose
4. The single-dose topical therapies should be reserved for mild VVC because of their slightly lower effectiveness.
5. Multiday regimens are more appropriate for moderate to severe VVC, and the use of a cream is preferred in the presence of vulvar symptoms.
6. Use of terconazole is more effective in non–*C. albicans* VVC.
7. The choice of an oral versus topical therapy can be based on the patient's preference.
8. Treatment of VVC in pregnancy should use one of the topical azoles, preferably for 7 days.[35]
9. Treatment of sexual partners is not indicated except in cases of symptomatic balanitis or penile dermatitis.
10. In recurrent VVC, it is necessary to assess for predisposing conditions and to confirm the diagnosis by culture. Evaluation should include a fasting glucose concentration in nonpregnant patients or a glucose tolerance test if the patient is pregnant.
11. Routine HIV testing is not indicated in patients without identifiable risk factors.[30]
12. An optimum treatment strategy for recurrent VVC has not been defined. For established diagnoses of recurrent VVC, maintenance therapy needs to be given frequently enough to prevent vaginal regrowth, but the optimal interval has not been established. A longer duration of initial therapy, 14 days for vaginal therapy and oral fluconazole every third day for three doses, has been suggested.[30]
13. Oral fluconazole, 150 mg, administered weekly for 6 months, is the first-line treatment for recurrent VVC.[30,36,37]

Life Span Considerations

VVC can occur at any point in a woman's reproductive life but is more common during pregnancy and among women who are obese, are immunocompromised, or have poorly controlled diabetes. Sexually active women who are experiencing vulvovaginal symptoms may be concerned about STIs, and sexually active adolescents may be uncomfortable discussing their symptoms with parents, especially if their parents are unaware they are sexually active. During the perimenopausal and postmenopausal years, VVC can occur in the setting of atrophy associated with estrogen deficiency. In addition, as women age they are at increased risk of type 2 diabetes, which is an independent risk factor for VVC.

Complications

Complications are uncommon. The most common are superficial lesions and skin fissures that may occur in the vagina and vulva. Severely immunosuppressed patients may develop systemic infection. Patients with type 2 diabetes who are taking oral hypoglycemic medications and are being treated with fluconazole are at increased risk for hypoglycemia. Fluconazole has many drug interactions. Practitioners should be aware of other medications women are taking before prescribing.

Indications for Referral or Hospitalization

- VVC rarely necessitates hospitalization.
- Referral may be indication for women who are severely immunocompromised, are infected with HIV, or have poorly controlled diabetes.

Patient and Family Education

Women should be reassured that most episodes of VVC resolve easily. If women self-treat with an OTC preparation and their symptoms do not improve, they should be evaluated at an office visit. The vaginal preparations are oil based and could potentially weaken latex condoms and diaphragms. Vaginal hygiene measures should be encouraged: cotton underwear, loose-fitting clothing, changing clothing after excessive perspiration or swimming, and avoidance of douching and scented vaginal sprays or perfumes. Overweight and obese women should be encouraged to decrease their weight, and women with diabetes will experience fewer episodes of VVC with tight glucose control.

ATROPHIC VAGINITIS

Pathophysiology

Atrophic vaginitis is caused by reduced endogenous estrogen levels—most commonly found in the postmenopausal patient, but lactation, antagonistic medications, and ovarian failure resulting from disease processes also induce hypoestrogenic states. The lower estrogen level causes the vaginal epithelium to become thin and fragile, with decreased glycogen content. There is an increased pH as a result of decreased lactic acid production, leading to an environment prone to an overgrowth of pathogenic organisms and to a lowered concentration of lactobacilli.[38] Despite these changes, symptoms will vary and some women with vaginal atrophy are not symptomatic.

Clinical Presentation and Physical Examination

Women with atrophic vaginitis often report vaginal soreness, pruritus, vulvovaginal dryness, occasional vaginal discharge, spotting, and dyspareunia. The vulvar skin is thin, with decreased subcutaneous tissue and variable pubic hair loss. The vaginal walls are pale with decreased or absent rugae. The vaginal tissue is often friable and can contain petechiae. Vaginal discharge can be thick, watery, or blood-tinged.[39]

Diagnostics

- The vaginal pH in atrophic vaginitis is usually 5.5 to 7.
- The saline wet mount typically reveals increased leukocytes and small, round epithelial cells with an absence of clue cells and negative amine test.

DIAGNOSTICS

Atrophic Vaginitis

INITIAL	OTHER DIAGNOSTICS
pH	Endometrial biopsy*
LABORATORY	
Wet mount	
Culture	

*If indicated.

- If unexplained vaginal bleeding is present, endometrial biopsy is necessary.
- If vulvar pruritus is present, a biopsy is indicated to exclude vulvar dystrophy or carcinoma.
- STI testing should be done as indicated based on history.

Differential Diagnosis

Although atrophic vaginitis is distinguished by the presence of a hypoestrogenic state, other potential diagnoses must be considered.

DIFFERENTIAL DIAGNOSIS

Atrophic Vaginitis

- BV
- VVC
- Trichomoniasis
- Chlamydia
- Gonorrhea
- Foreign body
- Physiologic discharge
- Contact dermatitis or hypersensitivity reaction

Management

The goal of treatment is to correct the hypoestrogenic environment through estrogen therapy. This causes maturation of the epithelium, reversing the changes that resulted in the vaginitis.[39]

- Treatment recommendations usually involve topical estrogen cream, tablets, or vaginal rings. Typical regimens include the following[40]:
  - Estradiol cream 0.1%, 2 to 4 g intravaginally every day for 1 to 2 weeks, then 1 to 2 g intravaginally every day for 1 to 2 weeks, then 1 g intravaginally one to three times per week for maintenance.
  - Conjugated estrogen cream, 2 to 4 g intravaginally every day for 1 to 2 weeks, then 2 to 4 g intravaginally every other day for 1 to 2 weeks. The conjugated estrogen cream is then tapered and discontinued.
  - A pill form of estradiol is also available and is used intravaginally every day for 1 to 2 weeks, then twice weekly for 2 to 4 weeks, then tapered and discontinued.
  - A vaginal estrogen ring is available that is placed in the vagina and remains in place for 90 days.
  - Ospemifene, an oral estrogen agonist-antagonist, 60 mg daily.[41]
- Women who use topical estrogen for more than 6 to 12 months should be monitored for abnormal vaginal bleeding. Although the risk of endometrial hyperplasia is far less with topical agents compared with systemic estrogen treatment, any abnormal bleeding should be investigated. Although there are no established guidelines for monitoring the endometrial lining, a pelvic ultrasound for endometrial thickness or endometrial biopsy can be considered if there are concerns about endometrial hyperplasia.
- Topical estrogen therapy can be used safely in many patients and does not have the same cardiovascular and oncogenic risk profile as systemic estrogen treatment.
- Patients with atrophic vaginitis who decline topical estrogen treatment or in whom the hypoestrogenic state is temporary (e.g., breastfeeding) may benefit from the use of a vaginal moisturizer (e.g., Replens), lubricants, or acidifying agents. These modalities will increase lubrication and moisture but will not improve tissue integrity or elasticity.

Life Span Considerations

Atrophic vaginitis exists in a hypoestrogenic state and therefore almost universally affects postmenopausal women. Although topical estrogen is the treatment of choice, some women may decline the use of hormones. Postmenopausal women should continue sexual activity if possible because this will help keep vaginal tissue pliable and elastic. Dyspareunia is a common complaint among women who have atrophic vaginitis, and comfort measures (use of lubricants, moisturizers, prolonged foreplay) should be encouraged. Atrophic vaginitis can also occur in women who are breastfeeding and have decreased estrogen levels, although this is temporary and resolves once lactation amenorrhea resolves.

Complications

Complications from atrophic vaginitis are rare. After prolonged estrogen deficiency vulvovaginal tissue can become thin and friable and susceptible to tearing and bruising from even mild trauma.

Indications for Referral or Hospitalization

Atrophic vaginitis does not require hospitalization.

- Referral to a gynecologist who specializes in menopause is indicated in cases of treatment failure.
- Postmenopausal women with unexplained vaginal bleeding should undergo endometrial biopsy.
- Gynecologic consultation is also indicated in cases with an unusual presentation or in which the cause is unknown or unclear.

Patient and Family Education

Women who are considering estrogen therapy need education about the actual risks of treatment. There is much confusion and misinformation surrounding the use of postmenopausal estrogen. Topical treatment does not carry the same risks as systemic treatment. Women using topical estrogen should be educated on expected treatment time, the weaning process, and the potential side effects. Women should also be instructed to report any abnormal bleeding or gynecologic concerns.

REFERENCES

For a full list of references, scan the QR code or visit http://booksite.elsevier.com/9780323355018

PART 15

Evaluation and Management of Musculoskeletal and Arthritic Disorders

CHAPTER 171

ANKLE AND FOOT PAIN

Joanne Sandberg-Cook

In the United States, foot and ankle problems are extremely common, with an incidence rate of 24% in middle-aged and older adults.[1] Sports injuries are often the cause, but even activities of daily living stress the foot and ankle. Walking alone puts up to 1.5 times the body weight on the foot. The average person logs roughly 1000 miles yearly. During 1 hour of strenuous exercise, feet cushion up to 1 million pounds of pressure.

Foot and ankle pain is more prevalent in women, people who are older and obese, and those with other lower extremity joint pain or deformity. However, children and adolescents are also commonly injured during sports activities. The specific functions of the ankle and foot predispose them to injuries and disorders that can result in chronic problems if they are not identified quickly and managed properly.

ANKLE SPRAINS

DEFINITION AND EPIDEMIOLOGY

The uniaxial ankle joint, or ankle joint, is the most primitive joint in the body and is crucial to walking, running, and the performance of all sports. The limited motion of the ankle gives it stability. The ankle joint consists of three major bones: the tibia, fibula, and talus. The tibia and fibula form the ankle mortise, and the talus fits into this mortise. The talus, which has no muscle or tendon attachment, gives the ankle its hinge motion. The talus also bears the entire weight of the extremity during walking. The deltoid, anterior talofibular, calcaneal fibular, and posterior talofibular ligaments hold the ankle bones in the mortise.

Ankle sprains occur at all ages and are common problems encountered by health care providers. A review of literature reveals that ankle sprain account for 15% to 20% of all sports injuries.[2] A sprain is a ligamentous injury caused by an abnormal motion, a sudden change in direction, or a misstep on an uneven surface. Even a minor ankle sprain can jeopardize joint stability. The severity of the physical findings determines the sprain category (Table 171-1), and the category defines the management of the injury. Previous ankle sprains can increase the potential for injury recurrence. Early diagnosis, treatment, rehabilitation, and subsequent ankle support during activity decrease the recurrence of a sprain in a previously injured ankle.

PATHOPHYSIOLOGY

Two types of injuries cause an ankle sprain. The most common is the inversion injury, in which the foot plantar flexes and internally rotates as the ankle inverts. The "roll" of the ankle injures the lateral ligaments and can also cause a lateral avulsion fracture. The less common eversion injury occurs when the ankle sustains an external rotation mechanism. Eversion stress injures the medial structures of the ankle, damaging the deltoid ligament or the syndesmosis.

CLINICAL PRESENTATION

The most common presentation of an ankle sprain is a swollen and painful joint. Ecchymosis and decreased range of motion are generally present. In many instances, weight bearing causes pain; some patients are unable to bear any weight on the affected joint.

In obtaining the history, it is important to determine whether the patient heard any audible sounds at the time of injury. An audible "snap" or "pop" indicates the potential for a more serious injury. Immediate swelling or ecchymosis raises the index of suspicion for a fracture or substantial amount of joint involvement. Patients also commonly report a sensation of lightheadedness, nausea, or diaphoresis immediately after the injury.

PHYSICAL EXAMINATION

With a sprain, the ankle joint is often swollen and ecchymotic, and the edema can create an illusion of deformity. Limited active and passive motion and point tenderness at the site of injury are common. Joint laxity is present in more severe sprains. Muscle spasm often prevents accurate testing of strength and stability. If the injury is not acute, swelling and ecchymosis at the lateral aspect of the foot and the toes are common. With severe ankle sprains, tenderness may extend up the extremity. The entire lower limb should always be palpated.

DIAGNOSTICS

DIAGNOSTICS

Ankle Pain

IMAGING
X-ray studies*
MRI*
CT*

*If indicated.

Although guidelines for radiography are controversial, plain radiographs are recommended for severe injuries, especially when instability is present or fracture is suspected. An x-ray study of the lower leg should also be performed if there is tenderness at the

TABLE 171-1 Classification and Treatment of Ankle Sprains

Grade 1	Grade 2	Grade 3
PATHOLOGY		
Stretching or minor tearing of ligament fibers	Partial tearing of ligament fibers	Complete tearing of ligament fibers
FINDINGS		
Minimum pain	Mild to moderate pain	Severe pain
Mild swelling	Moderate swelling	Significant swelling*
Mild ecchymosis	Moderate ecchymosis	Severe ecchymosis*
Full ROM	Painful, slightly limited motion and stability	Loss of motion and stability
Mild point tenderness	Point tenderness over joint	Severe pain (difficult examination)
Stable joint	Mild joint laxity with stress	Abnormal joint movement
Ability to bear weight	Painful to bear weight (may be unable to do so)	Inability to bear weight
TREATMENT		
RICE; active ROM exercises	RICE; active ROM exercises as tolerated	Referral to orthopedic surgeon (may require surgery)
Non–weight-bearing activity (swimming, stationary bike)	Partial weight bearing (crutches, cane) as tolerated Gradual progression to full weight bearing	Cast for 10-14 days Non–weight bearing activity Gradual progression to full weight bearing
Return to sports in 2-3 wk	Return to sports in 4-8 wk with semirigid ankle support	Rehabilitation before returning to sports with semirigid ankle support
SEQUELAE		
Tends to recur in first month if not fully rehabilitated	Recurrent sprains, joint instability, traumatic arthritis	Persistent instability (nonsurgical treatment), traumatic arthritis

*Occurs rapidly, usually within the first 30 minutes.
RICE, rest, ice, compression, and elevation; ROM, range of motion.
Modified from Peterson W, Rembitzki I, Koppenburg A, et al. Treatment of acute ankle ligament injuries: a systematic review. *Arch Orthop Trauma Surg* 133(8):1129-1141, 2013.

fibular head to rule out fracture. With less severe injuries, radiographs can be used to exclude an avulsion injury. More extensive radiologic examinations, such as stress films or computed tomography (CT) or magnetic resonance imaging (MRI) scans, are considered in consultation with an orthopedic surgeon, especially preoperatively.

DIFFERENTIAL DIAGNOSIS

Ankle injuries range from simple strains to severe injuries. The possibility of associated fibula fracture, stress fracture, avulsion fracture, or dislocation should be considered. Bursitis and tendinitis should be included in the differential diagnosis, especially if no distinct injury is recalled. Osteoarthritis, rheumatoid arthritis, and gouty arthritis are also common causes of ankle pain and swelling, especially in the older adult.

MANAGEMENT

The severity of the sprain dictates the management (see Table 171-1). Rest and protection, ice, compression, and elevation (RICE) are key first steps in providing pain relief and limiting swelling. Nonsteroidal anti-inflammatory drugs (NSAIDs) can help with pain management and may allow faster rehabilitation, although they can be associated with gastrointestinal (GI) side effects and in older adults should be used cautiously because of cardiovascular and renal concerns.[2] Topical NSAID gels are very effective at reducing pain and swelling and improving function in grade 1 and 2 sprains.[3] Thromboembolic deterrent (TED) hose provide support to the entire lower limb, aid in circulation, and are less bulky than ankle splints or braces for grade l and 2 sprains. Casting for 10 to 14 days has been shown to be effective in grade 3 sprains.[2] Semirigid supports used after

DIFFERENTIAL DIAGNOSIS

Ankle Pain

MUSCULOSKELETAL
- Infection
- Fracture
- Sprain and strains
- Bursitis (including retrocalcaneal bursitis)
- Dislocation or subluxation
- Tendinitis (including Achilles)
- Arthritis (inflammatory, reactive and degenerative)
- Gout or pseudogout

NEUROLOGIC
- Radiculopathy
- Peripheral neuropathy
- Tarsal tunnel syndrome

VASCULAR
- Peripheral vascular disease (arterial and venous)
- Foot ulcers

the acute injury has resolved may protect from subsequent sprains. All sprains require rehabilitation to restore the ankle to a stable and pain-free state. It is important for patients to understand that the treatment and recovery process will take weeks. Rehabilitation should begin as soon as possible after the injury and should include range-of-motion and strengthening exercises.[4,5] Even a severely swollen ankle can be mobilized with the simple exercise of "writing the alphabet" (active range of motion) with the affected foot. A program of active and passive resistive exercises progresses as range of motion and strength improve.

COMPLICATIONS

Ankle sprains can recur within the first month if the ankle has not been fully rehabilitated. Grade 2 and 3 sprains carry with them an increased risk of joint instability and traumatic arthritis. Recurrent sprains, which result in chronic instability, may require surgical repair.[5] A weak ankle joint is at risk for fracture when it is stressed.

INDICATIONS FOR REFERRAL OR HOSPITALIZATION

Fractures, dislocations, or subluxations and grade 3 sprains require an orthopedic referral. Physical therapy may also be indicated to promote rehabilitation and a safe return to sports or work-related activities.

PATIENT AND FAMILY EDUCATION

Patients need to understand the importance of RICE as well as the necessity of preventing weight bearing on the injured ankle. Patients and family members should also be instructed in medication doses and side effects, proper elastic bandage wrapping technique, cast care, and crutch use. The recuperative process and the risk of recurrence also require explanation.

ACHILLES TENDINOPATHY

DEFINITION AND EPIDEMIOLOGY

The Achilles tendon is posterior to the ankle joint and is responsible for flexion and extension of the ankle. It attaches the gastrocnemius and the soleus muscles of the calf to the calcaneus muscle and is palpable from the distal pole of the calf to the calcaneus. Disorders of the Achilles tendon include tendinosis, paratendonitis, insertional tendinosis, and frank rupture.

Achilles tendinitis manifests as pain with or without swelling around the Achilles tendon. Unlike other tendons, the Achilles tendon does not have a synovial sheath but instead has a paratenon, which, like a synovial sheath, functions to provide lubrication and vasculature to the tendon. Except for severe cases, true Achilles tendinopathy primarily affects the paratenon, resulting in inflammation, degeneration, and friability of the tendon.[6] A nodule of mucoid degeneration can form in the body of the tendon in severe or chronic Achilles tendinitis.[6]

PATHOPHYSIOLOGY

Achilles tendinopathy can occur in both adolescents and adults in both traumatic and nontraumatic settings. Aging, improper training, running up hills, or wearing shoes with soles that are too rigid can also contribute to the development of Achilles tendinopathy. Shoes or boots with a high back can irritate the tendon, causing pain and inflammation. Wearing of shoes with heels that maintain plantar flexion (high heels) for long periods can cause the tendon to shorten. Changing to flat or running shoes then increases stress on the tendon, causing pain. On occasion, Achilles tendinitis is caused by an anatomic abnormality, such as excessive foot pronation or tight hamstrings or gastrocnemius muscles.[6,7]

CLINICAL PRESENTATION

Patients with Achilles tendinopathy may have intermittent symptoms and may describe a pain that subsides during exercise but increases in severity while at rest. Pain can be located in the heel (insertional tendinopathy) or along the length of the tendon (tendinosis). Morning stiffness or severe pain on climbing stairs is also common. Most patients have an abnormal gait. Some limp, and some walk on their toes to avoid the heel-strike phase of walking.

PHYSICAL EXAMINATION

Localized swelling may be present around the tendon. There may be a bony prominence at the heel known as a Haglund deformity. Pain is often worse in the morning or after a period of inactivity and aggravated by shoe pressure. A palpable nodule, inflammatory signs, and crepitus may be present in severe or chronic cases.[7]

DIAGNOSTICS

Radiologic or laboratory tests are usually unnecessary, but the appropriate diagnostic tests should be guided by the history. Ultrasound is inexpensive and noninvasive and can be used to rule out rupture of the tendon. MRI is the gold standard but may not be needed in mild or straightforward cases. MRI is usually done if surgical intervention is a consideration.

DIFFERENTIAL DIAGNOSIS

Achilles tendinopathy causes primarily heel pain. Heel pain has varied causes. Retrocalcaneal bursitis, infection, fracture, plantar fasciitis, and partial tendon rupture should be considered in the differential diagnosis of Achilles tendinopathy. Posterior calf pain can also be caused by muscle strain, bruising, or thromboembolic disease.[8]

MANAGEMENT

Treatment of the acute phase of Achilles tendinopathy begins with the cessation of all sports activities and exercise. Tendon rest is imperative to avoid further injury. Severe inflammation may respond best to immobilization in a boot or cast. Crutches and partial weight bearing may be indicated. NSAIDs, either oral or topical, and an ice massage for 20 minutes three or four times a day help decrease inflammation and pain.[9] A simple shoe insert that raises the heel approximately 2 cm (¾ inch) also helps ease strain on the tendon. In more severe or chronic cases, ultrasound is an adjunct therapy used by physical therapists. Regular follow-up visits to assess progress and to discourage the patient from returning to activity prematurely are necessary. Resolution of acute tendinopathy can take 8 weeks or longer.[7] A program of stretching and strengthening begins when pain and swelling have subsided. Many patients can recover fully with exercise alone.[10] To prevent recurrence or rupture, it is essential that patients do stretching exercises before engaging in any exercise.

Severe cases unresponsive to conservative treatment may benefit from surgical debridement. In rare cases, tendon transplant to augment the strength of the damaged tendon may be necessary.[11]

COMPLICATIONS

Achilles tendon rupture is the most common complication of Achilles tendinitis. Frank rupture is best demonstrated by MRI of the area. Immobilization and/or surgery may be necessary for healing and return to function. Shortening of the tendon, chronic pain, chronic foot drop, and recurrent injuries as a result of the associated abnormal gait also may result from acute tendininopathy.[7]

INDICATIONS FOR REFERRAL OR HOSPITALIZATION

Patients with severe tendinitis or suspected tendon rupture require immediate referral to an orthopedic surgeon. In addition, patients who fail to respond to conservative therapy or who have significant tightness in the hamstrings or gastrocnemius require referral. Most patients will benefit from a referral to physical therapy for pain management and longer-term stretching and strengthening.

PATIENT AND FAMILY EDUCATION

Achilles tendinopathy can be a frustrating, slowly resolving, and recurrent problem. Patients with this condition need support during rehabilitation and need to be educated about proper retraining and stretching programs. During the rehabilitative phase, alternative activities such as swimming and cycling can be pursued as long as participation does not cause pain.

ACHILLES TENDON RUPTURE

DEFINITION AND EPIDEMIOLOGY

Achilles tendon rupture is a sudden event that results from a forced stretch on an already degenerating tendon; it is a soft tissue emergency. There is an increased risk for this injury in poorly conditioned athletes older than 30 years. In all, 80% of those injured are men; moreover, because most right-handed people begin their gait with the left foot, there is a higher incidence of left tendon ruptures.[9]

PATHOPHYSIOLOGY

Despite being the thickest and strongest tendon in the body, the Achilles tendon is the one most commonly ruptured, possibly as a result of underlying tendon degeneration or weakness that predisposes the tendon to rupture. In persons older than 30 years, there is a decreased blood supply to the area where the tendon most often ruptures. The offending event is often a jump, a sudden change in direction, or simply a push-off in stride. The pop of a tendon rupture is audible to others nearby.

CLINICAL PRESENTATION

The classic comment by patients with an Achilles tendon rupture is, "I thought I was shot in the calf." There is sudden weakness in the ankle. It is impossible to rise up on the toes, and most people limp; pain, however, is not common.

PHYSICAL EXAMINATION

There is a visible and palpable gap overlying the tendon where the rupture occurred, usually about 4 cm (1½ inches) above the calcaneal prominence. The definitive evaluation is the Thompson test, which is performed with the patient kneeling on a chair or prone with the knee in flexed position. The tendon is intact if the foot plantar flexes when the calf is squeezed (negative Thompson result). If there is no movement, the tendon is ruptured (positive Thompson result). The Thompson test result can be negative if the tear is partial.

DIAGNOSTICS

Radiologic examinations are not helpful because tendons are not radiopaque. Ultrasound or MRI will demonstrate the rupture and can be used if indicated.

DIFFERENTIAL DIAGNOSIS

The classic presentation and physical findings that characterize a ruptured Achilles tendon simplify the diagnosis. However, the diagnosis may be more complex with a partial tear. Achilles tendinopathy or retrocalcaneal bursitis is not usually associated with a sudden onset or audible pop.

MANAGEMENT

There are two accepted treatments of the ruptured Achilles tendon. The conservative, nonsurgical approach requires a long-leg cast with the foot in a plantar-flexed position. The cast stays on for approximately 6 weeks, allowing the tendon to heal by scar formation. Wearing of a heel lift for 2 months helps prevent undue stress on the new scar after casting. Unfortunately, this method has multiple disadvantages. The tendon heals longer in length, which weakens the calf muscle and the push-off power. Calf muscles also atrophy in a cast, which adds to the decreased strength and size and longer rehabilitation. In addition, 20% of the tendons allowed to heal in this manner rupture again once activities resume.[8] Patients with chronic pain who are not surgical candidates may benefit from an ankle-foot orthosis.

The second method of treatment for a ruptured Achilles tendon is surgical repair, usually by direct reapproximation of the two ends of the tendon. Tendon transplant may also be used to augment strength. The patient is in a long-leg cast for 6 weeks after surgery, then wears a short-leg, walking cast for an additional 4 weeks.[11] As in the nonoperative method, a heel lift is used to prevent undue stress on the tendon. Open surgical treatment of acute Achilles tendon ruptures significantly reduces the risk of rerupture compared with nonsurgical treatment but produces significantly higher risks of other complications, including wound infection, damage to the sural nerve, and deep venous thrombosis (DVT). Surgical complications may be reduced by performing surgery percutaneously.[12,13]

COMPLICATIONS

Weakened or atrophied muscles with resultant gait disorders are a common complication of tendon ruptures. Close attention to rehabilitation and muscle strengthening after the injury helps reduce the magnitude of these complications.

INDICATIONS FOR REFERRAL OR HOSPITALIZATION

An Achilles tendon rupture is a soft tissue emergency. Immediate referral to an orthopedic surgeon is required.

PATIENT AND FAMILY EDUCATION

The most important education for Achilles tendon rupture is prevention. Patients who are novice exercisers should be instructed to follow a simple, gentle stretching program beforehand. For example, patients can stand on a slanted board or on the edge of a step and let the heels drop below the level of the step. They hold this stretched position for 10 to 15 seconds, and then repeat the exercise for 10 to 15 minutes. If patients cannot feel a pull on the Achilles tendon, they are not doing the stretch properly. Bouncing is counterproductive.

OSTEOCHONDRITIS DISSECANS

DEFINITION AND EPIDEMIOLOGY

Originally defined as the nontraumatic development of loose bodies within a joint, osteochondritis dissecans is a joint disorder caused by a small fragment of bone underlying the articular cartilage that becomes avascular and necrotic.[14] Osteochondritis dissecans is seen more in adolescents and young adults and usually in males. This condition occurs most commonly in the knee but remains a significant source of ankle pain in the young athlete who participates in activities that place great stress on the ankle (ballet dancers, runners, basketball players). In the older adult, a loose body is typically the result of cartilage degeneration. The symptoms, including pain, joint instability, and inflammation, are the same in both groups.

PATHOPHYSIOLOGY

The cause of this condition is unknown. Several theories have suggested various causes, including trauma, nonunion of a fracture line, ischemic necrosis, and cartilage degeneration. Additionally noted are a familial tendency, certain skeletal abnormalities, and endocrine abnormalities.[14]

CLINICAL PRESENTATION

The usual presentation of osteochondritis dissecans is chronic pain and swelling that develops gradually over months. Activity increases the swelling and the pain, which intensifies as the ankle stiffens. Rest relieves the symptoms. On occasion, the athlete will recall a traumatic event.

PHYSICAL EXAMINATION

Range of motion is usually normal, and the joint is stable. Because the damaged area is within the joint, it is often difficult to palpate an area of tenderness, although there may be a palpable joint effusion.

DIAGNOSTICS

Radiologic examination alone provides the definitive diagnosis with direct visualization of the loose body. Plain x-ray films of the ankle occasionally reveal a loose bone fragment or an area of sclerotic bone. CT or MRI helps better define the lesion and stage the injury.

DIFFERENTIAL DIAGNOSIS

If trauma before the occurrence of symptoms is reported, fracture should be considered. Tendinitis and recurrent sprain should also be considered. Osteoarthritis of the joint must be considered in the older adult. Other types of inflammatory arthritis causing ankle pain include rheumatoid arthritis, gout, and spondyloarthropathies.

MANAGEMENT

Osteochondritis dissecans warrants close observation by an orthopedic surgeon. The painful area has decreased or no capacity to heal itself; therefore surgery is often necessary. In the younger child with a shorter duration of pain, immobilization in a cast for 4 to 6 weeks may resolve the problem. Older patients, patients with a longer duration of injury, or patients with a loose bone fragment that affects function may require surgery.[15]

COMPLICATIONS

Degenerative arthritis, decreased range of motion, and chronic pain with associated gait disturbance are potential sequelae of this condition.

INDICATIONS FOR REFERRAL OR HOSPITALIZATION

Osteochondritis dissecans is a potentially serious condition. Orthopedic consultation is recommended to prevent complications.

PATIENT AND FAMILY EDUCATION

The exact cause of osteochondritis dissecans is unknown. Therefore it is important that patients and families understand that any joint pain that occurs during exercise or interferes with normal activities of daily living requires medical assessment. Careful explanation of the potential sequelae of this condition, including degenerative arthritis, decreased range of motion, and chronic pain, is also necessary.

Other possible causes of ankle pain include osteoarthritis (see Chapter 184, rheumatoid arthritis (see Chapter 218, seronegative spondyloarthropathies (see Chapter 215, and gout (see Chapter 176.

PLANTAR FASCIITIS

DEFINITION AND EPIDEMIOLOGY

Plantar fasciitis is a painful disorder that involves the plantar aspect of the heel. It can be acute or chronic and is characterized by pain in the bottom of the foot, along the arch, and in the heel.[16] A dense fibrous tissue, the plantar fascia, extends from the calcaneal tuberosity to the metatarsal heads. The fascia can become irritated from overuse, trauma, or shoes with poor arch support. People with flat or cavus feet are especially vulnerable to this condition.

PATHOPHYSIOLOGY

The plantar fascia supports the arch and the sole of the foot. High impact or stress, such as running and jumping, increases the pressure exerted on the fascia by spreading the toes or flattening the arch; this tears the fascia. Four common causes of fascia tears or inflammation are a sudden turn that places increased pressure on the sole of the foot, shoes with inadequate support, shoes with stiff soles, and feet that pronate excessively. Other contributing factors include obesity, a job that requires standing for long periods, and excessive running. Patients commonly have heel spurs, although the relationship is unclear. The pain is gradual in onset and increases as the inflammation worsens or as the tear extends.[17]

CLINICAL PRESENTATION

Patients with plantar fasciitis complain of pain with weight bearing the first thing in the morning or after periods of rest. Pain can also be elicited with stretching of the fascia. High-impact activities, running, barefoot walking, standing for prolonged periods, and rising up on toes can aggravate the pain or make it unbearable. Patients occasionally limp or avoid planting the heel when walking.

PHYSICAL EXAMINATION

With plantar fasciitis, there is point tenderness at the insertion of the fascia to the calcaneus. The patient may have fullness along the arch and pain along the body of the fascia, at the medial and lateral aspects of the heel, or at the metatarsal heads. Plantar pain is common in obese patients, patients with pronated feet, or those with atrophy of the calcaneal fat pad.

DIAGNOSTICS

Weight-bearing x-ray studies are indicated to rule out any bone abnormality or other underlying causes, such as a foreign body. Radiographs commonly reveal a bone spur that points forward from the heel. In cases unresponsive to conservative treatment, ultrasound or MRI may help to rule out more serious issues.

DIAGNOSTICS

Foot Pain

IMAGING

X-ray studies*
Ultrasonography or MRI*

*If indicated.

DIFFERENTIAL DIAGNOSIS

A history of early morning heel discomfort that resolves after several minutes but returns later in the day is usually clinically diagnostic of plantar fasciitis. However, other causes of heel pain should be considered; these include calcaneal fracture, especially if associated with a history of trauma, retrocalcaneal or infracalcaneal bursitis, gout, infection of the calcaneal fat pad, arthritis, reactive arthritis, plantar warts, and tarsal tunnel syndrome, as well as neuropathy and peripheral vascular disease.

DIFFERENTIAL DIAGNOSIS

Foot Pain

HEEL PAIN

- Achilles tendinopathy
- Plantar fasciitis
- Calcaneal fracture
- Retrocalcaneal or infracalcaneal bursitis
- Gout
- Infection
- Reactive arthritis
- Tarsal tunnel syndrome

FOREFOOT PAIN

- Morton neuroma
- Fracture
- Infection
- Ganglion
- Ledderhose syndrome
- Arthritis (inflammatory or degenerative)
- Gout
- Flat feet
- Corn
- Bunion
- Peripheral neuritis or neuropathy
- Peripheral vascular disease

MANAGEMENT

A conservative approach to management of this condition begins with complete rest from high-impact activities. Walking barefoot or in flat shoes (i.e., flip-flops) should be avoided. All shoes should have good arch support, which can be achieved with commercially available arch supports. Some patients do well with a heel cup or heel pad that raises the heel approximately ¼ inch. NSAIDs and ice massage help reduce inflammation and pain. A key component of treatment is a program of exercises that stretch the heel cord and plantar fascia. Corticosteroid injection at the heel may be very helpful.

Second-tier treatment options may include night splints, a second steroid injection, prescription orthotics, immobilization, and formal referral to physical therapy. Extracorporeal shock wave therapy is often recommended when more conservative therapy fails to relieve symptoms. This form of therapy is delivered either in a series of low-intensity treatments, which can be mildly painful, or a single high-intensity treatment, which can be very painful and require pretreatment sedation. Shock wave therapy is thought to work by inducing microtrauma to the tissue, which then initiates a healing response that includes increased formation of blood vessels carrying nutrients to the area and inflammatory mediators out of the area.[17]

Plantar fasciotomy is reserved for cases that fail to respond to all other treatment.

COMPLICATIONS

Usually no complications are associated with plantar fasciitis. However, an alteration in gait can cause other musculoskeletal problems, such as hip or back pain. Plantar fasciitis can be a lingering problem that frustrates both the patient and the provider.

INDICATIONS FOR REFERRAL OR HOSPITALIZATION

Any patient who fails to respond to conservative therapies should be referred to an orthopedic surgeon or a podiatrist. Ultrasound treatment by a physical therapist helps in severe cases; some patients benefit from custom-made orthotics, whereas others require cortisone injections. In rare cases, the fascia is surgically released.

PATIENT AND FAMILY EDUCATION

Rest is the first treatment of plantar fasciitis. Patients are advised to keep weight off the foot until the inflammation resolves. Ice to the sore area for 20 minutes three or four times a day can be helpful to relieve symptoms. The health care provider often will prescribe nonsteroidal anti-inflammatory medication, such as ibuprofen. Custom orthotics or night splints that keep the foot in dorsiflexion can be helpful. A program of home exercises to stretch the Achilles tendon and plantar fascia is the mainstay for treatment of the condition and lessening the chance of recurrence.[18] Overweight patients should be advised to lose weight. Many public access websites that demonstrate stretching techniques are available.[19]

MORTON NEUROMA

DEFINITION AND EPIDEMIOLOGY

Morton neuroma is a result of perineural fibrosis of the plantar nerve at the point where the medial and lateral branches of the plantar nerve converge. This condition is seen primarily in middle-aged women, with the most common cause thought to be being pointed-toe or high-heeled shoes causing entrapment, although repetitive trauma, ischemia, impingement, and intermetatarsal bursitis are contributors.[20] This condition can also develop in people with claw toes and bunions.

PATHOPHYSIOLOGY

Compression of the interdigital plantar nerves causes repeated trauma, which in turn causes inflammation and fibrosis of the nerve sheath. Tight, pointed-toe shoes aggravate the irritation once the neuroma has formed.

CLINICAL PRESENTATION

Patients with Morton neuroma report severe pain and burning in the region of the third web space. Going barefoot and undergoing foot massages relieve the discomfort. Elevation of the foot aggravates the condition.

PHYSICAL EXAMINATION

The physical examination of a patient with Morton neuroma usually reveals point tenderness and often edema over the third web space, between the third and fourth metatarsals. Mulder sign is elicited if compression of the medial and lateral sides of the patient's foot with one hand and squeezing between the third and fourth metatarsal bones, or other web space, with the other results in a palpable or audible click. The patient may also feel acute pain radiating to the adjacent toes and upward along the foot.[20] On occasion, paresthesia occurs at the reciprocal surfaces of the toes. The examination findings are otherwise unremarkable.

DIAGNOSTICS

Ultrasound or MRI can aid in diagnosis in the absence of a clear-cut history and examination findings.[20]

DIFFERENTIAL DIAGNOSIS

The plantar surface of the foot should be smooth and nontender. Calluses and plantar warts on the ball of the foot may be tender, rough, and nodular. Ganglia are cystlike in appearance, whereas infectious processes classically have edema, erythema, warmth, and tenderness. Ledderhose syndrome, also known as *plantar fibromatosis,* is a disorder of fibrous tissue proliferation, characterized by a slow-growing nodular thickening, most often within the central band of the plantar aponeurosis. It is often associated with painless, thickened palmar fascia and with Dupuytren contracture (see Chapter 177 and Peyronie disease. Stress fractures, bursitis, or arthritic changes must also be ruled out.

MANAGEMENT

Conservative treatment using a stepwise protocol can resolve this condition. Patient education, wider-toed shoes, insole adjustments, separation of the toes with a small pad, and NSAIDs help reduce the inflammation. In persistent cases, injection with steroids, alcohol, or local anesthetic can be temporarily effective at relieving pain but offers no long-term solution. Finally, surgical excision may be indicated as a last resort.[21]

COMPLICATIONS

Chronic pain alters gait. Injections with sclerosing agents (alcohol) is commonly recommended but is not a permanent solution and is associated with injection site pain. Surgical removal of the neuroma may cause the toes to become permanently numb.

INDICATIONS FOR REFERRAL OR HOSPITALIZATION

If conservative treatment and steroid injections are not effective, a referral for excision of the neuroma is advised.

PATIENT AND FAMILY EDUCATION

Patients should be encouraged to wear properly fitting shoes that have adequate toe room, good arch support, and a low or flat heel. Shoes should be purchased at the end of the day, when feet are bigger, and should be replaced when support wears out. Shoes should be fitted to ensure proper size. Metatarsal arch pads, if used correctly, may ease the discomfort associated with Morton neuroma and metatarsalgia.

OTHER COMMON CAUSES OF FOOT PAIN

Bunions, bunionettes, corns, calluses, hammertoes, hallux rigidus, hallux valgus, plantar warts, ingrown toenails, and tarsal tunnel syndrome are discussed in Table 171-2, along with their differential diagnoses and management. Stress fractures of the metatarsals are common injuries in runners and others participating in running sports.

TABLE 171-2 Other Common Foot Problems*

Problem	Presentation	Examination and Diagnostics	Differential Diagnosis and Management
BUNION			
An inflammatory degenerative deformity of the first metatarsophalangeal (MTP) joint related to flat feet or laxity of the first toe and first metatarsal bone	Intense pain over the first MTP joint	Edema, deformity, and tenderness of the first metatarsal head; may have joint crepitus on palpation *Diagnostics:* If gout is suspected, uric acid levels and joint aspiration are considered; x-ray studies are not diagnostic	*Differential diagnosis:* Gout *Management:* Warm packs or soaks, NSAIDs, and well-fitted shoes with adequate toe space Podiatry referral indicated for custom-made protective shield or foot mold Orthopedic or podiatry referral necessary for surgical correction if conservative management does not control pain

Continued

TABLE 171-2 **Other Common Foot Problems*—cont'd**

Problem	Presentation	Examination and Diagnostics	Differential Diagnosis and Management
BUNIONETTE			
Pressure over the bone prominence on the fifth metatarsal head that results in bursa or ulceration	Painful, edematous lesion on the MTP joint of the fifth toe	Edema and erythema over the lateral aspect of the MTP of the fifth toe; may be accompanied by a cystlike, fluid-filled lesion	Properly fitting shoes with adequate toe room, bunion padding Filing down of hard lesions
CALLUS			
Hypertrophied area of skin on sole of foot related to excessive supination, pronation, or other abnormality	Usually asymptomatic	Dried, hypertrophied epidermal layer; may surround or protect a plantar wart or foreign body	Daily skin cream or lanolin, use of pumice stone by patient Debridement of painful calluses with a scalpel to relieve pressure Orthotic device as indicated For patients with diabetes or PVD, see Corn
CORN			
Hard corn (heloma durum): hyperkeratotic lesions caused by pressure or friction; usually found on the toes or other bone prominence Soft corn (heloma molle): macerated, interdigital, and painful; caused by pressure	Painful lesion between toes or on dorsal surface of toes	Erythematous, painful lesion; patient may also have hammertoes	Avoidance of tight-fitting shoes, use of corn pads to relieve pressure, routine paring of corns with file or scalpel Powder and lamb's wool or soft cotton between toes to prevent excessive moisture Referral to orthotic specialist for customized orthotic device Surgical repair for accompanying hammertoe or arthroplasty as needed Vigilant care for patients with diabetes or peripheral vascular disease (PVD) to prevent corns or calluses and ulceration or infection
HALLUX FLEXUS (HAMMERTOE OR CLAW TOE)			
Dorsiflexion of proximal joint of second toe while middle joint is plantar flexed	Painful corn the most common complaint	Dorsal flexion of first phalanx of second toe (either foot), with plantar flexion in second phalanx; may be accompanied by painful callus on metatarsal head or at nail end as well as painful corn on dorsal surface of the proximal interphalangeal joint	See Corn Referral to podiatrist or orthopedic surgeon for surgical repair
HALLUX RIGIDUS			
Inflexible great toe, usually a result of arthritic changes	Pain with ambulation, climbing stairs	Immobile, fixated first MTP joint; may be slightly edematous with accompanying irregularity of joint edges related to osteophyte formation; diminished active and passive range of motion caused by immobility and pain *Diagnostics:* x-ray study (anteroposterior and lateral views)	NSAIDs for pain Podiatry or orthopedic referral for surgical repair

TABLE 171-2 Other Common Foot Problems*—cont'd

Problem	Presentation	Examination and Diagnostics	Differential Diagnosis and Management
HALLUX VALGUS, HALLUX VARUS			
Hallux valgus: great toe laterally displaced toward other toes *Hallux varus:* great toe medially displaced away from other toes	Painful bunion of first MTP joint	*Hallux valgus:* great toe laterally displaced with possible accompanying bunion, hammertoe; may have extension of second toe over great toe *Hallux varus:* great toe medially displaced	Bunion care as described under Bunion Surgical or podiatry referral as indicated
ONYCHOCRYPTOSIS (INGROWN TOENAIL)			
Usually related to poor nail trimming or tight-fitting shoes	Pain and edema of great toe	Tender, edematous, erythematous area at corner of distal nail bed; lateral nail bed usually involved and obscured by hypertrophied tissue Evidence of purulent discharge Careful examination for lymphangitis and range of motion	For minimum ingrown toenail, wedge removal of nail edge to relieve discomfort If infection is present, patient is immunocompromised, or nail is severely ingrown, podiatry or surgical consultation for nail excision and possible matricectomy Treatment of infection with appropriate antibiotic; patient instructed to soak foot in warm water several times daily, to elevate foot, to apply bandage, and to wear open-toed shoes or soft slippers Further instruction regarding nail care
PLANTAR WARTS			
Warty growth on plantar surface caused by viral infection	May be asymptomatic or patient may report pruritic, painful lesion on sole of foot; increasing pain with weight-bearing activities	Callus possibly obscuring wart, which commonly is 1 mm to 1 cm in size Paring of callus revealing rough lesion with numerous small, black spots in center of lesion	*Differential diagnosis:* Porokeratotic lesion, foreign body *Management:* May resolve spontaneously For patients without diabetes or PVD: daily debridement with pumice stone, application of salicylic acid solution nightly to affected area, and gentle debridement of lesion each morning with an emery board Reminder to patients that lesions can spread, so debrided tissue must be carefully discarded Referral to podiatry indicated if conservative measures fail
TARSAL TUNNEL SYNDROME			
Compression of the tibial nerve	Pain, numbness, and tingling sole of foot	Tinel test Nerve conduction velocity studies	*Differential diagnosis:* Ankle arthritis, neuropathy *Management:* NSAIDs, orthotics, steroid injection, podiatry or surgical referral for decompression

*Because of the classic presentation of these disorders, diagnostic testing and differential diagnoses are noted only when indicated.

CHAPTER 172

BONE TUMORS

Henry Degroot III

DEFINITION AND EPIDEMIOLOGY

The term *bone tumor* is broadly used and encompasses a wide variety of bone lesions. Bone tumors may be benign neoplasms of the musculoskeletal tissues, such as osteoblastoma or chondroblastoma (CBMA); a sarcoma, which is a malignant tumor of mesenchymal or neuroectodermal origin such as osteosarcoma and Ewing sarcoma; a tumor of vascular, hematopoietic, or lymphoid tissues, such as hemangioma, multiple myeloma, or lymphoma; or a metastatic cancer, which is a secondary tumor that arises from a cancer elsewhere in the body, such as breast or prostate. In addition, the term *bone tumor* may apply to hamartomas, which are abnormal growths of normal tissues, such as osteochondroma, and to non-neoplastic lesions of uncertain cause, such as aneurysmal bone cyst (ABC) and pigmented villonodular synovitis. Tumor mimics, such as bone lesions caused by gout, arthritis, and metabolic diseases, can also have the appearance of a bone tumor. Because so many disparate bone lesions may be described as bone tumors, clinicians should take care when informing patients that they may have a bone tumor.

The most common malignant tumor that originates in bone is multiple myeloma, with an incidence of 6.1 per 100,000. Approximately 20,000 adults are diagnosed with multiple myeloma each year, and 10,000 will die of the disease. The median age at diagnosis is 70 years.

Myeloma, lymphoma, and leukemia are lymphoproliferative disorders characterized by excess production of abnormal lymphocytes. Primary lymphoma of bone is a rare type of lymphoma that accounts for approximately 7% of all malignant bone tumors. Cancers that originate in connective tissues such as bone, tendons, or muscles are classified as sarcomas. Osteosarcoma, the most common bone sarcoma, originates from primitive mesenchymal bone-forming cells. Ewing sarcoma originates from cells that arise in the embryonic neural crest. Chondrosarcoma (CHSA)develops in primitive mesenchymal cartilage-forming cells.[1] Primary cancers of the bone account for less than 0.2% of all cancers. Osteosarcoma is the most common sarcoma, with an incidence estimated to be 1 in 1 million. After osteosarcoma, CHSA and malignant fibrous histiocytoma are the most common varieties of sarcoma. Approximately 3000 primary bone sarcomas are diagnosed each year in the United States. In children and teenagers younger than 20 years, the incidence of malignant bone tumors is 8.7 per million.[2]

In adults older than 40 years, metastatic deposits in bone from cancers elsewhere in the body are the most common cause of bone tumors. Approximately 70% of patients with advanced breast or prostate cancer and 15% to 30% of patients with kidney, lung, uterine, thyroid, stomach, rectal, bladder, and colon cancer will develop metastatic cancer in the bones.[3] More than 350,000 people die with bone metastasis each year in the United States.[3] Breast cancer has been found to be the most common primary tumor type (n = 4041). In the Medicare cohort (mean age 75.6 years; standard deviation [SD] = 7.8), 6427 (0.495%) patients were identified with metastatic bone disease. Breast (n = 1798) and prostate (n = 1862) cancers were the most common primary tumor types. It is estimated that 279,679 (95% confidence interval, 274,579 to 284,780) U.S. adults alive on December 31, 2008, had had evidence of metastatic bone disease in the previous 5 years. Breast, prostate, and lung cancers accounted for 68% of these cases.[4]

The incidence of benign bone tumors is difficult to estimate because many are left untreated and others are never discovered. In children, osteochondroma, nonossifying fibroma, and fibrous dysplasia (FD) are the most common benign bone tumors. In persons aged 20 to 40 years, giant cell tumor (GCT) and enchondroma are the most commonly diagnosed bone tumors.[5] A recent study indicates that this incidence has not changed in past 30 years.[6]

PATHOPHYSIOLOGY

In most cases, bone tumors arise from the deletion, addition, or modification of the tumor cell DNA or DNA-associated proteins. Genetic alterations have been identified in both benign and malignant bone and soft tissue neoplasms. These genetic and epigenetic anomalies disrupt the orderly growth, division, or senescence of cells by a number of mechanisms. One type of tumorigenesis is linked to the creation of a novel "fusion" gene. Approximately half of the fusion genes that have been identified in sarcomas belong to the FET family of transcription regulation genes. More than one molecular or genetic abnormality may be necessary for the development of cancer. The identification of precise markers and mechanisms of tumorigenesis in the laboratory has now benefited the clinician at the bedside in the form of highly specific diagnostic tests and treatments. The identification of specific chromosomal abnormalities allows definitive diagnosis of certain sarcomas using DNA probes. In addition, treatments that inhibit critical molecular abnormalities in bone tumors are now a reality. Outside the laboratory, researchers are examining large epidemiologic and genomic databases, seeking to apply "big data" techniques to the understanding and treatment of bone cancers.

Some bone cancers arise from an inherited tumor gene such as the retinoblastoma *(RB1)* gene. The cells of normal individuals have two intact *RB1* genes on chromosome 13, and both genes must be defective for cancer to develop. Affected individuals inherit one defective copy of the *RB1* gene from a parent; the other mutates during fetal development. These children develop retinoblastoma in childhood and they are at high risk for osteosarcoma, small cell lung cancer, and synovial sarcoma as adults.[7]

A small number of malignant bone tumors are caused by chronic diseases. Approximately 5% of patients with widespread Paget disease of bone (see Chapter 182 develop sarcoma in the affected bones, usually osteosarcoma. Patients with longstanding infection in the bone (see Chapter 185 are at risk for development of a malignant tumor, including squamous cell carcinoma, at the site of the draining infection. The data on exposure to chlorinated dioxin contaminants in the herbicide Agent Orange have not provided consistent evidence of an increased cancer risk in exposed individuals.[8] Other factors, such as genetic polymorphisms, which are known to increase the risk of developing non-Hodgkin lymphoma, may play a role.[9]

CLINICAL PRESENTATION

Bone tumors are likely to be discovered in an ambulatory setting such as a primary care office. There are three distinct

BOX 172-1

Presentation of Bone Tumor

INCIDENTAL OR LATENT BONE TUMOR
Found on an imaging study performed for an unrelated reason or a minor injury. No pain before injury, and pain improving day by day. The pain is unrelated to the tumor.

ACTIVE BONE TUMOR
Manifests with months of mild, gradually increasing pain with no mass and minimal dysfunction. A minor injury may lead to a pathologic fracture of the involved bone.

AGGRESSIVE BONE TUMOR
Manifests with months of progressively severe pain and a mass or swelling near a joint. Constitutional symptoms are usually absent.

METASTATIC BONE TUMOR
Manifests in a patient older than 40 years with progressive pain in the back, hip, shoulder, or ribs. Patients with cancer of the breast, prostate, lung, thyroid, kidney, or gastrointestinal sites are at an increased risk for metastasis to bone. Approximately 25% of patients have no previous history of cancer.

patterns of clinical presentation depending on whether the tumor is latent, active, or aggressive (Box 172-1). Latent bone tumors, such as nonossifying fibroma in children and enchondroma in adults, do not grow appreciably over time and do not cause bone pain or symptoms. These tumors are usually discovered as incidental findings during an evaluation for a musculoskeletal injury. In latent bone tumors, the radiographs show that the lesion is not growing and is not causing any damage to the bone. A careful history and physical examination combined with the x-ray findings are often enough to verify that the injured ligament, bone, or tendon is the source of the pain, not the tumor. In general, no workup or treatment for the tumor is needed other than repeat radiographs in 6 to 12 months to verify that the lesion is not clinically significant. In some cases, latent bone tumors may be large enough to create a real or perceived risk of pathologic fracture. In these cases referral for risk assessment is recommended. Careful analysis of the radiographs and other imaging studies is used to calculate the risk of pathologic fracture and decide on the need for prophylactic fixation.[10]

Active bone tumors are usually (but not always) benign. These tumors grow slowly and will locally invade and weaken the bone. Examples of active tumors include ABCs and unicameral bone cysts (UBCs), CBMAs, chondromyxoid fibromas (CMFs), and FD in children; and FD, GCT, and ~~human~~ CHSA in adults. In the primary care setting, the patient reports months of mild, gradually increasing pain with minimal loss of function and no obvious abnormalities on physical examination. In these patients, pain after an injury may be the reason the patient visits the primary care provider (PCP), but a careful history will reveal that the pain was present and gradually increasing before the injury. This is an important distinction because it establishes that the tumor is the source of the pain, not the injury. In active bone tumors, the radiographs show that the tumor is slowly growing. There will be evidence of local damage and a corresponding response from the involved bone. Referral of these cases to a specialist is recommended. These patients will require a regional skeletal workup and a biopsy before treatment. Most of these tumors are benign, and as a result many can be treated by thorough curettage of the tumor cavity followed by packing with bone graft, bone cement, or other material to restore the bone integrity.

Aggressive bone tumors are likely to be malignant and typically are discovered after months of progressively severe pain and a mass or swelling of the limb or joint. Examples of aggressive bone tumors include osteosarcoma, lymphoma, Ewing sarcoma, and metastatic adenocarcinoma. Constitutional symptoms are unusual in aggressive bone tumors, but fever and leukocytosis may occur in Ewing sarcoma and lymphoma. In the early stages the pain may mimic a musculoskeletal injury or a sprained joint, but as time goes on the pain changes. The pain becomes less activity related and more constant and may occur at night. There is swelling or a mass near a large joint such as the knee, hip, or shoulder. In active bone tumors, the radiographs show a permeative lesion that has clearly been growing and has damaged the bone, invaded the soft tissues, and prompted a vigorous local response such as a periosteal reaction. Careful history taking will allow the clinician to distinguish the pain of an aggressive bone tumor from typical pain of musculoskeletal origin, even at a relatively early stage. Patients with chordoma, a type of sarcoma that has a predilection for the sacrum, may come to their health care provider with persistent low back pain, constipation, or difficulty with defecation. Digital rectal examination reveals a mass growing out of the sacrum, which can block the rectum. Patients with active bone tumors require prompt referral to a specialist. A complete workup, including computed tomography (CT) scan of the chest and a whole body bone scan, is required. These tumors have a significant risk of being malignant sarcomas, which are treated by combination therapy including aggressive surgery, chemotherapy, and occasionally radiation.

Adults who have been treated for cancers of the breast, prostate, lung, thyroid, kidney, or some gastrointestinal sites are at risk of bone metastasis, even years after the completion of the treatment. The metastasis may initially manifest as a musculoskeletal ache or stiffness in the back, shoulder, hip, or chest wall. These patients should receive regular follow-up monitoring for bone metastasis.

COMMON CLINICAL SCENARIOS

There are common clinical circumstances in which a primary care physician is called on to evaluate the potential for a bone tumor.

Patient with an Occult Fracture

In the majority of cases, occult fracture is caused by osteoporosis. Separating osteoporotic fractures from pathologic fractures caused by bone tumor is usually straightforward. Osteoporotic fractures typically manifest with a prodromal period of 1 to 4 weeks of gradually increasing pain followed by an acute exacerbation and abnormal x-ray findings. The patient's clinical and radiographic findings are usually indicative of advanced osteoporosis. Where uncertainty exists, a magnetic resonance imaging (MRI) scan is helpful to distinguish a bone tumor or marrow-replacing neoplasm from osteoporotic fracture. In contrast, patients with impending pathologic fractures may have had many weeks or months of prodromal pain. Pain caused by impending pathologic fracture is most common in the hip, femur, and axial skeleton. The pain is mechanical in nature and exacerbated by walking or standing. Later it becomes more constant, independent of activities, deep or boring in nature, and more likely to occur at night. Most but not all patients have a previous diagnosis of cancer, especially breast or lung cancer. A significant percentage of patients have an actual or impending pathologic fracture as their first symptom of malignancy. Evaluation of cancer risk factors, smoking status, and the adequacy of cancer screening examinations allows the clinician to accurately assess the risk of undiagnosed cancer. When there is pain present, the bone lesion will be readily visible on imaging studies; usually no more than plain radiographs are needed. Studies have shown that in most patients who ultimately sustain fractures, early symptoms were missed. Among patients with fractures, many report a period of 1 to 3 days of increased pain on top of their deep bone pain.

Patient with Bone Pain

Musculoskeletal pain is a ubiquitous complaint in primary care practice, and it may be difficult to differentiate pain originating from deep soft tissue elements from bone pain. Back pain, knee pain, and shoulder pain are the most common anatomic sites and comprise almost two thirds of the total painful anatomic sites. Differentiation of tumor pain and bone pain is discussed earlier.

Patient with an Abnormal Bony Deformity

Patients with an abnormal bony deformity after injury or seizure, plus all potentially neglected or dependent older adults, and all pediatric patients with an abnormal bony deformity should undergo prompt evaluation by an orthopedic specialist. The remaining patients with atraumatic bony deformity, in many cases, have periarticular bone joint enlargement associated with osteoarthritis. This can manifest as an enlargement of the proximal end of the clavicle or the bones of the knee, ankle, fingers, and feet as a result of degenerative changes in the articulations. A neoplasm or bone tumor can typically be ruled out by radiographs. Other possible causes include diffuse idiopathic skeletal hyperostosis (DISH).

MEDICAL HISTORY AND PHYSICAL EXAMINATION

The evaluation of a bone tumor begins with a thorough history and physical examination.[11] In addition to the general medical history, the patient's cancer risk factors and personal cancer history must be elicited. Tobacco use as well as the status of cancer screening examinations, such as prostate examination and breast self-examination and mammography, should be documented. Patients who were treated for cancer in the past may consider themselves cured, and as a result they may not volunteer their cancer history unless carefully prompted. A thorough health history is often the most efficient way to identify the origin of the bone tumor. In taking the history of present illness, the provider should endeavor to establish the precise chronology of the pain. Patients may ascribe the pain from a bone tumor to a minor injury or accident. However, closer questioning will often reveal that the pain was present before the injury.

The general physical examination may reveal a systemic condition that might be associated with bone tumors, such as a growth disturbance, anemia, or cachexia. The focused musculoskeletal examination should assess the entire region of the body involved in the problem, not just an isolated part. The shoulder, hip, and knee cannot be comprehensively examined with the patient's clothing left on, and an incomplete examination may contribute to delay in making the correct diagnosis. The examiner should look for the presence of warmth or inflammation, a mass, loss of full joint motion, or lymphadenopathy. Subtle abnormalities are easy to identify by comparing the findings in the affected region with those in the corresponding normal region. Even large lesions that are deep seated in the shoulder, pelvis, or thigh may be difficult to identify by palpation. However, they can be easily seen if the examiner visually compares the normal and the abnormal sides of the body from a short distance away.

DIAGNOSTICS

Screening laboratory examinations have a very limited role in the initial diagnostic evaluation of a patient with a suspected bone tumor. Specific diagnostic test-s are still very valuable. Laboratory tests are used in a targeted way (Table 172-1). For example, the widespread use of prostate-specific antigen (PSA) as a prostate cancer screening tool has been reduced or eliminated in favor of risk-adjusted screening by age. A similar targeted approach applies to all bone tumors. A patient with suspected multiple myeloma should have serum protein electrophoresis tested to identify secretion of tumor paraproteins. However, patients with high-grade sarcoma may have entirely normal laboratory findings. Bone lesions caused by infection are associated with an elevated or normal white blood cell count, an elevated erythrocyte sedimentation rate (ESR), and elevated C-reactive protein. In certain sarcomas, a definitive diagnosis can be made from pathognomonic molecular markers that can be identified by the pathologist in the biopsy material.

IMAGING STUDIES

After the history and physical examination have been completed, the best next step is a plain x-ray examination. Advanced imaging, such as MRI, CT, positron emission tomography (PET), and bone scans, may not be needed and should in most cases be coordinated with the specialist. For most bone tumors, a differential diagnosis can be constructed based on the features on the plain x-ray film. In some cases, no other studies are

DIAGNOSTICS

Bone Tumors

LABORATORY
- CBC
- ESR
- C-reactive protein
- Alkaline phosphatase
- Calcium
- Phosphorus
- Uric Acid
- LFTs
- CA-125
- PSA

IMAGING
- X-ray examination, two planes
- CT or MRI
- PET scan
- Bone scan
- Bone biopsy

SPECIFIC BLOOD TESTS (USUALLY ORDERED BY SPECIALIST)
- 5-Hydroxyindoleacetic acid
- Carcinoembryonic antigen

CBC, complete blood count; LFTs, liver function tests.

TABLE 172-1 Diagnostic Tests for Bone Tumors

Method	Best for	Expected Result	Precautions
Plain radiograph	Evaluation of suspected tumor after physical examination and history	Benign: well circumscribed, sclerotic margin Aggressive: poorly circumscribed permeative destruction of bone	Soft tissue lesions not detected, no abnormality seen in early metastasis
Hematology: complete blood count (CBC), erythrocyte sedimentation rate (ESR), C-reactive protein	Differentiation of tumor from infection, evaluation of suspected hematologic malignant neoplasm (e.g., myeloma, lymphoma)	Lesions caused by infection: elevated white blood cell count, elevated ESR	Most benign bone tumors do not cause alterations in CBC, ESR, or C-reactive protein
Blood chemistry	Evaluation of prognosis (e.g., osteosarcoma), confirmation of diagnosis (e.g., Paget disease)	Elevated alkaline phosphatase and ionized calcium levels	Some bone tumors do not cause alterations in blood chemistry
Specific blood tests	Index of tumor activity in specific cancers (e.g., prostate-specific antigen [PSA] in prostate cancer)	Dependent on type of cancer (e.g., prostate cancer with metastasis will show abnormal PSA levels)	Not useful as an initial screening tool
Urinalysis	Confirmation of specific diagnostic entity (e.g., Bence-Jones protein for myeloma, hematuria in renal cell carcinoma)	Elevated secretion of tumor paraproteins	Not diagnostically useful for benign bone tumors
Technetium 99m (^{99m}Tc) bone scan	Determination of presence and location of multiple bone metastases in cancer	Abnormally elevated tracer uptake in areas of possible metastatic deposits in bone ("hot spots")	False-positive results from old fracture, arthritis, infection, and other nontumor causes
Computed tomography	Evaluation of lesions in complex bones, such as pelvis or spine	Extent of bone destruction, quantitative risk of pathologic fracture	Substantial radiation dose
Magnetic resonance imaging	Soft tissue lesions, hematologic malignant neoplasm (e.g., lymphoma), staging of lymph nodes	Tumors invisible on other imaging techniques (e.g., early metastasis from breast cancer)	False-positive results from injury, infection, smoking, and metabolic diseases
Positron emission tomography (PET)	Assessment of effectiveness of treatment for bone tumors	High absorption of tracer by cancer cells	Role in staging and diagnosis of bone tumors is not well defined, some tumors are PET negative

needed. A careful analysis of the plain radiographs by an experienced radiologist or orthopedic tumor specialist may be sufficient to confirm the diagnosis.

The behavior patterns of bone tumors, and thus their treatment and prognosis, can often be determined with some degree of certainty on the basis of the plain radiographs alone. Benign bone lesions with a latent behavior pattern are usually well circumscribed with a very sharp zone of transition between the lesion and the surrounding bone as well as a more or less prominent sclerotic margin. Enlarging bone tumors with an active behavior pattern are typically less sharply circumscribed, with a zone of transition between the lesion and the normal surrounding bone of a few millimeters or more. There may be expansion or even focal destruction of the bone cortex and even some expansion into the soft tissues. Bone tumors with an aggressive behavior pattern usually appear poorly circumscribed, with a wide or imperceptible zone of transition. There may be permeative destruction of the bone. The lesion may destroy the nearby cortex, or it may have permeated directly out of the bone into the soft tissue without destroying the cortex. A large soft tissue mass may be seen.

Advanced imaging should be coordinated with a specialist. CT scans are most helpful for lesions that form bone or lesions that occur in complex bones such as the pelvis and spine. CT scan is the best imaging modality to determine the extent of bone destruction and the exact extent of the bone lesion. Data from CT scans can be used to quantitate the risk of pathologic fracture from a lesion.[12]

MRI is the best imaging modality for visualization of soft tissue lesions or non–bone-forming bone tumors and for determination of the status of the nearby anatomy for surgical planning. MRI scans will detect bone tumors, such as early metastasis from breast cancer, that may be invisible on other studies. MRI scan is especially valuable for planning of surgery on bone tumors.

Technetium 99m (^{99m}Tc) bone scans are helpful for detection of lesions that may be invisible on plain x-ray studies. Whole-body ^{99m}Tc bone scans are not a useful diagnostic tool because nonspecific and abnormal findings may be caused by old fractures, arthritis, or other factors. Whole body bone scans are very useful as screening studies for patients with high risk of bone metastasis; to quantitate the locations of asymptomatic bone metastasis; and to follow the response to therapy for cancers with bone metastasis. For example, in non–small cell lung cancer patients with normal laboratory findings, bone scans can detect silent bone metastasis and avoid understaging and overtreatment errors. PET scans are often combined with CT scans (PET/CT) and may detect bone tumors that might otherwise be missed. PET/CT does not accurately predict the malignant potential of bone tumors. PET/CT scans can be used for cancer staging and to assess the effectiveness of chemotherapy for bone tumors. Ultrasound scans do not penetrate bone and cannot discriminate benign from malignant neoplasms. Ultrasound can be useful to guide needle biopsy procedures on bone lesions. Angiography was formerly used to locate and to diagnose bone tumors. However, angiography has been superseded by magnetic resonance angiography.

Role of Biopsy

Biopsy, by traditional incisional methods, by core needle methods, or by fine-needle aspiration methods, is the process of sampling the cells of the tumor for pathologic diagnosis. A biopsy should be the last procedure after all imaging studies, examinations, and other necessary investigations have been completed.

Biopsy of bone tumors has been associated with numerous complications including errors in diagnosis and prognosis; skin, soft tissue, and wound complications; and even erroneous amputation. Although biopsy is technically a straightforward procedure, the complications resulting from a poorly planned or poorly executed biopsy may have a profound impact on the patient's treatment and prognosis. Therefore, tumor specialists recommend that the biopsy of the bone tumor be performed only by the surgeon who will be performing the definitive surgical treatment of the lesion.[13]

The interpretation of bone tumor pathology is a complex and difficult task and typically referred to specialized pathologists who have sufficient experience in bone tumor diagnosis. It is essential for the bone tumor surgeon, the radiologist, and the pathologist to work together in a cooperative manner to properly diagnose a bone tumor.

DIFFERENTIAL DIAGNOSIS

The differential diagnosis is based on the patient's age, the history and examination findings, and the imaging studies. The laboratory examinations may help narrow the field. Once a short list of possibilities has been formulated, a biopsy is performed. After the biopsy a culture of the material found in the lesion is often performed. In children and adults, osteomyelit is and tuberculosis can cause localized bone or joint destruction, swelling, and pain, which makes them difficult to distinguish from bone cancer. Lesions that mimic bone tumors may arise from metabolic diseases, such as diabetes, gout, and hyperparathyroidism. In addition, other lesions need to be considered, such as congenital, post-traumatic, and degenerative lesions.

MANAGEMENT

Benign Bone Tumors

Treatment of benign bone tumors depends on their behavior patterns (Table 172-2). Management of bone lesions with a latent behavior pattern, such as nonossifying fibroma,

TABLE 172-2 Management of Bone Tumors

Type of Tumor	Examples	Staging Workup	Biopsy Considerations	Surgical Management	Adjuvant Treatments	Follow-up Guidelines
Bone tumor with latent behavior pattern	Nonossified fibroma, enchondroma	History, physical examination, and plain x-ray studies	Necessary only if diagnostic workup reveals risk of pathologic fracture	Surgery often not required	None required	1-2 yr follow-up with plain x-ray examinations to verify lack of change
Bone tumor with active behavior pattern	Giant cell tumor, chondroblastoma	History, physical examination, plain x-ray studies, MRI, CT	Core needle or open incisional biopsy may be combined with surgical treatment	Most lesions treated with curettage and packing of the bone defect	Liquid nitrogen, phenol, or mechanical burr used to reduce recurrence	2-5 yr clinical and x-ray follow-up to verify lack of recurrence
Bone tumor with aggressive behavior pattern	Osteosarcoma, Ewing sarcoma, lymphoma, myeloma	History, physical examination, plain x-ray studies, MRI, CT, ^{99m}Tc bone scan, CT scan of chest	Core needle or open incisional technique after completion of all imaging	Resection with a wide surgical margin	Bisphosphonates, chemotherapy, and radiotherapy	5-10 yr clinical follow-up with intermittent imaging to verify lack of recurrence; intermittent chest CT to rule out metastasis
Metastatic bone tumor	Metastatic breast, lung, prostate, renal, thyroid, and gastrointestinal cancers are typical	History, physical examination, ^{99m}Tc bone scan, skeletal survey	If primary tumor is known, closed needle biopsy technique for confirmation	Surgical stabilization of bones at risk of pathologic fracture, especially long bones	Bisphosphonates (zoledronic acid), radiation appropriate for small tumors (strontium 89, samarium 153)	Dependent on cancer diagnosis; typical to follow with ^{99m}Tc bone scans

enchondroma, and FD, may require no treatment. These benign tumors do not represent a significant risk to the patient's health. Once a bone tumor specialist has examined these tumors and determined that there is no increased risk of pathologic fracture, the tumor may be observed without biopsy. X-ray studies to verify that the tumor is not growing or changing are recommended every 3 to 6 months for 2 or 3 years. In some circumstances, when there is a risk of pathologic fracture, the tumor is removed by curettage and the bone is strengthened with bone graft, with or without a metallic plate or intramedullary rod.

DIFFERENTIAL DIAGNOSIS

Bone Tumors

MUSCULOSKELETAL
- Arthritis (monoarticular and polyarticular)
- Avascular necrosis and bone infarcts
- Bursitis
- Heterotopic ossification
- Pigmented villonodular synovitis
- Paget disease

INFECTIOUS
- Tuberculosis
- Osteomyelitis
- Cellulitis

HEMATOLOGIC
- Gaucher disease
- Lymphoma
- Leukemia

NEUROGENIC
- Charcot joint

OTHER
- Ganglion and epidermoid cysts
- Stress fracture

Bone lesions with an active behavior pattern, such as GCT, CBMA, and CMF, require local treatment. After the workup and diagnosis, the lesions are removed by complete curettage. To reduce the chance of local recurrence, phenol, liquid nitrogen, or a mechanical burr may be used to additionally treat the site of the tumor and to remove or kill any residual cells. The bone defect is filled with acrylic bone cement or bone graft, and a plate or screws may be added according to the surgeon's preference. Bone lesions with an aggressive behavior pattern are treated according to the type of tumor.

Malignant Tumors and Sarcoma in Bone

Multiple myeloma is treated by multidrug chemotherapy or autologous stem cell transplantations, irradiation, maintenance of fluid and electrolyte balance, orthopedic stabilization of pathologic fractures, and bisphosphonates. (See Chapter 241) Monitoring for hypercalcemia, anemia, dehydration, and infection is necessary. Intravenous therapy with pamidronate or zoledronic acid reduces the number of skeletal complications in myeloma and is recommended for all patients with multiple myeloma who have identifiable lytic bone lesions. For painful vertebral compression fractures, vertebroplasty can provide rapid and long-lasting relief of pain.

The treatment of malignant bone tumors and sarcomas varies by tumor type and stage. Low-grade malignant tumors and some sarcomas, such as many CHSAs, adamantinoma, and epithelioid hemangioendothelioma, may be treated by surgical removal with a wide margin only. Chemotherapy and radiotherapy may not be required. The goal of surgery in these cases is to remove the entire tumor, including a cuff of surrounding normal bone and soft tissue to ensure that there is no local recurrence. The resulting bone defect may be reconstituted with an allograft bone, a metallic prosthesis, or a combination of these.

High-grade malignant sarcomas, such as osteosarcoma and Ewing sarcoma, are treated with multimodality treatment, which combines surgery, preoperative and postoperative chemotherapy and radiotherapy, and bisphosphonates, according to the type and location of the tumor. In Ewing sarcoma, if the surgical treatment does not result in a wide margin, radiotherapy is used to reduce the risk of local recurrence. Bisphosphonate medications, such as pamidronate and zoledronic acid, are widely used to prevent unnecessary loss of bone mineral mass and fractures during treatment. Prolonged use of bisphosphonates in cancer patients carries a risk of osteonecrosis of the jaw and pathologic fractures.[14]

Metastatic Cancers in Bone

The management of patients with bone metastasis is focused on reducing the incidence of new metastatic tumor deposits in bone, hypercalcemia of malignancy, cord compression, pathologic fracture, radiation to bone, and surgery to bone, collectively known as skeletal-related events (SREs). Bisphosphonates and denosumab are most commonly used. Zoledronic acid is the most commonly used bisphosphonate, and it has been shown to prevent, minimize, and delay the onset of SREs. Denosumab, a new monoclonal antibody, also reduces the risk of SREs in metastatic cancer. Denosumab inhibits RANKL, which is a primary signaling protein in bone loss. Metastatic tumors in the skeleton are treated on the basis of location, symptoms, and tumor type. Estimation of the patient's ability to withstand the surgery and of the overall duration of survival helps guide the selection of treatment but is prone to error and should be used with caution. Most patients with cancer metastasis in bone cannot be cured, but function, pain control, and quality of life (QOL) can be enhanced by prompt and appropriate surgical treatments. Orthopedic stabilization of metastatic lesions will help maintain the patient's independence, dignity, and self-worth and minimize dependency, need for institutional care, and dependency on narcotic drugs. Patients with known metastatic lesions in bone should be systematically monitored for additional metastatic lesions so that they may be treated before they become advanced and cause complications.

Once a lesion is discovered, it should be evaluated by an orthopedic surgeon to estimate the risk of pathologic fracture. Pathologic fracture probability calculation is based on the size, radiologic features, pain characteristics, and skeletal location of the lesions. Metastatic lesions in the intertrochanteric region of the proximal femur just below the hip have the highest risk of pathologic fracture.[10]

Orthopedic stabilization is indicated to maintain and to restore functional ability and to relieve pain from impending or actual pathologic fractures in long bones such as the humerus, femur, and tibia. Stabilization of impending fractures before actual pathologic fracture results in easier treatment and more rapid recovery for the patient. The weakened or fractured bones are usually stabilized with orthopedic plates or rods, combined with polymethyl methacrylate cement. After orthopedic stabilization, radiation may be recommended to prevent or to delay local recurrence and local progression of the tumor in a dose-dependent fashion. For metastatic lesions in the small bones or non–weight-bearing bones, such as the hands, feet, ribs, and scapula, radiation therapy is preferable to surgery. Patients with metastatic deposits in the bones should be given intravenous pamidronate or zoledronic acid. This treatment has been shown to decrease bone mineral loss associated with treatment, as well as to prevent or delay the onset of additional SREs in cancer patients with bone metastasis.[14,15]

Pain Management

Patients with bone tumors require a comprehensive pain management program. Benign bone tumors typically cause moderate pain, and surgical treatment results in a temporary increase in pain that may be managed with conventional modalities.

Patients with malignant or metastatic tumors in bone require more advanced pain management. Long-acting opioid pain medicines, transdermal delivery systems, pain medicine pumps, and multidrug protocols using controlled-release narcotics coupled with short-acting narcotics for breakthrough pain have been successfully used in the management of cancer pain. Pain management should be monitored to prevent overtreatment or undertreatment. External beam radiation is effective in controlling pain in the majority of patients. The radionuclides strontium 89 and samarium 153 have been shown to be effective for generalized bone pain in patients with widely disseminated metastatic deposits.[15]

Bisphosphonates should be considered for all patients with painful bone lesions. Bisphosphonate medications can decrease pain by preventing the growth and development of new and existing bone lesions. Although it is tempting to place patients with metastatic bone lesions on activity restriction to prevent pain, this may unintentionally accelerate bone damage because of disuse atrophy and calcium loss. Maintenance of normal activity levels should be the goal wherever possible. Patients with metastatic cancer in the vertebra may develop compression fractures leading to severe back pain. Vertebroplasty, which involves the injection of bone cement to stabilize the vertebral body, may be indicated in these patients. Vertebroplasty is a minimally invasive procedure and may result in substantial pain relief. Complications such as infection, paraplegia, and cement embolism can occur.[16]

Postsurgical pain and phantom limb pain can be significant challenges in sarcoma patients. Gabapentin, amitriptyline, and benzodiazepine drugs as well as physical therapy, counseling, and counterirritant therapy, such as transcutaneous electrical nerve stimulation (TENS) units, are helpful adjuncts in complex pain control situations. Severe or chronic postoperative or post-cancer pain is often managed by pain control specialists.

PROGNOSIS AND SURVIVAL

Primary Benign and Malignant Bone Tumors

Most latent bone tumors have no impact on patient prognosis or survival. Active bone tumors may locally damage bones and joints and result in loss of mobility or function. Some multifocal bone tumors, such as hereditary multiple exostosis and polyostotic FD, can lead to severe limitation of mobility, deformity, and chronic pain.

The prognosis for malignant sarcoma in bone is strongly related to the stage of the tumor rather than the cell type of the tumor. Patients with localized sarcoma have an 83% survival rate at 5 years. If regional metastasis has occurred, the 5-year survival rate drops to 54%; and if distant metastasis has occurred, 5-year survival is 16%. The 10-year survival rate is only slightly worse than the 5-year rate.[2] Survival in high-grade sarcoma has not changed dramatically in the past few decades, despite enhanced diagnostic and therapeutic modalities, new chemotherapeutic agents, and new surgical techniques.[17]

Multiple myeloma, a disease primarily affecting older adults, has improved prognosis and survival in the past 10 years because of new active chemotherapy agents, autologous stem cell transplantation, and the use of bisphosphonates. Median survival is more than 5 years, and 3-year survival is 75% to 80%. Important prognostic variables include age, disease stage, renal function, and performance status, as well as the presence of specific DNA abnormalities in the tumor cells.

Metastatic Bone Tumors

Increased use of bisphosphonates and denosumab, combined with targeted chemotherapy, radiation, and surgery, has contributed to a decrease in overall mortality for breast, lung, colon and rectal, and stomach cancers; leukemia; non-Hodgkin lymphoma; and cancers of other sites.[18] Aggressive treatment of metastatic bone disease can lead to prolonged survival, and the number of patients living with metastatic cancer continues to grow.[19] Patients' QOL and performance status can be maintained despite the presence of skeletal metastasis. Treatment of skeletal-related events (SREs) in patients with metastatic cancer, including treatment and stabilization of fractures, should not be withheld as long as there is a reasonable chance that the patient would benefit, even palliatively. Physicians' predictions of survival time for patients with advanced cancer are known to be inaccurate.[20] Surgery for bone metastasis is most commonly used to treat impending or actual pathologic fractures and intractable bone pain. Cancer of the breast, prostate, kidney, and lung and myeloma account for approximately 80% of cases requiring surgical treatment of bone metastasis.[19]

After years of slowly increasing, breast cancer death rates began decreasing in 2007, especially among younger women. Currently, 5-year survival for patients with breast cancer and bone metastasis (stage IV) is 22%. Mean survival time for these patients is 24 to 34 months. Locoregional treatment for patients with breast cancer who have metastasis to bone at the time of presentation does not seem to improve overall survival.[21] Chemotherapy in advanced breast cancer with metastases does not improve survival but can lengthen life and improve QOL.[22] Approximately 17% of breast cancer patients with painful skeletal metastasis will need surgical treatment. The majority of surgical procedures for metastatic breast cancer are performed on the spine and the proximal femur.

Prostate cancer survival after the advent of bone metastasis depends on whether the metastatic deposits are local or distant to the prostate. Current smokers with stage IV prostate cancer have worse survival than former smokers and men who never smoked.[23] Zoledronic acid treatment of patients with metastatic prostate cancer leads to slower onset of biochemical recurrence.[24] In patients with widespread metastatic disease, bone-targeting radiopharmaceuticals can be used to treat bone pain and prolong life.[25]

Renal cell carcinoma with metastasis has a median survival of 10 to 12 months and a 5-year survival rate of 8%. However, surgical resection of isolated bony metastasis and nephrectomy can increase the median survival for these patients.[26]

Bone metastasis is common and debilitating in lung cancer, affecting 30% to 40% of patients.[27] The 5-year survival of patients with metastatic (stage IV) lung cancer is just 1%. Early detection of SREs in lung cancer results in improved QOL and performance status. SREs in lung cancer can be delayed or prevented by denosumab.[28]

LIFE SPAN CONSIDERATIONS

Benign bone tumors are uncommon in children younger than 10 years. Between the ages of 10 and 20 years, osteochondroma, osteoid osteoma, Langerhans cell histiocytosis, and FD are common benign bone tumors. In adults aged 20 to 40, enchondroma and GCT are commonly seen benign bone tumors.

Bone cancers have a strong predilection for certain age ranges. Children younger than 5 years are at risk for metastatic neuroblastoma in the bone. After the age of 8 years, the risk of Ewing sarcoma and osteosarcoma increases, especially around the time of the child's growth spurt. In young to middle-age adults, lymphoma of bone may be the most common malignant tumor of bone. Adults older than 40 years are at increasing risk of adenocarcinoma with metastatic deposits in the bone. Finally, age 50 through 70 is the time of life when multiple myeloma and CHSA are most likely to occur.

INDICATIONS FOR REFERRAL OR HOSPITALIZATION

The number of possible bone tumors and the complexities of their treatment present a challenge for health care providers. Early and prompt referral of these patients to a pediatric orthopedic surgeon or orthopedic oncologist for evaluation, diagnostic workup, and possible treatment is recommended. It is preferable to refer patients before advanced imaging studies have been performed or to schedule the advanced imaging studies in cooperation with the orthopedic specialist. In this way, necessary imaging studies can be performed in a timely fashion, and wasteful and unnecessary tests can be avoided. Biopsy should be performed only by the surgeon or team who will be performing the definitive tumor treatment. The following are criteria for referral to an orthopedic specialist:

- Musculoskeletal pain that lasts more than 6 months despite appropriate activity or occupational modifications
- Musculoskeletal pain in the setting of a history of cancer
- Unexplained deformity or mass
- Significant pain that occurs at night or that requires narcotic analgesic medications in patients without biopsychosocial factors

Delay in diagnosis of bone cancer and bone tumors has been the cause of a significant amount of malpractice litigation against physicians and health care providers of all types.[29] Many factors contribute to delay in diagnosis. The patient may fail to appear in a timely fashion for an evaluation or may miss a scheduled follow-up appointment. The physician or health care provider may fail to appreciate the significance of the patient's complaints, may perform an incomplete examination, or may fail to schedule tests in a timely manner. Bone tumors may occur in vigorous, active individuals whose symptoms mimic minor musculoskeletal injuries, leading to delay and an incorrect initial diagnosis. The common perception that patients with bone cancer have cachexia, night pain, weight loss, or other severe systemic symptoms is false and misleading. A complete history, a careful examination, plain radiographs, and appropriate follow-up are usually sufficient to distinguish patients with bone tumors from patients with common musculoskeletal ailments.

PATIENT AND FAMILY EDUCATION

Because the discovery of a bone tumor always brings the specter of bone cancer, the patient and family should receive complete and comprehensive information about the condition as soon as it is available. Informing a patient about a new cancer diagnosis must be handled carefully. If the referring health care provider is not able to determine the prognosis and health risk associated with the tumor, it is preferable not to speculate. Partial or incomplete information may promote more anxiety and stress. The initial diagnosis can be emotionally devastating to the patient and to a family; compassion, support, and excellent communication are necessary. The physician should wait until the diagnostic and staging process is complete before giving an opinion about the treatment and the prognosis. The impact of the discussion in which a diagnosis of cancer is given has been shown to lead to poor recall of the information presented.[30]

The treatment of benign and malignant bone tumors may have a significant impact on the patient's QOL or function. As a result, the patient and family should participate in selecting the appropriate treatment. Complete information about available treatment options and alternatives should be given, including benefits and potential complications. This allows the patient and family to understand the process and to come to a shared decision about the best treatment based on individual circumstances and preferences. Having the family participate increases their "buy-in" and enhances their support of the patient as well as their commitment to seeing the treatment through. Patients with cancer who have a strong support network have been shown to have better survival rates than patients who are isolated and lack support.[31] The patient and family should be encouraged to maintain close and frequent interaction, join a support group, or participate in family or individual counseling to whatever extent is needed.

CHAPTER 173

BURSITIS

Wendy L. Halm

A bursa is a sac lined with synovial fluid, which provides lubrication and facilitates smooth movement between tissues of an extremity. Bursitis is a pathologic inflammatory disorder of the bursa caused by varied acute or insidious processes. These processes may include trauma or repetitive injury, autoimmune diseases, crystal deposits, and infection.[1,2] Bursitis can result in mild pain or become a disabling condition. There are numerous bursae throughout the body, but only a few ever cause problems; these include bursae in the shoulder, hip, knee, elbow, and heel.

A diagnosis of bursitis is usually suspected on clinical grounds. Common features may include pain at motion and at rest; regional loss of range of motion; visible local swelling, especially if the affected bursa lies close to the surface; erythema and warmth over site; and tenderness to palpation.

SHOULDER BURSITIS

DEFINITION AND EPIDEMIOLOGY

The four major bursae around the shoulder are the subacromial (subdeltoid), subcoracoid, subscapular, and scapular bursae. The subacromial bursa is located between the deltoid muscle and rotator cuff and extends under the acromion and coracoacromial arch. Subacromial bursitis is the most common type of bursitis.[1,3] The overhead athlete is at risk for shoulder injury because of the mechanics associated with rapid shoulder elevation, abduction, and external rotation. If it is left untreated, the condition can progress to an irreversible impingement condition.[4]

CLINICAL PRESENTATION AND PHYSICAL EXAMINATION

Anterior or lateral shoulder pain with acute or insidious onset is the most common presenting complaint of patients with shoulder bursitis (see Chapter 187). The pain is exacerbated by overhead activities, and there may be a deep aching that interrupts sleep at night. Increased pain with active abduction and internal rotation of the arm plus tenderness below the acromion is demonstrated. Weakness can often be established with internal rotation. A complete neuromuscular examination with careful palpation and passive and active range of motion should be performed. In addition, a quick cervical spine examination can help rule out cervical pain with radiculopathy as the cause of the shoulder pain. The Neer and Hawkins impingement signs are the most sensitive and specific for subacromial bursitis. They indicate inflammation of the subacromial bursa and potentially the rotator cuff (Box 173-1).[5,6] Clinicians should be aware of significant clinical diversity regarding the sensitivity and specificity of shoulder diagnostic tests.[7-9]

DIAGNOSTICS

Initial diagnostics should include plain radiography to exclude foreign body penetration, presence of arthritis (and to determine its extent), or fracture.[5-7]

- Plain radiography may demonstrate a hooked acromion, calcification of the supraspinatus tendon, osteopenia of the humerus greater tuberosity, and a distance of less than 5 mm between the acromion and humerus.[6,10,11]

  Other diagnostics may include the following:
  - Ultrasonography can be useful in the diagnosis but is operator dependent and more useful for the identification of rotator cuff pathology.[12]
  - Magnetic resonance imaging (MRI) is now considered the gold standard and is widely used.

If the condition is related to an autoimmune or inflammatory process, serologic tests may reveal an elevated erythrocyte sedimentation rate (ESR), rheumatoid factor, or antinuclear antibodies. If a septic cause is suspected, a white blood cell count as well as a Gram stain and culture of the bursa fluid should be obtained.[11] If an aseptic condition is the cause of the bursitis, crystals may be observed in the bursa aspirate (Box 173-2).[13,14]

The impingement injection test is one method of differentiating between impingement and other shoulder disorders.[3,4] With this test, 10 mL of 1% lidocaine (Xylocaine) is injected into the subacromial space; after 5 to 10 minutes, the maneuvers for the impingement signs are repeated. If the pain is reduced 50%, the shoulder pain is secondary to subacromial bursitis and tendinitis.

BOX 173-1

Neer and Hawkins Impingement Signs

NEER IMPINGEMENT SIGN

- Raise and pull on straightened arm forcibly from the side to full abduction above the head.
- The maneuver causes pain in patients with impingement.

HAWKINS IMPINGEMENT SIGN

- Flex the elbow to 90 degrees and raise the upper arm to 90 degrees of abduction (parallel to the floor). Then rotate the arm internally across the front of the body, causing compression of the rotator cuff and subacromial bursa between the head of the humerus and coracoacromial ligament.
- The maneuver causes pain in patients with impingement.

Data from Neer CS: (1983). Impingement lesions. *Clin Orthop Relat Res* 173:70-77, 1983; and Hawkins RJ, Kennedy JC: Impingement syndrome in athletes. *Am J Sports Med* 8(3):151-157, 1980.

DIAGNOSTICS

Bursitis

LABORATORY
Complete blood count and differential*
ESR*
Rheumatoid factor*
Uric acid*
Antinuclear antibody*
Culture and sensitivity (of bursa fluid)*
Gram stain (of bursa fluid)*
Analysis of bursa aspirate for crystals*

IMAGING
X-ray studies
Ultrasound
MRI

OTHER DIAGNOSTICS
Joint aspiration

*If indicated.

DIFFERENTIAL DIAGNOSIS

The differential diagnosis includes fracture, dislocation, trauma, arthritis, adhesive capsulitis, rotator cuff tendinitis or tear, muscle strain, and referred pain. Causes of referred pain to the shoulder can include disorders of the cervical spine, chest cavity, breasts, axillary area, and abdomen.[6]

DIFFERENTIAL DIAGNOSIS

Shoulder Bursitis

- Fracture or dislocation
- Trauma
- Arthritis (osteoarthritis or rheumatoid arthritis)
- Adhesive capsulitis
- Rotator cuff tendinitis or tear
- Strain
- Referred pain
- Subacromial spur
- Neoplasm
- Cervical radiculopathy

BOX 173-2

Guidelines for Joint and Bursa Aspiration and Injection

PURPOSE

Bursa aspiration and injection are performed to obtain bursal fluid for evaluation to determine the cause of the inflammation and for drainage of abnormal fluid accumulation to relieve pain. Local anesthetics, such as lidocaine and corticosteroids, may be introduced into the bursa for symptomatic management of inflammation. Subacromial, trochanteric, anserine, and prepatellar bursitis are conditions that improve with local injection of corticosteroids.

CONTRAINDICATIONS

Contraindications to aspiration and injection include cellulitis at the injection site, primary coagulopathy or uncontrolled anticoagulant therapy, septic effusion of a bursa or periarticular structure, more than three previous injections at the same site in the previous 12 months or lack of improvement after two prior injections, suspected bacteremia from another site, unstable joints (for corticosteroid injection), tumors, fractures, joint prosthesis, and inaccessible joints.

PATIENT EDUCATION AND CONSENT

Patient education and consent are necessary before the procedure. The risks and benefits of bursa aspiration should be explained. Adverse effects of introducing a needle into the bursa include infection, bleeding, and pain. Potential complications of corticosteroid therapy include postinjection flare (increased pain for 1 or 2 days), arthropathy, tendon rupture, facial flushing, skin atrophy and depigmentation, transient paresis, transient elevations in blood sugar (if steroid is injected), hypersensitivity reaction, pericapsular calcification, and acceleration of cartilage attrition.

TECHNIQUE

Aseptic technique for bursa aspiration and injection begins by preparing the site for aspiration or injection with povidone-iodine and draping accordingly. The appropriate needle for the procedure is selected: an 18- or 20-gauge needle for aspiration, and a 22- or 25-gauge $1\frac{1}{2}$-inch needle for injection. A 5- or 10-mL Luer-Lok syringe is recommended. Figures 173-1 to 173-7 demonstrate techniques for aspiration and injection of the more commonly problematic bursae.

A variety of corticosteroid preparations are available in different potencies. The three common corticosteroid local injection therapies for bursitis are hydrocortisone acetate, 25 or 50 mg/mL, which is short acting; triamcinolone acetonide, 40 mg/mL, an intermediate-acting preparation; and long-acting dexamethasone sodium acetate, 8 mg/mL. The typical injected volume will vary from small to large joints.

Lidocaine is combined with the steroid of choice to disperse the steroid at the injection site and reduce procedure-associated pain. A history of lidocaine allergy must first be obtained. Lidocaine, 5 mL, is combined with the steroid for subacromial, trochanteric, or calcaneal bursae. For smaller bursae, such as the olecranon and prepatellar bursa, up to 3 mL of lidocaine combined with the chosen steroid is recommended.

FOLLOW-UP

Procedure aftercare includes applying a bandage over the aspiration-injection site and explaining to the patient that the procedure is provided in addition to other conservative measures and is not a cure in itself. Oral nonsteroidal anti-inflammatory drugs are continued if there is no contraindication. Symptoms of infection should be reported immediately.

Data from Monseau AJ, Singh Nizran P: Common injections in musculoskeletal medicine. *Prim Care* 40(4):987-100, 2014.

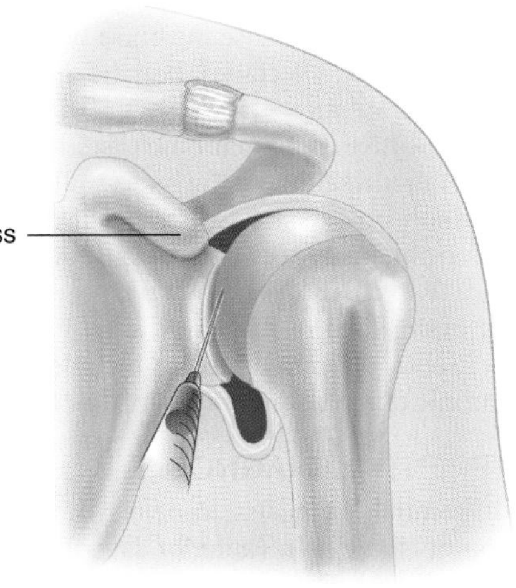

FIGURE 173-1 Injection of subacromial bursa and rotator cuff tendons. (From Lawry G, Kreder H, Hawker G, et al: *Fam's musculoskeletal examination and joint injections techniques,* ed 2, St Louis, 2010, Mosby.)

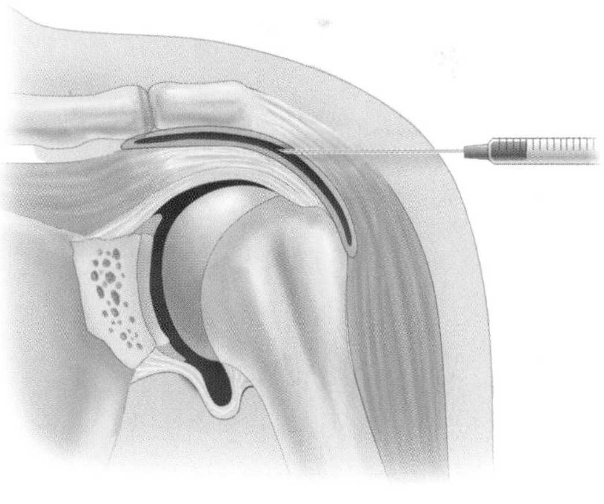

FIGURE 173-2 Aspiration and injection of subacromial bursa. (From Lawry G, Kreder H, Hawker G, et al: *Fam's musculoskeletal examination and joint injections techniques,* ed 2, St Louis, 2010, Mosby.)

MANAGEMENT

Orthopedic specialist referral is indicated for a demonstrated rotator cuff tear, for subacromial fibrosis, to assist in treatment of septic bursitis, or for excision of chronic enlarged bursa when indicated. A rheumatology consultation may be indicated for patients with underlying rheumatoid arthritis who have bursitis.

Immediate emergency department referral is indicated for patients with symptoms consistent with septic bursitis or difficult-to-treat pain. Fever, erythema, warmth, and fluctuance (especially in conjunction with a patient history of diabetes, alcoholism, or impaired skin integrity) should heighten the clinician's suspicion of septic bursitis.[14]

The primary goals of treatment are the reduction of pain and improvement of range of motion. Except for autoimmune and

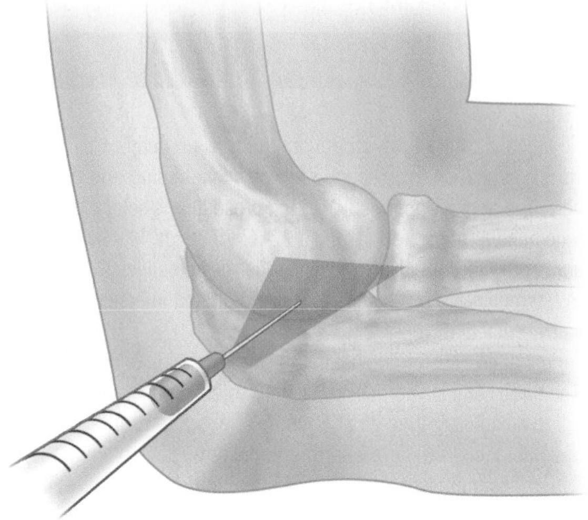

FIGURE 173-3 Aspiration and injection of the elbow joint. (From Lawry G, Kreder H, Hawker G, et al: *Fam's musculoskeletal examination and joint injections techniques,* ed 2, St Louis, 2010, Mosby.)

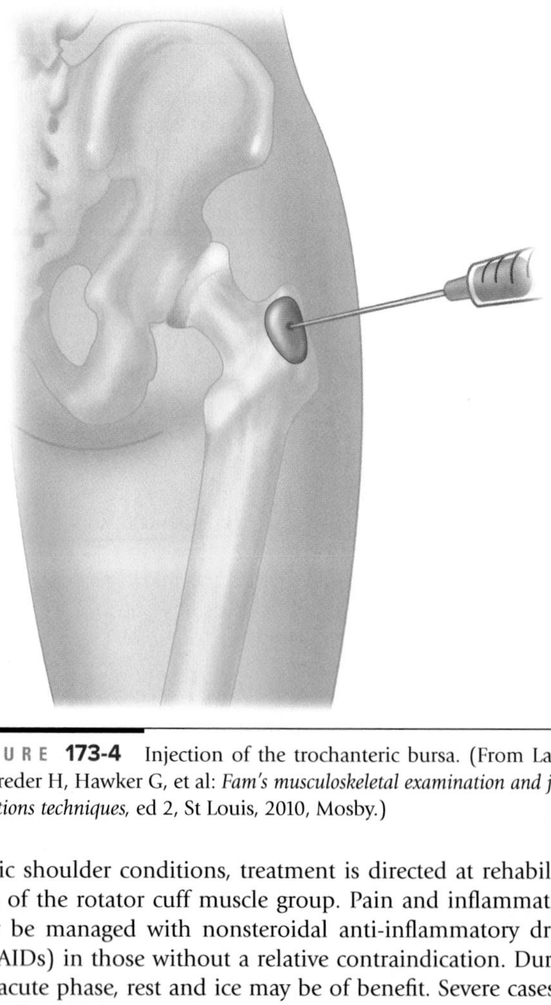

FIGURE 173-4 Injection of the trochanteric bursa. (From Lawry G, Kreder H, Hawker G, et al: *Fam's musculoskeletal examination and joint injections techniques,* ed 2, St Louis, 2010, Mosby.)

septic shoulder conditions, treatment is directed at rehabilitation of the rotator cuff muscle group. Pain and inflammation may be managed with nonsteroidal anti-inflammatory drugs (NSAIDs) in those without a relative contraindication. During the acute phase, rest and ice may be of benefit. Severe cases of shoulder bursitis may be managed with corticosteroid injections, guided by ultrasound or clinical landmarks. Injections should be limited to three or four injections per 12-month period, no less than 30 days apart.[15] Additional therapeutic options may include physical therapy, ultrasound, electrical

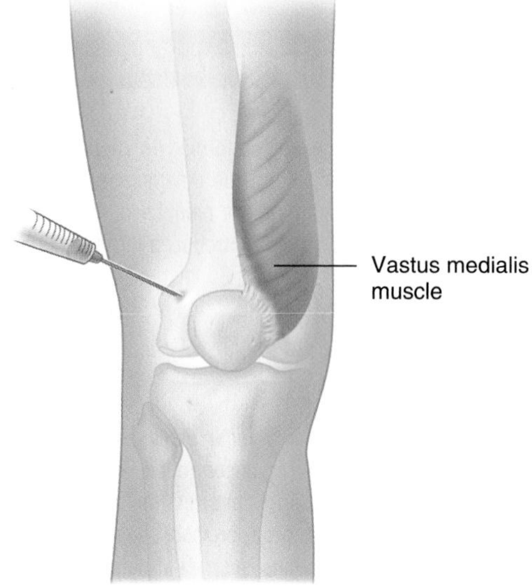

FIGURE 173-5 Injection of the knee. (From Lawry G, Kreder H, Hawker G, et al: *Fam's musculoskeletal examination and joint injections techniques,* ed 2, St Louis, 2010, Mosby.)

stimulation, acupuncture, or surgical intervention. Immobilization should be avoided because it may worsen the condition by causing adhesions.

ELBOW (OLECRANON) BURSITIS

Located on the extensor aspect of the elbow, overlying the olecranon process, olecranon bursitis (see Chapter 175) is the most common type of elbow bursitis. Visible posterior elbow swelling is easily recognized because the bursa lies close to the skin on a bone prominence. Olecranon bursitis may be acute or chronic and septic or aseptic.[9] Most cases result from acute trauma or chronic repetitive injury; chronic cases related to repetitive injury result in thickening of the bursa wall. One third of all cases of olecranon bursitis are septic, and if this is suspected, fluid should be obtained for culture and antibiotics should be started empirically to cover *Staphylococcus aureus,* the organism that accounts for the majority of septic cases.[16] Risk factors for development of septic olecranon bursitis include diabetes, alcoholism, and chronic obstructive pulmonary disease (COPD).[14]

DIFFERENTIAL DIAGNOSIS

The differential diagnosis can be narrowed based on anatomic location of elbow pain (anterior, lateral, medial, or posterior). Posterior elbow pain differential diagnoses include fracture, arthritis, impingement, and triceps tendinopathy.[16]

DIFFERENTIAL DIAGNOSIS

Elbow (Olecranon) Bursitis

- Septic bursitis
- Gout
- Arthritis (osteoarthritis or rheumatoid arthritis)
- Tendinitis
- Effusion
- Fracture
- Epicondylitis
- Sprain
- Trauma
- Triceps strain

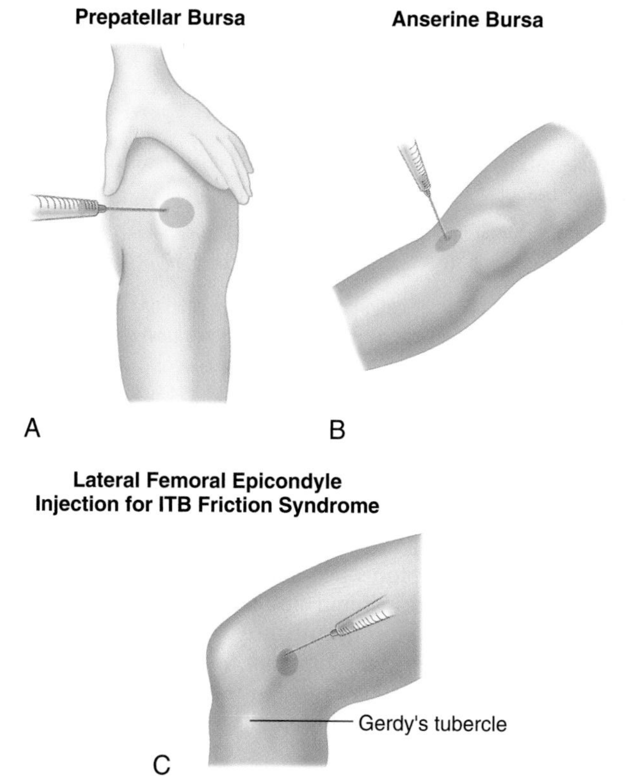

FIGURE 173-6 Injection of the prepatellar bursa (A), the anserine bursa (B), and the lateral femoral epicondyle (C). (From Lawry G, Kreder H, Hawker G, et al: *Fam's musculoskeletal examination and joint injections techniques*, ed 2, St Louis, 2010, Mosby.)

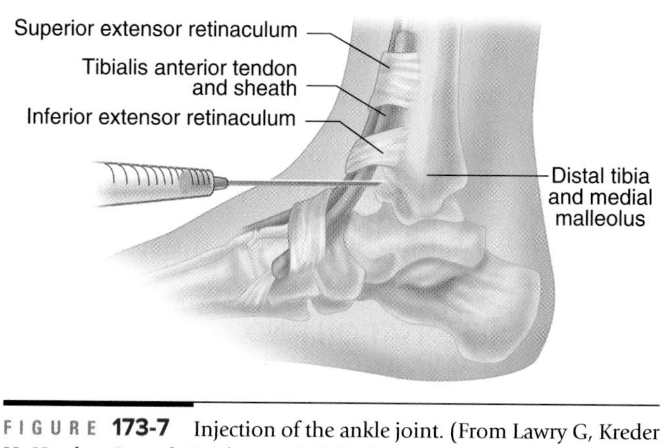

FIGURE 173-7 Injection of the ankle joint. (From Lawry G, Kreder H, Hawker G, et al: *Fam's musculoskeletal examination and joint injections techniques*, ed 2, St Louis, 2010, Mosby.)

MANAGEMENT

Orthopedic specialist referral is indicated to assist in treatment of septic bursitis or for excision of chronic enlarged bursa when indicated.

Immediate emergency department referral is indicated for those with symptoms consistent with septic bursitis or difficult-to-treat pain. Fever, erythema, warmth, and fluctuance (especially in conjunction with a patient history of gout, diabetes, alcoholism, or impaired skin integrity) should heighten the clinician's suspicion of septic bursitis.[14]

The primary goals of treatment are the reduction of pain and improvement of range of motion. Except for autoimmune and septic elbow conditions, treatment is directed at rehabilitation of the elbow.

- Pain and inflammation may be managed with NSAIDs in those without a relative contraindication.
- During the acute phase, protection with elbow pads, rest, and ice may be of benefit.
- Physical or occupational therapy referral for education regarding joint protection and avoidance of repetitive activity should be considered.
- Aspiration of bursae should be performed only when the diagnosis is uncertain or to relieve symptoms in refractory cases.[16]
- Injection of a steroid into the bursal sac may be used with caution after the chance of infection has been eliminated.[17]
- Surgical excision of the bursal sac in presence of an olecranon spur or when compressive treatment fails is recommended only in cases of chronic pain and is done very rarely.[17]

HIP BURSITIS

DEFINITION AND EPIDEMIOLOGY

Hip bursitis (see Chapter 179) is a common disorder that results from trauma, musculotendinous overuse, degenerative changes, biomechanical abnormalities, or systemic disease. The trochanteric, iliopsoas, and ischiogluteal groups are the major structures of bursae around the hip. Trochanteric bursitis is the most common bursitis, affecting women more than men, running athletes, and patients who have undergone a total hip replacement (Table 173-1).[18]

CLINICAL PRESENTATION AND PHYSICAL EXAMINATION

Hip bursitis is characterized by pain over the affected bursa. The pain may be sudden or gradual in onset and results from overuse or trauma. Depending on which bursa is inflamed, the pain can have a pseudoradicular quality with radiation down the lateral thigh to the knee or anteriorly to the groin. Pain is often worse at night.[18] Pain on palpation that is well localized over the greater trochanter or ischial spines (point tenderness) and possibly accompanied by redness, warmth, and swelling may indicate bursitis. The hip examination should include the hip, back, abdomen, and vascular and neurologic systems. A gait analysis and stance assessment followed by evaluation of the patient in seated supine, lateral, and prone positions should be completed. Hip flexion and rotation may exacerbate the pain. Passive joint motion is usually not affected, although guarding may limit active motion.[19]

DIFFERENTIAL DIAGNOSIS

The differential diagnosis can be narrowed when age is considered. In older adults with hip pain, fractures and degenerative arthritis should be considered first.[19] Bursitis of the hip can be confused with radicular pain originating in the spine or hip joint or a pathologic change or tenosynovitis of the hamstring (see differential diagnosis box).

TABLE 173-1 Hip Bursitis

	Hip Bursae		
	Trochanteric	**Ischiogluteal**	**Iliopsoas**
Location of pain	Lateral hip to lateral thigh and buttock	Ischial tuberosity into posterior thigh; worse with sitting; cannot sleep on affected side	Groin, with radiation to anterior hip
Examination	Pain worse with hip rotation; may be soft tissue swelling	Tenderness over the ischial tuberosity	Pain worse with resisted hip flexion and hyperextension
Diagnostics	X-ray studies are usually normal and noncontributory for hip bursitis; a bone scan may be helpful only in refractory conditions	X-ray studies may show calcification of the bursa and associated structures consistent with chronic inflammation	X-ray studies may show degenerative changes, effusion, or calcification
Differential diagnosis*	Fracture of the greater trochanter	Fracture	Hip arthritis

*Consider herniated disk, avascular necrosis, or systemic disease.
Data from Waldman S: *Pain management*, ed 2, St Louis, Saunders, 2011.

DIFFERENTIAL DIAGNOSIS

Hip Bursitis

- Arthritis (osteoarthritis and rheumatoid arthritis)
- Sciatica
- Aseptic arthritis
- Fracture
- Peripheral neuropathy
- Avascular necrosis
- Referred pelvic pain
- Trauma
- Lumbar radiculopathy
- Thrombophlebitis
- Sacroiliitis
- Neoplasm
- Tendinitis

MANAGEMENT

Orthopedic specialist referral is indicated to assist in treatment of septic bursitis or for excision of chronic enlarged bursa when indicated. Rheumatology consultation is recommended for patients who do not respond to intrabursal steroids or have recurrent bursitis.

Immediate emergency department referral is indicated for those with symptoms consistent with septic bursitis or difficult-to-treat pain. Patients who have a history of trauma and clinical findings of a potential hip fracture, such as pain with internal rotation of the hip or pain in the groin, should be referred to the emergency department for further workup.

Except for autoimmune and septic bursitis, the primary goals of treatment are the reduction of inflammation, gait correction, and prevention of recurrence.

- Pain and inflammation may be managed with NSAIDs in those without a relative contraindication.
- During the acute phase, rest, ice, and elevation may be of benefit.
- Additional therapeutic options may include physical therapy, ultrasound, electrical stimulation, or acupuncture. Stretching and strengthening of the gluteus medius muscle and iliotibial band can be beneficial for trochanteric bursitis.
- Uncomplicated hip bursitis may respond favorably to local glucocorticoid injection if conservative treatment is unsuccessful.[20]
- Surgery is rarely performed for this condition.
- Patients with symptoms persisting for 6 to 8 weeks despite basic care measures should be reevaluated for underlying causes, including a gait disturbance.
- Older adult patients with hip pain for more than a month or who have concerning historical features, signs, or symptoms should undergo additional diagnostic imaging.[21]

KNEE BURSITIS

DEFINITION AND EPIDEMIOLOGY

Knee bursitis occurs usually in the prepatellar or the pes anserine bursa. The prepatellar bursa is located between the skin and the patella and can be susceptible to an infectious septic bursitis because of its superficial location. Prepatellar bursitis is sometimes referred to as housemaid's knee and commonly results from activities that require excessive kneeling, such as carpentry, gardening, roofing, wrestling, and carpet laying.[22]

Pes anserine bursitis is commonly seen in the obese, those with degenerative or inflammatory joint disease, the middle-aged, and older female long-distance runners.[13] Pain is located in the anterior and medial knee area just below the joint line. Pain may worsen with the use of stairs and is commonly prevalent at night.

CLINICAL PRESENTATION AND PHYSICAL EXAMINATION

Except in infectious cases, severe pain is unusual in prepatellar bursitis, although it is common in anserine bursitis, especially at night. There is tenderness over the anterior knee in prepatellar bursitis that is accompanied by localized edema over the lower half of the patella and upper body of the patellar tendon (prepatellar bursitis) or on both sides of the patellar tendon (infrapatellar bursitis).[23] There is often bursa thickening that feels rough, like nodules or bone chips. Although the inflamed bursa causes swelling, the edema is different from that noted when there is fluid in the knee joint or effusion (see Chapter 181). The ballottement test may be used to evaluate for knee effusion and help in differentiating prepatellar bursal swelling from true knee effusion. The test is performed by applying firm downward pressure to the patella (Fig. 173-8). If a click is felt when the patella reaches the femoral condyle, a joint effusion is likely to be present. A ballottement test result will be negative (see

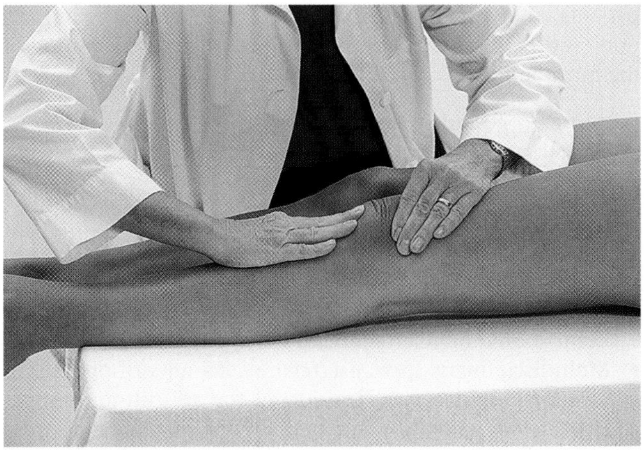

FIGURE 173-8 Technique for testing for knee joint effusion. (From Swartz M: *The musculoskeletal system*, ed 7, St Louis, 2014, Saunders.)

Fig. 173-8) if the problem is bursitis. A septic prepatellar bursitis may appear cellulitic.[24]

DIFFERENTIAL DIAGNOSIS

It is necessary to obtain bursa aspirate to exclude a septic cause of prepatellar bursitis. Loss of full extension of the knee or resistance to full flexion may indicate infection. If the test result is positive for septic bursitis, culture and sensitivity are performed to guide appropriate antibiotic treatment.

DIFFERENTIAL DIAGNOSIS

Knee (Prepatellar) Bursitis

- Effusion from internal derangement
- Arthritis (osteoarthritis or rheumatoid arthritis)
- Fracture
- Gout
- Sprain
- Retropatellar bursitis
- Pes anserine bursitis
- Osteochondritis dissecans
- Referred pain (usually from hip or spinal disease)
- Overuse syndrome
- Chondromalacia
- Patellofemoral joint instability
- Trauma
- Septic bursitis

MANAGEMENT

Specialist referral is indicated to assist in treatment of septic bursitis or for excision of chronic enlarged bursa when indicated. Classic signs of infection may not be present; therefore bursal fluid should always be sent for laboratory analysis.

Immediate emergency department referral is indicated for those with symptoms consistent with septic bursitis or symptoms that have not improved in 36 to 48 hours despite aspiration. Pyogenic prepatellar bursitis is common in children. Aspiration, immobilization, and antibiotic coverage are indicated.

The primary goals of treatment are the reduction of pain and improvement of range of motion. Except for autoimmune and septic knee conditions, treatment is directed at rehabilitation of the knee.

- Pain and inflammation can be managed with oral or topical NSAIDs in those without contraindications.
- Protection, rest (plus immobilization), ice, compression, and elevation, in combination or separately, may be helpful. Elastic compression dressings should be applied for a minimum of 3 days.[22,24]
- Aspiration of a significant effusion may aide with diagnosis, especially if crystal disease or infection is suspected.[22]
- A steroid injection, after sepsis has been ruled out, may bring significant, if temporary, relief.
- Physical therapy may be beneficial to assist with stretching and strengthening exercises and to provide education about joint protection and avoidance of repetitive motion injury.
- Septic bursitis often responds well to immobilization, one or two daily aspirations, and antibiotic coverage for staphylococci.[24]
- Surgery is reserved for refractory cases and is rarely needed. However, complete excision of the bursa may be necessary if healing fails to occur after simple drainage.[2]

HEEL (CALCANEAL) BURSITIS

DEFINITION AND EPIDEMIOLOGY

There are two clinically significant bursae in the posterior heel (see Chapter 172). The retrocalcaneal bursa lies between the calcaneus and the Achilles tendon. The posterior calcaneal bursa is located between the Achilles tendon and the skin. Calcaneal bursitis is the result of local mechanical irritation to the posterior heel and affects ice skaters (primarily female) and long-distance runners.[25]

CLINICAL PRESENTATION AND PHYSICAL EXAMINATION

The usual presentation of calcaneal bursitis includes a history of poorly fitting shoes. This causes the heel to rub on the back of the shoe and results in heel pain. Physical findings include erythema at the affected area or a palpable, swollen bursa that is tender at the Achilles tendon insertion site at the posterior heel.[25] In addition, there can be pain radiating to the Achilles tendon that is increased by squeezing the bursa just anterior to the Achilles tendon and compressing the bursa from side to side. Bursitis may also occur in association with both Achilles tendinitis and Haglund disease (abnormal prominence of the posterior calcaneal tuberosity) (see Chapter 172).

DIFFERENTIAL DIAGNOSIS

The differential diagnosis should include stress fracture, the symptoms of which may mimic Achilles bursitis and tendonitis. The Achilles tendon is susceptible to repetitive motion injury, and running is often implicated as an inciting factor.

DIFFERENTIAL DIAGNOSIS

Heel (Calcaneal) Bursitis

- Achilles tendinitis or rupture
- Plantar fasciitis
- Rheumatoid arthritis
- Bone lesions; including fracture, infection, or neoplasm
- Seronegative spondyloarthropathies
- Gout

MANAGEMENT

Specialist referral is indicated for patients whose symptoms do not improve within 4 to 6 weeks. **Orthopedic specialist referral** is indicated for patients who have not improved with conservative management.

Immediate emergency department referral is indicated for patients with acute onset of pain or in conjunction with a traumatic event. A patient history of a snap or audible pop followed by acute pain should raise the clinician's suspicion of an acute Achilles tendon rupture. History of quinolone use has been associated with rupture of Achilles tendon in the elderly and patients using corticosteroids.[26]

Initial goals of the treatment of patients with retrocalcaneal bursitis are to control pain and attempt to allow the patient to return to normal function and activity. Pain and inflammation may be managed with NSAIDs in those without a relative contraindication.

Transdermal nonsteroidal patches or gel as well as lidocaine patches may be helpful.

During the acute phase, rest, ice, and elevation may be of benefit.

Activity modification and bracing (CAM walker) may be helpful in cases that are recalcitrant to conservative management.[27]

Open-heeled shoes (clogs), bare feet, sandals, heel lifts, or U-shaped pads may help to minimize pressure on the bony ridge of the ankle.[25,26]

Cortisone injection should be used cautiously to prevent rupture of the Achilles tendon.[25,27]

Surgical treatment (rare) may be required to remove inflamed bursa and associated bony prominence. This can be completed through open surgery or endoscopically.[25,27]

LIFE SPAN CONSIDERATIONS

When considering medication treatment for the older adult, clinicians should consider potentially inappropriate medications as well as potential medication interactions. NSAID use in older adults has been associated with increased risk of gastrointestinal bleeding and peptic ulcer disease in high-risk groups, including those older than 75 or those taking oral or parenteral corticosteroids, anticoagulants, or antiplatelet agents.[28] Topical NSAIDs or lidocaine patches may be a better option for this age group. Invasive treatment options (such as aspiration and injection) should be carefully considered to prevent iatrogenic illness.

COMPLICATIONS

The pain of bursitis can be disabling for many patients. Some patients with shoulder or elbow bursitis stop using the affected extremity, resulting in weakness and increased disability; others do not bear weight on the affected extremity to avoid pain. Unfortunately, recurrent episodes of acute bursitis can progress to chronic bursitis. The adjacent tissue may be compromised in cases of severe bursal swelling, and it may be difficult to determine the true cause of the patient's discomfort, as occurs in shoulder bursitis. Infection of the bursa or surrounding tissue is not uncommon, and providers must always maintain an index of suspicion and rule out a possible infection as the cause of a bursitis. Oral antibiotic therapy may be sufficient for some patients with septic bursitis, but many patients require intravenous antibiotic therapy, hospitalization, and daily aspiration of the bursa fluid.

INDICATIONS FOR REFERRAL OR HOSPITALIZATION

In general, patients with bursitis do not need further specialist referral or hospitalization.

- Patients with suspected septic bursitis should be referred to a physician or orthopedic specialist expediently.
- Patients with an acute onset of pain or a recent traumatic event should be referred to the emergency room.
- Multidisciplinary specialist referrals to an orthopedist or rheumatologist can be considered for difficult-to-treat patients or for patients with an underlying rheumatic disorder who do not respond to conservative measures within a reasonable period.
- Referrals to a physical or occupational therapist may expedite recovery time and assist with stretching and strengthening exercises as well as joint protection techiques.
- Indications for hospitalization are limited and usually are related to the need for intravenous antibiotics or inability to control pain, or for patients with comorbid conditions, such as diabetes or immunosuppression.

PATIENT EDUCATION

Bursitis is related to repetitive activities, and recurrence is possible. Patients should understand this and try to modify or avoid activities that may exacerbate the disorder and should protect joints from further trauma whenever possible. Patients with prepatellar bursitis, for example, should use knee pads. Rest is indicated during the acute process, but gentle stretching and range-of-motion exercises should begin as soon as possible to prevent stiffness and to maintain mobility. Ice and heat plus NSAIDs help decrease joint inflammation. A joint that becomes erythematous, tender, and edematous with associated fever requires immediate assessment by a health care provider. If corticosteroid injections are necessary, the risks and benefits should be discussed before injection.

CHAPTER 174

ELBOW PAIN

Denise A. Vanacore-Chase

DEFINITION AND EPIDEMIOLOGY

The elbow is a hinged joint that is a three-joint complex formed by the humerus, radius, and ulna.[1] It allows flexion and extension of the elbow. Microtears of the muscles, ligaments, and tendons from inflammation and trauma are common causes of acute and chronic elbow pain.

Most elbow injuries result from overuse during high-force or repetitive motion activities. Two groups of people seem to be at increased risk for elbow disorders. The first is high-performance athletes, especially in racket and throwing sports such as baseball, tennis, racquetball, golf, and basketball. The second group includes those with jobs that require forceful or repetitive wrist and elbow rotation, lifting, gripping, or torqueing motions. High-risk occupations include factory workers, laborers, carpenters, and grocery checkers. The prevalence of occupational lateral epicondylitis is as high as 5.2% and the prevalence of medial epicondylitis is 1.5%.[1] In the general population, injuries may occur from pursuing recreational hobbies. Improper preparation, lack of strength or conditioning, and overzealousness can all contribute to elbow pain. The lateral side is affected 7 to 10 times more often than the medial.[1]

The elbow is also vulnerable to inflammatory arthritides, including rheumatoid arthritis and the spondyloarthropathies.

It is critical that the elbow joint be fully functional for an individual to have full hand and wrist movement.

PATHOPHYSIOLOGY

The elbow is formed by the articulations of the humerus, radius, and ulna. The humeroulnar articulation is a hinge joint and allows flexion and extension of the elbow and flexion, extension, pronation, and supination of the wrist.[1] The humeroradial and radioulnar articulations are partially ligamental; their flexibility allows rotation of the radius and pronation-supination of the forearm. This inhibits the amount of excessive motion in the joint and limits the joint to operating as a hinge.

Stability of the elbow is accomplished through bones, ligaments, and muscles. The humeroulnar joint is the main stabilizer for flexion and extension of the elbow. Rotational stability is divided into valgus and varus stabilizers. A valgus stress is a force on the medial elbow from throwing or axial compression. Primary valgus stabilizers are the medial (ulnar) collateral ligaments and their supporting muscles. A varus stress is a force on the lateral elbow. The lateral (radial) collateral ligaments stabilize for varus stress.

Elbow injuries may be classified as acute or chronic. Acute injuries result from a single high force, such as a fall or direct blow, that is greater in strength than the tendon, ligament, or bone affected. However, most injuries are chronic. Chronic injuries occur from repetitive, submaximal forces that overload the elbow's ability to adequately heal, causing recurrent pain.[2]

CLINICAL PRESENTATION

Elbow pain may be traced to a specific activity or chain of events or may appear insidiously, with no identifiable trigger. The pain may or may not radiate into the shoulder or into the wrist. The patient may experience weakness in the hand, wrist, or elbow.[1] Once an injury has occurred, everyday activities such as picking up groceries, reaching, or pulling can cause pain. A thorough history, including occupational and recreational activities and any prior elbow injury, is essential. An assessment of the onset and type of pain is also important.[3] Pain can be described as sharp, intermittent, and usually in the vicinity of the lateral or medial epicondyle.

A history of falls, a direct impact to the elbow, or a history of other joint pain or swelling is also needed to exclude fracture, rheumatoid arthritis, seronegative spondyloarthropathy, crystal arthropathies, or other systemic diseases.

PHYSICAL EXAMINATION

Physical examination of both elbows is performed to assess for alteration in carrying angle, posture, strength, and range of motion. Bone and soft tissue landmarks should be assessed for asymmetry, malalignment, erythema, swelling, and tenderness. Bone landmarks to be examined are the medial and lateral epicondyles of the humerus and the olecranon process of the ulna. Range-of-motion testing includes flexion and extension and pronation and supination. Normal flexion and extension are 0 to 135 degrees. The elbow can rotate from 0 to 180 degrees. Normal range of motion effectively rules out involvement of the elbow joint itself. Functional range of motion for normal activities of daily living is 30 to 130 degrees of flexion, with the greatest strength and greatest stress on the elbow at 70 degrees.[1] Extra-articular pathologic conditions, including epicondylitis and olecranon bursitis, rarely affect elbow range of motion.[4]

The extensor tendons at the lateral epicondyle and the flexor tendons at the medial epicondyle are palpated for tenderness. Several confirmatory tests or maneuvers may be helpful. Resisted wrist extension or flexion may help diagnose lateral or medial epicondylitis, respectively. A local anesthetic block can be placed near the suspected involved tendon. Relief of pain with this injection is confirmatory.[1]

Posteriorly, the olecranon bursa overlies the olecranon process. The olecranon bursa is inspected and palpated for redness, swelling, tenderness, or chronic thickening.

The ulnar nerve sits in a groove between the medial epicondyle and the olecranon process.[4] The Tinel sign is present when tapping over the ulnar groove reproduces pain or numbness felt in the fourth and fifth fingers. Muscles for wrist flexion and pronation originate through tendons from the medial epicondyle and then spread out along the palmar surface of the forearm.

Physical examination should include the wrist, shoulder, and neck because pathologic conditions at these sites may cause referred pain to the elbow. Location and radiation of the pain are critical for accurate assessment. Lateral elbow pain with passive wrist flexion and active wrist extension usually indicates lateral epicondylitis, and medial epicondylitis is indicated by pain with resisted wrist flexion and forearm pronation and passive wrist extension.[5]

DIAGNOSTICS

Testing is based on the mechanism of injury or duration of symptoms. X-ray studies of the elbow are the most commonly ordered tests. Standard x-ray studies include an anteroposterior film with the elbow fully extended and supinated and a lateral view with the elbow flexed at 90 degrees and the forearm

DIAGNOSTICS

Elbow Pain

LABORATORY
CBC and differential
ESR*
Rheumatoid factor*
Antinuclear antibodies*
Uric acid level
Lyme titer*

IMAGING
X-ray studies* (anteroposterior, lateral, and oblique)
MRI*
Diagnostic musculoskeletal ultrasound*
Angiogram*

OTHER DIAGNOSTICS
Joint aspiration*

*If indicated.

supinated. Oblique views may be needed to better study the radial head and shaft, the humeral condyles, and the coronoid process of the ulna.[6] Laboratory testing is based on the clinical history. A complete blood count (CBC), erythrocyte sedimentation rate (ESR), rheumatoid factor, antinuclear antibody test, Lyme titer, or elbow joint or bursal aspiration may be indicated to exclude infection or systemic disease. Joint aspirate should be evaluated with a culture and Gram stain and examined for crystals.[7] Magnetic resonance imaging (MRI) is the diagnostic tool of choice to examine the joint for loose bodies, ligament injury, stress fractures, or osteochondral lesions. Ultrasound is being used more frequently to determine the loss of the tendon's normal fibrillar pattern and neovascularization.[1] Ultrasound is best reserved for patients with atypical presentations or poor response to treatment.

DIFFERENTIAL DIAGNOSIS

The most common causes of elbow pain are sprains, fractures, bursitis, and epicondylitis. Lateral epicondylitis is called *tennis elbow;* medial epicondylitis is called *golfer's elbow.* Medial collateral ligament instability and ulnar neuritis can also cause pain (Table 174-1). Elbow pain is often caused by local injury but may result from a referred, external condition. Based on the history, the differential diagnosis for referred pain should include cervical disk or nerve root problems; thoracic outlet or brachial plexus disease; radicular pain from shoulder, neck, or wrist overuse injuries; diabetes; cardiovascular disease; and peripheral nerve entrapment syndromes.[4,6] Acute injuries are most often related to overuse, direct trauma, or fractures. Systemic diseases that may cause elbow pain, such as rheumatoid arthritis (Chapter 221), osteoarthritis (Chapter 183), psoriatic arthritis (Chapter 218), Lyme disease (Chapter 236), and infection, should also be considered. On the basis of the examination and neurologic findings, electromyography and nerve conduction studies may be indicated to rule out nerve entrapment.[4,6,8]

DIFFERENTIAL DIAGNOSIS

Elbow Pain

- Arthritis (inflammatory or degenerative)
- Brachial plexus disease
- Bursitis
- Cardiovascular disease
- Cervical disk disease
- Cubital tunnel syndrome
- Diabetes
- Digital biceps tendon rupture
- Dislocation
- Epicondylitis, lateral (tennis elbow)
- Epicondylitis, medial (golfer's elbow)
- Fracture
- Gout or pseudogout
- Impingement
- Lyme disease
- Osteochondrosis
- Osteophytes
- Overuse injuries
- Peripheral nerve entrapment
- Psoriatic arthritis
- Radicular pain
- Sepsis
- Sprain
- Tendinitis
- Thoracic outlet syndrome
- Triceps rupture
- Ulnar neuritis
- Ulnar collateral ligament injury

MANAGEMENT

Ideally, treatment begins before injury occurs. Injury prevention strategies include flexibility, strength, and endurance training; warm-up and cool-down stretching exercises; and avoidance

TABLE 174-1 Common Elbow Ailments

Ailment	Presentation	Examination	Differential Diagnosis and Management
EPICONDYLITIS			
Inflammatory condition characterized by pain at tendon origin of muscle groups at medial (golfer's elbow) or lateral (tennis elbow) aspects of elbow; usually self-limited but may take several months for full recovery	Gradual or acute onset of pain along affected epicondyle, with or without radiation; possible history of heavy lifting, hammering, screwing, or gripping	Local tenderness over or just distal to affected epicondyle; possible tenderness of flexor and extensor muscles; ROM and distal neurovascular examination findings within normal limits *Lateral epicondylitis:* Pain at or around lateral epicondyle reproduced by resistive wrist extension (examiner applying pressure to force wrist into flexion while patient extends wrist) *Medial epicondylitis:* Pain exacerbated by resistive wrist flexion	*Differential diagnosis:* Cubital tunnel syndrome, cervical radiculopathy, rotator cuff tendinitis, lateral or medial collateral ligament sprains, osteoarthritis, or avulsion fracture *Management:* Conservative treatment: oral or topical NSAIDs, tennis elbow splint, "palms-up" lifting, toning exercises of wrist extensors; steroid injection if conservative treatment fails; orthopedic referral for surgical evaluation if treatment fails[8]
SPRAINS (SEE CHAPTER 188)			
Tearing or stretching of lateral or medial collateral ligaments from varus or valgus stretch	Pain after throwing, overhead, or weight-bearing activity (medial) or fall onto extended elbow (lateral)	Tenderness of overlying affected ligaments; medial tenderness a maximum of 2 cm (⅘ inch) distal to epicondyle, with pain or instability with valgus stretch at 30 degrees of elbow flexion; lateral tenderness vague, reproduced only with arm extended and supinated	*Differential diagnosis:* Epicondylitis, radial or ulnar nerve irritation, avulsion fracture, or ligament tear *Management:* PRICE; may use sling and splint for 48 hours if significant pain and swelling; oral or topical NSAIDs or analgesics

TABLE 174-1 Common Elbow Ailments—cont'd

Ailment	Presentation	Examination	Differential Diagnosis and Management
RADIAL HEAD FRACTURES			
Usually caused by fall onto outstretched hand; commonly involves superior portion of radial bone	Affected arm usually cradled at 90 degrees; pain decreasing 30 minutes after injury, then recurring several hours later because of bleeding in joint	Local or diffuse edema; tenderness over radial head; ROM limited, rotation quite painful; grasp strength diminished; intact radial pulse and normal neurologic examination of hand and wrist	*Differential diagnosis:* Acute lateral epicondylitis, capsular tears, cartilage injury, subluxation or dislocation of radial head, fracture of olecranon or humerus *Management:* PRICE immobilization with posterior splint or sling with elbow flexed at 90 degrees; orthopedic referral recommended; surgical repair often required for displaced or complicated fractures
ULNAR NEURITIS			
Also called *cubital tunnel syndrome* Compression of ulnar nerve causing numbness or tingling in nerve's distribution	May be complication of rheumatoid arthritis, ganglion, elbow fracture, repeated irritation, or medial ligament sprain; pain usually localized to medial elbow; may radiate down forearm or cause clumsiness of hand; numbness and tingling replacing pain in severe cases	Tenderness of ulnar groove; sensory loss of fifth digit; diminished motor strength of fourth and fifth digits; presence of Tinel sign (tingling sensation down forearm and hand in ulnar distribution when tapping over ulnar groove); in severe cases may be forearm motor weakness and muscle atrophy *Diagnostics:* electromyographic studies	*Differential diagnosis:* Medial epicondylitis, cervical disk disease, thoracic outlet syndrome *Management:* PRICE, elbow pads, wrist-elbow splint, support in neutral position, oral or topical NSAIDs, physical therapy; conservative treatment rarely effective; referral to orthopedics or neurology appropriate
OLECRANON BURSITIS (SEE CHAPTER 175)			
Swelling of bursal sac overlying olecranon process; may be acute, chronic, septic, or aseptic and/or associated with history of trauma, rheumatoid arthritis, or crystal arthropathy	After acute injury, development of painful, edematous elbow; in chronic inflammation, soft, edematous nontender elbow; ROM often intact	Edema, possible tenderness over posterior elbow; full ROM and normal neurologic examination findings; in chronic bursitis, rough nodular consistency noted; if secondary infection, fever, warmth, erythema, and tenderness present	*Differential diagnosis:* Consider tendinitis; synovitis if edema is diffuse with limited elbow extension; infection; fracture with history of trauma; gout if extremely tender and erythematous; osteophytes; osteochondrosis *Management:* X-ray studies if indicated; aspiration of bursal fluid for diagnosis; hospitalization may be recommended if infected for periodic aspiration or intravenous antibiotics; otherwise, oral or topical NSAIDs, elbow pads, avoidance of direct pressure; oral antibiotics if indicated; steroid injection after infection ruled out; orthopedic referral if signs of infection, joint involvement, or decreasing ROM

NSAIDs, nonsteroidal anti-inflammatory drugs; PRICE, protection, rest, ice, compression, elevation; ROM, range of motion.

of fatigue by limiting total activity time. Proper equipment, body mechanics, and ergonomics are also important to prevent injuries.[9]

Once injury occurs, general goals of treatment are summarized by the mnemonic *PRICEMM* (protection, rest, ice, compression, elevation, medication, modalities); joint protection should be initiated to protect the elbow from further injury, promote healing of microtears, and reduce pain and swelling, along with rest, ice, compression, and elevation.[9] Nonsteroidal anti-inflammatory drugs can be used to reduce pain and tissue inflammation. After 2 weeks of conservative treatment, and after infection has been ruled out, corticosteroid injection may be considered to provide further improvement of the condition.[8,10]

Steroid injections may provide temporary relief that allows the patient to fully participate in rehabilitation activities (see Fig. 171-3).[10] Splinting that keeps the wrist in 30 to 45 degrees of extension may be useful for lateral epicondylitis.[2] Physical therapy with ultrasound or electrical stimulation can be used acutely, followed by rehabilitation exercises and a gradual return to activity. Changes in technique, equipment, and ergonomics should also be implemented to prevent injury recurrence.[2]

Management of arthritis includes anti-inflammatory medications (for short periods and with close monitoring of side effects), balanced rest and exercise, joint conservation techniques, and avoidance of pain-generating activities. Occupational therapy can be helpful to these patients.[7]

COMPLICATIONS

Recurrent epicondylitis or tendinitis may cause cumulative weakening of those tissues, resulting in impairment of grip function or lifting ability and nerve entrapment of the arm.[6,7] Limitation of elbow range of motion, arthritis, and chronic elbow pain may be caused by improper diagnosis or failure to treat the underlying elbow disorder. Repeated steroid injections may cause weakness or even rupture of the tendon and should be limited to three injections per year.[11]

CONSIDERATION FOR REFERRAL

Patients with acute trauma resulting in fracture, dislocation, and vascular or neurologic clinical findings should be referred to an orthopedist. Patients with recurrent injury, failure to improve with basic management, chronic pain with activity, arm weakness, or pain or swelling in other joints should also be referred. Both physical and occupational therapists can be extremely helpful with both treatment and education. Vocational counseling may be indicated for patients with repetitive stress injuries causing elbow pain and disability.

PATIENT EDUCATION

Injury prevention and early recovery are assisted by teaching about proper stretching and conditioning exercises, need for rest at the earliest symptoms of pain, use of ergonomic redesign (e.g., in rackets, workplace, power tools), and proper body mechanics for sports and repetitive motion activities. Individuals with recurrent injury or any change in elbow function or mobility should be advised to seek prompt medical attention to minimize complications.

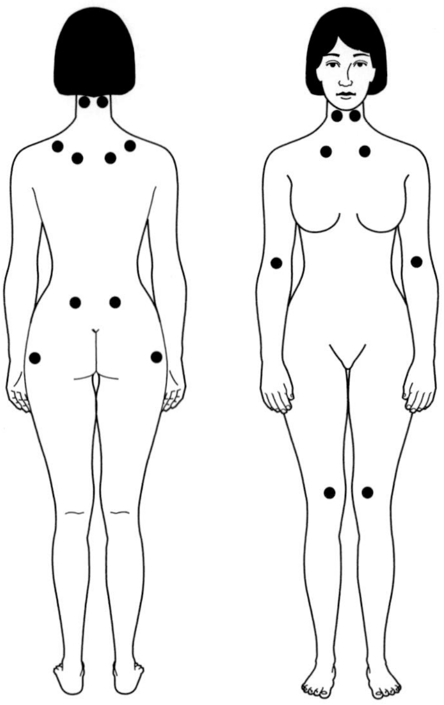

FIGURE **175-1** Tender point locations for the 1990 classification criteria for fibromyalgia. (From Wolfe F, Smythe HA, Yunus MB, et al: The American College of Rheumatology 1990 criteria for the classification of fibromyalgia: report of the Multicenter Criteria Committee, *Arthritis Rheum* 33[2]:160-172, 1990.)

CHAPTER 175

FIBROMYALGIA AND MYOFASCIAL PAIN SYNDROME

Lin A. Brown

DEFINITION AND EPIDEMIOLOGY

Fibromyalgia syndrome (FMS), a disorder usually included with rheumatologic conditions, is characterized by symptoms of widespread musculoskeletal pain, fatigue, nonrestorative sleep, depression, headaches, and gastrointestinal complaints (irritable bowel syndrome). FMS gained acceptance as a disorder in 1990 after the American College of Rheumatology developed classification criteria for the disorder.

Fibromyalgia as defined in 1990 included more than 3 months of musculoskeletal pain present above and below the waist bilaterally, associated with pain on palpation of specific tender points (Fig. 175-1). No other source of pain is identified, although there may be so-called drivers of pain such as painful joints from rheumatoid arthritis that can be complicated by fibromyalgia. The pain is usually accompanied by profound fatigue and sleep disturbance (nonrestorative sleep). Most patients with chronic fatigue syndrome also meet diagnostic criteria for FMS. Myofascial pain syndrome is a more limited expression of the same condition (e.g., pain limited to the shoulder and neck, upper back).

In 2010, the American College of Rheumatology put forth a new set of classification criteria that eliminated the tender point examination and replaced it with a report of pain surveyed in 19 areas as well as severity of symptoms associated with fibromyalgia (Box 175-1).

FMS is diagnosed eight to nine times more often in women than in men of all age groups, with an onset in general at 40 to 50 years of age. FMS rarely begins after the age of 55 years. FMS affects approximately 5 million Americans, accounting for 2% of all primary care visits, 10% of all internal medicine referrals, and up to 20% of rheumatology referrals.[1] Symptoms start gradually in adulthood or, rarely, in childhood and wax and wane in intensity.[1]

PATHOPHYSIOLOGY

Although the cause of FMS is unclear, research has implicated central nervous system dysfunction and not muscle disease, autoimmune disease, or viral disease. Pain beginning in the periphery is processed in the spinal cord and transmitted to the brain. For unclear reasons, some pain becomes "louder" at the level of the spinal cord and brain, a condition called central sensitization. The brain responds with pain recognition at a lower threshold and over a wider area than that originally involved.[2,3] In addition, neuroendocrine disturbances at the level of the hypothalamus or pituitary, involving decreased levels of growth hormone (GH), insulin-like growth factor (IGF), and possibly prolactin, have been found in FMS patients.[4] These hormones are released during the stages of sleep, specifically

BOX 175-1

Fibromyalgia Diagnostic Criteria

A person satisfies diagnostic criteria for fibromyalgia if the following three conditions are met:

1. Widespread pain index (WPI) score ≥7 and symptoms severity (SS) scale score >5 *or* WPI score 3-6 and SS scale score ≥9.
2. Symptoms have been present at a similar level for at least 3 months.
3. The patient does not have a disorder that would otherwise explain the pain.

ASCERTAINMENT

1. WPI Score

Note the number of areas in which the patient has had pain over the last week. In how many areas has the pain had pain? Score will be 0 to 19.

Shoulder girdle, left
Should girdle, right
Upper arm, left
Upper arm, right
Lower arm, left
Lower arm right
Hip (buttock, trochanter), left
Hip (buttock, trochanter), right
Upper leg, left
Upper leg, right
Lower leg, left
Lower leg, right
Jaw, left
Jaw, right
Chest
Abdomen
Upper back
Lower back
Neck

2. SS Scale Score

Cardinal symptoms:

- Fatigue
- Waking refreshed
- Cognitive symptoms

For each of these three symptoms, indicate the level of severity over the past week using the following scale:

0 = no problem
1 = slight or mild problems, generally mild or intermittent
2 = moderate, considerable problems, often present and/or at a moderate level
3 = severe: pervasive, continuous, life-disturbing problems

Considering somatic symptoms in general*, indicate whether the patient has the following:

0 = no symptoms
1 = few symptoms
2 = a moderate number of symptoms
3 = a great deal of symptoms

The SS scale score is the sum of the severity of the three cardinal symptoms plus the extent (severity) of somatic symptoms in general. The final score will be 0 to 12.

*Somatic symptoms that might be considered: muscle pain, irritable bowel syndrome, fatigue or tiredness, thinking or remembering problems, muscle weakness, headache, pain or cramps in the abdomen, numbness or tingling, dizziness, insomnia, depression, constipation, pain in the upper abdomen, vomiting, heartburn, oral ulcers, loss of or change in taste, dry eyes, shortness of breath, loss of appetite, hair loss, frequent urination, painful urination, and bladder spasm.

From Wolfe F, Clauw D, Fitzcharles MA, et al: The American College of Rheumatology preliminary diagnostic criteria for fibromyalgia and measurement of symptom severity, *Arthritis Care Res (Hoboken)* 62(5):600-610, 2010.

GH in stage 3 and stage 4 of non–rapid eye movement (REM) sleep. In sleep studies, patients with FMS have disturbances with non-REM sleep and difficulty in progressing to stage 3 and stage 4 sleep, resulting in morning fatigue. One third of FMS patients have low IGF, an indication of low GH secretion, lending credence to disturbed stage 4 sleep as important in FMS. Treatment with GH increases IGF levels, improves pain and sleep, and reduces overall symptoms, although the cost is prohibitive.[2,3]

Other neuroendocrine abnormalities include elevation of cerebrospinal fluid substance P levels and dysregulated cortisol production. FMS patients have three times the levels of substance P, which is significant because this neurotransmitter plays a role in enhanced pain perception. This may be the reason for the heightened pain perception experienced by fibromyalgia patients. Alteration in the hypopituitary-adrenal axis with low production of cortisol, perhaps secondary to chronic stress response, contrasts with depression, in which high production of cortisol is found. These results suggest that part of the cause of FMS may be a product of disturbances in the autonomic and endocrine stress response systems.[2] In addition, serotonin levels are low in the brain and in the platelets of patients with fibromyalgia.

Although these theories explain part of the pathogenesis of FMS, the primary cause of the central dysregulation is unknown. FMS frequently follows physical or mental trauma, viral illness, and stress.

CLINICAL PRESENTATION

Persistent widespread pain is the hallmark of the syndrome, along with chronic fatigue. Patients have a variety of other somatic complaints: nonrestorative sleep; cognitive difficulties; auditory, vestibular, and ocular complaints; chronic rhinitis or "allergies"; migraines; palpitations; irritable bowel syndrome; subjective sense of joint swelling; and mood disorders.[4] With such generalized complaints, it is clear how the patient's complaints can be confused with an autoimmune disease such as lupus.

PHYSICAL EXAMINATION

With fibromyalgia, muscle strength is normal (although effort may be affected by pain and judging pain may also be difficult), and there is no evidence of synovitis or soft tissue inflammation. Making the diagnosis depends on findings from the history and physical examination. FMS should be considered with any musculoskeletal pain not explained by a clearly defined anatomic lesion.

The American College of Rheumatology recently revised the criteria for FMS symptoms[5] (see Box 175-1). The previous pressure point evaluation of sites has been supplanted by patient report of widespread pain present in up to 19 areas plus the severity of other symptoms including fatigue, disordered sleep, bowel complaints, and others (see Box 175-1).

DIAGNOSTICS

An in-depth history and physical examination reduce the need for extensive and expensive objective tests. Laboratory values and electromyography findings are typically normal. Complete blood count, erythrocyte sedimentation rate or C-reactive protein (CRP), vitamin D level, and thyroid-stimulating hormone level are of value in excluding underlying disorders. Antinuclear antibody (ANA), rheumatoid factor, and anti–citrullinated protein antibody (ACPA) testing should be ordered only in the setting of synovitis on examination or other findings suggestive of lupus or rheumatoid arthritis. Sleep studies may be warranted for some patients, especially those with characteristics of obstructive sleep apnea. Obstructive sleep apnea is characterized by daytime sleepiness as opposed to daytime fatigue. Radiographs are not recommended unless a secondary disorder such as degenerative arthritis as a driver of fibromyalgia is suspected.

DIFFERENTIAL DIAGNOSIS

Symptoms of fibromyalgia often overlap with those of myofascial pain syndrome, chronic fatigue syndrome, hypothyroidism, bursitis or tendinitis, depression, and anxiety. Connective tissue diseases that should be included in the differential diagnosis include rheumatoid arthritis, systemic lupus erythematous, polymyalgia rheumatica, and polymyositis.

DIFFERENTIAL DIAGNOSIS
Fibromyalgia

- Hypothyroidism
- Hypovitaminosis D (<30 ng/mL)
- Bursitis
- Tendinitis
- Depression
- Anxiety
- Rheumatoid arthritis
- Systemic lupus erythematous
- Polymyalgia rheumatic
- Polymyositis

MANAGEMENT

Treatment of FMS does not conform to a specific algorithm or paradigm and is as much an art as a science. The goal of therapy should be to empower patients to control their own pain, to enhance sleep, and to maintain function. Education allows the patient opportunities to individualize treatment and to reduce symptoms. Treatment may incorporate pharmacologic therapies, cognitive behavioral therapy, exercise, and alternative therapies.[6]

Pharmacology

Low doses of tricyclic drugs have been studied, particularly amitriptyline, 10 mg taken 2 to 3 hours before bedtime, allowing peak sedative effect and reducing sedation on awakening. Cyclobenzaprine, also a tricyclic, can be used as well at 5 to 10 mg at night (Table 175-1). Doses should start low and increase slowly. Selective serotonin reuptake inhibitors, such as fluoxetine (Prozac) 20 mg, have also been studied, but duloxetine (Cymbalta) and milnacipran (Savella), both dual serotonin-norepinephrine reuptake inhibitors, may work better and are approved by the Food and Drug Administration for treatment of fibromyalgia.

Other medications that have proved helpful for pain include gabapentin (Neurontin) and pregabalin (Lyrica). Trazodone (Desyrel) and zolpidem (Ambien) may help sleep but do not increase time spent in stage 4. Nonsteroidal anti-inflammatory drugs (NSAIDs) and acetaminophen can be tried and are commonly prescribed, although NSAIDs have not been proved effective for the pain of fibromyalgia. Identification of pain generators, such as osteoarthritis of the knee, spinal stenosis, restless leg syndrome, and diabetic neuropathy, can result in treatment of these conditions, which may play a role in reducing sleep disturbances and hence pain and fatigue.[4,6,7]

Chronic Opioid Analgesic Therapy

Chronic opioid analgesic therapy should be used only after all other pharmacologic and nonpharmacologic therapies have been tried. If it is used, patients need to be aware of the high dependency possibility and be closely monitored.[6] The provider should sign a contract with any patient prescribed a

TABLE 175-1 Pharmacologic Therapy for Fibromyalgia

Medication	Proposed Action
Amitriptyline, 10-20 mg at bedtime; may increase if needed	Restoration of restorative sleep
Cyclobenzaprine, 5-10 mg at bedtime	Pain relief
Fluoxetine (Prozac), 20-40 mg per day	Antidepressant and pain relief
Milnacipran (Savella), 50 mg twice per day	Antidepressant and pain relief
Duloxetine (Cymbalta), 20-60 mg per day	Antidepressant and pain relief
Venlafaxine, 75 mg 2-3 times per day	Augment central adrenergic response to decrease pain
Gabapentin, 300 mg 3 times per day	Pain relief
Pregabalin (Lyrica), 75 mg twice per day	Pain relief
Trazodone, 50 mg daily at bedtime	Improve sleep
Zolpidem tartrate (Ambien), 5-10 mg daily at bedtime	Improve sleep
Lidocaine 1%, 2-3 mL equal parts intramuscularly in tender point areas	Pain relief for recalcitrant tender point pain

narcotic medication so that continued treatment can be tied to functional improvement, and dysfunctional behavior can be avoided.

Cognitive Behavioral Therapy

Cognitive behavioral therapy uses different approaches to integrate coping skills, relaxation training, activity pacing, visual imagery techniques, and goal setting to allow the patient control to improve function and pain.[4,6] It has been shown in multiple studies to be effective in treating FMS by reducing pain and increasing a sense of well-being.[7,8]

The Arthritis Foundation (www.arthritis.org) and the American College of Rheumatology (www.rheumatology.org) as well as other organizations can help direct patients to self-help books and classes. Many pain clinics and psychiatry departments provide cognitive behavioral therapy.

Exercise

Aerobic exercise can improve pain and have an antidepressant effect.[9] Usually, patients with fibromyalgia have not been active physically and experience increased pain when they begin an aerobic exercise program. Hence, the exercise prescription should begin at a low intensity and for short duration. The duration and intensity should increase over time as the patient is able to do so. To be beneficial, the exercise needs to be consistent and aerobic. Some experts recommend thinking of exercise as a drug with the ability to be overdosed and misused. However, used correctly, exercise clearly works to improve pain, sleep, and function. Gentle stretching and yoga are useful adjuncts before engaging in a low-impact activity such as biking, swimming, and walking. Massage aids in relaxation and produces physiologic benefits as well, but neither stretching nor massage is a substitute for aerobic exercise. Encouragement to continue the exercise program is needed to combat the continued muscle wasting often associated with fibromyalgia as well as to alleviate the patient's perception that pain is inevitable. Postexercise pain should be distinguished from fibromyalgia pain; it may respond to heat, ice, or NSAIDs. Patients should consider a one-on-one therapist or exercise partner for any program to improve success.[9]

Exercise and cognitive behavioral therapy are clearly beneficial and should form the cornerstone of any other therapy for fibromyalgia.

Alternative Therapies

Acupuncture has produced mixed results in fibromyalgia, although it has been found to be useful in other painful conditions. Massage therapy likewise has preliminary support; some studies show a positive response. Chiropractic manipulation, hypnosis, biofeedback, and magnet therapy all show insufficient evidence for effectiveness to be recommended as treatments.[10] Trigger point injections have been studied and are reported to be effective adjuncts to a treatment regimen. The judicious use of trigger point injections with lidocaine (Xylocaine) or bupivacaine (Marcaine) is often tried for symptoms not controlled with oral medications, with some success.[11] Any treatment that is not effective should be discontinued.

Multidisciplinary Approach

Group therapy programs are based on cognitive behavioral therapy approaches for living day to day effectively and increasing endurance and strength. These programs often include care from a rheumatologist and a physical therapist as well as group exercise programs, pain and stress management lectures, and even massage therapy. They are clearly effective compared with usual treatment with a family physician.[12]

COMPLICATIONS

Fibromyalgia does not result in damage to muscle, joints, or vital organs, and this is important for patients to understand. They hurt, but the pain is not indicative of tissue damage or a shortened life expectancy. Disability, however, is frequently perceived, and this is a difficult issue in FMS because disability is often difficult to document or to compensate for. Other complications include depression, insomnia, muscle atrophy, misdiagnosis, and drug-seeking behavior.

INDICATIONS FOR REFERRAL OR HOSPITALIZATION

FMS patients should be managed in primary care, where there is a partnership and willingness for creativity in treatment plans, perhaps including alternative treatments.[13,14] Pain management clinics for pain control have been effective for chronic pain. Psychologists, physical therapists, and chiropractors may aid in symptom control. Hospital admissions are not required.

PATIENT AND FAMILY EDUCATION

Education is imperative for improved patient understanding of fibromyalgia and the development of individual strategies to cope with the pain, fatigue, and chronic nature of the syndrome. The importance of regular exercise and adequate rest should be emphasized. Family members are affected and should be involved in education to understand the disorder and to maximize support for these patients. Support groups can be invaluable. Information abounds on the Internet, so careful evaluation is required. Available resources include the following:

The American College of Rheumatology
www.rheumatology.org

Arthritis Foundation
1330 West Peachtree St., Suite 100
Atlanta, GA 30309
404-872-7100
www.arthritis.org

National Institute of Arthritis and Musculoskeletal and Skin Diseases
National Institutes of Health
www.niams.nih.gov

Fibromyalgia Network
PO Box 31750
Tucson, AZ 85751
800-853-2929
www.fmnetnews.com

HEALTH PROMOTION

FMS is a syndrome that requires providing patients with the tools needed to improve activities of daily living and manage pain. Healthy diet, exercise, weight control, support systems, stress reduction through meditation or counseling, and improved self-esteem are all within the patient's control and will result in reduced pain and improved function.

CHAPTER 176

GOUT

Naomi Schlesinger

DEFINITION

Gout is a systemic metabolic disease. Humans do not express the enzyme urate oxidase (uricase), which converts urate to the more soluble and easily excreted compound allantoin. This may lead to hyperuricemia. Gouty arthritis has four clinical stages[1]: asymptomatic hyperuricemia, acute gouty flares, intercritical gout (intervals between acute flares), and chronic tophaceous gout. Acute flares in patients with gout are caused by inflammation from monosodium urate (MSU) crystal deposition as a result of chronically elevated levels of urate in plasma and extracellular fluids.

Gout is a common inflammatory arthritis. An estimated 8.3 million adults in the United States (prevalence of 3.9%) have gout.[2] The prevalence of gout is increasing. This is occurring because of increasing life expectancy and increases in prevalence of risk factors for gout such as greater use of diuretics and low-dose aspirin (acetylsalicylic acid) as well as an increase in prevalence of comorbidities such as obesity, renal disease, hypertension, and the metabolic syndrome.[3]

In the asymptomatic hyperuricemia stage, the patient has elevated levels of serum urate (SU) but no previous acute flares. During this phase, however, MSU crystals may "silently" be deposited in the tissues and joints and possibly other organs and result in "hidden damage," which can occasionally occur over time even in the absence of clinically apparent gout. Hyperuricemia is often present for many years in the absence of clinical signs of gout. Acute flares occur as a result of the deposition of MSU crystals and activation of an inflammatory response leading to intense pain and other signs of inflammation, such as swelling, redness, and warmth of the involved joints. Over time, or with the help of drugs to terminate the acute flare, the flare will subside. At that point, even though the patient is not experiencing a flare, he or she is still considered to have gout and is in the intercritical stage until another flare occurs. Uncontrolled hyperuricemia and resultant gout can eventually evolve into the destructive chronic tophaceous gout.

The SU level is the single most important risk factor for development of gout.[4] The SU level is elevated when it exceeds 6.8 mg/dL, the limit of solubility of MSU in serum at 37° C (98.6° F). A sustained elevation of SU is virtually essential for the development of gout but by itself is insufficient to cause the disease. In fact, most patients with hyperuricemia never develop gout.

It is now suspected that hyperuricemia may be a risk factor for cardiovascular disease as well as for hypertension, renal insufficiency, and nephrolithiasis.

EPIDEMIOLOGY

Prevalence

Gouty arthritis is the most common inflammatory arthritis in adults. An estimated 8.3 million adults in the United States have gouty arthritis, corresponding to a prevalence of 3.9%.[2] Prevalence increases with age, peaking at about 10% among men aged 70 to 79 years, and 6% in women aged 80 years or older.[2] With the aging of populations in most developed countries, various studies have reported that the incidence of gout is increasing[2,3]; this is probably driven not only by the increasing life expectancy in most countries but also by increases in the prevalence of risk factors for gout, including greater use of diuretics and low-dose aspirin (acetylsalicylic acid), and the increasing prevalence of comorbidities such as obesity, renal disease, hypertension, and metabolic syndrome.

PATHOPHYSIOLOGY

Uricase, an end product of purine metabolism, is an enzyme that converts uric acid to allantoin, the soluble form. Its gene is silent in humans. The solubility of MSU crystals is related to temperature. At 37° C (98.6° F), the maximum solubility of urate in physiologic saline is 6.8 mg/dL; but at 30° C (86° F), it is only 4.5 mg/dL. If SU concentration is increased for a sustained period, MSU will come out of solution to form crystals. Microtophi may subsequently form, particularly in the cooler parts of the body as well as at points of mechanical pressure, such as fingers and toes, olecranon bursae, and ears. Sustained hyperuricemia is a risk factor for gout; however, most patients with hyperuricemia will never have a gout flare, and current guidelines suggest that no treatment is required, although it is prudent to determine the cause of hyperuricemia and to correct it if possible.

Uric acid production is increased in males after puberty and in females after menopause. The predominant cause of hyperuricemia in most patients is undersecretion of urate by the kidneys. Lower clearance of urate is seen in all gout patients compared with normal controls; it is therefore not surprising that up to 73% of all gout patients have mild to severe renal insufficiency.[5]

CLINICAL PRESENTATION

Acute gout is characterized by a rapid onset and buildup of pain. The first flare often begins at night and wakes the patient from sleep. During an acute gouty flare, the patient experiences exquisite pain associated with warmth, redness, swelling, and decreased range of motion of the affected joint or joints. The initial episode is usually monoarticular in men. The first metatarsophalangeal (MTP) joint is the initial one involved in approximately half the patients. Acute synovitis of the first MTP joint of the big toe is referred to as *podagra*. Other joints involved (in decreasing order of frequency) are insteps, heels, knees, wrists, fingers, and elbows.[6]

In his classic description of the onset of an acute flare, Thomas Sydenham (London, 1683), a long-time sufferer from gout, wrote, "The victim goes to bed and sleeps quietly. About two in the morning he is awakened by a pain in the great toe; rarely in the heel, ankle or instep. The pain resembles that of a dislocated bone… [It] becomes so exquisitely painful as not to endure the weight of clothes nor the shaking of the room by a person walking in."[7]

Systemic symptoms and signs of fatigue, fever, and chills may accompany the acute arthritis because of increased production of proinflammatory cytokines such as interleukin-1. The natural course of the untreated flare lasts several hours to several weeks.

Chronic tophaceous gout usually develops after 5 to 10 years of acute intermittent gout, although rarely patients have tophi as their initial manifestation of the disease. *Tophus* means "chalk stone" in Latin. Tophi appear as firm swellings. They may appear at any site. The most common sites for the tophi to appear are the digits of the hands and feet and in the olecranon bursa. Tophi of the helix or antihelix of the ear are classic but less common. Tophi may be associated with a destructive deforming arthritis and may rarely ulcerate, in which case secondary infection may be a problem.[8] Local trauma and binges of alcohol, overeating, or fasting have been implicated as factors that precipitate an acute flare. Use of diuretics may also increase the risk of gout flares. In the hospital setting, acute flares of gout often occur postoperatively or are associated with severe acute medical illnesses. Changes in the body's total uric acid pool also can precipitate a disease flare because homeostatic mechanisms mobilize the deposited MSU crystals. This is commonly seen in patients newly initiated on urate-lowering therapy (ULT) and can be mitigated by slow titration of the dose upward and the addition of concomitant prophylactic therapy, such as nonsteroidal anti-inflammatory drugs (NSAIDs) or colchicine.[8] Finally, seasonal factors have been noted to relate to acute flares—for example, increased gout flares in the spring.[9]

DIAGNOSTICS

A definitive diagnosis of gout is achieved by needle aspiration of the acutely inflamed joint or suspected tophus. Even when clinical appearance strongly suggests gout, diagnosis has to be confirmed by needle aspiration.[10] MSU crystals can be observed in more than 95% of patients experiencing attacks of acute gout.[11] However, this method is invasive and diagnosis is not always possible.

The typical clinical history includes sudden (reaching its pain peak within 2 to 4 hours) and severe, exquisite pain in a joint, most classically the first MTP joint (toe), that may wake the patient. The patient may have renal disease or be taking medications that can elevate SU. Elevated SU level, however, in up to 49% of patients may be normal during the acute flare.[12]

Advanced radiology can help with the diagnosis of gout. On ultrasonography, the double-contour sign or urate icing is highly specific for diagnosis of gout.[13] The double-contour sign is observed on ultrasound examination as a hyperechoic band over anechoic cartilage and is believed to be indicative of MSU crystals overlying articular cartilage. Dual-energy computed tomography (DECT) is an advanced imaging modality that enables visualization of MSU crystal deposits by analysis of the chemical composition of the scanned materials. DECT provides good diagnostic accuracy for detection of MSU deposits in patients with gout. However, sensitivity is lower in patients with recent-onset disease.

DIFFERENTIAL DIAGNOSIS

Difficulties in the clinical diagnosis of gout occur because the disease can be polyarticular and chronic, especially in the elderly. Atypical joint involvement can also occur, such as in Heberden nodes, especially in elderly women. It can cause diagnostic confusion with rheumatoid arthritis. However, gout tends to be less symmetric than typical rheumatoid arthritis. Tophi sometimes tend to be confused with rheumatoid nodules, and therefore, when in doubt, the provider should perform needle aspiration to look for MSU crystals. It is sometimes difficult to determine whether the patient with acute arthritis has gout or pseudogout. Almost half of acute attacks of calcium pyrophosphate deposition disease (CPPD) affect the knees, but the wrists, metacarpophalangeal joints, elbows, and shoulders may be involved. However, under compensated polarized light, the difference between the two types of crystals is evident, and the correct diagnosis can be made. The CPPD crystals are rhomboid and have weakly positive birefringence.

DIFFERENTIAL DIAGNOSIS

Gout

- Pseudogout
- Calcium apatite deposition disease
- Calcium oxalate deposition disease
- Rheumatoid arthritis
- Septic arthritis
- Lyme arthritis
- Psoriatic arthritis
- Reactive arthritis
- Cellulitis
- Bursitis
- Tenosynovitis
- Joint injury
- Soft tissue injury
- Fractures
- Dislocations

MANAGEMENT

There are three types of therapies in the management of gout: (1) treatment of the acute flare; (2) lowering of the total body uric acid pool to prevent tissue deposition of MSU crystals; and (3) anti-inflammatory prophylaxis to prevent acute flares, especially when ULT is started.

Nonpharmacologic Management

Gout is a metabolic disorder. It is influenced by dietary factors (including overeating, obesity, alcohol abuse, and hyperlipidemia) and insulin resistance syndrome. Avoidance of factors that may contribute to the development of gout among asymptomatic hyperuricemic patients may reduce gouty flares. This includes avoiding diuretics when possible, controlling weight, and limiting alcohol consumption.

The traditional gout prevention diet has been a low-purine, low-protein, alcohol-restricted diet; however, this diet is hard to follow. This is opposed to a diet focused on weight reduction with unlimited purines, which limits calories and restricts carbohydrates but increases proportional intake of protein and unsaturated fat. In an observational study monitoring patients with gout on a diet moderately decreased in calories and increased in protein, the mean SU level decreased by 18% after 4 months of dietary intervention.[14] This was accompanied by a 67% reduction in monthly gouty attack frequency. Therefore the authors advocate the limitation of carbohydrate intake, an increased proportional intake of protein, and the use of unsaturated fat, because they all enhance insulin sensitivity and therefore may promote a reduction in SU.

An alcohol-restricted diet in patients with gout is of importance because alcohol consumption is closely associated with hyperuricemia and gout. It is estimated that half of individuals with gout drink alcohol excessively.[15]

It has been shown that low-fat dairy products have a protective effect on SU levels. A significant inverse association was noted between the intake of dairy and SU level in the Third National Health and Nutrition Examination Survey (NHANES III) (odds ratio [OR] 0.66; 95% confidence interval [CI] 0.48-0.89).[16] The dairy proteins casein and lactalbumin were thought to lower SU level by inducing urinary excretion of uric acid.[17] Studies suggest that cherry juice concentrate reduces the incidence of acute flares when it is consumed over a period of 4 months or more. Cherry juice concentrate appears to have anti-inflammatory properties and some reports suggest that it may be useful as prophylaxis for gout.[18]

Joint motion may increase inflammation, whereas rest of affected joints may aid in its resolution.[19] Less medication is needed if the patient can rest the affected joint for 1 or 2 days.[20] Cold applications may also be a useful adjunct to treatment of acute gouty flares.[21]

Pharmacologic Management

Treatment of Acute Gout. The current options available for the treatment of acute gouty flares are NSAIDs, colchicine, corticosteroids (oral, intravenous, intramuscular, and intra-articular), and adrenocorticotropic hormone (ACTH). In a patient without comorbidities, NSAIDs are the mainstay of therapy (Box 176-1).

Guidelines and recommendations by the American College of Rheumatology (ACR) Task Force Panels (TFPs) may help physicians in the treatment of gout. The ACR TFP recommended oral colchicine and/or NSAIDs as first-line treatment for acute gout and combinations of these medications in severe or refractory attacks. The ACR guidelines for the treatment of acute gout recommended initiating drug therapy within 24 hours of the onset of the acute attack (based on the consensus that early treatment leads to better outcomes). It is proposed that during the acute attack, ULT be continued without interruption.[22]

The most important determinant of therapeutic success is not which NSAID is chosen, but rather how soon NSAID therapy is initiated at the appropriate dose and duration of therapy. In more than 90% of patients, the attack completely resolves within 5 to 8 days of initiation of therapy. Unfortunately, the use of NSAIDs is limited by side effects and comorbidities. NSAID therapy should be avoided in patients with peptic ulcer disease, impaired renal function, liver disease, and poorly compensated congestive heart failure and in patients receiving anticoagulation therapy. Side effects of NSAIDs are also more pronounced in elderly patients.

BOX 176-1

Treatment of Acute Gout

- Ideally, confirm diagnosis by joint aspiration: intracellular monosodium urate crystals in synovial fluid. (This can be difficult in the primary care setting, especially when access to rheumatologists is limited or nonexistent.)
- Initial treatment is with NSAIDs unless there are risk factors for their use: age older than 65 years (relative risk), creatinine clearance less than 50 mL/min, poorly controlled congestive heart failure, history of or active peptic ulcer disease, anticoagulant therapy, or hepatic dysfunction. NSAIDs should be used early in the attack. Higher doses need to be used in the first 24-48 hr It does not matter which NSAID is used.
- In a severe oligoarticular or polyarticular gouty attack or when NSAIDs are not tolerated or are contraindicated, use systemic corticosteroids (7- to 14-day taper). Parenteral, intramuscular, or intravenous (corticosteroids or adrenocorticotropic hormone) medications may be helpful, especially in patients with renal failure.
- Oral colchicine should be used within 36 hr of onset of an acute attack. Colchicine should be used cautiously because of its toxicity. If one or two joints are involved, intra-articular corticosteroid treatment may be beneficial.
- Do not start or stop urate lowering therapy during the acute attack.

Oral colchicine has been used for many years but was not approved by the U.S. Food and Drug Administration (FDA) until recently.[23] The FDA-approved dose of oral colchicine (Colcrys) for the treatment of acute gout attacks is 1.2 mg followed by 0.6 mg in 1 hour (total 1.8 mg). It is most effective during the first 12 to 24 hours of an attack, and its effectiveness may decline with the duration of inflammation. Colchicine is primarily eliminated by the hepatobiliary tract. Renal excretion accounts for 10% to 20% of colchicine elimination in patients with normal renal function. Colchicine should not be used if the glomerular filtration rate (GFR) is less than 10 mL/min, and the dose should be decreased by at least half if the GFR is less than 50 mL/min. A clinical response to colchicine is not pathognomonic for gout; it can also be seen with pseudogout, sarcoid arthropathy, psoriatic arthritis, and calcific tendinitis.

Intra-articular corticosteroids are currently accepted as practical and beneficial when only one or two joints are actively inflamed.[1] Patients with polyarticular gout who demonstrate suboptimum or delayed response to oral NSAIDs or who have contraindications to the usual NSAIDs may also benefit from adjunctive corticosteroid injections into joints with persistent synovitis.[1] It is particularly important to ensure that the joint is not infected before corticosteroids are injected intra-articularly.

Corticosteroids can be given to patients who cannot use NSAIDs or colchicine. Steroids can be given orally, intravenously, intramuscularly, intra-articularly, or indirectly by ACTH. Corticosteroid treatment is particularly useful in patients with moderate to severe chronic kidney disease. A study by Janssens and colleagues[24] of 120 patients compared oral prednisolone with naproxen. The latter demonstrated equivalent efficacy for oral prednisolone and naproxen. Both therapies were well tolerated, with 66% (prednisolone) and 63% (naproxen) of patients reporting no adverse effects. Prednisone can be given at a dose of approximately 30 to 40 mg for 1 to 3 days and then tapered during 1 to 2 weeks. Tapering more rapidly can result in a rebound flare.

Randomized long-term prospective, placebo-controlled trials are needed to evaluate the therapeutic role of colchicine versus NSAIDs as well as that of corticosteroids and ACTH in the treatment of acute gout flares.

Treatment of Chronic Gout. The goal of treatment is to achieve resolution of MSU crystals by reducing the SU level to lower than the saturation threshold to permit spontaneous dissolution of MSU crystal deposition in the tissue (Box 176-2). Maintenance of the SU level at less than 6 mg/dL and not just within the "normal range" helps ensure resolution of tophi and eventual cessation of acute gouty flares.

The evidence on when to start ULT is conflicting. Cost-effectiveness of ULT has been studied, with the conclusion that therapy is cost saving in patients who have two or more attacks a year.[25] However, whether ULT should be initiated after the first gout flare has been questioned.

It has been suggested that ULT should not be started during an acute gouty flare because it could lead to a more intense and prolonged flare. Typically, ULT should be started 6 to 8 weeks after the flare has resolved. ULT should be started at low doses and increased slowly every 4 to 6 weeks to reach SU levels (<6 mg/dL) or the maximum tolerated or maximum doses advised.

ULT includes the uricostatic drugs, which are xanthine oxidase inhibitors that decrease uric acid synthesis (allopurinol,

BOX 176-2

Treatment of Chronic Gout

- Start urate-lowering therapy in patients who have two or more attacks a year, although in some patients it may be appropriate to start ULT after one flare.
- It is better not to start urate-lowering therapy during an acute attack.
- Uricosuric drugs and febuxostat are the urate-lowering therapies of choice in allopurinol-allergic patients, underexcretors with normal renal function, and patients with no history of urolithiasis.
- Use allopurinol in patients with renal calculi, renal insufficiency, concomitant diuretic therapy, cyclosporine therapy, or urate overproduction.
- Use concomitant colchicine prophylaxis until serum urate (SU) has been at the desired level (5-6 mg/dL) for some months and no recent gouty flares have occurred (6-12 months).
- Monitor SU level and aim for SU <6 mg/dL. Check SU level every 3-6 months and adjust the urate-lowering therapy dose accordingly.

febuxostat); the uricosuric drugs, which inhibit uric acid reabsorption in the proximal tubule (probenecid; benzbromarone, which is not available in the United States and is off the market in most countries secondary to liver toxicity); losartan and fenofibrate, which have a small uricosuric effect; and the uricolytic drugs, such as pegloticase, which catalyzes conversion of uric acid into allantoin.

Allopurinol is the most commonly prescribed ULT, primarily because of its once-a-day administration and its great efficacy.[26] It can be given in a single morning dose of 100 mg up to 300 mg initially and increased to 800 mg if needed. The ACR TFP recommended[26] that allopurinol be started at 100 mg/day (50 mg/day in CKD 4 or worse) or febuxostat at 40 mg/day. If SU exceeds 6 mg/dL, allopurinol is increased by 100 mg/day or febuxostat to 80 mg/day. If the SU target is not achieved with one xanthine oxidase inhibitor, combination therapy with another can be used or a uricosuric drug can be added.[26] It was recommended that SU levels be monitored every 2 to 5 weeks after initiation of ULT until they reach less than 6.0 mg/dL. Dosage adjustments are necessary in patients with impaired creatinine clearance.[27,28]

Febuxostat is an oral, nonpurine, once-daily medication, an inhibitor of xanthine oxidase. In clinical studies, febuxostat at a daily dose of 80 mg was more effective than allopurinol at the commonly used fixed daily dose of 300 mg in lowering SU level below 6 mg/dL. Febuxostat may be of most immediate value in patients with allopurinol hypersensitivity and in patients with renal disease. In a study of subjects with impaired renal function, the ability of febuxostat to lower SU levels was not altered in patients with mild to moderate renal insufficiency.[29]

Probenecid is the most widely used uricosuric agent available in the United States; however, its use is limited in patients with moderate renal function impairment. The maintenance dose of probenecid ranges from 500 mg to 3 g/day, administered twice or three times daily.

Use of recombinant uricase in patients with chronic gout is limited by the need for parenteral administration, potential antigenicity, production of antiuricase antibodies, and declining efficacy, as well as by price. However, it is a very effective ULT and is an important therapy in patients with severe tophaceous gout.

Prophylaxis

Prophylaxis refers to the continuous use of anti-inflammatory drugs to prevent gout flares. Prophylaxis is particularly relevant when ULT is initiated because this period is frequently associated with gout flares. In the absence of prophylaxis, up to three quarters of patients will have a gout flare soon after ULT is started.

The ACR TFP recommended use of either low-dose oral colchicine (0.5 mg or 0.6 mg once daily [qd] or twice daily [bid]) or NSAIDs with a proton pump inhibitor or low-dose prednisone (≤10 mg/day). The Panel advised that these drugs be initiated when ULT is started.[22] Maintenance of the SU level below 6 mg/dL is what ultimately decreases the incidence of gouty flares.

Studies are needed to assess appropriate length of prophylaxis. Prophylaxis usually is continued until the SU value has been maintained at less than 6 mg/dL and there have been no acute attacks for 3 to 6 months. It is important to warn patients that discontinuation of the prophylactic medication may be followed by an exacerbation of acute flares and to advise them what to do should this occur.

COMPLICATIONS

Nephrolithiasis occurs in up to approximately 27% of patients with primary gout.[30] The solubility of uric acid crystals increases as the urine pH becomes more alkaline. Acidic urine saturated with uric acid crystals may result in spontaneous stone formation. Other types of stones may also develop because uric acid can act as a nidus for calcium oxalate or phosphate stones.

Long-term deposition of crystals in the renal parenchyma can cause chronic urate nephropathy. The formation of microtophi causes a giant cell inflammatory reaction. This results in proteinuria and inability of the kidney to concentrate urine.

It is suspected that gout may lead to cardiovascular disease, hypertension, and renal insufficiency, as well.

Other complications may be related to therapy. Severe side effects of colchicine include bone marrow suppression, renal failure, alopecia, disseminated intravascular coagulation, hepatic necrosis, diarrhea, seizures, arrhythmias leading to complete heart block, and death. Neuromuscular toxicity related to colchicine therapy is also a well-recognized complication. Acute rhabdomyolysis with myoglobinuria and renal failure is most commonly seen in individuals concomitantly taking a 5-hydroxy-3-methylglutaryl-coenzyme A [HMG-CoA] reductase inhibitor (statin) or cyclosporine had adverse events due to allopurinol are not uncommon.

About 20% of patients who take allopurinol report side effects; 5% of patients discontinue the medication. More common side effects include gastrointestinal intolerance and rashes. Other adverse reactions include fever, toxic epidermal necrolysis, alopecia, bone marrow suppression with leukopenia or thrombocytopenia, agranulocytosis, aplastic anemia, granulomatous hepatitis, jaundice, sarcoid-like reaction, and vasculitis. The most severe reaction is the allopurinol hypersensitivity syndrome, which consists of a constellation of findings that may include fever, rash, eosinophilia, hepatitis, progressive renal insufficiency, and death. This is most likely to develop in individuals with preexisting renal dysfunction and those taking thiazide diuretics.

INDICATIONS FOR REFERRAL OR HOSPITALIZATION

A rheumatologist should be consulted to establish the diagnosis of gout by joint aspiration and MSU crystal identification. If the treatment is effective but drug toxicity or intolerance occurs, a rheumatology consultation is warranted as well. This could occur if the patient is still having acute flares with the maximum tolerated treatment, the diagnosis is in doubt, or the patient is unable to use or to tolerate his or her medication.

Hospitalization is rarely necessary unless there is confirmed or suspected bacterial arthritis in a patient suspected of having gout, a severe drug reaction occurs (such as allopurinol hypersensitivity), or drug therapy worsens a comorbidity (e.g., such as when a patient with diabetes mellitus is given corticosteroids and blood glucose levels are difficult to control).

PATIENT AND FAMILY EDUCATION

Health care providers should educate patients with gout and their families on the following points:

- Gout can be accurately diagnosed by identification of the characteristic crystals.
- There are three types of treatment for gout: medications to control the flares of joint pain (e.g., NSAIDs, colchicine, and corticosteroids); medications to prevent further attacks (e.g., colchicine and NSAIDs); and medications that will help lower the level of uric acid in the body over time so that the flares occur less frequently or not at all.
- People with chronic gout require lifetime treatment with drugs to lower the uric acid body pool.
- Lifestyle changes, such as controlling weight, limiting alcohol consumption, limiting meals with meats and fish rich in purines, increasing low-fat dairy consumption, and consuming cherries, are helpful in controlling gout.

RESOURCES

American College of Rheumatology: www.rheumatology.org/practice/clinical/patients/diseases_and_conditions/gout.asp
Arthritis Foundation: www.arthritis.org
National Institute of Arthritis and Musculoskeletal and Skin Diseases: www.niams.nih.gov
Men's Health Network: www.menshealthnetwork.org
Gout and Uric Acid Education Society: http://gouteducation.org

CHAPTER 177

HAND AND WRIST PAIN

Wendy L. Halm

DEFINITION AND EPIDEMIOLOGY

Hand disorders may result from recreational or work-related activities or from inflammatory or degenerative disease. Acute wrist pain from fractures, contusions, strains and sprains, and instability is a common presentation. Incidence of scaphoid fracture peaks at age 15, and such fractures are infrequent in the older adult.[1] Trauma or injury to the wrist may lead to the development of a ganglion cyst. Chronic wrist pain may be caused by arthritis of the hands and fingers, overuse, old injuries, or neurologic disorders. Job specialization, repetitive tasks, and workplace demographics have contributed to an increased incidence of cumulative hand and wrist injuries. Musculoskeletal-related ergonomic injuries accounted for 34% of all workplace injuries and illnesses and resulted in a median of 9 days away from work in 2012.[2] These injuries, which are also known as *cumulative trauma disorders*, are defined as muscle, tendon, osseous, or neurologic conditions produced or exacerbated by repetitive movements.[3,4] Many other factors, including sports activities, age, and various medical conditions, contribute to the development of hand and wrist pain.

PATHOPHYSIOLOGY

Acute hand and wrist injuries stemming from sports-related activities are common, including injuries to the palm from swinging a baseball bat or golf club and the classic injury to the thumb from the strap of a ski pole. Fractures of the scaphoid bone can occur during a fall onto an outstretched hand. Excessive physical activity (such as gardening or painting), may initiate or worsen existing chronic hand conditions, causing an acute pain flare. Ganglion cysts are fluid-filled sacks that can appear, disappear, and change size. Their cause is unknown.

Wrist pain in the presence of systemic symptoms, such as fatigue, fever, or bilateral hand pain, suggests a systemic issue, such as Lyme disease, rheumatoid arthritis, systemic lupus erythematosus (SLE), or malignancy. Chronic wrist pain from cumulative trauma disorders usually results from repetitive microtrauma that over time affects the tendons, tendon sheaths, and connective tissues. The exact pathologic mechanism is not clearly understood.[3]

Carpal tunnel syndrome (CTS) is caused by compressive neuropathy of the median nerve. A bony canal bordered by the carpal bones on the radial, ulnar, and dorsal sides is roofed by the transverse carpal ligament. This canal provides a passage for the nine digital flexor tendons, the blood vessels, and the median nerve of the hand. Repetitive motion and overuse have often been thought to cause the syndrome, but recent studies may present differing conclusions. As the tendons swell, the cross-sectional area in the tunnel decreases. The resultant pressure in the small tunnel causes pressure on the median nerve. Nerve conduction is impeded, muscle strength is decreased because of the disturbance in motor fibers, and pain and paresthesia occur because of the disturbance in the sensory fibers.[5] Common risk factors for development of CTS include repetitive maneuvers, obesity, pregnancy, diabetes mellitus, hypothyroidism, and female gender.[4]

CLINICAL PRESENTATION

Localized pain, numbness, tingling, weakness, and immobility are the common reasons that patients with hand or wrist disorders seek care. The symptoms may be intermittent or constant and often affect quality of life. Onset, duration, and location of all symptoms related to wrist pain should be noted. Age, sex, hand dominance, occupation, and hobbies or sports should also be documented. Past medical history should be explored for previous hand or wrist injury and any condition that might compromise nerve function, including pregnancy. Patients with a traumatic hand or wrist injury should be evaluated for fracture.

Ganglion Cyst

Fluid-filled ganglion cysts commonly occur at the dorsal or volar or /radial aspect of the wrist and may cause pain during activity or with pressure over the area.[6,7] Cysts may be asymptomatic and fluctuate in size.

Trigger Finger

Trigger finger, or stenosing tenosynovitis, is a disorder of the flexor tendons of the fingers or thumb. This condition, which may be more prevalent in patients with diabetes, gout, or rheumatoid arthritis, occurs most commonly when a nodule or thickening in the tendon catches on the edge of the A1 pulley of the finger as the tendon attempts to glide during movement.[6,7] This thickening narrows the fibrous canal, which impedes tendon movement. The pulley action is impaired, causing a painful locking or triggering of the affected digit or thumb during extension. Although any digit may be affected; the middle or ring finger is most commonly involved.[5]

Tenosynovitis

Chronic stenosing tenosynovitis (de Quervain tenosynovitis) is a condition that causes pain at the thumb base and into the distal radius.[1] Women 30 to 59 years of age are more likely to have this condition.[1,5] Activities requiring excessive repetitive motions (e.g., knitting) may aggravate this problem. It is also seen in new parents who frequently lift their child using wrist strength alone. Pain is noted with ulnar deviation under stress. Pouring from a pitcher or carton often reproduces pain.

Palmar Fibrosis

Dupuytren contracture, or palmar fibrosis, may be a hereditary process that initially develops as a painless nodule on the palmar fascia at the base of a digit.[8] An inflammatory fibrosis subsequently expands into a bandlike cord under puckered skin and can lead to a flexion contracture. Although any finger (and both hands) may be affected, the resultant contracture most often affects the ring finger. The little finger may also be involved. The index finger is the least commonly affected digit for Dupuytren disease.

Carpal Tunnel Syndrome

CTS results from compression of the median nerve in the carpal tunnel of the wrist. Patients may have intermittent wrist pain and numbness and tingling that radiates from the palm to the thumb, index finger, middle finger, and medial aspect of the ring finger. In addition, the patient may report intermittent nocturnal paresthesia, pain and tightness at the wrist and forearm that increases with activity, and an inability to hold objects or a tendency to drop things.[9] A tendency for symptoms to occur while driving, speaking on the telephone, or performing hygiene activities (brushing teeth, washing hair) may be reported. If the compression continues, the motor component of the median nerve is affected, and the ability to grasp with the thumb and index finger may be compromised.[9]

Trapeziometacarpal Arthritis

Arthritis is a common cause of hand and wrist pain. The trapeziometacarpal or basal joint area is a common site of osteoarthritis. Complaints include pain at the base of the thumb and weakness and pain with pinching or grasping. Arthritis in the hand can also be seen with osteoarthritis of the distal interphalangeal (DIP) and proximal interphalangeal (PIP) joints. Nodules are often seen at the DIP and PIP joints and are referred to as Heberden (DIP) and Bouchard (PIP) nodes, respectively (see Chapter 183). Rheumatoid arthritis commonly involves the metacarpophalangeal joints and the wrist in a bilateral and symmetric fashion, causing pain, inflammation, and deformity (see Chapter 221).

In the case of a history of fall or other trauma, especially in the older adult, fracture is always a consideration until it is ruled out with x-ray examination.

PHYSICAL EXAMINATION

Complex anatomy and proximity of structures can make examination of the hand and wrist difficult. The physical examination should begin with inspection, noting any muscle wasting, localized swelling or masses, skin discoloration, hair loss, or deformity.[7] Individual carpal bones should be palpated, passive and active range of motion should be assessed, and grip strength should be tested. Palpation of the anatomical snuff-box is necessary to exclude the possibility of scaphoid fracture. Motor function and sensory testing are also necessary. Additional provocative maneuvers and specific tests may be indicated. Physical findings seen in common causes of hand and wrist pain are described in the following paragraphs.

Ganglion Cyst

Most cysts will be smooth and will transilluminate with light. Pain may or may not be present with palpation. Numbness, tingling, or weakness may be present if the mass is compressing the median or ulnar nerve at the wrist.[6]

Trigger Finger

Edema at the distal palm may be noted. The finger is fully flexed with the examiner's finger on the metacarpophalangeal joint. The patient slowly extends the digit, and a "pop" is felt as the tendon slides back through the affected pulley. This maneuver is occasionally painful to the patient. Trigger thumb is examined in a similar manner. The patient will feel that the interphalangeal joint of the thumb is the culprit, but it is in fact the A1 pulley at the base of the thumb. Regardless of finger, there is often a palpable, tender nodule at the base of the affected digit.[7]

Tenosynovitis

On inspection, there may be a visible nodule at the radial base of the thumb. Edema and tenderness may be present over the radial stylus. The Finkelstein test is conducted when the patient folds the thumb across the palm and flexes the fingers over the thumb, and then the clinician deviates the hand in the direction of the ulna; the test result is positive if pain is reproduced over the radial stylus. Grip and pinch strength should also be assessed.[7]

Palmar Fibrosis

Skin changes can be the earliest manifestation. Skin may pucker with passive extension of the affected finger(s). Nodes or knuckle pads may form over the dorsum of the hand. Contracture may be evident on one or both hands as well as on the feet (Ledderhose disease) and on the penis (Peyronie disease). Painless edema along the nodule may also be present.

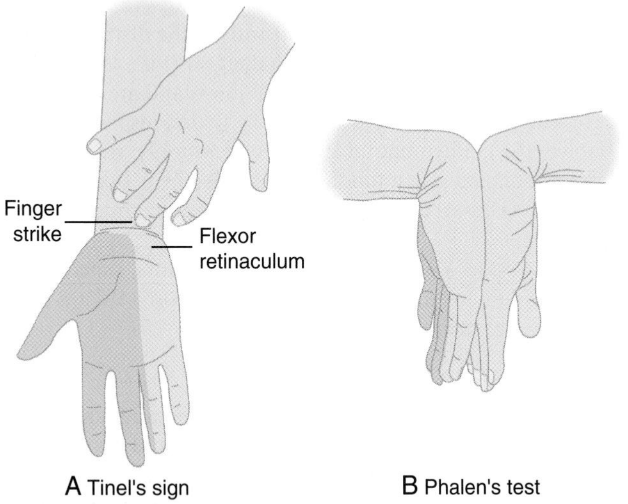

FIGURE 177-1 Clinical examination for carpal tunnel syndrome includes tests for Tinel sign (A) and Phalen sign (B). (From Black JM: *Medical-surgical nursing: clinical management for positive outcomes,* ed 8, St Louis, 2009, Saunders.)

Carpal Tunnel Syndrome

Atrophy of the thenar eminence may be evident in chronic cases, but edema is generally not present.[6] Tenderness, motor strength (including grip and pinch), and sensory deficits must be determined. A two-point discrimination test can be performed with a caliper. The Phalen maneuver and Tinel sign may reproduce symptoms (Fig. 177-1).

Trapeziometacarpal Arthritis

Pain at the base of the thumb is usually present. Pain can be elicited by adducting the first metacarpal and hyperextending the first metacarpal phalanx. The grind test will also elicit pain and may be remarkable for crepitus.[6] This is a degenerative form of arthritis and is often seen with other manifestations of degenerative arthritis of the hands.

DIAGNOSTICS AND DIFFERENTIAL DIAGNOSIS

- Diagnostic tests may be indicated after localizing the source of pain and narrowing the differential diagnosis.
- Initial diagnostic tests may include radiographic evaluation to rule out bone abnormality.
- Laboratory studies are rarely necessary. However, serum glucose concentration, thyroid-stimulating hormone (TSH) concentration, erythrocyte sedimentation rate (ESR), antinuclear antibody (ANA) testing, and rheumatoid factor may be indicated. Anti–citrullinated protein antibodies (ACPAs), a serologic marker for rheumatoid arthritis, may be helpful in the differential diagnosis to determine whether the patient's symptoms are related to rheumatoid arthritis or another autoimmune disorder.[10]
- Electromyography (EMG) may be ordered by a specialist.

Ganglion Cyst

Diagnosis may be made with history and physical examination findings. Underlying bony pathology can be confirmed with x-ray studies. Ultrasound imaging can be used to confirm the diagnosis. The differential diagnosis includes tumor and arterial aneurysm.[6]

Trigger Finger

Diagnostic tests are not indicated unless associated conditions are suspected. The differential diagnosis should include joint arthrosis, rheumatoid arthritis, flexor tendon rupture, tendon sheath cysts, and Dupuytren contracture. Associated conditions include diabetes, rheumatoid arthritis, and occupational or recreational vibration exposure.

Tenosynovitis

Diagnosis may be made with history and physical examination findings. Radiographs may be indicated to exclude fracture or arthritis. Complete blood count (CBC), ESR, ANAs, ACPAs, and rheumatoid factor may also be measured if rheumatoid arthritis is suspected. The differential diagnosis includes stenosing tenosynovitis of the thumb, fracture, and arthritis.

Palmar Fibrosis

Diagnosis may be made with history and physical examination findings, because Dupuytren contracture has a classic appearance. Differential diagnosis may include soft tissue tumor or tendon cyst.

Carpal Tunnel Syndrome

Diagnosis may be made with history and physical examination findings. Electrodiagnostic studies, such as EMG and nerve conduction studies (NCSs), can be helpful to confirm or exclude CTS. The differential diagnosis includes cervical radiculopathy, basal joint arthritis of the thumb, thoracic outlet syndrome, and polyneuropathy.[11]

Trapeziometacarpal Arthritis

X-ray studies are indicated to exclude fracture and to determine the stage of the disease. The differential diagnosis should also include infection, radial bursitis, tenosynovitis, and sprain.

DIAGNOSTICS

Hand and Wrist Pain

LABORATORY
Serum glucose*
TSH*
ESR*
ANAs*
Rheumatoid factor,* CRP,* ACPAs*

IMAGING
X-ray studies*
Ultrasound*

OTHER DIAGNOSTICS
EMG*

*If indicated.
CRP, C-reactive protein.

DIFFERENTIAL DIAGNOSIS

Hand and Wrist Pain

MUSCULOSKELETAL
- Fracture
- Sprain
- Strain
- Ganglion
- Stenosing tenosynovitis
- de Quervain disease
- Dupuytren contracture
- Carpal tunnel syndrome
- Cubital tunnel syndrome
- Trapeziometacarpal arthritis
- Rheumatoid arthritis
- Osteoarthritis
- Raynaud syndrome
- Gouty tophi

MANAGEMENT

Orthopedic physician consultation is indicated for patients in whom conservative treatment fails or in those who may benefit from surgical intervention.

Immediate emergency department or same-day orthopedic referral is indicated for patients with known or suspected fractures of the hand or wrist.

Reduction of risk factors, prevention of further injury, management of pain, restoration of function, and strengthening of muscle should be the primary goals of treatment.[3,4,11,12] Patients with mild symptoms are likely to respond to conservative management, including lifestyle modification, rest, splinting, and use of nonsteroidal anti-inflammatory drugs (NSAIDs). Treatment should be expedient and interdisciplinary to avoid prolonged disability. Referral to physical and occupational therapists can be extremely helpful. An early return to work and job retention are key to a full psychological as well as physical recovery. Vocational counseling may be needed in work-related injury cases.

Ganglion Cysts

Cysts may fluctuate in size and may resolve on their own. Aspiration or injection may be beneficial for dorsal ganglia or volar retinacular cysts. Clinicians should refrain from aspirating or injecting ganglia over the volar wrist aspect, because the radial artery is in close proximity.[7] Surgical excision of the ganglia may be indicated for symptomatic wrist ganglia.

Trigger Finger

Immediate orthopedic referral is indicated if the finger cannot be passively extended. Treatment of an associated condition, rest, NSAIDs, and splinting of the PIP joint of the affected finger are appropriate interventions.[6] A thumb spica splint should be applied to affected thumbs. If there is no improvement after 2 weeks, an orthopedic evaluation is indicated for possible corticosteroid injection or surgical release of the tendon.[7]

Tenosynovitis

Ice, NSAIDs, and continuous immobilization in a padded gutter splint are initially indicated; cortisone injection of the nodule may offer the greatest relief. An orthopedic referral is necessary if there is no improvement after 2 weeks.[6,13]

Palmar Fibrosis

Treatment depends on severity of disease. If contractures are interfering with function, a referral to a hand specialist for surgical excision of the fascia may be warranted. Goniometric measurements of the contracture (if present) should be noted. Patients with any contracture of more than 30 degrees should be referred to a hand specialist. Passive extension, NSAIDs, and cortisone injections have had less than impressive results and are not recommended.[8]

Carpal Tunnel Syndrome

Treatment consists of neutral wrist splints, NSAIDs, ice, and work-home modification (Box 177-1). Occupational therapy referral may be helpful for splint fabrication or workplace modification. If there is no improvement in 2 to 7 weeks, a referral to a hand specialist is indicated for steroid injection or surgical evaluation.[6,14]

BOX 177-1

Treatment of Carpal Tunnel Syndrome

- Rest or reduced activity
- Ice or cold packs to affected area
- NSAIDs (if no contraindications)
- Splinting at night
- Physical or occupational therapy
- Orthopedic, neurosurgical, or plastic surgery referral, if persistent symptoms
- Ergonomic adaptations to the work environment

Trapeziometacarpal Arthritis

The use of splinting and NSAIDs for 3 weeks is appropriate initially.[7] If relief is not achieved, a referral to an orthopedist for steroid injection is warranted.

LIFE SPAN CONSIDERATIONS

Older adults are at risk for hand and wrist pain from arthritis and fractures. Distal radius fractures are common, given the increased risk of falls and the prevalence of osteoporosis. An age-associated increase in the concentration of PTH may interfere with serum calcium concentration.

COMPLICATIONS

Contractures, deformity, and pain are significant complications of hand and wrist disorders. In addition, nerve compression can jeopardize the sensory function, motor function, and reflexes of the affected hand. These problems affect quality of life, work, and recreational activities. Although surgery may be indicated for hand disorders that are not responsive to conservative therapies, there is an inherent risk in any surgical procedure. Continued symptoms, reflex sympathetic dystrophy, nerve damage, and disfigurement are additional hazards associated with any surgical procedure of the hand or wrist.

INDICATIONS FOR REFERRAL OR HOSPITALIZATION

Hand and Wrist Pain

In absence of acute injury or pain, wrist pain may be managed by primary care clinicians if patients respond well to conservative treatment.

- Orthopedic referral is indicated for patients in whom conservative treatment fails or who may benefit from surgical intervention.
- Patients with a finger locked in flexion should receive a same-day referral to orthopedics.
- Immediate emergency department or same-day orthopedic referral is indicated for known or suspected fractures of the hand or wrist.

EDUCATION AND HEALTH PROMOTION

Patients should understand the importance of hourly 10-minute rest periods during activities that require repetitive hand movements. Splints that keep the wrist straight or slightly extended should be worn at night and, if necessary, during the day. Careful explanation of splint use is important because patients often remove the splint during activity, which results in further inflammation and a prolonged recovery period. Wrist splints can also be worn while sleeping to relieve discomfort during the night.

The use of cold packs and NSAID therapy should also be explained. Hand weakness, symptoms that increase in severity, or symptoms not relieved by conservative therapies should be reported to the health care provider.

Avoidance of overexertion and repetitive motions of the hand and wrist can prevent many cases of injury. Warming up and stretching of these muscles before activity may help decrease the risk of injury.[14] The use of proper body mechanics may also reduce the risk of injury. It may be necessary to arrange the work environment to allow more comfort and less strain on the body.[3] Taking frequent rest breaks during repetitive activities and doing strengthening exercises may help as well. Joint protection and energy conservation techniques and the use of adaptive equipment may be necessary for painful or arthritic hands.

CHAPTER 178

HIP PAIN

Ann S. Bruner-Welch

DEFINITION AND EPIDEMIOLOGY

Hip pain is a common complaint in primary care. It is a major source of discomfort and functional limitation, particularly in older patients, with a long list of potential causes.[1-3] It is helpful, therefore, to consider hip anatomy, patient age, and preceding history in teasing out the problem.[4] An accurate diagnosis and appropriate management are important in reducing the burden for both the patient and the family.

Hip pain may be broadly defined as any sensation of pain immediately surrounding or within the pelvic girdle. Limitations in range of motion are not uncommon, and activity or weight bearing frequently increases symptoms.[5]

Because hip pain is a symptom and not a specific disease entity, there is no epidemiologic pattern that describes the prevalence and incidence. Major causes of hip pain differ across age groups and may be categorized as traumatic or nontraumatic (Table 178-1).

Orthopedic consultation is indicated for patients with suspected hip dislocation, fracture, sepsis, end-stage degenerative joint disease that is failing to respond to conservative treatment, or osseous abnormalities that are seen radiographically.

PATHOPHYSIOLOGY

A review of hip and pelvic anatomy is the key to understanding the potential source of pain. The hip, like the shoulder, is a diarthrodial ball-and-socket synovial joint. The ball and socket of the hip joint is made up of the head of the proximal femur and the acetabulum or socket of the pelvis.[6] The acetabulum is composed of the ischium, pubis, and ilium within the pelvis. A cartilaginous labral lip makes the socket of the acetabulum deeper for stability but maintains flexibility for greater range of hip motion. Strong fibrous, stabilizing ligaments form the capsule that covers the entire hip joint. Articular cartilage covers the bone ends. Completely lining the capsule and extending down to the neck of the femur is the synovial membrane; it secretes synovial fluid, which provides lubrication for motion. Fluid-filled sacs (or bursae), found in spaces among the tendons, ligaments, and bones, reduce friction over bone prominences and permit ease of motion.[6]

The primary functions of the hip are weight bearing and locomotion. The muscles of the hip are essential in maintaining upright stability and gait. The muscles of the hip may be classified into five functional groups according to their action: abductors, flexors, adductors, extensors, and rotators. Musculotendinous pain of the hip may contribute to distortions of gait, producing a limp.

Any one of these structures may become inflamed, stretched, torn, infected, or worn out, causing pain. Crystalline deposits within the joint or surrounding tissues may also cause tissue destruction and pain.[7] In growing children, changes, injury, or irritation at growth plates can also cause pain.[7,8] The underlying cause of the pain is the result of the actual pathophysiologic process.

Active individuals can stress the bone and supporting soft tissue. Muscle, tendon, or ligament strains and sprains are common in more active individuals. Labral tears also typically occur in active individuals. Very active individuals can develop stress fractures.[9] Modulation in activity may be necessary for the joint to heal and the pain to resolve.

Bursitis (see Chapter 173) is an irritation and inflammation of the bursa, usually over bone prominences such as the greater

TABLE 178-1 Causes of Hip Pain and Age Groups Commonly Affected

Age Group	Traumatic Cause*	Nontraumatic Cause
Adolescents and young adults	SCFE† Stress fracture Sprains, strains	SCFE Juvenile arthritis, infectious arthritis
Adults	Stress fracture Sprains, strains	Bursitis or tendinitis, infectious arthritis Neuropathy, fasciitis, rheumatoid arthritis, osteoarthritis, sacroiliac joint dysfunction, piriformis syndrome, femoroacetabular impingement syndrome
Older adults	Hip fracture Dislocation	Osteoarthritis, bursitis, tendinitis, neuropathy, fasciitis Spinal stenosis, sacroiliac joint dysfunction, piriformis syndrome

*Avascular necrosis should always be ruled out for hip pain caused by trauma.
†Slipped capital femoral epiphysis (SCFE) may occur with or without trauma.

trochanter. It is common in individuals with lateral hip pain on ambulation and at night.[1-3,10] Osteoarthritis (OA) (see Chapter 184) is a breakdown or degeneration of the cartilage within the joint, causing bone ends to rub.[1-3,11] Rheumatoid arthritis (RA) (see Chapter 218) is an inflammatory, autoimmune, destructive joint process that frequently affects multiple joints and causes synovitis, pain, and stiffness.[1-3,12] The joint involvement in RA is often symmetric; therefore both hips may be painful. Psoriatic arthritis (see Chapter 215) is more common in men than in women and should be considered in individuals diagnosed with psoriasis.[5] Gout and pseudogout (see Chapter 176) leave crystalline deposits within the joint, leading to joint inflammation, acute-onset pain, and eventual cartilage destruction.[7]

Avascular necrosis is loss of blood supply and subsequent death of subchondral bone tissue; it is often related to trauma, alcohol intoxication, sickle cell anemia, or corticosteroid use.[1-3,13] Protease inhibitors, RA, or systemic lupus erythematosus (see Chapter 219) can also be causative. Avascular necrosis can occur in a number of sites in the body, including the femoral head, and can be bilateral. The cartilage remains intact; however, the bone beneath it becomes flattened and misshapen.[13]

Fractures and hip dislocations in younger to middle-aged people are most commonly associated with significant trauma, such as motor vehicle accidents or significant falls. They may be followed in primary care once they are stabilized. Low-impact trauma should not produce a significant fracture in young healthy adults. Fragility fractures at any age should prompt further bone density testing and endocrinology evaluation, including looking for secondary causes of osteopenia or osteoporosis (see Chapter 182), such as vitamin D deficiency, hyperparathyroidism, anorexia nervosa, female athlete triad, or other reversible causes of brittle bones.[1-3,14] Hip dislocations should be considered if there is a history of hip replacement surgery or congenital hip dislocation.

Infection (see Chapter 179) is uncommon but can be a devastating cause of rapid-onset hip pain and fever.[1-3,15] It can become indolent and recurrent, particularly with more virulent microbes. Recent dental work, skin infection, endocarditis, and intestinal procedures are frequent sources, particularly if a prosthesis is in place. In the adolescent and young adult, *Neisseria gonorrhoeae* is the most common causative organism.[15] In adults of all ages, *Staphylococcus aureus* is the usual source of infection, although other pathogens may be implicated. Methicillin-resistant *Staphylococcus aureus* (MRSA) is becoming a more common pathogen.[15]

Neoplasms can originate in the bone or metastasize to it and can cause anything from odd bone growths along the cortex to benign or destructive cystic lesions to complete bone destruction. All patients with questionable x-ray findings should be referred to a specialist promptly for further evaluation.[1-3,16] Multiple myeloma and osteosarcoma are the most common primary metastatic tumors (see Chapter 172).[16] These tumors frequently manifest as pathologic fractures. Benign bone tumors are frequently found incidentally on x-ray examination.[14]

Hip pain can also be referred from the back or sacroiliac joint. This cause can frequently be teased out during evaluation because hip motion does not affect the discomfort, but back or sacroiliac mobilization does.[1-6] Inguinal hernias can also cause hip pain and can be discovered during examination.[1-6] This anterior hip or groin pain or bulging usually increases with bearing down or lifting of heavy objects and is frequently associated with a history of straining before onset of pain.

Femoroacetabular impingement (FAI) syndrome is becoming recognized as a frequent cause of hip pain. Bone spurs develop along the edges of the acetabulum or femoral head, causing it to deform and become irregularly shaped, or the socket becomes deeper than it should be, or angled more posteriorly than normal. Any of these changes from normal increases friction between the socket and the femoral head or neck, and the shape mismatch increases cartilaginous wear and tearing of the labrum seal around the joint.[1-3,17,18] There are three types of impingement, depending on whether there is a cam action or pinching of the rim of the acetabulum, irritation of the femoral head or neck, or both. When symptoms develop, it usually indicates that damage to either the labrum or cartilage has occurred.[17,18]

Hip pain is much less common in children than in adults.[7,8] Congenital hip dislocation should be considered in infants and subsequent hip dysplasia in young children.[1-3,7,8] Apophysitis is a tendinitis in the growing skeleton found in childhood through young adolescence.[7,8] Legg-Calvé-Perthes disease is avascular necrosis of the femoral head found mostly in 4- to 8-year-old boys.[7,8]

Transient synovitis, a benign, self-limiting, but painful condition, is the most common cause of pain during childhood.[7,8] It can occur in growing bones, and the incidence typically decreases by age 12. Age 2 to 5 is most commonly affected age group. Causes can include allergic, traumatic, viral, or poststreptococcal toxic synovitis. Fever is rare. Restricted hip abduction is the most sensitive range of motion limitation.[6] Pain is worse in the morning and eases with activity.[7,8] Ruling out juvenile arthritis and sepsis is especially important, and following closely for the possible development of Legg-Calvé-Perthes disease is clearly indicated.

Slipped capital femoral epiphysis (SCFE), in which the growing femoral head and growth plate slip in relation to the remainder of the head and femoral neck, is most common in 11- to 14-year-olds and in boys more than girls. It can be traumatic or atraumatic. It is more common during periods of rapid growth, is associated with obesity, and can be bilateral.[1-3,7,8]

CLINICAL PRESENTATION

A careful history must be obtained from the patient, with particular attention to the history of the present illness. Any history of joint replacement and recent or old trauma to the hip and lower back or history of cancer should be sought. Pertinent questions related to age, location, onset, duration, severity, setting, timing, associated symptoms, and aggravating or alleviating factors will be useful in narrowing the diagnosis. Recent activity (vocational or recreational), skin problems (rashes, cuts, or abrasions), social habits, medications, procedures, surgery, trauma, or history of cancer may also prove helpful.[1,4]

Most patients with hip pain experience increased pain with activity. Pain with hip motion is more likely to be caused by hip disease, whereas painless hip motion is probably originating from another area, such as the back. Pain at rest may indicate inflammatory, infectious, or neoplastic disease.

Soft tissue sprains and strains are usually directly relatable to an activity such as sports, heavy lifting, or an unusual increase in physical activity and frequently include a report of sudden acceleration or deceleration, impact, movement, twist, stop in motion, drop of something, or similar anecdote.[9] Labral tears manifest similarly and may include popping, catching, or a sense of hip instability or giving way.[17]

Bursitis manifests with point tenderness and focal pain over the bursa. Any of the three major bursae surrounding the hip may be affected. Trochanteric bursitis is the most common form, with complaints of pain in the lateral hip over the greater trochanter.[10-12] The discomfort can also be posterior to the greater trochanter with radiation down the lateral thigh to the knee.[10-12] Ischiogluteal bursitis causes pain over the ischial tuberosity with radiation to the posterior thigh and is common in people who sit a lot or who have fallen. Pain in the groin with radiation to the anterior thigh may indicate iliopsoas bursitis. Pain will be aggravated with walking (see Chapter 173).

OA (see Chapter 184), or degenerative joint disease, affecting the hip will result in progressively worsening pain with activity and improvement with rest. Pain can be felt in the groin, buttock, or anterior thigh.[10,11] Often the patient is not able to determine the exact location of the pain as synovitis, muscle spasm, and capsular contracture progress. The pain is often accompanied by stiffness on first arising in the morning and after long periods of inactivity (gel phenomenon).[10,11] The duration of stiffness with OA is usually short, lasting only 5 to 30 minutes. Walking or prolonged standing will tend to aggravate the pain, and rest relieves it. When OA is the cause, pain or joint deformity may also be present in other joints of the body, especially the knees and the joints of the hands.[11]

The patient with septic or infectious arthritis of the hip will have a high fever, excruciating pain, and limited range of motion (see Chapter 179). It is important to obtain consultation as soon as a joint infection is suspected. Culture specimens should be obtained before any antibiotics are started because it can be tricky or impossible to find the pathogen once antibiotics have been given.[15]

In avascular necrosis, also called osteonecrosis, patients report a gradual onset of dull aching or throbbing pain in the groin or occasionally the lateral hip or buttock.[13] The condition can manifest 3 to 4 months after a nonsurgical hip fracture if the blood supply to the femoral head was disrupted.[13,19-21]

Adolescence should suggest other pathologic considerations. SCFE can manifest suddenly or with the insidious onset of moderate to severe hip, thigh, or knee pain associated with a limp, especially in an 11- to 14-year-old adolescent.[8] SCFE is also associated with obesity; more than half of affected adolescents exceed the 95th percentile for weight and age.[7,8] Delayed sexual maturity may also be evident.

Other considerations for the younger patient should include Legg-Calvé-Perthes disease in the 4- to 8-year-old with progressive groin pain with limp.[7,8] Avascular necrosis of the femoral head develops as the disease progresses. Apophysitis is a tendinitis within a growing skeleton and is not uncommon among athletic youth.[7,8] Transient synovitis should be considered in growing children as well. These children will have a history of recent growth spurt, injury, viral infection, or poststreptococcal infection. RA should be considered for chronic hip pain. RA is usually symmetric, affecting multiple small and large joints.[12]

PHYSICAL EXAMINATION

The back, sacroiliac joints, hips, knees, and ankles should be examined. The examination should include general observation and vital signs; and for each area examined, inspection, palpation, range of motion, strength, and stability should be assessed. Two tests of hip function during physical examination are essential: gait and range of motion. A good neurologic examination is also important.

With true hip joint disease, the gait may be affected by a limp (antalgic gait) that is characterized by an exaggerated swaying motion of the upper body toward the painful hip while walking (Trendelenburg gait).[2,5] Motion restrictions of abduction and internal rotation are usually more pronounced than restriction of adduction and external rotation. Pain, muscle spasm, and guarding are noted with passive and active range of motion. Inspection may reveal a flexion contracture of the hip and atrophy of the musculature of the buttocks. Crepitus of the joint may be felt or heard with palpation and movement. Infection may also manifest with fever, limited motion, and exquisite pain with motion.

Bursitis, particularly over the greater trochanter, typically manifests with point tenderness over the lateral prominence.[10] Hip flexion and internal rotation may exacerbate the pain. Stress fractures (usually of the femoral neck) will cause pain in the groin of anterior thigh with (usually) a pronounced limp.[9]

In the older patient, fracture should be suspected if there is a history of a fall or rotational injury to the hip.[14,21] The patient will report hip, groin, or thigh pain and will be unable to bear weight or to move the leg well. The affected extremity will often be shortened and externally rotated.[20,21]

In the adolescent patient with SCFE, significant muscle spasm and restricted internal rotation will be evident.[7,8] With transient synovitis, patients will be able to bear weight; however, they will have restricted abduction.[7,8]

DIAGNOSTICS

The diagnosis of hip pain is made initially on the basis of history and clinical examination of the patient. X-ray examination is typically the next step in assessing the hip if something more than soft tissue disease is suspected. X-ray studies should include an anteroposterior (AP) view of the pelvis and frog-leg and lateral views of the hip. Two views of the lumbosacral spine can be added if the examination findings suggest back disease. Weight-bearing films are important to assess the extent of joint degeneration and joint space narrowing when fracture is not suspected. The x-ray findings for transient synovitis will be normal.[8,22]

If inflammatory causes are suspected, a complete blood count (CBC), erythrocyte sedimentation rate (ESR), C-reactive protein (CRP) level, anti–cyclic citrullinated protein (anti-CCP) antibodies, and rheumatoid factor should be obtained.[10,12,22] Uric acid is added if gout is suspected.[7] If there

DIAGNOSTICS

Hip Pain

LABORATORY*
- CBC and differential
- ESR
- Rheumatoid factor, anti-CCP antibodies
- CRP
- Uric acid

IMAGING
- X-ray examination
- MRI*

OTHER DIAGNOSTICS
- Joint aspiration for culture and sensitivity, crystalline deposits, and cell count*

*If indicated.

is radiographic evidence of effusion, joint aspiration performed under fluoroscopic guidance is indicated. Aspirate is sent for culture and sensitivity, cell count with differential, and identification of crystalline deposits.

If avascular necrosis is suspected, magnetic resonance imaging (MRI) is the diagnostic test of choice. MRI is not as sensitive in identifying cartilaginous changes of the joint as computed tomography (CT).[13] If rheumatic causes are suspected, a rheumatoid panel is added.[13,22] Nerve conduction studies should be considered to rule out neuropathy if indicated, and a bone density test should be done in the case of fragility fractures.[14,21]

DIFFERENTIAL DIAGNOSIS

It is helpful to consider the patient's age, the location of the pain, and the preceding activities to determine the most likely source. Although the most common cause of hip pain in the older adult is OA, other diagnostic possibilities should be considered, especially if there is no relief of symptoms with standard treatment and the medical history points in other directions. Fractures, dislocations, inflammatory arthritis, infections, metastases, and avascular necrosis are other important causes of hip pain.[5]

Minimum force applied to the hip joint may produce a fracture, especially in the older woman with osteoporosis. Vitamin D deficiency is a growing concern for fragility fractures in younger patients. In patients who are runners or who participate in sports, a femoral stress fracture should also be considered as a cause of hip pain.[9]

Traumatic dislocations are more often seen in young patients who engage in activities with a risk for violent injury. Atraumatic hip dislocations should be considered in patients with sudden hip pain if they have undergone prior hip replacement surgery.[19,20] Infection should be considered if fever is present with hip pain.[15] Avascular necrosis should be considered if pain is subacute or chronic, especially if there is a history of trauma, autoimmune disease, or steroid use.[5,13,]

Extra-articular causes of hip pain include referred pain from degenerative disks, spinal stenosis, sacroiliac dysfunction, leg length discrepancies, bursitis, malignant neoplasms, Paget disease, and osteomyelitis.[5] Neuropathic pain of diabetes, alcoholism, and vitamin B_{12} deficiency as well as vascular diseases such as atherosclerosis, diabetes, and vasculitis need to be considered when systemic disease is present or with atypical findings.[5,23]

Infection of the hip joint is rare in adults, although this should be considered in children or adults with a prosthetic hip and new-onset hip pain and fever. Patients in whom septic arthritis of the hip develops are typically immunocompromised because of corticosteroids or chemotherapeutic agents. Injection drug users are also at increased risk for joint infection. Antibiotic-resistant microorganisms such as MRSA are becoming a community-acquired phenomenon in addition to nosocomial infection.

In children, transient synovitis is the most common cause of hip pain, but other causes including congenital hip dysplasia or Legg-Calvé-Perthes disease should also be considered for indolent pain. An important cause of hip pain in the adolescent is SCFE, which may or may not be associated with trauma. Although the underlying cause is unclear, SCFE is most likely to be seen during the growth spurt at age 10 to 15 years. The typical patient is an obese male adolescent. Juvenile arthritis is another important consideration in children or adolescents because it can lead to complete joint destruction with the need for hip replacement in early adulthood.[12]

> **DIFFERENTIAL DIAGNOSIS**
>
> **Hip Pain**
>
> - RA
> - OA
> - Septic arthritis
> - Joint infection
> - Malignant neoplasm
> - Sprain
> - Strain
> - Fracture
> - Traumatic dislocation
> - Bursitis or tendinitis
> - Fasciitis
> - Septic sacroiliitis
> - Osteomyelitis
> - Cellulitis
> - Gout
> - Pseudogout
> - Sickle cell disease
> - Avascular necrosis
> - Osteoporosis
> - Paget disease
> - Neuropathy
> - Vascular disease with claudication
> - Transient synovitis
> - Femoral acetabular impingement

MANAGEMENT

Hip pain is a symptom of an underlying pathophysiologic process. Although hip pain itself has the potential to produce functional limitations and to impair quality of life, the management should be directed toward identification and treatment of the underlying cause of the pain. Evidence-based practice in treating the adult patient with hip pain is focused on the various causes of the hip pain reviewed earlier.

Pain management is a major issue for patients with OA involving the hip. Although most randomized controlled trials have focused on OA of the knee, some have demonstrated benefits of using nonsteroidal anti-inflammatory drugs (NSAIDs) and acetaminophen analgesics for relief of hip pain.[11] There is no clear evidence that either class of analgesic is superior; however, acetaminophen may be better tolerated by older adults and is the first-line recommendation.[11] NSAID gels and patches are promising. Lidocaine patches are helpful to some patients. Capsaicin, an over-the-counter topical analgesic, has also been shown to provide short-term pain relief and has fewer side effects than oral agents.[24,25] The adverse effect most commonly reported for topical agents is local skin irritation. For pain related to bursitis, tendinitis, or traumatic injury, NSAIDs will likely be more effective in controlling the pain and promoting mobility.[11] Adding glucosamine or glucosamine chondroitin, or other alternative dietary supplements such as *S*-adenosylmethionine (SAM-*e*) or methylsulfonylmethane (MSM), may be helpful for some patients.[24,25]

Fluoroscopically guided intra-articular injection of corticosteroids may be helpful for arthritis patients; however, the effects wane as disease progresses. Corticosteroids leave deposits within the joint and can cause further joint degradation; thereby the frequency with which they are administered should be limited to three times a year or less. These agents should be given only with the guidance of an orthopedic or rheumatologic specialist or an interventional radiologist.

Nonpharmacologic measures are aimed at restoration and maintenance of function of the joint as an adjunct to pharmacologic therapy.[11,23] Recommendations for complete rest or inactivity of the joint should be given only after careful weighing of the risk versus benefit. Muscle atrophy, weakness, and generalized deconditioning may result and contribute to the primary problem. This is especially true in the older population. Evidence for benefit does exist for exercise and education for reducing pain, with the strongest evidence pointing to the benefits of exercise.[23] Exercise also improves functional status and provides a sense of well-being. Physical therapists can be helpful in developing an appropriate exercise regimen. Range of motion and low-stress, low-impact exercises should be prescribed. An aquatic exercise program may promote mobility while relieving mechanical weight bearing on the joint.[23] The use of heat before and ice after exercise can also alleviate pain.

Ultimately, surgery may be the best option for relief of pain and restoration of function. Total joint replacement is an extremely effective intervention for patients with painful OA or avascular necrosis, even in the older adult.[19,20] Surgical intervention may also be indicated for septic arthritis, instability, and FAI.[9,17-20] Of course, surgical repair of hip fracture is performed in almost every instance. Consultation with an orthopedic surgeon is needed whenever surgery is considered.

COMPLICATIONS

Complications of hip pain depend on the cause. Osteoporosis of the hip may result in a fracture with or without trauma. Chronic pain accompanied by loss of function and mobility may result in deconditioning and falls with injury. Older patients in particular should be monitored for gastrointestinal and renal side effects if they are taking NSAIDs. An adolescent with SCFE has a guarded long-term prognosis for repeated injury, contralateral disease, and complications.[7] Avascular necrosis of the femoral head may occur in approximately 30% of patients with SCFE.[7,19,20] Premature development of degenerative arthritis may occur with or without avascular necrosis.[13,19,20] Congenital hip dislocations can lead to chronic pain, gait impairment, early onset arthritis, and need for surgical intervention at a young age if not screened for and treated early.[19,20]

INDICATIONS FOR REFERRAL OR HOSPITALIZATION

Hip pain requires an ongoing assessment of the patient's functional capabilities and relief of painful symptoms. A multidisciplinary approach involving a physical therapist and an occupational therapist is indicated. Physical therapy improves joint mobility and prevents the complications of joint disuse. Occupational therapists may assist patients with limitations of function by adapting activities of daily living and providing assistive devices for optimum independence. Referral to an orthopedic surgeon for consideration of surgery is indicated for patients with late- to end-stage OA, joint infection, or avascular necrosis and for those with progressive loss of function or refractory pain. Urgent referral is required for patients with infection, hip fracture, and dislocation.

PATIENT AND FAMILY EDUCATION AND HEALTH PROMOTION

Chronic joint pain can be mentally and physically wearing on patients and family. A multidisciplinary approach to care with the patient as an active participant in the decision-making process may prove more satisfactory for everyone in the long term. The patient is entitled to an explanation about the source of the pain and whether it is likely to be temporary or chronic. Facilitating the patient's understanding of anticipated outcomes and prognosis is extremely beneficial in strengthening the patient-provider relationship.

Health-promoting activities should be directed toward maintenance and preservation of function of the joint. The management of a painful hip may include range-of-motion and muscle-strengthening exercises as recommended by the physical therapist. Maintenance of optimum weight should be encouraged because excess weight places tremendous stresses on the hip. The patient taking NSAIDs should take these medications with food and be knowledgeable of the signs and symptoms of gastrointestinal irritation. Renal function should be monitored, particularly in older patients. Alternative or herbal supplementation with glucosamine and glucosamine chondroitin appear to be effective in some patients and can be encouraged, although evidence is lacking.[24,25] Assessment of the home environment and the need for ambulatory assistive devices is warranted to reduce the risk of falls, especially in older or frailer patients.

CHAPTER 179

INFECTIOUS ARTHRITIS

Kevin D. Kerin

A septic joint is a medical emergency.

DEFINITION AND EPIDEMIOLOGY

Inflammation of a joint is called arthritis and is an observable finding, whereas pain in a joint is called arthralgia and is a subjective description. One important type of arthritis is infectious arthritis, considered to be a medical emergency. Infectious arthritis can be caused by a large number of organisms, including bacteria, fungi, viruses, and filariae. The term *septic arthritis* is most commonly used to describe arthritis caused by a bacterial pathogen. An infectious cause of joint inflammation needs to be considered even when a noninfectious type of inflammatory arthritis (rheumatoid arthritis, gout) has been previously diagnosed. Bacterial and viral arthritides usually manifest acutely with systemic and articular symptoms. In contrast, Lyme disease and mycobacterial, fungal, filarial, and some bacterial arthritides (*Neisseria gonorrhoeae, Neisseria meningitidis*) may be subacute or chronic and relatively indolent. Infectious arthritis is seen in all age groups, although the highest incidence is in children and the elderly.

PATHOPHYSIOLOGY

Synovial joints such as the knee and hip are particularly vulnerable to infection. Abnormal synovial joints, such as those previously damaged by other traumatic, inflammatory, or degenerative processes, are especially susceptible to infection. One explanation is that synovial tissue is highly vascularized, lacks a basement membrane, and is thus susceptible to the hematogenous spread of infectious organisms from a locus of infection.[1] Other avenues of infection of the joint space include extension of infection from osteomyelitis or adjacent soft tissue infection and direct inoculation from penetration of a foreign body. A joint infection is a medical emergency and can be a rapid, severely destructive process. Once a bacterial infection is established in a joint space, a complex cascade of events follows: changes in synovial tissue; migration of acute and chronic inflammatory cells to the joint space; release of inflammatory cytokines, proteases, and collagenases; changes in intra-articular fluid volume and pressure; and chondrocyte changes.[2]

Staphylococcus aureus is the most common cause of acute bacterial arthritis across all age groups.[2] Its affinity for joints can be explained in part by the structure of the microbe, which elaborates certain surface and secreted proteins that may facilitate colonization of tissue. This organism also has receptors for glycoproteins found in joints and has frequent access by hematogenous seeding from minor wounds and abrasions because of its presence as normal skin flora. Streptococci are also considered to be normal skin flora, and are second only to *S. aureus* as causative agents of infectious arthritis. *N. gonorrhoeae* is the most common cause of infectious arthritis from a sexually transmitted bacterium and is most frequently seen in sexually active adults younger than 30 years.[3] This is not unexpected, given the ease with which *N. gonorrhoeae* invades the bloodstream during menses or parturition and after acute urethritis. Gram-negative bacilli cause approximately 10% of cases of septic arthritis, often in older adults and neonates, and are associated with a better outcome than gram-positive infections.[4] In a community-based study of septic arthritis in native joints, older age and limited range of motion were predictors for gram-positive cocci as the cause, whereas diabetes mellitus with end-organ damage and malignant change were predictors for gram-negative bacteria.[4] Anaerobes are an uncommon cause of infectious arthritis and are associated with human bites, intra-abdominal abscesses, and periarticular decubitus ulcers.[5] Alphavirus infection, after initial febrile illness, may progress to cause a polyarticular inflammatory arthritis that bears similarity to seronegative rheumatoid arthritis. Chikungunya viral arthritis (transmitted by mosquito) is an example of an alphavirus and appeared in the United States in 2014.[6,7]

CLINICAL PRESENTATION

Septic arthritis usually manifests with the acute onset of a painful, red, swollen joint that is warm to the touch. An important historical point that helps distinguish septic arthritis from sterile inflammation is that the affected joint is painful at rest as well as with motion and weight bearing. The rapid accumulation of fluid volume and rise in intra-articular pressure are prime contributors to rest pain. The affected joint will be held in a position that allows maximum intra-articular volume. The pain of arthritis from other causes usually is relieved with rest. Fever in a patient with septic arthritis is usually present but may be low grade or absent (especially in older adults); rigors caused by bacteremia may also be present. Fever and rigors have low sensitivity and specificity in the diagnosis of septic arthritis because these findings may also be seen in acute crystal-induced arthritis. Any joint may be involved in infectious arthritis, yet the knee and hip are the most commonly affected. Septic arthritis in an unusual location, such as the sternoclavicular or sacroiliac joint, should raise the suspicion of injection drug use.[8] The sudden onset of monoarticular arthritis is the usual presentation of nongonococcal arthritis, although a polyarticular presentation is not unusual. A polyarticular septic arthritis is sometimes seen with streptococcal or staphylococcal infections but usually affects only two or three joints (pauciarticular).

Infectious arthritis occurs more commonly in patients with an impaired immune system and in those with preexisting joint abnormalities, such as rheumatoid arthritis, gout, osteoarthritis, or a prosthetic joint. It is important to consider infection as a cause of an acute monoarticular or pauciarticular flare, even in those with an established diagnosis of a chronic rheumatologic condition. The fever and joint inflammation are less striking in gonococcal arthritis, which is characterized by a migrating polyarticular course.[9] Human immunodeficiency virus (HIV) infection with the associated immunosuppression is a special situation in which septic arthritis is uncommon; however, when it is seen, it may be a result of atypical organisms, such as *Mycobacterium tuberculosis, Sporothrix schenckii,* and *Candida albicans,* in addition to more common organisms such as *S. aureus* and *N. gonorrhoeae.*[10]

PHYSICAL EXAMINATION

The manifestations of inflammation were vividly described by Celsus in the first century AD as rubor, tumor, calor, and dolor (redness, swelling, heat, and pain). The inflamed joint is erythematous, warm to the touch, swollen, and painful, with passive and active range of motion. Synovial effusion is usually present, although it is less obvious in certain joints, such as the hip and shoulder. A large effusion creates an asymmetry in size with loss of anatomic landmarks. A smaller effusion in the knee may be detected by a "bulge sign" (the examiner presses on the medial aspect of the knee to displace fluid toward the suprapatellar region and then looks for a small bulge in this area after applying pressure on the opposite side of the knee) or patellar ballottement (see Fig. 173-8) (the examiner taps on the patella while applying pressure to the suprapatellar area to try to elicit a "click," signifying synovial fluid beneath the patella).

Decreased range of motion, muscle spasm, and apprehension to joint examination are prominent features of the examination. The proximal lymph node may be enlarged and tender, indicative of proximal lymphangitic spread of infection. An original source of infection, such as an abscess, cellulitis, gonococcal urethritis, pneumonia, urinary tract infection, or endocarditis, should be sought. Distinct clinical presentations are seen in special situations, which are discussed in the following sections.

Gonococcal Arthritis

Disseminated gonococcal infection (see Chapter 153) is the most common cause of septic arthritis in sexually active adolescents and young adults.[11] There appear to be two distinct clinical presentations. One has been called the arthritis-dermatitis syndrome and reflects a bacteremic stage; the other is a localized septic arthritis.[11] The classic triad of clinical findings in disseminated infection is dermatitis, tenosynovitis, and a migratory polyarthritis. The first group is distinguished by tenosynovitis and dermatitis. Skin lesions are present in countable numbers and multiple stages; these lesions are most often maculopapular but are sometimes necrotic, pustular, or vesicular. The lesions are painless and nonpruritic and typically spare the face and scalp. The lesions resolve in several days without scarring.[12] An asymmetric migratory polyarthralgia that affects knees, elbows, wrists, ankles, metacarpophalangeal joints, and associated tendon sheaths is the presentation more common than actual polyarthritis. Synovial fluid cell counts are lower than those commonly seen in bacterial arthritis, and the synovial fluid culture is often negative. The blood culture may be positive. Only 25% of patients have genitourinary symptoms of gonorrhea.[3]

The more focal septic arthritis seen in the second group may occur after a migratory polyarthritis, tenosynovitis, or dermatitis, with the arthritis now settled in one or two joints. The synovial fluid is more purulent, and the culture is more likely to be positive. Blood cultures are typically negative. Taken as a group, cultures of the pharynx, cervix, urethra, and rectum are positive in up to 80% of patients if specimens are obtained early on selective media (e.g., Thayer-Martin).[3] Synovial fluid culture specimens should be plated directly onto chocolate agar.

There may be clinical uncertainty about the diagnosis, especially in the context of a wide range of synovial fluid leukocyte counts and negative blood cultures. In this situation, ceftriaxone, 1 g/day intravenously for 24 hours, can be a valid diagnostic and appropriate therapeutic strategy.

Prosthetic Joint Infection

Millions of people have prosthetic joints, and it is estimated that approximately 4 million knee or hip arthroplasties will be performed annually by the year 2030.[13] Although the rates of infection after hip or knee arthroplasty have declined significantly to approximately 1%,[14] the large number of current and projected prosthetic joints makes this a relatively common problem. It is a serious, potentially devastating problem and is associated with major disability and cost. In most cases, in patients not considered to be too frail or poor surgical candidates, the prosthetic joint needs to be removed, and the patient will require up to 6 weeks of intravenous antibiotics (with or without an antibiotic-impregnated cement spacer), followed by reimplantation of a new prosthetic joint once infection has been eradicated.[15] Biofilms, complex microbial communities formed by bacteria causing prosthetic joint infections, contribute to antibiotic resistance.[16] Coagulase-negative staphylococci are common in this clinical setting and produce an indolent course. Hematogenous seeding at the bone-cement interface with *S. aureus* or group A streptococci may manifest more acutely with sepsis or toxic shock, which is characteristic of these more virulent organisms.[16]

Infections in older patients with underlying disease may include gram-negative bacilli (15% to 20%) and anaerobes (7%).[17]

One way to classify prosthetic joint infections is by the amount of time elapsed since joint surgery: early (within 3 months), delayed (3 to 24 months), and late (>24 months). Early and delayed infections have their origin at the time of prosthetic placement, whereas late infections are caused by hematogenous seeding of bacteria. Infection in a prosthetic joint is often difficult to diagnose, and clinical manifestations may vary by the timing of the infection in relation to the surgery. As a rule, most patients have joint pain with or without radiographic evidence of loosening of the prosthesis. A minority of patients have fever, joint swelling, or sinus track drainage. It may be difficult to differentiate a delayed-onset infection of a prosthetic joint from a noninfectious inflammation, such as a reaction to components of the prosthetic joint or a mechanical problem with the hardware (e.g., loosening, dislocation, hemarthrosis, and malposition).[18] A helpful observation is that mechanical problems are painful during motion, weight bearing, and pivoting but are comfortable while at rest. Constant joint pain suggests an infection.

Laboratory tests such as acute-phase reactants (erythrocyte sedimentation rate [ESR], C-reactive protein [CRP]) and leukocyte count are not especially helpful because a number of inflammatory conditions can cause elevated levels in any of these tests, and normal values do not rule out infection. Plain radiographs may be helpful, especially if serial studies are available for comparison. Classic radiographic findings of infection include lucencies along the bone-cement interface, migration of the prosthesis, and periosteal reactions. These findings are not present in acute or early infections and are difficult to differentiate from mechanical complications in those with delayed-onset infections. A technetium bone scan may take up to 1 year to become normal after surgery[19] because of bone remodeling, yet a normal bone scan provides strong evidence against an infected prosthetic joint if the timing is right. Other radiologic techniques, such as sequential bone and gallium scanning or combined leukocyte-marrow scintigraphy, have shown greater accuracy in the diagnosis of a prosthetic joint infection, but are costly, time-consuming, and not widely available. Ultimately, the diagnosis of a prosthetic joint infection relies on aggressive attempts to isolate an organism by obtaining joint fluid or tissue.

The recommendations to patients with prosthetic joints about antibiotic prophylaxis for dental procedures are debated and confusing, with conflicting recommendations over the years. Currently, the American Academy of Orthopaedic Surgeons recommends that clinicians consider antibiotic prophylaxis for essentially all patients with prosthetic joints before dental procedures.[20] A case-control study concluded, however, that dental procedures are not risk factors for infection of knee or hip prosthetic joints.[21]

Lyme Disease

The clinical manifestations of Lyme disease can be separated into early localized disease (1 to 30 days), early disseminated disease (days to 10 months), and late disease (months to years) on the basis of the elapsed time from tick exposure to symptoms (see Chapter 234). Only 30% of patients with Lyme disease recall a tick bite, but in the setting of known tick exposure, 80% of patients with early, localized Lyme disease experience arthralgias or migratory arthritis.[22] During this stage, the characteristic rash (erythema chronicum migrans) appears with an expanding red border and central clearing, occasionally creating the classic bull's eye appearance. Fever, headache, myalgias, arthralgias, and lymphadenopathy may be more noticeable than the skin lesions, which are usually painless.

The manifestations of early, disseminated Lyme disease include multiple systemic features: cardiac problems (pericarditis, atrioventricular nodal heart block, and myopathy), neurologic problems, and musculoskeletal problems (migratory polyarthralgias or polyarthritis) in 50%.[22] More prolonged attacks of true arthritis develop in a few joints. In late Lyme disease, about 60% of patients have a migratory polyarthritis and 10% of patients develop a chronic arthritis that settles in one or two large joints, usually the knees.[23]

In Lyme disease, the causative spirochete, *Borrelia burgdorferi*, is difficult to culture from synovial fluid, but sensitive methods of antigen detection, such as enzyme-linked immunosorbent assay (ELISA) and polymerase chain reaction (PCR), can reveal its presence. Having a high index of suspicion in the right clinical setting is essential to establishing the diagnosis. In the wrong clinical setting (without sufficiently high pretest probability), serologic tests for Lyme disease are misleading because of the high false-positive rate; therefore, such tests should not be ordered indiscriminantly.[22] All patients with true arthritis attributed to early, disseminated, or late Lyme disease should have a positive response on the Lyme ELISA, subsequently confirmed by Western blot.

The outcome is better if diagnosis and treatment are rendered early in this form of infectious arthritis. Medical therapy fails in approximately 50% of patients with late Lyme disease arthritis; progressive joint destruction may then merit synovectomy or total joint arthroplasty.[23]

Injection Drug Use

Infectious arthritis in unusual or axial locations (e.g., sacroiliac joint, sternoclavicular joint, symphysis pubis) should raise suspicion of injection drug use. Similarly, the presence of unusual organisms—*Pseudomonas aeruginosa, Serratia marcescens,* and *Candida* species—in joint fluid should lead to open-ended and nonjudgmental queries about recreational drug use. Still, most of the joint infections in these joints are caused by *S. aureus* with or without injection drug use.[24] Methicillin-resistant *Staphylococcus aureus* (MRSA) is the most common pathogen.[25] In patients who use injection recreational drugs, disseminated gonococcal disease, HIV infection, and syphilis should also be considered in the differential diagnosis.

Septic Sacroiliitis

Septic sacroiliitis can be an elusive diagnosis for health care providers because of the nonspecific nature of presenting symptoms. Patients may have fever and low back pain or gluteal region pain that is intensified by ambulation.[26] The physical examination alone is inadequate in distinguishing sacroiliitis from muscle pain, intervertebral disk disease, femoral nerve entrapment in the buttocks (piriformis muscle syndrome), or bursitis. Certain physical examination maneuvers have been devised to try to isolate and stress the sacroiliac joints. Plain radiographs are not helpful in early diagnosis. Focal pain that occurs when shear forces are applied to the sacroiliac joint may indicate septic sacroiliitis, in which case the patient should be referred immediately for a computed tomography (CT) scan or magnetic resonance imaging (MRI). MRI is uniquely suited to this difficult diagnosis because it alone has the potential to define fluid in the sacroiliac joint, adjacent bone marrow inflammation, and soft tissue abscesses that may extend into the abdominal cavity and the psoas, iliac, and piriform muscles. Because of the complexity of the involved joints and difficult access, these collections need pigtail catheter drainage or surgical debridement.[26]

DIAGNOSTICS

In patients with infectious arthritis, increases in the peripheral white blood cell (WBC) count, ESR, and CRP level are frequent but nonspecific findings. Peripheral blood cultures are positive in 40% of cases and are the only sources of microorganisms in 10% of cases.[27] Younger patients suspected of having gonococcal arthritis should have pharyngeal, rectal, and cervical or urethral cultures on specialized gonococcal media.[3] The most important examination for the diagnosis of infectious arthritis is synovial fluid, not only for culture but also for cellular and chemical analysis. Aspiration of inflamed joints provides three important pieces of information: diagnosis of crystal-induced arthritis, degree of inflammation (cell count), and specimen for Gram stain and culture. Any joint suspected of infection should be aspirated without delay because the outcome of infectious arthritis depends on early diagnosis and treatment. Sterile technique should be used, and the provider should avoid entering the joint through an area of skin that may be infected. It is important to send blood and synovial fluid culture specimens for analysis before antibiotics are started.

The most useful component of synovial fluid analysis consists of evaluation for crystals, cell count and differential, protein, Gram stain, and cultures (aerobic and anaerobic). Synovial fluid WBC and granulocyte percentage are especially useful in determining likelihood of septic arthritis before Gram stain and cultures have been completed.[28] Synovial fluid protein and glucose concentrations are less useful diagnostic tests. Synovial fluid protein is significantly elevated in both infectious arthritis and other forms of inflammatory arthritis. Synovial fluid glucose concentration of less than 40 mg/dL or less than 50% of a simultaneous blood glucose concentration is supportive evidence for bacterial arthritis. Synovial fluid lactic acid has high negative predictive value for bacterial arthritis yet is not widely used.[2] With chronic synovitis, fungal and mycobacterial culture specimens are also sent for analysis, and special stains for acid-fast bacteria and fungi are performed. Synovial fluid WBC counts may be very high (Table 179-1); cell counts in the 100,000/mm^3 range are considered to indicate infection until proven otherwise.[28] There is a considerable overlap in synovial WBC counts among infectious and noninfectious causes of arthritis. Gout, reactive arthritis, and rheumatoid arthritis may cause high cell counts normally associated with sepsis, whereas early infectious arthritis or established gonococcal arthritis may cause relatively low cell counts. The predominance of

TABLE 179-1 Synovial Fluid Analysis

Characteristic	Normal	Noninflammatory (Osteoarthritis)	Inflammatory (Rheumatoid)	Septic (Infection)
Volume	<3.5 mL	>3.5 mL	Large	Large
Clarity	Clear	Transparent	Translucent	Opaque
WBCs/mm^3	<200	200-2000	2000-75,000	50,000-100,000
Polymorphonuclear leukocytes	<25%	<25%	>50%	>75%
Culture	Negative	Negative	Negative	Positive
Glucose concentration	Equal to blood	Equal to blood	>50% blood glucose	<50% blood glucose
Protein level	1.7 g/dL	<3 g/dL	>3 g/dL	>3 g/dL

polymorphonuclear leukocytes in synovial fluid is a clue, but it is specific only if it exceeds 85%. Intracellular crystals and the profusion of polymorphonuclear cells suggest gout or pseudogout, but free-floating crystals are sometimes seen in infectious arthritis. Synovial fluid PCR may be used to diagnose gonococcal arthritis and Lyme disease arthritis.

Radiographs are not useful in the initial diagnosis of a septic joint. It may take 2 weeks for joint space narrowing and marginal erosions to be demonstrated, too late to salvage a functional joint. Radiographs are useful in identifying underlying arthritis or osteomyelitis. A three-phase technetium bone scan is helpful in differentiating cellulitis, infectious arthritis, and osteomyelitis.[29] Musculoskeletal ultrasound is an increasingly popular imaging technology and can identify small amounts of fluid and inflammatory changes in the articular and periarticular structures. However, arthrocentesis is a better diagnostic tool. Bone scan, gallium scan, and indium leukocyte scan are of little practical value. A CT scan or MRI is advantageous in difficult diagnostic situations (e.g., sternoclavicular or sacroiliac joint involvement) and as a guide to joint aspiration and anatomic definition of an infected hip.[30]

DIAGNOSTICS

Infectious Arthritis

LABORATORY
Complete blood count and differential
ESR
CRP
Blood cultures
Rectal, cervical, urethral, or pharyngeal cultures*
Lyme ELISA, Western blot test*

IMAGING
X-ray studies
CT scan, MRI*

OTHER DIAGNOSTICS
Joint aspiration of synovial fluid for crystals, culture, cell count, and Gram stain

*If indicated.

DIFFERENTIAL DIAGNOSIS

A synovial fluid leukocyte count of more than 2000/mm^3 is considered inflammatory, and a cell count of more than 50,000/mm^3 is considered septic until proven otherwise by Gram stain and cultures.[31] There is a significant overlap in synovial fluid leukocyte counts in inflammatory conditions from infectious and noninfectious causes. Other types of inflammatory arthritis are distinguished from infectious arthritis by culture and Gram stain; however, gout, reactive arthritis, and rheumatoid arthritis may accrue cell counts in the infectious arthritis range. In such situations, antibiotics should be initiated until cultures are finalized.

DIFFERENTIAL DIAGNOSIS

Rheumatic Disorders

- Bursitis
- Gout
- Pseudogout
- Rheumatoid arthritis
- Reactive arthritis
- Rheumatic fever
- Osteoarthritis
- Osteomyelitis
- Cellulitis

Cellulitis, bursitis, and acute osteomyelitis should be distinguished by their greater range of motion and less than circumferential swelling. Polyarticular infectious arthritis is sometimes seen with staphylococci and streptococci but may also suggest metastatic foci resulting from subacute bacterial endocarditis. Polyarticular noninfectious arthritis is seen with rheumatic fever or poststreptococcal reactive arthritis. In either case, the joint is not the focus of the streptococcal infection. The arthritis of rheumatic fever is migratory and resolves spontaneously in 1 month. Another form of acute reactive arthritis, previously called Reiter syndrome and now known as reactive arthritis, may be accompanied by urethritis, conjunctivitis, and enthesopathy (i.e., inflamed tendon insertions) (see Chapter 215).

DIFFERENTIAL DIAGNOSIS

Infectious Arthritis

- S. aureus and streptococci
- Gram-negative organisms (injection drug use, neonatal, older adults)
- Gonococcal arthritis
- Prosthetic joint (coagulase-negative staphylococci)
- Lyme disease
- Septic sacroiliitis
- Viral infection
- Mycobacterial or fungal infection

MANAGEMENT

Early initiation of antimicrobial therapy and drainage is required treatment of infectious arthritis. If this condition remains undiagnosed or untreated longer than 5 to 7 days, the prognosis for a functional joint is poor. The initial choice of antibiotic should be sufficiently broad to cover likely sources of infection for an individual, and then the antibiotic may be changed on the basis of the results of the Gram stain and culture. Older children and adults do well with nafcillin, oxacillin, or cefazolin, especially if the Gram stain suggests *S. aureus* and the risk of MRSA is low. For patients at high risk for gram-negative septic arthritis (elderly, immunocompromised), cefepime should be considered as an initial broad-spectrum antibiotic.[2] For coverage of gonococcal arthritis, sexually active young adults should receive ceftriaxone, 1 g intravenously daily for 7 to 10 days.[3] Pending culture results, infectious arthritis in a prosthetic joint after recent surgery or in other individuals at risk for MRSA (hemodialysis patients, those with diabetes mellitus, nursing home residents) may require empirical vancomycin to cover the possibility of coagulase-negative staphylococci or MRSA. Aminoglycosides and antipseudomonal β-lactams are sometimes added for synergism in patients who are infected with *S. aureus* or injection drug users in whom *P. aeruginosa* is suspected. Linezolid, daptomycin, and pristinamycin have shown some promise in the treatment of MRSA septic arthritis.[2]

Duration of therapy is 2 weeks for *Haemophilus influenzae* and streptococci and 3 weeks for staphylococci or gram-negative bacilli. Shorter courses and oral regimens are often effective in children. Gonococcal arthritis responds quickly and may be treated entirely on an outpatient basis with 2 or 3 days of intravenous ceftriaxone, followed by early conversion to oral cefixime, 400 mg twice daily, or ciprofloxacin, 500 mg twice daily, to complete a 10- to 14-day course. Patients with underlying rheumatoid arthritis and virulent organisms should be treated for 4 weeks.[2] Newer fluoroquinolones such as gatifloxacin, moxifloxacin, levofloxacin, and trovafloxacin have improved gram-positive coverage. Intravenous and oral antibiotics have ready access to inflamed joints and should not be given by intra-articular injection or added to solutions for irrigating joints. Antibiotics injected directly into joints may initiate chemical synovitis and prolong postinfectious arthritis.

An infected joint is similar to an abscess that needs daily drainage until the inflammation has resolved.[32] Reactive oxygen species and proteolytic enzymes, which destroy cartilage, are produced by activated leukocytes. Therefore it is important that purulent material and bacterial toxins be removed to preserve cartilage. This is accomplished equally well with either daily arthrocentesis or arthroscopic lavage with placement of drains. Daily arthrocentesis is less expensive and is not complicated by instrumentation morbidity; it also offers the possibility of serial culture and cell counts of synovial fluid to gauge response to therapy. Arthroscopic lavage with debridement and placement of drains or open arthrotomy is appropriate if there is persistence of recurrent effusion and elevation of cell counts after several days of daily arthrocentesis or if loculated fluid is suspected. Hips should be surgically drained at the outset because of their anatomic complexity.[32]

An infected prosthetic joint usually requires drainage and debridement and may require removal of all prosthetic components and cement. A definitive approach is a two-step procedure, with removal of prosthesis and cement and 6 weeks of antibiotics followed by revision arthroplasty. An antibiotic-impregnated spacer may be used to maintain the joint space to prevent contracture pending reimplantation of a permanent prosthesis. Historically, even with sensitive organisms, retention of the prosthesis and antibiotic therapy with limited surgical debridement is often unsuccessful. In light of some studies reporting increasing rates of success in the retention of infected prosthetic joints with appropriate antibiotic therapy, there has been growing interest in this surgical approach.[33] Risk factors predicting treatment failure of this approach include sinus tract presence and symptom duration of 8 days or longer. If revision arthroplasty is to be done, 6 weeks of intravenous antibiotics are crucial to achieve the 90% success rate.[17,33]

LIFE SPAN CONSIDERATIONS

Mortality is low when infectious arthritis is diagnosed and treated appropriately. However, the associated infection carries significant mortality in older or immunocompromised patients.

Toxic shock or a continuing infectious syndrome despite a sterile blood culture is attributable to toxin production by small residual foci of staphylococci or streptococci around dead cartilage or prosthetic joints. There should be no delay in prosthetic joint removal and surgical debridement in the setting of toxic shock or sepsis syndrome because death may result. Surgery should not be delayed because the problem is typically an abscess, which is unlikely to respond to a continued course of antibiotics.

COMPLICATIONS

Progressive loss of joint function develops in 25% to 50% of patients.[31] A relapse of infectious arthritis may occur if the selection or duration of the antibiotic therapy is inappropriate. Recurrent aseptic joint effusion is common and is referred to as postinfectious synovitis. Minor trauma may exacerbate such synovitis. More immediate complications include an associated abscess or bursa infection, which must be drained, and associated osteomyelitis. Ankylosis (fusion), ligamentous instability, and joint contracture are consequences of delayed diagnosis. A total joint arthroplasty can restore mobility in such joints but cannot reverse ligamentous instability or joint contracture. Secondary osteoarthritis is a delayed complication that may require eventual arthroplasty. Some factors that determine outcome are listed in Box 179-1.

BOX 179-1

Factors Affecting Outcome in Infectious Arthritis

- Delay in diagnosis and treatment beyond 7 days
- Persistently positive culture and effusion after 5 days of treatment
- Prior arthritis, especially rheumatoid arthritis
- Compromised host and older patients
- Virulence of organism: *S. aureus* versus coagulase-negative staphylococci
- Specific joint involved: hips worse than knees
- Injection drug use: good prognosis with aggressive organisms
- Appropriate antibiotics
- Effective drainage and debridement
- Physical therapy: initially non–weight bearing, early mobilization, splint contractures

INDICATIONS FOR REFERRAL OR HOSPITALIZATION

A joint infection is a medical emergency. All patients with infectious arthritis should be hospitalized initially because they need to adhere to strict non–weight-bearing activities to preserve cartilage, may require daily aspiration, or will need initial surgical drainage. For patients who have been prescribed bed rest, early mobilization with a passive mobilization device helps prevent adhesions and contractures. Infectious disease, rheumatology, and orthopedic consultations are obtained when the patient is hospitalized. A physical therapist should be part of the care team because early mobilization and eventual weight bearing are important. Cartilage has no blood supply and is in part dependent on intermittent compression for nutritional requirements and integrity of structure. It is thus important to try to achieve early mobilization. When the effusion has subsided, early discharge with home intravenous therapy or oral antibiotics is feasible.

Gonococcal arthritis may, in some cases, be managed on an outpatient basis. However, gonococcal arthritis may be confused with reactive arthritis (occasionally referred to as Reiter syndrome)—a triad of urethritis, conjunctivitis, and arthritis.[34] In the appropriate clinical setting (adequate pretest probability) and if cultures are negative, a rapid response to intravenous ceftriaxone may be considered diagnostic of gonococcal arthritis.

PATIENT AND FAMILY EDUCATION

To remove potential sources of bacteremia, patients should be instructed to be certain that any necessary extensive dental work is done and wounds or ulcers are healed before undergoing a total joint arthroplasty. Antibiotic prophylaxis before surgery for total joint arthroplasty is advised to prevent postsurgical infectious arthritis. Lifelong antibiotic prophylaxis before urologic, intestinal, or dental procedures for patients who have undergone a joint replacement is advised by the American Academy of Orthopaedic Surgeons unless otherwise indicated by the patient's health status. Other societies have differing opinions, which complicates these decisions.[35] Patients with rheumatoid arthritis, especially those taking immunosuppressant medications such as prednisone, methotrexate, and biologic disease-modifying antirheumatic drugs (DMARDs), should be aware that superimposed infectious arthritis is possible. They should disclose any monoarticular flare to their physician for early diagnostic arthrocentesis. Cellulitis, wounds, and ulcers should receive prompt medical attention to prevent bacteremia. Patients recovering from infectious arthritis must be instructed in home physical therapy to prevent contracture and to advance weight bearing after inflammation has subsided. The potential side effects of antibiotics need to be explained, antibiotic-associated diarrhea should be anticipated, and patients with indwelling central lines must be instructed in line care and signs of line infection.

CHAPTER 180

KNEE PAIN

Wendy L. Halm

DEFINITION AND EPIDEMIOLOGY

Knee pain is a common problem that can originate in any of the bony structures of the knee joint (femur, tibia, fibula), the kneecap (patella), or the ligaments and cartilage (meniscus) of the knee. In addition, soft tissue structure surrounding the knee joint (muscle, tendons, bursae) surrounding the knee can also be a source of pain. Knee pain can affect people of all ages and can be attributed many causes.

The multiple structures within the knee make it vulnerable to various types of injuries and degenerative change. Many injuries can be treated conservatively; others require surgery. There also are many extra-articular structures that can become inflamed or injured, causing knee pain.

Knee pain is often classified according to cause and longevity of symptoms. Knee pain can also be a result of an acute injury, trauma, or a particular athletic move. Knee pain related to chronic and or inflammatory disease, such as bursitis, osteoarthritis, rheumatoid arthritis, or gout, is discussed in other chapters.

Knee Pain

The knee is a modified hinge joint that flexes and extends and has some rotational mobility. The knee joint contains three bones, three articulations, five major tendons, four major ligaments, two menisci, and 12 bursae. The lateral and medial articulations are between the femoral and tibial condyles. The intermediate articulation is between the patella and the femur. A relatively weak joint, the knee gains its strength from the strong ligaments that attach the femur to the tibia. Five intrinsic ligaments assist in strengthening the articular capsule. The cruciate ligaments connect the femur and tibia within the articular capsule, crossing each other in the form of an X.[1]

As a major weight-bearing joint, the knee is susceptible to many injuries. Torsion is limited in the joint, and any motion that extends beyond the defined range results in a ligamentous injury. Because the knee depends on the integrity of the ligaments to provide its stability, a knee injury can be a calamitous event.

The approach to knee pain begins with a careful history and review of symptoms, focusing particularly on the presence of trauma, mechanism of injury, and limitations. Patients with any penetrating injury, especially if there is joint involvement, should be referred to the emergency department. Patients with a history of a traumatic event with presence of effusion or swelling, fever or other systemic illness, erythematous and swollen knees, knee pain in conjunction with sexually transmitted infections, or cellulitis over or adjacent to the affected knee or who have a history of bleeding disorders or anticoagulation are particularly concerning and should be managed with same-day orthopedic consultation.[2]

Physical examination of the knee can be frustrating to novice providers and requires both practice and patience. Ideally, the provider's physical examination skills are honed under the guidance and critique of an experienced colleague. A systematic approach that includes elements of inspection, range of motion, palpation, sensation, and special tests to evaluate stability is critical to correct diagnosis of knee pain.[2,3]

Collateral Ligament Sprains

There are two collateral ligaments: the medial collateral ligament (MCL) and the lateral collateral ligament (LCL). The MCL attaches to the medial condyle of the femur and the tibia. The LCL attaches to the lateral femoral condyle and extends to the lateral tibial plateau.[2] The purpose of the collateral ligaments is to provide support to the inner and the lateral portions of the knee. The MCL and the LCL are injured when valgus or varus stress to the joint extends beyond the normal range of motion. MCL injuries are more common in athletic males and often include an injury to the medial meniscus.[4] Football players and skiers are more prone to ligamentous injuries, but they can occur just as easily on the dance floor or in the bathroom.

PATHOPHYSIOLOGY

An external rotational wrenching motion of the knee or a blow to the lateral side of the knee with a firmly planted foot causes injury to the MCL. LCL injuries occur with an internal rotation or a blow to the medial side of the knee with a firmly planted foot.[2,5] The injuries are graded as first-, second-, or third-degree sprains (Table 180-1).

CLINICAL PRESENTATION

Patients with an MCL injury will typically have medial knee pain. Swelling and instability are uncommon and may signify more serious injury, such as a tear of the medial meniscus. LCL injuries manifest with acute lateral knee pain and may have associated instability and peroneal nerve palsy (commonly manifesting as a drop foot).[2]

PHYSICAL EXAMINATION

An examination immediately after the injury is more accurate and helps ascertain the severity of the injury.[2] Examination of the knee is more difficult in the presence of edema and muscle

TABLE 180-1 Collateral Ligament Sprains

First Degree	Second Degree	Third Degree
PATHOLOGY		
Ligament fibers attached	Partial avulsion of fibers from femoral condyle	Complete rupture of ligament (often associated with anterior or posterior cruciate ligament tears or tibial plateau fractures)
FINDINGS		
Tenderness along body of ligament	Pain at joint line of ligament insertion	Significant pain at ligament insertion and joint line
Minimum or no swelling	Swelling with tenderness localized to attachment point	Significant swelling with ecchymosis
No joint widening with ligament stress	Slight to moderate increase in joint widening with stress	Increased joint widening with minimum stress

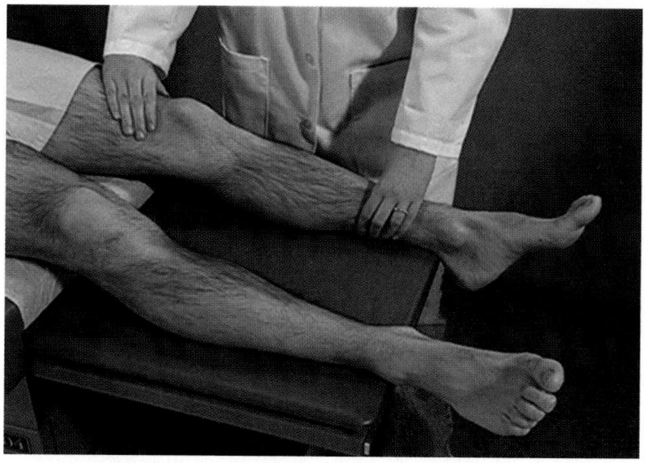

FIGURE 180-1 Valgus stress test of the knee. (From Ball JW, Dains JE, Flynn JA, et al. *Seidel's physical examination handbook*, ed 8, St Louis, 2014, Elsevier.)

spasm. The examination should include observation; palpation; assessment of range of motion, motor strength, sensation, and vascular structures; ligamentous testing and stability assessment; and provocative maneuvers. The normal knee should be tested first to establish a baseline. Both knees should be observed for swelling, deformity, muscle atrophy, and patella placement. Fluctuance should be determined with the patient first standing and then supine. Tenderness and bone landmarks should be ascertained as well. In the suspected collateral ligament sprain, there is tenderness along the body of the ligament, and point tenderness at the attachment site is commonly present. With MCL injury, there may be tenderness at the medial joint line because the MCL attaches to the medial meniscus. Pain at the lateral joint line can be indicative of an internal joint injury.

Valgus stress on the knee joint determines MCL laxity (Fig. 180-1). If the clinician identifies significant valgus laxity with the knee in full extension, an injury involving the entire MCL complex or the anterior cruciate ligament (ACL) should be suspected.[5] Varus stress on the knee joint determines LCL laxity (see Fig. 180-1). Laxity at 30 degrees of flexion indicates injury to the LCL.[2] Active range of motion in extension and flexion should be assessed. If active range of motion is not possible, passive extension and flexion should be determined.

DIAGNOSTICS

Initial diagnostics should include plain radiographs to exclude fractures and dislocations. More extensive radiologic examinations, such as magnetic resonance imaging (MRI), should be considered in consultation with an orthopedist.

DIAGNOSTICS

Knee Pain

IMAGING
X-ray studies (anteroposterior, lateral, sunrise)
MRI, CT scan, ultrasound*

OTHER DIAGNOSTICS
Joint aspiration (e.g., for cell count) if inflammatory, crystal, or infectious cause is suspected*

*If indicated.
CT, computed tomography.

DIFFERENTIAL DIAGNOSIS

As with any joint injury, a fracture or dislocation must be considered. In the knee, injury to the ACL, posterior cruciate ligament (PCL), or articular cartilage or patellar dislocation should be considered.

DIFFERENTIAL DIAGNOSIS

Knee Pain

- Abscess
- Arthritis
- Bursitis
- Chondromalacia patellae
- Collateral ligament sprains
- Cruciate ligament injury
- Dislocation
- Effusion
- Fracture
- Hemarthrosis
- Meniscus injuries
- Ruptured muscle
- Synovitis

MANAGEMENT

Orthopedic physician consultation is indicated for chronic MCL tears, acute MCL tears with other ligamentous injuries, and LCL or posterolateral corner injuries.

Immediate emergency department referral is indicated for severe sprains, tears, or suspected fractures.

Conservative treatment of isolated first- and second-degree sprains is recommended.[4]

If the knee is unstable on examination, an MCL-stabilizing brace is worn at all times. Pain and inflammation can be treated with nonsteroidal anti-inflammatory drugs (NSAIDs) or acetaminophen. The patient should avoid bearing weight on the affected knee. Simple straight leg raises and quadriceps-tightening exercises as well as simple hamstring-strengthening exercises can be done easily right in the brace. Once pain and swelling have subsided, the patient should be referred to physical therapy for more progressive rehabilitation.[5] Adjunctive therapy may include ultrasound or electrical muscle stimulation.[5] Surgical repair may be indicated for certain grade III injuries.[4,5]

LIFE SPAN CONSIDERATIONS

When considering medication treatment for the older adult, clinicians should consider potentially inappropriate medications. The use of NSAIDs in the older adult has been associated with increased risk of gastrointestinal (GI) bleeding and peptic ulcer disease in high-risk groups, including those older than 75 years, or in patients who are taking oral or parenteral corticosteroids, anticoagulants, or antiplatelet agents.[6]

COMPLICATIONS

Without accurate diagnosis and treatment, the injury can extend, jeopardizing the joint's stability and other structures. The incompletely rehabilitated knee will be weak and potentially unstable. Traumatic arthritis can be a sequela of any joint injury.

INDICATIONS FOR REFERRAL OR HOSPITALIZATION

- All patients with severe sprains, tears, and fractures should be referred to the emergency room or for same-day orthopedic consultation.
- Referral to a physical therapist should be considered to assist in complete rehabilitation.

PATIENT AND FAMILY EDUCATION

Explanation of the importance of adherence to the rehabilitative process is imperative. In some instances, a knee support for sports is necessary. Pain and swelling are indicators that the knee is being overstressed or has been reinjured.

CRUCIATE LIGAMENT INJURIES

DEFINITION AND EPIDEMIOLOGY

Resembling an X, the cruciate ligaments crisscross within the joint capsule but are extrasynovial. There are two cruciate ligaments: the ACL and the PCL. The ACL attaches to the anterior part of the intercondylar area of the tibia, posterior to the medial meniscus, and rises superiorly, posteriorly, and laterally to attach to the posterior section of the medial side of the lateral condyle of the femur.[1] The ACL restrains the anterior to posterior alignment of the knee, keeping the proper relationship of the femur to the tibia. It is loose with the knee in flexion and tight when the knee is fully extended. It is the weaker of the two cruciate ligaments.

The PCL originates at the posterior part of the intercondylar area of the tibia. It crosses superiorly and anteriorly on the medial side of the ACL and attaches to the anterior part of the lateral surface of the medial femoral condyle. The PCL is tight with the knee in flexion. The PCL restrains the posterior to anterior alignment of the knee.

A cruciate ligament injury can be a sprain, a partial tear, or a complete disruption of the ligament. Physical examination and radiologic tests as indicated are used to determine the degree of the injury. The ACL is the most commonly involved structure in severe knee injuries. Female gender and intensity of play increase the risk of ACL tear.[7] The PCL is less often injured.

PATHOPHYSIOLOGY

The PCL is the stronger ligament and is usually injured through trauma to the anterior surface of the proximal tibia (as in hitting the dashboard) or falling onto the tibial tubercle with the knee flexed.[2,4] The ACL is typically injured in sports during rapid deceleration or on quickly changing directions. The ACL can also be torn with a direct blow to the lateral portion of the knee.[7]

The ACL injury often occurs in combination with ruptures of the MCL and the medial meniscus. Once the ligament is torn, the knee is unstable. Swelling occurs rapidly in an ACL or PCL injury because of bleeding from the ligament tear.[7]

CLINICAL PRESENTATION

The patient with an acute ACL injury may recall hearing a "pop" or feeling the knee "snap" and has an instantaneous sensation of something being "terribly wrong."[5] Patients with an MCL injury may not remember the exact mechanism of injury. Pain from the injury prevents a return to the activity. Patients report a distrust of the knee during activities and that the knee "gives out," especially during exertion.

PHYSICAL EXAMINATION

Swelling and pain in the acutely injured knee often prohibit a thorough examination. The knee is swollen, and the patient is unable to fully flex or extend the knee. Hamstring spasms and the posterior horn of the meniscus can stabilize the knee, falsely indicating a stable joint; thus it is important for the patient to relax. The normal knee should be examined first to allay anxiety and to establish a baseline because most people have some degree of laxity in the ligaments.

The Lachman test is used to assess the ACL. The knee should be flexed to about 15 to 30 degrees. One hand is placed just below the knee joint on the posterior aspect of the tibia-fibula. The other hand is placed on the anterior aspect of the femur just above the joint. The examiner lifts up the lower leg while pushing down on the upper leg. If the ACL is intact, after a few millimeters of movement, the examiner should feel a "knock" or a firm "stop" as the ACL prevents the tibia from sliding forward. In the absence of a firm end point, a ligament tear should be suspected.[7]

The anterior drawer test also is used to assess the ACL (Fig. 180-2). The knee should be flexed to about 90 degrees, with the foot kept flat on the examination surface. The examiner sits on the patient's foot and firmly grasps the lower leg, placing the fingers below the popliteal space and the thumbs on the tibial tuberosity. The examiner pulls gently but firmly on the tibia, attempting to slide the tibia forward. A "soft" or absent end point indicates a tear.[7]

The posterior drawer test also is used to assess the PCL (see Fig. 180-2). With the patient positioned the same as for the

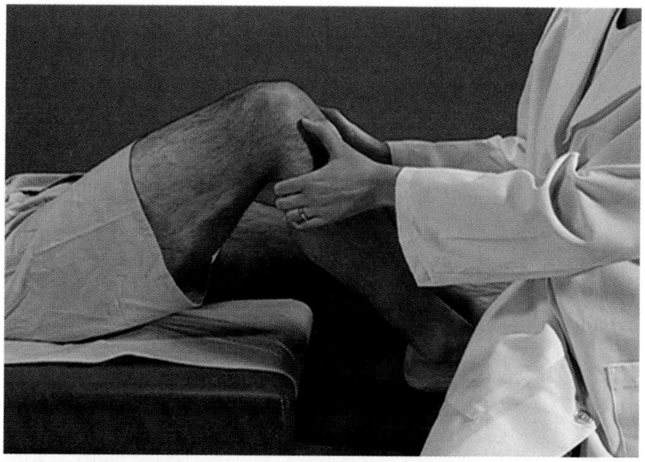

FIGURE 180-2 Drawer test for anterior and posterior stability of the knee. (From Ball JW, Dains JE, Flynn JA, et al. *Seidel's physical examination handbook,* ed 8, St Louis, 2014, Elsevier.)

anterior drawer test, the examiner pushes posteriorly on the tibia. A torn PCL allows the tibia to slide backward.[4]

DIAGNOSTICS

Initial diagnostics should include x-ray studies of the knee. Plain films demonstrate effusions and alignment, determine skeletal maturity and the presence of loose bodies or avulsion fractures, and can be used to identify degenerative changes in the middle-aged to older patient. The Segond fracture, an avulsion of the lateral aspect of the tibial plateau, is pathognomonic of an ACL tear. MRI provides a definitive evaluation of the ligaments.

DIFFERENTIAL DIAGNOSIS

As with any knee injury, damage to other intra-articular structures must be considered. Fracture-dislocations are included in the differential diagnosis.

MANAGEMENT

Orthopedic physician consultation is indicated for patients with a suspected ACL or PCL tear.

Immediate emergency department referral is indicated for severe sprains, tears, or suspected fractures.

Initial treatment measures are directed at restoring painless range of motion and preserving quadriceps strength. The degree of the tear with or without instability guides the treatment plan.

Partial tears and tears without a concurrent fracture or meniscus tear can often be managed conservatively. Grade 1 and 2 PCL tears are usually treated conservatively.[4] Physical therapy is beneficial. The quadriceps muscle begins to atrophy quickly with inactivity; therefore, strengthening exercises should begin as tolerated, starting with the simple straight leg raise. The quadriceps muscles are adjunct stabilizers to the ACL, and rehabilitation by physical therapy should stress regaining of full range of motion and strength.[2]

A derotational brace may be useful for unstable knees, but bracing with an immobilizer is controversial. Weight bearing on the affected knee should be avoided. Surgical reconstruction may be indicated, especially in athletes and younger patients, after the swelling and inflammation have decreased, usually 3 to 4 weeks after injury. Extensive rehabilitation is expected.[5,7]

LIFE SPAN CONSIDERATIONS

Patients who do not participate in active sports or older patients may be managed more conservatively with muscle strength training.

COMPLICATIONS

The patient with an unstable knee is in jeopardy of fracture, aggravation of the initial injury, or falls as a direct result of the instability. A knee that has sustained severe trauma is susceptible to degenerative changes of the articular surface, development of arthritis, and chronic pain.

INDICATIONS FOR REFERRAL OR HOSPITALIZATION

- All persons who have sustained an acute injury to the cruciate ligaments require an evaluation by an orthopedic surgeon.
- All persons with PCL or ACL injuries should be referred to physical therapy to focus on hamstring strength and core stability.

PATIENT AND FAMILY EDUCATION

Resumption of activity generally occurs at 6 to 9 months. The patient should have full and equal strength and range of motion before returning to athletics.[5,7]

MENISCUS INJURIES

DEFINITION AND EPIDEMIOLOGY

The menisci are crescent-shaped fibrocartilaginous structures on the articular surface of the tibia. They act as shock absorbers for the knee and help control normal knee motion.[1] Meniscus tears are the third most common of all knee injuries. The medial meniscus is injured or torn more often than the lateral meniscus because of its structure, mobility, and attachment.[8] Meniscal injuries are more common in males and are often associated with an ACL tear in the athletic population.[9] Older patients may have minimal or no known trauma associated with degenerative tears.[9]

PATHOPHYSIOLOGY

The menisci maintain the space between the bones in the knee joint. They are injured when the weight-bearing knee is twisted while it is in the flexed position. The femur compresses against the tibia and grinds against the meniscus. This grinding motion tears the meniscus as the force exceeds the strength of the fibrocartilage. Once torn, the menisci cannot heal. Menisci tear as a direct result of injury or indirectly as a result of the normal wear and tear on the knee.

CLINICAL PRESENTATION

In an acute injury, joint effusion is usually present. There is tenderness along the joint line, and the person often has a sense of instability. Those with a degenerative tear will complain of joint line discomfort and a sense of locking or giving

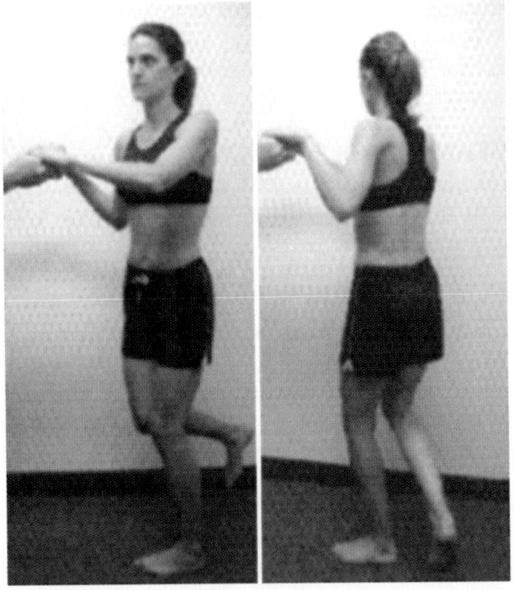

FIGURE 180-3 The Thessaly test for meniscal integrity at 20 degrees of flexion. (From Cleland J, Koppenhaver S: *Netter's orthopaedic clinical examination: an evidence-based approach*, ed 2, Philadelphia, 2011, Elsevier.)

way, especially while descending stairs or walking on uneven surfaces.

PHYSICAL EXAMINATION

The physical examination should include palpation of the joint line, assessing for tenderness and presence of an effusion. The examination findings may be unremarkable owing to the type and location of the tear. The Thessaly test (Fig. 180-3) is the most sensitive. To perform the Thessaly test, the provider holds the outstretched hands of the patient for support. The patient flexes the affected knee to 5 degrees while flexing the unaffected knee and lifting the foot off of the floor so that all of the body weight is on the affected knee. The patient twists on the affected knee three times. Those who have meniscal tears experience joint line pain and may also have a locking sensation. The test is then repeated at 20 degrees of flexion.

The McMurray test helps ascertain a tear in the cartilage. To perform the McMurray test, the examiner has the patient lie supine with the legs straight. The examiner firmly grasps the heel or ankle with one hand and places the other hand on the knee joint, with the fingers on the medial side and the thumb at the lateral side. The examiner flexes the knee while rotating the tibia internally and externally on the femur. This maneuver will loosen the joint. Then, while flexing and externally rotating the leg, the examiner applies valgus stress to the lateral side of the knee. The examiner holds the valgus stress on the joint while extending the leg and palpating the medial joint line. If a click or pop is heard or felt, the medial meniscus is torn.[8]

The McMurray test can also be performed with the patient in a sitting position and the knee flexed to 90 degrees (Fig. 180-4). The patient should internally rotate the affected leg while the practitioner slowly extends the leg. While performing the maneuver, the practitioner should apply resistance to the knee medially to test the medial meniscus. The practitioner should repeat the maneuver, applying resistance to the knee laterally to test the lateral meniscus. The test result is positive if the knee cannot be extended.

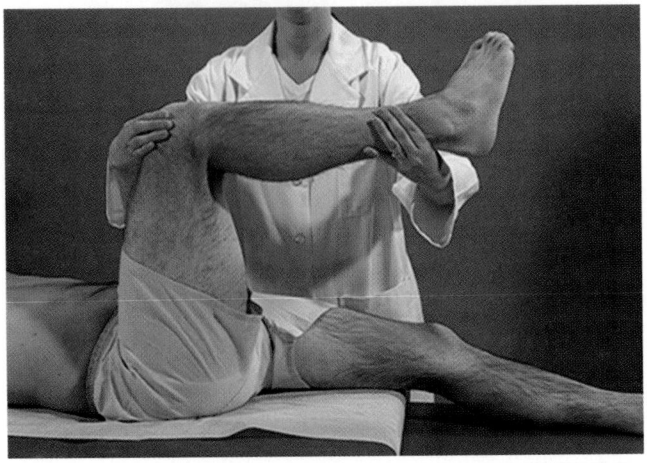

FIGURE 180-4 McMurray test of the knee. (From Ball JW, Dains JE, Flynn JA, et al. *Seidel's physical examination handbook*, ed 8, St Louis, 2014, Elsevier.)

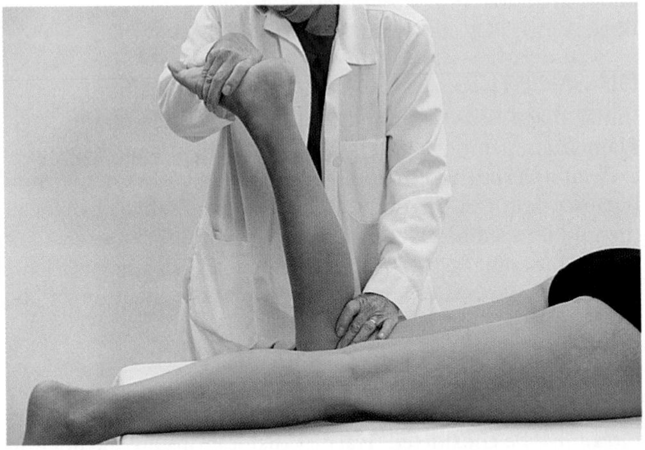

FIGURE 180-5 Apley assessment of the knee. (From Cleland J, Koppenhaver S: *Netter's orthopaedic clinical examination: an evidence-based approach*, ed 2, Philadelphia, 2011, Elsevier.)

In addition to the McMurray test, a simpler test is the Apley compression test (Fig. 180-5). This test should be done with the patient prone and the affected leg flexed to 90 degrees. The examiner places his or her knee on the patient's posterior thigh to stabilize it, grabs the foot firmly, leans on the heel to squeeze the menisci between the femur and the tibia, and rotates the tibia. If pain is elicited, there is a tear in the meniscus. The patient should be asked to describe the location of the pain to distinguish a medial meniscus tear from a lateral meniscus tear.

DIAGNOSTICS

Initial diagnostics should include an x-ray examination to identify joint space narrowing, early osteoarthritis changes, or loose bodies. The best diagnostic test is MRI.

DIFFERENTIAL DIAGNOSIS

Diagnosis can be difficult because the menisci are avascular and have no nerve supply on their inner two thirds.[3] The patient often has a sense of joint instability in addition to joint line tenderness; thus the potential for fracture or other structural injury must be considered. Meniscal tears are often concomitant with tears of the ACL.

MANAGEMENT

Orthopedic consultation is indicated for patients with persistent symptoms that limit activity.

Immediate emergency referral is indicated if the patient's knee is locked and cannot be extended or flexed.

Certain tears and chronic degenerative meniscal injury are generally treated conservatively. RICE is recommended acutely, with activity modification maintained for 6 to 12 weeks. Pain and inflammation can be treated with NSAIDs or acetaminophen. Intra-articular injections of corticosteroids should be limited to patients with concomitant osteoarthrosis.[2] Crutches or a walker for older adults may be helpful if pain is severe, and limiting weight bearing is helpful.

Rehabilitation to improve the strength of the quadriceps and hamstring muscles is imperative. Straight leg raises with the knee in extension, but not locked, can be started immediately, and weight bearing is gradually increased. Non–weight-bearing activities, such as swimming and riding a stationary bicycle, are excellent for increasing range of motion and strength.

Surgical intervention may be considered for complex tears, tears associated with ACL rupture, ongoing symptoms that affect daily life, select physical findings, or a failure to respond to nonsurgical treatment.[9] Arthroscopy may be performed by the orthopedic surgeon to accurately diagnose a meniscal tear but has not been helpful in alleviating symptoms.

LIFE SPAN CONSIDERATIONS

Older adults may be treated more conservatively. Physical therapy for chronic meniscal injury is beneficial. Patients with persistent effusion and recurrent mechanical dysfunction will need to be evaluated by an orthopedic surgeon.

COMPLICATIONS

Articular damage from the meniscus tear may result in long-term stiffness or osteoarthritis (see Chapter 184.[2] Because the menisci are stabilizers for the knee, loss of their integrity can lead to more extensive injuries.

INDICATIONS FOR REFERRAL OR HOSPITALIZATION

- Same-day orthopedic referral is indicated for patients with a locked knee that they cannot fully extend.
- Routine orthopedic referral is necessary for patients with persistent locking or swelling in the knee, or when symptoms do not respond to conservative measures.

PATIENT AND FAMILY EDUCATION

Maintaining quadriceps and hamstring strength, in addition to hip flexor and abductor range of motion, is essential to minimize the disabilities associated with this injury. Although the knee may not be 100% normal, participation in sports with proper warm-up and equipment can be enjoyed. Achiness and swelling after a particularly strenuous workout or game can be normal. Ice and NSAIDs can help control the symptoms. A patient with persistent swelling, pain, or episodes of instability should be reevaluated.

PATELLOFEMORAL PAIN SYNDROME

DEFINITION AND EPIDEMIOLOGY

Patellofemoral pain syndrome (PFPS) is one of the most common overuse injuries of the knee. It refers to knee pain that is localized to the anterior portion of the knee. Other common names for PFPS include runner's knee, chondromalacia patellae, retropatellar pain syndrome, and anterior knee pain.

PATHOPHYSIOLOGY

The cause of PFPS is poorly understood. It is likely that the syndrome results from abnormal lateral tracking of the patella resulting from weak quadriceps muscles, poor flexibility, patellar hypermobility, a tight iliotibial band, anatomic malalignment, or overuse.[9,10]

Women are more likely to experience abnormal lateral tracking because of an anatomically wider pelvis and the resultant slight angle of the femur as it meets the knee.

CLINICAL PRESENTATION

Patients report knee pain that is often bilateral and is largely limited to the anterior portion of the knee, around and behind the patella. PFPS is exacerbated by sporting activity, squatting, kneeling, climbing stairs, or descent and hill running.[9,10] Patients may report a feeling that the knee is "giving out" or that they have pain with prolonged sitting with the knees flexed (the "theater sign"). Rarely, patients may complain of an effusion, which should be further evaluated for other causes.[10]

PHYSICAL EXAMINATION

A complete examination of the knee, including gait observation, is critical to establish a diagnosis and to rule out other causes. Clinicians should assess for symptoms of patellar dislocation.[10] Anterior knee pain with quadriceps contraction, pain during squatting, and pain on palpation of the posteromedial or posterolateral border of the patella should be assessed.[9] The provider may notice a lateral tracking of the patella when the patient is in a seated position. Rocking of the patella in the patellar groove while the leg is fully extended may elicit pain. The patient may also demonstrate weak or tight quadriceps muscles or a tight iliotibial band.

DIAGNOSTICS

Diagnostic tests are usually not indicated. A positive history in conjunction with positive clinical findings on examination is usually sufficient for diagnosis. Plain radiographs may be useful in identifying other causes of knee pain, such as osteoarthritis or loose bodies. Diagnostic studies are indicated when the patient is not responding to therapy.

DIFFERENTIAL DIAGNOSIS

Patellar tendonitis, bursitis, patellofemoral arthritis, and patellar subluxation should be considered.[9] There are several other rare causes of anterior knee pain that can be explored in conjunction with a referral to orthopedics, rheumatology, or sports medicine if the patient does not respond to therapy. Any effusions or complaints of joint locking require further evaluation.

MANAGEMENT

Orthopedic physician consultation is indicated for patients who do not respond to conservative treatment.

Emergency department referral is indicated for patients with joint locking, obvious patellar dislocation, or severe pain.

Primary management of PFPS is generally nonoperative and focused on symptom management.

RICE should be used acutely to reduce swelling and alleviate pain Activity modification should limit flexion (e.g., reduction of jumping and squatting, reduction of climbing activities).[11] Pain and inflammation can be treated with NSAIDs or acetaminophen. Immobilization with a patellofemoral brace or patellar taping may be of benefit.

Rehabilitation to strengthen muscles supporting the knee is the cornerstone intervention. Orthotics, steroid injections, and viscosupplementation (see Chapter 184) may also provide pain relief.[10] Surgery is rarely indicated.

INDICATIONS FOR REFERRAL OR HOSPITALIZATION

- Patients who do not respond to conservative management and rehabilitation should be referred to orthopedics.
- Patients with persistent effusion, pain, or episodes of instability should be reevaluated.

LIFE SPAN CONSIDERATIONS

Older patients who have arthritis affecting the patellofemoral joint may be at risk for developing PFPS.

COMPLICATIONS

PFPS rarely results in complications, although it can contribute to deconditioning and further weakness of the quadriceps muscles. Surgical interventions have mixed outcomes.

PATIENT AND FAMILY EDUCATION

The cornerstone of management is relative rest and physical therapy; it is important to remind patients of the importance of adhering to the rehabilitation plan.

INFLAMMATORY AND DEGENERATIVE DISORDERS

As people age or become deconditioned as a result of chronic injury or disease, knee pain can be caused by a variety of inflammatory or extra-articular conditions and by age-related degeneration. Anserine bursitis (see Chapter 173) is commonly seen in middle-aged women with osteoarthritis of the knee and a valgus deformity. This disorder produces pain and tenderness over the medial aspect of the knee about 5 cm (2 inches) below the joint line. Obvious swelling is not uncommon. Anserine bursitis is treated conservatively with ice and NSAIDs, but steroid injections may be necessary to alleviate pain in particularly severe cases.

Prepatellar bursitis (housemaid's knee) manifests as a swelling superficial to the patella. This condition results from trauma such as that occurring with frequent kneeling and is seen commonly in persons who work on their knees, such as floor or carpet layers. Pain is mild unless direct pressure is applied over the bursa, and there is no pain with weight bearing or range of motion of the knee. The condition is treated with rest, ice, and NSAIDs and is prevented by protecting the knee from repeated trauma.

Inflammatory arthritis including rheumatoid arthritis (see Chapter 218), psoriatic arthritis (see Chapter 215), reactive arthritis (see Chapter 215), gout (see Chapter 176), and pseudogout (see Chapter 176) can cause acute pain and swelling of the knee that can progress to cartilage degeneration and the eventual need for joint replacement surgery.

Popliteal cysts (Baker cysts) are commonly seen in conjunction with rheumatoid arthritis, osteoarthritis, or internal derangements of the knee. Initially, a cystic swelling in the popliteal space may be the only finding. As the cyst increases in size, the possibility of rupture increases. A ruptured cyst will drain into the calf, causing pain, erythema, and swelling, mimicking phlebitis. An ultrasound examination will provide a location and extent of the cyst.[12]

Osteoarthritis is probably the most common cause of knee pain in the older adult (see Chapter 184). Pain, stiffness, and decreased function are cardinal signs. Pain is generally insidious in onset and characterized as mild to moderate. Resting the knee usually alleviates the pain. Osteoarthritis is progressive, and the cartilage damage is permanent. However, conservative treatment, including muscle strengthening, weight loss, analgesics, and NSAIDs, is often effective. Injections of steroids or hyaluronan may provide temporary relief. Severe disease, manifesting with resting or night pain and increasing difficulty with ambulation, may require joint replacement surgery.[13]

Referred pain syndrome can originate with problems of the low back, sacroiliac, or hip joint. Pain from any of these areas can be referred to the knee, resulting in pain. Referred pain should be considered when findings of examination of the knee joint are relatively normal without swelling or local tenderness and with normal range of motion.

CHAPTER 181

LOW BACK PAIN

Lindsay Ramey • Zacharia Isaac • Sharon Alzner

DEFINITION AND EPIDEMIOLOGY

Low back pain is the most common musculoskeletal problem worldwide and is estimated to affect up to 85% of the population at some time in a person's life. It has an estimated yearly prevalence of 38% and occurs most frequently in females and those aged 40 to 80 years.[1] In the United States, back pain is the second most common reason for visits to a physician. It is also a leading cause of hospital admissions and subsequent surgery.

Low back pain is commonly classified by symptom duration as acute, subacute, or chronic (Table 181-1). Approximately 30% to 60% of people with acute low back pain recover within 1 week, and 80% to 90% recover within 6 weeks.[2] However, recurrence rates are high, with up to 50% reporting recurrence of pain within 6 months.[2] Although low back pain is typically transient, if it persists and becomes subacute, there is an

TABLE 181-1 Classification of Low Back Pain

By Symptom Duration	By Pathophysiology	By Symptom
Acute: Less than 6 weeks	Mechanical	Axial low back pain
Subacute: 6 weeks to 3 months	Systemic medical (nonmechanical)	Radicular pain
Chronic: More than 3 months, with symptoms more than half the days in the last 6 months		

increased risk for developing chronic low back pain. The average prevalence of chronic low back pain is approximately 15% in adults and 27% in the elderly and has been shown to be increasing as the population ages.[3]

Risk factors for development of low back pain are broad. Age older than 65 years is a prominent risk factor for the development of musculoskeletal impairment, with a majority of these cases involving the back. Genetic disposition, obesity, and smoking have also been linked to accelerated degenerative disk disease, increasing the risk of low back pain.[3] Studies of identical twins support the strong influence of genetic factors on the development of degenerative disk disease. Jobs involving heavy lifting, pulling, pushing, prolonged walking or standing, and vehicular driving have been found to be predictors of future low back pain.[4] Preexisting psychological conditions such as anxiety, depression, or somatization disorder, in addition to maladaptive coping strategies, lower socioeconomic status, and poor general health, are risk factors for chronic low back pain.[5] In fact, these factors are stronger predictors of long-term disability than any anatomic findings on imaging.

The total cost of low back pain in the Unites States exceeds $100 billion annually, most of which is spent on those who develop chronic, disabling low back pain. Fewer than 5% of back pain patients account for 75% of the total costs.[6] In addition to the financial burden, chronic low back pain can have a significant impact on quality of life, with 60% of patients reporting inability to perform daily activities and 25% being unable to work.[7] Given the significant socioeconomic burden of chronic low back pain, it becomes pertinent to understand the natural course of low back pain and risk factors for developing chronic pain to help direct diagnostic and treatment decisions.

PATHOPHYSIOLOGY

The lumbar spine consists of five lumbar vertebrae that increase in size caudally. Each vertebral body is separated by shock-absorbing intervertebral disks, consisting of a gelatinous nucleus pulposus surrounded by the fibrous rings of the anulus fibrosus. The nucleus pulposus consists of water, proteoglycans, and collagen; it is 90% water at birth and desiccates with time as part of the degenerative cascade. The neural arch is formed laterally by the pedicles, which connect the posterior elements to the vertebral bodies, and encloses the central canal where the spinal cord and cauda equina reside. The posterior elements consist of the laminae, spinous processes, and articular processes that form the facet joints. The space between adjacent pedicles forms the foramen through which spinal nerve roots may enter and exit the spinal canal. In addition, there are ligamentous structures supporting the lumbar spine. Pain can arise from the innervated intervertebral disks, facet joints, ligaments, or spinal nerve roots.

The lumbar spine is supported by various muscles that help provide dynamic stabilization to the spine and pelvis. Posteriorly, the paraspinal muscles consist of the erector spinae, multifidi, psoas, and quadratus lumborum. Anteriorly, the abdominal musculature, including the transversus abdominis, plays a critical role in supporting the lumbar spine. There is evidence to support that the structure and function of these spinal stabilizers are altered in patients with low back pain.[8] In addition, these muscles can be a potential source of myofascial low back pain.

Low back pain has been classified based on pathophysiology as either mechanical or the result of a systemic medical illness. Medical causes of low back pain include inflammatory, infectious, neoplastic, and visceral sources. Systemic medical causes of low back pain are rare but frequently associated with the need for time-sensitive treatment. If no primary systemic source is identified, the pain is classified as mechanical pain. Mechanical causes of low back pain include direct injury, deformity, imbalance, or overuse of identifiable structures in the lumbar spine, but are most commonly degenerative in nature. Structural sources of mechanical low back pain include the intervertebral disks, facet joints, vertebral bodies, nerves and nerve roots, ligamentous structures, paraspinal muscles, and sacroiliac joints. For example, wear and tear of the spine with aging can lead to intervertebral disk degeneration and herniation, facet and uncovertebral arthritis, osteophyte formation, ligamentous and capsular hypertrophy, and spondylolisthesis at various rates, which can be sources of pain independently or can lead to nerve root compression with resulting pain. When nerve root injury is contributing to low back pain, it can produce symptoms radiating down the leg including pain, weakness, paresthesias, and altered reflexes in a specific dermatomal or myotomal distribution, termed radiculopathy. Radiculopathy is reported in approximately 7% of patients with low back pain.[2]

Radicular pain is commonly attributed to direct compression of the spinal nerve roots with resulting structural, biochemical, and vascular changes in and around the spinal nerve. In addition, mechanical stimulation of the lumbar spinal nerve roots has been shown to increase the production of the pain-generating neuropeptide substance P.[9] Studies have shown that disk herniations and tears in the anulus fibrosus can produce increased inflammatory mediators, such as phospholipase A_2, cyclooxygenase 2, nitric oxide, cytokines, interleukins, and immunoglobulins, which can lead to local swelling and swelling of the spinal nerve roots.[9]

Pain can be further classified as nociceptive or neuropathic. Nociceptive pain is associated with tissue damage. Neuropathic pain is associated with minimal or no tissue damage and is more related to a dysfunction of the pain regulatory function of the central and peripheral nervous system. Why damage to specific anatomic locations produces severe pain in some but no pain in others is quite complicated and not fully understood but relates to numerous factors including local inflammation, biomechanical factors, muscular strength and flexibility deficiencies and imbalances, and centrally mediated pain regulatory systems that are influenced by mood, sleep, cardiovascular health, and psychosocial context.

CLINICAL PRESENTATION

Symptomatically, mechanical lumbar spine disorders can be classified as axial or radicular pain. Axial low back pain is typically isolated to the back at the lumbar spine or lumbosacral junction with varying degrees of gluteal symptoms. New, acute low back pain typically is axial pain only but can be severe, disrupting sleep, work, and activities of daily living. It is often exacerbated by prolonged sitting, standing, leaning, or bending and is mitigated by frequent positional shifts. Extension typically worsens pain mediated from the posterior elements, whereas flexion typically worsens pain mediated from anterior elements. The seated position, forward flexion, and Valsalva maneuver can increase intradiskal pressure, worsening disk-mediated low back pain. Facet loading may worsen facet-mediated pain.

Patients with the syndrome of lumbar radiculopathy will often have leg and thigh pain greater than low back pain. Pain can be severe even in the absence of neurologic deficit. Neurologic symptoms of numbness, tingling, weakness, reflex changes, and root tension signs may be seen on examination. Symptoms are exacerbated by prolonged sitting, coughing, sneezing, Valsalva maneuver, and bending. Pain is often mitigated by frequent positional shifts and walking. Pain radiating past the knee and into the calf or foot is typically radicular and represents nerve root or peripheral nerve injury. However, pain in the buttocks and thigh is not always radicular and can come from anatomic locations outside of the spine. It can be referred from adjacent bone, ligament, or muscle structures, making it important to evaluate the hip, pelvis, and surrounding musculature to rule out any other contributing pathology before attributing this type of pain to the lumbar spine.

Other specific causes of low back pain have a more identifiable presentation. Patients with lumbar spinal stenosis, narrowing of the spinal canal with or without compression of the spinal cord, typically have back pain and neurogenic claudication. Patients often describe their legs as feeling heavy or wooden. Neurogenic claudication is defined as thigh and calf pain worsened by standing or walking and alleviated with sitting. This can be differentiated from vascular claudication in that patients with vascular claudication may have altered peripheral pulses, more difficulty with uphill walking, no symptoms with standing alone, and a steady degree of symptomatic severity from day to day. In contrast, patients with neurogenic claudication have significant day-to-day variability, and symptoms with standing still. Walking with a shopping cart is often better tolerated in neurogenic claudication because the patient is flexed forward, thus expanding the spinal canal diameter. Neurologic changes are usually more subtle, with vibratory loss in the distal lower extremities, increased pain with lumbar extension, absent root tension signs, mild balance deficits, and largely normal strength on examination.

In conus medullaris and cauda equina syndromes, saddle anesthesia, urinary retention or incontinence, lower extremity weakness, and recent-onset erectile dysfunction can be seen. Cauda equina syndrome involves compression of multiple lumbosacral nerve roots below the termination of the spinal cord, called the cauda equina, leading to the aforementioned symptoms and hyporeflexia in the lower extremities. This syndrome can be caused by several conditions, including trauma, tumors, spondylolisthesis, and direct compression secondary to severe spinal stenosis or a large disk herniation. It is a very rare but serious neurologic condition, and urgent surgical referral is recommended.

Other conditions to consider are the seronegative spondyloarthropathies, spinal tumors, vertebral fractures, and spinal infections. Seronegative spondyloarthropathies (see Chapter 215) typically are seen in younger patients with symptoms of pain, stiffness, and reduced range of movement in the morning that improves with activity. Family history and additional joint symptoms should be explored. Tumors of the spine may occur in patients with prior history of malignant disease; localized pain is frequently reported to increase in the supine position and at night. Although classically taught "red flags" for tumor include age older than 50, weight loss, and failure to improve after 1 month, there is low diagnostic accuracy for any of these factors independently.[10] In patients with recent spinal surgery, recent skin or urine infections, history of intravenous drug abuse, or immunocompromised states, infection should be considered. Although fever is commonly sited as a red flag for spinal infection, this finding has low sensitivity and lack of fever does not rule out infection. Vertebral fracture should be considered in the differential if there is a history of significant trauma, older age, or corticosteroid use.[11] Among all primary care patients with low back pain, fewer than 5% have a serious systemic pathology. However, given the important clinical implications, it is paramount to screen for these diagnoses.

PHYSICAL EXAMINATION

Physical examination starts with careful observation of the patient; the examiner looks for discomfort or frequent change of positions and evaluates the patient's affect. Spinal examination then begins with observation of the lumbar spine, looking for any asymmetries or abnormal curvature. Palpation and percussion of the spinous processes should be performed to evaluate for osseous pain and spinal infection. The range of motion of the lumbar spine should be assessed in flexion, extension, lateral flexion, and rotation to evaluate for changes in symptoms throughout the movements. The normal range of motion of the lumbar spine is 40 to 60 degrees of forward flexion, 20 to 35 degrees of extension, 15 to 20 degrees of lateral flexion, and 3 to 18 degrees of rotation. Pain with movement in specific directions should be noted. As previously explained, anterior sources of pain tend to worsen with forward flexion and posterior sources of pain tend to worsen with extension. Although limitations in range of motion may not permit identification of the specific source of pain, assessment of range of motion can provide an index for future comparison to assess therapeutic response. Facet loading can be performed by placing the patient in hyperextension with a slight rotation toward each side to help identify facet-mediated pain.

Anatomic alignment during neutral standing should be noted. Romberg testing should be performed to test balance. Gait should be examined to look for antalgia, footdrop, spastic or mechanical movement, Trendelenburg gait, and widened or narrowed steps. The skin and lower extremity pulses should be examined to look for vascular insufficiency as a potential cause of thigh or calf symptoms. In addition, if patients are describing symptoms of cauda equina syndrome, rectal examination should be considered to evaluate for loss of rectal tone.

Neurologic examination should be undertaken, assessing the symmetry of the patient's strength in hip flexion, knee extension, knee flexion, ankle dorsiflexion, ankle plantar flexion, foot

TABLE 181-2 Lumbar Dermatomes

Root	Muscle Group Affected	Dermatome	Reflexes	Special Maneuvers
L1	None	Back, groin	None	None
L2	Hip flexors, hip adductors	Anterolateral upper thigh	None	Femoral stretch
L3	Hip flexors, quadriceps, hip adductors	Anterior lower thigh, medial knee	± Patellar	Femoral stretch
L4	Quadriceps, ankle dorsiflexors	Medial lower leg	Patellar	Femoral stretch
L5	Extensor hallucis, ankle dorsiflexors, hamstrings, hip abductors, peroneals	Lateral lower leg, dorsal medial three toes	Medial hamstring	Straight leg raise
S1	Ankle plantar flexors, gluteals, hamstrings, peroneals	Posterior thigh, lateral toes, sole of foot	Achilles	Straight leg raise

eversion, great toe extension, and hip abduction bilaterally. In addition, the patient should be observed walking on heels and toes to assess for functional strength in L5 and S1, respectively. It may be difficult for the examiner to overcome the quadriceps, even if there is some weakness. The examiner should have the patient perform single-legged sit-to-stand testing bilaterally, with examiner support for balance, to pick up mild quadriceps weakness. Because plantar flexion weakness may be difficult to detect, it is recommended to test the S1 myotome with repeated standing calf raises on each leg to elicit any mild weakness or muscular atrophy. Sensation to both light touch and pinprick should be checked for sensory deficits throughout the dermatomes listed in Table 181-2. Bilateral reflexes should also be elicited at the patella (L4 nerve root), and Achilles (S1 nerve root). Babinski examination and evaluation for clonus, muscle spasticity, or increased tone can help assess for upper motor neuron involvement. Because disk herniations are most common at L4-L5 and L5-S1, clinical changes in these myotomes and dermatomes should be thoroughly assessed.

If the patient's symptoms are radicular in nature, root tension signs can help identify irritation of the lumbar nerve roots. The straight leg raise test is performed to assess for damage to L5-S1. With the patient in the supine position, the examiner raises the straight leg to approximately 70 to 90 degrees of hip flexion. If the patient's typical pain or paresthesias are reproduced at any point when the leg is in 20 to 70 degrees of hip flexion, the test result is positive and indicates that a nerve root impingement from a herniated disk is likely contributing, referred to as sciatica. Studies have reported a high sensitivity but low specificity of the straight leg raise.[12] If the unaffected leg is tested and symptoms are reproduced in the symptomatic leg, this is called a positive crossed straight leg raise and has increased specificity for disk herniation.[12] A modification to the straight leg raise can be performed in the seated position and is referred to as the seated slump test. The patient is asked to slump forward, allowing the thoracic and lumbar spine to collapse into flexion, and then to fully flex the cervical spine toward the chest. The patient is then asked to extend each leg fully and dorsiflex the ankle to see if there is reproduction of symptoms down the leg.[13] Another root tension sign, the femoral nerve stretch test, is used to look for an upper lumbar radiculopathy in L2-L4 distribution. With the patient in the prone position, the leg is flexed at the knee and the hip is brought into extension. The test result is considered positive if a reproduction of typical pain in the anterior thigh occurs.

DIAGNOSTICS

The most recent guidelines from the American Academy of Family Physicians, American College of Physicians, and American Pain Society do not recommend routine imaging for patients with acute or nonspecific low back pain, because this does not improve clinical outcomes and exposes patients to unnecessary radiation.[14,15] A systematic review and meta-analysis of six trials comparing immediate imaging with usual care for patients with acute and subacute low back pain, without suspicion for infection or malignancy, found no significant difference in short- or long-term outcomes for pain or function.[16] However, if a patient has certain red-flag symptoms, described earlier, or if clinical improvement has not occurred in 4 to 6 weeks, plain radiographs of the lumbar spine are the preferred initial diagnostic tool.[14] Typically, anterior-posterior and lateral views are sufficient. Oblique views can also be obtained to visualize the pars interarticularis but are not routinely recommended. Because plain radiographs have low sensitivity and specificity,[15] their diagnostic yield is limited; persistent pain or suspicious symptoms may prompt additional imaging.

The most widely used imaging modality to further evaluate low back pain and radiculopathy is magnetic resonance imaging (MRI). Its principal use is to evaluate the bone structures and soft tissues, and it can be helpful to look for degenerative disk disease, disk herniations, spinal stenosis, and cord or root compression. With the addition of gadolinium, it can be used to look for tumor or infection and can distinguish epidural scar tissue in postoperative patients. MRI, however, is an expensive diagnostic tool. Guidelines recommend MRI acutely only if patients have severe or progressive neurologic deficits or symptoms of a serious underlying condition.[14] MRI can also be considered for a patient with persistent low back pain with symptoms of nerve root impingement refractory to conservative treatment, for which interventional procedures are being considered. Although it is superior for identification of potential pain generators in the spine, MRI abnormalities do not always correlate with clinical complaints, and multiple studies have found common pain-producing degenerative findings in asymptomatic patients.[17] In cases where radiographic findings are consistent with clinical presentation, the magnitude of radiographic findings does not correlate with symptom severity or clinical outcome, and symptom improvement does not correlate with resolution of radiographic defects.[18] For this reason, physicians should focus on clinical presentation rather than radiographic abnormalities. Contraindications to MRI include pacemaker, retained metal fragments such as from a gunshot wound, and severe claustrophobia. Most currently used orthopedic metal does not preclude MRI imaging.

Other diagnostic tools used for low back pain are radionuclide bone scintigraphy and computed tomography (CT). Bone scintigraphy is helpful if the history and physical examination raise suspicion for osteomyelitis, bone neoplasm, or occult fracture. The addition of bone scan with single-photon emission computed tomography (SPECT) can identify recent pars fracture and facet osteoarthritis. CT can be helpful in assessing the bone architecture of the spine and can also provide helpful imaging in a postsurgical patient with excessive hardware or in those with contraindications to MRI. CT imaging can be used to assess for degenerative disorders such as spondylosis, spondylolysis, spondylolisthesis, and spinal stenosis as well as to show cortical irregularities in osteoarthritis. It can be used in combination with myelography to visualize the borders and contents of the dural sac and to evaluate for cord compression.

Other diagnostic workup may be considered on a case-by-case basis. Laboratory testing, such as erythrocyte sedimentation rate and C-reactive protein, can be helpful in a patient with constitutional symptoms to quantify systemic inflammation, as can be seen with infection, inflammatory spondyloarthropathies, or neoplasm. Neoplasm may also be associated with an abnormal complete blood count, alkaline phosphatase, or calcium level. Electrodiagnostic studies can be helpful in assessing neurologic changes associated with denervation caused by subacute and chronic radiculopathy. Electromyography may not be able to detect acute changes until approximately 3 to 4 weeks after the initial insult. The needle electromyographic portion of the examination can identify radiculopathy with high specificity; however, it is relatively insensitive to the clinical syndrome of radicular pain without motor or reflex changes.

The goal of diagnostic testing is to help guide management strategies and improve patient outcomes. Unless there is clear indication that testing can aid in this process, routine testing is not recommended, especially in a population with low clinical suspicion, because this can lead to false positives, unnecessary medical expenses, and avoidable patient anxiety. Many patients have come to expect imaging, so it is important for the clinician to educate the patient and provide reassurance. Imaging for reassurance has not been shown to improve outcomes. In one randomized trial, low-risk patients who received an educational intervention rather than radiography were equally satisfied with their care and had no difference in clinical outcomes.[19]

DIFFERENTIAL DIAGNOSIS

As described earlier, the majority of low back pain is mechanical pain and attributed to degenerative changes. Although this degenerative process is a common progression with aging and typically benign, it may cause compression or irritation of the spinal nerve roots or the spinal cord, leading to radiculopathy and myelopathy. In addition, other sources of low back pain requiring intervention should be considered, including fracture, inflammatory disease, neoplasm, infection, and other medical causes.

A thorough history including past medical, social, occupational, and family history as well as review of systems including constitutional symptoms, skin changes, abdominal or visceral pain, neurologic changes, and bowel or bladder complaints should be undertaken for a patient with low back pain. Other conditions that can mimic lumbar spine degenerative disorders include diabetic amyotrophy (radiculoplexus), vascular claudication, sacroiliitis and associated seronegative spondyloarthropathy, shingles with or without rash, pancreatitis, intra-abdominal or gynecologic pathology, renal colic, Lyme radiculopathy, epidural abscess or osteomyelitis, osteoporotic or malignant fractures, and malignant disease involving the spine and spinal canal. Red flags, discussed earlier, should be considered when forming the differential diagnosis. In addition, surrounding muscles and ligaments can be a source of pain, and adjacent bones or joints can elicit pain in similar distributions and should be considered in the differential diagnosis.

DIFFERENTIAL DIAGNOSIS

Low Back Pain

MECHANICAL CAUSES OF LOW BACK PAIN

- Diskogenic pain or disk herniation
- Facet-mediated pain
- Radicular pain from nerve root compression
- Lumbar spinal stenosis with or without radiculopathy or myelopathy
  - Cauda equina syndrome
  - Conus medullaris syndrome
- Spondylolisthesis
- Muscle strain
- Osteoporotic fracture

SYSTEMIC MEDICAL CAUSES OF LOW BACK PAIN

- Infection
  - Osteomyelitis, diskitis, epidural abscess, tuberculosis, shingles
- Neoplasm
  - Multiple myeloma, lymphoma and leukemia, spinal cord tumors, retroperitoneal tumors, osteoma
- Inflammatory disease
  - Ankylosing spondylitis, psoriatic arthritis, reactive arthritis (Reiter disease), enteropathy-associated arthritis
- Visceral disease
  - Intra-abdominal pathology (pancreatitis, cholecystitis, abdominal aortic aneurysm), gynecologic pathology (endometriosis, pelvic inflammatory disease), renal pathology (kidney stones, renal stones, perinephric abscess, kidney infection)
- Other
  - Hip or pelvic pathology
  - Fibromyalgia
  - Peripheral neuropathy

MANAGEMENT

Specialist referral is indicated for refractory back or radicular symptoms, neurologic weakness, consideration of interventional procedure, or diagnostic dilemma.

Immediate emergency department referral is indicated for significant neurologic compromise or cauda equina syndrome for consideration of surgical decompression.

The primary goal of treatment is to identify and treat any serious or systemic causes of low back pain early. If no serious or concerning source of pain is identified, the goal is to minimize pain and functional limitation and prevent chronic, disabling low back pain.

Physical Therapy Management of Low Back Pain

The physical therapy management of low back pain is most effective when a multimodal treatment approach with a combination of therapeutic exercise, manual therapy, modalities, and patient education is used. Early entry into a physical therapy program, within the first 6 weeks of symptom onset, has been shown to reduce risk of progression of psychosocial features associated with low back pain such as depression, somatic distress, and anxiety.[20,21] In addition, primary care referral of patients with low back pain to physical therapy performed within 14 days of onset was associated with decreased advanced imaging, additional physicians visits, major surgery, lumbar spine injections, and opioid medications compared with delayed physical therapy entry (more than 14 days).[22] Ultimately, the sooner the referral is made and physical therapy is initiated, the better the chance for a positive outcome. Once a referral to physical therapy is deemed appropriate, the physician should write a prescription noting the diagnosis, stating "evaluate and treat" with any specific treatment recommendations, a suggestion of the estimated frequency and duration of treatment, and relevant precautions. For most acute initial spine conditions, one to three visits per week for the appropriate time period required to rehabilitate the particular patient (typically 4 to 8 weeks) is appropriate. Chronic spinal conditions may require more than 8 weeks for rehabilitation, depending on the diagnosis.

Therapeutic Exercise. Although there is limited evidence to support the use of exercise therapy in acute low back pain, exercise therapy has been shown to be beneficial to patients with subacute and chronic low back pain, providing both short-term pain relief and longer-lasting functional improvement.[23,24] Therapeutic exercise interventions used in physical therapy include range-of-motion and stretching exercises, core stabilization and motor control exercises, strengthening, and general conditioning. Range-of-motion exercises are typically prescribed with a directional bias, such as flexion, extension, side-glide, or rotation, based on the patient's response during the examination, called mechanical diagnosis therapy. Specific lumbar spine diagnoses tend to result in directional preferences. For example, spinal stenosis tends to respond better to a flexion-based program, whereas disk herniations with accompanying radiculopathy tend to respond more favorably to extension-based programs. Individualized exercises prescribed to match the directional preference have been shown to decrease patients' pain and reduce medication use.[25,26]

Core strengthening includes strengthening of the abdominal, gluteal, hip girdle, and paraspinal musculature to promote lumbar stability by providing dynamic support. There are limited randomized controlled trials that show the benefit of core strengthening, but, given its low risk, it is used regularly. Lumbar core stabilization instruction can be individualized according to the patient's directional preference, with emphasis on appropriate recruitment patterns of the deep core spinal stabilizers, because these muscles have demonstrated altered recruitment patterns in patients with low back pain.[27] Rehabilitative ultrasound imaging is useful in assisting with assessment of aberrant motor recruitment patterns and in providing biofeedback for neuromuscular re-education of the deep lumbopelvic muscles, including the transversus abdominis, the internal and external obliques, and the multifidi.[27] Stretching of the hamstrings, hip flexors, piriformis, and gastrocnemius and soleus muscles along with other muscle tissues found to be tight may also be beneficial in relieving local myofascial symptoms.

Conditioning, such as cardiovascular fitness, is also an important component in the rehabilitation of the spine; studies suggest that people who are physically fit experience low back pain less frequently than do people who are not physically fit.[28] Exercise therapy has been shown to be more beneficial when it includes aerobic activity and cognitive-behavioral strategies that promote a gradual increase in daily activity. Aerobic conditioning is also an important part of the treatment of chronic pain conditions such as fibromyalgia, which can be a comorbid syndrome in patients with low back pain.

Manual Therapy. Manual therapy for the lumbar spine can include but is not limited to spinal manipulative therapy (SMT), spinal mobilization, and myofascial release. SMT is defined as the application of high-velocity, low-amplitude manual thrust to the spinal joints just beyond the joint range of motion. When manipulation is contraindicated, spinal mobilization techniques can be used to restore joint mobility to hypomobile joints. Spinal mobilization is the application of manual force to the spinal joints within the passive joint's physiologic range of motion without a thrust. Although individualized randomized controlled trials have shown variable results, two recent Cochrane reviews found that spinal manipulation was more effective than sham and comparable to other modalities for acute and chronic low back pain.[29,30] Similarly, Bronfort and coworkers[31] published a review supporting the use of SMT and mobilization for the treatment of chronic low back pain. Based on the current evidence, manipulation may be worth a trial in patients with interest and access. Contraindications to manipulation include direct trauma, unexplained weight loss, history of cancer, spinal fracture, unrelenting night pain, osteoporosis, severe spinal stenosis, cauda equina syndrome, and neurologic deficits with limb weakness.

Therapeutic Modalities. Modalities frequently used in physical therapy include the following.

- *Ice.* Patients are instructed to ice for 10 to 15 minutes several times a day for acute episodes of low back pain to help reduce edema, though research has produced insufficient data to show its benefit. Contraindications include cold sensitivity, Reynaud phenomenon, open wounds, and impaired sensation.
- *Superficial heat.* Heat is commonly applied during therapy, to help promote circulation to the area and possibly hasten healing, but also as a method to manage pain. Contraindications include malignant disease, active bleeding into a joint or muscle tissue, anesthesia or impaired sensation, and impaired mentation.
- *Ultrasound to treat tendon, ligament, and joint injuries.* Ultrasound, a form of deep heat, can be useful in treating muscle spasms, tendinopathy, or degenerative arthritis. Contraindications include malignant disease, laminectomy sites, fluid-containing cavities, unhealed joint fractures, and joint arthroplasty containing methylmethacrylate or high-density polyethylene.
- *Transcutaneous electrical nerve stimulation (TENS) for analgesia.* Contraindications to electrical stimulation include cardiac pacemakers and defibrillators, areas with metal close to the skin, anesthetic areas, incompletely healed wounds, and areas near the eyes, carotid sinus, or mucous membranes.
- *Traction.* Traction has been classically used for patients with radicular symptoms to help resolve neurologic deficits

and reduce pain. Studies addressing the efficacy of traction have been largely inconclusive. A recent systematic review found that traction provided no benefit in the short or long term for patients with low back pain with or without sciatica.[32]

Research on these modalities has provided inconsistent results regarding their benefit when compared with placebo, and there are insufficient data to recommend these strategies based on the current evidence. However, because these modalities have low risk, a trial may be warranted in specific cases if not contraindicated.

Medications

Medications can be a helpful strategy for pain management. A trial of nonsteroidal anti-inflammatory drugs (NSAIDs) or acetaminophen is the recommended first-line treatment for acute low back pain and acute exacerbations of subacute or chronic low back pain by the American College of Physicians, if the patient has no contraindications.[14] However, clinical trials have shown variable results with limited benefit from these medications and patients should be monitored for adverse effects. Additional medications can be used for short-term pain management if the pain is severe, including muscle relaxants. Centrally acting skeletal muscle relaxants, such as cyclobenzaprine, can be used to help reduce back spasms associated with mechanical low back pain and have been found to be more effective than placebo for short-term relief of acute low back pain.[33] Side effects, particularly sedation, can be limiting. There is insufficient evidence to determine if these medications are beneficial in subacute or chronic back pain management.

Although opioid analgesics are commonly prescribed, there are limited data to support their use for acute low back pain. Because of this, prescription becomes a matter of clinical judgement. If prescribed, their use should be restricted to the short term and patients monitored closely for adverse effects or signs of abuse. A 2013 systematic review found that opioids, compared with placebo, had short-term efficacy for pain relief and functional improvement in chronic low back pain. However, trials comparing opioids with NSAIDS or antidepressants found no significant difference between groups, and there were no trials evaluating the long-term use of opioids.[34] This suggests that opioids may be beneficial for short-term use in selected patients with acute exacerbations, but does not provide evidence to support the use of opioids for long-term treatment of chronic low back pain. Clinical trials have supported the use of tramadol, a nonopioid medication that acts on the opioid receptor, as an alternative to opioids.[34,35]

Other medications used for the management of chronic low back pain include tricyclic antidepressants and mixed norepinephrine-serotonin reuptake inhibitors. Although studies to support these medications have shown small and variable benefits, many patients with chronic low back pain have undiagnosed depression and may benefit from a trial of these medications if not responding to other treatment options. The clinician must monitor for medication side effects, particularly anticholinergic effects. Gabapentin has been shown to be beneficial for treatment of central pain syndrome as well as radiculopathy. Used anecdotally by many practitioners, systemic corticosteroids have not been shown to be more effective than placebo for treatment of low back pain with or without leg symptoms and are not recommended. More recently, glucosamine has been tested for management of low back pain with no evidence of benefit.

COMPLEMENTARY AND ALTERNATIVE MANAGEMENT

Complementary and alternative treatments of subacute and chronic low back pain have also been shown to be useful for some patients. Acupuncture or dry needling,[36] chiropractic manipulation,[36] and massage therapy are alternative therapies with limited side effects and research to suggest they may be more beneficial than placebo treatments for short-term pain relief. However, few of these therapies have been shown to be effective in the long term for chronic low back pain.[14] In addition, studies have shown that patient expectations of benefits may play a role in perceived benefits, particularly with regard to acupuncture, so patient selection should be considered.

PSYCHOLOGICAL HEALTH

Because psychosocial issues are a known risk factor for chronic low back pain, modification of maladaptive pain behaviors and cognitive processes associated with pain perception through use of behavioral therapy has been studied as a treatment adjunctive for chronic back pain. A 2010 Cochrane review found moderate-quality evidence supporting the benefit of behavioral treatment compared with standard care in the short term.[37] More recent studies have shown the benefit of a multidisciplinary approaching incorporating cognitive behavioral therapy with traditional exercise programs, with regard to patient-rated pain, disability, and fear-avoidance behavior, as well as overall quality of life, in both the short and long term in patients with and without preexisting mood disorders.[38,39] In addition, these studies have shown this to be a cost-effective management option.

SPINAL INTERVENTIONAL PROCEDURES

Another consideration for treatment of subacute and chronic low back pain is lumbar epidural corticosteroid injection. This typically requires referral to an interventional spine physician. Indications for epidural injections supported by the literature are symptoms of radiculopathy and spinal stenosis.[9] Although randomized trial results are varied, research suggests that these injections offer short-term symptom relief for patients with sciatica.[40] Further studies are needed to assess the efficacy of epidural injections for axial low back pain. Injections can also be performed into the facet joints or the nerves innervating the joint, with subsequent radiofrequency ablation of these nerves if beneficial, for symptomatic relief of facet-mediated pain. Trigger point injections performed into the muscles in the area of pain can also help in the short term and are of low risk when dry needling or injection of anesthetic without corticosteroid is performed. Studies on these later options have shown varied results and are ongoing. Other alternatives, such as prolotherapy, oxygen-ozone injections, Botox injections, and tumor necrosis factor-α injections, are currently being researched and have uncertain efficacy at this time.

COMPLICATIONS

Serious life-threatening complications of degenerative lumbar spine disorders are rare. If serious underlying conditions have not been discovered by thorough history, physical examination, and diagnostic workup, episodes of low back pain are typically self-limited. Special attention is warranted when significant neurologic weakness or cauda equina syndrome is occurring, and urgent referral to a spine surgeon is appropriate.

Substantial comorbid sequelae of chronic pain can occur. These include development of chronic pain syndrome and centrally mediated sensitization to pain, sleep disturbance, anxiety and depression because of chronic pain, disruption of activities of daily living, loss of work and wages, and disruption of interpersonal relationships.

INDICATIONS FOR REFERRAL OR HOSPITALIZATION

- Mechanical low back pain in the acute and subacute phases does not typically necessitate further specialist referral or hospitalization.
- Physical therapy referral may be a useful adjunct to conservative measures. Refractory low back pain lasting 4 to 6 weeks has classically been an indication for physical therapy referral. However, current research suggests that early referral within the first 2 weeks of presentation has shown improved outcomes, particularly in patients with psychosocial comorbidities, and should be considered in such patients.
- Referral to a spine specialist should be considered if the patient's pain is severe and refractory, functionally limiting, or persistent beyond the expected duration. A variety of specialties have concentrations in spine, including physical medicine and rehabilitation, anesthesia pain management, rheumatology, orthopedics, and neurology. Diagnostic studies, pharmacologic measures, activity and exercise recommendations, interventional procedures, and surgical interventions can be discussed with a spine specialist, as needed.
- Referral to an orthopedic spine surgeon or neurosurgeon should be made for a patient with progressive weakness or neurologic deficits for consideration of surgical decompression, if deemed appropriate by the surgeon. If the patient has symptoms of radiculopathy or spinal stenosis, surgical referral may be indicated if the patient fails to respond to conservative management. Surgical care has been shown to be superior to conservative care for patients with herniated disk–related radicular symptoms, spinal stenosis with pseudoclaudication, and degenerative spondylolisthesis.[41-43]
- Multidisciplinary pain management center referral should be considered for patients with chronic, refractory, debilitating low back pain without surgical indications.
- Radiculopathy with significant weakness or cauda equina syndrome with associated bowel or bladder incontinence, saddle anesthesia, and progressive weakness should be treated with emergent hospitalization for surgical evaluation.

LIFE SPAN CONSIDERATIONS

Once a patient has had an episode of low back pain, the chance of recurrence is 75% in the next 12 months. That patient is then at increased risk for recurrent episodes throughout his or her life span. Maintaining ideal body weight and aerobic exercise may decrease frequency of flares. If the patient has a disk herniation and radicular symptoms, although this disk material will likely be reabsorbed with time, the disk is at risk of reherniation, and persistence of chronic axial low back pain is common.

Spondylolysis often occurs in an athletic child or teen and may lead to spondylolisthesis in the older adult. Neurologic compression or traction from spondylolisthesis can result in back and radicular pain. Patients with ankylosing spondylitis usually are seen in late adolescence or early 20s, and these patients frequently develop thoracic kyphosis and low back pain with aging.

Age is a strong factor for development of degenerative disk disease and spinal stenosis. Age- and medication-related osteoporosis will increase the risk of vertebral compression fractures and resultant loss of height and development of kyphosis or scoliosis. One prospective study showed that 57% of asymptomatic patients over the age of 60 had abnormal MRIs, 36% with herniated disks and 21% with lumbar stenosis, despite their lack of symptoms. In fact, all but one patient had evidence of degeneration and bulging disks by the age of 60, supporting that spinal degeneration is a normal and expected change with age but can have variable clinical manifestations.[44]

PATIENT EDUCATION AND HEALTH PROMOTION

Patient education should start with reassurance and support. Explaining the natural history of mechanical low back pain and that most cases will resolve in a timely manner is critical. It is also important to educate the patient that pain may come and go, despite activity, and that recurrence is common after the first episode of low back pain. Because these episodes are not related to activity, activity avoidance should be discouraged. Exercise has been shown to help minimize recurrences and treat subacute and chronic low back pain, so regular daily activity should be advised. Maintenance of ideal body weight and proper body mechanics should be emphasized to help reduce the frequency of recurrence of episodes and improve pain tolerance. Encouraging frequent position shifting helps patients with many degenerative spinal issues. If a patient needs to return to a physically demanding job, a back school program may be helpful.

Risk factors for inflammation and disk degeneration, such as smoking and obesity, should be addressed. Treatment of underlying medical conditions such as osteoporosis should be considered, to lessen the risk of conditions such as compression fractures. In addition, if the patient has concomitant psychosocial factors, these should be addressed.

Patients need to understand red flags that would warrant urgent medical evaluation, including new limb weakness, change in bowel or bladder function, and constitutional signs. This will ensure that any dangerous systemic issues are addressed early and that the more urgent functional sequelae are treated on a timely basis, thereby avoiding permanent neurologic damage.

CHAPTER 182

METABOLIC BONE DISEASE: OSTEOPOROSIS AND PAGET DISEASE OF BONE

Alan Ona Malabanan

OSTEOPOROSIS

DEFINITION AND EPIDEMIOLOGY

Osteoporosis is characterized by increased bone fragility and increased susceptibility to fracture. This increased bone fragility results from decreases in bone mass and deterioration of bone microarchitecture that occur as the result of estrogen deficiency and aging. A variety of diseases, such as rheumatoid arthritis, and medications, such as glucocorticoids, may contribute to bone loss. Osteoporosis is the most common metabolic bone disease; more than 10 million Americans are affected, and an additional 33.6 million have low bone mass and are at high risk for development of the disease. An important responsibility of the primary care provider is the prevention, detection, and treatment of osteoporosis.[1]

Osteoporosis is also defined by the World Health Organization (WHO) as a bone mineral density (BMD) of 2.5 standard deviations (SDs) or less below the young normal mean (i.e., T-score ≤−2.5). The International Society for Clinical Densitometry (ISCD) has recommended that this definition be applied only to postmenopausal women and men older than 50 years.[2] In the absence of osteoporotic fracture, this densitometric definition is the most clinically relevant, but it should not be used as the sole criterion for treatment decision. Much as elevated cholesterol concentration is one risk factor for heart attack, osteoporosis is but one risk factor for osteoporotic fracture. There is no definitive BMD threshold at which osteoporotic fractures occur, only an increasing likelihood of fracture with decreasing BMD. Other risk factors, such as increasing age, family history of hip fracture, current cigarette smoking, prior osteoporotic fracture, glucocorticoid use, rheumatoid arthritis, and excessive alcohol intake, have an impact on this fracture likelihood independent of the BMD. The National Osteoporosis Foundation guidelines recommend the use of the WHO Fracture Risk Assessment Tool (FRAX) score to guide treatment in patients who have densitometric osteopenia but are at high absolute risk for fracture.[1]

PATHOPHYSIOLOGY

In addition to providing a supportive and protective framework for the body, bone serves as a large calcium reservoir. Calcium is necessary for proper neural, musculoskeletal, and cardiac function. Normal bone remodeling allows both access to the calcium reservoir and replacement or repair of old and damaged bone. Bone remodeling has two main phases: bone resorption and bone formation.

Bone resorption, which releases calcium into the circulation, is the removal of damaged or old bone by osteoclasts, cells derived from macrophages and monocytes. This process is rapid and occurs in a matter of days to weeks. Osteoblasts, in response to parathyroid hormone (PTH) and other cytokines, secrete RANK (receptor activator of nuclear factor κB) ligand and monocyte colony-stimulating factor, which cause monocytes and macrophages to differentiate into osteoclasts and to proliferate. Osteoclasts produce powerful degradative enzymes, such as cathepsin K, to break down bone, releasing calcium, phosphorus, and type I collagen cross-linked products into the circulation.

Bone formation occurs when osteoblasts lay down osteoid, an organic matrix composed of type I collagen and other proteins. Bone formation, occurring during months, is a slow process. It is estimated that the skeleton is completely replaced during approximately 4 years. Osteoblasts are also responsible for mineralization of the bone, depositing calcium and phosphorus into the osteoid. This process depends on the presence of adequate amounts of calcium and phosphorus and alkaline phosphatase activity. Poor bone mineralization leads to osteomalacia, a painful softening of the bone.

Normally, bone resorption and bone formation proceed at equal rates. In osteoporosis, however, the rate of bone resorption exceeds that of bone formation, producing a net loss of bone. This uncoupling of bone resorption and bone formation is a consequence of estrogen deficiency and is most pronounced in the first 5 to 10 years after menopause.

Glucocorticoid use is the most common cause of secondary osteoporosis. It causes osteoblast death, prolongs the life of osteoclasts, decreases levels of estrogen and testosterone, increases the metabolism of vitamin D, and decreases the intestinal absorption of calcium, although the evidence supporting a strong role for PTH and hypogonadism in glucocorticoid-induced osteoporosis is lacking. This increased bone resorption and decreased bone formation lead to a rapid loss of bone, the majority of which occurs in the first 6 months of glucocorticoid use. In addition, the bone quality is impaired, leading to a rapid increase in relative risk of fracture by as much as 75% within the first 3 months after initiation of glucocorticoids.[3] Other drugs, such as chronic opiates, immunosuppressants, anticonvulsants, heparin, excessive thyroid hormone, leuprolide, and cancer chemotherapeutics, lead to similar changes in bone metabolism.

Risk Factors

Risk factors, both unmodifiable and modifiable, increase the risk of bone loss or osteoporotic fracture. The WHO FRAX model includes the following risk factors: advanced age, female gender, a prior osteoporotic fracture (including morphometric vertebral fracture), femoral neck BMD, low body mass index, oral glucocorticoid use of 5 mg of prednisone or more per day for 3 or more months (ever), rheumatoid arthritis, secondary osteoporosis, parental history of hip fracture, current smoking, and alcohol intake of three or more drinks per day. The National Osteoporosis Foundation recommends use of these risk factors through the WHO FRAX (at www.shef.ac.uk/FRAX) to decide on treatment of densitometric osteopenia in postmenopausal women and men aged 50 years and older. There are many other risk factors not included in FRAX that may play a role in individual assessment of need for bone density testing or osteoporosis therapy (Box 182-1).

CLINICAL PRESENTATION

Unless an osteoporotic fracture is present, osteoporosis is clinically silent. Low BMD in the absence of osteoporotic fracture does not cause pain. If pain is present, the fracture should be

BOX 182-1

Risk Factors for Bone Loss or Osteoporotic Fracture

UNMODIFIABLE
- Advanced age*
- Female gender*
- White or Asian race
- Personal history of fracture*
- History of fracture in a first-degree relative*
- Dementia

MODIFIABLE
- Hypogonadism
- Current cigarette smoking*
- Excessive alcohol* or caffeine use
- Low calcium intake
- Low body weight (<58 kg [127 lb])*
- Inadequate physical activity
- Visual impairment
- Glucocorticoid* or anticonvulsant use
- Thyrotoxicosis
- Recurrent falls
- Poor health or frailty

*Included in FRAX calculations.

confirmed or a secondary cause of the low BMD, such as osteomalacia, ruled out.

The sine qua non of osteoporosis is an osteoporotic fracture, a fracture occurring with no or minimum trauma. The presence of a typical osteoporotic fracture in a postmenopausal woman is usually sufficient for the diagnosis of osteoporosis. The typical sites of fractures include the vertebrae, the distal wrist, the proximal femur, and the ribs. Unfortunately, even in the presence of a typical osteoporotic fracture, the diagnosis of osteoporosis is often missed and treatment is never initiated. Osteoporosis occurring in men and premenopausal or perimenopausal women should lead to a consideration of secondary causes of osteoporosis.

PHYSICAL EXAMINATION

Severe or established osteoporosis, that is, osteoporosis with fractures, is readily identifiable. The dowager's hump is a thoracic spine kyphosis that occurs with multiple vertebral compression fractures. Vertebral compression fractures may also lead to scoliosis and height loss. A wall-occiput distance greater than 0 cm and rib-pelvis distance less than 2 fingerbreadths suggest the presence of occult spinal fracture.[4]

The physical examination in osteoporosis should be directed toward finding signs of secondary osteoporosis. Band keratopathy may suggest a diagnosis of primary hyperparathyroidism. Exophthalmos or lid lag, goiter, tremor, warm moist skin, weight loss, or pretibial myxedema may indicate a diagnosis of hyperthyroidism. Dorsal fat, facial plethora, supraclavicular fat, hypertension, centripetal obesity, proximal muscle weakness, edema, or violaceous abdominal striae may suggest a diagnosis of Cushing syndrome. Gynecomastia, decreased facial or axillary hair, and testicular atrophy may suggest hypogonadism. Blue sclera or dentition as well as joint hypermobility may suggest a diagnosis of osteogenesis imperfecta.

Fall risk should be assessed in each patient with osteoporosis. Lower extremity strength, balance, gait, and postural reflexes should be carefully assessed. Poor visual acuity, weak grip strength, difficulty rising from a chair, Romberg sign, excessive body sway, and unsteady gait may all be signs of increased fall risk that may benefit from evaluation by a physical therapist or in a specialty fall clinic.

DIAGNOSTICS

Routine chemistry profiles (serum electrolyte values; fasting serum calcium and phosphorus levels; serum glucose, blood urea nitrogen [BUN], and creatinine concentrations) are usually normal in idiopathic osteoporosis. However, screening laboratory tests may be indicated to exclude underlying pathologic processes suggested by physical examination or presenting symptoms. Serum calcium concentration, PTH level, thyroid-stimulating hormone (TSH) level in those receiving thyroid hormone, and 24-hour urine calcium excretion may be the most cost-effective workup for identification of secondary causes of osteoporosis among postmenopausal women, although a study has suggested that TSH level alone is sufficient in the majority of postmenopausal women.[5,6] Vitamin D deficiency is common among women with osteoporosis.[7] Guidelines from the Institute of Medicine have supported a serum 25-hydroxyvitamin D level of 20 ng/mL as the threshold for vitamin D sufficiency for the general population,[8] although the Endocrine Society guidelines support a threshold of 30 ng/mL for individual patients without a history of sarcoidosis, who are susceptible to a vitamin D toxicity, with hypercalciuria and hypercalcemia.[9] The National Osteoporosis Foundation recommends intake of 800 to 1000 IU of vitamin D supplementation daily. A variety of regimens for vitamin D correction are available, but the greatest success in achieving a 25-hydroxyvitamin D level of 20 ng/mL appears to be linked to a total intake of at least 600,000 IU (i.e., 50,000 IU of vitamin D_2 three times weekly for 4 weeks).[10] A regimen of 50,000 IU of vitamin D_2 every other week appears to be safe and effective with up to 6 years of therapy.[11] There have been concerns that annual high-dose vitamin D regimens may increase the risk of falls among women.[12]

Biochemical markers are urine and blood tests that measure breakdown products of bone and collagen. A biochemical marker is an indirect measurement of bone turnover (i.e., bone resorption and formation). Bone resorption markers (N-telopeptides and C-telopeptides CTX) are used to evaluate osteoclast activity, and bone formation markers (bone-specific alkaline phosphatase, osteocalcin, procollagen I extension peptides) are used to evaluate osteoblast activity. High levels imply increased bone turnover. At this time, the role of bone markers in primary care is unclear, although specialists may use them. Bone resorption markers help identify response to antiresorptive drug treatment. Six-month intervals are the usual frequency for testing of bone markers.

Plain radiographs are useful primarily in confirming the presence of fracture. They are insensitive to decreases in bone mass. In the absence of fracture, the definitive method for diagnosis of osteoporosis is bone densitometry, by dual energy x-ray absorptiometry, of the hip and posteroanterior lumbar spine. The wrist may be used in very obese patients, uninterpretable hip and spine scans, and primary hyperparathyroidism. Indications for bone densitometry are listed in Box 182-2. Bone density assessment of other sites, such as the finger, wrist, and ankle, and the use of other technologies, such as ultrasonography, are useful in diagnosis of osteoporosis and predicting fracture risk (particularly in adults older than 65 years) but may not be as useful in ruling out osteoporosis. Vertebral fracture assessment, which may be obtained from some bone density services, offers information similar to that of thoracic and lumbar spine radiography, with much less radiation exposure. The presence of a vertebral compression fracture, which may be asymptomatic, in

BOX 182-2

Indications for Bone Densitometry

- In women age 65 and older and men age 70 and older
- In postmenopausal women and men older than 50-69, based on risk factor profile
- In postmenopausal women and men age 50 and older who have had a fracture in adulthood and who have low bone mass or bone loss

Data from Cosman F, de Beur SJ, LeBoff MS, et al: Clinician's guide to prevention and treatment of osteoporosis. *Osteoporos Int* 25(10):2359-2381, 2014.

the setting of osteopenia is sufficient for the clinical diagnosis of osteoporosis, particularly in the absence of or with minimal trauma. The ISCD recommends this testing when the T-score is below −1.0 and one or more of the following is present: women age 70 years or older; or men age 80 years or older; historical height loss of greater than 1½ inches; self-reported but undocumented prior vertebral fracture; and glucocorticoids therapy equivalent to 5 mg of prednisone or more or the equivalent per day for 3 months or longer.[2]

DIAGNOSTICS

Osteoporosis

LABORATORY
- CBC and differential
- Serum electrolytes
- BUN and creatinine
- LFTs
- Serum calcium with albumin
- Serum phosphorus
- 25-Hydroxyvitamin D
- Intact PTH
- TSH
- Serum and urine protein electrophoresis*
- 24-Hour urine calcium
- 24-Hour urine free cortisol*
- Urinary N-telopeptides, serum C-telopeptides*
- Serum testosterone*
- Tissue transglutaminase antibody*

IMAGING
- Bone densitometry
- Bone scan*
- X-ray studies*
- CT*
- MRI*

INVASIVE TESTING
- Bone biopsy*

*If indicated.
CBC, complete blood count; CT, computed tomography; LFTs, liver function tests; MRI, magnetic resonance imaging.

Bone densitometry provides three pertinent numbers. The first is the actual area density in grams per centimeters squared. This density is then compared with the reference database for young normal adults and age-matched adults. This comparison results in a T-score and a Z-score, respectively. The T-score is used in diagnosis of osteopenia (T score <-1.0 and >-2.5) and osteoporosis (≤ -2.5). The Z-score is ignored unless it is less than −2.0 or the patient is a premenopausal woman or man younger than 50 years, and then it is preferentially used.

Only bone densitometry of the posteroanterior lumbar spine and hip is recommended for monitoring of osteoporosis treatment efficacy, and it is generally performed at 1- to 2-year intervals, depending on the precision of the scan. In general, a 5% density change is considered significant and not caused by measurement statistical variation, but each bone density service should determine its least significant change, as recommended by the ISCD.[2] Some disease states, such as chronic glucocorticoid therapy and paraplegia, may lead to more rapid bone density changes. In these cases, assessment of bone density every 6 months to 1 year may be justified.

DIFFERENTIAL DIAGNOSIS

Osteoporosis is classified as primary or secondary. Primary osteoporosis includes bone loss arising from menopausal estrogen deficiency or aging. Secondary osteoporosis results from an acquired or inherited disease that interferes with bone remodeling or increases bone turnover.

Postmenopausal osteoporosis should be distinguished from secondary causes of osteoporosis (Box 182-3). Secondary causes of osteoporosis may be reversible. Suspicion of secondary causes of osteoporosis should be high in premenopausal and perimenopausal women, men, those with bone density Z-scores of less than −2.0, and those with bone pain in the absence of fracture.

The presence of a fragility fracture in the absence of low bone density should raise the concern of localized bone destruction, as with metastatic disease or plasmacytoma. Thoracic spine fractures caused by metastasis are more likely when they involve vertebrae above T7. Less common metabolic bone diseases, such as Paget disease and osteopetrosis, also may lead to pathologic fractures, despite normal or even high bone density. Further testing, which can include computed tomography (CT) scanning, magnetic resonance imaging (MRI), nuclear medicine bone scanning, or even tetracycline-labeled bone biopsy, may be indicated.

MANAGEMENT

Much of the bone loss of osteoporosis is irreversible, and prevention should be the major focus of health care providers. Ideally, efforts at preventing osteoporosis should begin before puberty and should consist of adequate calcium and vitamin D intake, adequate weight-bearing exercise, and maintenance of normal body weight. Avoidance of cigarette smoking and excessive alcohol intake should be stressed. These preventive efforts are also recommended in adults and in those in whom osteoporosis has already developed.

The National Osteoporosis Foundation recommends 1000 to 1200 mg of elemental calcium (3 to 4 cups of milk) daily and 800 to 1000 IU of vitamin D daily. Orange juice with

DIFFERENTIAL DIAGNOSIS

Osteoporosis

- Aging
- Estrogen or testosterone deficiency
- Diabetes mellitus
- Cushing syndrome
- Hyperthyroidism
- Hyperparathyroidism
- Hyperprolactinemia
- Acromegaly
- Hypercalciuria
- Chronic renal disease
- Renal transplantation
- Liver disease
- Malabsorption
- Eating disorders, malnutrition
- Malignant disease, including metastatic diseases, multiple myeloma, lymphoma, leukemia
- Medications
- Osteopetrosis
- Paget disease
- Rheumatoid arthritis
- Osteogenesis imperfecta
- Marfan syndrome
- Turner syndrome
- Klinefelter syndrome

BOX 182-3

Secondary Causes of Low Bone Mass

ENDOCRINE DISEASES
Diabetes mellitus
Growth hormone deficiency
Acromegaly
Hypercortisolism
Hyperparathyroidism
Hyperthyroidism
Premature menopause
Male hypogonadism
Hyperprolactinemia
Athletic amenorrhea
Turner and Klinefelter syndromes

GASTROINTESTINAL DISORDERS
Gastrectomy
Celiac disease
Inflammatory bowel disease
Liver cirrhosis
Chronic biliary tract obstruction
Chronic therapy with proton pump inhibitors
Cystic fibrosis
Malabsorption
Primary biliary cirrhosis

HEMATOLOGIC DISEASES
Myeloma
Monoclonal gammopathy of undetermined significance
Lymphoma, leukemia
Systemic mastocytosis
Disseminated carcinoma
Chemotherapy
Gaucher disease
Glycogen storage diseases
Porphyria
Hemochromatosis
Sickle cell disease
Thalassemia
Hemophilia

RHEUMATOLOGIC DISEASES
Rheumatoid arthritis
Ankylosing spondylitis
Systemic lupus erythematosus

CONNECTIVE TISSUE DISEASES
Osteogenesis imperfecta
Marfan syndrome
Ehlers-Danlos syndrome
Pseudoxanthoma elasticum
Homocystinuria

OTHER CAUSES
Anorexia nervosa
End-stage renal disease
Chronic metabolic acidosis
Multiple sclerosis
Sarcoidosis
Muscular dystrophy
Parental nutrition

DRUGS
Glucocorticoids
Heparin
Cyclosporine and tacrolimus
Anticonvulsants
Cancer chemotherapeutic drugs
Gonadotropin-releasing hormone analogues
Lithium
Methotrexate
Cigarette smoking
Excessive alcohol use
Excessive thyroxine
Chronic opiate use
Premenopausal tamoxifen use

Data from Cosman F, de Beur SJ, LeBoff MS, et al: Clinician's guide to prevention and treatment of osteoporosis. *Osteoporos Int* 25(10):2359-2381, 2014; and Hofbauer LC, Hamann C, Ebeling PR: Approach to the patient with secondary osteoporosis, *Eur J Endocrinol* 162:1009-1020, 2010.

calcium has roughly the same content as milk. Those who are unable to obtain their calcium from the diet may have to use calcium supplements, such as calcium carbonate and calcium citrate.[1] Vitamin D, although it is synthesized from sunlight exposure and available in some foods, may need supplementation for vitamin D sufficiency to be achieved.[13] In 2011, the Institute of Medicine updated its recommended daily allowance (RDA) for calcium and vitamin D (Table 182-1), targeting a serum 25-hydroxyvitamin D level of 20 ng/mL (50 nmol/L). The RDA of calcium for all adults aged 19 to 50 years is 1000 mg daily; for men 51 to 70 years, 1000 mg daily; and for men older than 70 years as well as women aged 51 years and older, 1200 mg daily. The RDA for vitamin D for adults aged 19 to 70 years is 600 IU daily and for those older than 70 years, 800 IU daily.[8] The Endocrine Society has supported these guidelines but recognizes that some patients may need at least 1500 to 2000 IU daily to maintain their 25-hydroxyvitamin D levels above 30 ng/mL; obese patients, those with malabsorption, and those taking medications affecting the metabolism of vitamin D require 3000 to 6000 IU daily. Sarcoidosis patients may need less.[9] Studies have raised concerns about an increased risk of cardiovascular events in women taking calcium or calcium–vitamin D supplements.[14,15] In the end, there has to be a balance between good bone health and good cardiovascular health, and patient-provider discussions will need to consider this to avoid extremes of too little calcium and vitamin D as well as too much.

Bone is a dynamic tissue that adapts to loading (i.e., weight-bearing exercise) with hypertrophy and increased strength. Exercise is an important part of any osteoporosis therapy, but it is most effective when it is used in a preventive capacity, particularly in children and adolescents. Unloading of the skeleton, as

TABLE 182-1 **Recommended Calcium and Vitamin D Daily Intake**

Age (years)	Calcium (mg/day)	Vitamin D (IU/day)
1-3	700	600
4-8	1000	600
9-13	1300	600
14-18	1300	600
19-30	1000	600
31-50	1000	600
51-70	1000 (male), 1200 (female)	600
>70	1200	800
14-18, pregnant or lactating	1300	600
19-50, pregnant or lactating	1000	600

Data from Institute of Medicine: *Dietary reference intakes for calcium and vitamin D*, Washington, DC, 2011, National Academies Press.

occurs with bed rest, space flight, and spinal cord injury, results in dramatic decrements in bone mass. Conversely, weight-bearing exercise and weight training may modestly increase bone density, and their effects are dependent on estrogen status. Exercise alone has not been shown to prevent early menopausal bone loss, and there is no evidence of a decrease in fracture risk with exercise alone. A Cochrane meta-analysis found a slight benefit of exercise for bone density and fracture risk (number needed to treat to prevent one fracture was 25) for postmenopausal women. The most effective exercise for femoral neck bone density is non–weight-bearing, high-force exercise such as progressive resistance strength training for the lower limbs, and for the spine bone density is a combination exercise program.[16]

Some exercise regimens, such as tai chi, lower limb strengthening, yoga, and balance training, may decrease risk of fall. Exercises to be avoided include high-impact loading, abrupt or explosive movements, resistive trunk flexion, twisting movements, and dynamic abdominal exercises. Referral to a physical therapist for guided exercise may be helpful.[17]

Walking is a good exercise. For women of average weight (143 pounds), walking 4892 steps daily at 2.2 mph is sufficient to maintain femoral neck bone density. Lighter women require more steps (18,568 steps daily at 115.5 pounds), and heavier women require fewer steps (1638 steps daily at 173.1 pounds). Walking faster requires fewer steps, and walking more slowly requires more steps.[18]

Hip protector pads have been shown in some studies to prevent hip fractures from falls, particularly in those with a fall history and low body mass index.[19] Noncompliance with hip protector pads may limit their efficacy. A meta-analysis by Sawka and colleagues[20] did not find evidence for significant hip fracture prevention in relatively low-risk community-dwelling populations, however.

In those with osteoporosis, preventive measures of calcium, vitamin D, and exercise alone are not sufficient to prevent osteoporotic fracture. For those with densitometric osteoporosis (T-score <−2.5), those with densitometric osteopenia (T-score <−1.0 and >−2.5) with multiple risk factors, and particularly those who already have osteoporotic fracture, pharmacologic therapy is imperative. The National Osteoporosis Foundation 2014 guidelines, which apply to postmenopausal women and men older than 50 years, recommend treatment for those with T-scores of −2.5 or lower at the femoral neck or the spine, those with typical fragility fractures, and those with a T-score that is higher than −2.5 and lower than −1.0 (i.e., osteopenia) with a FRAX score of 20% or higher for major osteoporotic fracture risk and 3% or higher for hip fracture risk. The FRAX calculator is accessible at www.shef.ac.uk/FRAX. The FRAX model has limitations in that it does not include lumbar spine or wrist T-score or fall risk.[1] All therapies should be reevaluated for risk/benefit ratio of ongoing treatment, and no pharmacologic therapy should be considered indefinite in duration.[1]

The only FDA-approved agents at this time that have been proved in prospective studies to prevent both vertebral and nonvertebral fractures are the bisphosphonates (alendronate, risedronate, zoledronic acid), teriparatide, and denosumab. Bisphosphonates, which are synthetic analogues of pyrophosphate, reduce bone resorption and bone loss by binding to bone and poisoning active osteoclasts. Four bisphosphonates are currently approved by the FDA for the prevention and treatment of postmenopausal osteoporosis: alendronate, risedronate, ibandronate, and zoledronic acid. Alendronate (Fosamax), risedronate (Actonel), and zoledronic acid (Reclast) are also approved for use in glucocorticoid-induced osteoporosis. Alendronate, risedronate, and zoledronic acid are approved for increasing bone mass in men as well as for treatment of glucocorticoid-induced osteoporosis. Risedronate and zoledronic acid are also indicated in the prevention of glucocorticoid-induced osteoporosis.

Studies with these agents have shown yearly bone density increases of 2% to 3% at the lumbar spine, which is the skeletal site most responsive to these agents. Contraindications to bisphosphonates include disorders of esophageal motility or active gastroesophageal bleeding (for oral bisphosphonates), hypocalcemia, untreated vitamin D deficiency, and renal disease (creatinine clearance <35 mL/min). There have been concerns about the risk of esophageal cancer with oral bisphosphonates,[21,22] although not seen in all studies,[23] and the presence of Barrett esophagus would be a relative contraindication. The recommended dose of alendronate for prevention is 5 mg/day (or 35 mg/wk). For the treatment of osteoporosis, the dose is 10 mg/day or (70 mg/wk). With risedronate, the prevention and treatment doses are the same: 5 mg/day, 35 mg once a week, 75 mg twice a month, or 150 mg once a month. Ibandronate is given at 2.5 mg/day, 150 mg once a month orally, or 3 mg by intravenous push every 3 months. Zoledronic acid is given at 5 mg intravenously every year for the treatment of osteoporosis and every other year for the prevention of osteoporosis. Oral bisphosphonates should be taken on an empty stomach, with 6 to 8 ounces of water, and 30 minutes before eating (60 minutes for ibandronate), taking other medications, or lying down. Taking bisphosphonates with food or coffee will reduce their absorption and potentially eliminate their benefit. To decrease gastrointestinal effects, it is important that patients be given explicit instructions on proper administration, because esophagitis can be a problem.

Bisphosphonates are potent antiresorptive agents and may potentially oversuppress bone turnover. Bisphosphonate-related osteonecrosis of the jaw is defined as exposed bone in the maxillofacial region for more than 8 weeks associated with current or previous bisphosphonate therapy, in the absence of radiation therapy to the jaw. It is rare in patients treated with bisphosphonates for osteoporosis, with a wide range of estimates from 1 in 1700 to 1 in 263,000. The cumulative incidence in cancer patients treated with high-dose potent intravenous bisphosphonates, such as pamidronate and zoledronic acid, is much higher at 0.8% to 12%. There is a higher risk with longer duration of action, increasing age, and dentoalveolar surgery including dental extraction, dental implant placement, periapical surgery, and periodontal surgery involving alveolar bone injury.[24] Good dental hygiene should be maintained during bisphosphonate therapy, and patients should be informed of the low but present risk. Development of osteonecrosis of the jaw may involve cessation of the bisphosphonate, but providers should also consider the increased risk of fractures that may result. Serum CTX, a marker of bone resorption, has been suggested as a test to assess risk for osteonecrosis of the jaw; however, there is limited evidence supporting its usefulness.[25] Denosumab use has also been associated with osteonecrosis of the jaw. Teriparatide may have a role in the treatment of osteonecrosis of the jaw.[26]

The American Association of Oral and Maxillofacial Surgeons has recently updated its guidelines for medication-related osteonecrosis of the jaw. The Association recognizes a very low risk for the problem, at a rate of 0.1% but increasing to 0.21% when patients have been on bisphosphonate treatment for longer than 4 years. The guidelines recommend pretreatment dental evaluation and care, which may decrease the risk of osteonecrosis of the jaw by 50%. For patients on long-term therapy, the recommendation is for consideration of a 2-month drug holiday before an invasive dental procedure. The guidelines do not offer any recommendations for denosumab therapy.[27]

Cases of unusual fractures, including subtrochanteric hip fractures and femoral shaft fractures, occurring with long-term bisphosphonate therapy and associated with low bone turnover have also been described. These fractures are typically associated with minimal if any trauma and characterized by simple transverse or oblique (<30 degrees) fracture with cortical beaking, diffuse cortical thickening, delayed healing, and evidence of stress reaction or fracture on the contralateral side. They are often preceded by prodromal thigh or groin pain for weeks to months before fracture. There is increased risk with concomitant glucocorticoid use.[28] An analysis of alendronate and zoledronic acid therapy data suggest a rate of 2.3 subtrochanteric or diaphyseal fractures per 10,000 patient-years of bisphosphonate treatment, which would also be associated with a prevention of 100 fractures.[29] Patients receiving long-term bisphosphonate therapy should be made aware of this rare complication and should be evaluated promptly if they develop unexplained groin or thigh pain. Consideration of cessation of bisphosphonates and switching to other osteoporosis therapies may be considered after 5 years of therapy for those at moderate risk for osteoporotic fracture and after 10 years of therapy for those at high risk. Bisphosphonates should be avoided in those at low risk for osteoporotic fracture.[30]

Raloxifene (Evista) is FDA approved for postmenopausal osteoporosis prevention and treatment at a dose of 60 mg/day. Raloxifene, a selective estrogen receptor modulator, acts as an estrogen receptor agonist on the skeleton but as an antagonist on breast and uterine tissue. Raloxifene has been shown to produce roughly a 1.5% to 3% increase in spine and femoral neck density after 3 years, with a 30% reduction in new vertebral fractures. No reduction in nonvertebral fractures has been shown. There is an increased relative risk of venous thromboembolic disease, fatal stroke, hot flashes, and leg cramps with raloxifene, and a patient's individual risk for these conditions should be considered carefully. Raloxifene is as effective as tamoxifen in preventing invasive breast cancer, with fewer thromboembolic events and cataracts, and is now indicated in reducing the risk for invasive breast cancer.[31]

Hormone replacement is FDA approved only for the prevention of osteoporosis, not for its treatment. Estrogen inhibits bone resorption, decreases bone remodeling, and enhances absorption of calcium. There are good data showing prevention of both vertebral and nonvertebral fractures, although the increased risk for coronary events, breast cancer, and thromboembolic disease may outweigh the benefits in many women.[32] A combination of conjugated estrogens and bazedoxifene acetate (a selective estrogen receptor modulator) has been approved for the treatment of moderate to severe menopausal vasomotor symptoms and prevention of osteoporosis.

Contraindications to the use of estrogen include undiagnosed vaginal bleeding, pregnancy, active thrombosis or thrombophlebitis, active liver disease, endometrial adenocarcinoma, breast cancer, and other estrogen-dependent tumors. Caution should be exercised with a medical diagnosis of endometriosis, uterine leiomyoma, gallbladder disease, or migraine headaches; a family history of breast cancer; or a history of thrombophlebitis. Once estrogen therapy is stopped, bone loss resumes at the same rate as in untreated women. With long-term use of estrogen, those at risk for breast cancer and those with a history of uncomfortable side effects should be monitored closely.

Subcutaneous PTH is an anabolic bone agent. Anabolic agents stimulate bone formation and increase bone remodeling rates. Intermittent PTH administration shows an anabolic effect, increasing bone mass, whereas continuous PTH administration leads to bone loss as in primary hyperparathyroidism. Teriparatide, a PTH analogue (PTH 1-34) administered subcutaneously, has been shown to increase bone density at the hip and spine by 2% and 8%, respectively, after 1 year of therapy, in postmenopausal women[33] and in both men and women receiving glucocorticoid therapy. It has been shown to decrease vertebral fractures by approximately 65% and nonvertebral fractures by 35%. It appears more effective than alendronate in treating glucocorticoid-induced osteoporosis.[34] It is contraindicated in those with hypercalcemia and those at increased risk for osteosarcoma (those with radiotherapy of bone, Paget disease, unexplained elevations of alkaline phosphatase, and open epiphyseal growth plates) because teriparatide use increased the risk of osteosarcoma in animals. It is approved for 2 years of use, and there is a rapid loss of bone density gains after cessation. Alendronate therapy after PTH use helps maintain and increase bone density.[35] Retreatment with PTH after alendronate therapy may provide additional bone density gains.[36]

Calcitonin is a peptide hormone that appears to slow bone loss and temporarily increase vertebral bone mass by decreasing osteoclastic activity. The drug's effect is more pronounced on trabecular bone. The nasal spray produces a 3% increase in vertebral bone only and is not as effective as estrogen and alendronate in forming new bone. Drug delivery is by injection or nasal spray; the recommended dose is 50 to 100 units/

day three times per week for the injection and 200 units/day, alternating nostrils, for the nasal spray. It is FDA approved for use in postmenopausal women (>5 years postmenopause) with osteoporosis. Supplementation with calcium and vitamin D enhances therapy. Most osteoporosis experts do not advise the use of calcitonin therapy alone in treating established osteoporosis.

Denosumab (Prolia) is a monoclonal antibody that inhibits RANK ligand and potently reduces bone resorption. It is given subcutaneously at a dose of 60 mg every 6 months. It has been shown to decrease vertebral and nonvertebral fracture and is approved for use in postmenopausal women with osteoporosis. It is contraindicated in patients with hypocalcemia. Adverse reactions are serious infections including skin infections, eczema and dermatitis, hypocalcemia (especially in patients with renal insufficiency), osteonecrosis of the jaw, and significant suppression of bone turnover.[37] Cessation of therapy leads to rapid loss of action and bone density gains, and the drug is not cleared by the kidney.

Combinations of therapies (e.g., bisphosphonates and estrogen, PTH and estrogen, and PTH and bisphosphonates) may have additive effects on bone density increases. It is not clear whether these bone density increases are associated with decreased fracture risk, and there may be additive effects on suppression of bone resorption. Studies of combination PTH and alendronate have shown no advantage over PTH alone. Sequential use of PTH first, followed by alendronate, appears to produce the best bone density increases.[38,39] This effect has also been seen in PTH combined with raloxifene.[40]

Work from the Denosumab and Teriparatide Administration Study (DATA) showed that the combination of denosumab and teriparatide produces additive gains, with a 9.1% spine density increase and a 4.9% total hip density gain after 12 months of therapy.[41] After 24 months, there was a 12.9% spine density increase and 6.8% total hip density increase.[42] In results from the DATA-Switch trial, sequential treatment with combination teriparatide and denosumab for 18 months followed by denosumab produced the greatest bone density gains—15.0% at the spine and 7.1% at the total hip.[43] Whether the improvement in bone density gains translates to fewer fractures remains to be established, and the significant expense may be a significant obstacle.

Two newer therapies on the horizon are odanacatib, a once-weekly oral antiresorptive that inhibits the enzyme cathepsin K, and the anti-sclerostin antibodies romosozumab and blosozumab, potent anabolic agents. Romosozumab, a once-monthly subcutaneous drug, has been shown to produce greater bone density gains than either alendronate or teriparatide.[44]

Co-Management with Specialists

Co-management depends on each patient's particular needs. Fracture management and pain control are the primary reasons for referral. Referrals may also be made to the following specialists:

- *Endocrinologists or rheumatologists* specializing in metabolic bone disease for patients with persistent fractures, patients with secondary osteoporosis, premenopausal women or children with osteoporosis, or those with osteoporosis who are intolerant of FDA-approved therapies
- *Pain specialist* to manage escalating chronic pain associated with debilitating bone and muscle changes associated with fractures
- *Physical therapist* for management of exercise for osteoporosis, spinal and posture strengthening, pain management, and fall and fracture prevention
- *Nutritionist* for balanced diet guidelines regarding calcium and vitamin D intake appropriate for the individual's age and activity level
- *Orthopedic surgeon* for surgical correction of bone fractures or consideration of bone biopsy
- *Interventional radiologist* for vertebroplasty or kyphoplasty for painful vertebral fractures

LIFE SPAN CONSIDERATIONS

Osteoporotic fractures, especially those of the hip, are associated with increased morbidity and increased mortality. In the first year after hip fracture, there is a 10% to 20% excess mortality. Mortality rates in men with hip fracture are higher because of comorbid conditions. In women with vertebral fractures, those with one or more fractures had a 1.23-fold greater age-adjusted mortality rate, with mortality increasing with greater numbers of vertebral fractures.

COMPLICATIONS

Eighty-four percent of those with clinically diagnosed vertebral compression fractures report having pain. The acute pain of vertebral fracture usually lasts between 2 weeks and 3 months. Chronic back pain from spinal changes, microfractures, and muscle spasms can develop. Patients may develop reduced exercise tolerance and pulmonary reserve. Abdominal protuberance because of loss of height at the lumbar spine may lead to early satiety and resultant weight loss. There is a loss of self-esteem and a distortion of body image.

Altered activity or inability to participate in activities of daily living because of pain may persist for a much longer period. In these patients, bed rest and decreased activity for a few days are warranted. The individual should be instructed in proper positioning, either lying supine or side lying with pillows positioned under the knees or between the knees. Medications for pain, such as muscle relaxants for spasms, nonsteroidals (cyclooxygenase 1 and 2 inhibitors), and acetaminophen for pain and inflammation, should be prescribed as needed. Narcotics should be used sparingly because of the potential for addiction and associated fall risk. Studies indicate that the use of both calcitonin and bisphosphonates is effective at reducing pain associated with osteoporotic compression fractures, not only by reducing the risk of fracture but also with a direct effect on bone pain.[45]

Moist heat or ice may help with pain relief. Moist heat is generally recommended for muscle spasms, and ice is recommended for bone inflammation or pain. The individual in acute pain may need to use a cane or walker to walk safely. Short-term use of a spinal support may be beneficial (Table 182-2). Also available is a posture training support designed to pull the shoulders back with weights as the muscles become stronger.

Chronic pain management may be enhanced with physical therapy. Modalities include transcutaneous electrical nerve stimulation, electrical muscle stimulation, ultrasound with healed fractures, iontophoresis, and heat or ice. Manual therapy, including joint mobilization, muscle energy techniques, myofascial release, and strain-counterstrain on trigger points in muscle, is beneficial in mobilizing soft tissue and improving muscle imbalance of the spine.

TABLE 182-2 Physical Therapy: Spinal Support

Area	Support
Thoracolumbar area	Body jacket clamshell brace Jewett three-point brace Boston brace
Lumbosacral area	Lumbosacral corset

BOX 182-4

Fall Prevention Measures

- Regular eye examinations and correction for inadequacies
- Hearing evaluation for sound detection
- Use of assistive devices (cane or walker) as needed
- Use of rubber-soled, flat-soled, fully enclosed shoes
- Use of handrails and steady pieces of furniture
- Use of grab bars, tub seats, and elevated toilets in the bathroom
- Walkways clear of objects and throw rugs
- Proper lighting in hallways and stairways

Vertebroplasty and kyphoplasty are minimally invasive techniques in which polymethyl methacrylate (PMMA) cement is injected into the fractured vertebra, thereby stabilizing it. The two techniques differ in that vertebroplasty uses a high-pressure injection system and kyphoplasty uses a balloon to expand the collapsed vertebra to produce a space for the PMMA. Vertebroplasty has a reported rate of success in pain relief of 70% to 90%; the rate for kyphoplasty is 90%, although two randomized placebo-controlled trials have raised questions about efficacy over placebo.[46,47] Kyphoplasty has the added benefit of significantly increasing vertebral height. Complication rates are low and include radiculopathy and cord compression. Cement leakage is common, particularly in vertebroplasty. This appears an effective therapy for pain relief of vertebral fractures, although the biomechanical effects on the adjacent nonfractured vertebrae are not yet clear.

INDICATIONS FOR REFERRAL OR HOSPITALIZATION

The treatment of fractures is primarily supportive and requires physician consultation. Hospitalization for severe pain or setting of fractures (e.g., hip fractures) requires consultation with a specialist. Monitoring for potential complications after hip fractures or for pain management is indicated.

PATIENT AND FAMILY EDUCATION

Patient education is essential for the prevention and treatment of fractures. Education encompasses nutrition, psychosocial issues, risk factor modification, proper body mechanics and positioning, safety, and fall prevention. Most accidents occur in the home and are related to poor vision, decreased hearing, slowed reflexes, impaired mental status, limited spinal flexibility, decreased lower extremity strength, and unsteady gait. These factors, coupled with decreased muscle and fat mass to cushion the fall, place the individual at jeopardy for injury. Education of individuals prepares them to take an active role in their care (Box 182-4). Family members should be informed of their risk of osteoporosis and encouraged to take preventive measures. Other educational resources can be accessed at the National Osteoporosis Foundation website at www.nof.org.

PAGET DISEASE OF BONE

DEFINITION AND EPIDEMIOLOGY

Paget disease is the second most common metabolic bone disease in older adults.

Traditionally, medical and surgical specialists have managed the various manifestations of the disease, but now, with more effective treatments available, the primary care team can provide complete management in most cases.

Paget disease is uncommon before the age of 40 years; however, by the age of 80 years, 1 in 10 persons is affected by the disease. Between 18% and 25% of the U.S. population have at least one family member with Paget disease. The most frequent genetic mutation linked to Paget disease is in the sequestosome 1 gene, found in 30% of patients with familial Paget disease, which may produce a more severe clinical picture. There has been some evidence supporting an etiologic role of paramyxoviruses and the measles viruses. Paget disease is common in England, western Europe, New Zealand, Australia, and the United States; it is uncommon in Asia, Africa, India, and Scandinavia.[48]

PATHOPHYSIOLOGY

Paget disease is characterized by a localized increase in bone turnover and blood flow. It can affect one or more sites (monostotic versus polyostotic). Once the disease is fully established, previously unaffected bones are usually spared. For reasons that are still not well understood, osteoclasts in the affected area are increased in number, size, and activity and cause breakdown of focal areas of bone at great speed. The osteoblasts, which are unaffected by the disease process, try to keep up with the bone degradation by laying down new osteoid as fast as they can. However, the newly formed bone is disorganized and lacks the architectural integrity of normal bone. This results in mechanically weak, highly vascular bone that is prone to deformity and fractures, especially if weight-bearing parts of the skeleton are affected.

CLINICAL PRESENTATION

Although Paget disease is usually asymptomatic, bone pain is the most common presenting symptom. The pain can be misinterpreted as part of the aging process or as part of another disease process. Patients may be misdiagnosed as having osteoarthritis. Failure to diagnose and to initiate early treatment of the disease can result in irreversible consequences and significant morbidity.

The degree and character of the bone pain vary with the location and activity of Paget disease. The most commonly involved sites are the pelvis, femur, tibia, spine, and skull. The hands and feet are only rarely involved. In general, the affected bone is moderately painful both at rest and during motion. Most patients describe the pain as a deep ache (like a toothache) that can become severe and sharp with weight bearing and when the area is warmed. Hot baths and even warm bedclothes can intensify the pain.

PHYSICAL EXAMINATION

On examination, the affected area is often tender to the touch and may be warm as a result of increased new blood vessel growth within the bone itself. There may be increased pulsatility in the area. The pagetic bone can be noticeably enlarged. Affected bones may be deformed in a bow shape either from the effects of gravity or from the tension of the attached musculature on the architecturally incompetent pagetic bone. When bones in the lower extremity become deformed, the patient will have an abnormal gait and, often, arthritic changes within the surrounding joints as a result of the mechanical stress. The head size may increase with skull involvement, and frontal bossing may be evident.

Nerve entrapments can occur with bone overgrowth, resulting in a variety of neuropathies, including cranial nerve palsies. Hearing loss may occur from sensory neuropathy or conduction impairment as a result of pagetic involvement of the ossicles of the inner ear. When the spine is involved, bone overgrowth can result in spinal stenosis with attendant radiculopathies or motor impairments.

DIAGNOSTICS

Diagnosis is confirmed by checking the serum alkaline phosphatase (SAP) or urinary N-telopeptide cross-links (NTX) level, both of which will be elevated in active disease. These levels correlate with the extent and activity of the disease. If a single bone is involved (i.e., monostotic disease), a serum bone-specific alkaline phosphatase, a serum amino-terminal propeptide of type 1 collagen (PINP), NTX, or β C-terminal telopeptide of type I collagen (CTX) may be more sensitive measures than SAP.[49] Radiographic studies of the affected areas usually show a classic mixed sclerotic-lytic (cotton-wool) pattern, cortical thickening, and bone enlargement. Bone scans show increased uptake in affected areas, but this pattern can be difficult to differentiate from other processes such as cancer and arthritis.

DIAGNOSTICS

Paget Disease

LABORATORY

Serum alkaline phosphatase (SAP)
Serum bone-specific alkaline phosphatase*
Serum amino-terminal propeptide of type 1 collagen (PINP)*
Urinary N-telopeptide
β C-terminal telopeptide of type I collagen (CTX)*

IMAGING

Plain radiographs of affected areas
Nuclear medicine bone scan
MRI (if neurologic symptoms)

*If indicated.

DIFFERENTIAL DIAGNOSIS

The symptoms and signs of Paget disease must be distinguished from those of several other conditions. When the joints are involved, the differential diagnosis includes osteoarthritis, gout, and pseudogout. Ironically, these three diagnoses can coexist with Paget disease, can be a complication of Paget disease, or can mimic the symptoms of Paget disease when it affects the bone adjacent to a joint.

Bone pain that occurs with an elevated SAP level and positive bone scan must be distinguished from malignant disease, most commonly a metastasis from a distant site. In early, active Paget disease, the initial wave of osteoclastic resorption can appear as lytic lesions on plain radiographs and thus may mimic such malignant neoplasms as multiple myeloma. However, in most cases, the radiograph will show changes pathognomonic of Paget disease.

DIFFERENTIAL DIAGNOSIS

Paget Disease

- Osteoarthritis
- Osteomalacia
- Gout
- Pseudogout
- Malignant disease

MANAGEMENT

The goals of treatment are to suppress osteoclastic activity, allowing the osteoblasts to catch up and lay down architecturally normal bone, which in turn reduces symptoms and prevents disease progression. Symptoms of bone pain, excessive warmth over bone, headache caused by skull involvement, low back pain caused by vertebral involvement, and some syndromes of neural compromise are the most likely to improve.[48] All patients with bone pain or neurologic impingements, patients with congestive heart failure, and patients who are at risk for complications because of the site of disease (femoral head, tibia, skull) should receive pharmacologic therapy (Box 182-5 and Table 182-3).[49] Presurgical treatment of Paget disease, when surgery of pagetic bone is planned, is suggested in decreasing intraoperative bleeding. Some controversy remains about whether to treat patients solely on the basis of an elevated SAP level, and results from the PRISM trial (The Paget's Disease Randomized Trail of Intensive vs Symptomatic Management) suggest that treatment on this basis is not justified.[50] Bone pain usually responds within 2 to 3 weeks of active drug treatment. Neuropathies, if detected early, may also respond, but arthropathy will not because it represents fixed-joint degradation. Efficacy of treatment is determined by the amount and duration of the reduction in SAP or NTX.

Bisphosphonates

Bisphosphonates are the most widely used agents for the treatment of Paget disease. They reduce bone turnover by inhibiting key cellular functions that govern osteoclastic bone resorption.

BOX 182-5

Indications for Drug Therapy in Paget Disease

- Bone or joint pain
- Pagetic lesions in weight-bearing sites
- Involvement of the skull
- Nerve entrapments
- Preparation for elective joint replacement or surgery on pagetic bone

TABLE 182-3 FDA-Approved Pharmacologic Treatment of Paget Disease

Drug	Dose	Side Effects
BISPHOSPHONATES		
Alendronate	40 mg PO per day for 6 mo	Nausea, esophageal ulcers
Risedronate	30 mg PO per day for 2 mo	Nausea, esophageal ulcers
Pamidronate	30 mg IV per day for 3 days or 60-90 mg IV once; repeated doses may be necessary for more severe disease	Mild fever, hypocalcemia, influenza-like symptoms, transient leukopenia
Zoledronic acid	5 mg IV during 15 min	Mild fever, hypocalcemia, influenza-like symptoms, transient leukopenia
Etidronate	5 mg/kg/day (max 400 mg) PO per day for 6 mo*	Nausea, osteomalacia
Tiludronate	400 mg PO per day for 3 mo	Back pain, diarrhea, nausea
CALCITONIN		
Salmon	100 IU SC per day for 3-6 mo, and then 50-100 IU every other day or 3 times per wk	Flushing, nausea, loss of efficacy

*Etidronate should be given cyclically with at least 6 months of no treatment between courses.

Etidronate (Didronel) was the first bisphosphonate available, although it is not used as commonly now. It is contraindicated in the presence of advancing lytic lesions in a weight-bearing bone.[48] Tiludronate is also approved for Paget disease but rarely used. Alendronate (Fosamax) at 40 mg daily for 6 months and risedronate (Actonel) at 30 mg daily for 2 months are the oral bisphosphonates of choice for treatment of Paget disease in the United States. Clear evidence from randomized controlled trials has shown that both achieve quick normalization of biochemical markers and reduction of pain. In addition, both have prolonged post-treatment effects and low relapse rates. However, all bisphosphonates are poorly absorbed from the gut, and absorption is further diminished when they are taken with food or any liquid other than water. Thus, oral bisphosphonates must be taken with plain water on an empty stomach at least a half-hour before a meal. Waiting longer will enhance absorption. The main side effects are stomach upset and, rarely, esophageal ulceration.

Intravenous bisphosphonates such as pamidronate (Aredia) and zoledronic acid (Reclast) are potent treatment options for those unable to tolerate oral agents. Studies of both agents have shown dramatic and long-lasting improvement in both markers and symptoms. Because of its rapid onset of action, intravenous administration is the route of choice for patients with impending fracture, neurologic impingements, hydrocephalus, or severe refractory disease. The side effects are generally minor, but transient hypocalcemia, leukopenia, and influenza-like symptoms can be seen. These therapies can worsen renal function in those with preexisting renal disease and cause profound hypocalcemia in those with vitamin D deficiency.[51] The Endocrine Society suggests 5 mg of zoledronic acid given intravenously as treatment of choice for Paget disease, provided there are no contraindications.[49]

Comparison studies between the most potent bisphosphonates, oral risedronate and intravenous zoledronic acid, have shown the latter to be more effective at normalizing alkaline phosphatase and maintaining a durable response.[52,53] Because of cost considerations and insurer guidelines, it may be most cost-effective to proceed with generic alendronate or intravenous pamidronate and then to consider risedronate or intravenous zoledronic acid if there are concerns about treatment failure or resistance.

As previously outlined, potent bisphosphonates have been associated with osteonecrosis of the jaw. There have been reports of osteonecrosis of the jaw in patients with Paget disease, although high doses of bisphosphonates were given for longer than typically prescribed.[54]

Calcitonin

Calcitonin, although not as potent or long lasting as the bisphosphonates, remains a well-tolerated treatment option. Pain typically remits after 2 to 3 weeks, and as treatment continues, lytic lesions fill in with new normal bone, vascularity decreases, and neurologic deficits (if any) improve. However, the effect of calcitonin wears off with time because of the development of antibodies (in the case of salmon or porcine calcitonin) and downregulation of calcitonin receptors. The effective dose of salmon calcitonin is 100 IU subcutaneously every day for 3 to 6 months, followed by injections every other day or three times a week as dictated by clinical symptoms and biochemical markers. Nasal salmon calcitonin (200 IU) can be used in a similar schedule but is not specifically approved for use in Paget disease. The main side effects of injectable calcitonin are transient flushing and nausea. Vomiting, diarrhea, and abdominal pain can also occur. Nasal calcitonin is generally better tolerated but can cause nasal irritation.

Other Therapies

Gallium nitrate and mithramycin are no longer used in Paget disease, having been supplanted by less toxic and more effective bisphosphonates. Denosumab, approved for osteoporosis, has been described as effective, off label, in an elder man with renal disease.[55]

Adjuvant Therapy

Nonsteroidal anti-inflammatory drugs can be useful adjuncts for patients with joint or bone pain. When pain is severe, opioids may need to be used until Paget disease is controlled. Assistive devices, including shoe lifts, walkers, and canes for equalizing leg length discrepancies, as well as physical therapy for joint symptoms, are often helpful. Calcium and vitamin D supplements are imperative for those with low dietary intake to ensure adequate bone mineralization and to prevent hypocalcemia.

Ongoing Monitoring

Patients with Paget disease need to be evaluated periodically. Those with asymptomatic disease in areas of the skeleton where there is little or no risk (e.g., the iliac crest) can be monitored less closely. Conversely, those with active disease in weight-bearing bones or the skull require aggressive follow-up care. Disease activity is monitored by biochemical markers (SAP or NTX), which are usually measured at 3- to 6-month intervals in active disease or yearly in inactive disease. In addition, pain, joint symptoms, neurologic function, and medication side effects need to be assessed at every visit.

LIFE SPAN CONSIDERATIONS

Although untreated Paget disease can cause pain and deformity, the life span is unaffected unless the patient develops osteosarcoma or severe flattening of the base of the skull with spinal cord compression. Indications for the use of bisphosphonates have been extended to include younger patients to prevent bone deformity of the limbs and the secondary osteoarthritis that is seen with these deformities.

The use of bisphosphonates is also recommended for older patients to prevent bone fragility and fracture.

COMPLICATIONS

Bone pain typical of Paget disease must be distinguished from other long-term consequences of untreated Paget disease, including neural compromise, fractures, joint deterioration, and sarcomatous transformation. Nerve compression is most common when the spine or skull is involved. Enlarging bone in the vertebrae can compress spinal nerve roots or even the spinal cord itself, resulting in neuropathic pain or myelopathies. Cranial nerves, which exit the skull through tiny foramina, can also be compressed, resulting in facial pain, paralysis, or deafness. Involvement of the base of the skull can result in hydrocephalus (often manifesting as dementia) or brainstem compression.

Pagetic fractures appear with sudden, severe knifelike pain. They may be traumatic or, if the pagetic bone is weakened by extensive lytic disease, can occur spontaneously. Until Paget disease is controlled, healing is difficult and slow. Pagetic arthropathy occurs when bone adjacent to joint surfaces (e.g., the femoral head or the acetabulum) is affected, resulting in abnormal joint architecture and subsequent degenerative arthritis.

The most dreaded consequence of long-term Paget disease is osteosarcoma. This is heralded by a sudden increase in pain intensity at a pagetic site. Although it is rare, osteosarcoma carries an extremely poor prognosis. The majority of patients die within 1 to 3 years.

INDICATIONS FOR REFERRAL OR HOSPITALIZATION

Medical management of straightforward cases can be easily handled by the primary health care provider. However, physical therapists are invaluable members of the management team because of their expertise in maximizing physical function and knowledge of assistive devices. Referral to a rheumatologist or endocrinologist specializing in metabolic bone disease is indicated if the patient's disease is unresponsive to usual treatment. Orthopedic referral is indicated when an associated arthropathy or spinal stenosis causes unremitting pain or loss of function.

Severe neurologic complications, such as hydrocephalus, require aggressive inpatient antipagetic therapy combined with neurosurgical intervention. Other causes of hospitalization include fracture, elective joint replacement, and spinal decompression.

PATIENT AND FAMILY EDUCATION

Patients and their families must understand the disease process and medical treatment to manage Paget disease optimally. First, they need to be informed about how to take their medications and what side effects could occur. Second, patients need to promptly report any worsening of their symptoms, which could herald disease progression, fracture, or sarcomatous transformation. Those with skull involvement need to understand what neuropathic symptoms to look for and the importance of prompt reporting. For example, progressive hearing loss should not be blamed on age.

In addition, family members should inform their own primary care team of their family history of Paget disease and should be cautioned to report bone pain or symptoms of nerve compression. Additional resources may be found on the Paget Foundation website at www.paget.org.

HEALTH PROMOTION

Patients should be encouraged to remain as physically active as possible. If the tibia or proximal femur is affected, heavy weight-bearing exercise should be avoided until the disease is in remission. Swimming, bicycling, and tai chi are excellent alternatives for patients with painful arthropathy. Adequate dietary (or supplemental) calcium and vitamin D are important to help maintain bone density.

CHAPTER 183

NECK PAIN

Zacharia Isaac • Sharon Alzner • María I. Bascarán

DEFINITION AND EPIDEMIOLOGY

Neck pain is a common complaint in primary care practices because most people are likely to have some degree of neck pain in their lifetime. The annual prevalence among adults exceeds 30%, and 33% to 65% of these patients are recovered at 1 year.[1] In addition, of those who experience neck pain, 50% to 75% will experience another episode 1 to 5 years later. Neck pain is the fourth leading cause of disability.[1] There are several identifiable sources of neck pain, including the bone, disks, joints, ligaments, fascia, muscles, and nerve roots. Pain can be experienced solely in the neck or can move into the head, shoulders, or arms and can start without an inciting event. If an episode of neck pain lasts longer than 12 weeks, it is typically defined as chronic neck pain.

Chronic neck pain can also occur after a hyperextension injury (whiplash), usually in a motor vehicle collision or sometimes during work or sporting events. In chronic whiplash injury, many structures may be involved, including but not limited to the intervertebral disks; facet joints; ligaments; and other cervical soft tissues. Risk factors for neck pain include manual labor occupations, female gender, headaches, smoking, poor job satisfaction, and poor biomechanics.

PATHOPHYSIOLOGY

The cervical spine is made up of seven cervical vertebrae, C1 through C7. The C2 through C7 bodies are separated by five intervertebral disks, giving this portion of the spine a natural cervical lordosis. Each intervertebral disk consists of a gelatinous nucleus pulposus, surrounded by the fibrous rings of the anulus fibrosus. The nucleus pulposus consists of water, proteoglycans, and collagen. At birth it is 90% water, and it degenerates with time. These disks allow dissipation of axial loading forces throughout various ranges of motion; with degeneration over time, they can cause mechanical bilateral or midline neck pain. The support of the cervical spine comes from the various ligamentous, articular, and muscular structures, which can also be pain-mediating structures. The uncovertebral articulation is an important structure in the cervical spine and represents an area of vertebral and disk articulation in the cervical neural foramen. The degenerative hypertrophy of this area and the resultant narrowing of the neural foramen commonly result in radicular pain.

Cervical sprains and strains can be caused by overstretching or tearing of spinal ligaments and muscles. In the acute phase of neck pain without neurologic symptoms, the diagnosis of cervical sprain and strain is often made without an inciting event, and the precise diagnosis is not evident. Cervical sprains and strains commonly occur after automobile accidents, trauma, or other injuries. In addition, motor vehicle accidents and associated whiplash injuries have been known to cause upper cervical facet joint–mediated pain. These occur most frequently as a result of rear-end or side-impact motor vehicle collisions. There are well-described sclerotomal referral patterns for neck pain arising from the facet joints, with the pain extending into the head and shoulders, either unilaterally or bilaterally.

Cervical radiculopathy can typically cause neck pain extending into the arm. The pain pattern is usually worse in the arm than in the neck with associated neurologic symptoms, such as weakness, numbness, and tingling. One common cause of radicular neck pain is a herniated cervical intervertebral disk (most commonly at the C6-7 followed by the C5-6 level). Herniated disk material has been shown to be inflammatory in nature and produces phospholipase A_2, a key mediator in the arachidonic acid cascade. Cervical spondylosis can also result from uncovertebral hypertrophy and is also a common cause of cervical radiculopathy. As the disks degenerate with time, there can be small herniations that calcify, causing disk osteophyte complexes to form. These complexes, combined with the ligamentous hypertrophy and loss of disk height that occur with aging, can cause impingement of nerve roots with resultant radicular pain.[2]

Cervical myelopathy caused by spinal cord compression is a possible complication of cervical spondylosis and can manifest with neck pain, radicular extremity pain, loss of manual dexterity, globally referred symptoms, gait instability, bowel or bladder dysfunction, and progressive weakness. Such symptoms warrant further diagnostic evaluation with magnetic resonance imaging (MRI) of the cervical spine if there is no contraindication.

CLINICAL PRESENTATION

A thorough history, including past medical, social, occupational, and family history, as well as a review of systems, including constitutional symptoms, skin changes, visceral pain, neurologic changes, and bowel or bladder complaints, should be performed. In addition, any history of previous trauma or whiplash should be elicited. Details surrounding the onset of pain, location and radiation of the pain, quality of pain over time, aggravating and alleviating factors, and associated symptoms such as headaches or systemic symptoms should be sought. Psychosocial elements including psychological and occupational history should also be evaluated to look for any confounding variables.

The location and radiation of pain can help elucidate the cause. Neck pain that remains in the neck region without radiation into the arms is typically referred to as axial neck pain. This pain can result from a cervical sprain or strain or be referred from the intervertebral disks or facet joints. Neck mobility may be limited from many of these causes; however, certain maneuvers can help elucidate the painful source. With axial neck pain, the motor strength and reflex examination findings are normal.

Radicular neck pain is usually described as pain greater in the arm than in the neck but commonly occurring in both. Neurologic symptoms, such as pain, weakness, numbness, and tingling, can also be found in the affected spinal nerve root distribution. The patient will likely report a relatively abrupt onset of pain that may worsen with particular movements, including cervical extension and ipsilateral rotation. In addition, a patient may have the arm in a position that decreases neural tension on the nerve root. This usually involves placing the upper arm closer to the head either in an overhead position or crossed in front of the throat. If the patient has any neurologic symptoms, such as weakness in the lower extremities, gait disturbance, bowel or bladder dysfunction, or sexual dysfunction, cervical myelopathy should be considered and immediately evaluated.

Facet joint pain is also a cause of axial neck pain and has been associated with whiplash injuries and headaches. Whiplash injury is experienced with an abrupt flexion-extension type of injury. Pain is typically off the midline, and although there are defined sclerotomes for referral, pain is usually worse in the neck. The pathophysiologic mechanism for whiplash syndrome is unclear; however, it is thought to be caused by soft tissue injury with local release of inflammatory mediators. The cervical zygapophyseal joints have been implicated as the major source of chronic pain after whiplash.[1] Significant biomechanical and psychosocial factors play a role, and severity of acute symptoms, comorbid depression, anxiety, and not being at fault for the accident are poor prognostic factors.

PHYSICAL EXAMINATION

Physical examination starts with careful observation of the patient, looking for cervical alignment, discomfort, and frequent position changes and evaluating the patient's affect. Gait should be examined for unsteadiness, spastic or mechanical movement, and widened or narrowed steps. The skin and vascular system should be appraised for medical causes of neck pain, including meningitis, dental or jaw pain, and malignant neoplasm.

Cervical range of motion should be determined. It should be noted whether the patient moves in a limited, guarded fashion or if there is an ease to the movement. The normal range of motion of the cervical spine is 90 degrees of rotation, 45 degrees of lateral tilt, 60 degrees of forward flexion, and 75 degrees of extension. The patient should be inspected for loss of cervical lordosis and atrophy of the paraspinal, periscapular, and arm muscles. Palpation of the paraspinal muscles and trapezius muscles should be performed to assess for the degree of tenderness, although positive findings of pain are nonspecific in nature and can be related to many causes of axial neck pain. The facet joints should also be palpated to reproduce the patient's typical symptoms.

Neurologic examination should include manual muscle strength testing, sensation, and reflexes and evaluation for upper motor neuron signs. Examination and manual muscle strength testing (shoulder elevation, abduction, and internal and external rotation; elbow flexion and extension; wrist extension and flexion; and hand and digit intrinsic muscles) may help define the involved dermatome (Table 183-1). In addition, sensation to both light touch and pinprick should be checked for deficits throughout the dermatomes. Reflexes should also be elicited at the biceps, triceps, and brachioradialis tendons bilaterally to look for asymmetry or hyperreflexia. The Babinski response and Hoffmann sign as well as evaluation for both clonus and muscle spasticity can determine if central nervous system involvement of the brain or spinal cord is occurring.

Provocative maneuvers such as the modified Spurling maneuver, when it is performed and the response is positive, can be suggestive of cervical spinal nerve root involvement (high sensitivity, low specificity). This test is performed by placing the head in extension, lateral flexion, and ipsilateral rotation. With placement of an axial load on the head, reproduction of typical symptoms down the arm can be specific for cervical radiculopathy.[3] The Elvey upper limb tension test is performed by turning the head contralaterally with the arm abducted and elbow extended; a positive test response is reproduction of arm symptoms.[3] The Lhermitte sign can also be elicited by rapidly flexing the neck while the patient is seated.[2] This can produce an electric shock sensation down the spine and into the limbs; the response is positive with cervical cord disorders such as compression, tumor, and multiple sclerosis.

In addition to cervical causes of neck pain, the provider should evaluate for other mimicking disorders. The Adson test for vascular thoracic outlet syndrome is done with the patient standing. The examiner palpates the radial pulse while moving the upper extremity in abduction, extension, and external rotation as the patient rotates the head toward the ipsilateral side with the breath held.[2] If the patient's pulse diminishes, this is considered a positive test result; however, this finding is often nonspecific. Mechanical shoulder disorders can also refer pain in a distribution similar to that of the cervical spine. Shoulder examination should also be performed to ensure that there is no shoulder disorder that is mimicking or contributing to neck pain symptoms.

DIAGNOSTICS

- Plain radiographs of the cervical spine are warranted if the patient has a history of cancer, recent trauma, long-standing corticosteroid use, osteoporosis, drug or alcohol abuse, or concerning constitutional or neurologic symptoms. When a patient visits the clinic with cervical spine pain after trauma or a motor vehicle accident, the Canadian Cervical Spine Rule, when used correctly, is helpful in identifying those patients who are at high risk for a cervical spine fracture and should therefore undergo cervical radiography.[4] The Canadian Cervical Spine Rule has been validated with high sensitivity using CT scan as the gold standard, is superior to the National Emergency X-Radiography Utilization Study (NEXUS) Low-Risk Criteria, and results in reduced rates of radiography.[5,6]
  - Lateral views can help demonstrate vertebral alignment and evaluate the normal cervical lordosis as well as evaluate for bone changes, such as a fracture or osteoarthritis. Flexion and extension views can additionally be taken to evaluate for segmental instability. Oblique views can help characterize any foraminal compromise and possible encroachment on the exiting nerves. However, routine x-ray examination was not helpful in demonstrating issues that changed clinical management and is therefore not recommended for routine episodes of neck pain.
- Radionuclide bone scintigraphy is another tool occasionally used for the diagnosis of neck pain. This is helpful if the history and physical examination findings raise suspicion for osteomyelitis, metastatic disease, or occult fracture. In addition, it can show increased uptake and activity in the axial and appendicular joints, which can be consistent with conditions such as osteoarthritis.
- If the patient has neurologic findings, symptoms concerning for medical causes of pain, occult fracture, or persistent pain after conservative treatment, further imaging is warranted. Computed tomography (CT) scans or MRI can be considered.
  - CT scans are better at identifying bone and degenerative changes and are typically performed acutely, such as in the case of a patient with a history of head trauma or cervical trauma and neck pain with high possibility of cervical fracture. However, CT scans expose the patient to a large amount of radiation and are not able to identify

TABLE 183-1 Cervical Dermatomes

Root	Muscle Group Affected	Dermatome	Reflexes
C5	Deltoid, biceps, supraspinatus, infraspinatus, rhomboids	Lateral arm	Biceps
C6	Biceps, infraspinatus, brachioradialis, pronator teres, triceps	Lateral arm and forearm, lateral digits (thumb)	Biceps, brachioradialis
C7	Triceps, pronator teres, wrist flexors	Posterolateral arm and forearm, middle digits	Triceps
C8	Finger flexors, thumb opposition, hand intrinsics	Medial arm and forearm, medial digits (pinky)	None

pathologic cord changes, such as spinal cord edema, demyelination, and intrinsic spinal cord tumors. CT scans can be performed with myelography in a patient with contraindication to MRI (e.g., pacemaker, shrapnel) to evaluate for nerve root or spinal cord compression.
  - MRI is the most widely used imaging modality to evaluate for neck pain and radiculopathy. Its principal use is to evaluate the bone structures and soft tissues, and it can be helpful in identifying degenerative disk disease, anular tears, disk herniations, spinal stenosis, and cord or nerve root compression. With the addition of gadolinium, it can be used to look for tumor or infection. Although it is superior at evaluating degenerative changes in the spine, there is a high likelihood that many findings are asymptomatic and may not be the source of the patient's pain. MRI studies have revealed that 19% of asymptomatic patients have anatomic abnormalities such as cervical disk herniations without any reported neck pain or radicular symptoms.[7]
- Other diagnostic workup can be included for more patient-specific situations.
  - Erythrocyte sedimentation rate and C-reactive protein can be helpful in a patient with constitutional symptoms as markers of systemic inflammation.
  - Neoplasm may be reflected in an abnormal complete blood count, alkaline phosphatase level, or calcium level.
- Electrodiagnostic studies can be helpful in distinguishing neurologic changes with denervation and reinnervation from subacute and chronic radiculopathy.[8] These studies will not show acute changes until approximately 3 to 4 weeks after the initial insult; however, needle electromyography (EMG) can highlight chronic changes with good sensitivity and high specificity.[8]

DIAGNOSTICS

Neck Pain

IMAGING	OTHER DIAGNOSTICS
X-ray examination*	EMG*
Radionuclide bone scintigraphy*	
CT scan or MRI*	

*If indicated.

DIFFERENTIAL DIAGNOSIS

The differential diagnosis of neck pain can be broad. The clinically common degenerative causes of neck pain are discussed earlier in the chapter. It is imperative to rule out serious sources of neck pain, including infection, fracture, inflammatory diseases, neoplasm, and other medical causes, with a thorough history and physical examination. Evaluation for any systemic signs, such as fevers, chills, weight loss, recumbency pain, headaches, and history of cancer, is important to rule out metastatic disease or infection. Diabetic neuropathy, Lyme disease, and herpes zoster can cause radiculopathy without cervical spondylosis. Thoracic outlet syndrome and brachial plexopathy should be considered in a patient with radicular symptoms. Other nondegenerative causes of neck pain include infectious or malignant causes involving the neck, referred pain from cardiac ischemia, intrathoracic disease from diaphragmatic irritation, and cervical dystonia or torticollis.

DIFFERENTIAL DIAGNOSIS

Neck Pain

MUSCULOSKELETAL
- Cervical spondylosis (degenerative disk disease)
- Cervical stenosis
- Cervicogenic headache
- Disk herniation or radiculopathy
- Dislocation, fracture, subluxation
- Whiplash, trauma
- Shoulder pathology

AUTOIMMUNE OR IDIOPATHIC
- Ankylosing spondylitis
- Fibromyalgia
- Juvenile rheumatoid arthritis
- Polymyositis
- Polymyalgia rheumatica
- Rheumatoid arthritis

REFERRED PAIN FROM
- Aortic aneurysm
- Heart, lung
- Gallbladder
- Meningitis
- Subarachnoid hemorrhage
- Cancer of the esophagus

RARE DIFFERENTIAL DIAGNOSES
- Paget disease
- Polio
- Tetanus
- Tuberculosis
- Syphilis (can cause osteitis and osteophytes)
- Infection of mandible teeth and temporomandibular joint pain

MANAGEMENT

Orthopedic spine surgeon or neurosurgery consultation is indicated for patients with progressive weakness or neurologic deficits.

Immediate emergency department referral is indicated for associated trauma or if diagnostic workup reveals fracture or instability of the cervical spine.

If the symptoms and examination findings are consistent with mechanical neck pain, the patient should be assured that a concerning underlying pathologic process is unlikely.

Physical modalities such as heat, ice, and massage can also be used by the patient if they are helpful. Appropriate posture and biomechanics should be encouraged, and ergonomic evaluation should be considered. Repetitive and heavy lifting of more than 10 pounds as well as positioning of the cervical spine in painful positions should be avoided. There should be no repetitive bending, upper extremity twisting, over-the-head movement, or exaggerated neck movements.

Manual or mechanical traction can be tried only after acute muscle pain has subsided and in patients without cervical stenosis or myelopathy. There is inconclusive evidence that continuous traction is any more effective than intermittent (manual).[9] Current literature does not show evidence to support the efficacy of continuous traction. It has not been shown to improve pain or function in patients with chronic neck pain with or without radiculopathy.[10] Intermittent traction may have some efficacy.

Activity levels should be increased slowly, and the patient should be aware that symptoms may wax and wane throughout the natural history of an acute flare of mechanical neck pain. If symptoms become more chronic and the neurologic examination shows the patient to be stable, activity and exercise should be encouraged to avoid further deconditioning.

PHYSICAL THERAPY MANAGEMENT OF CERVICAL SPINE PAIN

The physical therapy management of cervical spine pain is most effective when a multimodal treatment approach is used. Physical therapy interventions for the cervical spine can include a combination of therapeutic exercise, manual therapy, modalities, and patient education. Once a physical therapy referral is deemed appropriate, the physician should write a prescription, noting the diagnosis, stating "evaluate and treat," and suggesting the estimated frequency, duration of treatment, and relevant precautions. For most cervical spine conditions, one to three visits per week for the appropriate time period required to rehabilitate the particular patient, typically 4 to 8 weeks or more, depending on the severity and chronicity of symptoms, is appropriate.

The physical therapist will perform a thorough examination, assess the cause of the cervical spine pain or radiculopathy, come up with a differential diagnosis, and then devise a specific treatment plan or refer the patient to a physician if any red flags, indicating serious underlying pathology, are present. Several researchers have proposed strategies for the classification of patients with neck pain to improve the efficacy of treatment interventions.[11-13] These researchers have all created a decision-making algorithm that classifies cervical pain into clinical patterns, which helps in guiding treatment according to pattern-specific guidelines. Essentially, neck pain patients are categorized into the following clinical subgroups, as proposed by Childs and colleagues[12,13]:

- Mobility
- Centralization
- Exercise and conditioning
- Reduction of headache
- Pain control

The subgroups are matched, based on specific clinical characteristics, with the management strategy most likely to benefit the treatment-matched subgroup. The goal of the classification system is to improve the outcomes with the physical therapy treatment of neck pain.[11-13]

Therapeutic Exercise

Therapeutic exercise interventions are prescribed to help correct range-of-motion limitations, muscle imbalances, dysfunctional movement and motor control patterns, and poor posture; to improve muscle endurance; and to reduce muscle spasms, trigger points, and myofascial pain.

Physical therapy exercise prescription therefore includes the following:

- Range-of-motion exercises
- Flexibility (stretching) exercises
- Motor control and neuromuscular reeducation
- Strength and endurance exercises
- Postural exercises and education

Common dysfunctional postures in patients with neck pain include the following:

- Forward head posture
- Rounded forward and internally rotated shoulders
- Increased thoracic kyphosis
- Protracted scapulae

Dysfunctional postures contribute to cervical and thoracic pain, limited mobility, and impaired function.[11] Patients with dysfunctional postures, as well as patients falling into the conditioning and exercise subgroup mentioned previously, would benefit from therapeutic exercises.

Examples of some commonly prescribed exercises are as follows:

- Range-of-motion and flexibility exercises:
  - Can include but are not limited to active cervical movements into rotation, flexion, extension, side bend, and chin tucks. Chin tucks help restore upper cervical neck flexion within limits of pain.
  - Scapular retraction is helpful to promote thoracic spine extension and improve posture.
  - Upper trapezius, levator scapulae, pectoralis major muscle, and suboccipital muscle stretching are examples of flexibility exercises that may help alleviate tightness.
  - The pain control classification subgroup would benefit from gentle range-of-motion exercises and active exercises to tolerance.[12,13]
- Cervical muscle endurance training:
  - Deep neck flexor or craniocervical flexor muscle endurance was found to be impaired in patients with cervicogenic headaches and neck pain compared with control groups; therefore training the deep neck flexors through specific exercises has been shown to help alleviate cervicogenic headaches and chronic neck pain.[14-16]
  - Chin tucks in the supine position and chin tucks with a small head lift (more advanced) are commonly used to help train the deep neck flexors and cervicocranial flexor muscle group.
- Shoulder girdle and periscapular strengthening exercises:
  - These exercises help improve shoulder mechanics and alleviate stress on the cervical spine.
  - The exercises commonly prescribed include:
    - Rotator cuff strengthening exercises to reduce excessive loading of the upper trapezius muscles
    - Periscapular exercises such as scapular retraction with resistance as well as middle trapezius, rhomboid, lower trapezius, and latissimus dorsi muscle strengthening.
- Diaphragmatic breathing exercises can also help relax cervicothoracic muscles and retrain dysfunctional breathing patterns, which contribute to cervical muscle tightness.
  - The reduce headache subgroup would also benefit from the aforementioned interventions, particularly the deep neck flexor and craniocervical flexor muscle endurance training exercises, as well as postural exercises.[12,13]

Manual Therapy

Manual therapy for the cervical spine can include, but is not limited to, spinal manipulative therapy, spinal mobilization, muscle energy techniques, and myofascial release (MFR). Before any manual therapy is performed on the cervical spine, it is extremely important to rule out vertebrobasilar insufficiency (VBI), upper motor neuron involvement, and cervical spine instability.

The goals of manual therapy interventions are to:

- Restore joint mobility and correct joint dysfunctions
- Decrease muscle spasm/tightness
- Reduce stress on neurologic tissues
- Normalize joint mechanics

Spinal manipulative therapy is defined as the application of high-velocity, low-amplitude manual thrust to the spinal joints just beyond the joint range of motion.

Contraindications to manipulation include the following:

- Positive Hoffmann sign (indicative of upper motor neuron disease)
- Positive VBI test result
- Clinical signs of VBI (dizziness, diplopia, drop attacks, dysphagia, dysarthria)
- Direct trauma (see diagnostics section discussing the Canadian C-Spine Rule)
- Unexplained weight loss
- History of cancer
- Spinal fracture
- Unrelenting night pain
- Osteoporosis
- Severe spinal stenosis
- Neurologic deficits with limb weakness

When manipulation is contraindicated or unlikely to be beneficial, spinal mobilization techniques can be used to restore joint mobility to hypomobile joints, as long as mobilization is not also contraindicated. Spinal mobilization is the application of manual force to the spinal joints within the passive joint's physiologic range of motion without a thrust.[17] When a patient falls into the mobility classification subgroup mentioned earlier, then mobilization or manipulation of the cervical spine is the intervention of choice, provided there are no contraindications.

In randomized controlled trials, manual therapy consisting of spinal manipulation performed by a physical therapist was more effective in improving outcomes when compared with a physical therapy intervention that did not include a manual therapy approach, or a home exercise program.[12,18]

Muscle energy techniques involve a contract-relax technique that facilitates relaxation of muscle, improves range of motion, and enhances stretching of tight muscle tissue; it can be used as a form of neuromuscular reeducation.

MFR involves the application of manual sustained stretch to the skin, which will affect the underlying myofascial tissue. MFR assists in elongating and releasing tight and restricted tissue.

There is evidence to support the combined use of manual therapy and exercise for patients with cervicogenic headaches and mechanical neck pain with or without upper extremity symptoms compared with just spinal manipulation or exercise.[19]

The mobility, headache, and possibly pain control subgroups will benefit from some of the manual therapy interventions mentioned here.[12]

Modalities

Modalities frequently used in physical therapy for the cervical spine include ice, heat, ultrasound, electrical stimulation, and low-level laser therapy. Modalities are a helpful adjunct for the overall therapy program but are unlikely to be helpful long term when used in isolation.

Despite the limited evidence to support the use of modalities, they may be useful in treating patients who would fall into the pain control subgroup, as long as they are helpful for reducing symptoms. However, activity within tolerance is preferable to passive treatments, such as modalities.

Traction

Traction is usually indicated for patients with radicular symptoms to help resolve neurologic deficits, centralize radicular symptoms, and reduce pain. Studies addressing the efficacy of traction have been largely inconclusive; however one prospective study demonstrated that intermittent cervical spine traction (below 6 kg manual and up to 12 kg mechanical) was useful for reducing neck pain and radicular pain when used in conjunction with a multimodal approach, if symptoms have been present for less than 3 months.[20] Therefore, intermittent cervical traction may serve as an adjunct treatment option for nonchronic neck pain with or without radiculopathy. In addition, one retrospective study did support the use of home cervical traction and reported positive results.[12,20]

If a patient experiences centralization of cervical spine symptoms with application of manual traction, and the pain has been present for less than 3 months, the patient would be placed in the centralization subgroup and receive the most appropriate matched intervention, such as cervical spine mechanical or manual traction or chin tuck exercises to achieve the goal of pain reduction and centralization of symptoms.[12]

MEDICATIONS

1. Medications can also be a helpful adjunct through recovery. Oral over-the-counter (OTC) analgesics such as Tylenol and low-dose nonsteroidal anti-inflammatory drugs (NSAIDs) can be used if the patient has no medical contraindications. Higher anti-inflammatory doses of NSAIDs can be helpful.
2. A skeletal muscle relaxant, such as tizanidine, cyclobenzaprine, or baclofen, can also be used to help reduce muscle spasms associated with some cases of mechanical neck pain.
3. Opioid analgesics and tramadol are other options when used cautiously if patients do not have an adequate response to OTC pain medications. Careful reassessment should be performed if the patient has a history of drug abuse or has failed to respond after a reasonable treatment course.
4. For chronic neck pain, patients can be considered candidates for tricyclic antidepressants or mixed norepinephrine-serotonin reuptake inhibitors if they have no contraindications to these medications.
5. Gabapentin has also been shown to be beneficial for central pain syndromes and radiculopathy and can help restore sleep and function.
6. Complementary and alternative medicine treatments for subacute and chronic neck pain have also been shown to be useful for some patients. Acupuncture, cognitive-behavioral therapy, relaxation therapy, massage, reflexology, spa therapy, transcutaneous electrical nerve stimulation, and cold laser are reasonable to try and can provide short-term relief to patients. However, few of these therapies have been shown to be effective in the long term for chronic neck pain.
7. Other options to be considered for treatment of subacute or chronic neck and radicular pain include epidural corticosteroid injections.[21] This treatment typically requires referral to an interventional spine physician. Cervical epidural injections can be helpful to treat symptoms of radiculopathy as well as chronic neck pain.[22] In addition, injections can be performed into the facet joints or directly to the nerves supplying innervation to the joint for symptoms of facet syndrome.

8. Trigger point injections into the muscles in the area of pain can also help in the short term; however, studies demonstrate variable results.

COMPLICATIONS

Complications of an acute episode of mechanical neck pain are rare. If there is concern for instability or history of trauma, fracture and bone disease should be ruled out. If there are worrisome systemic features, more serious medical conditions should be ruled out. An episode of neck pain that follows a whiplash injury without traumatic fracture or other complications may continue to progress into chronic neck pain with associated headaches. If the patient has neurologic changes, further workup and appropriate imaging should be ordered to evaluate for radiculopathy or myelopathy. If neurologic symptoms change or worsen, surgical evaluation and referral should be initiated. Most episodes of acute neck pain are self-limited; however, there is the risk for continued pain and transition to chronic neck pain. Sequelae of chronic pain include mood disturbance, insomnia, opiate habituation, addiction, disturbance of interpersonal relationships and sexual relationships, loss of employment, and personal isolation.

INDICATIONS FOR REFERRAL OR HOSPITALIZATION

In general, mechanical neck pain does not need further specialist referral or hospitalization.

- If there was an associated trauma or if diagnostic workup reveals fracture or instability of the cervical spine, the patient should be referred immediately to an emergency department for further spine evaluation, monitoring, and treatment if necessary.
- Cervical myelopathy with associated gait disturbance, upper motor neuron signs, bowel or bladder incontinence, weakness in the upper or lower extremities, or incapacitating neck pain should indicate more urgent diagnosis and likely surgical intervention.
- For symptoms of mechanical or radicular neck pain, physical therapy referral can be a useful adjunct with conservative management and should be considered for patients to help with strength, endurance, and flexibility.
- Referral to an interventional spine physician can be considered if interventional procedures such as injections are appropriate.
- Referral to an orthopedic spine physician or neurosurgeon should be prompted by progressive weakness or neurologic deficits.
- If the patient has symptoms of chronic radiculopathy, surgical referral can be indicated if conservative management fails.
- Multidisciplinary specialist referrals to a pain physician or rehabilitation center can also be considered with chronic neck pain without surgical indications.

LIFE SPAN CONSIDERATIONS

After the initial episode of neck pain, the chances are high that pain will recur in the patient's lifetime. If the patient has a disk herniation and radicular symptoms, this disk material will likely be reabsorbed with time; however, the patient should be warned that the disk is at risk for reherniation. In addition, age can be a risk factor for development of degenerative disk disease and spondylotic changes. These can continue to progress and lead to recurrent episodes of neck pain as well as to chronic neck pain symptoms. Patients with diffuse idiopathic skeletal hyperostosis develop anterior osteophytes that can progress with age, causing stiffness and pain, and the osteophytes can become large and indent the esophagus and cause dysphagia.

Younger patients tend to have disk herniations, axial neck pain, myofascial pain syndrome, fibromyalgia, or whiplash-induced neck pain. Older patients tend to develop cervical stenosis with or without myelopathy, uncovertebral hypertrophy and resultant foraminal stenosis with radicular pain, disk herniations, axial neck pain, or whiplash-induced neck pain.

EDUCATION AND HEALTH PROMOTION

Patient education should start with reassurance and support. Explaining the natural history of mechanical neck pain and that most cases will resolve in a timely manner is important. Preemptive exercise and conditioning can help reduce the frequency of recurrence of episodes and should be communicated to the patient. Postural exercises and reminders should be provided to keep the neck in a neutral position in line with the thoracic spine or ear in line with the shoulder, with emphasis placed on keeping the shoulders back and chest forward. Recommending the use of lumbar support when sitting helps the patient maintain proper head and neck alignment and prevents slouching postures that can exacerbate neck pain. Ergonomic evaluation and sleeping position considerations should be mentioned to the patient. Overhead lifting and poor biomechanics while reaching should also be addressed, and proper body mechanics should be used at all times. Risk factors for disk degeneration, such as smoking, should be addressed, and the patient should be encouraged to quit smoking if possible. If the patient has concomitant psychosocial conditions, these should be addressed.

Patients should also be educated on the warning signs of potentially serious complications, including sudden or progressive limb weakness, bowel or bladder changes, and constitutional symptoms. Reporting of these symptoms on a timely basis can expedite urgent treatment.

CHAPTER 184

OSTEOARTHRITIS

Joanne Sandberg-Cook

DEFINITION AND EPIDEMIOLOGY

Osteoarthritis (OA) is a progressive degenerative joint process. It involves degeneration of the articular (hyaline) cartilage layer on the ends of bones at the joints as well as increasing thickness and sclerosis of the bone plate and subsequent involvement of joint protective mechanisms including ligaments and muscle. OA manifests as a monoarticular or polyarticular phenomenon and is often asymmetric. It can occasionally appear as a more generalized disease. OA is the most common type of arthritis, and it usually begins asymptomatically in the second or third decade of life. By the fourth decade, most people have some degree of pathologic (radiologic) change on articular weight-bearing surfaces. Symptoms typically begin to appear in the fourth through sixth decades of life. Some degree of symptomatic arthritis is extremely common by the seventh decade. OA occurs more commonly in women, at least in middle-aged and elderly persons. Risk factors include age, obesity, prior trauma, genetics, repetitive activities, metabolic disorders, neurologic diseases, and hematologic conditions.[1]

The carpometacarpal joints of the thumbs, distal interphalangeal joints of the fingers, first metatarsophalangeal joints of the feet, cervical and lumbar spine, and weight-bearing joints such as the hips and knees are most commonly affected. OA can also affect previously injured joints. Pain, stiffness, and limited range of motion are the most common reasons for seeking medical care. The degenerative effects of OA result in physical disability and can have a profound impact on the quality of life.[1,2]

PATHOPHYSIOLOGY

Initially, the cartilage softens and becomes overhydrated and boggy, with decreased quantity and size of proteoglycans within the matrix. Collagen also loses its stiffness, with fewer cells and loss of cross-links as degradation continues.[3,4] The surface layers fibrillate, and the cartilage loses its thickness, develops surface crevices, and then loses integrity. Loose cartilaginous fragments (known as loose bodies) can flake off, blocking range of motion and contributing to pain and disability.[4]

Chondrocytes proliferate with increased metabolic activity as the subchondral bone scleroses under the damaged areas. The bone thickens, stiffens, and then produces cysts, microfractures, and osteophytes at the joint margins,[4] findings that are often seen on imaging. The associated increased metabolic activity can be detected on a bone scan.

The cartilage surface is completely aneural, making the pathogenesis of pain from OA speculative. It is now thought to be a whole-joint disease with significant inflammatory soft tissues changes including synovitis as well as bone marrow lesions. Changes in joint nociceptors have been identified, and some researchers have suggested neuropathic pathways as contributors to pain.[4] Joint effusions are not uncommon, especially in the knee, causing stiffness and difficulty walking.

CLINICAL PRESENTATION AND PHYSICAL EXAMINATION

Insidious, progressive pain or stiffness of one or more joints may be the initial presenting complaint. Symptoms are most prevalent on arising, with a duration of less than 1 hour, and after a prolonged activity and are relieved by rest.[3] Weight-bearing activities, such as going up or down stairs, getting up from a sitting position, walking, prolonged standing, or changing activity level, can be particularly troublesome. The patient may also complain of crepitus (grinding), swelling, joint deformity, and gradual loss of motion as the disease progresses.[5]

When OA involves the cervical or lumbar spine, neuropathy and radiculopathy may develop as nerves are compressed. OA involving the hip manifests with groin or buttock pain that can radiate to the knee. The pain can cause the patient to "favor" the hip, which in turn can contribute to specific muscle weakness. The resultant gait is known as Trendelenburg gait. OA of the knee involves the medial joint compartment 70% of the time, leading to a varus deformity of the extremity. It can then progress to include the lateral joint compartment and patellofemoral articulations as well. Pain on palpation of the medial and lateral joint lines and joint effusions are often seen. Quadriceps muscle atrophy is common on the affected side.[5]

OA of the hands manifests as Heberden nodes (deformity of the distal interphalangeal joints) and Bouchard nodes (deformity of the proximal interphalangeal joints). A compression test as well as pain with palpation of the joint can detect OA of the carpometacarpal joint. Contracture, deformity, and even joint fusion are common as the disease progresses.[5] Fortunately, OA of the hands is seldom completely disabling.

DIAGNOSTICS

In the early stages of OA, radiographic findings may not be evident.[3] As the disease progresses and joint space is lost, radiographic changes become more prominent. Plain radiographs are often all that are needed to confirm the diagnosis. Magnetic resonance imaging (MRI) helps to identify changes in surrounding soft tissue. A bone scan may show increased metabolic activity within an arthritic joint.[4]

OA is a nonsystemic disease. There are no serologic markers for OA as yet, but serologic tests are commonly performed to rule out other disorders. Examination of the joint fluid may be helpful in ruling out crystalline, infectious, or inflammatory conditions. See the the diagnostics box for optional testing.

DIAGNOSTICS

Osteoarthritis

LABORATORY
- Rheumatoid factor*
- Cyclic citrullinated peptide*
- Antinuclear antibodies*
- CBC and differential*
- ESR*
- Uric acid*
- Joint aspirate for crystals, white blood cells*
- C-reactive protein*

IMAGING
- X-ray studies
- MRI*
- CT scan*
- Bone scan*

*If indicated by the presence of more systemic features such as fever, polyarticular pain, or abnormalities in blood chemistry values.
CBC, complete blood count; CT, computed tomography; ESR, erythrocyte sedimentation rate.

DIFFERENTIAL DIAGNOSIS

The differential diagnosis box lists other diseases that should be considered and excluded when appropriate. Other arthritic conditions, such as rheumatoid arthritis (see Chapter 218), gout and pseudogout (see Chapter 176), and psoriatic arthritis (see Chapter 215), are commonly seen with OA.[5]

DIFFERENTIAL DIAGNOSIS

Osteoarthritis

- Avascular necrosis
- Bursitis
- Fibromyalgia
- Fracture or dislocation
- Gout or pseudogout
- Lyme disease
- Malignant disease
- Osteomyelitis
- Osteonecrosis
- Paget disease
- Rheumatoid arthritis
- Tendinitis

MANAGEMENT

Pharmacologic Management

Acetaminophen. Acetaminophen remains the mainstay for initial treatment of early OA. The analgesic properties

can reduce discomfort without the additional risks of anti-inflammatory medications.[6,7]
- The current recommendation is 1 g three times daily.
- The maximum daily dose is 3 g/24 hr (650 mg every 6 hours) for adults.
- The maximum daily dose of acetaminophen in patients receiving warfarin therapy should not exceed 2500 mg orally. Hepatotoxicity is a concern, particularly if acetaminophen is used in conjunction with alcohol or with other products that use it in combination.
- Acetaminophen is found in a wide variety of over-the-counter and prescription products, such as sleep aids, cold remedies, and prescription pain medications.

Tramadol Hydrochloride (Ultram). Tramadol is a centrally acting pain reliever that is indicated for moderate to moderately severe pain.
- Tramadol is a nonopioid.
- Tramadol is not a nonsteroidal anti-inflammatory drug (NSAID).
- The package insert should be followed for dosage and precautions.
- Tramadol is also available as a combination drug with acetaminophen. The combination is synergistic and can be given in addition to NSAIDs.

Nonsteroidal Anti-Inflammatory Drugs.
- NSAIDs have long been part of the treatment regimen for OA.
- They are most beneficial for their analgesic rather than their anti-inflammatory properties.[7,8]
- Cyclooxygenase 2 (COX-2)–selective NSAIDs.
  - Designed to reduce the gastrointestinal toxicity of traditional NSAIDs.
  - Two of the three early COX-2 medications, rofecoxib (Vioxx) and valdecoxib (Bextra), were found to have serious side effects, including cardiovascular toxicity and an increased incidence of Stevens-Johnson syndrome.[9,10]
  - Per 2005 and revised 2010 guidelines, the U.S. Food and Drug Administration (FDA) requires all COX-2–selective as well as nonselective NSAIDs to carry the same cardiovascular risk warnings.
  - Celecoxib continues to be widely used and remains a good alternative for some patients, especially the following:
    - Those receiving warfarin
    - Those taking chronic steroids
    - Those who have gastrointestinal intolerance to traditional NSAIDs
- Meloxicam (Mobic), a preferential inhibitor of COX-2 but not a true COX-2 inhibitor, is well tolerated, with few side effects or drug-drug interactions.
- Patients at risk of stroke or myocardial infarction should continue to receive prophylactic aspirin.
- Traditional nonselective NSAIDs include ibuprofen, naproxen, diclofenac, and others.[11]
  - All have minimally increased cardiovascular toxicity.[12]
  - Caution is recommended with any NSAID.
  - The provider should monitor patients on NSAIDs closely for anemia and changes in renal function, liver function, and blood pressure.
  - NSAIDs should be avoided in patients with heart failure.[13]
  - Consideration may be given to prescribing gastrointestinal protective agents, such as H_2 blockers, prostaglandin E_2 inhibitors, or proton pump inhibitors, to reduce gastrointestinal intolerance.[8,9]
  - Older adults are especially vulnerable to the effects of NSAIDs. The American Collage of Rheumatology recommends that patients older than 75 years avoid oral NSAIDs in favor of topical alternatives.[7]

Intra-Articular Approaches to Treatment

Hyaluronan.
- Intra-articular injections of exogenous hyaluronan, most effective in mild to moderate OA, can help reduce the pain of OA of the knee and improve fluid viscosity within the joint.[14]
- It has been compared favorably to naproxen in efficacy in double-blind, placebo-controlled studies and has fewer adverse reactions.[14]
- It is injected once a week for 3 to 5 weeks, depending on the preparation, and it may provide benefit for 6 months or longer.[14]

Intra-Articular Corticosteroid Injections.
- Intra-articular corticosteroid injections can also provide significant pain relief for mild to severe disease, but the duration of benefit varies widely.
- Even in severe disease, injections are not recommended more often than every 3 to 4 months.
- Caution should be used with patients who are taking oral prednisone preparations or who have diabetes.
- All patients should be warned about transient increased pain, warmth, or redness of the joint after an injection. If these symptoms persist, the patient should seek follow-up care (see Chapter 173).[3,5]
- Triamcinolone acetonide (Kenalog) and methylprednisolone acetate (Depo-Medrol) are the preferred corticosteroid preparations because they remain in solution within the joint and do not leave behind crystalline particulate debris.
- Diabetic patients should be warned to expect a transient elevation in blood glucose levels for about 3 to 4 days.

Other Medications Helpful for Chronic Pain

- Low-dose, long-acting opioids may be prescribed.
  - They can be well tolerated and very effective in managing chronic pain associated with OA. The usual warnings of increased sedation, constipation, dependence, and abuse apply here as well.
- Gabapentin (Neurontin), selective serotonin reuptake inhibitors, and tricyclic antidepressants have also been used adjunctively in the management of chronic pain.
- Topical medications, including over-the-counter rubs and patches and lidocaine patches as well as topical NSAID gel (diclofenac), may also provide some temporary benefit and are now recommended as a first-line agent for patients older than 75 years.[7]

Nonpharmacologic Management

Exercise has a number of potential benefits for OA management including strengthening of supporting structure, improved range of motion, and decreased pain.
- Aerobic exercise can help with cardiovascular conditioning and weight reduction (if indicated).
- Physical and occupational therapy can improve muscle strength and allow the patient to maintain range of motion and functional capacity.[15,16]
  - Stretching programs may be provided to reduce contractures that lead to excess joint wear.

- Assistive devices, such as canes and walkers, can help reduce the load from lower extremity joints.
- Heat and ice may also provide symptomatic relief and improve exercise tolerance.
- Supportive, well-cushioned footwear with lifts or wedges can help adjust for angular deformities or leg length discrepancies.

Weight control may be indicated.

- Each pound of weight increases loading across the knee threefold to sixfold.[17]
- Losing weight will help reduce symptoms as it helps unload the joint.

The Arthritis, Diet, and Activity Promotion Trial (ADAPT) demonstrated that the combination of modest weight loss plus moderate exercise provides better overall improvements in self-reported measures of function and pain and in performance measures of mobility in older overweight and obese adults with knee OA compared with either intervention alone.[17]

Complementary Approaches

Acupuncture. Acupuncture has been shown to improve pain and physical function at both 8 and 26 weeks.[18]

Glucosamine with or Without Chondroitin. A study has supported the use of glucosamine with or without chondroitin for OA of the knees.[19] However, past multicenter double-blind studies have failed to demonstrate significant pain relief compared with placebo.[19] If patients wish to try this supplement, the recommended dosage is 500 mg of glucosamine sulfate three times daily for 3 to 6 months. If no improvement is noted, the supplement should be discontinued. There are few side effects or known drug-drug interactions. Glucosamine is a dietary supplement, not regulated by the FDA; potency and quality may not be consistent among brands.

Other Herbs and Dietary Supplements. Omega-3 fatty acids, bromelain, dimethyl sulfoxide (DMSO), ginger, methylsulfonylmethane (MSM), and S-adenosylmethionine (SAM-e) have all been used for the treatment of OA.

- Health care providers should be aware of any supplements being taken by their patients.
- The Arthritis Foundation has published a guide to many of the most commonly used supplements along with any associated study results.[20]
- The cycline antibiotics, including doxycycline, minocycline, and tetracycline, have been tested in randomized clinical trials; no measurable difference in pain or function was found.[21] Therapeutic magnets and copper have been used; there is limited scientific evidence to support their efficacy.

Surgery

Surgical consultation should be sought in the following situations:

- Failure to respond to all medical treatment
- Pain and disability that are compromising lifestyle

Total joint replacement may be recommended. Hip and knee replacement surgeries are highly successful operations that relieve pain and suffering for most.

Surgery is most likely to be successful when it is performed by a surgeon who does 35 or more such surgeries in a year and in an institution where such procedures are commonplace.[22,23]

The American Academy of Orthopaedic Surgeons recommends against the following:

- Needle lavage
- Arthroscopy with debridement
- Free-floating interpositional devices[24]

LIFE SPAN CONSIDERATIONS

OA is a disease of older adults that causes significant pain, disability, and loss of functional independence. Medications, especially NSAIDs, are more likely to cause cardiovascular, gastrointestinal, and renal toxicity in the older adult, and these patients should therefore be closely monitored. Joint replacement can offer improved function and pain control, but any surgical procedure is riskier in the older adult, with a higher incidence of postoperative complications and slower recovery. The primary goals of management, both conservative and surgical, are to improve the quality of life and to reduce pain.

COMPLICATIONS

Pain and immobility that affect the patient's functional capacity and quality of life are the main complications associated with OA. When patients hurt, they find it difficult to exercise or to control weight. This can have a detrimental effect globally on the patient's well-being and mood. The risk of falling is higher as a direct effect of a painful or immobile arthritic joint and weakened muscle. This can lead to fractures, dislocations, head injury, and increased immobility.

Other complications are directly related to the treatment of the disease, including medication side effects, infection or microfractures of damaged joints, and failure of prosthetic components.

INDICATIONS FOR REFERRAL OR HOSPITALIZATION

Orthopedic consultation is considered when conservative measures fail or the patient's quality of life is significantly diminished. Frequent or constant disabling pain, especially pain at rest, and functionally limiting symptoms are the most important criteria for orthopedic consultation and surgery.

A number of pain-relieving procedures, including conservative measures such as intra-articular corticosteroid injections and bracing, can be done in the primary care office.[25] Advanced techniques and technologies have revolutionized joint replacement surgeries, making this an option for younger patients with painful arthritis.

Once a patient has undergone total joint replacement, long-term management may include prophylactic antibiotics for dental work or endoscopy. Annual x-ray examinations to evaluate the position and fixation of prosthetic components may also be recommended.

FUTURE DIRECTIONS

Current research is moving in the direction of disease-modifying agents that are designed to alter the course of OA rather than to cover its symptoms. Cartilage cell replacement, stem cell transplantation, gene therapy, and implantable gene chips are proving to be exciting new directions for researchers.[26] Use of growth factors to alter disease progression is also being researched, although it is not yet recommended.[26] Newer medications and advances in prosthetic components to help manage symptoms continue to be explored as well.

PATIENT AND FAMILY EDUCATION

The treatment of OA should begin with a clear explanation of the disease process and likely progression of the disease.

Instruction on methods to protect the painful joint should include workplace or lifestyle modifications including weight reduction. The use of assistive devices, such as a cane, crutches, or a walker, can be helpful. Patients are encouraged to be realistic about their limitations to avoid exacerbations of symptoms.

HEALTH PROMOTION

Obesity and repetitive stress or trauma are specific modifiable risk factors for the development of OA; reduction in one or both may substantially reduce symptoms and disease progression. Maintaining an active lifestyle including low-impact, moderate-intensity exercise and weight control can significantly improve the quality of life for these individuals.[27] Policies and interventions to reduce musculoskeletal injuries in all settings should be implemented and enforced. This includes the prevention of athletic injuries in schools, interventions for workplace injuries, and training and education to reduce injuries related to falls.[28]

CHAPTER 185

OSTEOMYELITIS

Ruta M. Shah

DEFINITION AND EPIDEMIOLOGY

Osteomyelitis is inflammation of the bone caused by infection. It is one of the most difficult-to-treat infectious diseases. It can lead to progressive destruction of bone and formation of sequestra, making it difficult to cure in many cases. Infection of bone has been classically divided into three groups: (1) hematogenous osteomyelitis, seeded from bacteremia; (2) osteomyelitis associated with a contiguous focus, such as a puncture wound, foreign body, or adjoining soft tissue infection; and (3) osteomyelitis associated with peripheral vascular disease, such as diabetic foot infections or other vascular insufficiency.[1]

These groups may be further divided into acute and chronic varieties. Acute osteomyelitis is generally defined as infection before the development of bone necrosis; chronic osteomyelitis indicates the presence of osteonecrosis, and its removal often requires surgical debridement.[1] Clinically, acute disease can manifest as the sudden onset of inflammation, warmth, redness, and edema. Hematogenous osteomyelitis in the young is most likely to be seen acutely, usually with a single organism seeding the medullary cavity, and a good prognosis can be predicted. This entity is most commonly seen in children (50% of cases occur in children younger than 5 years), with a second peak occurring in older adults. In contrast to acute disease, chronic osteomyelitis develops during long periods, often months or longer.[1] Osteomyelitis with vascular insufficiency in older adults is an example of these more indolent infections. In this situation, an external focus erodes into the superficial periosteum. Formation of sinus tracts is also a potential feature. The flora is usually mixed, and the prognosis varies greatly with factors such as the extent of bone involvement, the presence of sequestra, areas of denuded dead bone, the type of organism, and host conditions. Acute osteomyelitis that is not diagnosed or that is inadequately treated may advance to chronic osteomyelitis, resulting in a more complicated clinical picture.[2]

Two major classification schemes exist for osteomyelitis. The Waldvogel classification system is based on the cause of the infection (hematogenous versus a contiguous focus of infection) and duration of illness (acute versus chronic) but does not provide information about specific therapeutics.[2] The classification scheme by Cierny and colleagues takes into consideration the extent of anatomic involvement (anatomic stage) and host factors (physiologic class), providing a guide to determination of the prognosis, extent of surgical intervention, and antibiotic treatment required.[3] Depending on the anatomic stage, further surgical resection, revascularization, muscle flaps, skin grafts, management of dead space, and bone grafts may be required (Table 185-1). Physiologic class is divided by characteristics of hosts classified as A, B, or C (Box 185-1).[4] A favorable prognosis accompanies A hosts, who have normal vasculature and metabolic factors and a normal immune system. B hosts carry a worse prognosis by virtue of local or systemic compromise. Systemic factors, such as diabetes, smoking, malnutrition, hypoxia, immunosuppression, or immunodeficiency, and local factors, such as lymphedema, venous stasis, arterial

TABLE 185-1 Anatomic Classification of Adult Long Bone Osteomyelitis (Cierny-Mader Syndrome)

Stage and Description	Etiology	Treatment
I. Medullary: Necrosis limited to medullary contents and endosteal surfaces	Hematogenous infection	**Pediatric:** Antibiotics; host alteration (e.g., nutritional support) **Adult:** Unroofing; intramedullary reaming
II. Superficial: Bone necrosis limited to exposed surface	Contiguous soft tissue infection	**Pediatric:** Antibiotics; host alteration **Adult:** Superficial debridement; local or microvascular flap coverage; possible ablation
III. Localized: Full-thickness cortical sequestration; infection well marginated, and bone stable before and after debridement	Trauma; evolution of stage I or II; iatrogenic	Antibiotics; host alteration; debridement; dead space management; temporary stabilization; bone graft optional
IV. Diffuse: Circumferential or permeative infection; bone unstable before or after debridement	Trauma; evolution of stage I or II; iatrogenic	Antibiotics; host alteration; debridement; dead space management; stabilization (internal or external fixation); possible ablation

BOX 185-1

Physiologic Classification of Hosts with Osteomyelitis (Cierny-Mader System)

A. Normal hosts with osteomyelitis

B_S. Systemic compromise
- Diabetes mellitus
- Extremes of age
- Hypoxia (chronic)
- Immunosuppression
- Immunodeficiency
- Malignant disease
- Malnutrition
- Renal failure
- Hepatic failure

B_L. Local compromise
- Arteritis
- Extensive scarring
- Sensory loss
- Lymphedema
- Major vessel compromise
- Small vessel disease
- Venous stasis
- Tissue irradiation
- Tobacco abuse

C. Fragile host; treatment worse than osteomyelitis

insufficiency, or sensory deficits, may require attention during treatment. C hosts represent a group for which treatment of the osteomyelitis may be worse than the disease itself. The Cierny-Mader staging system is important to medical and surgical management but also guides prognosis and education.

PATHOPHYSIOLOGY

Pathogenesis of osteomyelitis is affected by the organism and its virulence, age of the patient, immunocompromise and comorbidities, and type of bone affected. In children, hematogenous spread is the most common route of infection, most commonly affecting the long bones. This may also extend into the joint space, causing septic arthritis. Acute inflammation contributes to destruction of bone. This inflammation then compromises blood flow and leads to further bone destruction and the formation of sequestra. Antibiotics penetrate these areas poorly, often leading to an inadequate response to treatment with antibiotics alone. The periosteum can thicken and surround this area of dead bone, forming an enclosed capsule (involucrum). Surgical intervention is often needed to debride necrotic tissue.[2] In children, Brodie's abscess is an example of this type of enclosed infection commonly found in the metaphysis.

Infecting organisms also differ according to the patient's age and condition and whether the focus is contiguous or hematogenous. *Staphylococcus aureus* is the most commonly isolated pathogen overall (isolated in 70% of culture-positive cases), and there has been a significant increase in methicillin-resistant *Staphylococcus aureus* (MRSA) infection.[5,6] A single organism is the norm for hematogenous osteomyelitis. Infants most often harbor *S. aureus, Streptococcus pyogenes,* and gram-negative enteric organisms. With the advent of *Haemophilus influenzae* type b (Hib) conjugate vaccine, *H. influenzae* is now uncommon in children older than 1 year. Salmonella can cause infection in patients with sickle cell disease.[7] Patients with sickle cell disease are a unique subset of patients, and microbiologic data are essential to determining the appropriate antibiotic regimen.

In adults, *S. aureus* is also the dominant pathogen in both hematogenous and contiguous osteomyelitis. However, practitioners should be aware that in patients with chronic ulceration and vascular insufficiency, mixed infection is more commonly present. Organisms such as *S. aureus,* streptococci, anaerobes, and gram-negative bacilli are involved.[8] Again, the prevalence of MRSA, including community-acquired strains, continues to be on the rise. This pathogen must therefore be considered in all patients with osteomyelitis, not only those with health care exposures.[7] Some of these MRSA isolates harbor the Panton-Valentine leukocidin *(PVL)* gene, which has been associated with more aggressive soft tissue and multifocal infection, as well as protracted fever and bacteremia. The need for surgical drainage is also more common in these patients.[7]

CLINICAL PRESENTATION

Osteomyelitis is largely a clinical diagnosis with supportive data from imaging and cultures. Patients can have a variety of symptoms. In children, symptoms may include fever, decreased range of motion, and pain and may evolve during a few days to weeks. However, the onset can be insidious, which may delay diagnosis.[6] Chronic osteomyelitis can develop after inadequately treated osteomyelitis and can manifest in the patient with a history of osteomyelitis as recurrence of pain, swelling, and a draining sinus.[1] In adults, acute osteomyelitis is less commonly hematogenous, and when it is, it usually affects the vertebrae. Osteomyelitis can also occur by direct inoculation from trauma or surgery or in diabetic patients with vascular insufficiency and skin ulceration. Patients can manifest local symptoms such as fever, pain, erythema, and swelling. However, more commonly, patients may have a subacute presentation, with nonspecific pain and vague symptoms being the norm. Chronic osteomyelitis may manifest with a draining sinus tract. Adjacent ulcer and soft tissue cellulitis may mask bone tenderness.[9] In such a situation, the diagnosis of chronic osteomyelitis can be difficult. Large diabetic foot ulcerations and exposed bone or probing to the bone predict a high likelihood of osteomyelitis. Chronic osteomyelitis is seldom associated with fever or leukocytosis, and inflammation markers can also be normal. Subacute presentation of osteomyelitis may challenge health care providers caring for patients with fever of unknown origin.

PHYSICAL EXAMINATION

Physical examination may elicit bone tenderness. Ulcers with visible bone or sinus tracts that probe to bone are usually diagnostic of osteomyelitis.[10] In these circumstances, specific diagnostic imaging tests may not be necessary.

Special situations and clinical syndromes are important to recognize and are briefly discussed here.

Vertebral Osteomyelitis

Low back pain is a common problem for which a precise source may not be discovered in a large number of patients. Health care providers should be aware of warning signs that should lead to further investigation (Box 185-2). Back pain is the most common initial symptom for vertebral osteomyelitis. Fever and leukocytosis are absent in 50% of cases, and tenderness of the spine to palpation is also not invariably present.[11] Therefore, diagnosis is often delayed, and a high level of clinical suspicion must be maintained. Pyogenic vertebral osteomyelitis is usually hematogenous and therefore commonly a complication of initial primary infection. This primary source is elucidated in about 50% of cases.[12] An example is infective endocarditis. A high rate of infectious endocarditis and spontaneous vertebral osteomyelitis has been reported (27% to 31%).[12] Early diagnosis of infectious endocarditis in patients with a diagnosis of vertebral osteomyelitis is critical because surgical or other specific interventions may be required. Clinical features that may

BOX 185-2

Thoracic and Low Back Pain: Warning Signs Suggestive of Malignant Disease or Osteomyelitis

- Previous cancer
- Weight loss
- Elevated erythrocyte sedimentation rate
- Fever, other constitutional symptoms
- Localized tenderness over vertebral body
- Lack of positional relief
- Lack of improvement over time
- Distant foci of infection (endocarditis)
- Indwelling intravenous catheters
- Injection drug abuse
- Neurologic signs (weakness, sensory loss, asymmetric reflexes, loss of bowel or bladder function)
- Thoracic pain

raise concern for infectious endocarditis in a patient with vertebral osteomyelitis include a predisposing cardiac condition or valve replacement, bacteremia with a gram-positive organism (e.g., *Streptococcus, Enterococcus,* and *Staphylococcus* species) as opposed to a gram-negative organism, and poorer prognosis.[12]

Osteomyelitis may be recognized by a radiologic process that involves both sides of the vertebral disk and adjacent vertebrae symmetrically. Malignant disease does not cross the disk to involve adjacent vertebrae.[13] Early recognition is important because posterior extension causes epidural abscess and cord compression. Severe and lancinating back pain may be suggestive of epidural abscess.[14] Collapsed vertebrae may also threaten the spinal cord. The course may be complicated by paravertebral, epidural, and psoas abscesses, all of which must be drained.[15]

Pyogenic vertebral osteomyelitis is primarily a disease of adults and is usually hematogenous and insidious in onset. Pain evolves gradually during weeks to months. Fever and leukocytosis are absent in 50% of cases. Although *S. aureus* is the predominant organism, gram-negative organisms can also cause vertebral osteomyelitis. The most common sources are urinary (32%) and abdominal (25%). In a significant percent, the source remains occult.[15] In young patients with injection drug use, organisms such as *Pseudomonas aeruginosa, Candida* species, and *S. aureus* (including MRSA) must be considered. A patient history for potential environmental exposures, which may suggest exposure to a particular endemic pathogen, should also be obtained. The possibility of unusual pathogens, such as *Candida* species, other fungi,[16] mycobacteria, and gram-negative organisms, emphasizes the need to make a causative diagnosis whenever possible if treatment is to be successful.

Diabetic Foot

A diabetic foot ulcer is the classic example of contiguous focus osteomyelitis in an area of vascular insufficiency. Arterial insufficiency and revascularization are important considerations and often require vascular surgical consultation. In patients with diabetes, the risk of amputation is increased. It is critical that health care providers promote prevention, monitoring and early recognition, and adequate care of diabetic foot ulcers.

Recognition of osteomyelitis in a diabetic foot may be difficult. Patients may have classic signs of infection such as swelling, odor, drainage, tenderness, and a poorly healing wound with necrotic tissue, but, alternatively, classic signs and systemic toxicity may be absent.[17] Probing to bone also makes osteomyelitis likely.[10,17] Plain radiography is recommended in patients with diabetic foot infection, looking for bony abnormality or soft tissue changes. Further imaging with magnetic resonance imaging (MRI) can be performed in patients who require more specific diagnosis or in whom abscess is a concern. Bone scans and tagged white cell scans are alternatives but can be problematic owing to their low specificity.[17] Biopsy of bone or debridement culture (when indicated) is the definitive diagnostic study and supplies good microbiologic evidence to direct antibiotic treatment.[17] However, poor healing at the biopsy site may further compromise the foot. Thus, empirical therapy is often undertaken unless debridement is indicated by anatomic criteria. Failure of therapy in later stages may necessitate chronic suppression with oral antibiotics or amputation.

Pseudomonas Infection

Pseudomonas osteomyelitis of the foot is a unique form of infection that follows a puncture wound, such as a nail through the shoe. Sneakers provide a wet, fertile environment for *P. aeruginosa. Pseudomonas* organisms also may be associated with injection drug abuse and may involve unusual sites, such as sacroiliac, sternoclavicular, and pubic joints and contiguous bone.[1]

Sickle Cell Disease

Patients with sickle cell disease (see Chapter 237) are at high risk for osteomyelitis, especially in areas where decreased blood flow has led to infarcted bone.[18] Bowel ischemia, a result of intravascular sickling, encourages enteric flora to enter the circulation. *S. aureus* is most common, but enteric gram-negative organisms, especially *Salmonella* organisms, are often encountered.[7] Osteomyelitis may be difficult to distinguish from bone infarction because it can have similar signs and symptoms. Sequential bone marrow and bone scans may help differentiate between the two entities.[19]

DIAGNOSTICS

Given the spectrum of disease and varied microbiologic characteristics of osteomyelitis, cultures of bone and blood are essential to diagnosis and management. Cultures from sinus tracts or ulcers may not be indicative of organisms in underlying bone. However, they can be of benefit in identification of resistant organisms and in identification of *S. aureus* because cultures of this organism from sinus tracts frequently correlate with deeper infection.[20] Blood cultures are positive in 40% of cases of acute osteomyelitis but are rarely positive in chronic osteomyelitis. In adults with contiguous focus chronic osteomyelitis, deep tissue culture specimens or specimens from surgical debridement of bone and soft tissue are preferred to help aim antibiotic therapy.[17]

Leukocyte counts may be normal or elevated. Erythrocyte sedimentation rate (ESR) and C-reactive protein (CRP) are usually elevated in acute disease and should be monitored for response to therapy.[21,22] CRP may be more valuable in monitoring the response to therapy because it changes more rapidly than the ESR does. ESR and CRP may be normal in chronic osteomyelitis. Visible bone or sinus tracts that probe to bone are usually diagnostic of chronic osteomyelitis.[10,17]

Radiologic tests are frequently used to diagnose osteomyelitis. Plain films usually begin to demonstrate destructive processes within 2 weeks of onset in acute osteomyelitis and are recommended in patients with new diabetic foot infection.[17] They are inexpensive and may be helpful in determining extent and activity in chronic osteomyelitis but may be difficult to interpret in the diabetic foot, in which neuropathic osteoarthritis is common.[23]

In cases in which conventional radiography is ambiguous (i.e., at less than 2 weeks in acute osteomyelitis or with confounding bone disease in chronic osteomyelitis), radiographs may be followed by other radiologic tests. The sensitivity and specificity of MRI are among the highest reported for any radiologic test used for the diagnosis of osteomyelitis, detecting acute osteomyelitis at as early as 3 to 5 days.[24] MRI also has great negative predictive value. MRI can be useful in determining the extent of infection and is the preferred imaging modality in vertebral osteomyelitis and evaluation of diabetic foot osteomyelitis.[10] Especially when surgery is contemplated, MRI can best define sequestra, anatomic stage, and associated abscess. Both computed tomography (CT) and MRI imaging are capable of identifying an abscess and allow guided needle aspiration of bone. Among the disadvantages of MRI are its expense and the fact that young children may require sedation to undergo an examination. In addition, bone marrow edema, as seen on MRI, can be present in other conditions, such as trauma, fracture, surgical change, Charcot arthropathy, and osteonecrosis, making the interpretation challenging at times.[24] CT and MRI are both disturbed by metallic joint prostheses or internal fixation hardware.

Three- or four-phase bone scans become abnormal in as little as 48 to 72 hours and can differentiate between bone and soft tissue involvement.[23] These tests have a relatively high sensitivity, although their specificity is generally lower because of their inability to distinguish fracture, osteoarthritis, tumor, gouty tophi, and neuropathic bone formation from infection.[23]

DIAGNOSTICS

Osteomyelitis

LABORATORY
Complete blood count and differential
Blood cultures
ESR

IMAGING
X-ray examination
MRI or CT scan*
Bone scan*
Gallium or indium scan*

OTHER DIAGNOSTICS
Open bone biopsy or needle aspiration of bone with culture and sensitivity*

*If indicated.

DIFFERENTIAL DIAGNOSIS

Osteomyelitis at the metaphysis of long bones approximates the joint and must be distinguished from septic arthritis (see Chapter 179). Examination for joint effusion and arthrocentesis will diagnose a septic joint, and the bone will be radiologically normal. Gout may cause cystic erosion in bone associated with a draining tophus (see Chapter 176). Although cultures are often positive for skin flora, the drainage is laden with crystals rather than neutrophils. Tophaceous gout is antibacterial and unlikely to be infected. Bone infarcts in hemoglobinopathy are multiple and recurrent, unlike unifocal osteomyelitis. Post-traumatic periosteal reaction may mimic early osteomyelitis radiologically or may serve as a site for osteomyelitis secondary to recent trauma. Nonspecific periosteal or cortical change caused by adjacent bursitis, abscess, or ulcer is difficult to distinguish from contiguous focus osteomyelitis. Tumor may or may not have distinguishing features on plain films and must be considered in the differential diagnosis. Old, inactive osteomyelitis may be indistinguishable from active infection radiologically. Finally, a focus of osteomyelitis secondary to subacute bacterial endocarditis must be considered if blood cultures are positive and a new cardiac murmur is appreciated.

DIFFERENTIAL DIAGNOSIS

Osteomyelitis

- Septic arthritis
- Gout
- Post-traumatic periosteal reaction
- Bursitis
- Abscess
- Ulcer
- Tumor
- Subacute bacterial endocarditis
- Hemoglobinopathy (bone infarction)

MANAGEMENT

Specialist Consultation

- Infectious disease consultation is recommended for the management of long-term antibiotics, for patients with resistant organisms, or for complex wound infection.
- Surgical consultation is necessary in patients with vascular insufficiency and/or debrideable or drainable infectious focus.
- Consultation with a wound care specialist should be done early for patients with progressive or chronic wounds.
- Neurosurgical consultation should be sought for any patient with suspected epidural abscess.

Immediate Emergency Department Referral

- Indicated for patients with neurologic symptoms
- Severe back or joint pain associated with fever
  - Sepsis symptoms related to infected bone or joint focus
  - Severe cellulitis or suspected abscess
- Patients with severe diabetic foot infections, those who have poor social support, or those in whom outpatient therapy is failing may also need to be hospitalized.

Antibiotics alone often manage acute hematogenous medullary infection in children. Later stages with involucrum need to be surgically unroofed. All more destructive stages require surgical intervention as defined in Table 185-1 as well as prolonged antibiotic therapy based on the sensitivity of organisms obtained by culture of bone at surgery. In stage IV disease, extensive removal of infected bone may require orthopedic rod internal fixation, external fixation, bone graft, and dead space management with antibiotic-impregnated beads and two-phase joint replacement. Plastic surgery may be required to bring skin grafts or tissue flaps over bone to fill defects and to revascularize. Vascular surgery may be required to revascularize with bypass grafts or to reroute major vessels away from infected areas.

Most often, osteomyelitis is treated with 4 to 6 weeks of intravenous antibiotic therapy through a central line, most

TABLE 185-2 Empirical Therapy for Osteomyelitis in Adults

Classification	Organism	Empirical Antibiotic
Acute hematogenous osteomyelitis	*Staphylococcus aureus*, streptococci	Nafcillin, oxacillin, cefazolin*
Contiguous focus vascular insufficiency, diabetic foot, neuropathic ulcer	*S. aureus*, streptococci, gram-negative bacilli, anaerobes	Ampicillin-sulbactam, piperacillin-tazobactam, imipenem-cilastatin*
ADDITIONAL CONSIDERATIONS IN SPECIAL HOSTS		
Injection drug abuse	*S. aureus, Pseudomonas, Serratia, Enterobacter* organisms	Depends on pathogen
Hemoglobinopathies	*Salmonella* organisms	Depends on sensitivity
Immunosuppression	*Enterobacter* organisms, mycobacteria, fungi	Other

*Vancomycin, linezolid may be substituted or added if the patient is at risk for or prior cultures indicate presence of MRSA.
Modified from Mader JT, Calhoun J: Long-bone osteomyelitis diagnosis and management, *Hosp Pract (Off Ed)* 29(10):71-76, 1994.

commonly a peripherally inserted central catheter (PICC).[25] Two meta-analyses concluded, however, that no definitive recommendation can be made about the best mode of administration, drugs, or length of treatment for osteomyelitis.[26] A Cochrane review based on eight small randomized trials looking at the use of antibiotics for treatment of chronic osteomyelitis was unable to find a difference among methods of antibiotic administration. However, there was insufficient evidence, and the lack of newer trials addressing this topic made it difficult to infer an optimal duration of antibiotics.[26]

Sensitive organisms may respond to oral antibiotics that are highly bioavailable. The quinolones and linezolid are a good oral option for treatment of osteomyelitis with a sensitive organism.[27] A meta-analysis comparing fluoroquinolones and β-lactam (intravenous)–based regimens showed no difference in efficacy, infection relapse, superinfection, and adverse events. However, their use is limited in *S. aureus* osteomyelitis because of increasing resistance and the development of resistance with therapy.[27,28] Trimethoprim-sulfamethoxazole, linezolid, and rifampin have been used orally to treat osteomyelitis, although rifampin should not be used as a single agent because of rapidly emerging resistance to this agent when it is used alone.[29] Children with acute osteomyelitis may be successfully treated with 2 to 5 weeks of oral antibiotics, after responding to 1 to 2 weeks of parenteral antibiotics.[30] The doses of oral penicillins and cephalosporins are higher than doses used for common infections.

Vertebral osteomyelitis is usually treated with intravenous antibiotics that are appropriate for the isolated organism for a minimum of 6 weeks, although longer courses (12 weeks) are frequently used. Surgery is now infrequently required and is usually reserved for cases with cord compression or spinal instability or cases in which the disease progresses despite adequate therapy.[1] As opposed to vertebral osteomyelitis, in which hematogenous focus yields a single organism, diabetic contiguous focus osteomyelitis yields mixed flora. Coagulase-positive and coagulase-negative staphylococci, streptococci, anaerobes, and gram-negative bacilli are predictably present in necrotic tissue. An accompanying cellulitis is usually a result of streptococci or staphylococci and may be treated with nafcillin or cefazolin alone.[21] However, to treat the ulcer or underlying osteomyelitis, coverage of all organisms is necessary (e.g., ampicillin-sulbactam, piperacillin-tazobactam, or imipenem-cilastatin). Presence or suspicion of *Pseudomonas* organisms will necessitate the addition of an antipseudomonal antibiotic, such as piperacillin, ceftazidime, or ciprofloxacin (Table 185-2). Aminoglycosides have poor penetration into bone and do not work well in abscesses, where pH is low.

With the increase in incidence of MRSA infections, questions have arisen about the best agents for treatment of osteomyelitis caused by this organism. Intravenous vancomycin is generally used as empirical therapy when this organism is suspected, although failure rates for this antibiotic in *S. aureus* osteomyelitis are considerably higher than for β-lactam antibiotics in sensitive infection. Higher levels of vancomycin are usually needed to optimize penetration of this agent into the infected bone.[30] Daptomycin and linezolid have shown promise in the treatment of MRSA and gram-positive osteomyelitis.[31,32] Linezolid has excellent oral bioavailability and hence can be taken orally with excellent efficacy. Important adverse reactions may limit longer durations (longer than 2 or 3 weeks) of therapy, including hematologic disorders (neutropenia, thrombocytopenia, anemia).[33] Practitioners should be aware that development of resistance to these newer medications, although uncommon, has been reported.[34]

The health care provider must monitor the patient for allergic reaction and toxicity of antibiotics, diarrhea caused by *Clostridium difficile* (see Chapter 232), thrombosis and infection of central lines, and response to therapy. Central lines should be removed soon after completion of antibiotics to avoid providing a focus for further infection. Health care providers should also address nutrition, control of diabetes, reduction of immunosuppressive drugs, rehabilitation for alcohol and substance abuse, smoking cessation for those with vascular insufficiency, treatment of ulcers, and monitoring for patients who are at high risk for development of foot infection. Regular visits to a podiatrist may provide nail care, attention to footwear, wound care, and prophylactic surgery.

LIFE SPAN CONSIDERATIONS

Osteomyelitis is usually not a fatal infection, but associated sepsis may be life-threatening. Persons of any age can develop a bone infection, although it is more common in children and persons older than 50 years.

COMPLICATIONS

Failure of aggressive therapy and relapse are common in patients with diabetes or vascular insufficiency or in compromised hosts. *S. aureus* is noted for associated cellulitis, sepsis, and metastatic foci of infection that may be distant from the site of the osteomyelitis. Fracture through advanced anatomic disease should be preventable by orthopedic evaluation. Sinus tracts, abscesses, and hematomas need to be diagnosed and drained. Infection may threaten adjacent vessels, tendons, and nerves. Chronic osteomyelitis can cause squamous cell carcinoma at the site of chronic drainage.[35] Amyloidosis has been caused by the systemic response to chronic osteomyelitis.[36] Long-term antibiotic use may be associated with a number of complications, including line infections or thrombosis, adverse drug reactions, and the development of resistant organisms.

Amputation is a consequence that may necessitate physical therapy, prosthetics, vocational counseling, and psychiatric counseling. Chronic use of a suppressive antibiotic is an option if the surgery is too life-threatening or amputation is being contemplated with understandable reluctance. The patient's quality of life is certainly altered by amputation. However, health care providers may need to provide information about below-the-knee amputation and a prosthesis, which may be more functional than a chronically draining site of osteomyelitis in a foot with marginal blood flow.

PATIENT AND FAMILY EDUCATION

In addition to receiving an explanation of the various diagnostic and therapeutic options, patients should understand that "cure" is an elusive concept in this disease. Acute osteomyelitis may relapse years after treatment, and chronic osteomyelitis may smolder indefinitely in a subacute fashion with intermittent drainage. Stating that osteomyelitis is arrested rather than cured is usually appropriate. Patients with extensive bone defects must take precautions against fracture. Patients need to be educated about prolonged therapy, central venous lines, relapses, antibiotic complications, amputation, and suppression. Preventive measures include teaching daily foot inspection to patients with diabetes, arthritis, vascular insufficiency, or neuropathy because these patients are particularly susceptible to infections in the feet. Diabetic and neuropathic ulcers require prompt medical attention. Insensate feet must be protected from heat, cold, and trauma. Control of diabetes, management of edema, good nutrition, and smoking cessation are all important.

CHAPTER 186

SHOULDER PAIN

Kathy J. Fabiszewski

DEFINITION AND EPIDEMIOLOGY

Shoulder pain and dysfunction are among the most common musculoskeletal complaints encountered in primary and acute care settings, responsible for approximately 16% to 20% of all musculoskeletal encounters.[1,2] Shoulder pain is second only to low back pain in patients seeking care for musculoskeletal symptoms in primary care,[3] with approximately 1% of adults older than 45 years consulting a primary care provider for new shoulder pain annually.[4] An estimated 20% of the population will have shoulder pain during their lifetime.[3,4] Shoulder pain encompasses a diverse array of pathologies and can affect up to one fourth of the population, depending on age and risk factors.[4] Shoulder pain is most often caused by an intrinsic disorder of the shoulder resulting from acute or chronic trauma, injury, and overuse or inflammation of the shoulder girdle and the surrounding articular surfaces, ligaments, tendons, and periarticular structures. Injury coupled with pain predisposes the individual to functional impairment or disability. The primary health care provider can, in most cases, diagnose and treat shoulder pain without specialty consultation.

PATHOPHYSIOLOGY

The shoulder is the most movable joint in the body and is composed of four separate joints or articulations that are made up of only three bones: the scapula, clavicle, and proximal humerus. The shoulder, or glenohumeral joint (the articulation of the humerus and the glenoid fossa of the scapula), is a closely fitted, shallow, complex ball-and-socket joint that is capable of a wide, almost global, range of motion. Adjacent to the glenohumeral joint are the acromioclavicular joint (the articulation between the acromion process and the clavicle) and the sternoclavicular joint (the articulation between the manubrium of the sternum and the clavicle), which form the shoulder girdle. At the scapulothoracic articulation, the scapula is suspended from the posterior thoracic wall by muscle attachments to the ribs and spine.[5] Normal shoulder motion depends on the smooth, integrated movement of these four articulations.

The primary movers of the glenohumeral joint are the pectoralis major and minor (adduct the shoulder), deltoid (abducts the shoulder), teres major, and latissimus dorsi.[5] The trapezius muscles elevate and rotate the scapula. The shoulder joints are stabilized by the soft tissues of the shoulder girdle, including the joint capsule, glenoid labrum (a fibrocartilaginous ring attached to the outer rim of the glenoid that provides depth and stability), muscles of the rotator cuff, long head of the biceps, and scapular stabilizers. The shoulder socket (glenoid) is shallow and, because of the wide range of motion of the glenohumeral joint, inherently unstable; it is, in fact, the most unstable ball-and-socket joint in the human body. This anatomic arrangement provides for greater mobility but is accomplished by compromise of some stability (the maintenance of the humeral head properly positioned within the glenoid cavity), making the shoulder one of the most commonly dislocated joints in the body.

The rotator cuff consists of the musculotendinous attachments of four muscles—the supraspinatus, infraspinatus, teres minor, and subscapularis muscles—that come together and form a cuff around the head of the humerus, attaching to the greater and lesser tuberosities. The rotator cuff compresses the humeral head in the glenoid fossa against the labrum and acts as the primary dynamic stabilizer to the glenohumeral joint. The chief function of the rotator cuff is the maintenance of stability during movements.[6]

The greater tuberosity of the humerus, the tendons of the rotator cuff muscles that elevate the arm, and the subacromial bursa move back and forth through a tight archway of bone and ligament known as the coracoacromial arch. When the arm is raised, the archway becomes smaller, causing these structures to impinge on one another and making them prone to inflammation and degeneration.

CLINICAL PRESENTATION

Shoulder pain symptoms may be acute or chronic, specific or vague, persistent or recurrent. The patient with a shoulder problem typically reports shoulder pain that is aggravated by movement and is often accompanied by limitation of movement. There may or may not be a history of trauma or overuse. Surprisingly, many individuals fail to recollect an episode of trauma unless specifically asked. Patients younger than 40 years with a history of trauma are more likely to have shoulder dislocation or subluxation, whereas rotator cuff tear is more common after trauma in those older than 40 years.[1]

Patients often report difficulty with activities of daily living, such as bathing, combing their hair, or dressing, as well as with driving, carrying groceries, and exercising. Loss of range of motion is associated with adhesive capsulitis and glenohumeral arthritis.[1] Other symptoms may include stiffness, crepitation, instability, and aching discomfort related to vigorous or sustained use. Most shoulder disorders hurt more when the shoulder is elevated, whereas many cervical radiculopathies feel better with the shoulder in an elevated position.[6] Numbness, tingling, and pain radiating distal to the elbow suggest a cervical cause of the symptoms and are seldom indicative of shoulder disease.[1] Weakness is associated with rotator cuff disorders and glenohumeral arthritis.[1] Anterior-superior shoulder pain is associated with acromioclavicular joint disease.[1] Diffuse shoulder pain is associated with rotator cuff disorders, adhesive capsulitis, or glenohumeral arthritis.[1]

Inquiry about hand dominance, occupational activities (e.g., lifting, chronic stress on joints, safety precautions), exercise and recreational activities (extent, type, and frequency), and self-care capacity facilitates identification of contributing factors, potential causes, and the functional impact of the symptoms. A history of collision sports (football, hockey) or weightlifting makes instability or acromioclavicular arthritis more likely, whereas overhead sports (baseball, softball, tennis) make rotator cuff disease more likely.[1] Superior labral tears, including superior labrum anterior and posterior (SLAP) injury, may occur during a motor vehicle accident; a fall onto an outstretched arm; forceful pulling of the arm, such as when trying to catch a heavy object; or forceful movement of the arm when it is above shoulder level.[7] Identification of any history of recent or remote trauma, including the details of injury, is vital. Determination of previous diagnostic studies, hospitalizations, surgeries, or therapies guides diagnostic evaluation. A detailed medical history is also important because adhesive capsulitis is associated with diabetes mellitus and thyroid disorders,[1] and humeral fractures are a consideration in the older adult with osteoporosis or cancer.

Because nonextrinsic shoulder pain may be caused by either intrinsic shoulder disorders or referred pain, it is also critical to ascertain the exact location and distribution of the pain. It is unusual for pain originating in the shoulder, for example, to radiate below the elbow.[1] Vague, poorly localized pain is often extrinsic in origin. Pain involving other joints is suggestive of a generalized arthritic process. Characterization of the type, intensity, timing, and duration of pain as well as identification of ameliorating and exacerbating factors is also essential. The American Shoulder and Elbow Surgeons standardized form for assessment of the shoulder incorporates a synopsis of both patient self-evaluation data and physical examination parameters and is useful in organizing a primary care approach to shoulder pain (Fig. 186-1).

PHYSICAL EXAMINATION

Physical examination of the shoulder should be performed in a systemic manner beginning with careful visual inspection of the shoulder. Anterior and posterior examination for surgical scars, displacement of bone prominences, warmth, swelling, changes in skin color or texture, suprascapular or infrascapular muscle atrophy, and winging of the scapula is necessary. Asymmetry with the contralateral shoulder should be noted. Classically, there is focal tenderness that may or may not reproduce the presenting complaint. Before any shoulder movement is initiated, the examiner should palpate each shoulder for tenderness in the sternoclavicular joint, the acromioclavicular joint, and the shoulder itself. Palpation of both shoulders simultaneously allows the examiner to compare the affected shoulder with the unaffected shoulder. Palpation of bone landmarks is especially valuable in excluding a joint disorder; palpation of the muscle structures is useful in excluding spasm. A simple shoulder examination checklist is provided in Box 186-1.

Active range of motion should be assessed first to determine the integrity of the rotator cuff and to ascertain the location of the pain. Active range of motion of each shoulder should be measured, including forward flexion (normal is 180 degrees), extension (normal is 70 degrees), external rotation (normal is 45 degrees), internal rotation (normal is 60 degrees), abduction (normal is 180 degrees), and adduction (normal is 180 degrees). Any clicks or crepitation suggestive of impingement should be noted. Passive range of motion should be compared with active range of motion and is particularly useful in determining whether adhesive capsulitis (frozen shoulder) is present. A person with adhesive capsulitis can typically still abduct the arm 60 degrees. Patients with a rotator cuff tear seldom lose passive shoulder motion.[8]

BOX 186-1

Shoulder Examination

INSPECTION

Visual inspection comparing the affected shoulder with the uninvolved shoulder

Range of motion of the cervical spine

Active range of motion of the shoulder
- Wall push (look for winging)
- Forward elevation, flexion
- Extension
- External rotation
- Internal rotation
- Abduction
- Adduction

Passive range of motion of the shoulder
- Impingement test

Strength testing of all major muscle groups
- Flexor-extensor of the wrist
- Biceps
- Triceps
- Supraspinatus isolation
- Internal rotators
- External rotators
- Deltoid

Deep tendon reflexes

Peripheral pulses (check for bruits)

PALPATION

Supraclavicular fissure
Sternoclavicular joint
Acromioclavicular joint
Glenohumeral joint
Biceps tendon insertion
Muscle structures

SHOULDER ASSESSMENT FORM
AMERICAN SHOULDER AND ELBOW SURGEONS

Examiner:

Name:	Date:
Age: Hand dominance: R L Ambi	Gender: M F
Diagnosis:	Initial Assessment? Y N
Procedure/data:	Follow-up: Y N

PATIENT SELF-EVALUATION

Are you having pain in your shoulder? (Circle the correct answer)	Y	N

Mark where your pain is

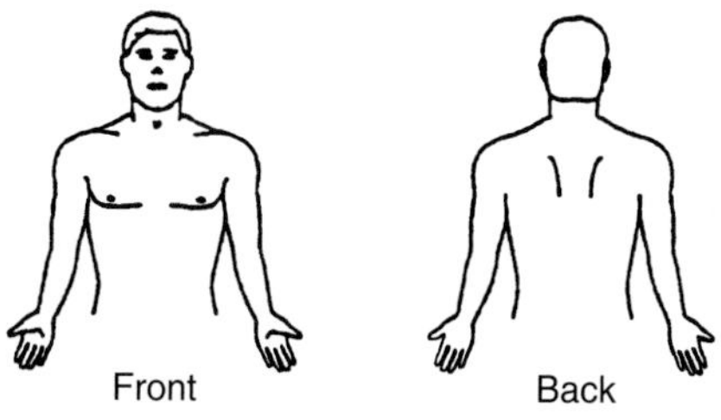

Do you have pain in your shoulder at night?	Y	N
Do you take pain medication (aspirin, Advil, Tylenol, etc.)?	Y	N
Do you take narcotic pain medication (codeine or stronger)?	Y	N
How many pills do you take each day (average)?	______ pills	

How bad is your pain today (mark line)?

0 |—|—|—|—|—|—|—|—|—|—| 10
No pain at all — Pain as bad as it can be

Does your shoulder feel unstable (as if it is going to dislocate)?	Y	N

How unstable is your shoulder (mark line)?

0 |—|—|—|—|—|—|—|—|—|—| 10
Very stable — Very unstable

Circle the number in the box that indicates your ability to do the following activities: 0 = unable to do; 1 = very difficult to do; 2 = somewhat difficult; 3 = not difficult

Activity	Right Arm	Left Arm
1. Put on a coat	0 1 2 3	0 1 2 3
2. Sleep on your painful or affected side	0 1 2 3	0 1 2 3
3. Wash back/do up bra in back	0 1 2 3	0 1 2 3
4. Manage toileting	0 1 2 3	0 1 2 3
5. Comb hair	0 1 2 3	0 1 2 3
6. Reach a high shelf	0 1 2 3	0 1 2 3
7. Lift 10 lb above the shoulder	0 1 2 3	0 1 2 3
8. Throw a ball overhand	0 1 2 3	0 1 2 3
9. Do usual work–List:	0 1 2 3	0 1 2 3
10. Do usual sport–List:	0 1 2 3	0 1 2 3

FIGURE **186-1** The American Shoulder and Elbow Surgeons standardized form for assessment of the shoulder. (Reprinted with permission of the American Shoulder and Elbow Surgeons.)

Strength testing of the individual rotator cuff muscles is then performed with use of resisted movements. An important component of the physical examination of the shoulder involves tests to detect pathology.[9] Table 186-1 summarizes special tests of shoulder function and their associated disorders. Although many of these clinical tests have variable accuracy for elucidating the exact cause of shoulder pain,[10] they may be used to confirm a suspected diagnosis, provide a differential diagnosis, or differentiate among various structures or to better understand the cause of unusual signs or symptoms. Complete neurovascular assessment of the associated shoulder structures should also be performed to identify other underlying sources of pain or dysfunction. Sensory, motor, deep tendon reflex, or circulatory impairment should be documented. The spine and peripheral joints are examined for evidence of coexisting joint disease.

Evaluation of a painful shoulder is challenging because the problem is often dynamic, with pain occurring only with specific activity. It is necessary to determine whether the discomfort and immobility are articular (bone) or periarticular (soft tissue structure). With inflammatory bursitis, erythema or bulging in the anterior shoulder may be seen. With bursitis or adhesive capsulitis, both active and passive range of motion will be limited. Marked weakness in abduction and external rotation suggests rotator cuff tear.[6]

DIAGNOSTICS

Diagnostic tests should be used judiciously to confirm or to refine suspected clinical diagnoses. It is unwise to base a diagnosis on a radiologic test alone because x-ray studies can be misleading or unrevealing. Findings on radiography and even magnetic resonance imaging (MRI) are often normal in soft tissue problems in the young athlete. Most conditions seen in primary care do not have specific radiographic findings.[6] A thorough history and targeted musculoskeletal examinations are most critical in providing clues to the diagnosis.

TABLE 186-1 Tests of Shoulder Function

Test	Technique	Interpretation
Apprehension test	Abduct to 90 degrees and slowly externally rotate patient's arm to a position where it might easily dislocate.	Impending dislocation or glenohumeral instability is signaled by noticeable look of apprehension on patient's face, with patient resisting further motion.
Drop arm test	Have patient hold affected extremity in a fully abducted position, then ask patient to slowly lower arm to side.	Rotator cuff tearing or supraspinatus tearing is suggested if patient's arm drops to side (as opposed to being slowly lowered to the side) from a position of 90 degrees of abduction.
Empty can test	Have patient hold out affected arm as if offering examiner a can of soda (abduction to 90 degrees), and then have patient turn arm to empty the contents (internal rotation).	Rotator cuff tendinitis or tear is suggested if pain is produced or weakness noted by maneuver of "emptying the can."
Impingement test	Have patient elevate arm slowly into overhead position.	Rotator cuff strain, tendinitis, or tear is suggested if patient experiences sharp "catches" of pain or impingement with this maneuver.
Yergason test	Have patient fully flex elbow (90 degrees). Grasp the patient's flexed elbow in one hand while holding patient's wrist in other hand; to test stability of biceps tendon, externally rotate the patient's arm as patient resists and, at same time, pull downward on patient's elbow.	Pain with this maneuver suggests that the biceps tendon is unstable in the biceps groove; no pain is experienced with a stable tendon.
Modified dynamic labral shear test	Have patient stand with arm flexed 90 degrees at the elbow, abducted in the scapular plane more than 120 degrees, and externally rotated to tightness. Stand behind patient and guide the involved upper extremity into maximal horizontal abduction. Apply a shear load to the joint by maintaining external rotation and horizontal abduction and lowering arm from 120 degrees to 60 degrees of abduction.	Reproduction of pain and/or painful click or catch in the posterior joint line between 120 degrees and 90 degrees abduction suggests labral tear.[10]
Sulcus sign	Have patient stand with arm at the side. Apply traction through the patient's arm in the inferior direction.	Indicates glenohumeral laxity or instability.
Hawkin test	Forward flex the shoulder and elbow to 90 degrees. Apply force to the forearm to internally rotate the shoulder.	Elicitation of subacromial pain indicates supraspinatus tendinitis.
Cross-body adduction	Elevate shoulder to 90 degrees. Horizontally adduct the shoulder and arm across the body.	Pain at the acromioclavicular joint suggests acromioclavicular joint arthritis.
Spurling test	Have patient flex cervical spine laterally toward the ipsilateral shoulder. Apply a downward axial force on the head.	Pain radiating toward the shoulder and arm may indicate nerve root compression, implicating the cervical spine as the source of shoulder pain.

Radiographs are usually the initial imaging test performed for most suspected abnormalities in the shoulder and will often suffice to diagnose or exclude an abnormality, or will guide further imaging.[11] Plain x-ray films may help diagnose massive rotator cuff tears, calcific tendinitis, shoulder instability, and shoulder arthritis. Shoulder films are recommended for a history of trauma, with reduced range of motion, or if arthritis or neoplastic disease is a consideration. With all significant trauma, it is imperative to obtain the appropriate x-ray studies, including standard anteroposterior views of the glenohumeral joint with the arm at 30 degrees of external rotation, axillary lateral views, and scapula Y views that detect dislocation not seen on standard views. On occasion, in atraumatic presentations, calcifications from previous or chronic injuries can be seen. In cases of recurrent rotator cuff tendinitis or subacromial bursitis, x-ray studies may be helpful in looking for spurring of the acromial process or inferior acromioclavicular osteophytes. Loss of articular cartilage between the humeral head and the glenoid may confirm suspected glenohumeral joint arthritis. Osteophytes consistent with osteoarthritis may also be seen. X-ray studies of the cervical spine are indicated if cervical radiculopathy is suspected.

When the diagnosis of shoulder pain remains unclear or when the outcome would affect management, additional testing with the use of imaging techniques should be performed. MRI is the preferred imaging modality for evaluation of the soft tissue structures of the shoulder including the rotator cuff, biceps muscles, tendons, and bursa. MRI should be performed only for a valid medical reason and after careful consideration of alternative diagnostic techniques.[11] In many cases of shoulder pain in the primary care setting, however, MRI findings are rarely helpful initially, with the exception of a significant trauma history, and are unlikely to alter management. In addition, the frequency of nonspecific MRI findings often found in asymptomatic individuals is such that unless the clinician knows of the specific abnormality to be corroborated by MRI, its ordering should probably be left to a specialist. Although MRI is one of the most sensitive diagnostic tests for detecting anatomic abnormalities of the shoulder, the findings may be misleading if not closely correlated with other imaging studies, the patient history, physical examination, and tests of shoulder function.[11] Collaboration between the ordering clinician and the radiologist is often of benefit in interpreting radiologic findings in the context of the clinical picture. Diagnostic imaging studies, which also include ultrasonography and computed tomography (CT) scans as well as invasive studies such as MRI arthrography, are best ordered in consultation with a specialist, particularly when there may be a need for surgical intervention.

Laboratory studies are seldom indicated. However, complete blood count (CBC), erythrocyte sedimentation rate (ESR), uric acid level, and serologic tests for rheumatologic diseases should be performed in accordance with the history and examination findings.

DIAGNOSTICS

Shoulder Pain

LABORATORY
CBC and differential*
ESR*, CRP*
Serologic tests for rheumatologic disease*

IMAGING
X-ray studies*
Anteroposterior views
Axillary lateral views
Scapula Y view
MRI*
CT scan*
Ultrasound*
Arthrography*
Arthrocentesis*

*If indicated.
CRP-C-reative protein.

DIFFERENTIAL DIAGNOSIS

The ability to correlate the history and physical examination with a functional knowledge of anatomy, an understanding of the mechanism of injury, and the reproduction of symptoms clinically will often lead to diagnosis of the problem.[12] Common patterns of shoulder pain also guide the differential diagnosis. Shoulder disorders can be categorized as acute (less than 2 weeks' duration) or chronic and traumatic or atraumatic. The diagnosis of shoulder pain is simplified when there is a history of trauma (Box 186-2). If the duration of pain is less than 2 weeks, the patient may recall an injury or fall. The diagnosis of subacute or chronic shoulder pain with an onset weeks to months after the incident or injury is much more challenging. Common causes of chronic shoulder pain include rotator cuff disorders, adhesive capsulitis, shoulder instability, tendinitis, and arthritis.[1]

It is important to understand the concept of instability. The extreme of instability is a frank shoulder dislocation caused by trauma, for which the patient usually goes to the emergency department. Shoulder subluxation, whereby the humeral head is pulled out of the glenoid cavity partially or totally but reduces itself spontaneously, is often a transient instability considered less extreme than a dislocation. More subtle degrees of instability seen in primary care settings include dysfunction of the rotator cuff that can lead to minor degrees of instability, which can then lead to impingement of the rotator cuff against the underside of the coracoacromial ligament of the acromion itself.[6] This leads to the pain often referred to as *impingement syndrome* or *subacromial bursitis* or *tendinitis*.[6]

Red flag indicators to consider in the individual with atraumatic shoulder pain include significant sensory or motor deficits suggestive of neurologic lesion and/or a history of cancer, especially breast or prostate, with atraumatic deformity or mass that may represent a tumor metastasis.

Although sports injuries from overuse ("muscular strain"), shoulder separation caused by a sprain of the acromioclavicular ligaments, and subluxation of the glenohumeral joint are most common in teenagers and young adults,[8] trauma followed by shoulder immobilization or gradual onset of shoulder pain on the nondominant side of a middle-aged woman is more likely adhesive capsulitis. Calcific tendinitis of the rotator cuff tendons

BOX 186-2

Acute Shoulder Injury

Fracture (clavicle, proximal humerus)
Glenohumeral dislocation
Acromioclavicular sprain or dislocation
Rotator cuff tear
Labral tear
Bursitis (subacromial or subdeltoid)

typically manifests as activity-related shoulder pain.[13] Shoulder pain in middle-aged and older adults more often develops with rotator cuff lesions, such as supraspinatus tendinopathy and partial- or full-thickness tendon tears.[14] Severe acute shoulder pain with restricted movement in a laborer or athlete is likely acute calcific tendinitis.[8] Shoulder pain aggravated by reaching, by overhead activities, or with internal rotation movements such as reaching toward the low back is likely caused by rotator cuff impingement. Pain in the shoulder at night that makes sleeping on the affected arm impossible is rotator cuff disease until proven otherwise. Pain in the shoulder with repetitive overhead activity also suggests rotator cuff disease. Pain at rest should suggest that the problem is extrinsic to the shoulder girdle, although acute inflammatory conditions often cause night pain. Erythema and fever with shoulder pain suggest septic arthritis or pseudogout. Pain associated with a throwing motion may be secondary to instability. Pain in the supraclavicular area and toward the vertebral border of the scapula is often referred pain from the neck. Shoulder pain from tendinopathy often radiates to the midarm but not lower. Morning stiffness lasting more than 1 hour, rest pain that improves as the day wears on, and bilateral shoulder pain in an older adult are symptoms of inflammatory conditions including rheumatoid arthritis, polymyalgia rheumatica, and pseudogout.

DIFFERENTIAL DIAGNOSIS

Shoulder Pain

- Dislocation, instability, and subluxation
- Adhesive capsulitis
- Localized shoulder pathology
- Acute calcific tendinitis
- Rotator cuff disease
- Impingement syndrome
- Bursitis
- Tendinitis
- Noninflammatory arthritis
  - Acromioclavicular osteoarthritis
  - Glenohumeral osteoarthritis
- Inflammatory arthritis
  - Polymyalgia rheumatic
  - Pseudogout
  - Psoriatic arthritis
  - Rheumatoid arthritis
  - Septic arthritis
- Acromioclavicular joint separation
- Fractures
- Referred shoulder pain
  - Reflex sympathetic dystrophy
  - Thoracic outlet syndrome
  - Cardiovascular causes (pericarditis, ischemia or angina, dissecting aortic aneurysm)
  - Gastrointestinal causes (hepatic inflammation or congestion, cholecystitis, pancreatitis)
  - Pulmonary causes (pleurisy, Pancoast tumor)
  - After laparoscopic surgery
- Malignant disease or metastasis

Tendinitis

Tendinitis occurs when the tendons or surrounding tissue become inflamed, swollen, and tender. Supraspinatus tendinitis is a very common cause of shoulder pain and is usually caused by degenerative changes in that tendon with advancing age.[8] Other common causes of tendinitis include overhead or repetitive activity, weakened rotator cuff (usually in combination with overhead activity), heavy lifting activities, and muscle strain. In rotator cuff tendinitis, abnormal repetitive stresses cause a mechanical irritation of the structures below the acromial bursa. With calcific tendinitis, calcific deposits form in the rotator cuff tendon, causing local mechanical irritation. Biceps tendinitis, which can result from overuse activities above the head, can lead to subacromial impingement, particularly in internal rotation. Elbow flexion against resistance usually reproduces pain located over the anterior aspect of the shoulder and upper arm.

Tendinitis often has no isolated precipitating event. Most patients report a deep ache in the shoulder, with increasing pain on abduction and internal rotation. Determination of what position or posture causes pain is diagnostic. Pain with arm elevation, for example, is suggestive of rotator cuff tendinitis or subacromial bursitis. Point tenderness is often localized to the vicinity of the greater tuberosity below the acromion and along the lateral aspect of the humeral head. The reflexive shrug will be noted as the patient tries to abduct the arm. The shrug helps reduce the pain caused by impingement on the acromion.

Generalized muscle weakness on manual muscle testing, especially with internal and external rotation, is characteristic of rotator cuff tendinitis.[15] Also, the empty can test and the impingement test are useful in validating the clinical diagnosis (see Table 186-1).

Bursitis

Bursitis occurs when the bursa becomes inflamed and painful as surrounding muscles move over it. The bursa's primary function is to maintain a gliding surface between muscles and ligaments (see Chapter 173). The most common cause of bursitis is overuse. Pitching, tennis, swimming, or repetitive use of the arm at or above shoulder level can cause subacromial bursitis.

The calcific deposits in tendinitis may occasionally extend the inflammatory process into the subacromial bursa, producing inflammation in the wall of the bursa.

Symptom onset in bursitis is usually abrupt, with pain often felt at the tip of the shoulder or along the upper third of the humerus. The pain is referred down the deltoid muscle into the upper arm. It occurs when the arm is lifted overhead or twisted. In extreme cases, pain will be present continuously and may disrupt sleep.

Rotator Cuff Tear or Rupture

Rotator cuff problems are a very common source of shoulder pain, accounting for more than two thirds of all cases.[4] In rotator cuff diseases, the supraspinatus tendon is the most commonly injured tendon because the tracking of the tendon is directly under the anterior edge of the acromion.[6] There is significant association between increasing age and tears in the rotator cuff,[16,17] with risk for tear progression with advancing age, beginning with microscopic tears, progressing to partial-thickness tears, and then on to full-thickness tears.[6] Rotator cuff disease is classified or graded to reflect progressively worsening symptoms and functional impairment. Grade I disease of the rotator cuff, which is most common in young adults, involves acute inflammation and edema resulting from either acute trauma or repetitive overhead activity. Grade II disease, which is seen in middle-aged adults, is characterized by chronic degenerative changes without actual tear. Grade III disease, commonly observed in older adult populations, represents disruption of tendon integrity (a tear).

Excessive use of the shoulder involving repetitive, stressful movement and injury or repeated injuries will produce this partial or complete rupture or disintegration of the rotator cuff. A weakened rotator cuff at the supraspinatus tendon may tear spontaneously as a result of minimum trauma, such as a fall. Tears tend not to be painful. Muscle atrophy often accompanies rotator cuff tears. Although the rotator cuff is not easily palpable, point tenderness to manual palpation is maximum just below the greater tuberosity of the humerus. Incomplete ruptures produce chronic thickening of the subacromial bursa and impingement syndrome. There is little chance for spontaneous healing of a torn rotator cuff.

The patient with rotator cuff tear typically reports shoulder pain aggravated by movement, especially overhead activity, and radiating to the anterior aspect of the arm. Abduction is painful and weak, and tenderness may be elicited over the insertion of the greater tuberosity. On examination, the patient will be unable to abduct the arm, instead producing a characteristic shoulder shrug. Passive range of motion may be unaffected. The drop arm test and the empty can test assess the integrity of the rotator cuff, and results are positive with significant tears (see Table 186-1).

Labral Tear (SLAP Lesions)

Symptoms suggestive of a labral tear or SLAP lesion include deep shoulder pain with specific shoulder positions, pain during overhead maneuvers such as in tennis, swimming, or throwing sports, a catching sensation, a sense of loss of shoulder strength, instability, and crepitus. Employed when a SLAP lesion is suspected, the modified dynamic labral shear test (Table 186-1) helps establish a causal relationship between the patient's symptomatology and labral pathology.

Subacromial Impingement Syndrome

The tendons composing the rotator cuff can be worn down by repetitive excursion between the greater tuberosity of the humerus and the acromion and the acromioclavicular ligament.[16] This repetitive trauma can lead to compression of both the tendons and the subacromial bursa, resulting in edema, hemorrhage, inflammation, and ultimately fibrosis. Impingement occurs as a result of acute trauma, repetitive overhead activities, pushing and pulling activities, subtle or overt instability of the glenohumeral joint, and degenerative and inflammatory disorders of the tendons and bursa.[16]

Shoulder Instability, Dislocation, and Subluxation

Shoulder dislocation predisposes the patient to recurrent instability. Instability results from post-traumatic capsular tear or stretch. Athletes are subject to numerous repetitive loads that can lead to symptoms of instability.[6] There are two primary types of shoulder instability: traumatic, unidirectional instability; and atraumatic, multidirectional, bilateral, inferior capsule shift, which is often more responsive to rehabilitative efforts. Dislocation is much more common in young adults, with the likelihood of redislocation decreasing with advancing age. In older adults, rotator cuff tears commonly occur with dislocation. A history of traumatic dislocation and medical or surgical reduction is a powerful risk factor for instability. The patient will simply complain of the shoulder's "giving out." Dislocation results from trauma to the shoulder while it is hyperextended. Dislocations are often anterior and are characterized by loss of the shoulder's rounded appearance. The patient typically is seen with the hands held to the side. There is prominence of the acromion, painful limitation of movement, and displacement of the humerus away from the trunk.

The apprehension test detects chronic shoulder dislocation (see Table 186-1). The Yergason test for long head of the biceps tendon stability determines whether the biceps tendon is stable in the occipital groove[10] (see Table 186-1). A palm-up hand position is used to rule out posterior dislocation.

Arthritis

Arthritis of the glenohumeral joint is a gradual, progressive mechanical and biochemical breakdown of the articular cartilage and other joint tissues including bone and joint capsule. It is a common cause of debilitating shoulder pain, affecting up to one third of patients older than 60 years.[17] It may be secondary to inflammatory arthritis or osteoarthritis. In patients older than 50 years, the distinguishing features of shoulder arthritis are the gradual onset and progression of pain at rest, aggravated by movement, and loss of motion.[1] The patient reports a grinding or clicking sound with motion. Examination may reveal muscle wasting, crepitation, effusion, and decreased range of motion.

Although the shoulder may undergo arthritic changes from a number of causes, these changes are much better tolerated than arthritic changes occurring in the weight-bearing joints. A hot, red, swollen, and painful shoulder accompanied by fever and chills is suggestive of septic arthritis (see Chapter 179).

Shoulder Trauma

With severe shoulder trauma, the differential diagnosis includes acromioclavicular separation (crepitus and elevation at the acromioclavicular joint), fractures of the clavicle or proximal humerus, strains, sprains, subluxation, and dislocation. Severe shoulder trauma not promptly responsive to conservative treatment warrants orthopedic referral. Red flag indicators to consider in the individual with shoulder pain after trauma include shoulder deformity and loss of rotation, which may represent fracture, unreduced dislocation, or signs of an acute rotator cuff tear.

Extrinsic Shoulder Disorders

Shoulder pain may be specific to the shoulder girdle area or may be referred from another anatomic location. Referred pain should be suspected when passive shoulder motion shows a painless complete arc, no specific periarticular shoulder tender point is identified, muscle strength is within normal limits, or pain cannot be reproduced with various tests of the shoulder muscles.

Referred pain may be neurologic in origin (cervical nerve root compression, supraspinatus nerve compression, cervical spine disease) or cardiovascular in origin (myocardial ischemia or infarction, thoracic outlet syndrome). Because the shoulder is located in the thoracic dermatome area, pain can be referred from several intrathoracic or abdominal organs (pneumonia, pulmonary embolus, hepatobiliary disease) innervated by the same nerves. Shoulder symptoms may also be related to diaphragmatic irritation, which shares the same root innervation (C5, C6) as the dermatome covering the shoulder's summit.

Cervical spondylosis, herniated cervical disk, cervical trauma, or other neck problems may also cause pain radiating to the shoulder, scapula, or upper back (see Chapter 183). This pain is often felt at the superomedial angle of the scapula and may be verified by the Spurling test, in which radicular pain is reproduced with head compression.[10] The Spurling test is a useful tool in differentiating shoulder pathologic conditions from cervical radiculopathy.[18] For the Spurling test, the patient should extend the neck and laterally tilt the head to the affected side. The examiner should apply downward force to the top of the head. If the test result is positive, the radicular pain or paresthesia will be evident. This is because of narrowing of the foramina against the inflamed nerve root or spinal cord from a ruptured disk. Sometimes a spinal fracture, in addition to causing local pain, may radiate pain to the shoulder along the course of any muscle affected by the fracture (see Table 186-1).

Reflex sympathetic dystrophy after myocardial infarction, cerebrovascular accident, or trauma can also cause shoulder pain. The characteristic features are persistent burning pain, diffuse tenderness, immobilization of the shoulder, and vasomotor changes in the hands. Gallbladder disease can cause scapular pain as well as right upper abdominal pain and tenderness. Pain caused by bone malignant neoplasm is usually gnawing, constant, and unrelated to movement.

MANAGEMENT

Immediate emergency department referral or orthopedic consultation is indicated for patients with suspected shoulder dislocation or fracture.

Specialist consultation is indicated for patients with acromioclavicular separation, sternoclavicular subluxation, and functionally significant rotator cuff tears.

Although neither national specialty guidelines nor evidence-based practice guidelines are available as templates for approaching the management of shoulder pain, certain general principles of management apply to most presentations. The cornerstone of treatment is the achievement of pain control that permits a return to normal functional use of the shoulder.[4] Goals of treatment center on maximizing physical comfort and preserving shoulder joint mobility and function. Treatment includes both pharmacologic and a variety of nonpharmacologic approaches, including the triad of activity modification, ice packs or cold for the first few days followed by heat, and graded exercise. Other appropriate therapeutic modalities include physical therapy, nonsteroidal anti-inflammatory drugs (NSAIDs) or acetaminophen, and intra-articular corticosteroid injections.

In persons with acute post-traumatic tear, orthopedic referral and early surgical options are warranted.[19] Activity modification is prescribed to reduce acute shoulder pain, with specific recommendation based on the underlying diagnosis.[3] In general, the patient avoids any activity that precipitates symptoms and especially the offending or "abusive" activity. Although a sling is useful in some situations, immobilization is recommended only when instability is apparent and never for more than 3 or 4 days. Sports and job modifications may be beneficial.[2]

Applications of ice or heat may provide relief. Ice reduces edema and bleeding and is most often recommended after trauma. Both heat and cold have been demonstrated to reduce muscle spasm and pain. Ice applied topically to the affected joint for 30 minutes three or four times a day, particularly after any activity that involves use of the affected extremity, may reduce inflammation and swelling and promote comfort. Ice massage may also be of therapeutic benefit.

Restoration of normal shoulder function should begin as soon as acute pain has subsided. The overall goals of any therapeutic exercise program include maintaining or restoring full range of motion, decreasing inflammation (with ice, NSAIDs, and deep friction massage), and strengthening the rotator cuff musculature. Range-of-motion exercises, including the pendulum swing and the wall climb (in which the patient "walks" his or her fingers up a wall), can be performed two or three times daily for 5 to 10 minutes and are helpful in preserving functional mobility. Strengthening exercises with weight or resistance and stretching-strengthening exercises with TheraBand are indicated only after the pain has subsided.

After trauma or surgery, shoulder rehabilitation including a supervised exercise program under the direction of a physical therapist is recommended to improve outcomes Physical rehabilitation programs use anatomy, biomechanics, and knowledge of tissue response to trauma to restore range of motion, to strengthen the shoulder girdle, to maximize functional ability, and to resolve symptoms.

Physical therapy plays a key role in the nonsurgical treatment of rotator cuff disease as well by strengthening and retraining the rotator cuff muscles and the scapular stabilizing musculature to pull the humerus down in the joint, decreasing further impingement. Physical therapy can also guide in ergonomic adjustment to strengthen rhomboids to decrease slouching, making the acromion less likely to impinge with humeral movement, and in modification of daily routine to avoid offending repetitive arm movements. Adjunctive physical therapy modalities, such as local heat application, electrogalvanic stimulation, ultrasound, and transverse friction massage, may promote tissue extensibility and joint function in chronic situations.

In shoulder impingement syndrome (SIS), physical therapy and corticosteroid injections are similarly effective, but physical therapy might be less costly to the health care system in the year after treatment.[20]

In adhesive capsulitis, a combination of manual therapy and exercise may not be as effective as glucocorticoid injection in the short term.[4]

Acupuncture, when it is combined with mobilization, may confer short-term analgesic effects in chronic shoulder conditions, including adhesive capsulitis, rotator cuff disease, and osteoarthritis.[21]

Pain-relieving medications may be indicated and are often necessary to allow progression of treatment.[3] The drugs of choice include NSAIDs and acetaminophen. Acetaminophen may be recommended for milder analgesia or for patients for whom NSAIDs are contraindicated. Oral NSAIDs may be effective and are likely to be beneficial in the short term in those with acute tendinitis or subacromial bursitis or both.[19] Topical NSAIDs may be helpful for some patients and preferred for older adults who tolerate oral NSAIDs less well. Although acetaminophen has no anti-inflammatory activity, its analgesic effect is comparable to that of ibuprofen and naproxen with fewer side effects.[22]

Patients should be instructed to use anti-inflammatory medication as prescribed, not just when pain is severe. In addition, they should be counseled about the medication's action, dosage, potential adverse effects, and drug-drug interactions. Certain NSAIDs are available over the counter, and these should be discontinued if a prescription-strength product is recommended.[22]

Alternative pharmacotherapeutic options for the treatment of shoulder pain include short-term, low-potency oral opioids, such as acetaminophen with codeine, and nonopioids, such as tramadol (Ultram). The risks and potential side effects of each agent prescribed must be examined for each patient. The effectiveness of topical anti-inflammatory drugs (NSAIDs), oral acetaminophen, or oral corticosteroids in improving shoulder pain has not been formally studied and is therefore not evidence based, but all are widely used for individual patients.[19]

Corticosteroid injections may reduce pain and expedite functional recovery in patients with inflammatory conditions such as bursitis and tendinitis as well as in rotator cuff impingement that does not improve with conservative therapy (see Chapter 173). In SIS, the application of the lidocaine-tetracaine patch has been shown to reduce pain and restore more normal range of motion to the same extent as a single corticosteroid injection.[23]

The body of evidence supporting the intra-articular injection of sodium hyaluronate for shoulder pain secondary to glenohumeral arthritis, rotator cuff tears, and adhesive capsulitis is conflicting, with many studies showing no significant difference between these and corticosteroid injections when relief of pain and improved mobility are the expected outcome. However, corticosteroid injections, if repeated frequently, potentially cause tendon degeneration and long-term loss of function. Hyaluronans are large polysaccharide molecules found naturally in synovial fluid that help foster a viscous environment, cushioning joints and preserving joint function.[24]

Health-promoting behaviors, such as protecting joints, balancing rest and exercise, and maintaining an optimistic attitude, can improve outcomes, as can attention to athletic and occupational considerations (e.g., workplace design, worker training, conditioning).[25]

LIFE SPAN CONSIDERATIONS

Children rarely have rotator cuff tears but commonly have shoulder joint instability (subluxations or dislocations of the glenohumeral joint) because of overuse or sports injuries. In adolescents and young adults, acromioclavicular sprain and tendinitis are common causes of shoulder pain, but tears in the rotator cuff are rare. In patients younger than 40 years, glenohumeral instability typically is accompanied by a history of subluxation or dislocation events.[1] Middle-aged and older patients rarely have problems with instability; but because the rotator cuff apparatus undergoes significant age-related changes, middle-aged and older adults commonly are seen with rotator cuff lesions (tendinitis, tears, and impingement syndromes), glenohumeral joint problems (adhesive capsulitis and osteoarthritis), and subacromial bursitis.

Musculoskeletal disease is a leading cause of functional disability in the older population. Rotator cuff tears often go unrecognized in the older adult or are clinically confused with degenerative tendinitis or other forms of shoulder disease in older adults. One study focusing on the repair of rotator cuff tears in patients older than 65 years who did not respond to conservative treatment found excellent 5-year outcomes after isolated supraspinatus tendon repairs, suggesting that withholding surgical intervention because of age may not be justified. Acute pain after trauma may suggest a fracture of the neck of the humerus in an older patient.

COMPLICATIONS

The most common and worrisome complication of chronic shoulder pain is adhesive capsulitis (frozen shoulder). Adhesive capsulitis is characterized by a gradual, progressive decline in shoulder mobility, often resulting from prolonged joint immobilization after a painful episode. Diffuse aching pain and limited mobility are common. Pain is related to the stretching of the restricted joint capsule. Both active and passive range of motion of the glenohumeral joint and scapula is limited. Patients may have difficulty with activities of daily living, including dressing, toileting, and even feeding themselves. Treatment includes corticosteroid injections and physical therapy using modalities, mobilization, manipulation, and stretching exercises.[26]

INDICATIONS FOR REFERRAL OR HOSPITALIZATION

In general, shoulder pain in the acute or subacute phases does not require further specialist referral or hospitalization.

- A referral to an orthopedist may be indicated for more aggressive diagnostic testing, including radiography to assess for calcifications, spurs, or arthritic changes and MRI, arthrography, ultrasonography, or electromyography for continued muscle weakness.
- Arthroscopic acromioplasty may be required for debridement of bursa, subacromial decompression, repair of ligaments, and repair of tendons if a tear is present.
- Total shoulder replacement may be necessary for end-stage arthritic conditions of the glenohumeral joint.
- Failure to respond to conservative, nonoperative therapy or escalating symptoms despite conservative therapy; shoulder dislocation or instability; rotator cuff tear or rupture; severe disabling arthritis; and infection are among the definitive indications for referral.
- In cases in which arthrocentesis or arthroscopy is indicated, referral to a rheumatologist or an orthopedist may be indicated.

PATIENT AND FAMILY EDUCATION

Teaching patients about strategies to preserve musculoskeletal function and to prevent injury is important. Recovery takes time and requires a multidisciplinary approach, including patient participation. If exercise programs are not taken seriously, chronic or recurrent pain and loss of function may result. Recovery from shoulder injury and pain can be an excruciatingly slow process, requiring 6 weeks to 6 months. Education about the healing process and the factors that affect healing, including patient motivation, adherence to interventions, social support, nutrition, lifestyle behaviors, exercise, age, occupation, mental status, depression, and comorbidities, is necessary.

In addition, the importance of exercise and warm-up and stretching before activities should be stressed. Avoidance of repetitive movements and overuse should be carefully explained. For chronic conditions, patients should understand that although the pain may resolve, the condition can recur. Reinforcement of the need for modification of activities, adherence to exercise regimens, ice packs, medications, and gradual resumption of activities is also necessary.

CHAPTER 187

SPRAINS, STRAINS, AND FRACTURES

Christine M. Wilson • Mary E. Farrell • Nicole C. Bove • Susan E. Bove

DEFINITION AND EPIDEMIOLOGY

Common musculoskeletal injuries include sprains, strains, dislocations, and fractures. Sprains result from a stretching and/or tearing of the ligaments that bind the joint (bone to bone) as the joint is forced beyond its normal range of motion. Strains result from the overstretching or overuse of muscles and/or tendon (muscles to bones). Dislocations occur when a bone is displaced at the joint so that the articulating surfaces of the bones detach. Partial displacements are called subluxations. A fracture is a break in the cortex of bone. Fractures may be classified as closed or open. A closed (simple) fracture has no associated disruption in the continuity of the overlying skin. An open (compound) fracture has an associated disruption through the skin to the environment.

Immediate emergency department referral or physician consultation is indicated for any patient with compound fractures or neurovascular compromise of an extremity.

Strains and sprains are often cared for in private physician offices, clinics, and athletic training centers or simply at home. This makes statistical tracking of these types of injuries impossible. Although insurance companies' billed diagnosis codes offer a means of data collection if patients are treated at a medical facility, many of these injuries are managed at home.[1]

PATHOPHYSIOLOGY

Strains, sprains, and fractures are common musculoskeletal injuries. Strains are minor injuries that result when a muscle is overstretched. No actual muscle damage occurs with a muscle strain. A sprain involves actual injury to the supporting structures of the affected joint and is described in three grades of severity. The degree of damage to these structures depends on the amount of tissue and fiber shearing and tearing that occurs. A grade 1 sprain usually involves minimal injury with stretched fibers or a few microscopic tears of a ligament resulting from overstretching and causes only pain and edema. A grade 2 sprain is an incomplete tear of a ligament and also includes some functional impairment, ecchymosis, and discomfort or pain with weight bearing. A grade 3 sprain is a full or complete tear of the ligament with loss of ligament integrity. Grade 3 sprains of the lower extremities result in severe weakness loss of function produced by the detached muscle.[2]

Bone injuries can result in fractures, avulsion fractures, stress fractures, and dislocations. A fracture is a break in the bone. An avulsion or osteochondral fracture occurs when the ligament pulls away from the bone, bringing fragments with it, usually after a forceful injury. The pulling or pushing of a bone out of its normal position in the joint results in dislocation, which can be complete or incomplete. Stress fractures are small cracks in bone that initially may not be seen on x-ray examination. Repeated x-ray studies after 2 weeks or more may show new bone formation at the fracture site. The Ottawa Ankle Rules (OARs) were introduced for determining the need for radiographs of the acutely injured ankle or midfoot.[3] However there are now data questioning their usefulness.[4]

CLINICAL PRESENTATION

Strains cause local pain and, if severe, palpable swelling or muscle spasm. Sprains may demonstrate swelling, discoloration, and pain with movement. Fractures usually manifest with an area of pinpoint pain. There may or may not be associated swelling, discoloration, and decreased range of motion with a fracture. Dislocations involve the joint and often produce a visible deformity. Patients often experience more pain with dislocations than with fractures, as the nerves, tendons, and vessels crossing the joint are disrupted. Injuries that occur as a result of crushing or compression should be evaluated immediately because they can lead to neurovascular compromise and permanent tissue damage. It is difficult if not impossible to exclude a fracture without x-ray studies.

PHYSICAL EXAMINATION

In any trauma, it is essential to exclude or to stabilize any life-threatening injuries first. A good musculoskeletal examination includes an in-depth history, which should explore the mechanism of injury with a focus on the physical forces incurred by the patient. Often, this assessment is simplified by asking the patient to use the opposite extremity to reconstruct the exact motion of the affected side during the injury.

A good history of the mechanism of injury will also provide vital information about the presence of a compression injury. This will permit accurate diagnosis of these injuries and allow correct treatment and ongoing monitoring. A past medical history of arthritis, birth defects, or past injuries or surgery that resulted in deformity must be elicited.

Physical examination includes observations of the patient's favoring or guarding of the affected area. Pain, swelling, discoloration, deformity, or open wounds should be noted. The joint above and below the injury should also be examined for injury. Circulatory, motor, and sensory function must be assessed. Palpation for joint laxity can be deferred until a fracture is ruled out.

In an elbow injury, the arm is usually flexed at the elbow with the palm toward the chest. From this position, the patient should be asked to move only the lower arm away from the body so that the hand is pointing straight ahead. If elbow pain is elicited, this is indicative of a radial head fracture.

Wrist fractures are quite common in the older adult who has fallen on an outstretched arm. Colles fractures (extension fracture of the distal end of the radius) and Smith fractures (flexion fracture of the distal end of the radius) are the most commonly seen types.

When evaluating fractures in adolescents or children, it is important to recall the classification method developed by Salter-Harris. There are five major types (and more subdivisions) of Salter-Harris fractures, all involving the growth plate of the immature skeleton.[5]

Ankle fractures with tenderness through the mortise of the ankle can indicate an associated knee fracture. This indirect fracture of the knee is easily missed on the initial examination; therefore care should be taken to palpate the areas of the upper tibia and fibula and the knee.

DIAGNOSTICS

Because of the difficulty in determining the type of musculoskeletal injury based on presenting symptoms alone, radiologic examinations are often ordered. Radiologic examinations help diagnose fractures versus soft tissue injury. A history of trauma followed by immediate signs or symptoms of pain, swelling, discoloration, limited range of motion, or decreased strength is an indication for x-ray studies. Injuries associated with the ability to bear weight or the absence of swelling, however, may still require x-ray evaluation to rule out fracture.

Fractures are diagnosed when a break in the bone cortex is visible on two radiographic views. Angulated fractures refer to either open or closed fractures, usually with more than 30 degrees of angulation. A transverse fracture is straight across the bone. Oblique fractures are seen diagonally on x-ray films. Spiral fractures are seen as wrapping around the bone. A greenstick fracture is diagnosed when the bone tears as if a fresh twig were being bent in two. This is commonly seen in children because they have a more porous cortex, which makes the bone more flexible. An impacted fracture occurs when both pieces of the broken bone are crushed into each other. A comminuted fracture is observed when the bone ends shatter with multiple fragments.

Other Types of Fractures

Stress fractures occur from overuse and continued pounding to the bone, which causes it to fracture. They are often seen in athletes who run on hard surfaces. Impaired healing results from repeated injury and pounding on pavement. In the athlete younger than 15 years, the growth plate is still open, and overuse alone may cause a stress fracture in the elbows, knees, tibias, fibulas, heels, and foot.[6] Jones fractures involve a fifth metatarsal stress fracture. The fracture itself is distal to the proximal tuberosity and tends not to heal without prolonged immobilization or internal fixation.

Three common clinical presentations require consideration of additional radiographic views. These are injuries to the navicula, patella, and acromioclavicular joint. Although it is possible to miss a navicular fracture with only a wrist series, the addition of an ulnar deviation view allows more complete assessment of this injury. This view is especially important in the presence of snuffbox tenderness. An injured patella may be better assessed with the sunrise view, which will clearly identify joint effusion and patella fracture. X-ray views taken of a tender acromioclavicular joint while the patient is weight bearing will confirm acromioclavicular separation and allow grading. Hip x-ray examination usually requires a frog-leg view.

Foot fractures of the talus and calcaneus have been misdiagnosed as ankle sprains. A foot fracture must be carefully considered in the differential diagnosis if the patient reports a twisting injury or severe fall and is walking with an antalgic gait (manner of walking so as to minimize pain in a limb).[7] Talar dome fractures at any age may not be visible on x-ray films for 2 to 4 weeks after injury. In an elbow injury, the arm is usually flexed at the elbow with the palm toward the chest. From this position, the patient should be asked to move only the lower arm away from the body so that the hand is pointing straight ahead. If elbow pain is elicited, this is indicative of a radial head fracture.

DIAGNOSTICS

Sprains, Strains, and Fractures

IMAGING

X-ray studies*

*If indicated.

Compression fractures of the vertebra are seen in older adults with osteoporosis (see Chapter 182), patients on chronic steroids, and those with certain metabolic diseases.

DIFFERENTIAL DIAGNOSIS

Presentation of any musculoskeletal injury requires exclusion of sprains, strains, fractures, dislocations, subluxations, and ligamentous or muscle tears. A large muscle rupture may initially be seen as a convex or concave area with decreased range of motion and pain. Once traumatic injury has been excluded, local and systemic causes, such as various forms of arthritis, autoimmune diseases, infection, phlebitis, and tumor, must be considered.

DIFFERENTIAL DIAGNOSIS

Sprains, Strains, and Fractures

- Sprain
- Strain
- Dislocation
- Muscle or ligament tear
- Arthritis
- Infection
- Phlebitis
- Tumor
- Autoimmune disorder
- Fracture
  - Angulated
  - Transverse
  - Oblique
  - Spiral
  - Greenstick
  - Impacted
  - Comminuted
  - Stress
  - Avulsion

MANAGEMENT

Care of a fracture, strain, or sprain follows these initial guidelines. If appropriate, blood and body fluid precautions should be observed. All jewelry must be removed from the affected limb. Irrigation with normal saline should be considered for any open wounds; the area should then be dressed and bandaged. Impaled objects must be stabilized. If a compartmental or crush injury is suspected, any restrictive dressing or clothing should be removed. Although all orthopedic injuries require assessment of neurovascular function distal to the injury, it is imperative that this function be closely monitored with a compartmental or crush injury or if the patient is diabetic.

If radiographic findings are negative for fracture or dislocation, most acute orthopedic injuries will respond to rest, ice, compression, and elevation (RICE); immobilization or protection, rest, ice, compression, and elevation (PRICE); or protection, optimal loading, ice, compression, and elevation (POLICE).[8]

In uncomplicated soft tissue injuries, the extremity should be elevated above the level of the heart for the first 24 hours to reduce swelling. This implies that the more distal joint should be higher than each preceding proximal joint.

If ice is used, it should be applied in 20-minute intervals as often as tolerated, allowing the skin to return to room temperature between applications. Instructions should include placement of a cloth between the ice and the skin to prevent cold injury to the skin. Ice therapy can be continued unless muscle spasm occurs, at which time a switch to moist heat is recommended. In minor injuries, nonsteroidal anti-inflammatory drugs (NSAIDs) are recommended for pain relief and reduction of inflammation if no contraindications to this medication exist. Acetaminophen up to 3 g/day in divided doses can be helpful for those who should not take NSAIDs. Severe injuries mandate consideration of narcotic analgesic agents.

If there is no joint involvement and pulses are palpable distal to the injury, the area should be splinted, immobilized, or supported as needed. However, the use of compression has been found to have more negative outcomes including irritation than lace-up ankle braces in ankle injury. If there is no palpable pulse and no joint involvement, gentle traction should be applied distally along the long axis until the pulse is palpable. The extremity should then be immobilized. Extremity injuries require constant monitoring of the neurovasculature to prevent complications. Slings, elastic wraps, air casts, splints, and plaster can be used to support injured extremities. Wrapping a pillow around an injured ankle and securing it with tape is acceptable for comfort until x-ray films are obtained. A sling and swathe can easily splint shoulder injuries. The exception to this is an anterior dislocation of the shoulder, which places the arm in abduction and requires splinting in this position. Finger fractures not involving the fingertip should be splinted in the "safe" position, with the metacarpophalangeal joint in 70 degrees of flexion and the proximal interphalangeal joint in 20 degrees of flexion. This position minimizes shortening of the collateral ligaments and subsequent loss of hand function.

Minor sprains or strains may be supported with a simple elastic wrap. An air splint is an appropriate choice for an ankle with an inversion or eversion injury. However, a grade 3 ankle sprain may need an air cast, plaster casting, or surgery. With a knee injury, a knee immobilizer should be used to prevent compression on the plexus located in the popliteal space. If an immobilizer is unavailable, a 6-inch elastic bandage may be substituted. Clavicular fractures with displacement rarely result in injury to the brachial plexus and adjacent vessels. Clavicular fractures heal well, usually within 2 months. If the fracture does not involve injury to surrounding structures, it is easily managed by making the patient comfortable in a clavicular splint. Although this figure-of-eight bandage will not reduce a clavicular fracture, it affords great comfort for the patient.

If the back is strained, bed rest can increase pain and decrease rate of return to functional activity and is not recommended routinely (see Chapter 181). Functional movements are encouraged quickly with gentle reconditioning to allow a rapid return to other activities. Long-term bracing of back muscles is not recommended because it can cause weakness.

RICE has been the standard of care for most sprains and strains for decades and is cited in the patient education information of many national governmental and private organizations.[9-13] Because it is such a well-accepted practice, the need for randomized clinical trials to provide the evidence needed for practice has been slow in coming. There are limited data to evaluate the use of ice versus heat, so the psychological effects of each must be considered when therapy is being chosen. Cryotherapy reduces pain, muscle spasm, metabolic demand, swelling, inflammation, muscle spasm, and circulation. Heat therapy will provide pain relief as a result of increased elasticity of tissues, circulation, and metabolism.[14]

Some research has suggested that RICE may not be as beneficial as once thought for lateral ankle sprains except if used with (1) exercise therapy for edema versus use of heat or (2) if used intermittently for short-term pain relief rather than continuous application. Data from one study demonstrated continued vasoconstriction after area rewarming with use of four different U.S. Food and Drug Administration (FDA)–approved continuous cryotherapy devices.[15] However; RICE still remains the clinical approach for minor ankle sprains and strains. The use of the economical elastic bandage is clinically supported because the ankle does not have the exposed plexus of nerves and arteries so easily compressed with an elastic bandage application to the knee, nor does the ankle elastic bandage tend to roll onto itself, causing uneven compression as with the knee. Although intuitively the 90-degree angle of the ankle does not allow a cylindric elastic bandage to contour to the anatomy, it is still the standard of care for ankles despite the concerns that it may act as an anterior compression band and does not prevent inversion or eversion. A stronger mechanical support may actually increase the risk to other joints by transference of the load to the second joint. The knee is still best supported by a knee immobilizer.

NSAIDs have demonstrated some efficacy without adverse side effects; however, prolonged use will slow bone and tendon healing.[13] In addition to RICE, one study found that low-level laser treatment may decrease edema in grade 2 ankle sprains.[16] A patent is currently pending on a system and method for use of vacuum for promoting the healing of sprains by increasing tissue perfusion.[17]

What is clear is that in the age of evidence-based practice, this treatment regimen (RICE) needs to be examined in randomized trials focusing on various body parts until a statistically significant advantage can be demonstrated. Until then, RICE remains a standard treatment.

COMPLICATIONS

Complications may occur as a direct result of the injury or as a consequence of treatment provided, and they may be seen within the first hours of injury or weeks after trauma. Critical neurovascular structures lie close to the skeleton; thus, disruption of the bone may lacerate, entrap, impale, or compress nerves and vessels at the fracture site. Finger fractures through the volar plate require splinting in extension for 6 weeks. Otherwise, the injury to the extensor tendon will cause a "mallet finger," an inability to actively extend the end of the finger.

Long bone fractures of the lower extremities at any age require close monitoring. These fractures may have associated blood loss of up to 2 L and may induce hypovolemic shock. Compartment syndrome may occur with any musculoskeletal injury that results in decreased vascular flow to the compartment, thereby causing muscle ischemia and necrosis. The term *compartment* refers to an area where fascia wraps around a muscle group and its supplying arteries, veins, and nerves. When the intracompartmental pressure becomes greater than the vascular perfusion pressure, the tissue, vessels, nerves, and muscles become ischemic within the tight area. Because the fascia is inelastic, anything that increases compression, such as elastic bandages, casts, constrictive jewelry or clothing, bleeding into an area, or peripheral vascular disease, can potentiate this risk. The initial compression results in histamine release, which causes increased swelling and capillary dilation. This secondary swelling and dilation increase compression, which leads to further histamine release and more compression. The cyclic process continues, and irreversible muscle and nerve damage occurs in 2 to 4 hours. In 24 to 48 hours, complete limb function is lost, and permanent deformity results. The presenting symptoms of this syndrome may include pain, paresthesias, pallor, pulselessness, or paralysis. Nonsurgical treatment includes stopping or decreasing activity to an asymptomatic level.[18] Cooling and elevation may slow or prevent this process. However, surgical intervention may be required to relieve pressure.

Volkmann contracture is an example of compartment syndrome usually associated with a supracondylar fracture of the elbow. Many different names and descriptions are used to label compartment syndrome. It is essential that presenting signs and symptoms be identified quickly to enable successful intervention.

Acute infection resulting from an open fracture usually occurs within the first 24 to 48 hours. Gas gangrene, a rare occurrence, manifests in a contaminated open fracture approximately 72 hours after injury. Osteomyelitis, a chronic infection, is seen weeks later (see Chapter 185).

After long bone, pelvic, or multiple fractures, fat embolism syndrome may occur within the first 48 to 72 hours. This manifests with the sudden onset of respiratory distress and extreme arterial hypoxia. Pulmonary emboli are a later complication, generally occurring approximately 2 weeks after the fracture.

Delayed union refers to a fracture that is able to heal but in a longer time frame than expected. Nonunion occurs if the fracture does not heal sufficiently to support normal limb function and pain continues. Malunion is defined as healing with a poor functional or cosmetic outcome; this generally requires surgical intervention. To protect the fracture site, a cast or brace may be used if complete union fails to occur.

Additional complications include joint stiffness, post-traumatic arthritis, implant failure, and osteochondrosis (avascular necrosis). Reflex sympathetic dystrophy is a neurologic syndrome that should be suspected if a patient is seen with prolonged, increasing pain extending beyond the anticipated period for healing along with discoloration and temperature changes of the limb. It is also known as reflex sympathetic dystrophy syndrome and complex regional pain syndrome.[19]

Fracture blisters, histologically comparable to second-degree burn blisters, result from a separation of the dermis from the stratified squamous epithelium because of edema. They occur in 6% to 7% of ankle fractures[20] and are most commonly seen with fractures caused by severe twisting but may appear with other joint or limb trauma. Fracture blisters typically emerge on parts of the body with minimum soft tissue between the skin and bone, such as the elbow, ankle, foot, and shin.[20]

INDICATIONS FOR REFERRAL OR HOSPITALIZATION

If a fracture or dislocation is confirmed on x-ray examination, an orthopedist must be consulted. Compartment syndrome requires immediate orthopedic referral. The orthopedist will provide instructions for management and hospitalization.

Some primary care practices have guidelines for minor dislocation treatments, such as finger dislocation reductions. The orthopedist is consulted only if the reduction fails. Other types of dislocations, such as of a shoulder, require premedication and are usually referred to emergency department physicians or orthopedists. Any injury that does not resolve in the typically expected time frame should be referred as well.

Physical therapy or occupational therapy referral should be considered for any injury not expected to resolve spontaneously in 10 days. Physical therapists may also be consulted to evaluate ambulation and to teach the patient proper use of ambulatory assistive devices. Occupational therapy can be helpful with the appropriate splinting of hand and finger injuries and subsequent rehabilitation.

LIFE SPAN CONSIDERATIONS

In the evaluation of fractures, especially in adolescents or children, it is important to recall the classification method developed by Salter-Harris. A type I Salter-Harris fracture occurs when trauma causes complete epiphyseal separation only, without any bone fracture. A type I fracture is diagnosed by clinical examination even if it cannot be confirmed by radiologic examination. Types II to V are diagnosed by radiography. The most common Salter-Harris fracture is type II.

A type II fracture runs along the epiphysis with an associated triangular break in the metaphysis of the bone. Type III and type IV fractures are intra-articular. Type III fractures are uncommon and involve the joint surface as well as the epiphyseal plate and its periphery. Type IV fractures involve the joint surface, epiphysis, epiphyseal plate, and metaphysis. The prognosis for growth is poor in type IV fractures unless reduction and maintenance are flawless.[21] Type V fractures occur when a crushing trauma causes the epiphysis to compress the physis, leading to growth retardation.[5] The diagnosis of Salter-Harris type I navicular fracture is made if the clinical examination demonstrates tenderness on palpation at the snuffbox.

The risk of falling and therefore fractures increases in patients older than 65 years. Fractures of any type in the older adult increase mortality, which after a hip fracture especially persists for years.[22] Osteoporosis, poor physical conditioning, balance issues, environmental risks related to poor vision such as scatter rugs and poor lighting, comorbidities, polypharmacy, and general frailty exacerbate this risk. Osteoporosis fractures are more common than heart disease or stroke and are a leading cause of disability and nursing home placement in this population (see Chapter 13).

EDUCATION AND HEALTH PROMOTION

The patient should be instructed in how to check for paresthesias, pallor, pulselessness, decreasing circulation, and paralysis in the injured extremity. Education should address the fact that pain is expected to gradually decrease and that any pain that continues, increases, or is not relieved by medication must be reported to the practitioner.

Elastic bandages need to be removed every 2 to 3 hours for 15 minutes and then reapplied to be snug but not constricting. If a splint or immobilizer is used, specific idiosyncrasies of that particular apparatus should be explained. Patients with casts should be diligent about elevation and neurovascular assessment. Patients should also be encouraged to wiggle their fingers or toes to prevent swelling. A cast will conduct cold. Ice contained in a plastic bag is wrapped in a thin cloth to absorb condensation and protect the cast from moisture. The cold will be conducted to the injury, which reduces swelling. Casts should be kept clean and dry. To prevent skin breakdown under or around the edges of the cast, foreign objects such as cast fragments, liquids, lotions, powders, or any device intended to relieve itching should be avoided. Instructions also need to include recommendations for weight bearing, bathing, and follow-up care.

Home, yard, and workplace safety checks as well as medication reviews and vision checks should be performed on a regular basis, especially for older adults as part of a routine fall-risk assessment. Poor lighting or outdoor activities at night also account for many injuries. Seasonal issues, including ice and wet surfaces, should be addressed before accidents occur. Warm-up stretches and exercises for any sport are essential. Patients should have yearly physical examinations and ask specifically if their health and physical stature are compatible with the desired sport. Providers should then instruct the parents and children about specific risks and ask about risky behaviors. Coaches should be instructed regarding safe play and pediatric risks involved with their sport and then should ensure that children understand and follow the rules. Training programs and instructional programs for both coaches and sports enthusiasts are essential. No sports activity should begin before warm-up and stretching exercises, and no sport should be undertaken if the individual is not conditioned for the physical component involved. Safety gear should be checked for fit and worn at all times, and spotters should be used. Properly fitting shoes or protective footwear should be considered in activities that could cause stress injuries to ankles and other joints. First aid equipment and trained personnel should be available during any organized sport to provide immediate care of injuries. Pain needs to be acknowledged as a warning sign, and activity should be stopped. The health care provider caring for an injured patient should determine when it is safe for the patient to return to previous activity levels.

REFERENCES

For a full list of references, scan the QR code or visit http://booksite.elsevier.com/9780323355018

PART 16

Evaluation and Management of Neurologic Disorders

CHAPTER 188

NEUROPSYCHOLOGICAL EVALUATION

Laura A. Rabin

Mr. B., a 62-year-old man, visits his primary care practitioner with concern about his memory and concentration abilities, disrupted sleep, and low energy level. He began to notice these problems about 6 to 8 months ago, and he feels they have been worsening. His cognitive problems are interfering with his ability to be productive in his professional art studio. For example, he misplaces art supplies and cannot settle into reading a book as he used to because his mind wanders. He has also lost interest in socializing. Mr. B. has a history of hypertension and hypercholesterolemia, both well controlled with medication. He and his spouse of over 30 years divorced 2 years ago, and his two grown children, with whom he reportedly is close, live in other parts of the country. On the Folstein Mini-Mental State Examination (MMSE), Mr. B. was fully oriented, aware of his circumstances and current events, and scored a 28/30. His only errors were the inability to recall one of three words after a brief distractor task and misstating the floor of the clinic (reporting "second" instead of "third"). He reportedly lives alone and carries out all complex activities of daily living without assistance.

Many individuals visit primary care practitioners with complaints about aspects of cognition. With rapid advances in medicine and technology, in particular the proliferation of sophisticated neuroimaging techniques, one may question the usefulness and added value of a neuropsychological assessment with its paper-and-pencil tests, questionnaires, and comprehensive test reports. In today's complex health care environment, in which meeting patient needs often requires the work of interdisciplinary teams of health care professionals, what role does the neuropsychologist play? This chapter attempts to answer these and other questions related to the role of neuropsychological assessment in primary care settings. The chapter begins with brief overview of the field of clinical neuropsychology, its evolution as a health care specialty, and the role of its practitioners in collaborative practice efforts. It also addresses the expertise and unique perspective on patient care that neuropsychologists bring to the treatment of patients with a range of psychological, cognitive, behavioral, and medical issues. We return to Mr. B. later in our discussion.

OVERVIEW OF CLINICAL NEUROPSYCHOLOGY

Clinical neuropsychology is an applied science concerned with the behavioral expression of central nervous system dysfunction.[1] The field of neuropsychology has strong interdisciplinary ties to clinical psychology, neuroscience, and medicine, especially behavioral neurology and psychiatry. Neuropsychology emerged in the 20th century, combining information about neurologic patients with psychological techniques, such as the objective observation of behavior and the use of standardized assessment instruments to characterize and quantify cognitive impairment and its behavioral consequences. Initially, the primary goals of neuropsychological assessments were to localize, lateralize, and detect the site of lesions in patients with brain damage through noninvasive, standardized techniques and to aid in diagnosis and quantification of the cognitive deficits associated with specific neurologic disorders. With the advent of neuroradiologic procedures (e.g., computed tomography [CT], positron emission tomography [PET], magnetic resonance imaging [MRI] and functional magnetic resonance imaging [fMRI]), the objective of neuropsychological evaluations expanded to include analysis of patients' neurocognitive strengths and weaknesses, description of the functional consequences of brain dysfunction, prediction of risk of future cognitive decline, remediation of neurocognitive impairment, and introduction of compensatory interventions to maximize remaining abilities.[1-4]

Neuropsychology has undergone tremendous growth in recent decades. There are likely more than 2000 neuropsychological tests available, although a much smaller number (approximately 50 to 100) receive widespread and regular use by neuropsychologists. In addition, there are national and international scientific and professional organizations, books and journals that distribute basic and applied research, doctoral and postdoctoral training programs, and board certification procedures. Ongoing efforts to advance neuropsychology have included collaborations with medical and governmental agencies to establish billing codes and reimbursement guidelines for services, the facilitation of multicultural assessment practices, the establishment of honors to acknowledge excellence in the field, and the development of national and international conventions and conferences.[1-4]

PROFESSIONAL FUNCTIONS AND ROLES

Most neuropsychologists possess a doctoral degree in clinical psychology with a specialization in neuropsychology gained through advanced coursework and training at the doctoral, internship, and postdoctoral levels in basic and applied neuroscience, neuroanatomy, research methods, and psychometry. In addition to being licensed psychologists (a minimum requirement for all practicing neuropsychologists), neuropsychologists increasingly seek board certification through the American Board of Clinical Neuropsychology (ABCN) or the American Board of Professional Neuropsychology (ABPN).[5,6]

Neuropsychologists address important clinical problems through the application of knowledge about brain-behavior relationships. Clinical work consists primarily of cognitive assessment, diagnosis, and treatment of neurologic, psychiatric, and general medical conditions.[1,4,7] Because psychological states are inextricably connected with cognition and functional status, neuropsychologists are also trained to examine emotional and personality functioning. In addition, neuropsychologists increasingly receive specialized training in the use and interpretation of neuroimaging data.[8] Even with the widespread use of sophisticated techniques to image the structure, function, and pharmacology of the brain, traditional neuropsychological assessment continues to play a key role in diagnosis and characterization of the behavioral sequelae of brain dysfunction. Indeed, many neurologic and psychiatric disorders result from brain changes not visible on even high-resolution scanners (e.g., transient ischemic attacks, mild concussions, attention and learning disabilities). Furthermore, the location and extent of structural lesions may not accurately predict subsequent cognitive and behavioral changes; individuals with brain lesions that appear similar on imaging studies may have vastly different neuropsychological profiles.[8] Thus, detailed characterization of cognitive and functional capacities may be as important to patient care as quantification of structural and functional brain abnormalities.

ASSESSMENT TOOLS AND APPROACHES

Concomitant with the expansion of neuropsychological services has been the development of a large collection of objective instruments to evaluate capacities such as intelligence, academic achievement, verbal and language skills, processing speed, attention and working memory, learning and memory, executive functioning, reasoning and problem solving, visuospatial and visuoconstructive abilities, perception, sensory and motor skills, mood, and personality.[1] There are also numerous well-validated cognitive effort tests available to identify cases in which patients are motivated (either consciously or unconsciously) to present themselves as more impaired than is actually the case. If a test taker's effort or level of motivation is suboptimal, then the validity and reliability of the entire assessment may be called into question.[4,9]

Box 188-1 presents a sample of some commonly used neuropsychological tests. Whenever possible, testing measures are published, standardized, well normed, up-to-date, and accepted as reliable and valid tools in the field. Many instruments in common use today are adaptations of techniques that have been used for decades. For example, the most widely used intellectual and memory assessment batteries (i.e., Wechsler Adult Intelligence Scale, Fourth Edition [WAIS-IV] and Wechsler Memory Scale, Fourth Edition [WMS-IV]) are similar in overall content to the original versions developed in 1955 and 1947, respectively. In many cases, revisions reflect changes made to accommodate advances in the quality of normative data, the effects of cultural and educational factors on test scores, and empirical findings that guide interpretation of test performance.[1,10,11]

In addition to paper-and-pencil tests, neuropsychologists routinely use subjective rating scales, questionnaires, and tests of personality and emotional functioning. Direct observations of individuals in their natural environments and performance-based tests of everyday activities provide more direct and face-valid assessments of individuals' functional capacities but are associated with drawbacks that limit routine use.[7] Computerized cognitive tests and test batteries are increasingly discussed in the literature, although actual use of computerized instruments has not matched expectations.[12,13] Currently there are two

BOX 188-1

Commonly Used Neuropsychological Instruments

MENTAL STATUS SCALES AND GENERAL COGNITIVE SCREENING INSTRUMENTS
- Montreal Cognitive Assessment
- Repeatable Battery for the Assessment of Neuropsychological Status
- Dementia Rating Scale

INTELLIGENCE
- Wechsler Adult Intelligence Scale, Fourth Edition

ACHIEVEMENT
- Wide Range Achievement Test, Fourth Edition
- Woodcock-Johnson Tests of Achievement, Third Edition

MEMORY
- Wechsler Memory Scale, Fourth Edition
- California Verbal Learning Test, Second Edition
- Brief Visuospatial Memory Test, Revised

ATTENTION AND CONCENTRATION
- Digit Span Task
- Trail Making Test

EXECUTIVE FUNCTIONS
- Wisconsin Card Sorting Test
- Delis-Kaplan Executive Function System
- Category Test

LANGUAGE
- Boston Naming Test
- Verbal Fluency Test

PERCEPTUAL ORGANIZATION AND VISUOSPATIAL SKILLS
- Rey-Osterrieth Complex Figure
- Hooper Visual Organization Test

PSYCHOMOTOR AND SENSORY FUNCTIONS
- Grooved Pegboard Test
- Finger Tapping Test
- Tactual Performance Test

SYMPTOM VALIDITY AND EFFORT
- Test of Memory Malingering
- Victoria Symptom Validity Test
- Recognition Memory Test

Note: This box presents a very small sample of instruments used routinely by neuropsychologists. For more comprehensive listings, the reader is referred to various test compendiums.[1,10,11,15] In addition, cognitive capacities are complex and multidimensional, and performance on a given task will rely on multiple abilities. Thus, although tests are classified according to their primary domain, it is generally not possible to create "pure" tests of attention, memory, or executive functions, for example, or to designate tasks as falling within a single neuropsychological ability area.

main approaches to computerized testing: (1) the adaptation of existing examiner-administered instruments to computerized administration and/or scoring formats; and (2) the development of new computerized tests and test batteries that measure aspects of cognition not easily captured through paper-and-pencil tasks. This may include tests designed to assess domains such as attention, vigilance, and speed of information processing or the use of video and computer graphics to provide realistic simulations of the cognitive tasks performed in everyday life.[12,13] A comprehensive review of computerized neuropsychological instruments and their advantages and limitations is beyond the scope of this chapter, but it is crucial that such evaluations be conducted in accordance with American Psychological Association guidelines concerning reliability and validity of tests, normative data, and user qualifications.[14]

With regard to test selection, a flexible battery composed of variable but routine groupings of tests for different types of patients is preferred. Tests are selected on the basis of hypotheses generated through a clinical interview, observation of the patient, and review of medical records. The flexible approach has the advantage of preventing unnecessary testing. Because patients often find neuropsychological testing stressful and fatiguing, which can negatively influence performance, advocates of the flexible approach argue that tailoring of test batteries to particular patients can provide more accurate information. Far fewer neuropsychologists opt for a completely flexible approach, based on the needs of the individual case, or a fixed or standardized battery, which uses the same grouping of tests for all patient types and referral questions.[1,4,15]

NEUROPSYCHOLOGY WITHIN PRIMARY CARE SETTINGS

Box 188-2 presents common neuropsychological assessment goals.

As part of the normal aging process, individuals may experience declines in certain cognitive abilities, such as encoding new information, word retrieval (e.g., recalling names), speed of information processing, complex attention, working memory, and executive functioning (e.g., less efficient novel problem solving, multitasking, and inductive reasoning). Cognitive complaints are common in older adults, and questions often arise in primary care settings as to the nature and underlying cause of any perceived or observed cognitive dysfunction. This is an important issue, because the presence of cognitive decline is associated with increased morbidity and mortality; even mild dysfunction may have a significant impact on older adults' quality of life and ability to provide for their own needs independently. In addition, for older adults with psychiatric or chronic medical disorders, existing cognitive deficits may be exacerbated by normal age-related changes.[16,17]

Research has focused on differentiation of benign or stable cognitive difficulties from those associated with neurodegenerative disorders such as Alzheimer disease. Specific neuropsychological profiles (including patterns of cognitive deficit and preservation) can help distinguish Alzheimer disease from other neuropathologically distinct neurodegenerative disorders such as vascular dementia, dementia with Lewy bodies, frontotemporal dementia, and Huntington disease. Neuropsychological findings can inform diagnosis, treatment, and disease monitoring as well as complex issues related to capacity to consent to treatment or to make important medical and financial decisions. Neuropsychological testing can also identify particular deficits occurring in the earliest (or prodromal) stages of dementia that distinguish these conditions from normal aging and can predict the likelihood of subsequent decline.[16-18] Neuropsychological assessment is particularly indicated in the evaluation of high-functioning individuals who may perform at ceiling on brief cognitive screens despite actual deficits. Finally, although cognitive complaints may indicate actual neuropsychological deficit, they may also reflect affective symptoms, personality characteristics, metabolic dysfunction, demographic factors, or even medication side effects. Subtleties in neuropsychological performance, taken in the context of the clinical

BOX 188-2

Neuropsychological Assessment Goals

- Objectively measure complaints of cognitive difficulties
- Establish a baseline level of neuropsychological functioning
- Monitor changes in cognition over time (document recovery or progression of symptoms)
- Assist in differential diagnosis and determination of the severity of a condition
- Test the effects of medication, remediation, or other intervention on cognition and function
- Characterize the cognitive capacities of brain-injured patients to determine rehabilitation goals, placement, and return-to-work options and to make recommendations for independent living
- Monitor the cognitive status of patients who have undergone medical or surgical intervention for neurologic disease (e.g., drug therapy for Parkinson disease patients, tumor resection)
- Assist in identifying neurobehavioral or developmental disorders that may influence cognitive and behavioral functions (e.g., dyslexia, attention-deficit/hyperactivity disorder [ADHD], autism spectrum disorders, mental retardation)
- Assess subtle deficits in disorders with known neurocognitive sequelae (e.g., multiple sclerosis, sleep apnea, hepatic or renal dysfunction)
- Evaluate cognition in situations in which findings of neurodiagnostic procedures are normal but history indicates that brain injury is likely (e.g., mild closed head trauma, early human immunodeficiency virus [HIV]–related dementia)
- Answer questions about decision-making capacity: for example, financial decision-making, medical decision-making, capacity to prepare a will, capacity to enter into a contract
- Determine the extent to which pain problems interfere with cognitive functioning
- In medicolegal situations, address claims of brain injury frequent in plaintiffs who have sustained head trauma in motor vehicle accidents, through exposure to toxic chemicals or carbon monoxide, by electrical injury, and the like
- Address the role and likely contribution of emotional, personality, or drug and alcohol factors in cognitive difficulties
- Describe the implications of cognitive deficits for everyday functioning (e.g., capacity to comply with medication regimen, drive, work in a competitive or sheltered capacity, attend school)
- Conduct presurgical workup of patients undergoing brain tumor resection, epilepsy surgery, or deep brain stimulator implantation for movement disorders; may involve baseline characterization of cognitive and emotional function with postsurgical follow-up or Wada testing and intraoperative cortical mapping conducted in concert with neurosurgical team

history, may help discriminate among possible causes for cognitive complaints in older adults.[16]

In addition to overtly neurocognitive disorders such as dementia, many neuropsychiatric conditions are associated with neuropsychological impairment including schizophrenia, severe mood disorders, traumatic brain injury, attention-deficit/hyperactivity disorder, seizure disorders, neurotoxic exposure, and substance abuse. Medical conditions such as diabetes, respiratory disorders, cerebrovascular disorders, infectious diseases, nutritional deficiencies, cancer, movement and demyelinating disorders, thyroid dysfunction, and chronic pain may be accompanied by modest to profound neuropsychological changes. Cognition also might be affected by surgical interventions for cardiovascular diseases and radiation therapy and chemotherapy for cancer. Neuropsychological assessment can be used to detect and characterize these cognitive changes, address their impact on daily functioning, make treatment recommendations, and monitor cognition over time. Testing can also help predict disease course and prognosis, treatment effectiveness, and outcome of psychiatric interventions.[19,20]

Patients' cognitive dysfunction may result from various forms of brain injury, psychological disorders, or interpersonal disruptions. For example, reading problems in an otherwise healthy 25-year-old graduate student may be the result of a previously undiagnosed reading disability. Alternatively, problems with attention, concentration, or verbal short-term memory or slowed processing caused by emotional disruption may better account for the observed difficulties. Moreover, disrupted cognition can signify many problems, in much the same way that pain or sleep disturbance can be caused by various medical conditions. Cognitive abilities are also highly interrelated, and performance on any test is dependent on the integrity of many different abilities and overall levels of alertness and effort. Determination of the exact nature of the deficit is important for accurate diagnosis and effective treatment.[1,11,20]

WHEN TO REFER

Neuropsychological evaluations can provide important information about patients' current mental status, identify areas of cognitive strength and weakness, and contribute to differential diagnosis and treatment planning. Patient characteristics that signal the need for an evaluation may include repetitive speech, missing or confusing the dates of appointments, problems complying with medical recommendations, declines in social grace or hygiene and appearance, changes in driving skills, and medication mismanagement. Many patients report difficulties with cognition to their providers. It may be difficult without a formal neuropsychological evaluation to discern the validity of these complaints, the nature and severity of any cognitive dysfunction, and the cause. The timely detection of cognitive impairment provides important information that can inform the treatment of potentially reversible conditions, educate the patient and family about the functional consequences of cognitive difficulties and their management, and guide future planning. It is therefore important for primary care clinicians to ask patients and available significant others about the nature of the reported cognitive symptoms, frequency and severity, onset and course, and degree to which they interfere with regular activities.[17,20]

Referral for evaluation often follows from brief mental status or cognitive screening tests carried out in the primary care office, which can identify patients most likely to benefit from more comprehensive assessment. Brief screens (e.g., MMSE, 7-Minute Screen, Montreal Cognitive Assessment [MoCA]) provide useful information about patients' general cognitive abilities and areas of weakness or deficit, but they lack diagnostic precision. Brief cognitive screens also are prone to false-positive results for those with low levels of education, illiteracy, low premorbid intelligence, poor knowledge of English, poor cooperation and motivation, or sensory impairment.[20] They are also limited by ceiling effects, particularly in cases of mild dysfunction and in high-functioning individuals who may perform well despite cognitive impairment, resulting in high false-negative rates. False-negative screening results pose a strong concern because they can deprive patients of further diagnostic assessment or early pharmacologic intervention. The accuracy of screening assessments in the primary care office can be improved by supplementing them with structured informant report questionnaires or interviews. The clinician may then be in a good position to determine which patients warrant referral for more extensive cognitive assessment.[1,20] Because screening results provide an objective basis for recommending comprehensive testing, they may also increase the likelihood of gaining approval and payment for such services by insurance companies.

OVERVIEW OF THE ASSESSMENT PROCESS

The neuropsychological assessment can be viewed as an extension of the mental status screen with comprehensive assessment of cognitive functioning and subsequent description of how the brain processes information in the context of normative factors such as age, education, and gender. In referring a patient for an assessment, it is important for the primary care practitioner to be as specific as possible about the referral question to increase the likelihood of obtaining information of value and relevance to the case. It is also helpful, with the patient's consent, to send relevant medical records to the neuropsychologist, including laboratory test and neuroimaging results.[1,11,21]

The neuropsychological evaluation typically commences with an in-depth clinical interview that covers the reason for the evaluation; presenting symptoms; social, educational, and occupational background; information about the patient's birth and early development; medical, neurologic, and medication history; substance abuse history; psychiatric and behavioral health history; previous neuropsychological assessments; family medical and psychiatric history; and the patient's perspective on the problem. Collateral information should be gathered whenever possible—from a patient's spouse or child, close friend, or teacher or employer—and ideally should include information about the course and history of cognitive symptoms, the impact on daily functioning, and relevant medical and psychiatric history.[4,21] Another important function of the interview is that it provides insight into a patient's level of motivation and cooperation so that any accommodations or modifications to the evaluation can be made. Finally, the interview is an opportunity for the patient to ask questions or raise concerns about the assessment process.[4]

The interview is followed by administration of standardized measures of cognition and mood. Standardization (i.e., prescribed verbal instructions and formalized administration routines) is crucial because it ensures that measurement of cognitive functioning is carried out in an objective and reliable manner. In cases that deviate from a standardized testing environment, these deviations must be documented in the test report because they compromise the validity of the evaluation. Although a comprehensive review of psychometric properties of tests is beyond the scope of this chapter, issues of reliability and validity are crucial to the test development and assessment processes. In addition, the competent use of neuropsychological tests demands a solid working knowledge of the standards and psychometric properties of each test administered.[1,10,15]

The duration of the evaluation and length of the test battery will vary according to setting, referral question, patient characteristics, practitioner preferences, and reimbursement considerations. The assessment may last anywhere from approximately 1 to 6 hours. Typically, a battery will include more than one test within each cognitive domain of interest (e.g., verbal memory) to ensure sufficient data about the ability level in that area. Tasks are presented in multiple modalities (e.g., orally, visually, and occasional with tactile or olfactory stimulation), depending on the referral question and purpose of the examination. It is important for the examiner to ensure a professional, comfortable, and distraction-free environment that permits patients to put forth the best performance possible. Therefore tests are usually administered one-on-one in a quiet office with the examiner sitting across from the patient. Because patients may become anxious or frustrated during testing, evaluators provide redirection, reassurance, and breaks as needed. Lengthy test batteries are often divided into two or three shorter sessions that may occur within a single day or across several days. In some settings, the neuropsychologist will administer the tests; in other settings, a graduate student or highly trained technician (psychometrist) will administer and score tests under the supervision of a licensed neuropsychologist. In all cases, the neuropsychologist should conduct the clinical interview, interpret the data, and prepare the test report.[1,15]

SCORING AND INTERPRETATION OF NEUROPSYCHOLOGICAL TEST DATA

Neuropsychological data are scored according to set procedures, detailed in test manuals, and interpreted with regard to normative data that provide an objective reference against which to compare an individual's current test performance. In general, norms enable neuropsychologists to determine where an individual's test performance falls relative to the general population of "normal" individuals who share key social, educational, cultural, and generational backgrounds with the patient. For example, a patient's scores can be characterized as below average, average, high average, and the like. In some cases, the goal is to determine whether impairment in function has occurred (i.e., whether current performance represents a change from the individual's baseline functioning, suggestive of an underlying brain disease process). In such cases, the reference standard is the premorbid status of the individual and degree to which observed performance differs from expected levels. A patient's scores can be characterized as moderately impaired, mildly impaired, or within normal limits. Sometimes the neuropsychologist will adjust norms for demographic factors known to affect test performance (e.g., age and level or quality of education) to increase the specificity or probability of the test to correctly classify performance as normal or abnormal. An important issue is the quality of the norms, which relates to the selection of the normative sample, how representative the data are with regard to the particular patient, and approach used to develop the data.[15,22]

Whereas normative data provide an important starting point for the interpretive process, neuropsychologists do not rely solely on test scores when forming clinical judgments. Interpretation must account for other relevant information: patient behavior during the assessment (e.g., level of motivation and engagement, expectations regarding the examination); presenting symptoms; medical, psychiatric, and educational or vocational history; risk factors for cognitive dysfunction; current life circumstances; and aspects of mood and personality. Qualitative aspects of a patient's performance are crucial because low test scores can result from true dysfunction or another factor, such as poor effort, confusion about task instructions, sensory or motor deficits, or deliberate failure (i.e., malingering). The neuropsychologist will use all relevant quantitative and qualitative data, including types of errors made and pattern of functioning across tests measuring different abilities, to arrive at an accurate understanding of a patient's neuropsychological profile.[1,9,15]

After evaluation, interpretation, and integration of the various sources of information, a written report is prepared. The report will include a summary of the patient's history and reason for referral, behavioral observations, test results, summary, and recommendations. In general, the report should provide a comprehensive picture of the patient's cognitive strengths and weaknesses and address issues raised by the referring clinician, such as differential diagnosis, determination of factors primarily responsible for cognitive complaints, patient's employability or competence in handling various daily functions, and ability to live independently. The report may also address possible remedial techniques, compensatory strategies, or accommodations that should be made in the home or in employment or educational settings. Test scores are often included in the reports to minimize confusion about how interpretations were made. The inclusion of test scores (including raw scores or percentiles and standard scores with accompanying descriptors, such as "mildly impaired range") is critical for comparing the results of initial evaluations with subsequent ones. The report should also mention adjustments for demographic factors in each test.[4,15]

Depending on the nature of the referral and approach to medical care, the neuropsychologist may give direct feedback to the patient or to the referring physician, who in turn will provide feedback to the patient. In either case, it is important that the patient (and any significant others) gain complete understanding of condition diagnosis, possible interventions, and future expectations.[11,15,17]

ADDITIONAL CONSIDERATIONS IN NEUROPSYCHOLOGICAL ASSESSMENT

Issues of diversity pose challenges for neuropsychologists, who are frequently asked to evaluate patients from varied ethic or racial, socioeconomic, cultural, and linguistic backgrounds. As an example, geriatric specialists frequently encounter older adults who came to the United States at a young age and later informally learned English. Such individuals may achieve low scores on naming tests, despite acquired fluency, because of limited education and exposure to certain words. Failure to account for such cultural differences may lead to erroneous identification of a language deficit. Important ongoing issues within the area of cultural neuropsychology are development of instruments valid for use with individuals from diverse backgrounds; establishment of normative data sets for existing tests that account for factors such as racial and ethnic background, level of acculturation, quality of education, and bilingualism; the need for referral sources for diverse clients; and the need to provide adequate exposure to cultural neuropsychological issues for current and future trainees.[23,24]

Certain limitations are associated with the neuropsychological examination. As noted before, patients may not always put forth their best effort, leading to underestimation of true abilities. In addition, the standard neuropsychological examination, with its highly structured setting and individually administered tests, provides a degree of structure that is generally unavailable in the real world. Some patients may find themselves capable of inhibiting inappropriate behaviors or giving adequate responses to questions because the evaluation setting introduces an external structure sufficient to suppress difficulties. Thus the real-world deficits of these patients may not be reflected on formal testing.[1] Finally, neuropsychological assessment can prove to be costly. However, it is generally reimbursable by third-party payers when deemed medically necessary with precertification or authorization. The specifics will vary by diagnostic codes used, geographic location of the examiner, and patient population (e.g., older adults tend to be insured by Medicare, which covers neuropsychological services); managed care plans often require use of providers on the plan.

CASE STUDY

We now return to the case of Mr. B. Although Mr. B.'s MMSE score of 28/30 was well within normal limits, his primary care practitioner was aware of the drawbacks associated with brief cognitive screening tools (reviewed earlier). Mr. B. was referred for neuropsychological evaluation to assess for neurocognitive deficits and help determine whether his reported difficulties were attributable to a neurodegenerative process or some other cause. Mr. B. underwent a 4-hour evaluation, which revealed mild deficits in psychomotor speed, attention, and verbal learning (relative to estimates of his baseline functioning) and preservation of general cognition and all other neuropsychological abilities assessed, including memory for learned information, visuospatial skills, expressive and receptive language, working memory, reasoning and problem solving, verbal fluency, and praxis. His overall cognitive profile and evidence of functional independence were inconsistent with a progressive neurodegenerative process. The most prominent feature of Mr. B.'s examination was a moderate to severe level of depression, including sadness, loss of pleasure and interest, fatigue, and loss of appetite, to which observed cognitive deficits were thought to be attributable.

Research suggests that late-life depression is associated with a number of neuropsychological sequelae and that timely treatment can facilitate partial or complete remission of mood symptoms, enhance overall well-being, and minimize cognitive dysfunction. Therefore, Mr. B.'s neuropsychologist recommended a comprehensive treatment approach that included psychotherapy aimed at decreasing depressive ideation and increasing opportunities for meaningful social interaction, pharmacologic consultation, and introduction of compensatory strategies that Mr. B. can use when he experiences cognitive difficulties. For example, while working in his art studio, Mr. B. now breaks complex tasks into small, manageable pieces, which he undertakes one at a time rather than simultaneously. In addition, before sitting down to work he creates a quiet, distraction-free area and allows himself ample time to complete each task. Although Mr. B.'s assessment was not consistent with a neurodegenerative disorder, he had cerebrovascular risk factors. Therefore neuroimaging was recommended in addition to repeat neuropsychological testing in approximately 2 years, or sooner if Mr. B. or those close to him perceive a significant decline in one or more cognitive or functional domains.[25] Finally, the neuropsychologist highlighted Mr. B.'s areas of intact cognition, addressing the potential for improved cognitive efficiency with treatment of his depression. Mr. B. was strongly encouraged to re-engage in long-standing intellectual and leisure activities and to seek out additional structured activities (e.g., volunteer work, arts classes) to maximize social and cognitive stimulation.

SUMMARY

Survey research has indicated that primary care physicians are the least likely medical specialists to use neuropsychological services, in part because of unfamiliarity with what this testing has to offer. Most of the respondents who had used neuropsychological services, however, were very satisfied with the results.[26]

The neuropsychological examination can serve as an important supplement to an initial primary care visit.[21] Because the standard of care for many chronic or irreversible diseases involves stabilization rather than cure, early identification is imperative; cognitive loss cannot be reversed. Many neurologic diseases (e.g., multiple sclerosis, brain tumors, stroke) have associated cognitive and behavioral changes, and the neuropsychological examination can helpfully distinguish neurologic from psychiatric disease. Other patients who may benefit include those with developmental disorders, learning disabilities, attention deficits, substance abuse problems, and severe mental illness. Patients with acquired brain injury (e.g., motor vehicle accidents, sports-related concussions, toxic exposure) may be assisted by characterization of their baseline functioning and documentation of recovery, cognitive strengths and weaknesses, and resulting psychiatric difficulties. In working with older adults, it is often important to discriminate between normal age-related changes in cognition and disease-associated decline. Furthermore, when litigation accompanies injury, the neuropsychological evaluation can help distinguish exaggeration of cognitive symptoms, or malingering, from true deficit. Finally, the "difficult patient" may actually have cognitive dysfunction that interferes with the ability to follow medical directions.[27]

Neuropsychological consultation uses a standardized normative approach to measure and to describe cognition and other aspects of functioning in an objective manner. Whereas primary care practitioners focus on treating patients' physical complaints and ailments, the nature of their practice and expertise places them in an ideal situation to identify early signs of cognitive dysfunction. In this regard, primary care practitioners and neuropsychologists can work together to ensure comprehensive assessment of cognitive functioning that leads to better outcomes for patients. Moreover, the emerging emphasis on the functional relevance of cognitive deficits will enable clinical neuropsychologists to make unique contributions within primary care settings through a combination of diagnostic and treatment services for cognitive health.

CHAPTER 189

AMYOTROPHIC LATERAL SCLEROSIS

Stephanie Cassone

DEFINITION AND EPIDEMIOLOGY

Amyotrophic lateral sclerosis (ALS) is the most common of the progressive motor neuron diseases. It is also often referred to as *Lou Gehrig's disease*, after the New York Yankee baseball player who was diagnosed with the disease in the late 1930s. Classified as a neurodegenerative disorder, it is an incurable disease that produces progressive muscle weakness and ultimately death.[1]

ALS is a progressive motor neuron disease characterized by dysfunction of both upper motor neurons (UMNs) and lower motor neurons (LMNs) in the corticospinal and corticobulbar tracts, anterior motor horn cells, and bulbar motor nuclei. Most cases (90% to 95%) of ALS are sporadic, appearing at random with no clearly defined risk factors. Approximately 10% are familial, with about one third thought to be caused by a defect in the gene known as *C9orf72*, and another 20% of familial cases from mutations in the superoxide dismutase 1 *(SOD1)* gene.[1] There are also a variety of clinical variants, including progressive muscular atrophy and progressive bulbar palsy, affecting LMNs in limb and bulbar muscles, respectively. Primary lateral sclerosis and progressive pseudobulbar palsy affect UMNs in limb and bulbar muscles. Although these clinical variants may manifest differently early on, they all eventually affect both LMNs and UMNs.[2] Symptoms of autonomic, ocular movement, sensation, and cognitive dysfunction may also occur from degenerative involvement of other cortical areas.[2] The prevalence rate of ALS in the United States is 3.9 cases per 100,000 population.[2]

Neurology consultation is indicated for all patients with suspected ALS.

PATHOPHYSIOLOGY

The cause of ALS remains unknown, although the recent literature suggests several major hypotheses. There are rare familial cases of ALS (5% to 10% of cases) in which mutations in the *SOD1* gene have been discovered. Many cases of ALS, however, are sporadic, not familial, and several theories of cause are postulated. The first describes excitotoxic stimulation as a result of accumulation of glutamate in the central nervous system. It appears that the excess glutamate is toxic to motor neurons. The second hypothesis suggests an autoimmune process with autoantibodies to the calcium channels in motor neurons. The third is a familial hypothesis that neuronal injury is secondary to altered function of the enzyme SOD1 and subsequent accumulation of free oxygen radicals.[3]

There is evidence that this oxidative stress, mediated by free radicals, is important in the initiation of the disease. The role of abnormal protein aggregation has also been gaining recognition in neurodegenerative diseases including ALS. Research into the role of environmental exposures and viral agents as risk factors for the disease continues.[3]

The proposed causative mechanisms all lead to neuronal damage of both UMNs and LMNs. The UMNs are initially altered in the motor cortex, thereby affecting the corticospinal and corticobulbar tracts. The LMNs are affected at the anterior motor horn cells in the spinal cord and at the respective motor nuclei in the brainstem. Death of the motor neurons in the brainstem and spinal cord leads to denervation and atrophy of muscle fibers.

CLINICAL PRESENTATION AND PHYSICAL EXAMINATION

A precise documentation of the history of symptoms and a complete physical examination highlighting the neurologic examination are essential. Early LMN cell death leads to an insidious onset of asymmetric weakness that is evident initially in the limbs, usually in the arms. Early findings include foot drop, difficulty walking, and weakness with lifting arms.[4] It is important to assess UMNs and LMNs as well as bulbar signs and symptoms.

UMN dysfunction may manifest as hyperreflexia, spasticity, Babinski signs, incoordination, and weakness. LMN dysfunction may manifest as weakness, muscle atrophy, and fasciculations (spontaneous twitching). Fasciculations may be focal, multifocal, or diffuse. Fasciculations are accompanied by UMN signs and weakness in patients with ALS. Bulbar signs and symptoms include dysarthria, dysphagia, sialorrhea, tongue atrophy, and tongue fasciculations. Bulbar presentation is often closely related to reduced vital capacity resulting from difficulty in speaking and swallowing and carries a poor prognosis compared with limb onset.[5]

As the disease progresses, both UMN and LMN involvement becomes evident, with a more symmetric distribution of the disease. Yet even in the late stages of disease, sensation and bowel and bladder function are spared. There is a known link between ALS and executive dysfunction of the frontal and temporal lobes that may manifest as subtle cognitive dysfunction or, in about 15%, as frontotemporal dementia.[4]

DIAGNOSTICS

The diagnosis of ALS is usually made when there are widespread UMN and LMN signs in the absence of any electrophysiologic and pathologic signs of other disease processes as well as absence of neuroimaging evidence of other disease processes. In 1994, the World Federation of Neurology presented diagnostic criteria for ALS. These were subsequently revised in 1998 and renamed Airlie House criteria. Awaji-Shima criteria were introduced in 2008, which improved diagnostic sensitivity without increasing false positives.[2] These criteria include signs of LMN degeneration by clinical, electrophysiologic, or neuropathologic examination; signs of UMN degeneration by clinical examination; and progression of the motor syndrome within a region or to other regions. The four regions are bulbar, cervical, thoracic, and lumbosacral.[2]

There are no specific biochemical or laboratory markers for ALS. Laboratory and other diagnostic studies are considered to exclude other disorders in the differential diagnosis. Electrodiagnostic evaluation with electromyography (EMG) and nerve conduction studies are indicated for all patients with suspected ALS. Magnetic resonance imaging (MRI) may reveal changes consistent with UMN dysfunction. Routine laboratory studies, lumbar puncture, Lyme titer, and additional serologic studies may be necessary to exclude other disease processes.[1]

DIAGNOSTICS

Amyotrophic Lateral Sclerosis

LABORATORY
CBC and differential
ESR
Serum electrolytes
BUN
Creatinine
Serum glucose
TSH
Lead levels
Calcium
Lyme titer
Vitamin B_{12}
Folate
Creatine kinase
Liver function tests
ANA testing
RF
HIV
Serum paraprotein
Cerebrospinal fluid culture
Screening for hereditary disorders*

IMAGING
MRI (head, foramen magnum, and cervical spine)

OTHER DIAGNOSTICS
EMG, nerve conduction studies
Lumbar puncture

*If indicated.
ANA, antinuclear antibody test; BUN, blood urea nitrogen; CBC, complete blood count; EMG, electromyography; ESR, erythrocyte sedimentation rate; HIV, human immunodeficiency virus; MRI, magnetic resonance imaging; RF, rheumatoid factor; TSH, thyroid-stimulating hormone.

DIFFERENTIAL DIAGNOSIS

Differentiation of ALS from treatable neurologic disorders is important now that there are specific treatments available. It is also important to diagnose ALS early and initiate the appropriate medical therapy. Atypical features that should alert the practitioner to a disease other than ALS include restriction of the disease to just UMNs or LMNs, involvement of neurons other than motor neurons, and EMG findings not consistent with ALS. The two conditions most commonly are mistaken for ALS include motor neuropathy with conduction block, and cervical spondylotic myelopathy.[2]

MANAGEMENT

Symptom management continues to be the cornerstone of treatment. As more is discovered about the mechanisms of this disease, more treatment options become available. Riluzole (Rilutek) is the only pharmacologic agent approved by the U.S. Food and Drug Administration (FDA) that has demonstrated an impact on ALS survival. The clinical benefits are minimal, extending the ventilator-free survival period by approximately 2 months. Riluzole is an antiglutamate that appears to slow progression of ALS and may improve survival in patients with early bulbar involvement.[3] The most common side effects described with riluzole are asthenia, dizziness, gastrointestinal distress, neutropenia, and elevated liver enzymes. Therefore it is recommended that the patient be regularly monitored for neutropenia and that liver function tests be performed at the onset of treatment, monthly during the first 3 months of therapy, and every 3 months thereafter.[4]

The primary goal of treatment is supportive care, including with use of riluzole, and the following symptom management[4-6]:

- Depression and anxiety: selective serotonin reuptake inhibitors (SSRIs), serotonin-norepinephrine reuptake inhibitors (SNRIs), and/or benzodiazepines
- Cramps: benzodiazepines
- Spasticity: baclofen, benzodiazepines, or tizanidine (Zanaflex)

DIFFERENTIAL DIAGNOSIS

Amyotrophic Lateral Sclerosis

NEUROLOGIC
- Benign fasciculations
- Primary lateral sclerosis
- Parkinson disease
- Huntington disease
- Progressive bulbar palsy
- Myasthenia gravis
- Familial ALS
- Motor neuron syndromes in malignant diseases
- Sporadic ALS

IMMUNOLOGIC/INFECTIOUS
- Herpes zoster
- Poliomyelitis
- Lyme disease
- Tetanus
- LMN axonal neuropathy
- Multifocal motor neuropathy with conduction block

STRUCTURAL
- Tumor
  - Foramen magnum
  - Parasagittal tumor

MUSCULOSKELETAL
- Cervical spine compression
- Cervical spondylotic myelopathy

METABOLIC
- Chronic aluminum or lead poisoning
- Drug intoxication (phenytoin or strychnine)
- Vitamin deficiency or malabsorption syndrome
- Thyrotoxicosis

- Sialorrhea: atropine sulfate ophthalmic drops, diphenhydramine (Benadryl), or hyoscyamine (Levsin). (Providers should take care to not overly dry out secretions, which could thicken phlegm.)
- Urinary urgency: oxybutynin (Ditropan) or tolterodine (Detrol)
- Sleep disturbance: trazodone, amitriptyline (Elavil), or mirtazapine (Remeron)
- Fatigue: methylphenidate (Ritalin) or modafinil (Provigil)
- Brain-computer interface—used for communication

Other treatments are being investigated. The current clinical drug trials for ALS can be found on the ALS Association website, www.alsa.org.

LIFE SPAN CONSIDERATIONS

According to the ALS Association, some patients with ALS will live for 10 to 20 years, but on average the life expectancy after diagnosis is 2 to 5 years. The variability and rapid progression can make it difficult to predict survival time. Most patients die of respiratory failure or infection. The two factors that most influence survival are patient age and the presence or absence of bulbar symptoms at the time of diagnosis. Patients with bulbar symptoms at the onset of disease have a poorer prognosis and shorter duration of survival, as do older patients.[4]

COMPLICATIONS

Anxiety and depression are common, so it is important to identify and treat these symptoms to ensure the best quality of life for the patient. Depression can be a component of the ALS disease process and should be explained to the patient and caregiver. Caregiver depression also needs to be considered, along with the interaction between the patient and the caregiver. An SSRI is a reasonable choice for treatment of depression in patients with ALS. The pseudobulbar effect of laughing and crying inappropriately needs to be differentiated from depression.

It is also important to recognize existential despair in some patients. These patients are not just depressed, but may be experiencing overwhelming feelings of demoralization, hopelessness, and lack of meaning as they face their own mortality. They are more likely to consider suicide and require close follow-up and psychosocial support.[6]

Preventing malnutrition in ALS can positively affect quality of life and length of survival. Malnutrition can impair respiratory and immune system function and can exacerbate generalized muscular weakness. The American Academy of Neurology (AAN) recommends a nutrition consultation every 3 months for patients with ALS. In the initial stages of dysphagia and ALS diagnosis, there should be a collaboration between the dietitian and the speech language pathologist to determine appropriate food and fluid consistency, especially if bulbar symptoms are present.[7] As dysphagia progresses, percutaneous endoscopic gastrostomy (PEG) tube placement may be indicated if this aligns with the patient's goals for care. The AAN ALS Practice Parameters suggest PEG placement while the patient's forced vital capacity (FVC) is greater than 50% of the predicted value or when there is dysphagia and/or a nutritional status decline, which can be indicated by a 5% to 10% loss of body weight. Before feeding tube placement, a discussion with the patient and caregiver is necessary to discuss the risks and benefits of the procedure, the daily management of the tube feedings, and the appropriate timing of the tube placement with regard to the disease process. A referral to a gastroenterologist and discussion with palliative medicine providers would be warranted for further discussion of gastrostomy tube placement.[7]

Management of respiratory dysfunction in ALS consists of pulmonary function monitoring (e.g., FVC), respiratory therapy, incentive spirometry, and noninvasive positive-pressure ventilation (NIPPV) as needed. Initiation of NIPPV when the patient first demonstrates difficulty with ventilation (i.e., FVC <50% of predicted value) can provide significant relief of sleep disturbance, which can cause daytime sleepiness, morning headaches, dyspnea, and orthopnea. Serial pulmonary function tests will provide objective evidence of respiratory decline.[2,4] Respiratory musculature weakness can result in aspiration and pneumonia. Only 4% to 6% of patients with ALS elect to have a tracheostomy and invasive ventilation, making a clear distinction between noninvasive ventilation as a way of relieving respiratory symptoms and invasive ventilation as a clear life-extending procedure that requires 24-hour supervision.[3] Diaphragm pacing with surgically attached electrodes to the phrenic nerve provides low-frequency stimulation to help maintain diaphragm strength.[3] An assisted cough device, suction machine, expectorants, mucolytics, antibiotics, and theophylline can also help relieve respiratory symptoms. Patients who refuse NIPPV or whose symptoms are not fully controlled may benefit from morphine, a safe and effective therapy in managing dyspnea.[6]

It is important to keep patients as functional as possible, to anticipate problems, and to ensure patient awareness before problems occur. Cramping, spasticity, and pain are common complaints and should be treated with appropriate pharmacologic agents. It is also important to vaccinate against pneumococcal infection and influenza.[4]

INDICATIONS FOR REFERRAL OR HOSPITALIZATION

The primary health care provider is responsible for the collaborative care of the patient in addition to identifying and treating any psychosocial issues as they appear. Early diagnosis and management by a team that specializes in ALS positively affects quality of life and prolongs survival.[8]

If a motor neuron disease is suspected, it important to make appropriate referrals to specialists for further follow-up. A prompt referral to a neurologist or neuromuscular clinic is warranted. This will likely shorten the time to diagnosis.[8]

- If ALS is diagnosed, referrals for supportive care by a multidisciplinary team are necessary. The collaborative team should include physicians, nurses, physical therapists, occupational therapists, speech therapists, dietitians, social workers, pulmonology and palliative medicine specialists, and the local ALS resource group.[1] In some areas there are ALS clinics that provide a multidisciplinary approach to patient care at each visit. This team can also help clarify the patient's wishes about artificial feeding or hydration, resuscitation, intubation, treatment of infection with antibiotics, and even hospitalizations.[4]
- Hospitalization is indicated when symptoms become emergent and is based on the patient's goals for care. Hospitalization is warranted when symptoms are unstable or if there is an inability to swallow, respiratory compromise, rapid loss of limb function, or failure to thrive.[5]

PATIENT AND FAMILY EDUCATION

ALS is a physically, mentally, and financially debilitating disease. It is important to educate patients and families about its natural history. Discussion topics must include the use of medications, assistive devices, home modifications, and in-home support. Discussions about goals of care are important to address advance directives, gastrostomy tube placement, ventilatory support, and hospice care to provide additional support for patients in home, with the goal of honoring their wish to stay out of the hospital.

Patients, family, and friends may be experiencing a great deal of distress. A consultation with palliative care providers at the time of diagnosis can be beneficial for determining the goals of care and end-of-life wishes. Patients should be encouraged to appoint a health care proxy and openly discuss advance directives with their proxy and others who will be involved in their care. Many patients will elect not to have a gastrostomy tube placed and will refuse ventilatory support.[9] Palliative care and hospice services are options that will allow patients to maintain independence and quality of life for as long as possible and in a manner that respects their wishes and provides symptom relief. Patients and caretakers should be referred to local ALS foundations, support groups, and resources to assist with care and provide educational information. Caring for ALS patients and their families requires a multidisciplinary team that is physically, psychologically, emotionally, and spiritually supportive.

CHAPTER 190

BELL PALSY

Wanda J. Handel

DEFINITION AND EPIDEMIOLOGY

Defined as an acute, unilateral weakness or paralysis of the facial nerve with an onset of less than 72 hours and unknown cause, Bell palsy is the most commonly diagnosed peripheral facial nerve condition.[1] Although the condition is typically self-limiting, some patients have persistent facial paralysis and are at risk for eye injury.[1] People of all ages are affected, but incidence is most common in young and middle-aged adults (ages 15 to 45), with an even distribution between men and women and an annual incidence of 11 to 40 cases per 100,000.[2-4] Either side of the face may be affected.[4] Incidence is higher during pregnancy, particularly in the last trimester, in the first week postpartum, and in women with preeclampsia. Other risk factors that increase incidence include diabetes, hypothyroidism, recent upper respiratory infections, obesity, family history, and hypertension.[1,5]

PATHOPHYSIOLOGY

The facial nerve (cranial nerve [CN] VII) is mixed: afferent fibers from the anterior two thirds of the tongue and the external auditory canal; efferent fibers to the facial muscles; and parasympathetic fibers to the lacrimal, sublingual, and submandibular glands. Knowledge of the topographic anatomy of the facial nerve can provide clinical clues to sites of injury. Sparing of the forehead muscles typically suggests an upper motor neuron or central lesion because the forehead is bilaterally innervated.[3] The typical unilateral facial paralysis of Bell palsy is assumed to be initiated by a triggering event that places physiologic stress on the body (e.g., an upper respiratory tract infection or ischemia to the nerve). This stressor promotes the body's protective inflammatory response with its release of acute-phase reactants. The intraneural inflammatory response results in edema of the facial nerve. If the edema is not alleviated, there is ischemia of the nerve, with resulting axonal demyelination and inevitable nerve degeneration. Varying degrees of motor control loss become obvious about 3 days after nerve demyelination.[5]

Although the cause of Bell palsy remains idiopathic, and causative factors such as genetic, vascular, nerve compression, infectious, and metabolic changes have been discussed, the two most accepted hypotheses are a viral and an autoimmune pathomechanism. Viruses such as human herpes simplex virus type 1 (HSV-1) and type 2 (HSV-2) and varicella-zoster virus (VZV) all have the ability to cause latent infections in a single peripheral nerve distribution for the life of the host.[3] Reactivation of any one of these viruses could cause Bell palsy in an individual. However, current polymerase chain reaction testing can only confirm that the virus exists within the nerve; it cannot delineate whether the virus is in a latent or active state.[6] Lyme disease has also been implicated. Immunologic theory is the peripheral demyelination of Bell palsy is a cell-mediated response such as the demyelination in Guillain-Barré syndrome,[3] Bell palsy remains a diagnosis of exclusion, meaning a complete history and thorough physical examination are needed.

CLINICAL PRESENTATION

The typical onset is acute and progressive; maximum paralysis is attained in about half of the cases within 48 to 72 hours and in nearly all cases by day 5. Individuals may report pain behind the ipsilateral ear preceding the facial paralysis by 1 to 2 days. Typically, a smooth forehead, widened palpebral fissure, inability to close the eye, flattened nasolabial fold, and asymmetric smile are characteristic. Tearing, drooling, postauricular pain, tinnitus, and a mild hearing deficit may occur. Complaints of altered taste (dysgeusia) and an increased sensitivity to sound (hyperacusis) as well as hypoesthesia in one or more branches of the trigeminal nerve may also be present.[1,3,5] Timing of onset is key in the diagnosis; slowly progressive or relapsing courses suggest other entities.[1]

Other associated symptoms include a history of recent infections, especially viral illnesses such as chickenpox, mumps, mononucleosis, coxsackievirus, cytomegalovirus, human immunodeficiency virus (HIV), and influenza. The presence of chronic illnesses, such as diabetes mellitus, hypertension, or hypothyroidism, should be ascertained, and the patient should be queried about pregnancy, rashes or skin lesions, and insect bites. Any history of facial trauma should be carefully noted.[1]

PHYSICAL EXAMINATION

A complete physical and neurologic examination is warranted to rule out more serious central nervous system conditions such as stroke, tumor, and multiple sclerosis. The CN examination is key in identifying CN VII as the peripheral source of the facial weakness. The patient is asked to smile, show the teeth, puff out cheeks, raise eyebrows, and close eyes tightly. Any facial asymmetry is noted, paying close attention to whether the facial weakness is upper and lower or lower alone. Bell palsy causes a unilateral, full-face paresis or paralysis, with an ipsilateral source indicating a peripheral nerve problem. The patient is observed for lack of eyelid closure and absence of wrinkling of the forehead. Drooling and continuous tearing of the eye may also be present. A central nervous system lesion may manifest as a lower facial weakness with sparing of the forehead, and other deficits may be noted on full neurologic examination.[5,7,8] Attention to otologic and head and neck examination is warranted to assess for decreased hearing and vesicles on the face or in and around the external ear canal, which may indicate herpes zoster oticus (Ramsay Hunt syndrome), although absence of vesicles does not rule out zoster sine herpete.[5]

Special attention to the sensory and motor functions of the branches of the facial nerve is also necessary. Minor asymmetry of the lower face may be a normal deviation. The degree of facial weakness should be documented. A number of grading systems have been developed to objectively define the severity of the palsy. Clinicians may find the House-Brackmann tool helpful in gauging the severity of neural degeneration and in establishing objective measures of recovery.[1,9] A photographic record is also helpful in establishing the extent of facial muscle weakness and documenting progressive neural regeneration.

DIAGNOSTICS

Routine diagnostic tests and imaging are not recommended for new-onset Bell palsy. Diagnostic studies may be useful to exclude identifiable conditions such as Lyme disease in the

DIAGNOSTICS

Bell Palsy

LABORATORY

No routine laboratory testing or imaging for new-onset Bell palsy

Laboratory testing to rule out identifiable cause in patients with atypical presentation

Lyme titer for patients with tick exposure or in endemic areas

IMAGING

No routine imaging for new-onset Bell palsy

MRI with and without contrast to view the entire facial nerve (including internal auditory canal and face)

- For patients with atypical presentation (isolated paralysis of a branch of the facial nerve, recurrent paralysis, or paralysis with other cranial nerve involvement)
- For patients in whom paralysis fails to subside within 3-month time frame
- To rule out other suspected identifiable cause

OTHER DIAGNOSTICS

Electrodiagnostic testing offered to patients with complete facial paralysis approximately 7 days after onset to quantify the degree of nerve damage

MRI, magnetic resonance imaging.

differential diagnosis and to determine prognosis. Imaging is warranted in atypical presentation, such as bilateral facial nerve palsies.[1]

DIFFERENTIAL DIAGNOSIS

The list of conditions to be included in the differential diagnosis for unilateral facial paralysis is lengthy. Infectious, traumatic, neoplastic, immunologic, and metabolic conditions (e.g., otitis media, cholesteatoma, tumors, mastoiditis, Lyme disease, pregnancy, sarcoidosis, diabetes mellitus, and hypothyroidism) should be considered.

MANAGEMENT

Specialist consultation is indicated for patients with atypical presentation (with or without signs of central nervous system pathology), Bell palsy in pregnancy, signs and symptoms of corneal abrasion, persistent facial weakness or paralysis without improvement after 2 weeks, or need for surgery or botulinum toxin injection.

The primary goals of treatment are to decrease the inflammatory response and swelling, decrease nerve function recovery time, and protect the eye from complications. More than 75% of patients will recover some nerve function within the first 3 weeks, although another 30% will have persistent symptoms and an incomplete recovery.[10]

Steroids are highly effective and increase the probability of nerve recovery. Unless contraindicated (such as in diabetes), steroids are started in patients with new-onset Bell palsy within 72 hours of onset of symptoms. Prednisone or prednisolone is given at a dosage of 60 mg daily orally for 5 days followed by taper for 5 days.[1,7,10] A modest additional effect of 7% recovery is reported with the coadministration of steroids and an antiviral medication. Acyclovir, 400 mg daily orally for 7 days, or valacyclovir, 1000 mg orally three times per day for 7 days, may be used.[1,7,10] Administration of antivirals alone has not shown efficacy.[1,7,10]

Protection of the eye is the single most important goal of care for the patient with Bell palsy. Exposure keratitis can result in blindness, and the cornea must be protected from abrasion from dust and debris.

- Lubricating eye drops such as methylcellulose every 2 hours, with an ocular lubricant at bedtime, can help.[1]
- Protective eyeglasses and moisture chambers should be used.[1]
- Eyelids should be closed and taped at night to protect the cornea, but care must be observed to be sure that the patient understands the technique and does not cause a corneal abrasion.[1,5]
- Upper eyelid weights are another option for persistent lagopthalmos.[1,5]

Surgical decompression of the facial nerve is not routinely performed, but if desired requires quick planning within weeks 1 and 2 after onset.[1,5] Associated pain should be managed with nonsteroidal agents if they are not contraindicated.[11] Massage of weakened facial muscles may help preserve muscle tone and provide some comfort. Acupuncture and physical therapy may show some benefit, but more information is needed for treatment recommendations.[1]

DIFFERENTIAL DIAGNOSIS

Bell Palsy

NEUROLOGIC

Central Nervous System

- Stroke
- Tumor
- Multiple sclerosis

Peripheral Nervous System

- Bell palsy
- Lyme disease
- Guillain-Barré syndrome

HEAD, EYES, EARS, NOSE, AND THROAT

- Otitis media
- Mastoiditis
- Ramsay-Hunt syndrome
- Zoster sine herpete
- Parotid tumor
- Cholesteatoma

GYNECOLOGIC

- Pregnancy

ENDOCRINE

- Diabetes
- Hypothyroidism

IMMUNOLOGIC

- Sarcoidosis

OTHER CAUSES

- Trauma

COMPLICATIONS

Evidence of poor functional recovery can be seen in facial asymmetry as a result of muscle weakness and synkinesis. Loss of vision in the affected eye from corneal ulceration is among the worst possible outcomes. Hearing loss and permanent tinnitus are sequelae indicating damage to the auditory nerve. Physician consultation is indicated for patients with corneal abrasions or an eyelid that cannot close.

INDICATIONS FOR REFERRAL OR HOSPITALIZATION[1,5,7]

In general, new-onset bell palsy does not require referral or hospitalization.

- Patients with new ocular signs of itching, pain, irritation, or corneal abrasion should be referred to an ophthalmologist.
- Patients with severe lid symptoms or in whom supportive eye care has failed should be referred to an ophthalmologist for consideration of temporary options such as botulinum

toxin injections, temporary or permanent tarsorrhaphy, or a permanent surgical option of a lid weight.

- Patients in whom the provider suspects central nervous system involvement, such as stroke, tumor, or multiple sclerosis, and patients with an atypical presentation or with recurrence, progressive symptoms, or failure to improve should be referred to a neurologist.
- Pregnant individuals should be co-managed with the obstetrician.
- Patients with complete facial paralysis after day 7 from onset but before day 14 may be referred to a neurologist for electrodiagnostic studies, electroneurophysiologic testing, or facial electromyography to assist with prognosis.
- Referral to a neurosurgeon for decompressive surgery is controversial and should take place within a narrow window of after 7 days but before day 14 of onset and in patients with more than 90% nerve conduction loss on electroneurodiagnostic testing.
- Patients with persistent complete facial paralysis or failure to recover acceptable movement, patients with muscle spasms, and those with synkinesia should be referred to an otolaryngologist, plastic surgeon, or neurosurgeon for botulinum toxin injection or consultation for facial nerve grafting.

LIFE SPAN CONSIDERATIONS

Bell palsy occurs three times more often during pregnancy. An increase in vascular volume and pregnancy-induced hypertension may contribute to palsy of the facial nerve as a result of edema and entrapment. A viral cause cannot be excluded. For the health care provider giving prenatal care, it is recommended that the advice of an obstetrician be solicited and referral considered.[5] Children with new-onset Bell palsy show higher rates of spontaneous recovery, and no clear evidence exists to show potential benefit from corticosteroids. Clinician judgment and discussion with patient care provider should guide treatment.[1] Lyme disease is found in 50% of cases of facial palsy in children younger than 10 years. Serologic testing is warranted in this age group.[5]

EDUCATION AND HEALTH PROMOTION

Providing a full explanation of Bell palsy and its usual benign clinical course can allay the fright that patients experience from the onset of facial paralysis. The health care provider should caution the patient about corneal abrasion and instruct the patient in use of eye drops during the day and ocular lubricant at night. The provider should teach the patient about patching the eyelid closed at night, taking care to close the eyelid to protect the cornea. Patients should be encouraged to report any ocular pain, discharge, or drainage. The provider should be notified if symptoms worsen or recur. Providing information about medications, including the name, therapeutic effects, common side effects, dosage, and any other special considerations, will help engender compliance. The provider also teaches the patient to perform facial muscle exercises in front of a mirror two or three times a day and encourages follow-up care for evaluation of treatment, provision of emotional support, and documentation of recovery of facial muscle function.

CHAPTER 191

CEREBROVASCULAR EVENTS

John J. Graykoski

DEFINITION AND EPIDEMIOLOGY

A stroke is an interruption of blood circulation to the brain causing a neurologic deficit that reflects the area of the brain affected. A stroke can be ischemic or hemorrhagic.[1] Ischemic stroke is most prevalent. It is occlusive in nature. Lacunar strokes are seen more in older adults and diabetic patients. They affect smaller areas of the brain by closing off arterioles.

Hemorrhagic stroke has a lower incidence than ischemic stroke but is more deadly.

Transient ischemic attacks (TIAs) are neurologic deficits that resolve completely within a few hours but no more than 24 hours. A TIA is part of a spectrum ending in acute ischemic stroke, referred to collectively as an acute cerebrovascular syndrome (ACVS) which reflects the growing awareness that stroke can be the end result of TIA. More aggressive management of TIA, including neurologic consultation and hospitalization, can reduce the risk of more devastating stroke.[1]

Ischemic strokes tend to occur in older patients with other disease processes, whereas hemorrhagic strokes typically occur in healthy individuals between the ages of 40 and 60 years. Risk factors for ischemic stroke include hypertension, older age, cigarette smoking, male gender, family history, race, previous stroke or TIA, carotid stenosis of more than 80%, atrial fibrillation, and drug abuse. Other factors that may contribute are diabetes, obesity, sedentary lifestyle, and elevated serum cholesterol.

Stroke is now the fifth most common cause of death in the United States. This is an improvement from being the third most common cause only a few years ago. The decrease is in large part a result of how stroke is managed (see the Management section). Every year, 795,000 people in the United States have a stroke; stroke kills 130,000 per year.[2,3,4] There are racial disparities in stroke occurrence; both black men and black women are twice as likely as other races to have a first stroke, and more likely to die.[3] Stroke remains a leading cause of disability in the United States, with significant social and financial implications for families and society. The cost of stroke care is estimated to be $36.5 billion dollars annually. Stroke also represents a significant burden for long-term care. Fifty percent to 70% of stroke survivors regain functional independence, but 15% to 30% are permanently disabled. Institutional care is required by 20% at 3 months after onset.

PATHOPHYSIOLOGY

Ischemic Stroke

Ischemic stroke is the most common type of stroke. In a thrombotic event, a critical degree of atherosclerosis causes complete or relatively complete blockage of blood flow through a local area. In an embolic event, a clot forms elsewhere (e.g., a fibrillating atrium), breaks off, and travels through the arterial circulation until it lodges in a vessel and blocks the flow of blood distally. The effects of arterial occlusion on brain tissue vary, depending on the location of the occlusion in relation to available collateral and anastomotic channels and the degree and duration of the ischemia. The specific neurologic deficit relates to the location and size of the infarction or focus of ischemia. At the time of arterial occlusion, the viscosity of the blood and resistance to flow both increase, and there is sludging within the vessels. The tissue becomes pale. If the ischemia is prolonged, sludging and endothelial damage prevent normal reflow. Cellular breakdown and swelling occur.[5]

Hemorrhagic Stroke

Thirteen percent of all strokes are the results of brain bleeds.[5] There are two types of hemorrhagic stroke: subarachnoid and intracerebral. A subarachnoid bleed occurs in the subarachnoid space, the area between the tissue that covers the brain and the brain. These are usually caused by an aneurysm, arteriovenous malformation, or an inherited bleeding disorder. Risk factors include smoking, hypertension, connective tissue disorders, other known aneurysms, and polycystic kidney disease. Family history may play a role.[5]

Anticoagulation with warfarin and antiplatelet therapy increase the risk of brain bleed in individuals taking those medications, especially with head injury.

Intracerebral hemorrhage is caused by a weakened artery in the brain. Uncontrolled hypertension is the most common cause of the vessel weakening. Other contributing risks include smoking, obesity, high-fat diet, and drugs, including cocaine.[6]

In either embolic or hemorrhagic stroke, an area immediately surrounding the injury dies within a few minutes from lack of oxygen and the failure of the oxygen-dependent adenosine triphosphate (ATP) metabolic pathway. In a broader area of injury, referred to as the penumbra, the damage is more dynamic, extending for 12 to 24 hours. It is believed the release of intracellular calcium initiates the sequence of programmed cell death, or apoptosis.[6]

CLINICAL PRESENTATION

Patients with ACVS (TIA and strokes) have a similar presentation, although time is a major differentiating factor. The symptoms of cerebral ischemia are widely variable and depend on the vascular territory involved. When the carotid artery circulation is involved, the symptoms reflect ischemia to the ipsilateral eye or brain. The classic visual disturbance (amaurosis fugax) is a transient, painless loss of vision, often described as a shade descending over the visual field. Hemispheric brain ischemia usually causes weakness or numbness of the contralateral face or limbs. Language difficulties and cognitive and behavioral changes may also occur. Vertebrobasilar ACVS (TIA) and strokes may manifest with vertigo, nystagmus, diplopia, dysconjugate gaze, or deficits of cranial nerves III to XII.

Many signs and symptoms are common to strokes affecting both anterior (carotid) and posterior (vertebrobasilar) circulation. These include hemiparesis, hemisensory loss, visual field defects, ataxia (difficulty with balance and coordination), dysarthria (difficulty speaking), reflex asymmetry, and Babinski sign. Headache does not usually occur in ischemic stroke but is common in hemorrhagic stroke. When it is present, headache is not nearly as severe as in intracerebral or subarachnoid hemorrhage, and the neck is not stiff. ACVS (TIA) more commonly precedes ischemic stroke than hemorrhagic stroke.

In ischemic stroke, the patient usually has a single attack, and the entire illness evolves within a few hours. However, the stroke may occur in a "stuttering" fashion, with intermittent progression of neurologic deficits that extends for several hours, a day, or longer. A partial stroke may occur and even recede temporarily for several hours, after which there may be rapid progression to the full-blown stroke. The stroke may involve several parts of the body at once or only one part (e.g., a limb or one side of the face), with the other parts becoming involved in a stepwise fashion until the stroke is fully developed. The stroke may occur during sleep, with the patient remaining unaware until he or she tries to get up and discovers the paralysis.

In subarachnoid hemorrhage, the clinical presentation is usually heralded by the abrupt onset of a severe headache ("the worst headache of my life"), nausea and vomiting, signs of meningeal irritation, and varying degrees of neurologic dysfunction. Loss of consciousness at the time of the initial event is common but is usually short-lived. Nearly 50% of patients with aneurysmal subarachnoid hemorrhage give a history of atypical headaches occurring days to weeks before the definitive event. These sentinel headaches are characteristically sudden in onset and are often associated with nausea, vomiting, and dizziness, with or without neurologic dysfunction. Some hemorrhagic events may manifest with seizures.

Patients with hypertensive intracerebral hemorrhage may have no consistent warning or prodromal symptoms. In the majority of cases, the hemorrhage has its onset while the patient is up and active; onset during sleep is rare. The blood pressure is elevated in almost all cases. The neurologic signs and symptoms vary with the site and size of the extravasation of blood. The patient may lapse almost immediately into stupor and coma, with hemiplegia and steady deterioration to death during the next several hours. More often, the patient complains of a headache, followed within a few minutes by unilateral facial sag, slurred speech, weakness in an arm and leg, and eye deviation away from the paretic limbs. These events, occurring during a period of 5 to 30 minutes, strongly suggest intracerebral bleeding. More advanced cases are characterized by paralysis, aphasia, stupor, coma, deep and irregular respiration, dilated and fixed pupils, and, occasionally, decerebrate rigidity.

PHYSICAL EXAMINATION

Findings on physical examination correspond to the location of the vascular event and associated neurologic deficit. Initial attention should always focus on a patent and protected airway, a good respiratory effort, and a competent heart rate with good peripheral circulation (ABCs of advanced clinical life support). A complete neurologic examination to assess areas of deficit should quickly follow.

Because ACVS (TIA) precedes 7.1% of all strokes,[7] a risk stratification tool should be used to guide treatment for ACVS (TIA). The $ABCD^2$ score (Table 191-1) is valuable for this purpose.[8]

DIAGNOSTICS

Diagnostic studies are necessary to determine the type of stroke and the probable cause as well as to detect complications. Because management is vastly different, it is important to be able to quickly differentiate ischemic stroke from hemorrhagic stroke and to exclude disorders that may occasionally resemble stroke.

A head computed tomography (CT) scan is the most common initial imaging procedure. A noncontrast CT scan is better than magnetic resonance imaging (MRI) in discriminating between hemorrhagic and ischemic stroke. Patients who have

TABLE 191-1 **ABCD^2 Score for Acute Cerebral Vascular Syndrome (Transient Ischemic Attack)**

Criteria		Points if Positive
Age ≥60 years		1 point
Blood pressure ≥140 mm Hg systolic and/ or ≥90 mm Hg diastolic		1 point
Clinical presentation		
Unilateral weakness with or without speech changes		2 points
Speech changes, no unilateral weakness		1 point
Duration		
≥60 minutes		2 points
≤59 minutes		1 point
Diabetes		1 point
Guide		
ABCD^2 Score	**48-hour Stroke Risk**	**Comment**
1-3 points	1%	Obtain neurology consultation; possible outpatient treatment and evaluation
4-5 points	4.1%	Hospitalization justified
6-7 points	8.1%	Hospitalization beneficial

atypical presentations or who have unusual findings on noncontrast CT scans ought to have a CT scan with contrast enhancement or MRI to exclude tumor. CT can miss small subcortical or cortical infarctions or lesions in the posterior fossa. Among patients with ischemic stroke, the CT scan may be normal in the first few hours but will usually show abnormalities after 12 hours or more. In hemorrhagic stroke, the head CT scan will usually be abnormal at presentation to the emergency department. If the initial CT scan shows hemorrhage, other studies (e.g., arteriography) may be necessary to determine whether an underlying vascular malformation is present. In certified stroke centers, the time from presentation in the emergency department to CT is a measured statistic, with the goal of making a determination on the use of thrombolytics within the 3- to 4.5-hour window when most eligible candidates could benefit.

Other diagnostic studies include an electrocardiogram (ECG), chest radiography, pulse oximetry or arterial blood gas (ABG) assessment, complete blood count (CBC) with platelets, prothrombin time (PT), partial thromboplastin time (PTT), serum glucose concentration, creatinine level, blood urea nitrogen (BUN) level, and electrolyte values. Doing these tests should not delay the CT scan; time is of the essence, and in specialty stroke centers the clock is literally ticking. Depending on the clinical presentation, other tests may be necessary, including examination of the cerebrospinal fluid if central nervous system infection is suspected or when the clinical picture suggests subarachnoid hemorrhage but the head CT scan is normal. Electroencephalography (EEG) is indicated when the clinical picture suggests seizure. Carotid ultrasonography will assess patency of the carotid arteries. Carotid arteriography or magnetic resonance angiography should be done in patients with severe carotid stenosis on ultrasound evaluation who are considered candidates for endarterectomy. Transesophageal echocardiography and Holter monitoring may be performed if the presentation is suggestive of an embolic event originating from the heart. Other laboratory tests that may be indicated include serum cholesterol level, toxicology screening, erythrocyte sedimentation rate (ESR), hemoglobin electrophoresis, fibrinogen level, serum protein electrophoresis, antiphospholipid antibody level, serologic test for syphilis, protein C level, protein S level, antithrombin III level, lupus anticoagulant, anticardiolipin antibody level, and connective tissue disease screen.

The National Institutes of Health (NIH) Stroke Scale is now the basic neurologic assessment for stroke patients.[9] It identifies and quantifies deficits at baseline and provides a standardized scoring system to allow tracking of progression. This assessment should be done as soon as practical after the patient has arrived, and the results should accompany the patient throughout care.

DIFFERENTIAL DIAGNOSIS

A number of conditions may be mistaken for ACVS (TIA) and stroke including migraine and migraine equivalents, simple partial or complex partial seizures, subdural hematoma, brain tumor, syncope, demyelinating diseases, encephalitis conversion disorders, transient global amnesia, or toxic or metabolic encephalopathy, among others.

MANAGEMENT

Immediate emergency department referral or specialist consultation is indicated for all patients with suspected acute cerebrovascular accident.

Initial management depends on the acuity of presentation. In general, the patient who is seen days after a probable TIA but has no current signs or symptoms of neurologic dysfunction can be evaluated and treated in the outpatient setting. Identification of the most likely cause of the TIA is vital to proper management. For example, management of the patient with severe carotid stenosis will be different from that of the patient with atrial fibrillation. Treatment of all patients with TIA or stroke should include risk factor management.

The patient who is seen acutely with neurologic signs and symptoms compatible with TIA or stroke should be managed as a medical emergency. Risk stratification of TIA should be determined by use of the ABCD^2 score.

In the primary care setting, most management of stroke involves efforts at primary or secondary intervention including risk reduction to include blood pressure control, aspirin therapy, smoking cessation, and blood sugar and cholesterol management.

For acute stroke, time is of the essence. Educational efforts should be directed at patient and family to ensure that early signs of stroke prompt an immediate 911 call. A national education campaign stresses early recognition (see Box 191-1).

Community organization is critical in managing stroke. Integrated emergency medical services (EMS) and hospital systems are needed so that the appropriate care is available rapidly within the window of opportunity. The national coalition organized to advocate for rapid and appropriate care has established guidelines and protocols to create an integrated response.

DIAGNOSTICS

Cerebrovascular Events

INITIAL

Stat CT scan of head (noncontrast)
ECG
Pulse oximetry
National Institutes of Health Stroke Scale[9]
ABCD^2 risk stratification for ACVS (TIA)

LABORATORY

CBC and differential
PT, PTT, international normalized ratio
Serum electrolytes
BUN
Creatinine
Serum glucose
Toxic screen
Lumbar puncture (immediate if severe headache but negative CT to rule out subarachnoid hemorrhage)

OTHER DIAGNOSTICS

The following are tests to consider after emergency care, stabilization, and treatments.

Imaging

Transesophageal echocardiography
Chest x-ray studies*

Laboratory

Lipid profile*
ESR*
Hemoglobin electrophoresis*
Fibrinogen*
Serum protein electrophoresis*
Antiphospholipid antibody*
Fluorescent treponemal antibody absorption test or rapid plasma reagin*
Protein C, protein S*
Antithrombin III*
Lupus anticoagulant*
Anticardiolipin antibody*
Connective tissue disease screening*
ABGs*

Other Studies

Carotid ultrasound*
EEG*
Arteriography*
Holter or event monitoring*

*If indicated.

DIFFERENTIAL DIAGNOSIS

Cerebrovascular Events

NEUROLOGIC

- Migraine
- Seizures
- Subdural or epidural hematoma
- Tumor (primary, metastatic)
- Syncope
- Transient global amnesia
- Encephalopathy

METABOLIC OR ENDOCRINE

- Hypoglycemia
- Nonketotic hyperosmolar coma

CARDIAC (POST–CARDIAC ARREST ISCHEMIA)

- Cardiac arrhythmia
- Transient global amnesia
- Encephalopathy

PSYCHIATRIC

- Conversion disorder
- Hyperventilation
- Panic attack
- Drug overdose (cocaine, amphetamine)

IMMUNOLOGIC

- Infection (meningitis, encephalitis) or systemic infection
- Demyelinating disease

BOX 191-1

Stroke Symptoms Guide

- Sudden numbness or weakness of face, arm, or leg, especially on one side of the body
- Sudden confusion or trouble speaking or understanding speech
- Sudden trouble seeing in one or both eyes
- Sudden trouble walking, dizziness, loss of balance or coordination
- Sudden severe headache with no known cause

Acute stroke-ready hospitals are needed. These community hospitals will have trained stroke response personnel available in the emergency department and will use standard care protocols. They will use telemedicine for rapid consultation with neurologists. They will have the capacity to administer clot-busting drugs and to initiate rapid reversal of anticoagulation. EMS agencies serving the hospital will have training in stroke recognition and will trigger a stroke code similar to a response to heart attack. Rapid transfer to appropriate tertiary facilities is accomplished by interfacility agreement.[10]

Primary stroke centers are accredited hospitals that demonstrate consistent stroke response and measure outcomes including time from arrival to administration of thrombolytics and have a consistent level of care using accepted treatment algorithms.

Comprehensive stroke centers have neurosurgeons, neurologists, neurologic intensive care units, interventional radiologists, and extensive rehabilitation services. These tertiary facilities support the acute stroke-ready hospitals and primary stroke centers through education, streamlined transfer, and acute specialized treatment.

In the emergency department, initial management of suspected stroke includes assessment of the ABCs (airway, breathing, and circulation) and vital signs. The airway should be secured; oxygen administered by nasal cannula; a cardiac monitor, pulse oximeter, and sphygmomanometer attached; intravenous access established; a physical examination performed; and an emergent, noncontrast head CT scan obtained. In addition, a 12-lead ECG, portable chest radiograph, and laboratory tests (as described previously) are indicated. If hemorrhage has occurred, a neurosurgeon should be contacted. If ischemic stroke has occurred, a neurologist should be consulted and thrombolytic therapy should be rapidly administered if the patient meets the criteria.

Careful blood pressure management is necessary in the acute ischemic stroke setting. Patients who have a stroke commonly have elevated blood pressure after the acute event. The conscious stroke patient is usually anxious. The blood pressure will often fall when the patient is moved to a quieter room and allowed to rest after completion of the initial evaluation. There is evidence that an acute hypertensive response may represent a beneficial compensatory response to maintain cerebral perfusion.[11] If the brain is already ischemic, lowering of the blood pressure may only exacerbate hypoperfusion and injury. Therefore, except when the blood pressure is extremely high, it is best not to lower it during the first few days after an ischemic infarction. After that time, the blood pressure usually returns to the previous baseline value without additional treatment. More recent studies also demonstrate no difference in mortality or morbidity between patients whose blood pressure was lowered versus those who were not treated for elevated blood pressure at the time of the acute stroke.[12] Patients with a systolic blood pressure of more than 220 mm Hg or a diastolic blood pressure of more than 120 mm Hg and medical conditions requiring blood pressure control may require medical intervention.

If an antihypertensive drug is necessary, labetalol is currently one of several choices. The drug is given orally if the patient is not dysphasic, or intravenously.[11] Oral lisinopril has also been studied. Both are effective at lowering dangerously high blood pressure after stroke without significant risk of long-term adverse outcomes. Sublingual calcium antagonists should not be used because of their rapid absorption and sometimes precipitous decline in blood pressure. If antihypertensive therapy is necessary, blood pressure reduction should be gradual and gentle, and the patient should be carefully monitored. The therapy should be discontinued if there is any neurologic deterioration. In patients with subarachnoid hemorrhage, the blood pressure should be reduced to prestroke levels.

Thrombolytic Therapy

In June 1996, the U.S. Food and Drug Administration approved the use of intravenous recombinant tissue plasminogen activator (tPA) for treatment of appropriately selected patients with ischemic stroke if it is administered within 3 hours from the onset of symptoms. Despite an increased incidence of bleeding complications,[13] studies show a significant reduction in neurologic disability in patients treated with tPA compared with patients treated in the conventional manner.[14] The time to treatment is the most important determinant of success in treating ischemic stroke (the sooner thrombolytic therapy is started, the better the outcome). Inclusion criteria for use of tPA include age of 18 years or older, clinical diagnosis of ischemic stroke, and time of onset less than 180 minutes before tPA administration. The exclusion criteria list is much longer, focusing primarily on evidence of current bleeding or a risk of bleeding that is sufficient to outweigh potential benefits of tPA treatment. Because tPA is the only approved specific treatment of acute ischemic stroke and many patients do not fulfill the criteria for its use, the major goals of stroke management are to limit the size of the infarction, to prevent and to treat complications, and to prevent recurrences. Guidelines revised in 2009 now expand the window for administration of tPA to 4.5 hours. However, new exclusions have been added.[14] People receiving oral anticoagulation agents, those with a history of diabetes and previous stroke, those older than 80 years, and patients with an NIH Stroke Scale score of more than 25 are excluded from receiving tPA in the 3- to 4.5-hour expanded window.[15]

Surgery

Certain types of stroke may require urgent neurosurgical intervention. Neurosurgical consultation is indicated in cases of subarachnoid hemorrhage, intracerebral hemorrhage, and increased intracranial pressure causing neurologic compromise.

Carotid endarterectomy has been demonstrated to have a beneficial effect (compared with medical therapy alone) in patients with carotid stenosis of more than 70% to 80%, but the role of endarterectomy for patients with lesser degrees of stenosis has not been clearly established. The benefit of surgery must be weighed against potential perioperative morbidity and mortality.

Carotid endarterectomy is strongly indicated in patients with hemispheric ACVS (TIA) and in 70% to 99% of patients with ipsilateral carotid stenosis; it should be undertaken as soon as possible in these patients because of the high risk of a full stroke.[16] Surgery for intracranial or vertebrobasilar disease has not been shown to be of any benefit.

Subarachnoid hemorrhage can be treated by interventional radiology through introduction of a coil into the aneurysm, but time is critical in getting a patient to an appropriate center.

In intracerebral stroke, interventions can include placement of a ventriculostomy to measure intracranial pressure. Surgical intervention to relieve pressure may be indicated.

Antiplatelet Agents

Numerous studies have demonstrated a benefit of antiplatelet agents in reducing stroke risk in patients who have had ACVS (TIA) or minor stroke.[17] The relative benefit of antiplatelet therapy is remarkably constant regardless of age, gender, blood pressure, and the presence or absence of diabetes. Aspirin is the standard medical therapy for ACVS (TIA) and ischemic stroke prevention. The optimum dose remains somewhat controversial, but there is increasing evidence that lower doses are as effective as higher doses and have fewer gastrointestinal side effects. Currently prescribed regimens range from 85 to 325 mg every day. A meta-analysis of six major studies involving more than 94,000 people showed that the benefit of aspirin in preventing stroke is greater than any risk.[18]

Warfarin (Coumadin) is indicated for ACVS (TIA) and stroke prevention in patients at risk for cardiac embolism. This includes patients with chronic or paroxysmal atrial fibrillation, left ventricular dysfunction with congestive heart failure, and artificial cardiac valves.

A class of antiplatelet drugs, the thienopyridines, is modestly more effective than aspirin, but the degree of additional benefit is unclear. Two representative drugs from this class are clopidogrel (Plavix) and ticlopidine (Ticlid). Ticlopidine, however, has potential side effects, which can include diarrhea, thrombotic thrombocytopenic purpura, and neutropenia. These risks require hematologic monitoring. Ticlopidine should be reserved for patients who are intolerant of or allergic to aspirin therapy or who have failed to respond to aspirin therapy. Dipyridamole (Persantine) in combination with aspirin demonstrates rates of recurrence similar to those of clopidogrel.[18,19]

Reversal of anticoagulation must be initiated when a patient with a head bleed is on anticoagulation agents, including warfarin, the new generation of anticoagulants that do not require regular monitoring of bleeding time (direct thrombin inhibitors, novel oral anticoagulants), and antiplatelet drugs such as clopidogrel and aspirin.[20]

Vitamin K and 3- or 4-factor prothrombin complex concentrate are used to reverse the effects of warfarin. Clopidogrel and aspirin reversal may be aided by administration of platelets; however, the amount needed is significant.

Protamine can be administered for heparin and low-molecular-weight heparin products.

The lack of an antidote for newer agents such as dabigatran continues to be cause for concern. Hemodialysis and prothrombin complex are the only current options. Research is ongoing, and newer reversal agents and new anticoagulation agents that have unique reversal drugs may be emerging.[20]

LIFE SPAN CONSIDERATIONS

Pregnancy

Stroke during pregnancy is a major tragedy but fortunately rare. In a retrospective study of hospital admissions for delivery in the United Kingdom, the incidence was found to be 1.5 cases per 100,000 deliveries.[21] Risk factors include a history of migraine, gestational diabetes, and preeclampsia. The health care provider can best address this through pregnancy preparation counseling for all fertile women, stressing the need for early and complete prenatal care as well as risk identification and management. Extreme weight change, proteinuria, or elevated blood pressure in the gravid patient requires early intervention.

Geriatric Patients

Stroke will disproportionately affect older persons. In older adults, especially the very old and those with comorbid conditions, therapeutic interventions such as surgery and thrombolysis can be contraindicated. In these situations, comprehensive assessment of need will help determine where appropriate care can be provided. Some will retain sufficient capacities that they can return home with supportive services. Many others will require skilled nursing care.

Age is a direct predictor of both mortality and morbidity, with the oldest patients more likely to die and/or need extended care.[22] Death rates within the first year can be as high as 35% for white women older than 65 years.[23] It is critical that the health care provider know the patient's intentions regarding end-of-life care. It is not sufficient to know whether a patient desires intubation or defibrillation in case of respiratory or cardiac arrest. A clear statement about the use of feeding tubes or intravenous hydration can be extremely helpful in directing care. A surrogate decision maker must be identified, and his or her role defined through advance directives. More important, health care providers should learn what a patient values in life to help guide decisions when impairments may significantly affect those aspects that bring meaning. In this way, care can be tailored to the patient's desires. Ideally, stroke patients should be referred for palliative care consultation. This specialty addresses the issues of comfort, end-of-life decisions, community resources, family engagement, and education. Palliative care consultation also helps patients and families make informed decisions about ongoing care and the effectiveness and value of other interventions.

COMPLICATIONS

The complications of stroke affect virtually every organ system. Early complications of stroke include cerebral edema, increased intracranial pressure, pulmonary and urinary tract infections, sepsis, seizures, hypertension, hypotension, cardiac arrhythmias, myocardial ischemia and infarction, deep venous thrombosis, pulmonary embolism, dysphagia, dysarthria, pressure sores, depression, and extension or progression of the stroke. Later complications include permanent residual problems with mobility, activities of daily living, communication, nutrition, swallowing, behavior, continence, sexual function, limb contractures, and dementia.

A patient with an acute stroke should be admitted to the hospital, with management directed toward limiting, if possible, the amount of brain injury and preventing or ameliorating the constellation of potential complications. Complications in the hospitalized stroke patient include pneumonia, seizures, myocardial infarction, deep venous thrombosis, pressure ulcers, hyperglycemia, hypoglycemia, depression, limb contractures, and constipation. Awareness of these potential complications and specific therapies directed toward their prevention will dramatically reduce the stroke patient's morbidity and mortality. Of particular importance is physical, occupational, and speech therapy, which should be initiated as soon as the patient is medically stable and able to participate.

INDICATIONS FOR REFERRAL OR HOSPITALIZATION

All patients with suspected ACVS (TIA) or stroke should be referred to the hospital emergency department. Time is critical. Any patient seen in an outpatient setting with strokelike symptoms should be transported immediately for evaluation and CT scan and to a center with the ability to implement a tPA protocol. Clear survival benefit exists in those hospitals with dedicated stroke units. Stroke centers are expanding telemedicine to outlying community hospitals, which allows for faster specialist evaluation, expediting both diagnosis and treatment.

Depending on the type of neurologic injury, neurosurgery specialists may be consulted. After the patient has been stabilized, rehabilitation services including physical therapy, occupational therapy, speech therapy, and vocational counseling are employed. Counselors are consulted regarding patient and family issues surrounding a potentially life-altering diagnosis.

Palliative medicine may be helpful in clarifying goals of treatment with patients and family decision makers.

EDUCATION AND HEALTH PROMOTION

Two elements of patient education are paramount: (1) risk factor reduction and (2) stroke symptom recognition and emergency treatment. Hypertension is the most important independent and modifiable risk factor. It is imperative that patients with hypertension be educated about their disease and the importance of medical therapy and lifestyle changes for prevention of complications such as stroke. Cigarette smoking, obesity, diabetes, sedentary lifestyle, and hypercholesterolemia are other modifiable factors that require patient education and treatment.

Atrial fibrillation results in a four to five times greater risk of stroke, and treatment is essential to reducing this risk. Despite the rapid evolution of stroke care and exciting possibilities being investigated, the most important function for the health care provider is aggressive early identification and treatment of at-risk individuals, education for all patients, and appropriate early intervention for those with elevated blood pressure, glucose intolerance, obesity, smoking, and sedentary lifestyles.[24]

The public, particularly those individuals with risk factors, must be educated about the signs and symptoms of ACVS (TIA) and stroke. Public education campaigns urge those who feel they may be having a stroke or those with them to think about the acronym *FAST* (face, arm, speech, time) as a way of identifying the signs of a stroke and to call 911 immediately. The term *brain attack* can be used to convey the same sense of urgency that *heart attack* carries. Factors that have been shown to be associated with delay in treatment include lack of recognition of stroke signs and symptoms, calls made to the health care provider instead of the emergency medical number, living alone, onset while asleep, onset at home rather than at work, and milder severity of stroke. Patients at risk should be taught to recognize the signs and symptoms of a stroke and to call 911 as soon as symptoms occur.

Those patients who do survive have a wide range of physical and psychological impairments, including impairments of motor, sensory, perceptual, cognitive, and communication skills that may seriously interfere with social interactions and ability to engage in normal activities of daily living. The direct and indirect costs for the patient, family, and society are incalculable.

Rehabilitation services are essential to optimize stroke recovery and should begin within 48 hours of stabilization. The recovery stage of stroke requires significant adaptive training for the patient, family, and caregivers. The family itself will be stressed by the recovery process and will need access to counseling, peer support, and other community resources.

CHAPTER 192

DELIRIUM

Karen Dick

DEFINITION AND EPIDEMIOLOGY

Delirium is a serious and significant health problem for older adults and others and one that requires prompt recognition and treatment. Delirium is often the first and only indicator in older adults of underlying physical illness, such as infection, myocardial infarction, or drug toxicity, and it is the leading complication of hospitalization for older adults. Delirium persists in up to 25% of patients and is associated with worse clinical outcomes including higher in-hospital and postdischarge mortality, longer lengths of stay, greater probability of placement in a nursing facility, and the possibility of permanent cognitive impairment.[1]

According to the *Diagnostic and Statistical Manual of Mental Disorders,* Fifth Edition (DSM-5), delirium can develop from a general medical condition, substance intoxication or withdrawal, medications, or multiple causes (Box 192-1).[2] It is characterized by a disturbance in attention, consciousness, and cognition. The hallmark of delirium is a clouding of consciousness, with an inability to focus, sustain, or shift attention, as well as a change in cognition, including impairment in short-term memory, disorientation, and perceptual disturbances.[2] This syndrome can occur in elders at any point across the care continuum, from community and long-term care to acute care settings. Once thought to be transient, delirium symptoms can last weeks to months. Persistent delirium has been associated with worse long-term cognitive and functional outcomes than delirium that has resolved.[3]

BOX 192-1

Diagnostic Criteria for Delirium

A. A disturbance in attention (i.e., reduced ability to direct, focus, sustain, and shift attention) and awareness (reduced orientation to the environment).
B. The disturbance develops over a short period of time (usually hours to a few days), represents a change from baseline attention and awareness, and tends to fluctuate in severity during the course of a day.
C. An additional disturbance in cognition (e.g., memory deficit, disorientation, language, visuospatial ability, or perception).
D. The disturbances in Criteria A and C are not better explained by another preexisting, established, or evolving neurocognitive disorder and do not occur in the context of a severely reduced level of arousal, such as coma.
E. There is evidence from the history, physical examination, or laboratory findings that the disturbance is a direct physiologic consequence of another medical condition, substance intoxication or withdrawal (i.e., caused by a drug of abuse or a medication), or exposure to a toxin, or is a result of multiple etiologies.

Reprinted with permission from the Diagnostic and Statistical Manual of Mental Disorders, Fifth Edition, (Copyright 2013). American Psychiatric Association.

The incidence estimates for delirium in hospitalized patients range widely, from 11% to 82%, because of both sampling and diagnostic criteria.[1] Patients who have undergone hip fracture repair are particularly prone to delirium, with incidence rates ranging from 35% to 65%.[4] Delirium has also been described in patients at the end of life, particularly in patients with advanced cancer, and is very common in intensive care unit (ICU) patients. Delirium is also a common problem in long-term and subacute settings. It has been suggested that many patients who become delirious are never recognized as such and may be incorrectly labeled as having dementia, a psychiatric disorder, or unmanageable behavior.[1] Patients with an underlying dementia are at even greater risk for development of delirium in the setting of acute illness, which is known as delirium superimposed on dementia (DSD).[5]

The prevalence of DSD ranges from 22% to 89% in hospitalized individuals 65 years and older and warrants careful monitoring of patients at risk who enter the health care setting with an acute problem.[5] Eight percent to 17% of all older adults seen in the emergency room are delirious. This number rises to 40% for nursing home residents who come to the emergency room.[1]

Physician consultation is indicated for patients with delirium.

PATHOPHYSIOLOGY

The exact cause of delirium remains a topic of disagreement. Several mechanisms have been proposed that might explain the physiologic precipitant underlying the development of delirium[6-8]: (1) an insufficiency of cerebral metabolism as demonstrated by diffuse slowing on an electroencephalogram in a patient with delirium; (2) a central abnormality caused by an imbalance of central cholinergic and adrenergic metabolism; (3) the activation of cytokines; (4) a stress reaction as evidenced by abnormally high circulating corticosteroid levels and an abnormality in brain network connectivity and changes in inhibitory tone. All of these can contribute to the disruption of neurotransmission.

Despite the continuing disagreement as to the exact mechanism, the acetylcholine theory has drawn more attention of late. Patients with Alzheimer dementia have decreased acetylcholine because of loss of cholinergic neurons and are at high risk of delirium. Anticholinergic drugs are known to precipitate delirium, and certain metabolic abnormalities may decrease acetylcholine synthesis in the central nervous system and contribute to the development of delirium. There is also some evidence that even drugs used commonly in the elderly, such as digoxin, furosemide, prednisone, and theophylline, may have anticholinergic activity.[9] Increased levels of anticholinergic activity have been shown to correlate with the severity of delirium in some hospitalized elderly patients.

It is likely that several physiologic, psychological, and environmental variables, in combination with the known effects of the normal aging process, contribute to the development of delirium.

CLINICAL PRESENTATION

Delirium occurs acutely during hours to days and is characterized by fluctuations in mental status during the course of the day. This fluctuating presentation is problematic because patients may have periods of lucidity interspersed with inattention and high distractibility, motor restlessness, speech that is difficult to follow, and perceptual disturbances that range from misinterpretations of the environment to frank visual hallucinations. Memory, particularly in relation to recent events, is often impaired, and disorientation, most commonly to time (day of the week or time of the year) or place, is usually present. Patients may also exhibit affective signs of fear, anxiety, or anger. They may have a history of a fragmented and disordered sleep-wake cycle. Symptoms may be worse in the late afternoon or evening, which is labeled sundowning; however, it is not clear whether sundowning is a component of delirium or a separate clinical condition.[10] Patients with a history of dementia are at greatest risk for sundowning.

Clinical subtypes of delirium that have been identified include hyperactive, hypoactive, and mixed variants.[11] The hyperactive subtype, manifesting with agitation and restlessness, is often thought of as the typical presentation of delirium. Surprisingly, these cases account for less than 25% of all cases but have the worst outcomes, including nursing home placement or death within 1 month.[12] The hypoactive subtype includes patients who have decreased alertness, sparse or slow speech, lethargy, slowed movements, and apathy. These patients may be somnolent or stuporous. Because these patients are quiet and do not present increased demands for care or surveillance from family or nursing staff, the chance that these patients will not be identified as delirious is high. However, in one study of hip fracture patients that looked at both delirium severity and psychomotor types, patients with pure hypoactive delirium had better outcomes than did patients with hyperactive delirium, even after adjustment for severity.[12] The mixed variant subtype includes symptoms of both hyperactive and hypoactive delirium, with patients cycling between the two; this accounts for more than 50% of cases. These patients often are not identified as being delirious until they become agitated and confused with more symptoms of the hyperactive state.

Because the diagnosis of delirium is based on history, physical examination, or laboratory evidence of an underlying medical condition, careful attention to other symptoms and conditions is necessary. A careful history from family or caregivers is imperative, especially in community-dwelling older adults.

In long-term care, the nursing staff can provide invaluable information as to subtle changes in behavior, appetite, or functional status that may be the warning signs of an underlying problem. Urinary tract infection and pneumonia in the frail nursing home patient often manifest with an altered mental status as the only indicator of an underlying problem.

Polypharmacy and biologic vulnerability for adverse effects make the older person more prone to medication-induced delirium, and a thorough review of all medications, including prescription and over-the-counter preparations, is an essential part of the assessment process.[13] Anticholinergic medications have long been implicated as a risk factor for delirium, and although research results have been mixed as to the strength of the association and the relationship to severity of symptoms, these medications need to be discontinued whenever possible.[14] The patient's use of alcohol and other substances also needs to be evaluated and validated with family members when possible.

It is also important to assess psychosocial and sociocultural factors to better understand the patient's baseline personality and psychological functioning. For patients admitted to the hospital, information from family members or long-term care facilities can be critical in understanding premorbid behavior and function.

PHYSICAL EXAMINATION

In an attempt to identify the precipitating medical condition, a thorough review of systems and a comprehensive physical examination should be undertaken. This may be difficult, however, if the patient is unable to answer questions or to follow even simple commands. A detailed history from family members or other caregivers becomes critical in identifying the onset and development of symptoms and in establishing a sudden change in affect, cognition, or behavior. A neurologic examination is necessary to exclude trauma and focal signs suggestive of a central nervous system disturbance (e.g., traumatic brain injury, tumor, stroke, seizure).

Careful observation of the patient's gait, level of consciousness, speech, appearance, and interactions with others can be most helpful in establishing a diagnosis. Mental status testing is important to establish the degree of cognitive impairment but may have to be modified if the patient is unable to cooperate with the examination. Patients with delirium are often unable to pay attention well enough to answer questions on a standard cognitive screening examination. Assessment tools that have been developed specifically for the diagnosis of delirium include the Delirium Rating Scale–revised version[15] and the Confusion Assessment Method (Table 192-1).[16] Both are capable of assessing the complex features of delirium and of distinguishing delirium from dementia, and both are feasible for use in delirious patients. The Confusion Assessment Method is now the most widely used tool for evaluation of the presence of delirium. A delirium severity tool (CAM-S) has been developed and allows clinicians to monitor the patient's changing symptoms over time.[17]

DIAGNOSTICS

More than one medical condition may be contributing to the development of delirium, and multiple causes, including substance intoxication or withdrawal, should be considered. The

TABLE 192-1 The Confusion Assessment Method Diagnostic Algorithm

Feature	Assessment Finding
Feature 1: Acute onset and fluctuating course	Usually obtained from a family member or nurse and shown by positive responses to the following questions: Is there evidence of an acute change in mental status from the baseline? Did the abnormal behavior fluctuate during the day—that is, tend to come and go, or to increase and decrease in severity?
Feature 2: Inattention	Shown by a positive response to the following: Did the patient have difficulty focusing attention—for example, being easily distractible or having difficulty keeping track of what was being said?
Feature 3: Disorganized thinking	Shown by a positive response to the following: Was the patient's thinking disoriented or incoherent, such as rambling or irrelevant conversation, unclear or illogical flow of ideas, or unpredictable switching from subject to subject?
Feature 4: Altered level of consciousness	Shown by any answer other than "alert" to the following: Overall, how would you rate this patient's level of consciousness? Normal = alert Hyperalert = vigilant Drowsy, easily aroused = lethargic Difficult to arouse = stupor Unarousable = coma

The diagnosis of delirium requires the presence of features 1 and 2 and either 3 or 4.
From Inouye SK, van Dyck CH, Alessi CA et al: Clarifying confusion: the confusion assessment method, *Ann Intern Med* 113(12):941-948, 1990.

DIAGNOSTICS

Delirium

LABORATORY
CBC and differential
ESR
Platelet count
Serum electrolytes
Serum glucose
Calcium
Magnesium
Phosphorus
BUN
Creatinine
LFTs
Vitamin B_{12}
Folate
Thiamine
Ammonia
Thyroid function tests
Blood and urine toxic screens
Medication levels
Urinalysis and culture

IMAGING
Chest x-ray study

OTHER DIAGNOSTICS
ECG
Head CT or MRI*
Lumbar puncture*

*If indicated.
BUN, blood urea nitrogen; ECG, electrocardiogram; ESR, erythrocyte sedimentation rate; LFTs, liver function tests.

choice of specific diagnostic studies is guided by the history and physical examination and may include computed tomography (CT) or magnetic resonance imaging (MRI) of the head, lumbar puncture, and laboratory studies. A complete blood count (CBC), basic metabolic profile, thyroid function test, drug and alcohol levels, and urine culture and sensitivity should be checked. Although electroencephalography is rarely done, it can be helpful in confirming the diagnosis and will show a characteristic slowing of brain wave activity.[18]

DIFFERENTIAL DIAGNOSIS

DSM-5 diagnostic criteria for delirium mandate that the cause be specified. Specific causes include systemic diseases, primary cerebral disease, metabolic disturbances, intoxication with exogenous substances (drugs or poisons), and withdrawal from drugs or alcohol.[2]

Delirium must be distinguished from other organic and psychiatric syndromes, including dementia and depression. All three of these conditions have manifestations in common and can occur in the same patient at the same time; the interrelationships among them are complex. It is critical to establish the onset of symptoms because unlike depression and dementia,

DIFFERENTIAL DIAGNOSIS

Delirium

SYSTEMIC DISEASES
- Infections: urinary tract, pneumonia, subacute bacterial endocarditis, meningitis, Lyme disease
- Myocardial infarction, congestive heart failure, arrhythmias, pulmonary embolus
- Anemia

PRIMARY CEREBRAL DISEASE
- Cerebrovascular accident
- Transient ischemic attack
- Subdural hematoma
- Temporal arteritis
- Seizure

METABOLIC DISTURBANCES
- Dehydration
- Elevation or decrease in sodium, calcium, magnesium, potassium
- Acid-base imbalance
- Hypoxia
- Hypoglycemia
- Hepatic insufficiency
- Renal insufficiency
- Thyroid dysfunction
- Vitamin deficiencies

INTOXICATION
- Alcohol
- Anticholinergics
- Narcotics
- Sedative-hypnotics
- Antidepressants
- Nonsteroidals
- Heavy metal poisons

WITHDRAWAL
- Alcohol
- Benzodiazepines
- Sedatives and hypnotics
- Narcotics

delirium is acute in onset. A psychiatric referral may be necessary to establish a diagnosis.

MANAGEMENT

Treatment of delirium is both definitive and palliative. Current practice remains empirically based without consensus for evidence-based guidelines for diagnosis and management.[19] Definitive care is aimed at identification and treatment of the precipitating causes; palliative care is directed toward the management of symptoms, such as agitation, restlessness, and hallucinations.[13] Studies have suggested that an interdisciplinary, nonpharmacologic approach may be effective.[20,21] In general, nonessential medications need to be tapered or discontinued. The sleep-wake cycle needs to be regulated and sensory deficits corrected. The patient should be in a setting that provides necessary medical interventions and close behavioral monitoring and that maintains patient safety. Interventions such as frequent reorientation, reduced stimulation, and a calm and comforting approach can be helpful. Attention to hydration and toileting needs as well as frequent visits and short periods of ambulation can be helpful. Families can often provide a stabilizing presence and can assist with establishing a reassuring and familiar routine. Physical and chemical restraints should be avoided whenever possible.

Antipsychotic medications such as haloperidol and droperidol may be useful in controlling agitation and psychosis, although there is no compelling evidence that demonstrates improvement in the prognosis of delirium with their use. Dosage should be guided by the patient's initial response and by frequent reassessment. Typically the lowest effective dose is employed. Newer antipsychotics such as risperidone, quetiapine, and olanzapine may be used in small doses for behavior management in the short term when patient or staff safety is compromised. Benzodiazepines are useful in the treatment of alcohol and sedative withdrawal. The goals of treatment are to promote recovery, to prevent additional complications, to maintain the patient's safety, and to maximize function.

COMPLICATIONS

Delirium contributes to increased morbidity and mortality, longer hospital stays, functional impairment, and more permanent forms of cognitive impairment if it is not recognized and treated in a timely fashion.[1] It has been suggested that an episode of delirium may represent the unmasking of an unrecognized dementia in the setting of an acute illness. Patients who become delirious during a hospitalization have longer lengths of stay and higher rates of referral to skilled nursing facilities on discharge. Although it was once thought that delirium was transient, there is now evidence that functional impairment may persist for up to 6 months after treatment.[22] In a meta-analysis of patients diagnosed with delirium during hospitalization, the mortality rate after an average of 22 months of observation was 38% versus 27% for control patients.[23] Admission to long-term care was also higher for those who had been delirious, at 33% versus only 10 % of controls. Sixty-two percent of delirious patients went on to develop dementia, versus 8.1% of controls.[23]

INDICATIONS FOR REFERRAL OR HOSPITALIZATION

The need to identify, remove, or treat the underlying condition is critical to modification of the delirious state and prevention of subsequent morbidities and complications. Hospitalization is an additional stressor that contributes to delirium, and decisions for treatment should be based on an evaluation of the patient's overall functional status, the caregivers' ability to provide supportive care, and, most important, the patient's safety. Patients are often admitted to the hospital with a diagnosis of mental status change as the search for the underlying cause is actively pursued. Patients with persistent mental status changes may be discharged home from the hospital or rehabilitation settings and may have impaired cognitive functioning when seen by their primary care providers, making transitional care interventions essential.

PATIENT AND FAMILY EDUCATION

Patients who have experienced episodes of delirium report feelings of fear and anxiety and often describe vivid hallucinations. Patients and families need reassurance that the delirium is related to a medical condition and is not a sign that the patient is "crazy," is "losing his mind," or is becoming "senile." Patients also need an opportunity to reflect on the experience and to express their feelings.

Patients with advanced age, preexisting cognitive impairment, or severe, chronic illnesses as well as those taking psychoactive medication are most at risk for delirium.[13,24] Although many of these risk factors are not modifiable, it is important that all caregivers be able to recognize the risks and presenting signs and symptoms of delirium.

CHAPTER 193

DEMENTIA

Karen Dick

DEFINITION AND EPIDEMIOLOGY

Most people enjoy a fruitful and productive period during their later years. However, for 5% to 10% of the population older than 65 years and 45% to 50% of the population older than 85 years, these years are associated with a serious form of cognitive impairment known as dementia.[1] It is estimated that more than 5 million people in the United States—regardless of race, gender, or socioeconomic status—have the most common type of dementia, Alzheimer disease. The Alzheimer's Association estimates that nearly 16 million Americans will have dementia of the Alzheimer type by 2050 unless a cure is found.[1] Alzheimer disease is the sixth leading cause of death in the United States and the only cause of death among the top 10 in the United States that cannot be prevented, cured, or even slowed.[1]

Dementia is often the reason for institutionalization; it accounts for more than 50% of all nursing home admissions, and according to 2010 data, up to 50% of patients residing in nursing homes have dementia.[2] It has long been a common belief that memory loss is an inevitable and incurable part of the aging process, making any clinical intervention useless. However, with the recent advances in research, as evidenced by numerous clinical trials and new drug therapies, early detection, treatment, education, and support for families are even more critical.

The term *dementia* includes several symptoms, including a progressive loss of memory and behavioral changes, which together interfere with independence in activities of daily living. The *Diagnostic and Statistical Manual of Mental Disorders,* Fifth Edition, defines *dementia* under the heading of Major or Mild Neurocognitive Disorders and further divides by type; examples include the following:

- Neurocognitive Disorder Due to Alzheimer Disease
- Frontotemporal Neurocognitive Disorder
- Neurocognitive Disorder with Lewy Bodies
- Vascular Neurocognitive Disorder
- Neurocognitive Disorder Due to Traumatic Brain Injury
- Substance/Medication-Induced Neurocognitive Disorder

The diagnostic criteria for Alzheimer Disease and Vascular neurocognitive disorders are described in Boxes 193-1 and 193-2.[3] These are the two most common types of dementia and account for about 80% to 90% of all dementias in older adults.[4]

Mild Cognitive Impairment

Mild cognitive impairment (MCI) is thought to be a transitional state between normal aging and dementia. Patients may have one of two types: amnestic, characterized by deficits in memory; or nonamnestic, which involves impairments in other cognitive functions. Because it is believed that these patients may progress to dementia at a rate of 10% to 15% a year, MCI is considered a risk factor for all types of dementia, and these patients need close monitoring and follow-up.[5]

PATHOPHYSIOLOGY

Alzheimer Disease

Alzheimer disease is characterized by amyloid plaques and neurofibrillary tangles. Examinations of the brains of patients with Alzheimer disease show atrophy of the cerebral cortex that is usually diffuse but may be more pronounced in the frontal, temporal, and parietal lobes.[6] The degree of atrophy may not correlate with the degree of cognitive impairment. The amyloid hypothesis presumes a central role for abnormal amyloid processing and remains the most widely embraced causative theory.[6] Biochemically, there is disruption to the cortical pathways involved in catecholaminergic, serotonergic, and cholinergic transmission. There is a reduction of choline acetyltransferase, an enzyme found only in cholinergic neurons. Advances in genetic research have included the identification of apolipoprotein E, a protein involved in cholesterol transport linked to Alzheimer disease, and the identification of the β-amyloid gene on chromosome 21. Researchers continue to explore the role of inflammation and oxidative stress and their effects on neuronal health. Clinical trials are under way investigating the effects of antiamyloid therapies including antibody-stimulating vaccines and other drug compounds.

Vascular Dementia

Multiple areas of focal ischemic change characterize vascular dementia, formerly known as multi-infarct dementia. The defining lesion is the lacunar infarct. Lacunae are defined as gaps, missing areas, or holes.[7] The infarctions occur in tiny arteries deep in the brain. Patients with hypertension, diabetes, hyperlipidemia, or peripheral vascular occlusive diseases are at particular risk.[4] Patients may have a mixed dementia with both Alzheimer and vascular types.

BOX 193-1

Diagnostic Criteria for Major and Mild Neurocognitive Disorder Due to Alzheimer Disease

A. The criteria are met for major or mild neurocognitive disorder.

B. There is insidious onset and gradual progression of impairment in one or more cognitive domains (for major neurocognitive disorder, at least two domains must be impaired).

C. Criteria are met for either probable or possible Alzheimer's disease as follows:

For major neurocognitive disorder.

Probable Alzheimer's disease is diagnosed if either of the following is present; otherwise, *possible Alzheimer's disease* should be diagnosed.

1. Evidence of a causative Alzheimer's disease genetic mutation from family history or genetic testing.
2. All three of the following are present:
   a. Clear evidence of decline in memory and learning and at least one other cognitive domain (based on detailed history or serial neuropsychological testing).
   b. Steadily progressive, gradual decline in cognition, without extended plateaus.
   c. No evidence of mixed etiology (i.e., absence of other neurodegenerative or cerebrovascular disease, or another neurological, mental, or systemic disease or condition likely contributing to cognitive decline).

For mild neurocognitive disorder:

Probable Alzheimer's disease is diagnosed if there is evidence of a causative Alzheimer's disease genetic mutation from either genetic testing or family history.

Possible Alzheimer's disease is diagnosed if there is no evidence of a causative Alzheimer's disease genetic mutation from either genetic testing or family history, and all three of the following are present:

1. Clear evidence of decline in memory and learning.
2. Steadily progressive, gradual decline in cognition, without extended plateaus.
3. No evidence of mixed etiology (i.e., absence of other neurodegenerative or cerebrovascular disease, or another neurological or systemic disease or condition likely contributing to cognitive decline).

D. The disturbance is not better explained by cerebrovascular disease, another neurodegenerative disease, the effects of a substance, or another mental, neurological, or systemic disorder.

(Reprinted with permission from the Diagnostic and Statistical Manual of Mental Disorders, Fifth Edition, (Copyright 2013). American Psychiatric Association.)

Lewy Body Dementia

Lewy body dementia is characterized by the presence of Lewy bodies in the brain. These are proteins that enter neurons and cause cell degeneration and death. There is a loss of dopamine-producing neurons, similar to that seen in Parkinson disease, and a loss of acetylcholine, similar to that seen in Alzheimer disease.[8]

Pseudodementia

Depression in older adults can lead to memory loss, attention deficits, and problems with initiation, and is referred to as *pseudodementia.* Clinicians need to be aware that depression may go untreated, especially with patients not complaining of sadness

BOX 193-2

Diagnostic Criteria for Major or Mild Vascular Neurocognitive Disorder

A. The criteria are met for major or mild neurocognitive disorder.
B. The clinical features are consistent with a vascular etiology, as suggested by either of the following:
   1. Onset of the cognitive deficits is temporally related to one or more cerebrovascular events.
   2. Evidence for decline is prominent in complex attention (including processing speed) and frontal-executive function.
C. There is evidence of the presence of cerebrovascular disease from history, physical examination, and/or neuroimaging considered sufficient to account for the neurocognitive deficits.
D. The symptoms are not better explained by another brain disease or systemic disorder.

Probable vascular neurocognitive disorder is diagnosed if one of the following is present; othenwise *possible vascular neurocognitive disorder* should be diagnosed:
   1. Clinical criteria are supported by neuroimaging evidence of significant parenchymal injury attributed to cerebrovascular disease (neuroimaging-supported).
   2. The neurocognitive syndrome is temporally related to one or more documented cerebrovascular events.
   3. Both clinical and genetic (e.g., cerebral autosomal dominant arteriopathy with subcortical infarcts and leukoencephalopathy) evidence of cerebrovascular disease is present.

Possible vascular neurocognitive disorder is diagnosed if the clinical criteria are met but neuroimaging is not available and the temporal relationship of the neurocognitive syndrome with one or more cerebrovascular events is not established.

(Reprinted with permission from the Diagnostic and Statistical Manual of Mental Disorders, Fifth Edition, (Copyright 2013). American Psychiatric Association.)

BOX 193-3

Stages of Alzheimer Disease

EARLY-STAGE DEMENTIA

- Memory loss
- Time and spatial disorientation
- Poor judgment
- Personality changes
- Withdrawal or depression
- Perceptual disturbances

MIDDLE-STAGE DEMENTIA

- Recent and remote memory worsens
- Increased aphasia (slowed speech and understanding)
- Apraxia
- Hyperorality
- Disorientation to place and time
- Restlessness or pacing
- Perseveration
- Irritability
- Loss of impulse control

LATE-STAGE DEMENTIA

- Incontinence of urine and feces
- Loss of motor skills, rigidity
- Decreased appetite and dysphagia
- Agnosia
- Apraxia
- Severely impaired communication
- Possible inability to recognize family members or self in mirror
- Loss of most or all self-care abilities
- Severely impaired cognition
- Depressed immune system

or anxiety, which may lead to impairments in cognition. A complicating factor is that older adults with depression may be at increased risk of dementia. To complicate this more, depression may be a common early dementia presentation.[9] A therapeutic trial of antidepressants and subsequent reevaluation of mood and cognition should be pursued to appropriately diagnose one or both conditions.

CLINICAL PRESENTATION

Memory loss, personality changes, language disturbances, and problems with independent activities of daily living are common presenting symptoms of dementia. A concerned family member or friend typically makes the initial presentation to a health care provider. It may take months to years for family members to seek medical attention because subtle changes in cognition may be overlooked or attributed to old age. Patients with dementia do not typically worry about what is wrong with them. These patients often have little understanding of the seriousness of their symptoms or of safety concerns (e.g., driving, cooking). On the other hand, patients with depression or benign forgetfulness often appear to the health care provider to be overly concerned about minor symptoms (e.g., forgetting a name, misplacing keys). An anecdotal finding in primary care is that patients worried about memory problems often have only minor problems, whereas patients who seem unconcerned pose a major worry to providers.

Patients with Lewy body dementia may have visual hallucinations, motor impairments, postural instability, and sleep disturbances. They also show an increased sensitivity to neuroleptics; these are the patients who, when given drugs such as haloperidol for acute agitation, get worse.[8]

Alzheimer disease is commonly divided into three stages: early, middle, and late (Box 193-3). The initial symptom is typically short-term memory loss. The earliest stage is often accompanied by symptoms of anxiety and depression. Word finding and naming problems may emerge as symptoms progress. The second stage is characterized by a worsening of memory and language as well as judgment. Disorientation to time and place is common. There may be neuropsychiatric symptoms, including paranoia, hallucinations, and delusional thinking. Urinary incontinence may be a problem. The final stage is characterized by motor rigidity, prominent neurologic abnormalities including apraxia and agnosia, severe cognitive and language impairment, and death. The average duration of the disease from diagnosis until death is 9 years.[9] Staging of a patient's disease based on clinical presentation and examination can be helpful to patients and families in planning subsequent care and treatment.

PHYSICAL EXAMINATION

The basic components of an evaluation for dementia include a careful and detailed history from family members or caregivers and a complete physical and neurologic examination. A thorough review of all medications, including any over-the-counter products (sleeping medications; anticholinergic cold remedies; herbal, homeopathic, or nutritional supplements), should also be addressed. The use of alcohol or other substances should be carefully reviewed and documented. The physical examination should focus on neurologic signs; blood pressure; carotid bruits; and the assessment of cognition, mood, function, and behavior. Many screening tools are available. The Katz Index of Independence in Activities of Daily Living or the "get up and go" test can be used to evaluate function.[10,11] The Folstein Mini-Mental State Examination (MMSE), the Montreal Cognitive Assessment (MoCA), and the Mini-Cog are useful tools for evaluation of cognition.[12,13] The Mini-Cog combines the clock drawing test with three-item recall, and performance in diverse populations is comparable to that found with the MMSE.[12] The MoCA has consistently been found to be accurate in detecting minimal cognitive impairment.[14] Other tools include the General Practitioner Assessment of Cognition (GPCOG) and the Memory Impairment Screen (MIS).[15] The Geriatric Depression Scale (Short Form) has been shown to be both valid and reliable in clinical practice for assessment of mood.[16] One of the benefits of these tools is the ability to compare scores year to year to provide families with an objective description of disease progression. It is also important to assess and to monitor for changes in behavior, specifically anxiety, restlessness, aggression, delusions, visual or auditory hallucinations, and wandering. There are also a number of tools that can be completed by family members or caregivers; these tools collect observations that can be invaluable in adding to the comprehensiveness of the patient workup. Examples of common patient and informant tools can be found on the Alzheimer's Association website (www.alz.org) in the health care professionals section under "Cognitive Assessment Toolkit."[15]

DIAGNOSTICS

Because dementia has no single standard test and is a disease of exclusion, the diagnostic evaluation should determine whether the patient has a reversible condition that may be contributing to or causing cognitive decline. The most important tests include a complete blood count (CBC), thyroid-stimulating hormone (TSH) concentration, vitamin B_{12} and folate levels, and a metabolic screen. Medications that have measurable levels, such as digoxin, carbamazepine (Tegretol), theophylline, and divalproex sodium (Depakote), should be measured. Current research is centered on refining biomarkers for clinical diagnosis of preclinical disease, MCI, and dementia.

Imaging studies are useful in identifying mass lesions, vascular lesions, or infections but do not confirm a diagnosis of dementia. All guidelines recommend a baseline brain imaging study; a non–contrast-enhanced computed tomography (CT) scan is adequate. However, many providers prefer magnetic resonance imaging (MRI) because of its better resolution for patients with primary attentional or frontal temporal syndromes or if subcortical pathology or stroke is suspected.[9] Positron emission tomography (PET) and single-photon emission computed tomography (SPECT) may be useful in difficult-to-diagnose cases. Referral for neuropsychological testing can also be useful for differentiation between MCI and dementia and between dementia and depression.

DIFFERENTIAL DIAGNOSIS

Dementia has innumerable causes that cannot always be determined by diagnostic evaluation. Some dementia syndromes (e.g., Pick disease, Alzheimer disease) are characterized by a lack of neurologic signs; others are associated with a definitive neurologic disease, such as Huntington disease, diffuse Lewy body disease, and human immunodeficiency virus (HIV) infection. Delirium and depression are treatable conditions that may manifest with the same symptoms as dementia; however, errors on mental status testing will differ. Patients with dementia have a normal level of consciousness without inattention. Patients with depression often answer questions with "I don't know," whereas those with dementia may confabulate an answer.

Medical illnesses, drug overdoses, adverse effects of medication (especially anticholinergics or anxiolytics), sensory

DIAGNOSTICS

Dementia

LABORATORY
CBC
LFTs
TSH
Vitamin B_{12}
Folate
Serum electrolytes
BUN
Creatinine
Serum glucose
Drug and alcohol levels*

IMAGING
Non–contract-enhanced CT scan or MRI

*If indicated.
BUN, blood urea nitrogen; LFTs, liver function tests.

DIFFERENTIAL DIAGNOSIS

Dementia

- Alcoholic dementia
- Medication, organic toxin, heavy metal intoxication
- Medical illness
  - Liver disease
  - Hypothyroidism
  - Chronic hypoglycemia
  - Adrenal insufficiency
  - Cushing disease
- Vitamin deficiency
  - Thiamine
  - Vitamin B_{12}
  - Folic acid
- Neoplasm and paraneoplastic syndromes
- Trauma, subdural hematoma, hydrocephalus
- Infectious disease
  - HIV dementia
  - Viral encephalopathy, herpes simplex virus infection
  - Syphilis, Lyme disease, *Borrelia* infection
  - Toxoplasmosis, cryptococcosis, cytomegalovirus infection
- Depression
- Vasculitis
- Alzheimer dementia
- Vascular dementia
- Pick disease
- Diffuse Lewy body dementia
- Huntington disease
- Creutzfeldt-Jakob disease
- Shy-Drager syndrome
- Progressive supranuclear palsy
- Parkinson disease and other movement disorders

impairments, and nutritional deficits are all part of the differential diagnosis.

MANAGEMENT

Management of dementia depends on the stage of the disease. The family and community supports required are often the same for vascular dementia and Alzheimer disease. The goal of management includes treatment of all correctable factors that may impair cognition to improve daily functioning and to delay disability. Activities that promote and enhance cognition and social engagement are to be encouraged.

It is important to address safety concerns, including driving competency, soon after the diagnosis is made. Laws regarding mandatory reporting of unsafe drivers vary from state to state and can be confirmed by calling the state department of motor vehicles. A kitchen safety evaluation alerts caregivers to possible problems with cooking. A health care proxy and durable power of attorney for health care can help prevent conflicts regarding intensity of medical care later in the course of the disease. A discussion of the patient's preference for resuscitation and technology should take place while the patient is still able to participate. Encouraging families to contact the local chapter of the Alzheimer's Association is an important step; through this association, caregivers can gain support, obtain reading material to promote understanding of the disease and behavior management, and determine the availability of respite care. Many websites and online support groups can help family members access and share information.

Although studies of vitamin E use in patients with Alzheimer disease have had mixed results, supplementation with 2000 IU of vitamin E daily is reasonable to consider in appropriate patients.[17]

Two classes of drugs are currently approved by the U.S. Food and Drug Administration to treat the cognitive symptoms of dementia: the cholinesterase inhibitors and *N*-methyl-D-aspartate (NMDA) receptor antagonists. The cholinesterase inhibitors include donepezil (Aricept), rivastigmine (Exelon), and galantamine (Razadyne). These drugs can be used for the treatment of mild to moderate dementia for both Alzheimer disease and for patients with vascular dementia. The choice between them is based on cost, mode of delivery (patch, pill, or liquid), individual patient tolerance, and provider experience; efficacy appears to be similar. Memantine (Namenda) is an NMDA receptor antagonist that can be used in combination with a cholinesterase inhibitor for those with moderate to severe disease. Although these medications do not alter the course of dementia, they have been shown to delay or to slow worsening of symptoms.[17] Patients with vascular dementia should continue with optimal treatment of risk factors (e.g., hypertension, hyperglycemia, smoking, hyperlipidemia, diet) that may delay progression.

Patients with a dementia may develop social withdrawal, sleep impairments, and malaise, which are thought to be related to depression but may be entirely caused by cognitive deficits. Depressive symptoms have traditionally been treated with antidepressants, even if the patient does not meet the criteria for major depression. In general, selective serotonin reuptake inhibitors (SSRIs) are preferred as the class of medications to use. Citalopram has been shown to improve other neuropsychiatric symptoms such as agitation and may be useful at doses not exceeding 20 mg/day.[18] It should be avoided in patients at increased risk of arrhythmias. Depression in persons with dementia can often be improved with nonpharmacologic approaches such as exercise and participation in pleasurable activities. Cognitive behavioral therapy may be useful for patients with mild to moderate dementia. Because management may differ, determination of which form of dementia is present is important. In addition, behavior management needs to be individualized. Certain behavioral problems may be amenable to medication or to family education about the avoidance and management of difficult situations.

Providers should avoid use of any antipsychotics, both typical and atypical, for noncognitive symptoms or challenging behaviors unless patients are at risk of harm to themselves or others. An increased risk of cerebrovascular events and a small increased risk of death in patients with dementia have led to "black box" warnings for risperidone, olanzapine, and aripiprazole. Risks and benefits must be discussed with patients and caregivers before use of any of these drugs, and they should be used for the shortest possible duration and at the lowest effective dose.[19]

COMPLICATIONS

Dementia has many complications that vary with the stages of illness. In the early stages, getting lost or having a motor vehicle accident puts patients (and others) at risk. In the middle stage, falls, incontinence, and sleep disturbances may cause further problems. Contractures, pressure ulcers, urinary tract infections, and pneumonia, all a result of immobility, are common in late and final stages of the disease. Deconditioning and nutritional deficits are also commonly seen. Patients may develop apraxia and forget how to chew and swallow. Weight loss becomes inevitable. An inability to communicate as a result of aphasia and an inability to tell caretakers about symptoms lead to further frustration and difficulty in diagnosis of complications. Death is often the result of infectious complications.

INDICATIONS FOR REFERRAL OR HOSPITALIZATION

Many patients with dementia are frail, older adults with multiple medical, nursing, and social service needs. Involvement of other disciplines is helpful for patients, families, and providers. Physical therapists can optimize function by evaluating and recommending exercises or the appropriate adaptive equipment. Driving evaluations and kitchen and home safety evaluations can be performed by occupational therapists. These therapists can also recommend equipment to help with feeding. Speech therapy may be necessary for swallowing or dysphagia assessments in the later stages of dementia. A neurology consultation is often helpful for patients with an unclear clinical picture. A neuropsychologist or geropsychiatrist may be able to differentiate unusual presentations of dementia, especially if depression is present.

Patients with end-stage dementia are eligible for referral to hospice under the Medicare hospice benefit but must meet criteria related to bed-bound status and stage of disease. These hospice services can be provided in the home or in long-term care facilities.

PATIENT AND FAMILY EDUCATION

The focus of patient education is to maintain independence by emphasizing patients' strengths and allowing them to continue normal activities. A woman who is no longer able to follow a recipe may still be able to knead dough and make a loaf of her special bread with help. A grandmother unable to be left alone with her grandchild is still able to rock an infant to sleep and sing a lullaby she once heard as a child. A carpenter may no longer be able to operate electrical shop tools but may still be able to hammer and glue pieces of furniture that have been precut. Feeling robbed of self-esteem is a major detriment to function; education for families is essential. Behavioral guidance, social supports, and recognition of the difficult caregiver role will benefit both patient and caregiver and may prevent illness or injury.

Families need guidance and suggestions regarding the appropriate settings and activities for their loved ones. The decision about nursing home placement is always difficult and usually comes after community services and family support have been maximized. An acute illness or injury often precedes nursing home placement. Adult day care and group homes are appropriate in the early to middle stages of the disease; special care units are used during the middle stages of dementia. These units represent a wide variation in philosophies, goals, and design. Although many families are reluctant to enroll their relative in a program or living arrangement specifically for people with dementia, the focus of activities is at an appropriate level so that patients can participate and enjoy them. The frustration of not being able to participate in activities that are too difficult is minimized. Staff members are specifically trained to handle behavioral problems in nonpharmacologic ways. Persons with late-stage dementia who are unable to participate in activities are often cared for on the general units of a nursing home.

Families also need to be able to recognize the symptoms of medical illness in a person with dementia; families should understand patients' increased susceptibility to delirium (see Chapter 192). Pneumonia without a fever or cough, a myocardial infarction without chest pain, and a urinary tract infection with no urinary symptoms are typical. A change in behavior that is noticeable only to those who know the patient well may be the only sign of illness. Families need to be given resource information about support groups, financial and legal matters, and how to tell family and friends about the diagnosis.

Caregivers can find information and resources at the Alzheimer's Disease Education and Referral (ADEAR) Center website at www.nia.nih.gov/alzheimers.

The Alzheimer's Association (www.alz.org) has state and local chapters and maintains a 24-hour help line at 800-272-3900. Providers can find guidelines for the evaluation and treatment of dementia developed by the American Academy of Neurology, the American Psychiatric Society, and the U.S. Preventive Services Task Force at www.guideline.gov.

Many believe that the future holds great promise in the way we identify and treat patients with dementia. Researchers are looking for ways to detect it at its earliest stages with biomarkers such as blood and cerebrospinal levels and brain imaging; these kinds of diagnostics could identify those at risk so that preventive therapies could be put in place. There are hundreds of clinical trials under way, and patients and families should be encouraged to explore possibilities of participation; information about these can be found on the Alzheimer's Association website.

CHAPTER 194

DIZZINESS AND VERTIGO

Nancy McQueen Le • Katie McCabe

DIZZINESS

DEFINITION AND EPIDEMIOLOGY

It is estimated that dizziness affects 20% to 30% of people in the general population.[1] Dizziness is a common, nonspecific term used to describe a variety of subjective states with varied causes. Clinically, it is helpful to classify dizziness into the categories of vertigo, presyncope or syncope, and disequilibrium. Differentiation of the type of dizziness experienced will dictate the direction of evaluation and treatment.

Vertigo is the illusion of movement of either oneself or the environment—spinning, tilting, or moving back and forth. Vertigo can be related to a peripheral or central disorder. Peripheral causes may include benign paroxysmal positional vertigo (BPPV), vestibular neuronitis, acute labyrinthitis, Meniere disease, ototoxicity, and head trauma. Central disorders include brainstem or cerebellar ischemia or hemorrhage, tumors, multiple sclerosis, and a migrainous syndrome.

Presyncopal lightheadedness is often referred to as a sense of wooziness or impending faint. However, lightheadedness is not exclusive to a presyncopal episode and can be a feeling that manifests in some states of disequilibrium or vertiginous conditions. Cardiac conditions associated with lightheadedness or syncope include arrhythmias, sick sinus syndrome, mitral valve prolapse, aortic stenosis, and heart block. Dehydration, hypotension, and cough or Valsalva-related syncope are common causes of vascular-related syncope or presyncope.

Disequilibrium is a sense of insecurity or imbalance, and/or unsteadiness in walking. Although this feeling is described as dizziness, it often occurs in the absence of abnormal head sensations. Disequilibrium may result from Parkinson disease, peripheral neuropathy, vision disorders, musculoskeletal disorders, or cerebrovascular insults.

The lifetime prevalence estimates of significant dizziness range from 17% to 30%, and for vertigo, 3% to 10%.[2] It has been noted that less than half of patients complaining of dizziness actually have vertigo. Even after evaluation, the largest diagnostic group is represented by dizziness of uncertain cause.

PATHOPHYSIOLOGY

Vertigo is caused by an imbalance in the vestibular system that may result from lesions in the inner ear, vestibular nerve, brainstem, or cerebellum. Less commonly, vertigo may result from lesions in the subjective sensory pathways of the thalamus or cortex or stretch receptors in the neck.[3]

Lightheadedness or presyncope or syncope is most commonly a result of a cardiovascular problem. Causes include orthostatic hypotension, vasovagal episodes, hyperventilation, and decreased cardiac output. Less common causes of lightheadedness are hypoglycemia and seizure activity. It is rarely a manifestation of impending stroke.

Disequilibrium may result from visual impairment, bilateral or unilateral vestibular loss, proprioceptive loss, impaired cerebellar function, or involvement of motor (frontal and basal ganglia) centers. Multisensory disequilibrium describes a syndrome of impaired balance caused by some degree of combined dysfunction in the areas of vestibular, visual, and proprioceptive sensation.[3]

CLINICAL PRESENTATION

Dizziness is an intensely subjective sensation that may be difficult to describe. However, a thorough history will often differentiate the type of dizziness being experienced. It is helpful to start by eliciting a description of the dizziness in the patient's own words, making note of how precise or vague the details are. This description can be further guided through specific questioning and the suggestion of some varied descriptors, especially if the individual is having difficulty articulating his or her sensory experience. Further history is then directed toward defining the characteristics of the dizziness, the time course of individual episodes, the pattern of recurrences, the precipitating and relieving factors, and any associated symptoms. A general medical history must be included, with special focus on neurologic and cardiovascular systems, medication history, and functional history.[3,4]

True vertigo is such a striking phenomenon that it is usually readily and precisely described as a clear sensation of spinning, tilting, rotating, or swaying. Lack of spinning sensation cannot be used to exclude vestibular disease.[5] Associated symptoms can include nausea, vomiting, diaphoresis, disequilibrium, nystagmus, and blurry vision. Ear symptoms, including pain or pressure, tinnitus, and altered hearing, may be present.

Lightheadedness is classically described as a sense of wooziness or impending faint. It is often accompanied by diaphoresis, apprehension, nausea, and, in the extreme, an actual transient "blackout" with diminished vision but with persisting vague awareness of one's surroundings. In these patients, it is important to ask about heart palpitations, chest discomfort, and dyspnea.

Disequilibrium is described as a sense of imbalance or insecurity on rising or when walking. Patients often say they are dizzy when they are not in fact vertiginous or presyncopal but rather "off-kilter." They may have begun to use a cane or "furniture walking" for unclear reasons. The sense of imbalance may be worse in the dark or may be accompanied by changes in gait characterized by a shortened step length and widened base of support.[4,6] When the description elicited is vague or ill defined, it may reflect multifactorial issues. A specific sensory experience in multisensory disequilibrium may be difficult to describe.

Dizziness can also be related to psychogenic causes, such as anxiety states or agoraphobia. Nonspecific dizziness can be caused by hyperventilation; however, if associated with nystagmus, a vestibular cause cannot be excluded. Anxiety and apprehension often accompany physiologic dizziness, so complaints of "dizziness" should not be automatically attributed to a psychogenic cause.

PHYSICAL EXAMINATION

The physical examination in any complaint of dizziness should always include a general medical review as well as a review of medications, including herbals and over-the-counter drugs. This information will guide a more focused examination.

The neurologic examination should include a cognitive screen. Cranial nerves are assessed with particular emphasis on visual acuity, eye movements, and nystagmus. Motor examination should include evaluation of power, muscle tone, coordination, and deep tendon reflexes. Sensory examination emphasizes basic vision and hearing assessments as well as testing of primary sensory modalities. Gait and balance evaluation includes observation of stride, arm swing, tandem gait with eyes opened and then closed, and Romberg sign. Otologic evaluation includes otoscopic examination and hearing assessment including the Weber and Rinne tests.

Cardiovascular evaluation includes cardiac rate and rhythm, auscultation of heart sounds and carotid bruits, and blood pressure measurement. Orthostatic vital signs, both blood pressure and heart rate, should also be determined.

A neuro-otologic examination refers to a number of special examination procedures considered when problems related to vertigo or disequilibrium are suspected, which may be performed in a specialty clinic setting. These procedures specifically assess the vestibulo-ocular and vestibulospinal systems and help distinguish between peripheral disorders and central disorders. They may include evaluation for nystagmus, position testing (Hallpike-Dix maneuver; Box 194-1), head-fixed/body-turn maneuvers, postural sway on a foam surface, and stepping test (marching in place with the eyes closed).[4]

DIAGNOSTICS

If a vestibular lesion is suspected, the Hallpike-Dix positioning maneuver would be performed (see Box 194-1). Further examination might be pursued in consultation with an ear, nose, and throat (ENT) or neurology specialist, including vestibular laboratory testing, an audiogram, or neuroimaging. Vestibular laboratory testing can help differentiate peripheral from central lesions, confirm lateralization of a documented abnormality, and allow serial evaluation for monitoring purposes.[2,4] Furthermore, it can give valuable functional information and help guide physical therapy interventions. Vestibular laboratory studies include electronystagmography, rotational testing, and posturography.

Audiology evaluation, including the Weber and Rinne tests, may have an important adjunctive role in helping establish or confirm a suspected diagnosis. Many disorders resulting in vertigo have associated hearing involvement. The presence or absence of specific hearing findings can help confirm or exclude some conditions, and differentiate a central versus a peripheral cause. Hearing loss is defined as conductive or sensorineural on the basis of the cause.

Neuroimaging may be considered when central (brain) or structural (bony labyrinthine, internal auditory canal) lesions are amenable to visualization. Either a computed tomography

BOX 194-1

Positional Nystagmus Testing (Hallpike-Dix Maneuver)

1. Check the patient for spontaneous nystagmus while he or she is seated on the examining table.
2. Bring the patient quickly back to the recumbent or supine position with the head extended back 30 to 45 degrees over the end of the bed or table and the head tilted 30 to 45 degrees to one side (i.e., one ear down toward the floor).
3. Repeat the previous step two times, once with the head tilted to the left, and then again with the head tilted to the right.
4. Observe the patient for latency, duration, direction, and fatigability of nystagmus, both while positioned down and as helped to upright position.

(CT) scan or magnetic resonance imaging (MRI) is appropriate, depending on what is suspected. Magnetic resonance angiography is used when vertebrobasilar insufficiency is a concern.

If cardiac issues are suspected, evaluation routinely begins with electrocardiography (ECG). Holter monitoring or telemetry may also be indicated if an arrhythmia is suspected. Serial orthostatic vital signs in conjunction with these studies can provide important data. Echocardiography may be indicated to further evaluate cardiac status.

When multisystem disequilibrium is suspected or must be excluded, formal ophthalmologic evaluation is necessary. Assessment of peripheral nerve function by electromyography and nerve conduction velocity in these instances can be definitive.

Electroencephalography may be considered to exclude seizure activity (see Chapter 201). Vertigo, disequilibrium, and lightheadedness are not common manifestations of seizures, and thus such testing is commonly under the guidance of a neurologist.

The choice of laboratory diagnostic studies should be guided by presentation and examination. A basic laboratory review usually includes thyroid-stimulating hormone (TSH) concentration, complete blood count (CBC), electrolyte values, serum glucose concentration, blood urea nitrogen (BUN) concentration, creatinine concentration, vitamin B_{12} level, and rapid plasma reagin (RPR), as indicated.

DIAGNOSTICS

Dizziness and Vertigo

VESTIBULAR DISORDERS
- Audiogram
- CT scan, MRI, magnetic resonance angiography (with gadolinium)*
- Vestibular laboratory testing*
- Electronystagmography
- Posturography

CARDIAC DISORDERS
- ECG
- Holter or event monitor
- Echocardiogram

LABORATORY
- Basic metabolic screen
- Electrolytes
- CBC and differential
- BUN, creatinine
- Serum glucose
- TSH
- Vitamin B_{12}
- RPR*

*If indicated.

DIFFERENTIAL DIAGNOSIS

Clarifying the diagnosis of dizziness begins with differentiating vertigo, lightheadedness, and disequilibrium.

Vertigo is a phenomenon resulting from a vast array of causes. Anatomically and neurologically, it is helpful to start by determining whether the vertigo is caused by a peripheral or central lesion. Peripheral problems refer to problems of the inner ear or cranial nerve VIII. Peripheral lesions include vestibular neuronitis, labyrinthitis, benign positional vertigo, Meniere disease, post-traumatic vertigo, acoustic neuroma, and ototoxic drug–induced conditions.[4] The general hallmarks of these conditions include a higher likelihood of associated nausea, normal neurologic examination findings, and symptoms that are position related. Central or brain disorders usually involve the brainstem or cerebellum and include vertebrobasilar insufficiency or infarction, multiple sclerosis, posterior fossa tumor, basilar migraine, and central nervous system infection (syphilis).[4] Hallmarks of a central cause include associated neurologic findings and vertigo and nausea that are not position related.

Lightheadedness is most commonly related to cardiovascular issues. Diagnostic evaluation should exclude cardiac arrhythmias, critical aortic stenosis, vasovagal response, and orthostatic hypotension (autonomic insufficiency, volume depletion with anemia, drug-induced condition). When a psychogenic cause is suspected, it must be considered only in the context of excluding atypical manifestations of other causes. Possible causes to be considered in the evaluation process include anxiety reactions, agoraphobia, hyperventilation, and depression.

Disequilibrium is sometimes clear from the history. In many cases, the descriptions elicited are imprecise or vague yet seem to suggest balance problems rather than actual dizziness. When a description of balance impairment in the absence of dizziness is clear, the focus turns to evaluation of multisystem impairment, particularly vision and peripheral sensory function. Disequilibrium should be distinguished from complaints that may be based on visual problems or related to psychogenic conditions. Diabetes mellitus is a common cause of a multisystem disequilibrium state. However, a number of other conditions should be considered, including cerebellar disorders, extrapyramidal system disorders, drug toxicity, and posterior fossa tumors.[3]

DIFFERENTIAL DIAGNOSIS

Dizziness and Vertigo

VESTIBULAR DISORDERS

Peripheral
- Benign paroxysmal positional vertigo
- Vestibular neuronitis
- Bacterial labyrinthitis
- Meniere disease
- Nerve damage
  - Ototoxic drugs
  - Head trauma
- Acoustic neuroma
- Perilymphatic fistula
- Physiologic
  - Motion sickness
- Height vertigo

Central
- Vertebrobasilar insufficiency
  - Transitory ischemic attack, cerebrovascular accident
- Multiple sclerosis
- Tumor in posterior fossa
  - Cerebellar pontine angle
  - Brainstem
  - Cerebellar
- Migraine syndrome
- Central nervous system infection
- Cervical dizziness
  - Drop attacks

SYNCOPE
- Cardiac arrhythmias
- Critical aortic stenosis
- Medication effects
- Systemic illness
  - Infection
  - Vasculitis
  - Endocrine (in diabetes)
- Volume depletion
- Valsalva-related syncope
- Hypotension
- Hypoxia
- Severe anemia
- Hyperventilation
- Hypoglycemia
- Psychogenic (anxiety, depression)

DISEQUILIBRIUM (WITHOUT VERTIGO)
- Bilateral vestibular loss
- Sensory ataxias
  - Vitamin B_{12} deficiency
  - Tabes dorsalis
  - Peripheral neuropathy
  - Myelopathy
  - Multisystem disequilibrium
- Cerebellar degeneration syndromes
- Apractic syndromes (frontal lobe syndromes, hydrocephalus, multi-infarct state)
- Extrapyramidal syndromes (Parkinson disease, progressive supranuclear palsy)

MANAGEMENT

Specialist referral is indicated when (1) there are positive neurologic signs, (2) an underlying cardiac disorder is suspected, (3) the diagnosis remains unclear, or (4) there is a lack of response to standard treatments.

Immediate emergency department referral is indicated for patients with acute focal neurologic symptoms or in whom a serious medical condition is suspected. Acute labyrinthitis accompanied by a fever always requires urgent referral and treatment.[3]

The primary goals of treatment are as follows:

- Treat underlying diagnosed conditions.
- Manage the symptoms, which may include medication management as well as physical and vestibular rehabilitation.

COMPLICATIONS

The risk of falling is greatly increased in the patient with dizziness. This is especially problematic in older patients, in whom the risk of fracture is the highest. Intractable nausea or vomiting associated with dizziness, although rare, can be disabling. Side effects of medications, especially anticholinergics or antihistamines, can include drowsiness, urinary retention, and confusion (especially in older patients). Benzodiazepines should be used cautiously because of the side effect profile and the potential for dependence. Other complications are related to the specific cause of the dizziness and may include visual disturbances, tinnitus, decreased hearing, and balance and gait disorders.

EDUCATION AND HEALTH PROMOTION

Patient education should always include information about the diagnostic evaluation and, once a diagnosis is determined, specific information regarding the prognosis, treatment options, and complications. If an exercise program for vestibular compensation is initiated, patients should be told that they may initially feel worse, but as they continue the program, symptoms will subside. Specific aspects of their program should be reinforced. Other teaching emphasizes how medications can be used to relieve symptoms and the potential side effects of these agents.

The Vestibular Disorders Association is a national organization dedicated to providing information and support to people with dizziness and balance disorders. Patients can be encouraged to contact them at 1-800-837-8428 or online at www.vestibular.org.

BENIGN PAROXYSMAL POSITIONAL VERTIGO

DEFINITION AND EPIDEMIOLOGY

BPPV is a syndrome that may be a manifestation of several varied inner ear conditions. In more than half the cases, no certain cause is determined. When a cause can be identified, the two most common are head trauma and a prior viral inner ear infection. In older adults, BPPV is the most common vestibular disorder.[7] It is characterized by a sensation of spinning, whirling, or tilting with movement or position change. It is estimated that about 15% of patients with BPPV will have at least one recurrent episode within 1 year after a remission.[8]

PATHOPHYSIOLOGY

Otoconia refers to debris in the inner ear made up of small crystals of calcium carbonate. With certain position changes, these crystals shift and disperse within the semicircular canal, sending false signals to the brain.

CLINICAL PRESENTATION

Symptoms of BPPV are precipitated by a change in head position. The most characteristic description is vertigo, which may be a sensation of spinning or whirling of oneself or the environment. Common movements that precipitate this vertigo are rolling over in bed, arising or turning abruptly, or first lying back on the bed. The symptoms are usually intermittent.

The nystagmus associated with BPPV is characteristic, and any deviation from the typical profiles should suggest a central lesion. The nystagmus is observed by use of the Hallpike-Dix maneuver (see Box 194-1). If it is vertical or torsional in nature and lasts less than 30 seconds, it is consistent with a posterior semicircular canal variant. If the nystagmus is direction changing and horizontal (beating toward the ground) and lasts about 1 minute, it is consistent with a horizontal canal variant. Both types should show fatiguing with repeated positioning.

Vertigo that is spontaneous (not position related) and the presence of focal neurologic findings suggest a central cause. Significant nausea or imbalance is not typical.

PHYSICAL EXAMINATION

With any new complaint of dizziness, a careful history and physical examination as outlined previously are always recommended. The Hallpike-Dix maneuver can be diagnostic of BPPV if the nystagmus is of the characteristic profile previously described. The dizziness and vertigo will be elicited with the affected ear down. In some cases, the history is compelling for BPPV, but at the time of the examination, position testing does not produce the dizziness or nystagmus (probably because of the intermittent nature of BPPV). The remainder of the neurologic examination findings should be normal.

DIAGNOSTICS

The diagnosis may be confirmed by history and a positive Hallpike-Dix test result. Further testing is warranted if there are positive neurologic findings, any associated features beyond the vertigo and a mild imbalance, or any symptoms or findings that are not movement or position related. If the history is compelling but position testing is not confirmatory, electronystagmography may be helpful.

DIFFERENTIAL DIAGNOSIS

The symptom of vertigo is differentiated from syncope or disequilibrium through a careful history. Vertigo can be a manifestation of peripheral or central disorders of the vestibular system. If there are more symptoms or findings than the vertigo, a mild associated imbalance, and a positive Hallpike-Dix test result, further diagnoses should be pursued.

MANAGEMENT

Specialist referral—ENT or neurology—is indicated if the patient is not responding to canalith repositioning procedures, such as Epley maneuvers, or vestibular rehabilitation.

Immediate emergency department referral is not indicated in a patient with BPPV.

- BPPV may remit in a few days or weeks without any treatment.[8]
- The canalith repositioning procedure is a specific positioning exercise that is designed to move ear crystal particles from the semicircular canal. If BPPV is confirmed, this is the first-line treatment rather than the commonly prescribed vestibular suppressant meclizine. The classic Epley maneuver involves moving the patient from one head-hanging position to another. This presumably rotates the particles out of the semicircular canal and into the utricle of the inner ear, where they are cleared through the endolymphatic duct and no longer affect the dynamics of the semicircular canals. The patient must then not lie flat for 48 to 72 hours to prevent the particles from reentering the posterior canal. The vertigo may recur in a week or two in 10% to 20% of patients, in which case the maneuver should be repeated. Patients can be taught to do the maneuver at home.[9]
- Vestibular rehabilitation may facilitate a quicker and often more prolonged remission. Such therapy consists of habituation exercises designed to train the brain to react less to the confused signals sent from the inner ear. This occurs most effectively if the patient continues with normal head movements despite their causing vertigo. Some exercises can facilitate compensation, such as lying or rolling in a position that will precipitate the vertigo and staying in that position until the vertigo subsides or for 30 seconds. These exercises should be repeated twice a day until the vertigo is gone.[10]
- Medications such as meclizine may be used as a vestibular suppressant if vertigo is severe. However, in BPPV, the acute attacks are not suppressed by medications, and canalith-repositioning maneuvers are more effective in controlling the condition.[10] Medications that cause vestibular suppression slow recovery because they slow compensatory mechanisms. It should be noted that these medication only suppress symptoms, so they should not be heavily relied on or used as monotherapy management for BPPV.
- In rare refractory cases, canal-plugging surgery may be considered.[10]

COMPLICATIONS

As its name implies, BPPV is a benign condition. Associated or indirect complications could include risk of falling and the risks inherent in self-imposed decreased mobility (common because of fear of precipitating the vertigo). Safety issues related to driving should be addressed, if head turning precipitates the vertigo. The condition may interfere with work.

EDUCATION AND HEALTH PROMOTION

The experience of acute vertigo can be frightening. Information about the evaluation, prognosis, and treatment options will help alleviate fears of a more serious condition. It is important to emphasize that the most effective treatment (vestibular therapy and exercises) may initially cause increased symptoms, but the treatment must continue for the symptoms to subside. The Vestibular Disorders Association website (www.vestibular.org) has helpful information for patients as well as for providers and provides extensive specialty referral resources throughout the United States.[10]

CHAPTER 195

GUILLAIN-BARRÉ SYNDROME

Seth Kolkin

DEFINITION AND EPIDEMIOLOGY

Guillain-Barré syndrome (GBS) is a group of acute monophasic immune-mediated peripheral neuropathies. Initially GBS referred only to a demyelinating neuropathy, but now acute inflammatory demyelinating polyradiculoneuropathy (AIDP) accounts for 85% to 90% of GBS in North America and Europe. Other subtypes include the Miller Fisher syndrome (MFS), in which oculomotor nerve myelin is affected, or axonal variants in which the axon rather than the myelin sheath is targeted. Axonal variants of GBS are more common in some populations around the world—for example, nearly 40% of GBS in Japan and Mexico and 75% in China.[1-6] Although the syndrome was initially described by Landry in 1859 and then Strohl, Barré, and Guillain in 1916, awareness was heightened when a cluster of cases followed mass vaccinations for swine influenza in 1976. There has not been a clear association between subsequent vaccination programs and GBS.[7]

Patients with GBS usually develop weakness over several days to weeks, and when weakness is accompanied by respiratory weakness and/or autonomic instability, patients can become critically ill. Up to 5% die despite intensive care unit (ICU) care, and about 20% of patients have residual weakness a year later.[1] The incidence of GBS is between 1 and 2 per 100,000.[5] Relapses occur in 5% to 10% of patients, on average 7 years after the initial attack.

PATHOPHYSIOLOGY

Two thirds of the time, GBS follows an upper respiratory or gastrointestinal infection by 1 to 4 weeks. The most commonly identified viruses are cytomegalovirus (CMV) and Epstein-Barr virus, and bacteria include *Campylobacter jejuni* (23% to 45%), *Mycoplasma pneumoniae* (5%), and *Haemophilus influenzae*. However, the risk of GBS after *C. jejuni* infection is less than 1 : 1000, and between 1 and 2 per 1000 after CMV, so host factors are presumed to play a role as well.[5] Molecular mimicry—the immune system's antibody response recognizing components of the host's peripheral nerve—is thought to be the cause of GBS. This has been best characterized in some acute motor axonal neuropathy (AMAN) patients with *C. jejuni* infection in which antibodies directed at the lipo-oligosaccharide coating of the bacteria cross-react with gangliosides (GM1 and GD1a) on the axon in the node of Ranvier.[6] In addition, patients with MFS have antibodies directed against the GQ1b ganglioside, which is in spinal nerve root and cranial nerve paranodal myelin.[8] Most recently, serum autoantibodies against moesin (membrane-organizing extension spike protein) on the myelinating Schwann cells have been identified in AIDP patients after CMV infection.[9] Once bound, those antibodies cause an influx of T lymphocytes and macrophages and activate membrane attack complex, thus damaging the nerve myelin or axon.

CLINICAL PRESENTATION

Patients develop the onset of relatively symmetric paresthesias and/or weakness, typically starting in the lower extremities and evolving over hours to days. Frequently there is a history of an antecedent infection. They often have back pain but do not have bowel or bladder dysfunction early in the course. The weakness can spread to involve the upper extremities then the respiratory muscles and finally can progress to complete paralysis. The weakness typically peaks in about 3 weeks, at which point 25% of patients have respiratory insufficiency and two thirds are unable to walk independently.

Patients with AMAN, as opposed to AIDP, can have preserved reflexes and tend not to have pain.

Patients with MFS will have ophthalmoplegia, ataxia, and areflexia and can also have distal paresthesias. Their syndrome peaks in 1 week, and these patients tend to recover more quickly and completely.[8]

PHYSICAL EXAMINATION

Even though sensory symptoms are typical, sensory findings on examination are usually absent. Progressive weakness, almost always with an evolving loss of deep tendon reflexes, is typical of GBS. Patients with respiratory muscle weakness have decreased breath sounds and a weakened cough, reduced vital capacity on bedside spirometry, and neck muscle weakness. In addition, autonomic instability can cause wide fluctuations in pulse rate and blood pressure, urinary retention, and bowel dysmotility.

On examination, MFS patients have incoordination in the extremities and weakness of eye movements with double vision.

DIAGNOSTICS

After the presence of true weakness has been confirmed, the neurologic examination is essential to determine which component(s) of the nervous system are involved—brain, spinal cord, peripheral nerve, neuromuscular junction, and/or muscle.

- Lesions in the brain usually cause unilateral weakness and are often associated with other neurologic signs and symptoms (e.g., involving the cranial nerves or cognition).
- A sensory level on the torso, bowel or bladder involvement, increased deep tendon reflexes, and/or a Babinski sign would suggest spinal cord pathology rather than the peripheral nerve dysfunction of GBS.

Screening for a systemic infection or organ dysfunction is based on the history and accompanying abnormalities on the general physical examination, complete blood count (CBC), and complete metabolic profile (CMP). Liver transaminases are elevated in 40% of patients and, because of syndrome of inappropriate antidiuretic hormone (SIADH), serum sodium is reduced in 25%.[1]

If GBS is suspected, lumbar puncture is the most important confirmatory laboratory test.

- Classically, there is albuminocytologic disassociation—that is, an elevated cerebrospinal fluid (CSF) protein with minimal if any increase of mononuclear CSF white blood cells (<10/mL^3). However, that pattern might not be seen during the first week of illness.[1-4]
- Acutely, the spinal fluid might show polymorphonuclear leukocytes (PMNs) without an elevated protein level but often converts to the typical pattern in a few days.

Nerve conduction studies and electromyography are not necessary for the diagnosis of GBS, which often does not evolve into a diagnostic axonal or demyelinating pattern until several weeks into the illness. Therefore, although these modalities can have significant prognostic significance, they do not usually play a role in acute diagnosis and management.

Magnetic resonance imaging (MRI) is typically not necessary. However, if there is concern for spine pathology, MRI might be done. In GBS there can be gadolinium enhancement of the nerve roots reflecting inflammation and their involvement as part of the peripheral nervous system.

DIFFERENTIAL DIAGNOSIS

Rapidly evolving bilateral weakness accompanied by bowel or bladder dysfunction, increased reflexes, a Babinski sign, or a sensory level over the torso should prompt an investigation for spinal cord or cauda equina pathology. MRI of the appropriate spinal level, depending on the distribution of signs and symptoms, might reveal compression from a herniated disc or mass lesion or inflammation within the spinal cord itself—a transverse myelitis. It would be rare for a brainstem or cortical brain lesion to cause bilateral weakness without cranial nerve dysfunction or impaired consciousness.

"Red flags" (Table 195-1) indicating acute weakness resulting from peripheral nervous system dysfunction other than GBS include retained reflexes, limited sensory symptoms, pleocytosis in the spinal fluid, abnormal pupil light reflexes, and ptosis or other extraocular muscle weakness.[2] In addition, it is important to check for any recent history of potential toxic ingestions (e.g., botulism and seafood toxins) or exposures (e.g., organophosphates).

If the onset of weakness is subacute occurring over weeks or longer, other peripheral nerve, muscle, or neuromuscular junction causes should be considered.

MANAGEMENT

Specialist consultation is indicated for rapidly evolving bilateral weakness that can be confirmed on physical examination.

Immediate emergency department referral is indicated if screening for a systemic cause cannot be done immediately in the outpatient setting or if a systemic cause that can be corrected on an outpatient basis cannot be confirmed.

- If GBS is suspected, hospitalization to monitor progressive weakness, provide supportive care, and manage potential complications is necessary in all but the mildest cases.
- When initiated within the first 2 weeks of illness, treatment of GBS with intravenous immune globulin (IVIG) or plasma exchange (PE) reduces the duration of mechanical ventilation and hastens recovery from GBS.[10-12]

TABLE 195-1 Potential Guillain-Barré Mimics

Red Flag	Alternative Considerations
Limited sensory symptoms	Tick paralysis
Abnormal pupil response	Botulism Tick paralysis Organophosphate poisoning
CSF pleocytosis (>10/mL^3)	West Nile virus Lyme disease HIV
Ptosis and extraocular muscle weakness	Myasthenia gravis

- IVIG is given as a daily infusion for 5 days (total dose 2 g/kg) but can be limited by availability of the medication and is contraindicated in the presence of a selective immunoglobulin A (IgA) deficiency.
- PE is done with five exchanges over 2 weeks and is limited by available resources, logistics, and hemodynamic stability.
- Corticosteroids are not indicated for the treatment of GBS.[13]

- Imaging studies are not usually necessary for GBS, but may be required to exclude alternative diagnoses and assess comorbidities (e.g., pneumonia).
- Strength must be evaluated frequently and is most conveniently tracked with use of a table that records muscle power using the 5-point Medical Research Council (MRC) scale in representative proximal and distal muscles in all four extremities, plus neck flexion and extension.
- Bedridden patients need prophylaxis against deep vein thrombosis and monitoring for pulmonary emboli.
- Physical, occupational, and speech therapy are each important at various stages of the disease to maintain joint range of motion, compensate for weakness, and maximize safe swallowing.
- Respiratory weakness and dysphagia increase the risk of respiratory insufficiency and pneumonia and need to be monitored by evaluating speech, breath sounds, and bedside spirometry findings, especially the vital capacity (VC). The frequency of monitoring depends on the level of respiratory compromise.
- Intubation and mechanical ventilation are typically necessary as the VC approaches 1 L. Some clinicians consider the "20/30/40 rule"—VC 20 mL/kg, negative inspiratory force 30 cm H_2O, and/or maximum expiratory pressure 40 cm H_2O—as a threshold for artificial ventilation.[14]
- Dysfunction of the autonomic component of peripheral nerves is common and, after respiratory insufficiency, needs the most attention to avoid life-threatening complications.[14]
  - Cardiac telemetry is needed to monitor for potentially dramatic swings in heart rate that can require a temporary pacemaker.
  - Blood pressure and fluid management is needed for hemodynamic fluctuations and compromise.
  - Urinary retention can cause discomfort, exacerbate hemodynamic instability, and result in infection. Indwelling urinary catheters are usually necessary.
  - Bowel dysmotility can lead to ileus and perforation. Repeated abdominal examination and bowel management are essential.

COMPLICATIONS

Despite treatment, careful ICU monitoring, and management of weakness, autonomic dysfunction, and infections, up to 5% of patients with GBS die. In addition to fatigue, residual weakness is present in 10% to 20% of patients a year later.

INDICATIONS FOR REFERRAL OR HOSPITALIZATION

All but the mildest cases of GBS necessitate hospitalization to monitor evolving weakness until they have reached a nadir. Rehabilitation services will be needed to assist in full recovery of strength and function. Vocational counseling may be needed for those left with residual impairment.

LIFE SPAN CONSIDERATIONS

GBS tends to be milder with less residual effect in the pediatric population. After the age of 50 the incidence is approximately twice that of the younger population, and with increased age recovery can be less complete.[5]

EDUCATION AND HEALTH PROMOTION

The patient and family should be educated about the course of the disease, what symptoms to alert the caregivers about, and long-term expectations. Individuals should be encouraged to continue with annual influenza prophylaxis because the risk of mortality and morbidity from influenza is much higher than any potential risk of GBS. Education and support can be obtained through the GBS/CIDP Foundation International, The Holly Building 104½ Forrest Avenue, Narberth, PA 19072 or at www.gbs-cidp.org.

CHAPTER 196

HEADACHE

Jillian Belmont

DEFINITION AND EPIDEMIOLOGY

Headache is experienced by 90% to 95% of the population and is one of the 10 most common complaints in the outpatient setting.[1] Many people with headache are never diagnosed by a physician. Some individuals treat headaches at home with over-the-counter (OTC) medications and home remedies such as ice packs and rest. Research has shown that even with the development of newer medications, up to 57% of patients with headaches use OTC medications, and many do not seek care for their headaches because they do not believe that satisfactory treatment is available.[1] It is essential to differentiate secondary from primary headaches because secondary headaches can be harbingers of a potentially more serious medical problem than the benign, primary headaches usually seen in the office setting. Secondary headaches are less common and are usually the result of an underlying disease or condition, such as aneurysm, tumor, hemorrhage, temporal arteritis, or meningitis.[1] Once the primary problem has been identified and treated, secondary headaches may dissipate.

Primary headaches are more common and are not symptomatic of another medical condition. These are distinct disorders that result from pathophysiologic mechanisms. Types of primary headaches include migraine with and without aura, chronic or episodic tension-type headaches, and chronic or episodic cluster headaches.[1]

Primary headache disorders affect people of all ages, races, income levels and geographic areas and have an estimated lifetime prevalence of 47% in adults worldwide.[2] These headaches may range in intensity from mild to severe but cause considerable distress, expense, and loss of work time. In general, migraine varies by age and sex, increasing in frequency to about the age of 40 years and declining thereafter in both men and women. Women experience migraine three times more often than men do. Similarly, tension-type headache is seen more in women than in men, with a male-to-female ratio of 4:5.[3]

Cluster headache, on the other hand, is more common in men than in women; attacks usually begin between the ages of 20 and 40 years.[3]

Clinical and research evidence has demonstrated a relationship between migraine and other disease processes, including epilepsy, major depression or panic disorder, and cardiac shunting. The neurotransmitter serotonin has been suggested as a basis for both migraine and major depression. Knowing that a co-occurrence exists helps in the treatment of each disease and provides clues to the pathophysiologic mechanism of migraine.[4]

PATHOPHYSIOLOGY

The exact mechanism of a headache is still debated. Previously, headaches were thought to be caused by increased blood flow to the head, resulting in distended vessels and pressure on the nerve fibers of the brain.[5] This "vascular theory" was popular for many years until the 1930s, when Harold Wolfe determined that migraine, specifically, was caused by both vascular and chemical changes within the brain.[5]

Many theories have since identified several neurochemicals as key elements in migraine development. Serotonin (5-hydroxytryptamine [5-HT]), a powerful vasoconstrictor, sensitizes the blood vessel walls to painful dilation. Other neurochemicals, such as dopamine, substance P (a polypeptide), and calcitonin gene–related peptide, may alter the excitability of the brain and mediate the vasoconstriction or vasodilation of blood vessels.[1] Neurogenic inflammation is responsible for the pain of migraine.[5]

In review of the various theories, it is clear that during a headache, changes occur in the vasculature of the brain and in the neurochemicals found within the body. These changes are a result of a brain response to a stimulus, or trigger. Vasodilation and vasoconstriction subsequently cause the release of neurochemicals, which may be responsible for the headache and for the feelings of impending doom or fatigue that can occur before and after an attack.

CLINICAL PRESENTATION

The International Headache Society has developed criteria for various types of headache disorders. The criteria can be tedious to use and are not applicable in many primary care settings, but the information may allow the provider to quickly differentiate the various types of primary headache conditions.[6]

Migraine

The two major types of migraine are migraine with aura and migraine without aura. Migraine without aura is the more common of the two. In general, the patient complains of an ipsilateral headache. The pain is described as pounding or throbbing, is moderate to severe in intensity, and is aggravated by physical activity. This headache, which is episodic, lasts 4 to 72 hours and may be associated with nausea, vomiting, photophobia, and phonophobia. These patients usually retreat to a dark, quiet room until the attack is over. They often can identify a trigger that will precipitate the attacks. Triggers are an individual characteristic and may be difficult to identify because they may not always stimulate a headache. Common triggers include medication overuse, obesity, depression, stressful life events, sleep problems including snoring, weather changes, foods (cheese, chocolate), alcohol, change in altitude, delay or skipping of a meal, and hormonal changes.[1,7]

In migraine with aura, the aura usually occurs before the onset of head pain, although it can sometimes extend into the period of headache. The classic aura, or "fortification spectrum," occurs in about 10% of patients and is described as jagged lines similar to the stone fortifications found around a fort.[1] Visual auras can also be characterized by spots, shimmering bright lights, or areas of visual loss (scotomas). Somatosensory-type auras can also occur, with tingling or numbness of the fingers, motor disturbances such as hemiparesis or monoparesis, and cognitive disorders.[1] These visual and somatosensory disturbances usually last seconds but can last as long as 20 minutes. The patient then experiences head pain and features similar to those of migraine without aura.

A prodrome can be part of a migraine.[8] Several days before the aura or start of the head pain, the person may have feelings of doom or fatigue. During this period, increased irritability, decreased energy, and food cravings are common complaints. This can often be an early signal that a severe headache is coming and may enable the patient to use both pharmacologic and nonpharmacologic modalities in the hope of aborting the attack.

Tension-Type Headache

Acute tension-type headaches are described as feeling like there is a tight band around the head. Nausea and vomiting are not present, and the pain can be mild to moderate in intensity. This headache can last minutes to hours. It usually is not exacerbated by physical activity, but a common trigger is stress. Overall, the acute tension-type headache is a nagging headache that occurs fewer than 15 days per month, is present most of the day, and may start after the person wakes up. It rarely awakens the person. Chronic tension-type headache is similar in presentation to the acute type but occurs more often than 15 days per month.[9]

Cluster Headache

The patient with cluster headache, acute or chronic, is usually awakened during the night with severe unilateral, retro-orbital pain. A cluster headache reaches maximum intensity in about 15 minutes and usually lasts about 90 minutes, although some can last 3 hours.[6,10] These attacks can occur several times per day. The pain is described as agonizing, and unlike migraineurs, these patients often cannot sit still. The severe intensity of cluster pain causes restlessness, moaning, crying, and often pacing. Patients may indulge in self-hurting behavior and may have thoughts of suicide.[11] Other features of cluster headache include ipsilateral injection of the conjunctiva, lacrimation, rhinorrhea, and partial Horner sign. For the patient with acute cluster headache, attacks occur in groups (or clusters) lasting days to weeks and then subside until the next attack. Years can pass between attacks, and the event often occurs at the same time each year. The patient with chronic cluster headache has the same presentation as the patient with the acute type but does not experience any remission longer than 1 month for at least 1 year. These headaches are also relatively resistant to therapy. Although it is well tolerated between attacks, alcohol will often precipitate an attack in patients with acute or chronic cluster headache.[6,11]

PHYSICAL EXAMINATION

The history is the most important part of the evaluation. With most primary headache disorders, the diagnosis can be made on the basis of the history alone.[12] It is important that the patient characterize the headache by describing the duration, quality, and location of the pain. The presence or absence of any precipitating factors, or triggers, and the age at onset should be established. The presence of associated symptoms, such as nausea, vomiting, and photophobia, should be explored. Can the patient be active during these headaches, or does the patient need to lie still in a dark room? How does the patient describe his or her sleep and energy? Sleep is usually labile in the person with headache, and energy may be poor. A medication profile is essential and should include medications that have been tried in the past for headache control. If OTC medications are taken, the number used per month should be identified because patients may not view OTC drugs as medications. Migraine is known to be familial; therefore, it is important to determine whether any family member has had headaches that might have been called sinus headaches or sick headaches or headaches that were disabling. Asking about the presence of any physical abuse is important because it has been shown that a history of abuse contributes to refractory headaches.

A targeted physical examination is important in ruling out harmful secondary headache pathologies and confirms any information given in the history.[12] The examination findings in primary headache disorders are usually within normal limits. Key aspects of the physical examination include a cardiopulmonary and complete neurologic assessment with a major focus on the following:

- Funduscopic and pupillary assessment
- Auscultation of the carotid and vertebral arteries
- Mental status examination
- Palpation of the head, neck, and temporal arteries
- Evaluation for any neck stiffness, focal weakness, sensory loss and gait
- Vital signs

Many patients with tension-type headaches or migraines have tight cervical musculature. Painful biceps insertions, along with general aches and pains along the back, hips, and knees, may herald the beginning of fibromyalgia (see Chapter 175), a condition commonly seen in migraineurs. Pain and pressure on palpation of the sinuses accompanied by purulent nasal discharge may be indicative of sinusitis. The temporomandibular joints may click and pop when the mouth is opened and closed, but rarely is this the cause of a headache. Tension is often exhibited in the musculature surrounding this joint, and the subsequent bruxism may potentiate pain in this area.

Serious symptoms and findings include a headache accompanied by a stiff neck; fever; malaise; nausea or vomiting; and the presence of any aphasia, weakness, or poor coordination. Other danger signs include the following[1,12]:

- Onset of headache after the age of 50 years
- Asymmetry of pupillary responses
- Decreased deep tendon reflexes
- Headache described as "the worst ever experienced"
- Personality change
- Onset of a new or different headache
- Onset of a headache that progressively worsens
- Papilledema
- Painful temporal arteries

Further investigation and referral to a specialist or hospital would be warranted with any of these signs. Positive neurologic findings on examination are indicative of a central nervous system problem and should not be attributed to migraine unless a prior pattern has been documented with serious findings previously excluded.

DIAGNOSTICS

The use of diagnostic studies depends on the results of the history and physical examination. Most diagnostic studies in the patient with primary headache are unrevealing. If the diagnosis is not clear or the history or physical findings are cause for concern, diagnostic studies should be used to distinguish primary headache from a secondary condition.

Blood tests are usually not indicated, although exceptions, based on history and physical examination findings, may include a complete blood count (CBC) to exclude anemia or an infectious process, erythrocyte sedimentation rate (ESR) or C-reactive protein (CRP) to help exclude temporal arteritis, and thyroid function tests to identify thyroid dysfunction. Lyme titer or rheumatoid factors may also be indicated in some situations.

Practice guidelines developed by the U.S. Headache Consortium advocate three principles for diagnostic testing: (1) testing should be avoided if it will not change the management of the patient, (2) testing is not indicated if the patient is not significantly more likely than the general public to have an abnormality, and (3) testing may make sense in a patient who is excessively concerned that he or she has a serious problem that is causing the headaches.[13] Neuroimaging should be considered when any serious signs or symptoms are present during the physical examination, but it is not indicated if the patient has had these headaches for years, if there are no focal neurologic signs, and if the headache improves without the use of analgesics.

DIAGNOSTICS

Headache

LABORATORY
CBC and differential*
ESR*, CRP
Thyroid function tests*
Lyme titer*
Rheumatoid factor*
CSF cell count, protein, glucose*

IMAGING
CT scan, MRI*

*If indicated.
CSF, cerebrospinal fluid; CT, computed tomography; MRI, magnetic resonance imaging.

DIFFERENTIAL DIAGNOSIS

The history and physical examination will aid in excluding potential diagnoses. The differential diagnosis includes fever, meningitis, pseudotumor cerebri, hemorrhage, rheumatologic disorders (e.g., lupus erythematosus, rheumatoid arthritis), Lyme disease, temporal arteritis, trigeminal neuralgia, thyroid dysfunction, sleep apnea, tumor, aneurysm, and pheochromocytoma, among many others. Headache is a feature of many disease processes (see the differential diagnosis box).

MANAGEMENT

Physician consultation is indicated for patients with suspected temporal arteritis, change in mental status, nuchal rigidity, neurologic deficit, or new onset of headache, especially over the age of 50.

Immediate emergency department referral is indicated for abrupt onset "thunderclap headache," trauma, or headache with associated neurologic abnormalities on physical examination.

DIFFERENTIAL DIAGNOSIS
Headache

PRIMARY HEADACHE
- Migraine
- Cluster headache
- Tension-type headache
- Secondary Headache

Infectious or Inflammatory Causes
- Fever
- Meningitis
- Temporal arteritis
- Lyme disease
- Trigeminal neuralgia
- Rheumatoid arthritis
- Systemic lupus erythematosus
- Sinusitis

Ear, Nose, and Throat Causes
- Eye disorder
- Abscess
- Earache

Structural Causes
- Tumor
- Hemorrhage
- Aneurysm
- Subdural hematoma

Metabolic Causes
- Thyroid dysfunction
- Pheochromocytoma
- Sleep apnea

Other Causes
- Pseudotumor cerebri
- Trauma

The U.S. Headache Consortium has developed evidence-based practice guidelines for migraine that cover both nonpharmacologic and pharmacologic modalities, with the goals of reducing the frequency of attacks, improving the response to therapy, and restoring the patient to normal functioning. Control can be achieved after a proper diagnosis is made and proper treatment is prescribed. Currently, no cure exists for primary headaches, although control is possible for most patients.[14]

Nonpharmacologic Management

Nonpharmacologic measures attempt to control the headache without medication. These methods include behavior modification, biofeedback, acupressure, management of headache triggers, and a wellness program.

- Behavior modification uses several methods, such as relaxation through tapes and stress management, as well as modification of daily activities.
- Biofeedback involves the use of instrumentation to bring under voluntary control physiologic processes of which the individual is normally unaware. For example, during a migraine attack, vasoconstriction of the periphery causes cold hands. Biofeedback training teaches migraineurs to raise hand temperature and thereby prevent an attack.
- The area between the thumb and the first finger (or other acupressure areas) can be depressed during a headache to offer some relief. It is thought that this pressure causes the release of endogenous endorphins and adrenocorticotropic hormones, which aborts the headache in some people.[1]
- A wellness program consisting of balanced meals, regular exercise, and adequate sleep can also be helpful in controlling headache bouts. Overall, nonpharmacologic approaches may help patients avoid triggers that might be initiating headaches.
- Another important nonpharmacologic measure is having the patient keep a headache diary. The diary documents the number of headaches, triggers, and treatment successes and failures. The patient should keep this record daily because attempting to fill it in before a follow-up appointment may be less accurate. It is important for the patient to bring the diary to office visits so information can be shared and the treatment plan adjusted if necessary.[15]

Pharmacologic Management

Pharmacologic treatment can be divided into two areas: abortive and preventive. Management should match the level of therapy to the intensity of the headache. If the attack is severe, early intervention is in the patient's best interest. Providers need to supply education and a range of treatment modalities, allowing the patient to select the most effective treatment.

Preventive Therapy. Preventive therapy is appropriate for patients if they are unable to deal with their attacks, they experience more than four headaches a month, or the attacks are prolonged and refractory to medicine. Preventive therapy is given daily and, if successful, will decrease headache intensity and frequency. When choosing preventive treatment, the provider must consider the patient's history, including any comorbid conditions.

- For example, a connection has been shown between epilepsy and migraine; therefore anticonvulsants, such as divalproex sodium (Depakote), gabapentin (Neurontin), and topiramate (Topamax), can be used to control migraine.
- A patient with cold hands, Raynaud phenomenon, or hypertension may do well with calcium channel blockers, such as diltiazem (Cardizem) and amlodipine (Norvasc), which cause vasodilation and decrease blood pressure.
- A beta blocker, such as propranolol (Inderal) or atenolol, may be chosen for the patient with palpitations caused by mitral valve prolapse or panic disorders and should be avoided in those with asthma.
- If sleep is a problem or if chronic pain persists in the shoulders, a tricyclic antidepressant, such as amitriptyline (Elavil), may facilitate sleep and also decrease the sensation of pain.[12,16]

The mechanism of action for both beta blockers and calcium channel blockers is not fully understood.

- Calcium channel blockers prevent calcium from entering the cells and therefore decrease their excitability. This may in turn prevent vascular spasm and headache.
- Beta blockers affect the $beta_1$-adrenergic receptors and inhibit the usual adrenergic responses.[15] Beyond these mechanisms, it has been theorized that either may have an effect on the serotonergic system within the brain and the vascular system.

Both migraine and tension-type headache may result from an imbalance of neurochemicals. Adjustment of these neurochemicals to a more normal level may decrease the number and frequency of headaches.

- The tricyclic antidepressants and the selective serotonin reuptake inhibitors (SSRIs), such as sertraline (Zoloft), modulate the levels of serotonin in the brain. Both the tricyclic antidepressants and the SSRIs have an extensive side effect profile. Weight gain and sexual dysfunction may not be acceptable to patients, although the starting dose for many of the medications can be low. The SSRIs are better tolerated, but they might not be as effective as the tricyclic antidepressants for headaches.[14,16]

Abortive Therapy. Abortive therapy is used to treat the intensity and duration of pain during an attack and to manage associated symptoms, such as nausea and vomiting. It is important to prescribe an adequate amount of medication. Patients also need to be instructed to take an appropriate amount initially to abort the headache. The appropriate medicine depends on the prior response to treatment, the presence of nausea or vomiting, and the interval between headache onset and peak intensity. A patient with a severe migraine or cluster attack that peaks to full intensity within 15 minutes will most likely benefit from parenteral or nasal therapy rather than oral medication. For many patients, the pain of the headache is severe, but the associated nausea and vomiting are incapacitating. During a migraine attack, gastric emptying is slowed, causing gastric stasis. Medications that "turn the stomach back on," such as metoclopramide (Reglan), will augment the availability of the abortive therapy, enhance gastric motility, and decrease the nausea.[1] Rectal formulations can also be used when abortive therapies are prescribed.

Many of the abortive medications are powerful analgesics. When these medications, including acetaminophen (Tylenol), aspirin, and ibuprofen (Advil), are taken frequently, a condition called analgesic rebound can develop in a headache-prone individual.[17] The medications prescribed to abort a headache will essentially potentiate the headache and make it a daily condition. Strict guidelines on the use of all abortive medicine as well as limitations on medication refills need to be reviewed with the patient to prevent dependency and possible rebound.[1,17] Patients should be instructed to limit abortive use to 2 days per week or less. Table 196-1 reviews the most common abortive therapies for headache control.

- Simple analgesics, such as acetaminophen and aspirin, can represent first-line treatment in the management of mild to moderate headaches.[18] Caffeine combinations (Excedrin, Anacin) can potentiate their absorption and analgesia. When simple analgesics are ineffective, combining them with a short-acting barbiturate, such as butalbital (Fioricet, Fiorinal, Esgic), may be effective.
- Nonsteroidal anti-inflammatory drugs (NSAIDs) are helpful in treating an acute attack. Naproxen sodium (Anaprox DS, Aleve) has a longer half-life and a better safety profile than some of the other NSAIDs. The addition of metoclopramide to many of the NSAIDs when nausea is present will facilitate their absorption and potentiate their effect.
- Ergot derivatives are effective in the treatment of moderate to severe attacks that might not have responded to simple or combination analgesics. Two forms are currently in use: ergotamine tartrate (Cafergot) and dihydroergotamine. Ergotamine tartrate is available in both rectal and oral forms, but the rectal dose is more potent than the oral preparation.[1,19,20] Dosage regimens need to be reviewed with the patient and adjusted to achieve pain relief without vomiting. Dihydroergotamine is available in both an injectable form and a nasal spray. The injectable form (D.H.E. 45) can be given by the parenteral, subcutaneous, or intramuscular route. The nasal form (Migranal) is easily administered and much more convenient. Because all forms of the ergots can cause nausea and vomiting, premedication with an antiemetic, such as promethazine (Phenergan) or prochlorperazine (Compazine), is necessary. Ergot derivatives may have a high potential for overuse and subsequent rebound headaches; patients need to be made aware of the risk for rebound headaches when this medication is prescribed. With the development of triptans, the use of ergot derivatives is no longer considered first-line therapy, although they are effective and less expensive than a triptan.[20]
- Corticosteroids (dexamethasone [Decadron], prednisone) are often used when the patient is unable to abort an attack and the attack continues for several days. The side effects with the extended use of corticosteroids are serious and include elevated blood sugar and blood pressure, cataracts, aseptic necrosis of the hip and gastrointestinal bleeding; therefore, frequent use is not recommended.
- Triptans, developed approximately 20 years ago, have given many migraine and cluster headache patients relief within a short time.[19,21] The triptans target specific receptors (5-HT) in the brain that are believed to generate headache. Relief can be almost complete, allowing a return to normal daily activities with few side effects. These medications are arterial constrictors and should be used with caution in the presence of known cardiac disease. Many forms of triptans are available: oral, "quick melt," transnasal, injectable, and a transdermal preparation (see Table 196-1). The brands of each medication have slight differences; if one triptan is ineffective, another may prove to be effective for a patient. As with most abortive medications, the goal is to take the dose of medication required to stop the headache before it becomes severe.

Patients with cluster headache use many of the same medications and treatment regimens as do patients with migraine or tension-type headache.[22] The cluster attack has such a rapid onset that preventing the attacks may be the key to successful treatment. Preventive therapy includes verapamil and lithium as first-line options.

- Verapamil is usually well tolerated and does not require the close monitoring necessary with lithium. Calcium channel blockers may prevent the vasospasm that occurs during a cluster attack by blocking the flow of calcium.
- Lithium, long used for bipolar disorder, also controls cluster headaches. Levels should be monitored, and patient education about the signs and symptoms of lithium toxicity is important. Therapy should be slowly titrated upward.

With both regimens, therapy is continued until the patient is free of any attacks for several weeks. Patients are then slowly weaned from the medication.

Because of the rapid onset of the cluster headache, abortive therapy needs to be in either a parenteral or a nasal form.

- Oxygen can be effective in as many as 75% of patients and should be delivered at a rate of 10 to 15 L/min through a non-rebreather face mask.[23] The oxygen should be inhaled at the start of an attack. If this is effective, an oxygen tank should be readily available at all times.
- The triptans are effective treatment options for the patient with cluster headache, although overuse may be a concern in patients with chronic cluster headache.

The abortive management of tension-type headaches involves many of the same medications as for migraine, and the same principles should be applied in choosing treatments for these patients.

- For mild attacks, NSAIDs may be helpful. Because there usually is no nausea, antiemetics may not be necessary.
- Muscle relaxants such as metaxalone (Skelaxin) and carisoprodol (Soma), used cautiously, have been helpful with mild to moderate attacks.
- Triptan drugs may abort a severe tension attack as well. As with migraine, the use of these medications should be limited to 2 days a week or less to prevent rebound headaches.

TABLE 196-1 Abortive Therapies for Headache

Medications	Route	Dosage	Considerations
NSAIDS			
Ibuprofen (Advil, Motrin)	PO	1200 mg × 1, repeat 600 mg q 4 hours × 2	As with all NSAIDs, side effects include dyspepsia, heartburn, bleeding, and nausea or vomiting; contraindicated in patients with history of ulcer; will have better effect if taken on an empty stomach but might not be well tolerated by patient.
Naproxen sodium (Anaprox DS)	PO	Initial 875 mg, repeat 220-550 mg 8 hours max 1.5 g/day	
Indomethacin (Indocin)	PO, PR	25-50 mg tid prn	Indomethacin suppositories are not available in the United States but can be compounded by a pharmacist.
Ketorolac (Toradol)	IM	30-60 mg × 1 prn, may repeat 15-30 mg q6h	Most often used in an emergency department setting. Do not exceed 5 consecutive days of use.
GLUCOCORTICOIDS			
Dexamethasone	PO	10-12 mg/day × 1-2 days	Should be limited to less than one treatment per month; hold NSAIDs while administering glucocorticoids; use when usual treatments have not aborted headache and it continues for several days.
Prednisone	PO	40-60 mg initially taper over 7 days	
MUSCLE RELAXANTS			
Carisoprodol (Soma)	PO	350 mg, ½ or 1 tablet PO up to 4 times per day prn	Encourage patient to start with lowest dose and increase as needed to take away muscle tightness; this may often abort a migraine; used on headaches described as "tight" or "pressure"; used frequently with tension-type headaches; caution patient about sedation.
Metaxalone (Skelaxin)	PO	400 mg, 1 or 2 tablets 3 or 4 times per day	
NARCOTIC ANALGESICS			
Meperidine (Demerol)			no longer recommended for the treatment of acute migraine
COMBINATION ANALGESICS			
Butalbital combination (Fioricet, Fiorinal)	PO	2 tablets PO stat at headache onset; may repeat 1 tablet q4h prn, max 5 tablets/day or 15 tablets/mo	Take full dose right at start of headache; adding metoclopramide to these may facilitate absorption; because of risk of rebound headache, limit to 2 days per week.
ASA plus caffeine (Excedrin)	PO	1 or 2 tablets PO stat at headache onset; may repeat q4h prn	
OTHER			
Acetaminophen	PO, PR	650-1000 mg (not to exceed 3 g in 24 hr)	Best used early as abortive therapy; rectal preparation better tolerated when nausea or vomiting a prominent feature.
Isometheptene mucate, dichloralphenazone, and acetaminophen (Midrin)	PO	2 caplets stat, and then repeat with 1 caplet q1h up to 5 caplet in 12 hr	May cause sedation; maximum dose: 5 caplets/12 hr.
Metoclopramide (Reglan)	PO	10 mg twice per day prn	May facilitate absorption of many abortives; watch for akathisia.
Prochlorperazine (Compazine)	PO PR	5-10 mg q8h 25 mg q12h	

- For many of these patients, stress may be triggering the attack, so nonpharmacologic measures are often helpful.[24]

LIFE SPAN CONSIDERATIONS

As patients age, headaches often decrease. It is uncommon for headaches to appear after the age of 50 years. When an older patient is seen with a history of daily headache, analgesic rebound is often the cause; however, secondary processes need to be excluded. Triptans, and DHE pose a risk to the elderly secondary to their vasoconstrictive properties, and therefore headaches in these patients should be treated more conservatively with divalproex sodium, metoclopramide, or intravenous magnesium and at home with naproxen or hydroxyzine.[12]

During pregnancy, the headache pattern can change. Many women experience a decrease in headaches during the second and third trimesters, although some see no change in the pattern. For the pregnant woman, headache control is usually

TABLE 196-1 Abortive Therapies for Headache—cont'd

Medications	Route	Dosage	Considerations
ACUTE ABORTIVES			
Triptans			
Sumatriptan (Imitrex)	PO	Initial 25 mg, repeat 25-100 mg q2h prn, max 300 mg/day	**Separate all triptan doses by at least 2 hours;** common side effects are sensations of flushing, tingling, chest tightness, and throat tightness that will subside after 10-20 min; first dose should be administered under medical supervision; contraindicated in presence of hypertension, coronary artery disease, history of myocardial infarction, hepatic or renal dysfunction, or pregnancy.
	Nasal	20 mg for adults, 1 spray in 1 nostril twice per day prn	
	SC	6 mg SC twice per day prn	
Zolmitriptan (Zomig)	PO	2.5-5.0 mg twice per day prn; limited to three attacks per month; max 10 mg/day	
	Nasal		
	Fast-melt pill		
Naratriptan (Amerge)	PO	2.5 mg q2h prn, max 10 mg/day; limited to four attacks per month	
Rizatriptan (Maxalt, Maxalt-MLT)	PO	5-20 mg; max 30 mg/day	MLT no faster than PO, but useful when nausea or vomiting present.
Eletriptan (Relpax)	PO	40 mg, may repeat dose in 2 hr; max 80 mg/day	Should not be used within 3 days after ketoconazole, clarithromycin, or other CYP3A4 inhibitors.
Almotriptan (Axert)	PO	6.25-12.5 mg, may repeat in 2 hr; max 2 doses in 24 hr	Contains sulfa, therefore contraindicated in allergic patient.
Frovatriptan (Frova)	PO	2.5 mg, may repeat in 2 hr; max 7.5 mg/day	
Ergotamines			
D.H.E. 45, 1 mg/mL Migranal, 4 mg/mL	SC	1 mg, may repeat q1h; max 3 mg/24 hr	Effective therapy that can last all day but can cause nausea and vomiting; should premedicate with antiemetic, such as promethazine, before administration; leg cramping is common and usually responds to dose reduction.
	Nasal	1 spray in each nostril, may repeat in 15 min × 1	Max use 2 times per week.
Ergotamine and caffeine (Cafergot)	PO	2 tablets stat at onset, may repeat q30min; max 6 tablets/day or 10 tablets/week	May be more effective if metoclopramide is added; can lead to ergotamine-dependency headaches; its use should be limited to 2 days per week.
	PR	2-mg suppository cut into fourths; repeat ¼ suppository q30min until headache abates; limit to 2 suppositories per attack	Causes severe nausea, and dose must be titrated to a subnauseating dose; premedication with an antiemetic is key to success; may not be tolerated by many patients because of severe nausea and vomiting.

ASA, aspirin; NSAIDs, nonsteroidal anti-inflammatory drugs

Data from: Hale N, Paauw, D: Diagnosis and treatment of headache in the ambulatory care setting. *Med Clin North Am* 98:505-527, 2014; and Moses S: *Migraine abortive treatment.* Available at www.fpnotebook.com/legacy/Neuro/Headache/MgrnAbrtvTrtmnt.htm. Accessed August 1, 2014.

limited to abortive medications only, and preventive therapy should be tapered immediately. Acetaminophen at doses within normal parameters can be safely used during pregnancy. Meperidine is a pregnancy class C drug and has no known association with birth defects but can cause drowsiness and respiratory distress in the newborn if used during labor and delivery.

COMPLICATIONS

Misdiagnosis is the most serious complication. For this reason, all patients who report headache require a careful history and physical examination. Patients with positive physical findings require appropriate and timely referral. Other complications of headache include status migrainosus; dependency on narcotics, barbiturates, tranquilizers, or other agents; side effects of medication; inadequate treatment; and interruption of the activities of daily living.

INDICATIONS FOR REFERRAL OR HOSPITALIZATION

Most patients with headache can be managed within the primary care setting. Indications for referral to a specialist, a headache clinic, or a neurologist include the following:

- The headache is not easily controlled by routine headache medicines.
- Rebound headaches or habituation limits outpatient therapy.
- Headache is new and progressively worsening.
- Headache is described as the "worse headache of my life."
- Headache is affecting the patient's quality of life.
- Headache is accompanied by neurologic symptoms that last longer than 30 minutes or is accompanied by numbness or hemiparesis.

Hospitalization of the patient with headache may be appropriate in some situations. Headaches that are resistant to treatment may be rebound headaches and require intravenous medication to help abort the headache. Referral to a headache specialist or neurologist for consultation may be advantageous.

PATIENT AND FAMILY EDUCATION

Knowledge and education are important aspects of patient care. Education allows patients and families to make choices and may enable them to regain control. During the initial examination and subsequent treatment, open communication and reassurance are necessary because many patients believe that they have a life-threatening condition. It is important they realize that their physical examination findings are normal and that the information received during the history indicates a primary headache disorder. Family members should be included in the treatment plan because headache affects both the patient and the family members.

Educational materials on headaches are widely available. Pharmaceutical companies and national groups such as the American Headache Society Committee for Headache Education (www.achenet.org), the Migraine Action Association (www.migraine.org.uk), the World Headache Alliance (www.w-h-a.org), and the National Headache Foundation (www.headaches.org) have developed written information about headaches and their history, pathophysiology, treatment, and prevention. The brochures and videos are available to the public, either free of charge or at a nominal cost. These national groups encourage headache patients and their families to join for support and information. Websites also provide information and support.

HEALTH PROMOTION

As reviewed in the section on management, the nonpharmacologic measures are an important part of headache treatment. This can include the modalities reviewed there but also involves encouraging patients to lead a "regular lifestyle" of going to bed at the same time, getting up at the same time, eating three meals a day, limiting alcohol and caffeine intake, and including exercise as part of the daily routine. This wellness program may abort an attack or prevent triggers from initiating an attack. Being able to identify one's triggers through a daily diary can encourage the headache patient to modify behavior, eating habits, or lifestyle.

CHAPTER 197

INFECTIONS OF THE CENTRAL NERVOUS SYSTEM

Daniel W. O'Neill • Robyn M. Jennings

DEFINITION AND EPIDEMIOLOGY

Infections of the central nervous system (CNS) consist primarily of meningitis (inflammation of the meninges) and encephalitis (inflammation of the brain) and are caused by a variety of pathologic microorganisms. The high morbidity and mortality rates of bacterial meningitis make diagnosis and early treatment a high priority in the primary care setting. Bacterial meningitis is most common in children younger than 2 years, with a peak incidence at 3 to 8 months of age; however, it does occur throughout the life span, with *a second peak incidence after 60 years of age*. In the United States, the annual overall incidence rate is 1.3 to 2 per 100,000 persons.[1] Despite the use of effective antimicrobial therapy, annual mortality rates remain at 17% to 30%, with up to 50% of survivors having some long-term neurologic sequelae.[2]

Encephalitis is caused primarily by herpesviruses (most common in the United States), arboviruses (transmitted by insects), and enteroviruses.[3] An increase in encephalitis caused by cytomegalovirus, Epstein-Barr virus (EBV), and human herpesvirus is occurring because of an increase in immunocompromised states, including human immunodeficiency virus (HIV) infection, organ transplantation, and chemotherapy. Viruses cause CNS infection by direct spread of cranial nerve or olfactory tract infections, reactivation of a latent virus within the CNS, or viremia followed by spread across the blood-brain barrier.[3]

Meningitis is defined as either aseptic or septic, depending on the identification of bacteria on the Gram stain or culture. Aseptic meningitis is caused mostly by enteroviruses, for which there is a good prognosis and no specific therapy. Bacterial meningitis is usually spread hematogenously from another primary source (predominantly the respiratory tract) or by contiguous spread from sinusitis, mastoiditis, or otitis media. The pathogens in meningitis are age specific: group B streptococci and *Escherichia coli* are most common in children younger than 1 month; *Listeria monocytogenes* is more common in the very young (younger than 1 month) and adults older than 50 years; and *Streptococcus pneumoniae* and *Neisseria meningitidis* are the most common causes in children and adults, with the latter seen in epidemics involving young adults.[4] *Haemophilus influenzae* used to be the leading cause of meningitis in young children until the advent of universal vaccination.[1] Because of the widespread overuse of oral antibiotics, there has been a dramatic rise in multidrug-resistant *S. pneumoniae*.[4] *N. meningitidis* can occur in epidemic outbreaks in young adults. Elderly adults have a notably higher percentage of infections with *L. monocytogenes.* Staphylococci and gram-negative bacilli are seen in meningitis associated with neurosurgery and trauma.[1] In 2012, 158 cases of iatrogenic fungal meningitis were reported in the United States in patients who received contaminated epidural steroid injections.[5]

Risk factors for bacterial meningitis are previous basilar skull fracture or neurosurgery, sickle cell disease, complement deficiency, asplenia, alcoholism, immunodeficiency (HIV infection or organ transplant recipient), recent travel to an endemic area, and exposure to a community outbreak. Once the pathogen gains access to the cerebrospinal fluid (CSF), where there is little natural host defense, it replicates and releases bacterial cell wall proteins, which stimulate cytokine release and capillary leak. This leads to the accumulation of protein and leukocytes, cerebral edema, microvascular thrombosis, and, ultimately, cerebral ischemia and hypoxia.

CLINICAL PRESENTATION

The onset of symptoms of CNS infection can be either acute or subacute, with progression during several days. The classic adult presentation of bacterial meningitis is fever, headache, and stiff neck (meningismus); however, this is seen in only 44% of cases.[6] Altered levels of consciousness, seizures, and hypotension predict a poor outcome. Nausea, vomiting, and photophobia are more common but can also be seen with migraine. Ear, sinus, or lung infections may precede pneumococcal meningitis. In fact, older adult patients on presentation may lack fever or meningismus but may be confused or even obtunded, often after an antecedent infection such as bronchitis, pneumonia, sinusitis, or urinary tract infection.[7] Encephalitis manifests with signs and symptoms similar to those of meningitis but with more prevalent alterations in consciousness, focal neurologic signs, seizures, and autonomic and hypothalamic disturbances.[3]

PHYSICAL EXAMINATION

Nuchal rigidity, Kernig sign, and Brudzinski sign have low sensitivity but a moderate positive predictive value for meningitis in adults.[8] In older adults, nuchal rigidity has an even lower sensitivity and specificity. Kernig sign is present if a patient in the supine position resists passive knee extension when the hip is fully flexed on the abdomen. Brudzinski sign is present if a patient in the supine position actively flexes the hips when the neck is passively flexed. Jolt sensitivity (observing a worsening of headache when a patient moves his or her head twice horizontally) is another test for meningitis with low sensitivity but may be used as an adjunctive test.[8,9] Purpura and petechiae are often associated with rapidly progressing meningococcemia but can be seen with other infections or can be a sign of disseminated intravascular coagulopathy. In patients with meningitis, a careful neurologic examination may reveal focal deficits suggestive of brain abscess, cranial nerve inflammation, thrombosis, ischemia, or cerebral edema.[1] Meningitis can lead to increased intracranial pressure (ICP), which manifests as depressed consciousness, sluggishly reactive or dilated pupils, ophthalmoplegia, respiratory depression, bradycardia, hypertension, posturing, hyperreflexia, and spasticity. With clinical presentation alone, it is difficult to distinguish aseptic meningitis from bacterial meningitis or encephalitis.

DIAGNOSTICS

- Blood cultures (positive in 19% to 70% of patients with bacterial meningitis[6]), complete blood count (CBC) with differential, and serum glucose concentration should be obtained immediately. Erythrocyte sedimentation rate (ESR) and C-reactive protein (CRP) can be useful for following the course of the illness.
- Lumbar puncture (LP) must be performed in all patients with suspected meningitis or encephalitis.
- The following are contraindications for LP: cardiorespiratory compromise, shock, evidence of increased ICP, or cellulitis over the LP site. Thrombocytopenia, coagulopathies, and use of anticoagulants are relative contraindications.[6]
- Opening CSF pressures should be measured.
- A sample of the CSF should be sent for protein level, glucose concentration, Gram stain, culture, and cell count with differential. A positive Gram stain examination of CSF has nearly 100% specificity, but a negative Gram stain cannot rule out bacterial disease.[1] Rapid testing of the CSF for antigens of several common pathogens is widely available but not routinely used except in cases of prior antibiotic therapy.
- Extra tubes of CSF should be held for special studies, if indicated.
  - Interpretation of CSF values is helpful in distinguishing viral from bacterial infections (Table 197-1). Further testing of the CSF with viral cultures, polymerase chain reaction, specialized stains, and cultures may be indicated.
  - Measurement of serum CRP concentration may be helpful in patients with CSF findings consistent with meningitis but for whom the Gram stain result is negative. Serum CRP greater than 20 to 40 mg/L is highly sensitive for bacterial meningitis, especially in children.[6]
  - CSF lactate helps to distinguish between viral and bacterial meningitis; it has 93% sensitivity and 97% specificity for the latter.[6]
- If there is evidence of increased ICP or focal neurologic deficits, an immediate computed tomography (CT) scan must be performed before the LP to prevent uncal or cerebellar tonsillar herniation. One exception is for HIV patients in low-resource settings when the risks associated with delay in diagnosis and treatment of life-threatening infections outweigh the risk of herniation.[6]
- In all cases of suspected meningitis, the first dose of antimicrobials should be administered before the CT scan and LP to avoid critical delays in treatment. The CSF culture can

TABLE 197-1 Cerebrospinal Fluid Findings in Acute Meningitis

Findings	Normal	Bacterial Meningitis	Viral Meningitis
Opening pressure (mmH_2O CSF)	50-195	>180	WNL or mildly increased
Cell count ($cells/mm^3$)	<5 (15% neutrophils)	Up to 100,000 (>80% neutrophils)	10-10,000 (mostly lymphocytes)
Protein (mg/dL)	15-50	100-500	50-100
Glucose (mg/dL)	45-80	<40	WNL or 20-40
CSF/serum glucose ratio	>0.5	<0.4	WNL

WNL, within normal limits.

still yield bacteria 1 to 2 hours after the first dose of antibiotics.
- In suspected viral encephalitis, temporal and orbitofrontal hyperintensity T2 and fluid-attenuated inversion recovery (FLAIR) MRI is consistent with herpes simplex virus (HSV) infection. Electroencephalography will also show epileptiform changes with HSV.[3]

DIAGNOSTICS

Infections of the Central Nervous System

LABORATORY
CBC and differential
Blood cultures—two sets
Serum glucose
ESR and CRP

IMAGING
CT scan*
T2 and FLAIR MRI†

OTHER DIAGNOSTICS
LP (for CSF protein, glucose, cell count and differential, Gram stain, and culture; lactate, hold extra tubes for special studies)
Electroencephalography†

*If indicated.
†If encephalitis is suspected.[3]

DIFFERENTIAL DIAGNOSIS

Infections of the Central Nervous System

COMMON CAUSES OF BACTERIAL MENINGITIS
- *Streptococcus pneumoniae*
- *Neisseria meningitidis*
- *Haemophilus influenzae*
- *Listeria monocytogenes*
- Aerobic gram-negative bacilli (after trauma or neurosurgery)

COMMON CAUSES OF VIRAL ENCEPHALITIS
- West Nile virus (most recent outbreak was in 2009),
- Herpesvirus (HSV types 1 and 2 and varicella-zoster virus)
- Mumps virus
- Influenza virus
- Lymphocytic choriomeningitis virus
- EBV
- Rabies
- Measles virus
- Dengue fever
- HIV

OTHER INFECTIOUS CAUSES OF ENCEPHALITIS AND MENINGITIS
- Tuberculosis (usually a more indolent course with CSF lymphocytosis and hypoglycemia)
- Spirochetes (e.g., syphilis, Lyme disease, leptospirosis)
- Rickettsiae (e.g., Rocky Mountain spotted fever, typhus)
- Protozoa (e.g., malaria, Chagas disease, or amoebas)
- Fungal organisms
- Prion disease

CAUSES OF CNS INFECTIONS IN AIDS PATIENTS
- *Toxoplasma*
- *Cryptococcus*
- *Histoplasma*
- *Nocardia*
- Tuberculosis
- Cytomegalovirus
- Papovavirus

NONINFECTIOUS CAUSES OF ENCEPHALITIS AND MENINGITIS
- Carcinoma
- Vasculitis
- Multiple sclerosis
- Intravenous immune globulin therapy
- Drug reactions (e.g., nonsteroidal anti-inflammatory drugs)
- CNS hemorrhage
- Postvaccination aseptic meningitis

DIFFERENTIAL DIAGNOSIS

Although most cases of community-acquired, new-onset meningitis and encephalitis are bacterial and viral in origin, respectively, certain clinical or community factors warrant consideration of less common causes, including nonresponse to empirical treatment.

MANAGEMENT

Immediate emergency department referral or referral to a physician experienced in the treatment of CNS infections is indicated for all suspected CNS infections.

If bacterial meningitis is suspected, immediate empirical bactericidal therapy is directed against presumptive pathogens tailored to the patient's age, immune status, and setting of acquisition. If antibiotics are given within 6 hours, the case fatality rate has been shown to be 4% to 5%, compared with a 75% case fatality rate if antibiotics are not started for 8 to 10 hours.[1] Important factors to consider include antibiotic sensitivities and community acquisition versus nosocomial acquisition. A common combination used for community-acquired bacterial meningitis in children and adults in response to the development of penicillin-resistant pneumococcus is vancomycin (15 to 20 mg/kg intravenously every 8 to 12 hours; maximum dose 2 g at once or 60 mg/kg/day) plus a third-generation cephalosporin (cefotaxime, 2 g every 4 hours; or ceftriaxone, 2 g intravenously every 12 hours).[1] Other clinical factors and findings on Gram stain and culture will direct the narrowing of subsequent specific antimicrobial therapy. In patients at risk for *L. monocytogenes*, specifically those older than 50 years and those who are immunocompromised, empirical therapy should also include ampicillin (2 g every 4 hours).[1] Post-traumatic, neurosurgical, or CSF shunt patients should be empirically prescribed ceftazidime (2 g every 8 hours) plus vancomycin (1 to 2 g intravenously every 12 hours) to cover gram-negative enteric bacilli.[1] In patients with bacterial meningitis who have responded appropriately to antimicrobial therapy, repeated CSF analysis to document CSF sterilization and improvement of CSF parameters is not routinely indicated but should be performed for any patient who has not responded clinically after 48 hours of empirical antimicrobial therapy.[6] Adjunctive dexamethasone therapy (10 mg intravenously every 6 hours for 4 days) started before or with the first dose of antibiotics should be routine in cases of suspected bacterial meningitis to minimize damaging inflammation from bacteriolysis and long-term morbidity.[4,10] This is safe and most effective for pneumococcal meningitis without underlying comorbidities. Maintenance fluids should be used cautiously in the absence of hypovolemia. Measures to decrease ICP (elevating head 30 degrees, hyperventilation, mannitol) are initiated if necessary. Patients with bacterial meningitis require 24 hours of respiratory isolation and close monitoring, possibly in an intensive care unit.

Treatment of viral encephalitis is mostly supportive: optimization of fluid balance and electrolytes; symptomatic treatment of headache, fever, and nausea; airway protection; management of ICP; and management of seizures.

If HSV or varicella-zoster virus (VZV) encephalitis is suspected, intravenous acyclovir (10 mg/kg every 8 hours) should be initiated. Steroids may also benefit these patients.[4]

Consultation with specialists in infectious disease, critical care, neurology, or neurosurgery should be obtained if indicated. Neuropsychiatric testing, rehabilitation specialists, audiologists, psychiatrists, and other counselors may be needed in follow-up care.

COMPLICATIONS

Complications of bacterial meningitis include dehydration, septic shock, hemodynamic compromise, cerebral edema, disseminated intravascular coagulopathy, myocarditis, hyponatremia, seizures, and death, 5% to 18% of these patients still die despite antibiotic treatment.[11] Long-term sequelae are seen in up to 50% of survivors and consist of learning disability, hearing impairment, seizure disorder, and other neuropsychological impairment. Permanent neurologic damage is seen in up to 90% of patients with HSV-1 encephalitis, as well as in those with encephalitis from other causes.[3]

INDICATIONS FOR REFERRAL OR HOSPITALIZATION

Immediate emergency department referral and/or referral to a physician experienced in the treatment of CNS infections is indicated for all suspected CNS infections because early treatment reduces morbidity and mortality.

LIFE SPAN CONSIDERATIONS

In adults, age has been shown to correlate with mortality after bacterial meningitis.[11] In older adults, consideration should always be given to atypical presentations of CNS meningitis and *L. monocytogenes* as a causative organism. For all adults, use of adjunctive steroid therapy with meningitis has been shown to decrease long-term mortality.

EDUCATION AND HEALTH PROMOTION

Prevention is a valuable strategy to reduce the morbidity and mortality of bacterial meningitis. The *H. influenzae* type B and pneumococcal vaccines have proved to be effective in lowering the attack rate in all ages; they should be strongly encouraged for infants. The 23-valent polysaccharide pneumococcal vaccine should be administered to eligible candidates, including all patients older than 65 years, patients who are immunocompromised, patients with chronic disease, patients without a spleen, and patients in long-term care facilities. The quadrivalent meningococcal conjugate vaccine (MCV4) is routinely given to children 11 or 12 years old. A booster is given at age 16 because protection wanes after 5 years, and rates of meningitis peak at ages 16 to 21. Adolescents with HIV should receive two MCV4 shots 2 months apart with a booster at 16. High-risk adults younger than 56 and children age 2 to 10 can also receive the conjugate vaccine; adults older than 56 receive the meningococcal polysaccharide vaccine (MPSV4).[12] High-risk adults include those living in college dormitories, military recruits, those with complement deficiency or asplenia, those spending time in endemic areas, and scientists working with the causal organism.[13] For control of community outbreaks, chemoprophylaxis with rifampin (600 mg twice daily for 2 days), ceftriaxone (one dose, 250 mg given intramuscularly), or ciprofloxacin (a single dose of 500 mg) is indicated for close contacts of patients with *N. meningitidis* or *H. influenzae* infection.

For prevention of vector-borne diseases, including West Nile virus (see Chapter 236) and eastern equine encephalitis, designated resources in local and state public health departments are necessary, such as public education about mosquito control and the prevention of mosquito and tick bites.

CHAPTER 198

MOVEMENT DISORDERS AND ESSENTIAL TREMOR

Nancy McQueen Le • Katie McCube

DEFINITION AND EPIDEMIOLOGY

Movement disorders include a variety of neurologic conditions that cause alteration in normal movement or unnatural movements. These can be further categorized as excessive movements or hyperkinesis and decreased amplitude or range of movement or hypokinesis. Additional definitions can be found in Box 198-1.

The most common hyperkinetic movement disorders include essential tremor, restless legs syndrome, dystonia, and Tourette syndrome. Less common are hemifacial spasms, blepharospasm, ataxias, and Huntington disease.[1]

The most common hypokinetic movement disorder is Parkinson disease. Less common are progressive supranuclear palsy and multisystem atrophy.[1]

PATHOPHYSIOLOGY

Voluntary movement requires complex interactions between the pyramidal tracts, cerebellum, and basal ganglia to produce smooth, decisive movement without extraneous muscular contractions.[2] Many abnormal movements are associated with

BOX 198-1

Definitions

Akathisia: A sense of inner general restlessness reduced or relieved by moving about.

Asterixis: A brief flap of outstretched limb, transient inhibition of the muscles of posture.[1]

Ataxia: An unsteady or swaying motion. Movements may appear irregular or clumsy.

Athetosis: A slow, writhing, continuous, involuntary movement.

Chorea: An involuntary, irregular, nonrhythmic movement that seems to flow from one body part to another. The movements are unpredictable in timing, direction, and body part affected.

Dyskinesia: A general term for any abnormal involuntary movement. Paroxysmal dyskinesias are abnormal movements that occur only at certain times; hypnogenic dyskinesias typically occur during non–rapid eye movement (REM) sleep. Tardive dyskinesia refers to movements induced by dopaminergic agents, most commonly neuroleptics and metoclopramide.

Dystonia: A sustained involuntary muscle contraction that results in twisting movement and posture, often patterned and repetitive.

Myoclonus: Sudden, irregular, involuntary jerking of the muscles.

Myokymia: A fine quivering or rippling of muscles. Common and benign in facial muscles.

Stereotypy: A coordinated movement that repeats continually and identically. Compulsion.

Tics: Sudden, repetitive, nonrhythmic motor movement or vocalization. A habitual spasmodic involuntary muscle contraction.

Tremor: An oscillation, usually rhythmic and regular, affecting various body parts, such as limbs, neck, tongue, chin, or vocal cords. Can be classified as resting, postural, or action or intention tremor.

pathologic alterations within these structures and their connections, whereas others can arise from elsewhere in the central nervous system (CNS), such as the cerebral cortex or the spinal cord. The peripheral nervous system can also give rise to abnormal movements, such as restless leg syndrome.

In some movement disorders, such as Parkinson disease, the underlying complex pathology is becoming better understood, but for many movement disorders much of the cause remains unclear.

CLINICAL PRESENTATION

The presentation of movement disorders will depend on the underlying cause, so establishing a careful history specific to the patient's complaint is important (Box 198-2). The primary complaint may not be the abnormal movement, but the functional limitation it imposes on the patient's activities of daily living. Movement disorders primarily fall into several categories.

It is important to ascertain which category the movement disorder falls into by obtaining a careful history. This includes the age at onset, the regions of the body affected, progression of symptoms, the quality of movements and dysfunction, the factors that make symptoms better or worse, and the timing. A family history of movement disorder should be noted as well. A medication, alcohol, and drug history is necessary and should include prescription, over-the-counter, and illicit drug use. Alcohol, drugs, and/or medications can exacerbate or even mask underlying conditions or symptoms.

PHYSICAL EXAMINATION

The examination should be approached in a systematic fashion. Make note of observations throughout the examination visit. The examination should include a complete neurologic examination and general physical assessment. Subtle findings in movement may differentiate some of the disorders. All aspects of the neurologic examination may provide clues to assist in ruling in or out different movement disorders. A neurologic examination should include evaluation of cognition, cranial nerves, motor function (strength, tone, and coordination), sensor function, deep tendon reflexes (DTRs), and gait. The goal is to define the characteristics of the movement, determine which definition fits, and eliminate those that do not.

First look at obvious features. These include rhythm, duration, and continuity of contractions; type of oscillations (rapid or slow); and amplitude (fine or coarse). Note whether the movements occur at rest or during action and are patterned or random and whether there is a combination of movements. Also evaluate other factors such as speed, force, complexity of the movement, and any associated sensory symptoms.

BOX 198-2[3]

Categories of Movement Disorders

INSUFFICIENT MOVEMENT

- Akinetic, hypokinetic, or bradykinetic syndromes

TOO MUCH MOVEMENT

- Jerky
  - Myoclonus, chorea, and tic disorders
- Nonjerky
  - Dystonia and tremor

DIAGNOSTICS

Initial diagnostic studies to consider would be basic laboratory studies to rule out medical or metabolic abnormalities. If there is reason to suspect infection or alcohol or drug use, additional focused workup would be warranted. Neurologic imaging, often in conjunction with a neurologic referral, may be warranted if there are specific neurologic findings.

DIAGNOSTICS

Movement Disorders

Complete blood count (CBC) with differential
Basic metabolic profile (BMP)
Liver function tests (LFTs)

FOCUSED WORKUP

Infection workup (CBC, urinalysis, chest x-ray study)
Drugs or alcohol (toxicology screen, ammonia level, LFTs)

IMAGING

Computed tomography scan

DIFFERENTIAL DIAGNOSIS

Determining a differential diagnosis first requires defining the type of movements that are occurring, as described in Boxes 198-1 and 198-2.

DIFFERENTIAL DIAGNOSIS

Movement Disorders

HYPOKINETIC MOVEMENT SYNDROMES

- Parkinson disease
- Depression
- Hypothyroidism
- Slowing caused by musculoskeletal conditions

HYPERKINETIC MOVEMENT DISORDERS

Jerky Disorders

- Myoclonus
- Encephalopathy
- Essential or idiopathic disorder
- Epileptic
  - Startle reactions
- Chorea
  - Huntington disease
  - Hemiballismus
- Tics
  - Tourette syndrome
  - Periodic limb movement disorder
  - Complex partial seizures
  - Hemifacial spasms

Nonjerky Disorders

- Essential tremor
- Metabolic disorders
- Medications
  - LSD, dopamine antagonists and agonists, CNS stimulants, typical and atypical
  - antipsychotics
- Cerebellar tremor (stroke, MS, tumor)
- Dystonia
- Cervical (spasmodic torticollis)
- Blepharospasm
- Writer's cramp
- Genetic

Brain Injury

- Infections
- Stroke

MANAGEMENT

Specialist referral, likely a neurology referral, is indicated when (1) the diagnosis is uncertain, (2) the patient is not responding to standard treatment, or (3) the patient's condition is deteriorating.

Emergency department referral is indicated if the patient has acute focal neurologic symptoms or is suspected to have a serious medical condition.

The primary goals of treatment are as follows:

- Treat underlying conditions.
- Manage the symptoms, which may include medication management as well as physical and occupational therapy.

COMPLICATIONS

Most movement disorders can be placed on a continuum with symptoms ranging from mild to severe. Therefore, complications will vary.

Complications may include medication side effects, functional impairments such as diminished independence and activities of daily living, and balance and safety issues. Psychosocial issues include depression, difficulty with communication, self-consciousness, and issues with employment.

LIFE SPAN CONSIDERATIONS

Different movement disorders are more prevalent at certain ages, which may help guide the diagnosis. When medication management is warranted, geriatric patients may be more sensitive to treatment. Depending on the condition, some movement disorders may lead to social and employment issues in younger people.

EDUCATION AND HEALTH PROMOTION

Patient education should include information about the diagnostic evaluation and, once a diagnosis has been determined, specific information regarding the prognosis, treatment options, and complications. The provider should help patients and families by providing specific information about their conditions. This can include Web-based or written information and referrals to support groups. If the provider sends a patient to a website, the patient should bring materials or discuss what he or she has learned, to monitor for accuracy. Teaching should also emphasize how medications can be used to relieve symptoms and the potential side effects of these agents.

The International Parkinson and Movement Disorder Society website (www.movementdisorders.org) is a good resource for patients with movement disorders. This is a professional society that offers links to multiple other organizations and foundations for both patients and medical professionals.

ESSENTIAL TREMOR

DEFINITION AND EPIDEMIOLOGY

Essential tremor is a benign, chronic neurologic condition that involves symmetric, rhythmic trembling of the upper extremities, head, or voice. The legs are less commonly involved. The only clinical finding is the tremor, which may be present at rest and usually progresses over time.[3,4]

Oscillations are present throughout voluntary movement and are accentuated as the hand approaches a given target.[5] Emotional stress will also increase the symptoms, whereas alcohol or rest will diminish them.[3,5] Known as benign, familial, hereditary, or senile tremor,[3] this is the most common of the movement disorders. Men and women are affected equally, with a mean age at onset of 45 years. The condition can begin as early as adolescence but most often begins in the sixth or seventh decade of life. An estimated 10 million people in the United States have this condition. If more than one person in a family group has the condition, the tremor is termed familial or hereditary tremor. An autosomal dominant inheritance pattern can be identified in more than 50% of cases. If the tremor begins in old age, it is commonly termed senile tremor.[3,4]

PATHOPHYSIOLOGY

Although essential tremor is a neurologic disorder, little is known about its cause. To date, no structural defects have been identified on autopsy, and diagnostic study results are typically normal. It is believed to be caused by focal oscillatory activity within the CNS.[4] Positron emission tomography (PET) scan studies have found changes in regional blood flow in the cerebellum and inferior olivary nuclei of patients with essential tremor compared with matched control subjects.[4] It is unclear at this time if those changes are specific to essential tremor alone or are also found in other tremors. Because of the autosomal dominant inheritance, a thorough family history may prove helpful in establishing the diagnosis.[3,4] There is high variability in the rate of development of this disease.

CLINICAL PRESENTATION

For essential tremor, the patient's only complaint is that of tremor; any additional neurologic deficits should prompt consideration of an alternative diagnosis.[4] The patient typically reports a tremor at rest. The tremor becomes worse when the patient tries to move his or her hand or fingers in a purposeful manner. Furthermore, the amplitude of the tremor increases as the patient approaches his or her desired target.[5]

The patient may have difficulty in writing, eating, or performing other fine motor tasks. The head may nod ("yes" movements) or shake ("no" movements). Eyelid and facial tremor is also common.[4] The voice may quiver or shake. The tremor may be continual; however, it may also be episodic, sporadic, or intermittent. In general, the tremor disappears during sleep. A careful history of food, coffee or caffeine, antihistamines, medications, or illicit drug intake as well as of other symptoms is helpful in excluding other causes of the tremor.[5]

Patients often complain that the tremor is worse during periods of increased emotional stress or when they are trying to hurry. The tremor decreases with rest and alcohol; for this reason, a careful inquiry about alcohol consumption should be performed.[5,6]

The patient will not have problems with weakness or changes in muscle tone, nor will there be problems with coordination despite the tremor. The tremor generally does not affect the lower extremities.

The patient may have had the tremor for several years. A disabling disease progression may be what has brought the patient to the health care provider's attention. A careful history, including the age at onset, rate of progression and symmetry of the tremor, and exacerbating or alleviating factors, should be taken.

PHYSICAL EXAMINATION

An upper extremity tremor that cycles 6 to 10 times per second is obvious. The amplitude of this tremor increases with voluntary movement, particularly as the patient approaches a specific target.[5] The rate of cycles per second should remain unchanged. The fingertip-to-nose test is particularly helpful in eliciting this phenomenon.[7] The patient may have difficulty in writing or grasping small objects. Examination should include having the patient draw a circle; this is a useful marker for disease progression as well as for monitoring of treatment efficacy. The drawing should be included in the medical record. The patient's voice may quiver, and the head may shake or nod rhythmically. The eyelids and facial muscles may also twitch. All findings should be documented and updated at subsequent visits.

Muscle tone, gait, and posture should all be normal. The lower extremities should be tremor free. The arm swing with walking should be relatively normal. DTRs should also be normal; there should be no clonus.[5] Other findings suggest an alternative diagnosis.

DIAGNOSTICS

In general, the diagnosis is based on the history and examination findings. Laboratory or diagnostic testing should be considered when findings other than an isolated, generally symmetric upper extremity tremor are noted.[5]

DIFFERENTIAL DIAGNOSIS

Tremors may originate in the CNS, arise from metabolic abnormalities, or be induced by medication or alcohol. CNS tremors may be caused by Parkinson disease (see Chapter 200), Huntington chorea, or Sydenham chorea (secondary to streptococcal infections), or they may be cerebellar in nature. Metabolic tremors may be related to a thyroid abnormality, pheochromocytoma, or liver disease.[8]

DIFFERENTIAL DIAGNOSIS

Essential Tremor

- Parkinson disease
- Cerebellar tremor
- Drug-induced tremor
- Dystonic tremor
- Enhanced physiologic tremor
- Fragile X–associated tremor-ataxia syndrome (FXTAS)
- Holmes tremor
- Primary writing tremor
- Orthostatic tremor
- Psychogenic tremor
- Wilson disease

MANAGEMENT

Specialist referral, likely a neurology referral, is indicated when (1) the diagnosis is uncertain, (2) the patient is not responding to standard treatment, or (3) the patient's condition is deteriorating.

Emergency department referral is indicated if the patient has acute focal neurologic symptoms or is suspected to have a serious medical condition.

Reassurance may be all that is necessary.[5] If the tremor is functionally or socially problematic, medication may be used. Persistent trials and evaluations may be required to find the medication that is most effective but has minimal side effects. The American Academy of Neurology (AAN) published guidelines, updated in 2011, provide the most current approach to medication selection.[9] Medications used to manage essential tremor fall under several different categories.

Initial medical therapy is usually propranolol or primidone.

- Beta blockers: The most commonly prescribed medication for this condition is propranolol (Inderal).[9] The patient should be started at a low dose and may need frequent titrations to an effective dose. Symptoms and medication tolerance should be reevaluated after 1 to 2 weeks. Consultation with cardiology specialists is recommended in patients with cardiac disease.
- Anticonvulsants: When beta blockers are not effective or tolerated, primidone (Mysoline) is the next option. Like propranolol, primidone reduces the amplitude but not the frequency of the tremor. Both gabapentin and topiramate have been shown to possibly reduce tremor, but the evidence is not as strong.
- Combined therapy: The use of propranolol and primidone together may be considered if there is some benefit from one agent alone but that benefit is suboptimal. The combined use of these drugs is possibly more effective than either drug alone.
- Benzodiazepines: Medications such as alprazolam and clonazepam are considered possibly effective. However, caution should be used because of side effects and possibility of misuse.
- Alcohol: Although alcohol has long been known to alleviate essential tremor, few formal studies have been completed to demonstrate its efficacy. Regular use of alcohol is not recommended as a long-term management strategy.[9]

COMPLICATIONS

Complications may include medication side effects and functional impairments such as diminished independence and activities of daily living, and balance and safety issues. Psychosocial issues include depression, self-consciousness, and issues with employment.

LIFE SPAN CONSIDERATIONS

Although essential tremor is considered a benign condition, it may have a profound effect on the patient's quality of life. The tremor may be embarrassing, particularly in younger patients. The condition may cause the patient to withdraw socially.[4-6] Careful observation for depression, alcoholism, and suicidal ideation in younger patients is important. Antidepressants and counseling may be required to help patients cope with the disorder. When medication management is warranted, geriatric populations may be more sensitive to treatment.

Severe tremors can significantly interfere with activities of daily living. Basic fine motor activities, including eating and dressing, can be impossible for some patients. Treatment is aimed at control of the severity of the tremor to facilitate independence.[3-6]

EDUCATION AND HEALTH PROMOTION

The patient should be advised to avoid stimulants such as caffeine, soda, and coffee. Many over-the-counter allergy and cold preparations have stimulants in them that can also accentuate the tremors.

Careful education about the chronicity, progression, and prognosis of the disease is necessary. Although it is medically considered a benign condition, this disorder may have significant psychosocial implications, requiring frequent reevaluation and patient support. Patients also should understand that the condition is hereditary.

Health and quality of life can be improved if the patient understands the disease process and receives support as necessary. An appropriate diet and a good exercise program can also be beneficial. Alcohol abuse should always be a concern because consumption of alcohol is known to be effective at diminishing the tremor.[6]

CHAPTER 199

MULTIPLE SCLEROSIS

Barbara S. Bishop

DEFINITION AND EPIDEMIOLOGY

Multiple sclerosis (MS) is a chronic progressive inflammatory and neurodegenerative disease affecting the central nervous system (CNS). The hallmark lesion in MS, called a plaque, was first described in the 1800s.[1] Multiple lesions are seen in multiple locations, hence the name *multiple sclerosis.* On histologic examination, the lesions are characterized by inflammation, demyelination, axonal injury and transaction, axonal loss, and gliosis.[1-3] MS is thought to be a complicated interaction among the autoimmune system, genetic variables, and environmental factors.[1] Clues to the cause of MS come from the worldwide and nonrandom pattern of this disease, studies of structural and functional changes within the CNS, immunologic studies, and genetic studies (particularly studies of families and twins).[1-3] To date, no single causative factor has been identified. It has been postulated that low vitamin D levels, exposure to Epstein-Barr virus (EBV) in preadolescence, and smoking are significant contributing environmental factors in MS. More than 100 genes have been identified that are associated with MS.[4-6] Box 199-1 describes the types of presentation and clinical courses of MS. The onset of MS is likely to occur between 20 and 50 years of age. MS affects three times as many women as men. It can also occur in the pediatric and geriatric populations. MS affects up to 450,000[8] Americans and approximately 2.5 million persons worldwide. The worldwide pattern of MS shows that it is less common near the equator, and the highest incidence is across northern Europe, North America, and Australia. It occurs most commonly in Caucasians.[1,2] African Americans tend to have more aggressive disease courses.[7]

Specialist referral is indicated for all suspected cases of MS.

BOX 199-1

Clinical Courses of MS

Radiographically isolated syndrome (RIS): Presence of magnetic resonance imaging (MRI) lesions specific to MS that may meet the MRI diagnostic criteria for MS without clinical symptoms. Sixty-five percent of patients convert to MS in 5.3 years.

Clinically isolated syndrome (CIS): Acute or subacute focal neurologic event indicative of demyelination and often associated with clinically silent lesions on MRI. Up to 90% of MS patients have CIS on presentation.

Relapsing-remitting MS (RRMS): Course punctuated by clinical relapses (exacerbations) followed by periods of clinical remission; most common type; 85% of MS patients have RRMS at time of diagnosis.

Primary-progressive MS (PPMS): Accumulating disability from initial presentation without clearly defined relapses or remissions. Approximately 10% of MS patients have PPMS.

Secondary-progressive MS (SPMS): Thought to be the natural evolution of RRMS. It represents a progressive course with or without relapses. Natural history states that 50% of RRMS will convert to SPMS, and 90% after 25 years.

Progressive-relapsing MS (PRMS): Steadily progressive from onset, but also with acute attacks. Approximately 5% of MS patients have this type.

Benign: Expanded Disability Severity Scale (EDSS) score ≤3 for more than 10 years. This definition does not take into account domains of fatigue, cognition, mood, pain, social functional levels, and radiographic changes. Studies have supported decline in all aforementioned domains. In addition, approximately 50% of patients with "benign" MS progress to having EDSS scores ≥6.0 or progress to SPMS within 20 years.

Data from Compston A, Coles A : Multiple sclerosis *Lancet* 372:1502-1517, 2008; Moses H Jr, Picone M, Smith V: *Clinician's primer on multiple sclerosis: an in-depth overview,* Denver, CO, 2008, Consensus Medical Communications; Okuda DT, Mowry EM, Beheshtian A, et al: Incidental MRI anomalies suggestive of multiple sclerosis: the radiologically isolated syndrome. *Neurology* 72(9):800-805, 2009; Leahy H, Garg N: Radiologically isolated syndrome: an overview. *Neurol Bull* 5:22-26, 2013; and Costella K, Halper J, et al: *The use of drug modifying therapy in multiple sclerosis: principles and current evidence.* Denver, 2014, Consortium of Multiple Sclerosis Centers (CMSC). www.mscare.org.

PATHOPHYSIOLOGY

MS has historically been thought of as an inflammatory disease of the white matter of the CNS. This paradigm has changed. It is not only inflammatory but also neurodegenerative and involves not only the white matter but the gray matter as well.

The sequence of events has become better clarified but is still not thoroughly understood. Presently, it is believed that a triggering event, most probably from the environment, activates the inflammatory process outside the CNS. This inflammatory process includes T- and B-cell activity, macrophages, natural killer cells, and others, demonstrating a complex and encompassing immune response from both the innate and adaptive immune systems. There is degradation of the blood-brain barrier, allowing the proinflammatory cytokines to penetrate the CNS. Once the proinflammatory cytokines are in the CNS, reactivation of the inflammatory process occurs, leading to demyelination and axonal destruction. Both the inflammatory and degenerative processes are seen early and simultaneously and often are felt to be interrelated. There is some support that they may also be independent of each other.[8] Regardless of the process, as the disease progresses, inflammation downregulates and neurodegeneration escalates. The process by which this occurs is not fully understood at this time.[2,3,9]

Recovery in early disease occurs because of the capacity of the CNS to functionally reorganize, compensate for axonal loss, and remyelinate. Remyelination is often incomplete and variable, and over time, axonal degradation becomes significant. Compensation is no longer possible. Permanent disability develops. It is believed that axonal degradation is responsible for permanent disability.[1-3,9,10]

CLINICAL PRESENTATION

There are four clinical courses of MS (see Box 199-1): relapsing-remitting (RRMS), primary-progressive (PPMS), secondary-progressive (SPMS), and progressive-relapsing (PRMS). RRMS is the most common form of MS. Natural history of the disease shows that 50% of MS patients will progress to SPMS within 11 to 15 years.[1,8]

At presentation, patients often have what is now referred to as a clinically isolated syndrome (CIS) or first clinical episode.

Patients typically have a focal neurologic deficit such as the eye pain or visual disturbances seen with optic neuritis. Sometimes the initial presentation is multifocal.[1,11] Magnetic resonance imaging (MRI) demonstrates multiple lesions consistent with MS. This is important, because it is now possible to treat patients at this very early stage of the disease process.[6,12] Radiographically isolated syndrome (RIS) is now reaching the literature. It is defined as the presence of MRI lesions specific to MS and may meet the MRI diagnostic criteria for MS; however, no clinical symptoms consistent with MS can be identified in the patient's history. Often these patients are undergoing MRI for some unrelated issue such as trauma or migraines. Currently, patients with RIS are not routinely being treated with disease-modifying therapy (DMT). Data to date suggest that 65% of patients will convert to MS within 5.3 years and 88% will convert in 14.1 years. Median time to conversion to CIS is 5.4 years.[13,14]

The most common presenting symptoms include visual disturbances and eye pain that comes and goes, pain in the neck or back, paresthesias or weakness of the limbs, or facial pain along the course of the trigeminal nerve. Other symptoms commonly seen include sensory symptoms (paresthesias), diplopia (intranuclear ophthalmoplegia), nystagmus, unsteady gait, or bowel or bladder dysfunction. Associated findings that increase the likelihood of MS include unexplained excessive fatigue, temperature or heat sensitivity, history of bandlike sensations around the waist (commonly referred to as the "MS hug"), dysarthria, muscle spasms, cognitive disturbances, and sexual dysfunction.[1-3,15]

The initial presentation of MS can often go unrecognized or is attributed to other causes, especially if the presenting symptom is vague, such as sensory distortion, bowel or bladder dysfunction, or cognitive impairment. Initial symptoms are sometimes so vague, transient, or mild that the patient may not seek medical advice.

Symptoms of MS are unpredictable and variable. As the disease progresses, a variety of signs and symptoms will require ongoing management[15,16] (see Table 199-1).

PHYSICAL EXAMINATION

A complete neurologic examination is required for patients with MS or suspected MS. The findings on neurologic examination may be normal, especially in early disease the patient may report problems consistent with symptoms without true focal deficit. The examination may be variable over time because of the fluctuating nature of the disease process. Specific domains of the neurologic examination for MS evaluation are as follows:

- Mental status: Observe for general conversation, fluidity of speech, speed of thought processing, integration of complex ideas, and following of multistep or complex directions. Neuropsychiatric testing is sensitive in elucidating cognitive issues associated with MS. It can also serve as a baseline for comparison over time.
- Cranial nerves (CNs): Extraocular movements [EOMs] should be assessed for conjugate movement, nystagmus, and intranuclear ophthalmoplegia; these may cause symptoms of diplopia. Vertigo may be experienced with EOM testing. Ophthalmic examination may reveal disc pallor, often seen with optic neuritis. The trigeminal nerve may reveal allodynia, common in trigeminal neuralgia, and a central seventh CN deficit may reflect a CNS lesion. The remaining CNs should also be examined because deficit may be seen in any CN, with the aforementioned being the most common.
- Motor testing may reveal weakness of a limb or more subtle weakness—for example, clumsiness of the hand and decreased fine dexterity. In the lower extremities, subtle plantar flexion or dorsiflexion weakness may be seen. The patient may drag the foot or trip on it frequently with ambulation and complain of falls or loss of balance when in fact it is a result of weakness. Increased tone and clonus in muscles should be assessed with passive range of motion. Gait should be evaluated to include evidence of circumduction, spasticity, or ataxia.
- Timed 25-foot walk test (T25FW) is becoming commonplace as part of the MS evaluation.
- Sensory examination should focus on pinprick, proprioception, and vibration testing to determine long-tract involvement. Patients may also have a distinct sensory level indicating spinal cord involvement, especially if transverse myelitis is suspected.
- Cerebellar: Finger-to-nose and Romberg testing can identify cerebellar involvement. Often, the patient will have an ataxic gait as well.
- Reflexes are often brisk with upgoing toes, consistent with CNS involvement.

In a patient with known MS, having a documented neurologic and functional baseline is imperative for evaluation of response to treatment or possible exacerbation of the disease. New neurologic findings can be mild or subtle yet result in significant functional deficits. Functional areas to review or examine might include driving, falls and injuries, and difficulties in the work arena, interpersonal skills, financial capabilities, and activities of daily living (ADLs). The Expanded Disability Severity Scale (EDSS), Fatigue Severity Scale (FSS), 12-item MS Walking Scale (MSWS-12), and T25FW can help supply quantitative support for functional limitations.[17-20]

DIAGNOSTICS

MS is still a clinical diagnosis. There must be separation of time and space. Events must be at least two distinct episodes lasting more than 24 hours occurring at least 30 days apart (separation of time), and there must be evidence of at least two different locations (separation of space). Signs and symptoms need to be consistent with inflammatory demyelinating disease. No other pathologic process can be found for the clinical and paraclinical findings.[4]

Ruling out other pathologic processes is essential. Historically this has been done by clinical history, examination, and diagnostic studies. MRI has helped to revolutionize the diagnosis of MS and has become the gold standard for diagnosis of MS via the McDonald criteria.[4] The McDonald criteria were initially brought into use in 2001 and underwent revisions in 2005 and again in 2010.[4,21] Diagnostic studies such as visual evoked potentials, optical coherence tomography (OCT), spinal tap, and blood work are still useful when diagnosis is unclear or if MRI is not readily available.[1,2,21,22]

DIFFERENTIAL DIAGNOSIS

Because many neurologic conditions must be considered, the differential diagnosis is extensive.

Consultation with a neurologist, MS neurology expert, or MS center should be considered for confirmation of diagnosis.

TABLE 199-1 **Symptomatic and Rehabilitative Therapies for Multiple Sclerosis***

Symptom	Description	Treatment Modalities
Ataxia	Incoordination and disturbance of balance and gait Worsened by spasticity, weakness, and fatigue Falls common	Home evaluation necessary to assess safety and fall risk Rehabilitation services for gait and balance; may work with balance balls and other techniques Medications ineffective Avoid alcohol
Bladder	Bladder: hesitancy, urgency, frequency incontinence; reported rates 52%-97%	Bladder: avoid dietary irritants such as caffeine and spicy foods; use toileting schedule; refer to urologist for formal workup; screen for UTI; fluid restriction at bedtime; biofeedback and Kegel exercises; clean intermittent catheterization; botulinum toxin; nerve stimulation devices *Drug therapy:* anticholinergics, antimuscarinics, and alpha blockers
Bowel	Bowel: irregular bowel is common; constipation, loose stools; constipation may aggravate bladder issues; reported rates 35%-68%	Bowel: fiber, stool softeners, laxatives, glycerin suppositories; bowel training programs, diet counseling, exercise *Drug therapy:* anticholinergic or muscle relaxant properties, such as oxybutynin, tolterodine, propantheline, antidiuretic hormone; botulinum toxin injections
Cognitive dysfunction	40%-70% of MS patients have some degree of cognitive impairment; executive functioning and memory are most common Can be a source of disability	Neuropsychological evaluation is important to define problem areas and provide recommendations; compensatory and restorative methods can be helpful; brain exercises such as those on Lumocity.com and CogMed.com Treat underlying disorders that can contribute to problem, such as depression, anxiety, fatigue, sleep disorders Adherence to DMT; some have been shown to slow cognitive decline *Drug therapy:* acetylcholinesterase inhibitors have not been found effective in larger studies
Depression	Endogenous as a result of changes in brain chemistry; may also be exogenous; higher incidence (56%) and rates of suicide than in other chronic or neurologic diseases	Antidepressants Counseling
Fatigue	Rates reported to be 65%-97% Highly debilitating; often the reason for disability Cause unknown Aggravated by depression, anemia, hypothyroidism, sleep disorder, elevated core body temperature	OT for energy conservation techniques Cooling vest or cap Staying well hydrated and drinking ice-cold water to bring down core body temperature Avoidance of heat Treat underlying problems Consider changing DMT if severe; glatiramer acetate may have less effect on fatigue than interferons *Drug therapy:* amantadine, methylphenidate, modafinil, armodafinil , fluoxetine (even if depression is not present)
Pain and paresthesias	Reported rates as high as 85% Trigeminal neuralgia and other forms of neuropathic pain (burning, numbness, tingling), migraines, spasms, musculoskeletal pain	Pain from spasms relieved with antispasmodics (discussed previously) PT and assistive devices Yoga, Pilates, tai chi for musculoskeletal pain *Drug therapy:* neuropathic pain—carbamazepine, gabapentin, pregabalin, topiramate, lamotrigine, lidocaine patch, duloxetine, tricyclic antidepressants; musculoskeletal pain—gabapentin, lidocaine patch, duloxetine, NSAIDs, muscle relaxants
Sexual dysfunction	Up to 90% in men and 85% in women Lack of interest or arousal Changes in self-esteem Problems with intimacy Impotence, anorgasmia, vaginal dryness Decreased or altered sensations Functional difficulties: spasms, bladder control	Try to coordinate symptomatic treatments to sexual activity (antispasmodics, self-catheterization); increased stimulation using vibration can be helpful; counseling may be necessary *Drug therapy:* erectile dysfunction medications for men, such as tadalafil, vardenafil, sildenafil citrate; remove offending medications if possible, such as SSRIs

TABLE 199-1 Symptomatic and Rehabilitative Therapies for Multiple Sclerosis—cont'd

Symptom	Description	Treatment Modalities
Spasticity	Reported rates: 40%-85% Stiff, slow movements; spasms	PT and assistive devices Yoga, Pilates, tai chi *Drug therapy:* baclofen intrathecal pump implantation; botulinum toxin injection; baclofen (Lioresal), tizanidine, dantrolene (Dantrium), benzodiazepine, gabapentin, levetiracetam
Tremor	May involve UE, LE, trunk, head, and voice and may be incapacitating Very difficult symptom to manage	OT help with weighted equipment and environmental modification strategies Deep brain stimulation can be considered and can be very effective for controlling tremor but is not FDA approved for MS tremor at this time. *Drug therapy:* most drugs are ineffective for MS tremor; some drugs that have been tried with limited success include propranolol and other beta blockers, clonazepam, primidone, ondansetron, isoniazid, and glutethimide
Weakness	Focal limb weakness caused by underlying demyelination and axonal loss	Rehabilitation services for strength training and adaptive devices such as braces and ambulatory assistive devices Keep core body temperature down; heat disrupts conduction For footdrop, ankle-foot orthoses can be helpful; WalkAide and Bioness systems, functional electrical stimulation devices, have been beneficial *Drug therapy:* dalfampridine, a potassium channel blocker, has recently been approved by the FDA to improve walking in MS; it is the only drug in its class

*Many medications used for MS symptoms are used off label.

LE, lower extremity; NSAIDs, nonsteroidal anti-inflammatory drugs; OT, occupational therapy; PT, physical therapy; SSRIs, selective serotonin reuptake inhibitors; UE, upper extremity; UTI, urinary tract infection.

Data from Moses H Jr, Picone M, Smith V: *Clinician's primer on multiple sclerosis: an in-depth overview,* Denver, CO, Consensus Medical Communications, 2008; Bennett S, Coyle P: *The clinician's primer on the latest advances in improved quality of life for patients with multiple sclerosis,* Denver, CO, Consensus Medical Communications, 2010; Thompson H. Mauk K. Nursing management of the patient with multiple sclerosis: AANN, ARN, and IOMSN clinical practice guideline series. 2011. American Association of Neuroscience nurses, Association of Rehabilitation Nurses, and International Organization of Multiple Sclerosis Nurses. Available at: www.rehabnurse.org/uploads/cpgms.pdf. accessed)ct 13, 2015. Polman CH, Reingold SC, Edan G, et al: Diagnostic criteria for multiple sclerosis: 2010 revisions to the "McDonald Criteria," *Ann Neurol* 69:292-302, 2011; and Toosy A, Ciccarelli O, Thompson A: Symptomatic treatment and management of multiple sclerosis. In Goodin DS, editor: *Handbook of clinical neurology,* Vol 122, *Multiple sclerosis and related disorders,* Amsterdam, Elsevier B.V., 2014.

DIAGNOSTICS

Multiple Sclerosis

LABORATORY

Complete blood count with differential
Antinuclear antibodies
Erythrocyte sedimentation rate
Fluorescent treponemal antibody absorption test (FTA-ABS) or Venereal Disease Research Laboratory (VDRL) test
Human immunodeficiency virus (HIV) test
Antiphospholipid antibodies
Prothrombin time/partial thromboplastin time (PT/PTT)
Rheumatoid factor
Angiotensin-converting enzyme
Thyroid-stimulating hormone (TSH)
Vitamin D
Lyme titer
Vitamin B_{12} levels

IMAGING

MRI with gadolinium (Consortium of Multiple Sclerosis Centers [CMSC] protocol recommended)[22]
Brain, cervical spine, thoracic spine
lumbar spine*

OTHER DIAGNOSTICS*

Visual evoked potentials
OCT
Lumbar puncture with cerebrospinal fluid analysis:
- Tube 1: protein, glucose, VDRL, cell count and differential
- Tube 2: cryptococcal antigen, India ink; fungal cultures; acid-fast bacillus (AFB) stain
- Tube 3: Gram stain and culture; cell count and differential
- Tube 4: MS profile, Lyme titer

*If indicated.

MANAGEMENT

Neurologist and MS specialist consultations are recommended for initial evaluation and initial prescription of DMT; MS exacerbation; and difficult-to-manage symptoms.

Immediate emergency department referral is indicated for suspected cases of progressive multifocal leukoencephalopathy (PML), encephalitis, new-onset seizure, or symptomatic cardiac dysfunction.

The goals of management are both multifaceted and complex. They include management of the disease itself, management of the symptoms, and maximization of quality of life for the patient and the patient's family system.

A comprehensive approach is essential to the management of MS. This is accomplished through a partnership with the patient, the patient's family system, and a comprehensive care team (CCT). The CCT consists of a neurologist, advanced practice nurse, physician assistant, and/or a center that *specializes* in MS. Other members of the team may include the primary care physician, internists, urologists, gynecologists, orthopedists, ophthalmologists, physiatrists, nurses, social workers, physical therapists, occupational therapists, speech language pathologists, recreation therapists, psychologists, and neuropsychologists. Team members should be found who have a special interest or specialization in MS, if they are available. Referral to team members will be variable, depending on patient symptoms and needs and availability of resources within the community.[23,24]

The CCT works to empower the person with MS by encouraging an active role in developing and implementing the plan of care. The care plan focuses not only on what occurs within the health care arena proper, but also on the home, workplace, and community to maximize function and quality of life. This is a dynamic process, given the ever-changing landscape of persons with MS.[24]

Multiple networks offer a vast array of resources for care providers and patients, including current research, treatment and care guidelines, and educational programs.

Management includes the following:

1. Education—getting the patient to understand the diagnosis and the importance of early treatment with DMTs: All DMTs have three goals: to decrease the exacerbation rate, to decrease MRI activity, and to slow the progression of disability.
2. DMT initiation: DMT initiation starts as early as possible with the first presentation of, usually, CIS. DMTs are often grouped by method of administration: injectable, infusible, and oral. The injectable DMTs are frequently referred to as platform therapies. There is long-term experience with most of the injectable medications. Safety and efficacy over time have been well established. Injectable DMTs include the interferons (Betaseron, Extavia, Avonex, Plegridy, and Rebif) and glatiramer acetate (Copaxone). The interferons have a similar biologic activity and adverse event profile. Patients should be monitored for depression while receiving treatment. Liver enzymes and hematologic profiles also need to be monitored.[8,25-30] Glatiramer acetate (Copaxone) is a synthetic protein; there are no depression, liver, or hematologic concerns.[31]
   - Infusable DMTs include mitoxantrone (Novantrone) and natalizumab (Tysabri). Mitoxantrone (Novantrone), an antineoplastic agent, was approved in October 2000 for the treatment of SPMS, worsening RRMS, and PRMS. The administration of mitoxantrone requires careful cardiac evaluation and monitoring, even years after the medication has been discontinued. It also carries a lifetime accumulated dose limit because of the risk of cardiac toxicity.[32] Leukemia is also a serious side effect seen over time. Because of these issues, it is not commonly used.
   - Natalizumab (Tysabri) is a monoclonal antibody with immunosuppressant effect that appeared promising in active clinical trials. It was taken off the market in February 2005 after three reported cases (two fatal) of PML. After much study, the U.S. Food and Drug Administration (FDA), in March 2006, allowed it to return to market under strict monitoring guidelines. It is approved for first-line use by the FDA; however, in general, it is recommended for patients with inadequate responses to other first-line therapies with less aggressive risk profiles or patients unable to tolerate other MS therapies.[33,34]
   - There are now three oral therapies available for the treatment of MS: fingolimod (Gilenya), teriflunomide (Aubagio), and dimethyl fumarate (Tecfidera). All three work

DIFFERENTIAL DIAGNOSIS

Multiple Sclerosis

Structural or anatomic
- Tumors, especially lymphoma or glioma of brain or spinal cord
- Myelopathy

Psychiatric disorder

Toxin exposure

Vascular
- Cerebrovascular accident (CVA)
- Arteriovenous malformation (AVM)
- Cerebral autosomal-dominant arteriopathy with subcortical infarcts and leukoencephalopathy (CADASIL)

Metabolic
- Vitamin B_{12} deficiency, vitamin D deficiency
- Adrenoleukodystrophy
- Mitochondrial disorders

Genetic
- Friedreich ataxia
- Olivopontocerebellar atrophies
- Hereditary spastic paraparesis

Infectious
- Lyme disease
- Syphilis
- Progressive multifocal leukoencephalopathy
- Human T-lymphotropic virus 1 (HTLV-1) or HIV infection

Inflammatory
- Rheumatoid arthritis
- Systemic lupus erythematosus
- Sjögren syndrome
- Vasculitis
- Sarcoidosis
- Behçet's disease

Other MS variants
- Neuromyelitis optica (Devic disease)
- Acute disseminated encephalomyelitis
- Marburg variant of MS
- Baló concentric sclerosis

by reducing circulating inflammatory lymphocytes outside the CNS. Each works by a different mechanism of action (MOA) and carries its own set of risks and side effects that need to be evaluated on a patient-by-patient basis.
- Other agents and treatments that exert immunosuppressant or immunomodulating effects have been prescribed in MS; these include azathioprine (Imuran), methotrexate (Rheumatrex), rituximab (Rituxan), cyclophosphamide (Cytoxan), mycophenolate mofetil (CellCept), plasmapheresis, and intravenous immune globulin (IVIG). These are used off label and have varying degrees of reported efficacy.[10,15,35] Approaches for neuroprotection, remyelination, and neural stem cell transplantation remain a topic of interest and research.[10]
- Vitamin D has been of great interest. Current research indicates that therapeutic levels of vitamin D have a beneficial effect on MS. A definitive target level has still not been determined; it has been suggested that a midrange level of 60 to 80 ng/ml is reasonable, but this may change with continued research. A low-sodium diet and smoking cessation have been shown to have a positive effect on both progression and disease severity of MS.[4,5]

3. Treatment of an exacerbation: The goal is to minimize the duration of the inflammation to incur fewer lasting deficits. Exacerbation is defined as the acute onset of neurologic symptom(s), lasting longer than 24 hours, which are preceded by a period of at least 30 days of clinical stability or improvement and have no underlying cause such as infection.[19] Exacerbations produce sustained effects on disability.[18] Treatment typically involves use of high-dose intravenous steroids for a short period or adrenocorticotropic hormone (ACTH). Corticosteroids are used in MS for the management of acute exacerbations because they downregulate the inflammatory lymphocytes outside the CNS and have the capacity to close the damaged blood-brain barrier, subsequently reducing inflammation in the CNS. Steroids are typically administered during the course of several days and may or may not be followed by a slower oral taper of these drugs.[36,37]
   - ACTH (Acthar) is given as a daily injection (subcutaneous or intramuscular) for up to 21 days. It downregulates inflammation both peripherally and centrally through the corticosteroid-independent melanocortin pathway.[37,38]
4. Postexacerbation: After an exacerbation, a course of rehabilitation is undertaken to address any new deficits or functional loss as well as to improve and maintain overall physical fitness.[8,10,15]
5. Symptom management: Table 199-1 shows treatment options and rehabilitative therapies for some of the more common MS symptoms.

LIFE SPAN CONSIDERATIONS

In some situations, a diagnosis of MS is actually followed by relief, especially for patients who have spent years experiencing strange symptoms and have coped with vague diagnoses or even outright skepticism. For others, the diagnosis is difficult; the variable clinical course of MS leads to an uncertain and unpredictable future. Natural history studies show that many persons with MS are still capable of ambulation and regular employment 15 to 20 years after diagnosis, and the life span is shortened by approximately 7 years compared with that of the general population. All routine health screening and treatments should continue as recommended, and life planning such as retirement should continue after diagnosis. Several factors are associated with a favorable prognosis: female gender, age at disease onset younger than 40 years, sensory symptoms as presenting episode, optic neuritis as an isolated first symptom, minor abnormalities on the brain MRI at the time of diagnosis, complete or almost complete recovery after exacerbation, and long periods between exacerbations.[1,8]

Pregnancy seems to have a neuroprotective effect. Acute exacerbation is common up to 6 months after delivery. Research has demonstrated that this does not tend to affect long-term outcome.[39] Use of IVIG may decrease the risk of postpartum exacerbation.[40] Use of DMTs is not recommended during pregnancy or while breastfeeding. If possible, it is generally recommended for women to stop DMT treatment 3 months before actively trying to conceive. A 3-month washout is also recommended for men on teriflunomide and mitoxantrone.

Ambulatory dysfunction, fatigue, and cognitive impairment are the biggest contributors to loss of employment for patients with MS.[41]

Complications and indications for referral or hospitalization include the following:
- If MS is suspected or diagnosed, referral to a neurology practice, preferably one that specializes in MS, is recommended. The management of care in the long term may have the neurology specialist take the role of primary manager, with medical issues deferred to the primary care provider (PCP). In other cases, the PCP may remain the primary manager, with the neurology specialist having a more consultative role. Regardless, a team approach is needed to maintain quality of life and wellness for the MS patient and the entire support system.
- Most MS exacerbations are handled on an outpatient basis. Hospitalization may be necessary if significant self-care deficits arise or if there are complications or concomitant infection or illness needing further clarification and management.
- Patients with MS are at higher risk for development of other autoimmune diseases, such as thyroid disease, diabetes, and rheumatoid arthritis, as well as osteoporosis, sleep disorders, frequent urinary tract infections, pressure ulcers, obesity, substance abuse, and depression. These diseases and conditions should be screened for and treated as indicated.[17,18] Primary care has a strong role with the MS patient related to screening and management of these other disease processes.

PATIENT AND FAMILY EDUCATION

The diagnosis of MS can be overwhelming for patients and families. Considerable support and education about the disease process, its variability, and available therapies are essential. A message of hope and not disability should be conveyed, with an emphasis on maintaining quality of life. The PCP should emphasize the benefits of DMT: it delays disability, reduces the frequency of clinical exacerbations, and reduces MRI activity. Encouraging adherence to DMT regimens and symptomatic treatment can help optimize quality of life. This will have an immediate effect, offering symptomatic relief, improving functioning, and helping to define an internal locus of control. Long-term benefits of adherence include promotion of self-efficacy and decrease in disability progression. Realistic expectation of treatment along with management of side effects must also be emphasized.

Beyond DMT and symptomatic treatment, the health care provider should focus education on promotion of health, wellness, and safety. This includes regular preventive health care visits, exercise, diet, lifestyle modifications, smoking cessation, and avoidance of drug and alcohol abuse. Driving evaluations may be needed. Community support groups may also be helpful.

Comprehensive issues should include balancing "normalcy" with the demands and challenges of living with a chronic and ever-changing disease, family planning, coping skills, caregiver issues, family systems, and relationship issues. Concerns about confidentiality, insurance, employment, and disability issues should also be addressed.[15,26]

The family and patients should be reminded that MS is frequently likened to a marathon, not a sprint. They need information and support to help them make the best decisions for their futures. The future of MS is promising.

RESOURCES

MS Views and News
www.msviewsandnews.org
MS World
www.msworld.org
Multiple Sclerosis Association of America
www.msassociation.org,
800-532-7667
Multiple Sclerosis Foundation
www.msfocus.org
888-MSFOCUS
National Multiple Sclerosis Society
www.nationalmssociety.org
800-344-4867

CHAPTER 200

PARKINSON DISEASE

Brenda L. Jordan

DEFINITION AND EPIDEMIOLOGY

Parkinson disease (PD) is a slowly progressive neurodegenerative disease with an insidious onset of the cardinal features of asymmetric resting tremor, bradykinesia, and rigidity, commonly with postural changes. The prevalence of PD is thought to be 0.3% in the general population and 1% in those older than 60 years. Worldwide, approximately 5 million people have PD; the incidence is 8 to 18.6 new cases per 100,000 person-years.[1] Mean age at diagnosis is 70.5 years, with a rapid increase in incidence after the age of 65 years. PD is uncommon in those younger than 40 years. Studies show 50% more men with PD than women.[2] The risk for development of PD appears to double if a first-degree relative has PD compared with people in the general population (Box 200-1).[1,2]

Traditionally considered a motor system disorder, PD is now recognized to be a complex disorder with diverse features. Those who develop PD may be affected by neuropsychiatric and other nonmotor manifestations in addition to the cardinal motor features.[3] The specific mechanisms of the neurodegeneration of PD are not understood. It is most likely caused by a cascade of events between genetics and environmental factors,[4,5] with abnormalities in protein processing,[6] oxidative stress,[7] mitochondrial dysfunction,[8] inflammation and immune regulation, and other mechanisms. Purely genetic Parkinson varieties probably affect a small minority of people with the *parkin* gene on chromosome 6.[4]

BOX 200-1

Risk Factors for Developing Parkinson Disease

- Family history of PD—associated with specific genes and genetic loci[7]
- Exposure to pesticides[5]
- History of head trauma resulting in concussion[8]
- Living in urban or industrial areas with high release of copper, manganese, or lead[9]
- Exposure to hydrocarbon solvents, particularly trichloroethylene[10]
- Living in rural area, farming or agricultural work, use of well water[5]
- Milk consumption[11]
- High dietary intake of iron with high intake of manganese[12]
- Excess body weight[13]
- Higher level of education with history of anemia[14,15]

PATHOPHYSIOLOGY

PD develops after widespread depletion of dopamine in the substantia nigra and the nigrostriatal pathway to the caudate and putamen. Depigmentation, neuronal loss, and gliosis are most significant in the substantia nigra pars compacta and the pontine locus ceruleus. This dopamine depletion ultimately results in increased inhibition of the thalamus and reduced excitatory input to the motor cortex, which results in the cardinal features of PD: tremor at rest, rigidity, bradykinesia, and postural instability. Compensatory mechanisms, including the large number of acetylcholine-secreting neurons with excitatory signals that remain active in the presymptomatic phase of PD, mask the deleterious effects of dopamine depletion.[16]

CLINICAL PRESENTATION

The clinical features most suggestive of PD are asymmetric or unilateral tremor, rigidity, bradykinesia with freezing, and flexed posture with loss of postural reflexes. Some investigators have postulated that there are clinically defined subgroups or subtypes that may affect the rate of progression of PD. The subtypes are tremor dominant, akinetic-rigid, and postural instability and gait difficulty. The tremor dominant subtype is associated with slower progression and less neuropsychiatric impairment than in the other two groups.[17] Rest tremor in PD is present at rest, is usually unilateral at first, and characteristically disappears with action. Rest tremor of the hands, described as "pill rolling," increases with walking and may be an early sign when others are not yet present. Most often, patients with PD exhibit a slow, coarse tremor with a rate varying from two to five oscillations per second, usually averaging four or five oscillations per second when the hand is motionless and decreasing with postural changes. There is a clear distinction from essential or intention tremors, which appear only or primarily with deliberate, willed movement.[18]

Another classic sign is rigidity, an increased resistance to passive movement at a joint, which occurs in 90% of patients with PD. The increased resistance to passive movement is equal in all directions and usually manifests with a ratcheting or "cogwheeling" during the movement. Rigidity of the passive limb increases when another limb is engaged in voluntary active movement.[19]

The patient with PD often has a uniquely flexed posture involving the entire body. The head is bowed; the trunk is bent forward; the back is kyphotic; the hands are held in front of the body; and the elbows, hips, and knees are flexed. Deformities of the hands and feet may also be apparent. Lateral tilting of the trunk is common.[19]

Other features of PD are associated with slowness of movement (hypokinesia), loss of automatic movement (bradykinesia), and difficulty initiating movement (freezing) or an irresistible impulse to take much quicker and shorter steps, which creates an almost running pace (festination). Shuffling gait with a decrease in arm swing may be evident. Masked facies (a reduction in spontaneous facial expression) and decreased frequency of blinking are prevalent. Speech becomes soft (hypophonia), and the voice often has a monotonous tone with lack of inflection (aprosody of speech). Some patients are not able to enunciate clearly (dysarthria) or may experience repetition of syllables (palilalia). All of these features clearly respond to treatment with levodopa, which is considered both diagnostic and therapeutic.[19]

PHYSICAL EXAMINATION

Postural reflexes can be tested by giving a sudden, firm pull on the shoulders from behind, but the health care provider should be prepared to catch the patient. Rigidity, demonstrated by cogwheeling, may be tested by grasping the patient's elbow at the antecubital region and slowly flexing and extending the elbow or pronating-supinating the forearm. Walking can also be marked by festination, whereby the patient walks faster and faster with short steps, trying to move the feet forward under the flexed body's center of gravity.[19]

The freezing phenomenon, a motor block, is a transient inability to perform active movements. It most often affects the legs but can involve eyelid opening, speaking, and writing. The feet may appear to be glued to the ground. Because patients with PD exhibit an increased ability to perform intentional or conscious movement as opposed to automatic movement, freezing can be overcome by having patients intentionally raise their legs as if stepping over objects or cycling. Despite severe bradykinesia with marked immobility, patients with PD may rise suddenly and move normally for a short burst of motor activity when physically cued (kinesia paradoxa).[19]

DIAGNOSTICS

Diagnostic studies are usually not indicated. There are no physiologic tests or blood tests, and neuroimaging is most helpful in differentiation of PD from other neurodegenerative disorders but requires specific neuroimaging best identified by neurologic specialists. The "gold standard" for diagnosis is postmortem neuropathologic examination, especially noting midbrain Lewy bodies. Diagnosis of idiopathic PD is based on the clinical presentation and physical examination findings, with two of the three cardinal manifestations (tremor, bradykinesia, rigidity) present. A rest tremor with unilateral onset and excellent response to dopaminergic therapy are important criteria for the diagnosis of idiopathic PD.[20,21]

According to the 2006 American Academy of Neurology (AAN) systematic review and practice parameter, a number of clinical features in early-stage PD are probably useful in distinguishing other forms of parkinsonism from PD.[22]

DIAGNOSTICS

Features Suggesting an Alternative Diagnosis

- Falls at presentation or early in the course of the disease
- Poor response to levodopa
- Symmetric motor signs
- Rapid progression to Hoehn and Yahr stage 3 with mild to moderate disease and some postural instability, but physically dependent
- Lack of tremor
- Dysautonomia early in the disease course, manifesting with urinary urgency or incontinence and fecal incontinence, urinary retention requiring catheterization, persistent erectile failure, or symptomatic orthostatic hypotension

DIFFERENTIAL DIAGNOSIS

The signs and symptoms of idiopathic PD can occur in other neurodegenerative disorders, including dementia with Lewy bodies, corticobasal degeneration, multiple system atrophy, and progressive supranuclear palsy. Secondary parkinsonism is seen in the presence of drug reactions (neuroleptics), infections (postencephalitic), metabolic disorders (parathyroid disorders), post-traumatic conditions, neoplastic disorders, toxicity (carbon monoxide), and vascular disorders. As previously noted, the diagnosis of PD and other forms of parkinsonism is often based on the response to levodopa, although this is no longer recommended.[21] Bradykinesia and rigidity respond best, but lack of improvement does not exclude the diagnosis of PD. Tremor may never respond satisfactorily. Signs and symptoms that can be useful in identifying patients with parkinsonism other than PD are falls at presentation and early in the disease, poor response to levodopa, symmetry with onset of tremor, rapid progression of symptoms, lack of tremor, and dysautonomia.[20,21]

MANAGEMENT

Judicious selection of symptomatic treatment options can maximize functional ability, but none appears to slow the progress of the disease. Treatment is individualized because each patient has a unique set of signs and symptoms; the patient's response to medications and social, occupational, and emotional needs must be considered. The goal is to maintain independence and functional ability for as long as possible. The European Federation of Neurological Societies (EFNS) and the International Parkinson and Movement Disorder Society European Section (MDS-ES) have published a useful algorithm for the management of PD that includes pharmacologic, nonpharmacologic, and surgical treatment.[23] Drug treatment acts in one of two ways: to increase the functional ability of the underactive dopaminergic system or to reduce the excessive influence of the excitatory cholinergic neurons. The decision to initiate medical therapy is determined by the degree of functional impairment. Important factors include the effect of disease on the dominant hand and the degree of interference with work, activities of daily living, and social and leisure function.[24]

DIFFERENTIAL DIAGNOSIS

Parkinson Disease

NEURODEGENERATIVE
- Alzheimer disease
- Corticobasal degeneration
- Dementia with Lewy bodies
- Frontotemporal dementia
- Huntington disease
- Multiple system atrophy
- Parkinsonism-dementia-ALS complex of Guam
- Progressive supranuclear palsy
- Spinocerebellar ataxias

SYMPTOMATIC
- Drug induced (neuroleptics, other dopamine receptor agonists)
- Infectious (after encephalitis, Creutzfeldt-Jakob disease)
- Metabolic (Wilson disease, neurodegeneration with brain iron accumulation, hepatocerebral degeneration, parathyroid disorders)
- Neoplastic
- Post-traumatic
- Toxic (carbon monoxide, manganese, MPTP)
- Vascular

OTHER
- Essential tremor
- Normal-pressure hydrocephalus

ALS, amyotrophic lateral sclerosis.

Pharmacotherapy

Selegiline. Selegiline (Eldepryl), a selective monoamine oxidase type B inhibitor, may have neuroprotective properties and can be modestly effective in treatment. Selegiline may delay the destruction of the nigral neurons and inhibit the metabolic breakdown of dopamine. As monotherapy, it does not produce any functional benefit. Some randomly controlled trials have demonstrated the benefit of selegiline in delaying the need for levodopa an average of 9 months if it is used for patients with early PD.[24] Adverse side effects and contraindications to administration and monitoring of selegiline should be noted. When it is given concurrently with levodopa, selegiline can increase the dopaminergic effect and contribute to dopaminergic toxicity. A maximum dose is currently considered to be 5 mg twice daily. An oral disintegrating tablet is available with a slightly lower dosage schedule.

Levodopa. Levodopa is the most effective drug for the symptomatic treatment of PD. It is particularly effective for akinetic symptoms. Tremor and rigidity can respond to levodopa, but postural instability is less likely to respond. Levodopa treatment is aimed at restoration of the amount of dopamine reaching the basal ganglia. Unfortunately, dopamine does not cross the blood-brain barrier; thus its precursor, levodopa, must be given. Levodopa is metabolized both peripherally and centrally. The peripheral metabolism is responsible for the majority of side effects. Sinemet combines levodopa with carbidopa, which blocks peripheral metabolism, allowing much more of the levodopa to enter the brain than if it were given alone. Sinemet 25/100 contains 25 mg of carbidopa and 100 mg of levodopa. Treatment should begin with small doses, one half of Sinemet 25/100 two or three times a day with meals and titrated to the lowest levodopa dose that produces a useful clinical response. Absence of response to 1000 to 1500 mg/day of levodopa would be a strong suggestion that the original PD diagnosis is incorrect. The optimum dose of carbidopa is 100 to 150 mg/day, which should completely block peripheral metabolism of levodopa. Levodopa is associated with a higher risk of dyskinesia than dopamine agonists (DAs) are. Therapy should be initiated with immediate-release preparations so that initial response can be better evaluated. Slow-release forms of carbidopa-levodopa provide a longer half-life and a lower peak plasma level of levodopa, reducing clinical fluctuations. Once the patient's condition is stable, reassessment may be performed every 3 to 6 months.[24] Novel formulations including a transdermal product (rotigotine patch) are available in the United States and may offer more continuous drug levels.

Within 5 years of starting levodopa, up to 50% (10% of patients per year) will develop levodopa-induced complications.[25] Complications include motor fluctuations (wearing-off phenomenon), involuntary movements (dyskinesia), abnormal postures of the extremities and trunk (dystonia), and other complex motor fluctuations. Motor complications are more common in patients with young-onset PD (40 to 59 years at PD onset) compared with older-onset PD (70 years at PD onset).[25] Two randomly controlled trials found no evidence that modified-release levodopa reduced motor complications or improved disease control at 5 years compared with immediate-release levodopa monotherapy in people with early PD.[24] Later onset of motor fluctuations in PD is associated with initial treatment with pramipexole rather than with levodopa. Evidence exists that DA monotherapy and combination therapy reduce the incidence of irreversible motor complications of dyskinesia and fluctuations in motor response related to long-term levodopa treatment. The same long-term randomly controlled trial, however, found that levodopa monotherapy is slightly more effective in treating the disabling motor impairments of PD.[24]

Dopamine Agonists. DAs are a group of synthetic agents that directly stimulate dopamine receptors. These drugs are direct agonists and do not require metabolic conversion to move into the brain and do not depend on neuronal uptake or release. An additional advantage over immediate-release levodopa is their longer duration of action. DAs were initially used for adjunctive treatment of advanced PD complicated by reduced levodopa response, motor fluctuations, dyskinesia, and other adverse effects of levodopa. Some investigators, despite the lack of conclusive evidence, have advocated the early use of DAs as a levodopa-sparing strategy. This strategy is based on the unproven concept that the long-term duration of a patient's responsiveness to levodopa is finite. Given the potential that DAs are associated with fewer motor fluctuations and the evidence of a higher incidence of levodopa-related dyskinesia in young-onset PD, some experts suggest that DAs for initial treatment of young-onset PD (younger than 60 years) is appropriate, whereas the more effective levodopa is used in patients 60 years of age and older. Ropinirole (Requip), pramipexole (Mirapex), and bromocriptine (Parlodel) are DAs that can be effective adjuncts to levodopa in older-onset PD patients or as monotherapy in young-onset PD patients.[26]

The agonists tend to induce orthostatic hypotension when they are first introduced. The best starting regimen is a small dose at bedtime for the first 3 days and then a switch to daytime administration, with a gradual increase. Bromocriptine and ropinirole may induce psychosis and confusion, whereas pramipexole induces somnolence. Overall, however, all are less likely than levodopa to induce dyskinesias, which makes them useful to reduce the severity of "off" states. All DAs should be used cautiously in patients with cardiac disease. DAs require maintenance doses at least three times a day. Ropinirole is started at 0.25 mg three times a day, and then increased by 0.25 mg per dose each week for 4 weeks for a total daily dose of 3 mg. After week 4, the ropinirole dose may be increased weekly by 1.5 mg/day to a maximum daily dose of 24 mg. Most benefit occurs in the range of 12 to 16 mg/day. Pramipexole is started at 0.125 mg twice a day; then the dose is increased gradually by 0.125 mg per dose every 5 to 7 days. Most patients are managed within the range of 1.5 to 4.5 mg/day. Bromocriptine is started at 1.25 mg twice a day and then, at 2- to 4-week intervals, increased by 2.5 mg/day. Most patients are managed on 20 to 40 mg daily in three or four divided doses.

Adverse effects of DAs include nausea, vomiting, sleepiness, orthostatic hypotension, confusion, and hallucinations. DAs have also been associated with increased risk of impulse control disorders, including pathologic gambling, compulsive sexual behavior, and compulsive buying.[26]

Catechol *O*-Methyltransferase Inhibitors. Catechol *O*-methyltransferase (COMT) inhibitors, such as entacapone (Comtan), are ineffective if given alone, but they prolong and potentiate the effect of levodopa when they are given in conjunction with levodopa. COMT inhibitors are used to treat motor fluctuations in patients who are experiencing end-of-dose "wearing-off" periods. Tolcapone (Tasmar) and entacapone are the COMT inhibitors prescribed. The starting dose of tolcapone is 100 mg three times daily. Entacapone is given at 200 mg with each dose of levodopa up to maximum of eight doses per day.[24]

Anticholinergics. Dopamine and acetylcholine are normally in a state of electrochemical balance in the basal ganglia. In PD, dopamine depletion produces cholinergic sensitivity so that cholinergic drugs exacerbate PD and anticholinergic drugs improve PD. Centrally acting anticholinergic drugs, such as trihexyphenidyl (Artane) and benztropine (Cogentin), are more useful in controlling tremor and rigidity than bradykinesia but may also cause typical side effects. Anticholinergics should be used in younger patients in whom tremor is the predominant problem. The potency of anticholinergics seems to decrease over time, and side effects such as blurred vision, dry mouth, bowel and bladder problems, and cognition changes limit their usefulness. Evidence of benefit of anticholinergics is unclear. Trihexyphenidyl is started at 0.5 to 1 mg daily with gradual increase to 2 to 5 mg three times a day. Benztropine is more commonly used for the treatment of antipsychotic-induced parkinsonism with doses of 0.5 to 2 mg once daily.

Amantadine. Amantadine is an antiviral agent that has mild antiparkinsonian activity. The mechanism of action is uncertain, but it increases dopamine release, inhibits dopamine reuptake, and stimulates dopamine receptors, and it may even have a central anticholinergic effect. Controlled trials demonstrated that it was more effective than anticholinergic drugs for akinesia and rigidity. Individual patients with advanced PD who have motor fluctuations and dyskinesia can benefit briefly from the addition of amantadine to the regimen of levodopa. Amantadine is administered in two divided doses of 100 to 200 mg each.[26]

Surgery

Deep Brain Stimulation. Deep brain stimulation (DBS) is the most frequently performed surgical procedure for the treatment of advanced PD. Two prospective randomized controlled trials that compared DBS with best medical therapy have shown that bilateral DBS improves motor function in selected patients with advanced typical PD and motor fluctuations.[27] The rate of serious adverse events is significantly higher in the DBS patients (40%) than in the best medical treatment group (15%). The adverse events are directly related to the surgical procedure and include postoperative headache, pain, and infection at the surgical site. These two trials demonstrated that DBS of the subthalamic nucleus or globus pallidus is more effective than the best medical therapy for improvement of motor function and quality of life for patients with advanced PD, at least in the short term.[27]

INDICATIONS FOR REFERRAL OR HOSPITALIZATION

Collaboration with other health care providers is common in the treatment of patients with PD. It is important to consult a neurologist before committing patients to medications. Physician consultation is indicated when patients are not responding to treatment or when the disease is progressing. Also, if there are signs and symptoms of depression, referral to a psychiatrist should be considered. Neuropsychological documentation of the precise nature and prevalence of the cognitive deficit has important implications in medical and psychosocial management of patients with PD. Hospitalization may be considered for complications such as pneumonia, deep venous thrombosis, and pulmonary embolus. Physical therapy can improve mobility and strength, which may help maintain independence and prevent injury. Occupational therapy can be useful; adaptive equipment can be provided to the patient or caregivers, and assistance can be provided to adapt the home or workplace as disability progresses.

COMPLICATIONS AND COMORBID PROBLEMS

Psychosis and Hallucinations

Psychosis, a frequent complication of PD, is characterized by visual hallucinations and delusions, often paranoid. Hallucinations are most common and affect up to 40% of patients with PD, mostly in the advanced stages of PD. Although dose reduction of antiparkinsonian drugs often resolves hallucinations, stopping all the offending medications is usually not an option and not all hallucinations are drug related. Antiparkinsonian drugs can be reduced or stopped in reverse order of their potency and effectiveness; the sequence begins with anticholinergics then proceeds to COMT inhibitors, then DAs, and then levodopa if all else fails. Quetiapine in low doses can be used to manage psychotic symptoms in PD, but studies have failed to demonstrate its efficacy.[28]

Dementia

Even though dementias such as Alzheimer disease and vascular dementia can coexist with PD, it is increasingly recognized that dementia is a common feature of PD. An area of recent debate and research is the question of whether PD dementia and dementia with Lewy bodies are distinct disorders or different presentations of the same disease. In studies, the prevalence of dementia in PD has been found to be as high as 41%, with incidence rates as high as 78%. Older age, age at onset of PD older than 60 years, duration of PD, and severity of parkinsonism may contribute to the incidence of dementia in PD.[29,30]

Depression

Depression is the most common psychiatric illness seen in PD and is associated with negative impact on mobility and quality of life. There is no clear consensus regarding the use of antidepressants for depression in patients with PD, but there are two concerns about treatment with selective serotonin reuptake inhibitors in PD: (1) the possibility of increasing motor symptoms and (2) a possible adverse reaction with selegiline when it is used concurrently.[31] When these drugs are used, close monitoring is advised. Studies have demonstrated benefit over placebo with pramipexole, venlafaxine, and sertraline. Bupropion may be a very good option for PD patients with depression; however, studies need to be done. Cognitive behavioral therapy can be very helpful.

Daytime Sleepiness and Fatigue

Daytime sleepiness and fatigue are common problems in patients with PD. Sudden somnolence can be a hazard for PD patients if they are still driving. Fatigue appears to be an independent symptom of PD but can certainly overlap with depression and daytime somnolence.

PATIENT AND FAMILY EDUCATION

Education is essential to help the patient and family understand and gain some control over this chronic and progressive disorder. Cautious education of the newly diagnosed patient with mild symptoms and uncertain future should be the rule, but it is clear that patients with access to Internet resources will educate themselves, so focused discussions about symptoms and treatments may need to occur with each visit. Education about medication effectiveness and side effects and drug and diet interactions is important. Discussion about driving and when to stop are difficult but essential.

Normal reactions of anger, depression, and anxiety and social and economic concerns are common, so emotional, psychological, and socioeconomic needs of the patient and family must be addressed. Support groups are especially valuable to patients and families because they provide emotional support, access to resources, and educational information.

Answering questions and addressing concerns honestly are part of establishing a successful provider-patient relationship. Reassurance and encouragement complement medication. The patient should be encouraged to contact a PD support group and a local PD information and referral center. Internet resources are also available for patients with PD. The patient may find the following resources helpful:

American Parkinson Disease Association
135 Parkinson Avenue
Staten Island, NY 10305
800-223-2732
www.apdaparkinson.org

National Parkinson Foundation
1501 NW 9th Avenue/Bob Hope Road
Miami, FL 33136-1494
800-327-4545
www.parkinson.org

Michael J. Fox Foundation for Parkinson's Research
Grand Central Station
PO Box 4777
New York, NY 10163
212-509-0995
http://www.michaeljfox.org

National Institute of Neurological Disorders and Stroke
www.ninds.nih.gov

CHAPTER 201

SEIZURE DISORDER

Karen L. Secore

DEFINITION AND EPIDEMIOLOGY

Epilepsy, a syndrome of recurrent (unprovoked) seizures, is a common neurologic condition that currently affects nearly 2.2 million people in the United States, with more than 100,000 to 150,000 new cases reported annually. Although the onset of seizures can occur at any age, incidence rates peak in neonates and young children, plateau, then rise again in the older adult population. In the United States, the prevalence of seizures is approximately 5 to 10 cases per 1000 persons in the general population; the lifetime risk for development of epilepsy is 1 in 27 people.[1]

A single seizure may result from discrete, temporary abnormalities, such as a high fever in small children, hyperventilation (in susceptible patients), or alcohol withdrawal. Causes of a first seizure leading to epilepsy include genetic factors, vascular abnormalities (e.g., ischemic strokes, hemorrhages, arteriovenous malformations), significant head trauma, brain tumors, metabolic factors, and infections such as encephalitis and meningitis. Strokes are a common cause of epilepsy, particularly in the elderly. Changes in levels of various electrolytes, in particular hyponatremia and hypercalcemia, may cause isolated seizures. Also, hyperglycemia and hypoglycemia can be responsible for seizure activity, especially in patients with underlying brain injuries. A first seizure may occur in the form of status epilepticus (SE). SE is currently defined as more than 30 minutes of continuous seizure activity or two or more seizures without recovery of baseline consciousness between attacks. However, owing the risk of systemic and brain injury from prolonged seizures, efforts are being made to change the definition to 5 minutes' duration. This definition is already accepted accepted by the American Epilepsy Society.[2]

Genetic predisposition is strongest in generalized forms of epilepsy in which the entire brain is electrically unstable; however, the genetic and biochemical defects are only starting to be characterized. Childhood absence (petit mal) epilepsy, juvenile myoclonic epilepsy, and generalized convulsive epilepsy are syndromes with a genetic predisposition. Mutations in γ-aminobutyric acid (GABA) receptors and sodium channels have been implicated. These types of epilepsy account for approximately one third of all cases, with seizures and abnormalities on electroencephalography (EEG) affecting the entire brain. The remaining types of epilepsy are related to localization; focal electrical abnormalities are usually the result of a structural lesion. The occurrence of prolonged or complicated febrile seizures in infancy is strongly correlated with the subsequent development of temporal lobe epilepsy.[3]

Physician consultation is indicated for suspected central nervous system (CNS) lesions, SE, initiation of antiepileptic medications, treatment failures, and women with epilepsy who are contemplating pregnancy.

PATHOPHYSIOLOGY

Although the terms *epilepsy* and *seizure disorder* are often used interchangeably, they have two distinct definitions. A *seizure* can be defined as an isolated event in which a group of neurons produces excessive electrical discharges in the brain. Seizures occur when the balance between excitation and inhibition of the brain's electrical activity becomes abnormally altered in favor of excitation. Seizures can be caused by the excess production or release of an excitatory neurotransmitter, which stimulates neurons to discharge abnormally, or by a loss of inhibitory neuronal activity, which permits abnormal excitation and discharges of neurons to occur. Single or even recurrent seizures can be triggered by hypoxia or other metabolic factors, but they do not constitute epilepsy unless they recur in a habitual and unprovoked manner. A subset of acute symptomatic seizures are those that occur in the setting of an acute medical illness or metabolic crisis. These conditions include hypoglycemia; nonketotic hyperglycemia; hyponatremia; hypocalcemia; magnesium levels below 0.8 mEq/L; renal failure and uremia; hyperthyroidism; disorders of porphyrin metabolism; cerebral anoxia as a complication of cardiac or respiratory arrest, carbon monoxide poisoning, drowning, or anesthetic; withdrawal states (particularly alcohol and benzodiazepine withdrawal); and drug toxicity or intoxication.

Epilepsy is characterized by recurrent seizures and is divided into syndromes on the basis of various causes, seizure types, associated neurologic symptoms, anatomic correlates, age, and family history. For diagnosis and treatment, it is valuable to be able to identify both the type of seizure and the epileptic syndrome.

CLASSIFICATION OF SEIZURES, EPILEPSY, AND EPILEPTIC SYNDROMES

In 1981, a commission for the International League Against Epilepsy (ILAE) developed, revised, and adopted the international classification of epileptic seizures (Box 201-1).[4] Efforts were made in 2010 to revise the classification; however, the ILEA 1981 version is still widely accepted. The motivation for revising the classification is to reflect the advances being made in basic and clinical neuroscience and incorporate those advances into clinical practice.[5] The classification includes two broad categories of seizure types: focal or localization related, and generalized. Focal seizures begin within networks limited to one cerebral hemisphere and show localized abnormalities on EEG. Depending on the spread of electrical activity, the patient may have varying levels of consciousness. By definition, focal seizures without impairment of consciousness, formerly known as simple partial seizures, are the aura, or warning, that the patient experiences before a larger seizure. Focal sensory seizures may be purely subjective, and focal motor seizures may involve no impairment of consciousness. If the seizure activity spreads and involves the brainstem or both hemispheres, consciousness becomes altered and the seizure is classified as complex partial, or more recently referred to as a focal seizure with impairment of consciousness. Altered consciousness and aberrations of behavior, such as automatisms (automatic repetitive movements), are usually associated with this type of seizure. If such seizures spread bilaterally and involve the motor cortex, the patient may have a secondarily generalized tonic-clonic seizure, now called a bilateral convulsive seizure.[5,6]

In contrast, primary generalized seizures occur when the initial abnormal electrical activity begins in both cerebral hemispheres and involves bilaterally distributed neuronal networks. These seizures are usually seen with idiopathic or hereditary types of epilepsy. Consciousness is almost always impaired, and

BOX 201-1

International Classification of Epileptic Seizures

I. **Partial seizures.** Epileptic focus is in one hemisphere of the brain. Also called focal or local seizures.
   A. **Simple partial seizures.** Usually the aura of a complex seizure. Patient has no loss of consciousness.
      1. Motor: tonic or clonic activity of one arm or leg
      2. Sensory: such as an auditory, olfactory, visual hallucination
      3. Autonomic: such as the epigastric rising sensation
      4. Psychic: déjà vu, fear, indescribable feeling
   B. **Complex partial seizure.** Consciousness is altered. Patient may exhibit complex behaviors.
      1. Can begin with a simple partial onset
      2. Can begin with immediate alteration of consciousness
   C. **Partial seizure evolving to generalized.** Patient starts with a simple or complex partial seizure that evolves into a generalized tonic-clonic seizure.
II. **Generalized.** Epileptic focus is not lateralized to one hemisphere. Begins in both hemispheres of the brain simultaneously.
   A. **Nonconvulsive.**
      1. Absence (petit mal)
      2. Atonic: loss of muscle tone (drop attacks)
   B. **Convulsive.** Involves motor activity.
      1. Myoclonic: abrupt muscle twitches or jerks
      2. Tonic-clonic (grand mal): tonic, then clonic activity
      3. Tonic: involving increased muscle tone, rigidity
      4. Clonic: muscle contraction and relaxation movements

Modified from Commission on Classification and Terminology of the International League Against Epilepsy: Proposal for revised clinical and electroencephalographic classification of epileptic seizures, *Epilepsia* 22(4):489-501, 1981.

the seizure may be convulsive or nonconvulsive. Motor activity and electroencephalographic changes are bilateral. Nonconvulsive generalized seizures, such as absence (petit mal) seizures, may be brief, and the patient may initially be diagnosed as a "daydreamer." The electroencephalographic characteristics of generalized spike and wave patterns are crucial for the proper diagnosis of these types of seizures. Convulsive primary generalized seizures, such as tonic-clonic (grand mal) types, are rarely missed but can be confused with secondarily generalized tonic-clonic seizures. Being able to differentiate between these two types is helpful in prescribing the appropriate treatment because each type may respond differently to certain antiepileptic medications. In the case of secondarily generalized seizures, it is important to exclude an underlying structural lesion, such as a brain tumor.

For treatment to be tailored to the individual, it is essential that consideration be given to the seizure type as well as the epileptic syndrome to which it belongs. The International Classification of Epilepsy and Epileptic Syndromes (Box 201-2) was adopted by the ILAE in 1989 and allows the practitioner to categorize cases by seizure type, cause, precipitating factors, age at onset, and prognosis.[5] This has been further adapted to classify the cause of seizures as genetic, structural, metabolic, or unknown. Epileptic syndromes can be further classified by age of onset, cognitive and developmental antecedents, electroencephalographic features, triggers, and patterns of occurrence related to sleep.[6] Although epilepsy can develop at any age, certain syndromes are more age-related than others. A variety of epileptic syndromes develop in early childhood. More than 50% and perhaps as many as 70% of childhood epilepsies, particularly the benign partial epilepsies, remit at the time of puberty.[7] Idiopathic, generalized epilepsy usually manifests by 18 years of age. After the age of 18 years, focal brain processes should be suspected. Brain tumors are a prominent cause of seizures in adults, whereas strokes are often the cause of seizures that begin late in life.[8] Symptomatic focal epilepsy syndromes account for 30% to 35% of all cases of epilepsy.[1] Seizure manifestations can be helpful in identifying which lobe of the brain is involved. Table 201-1 outlines the general characteristics of partial seizures in relation to the region of seizure origin; however, not all seizures fit neatly into a particular syndrome. Surgical treatment is often possible if the epileptic focus is in a surgically accessible region of the brain.

CLINICAL PRESENTATION

An accurate and detailed history is important. It is essential to obtain history not only from the patient but also from parents, relatives, or friends who have witnessed the seizures. Complicated pregnancy or childbirth, delayed childhood development, childhood diseases such as meningitis and encephalitis, significant head trauma with loss of consciousness, and family history of epilepsy are among the significant risk factors for the development of epilepsy. New-onset seizures require the determination of any recent history of headache, illness, trauma, or focal neurologic deficit.

An accurate description is important in attempting to decide whether an event was a seizure. The patient should be questioned to determine whether there was a warning before the event. A gastric sensation or a feeling of déjà vu is characteristic of temporal lobe epilepsy. A history of incontinence, injury, tongue biting, postictal confusion, lateralized weakness, or severe headache should raise suspicion of a true epileptic event. A detailed seizure history can also suggest where the seizures are originating, define seizure characteristics and frequency, and determine how the seizures are interfering with the patient's life.

A first seizure may appear in the form of SE. Immediate emergency department referral or physician consultation is indicated for SE or new-onset seizures.

BOX 201-2

International Classification of Epilepsy and Epileptic Syndromes

1. Localization related (focal, partial)
   1.1. Idiopathic (benign childhood epilepsy with centrotemporal spikes)
   1.2. Symptomatic (e.g., temporal lobe epilepsy, frontal lobe epilepsy)
   1.3. Cryptogenic (cause unknown)
2. Generalized epilepsies
   2.1. Idiopathic (juvenile myoclonic, juvenile absence, grand mal on awakening)
   2.2. Cryptogenic (Lennox-Gastaut syndrome, West syndrome)
   2.3. Symptomatic
3. Undetermined (neonatal types, Landau-Kleffner syndrome)
4. Special situation related (febrile seizures, metabolic seizures)

Modified from Commission on Classification and Terminology of the International League Against Epilepsy: Proposal for revised classification of epilepsy and epileptic syndromes, *Epilepsia* 30(4):389-399, 1989.

PHYSICAL EXAMINATION

A general physical examination should be performed on all patients with epilepsy and should be directed toward specific disease processes and focal neurologic deficits. Skin and mucous membranes should be assessed to identify areas of injury that may be related to events that occurred while consciousness was altered. Tongue biting and cheek biting are common during tonic-clonic seizures; the tongue and cheek are usually bitten on just one side, but bilateral findings are not uncommon. If the tip of the tongue is bitten, it should give rise to the suspicion of a non-epileptic psychogenic seizure. Cardiovascular assessment is important because syncope and arrhythmias are included in the differential diagnosis of epilepsy. Postural vital signs will determine whether orthostatic hypotension is a consideration. Neurologic signs, such as lateralized weakness, papilledema, memory problems, or changes in reflexes, can signify a structural lesion in the brain. In general, a patient with epilepsy will have unremarkable physical examination findings.

DIAGNOSTICS

Clinical presentation, physical examination, and differential considerations guide diagnostic testing. A new seizure may signify a serious pathologic condition. If infection of the CNS is

TABLE 201-1 **Clinical Manifestations of Complex Partial Seizures**

Site	Aura	Clinical Characteristics	Percentage of Partial Cases
Temporal	Epigastric sensation Déjà vu	Altered consciousness Oral, hand automatisms Moderate postictal confusion	75-85
Frontal	Dizziness or fear	Abrupt onset, rapid clearing Frenetic behavior Sexual automatisms Most occur during sleep	10-15
Parietal	Sensory	With or without altered consciousness Often begins with numbness, tingling, or pain	Rare
Occipital	Visual	May begin with eye twitching May include visual hallucinations May include ictal blindness	5-15

suspected (see Chapter 197), a complete blood count (CBC) and differential and a lumbar puncture are indicated. A chemistry profile, including calcium magnesium and phosphate, is necessary to exclude hypoglycemia, electrolyte abnormalities, or renal failure. Liver function tests (LFTs) should be performed to exclude hepatic failure. Alcohol and drug levels may be indicated. Magnetic resonance imaging (MRI) or computed tomography (CT) scan is indicated if structural abnormality, tumor, trauma, or cerebrovascular accident is suspected. Electrocardiography (ECG) should be performed to ascertain the presence of arrhythmias or heart block.

Diagnosis and classification of epilepsy and seizure types require confirmation that the patient does indeed have epileptic seizures. To treat the disorder appropriately, the practitioner must attempt to determine the cause of the epilepsy and classify it according to syndrome. Appropriate diagnostic tests should be part of the initial evaluation.[9]

Sleep-deprived EEG is useful because a baseline recording of background brain waves may reveal epileptic abnormalities. The positive predictive value of EEG in most clinics is more than 80%, although sensitivity is only 30%.[10] Because the chance of a patient having a seizure during routine EEG is small, ictal information may not be obtained; however, interictal epileptiform abnormalities may give localizing information and suggest epilepsy. Many patients with focal epilepsy show no focal or generalized abnormalities on routine EEG. Therefore a normal recording does not exclude a diagnosis of epilepsy. In contrast to focal epilepsy, generalized types of epilepsy often produce abnormalities of spike and wave activity or generalized slowing on routine electroencephalographic recordings. Interictal electroencephalographic abnormalities—either focal or generalized—are not synonymous with seizure activity, and therefore electroencephalographic abnormalities should not be the only basis for treatment.

Although neuroimaging studies can be of great value in diagnosis, the absence of structural abnormalities does not exclude a diagnosis of epilepsy. CT scans are useful for identification of large mass lesions, bleeding, subdural fluid collections, and cerebral infarcts, but they often miss more subtle changes in brain structure. MRI provides extensive anatomic detail and is useful in distinguishing small low-grade tumors, scars, and neural migration disorders from one another and from normal variants in brain structure. Except in an emergency, when the immediate availability of a CT scan is an advantage, MRIs should be the primary imaging study in patients with epilepsy.[9] In the preoperative evaluation of patients who are candidates for surgery, single-photon emission computerized tomography (SPECT), positron emission tomography (PET), magnetic resonance spectroscopy (MRS), functional magnetic resonance imaging (fMRI), and magnetoencephalography (MEG) are other imaging methods that may be considered.[9]

If a diagnosis of epilepsy cannot be confirmed or excluded after an accurate history, EEG, or imaging study, patients should be referred to a comprehensive epilepsy center in which long-term video and electroencephalographic monitoring can be done. This type of monitoring is intended to capture an event on video with simultaneous electroencephalographic recording and is almost always successful in distinguishing epilepsy from nonepileptic events.

For patients in SE, a battery of laboratory tests is usually performed: CBC; electrolyte values; glucose, magnesium, calcium, blood urea nitrogen (BUN), and creatinine concentrations; LFTs; coagulation studies (prothrombin time, partial thromboplastin time); alcohol level, toxicology screen; anticonvulsant drug levels; urinalysis; and pregnancy test. These should be done concurrently with stabilization of the patient. Examination of the cerebrospinal fluid is required if meningitis or encephalitis is suspected. Viral encephalitis should be treated empirically with acyclovir until the results of diagnostic studies for herpes virus are available. Similarly, suspected bacterial meningitis should be treated with appropriate antibiotics until culture results are available.[11]

DIFFERENTIAL DIAGNOSIS

A variety of nonepileptic paroxysmal events can be confused with epileptic seizures. Psychogenic seizures, also called nonepileptic seizures or pseudoseizures, are often mistaken for epileptic seizures; if patients are treated with antiepileptic drugs (AEDs), this usually increases the seizure frequency. A careful history can help raise suspicion for psychogenic seizures. In such cases, seizures may be symptoms of conversion disorder and the stress of physical or sexual abuse, a part of post-traumatic stress disorder, attention-seeking behavior, or a means of achieving secondary gain. Treatment involves the patient's acceptance of the diagnosis of psychogenic seizures and the beginning of a comprehensive psychotherapy program.

The second most common disorder to be confused with epilepsy is syncope (see Chapter 36). Syncope manifests with loss of consciousness, and convulsive syncope secondary to cerebral ischemia may mimic epileptic seizures. Syncope is often vasovagal, but cardiac causes include heart block and cardiac arrhythmia, and it can be induced by stimuli such as carotid massage, paroxysmal coughing, and voiding. Orthostatic hypotension is a frequent cause of syncope in the elderly. Presyncopal symptoms such as vertigo, sensory disturbances, and tinnitus are sometimes mistaken for epileptic auras or minor seizures.

Other disorders in the differential diagnosis include tumors, cerebrovascular disease, arteriovenous malformation, trauma, CNS infection, migraines, hyperventilation syndrome, movement disorders, transient ischemic attacks, transient global amnesia, and toxic metabolic disturbances such as alcohol withdrawal seizures. On occasion, sleep deprivation may cause generalized tonic-clonic seizures.[11] This phenomenon is not associated with a pathologic disorder.

DIAGNOSTICS

New-Onset Seizure

LABORATORY
Alcohol, drug levels*
Serum electrolytes*
BUN*
Creatinine*
Serum glucose*
Serum prolactin*
Calcium*
Magnesium and phosphate*
CBC and differential*
LFTs*

IMAGING
MRI, CT scan*

OTHER DIAGNOSTICS
ECG*
Lumbar puncture*
EEG*

*If indicated.
BUN, blood urea nitrogen.

DIFFERENTIAL DIAGNOSIS

Seizure Disorder

CARDIOVASCULAR CAUSES
- Syncope
- Cardiac arrhythmias
- Transient ischemic attacks
- Cerebral vascular disease
- Arteriovenous malformation

NEUROLOGIC AND NEUROVASCULAR CAUSES
- Migraine
- Transient global amnesia
- Movement disorder
- Brain tumor
- Cerebral vascular accident (stroke)
- Head trauma or brain injury

METABOLIC CAUSES
- Toxin metabolic disturbance
- Alcohol use or alcohol withdrawal
- Hyperventilation

OTHER CAUSES
- Infections of CNS
- Febrile seizure
- Psychogenic seizure
- Sleep deprivation
- Idiopathic cause

INITIAL STABILIZATION AND MANAGEMENT OF ACUTE SEIZURES

In the acute setting, most seizures resolve spontaneously within a few minutes and require no specific treatment apart from close observation to ensure that patients do not harm themselves. However, SE is a medical emergency that requires simultaneous medical stabilization (airway, breathing, circulation, and medications to control the seizures) and a search for the underlying cause. The Epilepsy Foundation of America's Working Group on Status Epilepticus defines SE as a continuous seizure lasting 30 minutes or more or two consecutive seizures in a row without mental clearing.[12,13] Efforts have recently been made to change the definition from 30 minutes of continuous seizure activity to 5 to 10 minutes.[2] This is based on the duration of seizure activity that may produce permanent injury. Generalized convulsive status epilepticus (GCSE) is a medical emergency that can lead to transient or permanent brain damage. Early treatment is a key factor in the outcome and prognosis. Initial management should maintain homeostasis and provide respiratory support. If seizures persist beyond 30 minutes, a vicious circle of maladaptive physiologic responses occurs.[13] SE may be complicated by hypotension, hypertension, hyperthermia, hypoglycemia, hypoxemia, acidosis, arrhythmias, rhabdomyolysis, pulmonary edema, fractures, and dislocations.

Mortality and morbidity rates have been related to the cause of SE and the seizure activity duration from the onset until treatment has been initiated. In patients with known epilepsy, half of the hospital-reported cases of GCSE have been associated with subtherapeutic antiepileptic drug (AED) levels.[2] This usually results because patients have not taken their medication as prescribed. Other common causes of SE are meningitis, head trauma, eclampsia, and progressive neurologic and neurodegenerative disorders.[2] In a study by the Veterans Affairs Status Epilepticus Cooperative Study Group comparing four treatments (lorazepam, phenytoin, phenobarbital, and diazepam) for GCSE, lorazepam was more likely than phenytoin to be successful when used as the initial treatment.[13] Recommendations for treatment of acute episodes of SE are listed in Table 201-2. Patients with SE should be admitted to intensive care for ongoing stabilization and workup.

MANAGEMENT

The goal of management in epilepsy is to control seizures with minimum adverse effects. In more than 50% of patients with epilepsy, seizures are completely controlled with medication.[14] Another 20% to 30% of patients have improvement of their symptoms with medications, but they are not seizure free or may experience significant side effects.[14] The remaining 25% to 30% of seizures are considered medically intractable.[14] Determination of the appropriate medical or surgical treatment is based on a variety of factors. These include patients' perception

TABLE 201-2 Recommended Emergency Treatment and Timetable for Status Epilepticus

Time (min)	Action
0-5	Diagnose status epilepticus (SE). Give oxygen by nasal cannula or mask; consider intubation if indicated. Establish an intravenous line; obtain blood samples for glucose, serum chemistry, hematology screen, toxicology, and antiepileptic drug levels.
6-9	If hypoglycemia is established or blood glucose is unknown, administer glucose: Adults: Give thiamine 100 mg followed by 50 mL of 50% glucose intravenously. Children: Give 2 mL of 25% glucose per kilogram.
10-20	Administer either 0.1 g of lorazepam per kilogram at 2 mg/min or 0.2 mg of diazepam per kilogram at 5 mg/min intravenously (if diazepam used, also give phenytoin in follow-up).
21-60	IF SE persists, administer 15-20 mg/kg of phenytoin intravenously no faster than 50 mg/min in adults and 1 mg/kg/min in children.* Monitor electrocardiogram and blood pressure.
>60	If SE does not stop after 20 mg of phenytoin per kilogram, give 20 mg of phenobarbital per kilogram intravenously at 100 mg/min. If SE persists, consult anesthesiology for consideration of intravenous anesthetic drugs to induce coma.

*In most centers, fosphenytoin is replacing phenytoin. The dosage is determined in phenytoin equivalents, and it can be administered twice as fast. It also causes less damage if it infiltrates.
Data from Treatment of convulsive status epilepticus: recommendations of the Epilepsy Foundation of America's Working Group on Status Epilepticus, *JAMA* 270(7):856, 1993.

of how the seizures are interfering with their life goals, economic considerations, personal support from family and friends, and severity and complexity of the epilepsy in that patient.

Conservative Management

Depending on a number of variables, including the potential for seizure recurrence, first seizures are usually not treated with AEDs. Only about 30% of persons who have a single, unprovoked, generalized tonic-clonic seizure have a second one, whether they are treated with medications or not.[15] Medication may delay recurrence or somewhat reduce its likelihood. Factors that should be considered in the decision to treat or not to treat a first seizure include the following:

- The type of seizure that occurred—Complex partial seizures are more likely to be recurrent than generalized tonic-clonic ones.
- Environment and occupation—for example, dangerous work environment, such as construction.
- Results of imaging studies and EEG—Treatment is prudent if either is abnormal because recurrence is likely.

The decision of whether to treat a patient who has had a single seizure has provoked controversy because of the lack of randomized, unbiased studies. Most studies have combined multiple seizure types, which clouds interpretation of the data. In one randomized multicenter trial of 1847 patients, immediate treatment increased the time to second and third seizures and reduced the time to 2-year remission when compared with untreated patients, but long-term remission rates were similar.[15,16] Although these results demonstrate the effectiveness of antiepileptic medication, the recurrence rate even in untreated patients is low enough that most patients with first seizures are not treated.

The two most consistent predictors of seizure recurrence are an abnormal electroencephalogram and an underlying cause. In patients with an unprovoked seizure for which there was an underlying antecedent cause (e.g., a previous head injury, mental retardation, or cerebral palsy), the risk of recurrent seizures was double that of patients with an unprovoked seizure for which there was no antecedent cause. After a second seizure, the risk of recurrence increases to more than 80%.[17]

Most epilepsy specialists advocate making treatment decisions after consideration of the risks and benefits of the treatment for a particular patient. Elements of decision-making include the risk to the patient according to the severity, timing, and frequency of seizures; age at seizure onset; and social and cognitive considerations. In determining risk, it is obvious that patients with generalized tonic-clonic seizures are more at risk for injury than are those with simple partial seizures. The timing of seizures is also important. Seizures that occur primarily while the patient is awake pose less risk. Seizures that occur only in relation to special circumstances, such as alcohol consumption, sleep deprivation, or pregnancy, are sometimes better treated by avoiding those factors than by taking antiepileptic medication. Age and cognition can be factors in decision-making. An adolescent who has just learned to drive may be more tolerant of the side effects related to seizure control than a young adult who has just entered college.[16]

Pharmacologic Management

Treatment choices vary with individual differences in cause, seizure type, age, and psychosocial factors. Control of seizures with a single drug should be the goal. Each drug should be titrated slowly to determine how it is tolerated, and each drug should be given a fair trial. The principles of treatment are fairly simple. As a first-line drug, levetiracetam (Keppra) has enormous advantages. It can be loaded acutely with equivalent oral and parenteral doses, and it has a broad spectrum of efficacy, against both generalized and focal forms of epilepsy. It has the added advantages of not causing sedation, not being an inducer of liver enzymes (and therefore not interfering with the metabolism of other medications), and being an acceptable drug in pregnancy. Drawbacks include psychiatric symptoms such as agitation, anxiety, and depression.

Valproate (Depakote) is another first-line drug that is most effective against generalized forms of epilepsy. Convulsive seizures as well as petit mal staring spells respond very well to valproate, but side effects including weight gain, hair loss, polycystic ovarian syndrome, hepatotoxicity, and a relatively high rate of birth defects in children born to mothers taking it have led to its being used less often than formerly. Ethosuximide is highly effective in children with petit mal seizures, but less so for other seizure types. Lamotrigine (Lamictal), like levetiracetam, has a very wide spectrum of efficacy, and has become the favored drug for women with epilepsy because of its very low rate of associated birth defects. Drawbacks include lack of a parenteral formulation, and relatively high rates of allergic rash that can evolve into Stevens-Johnson syndrome.

For focal epilepsy and complex partial seizures, with or without secondary generalization, carbamazepine (Tegretol) remains probably the single most effective drug and has the great advantage of low cost. It can, however, make some forms of generalized epilepsy worse and has no parenteral formulation. Phenytoin (Dilantin) is equally effective and can be given parenterally but has a worse side effect profile, particularly for women, in terms of osteoporosis, hirsutism, and coarsening of facial features. It can also be used for primary generalized epilepsy.

Topiramate (Topamax) is not a first-line drug because of its cognitive side effects, which include somnolence and dysphasia, but it does have a broad spectrum of efficacy, is effective for migraine prophylaxis, and also promotes weight loss. These qualities make it a favored drug in some settings. Lack of a parenteral formulation is a drawback. Gabapentin (Neurontin) actually exacerbates primary generalized epilepsies and is a weak drug for focal and secondarily generalized seizures. Because of its usefulness in pain management, it is sometimes used in mild cases of focal epilepsy wherein the provider is also trying to treat pain.

If seizures are frequent, efficacy can be determined quickly. About 50% of patients with epilepsy respond completely or almost completely to the first drug tried.[18] When medications are changed, the new medication should be added to the existing regimen. When the new medication is well tolerated and an effective dose has been achieved, the first medication can be slowly reduced. If the patient's seizures remain intractable after a trial of two or three single drugs, rational combinations of medications should be tried. Drugs with different mechanisms of action and different side effect profiles usually combine well.

Phenytoin with phenobarbital has been a traditional combination, but there is probably better evidence for the combined use of lamotrigine and valproate. Almost any combination of drugs has been found to be effective for at least a few patients. Among the 50% of patients who are refractory to monotherapy, probably another 25% will have their seizures controlled with some combination of medications; the remaining 25% remain refractory.[18] Half of these are candidates for epilepsy surgery; a residual 10% to 15% of patients will continue to have frequent seizures no matter what is tried.

Side effects occur in approximately 30% to 40% of patients taking AEDs.[16] Side effects include CNS involvement (such as somnolence, dizziness, tremor, and cognitive impairments), potential rashes, mood changes, weight changes, gastrointestinal disturbances, and headache.[16,18] The side effects should be carefully monitored and the doses adjusted to minimize the adverse effects of the medication. Rarely, an idiosyncratic reaction can occur, which can be life-threatening.

Measurements of blood levels of AEDs are helpful in determining whether a therapeutic dose has been achieved. For a steady level of the drug to be maintained in circulation, dosage frequency should be determined by the half-life of the drug. Table 201-3 compares the most common AEDs in terms of dose, peak, half-life, side effects, indications, and special considerations.

However, it is most important to follow the patient's response to treatment, not only in terms of drug levels, but in relation to efficacy and side effects. With many patients, seizures are controlled with low doses and levels of medications, whereas other patients require and tolerate high levels. Some patients experience significant side effects, even when drug levels are within a normal range. In this case, it may be best to order free AED levels, especially if the drug is highly protein bound. Protein binding, absorption, and elimination pharmacokinetics are extremely important factors to consider in predicting side effects and drug-drug interactions. The provider should obtain a complete list of medications, including over-the-counter preparations, from the patient. Blood levels should be obtained at least yearly, and more often if the patient is having breakthrough seizures, increased side effects, or signs of drug toxicity. In addition, CBC, electrolyte determinations, and LFTs should be performed within a month of beginning a new AED and periodically thereafter.

In making a decision to discontinue AED therapy, the provider and patient should consider the risk/benefit ratio. The risk for relapse is 20% to 40% in the first year of drug withdrawal and remains at about 36% during a 30-year period.[19] In one study, the risk of relapse was 2.9 times greater in those coming off of medication than in those staying on. Patients with the highest risk for relapse are those with a seizure disorder onset during adolescence, an abnormal electroencephalogram, an underlying neurologic condition, a definite diagnosis of primary generalized epilepsy, or a history of previous failures at discontinuing AEDs. There is insufficient evidence to establish when to withdraw AEDs in patients who are seizure free. One evidence-based review of 52 class II studies recommended that removal of medications be considered only if the patient has been seizure free for 2 to 5 years, has a single type of partial seizure, and has a normal electroencephalogram and IQ and normal findings on physical examination.[19]

Surgical Management

Of all patients with epilepsy, 25% to 30% are refractory to medical management.[20] Of the 25% to 30%, approximately half have focal lesions that are responsible for their seizures; these patients are good candidates for epilepsy surgery. The most common form of epilepsy surgery is a temporal lobectomy. Almost 80% of partial seizures in adults begin in the temporal lobes; a portion of one of the temporal lobes can be removed if tests consistently indicate that the seizures originate in that area. After temporal lobe surgery, success rates (complete seizure control) range from 65% to 95%.[20]

The removal of tumors, abnormal collections of blood vessels, and congenital lesions is another surgical resection option. These conditions can be found anywhere in the brain, and the best results are obtained when both the lesion and the surrounding epileptogenic brain are removed. It is often necessary to perform intracranial electroencephalographic mapping to delineate the epileptic zone and to identify cortically important areas, such as the language and motor cortex, which must be avoided during surgery.

Another major type of epilepsy surgery involves dividing the corpus callosum. With this type of surgery, the nerve fibers that connect one side of the brain to the other are severed; no tissue is removed. This surgery is most helpful for secondarily generalized tonic-clonic seizures and atonic seizures. Although seizures are not completely stopped by this procedure, they are confined to one hemisphere. Impairment of consciousness, convulsive seizure activity, and falls are often eliminated or greatly reduced.

Other surgical interventions available include multiple subpial transections wherein the surgeon makes a series of superficial cuts across brain tissue, theoretically interrupting the abnormal electrical signals; vagus nerve stimulation; and use of a responsive neurostimulation device, wherein wires implanted in the area of the seizures fire an electrical current into the area to prevent a seizure.[20]

After surgery, patients continue antiepileptic medication for several years. Patients who are seizure free for several years can consider a medication taper; however, there is not sufficient evidence to determine whether seizures will recur.

LIFE SPAN CONSIDERATIONS

Although stigma, social isolation, and depression can affect all persons with epilepsy, special concerns are recognized in specific age groups. Many patients develop epilepsy in early adolescence. This diagnosis can have a profound effect on self-esteem and instill a sense of lacking control because of the unpredictability of seizures. Parental overprotection and preoccupation with the child can lead to problems within the entire family unit. Adolescents should be encouraged to take responsibility for their own care. Providing education and the forum for a trusting relationship is the initial goal for this group of patients. Factual information should be presented in a straightforward, individualized manner, and the young adult should be encouraged to be honest and open about seizure frequency and compliance issues. Collaboration between patient and provider ideally results in a better understanding of the importance of medication, which makes adherence to the treatment plan more likely.

In women with epilepsy, there are additional concerns about contraception, fertility, and sexuality. Pregnancy has unpredictable effects on seizure control. Female adolescents should be counseled about family planning and birth control options. Patients taking hepatic enzyme–inducing AEDs should be given a higher-dose oral contraceptive, one with an estrogen content higher than 50 μg.[21] Women with epilepsy should be encouraged to plan their pregnancies and optimize seizure control in the prepregnancy year. They should also be given at least 1 mg of folic acid supplementation per day in advance; some AEDs

TABLE 201-3 Antiepileptic Drug (AED) Chart

Drug	Dosage Range	Side Effect Profile	Half-Life (HL) and Peak Effect	Drug Levels	Considerations
Phenobarbital (Luminal)	60-250 mg/day PO in divided doses or single-dose IV, 100-300 mg (up to 600 mg to load)	Drowsiness but tolerance usually develops. May cause difficulties with memory and cognition. May exacerbate depression in adults.	*HL:* 96 ± 12 hr Peak: Oral: 20-60 min IV: 15 min	15-40 (levels may not stabilize for 3-4 wk)	Do not stop abruptly. May cause hyperactivity in children. Used in partial and generalized seizures. Effective for motor seizures.
Phenytoin (Dilantin)	300-600 mg/day Loading dose: 1 g IV in divided doses	Gingival hypertrophy. Mild sedation. Rash, nausea, vomiting. Lethargy, nystagmus, ataxia with high doses. Difficulty with concentration and memory.	HL: Oral: 22 hr IV: 10-15 hr *Peak:* 4-12 hr 7-10 days to reach optimum levels	10-20 Levels may stay therapeutic for 7-10 days after stopping. Free level is ordered if patient is also taking valproic acid (VPA).	Used in partial and generalized seizures. Intravenous phenytoin and fosphenytoin are effective for treating status epilepticus.
Carbamazepine (Tegretol)	600-200 mg in divided doses	Drowsiness, dizziness, nausea and vomiting, which decrease with time. Start titration slowly to avoid side effects. Diplopia when toxic.	*HL:* 12-17 hr *Peak:* 4-5 hr after regular and 3-12 hr after XR or Carbatrol preparation.	Normal ranges vary by laboratory: 4-12 or 8-12 Drug takes about 2 days to achieve therapeutic level.	Used in partial seizures. Not for absence types. Should be taken with food. Generics should be avoided in patients with intractable seizures.
Primidone (Mysoline)	Slowly titrate up by 125 mg until reaching 250 mg tid	Drowsiness, ataxia, and vertigo may occur, which usually decrease with time or dose reduction.	*HL:* 12 ± 6 hr	Levels reported as primidone and phenobarbital Primidone: 5-12 Phenobarbital: 15-40	Used in partial and generalized seizures. Effective for motor seizures. If patient is allergic to phenobarbital, there is cross-sensitivity.
Valproic acid (VPA; Depakote)	15-60 mg/kg/day Rarely exceeds 3500-4000 mg/day	Drowsiness, mood changes, dizziness. Instruct patient on side effects of tremor and possible weight gain.	*HL:* 6-16 hr *Peak:* 1-4 hr after dose	Normal range 50-100 Levels over 100 may be tolerated by some if well controlled.	Effective in generalized seizures. May increase free Dilantin epoxide; obtain free Dilantin levels if needed. Avoid use in pregnant women
Lamotrigine (Lamictal)	Without VPA: range: 300-500 mg With VPA: range: 100-150 mg Children: 0.15-1.0 mg/kg Administer bid	Rash, headache, dizziness, and blurred vision. Blurred vision may occur more often in patients taking carbamazepine.	*HL:* 12-27 hr (with VPA: 70 hr) Peak: 1.4-4.8 hr	2.0-4.5 or 3-18 depending on laboratory Lamictal elimination is more rapid in patients taking hepatic enzyme–inducing AEDs.	Used in partial and generalized seizures. Risk of rash is higher in patients also taking VPA. Titrated to effect, not a certain blood level.
Gabapentin (Neurontin)	900-3600 mg/day Titrate to 300 mg tid then increase by 300-mg increments	Somnolence, dizziness, ataxia, and fatigue. Usually side effects are short-lived. Reduced interactions with other AEDs.	*HL:* 5-9 hr *Peak:* 2-3 hr	Normal range 2-20 Neurontin is not appreciably metabolized and significance of levels is uncertain.	Used in partial seizures. Should be taken 2 hours apart from Maalox to avoid changes in bioavailability.

Continued

TABLE 201-3 **Antiepileptic Drug (AED) Chart—cont'd**

Drug	Dosage Range	Side Effect Profile	Half-Life (HL) and Peak Effect	Drug Levels	Considerations
Topiramate (Topamax, Trokendi, Qudexy)	200-400 mg/day Administer bid titrate weekly in 25 mg bid increments over 6 weeks	Somnolence, dizziness, psychomotor slowing, speech hesitancy, and mood disturbances. Also may cause weight loss. Males have increased risk of kidney stones.	*HL:* 21 hr *Peak:* within 2 hr after dose	Not completely metabolized, and need for levels is uncertain.	Used as an adjunct in partial seizure disorders. May decrease estrogen levels in those on oral contraceptives. Recommend increased fluid intake.
Tiagabine (Gabitril)	12-32 mg/day Titrate by 4 mg/wk	Somnolence, dizziness, headache, mild memory impairment, and abdominal pain.	*HL:* 5-13 hr *Peak:* 0.5-1.0 hr	Not established at this time.	Used in partial seizures as an adjunctive therapy. Dose should be adjusted if hepatic disease is present.
Felbamate (Felbatol)	600-3600 mg/day titrate dose over several weeks	Insomnia, weight loss, headache. Refer to boxed warning regarding aplastic anemia and hepatic failure.	*HL:* 20-23 hr	Monitor concomitant drug levels. Monitor frequent CBC and LFTs.	Multiple drug interactions with other AEDs; consult a drug text for details. Used in partial and generalized seizures.
Zonisamide (Zonegran)	100-400 mg/day dosed qhs or bid	Somnolence, dizziness, anorexia, irritability, rash, renal calculi.	*HL:* 63 hr HL will decrease with the addition of other AEDs	10-40 μg/mL	Weak carbonic anhydrase inhibitor If allergic to sulfa, cross-sensitivity may occur.
Levetiracetam (Keppra)	1000-3000 mg/day bid	Somnolence, asthenia, infection, incoordination, behavioral abnormalities.	*HL:* 7 ± 1 hr	3-37 μg/mL	Occasionally associated with increased upper respiratory infections.
Oxcarbazepine (Trileptal, Oxtellar)	600-2400 mg/day 8-10 mg/kg	Dizziness, somnolence, headache, ataxia, diplopia	*HL:* 8-10 hr	10-monohydroxyl metabolite 12-30 mg/L	Increases phenytoin, phenobarbital, and VPA levels. Observe for hyponatremia.
Pregabalin (Lyrica)	150-600 mg/day	Dizziness, somnolence, ataxia, weight gain, peripheral edema, blurred vision.	*HL:* 6 hr (half life is 6 hours for Lyrica)	Not established currently	May lower platelet counts. Not metabolized in liver; excreted through kidney.

have been shown to inhibit folate action, and folate deficiency is associated with an increased risk of neural tube defects. Overall, AEDs probably double the baseline rate of birth defects.[22] Decisions to continue or to stop taking medication during pregnancy are difficult and should be discussed with a neurologist on an individual basis. Women who continue to take AEDs during pregnancy should be enrolled in the AED pregnancy registry, which can be located through the Epilepsy Foundation of America. AED levels may fluctuate unpredictably, and dosage modifications may be necessary. AED levels should be checked monthly and free levels obtained whenever possible. Lamotrigine and levetiracetam have been associated with lower rates of birth defects than other drugs.[22]

Hormonal changes also have an effect on seizure control. Many women note that seizures tend to occur just before or during their menstrual cycle. This is most likely related to low progesterone levels. Progesterone has been shown to decrease neuronal excitability in animal models, and Depo-Provera may have some role as an antiepileptic medication.[21] Little is known about the relationship between epilepsy and menopause. Studies are generally done with small numbers of women and evidence is conflicting.

The onset of epilepsy in elders has increased during the past decade. This increase is related to an increase in cerebrovascular disease, brain tumors, and Alzheimer disease, all associated with older age. Special concerns for older adults include an increased risk of head injury from an incidental fall, injury or falls that occur during seizures, the effects of AEDs on cognition and mobility, and interactions among various medications. Monotherapy is most important for this population to reduce side effects and drug interactions.[23] Dosage changes should be made slowly because older adults are more sensitive than young patients to even minor changes. Among AEDs, levetiracetam is least likely to interact with other drugs.

COMPLICATIONS

Medication complications in patients with epilepsy are usually related to seizure events. Injuries that occur during seizures include falls, burns, motor vehicle accidents, and aspiration pneumonia. Risks can be reduced by making lifestyle changes at work and during recreation. Patient advocacy helps ensure safe environments at work and school and can discourage discrimination.

Recent evidence suggests that women and also men taking enzyme-inducing antiepileptic medications are at increased risk for osteoporosis and osteomalacia. This is related to bone metabolism and inadequate absorption of vitamin D.[24] All patients should be taking vitamin D and calcium supplements.

Convulsive or generalized tonic-clonic SE is a medical emergency that can lead to brain damage or even death.[13] Mortality and morbidity rates are related to the cause of SE and the time from the onset of SE until seizures are controlled. In patients with known epilepsy, half of the hospital-reported cases of GCSE have been associated with subtherapeutic AED levels.[13] Other causes of SE include brain infection, trauma, and stroke. Most cases of SE can be treated successfully with parenteral drug therapy, including lorazepam, phenytoin, and phenobarbital.

INDICATIONS FOR REFERRAL OR HOSPITALIZATION

The following conditions warrant consideration for admission: SE, incomplete recovery from a single seizure or prolonged postictal state, suspected illness that requires treatment, drug or alcohol withdrawal, febrile illness (adult), expanding mass lesion, history of recent head trauma, or focal signs on examination.

Patients with frequent seizures or patients who meet the criteria for SE should be hospitalized for stabilization, further evaluation, and medication adjustment. Patients with seizures that are refractory to conventional therapy should be referred to a neurologist or epileptologist for further evaluation. If adequate seizure control is not achieved, patients should undergo presurgical and diagnostic evaluation with electroencephalographic video monitoring at a comprehensive epilepsy center. Patients who are having difficulty tolerating medications should also be referred for a neurology consultation. Patients with structural lesions should be referred promptly to a neurosurgeon for further evaluation.

PATIENT AND FAMILY EDUCATION

Epilepsy provides unique teaching opportunities because it is a chronic condition that affects all aspects of a patient's life. Patient and family education about safety is vital. It is imperative that patients avoid high places such as rooftops and ladders, not operate dangerous equipment that could cause cuts or crush injuries, and not swim alone. Family members should be taught simple first aid measures such as turning the patient onto his or her side and not putting objects into the mouth during a tonic-clonic seizure.

Other key areas for patient instruction include the following:

- General information
- Diagnostic studies
- Treatment plan
- Medication information
- Alternative or adjunctive therapies
- Safety issues and first aid for seizures
- Support services available (e.g., support groups, centers for independent living and how to access them)

HEALTH PROMOTION

Issues related to driving and other behaviors that impose a great safety risk should be discussed. Each state has varied restrictions for individuals with epilepsy who wish to obtain a driver's license. Information about the laws of a particular state can be found by calling the department of motor vehicles. Issues surrounding employment and psychosocial functioning should also be addressed. Resources such as vocational rehabilitation programs, clinical social workers, centers for independent living, and epilepsy support groups should be used.

Overall, moderation should be encouraged. Adequate rest, stress reduction, proper nutrition, and avoidance of known seizure precipitants can improve seizure control. Some studies advocate a ketogenic diet as helpful in controlling seizures, especially in children whose seizures are incompletely controlled with medication alone. Adults find this diet difficult to maintain because of its restrictions. Several studies of modified Atkins diets seem to show the same beneficial results.[25]

Epilepsy is a challenging condition and requires a comprehensive approach to treatment. The goal is to treat the patient but not make the treatment worse than the disease. Efforts to understand the impact of epilepsy on patients will improve the health care provider's ability to treat appropriately and compassionately.

CHAPTER 202

TRIGEMINAL NEURALGIA

Wanda J. Handel

DEFINITION AND EPIDEMIOLOGY

Trigeminal neuralgia is a common and well-defined pain disorder affecting the sensory branches of the trigeminal nerve. It is also known as *tic douloureux,* from the French for "painful spasm," and affects 12 people per 100,000.[1] Women are affected slightly more often than men (3:2), and older adults more often than younger persons. The mean age at onset is 54 years; most cases occur in individuals 50 to 70 years of age. Cases occurring in patients younger than 40 years are unusual.[1]

PATHOPHYSIOLOGY

The fifth cranial nerve, the trigeminal nerve, is a large, mixed sensory and motor nerve that originates in the brainstem and travels in the cervical cord, with the sensory ganglion found in the Meckel cave in the middle cranial fossa. The peripheral branches form three sensory divisions—ophthalmic (V1), maxillary (V2), and mandibular (V3)—that conduct sensory impulses from the greater part of the face and head, from the cornea and conjunctiva, and from the nose and mouth. These impulses eventually terminate in the thalamus, where they are relayed to the appropriate cortical area for interpretation. The motor portion of the nerve supplies the muscles of the jaw and sphenoid areas.

Most primary cases of trigeminal neuralgia are thought to be caused by vascular compression and are considered classic trigeminal neuralgia.[2] Secondary trigeminal neuralgia is differentiated by the ability to demonstrate a structural cause, such as compression, trauma, or multiple sclerosis.[3] The location of one of the cerebral arteries and its branches is thought to be a factor by creating compression on the nerve as it exits the brainstem. Demyelination, vascular changes, and degenerative changes in the sensory (gasserian) ganglion are postulated to generate altered impulse transmission, allowing ephaptic transmission between adjacent nerve fibers mediating light touch and pain.[4]

CLINICAL PRESENTATION

The primary feature of this disorder is recurrent paroxysms of pain in the distribution of any branch of the trigeminal nerve. The pain is usually described as burning, stabbing, sharp, penetrating, or electric shock–like and usually is on one side of the face. Males may have unshaven faces or portions thereof. The index of suspicion for multiple sclerosis rises if the patient exhibits bilateral facial pain. The duration of each paroxysm varies from seconds to more than 15 minutes and involves V2 and V3 more often than V1; V1 is more frequently affected by postherpetic neuralgia.[5] Pain may recur once a month or several times per day. If the pain occurs frequently during the day, the patient may report unremitting facial discomfort between discrete episodes. Usually, a patient does not awaken from sleep during a paroxysm.

During an attack, the patient may cease talking, stop chewing, become very still, rub or pinch the face, avoid making facial expressions during conversation, grimace, or make movements of the face and jaw. Between attacks, the patient is free of symptoms except for fear of an impending attack.

PHYSICAL EXAMINATION

A characteristic feature of trigeminal neuralgia is the trigger zone, a small area of the skin or orobuccal mucosa that the patient can identify as the point that sets off an attack. Trigger points are generally in the distribution of the nerve branch experiencing the pain. Chewing, talking, facial movement, or touch may elicit a paroxysm. Drafts or cool breezes may also precipitate symptoms. The patient may be reluctant to allow examination of the face for fear of triggering an attack. All cranial nerves should be examined in detail. In secondary trigeminal neuralgia, the corneal reflex may be abnormal.[5] The remainder of the physical examination, including the neurologic component, yields normal findings.

DIAGNOSTICS AND DIFFERENTIAL DIAGNOSIS

The diagnosis of trigeminal neuralgia is usually made without difficulty from the history and the characteristic manner in which the patient relates the history (the patient is careful not to touch any trigger points or painful areas). Criteria for diagnosis put forth by the International Headache Society include the following[3]:

- Paroxysms of pain lasting from a fraction of a second to 2 minutes and affecting one or more divisions of the trigeminal nerve without radiation of symptoms
- Pain characterized as at least three events of intense, sharp, superficial, or stabbing nature and precipitated from trigger areas or trigger factors
- No clinically identified neurologic deficit
- Not attributable to another disorder

However, the classic case presentation of trigeminal neuralgia may not always be encountered. Because there are innumerable causes of facial pain, prudence dictates that alternative diagnoses be investigated and that the patient be reexamined at regular intervals. The differential diagnosis should include headache (particularly migraine), acoustic neuroma, trigeminal neuroma, meningioma, aneurysms, acute polyneuropathy, chronic meningitis, other neuralgias, and dental abnormalities. Trigeminal neuralgia is a common cause of pain in multiple sclerosis.

Results of laboratory tests are either normal or noncontributory. If alternative diagnoses are suspected, an autoimmune laboratory panel may be indicated. Trigeminal reflex testing has demonstrated that abnormal reflexes are associated with greater risk of secondary trigeminal neuralgia. Magnetic resonance angiography of the posterior fossa may be undertaken to differentiate vascular abnormalities and to rule out compression from tumor or vessels. Magnetic resonance imaging (MRI) can also corroborate the presence of multiple sclerosis.[5]

DIAGNOSTICS

Trigeminal Neuralgia

Diagnosis is based primarily on the patient history and physical findings and requires no initial diagnostic laboratory or imaging studies unless history and physical findings suggest secondary trigeminal neuralgia.

IMAGING

Magnetic resonance angiography*
MRI*
Electrophysiologic testing*

*If indicated.

MANAGEMENT

The treatment of trigeminal neuralgia has not changed much during the past decade. Regardless of the intervention adopted, symptoms may remit spontaneously and permanently. A stepwise approach, including co-management with a neurologist, is warranted.

- Anticonvulsants are the first-line pharmacologic therapy.[6]
  - When using anticonvulsant therapy, the provider should titrate to the maximum therapeutic dose necessary to provide pain relief, and then titrate down to the lowest effective dose.
  - Abrupt withdrawal of these agents should be avoided. A partial listing of more commonly used agents can be found in Table 202-1.
- Carbamazepine (CBZ) and oxcarbazepine (OXZ).[7]
  - Approximately two thirds of patients will respond to CBZ. OXZ may be better tolerated in some individuals.[6,7]

TABLE 202-1 **Pharmacotherapy for Trigeminal Neuralgia**

	Starting Dose	Maximum Dose	Adverse Drug Events (Not All Inclusive)
FIRST-LINE TREATMENT			
Carbamazepine	100-200 mg daily	200-400 mg 3 times per day	Aplastic anemia, agranulocytosis, ataxia, diplopia, Stevens-Johnson syndrome
Oxcarbazepine	300 mg 2 times per day	600-1200 mg 2 times per day	Nausea, vomiting, hyponatremia, Stevens-Johnson syndrome
SECOND LINE TREATMENT—ADD ON OR SWITCH TO THE FOLLOWING			
Baclofen	5-10 mg 3 times per day	30 mg 3 times per day	Sedation, dizziness, dyspepsia, cognitive changes
Lamotrigine	25-50 mg daily	150-200 mg 2 times per day	Rash, Stevens-Johnson syndrome
Phenytoin	100-300 mg daily	300-500 mg daily	Rash, dizziness, confusion, ataxia
FOR PATIENTS WITH MULTIPLE SCLEROSIS			
Gabapentin	100-300 mg daily	300-600 mg three times per day	Dizziness, sedation, decreased coordination
Misoprostol	200 μg three times daily	600 μg per day	Headache, nausea, diarrhea, contraindicated in pregnancy

Modified from Pfaul T, Brinkerson M, Treuhert T: Misoprostol as a therapeutic option for trigeminal neuralgia in patients with multiple sclerosis. *Pain Med* 13(10):1377-1378, 2012; and Obermann M: Treatment options in trigeminal neuralgia. *Ther Adv Neurol Disord* 3(2):107-115, 2010.

- When prescribing CBZ, care must be taken to monitor for liver damage and hematologic changes using complete blood count (CBC), serum sodium levels, and liver function tests at periodic intervals.[6,8]
- If the patient does not respond satisfactorily to medical management or has relief only at a dose that causes intolerable adverse effects:
  - Combination drug therapy may be started with another agent.
  - Second-line medications may be used, including baclofen, lamotrigine, and phenytoin.[8]
- In acute attacks, intravenous administration of fosphenytoin, injections of botulinum toxin or sumatriptan, or intranasal lidocaine may afford pain relief while oral doses are uptitrated.[8]
- In patients with multiple sclerosis, the long-acting prostaglandin E analogue misoprostol (Cytotec) or gabapentin have been useful.[9]
- Patients with refractory pain who do not tolerate medications or in whom pharmacologic management with three medications fails may be referred to a neurosurgeon for surgical assessment.[10]

DIFFERENTIAL DIAGNOSIS

Trigeminal Neuralgia

- Neurologic
- Headache
- Acoustic neuroma
- Trigeminal neuroma
- Meningioma
- Acute polyneuropathy
- Chronic meningitis
- Multiple sclerosis
- Tumor
- Migrainous neuralgia

HEAD, EAR, EYE, NOSE, AND THROAT

- Dental disorders
- Abscess
- Temporomandibular joint syndrome
- Sinusitis

VASCULAR

- Cerebral aneurysms
- Cerebral arteriovenous malformations

LIFE SPAN CONSIDERATIONS

Careful consideration must be paid to the elderly patient, who may have preexisting age-related physiologic changes that can affect pharmacokinetics, such as decreased blood flow, renal and hepatic impairment, risk of interactions from polypharmacy, and a less predictable capacity for protein binding of the drug.[5,7] Slow titration is encouraged. Comorbid conditions may also make a patient a poor surgical candidate.

COMPLICATIONS

Complications are usually related to pharmacologic management. Carbamazepine therapy may result in aplastic anemia, drowsiness, dizziness, and ataxia. Other medications listed can cause drowsiness, dizziness, and cognitive changes. Surgical complications include facial numbness and pain, recurrent neuralgia, or facial paralysis, in addition to the risks associated with any surgical procedure. Pain control may also be a significant factor, particularly if patients cannot tolerate the usually prescribed medications. In such an instance, additional management concerns may arise, including weight loss, dehydration, and poor dental hygiene if chewing, liquids, and oral care are triggers, as well as social isolation and depression. All of these concerns are potentially more significant in the elderly population.

INDICATIONS FOR REFERRAL OR HOSPITALIZATION

The primary care provider is often the initial practitioner to evaluate the patient with facial pain. After a thorough history and neurologic examination, a patient presumed to have trigeminal neuralgia should be referred to a neurologist for a more comprehensive physical and imaging examination. Medical treatment may be initiated by the specialist and managed by the primary care provider. Care consists of medication initiation, observations for adverse effects, and consultation with the neurologist regarding dose adjustments and response to therapy. Consultation with a specialist is beneficial to the patient and provider in identifying the most efficacious regimen when combination drug therapy is necessary.

Referral to a neurosurgeon is indicated after medical therapies have been exhausted. Surgery is considered when medical regimens do not provide pain relief or side effects of medications are intolerable. Among the surgical interventions that may be appropriate are glycerol rhizotomy, radiofrequency ablation, microvascular decompression, and stereotactic radiosurgery.[10] Major disadvantages of glycerol rhizotomy, radiofrequency ablation, and decompression surgery include loss of facial sensation, keratitis, facial muscle weakness, spontaneous pain (anesthesia dolorosa), dysesthesias, and recurrent neuralgia.[10]

Consultation with a psychologist or psychiatrist may also be indicated, depending on the patient's adaptation skills. Multidisciplinary team meetings may be valuable in planning an approach to care. Referral to a pain center may also be an option for individuals with chronic pain.

EDUCATION AND HEALTH PROMOTION

Significant education is necessary to explain the varied medication therapies, all of which are sedating. Caution about use of these medications in conjunction with use of alcohol and other medications is essential. Discuss the need to monitor laboratory studies when taking medications. For patients in severe pain or those who are fearful of the next attack, it is important to consider the patient's activities of daily living, including eating, sleeping, and socializing with others. Severe pain may restrict adequate calorie intake; advising the patient to use a straw for liquids may allow intake of nutritional supplements. Maintenance of dental hygiene may be challenging because brushing may elicit pain; use of a Waterpik to clean the teeth may be of benefit to some. A collaborative relationship with the patient enhances a tailored, well-informed approach toward high-quality care.

CHAPTER 203

INTRACRANIAL TUMORS

Melissa C. Davis • Camilo E. Fadul

Primary malignant and nonmalignant intracranial tumors represent a small fraction of all types of cancer, but they have a major physical, psychological, and financial impact on individual patients, families, and communities. Brain metastases from systemic neoplasm are equally devastating and significantly more frequent. Expedient diagnosis and treatment of brain tumors are essential to minimize potential complications and to maximize functional quality of life. As the first point of contact for patients when acute or subtle changes in health occur, primary care practitioners play an important role in the diagnosis and ongoing care of patients with brain tumors. The practitioner's knowledge of a patient allows the detection of subtle clinical changes, affording appropriate evaluation and timely diagnosis. Ongoing supportive care during treatment and follow-up of a patient with the diagnosis of a brain tumor is imperative and can be well managed by the primary care practitioner in collaboration with the specialist.

DEFINITION AND EPIDEMIOLOGY

The term *brain tumor* is defined as the growth of abnormal cells in the tissue of the brain. This includes neoplasms that arise from intracranial structures, such as the meninges, which are not a component of the nervous system. Brain tumors can be nonmalignant or malignant, and can be primary or metastatic. Tumor nomenclature and grading are based on the histologic characteristics of the tissue. Whereas primary brain tumors arise from structures of the nervous system, brain metastases are thought to arise from the hematogenous spread of circulating tumor cells that migrate into the perivascular space after disruption of the basal membrane. For primary brain tumors, the World Health Organization (WHO) grading system provides a means to prognosticate the biologic behavior of the tumor. It is based on the tumor's proliferative potential, nuclear atypia, mitotic activity, and presence of necrosis (Table 203-1). Although prognosis correlates with WHO grade, immunohistochemistry and genetic profiling provide additional information that allows for more accurate brain tumor characterization. The combination of histology and genetic characteristics guide individualized treatment.

Tumors with glial characteristics, called gliomas, are the most frequent type of primary malignant brain tumor. Based on the cell of origin, gliomas are further classified into astrocytomas, oligodendrogliomas, mixed oligoastrocytomas, and ependymomas.[1] The hallmarks of high-grade malignant gliomas (anaplastic gliomas and glioblastoma) are neovascularization, high mitotic rate, infiltration into surrounding tissue, and presence of necrosis.

The cause of primary brain tumors is unknown. Previous cranial irradiation has been associated with the development of meningiomas. The incidence of meningioma also seems to be higher in women with a history of breast cancer, probably related to the expression of hormone receptors by these tumors. There are familial cancer syndromes that have a high incidence of brain tumors. For example, the Li-Fraumeni syndrome, caused by the mutation of the tumor suppressor gene *p53*, is associated with

TABLE 203-1 Classification of Central Nervous System Tumors

Tumor Type (Frequency)[3]	WHO Grade*
Astrocytoma (21.9%)	Grade I: Pilocytic astrocytoma Grade II: Diffuse astrocytoma Grade III: Anaplastic astrocytoma Grade IV: Glioblastoma
Oligodendroglioma (1.7%)	Grade II: Oligodendroglioma Grade III: Anaplastic oligodendroglioma
Mixed oligoastrocytoma (0.9%)	Grade II: Oligoastrocytoma Grade III: Anaplastic oligoastrocytoma
Ependymoma (1.9%)	Grade I: Subependymoma, myxopapillary ependymoma Grade II: Ependymoma Grade III: Anaplastic ependymoma
Meningioma (35.8%)	Grade I: Meningioma Grade II: Atypical meningioma Grade III: Malignant meningioma

*World Health Organization (WHO) classification.

a high incidence of brain tumors. Primary central nervous system (CNS) lymphoma occurs more frequently in patients who are immunosuppressed after transplantation or in patients with acquired immunodeficiency syndrome (AIDS) in association with Epstein-Barr virus infection. In patients who are not immunocompromised, the cause is uncertain.

In 2014, primary nervous system tumors will account for approximately 1.4% of all new cancer diagnoses.[2] In the United States, the estimated incidence of malignant and nonmalignant brain tumors is 21.03 cases per 100,000 person-years, with approximately 66,240 new cases per year. Meningioma, usually a nonmalignant brain tumor, accounts for 35.8% of all cases, followed by glioblastoma, a malignant brain tumor, which accounts for 15.6% of cases.[3] Survival rates vary significantly based on histology and grade. The 5-year relative survival rate for a grade I meningioma is 82%.[4] Conversely, the 5-year relative survival rate for glioblastoma (grade IV glioma) is less than 5%.[3]

The incidence of brain metastases varies significantly based on primary malignancy. Although melanoma and small cell lung cancer (SCLC) have the highest predilection to metastasize to the brain, the prevalence of brain metastases is higher from non-SCLC and breast cancer, given the frequency of these malignancies. It is expected that the incidence will increase as imaging techniques become more accessible, particularly brain magnetic resonance imaging (MRI). The incidence of brain metastases is also expected to increase as systemic therapy, which often does not cross the blood-brain barrier, improves survival.[5] Prognosis is influenced by primary malignancy, age, performance status, and number of brain metastases. Median survival after diagnosis of brain metastases ranges from 4.9 months for SCLC to 13.8 months for breast cancer.[6] The prognosis has improved in recent years, and the number of long-term survivors is increasing.

CLINICAL PRESENTATION

Brain tumors cause symptoms by infiltrating, expanding, and displacing healthy brain tissue. In addition to the infiltration of normal tissue, brain tumors can increase the permeability of blood vessels, leading to edema that dislodges and compresses normal structures. As the brain tumor volume and resulting edema move normal structures, patients can sustain ischemic strokes from blood vessel occlusion and herniation from displacement of brainstem structures. In addition, tumors can cause injury to normal neurons, resulting in increased excitability of the neurons and seizures. Tumors involving the hypothalamic-pituitary axis can cause a variety of endocrinologic syndromes.

A meticulously taken history and thorough examination are essential to the diagnosis of a brain tumor. The growth pattern and location will determine the symptoms. Fast-growing tumors such as glioblastoma tend to produce subacute symptoms, whereas slow-growing tumors such as meningiomas can become very large before producing symptoms. The clinical presentation of brain metastases is usually more abrupt, related to rapid tumor growth and associated edema. On occasion, brain tumors can have an acute presentation as the result of intratumoral bleeding or a seizure. In children, tumors are usually in the posterior fossa and most frequently manifest with signs of increased intracranial pressure.

There are three neurologic syndromes (combination of symptoms and signs) caused by an intracranial neoplasm, categorized as nonfocal, localizing (focal), and seizures. These syndromes vary according to tumor location, size, and growth rate. Nonfocal syndromes may include symptoms caused by increased intracranial pressure and brain herniation, personality changes, gait disorder, and endocrine dysfunction. Localizing symptoms are usually focal and specific to the area of the brain involved, and may include motor, sensory, language, or visual impairments. Approximately 30% of patients will experience a seizure at some point during the course of the illness. Seizures can be focal or generalized. Focal seizures involve one hemisphere of the brain and typically manifest as sensory or motor symptoms. Generalized seizures occur when there is abnormal electrical activity in both cerebral hemispheres[7] (see Chapter 201).

PHYSICAL EXAMINATION

The examination needs to be thorough, albeit focused on eliciting findings that provide the best diagnostic yield. A mini-mental examination should be included, given that alteration in mental status is frequently observed in nonfocal syndromes. Examination of the optic fundi is also crucial because papilledema may be the only finding to indicate increased intracranial pressure.

Components of the neurologic physical examination allow for localization to a particular brain region. Visual field testing by confrontation can localize involvement of the optic nerve pathway, as well as the occipital or parietotemporal lobes. Abnormalities of ocular movement can occur from compression of the oculomotor nerves or involvement of the brainstem. Motor and sensory abnormalities correlate with frontal or parietal involvement. Aphasia can be seen with damage to the dominant frontal or temporal lobes. Of note, focal speech disorders can be erroneously diagnosed as confusion (nonfocal). Gait, tone, and coordination examinations are fundamental for posterior fossa brain tumors. Examples of the signs most frequently elicited on presentation of intracranial tumors are included in Table 203-2. In the case of seizures, patients may initially have focal

TABLE 203-2 Physical Findings

Syndrome		Symptom or Sign
Nonfocal		Increased ICP: headache, confusion, papilledema, vomiting Herniation: cingulate, tentorial, tonsillar, CN III, CN VI Personality changes: dementia, anger, passivity, memory Gait disorder: ataxia Endocrine disorder: diabetes insipidus
Localizing	Frontal	Abulia, personality and behavioral changes, hemiparesis, aphasia
	Temporal	Aphasia, memory loss, superior quadrantanopsia
	Parietal	Sensory loss, quadrantanopsia or hemianopsia, visual spatial difficulties, dressing apraxia
	Occipital	Homonymous hemianopsia
	Cerebellar	Ataxia, dysmetria

CN, cranial nerve; ICP, intracranial pressure.
Data from Arrillaga-Romany IC, Lee EQ, Wen PW: Diagnosis of brain tumors: clinical and radiographic. In Packer RJ, Schiff D, editors: *Neuro-oncology*, Hoboken, NJ, 2012, John Wiley & Sons.

findings on examination that disappear once the patient has recovered from the postictal state.

DIAGNOSTICS

MRI with contrast enhancement is the preferred study for diagnosis of a brain tumor. Head computed tomography (CT) scan is frequently used, particularly in patients who are seen acutely in the emergency department, but MRI is more sensitive, especially in the posterior fossa. Nevertheless, the images are not specific for the type of tumor, and pathologic examination is required in most cases for definitive diagnosis.

If there is concern for metastases, CT scan of the chest, abdomen, and pelvis may be warranted. On the basis of the patient's presentation, further staging studies may be used to help define location of the primary cancer and extent of disease. These may include positron emission tomography (PET) scan and blood tests based on tumor origin. In general, lumbar puncture is contraindicated owing to concern of causing brain herniation.

Pathology examination is required in most cases to establish the diagnosis and to render treatment recommendations, the exception being when there is a history of metastatic cancer with typical radiologic appearance.

DIAGNOSTICS

Intracranial Tumors

IMAGING

Brain MRI with contrast
Head CT
PET/CT scan (if indicated)

DIFFERENTIAL DIAGNOSIS

The differential diagnosis is broad, but neoplasm should be considered in any patient with neurologic symptoms. A timeline of symptoms is useful in distinguishing an intracranial tumor from other entities. Cerebrovascular disease, in contrast to brain tumors, usually has an acute onset. Nevertheless, the possibly of an intratumoral bleed should be entertained in patients with intracerebral hemorrhage. Past medical history of neurologic symptoms that improve spontaneously provides clues to differentiate "tumefactive" multiple sclerosis from tumor. Brain abscess can be difficult to differentiate clinically and by imaging studies. Constitutional symptoms and infection outside the nervous system, albeit not always present, are helpful clues for the diagnosis of brain abscess. Other entities that can be included in the differential diagnosis are listed in the differential diagnosis box.

DIFFERENTIAL DIAGNOSIS

Intracranial Tumors

ONCOLOGIC

- Primary brain tumor, including primary CNS lymphoma
- Brain metastases

INFECTIOUS

- Abscess
- Meningitis
- Viral encephalitis, including herpes simplex encephalitis
- Lyme disease
- Syphilis
- Progressive multifocal leukoencephalopathy (PML)

VASCULAR

- Cerebral hemorrhage
- Cerebral infarction
- Aneurysm

INFLAMMATORY

- Multiple sclerosis
- Sarcoidosis
- Vasculitis
- Systemic lupus erythematosus (SLE)

MANAGEMENT

Oncologic management of primary brain tumors is based on tumor location, pathologic diagnosis, and patient performance status. The backbone of treatment consists of surgery, radiation therapy, and chemotherapy. As patients with brain tumors experience greater longevity, it is necessary to weigh the acute and long-term sequelae of treatment before initiation of therapy to minimize functional impairment. Clinical trials should be considered whenever possible.

1. The most effective treatment of brain tumors is surgical resection. The extent of resection will depend on location and functional areas of the brain affected.[1] Tumors such as meningiomas can be cured with complete surgical resection. When the location or cause of a brain tumor prohibits surgical resection, a biopsy is performed to obtain tissue for pathologic diagnosis.
2. Radiation therapy may be used as a primary, adjuvant, or palliative therapy to treat primary brain tumors. Radiation may be localized to the area of disease or may involve the whole brain. Radiation is delivered on a fractionated schedule, usually in the range of 30 to 60 Gy. Doses are based on tumor radiosensitivity and tolerance of normal surrounding tissue. Radiation is often recommended for patients with intermediate-grade meningioma that is subtotally resected, high-grade meningioma, low-grade glioma with high-risk features or progressive disease after surgical resection, or high-grade glioma. In the case of brain metastases, radiation options depend on the number and size of the metastases and include whole-brain radiation and/or radiosurgery.
3. Chemotherapy may also be used as a primary, adjuvant, or palliative treatment of brain tumors. Chemotherapy agents are limited because most do not effectively cross the blood-brain barrier. Chemotherapy decisions are based on tumor histology, grade, and chemotherapy mechanism of action. Temozolomide, an alkylating agent, is the most commonly used drug because of tumor sensitivity and the drug's ability to cross the blood-brain barrier. In glioblastoma, radiation therapy in combination with temozolomide has been shown to significantly prolong survival.[8] Primary CNS lymphoma is usually treated with high-dose methotrexate–based chemotherapy regimens; surgery is used only for diagnostic biopsy. Biologic therapies include targeted agents directed at blocking specific cellular pathways, thus impeding tumorigenesis.[9] An example is bevacizumab, which is a monoclonal antibody that interferes with angiogenesis.

Supportive Therapies

Supportive treatments are an integral part of the management of patients with brain tumors. Therapies are directed at symptoms related to the brain tumor, as well as to acute and late side effects of treatment. Steroids are used primarily for their anti-inflammatory effect. Dexamethasone is the most commonly used corticosteroid, and it is tapered as soon as clinically possible to minimize side effects.[9] Steroids are avoided before biopsy, when feasible, in patients thought to have primary CNS lymphoma because steroids may affect the pathologic diagnosis.

Venous thromboembolism (VTE) occurs in a high proportion of patients with high-grade gliomas and meningiomas, especially in the postoperative period.[10] Patients are monitored for symptoms of deep vein thrombosis and pulmonary embolism. Appropriate diagnostic studies should be obtained if there is clinical suspicion of a VTE. Low-molecular-weight heparin is the preferred pharmacologic treatment of VTE in patients with cancer.[10]

Seizure management and pharmacologic selection of anticonvulsant are based on the type of seizure. Non–enzyme-inducing antiepileptic agents are preferred because they do not interact with oncologic treatment. Some patients require multiple agents to control seizure activity. Referral for management to an epileptologist is appropriate when seizures are intractable (see Chapter 201).

Depression is frequently seen in patients with brain tumors and should be assessed with every patient encounter.[9] Selective serotonin reuptake inhibitors are the most frequently used agents. Bupropion is avoided in patients with seizures because it lowers the seizure threshold. Whenever possible, nonpharmacologic therapies, including counseling, massage, and exercise, should be used in conjunction with pharmacologic therapy.

Fatigue, secondary to both the brain tumor and treatment, is common. It can persist for more than a year after completion of therapy. Energy conservation, adequate nutrition, and regular activity are recommended as first-line treatment. If there is significant functional impairment of activities of daily living, methylphenidate and modafinil are sometimes considered because they may improve cognition, memory, and other functional markers.[11,12]

Dietary recommendations are important because patients may experience weight gain or weight loss as a result of disease and treatment. In general, a well-balanced diet with all food groups should be recommended, and early referral to a dietitian is advised for evaluation of weight and comorbid disease considerations.

Cognitive and functional impairments are often distressing to patients and family members. Rehabilitation should be directed toward maximizing functional performance and may include physical, occupational, speech, and/or cognitive therapy. Formal neuropsychological testing is useful to assess memory, attention, and initiation, and provides a means to measure changes over time (see Chapter 188). Assistive devices to accommodate mobility, communication, and hearing and visual losses are also readily available.

COMPLICATIONS

Complications from brain tumors may be related to the tumor or may occur as a result of treatment. Injury of nervous and vascular tissue, inflammation, and metabolic dysfunction by the tumor may have consequences that include cerebral hemorrhage, thrombosis, hydrocephalus, herniation, coagulopathies, paraneoplastic syndromes, endocrinopathies, and cerebral edema with mass effect. Treatment-related complications, which are described as acute (within the first 6 months) or late (after 6 months) effects, may include leukoencephalopathy, immunosuppression, cerebral hemorrhage, thrombosis, myelopathy, and neuropathy.

INDICATIONS FOR REFERRAL OR HOSPITALIZATION

When a brain tumor diagnosis is suspected in the primary care setting, appropriate diagnostic studies related to the differential diagnosis should be performed.

- After initial evaluation, referral to an oncology specialist is recommended. This specialist may be a neurosurgeon, neuro-oncologist, pediatric oncologist, or general oncologist.
- Partnering of the primary care provider with the referral specialist throughout the patient's course of disease is critical to ensure effective communication and treatment of the patient's symptoms or worsening disease.

LIFE SPAN CONSIDERATIONS

Brain tumors are the most frequent solid tumor in the pediatric population. The most common histology in children ages 0 to 4 years is embryonal tumor. From the ages of 5 years to 14 years, the most common histology is pilocytic astrocytoma, a grade I glioma. In adulthood, the rates of primary brain and CNS tumors increase with age. With meningioma, adults aged 55 to 64 years have an incidence of 14.13 cases per 100,000 person-years. For adults aged 85 years or older, the incidence increases to 48.93 cases per 100,000 person-years. The incidence of glioblastoma peaks at 75 and 84 years, with 14.64 cases per 100,000 person-years.[3] All age groups are at risk for metastatic brain tumors and neurologic complications of systemic cancer therapies.

Treatments vary based on age. For example, radiation therapy is avoided, whenever possible, in very young patients because of long-term neurotoxicity. During childbearing age, referral to a fertility specialist is recommended owing to treatment-related infertility. In older adults, treatment can cause greater toxicity than in younger adults. There is no standard of care for glioblastoma patients older than 70 years. Depending on functional status and age, some patients receive abbreviated courses of radiation and/or receive radiation or temozolomide alone, rather than concurrently.[13]

EDUCATION AND HEALTH PROMOTION

Communication with and education of patients with brain tumors and their families are vital components of any treatment program. It is important to provide information on the disease, treatments, side effects, and specific limitations in daily activity. Common limitations are related to safety, supervision, driving restrictions, and work limitations. Instructions and recommendations should be given verbally and in writing because of cognitive impairment. Ideally, advance directives are discussed soon after diagnosis. Although the need for palliative and hospice services may not arise for some time after diagnosis, early introduction to patients and families affords an easy transition to services when they are required. Referral to local support groups and local and national brain tumor associations should also be made at the time of diagnosis.

Patients with brain tumors can live for many years, particularly those with low-grade malignancies. Therefore, it is important to maintain and to encourage health promotion activities during treatment, follow-up, and survivorship. Health maintenance screening may include mammography, Papanicolaou (Pap) smear, colonoscopy, and bone density scan, as well as monitoring for chronic illness and risky behaviors.

Therapy for brain tumors can put patients at risk for conditions that bear monitoring and treatment. Potential problems depend on specific treatments the patient has received, tumor location in the brain or spinal cord, and supportive therapies used during treatment. The American College of Surgeons Commission on Cancer has mandated that by 2015, institutions seeking accreditation must be using treatment summaries (TSs) and survivorship care plans (SCPs). The TS and SCP are formulated by the oncology team and are given to patients and primary care providers. The documents outline characteristics of the tumor and treatment, monitoring recommendations for tumor recurrence and persistent or late effects, and who is responsible for monitoring. Barriers to such documents include time constraints, fragmented care across multiple institutions, difficulty obtaining data from medical records, lack of clarity as to which patients should have a TS and an SCP, and lack of standards for adult survivorship surveillance. Controversy remains regarding how to best provide care to cancer survivors.[14]

REFERENCES

For a full list of references, scan the QR code or visit http://booksite.elsevier.com/9780323355018

PART 17

Evaluation and Management of Endocrine and Metabolic Disorders

CHAPTER 204

ACROMEGALY

Alan Ona Malabanan

DEFINITION AND EPIDEMIOLOGY

Acromegaly is a rare, chronic, and insidious disease that results from prolonged excessive secretion of growth hormone (GH). This manifests as excessive bone and soft tissue growth. Untreated or partially treated patients with acromegaly have double the expected mortality rate of age-matched healthy subjects. The increased prevalence of hypertension, diabetes mellitus, and sleep apnea increases cardiovascular morbidity and mortality. Motor vehicle accidents from daytime somnolence and sleep deprivation also contribute to the overall mortality risk. In addition, patients with acromegaly have an increased risk for malignant disease, particularly of the colon. Morbidity also results from arthropathies. When GH excess occurs in children, gigantism results because the epiphyseal plates have not yet closed.

Acromegaly is rare, but the diagnosis is commonly delayed or missed. Many studies have suggested a prevalence of 40 to 130 per million persons with an incidence of 3 to 4 cases per million per year.[1] Other studies have seen a higher prevalence, including a study with a prevalence of 97 cases per million in a highly polluted area.[2] One study in Germany of serum insulin-like growth factor 1 (IGF-1) levels in a 6773 unselected general primary care patients suggest an incidence as high as 1034 per million patients.[3] Acromegaly is usually diagnosed in middle age; the mean age at diagnosis is 40 years in men and 45 years in women.

Physician consultation is indicated for all patients with suspected acromegaly.

PATHOPHYSIOLOGY

GH is secreted by somatotroph cells in the anterior pituitary gland. Its secretion is regulated by two hypothalamic hormones, growth hormone–releasing hormone (GHRH) and somatostatin (SS). GHRH stimulates both GH production and secretion, whereas SS inhibits GH secretion. GH secretion is pulsatile, with brief surges followed by long periods of inactivity. Many physiologic stimuli affect GH secretion, including stress (increased), sleep (increased), meals (increased or decreased), and aging (decreased). The variable nature of a random serum GH level limits its usefulness in diagnosis of acromegaly. IGF-1, or somatomedin C, is a GH-dependent protein produced in the liver. Its serum level is directly proportional to the 24-hour integrated serum GH level, and it is a much better indicator of GH excess than a random serum GH level. IGF-1 and GH increase during puberty and late adolescence and decline throughout adulthood.

The bone and soft tissue growth in acromegaly is a direct result of the effects of GH and IGF-1. In addition, GH has several other metabolic effects, including insulin antagonism, lipolysis, and protein anabolism, which in excess results in glucose intolerance, decreased fat stores, and increased muscle mass.

The most common cause of GH excess is a GH-secreting pituitary adenoma in more than 95% of cases; 25% of GH adenomas co-secrete prolactin.[4] Rare (<1%) causes include GHRH-producing tumors such as hypothalamic tumors, bronchial carcinoid, and pancreatic islet cell tumors. Ectopic production of GH has been described in pancreatic islet cell tumors and other rare tumors. Acromegaly may be associated with familial syndromes such as multiple endocrine neoplasia type I—a triad of pituitary tumor, hyperparathyroidism, and pancreatic tumor—and McCune-Albright syndrome, a genetic disease associated with polyostotic fibrous dysplasia, café au lait spots, and endocrine hyperfunction.

CLINICAL PRESENTATION

Acromegaly develops insidiously; many patients have symptoms for more than 10 years before diagnosis. Symptoms result from the effects of GH excess or from the effect of the pituitary mass on surrounding brain structures. An evaluation of 324 consecutive patients with acromegaly from 1981 to 2006 continued to show marked clinical manifestations of acromegaly at diagnosis, suggesting that it remains underdiagnosed until later stages, even with more advanced diagnostic tools over time.[5] Signs and symptoms at diagnosis included enlargement of facial features or hands and feet, joint pain, excessive sweating, headache, menstrual irregularity, snoring, macroglossia, increased spacing between teeth, vision problems, weight gain, deepening voice, paresthesias, acne, hirsutism, and mood instability. At time of diagnosis in patients in whom acromegaly was diagnosed early (within 5 to 9 years of symptom onset), 37% of patients had hypertension, 24% had carpal tunnel syndrome, 18% had diabetes mellitus, and 13% had sleep apnea.[5] Rates of these and other comorbidities are further increased with delay in diagnosis. Visual field disturbances and amenorrhea may also be presenting complaints. Acromegaly can be found incidentally in a workup for a pituitary mass, and primary care physicians are most likely to initiate workup.[6] The Endocrine Society suggests consideration of acromegaly in patients without the typical manifestations but who may have several associated conditions: sleep apnea, type 2 diabetes mellitus, debilitating arthritis, hyperhidrosis, and hypertension.[7]

PHYSICAL EXAMINATION

The earliest and most common physical changes occur in the skin and extremities. The growth of the soft tissues produces facial puffiness, broadening of the nose, furrowing of the brow, and skin thickening (bogginess) of the hands and feet. Enlargement of the tongue, uvula, and soft palate leads to sleep apnea. Vocal cord thickening results in a deeper and coarser voice. Skin tags (acrochorda) are more common in patients with acromegaly, as are colonic polyps. Patients may also have oily skin and excessive sweating (hyperhidrosis).

Facial bone growth leads to coarsened facial features, which are usually recognizable only when they are severe after years of change or after review of the patient's old photographs. The ubiquity of smartphones has greatly facilitated access to old photographs. These changes include growth of the calvaria and mandible, producing a prominent brow, an enlarged jaw, and dental malocclusion. With growth of the jaw, there is also widening of the spaces between the teeth. Excessive rib growth produces a barrel-shaped chest. Glove and shoe size changes result from bone growth in the hands and feet. Loss of lateral visual fields (bitemporal hemianopia), papilledema, extraocular palsy, or even rhinorrhea may result from impingement of the pituitary tumor on surrounding structures.

Enlarged organs (visceromegaly) may also occur in acromegaly. Macroglossia, enlargement of the tongue, may be present. The thyroid may be enlarged, possibly leading to a multinodular goiter. There is an increased association of thyroid cancer with acromegaly. Rarely, the liver and spleen will be enlarged on physical examination.

DIAGNOSTICS

Random serum GH levels are not useful in the diagnosis of acromegaly because GH secretion is pulsatile and levels can be affected by coexisting disease states, exercise, sleep patterns, and other factors. IGF-1 level is a good screening test and, as mentioned previously, is a reflection of the previous day's GH secretion, and it does not vary as GH does. There are normative reference ranges for IGF-1 that are gender and age adjusted; GH secretion and therefore IGF-1 level decline throughout adulthood. IGF binding protein 3, which is also GH dependent, can be measured and will be high in patients with acromegaly, although measurement of IGF-binding proteins usually does not confer additional information.[8,9] Unfortunately, normal and abnormal values for all of these tests may overlap.

The dynamic test of choice for diagnosis of acromegaly is the oral glucose tolerance test (OGTT), which most clearly demonstrates pathologic GH secretion. Of note, this test is contraindicated in patients with poorly controlled diabetes mellitus. An OGTT is performed after an overnight fast. Blood is drawn at baseline for serum glucose concentration and GH level. Then 75 g of oral glucose is given. Samples for serum glucose and GH are then taken at 60-minute intervals for a total of 120 minutes after the glucose load. In a normal individual, GH secretion is suppressed by an oral glucose load and should be suppressed to less than 1 ng/mL by the current immunoassays.[10] With the use of newer ultrasensitive assays, acromegaly may be missed in a quarter of patients with a cutoff value of 1 ng/mL; suppression to a level of less than 0.3 ng/mL may better distinguish those with and without acromegaly.[4] However, it is important to understand the assay being used and its characteristics in interpreting these data.

Results of the OGTT should always be evaluated together with the IGF-1 measurement. Acromegaly can be diagnosed with failure to suppress GH appropriately during an OGTT with an elevated age- and gender-matched IGF-1 level.[9] Studies have shown, however, that failure to suppress GH on OGTT in the setting of an elevated IGF-1 level does not rule out acromegaly.[11,12]

DIAGNOSTICS

Acromegaly

LABORATORY	IMAGING
Serum IGF-1 level	MRI
OGTT for GH suppression	CT (if MRI contraindicated)
Plasma GHRH*	

*If indicated.
CT, computed tomography.

After the biochemical diagnosis of acromegaly, magnetic resonance imaging (MRI) of the pituitary gland should be performed. If no pituitary tumor is seen or if generalized pituitary hyperplasia is seen, the possibility of ectopic GHRH production should be considered. A plasma GHRH determination may be helpful, and further abdominal and chest imaging may be pursued to look for the source. Also, more than 10% of normal individuals may have an incidental pituitary adenoma that is nonsecreting.

DIFFERENTIAL DIAGNOSIS

The primary differential diagnostic consideration in acromegaly is an etiologic one: What is the cause of the GH excess? A few other clinical situations, however, should be examined. Pseudoacromegaly is a syndrome characterized by acromegaloid features and severe insulin resistance without elevated GH or IGF-1 levels. Benign familial prognathism may prompt evaluation for acromegaly, but GH and IGF-1 levels are normal. Paget disease of bone can cause bone deformities, particularly in the skull, and GH and IGF-1 levels are also normal in this condition. Although the OGTT is the standard test for the diagnosis of acromegaly, GH secretion fails to be suppressed after a glucose load in some conditions. Among these are severe liver or renal disease, uncontrolled diabetes mellitus, malnutrition, anorexia nervosa, heroin addiction, and levodopa ingestion. Oral estrogen therapy may lower IGF-1 levels by decreasing the liver's response to GH.

DIFFERENTIAL DIAGNOSIS

Acromegaly

- Pseudoacromegaly
- Benign familial prognathism
- Paget disease of bone
- Severe liver disease
- Severe renal disease
- Uncontrolled diabetes
- Malnutrition
- Anorexia nervosa
- Heroin addiction
- Levodopa ingestion

MANAGEMENT AND CO-MANAGEMENT WITH SPECIALISTS

Acromegaly should be co-managed with an endocrinologist experienced in managing acromegaly and hypopituitarism. Early diagnosis is crucial in curing this disease because the success of surgical therapy, the therapy of choice, depends on tumor size. Disease control (post-treatment remission of acromegaly) is defined as a reduction in IGF-1 to the age-adjusted normal range. Also, suppression of GH after an OGTT to less than 0.4 ng/mL may define control.[9]

Transsphenoidal pituitary surgery, either endoscopic or microsurgical, is the treatment of choice for most microadenomas (<10 mm) and macroadenomas (>1 cm). Macroadenomas with invasion into the cavernous sinus or those compressing the optic chiasm may require debulking followed by further therapy (see later). The mortality rate for transsphenoidal surgery in acromegaly is less than 1% with experienced neurosurgeons. In patients with microadenomas that are well localized, the rate for control and IGF-1 normalization is approximately 75% to 95% at major neurosurgical centers.[13] The cure rate decreases to less than 40% to 68% for noninvasive tumors larger than 10 mm (macroadenomas).[13] The rate of biochemical cure has been found to correlate with initial tumor size, GH level, and tumor invasion characteristics.[14] A random GH level below 1 µg/dL 12 to 24 hours after surgery is predictive of surgical remission. If the level is higher than 1 µg/dL, a GH after OGTT is recommended.[7,15] Biochemical testing with IGF-1 and GH after OGTT, as well as an MRI, are recommended 12 weeks postoperatively.[7]

For patients who are not surgical candidates and for those with postsurgical recurrence, two alternatives exist: medical therapy and pituitary irradiation. SS analogues (octreotide and lanreotide) and dopamine agonists (bromocriptine and cabergoline) are the two most commonly used medical therapies. A GH receptor antagonist (pegvisomant) can be used when acromegaly is nonresponsive to other medical therapies.

Octreotide is given as three daily subcutaneous injections (100 to 250 µg per dose), or, with use of octreotide LAR, a long-acting formulation of the SS analogue, it can be given as 20 mg intramuscularly monthly; both are uptitrated if the serum IGF-1 level does not normalize. Lanreotide Autogel (LAN), another formulation of octreotide LAR, also has a depot form that is given every 4 weeks subcutaneously. A recent review of five studies comparing LAN with LAR found no significant differences in their control of biochemical end points.[16] LAR was found to normalize IGF-1 levels in 44% of patients and to reduce GH levels to less than 2.5 ng/mL in 34% of 98 patients studied with use of LAR for primary therapy. Multiple other long-term studies with more preselected populations show a higher rate of IGF-1 normalization and GH suppression with LAR.[17]

Cabergoline is the dopamine agonist of choice in treatment of acromegaly. When it is used as monotherapy, cabergoline may be effective in less than 10% of patients[13]; therefore it is rarely used by itself. Cabergoline, used in dosages of 1 to 4 mg/wk, has shown more promise in tumors co-secreting prolactin and as an adjuvant to SS therapy.[18] The Endocrine Society recommends medical therapy with dopamine agonist for milder disease.[7]

Pegvisomant, a GH analogue, selectively binds to GH receptors in the periphery, thus preventing endogenous GH binding to receptor. Indications for its use include patients who continue to have persistently elevated IGF-1 levels despite maximal therapy with other treatment modalities.[13] Pegvisomant can be used as monotherapy or in combination with an SS; it has been shown to improve quality of life when added to SS in patients who had normalized IGF-1 levels.[19] Because pegvisomant binds to GH receptors, this causes loss of negative feedback in the axis, and GH levels may increase. However, this does not cause a worsening of the acromegaly.

Common side effects of octreotide include diarrhea, abdominal discomfort, sinus bradycardia, and gallstones. Cabergoline can cause nausea, headache, and gastrointestinal cramping. Higher doses of cabergoline have been implicated in valvular heart abnormalities, although this was seen at higher doses than those typically used for acromegaly. Pegvisomant can lead to diarrhea and nausea, and liver function test results need to be monitored.

Radiation therapy is generally indicated in patients who have recurrence of disease with either resistance or intolerance to medical therapy, and it is a second- or third-line treatment.[13] Pituitary irradiation effects are delayed. Radiotherapy can normalize GH and IGF-1 levels in more than 60% of patients, but the maximum response is generally 10 to 15 years after pituitary irradiation.[13] There is a high risk of hypopituitarism (50%) over time, complicating this procedure. Various modalities of radiotherapy—stereotactic (proton beam, linear accelerator [LINAC], Gamma Knife) and conventional—are available. Stereotactic focused radiotherapy may be contraindicated if the tumor is within 5 mm (⅕ inch) of the optic nerve and chiasm.

LIFE SPAN CONSIDERATIONS

When GH excess occurs in children (before the closure of the epiphyseal plates), gigantism results. Acromegaly in younger patients tends to result from more aggressive tumors and may develop relatively rapidly.[4] In older patients, acromegaly develops insidiously during many years, and diagnosis is often delayed; most patients have symptoms for 10 years or more before diagnosis. Untreated or partially treated patients with acromegaly have double the expected mortality rate of age-matched healthy subjects, and a recent meta-analysis of 16 studies on mortality in patients with acromegaly found a standard mortality ratio (SMR) of 1.72 compared with the general population, even in patients who had transsphenoidal surgery (SMR of 1.32).[20]

COMPLICATIONS

The complications associated with advanced acromegaly are numerous and include diabetes, cardiovascular disease, hypertension, sleep apnea, osteoarthritis, peripheral neuropathies, and increased incidence of malignant disease, particularly of the colon. These conditions affect quality of life and increase mortality rates. All cases of acromegaly need to be co-managed in collaboration with an endocrinologist because many of the complications may not remit after treatment of the excess GH. Complications of surgical or radiation therapy include hypopituitarism and also require consultation with an endocrinologist.

INDICATIONS FOR REFERRAL OR HOSPITALIZATION

All patients thought to have acromegaly should be referred to an endocrinologist experienced in the evaluation and treatment of acromegaly, if possible. The rarity of this condition, its increased mortality rate, and the complexity of its manifestations make this critical. Patients with evidence of pituitary tumor mass effect or hemorrhage need urgent neurosurgical referral.

Advanced acromegaly may lead to neurologic or cardiovascular complications requiring hospitalization. Any patient with new symptoms of headache, visual disturbance, dyspnea, or chest pain should be promptly evaluated.

PATIENT EDUCATION AND HEALTH PROMOTION

The normalization of GH and IGF-1 levels is essential in the successful management of acromegaly and requires the patient's adherence to the prescribed medical therapy. Patients should realize that acromegaly is a chronic and progressive disease, resulting in a multitude of complications that may be avoided or delayed with prompt and appropriate therapy. Patients should be aware that the changes in physical appearance will likely not remit even with successful therapy but are likely to worsen if the condition is not treated. The provider should alert patients to the symptoms of sleep apnea, diabetes mellitus, heart disease, and hypopituitarism so that appropriate evaluation and therapy may be undertaken.

CHAPTER 205

ADRENAL GLAND DISORDERS

Marylou Virginia Robinson

DEFINITION AND EPIDEMIOLOGY

Adrenal gland disorders are conditions marked by inadequate or excessive amounts of glucocorticoid, mineralocorticoid, or androgen hormones as a consequence of changes in the adrenal gland itself, from hypothalamic or pituitary gland dysfunction, or through exogenous administration. The three most common types of adrenal gland disorders are discussed: Addison disease, Cushing syndrome, and pheochromocytoma.

Addison Disease (Primary Adrenal Insufficiency)

Once most commonly linked with bilateral adrenal destruction by tuberculosis (TB), Addison disease is now associated with autoimmune disturbances (70%) or significant physiologic stress. Recent increases in TB worldwide may alter these patterns. Prevalence is 4 to 11 cases per 100,000,[1] with 1 in 8000 European whites and twice as many women as men being affected.[2] More than 30% of acquired immunodeficiency syndrome (AIDS) patients develop adrenal insufficiency.[2] All three adrenal hormones can be unbalanced in Addison disease.

Cushing Syndrome

There is a spectrum of disorders associated with the overproduction of cortisol, the most familiar being Cushing syndrome. The term *Cushing disease* is reserved for pituitary-caused symptoms. It is estimated that 1% of all patients take glucocorticoid medications, which causes iatrogenic Cushing syndrome in a large number of patients. Endogenous cases can also be related to excess adrenocorticotropic hormone (ACTH) from pituitary tumors or adrenal gland hyperproduction.

Pheochromocytoma

Pheochromocytoma is a catecholamine-secreting tumor of chromaffin (pheochromocyte) cells. Ninety percent are found in the adrenal medulla; others arise intra-abdominally along the sympathetic ganglion chain.[3] The rare incidence of a primary malignant process occurs when the tumor spreads beyond chromaffin tissue. Pheochromocytomas are typically unilateral; however, bilateral involvement is common in the setting of polyglandular multiple endocrine neoplasia. Annual incidence is 2 to 8 cases per million, occurring primarily in the middle years. Ten percent are familial.[4]

PATHOPHYSIOLOGY

Hypothalamus-synthesized corticotropin-releasing hormone regulates the secretion of ACTH, which in turn regulates the production of glucocorticoids (cortisol). Cortisol adjusts the metabolic responses in the body to both physical and psychological stressors. These responses range from hepatic glucose production to inflammatory vascular reactions. Proinflammatory cytokines also increase cortisol secretion.[3] Normal circadian ACTH secretion is highest on waking and lowest at night. Men average 18 pulses of ACTH daily, but women have only 10.[1] Disrupted sleep-wake cycles of shift workers or travelers crossing time zones interrupt the pulses, which may result in changes in performance and behavior.

Primary underproduction disorders (Addison disease) stem from the destruction or dysfunction of the adrenal gland. Secondary disorders involve interruption of the hypothalamic-pituitary-adrenal (HPA) axis, pituitary tumors, or traumatic brain injury. Tertiary disorders are the sudden consequences of withdrawal of exogenous corticosteroids after high-dose use. Typically 90% of both adrenal glands is malfunctioning before clinically recognized insufficiency is present. Destruction by TB, adrenal hemorrhage (e.g., anticoagulant therapy or trauma), medications (rifampin, ketoconazole), and infections (meningococcemia, histoplasmosis) are rare causes. Inadequate production of cortisol in the context of severe sudden illness or trauma, particularly in chronic users of corticosteroids, is a more common manifestation.[1] Individuals with other pituitary dysfunction as well as septic shock, patients with critical illness,[5] childhood brain cancer survivors,[6] and patients sustaining traumatic brain injury[7] should be monitored long term for insufficiency symptoms.

Most cases of Cushing syndrome come from the suppression of pituitary ACTH production when steroids are administered in high doses for long periods. When use is for more than 10 to 14 days as part of the management of asthma, difficult dermatitis problems, malignant neoplasms, rheumatic diseases, and other disorders, careful monitoring is mandatory to detect early, persistent endogenous corticosteroid suppression. When long-term exogenous glucocorticoid therapy (>15 mg/day) is indicated, HPA axis suppression occurs. Alternate-day therapies have been suggested to alleviate symptoms but are not evidence based.[1] Steroid use for less than 3 weeks typically does not generate concern. The exception is frequent "burst" therapy in asthma and chronic obstructive pulmonary disease exacerbations, when natural return of adrenal function can be impaired. Timing of steroid doses is critical to reduce impact. Most of the administration should occur in the morning, as heavier doses at night suppress the morning pulse of ACTH more significantly. Recovery from iatrogenic suppression of cortisol production can take 6 to 9 months.[1]

Secondary Cushing syndrome results from ACTH-secreting tumors of the pituitary and occasionally (0.05%) from ectopic hormone secretion such as small cell lung carcinomas. Cortisol and ACTH levels are both elevated. Rarely, Cushing syndrome results from primary overproduction of cortisol by the adrenal gland (low levels of serum ACTH and high levels of serum cortisol).

Abnormal production of epinephrine and norepinephrine by a pheochromocytoma produces multisystem effects. Renal effects include sodium retention, increased renin secretion, and reduction of hydrostatic pressure. Cardiovascular effects involve peripheral vasoconstriction and increased cardiac contraction and workload from significant hypertension. Tissue oxygen consumption and gluconeogenesis are also increased.[4]

CLINICAL PRESENTATION

Addisonian presentations are nonspecific with chronic malaise, dizziness, nausea, chronic abdominal pain, muscle cramps, hyperpigmentation, decreased libido, weight loss, and salt craving. Decreased axilla and pubic hair with altered menses is linked to the disorder in women because of lowered androgens. Men produce most of their androgens in the testes, so they avoid most of this hair loss.[1] Depression, impaired memory, and agitation to include outright psychosis may occur in 20% to 40% of individuals. A patient with known Addison disease can exhibit an abrupt onset of vomiting, hypotension, and acute shock during a period of severe trauma, illness, or physical exertion when mineralocorticoid levels drop. Adrenal crisis can occur in patients normally well controlled with glucocorticoids.[1]

Cushing syndrome almost always manifests with chronic changes. Rapid weight gain, loss of menses, decreased libido, weakness, and bruising are all possible presenting symptoms. Many patients have hypertension, glucose intolerance, and insomnia. Memory and mental health disturbances occur in 50% of patients.[1] Depressed linear growth and excess weight gain are the most common presentations in pediatrics.[6]

Most adrenal tumors are incidentalomas, or the unexpected finding of a mass on computed tomography (CT) or magnetic resonance imaging (MRI) done for other reasons. Most (85%) of these masses are nonfunctional adrenal adenomas; the remainder are pheochromocytoma or metastasis from other organ cancers.[8] Symptoms of pheochromocytoma are episodic and include headache, diaphoresis, and palpitations, which may occur several times daily or only a few times a month. The symptomatic episodes last 15 to 30 minutes and may be precipitated by specific activities, such as position change, Valsalva maneuver, exercise, anxiety, or medications (e.g., anesthesia or metoclopramide).[4]

PHYSICAL EXAMINATION

Patients with Addison disease appear chronically ill. They exhibit weight loss, dehydration, and increased skin pigmentation on light-exposed skinfolds, a result of melanocyte stimulation by pituitary hormones. Darkened creases on the palms, elbows, knees, and lips commonly occur. Persons of color have darkened mucous membranes. Most discolorations resolve with adequate glucocorticoid therapy. Patients with secondary ACTH deficiency do not develop these skin changes.[1]

Patients with Cushing syndrome have a characteristic habitus similar to but subtly and importantly different from that of many patients with exogenous obesity. Central obesity, a moon face appearance caused by thickening of facial fat, the classically described buffalo hump dorsocervical fat pad (very common with all obesity), increased supraclavicular fat pads, hypertension, muscle weakness and wasting, hirsutism, red-purple abdominal skin striae of more than 1 cm in size, and acne can be associated signs. Emotional lability or depression, "senile" purpura on the hands, and other bruising can occur in all age groups.[1]

The hallmark of pheochromocytoma is a new onset of moderate to severe hypertension, with systolic pressures above 170 mm Hg. Arrhythmias, sinus tachycardia, or bradycardia may be present. The course is characterized by substantial variations in blood pressure measurements, palpitations, orthostasis, glucose intolerance, and diaphoresis, making "catching" it on a scheduled examination difficult. One third of patients have consistently normal blood pressure.[4] Cushing syndrome can be considered as a differential diagnosis for refractory hypertension.

DIAGNOSTICS

Addison Disease

Patients with Addison disease have an elevated serum ACTH concentration and suppressed levels of cortisol.

- Hyponatremia and hyperkalemia related to concurrent lost aldosterone production might be a serendipitous finding that suggests Addison disease in a previously undiagnosed patient.
- All diagnostics, including adrenal antibody studies to identify autoimmune disorders, should be ordered in concert with endocrinology.
- Screening is essential to exclude underlying TB.
- Patients with secondary insufficiency resulting from HPA axis issues have only glucocorticoid deficiency with intact aldosterone levels.[1]

Cushing Syndrome

Cushing syndrome is classically diagnosed by measurement of more than 100 μg of cortisol in the urine during a 24-hour period.

- This excretion study is thought to be more dependable than serum ACTH and serum cortisol testing; however, a single midnight (nadir) serum cortisol value above 7.5 μg/dL has nearly 100% specificity and 96% sensitivity.
- Suppression testing with ACTH is done in consultation with endocrine specialists to separate the physiology of obese and depressed patients from that of patients with true Cushing syndrome or to separate pituitary disorders from primary adrenal gland alterations.[1,2]

Pheochromocytoma

Elevated levels of fractionated metanephrines in a urine or plasma sample confirm the diagnosis of pheochromocytoma.[4]

- To increase accuracy, the collection must occur during a period of symptomatic episodes.
- Many medications alter the accuracy of the test (quinidine, theophylline, tetracycline, clofibrate, and disulfiram), including street drugs (LSD, cocaine) and over-the-counter substances (alcohol, pseudoephedrine), which can alter catecholamine levels.
- A careful medication review and specialist consultation regarding current test guidelines must occur before sampling.
- Abnormal test results should trigger an imaging search for a tumor.
- If a vascular mass is found in a hypertensive patient, the ratio of plasma aldosterone concentration to plasma renin activity (PAC/PRA) is determined to screen for primary aldosteronism.[9,10]

DIAGNOSTICS

Adrenal Gland Disorders

ADDISON DISEASE

Laboratory

Serum electrolytes
Blood urea nitrogen (BUN)
Creatinine
Serum glucose
Serum cortisol and serum ACTH
ACTH stimulation test (250 μg)

Other Diagnostics

Chest x-ray studies or purified protein derivative (PPD)

CUSHING DISEASE

Laboratory

Creatinine
24-Hour urine for cortisol
ACTH suppression test

PHEOCHROMOCYTOMA

Laboratory

Plasma free metanephrines
With 24-hour urine vanillylmandelic acid*
If hypertensive, random PAC/PRA

Imaging

CT scan or MRI*

*If indicated.

DIFFERENTIAL DIAGNOSIS

Both Addison disease and Cushing syndrome can be difficult to distinguish from normal physiology because both chronic and acute stresses affect adrenal hormone production. Mild addisonian symptoms can be mimicked by eating disorders, chronic fatigue syndrome, alcoholism, malnutrition, hyperthyroidism, diabetes, and the wasting effects of a chronic illness such as AIDS or metastatic cancer. Psychiatric symptoms, including apathy, confusion, and depression, are common with adrenal insufficiency presentations and often confound the clinical assessment. Most Cushing conditions are those associated with exogenous steroid use or abrupt withdrawal or inadequate steroid use in circumstances of stress. Cushing syndrome can be confused with depression, obesity, or polycystic ovary syndrome (PCOS).[11] The silver striae from rapid weight gain or pregnancy do not indicate adrenal dysfunction. Pheochromocytoma symptoms are commonly confused with anxiety or labile white coat hypertension; however, any issue that can induce a hypertensive spike should also be considered (e.g., stimulants, thyrotoxicosis, increased intracranial pressure).

DIFFERENTIAL DIAGNOSIS

Adrenal Gland Disorders

ADDISON DISEASE

- Eating disorders
- Alcoholism
- Malnutrition
- Hyperthyroidism
- Diabetes
- Chronic illness
- Psychogenic illness

CUSHING SYNDROME

- Obesity
- Depression
- PCOS

PHEOCHROMOCYTOMA

- Essential hypertension
- Anxiety
- Intracranial neoplasm or bleed
- Stimulant street drugs
- Medication withdrawal (clonidine, monoamine oxidase inhibitor)
- Thyrotoxicosis

MANAGEMENT

Specialist referral is indicated for patients with adrenal gland disorders.

Addison Disease

Acute adrenal crisis is best managed in the hospital, with intravenous corticosteroids and shock stabilization. Chronic adrenal insufficiency can be managed in an outpatient setting with oral hydrocortisone in divided daily doses (total, 20 to 30 mg) to allow restoration of a diurnal pattern.[2] Dosage is individualized, guided by the patient's symptomatic responses. Oral hydrocortisone is a fast-acting medication requiring multiple daily doses. Patients may do better on longer-acting steroids such as dexamethasone or prednisolone and subcutaneous hydrocortisone infusions to better simulate natural plasma fluctuations.[2]

Mineralocorticoid replacement in Addison syndrome with fludrocortisone (dose range, 0.05 to 0.2 mg/day orally) corrects the renal disturbance and hypotension. The need for replacement doses is monitored by frequent measurement of electrolytes, serum renin, serum ACTH, and judiciously timed serum cortisol levels.

Unless it is otherwise contraindicated, liberal use of salt may be encouraged in the face of resistant hyponatremia.

Cushing Syndrome

Management of Cushing syndrome depends on the source of the hypercortisolism. In Cushing disease, intentional P-450 cytochrome competition for processing steroids is used through daily ketoconazole administration, which mitigates the impact of cortisol.[12]

Pituitary tumor resection, when indicated, remains the first choice for therapy. Chemotherapy and radiation therapy may be used adjunctively.

Because chronic glucocorticoid levels are associated with osteoporotic tendencies, bone density measurements should be obtained, especially with concurrent conditions that have an impact on bone, such as thyroid replacement therapy and menopause.[1,2]

Pheochromocytoma

The management of pheochromocytoma is still based primarily on case reports and expert opinion.[4] Definitive treatment is surgical removal.

Presurgical antihypertensive therapy focuses on alpha-adrenergic blockade and attention to maintenance of adequate hydration. Beta or calcium channel blockers can be added if tachycardia or coronary artery vasospasm issues arise.[4,10]

Alternative Therapies

Advocates for alternative approaches believe science is not able to adequately measure the subtle changes in adrenal hormones that are depleted by chronic stress.[13] The term most commonly used is *adrenal fatigue,* a diagnosis not recognized by allopathic medicine. Adrenal fatigue is accelerated after a particularly stressful event, such as financial collapse, sustained emotional duress, illness, or suboptimal diets.[14]

Most alternative interventions center on the goal of improving energy, overcoming any iatrogenic impact of long-term steroid therapy, and combating the negative physiologic and psychological impacts of chronic stress and modern time-pressured lives. Energy-boosting herbals such as ginseng are classified by naturopathic healers as adaptogens—substances that help one adapt to stress.[14] When adaptogens are combined with substances that soothe excessive nervous system responses, such as skullcap *(Scutellaria)*, St. John's wort, and valerian, support is provided to overcome insomnia, irritability, and stress-induced hypertension. The negative impact of stress on the cardiovascular system is modulated with the use of antioxidants, fish oils, plant sterols, and the B-complex vitamins and avoidance of refined carbohydrates.[14] Sea salt is considered an essential ingredient to overcome the salt-wasting perceived to be the source of low energy. One or two 8-ounce glasses of water with ½ teaspoon of sea salt is encouraged by some websites.[13]

Licorice *(Glycyrrhiza)* is an ancient remedy for suppression of the fight-or-flight reactions associated with persistent stress.[14] Excess ingestion, however, is associated with resistant hypertension and can create havoc in patients taking digoxin. More recently, dehydroepiandrosterone (DHEA), an endogenous sex hormone precursor, has been suggested to be helpful[13]; however, high DHEA levels are linked with development of Cushing syndrome.[15]

COMPLICATIONS

Immediate life-threatening complications are, in general, confined to acute adrenal crisis. Sudden adrenal inadequacy can be mitigated with injectable hydrocortisone (Florinef) for home use. Addison disease and Cushing syndrome complications are prevented by giving careful attention to the side effects of exogenous steroids and to the patient's symptoms, emotional stability, and metabolic status. With Cushing syndrome, osteoporosis is a common complication, along with risk for infection, hypertension, and diabetes. Acute hypertensive crisis is a potential complication of pheochromocytoma.

INDICATIONS FOR REFERRAL OR HOSPITALIZATION

Consultation with endocrinology specialists is warranted if the diagnostic evaluation suggests either Addison disease or Cushing syndrome.

Referral and hospitalization are necessary for hypertensive crisis management and surgical intervention of pheochromocytoma.[4]

Management of an acute adrenal crisis requires immediate referral and hospitalization for fluid resuscitation and intravenous administration of hydrocortisone, 100 mg every 6 hours for an initial 24 hours, followed by careful dose tapering. Management of the associated hypotension, hypovolemia, and hypoglycemia is accomplished with careful monitoring in an intensive care setting. Patients who have been taking exogenous steroids at any time during the preceding year are at some risk for inadequate cortisol response when faced with the stress of any surgical procedure. These patients should be considered candidates for perioperative stress doses of hydrocortisone. Consultation with a provider comfortable with prescribing stress steroid doses is advised. In general, for patients with known adrenal insufficiency, hydrocortisone is added to intraoperative intravenous fluids and infused at a rate of 5 mg/hr. During the first 24 hours after surgery, a total of 150 to 200 mg is administered. The dose is then tapered by 50% per day if the postoperative period is without complications.[1,2]

PATIENT EDUCATION AND HEALTH PROMOTION

Careful explanation of the underlying disease processes and complications of chronic exogenous steroid dependency is an important component of patient and family education. Doubling of the hydrocortisone dose is required with fever and common illnesses. Patients and families must understand the risks of sudden withdrawal of corticosteroid medications and the need to alert medical personnel in the event of trauma, surgical procedure, or infection. Medical alert bracelets are vital to improve the recognition of emergency presentations of adrenal insufficiency. An emergency kit with syringe and directions on how and when to administer extraparenteral steroids should be carried at all times. Families need education on how to administer the medication intramuscularly. Health protection issues associated with potential hypertension, glucose intolerance, immune compromise, skin breakdown, and weight gain for steroid-dependent patients need to be emphasized. Quick access to the primary care provider should be an important goal of the provider-patient partnership.

CHAPTER 206

DIABETES MELLITUS

Mary E. Wood

DEFINITION AND EPIDEMIOLOGY

Diabetes mellitus is the most common metabolic disorder seen in primary care and a leading cause of cardiovascular disease (CVD), renal failure, blindness, and nontraumatic lower limb amputation. The American Diabetes Association (ADA) offers this definition:

> "Diabetes is a group of metabolic diseases characterized by hyperglycemia resulting from defects in insulin secretion, insulin action, or both."[1]

The World Health Organization states:

> "Diabetes is a condition primarily defined by the level of hyperglycemia giving rise to risk of microvascular damage (retinopathy, nephropathy, and neuropathy). It is associated with reduced life expectancy, significant morbidity due to specific diabetes-related microvascular complications, increased risk of macrovascular complications (ischemic heart disease, stroke, and peripheral vascular disease), and diminished quality of life."[2]

The total prevalence of diabetes in the United States as of 2012 was 29.1 million (9.3% of the population). Among adults aged 20 years and older, the prevalence of diabetes is slightly higher in men than in women (13.6% versus 11.2%). The prevalence of diabetes increases with age and is higher in Asian Americans (9.0 %), Hispanics (12.8%), non-Hispanic blacks (13.2%), and American Indians/Alaska Natives (15.9%) than in non-Hispanic whites (7.6%). Of the 29.1 million Americans with diabetes, 21.0 million have been diagnosed and 8.1 million remain undiagnosed.[3] An estimated 86 million Americans aged 20 and older have prediabetes, with

BOX 206-1

Screening for Diabetes in Asymptomatic Adults

Screen with fasting plasma glucose, 2-hr 75-g oral glucose tolerance test (OGTT), or hemoglobin A_{1c} (HbA_{1c}). Begin testing at age 45 years for all and at age 40-70 for those who are overweight (body mass index [BMI] ≥25 kg/m² [≥23 kg/m² in Asian Americans]) and/or have one or more of the following risk factors:

- Physical inactivity
- Family history of diabetes
- High-risk heritage (African American, Hispanic, Native American, Asian American, Pacific Islander)
- History of gestational diabetes or delivered a baby weighing >9 lb
- Hypertension (≥140/90 mm Hg or treated for hypertension)
- Dyslipidemia (high-density lipoprotein [HDL] <35 mg/dL and/or triglycerides >250 mg/dL)
- Presence of polycystic ovary syndrome
- Presence of acanthosis nigricans (indicative of insulin resistance)
- History of cardiovascular disease
- Previous HbA_{1c} ≥5.7% or history of prediabetes

If screening is negative, repeat every 3 years or earlier with a change in risk.

Data from American Diabetes Association: Standards of medical care in diabetes—2015, *Diabetes Care* 38 (Suppl 1):S10, 2015 and USPSTF level B recommendation, 2015.

BOX 206-2

Classification of Diabetes from the Expert Committee on the Diagnosis and Classification of Diabetes Mellitus

- In type 1 diabetes mellitus, insulin deficiency is caused by autoimmune beta cell destruction. The individual is dependent on exogenous insulin for survival and is prone to ketosis if insulin is withheld. Type 1 diabetes typically begins in childhood, adolescence, or young adulthood but may begin at any age. Accounting for only 5% to 10% of all diabetes in the United States, type 1 occurs after a viral or environmental trigger in genetically predisposed individuals. Onset is rapid and dramatic.
- Type 2 diabetes is the more common type of diabetes in the United States and is linked to obesity, in most cases. Type 2 diabetes can begin at any age, with a recent increase in onset during childhood and adolescence; it commonly runs in families. Type 2 diabetes is the result of insulin resistance and a relative deficiency of insulin. Exogenous insulin is not necessary for survival but may be an important part of the treatment as the disease progresses. Ketosis is rare in type 2 diabetes, except in the setting of severe illness or infection. Onset is insidious.
- Other specific types of diabetes include genetic defects of the beta cell, defects in insulin action, diseases of the exocrine pancreas (e.g., pancreatitis, cystic fibrosis), other endocrinopathies (e.g., Cushing syndrome, pheochromocytoma), and drug-induced hyperglycemia.
- Gestational diabetes mellitus (GDM) refers to glucose intolerance with onset or first recognition during pregnancy. Given the increase in women of childbearing age who have undiagnosed type 2 diabetes, the recommendation is now to identify glucose intolerance that antedates the pregnancy in high-risk women. If found, using standard criteria, the diagnosis of overt rather than gestational diabetes would be conferred. Women with GDM are at an increased risk for development of GDM with a subsequent pregnancy and type 2 diabetes within 5 to 10 years after delivery.
- Prediabetes is an intermediate stage in which the glucose levels are abnormal but do not meet the criteria for the diagnosis of diabetes. Prediabetes encompasses impaired fasting glucose (100 to 125 mg/dL) and impaired glucose tolerance (140 to 199 mg/dL 2 hr after 75-g glucose load). Individuals with prediabetes are at an increased risk for diabetes and cardiovascular disease. Progression to diabetes can be delayed or prevented with healthy diet, regular exercise, and weight loss.

Data from American Diabetes Association: Diagnosis and classification of diabetes mellitus, *Diabetes Care* 37(Suppl 1):S81-S09, 2014.

elevated glucose levels that do not meet the criteria for the diagnosis of diabetes. The prevalence of prediabetes is similar for non-Hispanic whites (35%), non-Hispanic blacks (39%), and Hispanics (38%).[3] Among individuals with prediabetes, healthy diet, regular exercise, and weight loss have been shown to prevent or delay the progression to diabetes.[4] Given this, an important focus of primary care is prevention of type 2 diabetes. Screening is recommended for early diagnosis (Box 206-1).

An estimated 90% to 95% of people in the United States with diabetes have type 2 diabetes (previously known as adult-onset diabetes, type II diabetes, or non–insulin-dependent diabetes mellitus). Fewer than 10% have type 1 diabetes (formerly known as juvenile-onset diabetes, type I diabetes, or insulin-dependent diabetes)[1,3] (Box 206-2).

Type 1 diabetes typically begins in childhood, adolescence, or early adulthood but can manifest at any age. Type 2 diabetes, which is strongly linked to obesity, was in the past diagnosed in middle-aged and older individuals but is now more commonly developing in childhood and adolescence. The incidence of both type 1 and type 2 diabetes is increasing, and the disease is occurring at an earlier age.[5]

The long-term complications of diabetes are a result of the microvascular and macrovascular damage to target end organs: the eyes, kidneys, heart, blood vessels, and nerves. Direct medical costs for diabetes care in 2012 were an estimated $17 billion. Indirect costs for disability and premature death were $69 billion.[3] To reduce the devastating effects of this disease, prevention, early detection, and aggressive treatment of the long-term complications of diabetes are essential.

PATHOPHYSIOLOGY

Type 1 and type 2 diabetes share the features of hyperglycemia and an increased risk for vascular and neuropathic complications. Physiologically, they are two distinct diseases. Type 1 diabetes is caused by the autoimmune destruction of the beta cells within the islets of Langerhans in the pancreas in a genetically predisposed individual. This results in insulinopenia and the lifelong dependence on exogenous insulin. Beta cell destruction is typically more rapid in infants and children and more gradual in adults. The majority of individuals with type 1 diabetes will test positive for the presence of antibodies (islet cell autoantibodies, insulin autoantibodies, GAD65 autoantibodies, or autoantibodies to tyrosine phosphatases IA-2 and IA-2β).[5] The surgical removal of the pancreas (e.g., Whipple procedure or pancreatectomy) results in type 1 diabetes with the added challenge created by the lack of glucagon secretion from the alpha cells. Insulin is required for most of the body's tissues to take up glucose as the preferred source of energy. Thus, insulin deficiency impairs the uptake of glucose, resulting in the search for energy elsewhere. Fats and proteins are broken down, and counterregulatory hormones trigger glycogenolysis. Inadequate insulin leads to hyperglycemia.

The pathophysiologic mechanism of type 2 diabetes is more obscure. Hallmarks of this disease have been called the "triumvirate" of decreased glucose uptake (insulin resistance), increased hepatic glucose production, and impaired insulin secretion. A new model of type 2 diabetes pathophysiology has been described by DeFronzo and called "the ominous octet," in recognition of the fact that there are eight mechanisms that contribute to type 2 diabetes.[6] The additional mechanisms include increased glucagon secretion, increased glucose reabsorption by the kidney, increased lipolysis, decreased incretin effect, and neurotransmitter dysfunction in the brain.

Fasting hyperglycemia results from increased hepatic glucose production in the impaired first phase of insulin secretion. Postprandial hyperglycemia is caused by the decreased uptake of glucose in the skeletal muscles. In response to the elevated blood glucose levels, the insulin pathways become resistant to hormonal impulses, resulting in hyperinsulinemia.

Insulin resistance by definition is the decreased sensitivity of tissue to glucose uptake with normal concentrations of insulin.[1] As hyperglycemia increases, so does insulin resistance. The body is able to adapt and to maintain homeostasis for a while, but as hyperglycemia progresses, diabetes occurs. As the degree of glucose intolerance advances, hyperglycemia results from the insufficient insulin produced by the beta cells.

The natural progression of type 2 diabetes includes normal glucose values as insulin resistance begins. Increased insulin secretion compensates for the resistance. As insulin resistance worsens, postprandial glucose values begin to rise. Later, insulin secretion begins to wane and fasting glucose levels start to climb. Placing the patient along this continuum will guide treatment decisions. For example, early in type 2 diabetes, treatment should aim to improve sensitivity to insulin. Later, treatment may require the enhancement of insulin secretion or endogenous insulin.

Primary insulin resistance, a defect in the target cells of insulin receptors and postreceptors, results in altered insulin action and sensitivity. The onset of insulin resistance can occur with hyperinsulinemia, in the fasting or fed state. The fed state is the time associated with insulin secretion after food intake to carbohydrate metabolism and synthesis of fat and protein. As insulin resistance proceeds, glucose transportation or use of glucose in the cell is altered. Secondary resistance is caused by hormones or abnormal physiologic states (e.g., puberty, pregnancy, advanced age). Other factors associated with the development of insulin resistance include a high-fat diet, sedentary lifestyle, smoking, and weight gain. Metabolic stress, as with illness and obesity, increases insulin resistance.

Many patients who have prediabetes or type 2 diabetes also have the metabolic syndrome. The metabolic syndrome is a group of metabolic components, synergistic in nature, that contribute to CVD. These components include abdominal obesity, insulin resistance and hyperglycemia, elevated triglyceride and low high-density lipoprotein (HDL) levels, hypertension, and a pro-inflammatory state. Weight loss, improved glycemic control, lipid management, and improved blood pressure may decrease the significance of this syndrome (see Chapter 212).

CLINICAL PRESENTATION

An individual with untreated type 1 diabetes will typically be seen after a brief period of profound symptoms. Polyuria, polydipsia, polyphagia, weight loss, blurred vision, and fatigue are overt signs of diabetes. Later, as the glycosuria increases, nausea, vomiting, abdominal pain, rapid shallow breathing, hypotension, and dehydration are signs of ketoacidosis (see the section Acute Complications of Diabetes). Medical care is essential.

The patient with type 2 diabetes may have no symptoms or only subtle symptoms that may persist for weeks, months, or even years before detection. Unfortunately, during this time, the vascular and neuropathic complications may begin to develop and progress before the diagnosis is made.[4] The symptoms include polyuria, polydipsia, blurred vision, fatigue, slowly healing wounds, and frequent infections. Some individuals may experience polyphagia and weight loss or numbness or tingling of feet and hands.

PHYSICAL EXAMINATION

At the time of diagnosis of diabetes, the physical examination focuses on dehydration, weight loss, and precipitating causes, such as illness, infection, or stress. The patient may appear dry and flushed. The skin, eyes, heart, and lungs should be assessed. The thyroid should be palpated because type 1 diabetes is associated with thyroid disorders. In patients with new type 2 diabetes, examination should be performed for early evidence of vascular and neuropathic complications as well as for persistent infections.

The purpose of periodic examination of patients with known diabetes is threefold: (1) to evaluate blood glucose control because poor control leads to end-organ complications; (2) to assess for the presence or progression of end-organ damage; and (3) to assess for associated diseases, such as other autoimmune disorders and cardiovascular risk factors.

Annual examinations are comprehensive. Periodic visits, every 3 months for patients with type 1 diabetes and those with type 2 diabetes who have one or more complications, should be conducted to assess end-organ involvement and glycemic control. Visits can be stretched to every 6 months if the individual with type 2 diabetes is stable and in control. Each examination should include weight and blood pressure measurements, a review of glycemic control, and evaluation of target end-organ damage[4] (Box 206-3).

DIAGNOSTICS

The diagnostic criteria for diabetes are based on the glucose threshold above which the risk of retinopathy is increased.[1] In a patient exhibiting significant symptoms of hyperglycemia, a random plasma glucose of 200 mg/dL or higher is diagnostic for diabetes. In an individual without symptoms, a second confirmatory test is recommended. In July 2009, an International Expert Committee recommended the use of hemoglobin A_{1c} (HbA_{1c}) as a diagnostic tool. An HbA_{1c} of 6.5% or higher, a fasting plasma glucose of 126 mg/dL or higher, or a 2-hour plasma glucose level of 200 mg/dL or higher during an oral glucose tolerance test fulfills the diagnostic criteria for diabetes[1] (Table 206-1).

HbA_{1c} is a nonfasting test and has the same relationship to risk of retinopathy as do the other tests. Because of the chance of laboratory error, this test should also be repeated in the absence of classic symptoms of hyperglycemia. HbA_{1c} results may

BOX 206-3

Physical Examination of Patients with Diabetes

Vital signs: Height, weight, body mass index (BMI), and blood pressure, including orthostatic measurements in a patient with long-standing diabetes and neuropathy.
Eye: Funduscopic examination for hemorrhages or exudates.
Oral cavity: Examine for gum disease, fungal infections, or lesions.
Neck: Palpate thyroid for enlargement or nodules.
Cardiac: Auscultate heart rate for rhythm, murmurs, clicks, or extra heart sounds.
Skin: Inspect for signs of irritation, infection, redness, ulcers, and acanthosis nigricans.
Feet: Palpate pulses for presence and quality, note presence of patellar and Achilles reflexes, perform monofilament examination to assess protective sensation.

Date from American Diabetes Association: Standards of medical care, *Diabetes Care* 38 (Suppl 1):S18, 2015.

TABLE 206-1 **Diagnostic Criteria for Diabetes and Prediabetes**

	Fasting Plasma Glucose*	Random Plasma Glucose	Oral Glucose Tolerance Test* (75-g Glucose, 2-hr Plasma Glucose)	HbA_{1c}*
Normal	<100 mg/dL		<140 mg/dL	<5.7%
Prediabetes	100-125 mg/dL		140-199 mg/dL	5.7%-6.4%
Diabetes	≥126 mg/dL	≥200 mg/dL with classic symptoms	≥200 mg/dL	≥6.5%

*Diagnosis must be confirmed with a second positive test result on a subsequent day.
Data from American Diabetes Association: Classification and diagnosis of diabetes, *Diabetes Care* 38(Suppl 1):S8-S16, 2015.

be inaccurate in patients with anemia or other hemoglobinopathies and during pregnancy.

If necessary, a C-peptide level can be helpful in distinguishing type 1 from type 2 diabetes. Markers of type 1 diabetes include islet cell autoantibodies, insulin autoantibodies, and GAD65 autoantibodies.

Delivering the diagnosis of diabetes to the patient should include not only the message that this is a serious disease for which there is no cure but also the positive encouragement that the patient will learn to manage the disease and be able to continue to work and to do the things that bring enjoyment. Inclusion of supportive family members or friends in this discussion is helpful.

DIAGNOSTICS

Diabetes

LABORATORY	*To distinguish Type 1 from Type 2 Diabetes*
Serum glucose (random or fasting)	C-peptide level
Oral glucose tolerance test	Insulin level
HbA_{1c}	1A autoantibodies

TABLE 206-2 **Glycemic Control Targets for Nonpregnant Adults**

HbA_{1c} level	<7%*
Premeal blood glucose level	80-130 mg/dL
Peak postmeal blood glucose level	<180 mg/dL

*Individualize HbA_{1c} target.
Data from American Diabetes Association: Standards of medical care in diabetes—2015, *Diabetes Care* 38(Suppl 1):S33-S40, 2015.

DIFFERENTIAL DIAGNOSIS

The diagnosis of diabetes is straightforward in a patient with polyuria and polydipsia. The differential diagnosis is limited to type 1 diabetes, type 2 diabetes, and diabetes insipidus. If hyperglycemia and glycosuria are absent and diabetes insipidus is excluded, consider hyperthyroidism (check triiodothyronine [T_3], thyroxine [T_4], and thyroid-stimulating hormone levels) or hyperparathyroidism (check parathyroid hormone and serum calcium levels). Secondary causes of diabetes should always be considered. These include excess of counterregulatory hormones (Cushing syndrome, pheochromocytoma, and acromegaly); significant hypokalemia caused by glucose intolerance; hyperaldosteronism or diuretic use; and destruction in the pancreatic islet from pancreatitis (caused by alcoholism or gallbladder disease), hemochromatosis, or drug-induced islet cell injury. In addition, infection or medication may cause glucose intolerance.

The differentiation between type 1 and type 2 is important for therapeutic purposes because patients with type 1 diabetes must receive insulin daily.

MANAGEMENT

Treatment of diabetes includes a healthy diet, regular exercise, medication, monitoring, self-care education, and periodic follow-up with the primary care provider and the diabetes care team. The combination of these therapies will aid the patient in achieving the best glycemic control possible without undue burden or adverse effects (Table 206-2).

Lifestyle Interventions

Nutritional therapy is essential in management of both type 1 and type 2 diabetes. A registered dietitian is crucial in helping to individualize a meal plan and to teach the patient and family about healthy nutrition.[7,8] The goal of nutritional therapy for diabetes and prediabetes is the development of the meal plan, balancing insulin with food intake and activity to achieve glycemic control. The nutrition goal for patients with type 1 diabetes is to promote normal growth and development during childhood, adolescence, pregnancy, and lactation; to balance energy intake and expenditure; and to achieve near-normal blood glucose levels. Matching insulin doses to carbohydrate intake is necessary. For patients with type 2 diabetes, the nutrition goals are the achievement and maintenance of a healthy weight, adequate blood pressure control and lipid levels, and good glycemic control (Box 206-4). To promote recovery from a severe illness, special dietary adjustments may be necessary and can be individualized with the help of a registered dietitian.

Exercise and physical activity have been shown to improve glycemic control.[9] Exercise causes increased glucose uptake in

BOX 206-4

Nutrition Guidelines for Patients with Diabetes

Recommend Dietary Guidelines for Americans[8] to achieve a healthy, balanced diet. In addition, for diabetes or prediabetes, the following are recommended:

Calories: Individualize to provide adequate amounts for weight control, growth and development, pregnancy, and lactation.
Portion control: For weight loss and maintenance.
Protein: Advise leaner protein and alternatives to meat.
Fat: Recommend unsaturated fat, rather than saturated fat; minimal intake of *trans* fat.
Carbohydrate: Identify foods that contain carbohydrates (e.g., fruits, starchy vegetables, milk, bread, cereal, pasta, rice, desserts).
Cholesterol: <200 mg/day.
Fiber: 20-35 g/day.
Sodium: Limit daily intake to 2300 mg.
Alcohol: Limit to one alcoholic beverage (12 oz beer, 5 oz wine, or 1½ oz distilled spirits) per day for women and two for men; ingest with food to reduce the risk of hypoglycemia.

Data from American Diabetes Association: Nutrition recommendations and interventions for diabetes, *Diabetes Care* 37(Suppl 1):S120-S143, 2104; and American Heart Association: Dietary Guidelines for Americans, 2010. *Sodium, blood pressure and cardiovascular disease.* Available at www.health.gov/dietaryguidelines/dga2010/DietaryGuidelines2010.pdf. Accessed January 5, 2015.

skeletal muscles as well as improved insulin sensitivity. All of the other benefits of exercise for the heart, lungs, and state of mind help reduce the risk of diabetes complications. It is important for the individual with type 1 diabetes to make appropriate adjustments in food intake and/or insulin doses to balance the effects of exercise. Postexercise hypoglycemia or hyperglycemia may occur. The exercise lag effect refers to the low blood glucose concentration that may happen many hours after exercise. To prevent hypoglycemia during exercise, the individual must balance activity with adequate food and appropriate insulin doses. High blood glucose levels after exercise may result from decreased circulating insulin and glucose uptake and increased hormonally regulated hepatic glucose. In the setting of exercise without adequate circulating insulin, ketosis is increased as fatty acids are broken down for energy, resulting in higher blood glucose levels and possible ketosis.[9]

In the individual with type 2 diabetes, exercise decreases insulin resistance and increases glucose uptake. Increased insulin sensitivity, contributing to the exercise lag effect, can last up to 48 hours after exercise. Thus, food intake and medication, especially insulin, need to be adjusted for the activity or exercise. A reduction in the insulin that is peaking at the time of exercise and perhaps the basal insulin as well may be necessary. In the patient with type 2 diabetes, it would be desirable to decrease the medication rather than increasing food consumption so as to promote weight loss.[9] Exercise has been shown to prevent or delay the progression from prediabetes to diabetes. Guidelines for exercise in diabetes are reviewed in Box 206-5.

Pharmacotherapy

Insulin, an anabolic hormone produced by the beta cells of the pancreas, plays a vital role in metabolism. Insulin therapy is the lifesaving treatment for type 1 diabetes. Insulin is also used by patients with type 2 diabetes who have persistent hyperglycemia despite lifestyle changes and oral and/or noninsulin injectable diabetes agents. An individual with type 2 diabetes who begins to take insulin does not then have type 1 diabetes. Rather, he or she now has insulin-treated type 2 diabetes.

BOX 206-5

Exercise Recommendations for Patients with Diabetes

TYPE 1 DIABETES

- Patients with well-controlled diabetes can enjoy exercise at all levels, from recreational activity to professional sports.
- Exercise should be avoided if the blood glucose concentration is >250 mg/dL and ketones are present in the blood or urine or if the blood glucose concentration is >300 mg/dL without ketones.
- Advise patients to delay exercise until carbohydrates are ingested if the blood glucose concentration is <100 mg/dL.
- Recommend that patients consume carbohydrates during and after intense or prolonged exercise.
- Teach about the exercise lag effect, which can cause hypoglycemia for many hours after exercise, particularly overnight.
- Modify exercise recommendations for patients with complications of diabetes.

TYPE 2 DIABETES AND PREDIABETES

- Individualize recommendations on the basis of diabetes complications, cardiac risk factors, and activity baseline. Advise patients to begin gradually and under supervision.
- Interrupt sedentary time with movement at least once every 90 min.
- Patients should perform at least 150 min/wk of moderate-intensity aerobic activity. This should be spread over at least 3 days in the week. More than 2 consecutive days without exercise should be avoided. More than this is associated with weight reduction and maintenance as well as greater reduction of cardiovascular disease risk.
- Patients should perform resistance exercise three times weekly.
- Patients who take insulin or insulin secretagogues must be prepared to treat hypoglycemia during and after exercise.

From Colberg, SR, Sigal, RJ, Fernhall, B, et al: Exercise and type 2 diabetes: the American College of Sports Medicine and the American Diabetes Association: joint position statement executive summary. *Diabetes Care* 33:2692-2696, 2010.

Physiologic secretion of insulin is biphasic: basal and prandial. The basal phase inhibits glycogenolysis and gluconeogenesis and maintains glucose in a steady state. The prandial phase controls the initial glucose load and reuptake. Early morning hyperglycemia caused by counterregulatory hormones (known as the dawn phenomenon) is controlled by basal insulin, and postmeal glucose spikes are controlled by prandial insulin. Insulin therapy should mimic this response.

There are a number of insulin products available that may be prescribed to tailor an individualized regimen for each patient, with the goal of optimal glycemic control while allowing a flexible lifestyle. Human insulin is derived synthetically from recombinant DNA (Humulin [Eli Lilly], Novolin [Novo-Nordisk]). Human insulin is available in regular, NPH, and 70/30, a premixed combination of 30% regular and 70% NPH. Humulin 50/50, pork-derived regular and NPH insulins, and Lente and Ultralente insulins are no longer available. The first inhaled insulin (Exubera) was briefly marketed but withdrawn by the manufacturer because of disappointing sales. A new insulin inhalation powder (Afrezza) received U.S. Food and Drug

Administration (FDA) approval in June 2014 and was initially marketed in early 2015. This is a rapid-acting insulin approved for use in adults. Individuals who use Afrezza must also take subcutaneous basal insulin daily. Side effects include hypoglycemia, cough, and throat pain. Inhaled insulin is not recommended for patients who smoke.

Five insulin analogues made of recombinant human insulin are available. Three are rapid acting (lispro, aspart, glulisine), and two are long acting or peakless (glargine and detemir). The three rapid-acting insulin products are used as prandial and correction insulin, and the peakless insulins provide true basal insulin coverage. Premixed insulin combinations are available for convenience. Individualized doses of basal and prandial insulin offer the best and most physiologic approach to tight glycemic control, with fewer episodes of hypoglycemia.

Insulin Therapy

Type 1 Diabetes. Individuals with type 1 diabetes are truly dependent on insulin for survival. Simplistically, type 1 diabetes is the absence of one hormone: insulin. The replacement of that hormone to mimic normal physiology is challenging. Individuals with type 1 diabetes are sensitive to insulin, with a dramatic response to too much insulin (hypoglycemia) or too little (hyperglycemia or diabetic ketoacidosis [DKA]). The patient must appreciate that daily insulin is essential.

The most physiologic regimen is basal/bolus insulin. This can be accomplished with multiple daily injections or with an insulin pump, also known as continuous subcutaneous insulin infusion. Exogenous insulin requirements vary from one patient to another and, for an individual, from day to day. Physiologic insulin secretion for adults who do not have diabetes is approximately 20 to 40 units/day.[10] Thus, most adults with type 1 diabetes will need to inject approximately this much insulin every 24 hours. One unit of any kind of insulin will cause the same reduction in blood glucose concentration in a given individual for the duration of that type of insulin. For example, 1 unit of a rapid-acting insulin may drop one patient's blood glucose level 60 mg/dL in 2 to 3 hours, and 1 unit of a long-acting insulin will reduce the glucose level 60 mg/dL for over 12-24 hours. A patient who is much more resistant to insulin will experience a drop of only 10 mg/dL in glucose concentration in 2 to 3 hours after 1 unit of rapid-acting insulin and a drop of 10 mg/dL for 24 hours after 1 unit of basal insulin.

When insulin treatment is initiated, body weight, morphologic development (obese versus muscular), age (adolescent versus elderly), and activity (sedentary versus athletic) must be considered. The type of insulin prescribed depends on the patient's needs and the provider's preference. Therapy should begin with conservative starting doses and continuously titrated to achieve the desired blood glucose levels. On the basis of the patient's weight, an initial total daily dose (TDD) may be calculated as 0.5 unit/kg. The TDD is then divided into basal and bolus doses. Fifty percent of the TDD is basal insulin, and 50% is divided among the mealtime doses. Frequent premeal and postmeal blood glucose monitoring will guide dose adjustments.

Glargine and detemir, true long-acting insulins, are typically given once daily, often at bedtime, and last for up to 24 hours, mimicking the basal secretion of insulin.[10] Basal insulin may be given at a different time of day, if it is more convenient for the patient, to maintain a consistent routine. Large doses may be divided into twice-daily injections given 12 hours apart. Some individuals notice a peak from their basal insulin, so they may split their dose into two daily injections to minimize this. The dose of basal insulin is not determined with a sliding scale, so as not to make a decision with 24-hour implications based on a single blood glucose value. Rather, the dose of basal insulin should be adjusted every 2 or 3 days until the fasting blood glucose level is less than 110 mg/dL. The basal insulin should be increased by increments of 2 to 5 units in an obese, insulin-resistant individual or by 1 to 2 units in an insulin-sensitive patient with a thin body frame or in patients with frequent episodes of hypoglycemia.[10] If the fasting glucose concentration is consistently lower than 80 mg/dL, the dose of basal insulin should be reduced.

To prevent high postprandial glucose levels, a rapid-acting insulin analogue should be injected just before, during, or immediately after the meal. A low premeal blood glucose level, unpredictable food intake, and delayed gastric emptying are common reasons for waiting until after the meal to inject the bolus dose. Most often, mealtime insulin is injected 10 minutes before eating. A bolus dose with meals allows more flexibility in mealtimes, prevention of postprandial hyperglycemia, and fewer episodes of hypoglycemia.[10] Initially, mealtime doses are $\frac{1}{6}$ the TDD, but they can later be fine-tuned on the basis of postprandial blood glucose monitoring. The best approach to determination of mealtime insulin doses is counting the amount of carbohydrate to be consumed and calculating the dose on the basis of an individualized carbohydrate-to-insulin ratio.

The goal of the diabetes plan is to attain glycemic control with appropriate insulin doses but without symptoms of hypoglycemia or hyperglycemia. Intensive insulin therapy is defined as four or more insulin injections each day or use of an insulin pump. This comprehensive strategy requires collaboration among the individual patient and family, the health care provider or diabetes specialist, and the diabetes education team of a nurse educator and dietitian. The more the patient knows about diabetes, the better and safer the diabetes management will be.

Hypoglycemia is the most serious side effect of insulin. Fear of hypoglycemia prevents some individuals from embracing intensive insulin therapy. To prevent both hypoglycemia and hyperglycemia, factors such as exercise and activity, meal composition, mealtimes, sleep patterns, illness, and psychological well-being must be considered in adjusting insulin doses. The most important tool for control of day-to-day variations and prevention of hypoglycemia is home blood glucose monitoring. For a patient using an insulin pump, co-management with an endocrinologist and diabetes care and education team is strongly recommended. Intensive insulin therapy is not appropriate for all patients, including those with hypoglycemia unawareness, those who are poorly motivated and unwilling to monitor their blood glucose levels frequently, older adults, and those who have a limited life expectancy.[10]

Basal/bolus insulin treatment is complex and more expensive than a twice-daily regimen of regular and NPH insulin or premixed insulin. This treatment regimen is an alternative for patients who cannot or will not take multiple daily injections. The patient using twice-daily insulin must eat meals on a schedule and be aware of the risk of nocturnal hypoglycemia. Regular insulin may be used as a less expensive alternative to a rapid-acting analogue but does not offer the immediate mealtime coverage, resulting in hyperglycemia postprandially and then hypoglycemia before the next meal. The four prepared insulin mixtures—Humalog 75/25, NovoLog 70/30, and mixtures of

BOX 206-6

Practical Insulin Tips

- Store unopened insulin vials and pens in the refrigerator.
- Once opened, clear insulin is good for 28 days at room temperature.
- Premixed insulins are good for 10 days at room temperature after opening.
- Contain used syringes, pen needles, and lancets in a sturdy plastic or metal container, such as a liquid detergent or bleach jug or a coffee can. Once it is full, tape the lid on tightly. Contact local landfill for disposal recommendations.

NPH and regular 70/30 (Novolin, Humulin)—offer ease and convenience for the individual. Dose adjustments, however, change both the short-acting and longer-acting insulin.

Insulin products are available in both a vial (to be drawn into a syringe) and a prefilled, disposable pen. A prescription for insulin must be accompanied by a second prescription for either syringes or insulin pen needles. Syringes are available in several different sizes, and needles come in several different lengths. NPH and regular insulin may be mixed in one syringe and injected together. Glargine and detemir cannot be mixed with another insulin (Box 206-6).

New concentrated insulin products, allowing the injection of a smaller volume, include Humalog U-200 and glargine U-300 (Toujeo). These are available only in pens, and doses are prescribed in actual units of insulin. Humulin Regular insulin U-500 has been available since 1997 and is known to behave differently than U-100 regular insulin. It is not yet available in a pen, so caution is necessary in prescribing to prevent errors (see later). Frequent glucose monitoring is recommended after a change in insulin concentration, because dose adjustments may be necessary.

Requirements for insulin increase during illness, surgery, and growth spurts and in patients with ketoacidosis. Insulin absorption from subcutaneous tissues varies about 25% among patients. The practitioner should be aware of a possible "honeymoon" phase in the patient with newly diagnosed type 1 diabetes with recovering beta cell function. Insulin requirements may decrease to 0.2 to 0.5 unit/kg body weight per day during this short-term phase.[4]

Type 2 Diabetes. Individuals with type 2 diabetes are not dependent on insulin but may require insulin for optimal glycemic control. This is common in a patient after several years of diabetes that has been well controlled with diet, exercise, and oral diabetes medications and may represent beta cell exhaustion. Patients must appreciate that this does not represent a "failure" on their part but rather is the natural progression of the disease. Encouragement to accept insulin as the most appropriate treatment of this phase of their diabetes, rather than to fear injections, is a useful strategy when insulin treatment is recommended (Box 206-7).

Insulin may be added to one or more oral diabetes medications or may replace oral medications. Because additional insulin may contribute to weight gain, it is essential that the patient understand that a healthy diet, regular exercise, and weight loss remain the cornerstones of diabetes treatment. The introduction of a medication does not take the place of lifestyle modification.

BOX 206-7

Management of Type 2 Diabetes

STEP 1

Present the diagnosis to the patient as a lifelong chronic condition that can be managed but not cured. Encourage lifestyle modifications of healthy diet, regular exercise, weight loss, and diabetes self-management education. Begin metformin.

If $HbA_{1c} > 7\%$, go to Step 2.

STEP 2

To metformin and lifestyle interventions, add one of the following:

- Basal insulin (most effective)
- Sulfonylurea (least expensive)
- Thiazolidinedione (no risk of hypoglycemia)
- Dipeptidyl peptidase 4 (DPP-4) inhibitor (few contraindications)
- Sodium-glucose cotransporter-2 (SGLT2) inhibitor (newest)
- Glucagon-like peptide 1 (GLP-1) receptor agonist (injection)

If $HbA_{1c} > 7\%$, go to Step 3.

STEP 3

In addition to metformin and lifestyle interventions, do the following:

- If basal insulin was inadequate, intensify the insulin regimen.
- If two agents were inadequate, begin basal insulin.

If $HbA_{1c} > 7\%$, go to Step 4.

STEP 4

While continuing metformin and lifestyle interventions, intensify the insulin regimen, including meal-time rapid-acting insulin. Reassure patients that the need for insulin does not represent a failure on their part but rather is the most appropriate treatment of the current phase of their disease.

Data from Inzucchi SE, Bergenstal RM, Buse JB, et al: Management of hyperglycemia in type 2 diabetes, 2015: a patient-centered approach. *Diabetes Care* 38(1):140-149, 2015.

As a first step, a single bedtime injection of intermediate- or long-acting insulin may be added to the oral medications to control fasting hyperglycemia and to provide basal insulin throughout the day. Basal insulin plus an insulin secretagogue for prandial glucose control works well for some. If the individual's glucose level remains above the targets after a few weeks, a rapid-acting insulin analogue can be added at mealtimes. Regular insulin may be used as an alternative but does not offer immediate mealtime coverage, so it may result in hyperglycemia postprandially, and then hypoglycemia before the next meal. Use of lispro, glulisine, or aspart before meals allows more flexibility, better coverage of hyperglycemia, and fewer episodes of hypoglycemia.[10] Initially, the analogue could be administered as a fixed dose with each meal or in different doses for low-carbohydrate and high-carbohydrate meals. When ready, the patient could be taught to count grams of carbohydrate and to calculate a more exact dose based on an individualized carbohydrate/insulin ratio.

Local reactions at the injection site are the most common form of allergic reaction to insulin. Delayed hypersensitivity may also occur but remains in the area of injection. The use of synthetic or purified insulin has decreased both local and systemic reactions. Occurrence of reactions may be secondary to improper injection technique, injection of cold insulin, or preservatives. If systemic reactions do occur, the individual may require desensitization (the process of slowly reintroducing the allergy-inducing insulin at minute doses until the body no longer has an allergic response).

Pramlintide (Symlin) is a synthetic analogue of human amylin and may be added to insulin treatment in both type 1 and type 2 diabetes. Amylin is a hormone produced in the pancreas and co-secreted with insulin. Amylin becomes deficient as beta cells are destroyed. Its role in diabetes treatment is to reduce the amount of glucose in the bloodstream by reducing the amount of food consumed. The release of amylin leads to a decrease in hepatic glycolysis and a slowing of gastric emptying into the small intestine, thereby increasing satiety. The results are decreased glucagon secretion and decreased postprandial glucose spikes. Available now only in a disposable, multidose pen, pramlintide is given by subcutaneous injection 10 to 15 minutes before meals, starting at a low dose of 15 to 60 μg (type 1) and 30 to 120 μg (type 2) and titrating slowly upward. The dose of mealtime insulin should be decreased by 30% to 50% and taken toward the end of the meal. Side effects include severe hypoglycemia, nausea, anorexia, and gastrointestinal distress. Therefore, it is important to titrate slowly, particularly if side effects are experienced. Severe hypoglycemia can occur from the mismatch of insulin timing with the postprandial glucose peak. Because of the delay in gastric emptying, pramlintide alters the postprandial glucose peak. If insulin reaches its peak before the peak in glucose concentration, postprandial hypoglycemia may occur, usually within 3 hours of pramlintide injection. Pramlintide is contraindicated in patients with gastroparesis.

Medications for Type 2 Diabetes

Treatment of type 2 diabetes includes management of dyslipidemia, hypertension, obesity, insulin resistance, and hypercoagulability as well as glycemic control.[11] The mainstays of therapy are education, diet, exercise, and achievement and maintenance of a desirable body weight. These therapies have no side effects, although they are difficult to sustain over time. Hyperglycemia may be reversed with weight loss of as little at 4 kg.[11] Early diagnosis and prompt initiation of treatment are associated with better sustained glycemic control and fewer long-term complications. Treatment of diabetes should be individualized to achieve an HbA_{1c} level as close to the nondiabetic range as possible, and a value of 7% or greater should be a "call to action."[11] This target should be modified for patients with a significant risk for dangerous hypoglycemia or with a limited life expectancy.

While recommendations for diet and exercise are being maximized, pharmacologic intervention should be considered. Consideration of the patient's place along the continuum of the natural progression of type 2 diabetes and the mechanisms[12] that are contributing to hyperglycemia, will guide the selection of medication(s). Individualization of medications should be determined on the basis of effectiveness, safety, tolerability, and cost. The reduction of risk for complications of diabetes has been shown to be related to the level of glycemic control over time rather than to the use of any single medication or combination.[11] Some agents used to improve glycemic control also have beneficial or detrimental effects on related conditions (e.g., obesity, elevated lipids).

The variety of diabetes medications to supplement lifestyle changes enables treatment individualization for improved glycemic control, targeting each patient along the continuum of type 2 diabetes. Agents with different mechanisms can be combined to achieve greater glucose reduction. Metformin (Glucophage), a biguanide, is commonly the first-line oral medication for type 2 diabetes. The mechanism of action is suppression of hepatic glucose production, which typically results in lower fasting glucose levels. A reduction of approximately 1.5% can be expected in the HbA_{1c} level. Side effects are typically mild and include temporary nausea and diarrhea. Metformin does not cause hypoglycemia and may promote weight loss. There is the rare but serious risk of lactic acidosis. For this reason, metformin must be held before the intravenous administration of contrast material and temporarily discontinued (up to 48 hours) after radiologic studies involving intravenous contrast dye. In addition, metformin should be discontinued if the serum creatinine concentration exceeds 1.4 mg/dL in women or 1.5 mg/dL in men. This creatinine threshold has been debated as being too conservative and thus restricts the use of metformin for many patients who might benefit. Use of the estimated glomeruler filtration rate (eGFR) instead has been recommended by professional societies and has been proposed to the FDA.[12]

Sulfonylureas help reduce blood glucose by stimulating insulin secretion and can also reduce the HbA_{1c} level by approximately 1.5%. The most common side effects are weight gain and hypoglycemia. *Persistent hypoglycemia is more frequent in older adults.* The second-generation medications in this class are glyburide (Micronase, DiaBeta, Glynase), glipizide (Glucotrol), and glimepiride (Amaryl). They are once- or twice-daily medications. Meglitinides (repaglinide [Prandin], nateglinide [Starlix]) are nonsulfonylurea insulin secretagogues. These are shorter-acting agents that must be taken with each meal and should be withheld if the patient is omitting a meal. The risk for weight gain exists, but these medications are less likely to cause hypoglycemia because of their shorter duration.

α-Glucosidase inhibitors (acarbose [Precose], miglitol [Glyset]) act in the small intestine, delaying the digestion of polysaccharides. The inhibition of starch and the sucrose enzyme causes lower postprandial glucose levels. To be effective, the pill must be taken with the first bite of a meal that contains carbohydrate. Alone, these medications will not cause hypoglycemia; but if they are used in combination with another medication and hypoglycemia occurs, glucose (not sucrose) is necessary for treatment. Sucrose would be blocked by the action of these agents, so patients are advised to carry glucose tablets or gel. Contraindications include inflammatory bowel disease, colonic ulceration, obstructive bowel disease, gastroparesis, and creatinine levels above 2 mg/dL. α-Glucosidase inhibitors typically result in a 0.5% reduction in HbA_{1c}.

The thiazolidinediones (TZDs) pioglitazone (Actos) and rosiglitazone (Avandia) are peroxisome proliferator-activated receptor γ (PPAR-γ) modulators. These agents improve the sensitivity of liver, fat, and muscle to both endogenous and exogenous insulin. Ultimately, this works to decrease insulin resistance, thereby improving insulin sensitivity and decreasing insulin levels. In addition, the TZDs reduce hepatic glucose output. Improvement of both fasting and postprandial blood glucose levels occurs over time and without stimulating insulin secretion. Side effects include weight gain and edema; thus, congestive heart failure is a contraindication. TZDs should not be used as first-line therapy if the patient is glucose toxic because it takes 4 to 8 weeks for the full effect. Advantages include the delay of beta cell exhaustion, decrease in insulin resistance, no hypoglycemia (if used alone), and improvement of triglyceride and HDL levels. Some studies have revealed a slight increase in low-density lipoprotein (LDL) levels with rosiglitazone. A disadvantage of this class is a possible increase in liver function enzymes. However, the recommendation is to monitor liver function test (LFT) results and to stop the drug if serum transaminase exceeds 2.5 times the upper limit of normal. LFTs should then be monitored until the results return to normal. Caution is to be exercised when TZDs are used with insulin because they may cause more peripheral edema and, in cardiac patients, congestive heart failure.

In July 2010, an FDA advisory panel reviewed evidence citing the increased risk of heart attack with rosiglitazone. The panel voted not to withdraw the drug but to continue to market it with additional restrictions and warnings. Subsequently, in response to the findings of the Rosiglitazone Evaluated for Cardiovascular Outcomes and Regulation of Glycemia in Diabetes (RECORD) trial, which showed no elevated risk of myocardial infarction (MI) or death in patients taking rosiglitazone compared with standard-of-care diabetes medications, the FDA lifted the restrictions.[13] The FDA has been conducting a safety review of a reported association between long-term pioglitazone exposure and bladder cancer. A history of bladder cancer is a contraindication to pioglitazone use.

The incretin mimetics glucagon-like peptide 1 (GLP-1) agonists are a class of noninsulin injectable medications indicated for treating type 2 diabetes that is inadequately controlled with healthy diet, regular exercise, and metformin. The GLP-1 peptide, produced in the small intestine, stimulates insulin secretion in the fed state. It acts to stimulate insulin secretion, to suppress glucagon secretion, and to slow gastric emptying. Gastrointestinal side effects are common and related to the effect on gastric motility. Weight loss is also common, but hypoglycemia is not.

Exenatide (Byetta) is given as a twice-daily subcutaneous injection 0 to 60 minutes before breakfast and dinner, starting with 5 μg and titrating to 10 μg after a month if needed. Liraglutide (Victoza) is a once-daily subcutaneous injection, taken without respect to mealtime. There are three once-weekly GLP-1 receptor agonists: exenatide (Bydureon), dulaglutide (Trulicity), and albiglutide (Tanzeum). The GLP-1 receptor agonists have been shown to contribute to weight loss and a reduction in systolic blood pressure, in addition to a reduction in HbA_{1c}. Combination therapy with insulin is an area of active investigation.

A higher dose of liraglutide is now marketed as Saxenda and is indicated as a treatment for weight loss, as an adjunct to diet and exercise. Side effects at the higher dose include nausea and hypoglycemia.

A related class of medications is the dipeptidyl peptidase 4 (DPP-4) inhibitors. They work to release insulin and to decrease glucagon levels by slowing the inactivation of incretin hormones. These medications help to regulate insulin by affecting both alpha and beta cells in response to elevated glucose levels. This process then helps decrease preprandial and postprandial glucose levels.

The newest class of oral agents to treat type 2 diabetes is the sodium-glucose cotransporter-2 (SGLT2) inhibitors. This class includes canagliflozin (Invokana), empagliflozin (Jardiance), and dapagliflozin (Farxiga). These once-daily pills cause increased excretion of glucose in the urine and thereby reduce plasma glucose concentration and may contribute to weight loss. The side effects include an increased risk for urinary tract infections (UTIs), genital infections in females, and hypotension.

If a single agent does not result in adequate glycemic control, a second agent may be added and then a third. Many different combinations have received FDA approval, and several two-medication tablets are available. The use of a combination tablet may reduce insurance copayments and may improve compliance because of the convenience. All medications have side effects, and many of the newer agents are expensive. An ADA position statement summarizes the current treatment recommendations.[12]

When a patient who is taking several diabetes medications in addition to medications for other conditions is not achieving the glycemic targets, insulin must be considered. Many patients find the switch from pills to insulin to be daunting. Thoughtful discussion of their concerns, reassurance, and a relaxed environment in which to practice injections can ease the transition. Insulin, given in adequate doses, can reduce any glucose level to the desired range. Individuals with type 2 diabetes may need large doses (1 unit/kg or more per day) to achieve desired glycemic control. An evening dose of intermediate-acting (NPH) or long-acting (glargine or detemir) insulin may be added to one or more oral medications. In some cases, other medications are discontinued and a split-mixed regimen of NPH and regular insulin or NPH and a rapid-acting analogue is recommended. Other patients will use basal/bolus insulin treatment alone. In addition to the insulin products used in type 1 diabetes, U-500 regular insulin may be used in type 2 diabetes. This is five times as concentrated as other insulins, allowing a patient with severe insulin resistance to inject a smaller volume. The use of U-500 insulin concentrate requires careful documentation and communication of the doses in actual units as well as in volume of insulin, to avoid overdosage or underdosage by a factor of five.

Insulin may be used as first-line treatment of the patient with type 2 diabetes in the following situations: HbA_{1c} level greater than 10% or glucose range above 250 mg/dL, severe illness with associated complications, gestational diabetes, and fragile older adults. However, the most common reason for use of insulin in type 2 diabetes management is failure to respond to the oral antihyperglycemic agents.

Combination therapy allows a more individualized regimen aimed at optimal glycemic control. Despite all the medications, however, a healthy diet and regular exercise remain the cornerstones of management of diabetes.

Blood Glucose Monitoring

Assessment of blood glucose levels is essential for achievement and maintenance of glycemic control. Because hyperglycemia is typically asymptomatic, monitoring is a valuable tool in the evaluation of one's status in real time. A handheld device and a drop of blood are all that is needed to measure the blood glucose level. Patients are encouraged to act on those results to adjust medications or to evaluate the effects of food and exercise. Monitoring is also used to assess for the acute complications of diabetes.

Many patients learn to adjust their own insulin doses. Fasting and premeal blood glucose levels give an overall view of basal control and should be between 70 and 130 mg/dL. Postmeal monitoring, 1 to 2 hours after a meal, helps to adjust meal-associated insulin doses. Results should be below 180 mg/dL.[4] Patients are encouraged to use the results of their blood glucose tests in real time, in addition to recording them for review with the provider at quarterly visits. A value lower than the target range may indicate hypoglycemia that requires immediate treatment. A value higher than the target range indicates hyperglycemia. Plenty of water and some exercise are indicated. Blood glucose results that are consistently higher than the targets should trigger a reevaluation of the treatment plan. A significantly elevated value may signal impending illness and should be followed carefully.

There are many different brands of glucose meters on the market, and insurance plans may favor a certain brand of meter and test strips. Prescriptions are required for reimbursement of the cost of meters, test strips, and lancets. All meters require a drop of blood from the fingertip, earlobe, or, in some cases, an alternate site. Newer products require very small drops of blood and provide the blood glucose result in as little as 5 seconds. Proper storage of test strips and appropriate coding of the meter when required are important for accurate results. To evaluate the range of glucose disparity between plasma and whole blood, a patient should have his or her blood tested with the home glucose meter and by the laboratory at the same time. If the difference is greater than 20%, another glucose meter should be used. Each meter has a toll-free number on the back for customer assistance. Home glucose meters cannot be repaired or recalibrated.

Follow-up Care

Diabetes is a chronic illness that requires periodic follow-up care. During visits, the health care provider evaluates glycemic control, the onset or progression of vascular complications, and the frequency and severity of hypoglycemic events. The patient's ability to understand and to manage his or her diabetes improves compliance and prevents acute complications. The frequency of visits depends on the level of glycemic control and the presence of complications. Each visit should include evaluation of blood pressure, weight and height (check against growth chart for age), eye and foot examinations, and review of the blood glucose log. Laboratory tests include an HbA_{1c} test every 3 months. A lipid profile is indicated yearly unless findings are abnormal or are being medically treated; then it is obtained every 4 to 6 months. Yearly screening for complications should include urinary microalbumin and urinalysis, blood urea nitrogen and creatinine levels, referral for an ophthalmologic examination, and, if indicated, a cardiovascular evaluation. Baseline electrocardiography is recommended after the age of 40 years. Exercise electrocardiography or peripheral vascular testing should be obtained when indicated. A discussion of results and goals for the next few months should occur at each visit.

Diabetes and Pregnancy

Pregnant women with preexisting diabetes and women with gestational diabetes mellitus (GDM) deserve special treatment considerations. GDM, a common complication of pregnancy, is defined as any degree of glucose intolerance with onset or first recognition during pregnancy.[14] Preexisting diabetes might be type 1 or type 2. Given the prevalence of undiagnosed type 2 diabetes, particularly among women of childbearing age, the recommendations for the screening and diagnosis of diabetes in pregnancy were revised in 2010.[14] The new screening strategy seeks to identify undiagnosed diabetes at the first prenatal visit as well as GDM later in the pregnancy (Box 206-8).

BOX 206-8

Diagnosis of Hyperglycemic Disorders of Pregnancy

At first prenatal visit, screen for preexisting diabetes in women with risk factors for type 2 diabetes. Measure fasting glucose, random glucose, or HbA_{1c} for high-risk women. If results indicate overt diabetes, initiate treatment for diabetes.

If results are not diagnostic but fasting plasma glucose concentration is 92 to 125 mg/dL inclusive, diagnose with GDM. If fasting plasma glucose is <92 mg/dL, screen for GDM at 24 to 28 weeks' gestation. At 24 to 28 weeks' gestation, screen for GDM with a 2-hr, 75-g oral glucose tolerance test (OGTT) performed after an overnight fast in all women not known to have type 1 or type 2 diabetes.

The diagnosis of GDM is made if one or more values are exceeded on a 75-g OGTT:

Fasting plasma glucose	92 mg/dL
1-hr plasma glucose	180 mg/dL
2-hr plasma glucose	153 mg/dL

The diagnosis of overt diabetes in pregnancy is made on the basis of the following:

Fasting plasma glucose	≥126 mg/dL
HbA_{1c}	≥6.5%
Random plasma glucose	≥200 mg/dL*

*Confirm with either fasting plasma glucose concentration or HbA_{1c} level.

Data from Dyer AR, Leiva A, Hod M, et al: International Association of Diabetes and Pregnancy Study Groups recommendations on the diagnosis and classification of hyperglycemia in pregnancy, *Diabetes Care* 33(3):676-682, 2010.

BOX 206-9

Maternal Complications of Diabetes

- Cesarean delivery
- Hyperglycemia, ketoacidosis
- Hypoglycemia
- Pregnancy-induced hypertension
- Pyelonephritis, other infections
- Polyhydramnios
- Preterm labor
- Spontaneous abortion
- Worsening of chronic complications (retinopathy, nephropathy, neuropathy, cardiac disease)

Data from American Diabetes Association: Management of diabetes in pregnancy. *Diabetes Care* 38(Suppl 1):S77-S79,2015.

Untreated or inadequately treated diabetes confers an increased risk of poor outcomes for the woman (Box 206-9) and her infant (Box 206-10). For the woman with preexisting diabetes, excellent glycemic control before conception is strongly recommended to reduce the risk of congenital anomalies. A discussion of preconception care should begin at puberty and recur annually for all women of childbearing potential (Box 206-11). Excellent diabetes care during the pregnancy is essential, as is care for the long-term health of both mother and baby.

Gestational Diabetes. The patient with GDM requires excellent glycemic control, rapidly achieved after diagnosis and sustained throughout pregnancy. Three percent to 10% of healthy pregnant women will develop GDM, with the higher

BOX 206-10

Neonatal Complications of Mothers with Diabetes

- Birth trauma
- Congenital anomalies (especially cardiac malformations and neural tube defects)
- Hyperbilirubinemia
- Hyperinsulinemia
- Hypertrophic cardiomyopathy
- Hypocalcemia
- Hypoglycemia
- Hypoxia
- Hypomagnesemia
- Left colon syndrome
- Macrosomia
- Neurologic instability, irritation
- Polycythemia
- Renal vein thrombosis
- Stillbirth

Data from Kitzmiller JL, Block JM, Brown FM, et al: Managing preexisting diabetes for pregnancy: summary of evidence and consensus recommendations for care, *Diabetes Care* 31(5):1060-1079, 2008.

BOX 206-11

Preconception Care for Women with Type 1 or Type 2 Diabetes

Beginning at puberty, all women of childbearing potential should be counseled to do the following:

- Achieve an HbA_{1c} level below 7% before conception to reduce the risk of anomalies (particularly anencephaly, microcephaly, and congenital heart disease) and miscarriage.
- Practice effective contraception until excellent glycemic control is achieved.
- Seek identification and treatment of chronic complications of diabetes before, during, and after pregnancy.
- Participate in perinatal care with a multidisciplinary obstetric and endocrine care team.

From American Diabetes Association: Standards of medical care in diabetes—2015, *Diabetes Care* 38(Suppl 1):S77-S79, 2015.

incidence in the same racial and ethnic groups that have a higher rate of type 2 diabetes.[3] Fetal complications of untreated and poorly treated GDM include birth injury, macrosomia, hypoglycemia, respiratory distress syndrome, and hyperbilirubinemia. Maternal complications include an increased incidence of cesarean delivery, preeclampsia, postpartum hemorrhage, and development of diabetes later in life.

Glucose intolerance is the cause of increasing insulin resistance during the latter half of pregnancy. Placental and counterregulatory hormones along with the stress of the growing fetus increase insulin resistance, thereby causing hyperglycemia.

Management of the patient with GDM is a priority because time is of the essence. Treatment begins with improvement of diet and exercise and may rapidly progress to medication if glycemic control is not achieved. Insulin therapy should be added to improve glycemic control when two or more glucose readings exceed the recommended target range. As the pregnancy progresses, insulin resistance caused by hormonal effects can supersede even strict dietary compliance, and insulin therapy becomes necessary. Higher doses of insulin may be necessary in the third trimester, when insulin resistance is the greatest.

Women who have had GDM carry a 40% to 60% chance for development of type 2 diabetes by the time their child is 5 to 10 years old.[3] There is the likelihood of GDM with a subsequent pregnancy and an increased risk of CVD.

Pregnancy in the Woman with Type 1 Diabetes. A generation ago, pregnancy was discouraged in women with type 1 diabetes. With proper planning, commitment, and the support of a diabetes and obstetric team, such a pregnancy is now encouraged. For a woman with type 1 diabetes, this is still considered a high-risk pregnancy that may result in life-threatening complications for both the mother (see Box 206-9) and the neonate (see Box 206-10). Therefore it is imperative that the woman with diabetes attain ideal glycemic control, including an HbA_{1c} level as close to normal as possible without excess hypoglycemia, before conception.[4] However, if an unanticipated pregnancy occurs, intensive glycemic control should be the immediate priority. There is a 1 in 10 chance of congenital anomaly in the growing fetus in the setting of poor maternal glycemic control.[15]

For the pregnant woman with diabetes, the metabolic changes that occur with the growing fetus can accelerate retinal and renal complications. Vascular complications of retinopathy, nephropathy, pregnancy-induced hypertension, and poorly controlled glycemia are strong risk factors for perinatal compromise. Pregnant women with type 1 diabetes are at high risk and need to be monitored closely by a team of specialists, including a high-risk obstetrician, endocrinologist, nephrologist, ophthalmologist, dietitian, and diabetes nurse educator.

Adjustments in insulin doses are needed for excellent glycemic control as pregnancy progresses. In the first trimester, insulin doses may be decreased because of hypoglycemia from the increase in fetal glucose transport and a loss of maternal amino acids. During the latter half of the second trimester, there is a rapid diversion to fat metabolism, resulting in higher concentrations of circulating glucose. The longer the duration of postprandial hyperglycemia, the more glucose is transported to the fetus, thus promoting fetal growth. During this time, there is also a degree of insulin resistance that occurs from the placental hormone (human placental lactogen), prolactin, and cortisol. Insulin requirements are increased during this stage and into the third trimester and then plateau around week 36 of gestation.

Dietary requirements, activity and exercise, blood glucose monitoring, and insulin doses must be adjusted for the pregnant state. Calorie requirements are increased and snacks are added, particularly during the first trimester, to prevent hypoglycemia and starvation ketosis. Multiple injections with changes in insulin type (NPH, regular, lispro, aspart, and detemir are FDA Pregnancy Category B; glargine and glulisine are Pregnancy Category C) or insulin pump therapy may be needed for better glycemic control. The advantage of the pump is that it allows frequent, small dose adjustments in basal rates and bolus doses with a rapid-acting insulin analogue. Safer and improved glycemic control can be achieved by more frequent blood glucose monitoring including fasting, preprandial and postprandial, bedtime, and middle of the night readings. Researchers have recently discovered the pathway that leads to the proliferation of beta cells during pregnancy.[16] Two hormones of pregnancy, prolactin and placental lactogen, trigger the expression of a gene in islet cells that causes increased production of serotonin by beta cells. The release of serotonin then results in increased beta cell mass. The process is reversed at birth, and beta cells return to their prepregnancy mass.

Pregnancy in the Woman with Type 2 Diabetes. For the woman with type 2 diabetes who is contemplating pregnancy, excellent glycemic control should be attained before conception to improve both fetal and maternal outcomes (see Box 206-11). Counsel the patient to delay conception until the HbA_{1c} level is less than 7%.[17] The literature on the use of oral agents at the time of conception and the concern for teratogenicity is limited. Metformin has been used for the treatment of polycystic ovary syndrome (PCOS) and in that instance is beneficial for improving the rate of ovulation. There has been no increase in anomalies in women who take metformin in the first trimester or throughout the pregnancy. The risk of teratogenicity of TZDs has not yet been determined. Women with PCOS, however, do not have hyperglycemia, so the risk may be different for women with type 2 diabetes. The conversion to insulin before conception is safe. Insulin requirements will diminish after delivery.

Later in the pregnancy, after organogenesis, resumption of oral medications may be considered. Discontinuation of a sulfonylurea before labor and delivery is recommended to reduce the risk of hypoglycemia after birth. Metformin, glyburide, and glipizide may be used during lactation.[15,18]

Pregnant women with diabetes should be referred for individualized medical nutrition therapy. The goals of medical nutrition therapy are adequate nutrition to support mother and baby, excellent glycemic control, appropriate weight gain, and development of lifelong healthy nutritional habits. For women without contraindications, 30 minutes of exercise or physical activity daily is recommended. Exercise will result in decreased weight gain, less fetal fat deposition, and improved glycemic control. The patient's ability to tolerate labor will also be enhanced by regular exercise. The patient should be taught the indications (dyspnea, chest pain, calf pain or swelling, vaginal bleeding, amniotic fluid leakage, or uterine contractions) to stop exercise and to seek medical help.[15] Monitoring of blood glucose concentration four or more times per day, including fasting and 2-hour postprandial blood glucose levels, is recommended.

In the pregnant woman with hypertension, the blood pressure target during pregnancy is 110 to 129/65 to 79 mm Hg. For pregnant women with type 2 diabetes, certain medications used to treat comorbidities are not safe during pregnancy or lactation and will have to be discontinued (e.g., angiotensin-converting enzyme [ACE] inhibitors, angiotensin II receptor blockers [ARBs], and statins).[17] Careful monitoring of blood pressure, renal and retinal status, glycemic control, and fetal well-being by a team of specialists is necessary throughout the pregnancy.

Co-Management with Specialists

Diabetes is a progressive disease requiring collaborative treatment from many specialties to prevent, to identify, or to slow the progression of end-organ complications. Specialists who care for patients with diabetes throughout the life span include endocrinologists, ophthalmologists, podiatrists, cardiologists, nephrologists, obstetricians, and vascular surgeons. Yearly visits to an ophthalmologist or an optometrist who is skilled in the care of patients with diabetes should begin at the time of diagnosis for patients with type 2 diabetes and for adults with type 1 diabetes. Prepubertal children with type 1 diabetes should begin to have annual eye examinations 5 years after diagnosis. The examination should include evaluation and treatment of diabetic retinopathy as well as of cataracts and retinal hemorrhaging. A patient with diabetes should be referred as needed to a podiatrist for treatment of ulcers, foot deformities, foot infections, callus removal, and nail care.

The patient with diabetes should be referred to a cardiologist for secondary prevention of CVD. Once microalbuminuria is present, a nephrology referral is indicated to prevent or to delay further renal disease. A vascular surgeon may be needed for treatment of peripheral vascular disease, nonhealing ulcers, or amputation.

Other referrals include consultation with a dietitian for medical nutrition therapy including carbohydrate-counting, calorie requirements, and weight loss; a diabetes educator to teach diabetes self-management; an exercise physiologist or physical therapist for exercise guidelines; and a social worker to help with the many occupational, financial, and emotional issues that are associated with living with diabetes.

A referral to a transplant center for consideration of pancreas transplantation should be provided for appropriate patients. Those with labile type 1 diabetes or those who have undergone renal transplantation and are already immunosuppressed would be good candidates. A patient who is morbidly obese and has multiple cardiac risk factors should be encouraged to consider bariatric surgery.

COMPLICATIONS

Psychological Complications

The diagnosis of diabetes, like that of any chronic illness, can be unexpected and potentially devastating. The emotional response to the diagnosis may range from denial to guilt to grief.[19] The support of family members and friends is important for the long-term acceptance of the disease and its progression. The diagnosis is often confirmed and presented to the patient in the ambulatory setting, where the adult patient is unaccompanied. The patient should be encouraged to share the diagnosis and to seek support from friends and family, as one would with the diagnosis of any life-changing disease.

Whereas 5% to 8% of the general population will experience a major depressive disorder sometime in their lifetime, there is a threefold to fourfold increase in the prevalence of depression in patients with type 1 or type 2 diabetes.[19] Without treatment, depression in the patient with diabetes can affect glycemic control. Depression may contribute to detrimental lifestyle habits such as overeating, inactivity, smoking, drinking alcohol, and medication noncompliance, all of which increase the risk for diabetes complications. Subclinical emotional distress can impede diabetes management, leading to poor glycemic control, poor self-image, confusion of treatment options, and progression of complications leading to a poor quality of life. Careful coordination of medical therapy and psychotherapy is needed. Treatment options include relaxation, education, support of family and friends, psychotherapy, and pharmacotherapy. The newer selective serotonin reuptake inhibitors are better choices for treatment than most other antidepressant agents because they do not cause hyperglycemia.

Another mental health issue that may complicate diabetes is an eating disorder. Omission of insulin in type 1 diabetes results in weight loss and is informally known as "diabulima." This method of weight loss is a significant risk for DKA. It is more common among young women and manifests as weight loss despite overeating and a decreased level of energy. Treatment requires collaboration between the diabetes care team and the eating disorder team.

Acute Complications of Diabetes

Hypoglycemia. Short-term, reversible complications of diabetes include the extremes of blood glucose concentration. Hypoglycemia, defined as a blood glucose level of less than 70 mg/dL, is caused by an imbalance of food, exercise, and insulin (Table 206-3). Initial symptoms are caused by the adrenergic response to a drop in the blood glucose concentration. When blood glucose levels are lower than 70 mg/dL (or perhaps higher in a patient with poor control), the hypothalamus senses the decreased blood glucose and triggers the sensation of hunger. This action stimulates the nervous system to increase gastric juices and stomach contractions. The adrenal medulla secretes epinephrine and cortisol, which stimulate glycogenolysis. This slows glycogenesis (the storage of glucose) and promotes gluconeogenesis (glucose formation from fatty and amino acids). As the blood glucose level decreases, cerebral function is altered. Neuroglycopenia occurs when the brain and central nervous system are not able to maintain normal function because of lowered glucose levels. The low glucose level is classified as mild, moderate, or severe based on neuroglycopenic symptoms and the individual's ability to treat himself or herself.[4]

The blood glucose level at which one feels symptoms of hypoglycemia differs among individuals and may vary for a given patient from one episode to the next. The sensation of symptoms may depend on factors such as the rapidity of the fall in glucose as well as preoccupation with other activities. Therefore, each individual must monitor blood glucose concentration when hypoglycemia is suspected, pay close attention to symptoms, and avoid delays in treatment.

The treatment of hypoglycemia is consumption of sugar. Mild to moderate hypoglycemia can be corrected with 15 g of carbohydrate. Twice this amount of carbohydrate may be needed to correct severe hypoglycemia. Liquids, such as juice or nondiet soda, can be consumed more quickly than solids. If the risk of aspiration exists, glucose gel may be applied between the cheek and the gum. All patients should be advised to keep a rapid-acting carbohydrate with them at all times, including next to the bed, to avoid a delay in treatment.

More is not better when treating a low–blood glucose reaction. Overtreatment or undertreatment of hypoglycemia can result in rebound hyperglycemia or an inadequate rise in glucose with continued or worsening symptoms, respectively. After the resolution of the hypoglycemic event, it can be useful for the patient to try to determine the cause of the event to help prevent future episodes.

Patients with diabetes should make certain that a family member or close friend knows how to recognize and to treat severe hypoglycemia by the intramuscular administration of glucagon or activation of emergency medical services.[4,20]

Hypoglycemia unawareness is the loss of autonomic symptoms that warn the individual of a low blood glucose level. Long duration of the disease, other neuropathic complications, and uncontrolled diabetes are risk factors for this dangerous condition. Frequent blood glucose monitoring, particularly before driving, is essential for those with hypoglycemia unawareness.[4] Raising the blood glucose target range is recommended to reduce the frequency of hypoglycemic episodes.

Intensive insulin therapy and near-normal glycemia can increase vulnerability to hypoglycemia. Health care providers must be aware of the influence of medications, food, and exercise on glucose control and be wary of nighttime moderate to severe hypoglycemia. The peakless basal insulin analogues are less likely to cause nocturnal hypoglycemia than is NPH. Older adults, those with type 1 diabetes, those with longer duration of diabetes, and patients with neuropathic complications are at greatest risk for hypoglycemia. Severe hypoglycemia, left untreated, can lead to seizure, coma, or death.

Fear of hypoglycemia may drive a patient to purposefully avoid tight glycemic control. It is important that providers and patients collaborate on a treatment plan that is safe and acceptable. A continuous glucose sensor measures glucose in the interstitial fluid every 5 minutes and will alarm to alert the patient

TABLE 206-3 Hypoglycemia

Condition	Signs and Symptoms	Treatment
Mild hypoglycemia	Blood glucose <70 mg/dL Shaking or trembling, sweating, hunger, tachycardia, weakness, lightheadedness, pallor, irritability, but no change in mental status; individual able to treat self.	Eat or drink 15 g of rapid-acting carbohydrate (avoid high-fat foods such as chocolate). Stop activity and check blood glucose in 10-15 minutes; if <70 mg/dL, take additional 15 g of carbohydrate. Once recovered, attempt to determine the cause so that similar episodes can be avoided in the future.
Plasma glucose <50 mg/dL	20-30 g of carbohydrate may be needed.	
Moderate hypoglycemia	Decreased thinking, increased emotions (anger, irritability), inability to complete tasks, some changes in mental status; individual may be able to treat self.	Take 15-30 g of rapid-acting carbohydrate and then follow aforementioned instructions.
Severe hypoglycemia	Confusion, drowsiness; may progress to unconsciousness; impaired neurologic function; individual requires assistance.	Take 30-45 g of simple-acting carbohydrate if able to safely swallow. If not, glucagon should be injected intramuscularly or subcutaneously (1 mg for adults; 0.5 mg for children <5 years; 0.25 mg for infants). Follow with snack or meal.

Data from Cryer PE, Davis SN, Shamoon H: Hypoglycemia in diabetes, *Diabetes Care* 26(6):1902-1912, 2003.

to a low or rapidly dropping blood glucose level. These devices are now available in noninvasive models (transdermal) that will alert the patient's mobile phone and call for help if the patient does not respond to the alert. This is a new supplemental tool to be used along with traditional fingerstick blood glucose monitoring.[4] Manufacturers of sensors advise confirmation of a glucose value before treatment with an insulin correction.

Hyperglycemia. Hyperglycemia is defined as a glucose level of 180 mg/dL or higher. Most patients will experience no symptoms at this glucose level, and some who have developed a tolerance for sustained hyperglycemia may report that they feel better in this range than at a normal glucose level. The symptoms of untreated diabetes (e.g., polyuria, polydipsia, blurry vision, fatigue) may accompany prolonged periods of hyperglycemia.

Treatment of intermittent hyperglycemia includes the administration of a correction dose of rapid-acting insulin if the patient has been advised to do so. Taking an additional dose of an oral diabetes medication is never recommended. Nonmedicinal strategies to reduce episodic hyperglycemia include drinking plenty of water and getting some extra exercise. Re-evaluation of the diet and exercise plan is also recommended.

Diabetic Ketoacidosis and Hyperglycemic Hyperosmolar State. If left untreated, hyperglycemia can progress to DKA or a hyperglycemic hyperosmolar state (HHS), previously called hyperglycemic hyperosmolar nonketotic coma. The new term recognizes that the patient may have altered sensorium without coma and may have a mild to moderate degree of ketosis.[21] These are medical emergencies that require immediate treatment and, in most cases, hospitalization.

DKA is caused by insulin deficiency and is characterized by hyperglycemia, ketonemia, and acidemia. The clinical presentation of DKA includes rapid development of abdominal pain, nausea and vomiting, Kussmaul respirations, and dehydration. Physical examination may reveal a fruity odor to the breath, tachycardia, hypotension, and changes in consciousness. Laboratory assessment includes arterial blood gas, electrolytes, glucose, anion gap, and β-hydroxybutyrate (serum ketones). Treatment of DKA includes fluid resuscitation, intravenous insulin administration, electrolyte monitoring and replacement, and investigation and treatment of an underlying illness or infection. Once the patient is stable, the cause of DKA should be determined and the patient should be counseled to prevent a recurrence. The most common causes include new-onset type 1 diabetes, omission of insulin, infection, illness, and major surgery.[21]

Hospitalization might be avoided with early detection and aggressive treatment of hyperglycemia and ketonuria. Fluids, insulin, and frequent blood glucose and ketone monitoring are essential (Box 206-12).

Prevention of DKA requires prompt attention to increasing hyperglycemia as well as home ketone monitoring (urine or blood) when indicated. Adherence to sick-day management guidelines (Box 206-13) will enable the individual with type 1 diabetes to actively participate in the prevention of ketoacidosis. Review of these guidelines with patients regularly, especially at the start of cold and influenza season, is recommended.

HHS is a medical emergency affecting the patient with type 2 diabetes. HHS is characterized by a relative deficiency of insulin that is inadequate to sustain normoglycemia but is adequate to prevent lipolysis and ketosis. This is most common in older adults, particularly nursing home residents, and in newly diagnosed individuals. Presenting symptoms include a gradual progression of polyuria, polydipsia, and altered level of consciousness. In patients living alone, treatment is often delayed because of altered sensorium, and this contributes to the significant mortality associated with HHS. On presentation, the patient is found to have significant hyperglycemia and profound dehydration. Seizures, tremor, hemiparesis, and disorientation may be present.

BOX 206-12

Ketone Monitoring

Teach all patients with type 1 diabetes when and how to test for ketones.

Test urine or blood ketones if:

- Blood glucose level unexplainably 250 mg/dL or higher
- Illness, infection, fever, stress present
- Positive ketones last test

Positive result indicates inadequate insulin.

- Drink plenty of water.
- Take correction insulin.
- Avoid exercise.
- Continue to monitor.
- Call provider for help.

BOX 206-13

Sick-Day Management for Patients with Diabetes

Rising blood glucose levels may be the first sign of impending illness. With unexplained high blood glucose levels or with illness, infection, or pain, the following general rules are recommended:

1. Monitor blood glucose at least every 4 hours with symptoms of nausea, anorexia, illness, or rising glucose levels.
2. If blood glucose level is higher than 250 mg/dL in type 1 diabetes, test for ketones.
3. With elevated blood glucose levels, supplemental rapid-acting insulin can be given every 2 to 4 hr. Advise a dose of rapid-acting insulin based on the correction factor. The increased insulin resistance of acute illness may necessitate higher doses.
4. Maintain adequate hydration by drinking 8 oz of calorie-free fluid hourly while awake. This can be alternated with a sodium-rich fluid, such as bouillon, consommé, or clear canned soups. If unable to eat a normal diet, alternate fluids containing carbohydrate, such as apple juice or regular ginger ale, with sugar-free fluids.
5. Continue to take diabetes medication, even if not eating. The most common cause of DKA is the omission of insulin when sick.
6. Antiemetics should be prescribed for those unable to tolerate fluids by mouth; monitor closely for dehydration. Intravenous fluid may be needed.
7. Contact health care provider for the following:
   - Difficulty breathing
   - Vomiting persisting more than 6 hr
   - Elevated blood glucose of 300 mg/dL or higher unresponsive to increased insulin after two doses
   - Moderate or high urinary ketones or blood ketones higher than 0.6 mmol/L
   - Questions or concerns

Precipitating causes include acute illness, infection or burns, medications, omission of insulin, new diagnosis of diabetes, and inadequate free water intake. Treatment includes reversal of dehydration and hyperglycemia and correction of any electrolyte abnormalities. The older adult patient should have a complete safety assessment before being discharged back to his or her current home.

Chronic Complications of Diabetes

The major morbidity and mortality associated with diabetes are results of the long-term, irreversible complications, a consequence of persistent hyperglycemia and other factors. Results from the Diabetes Control and Complications Trial (DCCT) in type 1 diabetes and the United Kingdom Prospective Diabetes Study (UKPDS) in type 2 diabetes revealed a significant reduction in the complications of retinopathy, nephropathy, and neuropathy when glycemic control was sustained in the HbA_{1c} range of approximately 7%.[4] Long-term follow-up of the DCCT cohorts demonstrated that the risk reduction effect of intensive glycemic control persists, even after some decline in glycemic control, as reported in the Epidemiology of Diabetes Interventions and Complications (EDIC) study.[4]

The benefits of intensive glucose management on the reduction of CVD for patients with type 2 diabetes must be individualized. The Action to Control Cardiovascular Risk in Diabetes (ACCORD) study, the Action in Diabetes and Vascular Disease (ADVANCE) study, and the Veterans Affairs Diabetes Trial (VADT) concluded that intensive therapy to normalize glycemic control did not result in fewer cardiovascular events among high-risk patients with type 2 diabetes and in fact was associated with an increase in mortality.[4] For patients with a shorter duration of diabetes, no significant CVD, and a reasonable life expectancy, an HbA_{1c} target of less than 7%, achieved without undue hypoglycemia, may result in a further reduction in risk of microvascular complications. For patients who have a limited life expectancy, with advanced diabetes complications or comorbidities, longer duration of diabetes, and a history of severe hypoglycemia, the HbA_{1c} target should be higher than 7%[4] (Box 206-14).

BOX 206-14

Prevention of Chronic Complications

- Glycemic control
- Blood pressure control
- Lipid control
- Smoking avoidance or cessation
- Weight control
- Aspirin*
- ACE inhibitor
- Early detection of chronic complications
  - Annual ophthalmology examination
  - Annual microalbuminuria evaluation
  - Foot examination to assess protective sensation
- Referral to specialists as needed
  - Ophthalmologist
  - Podiatrist
  - Nephrologist
  - Cardiologist

*There is not sufficient evidence to recommend aspirin for primary prevention in lower-risk individuals (e.g., men younger than 50 years or women younger than 60 years without other major risk factors).

Data from American Diabetes Association: Standards of medical care in diabetes—2015, *Diabetes Care* 38(Suppl 1):S49-S58, 2015.

Microvascular Complications

Diabetic Retinopathy. Nearly all patients with type 1 diabetes and 80% of patients with type 2 diabetes will have some form of retinopathy after 20 years of diabetes; 21% of type 2 patients have retinopathy at the time of diagnosis.[22] Left untreated, diabetic retinopathy may progress to vision loss and blindness. Therefore, annual screening for retinopathy with a dilated retinal examination by an ophthalmologist or optometrist skilled in recognizing retinopathy is recommended for all individuals with diabetes, beginning 5 years after diagnosis of type 1 and at the time of diagnosis for those with type 2. Patients are likely to experience no change in their vision until retinopathy is advanced. Routine examinations are essential for early detection, at a point at which the retinopathy is more successfully treated. Diabetic retinopathy is the leading cause of new-onset blindness in the United States.[22] Poor glucose control, hypertension, hyperlipidemia, nephropathy, anemia, sleep apnea, and smoking are all risk factors associated with the incidence and progression of diabetic retinopathy. Women with diabetes who are contemplating pregnancy are advised to have a thorough eye examination before conception and then each trimester during the pregnancy. A rapid progression of retinopathy during pregnancy is common.[15]

Nonproliferative retinopathy is treated by strict adherence to blood pressure and blood glucose control, smoking avoidance, and follow-up care by an eye specialist. Proliferative diabetic retinopathy (PDR) is treated with laser photocoagulation to halt the progression and to decrease the risk of severe vision loss. The earlier the treatment, the more positive the outcome, so regular dilated retinal examinations are essential because the patient is likely to have no recognizable change in his or her vision. Any new report of a sensation of "floaters" or "cobwebs" in the eye or a sudden, painless loss of vision should prompt an urgent referral to an ophthalmologist.

Other ocular conditions that are common in people with diabetes include cataracts that begin at a younger age and progress more rapidly than in people who do not have diabetes. Open-angle glaucoma is more common in diabetes. Individuals with diabetes may also experience blurred vision related to high or fluctuating blood glucose levels. This is temporary and will resolve with improved glycemic control.

Diabetic Nephropathy. Diabetes is the most common cause of end-stage renal disease (ESRD), necessitating dialysis or transplantation.[23] Nephropathy is present in 30% to 40% of patients with type 1 diabetes and represents the second leading cause of death for individuals with diabetes. Sixty percent of all patients with diabetes who ultimately require renal dialysis have type 2 diabetes.[4]

Diabetic nephropathy, also known as Kimmelstiel-Wilson syndrome, is characterized by proteinuria, hypertension, edema, and renal insufficiency. Chronic kidney disease progresses through five stages: (1) elevated glomerular filtration rate (GFR), indicating increased work of the kidney; (2) presence of microalbuminuria, with GFR elevated or back to normal; (3) proteinuria and hypertension with moderate reduction of GFR; (4) diminished GFR and rising blood urea nitrogen and creatinine concentrations; and (5) ESRD.

The GFR, which is usually elevated when a person is first diagnosed with diabetes, is directly related to the degree of hyperglycemia but is a poor measure of renal function because its elevation may ensue over a long "silent" period (about 15 years' duration) as histologic changes in the kidney progress. Serum creatinine, also an unreliable marker for renal disease, might not be elevated until more than 50% of function is lost and may be normal in older patients with renal damage because of decreased muscle mass.[23]

Because the earliest indication of renal damage from diabetes is the presence of microalbuminuria, all patients with diabetes should have this tested annually, beginning at the time of diagnosis of type 2 diabetes and 5 years after diagnosis of type 1 diabetes. There are typically no symptoms during the early stages of diabetic nephropathy, yet the presence of microalbuminuria is a harbinger of both renal failure and cardiovascular complications in diabetes.

Microalbuminuria analysis can be performed by an albumin/creatinine ratio, a random spot collection, a 24-hour collection, or a timed (e.g., 4-hour or overnight) collection. Microalbuminuria is diagnostic at more than 30 mg/24 hr excretion. Two of three positive collections in a 3- to 6-month period are necessary to confirm microalbuminuria. Ongoing monitoring of albumin excretion is useful to assess the response to treatment and the progression of the disease.

When microalbuminuria is confirmed, treatment with an ACE inhibitor or an ARB should be initiated. In individuals with type 1 diabetes, the use of an ACE inhibitor has been proven to slow the progression of nephropathy.[23] In those with type 2 diabetes, hypertension, and microalbuminuria, an ACE inhibitor or an ARB has been shown to delay the progression to proteinuria. In patients with type 2 diabetes who also have renal insufficiency, the progression of nephropathy can be delayed with the use of an ARB.[4] If one class of agent is not tolerated, it should be replaced with the other.

Control of blood pressure is the single most important intervention in the prevention and treatment of renal disease in the patient with diabetes. The ADA recommends a blood pressure target of 130/80 mm Hg. As with all treatment regimens, diet, exercise, weight loss, and smoking avoidance are vital. Restriction of protein intake is recommended for patients with kidney disease. Limiting protein intake to 0.8 to 1 g/kg body weight per day in the early stages of chronic kidney disease and to less than 0.8 g/kg body weight per day in the later stages is recommended to improve renal function.[4] Consultation with a nephrologist should occur when microalbuminuria (30 to 300 mg/24 hr), overt albuminuria (>2 mg/dL), or decreased GFR (<50 mL/min) is present. Consultation with a cardiologist or nephrologist is recommended if hypertension persists. The courses of diabetic retinopathy and diabetic nephropathy often parallel each other. Both are asymptomatic in the early stages, which supports the need for routine screening and interventions that have been shown to effectively delay progression.

Diabetic Neuropathy. Diabetic neuropathy affects 60% to 70% of individuals with diabetes. Nerve damage can occur in almost any nerve in the body. Duration of diabetes, glycemic control, blood pressure control, lipid control, smoking, and obesity are all factors that have an effect on nerve damage.[24] However, data from the EDIC study revealed that intensive therapy successfully improves glycemic control, resulting in a reduction in nerve damage that is sustained for years.[4]

Multiple mechanisms contribute to the pathogenesis of this complication. The onset of symptoms may be gradual or sudden, depending on the nerves that are affected. There are three major classes of diabetic neuropathies: peripheral or distal symmetric neuropathy, mononeuropathy, and autonomic neuropathy.

Peripheral neuropathy is the most common neuropathic complication. Distal numbness or impaired sensation is typically bilateral and can occur acutely or gradually as a complication of poor glycemic control. The feet and legs are typically affected first, and then the hands and arms may follow. Initially, sensations of tingling, burning, or prickling may be noticed, particularly at night. Patients may report an increased sensitivity to touch. There may be associated muscle weakness that affects the patient's gait. On clinical examination, there may be a loss of sensation as detected by the Semmes-Weinstein monofilament along with bilaterally absent knee or ankle jerk reflexes.

Progression of sensory deficits can cause destruction of cartilage in foot joints. This destruction results in loss of normal foot architecture, leaving the foot susceptible to deformities, such as hammertoes and Charcot joint. Charcot joint may be difficult to distinguish from active infection with cellulitis because both manifest with erythema and swelling. The presence of altered foot sensation makes the recommended daily foot inspection imperative, with guidance to seek professional care promptly for any abnormality.

Pain is present in about 25% of all patients with peripheral neuropathy.[24] Nonpharmacologic treatment of painful peripheral neuropathy is aimed at improvement of glycemic control; avoidance of alcohol; physical therapy; use of relaxation, acupuncture, or biofeedback techniques; or referral to a pain control clinic. Improvement in glycemic control may result in a temporary worsening of painful neuropathic symptoms, but pain will abate with the maintenance of good blood glucose levels.

Topical treatments include capsaicin and lidocaine patches. Pharmacologic options include γ-aminobutyric acid (GABA) analogues, tricyclic antidepressants, other types of antidepressants and anticonvulsants, and, in limited situations, narcotics.

The mononeuropathies occur in large nerves or nerve roots and produce radicular symptoms. Large nerve roots in the spinal cord, chest, or abdomen or even cranial nerves can be affected. Mononeuropathy involves both sensory and motor neurons, producing increased or decreased sensation, weakness, and pain. The pain produced by mononeuropathies can be severe and mimic degenerative disk disease, herpes zoster, carpal tunnel syndrome, Bell palsy, or intra-abdominal conditions. Oculomotor palsy, characterized by ptosis, pain, and sparing of the pupillary reflex, occurs in patients older than 50 years. Pain and oculomotor function improve gradually during several weeks, and full recovery usually occurs within 3 to 5 months.

Autonomic neuropathy affects both sympathetic and parasympathetic fibers. Although any organ system may be affected, the more common effects are found in the gastrointestinal tract, genitourinary tract, and cardiovascular system. Symptoms of gastrointestinal dysfunction include esophageal motility problems and gastroparesis with impaired gastric emptying. The gastroparesis affects food absorption, leading to erratic glycemic control. The delayed gastric emptying also produces early satiety, bloating, nausea, and vomiting. Bowel peristaltic dysfunction is evidenced by explosive diarrhea and altered small bowel motility. Chronic constipation is the most common of the gastrointestinal neuropathies. These symptoms may improve with control of hyperglycemia. Gastroparesis can be addressed through dietary modifications, careful timing of meal-associated rapid-acting insulin, and use of metoclopramide. Various modalities can be tried for control of diarrhea, including biofeedback, bismuth subsalicylate, loperamide, clonidine, and antibiotics.

Genitourinary symptoms usually consist of neurogenic bladder and sexual dysfunction. Bladder atony, characterized by a residual urine volume of more than 150 mL, may lead to recurrent UTIs and overflow incontinence. The occurrence of more than two UTIs per year indicates the need for further evaluation. Patients may mistakenly believe that their diabetes is in better control because they are urinating less frequently, in contrast to their previous polyuria. Timed and complete voiding is recommended. Bethanechol may be helpful as a conservative measure. The patient should be taught how to recognize and promptly report symptoms of a UTI.

Sexual dysfunction in women is characterized by decreased vaginal lubrication and decreased frequency of orgasm. Erectile dysfunction affects more than 50% of men who have had diabetes for more than 10 years.[3] Retrograde ejaculation is also common. Psychological, endocrine-related, and medication- or alcohol-induced impotence needs to be excluded before treatment recommendations are made. Men with diabetes may be successfully treated with a phosphodiesterase-5 (PDE5) inhibitor, although the efficacy is somewhat less than in men without diabetes.

Cardiovascular autonomic neuropathy has two major associated syndromes: orthostatic hypotension and cardiac denervation. Orthostatic hypotension may be pronounced, with an inability to tolerate abrupt rising from a supine to an upright posture. Cardiac denervation is characterized by a fixed heart rate in the range of 80 to 100 beats per minute, without regard for stress, exercise, or tilting. These patients may have myocardial ischemia or infarction without pain and are at risk for cardiac arrhythmias and sudden death. Significant exertion, aerobic exercise, and straining should be avoided. Because of the risk for hypoglycemia and potential cardiac arrhythmias, such patients are generally not candidates for intensive insulin therapy.

Hypoglycemia unawareness is also an autonomic neuropathy in which the individual no longer feels the adrenergic symptoms of a low blood glucose level. Neuroglycopenia occurs with no warning and is a significant safety risk. Patients who have experienced an unconscious hypoglycemic episode should be advised to maintain a slightly higher target blood glucose range, to monitor their blood glucose concentration frequently (particularly before driving), and to pay close attention to any symptoms of hypoglycemia. Friends and family members ought to be taught recognition and treatment of hypoglycemia.

Macrovascular Complications. The leading cause of death and disability in patients with type 2 diabetes is CVD. Diabetes significantly increases the risk of coronary, cerebrovascular, and peripheral vascular disease. This is associated with endothelial dysfunction, hypertension, and lipid abnormalities. In the setting of hyperglycemia, excess free fatty acids, and insulin resistance, there is greater oxidative stress that may damage the endothelium, and less nitric oxide is produced by the endothelium to decrease vasodilation. In addition, abnormalities in platelet function lead to greater activation and aggregation, increasing the risk for thrombosis.[25]

Individuals with diabetes have a twofold to fourfold increased risk for development of coronary artery disease (CAD). The risk for a patient with no history of CAD but with diabetes is equal to the risk of a patient who has had an MI. In patients with diabetes and known CAD, mortality is 45% after 7 years and 75% at 10 years. Diabetes patients with unstable angina are more likely to have an MI, and the MI is more likely to be fatal.[26] CAD in the patient with diabetes occurs earlier and more extensively than in patients without diabetes, and infarction may occur without the usual symptoms. Atypical symptoms of ischemia include dyspnea, fatigue, gastrointestinal distress, unexplained hyperglycemia, ketoacidosis, and congestive heart failure. Typical symptoms of exertional chest pain, chest tightness, and arm pain associated with activity or rest must be evaluated promptly. An initial or subsequent MI is more likely to precipitate long-term complications (e.g., heart failure or arrhythmia) or death in the patient with diabetes compared with the patient without diabetes.[26] Silent MIs are more common in patients with diabetes.

Congestive heart failure is twofold to fivefold more common in patients with insulin resistance.[27] The risk of stroke is increased twofold to fivefold in people with diabetes compared with those without.[28] Stroke-related mortality, repeated stroke, and dementia after stroke are also increased.[28] Slurred speech, intermittent dizziness, transient loss of vision, paresthesia, or weakness of an arm or leg suggests a transient ischemic attack (TIA) consistent with cerebrovascular disease. Because CVD is so common in type 2 diabetes, a carotid ultrasound study is important to evaluate possible episodes of TIA. Anticoagulant and antiplatelet medications may help prevent a recurrence of symptoms.

Peripheral vascular disease, or lower extremity arterial atherosclerosis, is two to four times more common among patients with diabetes.[26] Claudication, absent pedal pulses, and femoral bruits are typical manifestations. Revascularization procedures in patients with diabetes are challenging because of limited collateral vessel availability and frequent small-vessel disease.[26] Diabetes is the leading cause of nontraumatic amputation in the United States.[26] Although neuropathy is usually the cause of foot ulcers, poor blood flow is responsible for slow healing. Revascularization is indicated, if possible, for chronic ulcers.

Lower extremity amputation becomes necessary because of a combination of neuropathic and vascular damage. The precipitant is typically a small opening in the skin caused by stepping on a sharp object, a blister, or a nick from toenail clippers. If it is not noticed because there is no pain sensation, the injury is not treated. The injury then progresses to an infection that is difficult to heal. Daily foot care is essential for early detection of any lesion. A thorough visual inspection should be completed, and anything suspicious should be evaluated by a provider promptly. Patient education includes awareness of the signs and symptoms of an infection. Early and aggressive treatment of foot wounds is required to reduce the risk of severe infection and ultimately amputation.

Patients with diabetes should be aware that near-normal glycemia will reduce their risk for microvascular complications.[29] To reduce the risk of macrovascular complications, achievement of blood pressure and lipid targets along with healthy lifestyle habits is also necessary. Treatment must be modified over time to strive for optimal and safe risk reduction. Lifelong care to reduce cardiovascular events begins with disease prevention and early detection. Early identification of those patients requiring revascularization is essential. Patients with diabetes and CVD should be treated with ACE inhibitors, targeted blood pressure control, and lipid therapy. Individuals at high risk for CVD should be treated with daily aspirin if the risk for cerebrovascular and gastrointestinal bleeding is not excessive (Table 206-4). Their care should be managed in conjunction with a cardiologist.

Modification of all cardiac risk factors has been shown to reduce the risk of CVD.[29] Blood pressure, lipids, smoking, and lifestyle habits of all patients with diabetes should be assessed. C-reactive protein (CRP), as a measure of inflammation, is used as a primary prevention assessment in addition to measurement of cholesterol concentration. If CRP is elevated, in the absence of hypercholesterolemia, the risk of CVD is high. Patients with moderate or high CRP levels should be encouraged to modify lifestyle habits. Individuals with high CRP levels are at an increased risk for development of type 2 diabetes.[30]

Dyslipidemia in type 2 diabetes is characterized by hypertriglyceridemia, low HDL levels, and high LDL levels. A low-fat, low-cholesterol diet and aerobic exercise are essential treatment of dyslipidemia; however, most patients will also require medication. Statins are the first-line therapy to decrease LDL cholesterol. Fibrates reduce triglycerides and may raise HDL, but their role in preventing CVD is controversial, and recent studies have failed to show any benefit in diabetes compared with statins alone.[31] The LDL target remains less than 100 mg/dL for those without CVD and less than 70 mg/dL for those with overt CVD.[4]

Hypertension is associated with CAD, stroke, and peripheral vascular disease. Blood pressure should be treated to a target of less than 130/80 mm Hg. Lifestyle modification, including weight loss, low-sodium diet, physical activity, and moderation of alcohol consumption, is important. Pharmacologic therapy should be initiated to achieve the target, beginning with either an ACE inhibitor or an ARB. There is some evidence that a calcium channel blocker is the best second agent, although a diuretic is also a good choice. Most patients require more than two agents to achieve the blood pressure goal. Renal function and serum potassium concentration should be monitored carefully.

Aspirin is recommended as a strategy for primary prevention in those at increased risk for CVD and as secondary prevention for patients with a history of CVD. It is inexpensive, and in general the risk is low. Its efficacy is controversial.

The effect of a multifactorial intervention on mortality in type 2 diabetes (Steno-2)[32] study demonstrated decreased all-cause mortality and CVD mortality in the intensively treated cohort. There were 160 subjects with type 2 diabetes and microalbuminuria who were randomized to intensive or conventional treatment for 7.8 years. The effect was sustained for an additional 5.5 years of follow-up.

Three recent trials were designed to determine whether intensive glycemic control does reduce the risk of macrovascular complications. The ACCORD trial[33] enrolled more than 10,000 subjects with type 2 diabetes of approximately 10 years' duration, with a history of CVD or at least two CVD risk factors. The study's aim was to prevent MI, stroke, and CVD deaths by striving to achieve normal blood glucose control and blood pressure control and by employing combination lipid therapy. The intensive glucose control strategy was stopped early because there was a higher risk of death compared with standard glucose treatment. Intensive blood pressure treatment was found to reduce the risk of stroke by 40%, but this benefit was accompanied by a higher incidence of hypotension and hyperkalemia. Combination lipid therapy was found to be safe but did not show an improvement in the risk of CVD. The conclusion of the study was that for a high-risk group (longer duration of diabetes and existing CVD or high risk for CVD), intensive treatment adds risk without benefit. The results of this trial may not apply to those with a more recent diagnosis of diabetes or with a lower CVD risk.[34]

The ADVANCE[35] study, which randomized 11,140 patients with type 2 diabetes, and the VADT,[36] which enrolled 1791 patients, had similar findings for subjects with longer duration of diabetes and higher risk for CVD. Further analysis of the three trials suggests that there may be a benefit of intensive glycemic control for individuals with a shorter duration of diabetes, lower initial HbA_{1c} level, and no CVD at baseline.[4] For patients with a shorter duration of diabetes, no known significant CVD, and a longer life expectancy, a target HbA_{1c} level of below 7%, and even lower if it can be achieved without undue hypoglycemia, should be recommended. A less rigorous target should be advised for those with a history of severe hypoglycemia, advanced complications, significant CVD, longer duration of diabetes, advanced age, and limited life expectancy.[12] For all patients, other risk factors (blood pressure, lipids, lifestyle) should be treated according to the ADA and American Heart Association standards.[37]

The majority of investigations of screening and risk factor modification for CAD have been conducted in patients with type 2 diabetes. Patients with type 1 diabetes do have higher rates of CAD events than those without diabetes. This effect begins at a young age and increases with age.[37] The results of the EDIC study suggested that early and aggressive glycemic control reduces the risk of CAD in type 1 diabetes. The ADA and the American Heart Association recommend blood pressure and lipid control for patients with type 1 diabetes. An ACE inhibitor is indicated for anyone with type 1 diabetes and microalbuminuria, even if normotensive. Medication should be initiated if the blood pressure is above the 95th percentile or 130/80 mm Hg, whichever is lower. Pharmacologic treatment is recommended for patients with type 1 diabetes who have not achieved an LDL cholesterol concentration below 160 mg/dL with medical nutrition therapy. For those with an increased CVD risk, medication should begin if the LDL cholesterol concentration is not below 130 mg/dL. Patients who are overweight or obese may have a greater risk of CVD because of the atherogenic risk of insulin resistance.[37]

The morbidity and mortality rates for CVD in the United States have fallen markedly during the past 50 years. However, for individuals with diabetes, there has been an increase in CVD

TABLE 206-4 Aspirin Recommendation for Type 1 and Type 2 Diabetes

Patient's Risk for CVD	For Prevention of CVD
Adults with diabetes at low CVD risk	Aspirin not recommended
Adults with diabetes at increased CVD risk* (10 year risk >10%)	Consider low-dose aspirin (75-162 mg/day)

*Increased risk for CVD is defined as men older than 50 years and women older than 60 years with one or more of the following: smoking, hypertension, dyslipidemia, family history of CVD, and albuminuria.

Data from Neumiler JJ, White JR: Aspirin therapy in patients with diabetes: an update on current recommendations. *Diabetes Spectrum* 26(3):153-155, 2013.

during the same time span. Multivariate analysis in two time periods from the Framingham Heart Study demonstrated that risk factors for diabetes including hypertension, high cholesterol, smoking, and obesity are evident in the population up to 30 years before the onset of cardiovascular disease.[38] These findings underscore the importance of diabetes prevention and early and aggressive treatment of risk factors for all patients with diabetes.

INDICATIONS FOR REFERRAL OR HOSPITALIZATION

In addition to recommending that the patient be referred to specialists, referral to an endocrinologist or diabetologist should be considered in the following situations:

- New diagnosis of type 1 diabetes
- Poorly controlled type 2 diabetes, despite two or more oral diabetes medications
- Discovery of a diabetes complication
- After hospitalization
- Initiation of insulin pump or other intensive insulin therapy
- Contemplated or confirmed pregnancy
- Patient request

Based on the ADA recommendations,[20] the patient with diabetes requires hospitalization for the following:

- Acute metabolic complications
- DKA (blood glucose >250 mg/dL, arterial pH <7.30, and serum bicarbonate <15 mEq/L with ketonuria or ketonemia)
- HHS (impaired mental status, dehydration, serum osmolarity >320 mOsm/kg, and plasma glucose >600 mg/dL)
- Hypoglycemia with neuroglycopenia (blood glucose <50 mg/dL that does not respond to usual treatment) or coma, seizures or altered behavior, or persistent hypoglycemia caused by a sulfonylurea
- Uncontrolled diabetes
- Hyperglycemia with volume depletion
- Persistent hyperglycemia not responding to treatment and with metabolic deterioration
- Recurrent fasting hyperglycemia (>300 mg/dL or HbA_{1c} level more than twice the upper limit of normal) refractory to outpatient treatment
- Recurrent, severe hypoglycemia (<50 mg/dL) despite treatment
- Metabolic instability (glucose fluctuating between <50 mg/dL and >300 mg/dL)
- Recurrent DKA without infection or trauma as a precipitant
- Frequent absence from school or work as a result of psychosocial problems that lead to poor glycemic control
- Admission for complications of diabetes

Inpatient care may be appropriate in the event of the following:

- Newly diagnosed diabetes in young children
- Significant and sustained poor metabolic control that requires close monitoring
- Uncontrolled or newly diagnosed diabetes during pregnancy requiring insulin
- Severe, chronic complications of diabetes requiring intensive treatment

LIFE SPAN CONSIDERATIONS

Diabetes is a chronic and progressive disease with acute and chronic complications. It is present in individuals of all ages from infants to older adults. With each stage of development, there are issues regarding diabetes management, physical and emotional development, education and understanding, physical disabilities, nutrition, and financial, behavioral, and medical problems that will affect the diabetes treatment plan. Adolescents and older adults are at greatest risk for failure. Predictors that impede adherence to therapy include lack of practical knowledge, lack of control, vulnerability, lack of social acceptance, little or no family support, and fear of hypoglycemia. Other barriers include financial and occupational constraints. Consideration of all these issues is essential for optimal care.

Adolescents pose a particular challenge because metabolic and biologic changes affect glycemic control. Preadolescence or early adolescence (12 years of age), middle adolescence (13 to 15 years), and late adolescence (16 to 18 years) are marked by hormonal changes that often cause relative insulin resistance because of changing counterregulatory hormone responses and declining peripheral insulin action.

During adolescence, emotional and developmental issues emerge. The emotional stages of shock, denial, negotiation, anger, and acceptance can recur as the person ages. Developmental challenges of individual identity, sexual identity and exploration, the drive for independence and struggles with parents and authority, and peer acceptance can affect the ability of adolescents to manage their diabetes. Other concerns affecting diabetes management include athletic participation, recurrent ketoacidosis, inadequate nutrition, dieting and eating disorders, alcohol, drugs, and sexual activity. The health care provider's ability to communicate and to compromise without risking safety will foster the development of a trusting relationship. Education must be factual, specific, and consultative rather than directive and must be relevant to the adolescent's stage of development and emotional behavior. The treatment plan must be realistic and workable and agreed to by the patient and the provider. A written copy of the plan is helpful.

During young adulthood, developmental issues of career development, interpersonal relationships, self-image, health perception, and understanding of diabetes can influence glycemic control. As emotional ties to family decline, concerns related to marriage, pregnancy and children, employment, finances, and anticipation of complications can influence diabetes management. Health care providers must provide emotional support, updated information and resources, and re-evaluation of nutritional and pharmacologic therapies. Emphasis should be on blood glucose monitoring, appropriate physical activity, healthy nutrition, and medical intervention to prevent hypoglycemia and to maintain glycemic control. A collaborative relationship with the diabetes care team is essential, including evaluation and aggressive treatment of diabetes complications.

In middle-aged people with diabetes, the challenges include marriage and children, productivity, planning for retirement, and often caring for elderly parents. The comorbidities associated with diabetes may develop or progress. If the addition of insulin is required, there may be implications for the patient's occupation.

In older persons, concerns about loneliness, economics, and disease progression or failing health can affect diabetes management. Financial concerns can interfere with access to proper food, prescribed medications, blood glucose monitoring supplies, and medical care. Issues of weight loss, physical inactivity, failing vision or hearing, poor dexterity or amputation, memory impairment, gait disturbance or muscle weakness, sexual dysfunction, and physical and emotional isolation can affect glycemic control. A diminished sense of thirst may contribute to dehydration in the setting of hyperglycemia. As complications develop and health begins to falter, denial, anger, hostility, and depression can threaten the emotional well-being of the older patient with diabetes and influence diabetes management. Health care providers must offer resources and emotional support. The maintenance of function, independence, and general well-being as well as prevention of severe hypoglycemia and vascular compromise should take precedence over attaining optimum glycemic control. Insulin or sulfonylurea doses may need to be decreased at this time to reduce the risk of hypoglycemia and to prevent falls. It is essential that the older patient with diabetes understand and can follow the treatment plan. Frequent medical visits as well as simplified written instructions, in large print if necessary, are helpful for older adults with diabetes.

EDUCATION AND HEALTH PROMOTION

The goals of diabetes education are to promote optimal health, to improve quality of life, and to reduce the human and economic burden associated with poorly controlled diabetes.[37] The framework for diabetes education has shifted from content to outcomes. Rather than merely imparting information to patients, diabetes self-management education strives to guide patients in the setting of personal goals that result in changes in behavior leading to improved clinical outcomes.[39]

The ADA Education Recognition Program designates diabetes education programs that meet the national standards for diabetes self-management education. A listing of recognized programs can be found at http://professional.diabetes.org/ERP_List.aspx. A certified diabetes educator (CDE) is an individual from one of many disciplines (registered nurse, registered dietitian, pharmacist, physician, physician assistant, exercise physiologist, social worker, occupational therapist, physical therapist, clinical psychologist, optometrist, podiatrist, or health educator) who has met the requirements of the National Certification Board for Diabetes Educators. A listing of CDEs may be found at www.diabeteseducator.org/DiabetesEducation/Find.html.

Diabetes education is not a pamphlet, an appointment, or a class. It is a lifelong process through which the patient and family acquire the knowledge and practice the skills necessary to manage the patient's diabetes. As the individual passes through the stages of life, different information and resources are necessary. As new developments in diabetes treatment evolve, ongoing education is necessary to sustain self-care habits and to achieve the goal of excellent glycemic control. A variety of approaches to teaching should be offered because patients learn in many ways. Face-to-face instruction, group classes, written information, videos, and websites are common strategies. The patient's literacy level should be considered and appropriate materials provided.

At the time of diagnosis, the essential survival skills are taught to keep the patient safe until additional education can be arranged. Survival skills include understanding the basic pathophysiologic mechanism of the disease, understanding how and when to take medications, recognizing and treating hypoglycemia, and knowing when and whom to call for help. The next phase of diabetes education includes self-monitoring of blood glucose concentration, foot care, basic meal planning, and sick-day management.[4]

Advanced diabetes education offers guidance on counting carbohydrates, calculating insulin doses by use of carbohydrate/insulin ratios and correction factors, managing diabetes while traveling, and using preventive care.[37] Individualized education will be provided to those who wish to use an insulin pump or continuous glucose sensor.

Education for the family includes recognition and treatment of hypoglycemia (including glucagon administration), meal planning, and the provision of motivation and support. Patients and families are encouraged to learn all they can about diabetes to take control of their disease. Keeping abreast of new developments and staying motivated may be enhanced by reading magazines written for people who live with diabetes (e.g., *Diabetes Forecast, Diabetes Self-Management*) and participating in a diabetes support group.

Helpful websites for patients and families include the following:

- www.nutrition.gov (U.S. Department of Agriculture)
- www.choosemyplate.gov (U.S. Department of Agriculture)
- www.diabetesatwork.org (National Diabetes Education Program [NDEP] employment issues)
- www.diabetes.org (ADA)
- www.jdrf.org (Juvenile Diabetes Research Foundation)
- www.cdc.gov/diabetes/home (Centers for Disease Control and Prevention)
- www.ndep.nih.gov (NDEP)
- www.diabeteshealth.com
- www.diabetesmonitor.com

Helpful websites for health care professionals include the following:

- www.aace.com (American Association of Clinical Endocrinologists)
- www.diabeteseducator.org (American Association of Diabetes Educators)
- http://professional.diabetes.org (American Diabetes Association)
- www.diabetestechnology.org (Diabetes Technology Society)
- http://www.endocrine.org (Endocrine Society)
- http://diabetes.niddk.nih.gov (National Institute of Diabetes and Digestive and Kidney Diseases)

CHAPTER 207

HIRSUTISM

Michelle Freshman

DEFINITION AND EPIDEMIOLOGY

Hirsutism refers to excessive male pattern, terminal hair growth in women resulting from enhanced androgen-dependent sensitivity to increased levels of circulating androgens. Although areas of coarse, pigmented body hair are not unusual in women, concerns about abundance and distribution commonly arise. Thoughtful evaluation of the regions indicative of androgen excess helps discern a physiologic from pathologic cause. In each individual, regardless of gender or race, the number of hair follicles is predetermined (estimated to be 5,000,000); what differs are the pigmentation, thickness, phase duration, sebum production, and pattern of hair as driven by localized androgen responsivity[1] at the pilosebaceous unit. In addition to peripheral androgen metabolism, insulin and hormonal fluctuations are thought to contribute.[2] Hyperandrogenism may occur with or without ovulatory dysfunction or ovarian morphology abnormalities. When signs of virilism such as temporal balding or voice deepening accompany new-onset hirsutism, an ovarian, adrenal, or exogenous hormone source should be suspected, particularly in postmenopausal women as well as in those at increased risk of malignancy.

Millions of women worldwide are affected by hirsutism. In reproductive-age women, 3% to 15% are considered hirsute. Well over 80% of hirsute women have hyperandrogenism. The most common diagnosis associated with this finding is polycystic ovary syndrome (PCOS). In a publication of the Androgen Excess and PCOS Society involving 6281 women with PCOS, hirsutism was identified in 74.7%.[3] Mild cases are distinguished from clinically significant and progressive ones. In cases of isolated, mild hirsutism, approximately half appear to be unrelated to increased androgen levels, perhaps because of the limits of androgen detection or pilosebaceous level phenomena.[4] The degree of clinical hirsutism does not correlate directly with elevated androgen level. This incongruity between symptoms and signs is seen in cases of idiopathic hyperandrogenism (6% to 15%),[5] characterized by hirsutism in the setting of hyperandrogenism with normal ovulatory cycles and ovarian morphology as opposed to idiopathic hirsutism (4% to 7%),[5] characterized by hirsutism in the setting of normal androgen levels, menses, and ovaries, thought to arise from normal ethnic or familial hair pattern variations. In addition, 8% to 13%[3] of women report postmenopausal hirsutism, for which the pathophysiology is yet unclear.[1]

Polycystic Ovary Syndrome

PCOS affects 4% to 20% of menstruating women.[5,6] It is a heterogeneous syndrome, with varying contributions of excess androgens, luteinizing hormone (LH), follicle-stimulating hormone (FSH), and insulin resistance.[6] Most patients have a gonadotropin-dependent functional ovarian hyperandrogenemia, less often in conjunction with a mild adrenocorticotropic hormone (ACTH)–dependent functional adrenal hyperandrogenemia. Approximately 80% of patients are anovulatory[2]; 90% or more women with oligomenorrhea or amenorrhea have PCOS, and 95% of those with PCOS have oligomenorrhea or amenorrhea.[7] The combination of PCOS and amenorrhea is more likely to produce severe hyperandrogenemia.[7]

In the mildest form of PCOS, women have neither gonadotropin nor ovulatory abnormalities but still have decreased sex hormone–binding globulin (SHBG) from ovarian stimulation. In more severe cases, insulin resistance and menstrual cycle irregularities may drive up androgen levels both through increased LH pulse frequency and because free testosterone cannot bind to as many sites as a result of reduced levels of circulating SHBG. One unifying, possibly initiating component, is thought to be ovarian theca cell abnormality leading to increased testosterone and/or androstenedione production and amplification of pituitary LH, wherein the progesterone negative feedback loop is impaired and LH is overproduced.[6]

In 2013 the Clinical Guideline Subcommittee of the Endocrine Society appointed a task force to formulate PCOS guidelines with oversight from subject experts of both the Endocrine Society and the European Society of Endocrinology.[8] The resulting consensus requires two of the following: androgen excess (clinical or biochemical) and either ovulatory dysfunction (clinical) or polycystic ovaries (12 or more follicles 2 to 9 mm in diameter or >25 follicles per ovary and ovarian volume >10 mL in either ovary),[6,8] excluding prepubertal and postmenopausal women. In practice, both clinical and biochemical assessments are subject to limitations. Whereas hirsutism correlates well with hyperandrogenemia, acne, alopecia, acanthosis nigricans, and skin tags do not.[7] Cardiovascular risk indicators as well as metabolic disorders in hirsute women seem to correlate directly with androgen elevations.[2]

An important consideration for health care providers is deciding who is at risk for rare but potentially life-threatening conditions. Patients with PCOS are more likely to be obese, insulin resistant, and infertile[9] as well as face cardiac sequelae. Although many hirsute women have PCOS (72% to 82%,),[9] a minority (1.5% to 10%)[9-11] have hyperandrogenic insulin-resistant acanthosis nigricans (HAIRAN) syndrome, late-onset nonclassic congenital adrenal hyperplasia (NCCAH), prolactinemia, a thyroid disorder, or an androgen-secreting neoplasm. Tumors of the ovary or adrenal gland comprise fewer than 0.2% of women with hyperandrogenemia, half of which are malignant.[5,9]

Specialist referral is indicated for all patients with suspected hirsutism.

PATHOPHYSIOLOGY

Hair follicles exist in all regions of the body except the lips, palms, and soles. Starting several months after birth, hair may be vellus—short and soft—or terminal—thicker, stiffer, longer, and darker. Hair development follows a prescribed, repeating pathway of "growth, regression, and remodelling events,"[2] otherwise known as the anagen (active), telogen (static), and catagen (shedding) phases. Lengthening and thickening of vellus hair into terminal hair in androgen-sensitive but typically male-pattern regions of a woman's body heralds hirsutism. Testosterone prolongs the anagen phase of terminal hair but shortens this phase in scalp hair.[10] Vellus hair stems from undeveloped sebaceous glands.[2]

Distinguished from hirsutism is hypertrichosis. Despite an abundance of typically fine, short, unpigmented hair, androgens are not involved. This type of hair growth results from conditions such as anorexia nervosa, hypothyroidism, porphyria cutanea tarda, dermatomyositis and paraneoplastic syndrome, which causes hypertrichosis lanuginosa. Furthermore, cyclosporine, dexamethasone, diazoxide, minoxidil, penicillamine, phenytoin, and streptomycin are known contributors.[12] Body hair is often diffusely distributed about the midline, including the face and even the forehead in a nonsexual pattern. In familial constitutional hypertrichosis totalis (Ambras syndrome), genetic factors, rather than disease, dictate growth pattern. A diagnosis of hypertrichosis can be assessed by hair type and distribution.

Hirsutism and virilism result from greater testosterone activity. Testosterone activates the skin and hair follicles through enzyme type 1 5α-reductase, which converts testosterone to its potent metabolite, dihydrotestosterone (DHT). DHT converts vellus to terminal hair. This enzyme makes the difference, given similar androgen profiles, between a woman who is hirsute and one who is not. It is a process mediated by genetic variations.[5] Adrenarche, marked by terminal hair growth in the axillae and on the lower pubic triangle, arms, and lower leg, results from increasing dehydroepiandrosterone sulfate (DHEA-S) concentrations. Most centrally located terminal body hair responds to sex hormone production, especially the amount, duration of exposure, and genetics, which together determine the resultant density and diameter. The number of hair follicles is said to decline after the age of 40 years. Acne may surface during puberty with the increased production of androgens and sebum.

Adult women who develop hirsutism are clinically expressing hyperandrogenemia—that is, despite comparable total testosterone and DHT levels, they have different tissue-sensitive androgen metabolism. Terminal hair expression is ultimately controlled by follicular sensitivity to 5α-reductase. Serum testosterone and its immediate precursors—androstenedione, dehydroepiandrosterone (DHEA), and DHEA-S—are ultimately excreted through urine as 17-ketosteroids. These circulating androgens have a local influence at the pilosebaceous unit. DHEA-S mostly comes from the adrenal glands. The other two prohormones come from the peripheral conversion of circulating weaker androgens produced by the ovaries and adrenals.

Women with PCOS have abnormal adrenocortical secretion, although only 25% have absolute adrenal excess.[13] SHBG levels decrease because of suppressed liver production in response to one of several conditions: hyperinsulinemia, obesity, excess growth hormone (GH), or glucocorticoids. Hyperinsulinemia stimulates testosterone synthesis through ovarian thecal cells (hyperthecosis) acted on by LH. Hyperinsulinemia is also related to obesity (body mass index [BMI] >30 kg/m^2) and obesity-related disorders (see Chapters 206 and 212). The correlation among high BMI (>27 kg/m^2), PCOS, and androgen excess has been examined. Insulin resistance was more likely to occur in obese PCOS patients, but gonadotropins LH, androstenedione, DHEA, and DHEA-S were significantly higher in low-BMI PCOS patients than in weight-matched controls.[13] Moreover, testosterone level was independent of BMI.[13]

Androgen abnormalities causing hirsutism and occasionally virilism include those found in NCCAH, acromegaly (a rare nonandrogenic cause related to GH excess), and Cushing syndrome with or without virilization caused by tumor (see Chapters 204 and 205). Serum DHEA and DHEA-S levels are highest in adrenal carcinoma and lowest in adrenal adenoma. Serum DHEA level varies directly with ACTH excretion, so a decrease in ACTH corresponds with a decrease in DHEA. Cases in which the ACTH is high but the DHEA and DHEA-S are low are attributed to Cushing syndrome or ectopic ACTH syndrome, seen without adrenal growths. SHBG is also diminished in hypothyroidism, although hypothyroidism is more likely to lead to hypertrichosis (see Chapter 214).

In NCCAH an enzyme deficiency of 21-hydroxylase (21-OH), associated with the *CYP21A2* gene, causes an accumulation of 17-hydroxyprogesterone (17-OHP). Two other, rarer congenital adrenal hyperplasia (CAH) deficiency syndromes associated with virilization are 11β-hydroxylase (*CYP11B1* gene mutation) and 3β-hydroxysteroid dehydrogenase deficiency.[12]

CLINICAL PRESENTATION

Establishing a baseline is important because prior hair removal will render an objective assessment of hair growth pattern inaccurate. Furthermore, chronic skin irritation might lead to hair coarsening because of local changes at the pilosebaceous unit. Constitutional or familial hirsutism is common in individuals of Mediterranean or Middle Eastern descent but far less common in Asians. Inquiring about familial hair growth, acne, menstrual abnormalities, diabetes mellitus, hyperlipidemia, early-onset cardiac disease, maternal obesity, CAH, and a cancer diagnosis[3] as well as prior diagnosis or treatment of hirsutism will serve in the initial screening.

Gonadal abnormalities are indicative of elevated androgen levels and can be ascertained by a history of abnormal sexual development. Prepubertal androgenism or hermaphroditism might relate to CAH seen in early adrenarche or with adrenal tumors. Further workup is essential if signs of precocious puberty, clitoromegaly, fourchette development, or gonadal hypospadias are described. New-onset nipple discharge in a nonlactating woman is a key finding. A menstrual history and menopausal status should be elicited. Prepubertal or peripubertal stress causing an exaggerated adrenarche may be a contributing factor to cortisol overproduction and risk of PCOS.[11] Infertility may point to anovulation or oligo-ovulation. Irregular or intermenstrual bleeding may indicate the presence of endometrial neoplasm.

Exogenous hormone use may also play a role, whether for menstrual cycle control, acne management, or perceived competitive advantage among athletes. Thyroid replacement therapy can lead to manifestations of overtreatment, a rare cause of hirsutism. Hot or cold intolerance, sluggishness, tremors, hair thinning, weight gain, skin texture changes, and depression would suggest hypothyroidism. Hyperhidrosis; enlarged hands, feet, and face; and deepened voice might point to acromegaly.

Patients with PCOS or Cushing syndrome are likely to have lipid and insulin abnormalities to differing degrees, even metabolic syndrome. Cushing syndrome is evidenced by excess ACTH from unsuppressed androgen. Mood or sleep changes, weight gain, glaucoma, osteoporosis, increased susceptibility to illness, weakness of upper arms, and signs of steroid excess in facies or skin might be seen with Cushing syndrome. By contrast, excessive thirst or appetite might point to glucose intolerance. Dyslipidemia and hypertension are common in PCOS; depression, sleep apnea, and endometrial carcinoma have also been associated with PCOS. Visual changes or headache could relate to a pituitary tumor. Finally, surgical history related to endocrine or metabolic disease management may be relevant.

PHYSICAL EXAMINATION

Weight, height, and vital signs are especially pertinent given the profile of a significant proportion of patients with PCOS. Significant weight gain is important in consideration of ACTH excess. Obesity is seen in patients with PCOS or Cushing syndrome (see Chapter 206), although Cushing syndrome may show up as a mixture of the following, depending on severity: central obesity, extremity or muscle wasting, red striae, supraclavicular fat pads, moon facies, thin skin or bruising, and sometimes a buffalo hump. A rise in blood pressure and concomitant hirsutism could raise suspicion for excess ACTH in Cushing syndrome or acromegaly, although acromegaly is not commonly associated with hirsutism. Acanthosis nigricans, a pigmented patch on the back of the neck, elbows, knuckles, knees, or intertriginous regions, is seen commonly in obese women and is indicative of insulin resistance.

Thickened facial features, frontal bossing, prognathism, visual field defects, enlarged hands and feet, hyperhidrosis, or macroglossia may indicate the rare case of acromegaly. Thyroid enlargement or goiter should be noted and an abdominal examination performed to exclude masses.

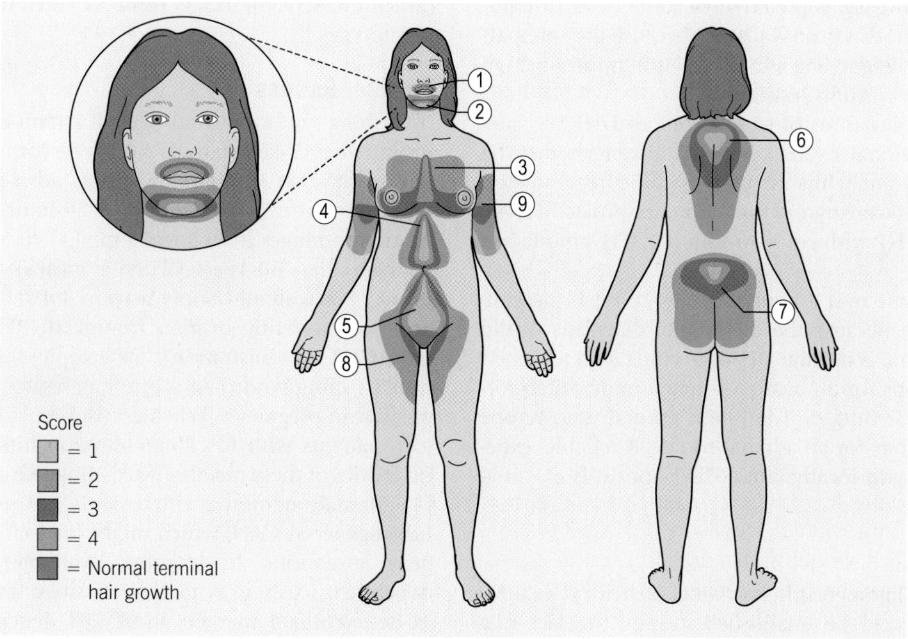

FIGURE 207-1 The modified Ferriman-Gallwey (mFG) hirsutism scoring system. In this system, nine body areas are evaluated for the amount of terminal hair growth. A score of 0 (no terminal hair growth) up to 4 (frankly virile) is given to each of the nine areas, and these are added together to compute a hormonal hirsutism score (mFG score). A total score below 3 is considered normal for East Asian and Native American females, whereas below 8 is considered normal in other populations. (From Bolognia, JL, Schaffer JV, Duncan KO, Ko CJ: *Dermatology essentials,* St Louis, 2014, Elsevier.)

Typically, androgen excess is thought to include hirsutism, acne, and male pattern alopecia. PCOS might include skin tags.[8] On the other hand, general hair loss might relate to hypothyroidism.

An essential component of the physical examination must include an objective measurement of hair growth pattern and quantity. Such an assessment has been captured by the standard Ferriman-Gallwey scoring system, originally established in 1961,[1] as well its modified form by others (the mFG; Fig. 207-1). The mFG serves to establish hirsutism clinically by rating nine body areas on a scale of 0 to 4 (upper lip, chin, chest, upper and lower back, upper and lower abdomen, arm, and thigh, excluding the original forearm and lower leg, which contribute less because these areas are overly androgen sensitive) (see Fig 207-1). Limitations of the mFG include poor inter-rater reliability and lack of sensitivity in the composite to heavily weighted areas that are particularly affected, such as on the face, lack of adjustments for racial variations, and the failure to assess the patient's perception of unwanted hair. A score higher than 8 in nonblack, non-Southeast or non–Far East Asians[3] indicates moderate hirsutism; a score higher than 15 indicates moderate to severe hirsutism and is an independent risk for PCOS.[9] Terminal hair on the upper back, shoulders, upper chest, cheeks, or upper abdomen delineates male pattern hair growth; masculinization involves huskiness of the voice, increased pectoral muscle mass, balding, mammary atrophy (defeminization), and, in cases of virilization, a fully deepened voice, changes in libido, and clitoromegaly.[14] Sexual ambiguity—such as downward placement of the urethral meatus or joining of posterior labial folds—may denote a congenital defect. A pelvic examination is performed to assess for the presence of ovarian masses. Pregnant women may need careful monitoring in the face of gestational hirsutism; postpartum patients and their newborns are observed for regression of virilization, once malignant causes have been excluded.[1]

DIAGNOSTICS

A hormonal evaluation in slow-onset, peripubertally hirsute, nonvirilized, normally menstruating patients should be deferred because the yield is low. Diagnosis in this population relies heavily on the physical examination and evidence of virilism. Newly developed, moderate hirsutism (Ferriman-Gallwey hirsutism score >15) in postpubertal women as well as hirsutism with virilization requires diligent investigation. Although methods of hair analysis include the weighing of plucked or shaved hair, and even microscopic observation and measurements of the shafts, the mFG is preferred in general.

Testosterone

Androgen measurements are subject to diurnal variation and other influences. Imprecise commercial assays may have inadvertently contributed to past misdiagnosis of idiopathic hyperandrogenism or idiopathic hirsutism.[2] Testing includes an early morning plasma total testosterone level followed by a free testosterone level should an abnormality arise. Although a normal testosterone level does not exclude hyperandrogenism, it is more leading for idiopathic hirsutism and the absence of malignant disease. Some use a free androgen index (FAI) or calculated free testosterone (CFT) level as part of a routine workup.[5] Lately, serum androgen levels are thought to be more sensitively measured through liquid chromatography with tandem mass spectrometry (LC-MS) or even immunochemiluminescence,[2] although they can be limited at the lower end of the range.[6] A CFT level from measurement of SHBG and total testosterone, rather than by direct assay, is preferred in some cases (if equilibrium dialysis methods are unavailable) because they are particularly helpful in diagnosing PCOS.[2,6] Furthermore, a high serum SHBG suggests insulin resistance.[2]

In cases of mild elevations of testosterone or DHEA-S, late-onset CAH or functional ovarian hyperandrogenism may be considered.[5] In moderately hirsute patients, if the free testosterone is 200 ng/dL or lower, thyroid function tests, prolactin level, and possibly a 17-OHP with corticotropin (ACTH) stimulation test should follow.

A testosterone value over 200 ng/dL (6.94 nmol/L) necessitates a serum DHEA because the differential diagnosis would include adrenal tumor. A normal DHEA-S with a high testosterone level is suspicious for an ovarian source tumor; an abnormal DHEA-S above 700 μg/dL (despite a normal testosterone level) is also suspicious for an adrenal source. A reliable, experienced laboratory, with locally established norms, is essential for accurate testing.

Ovarian Source

Documentation of oligomenorrheic or amenorrheic cycles from puberty onward should be established despite the fact that some patients will have regular but anovulatory cycles. Serum antimüllerian hormone might indicate PCOS, but this is controversial.[3,6] In the face of moderate to severe hirsutism, serum LH and FSH and an LH/FSH ratio of 2:1 or 3:1 can be helpful in supporting a diagnosis of PCOS. A midluteal serum progesterone level helps screen for anovulation.[8] Some specialists perform a 2-month gonadotropin suppression test to divide patients into gonadotropin-dependent (testosterone falls) versus gonadotropin-independent (testosterone does not fall) women with normal BMI.[13] This can delineate an ovarian versus adrenal source in an otherwise difficult-to-diagnose group.[13]

Ultrasound can be helpful in establishing the number of ovarian follicles (12 or more) and ovarian volume (2 to 9 mm or over 10) in order to establish PCOS (although this is still controversial) unless there is reason to suspect a tumor.[2] The presence of a pelvic mass warrants a pelvic computed tomography (CT) scan.

Adrenal Source

DHEA-S is seen as a screen for adrenal gland production to help distinguish tumors of adrenal origin in the face of virilization and a high testosterone level. Values above 700 μg/dL (13.6 mmol/L) are suggestive of adrenal hyperandrogenemia. With an abnormal free testosterone level, a transvaginal or adrenal ultrasound examination or adrenal CT study is needed. An elevated DHEA-S level should be followed by an adrenal ultrasound study or CT scan. Serum testosterone concentration would be high in patients with Cushing syndrome caused by an adrenal adenoma or carcinoma. A cushingoid appearance may result from an adrenal mass larger than 6 cm.[10]

Further testing for 21-OH–deficient NCCAH can be determined by high basal 17-OHP (>200 ng/dL or 6 nmol/L) in the early-morning follicular phase. If the 17-OHP levels are between 300 and 1000 ng/dL, then an ACTH stimulation test yielding a poststimulation 17-OHP value higher than 1000 ng/dL leads to a diagnosis of NCCAH or late-onset CAH; 21-OH deficiency values of 1000 ng/dL or lower may indicate a heterozygous 21-OH deficiency carrier.[9] Because the more severe form is discovered in infancy, a serum 17-OHP has become a required newborn screening test in the United States. Clinically it can be difficult to separate PCOS from NCCAH; there are overlapping phenotypes.[11]

Cortisol Excess

If Cushing syndrome is suspected, an initial 24-hour urine collection for 17-ketosteroids and free cortisol or an overnight dexamethasone suppression test is advised in the setting of rapid hirsutism or virilization. A 24-hour 17-ketosteroid concentration ranges from 5 to 15 mg (17 to 52 mmol) in women younger than 30 years (when it peaks). A positive 24-hour urine 17-ketosteroid study screens for adrenal androgens, an androgen-secreting ovarian tumor, an ACTH-secreting tumor (or ACTH administration), an ectopic androgen-secreting tumor, Cushing syndrome, a pituitary source, or PCOS. It may be positive in pregnancy. When cortisol replacement levels are too low, patients with CAH may develop hirsutism.[2] The relative quantities of these metabolites distinguish among three entities: (1) adrenal carcinoma with or without Cushing syndrome, (2) heterogeneous CAH, which might carry *CYP11B1* and *CYP21A2* gene mutations (genotyping available), and (3) ACTH-dependent Cushing syndrome. Positive testing for 17-OHP or 11-deoxycortisol markers in 21-OH deficiency of NCCAH or late-onset CAH, as guided by community prevalence,[2] as well as 3β-hydroxysteroid dehydrogenase deficiency,[12] accounts for 2% to 4% cases of hirsutism.[9]

Insulin Excess

HAIRAN, the combination of hyperandrogenism, insulin resistance, and acanthosis nigricans, is diagnosed with a fasting basal insulin level or an insulin level during a tolerance test.[4] A glucose tolerance test and lipid profile are valuable if dyslipidemia, insulin resistance, hyperinsulinemia, or diabetes mellitus is suspected. High circulating insulin levels affect the thecal cells of the ovaries. A spectrum of dermatologic signs—seborrhea, acne, hirsutism, and acanthosis nigricans—may feature in HAIRAN or reflect other causes of hyperandrogenemia, including hyperprolactinemia.[14] Because obesity is a contributing factor, BMI, cholesterol level, and blood pressure are pertinent.

Prolactin Excess

In the absence of testosterone, DHEA-S, cortisol, or 17-hydroxyhydrolase abnormalities, amenorrhea and hirsutism can occur in the setting of a prolactin tumor. Galactorrhea warrants measurement of a prolactin level; increased levels are indicative of hyperprolactinemia and possible thyroid dysfunction, although this is rare. In these cases, thyroid-stimulating hormone (TSH) and FSH are also measured. The pituitary is imaged by magnetic resonance imaging (MRI) to search for a prolactinoma.

Pituitary Source

Somatomedin C (insulin-like growth factor 1 [IGF-1]) testing is the most sensitive for acromegaly when clinical signs are leading, including vision changes, vision loss, and headaches, depending on the location of the tumor. IGF-1, a GH byproduct of the liver, may also lead to elevated insulin, lipid, and thyroid hormone levels. Another GH effect is hypogonadism. IGF-1 elevation warrants pituitary MRI to assess for adenoma. Untreated or unsuccessful treatment of acromegaly can lead to sleep apnea, diabetes (insulin resistance, increased lipid levels), hypercalciuria, colonic polyps or colorectal cancer, osteoporosis, hypertension, cardiomyopathy, arrhythmias, and cardiovascular disease (see Chapter 204).

Thyroid-Stimulating Hormone Excess

Hypothyroidism may result in hypertrichosis (see Chapter 214).

5α-Reductase Excess

No specific test exists for 5α-reductase excess, the effects of which are appreciated clinically. It may be that an otherwise idiopathic presentation of hirsutism relates to local mechanisms at the level of the pilosebaceous unit. Typically, there are no adverse sequelae, if the results of all other testing are normal.

Amenorrhea

Absent any other cause of hypothalamic-pituitary-adrenal, ovarian, pancreatic, thyroid, or metabolic (carbohydrate and lipid) dysfunction, a pregnancy test is indicated.

Pregnancy

Normal physiologic changes during pregnancy lead to increasing testosterone because of increasing serum SHBG, along with other androgens, which may result in hirsutism. Benign and malignant ovarian tumors may contribute to maternal and fetal virilization. Persistent corpus luteum of pregnancy requires imaging to diagnose.[14]

DIAGNOSTICS

Hirsutism

LABORATORY

- Total testosterone
- Free testosterone*
- DHEA*
- DHEA-S*
- LH*
- FSH*
- LH/FSH ratio*
- 24-Hour urinary excretion test for 17-ketosteroid*
- Early morning serum 17-OHP or serum 11-deoxycortisol with before and after ACTH stimulation for 21-OH deficiency of NCCAH*
- Prolactin*
- TSH*
- Glucose tolerance test*
- Fasting basal insulin*
- Free cortisol*
- Lipid profile*

IMAGING

- Pelvic ultrasound, pelvic CT scan*
- Abdominal ultrasound, CT scan*
- Adrenal CT scan*
- Abdominal MRI*

OTHER DIAGNOSTICS

- ACTH stimulation test*
- Dexamethasone suppression test*
- 24-Hour urinary excretion test for cortisol*
- Serum IGF-1*
- Genotyping*

*If indicated.

DIFFERENTIAL DIAGNOSIS

The onset of hirsutism most often corresponds to a variety of circumstantial or underlying medical conditions: initiation of virilizing drugs, progestins, steroids, or the antiseizure medication valproic acid; discontinuation of oral contraceptives; recent weight gain; ovarian or insulin disorders; and the onset of puberty or menopause. Medications intended to address sexual dysfunction or to promote athleticism are easy to link to signs of androgen excess, and prompt discontinuation should reverse hirsutism in the absence of occult disease. Oral contraceptives that serve to increase SHBG may be suppressing increased testosterone production until they are withdrawn. Progestins or steroids promote androgen production, as does hyperinsulinemia.

An investigation into conditions of insulin resistance is warranted with hirsute patients because hyperinsulinemia correlates inversely with SHBG concentrations. For patients with PCOS, the constellation of oligomenorrhea, amenorrhea, acne, seborrhea, alopecia, obesity, and ovarian cysts is often seen in conjunction with hirsutism. Normoandrogenic hirsutism is the second most commonly diagnosed condition after PCOS and is referred to as idiopathic hirsutism, in which ovulation and androgen hormone levels are normal and ovaries are not polycystic. However, some researchers believe that this categorization is imprecise, pointing to a subset of 40% of clinically hirsute patients who prove to be anovulatory with careful testing (luteal phase progesterone levels below 3 to 5 ng/mL) and actually have PCOS.[15] A significantly rarer consideration is CAH detected either in vivo or early in life and its milder form, NC-CAH, indicated by excess cortisol precursors after an ACTH hormone challenge. CAH is an autosomal recessive trait that appears in 1 in 1000 to 2000 individuals[11]; it is evidenced by mixed genitalia and salt wasting at birth, a positive family

DIFFERENTIAL DIAGNOSIS

Hirsutism

CONGENITAL

- CAH (classic CAH)
- Congenital late-onset adrenal hyperplasia, nonclassic (NCCAH)—21-OH or 11β-hydroxylase deficiencies)

ENDOCRINE

- Acromegaly†
- Androgen-secreting adrenal tumor†
- Androgen-secreting pituitary tumor†
- Ectopic ACTH-secreting tumor†
- HAIRAN (hyperandrogenism, insulin resistance, acanthosis nigricans)†
- Hyperprolactinemia†
- Hypothyroidism (as single presenting factor)†
- Insulin resistance, severe
- Morbid obesity

IDIOPATHIC

- Idiopathic hirsutism
- Idiopathic hyperandrogenism

PHARMACOLOGIC

- Iatrogenic hirsutism (bimatoprost, interferon alfa, mycophenolate, tacrolimus, progestins, psychiatric medications, among some rare others)
- Steroid use (anabolic and androgenic)

REPRODUCTIVE

- Androgen-secreting ovarian tumor (arrhenoblastoma-Sertoli-Leydig cell tumors—large; lipoid tumor—small; hilus cell tumor—small); ovarian hyperthecosis
- Gestational androgen excess of pregnancy (persistent corpus luteum or tumors)
- PCOS*

*Most common.
†Rare causes.

history, and Ashkenazi Jewish (3% to 4%), Hispanic, or Slavic descent. NCCAH might manifest as prepubertal hirsutism, early-onset puberty, irregular menses, or delayed menses. NC-CAH is said to affect 1 in 100 to 1000 women in the United States and can lead to serious complications In the presence of elevated ACTH levels, the differential diagnosis should include Cushing syndrome, glucocorticoid resistance, and anabolic steroid use. Urgent consideration is advised in the condition of hirsutism with concomitant virilism. Adrenal tumors (benign or malignant), enzyme deficiencies, and endocrinopathies are considerations if virilization accompanies hirsutism. Nonmalignant hyperthecosis of the ovary usually occurs in premenopausal women. Sertoli-Leydig cell tumors of the luteinized thecal cells of the ovary can be present in patients aged 20 to 40 years, sometimes in conjunction with HAIRAN. In these cases, removal of the often unilaterally affected ovary returns testosterone levels to normal and reverses signs of virilism. Other ovarian tumors include arrhenoblastomas and hilar cell tumors, which can lead to excess testosterone levels. A panel of androgen hormones (testosterone, androstenedione, DHEA, and DHEA-S) and imaging studies guide the diagnosis of pituitary, adrenal, or ovarian tumors.

MANAGEMENT

The causes of central hair growth are most often benign and can be managed effectively with a combination of medical therapy and mechanical hair removal. Because a woman's appraisal of her appearance is influenced by cosmetic and cultural standards, in cases of normal hair growth, reassurance is essential.

A commonly accepted, primary nonpharmacologic strategy is weight reduction in the overweight or obese patient. Decreasing weight lowers insulin resistance and reduces hyperandrogenism. There may also be cardiac and insulin resistance benefits to weight loss. A loss of 5% can restore regular menses or ovulation in some patients with PCOS.[6] Furthermore, smoking cessation is also critical to mitigate vascular embolic risk, particularly in patients on hormonal therapy, and especially in patients older than 35.

Cosmetic measures are advisable in all patients who desire temporary or permanent removal of unwanted hair. A temporary method is depilatory cream, which dissolves hair but may lead to skin irritation, allergic dermatitis, or permanent skin damage. Although shaving (which may cause stubble to appear coarser and thicker) and plucking (which is uncomfortable and can stimulate hair growth, folliculitis, and scarring) can be used on small areas, waxing removes hair at the base of the pilosebaceous unit and is more effective as a short-term solution, although it may produce superficial burns and infection. Bleaching of the hair is also a temporary measure until these hairs are shed and new ones replace them.

Electrolysis requires the insertion of a fine needle into the base of a hair follicle and the administration of electric current to permanently destroy the follicle. It is a popular although costly procedure, and results vary because it is highly operator dependent. Galvanic electrolysis may yield better results, especially if paired with thermolysis, called "blended treatment."[2] Caution is advised if acne, skin infection, diabetes mellitus, epilepsy, ischemic heart disease, in situ pacemaker, or artificial joints are present. Although painstaking and expensive, it can be permanent because it destroys the dermal papilla. Thermolysis treats more follicles at a time, in a similar manner, with alternating current. Temporary skin irritation can follow.

Patients who choose waxing or electrolysis should be instructed to observe for possible signs of infection. Eflornithine hydrochloride 13.9% topical cream has been shown to slow hair growth by inhibiting ornithine decarboxylase, which regulates cell proliferation at the follicle,[12] although this is a temporary treatment, requiring 8 to 24 weeks of twice-daily application for maximum effect and indefinite use thereafter. It can be combined with combined oral contraceptives (COCs) for better efficacy.

Laser hair removal by ruby, alexandrite, diode, or neodymium:yttrium-aluminum-garnet (Nd:YAG) laser as well as broad-band intense pulsed light therapy with or without radiofrequency for light hair (all representing differing red to infrared wavelengths in nanometers) has been shown to produce long-lasting effects, even permanent hair reduction.[4] Best results of laser therapy generally occur in patients with dark hair and light skin, although some experience complications such as hyperpigmentation or hypopigmentation of the skin.

Medications are used to suppress androgen secretion in the ovaries and adrenal glands or to block testosterone and DHT. Of the varied pharmacologic options, a first-line approach includes oral estrogen-progesterone agents (COCs), which have the added benefit of treating acne and oligomenorrhea. Oral contraceptives suppress ovarian androgen by inhibiting gonadotropin and LH secretion from the pituitary gland. Contraceptives also decrease adrenal DHEA-S through negative feedback on the glucocorticoid receptor. Aiming for 30 μg of ethinyl estradiol and 1 mg of synthetic progestin is seen as effective,[1-3] particularly because third-generation progestins have no adverse impact on metabolic profile, although they have slightly greater vascular risk.[2] This strategy is particularly effective in mild hirsutism.

Androgenic oral contraceptive pills, such as levonorgestrel, should be avoided. Progestins with low androgenic activity, which produce an antiandrogenic effect, are preferable. Norgestimate, desogestrel, and gestodene have been available longer than drospirenone, amiodarone HCL, trimegestone, and dienogest.[3,10]

Ultimately, the practitioner may want to stop medications after 1 to 2 years to see if any regression has been achieved and to observe for return of ovulatory function in premenopausal women. Unfortunately, the evidence in support of oral contraceptives as a means to effectively reduce unwanted hair is relatively weak because of limited studies and poor design.[9] Research has not borne out the relative efficacies of various combinations,[2] so treatment requires individualization. Antiandrogens are contraindicated in pregnancy, and birth control should be used with monotherapy.

A second option for treating androgen excess male pattern hair loss is choosing an antiandrogen in addition to COCs, particularly in cases of moderate to severe hirsutism, or as monotherapy if there is a contraindication to COCs. Spironolactone, 50 to 100 mg twice daily, although better known as a potassium-sparing diuretic, serves along with cyproterone acetate (CPA) and flutamide as a competitive antagonist at the androgen receptor. Spironolactone inhibits pituitary gonadotropin secretion and in turn the binding of testosterone and DHT to the androgen receptor, thereby improving the metabolic clearance of testosterone. Side effects rarely compel patients to discontinue drug therapy; however, nausea, vomiting, abdominal discomfort, diarrhea, fatigue, mental confusion, headache, dizziness, decreased libido, and sun hypersensitivity may follow. Known teratogenicity would prevent its use by women considering pregnancy. Hyperkalemia and postural hypotension are risks. Although there is some controversy as to whether the addition of an antiandrogen to COCs improves hirsutism more than monotherapy,[7] patients who do not respond to oral contraceptives or spironolactone treatments and are using effective birth control may ask about one of several antiandrogen compounds with ethinyl estradiol, such as cyproterone acetate (CPA). CPA is a steroid derived from 17-OHP. It blocks gonadotropin release and progestogen by binding to the DHT receptor.[10] The dose can be as low as 2 mg with drospirenone (co-cyprindiol), a weak antiandrogen. A dose of 12.5 to 200 mg/day (typically 50 to 100 mg) for 10 days of each menstrual cycle has become a standard. CPA is used widely in Europe, Canada and Mexico but is commercially unavailable in the United States. There is a risk of hepatotoxicity and smaller risk of thrombosis.

Finasteride, which inhibits 5α-reductase, decreasing the peripheral conversion of testosterone to the more potent DHT, is not approved for this indication. However, a small study showed that spironolactone with finasteride was more effective than monotherapy.[2] Finasteride doses range from 2.5 to 7.5 mg daily. Fortunately, antiandrogen in combination with COCs may serve not only to regulate menses but also to reduce endometrial hyperplasia risk.[2,16] There are significant teratogenic risks associated with finasteride.

Flutamide, a nonsteroidal antiandrogen, has been of interest given its efficacy. However, studies have failed to show an advantage among flutamide,[6] finasteride, or spironolactone, although finasteride and spironolactone have been used together to yield a 51% reduction in hirsutism score but with significant liver toxicity concern.[10] The latest recommendations from the Endocrine Society uniformly reject the use of flutamide (owing to risk of liver failure) topical gonadotropin-releasing hormone (GnRH) preparations, GnRH agonists (except in severe forms of hyperandrogenism, such as in ovarian hyperthecosis, after a failed trial of an oral contraceptive), glucocorticoid therapy (except in classic CAH or NCCAH caused by 21-OH deficiency, titrated against 17-OHP concentration for virilizing forms of CAH),[12] or insulin-lowering medication in treating hirsutism.

COMPLICATIONS

When an endocrinologist prescribes finasteride (5 mg/day) or low-dose flutamide (currently not FDA approved in women), which have been seen to have a significant impact on hirsutism, liver enzymes should be monitored regularly.[10] The combination of finasteride and flutamide has not been shown to surpass the effects of flutamide alone, but the significant risk of hepatotoxicity makes this combination very risky.[10] Patients must not become pregnant while receiving corrective hormonal therapy. The use of glucocorticoids to reduce hirsutism and to induce ovulation in NCCAH risks suppression of the hypothalamus-pituitary axis and induction of cushingoid features. PCOS can also accompany endometrial hyperplasia or other fertility concerns, which is likely to require other specialty collaboration.

Failure to diagnose an adrenal or ovarian tumor that may be malignant is a serious complication of hirsutism. Surgical removal of ovarian or adrenal tumors is recommended, although postsurgical complications, such as adhesions, are possible. The associated diseases of hyperandrogenism—diabetes mellitus, hypertension, and the possibility of estrogen-related cancers—are often associated with PCOS and necessitate careful follow-up monitoring. Gestational hyperandrogenism has potential complications for mother and baby.

INDICATIONS FOR REFERRAL OR HOSPITALIZATION

- Patients may be referred to an endocrinologist for androgen study abnormalities. Referral to an endocrinologist is appropriate if hirsutism is accompanied by virilism, which suggests the need for further imaging, androgen, insulin, or dexamethasone studies. An endocrinologist is also consulted for treatment failure or persistent infertility. Women with elevated androgens, insulin resistance, subfertility or infertility, and central obesity in particular require further follow-up, regardless of normal terminal hair distribution.
- A nephrologist should evaluate patients with insulin resistance and nephropathy or renal failure.
- A surgical consultation is indicated for the evaluation of patients with pituitary, adrenal, or ovarian tumors. Consideration of bariatric surgery in grade II or III obese patients may hold promise.[3]
- Although adult-onset acromegaly is largely associated with benign pituitary tumors, it is associated with much higher morbidity and mortality when it is untreated. The medical and surgical management of this multisystem disease requires specialist or multidisciplinary center expertise (see Chapter 204). The psychosocial effects of increasing body hair may warrant a psychiatric consultation if the hair has become a consuming concern. A mental health referral will be useful if there is reason to suspect underlying gonadal abnormality, such as chromosomal mosaicism or, in rare cases, hermaphroditism.
- Genetic counseling, or even fetal testing, may be appropriate in some cases.

LIFE SPAN CONSIDERATIONS

Hirsutism is a sensitive issue for adolescent girls, whose desire for peer acceptance may heavily influence body image and resulting health behaviors. Eating disorders related to PCOS are not unusual. Any menstrual cycle irregularities are of concern if they are accompanied by acne, alopecia, and hirsutism as well as insulin resistance because this might be a presentation of PCOS. Excessive hair growth can accompany pregnancy but usually disappears postpartum, often without long-term effects to mother or baby if sinister causes are excluded.

EDUCATION AND HEALTH PROMOTION

Education about realistic expectations of cosmetic hair removal, hair loss, and hair growth suppression as well as a reminder that even a drug holiday will likely return the patient to her previous hirsute status is essential. It will take 6 to 18 months to see a new set-point in hair growth.

Because oral contraceptives provide essential treatment for PCOS patients, avoidance of the 19-nortestosterone derivatives, including levonorgestrel, is important; they block the estrogen-mediated increase in SHBG concentration and are mildly androgenic. Patients using third-generation oral contraceptives should be advised of the possibility of thromboembolic events. All patients taking oral contraceptives should be strictly advised to stop smoking. Use of anabolic steroids for muscle building is strongly discouraged, given further potential adverse effects, such as cardiomyopathy.

The provider needs to address increased levels of anxiety and depression in women with PCOS and to provide reassurance about fears of masculinization, ridicule or social rejection, and sexual or gender identity. Sexual ambiguity in forms of CAH would be a high-priority concern to address. For patients with PCOS, a diet high in fiber and low in refined carbohydrates is encouraged, as is weight loss. Individual or group psychological counseling can help with self-image and weight management.

Women should be adequately counseled about their concerns and realistic expectations for future fertility. Because pregnancy is contraindicated during hormone therapy, pregnancy plans should be discussed in advance. Discontinuation of antiandrogen therapy will likely yield a return of terminal hair growth.

CHAPTER 208 HYPERCALCEMIA AND HYPOCALCEMIA

Alan Ona Malabanan

DEFINITION AND EPIDEMIOLOGY

A stable extracellular calcium concentration and proper compartmentalization of calcium are vitally important to a number of physiologic and cellular functions. A high intracellular calcium level can lead to organellar damage, aggregation of amino and nucleic acids, alteration of the integrity of lipid membranes, and phosphate (i.e., adenosine triphosphate) precipitation.[1] Consequently, aberrations in calcium homeostasis may lead to neuromuscular, cardiac, nephrologic, endocrine, coagulatory, and gastrointestinal dysfunction as well as to cellular and organism death.

Hypercalcemia, a high level of serum ionized calcium (i.e., ionized calcium >5.3 mg/dL), is a disorder in which the calcium level exceeds the upper limit of the normal range (i.e., total corrected calcium >10.5 mg/dL). Conversely, hypocalcemia is a low level of serum ionized calcium (i.e., ionized calcium <4.4 mg/dL), with a total corrected calcium level below 8.5 mg/dL. Both disorders can be a manifestation of a serious illness, such as malignant disease, or can be detected incidentally by laboratory testing in an asymptomatic patient. The calcium imbalance may have varied causes, may be chronic or acute, and may exhibit variable effects.

Hypercalcemia in the outpatient setting, most commonly primary hyperparathyroidism, is common; it has been estimated to be as high as 0.2% in patients older than 60 years,[2] although reports have suggested an initial declining incidence of 21.6 per 100,000 person-years[3] and a subsequent peak to 101.2 per 100,000 person-years and decline between 1997 and 2010.[4] Among inpatients, hypercalcemia is common in those with cancer (occurring in as many as 20%)[2] but also in critically ill patients (15%)[5] Hypocalcemia is common in hospitalized patients (18%) and particularly those in the intensive care unit (ICU; 85%).[6]

Physician consultation is indicated for patients with serum corrected calcium levels of less than 8.5 mg/dL or more than 10.5 mg/dL.

HYPERCALCEMIA

PATHOPHYSIOLOGY

Ninety-nine percent of the body's roughly 1 kg of calcium is found in the bone as hydroxyapatite. The remaining 1% is found in the extracellular fluid and soft tissues. Approximately 50% of plasma calcium is in the ionized, biologically active form; 10% is complexed in nonionic form; and 40% is protein bound, predominantly to albumin. Roughly 500 mg of the bone calcium is released from the bone each day in normal bone turnover.[7]

Alterations in albumin levels may cause changes in total calcium concentrations, without altering ionized calcium levels. The serum calcium concentration can be corrected for alterations in albumin by the following formula:

$$\text{Corrected serum calcium} = \text{Measured total calcium (mg/dL)} + ([\text{serum albumin (g/dL)} - 4.0] \times 0.8)$$

Alterations in acid-base balance may also alter ionized calcium levels. Increased acidemia decreases calcium binding to albumin and increases ionized calcium. Conversely, increased alkalemia increases calcium binding to albumin and decreases ionized calcium.

Extracellular calcium homeostasis is regulated primarily by the interaction between the calcium-sensing receptor (CaSR), parathyroid hormone (PTH), and 1,25-dihydroxyvitamin D_3 (calcitriol). PTH and calcitriol exert their effects through feedback mechanisms on three major organ systems: the skeleton, the intestinal tract, and the kidneys.

A decrease in serum ionized calcium is detected by the CaSR and stimulates the production of PTH. PTH has a direct effect on calcium and phosphorus through increased osteoclast activity, leading to bone resorption. PTH also directly stimulates the kidney tubules to reabsorb calcium and to excrete phosphorus, leading to a rise in serum calcium and a fall in serum phosphorus. PTH also increases renal conversion of 25-hydroxyvitamin D, the major circulating vitamin D metabolite, into calcitriol, the active vitamin D metabolite, which increases intestinal absorption of calcium and phosphate. Increases in serum calcium and 1,25-dihydroxyvitamin D levels inhibit release of PTH, reversing the process.

Hypercalcemia can be categorized as either PTH dependent or PTH independent, depending on whether PTH is nonsuppressed or suppressed, respectively. PTH-dependent hypercalcemia is typically a result of primary hyperparathyroidism, and PTH-independent hypercalcemia is typically a result of hypercalcemia of malignancy. Primary hyperparathyroidism results when an autonomous parathyroid cell line develops.

There are three malignancy-associated hypercalcemia PTH-independent mechanisms: humoral hypercalcemia of malignancy, local osteolytic hypercalcemia, and calcitriol-induced hypercalcemia. Humoral hypercalcemia of malignancy is the most common (approximately 80%) and is caused by excessive secretion of parathyroid hormone–related protein (PTHrP), which activates the same PTH-1 receptor activated by PTH. This has been associated with squamous carcinomas and breast and renal carcinomas. Local osteolytic hypercalcemia accounts for 20% of malignancy-associated hypercalcemia and has been associated with breast and hematologic cancers with widespread skeletal involvement. Calcitriol-induced hypercalcemia has been associated with lymphomas that increase production of calcitriol. Malignancy-associated hypercalcemia has also been associated with authentic ectopic hyperparathyroidism (i.e., non–PTHrP-related hypercalcemia).[8]

Milk-alkali syndrome, a combination of hypercalcemia, metabolic alkalosis, and renal insufficiency, develops in response to the simultaneous ingestion of large amounts of calcium and absorbable alkali, such as calcium carbonate. This is the third most common cause of hypercalcemia.[9] Disorders involving vitamin D or vitamin A excess or increased vitamin D activation lead to increased bone resorption and intestinal absorption of calcium. Hypercalcemia may also result from common mechanisms but rare causes, such as mammary hyperplasia and pregnancy (increased PTHrP), granulomatous disease from silicone injections (increased calcitriol), and betel nut consumption with oyster shell (milk-alkali syndrome).[10]

CLINICAL PRESENTATION

The presence and severity of symptoms in hypercalcemia are influenced by the magnitude of hypercalcemia, rate of rise of calcium, acid-base balance, and presence of hypoalbuminemia. A very high level of calcium may be tolerated chronically, whereas a less elevated but abrupt increase may cause significant symptoms. In general, however, corrected serum calcium levels below 11.5 mg/dL are rarely symptomatic.

The symptoms of hypercalcemia of any cause typically involve neuromuscular, cardiac, and gastrointestinal depression. Neurologic changes can range from the subtle, such as an inability to concentrate, increased fatigue, depression, or increased sleep requirement, to the dramatic, with confusion, delirium, stupor, or coma. Cardiovascular manifestations can include bradycardia, hypertension, electrocardiographic abnormalities such as arrhythmias (especially on digitalis), bundle branch or atrioventricular blocks, and shortened QT interval as well as cardiac arrest with severe hypercalcemia. Gastrointestinal symptoms are common and include constipation, anorexia, nausea, and vomiting. Peptic ulcers and pancreatitis are less common and may be more common with type I multiple endocrine neoplasia and primary hyperparathyroidism.[11,12] Renal symptoms can range from polyuria and nocturia (from nephrogenic diabetes insipidus), which can lead to volume depletion and worsened hypercalcemia, to nephrolithiasis, nephrocalcinosis, and renal failure.

PHYSICAL EXAMINATION

The physical examination findings are often unremarkable. Cardiovascular examination may reveal irregularity of rate and rhythm. Band keratopathy, calcium deposition in the cornea, may be present regardless of the cause of hypercalcemia. The presence of a neck mass (parathyroid carcinoma or medullary thyroid carcinoma in type IIA multiple endocrine neoplasia) or breast mass (breast carcinoma) may suggest the cause of the hypercalcemia. Central nervous system depression is reflected in hyporeflexia, changes in sensorium, muscle weakness, tremor, lethargy, and ataxia. With severe hypercalcemia, stupor and coma may result. There may be flank tenderness if nephrolithiasis is a complication. On occasion, pseudogout (calcium pyrophosphate dehydrate crystal deposition disease) may cause joint swelling or inflammation.

DIAGNOSTICS

The diagnosis of hypercalcemia is usually made by measuring the serum total calcium level along with a serum albumin level, with calculation of the corrected calcium concentration. In patients who are critically ill[13] or have chronic kidney disease,[14] the ionized calcium level may be useful. Once hypercalcemia has been confirmed, determination of the cause is the next step. Whereas the serum phosphate level (low in primary hyperparathyroidism) and the serum magnesium level (high in familial hypocalciuric hypercalcemia) may be useful, the intact PTH assay, ideally performed fasting, is the best test to determine whether the hypercalcemia is PTH dependent (PTH nonsuppressed) or PTH independent (PTH suppressed). If the hypercalcemia is PTH independent, further testing with serum calcitriol level, serum protein electrophoresis, and PTHrP level would be useful. A high or inappropriately normal serum calcitriol level should lead to an evaluation for tuberculosis, sarcoidosis, or lymphoma as a potential cause. A careful history of nonprescription supplements, such as calcium-containing antacids and cod liver oil, may be helpful in identifying milk-alkali syndrome or vitamin A or D toxicity as a cause of the hypercalcemia.

DIAGNOSTICS

Hypercalcemia and Hypocalcemia

LABORATORY
Serum calcium and serum albumin
Ionized calcium*
Intact PTH levels*
Serum 25-hydroxyvitamin D and 1,25-dihydroxyvitamin D*
Serum and urine protein electrophoresis*
Alkaline phosphatase*
Creatinine
Magnesium*
Phosphorus*

IMAGING
X-ray studies*
Bone scan*

OTHER DIAGNOSTICS
ECG*
Purified protein derivative testing*
Chest x-ray study*
Bone marrow biopsy*

*If indicated.
ECG, electrocardiogram.

DIFFERENTIAL DIAGNOSIS

Primary hyperparathyroidism and malignant disease account for 90% of hypercalcemia cases; primary hyperparathyroidism is the most common in the ambulatory patient, and malignant disease is the most common in the hospitalized patient. Primary hyperparathyroidism tends to have a milder, asymptomatic presentation with mild hypercalcemia; hypercalcemia of malignancy tends to occur in advanced and overt disease. Once these two diagnoses are excluded, consideration of milk-alkali syndrome, sarcoidosis, tuberculosis, vitamin D or A toxicity, and granulomatous disease may be based on the history and laboratory findings.

DIFFERENTIAL DIAGNOSIS

Hypercalcemia

PTH DEPENDENT
- Hyperparathyroidism (common)
- Lithium
- Familial hypocalciuric hypercalcemia (rare)
- Ectopic PTH secretion (rare)

PTH INDEPENDENT
- Malignancy (common)
  - Humoral hypercalcemia from PTHrP (common)
  - Local osteolytic hypercalcemia
  - Calcitriol mediated (lymphoma)
- Milk-alkali syndrome (common)
- Sarcoidosis
- Granulomatous disease (tuberculosis, HIV)
- Thyrotoxicosis
- Vitamin A or D toxicity
- Thiazide diuretic use
- Drug toxicity (theophylline, estrogens or antiestrogens, androgens, aluminum, foscarnet)
- Renal failure
- Addison disease
- Pheochromocytoma
- Immobilization
- Total parenteral nutrition
- Rhabdomyolysis

HIV, human immunodeficiency virus.

MANAGEMENT

Immediate emergency department referral is indicated for symptomatic hypercalcemia, particularly when it is associated with nausea or vomiting or a corrected serum calcium concentration above 12.0 mg/dL.

Management of hypercalcemia is tailored to the severity and acuity of the hypercalcemia. The management of mild hypercalcemia, usually caused by primary hyperparathyroidism, generally involves maintenance of hydration and volume status as well as avoidance of drugs that may worsen hypercalcemia.

Severe hypercalcemia, particularly with a corrected serum calcium concentration above 14.0 mg/dL, is a medical emergency and may require ICU care. Because the only way to remove calcium from the body is through the urine, the first efforts at treatment should be directed at aggressive restoration of volume status with intravenous normal saline, sometimes requiring as much as 6 liters in 24 hours (i.e., 250 mL/hr). With the increase in sodium and fluid delivery to the kidney, there is a concomitant increase in urinary calcium loss. Other electrolytes, such as potassium and magnesium, may be lost, and their levels should be monitored and corrected carefully. Furosemide has been commonly used to enhance urinary calcium losses, but there is scant evidence for its effectiveness and it is being recommended less often in current practice.[15] Parenteral salmon calcitonin is useful at further enhancing urinary calcium losses and can very rapidly lower serum calcium levels, although tachyphylaxis may develop, limiting its efficacy after 24 hours.

Further management is dependent on addressing the cause of the hypercalcemia. Hypercalcemia caused by intractable primary hyperparathyroidism or parathyroid carcinoma may be improved with cinacalcet (Sensipar),[16,17] although surgery is the only cure. Excessive bone resorption caused by hyperparathyroidism or hypercalcemia of malignancy from any cause will respond to intravenous pamidronate (Aredia) or zoledronic acid (Reclast), with improvements in the serum calcium concentration occurring in 24 to 48 hours. Glucocorticoids may have some usefulness in treating hypercalcemia caused by hematologic malignant neoplasms, probably because of their antitumor effects, as well as hypercalcemia from vitamin D intoxication or calcitriol-induced hypercalcemia (tuberculosis should be ruled out as a cause before initiation of glucocorticoids). Rarely, hemodialysis, plicamycin, or gallium nitrate may be necessary for control of serum calcium concentration.[2] Denosumab has been used off label to treat hypercalcemia of malignancy in patients not responding to bisphosphonates[18] or who have renal failure.[19]

LIFE SPAN CONSIDERATIONS

Among those with mild primary hyperparathyroidism, there is increased morbidity and mortality,[20] as there is in those on chronic hemodialysis with hyperparathyroidism and hypercalcemia.[21] Hypercalcemia of malignancy is a sign of advanced disease indicating an expected median survival of less than 60 to 90 days, although absence of any of the following prognostic factors may indicate a longer median survival: corrected hypercalcemia above 11.32 mg/dL, hypoalbuminemia, presence of liver metastasis, and squamous cell carcinoma.[20] Elevated ionized calcium levels above 1.4 mmol/L(5.6 mg/dL) are associated with ICU and hospital mortality in critically ill patients.[22]

COMPLICATIONS

A variety of complications may result from hypercalcemia, depending on the cause. In addition to the neuromuscular, renal, cardiovascular, and gastrointestinal complications mentioned previously, osteoporotic fractures and bone pain may result from hypercalcemia arising from increased bone resorption. Untreated severe hypercalcemia may lead to death.

HYPOCALCEMIA

PATHOPHYSIOLOGY

A low level of ionized serum calcium results from either increased calcium loss from the circulation (deposition in tissue, increased urinary excretion, increased binding within the circulation) or decreased entry of calcium into the circulation (malabsorption, decreased bone resorption). The causes of hypocalcemia can further be divided into inadequate PTH or calcitriol production, PTH or calcitriol resistance, and miscellaneous causes such as intravenous bisphosphonate use. PTH resistance may result from pseudohypoparathyroidism, a rare genetic disorder, or more commonly from chronic kidney disease or magnesium deficiency. Hypocalcemia resulting from vitamin D deficiency tends to be a late complication of long-standing disease.

CLINICAL PRESENTATION

As with hypercalcemia, the severity of hypocalcemia, the rapidity of its development, and the albumin and acid-base status determine its manifestations. A fairly low serum calcium level may be tolerated well if it developed slowly or if hypoalbuminemia and acidemia are present. Clinical manifestations of hypocalcemia are primarily associated with neuromuscular and cardiovascular dysfunction. Patients may have muscle weakness and cramping as well as tetany. Seizures, depression, and altered mental status and sensorium have been described. Patients may have generalized fatigue and congestive heart failure. Bronchospasm and laryngospasm can be a fatal complication of hypocalcemia. Patients may develop cataracts. Basal ganglia calcification may lead to a Parkinson-like motor disorder.[23]

PHYSICAL EXAMINATION

The physical examination may reveal features of spontaneous neuromuscular irritability with hyperreflexia of deep tendons. Chvostek sign (contraction of the facial muscle in response to tapping of the facial nerve against the bone anterior to the ear) and Trousseau sign (carpal spasm occurring after occlusion of the brachial artery with a blood pressure cuff for 3 minutes) are usually readily elicited. A Parkinson-like tremor may be present. Cardiovascular examination may reveal hypotension, impaired cardiac contractility, and bradyarrhythmias. Adults with chronic hypocalcemia may display coarse hair, dry and brittle nails, and scaly skin. A shortening of the fourth and fifth metacarpals may be seen in pseudohypoparathyroidism, a rare genetic disorder of PTH resistance. Evidence of increased intracranial pressure (papilledema) may also be noted. Subcapsular cataracts can be seen with slit-lamp examination.[6,23]

DIAGNOSTICS

As with hypercalcemia, once hypocalcemia has been confirmed, an intact PTH assay will help delineate the cause. A fasting serum phosphate concentration is also helpful; it is high in hypoparathyroidism and low in vitamin D deficiency. Serum magnesium and 25-hydroxyvitamin D concentrations should be assessed in all patients with hypocalcemia to identify those with hypomagnesemia or hypermagnesemia or vitamin D deficiency as a cause. Further testing with a 1,25-dihydroxyvitamin D level may be useful in identifying those with vitamin D–dependent rickets types I and II. A 24-hour determination of urine calcium and magnesium may be helpful in assessing patients who may have CaSR mutations, such as in autosomal dominant hypocalcemia. A tissue transglutaminase antibody test may be useful in confirming a diagnosis of celiac disease. An electrocardiogram provides a rapid way of assessing the calcium status by measuring the QTc interval, which is prolonged in hypocalcemia.

DIFFERENTIAL DIAGNOSIS

Chronic hypocalcemia can be ascribed to several disorders associated with an absence of PTH or with its ineffectiveness. Possible causes include surgery that involves the parathyroid (hungry bone syndrome) or thyroid, idiopathic hypoparathyroidism, pseudohypoparathyroidism, vitamin D deficiency, malabsorption syndromes, severe renal or liver disease, alcoholism and poor nutritional intake, osteoblastic malignant disease, pancreatitis, and hypomagnesemia or hyperphosphatemia. Hypoparathyroidism may occur in 12% soon after thyroidectomy but persists in less than 1%.[24] The cause is distinguished by clinical criteria, including duration of illness, symptoms of associated disorders, detection of hereditary features, and history of malnutrition and alcoholism. Acute transient hypocalcemia can be associated with severe sepsis, burns, acute renal failure, extensive blood transfusions with citrated blood, medications (foscarnet, intravenous bisphosphonates, denosumab), and pancreatitis.

DIFFERENTIAL DIAGNOSIS

Hypocalcemia

PTH DEPENDENT
- Hypoparathyroidism
  - Parathyroid or thyroid surgery
  - Idiopathic hypoparathyroidism (autoimmune)
  - Radiation therapy
  - Hemochromatosis
- Hypermagnesemia
- CaSR-activating mutation (autosomal dominant hypocalcemia)

PTH INDEPENDENT
- Vitamin D deficiency
- Malabsorption syndromes (celiac disease, gastric bypass surgery)
- Chronic kidney disease
- Liver disease
- Alcoholism
- Malnutrition
- Pancreatitis
- Hypomagnesemia
- Hyperphosphatemia
- Severe sepsis
- Burns
- Medications (amphotericin B, foscarnet, omeprazole, furosemide, bisphosphonates, denosumab)
- Extensive transfusion with citrated blood
- Pseudohypocalcemia (gadolinium contrast interferes with total calcium assay)

MANAGEMENT

Immediate emergency department referral is indicated for symptomatic hypocalcemia, particularly when it is associated with muscle cramping or stridor or a corrected serum calcium concentration below 8.0 mg/dL.

All patients with symptomatic hypocalcemia must be treated. Severe, symptomatic hypocalcemia in the presence of tetany, arrhythmias, or seizures should be treated emergently with intravenous administration of calcium. The treatment of hypocalcemia is guided by the acuity and severity of the hypocalcemia and the associated signs and symptoms. In acute, life-threatening situations, 1 or 2 ampules of calcium gluconate are diluted in 50 to 100 mL of 5% dextrose, infused during 10 to 20 minutes, and followed by a maintenance infusion of 10 ampules of calcium gluconate in 1 L of 5% dextrose at 50 mL/hr, titrated to symptoms and serum calcium level. With less severe symptoms, a more dilute calcium solution is infused during a longer period. Serum calcium concentration should be monitored frequently and the infusion adjusted accordingly. Until calcium levels have been restored, life-threatening symptoms such as hypotension and arrhythmias are refractory to medical management.

Vitamin D is the cornerstone of therapy for chronic hypocalcemia. Calcitriol is recommended (0.25 to 0.5 μg/day) with calcium supplementation as needed (500 to 1000 mg elemental calcium as calcium citrate or calcium carbonate two or three times daily with food, i.e., 200% to 300% of daily value). If renal function is intact, high-dose ergocalciferol (50,000 units daily) may be used, although the long-acting nature of this vitamin D preparation increases the risk for toxicity.[23]

Vitamin D and calcium can be varied independently. Higher doses of vitamin D allow more effective absorption of calcium from the intestinal tract. If intestinal absorption is inefficient, higher intakes of oral calcium permit adequate calcium assimilation. Dietary phosphate intake should probably be limited because excessive phosphate may lower serum calcium. The use of thiazide diuretics with sodium restriction in hypoparathyroidism lowers urinary calcium excretion, thus minimizing the risk for nephrolithiasis and allowing a lower dose of vitamin D and calcium supplementation. A low serum calcium level associated with a low serum albumin level does not require replacement. Serum pH, potassium, magnesium, and phosphorus levels should be monitored and corrected if necessary. This will usually correct hypocalcemia without further intervention.

LIFE SPAN CONSIDERATIONS

Chronic hypocalcemia can be managed by the patient's compliance with medications and close monitoring. Hypocalcemia may be associated with higher mortality among hemodialysis patients,[21] but this has not been shown in the general population.[25]

COMPLICATIONS

Complications of hypocalcemia include laryngospasm, airway obstruction, tetany, seizures, cardiac arrhythmias, coma, and death. Movement disorders, pseudotumor cerebri, and cataracts may also result from neurologic calcifications.

INDICATIONS FOR REFERRAL OR HOSPITALIZATION

Treatment of both hypocalcemic crisis and hypercalcemic crisis always requires hospitalization. Immediate intravenous correction of the imbalance, either through replacement of calcium in hypocalcemia or through fluid replacement and diuresis in hypercalcemia, with concurrent cardiac monitoring, possible intubation, laboratory analysis, and diligent observation is required until stabilization occurs. Referral to an endocrinologist and an experienced parathyroid surgeon may be necessary if primary hyperparathyroidism is diagnosed. Malignancy-induced hypercalcemia should be managed by an oncologist.

PATIENT AND FAMILY EDUCATION AND HEALTH PROMOTION

Patient and family education should emphasize lifestyle changes, including diet, hydration, and mobility. Patients should learn to identify foods that are high in calcium and adjust their diets according to their imbalance. Patients with hypercalcemia should be instructed to continue weight-bearing exercise to help maintain bone health and to ensure adequate fluid intake. Patients and families should also be taught to recognize early signs and symptoms of calcium imbalance and be instructed to seek medical assessment early. Early and mild manifestations may be treated without hospitalization; however, if it is neglected, a calcium imbalance can be life-threatening.

CHAPTER 209

HYPERKALEMIA AND HYPOKALEMIA

Joanne Sandberg-Cook

DEFINITION AND EPIDEMIOLOGY

The amount of potassium present in the average human body is approximately 50 mEq/kg. Of this, 90% is found in intracellular fluid, 8% in skin and bones, and 2% in extracellular fluid.[1-5] The maintenance of this relatively small amount of extracellular potassium is critical. Both hypokalemia and hyperkalemia are associated with an increased risk of complications, including cardiac arrhythmias and sudden death.

The definitions of hypokalemia and hyperkalemia are stated in terms of extracellular (or serum) potassium levels. Normal values for serum potassium levels depend on individual laboratories, but the usual range for normal values is approximately 3.5 to 5 mEq/L. Potassium imbalances can be defined as acute or chronic and can be further defined by the degree of severity.

Chronic hypokalemia and hyperkalemia develop in a minimum of weeks to months, and acute hypokalemia and hyperkalemia occur during hours to days. Mild hypokalemia occurs at serum levels of 3.5 to 4 mEq/L; moderate hypokalemia, 3 to 3.5 mEq/L; and severe hypokalemia, below 3 mEq/L. Mild to moderate hyperkalemia is defined as a serum level of 5.5 to 6.9 mEq/L, and severe hyperkalemia as a serum level of 7 mEq/L or higher.

Levels of potassium in the intracellular and extracellular fluids do not always correlate, as seen in diabetic ketoacidosis. Severe depletion of intracellular potassium (termed potassium deficiency) as a result of osmotic diuresis (which leads to increased renal loss of potassium), despite normal or even elevated extracellular (serum) levels of potassium, is caused by insulin deficiency.[6] Once exogenous insulin has been administered, clinical hypokalemia can develop rapidly.[6]

In most cases, hypokalemia is drug induced; approximately 30% of all patients who are treated with non–potassium-sparing diuretics develop low serum potassium levels.[5] Most cases of chronic hyperkalemia are caused by renal failure; however, the increased use of spironolactone after the publication of the Randomized Aldactone Evaluation Study has resulted in a marked increase in morbidity and mortality from hyperkalemia, with an estimated 50 excess hospital admissions per 1000 additional prescriptions for spironolactone.[7]

Specialist referral is indicated for serum potassium levels lower than 3 or higher than 6 mEq/L.

PATHOPHYSIOLOGY

Potassium balance is affected by intake, excretion, and internal potassium regulation.[1-3] The minimum daily requirement for potassium intake in the normal adult is approximately 40 to 50 mEq.[1-3] Excretion occurs primarily in the kidneys and gastrointestinal tract, with a small amount excreted in perspiration. Internal potassium regulation depends on acid-base balance, plasma insulin levels, plasma catecholamine levels, and aldosterone activity.[3]

Because the kidneys are normally able to conserve potassium efficiently, hypokalemia is rarely a result of inadequate intake. The main causes of hypokalemia are increased renal loss from exogenous drug administration; primary or secondary hyperaldosteronism; and internal shifting of potassium from the extracellular to the intracellular space, which can occur with insulin administration or catecholamine excess (Box 209-1). Although vomiting may cause hypokalemia, it is not because of a loss of potassium from the gastrointestinal tract but rather because of secondary hyperaldosteronism related to volume depletion[8] or, more rarely, metabolic alkalosis from loss of gastric secretions.[5]

BOX 209-1

Causes of Hypokalemia

MEDICATION INDUCED
- Non–potassium-sparing diuretics
- Beta-adrenergic agonists

VASCULAR
- Malignant hypertension
- Renovascular hypertension

ENDOCRINE
- Osmotic diuresis
- Primary hyperaldosteronism
- Secondary hyperaldosteronism
- Hypomagnesemia
- Exogenous insulin administration
- Catecholamine excess
- Renin-secreting tumor
- Thyrotoxic hypokalemic paralysis

GENETIC
- Liddle syndrome
- Bartter syndrome
- Gitelman syndrome
- Congenital adrenal hyperplasia
- 11β-Hydroxysteroid dehydrogenase deficiency

RENAL
- Type 1 renal tubular acidosis
- Type 2 renal tubular acidosis

OTHER
- Familial periodic hypokalemic paralysis
- Leukemia
- Trauma
- Excessive licorice ingestion

BOX 209-2

Causes of Hyperkalemia

PSEUDOHYPERKALEMIA
- Traumatic venipuncture
- Severe leukocytosis

TRUE HYPERKALEMIA

Renal
- Renal failure
- Type 4 renal tubular acidosis

Medication Induced
- Angiotensin-converting enzyme (ACE) inhibitors
- Potassium-sparing diuretics
- Nonsteroidal anti-inflammatory drugs (NSAIDs)
- Trimethoprim-sulfamethoxazole
- Heparin
- Beta blockers

Endocrine
- Hypoaldosteronism
- Adrenal insufficiency (Addison disease)
- Insulin deficiency
- Acidosis

Other
- Sickle cell anemia
- Systemic lupus erythematosus
- Familial hyperkalemic periodic paralysis
- Rhabdomyolysis
- Tumor lysis syndrome

The kidneys' ability to maintain potassium homeostasis is preserved until the glomerular filtration rate (GFR) falls below 10 mL/min.[8] Therefore, chronic hyperkalemia in patients with GFRs exceeding 20 mL/min is most likely caused by drug therapy, a defect in mineralocorticoid activity, or a lesion within the cortical collecting system.[2] Causes of hyperkalemia are listed in Box 209-2.

CLINICAL PRESENTATION

The prevention of clinically significant hypokalemia and hyperkalemia is essential. In the absence of early detection and treatment, hypokalemia can cause serious complications and even death. The major symptoms are associated with skeletal muscle.[2,4] Hypokalemia causes hyperpolarization, which decreases impulse conduction and muscle contraction.[2] Flaccid paralysis, beginning in the extremities and moving centrally, can eventually lead to respiratory paralysis. Possible cardiac complications include ventricular arrhythmias. Typical electrocardiographic findings include ST-segment depression, flattening and inversion of the T wave, and prominent U wave.[2,4] The appearance and severity of these electrocardiographic abnormalities do not correspond to the degree of hypokalemia, and they should not be used as a substitute for monitoring of serum levels.[4]

Clinical manifestations of hyperkalemia are chiefly cardiac, although neuromuscular complications can also occur.[2] Electrocardiographic changes associated with hyperkalemia include peaked T waves (often the first finding on electrocardiography [ECG]), ST-segment depression, widening of the QRS and PR intervals, and loss of the P wave.[2] A late sign on ECG is the appearance of a sine-wave pattern,[2,4] which usually indicates impending ventricular fibrillation and asystole.[2]

Although cardiac manifestations are obviously the most dangerous sequelae of hyperkalemia, neuromuscular complications, including paresthesias and fasciculations in the extremities, may be seen. Peripheral paralysis can occur, but paralysis of the respiratory muscles is rare.[2]

PHYSICAL EXAMINATION

A thorough history is the most important part of the physical examination. Any history of diuretic use, laxative use, vomiting, diarrhea, abnormal urinary output, diabetes mellitus, or hypertension, as well as a thorough diet and medication history, should be elicited. The physical examination should include a full assessment of vital signs (including orthostatic blood pressures); assessment of volume status[5]; and examination of the neuromuscular system, including assessment of muscle strength and reflexes.

DIAGNOSTICS

Diagnostics should assess the degree of the potassium imbalance as well as the cause. Serum electrolyte values, blood urea nitrogen (BUN) level, serum creatinine concentration, serum glucose concentration, 12-lead electrocardiogram, and urinary electrolyte values should be obtained.

Hypokalemia

Persons whose hypokalemia is not iatrogenic (i.e., drug induced) or the result of vomiting, diarrhea, alcoholism, or excessive licorice ingestion[9] should be evaluated to determine the underlying cause of the hypokalemia. To effectively organize the diagnostic evaluation, those with hypokalemia may be subdivided into three groups: those with increased renal potassium excretion (>20 mEq/L) and hypertension, those with increased renal potassium excretion but without hypertension, and those with normal or decreased renal potassium excretion.

With concomitant hypertension, plasma renin activity (PRA) and plasma aldosterone levels should be measured but only after the hypokalemia has been corrected. Primary hyperaldosteronism is suggested if the PRA is suppressed and the plasma aldosterone levels are elevated. Secondary hyperaldosteronism will result in both a high PRA level and a high plasma aldosterone level. Liddle syndrome will also cause hypokalemia and hypertension, but both PRA and plasma aldosterone levels will be suppressed.[10]

DIAGNOSTICS

Hypokalemia

LABORATORY
Serum electrolytes
BUN
Creatinine
Serum glucose
Serum magnesium
Plasma osmolality*
Urinary potassium, random
24-Hour urine collection for potassium*
Urine osmolality*
Early-morning urinary pH*
PRA*
Plasma aldosteronism*

OTHER DIAGNOSTICS
ECG*
Arterial blood gases (ABGs)

*If indicated.

DIAGNOSTICS

Hyperkalemia

LABORATORY
Serum electrolytes
BUN
Creatinine
Serum glucose
24-Hour urine collection for creatinine clearance*
Plasma aldosterone*
Cosyntropin stimulation test*

OTHER DIAGNOSTICS
ECG
Arterial blood gases (ABGs)*

*If indicated.

When blood pressure is normal, measurement of serum bicarbonate helps further the differential diagnosis. Low serum bicarbonate levels are consistent with diabetic ketoacidosis, metabolic acidosis, or renal tubular acidosis (RTA).[5] Hypokalemia associated with hyperchloremic metabolic acidosis is suggestive of type 1 RTA; morning urinary pH should be checked. Levels that are higher than 6 are consistent with type 1 RTA.

High serum bicarbonate levels in normotensive patients are consistent with Bartter syndrome.[11] Bartter syndrome will also result in high PRA and plasma aldosterone levels, but this is quite rare and is usually seen only in children or young adults. In addition to having the abnormal laboratory findings, patients with Bartter syndrome typically are of short stature, have muscle weakness, and are normotensive.[11]

Hypokalemia and normal serum bicarbonate levels in normotensive patients may also be caused by magnesium deficiency.[12] Individuals undergoing chemotherapy and those with a history of alcoholism and malabsorption syndrome are at risk for the development of magnesium deficiency.[12]

On occasion, hypokalemia is not the result of increased renal loss; these patients will have low urinary potassium (<20 mEq/L).[5] The differential diagnosis is fairly limited and typically involves some sort of gastrointestinal loss, through laxative abuse, villous adenoma, or severe diarrhea. Patients previously treated with non–potassium-sparing diuretics who are potassium depleted will also have low urinary potassium. Catecholamine excess, whether endogenous (as in acute myocardial infarction) or exogenous (as in beta-adrenergic agonist administration), may also cause transient hypokalemia because of an increased cellular uptake of potassium.[5]

If the cause of the hypokalemia is still unknown after thorough investigation of past medical history, medication profile, and evaluation, referral to an endocrinologist is indicated.

Hyperkalemia

In patients with hyperkalemia, renal status should be determined. Individuals with chronic renal failure who previously had normal potassium levels should undergo a 24-hour urine collection to assess for creatinine clearance and should be questioned thoroughly about any dietary changes, infection, trauma, and use of nonsteroidal anti-inflammatory drugs (NSAIDs), spironolactone, and other medications. Numerous cases of trimethoprim-sulfamethoxazole–induced hyperkalemia have been reported.[13] Individuals with preexisting renal impairment or disturbances in potassium excretion or with human immunodeficiency virus (HIV) infection (see Chapter 230) and those treated with angiotensin-converting enzyme (ACE) inhibitors, angiotensin receptor blockers (ARBs), and spironolactone appear to be most at risk.[13]

Persons without renal failure and with hyperkalemia should be assessed for adrenocortical insufficiency (Addison disease), which almost always results in hyponatremia, hypotension, hypovolemia, and renal insufficiency (see Chapter 205). An adrenocorticotropic hormone (ACTH; cosyntropin) stimulation test (with referral to an endocrinologist) should be performed if Addison disease is suspected. Hyperkalemia may also result from hypoaldosteronism and is twice as common in patients with diabetes mellitus.[14] PRA and plasma aldosterone levels are diagnostic. Secondary hypoaldosteronism can result from the prolonged use of heparin, but in general the hyperkalemia is mild.[14] ACE inhibitors and ARBs also decrease aldosterone levels and can cause hyperkalemia. Tubular unresponsiveness to aldosterone may also cause hyperkalemia and may be seen in patients with sickle cell disease, systemic lupus erythematosus, and amyloidosis.[14]

DIFFERENTIAL DIAGNOSIS

Hypokalemia and hyperkalemia are caused by a variety of disorders. Hypokalemia is usually related to one or more of the following: extracellular-to-intracellular potassium shift or renal and extrarenal potassium losses. Inadequate potassium intake is a relatively uncommon cause of hypokalemia. Hyperkalemia is related to inadequate potassium excretion (often related to impaired renal function), excessive potassium intake, or intracellular shift of potassium from tissue to serum.

DIFFERENTIAL DIAGNOSIS

Hypokalemia and Hyperkalemia

HYPOKALEMIA
- Inadequate dietary intake (uncommon)
- Extracellular-to-intracellular potassium shift
- Renal and extrarenal potassium loss

HYPERKALEMIA
- Inadequate potassium excretion (renal insufficiency)
- Excessive potassium intake
- Intracellular shift of potassium to serum

MANAGEMENT

The management of hypokalemia and hyperkalemia begins with identification of the underlying cause. Except for patients who are surreptitiously inducing vomiting or using large amounts of diuretics or laxatives, the cause of the potassium imbalance is usually readily apparent. Most cases are a result of either diuretic use or renal failure. Hyperkalemia can also be a pseudohyperkalemia, which may be caused by traumatic venipuncture or, rarely, leukocytosis in the setting of leukemia.[14]

All at-risk patients should be frequently screened by laboratory analysis. When diuretics are being prescribed, the patient's serum potassium concentration should be checked before initiation of treatment and then 1 and 4 weeks after the initiation of therapy.

In persons with chronic hyperkalemia, any use of ACE inhibitors, ARBs, NSAIDs, potassium-sparing diuretics, or salt substitutes (those containing potassium chloride) should be reassessed and most likely discontinued.

Acute Hypokalemia

The treatment of acute hypokalemia involves the administration of oral or intravenous potassium supplements. If life-threatening arrhythmias or neuromuscular symptoms are present, intravenous potassium supplementation should be initiated.[5] Intravenous potassium concentration should not exceed 40 mEq/L and is usually infused at a rate of less than 10 mEq/hr.[12] Cardiac monitoring and frequent serum potassium assessment (every 3 to 6 hours) are essential. Once all cardiac arrhythmias or neuromuscular symptoms have disappeared, the patient may be switched to oral replacement. The normal dosage for oral potassium is 20 to 40 mEq once to three times daily until serum potassium is normalized.[12]

Chronic Hypokalemia

The primary goal of treatment of chronic hypokalemia is identification of the underlying cause. In cases of drug-induced hypokalemia, the medication should be changed, if possible. If the clinical status prohibits this, then treatment depends on the degree of hypokalemia. Some controversy exists as to whether individuals with mild hypokalemia (3.5 to 4 mEq/L) should be aggressively treated; however, they can certainly benefit from dietary teaching. In patients with potassium levels lower than 3.5 mEq/L, oral supplementation should be given, with normal doses ranging between 20 and 80 mEq/day. Persons with hyperaldosteronism should be referred to an endocrinologist and may be successfully managed with spironolactone or eplerenone; eplerenone has been associated with fewer side effects because of its low affinity for sex hormone receptors.[15] If an aldosterone-secreting tumor is identified, surgical removal may be indicated.

Acute Hyperkalemia

Treatment of acute hyperkalemia with life-threatening symptoms (in general, seen at potassium levels ≥7 mEq/L) is accomplished by the intravenous administration of calcium.[2,4] The usual recommended dose is 10 mL of a 10% calcium solution such as calcium chloride. The electrocardiogram should be monitored while the calcium is administered. Calcium should be administered only when electrocardiographic changes such as a widening QRS have occurred.[4] Calcium does not correct the underlying hyperkalemia; it only counters the adverse neuromuscular effects of hyperkalemia.[4] Calcium infusion should always be followed by specific therapy aimed at lowering of the plasma potassium level (i.e., insulin and glucose infusion; see later).

The intravenous administration of glucose and insulin is the quickest way to treat acute hyperkalemia that has not yet resulted in life-threatening sequelae.[4,16] This results in a shift of extracellular potassium into the cell.[4] Care should be taken in diabetic patients with hyperkalemia because glucose infusion that is not accompanied by a matching infusion of insulin can actually result in increased hyperkalemia because of extracellular hyperosmolarity.[17]

When the individual is able to safely take medication orally and life-threatening sequelae have not developed, treatment with sodium polystyrene sulfate (Kayexalate) in sorbitol solution may be used. This may be the treatment of choice in outpatients who are stable but have potassium levels in the range of 5.5 to 6.9 mEq/L. In patients unable to tolerate oral administration, polystyrene sulfate may be given rectally.[16]

Sodium bicarbonate is occasionally used in the treatment of hyperkalemia, both to treat the acidosis that may accompany hyperkalemia and to correct the hyperkalemia itself by causing a pH-dependent shift of potassium from the extracellular to the intracellular space.[4] Sodium bicarbonate should be used with caution, and care should be taken not to cause sodium overload or metabolic alkalosis.

Chronic Hyperkalemia

The most common cause of chronic hyperkalemia is renal failure; therefore the most common method of management of chronic hyperkalemia is dialysis. It is rare for intake alone to account for hyperkalemia because renal excretion increases with increased intake in patients with normal renal function. Diet modification is essential, however, in persons with renal failure and chronic hyperkalemia. Referral to a dietitian can be helpful.

The treatment of chronic hyperkalemia caused by hypoaldosteronism may be accomplished with oral polystyrene sulfate or furosemide, but the preferred treatment is fludrocortisone acetate (Florinef).[17] If Addison disease is diagnosed, treatment with replacement hydrocortisone should correct the hyperkalemia. Potassium plays a significant role in regulating blood flow to the skeletal muscle. An increased concentration of potassium in the muscle during muscle activity causes vasodilation, which results in an increase in blood flow to the area. During states of hypokalemia, blood flow to the muscle is mitigated, resulting in a relative ischemia and muscle cramps. Decreased serum potassium can contribute to muscle dysfunction, and severe hypokalemia may cause muscle necrosis and rhabdomyolysis.[18] In addition, research supports a possible association between hyperkalemia and decreased cognitive performance.

COMPLICATIONS

Potassium abnormalities are potentially life-threatening. Cardiac conduction defects, arrhythmias, ileus, paralysis, muscle weakness, increased blood pressure, and renal injury are consequences of hypokalemia. Hyperkalemia also causes cardiac arrhythmias, heart block, ventricular fibrillation, muscle weakness, and paralysis.

INDICATIONS FOR REFERRAL OR HOSPITALIZATION

Any patients found to have an underlying metabolic disorder as a cause of hypokalemia or hyperkalemia and patients in whom the cause of the hypokalemia or hyperkalemia is unknown should be referred to an endocrinologist. Individuals with hyperkalemia and renal disease should always be referred to a renal specialist. All persons with life-threatening symptoms of hypokalemia or hyperkalemia should be evaluated for possible hospitalization. Also, those with hyperkalemia and acute renal failure should be urgently hospitalized.

PATIENT AND FAMILY EDUCATION

Patient education for hypokalemia or hyperkalemia should center on diet education and awareness of the importance of continued chronic supplementation therapy and laboratory monitoring. Education about potential drug effects on hypokalemia or hyperkalemia is also important. Chronic laxative use should be avoided because this has been associated with potassium loss. Individuals with chronic hypokalemia should avoid large amounts of licorice, which have also been associated with hypokalemia. Those taking potassium supplements should be advised not to crush the potassium tablets and to swallow the tablet with a large glass of fluid. If untoward effects of potassium occur, the patient should be advised to call or to see a health care provider.

HEALTH PROMOTION

Because hyperkalemia is usually secondary to renal failure and hypokalemia is usually the result of diuretic use, health promotion should focus on the prevention of renal failure and hypertension. When prevention is no longer possible, patient education about the need for monitoring and prevention of complications is paramount.

CHAPTER 210

HYPERNATREMIA AND HYPONATREMIA

Terry Mahan Buttaro

Specialist referral is indicated for serum sodium levels of less than 125 mEq/L or more than 155 mEq/L.

HYPERNATREMIA

DEFINITION AND EPIDEMIOLOGY

Hypernatremia affects people of all ages but is one of the more common electrolyte disorders seen in children and older adults.[1] Defined as a serum sodium level of more than 145 mEq/L, hypernatremia can be caused by a fluid volume deficit, excessive sodium intake, chronic renal disease, or other disorders.[2]

PATHOPHYSIOLOGY

Normally, water intake and water loss are balanced, but a disruption in water homeostasis can result in hypernatremia. When water loss exceeds water intake, serum osmolality rises, and thirst is stimulated. Water balance is achieved as water intake increases. Thirst receptors are stimulated when serum osmolality rises above the normal range of 290 to 295 mOsm/kg. Destruction of the thirst centers in the hypothalamus as a result of neoplasm, trauma, or vascular abnormalities leads to an inadequate thirst response and hypernatremia. In older adults, physiologic aging changes may increase susceptibility to electrolyte changes, but anyone unable to adequately express thirst, such as infants and those with a decreased sensorium, are also at risk for development of hypernatremia.

An excess of water loss in relation to intake leads to increased serum osmolality. In response to this rise in serum osmolality, antidiuretic hormone (ADH), or vasopressin, is secreted from the posterior pituitary gland. ADH increases the permeability of the renal collecting ducts to water. As a result, water is reabsorbed in the collecting ducts, and the urine becomes more concentrated. Patients with a deficit in the production of ADH or a diminished renal response to ADH will develop hypernatremia if water losses are not corrected. Older adults are especially at risk because of the diminished renal concentrating ability that occurs with aging.

Patients with diabetes insipidus develop hypernatremia when water intake is not enough to compensate for fluid loss. Also at risk for the development of hypernatremia as a result of losing large amounts of free water are patients who have osmotic diuresis because of hyperglycemia or the administration of osmotic diuretics such as mannitol.[1,2]

Hypernatremia also develops with an increase in insensible water losses. Normally, small amounts of fluids are lost from the skin, respiratory tract, and gastrointestinal tract. Conditions such as fever, tachypnea, diarrhea, vomiting, and burns increase the volume of insensible water loss. Hypernatremia results if these losses are not replaced. Patients who exercise vigorously and drink an insufficient amount of liquid and those with insufficient fluid intake in the setting of fever, vomiting, or diarrhea are at great risk for development of hypernatremia.[1,2]

Increased serum sodium is less often the result of excess sodium intake, including rapid intravenous administration of normal saline or high-solute tube feedings. However, the resultant sodium excess can cause an increase in serum osmolality and expansion of extracellular volume.[1,2]

CLINICAL PRESENTATION AND PHYSICAL EXAMINATION

The major clinical feature of hypernatremia is a central nervous system disturbance that results from dehydration and shrinkage of brain cells. The purpose of the history and physical examination is to determine the underlying cause of the increased serum sodium and guide diagnostics as well as treatment.[3] A recent history of fever, vomiting, diarrhea, polyuria, heat exposure, or surgery is significant. A careful review of medications (particularly a history of lithium or diuretic therapy), fluid intake and output during the previous 24 hours, and any intravenous therapy or tube feedings should be reviewed along with the past medical history.

Patients may report weakness, thirst, or lightheadedness or, if the hypernatremia is related to a hypothalamic lesion, be asymptomatic. Signs and symptoms of hypernatremia can be nonspecific and not develop until the serum sodium level becomes higher than 150 mEq/L. Agitation, irritability, confusion, and personality changes are early signs. Muscle twitching, tremor, spasticity, hyperreflexia, and lethargy may also be seen. Coma, seizures, and muscle weakness are later signs. Thirst is usually present unless the thirst receptors are nonfunctioning. Indications of volume depletion include hypotension, tachycardia, and abnormal postural changes in vital signs. Weight loss, flat neck veins, dry mucous membranes, and diminished skin turgor may also be seen, depending on the severity of the volume loss.[1,2]

Diminished urinary output is also a possible finding, except in patients with diabetes insipidus or osmotic diuresis as the underlying cause of the hypernatremia. Fever, flushing, and dry mucous membranes may also be present.[1,2]

Classification of the patient's fluid volume status is facilitated by evaluation of the patient's appearance, weight, postural vital signs, passive leg raising, and careful examination of the pulmonary, cardiac, and gastrointestinal systems.[4,5] Neurologic screening, including motor tone, strength, coordination, and cognitive and functional ability, is necessary to determine subtle neurologic changes.

DIAGNOSTICS

- Address patient fluid volume status (e.g., weight, vital signs, orthostatic changes when feasible, passive leg raising).
- Determine if the serum sodium elevation is a result of water loss, sodium gain, or a combination of both.[4] Initial diagnostic testing includes serum glucose, serum electrolytes, urea, calcium, blood urea nitrogen (BUN) concentration, creatinine level urinalysis, urine sodium, and urine osmolality.
  - Calculated serum sodium and osmolality are determined with this equation: (2[Na^+] + serum glucose/18 + BUN/2.8)
    - Serum sodium level above 145 mEq/L confirms hypernatremia.
    - Serum osmolality will likely be more than 300 mOsm/kg; hypovolemic hypernatremia is the most frequent type of hypernatremia.
  - Urine osmolality is increased to more than 600 mOsm/kg, except in patients taking diuretics or in those with diabetes insipidus or osmotic diuresis.
  - Urine specific gravity is not as precise as urine osmolality but is a quick test to determine urine concentration. The urine specific gravity of patients with hypernatremia is elevated, except in the cases noted previously.
  - Urine sodium levels can be elevated, normal, or decreased.
- Diabetes insipidus is associated with polyuria, low urine specific gravity, and low osmolality (less than 200 mOsm/kg).[6]
- Other diagnostics to consider include the following:
  - Complete blood count (CBC) and differential if an infection is suspected
    - Serum hematocrit and red blood cells will be elevated.
  - Serum lithium, when indicated
- Imaging studies (i.e., computed tomography [CT] scan or magnetic resonance imaging [MRI]) may be necessary to exclude a neurologic cause.[7]

DIAGNOSTICS

Hypernatremia

LABORATORY
Serum glucose
Serum electrolytes, calcium, and urea
BUN
Creatinine
CBC and differential
Urine sodium
Urine osmolality
Urine specific gravity

IMAGING
CT scan, MRI if indicated

DIFFERENTIAL DIAGNOSIS

It is important to determine the underlying cause of the sodium imbalance because treatment options vary with the cause. The patient with hypernatremia resulting from diabetes insipidus is treated differently from the patient whose imbalance is a result of excessive diarrhea caused by the use of lactulose.

DIFFERENTIAL DIAGNOSIS

Hypernatremia

- Water depletion with insufficient water intake
- Excessive sweating and increased insensible water loss
- Diarrheal conditions
- Viral illnesses
- Hepatic encephalopathy with use of lactulose
- Abnormal thirst mechanism
- Increased renal water loss with inadequate fluid intake
- Diabetes insipidus
- Nephrogenic diabetes insipidus
- Central diabetes insipidus
- Osmotic dieresis
- Glycosuria
- Mannitol use for dieresis
- Chronic renal failure
- Use of loop diuretics
- Water loss from peritoneal dialysis
- Excessive sodium intake with inadequate water intake
- High-solute tube feedings
- Rapid intravenous administration of normal saline
- Hyperactivity of the adrenal cortex
- Hyperosmolar hyperglycemic nonketotic coma

MANAGEMENT

The primary goal of treatment is the replacement of water loss and restoration of extracellular fluid volume.

- Hypernatremia may be managed on an outpatient basis if the degree of sodium imbalance is moderate and the patient is alert and able to drink sufficient amounts of fluids.
  - Oral water replacement is the safest, if the patient is:
    - Cognitively intact
    - Able to swallow safely
    - Mobile enough to obtain drinking water
- Patients with more severe hypernatremia will require treatment in an inpatient setting.
  - For patients who are hypovolemic as well as hypernatremic (serum sodium 150 to 170), fluid resuscitation with intravenous normal saline (0.9%) or Ringer's lactate is initially indicated.
  - Once vital signs are normalized and urine output is adequate, the serum sodium level can be corrected.

- If the hypernatremia is caused by sodium gain, loop diuretics and maintenance of fluid volume with intravenous therapy that is hypotonic to the patient's urine is indicated.[4]
- If the hypernatremia is caused by fluid loss, fluid volume must be replaced with a hypotonic intravenous fluid (0.45% NaCl) or 5% dextrose in water at 0.5 mEq/L/hr but not greater than 1 mmol/L/hr.[1,4]
- Acute hypernatremia (less than 48 hours) should be differentiated from chronic hypernatremia (greater than 48 hours), because correction of acute hypernatremia is more rapid (8 to 12 mmol/L/day, 2 to 3 mmol/L/hr) than the correction of chronic hypernatremia (no more than 8 to 10 mmol/L per day, 0.5 mmol/L/hr).[4] Patients diagnosed with acute-on-chronic hypernatremia also require a rapid decrease (8 to 12 mmol/L/day) in serum sodium.[4] The infusion rate is critical for patients with hypernatremia because a rate that is too slow or too rapid increases the risk for death.[3,4]
- Serum sodium, urine chemistry, and fluid volume status are monitored frequently (i.e., vital signs, intake and output, daily weight plus serum glucose, electrolytes, BUN, and creatinine; calculation of serum osmolality initially 2 hours after therapy is started, then periodically throughout the day in acute hypernatremia) while the patient is receiving intravenous therapy.[4]

- Electrolytes should be replaced as indicated.
- Diuretics and laxatives should be held until the deficit is corrected. The need for these medications should then be reevaluated, as some patients may need a diuretic to prevent fluid overload.
- Hypernatremia caused by central diabetes insipidus is treated with vasopressin or desmopressin acetate (DDAVP) to decrease renal water losses.[6]
- Nephrogenic diabetes insipidus is treated by discontinuing the offending agent and correcting electrolyte abnormalities.[6] Serum electrolyte levels and fluid status must be monitored closely.

LIFE SPAN CONSIDERATIONS

Aging is associated with a decreased ability to cope with environmental, disease-related, and drug-related stressors in sodium and water balance. Hypernatremia is commonly associated with fever, dehydration, warm environments, high-solute tube feedings, and diuretic or laxative therapy.

COMPLICATIONS

If hypernatremia is not corrected, cerebrovascular damage occurs from brain dehydration and shrinkage. Hypovolemic shock results when severe volume depletion is not corrected. If hypernatremia is not corrected carefully, patients may experience significant cognitive dysfunction.[4] Patients with cardiac disease should be monitored closely for signs and symptoms of congestive heart failure, which may occur if fluid is replaced too rapidly.[1,3]

INDICATIONS FOR REFERRAL OR HOSPITALIZATION

Hypernatremia may be managed on an outpatient basis if the degree of sodium imbalance is moderate and the patient is alert and able to drink sufficient amounts of fluids.

Older adults living alone or those at risk for development of congestive heart failure may best be managed in an inpatient setting.

Patients with severe hypernatremia (serum sodium >155 mEq/L) or severe volume depletion should be hospitalized.[1,3]

PATIENT AND FAMILY EDUCATION

Patients and families should understand that 1500 to 2000 mL of fluid should normally be consumed each day. Patients at risk for hypernatremia should understand the importance of maintaining proper fluid balance.

Older patients in particular need to be aware of the dangers of dehydration, especially in hot weather or if fever is present.

Patients who are taking diuretics or medications such as lithium and carbamazepine (Tegretol), which cause hypernatremia, need to be aware of this side effect. Patients who exercise regularly should be educated about the need for appropriate fluid intake when exercising. Patients with underlying conditions that put them at risk for hypernatremia need to be educated accordingly.[1,4]

HYPONATREMIA

DEFINITION AND EPIDEMIOLOGY

Hyponatremia is a common electrolyte disorder and a significant cause of morbidity and mortality, particularly in older adults.[1,7] The costs associated with hyponatremia can approach 3.6 billion dollars each year and are largely related to hospitalization.[8] Potential causes of hyponatremia include infections, traumatic brain injuries, malignant disease, endurance exercise, untoward medication effects, endocrine disorders, psychogenic polydipsia, syndrome of inappropriate antidiuretic hormone (SIADH), cerebral or renal salt wasting, acquired immunodeficiency syndrome (AIDS), and other illnesses.[9,10] Hyponatremia may be related to a dysfunction in the release of ADH (i.e., vasopressin) or renal insensitivity to the hormone, but is also associated with hyperglycemia, hypokalemia, adrenal insufficiency (primary or secondary to pituitary dysfunction), hypothalamic disorders, pregnancy, or other conditions that lead to excess water in relation to body sodium or cause salt loss in excess of water loss.[10]

Hyponatremia is defined as a serum sodium concentration of less than 135 mEq/L and can be an acute or a chronic condition. Acute hyponatremia sometimes develops in hospitalized patients after surgery and is often associated with fluid overload, but thiazide therapy and other medications can also cause hyponatremia. Chronic hyponatremia usually occurs outside the hospital, often is acquired over a longer period, and can cause falls, gait problems, cognitive changes, and osteoporosis.[10] This electrolyte disorder can affect more than 10% of outpatients and is associated with increased hospital length of stay and mortality.[8] Hyponatremia is one of the more common electrolyte disorders in older adults, but premenopausal women and children are also at risk.

Exercise-associated hyponatremia (EAH) is usually associated with female gender, environment (extreme heat or cold), smaller body weight, and prolonged exercise, but EAH also affects males and occurs even in shorter exercise events.[9] The incidence of EAH is variable, and those affected may often seem more asymptomatic than symptomatic.[9] The causes of EAH are associated with increased water intake, inappropriate vasopressin secretion, increased brain natriuretic peptide (BNP), sudden water absorption from the gastrointestinal tract, sodium loss associated with sweating, impairment of sodium store mobilization, and/or possibly medications such as nonsteroidals and selective serotonin reuptake inhibitors.[9,11] The Wilderness Medical Society practice guidelines were developed to assist in the prevention and management of EAH in the wilderness.[9]

Treatment of hyponatremia has always been challenging, and there has been increasing concern about how to treat patients appropriately.[8] It is a complex disorder, the causes are myriad, and treatments vary depending on the underlying pathology and patient age.[8] For example, treatment recommendations for children with hyponatremia differ significantly from treatment recommendations for adults and elders.[10] In recent years, the U.S. Expert Panel recommendations for diagnosis, evaluation, and treatment of hyponatremia and the European clinical practice guidelines on diagnosis and treatment of hyponatremia were released to assist health care providers in identifying and treating hyponatremia appropriately.[8,10] The European guidelines use a grading system to support the recommendations, but the U.S. panel determined that further research would be necessary to support a quality-of-evidence grading system.[8,10] Both sets of guidelines emphasize the difference between hypotonic hyponatremia and nonhypotonic hyponatremia and emphasize the importance of recognizing this disorder and treating it appropriately to avoid significant morbidity and mortality.[8,10]

PATHOPHYSIOLOGY

Sodium and other anions regulate body water and are determinants of serum osmolality. If serum sodium levels fall below normal limits, serum osmolality is decreased and extracellular water is permitted to seep into cells. This results in a hypotonic hyponatremia and the cerebral brain cell swelling that causes the neurologic features associated with hyponatremia. Normally, the body responds to an excess amount of water by diuresis. Renal mechanisms and vasopressin control body fluid volume and the composition of body fluids. An increase in serum osmolality above the normal 275 to 295 mOsm/kg stimulates the posterior pituitary to release vasopressin, which influences the distal tubules and collecting ducts in the kidneys to conserve water. As body fluid accumulates and serum osmolality becomes hypotonic, vasopressin is inhibited. In most circumstances, vasopressin release is affected by serum osmolality and blood pressure (i.e., baroregulation), but others factors can also affect vasopressin release and cause SIADH.[10] Medications and a person's genetic predisposition can also affect water output in the collecting ducts of the kidneys and thus decrease serum sodium.[10]

EAH is influenced by varied mechanisms. Primary causes include an overabundance of water intake or diminished vasopressin suppression, but increased levels of BNP during exercise may also affect some athletes.[9] Others may experience increased sodium losses associated with certain medications, sweat during exercise, increased water absorption from the gastrointestinal tract after exercise, or decreased mobilization of sodium stores.[9]

Psychogenic polydipsia, beer potomania (the association of severe hyponatremia with ingestion of large quantities of beer), and a reset osmostat have also been identified as precipitants of hypotonic hyponatremia with euvolemia. Psychogenic polydipsia can be related to angiotensin-converting enzyme (ACE) inhibitor or lithium therapy or to a biologic or psychiatric disorder; it may also be a compensatory mechanism for medications that cause dry mouth. Individuals with beer potomania derive most of their calorie intake from large quantities of beer, which contains relatively few solutes. The reduced solute delivery to the distal tubule restricts urine production and results in hyponatremia. The reset osmostat phenomenon, a type of SIADH, is found in patients with malignancy, malnutrition, debilitating conditions, and even pregnancy. Changes in cellular metabolism cause hypothalamic osmoreceptors to reset to maintain a lowered serum osmolality. The diagnosis of reset osmostat is complex. BUN and creatinine concentrations are usually normal, but urine sodium and osmolality are variable.[8]

Hyponatremia is also associated with other causes. The high glucose levels associated with hyperglycemia can cause intracellular fluid to shift into the extracellular compartment, causing a lower serum sodium because of the increase in extracellular fluid.[8] The solute changes that occur with hyperglycemia result in an isotonic or hypertonic hyponatremia.[8] Mannitol, surgical irrigants (e.g., glycine), and radiographic contrast agents act similarly and cause a hypertonic hyponatremia.[8] Significantly increased amounts of plasma proteins and lipids cause a factitious decrease in serum sodium and result in an isotonic pseudohyponatremia.[8]

CLINICAL PRESENTATION

Patient symptoms are often subtle, and the history may be inconclusive. Nonetheless, hyponatremia should be considered in the differential diagnosis of all individuals with headache, blurred vision, dizziness, lethargy, weakness, irritability, restlessness, impaired central nervous system function, history of falls, nonspecific gastrointestinal complaints (e.g., anorexia, nausea, vomiting), influenza-like symptoms, cardiac or respiratory distress, dysgeusia, unusual water-drinking behavior, or weight changes.[9,10] Stupor, seizures, psychosis, and coma are associated with sodium levels below 110 mEq/L.

The present and past medical history aids in identifying the cause of the lowered serum sodium and helps determine if the onset is acute or chronic. A thorough medication review including over-the-counter medications (e.g., nonsteroidal anti-inflammatory drugs [NSAIDs]) and diuretic or corticosteroid therapy is essential because numerous medications will precipitate this disorder. Other history should include history of alcohol use, allergies, any recent illness (e.g., vomiting or diarrhea) or surgery (particularly genitourologic), previous illnesses or psychiatric history, recent endurance exercise, and, in women, menstrual status and possibility of pregnancy.

PHYSICAL EXAMINATION

A complete examination, including weight, orthostatic vital sign changes, and determination of physical signs of euvolemia, volume depletion, or fluid overload (i.e., skin turgor, mucous membranes, presence of ascites or edema), is essential. The neurologic evaluation is particularly important and requires careful patient observation for mental status changes, gait abnormalities, and level of consciousness, as well as for signs of dehydration, heart failure, cirrhosis, or myxedema.[10]

DIAGNOSTICS

The patient's symptoms, history, physical examination, and diagnostic evaluation are critical in discerning the cause and subsequent management of the patient's volume status and hyponatremia. When possible, determining if the hyponatremia is acute (less than 48 hours' duration) or chronic (longer than 48 hours) is helpful, as is determining if the patient is moderately or severely symptomatic.

- Obtain spot urine sodium, urine osmolality, serum osmolality, serum glucose, electrolytes, uric acid, BUN and creatinine. If the serum glucose is elevated, correct the measured serum glucose (www.mdcalc.com/sodium-correction-for-hyperglycemia) to exclude hyperglycemia as the cause of the hyponatremia. Hyperglycemia results in an isotonic or hypertonic hyponatremia and does not cause brain edema.
- Exclude other causes of nonhypotonic hyponatremia: determine serum alcohol, lactate, urea, total protein, cholesterol, and triglycerides, which cause isotonic or hyperosmolar serum osmolality.
- Does the patient exhibit severe or acute symptoms, especially if hyperglycemia and other nonhypotonic hyponatremias have been excluded? If so, hospitalize for immediate treatment with hypertonic saline (3% NaCl).
- If patient does not have severe or acute symptoms and serum sodium is greater than 120 mmol/L, determine urine osmolality.[8] A urine osmolality of less than 100 mOsm/kg suggests an increase in water intake (i.e., beer potomania, low solute intake, or primary polydipsia).
- If the urine osmolality is greater than 100 mOsm/kg, check urine sodium concentration and serum sodium.
  - A urine sodium concentration below 20 to 30 mmol/L suggests decreased effective arterial volume as cause of the hypotonic hyponatremia.[8] The following should be considered:
    - Hyponatremia with expanded extracellular fluid: cirrhosis of the liver, heart failure, or nephrotic syndrome
    - Hyponatremia with reduced extracellular fluid: diarrhea, vomiting, third spacing, or diuretic therapy[8,10]
  - If the urine sodium concentration is greater than 30 mmol/L, evaluate fluid volume status. Is the patient taking diuretics or does he or she have kidney disease? If so, this may be the cause of the hypotonic hyponatremia. If the patient does not have kidney disease and is not taking diuretics and has reduced extracellular fluid volume, primary adrenal insufficiency, renal salt wasting, vomiting, cerebral salt wasting, and occult diuretics may be considered.[10] If the patient has a urine sodium concentration exceeding 30 mmol/L and is euvolemic, hypothyroidism (myxedema), secondary adrenal insufficiency, SIADH, or occult diuretics may be considered.[8,10] Patients with SIADH will have a urine osmolality exceeding 100 mOsm/kg, unless the SIADH is related to reset osmostat.[8]
  - Urine sodium can be misleading in some circumstances. Patients with SIADH may have a lower urinary sodium if they are anorexic or follow a low-sodium diet.[8] Also, diuretics can increase urinary sodium.

DIAGNOSTICS

Hyponatremia

LABORATORY

Spot urine sodium
Urine osmolality and urine sodium concentration
Serum glucose, electrolytes, BUN, creatinine
Serum osmolality
Serum alcohol
Serum lactate
Urea
Total protein
Liver function tests (LFTs)*
BNP* if heart failure suspected
CBC and differential*
Thyroid-stimulating hormone (TSH) (if signs of myxedema)*
Fasting lipid profile to exclude hyperlipidemia as a cause of isotonic hyponatremia*
Uric acid*
Cortisol level at 9 AM if adrenocorticotropic hormone (ACTH) deficiency is a consideration*
ACTH stimulation test (with recent steroid therapy)*

IMAGING

Chest x-ray examination (if congestive heart failure or malignancy is suspected)*
CT scan, MRI: to assess for malignancy or definitive neurologic problem*

*If indicated.

DIFFERENTIAL DIAGNOSIS

Endurance exercise must be differentiated from acute altitude illness, dehydration, or heat-related illness to prevent inappropriate and life-threatening treatment. Metabolic disturbances, severe illness, infection, medications (e.g., lithium, thiazides, desmopressin, vasopressin), depression, endocrine abnormalities, nutritional deficiencies, polydipsia, trauma, and cardiovascular and cerebrovascular accidents should be considered in the differential diagnosis. Identifying the cause of the hyponatremia (see differential diagnosis box) is crucial to ensure correct treatment. In addition, the differential diagnosis should include appropriate classification of the patient's hyponatremia as acute (<48 hours) or chronic (48 hours or longer); serum sodium as mild, moderate, or severe; and symptoms as acute or severe to determine if hospitalization is immediately indicated.[8,10] If the provider is unable to determine whether the hyponatremia is an acute versus a chronic event, the serum sodium correction guidelines for chronic hyponatremia should be followed.

MANAGEMENT

In primary care, the cause of hyponatremia is often medication related, because many medications cause a decrease in serum sodium. For that reason, it is essential to obtain a serum sodium level within 5 days (some patients will develop hyponatremia even sooner) after the initiation of a medication known to cause hyponatremia (e.g., carbamazepine, clofibrate, levetiracetam, thiazide diuretic, or selective serotonin receptor reuptake inhibitor) and/or to perform a careful medication review to determine if the patient is taking another medication that could be the cause of the decrease in serum sodium. A serum sodium level that is even slightly lower than normal should be concerning. The medication should be discontinued and the patient started on fluid restriction, and any salt restriction removed. Salty foods (e.g., pretzels) are also often recommended, particularly for exercise-associated hyponatremia.[12] Acute or symptomatic hyponatremia requires further diagnostic evaluation and treatment. Any medication that causes hyponatremia in a patient should not be restarted.

DIFFERENTIAL DIAGNOSIS

Hyponatremia

NONHYPOTONIC HYPONATREMIA

1. Pseudohyponatremia—serum Na^+ <135 mmol/L, plasma osmolality 280-295 mOsm/kg H_2O
   - Hyperlipidemia
   - Hyperproteinemia
2. Isotonic hyponatremia—serum Na^+ <135 mmol/L, plasma osmolality 280-295 mOsm/kg H_2O; or hypertonic hyponatremia*—serum Na <135 mmol/L, plasma osmolality >295 mOsm/kg H_2O
   - Glycine absorption related to gynecologic or urologic irrigating fluids used in surgery
   - Hyperglycemia
   - Mannitol
   - Radiographic contrast agents

HYPOTONIC HYPONATREMIA

Serum Na^+ <135 mmol/L, plasma osmolality <280 mOsm/kg H_2O

1. Hypovolemic hyponatremia (hypotonic hyponatremia with decreased extracellular volume—spot urine Na^+ <20 to 30 mmol/L; elevated uric acid, BUN, creatinine, and BUN/creatinine ratio
   - Diarrhea, vomiting (nonrenal sodium loss)
   - Diuretic induced (renal sodium loss): most often thiazide, but furosemide also
   - Transdermal sodium loss
   - Primary adrenal insufficiency
   - Cerebral salt wasting: related to head injury, cerebral hemorrhage, or neurosurgery
   - Kidney disease affecting renal reabsorption of sodium
   - Third spacing
2. Euvolemic hyponatremia (hypotonic hyponatremia with normal extracellular volume)—spot urine Na^+ ≥20 to 30 mmol/L†; normal uric acid, normal or low BUN
   - Exercise-associated hyponatremia
   - High water and low solute intake: anorexia nervosa, beer potomania, very-low-protein diet
   - Malignancy
   - Medications (e.g., thiazides, serotonin reuptake inhibitors, phenothiazines)
   - Myxedema
   - Nervous system disorders: acute intermittent porphyria, delirium tremens, Guillain-Barré syndrome, head trauma, infections, multiple sclerosis, Shy-Drager syndrome, tumors, vascular insults
   - NSIAD related to genetic mutation of *V2R*
   - Primary polydipsia
   - Pulmonary disorders: asthma, infections, cystic fibrosis, respiratory failure with positive-pressure breathing
   - Reset osmostat
   - Secondary adrenal insufficiency with resultant glucocorticoid deficiency
   - SIADH: urine Na^+ >20-30 mmol/L; urine osmolality >100 mOsm/kg; serum osmolality <275 mOsm/kg H_2O
   - Other causes: general anesthesia, hereditary causes, idiopathic condition, nausea, pain, stress
3. Hypervolemic hyponatremia (hypotonic hyponatremia with increased extracellular volume)—elevated brain natriuretic peptide; spot urine Na^+ <20-30 mmol/L
   - Acute renal injury
   - Chronic renal disease
   - Heart failure
   - Liver failure
   - Nephrotic syndrome

*Patients with hyperglycemia can become dehydrated as a result of the osmotic diuresis associated with hyperglycemia. Mannitol also can cause significant fluid and electrolyte disturbance as a result of the diuresis.

†Some patients with euvolemic hyponatremia may have secondary sodium depletion related to diet low in sodium. Patients on diuretic therapy with euvolemic hyponatremia may have elevated urine sodium. If euvolemic hyponatremia is strongly suspected but spot urine Na^+ is low, volume repletion with isotonic saline will possibly aid in determining actual diagnosis.

Isotonic Hyponatremia and Hypertonic Hyponatremia

- Pseudohyponatremia without plasma hypo-osmolality has been associated with hyperproteinemia, as well as with elevated cholesterol and triglycerides. In these disorders, partial displacement of the sodium-containing plasma by increased numbers of lipids or proteins causes falsely lowered sodium levels and is the result of a laboratory artifact.[13] Both conditions are isotonic hyponatremias associated with normal plasma osmolality and are treated with correction of the hyperproteinemia or hyperlipidemia.[8]
- Hyperosmolar pseudohyponatremia is related to conditions that elevate plasma osmolality (e.g., hyperglycemia, mannitol excess, and glycerol therapy). Increased serum glucose causes increased plasma osmolality, which shifts body water into the intravascular space and lowers serum sodium. Correction of plasma glucose concentration corrects the hyponatremia.[8]
- Pseudohyponatremia may also be caused by the absorption of isotonic irrigant solutions containing glycine or sorbitol after endometrial resection or a urologic procedure. The absorption of the irrigant lowers plasma sodium, but not usually plasma osmolality. Elevated serum osmolality with lowered serum sodium may occur in some cases. If an isotonic genitourinary irrigant is the cause of the hyponatremia, the irrigant should be discontinued.

Hypotonic Hyponatremia

Patients who are severely symptomatic with acute hypotonic hyponatremia require immediate hospitalization and treatment with an intravenous infusion of 100 mL of 3% NaCl over 10 minutes. Two repeated infusions of 100 mL of 3% NaCl, each over 10 minutes, are recommended if necessary to increase the serum sodium 4 to 6 mmol/L in an attempt to treat the brain edema causing the severe symptoms and avert cerebral ischemia, herniation, and neurologic injury.[8]

- Patients who are moderately symptomatic with acute hypotonic hyponatremia require hospitalization and a 3% NaCl infusion at 0.5 to 2 mL/kg/hr if there is even a small risk for brain herniation.[8]

- If there is doubt regarding whether the hyponatremia is acute as opposed to chronic, the correction of serum sodium should follow the treatment guidelines for chronic hyponatremia (see later).[8]
- Patients with severe chronic hyponatremia are at risk for osmotic demyelination syndrome (ODS) if the serum sodium is corrected too quickly. For this reason, patients with chronic hyponatremia should have the serum sodium corrected a maximum of 4 to 8 mmol/L/day if osmotic demyelination is not a serious concern, but only 4 to 6 mmol/L/day if osmotic demyelination is a more likely possibility (i.e., patient with history of advanced liver disease, alcoholism, malnutrition, hypokalemia, or serum sodium 105 mmol/L or less).[8] The 24-hour serum sodium goal for patients at great risk for ODS should not surpass 8 mmol/L/day.[8] For patients with average risk for ODS, the 24-hour serum sodium goal should not exceed 10 to 12 mmol/L/day.[8] Overcorrection should be prevented, and saline and/or vasopressin receptor antagonists (i.e., vaptan medications such as tolvaptan used in the treatment of SIADH) discontinued when the goal of therapy has been attained. Physician consultation is recommended to determine if free water, intravenous 5% dextrose in water infusion, or desmopressin therapy is indicated.[8]
  - The criteria for vaptan therapy require that the patient not have hypovolemic hyponatremia, nor should vaptan therapy be administered immediately after or concurrently with treatment with 3% NaCl or other therapies.[8] Physician consultation is indicated for patients who may benefit from vaptan therapy.
  - Repeat serum sodium levels are recommended at hours 1, 6, 12, and 24, with continued exploration of the cause if the patient is not improving.
  - Physician consultation is necessary for treatment of overcorrection of chronic hyponatremia and may be necessary for patients at risk of ODS (i.e., patients with advanced liver disease, alcoholism, hypokalemia, malnutrition, or serum sodium ≤105 mmol/L).[8]
- Acute hyponatremia with a serum sodium level of 130 to 135 mmol/L requires careful consideration and possibly treatment. The serum sodium measurement should be repeated, and any medications that cause hyponatremia should be discontinued and fluid intake limited.[10] Diagnostic testing is indicated if the repeat serum sodium measurement reveals hyponatremia. If the serum sodium has decreased more than 10 mmol/L, the patient should be hospitalized and should receive a single infusion of hypertonic saline (150 mL of 3% saline infused over 20 minutes).
- Determination of the underlying cause of the hyponatremia is essential. For example:
  - Hypovolemic hyponatremia requires fluid resuscitation with isotonic saline; or, if the serum sodium is less than 120 mmol/L, 3% NaCl is required for volume repletion.[8] Once the patient's fluid volume status has been restored (i.e., blood pressure normalization and clinical euvolemia), further determination of the cause of the hypovolemia should be pursued (e.g., diuretic therapy, gastrointestinal fluid loss, cerebral salt wasting, mineralocorticoid deficiency should be further investigated).
  - Hypervolemic hyponatremia requires fluid and dietary sodium restriction.[8]
  - In patients with heart failure–associated hyponatremia, fluid restriction* is initially indicated. Physician consultation is indicated for diuretic therapy, neurohormonal blockade, and/or vaptan therapy.
- In patients with cirrhosis-related hyponatremia, fluid restriction* in combination with diuretic therapy (i.e., spironolactone as well a loop diuretic) is recommended, as is a low-sodium diet and possibly paracentesis. Physician consultation is indicated for further treatments; demeclocycline and vaptan therapy is usually contraindicated.[8]
- Patients with nephrotic syndrome–related hyponatremia are best treated with fluid restriction,* although vaptan therapy can be considered in consultation with the physician.
  - Daily fluid restriction should be less than the patient's urinary output and insensible losses.
  - Vaptan therapy requires careful monitoring for liver dysfunction, is contraindicated in patients with liver disease, and is not indicated for long-term therapy (i.e., longer than 30 days).
- Euvolemic hyponatremia differs pathophysiologically from other types of hyponatremia, and identifying the cause and duration of the hyponatremia (i.e., acute versus chronic) directs treatment. Acute hyponatremia (symptomatic patients and less than 48 hours with low serum sodium [usually ≤120 mmol/L) necessitates hospitalization and emergent treatment with hypertonic saline.[8] Potential causes of and treatment considerations for euvolemic hyponatremia include the following:
  - Exercise-associated hyponatremia should always be part of the differential diagnosis if an athlete in a marathon or endurance event collapses or is symptomatic. Unfortunately, hyponatremic symptoms are not always evident immediately after athletic events, so athletes must be monitored for cognitive changes, coma, seizures, and severe dyspnea.[9] Patients with suspected endurance exercise–induced hyponatremia require oxygenation to maintain oxygen saturation at 95% (Grade 1C recommendation, American College of Chest Physicians [ACCP]) in addition to hospitalization for serum sodium analysis and intravenous therapy with the appropriate intravenous fluid. An accurate diagnosis of EAH versus acute altitude illness, dehydration, or heat-related illness is essential because the presentations are similar, but the treatments are quite different.[9] Until diagnostic evaluation and hospitalization are possible, fluid volume assessment and avoidance of hypotonic fluid are necessary[9] (Grade 1A recommendation [ACCP]). Fluid restriction is appropriate if the patient does not require intravenous support before hospitalization.[9] When the patient is hospitalized and EAH is confirmed by laboratory diagnosis, a 100-mL bolus of 3% hypertonic saline is appropriate, with two additional boluses at 10-minute intervals if necessary to increase the serum sodium by 4 to 5 mmol/L[9] (Grade 1A recommendation [ACCP]). If available, the initial bolus may be given on-site where the EAH occurred and, if necessary, repeated two more times.[8] Patients with acute hyponatremia that occurred over a short span of time (i.e., several hours) should improve with this treatment regimen and should not require further treatment other than monitoring.

- Nephrogenic syndrome of inappropriate antidiuresis (NSIAD) requires fluid restriction and possibly treatment with low-dose urea. Vasopressin receptor antagonist (vaptan) therapy is not indicated for this disorder.[14]
- Glucocorticoid deficiency should be excluded for all patients with euvolemic hyponatremia.
  - Measure serum cortisol and rapid cosyntropin-stimulation test results and, in consultation with physician, begin glucocorticoid therapy.[8]
  - Do not limit fluid intake.[8]
  - Monitor serum sodium carefully because rapid escalation of serum sodium is possible and will require possible treatment with intravenous dextrose and water, as well as desmopressin, requiring physician consultation.[8]
- Hypothyroidism: fluid restriction and thyroid replacement are usual therapies (see Chapter 214). Physician consultation is recommended for patients with myxedema.
- Low solute intake: improve nutritional intake of protein and electrolytes.
- Polydipsia
  - Primary polydipsia: fluid restriction, ice chips, hard candies to decrease thirst.[8]
  - Psychogenic polydipsia: fluid restriction, behavioral therapy, and medication therapy (possibly with clozapine) are recommended.[8] Rapid correction of hyponatremia is contraindicated in chronic hyponatremia.
- SIADH
  - Medications that cause SIADH should be discontinued.
  - The majority of patients with SIADH have chronic hyponatremia, but in some instances the low serum sodium may have an acute onset (48 hours or less), causing symptomatic hyponatremia (usually 120 mmol/L or less). In these circumstances, the treatment recommendations include 3% NaCl by bolus or intravenous infusion (not isotonic saline, which in patients with SIADH may cause further hyponatremia) to increase the serum sodium and prevent neurologic sequelae.[8]
    - Diagnostic testing should be initiated to confirm SIADH diagnosis.
    - Patients with chronic SIADH require fluid restriction (i.e., nonfood fluids 500 mL/day below the 24-hour urine volume) for several days. Sodium intake is not restricted, nor is protein intake restricted. If, however, the patient's urine reveals low electrolyte-free water excretion or the serum sodium fails to normalize with fluid restriction in the next 24 to 48 hours, vasopressin receptor antagonists (vaptans) or other pharmacologic interventions can be considered.[8]
    - Adequate fluid intake (not fluid restriction) is essential the first 24 to 48 hours after vaptan (i.e., conivaptan, tolvaptan) therapy is initiated, and serum sodium requires careful monitoring (every 6 hours for 48 hours).[8]
    - Stop vaptan therapy if water intake is not adequate or patient condition worsens, and monitor serum sodium more frequently.[8]
    - Patients with an elevated urine osmolality (>500 mOsm/kg water) do not as a rule respond to fluid restriction and will require pharmacologic therapy, as will patients with a low 24-hour urine volume (<1500 mL/day), patients whose combined urinary Na^+ and K^+ amounts are greater than the serum Na^+, and those in whom the serum Na^+ concentration fails to exceed 2 mmol/L/day after a fluid restriction of 1 L/day for 24 to 48 hours.[8]
    - Serum sodium is monitored every 4 to 6 hours until it is 125 mmol/L.

COMPLICATIONS

Brain damage or death from the encephalopathy that results from untreated hyponatremia is the most serious complication of hyponatremia. ODS (central pontine myelinolysis) is the untoward consequence of overcorrecting the serum sodium with intravenous hypertonic saline.[8,10] ODS can occur with rapid correction of serum sodium but has also been associated with slower correction of hyponatremia as well as with hypokalemia.

INDICATIONS FOR REFERRAL OR HOSPITALIZATION

Patients with acute hyponatremia, acute-on-chronic hyponatremia, and or moderate or profound symptomatic hyponatremia require hospitalization and consultation with a physician familiar with the treatment of hyponatremia. Patients with chronic hyponatremia recalcitrant to therapy should also be referred for specialist consultation.

PATIENT AND FAMILY EDUCATION

- Prevention of EAH
  - Fluid consumption should be judicious and based on thirst[9] (Grade 1C recommendation [ACCP]).
  - Weight gain during exercise is an indication that fluid intake should be curtailed until body weight is within 2% to 4% of the person's normal body weight[9] (Grade 1B recommendation [ACCP]).
  - Sodium supplements in exercise-related events lasting less than 18 hours have no known efficacy[9] (Grade 2B recommendation [ACCP]).
  - Education for runners and other athletes competing in endurance events should also include careful explanation of the early symptoms of hyponatremia and the importance of seeking medical attention to avoid the serious sequelae.
- Patients and caregivers (both family and professional) need to understand the nature of the hyponatremic disorder and recognize its associated neurologic symptoms as well as treatment side effects that necessitate health care provider notification (e.g., constipation).
  - Instructions regarding the importance of good oral hygiene, skin care, frequent weight measurements, dietary or fluid restriction, intake and output measurement, and medications (and their side effects) should be explicit and understandable.
  - Frequent follow-up care with continuous evaluation of the treatment plan is imperative.

CHAPTER 211

LIPID DISORDERS

Mary Young

DEFINITION AND EPIDEMIOLOGY

Lipid disorders are a significant risk factor in the development of atherosclerotic cardiovascular disease (ASCVD), which remains the leading cause of death in the United States. Adults older than 20 years in the United States have a 12.9% incidence of high total cholesterol, defined as total blood cholesterol above 240 mg/dL.[1]

The 2013 American College of Cardiology (ACC) and American Heart Association (AHA) guidelines on the assessment of cardiovascular (CV) risk[2] identify four groups of patients who will benefit from treatment with cholesterol-lowering 3-hydroxy-3-methylglutaryl-coenzyme A (HMG-CoA) reductase inhibitors (statins). This new guideline does not focus on goal treatment of low-density lipoprotein (LDL) levels. Rather, it focuses on the groups of patients for whom LDL lowering is proven most beneficial, including persons at risk of stroke. These new guideline recommendations replace the National Cholesterol Education Program Adult Treatment Panel III (NCEP ATP III) guidelines of 2003.[2-5]

Therapeutic lifestyle changes (TLCs), which include a heart-healthy diet, exercise, weight loss, and avoidance of tobacco, remain the first and most important intervention, followed by moderate- to high-intensity statin drugs to lower total cholesterol and low-density lipoprotein cholesterol (LDL-C), and to prevent coronary heart disease (CHD). Titrating statin drugs is no longer recommended to achieve goal levels of LDL.[2]

Lipid disorders are primarily caused by a combination of genetic, lifestyle, and nutritional factors. The primary goal of treatment is to decrease the lifetime and 10-year risk of ASCVD, based on risk calculations. The new guidelines support the initiation of statin drugs to lower overall risk, in conjunction with lifestyle changes. Four target groups for treatment with moderate- or high-intensity statin therapy have been identified[2]:

- Patients who have CV disease
- Patients with an LDL-C, or "bad" cholesterol, level of 190 mg/dL or higher
- Patients with type 2 diabetes who are age 40 to 75 years
- Patients with an estimated 10-year risk of CV disease of 7.5% or higher who are 40 to 75 years of age

These benefits affect both men and women, in all age ranges, including older adults.

PATHOPHYSIOLOGY

Fats and cholesterol are essential components of human cells and are synthesized by the liver. Additional cholesterol and a variety of other lipids are absorbed from the gastrointestinal tract during digestion and are transported through the bloodstream to the liver for processing.

Deposition of cholesterol into arterial and venous walls promotes atherosclerosis. This pathologic process is influenced by a number of factors, including toxins and inflammatory mediators within the bloodstream and in the vessel wall, and by the types and concentrations of the various lipoproteins. Lipoproteins are characterized by their density and include chylomicrons, very-low-density lipoprotein (VLDL), intermediate-density lipoprotein (IDL), LDL, and high-density lipoprotein (HDL). The progressive buildup of atheromatous plaque in the intimal arterial layer causes inflammation and narrowing of the vessel lumen. Gradually the atheromatous plaque enlarges and may rupture, causing coronary ischemia and infarction.

Low-Density Lipoprotein

LDL carries most of the cholesterol in the plasma and is the cause of atherogenic changes associated with the development of ASCVD. The principal function of LDL is to transport cholesterol to hepatic and extrahepatic cells. Although LDL particles are small, they carry approximately 70% of the circulating cholesterol in plasma. LDL is removed from the plasma by a single type of receptor located on the surface of many cells throughout the body: the LDL receptor. LDL's apolipoprotein B (apo B) binds to the LDL receptor when LDL is carried into the cells. One molecule of apo B is present for each LDL particle, but the quantity of cholesterol per particle can vary considerably. The ratio of LDL to apo B correlates with the size of the LDL particles. Low LDL-C/apo B ratios reflect small LDL particles. These smaller, denser LDL particles are more atherogenic than normal-sized LDL particles and are associated with insulin resistance, diabetes, hypertriglyceridemia, and low HDL levels, all of which are significant risk factors for ASCVD.

Elevation of lipoprotein(a) (Lp[a]) is significant in patients with known coronary artery disease (CAD) and elevated LDL, increasing the risk of CV events. Studies have indicated that the independent elevation of Lp(a) in persons without CAD may not be prognostic of CAD.[6]

High-Density Lipoprotein

HDL is an independent predictor of ASCVD risk. The role of HDL is significant; it lowers LDL by preventing oxidation of LDL within the arterial wall. In addition, when free cholesterol is released from cells into the plasma, it binds to HDL particles, resulting in a reverse cholesterol transport system. Cholesterol is returned to the liver, where it is excreted into bile, converted to bile acids, or reprocessed. There is an inverse relationship among VLDL remnants and small, dense LDL particles—known as atherogenic factors—and HDL. Because of the inverse relationship between levels of HDL and ASCVD risk, low levels of HDL (<40 mg/dL) have been identified as an independent risk factor for ASCVD regardless of the total cholesterol level. Higher high-density lipoprotein cholesterol (HDL-C) has a protective effect, and levels above 60 mg/dL are considered to be a negative risk factor, lowering the overall risk.

The ratio of total cholesterol to HDL-C is correlated to cardiac risk. A total cholesterol/HDL-C ratio of more than 4.5 is associated with increased cardiac risk. Apolipoprotein A-I (apo A-I) is the predominant lipoprotein in HDL, and measurement of apo A-I in addition to the apo B found in LDL may allow more accurate assessment of cardiac risk.

Physical activity increases HDL-C levels, emphasizing the importance of exercise in managing dyslipidemia. In addition, modest alcohol consumption (one or two drinks/day) increases HDL-C and appears to reduce cardiac risk. Excessive alcohol intake, however, increases triglycerides and detrimentally affects liver function.

Triglycerides

Hypertriglyceridemia is also associated with CAD, in conjunction with increased LDL and decreased HDL. Premature CAD associated with hypertriglyceridemia has a high correlation with familial hyperlipidemia, type 2 diabetes mellitus, and familial hypoalphalipoproteinemia. All of these are common in metabolic syndrome as well (see Chapter 212).

Obesity is a primary risk factor for hypertriglyceridemia, and central obesity correlated with insulin resistance contributes to dyslipidemia. Poorly managed diabetes, some medications, and alcohol consumption are risk factors for secondary hypertriglyceridemia. Triglyceride levels above 2000 mg/dL are most associated with secondary and familial causes.

Role of Lifestyle, Including Diet and Exercise

The sedentary lifestyle of many Americans has increased the incidence of obesity and hyperlipidemia, with a subsequent rise in ASCVD and diabetes. A consistently maintained program of improved nutrition, weight reduction, and exercise improves the lipid profile, decreasing LDL and raising HDL.[2-4]

Despite increased awareness of healthy lifestyle choices in the United States, obesity is an American epidemic affecting overall morbidity and mortality. Obesity increases triglyceride levels, total cholesterol, and LDL-C and decreases HDL-C.

Dietary cholesterol is derived from eating fatty meats and full fat dairy products. These food items are also high in saturated fats and calories and should be eaten in the lowest quantity possible.

There are three major types of dietary fats: saturated, monounsaturated, and polyunsaturated. Each subtype exerts different influences on lipid metabolism, with saturated fats being the most harmful. Saturated fats increase blood cholesterol levels significantly more than dietary cholesterol does. Reducing saturated fats in the diet from 14% to 7% of total calories can decrease total blood cholesterol levels by nearly 20 mg/dL. Unfortunately, the major sources of saturated fats in the American diet are meats, eggs, and dairy products, which are highly consumed by Americans. Certain vegetable oils, namely, tropical oils such as palm and coconut oil, are highly saturated and are most often found in commercially prepared cakes, muffins, cookies, and other baked goods.

Monounsaturated fats are derived from animal and plant oils. The main sources of monounsaturated fats in the American diet are peanuts, olives, avocados, and almonds. Monounsaturated fats do not by themselves raise or lower cholesterol levels but have been shown to help preserve baseline HDL levels when they are substituted for other fats. Their inclusion is a major feature of the popular Mediterranean diet.

Polyunsaturated fats are considered essential fatty acids because they cannot be synthesized by the body, unlike the saturated and monounsaturated fatty acids. Polyunsaturated fats are derived from vegetable oils consisting of omega-3 fatty acids or omega-6 fatty acids found in fish products. Dietary fish oils have been shown to lower total cholesterol and LDL levels while also increasing HDL levels.

Trans-fatty acids, from vegetable oils that have undergone extensive chemical processing or exposure to excess heat, have a detrimental effect on lipid levels. The most common sources in the American diet are margarine spreads, commercially produced baked goods, and deep-fried foods.

Insulin Resistance, Diabetes, and Metabolic Syndrome

Adult-onset diabetes is caused by a combination of factors, including progressive insulin resistance and inadequate insulin supply. Insulin resistance may or may not be associated with frank diabetes or even detectable high blood glucose levels. It is strongly influenced by genetic factors and is associated with abdominal obesity. Physical inactivity and a diet high in carbohydrates are major contributing factors. Insulin resistance, together with physical inactivity and obesity, often appears with other comorbidities, which include hypertension, high triglyceride levels, low HDL-C levels, and small, dense LDL particles, which are particularly atherogenic. Patients with these comorbid factors have metabolic syndrome (see Chapter 212), with a significantly increased risk for ASCVD.[7]

CLINICAL PRESENTATION

Persons with lipid disorders may be unaware of this, because signs and symptoms do not appear unless other comorbidities are associated with elevated lipids, such as heart disease. Physical signs and symptoms, such as xanthomas, are present only when the disease is severe and prolonged.

Initial clinical evaluation should include a complete medical and family history, with documentation of any known ASCVD, symptoms of exertional angina or claudication, hypertension, diet and exercise patterns, smoking, drug and alcohol history and use, obesity, and diabetes. Hypothyroidism and liver and renal diseases affect lipid metabolism and should also be evaluated. All cardiac risk factors, including a family history of premature ASCVD, should be reviewed with the patient. Assessment of lifetime risk of ASCVD is recommended, using published risk assessment tables available at http://my.americanheart.org/cvriskcalculator and www.cardiosource.org/en/Science-And-Quality/Practice-Guidelines-and-Quality-Standards/2013-Prevention-Guideline-Tools.aspx.2,6

PHYSICAL EXAMINATION

Accurate successive measurement of cardiac rate and rhythm, blood pressure, and height and weight, with determination of waist-to-hip ratio and body mass index, is important for all persons being evaluated for hyperlipidemia and ASCVD. Fatty deposits or xanthomas may be observed or palpated in persons with very high cholesterol levels from a familial hyperlipidemia. Xanthomas may be present on areas such as the Achilles tendon and on elbows, knees, and metacarpal joints. Deposits of cholesterol on the eyelids, called xanthelasma, may also be present. The presence of corneal arcus, an opaque white ring about the corneal periphery, should alert the provider to seek further evaluation, especially when it is observed in the young adult.

DIAGNOSTICS

Obtaining a fasting lipid panel, which includes total blood cholesterol, LDL-C, HDL, and triglycerides, is recommended for all adults older than 20 years, every 5 years. After the initiation of lipid-lowering drugs, a second panel should be obtained in 4 to 12 weeks to ensure adherence and efficacy. Thereafter, blood testing every 3 to 12 months is adequate, based on patient response and clinician assessment. An initial test of liver function is important before statins are initiated; this does not need to be repeated unless the patient is symptomatic of liver disease or has adverse effects of statin therapy. Monitoring of creatine kinase (CK) is not necessary unless the patient has muscle symptoms.[2]

DIAGNOSTICS

Lipid Disorders

LABORATORY

Fasting lipid panel every 5 years in adults older than 20 years:
- Total cholesterol below 200 mg/dL is optimal (high is above 240 mg/dL)
- LDL-C below 100 mg/dL is optimal (very high is above 190 mg/dL)
- HDL above 60 mg/dL is optimal (very low is below 40 mg/dL)
- Triglycerides below 150 mg/dL is optimal (very high is above 500 mg/dL)

Estimate 10-year ASCVD risk every 4 to 6 years.[2]

DIFFERENTIAL DIAGNOSIS

Before initiating medical therapy for dyslipidemia, the health care provider must consider other factors that may influence lipid metabolism. Diet, particularly excesses in overall calorie intake, and saturated fat may have an overall elevation effect on the lipid profile. Starvation states such as anorexia nervosa may cause an elevation in total serum cholesterol, whereas excessive intake of alcohol, poorly managed diabetes, or a familial tendency may elevate the triglyceride level.[8]

Other major causes of secondary dyslipidemia include adverse effects of some drugs, disorders of metabolism, and certain disease states. Drugs can affect lipid metabolism in a variety of ways. Glucocorticoids and estrogens may elevate triglyceride and HDL levels, whereas anabolic steroids can markedly reduce HDL levels. Thiazide diuretics elevate total cholesterol, triglyceride, and LDL levels. Alpha blockers may cause increases in HDL, whereas beta blockers can decrease HDL levels and increase triglyceride levels. Elevation of total cholesterol and triglyceride levels has been reported in individuals taking protease inhibitors to treat human immunodeficiency virus (HIV) infection.

The most common endocrine disorders associated with lipid abnormalities are hypothyroidism and diabetes. Screening for thyroid disease (thyroid-stimulating hormone concentration, T_3 and T_4) and diabetes (fasting blood glucose concentration and hemoglobin A_{1c} [HbA_{1c}]) must be completed when abnormalities in the lipid profile are evaluated. Stabilization to a euthyroid state should be achieved before initiation of lipid treatment.

DIFFERENTIAL DIAGNOSIS

Lipid Disorders

PRIMARY DISORDERS
- Familial disorders

SECONDARY DISORDERS
- Diet
  - High saturated fat intake
  - High cholesterol intake
  - Calorie excess
  - Very-low-calorie diet, as seen in anorexia nervosa
  - Excessive alcohol intake
  - High *trans*-fatty acid intake
- Drugs
  - Diuretics
  - Beta blockers
  - Anabolic steroids
  - Glucosteroids
  - Estrogens and androgens
  - Retinoids
  - Cyclosporine
  - Protease inhibitors
- Disorders of metabolism
  - Hypothyroidism
  - Obesity
  - Metabolic syndrome
  - Diabetes mellitus
- Other diseases
  - Obstructive liver disease
  - Nephrotic syndrome

In diabetics, achievement of adequate glycemic control will improve the lipid profile and is an integral component of therapy. Other disease states, such as nephrotic syndrome and obstructive liver disease, also contribute to lipid abnormalities and must be evaluated with a thorough medical history, physical examination, and laboratory tests, including urinalysis, blood urea nitrogen, creatinine, and liver function tests (LFTs).

MANAGEMENT

The primary goal of treatment is to lower the overall risk factors for ASCVD, reducing the morbidity and mortality associated with cardiac and vascular disease. Treatment with statins achieves a 20% to 30% reduction in CHD events.[2] Treatment with nonstatin lipid-lowering drugs is recommended only as an addition to statin therapy when goals are not achieved with high-intensity statin therapy, or when the patient cannot tolerate statins and has known CV disease. Nonstatin therapy for primary prevention is no longer recommended in patients intolerant to statins, because an increase in non-CV mortality has been found.[2]

Lifestyle modification, including a heart-healthy diet, exercise, reduction in body weight if BMI is higher than 24.9, and avoidance of tobacco products is recommended as primary treatment for patients unable to take statin drugs.[9,10] Patients with heart failure and those on dialysis do not have added benefit from statin therapy.[2]

Atherosclerotic Cardiovascular Disease Risk Assessment

The primary goal of treatment has shifted from lowering LDL-C to lowering overall lifetime risk and 10-year risk for CV events.[2-4,8] Risk calculators that focus on 10-year risk are recommended. The Framingham calculators have been revised to include stroke as a predicted outcome, but include other factors that may not be significant and is limited by an all-white population. The ACC/AHA risk calculator (Pooled Cohort Equations cardiovascular risk calculator) is applicable to African-American and non-Hispanic men and women ages 20 to 59 years. However, questions have been raised about accuracy.[8]

Lifestyle Modification

Despite increasing awareness of the importance of diet, exercise, and weight control, obesity in the United States persists as an epidemic and is a major risk factor for lipid disease and ASCVD.[11]

Diet. Heart-healthy diet recommendations per the ACC/AHA guidelines[2] are as follows. Based on a 2000-calorie/day diet, a heart-healthy eating pattern should include:
- Fruits: four or five servings a day
- Vegetables: four or five servings a day
- Whole grains, preferably high fiber: six to eight servings a day
- Fat-free or low-fat milk and milk products: two or three servings a day
- Lean meats, poultry, and fish: 6 or fewer ounces a day
- Nuts, legumes, and seeds: four or five servings a week
- Fats and oils: two or three servings of healthy oils per day, limit *trans* and saturated fat
- Limit sweets and added sugars

Maximum dietary therapy will typically achieve a reduction in LDL-C of 15 to 25 mg/dL, but a healthy balanced diet, exercise, and maintenance of an ideal body weight have additional benefits. This includes improved well-being and self-esteem and a decrease in the other comorbidities of obesity, hypertension, insulin resistance, and diabetes.

There is evidence that a very-low-fat diet (i.e., <10% of calories coming from fat) coming from whole-food and plant-based sources in conjunction with other lifestyle changes such as exercise, yoga, and meditation can reverse ASCVD.[12] Until recently, standard dietary recommendations were to limit total dietary fat to 30% of total calories and saturated fat to 10%. Newer dietary recommendations include a slightly more liberal limit on total fat of 25% to 35% of total calories, with increased restriction of saturated fat to less than 10%.[13] Saturated fats are primarily found in animal products, such as meat and dairy, but also are found in certain vegetable oils, such as palm and coconut.

Dietary fat should, whenever possible, be the unsaturated fat found in most vegetable oils and, in particular, the monounsaturated fat found in olive oil and nuts. Evidence for this dietary strategy comes from study of the Mediterranean diet. The consumption of saturated fats in this diet is lower, and there is a higher intake of monounsaturated fats from nuts, olives, and olive oil. This diet is found to increase HDL-C and to lower LDL-C, thus decreasing the risk for ASCVD.

Trans-fatty acids, which arise from excessive processing, are most atherogenic. *Trans*-fatty acids, found primarily in margarine spreads, commercially produced baked goods, and deep-fried foods, should be avoided whenever possible.

Replacement for fats in the diet should come from complex carbohydrates and by increasing fiber in the diet to 20 to 30 g/day. Whole-grain breads, pastas, and cereals and fresh fruits and vegetables are highly recommended.[12]

Food products in the United States are labeled with nutritional information, including the amount of total fat, saturated fat, cholesterol, and dietary fiber. This labeling and the increased awareness of nutrition in our society allow monitoring of dietary intake and foster adherence to dietary guidelines. For many patients, however, difficulties arise not only with food selection but also with cost, availability, and portion control. Referral to a qualified nutritionist can help patients understand nutrition and meet and maintain their dietary goals.

Exercise. The importance of physical activity should be stressed to all persons concerned about health, ASCVD, and lipid management. Regular aerobic exercise increases HDL-C; decreases total cholesterol, LDL-C, and triglyceride levels; and improves outcomes in other coexisting risk factors, such as obesity, hypertension, and insulin resistance.[7,11]

All patients with known CHD embarking on a new exercise regimen should have a recent exercise tolerance test and, based on the results, an appropriate, prescribed exercise program. Consideration for exercise testing in individuals with two or more CV risk factors should be based on the clinical evaluation and the level of exercise intensity to be performed. Low to moderate expenditure, such as moderate walking, can be safely recommended to most asymptomatic individuals without the need for or expense of an exercise test. Even low-level activity can have a dramatic impact on health when it is performed regularly. When a more intensive exercise program is being considered, an exercise test should be obtained, especially for those with multiple risk factors or individuals who have been sedentary. Patients should be encouraged to start slowly and to increase their intensity and duration of exercise gradually during several weeks, with the goal of doing moderate exercise for at least 30 minutes 5 days per week, with muscle-strengthening activities working all major muscle groups at least twice per week.[12]

Other Risk Factors. Smoking increases the overall risk of ASCVD, particularly when it is combined with familial history, dyslipidemia, hypertension, and diabetes. Elimination of use of tobacco products is essential to the prevention and treatment of disease. Referral to smoking cessation programs and the use of nicotine supplements (nicotine patch, nicotine gum), anti-anxiety medications, and counseling all support smoking cessation.

Refer to Chapters 15 and 16 for more detailed guidelines on lifestyle modification.

Pharmacotherapy

Statin drugs are the first choice when prescribing medications for hyperlipidemia. Moderate- or high-intensity dosage is recommended, based on risk factors and comorbidities. Titrating drugs for effect is not recommended except when the expected 30% to 50% reduction (LDL-C ≤100 mg/dL) in total cholesterol and LDL-C is not achieved. The dose may be increased in 4 to 6 weeks if the goal is not achieved with initial prescribing. Intensive use of atorvastatin 80 mg daily has been shown to reduce mortality in patients with acute coronary syndrome (ACS) and is recommended as first-line treatment during hospitalization. Of course, combination with lifestyle modifications is always recommended. For persons intolerant to statins, the first choice remains lifestyle changes. For secondary prevention in those unable to take statins, bile acid sequestrants, fenofibrate or niacin and ezetimibe should be considered. Referral to a specialist is recommended for these patients.[2-4] The usefulness of niacin in these patient has been questioned, with studies failing to demonstrate reduced CV events and showing significant complications of therapy.[14]

Several drugs available for the treatment of lipid disorders; they are listed in Table 211-1. The general drug categories are HMG-CoA reductase inhibitors, or statins; bile acid sequestrants, or resins; nicotinic acid (niacin); fibrates; cholesterol absorption inhibitors; and liposoluble antioxidants.

The first-choice and most effective drugs for lowering of LDL-C are the statins.[2-5] The statins currently available are atorvastatin (Lipitor), fluvastatin (Lescol), rosuvastatin (Crestor), lovastatin (Mevacor), pravastatin (Pravachol), pitavastatin (Livalo), and simvastatin (Zocor). This category of drugs also increases HDL-C and decreases triglyceride levels, remaining the first-line drug treatment of dyslipidemia.

Several large-scale randomized controlled trials have demonstrated dramatic reductions in morbidity and mortality from cardiac events with the use of statins.[2-4] There is a 1% incidence of hepatic inflammation; for this reason, the liver transaminases—aspartate transaminase and alanine transaminase—should be evaluated before initiation of treatment.[2] For elevations in the transaminases of 2 to 2½ times normal during therapy, treatment should be changed and sources of comorbid liver toxicity, such as alcohol, excluded.

A rare but serious adverse reaction to high-dose statins, particularly simvastatin, is drug-induced myopathy, which can range from mild myalgias to severe muscle breakdown or rhabdomyolysis with the potential for subsequent acute renal failure. In addition, there is an increased risk of myopathy when simvastatin is used in combination with certain medications. For patients taking amiodarone, amlodipine, diltiazem,

TABLE 211-1 **Expected Lipid-Lowering Effects and Side Effects of Currently Available Drugs**

Drug	Dose per Day	Total Cholesterol	LDL Cholesterol	HDL Cholesterol	Triglycerides	Side Effects	Patient Education
STATINS							
Lovastatin (Mevacor) Pravastatin (Pravachol)	20-80 mg 10-40 mg	↓15%-30% ↓15%-30%	↓20%-40% ↓20%-30%	↑5%-10% ↑5%-10%	↓10%-19% ↓10%-15%	Well tolerated as a class Increase in transaminases in 1% of patients.	Take with evening meal because most cholesterol is made in evening hours.
Simvastatin (Zocor)	5-80 mg	↓20%-30%	↓23%-40%	↑6%-12%	↓10%-20%	Rare episodes of myopathy with or without associated rhabdomyolysis.	Have regular laboratory measurement for efficacy and safety.
Fluvastatin (Lescol)	20-80 mg	↓20%-30%	↓20%-32%	↑7%	↓19%	Infrequent gastrointestinal upset, constipation, rash, headaches.	Call and report any unexplained muscle pains, tenderness, or weakness.
Pitavastatin (Livalo)	2-4 mg	↓23-31%	↓32-43%	↑8%	↓15-18%	Muscle pain, confusion, nausea, elevation in liver enzymes.	May be taken at any time of day without regard to meals.
Atorvastatin (Lipitor) Rosuvastatin (Crestor)	10-80 mg 5-40 mg	↓27%-40% —	↓36%-60% ↓45%-63%	↑7%-12% ↑8%-12%	↓17%-30% ↓10%-35%	Asian patients may experience a twofold elevation in median exposure to rosuvastatin; consider lower starting dose.	Avoid grapefruit juice.
CHOLESTEROL ABSORPTION INHIBITORS							
Ezetimibe (Zetia)	10 mg	↓13%	↓18%	↑1%	↓8%	Include liver enzyme abnormalities and myopathy.	May be taken with or without food and can be taken with a statin.
Ezetimibe and simvastatin (Vytorin)	10 mg/40 mg 10 mg/80 mg	↓38%	↓53%	↑7%	↓24%	Avoid in patients with severe hepatic impairment.	
FIBRIC ACIDS							
Gemfibrozil (Lopid)	600-1200 mg	↓6%	↓10%	↑10% (if HDL<35%, ↑25%)	↓35%	LFT abnormality, muscle aches, abdominal pain.	Take 30 minutes before breakfast and dinner. Have regular laboratory measurements of efficacy and safety. Avoid in patients with renal failure.
Fenofibrate (Tricor)	48 or 145 mg				↑30%		
Resins	4-24 g	↓10%	↓25%	None	10% of patients will have ↑	Indigestion, bloating, gas, constipation.	Mix with uncarbonated liquid.
Cholestyramine	4-16 g						Add high-fiber foods to diet. Drink plenty of fluids.
Colestipol	5-20 g						Start with lowest dose and advance as tolerated.

TABLE 211-1 Expected Lipid-Lowering Effects and Side Effects of Currently Available Drugs—cont'd

Drug	Dose per Day	Total Cholesterol	LDL Cholesterol	HDL Cholesterol	Triglycerides	Side Effects	Patient Education
Colesevelam	1.5-3.75 g	↓3.3%	↓10%	↑1.7%	↓8%	SE: Constipation. Other effects: reduction in HgbA1c in diabetics.	Take with 4-8 oz of fluid. Need to take resins 1 hour before or 4 hours after other medication.
Niacin	2-3 g	↓10%-25%	↓20%-40%	↑15%-30%	↓45%-50%	Flushing, itching, rash, gastrointestinal upset; increases in glucose, uric acid, and transaminases.	Predose with aspirin. Avoid taking with hot fluids and alcohol. Start with low dose and increase gradually during several weeks. Call if prolonged nausea occurs. Monitor with laboratory tests.

ranolazine, or verapamil, lower doses of simvastatin are required. Patients taking statins who report new muscle pain must have CK levels evaluated to determine muscle breakdown. If the CK level is elevated, the drug should be discontinued and the patient monitored for potential renal dysfunction. In the absence of symptoms, it is not necessary to routinely monitor CK levels. Combination therapy and higher doses of statins, particularly simvastatin in doses of 80 mg/day, increase the risk of myositis and rhabdomyolysis.[2] Higher doses of statins can also increase the risk of type 2 diabetes. Individual responses to medications must be considered.

Statin drugs should be administered in moderate- or high-intensity doses, based on ASCVD risk factors, and the presence of CHD. Bile acid sequestrants (resins) such as cholestyramine have been demonstrated to be safe and effective in lowering LDL modestly when they are used singularly and can further lower LDL in combination with HMG-CoA reductase inhibitors. They represent a safe alternative to statins in patients with liver disease or those who have had an adverse reaction.

Nonstatin drugs have not been shown to reduce CV events when added to statins and greatly increase the side effect profile. These drugs should be used primarily in patients who cannot tolerate statins or who have had an inadequate response to maximum statin doses.[2]

Nicotinic acid (niacin) demonstrates LDL- and triglyceride-lowering and HDL-raising effects, with doses as low as 1.5 to 2.0 g/day.[3] It may be added to statin therapy, as an adjunct to lowering LDL-C in patients with known coronary disease who have shown an inadequate to statins. Unfortunately, its use remains limited by unpleasant side effects, including flushing, itching, rash, and gastrointestinal upset. In rare cases, liver toxicity, hyperuricemia, and glucose intolerance have occurred, which may limit its usefulness.[14]

The fibric acids, which include gemfibrozil (Lopid) and fenofibrate (Tricor), are effective in lowering triglycerides and raising HDL-C, with modest decrease in LDL. They are used primarily to treat hypertriglyceridemia. A fasting serum triglyceride level of more than 400 mg/dL or the presence of pancreatitis necessitates treatment with this class of drugs. Fibrates decrease triglyceride values by 35% to 50% and increase HDL levels by 5% to 20%. Fibrates should not be administered to patients with severe hepatic or renal dysfunction, and when they are used in combination with statins, the risk of complications is higher.[2] Monitoring of LFT results is essential in prescribing fibric acids and combination therapy, to detect and to prevent liver damage.

Cholesterol absorption inhibitors (e.g., ezetimibe) are useful for patients who cannot tolerate statins or who would benefit from combination therapy in an effort to lower LDL-C in patients with known cardiac disease.[2]

Combination therapy is useful when single-drug use and lifestyle changes do not achieve goals for lowering cholesterol and LDL-C. The addition of a bile acid sequestrant to a statin can reduce LDL-C by an additional 10%. However, the combination of two systemic lipid-lowering drugs (e.g., niacin with a statin or gemfibrozil with a statin) can lead to increased frequency of side effects. LDL-C should be monitored every 6 months when therapy is initiated or doses are changed. Once goal LDL is achieved, monitoring every 6 to 12 months is reasonable.

Primary Prevention for Specific Populations

Young Adults. Persons aged 21 years or older with high LDL-C levels (>190 mg/dL) have a high lifetime risk of CV events. These individuals should be treated with high-intensity statin therapy, with the goal of reducing LDL-C levels by 50%. In addition, family screening is recommended, because very high LDL-C levels in the young population are most often familial.[2] Other causes of primary hyperlipidemia in young adults should also be evaluated, including excessive alcohol intake, diabetes, and albuminuria.

Screening for high cholesterol levels is also an opportunity for counseling about healthy lifestyle habits, including diet, exercise, weight control, and drug, alcohol, and tobacco use.

Consultation and collaboration with other health care providers, including exercise and nutrition specialists, is recommended when long-term therapy is being considered in younger adults.

Men. The benefit of lowering cholesterol in terms of lowering the risk for ASCVD has been most clearly demonstrated in men aged 35 to 65 years. Men in this age group also have a particularly high prevalence of obesity, hypertension, and tobacco use. They should be targeted for aggressive lifestyle modification, lipid screening, and drug therapy when appropriate.

Women. ASCVD has been perceived as a disease more prevalent in men, but half of all cardiac deaths occur in women, and CAD is the leading cause of death in women older than 50 years.[15] The main difference between the sexes is that the onset of ASCVD in women occurs on average 10 to 15 years later than in men and rarely before menopause. Women aged 45 to 75 years should be screened and treated for hyperlipidemia just as men should be treated. The absolute benefit of statin therapy to lower cholesterol and LDL-C is based on risk assessment and CV disease.

Older Adults. The evidence for lowering the risk of ASCVD and CAD events persists regardless of age. Lifestyle changes, including moderate exercise and a healthy diet, provide many benefits to the elderly and should be strongly encouraged, within individual limits. Overall morbidity and mortality must be considered, because the benefit of treatment of older adults with statins should outweigh the risks of adverse events and costs. Persons older than 75 years who have been taking and tolerating statins should continue therapy. Initiation of therapy in persons older than 75 must be individualized.[2]

Diabetes. Persons 40 to 75 years of age with diabetes should be treated with moderate-intensity statin therapy. High-intensity statin therapy is recommended for individuals with diabetes and a 10-year ASCVD risk of 7.5 or higher. This consideration recognizes that patients with diabetes are at a greater overall risk of ASCVD, CAD, and early death, regardless of race, sex, or ethnicity.[2-4]

Metabolic Syndrome. Patients with insulin resistance with or without diabetes and patients with the syndrome of abdominal obesity, physical inactivity, high triglycerides, and low HDL-C are at increased risk for ASCVD. It is essential to support and to encourage healthy lifestyle changes, including increased physical activity, dietary improvements, and weight loss. Achievement of good glycemic control must be a priority and will contribute to improvement in the lipid profile. Ten-year and lifetime risk assessment will guide treatment strategies.[7]

COMPLICATIONS

Elevated lipid levels for prolonged periods result in the progressive buildup of atheromatous plaque in the intimal arterial layer, causing narrowing of the lumen, which precipitates an immune and inflammatory process. Gradually, the atheromatous plaque enlarges and may occlude the lumen or rupture, causing ischemia and infarction and resulting in atherosclerotic CAD (see Chapter 120), peripheral vascular disease (see Chapter 125), cerebral vascular disease, and ACS or death. In addition, recognition of comorbid factors that may be life-threatening must be considered. This includes hypertriglyceridemia (>1000 mg/dL), pancreatitis, untreated thyroid disease, morbid obesity, and poorly managed diabetes.

INDICATIONS FOR REFERRAL

The treatment of lipid disorders for most individuals does not necessitate referral to a specialist, particularly with understanding and use of the revised 2013 ACC/AHA guidelines. However, for some patients, specialist consultation is essential to ensure positive outcomes:

1. A primary genetic lipid disorder is suspected.
2. The treatment plans are not successful in achieving treatment goals.
3. Comorbid conditions such as liver disease limit therapy.
4. Combination therapy is being considered.
5. Newly diagnosed comorbid conditions (e.g., diabetes and hypothyroidism) necessitate a collaborative approach to management.
6. Young adults in whom long-term therapy is being considered.

Immediate emergency department referral is indicated for patients who have severe hypertriglyceridemia and elevated liver and/or pancreatic enzymes, chest pain, respiratory difficulties, or rhabdomyolysis.

PATIENT EDUCATION

Patient education remains the single most important element of achieving lipid control. Lifestyle modification, including heart-healthy nutrition, weight loss, smoking cessation, and exercise are the primary treatment of lipid disorders, even when drug therapy is prescribed. In addition, many patients who start statin therapy do not continue after 1 year, despite education and support.

Referral to appropriate exercise, nutrition, and smoking cessation programs may aid in the collaborative effort to modify risk factors and lower ASCVD risk.[16] Use of support groups, patient teaching DVDs and handouts, and inclusion of family and friends in educational sessions is recommended to ensure success.

CHAPTER 212

METABOLIC SYNDROME

Donna Jenell Pease

DEFINITION AND EPIDEMIOLOGY

Metabolic syndrome is a cluster of disorders that was first introduced by Reaven[1] in 1988. It is characterized by insulin resistance with hyperinsulinemia; hypertension; abdominal (central or visceral) obesity; and dyslipidemia consisting of hypertriglyceridemia, low high-density lipoprotein (HDL) cholesterol, and increased small, dense low-density lipoprotein (LDL) particles. Characteristics that have been added more recently include elevated C-reactive protein (CRP) levels, increased plasminogen activator inhibitor 1 (PAI-1) levels, and microalbuminuria.[2]

Several organizations have developed simple criteria to diagnose metabolic syndrome.[3-6]

In 2009, a joint statement was issued by the International Diabetes Federation, the National Heart, Blood, and Lung

Institute, the American Heart Association, the World Heart Federation, the International Atherosclerosis Society, and the International Association for the Study of Obesity to standardize the diagnostic criteria for metabolic syndrome.[7] It includes the following:

- Elevated waist circumference: population- and country-specific definitions
- Elevated triglyceride levels: 150 mg/dL (1.7 mmol/L) or higher, or specific treatment for this lipid abnormality
- Reduced HDL cholesterol: below 40 mg/dL (1.0 mmol/L) in males and below 50 mg/dL (1.3 mmol/L) in females, or specific treatment for this lipid abnormality
- Elevated blood pressure: systolic 130 mm Hg or higher or diastolic 85 mm Hg or higher, or drug treatment of previously diagnosed hypertension
- Elevated fasting plasma glucose: 100 mg/dL or higher, or drug treatment for elevated glucose

Not all individuals with insulin resistance will develop all of the multiple components of this syndrome, but studies have found that the greater the number of associated characteristics an individual exhibits, the greater his or her risk for development of cardiovascular disease (CVD) or dying young. This syndrome has also been called the insulin resistance syndrome, Reaven syndrome, syndrome X, cardiovascular dysmetabolic syndrome, and deadly quartet.[2]

Metabolic syndrome often occurs in the general population, mostly in older individuals and in certain ethnicities. It is estimated that metabolic syndrome is present in approximately 22.9% of U.S. adults 20 years of age and older. The National Health and Nutrition Examination Survey (1999 to 2010) found that the prevalence of metabolic syndrome increased with age. Non-Hispanic black males were less likely than non-Hispanic white males to have metabolic syndrome, but non-Hispanic black and Mexican-American females were more likely than non-Hispanic white females to have it. Metabolic syndrome increased dramatically as body mass index (BMI) increased.[8]

Both genetic factors and environmental factors have been found to play a role in the incidence of metabolic syndrome. Studies have found a genetic predisposition to the syndrome and the associated cardiovascular risk factors in first-degree relatives of individuals diagnosed with type 2 diabetes. Researchers have also found that nonobese individuals with a family history of diabetes, hypertension, or obesity are genetically predisposed to the development of metabolic syndrome.[9]

Researchers have recently identified a genetic mutation in the gene *DYRK1B* that causes obesity related metabolic syndrome. The researchers found that *DYRK1B* inhibits pathways that keep glucose stable and promotes the production of fat on the body.[10]

An environmental factor involved with insulin resistance and obesity is the lifestyle typical of Western civilization, consisting of a high-fat diet and low levels of physical activity. High energy intake and low energy output have led to the increased prevalence of obesity seen today. Tissue sensitivity to insulin declines when an individual becomes overweight. The fat cells found in abdominal obesity are larger and are more insulin resistant. Abdominal fat is also more metabolically active, and fat lipolysis occurs more often, releasing excess free fatty acids that interfere with hepatic insulin clearance, thus resulting in higher levels of circulating insulin. It has been found that visceral or abdominal obesity may be one of the leading causes of insulin resistance. Visceral adipose tissue also releases cytokines, PAI-1, adiponectin, leptin, and resistin, which are potentially pathogenic and associated with higher CVD risk.[2]

Metabolic syndrome has been recognized as a side effect of several commonly used drugs, such as corticosteroids, antidepressants, and antipsychotics, that can predispose an individual to obesity and glucose intolerance.[11]

PATHOPHYSIOLOGY

Visceral or abdominal obesity leads to insulin resistance. Insulin resistance is defined as the impaired insulin-stimulated glucose uptake by skeletal muscle, adipose tissue, or liver. The mechanisms involved in insulin resistance may consist of abnormal insulin molecules, decreased number of insulin receptors, decreased glucose transporters, and defective postreceptor activity. Impairment at the receptor level is usually associated with decreased sensitivity to insulin, whereas postreceptor or cellular defects are associated with decreased responsiveness to insulin. When the cells become resistant to the insulin, the body compensates by producing more insulin to overcome the resistance and to maintain normal glucose levels. Fasting hyperinsulinemia occurs in response to elevated fasting plasma glucose. This hyperinsulinemia leads to the various other abnormalities associated with metabolic syndrome; they include hypertension, dyslipidemia, atherosclerosis, proinflammatory state, prothrombotic state, and microalbuminuria.[2]

Hypertension

Insulin resistance and visceral adiposity (central obesity) have been recognized as the main factors in the hypertension seen in metabolic syndrome. Insulin resistance and the resulting hyperinsulinemia induce blood pressure elevation by the activation of the sympathetic nervous system and the renin-angiotensin-aldosterone system, which causes urinary sodium excretion to decline. This increased sodium reabsorption causes expansion of the extracellular fluid volume and renal dilation and leads to hypertension, endothelial dysfunction, alteration in renal function, inflammation, and atherogenesis associated with metabolic syndrome.[12]

Dyslipidemia

The lipid abnormalities found in metabolic syndrome are elevated triglycerides, low HDL cholesterol, and increased small, dense LDL particles (referred to as pattern B, or atherogenic dyslipidemia). Obesity causes the adipocytes within the abdominal adipose tissue to become insulin resistant, thus impairing the adipocyte's ability to take up glucose and to store free fatty acids. The adipocytes release large amounts of free fatty acids into the systemic circulation. Muscle cells take up the large amounts of free fatty acid, become saturated with free fatty acids, and become insulin resistant as well. This results in diminished glucose disposal, hyperglycemia, and pancreatic beta cell stimulation to produce larger amounts of insulin (hyperinsulinemia). The free fatty acids that were unable to be absorbed by the muscle cells are diverted to the liver through the portal vein, where they impair normal insulin-mediated suppression of the hepatic glucose output and stimulate the synthesis, assembly, and secretion of lipoproteins that promote atherogenesis (raised triglycerides, low concentrations of HDL cholesterol, increased remnant lipoproteins, elevated apolipoprotein B levels, and small, dense LDL cholesterol). These adverse effects on lipoprotein levels increase the risk of atherosclerosis, ischemic heart disease, CVD, and overall cardiovascular mortality.

Individuals with metabolic syndrome are at increased risk for development of CVD and type 2 diabetes mellitus.[13]

Prothrombotic State

Studies have found that levels of PAI-1 correlate significantly with insulin resistance. Elevated levels of PAI-1 reflect impaired fibrinolysis, impaired endothelial function, and increased tendency toward acute arterial thrombosis. Insulin resistance also affects other coagulation factors, including platelet aggregability, platelet adhesion, levels of factor VII and factor VIII, tissue plasminogen activator, and fibrinogen.[14]

Proinflammatory State

Obesity is associated with a chronic inflammatory response characterized by abnormal adipokine production and the activation of proinflammatory signaling pathways. Inflammation plays a major role in atherogenesis. CRP is a marker of inflammation that has been found to be an independent CVD risk factor and an independent marker of insulin resistance. It has been found that CRP levels and cytokines (tumor necrosis factor-α and interleukin-6) are increased in patients with metabolic syndrome.[15]

Microalbuminuria

An association between microalbuminuria and metabolic syndrome has been found secondary to the effects of insulin on renal hemodynamics. Acute hyperinsulinemia causes renal vasodilation, resulting in increased plasma flow, increased glomerular hydrostatic pressure and gradient, and increased glomerular filtration rate. The localized elevated pressure in the glomerular vessels is involved in increased microalbumin secretion. Microalbuminuria is a strong predictor of cardiovascular morbidity and mortality.[16]

Other Pathophysiologic Effects

Several ongoing studies are currently investigating the association between metabolic syndrome and the following medical disorders: cognitive decline, sleep apnea and breathing disorders, polycystic ovary syndrome, low testosterone levels in men, cancer, and nonalcoholic fatty liver disease.

CLINICAL PRESENTATION

Because it is difficult to accurately measure insulin resistance, the diagnosis is usually clinical, based on a constellation of physical findings and laboratory characteristics. Insulin resistance can be suspected in the individual who is seen with abdominal obesity, increased triglycerides, low HDL cholesterol, and hypertension.

A physical sign that is suggestive of moderate to severe insulin resistance is the hyperkeratotic condition acanthosis nigricans. This is a diffuse, hyperpigmented, velvety thickening of the skin that is found in the neck and axillae. The onset is usually insidious, with the first visible change being darkening of the skin pigmentation so as to appear dirty. As the skin thickens, it becomes velvety, and the skin line is accentuated. The skin eventually becomes rugose and mammillated. The presence of skin tags in conjunction with acanthosis nigricans is also a sign of insulin resistance.[17]

PHYSICAL EXAMINATION

The physical examination consists of accurate measurement of the blood pressure, height and weight, and BMI or waist-to-hip ratio by the techniques described in the Diagnostics section. A patient with the clinical features of metabolic syndrome should be screened annually for hyperglycemia, glucose intolerance, and type 2 diabetes mellitus. Those who have a diagnosis of metabolic syndrome should also be screened for the cardiovascular complications that accompany the syndrome and managed appropriately. It is also important to obtain a thorough history during the assessment to determine whether the patient is at risk for development of insulin resistance secondary to genetic factors or family history.

DIAGNOSTICS

Several techniques are available for measurement of insulin resistance and sensitivity. The definitive test (gold standard) for determination of insulin resistance is the euglycemic insulin clamp technique. This technique is costly and performed in the laboratory setting. A more practical way of assessing insulin resistance in the clinical setting is through the measurement of the fasting plasma insulin concentration. High plasma insulin values with normal glucose levels are suggestive of insulin resistance.

A variety of measures of body mass and body fat exist that express different aspects of general obesity, fat distribution patterns, and fat percentage. BMI is calculated as weight divided by height squared and measures percentage of body fat or total adipose tissue. The ratio of waist and hip circumference is highly correlated with visceral adipose tissue. Waist circumference (often measured at the level of the umbilicus or the top of the iliac crest with the patient standing) or waist-to-hip ratio (the ratio of waist circumference to hip circumference measured at the iliac crest) correlates well with insulin resistance and metabolic syndrome. BMI and waist-to-hip ratio are the most routinely used anthropometric indexes because they are easy to use and have a high reliability.

Common laboratory tests can be used to screen for the various other features associated with metabolic syndrome. Impaired fasting glucose (IFG) is measured after an 8- to 12-hour fast; levels between 100 and 126 mg/dL are diagnostic of IFG. Impaired glucose tolerance (IGT) is measured by administration of a 75-g load of oral glucose; after 2 hours, if plasma glucose values are between 140 and 200 mg/dL, IGT can be diagnosed. HDL and triglyceride blood levels are measured after an 8- to 12-hour fast. Microalbumin is measured with a random urine test. An elevated plasma CRP level may indicate inflammation and an emerging risk factor for CVD.[3]

DIAGNOSTICS

Metabolic Syndrome

LABORATORY
- Glucose tolerance test, fasting blood glucose
- Fasting plasma insulin concentration
- Fasting lipid profile
- Urinalysis (for protein)
- CRP

DIFFERENTIAL DIAGNOSIS

The diagnosis of metabolic syndrome is based on clinical presentation, so it is important to rule out hypertension, dyslipidemia, or obesity without manifestations of insulin resistance. The differential diagnoses also include type 2 diabetes mellitus and IGT, which can be excluded with laboratory testing. Other diseases characterized by insulin resistance are polycystic ovary syndrome, Cushing syndrome, congenital adrenal hyperplasia, lipodystrophy and lipoatrophic diabetes, type A insulin resistance (insulin receptor mutations), and type B insulin resistance (anti–insulin receptor antibodies). Genetic syndromes (Down syndrome, Turner syndrome, or muscular dystrophies), neurodegenerative disorders (Werner syndrome and Friedreich ataxia), and excess hormonal antagonists such as glucocorticoids, growth hormone, and catecholamines are also characterized by insulin resistance.

DIFFERENTIAL DIAGNOSIS

Metabolic Syndrome

- Type 2 diabetes mellitus
- IGT, IFG
- Polycystic ovary syndrome
- Cushing syndrome
- Congenital adrenal hyperplasia
- Lipodystrophy and lipoatrophic diabetes
- Type A insulin resistance (insulin receptor mutations)
- Type B insulin resistance (anti–insulin receptor antibodies)
- Genetic syndromes

MANAGEMENT

It is imperative to treat the different components of metabolic syndrome appropriately to prevent or to lessen the risk of cardiovascular morbidity and mortality. Studies have found that the prevalence of coronary heart disease, myocardial infarction, and stroke is significantly increased with metabolic syndrome.[2,14,15] Methods to treat metabolic syndrome include both nonpharmacologic and pharmacologic measures.

Nonpharmacologic treatments for insulin resistance include healthy lifestyle changes in diet and exercise. Because many individuals with metabolic syndrome are overweight, dietary treatment should focus primarily on weight reduction. Weight loss lowers serum cholesterol and triglycerides, raises HDL cholesterol, lowers blood pressure and glucose, reduces insulin resistance, and decreases serum levels of CRP and PAI-1.

Weight reduction recommendation is a 10% decrease in body weight within 6 months. This can be achieved by a low-calorie diet (800 to 1500 kcal/day or a decrease of at least 500 kcal/day). General dietary recommendations include a low intake of saturated fats, *trans*–fatty acids, and cholesterol; reduced consumption of simple sugars; and increased intakes of fruits, vegetables, and whole grains. Dietary carbohydrates with a high glycemic index increase blood glucose levels more rapidly, whereas fiber-rich foods with a low glycemic index are digested and absorbed more slowly and can lower triglyceride and raise HDL cholesterol levels. Intake of soluble fiber has been shown to decrease postprandial glucose levels and concentrations of insulin. Plant-based foods, such as whole grains, fruits, and vegetables, can decrease systolic and diastolic blood pressures and reduce the incidence of coronary heart disease. A monounsaturated fat diet improves insulin sensitivity and the dyslipidemia associated with metabolic syndrome compared with a diet high in saturated fat. The treatment of the thrombogenic disorders (elevated plasma fibrinogen and factor VIII coagulant activity levels, raised PAI-1) can be improved with a low-fat diet and a high content of foods rich in complex carbohydrates and dietary fiber. "Crash diets" and "extreme diets," consisting of very low calories, high fat, and low carbohydrates, are not recommended because although initial weight loss is greater, the long-term weight loss is no more than that of the low-calorie diet, and they are seldom effective in producing long-term weight loss. Less than 7% of total calories should come from saturated fats, and less than 200 mg of cholesterol should be consumed per day. Plant stanols and sterols and soluble fibers such as cereal grains, beans, peas, legumes, fruits, and vegetables will lower LDL. Protein should not exceed 0.8 g/kg daily and should be lean or low fat. Following the DASH diet (Dietary Approaches to Stop Hypertension) can lower sodium intake.[18]

Exercise and physical training should include moderately intense cardiovascular aerobic exercise for 30 minutes 5 days a week or vigorously intense cardiovascular aerobic exercise for 20 minutes 3 days a week and 8 to 10 strength training exercises, 8 to 12 repetitions of each exercise twice a week. This could include brisk walking, bicycling, and swimming. The American Heart Association recommends 10,000 steps per day (5 miles). Suggestions also include adding multiple short bouts of activity (10 to 15 minutes), decreasing leisure-time sedentary activities such as watching television, using simple home exercise equipment such as treadmills, and self-monitoring of exercise. The exercise session should begin with a 10-minute warm-up consisting of light aerobic activity and stretching and end with a 5- to 10-minute cool-down period to lower the heart rate. If the individual is sedentary, a careful cardiovascular assessment may be needed before initiation of an exercise program. Exercise improves insulin resistance by increasing glucose use by the muscle. Glycogen synthase activity and the number of glucose transporters translocated to the cell surface increase after exercise. Glucose disposal by the skeletal muscle and insulin sensitivity continue for many hours after completion of the exercise. This improvement in insulin sensitivity may prevent the progression of the metabolic abnormalities. Regular aerobic training has also been shown to significantly decrease systolic and diastolic blood pressures. Physical training has been shown to decrease plasma levels of triglyceride by 15% to 30%. Exercise improves the removal of very-low-density lipoprotein (VLDL) and intermediate-density lipoprotein particles and decreases the levels of small, dense LDL associated with metabolic syndrome. An increase in HDL cholesterol may occur if exercise training is intense and prolonged. Regular physical exercise improves fibrinolytic activity and lowers levels of PAI-1. Exercise and calorie restriction can cause weight loss and a loss of intra-abdominal fat, which will decrease the insulin resistance associated with metabolic syndrome. Recommendations for exercise for individuals with metabolic syndrome are similar to those for individuals with type 2 diabetes (see Chapter 206).[19]

Although the Food and Drug Administration has not approved any drugs specifically for the treatment of metabolic syndrome, treatment of the individual risk factors associated with metabolic syndrome decreases CVD risk. Pharmacologic therapy would include antihypertensives, 3-hydroxy-3-methylglutaryl–coenzyme A (HMG-CoA) reductase inhibitors (statins), ezetimibe, fibric acid derivatives, aspirin therapy, the biguanide metformin, and weight loss medications.

Antihypertensive therapy includes a goal blood pressure of below 140/90 mm Hg. The classes of antihypertensives that have been found to be effective in reducing blood pressure and increasing insulin sensitivity are alpha-adrenergic antagonists and the angiotensin-converting enzyme (ACE) inhibitors. Alpha-adrenergic antagonists play a beneficial role in the dyslipidemia found in metabolic syndrome. They improve lipoprotein metabolism by decreasing triglyceride and VLDL concentrations and increasing HDL cholesterol. ACE inhibitors and angiotensin II receptor blockers have been found to reduce the incidence of type 2 diabetes in patients with hypertension and CVD; they improve the lipid profile, can prevent or retard progression of renal disease, and also improve the microalbuminuria found in metabolic syndrome. Calcium channel blockers are effective in lowering blood pressure and decreasing adverse CVD outcomes and have no profound adverse effects on lipid or glucose metabolism. Beta blockers are cardioprotective in patients with established CVD.[20]

Dyslipidemia should be treated. Goals are as follows: triglyceride levels below 150 mg/dL, LDL cholesterol below 100 mg/dL, and HDL cholesterol above 40 mg/dL in men or above 50 mg/dL in women with metabolic syndrome. Statins may lower LDL cholesterol by 25% to 45%, raise HDL cholesterol by 5% to 10%, and lower triglycerides by 7% to 30%. Statins modulate endothelial function, stabilize plaque, and provide anti-inflammatory and antithrombotic effects that can further reduce CVD risk in metabolic syndrome. Ezetimibe inhibits cholesterol absorption and in combination with statins can reduce LDL 20% to 30%.[21] If the triglyceride level is very high (>500 mg/dL), it is recommended that a fibric acid derivative (such as gemfibrozil), fenofibrate, or nicotinic acid (niacin) be used, which may decrease triglyceride levels by 20% to 50%.[21] Gemfibrozil has been shown to improve insulin action and flow-mediated vasodilation as well as to increase HDL levels. Nicotinic acid in high doses can raise plasma glucose levels. Severe myopathy may occur with the combination of a statin plus gemfibrozil. Creatine kinase (CK) and transaminases should be monitored when these medications are used.[21]

Aspirin is beneficial in the reduction of myocardial infarction in diabetic and nondiabetic individuals. Aspirin can significantly reduce cardiovascular events including myocardial infarction. Low-dose aspirin modifies the prothrombotic-proinflammatory state found in metabolic syndrome. The American Heart Association currently recommends use of aspirin prophylaxis in patients with established arteriosclerotic CVD, provided it is not contraindicated and the risk/benefit ratio suggests an advantage (Class 1, Level A evidence).[22]

Metformin has been shown to reduce hyperinsulinemia and insulin resistance, to lower blood triglyceride levels, to assist in weight reduction, and to lower plasma PAI-1 levels. Metformin improves the sensitivity of cells to insulin, reduces hepatic glucose production, and increases glucose uptake in muscle and other peripheral tissues. Through these mechanisms of action, metformin has been found to reduce or to prevent macrovascular complications. Serum creatinine must be monitored while metformin is being used.[23]

The Diabetes Prevention Program was a randomized clinical trial conducted to evaluate the safety and efficacy of interventions that may delay or prevent development of diabetes in individuals at increased risk for type 2 diabetes. The study found that intensive lifestyle interventions, including at least 150 minutes of moderate-intensity exercise per week together with a healthy diet to achieve and to maintain a 7% loss of body weight, reduced the incidence of diabetes by 58%; the use of metformin, 850 mg twice daily, reduced the incidence of diabetes by 31%.[24]

The National Institutes of Health recommends consideration of pharmacologic treatment for individuals with a BMI of at least 30 kg/m^2. Pharmacologic agents available to treat excess adiposity include appetite suppressants and inhibitors of nutrient absorption.

- Phentermine, a sympathomimetic amine anorectic, is recommended for short-term use only owing to the cardiac side effects of palpitations, hypertension, and tachycardia.
- These agents are usually taken in the morning and lead to decreased appetite later in the afternoon and evening.
- Orlistat (Xenical) is an inhibitor of gastrointestinal and pancreatic lipases and prevents the absorption of approximately 30% of the ingested dietary fat from the stomach and small intestine. Side effects include flatulence and fecal urgency. A multivitamin supplement is required to counter the malabsorption of the fat-soluble vitamins A, D, and E.
- Phentermine and topiramate extended release is a sympathomimetic amine anorectic. It should be used in combination with a low-calorie diet and increased physical activity. Side effects include dry mouth, paresthesia, constipation, dysgeusia, insomnia and dizziness.
- Locaserin hydrochloride is an appetite suppressant that stimulates the satiety center and reduces hunger by the production of opiomelanocortin neurons in the hypothalamus. It should also be used in combination with a low calorie diet and increased physical activity. Side effects include headache, upper respiratory infection, nausea, dizziness and fatigue.[25]
- Successful surgical procedures to treat obesity include gastric bypass (Roux-en-Y), gastroplasty (vertical banded gastroplasty), biliopancreatic diversion, biliary intestinal bypass, ileogastrostomy, and jejunoileal bypass. Follow-up after these procedures includes monitoring of vitamin and hematologic status, adherence to specific postoperative dietary guidelines, and psychological issues.[26]

LIFE SPAN CONSIDERATIONS

Insulin resistance may occur at any age. Childhood obesity is epidemic, and data from the International Obesity Task Force indicate that the overall prevalence of metabolic syndrome is 11.9% among overweight and 29.2% among obese adolescents.[27] The criteria for metabolic syndrome in children (aged 10 to 16 years) are the same as those for adults, but include waist circumference above the 90th percentile for age, gender, and race.

Childhood obesity increases the risk for metabolic syndrome in childhood, adolescence, and adulthood. This risk can be reduced if an obese child reduces his or her relative weight through diet and exercise. The baseline assessment of and identification of obese children can possibly lead to the prevention of adult obesity, metabolic syndrome, and cardiovascular risk.

Parents require education on ways to promote healthy lifestyle, proper nutrition, weight loss, and increased physical activity in young obese children. These healthy lifestyle modifications must continue throughout the entire life span.

Individuals older than 65 years have increased risk for metabolic syndrome. The older adult may be at increased risk for development of insulin resistance secondary to increased obesity, decreases in physical activity, and changes in body mass because of muscle loss and increased adipose tissue. Older adults may need to be educated on exercise programs tailored to their needs or modified for the chronic illnesses they have. Exercise recommendations are the same for older adults as mentioned earlier in the guidelines for cardiovascular aerobic exercises and strength training exercises, but for persons at risk for falling, the recommendations are to perform balance exercises and to have a physical activity plan with a health care provider to manage risks and take therapeutic needs into account. A referral to a dietitian may be beneficial because dietary recommendations may need to be modified to provide for the older adult's nutritional needs.

COMPLICATIONS

The complications associated with the features of metabolic syndrome include CVD, atherosclerotic vascular disease, ischemic heart disease, coronary artery disease, myocardial infarction, and stroke.

Insulin resistance is the pathophysiologic hallmark of IGT and type 2 diabetes and may occur decades before the clinical presentation of these diseases. As the beta cell function deteriorates and is no longer able to compensate for the insulin resistance and as glucose levels rise, a transition from insulin resistance to IGT with mild increases in postprandial glucose levels occurs and eventually results in type 2 diabetes mellitus.

Very high triglyceride levels can provoke an acute episode of pancreatitis. Elevated PAI-1 may lead to clotting dysfunction and coagulation abnormalities, resulting in an acute cardiovascular event such as stroke or myocardial infarction.

INDICATIONS FOR REFERRAL OR HOSPITALIZATION

A physician consultation is necessary when the hypertension or dyslipidemia (associated with metabolic syndrome) is resistant to therapy. Referral to a dietitian may be beneficial to assist the individual with meal planning and weight loss. A health psychologist can provide psychological support as well as support with realistic goal setting, stress management, and behavior modification methods. An exercise physiologist or physical therapist can assist in the development of a safe and effective exercise regimen. Commercial weight loss programs can offer social support, oversight, and accountability.

PATIENT AND FAMILY EDUCATION

Education should focus on the pathology of metabolic syndrome and associated characteristics along with the complications and cardiovascular risks that accompany the syndrome. This instruction should address medication use, mechanism of action, and adverse effects. Education must be provided to the patient and the family members because meal planning and participation in a physical fitness program will benefit the patient and family members involved. Family support is necessary to assist the patient with the lifestyle changes needed to decrease the risks of complications involved in the syndrome. Explaining the benefits of healthy eating and exercise can empower and motivate the patient. The discussion should involve exploring the patient's feelings toward metabolic syndrome and the treatment regimen. The patient should be instructed on mode, frequency, and intensity of exercise. Preferably, an exercise program of the patient's choice will better ensure adherence. Smoking cessation and limited use of alcohol, including the effects on insulin resistance, triglyceride levels, and cardiovascular risks, should be discussed. Mutual goal setting before the initiation of treatment is necessary for the patient's success. Both written and verbal instructions must be given to the patient and reinforced at each visit.

HEALTH PROMOTION

Health care providers are in a unique position to intervene, motivate, and influence the patient's outcome and the family members through teaching, counseling, and health promotion. As discussed previously, insulin resistance and metabolic syndrome are now being found in children; therefore it is imperative to start promoting healthy lifestyles at a very young age. Promotion of weight loss in the individual who is moderately obese can prevent the development of insulin resistance and the complications associated with the syndrome. Practitioners can assist the patient in changing harmful health behaviors through counseling on nutrition and facilitating increases in physical activity. Weight management behavioral changes include improvements in eating habits, such as setting goals, planning meals, reading labels, eating regularly, reducing portion sizes, controlling social and environmental cues that encourage overeating, monitoring results, and avoiding binges. Disease prevention and health promotion before the occurrence of complications associated with metabolic syndrome are more cost-effective in terms of health care dollars and promote savings in human suffering. Through health promotion and early intervention, the occurrence and ramifications of metabolic syndrome can surely be decreased or possibly eliminated.

CHAPTER 213

PARATHYROID GLAND DISORDERS

Alan Ona Malabanan

DEFINITION AND EPIDEMIOLOGY

The four parathyroid glands, located in the neck next to the thyroid, sense serum levels of ionized calcium by the calcium-sensing receptor and regulate calcium through parathyroid hormone (PTH) release. PTH is an 84–amino acid peptide that raises serum calcium concentration in three ways: (1) by acting directly on bone to release calcium into the extracellular fluid; (2) by acting directly on the kidney to decrease renal loss of calcium; and (3) by acting indirectly on the intestinal tract, through the activation of vitamin D, to increase dietary calcium absorption. Parathyroid disorders cause dysfunction through their effects on bone, kidney, serum calcium, and phosphorus.

The two major categories of parathyroid dysfunction are hyperparathyroidism (the oversecretion of PTH) and hypoparathyroidism (the undersecretion of PTH). PTH levels must always be interpreted in the context of the corrected serum calcium level or serum ionized calcium level (see Chapter 208). Considered in this manner, primary hyperparathyroidism can be defined as the *inappropriate* secretion of PTH in the setting of hypercalcemia. Secondary hyperparathyroidism is an *appropriately increased* secretion of PTH in the setting of low or normal serum calcium concentration and can be caused by vitamin D deficiency or renal failure. Tertiary hyperparathyroidism is prolonged secondary hyperparathyroidism in which hypercalcemia develops; it is an initially appropriate secretion that later becomes inappropriate. Hypoparathyroidism is the inappropriately low secretion of PTH in the setting of hypocalcemia.

Automated chemistry measurements have allowed the routine detection of asymptomatic hypercalcemia, increasing the recognition of early primary hyperparathyroidism. The estimated incidence of primary hyperparathyroidism ranges from 1 in 500 to 1 in 1000, with the peak incidence in the sixth decade of life. The incidence in women is higher than that in men, approximately 3:1.[1] For unclear reasons, there was a declining incidence after the 1970s, although some consideration has been given to prior exposure to head and neck irradiation in the 1930s and 1940s as well as nuclear testing in the 1950s and 1960s as potential causes of the increased and subsequently decreased incidence.[2] Recent work has suggested another peak in incidence in 1998, coincident with the introduction of national osteoporosis screening guidelines.[2]

Secondary hyperparathyroidism is found commonly in patients with chronic kidney disease (CKD), often when the glomerular filtration rate (GFR) falls below 50 mL/min. Vitamin D deficiency and insufficiency, defined as serum 25-hydroxyvitamin D levels of less than 20 ng/mL and 30 ng/mL, respectively, are other important causes of secondary hyperparathyroidism, particularly in older adults and institutionalized patients, and have been estimated to occur in 40% to 100% of U.S. and European community-dwelling elders.[3] Secondary hyperparathyroidism may also occur in patients being treated with glucocorticoids or proton pump inhibitors, which cause decreased intestinal calcium absorption.

Hypoparathyroidism is primarily a consequence of thyroid and parathyroid surgery. The incidence of acute postsurgical hypoparathyroidism ranges from 0.6% to 17%, depending on the skill of the surgeon and the type of operation. A study has suggested that the rate of long-term hypoparathyroidism after thyroidectomy is actually low.[4]

Specialist referral is indicated for all suspected cases of parathyroid disorders.

PATHOPHYSIOLOGY

In 80% of cases of primary hyperparathyroidism, excess PTH is produced by a single parathyroid adenoma. In 15% to 20% of cases, it is produced by hyperplasia of all four glands, which may be associated with multiple endocrine neoplasia (MEN) type I or type II. Primary hyperparathyroidism is produced by a parathyroid carcinoma in less than 0.5% of cases.[1]

Excess PTH stimulates osteoclast-mediated bone degradation, releasing calcium and phosphorus into the extracellular space. As a result, prolonged exposure to excess PTH will erode bone, particularly cortical (dense) bone. Trabecular bone is relatively spared because of a concomitant increase in osteoblast-mediated bone formation. Skeletal sites with primarily cortical bone, such as the wrist and proximal radius, are particularly at increased risk for fracture.

PTH acts on the kidney to increase calcium reabsorption and to increase phosphorus losses. The rising serum calcium concentration gradually exceeds the kidney's ability to reabsorb the filtered calcium, thus increasing urinary calcium. Nephrocalcinosis, nephrolithiasis, and renal dysfunction may result. PTH receptors also exist on a variety of tissues, including brain, skin, and heart. The effects of PTH on these tissues are not yet well characterized.

Secondary hyperparathyroidism represents a compensation for decreased serum levels of ionized calcium. The kidney is important in calcium and phosphorus homeostasis, and renal insufficiency disturbs calcium metabolism in four ways. First, decreased phosphorus clearance, hyperphosphatemia, and increases in fibroblast growth factor 23 decrease serum ionized calcium and calcitriol production. Second, decreased renal activation of vitamin D decreases intestinal calcium absorption. Third, uremia produces PTH resistance, thus necessitating higher levels of PTH. Finally, uremia decreases the inhibitory effect of calcium on PTH release. As with primary hyperparathyroidism, excess PTH will erode bone. These derangements in mineral metabolism may also lead to extraskeletal and vascular calcification.[5] Prolonged stimulation of the parathyroid glands by hypocalcemia results in hyperplasia of the glands. On occasion, this leads to autonomous parathyroid function and hypercalcemia (tertiary hyperparathyroidism).

Vitamin D deficiency results in decreased intestinal calcium absorption. This, coupled with the daily loss of calcium in the urine and the feces, leads to a net loss of calcium. To prevent overt hypocalcemia, the parathyroid glands secrete more PTH, releasing calcium from the bone and thus preserving normal serum calcium levels. Long-standing vitamin D deficiency may lead to overt hypocalcemia if calcium stores in the bone are depleted.

Hypoparathyroidism results from the destruction of the parathyroid glands, whether the result of surgery, irradiation, infiltration (hemochromatosis, amyloidosis, hemosiderosis), malignant disease, or autoimmune disease. As may be expected, decreased PTH affects the renal conservation of calcium, the intestinal absorption of calcium, and the degradative release of calcium from bone. Hypocalcemia results from these effects. Of note, hypomagnesemia or hypermagnesemia may decrease PTH secretion or diminish PTH action on the bone and should be considered a potential cause of hypoparathyroidism.

CLINICAL PRESENTATION

Asymptomatic elevation of serum calcium is the most common presentation of primary hyperparathyroidism. The hypercalcemia may be masked by hypoalbuminemia or minimized by concomitant vitamin D deficiency and the PTH levels may fall, inappropriately nonsuppressed, within the normal range. This hypercalcemia is usually accompanied by a fasting hypophosphatemia. A preclinical state, called normocalcemic primary hyperparathyroidism, has recently been identified but is currently not well characterized.[6]

Some patients may report nonspecific neurocognitive symptoms, which vary with the magnitude of hypercalcemia: weakness, easy fatigability, depression, intellectual weariness, cognitive impairment, loss of initiative, anxiety, irritability, and insomnia, some of which they or their physician may attribute to normal aging. Cardiovascular manifestations may include hypertension, coronary artery disease, left ventricular hypertrophy, and cardiac or valvular calcifications, which are associated with higher levels of serum calcium.[6] Kidney stones are also a common presenting symptom of primary hyperparathyroidism, although some "asymptomatic" patients may have a history of unexplained hematuria, nocturia, and polyuria.

Often, primary hyperparathyroidism may be identified during the evaluation of osteoporosis, which typically affects predominantly cortical bone sites (radius, femoral neck) more than predominantly trabecular bone sites (lumbar spine). A severe form of parathyroid bone disease, osteitis fibrosa cystica (OFC), is associated with multiple lytic bone lesions and subperiosteal bone resorption. OFC may be found in conjunction with an acute hyperparathyroid crisis in which the hypercalcemia develops quickly, causing obtundation, volume depletion, and cardiac arrhythmias.

Hyperparathyroidism may occur as part of a familial disorder such as MEN. MEN type I includes hyperparathyroidism, pituitary tumors, and pancreatic tumors (insulinoma, gastrinoma). MEN type IIA includes hyperparathyroidism, pheochromocytoma, and medullary thyroid carcinoma. In these disorders, the hyperparathyroidism is caused by parathyroid hyperplasia.

Secondary hyperparathyroidism is typically found with CKD stages 3 to 5 and vitamin D deficiency. Patients may be initially seen with bone pain or a pathologic fracture. Risk factors for vitamin D deficiency include minimum sun exposure, inadequate vitamin D dietary intake, obesity, malabsorption, prior gastric surgery, and medications that may increase the metabolism of vitamin D (e.g., rifampin, ketoconazole, and anticonvulsants). Other factors, such as aging, sunscreen use, and heavily pigmented skin, decrease sunlight-mediated vitamin D synthesis in the skin.[3] Secondary hyperparathyroidism in CKD produces a host of metabolic derangements, including hypocalcemia, hyperphosphatemia, and low 1,25-dihydroxyvitamin D levels. This hyperparathyroidism may be associated with increased vascular disease and vascular or soft tissue calcification.

Hypoparathyroidism manifests as hypocalcemia accompanied by hyperphosphatemia. The presentation can range from symptoms of perioral and digital paresthesias to life-threatening cardiac arrhythmias, seizures, and laryngospasm. The severity of presentation depends on the rapidity of the development of hypocalcemia. It may also depend on the presence of acidemia, which increases ionized calcium, or alkalemia, which decreases ionized calcium. Chronic hypocalcemia can produce premature cataract formation or basal ganglia calcifications, at times with a reversible Parkinson syndrome.

PHYSICAL EXAMINATION

Physical clues to primary hyperparathyroidism include band keratopathy, a white cloudiness at the nasal and temporal borders of the cornea. It may be mistaken for arcus senilis and is not specific for hypercalcemia caused by hyperparathyroidism. On occasion, there may be bone tenderness, particularly of the sternum and tibia. Rarely, there may be a palpable neck mass that is indicative of parathyroid carcinoma or medullary thyroid carcinoma (in MEN type II).

The physical clues to hypoparathyroidism include the signs indicative of hypocalcemia. The Chvostek sign may be present in cases of hypocalcemia. This test is performed by tapping (the point of a triangular reflex hammer or a fingertip may be used) over the facial nerve (cranial nerve VII). Contraction of the facial muscles (seen at the corner of the lip and cheek) is a positive test result. The Trousseau sign may also be present in hypocalcemia. This test is performed by placing a blood pressure cuff around the biceps and inflating the cuff approximately 10 to 20 mm Hg above the systolic blood pressure. The cuff is left inflated, maintaining a constant pressure, for 3 minutes or until a positive result is elicited. The test result is positive if carpal spasm occurs (flexion at the wrist and extension of the fingers). The presence of Chvostek and Trousseau signs can be affected by abnormalities in acid-base balance, potassium level, and magnesium level. Bone tenderness over the sternum or tibia may be present in vitamin D deficiency.[3]

Pseudohypoparathyroidism type Ia, a resistance to PTH and notable for hypocalcemia with elevated PTH, may be associated with obesity, short stature, round facies, brachydactyly of hands or feet, shortened fourth and fifth metacarpals, mild mental retardation, and subcutaneous ossifications.[7]

DIAGNOSTICS

Laboratory testing is necessary for the diagnosis of parathyroid disease. The most useful PTH assay is the PTH second- or third-generation assay, which allows measurement of the intact PTH molecule.

Primary hyperparathyroidism requires the assessment of PTH, serum calcium, albumin, 25-hydroxyvitamin D, and fasting phosphorus. A bone mineral density assessment of a cortical bone site (e.g., radius), in conjunction with the standard lumbar spine and hip, is useful to assess the risk for osteoporosis; renal imaging (renal ultrasound) is useful in assessing the presence of nephrolithiasis, and renal stones would be indicative of symptomatic primary hyperparathyroidism. A 24-hour urine collection for calcium and creatinine is useful in the initial evaluation of primary hyperparathyroidism and if it is high, consideration may be given to a kidney stone risk profile.[6] Electrocardiography (ECG) may be useful in assessing hypercalcemic cardiotoxicity (QT shortening). Although it is not recommended for diagnosis, imaging with sestamibi scan or neck ultrasound has been useful for anatomic localization of the enlarged parathyroid glands, making minimally invasive parathyroidectomy possible.[8]

Secondary hyperparathyroidism and hypoparathyroidism also require assessment of PTH, serum calcium, albumin, and fasting phosphorus. A serum 25-hydroxyvitamin D level, if it is less than 20 ng/mL, is useful in establishing vitamin D deficiency as the cause of the hyperparathyroidism. A 24-hour urine collection for calcium and creatinine would be helpful in the assessment of secondary hyperparathyroidism to assess for hypocalciuria (as a sign of calcium malabsorption) or hypercalciuria as a cause. A serum magnesium level may also be useful in evaluating hypoparathyroidism. ECG can reveal hypocalcemic cardiotoxicity (QT lengthening).

DIAGNOSTICS

Parathyroid Gland Disorders

HYPERPARATHYROIDISM

Laboratory

- PTH (PTH immunoradiometric assay)
- Serum calcium
- Albumin
- Fasting phosphorus
- 24-Hour urine calcium
- Serum 1,25-dihydroxyvitamin D*
- Serum 25-hydroxyvitamin D

Imaging

- X-ray examination of abdomen*
- Renal ultrasound
- Bone mineral densitometry (distal radius)

Other Diagnostics

- ECG*

HYPOPARATHYROIDISM

Laboratory

- PTH
- Serum calcium
- Albumin
- Fasting phosphorus
- Serum 1,25-dihydroxyvitamin D
- Magnesium
- Serum 25-hydroxyvitamin D

Other Diagnostics

- ECG*

*If indicated.

The most recent Kidney Disease: Improving Global Outcomes (KDIGO) guidelines for CKD–metabolic bone disease suggest that serum calcium, phosphorus, and PTH be measured in adult patients in CKD stage 3 and in children in CKD stage 2.[5] The frequency of monitoring is dependent on the severity of the CKD and the metabolic bone disease but may range from every 1 to 3 months to every 6 to 12 months. In CKD stages 4 and 5, alkaline phosphatase, an indicator of PTH effect on bone, may be tested every 12 months or more frequently if PTH is elevated. Those patients in CKD stages 3 to 5 with hyperparathyroidism should be evaluated and treated for hyperphosphatemia, hypocalcemia, and vitamin D insufficiency.

DIFFERENTIAL DIAGNOSIS

By definition, the differential diagnoses for the parathyroid diseases overlap with those of hypercalcemia and hypocalcemia. With primary hyperparathyroidism, the most important diagnosis to exclude is familial hypocalciuric hypercalcemia (FHH), an autosomal dominant trait characterized by hypercalcemia and hyperparathyroidism. With FHH, a mutation in the calcium-sensing receptor gene causes a defective calcium-sensing receptor that requires higher levels of calcium to suppress PTH secretion. Patients with FHH do not have the usual sequelae of primary hyperparathyroidism and generally have a benign course. A history of lifelong hypercalcemia, a family history of hypercalcemia, and concomitant mild hypermagnesemia are important clues to FHH.

In FHH, the fractional excretion of calcium (FE_{Ca}) is typically less than 0.01%. For patients with primary hyperparathyroidism, the FE_{Ca} is more than 0.013%. The formula is as follows:

$$FE_{Ca} = (U_{Ca} \times P_{Cr})/(U_{Cr} \times P_{Ca})$$

where U is urine concentration (mg/dL) of a 24-hour specimen and P is plasma concentration (mg/dL) for calcium (Ca) and creatinine (Cr).

An FE_{Ca} should be calculated to rule out FHH before parathyroidectomy for hyperparathyroidism. An FE_{Ca} of less than 0.01% suggests FHH. If it is needed, genetic analysis for a mutation in the calcium-sensing receptor can be done to confirm the diagnosis. Of note, autoantibodies directed at the calcium-sensing receptor can cause an acquired, immune-mediated disease that resembles FHH.

Another clinical situation that produces a similar picture is lithium-related parathyroid disease. Lithium appears to raise the calcium set-point through unclear mechanisms.

For hypoparathyroidism, the most important diagnostic consideration is hypomagnesemia or hypermagnesemia. Consideration of rare causes of hypoparathyroidism, such as autosomal dominant hypocalcemia or acquired calcium-sensing receptor activation, might be suggested by hypermagnesuria.

Pseudohypoparathyroidism, an inherited resistance to parathyroidism, can be a consideration if long-standing hypocalcemia is present with elevated levels of PTH in the face of normal magnesium balance and normal renal function.

DIFFERENTIAL DIAGNOSIS

Parathyroid Gland Disorders

HYPERPARATHYROIDISM
- Primary hyperparathyroidism
- Familial hyperparathyroidism
- Familial hypocalciuric hypercalcemia
- Lithium-related parathyroid disease
- Adenoma
- Radiation-induced hyperparathyroidism
- MEN syndrome
- Parathyroid carcinoma
- Secondary hyperparathyroidism
- Chronic renal disease
- Vitamin D deficiency
- Thiazide-induced hypercalcemia

HYPOPARATHYROIDISM
- Idiopathic
- Iatrogenic
- Congenital
- Polyglandular autoimmune syndrome
- Metastatic cancer
- Hemochromatosis
- Amyloidosis
- Hypermagnesemia or hypomagnesemia
- Parkinson syndrome

MANAGEMENT

The only cure for primary hyperparathyroidism is surgery, and referral to an experienced parathyroid surgeon is important. In most instances, resection of the parathyroid adenoma or 3 3/4 of the four hyperplastic parathyroid glands corrects the hyperparathyroidism. However, the changing character of primary hyperparathyroidism, with early diagnosis and primarily asymptomatic patients, has led to an increasing role for medical therapy.

An increasing body of data regarding the long-term complications and benefits of parathyroidectomy in asymptomatic patients with primary hyperparathyroidism has led to revisions in the criteria for parathyroidectomy:

- Age younger than 50 years.
- Serum calcium level 1 mg/dL above the upper limit of normal.
- Vertebral fracture by radiography, computed tomography (CT), magnetic resonance imaging (MRI), or densitometric vertebral fracture assessment (VFA).
- 24-Hour urine for calcium greater than 400 mg/day (>10 mmol/day) and increased stone risk by biochemical stone risk analysis.
- Presence of nephrolithiasis or nephrocalcinosis by radiography, ultrasound, or CT.
- GFR below 60 mL/min/1.73 m^2 (i.e., CKD stage 3), although there is no evidence that parathyroidectomy improves GFR.
- In perimenopausal or postmenopausal women and men older than 50 years, a T-score of −2.5 or lower at the lumbar spine, femoral neck, total hip, or distal radius; in premenopausal women and men younger than 50 years, a Z-score of −2.5 or lower at the same sites.[6]

Successful parathyroidectomy may lead, in some patients, to improvements in neurocognitive symptoms but more consistently to improvements in bone density and perhaps reduction in fracture risk.[8-10] The risk for nephrolithiasis decreases with parathyroidectomy, whereas cardiovascular disease and mortality do not seem to change.[8]

Medical management of primary hyperparathyroidism involves close monitoring of serum calcium and creatinine (at least annually) and bone density (every 1 to 2 years) to see if surgical criteria are met as the primary hyperparathyroidism progresses. Adequate calcium and vitamin D intake should be continued, ensuring a 25-hydroxyvitamin D level of at least 20 ng/mL.[6] Calcium and vitamin D restriction can worsen the bone disease and lead to worsening hyperparathyroidism. Patients should be encouraged to maintain weight-bearing activity and adequate fluid intake to prevent the volume depletion that can worsen hypercalcemia. Bisphosphonates, estrogen, and raloxifene therapy may be useful in increasing bone density without significant change in calcium levels in patients with primary hyperparathyroidism. Cinacalcet has been found to normalize serum calcium and PTH levels without improving bone density and is now approved for the medical management of hypercalcemia caused by primary hyperparathyroidism in patients in whom surgery is indicated but not possible. None of these therapies is a suitable replacement for parathyroidectomy but may be helpful in minimizing complications for those patients who are not surgical candidates.[11,12]

The management of secondary hyperparathyroidism depends on the cause. For renal failure, renal transplantation usually corrects the hyperparathyroidism, but it may be refractory if it is long-standing. Those patients in CKD stages 3 to 5 with hyperparathyroidism should be evaluated and treated for hyperphosphatemia, hypocalcemia, and vitamin D insufficiency. Phosphate levels should be treated, preferably with phosphate binders that are not calcium or aluminum based to minimize the effects on vascular calcification and aluminum toxicity. Patients with CKD stages 3 to 5, not on dialysis, with PTH levels increasing or above the normal range may be treated with calcitriol or vitamin D analogues. Patients with CKD stage 5 with PTH levels more than two to nine times the upper limit of normal, or rising PTH levels, may be treated with calcitriol or vitamin D analogues, cinacalcet, or a combination. These therapies may be modified or adjusted according to the presence of hypercalcemia, hyperphosphatemia, or hypocalcemia. In patients with CKD stages 3 to 5 who do not respond to medical or pharmacologic therapy, parathyroidectomy is indicated.[5]

Hypoparathyroidism is difficult to treat. PTH must be given parenterally and therefore is not easily replaced. Therapy usually consists of vitamin D analogues and calcium supplements. Dairy products, which are high in phosphorus, should be avoided. Perhaps the safest medication is calcitriol, but it is also the most expensive. It is preferable to ergocalciferol (vitamin D) because it acts more quickly (days versus weeks) and has a shorter duration of action, which allows rapid titration. Hypercalciuria is the main limitation of calcitriol therapy. The absence of the PTH effect on renal conservation of calcium results in hypercalciuria as intestinal absorption of calcium increases. Calcitriol should be started at 0.25 μg orally every day and increased as necessary every 2 to 4 weeks to bring serum calcium concentration into the low-normal range without producing hypercalciuria. The judicious use of thiazides may decrease urinary calcium loss and allow the normalization of serum calcium concentration. PTH therapy may decrease calcium and calcitriol requirements, without changing serum or urinary calcium levels.[13] PTH therapy has recently been approved for this indication but is available only through a restricted program.

COMPLICATIONS

Complications may result from the parathyroid disease process or its treatment. In addition to osteoporosis and nephrolithiasis, surgery for primary hyperparathyroidism may cause hypocalcemia as a result of temporary hypoparathyroidism, vitamin D deficiency, or hungry bone syndrome. With hungry bone syndrome, calcium and phosphorus are rapidly incorporated into bone. This cause of hypocalcemia is more common in patients with higher preoperative serum calcium and alkaline phosphatase levels or more severe bone disease.

INDICATIONS FOR REFERRAL OR HOSPITALIZATION

All patients with parathyroid disorders should be referred to a physician or an endocrinologist experienced in the treatment of parathyroid disease. If surgical therapy is indicated, a referral to an experienced parathyroid surgeon is essential.

LIFE SPAN CONSIDERATIONS

Cardiovascular mortality may be increased in patients with severe and moderately severe primary hyperparathyroidism, and this may decline after parathyroidectomy. The mortality may be affected by severity of the hypercalcemia, lower with milder hypercalcemia.[6] Increasing serum phosphate level (with resultant parathyroid disease) is associated with increasing mortality and cardiovascular disease among those with CKD, although there are no data showing that phosphate-lowering treatment decreases mortality.[5]

PATIENT EDUCATION AND HEALTH PROMOTION

For patients with primary hyperparathyroidism, understanding the importance of adequate calcium and fluid intake as well as continued monitoring of bone and calcium status is important. Patients unable to maintain fluid intake because of nausea or vomiting should be instructed to seek prompt medical attention. Potential complications of parathyroid bone disease, such as wrist and hip fractures, should be carefully explained. For patients with secondary hyperparathyroidism, the importance of calcium and vitamin D supplementation should be stressed. For patients who undergo surgical therapy or who have hypoparathyroidism, it is essential that they recognize the symptoms of hypocalcemia and the consequences of nonadherence to therapy, including tetany, laryngospasm, cardiac arrhythmias, and seizures.

CHAPTER 214

THYROID DISORDERS

Jennifer C. Braimon • Suzanne M. Rieke

Thyroid disease in its various forms is widely prevalent in the general population. Perhaps 50% of the population have microscopic nodules, 3.5% have occult papillary carcinoma, 15% have palpable goiters, and 10% have abnormal thyroid-stimulating hormone (TSH) levels; 5% of women have overt hypothyroidism or hyperthyroidism.[1]

Hormones secreted by the thyroid gland influence a variety of metabolic processes in the body. Thyroid function is regulated by TSH, which is secreted by basophilic cells in the anterior pituitary gland in response to the secretion of thyrotropin-releasing hormone (TRH) from the hypothalamus. TRH secretion is regulated in a negative feedback fashion by the thyroid hormones. Low serum levels of thyroid hormones trigger TRH release from the hypothalamus, which in turn causes TSH release from the pituitary. TSH causes increased release of thyroid hormones until a normal serum level is reached. Within the thyroid gland, thyroid function is affected by glandular organic iodine content.

BOX 214-1

Physiologic Effects of Thyroid Hormones

- Affect fetal development; secreted in fetus from 11 weeks and facilitate normal fetal growth
- Promote basal metabolic function; regulate oxygen consumption and heat production
- Affect cardiovascular muscle contraction
- Stimulate bone resorption and, to some extent, bone formation
- Permit normal glucose metabolism, absorption, and storage
- Function in the synthesis and breakdown of lipids
- Affect the rate of metabolism of many hormones and drugs (depends on amount of thyroid hormones)

The synthesis of T_4 (thyroxine) and T_3 (triiodothyronine) requires that adequate quantities of iodine enter the thyroid gland. Iodine enters from the bloodstream and is a constituent of both T_4 and T_3. These hormones are transported in the bloodstream bound to plasma proteins. The majority of T_4 is bound; only a small portion is free. However, it is the free T_4 concentration in the serum that indicates thyroidal activity. Approximately 80% of serum T_3 is formed in the liver, kidney, and muscle from the deiodination of T_4; the remaining 20% is secreted directly by the thyroid.[2] Alterations in the regulation of hormone secretion can have varied effects on the body (Box 214-1).

Alterations in the function of the thyroid gland may result in hypersecretion and increased metabolism (hyperthyroidism) or hyposecretion and decreased metabolism (hypothyroidism). Enlargement of the gland may also occur and take the form of localized nodules or generalized goiter. Localized nodules may be benign or malignant and solitary or multiple; goiters may be mild or extensive.

THYROID FUNCTION TESTING

Thyroid function can be evaluated in the laboratory through the use of thyroid function tests (TFTs). Thyroid structure and function can be assessed through a variety of imaging techniques and through biopsy.

TSH is the most sensitive indicator of overall thyroid function. Small changes in serum T_3 and T_4 levels affect TSH secretion in an inverse log-linear relationship. Current techniques allow measurement of serum TSH concentrations as low as 0.01 μIU/ml (third-generation assay, immunometric dual-antibody assay). This is generally the best screening test for thyroid dysfunction. Exceptions include patients with pituitary or hypothalamic (secondary or tertiary) disease and patients immediately after treatment of hypothyroidism or hyperthyroidism (when the TSH response to therapy may lag behind). In addition, various medications and nonthyroidal conditions may affect TSH levels.

TSH measurements are usually sufficient to categorize patients into one of three groups: hyperthyroid (TSH <0.3 μIU/ml), hypothyroid (TSH >4 μIU/ml), and euthyroid (TSH 0.3 to 4 μIU/ml). In a review by Surks and Boucai,[3] TSH distributions were found to shift to higher concentrations with age and to vary according to race, with higher concentrations found in whites than in blacks or Hispanics.

Approximately 99% of circulating T_4 and T_3 is bound to serum proteins. It is the free, unbound T_4 that is maintained at a constant level and correlates most with the thyroid state. Free T_4 traverses cell membranes to exert its effects on body tissues. Direct measurement by equilibrium dialysis of free T_4 is available but is cumbersome and technically demanding and is not for routine use. More commonly, a free thyroxine or a calculated free T_4 index that corrects the total T_4 (TT_4) level for the concentration of thyroxine-binding globulin (TBG) is used to asses the thyroxine level.

TBG determinations are inaccurate in patients with congenital absence of TBG or familial dysalbuminemic hyperthyroxinemia (FDH). Patients with FDH have aberrant albumin that binds T_4 (not T_3) with increased affinity. In FDH, laboratory tests reveal increased TT_4, normal total T_3 (TT_3), normal TSH, and normal free T_4 by equilibrium dialysis. Circumstances that increase TBG include pregnancy, acute hepatitis, and inherited abnormalities and the use of estrogen, oral contraceptives, methadone, or heroin. Decreased TBG results from acromegaly, nephrotic syndrome, cirrhosis, and chronic debilitating disease and from treatment with glucocorticoids, androgens, aspirin, nonsteroidal anti-inflammatory drugs (NSAIDs), and some penicillins.

If the TSH level is abnormal, a free thyroxine or free thyroxine index should be obtained. A T_3 level should be obtained in the evaluation of hyperthyroidism. T_3 determination is useful in diagnosis of T_3 toxicosis (normal TT_4, decreased TSH, and increased TT_3). T_3 levels may also be abnormal in what formerly was called euthyroid sick syndrome. T_3 levels may be low in patients with nonthyroidal illness.

Autoantibodies to thyroglobulin or thyroid microsomes may be found in patients with autoimmune thyroid disease. Thyroid peroxidase (TPO) is the major microsomal antigen. Anti-TPO antibodies are found in patients with Hashimoto thyroiditis and in less than 85% of patients with Graves disease (autoimmune hyperthyroidism). Antithyroglobulin antibodies are found in 20% of patients with Hashimoto thyroiditis and less than 20% of patients with Graves disease. Up to 15% of individuals in the general population have antibodies to either of these antigens. Quantification of the antibody titers is not clinically useful, although some studies suggest that the severity of thyroid destruction in Hashimoto thyroiditis is proportional to the anti-TPO titer. These tests are particularly useful in the evaluation of patients with atypical manifestations of autoimmune thyroid disease (i.e., isolated ophthalmopathy without signs of hyperthyroidism). They are also predictive of postpartum thyroiditis and neonatal Graves disease.[2]

Thyroid Imaging

Thyroid scans are used to assess the cause of hyperthyroidism (i.e., Graves disease, toxic nodules, thyroiditis) or the functional status of a nodule, but they are not used to assess thyroid function. Iodine isotope scans (iodine 123 [^{123}I]) are preferred to pertechnetate (technetium Tc 99m, TcO_4^-) because of the ability of the isotope scan to distinguish between hot and cold nodules. Pertechnetate is concentrated but not bound by thyroid tissues. The scan is performed 20 minutes after the administration of TcO_4^-. Its advantages include low radiation exposure to the patient, availability, and power of resolution (approximately 5 mm). Rarely, there will be a false-positive result (i.e., "hot" or false uptake) in malignant tissues. Iodine isotopes (^{123}I, ^{125}I, and ^{131}I) are concentrated and bound by thyroid tissues. The scan is performed 4 or 24 hours after the administration of ^{123}I or ^{125}I and 48, 72, or 96 hours after the administration of ^{131}I when it is used to search for metastatic thyroid cancer.

Normally the isotopes are distributed evenly throughout the thyroid gland. Each thyroid lobe is approximately 3 to 4 cm (1⅕ to 1⅗ inches) long, 1 to 1.5 cm (⅖ to ⅗ inch) wide, and 1 cm in depth. The isthmus measures about 0.5 cm (⅕ inch) in height and 2 to 3 mm (0.08 to 0.12 inch) in depth. A mottled appearance is seen in Hashimoto thyroiditis or in recently treated Graves disease. An inhomogeneous uptake is also seen in multinodular goiters.

Nodules are classified as hot, warm, or cold according to the concentration of iodine isotope in the nodule in comparison with the rest of the thyroid gland. Hot nodules are usually but not always benign. Many cold nodules (solid or cystic) are benign; however, most malignant neoplasms also appear as cold nodules. The normal radioactive iodine uptake (RAIU) is approximately 30%. Radionuclide imaging cannot be performed for at least 4 weeks in patients who have recently received iodine-containing compounds (i.e., intravenous contrast material). The results may also be inaccurate (falsely low uptake) in patients who are following a high-iodine diet. Exuberant iodine supplementation is becoming more prevalent and may cause a falsely low RAIU. When ordering isotope scans, the health care provider can order RAIU alone or with a scan.

Ultrasonography is used to evaluate the anatomy of the thyroid gland and to differentiate solid from cystic nodules. It is useful in detecting abnormalities larger than 0.5 cm (⅕ inch) in diameter. It localizes the position and depth of lesions and can be used to guide fine-needle aspiration (FNA). In a study by Papini and colleagues,[4] ultrasound features of thyroid nodules predictive of malignant transformation included irregular margins (relative risk (RR), 16.83), intranodular vascular spots (RR, 14.29), and microcalcifications (RR, 4.97). Eighty-seven percent of cancers manifested as a hypoechoic solid nodule on ultrasound.[4] Ultrasound cannot be used to visualize substernal goiters because of interference from bone. Computed tomography (CT) and magnetic resonance imaging (MRI) are better suited to assessment of substernal goiters. Cervical lymph nodes are also well visualized on ultrasound. Benign lymph nodes tend to be thin and oval with an echogenic hilum, whereas malignant nodes tend to be round with an undefined hilum and may be vascular. In a retrospective study of the ultrasound appearance of lymph nodes in 63 patients with increased cervical lymphadenopathy, a cystic appearance of cervical lymph nodes was characteristic of metastatic papillary thyroid carcinoma: 70% sensitivity, 100% specificity, 100% positive predictive value, 88% negative predictive value, and 90% accuracy.[5,6]

Fluorine 18 (^{18}F) fluorodeoxyglucose positron emission tomography (^{18}F-FDG-PET) has the highest resolution for detection of aggressive metastatic thyroid cancer lesions. Radiolabeled glucose is injected intravenously, and the scanner produces images that visualize where glucose is used. It identifies differences in how quickly cells metabolize glucose. Cancer cells metabolize glucose more quickly than normal cells do. Nodules with increased uptake on PET scan have a higher risk of malignancy.[7]

Long-term management of patients with differentiated thyroid cancers includes surveillance for recurrence after initial surgery and radioactive iodine ablation of remnant thyroid tissue. In these patients, disease-free status is defined by negative whole-body scan *and* undetectable thyroglobulin levels in the absence of interfering antibodies while the patient is receiving thyroid hormone suppression. FDG-PET scanning is especially useful in evaluating patients with differentiated thyroid cancer with elevated thyroglobulin levels and negative ^{131}I whole-body scans for metastases.[8] The ability of metastatic thyroid lesions to concentrate ^{131}I is usually indicative of a well-differentiated phenotype.[9] Metastases that do not concentrate ^{131}I are typically more aggressive. Most rapidly growing thyroid neoplasms have high metabolic rates. Well-differentiated thyroid tumors were found to retain FDG poorly. FDG volume of more than 125 mL or standard uptake of FDG of more than 10 g/mL suggested a significantly reduced survival. Focal uptake of ^{18}F-FDG can also be seen, however, in inflamed lymph nodes, thyroiditis, and benign thyroid nodules.

Thyroid Cytology

A biopsy specimen is obtained for histologic examination of thyroid tissue (i.e., the architecture is preserved) by closed needle biopsy. FNA biopsy obtains material for cytologic examination only. It is simple and safe but should be performed only by experienced practitioners and is done using ultrasound guidance. Initially, there had been concern about an increased risk of cancer spreading along the needle track from FNA, but this has not been observed. In experienced hands and with ultrasound guidance, FNA biopsy can be very accurate accurate in excluding cancer.

GOITER (SIMPLE, NONTOXIC)

DEFINITION AND EPIDEMIOLOGY

Enlargement of the thyroid gland is referred to as goiter. It may be caused by hormonal or immunologic stimulation or may result from inflammatory, infiltrative, or metabolic conditions, including iodine deficiency or excess, neoplasia, Graves disease, and thyroiditis.

Nontoxic (simple) goiter occurs when the thyroid gland enlarges in response to inadequate thyroid hormone production. Iodine deficiency remains the most common cause in large areas of Africa, Asia, and South America. The scarcity of iodine in the diet results in the production of TRH, which causes TSH to be secreted in large amounts. The increased TSH has two effects: (1) the retention of all available iodine by the thyroid and (2) the growth of thyroid cells. It is this latter effect that results in thyroid enlargement.

In developed countries, iodine is available in supplemented products such as table salt, fertilizers, animal feeds, and food preservatives. Therefore the most common cause of nontoxic goiter in developed countries is chronic autoimmune thyroiditis.

PATHOPHYSIOLOGY

On pathologic examination, simple goiter initially demonstrates a uniformly hypertrophic, hyperplastic, and hypervascular gland. Later, fibrosis may lead to formation of multiple nodules to create a multinodular goiter. These nodules may be "hot" and concentrate iodine or "cold" and not concentrate iodine. When the nodules become autonomous, hyperthyroidism may occur, a condition known as toxic multinodular goiter.

Individuals with a nontoxic goiter may or may not have increased levels of TSH. When levels are normal, it is believed the gland enlarges as a response to impaired hormone synthesis by increasing thyroid mass and cellular activity. In individuals with elevated levels of TSH, the thyroid gland increases mass and activity in response to this stimulation.

CLINICAL PRESENTATION

Patients with simple goiter usually are seen with either diffuse or multinodular thyroid enlargement. Symptoms such as difficulty swallowing and neck pressure may be present. Undetected and continued growth may result in extension of the thyroid gland downward to a substernal location in the chest. Presentation may include symptoms that result from compression of the trachea, esophagus, and vasculature.

PHYSICAL EXAMINATION

Examination of the thyroid should begin with observation under a good examining light. The normal gland is rarely visible. It is useful to have the patient extend the neck fully to permit inspection of the gland over the trachea. It is also helpful to observe from the side to identify any enlargement between the cricoid cartilage and the suprasternal notch. Any prominence in this area should be measured with a ruler and recorded; a high likelihood of goiter exists if the prominence is larger than 2 mm (0.08 inch). Having the patient swallow a sip of water enhances visualization and palpation of an enlarged gland. Palpation may be performed either in front of or behind the patient (depending on the practitioner's comfort), and the texture is noted. The texture of the thyroid can range from extremely soft to relatively firm; the gland may be smooth or may contain palpable nodules. Prominent glands should be measured, and the size recorded. Thyroid size should be categorized as normal or goiter. A small goiter is considered to be one to two times the normal size, and a large goiter is more than twice normal size.

Pemberton sign is used for examination when substernal goiter is suspected. The patient is asked to elevate both arms until they touch the sides of the head. Flushing of the face, cyanosis, and respiratory distress may occur as a result of impingement of structures within the thoracic inlet. Distention of neck veins may also be apparent in these patients.

DIAGNOSTICS

Laboratory studies may show low or normal free T_4 and a high, low, or, most often, normal TSH level. Thyroid ultrasound examination allows identification of gland size and the number and size of any nodules. If necessary for diagnosis, FNA may be performed. Isotope scans are not indicated as the first imaging study in patients with goiters. See the later discussions of thyroid nodules and thyroid cancer and hyperthyroidism.

DIAGNOSTICS

Goiter

LABORATORY	IMAGING
TSH	Radionuclide scanning*
Free T4*	Thyroid ultrasound
Antimicrosomal antibodies*	
	OTHER DIAGNOSTICS
	FNA*

*If indicated.

DIFFERENTIAL DIAGNOSIS

Simple goiter must also be differentiated from chronic autoimmune thyroiditis and toxic multinodular goiter. A careful history of symptoms is important. Also, with chronic autoimmune thyroiditis, circulating antimicrosomal antibody levels will be elevated.

DIFFERENTIAL DIAGNOSIS

Goiter

Iodine deficiency or excess
Neoplasia (multinodular, malignant)
Graves' disease
Simple goiter
Thyroiditis
- Chronic autoimmune (Hashimoto's) thyroiditis
- Silent thyroiditis
- Subacute thyroiditis
- Postpartum thyroiditis

Genetic goiter

MANAGEMENT

Specialist consultation is indicated for large goiters causing compressive symptoms and if indicated consultation with a thyroid surgeon.

The majority of nontoxic goiters grow slowly for many years. The presence of a goiter with no accompanying symptoms or cosmetic concerns is not an indication for treatment. Treatment indications include venous flow obstruction, compression of the trachea or esophagus, progressive enlargement of the entire goiter or individual nodules, neck discomfort, and cosmetic concerns. Treatment options include the following:

1. Surgical treatment, usually bilateral subtotal thyroidectomy, is the preferred treatment in otherwise healthy, young patients, especially in the presence of goiters that grow substernally or continue to enlarge, causing compressive symptoms. There is little evidence that postoperative suppressive T_4 treatment prevents goiter recurrence; therefore, it should not be routinely used. Routine postoperative monitoring of TSH may reveal how much functioning thyroid is left and help define those who may need postoperative treatment.[10]
2. Levothyroxine treatment will suppress TSH, correct any hypothyroidism, and slowly reduce the size of the goiter. However, this therapy may have significant adverse effects, such as decreased bone mineral density, atrial fibrillation, and biochemical hyperthyroidism, if it is not monitored closely. The best candidates for this form of treatment are young patients with small diffuse goiters and a high-normal TSH level. T_4 therapy is not recommended for patients with any type of goiter or nodule and a low TSH level because this therapy may cause hyperthyroidism, especially in older adults.[10] Some sources recommend a trial of suppressive therapy for patients with a solitary and nonfunctioning nodule, negative fine-needle aspirates, and normal or elevated TSH levels with the goal of keeping TSH at low-normal levels. Such therapy may continue for 6 months to 1 year before reevaluation.
3. Nontoxic multinodular goiter may also be treated with radioiodine to reduce thyroid volume. Therapy with ^{131}I has been found to be an effective alternative with few side effects

and is used more commonly in Europe than in the United States.[11] This therapy is especially useful in older patients or those with cardiopulmonary disease.

COMPLICATIONS

Nontoxic goiter, even if it is multinodular, has few complications. Of particular concern is the potential for a multinodular goiter to develop autonomous function with ensuing hyperthyroidism. Close monitoring of TSH enables identification of this potential problem. Large goiters, especially those with substernal components, can cause compressive symptoms. Surgical patients with a nontoxic goiter may require special observation for airway maintenance and hormone supplementation if indicated.

INDICATIONS FOR REFERRAL OR HOSPITALIZATION

Patients who have any indication for treatment of their goiter may require an endocrinology referral for discussion of an appropriate treatment and a surgical referral if thyroidectomy is selected as the treatment of choice.

LIFE SPAN CONSIDERATIONS

In general, multinodular goiter increases in frequency with aging. Also, benign diffuse goiter and multinodular goiters do tend to increase in size with age.

PATIENT AND FAMILY EDUCATION AND HEALTH PROMOTION

It is important that patients understand the definition and cause of the nontoxic goiter. Patients need to participate in developing the care plan and understand its rationale. Those who live in inland areas or have seafood allergies should use iodized salt. Patients should understand that nontoxic goiter is a manageable, highly livable condition that will not affect their lives in a negative way if it is well controlled.

THYROID NODULES AND THYROID CANCER

DEFINITION AND EPIDEMIOLOGY

A thyroid nodule is a distinct lesion within the thyroid that is radiologically different from the rest of the thyroid. Some palpable lesions do not correspond to radiologic abnormalities. Nonpalpable nodules found on ultrasound or other imaging studies are referred to as incidental thyroid nodules or thyroid incidentalomas. By this definition, thyroid nodules include both solid nodules and cysts.

With ultrasonography, approximately 50% of all single, palpable nodules are found to be in a multinodular gland. In general, nodules larger than 0.5 to 1 cm (⅕ to ⅖ inch) are palpable. Thyroid adenomas are benign neoplastic nodules within a capsule.

The prevalence of thyroid nodules depends on the method of evaluation. Palpable thyroid nodules are found in 4% to 7% of the general adult population.[12] Autopsy and ultrasound studies have quoted a prevalence as high as 50%. The lifetime risk for development of a thyroid nodule is estimated to be 5% to 10%. Thyroid nodules are common, and only 3% to 5% of all thyroid nodules are malignant.[12]

PATHOPHYSIOLOGY

Thyroid nodules may be caused by adenomas, cysts, carcinomas, multinodular goiters, Hashimoto thyroiditis, and subacute thyroiditis. Less common causes of neck lumps include the effects of prior surgery or ^{131}I, parathyroid cysts or adenomas, thyroglossal cysts, nonthyroidal lesions, and lymphomas.

Thyroid adenomas are benign, monoclonal growths. Benign thyroid tumors include embryonal, fetal, follicular, Hürthle cell, and papillary adenomas. They are distinguished by their characteristic histologic appearance. Malignant thyroid tumors include papillary, follicular, medullary, and anaplastic carcinomas.

CLINICAL PRESENTATION AND PHYSICAL EXAMINATION

Thyroid nodules are usually asymptomatic and are identified as a lump by patients or by providers during routine thyroid examinations. Increasing numbers of thyroid nodules are being identified incidentally during carotid Doppler ultrasound or other neck imaging studies. Clinical features that increase the likelihood of cancer include history of head and neck irradiation, family history of thyroid cancer, age younger than 20 years or older than 60 years, male gender, and history of multiple endocrine neoplasia type II or medullary thyroid cancer. Familial thyroid tumors also occur in Cowden disease (multiple hamartoma syndrome), Gardner syndrome (development of multiple tumors with autosomal dominant inheritance), and familial polyposis.

An anaplastic tumor may manifest as an enlarging, painful mass associated with hoarseness, dysphonia, dysphagia, or dyspnea. Patients with anaplastic thyroid cancer may have pathologic fractures of the spine or hip or thoracic outlet syndrome. Patients with toxic nodules may show symptoms of hyperthyroidism.

Important features noted during the physical examination include nodule size, consistency, and mobility and the presence and consistency of associated lymphadenopathy. Supraclavicular, anterior cervical, and submandibular lymph nodes should be examined. Although most thyroid cancers feel firm or hard, they can be soft and fluctuant on examination. The presence of a new nodule or enlarging nodule while a patient is receiving T_4 therapy is a cause for concern.

DIAGNOSTICS AND DIFFERENTIAL DIAGNOSIS

The initial evaluation of thyroid nodules includes history, physical examination, and measurement of TSH to exclude hyperthyroidism or hypothyroidism. The routine measurement of serum calcitonin (to exclude medullary thyroid cancer) is not useful or cost-effective.[13] Elevated TSH levels have been associated with an increased risk of malignant transformation in a thyroid nodule, as well as more advanced stage of differentiated thyroid cancer.[14,15]

Thyroid ultrasound evaluation should be performed for all patients with a suspected (i.e., incidental) abnormality found on CT, MRI, or ^{18}F-FDG-PET or with known thyroid nodules.[12] High-resolution sonography can clearly distinguish between solid and cystic components. The risk of malignancy in ^{18}F-FDG-PET–avid nodules is approximately 33%, and these cancers tend to be more aggressive. Ultrasound characteristics associated with a higher likelihood of malignancy include increased vascular flow to the nodule, hypoechoic nodules, irregular margins, absent halo, microcalcifications, and shape taller than the width in transverse dimension.[6] There are also ultrasound appearances that are predictive of benign nodules. Simple cysts are unlikely to be malignant. In a study by Bonavita and coworkers,[16] only 1 of 360 malignant nodules demonstrated a spongiform appearance (aggregation of multiple microcystic components making up more than 50% of the nodule volume).

Historically, radionuclide imaging was the first diagnostic test used in the evaluation of solitary thyroid nodules. Although it is true that most malignant thyroid neoplasms appear as cold nodules, most cold nodules are benign. Radionuclide scanning is now used as an initial test if a hyperfunctioning nodule is suspected. It may also be useful in patients with multinodular goiters to target FNA of cold nodules.

According to the revised American Thyroid Association guidelines for patients with thyroid nodules,[12] FNA biopsy is the procedure of choice in the evaluation of thyroid nodules. It is safe and technically simple but requires an experienced operator and cytopathologist. False-negative and false-positive rates are less than 5% with experienced users. Cytologic results are sufficient in 85% of biopsies for diagnosis. Ultrasound-guided FNAs have a lower rate of nondiagnostic and false-negative biopsy findings. The revised American Thyroid Association thyroid cancer guidelines (2015) recommend FNA for nodules larger than 1 cm with high-risk history, for solid nodules larger than 1 cm that are hypoechoic, and for complex (solid and cystic components) nodules larger than 1.5 cm with any suspicious ultrasound features.[12]

DIAGNOSTICS

Thyroid Nodules and Thyroid Cancer

LABORATORY
TSH

IMAGING
Thyroid ultrasound
Radionuclide scan*

OTHER DIAGNOSTICS
FNA

Molecular markers*
- mRNA gene expression classifier (high negative predictive value)
- Mutational analysis (high positive predictive value)

*If indicated.

DIFFERENTIAL DIAGNOSIS

Thyroid Nodules and Thyroid Cancer

BENIGN
- Adenomas
  - Follicular
  - Hürthle cell (oxyphil)
  - Colloid adenoma (multinodular goiter)
- Hashimoto (chronic lymphocytic) thyroiditis
- Subacute thyroiditis
- Cysts (colloid, simple, hemorrhagic)
- Thyroglossal duct cysts
- Parathyroid cysts or adenoma
- Surgery or radiation effects

MALIGNANT
- Papillary carcinoma
- Follicular carcinoma
- Hürthle cell carcinoma
- Anaplastic carcinoma
- Medullary carcinoma
- Primary thyroid lymphoma
- Metastatic carcinoma (e.g., renal cell, breast)

FNA cytology result categories include Benign, Follicular Lesion of Undetermined Significance (FLUS), Follicular Neoplasm, Suspicious for Malignancy, Malignancy, and Nondiagnostic. Risks for malignancy in each of theses categories are below 5%, 5% to 15%, 20% to 30%, 50% to 75%, and over 90%. Further evaluation of FNA aspirates for molecular markers may be considered for patients with indeterminate cytology. The use of gene expression classifiers, with high negative predictive value, may help to avoid diagnostic surgery in patients with indeterminate thyroid cytology results.[17,18]

MANAGEMENT

Specialist consultation with an endocrinologist or interventional radiologist is indicated for ultrasound-guided FNA biopsy of thyroid nodules, and immediate referral to a thyroid surgeon is indicated if compressive symptoms are present.

Immediate emergency department referral is indicated for patients who exhibit respiratory compromise from invasive tumors.

Management of thyroid nodule(s) noted after complete history and physical examination and TSH measurement is as follows:

- If TSH is suppressed, free T_4 and TT_3 are checked and a radionuclide scan is ordered (^{123}I uptake and scan). Autonomously functioning nodules appear as hot nodules on radionuclide scan. These nodules are rarely cancer, and therefore FNA is not required. Patients with functioning nodules with thyrotoxicosis should be treated with radioiodine or surgery. Use of thioamides is an option to treat hyperthyroidism in patients who want to avoid or defer definitive therapy. Patients with subclinical thyrotoxicoses can be monitored or treated (radioiodine or surgery) depending on adenoma size. FNA biopsy should be performed on indeterminate (warm) nodules and cold (nonfunctioning) nodules.
- If TSH is elevated, free T_4 is checked, the patient is started on levothyroxine therapy as indicated, and thyroid nodule(s) are evaluated.
- If TSH is normal, thyroid nodule(s) are evaluated as follows.
  - Thyroid ultrasound should be performed on all patients.
  - Patient is referred to endocrinologist or interventional radiologist for ultrasound-guided FNA biopsy.
  - Cytology results:
    - Benign: No further immediate evaluation is necessary. A repeated FNA biopsy should be reserved for enlarging nodules, defined as more than a 50% change in volume or a 20% increase in diameter with at least a 2-mm increase in two or more dimensions. A follow-up ultrasound should be performed in 6 to 12 months. The American Thyroid Association task force strongly recommends against use of T_4 suppression.[12]
    - Nondiagnostic: FNA is repeated in 2 to 3 months
    - FLUS or follicular neoplasm: FNA is repeated 2 to 3 months, and use of molecular markers is considered.
    - Suspicious for malignancy, or malignancy: Patient is referred to an experienced surgeon. For solitary lesions smaller than 1 cm, lobectomy may be performed. Total thyroidectomy is indicated if there is a history of head or neck irradiation, the tumor extends beyond the capsule, or the lesion is larger than 1 cm. The American Thyroid Association task force recommends

against use of radioactive iodine ablation in patients with low-grade thyroid cancer (unifocal cancer <1 cm or multifocal cancer with cumulative size <1 cm) in the absence of higher-risk features. Postoperative radioactive iodine therapy is used to ablate remnant thyroid tissue, to ease early detection of recurrence based on thyroglobulin levels, and to diagnose and treat metastases. Although most studies demonstrate a reduction in recurrence and decreased mortality with remnant ablation, benefits appear to be limited to patients with more advanced stages of thyroid cancer.[12,19]

Differentiated thyroid cancer is managed as follows:

- Use of the American Joint Committee on Cancer (AJCC) and Union for International Cancer Control (UICC) classification based on TNM (*T* refers to tumor size, *N* refers to lymph notes, and *M* refers to metastases) and age is recommended for all patients with differentiated thyroid cancer because of its usefulness in predicting mortality and its requirement for cancer registries.[19]
- Remnant ablation with radioactive iodine if indicated in patients with known distant metastases, evidence of extrathyroidal extension on pathology, tumor size larger than 4 cm, and tumors 1 to 4 cm with high-risk features.
- Thyroid hormone therapy is required to prevent hypothyroidism and prevent TSH stimulation of thyroid cancer cells. Suppression therapy (TSH below 0.3) is indicated for patients with intermediate and high-risk disease. The TSH goal with low-risk disease is 0.3 to 2.0.
- Patients with differentiated thyroid carcinoma are followed closely for the first 5 years and then at 6- to 12-month intervals. Thyroglobulin levels are followed postoperatively as a marker for recurrence (in the absence of interfering antithyroglobulin antibodies). Whole-body scans are followed after radioiodine therapy and in high-risk patients. Neck ultrasound is performed to assess for recurrence and metastatic cervical lymph nodes.

Medullary thyroid cancer and anaplastic thyroid cancers are more aggressive than well-differentiated thyroid cancers and therefore are treated differently.

LIFE SPAN CONSIDERATIONS

The net mortality rate of papillary thyroid cancer is 10% to 20% during 20 to 30 years. Several factors increase the risk of death from cancer: extrathyroidal invasion (six times the risk), metastasis (47 times), age older than 45 years (32 times), and tumor larger than 3 cm ($1\frac{1}{5}$ inches; six times).[3]

Various scoring systems are used to stratify the prognosis of patients with well-differentiated and medullary thyroid cancer. The AJCC/UICC staging system is recommended for all patients with differentiated thyroid cancer because of its usefulness in predicting mortality and its requirement for cancer registries. In patients 44 years old or younger, stage I disease is defined as any tumor size, with or without lymph node metastases without evidence of distant metastases; stage II disease in this age group is defined by the presence of any metastases. In patients 45 years old and older, stage I disease is defined as primary tumor 2 cm or smaller without lymph node or distant metastases; stage II disease is defined as primary tumor 2 to 4 cm without lymph node or distant metastases; and stage III disease includes patients with tumors larger than 4 cm without lymph node or distant metastases.[19]

COMPLICATIONS

Complications of thyroid surgery include hypoparathyroidism and hoarseness from recurrent laryngeal nerve damage. Side effects of radioiodine include thyroid tenderness, dry mouth, altered taste, and nausea. Cumulative doses of more than 300 mCi may increase the risk of leukemia. Bone marrow suppression is seen with cumulative doses of more than 500 mCi. Other potential complications of radioiodine include pulmonary fibrosis and ovarian or testicular failure. Treatment doses range from 30 to 150 mCi.

INDICATIONS FOR REFERRAL OR HOSPITALIZATION

Patients should be referred to a practitioner experienced in FNA biopsies. If the cytologic test results are positive or suggestive, the patient should be referred to an experienced thyroid surgeon. After surgery, the patient should be referred to a thyroid specialist, who can coordinate and administer therapeutic radioiodine. Patients are maintained with suppressive doses of T_4.

Indications for hospitalization include respiratory compromise because of invasive tumors.

PATIENT AND FAMILY EDUCATION AND HEALTH PROMOTION

Patients should be given instructions about precautions after radioiodine treatment or scanning. These instructions include the following:

- No kissing, exchanging of saliva, or sharing of food or eating utensils for 5 days; dishes should be washed in a dishwasher.
- No close contact with infants, young children (<8 years of age), or pregnant women for 5 days; it is permissible to be in the same room.
- No breastfeeding.
- Flush toilets twice after urinating, and wash hands thoroughly.
- If a sore throat or neck pain develops, take acetaminophen or aspirin.
- Notify the physician if nervousness, tremulousness, or palpitations increase.

Patients should be taught how to perform a thyroid self-examination. An informative website for patients with thyroid cancer is www.thyca.org.

HYPERTHYROIDISM

DEFINITION AND EPIDEMIOLOGY

Hyperthyroidism is defined as a clinical syndrome caused by the excess production or release of thyroid hormone and its clinical manifestations. The term *hyperthyroidism* implies that the thyroid is the source of excess thyroid hormone; *thyrotoxicosis* refers to the syndrome produced by excess thyroid hormone regardless of its source (e.g., overingestion of iodine). Primary hyperthyroidism is independent of TSH. TSH-dependent hyperthyroidism is called secondary hyperthyroidism. TRH-dependent hyperthyroidism is referred to as tertiary hyperthyroidism.

Graves disease (autoimmune hyperthyroidism) is the most common cause of hyperthyroidism. There is a female-to-male

TABLE 214-1 Signs and Symptoms of Hyperthyroidism

	Symptoms	Signs
Eyes	Dry eyes, blurry vision	*NO SPECS* mnemonic (see text)
Neck	Diffuse goiter in patients with Graves disease	Goiter with thyroid bruit in Graves disease
Respiratory system	Shortness of breath	Labored respiration
Cardiac system	Palpitation, tachycardia, angina	Systolic hypertension, congestive heart failure, tachycardia, atrial fibrillation
Gastrointestinal system	Hyperphagia, hyperdefecation, weight loss, weight gain (rare), anorexia in older adults	Weight loss, weight gain (rare)
Reproductive system	Amenorrhea, menstrual irregularities, infertility	
Neuromuscular system	Proximal muscle weakness, heat intolerance, tremor	Proximal muscle weakness, hyperreflexia
Skin	Pruritus; hyperhidrosis; warm, moist palms; onycholysis (brittle nails, Plummer nails)	Smooth, velvety skin; warm, moist palms; onycholysis; pretibial myxedema (Graves disease)
Skeletal system	Osteoporosis	Thyroid acropachy (Graves disease)
Psychiatric problems	Anxiety, irritability, nervousness, sleeplessness	Visually manifested
Older adults	Anorexia, constipation, normal pulse, weight loss	

predominance of 7 : 1, and it is most common in women aged 20 to 40 years. Transient hyperthyroidism (thyroiditis) needs to be excluded. Toxic multinodular goiters are usually seen in women older than 55 years who have a long history of goiter. Multinodular goiters with autonomy are more susceptible to iodine-induced hyperthyroidism. Iodine sources include topical povidone-iodine (Betadine), intravenous contrast medium, and iodine-containing drugs. Postpartum thyroiditis (painless) occurs in approximately 5% to 9% of all pregnant women, 25% of pregnant women with type 1 diabetes, and 75% of women with high microsomal antibody titers before pregnancy.[20]

TABLE 214-2 Thyroid Function Tests in Hyperthyroidism

	T_3	T_4/Free T_4 Index	TSH
Graves disease	Increase	Increase	Decrease
T_3 toxicosis	Increase	Normal	Decrease
T_4 toxicosis	Normal	Increase	Decrease
Subclinical hyperthyroidism	Normal	Normal	Decrease

PATHOPHYSIOLOGY

Graves disease is an autoimmune disorder in which thyroid-stimulating antibodies or immunoglobulins (TSIs) compete with TSH for TSH receptors on the thyroid and activate the production of cyclic adenosine monophosphate; this increases the synthesis and release of thyroid hormones. In white individuals, there is an increased prevalence of certain human leukocyte antigens (HLA-B8 and HLA-DR3).[21]

Subacute thyroiditis is a postviral illness. The thyroid gland is tender, and there is evidence of multinucleated giant cells on microscopic evaluation. Silent thyroiditis (painless) is believed to be an autoimmune disorder. On microscopic examination, there is evidence of lymphocytic infiltration that may mimic Hashimoto thyroiditis.

CLINICAL PRESENTATION AND PHYSICAL EXAMINATION

Because thyroid hormone acts on all organs, the clinical presentation is variable. The symptoms of hyperthyroidism are secondary to increased sympathetic activity and increased catabolism. Apathetic hyperthyroidism refers to patients who lack these symptoms. It is useful to describe the symptoms by organ system as shown in Table 214-1.

Lid lag may be seen with thyrotoxicosis, regardless of the origin of thyroid hormone. This symptom is caused by increased sympathetic activity. The other eye changes associated with Graves disease are caused by the action of TSIs on the connective tissue behind the eye. The *NO SPECS* mnemonic is used to describe the eye changes in association with Graves disease, as follows:

- *N*o signs or symptoms
- *O*nly signs, no symptoms
- *S*oft tissue swelling
- *P*roptosis
- *E*xtraocular muscle paresis
- *C*orneal involvement
- *S*ight loss (optic nerve involvement)

With subacute thyroiditis, the thyroid gland is tender, and patients often note a recent viral illness.

DIAGNOSTICS

TSH is the best screening test for primary hyperthyroidism. With primary hyperthyroidism, TSH levels will be low or undetectable. If TSH is suppressed, a T_3 update (T_3U) test (or any test of binding proteins) and T_4 levels should be obtained to determine the degree of hyperthyroidism. Alternatively, a free T_4 level can be obtained. TSH levels will remain suppressed for up to 3 months after treatment, and therefore the free T_4 or free T_4 index must be followed. See Table 214-2 for laboratory results in different types of hyperthyroidism.

BOX 214-2

Radioiodine Uptake in Different Forms of Hyperthyroidism

DECREASED OR ZERO RADIOIODINE UPTAKE

- Thyroiditis (subacute, painless)
- Iodine-induced hyperthyroidism
- Exogenous cause of hyperthyroidism
- Struma ovarii
- Metastatic thyroid cancer after thyroidectomy

NORMAL OR HIGH RADIOIODINE UPTAKE

- Graves disease
- Toxic nodule
- Toxic multinodular goiter
- TSH-induced hyperthyroidism
- Human chorionic gonadotropin–induced hyperthyroidism

Abnormal liver function test results are common in patients with hyperthyroidism. Elevations in alkaline phosphatase, alanine aminotransferase, aspartate aminotransferase, γ-glutamyltransferase, and total bilirubin levels can be seen.

As shown in Box 214-2, radioiodine uptake is useful in distinguishing Graves disease from thyroiditis.

A scan is useful in identifying a toxic multinodular goiter or solitary nodular goiter. In patients with a diffusely enlarged gland and obvious signs of eye disease, this test is not necessary for diagnosis of Graves disease but is needed for calculation of the radioiodine dose necessary if iodine ablation therapy is chosen. The erythrocyte sedimentation rate (ESR) will be increased in subacute thyroiditis. A careful review of iodine-containing medications is necessary in the evaluation of hyperthyroidism. With TSH-induced (secondary) hyperthyroidism, TSH is inappropriately elevated in the setting of increased T_4 index. Pituitary adenomas are best visualized on MRI. With TSH adenomas, there is an increased ratio of TSH alpha subunit/TSH.

DIAGNOSTICS

Hyperthyroidism

LABORATORY

TSH
T_4, free T_4
Total T_3
Thyroid-stimulating hormone receptor antibody*
Baseline complete blood count and liver function tests should be checked before initiation of treatment with thioamides*
ESR

IMAGING

Radioiodine uptake scan*
MRI*

*If indicated.

DIFFERENTIAL DIAGNOSIS

Differential diagnoses are described in the differential diagnosis box. Another consideration, "hamburger thyrotoxicosis," refers to an epidemic of thyrotoxicosis in the Midwest that was eventually traced to the ingestion of hamburger meat that included the strap muscles of slaughtered cattle (including thyroid tissue). The U.S. Department of Agriculture now prohibits the use of this material.

DIFFERENTIAL DIAGNOSIS

Thyrotoxicosis

NORMAL OR ELEVATED RADIOACTIVE IODINE UPTAKE

- Graves disease
- Toxic adenoma or toxic multinodular goiter
- TSH-producing pituitary adenoma
- Resistance to thyroid hormone
- Trophoblastic disease
- Hyperemesis gravidarum
- Thyroiditis
  - Silent (lymphocytic) thyroiditis (Hashimoto, postpartum)
  - Subacute thyroiditis
  - Amiodarone-induced thyroiditis
  - Acute thyroiditis
- Struma ovarii
- Exogenous (factitious) hyperthyroidism
- Iatrogenic causes
- Metastatic follicular thyroid carcinoma
- After thyroidectomy

MANAGEMENT

Specialist consultation with an endocrinologist is indicated for patients with Graves ophthalmopathy and for patients to be treated with radioiodine therapy. An ophthalmologist should see all patients with Graves ophthalmopathy.

Immediate emergency department referral is indicated for patients with thyroid storm, thyrotoxic crisis, and rapid atrial fibrillation.

The treatment of hyperthyroidism or thyrotoxicosis depends on the cause of the disease and the patient's age. Primary health care providers can perform the initial evaluation for hyperthyroidism. Laboratory confirmation of hyperthyroidism and radioiodine scans (if indicated) should be obtained. Thioamides can be administered by practitioners who are experienced with their use. Treatment options should be reviewed with patients.

Graves Disease

- Beta blockers should be initiated to alleviate the alpha-adrenergic symptoms of hyperthyroidism (tremor, tachycardia); the dose is adjusted to keep the heart rate at 60 to 90 beats per minute and to treat symptoms. Propranolol (Inderal) can be used at doses of 10 to 40 mg orally every 6 hours, or atenolol at 25 to 100 mg daily. These drugs must be used with caution in patients with congestive heart failure and bronchospasm, and they should be avoided in pregnant women because of untoward effects on the fetus.
- Thioamide therapy includes methimazole (MMI, Tapazole) and propylthiouracil (PTU).
  - Medical therapy is the treatment of choice for patients younger than 20 years old, for pregnant women, for those with a high likelihood of remission (mild disease, small goiters), and for those with active Graves orbitopathy. Baseline complete blood count and liver function test results should be checked before initiation of treatment. Thioamides inhibit thyroid hormone synthesis by blocking organification. PTU also inhibits the peripheral conversion of T_4 to T_3. PTU should not be used as a first-line

TABLE 214-3 Thioamide Therapy

	Methimazole	Propylthiouracil
Dose	5-20 mg PO q8h, or 15-60 mg/day PO	50-100 mg PO q6-8h
Tablets	5 mg, 10 mg	50 mg
Protein binding	0%	75%
Half-life	4-6 hr	75 min
Placental passage	High	1:1
Breast milk concentration	High	Low
Advantages	Long half-life	Inhibits conversion of T_4 to T_3; used during first trimester of pregnancy only

BOX 214-3

Side Effects of Thioamides

- Agranulocytosis occurs in 0.2%-0.5% of patients; it is usually reversible with discontinuation of medication.
- Baseline CBC and differential and liver function tests should be performed before initiation of treatment. Patients should be instructed to discontinue medications and to call if there are symptoms of infection (e.g., fever, pharyngitis); a CBC and differential should be obtained.
- Rash, arthralgias, myalgias (lupus-like reaction), and fever (3%-5% of patients) may occur.
- Nephrotic syndrome (methimazole) is rare.
- Aplastic anemia and thrombocytopenia are rare.
- PTU has been associated with severe PTU-related liver failure and should not be used as a first-line treatment.

drug in children or adults because of reports of severe PTU-related liver failure. In the past, PTU was considered the drug of choice throughout pregnancy because of possible teratogenic effects of MMI. PTU should be limited to the first trimester, and MMI should be used during the second trimester once organogenesis has been completed.[22] Thioamide therapy is described in Table 214-3 and Box 214-3. Side effects of thioamides include pruritic rash, jaundice, arthralgias, and low risk of agranulocytosis. Patients should be advised to contact their physician if they develop these symptoms; they should stop the medication in the setting of temperature above 102° and jaundice and should contact the physician immediately.

- Patients with small goiters and mild hyperthyroidism can be started on methimazole, 5 to 10 mg daily. Starting doses of 20 to 30 mg daily should be used in those with severe hyperthyroidism and large goiters. Starting doses of PTU are 50 to 100 mg three times daily. As noted, because of reports of PTU-related liver failure, PTU use is limited to the first trimester of pregnancy and in those intolerant of methimazole.
- After 6 to 12 months of treatment with thionamides, approximately 30 % of patients go into remission. Definitive therapy with radioiodine ablation is typically recommended if relapse occurs.
  - White blood count and TFT results are monitored every 4 to 6 weeks until the results are stable. TSH levels may remain suppressed for months, and therefore free T_4 should be monitored. In pregnant women, free T_4 levels should be kept at the high-normal range because of the thionamide effect of inhibiting the fetal thyroid gland.
- Radioiodine therapy is the treatment of choice in the United States for patients older than 20 years and for those for whom thioamide therapy has failed (through noncompliance or a relapse after treatment). It is contraindicated during pregnancy and should be avoided in patients with Graves ophthalmopathy because of the increased risk of exacerbation of eye symptoms after treatment. There is no evidence of increased incidence of long-term malignant neoplasms. Because of the high incidence of post-treatment hypothyroidism, TFT results should be monitored closely. Approximately 4 to 6 weeks after treatment, the T_4 index should be checked, and the patient should be reevaluated. If there is no evidence of hypothyroidism at that time, TSH and T_4 index should be monitored monthly for 3 to 4 months and then periodically.
- Thyroidectomy is recommended for pregnant women who cannot be managed with thioamides or who develop side effects, for patients who refuse radioiodine and cannot tolerate thioamides, and for patients with an obstructive goiter. Complications include hypothyroidism, hypoparathyroidism, and hoarseness (recurrent laryngeal nerve damage).

No studies to date have demonstrated any of these treatment options to be superior to any others. Other much less commonly used medications include cholestyramine (which decreases enterohepatic circulation of thyroid hormone), organic iodides (amiodarone and ipodate, which block T_4 to T_3 conversion), lithium and iodides (which block hormone release), and glucocorticoids (which block T_4 to T_3 conversion).

Subclinical Hyperthyroidism

Subclinical hyperthyroidism is defined as suppressed TSH with normal serum T_4 and T_3 levels. The cause of subclinical hyperthyroidism is the same as for overt hyperthyroidism. The majority of cases are the result of autonomously functioning thyroid nodules and multinodular goiters. Most elderly patients with subclinical hyperthyroidism have a multinodular goiter. Indications for therapy are based on the known skeletal and cardiovascular consequences of untreated hyperthyroidism. Postmenopausal women with exogenous subclinical hyperthyroidism have been found to have decreased bone density, but not premenopausal women.[23] The risk of atrial fibrillation has been shown to be related to the degree of TSH suppression. The cumulative incidence was 28% in patients with TSH levels of less than 0.1 μIU/mL, 16% when TSH levels were between 0.1 and 0.4 μIU/mL, and 11% in those with normal TSH levels.[21]

Treatment of subclinical hyperthyroidism should be considered for the following:

- Patients with endogenous subclinical hyperthyroidism with a TSH level of less than 0.1 μIU/mL as a result of Graves or nodular thyroid disease, especially patients older than 60 years and those at increased risk for heart disease, osteopenia, or osteoporosis. In those with TSH levels of 0.1 to 0.5 μIU/mL and low risk of complications, follow-up monitoring alone is appropriate.

- Patients high risk of complications with TSH level of 0.1 to 0.5 μIU/mL, especially if bone density is low.

Thyroiditis

Thyroiditis may be subacute or painless or may be a result of a toxic nodule or toxic multinodular goiter. Hyperthyroid findings may result.

Subacute Thyroiditis

- Symptomatic treatment with beta blockers can be used during the hyperthyroid phase.
- For pain relief, anti-inflammatory agents are used.
    - NSAIDs (1200 to 3200 mg daily in divided doses) or aspirin (2600 mg daily) is used first. If no pain relief has occurred in 2 to 3 days, these agents are discontinued and the patient is treated with prednisone (40 mg daily). Prednisone is continued until pain subsides and then is tapered by 5 to 10 mg every 5 days. Hyperthyroidism lasts for weeks to months and is followed by hypothyroidism (which lasts for months). TFTs should be performed every 2 to 8 weeks. Most patients become euthyroid, although 30% may remain hypothyroid. Recurrences are rare.

Painless Postpartum Thyroiditis

- Symptomatic treatment with beta blockers can be used during the hyperthyroid phase. Beta blockers are concentrated in breast milk and must be used with caution.
- Thyroid hormone therapy can be initiated if the hypothyroid phase is severe. TFT results should be monitored closely. Although most patients become clinically euthyroid, up to 30% remain hypothyroid. This condition tends to recur with subsequent pregnancies.

Toxic Nodule

- Radioiodine ablation is the treatment of choice after beta blocker therapy.
- Some studies have demonstrated effective therapy with alcohol ablation through repetitive percutaneous injections under ultrasound guidance. Surgical excision is another option, especially in patients with a large adenoma.

Toxic Multinodular Goiter

- Radioiodine ablation is the treatment of choice after beta blocker therapy. Other nodules may become toxic in the future and may require repeated doses of ^{131}I.
- Other treatment options include antithyroid drugs followed by subtotal thyroidectomy.

LIFE SPAN CONSIDERATIONS

Older patients may have apathetic hyperthyroidism (anorexia, weight loss, weakness) on presentation. There is an increased risk of atrial fibrillation and osteoporosis in patients with untreated Graves disease. Patients usually have symptoms of weight loss despite increased appetite. It is important to counsel patients on decreasing their food intake with treatment of hyperthyroidism to avoid significant weight gain with treatment. Patients should be counseled to avoid strenuous exercise and activity until adrenergic symptoms are controlled. Bone density should be checked in postmenopausal women. Smoking is a risk factor for Graves ophthalmopathy, and therefore patients should be counseled on smoking cessation.

COMPLICATIONS

Untreated Graves disease can lead to atrial fibrillation, congestive heart failure, angina, and osteoporosis. Thyroid storm is a rare, life-threatening form of hyperthyroidism that leads to systemic decompensation. The incidence has declined during the past few decades because of advances in medical management, but thyrotoxic crises account for approximately 1% of all hospitalizations for hyperthyroidism. Although it more commonly occurs with Graves disease, it can be found in conjunction with other causes of hyperthyroidism.

INDICATIONS FOR REFERRAL OR HOSPITALIZATIONS

Primary health care providers can perform the initial evaluation of hyperthyroidism as noted earlier. Referral to an endocrinologist is indicated if the primary care provider is not experienced with use of thionamides, for pregnant women, for patients interested in treatment with radioiodine, and for those with Graves eye disease. Patients with Graves ophthalmopathy should be referred to an ophthalmologist. Patients with thyroid storm require hospitalization and should be evaluated by an endocrinologist or by a physician familiar with its treatment. Thyroid storm requires aggressive inpatient management. The diagnosis is based on clinical findings: temperature of 102° F to 105° F, profuse sweating, pulse above 120 to 140 beats per minute, atrial fibrillation, restlessness, confusion, agitation, and coma. Gastrointestinal symptoms may include severe vomiting, diarrhea, and hepatomegaly with jaundice. The goals of therapy are to inhibit thyroid hormone formation and release, to provide alpha-adrenergic blockage, to provide supportive therapy, to identify and to treat any precipitating illness, and to initiate long-term therapy for prevention of further episodes of thyroid storm.

PATIENT AND FAMILY EDUCATION

Patients should understand the symptoms and treatment of hyperthyroidism and should be instructed in the "danger signs" of thyroid storm. If receiving beta blockers, they are instructed to monitor their pulse and to contact their health care provider if the pulse is less than 50 (or 40 if baseline heart rate is low) or more than 120 beats per minute.

Patients receiving thioamides should be cautioned about the rare but serious effects of agranulocytosis. They should discontinue thioamide therapy if they have signs of infection and a temperature higher than 38.3° C (101° F). Patients should be advised to call the health care provider and to have a CBC and differential performed to exclude agranulocytosis. Patients taking PTU should consider changing to MMI. If this is not an option, the patient should be told to contact the provider and to discontinue the medication if malaise, nausea and vomiting, jaundice, dark urine, or light-colored stool develops. TFT results should be monitored closely during pregnancy. Women with Graves disease who have received radioiodine ablation in the past should be advised that TSIs could still cross the placenta. They should inform their obstetricians that they have Graves disease so that the fetal thyroid and heart rate can be closely monitored.

HYPOTHYROIDISM

DEFINITION AND EPIDEMIOLOGY

Hypothyroidism is a condition resulting from the synthesis of thyroid hormone that is insufficient to meet the body's needs. It is the most common disorder of the thyroid gland.

This condition usually occurs in the setting of primary hypothyroidism, whereby diseases or treatments destroy thyroid tissue or prevalent conditions interfere with thyroid hormone biosynthesis. Rarely, it is caused by inadequate thyroidal stimulation by TSH, which is referred to as central or secondary hypothyroidism.

If hypothyroidism is congenital or occurs during infancy or childhood, growth and development are slowed and may result in mental retardation, a condition known as cretinism. In adulthood, untreated hypothyroidism results in decreased metabolic function and in the deposition of hydrophilic mucopolysaccharides in the skin and other tissues, which results in fluid and sodium retention and impairment of blood circulation and lymphatic drainage. Progressive and severe hypothyroidism with skin thickening and cardiovascular and renal manifestations is known as myxedema.

Hypothyroidism is found in 2% of women and 0.2% of men. The prevalence increases with age, with 6% of women and 2.5% of men older than 60 years having this condition. Subclinical hypothyroidism may occur in as many as 15% of persons 60 years of age or older. It has been found that in 20% to 40% of patients, subclinical hypothyroidism progresses to overt hypothyroidism within 4 years.[22,24]

Appropriate thyroid hormone biosynthesis depends on dietary intake of iodides and on various geographic and environmental factors that may affect a population's ability to obtain the recommended daily allowance of iodine. In the United States, adequate dietary sources of iodine have been established to prevent iodine deficiency disorders, which may manifest as hypothyroidism or goiter.

Previous irradiation for head and neck cancers may put a patient at increased risk for development of hypothyroidism. Radioactive treatment with ^{131}I for hyperthyroid disorders results in hypothyroidism in most cases. Subtotal or total thyroidectomy will render a patient hypothyroid.

The most common cause of primary hypothyroidism is chronic autoimmune thyroiditis. This may take atrophic or goitrous forms. When autoimmune thyroiditis coexists with a goiter, the condition is called Hashimoto thyroiditis. It is believed to be a familial autoimmune condition in which the lymphocytes become sensitized to an individual's own thyroid antigens, resulting in the formation of autoantibodies. The autoantibodies react with the thyroid antigens and destroy functional tissue. This manifests as an increase in TSH and the presence of antithyroid antibodies, including antimicrosomal, anti-TPO, and antithyroglobulin antibodies. Eventually there is a drop in serum T_4 and then T_3. Younger patients most often are seen with goiter, whereas older patients may have more severe disease and a small (atrophic) gland.

Transient primary hypothyroidism may be encountered during the postpartum period, 2 to 6 months after delivery. This condition may be preceded by a brief period of hyperthyroidism and can result in permanent thyroid failure. Postinfectious thyroiditis may follow a similar course. A sentinel viral upper respiratory tract infection followed by an inflamed, large tender thyroid gland, and transient hyperthyroidism followed by transient or permanent hypothyroidism, is the usual observed sequence of events.

Drugs with antithyroid action such as lithium, amiodarone, iodine, tyrosine kinase inhibitors, and radiographic contrast material may cause hypothyroidism. The drug effect may be transient during the period of use or may result in permanent thyroid failure. Patients with underlying chronic autoimmune thyroiditis living in iodine-sufficient geographic areas are more susceptible to hypothyroidism when taking iodine or iodine-containing drugs.

Pituitary (or secondary) causes of hypothyroidism are not common and are usually associated with other signs of pituitary hormone insufficiency. Patients with a history of pituitary disease or tumor may be at risk for thyroid hyposecretion.

PATHOPHYSIOLOGY

Thyroid hormone deficiency has many effects. Cardiac and metabolic consequences include impaired myocardial contractility, cardiomegaly, impaired lipid metabolism with accelerated atherosclerosis, hypertension, depressed ventilatory drive and fatigue, impaired energy use, and weight gain. Altered kidney and gastrointestinal performance includes a reduction in glomerular filtration rate and hyponatremia, hypomotility, and constipation, respectively. Musculoskeletal effects include an increased volume of muscle and slowness of contraction leading to myopathic disorders and connective tissue thickening. This can lead to entrapment neuropathies such as carpal tunnel syndrome. In children, delayed skeletal maturation may cause growth retardation. Impaired cellular function in the brain may cause depression or psychiatric disability, and diminished erythropoiesis results in anemia.

Characteristic myxedematous changes seen in untreated advanced disease are largely a result of deposition of hydrophilic mucopolysaccharides, especially hyaluronic acid, in the interstitial tissues. The hydrophilic nature of the mucopolysaccharides and increased capillary permeability to albumin create interstitial edema of heart muscle, striated muscle, and skin.

CLINICAL PRESENTATION

Presentation may range from subclinical hypothyroidism (with an asymptomatic TSH elevation) to overt myxedema (with slowed mentation and visible symptoms). The most common presenting symptom is fatigue. There may also be increased sensitivity to cold, weight gain, hoarseness, puffiness of the face and hands, heavy and irregular menstrual periods, dry skin, dry and brittle hair, depression, paresthesias, muscle aches, and constipation. A careful history will elicit the severity and duration of these symptoms. Goiter may or may not be present. Women are five to seven times more likely to be affected than are men, and more women are seen with goiter.

Symptoms may be more vague and subtle in older adults and include deafness, confusion, dementia, and ataxia.

PHYSICAL EXAMINATION

The physical examination should focus on the patient's general appearance and degree of energy and animation. Mentation may be slowed, and the patient may appear lethargic and expressionless. On occasion, severe depression or agitation results. Assessment of physical appearance includes texture, color, and general appearance of the skin. Facial expression and the texture and thickness of the hair should be noted; the patient's voice, which may be deepened, and pulse, which may be slowed, should also be assessed.

The thyroid gland may be large or small on examination and should be evaluated carefully for the presence or absence of nodules. Tenderness of the gland is suggestive of a subacute thyroiditis, whereas a nontender gland is more suggestive of chronic autoimmune thyroiditis. A rubbery, firm, symmetric goiter is characteristic of Hashimoto thyroiditis. Deep tendon reflexes should be evaluated. Any delay in the relaxation phase, which may be most noticeable in the Achilles tendon, should be noted. The patient's weight should be documented and compared with previous weights to determine if there has been any weight gain. Heart rate and respiratory rate should also be noted and documented. Diastolic blood pressure may be elevated. Respirations may be slow and shallow with advanced disease. Bowel sounds may be diminished.

The presence of headache or visual impairment may suggest secondary hypothyroidism, as may any other features of pituitary hormone excess or deficiencies. Postural hypotension may indicate coexistent endocrine deficiencies such as autoimmune adrenal insufficiency, as seen in Schmidt syndrome.

DIAGNOSTICS

TSH is the most appropriate first diagnostic test. If the TSH is elevated, free T_4 should be checked. Laboratory tests reveal an elevated TSH level, which may precede symptoms or decreases in T_4 and T_3. This condition is referred to as subclinical hypothyroidism (elevated TSH and normal free T_4). More advanced hypothyroidism shows not only elevated TSH but also low serum levels of free T_4 and a low free T_4 index. If pituitary or central hypothyroidism is suspected, the most appropriate test is a free T_4 assessment; TSH will not be useful in central hypothyroidism. Anti-TPO antibody levels will be elevated in patients with chronic autoimmune thyroiditis. Patients often demonstrate a mild normocytic, normochromic anemia. If menstrual periods are heavy, the anemia may be microcytic. If vitamin B_{12} deficiency is present, the anemia may be macrocytic. Hypercholesterolemia may also be present.

Imaging studies are unnecessary for chronic autoimmune thyroiditis. If imaging is used, the findings may be misleading. The pattern of uptake with goitrous autoimmune thyroiditis may be variable, whereas uptake may be low with atrophic thyroiditis. An ultrasound examination may be indicated to verify the presence of a suspected nodule. FNA biopsy may be necessary to evaluate a suspicious nodule or rapidly enlarging goiter. In severe hypothyroidism, other diagnostic tests may be needed to assess cardiac status, and electrocardiographic examination may reveal low-voltage QRS complexes and P and T waves as well as cardiac enlargement. This may result from both dilation and pericardial effusion. Bradycardia is usually present in severe hypothyroidism.

DIAGNOSTICS

Hypothyroidism

LABORATORY
TSH
Antimicrosomal antibodies*
Serum free T_4
Free T_4 index*

IMAGING
Thyroid ultrasound*

OTHER DIAGNOSTICS
FNA*

*If indicated.

DIFFERENTIAL DIAGNOSIS

DIFFERENTIAL DIAGNOSIS

Hypothyroidism

- Chronic autoimmune thyroiditis
- Postpartum thyroiditis
- Radiation-induced thyroid damage
- Postinfectious thyroiditis
- Medication-induced hypothyroidism (amiodarone, lithium, iodide, sunitinib, sorafenib)
- Post-thyroidectomy dysfunction
- Congenital absence of the thyroid
- Pituitary tumor
- Hypothalamic dysfunction
- Nephrotic syndrome
- Chronic nephritis
- Depression

MANAGEMENT

Specialist consultation is indicated in cases of central hypothyroidism and in severe primary hypothyroidism.

Immediate emergency department referral is indicated for myxedema coma.

- Hypothyroidism is treated with levothyroxine orally in amounts that return TSH to normal levels.[25]
- The desired amount is determined by the measurement of TSH for primary hypothyroidism and by the measurement of free thyroxine for central hypothyroidism.
- The dose necessary to achieve metabolic homeostasis is usually 1.7 μg/kg/day.
- In the United States, 12 different color-coded tablet strengths are available. Supplementation may begin with an initial dosage of 50 μg/day, with the dosage increased at 4- to 6-week intervals to 100 μg/day. In patients younger than 30 or 40 years with no history of other medical problems, the initial dose of T_4 can be 100 μg/day. Patients with ischemic heart disease or atrial fibrillation (and older patients in whom these conditions may become apparent with treatment) should start at 12.5 to 25 μg/day and increase by 25 μg/day every 8 weeks.
- A euthyroid effect is usually achieved 4 to 6 weeks after the onset of full-dose therapy, which can be adjusted, if necessary, according to TSH determinations.
- This daily dose is then monitored once or twice a year to maintain a mid-normal TSH level.
- Estrogen administration leads to an increase in TBG levels and thus may increase T_4 requirements in patients with hypothyroidism. If estrogen therapy is initiated in patients with hypothyroidism treated with levothyroxine, TSH should be rechecked in 12 weeks.
  - Serum L-triiodothyronine (L-T_3) is not routinely used to treat hypothyroidism. There are wide fluctuations in serum L-T_3 because of its short half-life (approximately 1 day). Slow-release formulations of L-T_3 are not currently commercially available. The role of L-T_3 replacement in hypothyroidism remains controversial.
  - Desiccated bovine thyroid is available, which contains a mixture of T_3 and T_4. One grain (60 mg) of Armour Thyroid contains about 44 μg of T_4 and 9 μg of T_3 and is bioequivalent to 75 to 88 μg of levothyroxine.

- Despite almost a dozen randomized studies, combination therapy with levothyroxine and triiodothyronine does not appear to be superior to levothyroxine monotherapy for treatment of hypothyroidism.

A study by Hennemann and colleagues[26] showed that treatment of hypothyroid rats with a combination of T_4 plus slow-release T_3 led to an improvement in both T_3 and T_4 levels, T_4/T_3 ratios, and serum TSH compared with treatment with levothyroxine alone. Human studies of slow-release T_3 preparations in combination with T_4 are necessary for clinical validation.

Subclinical Hypothyroidism

Subclinical hypothyroidism is defined as an elevated TSH level in the presence of normal thyroid hormone levels. The major causes of subclinical hypothyroidism are the same as for overt hypothyroidism; about 50% is caused by autoimmune thyroiditis, 40% is found in patients with a history of ablative therapy for Graves disease, and it is also commonly seen with inadequate T_4 replacement for overt hypothyroidism. Two population-based studies concluded the prevalence of subclinical hypothyroidism to be approximately 8% in women and 3% in men. However, in women older than 60 years the prevalence was 15%, whereas in elderly men the prevalence was 8%.[24]

Patients with type 1 diabetes mellitus or other autoimmune diseases have a higher rate of subclinical hypothyroidism. The development of overt hypothyroidism depends on the value of TSH and the presence of high thyroid antibody titers. Studies have shown that elderly patients with an initial TSH level above 20 μIU/ml and 80% of those with serum antithyroid microsomal antibody titers of 1:1600 or higher developed overt hypothyroidism. Other patients likely to progress to overt hypothyroidism are those with autoimmune thyroid disease and patients who have received radioiodine therapy or radiotherapy. Normalization of serum TSH is more likely to occur in patients with TSH levels of less than 10 μIU/mL and negative antithyroid antibodies.

Several reports suggest that subclinical hypothyroidism is associated with neuropsychiatric disease. Patients with depression and subclinical hypothyroidism have a higher prevalence of associated panic disorder and poorer response to antidepressant therapy than euthyroid patients do. A cross-sectional study of randomly selected subjects older than 65 years reported an increase in the prevalence of coronary heart disease in patients with serum TSH values above 10 μIU/L but not in patients with lower serum TSH concentrations.

In recommendations for treatment, there is not one level of TSH at which clinical action is indicated or contraindicated. However, for those individuals with TSH levels above 10 μIU/mL, treatment is more compelling because it improves cardiac contractility and serum lipid concentrations and secondarily reduces the risk of atherosclerosis. Treatment will also prevent growth of goiter and improve symptoms related to hypothyroidism. In patients with TSH levels of 4.5 to 10 μIU/mL, treatment can be considered if patients have typical hypothyroid symptoms that could benefit from T_4. The potential risk of treatment is the development of subclinical hyperthyroidism. If patients are not treated, regular follow-up is indicated. Patients with subtle symptoms such as infertility, menstrual cycle irregularities, depression, and fatigue may also benefit from replacement therapy. Patients without any of these symptoms and with a TSH level of less than 10 μIU/mL may be monitored at yearly intervals with TSH measurement for progression of thyroid failure.[27]

COMPLICATIONS

Myxedema coma, a hypothermic stuporous state that may be characterized by respiratory depression and eventually death, results from untreated hypothyroidism. It may be triggered by environmental stressors such as cold exposure or trauma and by internal stressors such as infection or medications that depress the central nervous system. These patients may require intravenous levothyroxine and glucocorticoid therapy for any coexistent adrenal insufficiency. Warming for the hypothermia, ventilatory support for the respiratory depression, and treatment of any renal and electrolyte imbalances are necessary.

In patients with underlying coronary disease, angina and arrhythmias may be a complication of therapy and a cause for concern. Some patients also experience palpitations after starting levothyroxine, especially if other medications are added. This is particularly true of stimulants such as caffeine and pseudoephedrine.

Long-term, marked overtreatment with T_4 can result in symptoms of hyperthyroidism. It can also result in bone resorption with significant decreases in bone mineral density.

INDICATIONS FOR REFERRAL OR HOSPITALIZATION

Referral to a surgeon may be necessary for a large goiter that is obstructive. Referral to an endocrinologist may be necessary if there is a solitary nodule requiring biopsy or if regulation of medication is difficult. Persistent symptoms and a normal TSH level or suspicion of secondary hypothyroidism should also prompt an endocrine referral. Hospitalization may be warranted if any of these conditions is severe. Usually, clinical or subclinical hypothyroidism can be managed on an outpatient basis.

LIFE SPAN CONSIDERATIONS

Older adults and those with known heart disease should be started at 12.5 to 25 μg of levothyroxine per day, which is increased gradually. This careful administration prevents arrhythmias, angina, and the other cardiac symptoms that may be precipitated by starting at a full daily dose. After the dose has been stabilized, annual TSH measurements are desirable. Patients should understand that supplementation is lifelong, not short term. Given the high prevalence of hypothyroidism in women older than 60 years and the presence of subtle symptoms, TSH screening is recommended in this age group.

Patients with known hypothyroidism require close monitoring during pregnancy. TSH should be measured during the prenatal evaluation and in every trimester thereafter. Most often, thyroid hormone requirements increase during pregnancy, and close monitoring will ensure appropriate levothyroxine replacement doses. Evidence has emerged that intrauterine fetal development can be adversely affected by untreated hypothyroidism.

Smoking has been found to impair both thyroid hormone secretion and thyroid hormone action. It may contribute to the incidence of subclinical hypothyroidism and may aggravate the clinical manifestations of overt hypothyroidism; therefore, smoking cessation is advised.

The consequences of untreated subclinical hypothyroidism are cardiac dysfunction (including atherosclerotic heart disease), elevations in total and low-density lipoprotein cholesterol levels, systemic hypothyroid symptoms, neuropsychiatric dysfunction, and progression to overt hypothyroidism.

PATIENT AND FAMILY EDUCATION AND HEALTH PROMOTION

The most important aspect of education is communicating to the patient and the family that levothyroxine replacement is a permanent and necessary treatment that cannot be discontinued. Patients should be encouraged not to increase their daily dose without medical supervision, informed not to double the next dose if one is skipped, and advised that atrial fibrillation and osteoporosis are possible consequences of persistent excessively high doses of levothyroxine. They should also understand that annual or biannual monitoring of TSH helps ensure that the medication dose remains accurate.

NONTHYROIDAL ILLNESS

Abnormalities in TFT results can occur in nonthyroidal illness. In the past this was referred to as the euthyroid sick syndrome (sick euthyroidism). A critically ill patient in an intensive care unit setting would be likely to have this abnormality. It is characterized by hypothalamic suppression of TSH release, acute inhibition of peripheral conversion of T_4 to T_3, and increased conversion of T_4 to rT_3. This results in low TSH levels, decreased levels of T_3, and increased levels of rT_3. Euthyroid sick syndrome is seen during carbohydrate restriction, liver disease, or severe acute or chronic illness. Patients with the low free T_4 levels in addition to low T_3 levels are severely ill and have an increased mortality rate. TT_4 levels can be decreased initially because of the liberation of fatty acids from ischemic or injured cells, which inhibits the binding of T_4 to TBG. A summary of laboratory tests during acute illness is provided in Table 214-4. These abnormalities resolve when the patient recovers. The TSH level rises to normal or higher-than-normal levels during the recovery phase; the changes are thought to be a protective adaptation to severe illness. Therapy with T_4 or T_3 has not been shown to improve outcomes and may actually worsen the situation. Given this syndrome, TFT results should not be checked in critically ill patients unless thyroid dysfunction is strongly suspected. If TFT results are checked, TSH alone does not suffice. TFT values should be interpreted in context of the current clinical scenario and time frame of illness.

DRUGS AND THE THYROID GLAND

Pharmacologic agents may cause thyroid dysfunction or abnormalities in TFT results. The most important examples are discussed in this section.

Amiodarone is an iodine-rich pharmacologic agent used in the management of refractory ventricular arrhythmias. It is highly lipophilic and concentrates in the thyroid gland, heart muscles, and adipose tissue. It has a very long half-life, and therefore its effects on the thyroid gland can be seen up to 2 to 3 years after discontinuation of the drug. Like iodine or radiographic contrast material, its effects on the thyroid gland can be variable, depending on the presence of underlying autoimmune disease and the geographic iodine availability. Individuals who have chronic autoimmune thyroiditis or are living in iodine-sufficient areas are more likely to develop hypothyroidism when exposed to iodinated agents, whereas patients with a multinodular goiter or those residing in iodine-deficient areas may be more likely to develop hyperthyroidism. The risk of either thyroid dysfunction is less likely when lower doses are used. In a meta-analysis of four randomized trials, the incidence of thyroid disease was 3.7% after a minimum of 1 year of low-dose therapy.[28,29]

Hypothyroidism is the more common thyroid disorder in patients taking amiodarone in the United States. Symptoms can develop as soon as 2 weeks and as late as 39 months after the initiation of amiodarone therapy. Clinical manifestations and diagnosis of amiodarone-associated hypothyroidism are similar to those of hypothyroidism of any cause. This condition is effectively treated with levothyroxine replacement therapy. It does not necessitate the discontinuation of amiodarone unless this therapy fails to correct the underlying arrhythmia. Goals of therapy include the establishment of a high-normal TSH level and a mid- to low-normal free T_4 level. A larger-than-normal dose may be required because of the effect of amiodarone on T_4 and T_3 production and action.

About 3% of patients treated with amiodarone in the United States become hyperthyroid. This usually occurs between 4 months and 3 years after the start of therapy. It is more common in iodine-deficient areas of the world. The clinical manifestations of amiodarone-induced hyperthyroidism (AIT) are often masked because its beta-blocking activity minimizes many of the adrenergic effects of thyroid hormone excess. Common symptoms include redevelopment of atrial arrhythmias, exacerbation of ischemic heart disease or congestive heart failure, restlessness, and low-grade fever. When thyrotoxicosis develops in the setting of amiodarone, it could be caused by overactivity of the thyroid gland (type 1) or destructive thyroiditis (type 2), in which there is inflammation of the thyroid gland (Table 214-5). A study by Tomisiti and colleagues showed that the onset of hyperthyroidism after initiation of treatment with amiodarone helps distinguish between type 1 and type 2 AIT. Thyrotoxicosis developed earlier in patients with type 1 AIT (3.5 months) versus 30 months with type 2 AIT. Most of the patients with type 2 AIT developed thyrotoxicosis after amiodarone withdrawal.[29] Amiodarone does not necessarily need to be discontinued immediately, and given its persistence in the system, discontinuation would not affect treatment. Treatment ultimately depends on the nature of the disease; such cases can be diagnostically challenging and difficult to manage. The differentiation of these two types can be attempted with the evaluation of cytokines, thyroid antibodies, 24-hour radioiodine uptake, and thyroid ultrasound. Type 1 hyperthyroidism is treated with antithyroid drugs, and type 2 thyroiditis is treated with oral steroids. If the mechanism of hyperthyroidism is uncertain, a combination of oral steroids and antithyroid drug is a prudent initial approach.

TABLE 214-4 Nonthyroidal Illness

	T_3	T_4	Free T_4	rT_3	TSH
Nonthyroidal illness	Decreased	Normal or decreased	Normal or decreased	Increased	Low

TABLE 214-5 Comparison of Type 1 and Type 2 Amiodarone-Associated Hyperthyroidism

	Type 1	Type 2
Cause	Overproduction of thyroid hormone because of Jod-Basedow effect (iodine load) in patients with underlying thyroid disease (nodular goiter, Graves disease)	Destructive thyroiditis from amiodarone, causing release of T_3 and T_4 but not increased production
Physical examination	Diffuse or nodular goiter often present	Normal thyroid
Thyroid antibodies	Present	Absent
24-Hour radioiodine uptake	Normal or increased	Low or absent
Color flow Doppler	Normal or increased	Low
Interleukin-6	Normal	May be elevated up to twofold
Treatment	Thioamides Perchlorate Thyroidectomy if refractory to medical treatment	Prednisone (approximately 40 mg/day) Thyroidectomy if refractory to medical treatment

Ultimately, thyroidectomy may be necessary if hyperthyroidism is refractory to medical intervention.

Ideally, before recommending amiodarone therapy, the health care provider should obtain baseline TFT results and determine the presence of thyroid antibodies. Underlying thyroid disease and family history of thyroid disorders should be noted; this would place the patient at an increased risk of thyroid dysfunction with this drug and would alert clinicians to this possibility. TFTs should be performed at 3-month intervals after the medication is started and for at least 1 year after it is discontinued.

Interferon alfa is used in the treatment of hepatitis B and C or malignant disease. Use of this agent can induce the production of thyroid antibodies, resulting in hypothyroidism or thyrotoxicosis or a biphasic thyroiditis. With discontinuation of this agent, these antibodies often disappear.

Lithium, as used in the treatment of psychiatric conditions such as bipolar depression, can induce thyroid dysfunction. It blocks the uptake of iodine and the release of thyroid hormone and can induce chronic autoimmune thyroiditis. Clinical or subclinical hypothyroidism or a goiter in a euthyroid patient is within the spectrum of lithium-induced thyroid disease. TFT abnormalities, including low TSH, low TT_3, and elevated rT_3, are noted in patients receiving steroids and pressor agents. Similar abnormalities in T_3 and rT_3 are noted with amiodarone. Much as in euthyroid sick syndrome, these agents block the formation of T_3 from T_4, and most of T_4 is shunted into the formation of rT_3.

Tyrosine kinase inhibitors (e.g., sunitinib, sorafenib, imatinib) are used to treat renal cell carcinoma and gastrointestinal stromal tumors. The development of hypothyroidism has been seen in 50% to 70% of patients treated with these agents.[30] Possible mechanisms of action include capillary regression, destructive thyroiditis, impaired iodine uptake, and increased type 3 deiodination (resulting in increased metabolism of thyroid hormones). It is most commonly seen with sunitinib, but it is thought to be a class effect. Hyperthyroidism has also been described.[30,31] Symptoms of hyperthyroidism and hypothyroidism may incorrectly be attributed to the primary malignancy or side effects of antineoplastic agents. Routine testing for thyroid abnormalities is recommended in these patients.

THYROID DISEASE IN PREGNANCY

Thyroid disease during pregnancy is evaluated and treated like that in nonpregnant women, but it presents some obstacles.[32] Changes in thyroid physiology to meet the increased metabolic demands in pregnancy include an increase in TBG concentration and cross-reactivity of human chorionic gonadotropin (hCG) with the TSH receptor. Estrogen stimulates TBG production and TBG sialylation, resulting in decreased TBG clearance. TBG concentration increases up to twofold, and, to maintain adequate free T_4 levels, T_4 and T_3 production increases. hCG, which is a weak thyroid stimulator, may cause hyperthyroidism during pregnancy. This has been described as "transient subclinical hyperthyroidism" or gestational transient hyperthyroidism." It occurs in 10% to 20% of normal pregnant women during the period of highest hCG concentrations, lasting from fertilization to about 11 weeks' gestation.[32] Because of changes in thyroid physiology in pregnancy, American Thyroid Association guidelines recommend trimester-specific reference ranges for TSH: first trimester, 0.1 to 2.5; second trimester, 0.2 to 3.0; and third trimester, 0.3 to 3.0.[33]

Overt hyperthyroidism, defined by TSH below 0.01 and elevated free T_4 and/or T_3 level, is rare and occurs in less than 0.4% of all pregnancies. Graves disease and hCG-mediated hyperthyroidism are the most common causes of hyperthyroidism during pregnancy.[32] Thyroiditis, toxic adenomas, and toxic multinodular goiters are less common causes of hyperthyroidism in pregnancy. Examples of hCG-mediated hyperthyroidism include transient subclinical hyperthyroidism, hyperemesis gravidarum, and trophoblastic hyperthyroidism. Women usually become euthyroid when the hyperemesis resolves and usually do not require antithyroid treatment. Trophoblastic hyperthyroidism occurs in approximately 60% of women with a hydatidiform mole or choriocarcinoma. The hyperthyroidism can be severe and is treated by removal of the mole or therapy against the choriocarcinoma. Graves hyperthyroidism is the most frequent cause of hyperthyroidism in pregnancy. It usually becomes less severe during the later stages of pregnancy. This is likely mediated by a change in the activity of the TSH receptor antibodies from stimulatory to blocking. Consequences of poorly controlled hyperthyroidism include increased risk of spontaneous pregnancy loss, premature labor, low birth weight, stillbirth, and preeclampsia.

The diagnosis of hyperthyroidism may be challenging. A TSH value of less than 0.01 μIU/mL and also a high serum free T_4 value are indicative of hyperthyroidism.[28] Because radioiodine is contraindicated during pregnancy, it is often impossible to decipher the cause of the hyperthyroidism. Clinical features of goiter, ophthalmopathy and pretibial myxedema are supportive of Graves disease. Adrenergic symptoms are difficult to assess during pregnancy. TSH receptor antibody TSHRAb) levels are elevated in 95% of patients with Graves disease. Treatment of pregnant women with overt hyperthyroid is limited because treatment can be harmful to the fetus. The goal is to maintain maternal T_4 in the high-normal range by use of the lowest dose of drug possible to prevent fetal hypothyroidism.

HYPERTHYROIDISM IN PREGNANCY

Diagnostics

- Physical examination: note pulse; assess for goiter, ophthalmopathy, and pretibial myxedema
- TSH, free T_4, TT_3
- Consider TSHRAb levels
- Consider thyroid ultrasound

Management

Thioamides are the mainstay of treatment for women with moderate to severe hyperthyroidism complicating pregnancy.

- PTU is used during the first trimester because of increased teratogenicity of methimazole (aplasia cutis).
- Methimazole is started and PTU is discontinued after the first trimester because of its increased hepatotoxicity.
- Free T_4 and TSH levels are monitored monthly to keep free T_4 levels in high-normal range and TSH levels in the low-normal range.
- Beta blockers can be used in women with moderate to severe hyperthyroidism with hyperadrenergic symptoms. Risks to the fetus include fetal growth restriction, hypoglycemia, and bradycardia.
  - Atenolol (25 to 50 mg daily) or propranolol 10 to 20 mg three or four times daily are preferred agents.
  - The goal is to wean the patient off beta blockers as soon as hyperthyroidism is controlled by thionamide.
- Fetal heart rate and growth should be monitored to watch for rare fetal hyperthyroidism.

Hypothyroidism during pregnancy is less frequent because many women with hypothyroidism are anovulatory or have high rates of first-trimester miscarriages. Hypothyroidism during pregnancy has been associated with early pregnancy loss, preeclampsia, placental abruption, low birth weight, perinatal mortality, and neuropsychological dysfunction. Thyroid hormone requirements increase by approximately 29% in pregnant women with preexisting hypothyroidism because of estrogen-induced elevations in TBG, increased volume of distribution of thyroid hormone, and increased placental transport and degradation of thyroid hormone. For this reason and because of the significance of maternal euthyroidism for normal fetal growth, it is recommended to increase the prepregnancy thyroid hormone dose by 30% as soon as pregnancy is confirmed. Serum TSH concentration should be measured 4 to 6 weeks after conception, 4 to 6 weeks after any change is made in the dose of T_4, and at least once each trimester. The TSH goal before conception and during pregnancy is approximately 0.5 to 2.5 μIU/L. A pregnant woman found to have a thyroid nodule should be evaluated in the same way as other patients are, except that radioiodine scanning is contraindicated.

HYPOTHYROIDISM IN PREGNANCY

- The TSH goal prior to conception is 0.5 to 2.5.
- With a positive pregnancy test result, the thyroid hormone dose is increased by 30%.
  - For example, if the prepregnancy levothyroxine dose was 100 μg daily, 1 tablet is taken daily Monday through Friday and 2 tablets daily are taken on Saturday and Sunday (an increase from 7 tablets per week to 9 tablets per week).
- TSH and free T_4 are monitored every month for the first half of pregnancy and then at least every trimester. The dose is adjusted in 12- to 25-μg increments.
- Postpartum patients are advised to start back on the prepregnancy levothyroxine dose—that is, if the patient was taking 100 μg daily preconception and the dose was increased, she should cut back to 100 μg daily postpartum. TSH and free T_4 are checked 6 weeks postpartum.

REFERENCES

For a full list of references, scan the QR code or visit http://booksite.elsevier.com/9780323355018

PART 18

Evaluation and Management of Rheumatic Disorders

CHAPTER 215

ANKYLOSING SPONDYLITIS AND RELATED DISORDERS

Carey Field

ANKYLOSING SPONDYLITIS

DEFINITION AND EPIDEMIOLOGY

The seronegative spondyloarthropathies are a group of inflammatory arthritides sharing many clinical, radiographic, and genetic features. They include ankylosing spondylitis (AS), reactive arthritis (ReA, formerly called Reiter syndrome), psoriatic arthritis (PsA), enteropathic arthritis associated with inflammatory bowel disease (IBD-SpA), and undifferentiated spondyloarthritis (uSpA). These illnesses are characterized by the presence of inflammatory back pain, sacroiliitis, inflammation of the bone insertions of ligaments and tendons (enthesitis), peripheral joint inflammation, and often eye inflammation and skin disease. AS is the prototype of the seronegative spondyloarthropathies.

AS has an estimated prevalence of 0.3% in North America.[1] It tends to be familial, and the incidence and prevalence of AS generally mirror the frequency of human leukocyte antigen HLA-B27 within the population. Worldwide, the male-to-female ratio ranges from 1.2:1 to 7:1, and the disease may be more severe in men.[1] The disease usually begins in the third or fourth decade of life, and rarely after the age of 45.[1]

PATHOPHYSIOLOGY

A strong association exists with the genetically determined histocompatibility antigen HLA-B27. Of note, however, HLA-B27 by itself is neither necessary nor sufficient for development of disease.[2] The association with HLA-B27 is the highest for AS, in which it is present in more than 90%; but overall, only 5% to 6% of HLA-B27–positive individuals develop AS[3] and the overall contribution of HLA-B27 to AS inheritance is only 23%. Several mechanisms have been proposed to explain the role the *HLA-B27* gene plays in the pathogenesis of the spondyloarthropathies; however, the exact mechanism remains unclear.[4]

The pathognomonic features of AS are inflammation of the bone insertions of ligaments and tendons (entheses), known as enthesitis or enthesopathy, bone destruction, and new bone formation. The pathophysiologic process of this disease begins with ligamentous inflammatory granulation tissue that is gradually replaced by fibrocartilage and then ossifies.

CLINICAL PRESENTATION

Low back pain caused by involvement of the spine or sacroiliac (SI) joints (caused by spondylitis or sacroiliitis) is the initial complaint of approximately 70% to 80% of patients.[3] Spondylitis begins in the lumbosacral spine, but as the disease progresses the upper portions of the spine become involved. The back pain of AS is inflammatory and can be distinguished clinically from back pain of other causes. It is usually insidious in onset; it is chronic, lasting for more than 3 months, with periods of exacerbation and remission. It is diffuse, poorly localized, and described as a deep ache or nagging discomfort. As in other types of inflammatory joint pain, the inflammatory back pain of AS worsens with bed rest and improves with exercise. Sleep disturbance is common, and patients may describe having to get up in the middle of the night to "walk the pain off." The back pain is worse in the morning and is associated with morning stiffness that is inflammatory in nature (i.e., lasts longer than 30 minutes).

AS patients may describe low back pain, buttock pain, or hip pain that may be suggestive of SI joint involvement. One third of AS patients develop hip pain (typically manifesting as groin pain that may refer to the thigh or knee).[5]

Patients may have significant peripheral joint involvement, and the diagnosis of AS can be made with only minimal sacroiliitis. Peripheral joint involvement is usually asymmetric, often involving large joints (often shoulders, hips, and knees), and is most frequently found in the lower limbs. Up to 50% of patients will develop peripheral arthritis at some point during their disease,[3] and some will develop chronic peripheral joint arthritis. Involvement of the hip joint can be an early manifestation in AS. Other areas of inflammatory enthesopathic (at ligament and tendon insertions) involvement peculiar to AS are the sternoclavicular joint, the costochondral joint, the Achilles tendon, the plantar fascia, and along the superior iliac crest. Whereas dactylitis (diffuse swelling of toes or fingers) is more commonly seen in the other seronegative spondyloarthropathies such as PsA, it has been seen in up to 8% of AS patients at some point during their disease.[6,7] Small joints of the hands and feet are infrequently involved, unlike in rheumatoid arthritis.

Extra-articular manifestations of the disease include low-grade fever, fatigue, and weight loss. In addition, patients may develop eye, bowel, skin, cardiac, and pulmonary disease. Inflammatory eye disease, usually acute anterior uveitis, manifests as a painful and often red eye with blurring of vision. It often recurs but seldom leads to permanent impairment of vision. Acute anterior uveitis occurs in up to 30% of patients during the course of their disease.[8] The inflammation is acute in onset 90% of the time, and in approximately 95% of patients, the uveitis is unilateral or unilateral-alternating.[3,9] The activity and severity of the eye disease does not correlate with the activity and severity of the articular disease of AS. It is more likely to occur later in the course of disease and is more common in HLA-B27 positive patients. Whereas ileal or colonic mucosal inflammation is detected histologically in up to 60% of patients with AS, symptomatic inflammatory bowel disease (IBD) develops in only 5% to 10% of patients.[10] AS patients are also at increased risk to develop psoriasis, which can be seen in up to 25% of patients.[10] Cardiac involvement may include aortic root dilation, aortic valve insufficiency, aortitis, conduction abnormalities, and accelerated atherosclerosis. Conduction abnormalities are the most common, seen in up to 33% of patients, whereas aortic root or valve involvement is seen in up to 10% of patients.[10] As in other inflammatory arthritides, AS patients are at increased risk for developing atherosclerosis leading to increased morbidity in the form of myocardial infarction and stroke.[11,12] Pulmonary manifestations may include restrictive lung disease caused by the musculoskeletal disease's impact on the chest wall, or parenchymal disease (as detected by high-resolution computed tomography [CT] scan) in the form of apical pulmonary fibrosis and interstitial lung disease.[12]

PHYSICAL EXAMINATION

Examination of the spine will show loss of the normal lumbar lordosis. Palpable muscle spasm of the paraspinal muscles is frequently present. Spine mobility is decreased in most patients and can be documented by the modified Schober flexion test of the lumbosacral spine, the Moll lateral flexion test of the thoracic spine, or measurement of chest expansion.[4] The modified Schober flexion test measures lumbosacral flexion. The patient stands erect, and two points are marked in the midline of the spine—one at the level of the dimples of Venus, and one 10 cm above the level of the dimples of Venus; the patient is then asked to bend forward, reaching for the floor as far as possible. Normal flexion is defined as an increase in the distance between the two points of 5 cm or more in a patient younger than 50 years.[13] The Moll lateral flexion test measures lateral thoracic spine flexion. The patient stands erect with the hands behind the head, and one mark is placed in the midaxillary line at the iliac crest, and another mark is placed 20 cm above the iliac crest; the patient is asked to tilt, bending the trunk to the opposite side as far as possible, and the distance between the two marks is measured. Normal thoracic spine tilt or lateral flexion is 3 cm. Chest expansion is measured with the patient standing erect with the hands on the head; with a centimeter tape wrapped around the chest at the nipple line, the patient is asked to first maximally expire and then maximally inspire. The chest circumference should be measured at both maximum expiration and maximum inspiration, and the measurement should normally increase by at least 5 cm with full inspiration.[13]

Extra-articular manifestations can produce physical findings such as the heart murmur of aortic valve insufficiency or the red, inflamed eye associated with acute iritis.

DIAGNOSTICS

The modified New York criteria from 1984 or the Assessment of SpondyloArthritis International Society (ASAS) criteria from 2009 can be used to diagnose AS. The modified New York criteria are useful for patients with evidence of radiographic AS, whereas the ASAS criteria are more useful for patients without radiographic evidence of disease (Boxes 215-1, 215-2, and 215-3).

BOX 215-1

Modified New York Criteria for Ankylosing Spondylitis (1984)

Define AS if the patient meets at least one clinical criterion and one radiologic criterion.

CLINICAL CRITERIA

- Low back pain and stiffness for more than 3 months that improves with exercise, but is not relieved by rest
- Limitation of motion of the lumbar spine in the sagittal and frontal planes
- Limitation of chest expansion relative to normal values correlated for age and sex

RADIOLOGIC CRITERION

- Sacroiliitis grade ≥2 bilaterally or grade 3 or 4 unilaterally

Modified from Sieper J, Rudwaleit M, Baraliakos X, et al: The assessment of SpondyloArthritis International Society (ASAS) handbook: a guide to assess spondyloarthritis. *Ann Rheum Dis* 68(Suppl 2):1-44, 2009.

BOX 215-2

Assessment of SpondyloArthritis International Society (ASAS) Classification Criteria for Axial Spondyloarthritis (SpA) in Patients with Back Pain for Three Months or Longer and Age at Onset Younger than 45 Years

Sacroiliitis on imaging plus ≥1 SpA feature	or	HLA-B27 plus ≥2 other SpA features

BOX 215-3

Features of Spondyloarthropathies

Spondyloarthritis (SpA) Features	Sacroiliitis on Imaging
Inflammatory back pain Arthritis Enthesitis (hell) Uveitis Dactylitis Psoriasis Crohn disease, colitis Good response to nonsteroidal anti-inflammatory drugs Family history of SpA HLA-B27 Elevated C-reactive protein	Active (acute) inflammation on magnetic resonance imaging is highly suggestive of sacroiliitis associated with SpA Definite radiographic sacroiliitis according to modified New York criteria

According to the modified New York criteria, presence of sacroiliitis on radiologic examination associated with one clinical criterion is considered to be diagnostic of definite AS.[13] Many patients will have normal findings on plain radiography because their disease has not been severe enough or of long enough duration to produce radiographic changes. Magnetic resonance imaging (MRI) is able to identify sacroiliitis earlier than standard plain x-ray studies.[14] As visualized on MRI, early sacroiliitis may produce bone marrow edema or osteitis on short T1 inversion recovery (STIR) and T1-weighted images. Sacroiliitis may also produce other inflammatory lesions identifiable on MRI, such as synovitis in the SI joints, capsulitis, and enthesitis, but the presence of concomitant SI bone marrow edema or osteitis is essential for defining active sacroiliitis by MRI.[14] More advanced sacroiliitis produces sclerosis, with the joint becoming indistinct and narrow over time. Complete bone fusion is seen late in the disease. Characteristic spine x-ray findings in AS include syndesmophyte formation, which leads to bone bridging from one vertebral body to the next, producing a "bamboo" spine appearance. Inflammatory changes can often occur early in disease before significant radiographic changes. X-ray changes in the hip occur in up to 50% of patients and are often bilateral and symmetric with uniform joint space narrowing in AS compared with osteoarthritis.[13]

Laboratory findings are generally nonspecific but may include an elevation in inflammatory serum markers including the erythrocyte sedimentation rate (ESR) or C-reactive protein (CRP) level. Occasionally, a normochromic, normocytic anemia of chronic disease may occur; however, anemia and elevated inflammatory markers are not necessary for the diagnosis. Rheumatoid factor and antinuclear antibodies are typically negative. Whereas up to 95% of patients of European descent with AS are HLA-B27 positive, HLA-B27 testing is inappropriate for screening of an asymptomatic population. The test result does not absolutely confirm or exclude AS, but it is important to note that in some cases it can be used in the ASAS criteria to assist the provider with making a diagnosis.[9]

DIAGNOSTICS

Ankylosing Spondylitis and Related Disorders

LABORATORY
Complete blood count (CBC) and differential
ESR
CRP
HLA-B27*
Rheumatoid factor, cyclic citrullinated peptide*
Antinuclear antibody*
Uric acid*
Enzyme-linked immunosorbent assay (ELISA) for *Borrelia burgdorferi* (Lyme disease)*

IMAGING
X-ray examination of spine, including SI joints
X-ray examination of small joints of hands and feet
MRI of SI joints

OTHER DIAGNOSTICS
Joint fluid analysis

*If indicated.

DIFFERENTIAL DIAGNOSIS

For patients with sacroiliitis or spinal disease, the principal diseases to consider are ReA (formerly Reiter syndrome), psoriatic spondylitis, and spondylitis of IBD, all of which are discussed later in this chapter. In the absence of axial involvement, the most common chronic inflammatory arthritides that can be confused with AS in the 20- to 40-year age group are seronegative rheumatoid arthritis (see Chapter 218) and Lyme arthritis (see Chapter 234). Rheumatoid arthritis is more likely to involve the upper extremity (especially small) joints, characteristically has hand involvement, and is symmetric. The presence of anti–cyclic citrullinated peptide antibodies, which are much more specific for rheumatoid arthritis, may be helpful in differentiating RA from AS. Lyme arthritis, which most commonly involves the knee, is usually monarticular or oligoarticular and is suggested by a history of tick exposure and of erythema migrans. The diagnosis of Lyme disease is established by enzyme-linked immunosorbent assay (ELISA) for *Borrelia burgdorferi* antibody confirmed by Western blot analysis.

DIFFERENTIAL DIAGNOSIS

Ankylosing Spondylitis and Related Disorders

- Amyloidosis
- Behçet syndrome
- Degenerative joint disease
- Disseminated idiopathic skeletal hyperostosis
- Familial Mediterranean fever
- Herniated intervertebral disk
- Lyme arthritis
- Polyarticular symmetric disease
- Psoriatic spondylitis
- ReA
- Seronegative rheumatoid arthritis
- Spondylitis of IBD
- Systemic sclerosis
- Vasculitis with abdominal involvement

Anatomic causes of noninflammatory (mechanical) back pain, such as a herniated intervertebral disk, and noninflammatory arthritis of the spine, such as degenerative joint disease or disseminated idiopathic skeletal hyperostosis, produce different pain, noninflammatory in nature, that is relieved by rest and aggravated by motion (see Chapter 181).

MANAGEMENT

The goals of treatment are to relieve symptoms, maintain the best possible functional capacity, prevent complications of the disease (e.g., flexion contractures), and minimize extra-articular manifestations (e.g., uveitis and aortic valve insufficiency). To achieve these goals, patient education, exercise, and medication management are all important. All patients should be strongly encouraged to perform exercises tailored for AS (through either a formal physical therapy or exercise program or a home-based practice). Various guide books and audio and video aids are available by mail or online through the Spondylitis Association of America and the Spondylitis Society in the United Kingdom; these aids can be used to perform exercises unsupervised at home if formal physical therapy is not possible.[15]

Nonsteroidal anti-inflammatory drugs (NSAIDs) are first-line therapy for all symptomatic patients with AS, unless contraindicated. Most patients with AS or other seronegative spondyloarthropathy typically respond symptomatically to NSAIDs; these medications can be used to help differentiate between inflammatory and noninflammatory back pain. NSAIDs help to reduce pain and stiffness and are able to reduce progression of structural damage to the spine if administered continuously. All NSAIDs (independent of their cyclooxygenase [COX] selectivity) are capable of reducing pain and stiffness in AS. Patients have variable responses to and tolerability for NSAIDs, and thus at least two NSAIDs (preferably from different classes) should be tried if the first one is found to be ineffective or causes intolerable gastrointestinal symptoms.[16]

Biologic anti–tumor necrosis factor (TNF) agents have been proved effective in the treatment of patients with AS.[17] Because of their cost and potential side effects, criteria for the use of these agents have been developed and were updated in 2010.[18] These criteria include fulfilling the diagnostic criteria for definite AS, as discussed previously (via the ASAS axial spondyloarthritis [SpA] or modified New York criteria for AS), and the presence of active disease for at least 4 weeks. All patients should have had an adequate therapeutic trial with at least two NSAIDs unless there is intolerability or a contraindication. Sulfasalazine and methotrexate, both considered disease-modifying antirheumatic drugs (DMARDs), have efficacy for those patients with peripheral arthritis,[19] and failure with one of these is recommended as a criterion for anti-TNF therapy. However, because neither sulfasalazine nor methotrexate has been shown to be significantly effective for axial disease, those patients do not require pretreatment with a DMARD and are candidates for anti-TNF therapy immediately after an unsuccessful NSAID trial.

Etanercept, infliximab, adalimumab, and golimumab are all currently approved for the treatment of AS. Studies with anti-TNF agents show rapid and sustained decrease in disease activity in AS.[20] There is reduction of spinal inflammation as assessed by MRI and, in some studies, sustained improvement in clinical measurements and in health-related quality-of-life indexes.[20] However, long-term data are not yet available regarding the impact of anti-TNF agents on the progression of disease. Patients who are more likely to respond to TNF antagonists include those with early disease, elevated CRP, and younger age. If patients fail to respond to a therapeutic trial of a TNF antagonist, attempting another is recommended. There is a suggestion that patients treated with etanercept or infliximab for AS have a decreased incidence of uveitis.[20]

Significant concerns and possible contraindications to the use of anti-TNF agents are similar to those for patients with rheumatoid arthritis and include active infection, untreated tuberculosis, heart failure, pregnancy, malignancy, and demyelinating disease. At this time, owing to conflicting results and an overall increased risk for malignancy in patients with inflammatory diseases, it is unclear whether or not patients with AS using anti-TNF agents are at increased risk for developing hematologic and solid tumors as compared with AS patients not using anti-TNFs. Thus, vigilance for the occurrence of lymphomas and other malignancies (including recurrence of solid tumors) is advised.[18,21] Side effects are rare but include infection and reactivation of latent tuberculosis or reactivation of hepatitis B virus infection, as in rheumatoid arthritis. In AS these drugs can be used as single agents without DMARDs or other immunosuppressive medication.

Use of systemic glucocorticoids is not recommended for long-term treatment of AS because there are limited data on their use in this setting, and their toxicities can be profound. However, one study has shown that systemic glucocorticoids used at relatively high doses in the short term may have some short-term benefit for pain control.[22]

Pain management is important to minimize spinal deformity and to allow patients to exercise. Patients stoop with pain, thereby increasing the likelihood of the spine's fusing in a kyphotic position. Analgesics such as acetaminophen and muscle relaxants can be beneficial adjunctive therapy. Patients often find the use of heat and massage helpful. Small doses of narcotic pain relievers used intermittently for short periods may be appropriate in selected situations. Local injections of corticosteroids can treat pain from enthesopathy, sacroiliitis, and peripheral arthritis.

LIFE SPAN CONSIDERATIONS

The prognosis with AS is variable. Death as a result of the disease itself is very unusual. Some patients have minimum symptoms that are limited to the low back and pelvis. Less commonly, patients may have progressive widespread disease with skeletal deformity and functional loss, requiring chronic medication and physical therapy. Chronic medical therapy can shorten the patient's life span as a result of medication side effects. Pregnancy in patients with AS does not improve symptoms, unlike what is observed in rheumatoid arthritis. The majority of women with AS have unchanged or temporarily aggravated disease activity during pregnancy. The disease has no effect on fertility, course of pregnancy, or delivery. However, the offspring of patients with AS have an increased risk for development of AS themselves.

COMPLICATIONS

Osteopenia is prevalent in patients with longstanding disease, and thus risk for vertebral fracture is increased. Osteopenia is difficult to detect by dual photon absorptiometry owing to the superimposed effect of syndesmophytes and periosteal bone formation, and thus lateral and volumetric lumbar dual-energy x-ray absorptiometry (DXA) or CT scanning of the spine is recommended in its place.[23] Visual loss secondary to inflammatory eye disease is a major cause of disability in this disease. A variety of neurologic complications of AS can be seen in long-standing disease. These include cord or spinal nerve compression secondary to spinal fracture of a fused spine or atlantoaxial subluxation. Amyloid deposition is a rare complication after years of inflammatory disease and can produce nephrotic syndrome or renal failure. Further possible complications, including cardiac and pulmonary complications, are discussed earlier in the extra-articular manifestations section of this chapter.

INDICATIONS FOR REFERRAL OR HOSPITALIZATION

A rheumatology referral is recommended to confirm diagnosis and to recommend a treatment plan. Referral to a physical therapist is appropriate to promote pain relief, to minimize deformity, and to maintain independent function. Referral to an orthopedic surgeon is indicated in patients who develop hip arthritis that is severe enough to produce night pain, rest pain, and pain on weight bearing, impairing the ability to walk. Immediate referral to an ophthalmologist is warranted for acute eye pain. Periodic ophthalmic monitoring is recommended when iritis has been a manifestation. Evaluation by a cardiologist is indicated in the presence of an aortic valve murmur. Known cardiac risk factors, such as hypertension, hyperlipidemia, and diabetes, should be evaluated and treated. Hospitalization is rarely indicated in patients with AS. Acute catastrophic neurologic complications, congestive heart failure and other cardiac events, and gastrointestinal bleeding resulting from NSAIDs are the most likely reasons for hospitalization.

PATIENT EDUCATION

Optimum management is enhanced when patients understand the chronic nature of the disease and their role in preventing disability and deformity. Exercise is an important component of management of AS. Regular physical activity and stretching, and practicing good posture are essential to maintaining flexibility and functionality and reducing pain from the disease.[15]

Ongoing attention to daytime and nighttime posture minimizes deformity; patients may practice prone lying to help with posture. Sleeping without a pillow under the head is also advised to prevent pain from overextension of the neck and spine. Because patients are more prone to spinal fractures, contact sports should be avoided; however, other forms of physical activity should be encouraged, especially swimming. Swimming is nonimpact and can provide excellent exercises for increasing and maintaining trunk and neck muscle strength. Swimming is recommended because it avoids excessive stressful weight bearing. The backstroke is particularly good for stretching anterior chest muscles and strengthening posterior chest and neck extensor muscles, thereby decreasing the tendency toward kyphosis.

REACTIVE ARTHRITIS (FORMERLY KNOWN AS REITER SYNDROME)

DEFINITION AND EPIDEMIOLOGY

ReA is an acute sterile inflammatory arthropathy that follows an infection in which there is no microbial invasion of the synovium or joint space and the prior infection is remote from the joint. Reiter syndrome, as first described by Hans Reiter in 1916, is a historic example of ReA defined by the classic triad of conjunctivitis, urethritis, and arthritis. Because as many as two thirds of patients are initially seen with an incomplete syndrome and do not fulfill all three criteria, *reactive arthritis* is a preferred and more general term. ReA has been observed after both sexually transmitted and dysenteric infection and can be initiated by a number of infectious organisms. The most common infectious agents associated with ReA are gastrointestinal and urogenital pathogens such as *Salmonella, Shigella, Yersinia, Campylobacter, Escherichia coli, Clostridium difficile,* and *Chlamydia* organisms *(Chlamydia trachomatis* and *Chlamydia pneumoniae)*.

ReA is a fairly uncommon disease. The exact prevalence of ReA in the general population is based on studies mostly done in the Scandinavian countries and is thought to be 30 to 40 cases per 100,000 adults.[24] The peak incidence of ReA is during young adulthood, in the third decade of life. Postvenereal ReA affects men more commonly, with male-to-female ratios ranging from 9:1 to 5:1. The dysenteric form of ReA affects males and females equally.

PATHOPHYSIOLOGY

Like AS, ReA has a strong association with the histocompatibility antigen HLA-B27 in Caucasian patients but not in patients from sub-Saharan Africa, where the HLA-B27 prevalence is lower. HLA-B27 is observed in 60% to 80% of patients with ReA and appears to be associated with increased disease susceptibility and severity of disease expression.[2] As in rheumatoid arthritis, there is inflammatory synovitis with infiltration of polymorphonuclear leukocytes, lymphocytes, and plasma cells. However, unlike in rheumatoid arthritis, production of synovial pannus is rare. As in AS, there is inflammation at the insertions of ligaments and tendons (enthesopathy). Erosions, bone proliferation, and periosteal new bone formation may occur.

The relationship between the antecedent infection and the development of ReA is not completely understood. The HLA-B27 molecule participates in binding of antigenic peptides and presenting them to CD8 T cells. That the disease does occur in patients with acquired immunodeficiency syndrome (AIDS), who presumably lack a full complement of functional CD4 T cells, suggests a role for CD8 cells in ReA.

CLINICAL PRESENTATION AND PHYSICAL EXAMINATION

ReA can occur without documented prior infection. When there has been an antecedent infection, arthritic symptoms tend to occur 1 to 4 weeks later. Less than 40% of patients are seen with the classic triad.[25] The eye and genitourinary tract features of the triad may take as long as 5 years to appear. Urethritis in men may be transient, and the genitourinary symptoms (cervicitis, cystitis, or mild urethritis) in women are often missed, occult, or not reported. The eye inflammation manifests classically as conjunctivitis, but blepharitis, keratitis, iritis, or uveitis can also be seen. The arthropathy of ReA is typically an asymmetric oligoarthritis, often in large joints of the lower extremities. Many patients have arthritis in the upper extremities including small joints of the hands. The axial spine and SI joints are less commonly involved.[25]

Patients may develop dactylitis as well as enthesitis of the Achilles or plantar fascia, anterolateral ribs, pubic symphysis, and iliac crest, which may manifest with pain or swelling in these areas.

Extra-Articular Manifestations

Patients may have constitutional symptoms such as malaise, fatigue, fever, headache, and weight loss. They may develop conjunctivitis and anterior uveitis; dermatologic manifestations including painless, shallow, lingual or palatal ulcerations; keratoderma blennorrhagica; circinate balanitis; and erythema nodosum. These tend to correlate with severity of disease. Keratoderma blennorrhagica is the most common dermatologic manifestation of ReA, appearing as painless papulosquamous lesions on the palms or soles.[25] The histopathology of keratoderma blennorrhagica is indistinguishable from that of pustular psoriasis. Circinate balanitis occurs in males and is seen as painless, asymptomatic, shallow, ulcerative lesions on the glans of the penis.

The course of the disease is highly variable; typical disease duration is 3 to 5 months. Some patients have recurrent acute attacks, often with disease-free intervals. A minority of patients may develop sustained disease activity with a chronic course. Chronicity and increased severity of disease are associated with HLA-B27 positivity.[24]

DIAGNOSTICS

For the most part, laboratory test results are nonspecific, consistent with an inflammatory process, and similar to those in AS. The ESR and CRP are elevated. There is often peripheral leukocytosis with thrombocytosis and a mild anemia. There is usually a synovial fluid leukocytosis, often with a polymorphonuclear leukocyte predominance that is suggestive of a septic arthritis, but cultures are negative. The x-ray studies of sausage digits, Achilles tendinitis, and plantar fasciitis may reveal the fluffy periosteal reaction of new bone formation. Periarticular demineralization or osteopenia is notably absent in ReA compared with rheumatoid arthritis. The syndesmophytes in the vertebral spine are not as fine as in AS, are nonmarginal and denser, and may be asymmetric and skip portions of the spine.

DIFFERENTIAL DIAGNOSIS

It can be difficult to distinguish between PsA and ReA because the arthritis is similar and the skin histology is identical. Only the finding of nail pitting, characteristic of PsA, differentiates the two. More important, ReA may be misdiagnosed as seronegative rheumatoid arthritis. ReA can have symmetric peripheral joint involvement like rheumatoid arthritis, but sacroiliitis is uncommon in rheumatoid arthritis. In rheumatoid arthritis, hip disease is a late sequela, and sausage digits, Achilles tendinitis, plantar fasciitis, and other presentations of enthesopathy do not occur. Dactylitis is not a feature of rheumatoid arthritis. Lyme disease often manifests as a chronic monarticular or oligoarticular arthritis, often with chronic knee arthritis, and can be differentiated from ReA by a positive *B. burgdorferi* antibody assay.

MANAGEMENT

In some patients, in particular those with genitourinary infection and some enteric infections, treatment of the infection that triggered the arthritis is indicated; however, the role of antibiotics in the treatment of the arthritis is under investigation, and they have not yet been proven to be of great benefit.[25] In treating the arthritis itself, treatment may differ based on the duration of symptoms. For symptoms that have been present for less than 6 months, NSAIDs are the recommended initial treatment. For patients who do not respond to NSAIDs or who have an allergy or intolerability, intra-articular steroid injections and systemic glucocorticoids may be used. For patients who have symptoms for longer than 6 months and are not responding to NSAID therapy, DMARDs are recommended. Sulfasalazine at a dose of 2 to 3 g/day has been found to be the most effective,[26] but methotrexate may be used as an alternative as well.

There are increasing data, but limited to case reports and case series, to suggest that anti-TNF therapy may be effective in patients with ReA[27] and may be an effective steroid-sparing therapy. Therefore, for patients in whom treatment with NSAIDs and DMARDs has failed, anti-TNF therapy may be considered.

COMPLICATIONS

The course of ReA is highly variable. Most patients' symptoms resolve within 6 to 12 months. However, some patients develop chronic, disabling arthritis for which they receive long-term treatment.

INDICATIONS FOR REFERRAL

Most patients with ReA can be managed by the primary care provider with initial diagnostic studies and management suggestions from a rheumatologist. In cases in which the skin disease or eye disease is prominent, referral to a dermatologist and/or an ophthalmologist respectively may be helpful. A physical therapist or occupational therapist should be consulted for suggestions about exercise regimens or teaching on joint protection and energy conservation.

PATIENT EDUCATION

Patient education should be directed toward management of the disease chronically, and patients should be counseled about the possible side effects of medications as they apply (including possible sterility, liver damage, risk for infection, and so on). In patients receiving NSAIDs, ulcer prevention with proton pump inhibitors or H_2 blockers may decrease the risk of gastrointestinal bleeding. Patients who receive sulfasalazine, methotrexate, or anti-TNF agents should be managed according to guidelines for patients with rheumatoid arthritis taking these medications, with regular screening.

PSORIATIC ARTHRITIS

DEFINITION AND EPIDEMIOLOGY

PsA is an inflammatory arthritis associated with the dermatologic condition of psoriasis. Approximately 20% to 30% of patients with psoriasis will develop inflammatory arthritis,[28] with men and women affected equally. However, axial disease occurs more frequently in men (3:1 ratio), and severe spinal involvement is more common in men who are positive for HLA-B27.[29] The most common age at onset is 30 to 40 years.

PATHOPHYSIOLOGY

Immune, genetic, and environmental factors influence disease expression. Genetically, PsA has been linked to HLA class 1 alleles, most notably the HLA-B27 and HLA-B39 alleles.[30] Patients have been known to have flares after trauma or after infections (bacterial or viral). An association with group A streptococcal infection has been proposed.[31] Immune mechanisms are suggested by a possible molecular similarity between streptococcal and epidermal components, which could allow T-cell clones directed against streptococci to initiate the skin disease.

CLINICAL PRESENTATION AND PHYSICAL EXAMINATION

PsA may occur before, concomitantly with, or after the onset of the skin disease.[31] Arthritis precedes the rash in 15% to 20% of patients.[29] In these patients, nail pitting is often present before rash—an early clue to the diagnosis. The arthritis is heterogeneous, with five different clinical presentations being recognized: oligoarticular asymmetric, 48%; spondyloarthropathy, 24%; polyarticular symmetric, 18%; distal phalangeal, 8%; and arthritis mutilans, 2%. The distal interphalangeal (DIP) joint and arthritis mutilans types are considered the most specific for PsA. Over time, patients typically develop overlapping forms of the disease. Other common features of PsA include enthesitis, tenosynovitis, and dactylitis. Arthritis mutilans is a destructive form of arthritis in which there is significant bone erosion with decreased bone length, producing redundant skin and opera-glass deformity (Fig. 215-1). Spondylitis can occur without sacroiliitis, be asymmetric, and skip portions of the spine.[32] Sacroiliitis in PsA is often asymmetric, in contrast to AS, in which bilateral SI involvement is more common. Systemic involvement is limited to eye inflammation (uveitis or conjunctivitis), which occurs in approximately 30% of patients.[9,33] Human immunodeficiency virus (HIV) infection in patients with PsA causes increased proliferation of the skin disease and is associated with rapidly progressive polyarticular joint involvement.[34]

DIAGNOSTICS

Laboratory test results are mostly nonspecific, as they are in the other seronegative spondyloarthropathies. The ESR and CRP level may be elevated in up to 40% of patients. Patients may have a normocytic anemia and/or leukocytosis. Test results for rheumatoid factor and antinuclear antibodies are typically negative but may be positive in a small percentage of patients.

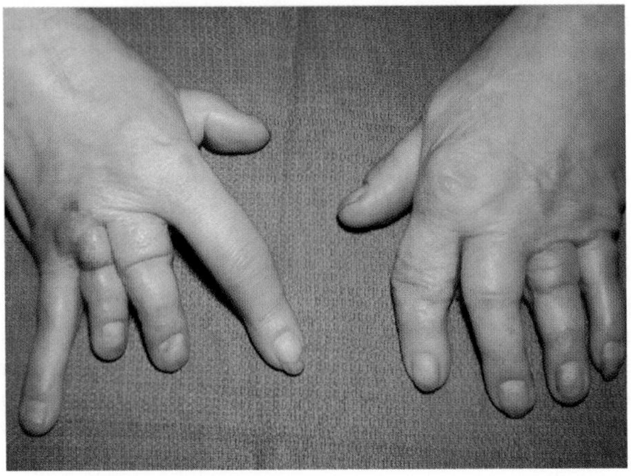

FIGURE 215-1 Arthritis mutilans (destructive arthritis) involving all digits. (From Harris E, Budd R, Firestein G: *Kelley's textbook of rheumatology,* ed 7, Philadelphia, 2005, Saunders.)

Hyperuricemia may result from the high purine turnover in psoriatic skin lesions. Psoriatic synovial histology is similar to rheumatoid synovial histology, with lymphocyte and plasma cell infiltration and microvascular changes.

The radiographic changes in hands and feet are distinctive.[30,32] Subchondral erosions and erosions with new bone formation, called proliferative erosions, are seen. In late disease, radiographs of the DIP joints may show whittling and a "pencil in cup" appearance, which is believed to be pathognomonic of PsA. Osteopenia is notably absent, and periosteal reaction can be seen along the bone shafts of sausage digits.

DIFFERENTIAL DIAGNOSIS

The differential diagnosis is broad, and PsA is often a challenge to diagnose when the arthritis precedes the skin disease. It may be difficult to distinguish between ReA and PsA. The skin lesions of both diseases are histologically similar. Both can manifest with eye disease. Nail pitting suggests PsA, whereas nail onycholysis can be seen in both diseases. Polyarticular symmetric disease can appear exactly like seronegative rheumatoid arthritis, and it may be impossible to differentiate the two. Antibodies against rheumatoid factor and cyclic citrullinated peptide, as well as antinuclear antibodies, can be found in a small proportion of patients, which may complicate the diagnosis as well. The monarticular arthritis of Lyme disease involving the knee can be differentiated from oligoarticular asymmetric PsA by *B. burgdorferi* antibody assay. DIP joints with degenerative changes may look similar to psoriatic DIP joints, but patients with PsA have morning stiffness for longer than 30 minutes, and other inflammatory symptoms and findings that distinguish it from primary degenerative joint disease.

MANAGEMENT

NSAIDs are first-line therapy for PsA; however, many patients have continued active disease despite these agents and require second-line therapy. DMARDs, including methotrexate, sulfasalazine, leflunomide, azathioprine, and others, are typical second-line therapies. Despite lack of robust evidence of its efficacy in PsA, methotrexate is the most widely used DMARD and has been the standard drug used in patients with erosive joint disease and aggressive skin disease. Recent studies have demonstrated that leflunomide is a very effective treatment for PsA.[28] Sulfasalazine may provide control of peripheral joint symptoms as well. Currently, five anti-TNF agents (etanercept, infliximab, adalimumab, golimumab, and certolizumab) have been shown to be effective in treating PsA.[28] As in rheumatoid arthritis and ankylosing spondylitis, the anti-TNF agents show sustained benefits in PsA with inhibition of radiologic progression and improvement in disability and quality-of-life indexes as well as improvement in the cutaneous lesions of psoriasis. Oral steroids are not recommended for the treatment of PsA because of the flare of skin disease that may occur on withdrawal of steroid medication.

A newer agent that has been approved for the treatment of PsA is ustekinumab, an interleukin 12 and 23 inhibitor. It has shown benefit for treatment of both the skin and the joint diseases.[28] Another potential drug on the horizon that may prove to be beneficial in patients with PsA is apremilast.[28]

Of note, suppression of the psoriatic skin disease is essential for the patient's comfort and appearance. It may also be important in the management of the associated arthritis because flares in the skin disease may correlate with flares in the joint disease.

COMPLICATIONS

Acute iritis can lead to loss of vision. Owing to potential side effects from medications used to treat PsA, (e.g., NSAIDs, DMARDs, anti-TNF agents), appropriate monitoring should occur. Patients with PsA, like those with rheumatoid arthritis and AS, appear to have an increased risk for cardiovascular disease.[35]

INDICATIONS FOR REFERRAL

Most patients with PsA can be managed by the primary care provider. In cases in which the joint or skin disease is disabling, referral to a rheumatologist or dermatologist for consultation may be helpful. As in other cases of inflammatory arthritis, referral to a physical therapist or occupational therapist for joint-protective exercise regimens as well as teaching in joint protection and energy conservation is very helpful. Patients disabled by joint disease may need vocational counseling.

PATIENT EDUCATION

Patients should be counseled about the chronic nature of this disease. Patients need to be aware of the possible side effects of medications as they apply (e.g., possible sterility, liver damage, risk for infection). Patients should understand the need for regular monitoring (including potential laboratory monitoring) while taking such medications. Appropriate forms of exercise may include range-of-motion and stretching exercises as well as swimming.

ARTHRITIS OF INFLAMMATORY BOWEL DISEASE

DEFINITION AND EPIDEMIOLOGY

The arthritis of IBD is an inflammatory arthritis associated with ulcerative colitis and with Crohn disease. Peripheral arthritis occurs in 15% to 20% of patients with IBD.[36] Axial joint involvement in the form of spondylitis and sacroiliitis occurs in approximately 10% to 36% of patients.[37] Approximately 27%

of patients with Crohn disease and ulcerative colitis will have radiographic evidence of sacroiliitis.[38] AS in Crohn disease and ulcerative colitis has an equal sex distribution.

PATHOPHYSIOLOGY

Arthritis is one of several extraintestinal manifestations associated with ulcerative colitis and Crohn disease. The mechanism of this association is not clearly understood; the arthritic manifestations of the disorder may be an immunologic phenomenon.

CLINICAL PRESENTATION AND PHYSICAL EXAMINATION

Two forms of arthritis occur in IBD: peripheral joint disease (a systemic manifestation of the IBD varying with bowel disease activity) and AS, which is unrelated to IBD activity. The peripheral arthritis is acute or subacute and is more common in the lower extremities than in the upper extremities. It tends to be associated with active IBD and flares when the bowel disease flares.[39]

The spondylitis seen in association with IBD is insidious and chronic and does not correlate with bowel disease activity. The joint involvement is identical to that of idiopathic AS. Patients may develop inflammatory eye disease, usually uveitis, which manifests as an acute, red, painful eye. SI joint involvement is strongly associated with acute uveitis. The clinical presentation of IBD may include complaints of joint pain, back pain, or morning stiffness. Mild abdominal pain with reports of bloody or mucous stools may antedate or occur with the joint disease, indicating a direct causal relationship between the two, but joint disease may be seen as the first symptom.

DIAGNOSTICS

Indicators of inflammation, including ESR and CRP, are often elevated. A mild hypochromic anemia is common. Joint fluid findings are consistent with inflammatory arthritis, showing cell counts of 1500 to 50,000 cells/mm.[40]

DIFFERENTIAL DIAGNOSIS

Inflammatory arthritis is seen in conjunction with gastrointestinal manifestations in a number of diseases, including vasculitis with abdominal involvement, systemic sclerosis complicated by motility dysfunction, amyloidosis, Behçet syndrome, familial Mediterranean fever, intestinal bypass, gluten sensitivity enteropathy, Whipple disease, and parasitic, bacterial, and viral infections.[39]

MANAGEMENT

NSAIDs, when tolerated, are useful for the control of joint pain. If symptoms are not controlled by NSAIDs or if NSAIDs are not tolerated, sulfasalazine is recommended. Sulfasalazine, which may be used to control the bowel disease, can be helpful in controlling the joint disease as well. Corticosteroids usually control both bowel and joint disease but are not desirable for long-term use because of drug toxicity. Methotrexate or azathioprine has been beneficial in patients whose disease is not controlled with sulfasalazine. The anti-TNF agents infliximab, adalimumab, and certolizumab are well tolerated and are approved for the treatment of Crohn disease and ulcerative colitis and are recommended for treatment of disease resistant to standard therapy. Both the gastroenterologic and arthritic manifestations of Crohn disease appear to respond to treatment with anti-TNF medications; however, etanercept has been shown to be effective only for the arthritis, and not the colitis.[3,41] The response of the arthropathy associated with ulcerative colitis to anti-TNF therapy has not been well studied.

COMPLICATIONS

Complications primarily arise with uncontrolled bowel disease. Abdominal pain and bloody diarrhea with weight loss can be severely disabling and may necessitate hospitalization. Corticosteroid-treated patients with IBD are at risk for steroid-induced osteoporosis and should be given appropriate calcium and vitamin D supplementation as well as prophylactic treatment with a bisphosphonate to prevent steroid-driven bone loss.

INDICATIONS FOR REFERRAL

Referral to a rheumatologist or a gastroenterologist is indicated for confirmation of the diagnosis or treatment suggestions. Referral to a physical or occupational therapist can be beneficial for patients dealing with severe joint disease. Dietary modifications may be helpful in controlling bowel disease, and referral to a dietitian may be useful.

PATIENT EDUCATION

Patients need to understand the chronicity of this disease and the relationship between their bowel disease and their arthritis. Unlike in PsA, there does not seem to be a correlation between the activity of the bowel disease and the joint disease. Total colectomy may provide a cure for patients with ulcerative colitis and effect remission of the associated arthritis. This is not necessarily true for patients with Crohn disease because the bowel inflammation can affect the remaining gastrointestinal tract even if the colon is removed. Patients need to understand their medication regimens and potential toxicities. Patients taking prednisone should be cautioned not to discontinue this medication abruptly. Dietary modifications may be crucial, and patients are often advised to adhere to a low-residue diet.

CHAPTER 216

POLYMYALGIA RHEUMATICA AND GIANT CELL ARTERITIS

Francisco P. Quismorio, Jr. • Dorothy K. Johnson

DEFINITION AND EPIDEMIOLOGY

Polymyalgia rheumatica (PMR) is a treatable, chronic systemic inflammatory condition of unknown cause seen in the elderly. Most patients are Caucasian, and, in general, PMR does not occur in patients younger than age 50. It is characterized by diffuse aching and stiffness of the shoulder girdle, neck, and pelvic girdle and is associated with elevated erythrocyte sedimentation rate (ESR) and/or C-reactive protein (CRP). There are no specific laboratory tests for PMR, and the diagnosis is made on clinical grounds and after exclusion of other inflammatory conditions.[1]

The incidence of PMR increases progressively with age, peaking 70 to 80 years. Women are affected two to three times more often than men. A population-based study in the United States found prevalence as high as 1 per 133 persons older than age 50 years.[2]

PATHOPHYSIOLOGY

The cause of PMR is not known; however, genetic, immune, and environmental influences are believed to be important factors. Human leukocyte antigen HLA-DRB1 genotypes and polymorphisms in genes involved in immunity, including those involved with tumor necrosis factor-α (TNF-α) and interleukin-1 (IL-1), are associated with increased susceptibility and/or severity of PMR. The higher incidence of PMR during winter months and the known variation in geographic distribution of the disease in the same country, including a higher prevalence in rural areas than in urban communities, implies a role for environmental factors.[3] The possible role of infectious agent(s) as a trigger of the disease has been suspected; however, no definite proof has been found.

CLINICAL PRESENTATION

The most remarkable features are the stiffness and aching of the shoulder girdle, pelvic girdle, and neck. Inflammatory in origin, the pain tends to be worse at night and may radiate distally to the elbows and the knees. Morning stiffness lasting longer than 1 hour and often all morning is common. The onset can be acute, such that the patient may remember the day and the hour of the onset. In most patients the onset is subacute and insidious. About half of patients experience systemic symptoms such as low-grade fever, depression, fatigue, malaise, and weight loss. About 25% of patients have inflammatory arthritis involving primarily the knees and wrists and less frequently the metacarpal joints. It can be mistaken for rheumatoid arthritis; however, in PMR the inflammatory arthritis is non-erosive, asymmetric, self-limiting, and highly responsive to systemic corticosteroids.[1,4] Tenosynovitis of the extensor tendons of the hands and feet can be seen in association with peripheral arthritis. Remitting seronegative symmetric synovitis with pitting edema syndrome (RS3PE) seen in 12% of PMR patients is characterized by pitting edema of the dorsum of the hands and wrists and sometimes on the dorsum of the feet.[1]

Physical examination reveals painful active motion of the shoulders and hips with limited range of motion. No signs of synovitis are present except in those with peripheral arthritis. True muscle weakness is absent; however, muscle strength is often difficult to assess because of the pain.

Classification Criteria

The American College of Rheumatology (ACR) and European League Against Rheumatism (EULAR) recently published classification criteria for PMR (Table 216-1).[4] Developed primarily for defining patient groups for clinical and epidemiologic studies, this criteria set is not intended for diagnosis in clinical practice. A patient 50 years or older with new-onset bilateral shoulder pain and elevated ESR and/or CRP is classified as having PMR in the presence of morning stiffness for longer than 45 minutes, new hip pain in the absence of peripheral synovitis, and negative rheumatoid factor (RF) and anti-CCP. When musculoskeletal ultrasound (MUS) findings are included in the criteria set, a score of 5 or higher has 66% sensitivity and 81% specificity for discriminating PMR from comparison patients.

TABLE 216-1 Classification Criteria for Polymyalgia Rheumatica

Clinical Feature	Points Without Ultrasound (0-6)	Points with Ultrasound (0-8)
Morning stiffness duration >45 minutes	2	2
Hip pain or limited range of motion	1	1
At least one shoulder with subdeltoid bursitis and/or biceps tenosynovitis and/or glenohumeral synovitis and one hip with synovitis and/or trochanteric bursitis	Not applicable	1
Absence of rheumatoid factor or anti-CCP antibodies	2	2
Absence of other joint involvement	1	1
Both shoulders with subdeltoid bursitis, biceps tenosynovitis, or glenohumeral synovitis	Not applicable	1

Diagnosis of PMR is made in the presence of the required criteria plus 4 points (without ultrasound findings) or plus 5 points (with ultrasound).[6]
CCP, cyclic citrullinated peptide.

DIAGNOSTICS

When PMR is suspected on clinical grounds, the following initial laboratory tests are recommended:

1. Complete blood count
2. ESR and CRP
3. Complete metabolic panel including blood urea nitrogen (BUN), creatinine, calcium, phosphate
4. Liver function tests
5. Serum protein electrophoresis
6. Rheumatoid factor and anti-CCP
7. Urinalysis
8. Thyroid-stimulating hormone
9. Chest x-ray examination

Laboratory abnormalities associated with active inflammation including elevated ESR, CRP, leukocytosis, thrombocytosis, mild normochromic anemia, and hypoalbuminemia are seen in the majority of patients. Low-titer rheumatoid factor may be seen in some patients; however, antinuclear antibody (ANA), antineutrophil cytoplasmic antibody (ANCA), and anti–cyclic citrullinated protein (anti-CCP) test results are generally negative.

Imaging

There are few controlled studies that address the role of imaging for the diagnosis and differential diagnosis of PMR.[5] MUS, magnetic resonance imaging (MRI), and positron emission tomography–computed tomography (PET/CT) can demonstrate the characteristic joint involvement in PMR including bilateral shoulder and hip bursitis, biceps tenosynovitis, as well as glenohumeral and hip synovitis. In clinical practice, MUS is the most commonly used imaging; MRI and PET/CT are not routinely done.

DIFFERENTIAL DIAGNOSIS

Nonrheumatic medical conditions that may mimic PMR in a patient aged 50 years or older include active malignancy such as lymphoma and multiple myeloma, active bacterial or viral infections, hypothyroidism, and drug-induced syndromes such as statin myopathy.[6]

Rheumatic diseases that should be in the differential diagnosis include elderly onset RA, late-onset seronegative spondyloarthropathies, late-onset systemic lupus erythematosus (SLE), inflammatory myopathies, calcium pyrophosphate arthritis, and chronic pain syndromes such as osteoarthritis of the neck and shoulders. Giant cell arteritis (GCA) may occur concomitantly with PMR (see later). Elderly onset RA differs from PMR with the presence of subcutaneous nodules, anti-CCP antibodies, and rheumatoid factor in the latter. Moreover, the clinical response to steroid therapy is more dramatic in PMR.

MANAGEMENT

Systemic corticosteroids remain the standard drug therapy, although there have been no placebo-controlled trials. Low-dose prednisone typically induces a rapid response within a few days of initiation of therapy. The usual starting dose is 15 mg to 20 mg of prednisone (or equivalent) daily. A higher dose of prednisone (60 mg daily) is used when there is evidence of concomitant GCA (see later).

The 2015 EULAR recommendations include an initial dose of 12.5 to 25 mgs of prednisone daily with strong recommendations against using doses higher than 30 mg/day. Begin tapering doses by 5 mgs a week after 4-8 weeks of therapy and continue using the lowest effective dose.[7] Nonsteroidal anti-inflammatory agents are not recommended.

There is no optimal corticosteroid regimen for every patient; thus the regimen should be flexible and individualized. There is variation not only in severity, but also in the presentation and course of the illness.

A marked overall clinical improvement within a week of corticosteroid therapy is expected, and laboratory abnormalities should improve within 4 to 8 weeks. The patient should be monitored for pain, morning stiffness, functional disability, osteoporosis risk, adverse drug reaction, and an alternative diagnosis. The majority of PMR patients are continued on low-dose corticosteroids for 1 to 2 years. PMR patients with concomitant GCA appear to require a longer duration of corticosteroid therapy.

COMPLICATIONS

Despite good clinical response to drug therapy, disease relapses are common and are seen in 50% of cases. Factors associated with high relapse rate include persistently elevated inflammatory markers, female sex, and rapid taper of corticosteroid dose.[8]

Adverse drug side effects including osteoporosis, fragility fractures, diabetes, hypertension, and cardiovascular events are not uncommon. Sixty-five percent of PMR patients treated with corticosteroid alone and 80% of those who receive corticosteroids and NSAIDS experience at least one adverse event.[9] Patients with long-standing PMR, especially those with high risk for corticosteroid side effects, should be maintained at the lowest dose possible. In addition, the use of a steroid-staring agent such as methotrexate, leflunomide, or azathioprine may be considered.

Bone protective measures (calcium, vitamin D, and bisphosphonates) are recommended for patients on chronic corticosteroid therapy.

The overall life survival of PMR patients appears to be better than that of the general population, and this may be in part a result of improved surveillance and medical follow-up.[10]

INDICATIONS FOR REFERRAL

Patients with PMR should be referred to a rheumatologist for definitive diagnosis and a prescription regimen. Follow-up can be managed by primary care providers with access to rheumatologists for questions or for patients not responding to usual regimens. Any patients with symptoms suggestive of temporal arteritis (see later) should also be referred to an ophthalmologist.

PATIENT EDUCATION

Patients with PMR should be educated about its association with GCA. Patients should be aware of the necessity to report immediately any new headache, change in vision, scalp tenderness, pain on chewing, or other new symptom.

Education about the risks of corticosteroid therapy is important. The patient should be informed of the potential life-threatening risk of sudden withdrawal of corticosteroids secondary to hypoadrenalism. Obtaining a medical alert bracelet indicating the use of corticosteroids should be recommended. Patients need to be aware of common steroid side effects and the importance of contacting their health care provider should they develop symptoms such as increased thirst, polyuria, and weight loss. Medications should be taken with food. Ulcer prophylaxis with proton pump inhibitors or histamine H_2 blockers should be considered for patients on corticosteroids. The patient should understand the risks of the development of corticosteroid-induced bone loss and the importance of behaviors such as daily weight-bearing exercise and adequate daily intake of calcium (1200 mg) and vitamin D (1000 international units), as well as the use of antiresorptive medication.

Association Between Polymyalgia Rheumatica and Giant Cell Arteritis

GCA is a systemic vasculitis of unknown cause that primarily involves large and medium-sized blood vessels. Both PMR and GCA affect the elderly and are well recognized to occur together more frequently than expected by chance. Sixteen percent to 21% of PMR patients develop GCA, and 40% to 60% of GCA patients have clinical features of PMR.[11,12] PMR can develop before, concomitantly with, or after the onset of GCA. A recent study in the United Kingdom concluded that the number of patients diagnosed with both PMR and GCA was 38 times greater than would have been expected if there was no association between the two diseases.[13]

Epidemiology of Giant Cell Arteritis

GCA, the most common primary vasculitis in adults, affect individuals aged 50 years and older, with a female-to-male ratio of 3:1 to 2:1.

The majority of patients are Caucasian, and the incidence rate increases with latitude in the Northern Hemisphere; the highest rates are found in Scandinavian countries and in North American populations of the same descent, with an incidence rate of more than 17 per 100,00 persons aged 50 years or older. The incidence rate increases with age and is highest at ages 70 to 79 years. GCA is less common among Asians and African Americans than among Caucasians.[14,15]

PATHOPHYSIOLOGY

The cause of GCA is not known. Multiple genes have been reported that confer disease susceptibility, including HLA-DRB1*04 allele and certain polymorphisms of the *IL-13* gene, vascular endothelial growth factor gene (*VEGF*) gene, and toll-like receptor gene (*TLR*). A possible relationship between GCA and infectious organisms including herpesvirus, parvovirus, and *Mycoplasma pneumoniae* has been suspected; however, to date, there is no definitive evidence to show that the disease is triggered by an infectious agent. The role of environmental agent(s) is suggested by seasonal fluctuation, geographic variation, and the cyclic pattern of the disease.

The classic pathology is that transmural inflammation involves all layers of the arterial wall and intimal hyperplasia and causes occlusion of the lumen. The hallmark lesion is characterized by a predominance of mononuclear infiltrates or granulomas with multinucleated giant cells. The inflammatory infiltrate consists of activated T cells, dendritic cells, and macrophages. The elastic lamina is fragmented and destroyed.

In addition to the carotid artery and its branches, GCA can involve the great arteries, especially the thoracic aorta and its branches. Stroke, blindness, and other clinical manifestations are caused by tissue ischemia as a consequence of the narrowing and occlusion of the lumen of the affected blood vessel.[11]

CLINICAL PRESENTATION

The clinical manifestations of GCA are protean and can be divided into four categories.[16,17] At initial presentation a patient may have one major complaint such as new-onset headache, or the presentation may have multiple clinical features.

Clinical manifestations caused by involvement of cranial arteries include headache, jaw claudication, visual impairment, scalp tenderness, prominent or tender temporal artery, tongue infarction, and strokes or neuropsychiatric symptoms.

New-onset headache, the most common symptom (seen in 70% to 80% of patients), is often the presenting complaint. Headache is severe and localized in the temporal region, although it can also be less defined. Scalp tenderness in the occipital and temporal areas is not uncommon. The temporal artery may be tender, swollen, or nodular.

Visual disturbances are present in 25% to 50% of patients; however, visual loss is reported in 6% to 10% of cases.[17] Sudden vision loss, diplopia, amaurosis fugax, and other visual complaints are considered a medical emergency; GCA should be identified and treated immediately to prevent blindness. The second eye is at risk if the disease is not treated aggressively and promptly. Anterior ischemic optic neuropathy caused by inflammation and occlusion of the posterior ciliary arteries is the most frequent ocular lesion.

Jaw claudication, reported by 30% to 40% of patients, is characterized by pain in the muscles of mastication that develops after a period of time chewing food and is relieved with rest.[14] Tingling or soreness of the tongue, ulceration, and loss of taste can be present. Strokes, deafness, and peripheral neuropathy are less common manifestations.

Systemic symptoms including fever, weight loss, anorexia, night sweats, and dry cough are reported in 30% to 60% of patients.[16] Depression and/or confusion may occur. Signs and symptoms of PMR are reported in 20% to 65% of patients.[16]

TABLE 216-2 American College of Rheumatology 1990 Classification Criteria for Giant Cell Arteritis

Criterion	Definition
1. Age at disease onset ≥50 yr	Development of symptoms or findings beginning at age 50 yr or older
2. New headache	New onset of or new type of localized pain in the head
3. Temporal artery abnormality	Temporal artery tenderness to palpation of decreased pulsation, unrelated to arteriosclerosis of cervical arteries
4. Elevated ESR	ESR ≥50 mm/hr by Westergren method
5. Abnormal artery biopsy	Biopsy specimen with artery showing vasculitis characterized by predominance of mononuclear infiltration or granulomatous inflammation, usually with multinucleated giant cells

For purposes of classification, a patient is said to have GCA if at least three of the five criteria are present. The presence of three criteria or more yields a sensitivity of 93.5% and a specificity of 91.2%.

Clinical features resulting from extracranial vessel involvement are seen in 5% to 20% and include claudication of the upper limbs and, rarely, aortic aneurysm or dissection.[16]

PHYSICAL EXAMINATION AND CLASSIFICATION CRITERIA OF GIANT CELL ARTERITIS

The diagnosis is made based on a constellation of symptoms and physical findings combined with laboratory tests including imaging. Physical examination should include palpation of the temporal arteries, examination of the scalp, auscultation of neck arteries, blood pressure measurement in both arms for evidence of vascular stenosis, and ocular funduscopy. The diagnosis is not difficult to make in the typical elderly patient with new-onset headache, temporal artery tenderness, jaw claudication, and systemic symptoms. However, a number of patients have minor or no features referable to the cranial arteries, so the diagnosis of GCA is not easily recognized.

Developed primarily for research and epidemiologic studies, the classification criteria of the ACR (Table 216-2) should not be used as diagnostic criteria. In clinical practice, the ACR criteria set is of limited value in evaluating an individual patient for GCA, with a positive predictive value of less than 30%.[5,17]

DIAGNOSTICS

Baseline laboratory tests are similar to those listed earlier for PMR. Elevated ESR (77% to 86% of patients), high CRP (95% to 98%), mild normochromic anemia, leukocytosis, and/or thrombocytosis are indicative of systemic inflammatory state.

Color Doppler ultrasound of the temporal arteries is frequently used as a diagnostic aid. Inflammatory edema of the blood vessel appearing as a hypoechoic vascular wall thickening (halo sign) has high sensitivity and specificity when the evaluation is performed by an experienced sonographer. The test is operator dependent and technique dependent, but with increasing experience and better ultrasound equipment, reliable and reproducible results can obtained. A negative color Doppler sonography finding, however, does not exclude the diagnosis of

occurs. Submersion of the patient's hand in ice water is not recommended. Physical examination of the digits can reveal dilated capillary loops at the base of the nail beds as a sign of secondary Raynaud phenomena. Nail fold capillaroscopy is performed by observing the capillary loops in the cuticle adjacent to the nail. Immersion oil or K-Y Jelly is helpful in making the keratin more translucent and therefore accentuating the capillary loops. Magnification can be achieved with an ophthalmoscope or with another magnifying instrument A DermLite can be especially helpful. Microvascular abnormalities such as tortuous or dilated capillary loops and capillary dropout are observed in secondary Raynaud phenomena. Other stigmata of connective tissue disease may be observed on physical examination, such as the sclerotic hidebound skin of scleroderma, rash, mechanic's hands dermatitis or polymyositis, and arthritis. Tissue breakdown and ulcerations, or pitted scars of former attacks, can also be present.

DIAGNOSTICS

The diagnosis of Raynaud phenomenon is based on a clinical history of the classic tricolor changes. Capillaroscopy of the nail fold allows direct visualization of the capillaries, helping to distinguish primary from secondary Raynaud phenomenon.[7] Antinuclear antibody (ANA) positivity is a predictor of progression to or association with a connective tissue disease.[8] In particular, the presence of an anticentromere antibody is associated with the development of CREST (the subset of scleroderma described earlier), whereas the anti–Scl-70 antibody is more often seen in scleroderma.[9] One source notes that 1% of patients with primary Raynaud phenomenon converted to secondary Raynaud phenomenon per year. However, 47% of patients with primary Raynaud phenomenon who had either ANA positivity or capillary changes progressed, compared with 80% if both were present (ANA and capillary changes).[10]

DIAGNOSTICS

Raynaud Phenomenon

INITIAL
Nail fold capillaroscopy

LABORATORY
Antinuclear antibody
Anti–Scl-70
Anticentromere antibody

DIFFERENTIAL DIAGNOSIS

The differential diagnosis of secondary Raynaud phenomenon is extensive and can be divided into several categories. These include occupational exposures (use of vibrating tools), drug exposures (amphetamines, beta blockers, cocaine, clonidine, ergot, interferon alfa, methysergide, nicotine, vinyl chloride, vinblastine, bleomycin, cisplatin, and cyclosporine), occlusive vascular disease, connective tissue disease, hematologic disorders (antiphospholipid syndrome, cryoglobulinemia, cryofibrinogenemia), cold agglutinins, and others.[1]

The presence of abnormal capillaroscopy findings and/or positive ANA increases the likelihood of Raynaud phenomenon associated with a connective tissue disease. Patients with primary Raynaud phenomenon tend to do well without medical intervention.

DIFFERENTIAL DIAGNOSIS

Raynaud Phenomenon

PRIMARY DISORDER
- Raynaud phenomenon

SECONDARY DISORDER
- Drug-induced condition
- Trauma (electric shock, frost bite, repetitive injury)
- Occupational injury or exposure (vibrating tool use)
- Connective tissue disease
  - Scleroderma
  - Systemic lupus erythematosus
  - Polymyositis
  - Dermatomyositis
  - Rheumatoid arthritis
- Hematologic disorders
  - Polycythemia
  - Cryoglobulinemia
  - Waldenström macroglobulinemia
  - Cold agglutinins
  - Cryofibrinogenemia
  - Myeloproliferative disorder
- Occlusive disease or disorder
  - Atherosclerosis
  - Thromboembolism
  - Thoracic outlet syndrome
  - Buerger disease (thromboangiitis obliterans)
  - Takayasu arteritis
- Neurologic disorder
  - Cervical disk disease
  - Tumor
  - Cerebrovascular accident
  - Poliomyelitis
- Pulmonary hypertension
- Reflex sympathetic dystrophy
- Chilblain

MANAGEMENT

In its most benign form, Raynaud phenomenon can be a mild inconvenience. Most patients have discomfort when Raynaud phenomenon is triggered but have no permanent damage. Environmental measures are the first line of management, including keeping the body core warm with vests, scarves, and hats; avoiding cold environments; using stress management; and strictly avoiding smoking. Nifedipine, a calcium channel blocker, may help prevent vasospasm.[11,12] If vasospasm is not controlled, other vasodilators, such as hydralazine and prazosin, can be added, provided the blood pressure is not adversely affected. Losartan, pentoxifylline, selective serotonin reuptake inhibitors, and sildenafil can also be used. No one treatment seems preferable to another, and several trials may be needed to find the optimal agent for each patient. Antiplatelet therapy with aspirin should be considered for all patients with secondary Raynaud phenomenon with a history of ischemic ulcers.[1]

Complementary and alternative medicine (CAM), commonly used by patients with Raynaud phenomenon as standard treatment, can be associated with adverse effects. The herbal *Ginkgo biloba* was studied in a double-blind placebo-controlled trial and was found to reduce the number of attacks by 56% compared with placebo, although the difference was not statistically significant.[13] However, a more recent randomized controlled trail found no significant effect from *G. biloba*.[14] To date, no other CAM treatment has been identified as effective, although there is some trend toward subjective improvement with fish oil, vitamin C, acupuncture, and laser treatment. More important, biofeedback, used for years as a treatment, was shown to be ineffective in a recent meta-analysis.[15,16]

Prostanoids and endothelin-blocking agents can be tried in severe digit-threatening disease. In severe Raynaud phenomenon, patients are hospitalized for intravenous administration of prostaglandin, such as prostaglandin E_1.[17] This therapy is reserved for those with secondary Raynaud phenomenon and severe digital ischemia. Oral and inhaled prostaglandin preparations are being studied in Japan, Europe, and the United States. So far, their usefulness is limited to patients with pulmonary hypertension. There have been mixed results with the treatment of Raynaud phenomenon.[3,13]

Patients should avoid estrogen, nicotine, beta blockers, and pseudoephedrine; these agents can exacerbate Raynaud phenomena.

In patients for whom standard medical therapy has failed and who are at risk for permanent ischemic damage, chemical ganglion sympathectomy can be considered. This can be achieved chemically with lidocaine blocks delivered locally or cervically or with injection of Botox (onabotulinumtoxinA). A vascular or hand surgeon can perform permanent digital sympathectomy if medical therapies fail. It is unclear whether the benefits of this procedure persist over time, and newer medical strategies may be more appropriate.[16]

COMPLICATIONS

In some patients, the protracted ischemia results in ulcerations that can become superinfected. Treatment of the infection can be challenging because local delivery of antibiotics is difficult, given the impaired blood flow. Rarely, ischemia can be so profound that loss of tissue and bone stock can occur, resulting in autoamputation of digits.

INDICATIONS FOR REFERRAL OR HOSPITALIZATION

Referral to a rheumatologist is necessary to exclude the presence of associated autoimmune disease. In severe cases, consultation with a vascular surgeon or anesthesiologist may be indicated. Patients who are in intractable pain or at risk for autoamputation of a digit or severe infection should be hospitalized under the care of a rheumatologist. A vascular surgeon should be consulted early if possible digit loss is suspected. Anesthesia can also be helpful in providing chemical ganglion sympathectomy for the relief of pain. Referral to an occupational therapist for evaluation and education can be helpful. Some patients have found biofeedback useful for management and reduction of Raynaud attacks, although recently studies have failed to demonstrate effectiveness.[18]

PATIENT EDUCATION

Patient education is crucial, and the potentially serious nature of this disorder should be emphasized. Patients should avoid exposing their hands to the cold if at all possible. Mittens, which are preferable to gloves, should be worn as soon as the weather begins to get cool. For some patients, mittens need to be worn when grocery shopping because reaching for food items in refrigerator or freezer sections can often trigger attacks. Keeping core temperature higher by wearing hats and layering clothing may also be of benefit. Sudden temperature changes should be avoided. For many patients, emotional stress can trigger episodes; relaxation techniques, behavioral modification, and biofeedback may play a role in limiting attacks. Most critically, patients should discontinue cigarette smoking if they are smokers. Medications to be avoided include decongestants, amphetamines, estrogen, and beta blockers.

If Raynaud phenomenon occurs with the use of vibrating machinery, such as jackhammers and chain saws, patients may need vocational counseling.

CHAPTER 218

RHEUMATOID ARTHRITIS

Dorothy K. Johnson • Francisco P. Quismorio, Jr.

DEFINITION AND EPIDEMIOLOGY

Rheumatoid arthritis (RA) is an autoimmune disorder characterized by symmetric inflammatory polyarthritis and varying degrees of extra-articular involvement. Most patients experience a chronic fluctuating course of the disease that may result in joint destruction, deformity, disability, and premature death. Major economic and emotional disabilities can result from RA and can have a significant impact on patients' families and loved ones. RA is a chronic disease and accounts for many more physician visits than in age-matched controls, although fewer hospitalizations and less disability over the past decade are the results of better treatment options and early disease remission objectives.

RA affects 0.6% of the adult population in the United States and may be declining.[1] Women are affected two or three times more often than men. The prevalence increases with age. Despite extensive research, the cause of RA remains unknown; however, most investigators believe that a combination of genetic, environmental, hormonal, and reproductive factors is important. RA probably occurs in a genetically susceptible person with an abnormal immune response to an undetermined antigen. Genetic studies have shown that RA is strongly linked to human leukocyte antigen HLA-DRB1 alleles, which encode similar sequences (shared epitope).[2] Other susceptibility genes, including T-cell receptor signaling, have recently been identified. Smoking, an environmental factor, has also been shown to increase risk for the disease.[2]

PATHOPHYSIOLOGY

The main target of inflammation is the synovial lining of diarthrodial joints. The earliest changes in the synovial membrane are seen in the capillaries and small blood vessels. There is proliferation of the lining cells and early infiltration by T lymphocytes. Later, there is diffuse infiltration with B and T lymphocytes, macrophages, and plasma cells. The synovial membrane undergoes hyperplastic thickening with the proliferation of lining cells and fibroblasts and formation of new blood vessels. This granulation tissue, called pannus, invades the cartilage and subchondral bone and is primarily responsible for the destruction of joint structures in RA.[3]

Immune complexes in the synovial tissue activate the complement system, which then participates in the inflammatory process. Kinins, prostaglandins, cytokines, and other mediators increase the permeability of blood vessels and attract leukocytes and lymphocytes into the joint. Neutrophils and macrophages ingest immune complexes and release enzymes that degrade articular cartilage and joint structures. Rheumatoid factor (RF), antibodies to citrullinated proteins, and possibly other autoantibodies produced locally in the synovium participate in the formation of pathogenic immune complexes.[2]

Autoimmunity activity appears to involve both B cells and T cells. T cells are the major infiltrating lymphocytes in the rheumatoid synovium. Many autoantigens are targeted by the immune system in RA, and some autoantigens are T-cell targets.

Activated T cells proliferate, expand, and stimulate monocytes, macrophages, and synovial fibroblasts to secrete cytokines, including interleukin-1 (IL-1) and tumor necrosis factor-α (TNF-α). Both cytokines stimulate mesenchymal cells to secrete matrix metalloproteinases that destroy cartilage and bone. Activated T cells stimulate B cells to produce immunoglobulins, including RF.[4]

Venules and small blood vessels become occluded by hypertrophied endothelial cells: fibrin, platelets, and inflammatory cells. The decreased circulation along with the increased metabolic demands of hypertrophy and hyperplasia results in hypoxia and metabolic acidosis. Acidosis stimulates the release of hydrolytic enzymes from synovial cells into the surrounding tissue, causing erosion of articular cartilage and inflammation of ligaments and tendons.[5]

CLINICAL PRESENTATION

The onset of RA is usually insidious, occurring during a period of several weeks or months, but in a small percentage of patients the onset is acute. The initial symptoms include general systemic manifestations of inflammation, weakness, weight loss, malaise, fatigue, anorexia, aching, and stiffness. Localized symptoms include painful, tender, swollen joints. Morning stiffness lasts for a minimum of 1 hour, sometimes all morning. The small joints of the hands (metacarpophalangeal and proximal interphalangeal joints), wrists, and small joints of the feet (metatarsophalangeal joints) are commonly affected initially. Joint involvement is bilateral and symmetric. The hips, knees, ankles, shoulders, and cervical spine may also be involved.

PHYSICAL EXAMINATION

A complete medical history should be obtained in a comfortable setting. Particular attention should be paid to the location, quality, quantity, course, and alleviating factors of the patient's pain. Functional activities, activities of daily living, instrumental activities of daily living, and social support should be assessed.

Physical examination of the peripheral joints and the axial skeleton is central to the evaluation of a patient with RA. The joints should be examined in an organized manner, and report of joint pain, tenderness, degree of swelling, range of motion, and deformity should be recorded. On palpation, the inflamed joint feels warm and tender and the synovial membrane feels thickened and boggy. The skin over the affected joint may look thin and shiny and have a ruddy color. During the joint examination, the examiner should support painful or weak joints.[6]

The physical examination should include evaluation for the presence of extra-articular manifestations. Subcutaneous nodules, which are present in 20% of patients with RA, are found over pressure areas, such as the extensor surface of the elbow and other areas of trauma. Rheumatoid nodules may occasionally be found on the cardiac valves, pericardium, pleura, lung parenchyma, and spleen. Other extra-articular manifestations of RA can include signs of vasculitis (mononeuritis multiplex, skin infarcts, and ulceration), ocular signs (Sjögren syndrome, episcleritis, and scleritis), respiratory symptoms (interstitial lung disease or pleurisy), cardiac involvement (pericarditis or valvular heart disease), and peripheral nerve entrapments.[7]

Sjögren syndrome, seen commonly in RA patients, is characterized by dry eyes (keratoconjunctivitis sicca) and dry mouth (xerostomia) and is caused by immune-mediated destruction of the salivary and lacrimal glands. Felty syndrome, an uncommon feature seen in long-standing RA, is characterized by skin ulcers, leukopenia, splenomegaly, and increased risk for bacterial infections.[7]

DIAGNOSTICS

The diagnosis of RA is primarily based on the clinical history and physical findings. Laboratory tests, including radiographs, are used to confirm the diagnosis, to exclude other conditions, and, more important, to predict the prognosis and to develop a treatment plan for the individual patient.

Because RA can affect many organs, it is important to obtain laboratory tests as a baseline evaluation and periodically during the course of treatment. Baseline evaluation should include a complete blood count (CBC); acute-phase reactants, including erythrocyte sedimentation rate (ESR) and C-reactive protein (CRP); serum creatinine; hepatic panel; urinalysis; RF; and anti–cyclic citrullinated peptide (anti-CCP) antibodies. Normocytic, normochromic anemia is common in RA. Evaluation of renal and hepatic functions is necessary because many antirheumatic agents have renal and hepatic toxicity and may be contraindicated if these organs are severely impaired.

RF in RA is an immunoglobulin M autoantibody that is directed against antigenic determinants in the immunoglobulin G molecule. Not all RA patients have a positive test result for RF at the time of diagnosis, but the result will become positive for 70% to 80% of patients during the course of disease.[8] RA patients with a high titer of RF tend to have more severe joint and extra-articular disease and a worse prognosis than RF-negative patients do. The titer of RF does not change rapidly with treatment, so frequent monitoring is not recommended. Compared with anti-CCP, RF has the same sensitivity for the diagnosis as RA (67% versus 69%); however, anti-CCP has significantly higher specificity for the disease (95% versus 85%).[9] RF can be seen in other rheumatic diseases as well as other nonrheumatic conditions such as chronic infections.

Acute-phase reactants are proteins that are synthesized rapidly by the liver in the presence of inflammation or tissue necrosis and include CRP, fibrinogen, complement proteins, and several other proteins. Measurement of serum concentration of CRP and ESR is widely used to assess the activity of the inflammatory process and to aid in monitoring of the response to therapy.[10]

Radiographs

Because the hands and feet are often involved in RA, x-ray studies of these and other affected joints help with the diagnosis and establish a baseline for future evaluation of the effectiveness of treatment. The radiographs of the joints and bones are often normal at the onset of the disease, but bone erosions can develop within the first years. Ultrasound and magnetic resonance imaging (MRI) are increasingly used to confirm the diagnosis of RA; bone marrow edema is a hallmark finding in early RA.[11] The American College of Rheumatology has established criteria for the classification of RA that can be used as guidelines for patient diagnosis and for research classification (Box 218-1).[12]

Synovial Fluid Analysis

Aspiration of an inflamed joint and examination of the synovial fluid are important to the diagnosis of RA. Normal synovial fluid is clear, viscous, and low in volume with a white blood cell count of 2000 cells/mm^3. In RA, the joint fluid is

BOX 218-1

American College of Rheumatology/European League Against Rheumatism 2010 Classification Criteria for Rheumatoid Arthritis

JOINT INVOLVEMENT (0-5)	
1 medium/large joint	0
2-10 medium/large joints	1
1-3 small joints	2
4-10 small joints	3
>10 joints (at least 1 small)	5
SEROLOGY (0-3)	
Neither RF nor ACPA positive	0
At least one test low positive	2
At least one test high positive	3
DURATION OF SYMPTOMS (0-1)	
<6 weeks	0
>6 weeks	1
ACUTE PHASE REACTANTS (0-1)	
Neither CRP nor ESR abnormal	0
Abnormal CRP or abnormal ESR	1

Score ≥6 = RA.
Subjects with bony erosions regardless of score = RA.
ACPA, anti–cyclic citrullinated peptide antibody.

DIAGNOSTICS

Rheumatoid Arthritis

LABORATORY
ESR
CRP
RF
Anti-CCP antibodies
CBC and differential count
Blood urea nitrogen (BUN), creatinine
Hepatic panel (alanine aminotransferase, aspartate aminotransferase, albumin, and alkaline phosphatase)
Urinalysis
Synovial fluid analysis
Hepatitis B and C panel

IMAGING
Radiography of selected involved joints
MRI
Ultrasound

inflammatory with poor viscosity and a high white blood cell count of more than 10,000 cells/mm^3 with a predominance of neutrophils.[10]

DIFFERENTIAL DIAGNOSIS

The differential diagnosis must include other causes of inflammatory arthritis. Initially, systemic lupus erythematosus, psoriatic arthritis, and seronegative spondyloarthropathies (see Chapter 215) may be indistinguishable from RA. Extra-articular manifestations of these disorders usually help establish the correct diagnosis. Although antinuclear antibodies may be present in RA patients' anti–double-stranded DNA (anti-dsDNA) and anti-Smith (anti-Sm) antibodies, the specific types of antinuclear antibody associated with systemic lupus erythematosus (see Chapter 219) are negative.

Soft tissue disorders such as fibromyalgia (see Chapter 175), tendinitis, bursitis, and, in older adults, polymyalgia rheumatica (see Chapter 216) may confound the diagnosis of RA early in the course of the disease. Viral infections, such as with human parvovirus, hepatitis viruses B and C, and human immunodeficiency virus (HIV), can cause symmetric polyarthritis and chronic arthralgia and should be considered in the differential diagnosis.

DIFFERENTIAL DIAGNOSIS

Rheumatoid Arthritis

- Fibromyalgia
- Osteoarthritis
- Viral syndrome
- Soft tissue syndromes
- Spondyloarthropathies
- Systemic lupus erythematosus
- Scleroderma
- Dermatomyositis and polymyositis
- Polymyalgia rheumatica
- Systemic vasculitis
- Lyme disease

MANAGEMENT

The standard goal of RA management is remission or low disease activity. This goal should be achieved as rapidly as possible after diagnosis. Management of RA is multifaceted. Nonpharmacologic measures, such as physical therapy, occupational therapy, and psychological interventions, aid in achieving the goal. Regular participation in dynamic and aerobic conditioning exercises improves joint symptoms, muscle strength, functional abilities, and psychological well-being.[13]

Assessing Cardiovascular Risk

There is an increased risk of cardiovascular (CV) disease in individuals with RA. The increased risk appears to result from an accentuation of traditional risk factors and the inflammatory burden.[14] Traditional risk factors include hypertension, dyslipidemia, smoking, older age, and female gender. In RA, it is recommended that the CV risk estimate be multiplied by 1.5 if at least two of the following three criteria are present: (1) disease duration of more than 10 years; (2) RF or anti-CCP positivity; or (3) presence of certain extra-articular manifestations.[15] CV risk should be assessed yearly by use of national guidelines, and risk assessment should be repeated when antirheumatic treatment has changed. There are several CV risk score calculators, such as the Framingham Score and the Systematic Coronary Risk Evaluation (SCORE) model, that the provider may find helpful.

Pharmacologic Agents

Choosing a pharmacologic agent for an individual patient is based on consideration of cost, efficacy, safety, and convenience. Pharmacologic therapy most often consists of combination therapy, synthetic and biologic disease-modifying antirheumatic drugs (DMARDs), nonsteroidal anti-inflammatory drugs (NSAIDs), and glucocorticoids (GCs). An assessment of the patient's prognosis should be made before the treatment regimen is selected (Box 218-2). Systematic monitoring of disease activity by composite measures should guide treatment decisions (Box 218-3).

Disease-Modifying Antirheumatic Drugs. The mainstay of treatment is synthetic or biologic DMARDs. New and highly effective DMARDs have continued to come to market, such as

BOX 218-2

Poor Prognostic Signs in Rheumatoid Arthritis

- Presence of extra-articular manifestations
- Increased ESR
- Joint bone erosions
- Presence of autoantibodies
- Functional limitations

BOX 218-3

Composite Outcome Measures Tools

- Disease Activity Scale (DAS28)
- Simplified Disease Activity Index (SDAI)
- Health Assessment Questionnaire (HAQ)
- Clinical Disease Activity Index (CDAI)
- Routine Assessment of Patient Index Data (RAPID)
- Rheumatoid Arthritis Disease Activity Index (RADAI)

agents that target TNF, IL-1 receptor, IL-6 receptor, B lymphocytes, and T-cell costimulation. Remission or low disease activity is the treatment goal that should be achieved as quickly as possible. Intensive medication strategies should be considered in every patient. Remission or low disease activity should be achieved preferably within 3 months and definitely by a maximum of 6 months. Treatment adjustment guided by careful monitoring should occur every 1 to 3 months to achieve low disease activity or remission.[16]

In general, treatment with DMARDs should be started as soon as the diagnosis of RA is established. Methotrexate (MTX) is a highly effective drug for disease modification. It is more effective at higher weekly doses (20 to 30 mg) than at lower doses and should be part of the first treatment strategy because it can be used as monotherapy, it increases the efficacy of biologic DMARDs when it used in combination, and it has a long-term safety profile.[17] MTX may induce hyperhomocysteinemia through depletion of folic acid levels. Therefore folic acid should be used in combination with MTX. If there are any contraindications to MTX, leflunomide, sulfasalazine, or parenteral gold salts could be prescribed. Added efficacy of antimalarial agents used in combination therapy is now being evaluated.[16]

If treatment goals are not met with MTX or other synthetic DMARD monotherapy or in combination therapy and if poor prognostic markers are present, a biologic DMARD, preferably a TNF inhibitor, should be used in combination with MTX.[18] In the absence of poor prognostic markers, DMARD combination therapy or switching to another DMARD should be instituted, or, in consultation with the patient, a biologic DMARD can be added. If the first TNF inhibitor in combination with MTX fails, the patient should be switched to a second TNF inhibitor.[18] If both TNF inhibitors fail, a switch to another DMARD, such as a B cell–targeted agent such as rituximab, could be tried.[19] DMARD-naive patients with poor prognostic markers should be considered for combination therapy with MTX plus a biologic agent as initial therapy.[18]

In patients with long-standing persistent remission, it is currently unclear how to continue or discontinue DMARD therapy. GCs should be tapered and discontinued first. In consultation with the patient, cautious titration of the synthetic DMARD dose could be considered. Assessment of the tapering process should be guided by rigorous monitoring.[20]

Glucocorticoids. GCs have been shown to have anti-inflammatory and disease-modifying properties.[21,22] GCs at low doses have been used successfully, but more rapid improvement may be achieved with the addition of GCs at higher doses for the short term.[22] Long-term or intermediate use of GCs can lead to adverse events. Therefore GCs should be used with caution for short periods.

Nonsteroidal Anti-Inflammatory Drugs. NSAIDs and cyclooxygenase 2 (COX-2) inhibitors are associated with an increased CV risk. Because of COX-2 inhibition, most but not all NSAIDs have prothrombotic effects. However, these medications improve pain and mobility in patients, which might counterbalance the prothrombotic effects as well as improve quality of life. There is also a possible interaction between some NSAIDs and aspirin. Some NSAIDs may impair aspirin's antiplatelet function, so patients using low-dose aspirin for CV disease should be counseled. Potential antithrombotic risk must be considered in prescribing these drugs with aspirin.

NSAIDs should be used cautiously in patients with CV disease or renal disease and those with a history of gastrointestinal bleeding. Acetaminophen is used preferentially in those cases.

Topical NSAIDs are very helpful for some patients and can be used with a lower of risk of adverse effects.[23]

Nonpharmacologic Treatment

Instruction in joint protection, conservation of energy, strengthening exercises, and a range-of-motion program is beneficial for all RA patients. Regular participation in dynamic and aerobic conditioning exercise programs improves joint symptoms, muscle strength, functional abilities, and psychological well-being. Consultation with occupational and physical therapists for assistive and adaptive devices and education about care of joints are recommended.[24]

Complementary and alternative therapy is of growing interest and use to RA patients. Many patients receiving conventional medical therapy are also using acupuncture, acupressure, herbs, and other complementary modalities although evidence of efficacy is lacking. Providers should always ask about the use of complementary and alternative therapies.[25]

Interdisciplinary Management

The rheumatologist should provide support and consultation to the patient and his or her health care provider. Because the level, training, and experience in the diagnosis and treatment of RA vary among health care providers, the responsibility for diagnosis, development of a treatment plan, and monitoring of therapy should be assigned to the rheumatologist. A general maintenance plan should be developed for the patient, with all health care providers participating.

LIFE SPAN CONSIDERATIONS

RA has a considerable impact on quality of life. Significant work disability has been identified in patients with RA; about half of patients who are working at the onset of disease become work disabled within 10 years,[26,27] Direct and indirect monetary costs of RA are enormous. Pregnancy should be avoided in RA patients taking immune-modulating medications. Women with RA are slower to conceive and have fewer children than age-matched controls.[28] Approximately half of the RA patients who choose to become pregnant will experience a temporary remission in disease activity for the duration of the pregnancy and a predictable flare of disease activity in the postpartum period.

Early death has been identified in RA patients, with the life span decreased by about 10 years primarily on the basis of CV disease.

COMPLICATIONS

Joint deformity, with the resulting sequelae of muscle, tendon, and ligament weakening or deconditioning and joint immobilization, is the most important complication. Small vessel vasculitis can cause neuropathy and skin ulcers. Cervical spine involvement can cause neck pain or abnormal neurologic findings because of myelopathy.[10]

Complications related to adverse reactions to medications include osteoporosis, osteonecrosis (avascular necrosis), retinal toxicity, gastrointestinal irritation and bleeding, and hepatic toxicity. Opportunistic infections, including the reactivation of tuberculosis, may develop with the anti–TNF-α agents, systemic corticosteroids, and other immunosuppressive agents.[29] It is well established that RA is associated with an increased risk of lymphoproliferative disorders. With the use of targeted biologic therapies including those that may interfere with innate tumor surveillance, there is concern for the development of other malignant neoplasms.[19,30]

INDICATIONS FOR REFERRAL OR HOSPITALIZATION

Referral to a rheumatologist for diagnosis and treatment of RA is strongly recommended. A rheumatologist should manage medication regimens and monitor for adverse drug reactions. Referral to an orthopedic surgeon specializing in joint replacement should be considered for end-stage joint disease. Quality of life is improved and pain relieved in most patients after joint replacement surgery. Physical and occupational therapists should be consulted for exercise programs and adaptive devices. A rheumatology nurse specialist can provide information about lifestyle changes, self-help programs, and community educational programs, such as those sponsored by the Arthritis Foundation. Because most patients experience a period of grief after diagnosis, referral to a clinical psychologist or social worker should be considered. Life role adjustments will frequently need to be made because of the disease, and many patients will benefit from psychological counseling through this transition.

PATIENT AND FAMILY EDUCATION

Patients should be educated about lifestyle modifications, such as increased rest for disease flare-ups, use of adaptive aids to facilitate function, prioritizing and planning of activities to accommodate fatigue, and use of splints for painful and swollen wrists and hands. Podiatric care for foot pain should be provided, along with special footwear and flexible orthotic devices. Education about the need for a regular aerobic and muscle-strengthening exercise program is essential to help reduce stiffness, to avoid joint contractures, and to prevent osteoporosis.

The health care provider should advise the patient about the benefit of warm showers in the morning and frequent position changes to alleviate stiffness. The use of pillows to position joints at night is contraindicated because this may predispose the patient to flexion deformities.

The health care provider should also educate the patient and family about medication use, restrictions, and side effects or adverse effects, including pregnancy and fetal effects. Warnings against stopping of certain medications without notifying the health care provider should be stressed. Instructions should be given about dietary restrictions or recommendations as they relate to medications.

Self-management programs, educational information, and exercise programs from the Arthritis Foundation are available to patients in print form and online at www.arthritis.org. Most material is available in Spanish and English.

CHAPTER 219

SYSTEMIC LUPUS ERYTHEMATOSUS

Francisco P. Quismorio, Jr • Dorothy K. Johnson

DEFINITION AND EPIDEMIOLOGY

Systemic lupus erythematosus (SLE) is a chronic multisystem inflammatory rheumatic disease that may cause diverse symptoms, such as fatigue, joint pain, rashes, seizures, edema, and chest pain.[1,2] SLE has a predilection for women, particularly during the prime childbearing age of 15 to 35 years. A wide variety of autoantibodies, including antinuclear antibodies (ANAs), are the most characteristic laboratory finding in SLE. SLE can damage many organ systems, notably the kidneys, lungs, heart, and brain, and may result in severe disability and even death.

SLE is not an uncommon rheumatic disease. The incidence and prevalence rates are difficult to measure with great precision; these rates vary by geographic distribution and by demographic characteristics. Data from recent American surveys suggest that the prevalence of SLE among whites ranges from 5.5 to 10 per 100,000 persons.[3] The reported incidence rates of SLE in the United States also vary from 1.8 to 7.6 cases per 100,000 persons per year. SLE is up to 10 times more common in women than in men.[3] The disease is more common in African-American women, among whom the prevalence may be as high as 1 in 500. The morbidity and mortality of SLE are increased among African-American and Hispanic patients compared with whites.[4] Epidemiologic data have suggested that the incidence of the disease may be increasing.[5]

The cause of SLE is unknown. Its association with certain genotypes, such as the C4 null allele and various HLA haplotypes, as well as the 25% rate of concordance in identical twins suggests that the disease is likely to be a result of an interaction between genetic makeup and one or more environmental triggers. Studies including genome-wide association analysis have identified several key susceptibility genes in SLE.[6] Because certain drugs can induce lupus-like syndromes, it is speculated that certain environmental agents may promote the development of SLE.[7] Other potential environmental triggers are a wide range of viruses (including the Epstein-Barr virus),[8,9] physical trauma, and emotional stress. Differences in the level and metabolism of estrogen, androgen, and other sex hormones may partly account for the female predilection for the disease.[9]

PATHOPHYSIOLOGY

The pathophysiologic hallmark of SLE is the development of antibodies directed against components of "self" tissues, particularly structures found within cell nuclei. The lupus erythematosus (LE) cell test, the first laboratory diagnostic test for the disease, described in 1948 by Hargraves, is predicated on the presence of ANAs specific for deoxyribonucleoprotein.[1] A wide variety of autoantibodies have since been reported in SLE, including antibodies directed against DNA and other nuclear constituents, red blood cells, platelets, white blood cells, and phospholipids. Autoantibodies form immune complexes in the circulation or in situ and become deposited in kidneys, skin, lungs, and other target organs. Circulating immune complexes are normally solubilized and cleared from the circulation by the reticuloendothelial system. In SLE, there is an aberrant clearance of immune complexes that may be related to defective solubilization of antigen-antibody complexes and abnormalities of complement and cell receptor functions. Individuals with genetic deficiencies of the early complement components C1q, C2, and C4 are at an increased risk for lupus-like autoimmune disease. Defective apoptosis (programmed cell death) with phagocytosis of cell debris allowing nuclear antigens to become antigenic, abnormalities in T- and B-cell functions, cytokines, innate immunity, and other immune mechanisms that promote self-tolerance all contribute to the development of autoimmunity in SLE.[9]

The deposition of immune complexes in tissues generates a local inflammatory response that may have organ-specific effects. Inflammation in blood vessels can cause vasculitis, which may result in vessel occlusion, ischemia, or infarction of the affected organ. Inflammation of serosal surfaces (lining of visceral organs) may result in pleurisy or pericarditis. The deposition of pathogenic immune complexes in the renal glomeruli can result in the development of lupus nephritis.

CLINICAL PRESENTATION AND PHYSICAL EXAMINATION

SLE is a systemic inflammatory disorder characterized by varied presentation, disease relapses, and remissions. The disease can develop acutely, with obvious severe manifestations that include arthritis, nephritis, serositis, and vasculitis, or it may become apparent in an individual who has had mild symptoms and subtle physical findings (e.g., fatigue, arthralgia, rashes) sporadically for many years. The disorder is often misdiagnosed because many of the early symptoms of SLE are nonspecific (e.g., fatigue, oral ulcers, joint pain) and the ANA test result is positive in approximately 5% of healthy persons. The American College of Rheumatology has developed and validated a set of criteria for the classification of SLE[10] (Box 219-1).

Malaise and fatigue, often profound, are common but nonspecific complaints. Anorexia and weight loss may be seen in patients with active disease, as can fevers, lymphadenopathy, tachycardia, and anemia. The malar (or butterfly) rash, one of the most recognizable features of SLE, is observed in only 35% of patients. This is a photosensitive erythematous rash on the cheeks and over the bridge of the nose that tends to spare the nasolabial folds. Discoid lupus rash is seen in 20% of patients with SLE. In a more benign clinical form of lupus, termed discoid lupus erythematosus, the disease is predominantly cutaneous with no or mild visceral involvement. Discoid lupus skin lesions are thick, round, erythematous plaques on the face, scalp, and extremities that heal with scarring, atrophy, depigmentation, and loss of hair. Mucous membrane ulcers are also common, occurring in the oral and nasal cavities. Discoid LE lesions can be disfiguring.

BOX 219-1

Revised Criteria for Classification of Systemic Lupus Erythematosus

1. Malar rash: Fixed erythema, flat or raised, over the malar eminences, tending to spare the nasolabial folds.
2. Discoid rash: Erythematous raised patches with adherent keratotic scaling and follicular plugging; atrophic scarring may occur in older lesions.
3. Photosensitivity: Skin rash as a result of unusual reaction to sunlight, by patient or physician observation.
4. Oral ulcers: Oral or nasopharyngeal ulceration, usually painless, observed by a physician.
5. Arthritis: Nonerosive arthritis involving two or more peripheral joints, characterized by tenderness, swelling, or effusion.
6. Serositis.
   a. Pleuritis—convincing history of pleuritic pain or rub heard by a physician or evidence of pleural effusion *or*
   b. Pericarditis—documented by electrocardiogram or rub or evidence of pericardial effusion
7. Renal disorder.
   a. Persistent proteinuria—more than 0.5 g/day or greater than 3+ if quantitation not performed *or*
   b. Cellular casts—may be red cell, hemoglobin, granular, tubular, or mixed
8. Neurologic disorder.
   a. Seizures—in the absence of offending drugs or known metabolic derangements (e.g., uremia, ketoacidosis, or electrolyte imbalance) *or*
   b. Psychosis—in the absence of offending drugs or known metabolic derangements (e.g., uremia, ketoacidosis, or electrolyte imbalance)
9. Hematologic disorder.
   a. Hemolytic anemia—with reticulocytosis *or*
   b. Leukopenia—less than 4000/mm^3 total on two or more occasions *or*
   c. Lymphopenia—less than 1500/mm^3 on two or more occasions *or*
   d. Thrombocytopenia—less than 100,000/mm^3 in the absence of offending drugs
10. Immunologic disorder.
   a. Anti-DNA antibody to native DNA in abnormal titer *or*
   b. Anti-Sm—presence of antibody to Sm nuclear antigen *or*
   c. Positive finding of antiphospholipid antibodies based on abnormal serum level of IgG or IgM anticardiolipin, positive test result for lupus anticoagulant, or false-positive serologic test result for syphilis known to be positive for at least 6 months and confirmed by fluorescent treponemal antibody absorption test or other specific treponemal antibody test.
11. ANA: An abnormal titer of ANA by immunofluorescence or an equivalent assay at any point in time and in the absence of drugs known to be associated with "drug-induced lupus" syndrome.

IgG, immunoglobulin G; IgM, immunoglobulin M.

Modified from Tan EM, Cohen AS, Fries JF et al: The 1982 revised criteria for the classification of systemic lupus erythematosus, *Arthritis Rheum* 25(11):1271-1277, 1982; and Hochberg MC: Updating the American College of Rheumatology revised criteria for the classification of systemic lupus erythematosus, *Arthritis Rheum* 40:1725, 1997.

Approximately one third of SLE patients experience Raynaud phenomenon, an episodic vasospastic phenomenon characterized by changes in blood flow to the extremities, accompanied by sequential color change of the digits, from white to purple to red, and often unpleasant tingling or painful sensations. Livedo reticularis is a purplish mottling or lacelike appearance of the skin, especially in the extremities, and is associated with antiphospholipid syndrome (see later). Cutaneous vasculitis may manifest as tender skin nodules, palpable purpura or skin infarcts, and ulcerations. Bruising or petechiae caused by immune thrombocytopenia may also occur.

Joint pain (arthralgia) occurs in 80% to 90% of patients with SLE, and inflammatory arthritis can be objectively documented in about 50% of patients.[1] The arthritis of SLE is typically milder than rheumatoid arthritis. It is nonerosive, and less than 10% of the patients will develop joint deformities, called Jaccoud arthropathy. Osteoporosis is common and is multifactorial in cause, including corticosteroid therapy, chronic inflammation, and physical inactivity. Metabolic bone disease related to vitamin D deficiency and secondary hyperparathyroidism may develop in those with chronic renal failure. Inflammatory myositis manifesting as proximal muscle weakness with elevated serum creatine kinase can be seen.

Chest pain is a common complaint and is often musculoskeletal in origin. More significantly, SLE can cause serious cardiopulmonary disease, including pleurisy, pericarditis, pneumonitis, interstitial lung disease, pulmonary hemorrhage, myocarditis, and valvular heart disease.

A subset of SLE patients develop antiphospholipid syndrome, characterized by hypercoagulability, recurrent venous or arterial thrombosis, repeated spontaneous abortions and fetal loss, and the presence of antiphospholipid antibodies as measured by anticardiolipin antibodies, anti–beta 2 glycoprotein 1, or lupus anticoagulant. These patients have an increased risk for pulmonary embolism, pulmonary hypertension, strokes, abortion and fetal loss, Libman-Sacks endocarditis, and valvular heart disease.

Lupus patients are at a greatly increased risk for development of ischemic heart disease, with a 1.5% annual incidence of a new coronary event and an overall prevalence of 6% to 10%. Compared with the general population, SLE patients are 5 to 10 times more likely to experience a coronary event.[11]

Accelerated atherosclerosis in SLE may relate to both traditional and nontraditional risk factors, including hypertension, alterations in lipid metabolism associated with nephrotic syndrome, long-term use of corticosteroids, and endothelial damage caused by chronic inflammatory process.[12] Hypertension is common and may be associated with underlying lupus nephritis, the use of corticosteroids, and possibly nonsteroidal anti-inflammatory drugs (NSAIDs) as contributing factors.

Mood changes, depression, and migraine headaches are common. SLE can cause wide-ranging neuropsychiatric abnormalities, the most common being cognitive dysfunction with impaired memory and concentration. Psychosis, seizures, altered consciousness, confusion, stroke, myelopathy, and neuropathies may develop. The pathogenesis of neuropsychiatric manifestations probably involves different mechanisms, including small-vessel vasculopathy, thrombosis associated with antiphospholipid syndrome, effects of complement split products, cytokines, and antineuronal antibodies.

Lupus nephritis develops during the course of the disease in 25% to 50% of patients.[1] Persistent proteinuria of more than 500 mg/day, cellular casts, and red blood cells in the urine sediment are observed. There is a spectrum of renal involvement ranging from mesangial lupus nephritis with increased cellularity and deposition of immune complexes limited to the mesangium to severe diffuse proliferative glomerulonephritis with involvement of all glomeruli. Evaluation and staging of renal disease in SLE require a kidney biopsy, and the histopathologic findings are useful in assessing renal prognosis and determining a therapeutic regimen. Hemodialysis or kidney transplantation becomes necessary in those who develop end-stage renal disease. Most patients who undergo kidney transplantation do relatively well because of the immunosuppression required to prevent graft rejection. SLE kidney transplant recipients have outcomes generally equivalent to those of nonlupus transplant recipients.

DIAGNOSTICS

During a disease exacerbation of SLE, laboratory tests reveal nonspecific evidence of systemic inflammation with an elevated erythrocyte sedimentation rate (ESR), C-reactive protein, and serum gamma globulins.[1,2] Anemia is common and may result from one or a combination of several mechanisms, including iron deficiency, chronic systemic inflammation causing an anemia of chronic disease, autoimmune hemolysis with a positive Coombs test result, bone marrow damage, and, in patients with renal insufficiency, inadequate erythropoietin response. Leukopenia, lymphopenia, and thrombocytopenia are characteristic hematologic features of the disease and appear to be mediated by organ-specific autoantibodies. Immune thrombocytopenic purpura may be the presenting manifestation of SLE and is associated with antiplatelet and antiphospholipid antibodies.

A urinalysis should always be obtained during follow-up visits because lupus nephritis can develop de novo in patients without previous kidney involvement. Blood urea nitrogen (BUN), creatinine, 24-hour urine protein excretion, or spot urine protein/creatinine ratio, and creatinine clearance should be monitored for changes indicating new nephritis or worsening renal function.

Although the "total" ANA test is the most sensitive diagnostic test, a positive ANA test result is not specific for SLE. In contrast, anti-Smith (anti-Sm) and anti–double-stranded DNA (anti-dsDNA) autoantibodies are more specific for the diagnosis of lupus (Table 219-1). Both types of autoantibodies are present in 30% to 40% of patients; thus, a negative test result for either anti-Sm or anti-dsDNA does not necessarily exclude a diagnosis of SLE.[9] The presence of anti-Ro/SSA and anti-La/SSB in 30% and 15% of patients, respectively, is associated with subacute cutaneous lupus, secondary Sjögren syndrome, and neonatal lupus syndrome (see Table 219-2).[1,2]

Antiphospholipid antibodies are a heterogeneous group of autoantibodies in SLE and are tested by immunoglobulin G (IgG) and IgM anticardiolipin antibodies, anti–beta 2 glycoprotein 1, and lupus anticoagulant. A prolonged activated partial thromboplastin time (aPTT) may suggest the presence of a lupus anticoagulant; however, the most commonly used assay for lupus anticoagulant is the dilute Russell's viper venom test (DRVVT). Antiphospholipid antibodies may sometimes cause a biologic false-positive test result for syphilis (Venereal Disease Research Laboratory [VDRL] or rapid plasma reagin); however, a syphilitic infection is excluded by negative specific antitreponemal test results.[13,14] Rheumatoid factor and other autoantibodies can be seen in SLE patients. Anti–cyclic citrullinated

TABLE 219-1 Clinical Significance of Specific Types of Antinuclear Antibodies in Systemic Lupus Erythematosus (SLE)

Antinuclear Antibody	Clinical Associations and Significance
Anti-dsDNA	Characteristic of SLE, useful in diagnosis; rising serum titer associated with disease activity, especially nephritis
Anti-Sm	Highly characteristic of SLE, useful in diagnosis; serum titer does not correlate well with disease activity
Anti-U1 RNP	Associated with mixed connective tissue disease
Anti-Ro/SSA and anti-La/SSB	Associated with risk for neonatal lupus syndrome, photosensitivity, subacute cutaneous lupus, and Sjögren syndrome
Anti-histone	Associated with drug-induced lupus; however, may also be seen in idiopathic SLE

DIAGNOSTICS

Systemic Lupus Erythematosus

LABORATORY

- Urinalysis
- CBC and differential
- BUN
- Creatinine
- ESR
- Rheumatoid factor
- C-reactive protein
- Total ANAs
- Serum gamma globulins
- Anti-dsDNA, anti-Sm, anti-Ro, anti-La, anti-ribonucleoprotein
- CH50*, C3, C4
- PT/PTT
- Lupus anticoagulant
- Anticardiolipin antibodies

*If indicated.

CBC, complete blood count; PT/PTT, prothrombin time/partial thromboplastin time.

peptide antibody, a characteristic finding in rheumatoid arthritis, has been reported rarely in SLE patients.

In contrast to other systemic rheumatic disorders, serum complement (C3 and C4) levels may decrease in SLE, indicating the activation and deposition of immune complexes in tissues. A drop in the serum concentration of C3 is associated with flares of nephritis. Complement can be activated in inflammation of other tissues, including the skin. Direct immunofluorescent test on a biopsy specimen of normal-appearing skin in SLE shows the presence of IgG, IgM, IgA, C3, and C1q deposits at the dermal-epidermal junction (lupus band test).

DIFFERENTIAL DIAGNOSIS

SLE can be mistaken for a number of diseases, particularly other systemic rheumatic conditions, including rheumatoid arthritis, mixed connective tissue disease, dermatomyositis, and primary systemic vasculitides, as well as fibromyalgia, multiple sclerosis, infections, and other nonrheumatic disorders. Individuals with fibromyalgia who have a low titer of ANA may be misdiagnosed as having SLE. Drug-induced lupus may develop in patients taking procainamide, hydralazine, quinidine, anticonvulsants, antithyroid medications, anti–tumor necrosis factor (TNF) agents, or other drugs.[7]

DIFFERENTIAL DIAGNOSIS

Systemic Lupus Erythematosus

- Fibromyalgia
- Mixed connective tissue disease
- Rheumatoid arthritis
- Dermatomyositis and polymyositis
- Primary Sjögren syndrome
- Systemic sclerosis (scleroderma)
- Primary vasculitides (e.g., Wegener granulomatosis, polyarteritis)
- Drug-induced lupus syndromes
- Multiple sclerosis
- Lymphoma and other malignant neoplasms
- Psychiatric disorders
- Infections

MANAGEMENT

Individuals diagnosed with SLE require guidance and education about the disease.[1] Avoidance of prolonged sun exposure is recommended because many patients are photosensitive, such that sun exposure may precipitate lupus rash and exacerbation of disease activity. Patients are advised to use sunscreen with a sun protection factor (SPF) of at least 30 and sun protective clothing to avoid excessive exposure. Modest physical exercise is considered helpful in maintaining cardiopulmonary fitness, avoiding obesity, and improving mood. Diet is important as a way to reduce risk factors including metabolic syndrome and atherosclerosis, but no specific food or diet has been shown to trigger lupus. Low-dose dietary supplementation with omega-3 polyunsaturated fatty acids (fish oil) has recently been shown to have a beneficial effect on disease activity and vascular function in SLE.[15] Many lupus patients, especially those with dark skin, have low vitamin D levels, raising a question of an association.

When indicated, statins can be safely prescribed to treat hypercholesterolemia in SLE patients. Because of the frequent occurrence of osteoporosis in these patients, attention should be paid to ensuring adequate calcium and vitamin D in the patient's diet. Regular health checkups by the primary care provider and with other specialists are important. Regular gynecologic care is important, considering an increased incidence of cervical dysplasia and human papillomavirus infection among SLE patients.[16] Issues regarding pregnancy and hormone replacement are complex in these patients and require communication among obstetrician-gynecologist, rheumatologist, and primary care provider. The patient with SLE will need dental consultation with consideration of antibiotic prophylaxis, given the risk for infective endocarditis, especially in those with valvular heart abnormalities.[17] When secondary Sjögren syndrome is present, accelerated problems with dental caries and gingivitis are often seen. Ophthalmologic monitoring is important to detect the onset of dry eyes (Sjögren syndrome) and to check for ocular side effects of hydroxychloroquine, chloroquine, and corticosteroids.

NSAIDs are typically used for the treatment of pain, particularly joint pain, fever, and serositis. Careful monitoring for NSAID toxicity is advised. Proton pump inhibitors are recommended for patients taking concomitant corticosteroids or aspirin. An unusual syndrome of aseptic meningitis can occur with the use of ibuprofen and other NSAIDs in SLE. All NSAIDs, including the cyclooxygenase 2 (COX-2)–selective NSAIDs, have effects on renal function that can exacerbate hypertension, edema, and renal insufficiency in patients with lupus nephritis. COX-2–selective NSAIDs should be avoided in patients with cardiovascular risk factors.

Hydroxychloroquine is widely prescribed and is effective in managing the musculoskeletal, cutaneous, and serosal manifestations of the disease (Table 219-2). It has been shown to be effective in allowing tapering of steroids, reducing flares of disease,[18] and reducing organ damage and as adjunctive therapy for antiphospholipid syndrome. Hydroxychloroquine has a better safety profile than chloroquine.

Corticosteroids remain the mainstay of drug therapy for SLE, and the dose depends on the severity and extent of the disease. For discoid and other lupus skin lesions, treatment with local corticosteroid cream, ointment, or local injection is often helpful. For patients with joint pain, fatigue, and milder disease that has failed to respond to hydroxychloroquine, low-dose corticosteroids (<10 mg/day) may improve the quality of life. For patients with major organ involvement (pericarditis, thrombocytopenia, autoimmune hemolytic anemia, nephritis, neuropsychiatric lupus) or multiorgan life-threatening disease, corticosteroids are given in higher dosages, ranging from 40 to 100 mg/day to "pulse" therapy of 1 g methylprednisolone intravenously every day for 3 days.

After the initial active disease begins to come under control, an immunosuppressive agent is added to help control disease and allow tapering of corticosteroids (steroid-sparing effect). The choice of immunosuppressive agent depends in part on the organ involvement. For diffuse lupus nephritis (class IV), studies have shown that the combination of intravenous cyclophosphamide and prednisone is associated with better renal outcome than is prednisone alone.[19] Mycophenolate mofetil has also been shown in controlled trials to be effective in lupus nephritis and has a better safety profile than cyclophosphamide.[20] For patients with severe persistent arthritis, methotrexate has been used. Azathioprine has shown efficacy in both renal and nonrenal lupus. Intravenous gamma globulin is efficacious in severe immune thrombocytopenic purpura and in other organ-threatening lupus.

Belimumab (Benlysta) a targeted, human monoclonal antibody that binds to soluble B lymphocyte stimulator (BLyS), has recently been approved as an adjunctive therapy of autoantibody-positive SLE patients with active disease who are receiving standard therapy. It is indicated primarily for mild to moderate disease such as arthritis, fatigue, constitutional symptoms, and skin lesions. It is not indicated for nephritis, neuropsychiatric lupus, vasculitis, or severe life-threatening organ involvement. Belimumab is an expensive medication; it is administered as a 1-hour intravenous infusion only and is given every 4 weeks after the loading course of three infusions at 2-week intervals.[21]

The treatment of antiphospholipid syndrome in SLE involves anticoagulation for thrombosis or pregnancy prophylaxis; however, certain aspects of therapy remain controversial.[13,14] Clearly, the patient who has experienced recurrent thrombosis or a major thrombotic event such as a pulmonary embolism or stroke should be treated with anticoagulation indefinitely. For pregnant SLE patients with antiphospholipid syndrome and prior fetal loss, subcutaneous low-molecular-weight heparin, low-dose aspirin, and hydroxychloroquine are recommended. Pregnant SLE patients with prior history of both obstetric and thrombotic complications are given a therapeutic dose of heparin, low-dose aspirin, and hydroxychloroquine. A pregnant SLE patient with moderate to high titer of antiphospholipid antibodies but without prior thrombotic or obstetric complications is given low-dose aspirin and hydroxychloroquine. Many rheumatologists also recommend low-dose aspirin daily and/or hydrochloroquine for SLE patients with moderate or high titers of antiphospholipid antibodies but without a previous history of thrombotic event or pregnancy loss; however, the value of the regimen remains to be validated.[14]

Patients with SLE who are at risk for osteoporosis require attention to bone health. Osteoporosis prophylaxis with calcium supplementation and vitamin D is appropriate.

TABLE 219-2 Drugs Used in Treatment of Systemic Lupus Erythematosus

Drug	Dose	Duration of Treatment
Hydroxychloroquine	200-400 mg/day 6.5 mg/kg lean body weight per day	6 months or longer
Prednisone (mild disease)	5-20 mg/day	Intermittent courses
Prednisone (moderate to severe; organ-threatening)	30-100 mg/day	Intermittent courses
Azathioprine	2 mgs/kgm/day Check level of thiopurine *S*-methyltransferase; patients with low enzyme activity may require lower dose of azathioprine.	6 months or longer
Mycophenolate	Up to 3000 mg/day Use lower dose in Asian patients.	6 months or longer
Cyclophosphamide IV	0.5-1 mg/kg/day	6 months or longer
Methotrexate with folic acid 1 mg/day	7.5-20 mg orally, once per wk	6 months or longer
Belimumab	Infusion 10 mg/kg at 2-wk intervals for 3 doses, followed by infusion once every 4 wk	>6 months

Measurement of bone density and implementation of osteoporosis therapy including bisphosphonates may be required, especially in patients receiving long-term steroid therapy. Avoidance of prolonged high doses of corticosteroids and use of steroid-sparing immunosuppressives may help limit steroid-induced bone loss.[22]

Optimum control of blood pressure is important because SLE patients are at increased risk for cardiovascular disease. High blood pressure increases the risk of kidney involvement or may result from kidney involvement. Systemic corticosteroids contribute to hypertension. Hypertensive patients with Raynaud phenomenon may benefit from the use of calcium channel blockers such as nifedipine or angiotensin receptor blockers.[23]

Many individuals with SLE have difficulty maintaining employment and household work roles.[23] The Americans with Disabilities Act may be able to support patients in efforts to obtain flexible work hours, placement of filters on fluorescent lights, or other accommodations to preserve employment or to enhance productivity. Methods of reducing the amount of energy expended in commuting, in doing household work, and in maintaining social activities should be explored. Women can be encouraged to adopt a manager rather than "doer" homemaker role; family counseling may help members manage family role changes necessitated by the disease.[24] The level of social support has been linked to health status, and studies have shown that persons with rheumatic diseases with higher levels of social support have better function.[24] Telephone counseling programs and more recently Internet support have been effective in reducing feelings of depression and anxiety as well as in improving function and providing support.[25,26] Some patients benefit from treatment with antidepressant medications.

Influenza vaccine should be administered yearly. Polyvalent pneumococcal vaccine should be considered, given evidence of splenic dysfunction and impaired immune response in these patients. Lupus patients are at increased risk for infective endocarditis and should receive antibiotic prophylaxis while undergoing invasive dental, genitourinary, and other invasive procedures.[2]

LIFE SPAN CONSIDERATIONS

The prognosis for patients with SLE has improved dramatically since its first description, when the disease was universally fatal. At present, more than 90% of patients with SLE live 10 years or longer after the onset of symptoms, although the survival rate for those with organ-threatening disease is somewhat lower.[1,2] Certain subsets of the population appear to experience worse disease. African Americans generally have more severe disease and a poorer prognosis.[4] The reasons for this are unclear but may relate, in part, to socioeconomic factors and reduced access to health care.

Pregnancy may be problematic for both mother and fetus, especially for women with antiphospholipid syndrome. Patients with SLE have increased fetal losses and are at increased risk for preeclampsia and premature rupture of membranes, resulting in prematurity, intrauterine growth retardation, and pregnancy loss. Maternal risks include disease flares during pregnancy, exacerbation of preexisting hypertension, worsening of renal status, and pulmonary embolism. Both prednisone and methylprednisolone can be safely used in pregnancy because they are inactivated by placental enzymes and do not affect the fetus. However, pregnancy-induced diabetes or hypertension can have effects on fetal well-being. The presence of maternal anti-Ro/SSA during pregnancy is associated with an increased risk for neonatal lupus syndrome in the baby characterized by congenital heart block and transient lupus rash. A high-risk obstetric service, when available, should observe pregnant SLE patients to monitor the progress of the pregnancy, including fetal heart rhythm.

Women who wish to avoid pregnancy should use birth control methods, at least during disease exacerbations, especially those with nephritis and those taking methotrexate, leflunomide, cyclophosphamide, mycophenolate, and other potentially teratogenic medications. Both injectable medroxyprogesterone (Depo-Provera) and progesterone-only minipills can be safely used, as can barrier methods. A recent systematic review showed that many women with SLE are good candidates for most contraceptive methods, including hormonal contraceptives; however, SLE patients with positive antiphospholipid antibodies should not be prescribed combined hormonal contraception.[27]

As young women with lupus live longer, the issue of hormone replacement at menopause becomes one of increasing concern. A controlled study showed that a short-term (12 months) hormone replacement therapy is associated with a small risk for lupus disease flares, but most of the flares were mild to moderate. The benefits of short-term replacement therapy in alleviating vasomotor symptoms in a menopausal woman with SLE should be considered on an individual basis. In a patient with high to moderate antiphospholipid antibodies, both estrogen and the selective estrogen receptor–modulating drug raloxifene should be avoided because of their association with hypercoagulability and venous thrombosis.[28]

COMPLICATIONS

Fever in SLE should always raise the question of whether it represents a lupus disease flare or an infectious process. In particular, fever in the absence of other signs of active SLE or fever associated with leukocytosis should prompt a search for an infection and appropriate culture. In patients taking corticosteroids or immunosuppressive agents, opportunistic organisms such as *Listeria monocytogenes, Pneumocystis jiroveci, Cryptococcus neoformans*, and others should be considered. Tuberculosis remains a significant infection in these patients. Fever with digital infarcts and joint pain could represent a flare of lupus but could also be caused by infective endocarditis. In evaluating these patients, the health care provider should promptly perform microbiologic cultures of blood, urine, cerebrospinal fluid, sputum, joint fluid, and other specimens, if available.

Previous sections have discussed some of the complications of lupus, including renal disease and renal failure, deep venous thrombosis and pulmonary embolism, stroke, coronary artery disease, and osteoporosis. Many of these complications are accelerated or worsened by corticosteroids. In particular, aseptic necrosis of bone (osteonecrosis), especially the femur, is an unfortunate complication. It can be seen in lupus patients who have not received corticosteroids but is much more prevalent among the steroid-treated patients.

Immunosuppressive agents are commonly used to limit corticosteroid-induced side effects (steroid sparing). However, these agents have toxicities of their own. Of note, cyclophosphamide is associated with sustained amenorrhea and premature ovarian failure, particularly in the patient who is older than 30 years. There is also an increased risk for cancer.[29]

Common causes of death from SLE are complications of infections, renal disease and its sequelae, premature atherosclerotic heart disease, thromboembolic events, neuropsychiatric lupus, and suicide. Early death results from complications of active disease, whereas later deaths are associated with accelerated atherosclerosis and other complications related to therapy.

INDICATIONS FOR REFERRAL OR HOSPITALIZATION

Patients with SLE should be referred to a rheumatologist at diagnosis for several reasons. Confirmation of the diagnosis of this serious illness is important because it is a life-altering chronic disease. Even patients with relatively mild or even asymptomatic lupus require periodic assessment of disease severity and activity, an evaluation best performed by a physician familiar with lupus. Given the myriad choices for management in this disease, the rheumatologist's involvement in patient care is important, even in mild cases. In uncontrolled disease with life-threatening organ involvement and in special complications such as pregnancy and antiphospholipid antibody syndrome, management by a rheumatologist is in the patient's best interest. Obviously, other specialists, such as a dermatologist, an ophthalmologist, a high-risk obstetrician, a nephrologist, a cardiologist, an orthopedic surgeon, and a hematologist, are often consulted to help manage specific problems related to SLE. Psychiatric or psychological consultation may assist the patient in dealing with the lifestyle changes wrought by this illness and in managing depression. An occupational therapist should design and teach methods of conserving energy and prescribe appropriate assistive technology. A physical therapist should be consulted to design an appropriate exercise regimen. Nutrition counseling is indicated for patients with obesity, diabetes, hyperlipidemia, or renal insufficiency.

PATIENT AND FAMILY EDUCATION

As with any chronic illness, education is essential to enable the patient with SLE to skillfully self-manage the disease on a day-to-day basis. Medication management, appropriate and disease-relevant health habits, and self-monitoring activities should be encouraged. Lower socioeconomic status is associated with poorer outcome in SLE, in part because of decreased adherence to complex treatment regimens and self-monitoring actions as well as a greater sense of learned helplessness.[4] These responses can be positively influenced by educational programs designed to enhance self-efficacy and self-management.[30]

The SLE self-help course, a group education and support program, has been developed to assist persons with disease-related self-management activities. Course evaluation has indicated improved feelings of self-worth and self-efficacy, increased enabling skills, and lowered uncertainty and depression in addition to increased knowledge about the disease.[31] The course is available through local chapters of the Arthritis Foundation (800-283-7800) or the Lupus Foundation of America (301-670-9292; 800-558-0121; Spanish: 800-558-0231).

CHAPTER 220

VASCULITIS

Simon M. Helfgott • Derrick J. Todd • Kevin Wei

DEFINITION AND EPIDEMIOLOGY

The vasculitides include a diverse group of uncommon disorders characterized by immune system–mediated inflammation and the destruction of blood vessel walls. Clinical signs and symptoms result from the subsequent impairment of blood flow through these damaged blood vessels to the distal tissues and organs. Patients with a vasculitic syndrome often have multiorgan dysfunction. Accordingly, these conditions are serious and often fatal if they are not recognized early and treated aggressively, usually with long-term immunosuppressive therapy. Although the specific vasculitides typically affect only certain organs, virtually any organ may be involved.

Because the vasculitic syndromes are uncommon and data on disease incidence are imprecise, conclusions about the epidemiology of these conditions are difficult to make. For most conditions, age at onset is variable, ranging from infancy to old age. Some vasculitides, however, affect only certain age groups; for example, giant cell arteritis (GCA, or temporal arteritis) does not occur in individuals younger than 50 years (see Chapter 216), Takayasu arteritis is virtually unknown in patients older than 40 years, and Kawasaki disease is a vasculitis of childhood. Ethnic differences among vasculitides are less distinct; GCA tends to affect individuals of northern European ancestry, whereas there appears to be a higher incidence of Takayasu arteritis in women of East Asian descent.

CLASSIFICATION OF VASCULITIC SYNDROMES

Ideally, classification of the vasculitides would be based on the underlying disease mechanisms of the various disorders. Our understanding of the immunopathogenesis of the vasculitides, however, remains far from complete. For this reason, vasculitides are often classified according to the size of the involved blood vessels (Box 220-1).[1] This classification scheme

BOX 220-1

The Vasculitides

LARGE VESSELS
GCA
Takayasu arteritis

MEDIUM VESSELS
Polyarteritis nodosa
Kawasaki disease
Primary angiitis of the central nervous system
Small to Medium Vessels*
Wegener granulomatosis
Microscopic polyangiitis
Churg-Strauss syndrome

SMALL VESSELS
Leukocytoclastic angiitis
Goodpasture syndrome
Henoch-Schönlein purpura
Cryoglobulinemic vasculitis
Drug-induced vasculitis
Behçet's disease
Relapsing polychondritis
Lupus vasculitis
Rheumatoid vasculitis
Sjögren syndrome vasculitis

*Antineutrophil cytoplasmic antibody–associated vasculitides.

does not necessarily account for disease mechanisms, but it is practical in that the clinical features of vasculitic syndromes that involve similar-sized vessels tend to affect common organ systems.

Large-vessel vasculitides include GCA, the most common of all systemic vasculitides, and Takayasu arteritis. These diseases typically involve the aorta or its major branches, including the carotid, vertebral, subclavian, mesenteric, renal, and iliac arteries. Clinically, these syndromes manifest as large-territory claudication or infarction of the involved vascular tree. The medium-vessel vasculitides include the antineutrophil cytoplasmic antibody (ANCA)–associated vasculitides Wegener granulomatosis (WG), Churg-Strauss syndrome (CSS), and microscopic polyangiitis (MPA) as well as polyarteritis nodosa (PAN) and Kawasaki disease. The last two conditions can cause aneurysms of the involved arteries, which may supply the heart, kidney, gastrointestinal tract, and gonads. The many types of small- and medium-vessel vasculitides cause ischemia at the level of the small arteries, arterioles, or capillaries and typically affect the skin, kidneys, lung, gastrointestinal tract, and nervous system as well as other sites that tend to be more disease specific.

PATHOPHYSIOLOGY

The pathophysiology of the vasculitides is varied. Multinucleated giant cells may be observed in biopsy specimens of the temporal artery in patients with GCA and are the hallmark of this diagnosis. Hepatitis B virus (HBV) surface antigen has been found in the serum of some patients with PAN, suggesting a role for this virus in the pathogenesis of PAN.[2] Infection with hepatitis C virus (HCV) can lead to the formation of cryoglobulins, which are immune complexes that are deposited in blood vessel walls and cause vascular inflammation and destruction.[2] The small- to medium-vessel vasculitides, WG, CSS, and MPA, are associated with the ANCA autoantibody. The role of ANCA, if any, in the pathogenesis of these conditions has not been fully elucidated. Necrotizing granulomas are a histologic feature of WG and CSS. Unique to CSS are the large numbers of circulating and tissue-based eosinophils.

Patients with a drug-induced vasculitis may have immune complex formation consisting of the foreign protein (offending drug) and its binding antibody.[3] In some instances, this may represent a true serum sickness reaction in which the patient's immune system generates antibodies against foreign protein (historically antisera). Alternatively, some medications (e.g., propylthiouracil [PTU], hydralazine, minocycline, and allopurinol) cause a vasculitis that is associated with positive ANCA serology, often in a very high titer. The contribution of ANCA in the pathogenesis of drug-induced vasculitis is unclear.

Patients with connective tissue diseases such as rheumatoid arthritis, systemic lupus erythematosus, or Sjögren syndrome may develop a small-vessel vasculitis, although it is not clear how the underlying disease process in these cases contributes to the systemic vasculitis.

CLINICAL PRESENTATION AND PHYSICAL EXAMINATION

Clinical manifestations of systemic vasculitis are protean, and therefore diagnosis and treatment are often delayed. In general, most vasculitic syndromes have characteristic clinical, laboratory, or pathologic features that allow their identification and classification.[1] A systematic approach to the vasculitides, based chiefly on clinical presentation and physical examination findings, can expedite the process.

Constitutional symptoms, including fever, malaise, fatigue, anorexia, weight loss, arthralgias, and myalgias, are almost uniformly present and therefore do not distinguish among the vasculitides. Their absence should call into question the diagnosis of vasculitis altogether. When fever is present, the temperature rarely exceeds 38.9 ° C (102 ° F), and it is not typically associated with rigors or chills.

GCA is the prototypical large-vessel vasculitis. It is the most common of all vasculitides, although it is found almost exclusively in patients older than 50 years (see Chapter 216).[4] The presentation of GCA is varied and includes the new onset of headache, scalp tenderness, cranial pain, visual disturbances, or jaw claudication in an older adult patient with constitutional symptoms. Arm claudication from subclavian artery stenosis can occur. Patients might report arm pain when brushing their hair, and a subclavian bruit may be present. Blindness is a dreaded complication of unrecognized GCA and, if it is not treated immediately, is often irreversible. Fever of unknown origin is a less common presentation. Aortic aneurysms occur, usually in the ascending thoracic aorta. Involvement of large vessels below the diaphragm (e.g., celiac, mesenteric, renal, and iliac arteries) is rare.

Approximately half of patients with known GCA also report diffuse shoulder and pelvic girdle achiness and carry the diagnosis of polymyalgia rheumatica.[5] On the other hand, GCA occurs in only about 10% to 20% of patients with known polymyalgia rheumatica.[6]

Takayasu arteritis is another large-vessel vasculitis that primarily affects women younger than 50 years.[7] Patients with this vasculitis classically do not have palpable pulses, and there may be signs of unequal blood pressures, arm claudication, or bruits in the neck or arms. Other presentations include cerebral vascular accident, heart failure, and ruptured aortic aneurysm. Because these are extremely unusual events in young persons, Takayasu arteritis should be considered in the appropriate clinical setting.

PAN is defined as a necrotizing arteritis that predominantly affects medium but also small arteries. Destruction of the blood vessel wall causes the development of aneurysms, which interfere with blood flow to affected organs. In addition to constitutional symptoms, common features of PAN include ulcerating skin lesions, hypertension from renal involvement, postprandial abdominal pain from mesenteric artery involvement, testicular or ovarian pain from gonadal artery involvement, and peripheral neuropathy (see later). Some patients with PAN have chronic infection with HBV.[8]

Kawasaki disease is a medium-vessel vasculitis of infancy and childhood classically causing high fever, bilateral conjunctivitis, tender cervical lymphadenopathy, desquamating rash, peripheral edema, and strawberry tongue. Affected children are at risk for coronary aneurysms, the major cause of death. Aspirin and intravenous immune globulin constitute the definitive therapy.

Primary angiitis of the central nervous system (PACNS) is a very rare vasculitic condition that exclusively affects the brain or spinal cord, usually of older adults.[9] Patients typically are seen with subacute dementia and personality changes. PACNS is often not recognized until late into the disease course, when stroke and coma occur. Brain biopsy is often required to confirm the diagnosis. Understandably, this condition is associated with significant morbidity and mortality.

WG, also known as granulomatosis with polyangiitis, is a small- to medium-vessel ANCA-associated vasculitis. Although it is varied in presentation, the classic triad of involvement is that of the upper airway, lower airway, and kidneys.[10] Disease of the ears, nose, and throat is common and can manifest as recurrent sinusitis, mucosal ulcerations, hearing loss, and epistaxis. Hemoptysis from pulmonary hemorrhage and stridor from subglottic stenosis often herald lower airway involvement, and both can be life-threatening. Renal involvement usually requires laboratory analysis to be identified (see later). Additional manifestations of WG can include palpable purpura, mononeuritis multiplex (defined later), central nervous system disease, and, less commonly, ocular, gastrointestinal, skeletal muscle, joint, or cardiac involvement. Overt joint swelling (i.e., arthritis) is uncommon. More often, patients complain of nonspecific arthralgias and myalgias.

CSS, also known as eosinophilic granulomatosis with polyangiitis (EGPA) is an ANCA-associated small- to medium-vessel vasculitis characterized by asthma and eosinophilia.[11] The condition should be suspected when a middle-aged or older adult patient develops new-onset asthma, which often precedes the vasculitis by up to 3 years. CSS vasculitis frequently affects the upper and lower respiratory tract, the peripheral nervous system as mononeuritis multiplex, and the heart as myocarditis or coronary arteritis. Other common involvement includes the central nervous system, gastrointestinal tract, skeletal muscle, joints, skin (palpable purpura), and kidney (glomerulonephritis).

MPA is a third ANCA-associated small- to medium-vessel vasculitis that has only recently been established as an entity distinct from PAN. Unlike WG and CSS, which cause granulomatous vasculitis, MPA is characterized by a necrotizing inflammation of involved vessels. Features of MPA include palpable purpura, glomerulonephritis, necrotizing alveolitis, mononeuritis multiplex, and gastrointestinal disease.

Certain medications and drugs may induce ANCA-associated vasculitis, including PTU, hydralazine, minocycline, and levamisole, a common adulterant found in cocaine. Symptoms from drug-induced ANCA-associated vasculitis include constitutional symptoms, arthralgias, and cutaneous vasculitis. Severe organ manifestations, including glomerulonephritis and alveolar hemorrhage, can also occur. Drug-induced ANCA-associated vasculitis is characterized by high-titer autoantibodies, including antibody to elastase or to lactoferrin. Providers who see patients taking these medications or toxins should be aware of the potential for the development of ANCA-associated vasculitis.[3]

Cutaneous vasculitis or leukocytoclastic angiitis typically involves the smallest blood vessels in the skin. In most cases, the skin is the only organ involved, although more widespread involvement may be observed in more severe cases. Patients are seen with palpable purpura of the lower extremities, but purpura may develop over the trunk and chest as well (see Chapter 63).

Henoch-Schönlein purpura (HSP) is a small-vessel vasculitis that may affect people of all ages, but usually from early childhood to middle age. Typically, there is involvement of the joints (with pain or swelling), skin (palpable purpura), gastrointestinal tract (abdominal pain, bleeding), and kidneys (microscopic hematuria, rising serum creatinine concentration). Although this is usually a benign disorder in children, it may be a more serious condition in adults, in whom renal involvement is more likely to lead to end-stage renal disease.[12]

Cryoglobulinemic vasculitis occurs in the setting of patients with serum cryoglobulins. Patients often have chronic infection with HCV, although cryoglobulins can occur in other settings (i.e., malignant disease, chronic infection, and systemic rheumatologic disease). Cryoglobulinemic vasculitis classically causes glomerulonephritis, arthralgias, palpable purpura, and peripheral neuropathy. Gastrointestinal and pulmonary involvement also occurs, although rarely.

In the evaluation of most small-vessel vasculitides, the presence of palpable purpura (see Chapter 63) is perhaps the most helpful physical examination finding (see Fig. 63-1). These lesions are usually multiple, more often seen in distal lower extremities. They occur as a result of extravasation of red blood cells and white blood cells outside of the destroyed blood vessel wall of the small arterioles. They vary in size from a few millimeters to 1 to 2 cm ($\frac{2}{5}$ to $\frac{4}{5}$ inch) in diameter. On occasion, they are pruritic. Other skin lesions, including livedo reticularis, nonpalpable purpura, and cutaneous ulcers, can also be seen.

The small- and medium-vessel vasculitides can involve a peripheral nerve, and a careful neurologic examination may detect these findings (e.g., sensory dysesthesia, motor weakness, optic neuritis). Classic findings include wristdrop, footdrop, or a facial droop. Vasculitic involvement of a single peripheral nerve is termed mononeuritis. Mononeuritis multiplex describes the cumulative involvement of multiple peripheral nerves over time and is highly suggestive of a vasculitis in the proper clinical setting.

DIAGNOSTICS

A high degree of clinical suspicion is required to establish the diagnosis of vasculitis because the multiorgan involvement can mimic many other conditions. Common diagnostic studies for all vasculitides should include a complete blood count (CBC) with differential, serum electrolyte values, blood urea nitrogen (BUN) and creatinine concentrations, liver function studies (LFTs), erythrocyte sedimentation rate (ESR), C-reactive protein (CRP) level, urinalysis with sediment, and chest x-ray examination. The CBC often shows anemia of chronic disease and reactive thrombocytosis. Eosinophilia supports CSS in the correct clinical setting. Elevated BUN and creatinine concentrations can occur in many of the vasculitides. Liver studies (albumin, transaminases, bilirubin, and alkaline phosphatase) can be elevated in some of the vasculitides, in particular GCA. ESR and CRP are markers of inflammation and are usually elevated. A fresh urine sediment should be carefully examined for red cell casts and dysmorphic red blood cells, which would suggest glomerulonephritis. The chest radiograph can show a variety of abnormalities, depending on the underlying vasculitic process. A widened mediastinum in a patient with large-vessel vasculitis raises the concern of a proximal (thoracic) aortic aneurysm. Pulmonary nodules, hemorrhage, or infiltrates can be seen in many of the small-vessel vasculitides. Of course, chest radiography can also show an infectious pulmonary process in patients with known vasculitis receiving immunosuppressive therapy. Patients should also have additional diagnostic testing for occult infectious and neoplastic processes as appropriate for their presentation.

In the specific evaluation of patients with suspected large-vessel vasculitis, a thorough history, physical examination, and basic studies as listed earlier are often enough for the diagnosis to be made. ESR and CRP are likely to be elevated and appear to correlate with disease activity in GCA. ESR is notoriously unreliable in patients with Takayasu arteritis, however. Additional laboratory testing is unlikely to be of diagnostic benefit.

Magnetic resonance arteriography (MRA) of the great vessels of the thorax can confirm suspected disease and reveal subclinical arterial stenosis as well. MRA is increasingly replacing traditional angiography, which is sometimes still used to determine central aortic blood pressures. Temporal artery biopsy showing granulomatous inflammation confirms the diagnosis of GCA. Noninvasive imaging with vascular ultrasound can be used to detect vessel wall inflammation or help guide temporal artery biopsy. Positron emission tomography (PET) has high sensitivity to detect inflammation in the walls of large arteries. However, the usefulness of PET scan for diagnosis of large-vessel vasculitis is still under investigation. In patients with suspected medium-vessel vasculitis, few additional laboratory studies are of value. In PAN, HBV surface antigen may be present, indicating chronic HBV infection. ANCA is occasionally positive, with a perinuclear antineutrophil cytoplasmic antibody (pANCA) pattern (described in next paragraph) and antimyeloperoxidase specificity. MRA may be helpful in the medium-vessel vasculitides, but involved vessels may be smaller than the limits of resolution of the study. Angiography can show characteristic aneurysms of involved arteries, confirming the diagnosis. On occasion, PAN can be detected fortuitously in a pathologic specimen after cholecystectomy, appendectomy, or orchiectomy.

In contrast to large- and medium-vessel vasculitides, for which few diagnostic laboratory tests have been developed, an armamentarium of blood tests exists to investigate suspected small-vessel vasculitis. These include ANCA, complements, anti–glomerular basement membrane (anti-GBM) antibodies, cryoglobulins, HCV serology, human immunodeficiency virus (HIV) serology, rheumatoid factor, and antinuclear antibodies. ANCA can show two patterns of staining: perinuclear (pANCA) and cytoplasmic (cANCA). In general, pANCA is associated with antimyeloperoxidase antibodies and can be found in MPA, CSS, or drug-induced vasculitis, whereas cANCA is associated with anti–proteinase 3 antibodies and is found in WG. Serum complements are low in some of the small-vessel vasculitides (e.g., HSP, cryoglobulinemic vasculitis, lupus vasculitis) but not in others. Although not truly vasculitic processes, anti-GBM disease and Goodpasture disease should be considered in the differential diagnosis of pulmonary-renal syndromes. Thus, anti-GBM should be measured if the diagnosis of small-vessel vasculitis is being considered.

Cryoglobulins, anti-HCV antibodies, and rheumatoid factor can each be seen in cryoglobulinemic vasculitis. Serum cryoglobulins must be obtained with great care because of the manner in which the specimen needs to be processed. If the specimen is allowed to cool below body temperature, cryoglobulins can precipitate prematurely, resulting in a false-negative test result. Thus, it is recommended that cryoglobulins be collected in a separate specimen tube. The tube should be maintained at body temperature (e.g., held in a warm hand or water bath) while being transported to the laboratory for immediate centrifugation. Measurement of antinuclear antibodies can occasionally be of benefit in patients with lupus vasculitis or Sjögren's vasculitis. Often these patients have significant involvement of their underlying connective tissue disease process.

Further imaging studies beyond a baseline chest radiograph should be tailored to disease involvement.[13] Sinusitis or other upper airway involvement necessitates a computed tomography (CT) scan of the head and neck. Chest CT should be performed in patients with significant pulmonary symptoms. Magnetic resonance imaging (MRI) of the brain with contrast enhancement can show a pattern consistent with central nervous system vasculitis. Electromyography can confirm the presence of peripheral nerve involvement by vasculitis.

Biopsy of involved organs is often necessary to confirm the presence of a small- to medium-vessel vasculitis.[13] Histologic evidence of blood vessel wall necrosis and inflammation establishes the diagnosis. Almost any organ can be sampled, but the simplest tissue to obtain for biopsy is the skin. Thus, any patient with a suspected vasculitis should be examined carefully for skin lesions that can be sampled for biopsy. Another useful biopsy site is the sural nerve, a purely sensory nerve that is easily accessible for biopsy. When this procedure is performed, the adjacent gastrocnemius muscle should also be sampled to increase the diagnostic yield. Often, it is necessary to obtain biopsy specimens of other organs, such as the lung, kidney, or even brain, depending on disease involvement. Successful lung biopsy generally requires that the procedure be done through an open lung approach or video-assisted thoracoscopy. Needle aspiration or biopsy through bronchoscopy is rarely diagnostic, and the same is true for biopsy of the bowel during endoscopic procedures. Neither is diagnostic because specimens do not contain arterioles, the vessels involved in the vasculitic process.

DIAGNOSTICS

Vasculitis

GENERAL ASSESSMENT
- CBC with differential
- Serum electrolytes
- BUN
- Creatinine
- LFTs
- ESR
- CRP
- Urinalysis
- Chest x-ray study

FURTHER EVALUATION OF LARGE-VESSEL VASCULITIS
- MRA of affected area
- PET computed tomography (CT)
- Vascular ultrasound
- Temporal artery biopsy
- Catheterization with angiography

FURTHER EVALUATION OF MEDIUM-VESSEL VASCULITIS
- HBV serology
- HIV serology
- Consider ANCA
- Catheterization with angiography
- Biopsy of affected tissue, if feasible

FURTHER EVALUATION OF SMALL-VESSEL VASCULITIS
- ANCA
- Complements (C3, C4, CH50)
- Anti-GBM antibodies
- Cryoglobulins
- HCV serology
- HIV serology
- Rheumatoid factor
- Antinuclear antibodies
- CT scan of involved area (head, neck, chest)
- Magnetic resonance imaging of brain with contrast if central nervous system is involved
- Electromyography of affected nerve
- Biopsy of affected tissue

DIFFERENTIAL DIAGNOSIS

The differential diagnosis of vasculitis can be very challenging because of the variable presentations. Many vasculitis "mimics" have been observed and broadly include infectious diseases, drug related disorders, malignancies, and other autoimmune diseases. Although often difficult to determine, an accurate diagnosis is essential to avoid treatment errors, which can lead to serious illness or death.

Cholesterol emboli syndrome can also mimic vasculitis. Affected patients are older and may be using an anticoagulant medication or have undergone some vascular manipulation, such as angiography, or sustained aortic trauma days to weeks

DIFFERENTIAL DIAGNOSIS

Vasculitis

- Autoimmune disease
  - Rheumatoid arthritis (RA)
  - Systemic lupus erythematosus (SLE)
  - Sjögren syndrome
  - Thrombocytopenia
  - Inflammatory bowel disease
  - Allergic angiitis
  - Antiphospholipid antibody syndrome
- Infectious diseases
  - Bacteremia
  - Infective endocarditis
  - Lyme disease
  - Rickettsial infection
    - Syphilis
  - Viral
    - HIV, HBV, HCV, herpes simplex virus
    - Viral endocarditis
  - Tuberculosis
- Malignancy
  - Lymphoma
  - Leukemia
  - Radiation-induced vasculopathy
- Medications
  - Antibiotics
  - Sulfonamides
  - Allopurinol
  - Nonsteroidal anti-inflammatories
  - Chemotherapeutic agents
  - Ergotamine abuse
  - Cocaine abuse
- Vascular
  - Arteroembolic vasculitis
  - Buerger disease
  - Vasospasm
  - Congenital coarctation of the aorta
  - Mycotic aneurysm
  - Atrial myxoma

From: Bateman H, Rehman A, Valeriano-Marcet J: Vasculitis-like syndromes. *Curr Rheumatol Rep* 11(6):422-429, 2009.

earlier. The presentation is characterized by fever, bilateral palpable purpura over the legs and feet, renal insufficiency, and eosinophilia.

MANAGEMENT

The choice of therapy in systemic vasculitis depends on the severity of the involvement. For example, drug-induced vasculitis may be treated successfully simply by withholding the offending agent. Patients with systemic disease of a more serious nature usually require high-dose corticosteroids either orally or intravenously. Oral doses in general are 0.5 to 1.0 mg of prednisone per kilogram per day, or the equivalent. For more serious disease, intravenous corticosteroid preparations (e.g., methylprednisolone) can be given for a faster mode of onset. Steroids are the mainstay of treatment for the large-vessel vasculitides, and few of the other agents discussed here show benefit in GCA.

Certain vasculitides, such as WG and MPA, warrant additional immunosuppressive therapy. Such is also the case for other vasculitides such as PAN, lupus vasculitis, and rheumatoid vasculitis when they affect the central nervous system, kidneys, heart, lungs, or other vital organs. Cyclophosphamide is traditionally the agent of choice to induce remission of vasculitis in any of these conditions. It has also been used to maintain remission. However, less toxic agents, such as methotrexate and azathioprine, may also show benefit in maintaining remission. Methotrexate and azathioprine can also act as a steroid-sparing agent in patients with disease refractory to corticosteroid therapy or in those who have developed serious corticosteroid-induced side effects (e.g., avascular necrosis). Less clear is the role of other drugs, such as mycophenolate mofetil. In several high-profile clinical trials, tumor necrosis factor-α antagonists did not show any benefit in GCA[14] or ANCA-associated vasculitis[15] and increased the risk of infectious complications in these patients. Rituximab, a B cell–depleting anti-CD20 monoclonal antibody, has shown promise in the treatment of ANCA-associated vasculitides.[16]

Because patients diagnosed with vasculitis typically require steroids for longer than 1 month, they should also be maintained with supplemental calcium, vitamin D, and, if necessary, a bisphosphonate to protect against bone loss. Blood pressure and blood glucose concentration should be monitored carefully. In addition, patients receiving high-dose steroids (>20 mg of prednisone per day) generally require prophylaxis against *Pneumocystis* pneumonia.[17] Trimethoprim-sulfamethoxazole is the agent of choice, although oral atovaquone or inhaled pentamidine can also be used in patients with sulfa allergies.

COMPLICATIONS

Serious complications from systemic vasculitis may often be life-threatening and include stroke, seizure, renal failure, pulmonary hemorrhage, myocardial infarction, thoracic aortic aneurysm, mesenteric infarct, and gangrene of distal extremities. The use of high-dose corticosteroids may predispose patients to the development of obesity, osteoporosis, hyperglycemia, hypertension, infections, and avascular necrosis. The use of other immunosuppressant agents can cause bone marrow suppression, may predispose to infections, and in the long term may also increase the risk for the development of malignant neoplasms.

INDICATIONS FOR REFERRAL OR HOSPITALIZATION

All patients thought to have a vasculitis should be referred to a rheumatologist for diagnosis and management because these conditions can be severe and life-threatening.

PATIENT AND FAMILY EDUCATION

Patients diagnosed with vasculitis must understand the potentially serious nature of their condition. Although some forms of vasculitis (e.g., drug-induced vasculitis or HSP) are a limited one-time event, most are chronic. Mortality resulting from vasculitis has been greatly reduced by earlier diagnosis and intervention with immunosuppressant therapies. Long-term survivors, however, are susceptible to complications of treatment or the disease process itself, including accelerated atherosclerosis and higher rates of infections and even malignant disease resulting from chronic immunosuppression.

Signs of worsening disease may include new rash, sensory loss, hemoptysis, hematuria, and proteinuria. A sudden headache or loss of vision should be reported immediately. Side effects of high-dose steroids, including hypertension, obesity, cataracts, skin thinning, and osteoporosis, should be reviewed with both the patient and family.

Given the potentially life-threatening complications of both the diseases and the treatment regimen, an open and accessible patient-provider relationship is essential.

REFERENCES

For a full list of references, scan the QR code or visit http://booksite.elsevier.com/9780323355018

PART 19

Evaluation and Management of Multisystem Disorders

CHAPTER 221

BAROTRAUMA AND OTHER DIVING INJURIES

Joel Dulaigh

The popularity of scuba diving has increased during the past several decades, along with the number of patients who are at risk for injuries sustained while diving. These injuries are diverse and vary in severity from the benign to the life-threatening. Many diving injuries require medical attention emergently. These include near-drowning, hypothermia, arterial gas embolism (AGE), decompression sickness (DCS), and marine animal bites or stings. Other diving injuries are not as serious, enabling patients to be seen by their own health care provider or at a nearby facility.

DECOMPRESSION SICKNESS AND BAROTRAUMA

PREDIVE PHYSICAL EXAMINATION AND DIAGNOSTICS

Because few health care providers are trained in sports or diving medicine, it may be necessary for the diver to assess injuries on-site and educate health care providers. The predive physical examination is an opportunity for both the diver and the health care provider to be aware of potential problems. A careful history is imperative.

Specific medical conditions to be aware of while acquiring the diver's medical history are those that would affect the air-filled spaces of the body, hemodynamics, cognitive function, and physical ability to self-rescue. A history of asthma that requires the use of inhaled medications for disease control is likely one of the most common diseases that both puts an individual at risk for air trapping[1] and is often overlooked by the provider. Many practitioners believe that if the disease is controlled with bronchodilators, the patient can dive without complication. This mistake is made when the provider does not understand the physics of gas laws as they relate to the risk of air trapping and pulmonary barotrauma. One factor commonly overlooked is the fact that cold, dry air commonly triggers bronchoconstriction. One must consider that the air coming from a scuba tank typically has much less than 1% humidity and is also cooler than the ambient air above the surface of the water.[2]

Diving is relatively contraindicated in any patient with a history of frequent ear infections, serous otitis, or chronic sinus infections. Pressure equalization (PE) tubes in the ears and chronic or intermittent aspiration suggesting an incompetent larynx are absolute contraindications, as are chronic lung disease, emphysema, and a history of spontaneous pneumothorax.[3] Known coronary artery disease, heart failure, certain dysrhythmias, and valvular disease are conditions that could affect the hemodynamics of the diver and are also contraindications. Immersion in water shunts approximately 700 mL of blood from the peripheral circulation to the body core. There is also an increase in right atrial pressure of up to 18 mm Hg and an increase of up to 100% in stroke volume and cardiac output. A patent foramen ovale (PFO) has been a controversial subject in diving medicine for years.[4] There is argument that a PFO increases the odds for development of DCS twofold to fivefold.[4] However, when the incidence of DCS is already at a rather low estimate of 1 to 35 cases per 10,000 dives, even a fivefold increase is still a very low risk. Arguably, the safest recommendation in the case of known PFO is to simply dive more conservatively.

Epilepsy and unstable diabetes are both contraindications to diving because of the possibility of loss of consciousness (LOC). LOC underwater results in the inability to protect one's airway and is nearly always fatal. Any condition that potentially results in LOC should be considered a contraindication to diving. Several cardiac conditions could predispose one to a decreased level of consciousness as well, most notably the presence of an implantable cardioverter-defibrillator (ICD). Although most of these devices themselves have been tested for pressure and may be suitable for a patient undergoing clinical hyperbaric treatments in a chamber, the ability to protect the airway is again the primary concern. A simple pacemaker, on the other hand, would not by itself be contraindicative. The provider would then need to evaluate the medical condition that required the device before clearing someone for recreational scuba diving. Obesity is a hazard in that it may reflect poor physical conditioning and may predispose a diver to DCS on the basis of nitrogen's lipid solubility.[5]

The physical examination should reveal a normal eye, ear, nose, and throat. The tympanic membrane should be intact, and each ear should be autoinflated by use of a modified Valsalva maneuver. A thorough neurologic examination is imperative. Normal neurologic examination findings with intact reflexes and strength are essential. The range of motion for all joints should be within normal limits. Lung and heart examination findings should be completely benign without rales, wheezes, murmurs, or extra sounds. Cardiac stress testing may be recommended for divers aged 45 years and older, as for any other activity requiring physical exertion. Older divers are at higher risk for chronic disease and should consider annual physical evaluation for diving fitness.[6]

Recommended studies before diving include a chest x-ray examination, electrocardiography, visual acuity testing, and pulmonary function tests. Bone and joint x-ray studies and periodic audiograms are required for commercial divers.[6]

PATHOPHYSIOLOGY

Most of the injuries sustained while diving stem directly from the differences in physical properties between liquids and gases.[7] A basic understanding of the laws of physics, particularly those laws that deal with pressure and density relative to liquids and gases, is important. The most pertinent of these are Boyle's, Dalton's, and Henry's gas laws. Barotrauma, the most common diving-related injury, develops when an air-filled body space fails to equilibrate its pressure with the environment when the pressures in that environment change. Barotrauma can occur during either descent or ascent.[7] Barotrauma of descent is also known as a "squeeze" and is most common in the middle ear and sinus spaces. Other air-filled spaces may also be affected, including dental or artificial spaces. Artificial spaces may be created by diving with ear plugs, using goggles rather than a mask that encompasses the nose, and using equipment such as a dry suit. Barotrauma of ascent is also referred to as a "reverse squeeze," and again affects the ears, sinuses, and dental air spaces. It is typically more severe because expanding gas volumes in a confined space can cause serious damage to tissues. The most severe of the ascending barotraumas is pulmonary barotrauma because of its life-threatening consequences.

Pulmonary barotrauma occurs when a diver ascends without exhaling or at a rate of ascent exceeding the rate at which expanding gas can exit through the tracheobronchial tree. Trapped air in the lungs expands and may rupture lung tissue, resulting in mediastinal emphysema, subcutaneous emphysema, or pneumothorax. AGE occurs as a result of pulmonary barotrauma when gas bubbles are released into the circulation. These bubbles are then carried to vital organs, causing life-threatening conditions or sudden death.[1] AGE is by far the most critical, life-threatening of all the diving-related illnesses.

DCS, also known as "the bends," is the result of bubble formation and growth from tissue inert gas supersaturation. During a dive, the body absorbs nitrogen from the breathing gas in proportion to the surrounding pressure. If the diver ascends too quickly, gas bubbles will form and grow in body tissue, causing symptoms of DCS. Studies have shown that the majority of divers bubble. One such study indicated that even after decompression diving using oxygen and 50% nitrox for decompression, 67% of divers showed evidence of venous gas emboli, yet only 7.8% had adverse effects of decompression.[8]

Nitrogen at higher pressures can also alter the electrical properties of brain function and cause nitrogen narcosis. The "martini law" suggests that every 33 feet of depth is the equivalent of about one alcoholic drink, causing many of the same impairments in judgment and coordination as alcohol intoxication.[7] The effects of nitrogen narcosis can have a more exponential effect at higher pressures.

The risk of DCS is most affected by depth and time. Rapid ascent, deeper and longer dives, repeated dives, and failure to follow appropriate decompression procedures increase these risks. Dive tables or decompression computers are used to calculate the rate of ascent based on the depth of the dive and are essential to safe diving. Following appropriate decompression procedures can reduce but not eliminate the risk of DCS.

The risk of DCS is also increased by air travel that occurs soon after a dive because the cabin pressure is typically less than sea level pressure. In 2002, the Divers Alert Network (DAN) posted specific guidelines for flying in a typically pressured cabin after a dive. Recommended wait times are 12 to 18 hours or more, depending on the depth and length of the dive.[8]

The term *dysbarism* has been used to describe these pressure-related injuries that result in tissue damage. *Barotrauma* refers to injury of compressible body spaces, most commonly the lung, middle or inner ear, sinuses, and gastrointestinal tract, or even air trapped under a dental filling, caused by pressure differences. *Decompression illness* is now the preferred term to describe an injured diver who has either AGE or DCS.[6]

CLINICAL PRESENTATION

DCS can manifest acutely, but delayed presentation is more frequent. In one clinical study, 98.9% of DCS patients had symptoms within 6 hours of surfacing from the dive, with an overall median latency of 62 minutes.[9] Cases of delayed onset of symptoms beyond 24 hours have also been reported. Altitude exposure, including commercial air travel, can precipitate DCS after an extended period of time. Individual differences in physical fitness, body weight, gender, fatigue, hydration, and age may make some divers more prone to DCS in spite of the use of appropriate decompression procedures.

Type I DCS is defined as pain in only one joint and can manifest with dull pain, especially in the upper extremities, with the shoulder being the most common.[10] Skin itching, rash, and localized swelling (lymphedema) are also common manifestations of type I DCS. The presence of pain in more than one location or any neurologic symptom is considered to indicate type II DCS. Type II DCS is more severe and is commonly characterized by neurologic or pulmonary symptoms, including chest pain and cough. Nervous system involvement most often manifests as patchy numbness or paresthesias, but paralysis can also occur. Headache, extreme fatigue, dizziness (including vertigo), urinary or anal sphincter disorders (usually urinary retention), or mental status and behavioral changes can also be seen. Hypovolemic shock can occur as a result of fluid shifts from intravascular to extravascular spaces.[9]

Pulmonary DCS, also known as "the chokes," and inner ear or vestibular DCS are both also classified as type II DCS.

PHYSICAL EXAMINATION

A careful history of the dive is essential. It is crucial to know where the dive took place, how deep the dive was, how much time was spent at specific depths, and the gas mixture the diver was breathing. If the diver was using a dive computer, it may be possible to download the dive profile to get a more accurate description of the dive details. Questions about the diver's predive condition, including hydration, travel schedule, and drug or alcohol intake, should be asked. Knowledge of first aid administered at the site is helpful. Multiple systems can be affected, but the neurologic and respiratory systems in particular must be carefully assessed. Disorientation, dizziness, fatigue, and joint pain with limited ability to move are common complaints. The joint pain of limb DCS can sometimes be relieved by inflating a blood pressure cuff around the affected joint, although this is not a reliable sign. This pain is often not affected by range of motion or palpation. Physical findings may also include skin blotching, weakness, ataxia, paresthesias, or paralysis. Hypotension, tachycardia, chest pain, and cough are common symptoms. A patient who collapses with LOC less than 10 minutes after the dive is considered to have an AGE until proven otherwise. The symptoms of AGE can mimic those of stroke, but a history of rapid or uncontrolled assent, especially in combination with symptoms of pulmonary barotrauma and strokelike symptoms, is highly indicative of AGE.

DIFFERENTIAL DIAGNOSIS

Many of the signs of DCS are identical to those of more common syndromes, including dehydration, electrolyte imbalance, viral syndromes, and exhaustion. The differential diagnosis for a patient with symptoms within 48 hours of a dive should always include decompression injury.[6] A central nervous system (CNS) lesion could certainly cause many of the neurologic symptoms discussed earlier. Sprains, strains, fracture, arthritis, and herniated disk can all cause musculoskeletal pain. Congestive heart failure and pulmonary edema can cause symptoms similar to those of pulmonary DCS. Dermatitis, allergic reactions, abrasions, contusions, or envenomation can lead to dermatologic symptoms, including cellulitis, rash, itching, and burning. Heat exhaustion or heat stroke can lead to muscle cramping or mental status changes. Deep venous thrombosis and thrombophlebitis can certainly be a cause of limb pain, but not usually joint pain.

MANAGEMENT

Medical stabilization at the nearest facility with rapid transport to the nearest recompression (hyperbaric oxygen) chamber (HBO chamber) is essential. This could include emergency care at the scene, with cardiopulmonary resuscitation and intubation if indicated. Injured divers are often hypovolemic, requiring aggressive intravenous hydration, but placement of the patient in the Trendelenburg position is contraindicated.[11] There is concern of potentiating hemorrhage in spinal cord and inner ear decompression illness, and therefore the routine use of aspirin in patients with neurologic DCS is not recommended.

DIFFERENTIAL DIAGNOSIS

Barotrauma

SYSTEMIC SYMPTOMS
- Dehydration
- Electrolyte imbalance
- Viral syndromes
- Exhaustion

NEUROLOGIC SYMPTOMS
- CNS lesions, cerebrovascular accident
- Heat exhaustion, heat stroke

MUSCULOSKELETAL SYMPTOMS (LIMB PAIN)
- Sprains, strains, fractures
- Arthritis
- Herniated disk
- DVT, phlebitis

CARDIAC OR PULMONARY SYMPTOMS
- Congestive heart failure
- Pulmonary edema
- Angina

DERMATOLOGIC SYMPTOMS
- Allergic reactions
- Abrasions
- Contusions
- Envenomations
- Cellulitis

For patients with limited mobility because of lower extremity weakness, low-molecular-weight heparin may be used to prevent deep vein thrombosis (DVT). Immediate treatment with inhaled 100% oxygen is the primary and most effective therapy in reducing symptoms while awaiting transport. The breathing of 100% oxygen increases the extraction of nitrogen from the tissues by reducing the partial pressure of nitrogen in the breathing gas. This change in pressure gradient aids in nitrogen elimination and can help reduce bubble size. Treatment of DCS with oxygen cannot be titrated based on pulse oximetry readings, because it is not the oxygen level that is of concern, but rather the displacement of the offending gas. However, this treatment does enhance oxygen delivery to ischemic tissues.[10] Even if the symptoms improve with 100% oxygen, the patient will still require recompression in an HBO chamber, although the number of recompression treatments may be decreased. Because preferred diving locations may be a great distance from home and require air travel, divers often are seen by health care providers several days after the onset of symptoms; even then, recompression in an HBO chamber may still be beneficial.[12]

Emergency management of AGE is the same as for DCS and includes on-site use of 100% inhaled oxygen therapy, medical stabilization, and transport to a recompression chamber. Keep vigilant watch for progression of life-threatening symptoms. Patients with mild presenting symptoms may relapse while undergoing recompression. This relapse may be on the basis of bubble interaction with blood vessel wall, causing an inflammatory response.[11] This response leads to blood vessel occlusion and cell damage, which can result in clinical deterioration or even death in spite of recompression treatments.[11] These patients are often observed in the hospital and discharged with careful instructions to return if symptoms increase. Persistent problems in maintaining adequate oxygen saturation may require hospitalization for chest tube placement and ongoing assessment of respiratory status.

LIFE SPAN CONSIDERATIONS

Children younger than 12 years are usually not certified to dive because they may lack the maturity to appreciate the inherent dangers and need for absolute adherence to the rules. Diving in pregnancy is not recommended because of risk to the fetus from the unknown effects of nitrogen diffusion across the placenta and decompression risk to the fetus. Older adults, who are more likely to have medical problems that could affect diving, should seek medical clearance before diving and thereafter annually or as health status changes.[13]

COMPLICATIONS

Complications of decompression illness include cardiac arrest, drowning or near-drowning, hypoxia, and permanent neurologic damage. Initial symptoms that appear minimal can worsen during the first few hours; thus it is recommended that patients with even mild symptoms be referred to a facility with a recompression chamber and medical personnel with knowledge of diving injuries. Typically, the sooner the onset of symptoms after diving, the more severe the case of DCS.

INDICATIONS FOR REFERRAL

All patients with DCS and pulmonary barotrauma (dysbarism) must be stabilized on-site and referred to the nearest recompression chamber facility. This referral can be made more than 24 hours after a dive with treatment success. Evaluation by a physician with board certification in undersea and hyperbaric medicine is preferred whenever possible. Patients with ear barotrauma may need to be seen and managed by an otolaryngologist, especially if they are not responding to conservative therapy. Those with potential round window rupture should be referred immediately.

PATIENT EDUCATION

All divers are required to complete a standard course in diving principles and first aid. Diving certification agencies have uniform standards established by the Recreational Scuba Training Council.[14] A basic life support certification is highly recommended. Extra training in the use of oxygen in an emergency is also recommended. Studies have found that exercising before diving and during decompression reduces the number of venous gas bubbles formed and may be protective against DCS.[9]

Divers should make every effort to avoid contact with marine life and wear protective clothing while diving. Venomous species are widespread throughout tropical, subtropical, and temperate waters, and the ability to visually identify these fish is advised. Appropriate gear in cold water will help prevent hypothermia. Recreational divers are encouraged to use dive tables and computers conservatively.[3] Immunizations, especially tetanus, should be current.

DAN is a nonprofit organization that provides expert medical information to the diving public and to medical providers treating diving-related injuries, promotes and supports diving research, and maintains a 24-hour emergency telephone line for diving accidents. DAN can provide medical providers with the location of the nearest recompression chamber. Health care providers who encounter patients with possible diving-related injuries can use DAN for both emergent and nonemergent consultations and questions, especially for cases in which decompression injuries are suspected. Duke Dive Medicine also provides direct consultation for providers by board-certified hyperbaric physicians and fellows. Duke Dive Medicine can be reached by calling 919-684-8111.

DAN can be contacted at Peter B. Bennett Center, 6 W. Colony Place, Durham, NC 27705; www.diversalertnetwork.org. Emergency medical numbers are as follows:

Diving emergency hotline (remember: call local emergency medical services [EMS] first, then DAN): 1- 919-684-9111 (accepts collect calls)

DAN medical information line: 1-919-684-2948

EAR BAROTRAUMA

Ear barotrauma was first described in 1897 and remains an important problem for both occupational and recreational divers. Again, the pathophysiologic process is related to an inability to equalize pressures during descent or ascent. The injuries can range from injury to the tympanic membrane (including rupture), to severe middle ear damage, to inner ear labyrinthine window rupture. Symptoms associated with these problems include dizziness, tinnitus, nausea, vertigo, ear pain, jaw or neck pain, and hearing difficulty.[15]

Examination of the ear canal may reveal bloody drainage and acute damage to the tympanic membrane. Inflammation of the eardrum or collection of fluid behind the eardrum may be seen. Nystagmus, hearing loss, and loss of balance may also be noted. The Weber and Rinne tests may be helpful in distinguishing conductive hearing loss (caused by middle ear barotrauma) from sensorineural hearing loss (implicating either inner ear barotrauma or inner ear DCS).[3]

MANAGEMENT

All patients must refrain from diving until symptoms have cleared. If symptoms are limited to the ear, referral to recompression centers is indicated only for treatment of inner ear DCS.[3] Systemic decongestants may provide symptomatic relief. Antibiotics may be necessary if purulent secretions are present. Topical anti-inflammatory, antibiotic drops may be helpful in alleviating the pain of otitis external. On occasion, mild systemic analgesics may be needed. Most tympanic membrane ruptures heal within 4 or 5 days.

Inner ear barotrauma with vertigo and tinnitus will require a period of bed rest, usually in the hospital, with medication to control vertigo and possibly sedatives to help the patient rest comfortably.[8] Surgical exploration to repair a round window rupture may be required. Referral to an audiologist for hearing evaluation may be necessary if hearing loss is severe or persistent.

Varying degrees of hearing loss, vestibular dysfunction resulting in chronic vertigo, balance disorders, and gait disorders are the most serious complications of ear barotrauma.[8] Permanent inner ear damage can be a contraindication to further diving.

SINUS BAROTRAUMA

Sinus barotrauma is associated with severe pain in the region of the sinuses and can occur during descent or ascent. The frontal sinus is most commonly involved. Epistaxis occurs in about half of cases.[3] This can be a problem for divers who have experienced it before and those with a history of chronic sinus problems.

MANAGEMENT

Topical and systemic nasal decongestants may provide both relief and prophylaxis for divers who are predisposed to this complication. Antibiotics may be indicated when infection is suspected. Patients who do not respond to conservative therapy should be referred to an otolaryngologist for ongoing management.[3]

PULMONARY BAROTRAUMA

Pulmonary barotrauma with AGE is second only to drowning as a cause of death in divers.[6] Trapped air in the lung expands and ruptures alveolar tissue, releasing air bubbles into the circulation. If a bubble lodges in the brain, stroke, seizures, paralysis, and unconsciousness can occur. Air bubbles traveling to the heart can lead to myocardial infarction or cardiac arrest. AGE can also cause minor symptoms, such as numbness, tingling, or weakness of a limb. Vision and hearing losses have also been seen, all without LOC.

The pathognomonic features of air embolism (AGE) include gas emboli in the retina and areas of pallor on the tongue, although this is rarely seen.[3] Pneumothorax can occur in conjunction with AGE or may occur in isolation and become evident at a later time. The patient may be in respiratory distress with mild to moderate pain. Tachypnea, pallor, decreased or absent oxygen saturation, and diminished breath sounds may be noted. Mediastinal air can track cephalad into the soft tissues of the neck and cause changes in the voice.[7] A chest x-ray examination will usually confirm the diagnosis, although computed tomography scans may be required.

MARINE ANIMAL BITES AND STINGS

The United States has 80,000 miles of coastline, and people are showing a greater interest in surfing, snorkeling, and scuba diving. A common source of injuries to divers is inadvertent contact with marine life. Bites and stings from sea creatures are common and range from the annoying to life-threatening. These injuries usually require immediate treatment, but patients who sustain multiple or deep wounds or serious systemic illness will require follow-up by health care providers. This discussion is limited to some of the more common or toxic species found in the Western Hemisphere.

CLINICAL PRESENTATION

It is often not possible to identify the marine animal that caused the injury. Coral scrapes are the most commonly seen injuries. The soft living material on the surface of rough coral is easily deposited into a cut or scrape. This can cause inflammation, infection, and delayed wound healing. Treatment consists of initially scrubbing the wound with soap and water, then flushing with copious amounts of water. Flushing of the wound with half-strength hydrogen peroxide and covering it with an antibiotic ointment and dry sterile dressing further ensure a clean wound.[16]

The envenomations of the stingray are notable for severe and painful reactions. The stingray partially buries itself in the sandy bottom, where it can be accidentally stepped on. The animal then lashes out defensively with a whip-like appendage that carries stingers. The venom has vasoconstrictive properties that can complicate the healing of more severe wounds.[17] Immediate symptoms may include nausea, vomiting, diarrhea, muscle cramps, headaches, seizures, hypotension, heart failure, respiratory distress, and death, although the number of confirmed human deaths from these encounters is much less than commonly believed.[17] Milder and delayed reactions can include regional lymphadenopathy, fever, malaise, nausea, vomiting, and delirium. The wounds inflicted are most commonly mild (erythema only) but often extremely painful. More severe encounters can result in vesicle formation, cellulitis, and necrotic breakdown. Recovery can take months, especially if the wounds are complicated by secondary infection.[16]

Immediate care of stingray envenomation involves rinsing with fresh water and removal of any foreign body. Soaking in warm water for 30 to 60 minutes may relieve the pain. The wound should then be washed gently in soap and water. Further monitoring of the wound for infection or bleeding with follow-up care is necessary.[16]

The sting of the sculpin, a common member of the scorpion fish family found off the coast of southern California, produces severe pain and occasionally nausea and vomiting. The venom produces protein that is rapidly broken down in the presence of heat. Treatment is immersion in water as hot as can be tolerated for 60 to 90 minutes. Once the pain is relieved, the wound should be flushed of debris, covered with a dressing, and monitored for infection.

Jellyfish have stinging cells called *nematocysts* that can continue to function even when they are separated from the organism or if the organism is dead. Jellyfish envenomation is quite painful, and the venom can cause cardiac, neurotoxic, or hemolytic reactions or necrotic skin wounds. Fatal anaphylaxis has been known to occur. First aid consists of removal of any adherent tentacles followed by a vinegar rinse. The wound is then washed with soap and water and treated with a topical hydrocortisone cream. Pain can be controlled with acetaminophen or ibuprofen. Antibiotics are usually not necessary.[16]

The Portuguese man-of-war, found in tropical and subtropical regions of the Pacific, in the northern Atlantic Gulf Stream, and in the Caribbean, is infamous for its painful sting and systemic manifestations. This animal has a "sail" that floats with the wind and often one or more tentacles that can extend 10 m (33 feet) or more and can be separated from the sail and drift invisibly toward the surface. Exposure to the tentacle and its powerful venom is what causes the injury.[18] Symptoms include severe pain, vomiting, and occasionally difficulty breathing. Anaphylactic shock is treated with epinephrine and other supportive measures. First aid generally consists of copious flushing with either sea or fresh water, removal of visible tentacles with tweezers or a gloved hand, and applications of ice to control pain. Rubbing should be avoided, and the application of vinegar, often helpful for other marine animal stings, is not recommended.[16]

MANAGEMENT

Good and immediate first aid is essential to uncomplicated healing. This should include immediate assessment of the patient's general status, especially if there is airway, breathing, or circulatory compromise requiring stabilization or resuscitation.[13] Gentle removal of visible spines, control of bleeding, analgesia, and transport to the nearest emergency department are recommended initial treatments.

In the emergency department, stings are managed immediately by removal of tentacles and spines (if this was not done at the dive site) and irrigation of the area. Local anesthesia should be used. Open wounds require careful and thorough irrigation and debridement of foreign bodies. Heat treatment by immersion of the affected limb into water no hotter than 45.4° C (114° F) can be effective with specific envenomations (see earlier).[10]

Wound care is then directed toward healing without secondary infection. Skin irritations and itching can be treated with warm or cool compresses and mild steroid creams. The patient's tetanus status should be ascertained and vaccine administered if more than 10 years have elapsed since the last immunization. The primary health care provider can manage bites and stings as long as wound healing is uncomplicated. Referral for surgical debridement may be necessary for nonhealing wounds.

CHAPTER 222

CHRONIC PAIN

Jennifer L. Culgin • Catherine M. Duffy

DEFINITION AND EPIDEMIOLOGY

Chronic pain is a complex, subjective, persistent, unpleasant sensory and emotional experience that affects more than 100 million people in the United States and has associated health care costs of up to $635 billion. Pain is a normal physiologic response to an actual or potential injury that prompts a useful protective response, but chronic pain may occur in the absence of injury, has no known physical benefit, and carries significant morbidity and mortality.[1] Chronic pain is defined by the International Association for the Study of Pain as "pain that persists beyond the expected time frame for healing." Any pain can be considered chronic if it continues 90 days past a reasonable healing time.[2] Chronic pain is self-perpetuating and influenced by factors that are both pathogenetically and physically remote from the originating cause.[3] Because complete pain relief is unlikely, control strategies for chronic pain extend from encouragement of local reparative processes to a more global management strategy of rehabilitation. Therapy focuses on promoting optimum functioning, coping, and quality of life with use of a full-dimensional approach of interdisciplinary care and community supports in decision-making and goals.[4]

Multiple conditions may result in the development of chronic pain, including headaches, low back pain, abdominal or pelvic pain, noncardiac chest pain, regional pain syndromes, and neuropathies and conditions that are vascular, cutaneous, musculoskeletal, cancerous, or psychological in nature.[4] The pain may be part of a broader clinical situation, such as a work-related injury, accident, trauma, or comorbid disease states. Patients with chronic pain typically seek a health care provider initially for headache, abdominal pain, musculoskeletal discomfort, or neurologic pain relief. Pain can also be related to other organic disorders, including diabetes, end-stage renal disease, alcoholism, and postherpetic syndromes.[5] There is also chronic pain syndrome. Both chronic pain and chronic pain syndrome can exist in the same patient, but the syndrome is complicated by physical, psychological, emotional, and social aspects.[2] Concomitant and well-known psychological sequelae to chronic pain include significant depression, anxiety, and anger. In 2010 the concept of mental defeat was introduced into the chronic pain literature. A psychological construct derived from work regarding torture and depression, it is described as an aspect of catastrophizing strongly associated with functional and psychosocial disability, emotional distress, self-reported pain interference, and sleep disturbance in patients with chronic pain. Treatment strategies aimed at prevention or reversal of mental defeat offer ways to reduce pain-related disability and to increase functionality.[6] Further studies on mental defeat in the Hong Kong chronic pain population found significant distress and disability among those seeking treatment for their pain, and it is thought that early identification of mental defeat can help with early intervention for depression and anxiety.[7]

This chronic pain state with its concomitant mood disorders results in negative alterations in daily activities, function, and personality.[5] Both chronic pain and its management can adversely influence respiration, mobility, and functional and mental status, with resulting disturbed sleep patterns, pneumonia, constipation, and venous thromboembolism. The adverse effects of chronic pain can be particularly deleterious in the elderly.[7]

PATHOPHYSIOLOGY

Pain is an unpleasant sensation unique to each patient. According to McCaffrey, "pain is whatever the experiencing person says it is, existing whenever the experiencing person says it does."[8] Chronic pain is caused by a "chronic pathologic process in somatic structures or viscera, or by prolonged and sometimes permanent dysfunction of the peripheral and central nervous system or both."[3] The physiologic, affective, and behavioral responses to chronic pain are quite different from the responses to acute pain. Pain is categorized pathophysiologically as either organic or idiopathic, and organic pain is further delineated as nociceptive (somatic or visceral) or neuropathic.

Somatic pain is caused by the activation of nociceptors in the peripheral tissues, including skin, bones, muscles, and soft tissue. It is usually described as being well localized and characterized as stabbing, aching, or throbbing. In contrast, visceral pain is usually poorly localized and often is not attributable to the involved organ (i.e., referred pain). It may be described as dull, crampy, or deep. Visceral nociceptive pain can be referred in a dermatomal distribution, because often the autonomic fibers innervate the organs or hollow viscera found in the dermatome.[9]

Organic neuropathic pain occurs as a result of injury or disease of the nervous system. Because it follows the distribution of peripheral nerves in a dermatomal pattern, neuropathic pain is most often described as burning, shooting, or tingling. Central neuropathic pain is caused by damage of the nerves in the central nervous system (CNS).[9] Idiopathic pain may not demonstrate any clinical evidence of an associated organic cause but might include additional psychological elements at the time of presentation. Nonetheless, as previously stated, the experience of pain is purely subjective. Subsequently, the reality of a patient's idiopathic pain is comparable to that of organic pain, and therefore it must be treated.

CLINICAL PRESENTATION

The clinical picture of chronic pain may be nonspecific and noted only in terms of a retrospective review, in which certain patterns may emerge. Both physical and psychological elements must be considered in a patient with chronic pain. As established, chronic pain is pain that continues for a prolonged period and beyond a reasonable healing time for a specific injury. The majority of patients with chronic pain in a recent study were being managed by their primary care physician, and few have ever seen a pain specialist.[10] Almost half of this study population had undergone radiographic tests in the prior 6 months, over three quarters were taking prescription medication for their pain, and half were using nonpharmacologic modalities in an attempt to manage pain.[10]

Patients who visit clinics with chronic pain often have additional issues such as depression, anxiety, sleep issues, overuse of medications, relationship issues, isolation, and low level of physical activity.[11,12] Adequate treatment may be complicated by a history of difficult patient-provider interactions in the past, financial barriers, and general lack of support. Despite the high prevalence of chronic pain, the varying results of studies in interdisciplinary approaches make it difficult to establish how to best treat these patients.

PHYSICAL EXAMINATION

Pain is frequently undermanaged because of poor clinical assessment. It is critical that pain assessment be integrated into a detailed history and physical assessment, with reassessment at each visit. An initial comprehensive clinical pain history should include past relevant health issues, psychiatric history, psychosocial factors, addiction risk, social and occupational functional assessment, goals of treatment, and pain beliefs. Previous treatments and outcomes, both traditional and alternative therapies, should be explored. A thorough review of current medications, including over-the-counter and complementary medications, should be included.[13] A referral to a behavioral specialist may be helpful.[14]

Pain assessment can be aided by the mnemonic *PQRST*.[15] *P* stands for provocative-palliative factors, such as specific positions or movement, temperature, or activities. *Q* stands for quality and includes the description of the pain, such as dull, boring, aching, or electrical. *R* stands for the region or site of pain, such as the torso, abdomen, back, or spine. *S* stands for severity and refers to how severe the pain is, measured by rating the pain over time. Most commonly, to quantify their pain, patients are asked to use a scale of 1 to 10, a scale of calm to distressed faces, or a scale of description of no pain to worst pain. No one scale applies to all patients; rather, the important issue is to choose one scale that is appropriate for a patient and use it consistently. *T* is for temporal or the timing of the pain during day or night, in which the pain is more constant or the duration longer. Box 222-1 offers sample questions for assessment.

The physical examination of a chronic pain patient should be thorough and multifactorial. It should include a general examination of appearance, gait, neurologic and mental status, cranial nerve testing results, motor and musculoskeletal strength, and reflexes and a full joint and myofascial examination.[16]

DIAGNOSTICS

No specific diagnostics are indicated for chronic pain. However, electrocardiography, x-ray studies, blood work or other diagnostic tests may be ordered to rule out other causes of the pain.

DIFFERENTIAL DIAGNOSIS

Because of the lack of specificity of the many symptoms associated with widespread pain, other diagnoses must be considered. Neurologic, non-neurologic, and psychiatric causes must be acknowledged and evaluated.

BOX 222-1

Questions for Assessment of Distress

- What is your day like?
- How does your pain interfere with your life?
- What are your expectations of pain relief?
- What are your past experiences of pain?
- How did you cope with pain in the past?
- How is this pain different?
- What is the meaning of pain?
- How are you coping with this pain?
- How has your life changed?
- Does culture or religion have any influence over expression of pain or pain management?

MANAGEMENT AND INTERDISCIPLINARY MANAGEMENT

Primary care providers often are managing chronic pain alone in a clinic, in addition to associated comorbidities that include insomnia, anxiety, and substance abuse.[17] The chronic physical and psychological components associated with chronic pain are most successfully managed with a multidisciplinary team approach. The primary goal is often to manage expectations, improve function, and maintain a therapeutic relationship with the patient.

1. Initiation of consultations with social workers, psychologists, and psychiatrists may be beneficial to assist in identifying coping mechanisms, introducing diverse interventions, and assisting with management of other mental health issues such as depression, anxiety, and anger.
2. If there is a history of substance abuse, a referral to a substance abuse counselor should be considered.
3. When pain is localized to a specific area, specialist consultation may be indicated (e.g., consultation with a gastroenterologist for chronic abdominal pain, a rheumatologist for joint pain, a neurologist for neuropathic pain, or an orthopedist for bone pain).
4. Referral to an inpatient or outpatient pain clinic or pain specialist, where available, may also be considered if the practitioner is uncomfortable managing opioids. It is important that one provider be responsible for all prescriptions. This will allow a systematic approach to pain medications, permit an adequate trial of medications before change, and avoid polypharmacy.

Pharmacologic Interventions

The decision to prescribe pain medication should begin only after assessment of patient goals, comorbidities, drug profiles, and drug-drug interactions.[17] Pharmacologic pain management incudes the guidelines of the three-step analgesic ladder for pain control developed by the World Health Organization and endorsed by the American Pain Society.[15] Although these guidelines were initially developed in 1986 as an approach to treatment of acute and cancer pain, they are relevant, effective, and recommended for chronic pain as well.[9,15]

Three-Step Analgesic Ladder

Step 1 Medications. Step 1 begins with the use of nonopioids and adjuvant medications. These include nonsteroidal anti-inflammatory drugs (NSAIDs), tricyclic antidepressants (TCAs), selective serotonin reuptake inhibitors (SSRIs), and adjuvants such as anticonvulsants.

NSAIDs are some of the most commonly prescribed nonopioid pain medications. They work to decrease pain and inflammation. Common examples of NSAIDs include ibuprofen (Advil, Motrin) and naproxen (Aleve, Naprosyn). Although NSAIDs are generally well tolerated in patients of varying ages, it is important to recognize the potential gastrointestinal and renal effects associated with this pharmacologic category. NSAIDs are also available in topical preparations, including patches and gels, which often are a better alternative for older adults.

TCAs are non-narcotic medications used in the treatment of chronic pain. In addition to pain relief, TCAs (e.g., amitriptyline, nortriptyline, and desipramine) mitigate the depression associated with chronic and physiologic nerve pain. TCA side effects drugs include dry mouth, constipation, and sedation. For this reason, older adults should be started on lower doses of TCAs. Treatment failure of one tricyclic medication does not indicate that a patient will not respond to a different TCA. Therefore it may be worthwhile at least to try a second agent in this class before discontinuing their use.

SSRIs (e.g., paroxetine [Paxil] and fluoxetine [Prozac]) can also be used in the treatment of chronic pain even if depression is not an issue, although maximum response may take several weeks. Common side effects include rash, urticaria, dizziness, and drowsiness.

Adjuvant medications, including anticonvulsants (e.g., carbamazepine, gabapentin, and pregabalin)[18] are also helpful in treating chronic pain, especially pain associated with neuropathy and paresthesias. The initial dose should be low and increased slowly. A common side effect is sedation, so scheduling a dose at night is helpful to avoid daytime drowsiness. Other potential side effects include headache, confusion, skin rash, nausea, and vomiting.

Step 2 Medications. Step 2 of the World Health Organization's three-step analgesic ladder includes mixed opiate products such as hydrocodone and acetaminophen (Vicodin, Lortab), oxycodone and acetaminophen (Percocet), codeine, acetaminophen and codeine phosphate (Tylenol No. 3), and tramadol (Ultram). These medications can be used alone or in combination with step 1 medications (do not exceed recommended acetaminophen dose of 3 g/day) to treat mild to moderate pain. Side effects of opioids include constipation (ensure patient is on a bowel regimen including laxative and stool softener, especially if long-term use of opioids is expected), sedation, nausea and vomiting, itching, and respiratory depression.

Step 3 Medications. Step 3 medications are recommended when step 2 drugs are not effective in relieving pain or when the pain is moderate to severe in intensity. These opiates should be considered only after all other reasonable attempts at analgesia have failed. Step 3 medications include pure opioid compounds such as morphine, fentanyl, oxycodone, methadone, and hydromorphone. Demerol (meperidine) was previously included in this class of medications. However, a high incidence of neurotoxicity severely limited its use, and it is no longer recommended for treatment of pain. Because of concerns about addiction, tolerance, and side effects (which are the same as with the step 2 medications), this group of medications is frequently underused. Continued patient and family education about the proper use of opioids in pain control is important.

Other Considerations. Access to and expense of prescription medications are essential considerations in the outpatient management of chronic pain. Insurance coverage varies considerably among commercial insurance and Medicare Part D plans. Although over-the-counter medications are relatively inexpensive, opioid and other pain medications can be expensive and require prior approval or letters of necessity. In addition, there is wide variability in terms of what medications are available in local pharmacies. Large-chain pharmacies may make it more difficult to access medications with 3-day ordering requirements.

Nerve Blocks. If medication management is unsuccessful or results in unwanted side effects, evaluation by an interventional pain specialist may provide alternative pain relief recommendations (e.g., nerve block—an anesthetic injected directly into a nerve to prevent painful conduction of pain at the nerve ending; and site point injection—a steroid injection at a trigger point area). Results from these procedures vary; however, many patients obtain some degree of pain relief for weeks or months, and these injections may decrease the need for medication or unwanted side effects associated with pain medications.

Nonpharmacologic Intervention

Patients often use traditional medicine in combination with complementary therapies; it is important to ask what (if any) therapies patients are presently using, because this information may affect the treatment plan.[19] Traditional and complementary therapies (e.g., nutritional and herbal supplements, spiritual healing, massage and therapeutic touch, meditation, acupuncture, biofeedback, and guided imagery) can be effective, particularly if practitioners collaborate (Table 222-1).[20]

TABLE 222-1 Nonpharmacologic Strategies

Strategy	Description	Examples
Cognitive-behavioral interventions	Pain often drains a person's focus and energy. Cognitive-behavioral interventions can temporarily raise the pain threshold, thereby allowing the patient's attention to be directed toward something other than the pain.	Relaxation, biofeedback, meditation, distraction, hypnosis, and support groups
Exercise	Exercise can improve general conditioning, thereby improving stamina and endurance. In addition, exercise can promote the production of endorphins, which are the body's natural pain relievers. Stress reduction is a secondary benefit of an exercise program and can assist in overall coping behaviors.	Physical therapy, occupational therapy, and exercise programs, including hydrotherapy
Complementary and alternative therapies	A process of manipulation of body parts and stimulation of healing through herbs and substances.	Chiropractic treatments, acupuncture, massage therapy, herbal preparations, and homeopathy
Transcutaneous electrical nerve stimulation (TENS)	In this process, a low-voltage electrical pulse is directed through the skin. The rationale for its use is to stimulate nerve fibers and interfere with the conduction of painful stimuli. It is often available through a physical therapist.	TENS units
Heat or cold therapy	Heat and cold act as counterirritants or reduce muscle spasm.	Heating pads, cooling blankets, gel packs

LIFE SPAN CONSIDERATIONS

Back pain is the leading cause of chronic pain, affecting 26 million people in the United States aged 20 to 60 years.[1] Older adults may underreport pain because they do not want to admit deficits, difficulties, diminished function, or cognitive changes. Some may report interference with nutrition, sleep, physical function, and social and recreational activities, all of which may be secondary to aches and pain. They may also describe depression and anxiety and exhibit greater need for health care use.[4,21] The 2011 National Health and Aging Trends Study found that bothersome pain affects over 50% of older adults, especially those with expected comorbidities of obesity, arthritis, osteoporosis, hip fractures, and mental health issues. In addition, pain was more common in older women and in older adults with lower levels of education and socioeconomic status.[22] Management of pain in older adults is complicated by their often multiple other health issues and the underprescribing of analgesics because of hesitancy on the part of both the prescriber and the patient. There is limited efficacy for nonpharmacologic treatments. Although a combination of prescription and nonpharmacologic interventions is recommended by the American Geriatric Society, only one third of older adults follow these guidelines, and of those who use prescription medication for pain, only one quarter reported regular use.[23]

Children can also experience chronic pain. Up to 16% of ER visits for children are attributed to chronic pain, and rates are increasing.[24,25] Just as in adults, chronic pain in children has psychological and social consequences, as well as physiologic effects, and up to 80% of children with chronic pain continue to have pain as adults. Studies reveal that children who experienced chronic pain in childhood have higher rates of suicidal or homicidal ideation; anxiety; and physical, sexual, and psychological abuse. Similar to the adult population, rates are higher in adolescent girls with concomitant anxiety and depression.[24,25] Management in general is based on analgesics, sleep management, and interventions to help with coping and restoring function, as well as pain education and psychological interventions.[26]

PATIENT AND FAMILY EDUCATION

The essential foundation for the management of chronic pain is patient access to information and education. Explicit instructions (in language the patient can understand) should be given to the patient and family and should include an explanation of the pathophysiologic changes of the affected body system, the pain cycle, the treatment plan, the medications prescribed, and their potential side effects. It is critical that the health care provider discuss realistic expectations for pain control—specifically, that the pain may not be totally eliminated but may, it is hoped, be reduced to a tolerable level, allowing improved activity, functioning, and quality of life. Proper education promotes a feeling of independence and empowerment for the patient, which can improve medication adherence and result in a willingness to accept necessary changes in treatment.

HEALTH PROMOTION

Health promotion activities for patients with chronic pain include strategies that promote activities of daily living and coping, with the goal of continued participation in their home, work, and social life. Educating a patient about using a comprehensive approach that focuses on both the physical and psychological dimensions of quality of life is often the most successful. It is important to explain the potential benefits that can be achieved with traditional medical management and complementary therapies. Medical management requires a systematic approach of appropriate treatment and education about the benefits and realistic outcomes. The use of complementary therapy requires a review of the patient's preferences regarding the various types of care. For patients not familiar with complementary therapies, it is important to provide information about how such therapies can enhance pain management and prevent dependency on medications.

CHAPTER 223

FATIGUE

Michelle Freshman

DEFINITION AND EPIDEMIOLOGY

Fatigue is a common complaint.[1] Over one third of community-based adults report fatigue[2] and 24% to 42% of primary care patients remark on significant fatigue, particularly those with concomitant inflammatory disorders.[2,3] In the United States, 10% to 15% of adults note that insomnia leads to daytime sleepiness and 30% are dissatisfied with their sleep quality.[4] Women are particularly at risk for insomnia, obstructive sleep apnea, and restless legs syndrome in addition to hormonal and psychosocial influences known to disrupt sleep.[3,4] Older adults seem to be more likely to identify fatigue as an issue.[5] In one sample including 754 nondisabled community-dwelling older adults, 31.1% of men and 42.1% of women reported fatigue severe enough to affect lifestyle. Fatigue was more common in the physically frail and those who also had depression.[5] Despite the preponderance of fatigue among older adults, it bears consideration in the context of chronic sleep-related complaints, which are prevalent in more than 50% of individuals older than 65 years,[6,7] as well as anemia, commonly seen in more than 50% of institutionalized older adults.[8] As the projected number of elders rises, the cost-effectiveness with which such information is captured and managed will be critical, as fatigue affects functional outcomes—physical, cognitive, mood, and social.[1] In fact, in a prospective study of 492 primary care patients aged 65 years or older, an affirmative answer to "Do you feel tired most of the time?" independently predicted 10-year mortality,[9] consistent with similar research in other countries.[10]

The subjective nature of this problem compels a practitioner to rely almost entirely on the patient's perception of diminished performance, despite ongoing efforts to establish standardized fatigue scales and identify useful biologic markers. Even the latest diagnostic rubric for fibromyalgia, commonly associated with fatigue, has evolved away from tender point examination to a previsit patient inventory of pain and illness.[11] More than 250 fatigue self-report tools exist; consensus on fatigue definition and method of assessment remains an ongoing challenge.[1] The Epworth Sleepiness Scale, Fatigue Symptom Inventory and Profile of Mood States, Multidimensional Fatigue Inventory, Pittsburgh Sleep Quality Index, and Visual Analog Fatigue Scale are notable.[2,12,13]

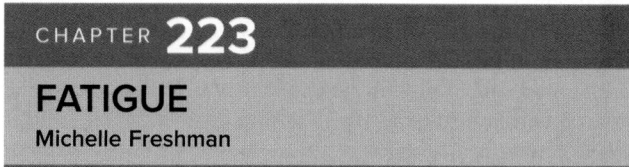

Conceptual differences exist among frequently interchanged terms. Fatigue is the "subjective lack of physical and/or mental energy that is perceived by the individual or caregiver to interfere with usual and desired activities."[12] Sleepiness is the inclination toward sleep usually despite an effort to avoid it. Insomnia signals trouble initiating or maintaining restorative sleep, which leads to tiredness.[14] Fatigue is considered akin to tiredness and exhaustion, and can in and of itself lead to more disabling symptoms than severe sleepiness alone; in fact, sleepiness lends itself better to objective measurement. Among sleep-related breathing disorder patients versus matched controls with similar levels of apnea, "high fatigue" contributed to more severe dysfunction than "high sleepiness."[12] Without adequate sleep, excessive daytime tiredness, neurocognitive impairment, metabolic irregularities, cardiac rhythm abnormalities, and affective disorders can arise.[4] It is helpful to establish acuity, chronicity, whether fatigue is a normal or abnormal response to situation or environment,[1] and whether it is tied to unique psychoneuroimmunologic[2] or possibly genetic factors and/or associated with precedent comorbidities. Cancer-related or cancer-treatment fatigue affects daily function and is considered disproportionate to a recent change in activity level, which is also influenced by common cofactors: insomnia, pain, depression, and loss of concentration.[14]

More objective measures, such as functional magnetic resonance imaging (MRI) and positron emission tomography, have contributed theoretically in helping to characterize the parts of the brain that may be activated to compensate for damaged processing regions. Transcranial magnetic brain stimulation is used in research to examine the excitability of central motor pathways and may have a future application in treating muscle-based fatigue and reducing chronic pain.[15] Given that fatigue is described in multiple ways, some concern exists that it may be underreported because what is expressed by the patient versus what is recorded by the provider may differ significantly, and some patients may believe that reporting fatigue may not be helpful or they may have adjusted expectations to a reduced energy level.[1] Although fatigue has been typified as having physical (neuromuscular), cognitive, and emotional components, the direction of the relationship among these domains and chronicity remain perplexing. For example, fatigue combined with irritability and depression is referred to as vital exhaustion and is implicated as a cardiovascular risk factor; by contrast, stroke has been associated with depression.[16] Whether fatigue is defined as a marked decrease in a patient's ability to exert himself or herself physically or mentally (whether lacking in initiating and sustaining movement)[17] during usual activities or fundamentally a lack of motivation or poor concentration more akin to depression and weighted further down by pain, researchers continue to search for a unifying concept. Sleep disorders (see Chapter 227) (obstructive sleep apnea, restless legs syndrome, periodic leg movement disorders, narcolepsy, somnambulism), which can be diagnosed by polysomnography and actigraphy, when adequately treated, actually improved overall fatigue in patients with multiple sclerosis (MS).[12]

PATHOPHYSIOLOGY

The pathophysiology of fatigue is entirely dependent on its cause. Given the subjective nature of this complaint, a careful review of symptoms and a physical examination are required. Fatigue researchers have focused on the neurobiology of immune activation and circadian dysfunction.[1] One increasingly well-recognized and reproducible phenomenon, considered adaptive in the face of infection or inflammatory disease, is called "sickness behavior." This incorporates "fatigue, depressive behavior, anhedonia, psychomotor slowing, anorexia, circadian alterations in sleep patterns and increased sensitivity to pain" and is associated with chronic fatigue syndrome (CFS) and other inflammatory states.[17,18] The notion that CFS results from an infection or chronic inflammatory illness continues to gain ground.[17] No definitive test exists for CFS, but researchers are tentatively pointing to environment, genetics, infections, adrenal function, biopsychosocial factors, aberrant inflammatory cytokines or deficient natural killer cell immunity, oxidative and nitrosative stress,[17,19] and mitochondrial and nutritional factors.[3,20]

Fatigue is the most often voiced complaint among cancer patients of all ages.[18] It is hypothesized that cancer-related fatigue represents alteration in circadian rhythms caused by some combination of hypothalamic-pituitary-adrenal hormonal (cortisol) disruption through monoamine pathways (monoaminergic, cholinergic, histaminergic) as well as associated neurotransmitters (orexin, serotonin, norepinephrine, dopamine, glutamine), involving tryptophan and inflammatory cytokines (interleukin [IL]-1β and tumor necrosis factor [TNF]-α) interacting with psychosocial influences.[14,18] Disruptions of the regular daily wake-sleep cycle are associated with cancer, dementia, and mortality in older adults, as well as fatigue, sleepiness, and depression.[18]

Another model of dysregulation comes from research related to MS and myalgic encephalomyelitis (ME)/CFS (more typically called CFS/ME). Authors Morris and Maes have built a compelling case for MS's biochemical, cytokine, cell-mediated immunologic, B-cell, autoimmune, and brain dysfunction triggers and symptom overlap with ME, while pointing to the few exceptions between the diagnoses.[19]

CLINICAL PRESENTATION

A symptom review should incorporate the effects of rest periods, such as bedtime sleep, naps, weekends, and vacation, on the perceived state of fatigue. Fatigue may accompany self-limited infection, persist for months, accompany repeated hospitalizations, or follow a precipitous decline in health status.

One common type of fatigue is physiologic, which arises from extraordinary demands on otherwise healthy individuals, such as poor sleep hygiene, peripartum status, and work or personal stress. Health-destructive practices, such as intentional sleep deprivation, a diet of nutritionally deficient foods, a sedentary lifestyle, and excessive intake of alcohol and caffeine or stimulant drugs, also result in protracted fatigue. Physiologic fatigue is generally manageable if the offending habits, disturbances, or exertional demands can be addressed.

Inquiry into sleep environment, habits, and mood may also be helpful. This intake should include typical sleep challenges (such as bedtime irregularity, noise, room temperature, lack of privacy or safety, partner-related issues, and sleeping pattern disturbance) and the more global psychological disruptors of generalized anxiety, loneliness, vegetative symptoms, change in circumstances (e.g., recent loss, a new job), anorexia, hopelessness, and suicidal ideation.

Recurrent, irresistible attacks of daytime sleepiness may indicate narcolepsy; seconds-long periods of expressionlessness might be explained as absence seizures. Obstructive sleep apnea can be associated with overweight status, anatomic abnormalities of the head and neck, tobacco and alcohol exposure, older age, and family history it may be associated with the triple hit of chronic obesity, diabetes, and cardiovascular illness including stroke, known as metabolic syndrome (see Chapter 212).

Concurrent central nervous system (CNS) illness or chronic pain produces fatigue. It is useful to know whether the patient has accompanying neurologic deficits such as dysphasia, weight loss, tremor, gait disturbance, or dysgraphia suggestive of Parkinson disease (see Chapter 200) or has sustained a traumatic brain injury. Commonly described in MS are paresthesias, muscle weakness, balance or gait disorders, vision loss, color perception loss, or eye pain (see Chapter 199).

Patients with rheumatologic diseases often report fatigue as a prominent symptom. If fatigue increases during the day but is relieved by rest, rheumatologic or other organic causes, such as occult cardiovascular illness, warrant consideration.

A family or personal history of malignant neoplasms, diabetes, anemia, or other chronic illnesses should also be gathered.

A medication inventory should include prescribed, over-the-counter, and self-prescribed remedies, including alcohol and nutraceuticals. Of particular concern is the use of caffeine, nicotine, amphetamines, cocaine, or CNS depressants. Among these are antipsychotics, cancer chemotherapy drugs (interferon alfa, high-dose corticosteroids, vincristine, cisplatin), cardiac drugs (calcium channel blockers, beta blockers, diuretics), phenobarbital, carbamazepine, H_1 and H_2 receptor blockers, antihistamines with anticholinergic effects, benzodiazepines, and sedative doses of tricyclic antidepressants. Moreover, long-term use of hypnotics and minor tranquilizers seems to perpetuate sleep disturbances rather than to solve them. One pernicious environmental toxin resulting from a workplace or residential heating unit malfunction is carbon monoxide. Initial carbon monoxide poisoning can manifest as fatigue, but substantial poisoning leads to coma and death (see Chapter 34). Screening for contacts with infectious agents or vectors, including pets and other animals, may point to viral or bacterial entities.

Psychosocial stressors contributing to fatigue can be overwhelming and clinically significant. Childhood trauma has been studied in association with low cortisol or adrenal dysfunction, which can be a component of chronic fatigue states, especially if inadequately managed in subset populations.[2] Any history of psychological illness or substance abuse and associated treatments is valuable.

Despite this, the cause of fatigue may be idiopathic, although this is the exception. Fatigue as a normal part of aging is increasingly debunked. Older adults are very likely to report fatigue and more likely to have other causes—subclinical disease, increased inflammation, physiologic dysregulation, or increased work in maintaining homeostasis—different from those of young adults or otherwise healthy elders.[5] However, fatigue often accompanies deconditioning after a prolonged illness or hospitalization, which is common in an older population.

Fatigue that has increased for months suggests potentially insidious disease, particularly in older adults.

PHYSICAL EXAMINATION

For patients with fatigue, the physical examination is an adjunct to a thorough history of the complaint. Initially, habitus including neck girth (a measure correlated with sleep apnea), speech, cognition, balance, and gait should be assessed. Measurements of temperature, postural blood pressure, and pulse, with attention to pulse character, may indicate postural hypotension or cardiac arrhythmia, which can precipitate fatigue. Skin should be examined for dryness, jaundice, pallor, petechiae, or lesions. Thinning hair, glossy tongue, poor skin turgor or wound healing, easy bruising, and body wasting can be signs of poor nutritional status. Thyromegaly and lymphadenopathy could be significant.

A complete examination of the cardiorespiratory system should be performed with attention to the presence of respiratory rales or consolidation determined by tactile fremitus and adventitious, irregular, or rapid breath sounds. Jugular venous distention, cardiac murmurs, or peripheral edema should be noted. The abdominal examination should carefully exclude ascites, bruits, organomegaly, and gastrointestinal bleeding. Neuromuscular coordination and movement, exertional strain, and joint function should be included to determine whether chronic disease, an inflammatory process, or acute infection exists.

DIAGNOSTICS

The judicious use of blood testing within appropriate time intervals speaks to the need to strike a balance between degree of clinical suspicion and risk of increased false-positive results, especially in cases of new, unexplained fatigue. Diagnostic investigation for chronic unexplained fatigue requires persistence because fatigue can be a manifestation of any number of organic diseases. Cancer-related anemia, cardiac output reduction, infection, hypogonadism, hypercalcemia caused by hypoparathyroidism, and renal insufficiency bear noting.[13,14] For patients with a suspected physical cause, generally useful laboratory studies are a complete blood count (CBC) with differential; chemistry profile including serum electrolyte values and serum glucose or glycosylated hemoglobin (HbA_{1c}), calcium, albumin, creatinine, and blood urea nitrogen (BUN) concentrations; liver enzymes; erythrocyte sedimentation rate (ESR); thyroid-stimulating hormone (TSH); urinalysis; and occult blood in stool. For patients thought to have CFS, a more targeted list to exclude other causes has been established (see Diagnostics, later).

Primary or secondary adrenal insufficiency would be implicated if peak cortisol and growth hormone responses after exogenous cortisol exposure are abnormal. Immunoglobulin levels, Lyme titer, rheumatoid factor, adrenocorticotropic hormone (ACTH), and serum creatine kinase muscle-brain fraction (CK-MB) might be added, depending on leading signs. Any abnormality requires follow-up.

In addition, if prompted by the history and physical examination, a pharyngeal culture, Monospot test, syphilis titer, hepatitis panel, human immunodeficiency virus (HIV) test, or tuberculosis screening might be necessary. A chest x-ray examination is ordered for suspected lung, cardiac, or disseminated disease. For patients in whom postpolio syndrome is suspected, a nerve conduction study and electromyography can differentiate myasthenia gravis from other neuropathies that are central as opposed to peripheral. Considering central neurologic disorders, a brain MRI with gadolinium contrast for suspected MS would help narrow the diagnosis from among 30 or so mimics, including low vitamin B_{12} (include serum methylmalonic acid), lupus, and ischemia. Sometimes a lumbar puncture is indicated for an infectious cause. A workup for sleep apnea requires overnight polysomnography and actigraphy to gauge the total number of apnea and hypopnea episodes per slept hour, and may be useful in capturing periodic limb movements;

DIAGNOSTICS

Fatigue

LABORATORY

CBC and differential*
Urinalysis*
BUN*
Creatinine*
Serum electrolytes (sodium, potassium, chloride, carbon dioxide)*
Serum glucose*
Calcium*
Phosphorus*
Albumin*
Globulin*
Total protein*
Liver function tests (alanine transaminase, aspartate transaminase, alkaline phosphatase)*
Thyroid function tests (TSH, free T_4)*
Antinuclear antibody*
Rheumatoid factor*†
C-reactive protein*
ESR
Iron studies† (lactate dehydrogenase, ferritin, transferrin saturation)
Vitamin B_{12} (and methylmalonic acid)
Vitamin D level
Folate
Fecal occult blood test
Throat culture
Monospot (heterophil antibody test)†
Purified protein derivative/tuberculin test†
HIV†
Hepatitis panel†
Rapid plasma reagin†
Lyme titer *(Borrelia burgdorferi)* or Western blot (may need cerebrospinal fluid)†
Immunoglobulins†
Immunoglobulin A (IgA) endomysial antibody†
IgA anti-tissue transglutaminase antibody†
ACTH†
Peak cortisol†
CK-MB, if time frame is appropriate†

IMAGING

Chest x-ray studies†
Abdominal or pelvic ultrasound, computed tomography†
Brain MRI with gadolinium†

OTHER DIAGNOSTICS

Echocardiography†
Electromyography†
Nerve conduction study†
Toxicology screen†
24-Hour urine collection†
Sleep study†

*Included in the workup for CFS as described by the Centers for Disease Control and Prevention (www.cdc.gov/cfs/disgnosis/index.html). Accessed February 2, 2015.
†If indicated.

however, it may not prove as useful in explaining symptoms of insomnia.[14]

All age- and history-appropriate cancer screenings, including breast, cervical, prostate, and colon, are recommended as well.

DIFFERENTIAL DIAGNOSIS

The differential diagnosis for fatigue can be divided into five categories: environmental, physiologic, physical, psychiatric, and situational. Prolonged fatigue is defined as persisting longer than 4 weeks; chronic fatigue persists more than 6 months. Physiologic fatigue results from adverse external influences, such as poor sleep hygiene (see Chapter 227), substance abuse (see Chapter 249), and medication side effects. Physical explanations include acute and chronic illnesses resulting from a host of systemic conditions, such as chronic anemia. For example, iron deficiency and ferritin elevation are associated with restless legs syndrome and may explain its predominance in women (13.9% female versus 6.1% male), suggesting the "iron dopamine hypothesis."[4] Any cardiac, pulmonary, hematologic, endocrine, rheumatologic, neuromuscular, skin, renal, immune, or CNS disorder may individually or collectively contribute to fatigue. Systemic disorders result from inflammation, malignant disease, infection, or environmental exposures such as noxious fumes or ingested poisons.

Fatigue accompanying cardiopulmonary, hematologic, and metabolic disturbances in most cases involves reduced oxygen intake, excess carbon dioxide retention, or poor perfusion resulting from pulmonary congestion or inelasticity or severe iron deficiency anemia. Malignant disease such as pancreatic cancer is known to manifest with marked fatigue and few other symptoms (see Chapter 143).

Morbid obesity can be a cause of fatigue, particularly in cases of sleep apnea, which may cause hemoglobin desaturation, leading to pulmonary hypertension. The decreased metabolic activity associated with hypothyroidism commonly produces sluggishness and depression, whereas hyperthyroidism in older patients can manifest with fatigue, weight loss, and apathy (see Chapter 214). Uncontrolled diabetes mellitus causes fatigue because of significant calorie and fluid depletion (see Chapter 206). Decompensated cirrhosis from fatty liver disease may lead to day/night sleep reversal.

In cases of acute or chronic infection, fever and lymphadenopathy often accompany fatigue. Fatigue is also associated with rheumatic diseases but is not usually the only symptom. Patients with MS commonly experience disabling fatigue—on the order of 53% to 92%.[19] Malignant neoplasms of the blood have been seen to predispose older adults to more role strain and fatigue; younger patients seem more vulnerable to psychosocial dysfunction and psychological distress.[5]

Another source of chronic fatigue is the phenomenon of postpolio syndrome, which affects possibly 25% to 40% of the approximately 1 million Americans who reported a history of poliomyelitis (www.ninds.nih.gov/disorders/post_polio/detail_post_polio.htm). Symptoms of postpolio syndrome arise four to five decades after initial infection and may lead to muscle weakness and atrophy in previously affected muscle groups, pain, and fatigue. Fortunately, polio has been nearly eradicated worldwide since the introduction and refinements of the 1955 vaccine.

Fibromyalgia, a diagnosis of exclusion based on self-reported generalized pain, fatigue, and cognitive symptoms, involves the joints, tendons, and muscles and is best treated in a multidisciplinary fashion (see Chapter 175).

Chronic fatigue accompanied by a 50% decrease in activity level (exclusive of all other medical and psychiatric explanations) warrants consideration of CFS/ME, chronic fatigue immune dysfunction syndrome, and postviral fatigue syndrome. CFS/ME is said to affect approximately 2 million people, women twice as often as men, usually between the ages of 30 and 40.[20] Prevalence ranges from 0.0007% to 2.8% of the general adult population.[21] The disorder takes an average of 5 years to diagnose, with low rates of improvement and much lower rates of cure.[3] The criteria for diagnosis include four of eight defining characteristics: unusual postexertional malaise, impaired memory or concentration, unrefreshing sleep, headaches, muscle pain, joint pain, sore throat, and tender lymph nodes (Box 223-1).[3] There is little recovery after rest, unlike in myasthenia gravis, with a component of physical symptoms. Muscle or joint pain, headaches, sore throat, enlarged and painful nodes, and mental dullness or confusion severe enough to affect routine activity are common.

Recognizing that inflammatory fatigue shares features with CFS/ME and fibromyalgia, it has been termed "cytokine-induced

BOX 223-1

Diagnostic Criteria for CFS: International CFS Case Definition (1994)

1. Severe chronic fatigue of 6 months or longer that is not explained by any medical or psychiatric diagnosis
2. The presence of four or more of the following eight symptoms:
   - Postexertional malaise lasting more than 24 hours
   - Unrefreshing sleep
   - Significant impairment in short-term memory or concentration
   - Muscle pain
   - Multijoint pain without swelling or redness
   - Sore throat
   - Tender lymph nodes
   - Headaches of a new type, pattern, or severity

From the Centers for Disease Control and Prevention: *Chronic fatigue syndrome (CFS): CFS toolkit—making a diagnosis.* Available at www.cdc.gov/cfs. Accessed February 2, 2015.

sickness behavior."[17] Depression can affect up to half of CFS patients, a rate much higher than in other chronic diseases,[20] and CFS may share features of other functional somatic disorders such as irritable bowel disease and multiple chemical sensitivity.[22] Myofascial conditions and fibromyalgia may be difficult to distinguish from CFS. Because fibromyalgia has no exclusionary considerations, it is diagnosed 10 times more often than CFS, on the order of 0.3% versus 3% of the population.[23] In fact, the controversy regarding labels mark fibromyalgia and CFS as overlapping in 20% to 75% of cases.[22] Myofascial pain syndrome involves painful, tender areas in muscles that twitch on palpation or produce an area of referred pain. This localized, short-term condition lacks systemic manifestations other than fatigue. Fibromyalgia, in contrast, has uniform trigger point associations; it shares pain and fatigue, as well as having other systemic features.

Fatigue often accompanies depression (see Chapter 248). Research on clinically diagnosed depression has established the contribution of neurotransmitters, including serotonin and norepinephrine. In addition, chronic anxiety or stress can lead to neck and shoulder muscle fatigue, irregular sleeping patterns, or irritable bowel symptoms. Clearly, anxiety, eating, and depressive disorders are among the mental illnesses that tax energy reserves. Somatoform disorders, in the absence of a medically identifiable entity, may also have a role. By the same token, depression is often identified along with fatigue-related illnesses. Poststroke fatigue affects more than one third of stroke survivors and has been strongly associated with depressive and possibly anxiety disorders, with indication that locus of control and coping difficulties may contribute to this, as with cancer and MS.[16] Persistent insomnia in women is linked to a fourfold greater risk of depression; reduction in sleep hours was associated with a 28% rise in the hormone ghrelin, which increased appetite and was correlated with weight gain among those with insomnia.[4]

Situational factors, such as increased stress (work, school, or relationship), unemployment, delayed effects of trauma, and bereavement, provoke fatigue.

MANAGEMENT

The patient with fatigue requires various degrees and types of support. The provider must acknowledge the fatigue as a valid complaint, worthy of further exploration. Behavioral, situational, and environmental contributions to sleep disturbance should be identified for optimal improvement. Treatment of primary, secondary, and chronic insomnia focuses on the sleep cycle and behavioral maladaptation. Some patients have restless legs syndrome or periodic limb movement, which causes undetectable sleep interruption with resultant unrefreshing sleep (see Chapter 198). For patients with restless legs syndrome, 80% of whom have periodic limb movement disorder[4] and many of whom have MS, optimizing sleep hygiene and healthful habits is key. In cases of deficiency, iron and vitamin C supplementation in addition to anti-inflammatory treatment is first-line treatment. Additional dopaminergic agents, benzodiazepines, and possibly anticonvulsants and/or clonidine may follow.[4,12]

For CFS, research has established what is not helpful—such as melatonin, methylphenidate, and citalopram—and what may be helpful including magnesium, possibly probiotics, low doses of antidepressants such as nortriptyline, anti-inflammatory and mild analgesics. In CFS/ME, the most strongly associated therapeutic benefit derives from graduated exercise and cognitive behavioral therapies.[17]

A patient with primary sleep disorder should be referred to a sleep disorder clinic. When poor sleep arises in the setting of clinically assessed depression, antidepressant medication might help both. When generalized anxiety disorder is identified, use of benzodiazepines other than on a short-term basis is discouraged in favor of buspirone, other antidepressants such as venlafaxine, and atypical antipsychotics, to avoid dependency. Cancer-related fatigue might respond to methylphenidate, 5 mg daily, or other psychostimulants, but the range of causes is wide and includes malnutrition, dehydration, electrolyte shifts, anemia, hypoxia, organ failure or insufficiency, emboli, cardiopulmonary compromise, and others such as adverse effects of treatment, physical limitations caused by disease and/or pain, and psychosocial effects (Table 223-1).[13] Within this complexity, any modifiable causes, such as anemia and anorexia-cachexia, should be identified and addressed (Table 223-2). Sometimes barriers to treatment reflect providers' lack of knowledge in treating cancer-related fatigue or overemphasis on pain management; the patient's own limited understanding of his or her fatigue may prevent the patient from asking for more help.[13]

Modafinil has been associated with improvement in poststroke and HIV-related fatigue[1] as well as in subsets of cancer patients with severe fatigue.[14,18] Pregabalin, a Food and Drug Administration–approved treatment of daytime somnolence in fibromyalgia patients, provides short-lived relief of fatigue, although preferred agents to treat the condition, with a focus on pain management, include tricyclic antidepressant compounds, low-dose naltrexone, gabapentinoids, serotonin norepinephrine reuptake inhibitors, and γ-hydroxybutyrate, with caution taken to avoid the ineffective anti-inflammatories, opioids (may potentiate hyperalgesia), and steroids.[11] A regimen of both muscle strengthening and aerobic exercise is thought to improve cardiovascular functioning, depth of sleep, and sense of well-being. For cancer-related fatigue, studies showed small to moderate improvements. One moderate- to high-intensity level aerobic and muscle strengthening exercise regimen of 150 minutes per week, using major muscle groups two or three times a week, showed a greater benefit to cancer patients than aerobic exercises alone, as did a supervised program as opposed to

DIFFERENTIAL DIAGNOSIS

Fatigue

ENVIRONMENTAL EXPOSURES

- Heavy metal toxicity (mercury, lead, nickel)
- Pesticides
- Pollutants
- Poisoning (carbon monoxide, ciguatera)
- Radiation exposure (nuclear reactor accident, cancer treatment)
- Vitamin B_{12} deficiency (could be secondary to disease)
- Vitamin D deficiency

PHYSIOLOGIC CAUSES

- Health-destructive behaviors
- Late-luteal phase of menses
- Medication side effects
- Menopause
- Perimenopause
- Peripartum and postpartum (particularly first and third trimesters)
- Poor sleep hygiene
- Postoperative (general anesthesia <6 months)
- Over-exercise syndrome[17]
- Substance abuse

PHYSICAL CAUSES

Cardiac

- Congestive heart failure
- Endocarditis
- Valvular disease

Endocrine

- Adrenal insufficiency (Addison disease)
- Diabetes mellitus
- Thyroid dysfunction

Gastroenterologic

- Chronic hepatitis C
- Cirrhosis, uncompensated
- Inflammatory bowel disease
- Primary biliary cirrhosis[17]

Hematologic and Oncologic

- Anemia of chronic disease
- Malignant disease (breast, cervical, lung, prostate, uterine)
- Radiation and/or chemotherapy

Infectious

- Acute or chronic
- HIV and acquired immunodeficiency syndrome (AIDS)
- Inherited febrile syndromes
- Lyme disease

Integumentary

- Burns[17]
- Psoriasis[17]

Nephrologic

- Renal insufficiency
- Nocturia

Neurologic or Neuromuscular

- CFS or myalgic encephalomyelitis
- Parkinson disease
- Periodic limb movement disorder
- Postpolio syndrome
- Restless legs syndrome
- Sleep apnea
- Stroke
- Traumatic brain injury

Rheumatologic

- Ankylosing spondylitis[17]
- Rheumatoid arthritis
- Sjögren syndrome
- Systemic lupus erythematosus
- Fibromyalgia

Pulmonary

- Congestive obstructive pulmonary disease
- Sarcoidosis

PSYCHOLOGICAL CAUSES

- Bipolar
- Chronic anxiety
- Depression
- Eating disorders
- Psychosis
- Schizophrenia
- Somatoform disorders

SITUATIONAL CAUSES

- Grief
- Low levels of daylight exposure (e.g., during winter months)
- Time zone travel
- Post-traumatic stress disorder
- Role stress
- Shift work schedule irregularity
- Unemployment

home-based exercise.[18] Lasting improvement in fatigue was demonstrated after 3 hours of aerobic exercise per week at 75% of maximal heart rate.[1] Individuals with chronic muscle fatigue and joint pain can influence the onset and toll of their illness by maintaining normal weight; avoiding exercising to the point of muscle pain; keeping body temperature warmer than air temperature (to avoid the muscle tension associated with cold); and using stress reduction, energy conservation, and time management techniques. The provider can empower the patient to have a sense of control over the situation by encouraging him or her to network, to read relevant publications, and to attend support group meetings.

CBT has also been used with success. Work on downplaying negative associations with fatigue is part of the treatment. In fact, overemphasis on making up lost sleep or focused effort on resting can cause hyperarousal.[14]

If the diagnosis is elusive, the patient is asked to keep a fatigue diary. Recording the time of onset, duration, severity, accompanying symptoms, relief measures, exercise, mood, diet, medications, alcohol and substance use, and stressors not only helps the health care provider but will also be helpful if future consultation is necessary.

For the subset of patients who are physically disabled by fatigue, employment considerations might require referral to a vocational counselor. A patient may wish to apply for up to 12 weeks of a temporary employment hiatus through the federal Family Medical Leave Act, workers' compensation for an employment-related injury, job reassignment, prepaid short-

TABLE 223-1 Examples of Possible Pharmacologic Interventions for Use in Cancer Patients Experiencing Fatigue

Cause of Fatigue	Possible Interventions
Anemia	If iron, folic acid, or vitamin B_{12} levels are low, use supplements (oral or intravenous) as appropriate. If hemoglobin levels are low, consider erythropoiesis-stimulating agents or whole blood or red blood cell transfusion.
Anticancer treatment	Consider reducing or delaying dose or stopping treatment (only if severe).
Dehydration	Rehydration with intravenous sodium chloride; depending on cause, possible interventions include discontinuation of diuretic, initiation of insulin treatment (if hyperglycemic), and treatments for fever or excessive sweating (e.g., clonidine, progestins, selective serotonin reuptake inhibitors, gabapentin if related to hot flashes).
Depression	Consider use of selective serotonin reuptake inhibitors.
Electrolyte disorders	Hypercalcemia: intravenous sodium chloride and bisphosphonates. Hyponatremia: fluid restriction and/or salt supplementation (oral or intravenous).
Other medications	Consider reducing dose or withdrawal of potential fatigue-inducing drugs (e.g., psychotropic drugs, anti-histamines, beta blockers).
Sleep disorders	Consider short-term short-acting benzodiazepine treatment if severe or unresponsive to nonpharmacologic intervention. Sedating anti-histamines, antidepressants, or antipsychotics may also be useful. Melatonin or methylphenidate may be beneficial if there is a disturbed day/night rhythm.
Tumor	Systemic anticancer therapy (e.g., chemotherapy, hormonal therapy, or targeted therapy).
Underlying symptoms	Pain or dyspnea can cause fatigue and should be treated appropriate (e.g., nonsteroidal anti-inflammatory drugs or opioids for pain, and morphine, corticosteroids, bronchodilators, or sedatives/anxiolytics for dyspnea).
Unknown	Psychostimulants (e.g., dexamphetamine, dexmethylphenidate or methylphenidate, modafinil) for symptomatic relief.
Weight loss	If there are metabolic abnormalities resulting from anorexia-cachexia syndrome, consider megestrol acetate or corticosteroids (depending on life expectancy).

Data from Koornstra RH, Peters M, Donofrio S, et al: Management of fatigue in patients with cancer—a practical review. *Cancer Treat Rev* 40:791-799, 2014.

TABLE 223-2 Examples of Possible Nonpharmacologic Interventions for Use in Cancer Patients Experiencing Fatigue

Nonpharmacologic Intervention	Examples
Complementary therapies	Relaxation therapy, massage, music, herbal remedies (e.g., American ginseng), yoga, and acupuncture may also provide relief.
Energy conservation	Help patients find a daily routine that balances activities and rest and that works for them based on their pattern of fatigue.
Other supportive care	Consultation with a dietician, physiotherapist, or occupational therapist as required.
Physical activity	Encourage physical activity and provide information on any available training and/or rehabilitation programs (supervised by a physical therapist if fatigue is severe).
Psychosocial support	This could include counseling or psychotherapy, cognitive behavioral therapy, and so on. Can be provided in the form of group therapy as part of a rehabilitation program or individually. Can also be sought through professional psychosocial oncology centers or through psychologists, counselors, and other sources. Inform patient about the possibility of spiritual care. Advise distraction (e.g., reading, listening to music, walking, gardening) if appropriate to patient.
Self-efficacy and self-management	Encourage positive patient factors such as self-efficacy, mastery, and learned resourcefulness.
Sleep therapy	Stimulus control, sleep restriction, and sleep hygiene may be beneficial.

Data from Koornstra RH, Peters M, Donofrio S, et al: Management of fatigue in patients with cancer—a practical review. *Cancer Treat Rev* 40:791-799, 2014.

and long-term disability through work, or government-administered long-term disability.

COMPLICATIONS

Complications of fatigue include daytime sleepiness, risk of injury or accident, poor performance, and cognitive and functional impairment in managing independent activities of daily living. A driving evaluation that includes a road test ensures the appropriateness of continued driving and protects both the driver and the public from accident or injury. In addition, individuals with chronic illnesses, including MS, fibromyalgia, and CFS, are especially vulnerable to depression, whether it is considered organic, disease driven, or situational. A depression inventory including questions about suicidal ideation and substance abuse is crucial because the risks are higher among these groups in particular.

INDICATIONS FOR REFERRAL OR HOSPITALIZATION

- Physician consultation may be helpful in the evaluation of the patient with fatigue when symptoms elude explanation or treatment.
- Specialist involvement is dictated by the suspected cause of the fatigue.
- Physical and occupational therapy referral for exercise programs and energy conservation techniques can be helpful.
- Specialty referral is also indicated for progressive symptoms, lack of response to therapy, or indications of life-threatening illness. It is important to consider services available to the patient with a chronic fatigue condition such as CFS or post-polio syndrome, which greatly affects the quality of life and work.
- When fatigue is associated with acute depression, psychosis, cardiomyopathy, congestive heart failure, chronic obstructive pulmonary disease (COPD) exacerbation, or obstructive sleep apnea resulting from morbid obesity or anatomic abnormality, patients should be referred to the appropriate specialist or acute care setting.
- A mental health referral or referral to support groups is helpful. CBT and intensive endurance rehabilitation have been effective for adult outpatients with CFS.
- Postpartum women with fatigue should be screened for anemia, thyroid and endocrine disorders, and urinary tract infections.
- Cancer-related fatigue calls for integrative treatment, multidisciplinary care coordination, and holistic, patient-centered care. Patients may be best served in a cancer center, where the needs of the patient and the patient's family are taken into account.

LIFE SPAN CONSIDERATIONS

A patient's age and life span stressors influence the evaluation for fatigue. Teenagers and newly independent young adults should be screened for deleterious health habits, given that they have a tendency toward experimentation with alcohol, drugs, irregular sleep, and poor nutrition. Transitions and losses resulting from changes such as marriage or the death of a loved one can be destabilizing. Situational depression or anxiety accompanies these developmental transitions and can cause fatigue.

Postpartum women are at risk for debilitating fatigue. Blood loss at the time of delivery coupled with sleep deprivation and the demands of caring for a newborn can contribute to profound fatigue. Concerned family members may be the first ones to approach the practitioner with concerns about a postpartum patient. Perimenopausal women may also complain of fatigue. Vasomotor symptoms can affect sleep, for which serotonin receptor blockers have helped; and in some cases, metrorrhagia can cause significant anemia, for which iron supplementation might help.

EDUCATION AND HEALTH PROMOTION

It is important to acknowledge fatigue as a legitimate symptom of various underlying illnesses. Fatigue in and of itself should be managed using traditional medical approaches as well as alternative therapies. The importance of proper nutrition, sleep, and exercise should be stressed to patients of all ages in concrete terms. This approach bolsters health, assists in maintaining an optimum quality of life, and protects against debilitating stressors and communicable illnesses. Consultation with a nutritionist, review of sleep hygiene, and an exercise tolerance test are recommended, when indicated.

Alcohol, illicit drug, tobacco, and caffeine consumption all have an adverse effect on restful sleep. Patients are advised to discontinue caffeine 4 to 6 hours before bed and to avoid late-night snacks and stimulants such as tobacco and alcohol. Regular sleep and wake times, minimum environmental stimuli such as noise and light, regulated ambient temperature, and early afternoon or morning exertion or exercise encourage good sleep hygiene.

Fatigue is not necessarily part of aging in the healthy adult. Because infectious, allergic, inflammatory, malignant, mood, or cognitive causes may be at root, fatigue concerns should be investigated, particularly if the fatigue is associated with lymph node enlargement or pain, weight loss, muscle aches, sore throat, headache, night sweats, or other troublesome constitutional symptoms.

CHAPTER 224

FEVER

Elizabeth A. Talbot • Laura E. Shevy

In primary care, a clinical encounter with a febrile patient can be challenging because of the many causes of fever, ranging from the familiar to esoteric infectious diseases to diverse noninfectious causes, and also because the causes of fever range in severity from self-limited to imminently life-threatening. This chapter defines fever, clarifies the types and patterns of fever, provides an approach to evaluation of the febrile patient within primary care, reviews special circumstances such as fever of unknown origin (FUO) and fever in young children, and provides principles for empiric management.

DEFINITION AND EPIDEMIOLOGY

Fever, or pyrexia, is a state of elevated core temperature resulting from a physiologic change in set point that is often part of the patient's defensive response. This response may be to the invasion of microorganisms or inanimate matter recognized as pathogenic or alien by the host.[1] A patient is often aware of being febrile because he or she feels either abnormally cold or warm, lethargic, and otherwise unwell; occasionally, however, the patient is asymptomatic and unaware of being febrile.

Diagnosis of a patient with fever is predicated on defining normal body temperature, appreciating inherent host variability, and accounting for limitations to accurate temperature measurement. Regarding normal body temperature, although most patients and providers believe that a core temperature of 37° C (98.6° F) is normal, research shows that 36.8° C (98.2° F) ± 1° C (1.8° F) is closer to normal for most healthy people.[2] In addition, a healthy person's body temperature fluctuates during the day. Diurnal variation may be as much as 1° C, with temperatures highest in the early evening and lowest in the early morning.[2,3] Normal body temperature also varies by sex and age. For example, compared with men, a woman's average temperature is 0.2° C higher and even 0.5° C higher while ovulating.[4] Elderly patients and those with certain illnesses, such as chronic kidney or liver disease, may have average body temperatures lower than those of healthy nonelderly populations.[2,5]

A clinician's ability to identify fever is affected by the accuracy of the device used, correct positioning of the device probe, choice of anatomic site for measurement, and age of the patient. Core body temperature can be measured in the axilla, rectum, mouth, tympanic membrane, and skin. There are excellent reviews describing which site is most appropriate for which population.[2] For an ambulatory adult the mouth is generally the preferred site for measurement of temperature, whereas for neonates the axilla may be best.

Fever is a distinct syndrome from hyperthermia, which is defined as an increase in body temperature that surpasses the body's ability to dissipate heat.[3] Hyperthermia can be precipitated by high environmental temperatures (as in heat stroke), strenuous physical exercise (exertional heat stroke), illicit drugs (cocaine, LSD, methamphetamine), and reactions to various prescribed medications.[3] Thyroid storm may be associated with hyperthermia and may manifest as delirium, seizures, coma, vomiting, diarrhea, jaundice, congestive heart failure, and cardiac dysrhythmias.[3] In further contrast, hypothermia is body temperature of 36° C (97° F) or lower, which can result from exposure to a cold environment, hypothyroidism, uremia, and overwhelming infection. The last scenario usually signifies a patient's inability to mount an appropriate fever, which is a poor prognostic sign.

Hyperpyrexia refers to a temperature in excess of 41.5° C (106.7° F). This life-threatening state is most commonly caused by central nervous system (CNS) hemorrhage and serious infections.[3] A temperature of 41° C (105.8° F) may lead to brain damage, whereas a temperature in excess of 43° C (109.4° F) is invariably fatal.

For noninfectious causes of elevated temperature, see Box 224-1.

BOX 224-1

Fever

Among noninfectious causes of elevated temperature, there are several characteristic clinical clues, as well as syndromic presentations.

- Heat stroke
  - Elevated temperature with lack of sweating in the appropriate context
- Exertional heat stroke
  - Elevated temperature in high environmental temperatures
- Nonexertional heat stroke
  - Medication effect
  - Iatrogenic diuresis with limited or no access to free water
  - Anticholinergic agents or anti-Parkinson medications
- Malignant hyperthermia
  - Autosomal dominant hereditary condition
  - Hyperthermia, muscular rigidity, and hemodynamic instability that occurs during general anesthesia
- Neuroleptic malignant syndrome
  - Withdrawal of CNS dopaminergic agents or receiving antidopaminergic agents
  - Hyperthermia, severe muscular rigidity, "lead pipe rigidity"
  - Mental status change, dysautonomia, hyporeflexia
- Serotonin syndrome
  - Serotonin toxicity
  - Fever, delirium, myoclonus, hyperreflexia

EVALUATING A FEBRILE PATIENT

Evaluation of a Patient with Fever Without a Clear Cause

As primary care clinicians know well, febrile episodes are often mild and self-limited. However, a minority are caused by serious conditions including infection, malignancy, adverse reactions to medication or blood products, connective tissue disease, and venous thromboembolic disease (to name just a few). The history and associated signs and symptoms often make the cause of these serious fevers obvious. But when the cause is not obvious, a broader differential diagnosis must be created by researching further information about both the patient and location-specific disease epidemiology.

The clinician should interview the patient to obtain a thorough history, including complete details of the fever pattern (Table 224-1) and associated symptoms. The fever pattern should be elucidated—when it began, how high it has been, and how it fluctuates during the day. Though rarely sufficient for a diagnosis, this history may provide key diagnostic clues.[6,7] For example, high fever with an evanescent rash and relative bradycardia may suggest typhoid fever, whereas an influenza-like febrile illness with relative bradycardia may prompt workup

TABLE 224-1 Fever Patterns

Fever Patterns	Description
Sustained or continuous	Constant elevation daily
Intermittent	Normal temperature at least once daily
Remittent	Temperature down but not to normal
Relapsing	Elevated temperature interspersed with long periods of normal temperature
Hectic	Widely fluctuating temperature
Relative bradycardia	Elevated temperature without expected elevation in pulse rate
Central fever	Elevated temperature related to CNS damage (malignancy, trauma, hemorrhage)
Factitious fever	False reporting of elevated temperature (report of fever by afebrile patient or intentionally caused infection manifesting true fever (Munchausen)

for leptospirosis in the right clinical context. A relapsing fever pattern may suggest an infection caused by *Borrelia* or *Streptobacillus* organisms. Cough, weight loss, and a hectic fever may raise consideration of tuberculosis (TB) or lymphoma.

Exposures to animals and animal products are often relevant within the story of a febrile patient. Rabies, cat-scratch disease (bartonellosis), pasteurellosis, toxoplasmosis, leptospirosis, anthrax, brucellosis, psittacosis, and rat-bite fever are febrile illness associated with animal or animal product exposure. Tick exposure is increasingly relevant as Lyme disease becomes epidemic in a wider geographic range. Babesiosis, ehrlichiosis, and Rocky Mountain spotted fever can also follow tick bites (see Chapter 234). Mosquito bites may herald febrile illness with the arboviruses, including West Nile virus, eastern equine encephalitis, chikungunya, and others. Arboviral disease is usually mandatorily reported, and specialized testing should be coordinated with the public health jurisdiction.

Discovery that a febrile patient has recently traveled to the tropics broadens the infectious disease differential diagnosis. Because most primary care clinicians do not routinely practice tropical medicine, such a differential diagnosis may be daunting. However, excellent surveillance data show that many of the classic tropical diseases, including Japanese encephalitis, Rift Valley fever, Ebola, Chagas disease, African trypanosomiasis, and yellow fever, are extremely unlikely in ill returning travelers.[8,9] Although rare in the United States in the summer, familiar and "unexotic" influenza circulates year-round in most of the tropics and may be the most common vaccine-preventable disease acquired during travel.[10]

A rational approach to fever in the returning traveler includes delineating in detail the clinical presentation, specifically detailing symptom onset in relation to the travel itinerary. This facilitates pathogen identification based on possible incubation periods. Further information should be sought, including a thorough history of pretravel vaccinations and immune status; malaria chemoprophylaxis and other medications used abroad; exposures abroad including animals, insect bites, and types of food and water consumed; as well as any unprotected intercourse. Because fever in the returning traveler is also potentially caused by pathogens acquired in the home country, details of exposure to illnesses at home since return should also be clarified.

The most important tropical disease in a febrile returning traveler is malaria, because it can be life-threatening. Dengue virus is more common than malaria but is usually self-limited.[11] A rapidly emerging global pathogen—chikungunya virus infection—should be considered even in primary care settings in a patient with acute onset of fever and polyarthralgia, especially in the traveler recently returned from areas with known virus transmission, such as Africa, Asia, Europe, India, and the Pacific Ocean islands. In late 2013, outbreaks of chikungunya virus were identified even in the Caribbean (see the Centers for Disease Control and Prevention [CDC] website at www.cdc.gov for the most updated epidemiology). Although chikungunya virus is not currently found in the United States, there is a very real risk that the virus will be imported by infected travelers (see Chapter 229). Typhoid fever, tularemia, extraintestinal amebiasis, and TB should also be considered for the patient with a clinically compatible febrile illness.

In an immunocompromised febrile patient, the differential diagnosis expands rapidly. Immunocompromised states include bone marrow transplantation, human immunodeficiency virus (HIV) infection, malignancy, or drug-induced immune dysfunction (such as chemotherapy or corticosteroid use).

The clinician must elicit any history of a recent surgical procedure or implantation of a foreign body, including joint prostheses and urinary or intravascular catheters, and their presence should direct the initial diagnostic investigation. A review of the patient's current immunizations, evaluations for latent TB infection (tuberculin skin test or interferon-γ release assay), and recent past infections can be helpful. For example, a history of otitis media, urinary tract infection, or pneumonia may signify progressive infections such as mastoiditis, renal abscess, or empyema, respectively.

A detailed medication history is vital in the evaluation of fever because many medications can cause fever either syndromically, as with neuroleptic malignant syndrome (see Box 224-1) NMS or serotonin syndrome, or as "drug fever."[11] Commonly implicated classes of medications that cause drug fever include antihypertensives, antiarrhythmic medications, antibiotics, thyroid medications, and antiepileptics. Drug fever occurs at any time from shortly after to years after initiation of a medication. Occasional clues to the diagnosis of drug fever are eosinophilia, rash, mild transaminitis, or elevated erythrocyte sedimentation rate (ESR), but more often drug fever is a diagnosis of exclusion. Stopping an implicated drug usually results in defervescence within 72 hours, and the fever resumes if the drug is restarted.

Physical examination signs that might suggest the cause of a fever should be diligently sought. Skin, sinus, nasal, ear, dental, and throat examinations are essential. Regional lymph node enlargement suggests a localized infectious process, whereas generalized lymphadenopathy may suggest systemic infection such as HIV infection or malignant disease such as lymphoma. Detection of a new or evolving heart murmur, especially in the setting of classic stigmata such as conjunctival hemorrhages, splinter hemorrhages, or Janeway lesions, is a valuable clue to endocarditis. Adventitious or asymmetric breath sounds may indicate pneumonia, pulmonary emboli, or pleural effusions. An abdominal mass, hepatosplenomegaly, or tenderness should prompt investigation for an abdominal source of fever. Calf tenderness with a palpable vascular cord is evidence of thrombophlebitis. An abnormal joint examination can suggest osteomyelitis, infectious arthritis, or autoimmune arthritis. Breast, pelvic, penile, and rectal examinations are indicated when infections or neoplasms are suspected.

Epidemiologic information about locally circulating illnesses and reported exposures to ill persons greatly informs the differential diagnosis of fever. Obviously, in the absence of travel or contact with a traveler, locally and seasonally prevalent diseases should be predominantly considered. For example, a normal host who develops a community-acquired prolonged febrile cough illness in the winter in New England should prompt testing for pertussis before testing for TB. The state, county, city, or local health department can serve as a resource for providers regarding local disease epidemiology. This is especially true of reportable diseases, but public health officials often are aware of outbreaks or the circulation of nonreportable diseases as well, such as the arrival of seasonal influenza, a school varicella outbreak, or the occurrence of summer enteroviral meningoencephalitis.

Diagnostic Evaluation of a Patient with Fever Without a Clear Cause

For a patient with fever without a clear cause, a reasonable initial diagnostic maneuver may include a complete blood count (CBC) with differential white count examination. Elevated numbers and proportion of neutrophilic granulocytes may indicate bacterial infection. Lymphocytes are classically elevated on the differential with some viral infections and, of course, with lymphocytic leukemia. Elevated monocytes can strongly suggest mononucleosis, but there are other infections and conditions in which monocytosis can be seen. Eosinophils classically suggest a parasitic infection, asthma, or allergy. Liver function tests, urinalysis, blood and other potential source cultures, and C-reactive protein (CRP) and ESR are also typical diagnostics to suggest diagnoses and to confirm a systemic process. The ESR is a sensitive but nonspecific test. However, when the patient's ESR is greater than 100 mm/hr, the possibility of osteomyelitis, endocarditis, temporal arteritis, or other rheumatologic diseases is increased. Serologic testing is reserved for when the history and physical examination suggest a particular diagnosis. Computed tomography and magnetic resonance imaging may be useful for detection of abscesses or mass lesions. Echocardiography is mandatory if there are cardiac findings, persistent bacteremia, or stigmata, which all may be consistent with endocarditis.

Evaluation of Fever of Unknown Origin

In contrast to simple fever without a recognized cause, there are clearly defined syndromes of FUO, with more specific varieties of nosocomial FUO, neutropenic FUO, and FUO associated with HIV infection.[11] The most common FUO in primary care settings is classic FUO, defined as temperature in excess of 38.3° C (101° F) persisting beyond 3 weeks for which intensive investigation fails to yield a diagnosis.[11] This intensive investigation is defined as 3 days of hospitalization, or three outpatient visits or 1 week of intensive outpatient investigations. Studies show that most causes of classic FUO in adults are atypical presentations of common diseases, rather than rare diseases.[12] Recent studies reported infectious causes (such as TB, occult abscesses, and bacterial endocarditis) to account for 15% to 30% of FUO; neoplastic processes (especially lymphoma, leukemia, and renal cell carcinoma), 10% to 30%; connective tissue diseases, 33% to 40%; miscellaneous (drug fever, hyperthyroidism, and factitious fever), 5% to 14%; and undiagnosed causes, 20% to 30%.[12,13]

In children, fever represents 10% to 25% of pediatric emergency department visits and is one of the most common reasons for a visit to the primary care provider. FUO in pediatric patients is more likely caused by infection than malignancy. Although most causes are self-limited viral illnesses, the incidence of other serious bacterial illnesses has been estimated at 6% to 10% in infants younger than 3 months and 5% to 7% in children 3 to 36 months of age.[14] Important noninfectious causes of FUO in the pediatric population are systemic onset juvenile arthritis and Takayasu arteritis. Hereditary periodic fever syndromes such as familial Mediterranean fever or hyperimmunoglobulin D syndrome can also cause fever in children and adults.[11]

Diagnostic Evaluation for Fever of Unknown Origin

During evaluation of a patient with FUO, hospitalization may be warranted to allow detailed history, physical examination, and diagnostic maneuvers. By the time a patient has met the definition for FUO, many standard laboratory evaluations and imaging studies have already been completed. More invasive evaluation, such as lumbar puncture, bone marrow, temporal artery, or liver biopsy, should be sought when clinical and laboratory findings implicate these systems as potential sources. Recent clinical data support the use of 18-fluoro-2-deoxygluocse positron emission tomography–computed tomography (FDG-PET/CT) in the workup of FUO but only when the patient has elevated ESR or CRP.[13,15] A recent meta-analysis reviewed 15 studies including 595 patients with FUO and elevated inflammatory markers and found that FDG-PET/CT had a diagnostic sensitivity of 85% according to a per-patient–based analysis. The false-positive rate was high, though (26% to 63%). Among pediatric patients, FDG-PET/CT substantively contributed to a diagnosis in 73%.[15] If applied early during the diagnostic algorithm, it was also cost-effective.[16]

LIFE SPAN CONSIDERATIONS

Fever is a common presenting complaint of children and infants seen in emergency departments. In 2003, the American College of Emergency Physicians updated its clinical policy for children coming to the emergency department with fever.[17] The policy applies to healthy full-term infants and children between the ages of 1 day and 36 months. Guidance that may be useful in primary care includes that febrile infants between the ages of 1 and 28 days should always be presumed to have a serious bacterial infection. The policy also clearly discourages a trial of antipyresis in clinical decision-making because a number of research trials have dispelled the misconception that response to antipyretic therapy indicates lower likelihood of serious bacterial infection.[18] A chest radiograph should be routinely obtained for febrile children younger than 3 months and for older children who have high temperatures (>39° C [102.2° F]) and a white blood cell count elevated above 20,000/mm^3. Empirical antibiotics may be appropriate for previously healthy, well-appearing children aged 3 to 36 months with temperature of 39° C or higher and a white blood cell count of 15,000/mm^3 or higher.[17]

Older adults are less likely to develop the high fevers of childhood; some seniors, even those with severe infections, may not be able to mount a febrile response at all. Hypothermia is common in this age group because of failing hypothalamic thermoregulatory systems.

MANAGEMENT

Treatment of the cause of a patient's fever is ultimately the best treatment for fever. Ideally, this treatment is directed, such as antibiotic therapy for an identified bacterial infection. In some circumstances, however, treatment must be empirical pending diagnosis. For example, there are many algorithms that guide the empirical treatment of neutropenic patients with fever.[19]

Surprisingly, though, there is no clear consensus as to whether fever itself should be suppressed with antipyretics. Fever is an adaptive response that has widely evolved among most members of the animal kingdom, strongly suggesting an adaptive role for fever.[2,3] Many experimental data suggest that fever is associated with improved outcome in infection, and some data suggest that suppression of fever may delay recovery from infection.[2]

In spite of some controversy, there are situations in which fever should definitely be treated. For example, any patient whose temperature exceeds 41° C (105.8° F) should immediately be treated with antipyretics and cooling measures to avoid brain damage.[3] Children are more susceptible to the harmful effects of elevated temperatures, manifesting seizures particularly at younger ages (3 months to 5 years). Patients with underlying cardiovascular disease may not tolerate the increased metabolic demands of prolonged high fever: an increase of 1° C (1.8° F) in temperature increases the basal metabolic rate by more than 10%.[3] In many settings of fever and identified infection, antipyretics can be given at regular intervals for symptomatic relief.

Antipyretic drugs include steroids, aspirin and other nonsteroidal anti-inflammatory drugs, and acetaminophen. Acetaminophen is usually the first line of treatment for fever. The risk of

Reye's syndrome makes aspirin contraindicated in children. Physical methods, such as sponging with cool water or alcohol and applying cold packs or cooling blankets, may be effective but are generally not considered first-line interventions.

In the absence of increased water intake, fever produces dehydration. It can cause confusion, delirium, and seizures and be associated with anorexia. Therefore, treatment for fever should also include close attention to maintenance of hydration and nutrition.

INDICATIONS FOR REFERRAL OR HOSPITALIZATION

Hospitalization may be indicated if the patient is unable to maintain hydration, is hemodynamically unstable, or has a suspected infection that can lead to rapid clinical deterioration, such as endocarditis, necrotizing fasciitis, or bacterial meningitis.

PATIENT AND FAMILY EDUCATION

Patients should be advised to call the health care provider for temperature that is higher than 38.6° C (101.5° F) for more than 24 hours. Immunosuppressed patients, including those with acquired immunodeficiency syndrome (AIDS) and those taking chemotherapeutic drugs, should be brought to medical attention if they have a temperature above 37.8° C (100° F). Parents should be especially cautioned against the use of aspirin in their febrile children because of risk of Reye's syndrome.[3]

CHAPTER 225

IMMUNODEFICIENCY

Nancy B. Kuemmerle

DEFINITION AND EPIDEMIOLOGY

Our immune system is the result of millions of years of evolution all leading to one overarching goal: to protect us from our environment. When working properly, immunity enables us to conduct all the normal affairs of running the human body, such as taking in nutrients, breathing air potentially contaminated with microorganisms or pollutants, and eliminating organisms that could potentially do us harm. When immunity develops abnormally (primary or inherited immunodeficiency) or later becomes compromised by any mechanism (secondary or acquired immunodeficiency), the result can prove catastrophic for the affected individual.

One need only recall the images of David Vetter, also known as the Bubble Boy, who lived with severe combined immunodeficiency disease (SCID) for almost all of his 12 years in a sterile enclosure, to understand the precarious situation caused by lack of a functional immune system. Fortunately, conditions such as David Vetter's are uncommon, probably affecting fewer than 1 in 100,000 live births, although the exact incidence is unknown.[1] More common primary immunodeficiencies, such as isolated immunoglobulin (Ig) A deficiency, can affect 1 in 500 to 1 in 300 individuals.[2] All told, immunodeficiency is seen in around 1 in 1200 live births in the United States; of these individuals, about 1 in 2000 are diagnosed before the age of 18.[1,2] More than 180 primary immunodeficiencies have been described since Colonel Ogden Bruton first discovered agammaglobulinemia in 1952.[2,3]

Acquired immunodeficiencies tend to be more common than inherited forms, and even the newest health care practitioner understands the toll that human immunodeficiency virus (HIV) and acquired immunodeficiency syndrome (AIDS), the most common secondary immunodeficiency in the United States, can take on patients, families, and the health care system. Acquired immunodeficiency is discussed in Chapter 230 and is not covered in detail here.

In general, whether inherited or acquired, most immunodeficiencies manifest as an unusual susceptibility to infection. The complications of immunodeficiency include, in addition to infection, autoimmune processes, unregulated inflammation, malignancies, and the complications of pharmacologic or other therapeutic interventions.[4] The type of infection can often provide a clue to the underlying mechanism of disease and to its potential treatment.[5] Although recurrent infections can frequently be masked with antibiotics, other allergic or autoimmune symptoms can also be clues that the patient may have an underlying deficiency. Consultation with an allergist or clinical immunologist is indicated for all patients with suspected immunodeficiency disorders.

PATHOPHYSIOLOGY

Primary immunodeficiencies are by definition congenital, and many arise from single-gene defects, although others come under the influence of multiple genes. As more is learned about the processing and maturation of cells of the immune system, it becomes apparent that mutations in any of a number of genes along a specific pathway can effect an immunodeficiency.[6] Immunodeficiencies can be linked to sex chromosomes, or they can be caused by mutations in somatic genes, in which case they are usually recessive; however, germline mutations can also be dominant acting.[6] Most appear by the age of 6 years, but milder forms may never cause enough morbidity to facilitate diagnosis or are discovered serendipitously.

Understanding how the immune system is structured can provide clues to the underlying mechanisms of a suspected immunodeficiency as well as allow its classification. The immune system is composed of two main divisions. The innate immune system is the section that provides nonspecific defense. Examples of innate immunity include physical barriers such as intact skin and mucus in the lungs, which block entry of harmful bacteria, viruses, and fungi; immune cells (macrophages, neutrophils), which recognize and target primitive protein sequences common to most nonself organisms; and finally protein components (such as complement or cytokines), which circulate throughout the blood, ready to latch onto foreign proteins. Whether a lowly snail or a sprinting cheetah, all living organisms, including humans, possess some of these innate tactics for fighting off the environment.

The adaptive immune system, on the other hand, is an evolutionary advance that we share only with fellow vertebrates. Here, foreign proteins (antigens) are recognized and processed by immune effector cells. This process, called immune priming, induces changes in the development and maturation of other cells (B and T cells), which then specifically target subsequent invaders for destruction. The respective cell lines produce antigen-specific antibodies (through B cells, or humoral immunity) or target the antigen for cell-mediated destruction (through T cells, or cell-mediated immunity).

Both these divisions are complex and are further regulated by added levels of intricacy. Failure of just one protein in one pathway can subsequently lead to partial or total deficiency of immune function. This is the pathophysiologic underpinning of immunodeficiency. Deficiencies in the innate immune system include barrier disorders (such as cystic fibrosis), neutrophil or phagocyte defects, and complement deficiencies. Disorders of the adaptive immune system usually manifest as B- or T-cell defects, antibody deficiencies, or SCIDs.

Relative frequencies of various immune disorders can also help guide diagnosis. The most common disorders are antibody deficiencies (50%), followed by combined B- and T-cell deficiencies (20%), phagocytic defects (18%), cellular defects (10%), and complement deficiencies (2%).[7]

CLINICAL PRESENTATION

Immunodeficient patients are usually vulnerable to repeated, chronic, or unusual infections. Findings suggestive of immune dysfunction include the following[8]:

- Recurrent, unusual, or difficult-to-treat infections
- Poor growth or loss of weight
- Recurrent pneumonia, ear infections, or sinusitis
- Multiple courses of antibiotics, or intravenous antibiotics necessary to clear infections
- Recurrent deep abscesses of the organs or skin
- A family history of primary immunodeficiency disease (PIDD)
- Swollen lymph glands or an enlarged spleen

In addition, serious or repeated infections with normally nonpathogenic organisms are a clue that immune dysfunction is a consideration.

Knowing how the immune system is organized and how shortages of its various components will manifest clinically can often provide clues to the health care practitioner of an immunodeficiency. For example, recurrent sinopulmonary infections with encapsulated bacteria such as *Streptococcus, Staphylococcus,* or *Haemophilus* organisms can be suggestive of an antibody deficiency or B-cell disturbance because humoral immunity is generally responsible for dispatching these types of pathogens. However, wide use of antibiotics can mask or cloud the diagnosis of a specific immunodeficiency. Thus it is sometimes important to watch for common associations seen in these diseases. Common related conditions include chronic diarrhea, eczema, hepatosplenomegaly, hematologic disorders, autoimmune diseases, and failure to thrive in infants and children.

An example is Wiskott-Aldrich syndrome (WAS), which like other humoral deficiencies, is characterized by recurrent infections with pneumococci. WAS is also associated with platelet maturation anomalies through the underlying genetic defect and thus could manifest with prolonged bleeding, easy bruising, and eczema. There is also a tendency in WAS for later development of T-cell anomalies.

Primary T-cell disorders manifest as unusual sensitivity to viruses, fungi, some parasites, and other bacteria that are the targets of this class of cell. Common T-cell mutations can affect the manner in which T cells mature or become activated. However, cell-to-cell communication can also be impaired—that is, there can be defects in their receptors or cytokines.

Even more severe are combined immunodeficiency disorders (CIDs) or SCIDs, which may knock out multiple immune cell pathways, usually as the result of an enzyme or early maturation defect. Both B- and T-cell lines can be affected, leading to early and devastating infections. Without prompt recognition and subsequent treatment with bone marrow transplantation or, more recently, gene therapy, these children's lives are usually measured in days to months rather than years.

Secondary immunodeficiencies are acquired or associated with underlying disorders and are not caused by intrinsic abnormalities in the development and function of the immune system. HIV and malnutrition are the most common causes of secondary immunodeficiency.[8] Other causes include malignant disease, immunosuppressive agents, and systemic inflammatory diseases such as rheumatoid arthritis and systemic lupus erythematosus.[9] Obesity may also compromise the pathways of immune surveillance.[10] There is some decrease in immunity that occurs with normal aging. Fewer T cells are produced; therefore, fewer are available to respond. Of course, malnutrition, common in the older adult, impairs immune responses.[8] Secondary immunodeficiencies must be considered in the differential diagnosis of patients with multiple or recurrent infections.

PHYSICAL EXAMINATION

A careful history usually provides evidence that identifies the nature of the immune system defect. The history should include a detailed description of infections, including age at onset, sites, patterns of recurrence, response to treatment, and pathogens if known. More severe immunodeficiency disorders such as SCID, characterized by deficits in both B and T cells, can manifest with life-threatening infections in the first few weeks of life.[2] Associated symptoms such as eczema, diarrhea, and arthritis should be noted. Risk factors for HIV should be assessed. A history of weight loss, enlarged lymph nodes, night sweats, fever, ecchymosis, pruritus, or epistaxis should be obtained. The past medical history should determine childhood illnesses, including developmental delay or failure to thrive, recurrent infections, autoimmune diseases, cancer, and history of splenectomy. A family history of unexplained death from infection may be significant. The patient's immunization history and response to immunizations should be assessed. A history of normal response to smallpox vaccination or contact dermatitis from poison ivy suggests an intact cellular immunity.

A complete physical examination should be performed with the goal of identifying the site and source of infection and any chronic indicators of immune dysfunction. It is important to review the growth parameters, such as height and weight, because failure to thrive is one of the more common features of adaptive immunodeficiency. Findings of ocular telangiectasia, tympanic membrane scarring, tonsillar absence, lymphadenopathy, periodontitis, dental erosions, gingivostomatitis, mucocutaneous candidiasis, eczema, vitiligo, oculocutaneous albinism, hepatosplenomegaly, clubbing or fungal infections of the nails, petechiae, and pallor can be associated with various immunodeficient states.[5,7] Also, the tendency for immunodeficiency to be part of other congenital syndromes should cause the practitioner to look for body dysmorphisms. Examples of these include micrognathia, short philtrum, and ear abnormalities seen with DiGeorge syndrome; short-limbed dwarfism associated with some T-cell disorders; and prominent forehead, deep-set eyes, broad nasal bridge, and prognathism associated with hyperimmunoglobulinemia E syndrome.[8] A full neurologic examination should also be performed. Broad-based gait in a young child could be the first sign of ataxia-telangiectasia before immunodeficiency becomes apparent.[11]

DIAGNOSTICS

When an immunodeficiency disorder is suspected, initial laboratory work should include studies that are broadly informative, readily available, and cost-effective. A complete blood count (CBC) with differential is important for detection of neutropenia and relative levels of various leukocytes. A peripheral smear should be done concurrently to look for abnormal cell morphologies. These can help exclude neutropenia and lymphopenia. Thrombocytopenia can be consistent with WAS. Metabolic profiles can be helpful to exclude potential immune-modulating diseases such as diabetes mellitus. HIV testing should be performed. When possible, it is important to identify all organisms infecting the patient. To this end, blood, urine, sputum, and wound cultures as well as consultation with a serologist can be helpful. An erythrocyte sedimentation rate (ESR) and C-reactive protein level should be assessed for evidence of inflammation or lack thereof. Pulmonary function tests (PFTs) should be considered when the patient's symptoms have a chronic respiratory component because immunodeficiencies can alter lung function over time.

Immune testing should also begin broadly, but clinical symptoms can help guide which tests are ordered. Primary health care practitioners should obtain quantitative serum immunoglobulins as part of the initial screening because antibody disorders are the most common immunodeficiencies.

Other specialized immune testing can be ordered and performed by the clinical immunologist. This includes examination of antibody production (e.g., IgE levels, antibody responses to protein or polysaccharide antigens, isohemagglutinins, IgG subclasses), T cells (functional assessment, quantification of T-cell subtypes), phagocytic function (nitroblue tetrazolium test, flow cytometry for diseased cell markers such as CD18), and complement deficiencies (complement levels C3, C4, CH50).[5,7,12,13] Checking of sweat chloride and cystic fibrosis transmembrane regulator gene assays can help exclude cystic fibrosis. Further evaluations, including enzyme measurements, genetic and chromosomal studies, chemotaxis assays, and surgical biopsies (e.g., lymph nodes, colon) may also be considered by the clinical immunologist.[7]

Delayed-type hypersensitivity (DTH) skin testing is a common test of T-cell function, and positive reactions to common antigens such as *Candida* organisms, tetanus, and mumps can help rule out T-cell disorders in 85% of adults.[7] There is more controversy in the use of DTH testing in infants and young children, who have not yet developed an exposure history adequate enough to turn a skin test result positive. Although some practitioners perform skin testing in children, there seems to be no usefulness in testing children younger than 1 year.

DIAGNOSTICS

Immunodeficiency

LABORATORY	OTHER DIAGNOSTICS
CBC and differential	Nitroblue tetrazolium test*
ESR	Skin testing (mumps)
Serology and cultures	QuantiFERON or purified protein derivative (PPD)
HIV	PFTs*
Qualitative immunoglobulin panel	
CH50	
Fasting glucose	
C-reactive protein	
Quantitative immunoglobulins	

*If indicated.

DIFFERENTIAL DIAGNOSIS

The differential diagnosis should include primary and secondary causes of immune dysfunction. Both B- and T-cell deficiencies can occur in association with secondary immunodeficiencies. Categories of secondary immunodeficiencies include infectious diseases (specifically HIV/AIDS), malignant neoplasms, immunosuppressive agents, malnutrition, hereditary metabolic defects, and chromosomal abnormalities. For newborns, practitioners should also consider congenital TORCH (toxoplasmosis, other infections, rubella, cytomegalovirus, or herpes simplex) infections.

MANAGEMENT

Immediate emergency department referral is indicated for fever greater than 38° C or 100.4° F or signs or symptoms of infection or infectious disease. Cultures should be obtained and broad-spectrum antibiotics started expeditiously.

There are two goals of treatment in providing care for a patient with a primary immunodeficiency: (1) to minimize the occurrence of infections and their impact on the overall health of the individual and (2) to replace the defective component of the immune system by passive transfer or transplantation when possible.[14-17]

- Immunodeficient patients should receive appropriate immunizations as recommended by the Centers for Disease Control and Prevention, with the exception of live vaccines.[18,19]
- They should receive antibiotic and antifungal prophylaxis.
- Patients with CIDs or SCIDs or B-cell disorders, and sometimes those with innate disorders, should receive immunoglobulin monitoring and replacement on a regular basis.
- CID or SCID patients, in particular, need prompt and aggressive management of infections.
- Patients with chronic granulomatous disease require cytokine replacement (e.g., interferon-γ [IFN-γ]).
- Some patients may need support with growth factors (e.g., granulocyte-macrophage colony-stimulating factor [GM-CSF]).
- In general, patients with immunodeficiencies need to be monitored for malignancy and comorbidities.

DIAGNOSIS

Immunodeficiency[12]

Replacement of defective immune components can be achieved by a variety of means, depending on the component in question. These include administration of exogenous immunoglobulins, cytokine therapy, enzyme replacement, plasma infusion, growth factors, and reconstitution of stem cells by transplantation or gene therapy (Box 225-1).

Intravenous immune globulin (IVIG) and subcutaneous IgG are used in a variety of humoral and cellular deficiencies, including X-linked agammaglobulinemia, common variable immunodeficiency (CVID), hyper-IgM syndrome, WAS, and SCID.[8,14,16,17] The rationale for this treatment is to replace absent or dysfunctional antibodies with normal components. There is long-standing evidence to show that this treatment can be helpful in the aforementioned conditions.[16,17] The use of IVIG in patients with IgA deficiency and some forms of CVID (those

BOX 225-1

Causes of Immunodeficiency

PRIMARY
- Congenital

SECONDARY
- Malignant neoplasms
- Immunosuppressive agents
- Malnutrition
- Infectious diseases

without detectable IgA) is complicated by the fact that some of these patients' IgA deficits are caused by the presence of anti-IgA antibodies. Because IVIG can contain trace amounts of both IgA and IgM, giving a patient with these autoantibodies a large infusion of IVIG could cause anaphylaxis. Accordingly, testing to identify the presence of anti-IgA antibodies can be done and special preparations of IVIG without IgA obtained.[7,15]

Administration of IVIG is usually initiated at 200 to 800 mg/kg per month and then subsequently titrated monthly based on trough levels. Trough levels are drawn after 4 weeks of treatment, and the recommended goal is to keep trough levels above 500 mg/dL.[5,7] There is some evidence to suggest that keeping trough levels above 600 mg/dL can be beneficial.[5] Adverse reactions to IVIG often occur on or near the infusion day and may be ameliorated by slowing of the infusion rate, attempting to control any concurrent infections, or switching manufacturers.[5,7] Common reactions include fever, chills, nausea, emesis, and myalgias. Uncommon and more severe adverse effects consist of anaphylactic symptoms of hypotension, respiratory distress, and flushing. These constitute a medical emergency and require immediate evaluation and resuscitation. If anaphylaxis occurs and the patient absolutely needs this replacement, the clinical immunologist may consider slow infusions with the subcutaneous form of the drug and pretreatment with diphenhydramine, acetaminophen, and/or corticosteroids.

The definitive treatment of SCID or CID is reconstitution of stem cells by stem cell transplantation (SCT) or gene therapy.[8,16,17] Pluripotent stem cells have the ability to become any leukocyte within the white blood cell milieu. By infusing these healthy predecessor cells after native cells have been destroyed by chemotherapeutic means, the practitioner should be able to completely replace diseased cells with healthy ones. SCT has been successful in stem cell deficiencies, almost all SCIDs, and a variety of other conditions, such as DiGeorge syndrome, leukocyte adhesion deficiency, and WAS.[13,16,17] SCT is most successful when HLA-identical sibling bone marrow donors are used. The adverse effects of the SCT process are numerous and primarily related to effects of conditioning chemotherapy and/or graft-versus-host disease.[16,17]

Gene therapy has been shown to reconstitute functionality to native immune cells in two SCIDs, common gamma-chain deficiency and adenosine deaminase (ADA) deficiency.[20] Briefly, copies of healthy genes are added to delivery vectors that insert the healthy gene into diseased cells, thereby using the cell's own machinery to then produce normal gene products. Although gene therapy holds promise, these techniques are still in the early stage. Given that several of the patients with ADA deficiency treated with gene therapy have later developed lymphoma, some further modifications are probably needed before this treatment could become widely available.[21]

Other modalities of immune function replacement are tailored to the specific pathophysiologic mechanism of each disease. Apart from SCT, patients with DiGeorge syndrome can also be treated with the thymic hormone thymosin or with transplantation of fetal thymic tissue with the goal of restoring T-cell function. ADA deficiency has also been treated with replacement of the ADA enzyme by use of a polyethylene glycol formulation.[7] Complement deficiencies can be treated with blood factor–rich fresh-frozen plasma. Replacement with the cytokine IFN-γ is used to treat patients with chronic granulomatous disease.[7] Progenitor cell growth factors such as GM-CSF are used to stimulate white blood cell proliferation in the presence of neutropenia.

LIFE SPAN CONSIDERATIONS

Some immunodeficiencies are mild and may even go unnoticed throughout a person's life. Such can be the case with isolated IgA deficiency, which affects 1 in 500 Americans and at one end of the spectrum can be asymptomatic. Approximately two thirds of immunodeficient patients will live to adulthood. However, many will have a shortened life span because of their disease. Death can result from overwhelming infections, chronic stigmata, or complications of the disease and some of the treatment modalities themselves. Frank discussion with patients and their families are important to help them anticipate potential deterioration of health, and the use of community or mental health resources can be helpful for patients and their families.

COMPLICATIONS

Complications associated with immunodeficiency or its management depend on the specific disease entity. In general, the complications of poorly controlled chronic or recurrent infections are common (e.g., bronchiectasis with recurrent pulmonary infections). Some patients' diseases have a tendency to worsen over time. Some patients may even be at greater risk for malignant or autoimmune diseases. For example, patients with CVID are at greater risk for development of lymphoma. Complications can also occur secondary to treatment.

INDICATIONS FOR REFERRAL

All patients should be referred to a clinical immunologist when the diagnosis of an immunodeficiency disorder is suspected, unless that disorder is already know to be secondary, and thus other specialists may be better suited to caring for the patient. For example, AIDS/HIV patients are now often cared for by infectious disease consultants or specialists in HIV medicine.

Once a definitive diagnosis of primary immunodeficiency is made and the care plan is developed by the clinical immunologist, the patient can be monitored in a collaborative fashion. Infections can be diagnosed and managed by the primary care practitioner. Patients should be closely monitored for the development of autoimmune diseases and malignant neoplasms. The majority of malignant neoplasms are seen in patients with ataxia-telangiectasia, WAS, and CVID.[16] Those requiring specialized therapy, such as immunoglobulin replacement therapy, bone marrow transplantation, or SCT, should receive this care under supervision of a clinical immunologist. Relatives of affected individuals should be referred for genetic testing and counseling as appropriate. It is especially important to screen for carrier status all female relatives of patients with X-linked disorders and both parents of a patient suspected to have an autosomal recessive inheritance pattern. Intrauterine diagnosis of some primary immunodeficiencies is possible for those with known familial disorders.[12]

PATIENT INFORMATION AND HEALTH PROMOTION

Patients with primary immunodeficiency disorders should understand the importance of avoiding contact with individuals with known contagious diseases, and they should be able to identify and report signs and symptoms of infection. It is essential that these patients seek care at the first sign of infection. Good personal hygiene and adaptation of health behaviors such as regular exercise and stress management should be recommended to promote good health and support immune function. Social service providers can help with affordability issues, and national organizations such as the Immune Deficiency Foundation (www.primaryimmune.org) and the Jeffrey Modell Foundation (http://www.info4pi.org/) can provide specific educational and support materials to patients, families, and practitioners.

Patients with congenital immunodeficiencies should have current childhood, adolescent, and adult vaccinations as recommended by the National Immunization Program of the Centers for Disease Control and Prevention.[18,19] Recommendations in the 2014 guidelines were as follows. Infants and children should be vaccinated for tetanus (DTaP), polio (IPV), *Haemophilus influenzae* (Hib), pneumococcus (PCV7), pneumococcus (PPV23), and hepatitis A (if indicated). The recommendations for adults are similar, with the addition of hepatitis B if indicated. Anthrax, polio (IPV), rabies, and inactivated typhoid can be used if indicated. In general, live attenuated vaccines (BCG, influenza LAIV, typhoid Ty21a, vaccinia, MMR, Zostavax, and yellow fever) are contraindicated because of the risk of vaccine-induced infection. There are two exceptions to this recommendation. First, the live attenuated form of the influenza vaccine (LAIV) cannot be used, but the inactivated form can be given to adults and children with primary immunodeficiency. Second, varicella vaccine is contraindicated in patients with T-cell involvement, but patients with humoral deficiency may be given the vaccine. For current guidelines, practitioners should check with their local or national health agency in charge of vaccine recommendations.

Practitioners should also keep in mind that the impairment in antibody responses seen in patients with humoral immunodeficiencies can make it difficult or impossible to achieve full protection by vaccination, even after repeated inoculations.[22] Even T-cell disorders, whether occurring alone or mixed with B-cell abnormalities, may not respond to vaccination.

Transfusions of whole blood are contraindicated in immunodeficient patients because the donor blood my contain lymphocytes that could induce a graft-versus-host rejection. Appropriate preparation of blood products before transfusion should include means such as irradiation to minimize the risk of infection, especially with viruses such as cytomegalovirus and the hepatitides.

The use of surgical treatments for immunodeficient patients is by and large controversial and untested. In general, there are no indications for tonsillectomy, adenoidectomy, or splenectomy in these patients. In fact, these procedures should be limited to certain circumstances, such as to control bleeding secondary to WAS-induced thrombocytopenia. Some proponents have recommended tympanostomy tube placement for those with recurrent otitis, but evidence is lacking on whether this provides significant advantage for this population. Further studies with regard to surgical interventions are needed.

CHAPTER 226

LYMPHADENOPATHY

Michelle Freshman

DEFINITION AND EPIDEMIOLOGY

Lymphadenopathy refers to lymph nodes that have enlarged or changed in consistency. Lymph nodes typically vary from 0.5 to 2.5 cm (⅕ to 1 inch) in diameter, averaging about 1 cm,[1] and are characterized by number, size, shape, texture, mobility, tenderness, and surrounding skin involvement. Three quarters of patients with enlarged lymph nodes have localized findings, half of which are in the head and neck.[1] Nodes located above the clavicles account for the largest palpable field; axillary and inguinal regions represent far fewer. Three or more noncontiguous groups of node enlargements constitute generalized lymphadenopathy. Lymphadenitis is defined as tender, warm, erythematous nodes, and suppurative lymphadenitis includes fluctuance.

On routine physical examination, generalized lymphadenopathy is a common incidental finding. A community-based sample of 2556 Dutch respondents revealed that 0.6% had unexplained lymphadenopathy, three quarters of which was localized and treated without further workup.[2] Whereas the majority of neck masses in younger patients are associated with infection and are self-resolving, congenital malformations and neoplasms manifest similarly. Nodes vary in size depending on location. Epitrochlear nodes larger than 0.5 cm or inguinal nodes larger than 1.5 cm are thought to be aberrant; nodes larger than 2 cm warrant prompt investigation, although most are infectious.[1] However, these enlargements become more suspicious in older patients. Malignant disease has been reported to occur in less than 1% of primary care cases of unexplained lymphadenopathy.[1] The commonly cited "rule of 80s" refers to patients older than 40 years who are seen with a neck mass: 80% of all nonthyroid neck masses are malignant, and 80% of those are metastatic. Among asymptomatic cervical lumps, about 12% are head and neck cancer cases, and of these cancers, approximately 80% are squamous cell carcinoma.[1] Diffuse lymphadenopathy in at-risk individuals of any age should prompt consideration of human immunodeficiency virus (HIV) infection (see Chapter 230).

PATHOPHYSIOLOGY

The lymph nodes are integral to the lymphatic drainage system and provide filtration of foreign substances through the action of lymphocytes, monocytes, and macrophages. Lymph fluid intermediates between blood and tissue. Lymph nodes are located in clusters around the lymphatic veins, where excess interstitial fluid is accumulated, processed, and returned to the bloodstream. The role of the lymphatic system in maintaining fluid balance, processing lipids and fat-soluble substances from intestinal lymph, and serving as a host defense has been a focus of therapeutic interest.[3,4]

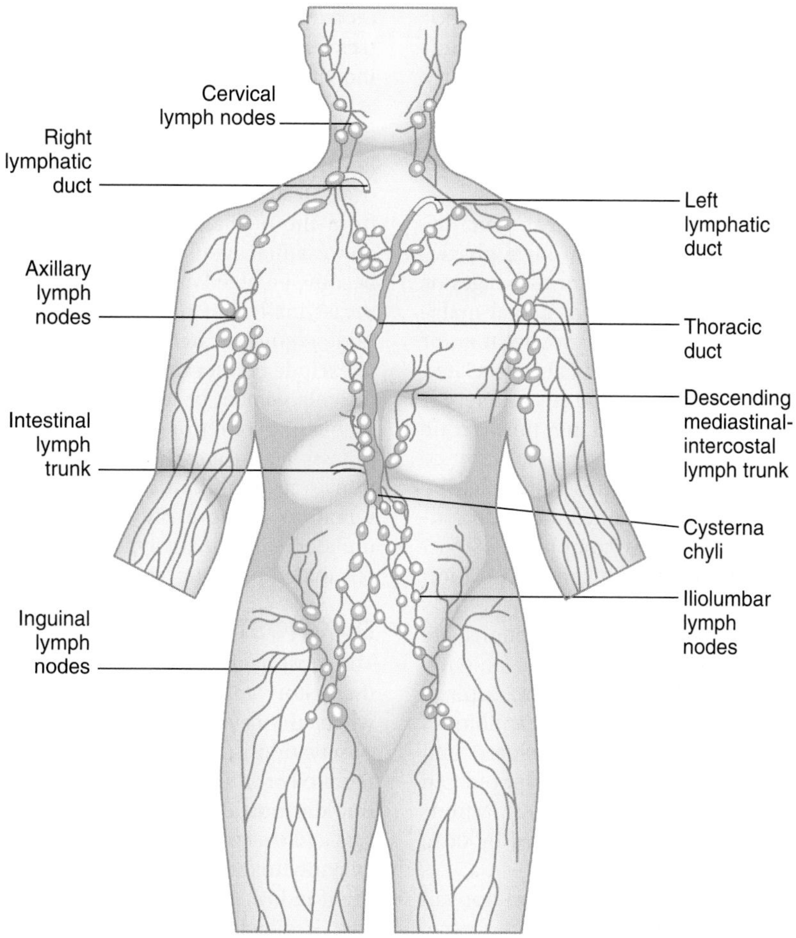

FIGURE 226-1 Major anatomic pathways and lymph node groups of the lymphatic system. (From Townsend CM Jr, Beauchamp RD, Evers BM, Mattox KL: *Sabiston textbook of surgery,* ed 18, St Louis, 2007, Elsevier.)

More than 600 lymph nodes exist in the human body. Tonsils, adenoids, the spleen, thymus, and Peyer patches of the ileum are also involved in immune surveillance and activation. The lymphatic system is made up of head and neck (internal and external drainage), supraclavicular, deltopectoral, axillary, epitrochlear, inguinal, and popliteal regions (Figure 226-1).

Because development of the lymphatic system is linked to venous development, the lymphatic ducts run along venous tracts. Lymph fluid ultimately reaches one of two large ducts in the thorax. The right lymphatic duct drains lymph from the right upper body—mediastinum, lungs, and esophagus—and into the right supraclavicular vein; the thoracic duct drains lymph from the rest of the body, including the abdominal cavity (stomach, gallbladder, and pancreas) and urogenital organs, into the left supraclavicular vein.

Lymph nodes swell in response to antigens. Afferent vessels carry the antigen-laden lymph fluid into the sinus of the node; efferent vessels carry the immune-mediated fluid away. Nodal swelling is caused by the proliferation of monocytes (the precursors to macrophages). Along with the lymph nodes, other lymphoid organ tissues—including the bone marrow, tonsils and adenoids, and spleen—may become disturbed or enlarged in the presence of antigen. Splenomegaly associated with lymphadenopathy may reflect lymphocytosis generated by infection, various types of immune hyperplasia, macrophage proliferation, or a tumor. Generalized lymphadenopathy may indicate systemic disease or malignant disease because the lymph system can be infiltrated by malignant cells and other cells not normally present in the nodes. Researchers suspect that if malignant cells were prevented from entering the lymphatic system or if their microenvironment were disrupted, lymph-based cancer cells might not circulate and metastasize.[3,5]

In summary, lymph nodes enlarge as a result of allergy or hypersensitivity to drug or environmental pollutants, tissue injury, autoimmune disease, infection, lymphoproliferative or myeloid abnormalities of bone marrow, and other malignancies or solid tumors.

CLINICAL PRESENTATION

Key factors to consider in the evaluation of the patient with lymphadenopathy are the age of the patient, the location of the swollen glands, and any associated symptoms.

A thorough symptom analysis should reveal infectious contacts or exposures (e.g., deer ticks, bird droppings, and cat or rat feces), foreign travel, travel to endemic infectious areas, or foreign birth. Patients should be asked about possible occupational exposure to chemicals, livestock, asbestos, silica (silicon dioxide), or beryllium. Sexual behaviors should be noted. Patients should also be asked about past medical or surgical history of abdominal, thoracic, breast, head and neck, pelvic, reproductive organ, or lower extremity malignant neoplasms including those associated with acquired immunodeficiency syndrome (AIDS), surgery, or injury; implanted silicone products (e.g., breast) or prosthetics; tattoo dyes; exposure to ultraviolet radiation; personal or family history of cancer, particularly lymphoma; irradiation; and chemotherapy.

A review of systems should include all areas of the skin for irregular or nonhealing lesions. A history of scalp pruritus (e.g., seborrheic dermatitis, scabies infection), conjunctivitis, eye pain, photophobia, visual complaints, unilateral ear pain, difficulty hearing, nose or throat pain or discharge, odynophagia, impaired swallowing, acidic food intolerance, vocal changes or persistent hoarseness, mastoid swelling or pain, dental maladies, dental malocclusion, facial paralysis, and muscle strain of the head or neck should be obtained elicited. Pain associated with the rapidly growing node is usually a good sign because it points to infection but may represent bleeding into the necrotic center of a malignant node.[6]

Breast changes, especially with axillary adenopathy, can be ominous. Lactation status should be ascertained. Gastrointestinal symptoms suggestive of malabsorption, complaints of diarrhea or constipation, or back pain with relief in the fetal position can suggest a malignant intra-abdominal process.

New medications as well as long-term prescriptions are worth reviewing for potential drug hypersensitivities. Drug hypersensitivity to phenytoin sodium, carbamazepine, aspirin, hydralazine (a lupus-like mimic), allopurinol, or antibiotics (including erythromycin, penicillin, and sulfa products) and serum sickness from vaccinations to smallpox or typhoid can result in generalized lymphadenopathy. Typically drug reactions produce generalized lymphadenopathy, accompanied by rash, fever, and joint pain.[1]

Inquiry into the incidence and frequency of blood transfusions, sexually transmitted diseases, smoked or chewed tobacco, and illegal drug or alcohol abuse is also necessary. Use of tobacco and alcohol together increases the risk of head and neck cancer substantially.

Any signs of external or internal bleeding, such as hemoptysis, hematuria, melena, or menorrhagia, should be pursued to exclude malignant disease.

PHYSICAL EXAMINATION

The history and location of the lymphadenopathy guide the physical examination (see Figure 226-1). Differentiation of normally palpable periauricular, cervical, axillary, and inguinal lymph nodes from enlarged nodes can be subtle.

The nodes should be characterized by size, distribution, degree of fluctuance, firmness, matted or shoddy quality, mobility or immobility, and tenderness or nontenderness. Unilateral or bilateral involvement, hard and fixed position, and symmetry or asymmetry may indicate or exclude malignant disease. Node characteristics, whether symptomatic or painful, may not initially reveal the diagnosis, even in cases of cancer.

A swollen node that is warm, tender, and rapidly enlarging may represent lymphadenitis and is suggestive of an infection at the drainage terminal. Lymphedema is an interruption of and blockage in drainage and may result from a variety of causes. Primary lymphedema refers to congenital malformations; secondary lymphedema refers to traumatic injury resulting from cancer obstruction, irradiation, recurrent infection, or surgery.

Evaluation of cervical nodes requires complete muscle relaxation and neutral positioning. Both anterior and posterior cervical node enlargement can indicate infection or carcinomas of the head or neck. The presence of posterior cervical adenopathy more often suggests an infectious cause. A supraclavicular node (sentinel node) can be elicited by the Valsalva maneuver in thin individuals. The Virchow node is the left supraclavicular node, at the base of most of the body's lymphatic drainage via the thoracic duct; an enlarged one poses significant concern for malignant disease of the stomach, gallbladder, kidney, pancreas, ovary, testes, or prostate. The right supraclavicular node drains from the mediastinum, lungs, and esophagus. Axillary nodes are terminal lymph drains for the upper extremities and can become enlarged as a result of cellulitis of the arm or hand or breast malignant neoplasms. Women with a positive axillary node require a careful breast examination and mammography to exclude breast cancer. Liver and spleen examinations looking for enlargement or tenderness are essential.

Inguinal or retroperitoneal nodes may be difficult to palpate unless they are grossly enlarged. Unilateral or bilateral presentation is an important consideration because the unilateral presentation is more often malignant. Men can be seen with unilateral malignant lymphedema of the leg in cases of disseminated prostate cancer.

DIAGNOSTICS

The most likely cause of lymphadenopathy is often revealed by the history and physical examination. However, in those cases where the cause is not evident, a period of 3 to 4 weeks of observation is recommended. Often during this time a cause is revealed or a direction for further investigation is apparent. Routine diagnostics to exclude infectious disease may lead the investigation: complete blood count (CBC) with differential and enzyme-linked immunosorbent assay or Western blot HIV testing if indicated by history. Further testing, which can be extensive, is directed by the results of initial screening and by the history and physical examination findings. The diagnostics box provides a comprehensive list of studies that may be ordered, usually in consultation with a specialist.

Splenomegaly with lymphadenopathy is an unusual and more ominous finding that might correlate with an abnormal CBC. Thyroid studies are warranted in suspected cases of thyroiditis, goiter, or carcinoma. Inguinal node enlargement most often has an infectious cause, and a host of sexually transmitted diseases would be part of the workup, including herpes simplex virus, gonorrhea, syphilis, chancroid, lymphogranuloma venereum, HIV, and reproductive organ cancers.

A chest radiograph is necessary to rule out tuberculosis (especially in HIV/AIDS patients or those born outside the United States), sarcoidosis, infection, and local or disseminated malignant disease. A mammogram is recommended when there is a persistent axillary node enlargement without other explanation. Ultrasound is thought to be a necessary tool to assess cervicofacial lymph nodes; in fact, it is considered superior to computed tomography (CT) scan in detecting small nodes and can differentiate between solid and less concerning cystic lesions.[7] CT, magnetic resonance imaging (MRI), and positron emission tomography (PET) may also contribute to diagnosis, biopsy precision, and tumor staging, particularly in the abdomen, pelvis, and chest.[1]

Biopsy should be considered when lymphadenopathy has persisted for more than 1 month without explanation or when malignant disease is suspected. The algorithms for selection of fine-needle aspiration cytology (FNAC) and high-tech imaging have become increasingly complex. Fine-needle aspiration (FNA) biopsy can be both highly sensitive and specific. Other

DIAGNOSTICS

Lymphadenopathy

LABORATORY

CBC and differential
Peripheral blood smear
Heterophil antibody (Monospot)*
HIV polymerase chain reaction (PCR)*
Herpesvirus PCR*
Varicella zoster virus PCR*
Rapid plasma reagin or Venereal Disease Research Laboratory (VDRL) testing*
Throat culture*
Nasal swab culture*
Purified protein derivative (PPD) or tuberculin skin test*
Sputum culture*
Liver function tests (LFTs)*
Hepatitis panel*
Epstein-Barr virus serology*
Rubella serology*
Cytomegalovirus PCR (urine, saliva culture or serology)*
Toxoplasma serology*
Histoplasma serology*
Cryptococcus serology*
Brucella serology*
Schistosoma serology*
Tularemia serology*
Trypanosoma serology, possible cerebrospinal fluid*
Typhoid fever blood culture*
Yersinia serology*
Lyme titer*
Urinalysis*
Blood urea nitrogen (BUN), creatinine*
Thyroid-stimulating hormone (TSH)*
Erythrocyte sedimentation rate (ESR)*
Antinuclear antibodies*
Rheumatoid factor*
Serum creatine kinase*
Monoclonal proteins in serum or urine*
Serum angiotensin-converting enzyme*
Serum complement level*
Immunoglobulins*

IMAGING

Chest x-ray examination*
Mammogram
CT scan*
Ultrasound*
Bone scan*
MRI*
F-18 fluorodeoxyglucose PET (^{18}F-FDG-PET)*

OTHER DIAGNOSTICS

Cat-scratch disease *(Bartonella henselae)* and Sjögren syndrome: skin and lip biopsies*
FNA cytology*
Lymph node biopsy*
Lesion biopsy*
Bone marrow biopsy*
Dermatomyositis: muscle biopsy*
Electromyography*

*If indicated.

techniques include ultrasound-guided FNAC and endobronchial ultrasound-guided transbronchial needle aspiration for hilar lymphadenopathy or transesophageal ultrasound-guided FNAC. Core needle biopsy may be preferable to FNAC, if it can be guided by ultrasound or CT. Surgical biopsy rather than ultrasound guided FNAC, may help with suspected lymphomas of the head or neck, given the architectural complexity of those cancerous nodes.[8] Inguinal nodes have the lowest yield; supraclavicular nodes have the highest.[6] With a plethora of immunohistochemical staining, flow cytometry, cytogenetics, and molecular genetic techniques available, refined diagnosis and management is ever more possible, particularly of the hematologic malignancies. Laparoscopic lymph node biopsy is preferred to all percutaneous sampling.[6] Sentinel node biopsy with blue dye and radioisotope in breast cancer is considered indispensable. Typing, clinical staging, and initial management of leukemias (see Chapter 239), lymphomas (see Chapter 240), and solid tumors require a specialist.

DIFFERENTIAL DIAGNOSIS

The mnemonic *CHICAGO* (cancers, hypersensitivities, infections, connective tissue disease, atypical lymphoproliferative disorders, granulomatous lesions, and other unusual causes) can offer an efficient framework.[2] Drugs specifically known to produce lymphadenopathy are described earlier, although drug hypersensitivities may include others not commonly reported.

Most infectious processes that occur with lymphadenopathy last less than 2 weeks and, in younger patients, are likely to be a benign form of reactive lymphatic hyperplasia, histiocytosis. More troublesome is lymphadenopathy lasting longer than 2 weeks; however, enlarged lymph nodes lasting more than 1 year without a change in size are likely to be benign. Head and neck area lymphadenopathy coupled with a history of tobacco or alcohol use should suggest cancer if it is accompanied by hoarseness, hemoptysis, otalgia or hearing loss, facial nerve deficits, nasal obstruction or bleeding, throat pain or difficulty swallowing, or nonhealing ulcers. Squamous cell carcinoma and variants comprise over 90% of laryngeal cancers, which are most often associated with alcohol and tobacco exposure, which likewise places other exposed structures at risk for carcinoma.[9]

Parotid swelling, or less commonly salivary gland enlargement, might signal the onset of mumps, known to be more severe in adults and teens. Secondary to infection, a malignancy is the most common cause of a head or neck lymph node enlargement.[10]

The Virchow node, a pathologic left anterior supraclavicular node, portends an abdominal neoplasm; the right anterior supraclavicular node points to a thoracic neoplasm; the Delphian node, at the midline prelaryngeal level, is considered a sinister sign of thyroid or laryngeal cancer.[2,10] In patients older than 40 years, supraclavicular lymphadenopathy is likely to be cancerous in 90%; in patients younger than 40, the risk goes down to 25%.[1]

Axillary node enlargement suggests infection but may represent breast neoplasm, melanoma, Hodgkin disease, or non-Hodgkin lymphoma. Other axillary involvement may stem from an arm and hand infection or even a metastasized gastric cancer, known ominously as the Irish node.[10] A palpable epitrochlear node may signal an infection such as secondary syphilis, lepromatous leprosy, leishmaniasis, connective tissue disorder, lymphoma, or leukemia, especially if other nodes are involved.[5]

Hilar or mediastinal nodes seen on chest radiographs or CT scan may be calcified or not and can result from a host of infectious, autoimmune, neoplastic, or injurious causes. Careful review of past radiologic studies and judicious chemistry, hematology, and microbiology testing should lead to a working diagnosis before ordering of bronchoscopy and mediastinoscopy. Bacterial pneumonia; tuberculosis; sarcoidosis; fungal infections (histoplasmosis, coccidiomycosis) and other infections (pertussis); lymphoma; and lung, breast, and metastatic adenocarcinoma are among the more common culprits. Amyloidosis is less common. Distinction is made among single or bilateral or calcified hilar nodes.[10]

A Sister Mary Joseph node, seen bulging in the periumbilical region, may be a sign of intra-abdominal or pelvic malignancy. Inguinal lymph nodes run in horizontal and vertical clusters. Inguinal lymphadenopathy may be confused with hernia if large enough; vessel malformations; lipomas; or ectopic endometrial, testicular, or splenic tissue. The node of Cloquet is the femoral node below the inguinal ligament and is associated with anal, vulvar, and penile cancers, including melanoma.[10]

An asymptomatic unilateral node enlargement in the inguinal area suggests a malignant neoplasm or lymphoma, although sexually transmitted disease may be suspected based on patient history. Splenomegaly may corroborate infectious mononucleosis or one of the lymphomas or leukemias, especially with generalized lymphadenopathy. Fever, weight loss (10% in 6 months), night sweats, and pruritus—known as the B symptoms—are known to occur in both Hodgkin and non-Hodgkin lymphomas.

DIFFERENTIAL DIAGNOSIS

Lymphadenopathy

INFECTIOUS CAUSES
- Mononucleosis-type syndromes
- Epstein-Barr virus*
- Toxoplasmosis*
- Cytomegalovirus*
- Initial stages of HIV infection*
- Cat-scratch disease
- Pharyngitis caused by group A streptococci, gonococci
- Tuberculosis lymphadenitis*
- Secondary syphilis*
- Hepatitis B*
- Lymphogranuloma venereum
- Chancroid

AUTOIMMUNE AND ALLERGIC CAUSES
- Chronic fatigue syndrome
- Kawasaki disease
- Systemic lupus erythematosus*
- Serum sickness

MALIGNANT CAUSES OF LYMPHADENOPATHY
- Lymphoma*
- Myelodysplastic syndromes (including acute myelodysplastic leukemia)
- Leukemia*

LESS COMMON CAUSES
- Lyme disease*
- Measles*
- Rubella*
- Tularemia
- Brucellosis*
- Plague
- Typhoid fever*
- Still's disease*
- Dermatomyositis*
- Amyloidosis*

*Causes of generalized lymphadenopathy.

MANAGEMENT

Symptomatic treatment of viral infections and appropriate antibiotic therapy for bacterial, mycobacterial, fungal, parasitic, rickettsial, and chlamydial infections are indicated if the pathogen is known. Congenital or benign growths, such as lipomas or pilar cysts that have led to cervical adenopathy, can be surgically removed. Abscesses and other deep structure infections are treated in the hospital and may require surgery for drainage.

Autoimmune diseases are mostly managed in the outpatient setting, unless complications or late-stage developments require more complex care. Atypical lymphoproliferative disorders, whether clonal or polyclonal type, such as Castleman disease, lymphomatoid granulomatosis, and papulosis, have the potential to develop into cancer and bear watching with an eye toward biopsy. Evidence of malignancy requires referral to the appropriate specialist. Patients with lymphadenopathy of unclear cause also require physician consultation, although sometimes the tincture of time with close follow-up reveals the diagnosis. Corticosteroid or indiscriminate antibiotic use is not recommended, especially because this will confound biopsy results.

Interdisciplinary Management

Chronic autoimmune illnesses such as lupus erythematosus, Sjögren syndrome, rheumatoid arthritis, sarcoidosis, and HIV/AIDS may require specialty consultation and management. Because HIV infection has been associated with Kaposi sarcoma, Castleman disease, Hodgkin and non-Hodgkin disease, and multidrug-resistant tuberculosis, specialty practices may be more likely to identify these complications. Similarly, Sjögren syndrome has been associated with a high risk for non-Hodgkin lymphoma, often in the salivary gland (see Chapter 96). For patients with malignant neoplasms, continued primary care surveillance to monitor further physical and psychosocial complications is essential. Lymphadenopathy may follow prior cancer treatment or radiation therapy and suggest a recrudescence of disease. It is also important that patients receive drug level monitoring, counseling, and weight management guidance during chemotherapy (see Chapter 245). Fortunately, monoclonal antibodies coupled with radiation therapy have significantly improved head and neck cancer survival rates.

LIFE SPAN CONSIDERATIONS

Age is a most important consideration in evaluation of these patients. In patients younger than 40 years, lymphadenopathy is often benign. In individuals older than 40 years, lymphadenopathy can represent a malignancy more often.

Lymphoma diagnosed in later life represents a growing group of cancers on the rise, especially as the population ages and survives longer. Older patients diagnosed with life-threatening infections or malignant neoplasms may decline treatment, especially if they have comorbidities. Patients and their families will certainly need guidance and support through these difficult decisions (see Chapter 13).

COMPLICATIONS

Complications may arise as a result of the disease process or clinical management. Mistaken identification of a malignant node as benign can result in local or generalized metastasis. Untreated or inadequately treated group A β-hemolytic streptococcal infection may lead to rheumatic heart disease and glomerulonephritis. Complications related to prescribed drugs, especially antibiotics and chemotherapeutic agents, are common. Fortunately, the sensitivity and specificity of radiologic and immunohistologic and DNA specific testing continue to improve diagnostic speed and precision, including for those entities that may develop malignant features.

INDICATIONS FOR REFERRAL OR HOSPITALIZATION

- Patients with unusual infectious diseases (e.g., those resulting from foreign travel or communicable illnesses), cases of rare animal or environmental exposure, chronic inflammatory diseases, or a diagnosis of malignant disease should be referred to the appropriate specialists for guidance on the latest treatment protocols. The crucial decision point for health care providers is when to perform biopsy of a node for a definitive diagnosis.
- A referral to an otolaryngologist or general surgeon might precede a visit to the oncologist. Immunosuppressed patients with AIDS, malignant disease, or other illnesses may require hospitalization for intensive nutritional, anti-infective, and chemotherapeutic support.
- Rheumatology, nephrology, gastroenterology, pulmonary, or allergy specialists are essential to autoimmune disease management, with attention to associations with unusual lymphomas.
- Oncologists provide a critical role when malignancies are identified. They may collaborate with medical and radiology oncology colleagues and use a multidisciplinary approach to whole-patient care.

PATIENT AND FAMILY EDUCATION

Patients with lymphadenopathy need reassurance that many cases are benign and require only watchful waiting. Nodes that persist for more than 4 weeks require further investigation. Ongoing cancer screening for early cancer detection significantly increases the odds for survival. Patients and family should receive support for psychological distress that may result from personal and family-related role changes as well as hair loss and other cosmetic changes from chemotherapy. Advance directives are often most comfortably discussed with health care providers and communicated to the consultant. End-of-life care may be best managed at home with the help of the family, community volunteers, and hospice services.

HEALTH PROMOTION

Because a number of diseases resulting in lymph node enlargement in otherwise healthy adults are sexually transmitted, patients should be well informed of this health risk and strategies for prevention. Frank discussion with patients and instruction about condom use are essential in preventing sexually transmitted diseases. Cancer prevention strategies include eliminating all forms of tobacco, reducing alcohol consumption, and protecting skin from ultraviolet radiation and occupational hazards. Cancer screening tests should be recommended and completed on the recommended schedule. Health behaviors that fortify the immune system, such as proper nutrition, sleep, exercise, emotional support, and stress management, are most likely to promote health and to assist recovery. Patients are often able to find educational and social support in local or state chapters of national disease foundations (see Chapter 16).

CHAPTER 227

SLEEP DISORDERS

Glen P. Greenough • Brooke G. Judd

Sleep disorders are associated with major functional impairments, including loss of productivity, work-related and vehicular accidents, social impairment, and cognitive and mood disturbances, as well as morbidity and mortality as a result of cardiovascular, endocrine, and immune disturbances. Given the significance of these disorders, it is incumbent on primary care providers to recognize the symptoms of sleep disorders, to make accurate diagnoses, to initiate sound referrals, and to develop successful treatment plans in collaboration with sleep medicine specialists.

In this chapter, an overview of normal sleep is presented along with a description of the most common disorders of sleep. The most recent edition of the *International Classification of Sleep Disorders*[1] (ICSD) organizes the conditions into seven major categories: insomnias, sleep-related breathing disorders, central disorders of hypersomnolence (excessive sleepiness not related to other sleep disorders), circadian rhythm sleep-wake disorders, sleep-related movement disorders, parasomnias (abnormal behaviors or events arising from sleep), and other sleep disorders. These categories, which are largely symptom based (e.g., insomnia or hypersomnias), serve as a guide to obtaining a detailed history and initiating essential diagnostic procedures.

From a practical standpoint, fundamental assessment of sleep, which should be part of any complete patient history, can begin with three basic questions: How are you sleeping at night? Are you excessively sleepy during the daytime? Are there any unusual events or problems with your sleep, especially heavy snoring? More detailed aspects of assessment are included in individual sections within this chapter.

NORMAL SLEEP

DEFINITION AND PHYSIOLOGY

Sleep is an active, dynamic physiologic process. Normal human sleep consists of two major states of consciousness: non–rapid eye movement (NREM) sleep and rapid eye movement (REM) sleep. NREM sleep is further divided into three stages from lightest (N1) to deepest (N3, also referred to as slow-wave or delta sleep). These stages unfold in a predictable, repeated cycle. In young adults, NREM sleep occupies about 75% of the night and REM the remaining 25%. Delta sleep is most prominent in young children and gradually diminishes through the life cycle. REM sleep (or its ontogenetic precursor) is seen in very high percentages in neonates and infants but diminishes rapidly in the first years of life and remains fixed at about 25% thereafter. Normal total sleep time varies considerably with age.[2] Although young children require longer sleep times, total sleep time begins to decline by the second decade, remains relatively stable from the third decade through the fifth decade, and falls off more dramatically after the age of 70 years. It remains unclear to what extent the decline in nocturnal sleep in older individuals is a function of diminished sleep need as opposed to decreased ability to sleep. Time to fall asleep (sleep latency) and wake time after sleep onset are increased in older adults, as is daytime napping, although much of this may be related to factors that often accompany aging as opposed to the aging process itself.

NREM sleep is associated with a decline in respirations, heart rate, and blood pressure; muscle relaxation; and diminished cognitive activity. Sleep starts (sudden muscle contractions involving part or all of the body) may occur during wake-sleep transitions. REM sleep is marked by pronounced changes in physiology, including skeletal muscle atonia; increased variability in heart rate, blood pressure, respiration, and autonomic function; REM; and heightened cognitive activity associated with dreaming. Ventilatory drive to hypoxia and hypercapnia is decreased during NREM sleep and reaches its lowest point in REM sleep.

Current theories of sleep regulation focus on the two-process model.[3] This model suggests that sleep is regulated by two factors: homeostatic sleep drive, which increases progressively during wake time; and circadian wake drive, which is based on the oscillating 24-hour rhythm of the major circadian clock, located in the suprachiasmatic nucleus of the hypothalamus. Thus, the timing and amount of sleep are influenced by complex interactions between the biologic rhythms and the length of time since the last sleep period. Average human circadian cycles naturally run slightly longer than 24 hours (about 24.2 hours) but are reset daily (entrained) to a 24-hour rhythm by a variety of environmental cues, the most important of which is exposure to light. Sleep-wake rhythms are normally synchronized with myriad other clock-regulated physiologic functions, including endocrine-metabolic, immune, and cardiovascular.

INSOMNIA AND NONRESTORATIVE SLEEP

DEFINITION AND EPIDEMIOLOGY

Current epidemiologic data indicate that about 30% to 35% of individuals in Western society report at least occasional insomnia.[4] Multiple studies place the prevalence of chronic insomnia at about 10%.[4] Insomnia is a complex condition that may represent a final common pathway with numerous contributing factors. Acute or transient insomnia (days to a few weeks) is an almost universal problem that is typically related to an acute stress or time zone shift (i.e., jet lag) and is usually self-resolving. Good sleep hygiene and, for some patients, short-term sleep medications are usually adequate. A potential complication of short-term insomnia is that some patients will begin to exhibit cognitions and behaviors that establish a foundation for development of a chronic insomnia problem.

PATHOPHYSIOLOGY

A widely accepted model of chronic insomnia suggests that it is a function of predisposing, precipitating, and perpetuating factors. Little is known about predisposing biologic or psychological factors, although it does seem clear that certain persons are at greater risk than others for the development of a chronic insomnia problem. Precipitating factors (which are sometimes referred to as causes of chronic insomnia) are identified in Box 227-1 and are discussed in greater detail later.

BOX 227-1

Some Key Precipitants of Chronic Insomnia

PSYCHIATRIC DISORDERS

Adjustment disorders
Mood disorders
- Major depressive disorder
- Bipolar disorder
- Dysthymic disorder

Anxiety disorders
- Generalized anxiety disorder
- Post-traumatic stress disorder
- Panic disorder

Psychotic disorders
Personality disorders

SUBSTANCES AND MEDICATIONS

Alcohol
Stimulants
- Amphetamines, methylphenidate, modafinil, cocaine, ecstasy (MDMA, or 3,4-methylenedioxymethamphetamine), or caffeine
- Steroids
- Bronchodilators
- Some antihypertensives

Some antidepressants
Cholesterol-lowering agents

MEDICAL AND NEUROLOGIC DISORDERS

Degenerative neurologic diseases
Stroke
Recurrent nocturnal headache
Traumatic brain injury
Chronic obstructive pulmonary disease, nocturnal dyspnea, cough
Nocturnal angina
Gastroesophageal reflux disease, other nocturnal gastrointestinal disturbance
Pain from any source
Nocturia
Endocrine disorders

OTHER SLEEP DISORDERS

Obstructive or central sleep apnea
Restless legs syndrome, periodic limb movements
Nightmare disorder
Circadian rhythm disorders

A unifying concept in the pathophysiology of chronic insomnia is that of hyperarousal.[5] Data indicate that patients with this condition exhibit evidence of both physiologic and cognitive hyperarousal, in the form of increased 24-hour metabolic rate, increased temperature, muscle tension, sleep electroencephalogram frequency, overactivity of the hypothalamic-pituitary-adrenal axis, and cognitive activity. It remains unclear how this hyperarousal develops, although preliminary data suggest that it is, at least in part, acquired and is amenable to change with therapeutic interventions such as cognitive behavioral treatment.

CLINICAL PRESENTATION

Psychiatric disorders, especially major depression, are the most common precipitating factors. Generalized anxiety, panic, and post-traumatic stress disorders are also associated with elevated rates of insomnia. Substance abuse or dependence, including alcohol, sedative-hypnotics, stimulants, and opiates, frequently manifests with insomnia, which may persist even after discontinuation of the substance. Excessive use of caffeine or even moderate use later in the day may also be problematic.

Circadian disorders, especially shift work and delayed sleep-wake phase disorder, are commonly associated with sleep complaints. Significant percentages of night shift workers experience abnormal sleep, with reduced total sleep times and poor quality of sleep. This pattern does not tend to improve during long periods of night work for most shift workers. As a result of circadian misalignment and sleep disturbances, shift workers are at increased risk for a number of medical disorders (ulcer disease, breast cancer among female shift workers, and cardiovascular disease) as well as accidents. Delayed sleep-wake phase disorder occurs most commonly in adolescents and younger adults and is characterized by an inability to sleep at normal clock times, with normal sleep onset occurring late (e.g., 4 AM), and subsequent inability to arise at conventional times (e.g., noon awakening). Sleep is otherwise restorative and normal, but the schedule is clearly inconsistent with meeting of normal school or work times. Advanced sleep-wake phase disorder is a less common circadian rhythm disorder, with normal sleep quantity and quality occurring early in the 24-hour day (e.g., 7 PM to 3 AM). It appears to be most common in older adults.

Medical conditions and medications may contribute to sleep disturbance. Among the most common are those associated with nocturnal pain, chronic lung disease, end-stage organ failure, endocrine disorders and other metabolic conditions, and especially neurodegenerative diseases. Likewise, many medications may aggravate sleep, most notably steroids, methylxanthines, some antihypertensives, stimulants, and certain antidepressant medications.

Other physiologic sleep disorders may result in an insomnia problem. The patient with restless legs syndrome (RLS) reports distressing, "creepy-crawly" sensations in the legs or, less commonly, arms. The sensation is associated with an irresistible urge to move the extremities. The sensations may interfere with sleep onset. RLS is often associated with periodic limb movements (PLMs), which are characterized by repetitive, periodic (every 20 to 40 seconds) limb movements, often resulting in arousals that the sleeper is unaware of (much as in obstructive sleep apnea [OSA]). RLS is discussed in greater detail in the section on movement disorders.

Although OSA is most often associated with complaints of daytime sleepiness rather than with insomnia, these patients may have clinically significant complaints of insomnia. This association may be more prevalent among women with OSA. Therefore OSA must also be considered in the differential diagnosis, particularly in obese patients and those with heavy snoring.

The essential features of chronic insomnia according to the ICSD-3 are frequent and persistent difficulty initiating or maintaining sleep with a daytime consequence. An important subtype of chronic insomnia is psychophysiologic insomnia (PPI), a conditioned arousal in response to efforts to sleep and negative expectations regarding the ability to sleep. Individuals with PPI may be able to sleep better when they are not trying to fall asleep or in settings other than their own bedroom. Symptoms may include difficulty getting to sleep as well as trouble returning to sleep after awakening. This type of insomnia exists commonly as a disorder in its own right. However, the hyperarousal and negative conditioning that occur in this disorder are frequent complicating factors in insomnia that is associated with the numerous precipitating factors described earlier. Often, when an initial precipitating factor (e.g., a major depression, acute stress, or medical illness) resolves, it is these conditioned psychophysiologic elements that serve as the perpetuating factors noted earlier in this chapter.

DIAGNOSTICS

The essential element in the evaluation of an insomnia complaint is the history. The nature of the onset, course, complications, and treatments of the condition must be elicited in detail. Sleep-wake schedule, including napping, is critical to assessment. Sleep logs, usually conducted for 1 or 2 weeks, can be a helpful adjunct to history. The log should contain the following information for each night: time of getting into bed, time lights are actually turned out (e.g., after television, reading), estimate of sleep latency (time to fall asleep after lights out), estimate of the number of awakenings and total awake time across the night, time of final awakening, and time of actual arising. Evidence of other sleep-related symptoms (e.g., snoring and observed pauses in breathing, limb movement or restless legs, nightmares, behavioral disturbances, headaches, pain, gastroesophageal reflux) must be sought from the patient and, whenever possible, the bed partner. Daytime consequences, particularly evidence of significant sleepiness, should be assessed. Medical, neurologic, and psychiatric evaluations as well as pertinent physical examination and appropriate laboratory procedures are essential.

Polysomnography (PSG), overnight sleep recording, contributes little to the diagnosis of most insomnia presentations and is usually reserved for those cases in which demonstrable physiologic disturbances are suspected, typically breathing disorders, hypersomnias, and some parasomnias. PSG may also be appropriate for patients with treatment-refractory insomnia.

DIFFERENTIAL DIAGNOSIS

DIFFERENTIAL DIAGNOSIS

Insomnia

- Chronic insomnia disorder
- Excessive time in bed
- Circadian rhythm disorders (shift work, delayed or advanced sleep phase)
- Short sleeper
- Other primary sleep disorder (RLS, periodic limb movement disorder, sleep-related breathing disorder)
- Short-term insomnia disorder

MANAGEMENT

The management of insomnia begins with careful identification of the contributing factors. Treatment is tailored based on those factors. When clear precipitating causes are present (e.g., major depression or RLS), specific therapies appropriate to those factors must be instituted (e.g., antidepressant medication or dopamine agonists for RLS). Attention must also be directed to substances or medications that may be disturbing sleep. Sleep hygiene education is an essential component for management of any insomnia problem but is typically not sufficient treatment in its own right.

Treatment of circadian rhythm sleep disorders is often complex and in many cases is best administered by sleep medicine specialists. Bright light therapy and melatonin have demonstrated therapeutic benefit in certain patients with sleep-wake schedule disorders. Chronotherapy (planned behavioral adjustments of schedule) involving progressive phase delay has also been used for patients with delayed sleep phase disorder.

1. Once precipitating factors have been evaluated and treated, additional therapeutic approaches lie largely in the pharmacologic and behavioral realm.
2. The most commonly employed hypnotic medications are benzodiazepine receptor agonists, so called because they act selectively at the benzodiazepine receptor. This category includes standard benzodiazepines and newer agents such as zolpidem (Ambien), zaleplon (Sonata), and eszopiclone (Lunesta), which bind at the benzodiazepine receptor. In addition to the benzodiazepine receptor agonists, the very-short-acting melatonin agonist ramelteon (Rozerem) is approved for treatment of sleep initiation problems.
3. The benzodiazepine receptor agonists and ramelteon have comparable efficacy and, like the benzodiazepines themselves, differ primarily with respect to the clinical duration of action. Although hypnotic medications have been indicated only for short-term use until recently, emerging data have demonstrated safe and effective long-term use of some benzodiazepine receptor agonists, without dosage escalation or evidence of dependency in controlled settings.[6] However, a clear algorithm for long-term use of pharmacologic therapies and the interaction of these therapies with nonpharmacologic approaches has yet to be elucidated.
4. Cognitive behavioral therapy for chronic insomnia (CBT-I), particularly PPI, is brief and produces sustained benefit.[7] Compared with short-term courses of medication, CBT-I produces durable improvement, whereas improvements seen with time-limited courses of hypnotics tend to dissipate rapidly after drug discontinuation. Behavioral therapies include sleep restriction therapy, stimulus control, and relaxation training (Table 227-1). These therapies are often combined on a case-by-case basis. The common component of the most successful therapeutic approaches is marked reduction of the time spent in bed awake. In addition to the behavioral components, successful CBT regimens also include cognitive restructuring to identify and to alter the distorted cognitions that are often so much a part of the fabric of insomnia.
5. Access to CBT-I by skilled and experienced clinicians can be problematic, particularly in primary care settings outside of larger centers. Training in behavioral therapy for insomnia is available to primary care providers in brief continuing education courses, and a referral to a psychologist familiar with the use of these therapies should be readily available in most urban communities. Internet-based CBT-I programs are currently evolving and offer promise of delivery of this much-needed therapy to larger populations of patients.

TABLE 227-1 Common Behavioral Therapies for Chronic Insomnia

Sleep restriction	Maintain a sleep log and determine the mean TST for the baseline period (e.g., 1-2 wk). Set bedtime and wake-up times to approximate the mean TST to achieve >85% sleep efficiency (TST/TIB × 100%) during 7 days. The goal is for the total TIB (not <5 hours) to approximate the TST. Make weekly adjustments: 1. For sleep efficiency (TST/TIB × 100%) >85%-90%, TIB can be increased by 15-20 min. 2. For sleep efficiency <80%, TIB can be further decreased by 15-20 min. Repeat TIB adjustment every 7 days.
Stimulus control	Go to bed only when sleepy; maintain a regular schedule; avoid naps; use the bed only for sleep. If unable to fall asleep (or back to sleep) within 20 minutes, remove yourself from bed—engage in relaxing activity until drowsy, then return to bed; repeat this as necessary.
Relaxation therapy	Progressive muscle relaxation training involves methodical tensing and relaxing of different muscle groups throughout the body. Specific techniques are widely available in written and audio form.

TIB, time in bed; TST, total sleep time.

LIFE SPAN CONSIDERATIONS

Advanced sleep phase syndrome, which may lead to sleep maintenance issues, is most common in older adult populations.

COMPLICATIONS

Insomnia is associated with mood disorder.

INDICATIONS FOR REFERRAL AND HOSPITALIZATION

Patients with insomnia that is persistent and causing impairment in daytime activities should be referred to a sleep specialist.

PATIENT AND FAMILY EDUCATION

Tips for good sleep hygiene from the National Sleep Foundation (http://sleepfoundation.org/ask-the-expert/sleep-hygiene) are as follows:

- *Avoid napping during the day.* It can disturb the normal pattern of sleep and wakefulness.
- *Avoid stimulants such as caffeine, nicotine, and alcohol too close to bedtime.* Although alcohol is well known to speed the onset of sleep, it disrupts sleep in the second half as the body begins to metabolize the alcohol, causing arousal.
- *Exercise can promote good sleep.* Vigorous exercise should be taken in the morning or late afternoon. A relaxing exercise, such as yoga, can be done before bed to help initiate a restful night's sleep.
- *Food can be disruptive right before sleep.* Stay away from large meals close to bedtime. Also, dietary changes can cause sleep problems; if someone is struggling with a sleep problem, it is not a good time to start experimenting with spicy dishes. And, remember, chocolate contains caffeine.

- *Ensure adequate exposure to natural light.* This is particularly important for older people, who may not venture outside as frequently as children and adults. Light exposure helps maintain a healthy sleep-wake cycle.
- *Establish a regular relaxing bedtime routine.* Try to avoid emotionally upsetting conversations and activities before trying to go to sleep. Do not dwell on your problems or bring them to bed.
- *Associate your bed with sleep.* It is not a good idea to use your bed to watch TV, listen to the radio, or read.

SLEEP-RELATED BREATHING DISORDERS

DEFINITION AND EPIDEMIOLOGY

The sleep-related breathing disorders encompass a number of disorders, including the OSA disorders, central sleep apnea (CSA) syndromes, and the sleep-related hypoventilation disorders.

OSA is the most common sleep-related breathing disorder. Clinically significant OSA occurs in at least 2% to 4% of women and 4% to 10% of men in North America.[8] The predominant physiologic derangement in OSA is repetitive upper airway narrowing or closure, which occurs during sleep. The closures (or near-closures) can occur many times a night, leading to significant sleep fragmentation and poor-quality sleep.

CSA is less common than OSA, although increasingly recognized. The CSA syndromes are characterized by reduced or absent airflow because of decreased or absent respiratory effort. As with OSA, CSA events often recur many times a night and can be associated with sleep fragmentation and poor-quality sleep. Many patients have a combination of OSA and CSA.

PATHOPHYSIOLOGY

OSA is characterized by repetitive episodes of complete upper airway occlusions (known as apneas) or partial upper airway occlusions (known as hypopneas) during sleep. These partial or complete airway closures lead to increased efforts to breathe, finally terminating in a brief central nervous system (CNS) arousal from sleep to reestablish patency of the upper airway. These events are often, although not always, associated with transient reductions in blood oxygen saturation. The cause of the upper airway narrowing may be related to craniofacial structure predisposing to a narrowed airway, as well excessive soft tissue bulk impinging on upper airway (excessive fat deposition in the tongue, soft palate, and lateral pharyngeal walls). The airway is kept patent by the pharyngeal dilating muscles. The activity of these muscles decreases with sleep onset, although it is normally adequate to maintain patency of the airway. In patients with OSA, however, the activity of the pharyngeal dilator muscles during sleep is not adequate to maintain full patency, and partial or complete obstruction ensues. With each brief arousal, the muscle activity returns to wakefulness levels and patency is reestablished.

In CSA, the primary derangement is altered CNS respiratory drive, such that the patient does not receive the usual metabolic feedback to the CNS during sleep to drive the breathing in its normal pattern. This leads to repetitive cycles characterized by cessation of airflow because of lack of respiratory effort, which terminates once the metabolic trigger to breathe (usually blood carbon dioxide levels) increases sufficiently to drive respiratory output from the CNS. As with OSA, there are often brief CNS arousals associated with these events, leading to fragmented sleep.

CSA has a variety of causes, the hallmark of all of them related to processes that affect chemoresponsiveness and respiratory pattern stability. The more common causes of CSA include underlying significant cardiac or neurologic disease, such as atrial fibrillation or flutter, congestive heart failure, stroke, or brainstem disorders. These illnesses are often associated with a type of CSA known as Cheyne-Stokes breathing. This pattern is characterized by recurrent central apneas alternating with a waxing and waning pattern of airflow. Another, more common cause of CSA is the use of opioid medications, particularly the long-acting opioids, which affect respiratory drive.

CLINICAL PRESENTATION

A history of OSA is most often suggested by loud, disruptive snoring, with or without witnessed apneas, nocturnal gasping, or choking. Patients may report frank excessive daytime sleepiness (EDS), daytime fatigue and tiredness without unintentional sleep, or even vague depressive symptoms. They are often not aware of fragmented sleep because the respiratory-related arousals are often too brief to be consciously registered during the night. In fact, patients not uncommonly report that they sleep well through the night and are puzzled by their daytime sleepiness. Nocturia is a frequent complication of the disorder.

The most common risk factor for OSA is obesity, and patients may be able to relate the onset of their symptoms to weight gain. The disorder is more common in men, although the prevalence rate in postmenopausal women approaches the same level as in men. A substance history is helpful in that particular substances may alter airway muscle tone and further increase risk for obstructive respiratory events. This includes the use of alcohol, opiates, or muscle relaxant medication such as the benzodiazepines in the evening. It is also helpful to elicit other medical history, such as heart disease, hypertension, or stroke, because these disorders may be seen with OSA. On physical examination, the presence of obesity and a crowded oropharynx may be suggestive of OSA in a patient with symptoms associated with the disease.

In addition to leading to EDS and impairment of daytime functioning, untreated OSA has been found to have associations with a variety of longer term health consequences. There is substantial convincing evidence that untreated OSA is an independent cause of systemic hypertension, other cardiovascular disease, and stroke.[9,10] In addition, there is mounting evidence of an association with metabolic syndrome and type 2 diabetes mellitus.[11] Individuals with CSA may be noted by their bed partner to have pauses in their breathing, which may or may not be followed by a period of more rapid breathing. They typically will not, however, have a history of snoring. These patients may also have complaints of EDS or daytime fatigue because the central apneic events disrupt sleep in a way similar to OSA events. Risk factors for CSA include decompensated congestive heart failure and the use of opioid medications, particularly the long-acting opioid medications such as methadone.

DIAGNOSTICS

Overnight Sleep Testing

- Full overnight PSG is the gold standard for the diagnosis of sleep-related breathing disorders.[12]

- Unattended out-of-center sleep testing (OCST) is increasingly being used for the diagnosis of OSA. OCST is typically performed at home and assesses fewer biometric measures than full PSG. OCST is more accessible and cost-effective than full PSG, although it is crucial to understand the limitations of the usefulness of OCST and potential pitfalls.[12] OCST is indicated for patients with moderate to high pretest probability of OSA and no significant comorbidities or use of medications that increase risk for other breathing disorders, such as CSA or hypoventilation. It is also important to understand that OCST generally underestimates the number of obstructive respiratory events, and full PSG should be considered if the OCST result is negative in a patient with significant OSA risk factors or reported symptoms.
- Overnight pulse oximetry is not sufficiently sensitive to be used as a reliable screening test for sleep apnea.

DIFFERENTIAL DIAGNOSIS

Sleep-related breathing disorders often overlap and cannot be distinguished by clinical history alone. Nocturnal breathing disorders may also occur as a symptom of other underlying cardiopulmonary disorders. It is important to identify whether the nocturnal disorder is related to other concurrent disease (such as chronic obstructive pulmonary disease [COPD] or congestive heart failure).

Other causes of sleep fragmentation and/or EDS should also be considered (see separate sections on insomnia and hypersomnia for list).

MANAGEMENT

Obstructive Sleep Apnea

- Continuous positive airway pressure (CPAP).
  - This is the most common and effective treatment, with efficacy rates of 95%. It is also essentially free of dangerous side effects.
  - The major impediments to successful CPAP therapy are comfort and acceptance. Careful counseling and initial attention to equipment fit can go a long way toward ensuring patient adherence with the device.
- Weight loss may also be helpful in the overall management strategy, although this should not be used as the sole treatment modality in patients with anything more than mild OSA.
- Custom-fit oral appliances.
  - Designed to increase posterior airway dimensions.
  - May be effective for milder OSA; not as effective as CPAP.
- Upper airway surgical procedures.
  - Standard procedures are designed to remove excessive upper airway tissue. These modalities, however, are less effective than CPAP, and success cannot be predicted before treatment. Less commonly, appropriate treatment choices may include tracheotomy or, in patients who have undergone a careful preoperative evaluation and failed to respond to less-invasive therapies, more extensive maxillofacial surgery.

Central Sleep Apnea

- If possible, tapering or discontinuation of medication that may be causing CSA.
- If CSA is related to decompensated or unstable cardiovascular process, the CSA may improve with improvement in the cardiovascular process.
- Positive airway pressure (PAP).
  - CSA may improve with CPAP, although there are newer PAP devices that are able to vary ventilatory support and rapidly adapt to changes in respiratory drive to alleviate the CSA events in patients in whom CPAP therapy fails.

LIFE SPAN CONSIDERATIONS

OSA may occur at any age, although it is most common between young adulthood and middle age. OSA does occur in older adults, although development of OSA does not necessarily increase with age.

COMPLICATIONS

As discussed earlier, substantial evidence implicates untreated OSA as a risk factor for multiple cardiovascular diseases, including systemic hypertension, coronary artery disease, congestive heart failure, and stroke. There is also accumulating evidence linking OSA to various arrhythmias, as well as increased risk for development of type 2 diabetes mellitus. OSA may also increase the severity of depression. Risk of motor vehicle accidents is significantly increased among those with OSA.

As opposed to OSA, CSA has not been identified as an independent risk factor for increased morbidity or mortality, although it can cause sleep fragmentation with associated hypersomnia, insomnia, or both.

INDICATIONS FOR REFERRAL OR HOSPITALIZATION

In general, sleep-related breathing disorders are managed in an outpatient setting by sleep medicine specialists.

PATIENT AND FAMILY EDUCATION

Patients should be educated about the impact of obesity on OSA, and weight loss should be encouraged. They should also be educated about the risks of untreated OSA and the importance of adhering to PAP treatment. They should understand that they should speak with the sleep provider if they are having problems tolerating PAP, because adjustments can be made to increase tolerance and acceptance.

CENTRAL NERVOUS SYSTEM HYPERSOMNIAS

DEFINITION AND EPIDEMIOLOGY

The primary disorders of hypersomnolence are characterized by an intrinsic CNS deficit resulting in a sleep-wake system that is inadequate for maintaining wakefulness or overactive in promoting sleep. The predominant clinical characteristic of these syndromes is EDS not caused by disturbed nocturnal sleep or misaligned circadian rhythms.

The primary hypersomnias include narcolepsy, idiopathic hypersomnia, and post-traumatic hypersomnia. Narcolepsy, the best defined of the primary hypersomnias, is characterized by EDS and inappropriate manifestations of REM sleep. These include such phenomena as cataplexy (sudden onset of REM-related muscle atonia precipitated by emotion during wakefulness) and hallucinations and paralysis occurring at sleep onset (hypnagogic) or offset (hypnopompic) related to inappropriately timed REM. The EDS and the REM-related symptoms can be extremely disabling and potentially dangerous, depending on when they occur.

Idiopathic CNS hypersomnia also involves CNS sleep system dysfunction, which results in profound EDS. However, with idiopathic CNS hypersomnia, there is no known disease of the REM system, and other symptoms present in narcolepsy are absent. Post-traumatic hypersomnia is not readily distinguishable from idiopathic hypersomnia, other than that the symptoms follow head injury or another CNS insult such as an infection.

CLINICAL PRESENTATION

Assessment of the patient with EDS usually begins with either the patient or a family member complaining of sleepiness or unintentional sleep in undesired situations. This may include falling asleep unintentionally while watching television or reading, in noisy gatherings, at work, in conversation, or even while driving. Information obtained from a family member can be essential to accurate diagnosis because patients with EDS may not recognize or may minimize the severity of their symptoms. It is important to obtain a full sleep history, including 24-hour sleep-wake schedules, time and duration of naps, and associated symptoms that may point to the underlying cause of the EDS symptoms.

The key clinical feature of narcolepsy is EDS. Cataplexy, hypnagogic or hypnopompic hallucinations, sleep paralysis, and fragmented, disturbed nocturnal sleep may be present, but not all are required for the diagnosis. Cataplexy is seen almost exclusively in narcolepsy and is characterized by sudden episodes of muscle atonia during wakefulness. Cataplexy is often brought on when the patient is experiencing a strong emotion, particularly laughter. Such episodes may pose potential danger, depending on when and where they occur. They are often only seconds in duration but can last for minutes or longer in some cases. The sleep paralysis involves REM-related atonia (excluding the ocular muscles and diaphragm) and is often described as terrifying by patients. The hypnagogic or hypnopompic hallucinations are dreamlike and often frightening fragments that occur near sleep onset or offset and typically involve the patient's confusion about whether he or she is awake or asleep. The typical onset of narcolepsy symptoms is in the second or third decade, although it can occur earlier or later in life. There is no gender predominance. There are no features on physical examination that are particularly helpful in identifying narcolepsy.

The diagnosis of idiopathic CNS hypersomnia is most often a diagnosis of exclusion. Patients typically have complaints of EDS despite adequate or prolonged total sleep time, and they do not have the symptoms that otherwise characterize narcolepsy. A careful history should be obtained regarding possible CNS insult from infection or trauma.

In addition to using the history to identify these disorders, the health care provider should also question the patient for symptoms suggestive of RLS or periodic limb movement disorder (PLMD; discussed in further detail later in this chapter). The patient's sleep-wake schedule should also be evaluated to make certain that insufficient sleep is not playing a role, and a complete medication and substance history should be obtained because many medications and drugs may cause sleepiness as a side effect.

DIAGNOSTICS

Overnight PSG is generally employed in assessing the primary hypersomnias. The purpose is to exclude other underlying causes of the patient's sleepiness symptoms, such as an occult sleep-related breathing disorder. If no cause of EDS is identified on overnight PSG, the next step is to perform a multiple sleep latency test (MSLT).[13] The MSLT is used to determine one's propensity for daytime sleep. The subject is given multiple opportunities to nap under standardized conditions, and a mean sleep-onset latency (i.e., time to fall asleep) is determined and compared with normative values. This is the most objective means of determining EDS, although daytime continuous PSG can confirm findings. The presence of sleep-onset REM episodes on the MSLT is a required diagnostic finding for narcolepsy.

DIFFERENTIAL DIAGNOSIS

See differential diagnosis box.

DIFFERENTIAL DIAGNOSIS

Excessive Daytime Somnolence

- Insufficient sleep
- Sleep-wake system deficit
- Narcolepsy
- Idiopathic CNS hypersomnia
- Post-traumatic hypersomnia
- Sleep fragmentation
- OSA or CSA
- PLMD
- Circadian rhythm disorder
- Substances, medication, or primary medical or neurologic disorder

MANAGEMENT

EDS as a result of CNS-based disorders has historically been treated with psychostimulants (e.g., dextroamphetamine or methylphenidate). The non–habit-forming stimulant modafinil is increasingly used. Cataplexy is treated by use of REM-suppressing medications. Most commonly, these have included the tricyclic antidepressants and the selective serotonin reuptake inhibitor–type antidepressants. More recently, γ-hydroxybutyrate has become available as a therapy for cataplexy.

SLEEP-RELATED MOVEMENT DISORDERS

DEFINITION AND EPIDEMIOLOGY

Sleep-related movement disorders are conditions in which patients have simple stereotyped movements or other sleep-related monophasic movements that disturb sleep. Sleep-related leg cramps, sleep-related rhythmic movement disorder, PLMD, and sleep-related bruxism are disorders that fall into this category. RLS, because of its association with PLMs, is included in this category. Because RLS is so common (5% to 10% in populations derived from Western Europe),[1] this will be the focus of this section.

Restless Legs Syndrome

The prevalence of RLS increases with age, but symptoms may start in childhood. RLS is seen more commonly in women. RLS is an uncomfortable sensation, usually in the legs, associated with a strong desire to move the legs. Because this discomfort occurs primarily in the evening, it may lead to sleep-onset difficulties.

PATHOPHYSIOLOGY

The pathophysiology of RLS is unclear. RLS may occur in association with a wide variety of conditions. Pregnancy, renal failure, and ferritin levels below 50 µg/L have the best-established associations. Peripheral neuropathy and Parkinson disease may also be associated with RLS. A number of widely used medications, including most antidepressants, sedating antihistamines, and dopamine antagonists, may cause or exacerbate RLS.[1] RLS, however, is often idiopathic or familial. Given the efficacy of dopaminergic agents in treating RLS, a CNS dysfunction in a dopaminergic system has been postulated as a cause of this syndrome.

CLINICAL PRESENTATION

Patients with RLS may visit their health care provider because they find the discomfort bothersome or possibly because of sleep-onset problems caused by the discomfort. RLS has four principal diagnostic criteria. The first is an urge to move the legs, usually accompanied or caused by an uncomfortable sensation in the legs. The second and third criteria are that this urge begins or worsens during inactivity or rest and is at least partially ameliorated by activity or movement, such as stretching or walking. The final criterion is that the urge or sensations are worsened or occur exclusively in the evening or at night. A family history is supportive of the diagnosis. A therapeutic response to levodopa or a dopamine agonist would also be supportive of the diagnosis of RLS.

PHYSICAL EXAMINATION

The findings on physical examination are normal unless the RLS occurs in the setting of an associated medical condition (e.g., peripheral neuropathy, Parkinson disease).

DIAGNOSTICS

RLS is a clinical diagnosis, but PSG can sometimes be helpful because it may offer information supportive of the diagnosis or RLS. PLMs are triple flexion (hip, knee, and ankle flexion) responses of the legs that occur every 5 to 90 seconds during sleep. PLMs are present on PSG in up to 90% of people with RLS. The presence of PLMs would then be supportive of the diagnosis of RLS. PLMs, however, can occur in association with other sleep disorders, such as sleep-disordered breathing, narcolepsy, and REM sleep behavior disorder. PLMs can also be seen in patients without sleep disorders as an incidental finding. PLMs in the absence of RLS are not labeled as a disorder (PLMD) unless they lead to disturbed sleep. PLMD is probably rare. PSG is useful in assessing for the presence of PLMs but is not necessary for the diagnosis of RLS. Assessing a patient's iron status may also be prudent in patients with RLS. Ferritin levels lower than 50 ng/mL have been associated with RLS. Patients with ferritin levels below 50 ng/mL may improve with iron replacement.

DIAGNOSTICS

Restless Legs Syndrome

LABORATORY	OTHER DIAGNOSTICS
Serum ferritin	PSG

DIFFERENTIAL DIAGNOSIS

RLS must be distinguished from other forms of lower extremity discomfort, such as arthritis, neuropathy, and vascular disease. The response of RLS to dopaminergic agents and the irresistible urge to move the legs in RLS can help distinguish it from these other disorders. Leg cramps can be distinguished from RLS in that typical leg cramps involve a specific muscle, which often visibly hardens. Stretching of the specific muscle improves the condition. In patients with suspected RLS, screening for the associated conditions listed previously (e.g., ferritin level) is prudent.

DIFFERENTIAL DIAGNOSIS

Restless Legs Syndrome

NEUROLOGIC
- Peripheral neuropathy

MUSCULOSKELETAL
- Arthritis
- Leg cramps

PSYCHIATRIC
- Anxiety

VASCULAR
- Claudication

MANAGEMENT

The primary goal of treatment is resolution of the lower extremity discomfort and associated sleep difficulties.

1. Mild forms of RLS can potentially be addressed with good sleep hygiene, massage, hot baths, or exercise.
2. If medication is desired, the dopaminergic agonists such as pramipexole, rotigotine, and ropinirole are the best-studied agents.[14]
3. Carbidopa-levodopa was commonly used for this disorder in the past, but because of rebound symptoms and augmentation (appearance of symptoms earlier in the day), it has been largely replaced by the dopamine agonists.
4. Rebound and augmentation may still be an issue with the newer dopamine agonists. Use of low doses of the dopamine agonists may help avoid rebound or augmentation.
5. Other options for the treatment of RLS include opioids, gabapentin enacarbil, gabapentin, pregabalin, carbamazepine, and clonidine.
6. Supplemental iron may be useful in patients with reduced ferritin levels.[15]
7. Reduction in the dose or discontinuation of a medication known to cause RLS may also offer relief.
8. PLMs as part of RLS or PLMD are often treated with the same medications as RLS alone.

COMPLICATIONS

Because of the timing of the leg discomfort in RLS, insomnia is often a complicating factor in RLS.

INDICATIONS FOR REFERRAL

Patients with difficult-to-manage RLS or RLS in the setting of significant medical comorbidities may merit referral to a sleep medicine specialist.

LIFESPAN CONSIDERATIONS

Onset of RLS may occur from childhood through late adulthood. Mean age of onset for familial RLS is in the third or fourth decade, with onset before the age of 21 in about one third of cases.[14] Early-onset (before the age of 45) RLS tends to be a more slowly progressive disorder, and some patients may have stable symptoms over time. Late-onset RLS (after the age of 45) tends to be more rapidly progressive.[14]

EDUCATION AND HEALTH PROMOTION

Patients and family should understand that this is generally a progressive and persistent disorder in its idiopathic form. Medication can be used to ameliorate the symptoms. Secondary forms of RLS may improve with treatment or resolution of the primary disorder.

PARASOMNIAS

DEFINITION AND EPIDEMIOLOGY

Parasomnias, as defined by the ICSD, are undesirable physical events or experiences that occur during entry into sleep, within sleep, or during arousals from sleep.[1] The pathophysiology of this heterogeneous group of disorders is variable and depends in part on the stage of sleep from which they arise. In the case of disorders of arousal from NREM sleep (e.g., sleepwalking, sleep terrors, confusional arousals), the mechanism is an abrupt and abnormal arousal from delta (stage N3) sleep. Any factor that increases delta sleep (e.g., prior sleep deprivation) or leads to fragmentation of delta sleep (e.g., OSA, biopsychosocial stress) could predispose the person to this group of disorders, although genetic predisposition may be an important factor for many affected individuals. This group of disorders most often occurs in children but can occur in adults.

REM sleep behavior disorder (RBD) and nightmare disorder are the most prominent REM-related parasomnias. RBD results from the loss of normal REM muscle atonia, typically in men older than 50 years. In this disorder, the patient enacts dreams, often in a potentially dangerous fashion. Nightmare disorder is a distinct disorder from RBD. Nightmares are terrifying dreams that often result in awakening. They are common on an occasional basis among adults and children. When nightmares occur repeatedly and are associated with significant distress or impairment, nightmare disorder should be considered. Nightmare disorder may result from psychological factors, inherited factors, prior sleep deprivation, or the use or withdrawal of certain medications. Specifically, the cessation of most types of antidepressant medications will predispose the patient to a transient increase in nightmares. Nightmares are especially common in post-traumatic stress disorder patients.

CLINICAL PRESENTATION AND DIAGNOSTICS

Patients may be initially seen with a chief complaint of disturbing behaviors during sleep. A careful history is helpful in distinguishing NREM from REM parasomnias. The disorders of arousal from NREM sleep (confusional arousals, sleepwalking, and sleep terrors) arise from slow-wave sleep, which occurs primarily in the first third of the night. There is often a family history of a disorder of arousal from NREM sleep. Features common to the disorders of arousal from NREM sleep according to the ICSD[1] include the following: (1) inappropriate or absent responsiveness to the intervention of others, (2) limited or no associated dream imagery, and (3) partial or complete amnesia for the event. Additional features can help distinguish the precise type of parasomnia. Confusional arousals consist of mental confusion precipitated by an arousal from sleep but without ambulation outside the bed and with no signs of terror or autonomic arousal. Sleep terrors consist of episodes in which the patient sits up and screams with a terrified expression. There are accompanying signs of autonomic arousal (mydriasis, tachypnea, and tachycardia). Patients will be amnestic or recall an image but not a complex dream, as would be the case with a nightmare. The episodes last 30 seconds to 3 minutes typically. Sleepwalking (somnambulism) consists of walking and automatic behaviors without awakening, usually for less than 5 minutes. Complex behaviors, such as eating and driving, may occur. The subject may be violent, particularly if an attempt is made to awaken him or her.

Disorders of arousal from NREM sleep are typically diagnosed by history. PSG can be helpful in detecting precipitating or associated disorders, such as OSA, and may also reveal an increase in slow-wave sleep percentage. The physical examination is usually unremarkable in these conditions.

In RBD, enactment of an often violent dream occurs. The patient and bed partner are at risk for injury during these events. Unlike in the disorders of arousal in NREM sleep, there is typically an associated dream with a coherent story line. PSG in patients with this disorder may reveal elevated muscle tone in REM sleep and PLMs. RBD may be idiopathic or may be associated with other neurologic disorders, making further neurologic assessment in newly diagnosed RBD patients a necessity. The strongest association is with the α-synucleinopathies (Parkinson disease, dementia with Lewy bodies, and multiple system atrophy). There may be a latency of years from the development of RBD until the onset of the parkinsonism. PSG is required to diagnose RBD definitively.

Nightmare disorder is characterized by awakenings from sleep associated with recall of a disturbing dream. In general, the patient is fully alert on awakening with clear recall of the dream. The patient may be so distressed as to have a delay in the return to sleep. Events typically occur in the second half of the night when REM sleep is most common. As one would expect, physical examination findings are typically normal, and PSG is not required to make the diagnosis.

DIFFERENTIAL DIAGNOSIS

Some disorders present during waking hours may also occur during sleep. Up to 50% of patients with panic disorder experience panic attacks at some point in their lifetime that arise out of sleep, typically NREM sleep.[15] Nocturnal seizures are another group of disorders that may arise from sleep. Certain types of nocturnal seizures, especially nocturnal frontal lobe epilepsy (NFLE), may arise exclusively from sleep. The sometimes bizarre nature of seizures in NFLE may make diagnosis a challenge.

DIFFERENTIAL DIAGNOSIS

Parasomnias

- Arousals secondary to sleep fragmentation from sleep apnea or other factors
- Confusional arousals
- Sleepwalking
- Sleep terrors
- Post-traumatic stress disorder
- Nightmares
- RBD
- Dissociative disorder
- Nocturnal panic attacks
- Nocturnal seizures
- Other

TABLE 227-2 Distinguishing Seizures in NFLE from NREM Parasomnias

	NREM Parasomnia	Seizure in NFLE
Episodes per month	<1 or a few	Usually >10
Episodes per night	1	>1
Type of episode	Nonstereotyped	Stereotyped
Episode duration	Minutes	Seconds

Modified from Malow BA, Plazzi G: Nocturnal seizures. In Chokroverty S, Hening WA, Walters AS, editors: *Sleep and movement disorders,* Philadelphia, 2003, Butterworth-Heinemann.

Clinical features can help distinguish NFLE from NREM parasomnias (Table 227-2), although overnight PSG or video-electroencephalographic monitoring is often required.

MANAGEMENT

Sleep medicine consultation is indicated for parasomnias during which violent or dangerous behavior is exhibited or parasomnias in the context of suspicion for other sleep disorders (such as OSA).

The primary goal of treatment is to keep the patient and others safe.

1. Many disorders of arousal from NREM sleep do not require pharmacologic treatment.
2. Reassurance of the patient or parents, coupled with attention to safety issues, may be sufficient.
3. Addressing predisposing factors, such as sleep deprivation, medications, and stress, may be helpful.
4. Benzodiazepines and tricyclic antidepressants have been successfully used in sleepwalking and night terrors. Sedating medications, however, may also precipitate confusional arousals, because they make it more difficult for the patient to awaken.
5. RBD responds to clonazepam in the majority of cases.[16] Administration is begun with 0.5 mg at bedtime and is titrated upward as needed, generally to a maximum dose of 2 mg at bedtime. Alternatives to clonazepam include melatonin 1-3 mg (more if prescribed by a sleep specialist) and pramipexole.
6. Image rehearsal therapy (IRT), systemic desensitization, progressive deep muscle relaxation training, lucid dreaming therapy, and self-exposure therapy all have been reported to be of help in treating nightmares, with IRT having the most evidence to support its use.[17]

LIFE SPAN CONSIDERATIONS

Disorders of arousal from NREM sleep are most commonly seen in children and typically resolve in adolescence. RBD is most commonly seen in men over the age of 50. Nightmare disorder can occur at any age.

COMPLICATIONS

Given the lack of awareness during disorders of arousal from NREM sleep, injury is possible. Patients with this disorder should keep their bedrooms clear of obstacles, consider child safety locks on windows, remove all dangerous objects from the bedroom (e.g., pills, knives), and consider a door alarm on the bedroom door. Because of the violent nature of the dream enactment, patients with RBD may injure themselves or their bed partners.

INDICATIONS FOR REFERRAL AND HOSPITALIZATION

Parasomnias do not usually require hospitalization to manage. Dangerous parasomnias or suspicion for RBD should generate a referral to a sleep medicine specialist. If there is suspicion for a concomitant sleep disorder such as sleep apnea that might act as a trigger for the parasomnia, evaluation along those lines should be considered.

PATIENT AND FAMILY EDUCATION

Families of children with disorders of arousal from NREM may require reassurance. Keeping the bedroom environment safe is essential. If a sleepwalker is encountered, he or she should be gently guided back to bed. Avoidance of triggers for parasomnias such as sleep deprivation is important. Patients with RBD and their families should be reassured that the violent dream enactment does not mean the affected individual has violent tendencies. Treatment is important to keep the patient and bed partner safe.

CHAPTER 228

UNINTENDED WEIGHT LOSS

Michelle Freshman

DEFINITION AND EPIDEMIOLOGY

Although not all involuntary weight loss is ominous, an unintentional loss in excess of 5% of body weight during a period of 6 to 12 months typically warrants further investigation.[1,2] With a weight loss of 10% of body weight over 12 months, the effects of protein-energy malnutrition and poor health outcomes are substantial.[3] By contrast with intentional weight loss, which has been associated with a decreased mortality rate up to a decade later, unintentional weight loss has been associated with a 30% increase in mortality.[1] The percentages of underweight men and women (because of loss of appetite or reduced intake) older than 65 are 25% and 30%, respectively.[4] Among older adults, involuntary weight loss may result from a broad spectrum of physiologic or psychosocial factors.

Unintentional weight loss and *involuntary weight loss* are synonymous terms. Many studies have pointed to the significance of a 5% to 10% weight loss within a year as a salient measure of decline in health, often incorporated in more global measures of frailty. Frailty, in particular, results from a condition of reduced physical ability and unintentional weight loss. In patients older than 70 who are chronically ill, frailty and subsequent vulnerability to adverse health events (disability, falls, hospitalizations, and death) is a significant risk.[5-7] In the Systolic Hypertension in the Elderly Program (SHEP) study of over 4700 people, subjects aged 60 years or older who had a weight loss of 1.6 kg/yr had a fivefold greater death rate; those with a low initial weight and a greater than 1.6 kg/yr weight loss had a 20-fold increased mortality compared with those without a weight change.[8] As many as 50% of hospitalized older adults are undernourished, and community-dwelling older adults who are undernourished are more likely to be frail.[6]

The definition of frailty expands on the condition of unintentional weight loss and takes into account an individual's risk for developing increased physical dependency and/or mortality when exposed to a stressor.[7] Frail older adults, in particular, are seen to be at greater risk for poor health outcomes, including death, beyond those expected for same-aged peers. To support aging in place for as long as possible, cross-disciplinary consensus work supports frailty as a medical condition, which can improve in response to early interventions to prevent both weight loss and dependency among predisabled elders.[7] Even with a thorough workup and the progression of time, weight loss may remain unexplained. In fact, as well known as the association of unexpected weight loss is with poor outcomes, malnutrition rates remain high, leading researchers to suspect that there exists a threshold before which the opportunity for medical intervention is more likely to be beneficial.

PATHOPHYSIOLOGY

Human weight homeostasis is a complex interaction of cytokines, neurons, adipose tissue hormones, gut peptides, and hypothalamic input, as influenced by psychosocial cues.[1] Satiety is driven by gastric distention neurons and release of cholecystokinin, peptide YY, glucagon-like peptide 1, and amylin; hunger is driven by ghrelin, whereas leptin, released from adipocytes affecting hypothalamic receptors, provides a negative feedback loop on food intake.[1] With aging, the speed of the responsiveness of visceral neurons and diminished sensitivity to the action of gut distention are attributed to early satiety; changes in ghrelin and other androgens as well as an increase in the appetite-suppressant leptin, particularly in women, have been associated with other reduced gastric emptying mechanisms suspected in the setting of circulating satiation hormones, including postprandial insulin and inflammatory cytokines.[3] Weight loss is thought to follow from one or more of the following: decreased calorie or fluid volume intake, decreased calorie absorption, or increased metabolic demands.

Decreased calorie intake may result from a behavioral adaptation to what is an unsatisfactory eating experience. Weight loss caused by functional anorexia may result from apathy, mechanical obstacles to mastication, depressed sense of taste and smell, delayed gastric emptying time, or pain with elimination. Decreased calorie absorption results from malabsorption, vomiting, diarrhea, and urinary frequency, which may tip the balance to decreased calorie intake. Increased metabolism occurs with infection, hyperactivity, hyperthyroidism, and tumor growth through neurohormonal mechanisms. A pathophysiologic connection exists between weight loss and infection through the diminished capacity of cell-mediated and humoral immune systems to mount an adequate response. Circulating gut hormones as well as proinflammatory cytokines contribute to anorexia and cachexia.[2,4]

The body's composition changes with aging. After age 30, lean body mass is incrementally replaced by gains in fat mass until about 65 or 70, when incremental weight loss of 0.1 to 0.2 kg/yr (0.2 to 0.4 lb/yr) or 0.5% per year[1,3] occurs, with a peak weight around age 60.[2] Protein-energy malnutrition occurs when the supply of proteins or calories is inadequate to maintain weight. A combination of the conditions marasmus (insufficient calories) and kwashiorkor (protein deficiency) occurs, as evidenced by changes in body composition, systemic weakness, and laboratory abnormalities. Although not specific to involuntary weight loss, sarcopenia refers to reduced muscle mass (more than two standard deviations from young adults of the same sex and ethnicity) and loss of muscle strength.[1] Sarcopenia contributes to frailty. Weight loss resulting from anorexia will cause muscle wasting; respiratory, immune, and gut consequences; hypoalbuminemia; a rise in C-reactive protein; decreased coagulation; and tissue damage, which often affects endurance, gait, and mobility.[4] Both of these conditions are flags for frailty and taken together point to cachexia.

Many chronically ill adults and elders, particularly nursing home patients, have weight loss–driven protein-energy malnutrition owing to medical, social, and psychological factors, all of which may be amenable to improvement; this may include conditions that produce cachexia from increased metabolic demands.[3] Cachexia is characterized by muscle wasting, following weight and fat loss, with underlying proteolytic disease, often confounded by anorexia. One definition calls for weight loss of 5% or greater over 12 months or less and three to five of the following: abnormal laboratory test results (increased inflammatory markers, anemia, and hypoalbuminemia), anorexia, decreased muscle strength, fatigue, and/or low fat-free mass index.[1] If cachexia has developed, it may disproportionately affect skeletal and cardiac muscle and is no longer a reversible process.[1] Cachexia and malnutrition are overlapping but distinct states, wherein cachexia results from a greater percentage (>5%) of weight loss over the previous 6 months. Precachexia refers to early clinical warning signs, developed in an effort to improve on a lack of staging of cachexia, when rapid intervention might forestall further wasting.[9] Defined as (1) underlying chronic disease, (2) unintentional weight loss of 5% or less of usual body weight during the last 6 months, (3) chronic or recurrent inflammatory response, and (4) anorexia or anorexia-related symptoms, precachexia is commonly associated with cancer, chronic obstructive pulmonary disease (COPD), chronic heart failure, renal or liver failure, acquired immunodeficiency syndrome (AIDS), or rheumatoid arthritis.

CLINICAL PRESENTATION

Patients may be unaware of weight changes. In the absence of consistent health records, they may only recall the observations of others or notice loose-fitting clothing as evidence of weight loss. In fact, many older patients may note a weight loss with pleasure, believing that lower weight is desirable. Obtaining a history of the quantity, quality, and regularity of food and fluid intake as well as of physical activity, mood, and cognition is of utmost importance.

For those who report polyphagia or polydipsia and appear to have lost weight, a set of endocrine disorders should be considered in the differential diagnosis; these include hypothyroidism, hyperthyroidism, diabetes mellitus, diabetes insipidus, hyperparathyroidism, pheochromocytoma, and adrenal insufficiency.

Symptoms associated with decreased intake, such as fever, night sweats, dyspnea, and mental status changes, suggest underlying infection, malignant disease, or possible neurologic impairment. In those with Parkinson disease or advanced Alzheimer dementia, tremor, forgetfulness, mental confusion, and apathy may inadvertently lead to meal skipping or reduced intake at meals.

Swallowing difficulties may cause a patient to adjust the types or amounts of food eaten. Common reasons for decreased intake include dysgeusia or ageusia, sticking or choking sensation, pain with chewing, dry mouth, unpleasant smell of food, heartburn, and gastric pain before or after eating or associated with eating of fatty or acidic foods. Older adults experience diminished senses of taste, smell, and thirst because of physiologic changes of the tongue and olfaction, which blunt the palatability of food and possibly slow transit time as a result. Severe gastroesophageal reflux, nausea, vomiting, abdominal bloating, flatulence, constipation, and diarrhea affect intake. Individuals may also try to prevent diarrhea by avoiding food. Milk products associated with these complaints might signal lactose intolerance. Gluten intolerance or sensitivity (celiac disease), now more commonly diagnosed than in the past, may cause diarrhea and lead to weight loss. Bloody, painful, or urgent stool can indicate hemorrhoids, inflammatory bowel disease, or malignant disease. Fatty, odorous stool can point to gallbladder disease or malabsorption syndromes. Paroxysmal, sustained, midabdominal pain, potentially indicative of pancreatic disease, can lead to malabsorption. A history of chronic diarrhea, whether secondary to bacterial or parasitic exposure or a result of underlying illness or recent hospitalization, should be elicited, as should erratic, severe abdominal pain associated with intestinal pseudo-obstruction. A review of genitourinary symptoms and musculoskeletal, dermatologic, and lymph node enlargement should be elicited. Situational stress or anxiety sometimes contributes to unintentional weight loss, as can changes in mood, affect, or coping.

Premorbid health conditions can tax a patient's reserves to a degree that interferes with adequate nutrition and hydration. Fatigue, shortness of breath, or impaired mobility may make the duration of a meal exhausting, resulting in decreased intake. It is critical to obtain a smoking, alcohol, and drug history. Patients who abuse alcohol may substitute it for food, leading to vitamin deficiencies and subsequent malnutrition. A history of risky sexual and self-harm behaviors, which put people at risk for debilitating infectious diseases including human immunodeficiency virus (HIV) and AIDS, should be elicited along with a history of eating disorders. Immunocompromised states can coexist with wasting syndrome.

Surgery can take a toll on health status. Surgical repair or resection of the intestine may place patients at risk for bowel torsion or obstruction owing to adhesion, leading to constipation, nausea, vomiting, and subsequent anorexia and weight loss. In these cases, small intestinal bacterial overgrowth is also of potential concern.

A review of medications is essential, especially if the patient is taking multiple medications. Amphetamines, benzodiazepines, decongestants, metformin, nicotine, and selective serotonin reuptake inhibitors (SSRIs) can cause anorexia.[2] Other medications can cause nausea, altered taste or smell, or dry mouth, although there is significant overlap among them (Box 228-1). Excessive use of diuretics or laxatives should also be explored.

A family medical history that includes gastrointestinal illness, celiac disease, cancer, or psychiatric illness may be relevant.

An inquiry into food affordability, availability, preparation, and safety and social isolation is essential. An older patient with early dementia may have trouble sequencing the steps necessary to procure and prepare food, aside from having physical limitations in manipulating containers. Recent adoption of new food practices, such as veganism, gluten-free diets, or religious fasting, coupled with inadequate education can lead to unintentional weight loss. Eating disorders cause severe malnutrition through ketosis and further weight loss vulnerability. Anorexia and bulimia nervosa are psychiatric disorders characterized by excessive concern for body shape and weight. Serious medical consequences including anemia, electrolyte imbalances, reduction in bone density, cessation of menses, and ECG disturbances may arise as a result of the behavioral manifestations of the illness. These disorders primarily affect young women and adolescents but men and older adults can also be affected. Risk factors are not fully understood. Patients frequently exhibit denial regarding the seriousness of their reduced weight. Many are depressed. Patients with bulimia often feel shame and embarrassment.

Management is multidisciplinary and communication with patients and team members is crucial. Medical stability is the first goal with progressive caloric intake as tolerated. Targeted weight gain of 0.5 to 1 pound a week is optimal. Careful monitoring of vital signs, electrolytes, and signs and symptoms of fluid overload is critical during refeeding. Physical and psychological comfort is assessed frequently. Patients suspected of suffering with eating disorders should be referred to specialists in this area. Excess alcohol can suppress appetite. Exotic travel and environmental, residential, or work exposures to infection or toxins may be risk factors.

BOX 228-1

Examples of Medications That Can Potentially Cause Weight Loss

CARDIAC
- Digoxin
- Aspirin
- Angiotensin-converting enzyme inhibitors
- Calcium channel blockers
- Hydralazine
- Loop diuretics
- Hydrochlorothiazides
- Spironolactone
- Statins
- Nitroglycerin

NEUROLOGIC AND PSYCHIATRIC
- SSRIs
- Tricyclics
- Neuroleptics
- Benzodiazepines
- Anticonvulsants
- Lithium
- Levodopa
- Dopamine agonists
- Donepezil
- Memantine

BONE AND JOINT (INCLUDING PAIN MEDICATIONS)
- Bisphosphonates
- Nonsteroidal anti-inflammatory drugs (including cyclooxygenase 2 [COX-2] inhibitors)
- Opiates
- Allopurinol
- Colchicine
- Gold
- Hydroxychloroquine

ENDOCRINE
- Levothyroxine
- Metformin

OTHER MEDICATIONS
- Anticholinergics
- Antibiotics
- Decongestants
- Antihistamines
- Iron
- Potassium
- Alcohol
- Nicotine

PHYSICAL EXAMINATION

General appearance, habitus, affect, speech, cognition, and recall provide basic information. Weight loss can be determined if a previsit weight is available and should be calculated as a percentage change from baseline. Serial skinfold measurement may be helpful to determine the percentage of body fat. Some assessment tools, such as the Mini Nutritional Assessment (MNA), focus on body mass index (BMI), calf and midarm circumference, and other measures, and delineate who is at greater risk for a host of hospital-based delays and complications, including death.[6] The short-form version (MNA-SF) includes 18 items, with a score below 9 indicating risk for both undernutrition and frailty in hospitalized patients.[6] Muscle wasting at the temples and intercostal spaces, which is more commonly seen in older adults, should be assessed in context.

Vital signs may indicate orthostasis or arrhythmias, suggestive of underlying cardiac disease and disability. Pallor, jaundice, rash, skin texture and turgor, hair consistency and distribution, and poor wound healing should be noted. Hyperpigmentation of the joints, waist, mouth, and palmar creases is associated with adrenal insufficiency.

Exophthalmos can be a hallmark of hyperthyroidism. An oropharyngeal examination is essential for glossitis, ulcers, exudates, masses, ill-fitting or odorous dentures, tooth or gum decay, and missing teeth. The temporomandibular joint should be palpated and gently extended to assess pain or crepitation. Lymphadenopathy, neck masses, and a diminished swallow reflex may warrant further studies. Thyroid enlargement requires further testing for thyroid dysfunction.

Dyspnea, arrhythmias, diminished breath sounds, jugular venous distention, wheezing, and ankle edema suggest cardiopulmonary problems that may interfere with appetite or energy demands.

Breast examination is important, given the rising incidence of cancers associated with aging. An abdominal examination that is positive for acute rigidity, masses, hepatomegaly, midepigastric tenderness, or ascites may indicate problems with digestion, absorption, or vascular flow; liver disease; or gastrointestinal tumor. Rectal ulcers, rectal lesions or fissures, hemorrhoids, swollen prostate or nodule, and painful defecation resulting from underlying disease processes may be seen on examination or follow-up studies. Pelvic and bimanual examination for cervical and ovarian cancer screening should be included, with follow-up imaging as indicated.

Finally, frailty is associated with slow ataxic gait, strength loss, a history of frequent falls and fear of falling, poor appetite, cognitive decline, and depressed affect. It is also correlated with sarcopenia, osteopenia, and immunologic markers, such as catabolic cytokines and coagulopathy.[10]

DIAGNOSTICS

Thyroid function studies to exclude hyperthyroidism are warranted in those who have signs of increased metabolism, including tachycardia (see Chapter 214) and weight loss. A complete blood count (CBC) with differential is helpful in determining the presence of infection or malignant disease. Detection of anemia should be followed by evaluation of serum iron, ferritin, thiamine, vitamin B_{12}, and folate levels (see Chapter 237). A chemistry profile, including calcium, potassium, alkaline phosphatase, liver biochemical studies, serum electrolytes, serum glucose, serum albumin (which is sensitive to hydration status), blood urea nitrogen (BUN), and creatinine, would suggest nutritional deficiencies or other underlying diseases. A urinalysis can reveal infection or unmask proteinuria or uremia associated with early anorexia of kidney disease. Hemoglobin A1c (HbA_{1c}) is warranted if diabetes is suspected. A chest x-ray examination is helpful if a pulmonary pathologic condition is suspected. Age- and history-appropriate cancer screenings should be recommended.

Although a stool evaluation for occult blood is indicated if a rectosigmoid source is suspected, testing for ova and parasites, culture, or fat content is based on history, clinical presentation, and physical signs. If the patient's history suggests a possible esophageal stricture or gastric or duodenal ulcer, several tests are available. An upper gastrointestinal series with or without small bowel follow-through, endoscopy, or barium swallow may help clarify symptoms in the setting of food-sticking sensation, low hematocrit, positive *Helicobacter pylori* status, or chronic diarrhea. Ultrasound examinations (pelvic, renal, and abdominal), echocardiography, and lung studies should be reserved for confirmation of suspected abdominal, renal, gynecologic, cardiac, or pulmonary causes of weight loss. Sigmoidoscopy or colonoscopy, Doppler flow ultrasonography, and magnetic resonance angiography are appropriate for a high suspicion of intestinal or mesenteric arterial disease.

Finally, a low score (<24) on the Mini-Mental State Examination or other tests for cognitive functioning should raise the question of dementia with poor functional capacity. A positive depression inventory is necessary to further explore situational or psychological diagnoses.

DIAGNOSTICS

Weight Loss

LABORATORY

Albumin
Blood, urea, nitrogen (BUN)
C-reactive protein*
Calcium
CBC and differential
Cholesterol (or lipid panel)*
Creatinine
Electrolytes (sodium, potassium, chloride, carbon dioxide)
Erythrocyte sedimentation rate*
Fecal occult blood test
Glucose
HIV*
Immunoglobulin A (IgA) and IgG endomysial antibodies*
IgA transglutaminase antibodies*
Lactate dehydrogenase*
Liver biochemical tests (alanine transaminase, aspartate transaminase, alkaline phosphatase)
Prostate-specific antigen
Stool for ova and parasites*
Stool for fecal fat*
Stool for culture*
Thyroid-stimulating hormone

IMAGING

Ultrasound (abdominal, pelvic, renal)
Computed tomography scan*
Magnetic resonance imaging*
Chest x-ray studies
Upper gastrointestinal tract imaging*

OTHER DIAGNOSTICS

Endoscopy*
Barium swallow*
Gastric emptying scan*
Colonic transit study*
Colonoscopy*
Echocardiography*

*If indicated.

DIFFERENTIAL DIAGNOSIS

Often, unintentional weight loss is a result of cancer. A rubric to predict malignancy proposed by Hernandez and colleagues includes age older than 80, white blood cell count higher than 12,000, alkaline phosphatase above 300 IU/L, and lactase dehydrogenase above 500 IU/L. The Hernandez rubric suggests that malignancy is less common when the albumin is higher than 3.5 g/dL. Others looked at inflammatory markers in younger patients, but involuntary weight loss is not yet an independent marker for malignancy in that group.[1] Some cancers cause a slow decline in weight, whereas gastrointestinal and head and neck cancers are more likely to cause a precipitous decline.[1] The notion that the reason for weight loss in malignancy is "competition" for calories between the tumor and the host is outdated. Newer research suggests that weight loss in malignancy is a metabolic reaction unrelated to the size of the tumor, more similar to a paraneoplastic syndrome.[11]

Nonmalignant gastrointestinal disease (9% to 19%) is another important cause of unintended weight loss, followed by psychiatric causes, including depression and dementia (9% to 24%).[2] Gastroenterologic or psychiatric illness leading to weight loss can result from a multitude of other organ system illnesses: cardiac, respiratory, endocrine, rheumatologic, and immunologic. Infections contribute a smaller percentage. Cases of unknown cause remain a high percentage of the total and may require additional workup to gain another 10% to 20% in diagnostic yield.[1]

DIFFERENTIAL DIAGNOSIS

Weight Loss

DECREASED CALORIE INTAKE
- Alcoholism
- "Anorexia of aging"—fullness, early satiety, tendency to snack less and eat smaller meals—can be associated with loss of physical independence
- Anorexia nervosa
- Anxiety
- Bulimia
- Cocaine use (appetite suppression)
- Cognitive impairment from multiple sclerosis, stroke
- Decreased access to food
- Decreased smell or taste
- Dementia, stroke
- Depression, decreased enjoyment of food
- Dieting
- Drug side effects
- Dry mouth
- Functional obstacles to eating
- Gastrointestinal or bowel distress
- HIV/AIDS or infectious diseases
- Hypomania
- Malignant neoplasms
- Poor nutrition
- Poor dentition, difficulty chewing
- Situational stress
- Social isolation
- Swallowing dysfunction

DECREASED CALORIE ABSORPTION
- AIDS wasting syndrome
- Alcoholism
- Chronic liver disease
- Diabetes mellitus, uncontrolled
- Diarrhea from illness or chemotherapy
- Gallbladder disease
- Post–gastrectomy surgery
- Protein-losing enteropathies
- Renal disease
- Skin wounds, infected or healing
- Small bowel disease
- Vomiting from illness or chemotherapy

INCREASED METABOLIC DEMANDS
- Adrenal insufficiency
- Cardiac cachexia with advanced congestive heart failure
- Chronic infections (HIV/AIDS, tuberculosis)
- Chronic respiratory disease
- Fever
- Hyperthyroidism
- Hypopituitarism
- Infection
- Inflammatory bowel disease
- Malignant neoplasms
- Mania
- Parkinson disease

As noted earlier, among those with unintentional weight loss, a psychiatric diagnosis is common. Adult-onset situational or chemical depression, late-stage Alzheimer dementia, schizophrenia, hypomania, and food-related or substance abuse disorders, even in later life, can take a toll.

Some cases of weight loss may defy diagnosis. Follow-up evaluation and support are useful in these patients. Fortunately, for those individuals with an elusive diagnosis, the prognosis tends to be relatively better than for those diagnosed with a specific reason for their weight loss.[1]

MANAGEMENT

The primary goals in managing involuntary weight loss are to provide adequate energy, protein, and micronutrients and to treat the underlying disease or, at least, any reversible illness. Medications are used to reverse nausea, to increase appetite, or both, including progestin, megestrol acetate, and the cannabinoid dronabinol, although there are a significant side effects with the last.[2] Medical marijuana is now legal in 24 states, with cachexia and wasting secondary to AIDS being two of many indications for its use. Studies are lacking as to efficacy.

Megestrol acetate, with the dosage goal of 800 mg/day, in some studies did improve appetite (possibly through neuropeptide Y stimulation).[1] This medication is used in patients with HIV, COPD, cystic fibrosis, or cancer and in older adults for weight enhancement without effect on quality of life.[1] However, there are continuing concerns about thromboembolic events, hypertension, and adrenal insufficiency.[10] There are no conclusive data on the efficacy of megestrol, cannabinoids, and nutritional or enteral feeding programs if the cause of involuntary weight loss is unknown.[2] Protein-rich nutritional supplements had a beneficial effect on underweight community-dwelling adults older than 65, resulting in reduced complications and readmissions, improved grip strength, and better protein stores and energy without a compromise in baseline food intake.[3] Mirtazapine, a serotonin antagonist, is used to promote appetite and improve depression, although orthostatic hypotension and dizziness are potential side effects.[2]

Eicosapentaenoic acid, an anti-inflammatory fatty acid found in fish oil, is promising for patients with advanced cancer because it may inhibit proteolytic activity arising from tumors.[12] Thalidomide, is approved by the Food and Drug Administration for the treatment of AIDS wasting, although it is seldom used due to severe teratogenisity. Corticosteroids (prednisone, methylprednisolone, dexamethasone), which are somewhat effective in cachexic patients, are effective for reasons that are not fully understood.[13] When taken for several weeks, corticosteroid preparations (equivalent to methylprednisolone 20 to 50 mg) can have a positive impact on anorexia, chronic nausea, fatigue or asthenia, performance status, and quality of life or well-being.[13]

The antidopaminergic metoclopramide, 10 to 15 mg, taken 30 minutes before meals and at bedtime, serves as an antiemetic with gastrointestinal prokinetic properties.[13] Some research suggests that appetite stimulation may be of limited usefulness but that its positive effects on reducing early satiety and nausea are beneficial.

Smaller food portions offered frequently and a calorie-rich breakfast may enhance nutritional intake. Calorie-dense foods and nutritional drinks can improve intake. With severe wasting or when oral feeding is not safe or desirable, enteral tube feedings (if the gastrointestinal tract is functional) or parenteral feedings can supplement or supplant oral feedings if acceptable to the patient. Protein quality has been a focus. The Recommended Daily Allowance (RDA) for protein is 0.8 g/kg/day for the general population, but elders show reduced anabolic response to protein and are thought to benefit from 1.0 to 1.3 g/kg/day spread over the day for maintenance.[4] An optimal assortment of essential amino acids have an effect on body weight; and on protein synthesis and oxidative stress protection.[5] A study of 2108 women in 35 prefectures of Japan revealed that type of protein (animal or vegetable) was less important than the amount of protein in the diet; this was also inversely associated with frailty.[5] Exercise (resistance and aerobic) may have dual benefits in bone and muscle preservation along with preventing falls in older adults. Exercise along with food support and reduced polypharmacy helps to restore physical function and may improve appetite.[7] Exercise may be the most beneficial intervention in frail elders, in whom nutritional interventions are less reliable.[14] Reduced energy expenditure in elders may lead to reduced appetite and weight. Sometimes regaining lost weight after an inadvertent weight loss (after illness or surgery) can be challenging because the older individual may not be inclined to eat enough to make up for the loss.[3]

Finally, to address the psychosocial and situational stress drivers of unintentional weight loss, one must consider increasing older age, loss of spouse, disability, and previous hospitalization as risk factors,[1] suggesting the necessity of psychosocial support.

INDICATIONS FOR REFERRAL OR HOSPITALIZATION

- If available, the services of a dietitian or nutritionist are invaluable. Occupational, physical, or speech therapists can also help. A social worker is critical to the team.
- Medical specialists, including geriatricians, gastroenterologists, cardiologists, pulmonologists, nephrologists, neurologists, oncologists, psychiatrists, and psychologists, should be consulted when necessary.
- A patient with severe anorexia associated with a weight loss in excess of 35% of ideal body weight, hypokalemia, hypotension, or prerenal azotemia related to dehydration requires immediate hospitalization.
- Patients with frailty in addition to cancer, HIV/AIDS, heart failure, renal failure, or diabetes or who are undergoing surgery are at particular risk[7] and may require hospitalization for nasal or gastric tube placement and feedings or parenteral nutrition, depending on patient wishes and treatment goals.
- Weight loss is a frequent finding in late-stage dementia; however, enteral feedings have not been shown to extend life or to prevent aspiration and are associated with infection, discomfort, increased use of physical restraints, and increased confusion and are not recommended in this population.

COMPLICATIONS

Patients who are at risk for malnutrition and weight loss require nutritional evaluation and support, whether in acute hospital, rehabilitative, or home settings. Complications of significant weight loss include severe malnutrition, weakness, loss of muscle mass, orthostatic hypotension, falls, immobility, and death. Immunocompromised patients and older adults are at special risk for weight loss–related complications.

Reversible complications such as community-acquired or nosocomial infections, community- or facility-acquired *Clostridium difficile* colitis, incontinence leading to skin breakdown, skin ulcers caused by low albumin in the setting of bed confinement, dental caries or denture complaints, poor pain control, and poor conditioning from repeated hospitalizations should be attended to as early as possible to preserve energy stores otherwise taxed by the disease and poor intake.

LIFE SPAN CONSIDERATIONS

Involuntary weight loss at any age should include screening for eating disorders. As older adults experience the physiologic changes that uniquely predispose them to weight loss, it is important to monitor weight and nutrition before weight loss occurs. Body mass peaks in men during their 40s and in women during their 50s, although the peak may be delayed by a decade. This peak results from shifts in muscle and fat stores and fat atrophy, causing a 1- to 2-kg (2.2- to 4.4-pound) decrease per decade. Diminished smell and taste sensations, which otherwise enhance the pleasurable experience of eating, are associated with aging.

Because older age brings limitations in physical abilities and the potential for social isolation, a thorough evaluation of functional independence and safety may uncover meal-related problems. Weight loss that is related to a disease process, acute illness, or depression may resist recovery, particularly in older adults, so optimal management requires a team effort, with a focus on maximizing abilities and interests. This is particularly true in institutional settings, where contributing factors such as dependency and illness can be assessed and addressed more easily. Anticipating malnutrition and weight loss during episodes of acute illness is likely to be crucial to the care of the vulnerable patient because catching up later is difficult. Older adults with advanced dementia commonly experience feeding and eating difficulties leading to weight loss. In spite of an increasing body of research demonstrating that feeding tubes do not extend life or improve quality of life in these patients, many institutionalized older adults with late-stage dementia are being fed enterally. The majority of nursing home residents do not have orders documenting their wishes in this situation, leaving family members in the difficult position of deciding to insert a feeding tube or to continue with hand feeding without adequate knowledge or education. This lack of clarity can be addressed before the situation reaches a decision point by addressing the patient's wishes and educating families in the office while the patient still possesses decisional capacity. "Comfort feeding only" orders can be written as part of an overall feeding care plan that directs all care efforts toward the comfort of the older patient.[15]

EDUCATION AND HEALTH PROMOTION

Teaching patients simple nutritional concepts and encouraging them to keep a food diary may be helpful. Suggestions for increasing meal attractiveness include flavor enhancement through polyunsaturated butters, oils, dressings, jellies, and creamers. Increased fiber and increased fluid content should be encouraged. Because zinc deficiency can lead to dysgeusia, adding a multivitamin along with protein-rich snacks and nutritional supplements may significantly improve appetite and intake.

Facilitating food procurement with prepackaged meals or home-delivered foods can make a difference. Increasing activity, social engagement, and a sense of functional capability in the face of dysfunction or physical limitation also improve quality of life. Appetite may also be improved with a simplified regimen that optimizes the number of medications taken.

Because weight loss can be a late sign of pulmonary, renal, or cardiac disease, it is important to encourage patients or their advocates to look for medical guidance to optimize their quality of life. Ultimately, a discussion of palliative care may be the most humane approach to comfort severely cachexic individuals and their families.

Primary prevention of weight loss includes promoting activities that support safe access to food, medical and dental services, and socialization for those at social or financial risk of decreased intake.

Preventing communicable diseases such as hepatitis A and B, diphtheria, and pertussis; receiving scheduled Pneumovax and influenza vaccines; managing sleep requirements; and making adjustments in diet for tastes and preferences all help safeguard nutritional status. Screening at-risk individuals for chronic mental illness and substance abuse, including situational depression and prolonged grieving—especially among the elderly, who face disproportionate loss and isolation—will help guide early intervention.

Other important strategies that enhance the eating experience are to manage side effects such as constipation, nausea and vomiting, and gas; to focus on the favorite meal of the day; and to choose easy-to-prepare foods with adequate flavorings. Malnutrition is better prevented than treated because significant weight loss can become irremediable.

REFERENCES

For a full list of references, scan the QR code or visit http://booksite.elsevier.com/9780323355018

PART 20

Evaluation and Management of Infectious Diseases

CHAPTER 229

EMERGING AND REEMERGING INFECTIOUS DISEASES

Lisa V. Adams • Elizabeth A. Talbot

Terms such as "emerging" and "reemerging" diseases increasingly appear in the clinical and even public parlance. Our patients are regularly bombarded by media stories about and images of these diseases and consequently often have questions (or even fears) that they might present to us. Because primary care providers are frequently on the front lines of the global battle to control these pathogens, this chapter intends to provide an overview of this category of diseases to improve our understanding and thereby our preparedness.

DEFINITIONS

Emerging infectious diseases result from newly discovered and previously unknown infections that threaten public health. Increased international travel and trade, deforestation and changing ecosystems, and rapid adaptation of microorganisms have contributed to this problem (Box 229-1).[1] For example, the 2009-2010 influenza A pandemic that was caused by a novel influenza A H1N1 virus spread within months from Mexico and other countries in the Southern Hemisphere to become the predominant influenza virus circulating in most countries.[2]

BOX 229-1

Pathogenesis of Emerging and Reemerging Infectious Diseases: Global Problem

- Global travel allows rapid dissemination of new pathogens.
- Urbanization as rural populations move to cities creates overcrowding and poverty.
- Civil wars and ethnic cleansing create displaced populations without health care.
- Irrigation, deforestation, and reforestation all upset ecosystems of vectors and animals.
- Living in ecozones and population migration increase contact with insects and animals.
- Infrastructure deterioration caused by poverty or natural disasters deters health care delivery.
- Injection drug abuse, relaxed sexual mores, and sexual tourism facilitate pathogen spread.
- Inappropriate use of antibiotics or antibiotic use in animal feed spawns resistance.
- Contagion spreads via bioterrorism.

Reemerging infectious diseases are those that had formerly caused so few infections that they were no longer considered a public health threat but have recently reactivated.[1] Dengue fever (DF) is an example of a reemerging infectious disease; its vector, the *Aedes aegypti* mosquito, has distributed it from Africa throughout the Americas via expanding world commerce. In addition, the gradual discontinuation of yellow fever mosquito control programs has allowed the *A. aegypti* mosquito to expand its geographic distribution in South America, the Caribbean, and now the southern United States, where cases of DF are more prevalent and more severe than in the past.

RISK FACTORS FAVORING EMERGENCE OF PATHOGENS

Our recent history has witnessed a rapid succession of newly identified pathogens—reemergent and now resistant bacteria, reemergent diarrheal illnesses (see Chapter 232) in developing nations, new respiratory pathogens, and vector-borne illnesses. Reasons for the emergence of infectious diseases are outlined in Box-229-1.

Central to the epidemiology of emerging and reemerging pathogens is the concept of globalization. Never before in human history have we been as vulnerable to diseases that were previously geographically contained. With the ease of global transport of people, animals, insect vectors, food, and goods, there is real and imminent risk of the introduction of new diseases that might be seen in primary care. Our interconnected world allows well-known pathogens rapid access to new, immunologically naive populations and facilitates the spread of novel pathogens and antimicrobial resistance. The following are some recent examples:

- Human immunodeficiency virus (HIV) (see Chapter 230) emerged when the simian immunodeficiency virus jumped species from African green monkeys to human populations, and then rapidly spread throughout the world.
- Widespread outbreaks of *Salmonella, Cyclospora,* and *Escherichia coli* O157:H7 diarrheal illnesses are directly related to the globalization of our food supply.
- The 2009 influenza A H1N1 pandemic spread from Mexico worldwide within months and became the predominant influenza virus circulating in most countries.
- Exotic pet aficionados have introduced previously geographically constrained pathogens into the human population. One such example is a human monkeypox outbreak linked to keeping Gambian giant pouched rats as pets.

In addition to globalization, changes in our societies and lifestyles have also been permissive for emergence and reemergence of certain infectious diseases. For example:

- Tuberculosis (TB) (see Chapter 235) has been an historic plague of humans, but trends toward urbanization and overcrowding have been linked to outbreaks of multidrug-resistant tuberculosis (MDR-TB).

- Epidemics of injection drug abuse have contributed to the HIV and hepatitis C epidemics.
- Rampant counterfeit drug sales and absent regulatory controls in Southeast Asia have contributed to the emergence of malaria species resistant to artemisinin-based therapy less than 10 years after it became the preferred therapy.
- Reforestation of farmlands, reemergence of deer herds, and our desire to live in ecozones (edge areas) have contributed to the rapid emergence of Lyme disease in the United States.
- Prescribing practices and antibiotic use in animal feed have contributed to the emergence of drug-resistant enteric pathogens, including vancomycin-resistant enterococci, methicillin-resistant *Staphylococcus aureus* (MRSA), and penicillin-resistant *Streptococcus pneumoniae.*
- Close contact exposes bird farmers and open market visitors to novel respiratory viruses such as avian influenzas or coronaviruses (e.g., severe acute respiratory syndrome [SARS], Middle East respiratory syndrome coronavirus [MERS-CoV]).

Natural disasters and infrastructure deterioration have also contributed to emergence and reemergence of certain pathogens:

- Resistant *Salmonella* and *Campylobacter* organisms in tsunami- or monsoon-stricken Southeast Asia
- Cholera in postearthquake Haiti

PATHOGENS

For this discussion, major emerging pathogens are categorized by their syndromes (e.g., respiratory, gastrointestinal), their mechanism of transmission (e.g., vector, zoonotic), and their threat through emerging antibiotic resistance. This discussion is intended to prepare the primary care clinician for expanding differential diagnoses and appropriate referral.

Acute Respiratory Diseases

Coronaviruses. Coronaviruses are pathogens in animals and humans, well known as a cause of the common cold. SARS is a coronavirus that emerged in 2002 from Guangdong Province, China.[3] It caused a severe and often fatal pneumonia, with prominent systemic symptoms. An incubation period of 4 to 7 days was followed by fever, an influenza-like illness, and, a few days later, symptoms of pneumonia, diarrhea, leukopenia, thrombocytopenia, and characteristically lymphopenia. Laboratory diagnosis was best made by detection of antibody, which appears about 10 days into the illness, or reverse transcriptase polymerase chain reaction (RT-PCR) on bronchial secretions.[4] About 25% of patients developed severe pneumonia complicated by acute respiratory distress syndrome (ARDS). Mortality was as high as 50% in older patients and hosts with underlying disease,[3] and survivors had significantly reduced exercise capacity and health status compared with the general population.[5]

The intrigue of SARS lies in its abrupt emergence as a new human pathogen. A coronavirus from a palm civet and/or a ferret badger in the live animal markets jumped species into humans and spread rapidly from person-to-person locally and then internationally via air travel. SARS also had high morbidity and mortality rates associated with spread in naive populations, with more than 8000 cases and 780 deaths reported from 29 countries before the outbreak ended in June 2003. We have not seen another case to date, but concern lingers because SARS coronavirus has been isolated from open-market animals and could still be circulating in animals only to reemerge as a human pathogen.[6]

Middle East Respiratory Syndrome. MERS is an emerging illness cause by a previously unknown coronavirus called Middle East respiratory syndrome coronavirus. The first case, reported in a 60-year-old man who lived in Saudi Arabia, had a fatal outcome.[7] At the time of this writing, all cases have been linked directly or indirectly to countries in the Arabian Peninsula, most notably Saudi Arabia, Qatar, Jordan, and the United Arab Emirates.[8] Transmission to health care workers caring for MERS patients has been documented, providing an important reminder to primary care clinicians to screen patients with consistent symptoms for any relevant travel history in order to institute appropriate infection control practices.[9]

After a 2- to 14-day incubation period, MERS patients typically develop fever, cough, and shortness of breath. Some will have gastrointestinal symptoms including diarrhea and/or nausea and vomiting. As with SARS, most patients progress to ARDS with multiorgan system failure. The mortality rate is approximately 55%.[8,10]

Those advising patients traveling to the affected region should check the website of the Centers for Disease Control and Prevention (CDC) for any updates on travel advisories. The current recommendations to travelers include fastidious adherence to routine measures to prevent respiratory illnesses, including washing hands, avoiding personal contact such as kissing and sharing eating utensils with ill individuals, and disinfecting frequently used surfaces such as doorknobs.[11]

Human Metapneumovirus. Human metapneumovirus (hMPV) is an example of a pathogen that has probably been causing respiratory tract illness for many years but is considered emerging because it has only recently been recognized. Discovered in 2001 by researchers applying molecular polymerase chain reaction (PCR) techniques to children with previously unexplained pneumonia, hMPV is now recognized to cause at least 5% to 10% of pediatric hospitalizations for lower respiratory tract illness in the United States.[12] Given how many children are hospitalized each year with lower respiratory tract illness, hMPV represents an important cause of morbidity and mortality. Serologic studies demonstrate antibodies to hMPV in virtually all children by the age of 5 years.[12] Although primarily recognized as a pediatric disease, hMPV has also recently been recognized in adults, most clearly as a major cause of severe lower respiratory tract illness in immunocompromised adults and elders.

HMPV causes a spectrum of illness ranging from upper to lower respiratory tract illness and is clinically indistinguishable from the more familiar respiratory syncytial virus (RSV) infection. hMPV is often milder and affects a slightly older group of children (6 to 12 months of age) in contrast to RSV, which often affects infants before 2 months of age.[12,13] Like RSV and influenza, hMPV circulates predominately in winter months, which is when it should be especially considered in the differential diagnosis. Because influenza, RSV, and hMPV share common seasonality and hosts, vigilance toward diagnosing coinfections should be maintained.

Diagnosis is best made with real-time PCR on bronchial secretions. The virus is difficult to grow, and serologic tests are yet to be standardized. No vaccine or antiviral therapy is available, but studies show that ribavirin and intravenous immune globulin inhibit hMPV in vitro. Repeated episodes of asymptomatic infection or with common cold symptoms maintain immunity in adults.[13]

Influenza A. See Chapter 231. Pandemic influenza A by definition is an emerging pathogen, which can cause staggering human morbidity and mortality, and an accompanying massive resource expenditure. Pandemic flu classically arises through an antigenic shift, which is a rearrangement of animal influenza genes into a human influenza virus. But we now also know that lesser changes ("antigenic drift") can sometimes cause pandemics, as was shown by sequencing the 1918 pandemic influenza virus, which killed as many as 30 million people worldwide.[14]

Influenza A impels us toward improved understanding of zoonotic viruses, continued surveillance in human and animal populations through international networks, and development of an influenza vaccine that offers broad protection against different viral variants. One vivid example of a recently emerged influenza virus is the 2009-2010 influenza pandemic. International air travel rapidly disseminated a new influenza A virus globally: within 6 months after the virus's emergence was recognized in Mexico, the World Health Organization (WHO) declared that the criteria for a pandemic had been met.[2,15,16] Global initiatives enabled public health jurisdictions to implement diagnostic and clinical management algorithms and international networks for surveillance and research, to track the virus and its evolution, and to optimize clinical outcomes.

We now know that the causative H1N1 influenza A virus is antigenically distinct from the preexisting seasonal human influenza virus and resulted from the reassortment between two influenza A (H1N1) swine viruses that themselves were the products of several independent avian to mammalian cross-species transmissions and prior reassortments among avian, human, and swine viruses.[17] Like the viruses responsible for the influenza pandemics of 1957 and 1968, the 2009 H1N1 virus is a descendant of the 1918 pandemic virus.[18] Unlike with seasonal influenza, children and young adults rather than elders experienced the highest attack rates from influenza A (H1N1) because most adults older than 60 years had protection from cross-protective antibodies they had developed from prior exposure to antigenically related influenza viruses.[19]

Clinical features, diagnostic approaches, treatment, and prevention of influenza A (H1N1) are discussed in Chapter 231.

Avian Influenza A (H5N1). Avian influenzas are always circulating among birds but do not usually "jump species" to infect mammalian cells. In 1997, a small outbreak of avian influenza A (H5N1) occurred within the live poultry markets of Hong Kong. This outbreak was unique in that the virus jumped from birds to humans and caused severe illness in 18 previously healthy adults, six of whom died. There was no human-to-human transmission, and an unprecedented culling of the entire poultry population of Hong Kong contained the outbreak. But in 2003, the same virus reemerged as the cause of a massive poultry outbreak across Asia. Human cases of H5N1 have followed in parallel to the geographic spread of the poultry pandemic. Most human cases had direct exposure to diseased birds. Although there have been family clusters, human-to-human transmission remains limited and unsustained.[20]

Primary care clinicians have a paramount role in providing their patients with seasonal influenza vaccination. The seasonal influenza vaccine will not protect us from avian influenza (H5N1), but 30,000 to 50,000 die each year in the United States from current endemic influenza strains, and immunization will prevent other influenza illnesses from being confused with avian influenza should human-to-human transmission become more facile. In 2013, the Food and Drug Administration approved the first adjuvanted vaccine to prevent avian influenza.[21] This vaccine could prove very useful if the H5N1 virus develops the capability for efficient human-to-human spread, which could lead to the next human pandemic.

Acute Diarrheal Illnesses

Vibrio cholerae. Cholera epidemics (see Chapter 232) characteristically emerge, decline, and reemerge throughout human history, brought on by natural disasters, civil war, and displaced populations. Six pandemics, caused by the classic biotype *Vibrio cholerae* O1, occurred before 1926, originated in Asia and India, and traveled in infected patients to Europe and the Americas. The seventh and current pandemic is caused by a new classic biotype, El Tor, first isolated in Egypt. It causes milder disease, which remained sporadic and endemic throughout Africa, Europe, and Asia for many years. Emergence of a new strain, *V. cholerae* O139, began in India and Bangladesh in 1992. Past exposure to *V. cholerae* O1 offers no immunity to *V. cholerae* O139, which has also been noted to be resistant to trimethoprim-sulfamethoxazole.[22]

V. cholerae is naturally found in water, attached to algae, crustaceans, and plankton. Warmer-than-usual waters (e.g., because of El Niño) facilitate its growth by changes in nutrients and salinity (e.g., from monsoons, tsunamis, and typhoons).[23] In this activated state, humans are more likely to become infected and transmit infection through fecally contaminated food or water. Direct person-to-person spread is unlikely because of the large inoculum required for infection. Infants and young children bear the brunt of epidemics in resource-limited nations, where 80% of all diarrheal deaths occur in children younger than 5 years.[24]

Disasters provide ready availability of contaminated water and food. In a recent tragic example of this reality, the catastrophic January 2010 earthquake in Haiti killed over 200,000 people and displaced over 1 million. Ten months after the earthquake, the Haitian Ministry of Public Health and Population was notified of a sudden increase in patients with watery diarrhea and dehydration. On October 21, 2010, the Haiti National Public Health Laboratory identified the pathogen as *V. cholera.* The first cholera outbreak in Haiti in at least a century was announced, and, at the time of this writing, over 470,000 cases of cholera have now been reported in Haiti, with 6631 attributable deaths. This marks the worst cholera outbreak in recent history, as well as the best-documented cholera outbreak in modern public health.[25]

Severe dehydration, electrolyte imbalance, renal failure, and metabolic acidosis can be fatal complications of cholera, and oral or intravenous rehydration is the most important intervention to avert death. Mortality is as high as 10% in epidemic settings without adequate health care support but 3% or less in centers versed in simple hydration techniques. Antibiotics are secondary in importance to hydration. One 300-mg dose of doxycycline, 1 g of ciprofloxacin, or 1 tablet of trimethoprim-sulfamethoxazole twice daily for 3 days is effective treatment if the organism is sensitive. Emerging antibiotic resistance is a problem for developing nations. Fortunately, cholera is a predictably reemergent disease most likely to be encountered after natural disasters, in refugee camps, and in urban slums where it is endemic. Simple measures to dispose of human waste, to avoid contaminated water, and to provide a potable water supply are critical public health priorities in these situations. Travelers intending to work or volunteer in such settings should be appropriately counseled about prevention methods, symptoms, and the need for prompt fluid replacement, and considered for emergency standby treatment.

***Escherichia coli* O157:H7.** *E. coli* O157:H7 was first recognized as a food-borne pathogen in the United States in 1982. Outbreaks occurred through distribution of contaminated hamburger meat, and enterohemorrhagic *Escherichia coli* (EHEC) soon became a common cause of bloody diarrhea. From January 2009 to December 2010, the CDC estimated 29,444 food-borne illnesses annually in the United States, resulting in 1184 hospitalizations and 23 deaths. Shiga toxin–producing *E. coli* caused 16% of the food-borne illnesses, and 22 of the 23 deaths.[26] See also Chapter 232.

Association of *E. coli* O157:H7 diarrhea with childhood hemolytic-uremic syndrome (HUS) exemplifies how a pathogen can evolve and cause increased, unexpected pathology. HUS was previously an unexplained illness, defined by hemolysis, thrombocytopenia, and acute renal failure, often in children. We now know that EHEC evolved to acquire a symbiotic relationship with a bacteriophage that encodes a Shiga-like toxin (SLT), a toxin also present in *Shigella dysenteriae.* SLT attaches to a receptor, globotriaosylceramide (GB), on enterocytes in the gut. GB receptors also exist on endothelial cells of glomerular capillaries and other small capillary beds. Damage to these capillary beds by circulating SLT explains the occurrence of acute renal failure, microangiopathic hemolytic anemia, and thrombocytopenia, which define HUS.[27] Further investigation demonstrates that HUS is the most common cause of acute renal failure in children. Elders are also vulnerable to *E. coli* O157:H7 because neutralizing antibodies to SLT decline as a person ages. *E. coli* O157:H7 has emerged as a common cause of HUS, a disease not previously recognized as infectious.[28]

Treatment of EHEC diarrhea is hydration and correction of electrolyte imbalance. Antibiotic treatment induces release of SLT and had been thought to worsen the risk of HUS, although a recent systematic review did not show an increased risk.[29] Practically, though, by the time HUS appears, the acute diarrhea has already subsided, so antibiotics are not likely to help. *E. coli* O157:H7 is also mandatorily reported to health departments.

Vector-Borne Diseases

Two important emerging vector-borne diseases, Lyme disease and West Nile virus, are discussed elsewhere. Lyme disease is discussed in detail in Chapter 234, and West Nile virus is covered in Chapter 236.

Dengue Fever. DF is a classic illustration of an infectious disease that is reemerging owing to human activities. The disease was held in check after World War II by mosquito control programs designed to eradicate yellow fever. With the gradual discontinuation of those programs, but also expanding world commerce and global warming, the dengue vector, the *Aedes* mosquito, has spread from Africa throughout the Americas, even into the southern United States.

The global distribution and impact of DF is now similar to that of malaria. With more than one third of the world's population living in areas at risk for DF, dengue virus is a leading cause of illness and death in the tropics and subtropics. There are an estimated 50 to 100 million cases occurring annually across 100 countries.[30,31] Reports of cases among U.S. travelers to dengue-endemic destinations are also increasing, and DF is now the most common acute febrile illness in travelers returning from the Caribbean, South America, and Asia.[31] DF can also be locally acquired in the United States, with cases reported sporadically along the Texas-Mexico border and an outbreak of 27 cases reported in 2009-2010 in Key West, Florida.[31]

DF is caused by four related viruses (designated DENV-1, DENV-2, DENV-3, and DENV-4). Immunity to one dengue virus serotype does not provide protection to the other three. DF is spread most commonly by the *A. aegypti* mosquito but also by the more adaptable *Aedes albopictus.*[30] Clinical DF develops after an incubation period of 3 to 7 days with the sudden onset of chills, fever, headache with characteristic retro-orbital pain, severe musculoskeletal pain, abdominal tenderness, back pain, and hyperesthesia of skin. The classic "saddleback" fever pattern may occur, with a lowering of fever around the third day followed by a recurrence on the fourth or fifth day.[30] As fever resolves, a maculopapular rash appears, which may be scarlatiniform or petechial. The illness may be biphasic, with acute illness followed by prolonged weakness, fatigue, and depression.

Leukopenia, neutropenia, thrombocytopenia, transaminitis, and severe musculoskeletal symptoms may help distinguish DF from other viral illness or typhoid fever in a returning traveler. Viremia reaches high levels, and viral blood culture, PCR, and serum immunoglobulin M (IgM) may all be used to make the diagnosis. IgM can be detected as early as 4 days after the onset of fever and can be used in patients with a clinical syndrome consistent with DF to establish a presumptive diagnosis from a single specimen or a confirmatory diagnosis if there is seroconversion between paired specimens.[30] Second exposures to dengue virus may be complicated by ARDS, hepatitis, myositis, rhabdomyolysis, or acute renal failure, which is more likely to be found in infants and older patients living in endemic or epidemic settings. Two of these more severe forms of dengue infection are dengue hemorrhagic fever (DHF) and dengue septic shock (DSS). DHF is characterized by hemorrhage, moderate to severe thrombocytopenia, and development of increased vascular fragility and platelet dysfunction.[30] Significant bleeding is rare in children with DHF, but skin and mucosal (gastrointestinal or vaginal) bleeding can occur in adults.[30] The mechanism for bleeding in DHF is unclear.[30]

There is no effective treatment other than supportive measures and fluid resuscitation for DSS.[30] Aspirin and anti-inflammatory drugs for analgesia and antipyretic effects should be avoided. Development of a dengue vaccine is recognized as an urgent global priority, and several promising candidates are being evaluated in clinical trials, including one tetravalent vaccine candidate advancing to human testing.[32,33] Dengue vaccine development is challenged by the need for a vaccine that induces immune responses against all dengue strains and by the fact that the mechanisms that provide protection against dengue infection and disease are poorly understood.[33] Consequently, it will likely be several years before a dengue vaccine is available for widespread use.

Chikungunya Fever. Caused by the mosquito-borne chikungunya virus (CHIKV), chikungunya fever was first reported in East Africa in the 1950s. The name *chikungunya* comes from the Kimakonde language of Tanzania and Mozambique and means "that which contorts or bends up."[34] This name was derived from descriptions of patients who assumed a typical stooped posture because of the severe arthritic symptoms. As with DF, *A. aegypti* is the main vector, with some transmission by *A. albopictus.* Global trade and migration have facilitated the spread of this virus from Africa to India through the islands of the Indian Ocean, and then throughout Southeast Asia and, most recently, in a northern region of Italy. The Italian outbreak is an important reminder that returning travelers who are ill can introduce pathogens into novel areas. In December 2013, local transmission of chikungunya fever in the Caribbean island of Saint Martin was reported by WHO.[35] Six months later, local transmission had been reported by more than a dozen Caribbean countries. It seems only a matter of time before local transmission will occur in the southern United States, where the mosquito vector is abundantly present.

CHIKV is primarily transmitted to humans through the bites of infected mosquitoes, predominantly *A. aegypti* and *A. albopictus.* The majority of people infected with CHIKV become symptomatic. After an incubation period of 3 to 7 days (range, 1 to 12 days), a patient develops an acute onset of high fever (typically >39° C [102° F]) and polyarthralgia. Other symptoms may include headache, myalgia, arthritis, conjunctivitis, nausea and vomiting, or maculopapular rash involving the trunk and extremities that may also involve the face, palms, or soles. Clinical laboratory findings can include lymphopenia, thrombocytopenia, elevated creatinine, and elevated hepatic transaminases.

Acute symptoms typically resolve within 7 to 14 days. Some patients have persistent or relapsing rheumatologic symptoms for months to years. Mortality is rare and occurs mostly in neonates, older adults, or those with comorbid conditions. Asymptomatic infection occurs in 3% to 25% of infected individuals.[34] As with DF, some patients have prolonged symptoms and a slow recovery phase lasting weeks to months. Vaccine development efforts have been stalled because of poor results and lack of funding.

Differentiation between DF and CHIKV fever can be challenging because of their overlapping presentations and common vectors. Table 229-1 provides a comparison of the clinical features of both diseases. Unlike with DF, anti-inflammatory agents can be used in CHIKV fever and are particularly helpful for the arthritis and arthralgias.

TABLE 229-1 Comparison of the Clinical Features of Chikungunya Fever and DF

Clinical Features	CHIKV Infection	Dengue Virus Infection
Fever (temperature >38.9° C)	+++	++
Myalgias	+	++
Arthralgias	+++	+/–
Headache	++	++*
Rash	++	+
Bleeding dyscrasias	+/–	++
Shock	–	+/–
Leukopenia	++	+++
Neutropenia	+	+++
Lymphopenia	+++	++
Thrombocytopenia	+	+++

The mean frequencies of symptoms were determined from studies in which the two diseases were directly compared among patients seeking care. Symbols indicate the percentage of patients exhibiting each feature: +++, 70%-100% of patients; ++, 40%-69%; +, 10%-39%; +/–, <10%; –, 0%.
*Headache was often retro-orbital.
From Staples JE, Breiman RF, Powers AM: Chikungunya fever: an epidemiological review of a re-emerging infectious disease, *Clin Infect Dis* 49(6):942-948, 2009.

Zika Fever. Zika virus is an emerging mosquito-borne virus first identified in 1947 in rhesus monkeys in Uganda. It was subsequently identified in humans in 1952 with recorded outbreaks in Africa, the Americas, Asia, and the Pacific.[35a] In May 2015, the Pan American Health Organization issued an alert regarding the first confirmed virus infection in Brazil. This outbreak led to reports of Guillain-Barre syndrome (see Chapter 195) and pregnant women giving birth to babies with severe birth defects. Since this first report, cases have been reported all over the Americas and the Caribbean Islands.

Zika virus is spread to people through the bite of an infected mosquito, mainly *Aedes aegypti*. This is the same mosquito that is responsible for both dengue fever and chikungunya virus infection (see previous discussion). The most common symptoms are fever, rash, joint pain, and conjunctivitis. The illness is usually mild and may be mistaken for a flu-like illness. Recently, however, a marked increase in the incidence of babies born with microcephaly in Brazil is thought to be related to the sharp increase in Zika infection.

There is no cure for Zika infection and currently no vaccine. Antivirals are not recommended. Prevention and control of the disease relies on reducing mosquitos and reducing contact between mosquitos and people. Recommendations include using insect repellent, wearing light-colored clothing the covers as much skin as possible, avoiding the outdoors when the mosquitos are most prevalent (daytime), and sleeping under mosquito netting. All sources of standing water should be removed.[35b]

Pregnant women are advised to postpone travel to areas where transmission is ongoing. Pregnant women can be infected in any trimester, and transmission to the baby had been documented throughout pregnancy.[35c] An association with microcephaly, a devastating birth defect that causes severe brain damage and disability, in affected infants has been noted. Several countries in affected regions are advising women to avoid pregnancy for up to two years, although this is not an official recommendation of the World Health Organization as of January 2016.

Tick-Borne Encephalitis. In the past 30 years, there has been a dramatic increase in tick-borne encephalitis (TBE) cases in Europe, with spread into new, previously unaffected regions. The geographic distribution of TBE has extended from central Europe and Scandinavia through the Eurasian continent to Far East Asia. The cause of this emergence of TBE is likely multifactorial: increased temperatures as a result of global warming (which favor both increases in the tick and reservoir rodent populations), changing ecology by increased forestation and garden cultivation, growing popularity of outdoor activities such as hiking and fishing and adventure travel, and declining socioeconomic status of some populations.[36]

TBE is caused by three antigenically related virus subtypes whose names correspond to their geographic origins: European, Siberian, and Far Eastern. The vector of the European subtype is *Ixodes ricinus,* whereas *Ixodes persulcatus* is the vector for the other two. TBE virus is transmitted within minutes of the tick bite; therefore, unlike in Lyme disease, early removal of ticks will not prevent disease.[37] Infections are most common in the early and late summer months when ticks and rodent hosts are most active. Transmission of TBE through consumption of unpasteurized milk produced by viremic livestock is responsible for a minority of cases.[38,39]

Asymptomatic TBE infections are common, occurring in roughly two thirds of those infected.[36,39] When symptoms do develop, onset is typically 8 days after the tick bite. One third of patients do not recall the tick bite. Those infected with the European subtype typically have a biphasic illness, beginning with a nonspecific febrile illness with myalgias, fatigue, and headache followed by a recovery period. One third will then progress to a neuroinvasive form of TBE, developing meningitis (50%), encephalitis (40%), or myelitis (10%).[36,40] Loss of consciousness, ataxia of the limbs, or acute flaccid paralysis of the upper extremities is also common. Treatment is supportive with fluids, analgesics, antipyretics (i.e., nonsteroidal anti-inflammatory agents), and ventilator support as needed. The benefit of corticosteroids has not been validated. Physical therapy of paralyzed limbs is also important to prevent atrophy.

Two inactivated TBE vaccines are licensed and available in Europe and Canada; however, they are not currently available in the United States.[36,40] Basic tick prevention practices (i.e., wearing long pants and socks when walking in wooded areas, use of repellents) are always advisable.

Zoonoses

Ebola Virus Disease. Ebola virus disease (EVD) is caused by a Filoviridae family virus, of the genus Ebolavirus. The virus was identified in 1976 during the first EVD outbreak near the Ebola River (hence the name) in then Zaire, now the Democratic Republic of Congo.[41] More recently, the highly fatal outbreak of EVD in 2013-2014 was concentrated in the three West African countries of Guinea, Liberia, and Sierra Leone.[42] Genomic sequencing and phylogenetic analysis revealed that the Ebola virus of this outbreak represented a new strain of Zaire Ebola virus.[42] Although the disease has been identified in gorillas, chimpanzees, and duikers as part of its sporadic epizootic cycle, the high mortality in these animals makes them unlikely natural reservoirs.[43] Recent evidence has implicated the fruit bat as the most likely reservoir host responsible for the enzootic cycle, and as the source of the 2013-2014 epidemic.[43] Human-to-human transmission occurs via contact with infectious body fluids such as urine, saliva, sweat, feces, vomit, breast milk, and semen.

EVD is characterized by the constellation of fever, fatigue, diarrhea, vomiting, headache, and anorexia. In a study of 37 patients with confirmed EVD in Conakry, Guinea, more than half had one or more of these symptoms, with fever present in 84%.[44] Onset of symptoms is typically abrupt. The mean incubation period during the 2013-2014 outbreak was 11 days, with 95% of confirmed EVD patients experiencing symptoms within 21 days of their last exposure (making this the recommended period for follow-up of contacts). The mean time for patients to seek care after the onset of their symptoms (a measure of the period of infectiousness in the community) was 5 days.[45] The median time from onset of symptoms to death was 8 days.[44] Overall mortality for EVD is approximately 70%, with lower rates for those who are hospitalized (43% to 64%).[44,45] Treatment outside of the United States has focused on fluid resuscitation (oral and intravenous), oxygen, and antibiotics (cephalosporins or fluoroquinolones).[44] In addition to these measures, patients treated in the United States during the 2013-2014 outbreak received a variety of experimental therapies including ZMapp, a combination monoclonal antibody antiviral drug made from tobacco plants, and blood transfusions from survivors of EVD.

In October 2014, the first U.S. citizen, a man who had recently returned to Texas from Liberia, was diagnosed with and subsequently died from EVD. This incident raised concerns about our preparedness for handling EVD. The subsequent transmission of EVD to two health care workers caring for that patient further revealed our own health system's vulnerabilities. In response, protocols were initiated to ensure that on presentation for care, all patients were screened for symptoms and relevant travel. Medical facilities were designated to receive and/or provide treatment to suspected or confirmed EVD patients by specially trained EVD care teams. The CDC produced necessary public health guidance, public education materials and a number of training videos to demonstrate the meticulous process for proper donning and doffing of personal protective equipment. Although most health care workers in the United States will never encounter a patient with suspected or confirmed EVD, it was imperative for facilities to develop the procedures and processes to prepare for this serious though unlikely event. The CDC's website remains the best resource for up-to-date information for health care providers.

At the time of writing, this unprecedented, emerging outbreak of EVD had spread to involve seven countries in West Africa, Spain, the United Kingdom, and the United States, with new cases being identified daily. Epidemic projections predicted there would be up to 1 million cases by January 2015.[46] Fortunately, the number of new cases slowed and resulted in a wordwide count of 28,650 cases, 11,316 deaths. Reports from Liberia suggested a slowing down in the number of cases, but at the same time a new cluster of EVD cases was being reported from Mali.[47,48] The international response garnered momentum, and novel drug and vaccine development research is under way. The outbreak has been controlled, representing an important historical event rather than an ongoing emerging infectious disease crisis.

Monkeypox. Traffic in exotic animals or exposure to pets or even laboratory animals can be harmful to your health. As suggested by its moniker, monkeys are affected by monkeypox, a disease similar to smallpox that circulates in central Africa. Important disease reservoirs are rodents and squirrels. Human transmission has been linked to animal exposures such as household rodent contact or preparation of bushmeat, both of which are common in areas where monkeypox is prevalent.[49] Human-to-human transmission is much less efficient than in smallpox but was reported in 12% of household contacts who had never received smallpox vaccination.[49] Historically, the smallpox vaccine was noted to incidentally prevent monkeypox. Now that smallpox vaccination is no longer required in any country and civil wars have increased dependence on hunting, human monkeypox has reemerged in central Africa. In 2003, there was an outbreak of monkeypox in the United States, with 72 cases reported from six Midwestern states. Investigation revealed that most cases followed the acquisition of a pet prairie dog, which became a reservoir for monkeypox after exposure to a shipment of infected wild rodents from Ghana.[49,50]

In contrast to smallpox, monkeypox usually produces severe adenopathy, does not effectively transmit person to person, and has a lower mortality rate of 10%.[49] Patients often defervesce on the day of or a few days after the onset of the classic pox rash, which often affects the face first.[49] Real-time PCR, IgG and IgM enzyme-linked immunosorbent assay, indirect fluorescent antibody assay, and viral culture are all helpful in diagnosis. Treatment is supportive. There are at least three promising compounds being investigated for antiviral activity against monkeypox including cidofovir.[49]

Antibiotic Resistance

Since their discovery in the middle of the 20th century, antibiotics have substantially reduced the threat posed by infectious diseases. Improvements in sanitation, housing, and nutrition as well as immunizations also contributed to a dramatic drop in mortality from infectious diseases. However, the recent emergence of antibiotic-resistant organisms threatens these gains, because infections caused by resistant organisms fail to respond to usual treatments, resulting in longer periods of infectivity and increased patient morbidity and mortality.

Resistance to antimicrobials has been attributed to the overprescribing of antibiotics, incomplete patient compliance with a prescribed course, and use of antibiotics as prophylaxis or growth stimulants in animal feed. Recommendations designed to combat antibiotic resistance are in place worldwide and consist in general of the following: education of prescribers and consumers as to the dangers of antibiotic overuse; attention to unnecessary veterinary antibiotic use; reduction of nosocomial transmission of such infections by improvement of hand hygiene in health care settings either with soap and water washing or the use of alcohol-based hand sanitizers; enhanced environmental cleaning; and surveillance policies.[51,52]

Methicillin-Resistant *Staphylococcus aureus*. MRSA has fully emerged as a common pathogen in our hospitals. Now we have also identified MRSA with resistance to vancomycin (intermediate [vancomycin-intermediate *Staphylococcus aureus;* VISA], or complete [vancomycin-resistant *Staphylococcus aureus;* VRSA]) in our hospitals.[53] The previously reliable health care association for MRSA infections is no longer valid, because an increasing number of patients with only community exposure have been identified with MRSA but have not had classic nosocomial exposures.[54] The emergence of community-associated methicillin-resistant *Staphylococcus aureus* (CA-MRSA) infections was documented as an outbreak in the Midwest in 1999, when a series of fatal cases of CA-MRSA infections occurred in Native American children who had no link to health care settings.[55] Today the community- versus health care–associated distinction is less important because patients can develop MRSA colonization in one realm and develop manifestations of infection in another. Community-onset, health care–associated methicillin-resistant *Staphylococcus aureus* (HA-MRSA) infections have been observed with increasing frequency among patients in community settings. CA-MRSA strains may also cause hospital-onset, health care–associated infections, because patients who become colonized with CA-MRSA strains in the community may require hospitalization and either transmit such strains to other hospitalized patients or develop infection while hospitalized (e.g., after surgery or insertion of an invasive device). In a 2011 review of MRSA cases nationally, fewer infections occurred in patients during hospitalization than in persons in the community without a recent health care exposure.[56]

CA-MRSA infections have been distinguished from HA-MRSA infections because they are associated with a gene that causes destruction of leukocytes and tissue necrosis; these strains have a predilection for skin and soft tissue infections as well as abscesses, necrotizing fasciitis, necrotizing pneumonia, and sepsis.[57] A clue to a toxin-producing strain of CA-MRSA is the early presence of a necrotic center, which sometimes leads to the misdiagnosis of recluse spider bite. Paradoxically, CA-MRSA is more likely to affect young, healthy outpatients, without the usual exposure to antibiotics and hospitals, and with higher morbidity and mortality than in HA-MRSA infections. A sensitivity pattern suggesting CA-MRSA in young, healthy outpatients with MRSA soft tissue infection might raise vigilance for more serious infection and complications, such as necrotizing fasciitis, metastatic abscess, pneumonia, empyema, or endocarditis.

Empirical treatment of MRSA—whether community or hospital acquired—should be guided by local epidemiology. Directed therapy should be based on the drug sensitivity pattern. Vancomycin is the most familiar first choice for the intravenous treatment of serious MRSA infections. Linezolid and daptomycin are useful when the patient is not tolerant of vancomycin or the minimum inhibitory concentration (MIC) to vancomycin is greater than 2 μg/mL. Linezolid is used frequently for MRSA lung infections. In a recent meta-analysis of randomized clinical trials comparing linezolid with vancomycin for hospital-acquired pneumonia, the two drugs were found to have similar efficacy and safety profiles.[58] Ceftaroline and ceftobiprole are newer cephalosporins that appear noninferior to comparator agents in the treatment of acute bacterial skin and skin structure infections and pneumonia.[59] Telavancin now has approval for treatment of hospital-acquired pneumonia.[59] Dalbavancin and oritavancin are intriguing options under development because they are administered once weekly and also appear noninferior to comparators.[59]

Macrolides, tetracyclines, and fluoroquinolones are commonly used oral agents for less serious MRSA infections. Unfortunately, resistance to these drugs can emerge under therapy, and treatment with trimethoprim-sulfamethoxazole and clindamycin has not been widely studied in serious CA-MRSA infections. Clindamycin is problematic because it is exported from the bacteria by the same inducible efflux pump (MLS_B) that renders the MRSA resistant to macrolides, and it should not be used if there is resistance to erythromycin or azithromycin. Recent data documenting emerging resistance of MRSA to linezolid and daptomycin are concerning and indicate the urgent need for continued vigilance of appropriate antibiotic use and new drug development to effectively combat this pathogen.[53]

Extensively Drug-Resistant Tuberculosis. In 2006, an outbreak of HIV infection–associated extensively drug-resistant tuberculosis (XDR-TB) was described among 53 patients in South Africa; 52 of the 53 died, with a median survival of 16 days from time of diagnosis.[60] This report brought XDR-TB into the spotlight in medical, public health, and lay communities. Subsequently, WHO and the CDC claimed XDR-TB a serious emerging threat to public health and international TB control efforts.

XDR-TB is defined as resistance to at least isoniazid and rifampin (which is the definition of MDR-TB) and any fluoroquinolone and to at least one of the three following injectable drugs used in TB treatment: amikacin, capreomycin, or kanamycin. Data show that XDR-TB numbers and rates are highest in countries of the former Soviet Union (especially Armenia,

Estonia, Latvia, Lithuania, Tomsk Oblast in Russia, and Azerbaijan).[61] Because of limited laboratory capacity to diagnose XDR-TB, the actual prevalence and distribution of XDR-TB cannot be firmly established.[61]

MDR-TB and XDR-TB are difficult to treat, requiring more costly and complex drug regimens of much greater duration than for drug-sensitive TB strains. In a meta-analysis of treatment outcomes among patients with XDR-TB, only 44% had favorable outcomes (i.e., were cured or completed treatment), whereas 21% died.[62] A review of MDR-TB outcomes yielded only slightly better results, with most studies reporting successful outcomes in the 50% to 60% range.[63] This illustrates that drug-resistant TB threatens to thwart the successes in international TB control achieved to date and to change the epidemiology of TB worldwide. Clearly, the need for inexpensive rapid diagnostics to detect extensive drug resistance and for new classes of drugs to treat TB has never been more urgent.

MDR-TB and XDR-TB treatment should be done in consultation with appropriate experts. It should begin with seeking support from your local or state health department and advancing to a regional consultation center if further support is needed. For the most complicated cases, National Jewish Hospital in Denver, Colorado, one of the leading facilities for treatment of drug-resistant TB, will provide consultation services including a physician-dedicated telephone line (further information is available at www.nationaljewish.org/professionals/referrals-and-consults/physician-line).

SUMMARY

Primary care clinicians are on the front lines of disease control. It is particularly challenging to maintain awareness of the recent succession of newly identified and reemerging pathogens such as new respiratory and vector-borne pathogens and newly introduced diarrheal illnesses in developing nations, as well as the emergence of antimicrobial resistance. Cooperation both locally and globally is needed for urgent control of these pathogens.

CHAPTER 230

HIV INFECTION

Bryan J. Marsh • Christina F. Martin

DEFINITION AND EPIDEMIOLOGY

Human immunodeficiency virus type 1 (HIV-1) is a member of the family of viruses known as retroviruses. HIV-1 was first isolated in 1985, at which time it was identified as the causative agent underlying the recently identified epidemic of acquired immunodeficiency syndrome (AIDS). HIV-1 is a zoonosis that was transmitted from chimpanzees to humans three or more times early in the 20th century. HIV-2 is a genetically distinct retrovirus that was transmitted from monkeys to humans; it also causes AIDS (although on average more slowly than does HIV-1) but is much less prevalent, both globally and in the United States, than HIV-1.

HIV infection presents a number of challenges for the health care provider. These include when to consider the diagnosis and to test for infection, when to initiate antiretroviral therapy (ART) and with which antiretrovirals (ARVs), and how to monitor disease progression and treatment efficacy. There is a need for close attention to avoid dangerous drug-drug interactions when patients are being treated with ART. The health care provider must also decide how to incorporate risk reduction counseling into clinical care to further reduce HIV transmission. Advice and support around family planning and pregnancy will be needed. When to recommend pre-exposure prophylaxis (PrEP) for those at high risk for acquiring HIV from an infected partner or postexposure prophylaxis after a possible exposure to HIV are other considerations.

The first AIDS case definition was developed by the Centers for Disease Control (CDC) in 1987 as a tool to aid in the study of the epidemiology of the AIDS epidemic. This definition encompassed a mixture of syndromes, primarily opportunistic infections and malignant neoplasms, associated with advanced immune dysfunction.[1] The AIDS case definition has subsequently been expanded several times and now requires that an individual have laboratory documentation of HIV infection and either (1) one of a broad spectrum of opportunistic infections, malignant neoplasms, and nonspecific syndromes or (2) a CD4 cell count of less than 200/mm^3.[2] Because AIDS is a clinical case definition used primarily for epidemiologic monitoring, once an individual is diagnosed with AIDS, that individual will always carry the diagnosis of AIDS, even after immune restoration such that the CD4 cell count is greater than 200/mm^3 and all complications of AIDS have resolved.

In addition to the AIDS case definition, several systems were used in the past to classify HIV-infected patients by degree of immune dysfunction, usually based on a combination of laboratory and clinical criteria, but these classification systems were developed before the dynamic nature of HIV infection became clear and before effective treatment became available. They have little usefulness for the clinician caring for HIV-infected patients.

Transmission of HIV can occur sexually, parenterally through either injection drug use or blood product transmission, and vertically from mother to child during pregnancy or through breastfeeding. The risk of sexual transmission varies by the nature of the sexual encounter but is generally in the range of 0.1% to 1% per episode of vaginal or rectal sex when no barrier protection is used. The risk of transmission through oral sex is markedly lower. Factors that increase the risk of transmission include other active sexually transmitted diseases (STDs) and a high HIV viral load. Transmission from blood products was virtually eliminated in the United States in 1985 when it became possible to screen blood donations for HIV. The risk of transmission from an untreated HIV-infected mother to child is 20% to 30% during pregnancy and delivery, with a subsequent risk of transmission through breastfeeding that is cumulative and depends on duration and consistency of breastfeeding.

The CDC estimates that more than 1.2 million people aged 13 or older were living with HIV infection in the United States as of the end of September, 2015 and that an estimated 50,000 people are infected annually.[3] Through 2012, the cumulative number of AIDS cases reported to the CDC was 1,155,792; this number also included 9905 children younger than 13 years.[3] Since 1997, the number of non-Hispanic African Americans living with AIDS has outnumbered the number of non-Hispanic whites. The three states reporting the highest number of cumulative AIDS cases were New York, California, and Florida. Total deaths through 2010 were 636,048, including 4961 children younger than 13 years.[3]

AIDS has been a reportable condition since 1987, but HIV infection has never been a nationally reportable disease, and consequently the understanding of U.S. epidemiology has been based primarily on AIDS cases. This has provided a picture of trends in the epidemic that is a number of years out of date and has become even less accurate more recently, with the introduction of therapy that can prevent progression of HIV infection to AIDS. On the basis of results from states in which HIV infection is a reportable condition, it is estimated that men who have sex with men (MSM) now account for 62% of all new HIV infections in the United States, followed by heterosexual transmission (28%). Among women with newly diagnosed HIV infection, however, almost 84% of cases are secondary to heterosexual transmission.[3] Important trends include a growing disproportion of cases in minorities, a growing proportion of cases in the southern states, and a resurgence of cases among MSM in at least some areas in the United States.

The extent of the HIV epidemic in the United States, the ongoing stigma associated with the disease, and the social and medical marginalization of some of those at highest risk of acquiring HIV infection have resulted in a relatively unsuccessful campaign to diagnose and bring HIV-infected people into care. Recent estimates suggest that as many as a quarter of all people living with HIV infection in the United States have not been diagnosed and that up to another quarter have been diagnosed but are not receiving care. Thus, there are as many as a half-million people with HIV infection who are at risk of disease progression and eventually life-threatening complications of AIDS and who also are likely to be at higher risk of transmitting HIV.

Because of the failure of the original approach to HIV testing, which relied on targeted testing of those identified as being at higher risk of HIV infection, in 2006 the CDC recommended that testing become universal. Opt-out HIV testing should now be offered at least once to all persons aged 13 to 64 years, regardless of risk, and repeated testing of persons with known risk should be performed annually. Testing should be performed in all health care settings and need not include prevention counseling.[4]

Because of the impact of this disease on public health, the Health Resources and Services Administration of the U.S. Department of Health and Human Services has provided dedicated federal funds through the Ryan White Comprehensive AIDS Resources Emergency (CARE) Act for HIV prevention and care services since 1990. In addition to HIV prevention services, allocated through each state, this act provides funding for both uninsured and low-income persons living with HIV infection to access primary and specialty HIV care, dental services, and case management as well as payment for their life-prolonging HIV medications. However, with the recent adoption of the Affordable Care Act, insurance coverage and payment for services are changing rapidly, thus causing confusion for patients. Lapses in insurance coverage lead to missed appointments and inconsistent adherence to therapy. Therefore it is important that all new HIV clients be provided a case manager to help them navigate insurance and other changing health care reimbursement options that may be available to them and to guarantee coverage without any lapses. Despite the high cost of HIV care, and ART in particular, HIV has had a relatively minor impact on U.S. health care and economy, but this is not the case in many economically disadvantaged countries. The Joint United Nations Programme on HIV/AIDS estimates that more than 35 million people worldwide were living with HIV/AIDS as of the end of 2012; of these, 32.1 million were adults, 17.7 million were women, and 3.3 million were children younger than 15 years.[5] Approximately 95% of people living with HIV infection now live in the developing world, and most of them still do not have access to any form of effective treatment for HIV infection and thus will likely die of AIDS. During 2012 alone, 2.3 million people became infected, and AIDS caused the deaths of an estimated 1.6 million people, including 210,000 children younger than 15 years.[5]

PATHOPHYSIOLOGY

Although some aspects of the HIV life cycle and HIV/AIDS pathophysiology still require further study, the general outline is well established. To infect a cell, HIV must attach to two cell surface proteins: first, CD4 and, second, one of two chemokine receptors, CCR5 or CXCR4, which are often referred to as coreceptors. The virus then fuses with the cell surface, followed by release of viral RNA and proteins into the infected cell. The viral RNA is then reverse transcribed to DNA (hence the name *retrovirus*), and this DNA is transported into the cell nucleus and incorporated into the cellular genome. Various cells, including monocytes-macrophages and dendritic cells, are susceptible to HIV infection, but the CD4 T lymphocyte is the primary target. A CD4 T lymphocyte that is infected by HIV can remain metabolically inactive with latent HIV infection, or it can be activated with resultant active HIV replication. Through mechanisms that are not entirely understood, with the replication of HIV in activated CD4 T cells and the resultant high-level viremia with the subsequent infection of more CD4 T cells, there is an inexorable decline in the total pool of CD4 T cells in the infected person. As the total number of CD4 T cells declines, as measured by the number of circulating CD4 T cells in peripheral blood (often referred to as the CD4 count or T-cell count), there is a steady decline in the functional capacity of the immune system. After sufficient damage, the infected person starts to develop complications of this immune dysfunction and eventually will develop one or more of the many complications of AIDS and die from the disease. With few exceptions, such as tuberculosis (TB), these AIDS-defining conditions seldom occur until the CD4 T-cell count drops below 200 cells/mm^3.

The rate of progression of immune dysfunction, monitored by the decline of the CD4 T-cell count in peripheral blood, varies significantly among individuals. Without ART, the average time from initial HIV infection until the development of a first complication of AIDS is about 8 years, and the average time from this first complication to death is another year. However, some individuals progress to AIDS in a few years (occasionally as short as 1 year), and some rare individuals (known as long-term nonprogressors or elite controllers) maintain a normal CD4 T-cell count indefinitely and never develop AIDS.

CLINICAL PRESENTATION

The clinical presentation of a person with HIV infection varies tremendously, but the spectrum of presentations is determined by the stage of disease and, most important, by whether the person is experiencing primary HIV infection (PHI), is in the period of clinical latency, or has progressed to AIDS. PHI refers to the time after infection but before the infected person has established a comprehensive immunologic response to infection—that is, the period when HIV can be identified in the person's blood but before standard serologic test results for HIV have become positive. This period before seroconversion (commonly referred to as the window period) typically lasts several weeks but rarely may be as long as 3 months. During this time, the infected person may experience a seroconversion illness, which is often described as influenza-like but is highly variable and most often consists of fever, myalgia, headache, and a pleomorphic rash.

During the years between PHI and AIDS, a person infected with HIV is typically asymptomatic; however, assorted clinical syndromes may occur during this period. It is important to be aware of these, both for management of a known HIV-infected patient and as indications to consider underlying HIV infection in as yet undiagnosed patients. On occasion, opportunistic infections occur at a CD4 range of more than 200 cells/mm^3; but in the United States, the more frequent although still rare severe complications at these higher CD4 counts are malignant neoplasms, the most important of which are lymphomas of various types (excluding the primary central nervous system lymphoma of advanced AIDS) and cervical and anal carcinoma. The most important severe infection that does occur at a higher rate in this CD4 range is TB. Less severe complications in this range include shingles, severe psoriasis, severe (particularly bacteremic) pneumococcal disease, recurrent oral and vaginal candidiasis, oral hairy leukoplakia, and idiopathic thrombocytopenia. The occurrence of any of these conditions in a patient without known HIV infection should result in assessment of risk for HIV infection and frequently in HIV serologic testing.

When a person infected with HIV has progressed to the severe immune dysfunction present in AIDS, he or she becomes at risk for all the potential complications thereof, and development of any one of these mandates testing for HIV infection. The risk for development of an HIV-associated complication increases steadily as the CD4 count drops below 200/mm^3. A few of the more common of the earlier complications are *Pneumocystis jiroveci* pneumonia (PJP), Kaposi sarcoma (KS, a primarily cutaneous malignant neoplasm that manifests as raised violaceous macules), cryptococcal meningitis, and esophageal candidiasis. At lower CD4 counts, especially below 50 cells/mm^3, additional complications may develop, including *Toxoplasma* encephalitis, disseminated *Mycobacterium avium-intracellulare* complex (MAC) infection, cytomegalovirus (CMV) retinitis, progressive multifocal leukoencephalopathy, AIDS dementia, primary central nervous system lymphoma, and AIDS wasting syndrome.

The evaluation of a person newly diagnosed with HIV infection is extensive. If the patient has an acute illness, whether from acute or chronic HIV infection, evaluation and management of that illness take priority; but whether the patient is ill or asymptomatic, the assessment needs to include a comprehensive history and physical examination and extensive laboratory evaluation and other testing. Aspects of the history that require particular attention include the following:

- Assessment of patients' understanding of the new diagnosis and of the implications for the future, both short and long term. In particular, it is important to define patients' emotional states and to ensure their safety, both from potential self-harm and from abuse by a partner, family, or others secondary to the depression and stigmatization often associated with a new diagnosis of HIV infection.
- The development of a trusting and therapeutic relationship with patients. A first medical appointment after a new diagnosis of HIV infection provides a unique opportunity for the health care provider to establish rapport with patients that is crucial for future health care. This requires the provider to balance the need to inquire about deeply personal, always emotionally intense, and sometimes shaming history with the importance of ensuring that patients understand that the primary purpose in collecting this information is to ensure comprehensive care. Successful negotiation of this encounter will facilitate future care, whereas an encounter that leaves the patient uncomfortable with or untrusting of the provider will affect the patient's willingness to return, to provide sensitive information, and to work productively with the provider. Depending on the patient's health and potential risk to others, it may be appropriate to defer some of this history and discussion for subsequent meetings. Should this be the case, it is often helpful to frame the subjects for future discussion so it is easier to return to them at the appropriate time.
- Medical history. This should be comprehensive but should also address in detail aspects of history that may give clues to possible exposures that increase the risk of certain opportunistic infections, including a detailed travel and exposure history. A history of prior STDs and exposure to TB is particularly important.
- Sexual history. This should include an attempt to define patients' sexual orientation; history of sexual behavior; prior use of condoms; ability to negotiate sexual activity and condom use (especially in a current relationship); and circumstances in which patients may be less able to constrain their sexual behavior because of peer pressure, concerns about safety, or loss of inhibition secondary to substance abuse.
- Substance abuse history. Details of the history and current use of illicit drugs, the use of alcohol, and the abuse of prescription medications aid in individual patient care, inform the choice of ART, and define the need for risk reduction interventions.
- Mental health. Because people living with HIV infection are more likely than the general population to experience mental health disorders and emotional distress, it is important to screen early for disorders such as depression, anxiety, posttraumatic stress disorder, sleep disturbance, alcohol and substance abuse, and suicidal or homicidal ideation. Many of these disorders can be exacerbated by the stresses of a new diagnosis of HIV infection, disclosing to loved ones, dealing with the death of a significant other, grappling with lifestyle changes, and living with a chronic illness. Furthermore, untreated mental health disorders may be exacerbated by some ARVs and may also adversely affect the high level of medication adherence that is required for effective ART.
- Alternative therapies. Because some alternative, herbal, or vitamin therapies are contraindicated in combination with some ARVs, the use of any of these therapies needs to be carefully defined and then researched for safety.

PHYSICAL EXAMINATION

The physical examination needs to be comprehensive, both for general health assessment and for detection of complications of HIV infection. Particular attention should be paid to the neurologic examination (for both focal and cognitive deficits) and the skin (for KS and assorted dermatitides), oropharynx (for thrush, oral hairy leukoplakia, periodontitis, KS), liver, and genitals (for STDs). If the patient has a CD4 count below 100/mm^3, the routine examination should always include a formal retinal examination (for CMV and other causes of retinitis).

DIAGNOSTICS

Diagnosis of HIV Infection

The diagnosis of chronic HIV-1 infection is established by the laboratory confirmation of the presence of antibodies to HIV-1, often referred to as serologic testing. From 1989 until 2014 the recommended algorithm for testing for HIV in the United States used two different diagnostic assays performed sequentially, and this algorithm remains widely in use. First, an enzyme-linked immunosorbent assay (ELISA) is performed as a screening test. The sensitivity of the HIV ELISA for diagnosing chronic infection is so high that almost no false-negative results occur, but as a consequence, the rate of false-positive results, especially in a low-risk population, is significant. A negative ELISA result thus excludes chronic HIV infection, and there is no role for additional testing. A positive ELISA result, however, must be confirmed by a second more specific test, either a Western blot or indirect immunofluorescence assay (IFA), which is performed automatically in the United States when a specimen is ELISA positive. Western blot testing identifies the presence of a number of discrete antibodies against HIV, and the results of the test are defined by the number of these antibodies (referred to as bands) that are present; the presence of no bands is defined as a negative test result, one band as an indeterminate result, and more than one band as a positive result. A negative Western blot result excludes chronic HIV infection (and thus establishes that the ELISA result was a false-positive secondary to nonsignificant cross-reacting antibodies), and a positive Western blot result definitively diagnoses chronic HIV infection.

An indeterminate Western blot result can have one of three causes: a cross-reacting antibody to one of the HIV-specific antibodies that are assayed by the HIV Western blot (i.e., a false-positive result); PHI, so soon after infection that the patient has made significant antibody against one HIV antigen but not yet against others; and HIV-2 infection, assuming the original Western blot was HIV-1 specific and not a combination HIV-1/HIV-2 Western blot. HIV-2 is very rare in the United States, so the important differential diagnosis is usually to distinguish between a false-positive test result and PHI. Depending on the estimate of likelihood of PHI, the workup of an individual with an indeterminate test result can be further approached in one of two ways:

- If there is a low likelihood of PHI, the serologic test is repeated 1 month after the initial indeterminate result. The majority of patients undergoing seroconversion will test positive. If serologic testing is repeated 3 months after the original indeterminate result, close to 100% of patients undergoing seroconversion will test positive and no further testing is needed. Viral load testing usually should not be obtained in this setting because the risk of a false-positive result and the added emotional distress and medical workup that this entails outweigh the low likelihood of obtaining a true positive result.
- If there is a significant likelihood of PHI, such as a recent potentially high-risk exposure to HIV or any recent risk and a syndrome suggestive of PHI, an alternative approach to confirming the diagnosis can be considered. In the setting of PHI, the degree of HIV viremia is exceptionally high, and a standard quantitative HIV assay (most commonly polymerase chain reaction [PCR] or branched chain DNA [bDNA]) will invariably be positive at very high titer. The advantages of the earlier diagnosis obtained with this approach, rather than waiting 1 to 3 months to repeat the serologic test, include less opportunity for loss to follow-up, the opportunity for referral to a research center or HIV specialist for consideration of treatment of PHI, and early intervention to reduce risky behavior and potential further transmission. This last advantage is of particular importance because the very high viremia associated with PHI results in a period of markedly increased transmissibility.

In 2014 the CDC published updated recommendations for routine HIV testing, which introduced the first significant change in HIV testing since 1989.[6] The new algorithm, along with the most significant changes and benefits, includes the following:

- Initial testing is with a new (fourth-generation) antigen/antibody combination immunoassay. The antibody assay detects both HIV-1 and HIV-2 antibodies, reducing the likelihood of missing the diagnosis of HIV-2, and the antigen assay detects p24 antigen. The p24 antigen is present in very high levels in early HIV infection and becomes detectable by this assay approximately 1 week earlier after initial infection than does the antibody assay, thus reducing the window period after initial infection to as short as 15 days.
- If the fourth-generation test is reactive, then the specimen should be retested with an HIV-1/HIV-2 antibody differentiation assay. Possible positive results from this are as follows: HIV-1 antibody positive, establishing HIV-1 infection; HIV-2 antibody positive, establishing HIV-2 infection; both HIV-1 and HIV-2 antibody positive, establishing coinfection with both HIV-1 and HIV-2. However, if neither HIV-1 nor HIV-2 antibody results are positive, this could be either because the initial fourth-generation assay was falsely positive and the individual is not HIV infected or because the initial test result was truly positive and the assay detected p24 antigen before the development of detectable HIV antibodies (i.e., diagnosing PHI).
- If the second step in the testing algorithm is negative, it is necessary to perform a third step to exclude PHI. The CDC algorithm recommends reflex testing with an HIV-1 nucleic acid test (NAT). In some laboratories it may not be practical at the time of initial testing to obtain the additional specimen required to perform the NAT, in which case it would be necessary to obtain an additional specimen from the patient for either an immediate HIV PCR (preferable if the patient is at high risk for recent HIV infection) or a 2- to 4-week delayed repeat fourth-generation assay (often preferable if the patient is deemed low risk).

HIV diagnostic testing is in a period of flux, and it is likely that there will be significant variability in the incorporation of the new algorithm into laboratories throughout the United States for the coming several years; providers should be aware of the specific algorithm that is being used by their laboratory and should have a low threshold for obtaining clarification of test results from the laboratory if there is any uncertainty about the interpretation (Fig. 230-1).

It is important to be certain that a patient entering care who reports a prior diagnosis of HIV infection truly is infected, so HIV serology should be repeated if an actual report of HIV

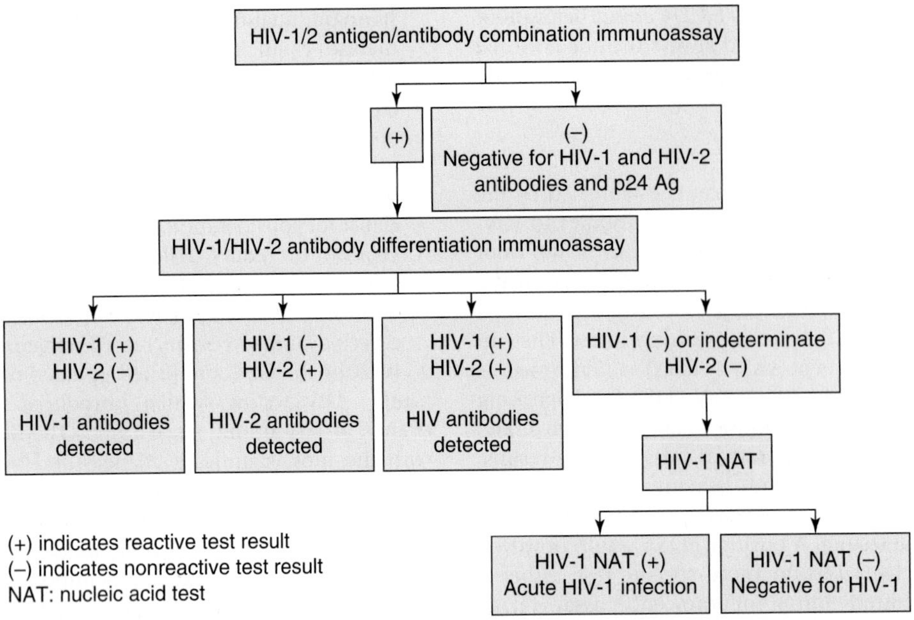

FIGURE 230-1 Algorithm for HIV testing. (From Centers for Disease Control and Prevention and Association of Public Health Laboratories: *Laboratory testing for the diagnosis of HIV infection: updated recommendations,* June 27, 2014. Available at http://stacks.CDC.gov/view/cdc/23447.)

serologic testing is not available. It is reasonable to make an exception to this if there is documentation of repeated positive results of viral load testing.

New patients whose serostatus is unknown or questionable should be counseled about the distinctions of anonymous versus confidential testing. Concerns about inadvertent disclosures or the reactions of insurance companies may result in a desire for anonymous testing, although this is not readily available in many locations.

An additional option for testing uses rapid HIV testing technologies. The currently available assays use either blood or oral fluid as the specimen and can provide results within minutes. These assays are all ELISAs, and results must therefore be interpreted as with a standard HIV ELISA: a negative result rules out chronic HIV infection, whereas a positive result must be confirmed with a second assay.

Laboratory and Other Testing of the Patient with Newly Diagnosed HIV Infection

When an individual is diagnosed with HIV infection, extensive additional testing should be performed. This is to determine the degree of immunosuppression and thus the strength of the indication for ART and other therapy, the HIV viral load and the extent of baseline resistance to ARVs, the presence of significant comorbid conditions, the need for appropriate immunizations, and the aspects of physiologic function that may affect the choice of ART.

The most important assay to establish current immunologic status is the determination of the CD4 count, which is reported as both the absolute number of $CD4^+$ lymphocytes/mm^3 of blood (normal range, 500 to 1700) and the percentage of all lymphocytes that are $CD4^+$ (normal range, 35% to 61%). In addition, quantifying the amount of HIV in the patient's plasma, known as the HIV viral load or viral burden, provides additional information about immune function (the higher the viral load, the more immunologically compromised the patient); but more important, it provides an estimate of the expected rate of immunologic decline (as measured by falling CD4 count). This is established at baseline because decline in viral load after starting of ART is the most important initial marker of efficacy of ART.

The plasma viral load can be measured by two technologies, reverse transcriptase PCR (RT-PCR) and bDNA. The results of these tests are reported as the number of copies of viral RNA per milliliter of plasma. During the chronic phase of HIV infection, the viral load is typically between 10,000 and 100,000 copies/mL; lower values are predictive of a slower than average rate of progression, and a higher viral load is predictive of more rapid progression. Finally, all patients with newly diagnosed HIV infection should undergo viral resistance testing, usually with an HIV genotype assay, to exclude the presence of infection with a virus resistant to one or more of the available ARVs.

Routine baseline testing should also include a complete blood count, comprehensive metabolic profile, amylase and lipase levels, and fasting lipid profile.

Some of the more important additional testing at baseline is performed to exclude latent infection with syphilis, *Toxoplasma gondii,* and CMV, all with standard serologic assays; and also coinfection with hepatitis B and C virus (HBV and HCV) and TB. Testing for the hepatitis viruses is performed through the same algorithm as for patients without HIV infection. Testing for TB, however, is more complex. The diagnosis of latent TB in a patient with HIV infection is complicated by the steady decline in the reliability of the purified protein derivative (PPD) test response as the CD4 count declines, to the point at which it is highly compromised if the CD4 count is less than 200/mm^3 and essentially worthless if it is less than 50/mm^3. Therefore, although it is always appropriate to perform PPD testing for newly diagnosed patients with HIV infection, this testing should always be repeated after patients with a nadir CD4 count of less than 200/mm^3 have been receiving ART long enough to suppress the HIV viral load and to raise the CD4 count above

200/mm^3. The definition of a positive PPD response in patients with HIV infection is induration of 5 mm or more. Testing for latent TB can also be performed with an interferon gamma release assay (IGRA), which is also useful in distinguishing a true-positive PPD response from a false-positive PPD response resulting from prior bacillus Calmette-Guérin (BCG) immunization, although the test characteristics have not been fully defined in HIV-infected patients. Because the risk for development of active TB in a patient with HIV infection and latent TB is exceptionally high (an annual risk of approximately 10%), treatment of latent TB is always indicated once active TB is excluded.

DIFFERENTIAL DIAGNOSIS

The differential diagnosis for a patient with a clinical syndrome consistent with a diagnosis of AIDS is fairly narrow. In the rare instances in which patients appear with such an illness, test negative for HIV on routine testing, and have no other evident cause of immunosuppression (such as an underlying malignant disease or treatment with a known immunosuppressing therapy), they should be immediately referred for expert consultation. There are many congenital immunodeficiency states, but most become evident in childhood (see Chapter 225). One interesting but exceptionally rare condition of unknown cause that mimics HIV infection and can first appear in adults is idiopathic CD4 lymphocytopenia; this is diagnosed in the presence of persistently low CD4 counts (<300/mm^3 or <20% of total lymphocytes) without laboratory evidence of HIV infection or other cause.

Measurement of the CD4 count should never be used as a surrogate for serologic diagnosis of HIV infection, especially in the setting of an acute illness. During an acute infectious illness of sufficient severity, it is not unusual for transient lymphopenia to develop with absolute CD4 lymphopenia that can even enter the AIDS range. In addition, the HIV viral load should not be used to diagnose HIV infection, except for the rare times when it is used to diagnose PHI.

MANAGEMENT

Physician consultation with an HIV specialist is indicated for any serious illness, any syndrome consistent with an opportunistic infection, or any other potentially infectious disease that cannot be readily diagnosed as a community-acquired infection.

Immediate emergency department referral is indicated for mental distress, suicidal or homicidal ideations, signs or symptoms suggestive of a severe opportunistic infection (OI) (e.g., delirium, focal neurologic deficit, rapidly progressive dyspnea, and visual loss).

The management of HIV infection includes highly active antiretroviral therapy (HAART), close attention to medication adherence, prevention of opportunistic infections with chemoprophylaxis, appropriate immunization, close monitoring for complications of HIV infection and its therapy, management of comorbid conditions, and attempts to minimize behavior that can result in HIV transmission. In addition, because HIV infection is now a treatable disease with a long life expectancy, all usual aspects of primary health care must also be provided. An excellent set of up-to-date guidelines for many aspects of HIV care is maintained at the U.S. Department of Health and Human Services AIDS information website (www.aidsinfo.nih.gov).

Treatment with HAART is one of the more complex areas of modern medicine. When it is done correctly, it can convert HIV infection from a progressive and inevitably fatal disease to a chronic disease with potentially normal life expectancy; but when it is done poorly, it can result in viral resistance to some or all antivirals and consequently the need for second-line therapies (more pills, more than once-daily administration, and more potential side effects) and eventually untreatable progressive disease. HAART should thus be prescribed only by clinicians with significant training and experience in its use.

Guidelines that address the initiation of HAART have always attempted to balance the obvious benefits of HAART with the disadvantages of treatment, which include the risk for development of resistance precluding future therapy, drug toxicities, and the medicalization of life in someone who may be clinically entirely well; however, as the benefits of therapy (even with a high CD4 count) have become more apparent and as first-line therapy has become safer, better tolerated, and easier to adhere to (as a result of minimizing pill burden, now often to one pill daily), the threshold for recommending treatment has fallen dramatically.[7,8] The consensus in the United States is that treatment should now be initiated in all individuals diagnosed with HIV regardless of CD4 count, with very few exceptions. These exceptions would include people who are elite controllers, those who have active OIs for which ART is delayed for a relatively brief period, and those who are unlikely to be able to adhere to ART because of psychological, socioeconomic, or other barriers. This recommendation is based on the efficacy, tolerability, and toxicity of current agents and on the results of retrospective cohort analyses and other clinical studies. The initiation of HAART in an asymptomatic patient, on the other hand, is never urgent, and there is usually time to educate the patient and to address other active problems that might adversely affect therapy, including depression related to the new diagnosis.

One of the absolute indications for HAART is the treatment of a pregnant woman to prevent mother-to-child transmission. Optimum HAART in a pregnant woman can reduce the risk of vertical transmission from approximately 25% to less than 2%, and recommended regimens have no known significant fetal toxicity.[9] This benefit is so significant that elective cesarean section is no longer indicated in the optimally treated pregnant woman.

There are now 25 ARVs (and nine formulations containing either two or three of these agents) approved for treatment of HIV infection in the United States, representing six different classes of agents: nucleoside analogue reverse transcriptase inhibitors (NRTIs), non-nucleoside reverse transcriptase inhibitors (NNRTIs), protease inhibitors (PIs), fusion inhibitors, CCR5 antagonists, and integrase strand transfer inhibitors (INSTIs). Despite the innumerable possible combinations of these agents, clinical trials and extensive experience have defined a few preferred regimens for first-line therapy, the easiest of which involves one pill once daily (see www.cdc.gov/hiv/basics/livingwithhiv/treatment), although many alternatives are based on patient-specific factors. First-line treatment usually consists of a combination of (1) two NRTIs and (2) a PI, an NNRTI, or an INSTI. The specific choice of agents is driven by the presence of antiviral resistance, a preferred schedule (once versus twice a day; with or without food; in the morning or before bed), drug interactions with other medications the patient is taking or may need to start, comorbid conditions, pregnancy or desire for pregnancy, baseline viral load, genetic contraindications (for abacavir), and patient concerns about specific possible adverse drug reactions.

The short-term goal of HAART is to suppress viral replication to such a degree that there is no detectable HIV in peripheral blood, most commonly measured by RT-PCR. When that is the case, the result of viral load testing is reported as below the lower limit of detection for the assay, which is currently less than 20 copies/mL and is often referred to as an undetectable viral load. The amount of time it takes to obtain an undetectable viral load after initiation of HAART depends on the baseline viral load, so the initial goal is to reduce the viral load by 10-fold to 100-fold within 4 to 6 weeks of initiation of therapy and to achieve complete suppression within 6 months. If that is not attained, the patient should be assessed for new viral resistance, medication adherence, and appropriateness of HAART. CD4 counts need not be measured soon after initiation of HAART, but with successful suppression of viral replication, the CD4 count should start to increase; typically, it increases 100 to 200/mm^3 in the first year after starting HAART.

When a patient is receiving stable HAART and has attained an undetectable viral load, it is crucial to monitor the patient carefully for ongoing efficacy (with viral load and CD4 testing), safety (with the specific laboratory testing determined by the given regimen), and adherence. If patients are less than 95% adherent, they run an unacceptably high risk for development of resistance to the agents in the regimen, demonstrated by virologic rebound after initial suppression to undetectable levels, with consequent need to change ARVs and—if repeated a few times—eventual loss of all effective therapy.

Historically, guidelines suggested monitoring the viral loads and CD4 count every 3 to 4 months after the viral load was suppressed and the patient was clinically well, but with the recognition of how well people do when they are highly adherent and the viral load is suppressed, these guidelines now allow for longer intervals.[8] In an individual who is clinically well and has a consistently suppressed viral load for at least 1 year, it is reasonable to consider monitoring the viral load every 6 months if the patient is also highly adherent to therapy, is reliably engaged in medical care, is not homeless, is not actively abusing alcohol or illicit drugs, does not have a mental health condition that might affect medical adherence, and is not participating in any high-risk activity. CD4 testing can be as infrequent as annually.

An often overlooked aspect of the care of patients receiving HAART is the danger of drug-drug interactions with many of the ARVs. These interactions can affect both the non-ARV, most often by decreasing metabolism (potentially to a life-threatening degree), and the ARV, of greatest concern by decreasing ARV concentrations to subtherapeutic levels and thus increasing the likelihood of resistance and failure. It is thus imperative that drug interactions be identified and discussed in consultation with the HIV specialist before starting or stopping any medication, whether prescription or over the counter.

When ART is not initiated, the patient should be evaluated in the clinic and by laboratory testing, primarily CD4 count and viral load, every 3 to 4 months. If other treatable comorbid conditions have been identified, such as hepatitis C or latent TB, this may be an appropriate time to address them.

Although HAART has the most profound impact on survival of all aspects of treatment of HIV infection, other components of care should not be forgotten. Chemoprophylaxis and immunizations should be provided when indicated, and routine health care should be provided. For a patient with AIDS who is starting HAART, primary chemoprophylaxis (the administration of a medication to prevent a first episode of an opportunistic infection) can reduce the risk for development of an opportunistic infection before adequate immune restoration; whereas for patients with AIDS for whom immune restoration will not occur (because of untreatable HIV infection secondary to the development of antiviral resistance or the patient's choice to defer ART), appropriate prophylaxis can provide a moderate prolongation of life expectancy. Decisions about when to start and to stop prophylactic medications will usually be made by the HIV specialist, but excellent guidelines for chemoprophylaxis and immunizations are readily available.[10]

After ART has been initiated, treatment interruptions should be strongly discouraged. Treatment interruption is associated with a risk of development of ART resistance, high rebound viremia with possible PHI-like illness, rapid CD4 decline, and an increased risk of death; as well as increased risk of HIV transmission through unsafe sexual and injection drug use (IDU) behavior. There may, however, be times when treatment interruption is appropriate or unavoidable, at which time the patient should be monitored closely both clinically and with CD4 and viral load testing.

In addition, a number of conditions require particularly careful monitoring and evaluation for people with HIV infection, no matter what the CD4 count.

- Latent TB. Given the high risk for development of active TB in a patient coinfected with HIV and TB, annual screening for latent TB, whether with PPD or IGRA, should be routine unless the risk of exposure is exceptionally low.
- Screening for human papillomavirus (HPV)–associated disease. Cervical carcinoma develops more frequently in HIV-infected women and requires close screening and aggressive management. As the result of a similar pathophysiologic mechanism, HPV-associated anal carcinoma occurs much more frequently in MSM with HIV infection; annual rectal examinations should be performed, as should workup of any consistent symptoms. Anal Papanicolaou smears are performed at some centers but are not currently standard of care.
- Screening for STDs. This is important both because many patients with HIV infection remain at risk for infection with STDs and because the presence of an STD increases the risk of HIV transmission.
- Management of chronic hepatitis B and hepatitis C. The leading cause of death for people coinfected with HIV and HCV in the United States is liver disease, so management of chronic hepatitis is an integral aspect of patient care. Until recently, because treatment of HCV was very poorly tolerated and not very effective, especially for those coinfected with HIV, few patients were treated. Contemporary treatment for HCV, however, is now highly effective and generally well tolerated (see Chapter 137), so all HIV and HCV coinfected patients should be considered candidates for treatment of HCV. There are challenges to treating HCV in a coinfected patient, most importantly drug interactions between the two sets of antivirals, so management of hepatitis C in a patient coinfected with HIV should be addressed by an HIV and HCV expert. The primary health care provider can play an important role by reinforcing the importance of alcohol abstinence and providing immunization for HBV and hepatitis

A virus for all nonimmune patients. There are fewer data on coinfection with HBV, but the issues are similar.

- Cardiovascular disease risk. Several ARVs, primarily PIs, increase the risk of cardiovascular disease, mediated primarily but not entirely by dyslipidemia and insulin resistance. It is thus important to address modifiable risk factors, to monitor lipids and glucose concentration, and to treat metabolic abnormalities when they develop.

Finally, it is important to recognize the impact of effective ART on the risk of HIV transmission, often referred to as "treatment as prevention," and the potential benefit of this effect on helping to control the HIV epidemic. Several clinical trials have demonstrated that the likelihood of HIV transmission, whether sexual or parenteral, is dramatically reduced when someone with HIV infection is on ART with an undetectable viral load; and mathematical modeling suggests that this could provide a significant benefit in helping to control the epidemic if a high enough proportion of people infected with HIV are on effective ART.

COMPLICATIONS

The most important complications for which a person with HIV infection is at risk are those that are secondary to immune dysfunction, as reflected in the CD4 count. These are discussed in the section on clinical presentation.

In addition to complications of immune dysfunction, it is important to monitor HIV-infected patients closely for complications of HAART. Antiviral therapy has a dramatic impact on life expectancy when it is prescribed appropriately, but these medications have a number of significant toxicities that must be actively monitored to reduce the risk of a spectrum of problems ranging from cosmetic to life-threatening. The potential toxicities vary according to the specific regimen, so appropriate monitoring is defined uniquely for every patient. A few general recommendations are warranted.

Metabolic Toxicities

The PI and, to a lesser degree, the NNRTI and NRTI classes of ARVs carry a risk of metabolic side effects that require monitoring. One of the most significant of these is dyslipidemia, which should be assessed by measuring a fasting lipid profile at baseline and then 1 to 3 months after any change in a pertinent medication. When ARV-induced dyslipidemia does develop, options for management include usual lipid-lowering therapy (diet, exercise, and medications) and change in ART if an equally effective alternative is available. A second complication is insulin resistance, which should be monitored at a minimum by appropriate interview at regular clinic appointments.

Lipodystrophy

Lipodystrophy refers to a change from baseline in the relative proportion of fat, whether centrally with intra-abdominal, breast, or dorsocervical fat accumulation or peripherally with limb and buttock subcutaneous fat atrophy. These toxicities have no clearly attributable risk of increased mortality but can be profoundly disfiguring. Because these changes are not readily reversible, they need to be watched for carefully and an appropriate medication change considered as needed.

Liver Disease

All but a few of the currently available ARVs are associated with one or more liver toxicities, ranging from otherwise asymptomatic hyperbilirubinemia to fulminant and potentially fatal drug-induced hepatitis to slowly progressive but also potentially fatal hepatic steatosis–lactic acidosis. It is thus important to define the nature of hepatotoxicity that is associated with a given regimen and to monitor appropriately, whether by interview or laboratory testing.

Drug Interactions

It cannot be overemphasized that there are innumerable potential drug interactions with almost all ART regimens, so any unusual symptom should always raise the concern of an adverse drug reaction to a new medication, whether it is prescribed, over the counter, herbal, or illicit, and a detailed history of the use of all medications and nutraceuticals should be obtained.

Immune Reconstitution Inflammatory Syndrome

A unique complication associated with ART is the immune reconstitution inflammatory syndrome (IRIS). When ART is initiated in a patient with a low CD4 count, there is a rapid improvement in the immune system's ability to produce an inflammatory reaction, which can result in an acute inflammatory reaction against both known and occult opportunistic infections. This typically occurs in the first several months after initiation of ART and produces symptoms based on the location of the infection. Two of the most common manifestations of IRIS are acute lymphadenitis as a reaction to MAC and acute uveitis to CMV. It is important to recognize IRIS because there may be significant associated morbidity (e.g., blindness with ocular CMV) and because management is very specific (a combination of antimicrobials, surgery, and corticosteroids).

INDICATIONS FOR REFERRAL OR HOSPITALIZATION

In general, all HIV-infected patients should be managed under the care of both a primary care provider and an HIV specialist. With a growing interest in finding a cure as well as the rapidly changing array of treatments, a specialist is in the unique position of providing the most up-to-date care. Other indications for referral include the following:

- Pregnancy in an HIV-infected woman or intention to become pregnant in serodiscordant couples
- HIV coinfection with hepatitis C or B or TB
- New symptoms in someone with immunosuppression (CD4 count ≤200), including:
  - Mental status changes
  - Severe headache
  - High fevers
  - Significant shortness of breath
- Opportunistic infections related to immunosuppression

All HIV-infected patients should be under the care of a primary health care provider and a clinician with HIV expertise, so referral to an HIV specialist should be recommended to all HIV-infected patients who enter care, whether they are newly diagnosed or are changing health care providers. Depending on the provider's expertise, the complexity and nature of the active medical issues, challenges of travel and other constraints on accessing care, and the patient's preferences, the division of responsibilities between the health care provider and the specialist can vary, so it is important to explicitly define their respective roles. Patients often wonder why they need to see a primary care provider when they are seen by an HIV specialist several times per year and so may need to be reminded that, given the long life expectancy that can now be anticipated for

HIV-infected patients, health maintenance and other aspects of primary care are as important to them as to the general population.

For HIV-infected patients who are in care, it is as important not to overreact to nonsevere acute illness as it is to be attentive to potential complications of HIV infection. In particular, most nonopportunistic infections can be managed just as they would be in an immunocompetent host, especially if the CD4 count is more than 200/mm^3. On the other hand, any more serious illness, any syndrome consistent with an opportunistic infection, or any potentially infectious disease that cannot be readily diagnosed as a community-acquired infection should prompt rapid consultation with an HIV specialist.

An important resource to help HIV-infected patients navigate the complex health care system may be the local AIDS service organization (ASO). ASOs are community-based organizations funded at least in part by the Ryan White CARE Act and are dedicated to assisting people living with HIV infection and their families by providing case management, support groups, transportation assistance, and emergency financial help for housing, food, and clothing. ASOs often provide additional services within their communities, including HIV prevention education and testing.

LIFE SPAN CONSIDERATIONS

The life expectancy of a patient newly diagnosed with HIV infection has steadily increased since the onset of the epidemic and continues to do so. The largest impact on life expectancy occurred in the mid-1990s with the introduction of HAART, but improvements in the safety and efficacy of available ARVs, the growing number of agents, and the growing sophistication in the management of people living with HIV infection have resulted in ongoing incremental improvements in life expectancy. The most important predictor of life expectancy is no longer the CD4 count and viral load at baseline but the patient's ability to tolerate and to maintain a high level of adherence to ARVs. Population statistics are not helpful in defining the prognosis for an individual patient, and the emphasis needs to be on the patient's idiosyncratic circumstances. Under ideal circumstances, though, it is reasonable to hope for a dramatic extension of and possibly even unaffected life expectancy.

Although HAART has dramatically improved the life expectancy and health of people living with HIV, there remain many unknowns about the impact of HIV infection on people living with HIV as they age. Some areas of concern and active research include bone pathology (osteoporosis and avascular necrosis), neurocognitive effects, risk of malignancies, frailty, and exacerbation of pain syndromes (e.g., from early ARVs). To whatever degree there is an association between HIV infection and any of these problems, it remains unclear what the predictors of risk for them might be, and whether earlier initiation of ART might minimize them.

Because life expectancy is long, it has become important to address long-term life plans and family planning with all patients infected with HIV. Discussions about desires and plans for children are particularly important. For an HIV-infected woman, the decision to become pregnant is usually complicated. If she has an uninfected male partner, the logistics of insemination are fairly straightforward, but the management of the pregnancy is intensive. When pregnancy is being considered, referral to an HIV specialist should be recommended for counseling about safe insemination, discussion of approaches to the prevention of mother-to-child transmission of HIV, and potential need to modify ART.

Adolescence is often a time for sexual debut and engaging in high-risk behaviors, including unprotected sex and experimentation with drugs and alcohol, which put the adolescent at risk for acquiring and transmitting HIV. It is therefore important to discuss the risks associated with such behaviors at every visit and to offer anticipatory guidance on abstinence, how to negotiate responsible sexual behaviors, and how to prevent pregnancy and HIV infection and other STDs through the use of contraception and condoms. Because hormonal methods of contraception will not prevent STDs, including HIV infection, it is important to ensure that adolescents understand the necessity of both consistent and proper use of condoms when engaging in sexual intercourse and also that they have access to an affordable condom supply.

EDUCATION AND HEALTH PROMOTION

Education for an HIV-infected patient needs to be extensive and ongoing. The initial diagnosis is often overwhelming, and basic education about HIV infection will often need to be repeated several times. The education needs to start by ensuring that the patient understands both the natural history of HIV infection and the potential immense benefit of current therapy, although it is a challenge to convey both the severity of the disease and the optimism that HAART can provide. The discussion of benefits needs to include not only the individual health benefits, but also the benefits of reduced risk of HIV transmission. This discussion often transitions into family planning and the need to discuss the nature of the risks associated with pregnancy. Initial discussions also need to define the nature of medical care for someone living with HIV infection, including the frequency of appointments, the significance of the CD4 count and viral load, the nature of medical therapy, the importance of strict adherence to ART when it is started, and any other pertinent aspects of care. In addition, initial education often needs to address misconceptions that the patient might have about HIV infection.

Further education needs to address both HIV-specific and usual aspects of general health maintenance. The patient should be informed about how to avoid exposure to infectious diseases, which includes discussion of food and water safety, pet hygiene, and international travel. The importance of patient-specific health maintenance issues should be addressed, including cigarette, alcohol, and other substance abuse. Nutritional counseling should be routinely provided.

The provider should also explicitly discuss the public health issues of HIV infection. This usually starts with a discussion of the mechanisms of transmission of HIV and how to prevent transmission. It might thus be necessary to instruct the patient on male or female condom use or on how to ensure that needles and other paraphernalia used for illicit drugs are sterile. This conversation also needs to address notification and testing of current and past partners, both sexual and needle-sharing partners, and of children born to an infected woman. It is thus important that the provider understand what resources are available for anonymous or confidential testing and for contact notification, which includes programs run by the department of health in every state.

Several clinical trials have demonstrated that the daily use of ARV medications by someone who is not HIV infected but who participates in ongoing high-risk behavior, usually referred to as pre-exposure prophylaxis, can significantly reduce the risk of HIV acquisition. Based on these trials, in 2012 the U.S. Food and Drug Administration (FDA) approved the daily use of Truvada, the coformulation of tenofovir disoproxil fumarate (TDF) 300 mg plus emtricitabine (FTC) 200 mg, for PrEP for the prevention of HIV acquisition. PrEP can be considered for all adults considered to be at very high risk for acquisition of HIV, including MSM; heterosexually active men and women, including HIV-discordant couples; and injection drug users. When delivered as part of a comprehensive set of prevention services, including risk reduction counseling, treatment for other STDs, and recommended use of condoms, PrEP been found to be both effective and safe in reducing the risk of acquiring HIV infection.[11] The efficacy of PrEP has been quite variable in these studies, and in fact not all studies have shown benefit; but in all cases, the higher the adherence to daily therapy, the greater the reduction in risk of HIV acquisition. Primary care providers will increasingly be asked to consider PrEP for their high-risk patients, and so it is essential to know for whom and how to prescribe this prophylactic treatment as well as to stress excellent adherence to the daily medication. A baseline HIV test must be performed before initiation of PrEP, to rule out acute or chronic HIV infection. Frequent monitoring for HIV acquisition and tests for other STIs and of renal function must be performed every few months.[11]

CHAPTER 231

INFLUENZA

Christina Martin

DEFINITION AND EPIDEMIOLOGY

Influenza is an acute infection of the respiratory tract caused by influenza virus type A or B. It is usually a self-limited disease that occurs in outbreaks, primarily during the winter months in temperate climates; it may occur year-round in the tropics. Influenza is highly contagious and occurs in all age groups. The rate of infection is highest among children; the rate of serious illness and death is highest among people 65 years old or older or those with underlying chronic medical conditions.[1] Influenza tends to occur in outbreaks, which can rapidly affect 10% to 40% of the population.[2] In 2009, the novel H1N1 (swine flu) virus emerged, infecting humans in pandemic proportion. It is now a regular human influenza virus that continues to circulate worldwide.

PATHOPHYSIOLOGY

Influenza is transmitted from person to person through respiratory secretions that contain virus. These respiratory secretions are spread in the form of droplets that are produced when a person talks, coughs, or sneezes. Virus is detectable and may be shed in respiratory secretions up to 24 hours before the onset of symptoms.

Once virus reaches the epithelium cells of the respiratory tract, it penetrates the cells and begins replication. This viral replication leads to cell death, which releases large amounts of virus that can infect adjacent cells. This quickly causes desquamation of the ciliated epithelium. Onset of the acute symptoms coincides with this desquamation.[2]

Influenza viruses evolve frequently owing to point mutations or recombination events that occur during viral replication. This is called antigenic drift. Previous exposure or vaccine may not confer immunity to these new virus variants, thus the reason for seasonal epidemics and the need for adjustment of vaccine every season.[1]

CLINICAL PRESENTATION

After an incubation period of 1 or 2 days, there is an abrupt onset of symptoms. These symptoms include fever, chills, headache, malaise, myalgia, and loss of appetite. Respiratory symptoms are also present but are usually overshadowed by the severity of the systemic symptoms. Respiratory symptoms include dry cough, nasal congestion with clear discharge, and sore throat. The cough is usually the most prominent of these respiratory symptoms.

The patient's temperature rises rapidly after onset, peaking at 37.7° C to 40° C (100° F to 104° F) in about 12 hours. The fever typically begins to decline on the second or third day but may last as long as 4 to 8 days. Systemic symptoms become less prominent as the fever decreases. A convalescent phase of 1 to 2 weeks follows the acute febrile stage. Cough, malaise, and fatigue, often extreme, are seen during the convalescent phase.[2]

Some patients have mild illness that resembles the common cold. Older adults, children under the age of 2 years, people with underlying chronic medical conditions, and pregnant women may experience a rapidly worsening course of influenza.

Symptoms caused by H1N1 are similar to those caused by seasonal influenza A or B.[3]

PHYSICAL EXAMINATION

Uncomplicated cases of influenza have minimal physical findings despite the severity of clinical complaints. At the onset of symptoms, the patient's face is often flushed, and the eyes may be watery and red. There may be fever. The skin may be hot and moist. Nasal passages can be inflamed, but pharyngeal erythema and exudates are not common.[4] Cervical lymph nodes may be enlarged and tender. The findings on chest examination are usually normal.

DIAGNOSTICS

Virus can be isolated from nose and throat specimens by nasal swabs or washings, sputum, and throat swabs. Of these, nasopharyngeal specimens are the preferred source. Ideally, samples should be collected within 12 to 36 hours of onset of illness.

The gold standard for influenza diagnosis is either conventional viral culture or reverse transcriptase polymerase chain reaction (RT-PCR) assays. Virus can be detected in cell cultures in 2 to 7 days. In situations wherein early diagnosis is crucial, there are several techniques to detect the presence of viral antigens in nose and throat specimens that yield results rapidly, in as little as 1 hour. These rapid tests may not be as sensitive as cell culture; however, they may be useful in the management of individual patients at high risk for serious complications from influenza, who may benefit most from early hospitalization, appropriate antiviral treatment, or prophylaxis for contacts.[5,6]

Infection with influenza virus can also be confirmed by at least a fourfold rise in antibody titer in convalescent serum taken 10 to 20 days after an acute serum sample.

Clinical diagnosis in the setting of a confirmed influenza outbreak is very accurate.

DIFFERENTIAL DIAGNOSIS

In the absence of a known outbreak of influenza, it may be difficult to distinguish an individual case of influenza from many of the other upper respiratory viral infections, such as the common cold or illness caused by respiratory syncytial virus. Other conditions to consider are *Mycoplasma pneumoniae* infection, bacterial pneumonia, and severe streptococcal pharyngitis.

DIFFERENTIAL DIAGNOSIS

Influenza Infection

HEAD, EYES, EARS, NOSE, AND THROAT
- Common cold
- Severe pharyngitis
- Epiglottitis (young children)

PULMONARY
- Respiratory syncytial virus (RSV)
- Bacterial pneumonia
- *Mycoplasma* pneumonia
- Parainfluenza
- Avian influenza
- Croup

SYSTEMIC
- Sepsis (infants)

BOX 231-1

Antiviral Influenza Chemoprophylaxis and Treatment Considerations

Antiviral treatment is recommended as soon as possible for any patient with confirmed or suspected influenza for the following high-risk groups:
- Any hospitalized person
- Anyone who has severe or complicated illness
- Persons at high risk for complications from influenza, including:
  - Children <2 years of age
  - Adults ≥65 years of age
  - Persons with chronic medical conditions in whom influenza will cause exacerbation or complications (e.g., pulmonary or cardiovascular disease, diabetes mellitus, or other metabolic, renal, hepatic, neurologic, or hematologic disorders)
  - Persons who have immunodeficiency
  - Institutionalized residents of nursing homes or other chronic-care facilities
  - Pregnant women (and up to 2 weeks postpartum)
  - Children receiving long-term aspirin therapy
- Unvaccinated household members or caregivers of persons at high-risk who may have been exposed to influenza

Data from Centers for Disease Control and Prevention (CDC): *Influenza antiviral medications: summary for clinicians, 2013-2014*. Available at www.cdc.gov/flu/professionals/antivirals/summary-clinicians.htm. Accessed July 23, 2014; and Fiore A, Uyeki T, Broder K, et al: Prevention and control of influenza vaccines: recommendations of the advisory committee on immunization practice (ACIP), 2010, *MMWR Recomm Rep* 59(RR-8):1-62, 2010.

MANAGEMENT

Specialist referral is indicated for persons with confirmed or suspected influenza infection who are at high risk of developing serious illness or complications. These include pregnant women, children younger than 2 years, patients aged 65 years or older, or persons with underlying chronic medical conditions, such as pulmonary or cardiac disease, diabetes mellitus, or immunosuppression.

Immediate emergency department referral is indicated for rapidly worsening symptoms, including cyanosis, dyspnea with oxygen requirement, confusion or listlessness, or exacerbation of chronic conditions such as pulmonary or cardiac disease, diabetes mellitus, or immunosuppression.

Treatment of influenza is primarily symptomatic. Patients should rest as much as possible and maintain an adequate fluid intake. Antipyretics and analgesics can be used to control fever and relieve headache and myalgia. Patients with influenza should not go to work or school.

In the United States there are currently four antiviral medications approved for the treatment of influenza. They are amantadine (Symmetrel), rimantadine (Flumadine), zanamivir (Relenza), and oseltamivir (Tamiflu). Antiviral treatment is recommended for patients at high risk for development of complications from influenza, those with severe illness, or for anyone requiring hospitalization for confirmed or suspected influenza. Resistance to antiviral medications may develop quickly, so clinicians should be aware of which strains of influenza are circulating in their community and consult the Centers for Disease Control and Prevention (CDC) website (www.cdc.gov/flu) for current recommendations on antiviral use; treatment recommendations change often.[3]

Antiviral drugs are most effective when they are started within 48 hours of the onset of symptoms; they can reduce the severity of the symptoms and the duration of symptoms by 1 to 2 days.[3] For high-risk patients in whom influenza is highly suspected, antivirals should be started as soon as possible, even if laboratory confirmation is not yet back (Box 231-1).

Prophylactic treatment with antivirals can be considered for those who are in close contact with persons at high risk for complications from influenza.[7] However, prophylaxis is not a substitute for vaccination; unvaccinated persons should be encouraged to be vaccinated to reduce the time for which prophylaxis is needed. Antiviral prophylaxis may be administered at the same time as the inactivated vaccine, but it should not be administered with the live attenuated influenza vaccine (LAIV) because the antivirals may interfere with the immune response to the LAIV.

COMPLICATIONS

The primary complications of influenza are pulmonary. The most notable pulmonary complications are primary influenza (viral) pneumonia, which is rare, and secondary bacterial pneumonia. Other pulmonary complications include croup in children and exacerbation of chronic pulmonary disease. Central nervous system complications such as Guillain-Barré syndrome and encephalitis occur rarely after influenza infection. The association of influenza infection and Reye syndrome in children prompted the recommendation that aspirin be avoided in the treatment of children with influenza. Other complications that have been associated with influenza infection are myositis, which is seen primarily in children, and toxic shock syndrome.[2]

INDICATIONS FOR REFERRAL OR HOSPITALIZATION

In a healthy person, influenza is usually a self-limiting illness, and a person should be able to recover at home within 1 to 2 weeks. However, the following are considerations:

- Patients who do not begin to gradually improve a few days after the onset of symptoms should be reevaluated and referred as appropriate.
- Hospitalization may be indicated for patients with underlying chronic medical conditions that can be complicated by the added stress of influenza infection.
- Anyone who is rapidly getting worse should be considered for hospitalization.

LIFE SPAN CONSIDERATIONS

Influenza can cause death in patients of any age group; however, mortality is highest in older people. In the United States, about 36,000 people die each year of influenza or its complications. People 65 years old or older account for more than 90% of these deaths. During the 2009 H1N1 (swine flu) pandemic, most deaths occurred in individuals 18 to 64 years old, with pregnant women among the most vulnerable.

Young infants with influenza infection may have clinical symptoms different from those in older children or adults. In the setting of influenza outbreak, clinicians should be aware that symptoms such as acute onset of high fever, irritability, runny nose, refusal to eat, or weakness may be the only signs of influenza in this young population.

PATIENT AND FAMILY EDUCATION

Patients and their families should be educated on the importance of receiving the influenza vaccine on a yearly basis. Basic personal hygiene measures, such as good handwashing and covering the mouth and nose during coughs and sneezes, staying at home when ill, and avoiding crowds during outbreaks, may help reduce the risk of acquiring and spreading influenza.

HEALTH PROMOTION AND PREVENTION

The influenza vaccine is the primary method of preventing influenza infection. Annual vaccination is recommended for all persons 6 months of age and older who do not have contraindications to vaccination.[1] To protect infants younger than 6 months or those who cannot receive the vaccine because of contraindications, it is even more important that the rest of the family or close personal contacts be vaccinated. The vaccine should be given each year beginning in the fall and continuing throughout the influenza season. International travelers anticipating travel during the fall or winter months in their destination countries should consider vaccination for influenza before their trip. Note that influenza season in the Northern Hemisphere is typically November to April, whereas in the Southern Hemisphere it is April to October; influenza season is year-round in the tropics and subtropics.[8]

There are several types of influenza vaccine currently available in the United States. Quadrivalent and trivalent inactivated influenza vaccines (IIV4 and IIV3, respectively) are commonly referred to as the "flu shot." The trivalent vaccines contain the same three strains of influenza virus—two influenza A subtypes (including H1N1) and one influenza B type—and the quadrivalent vaccines include an additional B type strain. IIV3 is approved for all people 6 months of age or older who do not have an egg allergy. IIV4 is approved in some cases for children as young as 6 months, but in others it is indicated only for persons 3 years of age or older. Therefore, it is important to know which vaccine is being offered and to check with the manufacturer for whom it is indicated. The quadrivalent LAIV (LAIV4, nasal spray) replaces the trivalent formulation of the past. LAIV4 is currently approved only for healthy nonpregnant people aged 2 to 49 years.[1] An intradermal vaccine (Fluzone) was made available for the 2011-2012 flu season for people ages 18 to 64 as an alternative to intramuscular and nasal vaccines.[9] There is now available an egg-free recombinant influenza vaccine for persons aged 18 to 49 years of age with severe allergy to eggs.[1]

Studies have shown that influenza vaccine effectiveness among children is more protective if the child receives two vaccine doses rather than one during the first season the child is vaccinated. Therefore the CDC now recommends that all children aged 6 months to 8 years who are being vaccinated for the first time receive two vaccine doses separated by at least 4 weeks.[1]

In 2010, a high-dose inactivated influenza vaccine was approved for use in people 65 years old and older. The high-dose formulation contains four times more hemagglutinin than the standard IIV. Older adult recipients of the high-dose vaccine had a better immunologic response than did recipients of the standard formulation. More local reactions were noted in recipients of the high-dose formulation.[1]

Each year, the U.S. Food and Drug Administration determines the three or four influenza strains to be included in the following year's vaccine on the basis of which viruses are most likely to cause epidemics in the coming winter.[1]

CHAPTER 232

INFECTIOUS DIARRHEA

Thomas H. Taylor

DEFINITION

Diarrhea is an alteration of normal bowel movement characterized by an increase in volume or frequency of stools. If the predominant symptoms are nausea and vomiting, viral gastroenteritis (i.e., noroviruses in adults and rotavirus in children) as well as food poisoning caused by the ingestion of preformed toxin (i.e., *Staphylococcus aureus* or *Bacillus cereus*) should be considered. If the predominant symptom is diarrhea, upper and lower bowel pathogens of the small intestine and colon, respectively, should be considered. Infections of the small intestine (upper intestinal diarrhea) cause less-frequent, small-volume, noninflammatory stools and are caused by enteric viruses, enterotoxic bacteria (e.g., enterotoxic *Escherichia coli*), and noninvasive parasites such as *Giardia* and *Cryptosporidium*. Small-volume diarrhea is the consequence of the great capacity of our colon to absorb water from the more proximally diseased small bowel.

Infections of the colon (lower intestinal diarrhea) are more likely to cause frequent, large-volume, inflammatory diarrhea, which is recognized by fever and mucus and blood in the stool, often referred to as dysentery. When dysentery is present,

TABLE 232-1 Noninflammatory, Inflammatory, and Penetrating Types of Diarrhea

Mechanism	Noninflammatory (adhesion, enterotoxin)	Inflammatory (invasion, cytotoxin)	Penetrating (invades lymphatics)
Location	Proximal small bowel	Colon	Distal small bowel
Illness	Small-volume diarrhea (gastroenteritis) Watery, large volume suggests a secretory mechanism (i.e., cholera)	Blood and mucus (dysentery) Larger volume Low abdominal pain Tenesmus	Enteric fever (typhoid fever) Rash (rose spots) Small-volume or no diarrhea
Stool examination	No fecal leukocytes	Fecal leukocytes	Fecal leukocytes
Examples	*Vibrio cholerae* (secretory) *Escherichia coli* (EAEC and ETEC) Norovirus Rotavirus Adenovirus Astrovirus *Giardia lamblia* *Cryptosporidium*	*Shigella* species *E. coli* (EIEC) *Salmonella* non-*typhi* species *Campylobacter* *Clostridium difficile* *Entamoeba histolytica* *Cyclospora cayetanensis* *Isospora belli* *Microsporidia*	*Salmonella typhi* *Salmonella paratyphi* *Yersinia enterocolitica*

EAEC, enteroadherent *E. coli*; EIEC, enteroinvasive *E. coli*; ETEC, enterotoxigenic *E. coli*.

Shigella, Salmonella, Campylobacter, Clostridium difficile, enteroinvasive *E. coli* (EIEC), and *Entamoeba histolytica* are likely pathogens. Dysentery is often associated with tenesmus, or pain and cramping in the rectum and left lower quadrant, with straining, spasm of the rectal sphincter, and ineffectual evacuation. Fecal leukocytes and stool Hemoccult smears are routinely tested to help differentiate inflammatory diarrhea from noninflammatory diarrhea. Watery diarrhea is a type of noninflammatory, small bowel diarrhea suggestive of a secretory mechanism. It is likely to be abrupt in onset, very large in volume, and associated with symptoms of acute loss of blood volume (shock); cholera is implicated. In this case, the capacity of the distal colon to absorb watery diarrhea produced in the small intestine is overwhelmed. Penetrating diarrhea refers to organisms that may cause a sometimes unrecognized inflammatory process, usually in the distal small bowel, with eventual invasion into the bloodstream associated with systemic manifestations referred to as enteric fever (i.e., *Salmonella typhi* or typhoid fever). Table 232-1 outlines the differences among noninflammatory, inflammatory, and penetrating diarrheas.

EPIDEMIOLOGY

Infectious diarrheal diseases are the second leading cause of morbidity and mortality worldwide. In the United States, each person experiences one or two bouts of diarrhea each year, or some 200 million to 375 million episodes of diarrheal illness occur each year, resulting in 3000 to 5000 deaths.[1] Infectious diarrhea is a problem for both industrialized and developing nations, but it is uniquely associated with high morbidity and mortality in developing nations. Inadequate food and water supplies lead to recurrent bouts of diarrhea in very young children, who are not able to maintain adequate hydration during acute episodes but, more important, have baseline malnutrition. Malnutrition sets them up for gastrointestinal infection, and recurrent infection worsens malnutrition. Recurrent bouts of diarrhea weaken bowel health in a fashion that leads to chronic diarrhea. The situation is worsened by the fact that infectious diseases such as measles remain rampant in developing nations and are often not survivable in malnourished children.

BOX 232-1

Epidemiologic Groups Susceptible to Inflammatory Diarrhea

- International travelers
- Infants in day care centers
- Adults in day care or nursing homes
- Malnourished patients
- Hospitalized patients
- Recent use of broad-spectrum antibiotics
- Immunocompromised patients
- Persons with acquired immunodeficiency syndrome (AIDS) and homosexuals
- Military personnel in areas of conflict
- Elderly or mentally incapacitated patients
- Institutionalized populations: prisons, basic training camps

Rotavirus, a common cause of childhood viral gastroenteritis even in the United States, shares this proclivity to cause death in malnourished children.

Fortunately, modes of transmission are well known and include three main routes: food-borne, water-borne, and person to person (fecal-oral). Non-*typhi Salmonella* species and *Campylobacter jejuni* are transmitted through food, but norovirus has become the most common food-borne diarrhea.[2] *Shigella* species are transmitted mainly person to person. *Giardia* and *Cryptosporidium* are principally water-borne. International health initiatives have made progress in reducing the global annual childhood mortality rate from 5 million to 1.5 million deaths per year by promotion of breastfeeding, measles and rotavirus vaccination programs, education about oral rehydration therapy (ORT), food distribution programs, and separation of drinking water from bathing and bathroom facilities. Residents of industrialized nations experience one or two bouts of diarrhea annually, compared with five or six in underdeveloped areas, but certain individuals may be affected more frequently and severely (Box 232-1).

PATHOPHYSIOLOGY

Viruses, bacteria, and parasites can all cause diarrhea. Viral infections usually occur on a year-round basis but peak in the winter months. Bacterial illnesses are more common in the summer or early fall. Acute infectious diarrhea may be categorized as noninflammatory, inflammatory, or penetrating and thus cause unique clinical scenarios. *E. coli* organisms have the potential to exchange plasmids and other transgenic virulence factors, which run the gamut of pathogenic mechanisms. Because *E. coli* is part of normal bowel flora, special techniques must be requested to discover pathogenic species. Distinct syndromes follow these four pathogenic mechanisms:

1. *Adherence.* The bowel is colonized with bacteria that are nonadherent and suppress overgrowth of more pathogenic bacteria. Pathogenic bacteria may adhere to the bowel wall and cause direct damage or more intimately expose cells to enterotoxins and cytotoxins—that is, enteroadherent *E. coli* (EAEC). Microvilli are effaced and enterocyte cytoskeleton is disrupted—that is, enteropathogenic *E. coli* (EPEC).
2. *Invasion.* Enteroinvasive organisms adhere to enterocytes and then invade the bowel wall, with ulceration, sloughing of tissue, blood, and mucus. Bacillary dysentery is the result, and *Shigella* (an organism that also produces a Shiga toxin) is the classic example. Other examples include EIEC, non-*typhi Salmonella* species, and *C. difficile.*
3. *Enterotoxins. Vibrio cholerae* is the classic example. Cholera toxin acts by a second messenger, cyclic adenosine monophosphate (cAMP), to phosphorylate chloride channels in apical epithelial cells to block sodium chloride absorption and in addition increases chloride secretion by crypt cells. Passive transport of water into the intestinal lumen follows the chloride and produces watery diarrhea. Intestinal mucosa remains intact, as do alternative, glucose-dependent absorption mechanisms. Thus, glucose and electrolyte ORT remains a viable treatment. Enterotoxigenic *E. coli* (ETEC) has a similar toxin-mediated mechanism.
4. *Cytotoxins. Shigella dysenteriae* produces the classic cytotoxin. Cytotoxins damage the mucosa by inhibiting cellular protein synthesis and producing an inflammatory colitis. This cytokine is immunologically and structurally related to cytokines produced by enterohemorrhagic *E. coli* (EHEC) and *Vibrio parahaemolyticus.* Shiga-like toxins (SLTs) also target vascular endothelial cells (verotoxin), which explains the hemolysis, hemorrhagic colitis, and glomerulonephritis seen with hemolytic-uremic syndrome (HUS). HUS accompanies *E. coli* O157:H7 diarrhea outbreaks from undercooked hamburger associated with some fast-food restaurants. *C. difficile, Clostridium perfringens,* and *Salmonella* strains also produce destructive cytotoxins.

CLINICAL PRESENTATION

A good medical history is most helpful in determining the cause of infectious diarrhea and directing the extent of diagnostic testing. The epidemiologic setting, clinical presentation, and laboratory features guide our empirical approach to a broad spectrum of pathogens. Given that most acute diarrhea in the United States is caused by noroviruses (50% to 80%),[2] which produce mild noninflammatory gastroenteritis with fewer than six low-volume stools per day, and that it is self-limited with resolution in 2 to 3 days, the health care provider should investigate and give antibiotics only for presentations not consistent with norovirus infection. The probability that this is not norovirus infection increases dramatically if there are epidemiologic clues: travel, antibiotic use, hospital-acquired infection, outbreak association, animal or pet contact, hiker drinking untreated water, shellfish ingestion, unpasteurized milk ingestion, uncooked eggs, and day care client or worker. The provider should consider bacterial causes (Table 232-2) if the clinical presentation is one of inflammatory diarrhea: fever, abdominal pain, tenesmus, large-volume diarrhea, more than six stools per day, and mucus or blood in stool. A search for the pathogen with empirical antibiotic treatment is in order.

The presence of chronic illness, chemotherapy, tube feedings, medications, immune deficiency, or human immunodeficiency virus (HIV) infection with low CD4 counts will prompt consideration of more severe manifestations of norovirus, rotavirus, adenovirus, or astrovirus infection and atypical presentation of bacterial and parasitic diarrhea. Chronic diarrhea, lasting more than 14 days, is suggestive of protozoan parasites: *Giardia, Cryptosporidium,* and *E. histolytica.* Systemic manifestations of fever, chills, rigors, night sweats, and weight loss suggest penetrating bacteria (i.e., *S. typhi* or *Yersinia enterocolitica*), and blood cultures are in order. Chronic or recurrent diarrhea is also suggestive of inflammatory bowel disease, such as ulcerative colitis or regional enteritis. Irritable bowel syndrome may be present in a diarrhea-predominant form, which has been recently related to idiopathic adult-onset bile malabsorbtion.[3]

Some bacterial pathogens and toxins may cause noninflammatory, self-limited disease in healthy people, but if they produce only norovirus-like illness, patients would not benefit from extensive laboratory tests or antibiotic treatment. Older adults or very young patients may develop complications from gastroenteritis or mild diarrhea and may benefit from hydration and admission, even if a pathogen search and antibiotics are

TABLE 232-2 Clinical Signs and Disease Probability

Clinical Signs	Disease
Nausea, vomiting, epigastric pain Small volume, short course	Norovirus, rotavirus, adenovirus, astrovirus *Escherichia coli* (EAEC and ETEC)
Blood or mucus in stool, low abdominal pain Large volume	*Shigella, Salmonella, Campylobacter* *E. coli* (EIEC), *Clostridium difficile, Entamoeba histolytica*
Watery stool, large volume, shock	Cholera, Shiga toxin–producing *E. coli* (STEC)
Rectal pain and tenesmus	*Shigella, Entamoeba histolytica*
Fever (temperature >101° F), chills, night sweats, weight loss	*Salmonella typhi, Yersinia enterocolitica*
Chronic diarrhea	*Cryptosporidium, Giardia, E. histolytica, Campylobacter, Yersinia*
HUS	*E. coli* O157:H7 or other STEC
Guillain-Barré syndrome	*Campylobacter jejuni*

withheld. A temporal association should be sought with medications related to diarrhea or food related to bacterial toxins, such as mayonnaise, cream pie, and potato salad (staphylococcal enterotoxin) or rice dish on the warming table (*B. cereus* food poisoning); an association that would ensure a good prognosis without need for antibiotics.

PHYSICAL EXAMINATION

The physical examination includes weight, temperature, and orthostatic vital signs (blood pressure and heart rate lying, sitting, and standing) to assess volume depletion (dry mucous membranes, decreased skin turgor, absent jugular venous pulsation). The patient's mental status should be noted along with a close assessment of skin color, temperature, and rashes. Signs of bowel perforation include an abdomen quiet to auscultation and rigid to palpation. Small bowel obstruction might include a tender abdomen, with distention and high-pitched bowel sounds, as opposed to the usual bowel rushes and scaphoid abdomen seen with diarrheal enteritis. Thyromegaly, tachycardia, and proptosis suggest hyperthyroidism as a cause of chronic diarrhea. Lymphadenopathy, especially cervical node, suggests lymphoma or bowel cancer as a cause of diarrhea. In the female patient with lower abdominal symptoms, a pelvic examination is imperative. In the geriatric patient, fecal impaction must be ruled out. All patients should now be tested for HIV infection, and diarrhea is a good indication.

DIAGNOSTICS

For the patient who has mild acute diarrhea or gastroenteritis, diagnostic evaluation is typically not indicated. This diarrhea is usually viral and considered benign. Symptoms commonly resolve within 1 week, often within 1 to 3 days, and a diagnosis is rarely helpful. Complete blood count (CBC), serum electrolyte values, and blood urea nitrogen (BUN) and creatinine concentrations are standard tests for evaluation of electrolyte derangement and dehydration. A stool sample for fecal leukocytes and occult blood should be taken for patients with a temperature above 38.8° C (102° F), bloody diarrhea, abdominal pain, or more than six unformed stools in a 24-hour period and for patients who are frail and elderly or immunocompromised.

Stool evaluation for occult blood and fecal leukocytes helps differentiate between inflammatory and noninflammatory diarrhea. Fecal leukocytes (or immunoassay for the neutrophil protein lactoferrin) are associated with *Campylobacter, Shigella, Salmonella, C. difficile,* and EHEC. If fecal leukocytes are present, typically in inflammatory diarrhea, the stool should be further evaluated by stool culture and perhaps for ova and parasites.[4] Diarrhea that develops after hospitalization is unlikely to represent infection with *Giardia* or *Cryptosporidium* and should not be tested for ova and parasites. Systemic leukocytosis is suggestive of *C. difficile* infection, and a stool sample for *C. difficile* toxin B is sent. The old enzyme-linked immunosorbent assay (ELISA), which required reflex testing for toxin, has been largely replaced by polymerase chain reaction (PCR) testing for toxin B gene.[5] This real-time test for the toxin B gene is more sensitive (98.7%) and specific (87.5%). It is not necessary to send more than one test sample for *C. difficile,* and the test should not be performed on formed stool.

Colonoscopy may differentiate inflammatory bacterial colitis, *C. difficile,* invasive *E. coli,* Shiga toxin–producing *E. coli* (STEC), or cytomegalovirus from inflammatory bowel disease, ischemic colitis, and irritable bowel disease.[6] There is some risk of bowel perforation, especially in the setting of pseudomembranous colitis. Computed tomography (CT) imaging is useful to discover mucosal thickening, hemorrhage, abscess, malignancy, and inflammatory colitis. Mucosal thickening and pericolonic stranding are signs of *C. difficile*–associated pseudomembranous colitis.

DIAGNOSTICS

Diarrhea

- CBC and differential
- Serum electrolytes
- BUN and creatinine
- Stool for occult blood and fecal leukocytes*
- Stool culture for *Salmonella, Shigella, Campylobacter, Escherichia coli* 0157*
- Stool for Shiga toxins, if culture negative bloody diarrhea (STEC)*
- Stool for *Clostridium difficile* PCR test for toxin B gene*
- Stool for ova and parasites, if diarrhea is chronic
- Blood culture (two times), with systemic symptoms (penetrating diarrhea)
- Norovirus PCR; available at Public Health Laboratories for outbreaks

*If inflammatory diarrhea.

DIFFERENTIAL DIAGNOSIS

A good history investigating epidemiology, clinical signs, and routine diagnostic tests allow consideration of broad categories: noninflammatory, inflammatory, and penetrating gastrointestinal illness. Noninflammatory illness suggesting gastroenteritis, norovirus, rotavirus, or traveler's diarrhea is differentiated from more inflammatory and penetrating disease; it requires only hydration and electrolyte replacement, without stool or blood culture or further diagnostic testing.

Noninflammatory Diarrhea: Acute Gastroenteritis

Norovirus, the most common cause of viral gastroenteritis or "intestinal flu" in older children and adults, is a member of the Caliciviridae family of small RNA viruses. Human caliciviruses cause disease year-round but are the most common cause of outbreaks of "winter vomiting syndrome"; they occur frequently in closed systems, such as cruise ships, hospitals, nursing homes, and military facilities. These viruses require low inocula, are highly transmissible, and are resistant to cooking and chlorine cleaners. Shellfish, such as clams and oysters, are filter feeders and readily concentrate organisms from contaminated water. Nonbacterial, food-related outbreaks are usually a result of these agents. The incubation period for various caliciviruses is only 1 or 2 days. Winter vomiting disease is characterized by abrupt onset of vomiting, diarrhea, and low-grade or no fever. The duration is also short, 1 to 3 days. Treatment consists of ORT, and antibiotics are not indicated.[7] Travelers are asked not to take antibiotic treatment, unless symptoms fail to subside within 24 hours.

Rotavirus is the most common cause of severe diarrhea in very young children. There is a seasonal pattern, from November to April in the United States. Fecal-oral transmission may occur through contaminated water, food preparation, and hands. Rotavirus invades small intestine villous enterocytes, causing malabsorption, and produces a viral enterotoxin, which induces a secretory diarrhea by stimulating chloride secretion but without cyclic nucleotide signaling (i.e., not a cholera toxin). Thus the diarrhea is watery and lasts 3 to 8 days, and it is cholera-like in its ability to dehydrate and to cause death in young malnourished children. Vomiting and fever may be prominent symptoms, as in other gastroenteritis. The incubation period is 4 to 7 days. Antibiotics are not warranted, and treatment is ORT. In the United States, 1 of 40 children will require admission for intravenous fluid resuscitation.[8] Although rotavirus is also associated with disease in winter months, rotavirus disease in older children and adults is mild, short-lived, and thus underreported.

Two vaccines, RotaTeq (RV5: three doses at 2, 4, and 6 months) and Rotarix (RV1: two doses at 2 and 4 months), have reduced infant mortality in developing nations and morbidity in developed nations. These live vaccines should be used with caution in immunocompromised children, but HIV positivity is not a contraindication.

Traveler's Diarrhea

A recent travel history decreases the probability of norovirus, but the type of diarrhea is still likely to be noninflammatory and of short duration. Fecal-oral contamination of food or water is implicated, and *E. coli* (EAEC or ETEC) organisms are the most likely pathogens. Traveler's diarrhea can occur during or up to 10 days after travel, affects 20% to 50% of travelers to developing countries, and in general lasts approximately 3 to 5 days. It is usually a self-limited illness, and the patient rarely develops complications. Treatment includes oral fluid replacement.[9] Loperamide (Imodium), 4 mg orally at onset and 2 mg after each loose stool up to 16 mg/day, can be helpful. A 3-day course of ciprofloxacin, 500 mg orally twice daily, or azithromycin as a single 1000-mg dose may be prescribed. Bismuth subsalicylate (Pepto-Bismol) has both antimicrobial and anti-inflammatory effects and may be taken as 2 tablets every 30 to 60 minutes up to eight doses per day.

Invasive bacteria such as *Campylobacter, Salmonella,* and *Shigella* are seen more in travel to southern Asia. The parasites *E. histolytica, Cryptosporidium,* and *Giardia* are a consideration if diarrhea persists beyond 1 week. Non–*E. coli* bacteria cause 10% to 20% of cases of traveler's diarrhea, but investigation should be undertaken only if diarrhea persists beyond 1 week or if clinical signs of inflammatory diarrhea ensue. The gastroenteritis viruses represent 10% to 20% but are also short-lived, and there is no benefit from extensive diagnostics or antibiotics. Travelers should take an antibiotic, usually ciprofloxacin, rifaximin, or azithromycin, only if diarrhea lasts more than 1 or 2 days or is associated with high fever.[10]

Prevention is the cornerstone of treatment. Traveler's diarrhea can be avoided by not using untreated water or ice cubes or unpasteurized milk and not eating raw fruits and vegetables and undercooked meat. Travelers must remember to drink only sealed or carbonated beverages. Benefit from chemoprophylactic agents, including bismuth subsalicylate and *Lactobacillus acidophilus,* is uncertain. Antibiotics are typically not prescribed as a preventive measure for travelers. Widespread antibiotic resistance to ampicillin, to trimethoprim-sulfamethoxazole (Bactrim DS), and, increasingly, to quinolones has made these agents less useful for the treatment of traveler's diarrhea. In addition, they are not effective against viral or parasitic infections and may provide a false sense of security.

Vibrio cholerae

Watery, large-volume, noninflammatory diarrhea is best exemplified by infection with *V. cholerae,* the prototype of enterotoxigenic, secretory diarrhea. Cholera is the most feared agent of epidemic and pandemic diarrhea because of its abrupt, severe dehydration and mortality in times of natural and artificial catastrophe. The organism is omnipresent because of its natural existence in marine algae and plankton, where reservoirs await the right conditions of flooding and water stagnation to activate from a dormant state and grow to appropriate inoculum size and find an appropriate vehicle (i.e., shellfish concentration, contaminated water supplies, and contaminated food). Cholera also has the capacity to remain endemic in certain regions where asymptomatic carriage and contaminated water remain problems. The pathophysiologic mechanism is noted for its simplicity. Enterotoxin activates adenylate cyclase, which increases cAMP in enterocytes in the distal small intestine. This classic second messenger (cAMP) blocks absorption of sodium and chloride by the microvilli and promotes secretion of chloride by the crypt cells. Water osmotically follows sodium chloride into the intestinal lumen, and massive secretory diarrhea ensues.[11] Electrolyte concentrations of stool are similar to those of plasma, and ORT is easily defined.

The incubation period is usually longer than 14 hours, a relatively short duration indicative of rapid in vivo toxin production. Watery stools contain diluted mucus (rice water stools) and are large volume and noninflammatory. The colon is not inflamed, and there is no cramping, abdominal pain, tenesmus, or fever. Fecal leukocytes, blood, tissue fragments, and mucous strands are absent. Complications include isotonic dehydration, hypovolemic shock, acute renal failure, metabolic acidosis (high anion gap), and electrolyte losses (potassium, sodium, and chloride). Antibiotics play a secondary role to ORT but may shorten the course. Emerging resistance to ampicillin, tetracyclines, azithromycin, trimethoprim-sulfamethoxazole, and recently fluoroquinolones complicates therapy.

Inflammatory Diarrhea

***Shigella* (*Shigella dysenteriae, Shigella flexneri, Shigella sonnei*).** *Shigella* infection is the prototype of inflammatory colitis diarrhea or bacillary dysentery. The small inoculation size allows easy fecal-oral transmission (children, day care centers, gay males), but summer prevalence might be accounted for by the potential for transmission via fly feet in outdoor settings with poor sanitation. *Shigella* causes an estimated 450,000 cases of diarrhea in the United States annually,[12] but this organism tends to be diagnosed and reported more than noninflammatory diarrheas. The incubation period is 12 to 72 hours, reflecting cytotoxin production. It is easily recognized by larger volume, frequent, bloody, foul diarrhea containing mucous and fecal leukocytes. Fever, cramps, and tenesmus are prominent symptoms. The need for ORT and possibly intravenous hydration should be recognized, and these measures implemented early.

Certain strains of *E. coli* (EIEC and EHEC) produce dysentery indistinguishable from shigellosis. SLTs also target vascular endothelial cells (verotoxin), which explains the hemolysis, hemorrhagic colitis, and glomerulonephritis seen with HUS accompanying *E. coli* O157:H7. Because of toxin production, antimotility agents should be avoided. Antibiotics had been thought to exacerbate HUS in *E. coli* O157:H7 disease because antibiotics fostered abrupt release of cytotoxin as bacteria were killed.[13] Shiga-toxin in *E. coli* is carried on bacteriophages. A meta-analysis did not show more HUS with antibiotic use, but antibiotics that damage DNA (fluoroquinolones and trimethoprim-sulfamethoxazole) convert lysogenic phage (integrated into cellular DNA) into lytic phage (replicative) and increase production of Shiga toxin.[14] Thus, many physicians still avoid use of these antibiotics if STEC is a consideration. Otherwise, *Shigella*, EIEC, and EHEC are causes of bloody diarrhea (dysentery), and all should be treated with antibiotics to improve morbidity and mortality. Some believe that mild disease is not lessened by antibiotics and does not require antibiotic treatment. However, the low inoculum size allows recovering mild cases to continue propagation of disease, and they should be treated for public health reasons. Antibiotics in infants and older adult patients with severe disease can be lifesaving. Ciprofloxacin (500 mg every 12 hours orally for 1 to 3 days in adults) and trimethoprim-sulfamethoxazole, azithromycin, and ceftriaxone are alternatives for children.

***Salmonella* (Non-*Typhi* Species).** Non-*typhi Salmonella* species are now the most common cause of inflammatory diarrhea in the United States, epidemiologically interesting, and more frequent in summer and fall.[15] Transmission is fecal-oral, and these organisms are responsible for most food-borne outbreaks in the United States. *Salmonella* species are widely disseminated in nature and are adaptable and virulent to humans; they frequently contaminate poultry, beef, eggs, and dairy products. Fresh produce (lettuce, tomatoes, cantaloupe), unpasteurized juices, and sprouts have been associated with recent interest in organic foods and *Salmonella* outbreaks. Pet turtles, snakes, iguanas, hedgehogs, outdoor cats, and petting zoos present a danger, especially to children. Raw milk and specialty cheeses are problematic. Dogs and children may be infected by chew products (e.g., dried pig ears). Beef jerky and summer sausage are the adult equivalents. Neonates are at high risk because of relative gastric achlorhydria and the buffering capacity of breast milk and formula. Human-to-human transmission may occur through food handling and contaminated water. Chronic carrier states (0.5%) are difficult to eradicate and present employment issues for food handlers and health care workers.[16]

Incubation periods of 12 to 48 hours reflect invasion of distal small bowel and colon mucosa. The inflammatory response is less severe than in shigellosis, but inflammatory diarrhea ensues. There is some propensity to multiply further in Peyer patches and to enter the circulation, as with enteric fever. Blood cultures are more likely to bear bacteria, and dissemination may occur with distant focal infection in meninges, heart valves, gallbladder, biliary tree, pancreas, mycotic aneurysm, and bone, leading to unusual complications.[17]

As with other inflammatory diarrhea, rehydration and electrolyte replacement are essential. Diarrhea is self-limited, antibiotic resistance is a growing concern, and antibiotic treatment may prolong the carrier state; thus, antibiotic treatment is usually deferred.[13] Exceptions include infants, older adults (50 years old or older), patients with sickle cell disease (bone infarcts become infected with *Salmonella*, causing osteomyelitis), immunocompromised patients, patients with valvular heart disease, and patients with vascular disease and endovascular stents or grafts (*Salmonella* has a propensity to settle on vascular plaques and to cause mycotic aneurysm).

***Campylobacter jejuni*.** *Campylobacter* is the second most common cause of inflammatory diarrhea in the United States.[15] Campylobacteriosis is a worldwide zoonosis; it is present in many animal species and enjoys a large natural reservoir, and thus we are regularly exposed from food and surface water. *Campylobacter*, like *Salmonella*, is susceptible to gastric acid and requires a relatively high inoculation dose. However, patients with alcoholism, cirrhosis, or diabetes and elders and neonates are more susceptible, and a dose as low as 500 organisms may be able to cause disease. *Campylobacter* offers variable production of cytotoxin, infects the terminal ileum and colon, and has a greater spectrum of disease, depending on host resistance and organism (i.e., *Campylobacter fetus* produces less dysentery than *C. jejuni* does). Disease may be subtle, chronic, acute, or full-blown dysentery. The organism is fastidious, so negative stool cultures do not rule it out. Wet preparation microscopic stool examination may show darting, comma-shaped organisms; and Gram stain of a stool specimen may reveal small, curved, gram-negative rods. Fecal leukocytes and stool Hemoccult slide test results are positive. Blood cultures are rarely positive, but *Campylobacter* is occasionally a cause of enteric fever. Like *S. typhi*, *Campylobacter* may cause more systemic disease than diarrhea.

For most healthy adults, *Campylobacter* produces a self-limited illness, and it is not clear that antibiotics shorten illness. Unlike *Salmonella*, the organism is not difficult to eradicate with antibiotics (i.e., antibiotics do not prolong the carrier state). Dysentery, prolonged colitis, bacteremia, enteric fever, and distant focal infections need to be treated with antibiotics. Macrolides have been the treatment of choice, but there is some resistance. In general, β-lactam antibiotics are not as effective, but fluoroquinolones, aminoglycosides, chloramphenicol, clindamycin, and tetracyclines are alternatives.

Because of the occasional insidious presentation of chronic colitis with bloody diarrhea and negative stool cultures, *Campylobacter* can be mistaken for ulcerative colitis. Postinfectious diarrhea or reactive arthritis may follow most forms of bacillary dysentery in human leukocyte antigen HLA-B27–positive individuals. Guillain-Barré syndrome is a unique but uncommon (1 in 2000) consequence of *Campylobacter* infection. Unfortunately, *Campylobacter* diarrhea is so common that 20% to 50% of cases of Guillain-Barré syndrome follow *Campylobacter* infections.[18]

***Escherichia coli* O157:H7.** *E. coli* O157:H7 was first recognized as a food-borne pathogen in the United States in 1982. Outbreaks occurred by distribution of contaminated hamburger meat, and EHEC soon became the most common cause of bloody diarrhea. The Centers for Disease Control and Prevention (CDC) estimates 73,000 illnesses annually in the United States, resulting in more than 2000 hospitalizations and 60 deaths.[15] *E. coli* O157:H7 is a zoonotic emerging pathogen that normally resides in the gut of healthy cattle. Early outbreaks of *E. coli* O157:H7–mediated disease were traced to unpasteurized apple cider made from fallen apples in orchards where cattle grazed, thus contaminating it with feces. Discovery of this relationship revealed the need to pasteurize apple cider. Improved cooking standards in fast-food restaurants have decreased the incidence of *E. coli* O157:H7 in ground beef foods, but the problem has shifted to water-borne and vegetable-associated disease. Our preference for organic foods, rejection of chemical fertilizer for cow manure, and contamination of water and vegetables with *E. coli* O157:H7 have introduced new sources of what used to be the hamburger disease.[19]

Another unique aspect of *E. coli* O157:H7 is the spectrum of disease this organism may cause, from mild diarrhea to severe hemorrhagic colitis. Antibiotic treatment causes release of SLT, a toxin that is also present in *S. dysenteriae* and that had been thought to worsen the risk of HUS, although a meta-analysis did not show an increased risk of HUS associated with antibiotic administration.[14] By the time HUS appears, the acute diarrhea has already subsided, so antibiotics are not likely to help.

Clostridium difficile. Antibiotic-associated diarrhea (AAD) has been with us since the advent of broad-spectrum antibiotics, which alter anaerobic and enteric bowel flora, allowing antibiotic-resistant *C. difficile* to grow and to produce AAD and more severe pseudomembranous colitis. There has been a gradual increase in *C. difficile*–associated disease during the past 15 years, but more urgent concern is raised by several recent studies showing both increasing rates and increasing severity of *C. difficile* colitis. The new epidemic is occurring in widespread geographic areas, causes disease in previously healthy patients, and is dominated by a previously uncommon strain of *C. difficile* that produces a binary toxin similar to the more virulent binary toxin of *C. perfringens*. The new strain also contains a mutation in the *tcdC* regulatory gene and consequently produces greater amounts of toxins A and B responsible for diarrhea. Interestingly, this strain is more resistant to the extended-spectrum fluoroquinolones. Recent overuse of fluoroquinolones may have selected out this particular strain of *C. difficile*, much like clindamycin selected out past strains of *C. difficile* and was more closely associated with AAD than other antibiotics.[20] The new epidemic strain of *C. difficile* is not resistant to either metronidazole or vancomycin.

Treatment of the new strain of *C. difficile* remains essentially the same as for past strains, but we need to be more alert to the increasing possibility of AAD and its increasing severity to prevent complications of toxic megacolon, colonic perforation, transverse volvulus, and protein-losing enteropathy. Broad-spectrum antibiotics should be stopped, if at all possible. Hydration and electrolyte replacement are of foremost importance. Although 10 days of oral metronidazole (500 mg three times daily) and oral vancomycin (125 mg four times daily) are equally effective in mild and moderate disease, metronidazole is preferred because of the greater cost of oral vancomycin and the possible selection of vancomycin-resistant *Enterococcus* (VRE) and more recently vancomycin-resistant *S. aureus* (VRSA). Oral vancomycin is preferred for severe cases of AAD. Severely ill patients must not be treated with intravenous vancomycin, because it does not get into the bowel lumen in significant concentrations. Vancomycin is not absorbed orally, nor does oral vancomycin progress to the colon in the setting of ileus. Such patients should be treated with intravenous metronidazole, which is excreted lower down through the bile duct and to some extent directly into the colon. In severely ill patients, liquid vancomycin may be placed into nasogastric tubes, high rectal tubes, and ostomies, in addition to intravenous metronidazole.[21] Surgical consultation should be obtained early in the course of severe disease because complications of toxic megacolon and colon perforation may require colectomy or diverting colostomy.

Recurrent *C. difficile* diarrhea follows a course of treatment in up to 20% of cases, and multiple relapses occur in at least 6%. Most cases of "recurrence" are simply a reflection of poor bowel health; it is expected to take 1 to 2 months for normal bowel habits to be recovered. Loose stools and urgency are to be expected and should not be treated. Repeated testing for *C. difficile* toxin should not be done because toxin and culture may remain positive in many improving patients. True relapses, defined as three large-volume diarrheal stools per day, fever, or leukocytosis, should be treated with another course of metronidazole, and a gradual weekly taper of dose (i.e., 500 mg three times daily, 500 mg twice daily, 500 mg every day, 500 mg every other day, 500 mg every third day) can be tried. Patients with multiple recurrences are prescribed metronidazole, the lowest dose that controls symptoms, for 2 to 3 months. Long-term use of metronidazole is discouraged because of effects of neuropathy and gastrointestinal intolerance. When bowel health has improved, another attempt at weaning may be tried. Long-term vancomycin use is fraught with expense and encourages colonization with VRE. Rifaximin and fidaxomicin are expensive new antibiotics that may reduce the relapse rate but should be used in consultation with infectious disease or gastroenterology specialists.[22] Biologic therapies include probiotics and fecal microbiota transplant (FMT). Probiotics decrease antibiotic-associated diarrhea but less clearly reduce recurrent *C. difficile*.[23] FMT is costly and shows encouraging promise, but lacks large randomized controlled trials to date to determine side effects and which patients are likely to benefit.[24] A recent phase III study found tolevamer, a toxin-binding polymer, inferior to both metronidazole and vancomycin and confirmed the superiority of vancomycin for severe AAD.[25]

Epidemic *C. difficile* places new emphasis on preventive measures. Antibiotic use should be limited to the shortest effective course and the narrowest spectrum antibiotic for each pathogen. Broad-spectrum empirical regimens should be narrowed as culture results return, and more specific diagnosis may allow early discontinuation. Isolation and cohort of multiple cases should be accompanied by gowns, gloves, and handwashing. It should be remembered that alcohol scrubs do not inactivate *C. difficile* spores, so soap and water are required to remove them from hands. Electronic thermometers should be replaced by disposable thermometers, and dedicated stethoscopes may be left in the room. Broad-spectrum antimicrobial use should be managed by hospital antibiotic stewardship programs, and outpatient use of clindamycin and fluoroquinolone antibiotics should be limited.

Genetic sequencing of hospital-associated *C. difficile* isolates has shown 45% to be genetically distinct, and thus inconsistent with hospital transmission. Distinct subtypes continued to be identified throughout the study period, suggesting a considerable reservoir unrelated to hospital contacts. Given genetically diverse sources, infection control techniques are likely to reduce but not eliminate *C. difficile* diarrhea.[26]

Food Poisoning: Bacterial Toxins

One to Six Hours After Ingestion

Staphylococcus aureus *Food Poisoning.* Summer picnics can be spoiled by foods that favor growth of *S. aureus* (cream pies, cream puffs, chocolate éclairs, chicken salad, mayonnaise) left too long in the warm sun. Incubation within food results in preformed staphylococcal enterotoxins. Short-incubation emetic syndrome produces intense nausea and vomiting within a few hours of ingestion. Long-incubation diarrhea syndrome causes severe abdominal cramps and diarrhea hours later. One feels as if death is imminent, but symptoms resolve completely within 12 hours, and treatment is for comfort only.

Bacillus cereus *Food Poisoning.* Short-incubation emetic syndrome is similar to the same syndrome caused by *S. aureus* enterotoxin, but it is caused by a preformed cereulide toxin capable of binding to gastric nerves. Diarrhea is mild and seen in only 33%. This syndrome is associated with fried rice held on warming tables for extended periods. Like staphylococcal food poisoning, this emetic syndrome resolves in 12 hours.

Eight to Fourteen Hours After Ingestion

Clostridium perfringens *Food Poisoning.* *C. perfringens* food poisoning follows ingestion of meat and gravies (beef and poultry). Up to 80% of these meats are contaminated with their own enteric flora in meat processing plants. Outbreaks occur in institutions and at banquets where large quantities of meat are precooked without ever reaching adequate internal temperatures to kill all contaminating bacteria and without reheating enough to kill incubating bacteria. In contrast to preformed enterotoxins seen in *Staphylococcus* and early-incubation *Bacillus* food poisoning, these enterotoxins are formed in vivo as the organism enters a vegetative state in the hostile environment of our intestines; hence the longer incubation period and action farther down in the intestine, mainly with abdominal cramps and diarrhea. Vomiting and fever are uncommon.

Bacillus cereus *Food Poisoning.* Long-incubation diarrhea syndrome is similar to *C. perfringens* food poisoning. It is caused by enterotoxin produced in vivo after ingestion. This explains the long incubation period and predominance of small intestinal cramps and diarrhea. There may be some nausea with both *C. perfringens* and long-incubation *B. cereus,* but vomiting and fever are rare. These two long-incubation syndromes are still limited to the life of their respective toxins and are usually resolved within 24 hours.

MANAGEMENT

Medications can be used for symptomatic relief of nausea and vomiting, abdominal cramping, and diarrhea. These are generally used in older children and healthy adults. Absorbents and antisecretory agents such as bismuth subsalicylate (Kaopectate, Pepto-Bismol) and antispasmodic-anticholinergic sedatives such as atropine sulfate, scopolamine hydrobromide, hyoscyamine sulfate, and phenobarbital are used to decrease abdominal cramping. Antisecretory agents such as bismuth subsalicylate also have an anti-inflammatory effect and are commonly used if vomiting and abdominal cramping are present. Bismuth subsalicylate may cause salicylate intoxication and should be used cautiously. Patients taking warfarin should be warned as well because anticoagulation will be affected. Concomitant use of bismuth subsalicylate with antibiotics may decrease the effectiveness of the antibiotics.

Antimotility agents will not shorten the duration of illness but may be used for convenience in noninflammatory diarrhea. Loperamide, diphenoxylate hydrochloride–atropine sulfate (Lomotil), and tincture of opium all decrease diarrhea. Loperamide is preferred in children, pregnant women, and immunocompromised patients. Crofelemer is a new chloride channel antisecretory drug approved for use in HIV patients with antiretroviral-associated diarrhea. It also reduces diarrheal events in patients with traveler's diarrhea.[27] If nausea is the main complaint, treatment with promethazine (Phenergan), prochlorperazine (Compazine), or another antiemetic is recommended. Antimotility agents should not be used in patients with bloody diarrhea, febrile diarrhea, or fecal leukocytosis. Antibiotics are used in only a small proportion of patients.

Treatment with antibiotics should be considered in the following situations: in the presence of fecal leukocytes without a confirmed positive stool culture; with occult blood; if the patient has fever with profuse, watery diarrhea (more than six stools per day), appears dehydrated, has had symptoms for more than 1 week, and is immunocompromised; or if hospitalization is considered. *Salmonella, Shigella,* or *Campylobacter* pathogens are the most likely cause of the infection in these cases. Ciprofloxacin or norfloxacin can be initiated until the stool culture results are verified but should not be used in children or pregnant or lactating women. If the diarrhea persists for longer than 2 weeks, *Giardia* organisms may be suspected and metronidazole can be initiated. Specific therapy is initiated once the pathogen is identified. Pedialyte, Enfalyte, Rehydralyte, and CeraLyte are commercial formulas for ORT. Rehydration therapies can be found on the internet at www.cdc.gov/cholera/treatment/rehydration-therapy.html or http://rehydrate.org/solutions/homemade.htm.

COMPLICATIONS

Complications from diarrhea are usually the result of dehydration. Regardless of the cause, attention should be directed toward fluid and electrolyte replacement. Electrolyte disorders, particularly hypocalcemia, hypomagnesemia, and hypokalemia, are common in persistent diarrhea. Continuous diarrhea can necessitate hospitalization for fluid and electrolyte replacement if the patient is unable to maintain hydration with oral fluid replacement. Sepsis and cardiovascular collapse are potential complications, and infants, older adults, and immunosuppressed patients are more susceptible to these complications. Refractory diarrhea is usually a symptom of a more serious illness and requires diagnostic evaluation and subspecialist consultation.

Association of *E. coli* O157:H7 diarrhea with childhood HUS has come to exemplify how a pathogen at one site can explain a disease at another, uninfected site. HUS was previously an unexplained illness defined by hemolysis, thrombocytopenia, and acute renal failure, often in children. EHEC has evolved by acquiring a symbiotic relationship with a bacteriophage that encodes SLT. SLT attaches to a receptor, globotriaosylceramide (GB), on enterocytes in the gut. GB receptors also exist on vascular endothelial cells of glomerular capillaries and other small capillary beds. Damage to these capillary beds caused by circulating SLT explains the occurrence of acute renal failure, microangiopathic hemolytic anemia, and thrombocytopenia, which define HUS. Neutralizing antibodies to SLT develop in most children before the age of 10 years and decline as they age. Thus, persons most severely affected by *E. coli* O157:H7 are the young and the elderly.

Joint inflammation, conjunctivitis, or urethritis that follows a bout of diarrhea by 7 to 10 days suggests reactive arthropathy after *Salmonella, Shigella,* or *Campylobacter* infection.[28] Sensory paresthesia followed rapidly by ascending motor weakness and loss of deep tendon reflexes implicates Guillain-Barré syndrome, often following *C. jejuni* enteritis.[18]

INDICATIONS FOR REFERRAL OR HOSPITALIZATION

If dehydration is severe or vomiting is protracted, intravenous fluids should be initiated. Children and older patients are especially vulnerable. Medical evaluation is indicated for children younger than 6 months or whose weight is below 8 kg; premature infants; children with chronic illness; infants with fever (temperature $\geq 38°$ C); and children with fever (temperature $>39°$ C), visible bloody stool, high-volume stool, and persistent vomiting. Signs of severe dehydration requiring admission for intravenous fluid administration include sunken eyes, dry mucous membranes, decreased skin turgor, lack of tears, decreased urine output (dry diapers), irritability, lethargy, tachycardia, and postural hypotension.[29] If symptoms of the illness persist beyond 3 weeks despite treatment measures, the provider should consider chronic lactose intolerance, parasites, malignant neoplasms, and disease states such as diabetes, thyrotoxicosis, lupus, HIV infection, inflammatory bowel disease, or irritable bowel syndrome, and consultation is indicated.

PATIENT AND FAMILY EDUCATION

Normal slow recovery of bowel health after a bout of *C. difficile* infection should be discussed to avoid overzealous treatment of recurrences. Avoidance of nonessential antibiotics in all patients, but especially after *C. difficile* infection, is an important discussion. Bacterial enteritis in children younger than 5 years may serve as a focus for bowel intussusception, which may occur in the 6-month period after enteritis.[30] Parents and providers should be aware. The following are some general recommendations that should be discussed with the patient and family:

- Practice good handwashing after each bowel movement to reduce the possibility of spreading disease to other family members.
- Immunocompromised patients are at greater risk of severe infection and should be diligent about proper safe food handling and preparation.
- Drink frequent, small sips of fluids (water, tea, bouillon, flat cola, flat ginger ale, or sports drink) to avoid dehydration.
- Avoid foods and let your stomach rest until bowel movements begin to return to normal or until you begin to feel better. Gradually add small amounts of food (e.g., crackers, toast, rice, bananas), avoiding those that may aggravate symptoms (e.g., dairy products, caffeine, high-fat or high-fiber foods, carbonated beverages, sugar-free products, and alcohol).
- It is better to avoid antidiarrheal products because most cases of diarrhea are self-limited.
- If symptoms persist or are accompanied by mental confusion, fever with temperature higher than 38.3° C (101° F), chills, vomiting, weakness (especially muscle weakness), dizziness, dry mouth, extreme thirst, little or no urinary output, severe abdominal discomfort, blurred vision, or black or bloody stools, immediately notify the health care provider.
- Children, day care workers, and food handlers should remain at home until diarrhea resolves.

PREVENTION

Therapy to reduce gastric acid has increasingly come under scrutiny because unsuspected side effects have come to light: osteoporosis, risk of hospital- and community-acquired pneumonia, and enteric infection such as *Campylobacter* and *Salmonella* enteritis.[31] Studies have linked chronic proton pump inhibitor use with *C. difficile* infection and relapse.[31] Physicians should offer other treatments for dyspepsia, prescribe shorter courses of proton pump inhibitors, and discontinue H_2 blockers and proton pump inhibitors in asymptomatic patients.

Prevention information for patients and providers includes the following:

- Handwashing remains the best preventive measure. Always wash hands after handling chicken or other raw meats. Wash cutting boards frequently. Change sponges and wash kitchen countertops frequently. Sponges may be disinfected by microwaving them on high or placing them in boiling water for 2 minutes.
- Use a meat thermometer to check temperature of roasts, chicken, and hamburger. When traveling, especially out of the country, drink and brush teeth with bottled water and eat only washed and then peeled fruits and vegetables. Avoid iced drinks, and never drink untreated water.
- Avoid high-risk foods, such as raw seafood, raw eggs, unpasteurized dairy products, and undercooked poultry and beef.
- Avoid foods that have sat out at room temperature for more than 2 hours.
- Defrost meats in the microwave or refrigerator, not at room temperature.
- Cook foods to the proper temperature.
- Avoid holding foods too long on steam tables or without refrigeration.

CHAPTER 233

INFECTIOUS MONONUCLEOSIS

Traci Alberti

DEFINITION AND EPIDEMIOLOGY

Infectious mononucleosis (IM) is an acute, self-limited, generally benign illness that occurs in both children and adults after primary infection with Epstein-Barr virus (EBV), cytomegalovirus (CMV), and other infectious agents. The classic manifestation of this syndrome includes fever, pharyngitis, lymphadenopathy, fatigue, and atypical lymphocytosis.[1]

In this chapter, the term *Epstein-Barr virus–associated infectious mononucleosis* (EBV-IM) is used to refer to IM caused by acute EBV infection. The term *non–Epstein-Barr virus–associated infectious mononucleosis* (non-EBV-IM) is used to refer to the clinical syndrome of IM that is caused by an agent other than EBV, such as CMV, *Toxoplasma gondii*, adenovirus, or hepatitis virus infection.[1] Non-EBV-IM illnesses account for approximately 10% of all IM cases. IM refers to the triad of fever, pharyngitis, and lymphadenopathy regardless of the infectious agent. This chapter deals primarily with the presentation, evaluation, and management of EBV-IM, the most common type of acute IM, which is seen, at least serologically, in 20% to 70% of adolescents and young adults.[2] EBV-IM occurs most often in adolescents and young adults, with the highest incidence occurring at ages 15 to 19 years In persons younger than 10 years and older than 30 years, the annual incidence of EBV-IM decreases dramatically to less than 1 case per 1000 persons, but mild infection in young adults may be underdiagnosed. It is most common in populations with many young adults, such as active-duty military personnel and college students, in whom the annual incidence ranges from 11 to 48 cases per 1000.[1] The chance for development of IM after EBV infection appears to increase from childhood to young adulthood; it is estimated that less than 10% of children develop IM after EBV exposure, but up to 78% of adolescents have a chance for development of EBV-IM after acute EBV infection.[3] IM is relatively uncommon in adults, accounting for less than 2% of adults who see their health care provider with a sore throat.[3]

PATHOPHYSIOLOGY

IM can be caused by a variety of infectious agents other than EBV, including CMV, herpesvirus 6, human immunodeficiency virus (HIV), adenovirus, hepatitis A virus, influenza A and B viruses, and rubella virus.[4] In addition, IM is also associated with some neoplasms. Transmission of IM varies, depending on the specific causative infectious agent. Transmission of EBV-IM occurs through exposure to oropharyngeal secretions, although blood products, genital secretions, and breast milk have also been reported as sources of transmission.[4] EBV is a relatively fragile DNA herpesvirus that cannot survive for long outside the host. The virus initially infects the oral epithelial cells and then spreads to the B lymphocytes, which then circulate through the reticuloendothelial system, causing a significant but time-limited immunologic response. Many of the signs and symptoms associated with the clinical presentation of EBV-IM are the result of this immunologic response. The incubation time of EBV-IM is usually 4 to 8 weeks. Hepatic involvement associated with EBV-IM varies in severity and increases with age, ranging from 10% in young adults to 30% in older adults.[3] Acute EBV infection stimulates the production of antibodies against EBV antigens, which remain present lifelong.

CLINICAL PRESENTATION

The classic triad of symptoms of acute IM includes fever, pharyngitis, and lymphadenopathy. The typical adolescent with EBV-IM is seen with sore throat, fever, and lymph node and tonsillar enlargement. Additional common presenting symptoms include pharyngeal inflammation and transient palatal petechiae. Older adults are less likely to have sore throat and adenopathy but more likely to have hepatomegaly and jaundice.[1] However, IM often manifests atypically, especially in young children and older adults, making diagnosis difficult. Pharyngitis is usually diffuse, with exudates present in approximately 30% of cases.[5] Lymphadenopathy usually affects the anterior and posterior cervical chain and may also be diffuse. Temperatures may be as high as 40° C (104° F), and the elevation may last as long as 2 weeks. Symptoms that may precede as well as persist throughout the acute phase of illness include malaise, anorexia, and fatigue. Symptoms of EBV-IM usually peak approximately 7 days after onset and become less pronounced during the next 1 to 3 weeks. Fatigue can persist for several months. Reports indicate that splenic enlargement occurs in 40% to 100% of cases and can be confirmed with ultrasound.[1,2]

Less common signs and symptoms of EBV-IM include upper airway compromise, abdominal pain, rash, hepatomegaly, jaundice, and eyelid edema. A rash, which occurs in approximately 5% to 10% of individuals, may be macular, urticarial, petechial, or erythema multiforme.[6]

PHYSICAL EXAMINATION

On physical examination, the patient may or may not appear ill, depending on degree of fever, associated signs and symptoms, and length of time since onset of symptoms. The classic clinical manifestation of fever, pharyngitis, and lymphadenopathy raises suspicion for EBV-IM. The anterior and posterior cervical chains should be assessed for lymphadenopathy, which may be diffuse. An abdominal examination identifies splenomegaly and hepatomegaly. Rash and jaundice should be noted because they are associated with EBV-IM, especially in older adults.

DIAGNOSTICS

A complete blood count (CBC) with differential will help identify absolute lymphocytosis, wherein more than 10% of cells are atypical. This is characteristic of IM, but not specific. The most useful laboratory test is the serologic test for heterophil antibodies. This will identify 85% of cases in older children and adults. It is possible for some infected persons to have a negative test result early in the illness, because circulating antibodies have not reached sufficient detectable levels. Repeat testing in 7 to 10 days is recommended if symptoms continue.[7] A positive test result may remain positive for up to a year after initial illness. Absolute lymphocytosis with a positive heterophil antibody test is diagnostic of acute infectious mononucleosis.

If the heterophil antibody test result is negative but EBV-IM is still highly suspected, further testing may be helpful. More sensitive tests have been developed that detect viral capsid antigen (VCA) immunoglobulins G (IgG) and M (IgM). When the results are negative, these tests are better than heterophil antibody tests in ruling out EBV-IM because they are better able to detect acute infection; but when the results are positive, the tests are similar in their ability to rule in disease.[5,8] VCA IgG and IgM results typically become positive within 1 to 2 weeks of infection, but VCA IgM becomes undetectable after 6 months. Antibody to Epstein-Barr nuclear antigen (EBNA) is not usually detectable until 6 to 8 weeks after the onset of symptoms but can help distinguish between acute and previous infections. If EBNA is positive in the presence of acute symptoms and suspected IM, then previous infection is suggested. A throat culture should be considered because 3% to 30% of patients with IM also have streptococcal pharyngitis. Liver function tests (LFTs) may also be considered; liver enzymes are elevated in approximately 80% to 90% of persons with IM.[1]

DIAGNOSTICS

Infectious Mononucleosis

LABORATORY
- Heterophil antibody
- VCA IgG and IgM*
- EBV nuclear antigen*
- CBC and differential*
- LFTs*

IMAGING
- Abdominal ultrasonography*

*If indicated.

DIFFERENTIAL DIAGNOSIS

The triad of fever, pharyngitis, and lymphadenopathy is associated with a number of diagnoses in addition to acute IM, including streptococcal pharyngitis and any one of several viral pharyngitides, acute CMV infection, and acute HIV infection.[1] The reported incidence of IM in patients with peritonsillar abscess ranges from 2% to 20%; therefore it is recommended that all patients with pharyngitis and peritonsillar abscess be fully assessed clinically and screened for IM.[9] If symptoms have been present for only a few days, group A β-hemolytic streptococcal pharyngitis or a viral upper respiratory tract infection should be considered. However, individuals with a positive streptococcal culture may also have acute IM. In individuals with a negative throat culture for group A β-hemolytic streptococci, symptoms that persist for more than a week are highly suggestive of acute IM.

DIFFERENTIAL DIAGNOSIS

Infectious Mononucleosis

INFECTIOUS CAUSES
- Bartonellosis (cat-scratch disease)
- CMV
- Corynebacterium diphtheria
- EBV
- Hepatitis A and B viruses
- HIV
- Human herpesvirus 6
- Lyme disease
- Malaria
- Meningococcemia
- Rubella
- Salmonella bacteremia
- Streptococcal pharyngitis
- Syphilis
- Toxoplasmosis
- Trichinosis
- Tuberculosis
- Viral pharyngitis

NONINFECTIOUS CAUSES
- Juvenile rheumatoid arthritis
- Kawasaki disease
- Lymphoma
- Sarcoidosis
- Systemic lupus erythematosus

DRUGS
- Dapsone
- Phenytoin
- Sulfonamides

Hepatitis A is another viral illness that occurs most frequently in children and adolescents, and although incubation routes are different, hepatitis A virus has an incubation period (15 to 45 days) similar to that of EBV (30 to 50 days).[10] Hepatitis A typically has an influenza-like onset occurring after a prodrome of myalgia, headache, fever, and malaise. Hepatitis A and IM can also occur concomitantly.

It may not be possible to distinguish clinically between IM caused by EBV infection and an IM-like syndrome caused by toxoplasmosis or CMV infection, and in fact the management of these syndromes is essentially the same. However, diagnostic testing to determine the cause is important in pregnant women because toxoplasmosis and acute HIV and CMV infections are associated with significant pregnancy complications. If acute HIV infection is suspected, a quantitative polymerase chain reaction test should be done.[1]

MANAGEMENT

Treatment of uncomplicated EBV-IM is primarily supportive, including adequate hydration, nonsteroidal anti-inflammatory drugs or acetaminophen for fever reduction and myalgias, throat lozenges or sprays, and gargling with a 2% lidocaine solution to relieve pharyngeal discomfort. Aspirin should be avoided because it has been associated with Reye syndrome in a few cases of acute EBV infection. Bed rest may be helpful during the acute phase of the illness, depending on the degree of fatigue. Individuals with splenomegaly should be encouraged to refrain from strenuous physical activity for 3 to 4 weeks to avoid the risk of splenic rupture before resolution of the splenomegaly.[11] Serial ultrasound studies starting at week 2 to 3 may be helpful in determining risk of rupture associated with splenomegaly. Studies revealed that neither corticosteroids nor acyclovir reduced the severity or duration of symptoms. Therefore, current management guidelines do not include the use of either of these agents in the treatment of acute uncomplicated EBV-IM, although corticosteroids may be useful in the treatment of several rare but severe complications associated with EBV-IM, such as airway obstruction, thrombocytopenia, or hemolytic anemia.[12] Most patients with EBV-IM recover uneventfully in approximately 2 to 4 weeks.

LIFE SPAN CONSIDERATIONS

Older individuals are at risk for misdiagnosis of EBV-IM because the disease is relatively uncommon in older adults, occurring in only 3% to 10% of those 40 years of age or older.[4] In addition, older adults with acute IM often manifest the disease differently; fever is present in more than 90% of individuals, but pharyngitis and lymphadenopathy are seen in less than 50% of patients.[4] The risk of EBV-associated liver disease is more common in older adults, and hepatitis, cholestasis, and hepatomegaly are seen in substantial numbers of older adults with EBV-IM. Jaundice is unusual, occurring in approximately 5% of EBV hepatitis.[3] Similarly, the risk of EBV-IM–associated hepatic failure and other complications increases with age. Nonetheless, the prognosis for EBV-IM is good even in older individuals.

COMPLICATIONS

Although the majority of individuals with EBV-IM recover uneventfully and without complications, a wide range of complications associated with EBV-IM has been reported. These complications include acute upper airway obstruction, hepatomegaly, splenomegaly, and splenic rupture.

Hepatitis involvement associated with EBV-IM occurs in approximately 10% of young adults and 30% of older adults.[3] EBV infections are often associated with mild hepatocellular hepatitis, but jaundice occurs in only 5% of individuals. Most cases go undetected and resolve spontaneously.

Patients with IM are likely to have splenomegaly, even if it is not detected on physical examination. Because splenomegaly increases the risk of splenic rupture, athletes should not compete in contact or collision sports for 3 to 4 weeks after onset of symptoms. Splenic rupture is estimated at 0.1% on the basis of retrospective studies.[11]

Hematologic complications, particularly thrombocytopenia (25% to 50%) and neutropenia (50% to 80%), are relatively common early in the course of illness.[1] Serious or even life-threatening hematologic complications include aplastic anemia, neutropenia, and thrombocytopenia.

A rash associated with antibiotic administration, particularly amoxicillin and ampicillin, has been documented in 80% to 100% of patients with IM for whom antibacterials have been prescribed.[13]

In 1% to 2% of cases, EBV-IM has been associated with neurologic complications, including cranial nerve palsies, Guillain-Barré syndrome, encephalitis, and peripheral neuropathies.[1]

- In rare cases, EBV-IM has been associated with fatal conduction abnormalities and myocarditis.
- IM is associated with an increased risk of multiple sclerosis irrespective of gender, age, and severity of infection, and the risk persists for at least 30 years after infection.[14]
- Various ophthalmologic problems have been associated with EBV-IM, including keratitis, uveitis, retinopathy, and periorbital cellulitis.
- Complications of EBV-IM can also result in a variety of renal pathologic conditions, including nephritic syndrome, hemolytic-uremic syndrome, and renal failure.
- Additional potential life-threatening complications of IM include epiglottitis with airway obstruction.

The association between EBV-IM and chronic fatigue has been controversial for some time. Transient fatigue is part of acute IM; however, the evidence for EBV-associated chronic fatigue is questionable given that virtually all adults, whether fatigued or not, have evidence of EBV infection. In fact, the Centers for Disease Control and Prevention (CDC) does not consider workup for EBV infection to be useful in the evaluation of individuals with chronic fatigue. More recent studies have implicated slightly increased parameters of inflammation and proinflammatory cytokines and impaired natural killer cell function as contributors to persistent fatigue. There is some evidence of viral persistence and inadequate containment of viral replication in patients with chronic fatigue.[15]

INDICATIONS FOR REFERRAL OR HOSPITALIZATION

IM caused by EBV is generally a self-limited disease of young adults. However, mild liver enzyme abnormalities are not uncommon, and hepatitis is a rare but well-recognized complication of EBV infection that generally resolves spontaneously. IM is rarely seen in older adults; however, the potential for complications appears to increase in the older population, and several cases of severe cholestatic jaundice and fulminant hepatitis associated with IM have been reported in this age group.[3] Abdominal imaging should be obtained in such cases to rule out a malignant extrahepatic biliary obstruction, and acute EBV infection should be considered in patients with cholestasis. Because this complication is rare, it is generally not established until more common causes have been eliminated and serology consistent with EBV infection has been obtained. The rate of peritonsillar abscess has been estimated to be as high as 23%.[7] Peritonsillar abscess can be a medical emergency, requiring surgical drainage and antibiotic therapy. Because of associated dysphagia and possible respiratory compromise, hospitalization may be indicated while treatment is initiated.

PATIENT AND FAMILY EDUCATION

Education about the nature of the illness and prognosis is important. Acute IM has been referred to colloquially as the "kissing disease," and it is important to communicate that transmission through oropharyngeal secretions occurs in a variety of ways other than kissing. Changes in routines and schedules during the first few weeks should be encouraged to allow sufficient rest. The fact that acute IM is usually an uncomplicated, self-limited illness is reassuring, especially during the first few weeks when the manifestations are most pronounced. However, education about the possible complications is important so that proper treatment can be initiated should any complications occur.

CHAPTER 234

TICK-BORNE ILLNESSES

Jodie Dionne-Odom

Ticks are excellent vectors for disease transmission. More than 800 species of these obligate blood-sucking creatures inhabit the planet. They are second only to mosquitoes as vectors of human disease, both infectious and toxic. Ticks can carry and transmit a remarkable array of pathogens, such as bacteria, spirochetes, rickettsiae, protozoa, viruses, nematodes, and toxins. A single tick bite can transmit multiple pathogens, a phenomenon that has led to atypical presentations of some classic tick-borne diseases.

Many, if not most, tick-borne illnesses have a specific geographic distribution. In the United States, ticks are the most common vectors of vector-borne diseases. The incidence of tick-borne and other vector-borne illnesses is increasing worldwide, probably on the basis of global warming, international travel and trade, deforestation, and increasing population density, especially in urban areas. The encroachment of human populations into previously uninhabited wilderness where ticks and their animal hosts live has led to the increased incidence of these illnesses, challenging infectious disease and public health experts worldwide.

LYME DISEASE

DEFINITION AND EPIDEMIOLOGY

Lyme disease is caused by the bacterium *Borrelia burgdorferi* and is transmitted to humans by the bite of a tick. It occurs in North America, Europe, and Asia and is now the most common vector-borne disease in the United States and Europe.[1] Although about 30,000 cases each year are reported to the Centers for Disease Control and Prevention (CDC; a significant increase over the past decade), an estimated 300,000 cases occur annually.[2] Illness usually occurs after a tick bite during the summer months and has a characteristic expanding skin lesion known as erythema migrans that appears at the site of the bite. If the rash goes unnoticed and treatment is not given, the spirochete may disseminate in days to weeks to other sites of the body, including the nervous system and the heart. All stages are usually curable with appropriate antibiotic therapy, but the ideal phase for diagnosis and treatment is in early infection.

PATHOPHYSIOLOGY

Lyme disease was initially recognized in 1976 as a separate entity when a cluster of children in Lyme, Connecticut, were thought to have juvenile rheumatoid arthritis and were later diagnosed with Lyme disease. Manifestations of illness had been previously reported in Europe as erythema chronicum migrans, Bannwarth syndrome, or acrodermatitis chronica atrophicans. In 1982, these syndromes were linked to the recovery of a previously unrecognized spirochete from a tick vector.[1]

The vector of transmission for Lyme disease is the *Ixodes* tick species, most commonly *Ixodes scapularis* in the United States. *Ixodes pacificus,* a less common vector, is found in the western United States, where the frequency of disease is low. The tick requires a blood meal at each stage of its life cycle (larval, nymphal, and adult stages). Horizontal transmission of *B. burgdorferi* occurs in the larval and nymphal stages and from certain rodents, particularly white-footed mice and chipmunks, found in the northeastern United States (from Maine to Virginia) and in the North Central states, including Wisconsin and Minnesota (Fig. 234-1). White-tailed deer are the preferred adult host but are not involved in the life cycle of the spirochete. Transmission of the spirochete to humans occurs only after an extended period of attachment (36 to 72 hours), a finding that has particular clinical importance in the diagnosis of illness associated with exposure.

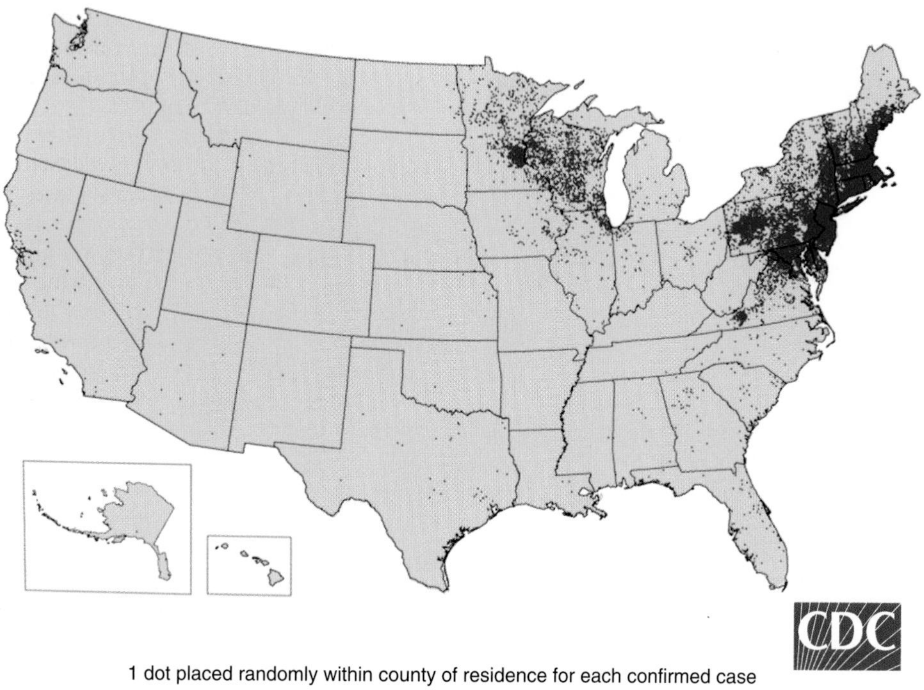
CDC
1 dot placed randomly within county of residence for each confirmed case

FIGURE 234-1 Reported cases of Lyme disease—United States, 2012. One dot is placed randomly within the county of residence of each confirmed case. Although Lyme disease cases have been reported in nearly every state, cases are reported from the county of residence, not necessarily the county of infection. (From Centers for Disease Control and Prevention [CDC]: *Lyme disease data and statistics*, 2012. Available at www.cdc.gov/lyme/stats/maps/map2012.html. Accessed July 25, 2014.)

CLINICAL PRESENTATION

The clinical characteristics of Lyme disease can be divided into three stages: early localized infection, early disseminated infection, and late persistent infection (Box 234-1). Stage 1 (early localized infection) is characterized by a pink-red spherical rash at the site of the tick bite called erythema migrans (Fig. 234-2). It occurs in 70% to 80% of patients and usually appears within 3 to 30 days of the tick bite. It often has a homogeneous appearance with evolution to a target-like lesion with central clearing. Patients often describe this lesion as burning, itchy, or painful, although it may be minimally symptomatic and go unrecognized owing to location. Erythema at the site of a tick bite can be located anywhere on the body but is most often found on the thigh, groin, axilla, or nape of the neck, given the propensity for ticks to attach to exposed skin (often the leg) and migrate to warm, moist areas of the body.

Stage 2 (early disseminated infection) occurs within several days to weeks of infection and may be associated with multiple annular secondary skin lesions. This stage is often accompanied by constitutional symptoms, including malaise, fatigue, headaches, fevers, chills, generalized achiness, and regional lymphadenopathy. If untreated, 15% of patients may develop neurologic abnormalities during a period of weeks to months, including unilateral cranial nerve VII palsy (Bell palsy), meningitis, encephalitis, motor and sensory radiculoneuritis, mononeuritis multiplex, cerebellar ataxia, and myelitis. Five percent of untreated patients may develop cardiac involvement, most commonly atrioventricular block, which often manifests as bradycardia and sudden death from Lyme carditis; this is very rare but has been reported.[3]

Stage 3 (late persistent infection) occurs months after disease onset and manifests as intermittent attacks of large joint pain and swelling in the context of strong cellular and humoral immune responses to *B. burgdorferi.* This may persist for years, but the natural history is complete resolution of symptoms and infection, even without specific therapy.

DIAGNOSTICS

Diagnosis of Lyme disease can be complicated, but testing is commonly performed; a study showed that large commercial laboratories in the United States performed 3.4 million Lyme disease tests in 2008.[4] Diagnosis of disease is predicated on three factors: presenting clinical characteristics, an epidemiologic link (possible tick exposure in an endemic area), and positive laboratory findings (an antibody response to *B. burgdorferi).* One exception to these rules is that early disease often occurs before the development of a detectable humoral immune response and thus requires a clinical diagnosis. For serologic testing, the CDC recommends a two-test approach of screening antibody testing followed by a more specific confirmatory test. Serum samples should be screened by enzyme-linked immunosorbent assay (ELISA), followed by confirmatory Western blot (WB) testing if results are positive or equivocal. For results to be called positive, an IgM WB must have two of the following three bands present: 23, 39, and 41 kDa. Careful interpretation of the results is essential and requires the clinician to take into account the history and clinical scenario, because the 23 and 41 kDa bands can be falsely positive. An immunoglobulin G (IgG) blot is considered positive if five of the following 10 bands are present: 18, 23, 28, 30, 39, 41, 45, 58, 66, and 93 kDa.[4]

Serodiagnosis is insensitive during the first few weeks of infection and only 30% of patients with erythema migrans will have detectable antibodies.[5] Approximately 70% of patients will have seroreactivity 2 to 4 weeks later. Patients without signs of acute illness and a persistently positive IgM and negative IgG

BOX 234-1

Manifestations of Lyme Disease

EARLY LOCALIZED STAGE 1 (DAYS TO WEEKS)

Erythema migrans
Regional lymphadenopathy
Minor constitutional symptoms

EARLY DISSEMINATED STAGE 2 (DAYS TO WEEKS)

Secondary annular lesions
Severe malaise or fatigue
Headaches
Fevers
Chills
Regional or generalized lymphadenopathy
Migratory arthralgias or arthritis
Neurologic abnormalities (meningitis, encephalitis, cranial neuritis, facial palsy, radiculoneuritis, mononeuritis multiplex)
Splenomegaly
Atrioventricular nodal block
Pancarditis
Conjunctivitis
Hepatitis
Sore throat
Cough
Microscopic hematuria or proteinuria

LATE PERSISTENT STAGE 3 (MONTHS)

- Acrodermatitis chronica atrophicans
- Localized scleroderma-like lesions
- Arthritis
- Ataxic gait
- Spastic paraparesis
- Chronic encephalomyelitis
- Subtle mental disorders
- Chronic axonal polyradiculopathy
- Keratitis
- Fatigue

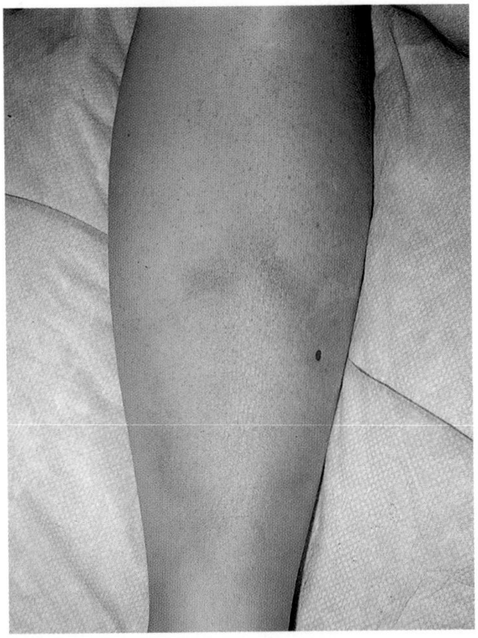

FIGURE 234-2 Erythema migrans. (From Habif TP: *Skin disease: diagnosis and treatment*, St Louis, 2001, Mosby.)

result months after a tick bite can be clinically assumed to have a false-positive IgM result or a persistent IgM response despite therapy. After antibiotic therapy, antibody titers decline slowly, although IgG and IgM responses may persist for years, complicating the diagnosis of subsequent reinfections with *B. burgdorferi*.[1]

One new test is the C6 ELISA, which appears to be more sensitive in early disease and performed well in patients who had been exposed to ticks in Europe, but it is somewhat less specific than the ELISA/WB testing and studies are ongoing.[6] Alternative diagnostics, such as polymerase chain reaction (PCR) assay of a skin biopsy sample or borrelial culture of skin or blood, are expensive to perform and are not currently recommended outside of a research setting.[7]

DIFFERENTIAL DIAGNOSIS

The differential diagnosis for Lyme disease varies according to the stage of disease. Erythema migrans may resemble an uninfected tick bite, and if it rapidly expands (>1 cm/day) then disappears, it is more likely to be an allergic reaction to the tick saliva. Secondary erythema migrans lesions may have the appearance of erythema multiforme. Facial palsies can also be seen with herpes simplex type 1 virus or varicella-zoster virus. Arthritis may be diagnosed as reactive arthritis in adults or pauciarticular juvenile rheumatoid arthritis in children. Some patients have nonspecific complaints, including chronic fatigue and weakness that occur for months to years after a tick bite. These individuals warrant an evaluation for untreated Lyme disease as well as other possible causes of their chronic symptoms.

MANAGEMENT

Treatment guidelines, as recommended by the Infectious Diseases Society of America, vary by stage of disease and extent of neurologic involvement. For early localized or disseminated infection, the treatment of choice is oral doxycycline, 100 mg twice daily for 14 days. Second-line treatment is amoxicillin, which is useful for children younger than 8 years and pregnant women, for whom doxycycline is contraindicated.[7] Third- and fourth-line treatments are cefuroxime and erythromycin, respectively. Duration of therapy and long-term outcomes in patients with early Lyme disease were assessed in a retrospective cohort study by Kowalski and coworkers.[8] Of the 607 patients who met the study inclusion criteria, 93% were treated with doxycycline; 17% were treated for less than 10 days, 33% were treated for 11 to 15 days, and 47% were treated for more than 16 days. Patients treated for less than 10 days had long-term outcomes similar to those of patients treated with longer courses, and treatment failure was exceedingly rare.[8]

About 15% of patients with disseminated infection experience a Jarisch-Herxheimer–like reaction with an increase in systemic symptoms with fever, malaise, and increased size or intensity of the rash during the first 24 hours of therapy.[2,7] Erythema migrans lesions usually resolve within 1 to 2 weeks after the initiation of antibiotic therapy, but systemic symptoms can take months to resolve.[2,7]

For patients with objective neurologic abnormalities, 2 to 4 weeks of intravenous ceftriaxone is advised.[9] Lyme carditis can be treated with oral or parenteral antibiotics, although syncope, dyspnea, chest pain, or evidence of second- or third-degree heart block probably warrant hospitalization, intravenous therapy, and continuous monitoring.[10] Temporary pacemakers may be required for advanced heart block but can be discontinued when the heart block resolves.[10] Lyme arthritis does not necessarily warrant parenteral therapy, but if symptoms persist, retreatment with a 4-week course of oral antibiotics or 2 to 4 weeks of parenteral ceftriaxone is advised. If symptoms improve but do not completely resolve, an additional 4-week course of oral antibiotics is favored. If patients have no resolution of symptoms despite parenteral therapy and if results of PCR testing of synovial fluid are negative, symptomatic treatment with nonsteroidal anti-inflammatory agents, intra-articular injections of corticosteroids, or disease-modifying antirheumatic drugs is recommended.[9]

PREVENTION

Prevention of Lyme disease is crucial until an effective vaccine is available and is best accomplished by avoidance of tick-infested areas. If this is not possible, protective clothing (long pants tucked into socks) and insecticides containing diethyltoluamide (DEET) or permethrin are effective at deterring ticks.[11] Inspection of the entire body for ticks is invaluable and should include moist parts of the body, such as groin and axillae. Removal of a tick within 24 hours of attachment is sufficient to prevent Lyme disease. Routine use of antimicrobial prophylaxis (doxycycline, 200 mg orally once) can be considered when all four of the following conditions are met: (1) the attached tick can be reliably identified as an adult or nymphal *I. scapularis* tick, and it has been attached for less than 36 hours on the basis of engorgement or certainty about the time of exposure; (2) prophylaxis can be started within 72 hours of tick removal; (3) ecologic information indicates that the local rate of infection of the ticks with *B. burgdorferi* is greater than 20%; and (4) there is no contraindication to the use of doxycycline.[11] There are no data to support the substitution of doxycycline with amoxicillin for prophylaxis.[10] Patients who have removed attached ticks should be monitored closely for signs and symptoms of tick-borne disease for up to 30 days.[12] This includes development or expansion of a skin lesion at the site of the tick bite or development of a viral-like illness.

The development of a Lyme disease vaccine has been challenging because *B. burgdorferi* spirochetes exploit tick proteins to establish an infection.[13] The former vaccine against Lyme disease was based on anti-OspA (anti–outer surface protein A). *Borrelia* organisms upregulate OspA while entering the tick and bind to the tick receptor for OspA, which allows them to remain inside the tick between blood meals. The OspA vaccine was approved by the U.S. Food and Drug Administration (FDA) in 1998.[13] It proved to be 80% protective against *B. burgdorferi* infection after three vaccine doses; however, high antibody titers did not persist long after vaccination, and additional boosters would have been required for immunity to be maintained. Therefore it was withdrawn from the market 4 years after it was released. Other vaccines are currently being investigated and include combining multiple *Borrelia* antigens and tick antigens to elicit a synergistic anti-*Borrelia* and anti-tick immune response. One such multivalent OspA candidate vaccine has been tested in 300 European participants in a phase I/II trial and was well tolerated with good levels of antibodies elicited.[14,15]

COMPLICATIONS

There has been much controversy over the incidence, prevalence, and pathogenesis of post–Lyme disease syndrome.[16] When these patients are evaluated, it is necessary to begin with objective evidence of having had *B. burgdorferi* infection with positive ELISA results and IgG on WB testing. Post–Lyme disease syndrome describes a small percentage of patients with ongoing pain, neurocognitive, or fatigue symptoms lasting more than 6 months, despite resolution of objective manifestations of infection with antibiotic therapy; it is often indistinguishable from chronic fatigue syndrome or fibromyalgia. Compared with patients with active Lyme disease, these patients describe more generalized or disabling symptoms, often with an impact on their quality of life.[17] There is no evidence to support the presence of an ongoing bacterial *B. burgdorferi* infection among patients who have completed the recommended treatment regimens for Lyme disease, although some people do continue to have ongoing symptoms, and this is an active area of investigation. One recent study showed elevated interleukin-23 (IL-23) levels and the presence of autoantibodies in a subset of these symptomatic individuals.[18] Further antibiotic treatment is not indicated for patients with chronic subjective symptoms, and long-term antibiotic therapy is associated with well-known risks of side effects, selection of antibiotic-resistant bacteria, and perturbation of normal flora.[19]

Unfortunately, many patients who have been treated for early Lyme disease subsequently become reinfected after the first episode has resolved. Reinfection is defined as "the development of a new tick-transmitted infection with Lyme *Borrelia* occurring after successful antimicrobial treatment of a prior episode of Lyme disease."[12] This is distinct from relapse, which is defined as "the presence of objective clinical and/or microbiological evidence of persistent infection with Lyme *Borrelia* after a non-curative course of antimicrobial treatment."[12] It has been well documented that reinfection occurs only after treatment of early Lyme disease (almost always erythema migrans) and not after manifestations of late infection. Reinfection is clinically evident by a repeated episode of erythema migrans, at a skin site different from the previous episode, occurring more than 1 year after the initial episode. In addition, reinfection occurs during months when the nymphal stage of the tick vector is abundant in the environment. The rate of recurrence is actually higher than the incidence of Lyme disease in the general population.[20] Proposed explanations for these findings include repeated tick bites (particularly in patients who live in endemic areas and who have low compliance with recommended preventive measures), immunologic factors (the immune response to erythema migrans is not fully protective), and microbiologic variation (evident by *Borrelia* strain variability as a means to circumvent host immune response). Furthermore, serologic testing is not useful in differentiating reinfection from initial infection, given the variability in IgM reactivity and potential for prolonged seroreactivity.[20]

Coinfection with other bacteria, specifically *Babesia microti* and *Anaplasma phagocytophilum*, may occur in patients with tick exposure in areas where these pathogens are endemic. Like *B. burgdorferi*, these organisms are also transmitted by the *Ixodes* tick species. Depending on the region, it has been reported that as many as 2% to 12% of patients with early Lyme disease may also have anaplasmosis and 2% to 40% may also have babesiosis, although the higher range of coinfection rates are limited to certain geographic locales.[21] Diagnostic testing for coinfection should be considered in patients whose symptoms are more severe than typical Lyme disease or who have high-grade fevers for more than 48 hours despite appropriate antibiotic therapy; in those who have symptoms resembling a viral infection that fail to improve or worsen despite resolution of the skin lesion; and in those with leukopenia, thrombocytopenia, or anemia.[7] These organisms will be further discussed in upcoming sections of the chapter.

BABESIOSIS

DEFINITION AND EPIDEMIOLOGY

Babesiosis is a zoonotic disease caused by protozoa of the genus *Babesia* that invade and eventually lyse erythrocytes. Young and healthy patients typically have a mild influenza-like illness, but babesiosis can develop into a life-threatening malaria-like syndrome in the immunocompromised host, specifically asplenic and older adult patients.

Although more than 100 species of *Babesia* infect vertebrate hosts, the majority of babesiosis in the Unites States can be attributed to *B. microti*, found mainly in the northeastern and upper Midwestern states.[22] Disease requires transmission of *Babesia* species organisms from a vertebrate reservoir to humans by the same *Ixodes* tick species that carries *B. burgdorferi*. Human infection is most commonly seen in the summer.[23] Babesiosis is limited to portions of the geographic areas where Lyme disease is endemic (see Fig. 234-1), but the prevalence of babesiosis is far lower than that of Lyme disease.[11]

Because infected patients can harbor circulating parasites for months to years without symptoms, patients may unknowingly transmit the organisms through blood transfusions.[22] According to the FDA, there have been an estimated 70 cases of transfusion-transmitted babesiosis since 1979 (most of which were reported in the past decade) and a total of nine deaths (eight of which occurred since November 2005).[24] In these fatal cases, the patients developed influenza-like symptoms within 2.4 to 7 weeks after having received a blood transfusion and later developed altered mental status, renal failure, or respiratory distress leading to death within 5 to 17 days after symptom onset.[24] All implicated donors had been asymptomatic at the time of donation but tested positive for babesiosis by peripheral blood smear or immunofluorescence antibody assay.[24] Unfortunately, *Babesia* species can survive blood-banking procedures such as refrigeration, leukoreduction, and filtration, and therefore babesiosis should be considered early in the evaluation of unexplained fever during the first few weeks after blood transfusion, especially in asplenic or immunocompromised patients.[24]

PATHOPHYSIOLOGY

I. scapularis ticks, primarily found in the northeastern United States, feed on white-tailed deer and white-footed mice and are responsible for the transmission of *B. microti* to humans. *Babesia divergens*–like organisms, found in the Midwest, originate from cottontail rabbits and are transmitted to humans by *Ixodes dentatus*. *Babesia duncani* is found on the West Coast and is thought to be transmitted to humans by *I. pacificus*.[23] Once the *Babesia* organisms invade erythrocytes, they undergo binary fission, forming a tetrad of merozoites classically known as a Maltese cross (seen on peripheral blood smear), which is diagnostic of *B. microti*.[23] As infection progresses, hemolytic anemia develops and tissue hypoxia may occur.[25]

The host immune response is required to control and to clear infected erythrocytes, but in the processes of doing so, it may contribute to disease progression.[25] In more severe infections, a stronger inflammatory response is required to contain infection, and this response often generates a sepsis-like syndrome or adult respiratory distress syndrome.[25]

CLINICAL PRESENTATION

There are three different syndromes of babesiosis based on the severity of disease: asymptomatic infection, mild to moderate viral-like illness, and severe disease resulting in death or a persistent relapsing course.[25] Healthy individuals who become infected with *Babesia* often remain asymptomatic during an incubation period that ranges from 1 to 6 weeks.[25] An epidemiologic study of babesiosis performed annual serosurvey of healthy residents of Block Island, Rhode Island and found that about one third of babesial infections were asymptomatic.[25]

In most cases of mild to moderate disease, symptoms of malaise and fatigue are followed by intermittent fevers, chills, sweats, headache, myalgia, arthralgia, anorexia, and cough.[25] In mild cases, symptoms abate without therapy within 2 weeks; however, fatigue and malaise may persist for months.[25] Fever is a prominent feature, and mild hepatosplenomegaly may be found on physical examination. Hemolytic anemia, thrombocytopenia, normal to low white blood cell count, and transaminitis may be evident on laboratory analysis.[23]

Severe disease is more often seen in asplenic patients, in those with coinfection with *B. burgdorferi* or human immunodeficiency virus (HIV), and in patients receiving immunosuppressive medications. Patients with more than one immunosuppressive condition have been shown to experience a prolonged relapsing course of illness.[23] Patients older than 50 years are more likely to experience severe disease. Complications of babesiosis more often occur in patients with severe disease and include acute respiratory failure, disseminated intravascular coagulation, congestive heart failure, liver and renal failure, and splenic infarct.[25] Death occurs in 5% to 9% of hospitalized patients.[23]

DIAGNOSTICS

Diagnosis of babesiosis requires strong clinical suspicion; it should be suspected in patients with a viral-like illness who have spent time outdoors in a babesial endemic area during the summer and early autumn months.[25] Babesiosis should also be considered in all patients with diagnosed Lyme disease or human granulocytic anaplasmosis because these are often simultaneously transmitted by the same tick, *I. scapularis*.[25]

Definitive diagnosis of babesiosis is made by identification of *Babesia* on Giemsa- or Wright-stained thick and thin blood smears. If parasitemia is low, multiple blood smears may need to be examined for a diagnosis to be made. *Babesia* may appear round, oval, or pear shaped. However, the ring form is the most common, and as a result, it can be confused with *Plasmodium falciparum*, except that it will lack hemozoin (brown pigmented deposits). The Maltese cross is diagnostic but rarely seen.

PCR assay is available and can be used in patients with symptoms suggestive of babesiosis who have negative blood smears. An indirect immunofluorescent antibody test for anti-babesial

IgG is available through the CDC. A titer greater than 1:64 is diagnostic of babesiosis. Titers greater than 1:1024 are indicative of active or recent infection, but titers are usually low during the acute phase of illness and do not correlate with symptom severity. Titers below 1:64 are generally reflective of past infection.[23]

MANAGEMENT

Treatment is not recommended for asymptomatic patients unless *Babesia* is persistently present on blood smear or by PCR analysis for more than 3 months. Symptomatic patients should be treated only if the blood smear or the result of the PCR assay is positive.[23] For mild to moderate infection with *B. microti*, the treatment of choice is atovaquone plus azithromycin for 7 to 10 days. Alternatively, clindamycin plus quinine can be used, but this combination has a much higher frequency of side effects, including tinnitus and gastroenteritis.[25] Clinical improvement usually occurs within 48 hours of initiation of therapy, and symptoms should resolve within 3 months of therapy. In patients with severe *B. microti* infection, 7 to 10 days of intravenous clindamycin plus oral quinine is recommended. In addition, partial or complete red blood cell exchange transfusion is recommended for all patients with parasitemia of more than 10% or for those with severe systemic illness. Hematocrit and parasitemia should be monitored daily in patients with severe infection until parasitemia is less than 5%.[23]

Immunocompromised patients are at risk for persistent relapsing babesial infection; therefore, therapy should be lengthened to a minimum of 6 weeks and at least 2 weeks after blood smear is negative.[23] If symptoms persist despite appropriate therapy, the possibility of coinfection with *B. burgdorferi* or *A. phagocytophilum* or both should be considered.[11]

PREVENTION

Prevention of infection requires avoidance of areas endemic for *I. scapularis* during the months of May through September. This is especially important for asplenic or immunocompromised patients. Individuals should wear protective clothing and use DEET- or permethrin-containing products on exposed skin. Tick checks of the entire body should be performed at the end of each exposure, and attached ticks should be removed as soon as possible. Unlike for Lyme disease, there are no data on the use of prophylactic antimicrobials in the prevention of babesiosis after a tick bite. To decrease transfusion-associated babesiosis, blood donation agencies prohibit individuals with a history of babesiosis from donating blood.

ANAPLASMOSIS

DEFINITION AND EPIDEMIOLOGY

Anaplasma is a genus of obligate intracytoplasmic bacteria belonging to the order Rickettsiales, family Anaplasmataceae (which includes the genera *Ehrlichia*, *Anaplasma*, and *Neorickettsia*). Until 1987, infections caused by members of the family Anaplasmataceae were known as veterinary diseases. The first case of anaplasmosis in the United States was in 1990 in a Wisconsin patient who died of a severe febrile illness 2 weeks after a tick bite. His peripheral blood smear was significant for clusters of small bacteria within neutrophils.[26]

Human granulocytotropic anaplasmosis (HGA) is caused by *A. phagocytophilum*, a gram-negative bacterium. HGA incidence tends to peak between June and December. The distribution of cases is identical to that of Lyme disease because it is transmitted by the same tick vector. It is estimated that 4% to 36% of patients with serologic evidence of *A. phagocytophilum* infection also have serologic evidence of *B. burgdorferi* or *B. microti* infection.[27]

PATHOPHYSIOLOGY

A. phagocytophilum is transmitted by the bites of the *I. scapularis* tick in the eastern United States, *I. pacificus* tick in California, *Ixodes ricinus* tick in Europe, and *Ixodes persulcatus* tick in Asia. The most common reservoir host is the white-footed mouse, but other hosts include squirrels, voles, wood rats, white-tailed deer, red deer, and roe deer. *A. phagocytophilum* is found predominantly within neutrophils and can disseminate to the bone marrow and the spleen.

CLINICAL PRESENTATION

Patients with HGA often have a nonspecific febrile illness, but symptoms can range from asymptomatic to fatal, depending on the age of the patient and comorbid conditions. After an incubation period of 5 to 21 days, patients often develop shaking chills, myalgias, and headache.[28] Less common symptoms include nausea, vomiting, diarrhea, cough, arthralgias, stiff neck, and confusion. A rash has been seen in about 6% of patients but is not associated with HGA and is, in fact, erythema migrans associated with *B. burgdorferi* coinfection.[27] HGA is usually a self-limited illness; untreated, the median duration of symptoms is 9 days.[29] Common laboratory findings include thrombocytopenia, leukopenia, mild anemia, and transaminitis. Neutropenia with a left shift and relative lymphocytosis may also occur.[29] These abnormalities often normalize by the end of the second week of illness.

DIAGNOSTICS

Diagnosis is made by the identification of morulae (clusters of bacteria) in the cytoplasm of peripheral blood neutrophils that have been Wright or Giemsa stained. Morulae are present in 20% to 80% of patients in the first week of illness. PCR amplification of *A. phagocytophilum*–specific DNA or isolation of *A. phagocytophilum* in culture can also confirm the diagnosis in the early stage of infection, but culture usually requires 1 week or more and is not routinely available. The most sensitive confirmatory test is the acute-phase and convalescent-phase indirect fluorescent antibody test for anti–*A. phagocytophilum* IgM and IgG. A fourfold rise in titer is definitive evidence of infection, but specific IgM tests are reactive only during the first 45 to 50 days of infection. Furthermore, antibodies can persist for months or years after infection and therefore should not be used to monitor treatment effectiveness.[28]

MANAGEMENT

Because of the potential for severe illness, all patients who have suspected or documented HGA should undergo treatment. The treatment of choice is doxycycline, 100 mg orally twice daily for 7 to 10 days. If the patient is at high risk for coinfection with *B. burgdorferi*, treatment should be extended to 14 days. Alternatively, in patients for whom doxycycline is contraindicated, rifampin can be used. Clinical improvement is usually seen within 24 to 48 hours of initiation of treatment. Furthermore, relapse or chronic infection has never been reported.[28]

PREVENTION

Prevention of anaplasmosis depends on avoidance of tick exposure. Individuals in endemic areas should wear protective clothing and use DEET- or permethrin-containing products to repel ticks. Tick checks should be performed regularly, and because *A. phagocytophilum* can be transmitted within 4 to 24 hours of a tick bite, attached ticks should be removed immediately.[28] There are no data to support the use of prophylactic antibiotics.[29]

COMPLICATIONS

There have been no reported cases of patients with active clinical illness persisting beyond 2 months. Overall long-term prognosis appears to be favorable. However, severe complications include septic or toxic shock–like syndrome, respiratory insufficiency, invasive opportunistic infections (both viral and fungal), rhabdomyolysis, pancarditis, acute renal failure, hemorrhage, and neurologic diseases such as brachial plexopathy and demyelinating polyneuropathy.[28] There have been eight reported deaths from HGA, mainly occurring in patients with factors known to suppress the immune system, including advanced age, immunosuppressive therapy, chronic inflammatory diseases, and underlying malignant disease.[11]

There have been reports of transfusion-transmitted anaplasmosis, but unfortunately, screening of donors for a recent history of tick bites would not identify high-risk donors because recollection of exposure is infrequent. Because *Anaplasma* is associated with white blood cells, leukoreduction techniques should reduce the risk of transfusion transmission through red blood cell components.[30]

EHRLICHIOSIS

DEFINITION AND EPIDEMIOLOGY

Human monocytotropic ehrlichiosis (HME) is a tick-borne illness caused by *Ehrlichia chaffeensis.* Unlike the previously described illnesses, *E. chaffeensis* is transmitted to humans by the Lone Star tick *(Amblyomma americanum)* and is most prevalent in regions where white-tailed deer and Lone Star ticks coexist. HME is seasonal and peaks between May and August; it has been documented in 47 states, particularly in the South Central, southeastern, and mid-Atlantic United States. It predominantly affects males, and 42% of cases necessitate hospitalization, with 17% being life-threatening cases.[26]

PATHOPHYSIOLOGY

After a tick bite, *E. chaffeensis* organisms enter the skin and invade cells of the hematopoietic and lymphoreticular systems, creating morulae within macrophages and monocytes. Morulae can also be found in bone marrow, hepatic sinusoids, lymph nodes, splenic cords, splenic sinusoids, splenic periarteriolar lymphoid sheaths, and cerebrospinal fluid macrophages and macrophages in perivascular lymphohistiocytic infiltrates in the kidney, appendix, and heart. The host immune response is responsible for the majority of clinical manifestations.[26]

CLINICAL PRESENTATION

After an incubation period of about 7 days, patients will develop symptoms of fever, chills, headache, myalgias, and malaise. Immunocompetent patients can have mild to severe multisystem illness lasting about 23 days. Symptoms may progress to include nausea, anorexia, vomiting, and weight loss. Less than half of patients (mostly children) will develop a maculopapular or petechial rash. Severely ill patients may have cough, diarrhea, confusion, and lymphadenopathy, and 17% develop complications of adult respiratory distress syndrome, acute renal insufficiency, meningoencephalitis, coagulopathy, gastrointestinal hemorrhage, and death. Cerebrospinal fluid analysis usually shows a lymphocyte-predominant pleocytosis and increased protein concentration. Laboratory evaluation often reveals thrombocytopenia, leukopenia, and transaminitis. Chest radiography will show infiltrates in almost half of all patients. Immunocompromised hosts and those with HIV infection usually have a more virulent form of HME associated with overwhelming infection, a toxic shock–like or sepsis-like syndrome, and death in 3% of cases.[26,31]

DIAGNOSTICS

The diagnosis of HME is largely based on epidemiologic and clinical factors, and it should be made early for empirical antiehrlichial treatment to be administered. The identification of morulae on blood smear is seen in less than 10% of patients with HME and mostly in immunocompromised patients with overwhelming ehrlichiosis. PCR assays to detect bacterial DNA have a sensitivity of 60% to 75% during active infection and before the presence of detectable serum antibodies.[31] The most sensitive confirmatory test is detection of seroconversion, or a fourfold change in antibody titer between the acute and convalescent phases.[31] Only 22% to 44% of sera tested within the first week of illness have a titer of 80 or higher (positive titer is greater than 64). Seroconversion is usually seen 4 weeks after onset of illness and peaks at 6 weeks.[26] Furthermore, IgG antibodies can persist for months to years without evidence of persistent infection, and there is a high seroprevalence rate among individuals in endemic regions.[31]

MANAGEMENT

Doxycycline remains the treatment of choice and should be started as soon as possible. In a retrospective cohort study to evaluate the relationship of early appropriate therapy to outcomes, 28 (60.9%) of 46 patients had a delay of more than 24 hours in initiation of therapy. As a result, these patients had significantly more complications during their hospitalization, including pulmonary complications, admission to the intensive care unit, mechanical ventilation, and the need for vasopressors. They also had a longer length of illness and longer hospitalization. Interestingly, these patients were also more severely ill at presentation, including abnormal findings on lung and neurologic examinations, abnormal chest radiographs, and elevated bilirubin levels, suggesting that clinicians may not recognize that ehrlichiosis can be associated with severe illness at presentation and that these patients would benefit most from early initiation of therapy.[32] The recommended duration of treatment is 7 to 10 days. *E. chaffeensis* has been shown to be susceptible to rifampin and resistant to fluoroquinolones in vitro, but there have been no clinical trials to support the use of rifampin for HME.[26]

Prevention of HME is dependent on avoidance of tick exposure, the use of DEET-containing insect repellent, careful tick checks of the entire body, and prompt removal of ticks.[26]

ROCKY MOUNTAIN SPOTTED FEVER

DEFINITION AND EPIDEMIOLOGY

Rocky Mountain spotted fever (RMSF) is a life-threatening disease first recognized in Idaho in the late 19th century by Edward E. Maxey, who described "a febrile disease, characterized clinically by a continuous moderately high fever, and a profuse or purpuric eruption in the skin, appearing first on ankles, wrists, and forehead, but rapidly spreading to all parts of body."[33] The infectious agent was later identified in 1919 as *Rickettsia rickettsii,* when it was found within endothelial cells. Rickettsiae belong to the spotted fever group and are obligate intracellular bacteria that reside in the cytoplasm or nucleus of host cells. The tick is the vector and the main reservoir, and therefore the pathogen is maintained in nature across several tick generations. The species of tick vector vary geographically: the American dog tick *(Dermacentor variabilis)* is found in the eastern two thirds of the United States and the Far West; the Rocky Mountain wood tick *(Dermacentor andersoni)* is found in the western states and Canada; and the brown dog tick *(Rhipicephalus sanguineus)* is found in Mexico and Arizona.[33]

RMSF originally occurred only in the western United States, but the prevalence of disease is currently higher in the South Atlantic states (Maryland, Virginia, North Carolina, and South Carolina) and in the South Central regions (Oklahoma, Tennessee, and Arkansas). Most cases occur in children younger than 10 years and adults aged 40 to 64 years. It is also more common in men and white individuals. Infection usually occurs between April and September.[33]

PATHOPHYSIOLOGY

Rickettsiae are transmitted to humans through the skin by a tick bite. The tick must be attached and feeding for 6 to 10 hours for transmission to occur. Humans can also be infected when they are exposed to infected hemolymph from the tick when it is crushed between the fingers during removal. There have also been reports of infection from inhalation of contaminated aerosol or parenteral inoculation of *R. rickettsii* in the laboratory setting; therefore, careful technique and the use of biohazard containment hoods, masks, and gloves are recommended. The rickettsiae then spread to the systemic and pulmonary circulation, where they attach to the vascular endothelium and induce phagocytosis and establish multiple disseminated foci of infection. Infection is spread from endothelial cell to endothelial cell, causing vascular injury, and the host immune and inflammatory responses, although needed to fight infection, contribute to further vascular damage.[34]

CLINICAL PRESENTATION

The incubation period varies from 2 to 14 days (median of 7 days) on the basis of inoculum size. Symptoms of RMSF vary greatly, but the classic clinical triad of fever, severe headache, and rash is seen in 60% to 70% of patients during the first 2 weeks after a tick bite.[35] Rash is seen in 88% to 90% of patients and is a major diagnostic sign. It usually appears within 3 to 5 days of fever onset and typically begins around the wrists and ankles, and in 36% to 82% of patients it involves the palms and soles.[36] It appears as small, blanching, erythematous macules that evolve during the first week, becoming maculopapular with central petechiae.[34] Skin necrosis and gangrene (seen in 4% of cases) can develop as a result of continued rickettsial damage to the microcirculation, ultimately necessitating amputation. Other accompanying symptoms include myalgias (abdomen, back, and legs), anorexia, nausea, vomiting, abdominal pain, and photophobia. Signs of meningitis or meningoencephalitis, such as focal neurologic deficits, transient deafness, meningismus, and photophobia, are indicators of a poor prognosis. Severe cases of RMSF include development of renal failure, ocular manifestations, skeletal muscle involvement, pulmonary involvement, and myocardial dysfunction. Death occurs 7 to 15 days after symptom onset if it is left untreated, but in fulminant RMSF, death occurs within the first 5 days. Fulminant RMSF occurs more often in black males with glucose-6-phosphate dehydrogenase deficiency as a result of hemolysis, and it is difficult to diagnose because the course is more rapid, the rash develops shortly before death, and antibodies have not had time to develop. Older age and alcoholism are also risk factors for a more lethal outcome. Laboratory findings that suggest the diagnosis of RMSF are a normal white blood cell count with increased numbers of immature bands, thrombocytopenia, transaminitis, and hyponatremia.[35]

DIAGNOSTICS

The diagnosis of RMSF is largely based on clinical findings and epidemiologic data, especially when the rash is absent. Isolation of *R. rickettsii* from blood is ideal, but few laboratories are able to perform this task because cultivation requires the use of living host cells or cell cultures. Serologic testing is used to confirm the diagnosis, but antibodies to *R. rickettsii* are usually not detectable until the convalescent stage of disease (7 to 10 days after disease onset). The indirect fluorescent antibody test is a highly sensitive test, but it cannot distinguish between *R. rickettsii* and other spotted fever group rickettsiae. A convalescent titer of greater than 1:64 is considered diagnostic. Immunohistochemical staining of rickettsiae antigens of tissue samples may be helpful during acute stages of disease, but the sensitivity and specificity of skin biopsy are 79% and 100%, respectively.[33] PCR amplification of *R. rickettsii* DNA is sensitive only late in the course of disease, when the number of circulating rickettsiae is higher.[36]

MANAGEMENT

Because of the fatal nature of this disease, the decision to treat should not be delayed for laboratory confirmation, and any patient with fever and rash should be considered for hospitalization and antimicrobial therapy. The treatment of choice for RMSF is doxycycline for 7 days or until the patient has been afebrile for at least 2 to 3 days. Chloramphenicol remains the treatment of choice in pregnant women.[33] Early initiation of therapy is critical for a favorable prognosis.[34]

No vaccine is currently available; the best means of prevention is avoidance of tick exposure, use of DEET-containing insect repellent and protective clothing, frequent tick checks, and prompt removal of attached ticks. The proper removal of ticks includes wearing protective gloves, grasping the tick as close to the point of attachment as possible, pulling the tick straight outward, and thoroughly disinfecting the bite wound. Prophylactic antimicrobial therapy is not indicated to prevent RMSF. Refer to Table 234-1 for a summary of the tick-borne illnesses reviewed in this chapter.

TABLE 234-1 **Comparison of Tick-Borne Illnesses in the United States**

	Lyme Disease	Babesiosis	HGA	HME	RMSF
Organism	*Borrelia burgdorferi*	*Babesia microti*	*Anaplasma phagocytophilum*	*Ehrlichia chaffeensis*	*Rickettsia rickettsii*
Tick vector	*Ixodes scapularis* *Ixodes pacificus*	*I. scapularis* *I. pacificus* *Ixodes dentatus*	*I. scapularis* *I. pacificus*	*Amblyomma americanum*	*Dermacentor variabilis* *Dermacentor andersoni* *Rhipicephalus sanguineus*
Distribution	Northeastern and North Central states	Northeastern and upper Midwestern states	New England, North Central and Pacific states	South and Mid-Atlantic, North Central and South Central states, isolated areas of New England	South Atlantic and South Central states
Incubation	3-30 days	7-42 days	5-21 days	5-14 days	2-14 days
Initial symptoms	Erythema migrans, fatigue, malaise	Fever, fatigue, malaise	Fever, headache, malaise, myalgia, vomiting	Fever, headache, malaise, myalgia	Fever, headache, myalgia, nausea, vomiting, anorexia
Rash	Erythema migrans (70%-80% of patients)	Usually erythema migrans from coinfection with Lyme disease	Rare	Maculopapular (<30% of adults and 60% of children)	Maculopapular or petechial involving palms and soles (50%-60% of adults and >90% of children)
Common laboratory findings	—	Leukopenia, anemia, thrombocytopenia, transaminitis	Leukopenia, thrombocytopenia, transaminitis	Leukopenia, thrombocytopenia, transaminitis	Thrombocytopenia, hyponatremia, transaminitis
Blood smear	—	Merozoites within erythrocytes	Morulae within neutrophils (20%-80% of patients)	Morulae within monocytes or macrophages (<10% of patients)	—
Treatment	Doxycycline	Atovaquone plus azithromycin *Or* Clindamycin plus quinine	Doxycycline	Doxycycline	Doxycycline
Case fatality	—	5%-9%	<1%	2%-3%	5%-10%

CHAPTER 235

TUBERCULOSIS

Patricia Polgar-Bailey

DEFINITION AND EPIDEMIOLOGY

Tuberculosis (TB) is an airborne infectious disease caused by *Mycobacterium tuberculosis,* an acid-fast aerobic bacterium that is capable of remaining alive outside the host for a relatively long time. In the United States, most cases of TB are caused by *M. tuberculosis,* also referred to as the tubercle bacillus. However, several closely related *Mycobacterium* species can cause disease in humans, including *Mycobacterium bovis,* the cause of TB in cattle; *Mycobacterium avium,* one of the causes of TB in birds; and *Mycobacterium africanum.* TB caused by these organisms was relatively rare in the United States until they were identified as the cause of opportunistic infections in patients infected with human immunodeficiency virus (HIV).

TB has been described as the greatest killer in history, claiming more lives than any other infectious disease.[1] Globally, TB transmission continues despite highly effective frontline combination therapy, a widely administered vaccine, intensive control efforts, and the allocation of tremendous resources to improve interventions.[2,3] There are an estimated 8.6 million new case of TB and 1.3 million deaths from the disease annually.[4] In 2014, globally approximately 480,000 people developed multidrug-resistant tuberculosis (MDR-TB) and more than half of these cases were in India, China, and the Russian Federation.[5] The increasing incidence and transmission of TB is largely a result of the spread of HIV in Africa and to the economic difficulties and associated decline in health infrastructure in eastern Europe and central Asia as well as increased reporting. Approximately 80% of all TB cases are found in 22 "high-burden" countries, most of which are in Africa and Asia. India has the highest rate of TB mortality, followed by China, where there are 150,000 TB-related deaths annually.[4]

Persons with active TB who receive no treatment can infect an average of 10 to 15 people annually.[6] Southeast Asia currently has the highest prevalence of TB, with one third of new cases occurring in this area every year, but the incidence per capita is highest in sub-Saharan Africa, where the presence of TB parallels the HIV and acquired immunodeficiency syndrome (AIDS) epidemic.

Two billion people have latent tuberculosis infection (LTBI), the presence of *M. tuberculosis* in the body without signs and symptoms or radiographic or bacteriologic evidence of TB; without treatment, approximately 5% to 10% of these individuals will progress to active disease at some point in their lifetime.[1,7] In the United States, approximately 9 to 14 million people have LTBI.[1]

During the mid-20th century, the United States benefited from relatively successful control of TB. From 1953 to 1985, the reported cases of TB in the United States dropped from 84,000 to 22,000.[8] From 1985 to 1992, there was an unprecedented resurgence of TB in the United States. Since 1993, the annual TB rate has decreased steadily. In 2013, the TB case rate in the United States was 3.0 cases per 100,000 (30 per million), decreased from 3.8 per 100,000 persons in 2009. Nine states and the District of Columbia reported case rates above the national average of 3.0 cases per 100,000.[9] Hispanics (29%) represented the largest percentage of total cases. Asians (28%) constituted the second largest percentage of cases, surpassing non-Hispanic blacks and African Americans. Foreign-born persons represent a disproportionate percentage (59%) of the national case total; in 2007, the TB case rate was more than 10 times as high among foreign-born as among U.S.-born residents.[10,11] Asians represent the largest percentage of foreign-born cases, and Asians born outside of the United States represent 44% of the TB cases in foreign-born persons and 26% of the national case total.

Although the annual incidence of TB has decreased, the percentage of primary drug-resistant cases increased to 1.2% in 2009 compared with 1.0% in 2008. Primary drug resistance is defined as no previous history of TB and resistance to at least isoniazid (INH) and rifampin, the most potent first-line antitubercular drugs.[1] MDR-TB emerged during the 1990s as a significant threat to TB control, both in the United States and worldwide, and remains a significant threat to TB control. MDR-TB treatment requires the use of second-line drugs that are less effective, more toxic, and costlier than first-line INH- and rifampin-based regimens. In addition, MDR-TB is associated with higher morbidity and mortality than non–drug-resistant TB.[1]

Historically, TB in the United States was a disease that affected primarily older adults; increasingly, younger adults and children are being affected, particularly foreign-born children and adolescents.[7,12] An estimated 11% of TB cases worldwide occur in children younger than 15 years. In TB-endemic areas, children are at increased risk of acquiring TB because of the increased likelihood of close contact and exposure to adults with TB. Progression from infection to disease (approximately 8% to 10% overall) is higher for children of all ages and highest for infants younger than 1 year (43%) and children aged 1 to 5 years (24%). Of additional concern are those children who do not progress from infection to active disease in childhood but who constitute a potential pool for disease in adulthood.[12]

Many factors have contributed to the increased incidence of TB, including the HIV epidemic and higher rates of poverty, homelessness, incarceration, and drug use. An increasing number of immigrants, many of whom live in crowded housing and have inadequate health care, and an increasing number of residents in long-term care facilities have also contributed to this public health problem. Deterioration in the health care infrastructure and reductions in TB outreach programs, which historically improved compliance with treatment regimens, have also contributed to the resurgence of TB.

Alcohol and illegal drug use increase the risk of TB transmission and act as barriers to TB control and prevention.[13] Substance abuse decreases the likelihood of seeking medical care and adhering to and completing therapy. In addition, the use of substances often takes place in enclosed crowded spaces with poor ventilation, which increases the risk of TB exposure and transmission. In the United States, approximately one of three U.S.-born persons aged 15 years with TB also abuses substances.

TB is largely a social disease, and homeless and incarcerated individuals are at increased risk of infection with TB.[14,15] TB control can be particularly problematic in correctional and detention facilities, in which persons from diverse backgrounds and communities live together for varying and sometimes extended periods. In July 2006, the Centers for Disease Control and Prevention (CDC) published guidelines for the prevention and control of TB in jails, prisons, and other correctional and detention facilities.[16] Providers working in these settings should familiarize themselves with the recommendations, which can be found in *Morbidity and Mortality Weekly Report* (MMWR) or on the Internet at www.cdc.gov/mmwr/preview/mmwrhtml/rr5509a1.htm.

Transmission of *M. tuberculosis* in health care institutions was a contributing factor to the resurgence of TB during the period from 1985 to 1992, and recommendations were developed to prevent transmission in these settings. However, the elevated risk among health care workers may be attributable to other factors (e.g., birth in a country with a high incidence of TB). A recent large multistate occupational survey indicated that health care workers, with the exception of respiratory therapists, do not have a higher risk for TB than the general population.[6]

The decelerating decline of the overall national TB rate, the persistent disparities in TB rates between U.S.-born and foreign-born persons and between whites and ethnic minorities, and the increase in MDR-TB cases all threaten progress toward the goal of eliminating TB in the United States.[8] Major challenges to successful control of TB in the United States include detection and treatment of TB in the non–U.S.-born population, elimination of delays in detecting and reporting cases of pulmonary TB and protecting contacts of TB-infected persons, and prevention of and response to TB outbreaks. In addition, there is a large reservoir of persons living in the United States with LTBI who are at risk for progression to TB disease. Finally, the successful control of TB depends on maintenance of clinical and public health expertise in TB management in an era of declining TB incidence.[6]

Treatment of TB benefits both the individual patient and the community as a whole. Therefore, any public health program or health care provider undertaking to treat a patient with TB is assuming a public health function that includes not only prescribing an appropriate medication regimen but also ensuring adherence to the regimen until treatment is completed.[17] According to a joint statement by the American Thoracic Society, CDC, and Infectious Diseases Society of America, the responsibility for successful treatment of TB is assigned to the public health program or private provider rather than to the individual with TB.[18]

Specialist referral is recommended for any patient suspected of having pulmonary or extrapulmonary TB.

PATHOPHYSIOLOGY

TB is spread primarily through direct infection (person to person), but it can also be spread indirectly by the airborne transmission of the tubercle bacilli, which can remain suspended in the air for several hours. Transmission, which may occur if these bacilli-laden sputum droplets (each containing one to three organisms) are inhaled, depends on three factors: the infectiousness of the person with TB, the environment in which the exposure occurred, and the duration of exposure. Although theoretically one organism implanted in the alveolus can initiate this process, 5 to 200 organisms are usually required.[19] Most of the larger inhaled particles become lodged in the upper respiratory tract, where infection is unlikely to take place. Infection begins if the droplet nuclei reach the alveolar macrophage and multiplication of the tubercle bacilli is initiated. A small number of mycobacteria spread through the lymph system to regional lymph nodes and through the bloodstream to more distant tissues and organs, including areas in which TB is more likely to develop, such as the apices of the lung, the kidneys, the brain, and the bone. Eighty-five percent of all TB cases involve the lungs; other common sites include the pleura, central nervous system (CNS), lymphatic system, genitourinary system, and bones and joints. TB can also become disseminated and then is referred to as miliary TB.

TB disease has two distinct epidemiologic patterns. Reactivation, or postprimary disease, is the most common clinical form of TB. Most symptomatic cases of TB arise in persons with a history of TB infection who were inadequately treated or not treated. The second epidemiologic profile, primary infection, does not usually appear as a symptomatic infection except in persons infected with HIV. More than 90% of persons with primary infection are entirely asymptomatic, and infection with TB is identified only by a positive reaction to a tuberculin skin test (TST).

Certain medical conditions and other factors increase the risk that LTBI will progress to active TB disease. The risk may be three times greater (as with coexistent diabetes mellitus) to 100 times greater (as with HIV infection) for persons who have these conditions compared with those who do not.[7] Medical conditions and other factors associated with progression from LTBI to TB disease are listed in Box 235-1.

BOX 235-1

Conditions and Other Factors Associated with Progression from LTBI to TB Disease

- HIV infection
- Chest radiographic findings suggestive of previous TB (in a person who receives inadequate or no treatment)
- Diabetes mellitus
- Silicosis
- Substance abuse (notably drug injection)
- Prolonged corticosteroid therapy
- Other immunosuppressive therapy
- Cancer of the head and neck
- Hematologic and reticuloendothelial diseases (e.g., leukemia and Hodgkin disease)
- End-stage renal disease
- Intestinal bypass or gastrectomy surgery
- Chronic malabsorption syndrome
- Low body weight (≥10% below the ideal)
- Recent TST converters (persons with baseline testing results who have an increase of 10 mm or more in the size of the TST reaction within a 2-year period. The risk of progression is greatest in the first 1 or 2 years after infection.)
- Infants and children under the age of 5 years who have a positive TB skin test result

From Centers for Disease Control and Prevention (CDC), National Center for HIV/AIDS, Viral Hepatitis, STD, and TB Prevention: *Latent tuberculosis infection: a guide for primary health care providers*, Atlanta, 2010, U.S. Department of Health and Human Services.

CLINICAL PRESENTATION

Persons who have been infected with *M. tuberculosis* but do not have active disease (LTBI) are completely asymptomatic. For the majority of persons, the only evidence of LTBI is an immune response against mycobacterial antigens, which is demonstrated by the Mantoux test or interferon gamma release assays (IGRAs). Two U.S. Food and Drug Administration (FDA)–approved IGRAs are commercially available in the United States: QuantiFERON-TB Gold In-Tube (QFT-GIT) test and T-SPOT.*TB* test.[20] There is no radiographic evidence of TB in persons with LTBI.

Symptoms of pulmonary TB (the most common site) include fatigue, anorexia, weight loss, night sweats, cough, chest pain, hemoptysis, irregular menses, and low-grade fever. Symptoms in adults are often subtle and may appear in conjunction with or simulate other illnesses and therefore are often not associated with TB. However, one third of persons with pulmonary TB are asymptomatic on initial presentation.[7]

Approximately 15% of cases of TB are extrapulmonary; common sites include the bones and joints, genitourinary system, lymphatic system, and CNS. The symptoms of extrapulmonary TB depend on the site affected. TB of the spine often causes back pain, whereas TB of the genitourinary system may result in hematuria or persistent dysuria.

PHYSICAL EXAMINATION

A complete physical examination is an essential part of the evaluation but cannot be used alone to confirm or to exclude TB. Even if the physical examination findings are entirely normal, it can provide useful information about the patient's overall condition. Certain findings, although not diagnostic of TB, may be suggestive of the diagnosis. Rales in the upper posterior portion of the chest, evidence of pleural effusion, lymphadenopathy, weight loss, and fever may increase the suspicion for TB. Confirmation of TB is based on the diagnostic evaluation presented in the next section.

DIAGNOSTICS

Screening is the first step in the diagnostic evaluation of TB and is performed to identify infected patients at high risk for TB who would benefit from preventive therapy as well as patients with TB who need treatment. If a person is infected with TB, a reaction to the TST is detectable 2 to 8 weeks after infection.[7] Because most patients infected with TB are asymptomatic, health care providers should administer the TST to all high-risk persons as part of their routine evaluation. Persons with any of the medical conditions or other factors listed in Box 235-1 should be screened annually unless there is prior documentation of a positive TST reaction. Other high-risk groups include close contacts of a person with infectious TB disease; foreign-born persons from areas in which TB is common (e.g., Asia, Africa, and

Latin America); the medically underserved and low-income populations, including high-risk racial and ethnic groups (e.g., Asians and Pacific Islanders, African Americans, Hispanics, and Native Americans), migrant farm workers, and homeless persons; residents of long-term care facilities (e.g., correctional facilities and nursing homes); and other groups identified as having a disproportionate prevalence of TB. Routine institutional screening is also recommended for health care workers and the staff of long-term institutional facilities who may have occupational exposure to TB or who would pose a risk to large numbers of susceptible persons if they developed active disease (e.g., staff member of an AIDS hospice).[7]

The standard and preferred method of screening for TB infection is the Mantoux test, which is administered by injection of 5 tuberculin units (0.1 mL) of purified protein derivative (PPD) solution intradermally into either the volar or the dorsal surface of the forearm. The injection should be made with a disposable tuberculin syringe with the needle bevel pointing upward. The injection should produce a discrete, pale elevation of the skin (a wheal) that is 6 to 10 mm (⅕ to ⅖ inch) in diameter and disappears within several hours. If a wheal is not produced, the injection was probably too deep and will likely result in a false-negative reading. In the absence of a wheal, the skin test should be repeated. The amount of induration, rather than the erythema, is measured. All reactions, even those classified as negative, should be recorded in millimeters of induration. If no induration is found, 0 mm should be recorded.

The skin test result is read within 48 to 72 hours. If the patient fails to show up for a scheduled reading within 72 hours, a positive reaction may still be measurable up to 1 week later. A TST must be repeated if the result was not measured and recorded in millimeters of induration.[7] TST results should be measured only by a trained health care professional. Patients or family members should not measure TST results. The TST should be repeated for all negative responses not documented within 72 hours.[1] The criteria to determine whether a skin test result is significant depends on a patient's risk for development of disease or ability to mount a reaction to the PPD. The criteria for a positive TST reaction are listed in Box 235-2. Once a patient has had a positive TST reaction, no subsequent tuberculin skin testing should be performed. The TST should never be performed on a person who has had a previous positive TST reaction or who has had treatment of TB disease.[7]

A variety of factors can cause a false-negative TST reaction, including the recipient's age, simultaneous administration of a live vaccine, concomitant infections, metabolic deficiencies, underlying disease, and improper placement or storage of the PPD solution. Live vaccinations such as the measles, mumps, rubella (MMR) and varicella vaccines may cause a false-negative response to the TST for up to 2 months after immunization. However, results of the TST performed simultaneously with inoculation of these vaccines are unaffected.[21] Other potential causes of false-negative test results are listed in Box 235-3.

Because there are many potential causes of a false-negative TST reaction, the absence of a positive reaction does not exclude TB disease or infection. Anergy, which is a decreased or absent delayed-type hypersensitivity response, can be caused by severe or febrile illness, miliary or pulmonary disease, and most of the factors listed in Box 235-3. Of all patients with TB, 10% to 25% have negative reactions to the TST. Approximately one third of patients with HIV infection and more than 60% of patients with AIDS have skin test reactions of less than 5 mm, even though

BOX 235-2

Criteria for a Positive TST Reaction

INDURATION ≥5 MM

Persons with HIV infection
Household or close contacts of persons with TB infection
Persons with fibrotic lesions or evidence of old, healed TB on chest radiographs
Organ transplant recipients
Patients who are immunosuppressed for other reasons (e.g., taking equivalent of ≥15 mg/day of prednisone for 1 month or more or those taking tumor necrosis factor-α (TNF-α) antagonists)

INDURATION ≥10 MM

Recent immigrants (within past 5 years) from countries with high TB prevalence
Residents or employees of high-risk congregate settings (prisons, jails, long-term care facilities for the elderly, hospitals and other health care facilities, residential facilities for patients with AIDS, and homeless shelters)
Medically underserved, low-income populations, including high-risk minority populations
Persons with clinical conditions and other factors listed in Box 235-1
Mycobacteriology laboratory personnel
Children younger than 4 years
Infants, children, or adolescents exposed to adults at high risk for TB disease

INDURATION ≥15 MM

Persons with no known risk factors for TB

From Centers for Disease Control and Prevention (CDC), National Center for HIV/AIDS, Viral Hepatitis, STD, and TB Prevention: *Latent tuberculosis infection: a guide for primary health care providers,* Atlanta, 2010, U.S. Department of Health and Human Services.

BOX 235-3

Potential Causes of False-Negative Tuberculin Test Reactions

- Age (>45 years, newborns)
- Immunosuppression (e.g., corticosteroids, chemotherapy, or other agents)
- Systemic viral, fungal, and bacterial infections
- Live virus vaccinations (e.g., MMR; trivalent oral poliovirus vaccine)
- Malnutrition, cachexia, or nutritional derangement (e.g., severe protein deficiency, zinc deficiency)
- Chronic renal failure
- Hematologic or lymphoreticular disorders (e.g., Hodgkin disease)
- Sarcoidosis
- Stress (e.g., burns, postoperative status, mental illness)
- Mechanical (injection too deep, inexperienced reader)
- Improper storage (exposure to light or heat)

Modified from American Thoracic Society: Diagnostic standards and classification of tuberculosis in adults and children, *Am J Respir Crit Care Med* 161(4 Pt 1):1376-1395, 2000. Available at www.thoracic.org/statements/resources/archive/tbadult1-20.pdf. Accessed September 21, 2015.

they have been infected with *M. tuberculosis.*[7] A negative TST result does not exclude LTBI in patients who are immunocompromised. The usefulness of anergy testing for immunocompromised individuals has not been consistently demonstrated and is no longer recommended.[7]

False-negative reactions to the TST can also result from a decreased or waning delayed-type hypersensitivity reaction over time, especially among older adults who may have been infected years before being screened for TB. Although they were previously infected with TB, their hypersensitivity to the PPD antigen has been blunted over time. Although they may not respond to the initial skin test, the skin test may stimulate or "boost" their ability to react to the tuberculin on a subsequent test. Therefore, skin testing is repeated in 1 to 3 weeks. A positive reaction to the second test probably represents a boosted reaction rather than a reaction to new infection. On the basis of this two-step testing, the patient should be classified as previously infected, and management should proceed accordingly. Guidelines to interpret the results of a two-step TST are included in Box 235-4.

IGRAs are blood tests that measure a person's immune reactivity to specific mycobacterial antigens. In a person infected with *M. tuberculosis,* the whole blood cells recognize simulated antigens and release interferon-γ (IFN-γ). Results are based on the amount of IFN-γ released.[7] When IGRAs are used for serial testing, there is no need for a second test because boosting does not occur.[7]

Many foreign countries vaccinate against TB by use of the bacillus Calmette-Guérin (BCG) vaccine. The BCG vaccine was first introduced in 1921 and continues to be the only vaccine used to prevent TB.[22] BCG has nonspecific immunologic effects and has been shown to be beneficial for other diseases. For example, BCG instillation into the bladder has been helpful in treating bladder cancer, and local application of BCG has been effective against common and genital warts. BCG is the most widely used vaccine worldwide. It has demonstrated efficacy in preventing miliary TB and TB meningitis in children but is not as effective in preventing pulmonary TB in adults.[22] BCG is used in many countries with a high prevalence of TB to prevent childhood tuberculous meningitis and miliary disease. It has not been generally recommended for use in the United States because of the low risk of infection with *M. tuberculosis,* the variable effectiveness of the vaccine against adult pulmonary TB, and the vaccine's potential interference with TST reactivity.[23]

Sensitivity to tuberculin varies significantly among persons who have received the BCG vaccination; this variance depends in part on the strain of BCG used and the person vaccinated. A history of BCG vaccination often confuses the diagnostic picture because there is no reliable way to determine whether a reaction to the TST is because of the BCG vaccine or infection with *M. tuberculosis.* Nevertheless, a prior history of BCG vaccination is not considered a contraindication to PPD tuberculin skin testing. A reaction to the TST is probably a result of infection with *M. tuberculosis* rather than the BCG vaccine if the induration is large, if significant time has elapsed since BCG vaccination, if the person has had recent exposure to someone with infectious TB, if there is a family history of TB, if the person comes from an area in which TB is endemic, or if the chest radiograph shows evidence of previous TB infection. Patients who have received the BCG vaccine should be screened, evaluated, and managed in a manner similar to those who have not been vaccinated with BCG.[7] Interpretation of the TST result is the same for persons who have had BCG vaccination.[7]

IGRAs can be used in all situations in which a TST is used. An advantage of IGRAs is that results are available 24 hours after blood collection, in contrast to the 2- or 3-day wait with tuberculin skin testing. In addition, a two-step TST is recommended in certain situations; but with IGRAs, two-step testing is neither necessary nor recommended. In addition, IGRAs eliminate the need for proper intradermal injection technique, whereas with the TST, lack of proper technique can result in the PPD solution's being "washed out," leading to a possible false-negative reaction. IGRAs are cost-effective and efficient in that they eliminate the need for a second visit for test reading and should lead to fewer false-positive results in populations that include many BCG-vaccinated people (e.g., many non–U.S.-born persons). Instructions for interpretation of IGRA results can be found in Box 235-5.

However, although IGRAs seem to have greater specificity, their sensitivity in detecting *M. tuberculosis* in young children and immunocompromised persons has not been determined. In addition, although IGRAs may save time for clinical staff, the labor and cost burden is shifted to microbiology staff, which needs to be figured into the cost of the tests. Finally, the difficulty of processing nonurgent blood specimens will be a barrier to use of IGRAs in some settings.

Advantages are that IGRAs require a single patient visit, do not cause a booster phenomenon, are less subject to reader bias than the TST, and are unaffected by BCG and most environmental mycobacteria.[7] Limitations of IGRAs are that blood samples must be processed within 8 to 16 hours and limited data exist on use in groups such as children younger than 5 years, persons recently exposed to TB, immunocompromised persons, and those who will be tested repeatedly (serial testing).

BOX **235-4**

Criteria for Interpretation of Two-Step TST Method

- If the first test reaction is positive, consider the person infected.
- If the first test reaction is negative, give second test 1 to 3 weeks later.
- If the second test reaction is positive, consider the person infected. If the second test reaction is negative, consider the person uninfected.

Modified from Centers for Disease Control and Prevention (CDC), National Center for HIV/AIDS, Viral Hepatitis, STD, and TB Prevention: *Latent tuberculosis infection: a guide for primary health care providers,* Atlanta, 2010, U.S. Department of Health and Human Services.

BOX **235-5**

Interpretation of IGRA Results

IGRA Test	Results Reported as
QuantiFERON-TB Gold In-Tube	Positive, negative, indeterminate
T-SPOT.*TB*	Positive, negative, indeterminate, borderline

Note: Laboratory should provide both quantitative and qualitative test results.
From Centers for Disease Control and Prevention (CDC), National Center for HIV/AIDS, Viral Hepatitis, STD, and TB Prevention: *Latent tuberculosis infection: a guide for primary health care providers,* Atlanta, 2010, U.S. Department of Health and Human Services.

According to the CDC, IGRAs are the preferred method of testing for groups of people who have a poor rate of returning to have the TST result read and for persons who have received the BCG vaccine.[7] The TST is the preferred method of testing for children younger than 5 years. Either the TST or an IGRA may be used without preference in other groups being tested for LTBI, but neither test plays a role in the diagnosis of active TB. Routine testing with both TST and IGRA is not recommended.

Persons with a positive tuberculin TST or IGRA reaction should have an anteroposterior chest radiograph to exclude active pulmonary TB and to detect fibrotic lesions, which may suggest an old TB infection or silicosis. Once these conditions have been excluded, no subsequent chest radiographs are indicated unless the person is symptomatic. In addition, anergic persons who have symptoms consistent with TB or have risk factors for TB should undergo a chest x-ray examination. Abnormalities in the apical and posterior segments of the upper lobe or in the superior segments of the lower lobe are those most often seen with pulmonary TB. Infiltrates without cavities and mediastinal or hilar lymphadenopathy may also be seen. HIV infection and other immunocompromising illnesses may result in unusual chest x-ray findings. Chest x-ray findings may be suggestive of TB but are never diagnostic. Nevertheless, they may be used to exclude the possibility of pulmonary TB.[7]

Persons thought to have pulmonary or laryngeal TB should have at least three sputum cultures performed to detect the presence of acid-fast bacilli (AFB). A positive smear is strongly suggestive but not diagnostic of TB because the AFB on a smear may be mycobacteria other than *M. tuberculosis.* It is also possible for those with TB to have negative AFB smears. Species of mycobacteria are identified by a variety of methods, including nucleic acid probes, liquid chromatography, and polymerase chain reactions. The diagnosis is confirmed by a positive culture of *M. tuberculosis* complex, *M. avium,* or *Mycobacterium intracellulare.* The mycobacterium isolates are then tested for drug susceptibility. Drug susceptibility is important to ensure appropriate treatment and should be repeated within 2 months if there has not been an adequate response to treatment.

New point-of-care diagnostic tests for TB are currently being developed. Several versions of mycobacterial lipoarabinomannan (LAM) antigen detection in urine are in development. Urine antigen tests will likely be particularly helpful in diagnosis of TB in HIV-coinfected persons.[24]

DIAGNOSTICS

Tuberculosis

INITIAL
PPD (*Note:* Patients with a previous history of a positive PPD reaction should not undergo this test again.)

LABORATORY
IGRA
Sputum culture for AFB × 3*

IMAGING
Chest x-ray studies*

*If indicated.

DIFFERENTIAL DIAGNOSIS

The differential diagnosis of TB varies by the type of TB and the site of involvement. The signs and symptoms associated with pulmonary TB are consistent with those of other respiratory illnesses, such as pneumonia, acute bronchitis, and carcinoma. Extrapulmonary TB can occur in any organ; therefore, persistent signs and symptoms in any organ should lead to consideration of TB.

DIFFERENTIAL DIAGNOSIS

Tuberculosis

- Pneumonia
- Acute bronchitis
- Carcinoma
- Sarcoidosis
- Wegener granulomatosis
- Lymphoma

MANAGEMENT

The management of TB depends entirely on the current clinical classification system of disease, which is based on the pathogenesis of the disease and the diagnostic results. The classification system is described in Table 235-1, and the official joint statement of the American Thoracic Society, CDC, and Infectious Diseases Society of America on the treatment of TB can be found in *MMWR Recommendations and Reports*[18] or on the Internet at www.cdc.gov/mmwr. Currently, there are six first-line drugs (INH, rifampin, rifabutin, rifapentine [RPT], pyrazinamide [PZA], and ethambutol) and nine second-line drugs

TABLE 235-1 Clinical Classification System for TB

Class	Type	Description
0	No TB exposure Not infected	No history of exposure Negative reaction to TST or QuantiFERON-TB test
1	TB exposure No evidence of infection	History of exposure Negative reaction to TST or QuantiFERON-TB test
2	TB infection No disease	Positive reaction to TST or QuantiFERON-TB test Negative bacteriologic studies (if done) No clinical, bacteriologic, or radiographic evidence of TB
3	TB Clinically active	*Mycobacterium tuberculosis* cultured (if done) Clinical, bacteriologic, or radiographic evidence of current disease
4	TB Not clinically active	History of episode(s) of TB *Or* Abnormal but stable radiographic findings Positive reaction to the TST or QuantiFERON-TB test Negative bacteriologic studies (if done) *And* No clinical or radiographic evidence of current disease
5	TB suspected	Diagnosis pending

From Centers for Disease Control and Prevention (CDC): *Interactive core curriculum on tuberculosis: what the clinician should know,* U.S. Department of Health and Human Services. Available at www.cdc.gov/tb/education/corecurr/pdf/corecurr_all.pdf. Accessed September 19, 2015.

(cycloserine, ethionamide, streptomycin, amikacin/kanamycin, capreomycin, *p*-aminosalicylic acid [PAS], levofloxacin, moxifloxacin, and gatifloxacin) approved by the FDA for treatment of TB. The long-term (more than several weeks) use of fluoroquinolones in children and adolescents has not been approved because of concerns about effects on bone and cartilage growth.[18]

Class 0 and class 1 TB require no treatment. Patients with class 1 TB (contacts of a person with infectious TB disease) should have another TST performed within 8 to 10 weeks when the initial TST or IGRA reaction is negative.[7] Children younger than 5 years and immunocompromised persons who have had contact with a person with infectious TB disease and who have had a negative reaction should have a chest radiograph. If it is normal, treatment should be started for LTBI and another test performed 8 to 10 weeks after contact has ended. If a repeated test reaction is positive, treatment should be continued. If a repeated test reaction is negative, treatment can be discontinued. However, for some contacts at high risk of infection with TB, a full course of LTBI treatment may be recommended even in the absence of a positive TST or IGRA result.[7] Local TB control programs can provide guidance about the medical management of such contacts. In the follow-up testing of contacts of persons with infectious TB, the retesting is not referred to as two-step testing. The second test is necessary to determine if infection occurred but was too early in onset to be detected at the time of the first test. If testing is repeated, the same type of test (TST or IGRA) can be used. Patients with class 2 TB have been infected with TB but do not have any evidence of clinically active disease. The main purpose of preventive therapy is to decrease the risk that LTBI will progress to clinically active TB disease. INH is most commonly used for preventive therapy and is highly effective when it is taken as prescribed. The usual preventive therapy regimen is INH, 5 mg/kg (maximum dose, 300 mg), daily for 9 months.[7]

INH is bactericidal, relatively nontoxic, inexpensive, and easily administered. The degree of protection conferred by INH varies according to the percentage of mycobacteria eradicated. INH has been shown to reduce the incidence of disease by 54% to 90%; the primary reason for this variation in efficacy appears to be the actual amount of INH taken during the year it was prescribed.

INH remains less widely prescribed in the United States than is indicated. Preventive therapy should be considered for persons younger than 35 years who have TST reactions of 10 mm or more and who have any risk factors for TB. Patients younger than 35 years with no known risk factors should be evaluated for preventive therapy if their reaction to the TST was 15 mm or more. Unless otherwise indicated, INH preventive therapy should be offered to individuals with class 2 TB (tuberculin positive), regardless of their history of BCG vaccination. High-priority candidates for TB preventive therapy, regardless of age, are listed in Box 235-6.

The major side effect of INH is hepatitis. Other problems associated with INH include peripheral neuropathy, gastrointestinal upset, and mild CNS effects. From 10% to 20% of patients prescribed INH develop mild abnormalities of liver function, which usually resolve even if INH therapy is continued.[7] Increased values of liver function tests (LFTs) can be accepted at five times the upper limit of normal for patients who have no symptoms of hepatitis if the serum bilirubin concentration is within the normal range.[7] Clinical hepatitis occurs in approximately 0.1% of people taking INH and is more common when INH is combined with other agents.[7] The risk for INH-induced hepatitis increases directly with increasing age; therefore, INH is recommended for patients older than 35 years only if they are at high risk for development of TB. Baseline and monthly LFTs and a monthly clinical evaluation should be performed for all persons undergoing INH therapy.[14] Alcohol consumption has also been identified as a contributing risk factor in the development of INH-induced hepatitis. Other drugs that increase the risk of INH-induced hepatitis include acetaminophen, phenytoin (Dilantin), steroids, methimazole (Tapazole), estropipate (Ogen, Ortho-Est), and metoclopramide (Reglan, Maxolon). INH administration increases the serum levels of certain drugs, including phenytoin, theophylline, carbamazepine (Tegretol), benzodiazepines, and anticoagulants. During INH administration, the serum levels of these drugs should be monitored more closely. Drugs that decrease the serum concentration of INH include antacids, corticosteroids, and laxatives. Symptomatic hepatitis associated with INH is rare in patients younger than 20 years but severe, and fatal cases have occurred. Therefore, younger patients taking INH should be monitored with the same precautions as for older individuals.[7]

BOX 235-6

High-Priority Candidates for TB Preventive Therapy

Preventive therapy should be recommended for the following persons with a positive skin test reaction, regardless of age (criterion for a positive reaction in millimeters of induration is listed in parentheses):

- Persons with known or suspected HIV infection, including persons who inject drugs whose HIV status is unknown (≥5 mm)
- Close contacts of persons with infectious clinically active TB (≥5 mm)
- Persons who have chest x-ray findings suggestive of previous TB and who have received inadequate or no treatment (≥5 mm)
- Persons who inject drugs and are known to be HIV negative (≥10 mm)
- Recent TST converters (≥10-mm increase within a 2-year period for those <35 years of age; ≥15-mm increase for those ≥35 years of age)
- Persons with medical conditions that increase the risk of TB, such as diabetes mellitus, prolonged corticosteroid therapy, immunosuppressive therapy, some hematologic and reticuloendothelial diseases, injection drug use, end-stage renal disease, and clinical situations associated with rapid weight loss (≥10 mm)

Peripheral neuropathy is associated with the administration of INH in less than 0.2% of people taking INH at conventional doses and most likely results from interference with pyridoxine absorption. It occurs more often in the presence of other conditions associated with neuropathy, such as diabetes, renal failure, HIV infection, alcoholism, and malnutrition.[7] It is recommended that pyridoxine (10 to 50 mg/day) be administered in conjunction with INH to patients with these conditions. In addition, pyridoxine should be administered to pregnant and breastfeeding women to prevent neuropathy and to patients with a seizure disorder who are undergoing INH therapy.

Three randomized controlled trials have shown that a new combination regimen of INH and RPT, administered weekly for 12 weeks as directly observed therapy (DOT), is as effective for

TABLE 235-2 Treatment Regimens for LTBI

Drug and Dose	Frequency and Duration (Doses)	Rating[*] (Evidence)[†] HIV Negative	HIV Positive
PREFERRED REGIMEN			
INH Adult: 5 mg/kg Children: 10-20 mg/kg Maximum dose 300 mg	Daily × 9 mo (270 doses)	A (II)	A (II)
ALTERNATIVE REGIMENS			
INH Adult: 15 mg/kg Children: 20-40 mg/kg Maximum dose 900 mg	Twice weekly × 9 mo[‡] (76 doses)	B (II)	B (II)
INH Adults: 5 mg/kg Children: Not recommended Maximum dose 300 mg	Daily × 6 mo (180 doses)	B (I)	C (I)
INH Adults: 15 mg/kg Children: Not recommended Maximum dose 900 mg	Twice weekly × 6 mo[‡] (52 doses)	B (II)	C (I)
Rifampin Adults: 10 mg/kg Children: 10-20 mg/kg Maximum dose 600 mg	Daily × 4 mo (120 doses) Daily × 6 mo (180 doses)	B (II)	B (II)

Note: In situations in which rifampin cannot be used (e.g., HIV-infected persons receiving protease inhibitors), rifabutin may be substituted.

*Strength of the recommendation: A = preferred regimen; B = acceptable alternative; C = offer when A and B cannot be given.

†Quality of the supporting evidence: I = randomized clinical trials data; II = data from clinical trials not randomized or from other population; III = expert opinion.

‡Intermittent regimen must be provided via DOT (i.e., health care worker observes the ingestion of medication).

From Centers for Disease Control and Prevention (CDC), National Center for HIV/AIDS, Viral Hepatitis, STD, and TB Prevention: *Latent tuberculosis infection: a guide for primary health care providers,* Atlanta, 2010, U.S. Department of Health and Human Services.

preventing TB as other regimens and is more likely to be completed than the U.S. standard of 9 months of daily INH without DOT.[25] This new INH-RPT regimen is considered an equal alternative to the 9-month INH regimen for otherwise healthy individuals aged 12 years or older who have LTBI and factors predictive for developing TB, including recent exposure to contagious TB, recent conversion from negative to positive on an indirect test for infection, and radiographic findings of healed pulmonary TB. RPT, like rifampin, is a rifamycin-class antibiotic that is approved by the FDA for treating TB disease; its use for treating LTBI is off label. RPT is microbicidal for susceptible *M. tuberculosis.* The drug has a long half-life, which allows for infrequent administration, and lends itself to DOT.

The choice between INH and INH-RPT depends on several factors, including the feasibility of DOT, ability to procure the drug, programmatic issues (e.g., feasibility of patient monitoring), and patient and provider preferences.[25] INH-RPT is not recommended for children younger than 2 years of age; HIV-infected patients receiving antiretroviral treatment, because drug interactions have not been studied; pregnant women because safety in pregnancy is not known; and patients with presumed INH or RPT resistance.

RPT dyes secretions red, including urine and tears, and can stain contact lenses. Uncommon adverse effects include neutropenia and elevated liver enzymes. RPT induces the metabolism of many medications, particularly those metabolized by cytochrome P-450 isoenzyme 3A; it should not be used with these medications, particularly medications having narrow therapeutic ranges (e.g., warfarin, methadone), unless monitored carefully.[25] Because missed doses or altered dosage intervals could significantly affect efficacy or safety of the INH-RPT regimen, DOT is recommended. At each encounter, in addition to receiving medication, patients should be instructed to seek medical attention immediately if they develop fever, yellow eyes, dizziness, rash, or aches or more than 1 day of nausea, vomiting, weakness, abdominal pain, or loss of appetite. If patients develop any of these symptoms, medication should be withheld while the cause of symptoms is determined. In addition, individuals receiving INH-RPT therapy should undergo monthly clinical assessments and physical examinations.

Additional treatment regimens for LTBI can be found in Table 235-2.

For persons who have had close contact with individuals with INH-resistant TB, preventive therapy with rifampin, 10 mg/kg daily for 4 months, should be considered.[7] Rifampin preventive therapy can also be considered for patients who are INH intolerant.

Rifampin is bactericidal and easily administered. The most common side effect is gastrointestinal upset. Other adverse reactions include rashes, hepatitis, and, rarely, thrombocytopenia and cholestatic jaundice. Hepatitis is more common when rifampin is combined with INH.[7] Rifampin is a cytochrome P-450 (hepatic microsomal enzyme) inducer that may increase the clearance of drugs metabolized by the liver, including oral hypoglycemic agents, glucocorticoids, estrogens, warfarin (Coumadin) derivatives, methadone, theophylline, antiarrhythmic agents (quinidine, verapamil, mexiletine), anticonvulsants, ketoconazole, and cyclosporine. By interfering with estrogen metabolism, rifampin may also interfere with the effectiveness of oral contraceptives.[18] Rifampin is contraindicated or should be used with caution in persons with HIV disease who are being treated with certain protease inhibitors or non-nucleoside reverse transcriptase inhibitors. In this situation, rifabutin may be substituted.[7]

On the basis of adverse event data, the CDC and American Thoracic Society revised their guidelines and in 2003 recommended against the use of rifampin and PZA for treatment of LTBI. A CDC cohort analysis in 2003 found the rates of severe liver injury and death related to the use of rifampin and PZA to be significantly higher than the rates of INH-associated liver injury in the treatment of LTBI.[18] On the basis of these findings, the American Thoracic Society and the CDC now recommend that this regimen in general not be offered to persons with LTBI unless the potential benefits of this regimen outweigh the risks for severe liver injury and death associated with rifampin-PZA. The CDC recommends that a TB and LTBI expert be consulted before rifampin-PZA is offered. In addition, patients should be asked about whether they have a history of liver disease or adverse effects from INH or other drugs, be informed of potential hepatotoxicity of the rifampin-PZA regimen, and be advised against the concurrent use of potentially hepatotoxic drugs (including over-the-counter drugs such as acetaminophen).[26]

Treatment of class 3 or clinically active TB requires multidrug therapy. The specific drug regimen should be developed in consultation with a specialist familiar with the management of TB. As previously mentioned, there are six first-line and nine second-line antitubercular drugs. The second-line antitubercular drugs, such as PAS, ethionamide, and cycloserine, tend to be less effective and more toxic than the first-line drugs previously discussed. They are generally used only in cases of drug-resistant TB or atypical mycobacterial infections. Research on newer antitubercular drugs continues to be of importance, especially in this era of emerging drug resistance.

Comprehensive guidelines for the treatment of active TB can be found in the official joint statement of the American Thoracic Society, CDC, and Infectious Diseases Society of America on the treatment of TB.[18] One of the purposes of therapy is to prevent the development of MDR-TB, and therefore the medication regimen is based on drug susceptibilities.

The antitubercular drug regimens used to treat extrapulmonary TB are similar to those used to treat pulmonary TB. Additional therapies, such as corticosteroid therapy or surgery, may be required, depending on the site of TB infection. The type of follow-up and bacteriologic evaluation required is determined by the site of infection.

The diagnosis of nonclinically active TB (class 4) is defined by a history of previous episodes of TB or stable radiographic findings in a patient with a positive TST reaction. Sputum cultures, if obtained, are negative, and there is no radiographic evidence of clinically active disease. Patients with class 4 TB may be treated in several ways, depending on TB risk factors and the coexisting medical conditions. Some patients may have completed a course of preventive therapy, and some may be receiving preventive therapy; for others, preventive therapy may not be indicated. Current, clinically active TB must be excluded before a patient can be assigned to class 4.

Patients are categorized as having class 5 TB while the evaluation for TB is still being done and the diagnosis of TB is pending. Patients remain in this class until all diagnostic studies have been performed but should not remain in this class for more than 3 months. If clinically active TB is strongly suspected, patients are prescribed multidrug therapy while the evaluation is still pending. If a diagnosis of clinically active TB (class 3) is confirmed, multidrug therapy is continued. If TB disease is excluded, the drug regimen is altered accordingly. For example, if a diagnosis is changed to infectious (class 2) TB, preventive therapy is continued if indicated. If active TB is highly possible, it is imperative to start multidrug therapy initially and to alter the regimen accordingly because progressing from single-drug therapy (e.g., INH) to multidrug therapy once a diagnosis of active disease has been confirmed increases the risk for spread of the disease and development of drug-resistant TB.

One of the most significant problems associated with TB control is adherence to antitubercular regimens. Treatment adherence is difficult to predict; many variables may affect a person's adherence to the medication regimen, including office-related variables (e.g., long wait times or inconvenient office hours), patient-related variables (misinformation, residential instability, poor access to health care, concomitant medical conditions, lack of financial resources, culture and language, and religious practices), and treatment variables (medication side effects, frequency of visits, and the process for obtaining refills).[7] Inconsistent or partial treatment has resulted in TB that is resistant to INH and rifampin (MDR-TB). MDR-TB is a particular problem in certain areas of the world, such as eastern Europe and central Asia, because of the breakdown in health system infrastructure and subsequent incomplete or inadequate treatments.[27] Although MDR-TB is treatable in general, the drug regimens required to treat it take longer and are considerably more expensive and toxic. Strategies to improve adherence, particularly with multidrug regimens, include providing education in the patient's primary language, reinforcing patient education at each visit, ensuring patient confidentiality, suggesting or providing medication reminders (e.g., a pill box or calendar), and collaborating with the local health department to provide DOT.[7]

In 1991, WHO introduced the DOTS (directly observed therapy short course) program, which includes five essential components: case detection by sputum-smear microscopy, government commitment to TB control, regular supply of TB drugs, supervised treatment, and reports on the progress of the health system. WHO has helped more than 180 countries implement DOTS, which is also used in the United States.[27] Cases of TB are subject to mandatory reporting in all 50 states, the District of Columbia, U.S. dependencies and possessions, and independent nations within the United States (e.g., Native American lands). TB in the United States is closely monitored by local, federal, and state health departments.[15] As part of DOT, a health care provider or other designated person directly observes the patient taking each dose of TB medication. DOT is routinely implemented in many areas, such as homeless shelters and institutional settings. Trained personnel can provide DOT daily or intermittently in the office, clinic, or field (patient's home, workplace, corner bar, or any site that is mutually agreeable).[17] Antitubercular regimens can often be prescribed to be taken two or three times weekly, making DOT less burdensome. DOT has been shown to be cost-effective when such intermittent regimens are used and is associated with a decrease in the acquisition and transmission of TB.[17,28] As a result, DOT is widely recommended and promoted for the management of patients with active TB. Universal DOT is credited with a decrease in the acquisition and transmission of resistant TB.[28]

The law in every state requires that a diagnosis of TB be reported to the local health department. All drug susceptibility test results should be forwarded to the health department. Reporting of TB is important for source and contact identification, epidemiologic surveillance, and the provision of resources for case management.

Interdisciplinary Management

Consultation with a specialist is required for the management of all patients requiring multidrug therapy, those with active clinical disease (class 3), and those for whom the evaluation is pending (class 5). In addition, consultation is indicated for patients with evidence of TB infection (class 2) and coexistent medical conditions, especially those that alter immune responsiveness, which may increase the risk for development of clinically active disease.

LIFE SPAN CONSIDERATIONS

One approach to improving TB detection and control has been to integrate tuberculin skin testing and LTBI treatment with services routinely accessed by clients, such as methadone maintenance clinics. Prenatal care offers another opportunity to see patients on a regular basis. Pregnant women should have a TST only if specific risk factors are present. If a TST or IGRA reaction is positive, a chest radiograph should be obtained with proper shielding.[7] Once TB disease has been excluded, treatment of LTBI should be considered for HIV-infected women or if there has been recent contact with a person with TB. In the absence of these risk factors, treatment should be deferred until after the woman has delivered. If treatment is started during pregnancy, INH daily or twice weekly (using DOT) is the preferred regimen. Supplementation with 10 to 25 mg of pyridoxine (vitamin B_6) daily is recommended. Pregnant women receiving INH should be monitored closely for hepatotoxicity because there is an increased risk during pregnancy and for 2 to 3 months postpartum. It is recommended that treatment of LTBI be delayed until 2 to 3 months postpartum unless there is a high risk of progression to TB disease.[29]

Breastfeeding is not contraindicated in women taking INH. Pyridoxine supplementation is recommended for nursing women. Pregnant women with clinically active TB (class 3) must receive adequate therapy as soon as TB is suspected because risk of transmission to the fetus is high. Untreated TB presents a much greater danger to a woman and her fetus than does treatment of the disease. The preferred initial drug regimen includes INH, rifampin, and ethambutol. These drugs do cross the placenta but have no demonstrated teratogenic side effects. A woman receiving antitubercular therapy should not be discouraged from breastfeeding; although small concentrations of the drug are found in breast milk, they do not cause toxicity in newborns.[30]

Older adults receiving antitubercular therapy must be monitored closely for drug side effects. Many of the adverse reactions increase with advancing age and decreased renal function.

COMPLICATIONS

Complications of TB can result from the disease process itself or can be secondary to drug therapy. The death rate of untreated pulmonary TB is approximately 60%, with a median time until death of 2½ years. Patients with miliary or disseminated TB often become ill before radiographic changes are apparent or a diagnosis of TB has been made. Without treatment, the prognosis for miliary TB is poor. However, miliary TB responds to the same drug regimens used to treat other forms of TB.

Persons taking antitubercular drugs need to be monitored closely for side effects and drug toxicities. Baseline laboratory evaluations and monthly examinations are indicated for most of the drugs used to treat TB.

TB and HIV/AIDS form a lethal combination because each disease speeds the progress of the other. Because HIV weakens the immune system, someone who is infected with HIV and TB is many times more likely to develop active TB than is someone infected with TB who is HIV negative. TB is the leading cause of death among people who are HIV positive and accounts for approximately 13% of AIDS-related deaths worldwide.[6]

Smoking and TB is thought to be another "lethal interaction," and smoking appears to be a risk factor for acquiring TB infection, developing active TB, having a more severe pulmonary TB, and being at increased risk of dying from the disease.[30] Even though smokers tend to have more innate immune cells and lymphocytes in their lungs, they seem to have an increased vulnerability to TB. The hypothesis is that immune cells and lymphocytes may be compromised in the presence of cigarette smoke, thereby compromising their effectiveness against TB.[31]

INDICATIONS FOR REFERRAL OR HOSPITALIZATION

Most patients with clinically active pulmonary TB should be considered for hospitalization during the first couple of weeks of therapy. After 2 weeks of multidrug therapy, the infectiousness of these patients is reduced significantly and they are no longer a threat to public health. Patients with extrapulmonary TB typically are much less infectious and can be managed as outpatients.

Persons with MDR-TB should be referred to an infectious disease specialist or a pulmonologist with expertise in the treatment of TB. Immunocompromised patients with active TB or any patients with disseminated disease should also be referred.

PATIENT AND FAMILY EDUCATION

Patient education is critical to controlling the resurgence of TB. The public must be educated about the role of TB screening and the need to identify persons infected with TB before active disease develops so they can benefit from preventive therapy. Bilingual and bicultural outreach staff workers are needed to work with immigrant individuals and communities to counter opposition to LTBI therapy based on cultural misunderstandings about its purpose and fears of stigmatization based on adherence to a long-term medication regimen. The importance of medication adherence must be carefully explained to patients receiving INH or multidrug therapy. Untreated TB can lead to reactivation of the disease in the future, progression of the disease, continued spread of the disease, and development of drug resistance. In addition, the potential drug side effects must be carefully discussed, and patients should be instructed to contact their health care provider as soon as any signs or symptoms associated with drug toxicity develop.

CHAPTER 236

WEST NILE VIRUS

Thomas H. Taylor

West Nile virus (WNV) is now the leading cause of epidemic encephalitis in the United States. During the past 10 years, the face of meningoencephalitis has changed from predominantly enterovirus and herpes simplex virus to a broad and more geographically varied spectrum of disease. The morbidity associated with more neuroinvasive forms of WNV is considerable, and ongoing neurologic deterioration may be related to viral persistence.

DEFINITIONS

WNV is an arboviral infection of the family Flaviviridae (from Latin *flavus,* "yellow"), which includes the prototype, yellow fever, as well as dengue fever, Japanese encephalitis (JE), St. Louis encephalitis (SLE), and tick-borne encephalitis (TBE). These viruses have a predisposition to cause acute febrile illness and central nervous system infections, encephalitis, and aseptic meningitis. West Nile fever (WNF) and West Nile encephalitis (WNE) are outcomes of WNV. All Flaviviridae may invade muscle, joints, and liver and thus give rise to complications of myositis, arthritis, and hepatitis. Encephalitis, meningitis, myelitis, and neuritis refer to inflammation of brain, leptomeninges, spinal cord, and nerve roots, respectively. Radiculitis refers to involvement primarily of the sensory nerve root, and acute flaccid paralysis (AFP) refers to a myelitis involving the anterior horn cells, or motor cells, of the spinal cord; both conditions may complicate WNV infection. Meningoencephalitis, or inflammation of both meninges and brain, is common in WNV infection.

Transmission of arboviral infection (*ar* for arthropod and *bo* for borne, or arthropod-borne viral infection) is predominantly by mosquitoes but sometimes by ticks. Birds are the WNV reservoir (and amplifying host). Horses and humans are susceptible but dead-end hosts. Many other vertebrates are susceptible to infection, but like humans, most do not sustain high-level viremias for long enough periods to become a reservoir or amplifying host.

EPIDEMIOLOGY

The evolution of WNV represents a true emerging infectious disease, with rapid spread throughout North America and now progressing to Central and South America, suggestive of what we might expect from the next influenza pandemic or acts of bioterrorism. WNV was first isolated from a febrile female patient in the West Nile district of Uganda in 1937 but was not associated with neurologic disease at that time. WNV did have close serologic identity with JE virus and SLE virus, two closely related and highly neurotropic viruses. For three decades, WNF, associated with fever, arthritis, and rash, circulated in Africa and the Middle East, with little neuroinvasive disease. The 1990s brought increasingly frequent and severe outbreaks of West Nile neuroinvasive disease (WNND) to Europe, Russia, and the Middle East, along avian migration routes. In 1999, WNV crossed the Atlantic and produced an outbreak of WNND in boroughs of New York City, epidemiologically associated with mosquito exposure.[1] The New World strain was closely related to a newly emergent clade 1a strain circulating in the Middle East and may have arrived via a febrile traveler, a transported mosquito, or a storm-blown avian host. Like its Middle East counterpart, this virus was neuroinvasive and rapidly spread from New York by bird migration routes along the entire East Coast and subsequently westward to involve all lower 48 states (not Alaska or Hawaii).[2] After emergence in the United States, WNV became the most common cause of neuroinvasive arbovirus disease, culminating in 9862 cases in 2003. A resurgence occurred in 2012 with 5674 cases, suggesting that WNV will follow a pattern of periodic outbreaks, as opposed to the more endemic pattern of other arboviruses circulating in the North America (Fig. 236-1).[3]

The virus is maintained in a bird-mosquito-bird cycle because wild birds develop high levels of viremia during long but relatively asymptomatic intervals, which facilitates transmission to many mosquitoes (amplification). Avian and mosquito

West Nile virus disease cases and deaths reported to CDC by year and clinical presentation, 1999–2013

Year	Neuroinvasive disease		Non-neuroinvasive disease		Total	
	Cases No.	Deaths No. (%)	Cases No.	Deaths No. (%)	Cases No.	Deaths No. (%)
1999	59	7 (12)	3	0 (0)	62	7 (11)
2000	19	2 (11)	2	0 (0)	21	2 (10)
2001	64	10 (16)	2	0 (0)	66	10 (15)
2002	2,946	276 (9)	1,210	8 (1)	4,156	284 (7)
2003	2,866	232 (8)	6,996	32 (<1)	9,862	264 (3)
2004	1,148	94 (8)	1,391	6 (<1)	2,539	100 (4)
2005	1,309	104 (8)	1,691	15 (1)	3,000	119 (4)
2006	1,495	162 (11)	2,774	15 (1)	4,269	177 (4)
2007	1,227	117 (10)	2,403	7 (<1)	3,630	124 (3)
2008	689	41 (6)	667	3 (<1)	1,356	44 (3)
2009	386	32 (8)	334	0 (0)	720	32 (4)
2010	629	54 (9)	392	3 (1)	1,021	57 (6)
2011	486	42 (9)	226	1 (<1)	712	43 (6)
2012	2,873	270 (9)	2,801	16 (1)	5,674	286 (5)
2013	1,267	111 (9)	1,202	8 (<1)	2,469	119 (5)
Total	**17,463**	**1,554 (9)**	**22,094**	**114 (<1)**	**39,557**	**1,668 (4)**

CDC

FIGURE **236-1** West Nile virus disease cases and deaths reported to the Centers for Disease Control and Prevention (CDC) by year and clinical presentation, 1999-2013. (From ArboNET, Arboviral Diseases Branch, CDC.)

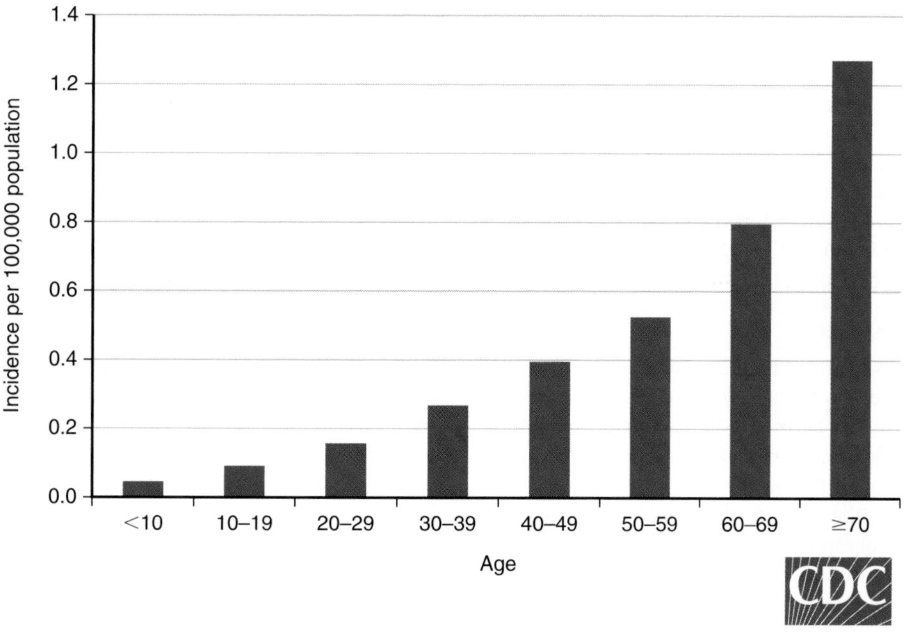

FIGURE 236-2 Average annual incidence of West Nile virus neuroinvasive disease reported to the Centers for Disease Control and Prevention (CDC) by age group, 1999-2013. (From ArboNET, Arboviral Diseases Branch, CDC.)

active surveillance is now recommended by the Centers for Disease Control and Prevention (CDC) to facilitate early warning of impending community outbreaks. *Culex* mosquitoes transmit the WNV to humans and horses, which are incidental hosts with low-level viremia of short duration (i.e., dead-end hosts). There has been no incidental human-to-human or other vertebrate-to-human transmission. However, transmission by transfusion, transplantation, laboratory inoculation, breast milk, hemodialysis, and in utero infection has occurred.[4] Most cases in North America have occurred in the late summer and early fall, in conjunction with high rates of mosquito WNV carriage. Children have high rates of infection but low rates of neuroinvasive disease, which is more likely to be aseptic meningitis as opposed to meningoencephalitis in adults.[5] Adults older than 65 years have higher mortality and 110 times the incidence of WNND compared with children[6] (Fig. 236-2).

CLINICAL PRESENTATION

As with SLE and JE viruses, most infection with WNV is asymptomatic. Serologic surveys indicate that only 20% of infected persons develop WNF, and less than 1% develop WNND.[7] Cases of neuroinvasive and non-neuroinvasive WNV reported to the CDC vary by year and state, but the total number of WNV infections can be estimated to be 50,000 annually (see Fig. 236-1).[3]

After an incubation period of 2 to 14 days, WNF is characterized by an influenza-like illness, fever, arthralgia, myalgia, rash, malaise, and headache. Gastrointestinal symptoms have included nausea, vomiting, and diarrhea. Generalized lymphadenopathy, splenomegaly, and hepatomegaly are common.[8] Rash appears early in 50% to 60% of cases and is a nonspecific maculopapular rash that most often begins on the trunk. Although WNV was confirmed serologically, the acute-phase serum tested negative at the time of rash in 57% of patients.[9] Convalescent serum is often needed to confirm the diagnosis in this early and nonspecific stage of illness.

Weakness is a prominent feature of WNF, and myelitis, caused by infection of motor anterior horn cells, may lead to AFP reminiscent of poliomyelitis.[10] As with poliovirus and more closely related JE and SLE viruses, a biphasic illness eventuates in aseptic meningitis (30%) and encephalitis (60%) as the second phase of illness after WNF.[6] Prominent findings in patients with encephalitis are movement disorders: tremor, parkinsonism, gait disturbances, myoclonus, and rarely seizure disorder. These motor disturbances appear early, have a pathophysiologic correlation with lesions seen on magnetic resonance imaging (MRI) in the basal ganglia and thalamus, and may resolve in ensuing months.[6] AFP can be recognized as progressive weakness, often asymmetric and suggestive of stroke, and loss of deep tendon reflexes. WNV infection is associated with Guillain-Barré syndrome (GBS), an autoimmune acute inflammatory demyelinating polyradiculopathy distinguished by preceding sensory paresthesias, symmetric ascending weakness, loss of deep tendon reflexes, and autonomic dysfunction (see Chapter 195). Sensory and autonomic nerve involvements are not seen with AFP. It is important to distinguish between AFP and GBS because AFP is associated with little long-term improvement but GBS is largely reversible over time.[7]

Aseptic (nonbacterial) meningitis and encephalitis commonly follow the symptoms of WNF by 4 to 7 days but may appear without a recognized prodrome as stiff neck (meningismus), headache, and sensitivity to light (photophobia). These symptoms may further proceed to encephalitis characterized by alterations in consciousness: lethargy, confusion, stupor, and coma. More focal encephalopathic signs include difficulty with word finding, speech, and memory, sometimes advancing to seizures, cranial neuropathy, upper motor neuron paralysis with hyperreflexia, and extensor plantar responses. The hypothalamic-pituitary axis may become involved and is associated with central nervous system–mediated fever, hyponatremia resulting from the syndrome of inappropriate antidiuretic hormone (SIADH), or diabetes insipidus (urinary water loss) caused by insufficient antidiuretic hormone.

Isolated acute febrile retinitis has recently been attributed to WNF. Fifty-two patients at a uveitis clinic had ocular symptoms after fever. Thirty-seven or 71% had at least two laboratory tests positive for WNV, and evaluation negative for other causes of retinitis. Visual acuity loss at final visit was common.[11]

PHYSICAL EXAMINATION

The general examination should include awareness of rash, arthritis, adenopathy, and splenomegaly. Photophobia is recognized by excessive reaction to bright light. Nuchal rigidity is recognized by passive flexing of the neck, which induces involuntary hip flexion (Brudzinski sign). More diffuse meningeal irritation is elicited by the Kernig sign: with hip flexed, attempts to extend the knee produce resistance and pain in the hamstring and back. Meningeal irritation in children may be recognized by tripoding, or sitting on the examination table supported by buttocks and both hands placed posterior, so as to maintain a rigid spine. Encephalitis is recognized by testing multiple areas of cognitive function, degree of alertness, speech, motor and sensory function, and cranial nerves. AFP may be recognized by abrupt onset of weakness and decreased deep tendon reflexes and may be distinguished from GBS by lack of autonomic or sensory nerve involvement.[7] Disease may progress rapidly, and frequently repeated examinations are required to assess the need for increasing levels of supportive care (Table 236-1).

DIAGNOSTICS

Serologic testing is the most effective method to confirm clinical suspicion of WNV infection. Enzyme-linked immunosorbent assay for detection of immunoglobulin M (IgM) in serum at 6 to 8 days or in cerebrospinal fluid (CSF) at 3 to 5 days is indicative of recent infection. Individuals recently infected with or vaccinated against related viruses, such as yellow fever, dengue fever, and JE, may have false-positive serologic results for WNV.[4] The problem of cross-reactivity with flaviviruses, including SLE virus circulating in the Northern Hemisphere, can be corrected by confirmatory testing with a plaque reduction neutralization assay. IgM antibody to WNV may persist for as long as 8 years after infection, which lessens the specificity of this test in serum and raises the possibility of persistant infection.[12] However, IgM does not cross the blood-brain barrier, and the presence of IgM in the CSF is strong evidence of local production and thus acute WNND infection.

Molecular amplification assays (e.g., polymerase chain reaction [PCR]) in serum are low yield (14%) because of the usually low levels and transient nature of viremia in acute infection of humans. PCR has moderate sensitivity (57%) for detection of WNV in CSF, but it disappears as CSF IgM antibody becomes positive. PCR is most useful in blood supply screening and active surveillance of bird and mosquito populations. Tissue samples from postmortem examinations may be tested by immunofluorescent antibody and viral culture.

Complete blood counts may be normal or moderately increased with a relative lymphocytosis, conversely, some patients may demonstrate lymphopenia. Hyponatremia may be indicative of SIADH, often seen with any encephalitis. The patient may have transaminitis consistent with a usually mild hepatitis. In such cases, serum amylase and lipase should be checked for concomitant pancreatitis. Muscle enzymes such as creatine kinase and myoglobin may be elevated to mild or severe degrees. Lumbar puncture should be performed and reveals a CSF pleocytosis in the range of cell counts often seen in aseptic meningitis (10 to 1000 cells/mm^3), with predominance of lymphocytes, mildly increased protein, and normal glucose concentration. There may be a predominance of neutrophils in early stages of encephalitis. Cerebral computed tomography (CT) findings are often normal. Cerebral MRI is more likely to reveal abnormalities such as enhancement of the leptomeninges or the periventricular areas, but it is diagnostic only of meningitis or encephalitis in general. MRI is the imaging procedure of choice, but it is possible to have clinical degrees of encephalitis without MRI abnormalities. T2-weighted images showing high-intensity signals in most commonly affected areas of the thalamus, basal ganglia, brainstem, and spinal cord may be early indications of encephalitis.[13]

Diagnostic tests for WNV are listed in Table 236-2.

TABLE 236-1 Type of Weakness Associated with WNV Infection Compared with Other Motor Neuron Diseases

Characteristic	AFP	GBS	WNV Weakness
Onset	With acute infection	1-8 weeks after infection	With acute infection
Fever	Present	Absent	Present
Leukocytosis	Present	Absent	Present
Distribution	Often asymmetric	Symmetric ascending	Generalized
Sensory	No sensory loss	Paresthesias, sensory loss	No sensory loss
Autonomic symptoms	No autonomic symptoms	Autonomic symptoms	No autonomic symptoms
Deep tendon reflex	Absent	Absent	Present
Central nervous system involvement	Encephalopathy common	Absent	Meningitis, encephalitis
Cerebrospinal fluid profile	Pleocytosis, protein elevated	No pleocytosis, protein elevated	Pleocytosis and protein if meningitis, encephalitis

TABLE 236-2 Diagnostic Tests for WNV

Diagnostic Test	Result
INITIAL DIAGNOSTICS	
Complete blood count with differential	Normal or moderately increased
Serum electrolytes, blood urea nitrogen, and creatinine	Fluid and electrolyte imbalance (e.g., hyponatremia [SIADH])
Liver function tests	Elevated transaminases
Amylase* and lipase*	Pancreatitis
CSF	Pleocytosis <1000 cells/mm^3, lymphocyte predominance Protein increased, but usually <100 mg/dL Glucose concentration normal
Serum or CSF IgM antibody	Positive: 50% on admission, 95% by day 10 of illness
Nucleic acid amplification (PCR)	Positive: 50% in CSF, but less in serum
IMAGING	
CT	Normal
MRI (preferred imaging technique)	Meningeal, periventricular, basal ganglia enhancement May be normal with clinical degrees of encephalitis

*If indicated.

DIFFERENTIAL DIAGNOSIS

Bacterial meningitis must quickly be distinguished from aseptic meningitis by a lumbar puncture, which identifies acute bacterial meningitis by a cell count of more than 1000 cells/mm^3, neutrophil predominance, and growth of common bacterial offenders. It is helpful clinically to distinguish between aseptic meningitis and encephalitis; but diagnostically, the same agents may affect both meninges and brain in varying degrees. Most causes of encephalitis are viral. Although the list is long, many viral causes of meningoencephalitis in North America are listed in the differential diagnosis box. Nonviral causes that should be considered include drug reactions, carcinomatous meningitis, vasculitis, Behçet syndrome, endocarditis, demyelinating diseases, postinfectious encephalitis, Lyme disease, leptospirosis, *Listeria*, cat-scratch disease, *Mycoplasma*, and various species of *Rickettsia*, *Ehrlichia*, and *Anaplasma*. Patients with acquired immunodeficiency syndrome (AIDS) have well-known opportunistic causes of encephalitis: toxoplasmosis, cytomegalovirus, mycobacteria, lymphoma, and progressive multifocal leukoencephalopathy (JC virus). Hypogammaglobulinemic patients may have encephalitis and myositis caused by chronic enterovirus infection. Patients with T-cell depletion, often from chemotherapy, exhibit unusual forms of encephalitis from various herpesviruses, inclusion body encephalitis from measles, and adenovirus.

Seasonal variation is helpful in identifying the arboviruses. Alphavirus, flavivirus, and bunyavirus groups are prevalent when mosquito vectors are active in late summer and early fall

DIFFERENTIAL DIAGNOSIS

Viral Causes of Acute Encephalomyelitis

ALPHAVIRUS
- Eastern equine
- Western equine
- Venezuelan equine

FLAVIVIRUS
- St. Louis
- West Nile
- Japanese
- Dengue
- Tick borne
- Yellow fever

BUNYAVIRUS
- Hepatitis A

ARENAVIRUS
- Lymphocytic choriomeningitis
- Machupo
- Lassa

REOVIRUS
- Colorado tick fever
- Rhabdovirus
- Rabies
- Lyssavirus species

FILOVIRUS
- Ebola
- Marburg

RETROVIRUS
- human immunodeficiency virus (HIV)

HERPESVIRUS
- Herpes simplex virus types 1 and 2
- Varicella-zoster virus
- Herpes B
- Cytomegalovirus
- Human herpesvirus 6
- Human herpesvirus 7
- Epstein-Barr virus

in North America. Tick vectors—TBE in Europe, analogous tick-borne Powassan viral encephalitis in North America, Lyme disease, and *Rickettsia*, *Ehrlichia*, and *Anaplasma* organisms—are active in late spring and early summer. Enteroviruses are a common cause of encephalitis in warm months, when fecal-oral and water spread is common, but enterovirus circulates at lower levels throughout the year. Herpesvirus infection and mumps occur more uniformly throughout the year. Lymphocytic choriomeningitis is most prevalent in late fall and winter, when rodents come into homes. Leptospirosis is most likely in summer, when rodents are about and urinating in bodies of water frequented by humans.

Geographic distribution and travel histories are important. The Flaviviridae viruses have distinct distribution patterns. WNV is now common in the Middle East, Eastern Europe, and North America and increasing in South America. Eastern equine encephalitis occurs in small outbreaks along the Atlantic and Gulf coasts and Great Lakes. SLE and La Crosse encephalitis occur in larger outbreaks, and they are now widely distributed in North America. The original names no longer reflect their present geographic distribution. TBE is found in the distribution of *Ixodes ricinus* and *Ixodes persulcatus* ticks in Eastern Europe and the adjoining Asian continent. JE manifests in large epidemics and is widespread over a third of the globe from Pakistan, India, Australia, and Asia to the eastern border of what once was the Union of Soviet Socialist Republics (USSR). Lyme disease encephalitis is concentrated in the Northeast and North Central/Midwest United States and in Europe.

MANAGEMENT

There is no specific antiviral drug for WNV infection, and treatment is supportive. All patients should be hospitalized and lumbar puncture performed to discern treatable bacterial meningitis, to rule out other treatable causes of encephalitis such as herpesvirus encephalitis, and to observe for progression of encephalitis and AFP. Prolonged periods of unconsciousness may be followed by remarkable periods of recovery, and the health care provider must ensure management of ventilators, bladder catheters, nutrition, intravenous lines, decubitus ulcers, aspiration pneumonia, urinary tract infection, line sepsis, venous thromboembolism, and seizures. Although steroids and osmotic agents have not been studied as adjunctive therapy, they may be used to manage acute cerebral edema. Ribavirin and interferon alfa showed limited effect against WNV in animal models and case reports, but a retrospective review of ribavirin use in Israel showed no effect on mortality and their use is currently not recommended.[14] Passive immunization with pooled human intravenous immune globulin (IVIG) was hypothesized to offer some cross-reacting antibodies from circulating antibody to WNV in North America. Studies in mice have shown pooled IVIG to have prophylactic and therapeutic efficacy. However, a phase I/II clinical trial of IVIG containing antibodies to WNV (Omr-IgG-am) for patients with WNV infection is complete and outcomes were not improved.[6]

LIFE SPAN CONSIDERATIONS

Most cases of WNV are asymptomatic; however, WNV causes encephalitis and paralytic syndromes much more commonly in elder patients, and meningitis more commonly in children. Most severe complications and deaths occur in elder or immunocompromised individuals.

There is often persistence of WNV-specific IgM antibody in cases of encephalitis, and persistence of WNV can be found in brain tissue in mice and monkey models of infection.[15,16] A cohort of patients with encephalitis detected WNV RNA in the urine of 5 of 20 patients 1.6 to 6.7 years into convalescence.[16,17] Individuals may have chronic symptoms or atypical progression,[18] which could be explained by persistent infection.

COMPLICATIONS

In addition to the chronic sequelae of severe encephalitis mentioned before, WNV may infect certain organ systems in a selective manner. Arthritis and myalgias are common, but frank myositis, with high serum myoglobin levels, may eventuate in rhabdomyolysis, and acute renal failure may ensue. Cardiomyopathy may be a further consequence of WNV predilection for muscle. As in other flavivirus-induced conditions, infection of the liver manifests as transaminitis, and progression to fulminant hepatitis has occurred. Pancreatitis may reflect infection of the pancreas and pancreatic duct. Acute pathologic conditions in the hypothalamic-pituitary axis may result in central hyperthermia, SIADH with hyponatremia, and diabetes insipidus. Acute myelitis causes AFP, which is often asymmetric and irreversible.[3] Basal ganglia pathologic conditions are reflected in chronic tremor, myoclonus, parkinsonism, and gait disturbances.[6]

Multifocal chorioretinitis is increasingly recognized as an ophthalmologic manifestation of WNV infection, but anterior uveitis, occlusive retinal vasculitis, and optic neuritis have all been reported.[3] Chorioretinitis occurs early in the course of WNF, and most patients have no ocular symptoms or have mildly reduced vision. The value of chorioretinitis as a specific marker of WNV was recognized early in the epidemic and is most common in patients with meningoencephalitis.[6]

Infection during pregnancy has generally favorable outcomes, although one in utero infection resulted in birth at 38 weeks' gestation of an infant with bilateral chorioretinitis and marked destruction of cerebral white matter. Birth outcomes after in utero infections in 72 pregnancies were investigated in 2003 and 2004. Seven had malformations, but none had conclusive evidence of a WNV cause, and only three had WNV infection during the time frame of organ development.[19]

INDICATIONS FOR REFERRAL OR HOSPITALIZATION

Patients with diagnosed WNF may be monitored in the primary care setting, but all patients with suspected WNND should be admitted to a hospital, where a lumbar puncture and MRI can be performed. Meningitis and encephalitis have nonspecific presentations, and an infectious disease expert should be consulted immediately to aid in differential diagnosis and to consider empirical treatment of bacterial meningitis or herpesvirus encephalitis pending confirmation of a specific diagnosis.

Patients need close monitoring for progression of encephalitis to stages of stupor and coma, at which point they should be in an intensive care unit, where a team from nursing, critical care, and pulmonary medicine will monitor for aspiration, airway protection, ventilator support, intravenous fluids, deep venous thrombosis, pulmonary embolism, and skin breakdown. A nutrition team may need to manage a long course of hyperalimentation. AFP may result in paralysis of respiratory muscles and need for various degrees of long-term respiratory support. Even without AFP, intensive physical and occupational therapy may be required because of chronic weakness from encephalopathy, tremor, Parkinsonism, and gait disturbances secondary to basal ganglia disease. Speech therapy may be needed to manage aspiration and speech issues. Depression is common and may have a physiologic origin in encephalitis, which will require psychiatric consultation and antidepressants before postencephalitis rehabilitation strategies can progress. A neuropsychologist may be required to perform more formal testing of cognitive function (see Chapter 188). Chaplain services and alternative spiritual leaders should be welcome.

Recovery from encephalitis and sequelae takes months to years, but higher levels of function may eventually ensue, and remarkable recoveries over time have occurred. Long-term rehabilitation care may be rewarding. Severely compromised patients, especially those with severe cognitive dysfunction, inability to eat, or inadequate airway protection, may not make a meaningful recovery, and withdrawal of support can be an option, with help from family, nurses, physicians, and chaplains and other spiritual leaders.

HEALTH PROMOTION

WNV is a disease for which an ounce of prevention is worth a ton of cure. Mosquito control and bite reduction can be accomplished individually and in coordination with regional vector control programs when an outbreak is imminent. Each of us should eliminate mosquito larva breeding sites, such as standing water in birdbaths, flowerpots, construction sites, and swimming pool covers. Insect repellents containing DEET (diethyltoluamide) in high concentrations (20%) are applied to skin. The insecticide permethrin is applied to clothing, mosquito nets, and tents. The combination of DEET on skin and permethrin on clothes is better than either agent used alone.

Watch for allergic skin reactions to DEET. Toxic encephalopathy may occur in young children, and DEET should not be used for children younger than 2 months. Older children, younger than 10 years, may use concentrations of DEET up to 10%. Avon Skin-So-Soft and citronella products are much less effective, so long-sleeved shirts, long pants, clothing insecticides, and mosquito nets should be the mainstay in young children. Avoid dusk and dawn exposure to mosquitoes because this is their preferred feeding time.[20]

Screening of the U.S. blood supply has been in effect since June 2003. This has greatly reduced but not eliminated the risk of blood product transmission, and it is estimated that screening for WNV is more cost-effective than screening for hepatitis C virus or human immunodeficiency virus (HIV).[21]

Although there is a vaccine for horses and human vaccine has been successfully tested in phase II trials, phase III testing is dependent on the next outbreak of WNV. A live attenuated chimeric vaccine, ChimeriVax-WN02, contains genetic material from WNV in a yellow fever virus vector.[22] Health care providers need to be aware of the clinical signs of WNF and WNND, including meningitis, encephalitis, and AFP, and patient guides for mosquito protection do exist (www.cdc.gov/ncidod/dvbid/westnile/repellentupdates.htm). The Kansas Department of Health implemented an extensive WNV education campaign, but follow-up evaluation demonstrated that media messages were not reaching targeted populations, and risk perception remained low.[23] Awareness of the dangers of mosquito and tick exposure, the diseases they transmit, protective measures, and early signs of specific disease is an educational goal, especially for those giving travel advice.[24]

REFERENCES

For a full list of references, scan the QR code or visit http://booksite.elsevier.com/9780323355018

PART 21

Evaluation and Management of Hematologic Disorders

CHAPTER 237

ANEMIA

Margaret M. Sennett

DEFINITION AND EPIDEMIOLOGY

Anemia is not a disease but rather a sign or symptom of an underlying disorder. Anemia is defined as a reduction in the number of red blood cells (RBCs), hemoglobin concentration, or hematocrit. In general, a hemoglobin concentration in adults below 13.6 g/dL for men or below 12 g/dL for women suggests anemia.[1] Although certain signs and symptoms are sometimes associated with anemia, the diagnosis is often based on laboratory data alone.

As one of the most common hematologic diagnoses, anemia affects people of every age group. Some types of anemia have a higher incidence in certain races and ethnicities. For example, sickle cell disease is most common in those of African ancestry, and thalassemia in people from the geographic regions of the Mediterranean, the Middle East, Southeast Asia, and parts of India and Pakistan.

PATHOPHYSIOLOGY

Anemia is a condition in which too little oxygen is being transported to the tissues. Inadequate supplies of oxygen in the tissues produce the symptoms of anemia. There are many types of anemia with a variety of different causes. Grouping them into the categories of (1) RBC production disorders, (2) RBC destruction disorders, and (3) anemia from blood loss enables a clear understanding of the pathophysiology of this disease.

Red Blood Cell Production Disorders

Erythropoiesis, the production of erythrocytes (RBCs), is limited to the axial skeleton and proximal ends of the long bones in the adult. The marrow is a special environment for hematopoietic development and consists of a matrix of reticular cells and fibers called the marrow stroma. It is here that stem cells are stimulated by colony-stimulating factors to grow and differentiate into the various blood cells including RBCs.[2]

The most common disorder related to inadequate RBC production is iron deficiency anemia (IDA; see later). Iron is critical for both erythrocyte proliferation and maturation and for hemoglobin synthesis. Under normal conditions, the turnover rate for erythrocytes is approximately 1% per day and erythrocytes survive 120 ± 20 days. Although, in response to hypoxia and anemia, marrow precursors may be seen in 2 to 3 days, an increase in the reticulocyte count will take several more days.[3] The most important factor in the body's ability to increase RBC production is iron. Without adequate iron stores, the marrow cannot increase erythropoiesis.[4]

Anemia of chronic kidney disease (ACKD) is also a result of inadequate RBC production. Erythropoietin is a glycoprotein hormone secreted by the kidney that induces erythroid precursor cells to differentiate, thereby increasing new RBC production. The control of erythropoiesis is dominated by the decreased concentration of hemoglobin in the blood. This leads to changes in tissue oxygen tension and in turn triggers receptors within the kidney to secrete erythropoietin. Chronic kidney disease can result in an undersecretion of erythropoietin, thereby suppressing an essential signal triggering RBC production.[4,5]

Other types of anemia caused by defects in RBC production include vitamin B_{12} and folate deficiency, anemia of chronic disease (ACD), and aplastic anemia, which is a result of bone marrow stem cell failure.[5]

Red Blood Cell Destruction Disorders

The mechanisms involved in the increased hemolysis or destruction of RBCs resulting in anemia include various hemoglobin disorders such as sickle cell anemia and thalassemia; RBC membrane defects as in hereditary spherocytosis and hereditary elliptocytosis; RBC enzyme defects as in glucose-6-phosphate dehydrogenase (G6PD) deficiency; and finally, autoimmune antibody production as seen in autoimmune hemolytic anemia.

Blood Loss

Acute blood loss resulting from situations such as trauma or severe menorrhagia may result in life-threatening anemia with significant symptoms of hemodynamic cardiovascular compromise. Anemia symptoms resulting from mild to moderate menorrhagia, chronic microscopic hematuria, or chronic occult gastrointestinal (GI) bleeding can be much more insidious because the body compensates for this type of slowly evolving anemia.

CLINICAL PRESENTATION

The presentation of anemia can be variable, depending on the acuteness of onset and the ability of the cardiopulmonary system to compensate. If the patient is healthy and the onset of anemia is gradual, there are few signs or symptoms until the hemoglobin value falls below 7.5 g/dL.[6] Patients may initially experience fatigue, malaise, headache, dyspnea, irritability, and a mild decrease in exercise tolerance. Further declines in hemoglobin concentration may be associated with a markedly reduced exercise capacity, resting tachycardia, and dyspnea requiring supplemental oxygen. Other nonspecific findings that can accompany long-term, moderate to severe anemia include wide pulse pressure, midsystolic or pansystolic murmur, confusion, lethargy, brittle nails, glossitis, angular cheilitis, and spoon-shaped nails.[4] Pallor of the mucous membranes, lips, conjunctivae, nail beds, and palmar creases is a common sign of anemia. When palmar creases are as pale as the surrounding skin, the patient usually has a hemoglobin value of less than 7 g/dL.[6]

PHYSICAL EXAMINATION

A head to toe physical examination is warranted in the evaluation of a patient with anemia. Overall appearance suggestive of decreased stamina and energy could suggest fatigue secondary to anemia, or anemia related to another chronic illness. A thorough cardiopulmonary examination including vital signs is essential. Increased heart or respiratory rate or the presence of a systolic murmur may be related to anemia. Special attention should be paid to characteristics of the integumentary system to evaluate for pallor, nail integrity, and signs of angular cheilitis. Also, symptoms of increased bruising may be a clue to a potential bleeding disorder contributing to blood loss and iron deficiency.

DIAGNOSTICS

Diagnostic evaluation of anemia initially should include a complete blood count (CBC) including platelet count, white cell differential, RBC morphology, reticulocyte count, and a peripheral blood smear. Evaluation of all blood cell lines is essential to confirm a sole anemia diagnosis, as opposed to a primary bone marrow disease such as aplastic anemia or an infiltrative process such as leukemia. Of the multiple indexes noted on a CBC report, the mean corpuscular volume (MCV) is the single most useful. Describing RBCs as microcytic, normocytic, or macrocytic based on the MCV determines what other testing is necessary to determine the cause of the anemia.

The reticulocyte count is the most easily accessible method of evaluating bone marrow production of RBCs (a direct bone marrow examination requires an invasive procedure). The reticulocyte count provides an assessment of whether the causative factor of anemia is related to either decreased production or increased loss. A normal reticulocyte count is 0.5% to 1.5% of the total RBCs. A normal absolute reticulocyte count (ARC) is 25,000 to 75,000/μL. Any value higher than 100,000/μL is considered a marrow that is responding normally to anemic conditions. Values below 75,000/μL are considered consistent with impaired (decreased) RBC production.[4] However, if reticulocytosis is associated with anemia, hemolysis needs to be ruled out by observing for hyperbilirubinemia (marker of hemoglobin catabolism) and increased serum lactate dehydrogenase (LDH), which is indicative of direct cellular injury. Also, a low serum haptoglobin value is a sign of intravascular hemolysis because haptoglobin binds the free hemoglobin that is released into the circulation as erythrocytes rupture. These hemoglobin-haptoglobin complexes are removed from the circulation by the reticuloendothelial system. Hemolytic anemias are complex to evaluate and diagnose; if they are suspected, referral should be made to a hematologist. A low reticulocyte count with anemia points to impaired erythropoiesis indicating a reduction in RBC precursors or ineffective production. Ineffective production is reported as erythroid hyperplasia on the bone marrow biopsy and aspiration report. This means the RBCs are being produced but are not viable and usually do not leave the marrow. Box 237-1 identifies conditions associated with either reticulocytosis or a decreased reticulocyte count.

A peripheral blood smear is critical in the evaluation of anemias. RBC size and shape variations as well as abnormal cell populations too small to change the indexes can be directly visualized. For example, as iron deficiency progresses, microcytic cells are noted on the smear long before the indexes change. Evidence of hemolysis as well as abnormal shaped cells (such as sickle shape or spherocytes) on the smear may offer additional clues as to the cause of the anemia.

BOX 237-1

Conditions That Can Influence Reticulocyte Counts

INCREASED RETICULOCYTE COUNTS

Hemolytic anemia
- Autoimmune hemolysis
- RBC enzyme deficiencies
- Traumatic or microangiopathic hemolysis
- RBC membrane problems (hereditary spherocytosis and elliptocytosis)

Three to 4 days after acute blood loss
Hemoglobinopathies
Toxin exposures
Hypersplenism
After treatment of anemias
- After adequate doses of iron to treat iron deficiency anemia
- After adequate doses of folate or vitamin B_{12} to correct a megaloblastic anemia

DECREASED RETICULOCYTE COUNTS

Iron deficiency anemia
Aplastic anemia
Untreated megaloblastic anemia
Radiotherapy
Marrow tumors
Myelodysplastic syndromes

Hemoglobin electrophoresis allows hemoglobin chains to be separated according to differences in the charges of their subunits. It is essential for accurate diagnosis of thalassemias and hemoglobinopathies.

Evaluation of the body's iron stores includes serum ferritin, serum iron, total iron-binding capacity (TIBC), and transferrin saturation percentage. The serum ferritin level reflects total body iron stores. It is the first laboratory value to become abnormal when iron stores are becoming depleted, even before IDA is reflected in RBC morphology. Ferritin concentrations less than 12 ng/mL indicate absence of iron stores. It is important to remember, however, that ferritin is an acute-phase reactant and may be elevated as a result of inflammation. Inflammation causes the release of tissue ferritins resulting from damage to the liver and other ferritin-rich tissues.[7] Serum ferritin levels are low in IDA and normal or elevated in ACD. Serum ferritin is also elevated in conditions unrelated to anemia, such as iron overload (either transfusion dependent or hereditary hemochromatosis), inflammatory disorders, and alcoholism.

The serum iron concentration reflects the amount of iron bound to transferrin, a plasma carrier protein that regulates iron transport in the blood. Normal values for serum iron are 65 to 165 μg/dL.[7] Transferrin is the transport protein for iron and is measured indirectly by the TIBC. The TIBC indicates the availability of binding sites on the protein for iron transport. Normal values for TIBC are 300 to 360 μg/dL.[7]

The percentage of transferrin saturation can be calculated from the TIBC and the serum iron values as follows:

$$\frac{\text{Serum iron}}{\text{TIBC}} \times 100$$

Normal values for percentage of transferrin saturation are 20% to 50%.[7]

Physician consultation is recommended for hemoglobin values of less than 10 g/dL in patients with known coronary artery disease and for any patient with postural vital sign changes or active bleeding. Physician consultation is also recommended for sickle cell crises, suspected aplastic anemia, or hemolytic anemia.

DIAGNOSTICS

Anemias

LABORATORY
CBC and differential
Peripheral smear
Reticulocyte count
Ferritin
TIBC*
Transferrin*
Serum iron*
Stool for occult blood × 3*
Hemoglobin electrophoresis*
Folate*
Vitamin B_{12}*
LFTs*
Thyroid function tests*
BUN*
Creatinine*
G6PD assay*
Erythropoietin level*
Serum homocysteine*
Methylmalonic acid*
Coombs direct and indirect tests*

OTHER DIAGNOSTICS
Bone marrow biopsy*

*If indicated.
BUN, blood urea nitrogen; LFTs, liver function tests.

DIFFERENTIAL DIAGNOSIS

Anemias are generally divided into three categories based on the size of the RBCs suggesting the underlying condition or disease. RBCs are normally uniform in size and shape, and deviations in their appearance can suggest a specific cause for the anemia. The degree of anisocytosis (variation in RBC size) is determined by looking at the RBC indexes on the CBC and at cell morphology on the peripheral smear. The most useful RBC index is the MCV. The MCV is a direct measurement averaging the RBC sizes in the sample. The RBC distribution width (RDW) is an indirect measurement that indicates the degree of homogeneity of the sample. For example, uniformly small RBCs will have a low MCV and a normal RDW, whereas a sample with mostly small RBCs but some normal RBCs can have a low MCV with an increased RDW, reflecting the heterogeneity of the sample. Based on the MCV, anemias are classified as microcytic (MCV <80 fL), normocytic (MCV 80 to 99 fL), or macrocytic (MCV >100 fL).[4] Variations in RBC shape (poikilocytosis) provide important diagnostic clues and in fact are often pathognomonic of underlying disease. Box 237-2 classifies commonly seen hematologic disorders according to RBC morphology.

BOX 237-2

Classification of Anemias Based on Red Blood Cell Morphology

SIZE

Microcytic (MCV <80 fL)
- Iron deficiency
- Thalassemia
- Anemia of chronic disease (occasionally)
- Sideroblastic anemia
- Hemoglobin E disease

Macrocytic (MCV >100 fL)
- Megaloblastic anemia (vitamin B_{12} or folate deficiency)

Normocytic (MCV 80-99 fL)
- Sickle cell disease
- Anemia of chronic disease
- Aplastic anemia
- Hemolytic anemias

SHAPE

Sickle
- Sickle cell disease

Targets
- Thalassemias
- Hemoglobin C
- Hemoglobin E

Spherocytes
- Hereditary spherocytosis
- Immune hemolysis

Elliptocytes
- Hereditary elliptocytosis

MICROCYTIC ANEMIA

IRON DEFICIENCY ANEMIA

IDA is the most common type of anemia in the world and the most common nutrient deficiency. In the adult population, IDA predominantly affects women of reproductive age and older adults. The most common cause is chronic blood loss, especially GI blood loss or menorrhagia.[4] Chronic GI blood losses should be suspected as a cause of IDA in adult men and postmenopausal women. Inadequate nutrition and increased requirements for iron are the principal causes of IDA in children and pregnant women. Box 237-3 lists additional causes of iron deficiency. The worldwide prevalence of anemia in pregnant women is 38%, and more than 50% of that is a result of iron deficiency. Daily prenatal use of iron has demonstrated improvement in maternal hemoglobin concentration and reduction in risk of having low-birth-weight babies.[8]

PATHOPHYSIOLOGY

Iron is an essential nutrient present in all living cells. The human body contains about 3 to 4 g of iron, with more than 70% contained within hemoglobin. The remainder of the body's iron is stored in the liver and marrow as ferritin and hemosiderin, and a small amount is bound to transferrin in the blood.[3] The normal man has a total body iron content of about 4000 mg. Women of childbearing age have about 2000 mg of total body iron, a significantly lower amount because of menstrual blood loss and lower dietary intake. The average adult normally loses approximately 1 mg of iron each day through the natural process of desquamation of cells from the skin, GI tract, and

BOX 237-3

Causes of Iron Deficiency

CONDITIONS LEADING TO MILD IRON DEFICIENCY*

Inadequate diet
Normal or heavy menses
Blood donation
Malabsorption
- Partial gastrectomy
- Malabsorption syndromes

Increased requirements
- Infancy and adolescence (periods of rapid growth)
- Pregnancy

Polycythemia vera treated with phlebotomy

CONDITIONS ASSOCIATED WITH MODERATE TO SEVERE IRON DEFICIENCY

Chronic blood loss
- GI conditions

Peptic ulcer disease
Varices
Malignant disease
Diverticulitis
- Severe menorrhagia

Severe malabsorption
- Gastrectomy
- Sprue and other malabsorption syndromes

*Usually no associated symptoms.

BOX 237-4

Factors That Influence Iron Absorption

SUBSTANCES THAT INHIBIT ABSORPTION

Soy protein
Bran
Dairy products
Tea and coffee
Calcium-rich antacids
Vegetable sources

SUBSTANCES THAT ENHANCE ABSORPTION

Ascorbic acid (vitamin C)
Citric acid
Meat, poultry, and fish sources
Other factors
- Low iron stores of individual
- Low iron content of meal

urinary tract. The adult woman loses an additional 1 mg through normal menstruation.

The recommended daily allowance of iron is 15 mg/day in the diet of nonpregnant women and 30 mg/day for pregnant women. Dietary iron is absorbed in the duodenum of the small intestine. The amount of iron absorbed from the intestine is determined by several factors, including the iron content of the meal, the form of iron being ingested, the individual's iron status, and the presence or absence of other substances that can enhance or inhibit iron absorption (Box 237-4).[9]

BOX 237-5

Laboratory Studies in IDA

- Hemoglobin: slight decrease to marked decrease
- Serum iron: decreased
- TIBC: increased
- Percentage of transferrin saturation: decreased (<10% in severe IDA)
- Serum ferritin: decreased

When iron requirements increase or intake declines, the small intestine increases absorption of iron to meet the increased demand. If there is no additional supply of iron to meet this increased demand, the body's iron stores begin to be depleted. At this point, several hematologic parameters are affected. The ferritin levels decline as body iron stores decrease. As body iron stores are depleted, the transferrin saturation decreases, leading to a reduced supply of iron to the RBC precursors, resulting in impaired (iron-deficient) erythropoiesis. At this stage, however, an overt microcytic anemia may not yet be present. Once the iron stores are truly depleted and no iron is available for erythropoiesis, an overt microcytic, hypochromic anemia is present, which manifests in the CBC by a low hemoglobin concentration. The RBC indexes are the last to change (decreased MCV, mean corpuscular hemoglobin [MCH], and mean corpuscular hemoglobin concentration [MCHC]). The peripheral smear will show hypochromia, microcytosis, mild anisocytosis, and poikilocytosis. Iron studies will show a low ferritin level and high TIBC.

CLINICAL PRESENTATION

Mild to moderate iron-deficient states are not associated with any clinical symptoms. Patients with severe IDA exhibit the same signs and symptoms of any type of severe anemia. Patients may complain of fatigue, decreased exercise tolerance, weakness, palpitations, irritability, and headaches. Complaints that are specifically related to iron store depletion include paresthesias, sore tongue, brittle nails, spoon-shaped nails (koilonychia), and pica for starch, ice, or clay.[5] In fact, a craving for ice (pagophagia) is a common symptom of women with IDA for unknown reasons.

PHYSICAL EXAMINATION

As the severity of the anemia increases, several physical changes may become evident. The patient may demonstrate a more forceful apical pulse, tachycardia with exertion, and a systolic flow murmur. Patients may also demonstrate pallor of the conjunctiva, mucous membranes, nail beds, and palmar creases. The characteristic spooning of the nails may also be present. In the older adult, signs of congestive heart failure may be present.

DIAGNOSTICS

IDA is commonly discovered incidentally during a routine CBC. Once IDA is diagnosed, the history may reveal factors that would cause iron deficiency, such as a recent hemorrhage, GI bleeding, menorrhagia, multiple pregnancies, or inadequate nutrition. Iron studies reveal a low serum iron level, decreased serum ferritin, increased TIBC, and decreased percentage of transferrin saturation (Box 237-5). Laboratory changes occur gradually as the iron stores are depleted. The earliest laboratory change is a fall in serum ferritin, reflecting depletion of iron stores. This change is followed by a decrease in serum iron and an increase in transferrin, producing a reduction in the percentage of transferrin saturation to less than 15% (this will drop below 10% as the severity progresses) and an associated increase in TIBC. The first change in the CBC is a drop in hemoglobin. Only with increasing severity and duration do the RBCs become microcytic and hypochromic.

The underlying cause of the iron deficiency must be identified. Blood loss by GI bleeding or repeated voluntary blood donation should be suspected until proven otherwise. Older adults with suspected IDA should be thoroughly evaluated for GI cancers, GI bleeding on the basis of nonsteroidal anti-inflammatory drug (NSAID) use, and alcohol abuse.

DIFFERENTIAL DIAGNOSIS

Only a few diseases need to be considered in the differential diagnosis of a microcytic hypochromic anemia. The thalassemias typically have a moderate to severe microcytosis with varying degrees of anemia but normal iron studies.

ACD presents a more common diagnostic dilemma. With long-standing chronic inflammatory illnesses such as rheumatoid arthritis, the defective iron supply can result in severe microcytic hypochromic anemia. Iron studies, especially the serum ferritin level, usually differentiate among true IDA, ACD, and thalassemia (Table 237-1). Both IDA and ACD are associated with low serum iron levels. The ferritin level is normal or increased in ACD and decreased in IDA. The TIBC is normal or low in ACD and increased in IDA.

Microcytosis can occur in patients with inherited sideroblastic anemias; however, these anemias are rare and are related to X-linked genes. Acquired sideroblastic anemias (idiopathic, secondary to drug or toxin exposure, myeloproliferative or myelodysplastic disease) can be microcytic but generally are macrocytic. These conditions are caused by defects in heme synthesis leading to accumulation of iron within bone marrow erythroid precursors and resulting in abnormal erythroid maturation. This anemia is characterized by ringed sideroblasts (erythroblasts with one third or more of the nucleus surrounded by ferritin deposits).[3] A bone marrow examination is necessary for diagnosis. The anemia tends to be severe (hemoglobin concentration of 6 g/dL) to moderate (hemoglobin concentration of 8 to 10 g/dL). Treatment of sideroblastic anemia consists of chronic transfusions and iron chelation therapy (to prevent or to treat the transfusion-dependent iron overload). Pyridoxine (vitamin B_6) therapy may sometimes partially correct the anemia in patients with hereditary sideroblastic anemia, leaving them with a milder anemia that does not require as many chronic transfusions.

DIFFERENTIAL DIAGNOSIS

Microcytic Anemia

- IDA
- Thalassemia
- ACD
- Sideroblastic anemia
- Lead poisoning, aluminum toxicity

MANAGEMENT

Treatment of IDA usually begins with an oral iron preparation. The usual adult therapeutic dose is 150 to 200 mg of elemental iron per day in divided doses until anemia is corrected. The pediatric dosing is 3 mg of elemental iron per kilogram, and liquid preparations are available. Administration should be continued empirically for 4 to 6 months or until the serum ferritin level exceeds 50 µg/L and then stopped. Common side effects of iron preparations are nausea, constipation, heartburn, upper GI discomfort, black stools, and diarrhea. Iron absorption is optimum when iron is taken 30 minutes before meals with ascorbic acid. Absorption can be reduced by as much as 40% to 50% if it is taken with meals; however, iron on an empty stomach can cause more side effects, leading to noncompliance with medication. GI upset, the most common side effect, may be avoided by starting with a single pill per day and slowly increasing to the recommended dose.

Once an adequate dose of iron is reached, changes in the hematologic markers should be seen in just a few weeks. The hemoglobin level should begin to rise within 1 to 2 weeks.

TABLE 237-1 Laboratory Values in Microcytic Anemias

Anemia	Hemoglobin*	MCV	MCHC	Serum Iron†	Serum Ferritin‡	TIBC§	Transferrin Saturation‖
Iron deficiency							
Early	N	N	N	N	N	N	N
Intermediate	N	N	N	↓/N	↓	High N	↓
Late	↓	↓	↓	↓	↓	↑	↓
Thalassemia minor	Low N/↓	↓	N/↓	N	N/≠	N	N
Chronic disease	Low N	N/↓	N/↓	↓	↑	↓	↑
Sideroblastic anemia	↓	↓	↓	↑	↑	N	↑

*N = 12-16 g/dL for women; 13.5-17.5 g/dL for men.
†N = 65-165 µg/dL for women; 75-175 µg/dL for men.
‡N = 12-150 µg/dL for women; 15-300 µg/dL for men.
§N = 240-450 µg/dL.
‖N = 20%-50%.
N, normal.

The MCV should correct within 1 to 2 months, reflecting the normalization of the erythrocyte size. Supplementation with oral iron should continue until the anemia is corrected, and until the underlying cause of the deficiency is corrected, or indefinitely if the cause of the deficiency is chronic.

If the anemia is severe, the patient has an iron malabsorption problem, or oral iron is not tolerated, replacement should be by parenteral (intramuscular or intravenous) administration of iron. Patients should be referred to a hematologist for intravenous administration of iron because it has traditionally been associated with adverse reactions. There are newer intravenous iron formulations (iron carboxymaltose and ferumoxytol) that appear to have a much safer profile. The novel structures of these preparations have been shown to reduce the risk of free iron reactions and result in lower immunogenicity. As a result, test doses are not necessary and much higher doses can be administered, thereby reducing the number of administrations necessary to replace iron stores.[10]

LIFE SPAN CONSIDERATIONS

Children require adequate iron intake to meet the increased demands of rapid growth. Nutritional iron deficits are especially common in children with excessive milk consumption at the expense of adequate intake of iron rich foods.

Teenage girls often become iron deficient as a result of menstrual blood loss, sometimes accompanied by poor diet in this age group.

Iron supplementation during pregnancy is almost always required. Pregnancy places a greater demand on iron stores, especially during the last two trimesters. The additional iron is needed to cover the needs of the developing fetus and placenta and to accommodate the increase in erythrocyte mass that normally occurs during the later stages of pregnancy. Many women enter pregnancy with inadequate iron reserves as a result of prepregnancy menstruation. Iron studies can be difficult to interpret in pregnancy because of the hemodilutional effects of the increase in blood volume during pregnancy, as well as the elevation of ferritin as an acute-phase reaction to the known inflammatory effects of pregnancy. Adequate maternal iron stores are essential to adequate brain development in the fetus.[11]

Older adults with suspected IDA should be thoroughly evaluated for GI cancers, even when their stools are negative for occult blood. Next to chronic disease, iron deficiency is the most common cause of a microcytic anemia in older adults.

COMPLICATIONS

Untreated IDA is especially worrisome during pregnancy. IDA may be associated with preterm delivery, low birth weight, and learning deficits. Untreated iron deficiency in all age groups can lead to severe anemia and may be associated with fatigue, falls, and cardiovascular compromise.

INDICATIONS FOR REFERRAL OR HOSPITALIZATION

Most patients with IDA are diagnosed and treated by their primary health care providers. Patients who are referred to a hematologist for any of the aforementioned reasons are generally referred back to the primary health care provider once the anemia has been corrected, or at least once an accurate diagnosis has been made and the patient is receiving stable iron replacement therapy.

Referral to a hematologist should be considered for the following reasons: nonadherence to or intolerance of oral iron replacement, persistent IDA necessitating parenteral iron therapy, and persistent microcytic anemia despite iron replacement and the exclusion of other conditions.

Other referrals may be required as evaluation for the cause of the iron deficiency progresses, such as referral to an internist or gastroenterologist to exclude GI blood loss or referral to an oncologist to treat any malignant neoplasms (either GI or gynecologic). Women of reproductive age may require referral to a gynecologist or a hematologist for evaluation of severe menorrhagia (the hematology referral may be helpful to rule out von Willebrand disease as a cause of the menorrhagia).

Healthy patients with IDA do not require hospitalization. Patients who are unable to adequately compensate for severe anemia may require hospitalization for cardiac or respiratory compromise that may occur.

PATIENT AND FAMILY EDUCATION

Patients should receive education about the use of iron supplements to ensure adequate treatment and an understanding of the prescribed regimen. Maximum absorption of iron occurs if it is ingested 30 minutes before meals. Substances that can enhance or inhibit iron absorption are listed in Box 237-4. Calcium can significantly inhibit iron absorption. Multivitamins with calcium or dairy products should be taken 1 to 2 hours after an iron supplement. Ascorbic acid may enhance absorption of iron; therefore, concurrent ingestion of foods rich in vitamin C, such as orange juice, should be encouraged.

Numerous iron supplementation preparations are on the market (Table 237-2), some with combinations of iron plus stool softeners, slow-release iron, or iron plus vitamin C. Patients who are intolerant of one preparation may find another that produces fewer or no side effects. The health care provider should therefore encourage patients to try various preparations before recommending parenteral iron.

HEALTH PROMOTION

Nutritional counseling is an important strategy to prevent further episodes of IDA and should include assessment of the patient's dietary intake. Assessment should also include the quantity and timing of iron ingestion and other substances that

TABLE 237-2 Common Iron Supplement Preparations

Preparation	Usual Dose	Amount of Elemental Iron in Dose (mg)
Ferrous sulfate		
Feosol	200 mg, 1-2 daily	65
Slow Fe	160 mg, 1-2 daily	50
Ferrous gluconate	324 mg 3 times a day	36
Polysaccharide-iron complex (Niferex)	150 mg, 1-2 tablets daily	150
Ferrous fumarate	150 mg, 1-2 tablets daily	50
Intravenous (Venofer) and intravenous or intramuscular (INFeD) preparations are also available.		

can interfere with iron absorption, such as tea, coffee, chocolate, dairy products, alcohol, and high-fiber foods. Strict vegetarians who rely on vegetable sources of iron instead of animal sources should be encouraged to supplement their diets with iron-fortified vitamins or to add iron-fortified foods to their diet. Patients whose IDA is secondary to other conditions should be encouraged to seek appropriate medical care.

THALASSEMIA

DEFINITION AND EPIDEMIOLOGY

Thalassemia is not a single disorder but rather a group of inherited blood disorders caused by variant or missing genes that affect how the body makes hemoglobin. The resulting anemia depends on the type of thalassemia inherited and varies from asymptomatic to severe hemolytic anemia. All of the thalassemias, except α-thalassemia of a silent carrier, produce some degree of microcytosis and hypochromia.

α-Thalassemia is most commonly found in people with ancestry from Southeast Asia, India, China, or the Philippines. β-Thalassemia is more frequent in those of Mediterranean, Middle Eastern, African, or Asian descent. Beta-thalassemia can be inherited concurrently with genes for the hemoglobinopathies, resulting in conditions such as sickle β-thalassemia (Sβ-thalassemia). Sβ-thalassemia severity is inversely proportional to the amount of β-globin produced. When no β-globin is produced ($S\beta^0$-thalassemia) the condition is almost identical to sickle cell disease.[12] Thalassemia affects males and females equally.

PATHOPHYSIOLOGY

The manifestations and severity of clinical symptoms depend on the number of chain deletions in the hemoglobin molecule. Normally, adult RBCs contain predominantly hemoglobin A_1 (96% to 97% of the cell's hemoglobin) and only small amounts of hemoglobin A_2 (2.5%) and hemoglobin F (<1%).[4] Thalassemia abnormalities produce changes in the normal amounts of adult hemoglobin. These quantitative changes are important in the diagnosis of thalassemia.

Inheritance of thalassemia occurs in a mendelian-recessive manner[12] (Fig. 237-1). The two main types of thalassemia are α (alpha) and β (beta), the two protein chains required to make normal hemoglobin. Four genes (two from each parent on chromosome 16) are involved in making α-globin. If one gene is affected, the person is called a silent carrier and usually has no symptoms. If two genes are affected, individuals are considered carriers and have mild anemia (α-thalassemia trait or α-thalassemia minor). People with hemoglobin H (α-thalassemia intermedia) disease have three genes affected and are moderately to severely anemic.[13] When all four genes are affected, the condition is called α-thalassemia major (hemoglobin hydrops fetalis), and most affected fetuses are born prematurely and stillborn or die shortly after birth.[13] The patients who survive will require lifelong transfusions and extensive medical care.

β-Thalassemia genes are located on chromosome 11; each parent provides one to an offspring. An individual is considered a carrier if one gene is affected; this is known as β-thalassemia

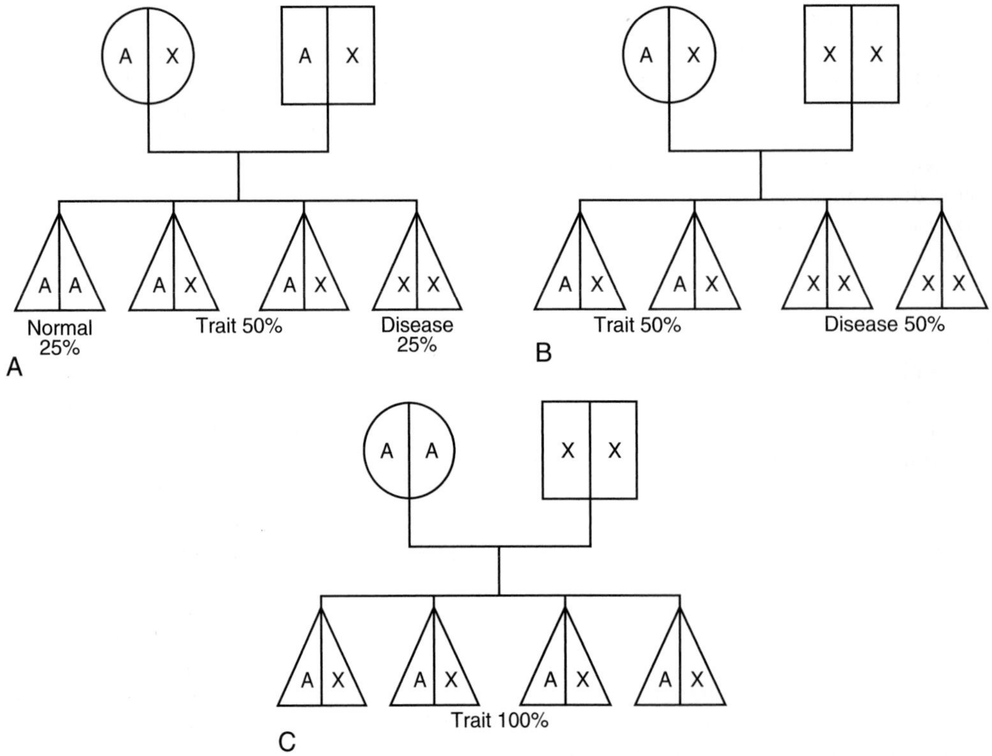

FIGURE 237-1 Inheritance patterns for autosomal genes. **A,** When both parents have a trait, offspring have a 25% chance of being normal, a 25% chance of having the disease, and a 50% chance of having the trait. **B,** When one parent has the disease and the other parent has the trait, offspring have a 50% chance of having the trait and a 50% chance of having the disease. **C,** When one parent has the disease and the other parent is normal, all offspring will have the trait. A, gene for normal hemoglobin; X, gene for abnormal hemoglobin (S, C, E) or thalassemia.

trait or minor. When both genes are affected, the condition is either β-thalassemia intermedia, causing moderate anemia, or β-thalassemia major (Cooley anemia) with severe anemia. Differentiation between β-thalassemia intermedia and major depends on the volume and frequency of transfusions.

CLINICAL PRESENTATION

The α- and β-thalassemias are classified as thalassemia minor (mild), thalassemia intermedia (moderate), or thalassemia major (severe) depending on the severity of the anemia. Throughout the world, the majority of patients have thalassemia minor. Patients with α- or β-thalassemia minor generally have either little or no hematologic effects or a mild microcytic hypochromic anemia that is often mistaken for IDA.[5]

Patients with thalassemia intermedia have a moderate microcytic and hypochromic anemia that is not transfusion dependent. Patients with thalassemia intermedia may require occasional transfusions during pregnancy or preoperatively. If patients with thalassemia intermedia begin to develop persistent clinical problems, such as abnormal facies, growth retardation, or pathologic fractures, they will require regular transfusions. At this point, these patients are given the diagnosis of thalassemia major.[14]

Patients with β-thalassemia major (also known as Cooley anemia) develop a severe, life-threatening anemia during their first year of life. This profound anemia is associated with developmental problems and decreased life expectancy. These patients require lifelong chronic RBC transfusions to maintain adequate hemoglobin levels and iron chelation.

PHYSICAL EXAMINATION

The physical examination findings are remarkable only in patients with thalassemia intermedia and β-thalassemia major. Patients can exhibit the characteristic physical changes of short stature and abnormal facies associated with cranial marrow expansion. In the United States, however, the facial abnormalities are seen primarily in patients with thalassemia intermedia because most patients with β-thalassemia major are hypertransfused to normal hemoglobin levels, thus preventing the marrow expansion.[5] Children can be diagnosed as early as 3 months of age, with findings of severe anemia, pallor, and jaundice and enlarged spleen, liver, or heart.

DIAGNOSTICS

Patients with thalassemia intermedia or major are diagnosed during the first few years of life. The diagnosis of β-thalassemia minor is based on a mildly decreased hemoglobin concentration, low MCV (<75 fL), normal iron studies, and normal hemoglobin electrophoresis with high levels of hemoglobin A_2. α-Thalassemia can be diagnosed at birth on a routine newborn screen. The hemoglobin electrophoresis will show evidence of Bart's hemoglobin in addition to fetal and normal adult hemoglobin and will be reported as French-American-British (FAB) classification. After the newborn period, α-thalassemia is more difficult to diagnose because a special test, α-globin DNA mutation analysis, is required, and only the largest of medical centers perform this test.

Patients with thalassemia intermedia who maintain adequate hemoglobin levels without requiring transfusions exhibit signs of a mild microcytic anemia with slightly low hemoglobin level and low MCV. Patients with β-thalassemia major who are hypertransfused have either low or low-normal hemoglobin level or relatively normal MCV (because they are receiving normal blood during transfusions). Peripheral smears of both patients with thalassemia intermedia and patients with β-thalassemia major have typical target cells present. Patients with β-thalassemia major who do not receive adequate iron chelation therapy reflect their state of overload with very high ferritin, very low TIBC, and percentage of transferrin saturation approaching 100%. Patients with thalassemia intermedia may have similar iron studies because they can develop iron overload as a result of iron hyperabsorption rather than from transfusions.

DIFFERENTIAL DIAGNOSIS

In most cases, the primary care provider needs to distinguish thalassemia minor from IDA. Both conditions are microcytic hypochromic anemias, but results of iron studies are normal in patients with thalassemia minor. In immigrants with Southeast Asian ancestry, the differential diagnosis of a mild microcytic anemia must differentiate between β-thalassemia minor and hemoglobin E disease.

Hemoglobin E is the second most common hemoglobin variant in the world (next to sickle cell disease). It is not a true thalassemia but rather a mild hemolytic anemia. It is characterized by a mild microcytic anemia with many target cells on the peripheral smear. It closely resembles the microcytic anemia of β-thalassemia minor, but hemoglobin E is found predominantly in people of Southeast Asian ancestry. Patients can also be double heterozygotes for hemoglobin E and sickle cell disease (ES), manifesting clinically as mild sickle cell disease or combined hemoglobin E and β-thalassemia, which results in a moderate to severe transfusion-dependent anemia that will be similar to β-thalassemia major.[14] Hemoglobin E is diagnosed by hemoglobin electrophoresis.

Often, patients with β-thalassemia minor or hemoglobin E are given a diagnosis of IDA because of their mild microcytic anemia and are prescribed a regimen of iron replacement. Failure to correct the anemia with iron supplementation should then lead the provider to suspect thalassemia minor (or hemoglobin E disease if the patient is of Southeast Asian ancestry).

MANAGEMENT

Patients with β-thalassemia minor do not require medical management but should be referred for genetic counseling if family planning is an issue. Patients with thalassemia intermedia can be adequately cared for in a primary care setting, with regular attention to any changes in their anemia. Patients with thalassemia intermedia who begin to develop persistent clinical problems, such as abnormal facies, growth retardation, or pathologic fractures, should be referred to a hematologist to begin chronic transfusion therapy. Patients with thalassemia intermedia who hyperabsorb iron and develop iron overload require chelation therapy.

In the United States, hematologists who are familiar with the disease manage most patients with β-thalassemia major and intermedia. Management consists of two equally important functions: (1) regular transfusions to maintain an adequate hemoglobin level to allow normal growth and development and (2) iron chelation therapy to prevent the complications of transfusion-dependent iron overload.

Regular transfusions of packed RBCs are the mainstay of therapy for β-thalassemia major. To maximize normal growth and development, transfusions are begun early in childhood to maintain an adequate hemoglobin trough level of typically around 10 g/dL, although this number can vary among institutions.[15] The frequency of the transfusions can vary among patients, but typically they are necessary every 3 to 5 weeks.[16]

Chelation therapy is standard for prevention of complications from iron overload. Complications of iron overload can be profound; deposition is concentrated in the liver and heart and is a major cause of death in patients requiring frequent RBC transfusions. The goal of chelation therapy is to reduce body iron stores and maintain a ferritin level of less than 1000 μg/L. However, ferritin is an acute-phase reactant and levels can fluctuate in the presence of body inflammation, and ferritin levels also do not predict cardiac iron loading accurately. Newer revolutionary magnetic resonance imaging (MRI) scanning techniques have allowed a much more accurate picture of the amount of iron overload in the body's organs, thereby helping providers determine the aggressiveness of the chelation therapy regimen.[16]

Deferoxamine is a chelating agent that removes iron from tissues and allows excretion of iron in urine and stools. Deferoxamine must be administered parenterally, in general through a subcutaneous needle, and delivered by slow infusion during at least 8 hours to effectively remove iron. The longer the infusion time, the more effectively the iron is removed. Parenteral therapy is administered 5 to 7 days a week for life. Chelation therapy given as only a single injection with blood transfusions is not effective in any setting. The normal subcutaneous dose is 25 to 40 mg/kg/day administered by continuous infusion during an 8- to 12-hour period.[16] If subcutaneous administration is not tolerated, intravenous therapy can be attempted but requires the use of an indwelling venous catheter. Deferasirox is the first oral iron chelator on the U.S. market. Recommended beginning daily doses start at 14 mg/kg, with adjustment every 3 months based on the monthly serum ferritin. If necessary, the dose can be escalated up to 40 mg/kg/day. This medication is a tablet dissolved in a large glass of water or juice and consumed on an empty stomach 30 minutes before meals. Taking the full amount may be difficult for young children. Patients with high liver iron overload may not respond to this medication, and it has not been shown to improve left ventricular ejection fraction. Renal toxicities have been reported, including proximal renal tubular dysfunction leading to electrolyte dysfunction (Fanconi syndrome).[16] Deferiprone is an oral agent that was approved by the U.S. Food and Drug Administration (FDA) for transfusion-dependent thalassemia patients who have not responded to other available therapy in 2011. This drug has shown effectiveness in removing iron from the heart, but the side effect profile includes neutropenia and possible liver toxicity.[16]

Bone marrow transplantation (BMT) is currently the only potential cure for β-thalassemia, but it is not without serious risks including graft-versus-host disease. Also, availability of donors is often a barrier for many patients. The success of transplantation is highest in children and those who are well chelated with minimal signs of iron overload including a normal liver and no cardiac complications.

Other therapies (including hydroxyurea and butyrate derivatives) are currently being investigated for their potential to induce fetal hemoglobin production.[17] Increasing fetal hemoglobin production may prove especially beneficial for patients with thalassemia intermedia as a way to avoid transfusions. Clinical trials in gene therapy are also beginning, and if successful will provide a cure for this disease.[18]

LIFE SPAN CONSIDERATIONS

Reproductive issues are a major concern. Well-chelated and well-transfused women may be fertile. Contraception counseling should be offered to all women with thalassemia who are sexually active with male partners. There are no restrictions as to the types of contraception available to women with β-thalassemia.

COMPLICATIONS

Many possible complications are associated with both transfusion regimens and chelation therapy, the most severe being diseases transmitted through the blood pool and iron overload.

Transfusions are usually well tolerated, but complications can occur. The development of alloantibodies can make it difficult to find suitable blood donors on a regular basis, requiring lengthy waiting periods of up to 48 hours, depending on proximity to regional blood centers. Viral infections such as human immunodeficiency virus (HIV) infection and hepatitis B and C have become less of an issue because of blood product screening; however, screening is not 100% accurate. Patients should receive hepatitis B vaccine and be screened for hepatitis B antibodies because immunity is not lifelong and may require boosters. Iron overload is the primary complication of chronic transfusions. Accumulation of excess iron leads to cirrhosis, heart failure, and endocrine problems such as diabetes mellitus, hypothyroidism, growth failure, and delayed sexual development.[16]

Chelation therapy can also be problematic. Chronic subcutaneous administration of deferoxamine can cause localized reactions such as scar tissue formation, itching, rash, and local irritation at the site of injection. There are also possible complications if a high dose of deferoxamine is given in the presence of low serum ferritin. These complications include toxic effects on the eye, such as cataracts, night blindness, and reduction of visual fields and acuity (these effects usually regress when deferoxamine therapy is stopped); hearing loss (high-tone deafness is irreversible despite cessation of therapy); and skeletal lesions, such as pseudorickets, metaphyseal changes, and short stature (these are also irreversible complications of deferoxamine therapy).[16]

Despite the availability of iron chelation therapy, complications of iron overload are common in patients with thalassemia who are older than 10 years. This may be a result of inadequate iron chelation early in life with resulting irreversible damage, insufficient chelation therapy, or poor compliance. Iron overload complications include endocrine, cardiac, and hepatic problems (Box 237-6). The presence of cardiac complications is an indication for continuous (24 hours a day, 7 days a week) iron chelation therapy. Combination therapy with multiple chelating agents is also being studied and is showing promise in patients with severe iron overload affecting organ function.[16]

Well-chelated patients with thalassemia who maintain a ferritin level of less than 1000 μg/L do not develop the major complications of iron overload. However, many of them have growth retardation and delayed puberty. Most people with β-thalassemia major are unusually short and may appear younger than their age. Young women are often amenorrheic. An endocrinology consultation may be indicated when the patient is nearing the age of puberty. Hormone replacement therapy (estrogen for

BOX 237-6

Complications of Iron Overload

ENDOCRINE PROBLEMS
- Growth retardation
- Diabetes mellitus
- Hypothyroidism
- Hypoparathyroidism
- Disturbed pubertal development

CARDIAC PROBLEMS
- Arrhythmias
- Pericarditis
- Cardiac failure

HEPATIC COMPLICATIONS
- Cirrhosis

girls or testosterone for boys) can be initiated to hasten maturation and sexual development.

INDICATIONS FOR REFERRAL OR HOSPITALIZATION

β-Thalassemia major is a chronic lifelong disease that requires constant attention by health care providers. Ideally, hematologists or health care providers familiar with the disease should manage these patients. Attention to issues of growth and development, compliance with transfusion and chelation therapy, reproductive issues, and assessment for the development of complications require frequent follow-up visits.

Even patients with β-thalassemia major who are well transfused and well chelated may experience considerable delays in puberty. These patients should be referred to a reproductive endocrinologist for possible hormone therapy.

Patients with thalassemia who receive chronic transfusion therapy and chelation therapy can lead relatively healthy lives. If they are not compliant, however, the complications of iron overload will eventually lead to increasing morbidity from liver disease and, especially, cardiac disease. When patients with β-thalassemia major are hospitalized for any reason, they should be transfused to maintain an adequate hemoglobin concentration and be maintained with chelation therapy. With adequate chelation therapy, the incidence of iron overload and its complications should be minimal.

PATIENT AND FAMILY EDUCATION

Patients with β-thalassemia major and their families assume a great deal of responsibility for their own health. Chelation therapy occurs at home, and patients must learn how to perform aseptic subcutaneous injections and use the infusion pump. Adherence to the chelation therapy schedule is essential. There are no signs and symptoms of iron overload until a fairly advanced stage; therefore it is difficult for young children and especially adolescents to understand the importance of a treatment for which they see no immediate need. Adolescents will have self-image issues. Delayed puberty, the need for daily medication infusions, and frequent trips to the hospital for transfusions will constantly remind them of being different from their peers. The daily (or usually nightly) requirement for infusions can interfere with a social life and complicate intimate relationships. The transfusion schedule can interfere with work or school, and most patients with β-thalassemia find that they require a flexible work or school schedule to accommodate their transfusion schedule.

HEALTH PROMOTION

Collaboration with patients and their families is important to promote patients' self-esteem and self-reliance. Patients who believe in the value of their own lives will be more likely to comply with the regular transfusion schedule and their daily chelation therapy.

MACROCYTIC ANEMIA: MEGALOBLASTIC ANEMIA

VITAMIN B_{12} AND FOLATE DEFICIENCY

Definition and Epidemiology

Vitamin B_{12} deficiency and folate deficiency are the primary causes of macrocytic anemia. Dietary sources of folic acid include fruits and vegetables, whereas cobalamin (vitamin B_{12}) is obtained primarily though meat protein and somewhat through dairy products and eggs. Both vitamins are essential for normal DNA synthesis, and tissues such as bone marrow are highly sensitive to any deficiency. Marrow precursors for all cell lines (erythroid, myeloid, and platelets) become larger than normal because they remain in the growth phase of the cell cycle. Because they are unable to properly synthesize DNA, they are not able to progress into the mitotic phase of the cell cycle and are therefore unable to complete normal growth and maturation, a condition referred to as megaloblastic bone marrow.[19] The resulting ineffective erythropoiesis causes the release of macrocytic RBCs into the circulation and worsening anemia.

Folate deficiency is found in the presence of decreased dietary intake, diseases associated with malabsorption, or increased requirements such as pregnancy. Alcoholism is a common cause of folate deficiency because of alcohol's interference with folate metabolism and the usual poor dietary habits related to alcoholism. Prolonged feeding of goat's milk to infants and fad diets can also be responsible for this disorder. In developing countries, malabsorption syndromes such as tropical and nontropical sprue are more common causes.[20] Folate deficiency is associated with neural tube defects in the fetus.

A long-term strict vegetarian diet can lead to a vitamin B_{12} deficiency, as can sole breastfeeding of an infant by a mother who has pernicious anemia.[20] Pernicious anemia is the most prevalent cause of vitamin B_{12} deficiency. It is a disease in which atrophy of the parietal cells of the stomach leads to a complete loss of intrinsic factor (IF). IF is necessary for the body to be able to absorb dietary sources of vitamin B_{12}.[19] It often coexists with other autoimmune disorders, GI disorders, type 1 diabetes, and thyroid disease. Chronic use of proton pump inhibitors and H_2 blockers can also possibly contribute, though studies are conflicting. Chronic gastritis can damage parietal cells, and partial or complete gastric resection results in loss of parietal cells and therefore loss of IF.[21] The onset of pernicious anemia usually occurs after the age of 50 years.

Pathophysiology

Dietary sources of vitamin B_{12} are found only in meat and meat byproducts. When vitamin B_{12} from food reaches the small bowel, it is bound to IF, a glycoprotein secreted by parietal cells of the stomach. The vitamin B_{12}-IF (cobalamin-IF) complex is then transported through the terminal ileum into the circulation. Vitamin B_{12} absorption cannot occur in the absence of IF.

Once it is in the circulation, vitamin B_{12} is bound to the transport protein transcobalamin II, which carries it to the liver, bone marrow, and other proliferating cells. A healthy adult receiving an adequate diet has a total body content of 2 to 5 mg of vitamin B_{12}, with at least 1 mg of that being stored in the liver.[20] Because the daily requirement of vitamin B_{12} is only 3 to 5 µg/day, most omnivorous individuals have no difficulty obtaining the necessary amounts from their diets as long as absorption is normal. Only strict vegetarians are at risk for a dietary deficiency, and it would take several years of a strict vegan diet for megaloblastosis to occur.

Dietary folate is readily available in most foods, especially green leafy vegetables; however, folate is heat labile and rapidly destroyed by prolonged cooking or food processing. Body stores are limited to approximately a 3-month reserve. It is possible that a prolonged inadequate diet may not provide sufficient amounts of folate for normal DNA production, especially for patients who are pregnant or have hemolytic anemias (high rates of cell turnover). Dietary folate deficiency is relatively uncommon because many foods, such as orange juice, are now supplemented. Folate deficiency is commonly associated with chronic alcoholism and can also be caused by the same malabsorption syndromes that lead to vitamin B_{12} deficiency (Box 237-7).

Clinical Presentation

A mild megaloblastic anemia produces few symptoms, and the CBC usually makes the diagnosis incidentally. A severe vitamin B_{12} deficiency includes signs and symptoms of marked anemia and neurologic deficits. Early neurologic symptoms include decreased vibratory sensation, loss of proprioception, peripheral neuropathy, and ataxia. Later involvement results in spasticity, hyperactive reflexes, and presence of Romberg sign. These neurologic symptoms result from the formation of a demyelinating lesion of the neurons of the spinal cord and cerebral cortex.[19] Neurologic symptoms may be evident in the absence of anemia and may not resolve with correction of the deficiency. Other classic symptoms of B_{12} deficiency include a sore mouth and loss of taste.

Folate deficiency is rarely associated with any symptoms, even in the severe state. Folate deficiency is not associated with neurologic or psychiatric disorders except those caused by neural tube defects.

BOX 237-7

Common Causes of Megaloblastic Anemia

INADEQUATE INTAKE
- Vegetarian diet devoid of animal proteins (vitamin B_{12})
- Chronic alcoholism (folate)

MALABSORPTION (VITAMIN B_{12} AND FOLATE)
- Lack of IF
- Gastric surgery
- Inflammatory bowel disease
- Sprue (tropical and nontropical)
- Celiac disease
- Intestinal tapeworm
- Hypothyroidism

INCREASED REQUIREMENTS (FOLATE)
- Pregnancy
- Hemolytic anemias

Physical Examination

The physical examination of a patient with severe megaloblastic anemia may reveal the classic changes associated with any severe anemia. The patient may also exhibit symptoms of weight loss or other symptoms consistent with malabsorption. Patients with severe vitamin B_{12} deficiency may have characteristic findings such as a beefy-red tongue and the aforementioned neurologic changes.[20]

Diagnostics

Findings on the CBC that suggest macrocytic anemia include low hemoglobin levels and MCV of more than 100 fL. Severe anemia may also be associated with leukopenia or thrombocytopenia. In addition, the reticulocyte count will be low. The peripheral smear is also helpful in diagnosis of megaloblastic anemia. Hypersegmented neutrophils and oval macrocytes are the earliest and most specific signs of megaloblastic anemia. Serum cobalamin (vitamin B_{12}), folate levels, and as well as the measurement of the vitamin B_{12} metabolites of methylmalonic acid and homocysteine, are essential to differentiate between vitamin B_{12} and folate deficiency. The normal range of serum methylmalonic acid is 70 to 270 nm/L, and the normal serum homocysteine level ranges from 5 to 14 nm/L.[20] Homocysteine is elevated in both vitamin B_{12} deficiency and folate deficiency. Methylmalonic acid is elevated in vitamin B_{12} deficiency and normal in folate deficiency.

It is important to distinguish vitamin B_{12} deficiency caused by malabsorption from that caused by lack of IF. Many of the medications now used to treat gastroesophageal reflux disease affect absorption. Long-term use of H_2 blockers inhibits release of IF; proton pump inhibitors can reduce absorption of protein-bound cobalamin and can eventually lead to malabsorption. The Schilling test has been the classic method to verify the diagnosis of pernicious anemia but is now rarely used. An assay for anti-IF or anti–parietal cell antibodies is the currently accepted method to verify the diagnosis of pernicious anemia. The presence of anti-IF antibodies is highly specific for pernicious anemia.

Differential Diagnosis

The differential diagnosis involves identification of the cause of the vitamin deficiency itself. It is important to accurately determine the cause of the macrocytic anemia because misdiagnosis can have extremely negative consequences. A vitamin B_{12} deficiency that is inappropriately treated with folic acid may result in permanent neurologic or psychiatric abnormalities.

It may also be necessary to distinguish the macrocytic anemia associated with vitamin B_{12} or folate deficiency from the macrocytosis caused by other conditions, such as drug or alcohol abuse, liver disease, hypothyroidism, myelodysplastic syndrome, exposure to chemotherapeutic agents, and hemolysis.[20] It is also essential to consider vitamin B_{12} deficiency in the differential diagnosis of any peripheral neuropathy, dementia, or other psychiatric disorder, especially in older adults.

DIFFERENTIAL DIAGNOSIS

Macrocytic Anemia

- Vitamin B_{12} deficiency
- Folic acid deficiency
- Myelodysplastic syndromes
- Liver disease
- Hypothyroidism
- Hemolysis
- Chemotherapeutic agents
- Hereditary disorder
- Alcoholism
- Drug reaction

Management

There are three basic stages to the management of megaloblastic anemia: (1) recognizing the anemia and classifying it as macrocytic; (2) differentiating whether it is a true folate deficiency, a vitamin B_{12} deficiency, or both combined; and (3) identifying the underlying cause.[20]

Initial management of a macrocytic anemia depends on the severity of the anemia. Patients with life-threatening anemia require slow transfusions of packed RBCs to correct the anemia. Treatment with both B_{12} and folate can be started until a definitive diagnosis is made. If the patient's cardiovascular system is unable to compensate for the degree of anemia, hospitalization is required until the patient's condition is stable.

Patients with asymptomatic anemia should not be treated until an accurate diagnosis is made. Treatment should then be targeted to replacement of the deficient vitamin and correction of the underlying disease, if possible. Some patients with B_{12} deficiency will be able to take oral vitamin B_{12} supplementation daily. Ideally, rapid correction of the deficiency is recommended. This can be accomplished with a protocol of vitamin B_{12}, 1-mg injections (subcutaneous or intramuscular) according to the following schedule: week 1, daily for 7 days; week 2, twice per week; weeks 3 to 6, once weekly; then monthly for life. Response to therapy is rapid with normal hematopoiesis and a much improved sense of well-being within 48 hours. Reticulocytosis begins in approximately 3 days and peaks in 7 to 10 days after the initiation of vitamin replacement. The anemia should resolve in 3 to 4 weeks.[20] It is important to note that even though the anemia will normalize, any advanced neurologic symptoms that have been ongoing for more than 3 months will remain permanent.[19,20] The recommended treatment of a macrocytic anemia resulting from folate deficiency is 1 mg of folic acid by mouth daily and correction of the underlying cause of the deficiency. Treatment should continue until at least a normal hemoglobin level is reached (usually in about 4 to 6 weeks) and should be continued indefinitely if the patient has an inadequate diet or if the underlying disease persists. Patients who have had partial or total gastrectomy, ileal resection, or any other evidence of gastric atrophy or intestinal malabsorption should receive prophylactic monthly parenteral vitamin B_{12} therapy and daily folic acid supplements.

Life Span Considerations

For any infant with macrocytic anemia, consumption of goat's milk or the possibility of pernicious anemia in the breastfeeding mother should be considered.

There is an association between folate deficiency and neural tube defects. Risk of neural tube defects is 1 to 5 per 1000 live births for the general population and approximately 10 times this risk among women with previous pregnancies involving neural tube defects. Women should take folic acid supplements before and during pregnancy to reduce the incidence of neural tube defects. The recommended intake is 0.4 mg/day either as a supplement or in the diet.

Annual screening for vitamin B_{12} deficiency is recommended for all older adults. Older adults with severe B_{12} deficiency can develop reversible cognitive change. Screening is also recommended for patients with hematologic, neurologic, or psychiatric abnormalities suggestive of vitamin B_{12} deficiency.

Complications

The complication of undiagnosed or mistreated vitamin B_{12} deficiency is irreversible neurologic damage. Manifestations of weakness, ataxia, and poor coordination may not completely resolve with therapy, depending on the duration of the deficiency and the extent of neurologic damage. Mental status changes can range from mild forgetfulness to severe dementia and psychosis. Patients with neurologic damage can have an almost normal blood count with normal indexes, which underscores the need to test for vitamin B_{12} levels in patients with unexplained neurologic deficits.

Indications for Referral or Hospitalization

A primary health care provider can easily manage patients who are receiving maintenance therapy for either vitamin B_{12} or folate replacement. These patients require regular visits for evaluation of therapy and, when indicated, monthly visits for vitamin B_{12} injections. Periodic evaluations should include a complete history and physical examination to look for the appearance or progression of any neurologic or psychiatric complications as well as continued assessment of the underlying disease causing the vitamin deficiency. Laboratory evaluations include CBC and serum cobalamin, methylmalonic acid, and folate levels. A hematologist should manage patients with refractory anemia.

Patients with severe macrocytic anemia should be referred to a hematologist for consultation and recommended therapy. Asymptomatic patients can be treated and monitored in an outpatient setting, either by a hematologist or by the patient's health care provider.

Patients with a severe, life-threatening anemia may require hospitalization for correction of the anemia. This is especially true for patients with a severe vitamin B_{12} deficiency, who require daily administration of parenteral vitamin B_{12} therapy to correct the vitamin deficiency.

Patient and Family Education

Patients with folate deficiency secondary to an inadequate diet require nutritional counseling to learn how to properly cook and prepare foods without losing their nutritional value. Daily folic acid supplementation may be required for patients receiving certain drugs, such as sulfasalazine and methotrexate (both used for certain inflammatory forms of arthritis or inflammatory bowel disease) and for patients with other hematologic diseases.

Patients with megaloblastic anemia secondary to vitamin B_{12} deficiency require monthly vitamin B_{12} injections. Patients or caregivers can easily be taught this injection technique so that injections can be administered at home. Parenteral vitamin B_{12} in the absence of pernicious anemia is not effective in increasing energy in older adults. Patients with conditions that require partial or total gastrectomy, ileal resections, and other small bowel removal need counseling on lifelong parenteral vitamin B_{12} and folic acid replacement.

Health Promotion

One preventive measure that health care providers can take to reduce the incidence of folate deficiency anemia is the early recognition and treatment of alcohol abuse. Lifestyle modifications include improving dietary sources of folic acid and vitamin B_{12} and taking vitamin supplements if necessary. Health care providers who see older patients should screen for cobalamin deficiency in cases of unexplained mental status changes or neuropathy and should begin therapy with vitamin B_{12} even before the anemia is noted.

NORMOCYTIC ANEMIA

SICKLE CELL DISEASE

Definition and Epidemiology

Sickle cell syndromes are the most common inherited hemoglobinopathies and include homozygous disease (hemoglobin SS), hemoglobin SC (also known as SC disease), Sβ-thalassemia, and conditions involving a variety of other rare, abnormal hemoglobins. Patients with sickle cell disease have mild to moderate hemolytic anemia that is generally well compensated for; however, over years this anemia can lead to chronic heart disease. The hallmark of sickle cell disease is the acute vaso-occlusive crisis that causes unpredictable, severe pain and organ damage.

Approximately 8% of African Americans carry the gene for sickle cell trait (hemoglobin AS), and about 1 in 400 are affected by the disease (hemoglobin SS).[22] Other types of sickle cell syndromes are found in Mediterranean, Middle Eastern, and Southeast Asian populations. People with only one gene for hemoglobin S are phenotypically normal (sickle cell trait). People who inherit one gene for hemoglobin S from each parent will have SS disease. People with either hemoglobin SC or Sβ-thalassemia have inherited one gene for hemoglobin S and the other gene for either hemoglobin C or β-thalassemia, respectively. In the case of Sβ-thalassemia, the hemoglobin S gene is combined with a thalassemia gene that makes a decreased amount of beta hemoglobin ($S\beta^{+}$-thalassemia) or a gene that make no beta hemoglobin ($S\beta^{0}$-thalassemia). The median life span of patients with SS and $S\beta^{0}$-thalassemia disease is 42 years for men and 48 years for women, and 15% of people born with sickle cell disease in the United States die by the age of 29 years. The life span is 60 to 70 years for patients with other types of sickle cell syndromes, including hemoglobin SC and $S\beta^{+}$-thalassemia.[5]

Pathophysiology

The hemoglobin defect occurs when valine replaces glutamic acid in the beta chain of hemoglobin, resulting in hemoglobin S.[23] Deoxygenated hemoglobin S tends to undergo irreversible polymerization, deforming the erythrocytes and giving them the pathognomonic sickle shape. The sickled cells are rigid and can be easily trapped in the microcirculation, causing obstruction, ischemia, and sometimes infarction. This process leads to the clinical consequences of severe pain and organ damage. These vaso-occlusive episodes, usually referred to as crises or pain crises, can occur anywhere in the body but commonly affect the joints, extremities, back, chest, abdomen, and lungs.

Clinical Presentation

Sickle cell trait has no clinical manifestations. Manifestations of sickle cell disease vary widely; some affected individuals have few painful vaso-occlusive crises or other rare complications, whereas many others are often hospitalized with painful crises or other complications. Patients with other types of sickle cell syndromes (hemoglobin SC or $S\beta^{+}$-thalassemia) are reported to have milder forms of disease, although this is not always true. For example, patients with hemoglobin SC can exhibit the same range of severity as patients with SS disease.

Physical Examination

Objective manifestations of moderate to severe hemolytic anemia include jaundice and a physiologic systolic flow murmur. Scleral icterus can range from mild to severe but often has no association with the severity of disease. The physiologic flow murmur secondary to anemia is often a grade 1 or 2 pansystolic murmur, which is heard best along the left sternal border. Cardiomegaly is routinely noted on the radiographs of adults with sickle cell disease and is also a compensatory manifestation of lifelong anemia.

Diagnostics

Accurate diagnosis of any sickle cell syndrome requires hemoglobin electrophoresis. Patients with sickle cell disease have evidence of hemolytic anemia: low hemoglobin, chronic reticulocytosis, chronic hyperbilirubinemia, and chronically elevated LDH levels. The peripheral blood smear shows mild to moderate anisocytosis and poikilocytosis with numerous sickle cells and Howell-Jolly bodies (evidence of the patient's functional asplenia).[5] Patients with sickle cell disease have target cells in addition to the sickle cells on their peripheral blood smears. Unfortunately, no laboratory tests are predictive or diagnostic of an acute painful crisis.

Differential Diagnosis

Most patients with sickle cell disease are diagnosed at birth. In fact, all states in the United States and many developed nations in the world currently have mandatory newborn screening for sickle hemoglobin. However, it is possible for persons who were not screened at birth and with very mild disease to go undiagnosed until they are in their adult years. These patients may have a mild hemolytic anemia (low hemoglobin concentration, slight hyperbilirubinemia with elevated LDH levels, and mild reticulocytosis). A history of occasional spontaneous painful events, usually abdominal or joint pains, should suggest a hemoglobinopathy. Accurate diagnosis requires hemoglobin electrophoresis to differentiate among the various forms of sickle cell disease. Other possible causes of hemolytic anemia include hereditary spherocytosis, hypersplenism, autoimmune hemolysis, and delayed hemolytic transfusion reaction.

Management

The frequency and severity of pain crises vary tremendously among patients and even in the same patient over time. Physical stresses including infection, change of weather (exposure to cold in particular), dehydration, fatigue, overexertion, or emotional stress may precipitate a crisis, but the majority of crises occur spontaneously with no obvious precipitating events.[23] The sites affected in an acute crisis vary among individuals, but crises tend to recur at the same sites for a particular person. The quality of the pain is usually similar as well. Most patients are able to distinguish a "typical" sickle cell pain crisis from other events, such as pyelonephritis or abdominal pain resulting from cholecystitis.

Most crises are mild to moderate in severity and can be managed at home with oral analgesics (either NSAIDs or oral narcotics), adequate hydration, rest, and local measures such as heat and gentle massage. Moderate to severe crises require treatment in an emergency department or a hospital-based outpatient treatment center with parenteral narcotic analgesics and hydration as well as the same local measures. Often, aggressive and early management of a crisis can prevent hospital admission. Hospitalizations for crises can last a few days to several weeks. Patients describe a severe crisis as the most intense pain they have ever experienced. Pain control often requires large quantities of narcotic analgesics. Initial dosage of parenteral narcotics in the hospital setting should take into account how much opioid the patient has been using at home, and this dose should be used as a starting point. Pain should be reassessed every 15 to 30 minutes, narcotics readministered as needed, and consideration given to escalating the dose by 25% until pain is under control.[24] Many adults with sickle cell disease have learned how to manage their pain without the behavioral signs that one would expect from someone experiencing severe pain. Therefore it becomes important in evaluating a sickle cell patient in crisis to believe the patient's report and to treat the pain quickly and appropriately.

DIFFERENTIAL DIAGNOSIS

Normocytic Anemia

- Sickle cell disorders
  - Sickle cell trait
  - Sickle cell anemia
  - Sβ-thalassemia
  - Sickle cell disease
- Hereditary spherocytosis
- Hypersplenism
- Autoimmune hemolysis
- Delayed hemolytic transfusion reaction
- Aplastic anemia

Hydroxyurea has become the standard of therapy for adult patients who experience three or more crises per year, have sickle cell–associated pain that interferes with daily activities, or have a history of severe or recurrent acute chest syndrome (ACS). In children older than 9 months, it should be offered regardless of clinical symptoms because it can reduce sickle cell disease–related complications.[24] Hydroxyurea induces hemoglobin F formation, thereby decreasing the total percentage of hemoglobin S in RBCs. This results in decreased sickling and hemolysis of RBCs and decreased veno-occlusion, the major cause of complications in this disease.[23,25] Hydroxyurea is started at a dose of 10 to 20 mg/kg/day. Patients must be monitored every 2 weeks for signs of toxicity (neutrophil count <2000/mm^3, platelet count <80,000/mm^3, or hemoglobin drop of 2 g/dL), in which case doses should be held until count recovery and then decreased 5 mg/kg/day below the dose at which the cytopenias occurred. When blood counts remain stable, the dose of hydroxyurea can be increased over a period of several months to a maximum dose of 35 mg/kg/day. If blood counts continue to be stable at this dose, patients should be monitored every 2 to 3 months.[24]

By definition, patients with sickle cell disease are anemic. The degree of anemia varies, but most have hemoglobin concentrations that range from 7 to 8 g/dL. Patients with hemoglobin SC tend to have hematocrit values in the high-20s to mid-30s. The baseline hemoglobin value tends to remain relatively stable in a given patient. Most patients are able to compensate for their level of anemia and do not require routine transfusions. In fact, transfusing patients to achieve hemoglobin concentrations above 10 g/dL can be dangerous because blood viscosity increases substantially at higher hematocrit levels and the increased viscosity can worsen the tendency to sickle by slowing transit time of the RBCs through low-oxygen regions of the circulation.[23] In general, transfusions in patients with sickle cell disease are indicated only before surgical procedures requiring anesthesia and in the circumstance of the severe complications of ACS, acute splenic sequestration, stroke, and aplastic crisis.

BMT is the only curative therapy for sickle cell disease and is becoming more widely used as a result of new reduced-toxicity conditioning regimens and other advances in transplant therapy. Some of the historical barriers to transplant have been the lack reliable prognostic factors for severity in this disease to determine the risk/benefit ratio; the lack of available donors in this minority population; and sickle cell–related organ damage (especially in older patients) increasing the risk of unsuccessful outcomes. Results from two international registries demonstrate 90% cure rate and very limited complications in patients with human leukocyte antigen (HLA)–identical sibling donors.[26]

Life Span Considerations

Pain crisis is the most common complication of sickle cell disease and occurs across all age groups. Appropriate management of pain crisis is reviewed earlier. An age-related complication in infants and toddlers is dactylitis. This is a painful swelling of the hands and feet as a result of bone marrow expansion from increased erythropoiesis. Another complication occurring most commonly in children is acute splenic sequestration. This is caused by trapping of RBCs in the splenic sinuses. This is a life-threatening emergency in children because it can progress to hypovolemic shock.[23]

Women with sickle cell disease can carry pregnancies to term but should be considered high risk because of the potential for obstetric complications such as preterm delivery, spontaneous abortion, thrombosis, preeclampsia, and pulmonary embolism after delivery.[24] The frequency of painful crises sometimes increases during pregnancy, but the crises are treated no differently from other crises, with narcotic analgesics and hydration. Pregnancy prevention and family planning options are the same for women with sickle cell disease as they are for other women. In fact, many women experience relief from menses-related crises with the use of oral contraceptives or other hormone contraception methods.

Pulmonary hypertension is one of the leading causes of mortality and morbidity in adults with sickle cell disease. Echocardiogram-based tricuspid jet velocity is a frequently used screening modality, and an increase in systolic pulmonary artery pressure is a poor prognostic factor.[23]

Sickle cell disease is a chronic condition that often leads to psychosocial difficulties as well as medical problems. Some patients experience frequent complications of their disease, making it almost impossible to participate in normal daily activities, to hold a regular job, or to attend school on a regular schedule.

Many of these patients can benefit from rehabilitation counseling and vocational training. Often, however, adults with sickle cell disease find that they are unable to work because of chronic pain or other multiorgan damage. These individuals are clearly disabled.

Complications

Chronic pain is a substantial problem for many children and most adults with sickle cell disease. The severity of the pain varies greatly among patients and can change over time. Some patients can manage their chronic pain with intermittent use of mild analgesics such as NSAIDs. Most patients, however, require frequent doses of oral narcotic analgesics. Often these patients become tolerant of narcotics, and the quantity of medication needed to control the pain can escalate over time. This physical tolerance should not be confused with psychological addiction and drug-seeking behaviors, which are uncommon in this population.

Splenic infarction caused by vaso-occlusion occurs very early in children, resulting in a functional asplenia. As a result, patients with sickle cell disease are immunocompromised and at risk of overwhelming sepsis from encapsulated organisms such as *Neisseria meningitidis, Haemophilus influenzae,* and *Streptococcus pneumoniae.* Patients are instructed to seek immediate medical evaluation including history, physical, CBC with differential, reticulocyte count, blood culture, and possibly urine culture for every fever of 38.5° C or higher.[24] Initiation of penicillin prophylaxis and immunizations specific to these organisms has helped to greatly decrease associated mortality.

The term *acute chest syndrome* is used to describe an acute pulmonary event in a sickle cell disease patient that can be either infectious or noninfectious in its cause. Fever, dyspnea, cough, pulmonary infiltrates on chest x-ray examination, and severe chest pain usually characterize the condition. Clinically, ACS is often more severe than pneumonia in the general population, with severe hypoxia and progressive multilobar involvement despite treatment with antibiotics. Typically the patient is hospitalized for a vaso-occlusive crisis and 1 to 3 days later develops respiratory distress. Causes of ACS include pneumonia, bone marrow fat embolism, infection, pulmonary infarct resulting from sickling, rib or sternal infarct, or pulmonary embolus.[23]

The most important step in the treatment of ACS is early recognition. Potential bacterial infections should be treated with appropriate antibiotics. Simple transfusions raising the hemoglobin concentration to 10 g/dL can be beneficial in patients with mild to moderate hypoxemia. Adequate ventilation is essential to recovery, and this can be achieved by using incentive spirometry in mild cases and mechanical ventilation in severe cases.[23]

Stroke in sickle cell disease is a medical emergency. The treatment of choice is an exchange transfusion followed by maintenance hypertransfusion and iron chelation therapy. It is recommended that children with sickle cell disease be screened by transcranial Doppler ultrasonography and that chronic transfusion therapy be started if results indicate a high risk of stroke.[23] Compliance with iron chelation therapy for prevention of future complications from iron overload is an essential component of chronic transfusion therapy.

Priapism is defined as a persistent, painful erection of the penis that can last several hours to several days. Priapism lasting more than 3 or 4 hours is a medical emergency because it can cause impotence. Referral to a urologist is recommended in this situation.[24] Treatment includes hydration, analgesia, and possibly evacuation of the blood from the corpus cavernosum.

There is a high risk of renal dysfunction or failure in adults with sickle cell disease. Renal failure results from the sickle cell–induced damage to renal microvasculature. Patients are monitored for proteinuria, and referral to a nephrologist is recommended when proteinuria is present. Often angiotensin-converting enzyme (ACE) inhibitor therapy is initiated for renal complications even in the absence of hypertension.[24] Renal dysfunction is typically diagnosed in the third or fourth decade and eventually progresses to renal failure. Subcutaneous erythropoietin or darbepoetin alfa to maintain appropriate hemoglobin levels is often helpful either to prevent or to reduce the need for transfusions in patients with renal insufficiency. Adults with renal failure usually require chronic transfusions and should be offered chelation therapy as necessary. Treatment of end-stage renal disease requires hemodialysis or kidney transplantation.

Skin ulcerations of the lower legs are the most common cutaneous complication of sickle cell disease, causing pain and physical disfigurement. The medial or lateral malleoli are more frequently involved, and ulcerations occur less commonly over the dorsum of the foot, near the Achilles tendon. The size of the ulcers varies from a few millimeters to large, circumferential ulcers that involve the entire ankle or foot. Lesions can extend into the dermis, the underlying subcutaneous tissue, and the underlying muscle fascia. These lesions are highly susceptible to infection and other complications. They are resistant to therapy and often exist for years (some patients report persistent ulcers for more than 10 years). Pain is the major problem and is often severe and unremitting, causing significant disability. Environment and geographic location influence the prevalence of leg ulcers, with great variability among the various regions of the globe. Age is also a factor; this problem is less common in younger patients.[27] The cause and pathogenesis of leg ulcers are not well understood. Clinical experience and epidemiology studies suggest a role for three factors: marginal blood supply to the skin of the lower extremities, local edema, and minor trauma.[23] The greatest risk factor for the development of leg ulcers is a history of previous ulcers.

Treatment is initially standard therapy consisting of debridement, wet to damp dressing, and topical dressings and agents.[24] Treatment of existing ulcers can be difficult and frustrating; healing is often only temporary. Zinc is important in wound healing. It is found in RBCs and is lost during hemolysis; therefore zinc deficiency is common in patients with sickle cell disease. There is some evidence that zinc supplementation benefits the healing of ankle ulcers. Other controversial treatments include chronic transfusions and skin grafting for ulcers that are resistant to more conservative therapy, but failure rates for both methods are high.[23]

Patients should be educated about the importance of preventing local trauma by wearing shoes that fit properly, using insect repellents to prevent bites, and promptly treating any minor cuts on the feet and ankles. Patients with a history of ulcers and leg edema are encouraged to wear compression stockings and to perform routine care of the skin with emollients, good local hygiene, and daily inspection for any minor trauma.

The bony skeleton is a common target of the consequences of sickling. Bone marrow necrosis, bone infarcts, avascular necrosis (AVN), and osteomyelitis are common complications. The heads of the femur and humerus are common sites for marrow infarction and necrosis. Infarcts can also occur in the spine, ribs, and sternum. Bone infarcts constitute a painful crisis that in general resolves in 1 to 2 weeks. Treatment does not differ from that of any other painful crisis and includes analgesia, hydration, and rest.

AVN commonly affects the hip and shoulder joints and is a more chronic condition than an acute bone infarct. Patients complain of severe chronic pain, limited range of motion, and pain with joint movement. Late stages are evident on plain radiographs, but MRI is much more sensitive in the identification of AVN in the early stages. Initially, NSAIDs and narcotic analgesics are the mainstay of treatment. In the earlier stages core decompression may be performed to attempt to increase blood flow and prevent further joint damage. Later stages are usually surgically corrected with joint replacement.

Retinopathy is a significant problem for patients with sickle cell disease. It is more common in patients with SC disease than in those with homozygous SS disease. The retinopathy resembles that seen in diabetes and is believed to be caused by ischemia to the retina. Lifelong management with an ophthalmologist is recommended.

Indications for Referral or Hospitalization

The chronic nature of sickle cell disease, the frequent need for acute treatment of painful crises, and the high risk for complications dictate that these patients are better cared for by specialists familiar with the disease. Many of the large urban hospitals in the United States have sickle cell centers where patients receive comprehensive care by multidisciplinary teams of physicians, nurse practitioners, physician assistants, nurses, psychologists, and social workers. These hospital-based centers allow prompt referral to other specialists such as neurologists, cardiologists, high-risk obstetricians, and ophthalmologists.

Most of the aforementioned complications require hospitalization for treatment. Patients with moderate to severe disease also have many admissions for intractable vaso-occlusive crises. These hospitalizations can last a couple of days to several weeks.

Consultation with a social worker is recommended for issues related to school, employment, housing, transportation, and medical billing issues.

Patient and Family Education

Patient education begins early in childhood and continues throughout life. Initially, parents are taught how to manage pain crises, to recognize signs of infection, and to administer daily medications. Coping with acute and chronic pain is a lifelong issue and involves learning both pharmacologic and nonpharmacologic interventions. Educating patients on the proper use of oral analgesics and management of painful crises is important and should occur at every opportunity. Patients need to be taught to seek prompt medical attention for any complication and not wait until they can speak to their health care provider.

The importance of preventive care must also be stressed. Routine care should include annual ophthalmologic, gynecologic, and dental examinations; periodic sickle cell clinic visits; and immunizations, including hepatitis A and B, annual influenza, pneumococcal, meningococcal, and *H. influenzae* vaccines. Also, regular screening such as transcranial Doppler for risk of stroke and echocardiogram for evaluation of pulmonary hypertension are recommended. A common cause of death in children with SS is *S. pneumoniae* sepsis. This susceptibility is a result of splenic malfunction and failure that begin in the first years of life and inability to make immunoglobulin G (IgG) antibodies to antigens. Prevention is vaccination and prophylactic penicillin. All infants with sickle cell disease should receive the complete series of the 13-valent conjugate pneumococcal vaccine beginning at 2 months of age. At 24 months of age, these children are given the 23-valent pneumococcal polysaccharide vaccine (PPV23). Although most children with sickle cell disease do not respond as well to the vaccine as non-SS children, a rise in IgG antibodies is noted. Prophylactic penicillin begins in the newborn period with oral penicillin V and continues until the age of 5 years, at which time the incidence of life-threatening infections from *Mycoplasma pneumoniae, Chlamydia*, parvovirus B19, and *Staphylococcus aureus* significantly decreases.[28] Parents must be taught to call and bring the child into the hospital for every fever. This is necessary so the child can be evaluated for sepsis. The evaluation involves drawing a blood culture and giving prophylactic intravenous antibiotic coverage until the results of the blood culture are known.

Health Promotion

Adequate hydration, regular exercise, and sufficient sleep play a role in helping patients manage their disease. Teaching children and young adults coping skills can be beneficial and can help them manage both the acute and chronic pain associated with their disease. Annual health screenings, ophthalmologic examinations, and vaccines are recommended but easily overlooked.

ANEMIA OF CHRONIC DISEASE

DEFINITION AND EPIDEMIOLOGY

ACD is a mild to moderate anemia that often accompanies inflammatory disorders, infection, or malignancy. It has also been referred to as anemia of inflammation. The RBCs are usually normochromic and normocytic and the hemoglobin is generally not less than 9 g/dL. This anemia has an insidious onset, is common in older adults, and is the most frequent type of anemia in hospitalized patients.[5]

PATHOPHYSIOLOGY

ACD is marked by low serum iron levels, but total iron stores are normal or elevated. Hepcidin, a liver-derived peptide that is a regulator of iron transport, is increased in inflammatory conditions, resulting in reduced transport of iron to erythroid precursors. Other possible mechanisms for ACD that have been suggested include a decreased RBC survival time, decreased use of reticuloendothelial iron for hemoglobin synthesis, and inflammatory cytokine inhibition of erythropoietin production.[5]

In ACKD there may be a relative deficiency of erythropoietin.[5] Erythropoietin is a renal hormone whose normal plasma levels increase logarithmically in response to decreased hemoglobin levels. Although serum erythropoietin levels may be increased, they are not elevated enough for the degree of anemia. The exact pathogenesis of ACKD is unclear but may include several factors, including a blunted erythropoietin response to anemia.

CLINICAL PRESENTATION

ACD is often mild and asymptomatic. Patients typically have symptoms that are associated with the underlying diseases rather than with the anemia itself. Progression of anemia results in the usual symptoms of advanced anemia, such as fatigue and poor activity tolerance.

PHYSICAL EXAMINATION

There are usually no changes in the physical examination findings associated with ACD. Any changes in the physical examination findings are a result of the patient's underlying disease.

DIAGNOSTICS

The CBC will usually reveal a normocytic anemia, but the anemia can occasionally be microcytic. Hemoglobin levels are generally 10 to 11 g/dL. There are no distinctive changes in RBC size or shape, but if microcytosis does occur, the RDW is slightly elevated. Iron studies reveal a low serum iron level, a normal or increased ferritin level, and a normal or elevated TIBC. Bone marrow examination, if it is done, reveals normal to increased bone marrow iron stores with decreased amounts of bone marrow sideroblasts. The reticulocyte count is normal.

No precise diagnostic criteria exist for ACD. ACD often coexists with IDA, but laboratory test results can be difficult to distinguish because frequent overlaps occur. The only true way to distinguish ACD from IDA is by assessment of iron stores (which are absent in IDA and normal or low in ACD) either by bone marrow aspiration and biopsy or by evaluation of the serum ferritin levels. Although bone marrow aspiration and biopsy are completed by the hematologist to exclude myelodysplastic syndromes and other diseases, they usually add nothing to an already negative serologic evaluation and physical examination findings that the less invasive procedure generates.

DIFFERENTIAL DIAGNOSIS

If the clinical picture is one of a mild microcytic anemia, the differential diagnosis is between ACD and IDA. Iron studies are the most useful to differentiate the two (see the differential diagnosis box in the section on iron deficiency anemia). ACD is a diagnosis of exclusion.

MANAGEMENT

After IDA has been excluded, mild anemia need not be treated unless it is symptomatic. The standard treatment for ACKD of renal insufficiency is recombinant human erythropoietin (rHuEPO) or darbepoetin alfa (novel erythropoiesis-stimulating protein [NESP]). Intermittent transfusions may be required with more severe anemias. As always, the underlying condition should be treated or optimally controlled. Treatment of the underlying disease will correct the anemia.

COMPLICATIONS

As long as the anemia is mild, the patient should have no complications associated with the anemia itself. Complications of the underlying disease should be managed appropriately.

INDICATIONS FOR REFERRAL OR HOSPITALIZATION

Once acute reasons for the anemia have been excluded and the diagnosis of ACD has been confirmed, patients should be monitored by the clinician who is managing the underlying medical condition. The anemia should be monitored with periodic CBCs and iron studies. Referral to a specialist may be necessary to initiate therapy with rHuEPO or NESP or if the anemia worsens and requires other interventions.

Given that ACD is associated with chronic medical conditions, it is possible that the patient may have an acute reason for anemia, such as a drug or transfusion reaction. ACD rarely requires hospitalization for management. If the cause of the anemia is uncertain, referral to or consultation with a hematologist is appropriate.

PATIENT AND FAMILY EDUCATION

Regular visits with the health care provider should include laboratory studies to monitor for anemia. Patients should be encouraged to contact their provider if they experience any increase in symptoms, such as fatigue, decreased exercise tolerance, or shortness of breath.

APLASTIC ANEMIA

DEFINITION AND EPIDEMIOLOGY

Aplastic anemia is a life-threatening condition resulting from bone marrow stem cell failure. It is characterized by a marked decrease in all hematopoietic precursors, resulting in pancytopenia. Aplastic anemia can affect people of all ages and both genders. It is a rare disorder with an estimated incidence of approximately 2 to 6 cases per million people per year.[29]

PATHOPHYSIOLOGY

In aplastic anemia, the damage to the bone marrow's ability to generate stem cells can be secondary to infection or exposures to toxins or medications, or it can be an immune mediated. Box 237-8 includes a few of the more than 500 medications that are associated with aplastic anemia.

BOX 237-8

Agents Associated with Aplastic Anemia

TOXINS

- Radiation
- Alkylating agents
- Insecticides
- Benzene and its derivatives
- Chemotherapeutic agents

MEDICATIONS

- Antibiotics (penicillin, chloramphenicol, cephalosporins, sulfonamides)
- Antidepressants (lithium, tricyclics)
- Anti-inflammatory drugs (gold salts, nonsteroidals, salicylates)
- Antimalarials
- Anticonvulsants

OTHER POSSIBLE CAUSES

- Viral: hepatitis C, HIV, Epstein-Barr virus
- Graft-versus-host disease
- Malignant neoplasm
- Pregnancy

CLINICAL PRESENTATION

Patients may be seen with abnormal bleeding, infection, and anemia. Onset is usually sudden without any other apparent illness. The history may reveal information about a recent viral infection, chronic disease, or exposure to an offending medication or toxin.

PHYSICAL EXAMINATION

The physical examination may reveal petechiae, ecchymosis, purpura, pallor of the skin and mucous membranes, and mild lymphadenopathy in the late stages. Early stages of aplastic anemia may show no significant changes on physical examination.

DIAGNOSTICS

A CBC will show pancytopenia with normocytic and normochromic RBC indexes and morphology. The reticulocyte count is also below normal, reflecting the lack of bone marrow activity. A bone marrow biopsy is essential for diagnosis. Severe aplastic anemia (SAA) is defined as a bone marrow cellularity of less than 25% and at least two of the following: absolute neutrophil count (ANC) less than 500/μL, ARC less than 20,000/μL, and platelet count less than 20,000/μL.[29]

DIFFERENTIAL DIAGNOSIS

Aplastic anemia is readily detected and easily distinguished from other forms of normocytic, normochromic anemia. Involvement of other cell types (myeloid, platelets) confirms the diagnosis.

MANAGEMENT

Any patient with symptoms suggestive of aplastic anemia should be referred to a hematologist for management. In patients with nonsevere aplastic anemia, observation and supportive care are the recommended treatment. Definitive treatment with either BMT or immunosuppressive therapy is reserved for SAA.[29] Use of blood products to correct the anemia should be minimized to prevent alloimmunization and to reduce the risk of graft failure after BMT. The decision to transfuse a patient with aplastic anemia should be made in consultation with the hematologist who will be treating the patient.

LIFE SPAN CONSIDERATIONS

The treatment of choice for aplastic anemia is based on the severity of the anemia and the age of the patient. BMT is more successful in younger patients and is the treatment of choice for children and adolescents if a suitable donor is available, or if they have not responded to immunosuppression therapy. Patients who are older than 40 years have a higher risk of transplant-related morbidity and mortality. Immunosuppression therapy is the treatment of choice for adults older than 40 years.[29]

COMPLICATIONS

Complications of untreated aplastic anemia include sepsis and death resulting from pancytopenia. Complications of BMT include graft failure, graft-versus-host disease, and a risk of secondary malignant neoplasms. Complications of immunosuppressive therapy include relapse and death resulting from pancytopenia or evolution of aplastic anemia to myelodysplasia or leukemia.[29]

INDICATIONS FOR REFERRAL OR HOSPITALIZATION

All patients who are thought to have aplastic anemia should be immediately referred to a hematologist for treatment. Patients with SAA require hospitalization for management of the pancytopenia and to begin treatment. Most patients who undergo BMT or immunosuppressive therapy should continue to be monitored by a hematologist or oncologist as necessary.

PATIENT AND FAMILY EDUCATION AND HEALTH PROMOTION

Aplastic anemia can be caused by exposure to toxins such as benzene and insecticides. Patients should be taught that proper handling of products such as paints and insecticides includes adequate ventilation of the work area and wearing of protective clothing, such as masks and gloves.

HEMOLYTIC ANEMIA

DEFINITION AND EPIDEMIOLOGY

All the hemolytic anemias are associated with an increased rate of RBC destruction. The clinical presentation varies according to the disease. Some patients are seen with chronic hemolytic states that are well compensated; others have acute, self-limited hemolytic episodes. The most common chronic hemolytic anemia is sickle cell disease (discussed previously). Most of the other hemolytic anemias (Box 237-9) are rare and are mentioned only briefly here.

G6PD deficiency is an inherited erythrocyte enzyme deficiency that can result in an acute hemolytic anemia. G6PD-induced hemolysis is usually precipitated either by infection or by ingestion of an oxidant drug or food.

G6PD is a sex-linked disorder; women are almost always carriers and males are affected. Phenotypes vary among various ethnicities, and patients with the Mediterranean variants typically experience severe hemolysis when exposed to inciting agents. The most common form of G6PD deficiency in the United States is a mild variant of the disorder that typically affects approximately 10% of African-American males. Other affected populations include Africans, Greeks, Sardinians, certain Jewish sects, and Southeast Asians.[5]

A mild chronic hemolytic anemia can also be caused by abnormalities in erythrocyte membrane protein composition.

BOX 237-9

Examples of Hemolytic Anemias

Hemoglobinopathies
G6PD deficiency
Membrane structural defects
- Hereditary spherocytosis
- Hereditary elliptocytosis

Autoimmune hemolysis
- Warm-reacting autoimmune hemolytic anemia
- Cold-reacting autoimmune hemolytic anemia

Hereditary spherocytosis and hereditary elliptocytosis are the best examples of this abnormality.[5] The prevalence of hereditary spherocytosis is approximately 1 in 2000 (mostly northern Europeans).[5] In the United States, the incidence of hereditary elliptocytosis is approximately 1 in 2000 to 5000, with one of the more common forms commonly seen in people of African-American and Mediterranean heritage.[5]

Autoimmune hemolytic anemia can be associated with conditions such as viral or bacterial infections, collagen vascular diseases, and lymphoproliferative disorders, or it can be idiopathic. Severity can range from mild to very severe, acute, and life-threatening. It is a very rare disease. The type associated with warm-reacting autoantibodies is seen in 80% to 90% of all cases of autoimmune hemolytic anemia, and the incidence of this type is 1 in 100,000.[5]

PATHOPHYSIOLOGY

Drugs associated with acute hemolysis in G6PD-deficient patients include aspirin and phenacetin, sulfonamides, nitrofurantoin, and primaquine. Ingestion of an offending drug can result in the denaturation of hemoglobin, leading to an acute hemolytic event.[5] Other precipitants of hemolysis include the ingestion of fava beans or mothballs and severe bacterial or viral infections.

The functional abnormality in hereditary spherocytosis and hereditary elliptocytosis results from defects in the structural proteins of the erythrocyte cytoskeleton, specifically a deficiency of the protein spectrin.[5]

In the autoimmune hemolytic anemias, the patient produces autoantibodies that react with the RBCs, causing premature erythrocyte destruction. Two types of autoantibodies are produced: warm-reacting autoantibodies and cold-reacting autoantibodies. Warm-reacting antibodies are reactive with cells at 37° C (98.6° F), and cold-reacting antibodies are reactive at temperatures below 37° C.[5]

CLINICAL PRESENTATION

Most hemolytic anemias are mild, well compensated for, and associated with few signs or symptoms. If the anemia is severe, the patient displays the usual symptoms of severe anemia, such as fatigue and exercise intolerance. Patients with G6PD deficiency may have minimum or no clinical signs. Often the first clue that a patient has the deficiency is the onset of an acute hemolytic anemia after ingestion of an oxidant drug. The hemolytic event is self-limited and usually mild. Patients with the Mediterranean form of G6PD deficiency are at risk for more severe hemolysis.[5]

Both hereditary spherocytosis and hereditary elliptocytosis are usually characterized by a mild hemolytic anemia that is well compensated for. Patients with hereditary spherocytosis, however, can have a severe hemolytic anemia, whereas patients with hereditary elliptocytosis rarely have a clinically significant hemolytic anemia. Splenomegaly, aplastic crises, and pigment gallstones can complicate severe hereditary spherocytosis.[5]

The anemia caused by autoimmune hemolysis ranges from mild and subclinical to severe and life threatening. Patients with a warm-reacting autoimmune hemolytic anemia can have splenomegaly and other symptoms of anemia such as jaundice if the hemolysis is moderate or severe. Patients also show signs and symptoms of the underlying disease. Box 237-10 gives examples of conditions associated with warm and cold antibody autoimmune hemolysis.

BOX 237-10

Conditions Associated with Autoimmune Hemolysis

CONDITIONS ASSOCIATED WITH WARM AUTOANTIBODIES

Infections
Collagen vascular diseases
- Systemic lupus erythematosus
- Rheumatoid arthritis

Lymphoproliferative disorders
- Leukemia
- Lymphoma

Drugs
- Quinidine or quinine
- Penicillin
- α-Methyldopa

Chronic renal disease
Idiopathic disease

CONDITIONS ASSOCIATED WITH COLD AUTOANTIBODIES

Malignant disease
M. pneumoniae infection
Viral pneumonia
Idiopathic disease

PHYSICAL EXAMINATION

Patients with hemolytic anemias have essentially normal findings on physical examination. The only remarkable evidence of hemolysis may be scleral icterus, especially in patients with chronic hemolytic anemias such as sickle cell disease.

DIAGNOSTICS

During a mild acute hemolytic event, serologic test results show a slight decrease in hemoglobin and the RBC count, elevated LDH level, and slight hyperbilirubinemia. Patients with chronic hemolytic anemias, even when they are well compensated for, have persistent reticulocytosis.

Assays for G6PD are useful and detect most deficient patients. In some milder variants of the disease, however, the screening test result may be negative for several weeks after an acute hemolytic event.

A positive family history and the presence of pathognomonic findings on the peripheral blood smear easily diagnose both hereditary spherocytosis and hereditary elliptocytosis. Patients with hereditary spherocytosis have a large number of microspherocytes on the peripheral blood smear and an elevated MCHC on the CBC. The RBCs of patients with hereditary elliptocytosis have a uniform elliptic (oval) shape.

The diagnosis of an autoimmune hemolytic anemia depends on laboratory findings of abnormal autoantibodies. The Coombs test (both direct and indirect) is used to screen for these antibodies. The direct Coombs test result is positive in most cases of autoimmune hemolytic anemia or transfusion reactions and in some cases of drug-induced hemolysis. The indirect Coombs test result is positive in cases of antibody formation from previous transfusions or pregnancy and in drug-induced hemolytic anemia.

DIFFERENTIAL DIAGNOSIS

In a patient demonstrating hemolytic anemia, the differential diagnosis should consider whether the anemia is acute or chronic and the severity of the anemia.

DIFFERENTIAL DIAGNOSIS

Hemolytic Anemia

- Sickle cell disease
- G6PD deficiency
- Hereditary disorders (hereditary spherocytosis, hereditary elliptocytosis)
- Autoimmune hemolytic anemia

MANAGEMENT

Management of a patient with a hemolytic anemia varies according to the individual disease state. Therefore, proper management begins with an accurate diagnosis. Patients who are able to compensate for their degree of anemia generally require little intervention. If the hemoglobin level begins to fall well below the patient's baseline, an occasional transfusion of packed RBCs may be necessary.

The acute, self-limited hemolysis in patients with mild G6PD deficiency rarely requires treatment. The resulting anemia is mild and resolves without intervention. Any patient who sees a health care provider because of an acute hemolytic event resulting from exposure to an oxidant drug should have serial CBCs to determine resolution of the anemia. The most important aspect of management of G6PD deficiency is ensuring the patient's awareness of the condition. All high-risk individuals should be screened, and information about what drugs and foods to avoid should be provided to all patients with the deficiency.

Patients with mild forms of hereditary spherocytosis or hereditary elliptocytosis maintain adequate hemoglobin levels and are in generally good health. Patients with severe hereditary spherocytosis may require a splenectomy to decrease the severity of the anemia.[5] These patients are also candidates for prophylactic cholecystectomy because of the high incidence of pigment gallstones (elective cholecystectomy should definitely be done if gallstones occur).

Patients with autoimmune hemolytic anemia are generally treated with some combination of corticosteroid therapy or immunosuppressive therapy, splenectomy, and transfusion with packed RBCs. The specific therapy varies according to the type and severity of the hemolytic anemia.

LIFE SPAN CONSIDERATIONS

Patients with G6PD deficiency, hemoglobinopathy, or a hereditary RBC membrane defect should be aware of the hereditary potential. Professional genetic counseling and screening should be offered to all patients who are considering pregnancy.

COMPLICATIONS

Most of the hemolytic anemias discussed here rarely cause complications, especially if the hemolysis is mild and self-limited or chronic but well compensated for. Patients with more severe forms of hemolytic anemia, especially autoimmune hemolytic anemia, are at risk for acute episodes of severe hemolysis, with the associated morbidity and mortality of a severe anemia.

INDICATIONS FOR REFERRAL OR HOSPITALIZATION

A referral to a hematologist is prudent when an acute hemolysis does not appear to be resolving or when the anemia is severe or does not respond to treatment. Acute hemolysis that occurs as a result of a mild form of hemolytic anemia does not require hospitalization for management. If the patient also has some other underlying condition or the anemia is severe, however, hospitalization may be required for management. As with any other type of anemia, the need for hospitalization depends on the patient's ability to compensate for the degree of anemia.

PATIENT AND FAMILY EDUCATION

Patients should understand the nature of their disorder well enough to be able to explain it to other health care providers. Patients with G6PD deficiency should be given a list of drugs and foods to avoid, including over-the-counter products that contain aspirin or phenacetin. Patients with drug-induced hemolysis should be made aware of the types of drugs to avoid. Those with autoimmune hemolytic anemias should be made aware of the types of situations and conditions that can aggravate their anemia. All patients should be instructed to contact their health care provider if there are any signs of increased anemia.

CHAPTER 238

BLOOD COAGULATION DISORDERS

Maura Malone • Laurel McKernan •
Leo R. Zacharski • Deborah L. Ornstein

DEFINITION AND EPIDEMIOLOGY

Coagulation is the process by which blood changes from the fluid phase that is needed for tissue perfusion to a cohesive gel that prevents blood loss. This transition is achieved through a complex process involving many different initiating and inhibiting proteins as well as certain cells, including platelets and white blood cells. The benefits of this mechanism are obvious and are taken for granted except in individuals who have an excess or deficiency of a coagulant or anticoagulant protein because they may bleed excessively or form pathologic clots. The normal coagulation mechanism may fail for numerous reasons. A quantitative deficiency or a qualitative abnormality in counterbalancing coagulant or anticoagulant participants may tip the balance toward either bleeding (coagulopathy) or clotting (thrombosis). Similarly, a defect at one point in the system can often be compensated for by therapy that targets a different point in the system. Disorders of coagulation factors may be inherited or acquired. Common inherited bleeding disorders include von Willebrand disease (vWD), hemophilia A, and hemophilia B. Acquired bleeding disorders most often result from medications (e.g., aspirin, nonsteroidal anti-inflammatory drugs [NSAIDs], or anticoagulants) or organ dysfunction that accompanies certain medical diseases (e.g., liver or kidney disease, cancer, or leukemia).

Determination of the correct diagnosis is required for appropriate management and can be challenging, particularly with mild bleeding disorders. Patients are often referred for medical evaluation because of one of the following: a bleeding or thrombotic episode, a positive family history, or an abnormal laboratory test result found, for example, during preoperative screening. The health care provider needs to determine, through clinical and laboratory assessment, whether these referral indicators reflect the presence of a coagulation disorder. Clinical and laboratory assessment go hand in hand, but it is all too common for patients with a clinical disorder to have no abnormality on routine laboratory testing.

An elaborate balance exists between substances in the blood that promote clotting (coagulation factors) and other substances that preserve blood in fluid form (anticoagulant factors). This balance is maintained until a blood vessel is injured. The blood coagulation mechanism is designed to interpret such injuries and to respond by developing a protective clot at the injury site to stop the flow of blood. Prevention of blood loss from the vasculature with injury is vital, and this process is referred to as hemostasis. The hemostatic mechanism is appropriately viewed as a complex system because a defect in any one of its many components can lead to malfunction of the entire system.

The normal hemostatic response proceeds in three phases.[1] In phase 1, blood vessels constrict, reducing blood flow from the site. In phase 2, platelets are activated and chemicals are released almost instantaneously, resulting in the formation of a platelet plug at the site of injury. Phase 3 begins within seconds after platelet activation. In this phase, tissue factor, a molecule present on cell surfaces, triggers a complex cascade involving more than a dozen coagulation factors. The end result of this cascade is the production of thrombin, a powerful enzyme that converts fibrinogen, which is present in solution in the blood, to fibrin. Fibrin is a durable, visible mesh that seals the injured vessel (the scab). Traditionally, this cascade is thought to consist of intrinsic pathways (entirely plasma derived) and extrinsic pathways (tissue factor initiated), and abnormalities of coagulation factors within their pathways can often be detected by common laboratory tests such as the activated partial thromboplastin time (aPTT) and the prothrombin time (PT). For example, prolongation of the aPTT is suggestive of an abnormality of a coagulation factor in the intrinsic pathway of coagulation, whereas a prolonged PT leads one to suspect an abnormality within the extrinsic pathway.

BLEEDING DISORDERS (COAGULOPATHIES)

PATHOPHYSIOLOGY AND CLINICAL PRESENTATION

The manifestations of bleeding disorders are determined by the type and severity of the defect. Important questions to ask when faced with a bleeding patient include the following: Is it a vascular disorder, platelet abnormality, or coagulation factor deficiency? Is it hereditary or acquired? These questions are answered through clinical and laboratory assessment.[2]

Patients with hereditary (congenital) bleeding disorders usually have a lifelong history of symptoms, such as easy bruising and prolonged bleeding with cuts, surgery, or other trauma. Severe deficiencies generally become evident when the affected individual becomes a toddler and is increasingly likely to sustain minor trauma. Although bleeding may occur spontaneously in individuals with moderate or severe bleeding disorders, mild hereditary deficiencies may go undiagnosed for years until significant trauma occurs or the individual undergoes surgery. In contrast, acquired disorders may become evident later in life in the absence of a history of abnormal bleeding. Clinical presentation of acquired bleeding disorders may include recent onset of increased bruising, bleeding with trauma, nosebleeds, or a recent change in platelet count or clotting test results. The type of bleeding reported by the individual under evaluation may indicate which pathway is involved. For example, excessive bruising, mucosal bleeding, and postsurgical hemorrhage are typical of platelet disorders, whereas a history of frank bleeding after surgery and hemorrhage into the joints and muscles are typical of a marked coagulation factor deficiency such as hemophilia A or B. However, there are no rigid distinctions between the types of defects and their clinical manifestations. Clinical symptoms are discussed further in the section on diagnosis.

PHYSICAL EXAMINATION

Bleeding disorders are usually diagnosed by the history and laboratory findings.[1] Physical examination may be unremarkable, especially with mild defects; however, a variety of findings, including bruises, petechiae, gingival bleeding, epistaxis, and hematomas, may be evident, especially in individuals with more severe defects. Some degree of bruising is common in the general population, especially in those with fair complexion, in whom bruises are seen more easily. However, bruises that occur on the trunk in addition to the extremities tend to be more significant.

DIAGNOSTICS AND DIFFERENTIAL DIAGNOSIS

The most valuable diagnostic test for a bleeding disorder is a careful, comprehensive bleeding history. The history should provide clues to the type of bleeding disorder that may be present and will direct the laboratory testing that is indicated for further evaluation. The hemostatic response to trauma or surgery elicited in taking of a bleeding history is generally a more sensitive test of hemostatic competence than are screening laboratory tests and is more useful for predicting whether an individual will have a bleeding complication after surgery.[3] There is no substitute for clinical experience in deciding whether a patient has a coagulation disorder.

The bleeding history has two major elements: the patient's history and the family history. The patient should be asked to describe each event in life that presented a hemostatic challenge. For example, descriptions should include the duration and intensity of bleeding with minor cuts and scratches, surgery, dental extractions, and menstrual periods. Spontaneous bleeding may occur in the form of joint or soft tissue bleeding, epistaxis, and bruising. Bruising without obvious trauma is more significant than bruising in response to trauma. It is particularly important to encourage the patient to quantitate the degree of bleeding. This may be done, for example, by estimating average bruise counts and location, duration of post-traumatic bleeding, or duration of menstruation and number of pads or tampons soaked. Menstrual blood is normally unclotted, and the passage of clots (e.g., with urination, defecation, or pad changes) may be significant. With practice, interviewers will refine their assessment skills and assist their patients in proper interpretations because what is "normal" bleeding to one person may be "heavy" to another. Box 238-1 gives examples of

BOX 238-1

Interview Questions for Evaluation of a Patient with a Suspected Bleeding Disorder

PATIENT HISTORY

Does the patient have ecchymoses, easy and frequent bruising?
- How many bruises are present at a given time—one or two, a half-dozen or dozen, more?
- Are they raised or flat?
- Are they on the chest and trunk or only on the limbs?
- Are there hematomas with injections?

Is epistaxis spontaneous, or does it occur with trauma?
- Is the bleeding one-sided or bilateral?
- Is it seasonal, or does it occur year-round?
- How many episodes occur in a month? How long do they last, and what measures do you use to stop them? Has medical attention been required to stop the bleeding?
- Do large clots form?

Are there any hemostatic challenges, such as injuries or lacerations?
- How long did the bleeding last—a brief moment or more prolonged duration (minutes, longer)?
- Did the laceration require sutures?
- Did the bleeding continue afterward? For how long? Did bleeding ever start up again after stopping?
- Have there been any fractures?

Have there been any dental extractions?
- Was there any excessive bleeding? For how long—an hour, half a day, a day, a week?

Has there been any prior surgery?
- What kind?
- Was there any reported excessive bleeding?
- Were any transfusions required?

Has there been any significant injury or other trauma that might challenge the coagulation mechanism?
- Is the bleeding immediate, platelet-type bleeding or delayed, with deep hematomas?

Obtain a detailed menstruation history when appropriate.
- How long does menstruation last?
- How heavy is it? What is heavy? In general, how many pads or tampons per day? Is there frequent flooding around the pad or tampon?
- Is there formation of large clots?

Has there been any recent illness? Are any medications, including over-the-counter medications (e.g., aspirin), currently being taken?

Was there any bleeding during pregnancy or delivery? Was a transfusion required?

FAMILY HISTORY

- Inquire about immediate family members—brothers, sisters, parents, children. Request documentation when appropriate.
- Inquire about extended family on the maternal and paternal sides—grandparents, aunts and uncles, cousins.
- Review a line of questioning similar to the patient history for clinical features, surgery, trauma, transfusions, and menstrual history.
- When questioning parents about their children, inquire about cephalhematomas, buccal mucosal bleeding, bleeding from the tongue or tooth extractions, bleeding with separation of the umbilical cord, bruising or hematomas with immunizations, and bruising with the onset of crawling and ambulation.

Note: A negative bleeding history in a young child may not rule out a bleeding disorder; rather, a hemostatic challenge has not yet been encountered.

interview questions for use in evaluation of a patient for a bleeding disorder.

The family history is critical in assessing coagulation disorders. The genetic defects in hemophilia A and B (factor VIII and IX deficiency, respectively) are inherited in an X-linked recessive pattern and affect only males. The defect is carried by females, however, who are usually (but not always) asymptomatic. Thus, a male patient's *maternal* grandfather, uncles, and cousins may have bleeding that provides a clue to the diagnosis of hemophilia A or B.

Although the bleeding history is of paramount importance in the evaluation for coagulation disorders, it is not without limitations. The accuracy of information reported largely depends on the interviewer's ability to elicit a description of previous hemostatic challenges. It is easy to miss events or to obtain an incomplete history. Mild bleeding disorders are difficult to identify, especially in the absence of a hemostatic challenge, as is often the case in young children. Spontaneous mutations commonly account for cases of hemophilia A and B; consequently, the family history may be negative.

In anticipation of the decision to refer the patient for specialized tests in the face of clinical suspicion, the provider should perform certain screening studies. The typical laboratory screen, available in most clinical laboratories, includes the platelet count, a peripheral blood smear review, PT, aPTT, thrombin time, fibrinogen level, and platelet function analysis (or bleeding time).[2,4] These studies provide basic information on the integrity of platelet function and coagulation factor pathways.

The platelet count is usually performed by automated counters. Low values can be confirmed by estimating the number of platelets present on the peripheral blood smear. Common causes of a low platelet count include immune destruction, acute and chronic infections (e.g., infectious mononucleosis, human immunodeficiency virus [HIV] infection, hepatitis C), medications, vasculitis, disseminated intravascular coagulation, and chemotherapy. On occasion, a low platelet count obtained by the automated counter is caused by formation of platelet clumps as a result of interaction with the anticoagulant (ethylenediaminetetraacetic acid [EDTA]) in the blood collection tube. Thrombocytopenia caused by platelet clumping is merely an in vitro phenomenon and readily discernible by review of the peripheral blood smear. Such "pseudo-thrombocytopenia" is not typically associated with clinical bleeding.

The bleeding time has been a useful screen for platelet disorders. The bleeding time, however, is a crude measure of hemostasis that is neither sensitive nor specific for identification of bleeding disorders and is subject to many variables that may lead to misleading test results. For these reasons, the bleeding time has been retired in many centers in favor of an automated platelet function analyzer, such as the PFA-100 system.[5] The PFA-100 is an automated system that emulates the platelet-dependent component of primary hemostasis. A blood specimen is collected from the patient by venipuncture into an anticoagulated tube and transferred to the PFA-100 instrument, where the time required to form a platelet plug after exposure to specially treated membranes (the closure time) is measured. The PFA-100 is simple to use, reproducible, and sensitive to vWD and some qualitative platelet disorders (including effects of medications, such as aspirin), but it suffers from a lack of specificity. Closure times with the PFA-100 are affected by many of the same variables that affect the bleeding time (e.g., thrombocytopenia [100,000/mm^3], anemia), but the test is less subject to operator error.

The PT measures the function of the extrinsic system and the common pathway of coagulation. It is sensitive to abnormalities of factors VII, X, V, and II and fibrinogen. The aPTT measures the function of the intrinsic system and the common pathway. It detects abnormalities of prekallikrein, high-molecular-weight kininogen, and factors XII, XI, X, IX, VIII, V, II and fibrinogen.

A prolonged PT or aPTT may be evaluated further by performing mixing studies, which incorporate different ratios of normal (control) and abnormal (patient) plasma.[4] "Correction" of the prolonged clotting time on addition of normal plasma suggests the presence of a coagulation factor deficiency; failure to correct the abnormality suggests the presence of an inhibitor, such as a lupus anticoagulant. The inhibitor in the patient plasma neutralizes the added normal plasma, which thus fails to correct the abnormal coagulation test result. Misinterpretation of the results of mixing studies is a common cause of a request for a coagulation consultation. Examples of causes of a prolonged PT or aPTT are noted in Box 238-2.

BOX 238-2

Interpretation of Abnormal Screening Coagulation Test Results

PROLONGED PT/INTERNATIONAL NORMALIZED RATIO (INR)

Mild liver disease
Early vitamin K deficiency or warfarin therapy
Factor VII deficiency
Inhibitor to factor VII
Variable effect of direct factor Xa inhibitors (e.g., rivaroxaban, apixaban, edoxaban)

PROLONGED APTT

Deficiency of intrinsic pathway factor (VIII, IX, XI, XII)
Severe vWD (with low factor VIII level)
Inhibitor to intrinsic pathway factor (most commonly, factor VIII)
Heparin
Variable effect of dabigatran

PROLONGED PT AND APTT

Multiple coagulation factor deficiencies
- Disseminated intravascular coagulation
- Advanced liver disease
- Severe vitamin K deficiency or warfarin therapy

Deficiency of or inhibitor to a common pathway factor (fibrinogen, II, V, X)
Treatment with direct thrombin inhibitor (hirudin, argatroban, bivalirudin)

If the patient has no personal or family history of bleeding with hemostatic challenges such as surgery or significant trauma, he or she is not likely to have a bleeding disorder, and laboratory evaluation is usually not helpful. If the patient has a negative bleeding history but has not had significant hemostatic challenges in life and has a positive family history for bleeding, screening tests may be advisable. Diagnosis may be important for planning future care, such as with invasive procedures or elective surgery. Patients may be able to avoid unnecessary blood transfusions if a bleeding disorder is diagnosed and appropriate prophylactic treatment provided.

If the patient has a negative bleeding history but abnormal blood test results, other factors need to be considered, such as effects of medications (e.g., aspirin, NSAIDs, anticoagulants, guaifenesin-containing over-the-counter cold remedies), allergies (rhinitis), or concurrent medical illness. Circulating anticoagulants are commonly found in patients with an unexplained prolonged aPTT and rarely cause clinical bleeding. Less commonly, individuals with a deficiency of factor XII, prekallikrein or high-molecular-weight kininogen may be identified after finding of an unexplained prolonged aPTT. These proteins do not appear to have a pivotal role in hemostasis in vivo; thus, although deficiencies result in prolongation of the aPTT, they do not result in a clinical bleeding disorder. Circulating anticoagulants may be distinguished from both hemostatic and nonhemostatic factor deficiencies by mixing studies.

If the patient has a positive bleeding history, it is essential to first exclude an anatomic explanation for the bleeding before proceeding to laboratory testing. Severe bleeding disorders are generally readily identified by screening laboratory tests. A positive history and abnormal laboratory screening test results suggest strongly that a bleeding disorder exists, and referral to a hematologist for further evaluation is needed to characterize the specific diagnosis. Unfortunately, screening coagulation tests are often relatively insensitive for detection of mild coagulation disorders. Examples of bleeding disorders that may be associated with normal screening test results include mild hemophilia, vWD, abnormal fibrinogens, factor XIII deficiency, and qualitative platelet disorders. A positive bleeding history in a patient with normal laboratory test results therefore also suggests the need for referral to a hematologist with specialty expertise in blood coagulation.

It is important to keep in mind that the quality of coagulation test results is highly dependent on the conditions under which the samples are obtained and on the experience and professional quality of the coagulation laboratory. Prompt specimen processing and proper plasma storage are mandatory. Certain tests, such as platelet aggregation studies, require immediate laboratory testing with specialized equipment by highly trained and experienced technicians. Ideally, patients undergoing evaluation for bleeding disorders should be free of medications for at least 2 weeks, and samples obtained preferably in the morning after overnight fasting. It may be

DIAGNOSTICS

Bleeding Disorders

PT and aPTT	Thrombin time
Platelet count and peripheral blood smear review	Fibrinogen level
	PFA-100 (or bleeding time)

inadvisable to make a critical diagnosis on the basis of results obtained from plasma samples after prolonged storage or shipment to a distant laboratory. Travel by the patient to the testing laboratory for blood sampling is optimum, and abnormal results should always be confirmed by repeated testing before a diagnosis of a bleeding disorder is conferred.

DIFFERENTIAL DIAGNOSIS

Bleeding Disorders

HEREDITARY
- Hereditary hemorrhagic telangiectasia (Osler-Weber-Rendu syndrome)
- Connective tissue disorder (e.g., Ehlers-Danlos syndrome)
- Benign joint hypermobility syndrome
- vWD
- Qualitative platelet disorders
- Congenital thrombocytopenia
- Hemophilia A and B
- Factor XI deficiency
- Rare coagulation factor deficiencies
- Fibrinolytic inhibitor deficiencies

ACQUIRED
- Vascular trauma
- Vitamin C deficiency
- Antiplatelet medications
- Acquired vWD
- Disseminated intravascular coagulation
- Uremia
- Immune thrombocytopenia
- Liver disease
- Vitamin K deficiency
- Anticoagulation
- Acquired coagulation factor inhibitors (especially factor VIII)

MANAGEMENT AND INDICATIONS FOR REFERRAL OR HOSPITALIZATION

Since 1975, hemophilia treatment centers (HTCs) in the United States have been federally funded to provide comprehensive, specialized care to persons with bleeding disorders. The value of HTCs was highlighted in one study in which it was shown that the risk of dying for male hemophiliacs who received care at HTCs was 40% lower than that for hemophiliacs who received care outside of an HTC.[6] Therefore, management of a patient with a congenital bleeding disorder by a primary health care provider should ideally be in conjunction with a hematologist with expertise in blood coagulation and with attention paid to guidelines put forth by the Medical and Scientific Advisory Council (MASAC) of the National Hemophilia Foundation.[7] Once the patient has been evaluated by a hematologist, a detailed care plan should be developed that includes the MASAC guidelines for management of bleeding episodes, trauma, or invasive procedures. Patients with a coagulation factor deficiency, such as moderate or severe hemophilia A or B, require replacement of the missing clotting protein. A variety of plasma-derived and recombinant coagulation factor concentrates are available, and the hematologist will assist in identifying the appropriate product and dose for the patient (Table 238-1).

In patients with defined bleeding disorders, it is better to overestimate than to underestimate the risk of bleeding and to treat prophylactically or as soon as possible after bleeding begins because hemostasis is more difficult to achieve once excessive bleeding has commenced. To ensure rapid and appropriate treatment, a local supply of the appropriate replacement product should be maintained. Most patients with congenital bleeding disorders learn to recognize bleeding episodes soon after they occur and may be trained in self-administration of the coagulation factor by the intravenous route. In general, any significant trauma will require coagulation factor replacement, and most invasive procedures, even a seemingly minor one such as a tooth extraction, may require pretreatment with a coagulation factor concentrate. Surgery in the patient with a bleeding disorder should be undertaken at a facility equipped with an on-site coagulation laboratory, a full range of treatment products, and expert hematology consultation.

Trauma or surgery often requires many days of coagulation factor replacement accompanied by laboratory monitoring to ensure that hemostatic levels of the deficient clotting protein are present. Mild versions of some bleeding disorders, such as mild hemophilia A and type 1 vWD, may be corrected temporarily by administration of desmopressin acetate (DDAVP), a synthetic analogue of vasopressin. This drug is given either intravenously or by high-concentrate nasal spray and increases blood levels of factor VIII and von Willebrand factor (vWF) by releasing them from their storage sites in vascular endothelial cells. Not all patients respond to desmopressin, so before desmopressin is used in an emergency or surgical setting, it is mandatory to have first demonstrated its effectiveness in each individual patient by administering the drug in a controlled setting (usually the medical office) and measuring coagulation factor levels after administration to document a rise in the deficient clotting factor. Box 238-3 illustrates important issues to consider in assessment of the type, degree, and treatment of a bleeding episode.

TABLE 238-1 Dosage Guidelines for Coagulation Factor Replacement Therapy for Patients with Hemophilia A (Factor VIII Deficiency) and Hemophilia B (Factor IX Deficiency)*

	Factor VIII	Factor IX[†]
Type of bleeding episode		
Minor	15-20 units/kg	20-40 units/kg
Major	20-50 units/kg	40-80 units/kg
Life-threatening	40-50 units/kg	80-100 units/kg
Coagulation factor recovery	*Concentration (plasma derived or recombinant):* 1 IU/kg raises factor level 2% % Correction × Weight (kg) × 0.5 = Dose (IU)	*Plasma derived:* 1 IU/kg raises factor level 1% % Correction × Weight (kg) = Dose (IU) *Recombinant:* 1.2-1.4 IU/kg raises factor level 1% (adults, children) % Correction × Weight (kg) × 1.2-1.4 = Dose (IU)

*Factor dose depends on type, location, and severity of bleeding episode. Single or multiple doses may be needed on the basis of severity of the bleeding episode.
†Recombinant factor IX may require increased dosage to achieve the desired circulating factor IX levels.

BOX 238-3

Important Considerations in Assessment of Bleeding Episodes

- Type of coagulation disorder
- Degree or severity of the disorder
- Presence of comorbidity associated with history of transfusion, such as hepatitis B, hepatitis C, HIV infection
- Site and extent of bleeding and number of treatments
- History of response to replacement product; history of circulating inhibitors
- Replacement product: choice, dose, half-life, risks, benefits
- Any adjunct therapies (e.g., oral antifibrinolytic agents) required

VON WILLEBRAND DISEASE

vWD results from a deficiency or abnormality in vWF and is the most common congenital bleeding disorder, occurring in up to 1% of the general population.[8] vWF functions as a bridging molecule that binds to receptors exposed on the platelet surface to link them both to one another and to the area of damage on the blood vessel wall. vWF also serves as the carrier protein for blood coagulation factor VIII and therefore plays a critical role in both platelet plug formation and fibrin thrombus synthesis. The diagnosis of vWD can be challenging because various conditions (e.g., medications, inflammation, stress, pregnancy) can elevate vWF from abnormally low levels into the normal range, thus masking a true deficient state. Moreover, the results of screening laboratory tests such as the PT and aPTT may be normal in vWD, leading to underdiagnosis. Epistaxis, menorrhagia, excessive bruising, and prolonged bleeding with cuts or dental extractions and in the intraoperative or immediate postoperative period are common manifestations of the bleeding phenotype in vWD.

There are three major types of vWD, all of which exhibit an autosomal inheritance pattern, thus affecting both males and females.[8] Type 1 vWD is a quantitative deficiency in vWF and is the most common type, representing 70% to 80% of symptomatic cases. Type 2 vWD is composed of four variants (2A, 2B, 2M, 2N); it is characterized by qualitative defects in vWF structure and represents about 20% to 30% of vWD cases. Type 3 vWD is a quantitative deficiency of vWF in which vWF is essentially absent; these cases are rare, fortunately, because patients with type 3 vWD have a severe bleeding disorder. Once vWD is diagnosed, it is important to identify the specific type of vWD that is present so that appropriate treatment can be prescribed. For example, desmopressin, which is the preferred treatment for most cases of type 1 vWD, is ineffective in most type 2 variants and may be harmful in type 2B vWD.

Screening laboratory test results may be normal in patients with vWD; thus those with suspected vWD and a compelling bleeding history should be referred to a hematologist for specialty evaluation. The tests that may be helpful in evaluating such a patient include the following:

- *Complete blood count (CBC):* generally normal; thrombocytopenia is present in type 2B vWD.
- *PFA-100 closure times, bleeding time:* generally prolonged; may be normal in mild cases.
- *PT:* normal.
- *aPTT:* generally normal; will be prolonged and correct in mixing study in patients with low factor VIII levels.
- *Fibrinogen, thrombin time:* normal.
- *vWF antigen:* quantitative immunoassay that measures the concentration of vWF protein in plasma. This is typically decreased in type 1, low to normal in type 2, and absent in type 3.
- *vWF activity (ristocetin cofactor activity [vWF:RCo]):* functional assay that measures the ability of vWF to interact with platelets and cause platelet agglutination through the antibiotic ristocetin. vWF activity is decreased in direct proportion to the decrease in vWF antigen in types 1 and 3 and disproportionately decreased in type 2 disease.
- *Factor VIII activity (FVIII:C):* because vWF functions as a carrier protein for factor VIII and enhances its stability in plasma, low vWF antigen levels typically result in proportionally low factor VIII activity. Factor VIII activity is disproportionately low, however, in type 2N vWD, in which the binding site for factor VIII on vWF is abnormal.
- *Low-dose ristocetin-induced platelet aggregation:* special test used to distinguish between type 2B and other subtypes of vWD.
- *vWF multimers:* this test is performed only after the preceding testing has identified vWD. vWF exists in the plasma in the form of multimers of various sizes. The large vWF multimers are biologically most active. Type 1 vWD is characterized by a decrease in all multimers; type 2 is characterized by a relatively selective decrease in the larger multimers. vWF multimers of all sizes are absent in type 3 disease.

A diagnosis of vWD must not be made on the basis of single test result to avoid falsely labeling a patient with a bleeding disorder. Factor VIII and vWF tests can be affected by methods of specimen collection and transportation, resulting in falsely low readings if scrupulous care is not taken to handle the blood specimen properly. Whereas many hospital laboratories perform screening coagulation tests, many fewer perform vWD-specific testing, thus necessitating that specimens be sent to outside reference laboratories. Specimens may be mishandled along the way, resulting in falsely low readings and leading to a misdiagnosis of vWD. Similarly, because plasma vWF levels vary from day to day depending on numerous extraneous factors, a single set of normal test results may not be sufficient to rule out the diagnosis. Accordingly, if a patient has a history suggestive of a bleeding disorder but normal (especially low-normal) vWD test results, the tests should be repeated at a point when the patient is clinically well and not experiencing physiologic or psychological stress, both of which may temporarily elevate vWF levels. The diagnosis of mild type 1 vWD can be difficult because overlap exists between vWF levels in healthy individuals and those in individuals with mild disease. For example, individuals with type O blood often have low or low-normal levels of vWF without evidence of a frank bleeding disorder. Determination of ABO type at the time of vWD testing may be helpful for interpreting the significance of vWD test results.

Once a diagnosis of vWD is confirmed, a treatment plan can be made, and this is best done in consultation with a hematologist. Most individuals with vWD do not require ongoing treatment with hemostatic agents but will require treatment for bleeding episodes and prophylaxis for invasive procedures. Many patients with type 1 vWD respond to desmopressin, but this response must be documented before use of the drug to prevent or to treat bleeding. Plasma-derived factor VIII concentrates that are rich in vWF are the current products of choice for vWD patients for whom desmopressin is not appropriate.[8]

HEMOPHILIA

Hemophilia is an X-linked recessive bleeding disorder characterized by low levels of factor VIII (hemophilia A) or factor IX (hemophilia B), resulting in defective fibrin clot formation. Minor injuries are sometimes associated with little immediate bleeding because platelet thrombus formation is normal. Hemophiliacs may experience delayed bleeding, however, as the platelet plug breaks down prematurely in the absence of a stabilizing fibrin clot. Joint and muscle hemorrhages are common in moderate and severe hemophilia. Recurrent hemarthroses result in hypertrophy and inflammation of joint synovial tissue, causing articular cartilage damage and ultimately leading to loss of joint function and long-term disability. Limb contractures are common, often requiring physical therapy for range of motion to be regained. Psoas muscle bleeding may cause vague hip pain or abdominal pain that is often confused with appendicitis or renal colic. Intracranial hemorrhage is a leading cause of death in hemophilia, and head trauma necessitates immediate coagulation factor replacement. This is the case even if the patient appears clinically stable and neurologically intact initially; delayed bleeding is common and may be catastrophic.

Hemophilia occurs in 1 in 10,000 male births and affects more than 400,000 males worldwide.[9] Hemophilia A is more common than hemophilia B, representing about 80% of cases. The diagnosis of hemophilia is usually straightforward, unlike that of vWD. The PT, thrombin time, and PFA-100 (or bleeding time) are usually normal, whereas the aPTT is usually prolonged. Patients with mild cases of hemophilia, however, may have a normal or minimally prolonged aPTT; thus, if the diagnosis is suspected, further evaluation is in order. The diagnosis of hemophilia requires demonstration of a low level of factor VIII in the case of hemophilia A or of factor IX in the case of hemophilia B. There are three categories of hemophilia—severe, moderate, and mild, in which the levels of the missing coagulation factor are less than 1%, 1% to 5%, and 6% to 40%, respectively. Patients with mild hemophilia may have severe bleeding only with trauma or surgery, whereas those with moderate and severe disease will often experience spontaneous bleeding.

Treatment of bleeding in a hemophiliac involves prompt, and occasionally prolonged, replacement of coagulation factors. Although patients with mild hemophilia A seldom bleed spontaneously, they will require coagulation factor replacement for significant injuries or surgery. Patients with moderate or severe hemophilia require infusions of coagulation factor concentrates to treat bleeding episodes, but mild hemophiliacs may respond, at least temporarily, to DDAVP,[9] which stimulates release of factor VIII from intracellular stores. Symptomatic head trauma requires immediate coagulation factor replacement and evaluation by a practitioner with expertise in neurologic injuries. Imaging studies should be performed to exclude intracranial bleeding, but coagulation factor concentrate infusions should be administered before any diagnostics are performed. Soft tissue hematomas may resolve with coagulation factor replacement if they are treated promptly; however, continued bleeding may result in compression of vital structures. In addition to treatment after bleeding is identified, preventive therapy must be administered before surgery or an invasive procedure. Regular prophylactic infusions of coagulation factor concentrates for children with severe hemophilia reduce the incidence of hemarthroses and prevent long-term joint damage,[10] and appear to maintain a beneficial effect for adults.[11] Coagulation factor concentrates are administered intravenously up to three times weekly for prophylaxis and up to two to three times daily for treatment of acute hemorrhage. The advent of recombinant coagulation factor products engineered to have extended half-lives promises to improve convenience and quality of life by reducing the frequency of infusions dramatically.[12] Gene therapy for the treatment of hemophilia is an active area of investigation.[13]

COMPLICATIONS

Bleeding resulting from coagulation disorders may produce a variety of complications. For example, the chronic, recurrent joint bleeding commonly experienced by patients with hemophilia may lead to joint immobility and limb contractures. Chronic bleeding can cause anemia as a result of iron deficiency. Bleeding into various organs can result in dysfunction of that organ. Such bleeding may be fatal if it occurs, for example, in the cranial cavity or the gastrointestinal tract. Antibodies or inhibitors to infused coagulation factor concentrates may develop, making it difficult to control bleeding even with minor injuries. Viral transmission via plasma-derived coagulation factor concentrates led to a substantial proportion of the hemophiliac population becoming infected with HIV and/or hepatitis C. With the development of efficient viral inactivation procedures for plasma-derived products and production of recombinant coagulation factors, the transmission of these viruses by coagulation factor concentrates has been essentially eliminated.

PATIENT EDUCATION AND LIFE SPAN CONSIDERATIONS

Education is an important and ongoing process. Patients should know the specific name of their bleeding disorder and be able to communicate this diagnosis to their health care providers. They should recognize the signs and symptoms of bleeding and know how to respond appropriately to ensure early and effective treatment. Each patient should have an emergency care plan that includes access to a dose of the appropriate coagulation factor concentrate because many hospitals do not maintain a supply of these products. Work and leisure activities should be reviewed for practices such as contact sports that present a risk for precipitation of bleeding episodes. Medications, such as aspirin and other NSAIDs, that aggravate bleeding tendencies should typically be avoided. Patients are advised to use medications that do not compromise hemostasis, such as acetaminophen, for mild discomfort. Medications must be reviewed periodically and new drugs evaluated for their potential to increase bleeding. For example, fish oil and selective serotonin reuptake inhibitors have antiplatelet activity and should be used with caution in patients with severe bleeding disorders. Wearing a medical alert bracelet or necklace is advised. The patient's coagulation status must be evaluated before dentist visits and surgical or other invasive procedures. Genetic counseling is recommended as a component of family planning.

THROMBOSIS DISORDERS (THROMBOPHILIA)

PATHOPHYSIOLOGY AND CLINICAL PRESENTATION

In the normal state, procoagulant enzymes trigger the formation of a blood clot (thrombus) to ensure hemostasis after injury. These procoagulant factors are balanced by inhibitory factors to ensure that excessive clotting does not occur and that the blood remains in the liquid state. When this equilibrium is disturbed, a hypercoagulable state results and thrombosis, the process by which an inappropriate thrombus forms in the living heart or vasculature, may occur. Thrombosis may occur in either the arterial or venous circulation, but risk factors for clot formation in the two circulations differ somewhat. For example, thrombi in arteries are commonly associated with atherosclerosis (hardening of the arteries), a condition that does not affect veins, and hereditary conditions leading to a hypercoagulable state increase the risk for formation of clots in veins but have little impact on arterial clot formation. Thrombophilia refers to a tendency to develop venous thrombosis and may result from acquired or hereditary factors, or often from a combination of both.

Thrombosis may occur in any vein in the body, but the majority of clots form in the deep veins of the lower extremities. This deep venous thrombosis (DVT) causes pain and swelling in the distal tissues. Segments may break off from thrombi in extremity veins and be transported to the right side of the heart, where they are then transmitted to the pulmonary arterial circulation in the form of pulmonary emboli (PE). It is estimated that 350,000 to 600,000 individuals in the United States experience venous thromboembolism (VTE), and up to 100,000 die of complications annually.[14]

Numerous conditions that may trigger VTE have been identified. For example, individuals with cancer, obesity, diabetes, or chronic inflammatory diseases are at increased risk. In addition, surgery, trauma, pregnancy, childbirth, immobilization, hospitalization, estrogen use, smoking, advanced age, extended travel, and acute medical illness are other well-established risk factors. Thrombosis may also occur in otherwise healthy individuals with no obvious explanation. These episodes are referred to as idiopathic and are frequently associated with a hereditary predisposition to venous thrombosis (i.e., thrombophilia).

The Virchow triad continues to define the pathogenesis of VTE, with changes in blood vessel walls, blood flow, and coagulability of the blood itself all contributing to risk. One example of an abnormality in the coagulability of the blood is activated protein C resistance (APCR). APCR is commonly caused by the presence of an abnormal coagulation factor V molecule resulting from a mutation in the factor V gene.[15] This abnormal factor V is known as factor V Leiden in honor of the city in the Netherlands where the mutation was identified. Factor V Leiden occurs in the heterozygous form in 3% to 8% of white individuals (affecting up to 60 million people worldwide) but is rare in individuals of African or Asian descent.[16] The mutated factor V enzyme resists breakdown by activated protein C, a protein that helps keep blood in the fluid state. Factor V Leiden is transmitted in an autosomal dominant inheritance pattern; thus both males and females are affected. A person with heterozygous factor V Leiden has about a threefold increased risk for development of VTE compared with the general population, which roughly translates to an increase in the absolute risk for development of VTE from 0.1% to about 0.3% annually in middle age. Homozygous factor V Leiden is less common than the heterozygous form, but is a stronger risk factor for VTE and increases the risk by about 18-fold. The majority of people with factor V Leiden are asymptomatic, however, and never develop VTE in their lifetimes.

Often, VTE results from additive risks factors, such as obesity, smoking, and estrogen-containing oral contraceptive use in the setting of a genetic predisposition. Aging is an overlooked risk factor for VTE and results in a doubling of risk for each decade of life. APCR resulting from factor V Leiden is the most common gene mutation leading to hereditary predisposition to VTE in white individuals. Sickle cell trait (see Chapter 237) occurs in around 1 of 12 African Americans and confers a twofold increased risk for DVT and a fourfold increased risk for PE.[17]

In addition to factor V Leiden and sickle cell trait, other genetic abnormalities that predispose individuals to VTE include the prothrombin gene variant (PT G20210A) and deficiencies of the natural anticoagulant proteins, protein C, protein S, and antithrombin (formerly known as antithrombin III).[15] Whereas factor V Leiden, PT G20210A, and sickle cell trait are relatively common and mild forms of thrombophilia, deficiencies of the natural anticoagulants are relatively rare and impart a more severe tendency to venous thrombosis. Inheritance of one abnormal factor V Leiden or PT G20210A gene results in an affected individual's being a heterozygote for the gene polymorphism. These gene polymorphisms are common enough that individuals with two abnormal copies of the genes (homozygotes) or one abnormal copy of each (compound heterozygotes) exist. The risk for VTE is higher in these individuals than in those who are simple heterozygotes for the polymorphisms, but most people remain asymptomatic unless other risk factors are present.

PHYSICAL EXAMINATION

Thrombi can form in both superficial and deep veins. Thrombi in the superficial veins manifest with localized tenderness at the site, redness, a feeling of warmth, and possible swelling of the affected limb. Because the vein is close to the surface, it may feel hard or ropelike when examined. The clinical features of DVT include pain, swelling, and erythema of the affected extremity. The Homan sign (pain with dorsiflexion of the foot) may also be present, but its absence does not exclude DVT. PE may be asymptomatic when accompanying DVT or may manifest with such symptoms as chest pain, shortness of breath, palpitations, syncope, or a vague feeling of doom. Physical examination is often neither sensitive nor specific for VTE, and further testing must be done when the condition is suspected.

DIAGNOSTICS AND DIFFERENTIAL DIAGNOSIS

D-dimer is a breakdown product of a fibrin clot that can be measured in the blood; it is virtually always elevated in a patient with an acute thrombosis. The D-dimer test is frequently the first test performed in patients with suspected VTE, but although it has a good sensitivity and negative predictive value for diagnosis of VTE, an abnormal test result is not specific and has a poor positive predictive value. That is, a negative D-dimer test result is helpful for ruling out VTE in patients with a low clinical probability of having VTE, but a positive test result does not rule it in, and further testing must be undertaken.[18] A Doppler ultrasound study is typically performed to evaluate for venous thrombosis in the limbs. It has excellent sensitivity for detection of proximal DVT but is relatively insensitive in the calf. Ascending venography, a radiologic procedure involving injection of contrast dye into the superficial and deep veins of the leg, permits diagnosis of DVT but is no longer commonly used. Computed tomography of the chest with intravenous administration of contrast material is increasingly the preferred test for evaluation of patients with suspected PE, replacing ventilation/perfusion scans in many institutions.

BOX 238-4

Some Causes of Hereditary Thrombophilia

- APCR caused by factor V Leiden
- Prothrombin gene variant, G20210A
- Protein C deficiency
- Protein S deficiency
- Antithrombin deficiency
- Homocystinuria
- Hyperhomocysteinemia
- Dysfibrinogenemia
- Factor XIII polymorphisms
- Increased plasma coagulation factors (fibrinogen; prothrombin; factors VIII, IX, XI)

Determination of the cause of VTE relies heavily on the history and physical examination, which focuses on identifying the presence of acquired risk factors as outlined before. Hereditary thrombophilia should be suspected in individuals with VTE that is unexplained, occurs at a young age (i.e., <50 years), occurs in an unusual location (e.g., mesenteric, cerebral circulations), is recurrent, or is associated with a family history of VTE in multiple first-degree relatives. Examples of common hereditary and acquired thrombophilia conditions are listed in Box 238-4.[19] Thrombophilic disorders are distinguished from one another primarily on the basis of the laboratory evaluation. The decision about which laboratory tests are indicated is determined by the medical history and clinical presentation. The goal of thrombophilia testing is to determine whether a defect is present that may be important for planning of future treatment and that may be sought in other family members who may or may not yet have had an episode of VTE. The results of thrombophilia testing rarely have implications for the acute treatment of VTE; thus, testing should be deferred until the end of the initial anticoagulation period to avoid falsely abnormal results from interference by anticoagulation, inflammation, or consumption of natural anticoagulants by the acute clot. Although genetic tests for thrombophilia can generally be accomplished at any time, optimal patient management involves genetic counseling and informed consent for the testing, which is best conducted in the office of the hematologist and not in the emergency department or the inpatient setting.

MANAGEMENT

Management of VTE should follow the American College of Chest Physicians guidelines for antithrombotic therapy for prevention and treatment of thrombosis.[20] The diagnosis of hereditary thrombophilia in itself is not an indication for treatment with anticoagulants, especially if thrombosis has not occurred. In general, VTE is treated the same in individuals with and without thrombophilia, and treatment is begun immediately with anticoagulants to prevent thrombus growth and subsequent pulmonary embolism.

Heparin has long been the initial treatment for VTE because its anticoagulant effect begins immediately. Heparin acts together with antithrombin to block coagulation factor enzymes, especially thrombin and activated factor X (factor Xa). Unfractionated heparin is administered intravenously, and the dose is adjusted according to the aPTT range established by each individual hospital laboratory. Care must be taken not to exceed the therapeutic aPTT range because this increases the risk for severe bleeding complications. Intravenous unfractionated heparin has largely been replaced by low-molecular-weight heparin (LMWH) for the treatment of acute VTE in most situations; however, LMWH also works with antithrombin but inhibits activated factor X to a much greater extent than thrombin. This ability of LMWH to block the clotting mechanism "upstream" accounts for many of the advantages of this drug. In randomized clinical trials, LMWH has been shown to be at least as effective and safe as intravenous unfractionated heparin for the initial treatment of both DVT and PE.[21] Compared with heparin, LMWH has a longer half-life, more consistent and complete absorption when it is injected subcutaneously, and fewer side effects including a lower risk for the potentially catastrophic complication of heparin-induced thrombocytopenia. LMWH is as effective when it is given in a fixed, weight-based subcutaneous dose as when it is given intravenously and does not require routine laboratory monitoring for dose adjustment.[22] These advantages permit management of many patients with DVT (and some low-risk patients with PE) entirely in the outpatient setting and also provide safe, outpatient control of thrombosis with self-administration should warfarin fail. Heparin and LMWH are biologic preparations extracted from animal intestines, usually pigs. A synthetic pentasaccharide molecule, fondaparinux, is also available for acute treatment of VTE. Its mechanism of action is like that of heparin and LMWH except that it inhibits activated factor X exclusively and has a longer half-life than LMWH, permitting once-daily subcutaneous administration. Like LMWH, it is administered in a fixed dose without laboratory monitoring, allowing convenient outpatient use. In randomized clinical trials, fondaparinux was equivalent in efficacy and safety to both LMWH and heparin for the initial treatment of VTE.[22]

Initial heparin or LMWH therapy is typically followed by treatment with a vitamin K antagonist, typically warfarin in the

DIFFERENTIAL DIAGNOSIS

Thrombophilia

HEREDITARY

- APCR caused by factor V Leiden
- Prothrombin gene mutation G20210A
- Protein C deficiency
- Protein S deficiency
- Antithrombin deficiency
- Homocystinuria
- Hyperhomocysteinemia
- Dysfibrinogenemia
- Factor XIII polymorphisms
- Increased plasma coagulation factors (fibrinogen; prothrombin; factors VIII, IX, XI)

ACQUIRED

- Active cancer or chemotherapy treatment
- Obesity
- Age
- Medications (estrogen, oral contraceptives)
- Autoimmune and inflammatory disorders (especially inflammatory bowel disease)
- Antiphospholipid antibodies
- Pregnancy or postpartum state
- Nephrotic syndrome
- Surgery and trauma
- Heparin-induced thrombocytopenia
- Myeloproliferative neoplasms
- Paroxysmal nocturnal hemoglobinuria
- Varicose veins
- HIV infection
- Wegener granulomatosis

United States, which is usually started concurrently with heparin or LMWH. Warfarin is administered orally and is absorbed from the intestine along with other nutrients, including vitamin K. Vitamin K is required for the production of coagulation factors II, VII, IX, and X in their fully active form by the liver. Warfarin competes with vitamin K, resulting in the production of incomplete, less active coagulation factors. This takes time, usually 5 days for coagulation factor synthesis to decrease and for previously activated coagulation factors to clear the circulation. During this period, heparin or LMWH and warfarin are given concurrently for full protection. When the warfarin becomes effective, as measured by laboratory testing (two consecutive international normalized ratio [INR] determinations in the therapeutic range at least 24 hours apart), heparin or LMWH is discontinued. Heparin or LMWH *must be* administered for a minimum of 5 days, however, irrespective of the rapidity with which a therapeutic INR is achieved. The patient is then maintained with warfarin on an outpatient basis for a minimum of 3 months after a first episode of VTE. In certain individuals at high risk for recurrence (e.g., those with idiopathic VTE, active cancer, or antiphospholipid syndrome), indefinite anticoagulation after a first event should be considered.[20]

Because warfarin and vitamin K are in competition, the effect of warfarin may be exaggerated when dietary vitamin K is inadequate. The effect of warfarin is also exaggerated with liver disease, and many different drugs increase or decrease the warfarin effects. Therefore it is important to identify any medications being used during anticoagulation therapy. When warfarin is stopped, the production of fully active coagulation factors gradually returns over several days. The amount of warfarin required to achieve an optimum degree of therapeutic anticoagulation varies among individuals and is determined by the PT, which is standardized by the INR calculation. Expression of the result as the INR is preferred because it eliminates variability among laboratories and reagents used to perform the PT measurement. The degree of warfarin anticoagulation required for maximum protection with minimum risk of bleeding depends on clinical conditions present at that time. The recommended target INR is 2.5 with a range of 2 to 3 for secondary prophylaxis to reduce the risk of recurrent VTE, and it is the same whether or not thrombophilia is identified.[20] Anticoagulation is best managed by dedicated anticoagulation clinics with use of validated dosage algorithms. The Anticoagulation Forum website (www.acforum.org) is an excellent resource for matters pertaining to management of acute and chronic anticoagulation.

Patients with active cancer benefit from long-term treatment with LMWH rather than with warfarin. A randomized clinical trial has established that 6 months of treatment with LMWH reduces the risk for recurrent VTE in cancer patients nearly 50% compared with warfarin, without an increased risk for bleeding when it is used for secondary prophylaxis.[23] Treatment with LMWH should therefore be considered for all cancer patients with VTE whenever feasible.

Although heparin, LMWH and warfarin are currently the mainstays of treatment and secondary prevention of VTE, a number of small-molecule, synthetic target-specific oral anticoagulants (TSOACs) have been available for some time in Europe and Canada and have recently been approved in the United States.[24] They have the advantages of being active orally in a fixed dose, not interacting with food or most other medications, and not requiring laboratory monitoring for dosage adjustment. In some cases, the TSOACs allow for an entirely oral treatment course for acute VTE, thus eliminating the need for painful LMWH injections.

Dabigatran is a direct inhibitor of thrombin (factor IIa), whereas rivaroxaban, apixaban, and others are direct inhibitors of activated factor X. Clinical trials have demonstrated equivalent efficacy of the TSOACs to LMWH-warfarin combinations for treating acute VTE and suggest a reduction in major bleeding complications.[24] Of theoretical concern with the use of TSOACs is the lack of an effective antidote in the event of an overdose or a major bleeding complication. Although warfarin effect is readily reversed with vitamin K or an infusion of a plasma-derived coagulation factor concentrate, TSOAC effect is irreversible for all practical purposes. The long half-life of warfarin (several days) makes having an antidote desirable, but the short half-lives of the TSOACs (hours) generally obviate the need for one.

Whereas TSOACs are appropriate for many people with acute VTE, there are some patient populations for which traditional anticoagulants may still be preferred. For example, patients with severe liver and/or kidney dysfunction may have impaired drug elimination pathways, leading to drug accumulation and an increased risk for bleeding. The TSOACs have not been studied in cases of massive PE or extensive DVT for which thrombolytic therapy is administered, nor have they been studied specifically in patients with severe thrombophilias such as cancer or antiphospholipid syndrome, and should be reserved for patients in these categories for whom traditional anticoagulation is otherwise not optimal. The safety of TSOACs in pregnancy is unknown; thus treatment and prevention of VTE in pregnancy are best accomplished with heparin or LMWH. Finally, although the TSOACs are safe and effective for stroke prevention in atrial fibrillation, they appear to be inferior to warfarin for prevention of mechanical heart valve thrombosis and should not be prescribed for that purpose.

COMPLICATIONS

Clot formation within intact vessels compromises the vascular supply to the affected areas. With venous thrombosis, the reduced flow of blood from the affected area of the body results in swelling and pain in that part. For example, a thrombus in the veins of the leg can result in swelling and discoloration of the foot and lower leg. When the obstruction is not relieved promptly, the swelling may become chronic and noticeable, especially after patients have been on their feet for a time. If it is not properly treated, DVT may result in venous valve damage, venous reflux, and ambulatory venous hypertension leading to the chronic, often debilitating complication of post-thrombotic syndrome (PTS). Below-the-knee compression stockings after acute DVT reduced the incidence and severity of PTS in older studies,[25] but their value has been questioned on the basis of more recent trials;[26,27] thus their use may be reserved for those with symptoms. Finally, if it is not promptly treated, a DVT may extend and break off, producing an embolus that may become lodged in the vessels of the lung (a pulmonary embolus). When such emboli are large or multiple, they can be life-threatening.

INDICATIONS FOR REFERRAL OR HOSPITALIZATION

Referral to a hematologist with experience in VTE and thrombophilia should be considered for patients with a history of unexplained or recurrent VTE, family history of VTE, or VTE at an early age or in unusual locations. Investigation for a hereditary predisposition to VTE may result in therapeutic or preventive measures for the patient or family members, but testing should be performed only after counseling of the patient about the potential implications of test results—both normal and abnormal—and only with the patient's informed consent. Test results should be discussed during a face-to-face meeting between the patient and a hematologist or genetic counselor, with the discussion tailored to the patient's specific circumstances.

Patients with DVT should be hospitalized when the clot is extensive or is accompanied by severe PE. Patients without sufficient outpatient support, who cannot inject themselves with LMWH, or who lack access to TSOACs should be hospitalized for initial treatment. In general, most patients with symptomatic PE should be hospitalized for initial treatment because the potential for life-threatening complications is high; however, protocols for risk stratification exist, and low-risk patients with PE may be considered for outpatient management. Often, hospitalization may be shortened when LMWH or TSOACs are used for initial anticoagulation because patients can self-administer these medications at home. Although LMWH and TSOACs make outpatient treatment a reality for many people with acute VTE, initial clinical follow-up should be no less diligent than if patients were hospitalized, given the potential for both clotting and bleeding complications early in the treatment course.

LIFE SPAN CONSIDERATIONS

Patients with a family history of coagulopathies may experience problems with pregnancy, especially miscarriage, and may benefit from genetic counseling. Pregnancy and the immediate postpartum period incur a higher risk of VTE. Oral contraceptives increase the risk of blood clotting, especially in smokers, so young women should be counseled appropriately. Hormone replacement therapy is also associated with increased risk of DVT and stroke and should be used for the shortest time possible. Older adults are more likely to have problems with blood clotting, especially if they also have an inherited coagulopathy.

PATIENT AND FAMILY EDUCATION

Patient education is an important component of safe and effective outpatient anticoagulation therapy. Patients need to be aware of their diagnosis and factors influencing anticoagulation treatment. Education focuses on the importance of keeping regular follow-up visits, monitoring anticoagulation doses, identifying signs of bleeding or clot progression, maintaining a consistent diet (if taking warfarin), noting changes in health and diet or medications, and avoiding hazardous activities such as contact sports. In addition, a regularly updated pharmacology resource should be consulted for medications that interact with warfarin, and information should be provided to patients with periodic updates.

Prolonged immobility is discouraged. When the at-risk patient is immobilized, such as while driving or flying, he or she should take frequent rest breaks for leg stretching or walking and consider wearing below-the-knee compression stockings. Patients at risk for VTE need information about the signs and symptoms of VTE and how to access appropriate care. Genetic counseling and risk management are essential for individuals with inherited disorders. Counseling about risk reduction is required and should include regular discussions of the role of weight loss, exercise, smoking cessation, and management of chronic medical conditions in reducing risk for recurrent VTE in individuals both with and without thrombophilia.

CHAPTER 239

LEUKEMIAS

Susan Brighton • Elizabeth Kimtis

Referral to a hematologist is indicated for all suspected cases of leukemia.

DEFINITION AND EPIDEMIOLOGY

Some of the most challenging and complex cancers to manage in the community setting are the leukemias, hematologic malignant neoplasms that affect the bone marrow and lymphatic tissue. There are four different types of leukemia, two acute and two chronic forms. The acute forms of leukemia are acute myelogenous leukemia (AML) and acute lymphocytic leukemia (ALL). Chronic myelogenous leukemia (CML) and chronic lymphocytic leukemia (CLL) are the two chronic forms of leukemia, with CLL being the most common form of leukemia.[1] Acute leukemias are distinguished by an abnormal production of immature white blood cells (WBCs), called blasts, and rapid disease progression over approximately 6 months, which results in limited life expectancy if left untreated. Chronic leukemias reveal an overabundance of more mature-appearing but ineffective WBCs. Disease progression is usually slower, over several years as opposed to months. The overproduction of leukemia cells displaces normal cells in the bone marrow and thus crowds out normal hematopoiesis, resulting in granulocytopenia, anemia, and thrombocytopenia. Depending on the type of leukemia, treatment may be as conservative as observation or as aggressive as bone marrow or peripheral blood stem cell transplantation. Consequences of the disease state and side effects of treatment represent a true challenge to the health care provider.

In 2015, there were estimated to be approximately 54,270 new cases of leukemia in the United States, with a slightly higher incidence of acute compared with chronic leukemia. The estimated number of deaths from leukemia in 2015 was approximately 24,450.[2,3] The exact cause of leukemia is unknown. Causes and risk factors for consideration are genetic factors and disorders, exposure to radiation, environmental factors, occupational exposures, drugs, viruses, and other bone marrow disorders.

Children with genetic disorders such as Down syndrome have an increased risk for the development of acute leukemia. Other conditions that are associated with a higher risk for developing leukemia include Ellis–van Creveld syndrome, Fanconi anemia, Klinefelter syndrome, Bloom syndrome, and ataxia-telangiectasia.

Exposure to ionizing radiation is the most conclusive predisposing factor associated with the development of leukemia. This became evident after World War II, when a large number of Japanese survivors of the atomic bomb demonstrated an increased incidence of AML and CML, usually 5 to 9 years after exposure.[2] Pioneer radiologists who were exposed to massive radiation also exhibited a high incidence of leukemia.[4]

Environmental factors such as hair dye, cigarette smoking, and sunbathing may also increase the risk for development of leukemia, although studies have been inconclusive.[5]

Occupational exposure to certain chemicals increases the risk for development of leukemia. Workers exposed to benzene (a hydrocarbon used in industry, such as rubber and shoemaking plants, and in unleaded gasoline), rubber cement, and cleaning solvents are at risk. Other occupations in which workers are at risk of contracting leukemia are those that expose workers to explosives, dyes, or paints including distilleries, pesticide manufacturing, and leather tanning industries.[5] Although the relationship between leukemia and viruses remains unclear, there does appear to be a correlation between retroviruses and T-cell leukemia and hairy cell leukemia.[6]

Antecedent hematologic disorders, such as polycythemia vera, aplastic anemia, myelodysplastic syndromes (MDSs), and other diseases of the bone marrow also appear to predispose individuals to leukemia. Intensive combination chemotherapy for patients with cancer has led to increased survival rates overall. However, these survivors must be continually evaluated for complications of the long-term cytotoxic treatment. One serious consequence is the development of a second cancer, especially myeloid leukemia. Therapy-related leukemia is typically a fatal disease. Treatment-related myelodysplastic syndrome (t-MDS) and treatment-related AML (t-AML) are the terms used to describe a clinical syndrome that is arguably the most serious unpredictable long-term complication of cancer treatment. In total, therapy-related myeloid neoplasms represent 10% to 20% of acute leukemias, MDSs, and myelodysplastic or myeloproliferative neoplasms.[7]

PATHOPHYSIOLOGY

All blood cells—WBCs, red blood cells and platelets—originate from the stem cell, which is predominantly found in the bone marrow. The stem cell's unique ability for self-renewal and differentiation is necessary to meet the body's requirements throughout a lifetime.[8]

Leukemia is a malignant disorder of the blood and blood-forming organs—the spleen, lymphatic system, and bone marrow. It is identified as acute or chronic by the onset of symptoms and the maturity of the blood cell. Leukemic cells are designated either myeloid or lymphoid, according to the type of cell that predominates, as identified by morphology of the cells in combination with flow cytometry, cytogenetics, and molecular markers.

There is a maturational arrest of immature leukocytes, or blasts, in acute leukemia. These blasts proliferate or accumulate uncontrollably, inhibiting normal hematopoiesis and contributing to organomegaly. In chronic leukemia, there is an accumulation of mature-appearing leukocytes that have lost their ability to function efficiently and to undergo apoptosis, or programmed cell death.

The accumulation of abnormal blood cells in the bone marrow and lymphatic tissue can result in organomegaly as well as abnormal hematopoiesis, causing anemia, neutropenia, and thrombocytopenia, as well as an impaired immune response.

CLINICAL PRESENTATION AND PHYSICAL EXAMINATION

Acute Leukemias

The presenting signs and symptoms of AML and ALL can be nonspecific, along with associated cytopenias. The patient may have fevers and/or recurrent infection owing to a low WBC count. Increasing weakness, progressive fatigue, pallor, or dyspnea, all related to anemia, is not uncommon. Unexplained or spontaneous bruising, oral bleeding, epistaxis, heavy menstrual periods, and excessive bleeding after minor dental or surgical procedures are all caused by thrombocytopenia. Rarely, patients may have chloromas, the collection of blast cells in the subcutaneous tissues. In addition, with AML, some patients have oral involvement manifesting with gum hypertrophy; therefore an oral examination may be helpful.

If leukemia infiltrates lymph nodes, spleen, and liver, diffuse lymphadenopathy and hepatosplenomegaly may be present on examination. Patients may also have bone pain as a result of a packed, expanding bone marrow. Younger patients may experience joint pain and swelling that resembles rheumatoid arthritis.

Ocular involvement is seen in both childhood and adult leukemia patients. Not all ocular lesions cause symptoms; therefore it is important to consider an ophthalmic examination at the time of diagnosis.[9]

Approximately 5% to 8% of patients have central nervous system (CNS) involvement at the time of initial diagnosis. Common signs and symptoms of leukemia that has invaded the CNS are headache, papilledema, vision changes such as diplopia, vomiting, mental status changes, and cranial nerve palsy. In AML, leukostasis occurs when the blast count exceeds 100,000 cells/mm^3, and the patient is at risk for a fatal cerebral hemorrhage.[10]

Physical examination findings such as lymphadenopathy, hepatosplenomegaly, and testicular involvement are more common in ALL than in AML.

Chronic Leukemias

Patients with CML and CLL are usually asymptomatic in the early stages of disease. There may be subtle changes in the WBC count and differential early in the course of disease. A cardinal finding on physical examination of patients with chronic leukemia is splenomegaly. The patient may report a mild sensation of fullness in the left upper quadrant or may have an obvious mass. Severe splenomegaly can compress surrounding organs, causing early satiety, weight loss, and peripheral leg edema related to compression of the splenic vein. As the disease progresses, other symptoms occur, such as bone pain, bleeding problems, infection, fatigue, pallor, adenopathy, fevers, and night sweats.[11]

DIAGNOSTICS AND DIFFERENTIAL DIAGNOSIS

Acute Leukemias

The key in making the diagnosis of acute leukemia lies with the evaluation of a complete blood count and bone marrow aspirate with biopsy, to study the morphology of the cells. Additional studies on these specimens should include immunophenotyping and cytogenetic analysis. Most patients initially have a combination of cytopenias, with striking abnormalities noted in the WBC count and differential. The parameters of the WBC count vary within a wide range, from 1000 to 100,000 cells/mm^3. Most patients have counts between 5000 and 30,000 cells/mm^3.[12]

Careful examination of the blood smear is essential. The significant finding on the blood smear is an increased population of blast cells and a decrease of granulocytes, red blood cells, and platelets. However, as many as 10% of all patients have normal blood counts even when the marrow has been replaced by leukemic cells; therefore bone marrow aspiration and biopsy are required for a definitive diagnosis. Auer rods (rod-shaped granules incorporated within the blast cells) are pathognomonic of AML.[12]

Additional laboratory studies should be performed to identify a wide range of metabolic and electrolyte abnormalities that can be seen in acute leukemia. Biochemical studies may reveal hyperuricemia. Hyperuricemia occurs because of the high turnover rate of proliferating leukemia cells resulting in rapid purine catabolism and elevations in serum uric acid. Electrolyte abnormalities are common, and an elevated lactate dehydrogenase (LDH) level can be seen in patients without change in other liver function test (LFT) parameters. The presence of any or all of these abnormalities is a reflection of the rate of growth and turnover of the leukemia cells.

Patients with excessive bruising or bleeding should undergo a coagulation panel to look for disseminated intravascular coagulation (DIC) or other coagulopathies. Any patient with an increased myeloblast count may be at risk for leukostasis. This condition primarily affects the lungs and brain, but any organ can be involved. Lowering of the blast count in a rapid fashion is necessary, usually with chemotherapy or leukapheresis. The differential diagnosis for ALL and AML includes lymphoma, although other infiltrative processes, such as solid tumors (e.g., breast cancer or small cell lung cancer), must be excluded. Some patients with fever and cytopenia who have a small number of circulating blast cells must be differentiated from those with reactions to tuberculosis, systemic lupus erythematosus, megaloblastic anemia, or aplastic anemia. Surface antigen and serologic studies can exclude viral infections such as infectious mononucleosis. AML needs to be distinguished from MDS or a myeloproliferative disorder, such as the transformation of CML in blast crisis.

Chronic Leukemias

At diagnosis, the WBC count in chronic leukemias may range from fewer than 10,000 to more than 200,000 cells/mm^3, with mature and predominantly myelocytic cells. In general, the red blood cell count is normal, but a slight degree of anemia may occur. Hypereosinophilia and hyperbasophilia are common. Increased levels of uric acid in the blood and urine are also found in patients with CML. Bone marrow biopsy reveals hyperplastic myeloid cells and storage cells similar to Gaucher cells scattered throughout the marrow. The striking biochemical abnormality in CML is the reduction or absence of leukocyte alkaline phosphatase. This, along with the positive test result for Philadelphia chromosome (Ph^1), the hallmark of CML, confirms the diagnosis. CML is the first cancer shown to be associated with a chromosomal abnormality.[11]

CLL is often discovered on a routine office visit when a CBC is ordered. The physical examination findings may be normal, but some patients have nontender adenopathy or splenomegaly. Patients may report fatigue, night sweats, occasional fever, or malaise. The majority of patients consult their health care provider because of a painless cervical lymph node that waxes and wanes but does not disappear completely.[11]

CLL is suspected whenever an absolute lymphocytosis in the peripheral blood occurs in an adult and is sustained over time. Lymphocytosis also occurs in infectious mononucleosis, pertussis, and toxoplasmosis; but in these conditions, the lymphocyte count returns to normal after a few weeks.

A peripheral smear may be adequate for the diagnosis of CLL; a bone marrow biopsy will always reveal lymphocytosis in cases of CLL. The lymphocyte count ranges from 10,000 to 150,000/mm^3. Because there may be a decrease in immunoglobulin (Ig) levels, serum protein electrophoresis should be performed; this test may reveal a marked decrease in levels of IgG and slight decreases in IgA and IgM levels.[12] A chest x-ray study may be helpful in detecting hilar and mediastinal adenopathy.

The differential diagnosis for CLL includes non-Hodgkin lymphoma, hairy cell leukemia, and a variety of other lymphoproliferative disorders.

DIAGNOSTICS

Leukemia

LABORATORY
CBC and differential
Peripheral blood smear evaluation
Serum electrolytes, including phosphorous level
Uric acid
LFTs
LDH
BCR-ABL polymerase chain reaction (PCR) for evaluation/monitoring of CML or Ph+ ALL
Urinalysis
Serum protein electrophoresis
DIC panel

OTHER DIAGNOSTICS
Bone marrow aspirate with biopsy
Lumbar puncture (if clinically indicated and for all patients with ALL)
Echocardiogram

DIFFERENTIAL DIAGNOSIS

Leukemia

- Lymphomas
- Solid tumors
- Systemic lupus erythematosus
- Megaloblastic anemia
- Aplastic anemia
- Lymphoproliferative disorders
- MDS
- Myeloproliferative disorders (i.e., CML in blast crisis)

MANAGEMENT

Acute Leukemias

Patients diagnosed with ALL and AML require aggressive chemotherapy to restore normal hematopoiesis. Given the abrupt onset, prompt evaluation and intervention are required in order to successfully eradicate the disease and improve the chance of survival. Treatment of AML involves two phases of therapy: induction therapy to induce a complete remission and consolidation therapy to secure the remission. Induction therapy usually requires a 1-month hospitalization during which patients are supported with blood product support and antibiotic therapy while normal hematopoiesis is restored. Treatment for ALL involves long-term use of chemotherapy in three phases: induction, consolidation, and maintenance therapy. The total time of therapy usually takes about 2 years.

Patients with AML may also undergo hematopoietic stem cell transplantation (HSCT). The increasing use of both autologous and allogeneic HSCTs will have a profound effect on the outcome of AML. The impact of these approaches continues to be researched. Management of these patients requires a multidisciplinary approach. Expertise in transfusion management, infectious disease, care of indwelling catheters, nutrition, chemotherapy and its side effects, and psychosocial counseling is required.[13]

Approximately 50% of patients with ALL who are younger than 15 years achieve a long-term, leukemia-free survival. Approximately 70% of all patients with AML who are younger than 60 years achieve a complete but short-lived remission; only 15% remain disease free for 5 years or more. The major cause of failure to achieve remission during induction therapy is death from hemorrhage and infection.[1]

Age, health, and other factors need to be taken into consideration when assessing treatment options. Older individuals or those in poor health may not do as well with intensive therapy.

Chronic Leukemias

CML has three phases: chronic phase, accelerated phase, and terminal blast crisis phase. The chronic phase has a duration of approximately 3 to 5 years; the durations of the other phases vary. In contrast, CLL is usually a long-term disease, with reported cases lasting 1 to 15 years.

Chronic leukemias are managed differently from acute leukemias. CML is treated initially with imatinib mesylate (Gleevec). The U.S. Food and Drug Administration approved Gleevec for CML treatment in May 2001. The translocation between chromosomes 9 and 22, or Ph^1, disappears in 75% of patients taking Gleevec by 18 months of therapy. Alternative treatments include the second-generation tyrosine kinase inhibitors dasatinib and nilotinib.[14] Allogeneic stem cell transplantation and clinical trials remain an option for patients who are intolerant of or refractory to tyrosine kinase inhibitors. Allogeneic stem cell transplant remains the only known cure for CML.

CLL and small lymphocytic lymphoma are the same disease, manifesting differently. They are treated identically, and the terms are commonly used interchangeably. Initiation of treatment should be individualized and based on prognostic information, including cytogenetic aberrations and stage of disease. Various treatment options exist, including enrollment in a clinical trial, purine analogs such as fludarabine, alkylating agents such as chlorambucil and bendamustine, and corticosteroids. Many of these drugs will be given in combination with other agents including monoclonal antibodies such as rituximab. For patients who have progressed in spite of having received first-line therapies, ibrutinib is the newest medication designed for treatment of patients with CLL. The drug is taken daily by mouth.

Patients diagnosed with leukemia who have undergone chemotherapy or perhaps HSCT are at risk for infection (bacterial, fungal, viral) and other long-term side effects of aggressive treatment. Patients with CLL are predisposed to several infectious complications that are related to the humoral immunocompromise associated with the disease process as well as to further immunosuppression from steroid therapy and cytotoxic therapy.[15] These patients benefit from monitoring of IgG levels and infusions of IVIG to replete their IgG levels and decrease their risk of infection. Periodic visits to the health care provider and the hematologist or oncologist are essential for close monitoring and support.

Patients who have undergone HSCT need close follow-up monitoring, which usually occurs in collaboration with the tertiary center that performed the HSCT. These patients are immunocompromised, and intervention in a timely fashion with antibiotics and antifungal agents when indicated will improve survival and quality of life. Continuing with routine health maintenance is also important when caring for this patient population.

BOX 239-1

Drugs Most Commonly Used to Treat Leukemias

ACUTE MYELOGENOUS LEUKEMIA
- Cytosine arabinoside IV
- Daunorubicin IV
- Idarubicin IV
- Azacitidine SC or IV
- Decitabine IV
- Tretinoin; ATRA
- Arsenic trioxide

CHRONIC MYELOGENOUS LEUKEMIA
- Busulfan PO
- Hydroxyurea PO
- Imatinib (Gleevec) PO
- Dasatinib (Sprycel) PO
- Nilotinib (Tasigna) PO

Advanced Stage
- Cytosine arabinoside IV

ACUTE LYMPHOCYTIC LEUKEMIA
- Vincristine
- L-Asparaginase IV
- Daunorubicin IV
- Prednisone PO
- Methotrexate PO
- Mercaptopurine PO

CHRONIC LYMPHOCYTIC LEUKEMIA
- Chlorambucil PO
- Corticosteroids PO

Advanced Stage
- Cyclophosphamide IV
- Doxorubicin IV
- Fludarabine IV
- Bendamustine IV
- Rituximab IV
- Ofatumumab IV
- Ibrutinib PO

Chemotherapy

Chemotherapy is the cornerstone of treatment for both acute and chronic leukemias. However, chemotherapy management for the leukemias varies (Box 239-1) depending on type. The goal of chemotherapy is to eradicate leukemic stem cells in acute leukemia and to decrease mature leukemia cells in chronic leukemia.

LIFE SPAN CONSIDERATIONS

Leukemia was once thought to be a childhood disease, but 90% of the newly diagnosed cases occur in adults. AML and CLL are the most common adult forms of the disease. ALL accounts for 80% of the childhood forms.[2]

COMPLICATIONS

Chemotherapeutic agents have many side effects, including bone marrow depression, gastrointestinal distress, nausea, vomiting, anorexia, stomatitis, diarrhea, constipation, rashes, alopecia, and fatigue. Specific agents have particular side effects. Daunorubicin may cause cardiotoxicity, vincristine may cause peripheral neuropathy, and asparaginase may cause elevated LFT values.

Complications of leukemia include possible sequelae from chemotherapy and HSCT (e.g., secondary malignant neoplasms, infection, fertility problems). Neuropathies and cardiopathies may develop and are usually related to the aggressive treatment regimen experienced by the leukemia patient. Despite the development of more effective antibiotics, granulocyte colony-stimulating factor, and granulocyte-macrophage colony-stimulating factor, bacterial and fungal infections continue to be a source of morbidity and mortality in patients with prolonged neutropenia.[15] Other syndromes that are potential complications are discussed next.

Tumor Lysis Syndrome

Tumor lysis syndrome is the most common of all the oncologic emergencies.[16]

Acute tumor lysis syndrome (ATLS) is most commonly seen in patients with AML and CML who are undergoing active treatment. ATLS occurs when patients with a high WBC count, heavy tumor burden, lymphadenopathy, and/or splenomegaly receive cytotoxic chemotherapy. Tumor cell membranes can rupture and release intracellular contents into the bloodstream.[16] ATLS is characterized by the development of acute hyperuricemia, hyperkalemia, hyperphosphatemia, and hypocalcemia, with or without acute renal failure.[16] Prevention and management of these metabolic complications require close monitoring. Renal function and chemistry values should be monitored daily. Fluid balance and electrolyte disturbances should be corrected with vigorous intravenous hydration and diuretics as indicated. The addition of sodium bicarbonate to maintain urinary alkalization is recommended, as is the use of allopurinol to decrease serum uric acid levels. If preventive measures are not effective, rasburicase can be used intravenously to rapidly break down serum uric acid. Monitoring with daily laboratory tests, weights, meticulous assessment of intake and output, and observation for signs and symptoms of fluid overload are critical in caring for this patient population. ATLS ordinarily resolves within 4 to 7 days if adequate renal function is maintained.

Disseminated Intravascular Coagulation

DIC is a hematologic disorder that occurs when there is an alteration in the blood-clotting mechanism. Acute promyelocytic leukemia (APL), the M3 subtype of AML, is most often associated with DIC. DIC can be acute or chronic and related to either the disease process or the treatment regimen. DIC is the most common serious hypercoagulable state that occurs in patients with cancer.[17] It is an event in which both clotting and hemorrhage exist simultaneously.

Acute leukemia, antineoplastic agents, infection, trauma, and hemolytic transfusion reactions interrupt normal body hemostasis and may initiate an episode of DIC. Spontaneous hemorrhage or the slow occult damage of multiple small clot formation within the lungs, organs of the CNS, or gastrointestinal tract may herald the presentation of DIC. Organ dysfunction from circulatory impairment leads to mental status changes, severe muscle pain, oliguria, and slowed gastrointestinal motility.[17] Symptoms may range from mild chronic episodes to acute and life-threatening incidents.

Abnormal laboratory findings suggest a diagnosis of DIC. A decreased platelet count, a prolonged prothrombin and partial thromboplastin time, and a decreased fibrinogen level with an elevation of fibrin degradation products confirm the diagnosis of DIC.[17]

Treatment of the underlying cause of DIC is vital. Hemorrhage is treated with replacement of fluids and blood component therapy; infection is treated with antibiotics; and cancer is treated with radiotherapy, chemotherapy, or surgery as indicated. Heparin therapy is more commonly used for the chronic DIC of malignant disease associated with thrombotic, thromboembolic, or necrotizing complications. Thorough, multiple system assessments in combination with patient and family education and involvement are necessary to prevent further injury and complications associated with DIC.

Leukostasis

The predominant cell in acute leukemia is undifferentiated or immature, usually a blast cell. In leukostasis, blood sludging or stasis occurs when the blood vessels become overcrowded with these blast cells. Individuals with high WBC counts and a large tumor burden are at risk for development of leukostasis. The small, delicate pulmonary and cranial vessels are the most susceptible. If leukostasis is left untreated, rupture and hemorrhage result in ischemia and infarct. Emergent treatment includes high-dose chemotherapy or cranial radiotherapy to decrease the number of circulating blast cells. Leukapheresis (the removal of WBCs from the plasma) may also be indicated.[1]

Pancytopenia

Regardless of the treatment regimen chosen, infection, bleeding, and symptomatic anemia are the most common side effects of leukemia and its therapy. The desired effect of treatment is severe myelosuppression, which puts the patient at risk for multiple complications. Prolonged periods of neutropenia leave the immunocompromised patient especially susceptible to infection. Until normal bone marrow function is restored, the leukemic patient lacks the normal host responses. Treatment with empirical antibiotics to prevent systemic or disseminated infection is indicated once infection is suspected. Prevention of infection must focus on providing meticulous care with any invasive treatment option and limiting unnecessary invasive procedures. Education empowers patients and their families to participate in their own health practices.

Fatigue is one of the most common symptoms associated with cancer and cancer therapies. Chronic low-grade anemia, stress, and alterations in sleeping, eating, and working are known to deplete energy levels. Fatigue can be one of the most disabling complications of cancer and chemotherapy treatments, perpetuating feelings of hopelessness and powerlessness. Supportive transfusion or erythropoietin therapies may be used to correct the anemia, exercise is encouraged, and many patients find support groups beneficial.[1]

INDICATIONS FOR REFERRAL OR HOSPITALIZATION

All patients with suspected leukemia should be referred to a hematologist or oncologist for evaluation and possible bone marrow aspiration and biopsy. Definitive diagnosis and treatment plans vary. In general, patients with acute leukemias are referred to a tertiary care center. Chronic leukemias are often managed in the community by a hematologist or oncologist. However, the primary health care provider plays a major role in the co-management of the leukemias. A hematology consultation is suggested before any invasive procedure, such as colonoscopy, cystoscopy, or surgery, whether minor or major.

PATIENT EDUCATION AND HEALTH PROMOTION

The educational goal for leukemia patients and their families is prevention of complications of the disease process and treatment, management of side effects, and access to community resources.

The bone marrow suppression of leukemia can be life-threatening. This may be a result of either the disease process itself or the chemotherapy instituted to treat the leukemia.

It is the health care team's responsibility to educate the patient and family about the numerous other effects of leukemia and its treatment, such as fever, headache, mucositis, nausea, vomiting, anorexia, diarrhea, constipation, pain, fatigue, insomnia, and depression. Patient self-care information is given in Box 239-2. After a leukemia diagnosis, patients will still require other cancer screening tests specific for age, including mammograms, Papanicolaou smears, prostate-specific antigen tests, and fecal occult blood testing. Other health-promoting activities include stopping smoking, maintaining normal weight, and getting adequate exercise.

BOX 239-2

Patient Education and Self-Care Strategies

LEUKOPENIA OR INFECTION

Cancer and cancer therapies can increase one's risk of infection by lowering the WBC count and altering the physical barriers of the skin and gastrointestinal mucosa, thereby allowing organisms to enter the body and cause infection.

Prevention and Management Strategies

- Stay away from people who are sick and crowds when your WBC counts are low.
- Wash hands with soap and water often. Use hand sanitizer when soap and water are unavailable.
- Maintain good mouth care and take good care of your skin.
- Serial monitoring of the WBC count throughout treatment and chemotherapy and the disease state may make your WBC count low, increasing the risk of infection.
- Wash raw vegetable and fruits well before eating them. Do not eat raw or undercooked fish, seafood, meat, chicken, or eggs.
- Take temperature twice daily and immediately report any signs or symptoms of infection, including temperature elevation above 100.5° F, shaking chills, productive cough, shortness of breath, redness, swelling, rash, headache, stiff neck, painful or frequent urination, or sinus pain or pressure.

THROMBOCYTOPENIA

Thrombocytopenia results from a low platelet count. Platelets are the cells that make your blood clot. Chemotherapy can lower the number of platelets by interfering with the bone marrow's ability to make them. Low platelets can result in increased bruising or bleeding.

Prevention and Management Strategies

- Brush your teeth with a soft toothbrush.
- Blow your nose gently.
- Use electric razors for shaving.
- Apply extra caution when using sharp objects.
- Avoid aspirin and nonsteroidal agents because they can interfere with the functioning of the platelet.
- Immediately report any signs or symptoms of thrombocytopenia including bruising, nosebleeds, bleeding gums, blood in the urine or stool, heavy bleeding during a menstrual period or a prolonged period, headaches or visual changes, or feeling very sleepy or confused.

ANEMIA

Anemia is a condition in which there are not enough healthy red blood cells to carry adequate oxygen to your tissues, resulting in excessive fatigue, lightheadedness, weakness, shortness of breath, and chest pain. Some types of chemotherapy cause anemia because they make it harder for the bone marrow to produce red blood cells. Anemia may also result from the disease overtaking the bone marrow, the factory of all blood cells.

Prevention and Management Strategies

- Get plenty of rest.
- Limit exercise and exertional activities. Take frequent rest periods.
- Eat a well-balanced diet.
- When moving from one position to another, do so slowly.
- Discuss whether blood transfusions or erythroid stimulating agents would be helpful.
- Immediately report any signs or symptoms of anemia, including lightheadedness, shortness of breath, ringing in the ears, pounding heart, increased heart rate, palpitation.

MUCOSITIS

Mucositis is the painful inflammation and ulceration of the mucous membranes lining the digestive tract, usually as an adverse effect of chemotherapy and radiotherapy treatment for cancer.

Prevention and Management Strategies

- Keep the mouth and lips moist.
- See the dentist regularly, ideally before cancer treatments begin.
- Perform good oral hygiene, brushing teeth with a soft toothbrush after meals; use only alcohol-free mouthwash.
- Rinse mouth with salt water (half teaspoon of salt in 8 ounces of water) after brushing and flossing.
- Eat a well-balanced diet including foods high in protein.
- Choose foods that are moist, soft, and easy to chew or swallow when your mouth is sore.
- Avoid hot, spicy, or acidic foods.
- Avoid alcohol and tobacco.
- Work with health care providers to control oral pain, bleeding, and infection.

CHEMOTHERAPY-INDUCED NAUSEA AND VOMITING

Chemotherapy-induced nausea and vomiting (CINV) continues to have a considerable effect on the physical and psychological well-being of patients with cancer. It can be classified as anticipatory (a conditioned response triggered when exposed to some stimuli), acute (occurring within 24 hours of chemotherapy administration), delayed (occurring after 24 hours and lasting up to 7 days), breakthrough (occurring despite prophylactic medications), and refractory (occurring because of a failure of prophylactic and breakthrough medications to control the symptoms).

BOX 239-2

Patient Education and Self-Care Strategies—cont'd

Prevention and Management Strategies

- Use antiemetics proactively at the first sign of nausea.
- Reduce food odors that might trigger nausea.
- Eat small, frequent meals composed of "comfort foods."
- Chew gum or suck on hard candies if you are experiencing taste changes.
- Stay well hydrated.
- Avoid foods that are too hot or too cold.
- Do not eat fatty, fried, spicy, or salty foods when nauseous.
- Use good oral hygiene, especially after meals.

DIARRHEA

Diarrhea is an abnormal increase in the liquidity and frequency of stools. Chemotherapy can cause diarrhea because it damages the healthy rapidly dividing cells that line the lower gastrointestinal tract. Left untreated, diarrhea can result in dehydration, weakness, weight loss, electrolyte imbalances, and poor nutrition.

Prevention and Management Strategies

- Stop taking laxatives and stool softeners.
- Take antidiarrheal medications as prescribed.
- Eat small frequent meals.
- Stay hydrated by drinking 8-12 cups of noncaffeinated beverages daily.
- Eat a low-fiber diet so as to not stimulate the motility of the bowel.
- Avoid caffeine, alcohol, and milk products, which can exacerbate the diarrhea.
- Avoid greasy, fried foods and foods that cause increased gas.

CONSTIPATION

Constipation is a condition in which there is difficulty in emptying the bowels, usually associated with hardened feces.

Prevention and Management Strategies

- Drink at least 8-10 glasses of fluids a day.
- Eat foods high in dietary fiber and avoid foods that are constipating.
- Stay active and exercise daily.
- Take laxatives and stool softeners as prescribed.
- Minimize, as possible, the use of medications that constipate, such as narcotics.
- If bowels do not move in 48 hours, call health care provider.

ALOPECIA

Alopecia is defined as loss of hair from the body. Some types of chemotherapy damage the cells that cause hair growth. Most of the time the hair on the head is lost first, but hair over the body can be lost as well. Hair loss is often a cause of great concern to the patient for cosmetic and psychological reasons but is a temporary side effect of chemotherapy. Hair loss can start 2-3 weeks after chemotherapy starts, and hair often grows back 2-3 months after chemotherapy is completed.

Prevention and Management Strategies

- Cut hair short before hair loss begins; this often makes it easier to manage.
- Avoid perming, dying, or chemically treating hair during chemotherapy, because this may irritate the scalp.
- Consider purchasing a wig or hair prosthesis.
- Protect scalp once hair falls out by applying sunscreen or wearing a hat or scarf.
- Keep the head warm; a great deal of body heat is lost through a bare scalp.
- Sleep on a satin pillowcase for increased comfort and less friction.
- Talk with others about your feelings.

FATIGUE

Fatigue is a common problem for patients during and after cancer treatment. It is a constant state of weariness that develops over time and diminishes your energy and mental capacity. Fatigue at this level affects your emotional and psychological well-being.

Prevention and Management Strategies

- Maintain good nutrition and hydration.
- Take a multivitamin supplement.
- Moderate daily exercise with rest periods.
- Improve sleep quality and quantity.
- Schedule activities for times of peak energy and focus.

INSOMNIA

Insomnia is a persistent disorder that can make it hard to fall asleep, hard to stay asleep, or both, despite the opportunity for adequate sleep. It can occur at times of higher-than-usual stress. With insomnia, you usually awaken feeling unrefreshed, which takes a toll on your ability to function during the day. Insomnia can sap not only your energy level and mood but also your health, work performance, and quality of life. Improving your sleep restores function of your body and mind, reduces other symptoms, and allows you to function and care for yourself and others.

Prevention and Management Strategies

- Keep to a consistent bedtime and wake time.
- Use bedroom for sleep and sexual activity only; avoid watching television or using the computer in bed because these activities are stimulating.
- Avoid sleeping excessively during the day. If a nap is needed, limit it to less than 1 hour.
- Get regular exercise.
- Avoid caffeinated beverages before bed.
- Seek treatment for conditions that can interfere with sleep, such as pain, hot flashes, anxiety, depression, shortness of breath, fever.

DEPRESSION

Depression is a mood disorder that causes a persistent feeling of sadness and loss of interest that affects how you feel, think, and behave and can lead to a variety of emotional and physical problems. You may have trouble doing normal day-to-day activities, and sometimes you may feel as if life isn't worth living. Most people with depression feel better with medication, psychological counseling, or both.

Prevention and Management Strategies

- Avoid alcohol, because it has a depressive effect.
- Discuss your feelings with your health care team.
- Consider joining a support group.
- Discuss pharmacologic interventions for depression and take as directed.
- Eat a well-balanced diet, exercise daily, and get plenty of rest.

Modified from Yarbro C, Wujcik D, Gobel BH, et al: *Cancer symptom management,* ed 4, Burlington, Mass, 2013, Jones and Bartlett.[18]

CHAPTER 240

LYMPHOMAS

Varghese Mathai

OVERVIEW OF LYMPHOMAS

Lymphomas are clonal disorders that arise from lymphocytes (B or T cells; rarely, natural killer [NK] cells). They are rare and extremely heterogeneous secondary to numerous histologic subtypes and variable clinical presentations. This heterogeneity has important prognostic implications on whether treatment is administered with curative intent. This focus of this chapter is twofold: (1) to enable an understanding of the diagnosis, staging, and initial evaluation of a lymphoma patient, and (2) to describe how the most common lymphoid malignancies are managed.

EPIDEMIOLOGY

The estimates from the Surveillance, Epidemiology, and End Results (SEER) Program for 2014 revealed that non-Hodgkin lymphoma (NHL) was the seventh most common type of cancer. NHL and Hodgkin lymphoma (HL) represented 5% percent of new cancer cases (NHL, 70,800; HL, 9190) and 3.5% of cancer deaths in 2014. The incidence of these disorders has increased approximately twofold over the last 30 years, with a slight male predominance.[1] The cause is unclear, but the increase is most significant in older patients with aggressive lymphoma. Many associate the increase in NHL with the human immunodeficiency virus (HIV), but with the widespread use of antiretroviral therapies the incidence of lymphoma has begun to decline.

ETIOLOGY AND RISK FACTORS

The many different forms of lymphoma have varied causes. The possible causes and associations with at least some forms of NHL include the following:

- Infectious agents
  - Epstein-Barr virus—associated with Burkitt lymphoma, HL, follicular dendritic cell sarcoma, extranodal NK–T-cell lymphoma[2]
  - Human T-cell leukemia virus—associated with adult T-cell lymphoma
  - *Helicobacter pylori*—associated with gastric lymphoma
  - Human herpesvirus 8 (HHV-8)—associated with primary effusion lymphoma, multicentric Castleman disease
  - Hepatitis C virus—associated with splenic marginal zone lymphoma, lymphoplasmacytic lymphoma, and diffuse large B-cell lymphoma (DLBCL)[3]
  - HIV infection[4]
- Chemicals: polychlorinated biphenyls (PCBs) diphenylhydantoin, dioxin, and phenoxy herbicides[5]
- Medical treatments, including radiation therapy and chemotherapy
- Genetic diseases, including Klinefelter syndrome, Chédiak-Higashi syndrome, ataxia-telangiectasia syndrome[6]
- Autoimmune diseases: Sjögren syndrome, rheumatoid arthritis, and systemic lupus erythematosus

CLINICAL PRESENTATION

The clinical presentation of HL and NHL varies and is dependent on the type of lymphoma and the area of involvement. Many patients have lymphadenopathy. In general, lymph nodes persisting for more than 4 weeks and lymph nodes larger than normal (up to 1.5 cm) will require intervention. In aggressive and highly aggressive NHLs, the lymphadenopathy increases quickly. Node size can wax and wane in more indolent lymphomas. "B" symptoms are often present in disseminated disease. These include fever higher than 38° C, drenching night sweats, and unintentional weight loss of more than 10% of body weight. See specific discussion later.

INITIAL EVALUATION

The initial evaluation includes the patient's history and a complete physical examination (including assessment of functional status using standardized scales such as the ECOG/Zubrod scale or the Karnofsky performance scale, both available online). A complete blood count (CBC), electrolytes, liver and renal function studies, lactate dehydrogenase (LDH), infectious disease panel (hepatitis B and C, HIV), and examination of the peripheral smear for the presence of atypical cells are initial diagnostics. Further diagnostics include a bone marrow biopsy and aspiration, positron emission tomography (PET), and computed tomography (CT) scan with intravenous and oral contrast.

MAKING THE DIAGNOSIS

After initial evaluation, proper histologic diagnosis and precise classification of the lymphoid neoplasm are the starting points for proper management. To allow for full assessment, an excisional biopsy is preferred when possible (versus core biopsy) to make the initial diagnosis of lymphoma. If a patient has already been treated for NHL or HL and a relapse is suspected, then core biopsy will suffice. The demonstration of monoclonality in biopsied tissue is diagnostic for lymphoma. The absence of monoclonality should make the underlying diagnosis questionable, and a repeat biopsy will likely be necessary.

CLASSIFICATION

Several classification systems have existed over the decades and continue to evolve. The latest, most comprehensive classification is the World Health Organization (WHO) classification developed in 2008.[7] The WHO classification is broken down by cell of origin (B, T, or NK) and by cell maturity.

The WHO modification of the Revised European-American Lymphoma (REAL) classification recognizes three major categories of lymphoid malignancies based on morphology and cell lineage: B-cell neoplasms, T-cell/NK-cell neoplasms, and Hodgkin lymphoma (HL). Both lymphomas and lymphoid leukemias are included in this classification because both solid and circulating phases are present in many lymphoid neoplasms, and distinction between them is artificial. Within the B-cell and T-cell categories, two subdivisions are recognized: precursor neoplasms, which correspond to the earliest stages of differentiation, and more mature differentiated neoplasms.[8]

STAGING

The Ann Arbor staging classification, modified at Cotswold's meeting in 1989 and initially used for HL, is also used for NHL (Table 240-1).

To complete staging, a bone marrow biopsy is performed. The bone marrow aspirate is less important, because it does not preserve morphology and may miss lymphoma. Bilateral biopsies increase the yield but change the stage in only a small number of patients. Lumbar puncture should be examined in highly

TABLE 240-1 Ann Arbor Staging System for Lymphoma

Stage*	Substage†	Definition
I	I	Single node region
	IE	Single extralymphatic site or involvement by direct extension
II	II	Two or more node regions on same side of diaphragm
	IIE	Single node region plus single localized extranodal site
	IIS	Spleen
	IIE+S	Extralymphatic site plus spleen
III	III	Involvement on both sides of diaphragm
IV	IV	Diffuse extralymphatic involvement

*Stages can be further classified as A (B symptoms absent) or B (B symptoms—fever, chills, night sweats, weight loss—present). A and B can be designated at any stage.
†Localized extralymphatic lesions with or without associated lymph node involvement are termed E (extranodal) lesions, and those involving the spleen are termed S.
From Cheson BJ: Hodgkin's disease and the non-Hodgkin's lymphomas. In Lenhard RE, Osteen RT, Gansler T, editors: *Clinical oncology,* Atlanta, Ga, 2001, American Cancer Society.

aggressive lymphomas (Burkitt and lymphoblastic) and with aggressive lymphomas with multiple extranodal sites, paraspinal disease, or testicular or paranasal sinus involvement.

HODGKIN LYMPHOMA

PATHOPHYSIOLOGY

HL, formerly called Hodgkin disease, arises from germinal center or post–germinal center B cells. HL has a unique cellular composition, containing a minority of neoplastic cells (Reed-Sternberg cells and their variants) in an inflammatory background[9] containing a variable number of small lymphocytes, eosinophils, neutrophils, histiocytes, plasma cells, fibroblasts, and collagen fibers. Morphologic features also determine the various subtypes of classical HL.

It is separated from the other B cell lymphomas based on its unique clinicopathologic features, and can be divided into two major subgroups based on the appearance and immunophenotype of the tumor cells:

Classical Hodgkin Lymphoma

The tumor cells in the classical HL group are also derived from germinal center B cells, but typically fail to express many of the genes and gene products that define normal germinal center B cells. Based on differences in the appearance of the tumor cells and the composition of the reactive background, classical HL is further divided into the following subtypes:

- Nodular sclerosis classical Hodgkin Lymphoma (NSHL)
- Mixed cellularity classical Hodgkin Lymphoma (MCHL)
- Lymphocyte-rich classical Hodgkin Lymphoma (LRHL)
- Lymphocyte-depleted classical Hodgkin Lymphoma (LDHL)

Nodular Lymphocyte-Predominant Hodgkin Lymphoma

The tumor cells in this subtype retain the immunophenotypic features of germinal center B cells.

CLINICAL PRESENTATION

Patients usually have painless adenopathy localized to the neck. The mediastinum is involved in the majority of patients (approximately two thirds), occasionally with large mediastinal masses. B symptoms are present in 20% to 25% of patients. Pruritus is common but is not a B symptom. On rare occasions, patients may experience pain in involved lymph nodes on ingesting alcohol—thought to be a result of alcohol-induced degranulation of eosinophils.

DIAGNOSTICS

The diagnosis of HL is made by the microscopic evaluation of involved tissue, usually obtained from a lymph node biopsy. Excisional biopsies are preferred, and large core needle biopsies may be adequate in select cases, but fine-needle aspiration (FNA) alone often does not provide enough tissue or information on the structural composition of the lymph node to enable an accurate diagnosis. Evaluation of the biopsy material should include both routine light microscopy and analysis of the immunophenotype with immunohistochemistry.

DIAGNOSTICS

Lymphomas

LABORATORY
- CBC and differential
- Serum electrolytes
- Liver function tests (LFTs)
- Blood urea nitrogen (BUN)
- Creatinine
- Serologic evaluation for Epstein-Barr virus
- HIV test
- Toxoplasmosis titer

IMAGING
- Chest x-ray examination
- CT scan of chest, abdomen, pelvis, head
- PET scan
- Gallium or thallium scan*

OTHER DIAGNOSTICS
- Lymph node biopsy
- Bone marrow biopsy

*If indicated.

DIFFERENTIAL DIAGNOSIS

Lymphadenopathy may be a primary or secondary sign of numerous disorders including infectious diseases, immunologic disorders, and malignancies (see Chapter 226). A patient with lymphadenopathy that is unexplained and persistent for 1 month should be referred for biopsy to rule out malignant disease.

DIFFERENTIAL DIAGNOSIS

Lymphomas

- Infectious process
- Viral syndromes
- Mononucleosis
- HIV infection
- Bacteremia
- Toxoplasmosis
- Autoimmune disease
- Other malignant disease

PROGNOSIS

Predicting the outcome is important to avoid overtreating patients with Hodgkin lymphoma and to identify others in whom standard treatment is likely to fail. Prognosticating outcome also helps patients and providers make often difficult treatment decisions. The Hasenclever Index for HL is commonly used.[10] Seven factors with similar independent prognostic effects were selected. The prognostic score was then defined as the number of adverse prognostic factors present at diagnosis. The prognostic score was used to predict rates of freedom from progression of disease (Fig. 240-1A) and overall survival (Fig. 240-1B). Figure 240-1 also presents freedom from progression of disease according to whether the prognostic score was 0 to 2, 3, or higher.

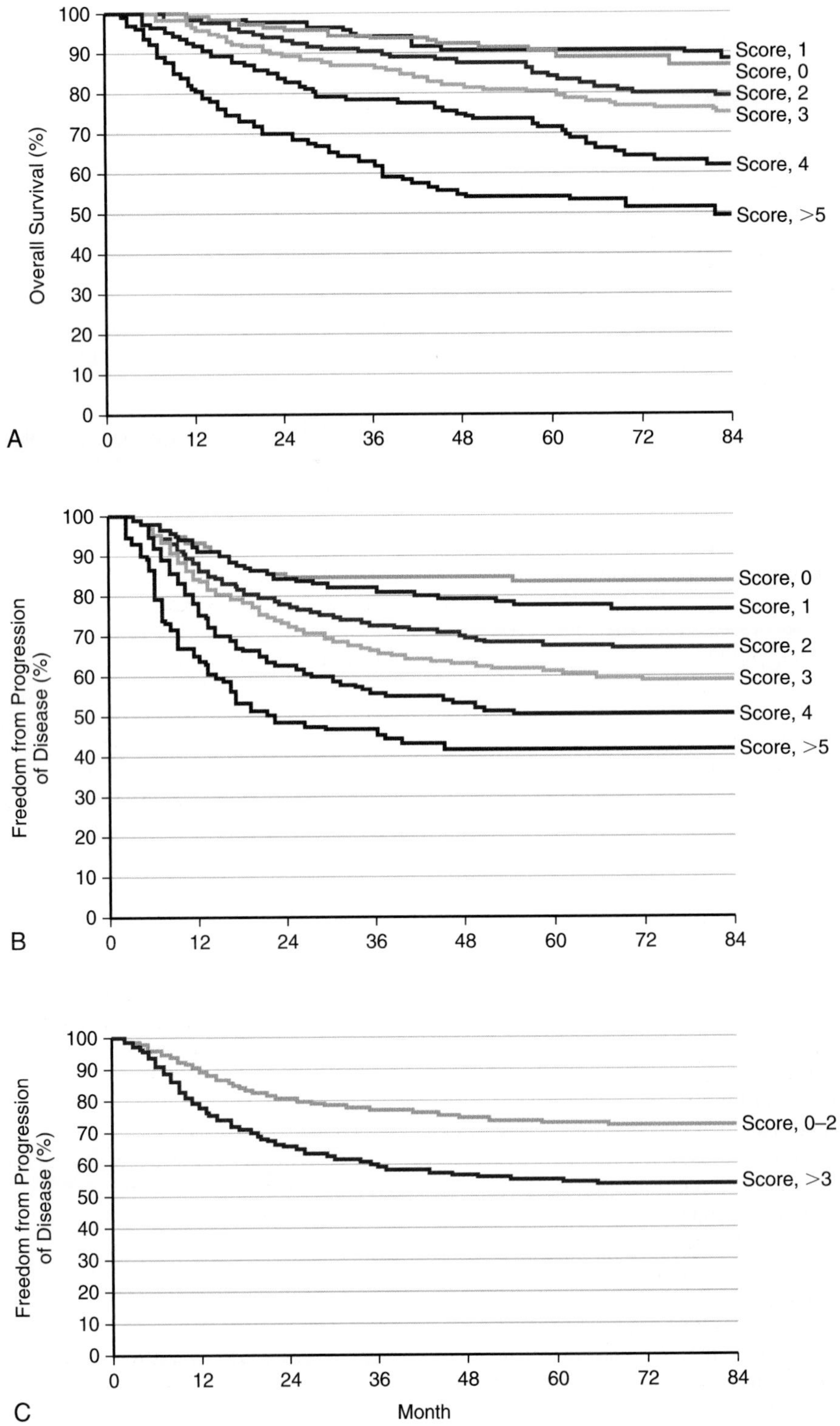

FIGURE 240-1 Prognostic scoring for Hodgkin lymphoma.

A score of 1 is given for each of the following risk factors present at diagnosis:

- Age older than 45 years
- Male gender
- Serum albumin below 40 g/dL
- Hemoglobin (Hb) below 10.5 g/dL
- Stage IV disease
- White blood cell (WBC) count higher than 15×10^9 per liter of blood
- Lymphopenia—fewer than 0.6×10^9 lymphocytes per liter of blood

MANAGEMENT

Over the past century, HL has been converted from a uniformly fatal disease to one that is curable in approximately 75% of patients worldwide. Although the majority of patients will be cured of their lymphoma, treatment-related toxicities have become a competing cause of late mortality. Accordingly, the selection of therapy must balance the desire to maintain a high rate of cure and the need to minimize long-term complications. Treatment has evolved such that patients with early stage disease can achieve long-term remission with less-intensive therapy, whereas more intensive therapy is reserved for patients with advanced-stage disease.

Combination chemotherapy is the cornerstone of HL treatment. ABVD (Adriamycin, bleomycin, vinblastine, and dacarbazine) combination chemotherapy appears to have the best overall efficacy with the least acute and chronic toxicity.

Selection of initial treatment for HL is usually based on presenting stage and prognostic factors. Most patients receive systemic chemotherapy either alone or as part of a combined modality treatment program with radiation. The need for proper staging is imperative because radiation therapy is not typically used in advanced-stage HL.

Advanced-stage HL refers to clinical stage III and IV disease, although many experts and clinical trials include patients with stage II plus bulky nodal disease.

Combination chemotherapy is the main treatment for patients with advanced-stage HL. Radiation therapy may be used for select patients as consolidation.

RELAPSING OR REFRACTORY DISEASE

High-dose chemotherapy with autologous hematopoietic stem cell transplant is the cornerstone of salvage therapy for patients with recurrent HL.[11]

Primary refractory (resistant) disease refers to patients who do not attain a complete remission after initial therapy. The incidence of primary refractory disease varies depending on the stage of disease at diagnosis and the treatment regimen used. Durable responses and remissions may be achieved in approximately half of these patients with second-line chemotherapy that incorporates drugs not used in initial treatment followed by high-dose chemotherapy and autologous hematopoietic cell rescue.[12]

Patients with HL relapse after prior treatment with chemotherapy are generally treated with either conventional chemotherapy combined with radiation therapy or high-dose chemotherapy and autologous hematopoietic cell transplantation (HCT) given with or without radiation therapy. The choice of therapy is usually based on prognostic features.

Salvage chemotherapy is administered in two phases: first a conventional-dose regimen to achieve major reduction in tumor bulk and promote mobilization of stem cell into the peripheral blood, followed by high-dose therapy with stem cell support.

About half of the patients destined to relapse will do so in the first year after treatment, and nearly all the relapses occur within 5 years of treatment. It is common to follow patients every few months for the first couple of years, gradually extending the interval between visits.

HL survivors are at risk of developing therapy-related complications that may manifest years after treatment, including second malignancies, cardiac disease, thyroid nodules, and radiation-induced hypothyroidism. Patients who have received mantle irradiation are at higher risk of cardiomyopathy, pericarditis, pneumonitis, and pulmonary fibrosis. These complications have surfaced as significant causes of increased mortality among survivors. Screening for some of these entities is advised in the hope that early detection may lead to better management.

NON-HODGKIN LYMPHOMA

DEFINITION

This disease category consists of some 40 different types of lymphomas with a predilection for older adults with a male predominance.

PATHOPHYSIOLOGY

The molecular biology research on NHL has begun to identify clues to the pathogenesis of some of these disorders. Basically these are tumors originating from lymphoid tissue, mostly B cells but occasionally T or NK cells.

CLINICAL PRESENTATION

The clinical presentation of NHL varies tremendously depending on the type of lymphoma and the areas of involvement. Some NHLs behave indolently, with lymphadenopathy waxing and waning over years. Others are highly aggressive, resulting in death within weeks if left untreated. In typical cases the following clinical presentations occur:

- Aggressive lymphomas commonly manifest acutely or subacutely with a rapidly growing mass, systemic B symptoms (i.e., fever, night sweats, weight loss), and/or elevated levels of serum LDH and uric acid. Examples of lymphomas with this aggressive or highly aggressive presentation include DLBCL, Burkitt lymphoma, adult T-cell leukemia-lymphoma, and precursor B and T lymphoblastic leukemia and lymphoma.
- Indolent lymphomas are often insidious, manifesting only with slow-growing lymphadenopathy, hepatomegaly, splenomegaly, or cytopenias. Examples of lymphomas that typically have indolent presentations include follicular lymphoma (FL), chronic lymphocytic leukemia or small lymphocytic lymphoma, and splenic marginal zone lymphoma.

DIAGNOSIS

Most patients with enlarged lymph nodes have a benign form of reactive lymphadenopathy often related to infection or inflammation. An unexplained enlarged node present for 1 month or longer should be investigated further Many centers use FNA as an initial screening test. When coupled with comprehensive immunophenotyping (typically flow cytometry), FNA is particularly useful at distinguishing reactive B-cell hyperplasias from clonal mature B-cell neoplasms. However, the general consensus is that accurate histopathologic evaluation of lymphomas requires a tissue biopsy, preferably an intact lymph node, and that FNAs suggesting the presence of a lymphoma should be followed up with a definitive tissue biopsy.[13]

FNA may provide enough information to confirm a recurrence in previously diagnosed patients.

The Ann Arbor staging system (Table 240-1) is also used for NHL to provide treatment, prognostic, and clinical trial data. Prognosticating outcomes has been a moving target over the past several years with the introduction of chemoimmunotherapy agents such as rituximab. As treatments improve, the hope for better individual prognostication will be realized.

The staging workup should also include PET scan, and CT scan of chest, abdomen, and pelvis. PET scans are now being used more frequently than CT because they can differentiate between active and necrotic tissue. In combination, these two scans changed the staging of the disease, which has also resulted in a change in the treatment choice.

MANAGEMENT

Indolent (Formerly Known as Low-Grade)

FL is the second most common subtype of NHL and the most common of the indolent NHLs, defined as those lymphomas in which survival of the untreated patient is measured in years. Treatment of FL depends on the stage of disease at presentation as evaluated by the Ann Arbor staging system.

Most patients with stage I or nonbulky stage II FL initiate treatment with radiation therapy rather than treatment with chemotherapy or an initial period of observation. This is principally based on the observation that some patients may have prolonged progression-free survival with radiation therapy. If significant morbidity is expected from radiotherapy based on the location of the tumor, or if the patient decides against radiotherapy, a management approach similar to that used for advanced-stage disease may be a reasonable alternative.

For patients with previously untreated advanced-stage FL who require therapy, we recommend treatment with an immunotherapy-based regimen or chemotherapy. A choice among the various regimens depends on patient characteristics and physician comfort. Bendamustine plus rituximab (BR) has been shown to improve the progression-free survival rates with less toxicity when compared with rituximab, cyclophosphomide, doxorubicon, vincristine, prednisone (R-CHOP).[14] R-CHOP may be preferred for patients with more aggressive histologic grade 3A disease.

Patients with asymptomatic recurrent FL do not require immediate treatment but should be followed closely for the development of symptomatic disease. Patients with symptomatic FL or those with an increase in disease tempo require treatment. Because relapse is common in indolent lymphoma, a biopsy should be conducted to rule out transformation to a higher grade lymphoma.

There is no standard therapy for patients with relapsed or refractory FL and practice varies widely; accordingly, patients should be encouraged to participate in clinical trials whenever possible. A choice among potential therapies must take into account characteristics of both the tumor and the patient as well as an evaluation of the initial response to treatment.

For most patients with relapsed or refractory FL, treatment with rituximab either alone or in combination with chemotherapy is the treatment of choice. The option between single agent rituximab and combination chemotherapy plus rituximab depends largely on the patient's tumor burden and performance status. For patients with a poor performance status and/or a clinically indolent course, single-agent rituximab may be an option because of its relatively low toxicity profile.

The decision of whether to proceed with HCT should be based on the patient's preference and condition and the expected disease course. For the disease course, there is no definitive score or metric. For eligible patients who relapse after a short initial response (i.e., <1 year) to chemoimmunotherapy and demonstrate chemotherapy-sensitive disease, allogeneic HCT should be considered.

Aggressive (Formerly Known as Intermediate or High Grade)

DLBCL is the most common histologic subtype of NHL. It is an aggressive NHL in which survival without treatment is measured in months. Advanced-stage DLBCL cannot be contained within one irradiation field, and this population accounts for 60% to 70% of patients with DLBCL.

For patients with advanced DLBCL, an anthracycline-based combination chemotherapy regimen plus rituximab is recommended—specifically, six to eight cycles of R-CHOP-21.[15] There is no role for the routine use of maintenance rituximab or high-dose chemotherapy with autologous hematopoietic cell rescue in first complete remission.

There is general agreement that patients with testicular, epidural, or sinus involvement are at increased risk of developing CNS disease. The evidence for an increased risk of CNS relapse is less strong for other scenarios that we still consider high risk, such as patients with breast or ovarian involvement, concordant bone marrow involvement, a high International Prognostic Index (IPI) score, or numerous extranodal sites of disease.

Relapsed or refractory DLBCL is treated with systemic chemotherapy with or without rituximab with plans to proceed to high-dose chemotherapy and autologous HCT in those with chemotherapy-sensitive disease.[16] The treatment of patients who are not candidates for HCT, who fail to respond to second-line chemotherapy regimens, or who relapse after HCT is generally palliative. Enrollment in a clinical trial can be an option.

Highly Aggressive

Burkitt lymphoma, or small noncleaved cell lymphoma, is a highly aggressive B-cell NHL characterized by the translocation and deregulation of the *c-myc* gene on chromosome 8. The standard of care has yet to be defined, and enrollment in a clinical trial may be the best option where available. However, for patients who are not candidates for such trials or for those who choose not to participate, intensive, short-duration combination chemotherapy with central nervous system (CNS) prophylaxis is indicated. Dose reduction should be avoided if at all possible, and therapy should be initiated quickly. Infusional chemotherapy with dose-adjusted etoposide, vincristine, doxorubicin, cyclophosphamide, and prednisone (EPOCH) plus rituximab is an acceptable alternative for patients who may not tolerate more aggressive regimens (e.g., older or less-fit patients).

Various intensive, short-duration combination chemotherapy regimens have been studied in patients with BL. These include CODOX-M (cyclophosphamide, vincristine, doxorubicin, high-dose methotrexate) with IVAC (ifosfamide, cytarabine, etoposide, and intrathecal methotrexate).

There is a paucity of data to guide the treatment of patients with recurrent or refractory BL. Whenever possible, patients should be encouraged to participate in clinical trials. Outside of a clinical trial, patients with refractory disease and those who relapse after an initial response to appropriate initial therapy have an extremely poor prognosis and should be considered for best supportive or palliative care. An important exception concerns the patient who did not receive appropriate initial therapy.

T-CELL LYMPHOMAS

The peripheral T-cell lymphomas (PTCLs) are a heterogeneous group of typically aggressive neoplasms that constitute less than 15% of all NHLs in adults. There is no general consensus regarding the optimal treatment regimen for these patients, and all patients should be encouraged to participate in clinical trials where available.

For most patients with newly diagnosed PTCL, induction combination chemotherapy with a CHOP (cyclophosphamide, doxorubicin, vincristine, prednisone)–based regimen rather than more intensive induction regimens.[17]

For patients younger than 60 years, the use of CHOP plus etoposide (CHOEP) rather than CHOP alone can be recommended.

Consolidation

After the completion of induction (first line or initial) chemotherapy, patients should be evaluated for the use of consolidation therapy with radiation therapy (localized disease) and/or autologous HCT.[18] Consolidation therapy is treatment that is given after cancer has disappeared following the initial (induction) therapy. Consolidation therapy is used to kill any cancer cells that may be left in the body. It may include radiation therapy, a stem cell transplant, or treatment with drugs that kill cancer cells. This is also called intensification therapy and postremission therapy. Those with limited-stage disease who achieve a partial response may attain a complete remission if consolidation radiation is administered. The use of auto-HCT in first complete response (CR) is principally based on the PTCL subtype and the IPI score.[19]

In relapsed T-cell lymphoma, there is no general consensus regarding the optimal treatment regimen, and all patients should be encouraged to participate in clinical trials where available. Patients who are not candidates for or choose not to participate in clinical trials are usually treated with combination chemotherapy regimens in an attempt to achieve a complete remission. At present, no single chemotherapy regimen is clearly superior to any other. Outside the context of a clinical trial, the selection of treatment should be based on expected toxicities, patient comorbidities, and preferences.

LIFE SPAN CONSIDERATIONS IN LYMPHOMAS OF ALL TYPES

After the completion of therapy, restaging, and documentation of complete remission, patients with all types of lymphoma are seen at periodic intervals to be monitored and assessed for possible relapse. The frequency and extent of these visits depends on the histologic subtype and comfort of both the patient and clinician. There have been no prospective, randomized trials comparing various schedules of follow-up. Any necessary radiologic and laboratory studies are usually performed by or can be coordinated with the patient's hematologist or oncologist to ensure adequate follow-up evaluation.

Relapsed disease can be suggested by changes on imaging studies or physical examination but can be confirmed only by biopsy. Accordingly, a biopsy should be performed to document relapsed disease before proceeding to salvage therapy.

Under some circumstances, gonadal dysfunction can affect quality of life after treatment. Transient and sometimes permanent male sterility may occur. Infertility may occur in at least 80% of women older than 25 years who receive nitrogen mustard, vincristine, procarbazine, or prednisone chemotherapy.[20] The newer, nonalkylating agent–containing regimens have a lower risk of infertility. However, sperm banking should be considered before treatment is initiated. Pregnancies occurring in patients or their partners do not appear to be associated with complications, congenital abnormalities, or spontaneous abortions.[20]

Improved treatment regimens and survival mean that many patients will return to primary health care providers for care and monitoring. Advance directives should be discussed with the patient, but with the understanding that some lymphomas can be treated successfully or have an indolent course. Patients are encouraged to prepare a living will and to appoint a health care proxy so that both the health care proxy and the health care provider understand their preferences for terminal care. Palliative care specialists have been shown to improve both quality of life and longevity.[21] Palliative care involves emotional and psychological care, support groups, pain and symptom management, family engagement, and general resources to support the patient and family. Any approach to cancer care should integrate palliative management from an early stage.

COMPLICATIONS IN ALL TYPES OF LYMPHOMA

Complications from lymphoma can occur during treatment, as a result of treatment, or from the disease itself.

During Therapy

Patients with cancer who undergo chemotherapy and radiotherapy are at risk of infection because of the immunosuppression from the cancer, the myelosuppression from chemotherapy, the break in skin barriers from the placement of Port-a-Caths and central lines, and the shifts in microbial flora. The myelosuppressive effect of chemotherapy can cause neutropenia. Absolute neutropenia is defined as fewer than 1000 neutrophils per cubic millimeter and bands in the bloodstream and is calculated by multiplying the total number of white cells from the CBC by the total percentage of neutrophils plus bands. The period of neutropenia after chemotherapy is relatively predictable; the lowest count of neutrophils occurs approximately 10 to 14 days after chemotherapy and recovers in about 3 to 4 weeks after chemotherapy. Although fever can be a presenting sign in a patient with lymphoma, fever in a patient after chemotherapy, especially in a neutropenic patient, may be a sign of life-threatening sepsis. Research shows that colony-stimulating factors can reduce the incidence of febrile neutropenia; however, these medications can be inconvenient and expensive and have toxicities, including bone pain. Guidelines for colony-stimulating factor administration have been issued by the American Society of Clinical Oncology, and the administration of these medications should be based on the recommendation of the treating hematologist or oncologist.[22]

Fatigue is a poorly understood phenomenon that affects the patient's quality of life. It can occur as a result of the treatment or the disease. It may be associated with anxiety or depression or with physiologic processes related to tumor necrosis factor and interleukin-1 and other cytokines. Physiologic conditions such as anemia in all types of lymphoma resulting from the chemotherapy and radiotherapy may also contribute to fatigue. A careful review of symptoms and CBC with differential is important. Current recommendations include education to relieve anxiety, activities that provide distraction, and participation in low-intensity exercise.[23] Packed red blood cell transfusion should be given to patients with severe anemia.

Post-Treatment Toxicities

A serious consequence of treatment is the increased risk of a second cancer, including acute myelogenous leukemia (AML). The risk of secondary AML can extend to 11 years after treatment. Radiotherapy with and without chemotherapy may contribute to increased risk of solid tumors in the radiation field. Solid tumors tend to occur in the second decade after treatment. Breast cancers in this population are often bilateral. Regular breast examination and mammography starting at an early age are recommended as part of routine post-treatment care.[24]

More than two thirds of patients who have undergone mantle irradiation develop thyroid disease, including hypothyroidism, Graves disease, silent thyrotoxicosis, and nodules, with a 2% risk of cancer. Mantle field irradiation also adds to the risk of cardiac toxicity.[25] This type of radiation is used less often than in the past, but previously treated patients remain at risk.

Other serious treatment complications are cardiotoxicity, which can be fatal, and pulmonary toxicity. High doses of doxorubicin can cause cardiomyopathy. It is unclear whether radiotherapy results in the acceleration of coronary artery disease.[25] Pulmonary fibrosis or restrictive disease has also been associated with bleomycin chemotherapy.

INDICATIONS FOR REFERRAL OR HOSPITALIZATION WITH LYMPHOMA OF ANY TYPE

A patient should be referred to a hematologist or oncologist with suspicion of or certainly after confirmation of the diagnosis of a lymphoma of any type. Patients with high-risk disease should be referred to a comprehensive cancer center whenever possible. These centers can often provide oncology care with access to the latest research treatments and clinical trials.

Patients with a diagnosis of lymphoma in remission should request that the hematologist or oncologist forward treatment records to the primary health care provider. Follow-up examinations should focus on both the presenting signs and symptoms of the disease and new symptoms or lymphadenopathy. The patient should be referred to the hematologist or oncologist if constitutional symptoms continue or recur or if suspicious nodes are found.

There is a high prevalence of depression among cancer patients. Patients who are depressed may find help through psychotherapy that involves social support, coping skills, emotional expression, and cognitive restructuring.[26] Antidepressants and psychostimulating medications may be beneficial as well. It is critical that pain be managed effectively because there is a direct relationship between unmanaged pain and increased levels of psychological distress. Referral to psychiatry or palliative medicine may be helpful.

The majority of treatments for lymphoma can be administered in an outpatient setting. The patient might be hospitalized for high-dose chemotherapy requiring careful monitoring of laboratory values and blood product support as well as for episodes of febrile neutropenia. Of course, induction chemotherapy preceding hematopoietic cell transplant requires hospitalization in a controlled environment.

PATIENT AND FAMILY EDUCATION FOR ALL TYPES OF LYMPHOMA

One of the most common reactions to the stress of a cancer diagnosis and treatment is anxiety and depression. Education about the disease, treatment, and prognosis can help relieve anxiety. Educational and social support resources for patients include American Cancer Society programs (www.cancer.gov/cancertopics/coping) and OncoLink (www.oncolink.org/coping).

Patients should be encouraged to remain active and engage in low levels of regular exercise. This will help to maintain strength and energy and improve mood.

Patients with neutropenia may be advised to avoid crowds and sick people and maintain a clean home environment including having rugs shampooed before treatment begins and moving live plants away from the patient. Care should be taken with pet waste, and whenever possible someone other than the patient should pick up pet waste or change litter boxes.

Nutrition education should begin at diagnosis to prevent complications caused by malnutrition and weight loss often associated with treatment. Dietary counseling should address the need for calorie- and protein-rich foods. Referral to a dietitian may be helpful. Avoidance of uncooked or unwashed foods is recommended. In general, alcoholic beverages should be avoided. Given the treatment-related pulmonary and cardiac toxicity, help with smoking cessation should be offered.

Many patients undergoing cancer treatment are taking oral medications new to them, including mild chemotherapeutic agents, antibiotics, antivirals, and antifungals. These need to be reviewed carefully with patients and families.

CHAPTER 241

MYELODYSPLASTIC SYNDROMES

Anna D. Schaal

DEFINITION AND EPIDEMIOLOGY

The myelodysplastic syndromes (MDSs) are a heterogeneous group of bone marrow disorders characterized by ineffective dysplastic growth of the hematopoietic precursors. MDS is not one disease but a diverse series of hematologic conditions that have variable clinical presentation, biologic activity, and prognosis.

There are three dominant features of this group of diseases. The first is impaired maturation of hematopoietic stem cells and increased cell death, or apoptosis. This is characterized by cytopenias. There also is a clonal expansion of the abnormal cell line, which manifests itself as progressive disease over time. Patients with MDS also have a variable risk of transformation to acute leukemia.

MDS is a relatively rare disease. It is primarily a disease of older adults, with the annual incidence rate rising to 4.6 per 100,000 persons per year in those 60 years old and older. Approximately 15,000 to 45,000 new cases of MDS are diagnosed each year in the United States. Males are affected about 1.5 to 2 times as often as females.[1]

Specialist referral is indicated for all suspected cases of MDS.

PATHOPHYSIOLOGY

The knowledge of pathophysiologic abnormalities that contribute to MDS is advancing at a remarkable pace. Defects in cellular differentiation, responsiveness to cytokines and growth factors, altered hematopoietic microenvironment, increased apoptosis, and abnormal DNA methylation are all pathways that lead to the ineffective hematopoiesis that is the trademark of MDS. This ineffective hematopoiesis results in peripheral cytopenias despite a packed, hypercellular bone marrow. In essence, the bone marrow produces cells that are not able to mature into functional red blood cells, white blood cells, and platelets.

The diagnostic classification of MDS has been a controversial topic for years. The World Health Organization has proposed a classification system. The acceptable categories include refractory anemia, refractory anemia with ringed sideroblasts, refractory cytopenia with multilineage dysplasia, 5q– syndrome, and myelodysplasia unclassifiable.[2] Each category of MDS behaves in a different manner and has different treatment implications.

The International Prognostic Scoring System–Revised (IPSS-R) is another useful classification system that is used to score the different variants of MDS (Table 241-1). The scoring is based on five factors: the percentage of blasts in the bone marrow, the specific karyotype or genetic abnormality risk group, hemoglobin, platelet count, and absolute neutrophil count (ANC). Corresponding scores that range from 0 to 6 help predict both survival and the risk of evolution to acute myeloid leukemia.[2] The IPSS-R is used to help with projecting prognosis and making treatment decisions.[3]

CLINICAL PRESENTATION AND PHYSICAL EXAMINATION

In general, the clinical presentation of MDS is related to symptoms of bone marrow failure or of the specific cytopenias that each patient is experiencing. If the red blood cells are the prominent lineage that is not maturing, then symptoms of anemia will be present. These may include fatigue, pallor, headaches, shortness of breath (or dyspnea) on exertion, and chest pains or palpitations. If the platelet count is low, easy bruising or bleeding will be the dominant presenting symptom. Frequent nose bleeds, petechiae, hematochezia, heavy menstrual bleeding, or large hematomas may encourage a patient to seek medical attention. Finally, if the white blood cells are not maturing, the main presenting symptoms will be of neutropenia, namely, frequent or severe infections. Splenomegaly is uncommon in MDS. Increasingly, more and more patients are being diagnosed incidentally from an abnormal complete blood count (CBC) done routinely in the primary care setting. In this case, patients feel well and have no subjective or physical examination findings that would make one suspect a myelodysplastic disorder.

DIAGNOSTICS

A number of specific diagnostic tests are required for the diagnosis of MDS. These include peripheral blood smear, bone marrow biopsy and aspirate with cytogenetic analysis, flow cytometry, and immunohistochemical staining.

The peripheral blood smear will often reveal erythrocytes with anisocytosis, poikilocytosis, or basophilic stippling. The

TABLE 241-1 The IPSS-R Parameters and Their Score Values

Prognostic Variable	0	0.5	1	1.5	2	3	4
Cytogenetics	Very good		Good		Intermediate	Poor	Very poor
BM* blast %	≤2%		>2% to <5%		5%-10%	>10%	
Hemoglobin	≥10		8 to <10	<8			
Platelets	≥100	50 to <100	<50				
ANC†	≥0.8	<0.8					

*Bone marrow.
†Absolute neutrophil (white blood cell) count.

Risk Group	Risk Score
Very low	≤1.5
Low	>1.5-3
Intermediate	>3-4.5
High	>4.5-6
Very high	>6

From Greenberg P, et al. Revised international prognostic scoring system for myelodysplastic syndromes. *Blood.* 2012;120(12):2454-2465.

granulocytes may be larger than normal and may lack normal granulation. Platelets may also be larger than normal.

The bone marrow biopsy almost always shows a hypercellular, packed marrow, which is in sharp contrast to the peripheral cytopenia. The hypercellular marrow often demonstrates defects in cellular maturation in all cell lines. For erythroid precursors, this includes megaloblastic cells, which are predominantly younger forms, and mature cells with distorted nuclei. Ringed sideroblasts will often be identified. These red blood cells are characterized by excessive cytoplasmic iron granules in a perinuclear distribution.[4] Megakaryocytes are the polynuclear cells responsible for platelet production. In MDS, the megakaryocytes are often smaller than normal and hypolobulated. The precursors for white blood cells may also have abnormal granulation and deformed nuclei.

Cytogenetic abnormalities play a role in prognosis. Cytogenetic abnormalities have been found in 50% to 60% of patients with de novo MDS and up to 80% of patients with therapy-related MDS.[5] Common abnormalities include 5q– syndrome, which is a good prognostic indicator, and monosomy 7, which is associated with a poor prognosis and an increased risk of transformation to acute leukemia.

DIAGNOSTICS

Myelodysplastic Disorders

LABORATORY	OTHER DIAGNOSTICS
CBC and differential	Bone marrow biopsy with cytogenetics, flow cytometry, and immunohistochemical staining
Peripheral blood smear	

DIFFERENTIAL DIAGNOSIS

Several disorders may mimic the morphologic changes of MDS and should be considered in the differential diagnosis. If anemia is the only presenting sign, common types of anemias must first be excluded, including folate and vitamin B_{12} deficiency, iron deficiency, anemia of chronic disease, renal failure, alcohol abuse, hereditary spherocytosis, and hemolysis. Infection, such as with human immunodeficiency virus (HIV), parvovirus, and Epstein-Barr virus, should also be ruled out. Drug toxicity or adverse reactions often imitate the cytopenias of MDS. Primary acute or chronic leukemia or a metastatic solid tumor with bone marrow metastasis should also be considered in the differential diagnosis. Other hematologic abnormalities often mimic MDS presentation, including aplastic anemia, Fanconi anemia, acute myeloid leukemia, myeloproliferative neoplasms and paroxysmal nocturnal hematuria. The bone marrow biopsy is the gold standard of diagnosis, because it often can exclude these disorders.

DIFFERENTIAL DIAGNOSIS

Myelodysplastic Disorders

- Vitamin B_{12}, folic acid, or iron deficiency
- Drug toxicity
- Alcohol toxicity
- HIV infection
- Irradiation
- Parvovirus infection
- Epstein-Barr virus infection
- Anemia of chronic disease
- Hemolysis
- Renal failure
- Leukemia
- Aplastic anemia
- Paroxysmal nocturnal hematuria
- Myeloproliferative neoplasms
- Fanconi anemia

MANAGEMENT

The clinical pathway of MDS and response to therapy vary significantly among individuals.

Because most individuals with MDS are older than 65 years, consideration should be given to a comprehensive geriatric evaluation of individuals before treatment is started as a way of predicting morbidity and mortality on the basis of age and comorbidities.[6]

The therapy for MDS ranges from supportive care to aggressive treatments. The goals of therapy include symptom management and improvement in quality of life while minimizing treatment-related toxicity and improving overall survival. These goals include decreasing the risk of progression to acute myelogenous leukemia (AML) (see Chapter 239).

A variety of agents are known to produce a response in MDS. Treatment decisions need to be tailored to the individual patient and should include consideration of age, functional status, and IPSS-R score. For those who are not good candidates for aggressive treatment strategies or who have failed to respond to such treatment attempts, supportive care becomes the foundation of therapy. This approach includes cytokine treatments and transfusion support, immunosuppression, and iron chelation. There is no evidence of any survival benefit from cytokine treatments; however, they may improve quality of life because they improve symptoms and decrease transfusion requirements. Cytokine treatment consists of erythropoietin (EPO), granulocyte colony-stimulating factor (G-CSF), and granulocyte-macrophage colony-stimulating factor (GM-CSF).[7]

EPO is a hormone that stimulates red blood cell production. Approximately 20% of patients will respond to EPO with an increase in hemoglobin. The patients who respond are usually those with low or no transfusion requirements.[8] Interestingly, the addition of G-CSF to EPO creates a synergy that improves the erythroid response in up to 50% of patients.[9] G-CSF and GM-CSF both stimulate white blood cell production. The absolute granulocyte count often increases with the use of these cytokines; however, the actual number of infections does not decrease.[10] Because of this, this therapy is typically not used routinely but more often when there is an active infection or an increased risk of infection.

Prophylactic antibiotic therapy is considered in patients with severe neutropenia, which is defined as an ANC of less than 500. It has been shown in a large meta-analysis that prophylactic treatment with fluoroquinolones in neutropenic patients can decrease the incidence of serious infections as well as reduce all-cause mortality.[11]

Most patients with MDS eventually become red cell transfusion dependent. Transfusions benefit patients by improving their symptoms of anemia; however, this is only a temporary improvement. The complications of chronic red blood cell transfusions include risk of infection, transfusion reactions, and iron overload necessitating chelation therapy. Platelet transfusion may be needed to prevent bleeding episodes in patients with thrombocytopenia. Quality-of-life issues emerge in the transfusion-dependent patient because of the time, resources, and support burden for patients who are required to go to a clinic for transfusions on a frequent basis.

In patients who are transfusion dependent, iron chelation becomes a consideration. Iron overload may contribute to both increased mortality and morbidity in early-stage MDS.[12] Once patients have received more than 20 red blood cell transfusions, patients become iron overloaded. For patients with serum ferritin levels greater than 2500 ng/mL, the goal is to decrease it to less than 1000 ng/mL.[7]

Immune suppression is also used for patients with MDS, with the primary goal of therapy being to improve quality of life. The use of antithymocyte globulin and cyclosporine has been found to be helpful by improving cytopenias and decreasing transfusion requirements. No benefit is noted in overall survival or time to leukemic transformation.[13]

A number of novel agents are now available or in clinical trial for MDS to prolong time to transfusion dependence. 5-Azacytidine, the first agent approved for the treatment of MDS, was approved by the U.S. Food and Drug Administration in 2004. 5-Azacytidine inhibits DNA methylation. Hypomethylation restores normal function of silenced growth genes that are responsible for differentiation and proliferation. A clinical trial supported its use, showing improvement in 24% of patients, with 66% of these responders becoming transfusion independent.[14] A phase III trial that compared 5-azacytidine and supportive care found that 60% of patients who received 5-azacytidine had hematologic response compared with only 5% in the supportive group arm. The median time of progression to AML or death was also significantly prolonged in the patients who received 5-azacytidine.[15] 5-Azacytidine is delivered in a subcutaneous injection for 7 days every 4 weeks. Its prominent side effects include myelosuppression, pain or skin reaction at injection sites, and nausea.

Decitabine, similar to 5-azacytidine, is also approved for the treatment of patients with MDS. It has been shown to be superior to supportive care alone, as evidenced by hematologic response rates, increased time to AML progression, and overall survival benefit, especially in high-risk patients.[16] In a recent study, median progression-free survival in older patients (older than 60) with higher risk disease was significantly improved as compared with patients receiving only supportive care.[17] Decitabine is also associated with serious side effects including fever, infection, and low blood counts. It is given intravenously for 3 consecutive days every 4 to 6 weeks.

Lenalidomide (Revlimid) is a 4-aminoglutarimide analogue of thalidomide that acts as an immunomodulatory agent. It is approved for the treatment of lower risk MDS. In a group of patients, 67% became transfusion independent and had a median rise in hemoglobin of 5.4 g/dL.[18] The major serious side effect is myelosuppression, which is dose dependent. Grades 3 and 4 neutropenia and thrombocytopenia occurred in 55% and 44%, respectively, which prompted dose modifications. Eighty-four percent of patients require a dose reduction. Interestingly, the cytopenias associated with this therapy seem to be predictive of a response. In other words, patients who had significant cytopenias and required dose reductions were more likely to become transfusion independent. Another serious adverse effect is an increased risk of thrombosis. It is recommended that patients taking lenalidomide be considered for anticoagulation therapy. Because lenalidomide is an analogue of thalidomide, a drug that has been associated with birth defects in the past, it is highly regulated and available only through specialty pharmacies and programs, because patients must consent to ensuring that no pregnancies develop while they are taking this medication. Other adverse reactions were uncommon and typically mild.[19,20]

Stem cell transplantation remains the only potentially curative treatment for MDS. This is preferred for a small number of patients with MDS, especially in those with high-risk disease and minimal comorbidities.[21,22] An allogeneic transplant, either human leukocyte antigen (HLA) identical related or unrelated, is indicated if the patient meets the rigorous transplantation requirements. Unfortunately, with the aged population of MDS patients, few meet this prerequisite. Stem cell transplantation should optimally be performed before disease progression. In patients with less advanced disease, 3-year survival rates of 65% to 75% are achieved. Among patients with advanced disease, the 3-year survival rate drops to 25% to 45%. The incidence of post-transplantation relapse is 5% to 35%, worsening with advanced disease.[23]

Reduced-intensity ("mini") stem cell transplantation allows more potential patients to meet the standards of transplantation. Mini-transplantation regimens are meant to treat the disease with a graft-versus-leukemia effect and do not depend on ablation of the patient's marrow. This type of transplant is better tolerated, and therefore more elderly patients and those with comorbidities may qualify. The disease-free progression after mini-transplantation is 60%. The 4-year probability of overall survival for patients with MDS is 49%. This therapy remains toxic, with a 20% risk of nonrelapse mortality.[24] Common causes of death included graft-versus-host disease and infections.

INDICATIONS FOR REFERRAL OR HOSPITALIZATION

Whenever MDS is suspected, patients are referred to a hematologist for both a review of the peripheral blood smear and a bone marrow biopsy. Hematologists will often observe patients long term with the help of primary health care providers to monitor disease progression and complications. For patients who have an MDS diagnosis, the following are indications for immediate referral to urgent or emergent care:

- In patients with an absolute neutropenia of less than 1000/mm^3, hospitalization for any febrile illness is warranted. Without prompt initiation of intravenous antibiotics, patients may quickly develop sepsis and require critical care.
- Any bleeding that does not resolve with 15 minutes of direct pressure requires an immediate CBC, with potential platelet transfusion to follow.
- Any trend of increasing peripheral blast population or worsening transfusion requirements is an indication for hematology follow-up to assess for transformation to acute leukemia.
- Nodular or flat diffuse rash could indicate transformation to acute leukemia and requires immediate laboratory review and consultation with dermatology specialists.
- Multidisciplinary team consultations including physical therapy for strength and conditioning, nutrition, social work, palliative care, and mental health are all helpful at different points along the MDS continuum.

COMPLICATIONS

The clinical course of MDS is inevitably progressive. The complications of MDS revolve around the offending cytopenias. Major bleeding episodes and infection are the most common reasons for hospital admissions. Transformation to acute leukemia ranges from 5% to 15% in low-risk groups to 40% to 50% in high-risk groups. This requires prompt intervention with induction chemotherapy if the patient is a candidate. Other, less-intense treatment regimens, such as oral melphalan, are also available.

Fatigue is another major complication of the disease itself. It is extremely common and can often become unrelenting. Patients often describe it as exhaustion. The fatigue can interfere with the patient's functional ability and can result in depression.

MDS is a heterogeneous group of bone marrow disorders that requires definitive diagnosis. Each patient must be evaluated and treated on his or her disease-specific symptom trajectory. Quality-of-life issues are paramount because both the disease and its treatments have the potential to disrupt normalcy. Caring support and social intervention can positively modify patients' experience with this disease as they encounter the different management strategies.

PATIENT AND FAMILY EDUCATION

The quality of life of those patients living with myelodysplasia is directly affected by both the disease and its accompanying treatments. The majority of patients who have this disease are elders, many with other comorbid conditions. This aging population will often have low physiologic reserves and a prolonged recovery from complications. Quality-of-life issues must be explored, and patients and families should be offered education in treatment choices, side effects, inconveniences, and cost in order to make informed decisions about their care. The patient's progress and response to therapies should be reevaluated and discussed with patients and family on a frequent basis.

It is also vital that neutropenic precautions be reviewed when necessary and that patients are aware of who to call and when to call if they develop fevers, chills, rigors, or persistent bleeding. Patients should also be educated on any clinical trials that may be available for their particular situation.

REFERENCES

For a full list of references, scan the QR code or visit http://booksite.elsevier.com/9780323355018

PART 22

Evaluation and Management of Oncologic Disorders

CHAPTER 242

COLLABORATIVE MANAGEMENT OF THE ONCOLOGY PATIENT

Jane Taylor Williams

Optimum cancer care depends on careful planning across multidisciplinary care settings to reduce the risk of fragmentation and to ensure a continuum of care. Many patients belong to managed care insurance plans that require the primary health care provider to maintain the gatekeeper role. Also, many oncology patients live hundreds of miles away from the cancer center and need qualified care close to home. It is important that the health care provider be viewed as a valuable member of the cancer care team, not as a resented intruder. Therefore it is necessary that all providers have a basic understanding of cancer-specific risk factors, presenting signs and symptoms, diagnostic tools, treatment options, prognosis, psychosocial issues, long-term survivor challenges, and available support systems.

CANCER RISKS

Approximately three fourths of all cancer risk factors are elements that individuals can control themselves. These include dietary habits, use of tobacco products or alcohol, sun exposure, lack of physical activity, and risky sexual behaviors. Emphasizing healthy lifestyle practices is a principal component of primary care, not only for cancer prevention but also for overall disease prevention. The American Cancer Society has recommendations for reducing the risks of cancer.[1]

SCREENING FOR CANCER

The American Cancer Society offers cancer-specific guidelines for screening of asymptomatic patients, and evidence-based screening guidelines can also be obtained from the National Cancer Institute.[1,2] These guidelines have changed over the last few years and are more conservative than previously. The health care provider still needs to be involved in high-quality screening activities as appropriate, which include the following comprehensive examinations: breast, gynecologic (women), genitourinary (men), colorectal, skin, and oral head and neck. Screening tests should be performed according to age-appropriate recommended guidelines and may include mammography, cervical smears, colorectal screening, and prostate screening. The new screening guidelines, such as for prostate cancer, recommend detailed discussions with the patient regarding pros and cons of screening. The health care provider will most likely be the one to detect cancer and will be the first source of information about diagnosis and possible treatment options before referring the patient to the oncologist or cancer center. Some cancers such as prostate cancer do not always require immediate treatment, and options may include active surveillance.

New information about genetic testing is widely available. Although only 5% to 10% of cancers are hereditary, providers must be diligent in obtaining accurate family histories to establish the possibility of a hereditary cancer syndrome. If this possibility does exist, the patient should be informed about the potential personal risk for cancer and about available surveillance and management strategies, including screening examinations, diagnostic tests, and cancer prevention strategies. Patients at high risk for certain cancers may need additional screening. For example, women suspected of being at risk for hereditary breast and ovarian syndromes are advised to have annual screening with magnetic resonance imaging in addition to mammograms beginning at an earlier age.[1] In addition, an annual CA-125 and transvaginal ultrasound screening for ovarian cancer is often advised.[2] Other high-risk guidelines can be obtained from the American Cancer Society and National Cancer Institute.[1,2] If indicated, a referral to a National Cancer Institute–designated comprehensive cancer center that offers genetic testing and counseling is appropriate.

PATIENT MANAGEMENT ISSUES

After a diagnosis of cancer, a timely referral for treatment increases the opportunity for optimum outcomes. In many cases, these outcomes include improved rates of cure, longer survival rates, and improved quality of life.

With shortened hospital stays, the management of cancer patients has moved from the hospital to the outpatient setting and often to the primary provider, especially in small or rural communities with no local oncologist. In such cases, collaboration with the oncology team in managing symptoms and monitoring for complications becomes essential. There needs to be clear communication with the oncology team regarding current treatment, including side effects and expected outcomes, current condition and prognosis, patient understanding, frequency of reports to and from the oncology team, and future treatment plans. Communication must clearly define areas of responsibility between the primary health care provider and the oncology team and should be task oriented. For example, if the health care provider agrees to monitor laboratory values for neutropenia, anemia, thrombocytopenia, kidney function, and liver function, he or she must be aware of critical laboratory parameters that require management by the oncology team or referral to a specialist. In addition, the primary health care provider can reinforce to the patient the signs and symptoms that indicate need for urgent evaluation, such as fever, mental status change, increasing pain, or persistent vomiting. The health care provider should recognize how treatment may affect blood glucose, blood pressure, thyroid function, kidney function, or liver enzymes and should be able to determine whether symptoms are related to cancer, cancer treatment, or other known or new conditions. Referral to the oncology team is required for symptoms that are difficult to manage, critical laboratory studies, and new suspicious findings. Oncologic emergencies requiring referral include spinal cord compression, hypercalcemia, tumor lysis syndrome, syndrome of inappropriate antidiuretic hormone, and superior vena cava syndrome (see Chapter 244). Cancer patients are also at increased risk of deep vein thrombosis (DVT) or pulmonary embolus (PE) resulting from the cancer itself or other factors such as certain medications, surgery, central venous catheters, and inactivity.

Febrile neutropenia—temperature above 38° C (100.4° F) and absolute neutrophil count below 500/mm^3—is a common complication of patients receiving chemotherapy and needs immediate attention. Standard procedures include hospitalization with chest x-ray examination, urine culture and sensitivity, blood cultures, and, if a central line is in place, culture of the line.

Cancer patients are also lured by the barrage of herbs and supplements lining the shelves of supermarkets, health food stores, and pharmacies. They also are influenced by magazines, television, and Internet advertisements. Health care providers should access credible websites to determine evidence of efficacy, toxicity, or potential interactions with chemotherapy, radiation therapy, or other medications and ensure their practice is evidence based.[3]

Long-term surveillance is important, especially for young survivors but also for the older population as more effective cancer treatments are developed.[4] Complications may affect the cardiovascular system, including increased risk of hypertension and hyperlipidemia from vascular endothelial injury and increased plasma renin and aldosterone levels.[5] Serious cardiovascular complications have been reported after cisplatin-based therapy. Peripheral neuropathy may occur with cisplatin or taxane therapies, and tinnitus and high-frequency hearing loss are related to peripheral neuropathy.[5] Bleomycin-related acute pulmonary toxicity is increased in cigarette smokers.[5] Young survivors may have problems with reproduction after radiotherapy or chemotherapy, and radiotherapy and chemotherapy may also increase the risk for additional primary malignant neoplasms in long-term survivors.[5] Other long-term effects include oral and dental problems, cognitive changes, electrolyte imbalances (e.g., hypomagnesemia), erectile dysfunction (men) and vaginal dryness or dyspareunia (women), and endocrine disorders.[3] Chronic fatigue and chronic pain syndromes are not uncommon, and depression, anxiety, and other psychological and social issues may persist for years.[4,5]

Caring for the cancer patient can place inordinate burdens on family and friends. Assessment of the caregivers' readiness and availability to care for the patient is imperative. The primary caregiver must be aware of the established support systems and the availability of additional community resources, such as various cancer-specific support groups, the United Ostomy Associations of America, I Can Cope, Candlelighters, Us TOO, and CanCare. The local American Cancer Society chapter is another excellent resource, and many communities have faith-based support services. Successful home care also depends on such factors as cultural beliefs, role delineation, and resolution of any existing interpersonal conflicts. In addition, personal values surrounding narcotic analgesic use and beliefs about death and dying should be explored.

ROLE OF THE PRIMARY HEALTH CARE PROVIDER

The primary health care provider is an essential resource between appointments with the oncologist, especially if the oncologist is in another city or if the health care provider is seeing the patient for management of other chronic conditions. If the provider is not receiving reports and updates from the oncologist, he or she should contact the oncologist and request to receive all vital information that will affect patient outcomes. This allows the primary health care provider to adequately monitor various symptoms, to answer the patient's questions about treatment side effects, and to reinforce information given by the oncologist. Establishment of a collaborative relationship between the oncology team and the health care provider ensures safe and continuous care, minimizes potential complications, and promotes patient and provider confidence.

Health care reform has redirected patient care from hospital-based to outpatient- or community-based care, and although improvements in cancer survival rates are encouraging, new challenges are emerging for the long-term survivor and the primary care provider. Both patients with cancer and cancer survivors are especially vulnerable to the risk of fragmentation of care when migrating from specialist to generalist or from hospital to home care. Consistent personnel who know the patient's situation are the key components for successful delivery of health care. It is the responsibility of the patient and all members of the multidisciplinary health care team to identify needs and form a collaborative plan so that outcomes of care can be optimized.

CHAPTER 243

BASIC PRINCIPLES OF ONCOLOGY TREATMENT

Leslie Lezell Levitan

Cancer treatment involves multidisciplinary team members including physician specialists, nurse practitioners, physician assistants, nurses, pharmacists, social workers, and several other health care professionals. Primary health care providers act as patient advocates and play a central role in coordinating care among all involved disciplines. Cancer treatment can be curative or palliative, depending on the patient's disease pathology and wishes for treatment. This chapter largely focuses on curative approaches to cancer treatment.

Using a combination of surgery, chemotherapy, radiation therapy, biotherapy, and hormonal and genetic therapy, the health care team can significantly lengthen disease-free intervals and achieve recognizable survival benefits for cancer patients. Surgery is the oldest treatment still used today and remains effective for cancer prevention, diagnosis, definitive treatment, rehabilitation, and palliation. In the early 1800s, elective surgery for visceral tumors was used in frontier America.[1] Radiation therapy and chemotherapy, historically used for palliative care,

are now used as adjunctive treatments for localized diseases and are even curative for some early-stage cancers.[2]

When considering cancer treatment, the tumor type is first evaluated by taking a tissue sample from the tumor for an accurate histologic diagnosis.[1] Once a diagnosis is established, the patient's disease is then staged to assess the extent of disease and to determine both prognosis and choice of therapy. Various cancer-staging systems are used for both individual and multiple cancers. The tumor, nodes, and metastasis (TNM) system is a widely used cancer classification system created by the American Joint Committee on Cancer and the International Union Against Cancer.[3,4] Common parameters in most staging systems include cell type, location of primary tumor, tumor grade, tumor size and number, lymph node involvement, and presence of metastases.[4]

In the earlier stages of disease (stage I or II), the tumor is typically localized, and the chances for cure are greater with the use of local or regional therapy. If the tumor stage is higher (stage III or IV), the cancer is no longer localized, and curative treatment may no longer be an option for the patient. The treatment plan is highly individualized to the patient and should take into account the risk/benefit ratio of the various options, the patient's performance status, the patient's willingness to consent to treatment, the availability of a treatment facility, financial restrictions, and the impact the treatment may have on the patient's quality of life.

RADIATION THERAPY

Radiation therapy is often used in combination with surgery, chemotherapy, and/or biologic therapies to eliminate or shrink tumors. Radiation therapy can also be given as sole treatment for patients with highly localized tumors that are histologically radiosensitive, or as an alternative to surgery for patients with a poor performance status who are medically unable to undergo surgery. When radiation treatment is used as an adjunct to treatment, the goal is to gain control of the disease, and the treatment may be delivered preoperatively or postoperatively. Preoperative radiation treatment can help to debulk the tumor to facilitate surgical resection. Postoperative radiation treatment may be chosen after surgical resection if there is a concern about local recurrence or if the resection margin remains suspicious for disease. Radiation may also be used in the palliative setting to address complaints of pain, bleeding, or brain metastasis or to control spinal cord compression by a tumor, thereby enhancing the patient's quality of life. Although treatment techniques and equipment may vary, the important principles of radiotherapy form a basis on which a course of treatment is decided.[2]

DNA is the critical target for the effects of radiotherapy. Ionizing radiation interacts directly with intracellular structures or indirectly through free radical formation when it combines with cellular water. These interactions may result in disruption of DNA, which ultimately can lead to cell death.[5] Factors that affect the response to radiotherapy include oxygen effect (well-oxygenated tumors have a greater response), vascularity of the tumor, linear energy transfer (the rate at which energy is lost from different types of radiation while traveling through matter), and use of bioreductive drugs (mitomycin [MMC], RSU 1069, and organic nitroxides).[6]

There are a variety of ways in which radiation therapy may be delivered in the treatment of cancer. The mode that is selected is dependent on the cancer histology, tumor location, patient's performance status, availability of technology, and expertise of the radiation oncologist. The goal of therapy is to optimize dose delivery to the tumor while minimizing damage to healthy tissue.

External Beam Radiotherapy

The most commonly used form of radiation therapy is external beam. Linear accelerators are used to generate high-energy x-rays, or photons, at varying energies, which penetrate the body and are directed at the tumor. The depth of photon penetration depends on the energy selected. Treatment delivered in this manner is accomplished with different combinations of energies, beam techniques, radiation shielding, and patient positioning. This form of treatment is used in a variety of cancers but is currently the gold standard for treatment of invasive breast cancers.[7]

Computed Tomography Simulation and Its Role in Radiotherapy

Once external beam therapy has been chosen, a simulation using computed tomography (CT) is then performed for radiation planning. During simulation, a planning CT scan is obtained so that the radiation oncologist can localize and define the tumor volume needed for treatment. Critical structures to be avoided are also identified at this time.[8] The treatment field is delineated, and marks corresponding to the area of treatment are subsequently made on the patient. These marks are used later during the treatment phase for proper patient alignment to the linear accelerator. Special immobilization devices, such as custom casts or molds, may be used during the simulation process to assist in the patient setup process.[9]

Fractionation

Once the CT simulation is completed and the goal and intent of treatment are decided, the dose of radiation to be prescribed is then determined. Fractionated radiation therapy is used to maximize the therapeutic benefit of radiation while minimizing the harmful effects of radiation on healthy tissue. The amount of radiation absorbed by tissue is expressed in the international unit gray (Gy): 1 Gy equals 100 rad (radiation absorbed dose); 1 cGy equals 1 rad. The total dose of radiation is typically spread out, or fractionated, into small treatments given during specific periods. Fractionation allows for repair of radiation damage to normal cells and their repopulation. It also gives an opportunity for reoxygenation of hypoxic tissue, thereby improving the effectiveness of radiation in subsequent fractions of treatment. Fractionated therapy also permits more time for cancer cells that were previously in a resistant part of their cell cycle to become more susceptible to the radiation effect during subsequent fractions.[5] The final dose and fraction scheme chosen will be a reflection of several factors that affect the radiation dose, including the goal of therapy, radiosensitivity of the tumor, cancer stage, and normal tissue tolerances of the different anatomic structures in the treatment field.[6]

Brachytherapy

Brachytherapy is another mode of radiation delivery, which involves placement of a radioactive source within the body or body cavity near the tumor site. It is used mainly in the treatment of prostate and cervical cancers; however, with advancements in diagnostic imaging, brachytherapy is now being used to treat other cancer sites as well.[10] Brachytherapy is often combined with external beam radiation and may be used preoperatively or postoperatively. Radioactive isotopes for brachytherapy application are contained in a variety of forms, such as wires, ribbons, tubes, needles, grains, seeds, and capsules. The radiation oncologist will determine the form based on the site being treated, the size of the lesion, and whether the implant is temporary or permanent. Brachytherapy is given at either a low-dose rate or a high-dose rate, which produces the same effect in a shorter period.[11]

Radiation Treatment Side Effects

Radiation treatment–related side effects can develop early in the course of therapy, or they may be delayed for several months to years after therapy. There are predictable side effects of radiation therapy for particular tumor types seen clinically, however. Factors that predict side effects include the body tissue treated, the daily dose and total dosage given, the particular method of radiation delivery, and individual factors (e.g., the patient's age and genetic makeup). Acute symptoms often develop 10 to 14 days into treatment and may not abate until 2 or more weeks after the treatments have completed.[2] Common side effects vary by the treatment site but may include fatigue, anorexia, mucositis, xerostomia, radiation caries, esophagitis, dysphagia, nausea, vomiting, diarrhea, tenesmus, cystitis, urethritis, alopecia, skin reactions, and bone marrow depression.[12] Delayed reactions to treatment can occur around 6 months after treatment but may not appear until several years after therapy. Delayed reactions may include fibrosis, fistula formation, and organ damage, and are thought to be the result of direct parenchymal damage or microvasculature damage.

Radiosurgery

Gamma Knife radiosurgery works by delivering extremely precise, high-dose beams of radiation directly to a tumor site in the brain, thereby avoiding healthy tissue. The most common use for radiosurgery is for the treatment of metastatic brain tumors.[13] Spinal oncologists now recommend use of radiotherapy for spinal metastases and metastatic epidural spinal cord compression as well.[14] The procedure is well tolerated by patients; it is less invasive than traditional neurosurgery and is usually done as a one-time therapy, completed in the same day, with minimal recovery.

Summary

Radiation oncology has come a long way since its beginnings in the 1800s. Intensity modulation and apparatuses for radiation therapy, image-guided and three-dimensional treatment planning for radiation therapy, particle therapy radiation, and advances in brachytherapy have allowed radiation oncologists more tools with which to treat cancer while reducing the toxicity of treatment.[5] The future holds promise for advances in cancer treatment, with radiation therapy continuing to play a major role in primary treatment and in combined modality approaches. The primary care provider's responsibility is to monitor for acute reactions during radiation therapy, to assess for delayed reactions during post-treatment surveillance, and to collaborate with the radiation oncologist in implementing a management strategy throughout the course of care.

CHEMOTHERAPY

The primary role of chemotherapy is to prevent cancer cells from multiplying, invading, and metastasizing, in order to prolong life.[15] Chemotherapeutic agents are classified by their mechanism of action, chemical structure, or biologic source. Alkylating agents were the first modern chemotherapeutic agents used in the clinical setting and were a product of the U.S. secret gas program in the two world wars. Exposure to mustard gas was shown to arrest bone marrow and lymphocyte tissue development. Therefore in 1942 a patient with lymphoma was treated with nitrogen mustard. In the same time period, another researcher observed that folic acid induced leukemic cell growth in children; this observation led to the development of folic acid analogues and later to the development of antimetabolites, a cornerstone in cancer treatment.[16]

Molecular genetic analysis of the DNA, RNA, and proteins of both normal and neoplastic cells has defined the mechanisms by which chemotherapy induces cell death. Understanding of how chemotherapy works and how molecular genetic changes can result in resistance to therapy has enabled newer types of treatment. These therapies combine molecular, genetic, and biologic strategies to increase the sensitivity of abnormal cells to treatment and to protect the normal tissues of the body from therapy-induced side effects, which may ultimately help patients with cancers that are resistant to standard therapies.[15,17]

Carcinogenesis, Cellular Kinetics, and Chemotherapy

Carcinogenesis is the process by which one or more normal cells undergo genetic changes, leading to malignant transformation. The direct exposure of DNA to a carcinogen may lead to irreversible genetic damage, allowing malignant transformation. The cell cycle is a sequence of steps through which both normal and abnormal cells grow and reproduce.[17,18] This process involves five phases: mitosis (M), which lasts about 30 to 60 minutes, when cell division occurs; resting phase (G_0), which is the largest variable in the cell cycle, when the cell is not active; first gap phase (G_1), which lasts 18 to 30 hours, when the cell manufactures enzymes to prepare for DNA synthesis; DNA synthesis (S), which can last 10 to 20 hours; and finally, second gap or premitotic phase (G_2), which can last 2 to 10 hours, when the cell produces ribonucleic acid, specialized proteins, and the mitotic spindle apparatus. The cell cycle then repeats again with the mitosis phase. Cell cycle kinetics can be altered when a cell becomes malignant. Chemotherapeutic agents are, therefore, classified according to the phase of the cell cycle in which they are active (Box 243-1).[17]

Role of Chemotherapy in Oncology

Chemotherapy can be used as induction treatment for advanced disease, as a primary treatment when no alternative treatment is superior, or for palliative treatment. It can be used as adjuvant therapy when alternative local therapies exist but are less effective alone (i.e., radiation therapy or surgery), and is often given first or even concurrently with local therapy, depending on the patient's clinical situation and cancer type. Chemotherapy helps with debulking the primary tumor or after the completion of local therapies, to eradicate micrometastases. Lastly, chemotherapy can be directly instilled into tumor sanctuary sites or perfused into specific regions of the body most affected by the cancer (e.g., the peritoneum or liver).[18] Administration of a combination of clinically effective antitumor drugs with nonoverlapping toxicities is the standard for a chemotherapeutic approach to most malignant neoplasms. This technique provides maximal cell kill for resistant cells, reduces

BOX 243-1

Cell Cycle Activity

CELL CYCLE PHASE: NONSPECIFIC AGENTS (DOSE DEPENDENT)

Classic alkylating agents (mechlorethamine, melphalan, busulfan, chlorambucil, cyclophosphamide, ifosfamide)
Anthracycline antibiotics (doxorubicin, daunorubicin, idarubicin)
Miscellaneous (dacarbazine, cisplatin, carboplatin)
Nitrosoureas (also G_0) (carmustine, lomustine, streptozocin)
Mitomycin C
Dactinomycin

CELL CYCLE PHASE: SPECIFIC AGENTS (SCHEDULE DEPENDENT)

S-Phase Agents

Antimetabolites

- Antifolates (methotrexate)
- Antipyrimidines (cytarabine, fluorouracil, gemcitabine, capecitabine)
- Antipurines (mercaptopurine, thioguanine, fludarabine, chlorodeoxyadenosine)
- Miscellaneous (hydroxyurea, procarbazine)
- Steroids (also G_1)

G_1-Phase Agents

Steroids
Asparaginase

G_2-Phase Agents

Bleomycin
Podophyllotoxins (etoposide, teniposide)

M-Phase Agents

Vinca alkaloids (vincristine, vinblastine, vinorelbine)
Taxanes (paclitaxel, docetaxel)

Data from Balmer CM, Valley AW, Iannucci A: Cancer treatment and chemotherapy. In DiPiro JT, Talbert RL, Yee GC, et al, editors: *Pharmacotherapy: a pathophysiologic approach,* ed 6, Burr Ridge, IL, 2005, McGraw-Hill.

the development of resistant cell lines, and minimizes toxicity (Box 243-2).[18]

Response to Chemotherapy

There is a wide range between therapeutic response and toxicity among patients receiving chemotherapy. The variability in this range can be attributed to differences in the characteristics of the patient, the chemotherapeutic agents given, and the type of tumor being treated. Patient factors include toxicity response, organ dysfunction, previous treatments, and age. Once toxicity occurs, a dose reduction or a treatment delay will most likely be indicated.[18]

The oncologist and primary health care provider often work collaboratively in managing common side effects from chemotherapy. Common symptoms include fatigue, anorexia, diarrhea, constipation, nausea and vomiting, cardiotoxicity, neurotoxicity, pulmonary toxicity, hepatotoxicity, hemorrhagic cystitis, nephrotoxicity, infertility, myelosuppression, mucositis, alopecia, and secondary malignant neoplasms. Adverse effects may vary depending on the combination of agents used.[15,17]

BOX 243-2

Chemotherapies Used for Specific Cancers

PRIMARY CHEMOTHERAPY (CANCERS IN WHICH CHEMOTHERAPY IS THE PRIMARY TREATMENT MODALITY)

- Acute leukemias
- Embryonal rhabdomyosarcoma
- Hodgkin lymphoma
- Germ cell tumor
- Myeloma
- Ovarian cancer
- Non-Hodgkin lymphoma
- Primary central nervous system lymphoma
- Small cell lung cancer
- Wilms tumor

PRIMARY CHEMOTHERAPY (CANCERS IN WHICH CHEMOTHERAPY HAS EXPANDING ROLE IN ADVANCED DISEASE)

- Bladder cancer
- Head and neck cancer
- Breast cancer
- Nasopharyngeal cancer
- Cervical cancer
- Non–small cell lung cancer
- Colorectal cancer
- Ovarian cancer
- Esophageal cancer
- Pancreatic cancer
- Gastric
- Prostate

NEOADJUVANT CHEMOTHERAPY (CANCERS IN WHICH NEOADJUVANT CHEMOTHERAPY IS EFFECTIVE IN ADVANCED DISEASE)

- Anal cancer
- Lung cancer
- Bladder cancer
- Ovarian cancer
- Breast cancer
- Osteogenic sarcoma
- Cervical cancer
- Rectal cancer
- Gastroesophageal cancer
- Soft tissue sarcoma
- Head and neck cancer

ADJUVANT CHEMOTHERAPY (CANCERS IN WHICH ADJUVANT CHEMOTHERAPY IS EFFECTIVE AFTER SURGERY)

- Anaplastic astrocytoma
- Melanoma
- Breast cancer
- Non–small cell lung cancer
- Colorectal cancer
- Osteogenic sarcoma
- Gastric cancer
- Pancreatic cancer

Data from DeVita V, Chu E: Principles of medical oncology. In DeVita VT, Lawrence TS, Rosenberg SA, editors: *Cancer: principles and practice of oncology,* ed 8, Philadelphia, 2008, Lippincott Williams & Wilkins.

TREATING THE CANCER PATIENT TODAY AND TOMORROW

Progress in molecular biology and biotechnology has had a major impact on the way patients with cancer are treated today. There is a greater understanding of the molecular nature of cancer and the immune system. At research centers across the United States and throughout the world, researchers are feverishly working to develop new treatments for cancer. Some of these include novel biologics, nanoparticle delivery mechanisms, and advance proton therapies that will hopefully prove successful and improve outcomes for cancer patients. Primary health care providers have multiple responsibilities to patients undergoing treatment for cancers including medical oversight and emotional and spiritual support. Accepting a patient's decision to discontinue or opt out of certain treatments is also an important part of managing the oncology patient.[19] Direct communication and collaboration between the oncology team and the primary care provider can assist with identification and recognition of subtle but potentially life-threatening changes in the cancer patient. Understanding the implications for different tumor types and monitoring for side effects are essential in caring for these patients, especially with the newer treatments coming down the pipeline.

CHAPTER 244

ONCOLOGY COMPLICATIONS AND PARANEOPLASTIC SYNDROMES

Jane Taylor Williams • Marilyn Kenebrew

An oncologic emergency is an acute, potentially life-threatening event that is directly or indirectly related to cancer or its treatment. If it is left unrecognized and untreated, significant morbidity or death may result. An oncologic emergency may also occur in an individual not previously diagnosed with cancer. Because cancer manifests in various ways, it must be considered part of the differential diagnosis of many complex medical events. In addition, because the nature of these entities is emergent and because treatment of the underlying cancer is required, all these syndromes require urgent referral to an oncologist.

Common structural emergencies are superior vena cava syndrome (SVCS) and spinal cord compression (SCC). Metabolic emergencies include hypercalcemia, syndrome of inappropriate antidiuretic hormone (SIADH), and tumor lysis syndrome (TLS). Other oncologic emergencies not discussed in this chapter include sepsis, disseminated intravascular coagulation, malignant pericardial effusions, and hyperviscosity caused by dysproteinemia or leukocytosis.

Immediate emergency department referral or specialist consultation is indicated for patients with angioedema, dyspnea, stridor, papilledema, seizures, and other signs of SVCS; patients with back pain accompanied by focal weakness, ataxia, or bowel or bladder dysfunction; patients with serum calcium levels of more than 12 mg/dL; patients with TLS; and patients with serum sodium levels of 125 mEq/L or less.

SUPERIOR VENA CAVA SYNDROME

DEFINITION AND EPIDEMIOLOGY

SVCS occurs when blood flow through the superior vena cava (SVC) is obstructed. Lung cancer is responsible in approximately 70% of SVCS cases.

PATHOPHYSIOLOGY

Any pathologic process that invades the lymphatics or structures of the superior mediastinum can encroach on the thin-walled, compliant SVC and cause obstruction of venous return to the heart. SVCS may result from external compression, direct invasion, or thrombosis of the SVC. The most common cause of SVC obstruction is malignant disease, usually lung cancer, particularly small cell lung cancer (SCLC), lymphoma, and metastatic breast cancer.[1] Furthermore, 80% of the tumors inducing SVCS originate in the right lung.[1] The most common nonmalignant cause of SVCS is thrombosis of the SVC associated with indwelling central venous catheters or pacemakers.[2]

CLINICAL PRESENTATION AND PHYSICAL EXAMINATION

SVCS is usually insidious in onset. The severity of presentation depends on the underlying cause, rapidity of obstruction, concurrent thrombosis, location of obstruction, and adequacy of collateral circulation. Swelling of the face, neck, or chest or orthopnea is the classic presenting complaint.[2] Other symptoms include headache, dizziness, visual disturbances, hoarseness, chest pain, and dysphagia. Physical findings include venous distention in the upper body, facial edema, cyanosis, arm and hand edema, telangiectasias of the chest and upper back, tachypnea, hoarseness, and stridor.[1,2] Neurologic abnormalities resulting from increased intracranial pressure include papilledema, agitation, lethargy, confusion, seizures, and coma.

DIAGNOSTICS

A chest x-ray examination commonly reflects a superior mediastinal mass or widening (64%), pleural effusion (26%), right hilar mass (12%), or adenopathy; however, 16% of patients may have normal radiographic findings.[1] Magnetic resonance imaging (MRI) or computed tomography (CT) scan of the chest is indicated to localize the level of SVC obstruction and to identify the presence of intrinsic or extrinsic obstruction, superimposed thrombosis, collateral circulation, mediastinal adenopathy, masses, and other sites of unrecognized disease in the chest. Because the underlying pathologic condition in many patients with new-onset SVCS is not identified, other diagnostic

DIAGNOSTICS

Superior Vena Cava Syndrome

IMAGING	OTHER DIAGNOSTICS
Chest x-ray examination	Biopsy
CT scan, MRI	

evaluations (biopsies) are almost always required before the definitive therapy can be administered.

DIFFERENTIAL DIAGNOSIS

With SVCS, idiopathic mediastinal fibrosis, tuberculosis, histoplasmosis, syphilis, and aneurysm of the aortic arch are among the differential diagnoses.[1,3] Other diagnoses to consider are constrictive pericarditis and thrombosis from indwelling catheters or pacemaker leads.

DIFFERENTIAL DIAGNOSIS

Superior Vena Cava Syndrome

- Idiopathic mediastinal fibrosis
- Tuberculosis
- Syphilis
- Histoplasmosis
- Goiter
- Aortic aneurysm
- Thrombosis
- Constrictive pericarditis

MANAGEMENT AND COMPLICATIONS

Treatment is directed at the underlying cause. The treatment of SVCS should be guided by the stage and histologic features of the primary process. Chemotherapy alone or in combination with radiotherapy is the treatment of choice for SVCS caused by SCLC and non-Hodgkin lymphoma, whereas non-SCLC is best treated with radiotherapy, endovascular stent placement, or both.[1,2,4] Temporary measures to alleviate discomfort include bed rest with elevation of the upper body, supplemental oxygen, and limited intravenous fluids. Venipuncture and intravenous lines should not be placed in the upper extremities. There may be temporary symptomatic improvement with diuretic therapy and reduced sodium diets, but dehydration may increase the risk for thrombosis and exacerbate the SVCS. The use of short-term corticosteroids to reduce the inflammation and edema associated with the tumor is controversial; however, corticosteroids and bronchodilators are indicated if stridor or airway compromise is present. Intubation or an emergency tracheostomy may be necessary. Patients with central nervous system (CNS) signs require high doses of dexamethasone to relieve increased intracranial pressure.[1] If the SVCS is a result of thrombosis, thrombolytic agents (urokinase or streptokinase) are effective if they are initiated within 7 days of symptom onset. Other, less-commonly used treatments include balloon angioplasty, caval stenting, and surgical bypass.[2] If left untreated, patients will develop marked venous distention, laryngeal edema, stridor, increased intracranial pressure, sagittal sinus thrombosis, and cerebral edema.

MALIGNANT SPINAL CORD COMPRESSION

DEFINITION AND EPIDEMIOLOGY

Neoplastic epidural SCC occurs in approximately 2.5% to 6%[5] of patients with cancer; two thirds of cord compression in adults arises from metastatic breast, lung, or prostate cancer. Other cancers that cause spinal cord metastases include non-Hodgkin lymphoma, melanoma, renal cell carcinoma, sarcoma, multiple myeloma, and unknown primary carcinoma. Approximately 20% of cases of SCC are seen as the initial manifestation of malignant disease.[6] Metastatic SCC is usually a symptom of advanced cancer.[7]

PATHOPHYSIOLOGY

SCC usually results when metastasis from a vertebral body extends into the epidural space or when a vertebral body collapses, resulting in a compression fracture. Direct extension of a paraspinous tumor through a vertebral foramen will also compress the spinal cord.[6] Rarely, a tumor may emanate from the epidural space without any bone involvement. The compression of the spinal cord impairs blood flow, resulting in spinal cord edema, ischemia, and infarction. The incidence of SCC is highest in multiple myeloma (8%), prostate cancer (7%), nasopharyngeal cancer (6.5%), and breast cancer (5.5%).[6]

CLINICAL PRESENTATION AND PHYSICAL EXAMINATION

The signs and symptoms of SCC depend on the area of spinal cord involved. The thoracic spine is involved most often (70%), followed by the lumbosacral (20%) and cervical (10%) vertebrae.[2] In 70% to 95% of patients, the presenting symptom is a constant, dull, aching back pain that is often worse when the patient is supine (opposite of the usual finding with a herniated disk).[6,8] The pain, which antedates the diagnosis of SCC by days to many months, is exacerbated by movement, sneezing, straining, or neck flexion.[5,6,8] Weakness, especially of the lower extremities, is the second most common symptom. It may be preceded or accompanied by sensory loss or paresthesia that ascends to the level of compression.[2] The loss of proprioception produces ataxia. Autonomic dysfunctions, such as urinary frequency, urgency, urinary retention, constipation, and sexual impotence, are late manifestations and are associated with a poor prognosis.[6] Physical findings may include tenderness on palpation of the involved vertebrae, hyperactive deep tendon reflexes, extensor plantar response, palpable bladder, and diminished rectal tone.[2]

DIAGNOSTICS

After an accurate neurologic history and physical examination, MRI is the preferred diagnostic test for SCC; MRI has a sensitivity of 93% and a specificity of 97%. A CT scan or myelography is reserved for patients who cannot undergo MRI (e.g., patients who have cardiac pacemakers or are claustrophobic).[6] Tumor biopsy may also be used to diagnose cancer in patients not previously diagnosed.[9] Patients with cancer who are seen with a new complaint of back pain should undergo an evaluation for SCC.

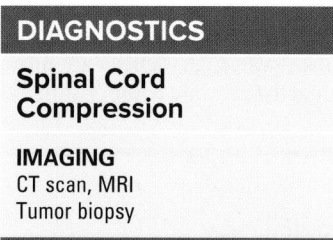

DIAGNOSTICS

Spinal Cord Compression

IMAGING
CT scan, MRI
Tumor biopsy

DIFFERENTIAL DIAGNOSIS

Other clinical situations may mimic SCC by causing motor or sensory deficits of the neck or upper and lower back or by causing pain. These situations include thoracic outlet syndromes, osteoarthritis of the spine, periarthritis of the shoulder, herniated disk, sacroiliitis, facet joint degenerative arthritis, spinal stenosis, irritation of the sciatic nerve, compression fracture from osteoporosis, epidural abscess, ankylosing spondylitis, leaking aortic aneurysm, and renal stones.

DIFFERENTIAL DIAGNOSIS

Spinal Cord Compression

- Thoracic outlet syndrome
- Osteoarthritis
- Periarthritis of shoulder
- Sacroiliitis
- Herniated disk
- Facet joint degenerative arthritis
- Spinal stenosis
- Sciatic nerve irritation
- Epidural abscess
- Leaking aortic aneurysm
- Renal stones
- Ankylosing spondylitis
- Compression fractures

MANAGEMENT

Clear indications of SCC in the cancer patient (e.g., focal weakness, ataxia, bowel or bladder dysfunction accompanied by back pain) demand an emergent evaluation and a referral. Immediate therapy with steroids (dexamethasone is most commonly used) may reduce vasogenic edema. The optimum loading dose and maintenance dose are controversial. An intravenous loading dose of 10 to 100 mg is given, followed by 4 to 24 mg every 6 hours. After 2 days, therapy is switched to 4 to 8 mg oral dexamethasone every 6 hours. Steroid doses are tapered every 4 days.[6,8] If neurologic decline results from dose reduction, the dose is maintained at effective levels during definitive treatment.

The decision to proceed with surgery, radiotherapy, or chemotherapy is based on the type of cancer. Radiotherapy alone is the definitive treatment for most patients.[2,5,6,8] Surgical decompression is indicated in the following situations: the histopathology of the cancer is unknown, neurologic deterioration develops during or after radiotherapy, the cancer is radiation resistant, a pathologic fracture causes compression by bone, or the spine is unstable.[2,5,6,8] Chemotherapy can be used for chemosensitive tumors (e.g., lung cancer, lymphoma) and is usually an adjunct to radiotherapy.[2,6]

COMPLICATIONS

If it is left untreated or undiagnosed, SCC can result in paraplegia, quadriplegia, or loss of bowel or bladder function. In most patients, motor function and sphincter control cannot be regained once they have been lost. Neurologic deficits are more likely to be reversed with a gradual than a rapid compression.[5,6,8]

HYPERCALCEMIA

DEFINITION AND EPIDEMIOLOGY

The most common metabolic emergency in patients with cancer is hypercalcemia, developing in 10% to 20% of patients with solid tumors.[10,11] The most common malignant neoplasms associated with hypercalcemia are lymphomas, multiple myeloma, and cancers of the breast, lung, kidney, head and neck, esophagus, thyroid, and prostate. Hypercalcemia develops when the rate of calcium mobilization from bone exceeds the renal threshold for calcium excretion. The serum calcium level is more than 11 mg/dL.[2,11]

PATHOPHYSIOLOGY

In ambulatory patients, 90% of cases of hypercalcemia are caused by either hyperparathyroidism or malignant disease; hyperthyroidism is also an important cause in the ambulatory population. The mechanisms involved in hypercalcemia of malignant neoplasms were thought to be related primarily to bone resorption resulting from metastatic bone lesions. Although bone metastasis results in hypercalcemia, recent evidence suggests that certain tumors secrete a variety of hormonal factors that stimulate osteoclast activity, resulting in the release of calcium from the bone. Several of these humoral factors are parathyroid hormone–related protein (PTHrP), osteoclast-activating factors, transforming growth factors, hematopoietic colony-stimulating factors, prostaglandins (E series), and 1,25-dihydroxyvitamin D.[5,11] Other phenomena that can contribute to and worsen hypercalcemia are immobility, dehydration, and renal insufficiency.[10,11]

CLINICAL PRESENTATION AND PHYSICAL EXAMINATION

Most patients with hypercalcemia see their health care provider with nonspecific symptoms of fatigue (70%), anorexia (60%), nausea, constipation (60%), weight loss (60%), bone pain (60%), polyuria, polydipsia, or dehydration.[2,11] The neurologic symptoms begin with vague muscle weakness, lethargy, apathy, and hyporeflexia and then progress to stupor and coma.[2,11] Ventricular extrasystoles and idioventricular rhythms can occur, especially in the presence of digoxin. The most important renal signs are nephrogenic diabetes insipidus and acute and chronic renal failure.[11]

DIAGNOSTICS

Because calcium binds to albumin, total calcium measurements can be greatly affected by changes in albumin concentrations. Hypoproteinemia is often seen in cancer patients; therefore the measurement of total serum calcium may understate the severity of the disorder. It is useful to obtain an initial measurement of ionized serum calcium; alternatively, total serum calcium can be adjusted for the level of serum protein by the following equation:

$$\text{Correlated calcium} = \text{Serum calcium} + 0.8\,(4 - \text{Serum albumin})$$

Other changes include a shortened QT interval on the electrocardiogram (ECG).[5,11]

If the corrected serum calcium level is greater than 3.0 mmol/L (0.6 mg/dL), treatment should always be considered.[12]

DIAGNOSTICS

Hypercalcemia

LABORATORY
Serum calcium
Serum phosphorus
Serum albumin
Total protein
Ionized serum calcium

OTHER DIAGNOSTICS
Electrocardiography

DIFFERENTIAL DIAGNOSIS

Other than neoplasia, causes of hypercalcemia to consider include primary or secondary hyperparathyroidism, acromegaly, adrenal insufficiency, sarcoidosis or other granulomatous disorders, Paget disease of bone, hypophosphatasia, familial hypocalciuric hypercalcemia, and renal failure. Other causes are immobilization, complications of renal transplantation, medication-induced hypercalcemia (thiazide diuretics, lithium), excessive intake of vitamin D or A, and milk-alkali syndrome (secondary to calcium ingestion for osteoporosis prevention or in some cases related to overuse of calcium carbonate in patients with peptic ulcer disease or gastroesophageal reflux).[11]

DIFFERENTIAL DIAGNOSIS

Hypercalcemia

- Primary or secondary hyperparathyroidism
- Acromegaly
- Adrenal insufficiency
- Sarcoidosis
- Granulomatous disease
- Paget disease of bone
- Hypophosphatasia
- Familial hypocalciuric hypercalcemia
- Renal failure or transplantation
- Medication-induced hypercalcemia
- Excessive vitamin D or A ingestion
- Immobilization
- Milk-alkali syndrome

MANAGEMENT

Oral or parenteral rehydration is recommended as initial therapy for all patients with hypercalcemia. The intravenous administration of normal saline is typically preferred for hospitalized patients, with infusion rates of 250 to 500 mL/hr in the initial hours.[2] Strict attention to adequate urinary output and fluid balance is critical. Furosemide is primarily used to prevent hypervolemia after euvolemia has been achieved with saline infusion. If renal function is normal, 20 to 40 mg of furosemide intravenously may be initiated after volume expansion has been achieved, with subsequent doses given if the urinary output is less than 150 to 200 mL/hr.[2]

Hospitalization is recommended for patients with a serum calcium level of 14 mg/dL or higher (3.5 mmol/L) for patients who have symptoms other than mild fatigue and constipation. For moderate to severe hypercalcemia, saline hydration alone does not typically reduce the serum calcium concentration, and antiresorptive drug therapy should be instituted within 24 hours. Third-generation bisphosphonates (pamidronate and zoledronate) are potent inhibitors of osteoclast activity. Compared with pamidronate, zoledronate showed superior results in terms of complete response rate (88% versus 70%) and response duration (32 versus 18 days). Moreover, zoledronate offers the convenience of a 15-minute infusion as opposed to a 2-hour infusion.[13] In patients with osteolysis mediated by PTHrP (epidermoid carcinomas) in which bisphosphonates may be inferior, treatment with gallium nitrate may be considered.

In addition, salmon calcitonin (4 IU/kg) reduces serum calcium concentration by inhibiting bone resorption and increasing renal calcium excretion. Given its rapid onset of action, serum calcium levels should be remeasured several hours after treatment. If the patient is found to be calcitonin sensitive, treatment may be repeated every 6 to 12 hours (4 to 8 IU/kg). A reduction in serum calcium concentration is achieved in 12 to 48 hours.[2,5,11] Ultimately, treatment of the underlying cancer will control the hypercalcemia.

COMPLICATIONS

Without treatment, symptoms progress to profound alterations in mental status, psychotic behavior, seizures, coma, and ultimately death. Prolonged hypercalcemia eventually causes permanent renal tubular abnormalities with renal tubular acidosis, glucosuria, aminoaciduria, and hyperphosphaturia. Sudden death from cardiac arrhythmias may occur when serum calcium concentration rises acutely.[11]

TUMOR LYSIS SYNDROME AND HYPERURICEMIA

DEFINITION AND EPIDEMIOLOGY

TLS is a metabolic imbalance that occurs with the rapid killing and lysis of neoplastic cells and the subsequent release of large quantities of intracellular potassium, phosphorus, and nucleic acids into the bloodstream. Patients with large tumor burdens of malignant neoplasms that are highly radiosensitive or chemosensitive, such as acute leukemia, high-grade lymphoma, and, to a lesser degree, solid tumors (e.g., breast cancer, SCLC, squamous cell carcinoma of the head and neck, hepatoblastoma, multiple myeloma) and myeloproliferative disorders, are at high risk for the development of this syndrome.[2,5,11,14]

PATHOPHYSIOLOGY

The metabolic consequences of cell death include the catabolism of nucleic acid purines by xanthine oxidase to produce uric acid. High levels of uric acid crystallize in the distal tubule of the nephron, with resultant acute obstructive uropathy and renal failure. The massive release of other intracellular products, such as potassium and phosphorus, may lead to life-threatening concentrations. This syndrome is characterized by hyperuricemia, uric acid nephropathy, hyperkalemia, hyperphosphatemia, hypocalcemia, and hyperazotemia. The severity of the syndrome depends on the extent of tumor burden and preexisting renal insufficiency.[2,5,11,14]

CLINICAL PRESENTATION AND PHYSICAL EXAMINATION

Although urate nephropathy with TLS is sometimes reported at the time of the initial cancer diagnosis, most cases develop within 1 or 2 days of the initiation of cytotoxic treatment. Patients develop rapidly progressive oliguria with signs of uremia. Edema, fluid overload, hypertension, congestive heart failure, and seizures may result. Acute hyperkalemia and hypocalcemia may result in cardiac arrhythmias, tetany, syncope, and sudden death. Hypocalcemia may cause mild muscle cramps, tetany, and seizures. Hyperphosphatemia may aggravate renal failure. Acidosis and anuria may result. These metabolic changes may occur individually or simultaneously.

DIAGNOSTICS

Serum electrolyte values and uric acid, phosphorus, calcium, and creatinine concentrations should be checked several times per day for 3 or 4 days after initiation of cytotoxic therapy. Hyperkalemia poses the greatest immediate threat; the elevation of serum potassium concentration often is the first sign of TLS. If hyperkalemia or hypocalcemia develops, an ECG should be evaluated and possible cardiac arrhythmia monitored.

DIAGNOSTICS

Tumor Lysis Syndrome

LABORATORY
Serum electrolytes
Uric acid
Phosphorus
Calcium
Creatinine

OTHER DIAGNOSTICS
ECG*

*if indicated.

Common changes on the ECG include peaked T waves and QRS widening.

DIFFERENTIAL DIAGNOSIS

Gout is the most common cause of hyperuricemia. Other causes of uremia include primary hyperuricemia from specific enzyme defects (Lesch-Nyhan syndrome, glycogen storage disease) and decreased renal clearance of uric acid secondary to intrinsic kidney disease.[11]

DIFFERENTIAL DIAGNOSIS

Tumor Lysis Syndrome

- Gout
- Enzyme defects resulting in primary hyperuricemia
- Decreased renal clearance of uric acid

MANAGEMENT AND COMPLICATIONS

Treatment is aimed at prevention by identifying patients at risk. Prophylactic measures include the initiation of allopurinol, a xanthine oxidase inhibitor, at 300 to 900 mg/day, starting 1 or 2 days before therapy and continuing until there is evidence of TLS. Dose adjustments should be made for patients with renal insufficiency. More rapid control and lower levels of plasma uric acid have been observed with the administration of rasburicase, a recombinant urate oxidase. Rasburicase is significantly more expensive than allopurinol and has been approved by the U.S. Food and Drug Administration for use in pediatric patients.[5,11] One should also avoid routine use of drugs that make the urine alkaline. Other prophylactic treatment includes vigorous intravenous hydration with approximately 3000 mL/day and diuresis with urinary pH of at least 7.0 before any chemotherapy or cytotoxic therapy is begun. The alkalinization of urine is a controversial topic; although it is recommended to avoid crystallization of uric acid, it may cause precipitation of calcium-phosphate complexes in the renal tubules.[5,11] The urine may be alkalinized by adding 100 mEq sodium bicarbonate to each liter of intravenous fluid. Hyperkalemia can be managed with an oral sodium-potassium exchange resin (sodium polystyrene sulfonate [Kayexalate], 15 g orally every 6 hours) or in combination with insulin-glucose therapy. Loop diuretics are also useful in the elimination of excess potassium. In the setting of hyperkalemia-induced cardiac arrhythmias, calcium gluconate offers immediate but transient benefits. In general, calcium replacement is not indicated because of the risk of producing acute nephrocalcinosis and increased renal failure by the precipitation of calcium phosphate in the kidney. Hyperphosphatemia can be controlled with the ingestion of aluminum hydroxide antacid. The hypocalcemia usually responds to the correction of hyperphosphatemia. Any of the previously mentioned imbalances may be severe enough to require temporary hemodialysis.[5,11]

SYNDROME OF INAPPROPRIATE ANTIDIURETIC HORMONE

DEFINITION AND EPIDEMIOLOGY

SIADH is a paraneoplastic syndrome that develops when excessive amounts of antidiuretic hormone (ADH) are present, causing excessive amounts of water retention. Ectopic ADH secretion has been noted in SCLC and in primary tumors with metastatic lesions to the brain and lung.[5,14]

PATHOPHYSIOLOGY

SIADH is characterized by excessive urinary loss of sodium and excessive retention of water by the renal tubules as well as by reduced levels of serum sodium and serum osmolality. Because the normal regulation of ADH release occurs from both the CNS and the chest through baroreceptors, any disorders affecting the CNS (structural, metabolic, psychiatric, or pharmacologic) or the lungs may cause SIADH. With excessive ADH secretion, excessive water is reabsorbed in the collecting ducts, and a dilutional hyponatremia occurs.

CLINICAL PRESENTATION AND PHYSICAL EXAMINATION

With mild hyponatremia, early manifestations include thirst, anorexia, mild nausea and vomiting, weight gain without edema, muscle cramps, headache, and mild lethargy.[5,14] Patients become more symptomatic as hyponatremia develops rapidly or as sodium levels fall below 115 mg/dL. Signs and symptoms include hyporeflexia, confusion, oliguria, seizures, and coma.[5,14]

DIAGNOSTICS

With SIADH, the serum sodium level is less than 135 mEq/L, plasma osmolality is less than 280 mOsm/kg, urine osmolality is more than 500 mOsm/kg, and urinary sodium is more than 20 mEq/L.[2] Creatinine should be measured. Thyroid and adrenal dysfunction may also need to be excluded.[10] A chest x-ray study and CT scan may be ordered to evaluate pulmonary or neurologic disorders that may cause excessive ADH production.

DIAGNOSTICS

Syndrome of Inappropriate Antidiuretic Hormone

LABORATORY
Serum electrolytes
Serum osmolality
Urine sodium
Urine osmolality
Blood urea nitrogen (BUN)
Creatinine
Thyroid-stimulating hormone (TSH)*

IMAGING
Chest x-ray examination*
CT scan*

*If indicated.

DIFFERENTIAL DIAGNOSIS

The differential diagnosis of hyponatremia includes liver disease, congestive heart failure, renal failure, hypothyroidism, adrenal insufficiency, psychogenic polydipsia, and idiosyncratic drug reaction (thiazide diuretics, angiotensin-converting enzyme inhibitors). Other causes include CNS infection (meningitis, abscess), CNS trauma (hemorrhage, stroke), and pulmonary infections (tuberculosis).[2,14]

DIFFERENTIAL DIAGNOSIS

Syndrome of Inappropriate Antidiuretic Hormone

- Small cell cancer of the lung
- Metastatic cancer to brain or lungs
- Liver disease
- Congestive heart failure
- Renal failure
- Adrenal insufficiency
- Medication-induced hyponatremia
- Pseudohyponatremia
- Hypothyroidism
- Polydipsia
- Reset osmostat
- Beer potomania
- CNS infection
- CNS trauma (stroke, hemorrhage)
- Pulmonary infection (tuberculosis)

MANAGEMENT AND COMPLICATIONS

Treatment of mild to moderate SIADH (serum sodium level of 120 to 134 mEq/L) with minimum symptoms consists of limiting fluid intake to 500 to 1000 mL/24 hr. If SIADH is refractory or if patients can be managed on an outpatient basis, demeclocycline, 600 to 1200 mg/day in divided doses, may be used.[2] Patients with significant neurologic impairments (coma, seizures) require hospitalization for treatment with 3% saline by slow infusion at a rate sufficient to increase the serum sodium level by 0.5 to 1.0 mEq/L/hr, not to exceed a rise of 20 mEq/L in serum sodium concentration during the first 48 hours to avoid development of central pontine myelinolysis.[14] During the correction period, serum sodium should be checked every 2 hours or at least every 4 hours to avoid overly rapid correction.[15] Untreated SIADH or too rapid an increase in serum sodium concentration may result in severe neurologic impairment or death.[2]

INDICATIONS FOR REFERRAL OR HOSPITALIZATION

All the complications discussed in this chapter are considered emergencies. Patients usually require hospitalization and are often sent to an emergency medical center. Because most of these complications are related to progression of the cancer, patients may need to be referred to an oncologist for further management.

PATIENT AND FAMILY EDUCATION

In any emergency, patients and families are frightened, but they also want honest explanations of their situation. Patients should be told possible causes of the symptoms being experienced and the possible plan of action, and they should be reassured that the oncologist is being notified immediately. Once treatment is initiated, the patient will benefit from reinforcement from the health care provider about instructions for medications, activities, and further warning signs that need to be reported.

CHAPTER 245

ONCOLOGY PAIN AND SYMPTOM MANAGEMENT IN PRIMARY CARE

Leslie Lezell Levitan

Primary care providers, in collaboration with the entire oncology team, play a key role in managing the symptoms experienced by patients undergoing treatment for cancer. In this chapter, specific recommendations for treating oncology patients, including pain control and managing symptoms commonly seen in cancer patients are extensively discussed. The goal of pain and symptom management should always focus on improving the patient's quality of life.

ONCOLOGY PAIN

DEFINITION AND EPIDEMIOLOGY

Experiencing pain and suffering is one of the most common fears that patients undergoing cancer treatment and their caregivers have. Despite this common fear, there remain many barriers providers encounter in their efforts to effectively manage oncology pain, including inadequate attention given to pain mechanisms and treatment modalities in most medical, nursing, and pharmacy program curricula; reluctance to prescribe opioids based on the prescriber's fear of addiction, abuse, diversion, and misuse; poor pain assessment, including discrepancies between perception of pain culturally and within one's gender; and patient nonadherence to a treatment regimen.[1] Other impediments include monitoring and regulatory controls, as well as potential insurance issues regarding payment for expensive medications, timely prior authorization paperwork, or phone calls by the provider.

The International Association for the Study of Pain defines pain as "an unpleasant sensory and emotional experience associated with actual or potential tissue damage, or described in terms of such damage."[2] Although pain is largely subjective by nature, there are both subjective and objective findings the provider can use to determine the severity of the oncology patient's pain perception. The impact of cancer pain, however, is unique to the individual and may be affected by a multitude of other symptoms that cancer patients concurrently experience.

PATHOPHYSIOLOGY

The key to treating pain effectively is to identify the underlying causes whenever possible. Cancer pain can be aggravated by factors such as infection, trauma, and tumor growth. Therefore, careful assessment and physical examination are essential. Factors such as inflammation and myofascial pain may also contribute to the overall pain perception.

Nociceptive pain is the most common type of pain and is a normal function of the central nervous system. Nociceptors respond to noxious stimuli and transmit a message through the peripheral nerves, to the spinal cord, and then up to the cerebral cortex, where the message can be interpreted. Some motor responses (e.g., withdrawal of an extremity from intense heat) are initiated from the spinal cord, whereas others are initiated by higher brain centers. Nociceptive pain is further differentiated as somatic (i.e., pain from soft tissue and musculoskeletal structures) or visceral (i.e., pain arising from the internal organs). Somatic pain is often described as dull, sharp, aching, crushing, or heavy, whereas visceral pain is often described as crampy.[3] There are fewer pain fibers in the viscera, and a convergence of visceral and cutaneous afferent fibers at the dorsal horn of the spinal cord; therefore, visceral pain can be referred to other areas. Cancer pain often exhibits a classic referral pattern, depending on the pathology of the cancer. For example, pain associated with cancer of the pancreas can be experienced as pain in the middle or upper back or as shoulder pain.

Neuropathic pain develops as a result of injury to the peripheral nerves, spinal cord, or brain tissue. Nerves can be injured or damaged by direct trauma (laceration, compression, stretching, crushing, burning, freezing, or exposure to toxic agents such as chemotherapeutic drugs or viruses), repetitive movements (typing), and diseases (polio, diabetes, multiple sclerosis). The result of the injury is a cascade of events that creates both anatomic and neurochemical changes in the neurons. Once the damage has occurred, the regeneration process of the nerve may result in incomplete healing, which can lead to chronic pain or reduced function.[3] Common examples of neuropathic pain syndromes that result in chronic pain include postherpetic neuralgia, phantom pain, post-thoracotomy pain, intercostal neuralgia, and peripheral neuropathy. Neuropathic pain is characteristically described as burning, numbness, tingling, shocking, electric, and jolting, and often has a delayed onset from the time of the precipitating injury. For example, postherpetic neuralgia can occur and persist months to years after the skin lesions of a herpes zoster virus (HZV) infection have completely healed. In that time, the perception of normally mild, nonpainful stimuli (e.g., touch or wearing clothing) can change to an exquisitely sensitive or painful sensation (allodynia or hyperesthesia). In moderate to severe cases, neuropathic pain may be accompanied by regional sympathetic dysfunction, whereby an injured nerve may develop an electrical or a chemical interaction with sympathetic nerve fibers, providing continuous painful stimuli to peripheral nerves.[2,3]

Many pain syndromes are accompanied by inflammation that either contributes to or is the primary underlying mechanism of the pain. The inflammatory response includes the release of prostaglandins and leukotrienes that sensitize peripheral nerves to painful stimuli. Associated swelling also causes pressure on the nerves or other sensitive structures, which will contribute to the severity of the pain.

CLINICAL PRESENTATION

The onset of cancer-associated pain can be acute and severe or may gradually progress from an awareness of discomfort to one of increasing intensity. Patients with chronic cancer pain that seems well managed for a long period of time may suddenly report worsening of pain or pain that is completely different in quality or location. Because it is possible for pain to be experienced before tumor detection, it is essential when treating someone with a history of cancer to rule out tumor growth from metastases, even if the patient has been disease free for some time. Patients who experience a sudden worsening of pain or a new pain might also fear relapse or a disease progression and may insist on referral back to the oncologist.

A careful and thorough history includes identification of the pattern, characteristics, severity, and impact of the pain. The provider should always ask the patient where specifically the pain is located, so that it is clear what is actually being treated. Providers should remember that cancer patients often have pain in multiple body areas from several sources; pain relief regimens need to accommodate this characteristic.

Because pain is subjective, a patient's report is the most reliable means of establishing the degree or intensity of the pain. The most convenient method, and one accessible to most patients, is the numeric rating scale (NRS) for pain. The patient rates his or her pain from 0 to 10, where 0 indicates no pain and 10 indicates the worst pain imaginable. Other scales can be used, such as the visual analog scale (VAS), the McGill Pain Questionnaire (MPQ), and the Wong-Baker Faces Scale. The Wong-Baker Faces Scale uses a series of faces depicting comfort level, which can be useful for children (3 years of age and older) and for patients with communication difficulties (e.g., a language barrier or difficulty with speech), because they can simply point to the face that matches how they feel.[4] It is important to use one scale consistently with the patient in order to develop a sense of the change in status or impact of interventions over time. While performing the pain assessment, it is also important to review other symptoms that may have an impact on a patient's pain level and treatment plan. Tools used to assess multiple symptoms include the Edmonton Symptom Assessment Scale (ESAS) and the MD Anderson Symptom Inventory (MDASI).

To interpret the ratings given by patients, providers must remember that these are subjective measures and therefore have no "normal" values. In general, ratings of 1 to 3 are considered to be mild pain; 4 to 6, moderate; and 7 or greater, severe.[4] A useful data point in a provider's assessment is to ask the patient what pain level can be tolerated, because this will help to establish the treatment goal. There is considerable individual variation in the way patients use these scales, so comparison among patients should be avoided except for aggregate analysis for research and quality assurance purposes.

Because pain is a subjective complaint, it can be influenced or distorted by delirium, somatization, and chemical coping. It is therefore imperative to assess not only the pain complaint but also the patient's cognitive status and coping mechanisms. Cognition can be assessed by standardized tools such as the Memorial Delirium Assessment Scale or Revised Delirium Rating Scale.[5] Somatization and chemical coping can be difficult to detect, but a careful medical history and patient interview can alert the provider to red flags, such as rapid opioid escalation, continuing complaints of severe pain despite aggressive titration, and history of substance abuse.

Objective findings also exist when determining a patient's level of pain. A nonverbal pain assessment is essential for those who are unable to effectively communicate, may be sedated, or even may be comatose. Some objective findings include facial grimacing (especially with movement), diaphoresis, shaking, restlessness, crying, moaning, fidgeting, hypertension, tachycardia, and tachypnea. Body language is also helpful with a nonverbal pain assessment. Additional nonverbal signs of pain include fists clenched, hitting, biting, kicking, guarding a sore area, and lying with the knees pulled to the chest or in fetal position.[6]

PHYSICAL EXAMINATION

Oncology patients can experience significant pain without giving the appearance of suffering. Coping abilities vary widely among individuals. With persistent pain, physiologic and psychosocial adaptations usually occur, which can be confusing on examination. The physical examination should focus initially on the reported painful areas to identify any lesions, inflammation, vascular changes, edema, or pain with palpation. Sensory changes in the affected part or new areas should also be carefully assessed. Changes between examinations may be related to new disease pathology or injury from other sources, such as chemotherapy or radiation therapy. Joint range of motion and muscle strength should also be assessed for changes in motor function. Providers should observe the patient during ambulation (whenever possible) to determine the impact of pain on movement and functional ability. Complaints of back pain with or without leg pain warrant a high suspicion of impending cord compression from primary tumor growth or metastases. Assessment questions for possible cord compression include a history of sensory changes (leg weakness, numbness, or tingling), autonomic dysfunction (loss of bladder or bowel control), and presence of severe back and/or leg pain (usually sudden onset).

DIAGNOSTICS

There are no specific imaging or laboratory techniques that a provider can order to directly study pain. The diagnostic evaluation should therefore be guided by the location and nature of the oncology patient's reports of pain, and understanding of the pathophysiology of the underlying disease. Relevant imaging is essential, however, and should be reviewed and repeated periodically. Computed tomography (CT) scans may be indicated to identify masses that involve the vital organs or lymphadenopathy. Bone scans and plain x-ray films should be obtained if bone metastases are suspected. A bone scan is a sensitive test used to image disease before it is visible on x-ray examination, but it is not specific and may be positive for other inflammatory processes. Because magnetic resonance imaging (MRI) can identify nerve root or spinal cord compression, patients with a history of tumors that tend to metastasize to the bone, especially breast, lung, renal, prostate, and unknown primary site, should promptly undergo MRI to exclude cord impingement with symptoms of back pain with or without leg pain. Spinal cord compression is a true medical emergency; the earliest possible intervention (steroids, surgery, and/or radiotherapy) is critical to preserve neurologic function. Electromyography (EMG) can detect nerve conduction problems not identified on a scan. Blood tests, including a complete blood count (CBC), can help evaluate for relapse of disease, particularly with cancers of the blood. Owing to rising health care costs and the limited information gained from some tests, the provider should always be mindful when ordering any test as to whether this will assist in decision making regarding the oncology patient's treatment.[7]

DIAGNOSTICS

Cancer Pain

IMAGING
Radiography*
CT*
MRI*
Bone scan*
EMG*

BLOOD TESTS
CBC with differential

*If indicated.

DIFFERENTIAL DIAGNOSIS

Pain is a significant problem for the majority of cancer patients at some point during the course of their disease and treatment. Researchers have found that 24% to 60% of patients undergoing active cancer treatment report pain, and 62% to 86% of patients with advanced cancer report pain.[8] Although oncology pain can occur at any time during the course of treatment, the incidence and severity of pain will often increase as the disease progresses. Common treatment-related cancer pain syndromes include those associated with surgery, chemotherapy, radiotherapy, and biologic therapy. For example, surgical patients may develop postmastectomy, post-thoracotomy, or phantom pain. Some chemotherapeutic agents can cause peripheral neuropathies, and extravasational agents can cause significant tissue and nerve damage. Radiation effects can be early (e.g., mucositis) or late (e.g., brachial plexopathy or osteoradionecrosis). Biologic agents such as interferon can cause peripheral neuropathy and joint pain, both of which can be transient or chronic in nature. Tumor-related pain can result from the compression of pain-sensitive structures by a mass (e.g., epidural cord compression), or it can be related to direct infiltration, especially of the nervous and musculoskeletal systems. Pain resulting from bone metastasis is one of the most severe and disabling types of oncology pain.

Oncology patients may experience pain that is unrelated to the oncologic problem, which the provider must also address in the treatment plan. Patients may have a documented, preexisting chronic pain problem, such as low back or neck pain, migraine headaches, or diabetic peripheral neuropathy. An infection can cause sudden and severe pain that is easily improved with appropriate antimicrobial medications. HZV can be contracted in immunocompromised oncology patients, manifesting with a localized rash following dermatomal distribution accompanied by sharp, burning, and/or aching pain that can resolve or persist. Obstruction, constipation, ileus, peptic ulcer disease, gallbladder disease, pancreatitis, diverticulitis, and appendicitis are examples of other diseases and conditions that can all cause acute or chronic abdominal pain and require intervention.[9]

DIFFERENTIAL DIAGNOSIS

Cancer Pain

- Tumor-related pain
  - Peripheral neuropathy
  - Cervical, lumbosacral, brachial
  - Bone metastasis
  - Epidural cord compression
- Treatment-related pain
  - Chemotherapy
  - Radiation therapy
  - Biologic therapy
  - Postsurgical
- Nonmalignant acute or chronic pain
- Preexisting pain syndromes
- Acute or chronic abdominal pain
- HZV (postherpetic neuralgia)
- Infection

MANAGEMENT

Effective pain management, particularly for the patient with advanced cancer, requires a comprehensive approach that often

BOX 245-1

Pain Management Pearls

Pain is a multidimensional experience that requires multidimensional assessment.
Pain and other symptoms can change rapidly. Regular and frequent assessment is necessary.
Reassure the patient and family that most pain can be relieved.
Reassure the patient and family about their concerns and fears regarding opioids.
Explain to the patient the differences among physical dependence, addiction, and tolerance.
Encourage normal activity to the fullest extent possible.
Treat pain promptly and aggressively.
Rational pain management tailors the regimen to the type and intensity of pain.
Regular around-the-clock administration with adequate breakthrough dosage and adjuvants as required plus proactive antiemetic and laxative regimens are the hallmarks of rational and effective pain management in cancer patients.
Opioid conversion tables are inexact; patients should be observed carefully whenever regimen changes are made.
Consider nonpharmacologic options to control pain, such as anesthetic and neurosurgical approaches, in intractable pain syndromes where the risk/benefit ratio favors benefit.
Beware of overzealous opioid use in the patient who is experiencing delirium and somatization.
Beware of the pitfalls of polypharmacy.
Treating the patient who has total pain (nociception, psychological distress, and spiritual distress) means treating the whole patient (body, mind, and spirit).

Modified from Reddy S: Pain management. In Elsayem A, Driver L, Bruera E, editors: *The M. D. Anderson symptom control and palliative care handbook,* San Antonio, 2003, University of Texas Health Science Center Printing Service.

involves the use of multiple modalities (Box 245-1). A thorough assessment, physical examination, and careful review of medical records are important to determine the type of pain and pathology of the pain, so an appropriate treatment plan can be established. Opioid pain medications and adjuvant treatments (e.g., muscle relaxants, NSAIDs, antidepressants, anticonvulsants, thermal modalities, relaxation techniques) are all used to improve the oncology patient's quality of life.[10,11]

Opioids, the preferred term for narcotic analgesics, are effective and well tolerated when used to relieve many forms of cancer pain. The most commonly used opioid medications for the treatment of cancer pain include morphine, oxycodone, oxymorphone, hydrocodone, hydromorphone, methadone, and fentanyl. Opioids are classified as pure agonists, mixed agonist-antagonists, or partial agonists. The pure agonists produce effective analgesia and (with the exception of meperidine [Demerol]) can be titrated to pain relief without having a ceiling effect (Box 245-2). Meperidine is not recommended for routine use in the cancer population. The metabolite normeperidine causes central nervous system excitability, which can lead to delirium, tremors, seizures, and even death. The risk of this side effect is increased in older adults and in those with renal insufficiency and hepatic impairment.[3,12]

The mixed agonist-antagonist opioids produce analgesia but can also reverse analgesia. These medications are also associated with a high incidence of psychotomimetic side effects and, like

BOX 245-2

Opioid Agonists Used for Cancer Pain

- Codeine (Tylenol No. 3 or No. 4*)
- Fentanyl (Actiq, Fentora, Duragesic†)
- Hydrocodone (Vicodin*, Lortab*, Zohydro†)
- Hydromorphone (Dilaudid)
- Oxymorphone (Opana, Opana ER†)
- Methadone (Dolophine)
- Morphine (MSIR, Roxanol, MS Contin†, Oramorph†, Avinza†, Kadian†)
- Oxycodone (Percocet*, Percodan‡, Roxicodone, OxyContin†)

Note: The following medications are not recommended for the relief of cancer pain: meperidine, mixed agonist-antagonists, partial agonists, and placebos.[3,6]
*Combination containing acetaminophen.
†Sustained- or controlled-release delivery system.
‡Combination containing aspirin.

meperidine, are not recommended for routine use in cancer patients. When agonist-antagonists are given to a patient who has been taking a pure agonist opioid, the agonist-antagonist acts as an antagonist by displacing the agonist from the opiate receptors, which precipitates withdrawal and reverses analgesia.[13] Withdrawal and exacerbation of pain reduce quality of life and pose a considerable risk to critically ill and debilitated patients. For these reasons, the injudicious use of naloxone, a pure opioid antagonist, should be avoided with cancer patients.

Unfortunately, pure agonist opioids remain underused and misunderstood by many providers. To use these opioids effectively, it is important to distinguish among key terms that are often misapplied in practice: addiction (a physical and/or mental need to use a substance), dependence (the use of a substance or thoughts about the substance that are increasingly important to the detriment of once important things), and tolerance (the need for higher doses of a substance to physically achieve the same response or a lesser response).[14] The phenomenon known as pseudoaddiction must also be recognized so patients can be properly educated about their treatment. Pseudoaddiction is a real and complex phenomenon in which patients may exhibit drug-seeking behaviors and appear aggressive when requesting to increase pain medications when, in fact, they are inadequately treated for their actual pain. These patients may be labeled as "difficult," "drug seeking," and "clock watchers." Although these actions may serve as warning signs to alert the practitioner to abuse, the adequacy of treatment must also be assessed before a judgment can be made.[15]

Patients may be reluctant to take opioid medications in the early stages of their cancer diagnosis owing to the belief that morphine is for "dying patients only." They may also report fears of becoming "immune" or that the drug will not work when it is "really needed." Although there are patients with stable cancer pain who may stay on the same dose of pain medication for years without a decreased efficacy, this is not the norm. Patients may develop tolerance to opioid medication with prolonged use, but dose escalation can counter this. Progression of the patient's disease is the most common reason for dose escalation, especially when a rapid increase is needed. Other causes of dose escalation can include delirium, somatization, and chemical coping. Opioid medications do not have a ceiling dose; therefore these medications can be continually titrated on the basis of the patient's need. The development of tolerance is often concerning to both prescribers and patients, especially when solely focusing on the total amount of medications the patient is taking daily.[1]

The World Health Organization (WHO) recommends a stepwise approach to managing cancer pain, which begins when the patient first experiences pain. Initially a nonopioid medication such as a nonsteroidal anti-inflammatory (NSAID) can be used for minor pain (1 to 3 on the pain scale of 1 to 10). If pain persists, initiation of a mild opioid is then indicated, followed by a stronger opioid. Titration of opioid medications is done until the patient experiences tolerable pain reduction, with the understanding that patients may never be truly "free" of pain. Throughout the step process, adjuvant medications (e.g., muscle relaxants, antidepressants, antianxiety agents, and anticonvulsant medications) are also used to help with fear and anxiety and to enhance pain reduction.[3,16,17]

The key principle for effective pain control with opioids is careful titration of the medication to achieve the desired comfort without adverse effects.[4,18] Considerable variability in dosage exists among patients. Tolerance will be seen with chronic administration of any opioid; however, this does not happen at the same rate for each patient.[13] Although some opioids (e.g., morphine and hydromorphone) are classified as strong and others (e.g., codeine and hydrocodone) are classified as weak, these opioids are all actually capable of producing equally effective analgesia when given in equianalgesic doses. Some weak opioids are combined with an NSAID or acetaminophen to enhance pain relief. Use of these combined medications is therefore limited by the risk of renal and hepatic problems related to the nonopioid drug.

There are numerous preparations widely available, allowing for different routes of administration of opioid medications. These include oral, sublingual, buccal, intravenous, subcutaneous, transdermal, rectal, and intraspinal (epidural and intrathecal).[11] The oral route of administration is the route of choice in most situations because of ease, comfort, and cost-effectiveness. The choice of route and drug depends on a variety of patient-related factors, including the pathology of the pain, functional status of the gastrointestinal (GI) tract, the abilities of the patient and caregiver to manage the regimen (e.g., cognitive function, psychomotor skills), side effects, the dosage forms, availability, and cost. More invasive routes of administration, such as parenteral and intraspinal, increase the risk for complications (e.g., infection and displacement of the needle) and are usually more costly. The subcutaneous, transdermal, and rectal routes can deliver excellent pain control in patients who cannot tolerate oral medications but want to be managed at home.

Short-acting opioids are clinically indicated to treat postoperative pain and for moderate isolated painful incidents. For the cancer patient, short-acting opioids can be especially helpful for breakthrough pain associated with activity, treatments, or other obvious factors. When an event or activity (e.g., ambulation) is known to provoke pain, the as-needed (prn) dose should be taken 30 to 45 minutes before that activity. For moderate to severe pain that is poorly managed, however, long-acting opioids should be administered around the clock, based on their expected duration of action. As-needed opioid administration with these patients can lead to greater peaks and valleys in analgesic blood levels between doses, especially if the patient waits until the pain is severe before taking the short-acting opioid. Moderate to severe cancer pain is best treated with a long-acting, scheduled opioid medication around the clock, and a short-acting opioid for breakthrough pain. The short-acting opioid dose should be 10% to 15% of the total daily dose of the long-acting opioid.[19] If two or three breakthrough doses are required routinely, the case can be made for the long-acting medication to be increased.

Some oncology patients with moderate to severe pain may require short-term or long-term use of parenteral or subcutaneous opioids. Patient-controlled analgesia pumps can be ideal for patients looking at end-of-life comfort care; these pumps provide continuously programmed opioid delivery. Pumps can also be very helpful with patients in an acute pain crisis, with the goal to ultimately wean off the pump and restart oral medications once the pain is more manageable. The on-demand patient-administered dose used as needed with or without a continuous (basal) infusion allows for individualized dosage and sustained analgesia. If the patient shows early evidence of delirium, somatization, or chemical coping, the on-demand patient-administered dose should be avoided because of the possibility of opioid-induced neurotoxicity.

Table 245-1 illustrates the relative equianalgesic doses for the most commonly used opioids. Morphine is often used for comparison with other opioids because it is the most widely used opioid and there is extensive existing research about its pharmacokinetics. The route of administration must be considered when calculating equianalgesic doses. For example, opioids administered through the GI tract are subject to a first-pass effect, whereby a portion of the drug is metabolized to nonanalgesic substances as it is routed through the hepatic circulation before being circulated systemically. If a patient is receiving adequate analgesia from 10 mg of morphine sulfate given parenterally, it takes 30 mg to achieve the same effect if it is given orally because approximately 20 mg is metabolized before reaching the systemic circulation. The parenteral-to-oral ratio also varies from drug to drug. In addition, the longer a patient is taking an opioid, the less accurate these relationships can be, because of cross-tolerance with similar substances. It must be noted that the relationship between different opioids is not absolute, so equianalgesic comparisons like the one in Table 245-1 are only rough guides. With opioid rotation, it is imperative to err on the side of caution because the risk of overdose does not outweigh the risk of transient discomfort.[3,19]

COMPLICATIONS

Vigilant oversight is critical to the successful treatment of patients with cancer pain. Side effects are among the most common reasons for opioid failure and premature abandonment of therapy. A patient who experiences nausea, sedation, or clouded thinking may be improperly labeled as allergic to opioids; however, a true allergy to opioid medications is actually quite rare. Some side effects, particularly nausea and sedation, are usually transient and improve once tolerance develops. Sedation from opioids can be from the medication itself or from sleep deprivation in patients who have experienced long periods of unrelieved pain. Sedation usually abates within 1 week on a stable dose of opioids and/or once sleep is restored.[3] Respiratory depression from opioids manifests with a rapid onset and can be very concerning to caregivers. Dose reduction is indicated until there is tolerance to the opioid. Most patients develop a tolerance to the emetic and sedating effects over several days. Pain also contributes to weight loss and cachexia because patients who are uncomfortable often have a decreased appetite.

Nausea and vomiting from opioids can be managed with antiemetics either scheduled or as needed, depending on the

TABLE 245-1 **Opioid Conversion Table**

Drug	Parenteral Dose (mg) Equivalent to 10 mg IV/SC Morphine	Oral Dose (mg) Equivalent to 30 mg Oral Morphine	Dosage Interval
Morphine	10	30	2-4 hr for immediate release; 8-24 hr for sustained release
Codeine	100	200	2-4 hr
Hydromorphone	1.5	7.5	2-4 hr
Oxymorphone	1	10	4-6 hr for immediate release 8-12 hr for sustained release
Methadone	1-10*	2-20*	8-24 hr
Oxycodone	N/A	20-30	2-4 hr for immediate release; 8-12 hr for sustained release
Fentanyl	0.1	N/A	4 hr for buccal administration

ORAL MORPHINE (MG/24 HR)	DURAGESIC PATCH EQUIVALENT (μG/HR); PATCH CHANGED EVERY 72 HR
60-134	25
135-224	50
225-314	75
315-404	100
405-494	125
495-584	150

Note: The equianalgesic table should be used as a rough guide only.
N/A, Not applicable.
*Not an exact dose.
Data from McPherson ML: Equianalgesic opioid dosing. In *Demystifying opioid conversion calculations: a guide for effective dosing,* Bethesda, Md, 2010, American Society of Health-System Pharmacists; and Narcotic analgesics and nonnarcotic analgesics. In Ko J, et al, editors: *MPR nurse practitioners' edition,* vol 21(2). New York, 2014, Haymarket Media.

severity. Nausea is often directly related to decreased bowel function, which may resolve once constipation is alleviated. Opiate drugs bind to receptors on the smooth muscle of the bowel, slowing intestinal motility and increasing fluid absorption. Unfortunately, patients do not develop a tolerance to the constipating effects of opioids, so most patients will need an aggressive bowel management program.[20] A patient who has not had a bowel movement in more than 3 to 5 days should be monitored for proper hydration and given a diet with foods rich in fiber. However, when patients are prescribed opioids for chronic use, they will likely need to routinely use stool softeners and occasional laxatives to maintain normal elimination. If this does not work, more aggressive therapies such as scheduled oral laxatives, rectal suppositories, and prepared enemas must be considered. In a refractory situation, laxatives and enemas may need to be repeated every 12 hours. Once proper bowel function has been restored, a prophylactic regimen is initiated with a combination of a senna laxative and stool softener.[20] In a sense, the bowel regimen is similar to the pain regimen with standard around-the-clock medications (laxative with stool softener) and more aggressive preparations (rectal suppository or enema) for breakthrough if no bowel movement occurs within 3 days. If at any time there is concern that an ileus or malignant bowel obstruction is present, the patient needs to be medically evaluated, including appropriate diagnostic tests (e.g., x-ray studies, CT).

All opioids have the potential to cause delirium, but patients are at a higher risk to develop delirium with rapid dose escalation, concomitant renal or hepatic failure, or underlying pathophysiologic causes of delirium. Other causes of delirium include polypharmacy, sepsis, electrolyte imbalances, dehydration, brain tumors, hypoxia, comorbid medical conditions, and paraneoplastic syndrome. Identification of the cause of the delirium and then reversal of it, if possible, is the appropriate treatment. If opioids are suspected to be the cause, an opioid rotation is required. See Chapter 192 for further discussion of delirium.

Less common opioid side effects include urinary retention and myoclonus (intermittent muscle jerking). Urinary retention is often transient and can be temporarily relieved with straight catheterization or rotation to another opioid. Myoclonus is usually seen at higher opioid doses and with long-term opioid use. It is important to monitor for myoclonus because it can lead to seizures if untreated.[21] If myoclonus persists, the opioid should be decreased or changed. Providers must watch for other complications such as GI bleeding with the prolonged use of NSAIDs, and hepatotoxicity with high doses of acetaminophen. The prescriber should always be aware of the amounts of these over-the-counter medications patients are taking daily, whether alone or combined with prescribed opioids.

INDICATIONS FOR REFERRAL OR HOSPITALIZATION

A pain management or palliative care specialist should be consulted when efforts to titrate a patient's opioid dose to desired effect or to manage the related side effects are not successful. Consultation is also appropriate whenever an invasive route of opioid administration is indicated and needs additional oversight. Referral to a pain center should be considered for procedures such as epidural steroid injections, trigger point injections, and nerve blocks. Hospitalization may be necessary if the patient's pain is so severe that despite all efforts the pain will not abate and high doses of intravenous opioid medication with close monitoring become necessary until the pain reduces.

PATIENT AND FAMILY EDUCATION

Education regarding side effects will help the oncology patient anticipate problems that may arise, and allow for active participation in care. Involving oncology patients in the care plan can promote optimal pain control.[1] Patients should be aware that most side effects from opioid medications will improve with tolerance and that treatment can be given without sacrificing pain reduction. General education about the differences between "around-the-clock" and "as-needed" administration also needs to be provided. Patients and caregivers should be instructed to contact the health care provider if medication regimens are no longer helping to keep the pain manageable, if constipation is poorly managed, or if there are signs and symptoms of opioid-induced neurotoxicity. Symptoms include sedation, delirium, hallucinations, and myoclonus; immediate dose reduction is required. Patients and caregivers should also be encouraged to discuss with the health care provider their concerns about pain management, including the fear of pain, the fear of addiction, and possible misconceptions about the management of oncology pain.

SYMPTOM MANAGEMENT IN THE ONCOLOGY PATIENT

In addition to pain, oncology patients experience many difficult symptoms related to treatments (including chemotherapy, radiation therapy, and surgery), medications, and disease progression (neoplasm, infection, obstruction, motility alterations, and malabsorption). The prevention of complications and early detection of lower grade toxic symptoms can lead to fewer and more easily managed sequelae and improve the cancer patient's quality of life. This section focuses on the most common problematic GI symptoms oncology patients may experience, which include nausea and vomiting, constipation and diarrhea, anorexia, and the oral manifestations of mucositis and xerostomia.

PATHOPHYSIOLOGY OF GASTROINTESTINAL DISTURBANCES

Chemotherapy-Induced Nausea and Vomiting

Nausea and vomiting are mediated centrally and occur when the vomiting center receives specific information (via neurotransmitters such as serotonin, acetylcholine, histamine, dopamine, and substance P) from the GI tract, the chemoreceptor trigger zone, the vestibular apparatus, or the cerebral cortex and limbic system. Chemotherapy-induced nausea and vomiting (CINV) is particularly common in the oncology patient and requires vigilant control for preservation of quality of life and prevention of complications (such as weight loss, dehydration, and electrolyte imbalances).[22,23] The three types of CINV are acute, delayed, and anticipatory. Acute nausea and vomiting occur within the first 24 hours of chemotherapy, whereas delayed nausea and vomiting occur more than 24 hours after chemotherapy. Anticipatory nausea and vomiting comprise a conditioned response resulting from the memory of emesis with previous chemotherapy administration.[22] Delayed and anticipatory nausea and vomiting can be more difficult to control, and both are more likely to happen if the acute phase is poorly controlled. Hence, optimum antiemetic control is essential from the first dose of chemotherapy.[22,23]

Some patient-related factors that affect the severity of CINV include gender, age, and alcohol intake. Females under the age of 30 years, or during menstruation, may have more nausea and vomiting than their male counterparts. Individuals with a high alcohol intake (more than five drinks daily) have better control of vomiting than those with low or no daily alcohol intake. Patients with a history of motion sickness or a propensity for nausea and vomiting (pregnancy, migraine headaches) may be more prone to delayed or anticipatory nausea and vomiting.[24] In addition to CINV, nausea and vomiting can result from localized radiotherapy therapy, medications (e.g., opioids, antimicrobials, iron), intestinal obstruction, fluid and electrolyte imbalances, metabolic alterations, constipation, tumor invasion of the GI tract, cytokine release from tumor, and brain metastasis (owing to increased intracranial pressure).[25]

Constipation

When stool is dry or hard, stool passage is infrequent or painful, or the feeling of incomplete evacuation occurs, constipation must be addressed.[20] It is important to consider the patient's usual pattern of defecation rather than a standard norm. The most common constipating chemotherapeutic agents are the vinca alkaloids, which result in autonomic nerve dysfunction and can lead to decreased peristalsis and paralytic ileus. CINV may contribute to constipation through decreased oral intake, fluid loss, and administration of 5-hydroxytryptamine type 3 (5-HT_3) antagonists. Cancer patients may also be prone to constipation from prolonged use of opioids, aluminum antacids, calcium, anticonvulsants, anticholinergic drugs, antispasmodics, diuretics, tricyclic antidepressants, anti-inflammatory drugs, and muscle relaxants. Primary or metastatic tumors of the bowel may result in extraluminal compression on the intestine itself, which can physically block the passage of stool, or interfere with the colon's neural innervation. Other contributors to constipation include fatigue and immobility (which reduce gastric motility), dehydration (hardening of the stool), altered mental status (inability to receive accurate cues with defecation), reduced time and privacy, and low residual diet.[20]

Diarrhea

Diarrhea is an intestinal disorder characterized by abnormal frequency and fluidity of fecal evacuations with stool volume amounts of more than 250 g/day.[26] In the clinical setting, however, it is typically diagnosed when stools are frequent, loose, and watery. Diarrhea is categorized as acute (lasting for 14 days or less), persistent (lasting more than 14 days), or chronic (lasting for 30 days or longer).[27] The most common causes of cancer-related diarrhea are abdominal irradiation, GI surgery, bone marrow transplantation, and chemotherapeutic agents, such as 5-fluorouracil, irinotecan, and docetaxel. In addition, diarrhea can be a manifestation of certain types of tumors (carcinoid), or it may be a side effect of certain medications or tube feedings. Patients who are immunosuppressed are more susceptible to infectious organisms, such as *Clostridium difficile ("C. diff")*, which causes excessive mucosal secretion of fluid and electrolytes by the bowel mucosa. Pseudodiarrhea may occur with an intestinal ileus or obstruction; therefore the provider needs to rule out whether there is a primary or secondary cause for the diarrhea.[26] An example of a secondary cause is liquid stool that is actually overflow stool from an occlusion of the colon by hard stool, allowing only liquid stool to pass. A careful history including the cancer patient's bowel patterns before the diarrhea started will help the provider identify the problem.

Anorexia

Anorexia is characterized by a decrease in appetite and food intake. The resulting weight loss could lead to cachexia, a syndrome of progressive wasting with a marked reduction of adipose tissue that may become irreversible and fatal.[28] Any interference with physiologic, psychological, and social stimuli can result in a decrease of food intake and nutritional status. Physiologically, appetite suppression results from the secretion of cytokines that act as anorexigenic agents. Physiologic factors that contribute to anorexia include nausea and vomiting, dysgeusia (taste alterations), constipation, dysphagia, odynophagia, fatigue, infection, and mucositis. Psychological factors include anxiety and depression. Social factors include personal or cultural preferences as well as loss of the patient's usual eating companions and change of atmosphere when hospitalized. Medical causes that contribute to anorexia can include tumors, bowel obstruction, fever, metabolic disorders (hepatic and renal dysfunction), and ectopic hormone production by tumors. Head and neck surgery may affect the ability to eat normally because of altered facial architecture. Radiotherapy can lead to glossitis, mucositis, esophagitis, and altered taste. Chemotherapeutic agents, antibiotics, antifungal agents, and pain medications may also reduce appetite.

Mucositis

Mucositis is the inflammation and ulceration of the mucous membranes in the GI tract as a result of destruction of the oral mucosal epithelium (and slow regrowth of tissue) caused by the effects of chemotherapeutic agents and/or radiotherapy.[29] All mucous membranes along the digestive tract (from the lips to the anus) can be affected by systemic chemotherapy, but the most common sites for mucositis are the oral cavity and the esophagus. The mucosa may become dry, inflamed, ulcerated, and often very painful. Pain is the major clinical problem with mucositis, because it can render the patient unable to practice adequate oral hygiene, eat or swallow properly, or speak clearly. The most common agents toxic to the mucosa are 5-fluorouracil, methotrexate, bleomycin, actinomycin D (dactinomycin), etoposide, cytarabine, cyclophosphamide, floxuridine, docetaxel, paclitaxel, vinblastine, doxorubicin, daunorubicin, mitoxantrone, chlorambucil, vindesine, thioguanine, amsacrine, and plicamycin.[25] Radiation therapy can also predispose tissue in the treatment field to mucositis. The risk for developing mucositis is not the same for all patients, nor is the severity of the inflammation similar; rather, it is a very specific experience with each cancer patient.

Xerostomia

Xerostomia is a decrease in the quantity and quality of saliva, resulting in thick, ropy saliva that interferes with nutrition, taste, and speech.[30] It can last for months or even years, and is often described as bothersome. Common causes include surgery or radiotherapy to the head and neck region, anticholinergic and opioid medications, oral infections, and dehydration.[25]

CLINICAL PRESENTATION OF GASTROINTESTINAL DISTURBANCES

When cancer patients experience significant GI disturbances, they will commonly report a reduced oral intake, have altered bowel functions, and are at high risk for dehydration and electrolyte imbalance. Constitutional symptoms such as fatigue, malaise, and weight loss are also common. A general overview of all organ systems provides the necessary information to narrow down the differential diagnosis. A thorough assessment of GI symptoms is essential; this includes quantification of the daily fluid and food intake and a description of the number and characteristics of bowel movements per day, the number and characteristics of recent emetic episodes, and any abdominal pain. Any significant symptoms should be further assessed by asking about the factors that exacerbate or relieve symptoms; the quality, severity, timing, and duration of symptoms; and the relationship to intake of food or medications. For example, dry mouth, dizziness, reduced urinary output, confusion, and hypotension may indicate dehydration.

PHYSICAL EXAMINATION OF GASTROINTESTINAL DISTURBANCES

The provider should assess for any weight loss in cancer patients but must be careful to note significant weight loss (>1% to 2% per week). Occasionally, weight loss can be the first sign of cancer relapse or exacerbation. In a patient with diarrhea, signs and symptoms of hypovolemia and hypoperfusion should be assessed. These include mental status changes, diaphoresis, tachycardia, orthostatic hypotension, and reduced skin turgor.[27] The oral cavity should be inspected for integrity of mucosa, ulcerations, thrush or exudate, erythema, and gingivitis. With a gloved finger and tongue depressor, the oral mucosa and oropharynx can be thoroughly examined. The abdomen should be inspected, auscultated, and palpated. Inspection is done first and may reveal striae, distention, and contour abnormalities. Jaundice can be detected by inspection of the skin and sclerae of the eyes. Auscultation of bowel sounds in all quadrants is done next, with palpation and percussion performed last. Rebound tenderness, visible peristalsis, distention, or altered bowel sounds may indicate obstruction. Paralytic obstruction or peritonitis is characterized by absent bowel sounds over 2 minutes.[9] Palpation can detect presence of stool, masses, hepatosplenomegaly, inguinal lymphadenopathy, and asymmetry of contour. Ascites can be detected by testing for a fluid wave or shifting dullness of the abdomen. Digital rectal examinations are avoided if the patient is neutropenic or thrombocytopenic or has received radiotherapy to the rectum, owing to bleeding and risk of infection. A guideline the provider can use to grade the severity of nausea and vomiting during examination can be found in Box 245-3.

DIAGNOSTICS FOR GASTROINTESTINAL DISTURBANCES

Laboratory tests are useful to alert the provider to potential complications that may arise in a cancer patient with altered GI function. A chemistry profile (including electrolytes, blood urea nitrogen [BUN], and creatinine) is used to evaluate for fluid and electrolyte imbalances.[31] Prolonged vomiting, diarrhea, and anorexia can cause dangerous shifts in electrolytes, and kidney function can deteriorate quite rapidly in a dehydrated patient who has received nephrotoxic chemotherapy. Additional

BOX 245-3

Severity Grading for Nausea and Vomiting

GRADE 1
- Loss of appetite with unchanged eating habits
- One or two episodes of vomiting in 24 hours

GRADE 2
- Reduced oral intake without significant weight loss, dehydration, or malnutrition
- Intravenous fluids indicated for less than 24 hours
- Three to five episodes of vomiting in 24 hours

GRADE 3
- Oral calorie or fluid intake is insufficient; intravenous fluids, tube feedings, or total parenteral nutrition (TPN) is indicated for 24 hours or more
- Six or more episodes of vomiting in 24 hours
- Hospitalization often indicated

GRADE 4
- Life-threatening consequences requiring urgent intervention

Modified from National Cancer Institute: *Nausea and vomiting PDQ*. Available at www.cancer.gov/cancertopics/pdq/supportivecare/nausea/HealthProfessional. Accessed August 8, 2014.

DIAGNOSTICS

Gastrointestinal Symptoms in the Oncology Patient

LABORATORY
Complete blood count (CBC) and differential
Serum electrolytes
BUN
Creatinine
Serum glucose
Serum calcium*
Serum magnesium*
Serum phosphorus*
Serum hCG*
Liver function tests (LFTs)*
Serum albumin and total protein*
Stool for occult blood and *Clostridium difficile* ("*C. diff*")*
Urinalysis*

IMAGING
Kidney, ureter, and bladder (KUB) study*

*If indicated.

chemistries include magnesium and phosphorus levels, which can decrease precipitously after chemotherapy that affects excretion (e.g., cisplatin and ifosfamide). An ileus can be caused by hypomagnesemia, hypophosphatemia, hypokalemia, and hypocalcaemia. A urinalysis is indicated if a urinary tract infection is the suspected cause of nausea and vomiting. Serum albumin, particularly prealbumin, can be useful in assessing nutritional status. A liver panel, including amylase and lipase levels, prothrombin time, and an albumin level should be ordered if hepatic dysfunction is suspected. Human chorionic gonadotropin (hCG) levels should always be included for females of childbearing age with nausea and vomiting, to exclude pregnancy.[31]

The previously discussed laboratory tests are commonly ordered in cancer patients with GI symptoms. Additional tests are warranted based on the patient's symptoms and physical examination. For example, testing a cancer patient's stool for occult blood (three sequential specimens) is necessary if GI bleeding is suspected. Testing stool for *C. difficile* is indicated for relentless diarrhea, particularly in a cancer patient who received broad-spectrum antibiotics or was recently hospitalized and is at high risk for a nosocomial infection. Additional stool studies, such as Gram stain and tests for leukocytosis and vancomycin-resistant enterococci (VRE), may also be indicated. Abdominal imaging (CT, MRI, or ultrasound) is necessary for suspicion of appendicitis, cholecystitis, or intestinal obstruction.[31]

DIFFERENTIAL DIAGNOSIS FOR GASTROINTESTINAL DISTURBANCES

It is important to recognize other conditions that cause symptoms resembling cancer-related GI symptoms (e.g., appendicitis, peritonitis, gastroenteritis, gastric reflux, hepatitis, pancreatitis, cholecystitis, peptic ulcer disease, ileus, obstruction, uremia, urinary tract infection, hypercalcemia, and psychogenic or anticipatory vomiting). These conditions should be considered when evaluating any patient with GI complaints. Other considerations may include anorexia nervosa, irritable bowel syndrome, increased intracranial pressure, spinal cord compression, vestibular disorders, acute myocardial infarction, and, in sexually active women of childbearing age, pregnancy. The patient's onset of symptoms, past medical history, risk factors for other diseases, and treatment side effects are essential elements in identifying the cause of the GI symptoms so that an appropriate treatment plan can be established.

DIFFERENTIAL DIAGNOSIS

Gastrointestinal Symptoms in the Oncology Patient

- Irritable bowel
- Gastroenteritis
- Hepatitis
- Pancreatitis
- Peptic ulcer disease
- Ileus
- Uremia
- Urinary tract infection
- Constipation
- Pregnancy
- Increased intracranial pressure
- Vestibular disorder
- Acute myocardial infarction
- Anorexia nervosa
- Psychogenic vomiting

MANAGEMENT OF GASTROINTESTINAL DISTURBANCES

Nausea and Vomiting

When the U.S. Food and Drug Administration (FDA) approved the 5-HT_3 antagonists in the early 1990s, this revolutionized antiemetic control with CINV. Further advancement was made, particularly with delayed emesis, after the class of antiemetics called neurokinin 1 (NK1) antagonists were developed. For an antiemetic regimen to be effective, it must interrupt the stimulation of the vomiting center. Therefore a combination of antiemetic agents is typically used to maximize prevention and control of both acute and delayed emesis.[23,32,33]

The best predictor of CINV is the emetic potential of the chemotherapeutic agent being used. Chemotherapy drugs are classified as having low, moderate, and severe emetic potential.

Age and gender can also predict CINV: patients younger than 50 and females are at particularly high risk.[23] Evidence-based studies continue to support the efficacy of 5-HT_3 antagonists, dexamethasone, and aprepitant in both acute and delayed emesis when they are given with chemotherapeutic agents with moderate or high emetic potential.[32,34] Palonosetron, a very-long-acting second-generation 5-HT_3 antagonist, provides superior control of delayed emesis, particularly with moderately emetogenic chemotherapy. In general, the 5-HT_3 antagonists are well tolerated with minimal side effects, although QT prolongation should be considered for patients with congenital or medication-induced QT prolongation.

When a cancer patient is not able to tolerate 5-HT_3 antagonists or the nausea and vomiting are not related to chemotherapeutic administration, antiemetic agents from another class are indicated. Metoclopramide is a dopamine receptor antagonist and, in combination with dexamethasone, is particularly beneficial for delayed emesis after chemotherapy. Phenothiazines (prochlorperazine) and butyrophenones (haloperidol, droperidol) are somewhat effective but less so than metoclopramide, and patients are at higher risk for extrapyramidal symptoms, especially in patients younger than 30 years. Benzodiazepines (lorazepam, clonazepam) and antihistamines (diphenhydramine, hydroxyzine) are useful adjunct medications for their antianxiety effect and prevention of the extrapyramidal reactions associated with some antiemetics but are not recommended for single-agent use for nausea and vomiting. Cannabinoids, both ingested and inhaled, have been found to have antiemetic benefits and also stimulate the appetite.[25,32,34]

Some cancer patients are able to interrupt the association of nausea and vomiting with chemotherapy through the use of behavioral interventions. Progressive muscle relaxation, hypnosis, guided imagery, biofeedback, and distraction can be valuable.[22] The provider should educate patients to remove or minimize any adverse sounds or smells that stimulate the vomiting center. Patients who experience sustained episodes of nausea and vomiting, even with treatment, are also encouraged to avoid eating their "favorite foods" so aversions to these foods can be avoided.

Constipation

The management of constipation should first address the most common precipitating factors, such as fiber, fluids, physical activity, and certain medications. Cancer patients should be educated to increase their fiber intake by consuming fruits (including figs, dates, and prunes), vegetables, and whole grains. When fiber is increased, it is important to also consume at least 1.5 liters of water per day.[20] Regular exercise should be encouraged for all patients. A physical therapist can be consulted for coordination of an exercise regimen for bed-bound patients and for those with physical limitations. Numerous medications cause constipation; however, for the cancer patient, some of these medications should not be stopped. Therefore it is important to identify patients at risk for constipation and initiate an appropriate bowel regimen.

Once constipation has occurred, fluid intake should be increased to 2 quarts per day.[20] If the constipation continues, an oral osmotic laxative (polyethylene glycol [MiraLax]) can be used. Methylnaltrexone bromide can be used subcutaneously to treat opioid-induced constipation; however, this is contraindicated in patients with known or suspected obstruction. Rectal agents should be avoided in cancer patients who are at risk for thrombocytopenia or leukopenia owing to risks of bleeding and infection. The patient should be given privacy and adequate time for defecation, and the use of a bedpan should be avoided if at all possible.

Diarrhea

The management of diarrhea begins with rehydration and dietary intervention. Bowel rest is not recommended because this can worsen diarrhea and lead to more severe dehydration.[27] Patients are educated to consume high-fiber, high-calorie, and high-protein meals. Identification and avoidance of aggravating foods, such as milk products and high-fat foods, can also help. Assess the patient's hydration status by evaluating vital signs, mucous membranes, and presence of postural hypotension.[26] Anticholinergic drugs, such as diphenoxylate plus atropine or loperamide, reduce gastric secretions and decrease intestinal peristalsis. Octreotide acetate, which is reserved for patients with excessive diarrhea, inhibits the release of intestinal hormones (including serotonin and gastrin), prolongs intestinal transit time, and increases intestinal water and electrolyte transport. Psyllium may be effective in controlling high-output diarrhea. Topical agents containing hydrocortisone or dibucaine are useful for perianal irritation. Glucocorticoid retention enemas can be helpful for radiation-induced proctitis. Antidiarrheal medications are contraindicated when a patient has a GI infection *(C. difficile)* or pseudodiarrhea that occurs with an ileus or partial small bowel obstruction.

Anorexia

Anorexia can be very difficult to manage in cancer patients. Treatment for anorexia focuses on patient education, behavioral changes, and pharmacologic intervention. Consultation with a nutritionist can be helpful for exploring high-calorie food options, supplements, appetizing recipes, and visually appealing foods. Increased physical activity and smaller, more frequent meals may also be helpful. Social interventions, such as having a family member share or prepare a meal, or using special table settings (e.g., having a sandwich on family china) may be helpful in stimulating the cancer patient's desire to eat.[28] Patients who develop dysgeusia may experience a metallic or bitter taste when eating, which stems from central nervous system involvement and will not simply decrease with use of plastic utensils. Identifying and avoiding food triggers can help reduce the patient's exposure to dysgeusia.[30]

Several pharmacologic agents have been helpful in managing anorexia. The most common, megestrol acetate (Megace), works well, but patients taking this have an increased risk of blood clots. Thus the provider must weigh the benefits and risks of use of this medication. Other agents include metoclopramide (which increases gastric emptying and is useful for patients with early satiety or delayed gastric emptying), dexamethasone (which stimulates appetite and induces a sense of well-being), and cannabinoids (which stimulate appetite and control nausea and vomiting). Patients who continue to have significant anorexia or weight loss may require formal nutritional support, such as enteral or parenteral feedings.[28]

Mucositis

Mucositis can develop anywhere along the mucous membranes (from the lips to the anus); however, the oral mucosa is most commonly affected in the cancer patient. Therefore, maintaining good oral hygiene is essential to the cancer patient's overall health and sense of well-being. It is important to assist the patient in developing a plan for oral care that includes daily plaque removal and mouth rinses after each meal and at bedtime. Soft toothbrushes and dental floss should be used regularly unless there is danger of mucosal injury or evidence of thrombocytopenia with active bleeding. Foam brushes can be substituted if needed. Nonirritating and nondrying mouth rinses, including normal saline and sodium bicarbonate peroxide, should be used. Hydrogen peroxide has an antifibroblastic effect and should be avoided because of the possible impairment of wound healing. The lips need extra lubrication to keep them moist and comfortable. Once the patient develops mucositis, topical formulations and cryotherapy (sucking on ice chips and popsicles) may help with painful oral lesions.[29] Opioid medications may be indicated for severe mucositis, which can cause moderate to severe pain. In general, patients should avoid all tobacco products, alcohol, and foods that cause irritation, such as hot, spicy, or rough foods.

Xerostomia

The thick, ropy saliva of xerostomia can cause food to form into a thick ball or stick to the teeth. Eating can be difficult and unpleasant because food needs to be lubricated enough to swallow it.[30] Oral care before meals may help freshen the mouth and reduce these symptoms. Increasing fluids during meals helps moisten food and aids in swallowing. Eating soft foods that are moistened with milk or gravy and avoiding dry, spicy, and acidic foods can also help xerostomia. Humidified air can help prevent mucous membranes from drying and cracking. Lubricating agents such as saliva substitutes are expensive and may or may not be helpful. Prolonged xerostomia can result in dental caries; regular dental checkups to assess for decay are required.

COMPLICATIONS OF GASTROINTESTINAL DISTURBANCES

Complications of GI symptoms can vary widely based on the patient's health, severity of symptoms, and grade of toxicity. For example, significant mucositis in the presence of neutropenia can be life-threatening and may require aggressive antibiotic management. Severe GI toxicities can create friable, edematous, and ulcerative mucosal insults, resulting in anorexia, malabsorption, malnutrition, dehydration, and intractable pain. Mechanical or paralytic obstruction of the bowel can be life-threatening if rupture is suspected and is often difficult to diagnose early in its presentation. Therefore any suspicion of obstruction should prompt an immediate referral to a GI specialist for surgical evaluation.

INDICATIONS FOR REFERRAL OR HOSPITALIZATION FOR GASTROINTESTINAL DISTURBANCES

Persistent or worsening GI symptoms may indicate a treatment complication or disease progression, and referral to a specialist or hospitalization may be warranted. A detailed history and physical examination will determine the differential diagnoses and the need for referral or hospitalization. Common causes of hospitalizations for treatment-related GI complications include acute or refractory nausea and vomiting, acute or refractory abdominal pain, GI bleeding, dysphagia, dehydration, orthostatic hypotension, intractable diarrhea, and severe constipation.[9]

PATIENT AND FAMILY EDUCATION FOR GASTROINTESTINAL DISTURBANCES

Oncology patients and their caregivers need to be educated on the importance of notifying a health care provider of the occurrence of GI symptoms, whether mild, moderate, or severe. Written instructions as well as verbal discussion of treatments for nausea, vomiting, diarrhea, constipation, and oral hygiene will help patients control problematic symptoms. A list of symptoms that indicate the need to call a health care provider should also be made available to the patient and family. Prompt recognition and reporting of GI symptoms, particularly when accompanied by fever, chills, or signs of dehydration, may help to avoid serious sequelae and increase the cancer patient's quality of life.[4,28,29]

OTHER ONCOLOGY SYMPTOMS

In addition to pain and GI disturbances, there are many other symptoms oncology patients experience during the treatment course. Some of these are physical conditions directly related to chemotherapy, radiation therapy, and surgeries associated with the cancer. These include neutropenia; fatigue; anemia; graft-versus-host disease; alopecia; cardiac, renal, side effects, and/or hepatotoxic chemotherapy; lymphedema; and surgical alterations to the body. Psychological symptoms include depression and anxiety associated with a cancer diagnosis and treatment. The psychosocial issues include sexuality, fertility, family dynamics, identity, and mortality. It is important that the primary care provider identify patient problems and coordinate care with the oncology team, because cancer patients will need medical, psychological, psychosocial, and spiritual support throughout their treatment.

CHAPTER 246

UNKNOWN PRIMARY CARCINOMA

Renato Lenzi

DEFINITION AND EPIDEMIOLOGY

Unknown primary carcinoma (UPC) is defined as the presence of documented metastatic cancer in the absence of an identifiable primary tumor site. It has been speculated that in patients with UPC, the tumor either remains below the limits of clinical or radiographic detection or regresses spontaneously.

Incidence rates of 1% to 15% have been reported, probably reflecting differences in referral patterns, demographics, and the type and extent of the evaluation performed. The overall incidence of UPC in the United States is estimated to be closer to 2% of the whole population of cancer patients.[1] It is estimated that in the United States the yearly incidence of UPC is 7 to 12 cases per 100,000 people per year.[2] UPC patients are heterogeneous in their clinical presentation and have widely varying clinical courses. As a group, these patients have a poor median survival of less than 1 year,[3-5] which has not significantly changed in the last decade despite the introduction over the years of chemotherapeutic and other agents with increased efficacy in the treatment of cancers of known primary sites. Except for a slight preponderance of male patients, the demographics (age and ethnicity) mirror those of the general population of cancer patients.[6]

PATHOPHYSIOLOGY

Overexpression of c-erbB2, c-myc, and Ras and multiple rearranged chromosome regions have been described.[7,8] Findings of chromosome 1 deletion, translocations, and gene amplification in UPC suggest that these tumors may rapidly progress to reach the ability to metastasize. It has been speculated that specific genetic changes of UPC may support metastatic but not local growth.[9] No molecular characteristics specific to UPC have been discovered, and molecular profiling shows strong similarities of a significant number of metastatic lesions of unknown primaries with cancers of known primary site.[10] Epidermal growth factor receptors (EGFR) family proteins, c-Kit/PDFGR, have been found to be overexpressed, presence in the circulation of tumor cells has been found to be common, and p53 overexpression has been reported in 50% of tumors studied.[11]

CLINICAL PRESENTATION

The clinical presentations of patients with UPC vary widely, probably reflecting the heterogeneous nature of the underlying malignant neoplasms. Subgroups of patients with similar clinical presentations have been identified as having disease that is responsive to therapy or longer survival times. These "favorable" subsets include women with peritoneal carcinomatosis and papillary histology, women with metastatic adenocarcinoma or carcinoma confined to the axillary nodes, patients with inguinal node metastases with histologic features of squamous cell carcinoma, patients with squamous cell carcinoma confined to lymph nodes in the high or middle neck, patients with midline metastasis of poorly differentiated carcinoma, men with elevated prostate-specific antigen (PSA) and bone metastasis, patients with one isolated resectable metastasis, and patients with neuroendocrine tumors. Moreover, it has been shown that patients initially seen with lymph node involvement have longer median survival times than do patients with lung, liver, or bone metastasis. Patients with multiple sites of metastasis, male patients, and those with poor performance status tend to have a worse prognosis.[12]

The tumor histology of 1109 consecutive UPC patients is summarized in Table 246-1. Glandular differentiation sufficient to permit a diagnosis of adenocarcinoma was identified in approximately 60% of patients with UPC. Nearly 30% of patients were diagnosed with carcinoma, and more than half of these had evidence of poorly differentiated or undifferentiated carcinoma. Squamous cell carcinoma and neuroendocrine carcinoma together accounted for 10% of patients and were associated with more favorable median survival times. Patients with carcinoma also had a longer median survival time (12 months) than that of patients with adenocarcinomas (9 months), but their survival advantage was not as pronounced as that of patients with squamous cell carcinoma (24 months) and neuroendocrine carcinoma (33 months).

PHYSICAL EXAMINATION

The initial evaluation should focus on signs and symptoms that could identify the primary site (e.g., blood in stool, persistent cough) and should include an inquiry about the family history of cancer. The physical examination should include a search for skin lesions, a careful breast and pelvic examination (for women), and a testicular and prostate examination (for men). Lymph node–bearing areas should be examined for adenopathy.

TABLE 246-1 Tumor Histology Distribution of 1109 Patients with UPC

Histology	Patients	% of Total
Adenocarcinoma	646	58.3
Well differentiated	14	
Moderately differentiated	45	
Poorly differentiated	220	
Mucinous	46	
No descriptor/other	321	
Carcinoma	317	28.6
Poorly differentiated	161	
Undifferentiated	21	
Large cell	9	
Small cell	14	
No descriptor/other	112	
Squamous	68	6.1
Neuroendocrine	48	4.3
Adenosquamous	7	0.6
Pathology not available for review/other	23	2.1

Unpublished data from Abbruzzese JL, Abbruzzese MC, Lenzi R, Houston, 2005, MD Anderson Cancer Center.

DIAGNOSTICS

A limited and focused evaluation that includes a pathologic review, careful physical examination, complete blood count (CBC), chemistry survey (SMA-20), chest radiography, computed tomography (CT) scan (of the chest, abdomen, and pelvis in all patients), PSA levels in men, and mammography in women has been shown to be effective in identifying the more treatable primary malignant neoplasms.[13] The baseline laboratory evaluation may provide important diagnostic cues (e.g., microcytic anemia suggests the possibility of an iron deficiency secondary to blood loss from a primary neoplasm in the gastrointestinal tract). Serum tumor markers are helpful in the differential diagnosis of cancer of unknown primary origin (CUP +). Alpha fetoprotein (AFP) is useful for the differential diagnosis of hepatocellular carcinoma and germ cell tumors. In association with the determination of human chorionic gonadotropin beta subunit (β-hCG), AFP is also indicated for the evaluation of patients with a midline tumor. CA-125, CA 15-3, carcinoembryonic antigen (CEA), and CA 19-9 are also commonly measured but are nonspecific and need to be considered in conjunction with other diagnostic information. PSA is useful in the evaluation of man with dominant metastatic bone disease with an adenocarcinoma histology.

Breast magnetic resonance imaging (MRI) should be done in women with axillary adenopathy if mammography and breast ultrasound examination findings are normal.[14] Positron emission tomography–computed tomography (PET/CT) scan has been evaluated in patients with cervical metastasis for the diagnosis of a primary neoplasm,[15] showing a high sensitivity and a low specificity.[15] PET/CT scan can be helpful to rule out additional sites of disease in those patients for whom the detection of additional unrecognized regional and distant metastatic lesions would alter the treatment strategy.[16] It can provide prognostic information by identifying UPC patients with distant, regional, or no disease spread.[17] Endoscopic procedures, such as triple endoscopy and endoscopic evaluation of the upper and lower gastrointestinal tract, are done as indicated on the basis of location of metastatic disease, symptoms, and results of biopsy material evaluation. Careful review of biopsy material is the most important single step in determining the primary site or identifying a unique histologic subset that is amenable to specific therapy.

Good communication between the primary health care provider and pathologist is needed to plan the optimum use of immunohistochemical staining or molecular studies for the evaluation of each patient. Carefully selected special studies can be extremely useful in diagnosis of the primary type in patients with morphologically undifferentiated or poorly differentiated neoplasms and in patients with well-differentiated carcinomas that cannot be further classified solely on morphologic criteria. Tumors testing cytokeratin (CK) 20^+/$CK7^-$/$CDX2^+$ are considered most likely to originate from the colon; and those testing thyroid transcription factor 1 (TTF-1)$^+$ and $CK7^+$, from the lung.[18,19] Useful markers in differentiating ovarian from breast carcinomas in the presence of positive progesterone or estrogen receptors are WT-1[20] and pax8.[21]

DIAGNOSTICS

Unknown Primary Carcinoma

PATHOLOGY

Review of biopsy material
- Morphology
- Immunohistochemistry
- Molecular studies

LABORATORY

CBC and differential
Complete chemistry profile
Serum tumor markers (AFP, β-hCG, PSA, CA-125, CA 15-3, CEA, CA 19-9) as indicated

IMAGING

Chest x-ray examination
CT scan of chest, abdomen, pelvis
Mammography, breast ultrasound
MRI for specific presentations
PET/CT scan as indicated

Note: Molecular profiling has been evaluated over the past 10 years as an additional tool to determine the tissue of origin of UPCs[22] procedures include real-time quantitative reverse transcription polymerase chain reaction (qRT-PCR),[23] microarray[24] and microRNA (miRNA)[25] techniques. Diagnostic molecular profiling for unknown primary cancer patients is available commercially. Although studies have shown consistency in molecular diagnosis, clinical features, responses to treatment, and outcomes,[26,27] molecular testing is currently not recommended for all patients with an unknown primary cancer in the absence of sufficient data from randomized trials.

DIFFERENTIAL DIAGNOSIS

At the beginning of the diagnostic evaluation, it is important to establish unequivocally whether the patient indeed has a neoplastic process. A small but significant percentage of the patients referred with a diagnosis of metastatic carcinoma of unknown primary were found on further evaluation not to have cancer.[6] In the majority of these cases, the diagnosis of neoplastic disease was made on the basis of radiographic studies only, and the initial evaluation did not include a biopsy. For example, a patient with osteoporosis and compression fractures of single or multiple vertebral bodies may be initially diagnosed as having metastatic bone lesions.

Clarification of the diagnosis is usually accomplished with a biopsy of the suspected metastatic site. Appropriate caution needs to be used in planning invasive diagnostic modalities because complications can result from the diagnostic procedure itself. For example, a liver biopsy may result in excessive bleeding if the liver lesion suspected of being neoplastic is actually a hemangioma. Additional imaging studies may need to be performed to better define a lesion for biopsy. In some cases, lesions that appear to be metastatic may indeed represent the primary cancer. For example, multiple liver lesions thought to be metastatic from an unknown site may represent a primary multifocal hepatocellular carcinoma.

DIFFERENTIAL DIAGNOSIS

Unknown Primary Carcinoma Conditions Responsive to Therapy

- Women with peritoneal carcinomatosis and papillary serous histology
- Women with isolated axillary node involvement
- Squamous cell carcinoma in high or middle neck nodes
- Squamous cell carcinoma in inguinal nodes
- Extragonadal germ cell syndrome

MANAGEMENT

The treatment of patients in whom the primary site or a unique histologic subtype (e.g., melanoma, lymphoma, sarcoma, neuroendocrine) has been identified should follow disease-specific guidelines.

The treatment of patients with adenocarcinoma and carcinoma histology and regional disease is based on the treatment used for patients with the most likely primary cancer to cause similar clinical features.

Patients with isolated involvement of head and neck or supraclavicular nodes are treated according to head and neck cancer guidelines. Patients with extensive adenopathy are often treated with systemic chemotherapy.

Male gender, age younger than 50 years, and rapidly growing and poorly differentiated carcinomas involving predominantly midline structures (mediastinum) are features of the extragonadal germ cell syndrome. A careful pathologic review may identify germ cell histology. In the absence of a specific pathologic diagnosis, these patients should be treated aggressively with chemotherapy regimens used for germ cell cancer; a non–small cell lung cancer (NSCLC) regimen is an option for patients 40 to 50 years of age. Patients 50 years or older are treated with regimens used for NSCLC.

In women, the most common cause of carcinomas confined to the axillary nodes is occult breast cancer. When a breast primary carcinoma is in the differential diagnosis, immunohistochemistry testing should include estrogen and progesterone receptors, human epidermal growth factor receptor-2 (HER-2), and gross cystic disease fluid protein.[21,28] If the pathologic findings are consistent with primary breast cancer, these patients should be treated similarly to patients with a known primary breast tumor of the corresponding stage. Overall, the survival rate appears to be similar to that of patients with breast cancer. Inguinal node metastases of unknown origin with histologic features of squamous cell carcinoma require careful inspection of the skin, anus, and distal genitourinary tract and a gynecologic examination in women. Patients in whom the primary tumor cannot be identified and who do not have additional sites of disease should be considered for lymph node dissection of the affected area and radiotherapy with or without chemotherapy.

Women with abdominal carcinomatosis and pathologic changes consistent with a müllerian primary are treated similarly to women with a diagnosed primary müllerian cancer of the same stage. The majority of patients with UPC, however, do not fit into one of the previously described subsets.

Chemotherapy with either investigational or standard agents should be offered to patients with adequate performance status. The chemotherapeutic agents studied for the treatment of these patients have included platinum compounds, 5-fluorouracil, taxanes, etoposide, gemcitabine, and irinotecan.[29-33]

Promising results with use of bevacizumab and erlotinib have been observed in patients with a poor prognosis.[34] Treatment targeted to the most likely primary neoplasm as determined by immunohistochemistry and molecular tumor profiling is supported for certain tumor types by preliminary data.[35] The introduction of biologic anticancer agents and of targeted therapy for the treatment of patients with unknown primary cancer represents the next step toward the goal of developing a more effective treatment model for these patients.

Interdisciplinary Management

The delivery of care to patients with UPC often requires a multidisciplinary team to provide adequate integration and planning of multimodality care. This care involves specialists in medical oncology, radiotherapy, surgery, and pain and symptom management.

LIFE SPAN CONSIDERATIONS

The median survival for patients with UPC is overall relatively short (less than a year). However, some of the patients belonging in the previously described favorable subgroups survive for several years, and a few patients with isolated lesions have survival of many years' duration and are probably cured. Patients belonging in the more treatable subsets need to be identified and treated accordingly. For all patients, a mandatory goal is timely administration of therapy without the undue delay of prolonged and unproductive testing. This can usually be accomplished if the limited and focused evaluation previously described is used. Prognostic parameters for these patients have been described, including sex, histology, number of metastatic sites, presence of liver metastasis, elevated lactate dehydrogenase levels, low serum albumin levels, performance status, and age; these can be of great help in formulating a prognosis and appropriate treatment planning.[36]

COMPLICATIONS

Like other patients with metastatic cancer, patients with UPC are at risk for a broad spectrum of complications. Complications directly related to the disease process include spinal cord compression from metastatic disease, hypercalcemia of malignancy, ureteral and biliary obstruction, pleural and pericardial effusions, and ascites. Complications related to treatment include chemotherapy-induced alopecia, nausea, vomiting, diarrhea, and mucositis as well as febrile neutropenia, anemia, and thrombocytopenia, which may require the transfusion of blood products. Narcotic analgesics are often necessary for pain control and may cause respiratory depression, hallucinations, somnolence, nausea, vomiting, and severe constipation.

Radiation treatment may cause fatigue and, depending on the anatomic area being treated, hair loss, esophagitis with dysphagia, gastritis, diarrhea, rectal pain or burning, and cystitis or dysuria.

Clinically significant anxiety and depression are often observed in these patients.

INDICATIONS FOR REFERRAL OR HOSPITALIZATION

Diagnostic evaluation and therapeutic decisions for patients with UPC are complex and require referral to a physician who specializes in the treatment of cancer patients. Hospitalization may be required for adequate management of symptoms and complications related to either the disease process (e.g., spinal cord compression, bleeding, hypercalcemia, intractable pain) or treatment side effects (e.g., intractable nausea and vomiting, febrile neutropenia, thrombocytopenia with bleeding). Hospitalization may also be required for the administration of chemotherapy or for procedures such as surgical stabilization of metastatic bone lesions or excision of limited metastatic disease.

PATIENT AND FAMILY EDUCATION

A diagnosis of UPC is a major challenge for patients and families. A higher prevalence of depressive symptoms (40%) and a higher frequency of somatization and anxiety have been reported in patients with unknown primary cancer compared with patients with metastatic and nonmetastatic cancer of known origin.[37] The lack of knowledge of the primary tumor results in diagnostic and therapeutic uncertainties and can generate anxiety in the health care provider and patient.[13] Although the primary site is not known, there are guidelines to help choose the most effective treatment for each patient. Patients need education about the side effects of chemotherapy and radiotherapy and need to be taught to recognize the complications that require immediate medical attention. It is also important to educate patients in the appropriate use of pain medications. Finally, it is often necessary to educate and communicate with these patients on emotionally charged topics, such as do-not-resuscitate status and the shift from chemotherapy to supportive care only. Training staff in these difficult aspects of patient communication will increase their confidence in dealing with these issues.[38]

REFERENCES

For a full list of references, scan the QR code or visit http://booksite.elsevier.com/9780323355018

PART 23 Evaluation and Management of Mental Health Disorders

CHAPTER 247

ANXIETY DISORDERS

Rene Love • Rose Vick

DEFINITION AND EPIDEMIOLOGY

Anxiety disorders are the most commonly occurring class of mental disorders per lifetime prevalence data.[1] Within anxiety disorders, specific phobias are the most common, with social phobias being the next most common. The least common of the anxiety disorders are obsessive-compulsive disorder (OCD) and agoraphobia without a history of panic disorder.[2] The development of anxiety disorders depends on several variables that affect the way the body responds to fear and anxiety, such as gender, age, culture, environment, qualities of the stressor, and genetics. In general, anxiety disorders typically begin much earlier than other mental disorders, and women are at higher risk than men.[2] More specifically, the onset of tic disorders and specific phobias begins in childhood with social phobias and OCD beginning in adolescence or early adulthood. The onset of post-traumatic stress disorder (PTSD) can vary; the disorder results from trauma exposure, which may occur at any point in life. Panic disorder, generalized anxiety disorder (GAD), and agoraphobia are the only anxiety disorders that have adult onset.

Fear can be healthy in our lives. Healthy fear warns us to get out of harm's way or motivates a person to take action. However, if a person's stress level becomes persistent, excessive, overwhelming, and disabling, then an anxiety disorder should be considered. There are several factors to take into account, such as culture, genetics, environment, and psychosocial issues, when diagnosing anxiety disorders.

In looking at the burden of anxiety disorders, women were found to miss more days from work as a result of anxiety disorders,[3] although both men and women with anxiety disorders were frequent users of all types of health care services, including emergency rooms. On the other hand, men but not women were more likely to visit a professional for either an emotional or substance use issue in the past year if they had an anxiety disorder. In considering cultural impact, European-American women were high health care users.[3] With regard to specific phobias, Asians and Latinos reported significantly lower rates than non-Latino whites.[4]

The *Diagnostic and Statistical Manual of Mental Disorders,* Fifth Edition (DSM-5) identifies the following anxiety disorders: Separation Anxiety Disorder; Selective Mutism; Specific Phobia; Social Anxiety Disorder (Social Phobia); Panic Disorder; Agoraphobia; Substance/Medication-Induced Anxiety Disorder; Anxiety Disorder Due to Another General Medical Condition; and Generalized Anxiety Disorder.[4] Also included are Posttraumatic Stress Disorder (PTSD) and Acute Stress Disorder (ASD).[4]

The following definitions of the more common anxiety disorders are adapted from the DSM-5. Separation anxiety disorder is developmentally excessive and inappropriate anxiety and distress regarding separating from attachment figures. Selective mutism is consistently failing to speak in situations in which the person is expected to speak, even though the person will speak in other situations, thereby interfering with the person's education and occupation. A specific phobia is extreme fear and distress about a specific object or situation such as snakes or heights. A social anxiety disorder is extreme fear and distress about social situations in which the individual is exposed to possible scrutiny by other people, which may cause the person to avoid social situations altogether. Panic disorder is characterized by recurring and unanticipated panic attacks. GAD is excessive anxiety that occurs more days than not about a wide variety of events or activities. PTSD occurs when a person is exposed to a trauma that causes intense psychological distress when he or she is exposed to either internal or external cues.[4]

PATHOPHYSIOLOGY

Fear is a normal response that promotes survival in the face of an actual environmental threat. For example, it is adaptive and beneficial to experience a fight-or-flight response via the sympathetic nervous system (SNS) when confronted by dangerous stimuli. Anxiety, on the other hand, is an unhealthy, exaggerated fear response that often occurs in the absence of a true environmental threat.[5] Physiologically, the body does not differentiate between anxiety and fear. Simply stated, blood flow is increased to the large muscle groups in preparation to flee or fight; the heart and legs are ready to take action, and the digestive system slows. However, the fear response is a complex process involving multiple organ systems, and therefore anxiety has many associated physical and psychological consequences. Subcortical (amygdala, hippocampus, brainstem, and hypothalamus) and cortical regions (insular cortex, orbitofrontal cortex, ventromedial prefrontal cortex, and anterior cingulate cortex) of the brain are involved in anxiety disorders.[6] The amygdala and hypothalamic-pituitary-adrenal (HPA) axis are two primary areas implicated in the neuropathology of anxiety. The amygdala is part of the limbic system and processes emotionally salient stimuli and initiates the appropriate behavioral response. The HPA axis functions as a hormonal feedback system and includes the hypothalamus, pituitary gland, and adrenal gland. Harmful stimuli undergo sensory processing, and information is relayed to the hypothalamus. The hypothalamus initiates the HPA axis by releasing corticotropin-releasing factor (CRF), which triggers the release of adrenocorticotropic hormone (ACTH) from the pituitary, which then triggers the release of glucocorticoids (including cortisol) from the adrenal gland.[5] When the system is functioning properly, it operates on a negative feedback loop:

the binding of glucocorticoids to glucocorticoid receptors inhibits further release of CRF and ACTH.[5] However, abnormalities in the HPA axis are implicated in individuals with anxiety disorders.[7]

It is well known that anxiety disorders have a strong familial link, and it is also understood that environmental factors contribute significantly to the development of anxiety disorders. Gene-environment (G × E) interactions related to anxiety have been demonstrated quite eloquently in rat studies, highlighting the significance of genetic and environmental influences as well as the concept of epigenetics.[8] During recent years, the serotonin transporter gene-linked polymorphic region (5-HTTLPR) has received a lot of attention in the literature owing to its association with increased vulnerability to psychiatric illness when combined with environmental stressors or adversity. There is evidence suggesting that individuals who are carriers of at least one short (S) allele and a history of adverse life events are at an increased risk for depression.[9] Experimental studies aimed at investigating the relationship between the 5-HTTLPR genotype and HPA axis reactivity in healthy individuals have produced inconsistent results. However, a recent meta-analysis demonstrated a small but significant association between the 5-HTTLPR genotype and HPA axis reactivity: specifically, individuals with the S/S genotype displayed increased cortisol reactivity compared with the S/L and L/L genotypes.[7]

Neurotransmitters including serotonin, norepinephrine, dopamine and γ-aminobutyric acid (GABA) have been well studied and are implicated in the pathophysiology of anxiety disorders. The involvement of these multiple neurotransmitter systems is complex and cannot be oversimplified as the presence of too much or not enough of a particular neurotransmitter. For example, serotonin pathways are involved in regulating mood states including anxiety and are also involved in the modulation of dopaminergic and noradrenergic pathways. Dopamine, serotonin, norepinephrine, and GABA have been linked to anxiety states and treatment for many years. Recent studies have investigated the role of glutamate, specifically the *N*-methyl-D-aspartate (NMDA) receptor, in the development and treatment of mood disorders and have led to efforts to develop novel psychopharmacologic treatments.[10] Clinical trials that expand our understanding of the role of glutamate in anxiety could change the way we treat anxiety disorders in the future. There remains much to learn about the development and management of anxiety disorders, but it is safe to stay that they involve complex interplay among genes, environment, culture, personality, and psychoneuroimmunologic factors.

CLINICAL PRESENTATION

Individuals with anxiety disorders often first are seen for treatment in primary care clinics and emergency departments. In addition to complaints of worry, anxiety, or fear, these individuals may also have numerous physical complaints. Anxiety disorders are highly comorbid with one another and other psychiatric illnesses including depression and substance use disorders.

Anxiety, by definition, is the anticipation of a future threat and is often associated with preparation for potential danger and/or avoidant behaviors.[4] Anxiety disorders differ from developmentally or situationally appropriate fears in that they are persistent (typically lasting 6 months or longer) and cause significant impairments in functioning.[4]

GAD is characterized by excessive anxiety and worry about a number of events or activities. The anxiety and worry are associated with three or more of the following six symptoms: (1) restlessness or feeling on edge, (2) easy fatigability, (3) difficulty concentrating, (4) irritability, (5) muscle tension, (6) sleep disturbance.[4] GAD is a chronic condition in which full remission rates are very low.[4] Children and adolescents tend to experience performance-focused worry and anxiety, whereas adults report more worry about their physical health or the well-being of their family.[4] In addition to worry, these individuals may also experience a variety of physical symptoms including tachycardia, shortness of breath, muscle tension and aches, trembling, twitching, sweating, dizziness, nausea, and diarrhea. Headaches and irritable bowel syndrome are two medical conditions frequently associated with GAD. In the United States, GAD causes significant functional impairment and disability and accounts for 110 million disability days per annum.[4]

Specific phobias are characterized by marked fear or anxiety about a specific object or situation. The phobic object or situation almost always provokes immediate fear, and the object or situation is either avoided or endured with intense fear or anxiety.[4] Specific phobias are coded based on the phobic stimulus (animal, natural environment, blood-injection-injury, situational, or other). Most people with specific phobias have more than one phobic stimulus, and functional impairment increases with the number of phobic stimuli. Blood-injection-injury phobias may cause individuals to neglect their physical health because of the anxiety associated with provider appointments. Fear of falling in the geriatric population can lead to reduced mobility and impairments in physical health and social functioning.[4] Social anxiety disorder or social phobia involves clinically significant anxiety about one or more social situations in which the individual is exposed to possible scrutiny by others (e.g., social interactions, eating, speaking in public).[4]

Panic disorder is characterized by recurrent unexpected panic attacks. A panic attack is defined as "an abrupt surge of intense fear or intense discomfort that reaches a peak within minutes"[4] and includes four or more of the symptoms listed in Box 247-1. Panic attacks can occur within the context of any other psychiatric disorder, and to reflect this the condition was added as a specifier in the DSM-5.

OCD consists of the presence of obsessions, compulsions, or both. Obsessions are defined as recurrent thoughts, urges, or

BOX 247-1

Symptoms of a Panic Attack

- Palpitations, pounding heart, accelerated heart rate
- Sweating
- Trembling or shaking
- Feeling of choking
- Chest pain or discomfort
- Chills or hot flashes
- Nausea or abdominal distress
- Feeling dizzy, unsteady, lightheaded, faint
- Derealization or depersonalization
- Fear of losing control or going crazy
- Fear of dying
- Numbness or tingling sensations

Data from American Psychiatric Association (APA): *Diagnostic and statistical manual of mental disorders*, ed 5 (text rev), Washington, DC, 2013, APA.

images that are intrusive and unwanted. Compulsions are repetitive behaviors or acts (e.g., checking, counting, praying) that the individual feels driven to perform and are aimed at reducing anxiety or a dreaded situation. Rates of OCD are higher in individuals with body dysmorphic disorder, trichotillomania, excoriation disorder, schizophrenia, schizoaffective disorder, bipolar disorder, eating disorders, and Tourette disorder.[4] Impairment is related to severity of symptoms and can affect interpersonal relationships, occupational and academic performance, physical health, and even successful treatment of the disorder.[4]

The DSM-5 was released in May 2013 and presents a new organizational system for some of the anxiety disorders. OCD is now located in the chapter Obsessive-Compulsive and Related Disorders, which includes OCD, Body Dysmorphic Disorder, Hoarding Disorder, Trichotillomania, and Excoriation Disorder. PTSD is now included with the Trauma- and Stressor-Related Disorders along with Acute Stress Disorder and Adjustment Disorder, among others. Separation Anxiety Disorder was previously included in Disorders Usually First Diagnosed in Infancy, Childhood, or Adolescence but is now applicable to adults and is included with the Anxiety Disorders. Another change to the DSM-5 is that individuals older than 18 with Agoraphobia, Specific Phobia, and Social Anxiety Disorder need not recognize that their anxiety is excessive or unreasonable, but the anxiety must be out of proportion to the actual threat.[4]

PHYSICAL EXAMINATION

It is not surprising that individuals with anxiety disorders often fear an underlying medical disorder, given the frequency of associated physical symptoms. Many of the physical symptoms of anxiety (chest pain, shortness of breath, dizziness, and gastrointestinal symptoms) could signal a serious medical illness. Therefore, medical causes must be explored and ruled out before a diagnosis of an anxiety disorder is made.

As with any physical examination, a thorough history is required. Some symptoms of anxiety disorders are preceded by recent events of interpersonal violence, accident, or natural disaster. The potential physical injuries that follow exposure to these events could include damage to any body system; thus a full physical examination is necessary. It is also important to inquire about psychosocial stressors and a remote history of traumas or abuse because these experiences increase risk for anxiety disorders. In a large study of women ages 65 and older, nearly 14% reported a lifetime history of physical assault, sexual assault, or both, and assaults were typically repeated events.[11] Women who had experienced a history of interpersonal violence were more likely to meet criteria for PTSD and other anxiety disorders than those who had not experienced interpersonal violence.[11] Providers need to ask specific questions regarding trauma history and be prepared to refer the individual for trauma-informed care.[11]

DIAGNOSTICS

There is no laboratory test, imaging modality, or physical examination finding that can definitively diagnosis an anxiety disorder. Like all mental health diagnoses, the symptoms must meet the criteria in the DSM-5, with the symptoms being at a moderate to severe level and affecting hygiene, relationships, employment, or education. Urine toxicologies are helpful to determine substance use that may contribute to the symptoms described by the patient. It is equally important to rule out other medical conditions through a physical examination and blood work to assess for infection, anemia, electrolyte imbalance, liver or kidney dysfunction, thyroid disease, hyperparathyroidism, and glucose intolerance. The importance of ruling out exposure to the anxiety-producing effects of caffeine is often missed, but caffeine may play a critical role in anxiety. Electrocardiograms may be obtained to rule out cardiac problems with a person experiencing panic attacks. The screening tool recommended for GAD in primary care settings for anxiety disorders is the GAD 7-item instrument (GAD-7).[12] The screening tool recommended for PTSD is the Primary Care PTSD Screen (PC-PTSD).[13] The Social Phobia Inventory (SPIN) Mini-SPIN Screening Tool has three items to assess for social phobias.[14] These scales will facilitate identification of patients who require additional assessment for a psychiatric disorder.

Side effects from medications and the physiologic effects of intoxication or withdrawal from substances should be taken into account when the symptoms of anxiety disorders are reviewed. Medications, other medical conditions, and other psychiatric conditions that mimic symptoms with anxiety disorders are included in the differential diagnosis box.

DIFFERENTIAL DIAGNOSIS

Anxiety Disorders

CARDIAC
- Arrhythmias
- Angina

RESPIRATORY
- Asthma
- Chronic obstructive pulmonary disease (COPD)
- Pulmonary emboli
- Hypoxia from any origin

ENDOCRINE
- Hyperthyroidism or hypothyroidism
- Hyperglycemia or hypoglycemia
- Menopause

NEUROLOGICAL
- Delirium
- Early dementia
- Migraines
- Epilepsy
- Traumatic brain injury

MEDICATIONS AND/OR SUBSTANCES
- Caffeine
- Cocaine
- Cannabis
- Steroids
- Nicotine
- Ephedrine and pseudoephedrine
- Amphetamines
- Anticholinergics
- Theophylline
- Digoxin
- Synthroid
- Antihypertensives

OTHER MENTAL HEALTH DIAGNOSES
- Substance intoxication
- Substance withdrawal
- Major depressive disorder
- Bipolar disorder
- Dementia
- Delirium
- Somatization disorder
- Eating disorder

MANAGEMENT

A mental health consultation is indicated for individuals who are not responding to or who have partial remission of symptoms with adequate doses of first-line pharmacologic interventions.

Immediate emergency department referral is indicated for individuals who are at risk of harm to themselves or others.

TABLE 247-1 **Pharmacologic Management of Anxiety Disorders: Indications and Considerations**

Medication	GAD	Panic Disorder	PTSD	Social Phobia	OCD	Advantages	Disadvantages
Benzodiazepines	✓	✓		✓		Rapid onset of action	Risk of dependence Drowsiness Increased fall risk in elderly
Buspirone	✓					No risk of dependence	Not well tolerated Limited evidence for efficacy
Tricyclic antidepressants	✓	✓	✓		✓	May also help with insomnia No risk of dependence	Slow onset of action Lethal in overdose
SSRIs or SNRIs	✓	✓	✓	✓	✓	First-line treatment Effective also for depression	Slow onset of action Side effects may influence long-term treatment adherence

SNRIs, serotonin-norepinephrine reuptake inhibitors; SSRIs, selective serotonin reuptake inhibitors.
Modified from Davidson JR, Feltner DE, Dugar A: Management of generalized anxiety disorder in primary care: identifying the challenges and unmet needs, *Prim Care Companion J Clin Psychiatry* 12(2), 2010.

In a review of several large samples of primary care patients, only one third to one half of the patients who met the criteria for GAD were diagnosed. Once diagnosed, at least one third were still not treated.[15] One potential reason for undertreatment is the perception of providers that this presentation of anxiety is a personality quality that will not respond to treatment.

Several consensus groups have published guidelines for the management of anxiety disorders, with varying motivations from cost containment to symptom reduction. Each contains different suggestions of measuring success, from service utilization costs and return to work to self-rated symptoms and satisfaction with mental health. These various guidelines, however, are centered on the same general goals of treatment: to reduce symptoms, to improve function, to treat comorbid conditions, and to achieve long-term remission.[15,16] Several classes of medications have been approved and are indicated for use in managing symptoms of anxiety disorders. There are very few research studies available to compare the efficacy of one class of medication with another in the management of an anxiety disorder; thus, selection of an agent is largely dependent on comorbid conditions, side effects, and history of previous treatments or predominant symptoms. Table 247-1 highlights medications indicated for the treatment of anxiety disorders as well as some advantages and disadvantages of each treatment that may influence prescription choice.

1. Antidepressants are considered first-line treatment for anxiety disorders. Selective serotonin reuptake inhibitors (SSRIs) and serotonin-norepinephrine reuptake inhibitors (SNRIs) have been demonstrated in multiple studies to be effective in managing symptoms of GAD, panic disorder, PTSD, social anxiety disorder, and OCD. In some cases, a dose higher than what is recommended for the management of major depressive disorder may be required for effective treatment of anxiety. There is variability in the half-life of these agents, which should be considered in review of a patient's ability to take a medication consistently (because missed doses may cause withdrawal symptoms) or of drug-drug interactions (because a medication with a longer half-life is more likely to affect the metabolism of other medications). Although SSRIs are generally well tolerated, their initial adverse effects, including headache, restlessness, increased anxiety, nausea, fatigue, and dizziness, paired with the delayed anxiolytic effect (2 to 4 weeks) may lead to discontinuation.[17] Individuals taking SNRIs should be monitored for increases in blood pressure and should also be aware of the risk of discontinuation syndromes when missing doses or stopping the medication abruptly.[17] Providers should also educate patients on the signs and symptoms of serotonin syndrome (mental status changes, autonomic instability, and neuromuscular changes), a potentially life-threatening side effect of SSRIs and SNRIs. Long-term side effects such as weight gain and sexual dysfunction may prove intolerable for some people.[17] "Starting low and going slow" can help to increase tolerability and thus improve adherence, particularly in the geriatric population.[17] Older adults are also more vulnerable to the less-common side effects of hyponatremia, hypercoagulation, reduced bone mineral density, and serotonin syndrome.[16-19]
2. Benzodiazepines should be used with caution and because of a short onset of action (within minutes) have efficacy in acute management of symptoms of panic, social anxiety, and GAD, presumably owing to their mechanism of action: increased GABA activity. Long-term use, however, is not recommended, especially if symptoms of depression are present. There are additional problems associated with this class of medications, including increased risk of falls, confusion, and memory problems, when they are used in older adults. The most common current use of benzodiazepines is in combination with SSRIs or SNRIs for short-term management of acute symptoms. Although benzodiazepines initially seem helpful for treatment of insomnia, they change the sleep architecture and are associated with marked rebound insomnia once the medication is stopped. Prescription of benzodiazepines includes a risk of respiratory distress, physiologic dependence, and tolerance. These risks are higher for people with current or previous substance use disorders; thus benzodiazepine use is typically contraindicated in this population.[17] Benzodiazepines may alter someone's ability to drive or to meet usual expectations and must not be stopped abruptly.[15,16]
3. Buspirone is a partial agonist at the 5-hydroxytryptamine 1A receptor and has been shown to be modestly effective in the treatment of GAD. It is not approved for use in any other anxiety disorder. It may exacerbate symptoms of depression, which excludes it from use with many people because

anxiety and depression have such a high comorbidity. It is also not well tolerated, with common side effects of nausea, fatigue, and dizziness.[15,19]

4. Tricyclic antidepressants (TCAs) and older monoamine oxidase inhibitors have indications for management of some of the anxiety disorders but are not considered first line because of tolerability. Clomipramine (Anafranil), a TCA, has a specific indication for OCD; however, it does not demonstrate any advantage over newer serotonin agents. TCAs carry a high risk of cardiac dysrhythmias and are lethal in overdose; thus they are contraindicated for patients with a history of or risk for suicide.[15,17,19]
5. Atypical antipsychotics may have a role in treating refractory anxiety symptoms, but this use is off label and not considered first-line treatment. Side effects of atypical antipsychotics include metabolic syndrome, extrapyramidal side effects, sexual dysfunction, and sedation.[17] Use of any atypical psychotic must be done with attention to the longer, more complex array of side effects, especially in older adults.[19]
6. Psychotherapy interventions have been widely investigated and reviewed for efficacy in the management of anxiety disorders. The most evidence supports cognitive behavioral therapies for GAD, PTSD, panic disorder, social phobias, and OCD. These interventions should be considered first-line treatment options in tandem with medications *or* as monotherapy and should be administered by trained psychotherapists. There is no medication that has been approved for the management of specific phobias, although SSRIs may be used in severe cases.[17] Exposure, systematic desensitization, and cognitive behavioral therapies are effective to extinguish these symptoms when they are offered in a skilled setting.[15,18,20] This intensive therapy is difficult to tolerate for some people with extreme symptoms, and there is generally a high dropout rate for these treatments. For those who complete treatment, only 50% will achieve full remission of symptoms, and data are unclear about the prevalence of relapse.[15]
7. Multiple studies have demonstrated clinical benefits of physical activity in the management of anxiety symptoms.[21] The positive effects of physical activity may be at least partially a result of anti-inflammatory and antioxidant mechanisms.[21] However, a recent meta-analysis found no significant benefit of aerobic exercise for individuals with anxiety disorders.[22] Exercise should be encouraged as an adjunctive treatment, given the overall physical and psychological benefits of exercise, but at this point does not have the evidence to support it as first-line treatment for anxiety disorders.[22] Although tai chi, acupuncture, and hypnosis have offered some relief for many people with anxiety symptoms, there are no large trials to support inclusion of these methods in evidence-based guidelines.[23-26]
8. The effectiveness of any management strategy is largely dependent on one's ability to remain consistent with the intervention or treatment. Psychoeducation related to anxiety disorders and a frank discussion with the patient about medication risks and benefits may increase adherence.[17] Once a medication has been initiated for anxiety, it should be continued for 6 to 24 months and discontinued only if most or all symptoms have resolved.[17] If a patient does not respond to an adequate dose of a medication after 4 to 6 weeks, the provider should switch medications or refer to a mental health provider.[17] The number of people with anxiety disorders who believe that their treatment needs are not being met has been noted to be as high as 70%. Additional barriers to effective treatment include worries about the cost of care, lack of awareness of resources or providers, and wait time to first appointments with specialists.[27,28]

COMPLICATIONS

Anxiety disorders are associated with severe impairments in numerous areas of functioning and use of primary care services.[29] Anxiety disorders commonly co-occur with substance use, other mental health disorders, and trauma or abuse. In addition to complications consistent with an increase in substance use and unhealthy lifestyle choices, declining physical health has been directly linked in clinical and statistic models to stressful events, anxiety, and fear.[30,31]

The experience of adverse events and symptoms of anxiety in childhood has been associated with an increase in obesity, smoking, physical inactivity, and depressed mood. For example, more than 50% of people with asthma have a diagnosable anxiety disorder. These individuals are more likely to be taking a significantly higher number of medications than are people with asthma without anxiety disorders.[32] Within populations of people with other well-defined medical issues (such as diabetes and heart disease), the presence of depression or anxiety symptoms is associated with increased morbidity and mortality.[33] For example, anxiety disorders are associated with poorer outcomes in individuals with established heart failure and may increase the risk of developing heart failure.[34] Individuals with anxiety disorders report lower scores in all areas of quality of life (physical, psychological, social, and environmental) when compared with matched controls.[35]

Suicidal ideation and the risk of completed suicides are higher for any person with mental health disorders compared with matched control samples of people who do not meet DSM criteria for a diagnosis. Specifically, for men in their 40s, women in their 20s, and women in their 60s, depression and anxiety were predictive of serious suicidal ideation.[36] Six percent of participants enrolled in a study evaluating risk factors for suicidal behavior in individuals with anxiety disorders attempted suicide at some point during the follow-up period.[37] In this sample, previous suicide attempt and mood disorders were the most powerful predictors of a future suicide attempt.[37] A guideline to assess the risk of suicide is reviewed in Chapter 245.

INDICATIONS FOR REFERRAL OR HOSPITALIZATION

Resources and access to behavioral health specialists will affect the timing of referrals to consultation outside of the primary care setting. There is an increasing number of mental health providers working alongside primary care providers in the same clinic across the nation, yet typically people with anxiety disorders are still being treated by their primary care provider initially. If the primary care provider is concerned for a person's personal safety or if the person has not responded to initial interventions, has complex medical problems, or is already receiving multiple medications, then a referral should be considered.

The primary care provider should obtain emergent care if the person is in danger of causing harm to self or others. Emergent care should also be sought if the person is gravely disabled (unable to provide for basic personal needs such as food, clothing, and shelter). Emergent care would also be required for severe side effects of medications such as serotonin syndrome, serotonin withdrawal, neuroleptic malignant syndrome, or lithium toxicity.

A referral to a specialist should also be considered if other psychiatric comorbidities are present, if the symptoms are not responding to initial treatments provided in primary care clinic, or to obtain psychotherapy, family education, or group therapy services.

LIFE SPAN CONSIDERATIONS

Mood and anxiety in late life tend to decline with age in the noninstitutionalized elderly but still remain common, especially in women, according to the National Comorbidity Survey Replication (NCS-R).[38] According to the NCS-R, 7% of older adults (age 65 or older) met criteria for an anxiety disorder in the previous 12 months, although it is highly unlikely that an older adult would develop new-onset anxiety. However, adults who have experienced anxiety throughout their lives are at higher risk for having mental and physical comorbidities, and the severity of the illness may be greater. Anxiety disorders in the elderly are frequently comorbid with cognitive decline and dementia.[39] Although the symptoms are expressed the same as in younger adults, anxiety disorders may be difficult to diagnose when cognitive decline is present.

Anxiety is one of the most common mental health diagnoses in children and adolescents and may lead to increased severity with development of other comorbidities in adulthood.[40] The largest epidemiology study involving surveys of adolescents in the United States revealed that 32% of the 10,000 children aged 13 to 18 years met symptom criteria for an anxiety disorder. Half of them began having symptoms before age 6.[41] The anxiety disorder in children and adolescents is often identified by the primary care provider because presenting complaints often include avoiding age-appropriate tasks or excessive physical complaints that are not substantiated by a physical examination.

EDUCATION AND HEALTH PROMOTION

It is important for family members of those having experienced a known trauma to be given education about the potential sequelae. Loved ones are encouraged to support and validate the survivor's experience of trauma, thereby increasing their protective factors by offering a safe environment where the experience can be discussed. There should also be an opportunity for the person to discuss the trauma and ongoing issues with a therapist. Trauma-Focused Cognitive Behavioral Therapy is the most effective therapy used for children and adolescents who have experienced a trauma.[42]

The most sophisticated studies demonstrating positive outcomes with people diagnosed with anxiety disorders use cognitive behavioral treatment.[43] Therapies may be offered if a person or parent of a child does not want to start medication, although studies using a combination of therapy and medications show the most promising results.[43] Cognitive behavioral treatment minimizes the likelihood of remission of symptoms. Families may engage in this process to better understand how to recognize warning signs of increased risk for distress and possible relapse. Behavioral therapy is recommended for persons with specific phobias or OCD.[43]

There are several Internet sites available for information and support for patients and families. They include the following:

National Alliance on Mental Illness: www.nami.org
National Institute of Mental Health: www.nimh.nih.gov/health/topics/anxiety-disorders/index.shtml
Anxiety and Depression Association of American: www.adaa.org
National Center for PTSD: www.ptsd.va.gov

Although people cannot change their genetic predisposition to mental illness, they can buffer the effects of stress and exposure to traumatic events. It is important to maintain good physical health, adequate nutrition, healthy weight and exercise routines, and appropriate sleep patterns, and to incorporate stress management techniques into the lifestyle. The primary care provider is in the privileged role of often being the first person to learn of a patient's anxiety or traumatic experience. Regardless of external pressures of time and schedule, the provider's response during this initial disclosure is critical. A validating, supportive, resourceful encounter enhances the patient's preexisting protective factors and ability to cope, thus supporting early intervention and treatment.

CHAPTER 248

MOOD DISORDERS

J. Nile Wagley

Normal variations exist in mood (emotional state) and affect (outward display of mood). Factors including age, personality development, and genetically predisposed temperament influence how any one person may interpret events, behave, and modulate his or her emotions. Specific criteria exist to separate these normal displays of personality and coping styles from episodes of diagnosable mood disorders that may benefit from treatment. Mood disorders, according to the fifth edition of the *Diagnostic and Statistical Manual of Mental Disorders* (DSM-5), are defined by mood episodes.[1]

A major depressive episode describes a condition in which a person has depressed mood or anhedonia (loss of interest or sense of pleasure) *and* four of the following symptoms: unintended change in weight, sleep disturbance, psychomotor agitation or retardation, fatigue, feelings of worthlessness or guilt, inability to concentrate, and recurrent thoughts of death or thoughts of suicide.

A manic episode is defined by a period of time (at least one week) during which a person's mood is abnormally elevated, expansive, or irritable in addition to at least three of the following symptoms: inflated self-esteem (grandiosity), decreased need for sleep without fatigue, pressured speech, racing thoughts, distractibility, psychomotor agitation, and excessive involvement in pleasure-seeking activities that may have high risk for undesirable consequences (excessive spending, sexual indiscretions).[1]

A mixed episode is present when symptoms of both major depressive and manic episodes are present nearly every day for a week or more and these symptoms are not related to a medication effect or substance. Like manic and major depressive episodes, a mixed episode can be diagnosed only when the symptoms cause marked impairment in one's ability to participate in usual activities and to function at previous expectations.[1]

A hypomanic episode describes symptoms of a manic episode that are shorter in duration and do not match the severity of a manic episode and thus are not associated with such marked impairment of function. Hypomanic episodes are not debilitating enough to warrant hospitalization or to lead to dangerous consequences.[1]

By use of the DSM-5 as a guide, diagnosis of a mood disorder includes consideration of psychosocial stressors. A major depressive or mood episode may follow a stressful event or traumatic experience. Often, family members and providers attribute some symptoms as appropriate coping in response to such an event. This bias, however, may delay access to treatment and result in additional complications in medical health, further coping, and overall prognosis. A person's response to the loss of a loved one is an example of this risk.

GRIEF AND BEREAVEMENT

Bereavement is currently not defined in DSM-5. The "V-Code" (which was established in DSM-IV to signify a condition that is the focus of clinical treatment but may not be a mental disorder) no longer exists in DSM-5. DSM-5 does refer to bereavement; it recommends that good clinical judgment be exercised in considering depressive symptoms when the loss of loved ones has occurred. Previously, a "bereavement exclusion" existed that prevented the diagnosis of certain depressive syndromes after the loss of a loved one. This has been removed in DSM-5 in acknowledgement that the loss of a loved one can precede or even precipitate severe depressive symptoms. DSM-5 contains Section III (Emerging Measures and Models), which lists Persistent Complex Bereavement Disorder under Conditions for Further Study but not as an official diagnosis. Although the DSM-5 seems to have carefully balanced its ability to provide standardized language for continuity of care with its desire to have continued usefulness as a billing tool, the underlying principles of bereavement and grief as part of our human experience have not changed. The International Classification of Diseases, Tenth Revision (ICD-10) classifies bereavement as a billable code: Z63.4. Both coding systems categorize grief as a condition that may be the focus of treatment; however, it is not considered a mental illness.[1,2] The terms *grief* and *bereavement* are used interchangeably in this section. Grief is associated with a wide range of emotions, including sadness, anger, guilt, and despair. Because no one is immune to loss, no age group or culture escapes the potential complications of grief.

According to the 2012 World Health Organization (WHO) data published in 2014, there were 56 million deaths globally, nearly one in nine deaths throughout the world was of a child younger than 5 years.[3] It is estimated that each death leaves an average of five people bereaved, resulting in almost 13 million people grieving each year in the United States alone.[4]

Grieving usually occurs after a person experiences the death of a family member, spouse, child, close friend, or pet. A grief response can also occur with other losses, such as a job or career loss, loss of physical health or abilities, miscarriage, divorce, financial loss, or the diminishing health of a spouse or loved one. The initial painful experience of disbelief, shock, loss, and sadness is often followed by a sense of emptiness, hopelessness, and loss of interest in usual activities, followed by a prolonged phase of restitution and recovery, which for many individuals represents a departure from the state of health and well-being to which they are accustomed.[5-7]

The length of the grief response varies. Elizabeth Kübler-Ross is credited with defining the five stages of grief that most people experience. She postulated that individuals experience periods of denial, anger, bargaining, depression, and acceptance.[8] The process of grieving is ongoing, does not follow a rigid order or time frame, and may vary or even skip stages. Not all of the stages of grief are necessarily obvious. They may be repeated many times and are often not completed before the process of moving through another stage.

Cultures have different ways of expressing and coping with grief. Some cultures expect and encourage expressions of grief, whereas in other cultures these expressions are suppressed. People of a certain heritage may have varying degrees of connection to traditional practices of their culture. The clinician should be cautious and not assume what may be a "normal" expectation of recovery or expression for any patient after a loss. The grieving patients themselves are the best source of information about cultural practices and beliefs around death. Only they can accurately represent how their values, traditions, and beliefs influence their grieving.

Gender and age differences in grief responses have been categorized and described in the literature. It has recently been suggested, however, that characteristics of coping style, preexisting mental health, and ability to provide help to others after the loss are more robust factors associated with recovery (absence of development of persistent depressive or anxiety symptoms).[5-9]

Physical complaints, which are often vague, are common during the grieving period. Office visits to the health care provider may become more frequent. Sleep and appetite disturbances are often reported. Women have been reported to have more illness and disability than men after the death of a family member.[10] If a person has been a caregiver to a loved one recently deceased, that person may have neglected his or her own personal health for months or years. The provider must be careful not to minimize somatic complaints during the period acutely following a loss.

Symptoms commonly associated with grief, such as sadness, low energy, and sleep and appetite disturbances, overlap with the symptoms of a major depressive episode as described earlier. Table 248-1 highlights some differences according to DSM diagnostic criteria for a depressed mood episode and symptom descriptions of grief.

The DSM-5 has proposed criteria for a Persistent Complex Bereavement Disorder with a unique constellation of symptoms. A 2009 paper reviewed the development and validation of symptom criteria, identifying Persistent Complex Bereavement Disorder as a distinct syndrome, separate from any mood or anxiety disorder described elsewhere in the text. The authors also suggested that identification of this disorder within 12 months of a loss has predictive value, citing the relative risk for development of comorbid anxiety and mood disorders or demonstration of marked functional impairment.[2]

Social support is critical after a loss. Providers should be aware of local resources for caregivers of patients with dementias or cancers, including support groups as well as therapists and social workers available for individual counseling. After a traumatic loss, however, social support may be so powerful as to mediate the effect of the loss and prevent symptoms that may lead to a diagnosis of post-traumatic stress disorder.

TABLE 248-1 Assessing Symptoms of Grief and a Depressive Mood Episode

Symptom	Common in Grief	Concerning for Depressive Mood Episode
Guilt	Specific to actions or behaviors at the time of death of loved one	Generalized and grandiose, not specific to one person or event
Thoughts of death	"Should have died with/instead of" the deceased	Pervasive and persistent with possible planning for self-injury
Sense of worthlessness	Helplessness specific to cause or circumstances of death	Pervasive and persistent sense of worthlessness and hopelessness
Psychomotor slowing	Limited time; days to weeks	Pervasive and persistent for more than 2 weeks
Functional impairment	Episodic; if consistent throughout all areas of function, limited to less than 2 months	Consistently impaired throughout all domains; inability to work, to engage with others, and to maintain basic self-care
Hallucinations	Only in relation to the deceased, such as hearing the deceased's voice or feeling as if the person were nearby	Not related to a specific person or event

Medication is commonly used for short-term symptom relief as indicated but should not be considered a first-line treatment when more effective therapies such as psychotherapy are available. Benzodiazepines (clonazepam, lorazepam, and alprazolam) prescribed in small doses for infrequent use may be helpful for symptoms of anxiety associated with grief, but the benefits gained may not be worth the side effects and inherent risk associated with these medications. Antidepressants may be indicated for some persons after a loss. If there is a previous history of a major depressive episode (before the loss) or additional history of trauma, a person may be more vulnerable to the development of a depressive disorder after the stress of the loss of a loved one. There is no evidence that normal bereavement requires professional intervention.[11] When considering treatment for complex bereavement, it has been demonstrated that psychotropic medication and supportive talk therapies have little impact. However, Complicated Grief Treatment (CGT) is a combination of cognitive behavioral interventions such as interpersonal psychotherapy and motivational interviewing that focuses on repeatedly revisiting and coming to terms with the loss while reengaging in life.[12] Prescribing practices should follow the guidelines described later in the section on management of depressive disorders.

Evidence is well established for the effectiveness of cognitive behavioral therapy in treating anxiety and depressive symptoms related to bereavement. Analyses continue to best determine who is most likely to benefit from this intensive therapy.[13] Primary care providers and family members can support recovery of the bereaved by supporting and encouraging completion of structured cognitive behavioral programs; the evidence suggests that if people are able to complete the program, they significantly benefit.[13]

Although loss indiscriminately affects people of all ages, ethnicity, and gender, many styles of coping exist. Because of this variation, characteristics of the bereaved are associated with different responses to treatment. Children may fear abandonment or the loss of others they love, and they may feel guilt or responsibility for the loss. They may begin to have behavioral problems at home or school. The loss of a parent in childhood is associated with more behavioral issues and psychosocial problems in adulthood. This may be related to the available coping skills of the child and the ability of remaining caregivers to be healthy supports. When children are included in the treatment of bereavement, such as with a family bereavement program, they have less-problematic symptoms related to the loss.[14]

Approximately 15% of pregnancies end in miscarriage; mothers and fathers often react differently, but both have high rates of persistent symptoms of bereavement that affect relationships, mood, physical health, and productivity months to years after the loss. Involvement in counseling sessions as a couple (as few as three sessions) can significantly reduce the prevalence of symptoms for both grieving parents.[15]

Older adults who lose their life partner are more at risk for complications in bereavement, including additional physical health problems and development of mental illnesses such as major depressive disorder (MDD) or PTSD. In a sample of nearly 300 bereaved elder adults, 16% met criteria for PTSD within 3 months of the loss and maintained this diagnosis for at least 18 months after the death of a spouse.[16] After a loss, people of all age groups are at higher risk for substance abuse and suicide.

DEPRESSIVE DISORDERS

DEFINITION AND EPIDEMIOLOGY

Major depressive disorder (referred to as MDD or depression throughout this chapter) is the most common of the depressive disorders and is diagnosed when all criteria are met for at least one major depressive episode, without history of manic or hypomanic behavior. Persistent Depressive Disorder (a consolidation of the DSM-IV–defined diagnoses Dysthymic Disorder and Chronic Major Depressive Disorder) describes a longer-term, persistent presentation of depressed mood accompanied by few or no episodes of positive mood or affect. The symptoms must not be better explained by any other medical or psychiatric condition, must cause marked impairment in function, and must be prominent for more days than not in a 2-week period for a diagnosis of MDD and a 2-year period for Dysthymic Disorder. The diagnosis Depressive Disorder Not Otherwise Specified (NOS) is used to describe patterns of symptoms that do not fit into these categories, yet for which depressed mood remains the predominant symptom.

WHO has developed a method for evaluating disease burden beyond mortality statistics. A report published in 2012, which reviewed statistics for 2014, analyzed causes of death and burden of injury and illness globally, by region, by gender, by age, and by national income. In this publication, WHO identified depression as the leading cause of disability in the world. Depression is already a major contributor to global disease burden. By 2020, it is estimated that depression will be the leading cause of overall disease burden across the globe (combining years of healthy life lost and mortality data), regardless of age, gender, or income.[3] In addition to lost work time and impairment in interpersonal and role functioning, people with MDD have been noted to use medical services at an increased rate. For example, a study of Medicaid recipients found that people with MDD receive the majority of their care in the general (primary care) setting. They cost the system more than twice (2.33) as much as someone without a diagnosable mental health problem in areas of general medical care and drug costs. Specialty care (mental health) was less used by those with MDD, and overall costs were surpassed only by those with diagnoses of bipolar disorder and psychotic disorders.[17]

Information on the epidemiology of MDD comes primarily from four large studies since the publication of the DSM-III in 1980. On the basis of these studies and the WHO data, the prevalence of lifetime depression in adults aged 18 to 65 years is 13% to 16%, with 5.3% to 8.6% of this population currently meeting criteria for the diagnosis.[18,19]

Women are approximately twice as likely as men to experience MDD in their lifetime. Adults aged 30 to 60 years have the highest rates of MDD, in samples of people younger than 65 years. The first diagnosed depressive episode was noted to occur at approximately 30 years of age, yet clinical reports and guidelines suggest that the first episode of MDD most often occurs at ages 18 to 22 years.[1] Of greater concern, treatment is often not sought until approximately 3 years after the onset of symptoms.

The National Comorbidity Survey (Replication) found that people identified as Hispanic or non-Hispanic black were less likely than non-Hispanic whites to have depression.[19] This differs greatly from the original reports of the 1980s and data from the original National Comorbidity Survey. Research consistently suggests no differences in prevalence of depression by education, urban versus rural, access to care, or geographic region; however, a disparity still exists in response to treatment, with those of a higher income status having better outcomes. The disparity is hypothesized to be related to the exposure to chronic stress in populations with less resources.[20]

Two specific populations have been omitted from these large-scale studies: (1) the elderly and (2) children and adolescents. Prevalence rates for these age groups vary widely, perhaps because of the complexity of changing roles, developing personalities, cognitive development or deterioration, and medical comorbidities. Several studies that screened adolescents for subclinical depression found rates as high as 30%.[21] Rates of diagnosed MDD are less clear, yet correlates of medical illness and impaired function match those of their adult counterparts. With control for the effects of medical illness, screening positive for probable depressive disorder was associated with poorer functioning in overall role activity and less educational achievement. Clinically, available interventions are offered when subclinical symptoms have been identified, thereby ideally reducing later complications of adult MDD.

In general, the prevalence of MDD has been noted to be slightly lower in older adults (>65 years) than in those 30 to 60 years of age. Although prevalence rates in older adults are 4% to 8%, the incidence (number of new cases in 1 year) has been noted to be as high as 15%.[22] Estimates of MDD in older adults vary widely by setting. Healthy older adults living in the community have an estimated prevalence of MDD of 3%. Of those who frequently access primary care services, rates increase to 17% to 37%, and 12% to 30% of those living in long-term care facilities meet diagnostic criteria for MDD.[23] Factors such as physical illness, hospitalization, death of a partner, and cognitive decline are more powerful predictors of MDD than is age alone. It is expected that as the retiring generation lives longer (women outliving men), with more medical problems, more hospitalizations, and less income, rates of MDD will continue to trend higher.

PATHOPHYSIOLOGY

With technologic advances allowing the evaluation of brain metabolism, neurotransmitter activity, and subtle differences in size of regions of the brain, literature related to the pathophysiology of neurologic disorders is abundant. Several theories have emerged for the biologic genesis of depression. Increased blood flow in the amygdala region and dysfunction in the limbic-prefrontal cortex communication systems have been identified in people with MDD.[24,25] Cortisol levels have been evaluated and explored as a potential measure for diagnosis of MDD. Studies have found increased basal levels of cortisol in people with depression as well as a general dysregulation of the stress response function that mediates cortisol. The hypothalamus-pituitary-adrenal axis is responsible for regulating the body's response to stress and is mediated by cortisol release. In people with MDD, it is slower to recover from stress stimuli.[26] Disruption of sleep patterns has been strongly associated with the occurrence of MDD, yet it remains unclear whether this is a risk factor or sequela of the disorder.[1]

The biologic theory that has the strongest implication for pharmacologic treatment involves the relationship between synaptic levels of neurotransmitters and MDD. Although norepinephrine and dopamine levels are implicated in symptom manifestation, the strongest research associates lower levels of serotonin with the diagnosis of MDD. Other studies suggest that rather than having a central role in the modulation of mood and sleep, serotonin levels may be more closely linked with the regulation of other neurobiologic systems in the brain designed to respond to stressful or emotional stimuli. Much of the research on serotonergic activity has been driven by the pharmaceutical companies and is therefore difficult to interpret at times. Advanced technology is now being used to explore the role of glutamate and melatonin and will have remarkable implications for predicting risk and future pharmaceutical interventions.[27]

Depression has a strong familial association; MDD is 1.5 to 3 times more common in first-degree biologic relatives of those with the disorder compared with the general population.[1] Environmental factors and personality development are closely linked with coping styles. Psychodynamic theories of the manifestation of mental illness include the need for mastery of developmental tasks, the healthy interpretation of events, and successful interpersonal interactions. Logically, children of parents with depressive symptoms are more inclined to develop difficulties with role functioning, including behavioral problems, substance abuse, and depressed mood.[1] Although some twin studies suggested a genetic predisposition, genetic variations have not been shown to increase the risk for depression.[28]

CLINICAL PRESENTATION

The majority of people with depressive disorders are seen by their health care providers for initial treatment, yet they may not identify the depressive symptoms as their chief complaint. Many patients may focus on vague somatic concerns rather than identifying or sharing emotions such as sadness or hopelessness. Family members or a provider who has established rapport with the patient may notice increased irritability. Irritability is likely to be the predominant symptom in children, whereas depressed mood and hopelessness are more apparent in adults, and somatic concerns dominate older adults' presentation. Loss of interest or pleasure in previously enjoyable events and social withdrawal are almost always present. Appetite is usually less than normal, and insomnia is prevalent yet may be missed because the person with depression may complain of fatigue or anergia without significant physical stimuli. Preoccupations with perceived personal deficits along with an exaggerated sense of guilt or worthlessness are also common. Impaired concentration, difficulty with decision-making, and mild memory impairment are possible and must not be confused with cognitive changes associated with dementia. Thoughts of death vary from "the world would be better off without me" to engaging in dangerous behaviors without concern for personal safety and to having specific plans for suicide.[1]

Depression is often a chronic condition. Depressive episodes may be separated by periods of partial or full recovery of varying lengths of time. Of people who have experienced one depressive episode, 60% are likely to have another; 70% of those who have had two depressive episodes are likely to have a third, and 90% of those who have had three episodes will have more. Five percent to 10% of people who have a depressive episode may later have a manic episode. Factors such as incomplete recovery, comorbid substance use, and personality disorders may have some predictive value in estimating the course of the illness, with these factors associated with more frequent episodes and increased severity of impairment.[29]

The presentation, communication, and interpretation of symptoms related to depressive disorders can be complicated by culture because research shows that the cultural background of the provider affects how those symptoms are interpreted. In the broadest of definitions, culture refers to the context in which one was raised and the norms with which one identifies. Family patterns, religious beliefs, societal and generational norms, and past experience all influence how symptoms of mental health problems are disclosed. A strong patient-provider relationship enhances the ability to detect and effectively manage mental health problems, regardless of cultural expectations or differences in subtle presentations of symptoms.

PHYSICAL EXAMINATION

During a clinical visit, the provider can elicit risk factors for depression through careful interview. Psychosocial stressors, sleep patterns, nutritional habits, and physical activity can be important indicators of a depressive disorder because many of these realms are often impaired when depression is present. Many people may come to the health care provider with vague somatic concerns. Even when depression is suspected, all other medical and psychiatric diagnoses must be explored through comprehensive history and physical examination. Many medical conditions and medications are associated with symptoms of depression, and complications of common medical conditions (including mortality) are greater in people who have also been diagnosed with MDD.[17,22]

DIAGNOSTICS

Currently, no laboratory tests or imaging studies can definitively diagnose MDD, in spite of the progress made in the exploration of biologic correlates of mental illness. Blood tests to evaluate nutritional, endocrine, and thyroid function are critical in ruling out medical, reversible causes for presenting symptoms. Imaging of the head and cardiac stress tests may also be helpful in considering ischemic disease, emboli, and traumatic injury as complicating factors.

MDD is diagnosed by interview, when criteria are met for a depressive episode and there is no history of manic or hypomanic behavior. A depressive episode is present when five of the following symptoms occur, more days than not, in a 2-week period and cause significant impairment in any realm of functioning: depressed mood, loss of interest or pleasure, significant unintended change in weight or appetite, significant change in sleep pattern, change in psychomotor activity (increased restlessness or psychomotor retardation), fatigue or loss of energy, feelings of worthlessness or guilt, impaired concentration or decision-making ability, and recurrent thoughts of death or suicide. At least one of the symptoms must be depressed mood (subjective or observed) or anhedonia (loss of pleasure), and symptoms must not be better explained by another medical or psychiatric disorder.[1]

Several structured interviews are available for the diagnosis of depressive disorders. The Structured Clinical Interview for DSM Disorders can be separated into modules for specific disorders. The Hamilton Depression Scale and the Beck Depression Inventory involve self-report of symptoms and do not require interviewer time. The Geriatric Depression Scale offers the ability to better assess the presence of depression that may be complicated by multiple physical conditions or medication effects common in the older population. The Primary Care Evaluation of Mental Disorders (PRIME-MD) is a tool designed for the use of health care providers in their daily practice, considering the pressures of time in the outpatient clinical setting.

Specifiers that further describe the characteristics of the disorder may be included but are more commonly diagnosed by a mental health provider. These include depression with the following characteristics:

- With or without psychotic features
- o: That is chronic
- i: With catatonic features
- c: With melancholic features
- m: With atypical features
- a: With postpartum onset
- p: That is a single episode or recurrent
- i: With seasonal pattern

The diagnostic criteria for MDD must be initially met, and the specifiers are used only to describe the pattern of onset or predominant symptom presentation.[1]

A diagnosis of Persistent Depressive Disorder (formerly know as Dysthymic Disorder) requires the presence of depressed mood (subjectively or reported by others) for more days than not during a 2-year period accompanied by two of the following: poor appetite or overeating, insomnia or hypersomnia, low energy, low self-esteem, poor concentration, and feelings of hopelessness. The presence of any specific mood episode must be excluded, and the symptoms must not be better accounted for by another medical or psychiatric diagnosis. Persistent Depressive Disorder is less common than MDD and often has an earlier onset. Children are more commonly seen with irritability rather than reporting depressed mood. The prevalence of Dysthymic Disorder is lower than that of MDD, with a lifetime community prevalence of 6%; however, Dysthymic Disorder may precede MDD. In these cases, the likelihood of full remission between episodes is decreased.[1]

Depressive Disorder NOS includes some symptoms of other depressive disorders, although full criteria for another diagnosis are not met because of duration of symptoms or severity of functional impairment. This category is also often used when medical or other psychiatric complications have not yet been fully explored, yet all symptoms for a major depressive episode are met.[1]

DIFFERENTIAL DIAGNOSIS

Patients with the following conditions may have sad mood, anhedonia, fatigue, and change in appetite: viral infection, hypothyroidism, hypoparathyroidism, hypoadrenocorticism, leukemia, lymphoma, cancer (pancreatic and others), cerebrovascular disease (transient ischemic attacks, stroke, vascular dementia), myocardial infarction, vitamin B_{12} deficiency, malnutrition, and concussion. When onset and intensity of depressive symptoms parallel the pattern of the medical illness yet persist in the context of optimum treatment for the medical condition, mood disorder resulting from a general medical condition with depressive features can be diagnosed.[1] Treatment options mirror those of MDD, and optimum treatment of depressive symptoms is associated with better overall prognosis.

DIFFERENTIAL DIAGNOSIS

Mood Disorders

MEDICAL CONDITIONS
- Traumatic or acquired injury (including spinal cord or head trauma, especially concussion)
- Seizure disorder
- Delirium
- Viral infection
- Hypothyroidism or thyrotoxicosis
- Hypoparathyroidism
- Hypoadrenocorticism
- Cancer (including lymphomas)
- Astrocytoma
- Encephalopathy
- Cerebrovascular disease
- Myocardial infarction
- Vitamin B_{12} deficiency
- Malnutrition

MEDICATIONS
- Cardiovascular drugs
- Antiparkinsonian drugs
- Antianxiety or sedative agents
- Anti-inflammatory medications
- Anti-infectives, antibiotics
- Stimulants
- Hormones
- Antihistamines

OTHER PSYCHIATRIC CONDITIONS
- Schizoaffective disorder
- Schizophrenia and other psychotic disorders
- PTSD
- Substance use disorders
- Other anxiety disorders and phobias
- Attention deficit disorders

Many medications cause side effects similar to depressive symptoms. Cardiovascular drugs such as clonidine and beta blockers may cause sedation and fatigue. Antiparkinsonian drugs such as levodopa and amantadine may be associated with psychomotor slowing. Antianxiety or sedative medications such as benzodiazepines may not be metabolized in the older person as quickly as expected, and accumulated metabolites may lead to general central nervous system depressive effects. Anti-inflammatory and antibiotic medications, stimulants, hormones, and antihistamines all may have an additional impact on the older adult. These potential medication effects must be considered and offending medications eliminated, when possible, to evaluate for a new diagnosis of MDD.

MANAGEMENT

Management begins with a therapeutic alliance and thorough assessment. Included in this assessment must be an evaluation of the patient's safety (see the section on suicide). Once symptoms have been assessed and other medical causes excluded or treated, the provider needs to consider the most appropriate setting for treatment. In the primary care setting, the provider must be able to follow indicators of recovery, the functional status of the patient with and without treatment, and the degree to which treatment is effective, as well as provide ongoing patient and family education. When the patient is referred elsewhere for psychiatric services, the primary care provider remains the central figure in managing and coordinating treatment.

Several classes of medications have emerged for the treatment of depression. Monoamine oxidase inhibitors (MAOIs) and tricyclic antidepressants (TCAs) were the standard of care until the first selective serotonin reuptake inhibitor (SSRI) was approved for use in the late 1980s. This was closely followed by the emergence of serotonin-norepinephrine reuptake inhibitors (SNRIs). Although these agents are relatively equal in efficacy of reducing symptoms of MDD alone, SSRIs and SNRIs offer a gentler side effect profile, have fewer drug interactions, and are less likely to be lethal in overdose.[30] MAOIs increase the level of tyramine, making it necessary for patients taking these drugs to restrict ingestion of tyramine-containing foods to avoid dangerous cardiotoxic effects. TCAs carry a risk of arrhythmia, are highly anticholinergic, and are lethal in overdose.[30] The newer, atypical agents (SNRIs) alter levels of norepinephrine in addition to serotonin with consistent efficacy in the management of depressive symptoms; however, they have some additional variations in side effect profile compared with the SSRIs.

Given equal efficacy among the general classes of medications, specific agents should be chosen on the basis of individual considerations of predominant symptoms, potential side effects, risk for interactions, and comorbid conditions.[30] Table 248-2 lists some of the adverse reactions to be considered in selection of an antidepressant. For example, an older adult woman with insomnia and decreased appetite may benefit from mirtazapine because it is likely to cause somnolence and to stimulate appetite. In this case, the individual or her caregivers must also be aware of the risk for hypotension with mirtazapine because it may increase her risk for injury related to dizziness or falls. Box 248-1 includes basic tips for prescribing antidepressant medications.

Once an agent has been selected, the initial dose should be maintained for 1 to 2 weeks before increasing to the target dose. Faster titrations are safe within an inpatient or supervised setting but may be associated with higher incidence of side effects. A trial of 4 to 8 weeks is necessary to determine effectiveness or response.[30] Once MDD is diagnosed and treated for the first time and symptoms are managed with an acceptable dose, medications should continue for 6 to 9 months. The likelihood

TABLE 248-2 Side Effects of Common Antidepressants

	Prevalence			
Adverse Reaction	**High (>30%)**	**Moderate (10%-30%)**	**Low (2%-10%)**	**Very Low (<2%)**
Drowsiness, fatigue, or sedation	Mirtazapine Trazodone Amitriptyline	Citalopram Fluoxetine Fluvoxamine Paroxetine Sertraline Venlafaxine	Duloxetine Escitalopram Bupropion Nortriptyline Desvenlafaxine	
Insomnia		Citalopram Fluoxetine Duloxetine Escitalopram Fluvoxamine Paroxetine Sertraline Bupropion Venlafaxine Desvenlafaxine (doses ≥100 mg)	Mirtazapine Trazodone Amitriptyline Desvenlafaxine	Nortriptyline
Excitement		Fluvoxamine Sertraline Bupropion Venlafaxine	Citalopram Fluoxetine Escitalopram Paroxetine Mirtazapine Nortriptyline Desvenlafaxine	Duloxetine Trazodone Amitriptyline
Confusion		Fluoxetine Amitriptyline Nortriptyline	Fluvoxamine Mirtazapine Bupropion Venlafaxine	Citalopram Duloxetine Escitalopram Paroxetine Sertraline Trazodone Desvenlafaxine
Headache		Citalopram Fluoxetine Escitalopram Fluvoxamine Paroxetine Sertraline Bupropion Venlafaxine Desvenlafaxine	Mirtazapine Trazodone Amitriptyline	Duloxetine Nortriptyline
Dry mouth	Mirtazapine Amitriptyline	Citalopram Fluoxetine Duloxetine Fluvoxamine Paroxetine Sertraline Bupropion Venlafaxine Desvenlafaxine Trazodone Nortriptyline	Escitalopram	

TABLE 248-2 Side Effects of Common Antidepressants—cont'd

	Prevalence			
Adverse Reaction	**High (>30%)**	**Moderate (10%-30%)**	**Low (2%-10%)**	**Very Low (<2%)**
Constipation		Duloxetine Fluvoxamine Paroxetine Mirtazapine Bupropion Venlafaxine Amitriptyline Nortriptyline	Citalopram Fluoxetine Escitalopram Sertraline Trazodone Desvenlafaxine	
Sweating		Citalopram Fluvoxamine Paroxetine Bupropion Venlafaxine Desvenlafaxine Amitriptyline	Fluoxetine Duloxetine Escitalopram Sertraline Mirtazapine	Trazodone Nortriptyline
Tremor		Fluoxetine Fluvoxamine Paroxetine Sertraline Bupropion Amitriptyline Nortriptyline	Citalopram Duloxetine Escitalopram Mirtazapine Venlafaxine Desvenlafaxine Trazodone	
Orthostatic hypotension or dizziness		Fluoxetine Paroxetine Sertraline Venlafaxine Trazodone Amitriptyline	Citalopram Duloxetine Escitalopram Fluvoxamine Mirtazapine Bupropion Nortriptyline Desvenlafaxine (dizziness)	Desvenlafaxine (orthostatic hypotension)
Electrocardiographic changes		Amitriptyline	Trazodone Nortriptyline	Citalopram Fluoxetine Duloxetine Escitalopram Fluvoxamine Paroxetine Sertraline Mirtazapine Bupropion Venlafaxine Desvenlafaxine
Nausea, diarrhea, or vomiting	Fluvoxamine Sertraline Venlafaxine	Citalopram Fluoxetine Duloxetine Escitalopram Paroxetine Bupropion Trazodone Desvenlafaxine	Mirtazapine Amitriptyline	Nortriptyline

Continued

TABLE 248-2 Side Effects of Common Antidepressants—cont'd

	Prevalence			
Adverse Reaction	**High (>30%)**	**Moderate (10%-30%)**	**Low (2%-10%)**	**Very Low (<2%)**
Rash			Fluoxetine Fluvoxamine Sertraline Bupropion Venlafaxine Amitriptyline	Citalopram Duloxetine Paroxetine Mirtazapine Escitalopram Trazodone Nortriptyline Desvenlafaxine
Weight gain	Mirtazapine Amitriptyline	Paroxetine	Citalopram Fluoxetine Escitalopram Sertraline Fluvoxamine Trazodone Nortriptyline	Duloxetine Bupropion Venlafaxine Desvenlafaxine
Sexual disturbance	Citalopram Fluoxetine Fluvoxamine Paroxetine Sertraline Venlafaxine	Mirtazapine	Duloxetine Escitalopram Amitriptyline Desvenlafaxine (0%-4% in men)	Bupropion Trazodone Nortriptyline Desvenlafaxine

Note: All medications that influence the serotonin system are associated with increased risk of bleeding, especially if they are used concomitantly with nonsteroidal anti-inflammatory or anticoagulation treatments.
Data from Work Group on Major Depressive Disorder: Practice guideline for the treatment of patients with major depressive disorder, ed 3, Washington, DC, 2010, American Psychiatric Association.

BOX 248-1

Prescribing Tips

- Some people will respond to antidepressants at initial doses.
- Higher doses of SSRIs and SNRIs may be more effective if there is a comorbid anxiety disorder.
- Reduce starting doses by 50% in older adults, people with impaired renal function, or those especially sensitive to side effects.
- Refer to package inserts for contraindications in people with severe renal or hepatic impairment and when switching to a new antidepressant (tapering and washout periods are necessary for some agents).
- Serotonin syndrome (confusion, hyperreflexia, myoclonus, fever) may occur when more than one serotonergic agent is prescribed.
- Serotonin withdrawal (influenza-like symptoms, anxiety) may occur when an SSRI is stopped suddenly.
- The risk for suicide is not necessarily reduced by antidepressant medication.

Data from Work Group on Major Depressive Disorder: *Practice guideline for the treatment of patients with major depressive disorder,* ed 3, Washington, DC, 2010, American Psychiatric Association.

of recurrent episodes increases if full remission of symptoms is not initially achieved. If there is an inadequate response to treatment after 6 weeks, the provider should conduct a thorough reassessment of the diagnosis, side effects, psychosocial stressors, and adherence to therapy recommendations. If treatment has thus far included medications alone, psychotherapy should be recommended. If symptoms persist beyond another 8 weeks with poor response to treatment, a referral may be made to a prescribing mental health provider to change agents, to consider augmentation strategies, or to review for additional treatment options. Once someone has experienced a third depressive episode, lifelong treatment with medications is recommended.[30]

Psychotherapy is effective at reducing symptoms of depression. If it is used alone, a longer course of treatment is expected before full remission of initial symptoms. Many studies suggest that a combination of medications and therapy offers the best odds for recovery.[30] Several types of therapy have demonstrated this effectiveness in clinical trials, including interpersonal therapy, cognitive therapy, behavioral therapy, combination cognitive behavioral therapy, and brief dynamic therapy. All psychotherapy requires a referral to a specialty provider.

Complementary agents available for the treatment of depressed mood include S-adenosylmethionine (SAM-e) and St. John's wort. The evidence for the efficacy of these interventions is not definitive. St. John's wort also affects the metabolism of other medications, thus risking additional drug-drug interactions and side effects.[30]

Nutrition plays a role in mood. Glycemic variability, vitamin deficiencies, and electrolyte imbalances may all be enhanced or stabilized with the benefit of improved mood. It is clear that adequate intake of good nutritional value has a role in the management and perhaps the prevention of mild to moderate symptoms of depression. Strategies of supplementation, however, are not validated in the literature for the treatment of MDD.

Bright light therapy has been researched for efficacy in the management of depression with seasonal and nonseasonal patterns. Although large clinical trials are still lacking, there is some evidence to suggest that it produces a modest improvement in symptoms of depressed mood, especially for people who also have sleep disorders or a seasonal pattern of depressed mood. It should also be considered for women who are pregnant and wish to avoid the risks of medications during pregnancy.

Electroconvulsive therapy (ECT) may be considered after resistance to pharmacologic interventions has been established. ECT requires management by a specialist team and often includes a brief inpatient stay. Although the number of recommended sessions may vary, evidence now suggests that efficacy can be predicted after the third session.[31]

New research on transcranial magnetic stimulation offers some promise for additional specialty procedures for the management of MDD that may be resistant to psychotropic medications; however, to date, not enough evidence exists to demonstrate its efficacy as first-line treatment or as an adjuvant to psychopharmacologic options.[30]

LIFE SPAN CONSIDERATIONS

In children and adolescents, an initial symptom of depression is often irritability rather than depressed mood and sadness. Randomized controlled trials suggest that combination treatment strategies (employing SSRIs and cognitive behavioral therapy) are as effective for children as for adults. A Food and Drug Administration "black box" warning now exists for the increased risk of suicidal thinking in children, adolescents, and young adults in the first few months of receiving SSRIs. In a meta-analysis, there was an increase in suicidal thoughts, with estimates that 1 to 3 of 100 individuals would demonstrate behaviors suggesting or directly endorsing increased suicidal thoughts. However, there has not been an increase in mortality from suicide within this group.[30]

MDD is rarely first diagnosed after the age of 65 years, although mood disorder caused by a general medical condition, with depressive features, is a diagnosis often made later in life. In the absence of a long-term relationship between an older adult and the provider, it may be difficult initially to distinguish between dementia and depression. Dementia is often slow in onset with a stable or steady decline in function, whereas depression may appear more rapidly with an inconsistent or fluctuating course. Somatic concerns, sad mood, difficulty concentrating, and disruptions to appetite and sleep patterns are more likely to be prominent in the presentation of MDD and concealed by the patient with dementia. An awareness of deficits and profound sadness and anergia are associated more with MDD, whereas patients with dementia may not seem quite as concerned about their inaccurate responses. Depression and dementia may coexist, and optimum treatment of both conditions is required to reduce functional impairment. Although suicidal thoughts are reduced within groups of older adults taking SSRIs, older white men have the highest rates of completed suicides among other age and ethnic groups.[30]

Treatment strategies for any depressive disorder in elders, once it is appropriately diagnosed, mirror those for healthy adults. Consideration of side effect profiles and possible drug interactions, however, becomes more critical. The initial dose should be half that of the adult starting dose, and titration that occurs more slowly will reduce the risk of complicating side effects or drug interactions. Older adults are specifically more vulnerable to the potential of hyponatremia as a side effect of SSRIs and SNRIs. Longer courses of treatment are often required for full remission of symptoms, yet prognosis is the same as for younger adults. Social support, however, plays a more influential role in reducing functional impairment when depressive symptoms are present in this population.

COMPLICATIONS

Depression has been researched both as a preexisting risk factor for people to develop cardiac disease and diabetes and as a postevent predictor of poorer outcomes (increased mortality and general decreased function). Strong associations have emerged suggesting that the rates of depression are higher when a co-occurring medical condition exists, and the presence of depression is an indicator of increased mortality. The prevalence of suicidal ideation is also increased for people with depression and a serious medical diagnosis.

Suicide

According to the Centers for Disease Control and Prevention, suicide is the second leading cause of death in Americans aged 25 to 35 years.[32] Men are four times more likely to complete a suicide attempt; however, the rate of attempted suicides is two to three times higher in women. For the 15- to 24-year age group, there are an estimated 100 attempts for every completed suicide; for individuals older than 65 years, only four attempts are made for every death by suicide. The rate of suicide in American Indian and Alaskan Native young adults and teens is nearly twice as high as the national average in this age group.[32]

Risk factors for suicide include unemployment, marital isolation, low socioeconomic status, family history of mental illness, family history of suicide, exposure to the suicidal behavior of others (including through media), family violence, personal history of physical or sexual abuse, alcohol or drug use, incarceration, and previous suicide attempts. Firearms are noted to be the method by which most men complete suicide, whereas poisoning is the method used by most women.[32]

Thoughts of death are common in people with depression. Given the risk of suicide in this population, anyone with MDD or subclinical symptoms must be carefully assessed. There are four components to a thorough suicide assessment (Box 248-2). First, it is important to understand the specific thoughts that someone may be having related to death. Hopelessness for the future—thoughts such as "The world would be better off without me" or "I wish I could go to sleep and not wake up"—must be explored further to determine level of risk. For example, the provider can say, "What you're telling me sounds incredibly difficult to manage. Has it been so bad that you've had thoughts of ending your own life?" If patients have not thought of suicide, they are likely to answer quickly and to volunteer reasons such as religious belief or family considerations. If they have thought of taking their own life, they are likely to answer more cautiously, wary of the potential reaction from the provider. Clinicians with less experience with psychiatry often fear that they will somehow contribute to the risk of suicide by asking the questions. This is a myth.

Once the patient has shared his or her suicidal ideation, the assessment must continue with an evaluation of specific plan, access to means, and intention to implement that plan. Many people who have thoughts of suicide and who have had ideas about a plan also have strong convictions about the circumstances under which they would or would not follow through with this plan. Others may have thought about ways to die yet

BOX 248-2

Assessing Risk for Suicide*

- Thoughts of suicide
- Plan to commit suicide
- Means to complete the plan
- Intention to follow through with the plan

*Consider impulsivity and the influence of substance use.

have not considered methods to access the means necessary for completion. Collaboration and consultation are critical in managing people with depression and thoughts of suicide.

"Contracting for safety" is a therapeutic intervention some specialty providers use. It is not a legal agreement, and even if it is in writing, it does not protect a provider from liability. It is a "promise" between the patient with suicidal ideation and the provider, reflective of a spoken or written commitment that the person will not act on his or her thoughts or carry out the plan for suicide. This is only as effective as the relationship between patient and provider and depends on the provider's commitment to the person with depression.

Suicidal ideation requires careful assessment. **Emergency psychiatric assessment for hospitalization** is indicated for anyone considered at high risk for self-harm.

INDICATIONS FOR REFERRAL OR HOSPITALIZATION

The majority of people with depressive disorders are treated in outpatient primary care settings. Concern for safety (suicide), lack of response to treatment, consideration of polypharmacy, and need for psychotherapy should prompt a referral to a specialty provider. It is advisable for health care providers to know the resources and systems to access mental health care in their area, to facilitate urgent referrals, and to provide accurate information to patients in need of those referrals. Box 248-3 highlights suggested referral criteria.

Screening tools and intensive case management services are structural interventions under exploration to enhance the management of MDD in the primary care setting. Many clinics also incorporate behavioral health specialists in the outpatient clinic to increase the ease of referral, to reduce the stigma of seeking services, and to enhance collaboration among providers of different specialties. Several studies are currently under way to evaluate the degree of improvement in treatment response and overall quality of patient care.

BOX 248-3

When to Refer to Mental Health Specialists

Emergent intervention is needed as soon as possible if:

- Patients are assessed as being at risk of harming themselves or others.
- Patients are so profoundly impaired by their symptoms that their own health is acutely suffering.
- Patients are experiencing symptoms of serotonin syndrome, serotonin withdrawal, neuroleptic malignant syndrome, or lithium toxicity.
- The provider is unsure of these risks.

Urgent intervention is needed within 1 week when:

- The patient is assessed as being at high risk for suicide yet is currently safe.
- Other psychiatric comorbidities are present, including substance use disorders.
- There is an indication for ECT.

Follow-up with specialty provider is needed within 1 month when:

- Recurrent symptoms are not responding to initial treatments provided in the primary care setting.
- Complications with medication management require frequent follow-up.
- Dementia is also present.
- Patients may benefit from psychotherapy, family education, or group support.

PATIENT AND FAMILY EDUCATION

Loved ones and family members may notice improvement in someone receiving treatment before the patient feels better. Depressed mood and hopelessness are often the last symptoms to respond to medications. During times of remission, the risk for suicide persists. Patients and families require education about the recurrent nature of depression and the risk for suicide. Information about the importance of complete remission of symptoms is also needed to improve prognosis and to prevent complications related to other medical illnesses. Social support may help identify warning signs of a recurring depressive episode and precipitate earlier treatment, which in turn predicts a better treatment response. Support groups or resources for families are often available through community mental health centers. A few national resources are listed here.

Grief Recovery Institute: www.grief.net

AARP grief and loss programs: www.aarp.org/families/grief_loss

Mental Health America: www.nmha.org

National Institute of Mental Health: www.nimh.nih.gov

American Psychiatric Association: www.psych.org

HEALTH PROMOTION

Regardless of predisposing factors, healthy lifestyle choices offer some protective value related to the onset of MDD given a particular stressor. Diets low in sugars and carbohydrates and high in omega-3 fatty acids and antioxidants have been associated with a generally stable and content mood. Mineral supplementation is not recommended as effective prevention for MDD. Exercise has been associated with acute improvements in mood as well as with deferral of the onset of additional medical comorbidities. As with most diseases and disorders, lifestyle modifications may reduce the risk of onset and deter the course of an illness, yet they may not fully mediate the impact of biologic influences.

BIPOLAR DISORDERS

DEFINITION AND EPIDEMIOLOGY

Bipolar affective disorders refer to constellations of symptoms that include a variation of moods that negatively affect one's ability to function. Bipolar I disorder is defined by one or more manic or mixed episodes during a patient's lifetime. Most often, a person who has experienced a manic or mixed episode has also had a major depressive episode, but the latter is not necessary for diagnosis. The diagnosis of bipolar II disorder is used when criteria for at least one major depressive episode are met in addition to at least one hypomanic episode. Bipolar Disorder Not Otherwise Specified is used when a clinician recognizes that a person has symptoms of a bipolar disorder, but full criteria (duration or level of impairment) may not be fulfilled. Cyclothymia refers to a milder form of bipolar disorder in which a person might have symptoms of mild depression and hypomania throughout a 2-year period. An additional specifier for bipolar disorders is rapid cycling. This is used when four or more distinct mood episodes occur in a single year.[1]

The prevalence of bipolar I disorder is approximately 1% of the population. In contrast to major depression, bipolar disorder affects men and women equally. Men are more likely to obtain the diagnosis after a manic episode, whereas women are more likely to acquire the diagnosis after a depressive episode.[1]

The prevalence of bipolar disorders does not have the variability across economic status or geography as noted with the prevalence of depression.[3] The age at onset for a bipolar disorder is generally between 15 and 30 years. Newly diagnosed mania rarely occurs in children or in adults older than 65 years. The initial episodes may be depressive; approximately 10% to 15% of adolescents with major depressive episodes are diagnosed with bipolar disorder later in life.[1]

Although bipolar disorders account for only 1% of the population, within this subgroup there is a dramatically higher burden of disease by measures of disability, health satisfaction, medical comorbidities, and cost of increased utilization of medical care. For example, in a retrospective analysis of claims through a large insurance carrier, people with bipolar disorders were more likely to have a metabolic comorbidity (37% versus 30%; $P > .0001$) than their healthy, age-matched control peers. The cost of care for the metabolic issues alone was twice that of individuals with metabolic disorders but without a bipolar disorder. Within this sample, overall use of medical services was higher, with higher costs of health care and medications in the group with bipolar disorders.[33]

PATHOPHYSIOLOGY

The pathophysiologic process of bipolar disorders is not well understood. As with depressive disorders, neuroimaging studies suggest that the thalamus, hypothalamus, amygdala, caudate, prefrontal cortex, and cerebellum are all involved, activated differently from healthy control groups. Although lithium has long been established as a standard treatment option, its mechanism of action is not known; however, advanced technology is beginning to allow researchers to look at the molecular impact that lithium has on glial and neuronal metabolism. These studies are still few, yet they suggest that lithium enhances glycolytic activity, stimulates the release of glutamate, and enhances lactate metabolism.[34] This evidence is preliminary and limited by the small groups and the inability to identify changes in the effect of the drug or neurobiologic changes over time.

Multiple studies have suggested a genetic link among mood disorders. The strongest evidence exists in the association of bipolar disorders and parents with either a bipolar or depressive disorder.[35] However, despite the evidence supporting a genetic link, a specific mode of genetic transmission has not yet been found.

CLINICAL PRESENTATION

The clinical presentation of bipolar disorder varies by the active mood episode. Symptoms of each mood episode in combination with a historical review for the presence or absence of previous episodes must be explored to confirm the diagnosis. As described previously, most people with depressive symptoms are seen first by their primary care provider and may have multiple somatic complaints. People with hypomania are not likely to complain of symptoms, because they often find that they enjoy the elevated mood and increased energy. In addition, in a manic episode, patients are most likely to be seen initially with a family member or at a family member's insistence, because insight into the potential negative sequelae of these symptoms does not often exist with a person's first experience of the episode. In addition to symptoms reviewed in the definitions of mood episodes, increased irritability and paranoia are common during manic episodes and are associated with increased social and interpersonal conflict. Based on findings in a large review of Medicaid patients with a diagnosis of a bipolar disorder, other medical or psychiatric conditions are diagnosed with an average of 6 months after initial Medicaid claims and a bipolar diagnosis.[36]

During acute mania, cognition and perception may become psychotic; delusions or hallucinations may be experienced. Persons in a manic episode experience racing thoughts and display tangential speech and inability to pay attention. Cognitive symptoms become obvious to others because of loose associations between ideas and, at times, the flight of ideas from one topic to another. Behavior can be bizarre and inappropriate and can seem disorganized.

Two thirds of people with bipolar disorders also have substance use disorders. When both of these diagnoses exist, there is an increased risk of perpetrating violent crime (independent of current episode, depressed or manic).[37] The course of an individual's illness may be influenced by high rates of comorbid alcohol or substance abuse. A person or a family member may seek assistance or come to medical attention because of the functional limitations of the substance use disorder before diagnosis of a bipolar disorder. Consistently, 32% of people with bipolar disorders are noted to have attempted suicide.[38]

PHYSICAL EXAMINATION

A person with bipolar disorder will not have complaints matching the symptoms of the disorder. The history is the most valuable part of the office visit for this diagnosis to be made. As with depressive disorders, a person may present with vague somatic complaints if he or she is in the midst of a depressive episode. If a manic or hypomanic episode is being experienced, the person may demonstrate rapid, tangential speech, irritability, and grandiosity and be easily distracted. The degree to which someone maintains energy for activities compared with the amount of sleep is the most discriminating factor in evaluating for a manic episode. Malnutrition and the consequences of risk-taking behavior may become evident during a physical examination. Patients who experience manic episodes are more likely to engage in behaviors such as drug use, unprotected sex, and dangerous driving. The effects of these behaviors may lead to further physical examination and testing for the adverse consequences of these actions (e.g., testing for hepatitis C, human immunodeficiency virus [HIV] infection). Because of the possibility that many symptoms have multiple differential diagnoses, including medical and psychiatric conditions, a thorough physical examination of all body systems is indicated.

DIAGNOSTICS

The accepted method of diagnosis of bipolar disorders incorporates the criteria outlined in the DSM-5, categorized by presence or absence of mood episodes as defined at the beginning of this chapter. As with other psychiatric disorders, once the symptom criteria are met, the person must also be determined to have a moderate degree of functional impairment from these symptoms, and not an underlying medical diagnosis or better-fitting psychiatric diagnosis. There are currently no laboratory values or genetic tests available for diagnosis of any mood disorder; however, several laboratory tests may be useful in excluding other medical disease.

DIFFERENTIAL DIAGNOSIS

Multiple other psychiatric conditions can co-occur with bipolar disorders; substance use disorders are the most common comorbidity. The presence of psychotic symptoms (hallucinations and paranoia) in a depressed or manic episode could confuse the diagnosis of bipolar disorder with schizophrenia or schizoaffective disorder. Validated history, confirmed by family members or prior medical records, will help in making this distinction. Symptoms of the following medical disorders may also resemble depressed mood or manic episodes and must be carefully explored before a psychiatric diagnosis is rendered.

Bipolar I disorder is distinguished from other mood disorders by matching the criteria for diagnosis with the patient's symptoms. It is distinguished from MDD by the presence of only one manic or mixed episode in the patient's lifetime. It is less easily distinguished from bipolar II disorder, in which the only difference is the presence of one or more manic or mixed episodes (bipolar I) as opposed to hypomanic episodes (bipolar II). Cyclothymic disorders also share similar criteria with bipolar I disorder and are differentiated by the duration and nature of symptoms. With cyclothymic disorder, the hypomanic and depressive symptoms are present but do not meet the criteria for manic episodes or major depressive episodes.[1]

MANAGEMENT

During any acute phase of a mood episode, the initial goal of the treatment is to assess and address issues of personal safety. As mentioned previously, more than 30% of people with bipolar disorders have attempted suicide. Bipolar disorder is a lifetime illness. There are times of remission from episodes of the mood disorder, but lifelong treatment is recommended to reduce the risks associated with future episodes of depressed or manic mood. Medications remain the first line of treatment for management, with augmentation strategies including psychotherapy and psychoeducation to optimize a person's ability to recognize triggers or early signs of the onset of an episode. These treatments may be additionally effective to address the functional lifestyle changes affiliated with bipolar disorder, effects of long-term medications, damage to social relationships, suicidal ideation, and risk for substance use disorders.

In 2004, treatment guidelines were published to represent the expert opinions of an international consensus group. At that time, lithium and lamotrigine were identified as having category 1 evidence (multiple randomized clinical trials with long-term follow-up) for use as first-line treatment in the management of bipolar disorders. Slightly weaker evidence supported the use of olanzapine or combination therapy of olanzapine and fluoxetine. Additions of valproate or other atypical antipsychotics and consideration for ECT are then discussed if symptoms are persistent and do not respond to initial treatment.[39]

It is estimated that 7% to 30% of patients with bipolar disorder switch from a depressed to a manic episode if they are treated with an antidepressant alone. Mood stabilization medications (lithium, lamotrigine, valproate) have been shown to have moderate effectiveness in long-term management of bipolar disorder. Lithium and olanzapine have some effectiveness in managing acute mania, whereas an olanzapine and fluoxetine combination has shown the most promising data for the management of bipolar depression.[40] The only research related to suicide risk reduction involves the use of lithium.[41] Researching the effectiveness of these medications is complicated in the population of individuals with a diagnosis of bipolar disorder. In addition to poor treatment compliance, there is little consistency in providers' adherence to the established guidelines.[36,40] The development of a team of multidisciplinary providers has the strongest evidence to influence outcomes for patients with bipolar disorders. The collaboration between a primary care provider and behavioral health specialists and case managers can improve both patient and provider adherence to treatment guidelines, reduce complications, and minimize functional impact of symptoms.[39]

Where access to psychiatric specialists may be limited, the primary care provider must begin treatment of an acute manic or depressive episode. The risks of suicide or harmful consequences of untreated symptoms increase with time if treatment is delayed. Therefore, the primary care provider is responsible for initiating treatment in many settings. Regardless of whether the treatment has been initiated by a primary care or behavioral health provider, monitoring for side effects, drug interactions, treatment adherence, and effectiveness of treatment often falls to the primary care provider. Table 248-3 summarizes some dosage and monitoring parameters of agents often used to treat bipolar disorder.

Before any medication is initiated, female patients should be screened for pregnancy because of the risk of teratogenic effects of these medications. The efficacy of birth control is also altered with some of these agents.

Whereas good evidence exists to support psychotherapy interventions for the management of depressive disorders, little is available about standardized psychotherapeutic approaches for people with bipolar disorders. Building a collaborative team remains the most salient approach to augment pharmacologic interventions.

LIFE SPAN CONSIDERATIONS

It is uncommon for people to be diagnosed with a bipolar disorder later in life. Because this is a lifetime illness, as patients age, additional consultation with a geriatric psychiatrist or mental health provider may prove especially valuable. Some literature suggests that the time between mood episodes decreases with age; thus, adherence to treatment is especially important. With age comes increased polypharmacy, and many of these agents used to treat bipolar disorder have multiple drug interactions and side effects that may increase over time. Because of these risks, ECT may be a stronger consideration in

TABLE 248-3 Prescribing or Monitoring of Medications Used in Bipolar Disorder

Medication	Baseline Testing	Dose Range or Serum Levels	Common Side Effects	Rare Side Effects	Ongoing Monitoring	Additional Considerations
Lithium	TSH Serum calcium	300-1800 mg/day 1-1.5 mEq/L for acute mania 0.6-1.2 mEq/L for maintenance	Nausea Vomiting Epigastric discomfort Dry mouth Metallic taste Diarrhea Weight gain	Diabetes insipidus Hyperparathyroidism Memory impairment Hair loss Arrhythmias Hyperthyroidism	Every 3-6 mo: urea and creatinine Every 6 mo × 2, then annually: TSH, serum calcium, weight	Lithium metabolism and concentration are commonly affected by other medications and electrolyte changes (sodium).*
Valproate	History of hematologic or hepatic disease	750-2000 mg/day (divided doses, titrate gradually) Maximum recommended dose 60 mg/kg/day	Nausea Vomiting Abdominal cramping Anorexia Diarrhea Sedation Tremor Transient hair loss Thrombocytopenia Elevated transaminase Elevated ammonia (may be asymptomatic)	Severe hepatic dysfunction Pancreatitis Extrapyramidal syndrome Hyperammonemic encephalopathy	Every 3 mo for a year, then annually: weight, full blood count, LFTs, menstrual changes, education related to bone health	
Carbamazepine	History of hematologic or hepatic disease	400-1200 mg/day for acute mania 200-400 mg/day for maintenance	Dry mouth Vomiting Diarrhea Anorexia Constipation Dizziness Headache Ataxia Drowsiness Blurred vision Diplopia Rash	Agranulocytosis Anemia Stevens-Johnson syndrome SIADH Arrhythmias Orofacial dyskinesias Hepatitis	Monthly: full blood count Every 3 mo × 1 year, then annually: LFTs, electrolytes, urea, and creatinine Frequently review effectiveness of oral contraceptives Provide advice on bone health Educate about potential for rash (requires emergent medical attention)	There is a high likelihood of influencing the metabolism of other medications, because carbamazepine has an impact on the cytochrome P-450 system.
Lamotrigine	None	50-200 mg/day Titrated slowly No serum monitoring	Dry mouth Nausea Vomiting Diplopia Headache Irritability Somnolence Tremor Insomnia Stevens-Johnson syndrome Arthralgia	Hepatic failure Blood dyscrasias Severe skin reaction Lupus-like reaction	Educate about potential for rash (requires emergent medical attention)	Starting at low dose and titrating slowly decreases risk of serious skin reaction. Adjust dose if it is used in combination with valproate or carbamazepine.

Continued

TABLE 248-3 **Prescribing or Monitoring of Medications Used in Bipolar Disorder—cont'd**

Medication	Baseline Testing	Dose Range or Serum Levels	Common Side Effects	Rare Side Effects	Ongoing Monitoring	Additional Considerations
Atypical antipsychotics	Family history of cardiac problems (abnormal QTc interval) Baseline lipids, glucose, and LFTs recommended for some agents	Olanzapine: 5-20 mg/day Risperidone: 1-6 mg/day Quetiapine: 200-600 mg/day Ziprasidone: 80-160 mg/day	Weight gain Dyslipidemia Hyperglycemia Hyperprolactinemia Tremor Akathisia Dystonia Constipation Dry mouth Blurred vision Urinary retention Sedation Increased appetite Nausea Peripheral edema Orthostatic hypotension Tachycardia Stroke or TIA (higher risk in older patients)	Jaundice Neuroleptic malignant syndrome Seizures Tardive dyskinesia Increased QTc interval SIADH Blood dyscrasias Cardiac arrest Lupus	Monthly × 3, then every 3 mo: weight Every 3 mo × 4, then annually: blood pressure, fasting glucose At 3 mo, then annually: fasting lipids Electrocardiogram, prolactin levels if indicated	Lower doses should be trialed with additional attention to drug interactions in older patients.
Antidepressants (SSRIs)	None	See Table 248-2	Nausea Diarrhea Dizziness Headache Insomnia Drowsiness Dry mouth Sweating Weight gain Sexual dysfunction	Sedation Confusion Tachycardia Hypotension Hyponatremia (SIADH) Elevated liver enzymes Hematologic complications Taste disturbance	Annually: weight	Refer to Tables 245-2 and 245-3.

These guidelines should not replace thorough review of package inserts or other references for prescribing or drug interactions.
*Symptoms of lithium toxicity include loss of balance, diarrhea, vomiting, weakness, ataxia, blurred vision, tremor, irritability, muscle twitching, agitation, tinnitus, polyuria, drowsiness, psychosis, and disorientation. Seizures, coma, and renal failure are additional risks of lithium toxicity. More frequent monitoring of serum lithium levels may be required if a person is taking multiple medications, starts a new medication, or has an acute illness that may deplete sodium or potassium stores.
LFTs, liver function tests; SIADH, syndrome of inappropriate antidiuretic hormone secretion; TIA, transient ischemic attack; TSH, thyroid-stimulating hormone.
Data from Malhi GS, Adams D, Berk M: The pharmacological treatment of bipolar disorder in primary care, *Med J Aust* 193:S24-S30, 2010.

management of bipolar disorders in older adults. There is less evidence to support clearer treatment guidelines for this age group.[40]

Early-onset bipolar disorders are associated with a more severe course of symptoms, increased complications, and comorbidities.[38] Because patients may be started on medications sooner, they are also at higher risk for complications related to extended duration of use of these agents. Additional genetics research may help identify a more individualized approach to treatment of younger patients and determination of risk. Presentation of symptoms may be more subtle; family and peers may not recognize when symptoms of bipolar disorder manifest outside of the realm of perceived "normal" variation in mood and behavior in adolescence. Close relationships among primary care providers, children, and families may help identify and assess this disorder early in its course. Because of the strong association with substance use disorders and the high risk of suicide in people with bipolar disorder, thorough assessment and patient and family education are critical.

COMPLICATIONS

The most concerning complication related to the diagnosis of bipolar disorder is suicide and suicidal ideation. Symptoms of mania may be associated with risky behaviors and additional threats to one's personal safety because of poor judgment of environment and inability to consider consequences of impulsive or disinhibited actions (sexual indiscretions, excessive spending, risk-taking sport, violence). Family relationships are often strained. Because of the familial link with the diagnosis, chances are that more than one family member may be struggling with bipolar disorder at a time, limiting the available support to any one patient.

Patients with bipolar disorder are also at high risk for co-occurring substance use disorders. This complication is likely to increase the risk of impulsive behaviors and suicide. Substance use also markedly compromises a person's ability to adhere to treatment recommendations, including medications. Alcohol and drug use will increase the side effects and toxicity of most medications, further complicating assessment and management strategies.

In addition to the complex side effects, the initiation of some medications for one mood episode may trigger the onset of another episode. For example, if a depressed episode is treated with an antidepressant alone, there is a likelihood of inducing a manic episode. Conversely, if a manic episode is treated with an older, typical antipsychotic alone, a depressive episode is likely to follow.[37]

In addition to the likelihood of a family member's also being affected by the symptoms of a mood disorder, the prevalence of depressed mood and suicidal ideation in the bipolar patient is associated with the general health of other family members.[42] As with many other disorders, there is also a higher risk for family members and caregivers to neglect their own health as the needs of the affected loved one increase.

INDICATIONS FOR REFERRAL OR HOSPITALIZATION

As with the management of any mood disorder, hospitalization may be required to ensure a person's ability to keep safe and to protect those around the person from harm. The same principles of referral and hospitalization apply for all mood disorders (see Box 248-3).

PATIENT AND FAMILY EDUCATION

Bipolar disorders require lifelong adaptations and treatment. Persons with the diagnosis and their family members can benefit from tracking how the symptoms affect the individual person. Some patients' symptoms may be triggered by lack of sleep, a stressful event, or a change in eating habits. Attention to and examination of these individual patterns may help patients and families avoid triggers to mood episodes or recognize early signs of the onset of a depressed or manic episode. Early recognition may help with reducing complications related to untreated episodes.

Patients and families would also benefit from additional counseling and support to address potential reluctance to accept lifelong pharmacologic treatment as well as the potential side effects of these treatments. Families are also a critical resource for providers because they recognize more subtle changes in personality and behavior that may suggest an approaching episode.

Many people with bipolar disorder tend to enjoy episodes of hypomania or the early symptoms of mania, as it comes as a relief to a depressive episode. People also find that during these times, they are productive and full of energy. This often delays treatment of the episode and therefore may lead to additional complications of mania. Families should be aware of this possibility and the reluctance that many patients may have to seek treatment.

CHAPTER 249

SUBSTANCE USE DISORDERS

J. Nile Wagley

DEFINITION AND EPIDEMIOLOGY

In 2013, 21.6 million persons aged 12 or older (8.2%) were classified as having had substance dependence or abuse in the previous year.[1] In adolescents, the statistics are equally alarming. For teenagers, a significant source of drugs and alcohol is the family home.[2] Illicit drugs are often associated with substance abuse, but alcohol, nicotine, and prescription painkillers are among the most widely abused substances in the United States.[3] The costs of drug, nicotine, and alcohol abuse to patients and society are staggering, associated with more than a half-million deaths and approaching a half-trillion dollars each year.[3] Yet substance abuse remains underdiagnosed and undertreated in primary care, even though human immunodeficiency virus (HIV) infection and cocaine, heroin, designer drug, methamphetamine, and prescription drug abuse and the recognition of the morbidity and mortality associated with substance abuse have increasingly brought this problem to the attention of health care providers.[2]

Patients with substance use problems have health, emotional, family, social, legal, and spiritual troubles that are vexing to the patient, the family, and the health care provider. Major hazards include overdose; withdrawal symptoms; violence and unintentional injuries; pregnancy and neonatal complications; social, economic, and family dysfunction; long-term health problems; and the complications of injection drug use (IDU). Substance use disorder is a constellation of cognitive, behavioral, and physiologic symptoms in which an individual continues using a substance despite the associated negative consequences.[3] The term *dependence* has psychological (cravings) and physiological components (tolerance and withdrawal). Not all patients who develop a physiologic dependence are "addicted." Physiologic dependence develops with the therapeutic use of several medications, such as opiates that are appropriately prescribed for chronic pain and corticosteroids that are prescribed for refractory inflammatory conditions. Although these patients may experience abstinence syndromes, they usually do not display addictive behaviors and should not be diagnosed with a substance use disorder on this basis alone.

The term *withdrawal* refers to the adverse physiologic syndromes that follow the removal of a drug on which one has become dependent. These symptoms can range from irritability to trouble sleeping, depending on the substance and level of dependence, and can last from a few days to several weeks. An individual who is abstinent is drug free, whereas an individual in recovery is in the long-term process of attending to the spiritual, physical, and psychosocial needs that have been affected by addiction. *Withdrawal* refers to the process of removal of the drug of dependence from the body, whereas *detoxification* refers in general to the administration of tapering doses of the same or cross-tolerant drugs to assist with withdrawal.

Tolerance refers to the need to increase the amount of drug to achieve the same effects. Because individuals who are tolerant have adapted to a certain level of drug use, they can experience both intoxication and withdrawal symptoms at the same time.

Relapse is the return to problem drug use after a significant period of abstinence; it may involve a drug different from the patient's original drug of choice.

Protracted withdrawal is the period of time, having been measured up to 2 years in long-term, heavy alcohol use, after abstinence has been achieved but while neurologic changes from drug use have not yet downregulated to pre–drug-use states. Common symptoms include anxiety, trouble sleeping, depressive symptoms, irritability, and impulse control.

Lastly, any untreated, precipitating conditions that existed before the substance use began may be present once abstinence has been achieved. For example, an individual with symptoms of anxiety may be more likely to use alcohol at unhealthy levels. Although alcohol reduces the immediately felt symptoms of anxiety, it will not resolve anxiety issues in the long run. The removal of alcohol may result in a return to original levels of anxiety.

In 2013, 2.8 million people in the United States older than 12 years tried illicit drugs for the first time in the previous month.[1] The National Survey on Drug Use and Health, conducted by the Substance Abuse and Mental Health Services Administration, estimated that in 2013, 2.5% of people in the United States aged 12 years and older abused prescription drugs (took prescription drugs not prescribed for them or took medication solely for pleasure or entertainment) in the month preceding the survey. Most people abused pain relievers, but a substantial number also abused tranquilizers, stimulants, and sedatives.[1]

PATHOPHYSIOLOGY

Addictive disorders are chronic relapsing conditions; the cause is probably the result of interactions among genetic and temperament susceptibility, psychosocial factors, availability of resources, and drug availability.[2] Both "brain reward" and avoidance of withdrawal contribute to addictive substance use. The science of brain reward continues to evolve; it is multifaceted, involving dopamine, norepinephrine, endogenous opioids (endorphins), γ-aminobutyric acid (GABA), serotonin, acetylcholine, and adrenergic systems.[4] Drugs act at various sites to stimulate brain reward, thereby reinforcing repeated use. Long-term alterations in brain reward pathways may explain persistent heightened vulnerability to drug effects and continued dependence long after the clinical physical dependence has resolved. Such alterations may in part explain the chronic relapsing nature of addiction.[5,6]

Major Drugs of Abuse

Drugs from one class can be used to enhance the desired effects or to attenuate the undesired effects of drugs from another class. Understanding the features of these drug classes should be tempered by the knowledge that addicted patients usually take drugs from more than one category at a time.

Central Nervous System Sedatives. GABA is the major inhibitory neurotransmitter that lowers cell excitability, and sedatives, in general, depress brain activity by boosting the GABA systems.

The major central nervous system (CNS) sedatives are alcohol, barbiturates, benzodiazepines, and other compounds that are similar to either barbiturates or benzodiazepines. γ-Hydroxybutyrate (GHB), synthesized in home laboratories, is a recreational drug that causes disinhibition, euphoria, and sedation. It is commonly used in "date rape."

Mild manifestations of sedative intoxication include tranquilization, fine lateral nystagmus, and slightly decreased alertness. Moderate intoxication manifests as ataxia, slurred speech, coarse nystagmus, and sedation. An overdose of these substances produces somnolence, staggering, and marked dysarthria; this can progress to coma, respiratory depression, and death. Depressant effects on the cerebral cortex may paradoxically cause stimulation, disinhibition, and excitement. The major hazards of sedative abuse include a dangerous abstinence syndrome, unintentional injuries, and overdose.

Alcohol, which has a ubiquitous and normative presence in human society, is by far the most commonly abused sedative-hypnotic drug. Ethyl alcohol acts as a CNS sedative; this effect is thought to be related primarily to its effects on the GABA system and possibly to alterations in cellular membrane fluidity.

Alcohol is absorbed from the stomach and small intestine, distributing to all body tissues in concentrations roughly proportional to their water content. Alcohol is metabolized in the liver by two principal pathways: (1) alcohol dehydrogenase (ADH) catalyzes degradation of alcohol to acetaldehyde, which is then metabolized by aldehyde dehydrogenase; and (2) the liver's microsomal ethanol-oxidizing system increases in activity with chronic exposure to alcohol. Both of these pathways reduce a cofactor, nicotinamide adenine dinucleotide (NAD), to NADH. Excess NADH produces a wide range of metabolic derangements, including fatty liver, hypertriglyceridemia, and hypoglycemia.[4]

It takes 1 hour for most individuals to oxidize 7.5 to 10 mL of alcohol, with the excess accumulating and causing toxicity. The effects of alcohol toxicity are roughly related to both the blood alcohol concentration (BAC) and the tolerance of the individual.[4] A level of 0.10% (100 mg/dL) is generally considered the BAC that results in clinical intoxication. Taking individual differences into account, a BAC of 50 mg/dL causes mild tranquilization; a BAC of 50 to 150 mg/dL causes impairment in coordination, speech, judgment, and concentration. BACs above 150 mg/dL cause delirium or stupor. Levels of consciousness decline at 300 to 400 mg/dL, leading to unconsciousness and, with increasing BAC levels, respiratory depression, cardiovascular collapse, and death.

Partial tolerance to alcohol develops and is associated with cross-tolerance to other drugs that affect the GABA system, such as benzodiazepines and barbiturates. Tolerance develops in several ways: intracellular adaptation; metabolically, such that the liver metabolizes alcohol more rapidly; and behaviorally, when the person changes his or her lifestyle to accommodate dependence. In patients who are alcohol dependent, an abstinence syndrome develops when alcohol levels decline. Pregnancy is perhaps the most important contraindication to alcohol use; a safe level of drinking during pregnancy has not been defined. The major manifestations of fetal alcohol syndrome are intellectual impairment and developmental delays, growth retardation, and characteristically abnormal facial features (short palpebral fissures, flattening of the midface, and a thin upper lip). More subtle behavioral and learning difficulties are termed *fetal alcohol effect,* but these cannot be diagnosed before the child reaches school age.

Barbiturates both enhance and mimic the effect of GABA, thus depressing all brain activity. They are classified by their onset and duration of action. Their prescribed use for sedation has largely been replaced by benzodiazepines, but phenobarbital is occasionally still useful for epilepsy, and butabarbital combinations are used for headaches. The therapeutic index of barbiturates is much narrower than that of benzodiazepines. Chronic use may cause slowed learning, impaired memory, sleep disturbances, and emotional lability. The short-acting (e.g., pentobarbital) and intermediate-acting (e.g., amobarbital) barbiturates have historically been the most often abused. Long-acting barbiturates (e.g., phenobarbital) are not considered intoxicating, but individuals with addiction often take them in high doses with alcohol, producing dangerous impairment and toxicity. The chronic metabolism of barbiturates induces hepatic enzymes that can speed the metabolism of other sedatives, phenytoin, and warfarin. Because tolerance to barbiturates is incomplete, chronic users are still vulnerable to overdose. The drugs methaqualone and glutethimide are synthetic compounds that are similar in toxicity and effect to barbiturates.

Benzodiazepines facilitate the action of GABA. They are often prescribed for relief of anxiety, insomnia, or muscle spasm or tension; for acute management of agitation; and for acute treatment of convulsions. Cross-tolerance and a wide therapeutic index make benzodiazepines good agents to assist with alcohol detoxification. In general, benzodiazepines have a wide margin of safety; however, their misuse is widespread among addicts and the potential for abuse is present for all patients. Their abuse potential seems to be associated with speed of onset and potency; rapidly acting drugs (e.g., diazepam, clonazepam, and alprazolam) have the greatest potential for abuse, and slower acting compounds (e.g., oxazepam) have the least. The high potency of clonazepam and alprazolam, with 1 mg roughly equivalent to 10 mg of diazepam, appears to contribute to their abuse potential and street value.

All benzodiazepines are metabolized to inactive compounds in the liver. Longer-acting benzodiazepines first require hepatic oxidation, which produces active drug metabolites. Zolpidem and zaleplon are short-acting synthetic hypnotics that are similar in action to the short-acting benzodiazepines.

Withdrawal from alcohol produces a similar range of manifestations, from mild emotional symptoms to life-threatening autonomic instability. Because the withdrawal syndrome develops when the BAC falls below the level to which the individual has adapted, highly tolerant individuals may experience the effects of abstinence even with a substantial level of alcohol in their systems. Within a few hours after the last drink, anxiety, headache, nausea, hypervigilance, tachycardia, and mild tremors develop. Diaphoresis, photophobia, hyperreflexia, a more rapid pulse, elevated blood pressure, more pronounced tremors, and hallucinations (auditory, visual, or tactile) constitute manifestations of more severe withdrawal. Some form of hallucination is common, and they persist in a small number of patients long after withdrawal. Tonic-clonic seizures, which are usually self-limited and short-lived, may occur during the first week of withdrawal and typically 12 to 48 hours after the last drink. With uncomplicated alcohol withdrawal, temperature does not usually rise to higher than 38.1° C (100.5° F). Major withdrawal can be dangerous because it may herald the development of delirium tremens (DTs), may aggravate a serious comorbid condition such as coronary artery disease or cerebrovascular disease, and may provoke status epilepticus.

DTs are a severe withdrawal syndrome characterized by deterioration of mental status and instability of the autonomic nervous system. DTs usually develop within 24 to 72 hours of the last drink. The development of disorientation, confusion, frank hallucinations, and elevated temperature in the setting of alcohol withdrawal should be considered an urgent situation. The mortality rate for DTs has been declining in recent years with better recognition and more aggressive treatment. Benzodiazepines have consistently been shown to be the safest and most effective drugs to assist with alcohol detoxification. Outpatient detoxification is labor-intensive and requires the patient to have good involved social support and the provider to have ready inpatient availability.

The severity of withdrawal from sedatives is generally proportional to the level and duration of use; barbiturates and rapidly acting, high-potency benzodiazepines produce the most severe syndromes. Restlessness, anxiety, and mild tremors usually develop approximately 12 to 24 hours after discontinuation of a short-acting drug. The onset may be delayed for several days if the primary drug is long acting. Chronic liver dysfunction may increase drug storage and thereby delay the manifestations of withdrawal. Escalating symptoms, increased tremors, dissociative and perceptual symptoms, increased pulse and blood pressure, and hyperreflexia develop. At this point, the patient becomes prone to convulsions, even if properly treated. If the patient is left untreated, withdrawal can progress to an acute psychosis that resembles DTs. Patients experiencing high-dose sedative withdrawal need to be treated on an inpatient basis with a long-acting sedative such as phenobarbital.

Acamprosate (Campral) is an anticraving medication used to help patients refrain from alcohol once they have stopped drinking.[7] It appears to reduce the activity of hyperactive glutamatergic neurons and to stimulate GABA transmission. Acamprosate is given three times per day after the patient achieves sobriety. The dose needs to be adjusted in patients with renal impairment and in those who weigh less than 60 kg. This medication is contraindicated in severe renal insufficiency. Patients treated with acamprosate seem to have decreased recidivism, although it has no superiority compared with naltrexone.[7]

Opioids. Opioids produce their effects by interacting with endogenous opioid receptors throughout the CNS and intestines. Morphine is the prototypical opioid, whereas heroin (diacetylmorphine) has historically been the form most often seriously abused. Pharmaceutical abuse has increased in recent years, making this the chief form of misused opiates.[1] Heroin is illegal in the United States and is sold on the streets as a white or brown powder, often diluted with sugar, talc, or quinine. Heroin may be insufflated (snorted), smoked, or dissolved and injected. Synthetic opioids include methadone, meperidine, and fentanyl. Tramadol is a mild synthetic with both mu and kappa opioid activity.

Opioids are useful for relief of pain and suffering, for cough suppression, and for their antidiarrheal effects. With a few individual differences, most opioids display similar pharmacologic actions and vary mostly in kinetics. Chronic administration inevitably produces some degree of physiologic dependence; the susceptibility to the development of addiction varies among individuals. Addiction, overdose, and premature labor are the most serious complications directly caused by opiates, with most other complications caused by IDU and hazardous lifestyles.

Aloofness, calmness, and mild sedation characterize opioid intoxication. A warm flush and sudden sensation of pleasure accompany injection, sometimes with mild nausea and vomiting. Individuals experience vague itching and characteristically scratch the nose. Opioid intoxication usually produces drowsiness and slowed movement but with less mental slowing than with sedative intoxication. Pupils constrict and respiratory rate and bowel motility decrease, effects that persist even if the individual has a high level of tolerance. Blood pressure and pulse are mildly decreased.

Stupor that progresses to coma, markedly slow and shallow respirations, and pulmonary edema characterize opioid overdose. Meperidine overdose or cerebral anoxia may produce dilated pupils; meperidine, tramadol, or propoxyphene overdose may produce seizures. Acute frothy pulmonary edema and eosinophilia are the prominent features of a hypersensitivity type of overdose. Naloxone, an intravenously administered pure opioid antagonist, reverses the stupor, usually precipitating an opioid abstinence syndrome. It is short acting, and the patient should be observed for at least 24 hours, especially if overdose with a long-acting opioid is suspected. Other toxic, neurologic, and metabolic causes should be sought when a patient who is stuporous does not respond to naloxone.

As blood levels decline, an abstinence syndrome develops. The timing of this syndrome varies with the duration of the drug's effect; withdrawal from long-acting opiates begins later and lasts longer. Severity is proportional to the size and duration of the habit. The syndrome starts with overwhelming fatigue and is followed by restlessness, pupillary dilation, temperature intolerance, general aches and arthromyalgias, increased respiratory rate and yawning, runny eyes and nose, piloerection, sweating, and hyperactive bowels. Nausea, vomiting, and elevated blood pressure and pulse may occur. Vital signs reveal little about withdrawal severity. The most reliable physical signs are pupillary dilation and constantly hyperactive bowel sounds. The patient is unable to sleep despite the administration of sedatives. Objectively, the syndrome resembles an acute episode of influenza that is accompanied by parasympathetic hyperactivity and intense drug craving. The syndrome can precipitate premature labor but otherwise is not dangerous. Protracted, low-level symptoms may persist for months or years.

Pharmacologic treatment of abstinence may include tapering doses of the long-acting opioid methadone or the mixed opioid agonist-antagonist drug buprenorphine. Clonidine is an alpha$_2$-adrenergic antihypertensive that attenuates some abstinence symptoms and, in combination with other medication for myalgias, abdominal cramps, and insomnia, can help withdraw patients from opioids.

Methadone is sometimes used to treat patients with chronic pain; but for more than 50 years, methadone maintenance programs have provided methadone and counseling to heroin-addicted individuals as a substitute for illicit opioids. Methadone maintenance is also the treatment of choice for heroin addicts who are pregnant. Their neonates are born physically dependent but can be safely withdrawn in the nursery. Although methadone is addictive, it was considered to be a safe alternative to heroin addiction because it could be maintained under supervision, it could be administered orally once daily, and it eliminated the dangers of intravenous needles. No drug is completely safe, however, and sudden cardiac death from Q-T interval prolongation and torsades de pointes has been associated with high-dose methadone, requiring both a careful history and continuous monitoring.[8]

Methadone detoxification is prescribed only through specially licensed drug treatment programs or for patients who are acutely hospitalized for a coexistent medical condition. Although patients remain physiologically dependent, these programs have demonstrated effectiveness in reducing illicit opioid use and the harm associated with opioid addiction.

Central Nervous System Stimulants. CNS stimulants encompass a wide array of drugs that increase alertness, cause excitation, and sometimes cause euphoria. Stimulant drugs include cocaine, amphetamines, and methylphenidate as well as several amphetamine-like psychotomimetic compounds.

Major stimulants are often used in combination with opioids or sedatives. Mild stimulant intoxication manifests with increased alertness, hyperactivity, anorexia, elevated blood pressure, and pulse elevation. Intoxication causes euphoric excitement, hyperstimulation, and grandiosity. Chronic stimulant users develop nervousness, irritability, insomnia, and often paranoia. Depression, hypersomnia, lethargy, poor concentration, and drug craving characterize stimulant withdrawal.

Cocaine hydrochloride has the properties of a CNS and peripheral nervous system stimulant and local anesthetic. The major methods of cocaine use are sniffing, injecting, and vaporization (smoking "crack"). Cocaine enhances the effects of dopamine, serotonin, and norepinephrine by elevating synaptic levels.

Restlessness, agitation, paranoia, and panic characterize acute intoxication. Blood pressure and pulse increase, and pupils dilate. Overdose can produce cardiac arrhythmias, including ventricular fibrillation and seizures. Vasospasm can cause myocardial, cerebral, or hepatic infarction, even in users with normal arteries. This also contributes to the premature separation of membranes when it is used during pregnancy. Cocaine effects vary by the route of administration. The onset is within minutes when it is inhaled nasally and within seconds when it is injected or smoked. The duration of effect is brief. The withdrawal syndrome appears quickly, reinforcing frequent administration and the accumulation of metabolites. Prostitution often accompanies crack cocaine addiction, making cocaine smoking an independent risk factor for sexually transmitted disease. The prenatal effects of maternal cocaine use may not be as drastic as originally feared, but the long-term ramifications may include cardiac, neurologic, and behavioral concerns.[9,10]

Amphetamine and amphetamine-like stimulants have effects that are qualitatively similar to those of cocaine, but their effects are more prolonged. The two most commonly abused forms of these substances are methamphetamine, which is synthesized in home laboratories, and methylphenidate, which is diverted from pharmaceutical supplies. The methods of methamphetamine use involve the oral route, sniffing, smoking, and injection. Tolerance develops rapidly, and users become sensitized and seizure prone. Chronic heavy use causes a paranoid psychosis that is difficult to manage, and it may cause long-term degeneration of dopaminergic neurons. Intravenous amphetamine use is associated with the development of vasculitis.[11] Burns and inhalation are common hazards of home methamphetamine synthesis.

Ecstasy, or 3,4-methylenedioxymethamphetamine (MDMA), has a chemical structure similar to that of amphetamines and mescaline and produces both stimulant and hallucinogenic effects. MDMA stimulates the release of serotonin, producing a feeling of empathy and closeness and an enhanced sense of pleasure, confidence, and endurance, with effects lasting several minutes to hours. Physical effects include muscle tension, teeth clenching, blurred vision, faintness, elevated blood pressure and pulse, and altered control of body temperature. The drug, which allows users to dance for extended periods, is usually used in crowded nightclubs, increasing the risk for hyperthermia, dehydration, and heart or kidney failure. The drug appears to cause long-lasting serotonin neuron loss and memory damage.[12]

Stimulant users who have persistent depression may benefit from antidepressant therapy, but no medication has been demonstrated to effectively treat stimulant withdrawal or drug craving. Sedation is often necessary during acute intoxication, and medications are often needed for detoxification from a coexisting dependence on sedatives or opioids.

Psychotomimetics and Hallucinogens. Psychotomimetics and hallucinogens are an informal category of drugs that alter perceptions and mimic psychotic or dissociative states. Included in this category are cannabinoids, lysergic acid diethylamide (LSD) and similarly acting hallucinogens, and phencyclidine (PCP). As with stimulant drugs, no medication has been demonstrated to effectively treat hallucinogen withdrawal or drug craving. Sedation is often needed during episodes of acute intoxication.

Cannabinoids, in the form of marijuana, are the active ingredients in the leaves or resin of the *Cannabis sativa* hemp plant; they are either smoked or taken orally. Marijuana is the most commonly abused illicit substance. Intoxication produces a mildly dissociated and dreamy mental state, an elevated pulse, dilated pupils, an increased appetite, and a characteristic odor. In high doses, it may produce hallucinations and, idiosyncratically, paranoia. Marijuana use is greatest in adolescence and young adulthood and possibly hinders emotional development and initiative. Heavy users appear to be prone to a mild abstinence syndrome that consists of nervousness, restlessness, and appetite and sleep disturbance.

PCP and the related compound ketamine are dissociative anesthetics whose action closely mimics schizophrenia. PCP is most commonly smoked but can be absorbed through any route. Individuals vary markedly in their responses. Mild intoxication induces giddiness, elation, expansiveness, and mild dissociation. Highly toxic individuals display disorientation, a bizarre affect, rotary nystagmus, ataxia, tachycardia, and a dissociative lack of concern with pain or the external world. These individuals are prone to self-mutilation and are difficult to contain despite sedation. Deaths from overdose are caused by hypertensive crisis, respiratory arrest, and status epilepticus.

The true hallucinogenic drugs are ergots (LSD), phenylalkylamines (mescaline), indolealkylamines (psilocybin), and the amphetamine-like drug MDMA (ecstasy). As with cannabis, young people are the main users of hallucinogens. LSD is the prototype and appears to produce its action by serotonin inhibition and dopamine stimulation. It is highly potent, and its effects are noted with oral ingestions of tiny fractions of a gram.

Tolerance to hallucinogens develops rapidly, sometimes after a single dose. Giddiness, visual and other sensory distortions, marked dissociation, widely dilated pupils, and peripheral vasoconstriction characterize intoxication. Patients may develop acute panic or psychosis. The effects last 8 to 12 hours; some patients report recurrent manifestations months to years later.

Inhalants. The term *inhalant* describes an informal grouping of differing substances that are used by inhalation of their vapors. Solvents (e.g., acetone, benzene, toluene), nitrous oxide gas, and volatile nitrites (e.g., amyl nitrite, butyl nitrite) are members of this group. Solvent inhalation produces a rapid sedative-like intoxication, including dizziness, drowsiness, slurred speech, and ataxia. Chronic complications include cerebral atrophy, peripheral neuropathy, toxic hepatitis, and bone marrow toxicity as well as the complications associated with lead poisoning and other impurities. Nitrous oxide is usually obtained from medical or laboratory supplies or from commercial aerosol sprays. It displaces CNS oxygen rapidly after inhalation, causing an acute euphoric state followed by a brief period of sedation; the major hazard is anoxia. The effect of the volatile nitrites is short-lived flushing, dizziness, euphoria, and hypotension. Chronic use can lead to methemoglobinemia, which is evidenced by cyanosis that does not respond to oxygen administration.

Anabolic Steroids. Anabolic steroids are synthetic derivatives of testosterone that are used to enhance athletic performance and to build lean muscle mass. Injection is the most common route of use, which makes the user susceptible to the hazards of unsterile injections. Intoxication is characterized by aggression, irritability, impulsiveness, and elation. Users also have disturbed hormonal cycles, acne, hair loss, excessive muscle growth, testicular atrophy or clitoral hypertrophy, breast enlargement or atrophy, liver toxicity, and elevated low-density lipoprotein. A common pattern of use is "cycling," which involves taking these drugs for weeks and then stopping them for short periods. Lethargy, restlessness, insomnia, and anorexia often occur with abstinence.

Injection Drug Use

IDU violates the first line of defense of the body, leaving the user vulnerable to infection, chemical impurities, and immediate drug toxicity. An annual average of 424,000 individuals inject drugs.[13] This method of use is obviously a greater hazard when injection equipment is shared. HIV-1 and hepatitis C virus have been found to remain viable in used syringes for weeks.[14]

Immunologic abnormalities include hypergammaglobulinemia, which may be related to repeated intravenous introduction of impurities, and hepatitis C. Chronic rheumatologic conditions are a consequence, as sometimes are false-positive serologic test results for syphilis. Neurologic complications include brain abscesses from endocarditis, cerebral anoxia, and transverse myelitis. Lung granulomas and abscesses can result from particles and pathogens that filter through the pulmonary circulation. Endocarditis may result from bacteria and fungi that settle in the endocardium. In the United States, IDU is the major means of transmission for hepatitis B and C viruses and has been linked to serious outbreaks of hepatitis D. Most injection drug users have serologic evidence of remote hepatitis virus B exposure. Renal disease may be the result of immune complex deposition, endocarditis, or nephrotoxic impurities. Vertebral osteomyelitis from hematologic seeding of the cancellous bone is the most common serious musculoskeletal condition associated with IDU. Cellulitis, subcutaneous abscesses, and fascial abscesses are a common result of injection infiltration outside of the vein. Phlebitis is common, particularly when irritating drugs are injected.

Poor venous access complicates the care of these patients, particularly when the management of comorbid conditions calls for frequent laboratory testing. Needle exchange and other "harm reduction" methods have been used with some success and much controversy to reduce the public and individual health hazards of IDU.

CLINICAL PRESENTATION AND PHYSICAL EXAMINATION

Patients may have no history of a recognized addictive disorder, may be actively addicted, may be in early recovery, or may have a history of addiction and be well established in recovery. Poor compliance and requests for disability testimony by an otherwise healthy patient should raise concerns about the presence of substance abuse. Behavioral problems appear first, and early manifestations of addiction are rarely apparent with routine examination. The time of the last substance use can be asked when medications are reviewed, and the temporal relationship between substance use and symptoms should be considered.

As a screening tool, the CAGE questionnaire—which focuses on Concern about drinking, being Annoyed by criticism about drinking, having Guilt about drinking, and taking an *Eye*-opener drink in the morning—can be woven into standard history taking.[15] These questions should be asked if the patient reports drinking or drug use when asked about medications or lifestyle. Two or more positive answers suggest an alcohol use disorder; but like any structured questionnaire, this should be interpreted contextually. A patient who answers yes to one question but is grossly tremulous is more likely to have a problem than a patient who scores a 4 but drinks only twice a year. Answers of yes to any question should be pursued by follow-up questions. Asking the following two questions may be as effective as CAGE, with the advantage of screening for both alcohol and drug concerns:

- Have you, in the past year, drunk or used more drugs than you meant to?
- Have you felt that you wanted or needed to cut down on your drinking or drug use in the past year?[16]

These questions can be woven into a standard history and should be asked if patients report drinking or drug use when they are asked about medications or lifestyle.

Health problems that suggest the presence of alcoholism include emotional difficulties, poor nutrition, trauma, seizures, unexplained tachycardia, refractory hypertension, dyspepsia, liver disease, pancreatitis, and peripheral neuropathy. Postural blood pressure and pulse changes may indicate gastrointestinal bleeding. The smell of alcohol strongly suggests alcohol dependence because even the heaviest drinkers will not drink before a primary care appointment.

Addiction-related causes of fever are endocarditis, acute retroviral syndrome–associated and HIV-associated infections, anticholinergic ingestion, and sedative withdrawal. Withdrawal from opioids will cause chills and sweats that are not accompanied by fever. Simultaneously elevated pulse and blood pressure often results from sedative withdrawal or stimulant toxicity. Weight may fluctuate because of an irregular diet, wasting infections, or chronic liver disease. Generalized edema may be a result of liver failure from chronic hepatitis, kidney failure from glomerulopathies, or heart failure from valvular insufficiency or cardiomyopathy. Overwhelming lethargy and fatigue accompany withdrawal from stimulants and very early opioid withdrawal. Varying degrees of lethargy are seen with coexisting vegetative depressions, chronic hepatitis, and kidney failure. Headaches commonly accompany alcohol and cocaine withdrawal. Sudden headaches may be related to cocaine-induced venospasms. Many addicts have a history of head trauma or brain abscess; therefore it is helpful if cranial nerve deficits are noted in initial examinations. Visual changes may be caused by retinal emboli from IDU or from several complications of HIV infection. Sedatives may cause diplopia. The sclerae should be examined for icterus. Opioid withdrawal or cannabis, stimulant, or hallucinogen intoxications dilate the pupils, and the use of opioids causes pupils to constrict. Sedative or alcohol intoxication causes nystagmus. Rotary nystagmus is a unique feature of PCP intoxication. Nasal heroin or cocaine use causes mucosal inflammation. Perforation of the nasal septum is caused by mucosal vasoconstriction and subsequent tissue ischemia with cocaine use. Inhalation of hot crack vapors can cause flaming pharyngitis and tonsillar swelling. In addition to well-known HIV-related adenopathy, injection drug users often have swollen lymph nodes in response to local injections. The cervical spine is a possible focus of osteomyelitis.

Because of hypersensitivity, nasal heroin use causes a bronchitis that resembles severe asthma. The bronchitis tends to get worse with each subsequent exposure and is difficult to control with steroids and bronchodilators if the patient continues to inhale heroin. Cocaine may make the heart hyperdynamic through its adrenergic effects, or it may slow myocardial impulses through its anesthetic effects. Ischemic chest pain can result from vasospasm that damages the intima and predisposes the patient to subsequent coronary artery disease. A variety of cocaine-induced arrhythmias can cause sudden death. Patients with endocarditis are usually febrile, with a new or changed murmur, petechiae, and possible signs of metastatic infections. A wide pulse pressure may represent secondary aortic regurgitation. The strain of acute sedative withdrawal may precipitate a serious cardiac event in a patient with preexisting cardiac disease.

Evidence of ascites should be determined in a patient with increasing abdominal girth. Mild tenderness in the right upper quadrant may be the only clinical manifestation of chronic hepatitis. The visceral pain and hyperactive bowel sounds from opioid withdrawal can be severe enough to mimic an acute abdominal emergency. Bleeding in the stool may be from alcohol-induced gastritis, liver congestion, coagulopathies, or hemorrhoids from opioid-related constipation.

The usual life of a patient with addiction leaves little time and energy for concern about regular Papanicolaou (Pap) tests and breast, testicular, rectal, and prostate examinations. In addition to neglecting these health maintenance examinations, addicts often exchange sex for drugs, adding to the concern about sexually transmitted diseases. Many addicts also have a history of sexual trauma and avoid genital examinations, which they can find frightening. The possibility of pregnancy is a consideration with all fertile female patients.

Vertebral tenderness raises the question of osteomyelitis or epidural abscess. Swollen and tender joints suggest septic arthritis from injected pathogens, gonorrhea, or syphilis. Arthromyalgias may be a prominent feature of opioid withdrawal. Arthromyalgias also commonly accompany polyarteritis syndromes, which are associated with intravenous amphetamine abuse and with hepatitis C.

Intoxication with alcohol or sedatives causes incoordination. Broad-based gaits are associated with alcohol-induced cerebellar degeneration. Intention tremors are the conspicuous physical sign of sedative withdrawal. Compression and trauma are the most common causes of mononeuropathy. Neuropathy of the ulnar or radial nerves sometimes follows prolonged periods of unconsciousness and results from compression of the nerves against the bone prominences. Peripheral manifestations of alcoholism or thiamine deficiency include proximally progressing decreased peripheral sensation and deep tendon reflexes. Symmetric hyperreflexia suggests stimulant drug toxicity or sedative withdrawal, whereas sedative toxicity causes reflexes to be sluggish. Seizure disorders are complicated by multiple drug use, head trauma, and past cerebral anoxia. Stimulant toxicity and withdrawal from sedatives or alcohol are the most common causes of drug-related convulsions. Substance abuse is the most common precipitant of psychiatric symptoms.

Edema of the hands without coexisting ankle or facial edema is usually a result of damaged veins. Needle marks from cocaine injection are usually multiple and recent, whereas those from heroin use are more deliberately tracked along large veins. Venous insufficiency and attendant complications are common, especially in older addicts. Palmar erythema suggests chronic liver disease. Patients often have scars from cigarette burns or wrist cutting.

Developing relationships with patients over time is the most useful way for the health care provider to understand the neurologic and psychiatric components of substance use disorder. This relationship also becomes the foundation by which change may begin to occur.

DIAGNOSTICS

The use of laboratory tests should be individualized and based on the clinical presentation. Toxicology testing is essential in evaluating many emergency situations. Drug screening may be useful in monitoring patients in treatment programs or receiving prescriptions for controlled substances. Most drugs concentrate in the urine, making urine tests generally better than serum tests for screening purposes. Because psychiatric symptoms are so often caused or influenced by substance use, toxicology tests may be most useful in evaluating refractory psychiatric symptoms.

Anemia and thrombocytopenia are often a result of liver disease or HIV infection. Liver function abnormalities are often caused by viral hepatitis or alcoholism. Hepatitis and syphilis serologic screening should be conducted at some point. Patients should be counseled and offered HIV testing in the office or given information about anonymous HIV test sites. Urine or blood human chorionic gonadotropin testing for pregnancy may be indicated and, if the result is positive, may be helpful in guiding the pace, intensity, and nature of treatment plans. Several laboratory values are altered by excessive alcohol use, although they are not sensitive or specific enough to be considered screening tests. Mean corpuscular volume is elevated from impaired folate use and probably from direct bone marrow toxicity. It may not return to normal for months, even with folate substitution. Affected liver enzymes include γ-glutamyl transpeptidase (GGT), alanine transaminase (AST), alanine aminotransferase (ALT), and alkaline phosphatase. All liver enzyme levels are nonspecific when interpreted in isolation. GGT returns to normal after approximately 3 weeks of alcohol abstinence and is useful for tracking abstinence. In contrast to chronic viral hepatitis, alcohol causes the AST level to rise in excess of the ALT level.

Baseline renal function tests are useful in detecting glomerulonephropathies associated with IDU. Baseline thyroid function tests are useful because sedatives and stimulants can mimic hypothyroidism or hyperthyroidism, respectively, whereas their abstinence syndromes cause the reverse effects. Patients usually need frequently neglected routine health maintenance screening tests such as Pap smears and lipid levels.

MANAGEMENT

As stated earlier, a trusting relationship is the foundation on which conversations about substance use can begin. Conveying a hopeful attitude is important. There is no way to predict when a single episodic encounter may be the time that the patient makes substantial progress. Because substance use disorders are often chronic conditions that progress slowly over time, health care providers address a patient's substance abuse problems, monitor progress, and provide regular supportive counseling. This provides the patient with a stable relationship during which reducing harm and keeping up with health maintenance can pay off in long-term benefits.

The primary care brief intervention format of (1) providing feedback of relevant data, (2) emphasizing patient responsibility and self-efficacy, (3) advising about recommended change, (4) providing a menu of helpful options, and (5) taking an empathetic approach is helpful whether or not the patient enters a formal treatment program.[17] Patients should be counseled about risk reduction strategies, such as using condoms, not sharing needles, and not driving while using. The provider should be familiar with local treatment, consultation, and case management services and have a handy referral list.

Although several studies have suggested that an inpatient detoxification is unlikely to affect the long-term course of addiction, it may be needed to stabilize the patient and to facilitate entry into longer-term treatment. Other treatment often is impossible without detoxification first. Individual motivated patients sometimes significantly reduce drug use after a brief detoxification without other services. A drug-related lifestyle may be a problem that is as big as or bigger than the direct effect of drug use.

Common formal treatment programs include outpatient methadone maintenance, long-term residential treatment programs, outpatient drug-free programs, individual counseling by a psychotherapist trained in modern approaches, and short-term inpatient rehabilitation programs. Acupuncture is effective for reducing craving in some individuals and may be a component of recovery. The most effective therapeutic approaches incorporate cognitive-behavioral therapy with specific components of motivational interviewing and harm reduction techniques. One of the most used treatment modalities is community-based 12-step programs, which have not demonstrated consistent good outcomes. Patients in longer-term recovery often benefit from insight-oriented therapy. Intensive outpatient or partial hospitalization programs for less-stable patients are designed to provide a daily therapeutic milieu while having the advantage of allowing patients to stay at home or even participate in the evening while working during the day. Long-term residential programs offer a drug-free therapeutic living environment that is staffed by counselors and usually other recovering addicts. The optimum duration of involvement in long-term residential treatment appears to be 6 months. These programs are especially helpful in supporting the recovery of addicts who are homeless and reintegrating them into society. Residential programs for these patients usually require a lengthier stay. Adolescent programs should include strong peer and family components.

The primary care provider may become a collaborative part of the treatment team or continue to treat the patient's medical conditions, to encourage continuing participation in the program, and to schedule follow-up visits after treatment termination to monitor progress and help prevent relapse. How to judiciously prescribe controlled substances is one of the major difficulties providers face in caring for these patients.

Drug-seeking patients may feign symptoms and request medications for longer than their medical conditions dictate. Medications that can be abused may reinitiate craving and addiction in patients who have achieved drug abstinence, whereas inadequately treated pain, depression, or anxiety may also be a trigger for relapse. Recognizing that symptom relief is a legitimate goal of care, the guidelines of the Drug Enforcement Administration (DEA) ask providers to consider the following when controlled substances are indicated: the severity of the patient's symptoms and ability to tolerate them, the patient's reliability in taking medications, and the addiction liability of the medication.[18]

Opiates, barbiturates, and stimulants are Schedule II drugs and have the highest potential for abuse. In general, prescribing opiates to treat opiate withdrawal is restricted to methadone programs and acute medical situations such as hospital admission. Schedule III and IV medications are considered by the DEA to have a lower potential for abuse. Prescriptions of controlled substances should be written only for recognized indications and for limited amounts, and they are usually recommended for finite periods. Recent research suggests that the nonmedical use of opioids is a predictable parallel phenomenon of their prescriptive availability and that the potential for and extent of diversion are directly related to the relative potency of the drug and the amount prescribed. The goal is to provide appropriate therapy to patients in pain but also to prevent drug abuse. Guidelines are available to assist the primary care provider treating patients with chronic noncancer pain, but it is also good practice to consult with addiction or pain specialists in prescribing controlled substances to patients with addiction or who might be at risk for addiction.[19] Antidepressant medications (usually selective serotonin reuptake inhibitors) may be useful for dysthymic states that persist after detoxification. The antidepressant trazodone is a useful adjunctive medication for persistent insomnia. It has a low potential for overdose and addiction, but its efficacy varies. When it is used to assist with sleep, trazodone is taken in a low dose approximately 30 to 40 minutes before going to bed.

Antagonist and aversive drugs are designed to block or to change the effect of the addictive drug and thereby help people avoid falling back into a pattern of abuse or dependence after discontinuing drug use. Disulfiram (Antabuse) has been used for years to help people refrain from drinking alcohol once they have stopped. This is helpful in very specific situations in which the individual is highly motived to stop drinking alcohol but feels powerless to do so in specific situations. Many are disappointed by the outcomes of using disulfiram because discontinued use of the prescription is always an option. Naltrexone is a narcotic antagonist that is sometimes used to treat people with opioid dependence. Naltrexone attaches to endorphin receptor sites throughout the brain and makes it impossible for opioids to exert their usual effects. There is less incentive to continue to use drugs because no high is experienced.[12] These drugs must be administered carefully because they have the potential to throw a person with an opioid addiction into serious withdrawal. Partial antagonists, which produce less-severe withdrawal symptoms, have also been used.

Discussion of substance abuse is usually better accepted when it is addressed in the context of the patient's overall health and quality of life. Patients may be susceptible to use of other substances, and this should be kept in mind. The provider's concerns about drinking and the evidence that supports these concerns should be shared and reinforced.

Brief interventions for heavy-drinking college students have been associated with reduction in drinking and in adverse consequences, although it is not clear how much improvement is attributable to the intervention and how much to the students' normal maturation.

Many patients with substance abuse disorders have been helped through the drug self-help movement. Related self-help programs have been developed for other substance-related disorders, including Narcotics Anonymous and Cocaine Anonymous, and for people who live and care for persons with substance abuse disorders, including Al-Anon and Alateen. Alcoholics Anonymous (AA) is the prototype community self-help group and for decades has provided millions of people with a foundation for alcoholism recovery. The focus and tone of individual meetings can differ, and patients may need to attend several before finding a meeting in which they feel comfortable. In brief, the 12 steps of recovery (12-step program) in AA ask that participants begin to acknowledge that they have a problem, that there is a spiritual dimension to life beyond their control, that personal relationships should be healed, and that recovering persons should use experiences and insight to help other alcoholics. These principles are the same at all AA and Narcotics Anonymous meetings, and the only requirement for attendance is a desire to stop using alcohol or mind-altering drugs. The advantage of the recommendation to attend "90 meetings in 90 days" is that it helps patients get into a routine of AA attendance, begin to understand that their problems are shared by others, and begin to establish a relationship with a member who has achieved successful sobriety. Some patients engage better with cognitive behavioral–oriented groups such as Rational Recovery; others may benefit simply from social engagement in non–drug-using communities or groups. Although AA has not been able to demonstrate consistent long-term outcomes, it seems to have been helpful to some in reducing alcohol use when other options are not available. In-depth, insight-oriented psychotherapeutic approaches have not been shown to be helpful in assisting with early recovery, but they may be helpful for patients who have established long-term sobriety.

Many self-help programs have expanded into residential treatment centers or therapeutic communities, where people with a history of substance abuse live, work, and socialize in a drug-free environment.[20]

Pharmacologic adjuncts include medications to prevent major withdrawal, drugs to reduce craving, antidepressants (usually selective serotonin reuptake inhibitors) for persistent dysthymia or coexisting depression, and disulfiram (Antabuse) as aversive therapy. Patients should also receive thiamine, multivitamins, and folic acid supplementation. Treatment for depression or mood stability may be helpful for some patients.

INDICATIONS FOR REFERRAL OR HOSPITALIZATION

Emergency department consultation should be considered for patients with unexplained fevers, delirium, overdose, severe sedative withdrawal, vital sign instability, severe headaches, chest pain, acute shortness of breath, acute abdominal pain and gastrointestinal bleeding, active suicidality, or a suspected recent head injury.

Referral to an inpatient or outpatient addiction program should always be discussed with actively addicted patients. Referral to the emergency department should be considered for patients with unexplained fevers, delirium, overdose, severe sedative withdrawal, vital sign instability, severe headaches, chest pain, acute shortness of breath, acute abdominal pain and gastrointestinal bleeding, or active suicidality. These patients often need to be stabilized and considered for hospitalization. Hospitalized substance abusers are notoriously difficult patients who are often unwelcome and sometimes undertreated for discomfort. In addition to assisting with the medical aspects of care, the health care provider collaborates with the inpatient team to help humanize the patient and help the hospital staff recognize and work with problem behaviors. Patients taking methadone should be kept on their usual dose and receive normal or slightly higher doses of pain medication as indicated by their medical conditions.

Medical clearance is often requested of the health care provider before a patient is admitted to a detoxification or rehabilitation program. A brief history and physical examination are necessary to identify and to stabilize acute health problems. It is helpful to know what resources are available at the program because it may or may not have medical support or medication on site. It should be clear, to both the patient and the program, that "medically clear" does not mean the patient does not have outstanding health problems that need future attention; it is simply an assessment that the patient is stable enough to enter a program.

Inpatient treatment should be considered for patients who have a history of severe withdrawal, who are drinking all day long, who are medically ill, or who are abusing other substances. Patients with repeated seizures, severe intoxication, or mental status changes that are not obviously attributable to intoxication, recent head trauma, fevers, postural hypotension or tachycardia, shortness of breath, chest pain, severe abdominal pain, severe vomiting, or diarrhea often need to be seen in the emergency department for stabilization and consideration for hospitalization. Pregnant women who are alcohol dependent should be referred for inpatient detoxification; this needs to be coordinated with the patient's obstetric team and often involves making arrangements for child care, and it should be done in conjunction with a treatment program that has experience with the treatment of pregnant women. If a patient does not yet have prenatal care, such care should be arranged urgently.

CHAPTER 250 OTHER MENTAL HEALTH DISORDERS

J. Nile Wagley

DEFINITION AND EPIDEMIOLOGY

Schizophrenia is a chronic, severe, and disabling brain disorder.[1] Schizophrenia interrupts a person's capacity to accurately perceive reality, to communicate and to relate to others, and to complete the usual activities of daily living, especially during acute phases of the illness. Schizophrenia affects approximately 1% of the population at similar rates across ethnic groups and is equal in prevalence in the genders. Onset of psychotic symptoms is usually between the ages of 16 and 30 years; young men experience a slightly earlier onset than women do. It is rare for this illness to occur in children and unusual for it to be diagnosed after the age of 45 years.[1] Diagnostic subtypes of schizophrenia have more historical significance than clinical usefulness. The most common subtype of schizophrenia, paranoid schizophrenia, is characterized by one or more delusions and frequent auditory hallucinations and may be persecutory.[2]

In addition to schizophrenia, there is an array of mental health disorders in which psychosis is a key feature, including dementia, brief psychotic disorder, schizophreniform and schizoaffective disorders, delusional disorder, and substance-induced psychotic disorders.

PATHOPHYSIOLOGY

The dopamine hypothesis of schizophrenic illness, which posits that the symptoms of schizophrenia result from altered and hyperactive dopaminergic functioning, has influenced pharmacologic development, yielding conventional first-generation typical antipsychotics and subsequent second-generation atypical antipsychotic therapies, which are discussed later in this chapter. However, the dopamine hypothesis is not enough to explain the pathophysiologic mechanism of this disease.[3]

Glutamate is the most abundant excitatory neurotransmitter in the brain; it is involved with learning and memory as well as the brain's plasticity, which helps in everyday interface with our environment. As in the dopaminergic pathways, dysregulations in glutamatergic pathways contribute to the psychotic symptoms of the illness, the "positive symptoms," as well as the cognitive dysfunctions, especially related to *N*-methyl-D-aspartate (NMDA) receptor hypofunctioning. γ-Aminobutyric acid (GABA) is the brain's major inhibitory transmitter, and there is evidence of alterations in GABA markers in schizophrenia. In addition, disturbances in serotonin function contribute to the so-called negative symptoms of the illness. Acetylcholine dysfunctions are also present, contributing to cognitive and memory problems as well as to the higher incidence of cigarette smoking in persons with schizophrenia.[3]

Postmortem studies have shown an enlarged third and lateral ventricle, which is not helpful diagnostically because other brain disorders, such as Alzheimer disease and hydrocephalus, show similar findings. There are not significant changes in the neuronal density of the hippocampus. The thalamus does show reduction in neuronal counts, especially in the projections to the dorsolateral prefrontal cortex, which is the functional area of the brain for problem solving, maintaining goals, and "paying attention."[2]

CLINICAL PRESENTATION

There is a characteristic "prodromal period" lasting, on average, 50 or more weeks before the psychotic presentation of the schizophrenic illness.[4] The patient or significant others may notice changes in grades, sleep, and mood, with particular complaints of anergia and reduced concentration, attention, drive, and motivation. Because some of these changes can also occur in the healthy teenager, it can be difficult to diagnose schizophrenia in teens, the usual age at onset of the illness. A combination of factors can predict schizophrenia in up to 80% of youth who are at high risk for development of the illness. These factors include the isolation of oneself and withdrawal from others, an increase in unusual thoughts and suspicions, and a family history of psychosis. Symptoms of schizophrenia fall into three main categories: positive, negative, and cognitive.[1]

Positive Symptoms

The so-called positive symptoms of schizophrenia are defined as symptoms "added" to the usual human experience. Psychotic symptoms of schizophrenia are the most recognizable to clinicians, patients, and families. Auditory hallucinations are the most common type of hallucination, with a 70% occurrence in patients with schizophrenia. Voices are the most common auditory hallucination, but other sounds, such as whispers, have been described. Frequently, the auditory hallucinations are profane, critical, and derogatory and can sometimes be command hallucinations.[2]

Visual hallucinations occur in approximately one third of patients, with animate objects, people, or parts of people being the most common hallucinations. Tactile hallucinations occur in 15% to 25% of patients; olfactory and gustatory hallucinations occur in a small number.[2]

Delusion, a fixed false belief, is another manifestation of the psychotic symptoms of schizophrenia. Delusions of persecution are the most common delusion, which 80% of hospitalized patients have experienced. Depending on the nature of the delusions, patients may act in ways that put them or others at risk.[2]

Negative Symptoms

The severity of the negative symptoms, which are a decrease or loss of normal functions, predicts long-term disability better than other symptom presentations do. The persistence of negative symptoms (Table 250-1) for 12 months, even present during periods of clinical stability and not related to any secondary causes, is predictive of the deficit syndrome in schizophrenia. The deficit syndrome is defined by lower quality of life, more hospitalizations, more symptomatic periods, and more social and physical anhedonia. Prevalence rates of deficit syndrome range from 10% to 30% in persons with schizophrenia. Deficit syndrome is marked by more disorganized behavior, progression of negative symptoms, and symptoms less responsive to medications and social skills training.[2]

TABLE 250-1 Negative Symptoms of Schizophrenia

Classic "A" Symptom	Dysfunctional Domain	Patient Presentation
Alogia	Communication	Talks very little with few words
Affect, blunted	Affect	Reduced range of expression and words and reduced recognition of emotions in others
Asocial	Socialization	Few friends; decreased interest in spending time with others; little sexual interest
Avolition	Motivation	Compromised ability to complete activities of daily living, especially hygiene
Anhedonia	Pleasure	No joy from past interests or pleasures

Cognitive Symptoms

There is increased awareness of the cognitive deficits related to schizophrenia. Problems include focusing and sustaining attention; monitoring and evaluating performance, especially in response to social cues; prioritizing; problem solving and setting and maintaining goals; problems with serial learning; and impaired verbal fluency.[3]

PHYSICAL EXAMINATION

A thorough physical examination is required for persons with psychotic mental changes before psychiatric treatment is initiated. Common hallucinatory presentations in psychosis may also be an indication of substance use disorders, drug toxicity, infection, or fluid and electrolyte imbalances. It may be necessary because of alterations in the patient's current mental status to obtain the history from family or significant others, or obtain information from other sources. The physical examination of an individual with a psychotic disorder requires more time and deliberateness because of disruptions in logical thought processes and reality testing. A simple explanation of what will be done during the examination can do much to obtain the patient's cooperation. If the patient is severely psychotic, a thorough physical examination may need to be postponed.

A mental status examination (MSE) is an essential assessment component for evaluation of schizophrenia or other psychotic disorders. The MSE assists the clinician in describing the individual's appearance, speech, behavior, and thoughts, serving as a baseline for diagnosis and future assessment (Table 250-2).[2]

DIAGNOSTICS

Whereas there are no definitive diagnostic tests for schizophrenia or psychotic disorders, it is essential to rule out organic causes of psychosis. Diagnostic tests should be directed at assessment for underlying medical conditions that may cause psychosis or mimic symptoms of psychosis. The completeness of diagnostic testing is outside the scope of this chapter, but it should at a minimum include blood chemistries, hepatic and renal studies, thyroid studies, complete blood count, syphilis and human immunodeficiency virus (HIV) infection screen, and alcohol and drug testing. Other laboratory testing should be conducted as indicated by the patient's history.[2]

Computed tomography (CT) or magnetic resonance imaging (MRI) is indicated with the initial presentation of psychosis to rule out structural or traumatic conditions that might account for the change in mental status. Imaging studies may identify

TABLE 250-2 Mental Status Examination

Appearance	Clothing, grooming, posture
Attitude toward examiner	Cooperative, friendly, defensive, guarded, evasive
Speech characteristics	Quantity, volume, rate
Behavior	Motor activity, mannerisms, tics, gestures
Mood and affect	Depressed, irritable, angry, euphoric, amount and range of facial expression
Perceptions	Hallucinations, illusions
Thought process and content	Rapid, slow, bizarre, goal directed, delusions, preoccupations, obsessions, compulsions, phobias, suicidality
Sensorium	Orientation, memory, attention, concentration, abstract thought
Insight	Understanding of illness and current situation
Judgment	Reasonableness of actions and decisions

Modified from Sadock B, Sadock V, Ruiz P: *Kaplan and Sadock's comprehensive textbook of psychiatry,* ed 9, Philadelphia, 2007, Lippincott Williams & Wilkins.

decreased activation of the frontal lobes and a reduced temporal volume of the hippocampus, amygdala, and parahippocampal gyrus characteristic of patients with schizophrenia.[2]

DIAGNOSTICS

Schizophrenia and Other Psychotic Disorders

- Blood chemistries
- Hepatic, renal, and thyroid function studies
- Complete blood count
- Syphilis and HIV infection screen
- Urine or serum drug screen
- Blood alcohol level
- Brain imaging (CT or MRI)
- Electroencephalography
- Heavy metal screen (lead, arsenic, iron, mercury)

DIFFERENTIAL DIAGNOSIS

In general, positive symptoms must be present for a minimum of 1 month, with some exceptions in the diagnostic criteria. There should also be significant social and occupational interruption that persists for a minimum of 6 months.[5] Medical conditions that may produce psychotic symptoms include neurologic, endocrine, metabolic, hepatic, renal, and autoimmune disorders.[2] A woman's risk of psychosis is highest during the postpartum period, for both initial and subsequent episodes, which should be considered.[6] Psychiatric conditions such as mania and severe depression may manifest with psychotic symptoms. Patients with schizophrenia have a high incidence of substance abuse (dual diagnosis), so toxicity from alcohol or drugs is screened.

In older adults, acute illnesses such as urinary tract infections can mimic a psychotic presentation (delirium), as can dementia associated with Alzheimer disease or vascular dementia, Parkinson disease, or HIV dementia.

TABLE 250-3 Conventional Antipsychotics

Generic Name	Trade Name
Chlorpromazine	Thorazine
Fluphenazine	Prolixin
Haloperidol	Haldol
Loxapine	Loxitane
Molindone	Moban
Perphenazine	Trilafon
Pimozide	Orap
Thioridazine	Mellaril
Thiothixene	Navane
Trifluoperazine	Stelazine

MANAGEMENT

In first-episode schizophrenia, there is increased treatment responsiveness and an increased sensitivity to medication adverse effects. Starting with lower doses is recommended, as is early intervention. Delays in entering care have tragically become the norm; it is imperative to have early detection and treatment to improve outcomes.[7] Schizophrenia and other psychotic disorders are treated with antipsychotic medications and nonpharmacologic care. The conventional antipsychotic medications (Table 250-3) are characterized by the psychomotor slowing, emotional quieting, and affective indifference that occur with the blocking of dopamine D_2 receptors in the mesolimbic dopamine pathway. The effects on the D_2 receptors make the conventional antipsychotics effective in managing the positive symptoms associated with schizophrenia.[3]

The blockage of the D_2 receptors by the conventional antipsychotics in the mesocortical dopamine pathway, however, can worsen the negative symptoms associated with schizophrenia and decrease cognitive function. Also, the D_2 blockade in the nigrostriatal tract prevents the benefits of dopamine in this pathway, producing abnormal movements similar to those seen in Parkinson disease, called extrapyramidal symptoms (EPSs), and tardive dyskinesia. The symptoms of tardive dyskinesia, sometimes irreversible, include movements such as a constant chewing, tongue protrusion, facial grimacing, and jerking movement of the extremities. D_2 receptor blockade in the tuberoinfundibular tract may cause a rise in prolactin with resultant hyperprolactinemia, affecting bone density and sexual performance. Last, the conventional antipsychotics also block muscarinic and cholinergic receptors, causing dry mouth, blurred vision, constipation, drowsiness, and weight gain, and alpha$_1$-adrenergic receptors, causing orthostatic hypotension.[3]

The second-generation antipsychotics, the atypical antipsychotic medications (Table 250-4), differ from the earlier class in that they not only work on positive symptoms but also improve the negative symptoms associated with schizophrenia and have a lower risk of EPSs. The atypical antipsychotics achieve these effects through their indirect effect on serotonin and dopamine interactions with diminished binding to the D_2 receptors in all tracts but the mesolimbic. Whereas this action does mediate some of the side effect profile of the conventional antipsychotics, the atypical antipsychotics have different

TABLE 250-4 Atypical Antipsychotics

Generic Name	Trade Name
Clozapine	Clozaril
Aripiprazole	Abilify
Olanzapine	Zyprexa
Quetiapine	Seroquel
Risperidone	Risperdal
Ziprasidone	Geodon

TABLE 250-5 Risk Factors Associated with Atypical Antipsychotics

Drug	Weight Gain	Cardiometabolic Risk*
Clozapine	+++	Definite risk
Aripiprazole	+/–	Limited data
Olanzapine	+++	Definite risk
Quetiapine	++	Definite risk
Risperidone	++	Intermediate
Ziprasidone	+/–	Limited data

*All carry the diabetes warning from the Food and Drug Administration.
Data from McEvoy JP, Meyer JM, Goff DC et al: Prevalence of the metabolic syndrome in patients with schizophrenia: baseline results from the Clinical Antipsychotic Trials of Intervention Effectiveness (CATIE) schizophrenia trial and comparison with national estimates from NHANES III, *Schizophr Res* 80(1):19-32, 2005; and Stahl S: *Stahl's essential psychopharmacology: neuroscientific basis and practical applications*, ed 3, Cambridge, 2008, Cambridge University Press.

significant risks. The atypical antipsychotics have been linked to increased cardiometabolic risk (weight gain, dyslipidemia, diabetes, and accelerated cardiovascular disease) and premature death (Table 250-5).[3,8]

Clozapine was the first atypical antipsychotic but is not considered a first-line treatment because of the potential adverse event of agranulocytosis, requiring enrollment in a registry and scheduled laboratory monitoring for life. Clozapine is indicated and effective for patients with persistent suicidal thoughts.[2] Clozapine is also indicated for the treatment of residual positive symptoms that have not responded to two adequate trials of other antipsychotic agents. An adequate trial of clozapine should be a minimum of 8 weeks (initially 12.5 mg PO twice a day with gradual titration up to a total daily dose of 300 to 800 mg/day) in collaboration or consultation with a psychiatrist. If the patient fails to respond to clozapine, clozapine blood level should be measured to learn if the serum level is above 350 ng/mL, and the dose is titrated as needed.[9]

The choice of antipsychotic medication should be based on individual preference, prior treatment response, side effect experience, adherence history, medical history and risk factors, and long-term treatment planning. Medication trials should be for 2 to 6 weeks to observe for response; when symptom relief is obtained, continuation of treatment for at least 1 year should be offered to reduce the risk of relapse.[9] For patients who have difficulty complying with needed medications, long-acting injectable antipsychotic medications can be used for maintenance treatment. The dosage of long-acting fluphenazine decanoate is 6.25 to 25 mg IM every 2 weeks; haloperidol decanoate, 50 to 200 mg IM every 4 weeks; and risperidone long-acting injectable, 25 to 50 mg IM every 2 weeks.[9]

For patients using first-generation antipsychotics, it is recommended to use prophylactic antiparkinson medications to reduce the EPS dystonia, which involves abnormal movements of the head and neck with spasms, impaired tongue and mouth movements, tongue protrusions, or deviated eye movements.[9] Young men are most at risk for this type of adverse event, especially African-American men.[2] Acute EPSs respond well to intramuscular benztropine (2 mg) or diphenhydramine (50 mg).

Tardive dyskinesia is a potential complication of typical antipsychotics, a movement disorder that is potentially irreversible. Use of atypical antipsychotics has helped decrease this adverse event but not eliminate it. Use of clozapine in patients with symptoms of tardive dyskinesia can help decrease these symptoms and still manage the illness of schizophrenia. Screening regularly for EPSs with a simple screening tool such as the Abnormal Involuntary Movement Scale (AIMS) should be done annually and after any antipsychotic medication changes.[2]

DIFFERENTIAL DIAGNOSIS

Schizophrenia and Other Psychotic Disorders

- Heavy metal exposure
- Medication or substance toxicity
  - Antiparkinson drugs
  - Digitalis
  - Steroids
  - Theophylline
  - Anticholinergics
  - Substance abuse
- Metabolic disorders
  - Hypoglycemia
  - Hypothyroidism
  - Hyperthyroidism
  - Porphyria
- Neurologic disorders
  - Brain lesion
  - Cerebrovascular accident
  - Encephalitis
  - Huntington chorea
  - Parkinson disease
  - Seizure disorder
- Nutritional deficiencies
- Psychiatric disorders
  - Bipolar disorder
  - Dementia
  - Major depression
  - Schizophrenia

Interdisciplinary Management

A collaborative relationship between the primary care and psychiatric providers is essential for optimal care of the patient with schizophrenia. Appropriate release of medical information forms should be submitted to all providers involved in the care of the patient to facilitate transfer of information. Having accurate medication reconciliation among all providers is of prime importance. Although primary care providers may or may not assume medication management, it is incumbent on the primary care provider to be familiar with side effects, drug interactions, and symptoms of toxicity of antipsychotic medications. As a diagnostic group, patients with schizophrenia have greater risks for comorbid illnesses that need ongoing assessment and intervention by the primary care clinician.

In addition, the primary care provider may be asked to coordinate care with the assistance of case management services. Case management assists the individual with budgeting, housing, and other facets of community living. Assertive community treatment (ACT) programs are beneficial in assisting individuals to live in the community. The key elements of ACT include a multidisciplinary team with a medication prescriber, shared case load among team members, direct service provision, high frequency of patient contact, low patient-to-staff ratios, and outreach to patients in the community. In fact, ACT significantly reduces hospitalizations and homelessness.[10]

Skills training in the patient's day-to-day environment yields the best results in improving activities of daily living. In addition, cognitive behavioral therapy (CBT) to treat negative symptoms and to increase effective coping is essential to care.[10] Nurse practitioners who care for persons with schizophrenia can coordinate these essentials of their care; the illness often prevents the patient from being his or her own advocate.

CBT is recommended in a group or individual therapy format of 4 to 9 months' duration. The focus is on identification of target problems and development of specific cognitive and behavioral strategies to cope.[9]

COMPLICATIONS

Type 2 diabetes mellitus has a 15% to 18% prevalence in persons with schizophrenia, compared with only 4% in the general population. Multiple risk factors that contribute to this grave disparity include poverty, urbanization, crowding, psychological stress, and the effects of antipsychotic medication.[2] Because of the pharmacologic treatments and other comorbidities, persons with schizophrenia are at risk for metabolic syndrome. Specific measurements for enlarged waist circumference based on gender and nationality are readily available. In addition, two of the following must be present: elevated triglyceride level of 150 mg/dL or higher; high-density lipoprotein concentration below 40 mg/dL in men and below 50 mg/dL in women; blood pressure of 130/85 mm Hg or higher or current medication treatment for hypertension; and fasting blood glucose concentration of 110 mg/dL or higher or prior type 2 diabetes mellitus diagnosis.[2]

The life expectancy of persons with schizophrenia may be 20 to 30 years shorter than that of the general population,[3] in part owing to the 10% suicidal death rate but also because of premature cardiovascular disease. The landmark Clinical Antipsychotic Trials of Intervention Effectiveness (CATIE) revealed increased prevalence of cardiometabolic risk factors in patients with schizophrenia.[11] Hypertension has an approximate prevalence of 15% in the general population, but persons with schizophrenia enrolled in the CATIE trials had a prevalence of 27%. Elevated triglyceride levels were found in 50.7% of the CATIE patients, and 48.9% had low high-density lipoprotein concentrations. The cardiovascular risks are also related to genetic factors; lifestyle factors such as smoking, unhealthy diet, lack of exercise contributing to diabetes, and obesity; and some of the antipsychotic medications.

Chronic obstructive pulmonary disease has a 22.6% prevalence in persons with schizophrenia, compared with 5% in the general population. In addition to a twofold increased incidence of cigarette smoking in persons with schizophrenia, they also have increased abdominal obesity and exposure to secondhand smoke.[2]

INDICATIONS FOR REFERRAL OR HOSPITALIZATION

The most dangerous adverse event from antipsychotic medications is neuroleptic malignant syndrome (NMS). The hallmark symptoms of this hypodopaminergic state are elevated core body temperature from modest to severe and severe muscle rigidity. Two or more of the following symptoms are also required for diagnosis: diaphoresis, tachycardia, elevated or labile blood pressure, dysphagia, incontinence, tremor, changes in level of consciousness, mutism, leukocytosis, laboratory evidence of muscle injures, and hepatic enzyme elevations. NMS is considered a medical emergency, requiring monitoring, intravenous fluids, dopamine agonists, muscle relaxants, and other measures delivered in a hospital setting.[2] Exacerbation of negative symptoms such as depression and suicidal ideation, exacerbation of psychotic symptoms, and increased agitation are potential reasons for referral for hospitalization.

PATIENT AND FAMILY EDUCATION

Recovery is the goal of mental health care and for care of persons with schizophrenia. Recovery is broadly defined as a process of healing and transformation, enabling a person with a mental health problem to live a meaningful life in a community of his or her choice while striving to achieve his or her full potential in safety. There are 10 fundamental components of recovery: self-direction, individualized and person-centered empowerment, holistic care, nonlinear perspectives, strengths-based interventions, peer support, respect, responsibility, and hope.[2] Family members experience significant distress, and family interventions have been found to decrease distress as well as to decrease the rates of relapse and hospitalization. Key elements of family-based services include illness education, crisis intervention, emotional support, and training on how to cope with schizophrenic symptoms and the related problems.[9]

HEALTH PROMOTION

Appropriate age-related recommendations for health screenings for individuals with schizophrenia should be completed. To monitor for metabolic syndrome, weight or body mass index and blood pressure are measured at each visit, with glucose and lipid concentrations monitored quarterly. In addition, monitoring should be conducted for prolactin elevation if patients are symptomatic or taking agents known to cause this adverse event.

Psychiatric advance directives are like other advance directives, allowing persons with schizophrenia to request how they prefer to receive care when exacerbations of their illness prevent them from acting on their own behalf. More information is available at the National Resource Center on Psychiatric Advance Directives website, with a state-by-state guide to providing this information for persons with schizophrenia.[12]

REFERENCES

For a full list of references, scan the QR code or visit http://booksite.elsevier.com/9780323355018

Index

Note: Page number followed by *f* indicated figures, *t* indicate tables, and *b* indicate boxes.

A

A wave, 517
ABC assessment, 226
ABCD Score, for transient ischemic attack, 1012*t*
Abdominal aortic aneurysm, 510-515
  clinical presentation of, 511
  complications of, 514
  definition and epidemiology of, 510-511
  diagnostics for, 511-512, 512*b*
  differential diagnosis of, 512, 512*b*
  indications for referral or hospitalization for, 514-515
  life span considerations with, 514
  management of, 512-513
  pathophysiology of, 511
  physical examination for, 511
  risk factors for, 510-511, 511*t*, 512*b*
  screening for, 148*t*-152*t*
Abdominal examination, for preparticipation sports physical, 186
Abdominal pain, 623-630
  with acute pancreatitis, 715
  causes of, 623
  definition and epidemiology of, 623
  location of, 623
  pathophysiology and clinical presentation of, 623
  type of, 623
Abortion, counseling for, 881-882
Abscesses
  anorectal, 634-635
  Bartholin gland cysts and, 803-805
  dental, 398-399
  peritonsillar, 411-413, 1254
  retropharyngeal, 412
  signs and symptoms of, 405
Absolute reticulocyte count (ARC), 1279
Abstinence, 1370
Acamprosate (Campral), 1371
Acanthosis nigricans, 1098
ACCORD trial, 1094
Accountable care organizations (ACOs), 1-2
ACE inhibitors, for heart failure, 564-565
Acebutolol, 576*t*-582*t*
Acetabulum, 936
Acetaminophen, 1034, 1199-1200
  for hip pain, 939
  for low back pain, 958
  N-acetylcysteine for, 226
  for osteoarthritis, 977-978
  for shoulder pain, 992
Acetyl-L-carnitine (ALC), 18
Achievement tests, 1000*b*
Achilles tendon
  rupture of, 900-901
  tendinopathy of, 899-900
Acid reflux, 670
Acid regurgitation, 671
Acid suppression therapies, for GERD, 675
Acid-fast bacilli (AFB), 1267
Aclidinium, 461
Acne inversa. *see* Hidradenitis suppurativa
Acne vulgaris, 249-252
  clinical presentation and physical examination for, 249-250, 250*b*
  complications of, 252
  definition and epidemiology of, 249
  diagnostics for, 250, 250*b*
  differential diagnosis of, 250, 250*b*
  indications for referral or hospitalization for, 252
  management of, 250-252
  pathophysiology of, 249, 249*f*
Acneiform lesions, 274*t*
Acquired immunodeficiency syndrome (AIDS)
  case definition of, 1232
  diarrhea and, 648
  service organization for, 1240
Acral-lentiginous melanoma, 248*f*
Acromegaly, 1071-1074
  clinical presentation of, 1071
  complications of, 1073
  definition and epidemiology of, 1071
  diagnostics for, 1072, 1072*b*
  differential diagnosis for, 1072, 1072*b*
  indications for referral or hospitalization for, 1073
  life span considerations with, 1073
  management and co-management with specialists for, 1072-1073
  pathophysiology of, 1071
  physical examination for, 1071-1072
ACTH (Acthar), 1049
Actinic keratoses, 242, 247-248, 248*b*
Activated charcoal, 210
Activated partial thromboplastin time (aPTT), 1298, 1300
  interpretation of, 1300*b*
Activated protein C resistance (APCR), 1304
Activities of daily living (ADLs), 84
Activity, physical, 537*t*
  abdominal aortic aneurysm and, 515
  aerobic, 131
  constipation and, 646
  and coronary artery disease, 540
  insufficient, of obesity, 111
  in lifestyle management, 134
  in pregnancy, 70
Acupuncture, for osteoarthritis, 979
Acute allergic conjunctivitis, 341-342, 341*f*
Acute cerebrovascular syndrome (ACVS), 1010. *see also* Transient ischemic attacks (TIAs)
Acute chest syndrome, 1292
Acute coronary syndrome (ACS), 537-538
Acute febrile retinitis, in West Nile fever, 1274
Acute flaccid paralysis (AFP), 1271-1272, 1274*t*
Acute lymphocytic leukemia (ALL), 1307, 1310*b*
Acute myelogenous leukemia (AML), 1307, 1310*b*
Acute myocardial infarction
  acute ST-segment elevation myocardial infarction. *see* Acute ST-segment elevation myocardial infarction
  echocardiography for, 547
  electrocardiography with, 545*f*-546*f*
  exercise tolerance testing for, 547
  management of, 550
  non-ST segment elevation myocardial infarction (NSTEMI). *see* Non-ST segment elevation myocardial infarction (NSTEMI)
  territory of, 545*t*
Acute respiratory diseases, 1226-1227
Acute respiratory failure (ARF), 466
Acute rheumatic fever (ARF), 413, 416
Acute ST-segment elevation myocardial infarction, 539
  clinical presentation of, 542
  diagnostics for, 545-547
Acute tumor lysis syndrome (ATLS), 1311
Acyclovir, 789*b*
  for Bell palsy, 1009
  for herpes simplex virus, 271, 271*t*
Adalimumab (fully human anti-TNF monoclonal antibody), 697
Adaptive immune system, 1200
Addiction, with oncology pain, 1335
Addison disease
  clinical presentation of, 1075
  definition and epidemiology of, 1074
  diagnostics for, 1075, 1076*b*
  differential diagnosis for, 1076, 1076*b*
  management of, 1076
  pathophysiology of, 1074
  physical examination for, 1075
Adenocarcinoma , esophageal, 676
Adenosine, 505*t*, 509
Adenovirus, in conjunctivitis, 340
Adhesions, 820
Adhesive capsulitis, in shoulder joint, 992
Adipocytes, 109
Adiposity, 112
Adjuvant therapy
  for chronic pain, 1188
  for Paget disease, 969-970
Adolescents
  challenges, 54
  cognitive development of, 55
  with diabetes mellitus, 1095
  dysmenorrhea in, 821
  emotional development of, 55
  health maintenance and health promotion for, 58-59
  health visit, 56-57
  issues, 54-59
  mental health, 57
  physical development of, 54-55
  physical examination of, 58
  resources for, 59*b*
  sexual activity and, 58
  sexual assault in, 229
  social development of, 55-56
  STIs and, 783
  three stages of, 54
  transition from, 54
Adoption, 882
Adrenal fatigue, 1076
Adrenal gland disorders, 1074-1077. *see also specific disorders*
  clinical presentation of, 1075
  complications of, 1077
  definition and epidemiology of, 1074
  diagnostics for, 1075, 1076*b*
  differential diagnosis for, 1076, 1076*b*
  indications for referral or hospitalization for, 1077
  management of, 1076-1077
  pathophysiology of, 1074-1075
  physical examination for, 1075
Adrenocorticotropic hormone (ACTH)
  acne and, 250*b*
  in adrenal gland disorders, 1074
Adson test, 972
Adults
  older, prevention of lipid disorders in, 1126
  young, prevention of lipid disorders in, 1125-1126
Advance care planning, 95-96
Advance directives, importance of, 86
ADVANCE study, 1094
Advanced cholesteatoma, 363
Advanced practice registered nurses (APRNs), compact license movement, 2
Advanced sleep-wake phase disorder, 1211
Adverse medical events, disclosure of errors and, 43-44
AED. *see* Automated external defibrillator (AED)
Aedes aegypti, 1225, 1228-1229

Aedes albopictus, 1228-1229
Aerobic activity, physical, 131
Affordable Care Act, 5, 1233
Afterload, 556-557
Aging/elderly
abuse of, 93
body's composition changes with, 1219
challenge of, 86
chronic pain in, 1189
cognitive impairment in, 87-88
dehydration, 88-89
with diabetes mellitus, 1095-1096
drivers counseling and, 85-86
evaluation of, 93*b*
failure to thrive, 91-93
falls in, 89-91
fatigue in, 1191
health screening for, 85, 85*t*
lipid disorder prevention in, 1126
pneumonia in, 487, 490
polypharmacy in, 87
sexual assault to, 229
skin associated with, 237
AIDS. *see* Acquired immunodeficiency syndrome (AIDS)
Air embolism (AGE), 1182-1185
Air travel
diving and, 1182
risks, 179
Airway hyperresponsiveness (AHR), 192, 422
Akathisia, 1040*b*
Alanine aminotransferase (ALT), 640-641
Albumin level, 182*t*
Albuterol, 435*t*-436*t*, 462*t*-463*t*
Alclometasone dipropionate, 244*t*
Alcohol
for essential tremor, 1043
gout and, 929
hypertension and, 570-571, 572*t*-573*t*
reducing energy intake and, 118
sleep and, 1212
Alcohol use, 1370
in college health, 172
screening for, 149*t*-152*t*
withdrawal from, 1371
Alcoholic hepatitis, 685-688, 690
Aldosterone antagonists, oral, for heart failure, 565
Alendronate (Fosamax), 858*b*, 969*t*
Aliskiren, 576*t*-582*t*
Alkalis, 209
Allergens
anaphylaxis-inducing, 194*b*
asthma and, 423
bronchospasm and, 192
environmental, 213-214
indoor, 385
inhaled, 194
outdoor, 385
in rhinitis, 384, 387-388
Allergic contact dermatitis (ICD), 266-267
Allergic rhinitis, 213, 379, 384-387
chronic rhinosinusitis and, comparison of, 378*t*
clinical presentation of, 384
complications of, 387
definition and epidemiology of, 384
diagnostics for, 385, 385*b*
differential diagnosis of, 385, 385*b*
indications for referral or hospitalization for, 387
management of, 385-387
pathophysiology of, 384
physical examination for, 384
Allergies, environmental. *see* Environmental allergies
Allergy immunotherapy, 215
Allopurinol, 1334
for gout, 931
Ally, definition of, 60
Alopecia, 252-255
clinical presentation of, 253
complications of, 255
definition and epidemiology of, 252
diagnostics for, 253, 253*b*, 254*t*
differential diagnosis of, 254, 254*b*
indications for referral or hospitalization for, 255
management of, 254-255
Alopecia *(Continued)*
pathophysiology of, 252-253
physical examination for, 253
Alopecia areata, 252-255, 254*t*
Alpha blockers, for hypertension, 576*t*-582*t*
Alpha fetoprotein (AFP), of unknown primary carcinoma, 1346
Alpha values, 10-11
Alpha-adrenergic agonists, 734
Alpha-adrenergic antagonists, for metabolic syndrome, 1129-1130
Alpha-beta blockers, for hypertension, 576*t*-582*t*
Alphavirus infection, 941
Alprazolam, 1043
ALS. *see* Amyotrophic lateral sclerosis (ALS)
Altered motility, 700-701
Alternaria, 213-214
Alternative therapies, 15-18
for adrenal gland disorders, 1076-1077
for common chronic conditions, 15-18
for HIV infection, 1234
Aluminum chloride hexahydrate, for hyperhidrosis, 289
Alvimopan, 646
Alzheimer disease, 1001-1002
neurocognitive disorder due to, 1020*b*
pathophysiology of, 1020-1021
stages of, 1021, 1021*b*
Amantadine, 1053
Amaurosis fugax, 333
Amblyomma americanum, 1260
Ambras syndrome, 1097
Ambrisentan, 498
Amenorrhea, 799-803, 1101
clinical presentation of, 799-800
complications of, 803
definition and epidemiology of, 799
with Depo-Provera, 834
diagnostics for, 800-801, 801*b*
differential diagnosis of, 801-802, 801*b*
indications for referral or hospitalization for, 803
life span considerations with, 803
management of, 802-803
pathophysiology of, 799
physical examination for, 800
primary, 801
secondary, 801-802
American Association of Oral and Maxillofacial Surgeons, 965
American Cancer Society, 479, 1326
American College of Cardiology (ACC), guidelines for noninvasive testing and markers for CAD, 504-505
American College of Cardiology/American Heart Association, guidelines for cardiac murmurs, 613-614
American College of Emergency Physicians, policy for febrile children, 1199
American Health Lawyers Association (AHLA), 44
American Nurses Association (ANA), 31
Americans with Disabilities Act, 170
Amiloride, for hypertension, 576*t*-582*t*
Aminophylline, 439
5-Aminosalicylic acid, 696
Amiodarone, 525
effects on thyroid gland, 1149, 1150*t*
Amitriptyline, 313-314, 926*t*, 1033, 1360*t*-1362*t*
Amlodipine, 576*t*-582*t*, 1033
Amnesia, retrograde, 220
Amoxicillin, 729*t*, 781*t*
for Lyme disease, 1256
for otitis media, 375*t*
for pharyngitis/tonsillitis, 415
Amoxicillin-clavulanate, 781*t*
Amphetamine, 1372
Amphetamine-like stimulants, 1372
Ampicillin, 874*b*
for endocarditis, 591*t*-595*t*
Ampicillin-sulbactam, for endocarditis, 591*t*-595*t*
Amputation
with diabetes mellitus, 1093
osteomyelitis and, 985
risk of, 317*b*
Amylin, 1084
Amyloid deposition, 1155
Amyloidosis, 657
Amyotrophic lateral sclerosis (ALS), 1005-1007
clinical presentation and physical examination for, 1005
complications, 1006-1007
definition and epidemiology of, 1005
diagnostics for, 1005, 1006*b*
differential diagnosis of, 1006, 1006*b*
indications for referral or hospitalization for, 1007
life span considerations with, 1006
management of, 1006
pathophysiology of, 1005
ANA. *see* American Nurses Association (ANA)
Anabolic steroids, 1373
acne and, 250*b*
Anaerobic bacteria, in epiglottitis, 406
Anagen effluvium, 254*t*
Anagen phase disturbance, 252-253
Anal fissure, 632-633
clinical presentation of, 632
complications and indications for referral or hospitalization for, 633
definition and epidemiology of, 632
differential diagnosis of, 633, 633*b*
life span considerations with, 633
management of, 633
pathophysiology of, 632
physical examination for, 632-633
Analgesics
for chronic pain, 1187-1188
for headaches, 1034, 1035*t*-1036*t*
nerve blocks as, 1188
three-step analgesic ladder, 1187-1188
Analysis of variance (ANOVA), 11
Anaphylaxis, 194-196
clinical presentation of, 195
complications of, 196
definition and epidemiology of, 194
diagnostics for, 192, 193*b*, 195, 195*b*
differential diagnosis of, 195, 196*b*
indications for referral or hospitalization for, 196
life span considerations with, 196
management of, 195-196
pathophysiology of, 194
physical examination for, 195
recognition and management of, 156
Anaplasma, 1259
Anaplasma phagocytophilum, 1259
Anaplasmosis, 1259-1260
Anasarca, in heart failure, 560*t*
Anatomic rhinitis, 388
Anatomic stress urinary incontinence, 731
Androgenetic alopecia, 254*t*
Androgenic hormones, in dry skin, 276
Androgens
in acne, 249, 251
acne and, 250*b*
hirsutism and, 1097
Anemia, 1278-1297, 1375
aplastic, 1294-1295, 1294*b*
of chronic disease, 1282, 1293-1294
of chronic kidney disease (ACKD), 1278, 1293-1294
classification of, 1280*b*
clinical presentation of, 1278-1279
definition and epidemiology of, 1278
diagnostics for, 1279-1280, 1280*b*
differential diagnosis of, 1280
hemolytic, 1295-1297
autoimmune, 1296, 1296*b*
clinical presentation of, 1296
complications of, 1297
definition and epidemiology of, 1295-1296
diagnostics for, 1296
differential diagnosis of, 1297, 1297*b*
examples of, 1295*b*
indications for referral or hospitalization for, 1297
life span considerations with, 1297
management of, 1297
pathophysiology of, 1296
physical examination for, 1296

Anemia *(Continued)*
iron deficiency, 1278, 1280
clinical presentation of, 1281
complications of, 1283
diagnostics for, 1281-1282
indications for referral or hospitalization for, 1283
laboratory studies of, 1281*b*
life span considerations with, 1283
management of, 1282-1283
pathophysiology of, 1280-1281
physical examination for, 1281
macrocytic, 1287-1290
complications of, 1289
differential diagnosis of, 1288, 1289*b*
indications for referral or hospitalization for, 1289
life span considerations with, 1289
management of, 1289
megaloblastic
causes of, 1288*b*
clinical presentation of, 1288
complications of, 1289
diagnostics for, 1288
differential diagnosis of, 1288, 1289*b*
indications for referral or hospitalization for, 1289
life span considerations with, 1289
management of, 1289
physical examination for, 1288
microcytic, 1280-1284
differential diagnosis of, 1282, 1282*b*
laboratory values in, 1282*t*
normocytic, 1290-1293, 1291*b*
normochromic, 588
pathophysiology of, 1278
patient education and self-care strategies in, 1312*b*-1313*b*
physical examination for, 1279
physician consultation for, 1280
screening for, 149*t*-152*t*
sickle cell disease and. *see* Sickle cell disease
thalassemia and. *see* Thalassemia
Anergy, 1265-1266
Anesthesia, classification in presurgery setting, 182*t*
Aneurysm, 605
abdominal. *see* Abdominal aortic aneurysm
Angiitis. *see* Vasculitis
Angina. *see also* Chest pain
equivalents of, 540-541
Angiodysplasias, 678
Angioedema, 195*f*, 274*t*
Angiography, 505*t*, 531. *see also specific modalities*
Angiotensin II blockers, for hypertension, 576*t*-582*t*
Angiotensin II receptor blockers, for coronary artery disease, 553
Angiotensin receptor blockers, for heart failure, 565
Angiotensin-converting enzyme (ACE) inhibitors
chronic cough and, 451-452, 455-456
for coronary artery disease, 537*t*, 553
for hypertension, 576*t*-582*t*
for metabolic syndrome, 1129-1130
for ST segment elevation myocardial infarction, 550
Animal bites, 255-258
clinical presentation of, 256
complications of, 257
definition and epidemiology of, 255
diagnostics for, 256, 256*b*
indications for referral or hospitalization for, 257
management of, 256-257
pathophysiology of, 255-256
physical examination for, 256
risk factors for, 255*b*
Animal exposures, fever and, 1197-1198
Anisocoria, 327
Ankle joints
aspiration and injection of, 917*f*
fracture of, 994
pain in, 897-903
sprains of, 897-899
classification and treatment of, 898*t*
clinical presentation of, 897
Ankle joints *(Continued)*
complications of, 899
definition and epidemiology of, 897
diagnostics for, 897-898, 897*b*
differential diagnosis of, 898, 898*b*
indications for referral or hospitalization for, 899
management of, 898-899
pathophysiology of, 897
physical examination for, 897
Ankylosing spondylitis, 1152-1156
clinical presentation of, 1152-1153
complications of, 1155
definition and epidemiology of, 1152
diagnostics for, 1153-1154, 1153*b*-1154*b*
differential diagnosis for, 1154, 1154*b*
indications for referral or hospitalization for, 1155
life span considerations with, 1155
management of, 1154-1155
pathophysiology of, 1152
physical examination for, 1153
Ann Arbor staging classification, 1314, 1315*t*, 1318
Anorectal abscess or fistula, 634-635
clinical presentation of, 635
definition and epidemiology of, 634-635
diagnostics for, 635, 635*b*
differential diagnosis of, 635, 635*b*
management, complications, and indications for referral or hospitalization in, 635
pathophysiology of, 635
physical examination for, 635
Anorexia, 1219
as oncology symptom, 1342, 1344
Anorexia nervosa
clinical presentation and physical examination of, 97
definition and epidemiology of, 96
diagnostics for, 97
differential diagnosis of, 97
in elderly, 96-98
management of, 97
pathophysiology of, 96-97
Anoro Ellipta, for COPD, 464
ANOVA. *see* Analysis of variance (ANOVA)
Anovulatory cycles, 821
Anserine bursa, 917*f*
Anserine bursitis, 952
Antagonist drugs, 1376
Antalgic gait, 938
Anterior epistaxis, management of, 381
Antiarrhythmic therapy, 524
Antibiotic resistance, 1231-1232
Antibiotics
for acne, 251
for acute bronchitis, 419
for Bartholin gland cysts and abscesses, 804-805
cholera and, 1227-1228
for COPD, 464-465
for dental abscess, 398-399
for epiglottitis, 405
for eyes, 350
immunodeficiency and, 1201
for infectious diarrhea, 1250
for infective endocarditis, 590, 591*t*-595*t*
for inflammatory bowel disease, 698
for otitis media, 375*t*
for parotitis, 410-411
for pharyngitis/tonsillitis, 415
for pneumonia, 490
for sinusitis, 391
for tympanic membrane perforation, 377
for UTIs, 779*t*, 781*t*
in wound management, 325
Anticholinergics
for asthma, 435*t*-436*t*, 441
for COPD, 461, 462*t*-463*t*
for nausea and vomiting, 712*b*
for Parkinson disease, 1053
Anticoagulants
for atrial fibrillation, 526
for heart failure, 567
Anticoagulation
for coronary artery disease, 553
for deep vein thrombosis, 607
Anticoagulation *(Continued)*
hemorrhagic stroke and, 1011
for pulmonary embolism, 495
Anticonstipation agents, 704
Anticonvulsants
for essential tremor, 1043
for headaches, 1033
sexual response and, 878*t*
for trigeminal neuralgia, 1064
Antidepressants, 113, 878*t*, 1352, 1352*t*, 1360*t*-1362*t*, 1367*t*-1368*t*
for parasomnias, 1218
Antidiarrheal agents, 704
Antidiuretic hormone (ADH), 1112, 1334
Antidopaminergic metoclopramide, 1222
Antiemetic medications, 711, 712*b*
Antiepileptic drug (AED), 1060, 1061*t*-1062*t*
Antiestrogens, 848
Antifungals
for seborrheic dermatitis, 309
solution, topical, 280-281
"Antigenic drift", 1227
Antigen-specific T cells, 214
Antihistamines
for itching, 278
for nausea and vomiting, 712*b*
for rhinitis, 386
for scratching, 276
for urticaria, 313
weight gain and, 113
Antihypertensives, 878*t*, 1014
for metabolic syndrome, 1129-1130
Anti-influenza agents, for acute bronchitis, 420
Antimicrobial therapy, for peritonitis, 628-629
Antimotility agents, 1250
Antimüllerian hormone (AMH), 852-853
Antineutrophil cytoplasmic antibody (ANCA), 1177-1179
Antinuclear antibodies (ANA), 1172, 1173*t*
Anti-outer surface protein A, 1257
Antiphospholipid antibodies, 1172-1173
Antiplatelet agents, for cerebrovascular events, 1014-1015
Antipsychotics, 878*t*, 1367*t*-1368*t*, 1379*t*-1380*t*
for anxiety disorders, 1353
for delirium, 1019
Antipyretic drugs, 1199-1200
Antirabies treatment, 257
Antiretrovirals (ARVs), 1237-1238
Antisecretory agents, 1250
Antispasmodics, 703-704
Antistreptolysin O (ASO) titer, 414
Antithrombin III, 1304
Antithrombotic therapy, for acute ST segment elevation myocardial infarction, 550
Anti-TNF therapy, for ankylosing spondylitis, 1154-1155
α_1-Antitrypsin (AAT)
COPD and, 458
deficiency of, 429-430
Antitussive therapy
for acute bronchitis, 419
for chronic cough, 455
Antiviral therapy
for herpes simplex virus, 271
for herpes zoster, 285
for herpetic whitlow, 292
for influenza, 1242
for myocarditis, 599
Ants, 197*t*
Anxiety
clinical presentation and physical examination of, 98
definition and epidemiology of, 98
diagnostics for, 98
differential diagnosis of, 98
in elderly, 98-99
heart failure and, 563
hypertension and, 572*t*-573*t*
indications for referral or hospitalization for, 98
management, 98
palliative care and, 98-99
pathophysiology of, 98

Anxiety disorders, 1349-1354
clinical presentation of, 1350-1351, 1350*b*
complications of, 1353
definition and epidemiology of, 1349
diagnostics for, 1351, 1351*b*
indications for referral or hospitalization for, 1353-1354
life span considerations with, 1354
management of, 1351-1353, 1352*t*
pathophysiology of, 1349-1350
physical examination for, 1351
Anxiolytics, 878*t*
Aorta, 510
Aortic dissections, and chest pain, 548*t*
Aortic regurgitation, 612*t*, 615-617
clinical presentation and physical examination of, 616
complications of, 617
definition and epidemiology of, 615-616
diagnostics for, 616-617
differential diagnosis of, 617
interdisciplinary management of, 617
management of, 617
pathophysiology of, 616
Aortic stenosis, 612*t*, 614-615
chest pain and, 548*t*
clinical presentation of, 614
complications of, 615
definition and epidemiology of, 614
diagnostics for, 614-615
differential diagnosis of, 615
in heart failure, 560*t*
interdisciplinary management of, 615
life span considerations with, 615
management of, 615
pathophysiology of, 614
physical examination for, 614
Aortic valve replacement, for aortic regurgitation, 615
Aortography, standard contrast, for abdominal aortic aneurysm, 512
Aortoiliac arteries, obstruction of, 600
Aphthous stomatitis, 409
Aphthous ulcers, 407
Apixaban, 607
Apley compression test, 950, 950*f*
Apocrine glands, 286
Apophysitis, 937
Appendicitis, 623-625
clinical presentation of, 624
complications of, 625
definition and epidemiology of, 623
diagnostics for, 624, 624*b*
differential diagnosis of, 624, 625*b*
indications for referral or hospitalization for, 625
management of, 624-625
pathophysiology of, 624
physical examination for, 624
Appendix testis, torsion of, 765, 767, 770
Apprehension test, 988*t*
Apremilast, 1158
Arboviral infection, 1272
Arcanobacterium species, 413
Arformoterol, 462*t*-463*t*
Arginine vasopressin, 557
Armour Thyroid, 1147
Arrhythmias, 515-529
categories of, 516
complications of, 528
definition and epidemiology of, 515-516
differential diagnosis of, 522-524, 523*b*
indications for referral or hospitalization for, 528
initial diagnostics for, 518, 519*b*
life span considerations with, 528
management of, 524-527
pathophysiology of, 516
physical examination, 517-518
referral to cardiologist, 528
referral to electrophysiology cardiologist, 528
syncope and, 231*b*
Arterial blood gases (ABGs), for pulmonary embolism, 494
Arterial insufficiency
acute, 604-605
clinical presentation of, 604
complications of, 605
definition and epidemiology of, 604
diagnostics for, 604-605, 605*b*
differential diagnosis of, 605, 605*b*
indications for referral or hospitalization for, 605
management of, 605
pathophysiology of, 604
physical examination for, 604
chronic, 600-604
diagnostics for, 602*b*
differential diagnosis of, 603*b*
physical examination for, 601*b*
peripheral, 599-600
clinical presentation of, 600-601
complications of, 603
definition and epidemiology of, 600
diagnostics for, 601-602
differential diagnosis of, 602-603
indications for referral or hospitalization in, 603-604
life span considerations with, 604
management of, 603
pathophysiology of, 600
physical examination for, 601
Arterial restenosis, 533-534
Arterial ulcers, 317-318, 321, 323-324
Arteriography, 604
carotid, for cerebrovascular events, 1012
Arthritis. *see also specific joints*
gonococcal, 941-942, 944-945
with gout. *see* Gout
infectious, 940-946
clinical presentation of, 941
complications of, 945
definition and epidemiology of, 940
diagnostics for, 943-944, 943*t*, 944*b*
differential diagnosis for, 944, 944*b*
indications for referral or hospitalization for, 945
life span considerations with, 945
management of, 944-945
outcome in, 945*b*
pathophysiology of, 940-941
physical examination for, 941-943
of inflammatory bowel disease, 1158-1159
psoriatic, 301-303, 1157-1158
reactive, 1156-1157
of shoulder joint, 991
with systemic lupus erythematosus, 1171*b*, 1172
trapeziometacarpal
clinical presentation of, 933
diagnostics and differential diagnosis for, 934
management of, 935
physical examination for, 934
Arthritis mutilans, 1157, 1158*f*
Articular cartilage, of hip joint, 936
Artificial tears, 348-349
Ascites
in heart failure, 560*t*
management of, 642, 642*b*
Ashkenazi Jewish, 37*f*
Aspartate transaminase (AST), 640-641
Aspergillus, 466
infective endocarditis and, 585
Aspiration/injection, of shoulder, 915*b*, 915*f*-917*f*
Aspirin, 549
for coronary artery disease, 550
for diabetes, 1094, 1094*t*
GI bleeding and, 680-681
for giant cell arteritis, 1163
for headaches, 1034
for heart failure, 566-567
for metabolic syndrome, 1130
Aspirin exacerbated respiratory disease (AERD), 423
Assessment of SpondyloArthritis International Society (ASAS) criteria, 1153, 1153*b*
Assisted reproductive technologies (ARTs), 849
Asteatotic eczema, 276*f*
Asterixis, 1040*b*
Asthma, 421-445
acute severe, 423-424
aspirin-induced, 423
with chronic cough, 454
chronic stable, 424
clinical presentation of, 423-424
complications of, 443
COPD and, 460
definition and epidemiology of, 421-422
development of, 422
diagnostics for, 428-429, 429*b*
differential diagnosis of, 429-430, 429*b*
environmental factors in, 423
exercise-induced, 423
financial impact of, 422
follow-up assessment for, components of, 426*b*
heart failure and, 563
home treatment for, 437*b*
hospitalization rates of, 422
indications for referral or hospitalization for, 443
initial assessment of, 424*b*-425*b*
life span considerations with, 442-443
management of, 430-431, 430*b*, 432*f*, 438*f*
interdisciplinary, 442
medications for, 431-442
long-term, 431-441, 433*t*-435*t*
quick-relief, 435*t*-436*t*, 441
morbidity and mortality of, 443
occupational, 167, 421
pathophysiology of, 422-423
pharmacotherapy for, 430
physical examination for, 424-428
in pregnancy, 74-75, 74*t*
reversibility and variability in, 428
risk factors and actions to reduce exposures in, 437*t*
severity of
classification by, 430, 431*f*
exacerbations of, 427*t*
monitoring therapy and, 441-442
socioeconomic status and, 443
Th1- type and Th2- type, 422
zone system for, 442
Asthma action plan (AAP), 442, 445
Astrocytoma, 1066*t*
Ataxia, 1040*b*
with multiple sclerosis, 1046*t*-1047*t*
Atenolol, 576*t*-582*t*
Atherogenesis, role of, in coronary artery disease, 504
Atherosclerosis
abdominal aortic aneurysms and, 629
chronic arterial insufficiency and, 600
with systemic lupus erythematosus, 1172
Atherosclerotic cardiovascular disease (ASCVD), 1120
risk assessment for, 1122
Athetosis, 1040*b*
Atopic conjunctivitis, 341-342
Atopic dermatitis (AD), 277-279
clinical presentation and physical examination of, 277, 277*f*
complications of, 278
definition and epidemiology of, 277
diagnostics for, 277-278, 278*b*
differential diagnosis of, 277-278, 278*b*
indications for referral or hospitalization for, 279
life span considerations with, 279
management of, 278
pathophysiology of, 277
Atopic diseases, 214
Atopy, 422
Atorvastatin (Lipitor), 1124*t*-1125*t*
Atresia (cell death and degeneration), 850
Atrial fibrillation, 520, 520*f*, 525-526
cardioversion for, 204*b*
defined, 203
mitral stenosis with, 622
Atrial flutter, 520, 525-526
cardioversion for, 204*b*
defined, 203
Atrial gallop, 542

Atrioventricular nodal blocks, 522-523
first-degree, 522
second-degree, 522
type I, 522-523, 523*f*
type II, 523, 523*f*
third-degree, 523
Atrioventricular nodal reentry tachycardia, 520
Atrioventricular reentry tachycardia, 520
Atrophic vaginitis, 856, 895-896
clinical presentation and physical examination of, 895
complications of, 896
diagnostics for, 895-896, 895*b*
differential diagnosis of, 896, 896*b*
indications for referral or hospitalization for, 896
life span considerations with, 896
management of, 896
pathophysiology of, 895
Atrophy, vulvovaginal, 855
Atropine, 534
for bradycardia, 527
Attention and concentration tests, 1000*b*
Atypical antipsychotics, 113
Audiogram, 365
for tympanic membrane perforation, 377
Audiology evaluation, 1025
Aura, 1031
Auricular disorders, 359-360. *see also specific disorders*
clinical presentation of, 359-360
complications of, 360
definition and epidemiology of, 359
diagnostics for, 360, 360*b*
differential diagnosis of, 360, 360*b*
indications for referral or hospitalization for, 360
life span considerations in, 360
management of, 360
pathophysiology of, 359
physical examination for, 360
Auscultation technique, 543*b*
Autoimmune diseases, lymphadenopathy and, 1208
Autoimmune hepatitis, 686
Autoimmune vasculitides, 379
Automated external defibrillator (AED), 206
Automatic technology, 48
Automaticity, cardiac, 516
Autonomic neuropathy, 1092-1093
Autosomal dominant disease, 68*t*
Autosomal recessive disease, 68*t*. *see also specific disorders*
Avascular necrosis, 937, 1293
Aversive drugs, 1376
Avian influenza A (H5N1), 1227
Axial low back pain, 954
Axillary nodes, 1206
enlargement of, 1207-1208
5-Azacytidine, 1323
Azathioprine, 1174, 1174*t*
for vasculitis, 1180
Azelaic acid, 251-252
Azelastine, 386
Azilsartan (Edarbi), 576*t*-582*t*
Azithromycin, 420, 789*b*
for pharyngitis/tonsillitis, 415

B

Babesia divergens, 1258
Babesia microti, 1258
Babesiosis, 1258-1259, 1262*t*
Bacillus Calmette-Guérin (BCG) vaccine, for tuberculosis, 1266
Bacillus cereus food poisoning
eight to fourteen hours after ingestion, 1250
one to six hours after ingestion, 1249-1250
Baclofen, 1065*t*
Bacteria
acute bronchitis and, 417
gram-negative, 487
gram-positive, 487
PID-related, 873
UTI-related, 778, 778*t*-779*t*, 781
Bacterial conjunctivitis, 341-342, 341*f*
Bacterial infections. *see specific pathogens and body parts*
Bacterial toxins, food poisoning of, 1249-1250
Bacteriuria, screening for, 149*t*-152*t*
Baker cysts, 952
Balanitis, 1156
Balloon mitral valvulotomy (BMV), 622
Balloon tamponade, for GI bleeding, 681
Ballottement test, 918-919
Bandages, elastic, 997
Barbiturates, 1370-1371
Bariatric surgery
defined, 123-124
indications and contraindications for, 123
monitoring after, 124
motivational interview before, 116
surgical techniques and outcomes, 123-124
Barotrauma, 1181-1184. *see also* Decompression sickness
clinical presentation of, 1182
complications of, 1183
differential diagnosis for, 1183, 1183*b*
ear, 1184
indications for referral for, 1183-1184
management of, 1183
pathophysiology of, 1182
physical examination for, 1182-1183
predive physical examination and diagnostics for, 1181-1182
pulmonary, 1184-1185
sinus, 1184
Barrett esophagus, 676
Bartholin gland
adenocarcinomas of, 841
cysts and abscesses, 803-805
clinical presentation of, 804
complications of, 805
definition and epidemiology of, 803-804
diagnostics for, 804, 804*b*
differential diagnosis of, 804, 804*b*
indications for referral or hospitalization for, 805
life span considerations with, 805
management of, 804-805
pathophysiology of, 804
physical examination for, 804
surgical treatments of, 805
Basal cell carcinoma (BCC)
definition and epidemiology of, 245-246
differential diagnosis of, 248*b*
physical examination of, 246, 247*f*
treatment of, 248
Basal ganglia, 1040-1041
Basal metabolic rate (BMR), 111
Baseline Dyspnea Index, 468
Baseline renal function tests, 1375
Basic life support (BLS), 207
Bath soaks, 244*t*
Beclomethasone dipropionate, 462*t*-463*t*
Bedbugs, 197*t*
Bedside Index of Severity in Acute Pancreatitis (BISAP), 715-716, 716*b*
Beer potomania, 1115
Bees, 197*t*
Behavioral therapies, for stress incontinence, 733-734
Belimumab (Benlysta), for systemic lupus erythematosus, 1174, 1174*t*
Bell palsy, 1008-1010, 1255
clinical presentation of, 1008
complications of, 1009
definition and epidemiology of, 1008
diagnostics for, 1008-1009, 1009*b*
differential diagnosis for, 1009, 1009*b*
indications for referral or hospitalization for, 1009-1010
life span considerations with, 1010
management of, 1009
pathophysiology of, 1008
physical examination for, 1008
Benign lymphoepithelial lesion of Godwin, 399-400
Benign multiple sclerosis, 1044*b*
Benign paroxysmal positional vertigo, 1027-1028
Benign prostatic hyperplasia (BPH), 738-740
clinical presentation of, 738-739, 739*t*
complications of, 740
Benign prostatic hyperplasia (BPH) *(Continued)*
definition and epidemiology of, 738
diagnostics for, 739-740, 740*b*
differential diagnosis of, 740, 740*b*
indications for referral or hospitalization for, 740
management of, 740
pathophysiology of, 738
physical examination for, 739
symptom index for, 739*t*
Benzamides, 712*b*
Benzathine penicillin, 789*b*
Benzodiazepines, 1352, 1352*t*
abuse of, 1371
for essential tremor, 1043
flumazenil for, 226
for grief and bereavement, 1356
for insomnia, 1212
for nausea and vomiting, 712*b*
for parasomnias, 1218
types of, 99*t*
Berberine, 17
Bereavement, 1355-1356, 1356*t*
"Bereavement exclusion", 1355
Beta blockers, 525-526, 551*b*
for acute ST segment elevation myocardial infarction, 550
classification of, 551
for coronary artery disease, 537*t*, 550-551
for essential tremor, 1043
for Graves disease, 1143-1144
for headaches, 1033
for heart failure, 566
for hypertension, 576*t*-582*t*
Beta$_2$-adrenergic agonist, 462*t*-463*t*, 464
Betahistine hydrochloride, 369
Betamethasone valerate, 244*t*
Betaxolol, 576*t*-582*t*
Bethesda System, 870*b*
Bilateral hilar lymphadenopathy (BHL), 501
Bile acid sequestrants, 1125
Bile salt malabsorption, diarrhea and, 656
Bilirubin levels, in neonates/infants, 80
Binge eating disorder (BED), defined, 117*t*
Biochemical marker, 961
Biofeedback training, 646
Bioidentical hormone therapy products, for menopause, 864-865
Bioimpedance analysis (BIA), 110
Biologic agents, in psoriasis, 303-304
Biologic threats, 136
Biologics (medications), 697-698, 697*t*
Biomarkers, in myocarditis, 598
Biopsy
of bones, 910
of GI tract, 695
of lymph nodes, 1206-1207
for myelodysplastic syndromes, 1322
for sarcoidosis, 501
of skin, 241-242, 241*f*-242*f*
in skin cancer, 246-247
small bowel, 652
of thyroid gland, 1137
for vasculitis, 1179
Bipolar disorders, 1364-1369
clinical presentation of, 1365
complications of, 1368-1369
definition and epidemiology of, 1364-1365
diagnostics for, 1366
differential diagnosis of, 1366
indications for referral or hospitalization for, 1369
life span considerations with, 1366-1368
management of, 1366, 1367*t*-1368*t*
pathophysiology of, 1365
physical examination for, 1365-1366
Birmingham eye trauma terminology, 356*t*
Bisacodyl, 646
Bisexual, definition of, 60
Bismuth subsalicylate (Pepto-Bismol), 179, 712*b*, 729*t*, 1250
Bisphosphonates, 858*b*
for bone tumors, 912
for osteoporosis, 964-965
for Paget disease, 968-969, 969*t*

Bite wounds, 255-257, 255*b*
animal and human, cellulitis and, 265
Bites and stings. *see* Insect bites and stings; Marine animal, bites and stings of
Bitolterol mesylate, 462*t*-463*t*
Bitter belching, 671
Biventricular pacing, 567
Black cohosh, for menopause, 860
Black widow spiders, 200
Bladder
cancer of, 794-795, 796*b*-798*b*, 797
multiple sclerosis and, 1046*t*-1047*t*
neck hypermobility in, 732
poor compliance in, 732
training for, 734-735
Blasts, 1307-1308
Bleeding disorders (coagulopathies), 1298-1303. *see also specific disorders*
assessment for, 1302*b*
complications of, 1303
diagnostics and differential diagnosis of, 1298-1301, 1300*b*-1301*b*
hemophilia in, 1303
history taking for, 1299*b*
management and indications for referral or hospitalization for, 1301
pathophysiology and clinical presentation of, 1298
patient education and life span considerations in, 1303
physical examination for, 1298
von Willebrand disease, 1302
Bleeding time, 1299-1300
Bleeding/hemorrhage, 247*t*
diverticular, 662-663, 663*b*
in eyes, 332*t*-334*t*
gastrointestinal, 677, 695
irregular, 854
Blepharitis, 332*t*-333*t*, 337-339
clinical presentation of, 337, 338*f*
complications of, 339
definition and epidemiology of, 337
diagnostics for, 338
differential diagnosis of, 338, 338*b*
indications for referral or hospitalization for, 339
life span considerations with, 339
management of, 338-339, 339*t*
pathophysiology of, 337
physical examination for, 337-338, 338*f*
Blinding, of subject and researcher, 8
Blister beetles, 197*t*
Blisters, fracture, 997
Blood clots. *see* Thromboembolism
Blood coagulation disorders, 1297-1307. *see also* specific disorders
Blood cultures, 590
Blood glucose monitoring, 1085-1086
Blood loss, 1278
quantification of, in hemoptysis, 472
Blood pressure
carotid stenosis and, 530
coronary artery disease and, 537*t*
reduction of, for hypertension, 584
screening for, 149*t*-152*t*
self-monitoring, 584
stroke and, 1014
test for, 146*t*-148*t*
Blood tests, 694
Blood vessels, 1176-1177, 1176*b*
BLS. *see* Basic life support (BLS)
Blue toe syndrome, 605
Body mass index (BMI)
calculations and classification, 116*b*
defined, 109-110
in pregnancy, 69*t*
Bone densitometry, indications for, 961-962, 962*b*
Bone lesions, 911
Bone marrow biopsy, for myelodysplastic syndromes, 1322
Bone marrow transplantation (BMT), 1286, 1291
Bone mass, causes of low, 963*b*
Bone mineral density (BMD), 857
test for, 146*t*-147*t*
Bone pain, 908
Bone resorption, 960
Bone scintigraphy, for low back pain, 956
Bone tumors, 906-913
benign, 910-912
clinical presentation of, 906-907, 907*b*
common clinical scenarios in, 907-908
definition and epidemiology of, 906
diagnostics for, 908, 908*b*, 909*t*
differential diagnosis of, 910, 911*b*
imaging studies of, 908-910
indications for referral or hospitalization for, 913
life span considerations with, 913
malignant, 911-912
management of, 910-912, 910*t*
medical history and physical examination for, 908
pathophysiology of, 906
prognosis of, 912-913
survival of, 912-913
Bony deformity, 908
Bordetella pertussis, acute bronchitis and, 417-419
Borrelia burgdorferi, 1254
Bosentan, 498
Bowel
multiple sclerosis and, 1046*t*-1047*t*
obstruction
life span considerations with, 106
in palliative care, 106
Bowman layer, 353
Brachytherapy, 1327-1328
Bradycardia/bradyarrhythmias, 201-203, 516
clinical presentation of, 202
definition and epidemiology of, 201
diagnostics for, 202, 202*b*
differential diagnosis of, 202, 202*b*, 522-524
disposition and referral for, 202
initial stabilization and management of, 202
management of, 527-528
pathophysiology of, 201-202
physical examination for, 202
prevention of, 203
Brain natriuretic peptide (BNP), 561
for pulmonary embolism, 494
Brain trauma, repetitive, 218
Brain tumor. *see* Intracranial tumors
Bravewell Collaborative, The, 15
BRCA risk assessment, screening for, 149*t*-152*t*
Breast and nipple evaluation
for cracked nipples, 83
for lactation/breastfeeding, 79
for pain, 808
Breast cancer, 833
in menopause, 858-859
preventive medications, screening for, 149*t*-152*t*
screening for, 146*t*-147*t*, 149*t*-154*t*
Breast disorders, 806-817
genetic testing of, 806-807
risk assessment models for, 806
risk factors for, 806
risk reduction of, 807
screening for, 807
Breast milk intake, 80*b*
Breast pain, 807-810
clinical presentation of, 808
complications of, 809
definition and epidemiology of, 807
diagnostics for, 808, 808*b*
differential diagnosis of, 808-809, 809*b*
indications for referral or hospitalization for, 809
management of, 809
pathophysiology of, 807-808
physical examination for, 808
Breast pumps, 83
Breastfeeding. *see also* Lactation
counseling for, 149*t*-152*t*
managing challenges to, 81-83
prenatal preparation for, 78-79
significant maternal and infant health benefits associated with, 79*b*
steps to successful, 79*b*
Breasts
engorgement of, 81-82
masses in, 814-816
clinical presentation of, 814-815
definition and epidemiology of, 814
Breasts *(Continued)*
diagnostics for, 815, 815*b*
differential diagnosis of, 815, 815*b*
indications for referral or hospitalization for, 815-816
life span considerations with, 815
management of, 815
pathophysiology of, 814
physical examination for, 815
Breath sounds, adventitious, 542
Breathing disorders, sleep-related, 1213-1214
Bright light therapy, 1362-1363
Bromelain, primary care and, 18
Bromides, acne and, 250*b*
Bromocriptine, 803, 1052, 1073
for infertility, 848
Bronchiectasis, 454
Bronchitis
acute, 417-420
clinical presentation and physical examination for, 417-418
complications of, 420
definition and epidemiology of, 417
diagnostics, 418, 418*b*
differential diagnosis of, 418-419, 418*b*
indications for referral or hospitalization for, 420
management of, 419-420
pathophysiology of, 417
chronic, 168, 419, 454, 456-457
occupational, 167
Bronchodilators, 461
short-acting, 441
Bronchogenic carcinoma, 474
Bronchoscopy
for chronic cough, 452
fiberoptic, for hemoptysis, 473
for sarcoidosis, 501
Bronchospasm
acute, 192-194
clinical presentation of, 192
definition and epidemiology of, 192
diagnostics for, 192
differential diagnosis of, 193, 193*b*
disposition and referral for, 193
initial stabilization and management of, 193
pathophysiology of, 192
physical examination for, 192
prevention and patient education for, 193-194
in asthma, 428
Brown recluse spiders, 198
Brudzinski sign, 1274
Bruits, 531
Bubble Boy, 1200
Budesonide, 433*t*-435*t*, 462*t*-463*t*
Buerger disease, 602
Building collaborative practice initiatives, 2
Bulla (bullae), 238*f*, 240, 274*t*
Bullous pemphigoid (BP), 258-259, 408
clinical presentation and physical examination of, 258
complications of, 259
definition and epidemiology of, 258
diagnostics for, 258, 258*b*
differential diagnosis of, 259, 259*b*
indications for referral or hospitalization for, 259
life span considerations with, 259
management of, 259
pathophysiology of, 258
Bullying, assessment in, 58*t*
Bundle branch block (BBB), 516, 523-524
hemiblocks, 524
left, 524
right, 524
Bunion, 903*t*-905*t*
Bunionette, 903*t*-905*t*
Bupropion, 1360*t*-1362*t*
Burkitt lymphoma, 1318
Burns, 259-261
center referral criteria for, 319*b*
classification of, 318, 319*b*
clinical presentation of, 260
complications of, 261
definition and epidemiology of, 259
diagnostics for, 260, 260*b*

Burns *(Continued)*
differential diagnosis of, 260, 260*b*
indications for referral or hospitalization for, 261
management of, 260-261, 322
pathophysiology of, 260
physical examination of, 260
as wounds, 317
Bursa aspiration/injection, 915*b*, 915*f*-917*f*. *see also specific joints*
Bursitis, 913-920, 936-937, 990. *see also specific joints*
Buspirone, 1352-1353, 1352*t*
Butenafine (Mentax), 281*t*

C
Cabergoline, 1073
Cachexia, 1219
in the elderly, 96-98
clinical presentation and physical examination of, 97
definition and epidemiology of, 96
diagnostics for, 97
differential diagnosis of, 97
in elderly, 96-98
management of, 97
pathophysiology of, 96-97
CAD. *see* Coronary artery disease (CAD)
Caffeine, 130
CAGE mnemonic for dietary assessment, 127*b*
Calcification, in coronary arteries, 508-509
Calcitonin, 858*b*
for osteoporosis, 965-966
for Paget disease, 969, 969*t*
Calcitriol, 1104, 1107
Calcium, 962-963, 964*t*
for hyperkalemia, 1111
for menopause, 860
Calcium channel blockers, 525-526
for coronary artery disease, 552-553, 553*b*
for dysmenorrhea, 824
for headaches, 1033
for hypertension, 576*t*-582*t*
for pulmonary hypertension, 498, 499*t*
for ST segment elevation myocardial infarction, 550
Calcium oxalate stones, 773, 776
Calcium stones, 775
Calculated free testosterone (CFT), 1099-1100
Calculi, urinary, 771-777
clinical presentation of, 773
complications of, 776
definition and epidemiology of, 771-772
diagnostics for, 774, 774*b*
differential diagnosis of, 774, 775*b*
indications for referral or hospitalization for, 776-777
life span considerations with, 777
management of, 774-776, 776*f*
pathophysiology of, 772-773
physical examination for, 773-774
recurrence rate for, 772
types of, 772-773
Callus, 903*t*-905*t*
Calorie intake, 130
Campylobacter, 1156
infection, 179
Campylobacter jejuni, 1028, 1248
Canalith repositioning procedure, 1028
Cancer. *see also oncology headings; specific tumors*
classification of, 1327
diarrhea and, 648
fatigue and, 1193, 1195*t*
female genital, 837
genitourinary, 794
lymphadenopathy and, 1207
in menopause, 858-859
risks of, 1325
of salivary gland, 400
screening for, 152-155, 1325
LGBTQ patient care and, 63
treatment of, 1330
unintentional weight loss and, 1221-1222
Cancer antigen 125 (CA-125), 840-841, 840*b*
Cancer-related checkup, 153*t*-154*t*
Candesartan, 576*t*-582*t*
Candida
infections, in intertrigo, 290-291
infective endocarditis and, 585
osteomyelitis and, 982
Candida albicans, 283, 293
oral infections from, 406
Candidiasis
oral, with inhalers, 464
skin, 283-284
clinical presentation and physical examination of, 283, 283*f*
complications of, 284
diagnostics for, 283*b*
differential diagnosis of, 283, 283*b*
indications for referral or hospitalization for, 284
management of, 283
treatments for, 281*t*
Cannabinoids, 712*b*, 1373
Cannabis sativa, 1373
Cantharidin, 316
Capsule endoscopy. *see* Wireless capsule endoscopy (WCE)
Captopril, 576*t*-582*t*
Carbamazepine, 1059, 1061*t*-1062*t*, 1367*t*-1368*t*
for trigeminal neuralgia, 1064, 1065*t*
Carbidopa-levodopa, 1216
Carbohydrates
dietary, 1129
reducing energy intake and, 118
Carbon dioxide laser therapy, 805
Carbon monoxide poisoning, 1191
Carbuncle, 262
Carcinogenesis, 1328
Cardiac arrest, 205-208
clinical presentation of, 206
complications of, 207
definition and epidemiology of, 205-206
diagnostics for, 207, 207*b*
differential diagnosis of, 207, 207*b*
disposition and referral for, 207
initial stabilization and management of, 207
pathophysiology of, 206
physical examination of, 206-207
prevention of, 207-208
Cardiac catheterization
for aortic stenosis, 614-615
for heart failure, 561
Cardiac diagnostic testing, 504-510
overview of, 504-509
Cardiac failure, 193
Cardiac implantable electronic device endocarditis, 586
Cardiac magnetic resonance imaging (cMRI), 497
Cardiac markers, 545*t*
Cardiac murmurs, 611-622, 612*t*
2014 American College of Cardiology/American Heart Association Guidelines for, 613-614
benign or innocent, 612*t*
cardiac arrhythmias and, 518
cause of, 613
continuous, 613
definition of, 611
diagnostics for, 615*b*
diastolic, 611-613, 617*b*
duration of, 613
evaluation of, 611
flow, 613-614
infective endocarditis and, 587
pansystolic, 542
systolic, 611, 615*b*
Cardiac resynchronization therapy, for heart failure, 567
Cardiac transplantation, for heart failure, 567
Cardiac ultrasound imaging, 507
Cardiomyopathy, 555-556
groups, 555
hypertrophic. *see* Hypertrophic cardiomyopathy
myocarditis and, 597
Cardio-oncology, 569
Cardiopulmonary resuscitation (CPR), 205
adult, 206*f*
Cardiovascular autonomic neuropathy, 1093
Cardiovascular disease (CVD)
with diabetes mellitus, 1093
HIV infection and, 1239
in menopause, 856
risk stratification in, 509-510
in women, diagnostic testing for, 509-510
Cardiovascular examination, of preparticipation sports physical, 186
Cardiovascular implantable electronic devices (CIEDs), 586, 590
endocarditis and, 588
Cardioversion
pharmacologic, 526
of unstable patients with tachycardia, 204*b*
Care management, 23
Care model, chronic, 19-21, 21*f*
Care transition, management of, in collaborative practice, 1
Career development, 14-15
collaborative research as strategy for, 15
Carotid angioplasty and stenting (CAS), 532, 534-535
complications of, 535
innovative approach to, 535
postprocedural care for, 535
procedure for, 534
traditional approach to, 534-535
Carotid artery disease, 529-536
clinical presentation of, 530-531
diagnostics for, 531
differential diagnosis for, 531-532
indications for referral or hospitalization for, 535-536
life span considerations with, 535
pathophysiology of, 529-530
physical examination for, 531
revascularization for, 532
Carotid endarterectomy, 532-534
for asymptomatic patients, 533
for cerebrovascular events, 1014
complications of, 533-534
periprocedural care for, 533
for symptomatic patients, 532-533
trials for, 532-533
Carotid sinus massage, 519
Carotid stenosis (CS), 529, 531, 534
Carpal tunnel syndrome
clinical presentation of, 933
diagnostics and differential diagnosis for, 934
management of, 935, 935*b*
physical examination for, 934, 934*f*
Carvedilol, 576*t*-582*t*
Case management, 23
of workers, 165-166
Cat bites, 255
Cataplexy, 1215
Cataracts, 326, 330, 335-337
clinical presentation of, 335-336
complications of, 336-337
definition and epidemiology of, 335
diagnostics for, 336
differential diagnosis of, 336, 336*b*
indications for referral or hospitalization for, 337
life span considerations with, 337
management of, 336
pathophysiology of, 335
physical examination for, 336, 336*f*
Catechol *O*-methyltransferase (COMT) inhibitors, 1053
Catecholamines, 557
Catheter or drain placement, for Bartholin gland cysts and abscesses, 805
Catheterization, clean intermittent, 735
Cauda equina syndrome, 602, 954
CD4 lymphopenia, 1237
CD4 T cells, 1233
Cefazolin, for endocarditis, 591*t*-595*t*
Cefdinir, for otitis media, 375*t*
Cefepime, for infectious arthritis, 944
Cefoxitin (Mefoxin), 874*b*
Cefpodoxime, for otitis media, 375*t*
Ceftaroline, 264

Ceftriaxone, 789*b*, 874*b*
for endocarditis, 591*t*-595*t*
for infectious arthritis, 944
for otitis media, 375*t*
Cefuroxime, 781*t*
for otitis media, 375*t*
Celecoxib, for osteoarthritis, 978
Celiac disease, 656
Celiac sprue, 689
Cell cycle activity, 1329*b*
Cellular kinetics, 1328
Cellulitis, 261-266, 332*t*-333*t*, 350-353
circumstances in, 265
clinical presentation and physical examination for, 262-263
definition and epidemiology of, 261-262
diagnostics for, 263
differential diagnosis of, 263, 263*b*
indications for referral or hospitalization for, 264-265
orbital. *see* Orbital cellulitis
pathophysiology of, 262
periorbital, 265
peritonsillar, 405, 411
preseptal. *see* Preseptal cellulitis
treatment of, 263-264
Centers for Disease Control and Prevention (CDC)
AIDS case definition by, 1232
guidelines for tuberculosis prevention and control in jails, prisons, and other correctional facilities, 1263
routine HIV testing, 1235
Vaccine Schedules App for Clinicians and Other Immunization Providers, 163
Centipedes, 197*t*
Centor criteria, for pharyngitis/tonsillitis, 414
Central nervous system (CNS)
depression, dysphagia and, 666*b*
effects of menopause in, 855-856
hypersomnias in, 1214-1215
infections of, 1037-1040. *see also specific infections*
clinical presentation of, 1038
complications of, 1040
definition and epidemiology of, 1037-1038
diagnostics for, 1038-1039, 1038*t*, 1039*b*
differential diagnosis for, 1039, 1039*b*
indications for referral or hospitalization for, 1040
life span considerations with, 1040
management of, 1039-1040
physical examination for, 1038
Central nervous system (CNS) sedatives, 1370-1371
Central nervous system (CNS) stimulants, 1372-1373
Central retinal vessel occlusion, 334*t*
Central sleep apnea (CSA)
causes of, 1213
management of, 1214
pathophysiology of, 1213
Central tendency, description of data and measures of, 10
Cephalexin, 781*t*
Cephalosporin
for gonorrhea, 789*b*
for pharyngitis/tonsillitis, 415
Cerebellum, 1040-1041
Cerebral emboli, in infective endocarditis, 587
Cerebrospinal fluid, findings, in acute meningitis, 1038*t*
Cerebrovascular disease
as causes of syncope, 231*b*
oral contraceptives and, 833
Cerebrovascular events, 1010-1016
antiplatelet agents for, 1014-1015
clinical presentation of, 1011
complications of, 1015
definition and epidemiology of, 1010
diagnostics for, 1011-1012, 1013*b*
differential diagnosis for, 1012, 1013*b*
in geriatric patients, 1015
hemorrhagic stroke, 1011
indications for referral or hospitalization for, 1015
ischemic stroke, 1010-1011
Cerebrovascular events *(Continued)*
life span considerations with, 1015
management of, 1012-1015, 1013*b*
pathophysiology of, 1010-1011
physical examination for, 1011, 1012*t*
in pregnancy, 1015
surgery for, 1014
thrombolytic therapy for, 1014
Cerumen impaction, 361-362
clinical presentation of, 361
complications of, 362
definition and epidemiology of, 361
diagnostics for, 361
differential diagnosis of, 361, 361*b*
indications for referral or hospitalization for, 362
life span considerations with, 362
management of, 361-362
pathophysiology of, 361
physical examination for, 361
Cervarix, 845, 871
Cervical cancer
clinical presentation and physical examination of, 869
HPV and, 868
pathophysiology of, 868
screening for, 146*t*-147*t*, 149*t*-154*t*, 869
vaccines for, 315
Cervical caps, 835
Cervical intraepithelial neoplasia (CIN), 844, 868-869
Cervical mucus testing, 837
Cervical muscle endurance training, 974
Cervical nodes, evaluation of, 1206
Cervical spine, 971
Cervical sponge, 835
Cervicitis, 784-791
Chalazion, 332*t*-333*t*, 337-339
clinical presentation of, 337, 338*f*
complications of, 339
definition and epidemiology of, 337
diagnostics for, 338
differential diagnosis of, 338, 338*b*
indications for referral or hospitalization for, 339
life span considerations with, 339
management of, 338-339, 339*t*
pathophysiology of, 337
physical examination for, 337-338, 338*f*
Chancre, 791, 791*f*
Chancroid, 785*t*-788*t*, 789*b*, 793
Chaperones, 52-53
Cheek biting, 1056
Chelation therapy, 1286
Chemical burn, 260
Chemical exposures, 208-211
chronic, 209
clinical presentation of, 208-209
definition and epidemiology of, 208
diagnostics and differential diagnosis of, 209-210, 209*b*
disposition and referral for, 210
initial stabilization and management of, 210
occupational, 166
pathophysiology of, 208
physical examination of, 209
prevention and patient education of, 210-211
red eye and, 332*t*-333*t*
in workplace, 208
Chemical injuries, in eyes, 345, 345*b*
Chemoreceptor trigger zone (CTZ), 709
Chemosis, 329, 335
Chemotherapy, 1310, 1328-1329
antiemetic for, 712*b*, 1341
for brain tumors, 1068
in oncology, 1328-1329
response to, 1329
for testicular cancer, 770
used for specific cancers, 1329*b*
Chemotherapy-induced nausea and vomiting (CINV), 1312*b*-1313*b*, 1341
Cherry juice, for gout, 929
Chest pain
cardiac, 484-485
congestive heart failure and, 481
Chest pain *(Continued)*
coronary artery disease and, 536-554
classification of, 541*b*
clinical presentation of, 540-542
diagnostics for, 542-547, 545*t*
differential diagnosis, 547, 548*t*
laboratory data for, 547
management of, 547-553
physical examination for, 542, 543*b*
GERD and, 671-672
noncardiac, 445-451
age considerations for, 449
causes of, 446*t*
clinical presentation of, 446-447
complications of, 449
definition and epidemiology of, 445-446
diagnostics for, 447, 447*b*
differential diagnosis of, 447-448, 449*b*
history taking for, 446, 446*b*
indications for referral or hospitalization in, 449, 450*b*
management of, 449, 450*f*
pathophysiology of, 446
physical examination for, 447
pulmonary, 448
with systemic lupus erythematosus, 1172
Chest radiograph
for cardiac arrhythmias, 518
for chronic cough, 452
for heart failure, 559-561
for lung cancer, 475
for pneumonia, 488
for presurgical clearance, 182*t*
Chewing (mastication), 664
Cheyne-Stokes breathing, 1213
CHICAGO mnemonic (lymphadenopathy), 1207
Chiggers, 197*t*
Chikungunya fever, 1228-1229, 1229*t*
Chikungunya viral arthritis, 941
Chikungunya virus infection, 1198
Children
chronic pain in, 1189
sexual assault to, 229
Chlamydia
clinical presentation of, 790-791
complications of, 791
definition and epidemiology of, 782, 790
diagnostics for, 791
management of, 785*t*-788*t*
pathophysiology of, 790
screening for, 149*t*-152*t*
treatment of, 789*b*
Chlamydia pneumoniae, 1156
Chlamydia test, 146*t*-147*t*
Chlamydia trachomatis, 785*t*-788*t*, 790, 872, 1156
Chlamydial conjunctivitis, 341-342
Chloramphenicol, for epiglottitis, 405-406
Chlorthalidone, 576*t*-582*t*
Cholecystitis, 635-639
acute, chest pain and, 548*t*
acute acalculous, 636, 636*b*
chronic, 636
clinical presentation of, 636-637
co-management of, with specialists, 638
complications of, 638-639
definition and epidemiology of, 635
diagnostics for, 637, 637*b*, 637*t*
differential diagnosis of, 637, 638*b*
gangrenous, 638-639
indications for referral or hospitalization for, 639
management of, 638
pathophysiology of, 636
physical examination for, 637
Cholecystostomy, 638
laparoscopic, 638
Cholelithiasis, 635-639
clinical presentation of, 636-637
co-management of, with specialists, 638
complications of, 638-639
definition and epidemiology of, 635
diagnostics for, 637, 637*b*, 637*t*
differential diagnosis of, 637, 638*b*
indications for referral or hospitalization for, 639
management of, 638
pathophysiology of, 636

Cholelithiasis *(Continued)*
physical examination for, 637
risk factors for, 636*b*
Cholesteatoma, 362-364
clinical presentation of, 363
definition of, 362-363
diagnostics for, 363, 363*b*
differential diagnosis of, 363, 363*b*
indications for referral or hospitalization for, 364
pathophysiology of, 363
physical examination for, 363
Cholesterol
abnormalities, screening for, 149*t*-152*t*
dietary, 1121
serum. *see also* Lipids, blood; *specific lipids*
routine screening of, 148*t*
test for, 146*t*-147*t*
Cholesterol absorption inhibitors, 1124*t*-1125*t*, 1125
Cholestyramine, 1124*t*-1125*t*
Cholinesterase inhibitors, for dementia, 1023
Chorea, 1040*b*
Chorioretinitis, 1276
Chromaffin cells, 1074
Chromosomal abnormalities, 68*t*
Chronic care model, 19-21, 21*f*
Chronic cyclic pelvic pain (CCPP), 823
Chronic disease, menopause and, 856-859
Chronic fatigue syndrome (CFS), 1190, 1193*b*
Chronic illness, in lifestyle management, 134
Chronic kidney disease (CKD), 531
categories of, 750*t*
classification of, 749
clinical presentation of, 751-752
complications of, 752*b*
diagnosis of, 749*t*
management of, 753-754
physical examination for, 752
Chronic lymphocytic leukemia (CLL), 1309, 1310*b*
Chronic myelogenous leukemia (CML), 1309, 1310*b*
Chronic obstructive pulmonary disease (COPD), 457-467
asthma and, 429
classification of, 459*b*
clinical presentation of, 458
complications of, 466
definition and epidemiology of, 457
diagnostics for, 459-460, 459*b*-460*b*
differential diagnosis of, 460, 461*b*
exercise training for, 465
heart failure and, 562-563
immunizations, 465
indications for referral or hospitalization for, 466-467
management of, 460-466
morbidity and mortality rates in, 457
nutrition of, 465
palliative care and hospice for, 466
pathophysiology of, 458
pharmacotherapy for, 461-465, 462*t*-463*t*
physical examination for, 458-459
psychological support for, 465
pulmonary rehabilitation for, 465
respiratory diseases and, 167
risk factors for, 457*b*
surgery for, 465-466
Chronic pain, 1186-1189. *see also* Pain
clinical presentation of, 1186-1187
definition and epidemiology of, 1186
diagnosis, establish, 51
diagnostics for, 1187
differential diagnosis for, 1187
evaluation of patient in, 50
fatigue and, 1191
life span considerations with, 1189
management of, 50-51, 1187-1188
nonpharmacologic intervention in, 1188, 1188*t*
pharmacologic interventions in, 1187-1188
pathophysiology of, 1186
physical examination for, 1187
Chronic Respiratory Disease Questionnaire, 468
Chronic respiratory exposure, 168
Chronic rhinosinusitis (CRS)
allergic rhinitis and, comparison of, 378*t*
clinical presentation of, 378
complications of, 379
definition and epidemiology of, 378
diagnostics for, 378-379
differential diagnosis of, 379, 379*b*
indications for referral or hospitalization for, 379
life span considerations with, 380
management of, 379
pathophysiology of, 378
physical examination for, 378
Chronic stable angina, 538
clinical presentation of, 540
diagnostics for, 542-543
electrocardiography for, 542
exercise tolerance testing for, 542-543, 543*b*
management of, 547
radiation symptoms in, 540
Chronic therapy, for chronic pain, 1188*t*
Chronic thromboembolic pulmonary hypertension (CTEPH), 496
Chronotherapy, 1212
Churg-Strauss syndrome (CSS), 1178
Chvostek sign, 1107
Ciclesonide, 462*t*-463*t*
Ciclopirox (Loprox), 281*t*
Cierny-Mader syndrome, 980*t*
Cigarette smoking. *see* Smoking
Cilostazol, 603
Cimetidine, 440*t*
Ciprofloxacin, 779*t*
Circadian disorders, 1211
Circinate balanitis, 1156
Circulating antineutrophil cytoplasmic antibodies (cANCAs), 397
Cirrhosis, 639-644
causes of, 639, 639*b*
clinical presentation of, 640
co-management of, 643
complications of, 643
definition and epidemiology of, 639-640
diagnostics for, 640-641, 641*b*
differential diagnosis of, 641, 641*b*
history in, 640
indications for referral or hospitalization for, 643
macronodular, 639-640
management of, 641-643, 689-690, 708
micronodular, 639-640
pathophysiology of, 640
physical examination for, 640
primary biliary, 640
process of, 686
Citalopram, 1360*t*-1362*t*
Clarithromycin, 729*t*
for pharyngitis/tonsillitis, 415
Classic orthostatic hypotension, 231
Classical Hodgkin lymphoma, 1315
Claudication, 600-601
Climacteric. *see* Menopause
Clindamycin
for otitis media, 375*t*
for salivary gland, 402
Clinical information systems, 19-20
design of, 23
Clinical significance, *versus* statistical significance, 11
Clinically isolated syndrome (CIS), multiple sclerosis, 1044*b*
Clobetasol, 884
Clobetasol propionate, 244*t*
Clomiphene, 848
Clonazepam, 1043
for REM sleep behavior disorder, 1218
Clonidine, for menopause, 865
Clopidogrel, 603, 1014
for coronary artery disease, 553
Closed fist injuries (CFIs), cellulitis and, 265
Closed globe injury, 356*t*
Clostridium difficile, 648, 656, 1156, 1249
colitis, 1223
in infectious diarrhea, 1246
Clostridium perfringens food poisoning, 1250
Clotrimazole (Lotrimin), 281*t*
Clozapine, 1380
Clubbing, digital, 472
Cluster headache, 1031
CNA HealthPro and Nurses Service Organization (CNA/NSO), 43
Coagulation, 1297
studies, for presurgical clearance, 182*t*
Coagulation factor replacement therapy, for hemophilia, 1301*t*
Coal tar preparations, 303
Coarctation of the aorta, 571, 572*t*-573*t*
Cocaine
abuse, in chronic rhinosinusitis, 379
use of, hypertension and, 572*t*-573*t*
Cocaine hydrochloride, 1372
Coenzyme Q10 (CoQ10), 16
Cognitive behavioral therapy (CBT)
for anxiety and depression, 1356
for chronic insomnia, 1212, 1212*t*
for chronic pain, 1188*t*
for dementia, 1023
for fatigue, 1194
for fibromyalgia syndrome, 927
Cognitive development, in adolescent, 55
Cognitive dysfunction, 1002
multiple sclerosis and, 1046*t*-1047*t*
Cognitive function, decline, in menopause, 857-858
Cognitive impairment. *see also* Dementia
with brain tumor, 1069
clinical presentation of, 88
definition and etiology, 87-88
in the elderly, 87-88
mild, 1020
Coinfection, in Lyme disease, 1257-1258
Colchicine, for gout, 930, 930*b*
Cold injury, 235-236
clinical presentation of, 235
complications of, 236
definition and epidemiology of, 235
diagnostics for, 235-236, 236*b*
differential diagnosis of, 236, 236*b*
indications for referral or hospitalization for, 236
life span considerations with, 236
management of, 236
pathophysiology of, 235
physical examination for, 235
Colesevelam, 1124*t*-1125*t*
Colestipol, 1124*t*-1125*t*
Colitis, *Clostridium difficile*, 656
Collaboration, 2
Collaborative practice
changing landscape of, 1-3
development, 14-15
models for, 6
new look of primary care, 2
opportunities to shape the landscape, 2-3
Collateral information, in neuropsychological assessment, 1002
Collateral ligament sprains, 946, 947*t*
College health, 170-173
for female students, 171
for male students, 171-172
resources for, 173
roles of providers, 170-171
screenings for, 173
topics in, 171-173
Colon
bleeding of, 680*b*
infections in, 1243-1244
polyps in, 726-727
tumors of, 726-727
clinical presentation of, 726
complications of, 727
definition and epidemiology of, 726
diagnostics for, 726-727, 727*b*
differential diagnosis of, 727, 727*b*
management of, 727
pathophysiology of, 726
physical examination for, 726
Colonoscopy, for inflammatory bowel disease, 695
Color Doppler ultrasound, for giant cell arteritis, 1162-1163

Colorectal cancer
menopause and, 859
screening for, 146*t*-154*t*
Colposcopy, 870
Combination therapy
for COPD, 464
for essential tremor, 1043
for psoriasis, 304
Combined immunodeficiency disorders (CIDs), 1201
treatment of, 1203
Common inheritance patterns, 37-38
Communication
with cancer patients, 1325-1326
patient, medical malpractice risk management strategies and, 45-46, 46*b*
Community resources, 21
Community-acquired pneumonia (CAP), 417-418
Community-associated methicillin-resistant *Staphylococcus aureus* (CA-MRSA), 1231
Community-based programs, 21
Compartment syndrome, 996-997
Compensatory mechanisms, in heart failure, 557-558
Complement activation, 1173
Complement system, 312
Complementary and alternative medicine (CAM), for Raynaud phenomenon, 1165
Complementary therapies
and alternative, for chronic pain, 1188, 1188*t*
for osteoarthritis, 979
Complete blood count (CBC)
for acute diarrhea, 650
for epiglottitis, 405
for immunodeficiency, 1202
for presurgical clearance, 182*t*
Complicated Grief Treatment (CGT), 1356
Component-resolved diagnostics (CRD) testing, 217
Comprehensive AIDS Resources Emergency (CARE) Act, 1233
Comprehensive care team (CCT), for multiple sclerosis, 1048
Compression fractures, 995
Computed tomography (CT)
for cerebrovascular events, 1011-1012
electron beam, 508-509
for hemoptysis, 473
for low back pain, 956
for neck pain, 972-973
for parotitis, 410
for seizures, 1056-1057
simulation, in radiotherapy, 1327
ultrafast, 508-509
Computed tomography angiography (CTA)
for abdominal aortic aneurysms, 512
for carotid artery disease, 531
for chronic stable angina, 543
for giant cell arteritis, 1163
in obese patients, 544
Computerized cognitive tests, 1000-1001
Condoms, 835
Condylomata acuminata, 315-316, 315*f*
Confidentiality, in college health, 171
Confusion Assessment Method, 1017, 1018*t*
Congenital anomalies, 68*t*
Congenital cholesteatoma, 363
Congestive heart failure (CHF)
with diabetes mellitus, 1093
infective endocarditis and, 587-588
Conjugate equine estrogen (CEE), 864
Conjunctiva, 329
hemorrhage, 330*f*
Conjunctivitis, 339-343
acute allergic, 341-342
bacterial, 341-342, 341*f*
clinical presentation and physical examination for, 340-341
definition of, 339
diagnostics for, 341
differential diagnosis of, 342, 342*b*
epidemiology of, 340
management of, 341-342
pathophysiology of, 340
referral for, indications for, 342-343
Conjunctivitis *(Continued)*
vernal and atopic, 341-342
viral, 340-341, 340*f*
Connective tissue diseases
bone tumors. *see* Bone tumors
with heart failure, 556*b*
osteoporosis and, 963*b*
Consent, informed, 46-47
Consolidation, in T-cell lymphomas, 1319
Constipation, 644-647, 1341, 1344
acute-onset, 645
chronic, 645
clinical presentation and physical examination for, 644-645
complications of, 646
definition and epidemiology of, 644
diagnostics for, 645, 645*b*
differential diagnosis of, 645, 645*b*
indications for referral or hospitalization for, 647
life span considerations with, 106, 646
management of, 645-646, 647*b*
medications associated with, 644*b*
in palliative care, 105-106
pathophysiology of, 644
in pregnancy, 72-73
Contact dermatitis, 266-267, 887-888
clinical presentation and physical examination for, 266, 887-888
complications of, 267, 888
definition and epidemiology of, 266
diagnostics for, 266-267, 266*b*, 888, 888*b*
differential diagnosis of, 266-267, 266*b*, 888, 888*b*
distribution diagnosis of, 267*t*
genital, 884
indications for referral or hospitalization for, 267, 888
life span considerations with, 888
management of, 267, 888
pathophysiology of, 887
Contact lenses, 330, 330*f*
Continuous positive airway pressure (CPAP), 1214
Contraception, 831
barrier methods of, 835-836
hormonal. *see* Oral contraceptives
hysteroscopic sterilization, 836
implantable, 834
injectable, 833-834
intrauterine, 836
natural family planning, 836-837
nonuse reasons for, 837
patch, 834
postcoital, 834-835
spermicidal, 835
sterilization, surgical, 836
vaginal ring, 836
Contraceptive therapy, for menopause, 861
Contusion, 356*t*
Convulsions. *see* Seizure disorder
Cooley anemia, 1285
Coombs test, 1296
COPD. *see* Chronic obstructive pulmonary disease (COPD)
COPD Assessment Test (CAT), 459, 459*b*
Copper IUDs, 836
Cor pulmonale, 440*t*, 466
Coral scrapes, 1185
Coral snakes, 200
Core needle biopsy, 1206-1207
Core strengthening, for low back pain, 957
Corn, 903*t*-905*t*
Cornea, 328-330, 355*b*
Corneal foreign body, in red eye, 332*t*-333*t*
Corneal surface defects, 343-345
clinical presentation of, 343
complications of, 345
definition and epidemiology of, 343, 343*f*
diagnostics for, 344, 344*b*, 344*f*
differential diagnosis of, 344, 344*b*
management of, 344-345, 345*b*
pathophysiology of, 343
physical examination for, 343-344
prevention of, 345
referral for, indications for, 345, 345*b*
Corns and calluses, 268-269
clinical presentation of, 268
complications of, 269
definition of, 268
diagnostics for, 268, 268*b*
differential diagnosis of, 268*b*
indications for referral or hospitalization for, 269
life span considerations with, 269
management of, 268-269
pathophysiology of, 268
physical examination for, 268
Coronary angiography, for variant angina, 544
Coronary Artery Calcium Score (CACS), 505-506
Coronary artery disease (CAD), 205, 536-554
clinical presentation of, 540-542
complications of, 554
definition and epidemiology of, 536-537
with diabetes mellitus, 1093
diagnostics for, 542-547, 545*t*
differential diagnosis of, 547
indications for referral or hospitalization in, 554
laboratory data for, 547
life span considerations with, 553-554
lipid guidelines for, 537-538
management of, 547-553
medications for, 537*t*
noninvasive assessment of, 504-510
pathophysiology of, 504, 538-540
relation of, to cardiac stress testing, 504
role of inflammation and atherogenesis in, 504
patient-related delays and initial treatment of, 536-537
pharmacologic therapy for, 550-553, 552*t*
physical examination of, 542, 543*b*
revascularization for, 507
risk factors for, 537
screening for, 155
secondary prevention of, 537*t*
statin therapy for, 538*t*
Coronary artery spasm, 539
Coronary Drug Project, 853
Coronary heart disease, 536
Coronary vasodilation, 551
Coronaviruses, 1226
Corticosteroids, 1222
acne and, 250*b*
for asthma, 431-441, 433*t*-435*t*
for brain tumors, 1068-1069
for contact dermatitis, 267
for COPD, 462*t*-463*t*, 464
for gout, 930
for headaches, 1034
inflammatory bowel disease and, 693*t*, 696-697
intra-articular injections of, for osteoarthritis, 978
for polymyalgia rheumatica, 1161
rectal use of, 697
for sarcoidosis, 502
for shoulder pain, 993
systemic, for asthma, 432-437, 435*t*-436*t*
for systemic lupus erythematosus, 1174
topical, 244*t*-245*t*, 245, 278, 303
for seborrheic dermatitis, 309
for vasculitis, 1180
Cortisol, 1074
hirsutism and, 1100
Costochondritis, 447, 456
chest pain and, 548*t*
Cough, 417
acute, 451
chronic, 451-457
bronchoscopy for, 452
characteristics of, 451*b*, 452
clinical presentation of, 452, 453*f*
complications of, 456
definition and epidemiology of, 451
diagnostics for, 452-454, 454*b*
differential diagnosis, 454-455, 455*b*
indications for referral or hospitalization for, 456, 456*b*
management of, 455-456
neural receptor in, 451-452
physical examination for, 452

Cough *(Continued)*
classification of, 451
lung cancer and, 475
postinfectious, 455
psychogenic, 455
Coughing. *see also* Cough, acute; Cough, chronic
asthma and, 423
Coumadin, GI bleeding and, 680-681
Counseling
and education, in pregnancy, 70
for unplanned pregnancy, 881-882
CPR. *see* Cardiopulmonary resuscitation (CPR)
Cracked nipples, 83
Crackles, 484
in heart failure, 560*t*
CRAFTT mnemonic, 57, 57*b*
Cranberry juice, 781
Cranial nerve III palsy, 328
Cranial nerve IV palsy, 328-329
Cranial nerves
fifth, 1063-1064
VII, 1008
C-reactive protein (CRP)
for neck pain, 973
for vasculitis, 1178-1179
Creams, 244, 244*t*
Creatine kinase (CK), in myocardial cell injury, 547
Creatinine, 751
Crisis pregnancy, 881-882
Crizotinib, 478
Crofelemer, 1250
Crohn disease (CD)
chronic diarrhea and, 653
definition and epidemiology of, 692
lesion in, 408
versus ulcerative colitis, 693*t*
Cromolyn, 437-439
Cromolyn/Nedocromil, 433*t*-435*t*
Cross-body adduction, 988*t*
Cruciate ligaments
anterior and posterior, 948
injuries, 948-949
Crusting, 247*t*
Cruveilhier-Baumgarten murmur, 640
Cryoglobulinemic vasculitis, 1178
Cryosurgery, of skin, 240
Cryotherapy, for warts, 316
Cryptorchidism, 764-765
Cullen sign, 715
Cultural competence, 4-5
Cultural diversity, in neuropsychological assessment, 1003-1004
Cultural issues, in college health, 173
Culturally responsive care, 29
Cultures, grief and, 1355
Curettage, of skin, 241
Cushing disease, 1074
Cushing syndrome
clinical presentation of, 1075
definition and epidemiology of, 1074
diagnostics for, 1075, 1076*b*
differential diagnosis for, 1076, 1076*b*
hypertension and, 571, 572*t*-573*t*
management of, 1076
pathophysiology of, 1074
physical examination for, 1075
Cutaneous herpes, 269-272
clinical presentation of, 270
complications of, 272
definition and epidemiology of, 269-270
diagnostics for, 270-271, 270*b*
differential diagnosis of, 271, 271*b*
indications for referral or hospitalization for, 272
life span considerations with, 272
management of, 271-272, 271*t*
pathophysiology of, 270
physical examination for, 270, 270*f*
Cyanosis, in dyspnea, 469
Cycle of abuse, violence perspectives and, 142
Cyclobenzaprine, 926*t*
Cyclooxygenase 2 (COX-2)-selective NSAIDs
for osteoarthritis, 978
for systemic lupus erythematosus, 1173-1174
Cyclophosphamide, 397
for systemic lupus erythematosus, 1174, 1174*t*
for vasculitis, 1180
Cyclosporine (Neoral), 303
Cyproterone acetate (CPA), 1102-1103
Cyst, 238*f*
Cystine stones, 776
Cystinuria, 773-774
Cytogenetic abnormalities, in myelodysplastic syndromes, 1322
Cytokines, 301-302, 1044
Cytotoxins, 1245

D

Dabigatran, 526, 607, 1306
Dacryocystitis, 332*t*-333*t*, 349-350
clinical presentation of, 349, 349*f*
complications of, 350
definition and epidemiology of, 349
diagnostics for, 349-350, 350*b*
differential diagnosis of, 350, 350*b*
indications for referral or hospitalization for, 350
management of, 350
pathophysiology of, 349
physical examination for, 349, 350*f*
Dairy products, gout and, 929
Dalbavancin, 264
Dallas criteria, for myocarditis, 597
Darifenacin (Enablex), 735
DASH diet, 132*t*-133*t*
Daytime sleepiness, 1190-1191
with Parkinson disease, 1054
D-dimer
levels, 606
in pulmonary embolism, 494
test, 1304
DDROPP mnemonic, 90
"Death rattle", 101-102
Debridement, in wound management, 321-322
Decision support, 20
Decision-making, vaccine administration, issues with, 155
Decitabine, 1323
Decompression sickness, 1181-1184
clinical presentation of, 1182
complications of, 1183
differential diagnosis for, 1183, 1183*b*
indications for referral for, 1183-1184
management of, 1183
pathophysiology of, 1182
physical examination for, 1182-1183
predive physical examination and diagnostics for, 1181-1182
Deep brain stimulation (DBS), 1053
Deep ulcer, 238*f*
Deep venous thrombosis (DVT), 1304, 1307. *see also* Thrombosis disorders (thrombophilia)
of lower extremity, 606-608
clinical presentation and physical examination of, 606
complications of, 608
definition and epidemiology of, 606
diagnostics for, 606
differential diagnosis of, 607
indications for referral and hospitalization for, 608
life span considerations with, 607-608
management of, 607
pathophysiology of, 606
patient and family education for, 608
pulmonary embolism and, 493
Defense of Marriage Act (DOMA), 61
Deferasirox, 1286
Deferiprone, 1286
Deferoxamine, 1286
Defibrillation, 212
for tachycardia, 204*b*
Degenerative disk disease, 953
Dehumidifiers, 216
Dehydration
clinical presentation of, 89
common causes of, 88*b*
definition and etiology of, 88
diagnostics for, 89
Dehydration *(Continued)*
differential diagnosis of, 89
education for, 89
heat-related illness and, 233
management of, 88*t*, 89
pathophysiology of, 89
prevention of, 89*b*
Dehydroepiandrosterone (DHEA), 250*b*, 757, 800, 1098
Dehydroepiandrosterone sulfate (DHEA-S), 1097-1098, 1100
Déjà vu, epilepsy and, 1056
Delayed sleep-wake phase disorder, 1211
Delayed-type hypersensitivity (DTH), 1202
Delirium, 1016-1019
clinical presentation of, 99, 1017
complications of, 1019
definition and epidemiology of, 99, 1016
diagnostics for, 99, 1017-1018, 1018*b*
criteria for, 1016*b*
differential diagnosis of, 99, 1018-1019, 1018*b*
in elderly, 98-100
indications for referral or hospitalization for, 1019
life span considerations with, 100
management of, 99-100, 1019, 1338-1339
pathophysiology of, 99, 1016-1017
physical examination for, 99, 1017
polypharmacy and, 88, 1017
subtypes of, 1017
superimposed on dementia, 1016
Delirium superimposed on dementia (DSD), 1016
Delirium tremens (DTs), 1371
Delivery system design, 20, 24-25
Delphian node, 1207
Delta sleep, 1209-1210, 1217
Dementia, 1019-1024
Alzheimer disease type of. *see* Alzheimer disease
clinical presentation of, 1021, 1021*b*
complications of, 1023
definition and epidemiology of, 1019-1020
diagnostics for, 1022, 1022*b*
differential diagnosis for, 1022, 1022*b*
indications for referral or hospitalization for, 1023
Lewy body. *see* Lewy body dementia
management of, 1023
with Parkinson disease, 1053
pathophysiology of, 1020-1021
physical examination for, 1021-1022
vascular, 1021
weight loss and, 1223
Demulcents, for chronic cough, 456
Dengue fever (DF), 1225, 1228, 1229*t*
Dengue virus, 1198
Denosumab (Prolia), 966, 969
Denosumab and Teriparatide Administration Study (DATA), 966
Dental abscess, 391, 398-399
clinical presentation of, 398
complications of, 399
definition and epidemiology of, 398
diagnostics for, 398, 398*b*
differential diagnosis of, 398, 399*b*
indications for referral or hospitalization for, 399
management of, 398-399
pathophysiology of, 398
physical examination for, 398
Dental caries, 149*t*-152*t*
Dental referral, of smell and taste disturbances, 394
Dependent rubor, 601
Depression. *see also* Major depressive disorder (MDD)
assessment of, 1356*t*
with brain tumor, 1069
clinical presentation and physical examination of, 100
definition and epidemiology of, 100
diagnostics for, 100
in elderly, 100-101
fatigue and, 1193
indications for referral or hospitalization, 101
life span considerations with, 101

Depression *(Continued)*
management of, 101
medication used for, 101*t*
in menopause, 854-855, 862*t*
multiple sclerosis and, 1046*t*-1047*t*
with Parkinson disease, 1053-1054
screening for, 149*t*-152*t*
Depressive disorders, 1356-1364
clinical presentation of, 1358
complications of, 1363-1364
definition and epidemiology of, 1356-1357
diagnostics for, 1358-1359
differential diagnosis of, 1359, 1359*b*
indications for referral or hospitalization for, 1364, 1364*b*
life span considerations with, 1363
management of, 1359-1363, 1360*t*-1362*t*, 1362*b*
pathophysiology of, 1357
physical examination for, 1358
Dermacentor andersoni, 1261
Dermacentor variabilis, 1261
Dermatitis herpetiformis, 656
Dermatitis medicamentosa, 273-275
clinical information resources for, 275
clinical presentation of, 273, 273*f*
complications of, 275
definition and epidemiology of, 273
diagnostics for, 273-274, 274*b*
differential diagnosis of, 274, 274*b*
indications for referral or hospitalization for, 275
management of, 275
pathophysiology of, 273
physical examination for, 273
Dermatographism, 239-240
Dermatologic disorders. *see* Skin, disorders of
Dermatologic manifestations, of reactive arthritis, 1156
Dermatologic therapy, 243-245
definition of, 243
medications of, 243-245
prescribing in, 243, 243*t*
topical corticosteroids in, 244*t*-245*t*, 245
vehicles in, 243-244, 244*t*
patient and family education in, 245
Dermatomes
cervical, 972*t*
lumbar, 955*t*
Dermatophyte infections, 279-282
clinical presentation and physical examination for, 279-280, 279*f*-280*f*
complications of, 281-282
definitions and epidemiology of, 279
diagnostics for, 280, 280*b*
differential diagnosis of, 280, 280*b*
indications for referral or hospitalization for, 282
management of, 280-281, 281*t*
oral medications in, 281
pathophysiology of, 279
Dermis, 235, 237
Dermoscopy, 239
Desiccated bovine thyroid, 1147
Desire, disorders of, 757
Desmopressin acetate (DDAVP), 1301
Desonide, 244*t*
Desoximetasone, 244*t*
Desvenlafaxine, 1360*t*-1362*t*
Detemir, 1082
Detrusor overactivity (DO), 731-732
Deviations, of nasal septum, 383
Dexamethasone, for brain tumors, 1068-1069
Dexamethasone elixir, for oral infections, 408
Diabetes insipidus, 1112
Diabetes mellitus, 1077-1096
aspirin recommendation for, 1094*t*
cataracts and, 336*f*
classification of, 1078*b*
clinical presentation of, 1079
complications of
acute, 1089-1091
chronic, 1091, 1091*b*
macrovascular, 1093-1095
microvascular, 1091-1095
psychological, 1088-1089
Diabetes mellitus *(Continued)*
coronary artery disease and, 537*t*
definition and epidemiology of, 1077-1078
diagnostics for, 1079-1080, 1080*b*, 1080*t*
differential diagnosis for, 1080
gestational, 76-77
glycemic control targets for, 1080*t*
indications for referral or hospitalization for, 1095
ischemic stroke and, 530
life span considerations with, 1095-1096
lipid disorders and, 1121
management of, 1080-1088
blood glucose monitoring in, 1085-1086
follow-up care in, 1086
insulin therapy in, 1082-1084, 1083*b*
lifestyle interventions in, 1080-1081, 1081*b*
pharmacotherapy in, 1081-1082
during pregnancy, 1086-1088, 1086*b*-1087*b*
with specialists, 1088
type 2, 1084-1085
nutrition guidelines for, 1081*b*
overview of, 128-129
pathophysiology of, 1078-1079
physical examination for, 1079, 1080*b*
screening for, 146*t*-152*t*, 1078*b*
sick-day management of, 1090*b*
skin and soft tissue infections in, 265
type 1, 1078-1079
insulin therapy for, 1082-1084
pregnancy and, 1087-1088
type 2, 1078-1079
insulin therapy for, 1083-1084, 1083*b*
medications for, 1084-1085
pregnancy and, 1088
UTIs and, 782
websites for, 1096
Diabetes self-management education (DSME) model, 24
Diabetic foot ulcers, 317, 317*b*, 320*t*, 324-325, 603, 982. *see also* Pressure ulcers
Diabetic nephropathy, 1091-1092
Diabetic neuropathy, 1092-1093
Diabetic peripheral neuropathy, 602
Diabetic retinopathy, 1091
Diagnostic and Statistical Manual of Mental Disorders, Fifth Edition (DSM-5), 1016
Diagnostic imaging. *see specific disorders and modalities*
Diaphragmatic breathing exercises, 974
Diaphragms (contraception), 835
Diarrhea, 1341-1342, 1344
acute, 1227-1228
diagnostics for, 650, 650*b*
evaluation of, 651*b*
chronic, 1245
diagnostics for, 650-652, 652*b*
evaluation of, 651*b*
from food and water, 179
infectious, microorganisms of, 696
lower intestinal, 1243-1244
noninfectious, 647-657
acute, 652-653, 654*b*-655*b*
chronic, 653-655, 654*b*-655*b*
clinical presentation of, 649
complications of, 656-657
definition and epidemiology of, 647
diagnostics for, 650-652, 650*b*, 652*b*
differential diagnosis of, 652-655, 654*b*-655*b*, 696
evaluation of, 651*b*
indications for referral or hospitalization for, 657
life span considerations with, 657
management of, 655-656
pathophysiology of, 648-649, 648*f*
physical examination for, 650
noninflammatory, 1244*t*, 1246-1247
small-volume, 1243
Diascopy, 239*b*
Diet. *see also* Nutrition
with brain tumor, 1069
for dysphagia, 668*t*-669*t*
gas-forming foods, 703*b*
Diet *(Continued)*
gout and, 929
for heart failure, 567-568
hypertension and, 570
with irritable bowel syndrome, 703
lipid disorders and, 1121-1123
for metabolic syndrome, 1129
weight loss and, 118-119, 130-131
Dietary Guidelines for Americans, 129
Dietary management, with renal failure, 754-755
Dietary supplements, 123
Diethylstilbestrol (DES), 828
Diethyltoluamide (DEET), 178
Diffuse large B-cell lymphoma (DLBCL), 1318
Diffusion-weighted magnetic resonance imaging (DW-MRI), 535
Diflorasone diacetate, 244*t*
Digoxin, 498, 525-526, 565-566
Dihydroergotamine, 1034
Dihydropyridine, 553, 576*t*-582*t*
Dihydrotestosterone (DHT), 738, 1097-1098
Dilated cardiomyopathy, 555
Dilation, 557
Diltiazem, 576*t*-582*t*, 1033
Dimethyl fumarate (Tecfidera), 1048-1049
Dipeptidyl peptidase 4 (DPP-4) inhibitors, 1085
Diphenhydramine, oral, 218
Dipyridamole, 505*t*, 509
for transient ischemic attack, 1014
Direct immunofluorescence (DIF) microscopy, in bullous pemphigoid, 258
Direct renin inhibitors, for hypertension, 576*t*-582*t*
Direct-to-consumer genetic testing, 31, 41-42
Disaster preparedness
evolution of emergency and, 188
in primary care, 188
primary patient care continues during, 189-190
Discharge instructions, for breastfeeding patients, 80
Discoid lupus rash, with systemic lupus erythematosus, 1171, 1171*b*
Disease management, population, 22
Disease-modifying antirheumatic drugs (DMARDs), 1168-1169
for psoriatic arthritis, 1158
Disequilibrium, 1024. *see also* Vertigo
Disseminated intravascular coagulation, 1311
Distress, assessment of, 1187*b*
Disulfiram (Antabuse), 1376
Diuretics
for hypertension, 576*t*-582*t*
oral, for heart failure, 565, 566*t*
for pulmonary hypertension, 498
Divalproex sodium (Depakote), 1033
Divers Alert Network (DAN), 1182
Diverse patient groups, address cultural variations among, 29-30
Diverticular bleeding, 662-663, 663*b*
Diverticular disease, 657-663
Diverticulitis, 660-662
clinical presentation of, 660
complications of, 662
definition and epidemiology of, 660
diagnostics for, 660, 661*b*
differential diagnosis for, 661, 661*b*
indications for referral or hospitalization for, 662
management of, 661-662
pathophysiology of, 660
physical examination for, 660
Diverticulosis, 657-660
clinical presentation of, 658
complications of, 659
definition and epidemiology of, 657-658
diagnostics for, 658-659, 659*b*
differential diagnosis for, 659, 659*b*
indications for referral or hospitalization for, 659
life span considerations with, 659
management of, 659
pathophysiology of, 658
physical examination for, 658
Diving injuries, 1181-1185
Dizziness, 1024-1028. *see also* Vertigo
clinical presentation of, 1025
complications of, 1027

Dizziness *(Continued)*
definition and epidemiology of, 1024
diagnostics for, 1025-1026, 1025*b*-1026*b*
differential diagnosis for, 1026, 1026*b*
management of, 1027
in Meniere disease, 368
pathophysiology of, 1024-1025
physical examination for, 1025
DMT initiation, for multiple sclerosis, 1048-1049
Dobutamine, 509
Documentation, in sexual assault, 228
Docusate sodium, 646
Dog bites, 255
DOMA. *see* Defense of Marriage Act (DOMA)
Domestic violence, clinical presentation and diagnoses of, 141
Donepezil (Aricept), 1023
Do-not-resuscitate (DNR), 96
Dopamine agonists, 1052-1053
for infertility, 848
Dopamine receptor antagonists, 712*b*
Dopaminergic agonists, for restless legs syndrome, 1216
DOTS (directly observed therapy short course) program, 1270
Dowager's hump, 961
Doxazosin, 576*t*-582*t*
Doxepin, 313-314
Doxycycline, 789*b*, 874*b*
for ehrlichiosis, 1260
for Lyme disease, 1256
for pneumonia, 489
Drawer test, 948, 949*f*
Dressings
for burns, 261
in wound management, 322
Dronedarone, 525
Drop arm test, 988*t*
Drospirenone, 833
Drug fever, 1198
Drug interactions, HIV infection and, 1239
Drug/alcohol testing, 165
Drug-induced liver injury (DILI), 686, 688-691
Drugs. *see* Medications/drugs
Dry eye, 332*t*-333*t*, 345-349
clinical presentation of, 346
complications of, 348
definition and epidemiology of, 345-346
diagnostics for, 347, 347*b*, 347*f*
differential diagnosis of, 347, 347*b*
indications for referral or hospitalization for, 348
life span considerations with, 348
management of, 348
pathophysiology of, 346, 346*f*
physical examination for, 346-347
Dry mouth. *see* Xerostomia
Dry skin (xerosis), 275-277
clinical presentation of, 276, 276*f*
complication of, 276-277
definition and epidemiology of, 275
diagnostics and differential diagnosis of, 276, 276*b*
indications for referral or hospitalization for, 277
management of, 276
pathophysiology of, 275-276
DSME. *see* Diabetes self-management education (DSME) model
Dual-energy x-ray absorptiometry (DXA), 857
Duke criteria, for endocarditis, 589, 589*b*
Duke's Treadmill Score (DTS), 543, 543*b*
Dukoral, 179
Duloxetine, 926*t*, 1360*t*-1362*t*
Dumping syndrome, 124
Dutasteride (Avodart), 735
Dysbarism, 1182
Dysentery, foods and water and, 179
Dysgeusia, Bell palsy and, 1008
Dyskinesia, 1040*b*
Dyslipidemia
alternative therapy for, 17
with diabetes mellitus, 1094
metabolic syndrome and, 1127-1128
treatment of, 1130
Dysmenorrhea, 821-825
clinical presentation of, 822-823
complications of, 824
definition and epidemiology of, 821
diagnostics for, 823, 823*b*
differential diagnosis of, 823, 823*b*
indications for referral or hospitalization for, 824-825
management of, 824, 824*b*
pathophysiology of, 821-822
physical examination for, 823
primary, 821
secondary, 821-822, 823*b*
Dyspareunia, 825-827
clinical presentation of, 826
complications of, 827
definition and epidemiology of, 825
diagnostics for, 826, 826*b*
differential diagnosis of, 826, 827*b*
examination of, 826
life span considerations with, 827
management of, 827
pathophysiology of, 825-826
Dysphagia
GERD and, 671
oropharyngeal, 663-669
aspiration and nonoral feeding in, 667-668
clinical presentation of, 665
complications of, 669
definition and epidemiology of, 663
diagnostics for, 665-666, 666*b*
differential diagnosis for, 667*b*
indications for referral or hospitalization for, 669
management of, 666-668, 668*t*-669*t*
medication-related conditions that cause, 666*b*
pathophysiology of, 664-665
physical examination for, 665
potential causes of, 664*b*
swallowing strategies and therapies for, 668, 668*t*-669*t*
Dysplastic nevi, 248*b*
Dyspnea, 467-471, 540-541
assessment of, 469*t*
associated symptoms in, 468-469
breathing pattern and body position and, 469
chronic, 460
clinical presentation of, 101-102, 467-469
complications of, 102
definition of, 101, 467
diagnostics for, 102, 470, 470*b*
differential diagnosis of, 102, 470, 470*b*
epidemiology of, 467
exposures in, 469
in heart failure, 562
indications for referral or hospitalization for, 102
intensity of, 468
life span considerations with, 102-103
management of, 102, 471
in palliative care, 101-103
pathophysiology of, 101, 467
physical examination for, 101-102, 469-470
quality of, 468
respiratory descriptions and causes of, 468*t*
scale for, 468, 468*t*
timing of, 468
Dystonia, 1040*b*

E

Ear barotrauma, 1184
Ear disorders. *see* Auricular disorders
Eardrum. *see* Tympanic membrane (TM)
Early disseminated infection, of Lyme disease, 1255, 1256*b*
Early localized infection, of Lyme disease, 1255, 1256*b*
Eastern equine encephalitis, 1040
Eating disorders, 117*t*. *see also specific disorders*
in college health, 171
Ebola virus disease, 1230
ECG. *see* Electrocardiography (ECG)
Echocardiography
with acute myocardial infarction, 547
with cardiac arrhythmias, 518
Echocardiography *(Continued)*
with color Doppler, 617
with dobutamine, 505*t*, 509
with exercise, 505*t*, 508
with heart failure, 558-559
with infective endocarditis, 588
M-mode, for mitral stenosis, 621
with myocarditis, 598
with non-ST segment elevation myocardial infarction, 544-545
three-dimensional and Doppler flow, 508
two-dimensional, 621
two-dimensional, comparison of myocardial perfusion imaging with, 508
with unstable angina, 544-545
with variant angina, 544
Eclampsia, 75*t*, 76
Econazole (Spectazole), 281*t*
Ecstasy, 1372-1373
Ecthyma, 262
Ectopic pregnancy, 828-831
clinical presentation of, 828
complications of, 831
definition and epidemiology of, 828
diagnostics for, 829, 829*b*
differential diagnosis of, 830, 830*b*
indications for referral or hospitalization for, 831
life span considerations with, 831
management of, 830
pathophysiology of, 828
physical examination for, 828-829
presentation and exam for, 73
Eczema, 888-889
clinical presentation and physical examination of, 889
complications of, 889
diagnostics for, 889, 889*b*
differential diagnosis of, 889, 889*b*
indications for referral or hospitalization for, 889
life span considerations with, 889
management of, 889
pathophysiology of, 888-889
Eczematous dermatitis. *see* Atopic dermatitis (AD)
Edema, 1375
in heart failure, 560*t*
scrotal, 763
Education
for chlamydia, 791
counseling and, in pregnancy, 70
in dehydration, 89
for genital herpes, 793
patient
acromegaly, 1073-1074
adrenal gland disorders, 1077
animal and human bites, 257-258
ankylosing spondylitis, 1155-1156
arthritis of inflammatory bowel disease, 1159
asthma, 443-445, 444*t*
Bell palsy, 1010
bleeding disorders (coagulopathies), 1303
breast pain, 809-810
carotid artery disease, 536
central nervous system infections, 1040
cerebrovascular events, 1015-1016
dizziness and vertigo, 1027
elbow pain, 924
fatigue, 1196
gastroesophageal reflux disease, 677
hand and wrist pain, 935-936
heel (calcaneal) bursitis, 920
hirsutism, 1103-1104
HIV infection, 1240-1241
hypertension, 584
incontinence, 736
infective endocarditis, 597
LGBTQ patient care and, 65
lipid disorders, 1126
low back pain, 959
lung cancer, 479
mastitis, 811
neck pain, 976
noninfectious diarrhea, 657
obstructive uropathies, 798
Paget disease of nipple, 814

Education (Continued)
parathyroid gland disorders, 1135
polymyalgia rheumatica, 1161-1162
prenatal care, 79b
Raynaud phenomenon, 1166
reactive arthritis, 1157
scuba diving, 1184
sexual dysfunction (male), 763
sexual dysfunction of female, 879
skin cancer, 248
sprains, strains and fractures, 997-998
testicular disorders, 771
trigeminal neuralgia, 1066
unintended weight loss, 1223-1224
unplanned pregnancy, 883
urinary calculi, 777
patient and family
abdominal aortic aneurysm, 515
Achilles tendinopathy, 900
Achilles tendon rupture, 900-901
acne, 252
acute arterial insufficiency, 605
acute bronchitis, 420
acute bronchospasm, 193-194
acute pancreatitis, 717
allergic rhinitis, 387
alopecia, 255
amenorrhea, 803
amyotrophic lateral sclerosis, 1007
anal fissure, 633
anaphylaxis, 196
ankle sprains, 899
anorectal abscess or fistula, 635
anorexia nervosa, 97-98
anxiety, 99
anxiety disorders, 1354
appendicitis, 625
atopic dermatitis, 279
atrophic vaginitis, 896
auricular disorders, 360
bacterial vaginosis, 893-894
Bartholin gland cysts and abscesses, 805
benign prostatic hyperplasia, 740
bipolar disorders, 1369
bone tumors, 913
bowel construction, 106
bradycardia/bradyarrhythmias, 203
breast masses, 816
bullous pemphigoid, 259
burns, 261
cachexia, 97-98
candidiasis, 284
cardiac arrest, 208
cardiac arrhythmias, 528-529
cataracts, 337
cellulitis, 265-266
cerumen impaction, 362
cervical cancer, 845
chemical exposure, 210-211
chest pain, 451
cholelithiasis and cholecystitis, 639
cholesteatoma, 364
chronic cough, 457
chronic pain, 1189
chronic pancreatitis, 720
chronic pelvic pain, 821
chronic rhinosinusitis, 380
chronic venous stasis, 609
cirrhosis, 643-644, 643b
cold injury, 236
colon tumors, 727
conjunctivitis, 343
constipation, 106, 647
contact dermatitis, 267, 888
COPD, 467
corns and calluses, 269
coronary artery disease, 554
cruciate ligament injuries, 949
cutaneous herpes, 272
dacryocystitis, 350
deep venous thrombosis, 608
delirium, 100, 1019
dementia, 1023-1024
dental abscess, 399
depression, 101

Education (Continued)
dermatitis medicamentosa, 275
dermatologic therapy, 245
dermatophyte infections, 282
diabetes mellitus, 1096
diverticular bleeding, 663
diverticulitis, 662
diverticulosis, 659-660
dry eye, 348-349
dry skin, 277
dysmenorrhea, 825
dyspareunia, 827
dysphagia, 669
dyspnea, 103, 471
ectopic pregnancy, 831
eczema and psoriasis, 889
electrical injuries, 213
endometrial cancer, 839
environmental allergies, 216
epiglottitis, 406
epistaxis, 382
esophagus tumors, 723
essential tremor, 1043
eyelid disorders, 339
fear, 99
fever, 1200
fibromyalgia syndrome, 927
food allergies, 217-218
gastrointestinal disturbances, 1345
gastrointestinal hemorrhage, 682
goiter, 1139
gout, 932
granulomatosis with polyangiitis, 397
Guillain-Barré syndrome, 1030
gynecomastia, 816-817
head trauma, 221
headache, 1037
hearing loss, 366-367
heart failure, 567, 569
heat-related illness, 235
hematuria, 749
hemoptysis, 474
hemorrhoids, 632
hepatitis, 691
herpes zoster, 286
herpetic whitlow, 292
hidradenitis suppurativa, 288
hip pain, 940
hypercalcemia and hypocalcemia, 1108
hyperhidrosis, 290
hyperkalemia and hypokalemia, 1112
hypernatremia, 1114
hyperthyroidism, 1145
hyponatremia, 1119
hypotension, 224
hypothyroidism, 1149
infectious arthritis, 945-946
infectious diarrhea, 1251
infectious mononucleosis, 1254
infertility, 849-850
inflammatory bowel disease, 699
influenza, 1243
insect bites and stings, 198
insomnia, 1212-1213
international traveler, 176-177
intertrigo, 291
intimate partner violence, 145
intracranial tumors, 1069-1070
iron deficiency anemia, 1283
irritable bowel syndrome, 705
jaundice, 709
knee pain, 948
leukemias, 1311-1312, 1312b-1313b
lichen planus, 886
lichen sclerosus, 884-885, 885b
lichen simplex chronicus, 887
lymphadenopathy, 1209
lymphomas, 1320
macrocytic anemia, 1289-1290
major depressive disorder, 1364
Meniere disease, 369
meniscus injuries, 951
metabolic syndrome, 1131
mitral stenosis, 622
Morton neuroma, 903

Education (Continued)
movement disorders, 1042
multiple sclerosis, 1049-1050
mumps, 411
myelodysplastic syndromes, 1324
myocarditis, 599
nasal trauma, 384
nasal tumors and polyps, 396
nasolacrimal duct obstruction, 350
nausea and vomiting, 105, 713
nipple discharge and galactorrhea, 813
obesity, 125
occupational respiratory diseases, 169
oncology complications, 1335
oncology pain, 1341
onychomycosis, 296
oral infections, 409
orbital cellulitis, 353
osteoarthritis, 979-980
osteochondritis dissecans, 901
osteomyelitis, 985
osteoporosis, 967
otitis externa, 372-373
otitis media, 376-377
ovarian cancer, 841
Paget disease of bone, 970
pain, 107
pancreatic pseudocyst, 722
Pap test abnormalities, 870-871
parasomnias, 1218
Parkinson disease, 1054
paronychial infections, 294
parotitis, 411
patellofemoral pain syndrome, 952
pelvic inflammatory disease, 875
peptic ulcer disease, 730
peripheral arterial insufficiency, 604
peritonsillar abscess, 413
pharyngitis/tonsillitis, 416
pinguecula, 355
plantar fasciitis, 902
pleural effusions, 483
pleurisy, 485
pneumonia, 491
pneumothorax, 493
poisoning, 226
preparticipation sports physical, 187
preseptal cellulitis, 353
presurgical clearance, 184-185
prostate cancer, 738
prostatitis, 743
proteinuria, 747
pruritus, 301
pruritus ani, 634
psoriasis, 304
pterygium, 355
pulmonary hypertension, 499-500
purpura, 307
renal failure, 756
reptile bites and scorpion stings, 201
rheumatoid arthritis, 1170
salivary gland diseases, 403
sarcoidosis, 503
scabies, 308
schizophrenia, 1381
seborrheic dermatitis, 310
seizure disorder, 1063
sexual assault, 230
sexually transmitted infections, 793
shoulder pain, 993
sickle cell disease, 1293
sinusitis, 392
sleep-related breathing disorders, 1214
sleep-related movement disorders, 1217
small intestine tumors, 726
smell and taste disturbances, 394
spider bites, 200
stasis dermatitis, 311
stomach tumors, 724
syncope, 233
systemic lupus erythematosus, 1176
tachycardia/tachyarrhythmias, 205
thalassemia, 1287
thrombosis disorders (thrombophilia), 1307
thyroid cancer and thyroid nodules, 1141

Education *(Continued)*
tinea versicolor, 282
tinnitus, 371
traumatic ocular disorders, 358
tuberculosis, 1271
tympanic membrane perforation, 377
unknown primary carcinoma, 1348
urinary tract infections, 782
urticaria, 314
vaginal cancer, 843
varicose veins, 609
vasculitis, 1180
venous stasis ulceration, 610
vestibular neuritis, 368
vitiligo, 298
vulvar cancer, 842
vulvar vestibulitis syndrome and vulvodynia, 892
vulvovaginal candidiasis, 895
warts, 316
wound management, 325
xerostomia, 103
Effortful swallow, 668*t*-669*t*
Eflornithine hydrochloride, 1102
Egocentrism, 55
Ehrlichia chaffeensis, 1260
Ehrlichiosis, 1260
Eicosapentaenoic acid, 1222
Elastase, 714-715
Elastin, 429-430
Elbow joint
aspiration and injection of, 916*f*
bursitis of (olecranon), 916-917, 922*t*-923*t*
differential diagnosis of, 916*b*
management of, 917
common ailments of, 922*t*-923*t*
fracture of, 994
golfer's, 922
injuries of, 921
pain in, 920-924
clinical presentation of, 921
complications of, 924
definition and epidemiology of, 920-921
diagnostics for, 921-922, 921*b*
differential diagnosis of, 922, 922*b*, 922*t*-923*t*
management of, 922-923
pathophysiology of, 921
physical examination for, 921
sprains of, 922*t*-923*t*
stability of, 921
tennis, 922
Elder abuse, 93
Electrical injuries, 211-213
alternating current (AC) and direct current (DC), 211
clinical presentation of, 211
definition and epidemiology of, 211
diagnostics for, 212, 212*b*
differential diagnosis of, 212, 212*b*
disposition and referral of, 212-213
initial stabilization and management of, 212
pathophysiology of, 211
physical examination for, 212
prevention and patient and family education of, 213
spectrum of, 211
Electrocardiography (ECG)
during asthma exacerbation, 429
for cardiac arrest, 207
for chemical exposure, 209
for chronic stable angina, 542
conduction abnormalities on, 518
for electrical injuries, 212
with exercise testing, 506
for heart failure, 559
for hypotension, 222-223
for myocarditis, 598
for non-ST segment elevation myocardial infarction, 544
with poisoning, 225
premature atrial contractions on, 522*f*
for preparticipation sports physical, 187
for presurgical clearance, 182*t*
for pulmonary embolism, 494
Electrocardiography (ECG) *(Continued)*
for seizures, 1056-1057
for ST-elevation acute myocardial infarction, 545, 545*f*-546*f*
for syncope, 232
for unstable angina, 544
for variant angina, 544
Electrocautery, of skin, 240-241
Electroconvulsive therapy (ECT), 1363
Electroencephalography (EEG), 232
for cerebrovascular events, 1012
for seizures, 1054
Electrolysis, 1102
Electrolyte values, for presurgical clearance, 182*t*
Electron beam computed tomography (EBCT), 508-509
Electronic health, health literacy of, 28
Electronic mail communication with patients, 48-49
Electronic medical records (EMRs), 2, 47-49
Electrophysiologic studies, in cardiac arrhythmias, 519
Elephantiasis, 765-768, 770-771
Elevation, 247*t*
Elliptocytosis, hereditary, 1296
Elvey upper limb tension test, 972
Embolectomy, 495
Embolic protective device (EPD), 534
Embolization, of vegetative material, 587
Emergency departments (EDs), 229
surge capacity and, 190
Emergency management, incident command system for, 188
Emergency medical services (EMS), 2
Emergency preparedness, and response in primary care, 188-191
Emotional development, of adolescent, 55
Emotions, unplanned pregnancy and, 881
Emphysema
changes related to, 168
defined, 457
Employment/work, pre-placement health evaluation, 164-165
Empty can test, 988*t*
Emulsion, 244*t*
Enalapril, 576*t*-582*t*
Encephalitis, causes of, 1037
Endarterectomy, carotid, for cerebrovascular events, 1014
Endocrine disorders/diseases. *see also specific disorders*
osteoporosis and, 963*b*
in pruritus, 300*b*
Endocrinology referral, of smell and taste disturbances, 394
End-of-life care, 94-108. *see also* Palliative care
Endoleak, 514
Endometrial cancer
in menopause, 858
screening for, 153*t*-154*t*
Endometrial intraepithelial neoplasia (EIN), 838
Endometriosis
management of, 827
pelvic pain, 817, 819-820
Endomyocardial biopsy (EMB), 597
for heart failure, 561
Endophthalmitis, 334*t*
Endoscopic variceal ligation, 681
Endoscopy, 695, 695*b*. *see also specific procedures*
for GI bleeding, 681
Endothelin receptor antagonists, for pulmonary hypertension, 499*t*
Endothelin-blocking agents, for Raynaud phenomenon, 1165
Endovascular stent grafts, for abdominal aortic aneurysm, 513-514
End-stage renal disease (ESRD), 743, 749, 755
Enemas, 646
Energy intake
obesity and, 111
and output
balance factors, 110
in obesity, 111
reduction of food intake, 110
reducing, 118
Entamoeba histolytica (amebiasis), 179
Enterococci, 585, 590
Enterotoxins, 1245, 1247
Environmental allergies, 213-216
clinical presentation and physical examination of, 214-215
common allergens, 213-214
complications of, 216
definition and epidemiology of, 213
diagnostics for, 215
differential diagnosis of, 215, 215*b*
management of, 215-216
pathophysiology of, 214
Environmental disorders. *see also* Occupational/environmental health
in pruritus, 300*b*
Enzyme-linked immunosorbent assay (ELISA), 1235
for bullous pemphigoid, 258
Enzymes, pancreatic, 713
Eosinophilic esophagitis, 671, 673
Eosinophilic granulomatosis with polyangiitis (EGPA), 1178
Ependymoma, 1066*t*
Epicondylitis, 922*t*-923*t*
Epidemics, 136
Epidermal growth factor, 275
Epidermal growth factor receptor (EGFR), gene mutations in, lung cancer and, 475
Epidermis, 237
Epidermoid cysts, 262
Epididymitis, 764-767, 768*b*, 770
Epiglottitis, 403-406, 412
in adult, 404*f*
clinical presentation of, 404
complications of, 406
definition and epidemiology of, 403
diagnostic and differential diagnosis for, 415
diagnostics for, 404-405, 405*b*
differential diagnosis of, 405, 405*b*
health promotion of, 406
indications for referral or hospitalization of, 406
life span considerations with, 406
management of, 405-406
pathophysiology of, 403-404
patient and family education of, 406
physical examination of, 404
Epilepsy. *see* Seizure disorder
Epinephrine
for anaphylaxis, 196
auto-injections, 196
dose, 196
for food allergies, 218
Epiphora, 335
Episcleritis, 332*t*-333*t*
Epistaxis, 380-382
clinical presentation of, 380
complications of, 381
definition and epidemiology of, 380
diagnostics for, 380-381, 380*b*
differential diagnosis of, 381, 381*b*
indications for referral or hospitalization for, 381
life span considerations with, 381-382
management of, 381
pathophysiology of, 380
physical examination for, 380
Epithelial salivary gland neoplasms, WHO classification of, 400*t*
Eplerenone, 1111
for hypertension, 576*t*-582*t*
Epley maneuver, 1028
Epoprostenol, 498
Eprosartan, 576*t*-582*t*
Epstein-Barr nuclear antigen (EBNA), 1252
Epstein-Barr virus, 413
Epstein-Barr virus-associated infectious mononucleosis (EBV-IM), 1251-1252. *see also* Infectious mononucleosis
Erectile dysfunction (ED), 756
cardiovascular risk factors in, 758
clinical presentation of, 759
complications of, 762
diagnostics for, 760, 760*b*
differential diagnosis for, 760, 760*b*
hormonal risk factors in, 758

Erectile dysfunction (ED) *(Continued)*
management of, 760-762
pharmacologic risk factors in, 758, 759*b*
physical examination for, 760
psychogenic factors in, 758
risk factors for, 758*b*
surgical risk factors in, 758
Ergot derivatives, for headaches, 1034
Ergotamine tartrate (Cafergot), 1034
Ergotamines, for headaches, 1035*t*-1036*t*
Eric Coleman's Care Transitions Intervention, 5
Erlotinib, 478
Eros Clitoral Therapy Device (Eros-CTD), 878
Erosion, 238*f*, 247*t*
Erysipelas, 262
Erythema migrans, 1255-1256, 1256*f*
Erythema multiforme, 274*t*
Erythema nodosum, 501
Erythrocyte sedimentation rate (ESR)
for neck pain, 973
for vasculitis, 1178-1179
Erythromycin, 789*b*
for infectious diseases of salivary gland, 402
Erythropoiesis, 1278
Erythropoietin (EPO), 1278, 1293, 1322
hypertension and, 572*t*-573*t*
Escherichia coli, 1156
characteristics of, 179
enteroadherent, 1245
meningitis and, 1037
O157:H7, 1228, 1248-1249
Esophageal spasm, 447-448
Esophageal varices, 678, 681
Esophagitis, 448
Esophagogastroduodenoscopy (EGD), 672
Esophagus
perforation of, 448
spasm of, 447-448
tumors of, 722-723
clinical presentation of, 722
complications of, 723
definition and epidemiology of, 722
diagnostics for, 722-723, 722*b*
differential diagnosis of, 723, 723*b*
management of, 723
pathophysiology of, 722
physical examination for, 722
Essential tremor, 1042-1043, 1043*b*
Essure (contraception), 836
Estimated date of delivery, 68
Estrogen
for amenorrhea, 802
for menopause, 861, 862*t*, 865, 865*t*-867*t*
in oral contraceptives, 831-832
for osteoporosis, 965
osteoporosis and, 857
replacement of
for incontinence, 734
for infertility, 848
Estrogen-progestogen therapy, for menopause, 862*t*
Ethacrynic acid, 576*t*-582*t*
Ethnic groups, STIs and, 782-783
Etidronate (Didronel), 969*t*
Euglycemic insulin clamp technique, 1128
Euthyroid sick syndrome, 1149
Evaluating key study parameters, of research, 8-11, 9*t*
Event monitor, 519
Evidence-based practice, in collaborative practice, 1
Exacerbate orthostatic intolerance, of hypotension, 223
Exacerbation, 1049
Exanthems, 274*t*
Excessive daytime sleepiness (EDS). *see also* Hypersomnias
differential diagnosis of, 1215*b*
Excision, for Bartholin gland cysts and abscesses, 805
Excitement, disorders of, 757-758
Excoriation, 238*f*
Executive function tests, 1000*b*
Exenatide (Byetta), 1085
Exercise, 1222-1223
for chronic pain, 1188*t*
for COPD, 465
Exercise *(Continued)*
for diabetes mellitus, 1080-1081, 1081*b*
for fibromyalgia syndrome, 927
as healthy lifestyle component, 131-134
for heart failure, 568
for hypertension, 571, 584
for incontinence, 734
in lifestyle assessment, 127
lipid disorders and, 1121, 1123
for low back pain, 957
for metabolic syndrome, 1129
for neck pain, 974
osteoporosis and, 963-964
Exercise myocardial perfusion imaging (EMPI), 505*t*
Exercise radionuclide angiography, 505*t*
Exercise tolerance testing, 506
for acute myocardial infarction, 547
for chronic stable angina, 542-543, 543*b*
comparisons of, 505*t*
for heart failure, 562
imaging adjuncts to, 506-509, 507*b*
with ischemia, 543
for non-ST segment elevation myocardial infarction, 544
sensitivity and specificity, 506
for unstable angina, 544
for variant angina, 544
Exercise-associated hyponatremia (EAH), 1114-1115, 1118-1119
Exercise-induced asthma, 423
Exertional heat stroke, 1197, 1197*b*
Exophthalmos, 1221
Experimental design
in research, 7
true, 7*t*
Exposure keratitis, 1009
Extensively drug-resistant tuberculosis, 1231-1232
External beam radiotherapy, 1327
Extracellular fluid volume, 1113-1114
Extracorporeal shock wave lithotripsy (ESWL), 775
Extraesophageal reflux (EER), 671
Extraesophageal symptoms, 671
Extrahepatic obstructive jaundice, 706
Extraocular movements, 328-329
Eye(s)
anterior segment of, 329-330, 330*f*
disease in. *see also* Ocular disorders
differential diagnosis of, 332*t*-333*t*, 333*b*
management of, 334*t*
signs and symptoms of, 331-335, 335*t*
evaluation of, 326-335
history of, 326-327
physical examination in, 327-331
screening recommendations for, 326
irrigation in, 345, 345*b*
movement, pain on, 335*t*
pain in, 334-335, 335*t*
posterior segment of, 330-331
reactive arthritis and, 1156
red, 331, 332*t*-333*t*
Eye opening, Glasgow Coma Scale, 219*t*
Eye wall, 356*t*
Eyelid disorders, 338*b*, 339*t*
Eyelid lesions, 332*t*-333*t*
Ezetimibe (Zetia), 1124*t*-1125*t*

F

Face
acromegaly and, 1072
pain in, 1064
Facet joint pain, 971
Facial nerve (CN VII), 393, 1008
Facilitatory techniques, for dysphagia, 668*t*-669*t*
Factor V Leiden, 1304
Failure to thrive (FTT)
causes of, 92*b*
clinical presentation of, 92
definition of, 91-93
management of, 92-93
pathophysiology of, 92
physical examination and diagnostics for, 92
Falls
in the elderly
clinical presentation of, 90
complications of, 91
Falls *(Continued)*
definition and etiology of, 89-90
diagnostics for, 90
management of, 90-91
pathophysiology of, 90
prevention of, 91*b*
risk for, 91*f*
prevention of, 967*b*
risk management, 51-52, 52*b*
Famciclovir, 789*b*
for herpes simplex virus, 271, 271*t*
Family history
genetic considerations in, 32-38
collection guidelines for, 35*b*
gathering, 34-36
interpreting, 36, 39*t*
tools, of genetic information, 39*t*
Family planning, natural, 836-837
Fanconi syndrome, 1286
Fat embolism syndrome, 997
Fatigue, 1189-1196
with brain tumor, 1069
chronic, 1190
clinical presentation of, 1190-1191
complications of, 1195-1196
definition and epidemiology of, 1189-1190
diagnostic criteria for, 1193*b*
diagnostics for, 1191-1192, 1192*b*
differential diagnosis for, 1192-1193, 1194*b*
indications for referral or hospitalization for, 1196
inflammatory, 1192-1193
life span considerations with, 1196
with lymphomas, 1320
management of, 1193-1195, 1195*t*
multiple sclerosis and, 1046*t*-1047*t*
with myelodysplastic syndromes, 1324
with Parkinson disease, 1054
pathophysiology of, 1190
physical examination for, 1191
prolonged, 1192
with systemic lupus erythematosus, 1171
Fats, dietary
reducing energy intake and, 118
types of, 1121
very-low-fat diet, 1123
Fatty diarrhea, 648
Fear
clinical presentation and physical examination of, 98
definition and epidemiology of, 98
diagnostics for, 98
differential diagnosis of, 98
in elderly, 98-99
of hastening death, 107
indications for referral or hospitalization, 98
management, 98
in palliative care, 98-99
pathophysiology of, 98
Febrile neutropenia, 1326
Febuxostat, for gout, 931
Fecal electrolyte composition, 648*f*
Fecal marker tests, for chronic diarrhea, 652
Felbamate (Felbatol), 1061*t*-1062*t*
Felodipine, 576*t*-582*t*
Femoral aneurysms, 605
Femoral arteries, obstruction of, 600
Femoral nerve stretch test, 955
Femoral veins, deep vein thrombosis of, 606
Femoroacetabular impingement (FAI) syndrome, 937
Fenofibrate (Tricor), 1124*t*-1125*t*
Ferriman-Gallwey scoring system, 1099, 1099*f*
Ferritin, 1279
Fertility control, 831-837. *see also* Contraception
definition and epidemiology of, 831
Fesoterodine (Toviaz), 735
Fetor hepaticus, 640
Fever, 1196-1200, 1197*b*
addiction-related causes of, 1374
definition and epidemiology of, 1196-1197
evaluation of, 1197-1199
indications for referral or hospitalization for, 1200

Fever *(Continued)*
in infective endocarditis, 587
life span considerations with, 1199
management of, 1199-1200
pattern, 1197, 1197*t*
with systemic lupus erythematosus, 1175
of unknown origin
diagnostic evaluation of, 1199
evaluation of, 1199
without clear cause
diagnostic for, 1198-1199
evaluation of, 1197-1198
Fiber, dietary, 645-646, 658, 703
Fibric acids, 1124*t*-1125*t*, 1125
Fibrin, 1298
Fibrinolytics, for pulmonary embolism, 495
Fibrocystic breast, 815
Fibromyalgia
chest pain and, 448
fatigue and, 1192
Fibromyalgia syndrome (FMS), 924-927
alternative therapies for, 927
clinical presentation of, 925
complications of, 927
definition and epidemiology of, 924, 924*f*, 925*b*
diagnostics for, 926
differential diagnosis of, 926, 926*b*
indications for referral or hospitalization for, 927
management of, 926-927
multidisciplinary approach of, 927
pathophysiology of, 924-925
pharmacology of, 926, 926*t*
physical examination for, 925-926
Fibrosis, 639
Filariasis, 765
Finasteride, 254, 735, 1103
Fine-needle aspiration (FNA) biopsy, 1206-1207, 1317-1318
of thyroid gland, 1137, 1140
Fine-needle aspiration cytology (FNAC), of salivary gland, 401
Fingertip unit (FTU), definition of, 243
Fingolimod (Gilenya), 1048-1049
Fire ant, 197*t*
First-degree burns, 260, 319*b*
Fissure, 238*f*
Fist injuries, closed, cellulitis and, 265
Fistulas, bowel to bowel, 692
Fitz-Hugh-Curtis Syndrome (FHCS), 872
Fitzpatrick sign, 239-240
Five wishes, 96, 96*b*
Fixed drug reactions, 274*t*
Flaviviridae, 1271-1272, 1275
Fleas, 197*t*
Flexibility exercises, for neck pain, 974
Flexor retinaculum, 934*f*
Flies, 197*t*
Floaters, in eyes, 331, 333
Flomax, 735
Fluconazole, 281*t*, 291
Fludrocortisone acetate (Florinef), for hyperkalemia, 1111
Fluid deprivation or excess, 88*b*. *see also* Hypernatremia; Hyponatremia
Flumazenil for benzodiazepines, 226
Fluocinolone acetonide, 244*t*
Fluocinonide, 244*t*
Fluorescein, 346-347, 349*f*
Fluorine 18 (^{18}F) fluorodeoxyglucose positron emission tomography (^{18}F-FDG-PET), of thyroid gland, 1137, 1139-1140
Fluoroquinolones, 781
Fluoxetine, 926*t*, 1360*t*-1362*t*
Flutamide, 1103
Fluticasone propionate, 244*t*, 462*t*-463*t*
Fluvastatin (Lescol), 1124*t*-1125*t*
Fluvoxamine, 1360*t*-1362*t*
Folate deficiency, 1287-1290
definition and epidemiology of, 1287
pathophysiology of, 1287-1288
Folic acid
antagonist, for ectopic pregnancy, 830
supplementation, 149*t*-152*t*
Follicle-stimulating hormone (FSH), 800, 850, 1097
Folstein Mini-Mental State Examination (MMSE), 1021-1022
Fondaparinux, 607
for pulmonary embolism, 495
Fontaine classification, for peripheral arterial insufficiency, 601
Food allergies, 216-218
definition and epidemiology of, 216-217
diagnostics for, 217
differential diagnoses of, 217, 217*b*
management and patient and family education, 217-218
pathophysiology of, 217
Food poisoning, 1249-1250
Food-or drink-related rhinitis, 389
Foods
anaphylaxis-inducing, 194*b*
for diet, 1129
quality, obesity and, 114
Foot (feet)
fractures of, 995
pain in, 897-903, 902*b*, 903*t*-905*t*
Foot care, for patients, with diabetes, 317*b*
Forced expiratory time, and COPD, 459
Forced expiratory volume (FEV_1), 428
Forced vital capacity (FVC), 428, 459
Forefoot tracing, 602
Foreign bodies
intraocular, 355
in ocular pain, 335*t*
ocular surface, 343-345
clinical presentation of, 343
complications of, 345
definition and epidemiology of, 343, 343*f*
diagnostics for, 344, 344*b*, 344*f*
differential diagnosis of, 344, 344*b*
management of, 344-345, 345*b*
pathophysiology of, 343
physical examination for, 343-344
prevention of, 345
referral for, indications for, 345, 345*b*
Formoterol, 441, 462*t*-463*t*
Fosfomycin tromethamine, 779*t*, 781*t*
Fosinopril, 576*t*-582*t*
Fractionation, 1327
Fracture Risk Assessment Tool (FRAX), WHO, 960
Fractures, 994-998. *see also* specific bones and joints
clinical presentation of, 994
complications of, 996-997
definition and epidemiology of, 994
delayed union of, 997
diagnostics for, 995, 995*b*
differential diagnosis for, 995, 995*b*
indications for referral or hospitalization for, 997
life span considerations with, 997
malunion of, 997
management of, 995-996
nasal, 383
nonunion of, 997
osteoporosis and, 965
pathophysiology of, 994
physical examination for, 994
stress, 994
vertebral compression, 961-962
Frailty, 91-93, 1218, 1221
Framing the question, intimate partner violence and, 144
Framingham risk score, 509-510
Freeze time, in cryosurgery, 240
Freezing phenomenon, 1051
Friction rub, 542
Frostbite, 235
Functional or transient incontinence, 732, 733*b*, 735
Functional status, tools for, 84
Fungal infections
with COPD, 466
superficial, 279-284
candidiasis in, 283-284, 283*b*, 283*f*
dermatophyte infections in, 279-282, 279*f*-280*f*, 280*b*, 281*t*
tinea versicolor in, 282, 282*b*
Furosemide, 576*t*-582*t*, 1334
Furuncles, 262
Fusobacterium species, 398

G

G6PD deficiency, 1295
Gabapentin, 926*t*, 1033, 1059, 1061*t*-1062*t*, 1065*t*
for low back pain, 958
for menopause, 865
Gadolinium, 512
Galactorrhea, 811-813
clinical presentation of, 811
definition and epidemiology of, 811
diagnostics for, 811-812, 811*b*
differential diagnosis of, 812, 812*b*
indications for referral or hospitalization for, 813
life span considerations with, 813
management of, 812-813
pathophysiology of, 811
physical examination for, 811
Galantamine (Razadyne), 1023
Gallbladder disease, 635
during pregnancy, 78
Gallium nitrate, 969
Galvanic electrolysis, 1102
Gamete intrafallopian transfer (GIFT), 849
Gamma Knife radiosurgery, 1328
Ganglion cyst
clinical presentation of, 933
diagnostics and differential diagnosis for, 934
management of, 935
physical examination for, 933
Gardasil, 845, 870
Gastric emptying scans, 672
Gastritis, bleeding and, 678
Gastroenteritis, acute, 1246-1247
Gastroesophageal reflux disease (GERD), 669-677
asthma and, 422-423
chest pain and, 548*t*
with chronic cough, 455
management of, 456
clinical presentation of, 671-672
complications of, 676
definition and epidemiology of, 669-670
diagnostics for, 672-673, 673*b*
differential diagnosis for, 673-674, 673*b*
indications for referral or hospitalization for, 677
life span considerations with, 677
management of, 674-676, 674*f*
acid suppression therapies in, 675
endoscopic therapies in, 675
lifestyle modifications in, 674, 674*b*
surgery in, 675-676
pathophysiology of, 670-671
physical examination for, 672
in pregnancy, 72
presurgical clearance and, 183
proton pump inhibitors for, 447
Gastrointestinal bleeding, prevention of, 642*b*
Gastrointestinal disorders. *see also specific disorders*
osteoporosis and, 963*b*
Gastrointestinal disturbances
clinical presentation of, 1342
complications of, 1345
diagnostics for, 1342-1343, 1343*b*
differential diagnosis of, 1343, 1343*b*
management of, 1343-1345
pathophysiology of, 1341-1342
physical examination for, 1342, 1343*b*
Gastrointestinal hemorrhage, 677-682
clinical presentation of, 678
complications of, 682
definition and epidemiology of, 677-678, 677*b*
diagnostics for, 679, 679*b*
differential diagnosis for, 679-680, 680*b*
indications for referral or hospitalization for, 682
life span considerations with, 682
management of, 680-682
interdisciplinary, 682
pathophysiology of, 678
physical examination for, 678-679
Gastrointestinal tract, tumors of, 722-727
colon, 726-727
esophagus, 722-723
small intestine, 725-726, 725*b*-726*b*
stomach, 723-724, 724*b*

Gay and Lesbian Medical Association (GLMA), 61
Gels, 244, 244*t*
Gemfibrozil (Lopid), 1124*t*-1125*t*
Gender
  abdominal aortic aneurysm and, 510-511
  coronary artery disease and, 553-554
  grief and, 1355
Gender expression, 60
Gender role conformity, 60
Gene therapy, 1203
General cognitive screening instruments, 1000*b*
General Practitioner Assessment of Cognition (GPCOG), 1021-1022
Generalized anxiety disorder (GAD), 1350
Generalized convulsive status epilepticus (GCSE), 1058
Genes, cervical cancer-related, 868
GENES acronym, 36
Genetic alliance, 42
Genetic Information Nondiscrimination Act (GINA), 31, 38-42
  overview of, 41*t*
Genetic/inherited disorders. *see also specific disorders*
  primary care and, 30-42
Genetics
  hypertension and, 571
  obesity and, 111-112
  testing used in, 30, 692-693, 806-807
    for cancer patients, 1325
    direct-to-consumer, 41-42
    screening and, 155
Genital herpes, 272, 785*t*-788*t*, 789*b*, 792-793
Genital tract cancers, 837-845
  cervical, 843-845
    clinical presentation and physical examination of, 844
    definition and epidemiology of, 843-844
    diagnostics and differential diagnosis for, 844, 844*b*
    indications for referral or hospitalization for, 844-845
    life span considerations with, 845
    management of, 844-845
    pathophysiology of, 844
  endometrial, 837-839
    clinical presentation and physical examination of, 838-839
    definition and epidemiology of, 837-838
    diagnostics and differential diagnosis for, 839, 839*b*
    indications for referral or hospitalization for, 839
    life span considerations with, 839
    management of, 839
    pathophysiology of, 838
    types of, 838
  ovarian, 839-841
    clinical presentation and physical examination of, 840
    definition and epidemiology of, 839
    diagnostics and differential diagnosis for, 840-841, 840*b*-841*b*
    indications for referral or hospitalization for, 841
    life span considerations with, 841
    management of, 841
    pathophysiology of, 839-840
  vaginal, 842-843, 843*b*
  vulvar, 841-842
    clinical presentation and physical examination of, 842
    definition and epidemiology of, 841
    diagnostics and differential diagnosis for, 842, 842*b*
    indications for referral or hospitalization for, 842
    life span considerations with, 842
    management of, 842
    pathophysiology of, 841-842
    types of, 841
Genital ulcers, 791-794
Genital warts. *see* Condylomata acuminata
Genitourinary examination, for preparticipation sports physical, 186
Genitourinary syndrome, of menopause, 855
Genitourinary tract disorders. *see also specific disorders*
  with diabetes mellitus, 1093
  infections in. *see* Urinary tract infections (UTIs)
  obstructions and tumors, 794-798
    clinical presentation of, 795
    complications of, 798*b*
    diagnostics for, 796*b*
    differential diagnosis of, 797*b*
Genome-wide association study (GWAS) data, 42
Genomics, 30. *see also* Genetics
Gentamicin, 874*b*
  for endocarditis, 591*t*-595*t*
Gerdy's tubercle, 917*f*
Geriatric Depression Scale, 1021-1022
Geriatric patients, cerebrovascular events in, 1015
Gestational diabetes mellitus (GDM), 76, 1086, 1086*b*
  screening for, 149*t*-152*t*
Giant cell arteritis, 1159-1164
  classification criteria of, 1162, 1162*t*
  clinical presentation of, 1162
  considerations for referral or hospitalization for, 1163-1164
  diagnostics for, 1162-1163
  differential diagnosis for, 1163
  epidemiology of, 1161-1162
  life span considerations with, 1163
  management of, 1163
    complications of, 1163
    monitoring treatment in, 1163
  pathophysiology of, 1162
  physical examination for, 1162
  polymyalgia rheumatica and, 1161
  in vasculitis, 1177
Giardia lamblia infection, 179
Gila monsters, 200
GINA. *see* Genetic Information Nondiscrimination Act (GINA)
Gingivitis, 407-409
Ginkgo biloba, for Raynaud phenomenon, 1165
Glargine, 1082
Glasgow Coma Scale (GCS), 219, 219*t*, 225
Glaucoma, 332*t*-334*t*
Gleason system, 736
Glenohumeral joint. *see* Shoulder joint
Glimepiride (Amaryl), 1084
Gliomas, 1066
Glipizide (Glucotrol), 1084
Global Initiative for Asthma (GINA), 424-426, 430
Global Initiative for Chronic Obstructive Lung Disease (GOLD) spirometry grading system, 459
Globus, 665
Glomerular filtration rate (GFR), 749, 1091-1092
Glomerular hematuria, 748
Glossopharyngeal nerve (CN IX), 393
Glucocorticoids, 1035*t*-1036*t*, 1074
  acne and, 250*b*
  for ankylosing spondylitis, 1155
  deficiency, 1119
  osteoporosis and, 960
  for rheumatoid arthritis, 1169
Glucophage (metformin), 1084
Glucosamine, with or without chondroitin, for osteoarthritis, 979
Glucose intolerance, 1087
  alternative therapy for, 16-17
Glucose tests. *see* Blood glucose monitoring
α-Glucosidase inhibitors, 1084
Glutamate, 1377
Gluten-sensitive enteropathy, 653
Glyburide, 1084
Glycemic control, 1080*t*
Goiter (simple, nontoxic), 1137-1139
  clinical presentation of, 1138
  complications of, 1139
  definition and epidemiology of, 1137
  diagnostics for, 1138, 1138*b*
  differential diagnosis for, 1138, 1138*b*
  indications for referral or hospitalization for, 1139
  life span considerations with, 1139
  management of, 1138-1139
Goiter (simple, nontoxic) *(Continued)*
  pathophysiology of, 1137-1138
  physical examination for, 1138
Golfer's elbow, 922
Gonococcal arthritis, 941-942, 944-945
Gonococcal conjunctivitis, 341, 341*f*
Gonococci, causing PID, 872
Gonorrhea
  clinical presentation of, 790
  complications of, 790
  definition and epidemiology of, 782, 784-790
  diagnostics for, 790
  management of, 785*t*-788*t*
  pathophysiology of, 790
  screening for, 149*t*-152*t*
  test for, 146*t*-147*t*
  treatment of, 789*b*
Gout, 928-932
  acute, treatment of, 930, 930*b*
  chronic, treatment of, 930-931, 931*b*
  clinical presentation of, 928-929
  complications of, 931
  definition of, 928
  diagnostics for, 929
  differential diagnosis of, 929, 929*b*
  epidemiology of, 928
  indications for referral or hospitalization for, 932
  management of, 929-931
    nonpharmacologic, 929-930
    pharmacologic, 930-931, 930*b*-931*b*
    prophylaxis in, 931
  pathophysiology of, 928
Gram stain, 239*b*
  infectious arthritis and, 944
Granuloma inguinale, 793
Granulomatosis with polyangiitis (GPA), 396-397
  clinical presentation of, 396
  complications of, 397
  defined, 396
  diagnostics for, 396-397, 397*b*
  differential diagnosis of, 397, 397*b*
  management and indications for referral or hospitalization for, 397
  pathophysiology of, 396
  physical examination for, 396
  in vasculitis, 1178
Graves disease, 1141-1142
  clinical presentation and physical examination for, 1142
  diagnostics for, 1143
  management of, 1143-1144
  pathophysiology of, 1142
Gravidity and parity, 68
Greater tuberosity, of humerus, 985
Grey Turner sign, 715
Grief and bereavement, 1355-1356, 1356*t*
Griseofulvin, 281*t*
Group A β-hemolytic *Streptococcus* (GAS), 413-414
Group B *Streptococcus*, 585
  in pregnancy, 72
Growth hormone (GH), 1071
Growth hormone-releasing hormone (GHRH), 1071
Guidelines for Adolescent Preventive Services (GAPS), 56
Guillain-Barré syndrome (GBS), 1028-1030, 1273, 1274*t*
  clinical presentation of, 1028-1029
  complications of, 1030
  definition and epidemiology of, 1028
  diagnostics for, 1029
  differential diagnosis for, 1029
  indications for referral or hospitalization for, 1030
  life span considerations with, 1030
  management of, 1029-1030
  mimics of, 1029*t*
  pathophysiology of, 1028
  physical examination for, 1029
Gut microbiota, 114
Guttate psoriasis, 302, 304
Gynecomastia, 816-817

H

H_1/ H_2 antagonists, 196
H_1 receptor antagonists, 313, 313*t*

H1N1 flu virus, 190-191
H_2 receptor antagonists, 313, 313*t*
HAECK organisms, 585, 591*t*-595*t*
Haemophilus ducreyi, 785*t*-788*t*
Haemophilus influenzae
acute bronchitis and, 417
conjunctivitis and, 341-342
in eyes, 351
meningitis and, 1037
osteomyelitis and, 981
pneumonia and, 487
type B (Hib), 403
Hair breakage, alopecia and, 254*t*
Hair growth pattern, 1099, 1099*f*
Hair loss, 1102-1103
Haiti, cholera outbreak, 1227
Halcinonide, 244*t*
Hallpike-Dix maneuver, 1025*b*, 1027
Hallucinations, with Parkinson disease, 1053
Hallucinogens, 1373
Hallux flexus (hammertoe or claw toe), 903*t*-905*t*
Hallux rigidus, 903*t*-905*t*
Hallux valgus/varus, 903*t*-905*t*
Halobetasol propionate, 244*t*
Hammertoe, 903*t*-905*t*
Hand, skin and soft tissue infections in, 265
Hand and wrist pain, 932-936
clinical presentation of, 932-933
complications of, 935
definition and epidemiology of, 932
diagnostics and differential diagnosis for, 934, 934*b*
indications for referral or hospitalization for, 935
life span considerations with, 935
management of, 935, 935*b*
pathophysiology of, 932
physical examination for, 933-934, 934*f*
Hand expression, 83
Hand-foot-and-mouth disease, 408
Hantavirus pulmonary syndrome (HPS), 488
Hard corn, 268
Hasenclever Index, 1315-1316
Hawkin test, 988*t*
Hazards, in workplace, 165
HBOC. *see* Hereditary breast and ovarian cancer (HBOC) syndrome
Head trauma, 218-221
clinical presentation of, 219
definition and epidemiology of, 218-219
diagnostics for, 220
differential diagnosis of, 220, 220*b*
disposition and referral for, 220-221
initial stabilization and management of, 220
minor, 220
pathophysiology of, 219
physical examination for, 219-220
Headache, 1030-1037
abortive therapy for, 1033-1035, 1035*t*-1036*t*
clinical presentation of, 1031
cluster, 1031
complications of, 1036-1037
definition and epidemiology of, 1030-1031
diagnostics for, 1032, 1032*b*
differential diagnosis for, 1032, 1033*b*
giant cell arteritis and, 1162
indications for referral or hospitalization for, 1037
life span considerations with, 1035-1036
management of, 1032-1035
nonpharmacologic, 1033
pharmacologic, 1033-1035
migraine. *see* Migraine headache
pathophysiology of, 1031
physical examination for, 1031-1032
preventive therapy for, 1033
primary and secondary, 1030
tension-type, 1031
Health administration, 170
Health care
barriers, 142
delivery, 3
disparities, 29
integrated for women, 78
outcomes, 27-28
Health care personnel
against influenza, practical resources for vaccinating, 163
vaccine recommendations for, 160-163
Health care providers
barriers, identification and treatment of, 142
for unplanned pregnancy, 881
Health care-associated endocarditis, 586
Health Information Technology for Economic and Clinical Health (HITECH) Act, 44-45
Health insurance, protection under GINA (legislation), 41*t*
Health literacy, 3-4, 27
assessment, 28-29
components, 28
and health care outcomes, 27-28
impact, measures to reduce, 29*b*
interventions, 29
low, risks associated with, 28*b*
resources, 29*b*
Health promotion
for abdominal aortic aneurysm, 515
for acne, 252
for acromegaly, 1073-1074
for acute arterial insufficiency, 605
for acute pancreatitis, 717
in adolescent issues, 58-59
for adrenal gland disorders, 1077
for amenorrhea, 803
for anaphylaxis, 196
for animal and human bites, 257-258
for anorexia nervosa, 97-98
for anxiety, 99
for anxiety disorders, 1354
for atopic dermatitis, 279
for auricular disorders, 360
for Bell palsy, 1010
for bowel construction, 106
for burns, 261
for cachexia, 97-98
for cataracts, 337
for cellulitis, 265-266
for central nervous system infections, 1040
for cerebrovascular events, 1015-1016
for cerumen impaction, 362
for chest pain, 451
for chlamydia, 791
for chronic pain, 1189
for chronic pelvic pain, 821
for chronic rhinosinusitis, 380
for cold injury, 236
for colon tumors, 727
for conjunctivitis, 343
for constipation, 106
for corns and calluses, 269
for coronary artery disease, 554
for cutaneous herpes, 272
for deep venous thrombosis, 608
for delirium, 100
for dental abscess, 399
for depression, 101
for dermatitis medicamentosa, 275
for diabetes mellitus, 1096
for diverticulosis, 659-660
for dizziness and vertigo, 1027
for dry eye, 348-349
for dry skin, 277
for dyspareunia, 827
for dysphagia, 669
for dyspnea, 103, 471
for epiglottitis, 406
for epistaxis, 382
for esophagus tumors, 723
for eyelid disorders, 339
for fatigue, 1196
for fear, 99
for fibromyalgia syndrome, 927
for gastrointestinal hemorrhage, 682
for genital herpes, 793
for GERD, 677
for Guillain-Barré syndrome, 1030
for hand and wrist pain, 935-936
for headache, 1037
for hearing loss, 367
for heart failure, 569
Health promotion *(Continued)*
for heat-related illness, 235
for hemolytic anemia, 1290
for hepatitis, 692
for herpetic whitlow, 292
for hip pain, 940
for hirsutism, 1103-1104
for HIV infection, 1240-1241
for hyperkalemia and hypokalemia, 1112
for hypertension, 584
for immunodeficiency, 1204
for infective endocarditis, 597
for inflammatory bowel disease, 699
for influenza, 1243
for intertrigo, 291
for intracranial tumors, 1069-1070
for iron deficiency anemia, 1283-1284
for irritable bowel syndrome, 705
for leukemias, 1311-1312, 1312*b*-1313*b*
in LGBTQ patient care, 65
in lifestyle management, 145
for low back pain, 959
for lung cancer, 479
for lymphadenopathy, 1209
for major depressive disorder, 1364
for megaloblastic anemia, 1290
for metabolic syndrome, 1131
for movement disorders, 1042
for mumps, 411
for nausea and vomiting, 105, 713
for neck pain, 976
for noninfectious diarrhea, 657
for obesity, 125
for obstructive uropathies, 798
for onychomycosis, 296
for oral infections, 409
for orbital cellulitis, 353
for osteoarthritis (OA), 980
for otitis externa, 372-373
for otitis media, 376-377
for Paget disease of bone, 970
for pain, 107
for Pap test abnormalities, 871
for parathyroid gland disorders, 1135
for paronychial infections, 294
for parotitis, 411
for peripheral arterial insufficiency, 604
for peritonsillar abscess, 413
for pharyngitis, 416
for pinguecula, 355
for pneumonia, 491
for preseptal cellulitis, 353
in presurgical clearance, 184-185
for prostate cancer, 738
for pruritus, 301
for psoriasis, 304
for pterygium, 355
for pulmonary hypertension, 500
for purpura, 307
for salivary gland diseases, 403
for schizophrenia, 1381
for seizure disorder, 1063
for sexual assault, 230
for sexual dysfunction
female, 879
male, 763
for sexually transmitted infections, 793-794
for sickle cell disease, 1293
for sinusitis, 392
for skin cancer, 248
for sleep-related movement disorders, 1217
for small intestine tumors, 726
for smell and taste disturbances, 394
for sprains, strains, and fractures, 997-998
for stasis dermatitis, 311
for stomach tumors, 724
for testicular disorders, 771
for thalassemia, 1287
for traumatic ocular disorders, 358
for trigeminal neuralgia, 1066
for unintended weight loss, 1223-1224
for urinary calculi, 777
for urticaria, 314
for West Nile virus, 1276-1277
in workplace, 164

Health promotion *(Continued)*
in wound management, 325
for xerostomia, 103
Health screening, 85, 85*t*
immunizations of, 155-163
issues with, 64
routine, 145-155
tests for men, 148*t*
tests for women, 146*t*-147*t*
Health-related quality of life (HRQL), 502
Healthy diet and physical activity counseling, screening for, 149*t*-152*t*
Healthy People 2010, LGBTQ patient care and, 60
Healthy People 2020, LGBTQ patient care and, 60
Healthy People initiative, 126
Hearing loss
associated with cerumen impaction, 361
clinical presentation and physical examination for, 365
complications of, 366
definition and epidemiology of, 364
diagnostics for, 365
differential diagnosis of, 365-366, 366*b*
indications for referral or hospitalization for, 366
life span considerations with, 366
management of, 366
pathophysiology of, 364-365
screening for, 149*t*-152*t*
Heart blocks, 528
Heart failure, 554-569
ACC/AHA classifications of, as guide to therapy, 563-564
advanced therapies for, 567
anxiety and, 563
asthma and upper respiratory tract infection and, 563
cardiac conditions, 562
and chronic pulmonary conditions, 562-563
classification of, 558, 561*t*
clinical presentation and physical examination for, 558, 558*b*
clinics for, 568
compensatory mechanisms in, 557-558
definition and epidemiology of, 554-556
diagnostics for, 558-563
differential diagnosis of, 562, 562*b*
emerging evidence for, 569
etiology of, 555-556
exercise or stress testing for, 562
indications for referral or hospitalization for, 568
laboratory evaluation of, 561, 562*t*
life span considerations with, 568-569
management of, 563-568
and neuromuscular disorders, 563
nonpharmacologic therapy for, 567-568
pathophysiology of, 556-558
pharmacologic therapy for, 564-567, 566*t*
pleural effusions and, 563
with preserved ejection fraction, 557
pulmonary embolism and, 563
readmission rates in, 568
recurrent acute decompensated, 557-558
with reduced ejection fraction, 556-557
revascularization for, 567
risk factors in, 556
signs of, 560*t*
symptoms of, 559*t*
types of, 554-555, 555*t*
Heart health, dietary influences on, 131
Heart murmurs. *see* Cardiac murmurs
Heart rate (pulse), exercise levels for, 131
Heart sound. *see* Cardiac murmurs
Heartburn, 671
Heat damage, 211
Heat stroke, 1197, 1197*b*
Heat therapy
for chronic pain, 1188*t*
superficial, for low back pain, 957
Heat-related illness, 233-235
clinical presentation of, 233-234
complications of, 234-235
definition and epidemiology of, 233
diagnostics for, 234, 234*b*
differential diagnosis of, 234, 234*b*
Heat-related illness *(Continued)*
indications for referral or hospitalization for, 235
life span considerations with, 235
management of, 234
pathophysiology of, 233
physical examination for, 234
Hedonic pathway, 110
Heel (calcaneal) bursitis, 919-920
clinical presentation and physical examination of, 919
complications of, 920
definition and epidemiology of, 919
differential diagnosis of, 919, 919*b*
indications for referral or hospitalization for, 920
life span considerations with, 920
management of, 920
Helicobacter pylori, 312, 626-627, 672, 678, 728-730, 729*t*
Hematemesis, 472, 678
Hematocele, 764-767, 770
Hematochezia, 678, 682
Hematologic disorders. *see also specific disorders*
osteoporosis and, 963*b*
in pruritus, 300*b*
with systemic lupus erythematosus, 1171*b*
Hematopoietic stem cell transplantation (HSCT), 1309-1310
Hematuria, 747-749
clinical presentation of, 747
common causes of, 747*b*
complications of, 749
definition and epidemiology of, 747
diagnostics and differential diagnosis of, 747-748, 748*b*-749*b*, 748*f*
indications for referral or hospitalization for, 749
management of, 749
pathophysiology of, 747
physical examination for, 747
Hemiblocks, 524
Hemochromatosis, 689
Hemodynamics, altered, in heart failure, 560*t*
Hemoglobin A_{1c} (HbA_{1c}), 128-129
chronic diarrhea and, 652
in diabetes mellitus, 1079-1080
targets for, 1080*t*
Hemoglobin defect, 1290
Hemoglobin E, 1285
Hemoglobin SS, 1290
Hemoglobinopathies, screening for, 149*t*-152*t*
Hemolytic anemias, 1279
Hemolytic jaundice, 706
Hemophilia treatment centers (HTCs), 1301
Hemoptysis, 456, 468-469, 471-474
clinical presentation of, 472
complications of, 474
definition and epidemiology of, 471-472
diagnostics for, 472-473, 473*b*
differential diagnosis for, 473, 473*b*
history and, 472
indications for referral or hospitalization for, 474
management of, 473-474
pathophysiology of, 472
physical examination for, 472
Hemorrhage. *see* Bleeding/hemorrhage
Hemorrhagic stroke, 1011
Hemorrhoids, 630-632
clinical presentation of, 630-631
complications of, 632
definition and epidemiology of, 630
diagnostics for, 631, 631*b*
differential diagnosis of, 631, 631*b*
indications for referral or hospitalization for, 632
internal, 630-631
life span considerations with, 631-632
management of, 631, 632*t*
pathophysiology of, 630
physical examination for, 631
in pregnancy, 72-73
thrombosed external, 631
Hemostatic response, 1298
Hemozoin, 1258
Henoch-Schönlein purpura (HSP), 1178
Heparin, 1305
in acute MI, 549
for deep venous thrombosis, 607
Hepatic encephalopathy, 643
Hepatic failure, management of, 643*b*
Hepatic jaundice, 705
Hepatitis, 683-692
alcoholic, 685-687
autoimmune, 686
chronic, 689-691
clinical presentation of, 687-688, 687*b*
complications of, 690-691
definition and epidemiology of, 683-686
diagnostics for, 688-689, 689*b*
differential diagnosis of, 689, 689*b*
drug-induced, 688
indications for referral or hospitalization for, 691
life span considerations with, 690
management of, 689-690
pathogenesis of, 686-687
physical examination for, 688
signs and symptoms of, 687*b*
viral, 683-685
features of, 683*t*
five main groups of, 683
high-risk groups for, 684*b*
Hepatitis A vaccine, 156-157, 161*t*-162*t*
Hepatitis A virus (HAV), 1253
definition and epidemiology of, 683
diagnostics for, 688
features of, 683*t*
pathogenesis of, 686-687
signs and symptoms of, 687*b*
Hepatitis B vaccine, 157, 160, 161*t*-162*t*
Hepatitis B virus (HBV)
definition and epidemiology of, 683
diagnostics for, 688
features of, 683*t*
HIV infection and, 1238-1239
pathogenesis of, 687
screening for, 149*t*-152*t*
signs and symptoms of, 687*b*
Hepatitis C virus (HCV)
diagnostics for, 688
features of, 683, 683*t*, 685
HIV infection and, 1238-1239
pathogenesis of, 687
screening for, 149*t*-152*t*
signs and symptoms of, 687*b*
Hepatitis D virus (HDV)
diagnostics for, 688
features of, 683*t*, 685
pathogenesis of, 687
signs and symptoms of, 687*b*
Hepatitis E virus (HEV)
diagnostics for, 688
features of, 683*t*, 685
pathogenesis of, 686-687
signs and symptoms of, 687*b*
Hepatobiliary disorders, in pruritus, 300*b*
Hepatocellular injury, 640
Hepatomegaly, in heart failure, 560*t*
Hepatorenal syndrome (HRS), 643
Hepatotoxic drugs, 642*b*
Hepcidin, 1293
Herbal therapies, for sexual dysfunction of female, 879
Herbs, for osteoarthritis, 979
Hereditary breast and ovarian cancer (HBOC) syndrome, 32
Hereditary hemorrhagic telangiectasia (HHT), 471-472
Hernia, scrotal-inguinal, 765, 767-768, 770
Herpes labialis, 271, 406-407
Herpes simplex virus (HSV), 269, 785*t*-788*t*
Bell palsy and, 1008
clinical presentation of, 270
complications of, 272
conjunctivitis and, 340
diagnostics for, 270-271
differential diagnosis of, 271
encephalitis and, 1039
frequent recurrences in, suppression of, 272
medications for, 271*t*
pathophysiology of, 270
physical examination for, 270, 270*f*
primary genital herpes, 272, 785*t*-788*t*
primary herpes labialis, 271

Herpes simplex virus (HSV) *(Continued)*
recurrent genital herpes, 272
recurrent herpes labialis, 271-272
types I and II, of oral infections, 406
Herpes zoster (shingles), 284-286
chest pain and, 448, 548*t*
clinical presentation and physical examination for, 284
complications of, 285
definition and epidemiology of, 284
diagnostics for, 284-285, 285*b*
differential diagnosis of, 285, 285*b*
indications for referral or hospitalization for, 286
life span considerations with, 285-286
management of, 285
ophthalmic zoster, 285*f*
pathophysiology of, 284
vaccine for, 157
Herpesvirus, culture for, 239*b*
Herpetic whitlow, 292, 292*b*
Hidradenitis suppurativa, 286-288
clinical presentation of, 286-287, 286*f*
complications of, 288
definition and epidemiology of, 286
diagnostics for, 287, 287*b*
differential diagnosis of, 287, 287*b*
indications for referral or hospitalization for, 288
life span considerations with, 288
management of, 287-288
pathophysiology of, 286
physical examination for, 287, 287*b*
High-density lipoproteins (HDLs), 1120
classification of, 128*t*
defined, 127-128
routine screening of, 148
High-efficiency particulate air (HEPA) filters, 216
High-grade malignant sarcomas, 911
Highly active antiretroviral therapy (HAART), 1237
Hilar or mediastinal nodes, 1208
Hip bursitis, 917-918
clinical presentation and physical examination for, 917
definition and epidemiology of, 917, 918*t*
differential diagnosis of, 917, 918*b*
management of, 918
Hip circumference, 1128
Hip joint
fractures and dislocations of, 937
pain in, 936-940
causes of, 936*t*
clinical presentation of, 937-938
complications of, 940
definition and epidemiology of, 936
diagnostics for, 938-939, 938*b*
differential diagnosis for, 939, 939*b*
indications for referral or hospitalization for, 940
management of, 939-940
pathophysiology of, 936-937
physical examination for, 938
Hip protector pads, 964
Hirschberg test, 328
Hirsutism, 1096-1104
clinical presentation of, 1098
complications of, 1103
definition and epidemiology of, 1096-1097
diagnostics for, 1099-1101, 1101*b*
differential diagnosis for, 1101-1102, 1101*b*
indications for referral or hospitalization for, 1103
life span considerations with, 1103
management of, 1102-1103
normoandrogenic, 1101-1102
pathophysiology of, 1097-1098
physical examination for, 1098-1099, 1099*f*
Histamine, in urticaria, 312
Histamine$_2$ receptor antagonists (H_2RAs), 675, 729
History
in bleeding disorders, 1298-1299, 1299*b*
for bone tumors, 908
for nausea and vomiting, 709-710
for STIs, 783*b*
History-taking skills
in angina, 540*b*
for bleeding disorders (coagulopathies), 1299*b*
History-taking skills *(Continued)*
collection guidelines for, 35*b*
with HIV infection, 1234
in pregnancy, 68-69, 68*t*
HIV. *see* Human immunodeficiency virus (HIV)
Hodgkin lymphoma (HL), 1314-1317
classical, 1315
clinical presentation of, 1315
diagnostics for, 1315, 1315*b*
differential diagnosis of, 1315, 1315*b*
management of, 1317
nodular lymphocyte-predominant, 1315
pathophysiology of, 1315
prognosis of, 1315-1317, 1316*f*
relapsing or refractory disease and, 1317
Holter monitor, 518-519
Home safety, 135
Hopelessness, 108
Hordeolum, 332*t*-333*t*, 337-339
clinical presentation of, 337, 338*f*
complications of, 339
definition and epidemiology of, 337
diagnostics for, 338
differential diagnosis of, 338, 338*b*
indications for referral or hospitalization for, 339
life span considerations with, 339
management of, 338-339, 339*t*
pathophysiology of, 337
physical examination for, 337-338, 338*f*
Hormodendrum, 213-214
Hormonal agents, sexual response and, 878*t*
Hormonal changes, seizure control and, 1062
Hormonal contraception, 831-835
Hormone replacement therapy (HRT), 802
in menopause, 861, 862*t*
for osteoporosis, 965
Hormone therapy, for menopause, 861-865, 862*t*
Hormones
amenorrhea and, 799
in dry skin, 276
energy hemostasis and, 111
in menopause, 851
Hornets, 197*t*
Hospital discharge, period after, 3
Household chemicals, 208
Housemaid's knee, 952
HPV vaccine, 871
5-HT (serotonin) receptor antagonists, 712*b*
Humalog, 1082-1083
Human bites, 255-258
clinical presentation of, 256
complications of, 257
definition and epidemiology of, 255
diagnostics for, 256, 256*b*
management of, 256-257
pathophysiology of, 255-256
physical examination for, 256
referral or hospitalization, indications for, 257
risk factors for, 255*b*
Human chorionic gonadotropin (HCG), 828-829
Human granulocytotropic anaplasmosis (HGA), 1259, 1262*t*
Human immunodeficiency virus (HIV)
emerging and reemerging, 1225
infection of, 1232-1241
algorithm for testing of, 1235, 1236*f*
clinical presentation of, 1233-1234
complications in, 1239
definition and epidemiology of, 1232-1233
diagnosis of, 1235-1236
differential diagnosis of, 1237
immediate ED referral for, 1237
indications for referral or hospitalization, 1239-1240
laboratory and testing for, 1236-1237
life span considerations with, 1240
management of, 1237-1239
pathophysiology of, 1233
physical examination for, 1234-1235
physician consultation for, 1237
psoriatic arthritis and, 1157
septic arthritis and, 941
LGBTQ patient care and, 63-64
screening for, 148*t*-152*t*
Human immunodeficiency virus (HIV) *(Continued)*
test for, 146*t*-147*t*
transmission of, 1232
type 1 (HIV-1), 1232
Human metapneumovirus, 1226-1227
Human monocytotropic ehrlichiosis (HME), 1260, 1262*t*
Human papillomavirus (HPV)
cervical cancer from, 870
LGBTQ patient care and, 63
oral infections from, 406
Pap test and, 868
screening for, 1238
vaccines for, 157-158, 161*t*-162*t*, 314-315
warts in, 314
Human weight homeostasis, 1219
Humerus, 985
Humidity, 385
Humulin, 1081-1082
Hungry bone syndrome, 1107
Hurley stages, 287, 287*b*
Hurricane Katrina, 188, 191
Hyaluronan, for osteoarthritis, 978
Hydantoins, acne and, 250*b*
Hydralazine, 576*t*-582*t*
for heart failure, 565
Hydrocarbons and metals, 209
Hydrocele, 764-767, 770
Hydrochlorothiazide, 576*t*-582*t*
Hydrocolloids, 311
Hydrocortisone, 244*t*
Hydronephrosis, 776
Hydroxychloroquine, for systemic lupus erythematosus, 1174, 1174*t*
Hydroxyurea, 1291
Hygiene hypothesis, 422
Hyperacusis, Bell palsy and, 1008
Hyperaldosteronism, primary, hypertension and, 571, 572*t*-573*t*
Hyperalgesia, 701
Hyperandrogenic insulin-resistant acanthosis nigricans (HAIRAN) syndrome, 1097, 1100
Hyperbilirubinemia, 706*b*, 707, 1279
Hypercalcemia, 1104-1106, 1332-1333
clinical presentation of, 1105, 1332
complications of, 1106, 1333
definition and epidemiology of, 1104, 1332
diagnostics for, 1105, 1105*b*, 1332, 1332*b*
differential diagnosis of, 1105, 1106*b*, 1332, 1333*b*
life span considerations with, 1106
management of, 1106, 1333
pathophysiology of, 1104-1105, 1332
physical examination for, 1105, 1332
Hypergammaglobulinemia, 501
Hyperglycemia, 1090
fasting, 1079
in pregnancy, 1086*b*
Hyperglycemic hyperosmolar state (HHS), 1090-1091
Hyperhidrosis, 288-290
clinical presentation of, 288
complications of, 289
definition and epidemiology of, 288
diagnostics for, 289, 289*b*
differential diagnosis of, 289, 289*b*
indications for referral or hospitalization for, 289-290
management of, 289
pathophysiology of, 288
physical examination of, 288-289
Hyperhomocysteinemia, and stroke, 530
Hyperinsulinemia, 117*t*
Hyperkalemia, 1108-1112
acute, 1111
causes of, 1109*b*
chronic, 1111
clinical presentation of, 1109
complications of, 1111
definition and epidemiology of, 1108
diagnostics for, 1110, 1110*b*
differential diagnosis for, 1110, 1110*b*
indications for referral or hospitalization for, 1112
management of, 1111

Hyperkalemia *(Continued)*
pathophysiology of, 1108-1109
physical examination for, 1109
with renal failure, 753-754
Hyperkeratotic condition acanthosis nigricans, 1128
Hyperlipidemia, overview of, 128. *see also* Lipid disorders
Hypernatremia, 1112-1114
clinical presentation and physical examination for, 1112-1113
complications of, 1114
definition and epidemiology of, 1112
diagnostics for, 1113, 1113*b*
differential diagnosis for, 1113, 1113*b*
indications for referral or hospitalization for, 1114
life span considerations with, 1114
management of, 1113-1114
pathophysiology of, 1112
Hyperoxaluria, 775-776
Hyperparathyroidism, 1131
clinical presentation of, 1132
diagnostics for, 1133, 1133*b*
differential diagnosis for, 1134, 1134*b*
management of, 1134
pathophysiology of, 1132
physical examination for, 1133
Hypersomnias, central nervous system, 1214-1215
Hypertension, 569-584
alternative therapy for, 16
clinical presentation of, 571-573
complications of, 583-584
definition and epidemiology of, 569-570
with diabetes mellitus, 1094
diagnostics for, 574, 574*b*
differential diagnosis for, 574, 574*b*
general treatment for, 575
nonpharmacologic, 575
pharmacologic, 575, 576*t*-582*t*
hypertensive crises and, 583-584, 583*b*
incidence of, 570
indications for referral or hospitalization for, 574-575
life span considerations with, 575-583
metabolic syndrome and, 1127
overview of, 128
pathophysiology of, 570-571
physical examination for, 573-574
in pregnancy, 75-76, 75*t*
prevalence of, 570
primary, 570-571
risk factors for, 570
secondary, 571, 572*t*-573*t*
severe, parenteral medications for, 583*t*
Hypertensive crises, 583-584, 583*b*
Hypertensive intracerebral hemorrhage, 1011
Hyperthermia, 1197
malignant, 1197*b*
Hyperthyroidism, 1141-1145
amiodarone and, 1150*t*
clinical presentation and physical examination for, 1142
complications of, 1145
definition and epidemiology of, 1141-1142
diagnostics for, 1142-1143, 1143*b*
differential diagnosis for, 1143, 1143*b*
indications for referral or hospitalization for, 1145
life span considerations with, 1145
management of, 1143-1145, 1144*b*, 1144*t*
pathophysiology of, 1142
physical examination of, 1221
in pregnancy, 77, 1151
radioiodine uptake in, 1143*b*
signs and symptoms of, 1142*t*
subclinical, 1144-1145
thyroid function tests in, 1142*t*
Hypertrichosis, 1097
Hypertriglyceridemia, 1120-1121
Hypertrophic cardiomyopathy, 555-556, 612*t*
Hyperuricemia, 1333-1334
Hyperuricosuria, 776
Hyphema, 332*t*-334*t*, 357, 357*f*
Hypnotic medications, for insomnia, 1212
Hypoactive sexual desire disorder, 878-879
Hypocalcemia, 1106-1108
clinical presentation of, 1106-1107
complications of, 1108
definition and epidemiology of, 1104
diagnostics for, 1107
differential diagnosis for, 1107, 1107*b*
indications for referral or hospitalization for, 1108
life span considerations with, 1108
management of, 1107-1108
pathophysiology of, 1106
physical examination for, 1107
Hypodermis, 237
Hypoglycemia, 1082, 1089-1090, 1089*t*, 1093
Hypokalemia, 1108-1112
acute, 1111
causes of, 1109*b*
chronic, 1111
clinical presentation of, 1109
complications of, 1111
definition and epidemiology of, 1108
diagnostics for, 1109-1110, 1110*b*
differential diagnosis for, 1110, 1110*b*
indications for referral or hospitalization for, 1112
management of, 1111
pathophysiology of, 1108-1109
physical examination for, 1109
Hypokinesia, Parkinson disease and, 1051
Hypomanic episode, 1355
Hyponatremia, 1114-1119
cirrhosis-related, 1118
clinical presentation of, 1115
complications of, 1119
definition and epidemiology of, 1114-1115
diagnostics for, 1116, 1116*b*
differential diagnosis for, 1116, 1117*b*
euvolemic, 1118-1119
exercise-associated, 1118
heart failure-associated, 1118
hypertonic, 1117
hypervolemic, 1118
hypotonic, 1117-1119
hypovolemic, 1118
indications for referral or hospitalization for, 1119
isotonic, 1117
management of, 1116-1119
nephrotic syndrome-related, 1118
pathophysiology of, 1115
physical examination for, 1115
Hypoparathyroidism, 1131
clinical presentation of, 1133
diagnostics for, 1133, 1133*b*
differential diagnosis for, 1134, 1134*b*
management of, 1135
pathophysiology of, 1132
physical examination for, 1133
Hypopyon, 329-330
Hypotension, 221-224
cardiopulmonary symptoms of, 222
clinical presentation and physical examination of, 222
definition and epidemiology of, 221
diagnostics for, 222-223, 223*b*
differential diagnosis of, 223, 223*b*
displaced, in heart failure, 560*t*
fundamental mechanisms of, 221
heat-related illness and, 233
indications for referral or hospitalization for, 224
life span considerations with, 224
management of, 223-224
pathophysiology of, 221-222
postprandial, 222
postural, 224
Hypothalamic obesity, 117*t*
Hypothermia, 235, 236*b*
Hypothyroidism, 117*t*, 1119, 1145-1149
amiodarone and, 1149
clinical presentation of, 1146
complications of, 1148
definition and epidemiology of, 1145-1146
diagnostics for, 1147, 1147*b*
differential diagnosis for, 1147*b*
indications for referral or hospitalization for, 1148
Hypothyroidism *(Continued)*
life span considerations with, 1148-1149
management of, 1147-1148
pathophysiology of, 1146
physical examination for, 1146-1147
in pregnancy, 77, 1151
screening for, 149*t*-152*t*
subclinical, 1148
Hypoxia, 440*t*
Hysteroscopic sterilization, 836

I

Ibandronate (Boniva), 858*b*
Ibuprofen (Advil), 1034
ICD. *see* Implantable cardioverter-defibrillator (ICD)
Ice
for low back pain, 957
for shoulder pain, 992
Idiopathic pain, 1186
Idiopathic rhinitis, 387-388, 388*b*
Ileal pouch-anal anastomosis (IPAA), 698
Image rehearsal therapy (IRT), for parasomnias, 1218
Imatinib mesylate (Gleevec), 1310
Imipenem-cilastatin, for endocarditis, 591*t*-595*t*
Imiquimod (Aldara), 316
Immigrants, 230
Immune priming, 1200
Immune reconstitution inflammatory syndrome, antiretroviral therapy and, 1239
Immune system, 1200
Immune testing, 1202
Immune thrombocytopenic purpura (ITP), 306
Immunization. *see also specific vaccines*
for adolescent, 59
in college health, 173
for COPD, 465
for international travelers, 177, 178*t*
vaccine-specific information and, 156-160
Immunoblotting, in bullous pemphigoid, 258
Immunodeficiency, 1200-1204
causes of, 1203*b*
clinical presentation of, 1201
complications of, 1203
definition and epidemiology of, 1200
diagnosis of, 1202-1203
diagnostics for, 1202, 1202*b*
differential diagnosis in, 1202
indications for referral for, 1203-1204
life span considerations with, 1203
management of, 1202
pathophysiology of, 1200-1201
physical examination for, 1201
Immunoglobulin A (IgA), chronic diarrhea and, 652
Immunoglobulin E (IgE), 384
serum levels, environmental allergies and, 215
Immunoglobulin G (IgG), 1252
blot, 1255
Immunoglobulin M (IgM), 1252
Immunologic disorder, with systemic lupus erythematosus, 1171*b*
Immunologic responses, 274
Immunomodulators, 433*t*-435*t*, 440-441, 697
Immunosuppressed patients, oral infections in, 408
Immunosuppressing therapy, 1237
Immunosuppression, dysphagia and, 666*b*
Immunotherapy, 386-387
Impaired fasting glucose (IFG), 16-17, 1128
Impaired glucose tolerance (IGT), 1128
Impaired hearing, 364-367. *see also* Hearing loss
Impetigo, 262
Impingement syndrome, 989
Impingement test, 988*t*
Implantable cardioverter-defibrillator (ICD), 206-207, 527, 567
In vitro fertilization (IVF), 848
Inborn leptin deficiency, 112
Incision and drainage, for Bartholin gland cysts, 805
Incontinence, 731-736
clinical presentation of, 732
complications of, 735

Incontinence *(Continued)*
definition and epidemiology of, 731, 731*b*
diagnostics for, 732-733, 733*b*
differential diagnosis of, 733, 733*b*
indications for referral or hospitalization for, 736
life span considerations with, 735
management of, 733-735, 733*b*
pathophysiology of, 731-732
physical examination for, 732
Incretin, 1085
Indacaterol, 462*t*-463*t*
Indapamide, 576*t*-582*t*
Indigestion, 671
Indirect immunofluorescence assay (IFA), 1235
Indirect immunofluorescence microscopy, in bullous pemphigoid, 258
Infections/infectious agents. *see also specific organisms and infections*
hip pain and, 937
HPV, 314
in mononucleosis, 413
from peripheral arterial insufficiency, 603
in pruritus, 300*b*
Infectious arthritis, 940-946
Infectious diarrhea, 1243-1251
clinical presentation of, 1245-1246, 1245*t*
complications of, 1250
definition of, 1243-1244
diagnostics for, 1246, 1246*b*
differential diagnosis of, 1246-1250
epidemiology of, 1244, 1244*b*
indications for referral or hospitalization for, 1250-1251
management of, 1250
pathophysiology of, 1245
physical examination for, 1246
Infectious diseases. *see also specific organisms and infections*
diarrhea. *see* Infectious diarrhea
emerging and reemerging, 1225-1232
definitions of, 1225
pathogenesis of, 1225*b*
in pruritus, 300*b*
of salivary gland, 400-401
worldwide mortality from, 178*t*
Infectious mononucleosis, 1251-1254
clinical presentation of, 412, 412*b*, 1252
complications of, 1253-1254
definition and epidemiology of, 1251-1252
diagnostics for, 1252, 1252*b*
differential diagnosis of, 1252-1253, 1253*b*
indications for referral or hospitalization in, 1254
life span considerations with, 1253
management of, 1253
pathophysiology of, 1252
physical examination for, 412, 412*b*, 414, 1252
Infectious rhinitis, 388
Infective endocarditis, 584-597
cardiac conditions associated with, 595*b*
cardiac findings, 587-588
with cardiovascular implantable electronic devices, 588
clinical presentation and physical examination of, 587-588
co-management of, with specialists, 590
complications of, 596
definition and epidemiology of, 584-586
diagnostics for, 588-589
differential diagnosis of, 589-590, 590*b*
fungal, 585
health care-associated, 586
indications for referral or hospitalization for, 596
in injection drug users, 586
life span considerations with, 597
management of, 590-596, 591*t*-595*t*
musculoskeletal findings in, 588
of native valves, 585
neurologic findings in, 587
ophthalmologic findings in, 587
pathophysiology of, 586-587
prevention of, 616*b*
primary prevention of, 595-596
prophylaxis for, 595*b*, 596*t*
of prosthetic valves, 585-586, 591*t*-595*t*
Infective endocarditis *(Continued)*
pulmonary findings in, 588
renal findings in, 588
right-sided *versus* left-sided, 586
splenic and dermatologic findings in, 588
Inferior vena cava (IVC) filter (IVCF), 495
Infertility, 845-850
clinical presentation of, 846
complications of, 849
definition and epidemiology of, 845
diagnostics for, 846-847, 847*b*
differential diagnosis of, 847-848, 847*b*
indications for referral or hospitalization for, 849
life span considerations with, 849
male and female factors in, 845
management of, 848-849
pathophysiology of, 845-846
pharmacologic therapy for, 848-849
physical examination for, 846
Infestations, in pruritus, 300*b*
Inflammation
in airway, 422-423
chronic, hemoptysis and, 472
in gastrointestinal tract, 693*t*
of liver, 686, 689
in purpura, 305
role of, in coronary artery disease, 504
Inflammatory arthritis, of knee, 952
Inflammatory bowel disease (IBD), 692-699
arthritis of, 1158-1159
clinical presentation of, 694
complications of, 698
Crohn disease *versus* ulcerative colitis, 693*t*
definition and epidemiology of, 692-693
diagnostics for, 694-695, 695*b*
differential diagnosis of, 695-696, 696*b*
genetic considerations in, 692-693
indications for referral or hospitalization for, 698
life span considerations with, 699
management of, 696-698
pathophysiology of, 693-694
pharmacotherapy for, 696-698
physical examination for, 694
Inflammatory cells, and asthma, 422
Inflammatory diarrhea, 1244*t*, 1247-1249
Inflammatory disorders. *see also specific disorders*
in pruritus, 300*b*
Inflammatory fatigue, 1192-1193
Inflammatory purpura, 306*b*
Infliximab (Remicade), 502, 697, 697*t*
Influenza, 1241-1243
chemoprophylaxis and treatment considerations for, 1242*b*
clinical presentation of, 1241
complications of, 1242
definition and epidemiology of, 1241
diagnostics for, 1241-1242
differential diagnosis of, 1242, 1242*b*
indications for referral or hospitalization for, 1243
injectable trivalent (TIV) vaccine, 161*t*-162*t*
life span considerations with, 1243
live attenuated vaccine, 161*t*-162*t*
management of, 1242
pathophysiology of, 1241
physical examination for, 1241
prevention of, 1243
Influenza A, 490
H1N1, 1225, 1227
pandemic, 1227
Influenza vaccine, 158, 160
Informed refusal, 47
Infrarenal aortic aneurysms, 605
Ingestions, harmful, 210
Inhalants, 1373
Inhaled allergens, anaphylaxis-inducing, 194*b*
Inhaled corticosteroids (ICSs), for asthma, 431-432, 432*f*, 439*t*
Inhaled glucocorticosteroid and bronchodilator therapy, combination of, for COPD, 462*t*-463*t*, 464
Inhalers, technique for use of, 445*b*
Inheritance patterns, common, 37-38
INH-RPT regimen, for tuberculosis, 1268-1269
Injectable contraception, 833-834
Injection drug use (IDU), 943, 1373
Injuries. *see also specific injuries*
burn. *see* Burns
chemical, 357
mechanical, 356
Innate immune system, 1200
Inner ear disturbances, 367-371
Meniere disease in, 368-369, 369*b*
tinnitus in, 369-371, 370*b*
vestibular neuritis in, 367-368, 367*b*-368*b*
Inotropic agents, for heart failure, 567
Insect bites and stings, 197-198
diagnostics for, 198, 198*b*
differential diagnosis of, 198, 198*b*
initial stabilization and management of, 198
prevention and patient education, 198
venom from, 194*b*
Insomnia, 1210-1213, 1211*b*
chronic, 1210
cognitive behavioral therapy for, 1212, 1212*t*
precipitants of, 1210*b*
in menopause, 856
nonrestorative sleep and, 1210-1213
primary care and, 18
psychophysiologic, 1211
Inspection technique, 543*b*
Instability, shoulder, 991
Institute of Medicine (IOM), 59-60
Insulin, 1081
hirsutism and, 1100
obesity and, 110
tips for use of, 1083*b*
Insulin resistance, 1079
lipid disorders and, 1121
measurement of, 1128
Insulin-like growth factor 1 (IGF-1), 1071
Integrated perspective, primary care and, 15-18
Integrative health care, 15-18
Intelligence tests, 1000*b*
Intent-to-treat table, 9*t*
Interdigital tinea pedis, 279-280, 280*f*
Interferon (IFN), 689-690, 1048-1049
Interferon alfa, 1150
Interferon gamma release assays (IGRAs), 1266, 1266*b*
International Classification of Sleep Disorders (ICSD), 1209
International normalized ratio (INR), 526
International Prognostic Scoring System-Revised (IPSS-R), 1321, 1321*t*
International traveler
air travel risks, 179
diarrhea from food and water, 179
health care of, 173-181
immunization and, 177
medications and prescriptions, 177-179
pre-travel preparation and patient education, 176-177, 177*b*
provider toolbox for travelers, 180*b*
resources for, 177*b*
travel documents needed, 177*b*
travel safety and, 179-180
International unit gray (Gy), 1327
Interpersonal relationships, stress management of, 135
Interprofessional Education Collaborative (IPEC), 2
Intersex, definition of, 60
Interstitial cystitis, pelvic pain, 817
Intertrigo, 290-291
clinical presentation and physical examination of, 290, 290*f*
complications of, 291
definition and epidemiology of, 290
diagnostics for, 290-291, 290*b*
differential diagnosis of, 291, 291*b*
indications for referral or hospitalization for, 291
life span considerations with, 291
management of, 291
pathophysiology of, 290
Interview, in neuropsychological assessment, 1002
"Intestinal flu", 1246
Intimate partner violence, 63, 140-145
barriers to identification and treatment, 142
clinical presentation of, 142-143

Intimate partner violence *(Continued)*
definition and epidemiology of, 140-142
health promotion of, 145
life span considerations of, 145
management of, 144-145
patient and family education of, 145
physical complaints of, 142-143
physical examination of, 143
psychosocial indicators of, 143
psychosocial intervention of, 144-145
screening for, 149*t*-152*t*
violence perspectives, 141-142
Intolerance, glucose , alternative therapy for, 16-17
Intra-articular corticosteroid injections, for osteoarthritis, 978
Intracerebral hemorrhage, 1011
Intracranial arterial occlusion, 531-532
Intracranial pressure (ICP), 219
Intracranial tumors, 1066-1070
classification of, 1066*t*
clinical presentation of, 1067
complications of, 1069
definition and epidemiology of, 1066-1067
diagnostics for, 1068, 1068*b*
differential diagnosis for, 1068, 1068*b*
indications for referral or hospitalization for, 1069
life span considerations with, 1069
management of, 1068-1069
supportive therapies in, 1068-1069
physical examination for, 1067-1068, 1067*t*
Intradermal testing, of environmental allergies, 215
Intraepithelial neoplasia, 890
Intrahepatic obstructive jaundice, 706
Intramuscular injections, needle length and injection site of, 156*t*
Intraocular foreign body, 356*t*
Intraocular pressure, 328
Intraoperative floppy iris syndrome (IFIS), 336-337
Intrauterine devices (IUDs), 836
Intravenous broad-spectrum antibiotics, for epiglottitis, 405-406
Intravenous immune globulin (IVIG)
administration of, 1203
for Guillain-Barré syndrome, 1030
use of, 1202-1203
Intrinsic sphincter deficiency (ISD), 731
Intrinsic sympathomimetic activity, 551
Intubation, for Guillain-Barré syndrome, 1030
Invasive fungal sinusitis, 391-392
Iodides, acne and, 250*b*
Ipecac, 210
Ipratropium bromide, 461, 462*t*-463*t*
Ipratropium HFA, 435*t*-436*t*
Irbesartan, 576*t*-582*t*
Iris, 330
Iritis, 331, 332*t*-334*t*
psoriatic arthritis and, 1158
Iron, 860
daily allowance of, 1281
Iron absorption, factors of, 1281*b*
Iron deficiency, causes of, 1281*b*
Iron overload, 1287*b*
Iron supplements, 149*t*-152*t*, 694
preparations, 1283, 1283*t*
Irregular bleeding, 854
Irrigation, in eye, 345, 345*b*
Irritable bowel syndrome (IBS), 699-705
alternative therapies for, 704
clinical presentation of, 701-702
comorbidities of, 702
complications of, 704
definition and epidemiology of, 699-700, 700*b*
diagnostics for, 700*b*, 702, 702*b*
diarrhea and, 648, 656
differential diagnosis of, 702, 703*b*
emergency "red flag" criteria of, 705*b*
indications for referral or hospitalization for, 704-705
life span considerations with, 704
management of, 703-704
pathophysiology of, 700-701
pelvic pain, 817
pharmacotherapy for, 703-704
Irritable bowel syndrome (IBS) *(Continued)*
physical examination for, 702
psychosocial factors in, 701
Irritant contact dermatitis (ICD), 266-267
Ischemia, exercise stress testing for, 543
Ischemic stroke, 1010-1011
Isoniazid (INH), 1268
acne and, 250*b*
Isotretinoin, 251-252
Isradipine, 576*t*-582*t*
ITCH acronym, 634
Itching, 278, 299. *see also* Pruritus; Scratching
in ocular pain, 335*t*
Itraconazole (Sporanox), 281*t*
Ivabradine, for heart failure, 566
Ivermectin, 308
Ixodes pacificus, 1254
Ixodes scapularis, 1254, 1258

J

Janeway lesions, 588
Jaundice, 705-709
breast milk, 81
causes of, 706*b*
classification of, 706*b*
clinical presentation of, 706
complications of, 708
definition and epidemiology of, 705, 706*b*
diagnostics for, 707-708, 707*b*
differential diagnosis of, 708, 708*b*
indications for referral or hospitalization for, 708
management of, 708
neonatal, 80-81
pathologic, 81
pathophysiology of, 705-706
patient and family education for, 709
physical examination for, 707
physiologic, 80-81
Jaw claudication, giant cell arteritis and, 1162
Jellyfish stings, 1185
Joint pain
primary care and, 18
with systemic lupus erythematosus, 1172
Joint United Nations Programme on HIV/AIDS, 1233
Jugular venous distention, in heart failure, 560*t*

K

Kansas Department of Health, extensive West Nile virus education campaign, 1277
Kaposi sarcoma, 1234
Kawasaki disease, 1177
Kegel exercises, 734
Keloid, 238*f*
Keratinization, 246
Keratitis, 332*t*-333*t*
Ketoacidosis, diabetic, 1090-1091
Ketoconazole (Nizoral), 281*t*
Ketone monitoring, 1090*b*
Kidney stones. *see* Urolithiasis
Kimmelstiel-Wilson syndrome, 1091
Kissing bugs, 197*t*
Klebsiella pneumoniae, 486
Knee
collateral ligament sprains in, 946, 947*t*
cruciate ligament injuries of, 948-949
inflammatory and degenerative disorders of, 952
injection of, 916*f*
meniscus injuries of, 949-951
pain in, 946-952
clinical presentation of, 946
complications of, 948
definition and epidemiology of, 946
diagnostics for, 947, 947*b*
differential diagnosis for, 947, 947*b*
indications for referral or hospitalization for, 948
life span considerations with, 948
management of, 947-948
pathophysiology of, 946
physical examination for, 946-947
Knee bursitis, 918-919
clinical presentation and physical examination of, 918-919, 919*f*
Knee bursitis *(Continued)*
definition and epidemiology of, 918
differential diagnosis of, 919, 919*b*
management of, 919
Koebner phenomenon, 302
Kübler-Ross, Elizabeth, 1355
Kwashiorkor, 1219
Kyphoplasty, 967
Kyphosis, 961

L

Labetalol, 576*t*-582*t*, 1014
Labral tear, 991
Labyrinthitis. *see* Vestibular neuritis
Laceration, 356*t*
Lachman test, 948
Lacrimal drainage system, 349
Lactase enzyme activity, 653
Lactation, 78-84. *see also* Breastfeeding
attachment and latch-on skills, 81
breast and nipple evaluation for breastfeeding, 79
breast pumps for, 83
breasts engorgement of, 81-82
discharge instructions of, 80
first few days and, 79-80
jaundice with, 80-81
let-down/milk ejection in, 82
low milk production with, 82
mastitis and, 810
prenatal lactation counseling, 78-79
weaning from, 83-84
Lactose intolerance, 653
Lactulose, 643, 646
Lamellar laceration, 356*t*
Lamotrigine, 1059, 1061*t*-1062*t*, 1065*t*, 1367*t*-1368*t*
Langerhans cells, 237
Language, of transitional care, 4-5
Language barriers, 30
Language tests, 1000*b*
Laparoscopic adjustable gastric banding (LAGB), 123
Laparoscopic lymph node biopsy, 1206-1207
Laparoscopy. *see also specific procedures*
for ectopic pregnancy, 830
Laparotomy, for ectopic pregnancy, 830
Laplace's law, 556-557
Large-scale disasters, critical role of primary care practices in, 189
Laser hair removal, 1102
Late gadolinium enhancement (LGE), 598
Late persistent infection, of Lyme disease, 1255, 1256*b*
Latent tuberculosis infection (LTBI), 1263
treatment regimen for, 1269*t*
Lateral collateral ligament (LCL), 946
Lateral femoral epicondyle, 917*f*
Lavage, gastric, 210
Laxatives, recommended, 105*t*
12-Lead electrocardiogram, for cardiac arrhythmias, 518
Leg cramps, 1216
Leg ulcers. *see under* Ulceration
Legal services or police, 229
Legg-Calvé-Perthes disease, 937
Legionella pneumophila, 486
Lenalidomide (Revlimid), 1323
Lens, 330
Lens, cataracts in, 335-336
Leptin, 110, 802
Lesbian, definition of, 60
Lesbian, gay, bisexual, and transgender (LGBT) population
in college health, 172
health disparities in, 29
Let-down/milk ejection, 82
Leukemias, 1307-1313
acute, 1307
clinical presentation and physical examination for, 1308
diagnostics and differential diagnosis of, 1308-1309
management of, 1309-1310

Leukemias *(Continued)*
chronic, 1307
clinical presentation and physical examination for, 1308
diagnostics and differential diagnosis of, 1309
management of, 1310
clinical presentation and physical examination for, 1308
complications of, 1310-1311
definition and epidemiology of, 1307-1308
diagnostics and differential diagnosis of, 1308-1309, 1309*b*
drugs for, 1310*b*
indications for referral or hospitalization in, 1311
life span considerations with, 1310
management of, 1309-1310
pathophysiology of, 1308
referral to a hematologist, 1307
Leukopenia, 1312*b*-1313*b*
Leukoplakia, 415, 415*f*
Leukostasis, 1311
Leukotriene modifiers, for asthma, 439-440
Leukotriene receptor antagonists (LTRAs), 313, 313*t*, 432*f*, 433*t*-435*t*
Leukotrienes, 439
Levalbuterol, 435*t*-436*t*, 462*t*-463*t*
Levetiracetam (Keppra), 1059, 1061*t*-1062*t*
Levodopa, 1052
Levofloxacin, 779*t*, 789*b*
Levonorgestrel (Norplant), 834
Levothyroxine, 1147-1148
Lewy bodies, neurocognitive disorder with, 1020*b*
Lewy body dementia, 1021
Lhermitte sign, 972
Lice, 197*t*
Lichen planus (LP), 885-886
clinical presentation and physical examination for, 885
complications of, 886
diagnostics for, 885, 885*b*
differential diagnosis of, 885, 885*b*
indications for referral or hospitalization for, 886
life span considerations with, 886
management of, 886
pathophysiology of, 885
Lichen sclerosus (LS), 883-885
clinical presentation and physical examination of, 883
complications of, 884
diagnostics for, 883-884, 884*b*
differential diagnosis of, 884, 884*b*
indications for referral or hospitalization for, 884
life span considerations with, 884
management of, 884
pathophysiology of, 883
Lichen simplex chronicus (LSC), 886-887
clinical presentation and physical examination of, 886
complications of, 887
diagnostics for, 886-887, 887*b*
differential diagnosis of, 887*b*
indications for referral or hospitalization for, 887
life span considerations with, 887
management of, 887
pathophysiology of, 886
Lichenification, 238*f*
Lichenoid lesions, 274*t*
Lichtenberg flowers, 212
Licorice *(Glycyrrhiza)*, 1077
Lidocaine, 926*t*
Life span considerations
with abdominal aortic aneurysm, 514
with acromegaly, 1073
with amenorrhea, 803
with amyotrophic lateral sclerosis (ALS), 1006
with anal fissure, 633
with anaphylaxis, 196
with ankylosing spondylitis, 1155
with anxiety disorders, 1354
with aortic stenosis, 615
with asthma, 442-443
with atopic dermatitis, 279
with atrophic vaginitis, 896
with auricular disorders, 360
Life span considerations *(Continued)*
with bacterial vaginosis, 893
with Bartholin gland cysts and abscesses, 805
with Bell palsy, 1010
with bipolar disorders, 1366-1368
with bleeding disorders (coagulopathies), 1303
with blepharitis, hordeolum, and chalazion, 339
with bone tumors, 913
with bowel obstruction, 106
with breast masses, 815
with bullous pemphigoid, 259
with cardiac arrhythmias, 528
with carotid artery disease, 535
with cataracts, 337
with central nervous system infections, 1040
with cerebrovascular events, 1015
with cerumen impaction, 362
with cervical cancer, 845
with chronic pain, 1189
with chronic pancreatitis, 720
with chronic pelvic pain, 820-821
with chronic rhinosinusitis, 380
with cold injury, 236
with constipation, 106, 646
with contact dermatitis, 888
with corns and calluses, 269
with coronary artery disease, 553-554
with cutaneous herpes, 272
with deep vein thrombosis, 607-608
with delirium, 100
with depression, 101
with depressive disorders, 1363
with diabetes mellitus, 1095-1096
with diverticulosis, 659
with dry eye, 348
with dyspareunia, 827
with dyspnea, 102-103
with ectopic pregnancy, 831
with eczema, 889
with endometrial cancer, 839
with epiglottitis, 406
with epistaxis, 381-382
with fatigue, 1196
with female sexual dysfunction, 879
with fever, 1199
with gastroesophageal reflux disease (GERD), 677
with gastrointestinal hemorrhage, 682
with goiter (simple, nontoxic), 1139
with Guillain-Barré syndrome (GBS), 1030
with hand and wrist pain, 935
with headache, 1035-1036
with hearing loss, 366
with heart failure, 568-569
with heat-related illness, 235
with heel (calcaneal) bursitis, 920
with hemolytic anemia, 1297
with hemorrhoids, 631-632
with hepatitis, 690
with herpes zoster, 285-286
with herpetic whitlow, 292
with hidradenitis suppurativa, 288
with hirsutism, 1103
with HIV infection, 1240
with hypercalcemia, 1106
with hypernatremia, 1114
with hypertension, 575-583
with hyperthyroidism, 1145
with hypocalcemia, 1108
with hypotension, 224
with hypothyroidism, 1148-1149
with immunodeficiency, 1203
with incontinence, 735
with infectious arthritis, 945
with infectious mononucleosis, 1253
with infective endocarditis, 597
with infertility, 849
with inflammatory bowel disease, 699
with influenza, 1243
with insomnia, 1212
with intertrigo, 291
with intracranial tumors, 1069
with iron deficiency anemia, 1283
with irritable bowel syndrome, 704
with knee pain, 948
with leukemias, 1310
Life span considerations *(Continued)*
LGBTQ patient care and, 64-65
with lichen planus, 886
with lichen sclerosus, 884
with lichen simplex chronicus, 887
in lifestyle management, 145
with low back pain, 959
with lung cancer, 479
with lymphadenopathy, 1208
with lymphomas, 1319
with megaloblastic anemia, 1289
with Meniere disease, 369
with meniscus injuries, 951
with metabolic syndrome, 1130-1131
with mitral regurgitation, 619
with mitral stenosis, 622
with movement disorders, 1042
with multiple sclerosis (MS), 1049
with myocarditis, 599
with nasal trauma, 383-384
with nasal tumors and polyps, 396
with nausea and vomiting, 105
with neck pain, 976
with nipple discharge and galactorrhea, 813
with noninfectious diarrhea, 657
with obesity, 125
with obstructive uropathies, 797
with occupational respiratory diseases, 169
with orbital cellulitis, 352
with osteoarthritis, 979
with osteomyelitis, 984
with osteoporosis, 966
with otitis externa, 372
with otitis media, 376-377
with ovarian cancer, 841
with Paget disease of bone, 970
with pain, 107
with Papanicolaou (Pap) test abnormalities, 869-870
with parasomnias, 1218
with parathyroid gland disorders, 1135
with paronychial infections, 294
with peripheral arterial insufficiency, 604
with peritonsillar abscess, 412
with pharyngitis/tonsillitis, 415-416
with pneumonia, 490
with pneumothorax, 493
with preseptal cellulitis, 352
with presurgical clearance, 183-184
with prostate cancer, 737-738
with prostatitis, 743
with pruritus, 301
with pruritus ani, 634
with psoriasis, 889
with pulmonary embolisms, 495
with purpura, 306
with renal failure, 755-756
with rheumatoid arthritis, 1169-1170
with salivary gland diseases, 402
with sarcoidosis, 502
in scuba diving, 1183
with seborrheic dermatitis, 310
with seizure disorders, 1060-1063
in sexual assault, 229
with sexual dysfunction, 763
with sexually transmitted infections (STIs), 784
with shoulder pain, 993
with sickle cell disease, 1291-1292
with sleep-related breathing disorders, 1214
with sleep-related movement disorders, 1216-1217
with smell and taste disturbances, 394
with sprains, strains, and fractures, 997
with systemic lupus erythematosus, 1175
with testicular disorders, 771
with thalassemia, 1286
with thyroid cancer, 1141
with thyroid nodules, 1141
with traumatic ocular disorders, 358
with trigeminal neuralgia, 1065
with tuberculosis, 1270-1271
with unintended weight loss, 1223
with unknown primary carcinoma (UPC), 1348
with unplanned pregnancy, 882
with urinary calculi, 777

Life span considerations *(Continued)*
with urinary tract infections (UTIs), 782
with vaginal cancer, 843
in vestibular neuritis, 368
with vulvar cancer, 842
with vulvar vestibulitis syndrome, 891
with vulvodynia, 891
with vulvovaginal candidiasis, 895
with West Nile virus, 1276
in wound management, 325
with xerostomia, 103
Lifestyle management, 125-136
assessment of lifestyle, 126-127
components of, 126
components of healthy lifestyle, 129-136
with diabetes mellitus, 1080-1081, 1081*b*
diagnostics for, 127-128
dietary influences on heart health, 131
life span issues, 129
lipid disorders and, 1121
menopause and, 859-860
related medical problems in, 128-129
Lifestyle modifications
for GERD, 674, 674*b*
with hypertension, 575
Li-Fraumeni syndrome, brain tumor and, 1066-1067
Ligament of Treitz, 680*b*
Light therapy, 1362-1363. *see also* Phototherapy
Lightheadedness, 1024
Lightning, 211
Linaclotide, 646
Lindane (Kwell), 308
Linezolid, for endocarditis, 591*t*-595*t*
LINX, 675
Lipid disorders, 1120-1126. *see also specific lipids*
clinical presentation of, 1121
complications of, 1126
definition and epidemiology of, 1120
diagnostics for, 1121, 1122*b*
differential diagnosis for, 1122, 1122*b*
indications for referral for, 1126
management of, 1122-1126
atherosclerotic cardiovascular disease risk assessment in, 1122
lifestyle modification in, 1122-1123
pharmacotherapy in, 1123-1125, 1124*t*-1125*t*
primary prevention for specific populations in, 1125-1126
pathophysiology of, 1120-1121
physical examination for, 1121
Lipids, blood. *see also* Cholesterol, serum
coronary artery disease and, 537*t*
Lipodystrophy, 1239
α-lipoic acid (ALA), 17-18
5-Lipoxygenase inhibitor, 433*t*-435*t*
Liquid nitrogen, 316
in cryosurgery, 240
Liraglutide, 1085
Lisinopril, 576*t*-582*t*, 1014
Listeria monocytogenes, meningitis and, 1037
Literacy, health, 3-4
Lithium, 1150, 1367*t*-1368*t*
acne and, 250*b*
for headaches, 1034
Liver, 683, 686
Liver biopsy, for cirrhosis, 639-641
Liver disease, from antiretrovirals, 1239
Liver function tests (LFTs), 688, 1252
for jaundice, 707
for presurgical clearance, 182*t*
for seizures, 1056-1057
Locaserin hydrochloride, 1130
Lok index, 641
Long bone fractures, 996-997
Long-acting inhaled beta$_2$-agonists (LABAs), 432*f*, 433*t*-435*t*, 441
Look AHEAD study, 119
Loop diuretics, 566*t*
Loop recorder, 519
Loperamide, 179, 1250
Lordosis, 818
Losartan, 576*t*-582*t*
Loss of consciousness (LOC), 218-219
Loss of protective sensation (LOPS), 317*b*
Lotions, 244, 244*t*
Lou Gehrig's disease. *see* Amyotrophic lateral sclerosis (ALS)
Lovastatin (Mevacor), 1124*t*-1125*t*
Low back pain, 952-959
ankylosing spondylitis and, 1152
classification of, 953*t*
clinical presentation of, 954
complications of, 958-959
definition and epidemiology of, 952-953
diagnostics for, 955-956
differential diagnosis for, 956, 956*b*
indications for referral or hospitalization for, 959
life span considerations with, 959
management of, 956-958
complementary and alternative, 958
medications for, 958
physical therapy, 957-958
osteomyelitis and, 981-982, 982*b*
pathophysiology of, 953
physical examination for, 954-955
psychological health and, 958
risk factors for, 953
spinal interventional procedures for, 958
Low-density lipoprotein (LDL), 1120
classification of, 128*t*
defined, 127-128
routine screening of, 155
Low-density lipoprotein cholesterol (LDL-C), 530
Lower esophageal sphincter (LES), 665, 670
pressure in, 666*b*
Lower extremities, weakness in, 1028-1029
Lower motor neurons (LMNs), 1005
Lower urinary tract symptoms (LUTS), 738-739
Low-molecular-weight heparin (LMWH), 1305
for pulmonary embolism, 495
Lubiprostone, 646
Ludwig's angina, 399, 405
Luliconazole (Luzu), 281*t*
Lumbar dermatomes, 955*t*
Lumbar epidural corticosteroid injection, 958
Lumbar spine, 953
Lung cancer, 474-479
clinical presentation and physical examination of, 475
complications of, 478
definition and epidemiology of, 474-475
diagnostics for, 475-476, 476*b*
differential diagnosis for, 477
indications for referral or hospitalization for, 478-479
life span considerations with, 479
management of, 477-478
small cell lung cancer, 478
stage I and II non-small cell lung cancer, 477-478
stage III non-small cell lung cancer, 478
stage IV non-small cell lung cancer, 478
in menopause, 859
metastasis of, 913
sites of, 475
pathophysiology of, 475
screening for, 149*t*-152*t*
signs, symptoms, and syndromes of, 476*t*
staging and treatment of, 477*t*
Lung transplantation, 500
for COPD, 465-466
Lung volume reduction surgery (LVRS), for COPD, 465
Lupus nephritis, 1172
Luteinizing hormone (LH), 799-800, 1097
Lyme carditis, 1257
Lyme disease, 942-943, 1254-1258, 1262*t*
clinical presentation of, 1255
complications of, 1257-1258
definition and epidemiology of, 1254
diagnostics for, 1255-1256
differential diagnosis of, 1256
emerging and reemerging, 1226
management of, 1256-1257
manifestations of, 1256*b*
pathophysiology of, 1254
prevention of, 1257
reported cases (map) of, 1255*f*
stages of, 1255
Lymph nodes
biopsy of, 1206-1207
distribution of, 1205*f*
physical examination of, 1206
structure and function of, 1204
swelling of, 1205
Lymphadenopathy, 1204-1209
clinical presentation of, 1205-1206
complications of, 1208-1209
definition and epidemiology of, 1204
diagnostics for, 1206-1207, 1207*b*
differential diagnosis of, 1207-1208, 1208*b*
indications for referral or hospitalization for, 1209
interdisciplinary management of, 1208
life span considerations with, 1208
management of, 1208
pathophysiology of, 1204-1205
physical examination for, 1206
Lymphatic system, 1204, 1205*f*
Lymphedema, primary, 1206
Lymphogranuloma venereum, 793
Lymphomas, 1314-1320. *see also specific lymphomas*
classification of, 1314
clinical presentation of, 1314
complications of, 1319-1320
post-treatment toxicities in, 1320
during therapy, 1319-1320
diagnosis of, 1314
epidemiology of, 1314
etiology and risk factors for, 1314
indications for referral or hospitalization for, 1320
initial evaluation of, 1314
in later life, 1208
life span considerations with, 1319
overview of, 1314
staging of, 1314-1315, 1315*t*
T-cell, 1319

M

Macroalbuminuria, 743
Macrolides, 440*t*
for acute bronchitis, 419-420
for dental abscess, 398-399
Macular degeneration, 333
Macule, 238*f*
Magnesium, 652-653
Magnesium ammonium phosphate stones, 776
Magnesium citrate, for chemical exposure, 210
Magnetic resonance angiography (MRA)
for abdominal aortic aneurysm, 512
for carotid artery disease, 531
Magnetic resonance arteriography, for vasculitis, 1178-1179
Magnetic resonance elastography (MRE), 641
Magnetic resonance imaging (MRI)
for abdominal aortic aneurysm, 512
breast, for unknown primary carcinoma, 1346-1347
for cerebrovascular events, 1011-1012
for chronic diarrhea, 652
for coronary artery disease, 505*t*, 508-509
for heart failure, 561
for low back pain, 955-956
for neck pain, 973
for parotitis, 410
for seizures, 1056-1057
Major depressive disorder (MDD), 1354, 1356-1364
clinical presentation of, 1358
complications of, 1363-1364
definition and epidemiology of, 1356-1357
diagnostics for, 1358-1359
differential diagnosis of, 1359, 1359*b*
life span considerations with, 1363
management of, 1359-1363, 1360*t*-1362*t*, 1362*b*
pathophysiology of, 1357
physical examination for, 1358
Malaise, with systemic lupus erythematosus, 1171
Malar rash, with systemic lupus erythematosus, 1171, 1171*b*

Malaria
emerging and reemerging, 1226
medications for, 177-179
in travel medicine, 177-179
Malassezia, in seborrheic dermatitis, 309
Malassezia furfur, 282
Male factor infertility, 845
Malignant hyperthermia, 1197*b*
Malignant melanoma (MM)
definition and epidemiology of, 245-246
differential diagnosis of, 248*b*
physical examination of, 246, 247*f*
treatment of, 248
Malignant neoplasms, in pruritus, 300*b*
Malignant otitis externa, 359, 372, 373*f*
Malignant spinal cord compression, 1331-1332, 1331*b*-1332*b*
Malnutrition, protein-energy, 1219
Maltese cross, 1258
Mandated reporting, in sexual assault, 229
Maneuvers
in swallowing therapy, 668*t*-669*t*
Valsalva. *see* Valsalva maneuvers
Manic episode, 1354
Manometry, esophageal, 673
Mantoux test, 1265
Manual therapy
for low back pain, 957
for neck pain, 974-975
Marasmus, 1219
Marijuana, 1373
Marine animal, bites and stings of, 1185
Marrow stroma, 1278
Marseilles-Rome classification system, 718
Marsupialization, 805
Mast cell stabilizers, 342
Mast cells
histamine and, 312
in rhinitis, 384
Mastalgia, 807-810
Mastication, 664
Mastitis, 83, 810-811
Mastodynia, 807-810
Material Safety Data Sheet (MSDS), on chemical exposure, 208
McDonald criteria, 1045
MCI. *see* Mild cognitive impairment (MCI)
McMurray test, 950, 950*f*
Mean corpuscular volume (MCV), 1279-1280
Measles, mumps, rubella vaccine, 158-160, 161*t*-162*t*
Mechanical circulatory support, for heart failure, 567
Mechanical obstruction, 379
Mechanical processes, syncope and, 231*b*
Mechanical ventilation, for Guillain-Barré syndrome, 1030
Meclizine, 368
for vertigo, 1028
Medial collateral ligament (MCL), 946
Medicaid, 61
Medical home, 21
patient-centered, 21, 22*b*
Medical record
documentation, 51
patient request to amend/make addendum to, 48
Medication analysis, 87*b*
Medication toxicity, in conjunctivitis, 341-342
Medications/drugs. *see also specific drugs and drug classes*
of abuse, in college health, 173
acne and, 250*b*
after bariatric surgery, 124
anaphylaxis-inducing, 194*b*
antiemetic, 711, 712*b*
associated with constipation, 644*b*
for asthma, 431-442
long-term, 431-441, 433*t*-435*t*
quick-relief, 435*t*-436*t*, 441
bullous pemphigoid and, 258
cardiac, 113
cardiac arrhythmias and, 518
cataracts and, 336-337
for chronic pain, 1187-1188
Medications/drugs *(Continued)*
for coronary artery disease, 537*t*
for dermatologic therapy, 243-245
for dermatophyte infections, 280-281, 281*t*
for diabetes, 113
diarrhea and, 649
for dry eye, 348
fatigue and, 1191
for fibromyalgia syndrome, 926, 926*t*
GERD and, 672
for grief and bereavement, 1356
high-liability clinical areas and, 50
hypertension and, 571, 576*t*-583*t*
for infectious diarrhea, 1250
by injection, 943
for international traveler, 177-179, 180*b*
lipid-lowering, 1124*t*-1125*t*
for neck pain, 975-976
osteoporosis and, 963*b*
pruritus from, 300*b*
purpura and, 307
for rhinitis, 386
safety, 4
samples, and dispensing, high-liability clinical areas and, 50
for scabies, 308
for seborrheic dermatitis, 310
for seizure, 113
sexual response and, 878*t*
sleep disorders from, 1211
for stress testing, 506
systemic, for psoriasis, 303
thyroid gland and, 1149-1150
for urticaria and angioedema, 313*t*
for warts, 316
weight loss from, 1220, 1220*b*
Medroxyprogesterone (Depo-Provera), 833-834
Megaloblastic anemia, 1287-1290, 1288*b*
Megestrol acetate, 1222
Meibomian gland, 337
dysfunction, 346, 346*f*
Melanocytes, 237, 296
Melatonin, for REM sleep behavior disorder, 1218
Meloxicam (Mobic), for osteoarthritis, 978
Memantine (Namenda), 1023
Memory Impairment Screen (MIS), 1021-1022
Memory tests, 1000*b*
Men, prevention of lipid disorders in, 1126
Menarche, 850
Mendelsohn maneuver, 668*t*-669*t*
Meniere disease, 368-369
clinical presentation of, 368
complications of, 369
definition and epidemiology of, 368
diagnostics for, 369, 369*b*
differential diagnosis of, 369, 369*b*
indications for referral or hospitalization for, 369
life span considerations with, 369
management of, 369
pathophysiology of, 368
physical examination for, 368-369
Meningioma, 1066*t*
Meningitis, 334*t*
bacterial, 1038*t*, 1275
causes of, 1037
cerebrospinal fluid findings in, 1038*t*
vaccine for, 1040
viral, 1038*t*
Meningococcal conjugate vaccine, 1040
Meningococcal polysaccharide vaccine, 1040
Meningococcal vaccine, 159, 161*t*-162*t*, 163
Meningoencephalitis, 1271-1272
Meniscus injuries, 949-951
clinical presentation of, 949-950
complications of, 951
definition and epidemiology of, 949
diagnostics for, 950
differential diagnosis for, 950-951
indications for referral or hospitalization for, 951
life span considerations with, 951
management of, 951
pathophysiology of, 949
physical examination for, 950
Menopause, 850-868
chronic disease and, 856-859
clinical presentation of, 854-856
definition and epidemiology of, 850-851, 851*t*, 852*f*
genital and sexual symptoms of, 861
hormones in, 851
implications for practice of, 868
management of, 859-860
nonpharmacological therapies for, 860-861
pharmacologic therapy for, 861-865
physical examination for, 859
physiology of, 851-853
prescription products for, 865*t*-867*t*
research and clinical trials of, 853-854
Menopause Decision-Support Algorithm, 861-862
Mental defeat, 1186
Mental health disorders, 1377-1381. *see also specific disorders*
in college health, 172
Mental health services, 229
Mental status
of adolescent, 57
assessment tools for, 84
examination for, 1379*t*
HIV infection and, 1234
scales, 1000*b*
testing, 1017
Mentorship, 15
Mesalamine, 693*t*, 696, 696*t*
Metabolic bone disease, 960-970
Metabolic disorders. *see also specific disorders*
diabetes mellitus. *see* Diabetes mellitus
in pruritus, 300*b*
Metabolic syndrome, 129, 1079, 1126-1131
clinical presentation of, 1128
complications of, 1131
definition and epidemiology of, 1126-1127
diagnostics for, 1128, 1128*b*
differential diagnosis for, 1128-1129, 1129*b*
indications for referral or hospitalization for, 1131
life span considerations with, 1130-1131
lipid disorders and, 1121
management of, 1129-1130
pathophysiology of, 1127-1128
physical examination for, 1128
Metabolic toxicities, 1239
Metamorphopsia, 333
Metaproterenol sulfate, 462*t*-463*t*
Metastases, brain, 1066
Metastatic cancers, in bone, 911-913
Metformin, 1084
for infertility, 848
for metabolic syndrome, 1130
Methacholine challenge, 453*f*, 454
Methadone, 1372
Methicillin-resistant *Staphylococcus aureus* (MRSA), 1231
care-associated, 488-489
osteomyelitis and, 981, 984
Methimazole, 1143-1144, 1144*t*
Methotrexate
for ectopic pregnancy, 830
for psoriasis, 303
for rheumatoid arthritis, 1169
for vasculitis, 1180
3,4-Methylenedioxymethamphetamine (MDMA), 1372-1373
Methylnaltrexone bromide, 646
Methylprednisolone, 433*t*-436*t*, 462*t*-463*t*
for vestibular neuritis, 368
Methylprednisolone acetate (Depo-Medrol), for osteoarthritis, 978
Methylxanthine, 433*t*-435*t*, 462*t*-463*t*, 464
Metoclopramide, antidopaminergic, 1222
Metolazone, 565, 576*t*-582*t*
Metoprolol, 576*t*-582*t*
Metronidazole, 251-252, 729*t*, 874*b*
MI. *see* Motivational interviewing (MI)
Miconazole (Monistat-Derm), 281*t*
Microalbuminuria, 743, 1092, 1128
Microcytosis, 1282
Microscopic polyangiitis (MPA), 1178

Microvascular angina, 538-539
clinical presentation of, 541
diagnostics for, 544
management of, 549
Middle East respiratory syndrome (MERS-CoV), 488, 1226
Middle-age, diabetes mellitus in, 1095
Migraine headache, 1031
sinusitis and, 391
visual loss and, 333, 334*t*
Mild cognitive impairment (MCI), 4, 1020
Military personnel/veterans, war-related exposures in, 166-167
Milk of magnesia, 646
Milk-alkali syndrome, 1105
Millipedes, 197*t*
Milnacipran (Savella), 926*t*
Mineral oil, 646
Minerals, for menopause, 860
Mini Nutritional Assessment, short-form version (MNA-SF), 1220-1221
Mini-Cog, 1021-1022
Minimize clinician bias, 30
Minipills, in oral contraceptives, 833
Minor burns. *see* Burns
Minor head trauma, 220
Minoxidil, 576*t*-582*t*
Mirtazapine, 1222, 1360*t*-1362*t*
Misoprostol, 1065*t*
Mithramycin, 969
Mitoxantrone (Novantrone), 1048
Mitral regurgitation, 612*t*, 617-619
clinical presentation and physical examination for, 618
complications of, 619
definition and epidemiology of, 617
diagnostics for, 618
differential diagnosis of, 618
in heart failure, 560*t*
interdisciplinary management of, 619
life span considerations with, 619
management of, 619
pathophysiology of, 617-618
Mitral stenosis, 612*t*, 620-622
clinical presentation and physical examination of, 621
complications of, 622
definition and epidemiology of, 620
diagnostics for, 621
differential diagnosis of, 621
indications for referral or hospitalization for, 622
interdisciplinary management and life span considerations for, 622
management of, 621-622
pathophysiology of, 621
Mitral valve prolapse, 612*t*, 619-620
chest pain and, 448, 548*t*
clinical presentation and physical examination of, 619-620
complications of, 620
definition and epidemiology of, 619
diagnostics for, 620
differential diagnosis of, 620
interdisciplinary management of, 620
management of, 620
pathophysiology of, 619
Mixed incontinence, 732, 733*b*, 735
Mixed oligoastrocytoma, 1066*t*
Modafinil, 1193-1194
Model for End-Stage Liver Disease (MELD), 640
Modified barium swallow (MBS), 665-666
Modified dynamic labral shear test, 988*t*
Moexipril, 576*t*-582*t*
Moll lateral flexion test, 1153
Molluscum contagiosum, 278, 340-341
Mometasone furoate, 244*t*, 462*t*-463*t*
Moniliasis, 283*f*
Monkeypox, 1230-1231
Monoamine oxidase inhibitors (MAOIs), hypertension and, 572*t*-573*t*
Monobenzone hydroquinone (MEH), 298
Mononeuropathies, 1092
Mononucleosis, infectious, 412, 412*b*, 414-415
Monosodium urate (MSU) crystal, 928
Monospot heterophile antibody test, for peritonsillar abscess, 412
Monounsaturated fats, 1121
Montelukast, 433*t*-435*t*, 439-440
Montreal Cognitive Assessment (MoCA), 1021-1022
Mood disorders, 1354-1369. *see also specific disorders*
chronic pain and, 1186
in menopause, 855-856
Mood disturbances, in unplanned pregnancy, 882
Moraxella catarrhalis, 486-487
in eyes, 351
Morbid obesity, fatigue and, 1192
Morbidity rates
in COPD, 457
obesity and, 114-115
Mortality rates
in COPD, 457
obesity and, 114-115
Morton neuroma, 902-903
Morulae
in anaplasmosis, 1259
in ehrlichiosis, 1260
Mosquitoes, 197*t*
Motility disorders, 649
Motivational interviewing (MI), 20, 25
Motor neurons, 1005
Motor response, 219*t*
Motor vehicle accidents, 180
Movement disorders, 1040-1043
clinical presentation of, 1041, 1041*b*
complications of, 1042
definition and epidemiology of, 1040, 1040*b*
diagnostics for, 1041, 1041*b*
differential diagnosis, 1041, 1041*b*
life span considerations with, 1042
management of, 1041-1042
pathophysiology of, 1040-1041
physical examination for, 1041
sleep-related, 1215-1217
Mucoactive agents, for COPD, 464
Mucosal injury, dysphagia and, 666*b*
Mucositis, 1312*b*-1313*b*, 1342, 1344-1345
Multidrug-resistant tuberculosis (MDR-TB), 1263
Multifocal atrial tachycardia, 520, 525
Multiple births, breastfeeding and, 83
Multiple diagnostic failures, 43
Multiple myeloma, 906, 911
Multiple sclerosis (MS), 1044-1050
clinical courses of, 1044*b*
clinical presentation of, 1044-1045
definition and epidemiology of, 1044
diagnostics for, 1045, 1047*b*
differential diagnosis for, 1045, 1048*b*
indications for referral or hospitalization for, 1049
life span considerations with, 1049
management of, 1048-1049
pathophysiology of, 1044
physical examination for, 1045
symptomatic and rehabilitative therapies for, 1046*t*-1047*t*
Multiple sleep latency test (MSLT), 1215
Multisystem disorders, evaluation and management of, 1181-1185
Mumps, 409
clinical presentation of, 410
complications of, 411, 411*b*
diagnostics for, 410, 410*b*
differential diagnosis for, 410, 410*b*
indications for referral or hospitalization for, 411
management of, 410-411
physical examination for, 410
Mumps paramyxovirus infection, of salivary gland, 402
Murmurs (heart sounds). *see* Cardiac murmurs
Murphy sign, 637
Muscle relaxants, 1035*t*-1036*t*
Musculoskeletal examination, for preparticipation sports physical, 186
Myalgias, infective endocarditis and, 588
Myalgic encephalomyelitis, 1190
Mycobacterium africanum, 1262
Mycobacterium avium, 1262
Mycobacterium bovis, 1262
Mycobacterium tuberculosis, 1262-1263
Mycophenolate, for systemic lupus erythematosus, 1174*t*
Mycoplasma pneumoniae, pneumonia and, 487
Mycotic aneurysms, infective endocarditis and, 587
Myelodysplastic syndromes, 1320-1324
clinical presentation and physical examination of, 1321
complications of, 1323-1324
diagnostics for, 1321-1322, 1322*b*
differential diagnosis of, 1322, 1322*b*
indications for referral or hospitalization for, 1323
management of, 1322-1323
pathophysiology of, 1321
quality-of-life issues in, 1322, 1324
specialist referral for, 1321
Myelopathy, cervical, 971
Myocardial infarction with nonobstructed coronary arteries (MINOCA), 539-540
Myocardial ischemia, 540
evaluation of, 559
Myocardial perfusion imaging (MPI), 505*t*, 507-508
comparison of, with two-dimensional echocardiography, 508
Myocarditis, 597-599
clinical manifestations of, 597-598
definition and epidemiology of, 597
diagnostics for, 598, 598*b*
differential diagnosis of, 598-599, 599*b*
management of, 599
pathophysiology of, 597
physical examination of, 598
prognosis and life span considerations for, 599
Myoclonus, 1040*b*
Myofascial pain syndrome, 924-927
Myoglobin, 547
Myokymia, 1040*b*
Myopathy
dysphagia and, 666*b*
from statins, 1123-1125
Myxedema coma, 1148

N

N-acetylcysteine for acetaminophen, 226
Nadolol, 527, 576*t*-582*t*
Nafcillin, for endocarditis, 591*t*-595*t*
Nail disorders, 292-296
dystrophies, 295*t*
herpetic whitlow, 292, 292*b*
onychomycosis, 294-296, 294*b*-295*b*, 295*f*
paronychial infections, 293-294, 293*b*
Naloxone for opioids, 226
Naltrexone, 1376
for infertility, 848
Narcolepsy, 1190-1191, 1215
Narcotic analgesics, 1035*t*-1036*t*
Narrow complex tachycardia, 520
Nasal congestion, discharge and, 378-380. *see also* Chronic rhinosinusitis (CRS)
Nasal heroin, 1374
Nasal septum, deviations of, 383
Nasal trauma, 382-384
clinical presentation of, 382
complications of, 383
definition and epidemiology of, 382
diagnostics for, 382-383, 383*b*
differential diagnosis of, 383, 383*b*
indications for referral or hospitalization for, 383
life span considerations with, 383-384
management of, 383
pathophysiology of, 382
physical examination for, 382
Nasal tumors and polyps, 394-396
clinical presentation of, 395
complications of, 396
definition and epidemiology of, 394-395
diagnostics for, 395, 395*b*
differential diagnosis of, 395, 395*b*
of geriatric, 396
indications for referral or hospitalization of, 396

Nasal tumors and polyps *(Continued)*
life span considerations with, 396
management of, 395-396
pathophysiology of, 395
pediatric, 396
physical examination for, 395
Nasolacrimal duct obstruction (NLDO), 349-350
clinical presentation of, 349, 349*f*
complications of, 350
definition and epidemiology of, 349
diagnostics for, 349-350, 350*b*
differential diagnosis of, 350, 350*b*
indications for referral or hospitalization for, 350
management of, 350
pathophysiology of, 349
physical examination for, 349, 350*f*
Natalizumab (Tysabri), 1048
National Cancer Institute, 1325
National Center for Advancing Translational Sciences (NCATS), 13
National Coalition for Health Professional Education in Genetics (NCHPEG), 42
National Heart, Lung, and Blood Institute (NHLBI), on asthma management, 430
National Institute for Occupational Safety and Health, 170
National Institutes of Health, National Human Genome Research Institute (NHGRI), 42
National Institutes of Health (NIH), on translational research definition, 11-12
National Institutes of Health (NIH) Stroke Scale, 1012
National Lung Screening Trial (NSLT), 479
National Practitioner Data Bank, 44
National Sleep Foundation, sleep hygiene from, 1212-1213
Native valve endocarditis, 585, 591*t*-595*t*
infectious organisms of, 585
risk factors for, 585
Nausea, in ocular pain, 335*t*
Nausea and vomiting, 709-713
chemotherapy-induced, 1341, 1343-1344
clinical presentation of, 709
complications of, 711
definition and epidemiology of, 709
diagnostics for, 710, 710*b*
differential diagnosis of, 711, 711*b*
history of, 709-710
indications for referral or hospitalization for, 711-713
management of, 711, 712*b*
in palliative care, 103-105
clinical presentation and physical examination of, 104
definition and epidemiology of, 103-104
diagnostics for, 104
indications for referral or hospitalization for, 105
life span considerations with, 105
management, 104-105
pathophysiology of, 104
pathophysiology of, 709
physical examination for, 710
in pregnancy, 72
severity grading for, 1343*b*
Neck pain, 970-976
clinical presentation of, 971
complications of, 976
definition and epidemiology of, 970-971
diagnostics for, 972-973, 973*b*
differential diagnosis for, 973, 973*b*
indications for referral or hospitalization for, 976
life span considerations with, 976
management of, 973-974
physical therapy, 974-975
medications for, 975-976
pathophysiology of, 971
physical examination for, 971-972
Neck veins, in cardiac arrhythmias, 517
Necrosis, of pancreas, 715
Necrotizing vasculitis, nasal, 396
Needle aspiration, for pneumothorax, 492-493
Neer and Hawkins impingement signs, 914, 914*b*
Neisseria gonorrhoeae, 341, 413, 784, 785*t*-788*t*, 872
infectious arthritis from, 941
Neisseria meningitidis, meningitis and, 1037
Nematocysts, 1185
Neonates/infants
born of diabetic pregnancies, 76
complications of mothers with diabetes in, 1087*b*
jaundice in, 80-81
Neoplasms, of hip, 937
Neoplastic disorders/diseases. *see also specific disorders*
in pruritus, 300*b*
of salivary gland, 401
Nephrogenic syndrome of inappropriate antidiuresis (NSIAD), 1119
Nephrolithiasis, with gout, 931
Nephrolithotomy, percutaneous, 775
Nephropathy, diabetic, 1091-1092
Nerve blocks, for chronic pain, 1188
Nervous system tumors, 1067
Neurally mediated syncope, 231
Neuritis
optic, 334*t*, 391
ulnar, 922*t*-923*t*
Neurocognitive disorders, 1002, 1020*b*
due to Alzheimer disease, 1020*b*
with Lewy bodies, 1020*b*
Neuroendocrine activation, 557
Neuroendocrine carcinoma, 1346
Neurogenic claudication, 954
Neurogenic orthostatic hypotension, 222
Neuroglycopenia, 1093
Neuroleptic malignant syndrome, 1197*b*, 1198
Neuroleptics, 99*t*, 113
Neurologic disorders
evaluation and management of, 999-1004
with systemic lupus erythematosus, 1171*b*
that interrupt sleep, 1210*b*
Neurologic examination, for low back pain, 954-955
Neurology referral, of smell and taste disturbances, 394
Neuromuscular disorders. *see also specific disorders*
heart failure and, 563
Neuromuscular examination, for preparticipation sports physical, 187
Neuromuscular junction blockade, dysphagia and, 666*b*
Neuro-otologic examination, 1025
Neuropathic pain, 953. *see also* Organic neuropathic pain
examples of, 1336
Neuropathy
alternative therapy for, 17-18
diabetic, 1092-1093
Neuropsychological disorders. *see also specific disorders*
assessment of
considerations in, 1003-1004
goals for, 1001*b*
process of, 1002-1003
tools and approaches for, 1000-1001, 1000*b*
case study on, 1004
evaluation of, 999-1004
professional functions and roles in, 999-1000
referral for, 1002
scoring and interpretation of test data in, 1003
Neuropsychologists, 999
Neuropsychology
clinical, 999
within primary care settings, 1001-1002
Neurotransmitters, 1350
enteric, 701
Neutropenia, febrile, 1326
Newest Vital Sign tool, 3-4, 28-29
Nicardipine, 576*t*-582*t*
Nicotine
addiction, genetics of, 136
effects of, 136
neurochemical, 136
withdrawal, 136
Nicotinic acid (niacin), 1124*t*-1125*t*, 1125
Nicotinic stomatitis, 409
Nifedipine, 576*t*-582*t*
Night shift workers, sleep disorders in, 1211
Nightmare disorder, 1217
Nipple
discharge from, 811-813, 1098
clinical presentation of, 811
definition and epidemiology of, 811
diagnostics for, 811-812, 811*b*
differential diagnosis of, 812, 812*b*
indications for referral or hospitalization for, 813
life span considerations with, 813
management of, 812-813
pathophysiology of, 811
physical examination for, 811
Paget disease of, 813-814, 813*b*-814*b*
eczema *versus*, 814*t*
Nissen fundoplication, 675-676
Nitrates
for coronary artery disease, 551-552, 552*t*
oral, for heart failure, 565
for ST segment elevation myocardial infarction, 550
tolerance, 552
Nitric oxide, for pulmonary hypertension, 498
Nitrite test, 780
Nitrofurantoin monohydrate, 779*t*, 781, 781*t*
Nitrogen narcosis, 1182
Nitroglycerin, 540
oral, 552
spray, 552
sublingual, 551-552
tablets, 552
topical, 552
N-methyl-D-aspartate (NMDA) receptor antagonists, 1023
Nociceptive pain, 953, 1186, 1335-1336
Nocturnal frontal lobe epilepsy (NFLE), 1217-1218, 1218*t*
Nocturnal seizures, 1217-1218, 1218*t*
Nodular lymphocyte-predominant Hodgkin lymphoma, 1315
Nodules, 238*f*
thyroid, 1139-1141
clinical presentation and physical examination for, 1139
complications of, 1141
definition and epidemiology of, 1139
diagnostics and differential diagnosis for, 1139-1140, 1140*b*
indications for referral or hospitalization for, 1141
life span considerations with, 1141
management of, 1140-1141
pathophysiology of, 1139
Noise trauma, 364
Nonadherent secondary dressing, for burns, 261
Nonalcoholic fatty liver disease (NAFLD), 686
Nondihydropyridines, for hypertension, 576*t*-582*t*
Non-Epstein-Barr virus-associated infectious mononucleosis (non-EBV-IM), 1251-1252
Nonerosive reflux disease (NERD), 675
Nonexertional heat stroke, 1197*b*
Nonglomerular hematuria, 748
Nongonococcal urethritis (NGU), 778. *see also* Urethritis
Non-Hodgkin lymphoma (NHL), 1314
aggressive (formerly known as intermediate or high grade), 1318
clinical presentation of, 1317
definition of, 1317
diagnosis of, 1317-1318
highly aggressive, 1318-1319
indolent (formerly known as low-grade), 1318
management of, 1318-1319
pathophysiology of, 1317
Nonimmunologic triggers, anaphylaxis-inducing, 194*b*
Noninflammatory purpura, 306*b*
Noninvasive positive-pressure ventilation (NIPPV), for ALS, 1007
Nonmalignant gastrointestinal disease, unintentional weight loss and, 1222
Nonpurulent skin and soft tissue infections
clinical presentation and physical examination of, 262-263
diagnostics for, 263
differential diagnosis of, 263

Nonpurulent skin and soft tissue infections *(Continued)*
pathophysiology of, 262
treatment of, 264
Non-rapid eye movement (NREM) sleep, 1209-1210
arousal from, 1217
Nonrestorative sleep, insomnia and, 1210-1213
Non-small cell lung cancer (NSCLC), 475
staging for, 475-476
treatment for
stage I and II, 477-478
stage III, 478
stage IV, 478
Non-ST segment elevation myocardial infarction (NSTEMI), 539
clinical presentation of, 541-542, 541*t*
diagnostics for, 544-545
echocardiography for, 544-545
electrocardiography for, 544
exercise tolerance testing for, 544
laboratory data for, 544
management of, 549-550
Nonsteroidal anti-inflammatory drugs (NSAIDs)
for ankylosing spondylitis, 1154
for arthritis of inflammatory bowel disease, 1159
for chronic pain, 1187
for dysmenorrhea, 824, 824*b*
GI bleeding and, 678
for gout, 930, 930*b*
for headaches, 1034, 1035*t*-1036*t*
for hip pain, 939
hypertension and, 572*t*-573*t*
liver injury from, 686
for low back pain, 958
for osteoarthritis, 978
for Paget disease, 969-970
peptic ulcer and, 728
for psoriatic arthritis, 1158
for rheumatoid arthritis, 1169
for sarcoidosis, 502
for shoulder pain, 992
for systemic lupus erythematosus, 1173-1174
Non-tetanus-prone wounds, 324*b*, 324*t*
Nonthyroidal illness, 1149, 1149*t*
Norelgestromin-ethinyl estradiol transdermal system (Ortho Evra), 834
Norovirus, 1246
Nortriptyline, 1360*t*-1362*t*
Nose disorders. *see also specific disorders*
congestion and discharge, 378-380
epistaxis, 380-382
nasal trauma, 382-384
tumors and polyps. *see* Nasal tumors and polyps
Nosebleed. *see* Epistaxis; Hemoptysis
NovoLog, 1082-1083
Nucleic acid test (NAT), 1235
Numeracy, health literacy of, 28
Numeric literacy, health literacy of, 28
Nurse practitioners
malpractice claims, 43
as member of transitional care teams, 1
as primary care providers, 19, 25*b*-27*b*
Nursing complaint, defending against board of, 44
Nursing home, managing risk in, 52
Nutrition
for COPD, 465
for diabetes mellitus, 1080, 1081*b*
for dysmenorrhea, 824
in healthy lifestyle components, 129-131
in lifestyle assessment, 126-127
obesity and, 114
with osteoporosis, 858*b*
pancreatitis and, 719
stroke and, 531
weight gain in pregnancy and, 69
Nutritional supplementation, after bariatric surgery, 124
Nystagmus, 1027
Nystatin (Mycostatin), 281*t*

O

Obesity, 109-125
blood pressure and, 570
clinical presentation with, 115
Obesity *(Continued)*
complications, social stigma, and discrimination, 114
coronary heart disease and, 530-531
definition of, 109-110
diagnostics for, 116
differential diagnosis of, 116, 117*t*
energy intake and, 111
energy output of, 111
environmental factors and, 113-114
epidemiology of, 109
fatigue and, 1192
genetics and, 111-112
increased morbidity and mortality in, 114-115
indications for referral or hospitalization for, 125
life span considerations with, 125
in lifestyle components, 126
lipid disorders and, 1121
management of, 116-124
maternal influences and, 112
monogenic causes of, 112
pathophysiology of, 110-115
peripheral arterial insufficiency and, 602
pharmaceuticals associated with weight gain, 112-113
physical activity, insufficient of, 111
polygenic, 112
prevalence of, 115
screening for, 149*t*-152*t*
Obscure bleeding, 677*b*
Obsessive-compulsive disorder (OCD), 1349
Obstetrics complications
bleeding, 73
constipation, 72-73
eclampsia, 75*t*, 76
ectopic pregnancy, 73
placental abruption, 73
preeclampsia, 75*t*
preterm labor, 73-74
Obstructive jaundice, 705
Obstructive processes, syncope and, 231*b*
Obstructive sleep apnea (OSA), 1190-1191, 1211, 1213
hypertension and, 571, 572*t*-573*t*
management of, 1214
obesity and, 114
pathophysiology of, 1213
Obstructive uropathies, 794-798
clinical presentation of, 795
complications of, 798, 798*b*
definition and epidemiology of, 794
diagnostics for, 796, 796*b*
differential diagnosis of, 797*b*
indications for referral or hospitalization for, 798
life span considerations with, 797
management of, 796-797
pathophysiology of, 794-795
physical examination for, 795-796
Occult bleeding, 677*b*
Occult fracture, 907-908
Occupational respiratory diseases, 166-169
complications of, 169
diagnostics for, 168*b*
indications for referral or hospitalization for, 169
life span considerations with, 169
management of, 169
Occupational Safety and Health Administration (OSHA)
on chemical exposure, 208
workplace surveillance of, 165
Occupational/environmental health
assessment of, 163-170
primary care role in, 164-166
regulatory agency and other requirements in, 169-170
Octreotide, 1073
Ocular alignment, 328-329
Ocular disorders. *see also* Visual disturbances
traumatic, 355-358
clinical presentation of, 357, 357*f*
complications of, 358
definition of, 355
diagnostics for, 357-358, 358*b*
differential diagnosis of, 358, 358*b*
Ocular disorders *(Continued)*
epidemiology of, 355-356
life span considerations with, 358
management of, 358
manifestations of, 355*b*
pathophysiology of, 356-357
physical examination for, 357
referral, indications of, 358
terminology of, 356*t*
Ocular pain, 334-335
Odynophagia, 671
Office emergencies
evolution of preparedness, 188
mitigation phase, 189
preparedness phase of, 189
preparing primary care office for small-scale emergencies and disasters, 188-189
primary care and, 190
recovery phase of, 189
response phase of, 189
surge capacity and, 190
Office Medication Administration Safety, 50
Ofloxacin, 779*t*, 789*b*
Ointments, 243-244, 244*t*
Olecranon. *see* Elbow joint
Olfactory nerve (CN I), 393
Oligoastrocytoma, 1066*t*
Oligodendroglioma, 1066*t*
Olmesartan, 576*t*-582*t*
Omalizumab, 432*f*, 433*t*-435*t*, 440-441
OMIM (Online Mendelian Inheritance in Man), 30
Oncologic emergency, 1325-1326, 1330
immediate ED referral or specialist consultation for, 1330
Oncology complications, 1330-1335
hypercalcemia, 1332-1333
hyperuricemia, 1333-1334
malignant spinal cord compression, 1331-1332, 1331*b*-1332*b*
superior vena cava syndrome, 1330-1331, 1330*b*-1331*b*
syndrome of inappropriate antidiuretic hormone, 1334-1335, 1334*b*-1335*b*
tumor lysis syndrome, 1333-1334, 1334*b*
Oncology pain, 1335-1341
clinical presentation of, 1336
complications of, 1339-1340
definition and epidemiology of, 1335
diagnostics for, 1337, 1337*b*
differential diagnosis of, 1337, 1337*b*
indications for referral or hospitalization for, 1340-1341
management of, 1337-1339, 1338*b*, 1340*t*
pathophysiology of, 1335-1336
physical examination for, 1337
Oncology patients
collaborative management of, 1325-1326
management issues in, 1325-1326
Oncology symptoms, patient management of, 1341-1345
anorexia, 1342, 1344
constipation, 1341, 1344
diarrhea, 1341-1342, 1344
mucositis, 1342, 1344-1345
nausea and vomiting, 1341, 1343-1344, 1343*b*
xerostomia, 1342, 1345
Oncology team, 1325-1326
Oncology treatment
basic principles of, 1326-1330
chemotherapy. *see* Chemotherapy
radiation. *see* Radiation therapy
Onychocryptosis (ingrown toenail), 903*t*-905*t*
Onychomycosis, 294-296
clinical presentation of, 294
complications of, 295
definition and epidemiology of, 294
in dermatophyte infections, 279-281
diagnostics for, 294, 294*b*
differential diagnosis of, 295, 295*b*, 295*f*
indications for referral or hospitalization for, 295-296
management of, 295
pathophysiology of, 294
physical examination for, 294

Oozing, 247*t*
Open globe injury, 356*t*
Open surgical repair, for abdominal aortic aneurysm, 513
Ophthalmic zoster, 284, 285*f*
Opiates, 1188
  agonist, for infertility, 848
  for chronic cough, 456
Opioid Risk Tool (ORT), 51
Opioids, 1371-1372
  for chronic pain, 1188
  conversion table for, 1340*t*
  defined, 1338
  fear of, 1338-1339, 1338*b*
  for fibromyalgia syndrome, 926-927
  for low back pain, 958
  naloxone for, 226
Optic disk, 331
Optic neuritis, 334*t*, 391
Oral cavity
  candidal infections of, 408-409
  carcinoma of, 408
Oral clotrimazole troches, 408
Oral communication, 28
Oral contraceptives
  androgenic, 1102
  for dysmenorrhea, 824
  hormones in, 831-833
  progestin-only (minipills), 833
  side effects of, 832
Oral glucose tolerance test (OGTT), 1079
  for acromegaly, 1072
Oral infections, 406-409
  aphthous ulcers, 407
  Candida albicans, 406
  clinical presentation of, 407
  complications of, 408-409
  definition and epidemiology of, 406
  diagnostics for, 407-408, 407*b*
  differential diagnosis of, 408, 408*b*
  indications for referral or hospitalization for, 409
  management of, 408
  pathophysiology of, 406-407
  physical examination for, 407
  stomatitis, 406
  viral, herpes simplex virus types I and II, 406
Oral route, loss of, in pain, 107
Oral therapy, for pelvic inflammatory disease, 874*b*
Orbital cellulitis, 265, 350-353
  clinical presentation and physical examination of, 351-352, 351*f*
  complications of, 353
  definition and epidemiology of, 350-351
  diagnostics for, 352, 352*b*
  differential diagnosis of, 352, 352*b*
  indications for referral or hospitalization for, 353
  life span considerations with, 352
  management of, 352
  pathophysiology of, 351
Orbital infection, 391
Orchitis, 764-767, 768*b*
Organic neuropathic pain, 1186
Organization centered interventions, 29
Organizational support, chronic care model and, 19
Orgasmic disorders
  female, 875-876
  male, 756-758
Oritavancin, 264
Orlistat (Xenical), 121, 1130
Orogastric lavage, 210
Orogenital contact, 409
Orthopedic stabilization, 911-912
Orthopnea, and heart failure, 563
Orthostatic hypotension, 221
  non-neurogenic causes of, 222
Orthostatic measurements, 222
Oseltamivir, 490
Osler nodes, 588
Osmotic demyelination syndrome (ODS), 1118
Osmotic diarrhea, 648, 648*f*
Osmotic laxatives, 646
Ospemifene (Osphena), for menopause, 865
Osteoarthritis (OA), 976-980
  clinical presentation and physical examination for, 977
  complications of, 979
  definition and epidemiology of, 976-977
  diagnostics for, 977, 977*b*
  differential diagnosis for, 977, 977*b*
  future directions in, 979
  of hip joint, 938
  indications for referral or hospitalization for, 979
  joints commonly affected by, 977
  of knee, 952
  life span considerations with, 979
  management of, 977-979
    complementary approaches in, 979
    intra-articular approaches in, 978
    medications in, 978
    nonpharmacologic, 978-979
    pharmacologic, 977-978
    surgery in, 979
  obesity and, 115
  pathophysiology of, 977
Osteochondritis dissecans, 901
Osteomyelitis, 980-985
  classification of, 980-981, 980*t*, 981*b*
  clinical presentation of, 981
  complications of, 984-985
  definition and epidemiology of, 980-981
  diagnostics for, 982-983, 983*b*
  differential diagnosis for, 983, 983*b*
  of frontal bone, 391
  immediate emergency department referral for, 983-984
  life span considerations with, 984
  management of, 983-984, 984*t*
  pathophysiology of, 981
  physical examination for, 981-982, 982*b*
  vertebral, 981-982, 984
Osteonecrosis
  of hip joint, 938
  of jaw, bisphosphonate-related, 964-965
Osteopenia, 1155
Osteoporosis, 960-967
  clinical presentation of, 960-961
  complications of, 966-967
  definition and epidemiology of, 960
  diagnostics for, 961-962, 962*b*
  differential diagnosis for, 962, 962*b*
  indications for referral or hospitalization for, 967
  life span considerations with, 966
  management of, 962-966
    with specialists, 966
  in menopause, 856-857
  nonhormonal agents for, 858*b*
  pathophysiology of, 960
  physical examination for, 961
  prevention and treatment interventions for, 858*b*
  risk factors for, 857*b*, 960, 961*b*
  screening for, 149*t*-152*t*
  with systemic lupus erythematosus, 1172, 1174-1175
Osteosarcoma, 906
Otitis externa, 371-373
  clinical presentation of, 371
  complications of, 372
  definition and epidemiology of, 371
  diagnostics in, 371, 371*b*
  differential diagnosis of, 372, 372*b*
  indications for referral or hospitalization for, 372, 373*f*
  life span considerations with, 372
  management of, 372
  pathophysiology of, 371
  physical examination for, 371
Otitis media, 373-377
  clinical presentation and physical examination for, 373-374
  complications of, 376
  definition and epidemiology of, 373
  diagnostics for, 374-375, 375*b*
  differential diagnosis of, 375, 376*b*
  indications for referral or hospitalization for, 376
  life span considerations with, 376
  management of, 375-376, 375*t*
  pathophysiology of, 373
Otoconia, 1027
Otolaryngology referral, of smell and taste disturbances, 394
Ototoxic antibiotics, for tympanic membrane perforation, 377
Outcomes, health, prenatal, 65
Out-of-center sleep testing (OCST), 1214
Outpatient parenteral antibiotic therapy (OPAT), for infective endocarditis, 596
OVA1, 841
Ovarian cancer, 839-841
  in menopause, 859
Ovary(ies), 800, 846, 850. *see also* Polycystic ovary syndrome (PCOS)
  hirsutism and, 1100
Overflow incontinence, 732, 733*b*, 735
Overnight sleep testing, 1213-1214
Overt bleeding, 677*b*
Ovulation, 847
Ovulatory dysfunctions, 846-848
Oxacillin, for endocarditis, 591*t*-595*t*
Oxcarbazepine, 1061*t*-1062*t*
  for trigeminal neuralgia, 1064, 1065*t*
Oxiconazole (Oxistat), 281*t*
Oxidative stress, 1005
Oxybutynin chloride (Ditropan), 735
Oxygen
  saturation. *see* Pulse oximetry
  supplemental
    criteria for, 460-461, 461*b*
    for dyspnea, 471
  therapy, with COPD, 460
Oxygenation, for chemical exposure, 210

P

p24 antigen, 1235
Pacemaker, temporary, 528
Paget disease
  of bone, 967-970
    clinical presentation of, 967
    complications of, 970
    definition and epidemiology of, 967
    diagnostics for, 968, 968*b*
    differential diagnosis for, 968, 968*b*
    indications for referral or hospitalization for, 970
    life span considerations with, 970
    management of, 968-970, 968*b*, 969*t*
    pathophysiology of, 967
    physical examination for, 968
  of nipple, 813-814
    clinical presentation of, 813
    diagnostics for, 813, 813*b*
    differential diagnosis of, 813, 814*b*
    eczema *versus*, 814*t*
    management of, 814
    pathophysiology of, 813
    physical examination for, 813
    referral for, indication for, 814
  vulvar, 842
Pain. *see also* Chronic pain
  ankle and foot, 897-903
  bone, 908, 912
  of cancer. *see* Oncology pain
  categories of, 1186
  chest. *see* Chest pain
  chronic, 1186-1189
  elbow, 920-924
  eyes, 334-335, 335*t*
  face, 1064
  hand and wrist, 932-936
  hip, 936-940
  joint, primary care and, 18
  knee, 946-952
  life span considerations with, 107
  management of, 107
    guidelines for, 51*t*
  multiple sclerosis and, 1046*t*-1047*t*
  neck, 970-976
  neuropathic, 1336
  nociceptive, 1186
  in palliative care, 106-107
  pancreas, 715, 719
  patellofemoral, 951-952
  pelvic, 817-821

Pain *(Continued)*
peripheral neuropathy, 1092
pleuritic, 481, 484
referred, 973*b*
scrotal, 763
shoulder, 985-993
spine, 1155
vulva, 889
Palliative care, 94-96
access to care, 95
definition and epidemiology of, 94
symptom management in, 96-108
underlying tenets of, 94*b*
web resources, 95*b*
Palliative sedation
for management of intractable symptoms in patients near death, 108
terminal delirium, 99*t*
Palmar fibrosis
clinical presentation of, 933
diagnostics and differential diagnosis for, 934
management of, 935
physical examination for, 933
Palpation technique, 543*b*
Palpitations, 516-517
Pamidronate (Aredia), 969*t*
Pancreatic insufficiency, chronic diarrhea and, 653
Pancreatic pseudocyst, 720-722
clinical presentation of, 721
complications of, 721
definition and epidemiology of, 720
diagnostics for, 721, 721*b*
differential diagnosis of, 721, 721*b*
indications for referral or hospitalization for, 721-722
interdisciplinary management of, 721
management of, 721
pathophysiology of, 720
Pancreatitis, 713-722
acute, 713-717
causes of, 713*b*
clinical presentation of, 715
complications of, 717
definition and epidemiology of, 713-714, 713*b*-714*b*
diagnostics for, 715-716, 716*b*
differential diagnosis of, 716, 716*b*
factors associated with, 714*b*
indications for referral or hospitalization for, 717
management of, 716-717
pathophysiology of, 714-715
physical examination for, 715
chronic, 717-720
causes of, 717, 718*b*
clinical presentation of, 718
complications of, 720
definition and epidemiology of, 717-718
diagnostics for, 718-719, 719*b*
differential diagnosis of, 719
indications for referral or hospitalization for, 720
life span considerations with, 720
management of, 719-720
pathophysiology of, 718
physical examination for, 718
surgical interventions of, 719-720
Pancytopenia, 1311
Panic attack, 1350*b*
Papanicolaou (Pap) test
abnormalities of, 868-871
clinical presentation and physical examination of, 869
definition and epidemiology of, 868
diagnostics for, 869
life span considerations with, 869-870
management of, 869, 870*b*
pathophysiology of, 868-869
HPV and, 868
techniques of, 869
Papillomas
inverted nasal, 395
oral infections from, 408
Papule, 238*f*
Paramyxovirus, and mumps, 409
Paraneoplastic syndromes, 1330-1335
Parasitic infestations, in pruritus, 300*b*
Parasomnias, 1217-1218, 1217*b*
Parathyroid gland disorders, 1131-1135
clinical presentation of, 1132-1133
complications of, 1135
definition and epidemiology of, 1131-1132
diagnostics for, 1133-1134, 1133*b*
differential diagnosis for, 1134, 1134*b*
indications for referral or hospitalization for, 1135
life span considerations with, 1135
management of, 1134-1135
pathophysiology of, 1132
physical examination for, 1133
Parathyroid hormone (PTH), 858*b*, 1104, 1131
Parathyroidectomy, 1134
Parent-adolescent communication, 882
Parenteral therapy, for pelvic inflammatory disease, 874*b*
Paresthesias, multiple sclerosis and, 1046*t*-1047*t*
Parietal pain, 623
Parkinson disease, 1050-1054
clinical presentation of, 1050-1051
complications and comorbid problems of, 1053-1054
definition and epidemiology of, 1050
diagnostics for, 1051, 1051*b*
differential diagnosis for, 1051, 1052*b*
dysphagia with, 665
indications for referral or hospitalization for, 1053
management of, 1051-1053
pharmacotherapy in, 1052-1053
surgery in, 1053
pathophysiology of, 1050
physical examination for, 1051
risk factors for, 1050*b*
Paronychial infections, 293-294
acute, 293-294
chronic, 294
clinical presentation and physical examination of, 293
complications of, 294
definition and epidemiology of, 293
diagnostics for, 293, 293*b*
differential diagnosis of, 293, 293*b*
indications for referral or hospitalization for, 294
life span considerations with, 294
management of, 293-294
pathophysiology of, 293
Parotid gland, 409
Parotid swelling, 1207
Parotitis, 409-411
acute suppurative, 409
clinical presentation of, 410
complications of, 411, 411*b*
definition and epidemiology of, 409
diagnostics for, 410, 410*b*
differential diagnosis for, 410, 410*b*
indications for referral or hospitalization for, 411
management of, 410-411
pathophysiology of, 409-410
physical examination for, 410
viral (mumps). *see* Mumps
Paroxetine, 865, 1360*t*-1362*t*
Paroxysmal nocturnal dyspnea, heart failure and, 563
Paroxysmal supraventricular tachycardia, 520, 525
Partial thromboplastin time (PTT), 607, 641
Partner education, for sexual dysfunction (male), 763
Paste, 244*t*
Patellofemoral pain syndrome (PFPS), 951-952
Patient adherence and compliance, 47
Patient barriers, identification and treatment of, 142
Patient care, LGBTQ, 59-65
access to care, 61
barriers to care, 61-62
cancer screening, 63
discuss with health care providers, 63*b*
goals of care, 60-61
human immunodeficiency virus, 63-64
Patient care, LGBTQ *(Continued)*
human papillomavirus, 63
issues with health screening, 64
life span considerations, 64-65
risky behavior and, 62
sexual reassignment intervention and, 64
specific health screenings, 62-64
Patient-centered care, 45
Patient-centered environment, 30
Patient-centered interventions, 29
Patient-centered medical home, 21, 22*b*
Patient denial of victimization, intimate partner violence and, 144
Patient dismissal, 47
Patient handoffs, 47
Patient portals, 48-49
Patient Protection and Affordable Care Act (PPACA), 21-22
Peak expiratory flow (PEF) measurements, in asthma, 428, 441
Peak flow meters, 445*b*
Pedigrees, 34-35
in AR disorders, 37
four-generation, 34*f*, 36*f*
fictitious, 37*f*-38*f*, 40*f*
history gathering for, 36
standardized symbol, 35*f*
systematic nature of, 35
Pegvisomant, 1073
Pelvic inflammatory disease (PID), 871-875
clinical presentation of, 872
complications of, 875
definition and epidemiology of, 871-872
diagnostics for, 873, 873*b*
differential diagnosis of, 873, 873*b*
indications for referral or hospitalization for, 875
management of, 873-875, 874*b*
pathophysiology of, 872
pelvic pain and, 817
physical examination for, 872-873
risk factors for, 872
Pelvic pain, chronic, 817-821
clinical presentation of, 818, 818*b*
complications of, 821
definition and epidemiology of, 817-818
diagnostics for, 819, 819*b*
differential diagnosis of, 819-820, 820*b*
indications for referral or hospitalization for, 821
life span considerations with, 820-821
management of, 820
pathophysiology of, 818
physical examination for, 818-819
populations risk of, 817-818
Penetrating injury, 356*t*
Penicillin G, for endocarditis, 591*t*-595*t*
Penicillins
for pharyngitis/tonsillitis, 415
for syphilis, 789*b*
Penile prosthesis, 762
Pentoxifylline, 603
Peppermint oil, 704
Peptic ulcer disease (PUD), 678, 682, 728-730
clinical presentation of, 728
complications of, 730
definition and epidemiology of, 728
diagnostics for, 728-729, 729*b*
differential diagnosis of, 729, 729*b*
indications for referral or hospitalization for, 730
management of, 729-730, 729*t*
pathophysiology of, 728
perforated. *see* Perforated peptic ulcer
physical examination for, 728
prevalence of, 626-627
Perception of dyspnea (POD), and asthma, 441
Perceptual organization tests, 1000*b*
Percutaneous nephrolithotomy (PCNL), 775
Perforated peptic ulcer, 626-627
clinical presentation of, 627
complications of, 627
definition and epidemiology of, 626-627
diagnostics for, 627, 627*b*
differential diagnosis of, 627, 627*b*
management of, 627
pathophysiology of, 627
physical examination for, 627

Perforating injury, 356*t*
Pericardial friction rub, 542
Pericarditis
chest pain and, 548*t*
with systemic lupus erythematosus, 1171*b*
Perimenopause, 850, 853, 868
Perindopril, 576*t*-582*t*
Periocular pain, 334-335
Periodic limb movements (PLMs), 1211, 1216
Periorbital cellulitis, 265
Peripheral arterial disease (PAD), diabetes and, 317*b*
Peripheral edema, peripheral arterial insufficiency and, 602
Peripheral neuropathy, 603, 1092
Peripheral vascular disease, 1093. *see also* Deep venous thrombosis (DVT)
Peritonitis, 628-629
clinical presentation of, 628
complications of, 629
definition and epidemiology of, 628
diagnostics for, 628, 628*b*
differential diagnosis of, 628, 628*b*
management of, 628-629
pathophysiology of, 628
physical examination for, 628
Peritonsillar abscess, 411-413, 1254
clinical presentation of, 411
complications of, 412
definition and epidemiology of, 411
diagnostics, 412, 412*b*
differential diagnosis for, 412
indications for referral or hospitalization for, 413
life span considerations with, 412
management of, 412
pathophysiology of, 411
physical examination for, 411-412
Peritonsillar cellulitis, 405, 411
Permethrin cream (Elimite), 308
Pernicious anemia, 1287
Persistent Complex Bereavement Disorder, 1355
Persistent proteinuria, 743
Personal history, genetic considerations in, 32-34, 33*b*
Personal preparedness, 135-136
Perspective on life, stress management of, 135
Perspiration. *see* Hyperhidrosis
Pertinent family health information, 36
Pertussis, 419
chronic cough and, 455
vaccination for, 159
Pessaries, 734-735
Petechiae, infective endocarditis and, 588
PFA-100 system, 1299-1300
Phalen's test, 934*f*
Pharmacologic agents, erectile dysfunction and, 759*b*
Pharmacologic rhinitis, 389
Pharmacologic stress testing, 509
Pharmacologic therapy
for hypotension, 223
for infertility, 848-849
for menopause, 861-865
Pharyngitis, 413-416
clinical presentation of, 413-414
complications of, 416
definition and epidemiology of, 413, 413*f*
diagnostics for, 414, 414*b*
differential diagnosis for, 414-415, 415*b*
health promotion for, 416
indications for referral or hospitalization for, 416
life span considerations with, 415-416
management of, 415
pathophysiology of, 413
physical examination for, 414
Phencyclidine (PCP), 1373
Phenobarbital, 440*t*, 1061*t*-1062*t*
acne and, 250*b*
Phenothiazines, 712*b*
Phentermine, 121, 1130
Phenylketonuria, screening for, 149*t*-152*t*
Phenytoin, 440*t*, 1059, 1061*t*-1062*t*, 1065*t*
acne and, 250*b*
Pheochromocytoma
clinical presentation of, 1075
definition and epidemiology of, 1074
diagnostics for, 1075, 1076*b*
differential diagnosis for, 1076, 1076*b*
hypertension and, 571, 572*t*-573*t*
management of, 1076
pathophysiology of, 1074-1075
physical examination for, 1075
Phlebitis, 606
Phlebotonics, 631
Phonophobia, 1031
Phosphodiesterase inhibitors, for pulmonary hypertension, 498, 499*t*
Phosphodiesterase type 5 (PDE5) inhibitors, 761, 761*t*
Phosphodiesterase-4 inhibitors, for COPD, 462*t*-463*t*, 464
Phosphorus, 754
Photochemotherapy, for vitiligo, 298
Photophobia, 1031
in ocular pain, 335*t*
Photopsia, 333
Photosensitivity, 274*t*
with systemic lupus erythematosus, 1171*b*
Phototherapy, for psoriasis, 303
Physical abuse, pelvic pain and, 817
Physical development, 54-55
Physical examination
of adolescent, 58
for dehydration, 89
for falls, 90
in lifestyle management, 127
with obesity, 115-116
in pregnancy, 66*t*-67*t*, 70
of preparticipation sports physical, 186-187
for presurgical clearance, 182
for workplace exposure, 168
Physical inactivity, stroke and, 531
Physical therapy (PT)
for incontinence, 734
for low back pain, 957-958
for neck pain, 974-975
for shoulder pain, 992
Physician consultation
in animal bites, 255
for preparticipation sports physical, 187
Physician Orders for Life-Sustaining Treatment (POLST), 86
Pigmentation changes. *see* Vitiligo
Pindolol, 576*t*-582*t*
Pinguecula, 332*t*-333*t*, 353-355
clinical presentation of, 353
definition and epidemiology of, 353
diagnostics for, 354, 354*b*
differential diagnosis of, 354, 354*b*
management of, 354
pathophysiology of, 353
physical examination of, 353-354, 354*f*
referral, indications of, 354-355
Pioglitazone, 1084-1085
Pirbuterol, 435*t*-436*t*
Pirbuterol acetate, 462*t*-463*t*
Piriform syndrome, 819
Pitavastatin (Livalo), 1124*t*-1125*t*
Pituitary gland, in acromegaly, 1071
Pituitary hormones, 799. *see also specific hormones*
hirsutism and, 1100-1101
Pityrosporum orbiculare, 282
Placebos, in research, 8
Placenta previa, 73
Placental abruption, 73
Plantar fasciitis, 901-902
clinical presentation of, 901-902
complications of, 902
definition and epidemiology of, 901
diagnostics for, 902, 902*b*
differential diagnosis of, 902, 902*b*
indications for referral or hospitalization for, 902
management of, 902
pathophysiology of, 901
physical examination for, 902
Plantar warts, 315-316, 903*t*-905*t*
Plaque, 238*f*
rupture of, 539
Plasma exchange (PE), for Guillain-Barré syndrome, 1030
Plasma viral load, 1236
Platelet count, 1299
Pleomorphic adenoma (PA), 400
Pleura, 479-480
Pleural biopsy, for pleural effusions, 482
Pleural effusions, 479-485
complications of, 483
congestive heart failure and, 481
definition and epidemiology of, 479-480
diagnostics for, 481-482, 482*b*
differential diagnosis, 482-483, 483*b*
exudative, 481
heart failure and, 563
indications for referral or hospitalization for, 483
malignant, 480-481
management of, 483
pathophysiology of, 480-481
physical examination for, 481
potential causes of, 480*b*
transudative, 481
Pleural friction rub, 484
Pleurisy, 479-485
clinical presentation of, 483-484
complications of, 485
definition and epidemiology of, 483
diagnostics for, 484, 484*b*
differential diagnosis for, 484-485, 484*b*
indications for referral or hospitalization for, 485
management of, 485
pathophysiology of, 483
physical examination for, 484
Pleuritic inflammation, pleurisy and, 484
Pleuritis, 483
with systemic lupus erythematosus, 1171*b*
Pneumococcal vaccine, 159, 161*t*-162*t*, 1040
Pneumocystis carinii pneumonia, 397
Pneumonia, 418, 485-491
atypical syndromes in, 487-488
bacterial syndromes in, 487
chest pain and, 548*t*
clinical presentation and physical examination of, 485
community-acquired, 485
epidemiologic characteristics related to, 486*t*
complications of, 490
definition and epidemiology of, 485
diagnostics for, 488-489, 489*b*
differential diagnosis of, 489, 489*b*
health care-associated, 485
hospital-acquired, 485
indications for referral and hospitalization for, 490-491
life span considerations with, 490
management of, 489-490
pathophysiology of, 485-486
patient and family eduction for, 491
recommendations for, 489
typical, 485-486
ventilator-associated, 485
Pneumothorax, 449, 491-493
chest pain and, 448, 548*t*
clinical presentation of, 491-492
complications of, 493
definition and epidemiology of, 491
diagnostics for, 492, 492*b*
differential diagnosis of, 492, 492*b*
iatrogenic, 491
indications for referral or hospitalization for, 493
life span considerations with, 493
management of, 492-493
pathophysiology of, 491
physical examination for, 492
secondary, 491, 493
Point of maximum impulse (PMI), 542
displaced, in heart failure, 560*t*
palpation of, 517
Poison control center personnel, on chemical exposure, 210
Poisoning, 224-226
clinical presentation of, 224-225
definition of, 224
diagnostics for, 225, 225*b*
differential diagnosis of, 225, 225*b*

Poisoning *(Continued)*
epidemiology of, 224
initial stabilization and management of, 225-226
pathophysiology of, 224
physical examination for, 225
prevention and patient education of, 226
POLICE therapy. *see* Protection, optimal loading, ice, compression, and elevation (POLICE) therapy
Polyarteritis nodosa (PAN), 1177
Polycarbophil (FiberCon), 646
Polycystic ovary syndrome (PCOS), 117*t*, 1088, 1097
Polydipsia, 1119
Polyethylene glycol (PEG), 646
Polygenic obesity, 112
Polymyalgia rheumatica (PMR), 1159-1164
classification criteria for, 1160, 1160*t*
clinical presentation of, 1160
complications of, 1161
definition and epidemiology of, 1159-1160
diagnostics for, 1160
differential diagnosis for, 1161
giant cell arteritis and, 1161
indications for referral for, 1161
management of, 1161
pathophysiology of, 1160
Polypharmacy
consequences of, 87
definition and etiology of, 87
delirium and, 1017
in the elderly, 87
management of, 87
pathophysiology of, 87
Polyps
in colon, 726-727
in nose, 394-397
Polyunsaturated fats, 1121
Popliteal aneurysms, 605
Popliteal cysts, 952
Population disease management, 22
Population health, 22
Population-based care
chronic care model in, 19-21, 21*f*
current challenges of, 19
solutions to, 19
management of, 21-23
preparing for primary care practice of future, 23-25
for primary care providers, 19-25
Portal hypertension, 640
Portuguese man-of-war, 1185
Positional nystagmus testing, 1025*b*
Positive airway pressure (PAP), 1214
Positron emission tomography (PET)
with fluorodeoxyglucose, 1137
for vasculitis, 1178-1179
Positron emission tomography-computed tomography (PET/CT) scan
for heart failure, 561
for unknown primary carcinoma, 1346-1347
Postabortion stress syndrome, 882
Postcoital contraception, 834-835
Posterior epistaxis, management of, 381
Posthepatic jaundice, 705
Postherpetic neuralgia (PHN), 284-286
Postinfectious cough, 455
Post-Lyme disease syndrome, 1257
Postpolio syndrome, fatigue and, 1192
Post-thrombotic syndrome (PTS), 495, 608, 1306
Post-traumatic stress disorder (PTSD), 1349
signs of, 44
Postural adjustments, for dysphagia, 668*t*-669*t*
Postural orthostatic tachycardia syndrome (POTS), 222
Posture
Parkinson disease and, 1051
pelvic pain and, 817-818
Postvoid residual (PVR), 733
Potassium, 1108
Potassium hydroxide (KOH)
microscopy preparation, 280
stain, 239*b*
Potassium-sparing diuretics, 566*t*, 576*t*-582*t*
Powder, 244*t*
Power analysis, in research, 10
Power and control, violence perspectives and, 141-142
PPACA. *see* Patient Protection and Affordable Care Act (PPACA)
PQRST mnemonic, 1187
Pramipexole (Mirapex), 1052
Pramlintide (Symlin), 1084
Pranlukast, 439-440
Pravastatin (Pravachol), 1124*t*-1125*t*
Prayer, stress management of, 135
Prazosin, 576*t*-582*t*
Precachexia, 1219
Prednicarbate, 244*t*
Prednisone/prednisolone, 433*t*-436*t*, 462*t*-463*t*, 464
for Bell palsy, 1009
for giant cell arteritis, 1163
for polymyalgia rheumatica, 1161
for systemic lupus erythematosus, 1174*t*
Preeclampsia, 75*t*
Pre-exposure prophylaxis (PrEP), for HIV infection, 1240-1241
Pregabalin, 926*t*, 1061*t*-1062*t*, 1193-1194
Pregnancy, 65-78
activity during, 70
in adolescent, 54
after bariatric surgery, 124
asthma in, 74-75, 74*t*
asthma management during, 443
cerebrovascular events in, 1015
common problems in, 70-73
constipation in, 72-73
crisis, 881-882
diabetes and, 1086-1088, 1086*b*-1087*b*
diagnosis of, 66-68
health history in, 68-69, 68*t*
hirsutism and, 1101
hypertension and, 75-76, 572*t*-573*t*
infections in, 71*t*
medical conditions in, 74-78
nutrition and weight gain in, 69, 69*t*
postpartum thyroiditis in, 1145
seizure disorders and, 1060-1062
with systemic lupus erythematosus, 1175
thyroid disease in, 1150-1151
unplanned, 879-883
care plan for, 882
clinical presentation of, 880
complications of, 882
counseling for, 881-882
definition and epidemiology of, 879-880
life span considerations with, 882
management of, 881-882
UTI treatment during, 781*t*
West Nile virus and, 1276
Pregnancy rhinitis, 379
Pregnancy test, for presurgical clearance, 182*t*
Prehepatic jaundice, 705
Prehypertension, alternative therapy for, 16
Premature atrial contractions (PACs), 521, 522*f*, 526
Premature junctional contractions, 522, 526
Premature ovarian failure, 851*t*
Premature ventricular contractions (PVC), 522, 522*f*
Prenatal care, 65-78
content and timing of, 66*t*-67*t*
delivery of, 66
goals of, 65
provider checklist for, 79*b*
use of, 66
Prenatal visit, content of, 66-70
Preoperative cardiac evaluation, in presurgical clearance, 184*t*
Preoperative management, after bariatric surgery, 124
Preparticipation physical evaluation (PPE), 58
Prepatellar bursa, 917*f*
Prepatellar bursitis, 952
Presbycusis, 364
Prescribe responsibly, practitioner's duty, 50
Prescription abuse, in college health, 173
Prescription Drug Monitoring Program (PDMP), 51
Prescription Pad Security, 50
Preseptal cellulitis, 350-353
clinical presentation and physical examination of, 351-352, 351*f*
complications of, 353
definition and epidemiology of, 350-351
diagnostics for, 352, 352*b*
differential diagnosis of, 352, 352*b*
indications for referral or hospitalization for, 353
life span considerations with, 352
management of, 352
pathophysiology of, 351
Pressure ulcers
clinical presentation of, 320
definition and epidemiology of, 317
differential diagnosis of, 321
management of, 322-323
staging of, 318, 318*b*
Presurgical clearance, 181-185
complications with, 183
diagnostics for, 182
differential diagnosis of, 182-183
indications for referral or hospitalization, 183
management of, 183
medication and fasting guidelines of, 183
physical examination for, 182
predictors of cardiac risk in, 184*t*
surgical or perioperative home, 185
tests for, 182*t*
Presyncopal lightheadedness, 1024
Presyncope, 1024
Preterm labor, 73-74
Prevention measures
for acute bronchospasm, 193-194
for cardiac arrest, 207-208
for chemical exposures, 210-211
for electrical injuries, 213
for insect bites and stings, 198
for poisoning, 226
for reptile bites and scorpion stings, 201
for syncope, 233
for tachycardia/tachyarrhythmias, 205
Prevotella species, 398
Priapism, 1292
PRICE therapy. *see* Protection, rest, ice, compression, and elevation (PRICE) therapy
Primary acquired cholesteatoma, 363
Primary adrenal insufficiency. *see* Addison disease
Primary angiitis of the central nervous system (PACNS), 1177
Primary biliary cirrhosis, 640
Primary care
challenges in, LGBTQ patient care, 62
culturally responsive, 27-30
obligations in, 29-30
current forces in, 1-2
in disaster situations, 188, 190
genetics considerations in, 30-42
resources of, 42
geriatric, 84-94
integrated perspective and, 15-18
in large-scale disasters, critical role of, 189
management, in sexual assault, 228-229
new look of, 2
nurse practitioner, 25*b*-27*b*
practice of future, 23-25
provider and, 15-18
routine. *see* Health screening
for small-scale emergencies and disasters, 188-189
and surge capacity, 190
vision of, 3
Primary health care provider, in cancer patients, 1326
Primary HIV infection (PHI), 1233-1234
serologic testing for, 1235
Primary spontaneous pneumothorax (PSP), 491
Primary-progressive multiple sclerosis, 1044*b*
Primidone (Mysoline), 1061*t*-1062*t*
Primordial germ cells (PGCs), 850
Prinzmetal angina, 539
Probenecid, for gout, 931
Probiotics, 646, 704
Prodrome, migraine and, 1031
Professional organizations, 170

Progesterone, 802
for menopause, 852, 865*t*-867*t*
Progesterone creams, for menopause, 860-861
Progestin, in oral contraceptives, 832-833
Progestin-only pills, in oral contraceptives, 833
Progressive-relapsing multiple sclerosis, 1044*b*
Proinflammatory state, 1128
Prolactin, hirsutism and, 1100
Prolactinemia, 799
Proliferative diabetic retinopathy (PDR), 1091
Prolonged fatigue, 1192
Prophylactic antibiotics. *see also specific antibiotics*
for infective endocarditis, 595*b*, 596*t*
for myelodysplastic syndromes, 1322
Propranolol, 576*t*-582*t*, 1033, 1043
Propylthiouracil (PTU), 1143-1144, 1144*t*
Prostacyclin synthase, for pulmonary hypertension, 498
Prostaglandins, dysmenorrhea and, 821
Prostanoids
for pulmonary hypertension, 499*t*
for Raynaud phenomenon, 1165
Prostate cancer, 736-738
clinical presentation of, 736
complications of, 738
definition and epidemiology of, 736
diagnostics and differential diagnosis for, 736-737, 737*b*
indications for referral and hospitalization for, 738
life span considerations with, 737-738
management of, 737
metastasis of, 912
pathophysiology of, 736
physical examination for, 736
screening for, 153*t*-154*t*
Prostate-specific antigen (PSA), 736-737
Prostatitis, 741-743
clinical presentation of, 741
complications of, 743
definition and epidemiology of, 741
diagnostics for, 741-742, 742*b*
differential diagnosis of, 742, 742*b*
indications for referral or hospitalization for, 743
life span considerations with, 743
management of, 742-743
pathophysiology of, 741
physical examination for, 741
Prosthesis, 762
Prosthetic joint infection, 942, 944
Prosthetic valve endocarditis, 585-586, 591*t*-595*t*
Protease inhibitors, 274
Protection, optimal loading, ice, compression, and elevation (POLICE) therapy, 995
Protection, rest, ice, compression, and elevation (PRICE) therapy, 995
Protein excretion, 743
Proteins, dietary, reducing energy intake and, 118
Proteinuria, 743-747
clinical presentation of, 744
common causes of, 744*b*
complications of, 746
definition and epidemiology of, 743-744
diagnostics and differential diagnosis of, 744-746, 745*f*, 746*b*
indications for referral or hospitalization for, 746-747
management of, 746
pathophysiology of, 744
physical examination for, 744
Proteus, 293
Prothrombin gene variant (PT G20210A), 1304
Prothrombin time (PT), 641, 1298, 1300
interpretation of, 1300*b*
Prothrombotic state, 1128
Proton pump inhibitors (PPIs), 447, 671, 673, 674*f*, 675
GI bleeding and, 681
Provocative maneuvers, cervical, 972
Provocative testing, tilt-table test, for cardiac arrhythmias, 519
Pruritus, 299-301
clinical presentation and physical examination of, 299
complications of, 301
Pruritus *(Continued)*
definition and epidemiology of, 299
diagnostics for, 299
differential diagnosis of, 299, 300*b*
of eyes, 335
indications for referral or hospitalization for, 301
life span considerations with, 301
management of, 299-301, 708
pathophysiology of, 299
in skin cancer, 247*t*
Pruritus ani, 633-634
clinical presentation of, 633
complications for, 634
definition and epidemiology of, 633
diagnostics for, 633-634, 634*b*
differential diagnosis, 634, 634*b*
indications for referral or hospitalization for, 634
life span considerations with, 634
management of, 634
pathophysiology of, 633
physical examination for, 633
Pseudoaddiction, 1338
Pseudoaneurysm, 510
Pseudodementia, 1021
Pseudohematuria, 747*b*
Pseudohyponatremia, 1115, 1117
Pseudohypoparathyroidism, 1133
Pseudomonas, 293
culture for, 239*b*
infection of, 982
Pseudomonas aeruginosa, 359, 586
Psoralens plus ultraviolet A (PUVA) light, 298
Psoriasis, 277, 301-304, 888-889
clinical presentation and physical examination of, 302, 302*f*, 889
complications of, 304, 889
definition and epidemiology of, 301
diagnostics for, 302, 889, 889*b*
differential diagnosis of, 302-303, 302*b*, 889, 889*b*
genital, 883
indications for referral or hospitalization for, 889
life span considerations with, 889
management of, 303-304, 889
of nails, 295, 295*f*
pathophysiology of, 301-302, 888-889
referral or hospitalization, indications of, 304
Psoriatic arthritis, 1157-1158
clinical presentation and physical examination of, 302
complications of, 304
definition and epidemiology of, 301
diagnostics for, 302
management of, 303
Psychiatric disorders/diseases
with chest pain, 448-449
that interrupt sleep, 1210*b*, 1211
Psychogenic cough, 455
Psychogenic polydipsia, 1115
Psychological health, low back pain and, 958
Psychological results, after bariatric surgery, 124
Psychological states, in pruritus, 300*b*
Psychological support, for COPD, 465
Psychomotor function tests, 1000*b*
Psychophysiologic insomnia (PPI), 1211
Psychosis, with Parkinson disease, 1053
Psychosocial stress, 114
Psychosocial stressors, fatigue and, 1191
Psychotherapy, for anxiety disorders, 1353
Psychotomimetics, 1373
Psychotropic agents, 704
Psyllium (Metamucil), 646
Pterygium, 332*t*-333*t*, 353-355
clinical presentation of, 353
definition and epidemiology of, 353
diagnostics for, 354, 354*b*
differential diagnosis of, 354, 354*b*
management of, 354
pathophysiology of, 353
physical examination of, 353-354, 354*f*
referral, indications of, 354-355
Ptyalism, 400, 402
Puberty, 54
PUD. *see* Peptic ulcer disease (PUD)
Pulmonary arterial hypertension (PAH), 496
Pulmonary barotrauma, 1184-1185
Pulmonary diseases, with heart failure, 556*b*
Pulmonary embolism, 449, 493-495
clinical presentation of, 494
complications of, 495
in deep venous thrombosis, 608
definition and epidemiology of, 493
diagnosis of, 494-495
diagnostics for, 494, 494*b*
differential diagnosis, 494*b*
heart failure and, 563
hemoptysis and, 473
infective endocarditis and, 588
life span considerations with, 495
management of, 495
pathophysiology of, 493
physical examination for, 494
Pulmonary embolization, acute bronchospasm and, 193
Pulmonary embolus, chest pain and, 548*t*
Pulmonary examination, for preparticipation sports physical, 186
Pulmonary function tests (PFTs), 168
for chronic cough, 453*f*
for presurgical clearance, 182*t*
for sarcoidosis, 501
Pulmonary hypertension, 496-500, 1291
chest pain and, 548*t*
clinical classification of, 497*b*
clinical presentation of, 496-497
complications of, 499
definition and epidemiology of, 496
diagnostics for, 497-498, 498*b*
differential diagnosis, 498
group 1, 496
group 2, 496
group 3, 496
group 4, 496
group 5, 496
indications for referral or hospitalization for, 499
management of, 498-499
pathophysiology of, 496
physical examination for, 497
therapies for, 499*t*
Pulmonary nodules, and lung cancer, 477
Pulmonary rehabilitation, 471
for COPD, 465
Pulse oximetry, 453*f*, 469
for COPD, 459-460
for pneumonia, 488
Pulse rate, exercise levels for, 131
Punch biopsy, 241, 241*f*
Pupil response, 327-328
Purpura, 274*t*, 304-307
clinical presentation of, 304-305
complications of, 306
definition and epidemiology of, 304
diagnostics for, 305, 305*b*
differential diagnosis of, 305-306, 306*b*
indications for referral or hospitalization for, 306
life span considerations with, 306
management of, 306
pathophysiology of, 304
physical examination of, 305, 305*f*
Purulent skin and soft tissue infections
clinical presentation and physical examination of, 262
diagnostics for, 263
differential diagnosis of, 263
pathophysiology of, 262
treatment of, 263-264
Pustule, 238*f*
Pyelonephritis
management of, 781-782
UTI-related, 779
Pyogenic vertebral osteomyelitis, 981-982
Pyramidal tracts, 1040-1041
Pyrexia. *see* Fever
Pyuria, 779

Q

Q waves, 545, 545*f*
Quality-of-life (QOL)
in myelodysplastic syndromes, 1322, 1324
in psoriasis, 301

QuantiFERON-TB Gold In-Tube (QFT-GIT) test, 1264
Quasi-experimental design, 7-8
Queer, definition of, 60
Questioning, definition of, 60
Quinapril, 576*t*-582*t*
Quinolones, 440*t*
Quinupristin-dalfopristin, for endocarditis, 591*t*-595*t*

R

Rabies, 255-257
rad (radiation absorbed dose), 1327
Radial head fractures, 922*t*-923*t*
Radiation therapy, 1327-1328
  for acromegaly, 1073
  for brain tumors, 1068
  side effects of, 1328
Radicular neck pain, 971
Radicular pain, 953
Radiculitis, 1271-1272
Radiculopathy, cervical, 971
Radioallergosorbent tests (RASTs), 385
Radiographically isolated syndrome (RIS), multiple sclerosis, 1044*b*
Radiography (x-rays)
  for inflammatory bowel disease, 694-695
  for rheumatoid arthritis, 1167
  for workplace exposures, 168
Radioiodine therapy, for Graves disease, 1144
Radioiodine uptake, 1143*b*
Radiologic tests, for osteomyelitis, 983
Radionuclide angiography, 505*t*
Radionuclide bone scintigraphy, for neck pain, 972
Radionuclide imaging, of thyroid gland, 1137, 1140
Radiosurgery, 1328
Radiotelemetry capsule, 673
Raloxifene (Evista), 858*b*, 965
Ramelteon, for insomnia, 1212
Ramipril, 576*t*-582*t*
Random selection, 7-8
Randomized clinical trials, in research, 8
Range of motion, cervical, 972
  exercises for, 974
Ranitidine, 729*t*
Ranolazine, 547
Ranson criteria (pancreatitis), 715-716
Rapid antigen detection test (RADT), 414
Rapid Estimate of Adult Literacy in Medicine (REALM) tool, 3-4
Rapid eye movement (REM) sleep, 1209-1210
Rasburicase, 1334
Rash
  in human granulocytotropic anaplasmosis, 1259
  in infectious mononucleosis, 1253
  in rickettsiae, 1261
Raynaud phenomenon, 1164-1166
  clinical presentation of, 1164
  complications of, 1166
  definition and epidemiology of, 1164
  diagnostics for, 1165, 1165*b*
  differential diagnosis for, 1165, 1165*b*
  indications for referral or hospitalization for, 1166
  management of, 1165-1166
  pathophysiology of, 1164, 1164*f*
  physical examination for, 1164-1165
RBC distribution width (RDW), 1280
Reactive arthritis, 1156-1157
Reading comprehension, health literacy of, 28
REALM. *see* Rapid Estimate of Adult Literacy in Medicine (REALM) tool
REALM-SF instrument, 28
Recommended Daily Allowance (RDA), 1222-1223
Recompression chamber, 1183
Reconciliation, high-liability clinical areas and, 50
Rectal bleeding, 695
Recurrent acute decompensated heart failure, 557-558
Red blood cell destruction disorders, 1278
Red blood cell production disorders, 1278
Red eye, 331, 332*t*-333*t*
5α-reductase, hirsutism and, 1101
Reentry mechanism, cardiac, 516
Referral
  for Achilles tendinopathy, 900
  for Achilles tendon rupture, 900
  for acne vulgaris, 252
  for acromegaly, 1073
  for acute arterial insufficiency, 605
  for acute bronchitis, 420
  for acute bronchospasm, 193
  for acute pancreatitis, 717
  for adrenal gland disorders, 1077
  for allergic rhinitis, 387
  for allergy, 394
  for alopecia, 255
  for amenorrhea, 803
  for amyotrophic lateral sclerosis, 1007
  for anaphylaxis, 196
  for animal and human bites, 257
  for ankle sprains, 899
  for ankylosing spondylitis, 1155
  for anorectal abscess or fistula, 635
  for anxiety, 98
  for anxiety disorders, 1353-1354
  for appendicitis, 625
  for arrhythmias, 528
  for asthma, 443
  for atopic dermatitis, 279
  for atrophic vaginitis, 896
  for auricular disorders, 360
  for bacterial vaginosis, 893
  for Bartholin gland cysts and abscesses, 805
  for Bell palsy, 1009-1010
  for benign prostatic hyperplasia, 740
  for bipolar disorders, 1369
  for bleeding disorders (coagulopathies), 1301
  for bone tumors, 913
  for bowel obstruction, 106
  for bradycardia/bradyarrhythmias, 202
  for breast masses, 815-816
  for breast pain, 809
  for bullous pemphigoid, 259
  for burns, 261
  for candidiasis, 284
  for cardiac arrest, 207
  for carotid artery disease, 535-536
  for cataracts, 337
  for cellulitis, 264-265
  for central nervous system infections, 1040
  for cerebrovascular events, 1015
  for cerumen impaction, 362
  for cervical cancer, 844-845
  for chemical exposure, 210
  for chest pain, 449, 450*b*
  for cholelithiasis and cholecystitis, 639
  for cholesteatoma, 364
  for chronic cough, 456, 456*b*
  for chronic pancreatitis, 720
  for chronic pelvic pain, 821
  for chronic rhinosinusitis, 379
  for chronic venous stasis, 609
  for cirrhosis, 643
  for cold injury, 236
  for conjunctivitis, 342-343
  for constipation, 106, 647
  for contact dermatitis, 267, 888
  for COPD, 466-467
  for corneal surface defects, 345, 345*b*
  for corns and calluses, 269
  for coronary artery disease, 554
  for cutaneous herpes, 272
  for dacryocystitis, 350
  for decompression sickness and barotrauma, 1183-1184
  for deep venous thrombosis of lower extremity, 608
  for delirium, 1019
  for dementia, 1023
  for dental abscess, 399
  for depression, 101
  for dermatitis medicamentosa, 275
  for dermatophyte infections, 282
  for diabetes mellitus, 1095
  for diverticulitis, 662
  for diverticulosis, 659
  for dry eye, 348
  for dry skin (xerosis), 277
Referral *(Continued)*
  for dysmenorrhea, 824-825
  for dyspareunia, 827
  for dyspnea, 102
  for ectopic pregnancy, 831
  for eczema and psoriasis, 889
  for elbow pain, 924
  for electrical injuries, 212-213
  for endometrial cancer, 839
  for epiglottitis, 406
  for epistaxis, 381
  for eyelid disorders, 339
  for fatigue, 1196
  for fear, 98
  for fever, 1200
  for fibromyalgia syndrome, 927
  for foreign bodies, ocular surface, 345*b*
  for gastrointestinal disturbances, 1345
  for gastrointestinal hemorrhage, 682
  for genital herpes, 793
  for GERD, 677
  for giant cell arteritis, 1163-1164
  for goiter (simple, nontoxic), 1139
  for gout, 932
  for granulomatosis with polyangiitis, 397
  for Guillain-Barré syndrome (GBS), 1030
  for gynecomastia, 816
  for hand and wrist pain, 935
  for head trauma, 220-221
  for headache, 1037
  for hearing loss, 366
  for heart failure, 568
  for heat-related illness, 235
  for heel (calcaneal) bursitis, 920
  for hematuria, 749
  for hemolytic anemia, 1297
  for hemoptysis, 474
  for hemorrhoids, 632
  for hepatitis, 691
  for herpes zoster, 286
  for herpetic whitlow, 292
  for hidradenitis suppurativa, 288
  for hip pain, 940
  for hirsutism, 1103
  for HIV infection, 1239-1240
  for hyperhidrosis, 289-290
  for hyperkalemia and hypokalemia, 1112
  for hypernatremia, 1114
  for hypertension, 574-575
  for hyperthyroidism, 1145
  for hypocalcemia, 1108
  for hyponatremia, 1119
  for hypotension, 224
  for hypothyroidism, 1148
  for immunodeficiency, 1203-1204
  for incontinence, 736
  for infectious arthritis, 945
  for infectious diarrhea, 1250-1251
  for infectious mononucleosis, 1254
  for infective endocarditis, 596
  for infertility, 849
  for inflammatory bowel disease, 698
  for influenza, 1243
  for insect bites and stings, 198
  for insomnia, 1212
  for intertrigo, 291
  for intracranial tumors, 1069
  for iron deficiency anemia, 1283
  for irritable bowel syndrome, 704-705, 705*b*
  for jaundice, 708
  for knee pain, 948
  in lactation guidance, 83
  for leukemias, 1311
  for lichen planus, 886
  for lichen sclerosus, 884
  for lichen simplex chronicus, 887
  for lipid disorders, 1126
  for low back pain, 959
  for lung cancer, 478-479
  for lymphadenopathy, 1209
  for lymphomas, 1320
  for macrocytic anemia, 1289
  for major depressive disorder, 1364, 1364*b*
  for mastitis, 810-811
  for Meniere disease, 369

Referral *(Continued)*
for meniscus injuries, 951
for metabolic syndrome, 1131
for mitral stenosis, 622
for Morton neuroma, 903
for multiple sclerosis (MS), 1049
for mumps, 411
for myelodysplastic syndromes, 1323
for nasal trauma, 383
for nasal tumors and polyps, 396
for nasolacrimal duct obstruction, 350
for nausea and vomiting, 105, 711-713
for neck pain, 976
for neuropsychological disorders, 1002
for nipple discharge and galactorrhea, 813
for noninfectious diarrhea, 657
for obesity, 125
for obstructive uropathies, 798
for occupational respiratory diseases, 169
for oncology complications, 1335
for oncology pain, 1340-1341
for onychomycosis, 295-296
ophthalmology, 345, 345*b*
for oral infections, 409
for orbital cellulitis, 353
for oropharyngeal dysphagia, 669
for osteoarthritis, 979
for osteochondritis dissecans, 901
for osteomyelitis, 983-984
for osteoporosis, 967
for otitis externa, 372
for otitis media, 376
for ovarian cancer, 841
for Paget disease
of bone, 970
of nipple, 814
for pancreatic pseudocyst, 721-722
for Pap test abnormalities, 870
for parasomnias, 1218
for parathyroid gland disorders, 1135
for Parkinson disease, 1053
for paronychial infections, 294
for parotitis, 411
for pelvic inflammatory disease, 875
for peptic ulcer disease, 730
for peripheral arterial insufficiency, 603-604
for pinguecula, 354-355
for plantar fasciitis, 902
for pleural effusions, 483
for pleurisy, 485
for pneumonia, 490-491
for pneumothorax, 493
for polymyalgia rheumatica, 1161
for preseptal cellulitis, 353
in presurgical clearance, 183
for prostate cancer, 738
for prostatitis, 743
for proteinuria, 746-747
for pruritus, 301
for pruritus ani, 634
psoriasis, 304
for pterygium, 354-355
for purpura, 306
for Raynaud phenomenon, 1166
for renal failure, 755
for reptile bites and scorpion stings, 201
for rheumatoid arthritis, 1170
for salivary gland diseases, 403
for sarcoidosis, 503
for scabies, 308
for schizophrenia, 1381
for seborrheic dermatitis, 310
for seizure disorder, 1063
for sexual assault, 229
for sexual dysfunction
female, 879
male, 762-763
for sexually transmitted infections, 793
for shoulder pain, 993
for sickle cell disease, 1293
for sinusitis, 392
for skin cancer, 248
for sleep-related breathing disorders, 1214
for sleep-related movement disorders, 1216
for smell and taste disturbances, 394
Referral *(Continued)*
for spider bites, 200
for sprains, strains, and fractures, 997
for stasis dermatitis, 311
for substance use disorders, 1376-1377
for syncope, 233
for systemic lupus erythematosus, 1176
for tachycardia/tachyarrhythmias, 205
for testicular disorders, 771
for thalassemia, 1287
for thrombosis disorders (thrombophilia), 1306-1307
for thyroid cancer, 1141
for thyroid nodules, 1141
for tinea versicolor, 282
for tinnitus, 371
for traumatic ocular disorders, 358
for trigeminal neuralgia, 1065-1066
for tuberculosis, 1271
for tumors of small intestine, 726
for tympanic membrane perforation, 377
for unintended weight loss, 1223
for unknown primary carcinoma, 1348
for unplanned pregnancy, 883
for urinary calculi, 776-777
for urinary tract infections, 782
for urticaria, 314
for vaginal cancer, 843
for vasculitis, 1180
for venous stasis ulceration, 610
for vestibular neuritis, 368
for vitiligo, 298
for vulvar cancer, 842
for vulvar vestibulitis syndrome and vulvodynia, 891-892
for vulvovaginal candidiasis, 895
for warts, 316
for West Nile virus, 1276
in wound management, 325
for xerostomia, 103
Referred pain, 623
sources of, 973*b*
Reflex sympathetic dystrophy, 992
Reflexes
as causes of syncope, 231*b*
cervical, 972*t*
vomiting, 709
Regional wall motion abnormalities (RWMAs), 598
Rehabilitation, for shoulder pain, 992
Rehabilitative ultrasound imaging, for low back pain, 957
Reinfection, of Lyme disease, 1257
Reiter syndrome. *see* Reactive arthritis
Relapse, 1369-1370
Relapsing or refractory disease, 1317
Relapsing-remitting multiple sclerosis, 1044*b*
Relative afferent pupillary defect (RAPD), 327-328
Relaxation response, 135
Relaxation therapy, for chronic insomnia, 1212*t*
Release of information, 48
Relizen, for menopause, 860
REM sleep behavior disorder (RBD), 1217
Remnant ablation, with radioactive iodine, for thyroid cancer, 1141
Renal artery stenosis, hypertension and, 571, 572*t*-573*t*
Renal cell carcinoma (RCC), 794-795, 796*b*-798*b*, 797
metastasis of, 912-913
Renal denervation, 575
Renal disorders. *see also specific disorders*
in pruritus, 300*b*
with systemic lupus erythematosus, 1171*b*
Renal failure, 749-756
acute renal failure, 750
cardiovascular management and complications of, 755
from chronic kidney disease, 749-750, 749*t*-750*t*, 752*b*
clinical presentation of, 751-752, 752*b*
complications of, 755
definition and epidemiology of, 749-750, 749*t*-750*t*
diagnostics for, 752-753
Renal failure *(Continued)*
differential diagnosis of, 753, 753*b*
hematologic management and complications of, 755
indications for referral or hospitalization for, 755
infective endocarditis and, 588
life span considerations with, 755-756
management of, 753-755
metabolic complications of, 755
pathophysiology of, 750-751, 751*f*
physical examination for, 752
psychosocial management and complications of, 755
sickle cell disease and, 1292
Renal hematuria, 748
Renal parenchymal disease, hypertension and, 571, 572*t*-573*t*
Renal tubular acidosis (RTA), 773
Renin, 570
Renin-angiotensin-aldosterone (RAAS) system, 557
Reperfusion therapy, for acute ST-segment elevation myocardial infarction, 550
Repetitive brain trauma, 218
Report, in neuropsychological evaluation, 1003
Reproductive hazards, 845-846
Reptile bites and scorpion stings, 200-201
clinical presentation of, 200
definition and epidemiology of, 200
diagnostics for, 200, 201*b*
differential diagnosis of, 200-201
disposition and referral of, 201
initial stabilization and management of, 201
pathophysiology of, 200
physical examination for, 200
prevention and patient education of, 201
Research
blinding of, 8
cause and effect in, 6-8
clinical significance *versus* statistical significance, 11
clinician-researcher partnerships in, 13
description of data and measures of central tendency, 10
descriptive studies and, 6
designs and data analysis methods, 6-8, 7*t*
distribution and error in, 10
evaluating key study parameters of, 8-11, 9*t*
experimental design in, 7, 7*t*
infrastructure, enhancing, 14
initiating collaborations in, 13
merging perspectives in, 13
methods for, 6
normal distribution graph in, 10*f*
placebos in, 8
power analysis in, 10
proposal development for, 14-15
protocol development for, 14-15
question development for, 14-15
random assignment in, 8
random selection, 7-8
randomized clinical trials in, 8
relationships between variables in, 6
standard deviation in, 10
statistical significance (alpha values) in, 10-11
statistics of differences and associations, 11
strategies to form collaborations, 13
translating into clinical practice, 11-13
type I and type II errors in, 9-10
understanding process in, 14-15
Resins, 1124*t*-1125*t*
Resnick's DIAPPERS mnemonic, 732*b*
Resource issues, 14
Respiratory diseases
diagnostics for, 168-169
inhaled noxious substances, 167
management of, 169
occupational, 166-169
complications of, 169
diagnostics for, 168*b*
indications for referral or hospitalization, 169
life span considerations of, 169
management of, 169
patient and family education, 169
Respiratory dysfunction, in ALS, 1007

Respiratory syncytial virus (RSV), 417, 1226
Responsive care, culturally, 29
Rest, ice, compression, and elevation (RICE) therapy, 898-899, 995
Restless legs syndrome (RLS), 1215, 1216*b*
insomnia problems in, 1211
management of, 1216
Reticulocyte count, 1279, 1279*b*
Retina, 330-331
Retinitis, acute febrile, 1274
Retinopathy, 574-575
diabetic, 1091
in sickle cell disease, 1293
Retrograde amnesia, 220
Retropharyngeal abscess, 412
signs and symptoms of, 405
Retrovirus, 1233
Revascularization, for heart failure, 567
Review of symptoms, 600*b*
Revised European-American Lymphoma (REAL), 1314
Rewarming in cold injury, 236
Rh incompatibility, 149*t*-152*t*
screening for, 149*t*-152*t*
Rheumatic disorders, evaluation and management of, 1152-1159
Rheumatoid arthritis (RA), 1166-1170
classification criteria for, 1168*b*
clinical presentation of, 1167
complications of, 1170
composite outcome measures tools for, 1169*b*
definition and epidemiology of, 1166
diagnostics for, 1167-1168, 1168*b*
differential diagnosis for, 1168, 1168*b*
of hip joint, 936-937
indications for referral or hospitalization for, 1170
life span considerations with, 1169-1170
management of, 1168-1169
assessing cardiovascular risk in, 1168
interdisciplinary, 1169
nonpharmacologic treatment for, 1169
pharmacologic agents for, 1168-1169
pathophysiology of, 1166-1167
physical examination for, 1167
poor prognostic signs in, 1169*b*
Rheumatologic diseases
fatigue and, 1191
osteoporosis and, 963*b*
Rheumatologic symptoms, with sarcoidosis, 501
Rheumatology referral, of smell and taste disturbances, 394
Rhinitis, 384-389
allergic. *see* Allergic rhinitis
anatomic, 388
food-or drink-related, 389
idiopathic, 387-388, 388*b*
infectious, 388
medicamentosa, 388-389
other causes of, 388-389
pharmacologic, 389
vasomotor, 387-388, 388*b*
Rhinitis medicamentosa, 379, 388-389
Rhinovirus, 417
Rhipicephalus sanguineus, 1261
Rhizoma coptidis, 17
Rib fracture, chronic cough and, 456
Ribavirin, 1275-1276
RICE therapy. *see* Rest, ice, compression, and elevation (RICE) therapy
Rice water stools, 1247
Rickettsia rickettsii, 1261
Rickettsiae, 1261
Rifampin, 440*t*, 1269
acne and, 250*b*
for endocarditis, 591*t*-595*t*
Rifaximin, 643
Right ventricular outflow tract (RVOT), 527
Right-sided heart catheterization (RHC), purpose of, 497-498
Rigidity, 1051
Riluzole, for ALS, 1006
Ringworm, 279, 280*f*
Rinne test, 365
Risedronate (Actonel), 858*b*, 969*t*
Risk assessment, genetic considerations in, 32, 33*f*
Risk management, 43-53
adverse medical events, disclosure of errors and, 43-44
chaperones, 52-53
curbside consultations and, 52
defending against board of nursing complaint, 44
electronic medical records, 47-49
falls, 51-52, 52*b*
high-liability clinical areas, 50-52
legal documents and, 49-50
managing risk in nursing home, 52
against medical advice, 50
medical malpractice risk management strategies, 45-47
National Practitioner Data Bank, 44
nurse practitioner malpractice claims and, 43
patient request for waiver, write-off or reimbursement of fees for services, 52
policies in, 53
scope of practice, 49
"second victim", 44
social media, 49
staff as patients, 52
surreptitious recording by patients, 49
Telemedicine, 44-45
third-party cases, 50
Risk stratification
in cardiovascular disorders, 509-510
preoperative cardiac, 513-514
Ristocetin cofactor activity, 1302
Rituximab, for vasculitis, 1180
Rivaroxaban, 607
Rivastigmine (Exelon), 1023
Rocky Mountain spotted fever, 1261, 1262*t*
Roflumilast, 464
Ropinirole (Requip), 1052
Rosacea, 250*f*, 251-252, 337-338
Rosenbaum near card, 327
Rosiglitazone, 1084-1085
Rosuvastatin (Crestor), 1124*t*-1125*t*
Rotarix, 1247
RotaTeq, 1247
Rotator cuff, 985
tear or rupture of, 990-991
Rotavirus, in acute gastroenteritis, 1246-1247
Roth spots, 587
Roux-en-Y gastric bypass (RYGB), 123
Rovsing sign, 624
Rupture, eye, 356*t*
Ruptured aortic aneurysm, 629-630. *see also* Abdominal aortic aneurysm
clinical presentation of, 629
complications of, 630
definition and epidemiology of, 629
diagnostics for, 629, 629*b*
differential diagnosis of, 630, 630*b*
management of, 630
pathophysiology of, 629
physical examination for, 629
Rutherford classification, for peripheral arterial insufficiency, 601

S

Sacral nerve stimulation, 646
Sacroiliitis, 1157
Safe administration, vaccine administration, issues with, 155-156
Safety assessment and planning, intimate partner violence and, 144-145
Safety issues
in female college students, 171
in home, 135
in lifestyle management, 135-136
in male college students, 172
medication, 4
occupational, 170
in sprains, strains and fractures, 997-998
travel, 179-180
Salivary gland diseases, 399-403
clinical presentation of, 400-401
complications of, 403
definition and epidemiology of, 399
diagnostics for, 401-402, 401*b*
differential diagnosis of, 402, 402*b*
Salivary gland diseases *(Continued)*
health promotion of, 403
indications for referral or hospitalization for, 403
life span considerations with, 402
management of, 402
pathophysiology of, 399-400
physical examination for, 401
Salivation, increased, dysphagia and, 666*b*
Salmeterol, 441
Salmeterol xinafoate, 462*t*-463*t*
Salmon calcitonin, 1333
Salmonella, 1156
infection, 179
non-*typhi* species, 1248
Salt intake, restriction in, for hypertension, 584
Salt sensitivity, 570
Sample walking program, in lifestyle management, 134*t*
Sarcoidosis, 500-503
clinical features of, 500*t*
clinical presentation and physical examination of, 500-501
complication of, 502, 502*b*
definition and epidemiology of, 500
diagnostics for, 501, 501*b*
differential diagnosis of, 501-502, 501*b*
indications for referral or hospitalization for, 503
life span considerations with, 502
management of, 502
pathophysiology of, 500
staging of, 501
Sarcoma, in bone, 911
Sarcopenia, 1219
Sarcoptes scabiei mite, 307
SARS-CoV, 488
Saturated fats, 1121
Scabies, 197*t*, 307-308
in atopic dermatitis, 278
clinical presentation and physical examination of, 307, 307*f*
complications of, 308
definition and epidemiology of, 307
diagnostics for, 307-308, 308*b*, 308*f*
differential diagnosis of, 308, 308*b*
indications for referral or hospitalization for, 308
management of, 308
pathophysiology of, 307, 307*f*
preparation, 239*b*
Scale, 238*f*
Scaliness, 247*t*
Scalp psoriasis, 303
Scar, 238*f*
acne and, 249-250
Schilling test, 1288
Schirmer test, 347
Schizophrenia
clinical presentation of, 1378
cognitive symptoms of, 1378
complications of, 1381
definition and epidemiology of, 1377
diagnostics for, 1378-1379, 1379*b*
differential diagnosis of, 1379, 1380*b*
indications for referral or hospitalization for, 1381
interdisciplinary management of, 1380-1381
management of, 1379-1381, 1379*t*-1380*t*
negative symptoms of, 1378, 1378*t*
pathophysiology of, 1377-1378
physical examination for, 1378, 1379*t*
positive symptoms of, 1378
Scissor excision, 242
Sclera, 329
Scleritis, 332*t*-333*t*
Sclerotherapy, endoscopic, 681
Scratch testing, of environmental allergies, 215
Scratching, 276, 299. *see also* Itching
Screening, health, issues with, 64
Screening Abdominal Aortic Aneurysms Very Efficiently (SAAAVE) Act, 511-512
Scrotal examination, 766*b*
Scrotal pain, 763
Scuba diving, contraindication for, 1181
Sculpin, sting of, 1185
Seated slump test, 955

Seborrheic dermatitis, 309-310
clinical presentation and physical examination of, 309
complications of, 310
definition and epidemiology of, 309
diagnostics for, 309, 309*b*
differential diagnosis of, 309, 309*b*
indications for referral or hospitalization for, 310
life span considerations with, 310
management of, 309-310
pathophysiology of, 309
patient and family education of, 310
Seborrheic keratoses, 240-241, 247-248, 248*f*
"Second victim", 44
Secondary acquired cholesteatoma, 363
Secondary immunodeficiencies, 1201
Secondary-progressive multiple sclerosis, 1044*b*
Second-degree burns, 260, 319*b*
Secretory diarrhea, 648, 648*f*, 653
Sedentary lifestyle, in lifestyle components, 126
Segmental limb pressures, 602
Seizure disorder, 1054-1063. *see also specific disorders*
acute, initial stabilization and management of, 1058
classification of, 1055-1056, 1055*b*-1056*b*
clinical presentation of, 1056, 1056*t*
complications of, 1063
definition and epidemiology of, 1054
diagnostics for, 1056-1057, 1057*b*
differential diagnosis for, 1057, 1058*b*
indications for referral or hospitalization for, 1063
life span considerations with, 1060-1063
management of, 1058-1060
conservative, 1059
pharmacologic, 1059-1060, 1061*t*-1062*t*
surgical, 1060
pathophysiology of, 1054-1055
physical examination for, 1056
Seizures, brain tumor and, 1067
Selective serotonin reuptake inhibitors (SSRIs)
for anxiety disorders, 1352, 1352*t*
for chronic pain, 1188
for headaches, 1033
for menopause, 865
weight gain and, 113
Selegiline (Eldepryl), 1052
Self-management support, 20-21, 24-25
techniques to encourage, 25
Self-neglect, chronic diarrhea and, 655
Senna, 646
Sensory function tests, 1000*b*
Sentinel node biopsy, 1206-1207
Septic arthritis, 940
of hip, 938
Septic sacroiliitis, 943
Seronegative spondyloarthropathies, 954
Serositis, with systemic lupus erythematosus, 1171*b*
Serotonin, 1031
Serotonin syndrome, 1197*b*, 1198
Serotonin-norepinephrine reuptake inhibitors (SNRIs)
for anxiety disorders, 1352, 1352*t*
for menopause, 865
Sertraline, 1360*t*-1362*t*
Serum testing, for cardiac arrhythmias, 518
^{99m}Tc sestamibi, 507
Severe acute respiratory syndrome (SARS), 417, 1226
Severe aplastic anemia (SAA), 1295
Severe combined immunodeficiency disease (SCID), 1200-1201
treatment of, 1203
Sex chromosomal abnormalities, 68*t*
Sex hormone-binding globulin (SHBG), 1097
Sexual abuse, pelvic pain and, 817
Sexual activity, 756, 759
adolescents/adolescence and, 58
in menopause, 856
in pregnancy, 70
Sexual and gender minorities (SGMs), 59
Sexual assault, 227-230
clinical presentation of, 227
definition and epidemiology of, 227
diagnostics for, 228-229
Sexual assault *(Continued)*
disabled adults and, 229-230
homeless or marginally housed, 230
immigrants, 230
indications for referral or hospitalization for, 229
life span considerations in, 229
male patients and, 229
to older adults, 229
physical examination for, 227-228
population specific, 229-230
Sexual dysfunction
clinical presentation of, 758-759
complications of, 762
definition and epidemiology of, 756-757
with diabetes mellitus, 1093
diagnostics for, 760, 760*b*
differential diagnosis of, 760, 760*b*
female, 875-879
clinical presentation of, 877
complications of, 879
definition and epidemiology of, 875-876
diagnostics for, 877, 877*b*
differential diagnosis of, 877-878, 878*t*
life span considerations with, 879
management of, 878-879
pathophysiology of, 876-877, 876*b*
physical examination for, 877
life span considerations with, 763
male, 756-763. *see also* Erectile dysfunction (ED)
management of, 760-762, 761*t*
medical conditions associated with, 876*b*
medications and, 878*t*
multiple sclerosis and, 1046*t*-1047*t*
pathophysiology of, 757-758
physical examination for, 759-760
referral for, 762-763
Sexual functioning, in menopause, 856
Sexual history, in HIV infection, 1234
Sexual Maturation Scale (SMS), 55
Sexual reassignment intervention, 64
Sexually transmitted diseases (STDs)
screening for, 1238
from sexual assault, 228
Sexually transmitted infections (STIs), 782-784. *see also specific infections*
clinical presentation of, 783, 783*b*
counseling for, 149*t*-152*t*
definition and epidemiology of, 782-783, 783*f*
diagnostics for, 784
history questions for, 783*b*
indications for referral or hospitalization for, 793
interdisciplinary management of, 784, 785*t*-788*t*
life span considerations with, 784
management of, 784, 789*b*
physical examination for, 783, 784*b*
Shave biopsy, 242, 242*f*
Shellfish, in acute gastroenteritis, 1246
Shiga-like toxins (SLTs), 1228, 1245
Shigella, 1156, 1247-1248
Shigella dysenteriae, 1245
Shigella infection, 179
Shingles. *see* Herpes zoster (shingles)
Short-acting inhaled beta$_2$-agonists (SABAs), 432*f*, 435*t*-436*t*, 441
Shoulder bursitis, 914-916
clinical presentation and physical examination of, 914, 914*b*
definition and epidemiology of, 914
diagnostics for, 914, 914*b*-915*b*, 915*f*-917*f*
differential diagnosis of, 914, 914*b*
management of, 915-916
Shoulder girdle and periscapular strengthening exercises, 974
Shoulder joint
anatomy of, 985
arthritis in, 991
aspiration and injection of, 915*b*, 915*f*-917*f*
bursitis of, 990
extrinsic disorders of, 991-992
instability, dislocation, and subluxation of, 991
tendinitis in, 989
trauma to, 991
Shoulder pain, 985-993
assessment form for, 987*f*
clinical presentation of, 986, 987*f*
Shoulder pain *(Continued)*
complications of, 993
definition and epidemiology of, 985
diagnostics for, 988-989, 989*b*
differential diagnosis for, 989-992, 989*b*-990*b*
indications for referral or hospitalization for, 993
life span considerations with, 993
management of, 992-993
pathophysiology of, 985
physical examination for, 986-988, 986*b*, 988*t*
referred, 991
Shoulder socket, 985
Sialadenitis, 409
Sialectasis, 399-400
Sialolithiasis, 399-400
Sialosis, 399-400
Sickle cell anemia, and chest pain, 448
Sickle cell disease, 982, 1290-1293
clinical presentation of, 1290
complications of, 1292-1293
definition and epidemiology of, 1290
diagnostics for, 1290
differential diagnosis of, 1290, 1291*b*
indications for referral or hospitalization for, 1293
life span considerations with, 1291-1292
management of, 1290-1291
pathophysiology of, 1290
physical examination for, 1290
Sickle cell trait, 1304
SIGECAPS mnemonic, 100*b*
Sildenafil (Viagra), 761, 761*t*
Silent myocardial ischemia, 538
management of, 547-549
Silvadene, 261
Silver nitrate, 805
Simvastatin (Zocor), 1124*t*-1125*t*
Single-photon emission computed tomography (SPECT), for low back pain, 956
Sinoatrial exit block, 522, 528
Sinus barotrauma, 1184
Sinus bradycardia, 522, 527-528
Sinus tachycardia, 520, 520*f*, 525
Sinuses
paranasal, 389
Sinuses, CT, 453*f*
Sinusitis, 379, 389-392
clinical presentation of, 389-390
complications of, 391-392
definition and epidemiology of, 389
diagnostics for, 390, 390*b*
differential diagnosis of, 390-391, 390*b*
health promotion of, 392
management of, 391
pathophysiology of, 389
physical examination of, 390
referral or hospitalization, indications of, 392
Sister Mary Joseph node, 1208
Six stages of change, in smoking cessation, 137*t*
Sjögren syndrome
defined, 400
with rheumatoid arthritis, 1167
Skin
assessment of, 237-240
history of, 239
physical examination of, 238*f*, 239-240
associated with aging, 237
disorders of, 237-240. *see also specific disorders*
definition and epidemiology of, 237
pruritic, 300*b*
examination technique, 239*b*
function of, anatomy, structures and, 237
normal flora on, 586
structure of, 243
Skin and soft tissue infections (SSTIs), 261-262
in diabetic patients, 265
of hands, 265
nonpurulent, 262-264
purulent, 262-263
Skin cancer
clinical presentation of, 246
definition and epidemiology of, 245-246
diagnostics for, 246-247, 247*b*

Skin cancer *(Continued)*
differential diagnosis of, 247-248, 248*b*, 248*f*
indications for referral and hospitalization for, 248
management of, 248
pathophysiology of, 246
physical examination for, 246, 247*f*-248*f*
screening for, 245-248
signs of, 247*t*
Skin cancer behavioral counseling, 149*t*-152*t*
Skin exposure, 210
Skin flora, 780
Skin lines, loss of, 247*t*
Skin prick test (SPT), 215
for food allergies, 217
Skin reactions, 274*t*
Skin tears, management of, 322
Skin testing, delayed-type hypersensitivity, 1202
Skin ulcerations, sickle cell disease and, 1292
SLAP lesions, 991
Sleep
in college health, 172
normal, 1209-1210
stress management and, 134-135
Sleep disorders, 1190, 1209-1218. *see also* Breathing disorders, sleep-related
central nervous system hypersomnias in, 1214-1215
with COPD, 466
insomnia and nonrestorative sleep in, 1210-1213
movement-related, 1215-1217
parasomnias in, 1217-1218
Sleep factors, 114
Sleep restriction, for chronic insomnia, 1212*t*
Sleepiness, 1189-1190
Sleepwalking (somnambulism), 1217
Slipped capital femoral epiphysis (SCFE), 937
Small bowel obstruction, 625-626
clinical presentation of, 625
complications of, 626
definition and epidemiology of, 625
diagnostics for, 626, 626*b*
differential diagnosis of, 626, 626*b*
management of, 626
pathophysiology of, 625
physical examination for, 626
Small cell lung cancer (SCLC), 475
management of, 478
Small intestine
bleeding of, 680*b*
infections in, 1243
tumors of, 725-726, 725*b*-726*b*
Smell and taste disturbances, 392-394
clinical presentation of, 393
complications of, 394
definition and epidemiology of, 392
diagnostics for, 393, 393*b*
differential diagnosis of, 393, 393*b*
of geriatrics, 394
indications for referral or hospitalization for, 394
life span considerations with, 394
management of, 393-394
pathophysiology of, 392-393
of pediatrics, 394
physical examination for, 393
Smell and taste specialist, referral to, of smell and taste disturbances, 394
Smoking cessation, 136-140
dyspnea and, 471
effects of nicotine, 136
incorporation of with primary care strategies, 139-140
for lung cancer, 479
modifying the approach, 138
motivation and strategies for, 138*t*
obesity and, 112
pharmacologic interventions, 138-139
pneumothorax and, 493
strategies to help patients quit, 136-140
Smoking/tobacco use, 136, 440*t*
abdominal aortic aneurysm and, 510-511, 515
carotid artery disease and, 530
chronic cough and, 451, 455-456
in college health, 172
Smoking/tobacco use *(Continued)*
COPD and, 457-458
cessation of, 460
coronary artery disease and, 537, 537*t*
hemoptysis and, 472
inflammatory bowel disease and, 693, 693*t*
lipid disorders and, 1123
lung cancer and, 474-475
obesity and, 112
with osteoporosis, 858*b*
pneumothorax and, 491
tuberculosis and, 1271
Snakes, venomous, 200
Snellen chart, 327
visual acuity with, 186
Social development, 55-56
Social media, 49
removal of post, 49
responding to negative comments, 49
threats on, 49
Social support, in grief, 1355
Sodium
in blood, 570
dietary restriction of, for heart failure, 567
serum, 1113
Sodium bicarbonate, for hyperkalemia, 1111
Sodium hyaluronate, for shoulder pain, 993
Sodium polystyrene sulfate, for hyperkalemia, 1111
Sodium-glucose cotransporter-2 (SGLT2) inhibitors, 1085
Soft corn, 268-269
Solifenacin (VESIcare), 735
Solutions, 244
Somatic pain, 1186
Somatomedin C, 1071
Somatostatin (SS), 1071
Sorbitol, for chemical exposure, 210
Sotalol, 527
Sour stomach, 671
Spasticity, multiple sclerosis and, 1046*t*-1047*t*
Specialist consultation
for environmental allergies, 215-216
for osteomyelitis, 983
Spermatocele, 764-767, 770
Spermicides, 835
Spherocytosis, hereditary, 1296
Spider bites, 198-200
definition and epidemiology of, 198-199
diagnostics for, 199, 199*b*
differential diagnosis of, 199, 199*b*
disposition and referral of, 200
history and physical examination, 199
initial stabilization and management of, 199-200
pathophysiology and clinical presentation of, 199
prevention and patient education of, 200
Spinal cord compression (SCC)., 1330
Spinal manipulative therapy (SMT), 957, 975
Spinal mobilization, 957, 975
Spinal support, 967*t*
Spine, pain in, 1155
Spiritual distress, in palliative care, 107-108
Spirometry, 168, 428, 453*f*, 470
Spirometry, with COPD, 459
Spironolactone, 833, 1102-1103
for hypertension, 576*t*-582*t*
Splenic infarction, 1292
Splenomegaly, 1206, 1208
infective endocarditis and, 588
Splinter hemorrhages, and infective endocarditis, 588
Spondylitis, 1157
Spondyloarthropathies, features of, 1153*b*
Spondylolysis, 959
Spontaneous bacterial peritonitis, 642-643
Sports and vehicular safety, 136
Sports physical, preparticipation, 185-187
diagnostics for, 187
history of, 185-186
medical clearance of, 187
physical examination for, 186-187
Sprains, 922*t*-923*t*, 994-998. *see also specific bones and joints*
cervical, 971
clinical presentation of, 994
Sprains *(Continued)*
complications of, 996-997
definition and epidemiology of, 994
diagnostics for, 995*b*
differential diagnosis for, 995, 995*b*
indications for referral or hospitalization for, 997
life span considerations with, 997
management of, 995-996
pathophysiology of, 994
physical examination for, 994
Spurling maneuver, 972
Spurling test, 988*t*, 991-992
Sputum
assessment of, in COPD, 460
in asthma, 429
characteristics of, in various pulmonary disorders, 452*b*
Sputum analysis, for pneumonia, 488
Squames, 237
Squamous cell abnormalities, cervical, 870*b*
Squamous cell carcinoma (SCC)
in auricle, 359
definition and epidemiology of, 245-246
differential diagnosis of, 248*b*
physical examination for, 246, 247*f*
treatment of, 248
in unknown primary carcinoma, 1346
Squamous cell hyperplasia, 886
ST segment, elevations in, 545-547, 545*f*-546*f*
Standard contrast aortography, for abdominal aortic aneurysm, 512
Standard deviation, in research, 10
Standardization, in neuropsychological assessment, 1002-1003
Standards for adult immunization practice, 155
Staphylococcus, 286, 293
culture for, 239*b*
Staphylococcus aureus
in atopic dermatitis, 278
in cellulitis, 262, 264
in conjunctivitis, 341
endocarditis and, 586, 589*b*
in eyelids, 337-338
in eyes, 351
food poisoning, 1249
in intertrigo, 290-291
joints and, 941
methicillin-resistant, 1231
osteomyelitis and, 981, 984*t*
Stasis dermatitis, 310-311
clinical presentation and physical examination of, 310, 310*f*
complications of, 311
definition and epidemiology of, 310
diagnostics for, 310, 311*b*
differential diagnosis of, 311, 311*b*
indications for referral or hospitalization for, 311
management of, 311
pathophysiology of, 310
Statin therapy, 603. *see also specific drugs*
high-intensity, 549-550
for lipid disorders, 1123, 1124*t*-1125*t*
Statistical significance (alpha values), in research, 10-11
Statistics, of differences and associations, 11
Status asthmaticus, 443
Status epilepticus, 1054, 1058, 1058*t*
Steatohepatitis, 686
Steatorrhea, 648
Stem cell transplantation (SCT), 1203
for myelodysplastic syndromes, 1323
Stensen duct, 409-410
Stereotactic body radiation therapy (SBRT), for lung cancer, 478
Stereotypy, 1040*b*
Sterile pyuria, 780
Sterilization, surgical, 836
Steroids
for Bell palsy, 1009
for brain tumors, 1068-1069
hypertension and, 572*t*-573*t*
intranasal, 386
topical, for seborrheic dermatitis, 309
Steroid-sparing effect, 1174
Stimulant laxatives, 646

Stimulators, for menopause, 861
Stimulus control, for chronic insomnia, 1212*t*
Stingray, envenomations of, 1185
Stomach, tumors of, 723-724, 724*b*
Stomatitis, 406
  aphthous, 409
Stone formation. *see* Calculi, urinary
Stool analysis, for chronic diarrhea, 650
Stool diary, 645
Stool tests, 694
Straight leg raise test, 955
Strains, 994-998. *see also specific bones and joints*
  cervical, 971
  clinical presentation of, 994
  complications of, 996-997
  definition and epidemiology of, 994
  diagnostics for, 995*b*
  differential diagnosis for, 995, 995*b*
  indications for referral or hospitalization for, 997
  life span considerations with, 997
  management of, 995-996
  pathophysiology of, 994
  physical examination for, 994
Stratum corneum, 237, 243, 275
STRAW +10 criteria, 851, 852*f*
Streptococcal species, native valve endocarditis and, 585-586
Streptococcus, 293
  culture for, 239*b*
Streptococcus anginosus, 398
Streptococcus bovis, 585, 589*b*
Streptococcus pneumoniae
  acute bronchitis and, 417
  in conjunctivitis, 341
  meningitis and, 1037
Streptococcus pyogenes, 413
  osteomyelitis and, 981
Streptomycin, for endocarditis, 591*t*-595*t*
Stress
  chronic diarrhea and, 655
  defined, 82
  in lifestyle components, 126-127
  management, in lifestyle management, 134-135
  psychosocial, 114
  signs of, 127
Stress fractures, 994
Stress incontinence, 731, 733-734, 733*b*
Stress testing, for cardiac arrhythmias, 518
Stressors, defined, 82
Stretta system, 675
Stroke, 334*t*, 529, 1010
  ischemic, 529
Struvite stones, 773, 776
Study of Women's Health Across the Nation (SWAN) trial, 850
Subacromial bursa, 915*f*
Subacromial bursitis, 989
Subacromial impingement syndrome, 991
Subacute thyroiditis, 1142
Subarachnoid hemorrhage, 1011
Subconjunctival hemorrhage, 332*t*-333*t*
Sublingual therapy, on environmental allergies, 216
Subluxation, shoulder, 991
Submandibular glands, 399-400
Substance abuse
  chronic diarrhea and, 655
  chronic pain and, 1187
  HIV infection and, 1234
Substance P/neurokinin$_1$ antagonists, 712*b*
Substance use disorders, 1369-1377
  clinical presentation and physical examination for, 1374-1375
  definition and epidemiology of, 1369-1370
  diagnostics for, 1375
  indications for referral or hospitalization for, 1376-1377
  major drugs of abuse, 1370-1373
  management of, 1375-1376
  pathophysiology of, 1370-1373
Sudden cardiac death, 207
Suicidal ideation, 1353
Suicide, 1363-1364, 1364*b*
  risk factors, 57*b*
Sulcus sign, 988*t*
Sulfasalazine, 1158
Sulfonylureas, 1084
Sunburns, 246, 248
Sundowning, 1017
"Super ACO", 2
Superimposed preeclampsia, 75*t*
Superior vena cava syndrome, 1330-1331, 1330*b*-1331*b*
Supersupraglottic swallow, 668*t*-669*t*
Supplements, dietary. *see also specific supplements*
  after bariatric surgery, 124
  for osteoarthritis, 979
Support stockings, 610, 610*t*
Supraclavicular node (sentinel node), 1206
Supraglottic swallow, 668*t*-669*t*
Supraventricular tachycardia with aberrancy, 520-521
Surge capacity, in disasters, 190
Surgery. *see also specific procedures*
  clearance for. *see* Presurgical clearance
  for inflammatory bowel disease, 698
  for osteoarthritis, 979
  weight loss and, 1220
Surgical office procedures, in skin, 240-242
  biopsy of, 241-242, 241*f*-242*f*
  cryosurgery of, 240
  curettage of, 241
  electrocautery of, 240-241
Surveillance, Epidemiology, and End Results (SEER) Program, 1314
Survivorship care plans (SCPs), for brain tumor, 1070
Suturing, recommendations for, 324*t*
Swallowing difficulties, weight loss and, 1219-1220
Sweating, 288-289
Sympathectomy, for Raynaud phenomenon, 1166
Sympathetic adrenergic activity, 557
Sympathetic nervous system, 570
Sympathomimetics, hypertension and, 572*t*-573*t*
Symptom validity and effort tests, 1000*b*
Syncope, 230-233, 1024, 1026*b*
  causes of, 231*b*
  clinical presentation of, 231-232
  definition and epidemiology of, 230
  diagnostics for, 232, 232*b*
  differential diagnosis of, 232
  disposition and referral of, 233
  heat-related illness and, 233
  initial stabilization and management of, 232-233
  pathophysiology of, 230-231
  physical examination of, 232
  prevention and patient education of, 233
  with seizures, 1057
  three main classifications of, 230
  true incidence of, 230
Syndrome of inappropriate antidiuretic hormone (SIADH), 1119, 1334-1335, 1334*b*-1335*b*
Syndrome X, 538-539
Synovial fluid analysis, 943*t*
  for rheumatoid arthritis, 1167-1168
Synovial membrane, 936
Syphilis
  clinical presentation of, 791-792
  complications of, 792
  definition and epidemiology of, 791, 791*f*
  diagnostics for, 792
  latent, 785*t*-788*t*
  pathophysiology of, 791
  primary, 785*t*-788*t*
  screening for, 146*t*-147*t*, 149*t*-152*t*
  secondary, 785*t*-788*t*
  stages of, 791*b*
  test for, 146*t*-147*t*
  treatment of, 789*b*
Systemic disorders/diseases
  alopecia and, 254*t*
  associated with pruritus, 300*b*
Systemic inflammatory response syndrome (SIRS), 715
Systemic lupus erythematosus (SLE), 1170-1176
  antinuclear antibodies in, 1173*t*
  classification of, 1171*b*
  clinical presentation and physical examination for, 1171-1172
Systemic lupus erythematosus (SLE) *(Continued)*
  complications of, 1175-1176
  definition and epidemiology of, 1170
  diagnostics for, 1172-1173, 1173*b*
  differential diagnosis for, 1173, 1173*b*
  indications for referral or hospitalization for, 1176
  life span considerations with, 1175
  management of, 1173-1175, 1174*t*
  organisms associated with, 1175
  pathophysiology of, 1170-1171
  Raynaud phenomenon with, 1172
Systemic therapy, in pruritus, 300-301
Systolic dysfunction, 556-557
Systolic Hypertension in the Elderly Program (SHEP), 1218

T

T cells, 1233
T_3 (triiodothyronine), 1136, 1149
T_4 (thyroxine), 1136, 1140, 1149
Tachycardia/tachyarrhythmias, 203-205, 515-516
  clinical presentation of, 203
  definition and epidemiology, 203
  diagnostics for, 203, 204*b*
  differential diagnosis of, 203-204, 204*b*, 520-522
  disposition and referral of, 205
  in heart failure, 560*t*
  heat-related illness and, 233
  initial stabilization and management of, 204
  management of, 524-525
  medication therapy for patients with, 205*b*
  pathophysiology of, 203
  physical examination of, 203
  prevention and patient education and, 205
Tacrolimus (Protopic), in atopic dermatitis, 278
Tadalafil (Cialis), 761, 761*t*
Takayasu arteritis, 1177
Takotsubo cardiomyopathy, chest pain and, 548*t*
Tamoxifen, 809
Tanner stages, 55
Tarantula, 198
Target-specific oral anticoagulants (TSOACs), 1306
Taste disorders, 392
tcdC regulatory gene, 1249
T-cell disorders, 1201
T-cell lymphomas, 1319
Team building, 14
Team leader, role of, 14
Team leading, 23-24
Tear duct, 349
Tedizolid, 264
Teenagers. *see* Adolescents
Telangiectasis, 338*f*
Telemedicine, 44-45
Telemedicine technology, for heart failure, 568
Telmisartan, 576*t*-582*t*
Telogen, 1097
Telogen effluvium, 254*t*
Telogen phase disturbance, 253
Temporal artery biopsy, for giant cell arteritis, 1163
Tendinitis, in shoulder, 989
Tenesmus, 694
Tennis elbow, 922
Tenosynovitis
  clinical presentation of, 933
  diagnostics and differential diagnosis for, 934
  management of, 935
  physical examination for, 933
Tension pneumothorax, 491, 493
  chest pain and, 548*t*
Tension-type headache, 1031
Terazosin, 576*t*-582*t*
Terazosin (Hytrin), 735
Terbinafine (Lamisil), 281*t*
Terbutaline sulfate, 462*t*-463*t*
Teriflunomide (Aubagio), 1048-1049
Teriparatide (PTH 1-34), 965
Terrorism, 226
Test batteries, 1000-1001, 1003
Test of Functional Health Literacy in Adults (TOFHLA), 3-4

Testicular disorders, 763-771. *see also specific disorders*
clinical presentation of, 765-766
complications of, 771
definition and epidemiology of, 763
diagnostics for, 767-768, 768*b*
differential diagnosis of, 768, 769*t*-770*t*
indications for referral or hospitalization for, 771
life span considerations with, 771
management of, 768-771
pathophysiology of, 763-765
physical examination for, 766-767
traumatic, 764-765, 767, 768*b*, 770
tumors, 764-768, 768*b*, 770
Testicular torsion, 764-767, 768*b*, 770
Testosterone, hirsutism and, 1097-1100
Tetanus, diphtheria, and acellular pertussis (Tdap) vaccine, 159-163, 161*t*-162*t*
Tetanus immunization, 322, 324*b*, 324*t*
Tetanus-prone wounds, 324*b*, 324*t*
Tetracycline, 729*t*
Thalassemia, 1284-1287
α-, 1284
β, 1284-1285
clinical presentation of, 1285
complications of, 1286-1287, 1287*b*
definition and epidemiology of, 1284
diagnostics for, 1285
differential diagnosis of, 1285
indications for referral or hospitalization for, 1287
inheritance of, 1284, 1284*f*
life span considerations with, 1286
management of, 1285-1286
pathophysiology of, 1284-1285
physical examination for, 1285
Thalidomide, 502, 1222
Thallium 201, 507
Theophylline, 433*t*-435*t*, 439, 462*t*-463*t*, 464
serum concentrations of, factors affecting, 440*t*
Therapeutic exercise
for low back pain, 957
for neck pain, 974
Thermal injuries, 233-236. *see also* Burns
cold injury, 235-236
heat-related illness, 233-235
Thermolysis, 1102
Thessaly test, 950, 950*f*
Thiazide diuretics, 566*t*
for hypertension, 576*t*-582*t*
Thiazide-like diuretics, for hypertension, 576*t*-582*t*
Thiazolidinediones, 1084-1085
Thienopyridines, 1014
Thioamide therapy, for Graves disease, 1143-1144, 1144*b*, 1144*t*
Third-degree burns, 260, 319*b*
Thirst, 1112
Thoracentesis, 482
Thoracic spine, pain in, 982*b*
Thoracoscopy, for pleural effusions, 482
Thornicroft's Translational Medicine Continuum, 12-13, 12*f*
Three-step analgesic ladder, 1187-1188
Thrombocytopenia, 1375
patient education and self-care strategies in, 1312*b*-1313*b*
Thromboembolism
in atrial fibrillation, 525
prevention of, 526
oral contraceptives and, 833
Thrombolysis in Myocardial Infarction (TIMI) risk score, 541-542, 541*t*
Thrombolytic therapy, 1014
Thrombophilia. *see also* Thrombosis disorders (thrombophilia)
causes of, 1305*b*
differential diagnosis of, 1305*b*
Thrombosis disorders (thrombophilia), 1303-1307
complications of, 1306
diagnostics and differential diagnosis of, 1304-1305
indications for referral or hospitalization for, 1306-1307
life span considerations with, 1307
Thrombosis disorders (thrombophilia) *(Continued)*
management of, 1305-1306
pathophysiology and clinical presentation of, 1303-1304
patient and family education in, 1307
physical examination in, 1304
Thrombus, 1303-1304
Thrush, 406
oral, 432
Thyroid cancer
biopsy of, 1137
clinical presentation and physical examination for, 1139
complications of, 1141
definition and epidemiology of, 1139
diagnostics and differential diagnosis for, 1139-1140, 1140*b*
indications for referral or hospitalization for, 1141
life span considerations with, 1141
management of, 1140-1141
nodules in, 1139-1141
pathophysiology of, 1139
patient and family education and health promotion for, 1141
Thyroid disorders/diseases, 1135-1151. *see also specific disorders*
hypertension and, 572*t*-573*t*
in pregnancy, 77-78, 1150-1151
Thyroid gland, 1135
cytology of, 1137
drugs and, 1149-1150
function testing of, 1136-1137, 1142*t*
imaging of, 1136-1137
Thyroid hormones. *see also specific hormones*
effects of, 1136*b*
therapy, for thyroid cancer, 1141
Thyroid peroxidase (TPO), 1136
Thyroid scans, 1136-1137
Thyroid storm, 1145, 1197
Thyroidectomy, for Graves disease, 1144
Thyroiditis, 1145
Thyroid-stimulating hormone (TSH), 1135
hirsutism and, 1101
in hypothyroidism, 1148
measurement of, 1140-1141
osteoporosis and, 961
testing for, 1136
Thyrotoxicosis, 1141, 1143*b*
Thyrotropin-releasing hormone (TRH), 1135
Thyroxine-binding globulin (TBG), 1136
Tiagabine (Gabitril), 1061*t*-1062*t*
Tic douloureux, 1063
Tick-borne encephalitis, 1229-1230
Tick-borne illnesses, 1254-1261. *see also specific illnesses*
comparison of, 1262*t*
Ticks, 197*t*, 198
Ticlopidine, 440*t*, 603, 1014
Tics, 1040*b*
Tilt-table test, for cardiac arrhythmias, 519
Tiludronate, 969*t*
Time management, stress management of, 135
Timolol maleate, 576*t*-582*t*
Tinea capitis, 254*t*, 279-280, 279*f*
Tinea corporis, 279-280, 280*f*, 281*t*
Tinea cruris, 279-280, 281*t*
Tinea lesions, in atopic dermatitis, 278
Tinea pedis, 279-280, 280*f*, 281*t*
Tinea unguium. *see* Onychomycosis
Tinea versicolor, 282, 282*b*
Tinel sign, 934*f*
Tinnitus, 369-371
clinical presentation of, 370
complications of, 371
definition and epidemiology of, 369
diagnostics for, 370, 370*b*
differential diagnosis of, 370, 370*b*
indications for referral or hospitalization for, 371
management of, 370-371
pathophysiology of, 370
physical examination for, 370
Tiotropium, 461
Tissue factor, 1298
Tissue plasminogen activator (tPA), 1014
TNF antagonists, for psoriasis, 303
Tobacco use counseling, 149*t*-152*t*
TOFHLA. *see* Test of Functional Health Literacy in Adults (TOFHLA)
Tolerance, 1369-1370
Tolterodine tartrate (Detrol), 735
Tongue biting, 1056
Tonic-clonic seizures (grand mal), 1055
Tono-Pen, 328
Tonsillectomy, 412
Tonsillitis, 413-416
clinical presentation of, 413-414
complications of, 416
definition and epidemiology of, 413, 413*f*
diagnostics for, 414, 414*b*
differential diagnosis for, 414-415, 415*b*
life span considerations with, 415-416
management of, 415
pathophysiology of, 413
physical examination for, 414
Topical medications
corticosteroids, 244*t*-245*t*, 245
for eyes, 350
for psoriasis, 303
Topiramate (Topamax), 1033, 1059, 1061*t*-1062*t*
Torsades De Pointes, 521
Torsemide, 576*t*-582*t*
Total daily dose (TDD), 1082
Toxic epidermal necrolysis, 274*t*
Toxic multinodular goiter, 1145
Toxic nodule, 1145
Toxicology testing, 1375
Toxoplasma gondii, 1251-1252
Tracer injection, 507
Traction
for low back pain, 957-958
for neck pain, 975
Tramadol hydrochloride (Ultram), for osteoarthritis, 978
Trandolapril, 576*t*-582*t*
Trans-catheter aortic valve replacement (TAVR), 615
Transcutaneous electrical nerve stimulation (TENS)
for chronic pain, 1188*t*
for low back pain, 957
Transcutaneous oxygen (T_{CPO2}), 602
Transdermal estrogen products, for menopause, 865*t*-867*t*
Transesophageal echocardiography (TEE)
for cardiac arrhythmias, 519, 526
for infective endocarditis, 588
Trans-fatty acids, 1121, 1123
Transferrin, 1279
Transgender, definition of, 60
Transient ischemic attacks (TIAs), 1010
ABCD Score for, 1012*t*
symptoms of, 529
Transient lower esophageal sphincter (LES) relaxations (TLESRs), 670
Transient proteinuria, 743
Transient synovitis, 937
Transitional care, 3-6
cognitive impairment of, 4
cultural competence and language of, 4-5
health literacy of, 3-4
medication safety of, 4
Transitional cell carcinoma (TCC), 795
Transjugular intrahepatic portosystemic shunt (TIPS), 681
Translational research, 11-12
Translational science spectrum, 13
Transtheoretical model (TTM), 25
Transthoracic 2D echocardiography, 614
Transthoracic echocardiogram (TTE)
for aortic regurgitation, 617-618
for mitral valve prolapse, 620
Transurethral resection of the prostate (TURP), 740
Trapeziometacarpal arthritis
clinical presentation of, 933
diagnostics and differential diagnosis for, 934
management of, 935
physical examination for, 934
Trauma, ocular. *see* Ocular disorders, traumatic
Traumatic brain injury (TBI), 218, 220

Travel medicine, 173
initial consultation, 175*f*-176*f*
providers services, 174*b*
Travel safety, 179-180
Travel vaccine, 178*t*
Travelers, fever in, 1198
Traveler's diarrhea, 1247
Trazodone, 926*t*, 1360*t*-1362*t*
Treadmill exercise, 505*t*
Treatment summaries (TSs), for brain tumor, 1070
Tremor, 1040*b*. *see also* Essential tremor
multiple sclerosis and, 1046*t*-1047*t*
Trendelenburg gait, 938
Treponema pallidum, 785*t*-788*t*
Treprostinil, 498
Triamcinolone acetonide, 244*t*
for osteoarthritis, 978
Triamterene, for hypertension, 576*t*-582*t*
Trichomonas vaginalis, 785*t*-788*t*
Trichomoniasis, in pregnancy, 71, 71*t*
Trichophyton, 294
Trichotillomania, 254*t*
Tricuspid regurgitation, in heart failure, 560*t*
Tricuspid stenosis, 612*t*
Tricuspid valve prolapse, 612*t*
Tricyclic antidepressants (TCAs), 113, 313, 313*t*
for anxiety disorders, 1352*t*, 1353
for chronic pain, 1187-1188
for headaches, 1033
for low back pain, 958
for parasomnias, 1218
Tricyclic drugs, for fibromyalgia syndrome, 926
Trigeminal nerve, 1063-1064
Trigeminal neuralgia, 391, 1063-1066
clinical presentation of, 1064
complications of, 1065
definition and epidemiology of, 1063
diagnostics and differential diagnosis for, 1064, 1064*b*-1065*b*
indications for referral or hospitalization for, 1065-1066
life span considerations with, 1065
management of, 1064-1065, 1065*t*
pathophysiology of, 1063-1064
physical examination for, 1064
Trigger finger
clinical presentation of, 933
diagnostics and differential diagnosis for, 934
management of, 935
physical examination for, 933
Trigger point, for fibromyalgia syndrome, 927
Trigger zone, of trigeminal neuralgia, 1064
Triggered activity (cardiac), 516
Triglycerides, 1120-1121
L-Triiodothyronine (L-T_3), serum, 1147
Trimethadione, acne and, 250*b*
Trimethoprim-sulfamethoxazole (TMP-SMX), 779*t*, 781
for vasculitis, 1180
Triptans, for headaches, 1034, 1035*t*-1036*t*
Trochanteric bursa, 916*f*
Tropical sprue, 179
Troponins, 547
True experimental design, 7*t*
True vertigo, 1025
Trypsin, 714-715
T-score, 961-962
TTM. *see* Transtheoretical model (TTM)
Tube thoracostomy, 492-493
Tuberculin skin test (TST), 1264-1265
false-negative reactions of, 1265, 1265*b*
positive reaction of, 1265, 1265*b*
two-step, 1266, 1266*b*
Tuberculosis (TB), 1262-1271
chronic cough and, 455
clinical classification system for, 1267*t*
clinical presentation of, 1264
complications of, 1271
definition and epidemiology of, 1262-1263
diagnostics for, 1264-1267, 1267*b*
differential diagnosis of, 1267, 1267*b*
emerging and reemerging, 1225
extensively drug-resistant, 1231-1232
factors associated with, 1264*b*
Tuberculosis (TB) *(Continued)*
indications for referral or hospitalization in, 1271
interdisciplinary management of, 1270
latent, 1238
life span considerations with, 1270-1271
management of, 1267-1270
occupational, 167
pathophysiology of, 1264
physical examination for, 1264
preventive therapy for, 1268*b*
screening for, 155
Tumor, nodes, and metastasis (TNM) system, 1327
Tumor lysis syndrome, 1311, 1333-1334, 1334*b*
Tumors. *see* specific site
23-valent pneumococcal polysaccharide vaccine (PPV23), 1293
Two-process model, of sleep regulation, 1210
Tympanic membrane (TM)
with cerumen impaction, 361
cholesteatoma and, 363
in otitis media, 374
perforation of, 377, 377*b*
Tyrosine kinase inhibitors, 1150
Tzanck test, 292*b*

U

Ubiquinone, 16
Ulceration
genital, 791-794
oral, 1171*b*
peptic. *see* Peptic ulcer disease (PUD)
in skin, 247*t*, 310-311
Ulcerative colitis (UC)
chronic diarrhea and, 653
Crohn disease *versus*, 693*t*
definition and epidemiology of, 692
Ulnar neuritis, 922*t*-923*t*
Ultrafast computed tomography, 508
Ultrasonography
for abdominal aortic aneurysm, 512
carotid, for cerebrovascular events, 1012
for ectopic pregnancy, 829
of thyroid gland, 1137
Ultrasound
duplex, for carotid artery disease, 531
for low back pain, 957
Ultraviolet B (UVB) light, 298, 353-354
Uncovertebral articulation, 971
Unfractionated heparin, for pulmonary embolism, 495
Universal screening, intimate partner violence and, 144
Unknown primary carcinoma (UPC), 1345-1348
clinical presentation of, 1346, 1346*t*
complications of, 1348
definition and epidemiology of, 1345-1346
diagnostics for, 1346-1347, 1347*b*
differential diagnosis of, 1347, 1347*b*
indications for referral or hospitalization for, 1348
interdisciplinary management of, 1348
life span considerations with, 1348
management of, 1347-1348
pathophysiology of, 1346
physical examination for, 1346
squamous cell carcinoma and, 1346
Unstable angina, 539
clinical presentation of, 541-542, 541*t*
diagnostics for, 544-545
echocardiography for, 544-545
electrocardiography for, 544
exercise tolerance testing for, 544
management of, 549-550
Upper airway cough syndrome, 454
Upper airway surgical procedures, for obstructive sleep apnea, 1214
Upper extremity arterial disease, peripheral arterial insufficiency and, 602-603
Upper intestinal diarrhea, 1243
Upper motor neurons (UMNs), 1005
Upper respiratory tract infection, 415
heart failure and, 563
Urate-lowering therapy (ULT), for gout, 930
Ureaplasma urealyticum, 785*t*-788*t*
Uremia, and infective endocarditis, 588
Ureteroscopy (URS), 775
Urethritis, 784-791
nongonococcal, 778, 785*t*-788*t*
treatment of, 789*b*
Urgency, urinary, 731-732
Uric acid stones, 773, 776
Uricase, recombinant, for gout, 931
Uricostatic drugs, for gout, 930-931
Uricosuric drugs, for gout, 930-931
Urinalysis, 182*t*
Urinary tract infections (UTIs), 777-782
clinical presentation of, 778-779, 779*t*
complications of, 782
definition and epidemiology of, 777-778
diagnostics for, 780
differential diagnosis of, 780-781, 781*b*
hematuria with, 747
indications for referral or hospitalization for, 782
life span considerations with, 782
management of, 781-782, 781*t*
pathophysiology of, 778, 778*t*, 779*b*
physical examination for, 779-780
in pregnancy, 70, 71*t*
risk factors for, 779*b*
Urinary tract obstruction, 794
Urinary urge incontinence (UUI), 731-732, 733*b*, 734-735
Urine culture, 780
and sensitivity , for presurgical clearance, 182*t*
Urine osmolality, 1113
Urolithiasis
definition and epidemiology of, 771-772, 794
differential diagnosis of, 774, 775*b*
Ursodeoxycholic acid, 638
Urticaria, 274*t*, 312-314
clinical presentation of, 312
complications of, 314
definition and epidemiology of, 312, 312*f*
diagnostics for, 313, 313*b*
differential diagnosis of, 313, 314*b*
health promotion of, 314
management of, 313-314, 313*t*
pathophysiology of, 312
patient and family education of, 314
physical examination of, 312-313
referral or hospitalization, indications of, 314
U.S. Preventive Services Task Force (USPSTF), 56*t*, 147, 479
Ustekinumab, 1158
Uveitis, 331, 332*t*-334*t*

V

V wave, 517
Vaccine. *see also* Immunization
acronyms, 155
administration, issues with, 155-156, 156*b*
adverse event reporting system, 156
contraindications to and precautions for, 161*t*-162*t*
for dengue, 1228
information, 178*t*
information statements, 155
for meningitis, 1040
provider toolbox, 180*b*
travel, 178*t*
Vaccine-specific information, 156-160
Vaginal estrogen products, for menopause, 865*t*-867*t*
Vaginal lubricants, 861
Vaginal moisturizers, 861
Vaginal ring, 836
Vaginismus, 825
Vaginitis, 892-896
atrophic, 856, 895-896
in pregnancy, 70-72
Vaginosis, bacterial, 892-894
clinical presentation and physical examination of, 892
complications of, 893
diagnostics for, 892, 892*b*
differential diagnosis of, 893, 893*b*
indications for referral or hospitalization for, 893
life span considerations with, 893
management of, 893

Vaginosis, bacterial *(Continued)*
pathophysiology of, 892
in pregnancy, 71*t*
Valacyclovir, 789*b*
for herpes simplex virus, 271, 271*t*
Valgus stress test, of knee, 947, 947*f*
Valproate, 1059, 1367*t*-1368*t*
Valproic acid, 113, 1061*t*-1062*t*
Valsalva maneuvers
for cardiac arrhythmias, 519
in eyes, 329
Valsartan, 576*t*-582*t*
Value-Based Purchasing (VBP), in collaborative practice, 1
Valvular heart disease, 611-622. *see also* Cardiac murmurs
definition, 611
progressive, stages of, 613*t*
Vancomycin, for endocarditis, 591*t*-595*t*
Vancomycin-resistant *Enterococcus* (VRE), 1249
Vardenafil (Levitra), 761, 761*t*
Varenicline, 139
Variant angina, 539
clinical presentation of, 541
diagnostics for, 544
echocardiography for, 544
electrocardiography for, 544
exercise tolerance testing for, 544
management of, 549
Varicella vaccine, 160, 161*t*-162*t*
Varicella-zoster virus (VZV). *see also* Herpes zoster (shingles)
Bell palsy and, 1008
encephalitis and, 1039
Varicocele, 763-768, 768*b*
Varicose veins, 609
clinical presentation and physical examination of, 609
complications of, 609
diagnostics and differential diagnosis of, 609
indications for referral or hospitalization in, 609
management of, 609
pathophysiology of, 609
patient and family education for, 609
primary, 609
secondary, 609
Varus stress, on knee joint, 947
Vascular dementia, 1021
Vasculitis, 1176-1180, 1176*b*
classification of, 1176-1177, 1176*b*
clinical presentation and physical examination for, 1177-1178
complications of, 1180
definition and epidemiology of, 1176
diagnostics for, 1178-1179, 1179*b*
differential diagnosis for, 1179-1180, 1180*b*
drug-induced, 305
indications for referral or hospitalization for, 1180
management of, 1180
pathophysiology of, 1177
Vasoconstrictor, in conjunctivitis, 340
Vasodilators
in cardiac testing, 509
for hypertension, 576*t*-582*t*
for pulmonary hypertension, 498
Vasomotor rhinitis, 387-388, 388*b*
Vasomotor symptoms, 854-855, 860-861
Vasopressin, dysmenorrhea and, 821
Vaughn-Williams classification, for antiarrhythmic medications, 524-525
Vector-borne diseases, 1228-1230
Vegetarian diet, 130
Vegetative material, embolization of, 587. *see also* Infective endocarditis
Venlafaxine, 926*t*, 1360*t*-1362*t*
Venous insufficiency, 310
peripheral, 605-606
diagnostics for, 606*b*
differential diagnosis of, 607*b*
Venous stasis, chronic, 608-609
clinical presentation and physical examination of, 608
complications of, 609
Venous stasis, chronic *(Continued)*
definition and epidemiology of, 608
diagnostics and differential diagnosis of, 608
indications for referral or hospitalization for, 609
management of, 609
pathophysiology of, 608
Venous stasis ulceration, 317, 609-610
clinical presentation and physical examination of, 610, 610*b*
complications for, 610
definition and epidemiology of, 609
diagnostics and differential diagnosis of, 610
indications for referral or hospitalization for, 610
management of, 610
pathophysiology of, 609-610
Venous thromboembolism (VTE), 1069, 1304. *see also* Thrombosis disorders (thrombophilia)
Ventilation/perfusion ($\dot{V}/\dot{Q}$) scan, for pulmonary embolism, 494
Ventricular fibrillation, 521
Ventricular gallop, 542
Ventricular hypertrophy, 557
Ventricular mural thrombi, 553
Ventricular outflow tract tachycardia, 521
Ventricular remodeling, in heart failure, 557
Ventricular septal defect, 612*t*
Ventricular tachycardia (VT), 202, 521, 521*f*, 527
Verapamil, 576*t*-582*t*
for headaches, 1034
Verbal response, 219*t*
Vernal conjunctivitis, 341-342
Verruca. *see* Warts
Vertebral tenderness, 1374
Vertebroplasty, 967
Vertical banded gastroplasty (VBG), 123
Vertigo, 1024-1028
benign paroxysmal positional, 1027-1028
clinical presentation of, 1025
complications of, 1027
definition and epidemiology of, 1024
diagnostics for, 1025-1026, 1025*b*-1026*b*
differential diagnosis for, 1026, 1026*b*
management of, 1027
pathophysiology of, 1024-1025
physical examination for, 1025
Very-low-calorie diets (VLCDs), 119
Vesicle, 238*f*
Vespids, 197
Vestibular disorders, 1026*b*
Vestibular Disorders Association, 1027
Vestibular laboratory testing, 1025
Vestibular neuritis, 367-368
clinical presentation of, 367
complications of, 368
definition and epidemiology of, 367
diagnostics for, 367, 367*b*
differential diagnosis of, 367-368, 368*b*
life span considerations with, 368
management of, 368
pathophysiology of, 367
patient and family education of, 368
physical examination of, 367
referral or hospitalization, indications of, 368
Vetter, David, 1200
Vibrators, for menopause, 861
Vibrio cholerae, 1227-1228, 1245, 1247
Vibrio parahaemolyticus, 1245
Victimization, patient disclosure of, intimate partner violence and, 144
Videofluoroscopic examination of swallowing (VFES), 665-666
Videofluoroscopy (VFS), 665-666
Violence
adolescence and, 57
domestic, clinical presentation and diagnoses of, 141
screening of, 57*b*
Viral capsid antigen (VCA), 1252
Viral conjunctivitis, 340-341, 340*f*
Viral infections. *see also specific pathogens and body parts*
oral, 406
Viral load
monitoring of, 1238
testing of, 1235
Viral rhinosinusitis, 391
Viral titers, 401-402
Virchow node, 1206-1207
Viridans streptococci, 398
Virilism, 1097-1098
Virtual colonoscopy, 695
Viruses
acute bronchitis and, 417
oncogenic, 314
pneumonia and, 488
Visceral hypersensitivity, 649
Visceral pain, 623
Visceral sensation, enhanced, 701
Visible myoglobinuria, 211
Vision loss
differential diagnosis of, 333*b*
management of, 334*t*
signs and symptoms of, 331-334
Visual acuity
physical examination of, 327
screening for, 149*t*-152*t*
Visual disturbances, visual loss and, 331-334
differential diagnosis of, 333*b*
management of, 334*t*
Visual fields, 329
Visual loss
ankylosing spondylitis and, 1155
giant cell arteritis and, 1162
Visuospatial skills, 1000*b*
Vital signs, of sports physical, preparticipation, 186
Vitamin B_{12} deficiency, 1287-1290
definition and epidemiology of, 1287
pathophysiology of, 1287-1288
Vitamin D
deficiency
hyperparathyroidism and, 1131
hypocalcemia and, 1107
osteoporosis and, 961, 964*t*
for menopause, 860
for multiple sclerosis, 1049
Vitamin D insufficiency, renal failure and, 754
Vitamin K, 1305-1306
Vitamins
for menopause, 860
Vitiligo, 296-298
clinical presentation of, 296-297
complications of, 298
definition and epidemiology of, 296
diagnostics for, 297, 297*b*
differential diagnosis of, 297, 297*b*
locations of, 297*b*
management of, 297-298
pathophysiology of, 296
physical examination for, 297
referral, indications for, 298
Vitreous humor, 331
Vocal cord dysfunction (VCD), and asthma, 429
Volkmann contracture, 997
Vomiting, in ocular pain, 335*t*
Vomiting center (VC), 709
Vomiting reflex, 709
Von Willebrand disease, 1302
VUCA mnemonics, 1
Vulvar disorders, 883-892. *see also specific disorders*
definition and epidemiology of, 883
Vulvar irritants, 888*b*
Vulvar pain, 889
Vulvar pruritus, 883
Vulvar vestibulitis, 825, 827
Vulvar vestibulitis syndrome (VVS), 889-892
clinical presentation and physical examination of, 890
complications of, 891
diagnostics for, 890, 891*b*
differential diagnosis of, 891, 891*b*
indications for referral or hospitalization for, 891-892
life span considerations with, 891
management of, 891
pathophysiology of, 889-890
Vulvitis, 825
Vulvodynia, 889-892
clinical presentation and physical examination of, 890

Vulvodynia *(Continued)*
complications of, 891
diagnostics for, 890, 891*b*
differential diagnosis of, 891, 891*b*
indications for referral or hospitalization for, 891-892
life span considerations with, 891
management of, 891
pathophysiology of, 889-890
Vulvovaginal atrophy (VVA), 855
Vulvovaginal candidiasis (VVC), 894-895
clinical presentation and physical examination of, 894
complications of, 895
diagnostics for, 894, 894*b*
differential diagnosis of, 894, 894*b*
indications for referral or hospitalization for, 895
life span considerations with, 895
management of, 894-895
pathophysiology of, 894
in pregnancy, 71*t*

W

Wagner Classification System, 318*t*
Waist circumference, 109-110, 1128
Walking, 964
Warfarin, 495, 526, 553, 607, 1014, 1305-1306
Warts, 314-316
clinical presentation and physical examination for, 315, 315*f*
complications of, 316
definition and epidemiology of, 314-315
diagnostics and differential diagnosis of, 315, 316*b*
management of, 316
pathophysiology of, 315
referral for, indications for, 316
Wasps, 197*t*
Watery diarrhea, 653
Weakness
associated with West Nile virus, 1274*t*
in Guillain-Barré syndrome, 1028-1029
multiple sclerosis and, 1046*t*-1047*t*
Weaning, 83-84
Weber glands, 411
Weber test, 365
Wegener granulomatosis. *see* Granulomatosis with polyangiitis (GPA)
Weight control remedies, hypertension and, 572*t*-573*t*
Weight gain. *see also* Obesity
after bariatric surgery, 124
coronary artery disease and, 537*t*
low infant weight gain, 82
pharmaceutical associated with, 112-113
in pregnancy, 69, 69*t*
from smoking cessation, 112
Weight homeostasis, human, 1219
Weight loss
with dehydration, 92
metabolic syndrome and, 1129
pharmaceutical options for, 120-123
resources for, 119-120
side effects of, 119
strategies for, 116-118
surgery for. *see* Bariatric surgery
unintended, 1218-1224
clinical presentation of, 1219-1220
complications of, 1223
definition and epidemiology of, 1218-1219
diagnostics for, 1221, 1221*b*
differential diagnosis of, 1221-1222, 1222*b*
indications for referral or hospitalization, 1223
life span considerations with, 1223
management of, 1222-1223
pathophysiology of, 1219
physical examination for, 1220-1221
Weight management, 109-125, 130
in college health, 171
Weight-bearing exercise, 858*b*, 963-964
WES. *see* Whole exome sequencing (WES)
West Nile virus, 1271-1277
clinical presentation of, 1273-1274
CNS and, 1040
complications of, 1276
definitions of, 1271-1272
diagnostics for, 1274, 1275*t*
differential diagnosis of, 1275, 1275*b*
epidemiology of, 1272-1273, 1272*f*
incidence of, 1272-1273, 1273*f*
indications for referral or hospitalization in, 1276
life span considerations with, 1276
management of, 1275-1276
Western blot testing, 1235
Wet dressing, 244*t*
WGS. *see* Whole genome sequencing (WGS)
Wheal, 238*f*
Wheezing
and asthma, 424-426
other causes of, 429
White coat hypertension, 574
Whole exome sequencing (WES), 31
Whole genome sequencing (WGS), 31
Wide-complex tachycardia, 520-521
Wilms tumor, 794-795, 796*b*-798*b*, 797
Window operation, 805
Window period, 1233-1234
Wireless capsule endoscopy (WCE), for GI bleeding, 681-682
Wiskott-Aldrich syndrome (WAS), 1201
Withdrawal, 1369
Wolf spiders, 200
Wolff-Parkinson-White Pattern, 520
Women
integrated health care for, 78
prevention of lipid disorders in, 1126
Women's Health Initiative (WHI), 853
Workers' compensation treatment, 165-166
Working mothers, breastfeeding and, 83
Workplace surveillance, 165
Work-related injuries, illnesses, exposures, treatment of, 166
Wound closure, 322
Wound management, 317-325
for acute wounds, 322
for chronic wounds, 322-325
classification of wounds in, 317-318
diagnostics for, 320-321, 320*b*
differential diagnosis for, 321
documentation of, 325*b*
pathophysiology in, 319-320
physical examination for, 320
principles of, 321-322
product selection, algorithm for, 323*f*
stages of, 319
surgical, 317, 325
tetanus immunization in, 324*t*
Wrist, fracture of, 994
Wuchereria bancrofti, 765

X

Xanthine derivatives, 439
Xanthinuria, 773
Xerostomia, 665, 666*b*, 1342, 1345
clinical presentation and physical examination, 103
defined, 400, 403
stepwise process for management of, 103
X-linked disorders/disease, 37-38, 40*f*, 68*t*

Y

Yellow jackets, 197*t*
Yergason test, 988*t*
Yersinia, 1156

Z

Zafirlukast, 439-440
Zanamivir, 490
Zika fever, 1229
Zileuton, 432*f*, 440
ZMapp, 1230
Zoledronic acid (Reclast), 858*b*, 964, 969*t*
Zollinger-Ellison syndrome, 670
Zolpidem tartrate (Ambien), 926*t*
Zones of injury, in burns, 260
Zonisamide (Zonegran), 1061*t*-1062*t*
Zoonoses, 1230-1231

Review

- APA guidelines for tx for UTI → AMCC
  → ANCP
- Tx of UTI
  - Keflex TID –
  - Amoxicillin 50mg/kg/Day for Day for UTI / Strep
    100mg/kg/Day for Day for otitis media

✓ Urine reflex

Flu

→ fever in flu wains in three day

→ fever continues for 3 days

→ Tamiflu → prevents virus from getting more severe. Reduces duration 12 hours to 1 day.
- N/V/D + Seizure
- high co-pay

Kimberly Pruett
857-230-0295